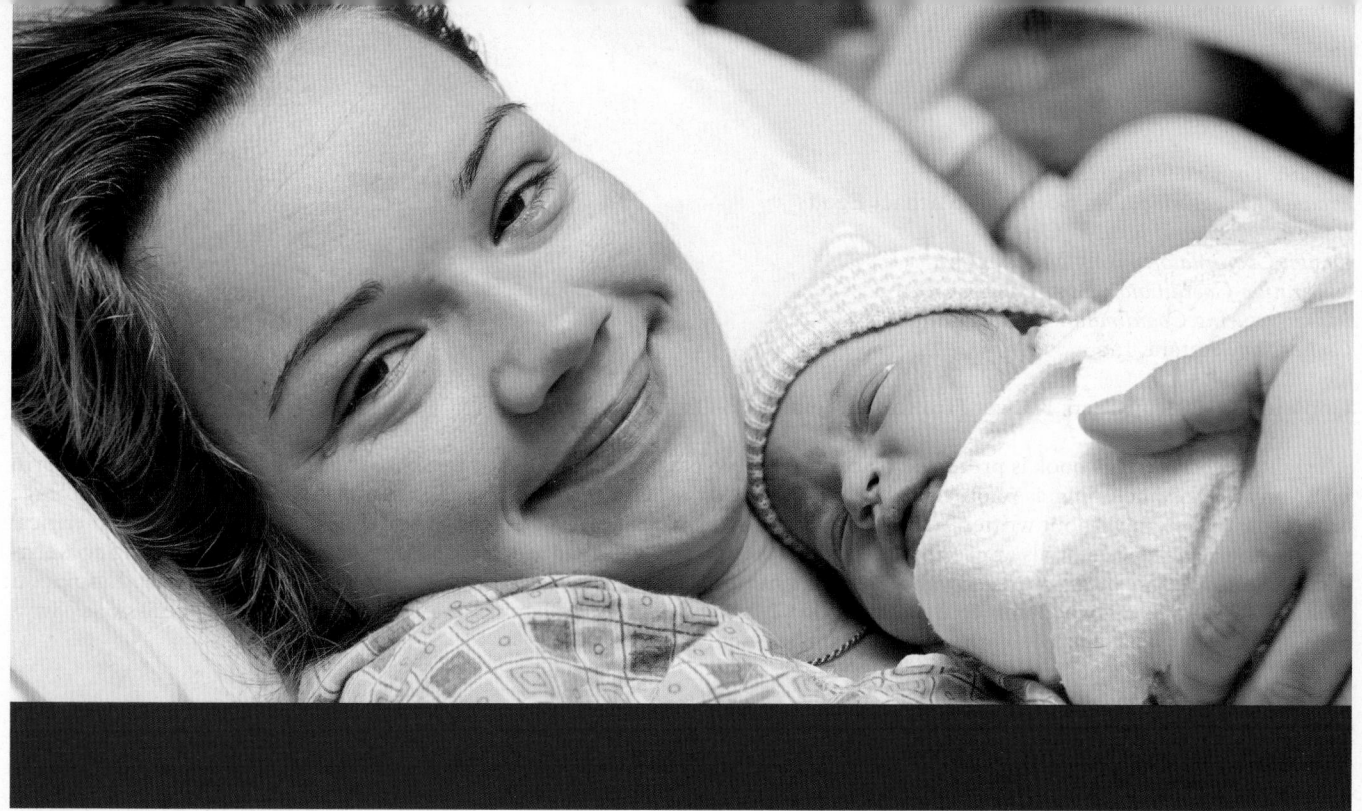

CANADIAN MATERNITY AND PEDIATRIC NURSING

Jean Chow, BN, MN, NM, RAc, PhD
Former faculty member, Faculty of Nursing
University of Calgary
Calgary, Alberta

Christine A. Ateah, RN, PhD
Associate Professor, Faculty of Nursing
University of Manitoba
Winnipeg, Manitoba

Shannon D. Scott, RN, PhD
Associate Professor, Faculty of Nursing
Canadian Institutes of Health Research,
    New Investigator
Alberta Heritage Foundation for Medical Research,
    Population Health Investigator
Assistant Professor (Adjunct), Department of
    Pediatrics, Faculty of Medicine & Dentistry
University of Alberta
Edmonton, Alberta

Susan Scott Ricci, ARNP, MSN, MEd
Nursing Faculty
University of Central Florida
Orlando, Florida
Former Nursing Program Director and Faculty
Lake Sumter Community College
Leesburg, Florida

Terri Kyle, MSN, CPNP
Director of Nursing
El Camino College
Torrance, California

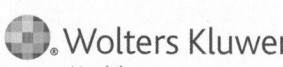
Wolters Kluwer
Health

Philadelphia · Baltimore · New York · London
Buenos Aires · Hong Kong · Sydney · Tokyo

Acquisitions Editor: Patrick Barbera
Product Managers: Laura Scott and Michael Egolf
Editorial Assistant: Jacalyn Clay
Design Coordinator: Holly McLaughlin
Illustration Coordinator: Brett MacNaughton
Manufacturing Coordinator: Karin Duffield
Compositor: Aptara, Inc.

9 8 7 6 5 4 3

Printed in China

Library of Congress Cataloging-in-Publication Data

Canadian maternity and pediatric nursing / Jean Chow . . . [et al.].
   p. ; cm.
  Includes bibliographical references and index.
  ISBN 978-1-4511-0223-9 (alk. paper)
  I. Chow, Jean.
   [DNLM: 1. Maternal-Child Nursing–Canada. 2. Women's Health–Canada.
WY 157.3]

  618.92′00231–dc23

2012020073

Care has been taken to confirm the accuracy of the information presented and to describe generally accepted practices. However, the authors, editors, and publisher are not responsible for errors or omissions or for any consequences from application of the information in this book and make no warranty, expressed or implied, with respect to the currency, completeness, or accuracy of the contents of the publication. Application of this information in a particular situation remains the professional responsibility of the practitioner; the clinical treatments described and recommended may not be considered absolute and universal recommendations.

The authors, editors, and publisher have exerted every effort to ensure that drug selection and dosage set forth in this text are in accordance with the current recommendations and practice at the time of publication. However, in view of ongoing research, changes in government regulations, and the constant flow of information relating to drug therapy and drug reactions, the reader is urged to check the package insert for each drug for any change in indications and dosage and for added warnings and precautions. This is particularly important when the recommended agent is a new or infrequently employed drug.

Some drugs and medical devices presented in this publication have Health Canada clearance for limited use in restricted research settings. It is the responsibility of the health care provider to ascertain the Health Canada status of each drug or device planned for use in his or her clinical practice.

LWW.com

This book is dedicated to my best teachers: students, women to whom I have provided care, and colleagues. The book is also dedicated to my loving husband Mike, who continually supports me in all my professional endeavours. My children, Diana, David, Geoffrey, and Arielle, have also been integral to my pursuits.

Jean Chow

This book is dedicated to my husband Curwood and our daughters Jaymie and Alexandra, my wonderful family, who always support, inspire, and encourage me in all that I do.

Christine A. Ateah

This book is dedicated to my children, Matthew, Alexander (Alex), and Sela, and to my partner and best friend Dwayne for providing unfailing love, support, and inspiration throughout this journey.

Shannon D. Scott

ACKNOWLEDGMENTS

I would like to thank so many people who have helped bring the exciting prospect of this textbook into being. My appreciation goes to Carrie Brandon for her ongoing leadership and Jean Rodenberger for approaching me with this project and believing that I could assist in achieving her vision. I would also like to especially thank Laura Scott for her editorial expertise and for her steadfastness to this project.

Also thanks to the many nurses and families for their participation in this book.

J.C.

We would like to express our sincere thanks and appreciation for the opportunity to author this textbook. We hope that our students and colleagues in pediatric nursing education and practice will find that this text is a useful resource to provide care to children and their families within the Canadian context. Thanks to Terri Kyle for the opportunity to adapt her original pediatric text. We acknowledge and greatly appreciate the immense effort to write the original version of such a complete and thorough work.

We would like to express our sincere appreciation for the support of Lippincott Williams & Wilkins (Wolters Kluwer Health). In particular we want to thank Laura Scott (Product Manager) who has worked with us from the beginning to plan and organize this adaptation and her ongoing patience and efforts to help us stay on track and meet deadlines. Thanks also to Patrick Barbera (Acquisitions Editor) for his ongoing support and commitment to this project, Jacalyn Clay (Editorial Assistant), Michael Egolf (Product Manager), Brett MacNaughton (Illustration Coordinator), Maureen McKinney, (Development Editor), and the rest of the editorial team. Special thanks to Stephen Wreakes, Medical Photographer, University of Alberta Hospital, Alberta Health Services, for his kindness in providing photos for several chapters.

We would also like to express our sincere and heartfelt appreciation to all of our pediatric nurse colleagues who contributed their wealth of knowledge and expertise to developing chapters for this book. This would not have been possible without all of you. We have been so impressed with your commitment to excellence, accuracy, and detail to help us make *Canadian Maternity and Pediatric Nursing* a reality!

C.A.A., S.D.S.

Jean Chow earned her Bachelor's and Master's degrees in nursing from the University of Calgary. She received her PhD in Nursing from the University of Colorado Health Sciences in Denver. She received her nurse-midwifery education from the State University of New York Stony Brook. She also earned a diploma in acupuncture from Grant McEwan University and facilitates the use of Chinese medicine for pregnant women. She has worked in labour and delivery as a RN and nurse midwife. Jean has taught in diploma, baccalaureate, and master in nursing programs. She believes that nurses need to be well educated in maternity, newborn care, and women's health to engage women and families in health promotion activities to build the foundation for healthy children, adults, and families.

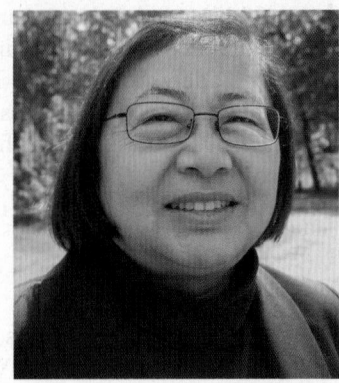

Dr. Christine A. Ateah holds a Diploma in Nursing (St. Boniface Hospital), Bachelor of Nursing (University of Manitoba), Master of Education (University of Alberta) and Interdisciplinary PhD (Family Studies, Nursing, Psychology, Community Health Sciences; University of Manitoba). Dr. Ateah has experience as a pediatric clinical nurse in medical, surgical, and community clinic settings. Over the past 20 years, she has taught undergraduate and graduate nursing education and conducted research in child and family health promotion, with a focus on parent education, child abuse prevention, and interprofessional education for health disciplines. In 2008, she was awarded the Excellence Award in Professional Nursing (Education) by the College of Registered Nurses of Manitoba.

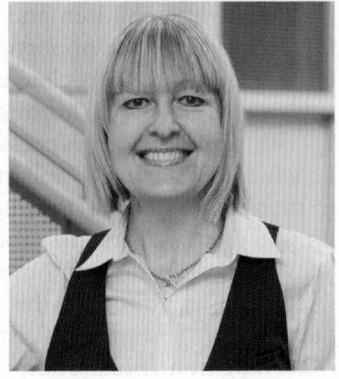

Dr. Ateah has conducted research on issues related to healthy child development including new parents' information needs, educational needs of parents of young children, experiences of and attitudes toward physical punishment across cultures, parent and infant bed-sharing practices, and pre-natal parent education intervention. She is a strong advocate for children's rights and is dedicated to helping parents promote the healthy development of their children.

Dr. Ateah has presented and published her research at the local, national, and international levels. She is a Scientist with the Manitoba Institute of Child Health and has co-authored a Canadian textbook on human development, now in its second edition, and has co-edited a book on family violence prevention.

Dr. Shannon D. Scott completed a Bachelor of Nursing, Masters of Nursing (both from the University of Manitoba), a PhD in Nursing (University of Alberta), and a Post-Doctoral Fellowship in the Department of Pediatrics, Faculty of Medicine and Dentistry from the University of Alberta. Dr. Scott worked as a pediatric nurse in medical/surgical and pediatric oncology areas. She has taught at the undergraduate programs of nursing at the University of Manitoba and currently at the University of Alberta in the undergraduate and graduate programs. For the past 20 years, Dr. Scott has been involved in the conduct of nursing research and currently has a large program of research called ECHO (translating Evidence into Child Health practice to enhance Outcomes). The research projects in Dr. Scott's program reflect her belief of the importance of the best available research evidence informing children's healthcare. Her research projects investigate the implementation of pediatric clinical pathways and guidelines. In 2010, Dr. Scott received prestigious *Population Health Investigator Award* from the *Alberta*

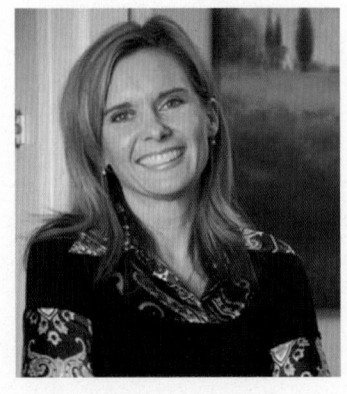

Heritage Foundation for Medical Research and a *New Investigator Award* from the *Canadian Institutes of Health Research* (2011). These awards allow her to dedicate her time to further develop her research program. Dr. Scott has a strong cohort of graduate students who lead many projects on research-based pediatric healthcare.

Dr. Scott has published more than 50 papers and has presented her research at local, national, and international venues. She is a member of the *Women and Children's Health Research Institute (University of Alberta)* and a member of the *International StarChild Risk of Bias Sub-committee* that is working to improve the conduct of research in children.

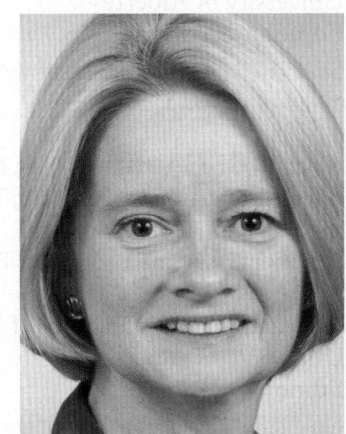

Susan Scott Ricci has a diploma from Washington Hospital Center School of Nursing, with a BSN, MSN, from Catholic University of America in Washington, D.C., and an M.Ed. in Counselling from the University of Southern Mississippi. She has worked in numerous women's health care settings, including labour and delivery, postpartum, prenatal, and family planning ambulatory care clinics. Susan is a women's health care nurse practitioner who has spent 30+ years in nursing education teaching in LPN, ADN, and BSN programs. She is involved in several professional nursing organizations and holds memberships in Sigma Theta Tau International Honor Society of Nursing, National Association of Ob/Gyn Nurses, Who's Who in Professional Nursing, American Nurses Association, and the Florida Council of Maternal-Child Nurses.

With Susan Scott Ricci's wealth of practical and educational experience, the time has come for her to concentrate on the "essential facts" of nursing instruction and reduce the amount of "nice to know" information that is presented to students. As an educator, she recognized the tendency for nursing educators to want to "cover the world" when teaching rather than focusing on the facts that students need to know to practice nursing. With this thought, Susan has directed her energy to the *birth* of this essentials textbook.

She recognizes that instructional time is shrinking as the world of health care is expanding exponentially. Therefore, with the valuable instructional time allotted, she has recognized the urgent need to present pertinent facts as concisely as possible to promote application of knowledge within nursing practice.

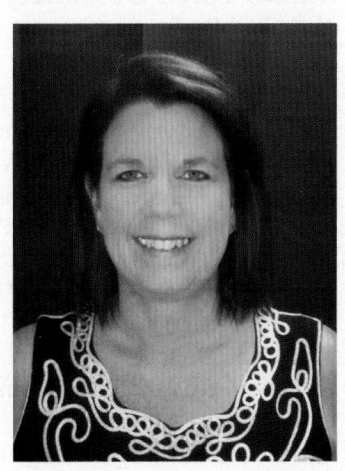

Terri Kyle earned a Bachelor of Science in Nursing from the University of North Carolina at Chapel Hill and a Master of Science in Nursing from Emory University in Atlanta, Georgia. She is a certified pediatric nurse practitioner and is currently enrolled in the Doctor of Nursing Practice program at the University of Florida. Practicing pediatric nursing for over 20 years, Terri has had the opportunity to serve children and their families in a variety of diverse settings.

She has experience in in-patient pediatrics in pediatric and neonatal intensive care units, newborn nursery, specialized pediatric units, and community hospitals. She has worked as a pediatric nurse practitioner in pediatric specialty clinics and primary care. She has been involved in teaching nursing for over 15 years with experience in both graduate and undergraduate education. Terri is a fellow in the National Association of Pediatric Nurse Practitioners and a member of the Sigma Theta Tau International Honor Society of Nursing, the National League for Nursing, the Society of Pediatric Nurses, and the Association of Camp Nurses.

With the limited time allotted in schools to the topic of maternity and pediatric nursing, Terri recognized the need for a textbook that "got to the point." She strongly believes in a concepts-based approach for learning nursing—that is, to teach the basics to students in a broad, contextual format so that they can apply that knowledge in a variety of situations. The concepts-based approach to nursing education is time efficient for nursing educators and fosters the development of critical thinking skills in student nurses.

CONTRIBUTORS TO THE FIRST CANADIAN EDITION

Keith E. Aronyk, MD, FRCSC
Divisional Director, Neurosurgery
Department of Surgery
University of Alberta
Edmonton, Alberta
CHAPTER 37 • Nursing Care of the Child with
a Neurologic Disorder

Mary E. Bauman, RN, BA, MN, NP
Nurse Practitioner, Pediatric Thrombosis
Stollery Children's Hospital
Adjunct Assistant Professor; Faculty of Medicine and
    Dentistry
Associate Faculty; Faculty of Nursing
University of Alberta
Edmonton, Alberta
CHAPTER 46 • Nursing Care of the Child with
a Hematologic Disorder

Angela Bayes, MN, NP
Nurse Practitioner, Pediatrics
Alberta Health Services
Calgary, Alberta
CHAPTER 33 • Nursing Care of the Child with
Special Needs

Susan Ruth Beischel, RN, BN, MN
Associate Professor
Mount Royal University
Calgary, Alberta
CHAPTER 20 • Nursing Management of Pregnancy at Risk:
Selected Health Conditions and Vulnerable Populations
CHAPTER 22 • Nursing Management of the Postpartum
Woman at Risk

Judy R. Bowie, RN, MN
Nursing Instructor
Red Deer College
Collaborative BScN Program
University of Alberta
Red Deer, Alberta
CHAPTER 11 • Maternal Adaptation During Pregnancy

Andrea Brandt, RN, BScN, MN
Professor
Georgian College
Staff Nurse
The Hospital for Sick Children
Barrie, Ontario
CHAPTER 17 • Newborn Adaptation

Lesa L. K. Chizawsky, RN, MN
Unit Manager
Stollery Children's Hospital
Edmonton, Alberta
CHAPTER 52 • Nursing Care During a Pediatric Emergency

Shelley Cobbett, RN, MN, Gnt, EdD
Assistant Professor
School of Nursing
Dalhousie University
Yarmouth, Nova Scotia
CHAPTER 8 • Cancers of the Female Reproductive Tract

Genevieve Currie, RN, MN
Associate Professor
Mount Royal University
Calgary, Alberta
CHAPTER 2 • Family-Centred Community-Based Care

Pia DeZorzi, BScN, RN, CPON
Professional Practice Leader, Nursing
British Columbia Children's Hospital
Vancouver, British Columbia
CHAPTER 47 • Nursing Care of the Child with
an Immunologic Disorder

Gwen Erdmann, BScN, RN
Manager, Medication Quality and Safety,
    Pharmacy Services
Alberta Health Services
University of Alberta
Edmonton, Alberta
CHAPTER 47 • Nursing Care of the Child with an
Immunologic Disorder

Kathleen Firth, RN, MN
Nurse Practitioner, Pediatric Orthopedics and Plastics
Stollery Children's Hospital
Edmonton, Alberta
CHAPTER 44 • Nursing Care of the Child with
a Musculoskeletal Disorder

Debbie Fraser, MN, RNC-NIC
Associate Professor
Advanced Nurse Practitioner Program
Centre for Nursing and Health Studies
Athabasca University
Athabasca, Alberta
CHAPTER 31 • Health Assessment of Children
CHAPTER 36 • Nursing Care of the Child with an Infectious
or Communicable Disorder

Jane Fryer, RN, BScN, MN
Nursing Instructor
Vancouver Career College
Abbotsford, British Columbia
CHAPTER 32 • Nursing Care of Children During Illness
and Hospitalization

Melanie Hamilton, RN, BN, MN
Nursing Instructor
Lethbridge College, Lethbridge, Alberta
CHAPTER 4 • Common Reproductive Issues

Elva Hammarstrand, RN, MN
Nursing Instructor
Red Deer College
Red Deer, Alberta
CHAPTER 1 • Perspectives on Maternal and Child Health Care

B. Nicole Harder, RN, MPA, PhD
Coordinator, Simulation Learning Centre
Faculty of Nursing
University of Manitoba
Winnipeg, Manitoba
CHAPTER 34 • Medication Administration, Intravenous Therapy,
and Nutritional Support

Lynne Harwood-Lunn, BScN, MN
Sessional Lecturer
York University
Toronto, Ontario
CHAPTER 23 • Nursing Care of the Newborn with Special Needs

Lois Hawkins, RN, BN, MN
Nurse Practitioner, Pediatric Cardiac Sciences
Faculty of Nursing
Stollery Children's Hospital
Associate Faculty
University of Alberta
Edmonton, Alberta
CHAPTER 40 • Nursing Care of the Child with
a Cardiovascular Disorder

Cindy Holland, RN, MN
Nurse Practitioner, Pediatric General Surgery
Winnipeg Children's Hospital
University of Manitoba
Winnipeg, Manitoba
CHAPTER 41 • Nursing Care of the Child with
a Gastrointestinal Disorder

Joan M. Humphries, RN, BSN, MN
Nurse Educator, Doctoral Student (Nursing)
Camosun College
University of Victoria
Victoria, British Columbia
CHAPTER 16 • Nursing Management During the
Postpartum Period

Sylvia M. Loewen
Senior Instructor
University of Calgary
Calgary, Alberta
CHAPTER 1 • Perspectives on Maternal and Child Health Care

Tara Loutit, RN, BSN
Faculty
British Columbia Institute of Technology
Burnaby, British Columbia
CHAPTER 18 • Nursing Management of the Newborn

Tracy Lynne Mackie, RN, MN, NP
Pediatric Nurse Practitioner
Sessional Instructor, University of Calgary
Nurse Practitioner, Unit 31 Pediatrics
Peter Lougheed Hospital
Calgary, Alberta
CHAPTER 45 • Nursing Care of the Child with
an Integumentary Disorder

Karen MacKinnon, RN, MScN, PhD
Assistant Professor
School of Nursing
University of Victoria
Victoria, British Columbia
CHAPTER 12 • Nursing Management During Pregnancy

Cyndee L. MacPhee
Associate Professor
Cape Breton University
Sydney, Nova Scotia
CHAPTER 14 • Nursing Management During Labour and Birth

Deborah Mansell, RN, MN
Assistant Professor
Mount Royal University
Calgary, Alberta
CHAPTER 15 • Postpartum Adaptations

Lenora Marcellus, RN, BSN, MN, PhD
Assistant Professor
School of Nursing
University of Victoria
Victoria, British Columbia
CHAPTER 10 • Fetal Development and Genetics
CHAPTER 18 • Nursing Management of the Newborn

Donna Martin, RN, PhD
Assistant Professor
Faculty of Nursing
University of Manitoba
Winnipeg, Manitoba
CHAPTER 43 • Nursing Care of the Child with
a Neuromuscular Disorder

Wilma McClure, RN
Former Nurse Coordinator, Dr. John Akabutu
  Comprehensive Centre for Bleeding Disorders
University of Alberta Hospital
Stollery Children's Hospital
Edmonton, Alberta
CHAPTER 46 • Nursing Care of the Child with a Hematologic
Disorder

Donna C. Meyer, RN, BScN, IBCLC
Public Health Nurse
Westview Public Health Nursing
Alberta Health Services
Edmonton, Alberta
CHAPTER 30 • Health Supervision

Pertice Moffitt, RN, BSN, MN, PhD
Senior Instructor of Nursing, Adjunct Professor
Aurora College
Yellowknife, Northwest Territories
CHAPTER 5 • Sexually Transmitted Infections

Susan Neufeld, RN, PhD
Sessional Instructor
Faculty of Nursing
University of Alberta
Edmonton, Alberta
CHAPTER 37 • Nursing Care of the Child with
a Neurologic Disorder

Deborah L. Olmstead, RN, MN
Clinical Nurse Specialist, Pediatric Respirology
Stollery Children's Hospital, Alberta Health Services
Edmonton, Alberta
CHAPTER 30 • Health Supervision

Shirley Perry, MN, RN
Nurse Practitioner, Pediatric Oncology
Stollery Children's Hospital
Edmonton, Alberta
CHAPTER 32 • Nursing Care of Children During Illness
and Hospitalization

Jannell A. Plouffe, RN, NP, BScN, MN, DNP
Director, Clinical Education
Health Sciences Centre
Adjunct Professor
Faculty of Nursing
University of Manitoba
Winnipeg, Manitoba
CHAPTER 39 • Nursing Care of the Child with
a Respiratory Disorder

Sherry Poncsak, RN, MN
Nursing Instructor
Red Deer College
Red Deer, Alberta
CHAPTER 19 • Nursing Management of Pregnancy at Risk:
Pregnancy-Related Complications

Margaret Quance, RN, PhD
Assistant Professor
Mount Royal University
Calgary, Alberta
CHAPTER 2 • Family-Centred Community-Based Care

Gwen R. Rempel, PhD, RN
Associate Professor; Alberta Heritage Foundation
    for Medical Research Population Health
    Investigator
Faculty of Nursing
University of Alberta
Edmonton, Alberta
CHAPTER 40 • Nursing Care of the Child with
a Cardiovascular Disorder

Susan Richards, RN, BScN, MN
Pediatric Otolaryngology Nurse Practitioner
Stollery Children's Hospital
Edmonton, Alberta
CHAPTER 38 • Nursing Care of the Child with
a Disorder of the Eyes or Ears

Cathy Ringham, RN, BSN
Doctoral Student
University of Victoria
Victoria, British Columbia
CHAPTER 24 • Nursing Management of the Newborn at Risk:
Acquired and Congenital Newborn Conditions

Doris Sawatzky-Dickson, MN, RN
Clinical Nurse Specialist
Health Sciences Centre
Lecturer
Faculty of Nursing
University of Manitoba
Winnipeg, Manitoba
Chapter 43: Nursing Care of the Child with
a Neuromuscular Disorder

Lisa Semple, RN, BN, MN
Assistant Professor
School of Nursing
Mount Royal University
Calgary, Alberta
CHAPTER 2 • Family-Centred Community-Based Care

Sarah Southon, MN, NP
Nurse Practitioner–Pediatric Spinal Deformities
Associate Faculty
University of Alberta
Stollery Children's Hospital
Edmonton, Alberta
CHAPTER 44 • Nursing Care of the Child with
a Musculoskeletal Disorder

Jennifer N. Stinson, RN, PhD, CPNP
Scientist, Child Health Evaluative Sciences
Nurse Practitioner, Chronic Pain Program
The Hospital for Sick Children
Assistant Professor
Lawrence S. Bloomberg Faculty of Nursing
University of Toronto
Toronto, Ontario
CHAPTER 35 • Pain Management in Children

Kala Streibel, RN, BScN
Nursing Instructor
Red Deer College
Red Deer, Alberta
CHAPTER 21 • Nursing Management of Labour and Birth at Risk

Julie Strong, RN, BN
Pediatric Transplant Coordinator
Transplant Manitoba—Pediatric Kidney Program
Children's Hospital, Health Sciences Centre
Winnipeg, Manitoba
CHAPTER 42 • Nursing Care of the Child with
a Genitourinary Disorder

Beverley Temple, RN, PhD
Assistant Professor, Researcher
St. Amant Research Centre
University of Manitoba
Winnipeg, Manitoba
CHAPTER 50 • Nursing Care of the Child with
a Genetic Disorder
CHAPTER 51 • Nursing Care of the Child with
a Cognitive or Mental Health Disorder

Jennifer E. Tyrrell, RN, MN
Clinical Nurse Specialist
The Hospital for Sick Children
Toronto, Ontario
CHAPTER 35 • Pain Management in Children

Mary Anne Venner, BScN, MN, NP
Pediatric Nurse Practitioner, Hematology Program
Stollery Children's Hospital
Alberta Health Services
Edmonton, Alberta
CHAPTER 46 • Nursing Care of the Child with
a Hematologic Disorder

Christina B. Whittaker, RN, MN
Nurse Educator and Patient Education Coordinator
Child Health Program
Health Sciences Centre
Winnipeg Regional Health Authority
Winnipeg, Manitoba
CHAPTER 48 • Nursing Care of the Child with
an Endocrine Disorder

Roberta L. Woodgate, RN, MN, PhD
Professor, Child Health and Illness
Faculty of Nursing
University of Manitoba
Winnipeg, Manitoba
CHAPTER 49 • Nursing Care of the Child with
a Neoplastic Disorder

REVIEWERS OF THE FIRST CANADIAN EDITION

Marion Alex, RN, MN, CNM
Associate Professor
School of Nursing
St. Francis Xavier University
Antigonish, Nova Scotia

Esther Aneke, RN, MSN, RM
BSN Faculty
Douglas College
New Westminster, British Columbia

Mandy M. Archibald, BScN, MN—PhD student
Research Assistant, Pediatric Registered Nurse
Stollery Children's Hospital
University of Alberta
Edmonton, Alberta

Joy Baker, BSN
Instructor of Nursing
University of Northern British Columbia—South
    Central Campus
Quesnel, British Columbia

Carol D. Banks, RN, BScN, MN(c), MBA
Professor of Nursing and Coordinator, Practical
    Nursing Program
Lambton College
Sarnia, Ontario

Jane Barnes, RN, BScN, MA
Nursing Faculty
Georgian College
Barrie, Ontario

Marisa E. Blahovich, RN, BScN, MScNEd
Partial Load Nursing Faculty
Institute for Applied Health Science—Mohawk College
Hamilton, Ontario

E. Gail Bremer, RN, BScN, BPE, MEd
Instructor
School of Nursing
Langara College
Vancouver, British Columbia

Mona Burrows, RN(EC), BScN, MSN, PHCNP
Professor
BScN Collaborative Program
St. Lawrence College/Laurentian University
Cornwall, Ontario

Natasha Bursey, RN, BN
Health Programs Instructor—BSN
Aurora College
Yellowknife, Northwest Territories

Ruth P. Chen, RN, MSN, PhD(c)
Assistant Professor
McMaster University
Hamilton, Ontario

Anu Chiarelli, RN, BA, MA
Instructor
Bow Valley College
Calgary, Alberta

Luisa Ciofani, RN, MSc(A), IBCLC, PNC(C)
Clinical Nurse Specialist—Obstetrics
McGill University Health Centre
Royal Victoria Hospital
Montreal, Quebec

Debra Clare, RN, BScN, MSN
Lecturer
Thompson Rivers University
Kamloops, British Columbia

Marianne Cochrane
Interim Co-Director, Collaborative BScN program
Durham College/University of Ontario Institute of
    Technology
Oshawa, Ontario

Lynn A. Cooze, MN, RN
Assistant Professor
School of Nursing
Memorial University of Newfoundland
St. John's, Newfoundland

Genevieve Currie, RN, BN, MN
Associate Professor
School of Nursing
Mount Royal University
Calgary, Alberta

Sally Dampier, RN, BScN, MMedSc(N)
Professor
Confederation College
Thunder Bay, Ontario

Arlene B. de la Rocha, RN, MEd, MScN
Professor
Collaborative BScN Program
Durham College
University of Ontario Institute of Technology
Oshawa, Ontario

Sharon Demers, RN, BN, CAE
Instructor
Assiniboine Community College
Winnipeg, Manitoba

Manjit Dhanoa-Yasi, RN, BScN, MN
Undergraduate Lecturer
Lawrence S. Bloomberg Faculty of Nursing
University of Toronto
Toronto, Ontario

Nancy A. Dower, BSc, PhD, MD, FRCPC
Medical Director of Pediatric Hematology
Co-Director of the Dr. John Akabutu Centre for
  Bleeding Disorders
Stollery Children's Hospital
Associate Professor of Pediatrics
University of Alberta
Edmonton, Alberta

M. Patrice Drake, BSc, BN, MN, RN
Clinical Nursing Instructor
School of Nursing
University of Prince Edward Island
Charlottetown, Prince Edward Island

Karen Driol, MS, BSN, RN
Faculty
School of Nursing
British Columbia Institute of Technology
Burnaby, British Columbia

Kerry Lynn Durnford, RN, BN, MN
Nursing Instructor
Health and Human Services Program
Aurora College
Yellowknife, Northwest Territories

Mary Elliott, RN, BScN, MEd
Professor
Humber Bachelor of Nursing Program
University of New Brunswick
Toronto, Ontario

Sheila Epp, BSN, MN, RN
Senior Instructor
School of Nursing
University of British Columbia (Okanagan Campus)
Kelowna, British Columbia

Katherine Fryer, EdD, MN, MBA, BScN
Lecturer
University of Windsor
Windsor, Ontario

Beverly Gaudet, RN, MN
Senior Instructor
Faculty of Nursing
University of New Brunswick
Fredericton, New Brunswick

Neghesti G. Gebru, RN, BScM, MN, PhD
Professor of Nursing
Cambrian College
Sudbury, Ontario

Wendy Gillespie, RN, NP, BScN, MN
Instructor
University of Calgary
Calgary, Alberta

Erin Glynn, RN, MN
Faculty
School of Nursing
Memorial University
St. John's, Newfoundland

Joanne Guatto
Professor of Nursing
George Brown College
Toronto, Ontario

Michelle Gulbransen, RN, BScN, MN
Professor
School of Nursing
St. Clair College
Windsor, Ontario

Mona Haimour, BScN, MN, RN
Faculty
Faculty of Health and Community Studies
Grant MacEwan University
Edmonton, Alberta

Melanie J. Hamilton, RN, BN, MN
Nursing Instructor
Department of Nursing Education & Health Sciences
Grande Prairie Regional College
Grande Prairie, Alberta

Elva Hammarstrand, RN, BN, MN
Instructor
Red Deer College
Red Deer, Alberta

Kathryn M. Hayward, MN, BScN, RN, IBCLC
Assistant Professor
School of Nursing
Dalhousie University
Halifax, Nova Scotia

Lisa Henczel, BSN, MSN, NP(F)
Family Nurse Practitioner
Professor/Lecturer
School of Nursing
University of British Columbia
Vancouver, British Columbia

Karen Hewson, RN, MN
Assistant Professor
College of Nursing
Southern Saskatchewan Campus
University of Saskatchewan
Regina, Saskatchewan

Nicole Irving, BN, RN
Instructor
Faculty of Nursing
University of New Brunswick
Fredericton, New Brunswick

Paul Jeffrey, RN (EC), BScN, MN, NP-Adult
Program Coordinator
Professor of Health Sciences, Nursing
Institute of Technology & Advanced Learning Faculty
   of Applied Health & Community Studies
Davis Campus
Sheridan College
Brampton, Ontario

Jennifer Anne Kane, RN, BSN, MEd
Faculty—BSN Program
Douglas College
Coquitlam, British Columbia

Paula Kelly, RN, BN, MN
Lecturer
School of Nursing
Memorial University of Newfoundland
St John's, Newfoundland

Siwon Kim, RN, BSN, MSN
Perinatal Faculty
British Columbia Institute of Technology
Burnaby, British Columbia

Amy Klepetar, RN, BA, BScN, MSPH
Assistant Professor
University of Northern British Columbia
Terrace, British Columbia

Sandra Kluka, RN, BN, MN, PhD
Program Coordinator
University of Manitoba
Winnipeg, Manitoba

Mary Anne Krahn, RN, BScN, MScN
BScN Program and Year Two Coordinator
Fanshawe College
London, Ontario

Roxanne Laforge, RN, MS, BSN, BA
Coordinator, Perinatal Education Program
Division of Continuing Professional Learning, College
   of Medicine
Continuing Nursing Education, College of Nursing
University of Saskatchewan
Saskatoon, Saskatchewan

Deborah Mansell, RN, MN
Instructor
Faculty of Nursing
University of Calgary
Calgary, Alberta

Lenora Marcellus, RN, BSN, MN, PhD
Assistant Professor
School of Nursing
University of Victoria
Victoria, British Columbia

Cathy Maser, RN-EC, BScN, MN, NP-Paeds
Lecturer
Lawrence S. Bloomberg Faculty of Nursing
University of Toronto
Nurse Practitioner
Division of Adolescent Medicine
The Hospital for Sick Children
Toronto, Ontario

Erin Miller, BScN
Faculty/Nurse Educator
Grant MacEwan University
Edmonton, Alberta

Kathy Mitchell, RN, BN
Professor
Faculty of Nursing
Algonquin College
Ottawa, Ontario

Jeanette Murray, RN, BScN, MA
Chairperson
School of Nursing
Thompson Rivers University
Kamloops, British Columbia

Marcella Ogenchuk, RN, PhD
Assistant Professor
College of Nursing
University of Saskatchewan
Saskatoon, Saskatchewan

Rebekah O'Neill, RN, BScN, MScN
Faculty of Health and Wellness (BScN Program)
Georgian College
Barrie, Ontario

Heather Ouellette, RN, BScN, MSc
Senior Laboratory Instructor
Clinical Lead, Paediatrics
School of Nursing
University of Northern British Columbia
Prince George, British Columbia

Pamela Pastirik, BN, MSN
Senior Nursing Instructor
Department of Nursing
University of New Brunswick
Saint John, New Brunswick

Chandra Pham, RN, BScN, MSN
Faculty
Douglas College
Coquitlam, British Columbia

Misty D. Reis, MN, NP, RN
Nurse Practitioner, Neonatal and Infant Follow
   Up Clinic
Glenrose Rehabilitation Hospital
Associate Faculty
Faculty of Nursing
University of Alberta
Edmonton, Alberta

Cathy P. Robinson, RN, BSN, MSN
Nursing Instructor
University of British Columbia—Okanagan
Kelowna, British Columbia

Shawna Rooke, RN, BSc, CCRN, MSc(c)
Advanced Nursing Practice Educator
The Hospital for Sick Children
Assistant Professor
University of Toronto
Toronto, Ontario

Frances Ross, RN, BScN, MScN
Professor
George Brown College
Toronto, Ontario

Kathryn Rousseau, BA, MScN, RN
Professor, Nursing
St. Clair College
Windsor, Ontario

Kerry Rusk, BScN, MN
Faculty Lecturer
Faculty of Nursing
University of Alberta
Edmonton, Alberta

Anna Schottner, RN, BN, MEd
Nursing Instructor
Medicine Hat College
Medicine Hat, Alberta

Stacey A. Sheets, RN, BScN, MScN
Professor of Nursing, Collaborative Nursing Program
St. Clair College of Applied Arts & Technology
Windsor, Ontario

Catherine Sheffer, MN, RN, PNC(C)
Lecturer
Dalhousie University
Halifax, Nova Scotia

Joanna Simmons-Swinden, RN
Nursing Instructor
Red River College
Winnipeg, Manitoba

Candy Sloboda, BN, MEd
Faculty Lecturer
University of Alberta
Edmonton, Alberta

Barbara Thompson, RN, BScN, MScN
Professor of Nursing
Sault College
Sault Ste. Marie, Ontario

Bev Valkenier
Lecturer
School of Nursing
University of British Columbia
Vancouver, British Columbia

Dale Wagner, RN, BSN, MS
Program Coordinator/Lecturer
School of Nursing
Thompson Rivers University
Kamloops, British Columbia

Janis Wegerhoff, RN, BScN, MN
Associate Professor and Chair of the Department of
    Advanced Specialty Health Studies
Mount Royal University
Calgary, Alberta

Wendy M. Wheeler, RN, BScN, MN
Instructor
Red Deer College
Reed Deer, Alberta

Colleen Wilkinson, RN, MS (N)
Academic Associate
Faculty of Health Sciences
University of Ontario Institute of Technology
Oshawa, Ontario

Jo'Anne Yearley, RN, MN, PNC(C)
Professor
Vancouver Island University
Nanaimo, British Columbia

CONTRIBUTING EDITOR AND REVIEWERS OF THE U.S. EDITION

CONTRIBUTING EDITOR

Susan Carman, BSN, MSN, MBA
Hubertus, Wisconsin

REVIEWERS

Virgie Barnes
Somerset Community College
Somerset, Kentucky

Kathleen Barta
University of Arkansas, Fayetteville
Fayetteville, Arkansas

Peggy Bozarth
Hopkinsville Community College
Hopkinsville, Kentucky

Marie Bright-Cobb
University of Akron
Akron, Ohio

Michele Brimeyer
University of Florida
Gainesville, Florida

Darlene Cantu
San Antonio College
San Antonio, Texas

Angelina Chambers
University of Texas Health Sciences, Houston
Houston, Texas

Patricia Coyne
Cochran School of Nursing
Yonkers, New York

Karen Davis
University of Arkansas Medical Sciences
Little Rock, Arkansas

Karen DeBoer
Macomb City CC Centre
Clinton Township, Michigan

Carol Deresz
University of Texas Health Sciences, San Antonio
San Antonio, Texas

Patricia DuClos-Miller
Capital Community College
Hartford, Connecticut

Linda Dunn
University of Alabama, Tuscaloosa
Tuscaloosa, Alabama

Bernadette Emerick
Indian River Community College
Fort Pierce, Florida

Mary-Margaret Finney
North Georgia College
Dahlonega, Georgia

Jamie Flower
University of Arkansas, Fort Smith
Fort Smith, Arkansas

Rosa Garces
University of Puerto Rico Medical Sciences
Mercedita, Puerto Rico

Susan Gauthier
University of Alberta
Edmonton, Alberta

Julie Greenawalt
Indiana University of Pennsylvania
Indiana, Pennsylvania

Teresa James
University of Texas Health Science Centre
San Antonio, Texas

Gloria Johns
Georgia Perimeter College
Clarkston, Georgia

Kathy Johnson
University of South Dakota
Sioux Falls, South Dakota

PREFACE

Many nursing curricula combine and teach maternity and pediatrics in tandem. This can be viewed as a *natural fit* of two content areas that belong together. Nursing education in general is founded upon the principle of mastering simpler concepts first and incorporating those concepts into the student's knowledge base. The student is then able to progress to problem solving in more complex situations. In today's education climate with reduced class time devoted to specialty courses, it is particularly important for nursing educators to focus on key concepts, rather than attempting to cover everything within a specific topic.

The intent of *Canadian Maternity and Pediatric Nursing* is to provide the nurse the basis needed for sound nursing care of women and children. The content in the book will enable the reader to guide women and children toward higher levels of wellness throughout the life cycle. The main objective of this adaptation of Susan Ricci and Terri Kyle's *Maternity and Pediatric Nursing* is to aid the students in building a strong knowledge base that reflects the Canadian context as well as to assist with the development of critical thinking skills. In addition, the focus of the textbook will allow the reader to anticipate, identify, and address common problems and provide timely, evidence-based interventions to reduce long-term sequelae.

This textbook is designed as a practical approach to understanding the health of women and children. The main objective is to help the student build a strong knowledge base and assist with the development of critical thinking skills. Women in our society are becoming empowered to make informed and responsible choices regarding their health and that of their children, but to do so they need the encouragement and support of nurses who care for them. This textbook focuses on women and children throughout their lifespan, covering a broad scope of topics with emphasis placed upon common issues. Maternity nursing content coverage is comprehensive, yet presented in a concise and straightforward manner. The pediatric nursing content presents the important differences when caring for children compared with caring for adults. A nursing process approach provides relevant information in a concise and non-redundant manner. The content covered in the text arms the student or practicing nurse with essential information to care for women and their families, to assist them to make the right choices safely, intelligently, and with confidence.

Organization

Each chapter of *Canadian Maternity and Pediatric Nursing* focuses on a different aspect of maternity and/or pediatric nursing care. The book is divided into eleven units, beginning with general concepts related to maternity and pediatric nursing care, progressing from women's health, pregnancy and birth, through child health promotion and nursing management of alterations in children's health.

Unit 1: Introduction to Maternity and Pediatric Nursing

Unit 1 helps build a foundation for the student beginning the study of the care of women, infants, and children. This unit explores contemporary issues and trends in maternity and pediatric nursing. Perspectives on women's health and pediatric nursing, use of the nursing process, family-centred and atraumatic care, communication, and community-based nursing are addressed.

Unit 2: Women's Health Throughout the Lifespan

Unit 2 introduces the student to selected women's health topics, including structure and function of the reproductive system, common reproductive concerns, sexually transmitted infections, problems of the breast, and benign disorders and cancers of the female reproductive tract. This unit encourages the student to assist women in maintaining their quality of life, reducing their risk of disease, and becoming active partners with their health care professional.

Unit 3: Pregnancy

Unit 3 addresses topics related to normal pregnancy, including fetal development, genetics, and maternal adaptation to pregnancy. Nursing management during normal pregnancy is addressed, encouraging application of basic knowledge to nursing practice. Nursing management includes maternal and fetal assessment throughout pregnancy, interventions to promote self-care and minimize common discomforts, and patient education.

Unit 4: Labour and Birth

Unit 4 begins with an explanation of the normal labour and birth process, including maternal and fetal adaptations. This is followed by content focusing on the nurse's role during normal labour and birth, which includes maternal and fetal assessment, pharmacologic and non-pharmacologic comfort measures and pain management, and specific nursing interventions during each stage of labour and birth.

Unit 5: Postpartum Period

Unit 5 focuses on maternal adaptation during the normal postpartum period. Both physiologic and psychological aspects are explored. Paternal adaptation is also considered. This unit also presents related nursing management, including assessment of physical and emotional status, promoting comfort, assisting with elimination, counselling about sexuality and contraception, promoting nutrition, promoting family adaptation, and preparing for discharge.

Unit 6: The Newborn

Unit 6 covers physiologic and behavioral adaptations of the normal newborn. It also delves into nursing management of the normal newborn, including immediate assessment and specific interventions as well as ongoing assessment, physical examination, and specific interventions during the early newborn period.

Unit 7: Childbearing at Risk

Unit 7 shifts the focus to at-risk pregnancy, childbirth, and postpartum care. Pre-existing conditions of the woman, pregnancy-related complications, at-risk labour, emergencies associated with labour and birth, and medical conditions and complications affecting the postpartum woman are all covered. Treatment and nursing management are presented for each medical condition. This organization allows the student to build on a solid foundation of normal material when studying the at-risk content.

Unit 8: The Newborn at Risk

Unit 8 continues to centre on at-risk content. Issues of the newborn with birthweight variations, gestational age variations, congenital conditions, and acquired disorders are explored. Treatment and nursing management are presented for each medical condition. This organization helps cement the student's understanding of the material.

Unit 9: Health Promotion for the Growing Child and Family

Unit 9 provides information related to growth and development expectations of the well child from newborn through adolescence. Although not exhaustive in nature, this unit provides a broad knowledge base related to normal growth and development that the nurse can draw on in any situation. Common concerns related to growth and development and client/family education are included in each age-specific chapter.

Unit 10: Foundations of Pediatric Nursing

Unit 10 covers broad concepts that provide the foundation for providing nursing care for children. Rather than reiterating all aspects of nursing care, the unit focuses on specific details needed to provide nursing care for children in general. The content remains focused upon differences in caring for children compared with adults. Topics covered in this unit include anticipatory guidance and routine well child care (including immunization and safety), health assessment, nursing care of the child in the hospital, concerns common to special needs children, pediatric variations in medication and intravenous fluid delivery and nutritional support, and pain management in children.

Unit 11: Nursing Care of the Child with a Health Disorder

Unit 11 focuses on children's responses to health disorders. This unit provides comprehensive coverage of illnesses affecting children and is presented according to broad topics of disorders organized with a body systems approach. It also includes infectious, genetic, and mental health disorders as well as pediatric emergencies. Each chapter follows a similar format in order to facilitate presentation of the information as well as reduce repetition. The chapters begin with a nursing process overview for the particular broad topic, presenting differences in children and how the nursing process applies. The approach provides a general framework for addressing disorders within the chapter. Individual disorders are then addressed with attention to specifics related to pathophysiology, nursing assessment, nursing management, and special considerations. Common pediatric disorders are covered in greater depth than less common disorders. The format of the chapters allows for the building of a strong knowledge base and encourages critical thinking. In addition, the format is nursing process driven and consistent from chapter to chapter, providing a practical and sensible presentation of the information.

Recurring Features

In order to provide the instructor and student with an exciting and user-friendly text, a number of recurring features have been developed.

Key Terms

A list of terms that are considered essential to the chapter's understanding is presented at the beginning of each chapter. Each key term appears in boldface, with the definition included in the text. Key terms may also be accessed on thePoint.

Learning Objectives

Learning Objectives included at the beginning of each chapter guide the student in understanding what is important and why, leading the student to prioritize information for learning. These valuable learning tools also provide opportunities for self-testing or instructor evaluation of student knowledge and ability.

WOW—Words of Wisdom

Each chapter opens with inspiring Words of Wisdom, which offer helpful, timely, or interesting thoughts. These WOW statements set the stage for each chapter and give the student valuable insight into nursing care of women, children, and their families.

Case Studies

Real-life scenarios present relevant woman, child, and family information that is intended to perfect the student's caregiving skills. Questions about the scenario provide an opportunity for the student to critically evaluate the appropriate course of action.

Watch and Learn Icon

A special icon **WATCH&LEARN** throughout the book directs the student to free video clips that highlight maternity nursing care, childhood growth and development, communication with children, and provision of nursing care to children in the hospital. These clips can be viewed on thePoint website.

Evidence–Based Practice

The consistent promotion of evidence-based practice is a key feature of the text. Throughout the chapters, pivotal questions addressed by current research have been incorporated into Evidence-Based Practice displays, which cite studies relevant to chapter content.

Teaching Guidelines

An important tool for achieving health promotion and disease prevention is health education. Throughout the textbook, Teaching Guidelines raise awareness, provide timely and accurate information, and are designed to ensure the student's preparation for educating women, children, and their families about various issues.

Drug Guides

Drug guide tables summarize information about commonly used medications. The actions, indications, and significant nursing implications presented assist the student in providing optimum care to women, children, and their families.

Common Laboratory and Diagnostic Tests

The Common Laboratory and Diagnostic Tests tables in many of the chapters provide the student with a general understanding of how a broad range of disorders is diagnosed. Rather than reading the information repeatedly throughout the narrative, the student is then able to refer to the table as needed.

Common Medical Treatments

The Common Medical Treatments tables in many of the nursing management chapters provide the student with a broad awareness of how a common group of disorders is treated either medically or surgically. The tables serve as a reference point for common medical treatments.

Nursing Care Plans

Nursing Care Plans* provide concrete examples of each step of the nursing process and are included in numerous chapters. The Nursing Care Plans summarize issue-or system-related content, thereby minimizing repetition.

Comparison Charts

These charts compare two or more disorders or other easily confused concepts. They serve to provide an explanation that clarifies the concepts for the student.

Nursing Procedures

Step-by-step Nursing Procedures are presented in a clear, concise format to facilitate competent performance of relevant procedures as well as to clarify pediatric variations when appropriate.

Consider This!

In every chapter the student is asked to *Consider This!* These first-person narratives engage the student in real-life scenarios experienced by their patients. The personal accounts evoke empathy and help the student to perfect caregiving skills. Each box ends with an opportunity for further contemplation, encouraging the student to think critically about the scenario.

Take Note!

The *Take Note!* feature draws the student's attention to points of critical emphasis throughout the chapter. This feature is often used to stress life-threatening or otherwise vitally important information.

Tables, Boxes, Illustrations, and Photographs

Abundant tables and boxes summarize key content throughout the book. Additionally, beautiful illustrations and photographs help the student to visualize the content. These features allow the student to quickly and easily access information.

Key Concepts

At the end of each chapter, Key Concepts provide a quick review of essential chapter elements. These bulleted lists help the student focus on the important aspects of the chapter.

References and Websites

References and websites that were used in the development of the text are provided at the end of each chapter. These listings enable the student to further explore topics of interest. Many online resources are provided as a means for the student to electronically explore relevant content material. These resources can be shared with women, children, and their families to enhance patient education and support.

---

*Nursing diagnoses within the care plans are from *Nursing Diagnoses: Definitions and Classification 2012–2014.* Copyright © 2012, 1994–2012 by NANDA International. Used by arrangement with Blackwell Publishing Limited, a company of John Wiley & Sons, Inc. In order to make safe and effective judgments using NANDA-I diagnoses, it is essential that nurses refer to the definitions and defining characteristics of the diagnoses listed in this work.

Chapter Worksheets

Chapter worksheets at the end of each chapter assist the student in reviewing essential concepts. Chapter worksheets include:

- **Multiple Choice Questions**—These review questions are written to test the student's ability to apply chapter material. Questions cover maternal-newborn and women's health content that the student might encounter on the national licensing exam (NCLEX).
- **Critical Thinking Exercises**—These exercises challenge the student to incorporate new knowledge with previously learned concepts and reach a satisfactory conclusion. They encourage the student to think critically, problem solve, and consider his or her own perspective on given topics.
- **Study Activities**—These interactive activities promote student participation in the learning process. This section encourages increased interaction/learning via clinical, on-line, and community activities.

Teaching–Learning Package

To facilitate mastery of this text's content, a comprehensive teaching/learning package has been developed to assist faculty and students.

Instructor's Resources

Tools to assist you with teaching your course are available upon adoption of this text on thePoint at http://thePoint.lww.com/Chow1e. Many of these tools are also included on the Instructor's Resource DVD-ROM. The following resources are provided with this Canadian adaptation:

- An **E-Book** on thePoint gives you access to the book's full text and images online.
- The **Test Generator** lets you put together exclusive new tests from a bank containing hundreds of CRNE-style questions to help you in assessing your students' understanding of the material. Test questions link to chapter learning objectives.
- **PowerPoint Presentations** that correspond to each chapter provide an easy way for you to integrate the textbook with your students' classroom experience, either via slide shows or handouts.
- An **Image Bank** provides access to photographs and illustrations from the text for use in your course.

In addition, the following materials from the U.S. textbook have been provided as additional resources:

- **Pre-Lecture Quizzes** are quick, knowledge-based assessments that allow you to check students' reading.
- **Guided Lecture Notes** walk you through the chapters, objective by objective, and provide you with corresponding PowerPoint slide numbers.
- **Discussion Topics** can be used as conversation starters or in online discussion boards.
- **Assignments** include group, written, clinical, and Web assignments for use in or out of class.
- A sample **Syllabus** provides guidance for setting up your maternity and pediatric nursing course.

Student Resources

An exciting set of free resources is available to help students review material. Students can access all these resources on thePoint at http://thepoint.lww.com/ Chow1e using the codes printed in the front of their textbooks.

- An **E-Book** on thePoint allows access to the book's full text and images online.
- **Multimedia Resources** appeal to a variety of learning styles. Icons in the text direct readers to relevant videos and animations.
- **And more!**

Contact your sales representative or visit www.LWW.com/Nursing for more details and ordering information.

CONTENTS

CHAPTER *9*
Violence and Abuse   254

CHAPTER *10*
Fetal Development and Genetics   279

CHAPTER *11*
Maternal Adaptation During Pregnancy   304

CHAPTER *12*
Nursing Management During Pregnancy   331

UNIT FOUR
LABOUR AND BIRTH 381

CHAPTER 13
Labour and Birth Process 383

CHAPTER 14
Nursing Management During Labour and Birth 408

UNIT FIVE
POSTPARTUM PERIOD 451

CHAPTER 15
Postpartum Adaptations 453

CHAPTER 20

Nursing Management of the Pregnancy at Risk: Selected Health Conditions and Vulnerable Populations 619

CHAPTER 21

Nursing Management of Labour and Birth at Risk 666

CHAPTER 22

Nursing Management of the Postpartum Woman at Risk 702

U N I T E I G H T
THE NEWBORN AT RISK 723

CHAPTER 23
Nursing Care of the Newborn with Special Needs 725

CHAPTER 24
Nursing Management of the Newborn at Risk: Acquired and Congenital Newborn Conditions 755

U N I T N I N E
HEALTH PROMOTION FOR THE GROWING CHILD AND FAMILY 799

CHAPTER 25
Growth and Development of the Newborn and Infant 801

CHAPTER 26
Growth and Development of the Toddler 833

CHAPTER 27
Growth and Development of the Preschooler 862

U N I T   E L E V E N
NURSING CARE OF THE CHILD WITH A HEALTH
DISORDER 1125

CHAPTER *36*
**Nursing Care of the Child with an Infectious or
Communicable Disorder 1127**

CHAPTER 42
Nursing Care of the Child with a Genitourinary Disorder 1422

CHAPTER 43
Nursing Care of the Child with a Neuromuscular Disorder 1466

CHAPTER 44
Nursing Care of the Child with a Musculoskeletal Disorder 1503

CHAPTER 45
Nursing Care of the Child with an Integumentary Disorder   1543

CHAPTER 46
Nursing Care of the Child with a Hematologic Disorder   1576
Hematology System Overview   1577

CHAPTER *47*

Nursing Care of the Child with an Immunologic Disorder 1617

CHAPTER *48*

Nursing Care of the Child with an Endocrine Disorder 1645

CHAPTER *49*

Nursing Care of the Child with a Neoplastic Disorder 1684

UNIT ONE

INTRODUCTION TO MATERNITY AND PEDIATRIC NURSING

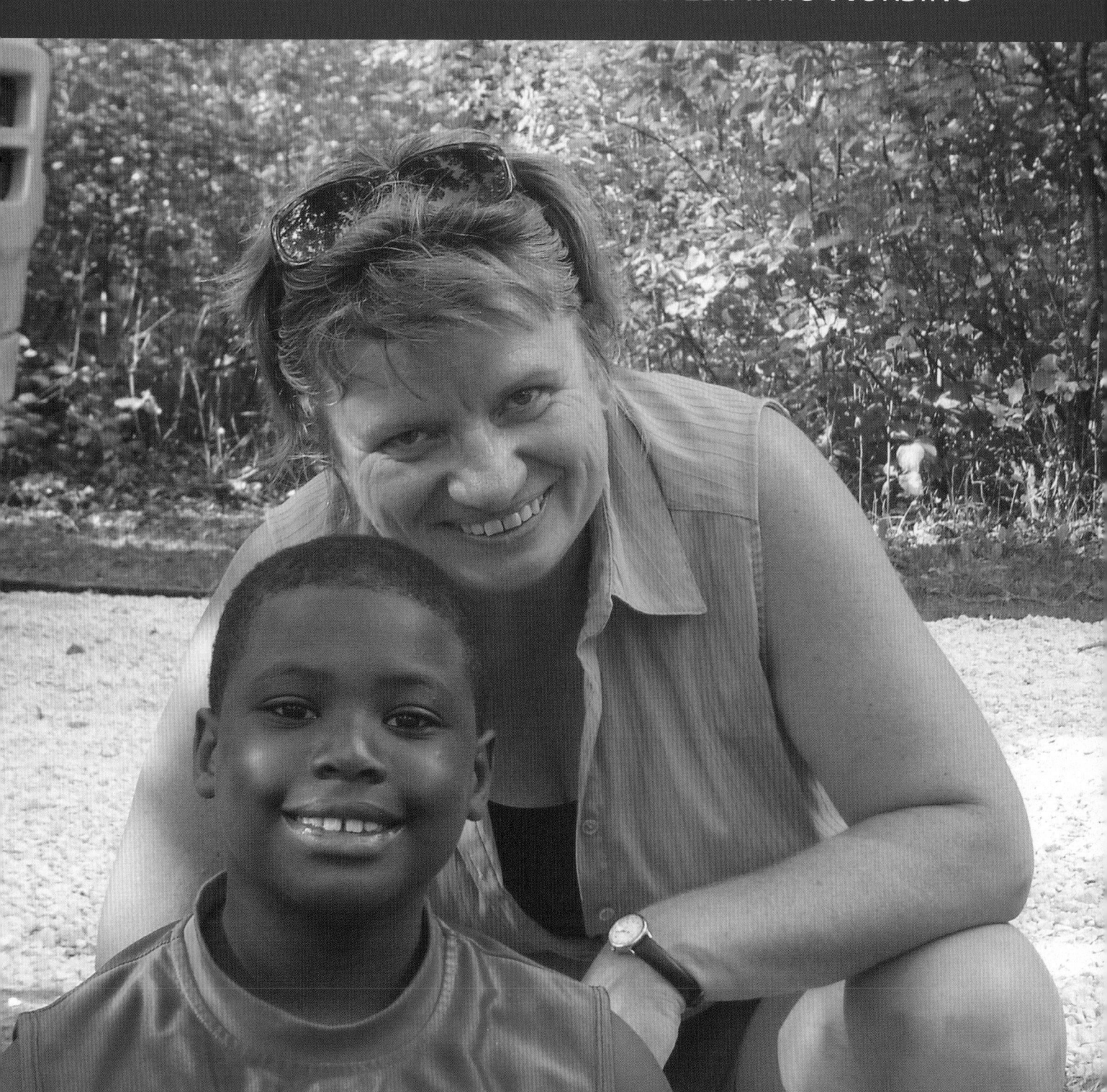

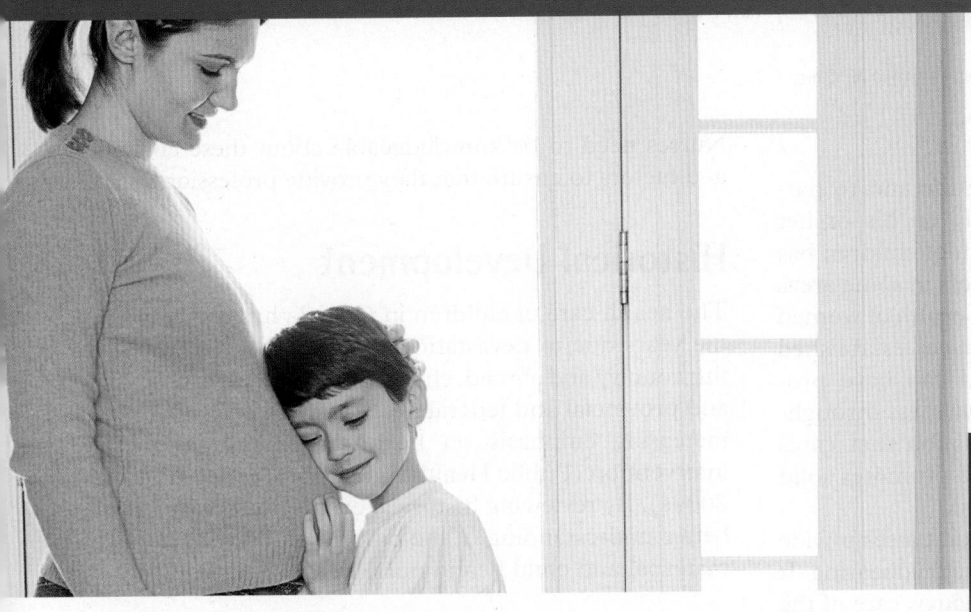

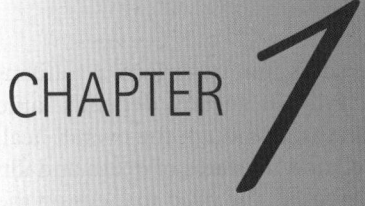

CHAPTER 1

Adapted by Elva Hammarstrand and
Sylvia M. Loewen

PERSPECTIVES ON MATERNAL AND CHILD HEALTH CARE

KEY TERMS

atraumatic care	evidence-based nursing	morbidity
case management	practice	mortality
childhood mortality rate	family	neonatal mortality rate
cultural safety	family-centred care	registered midwife
discipline	family structure	religion
doula	fetal mortality rate	social capital
emancipated minor	foster care	spirituality
ethnicity	infant mortality rate	
ethnocentrism	maternal mortality rate	

LEARNING OBJECTIVES

Upon completion of the chapter, the learner will be able to:

1. Identify the key milestones in the evolution of maternal and child health nursing.
2. Describe the major components, concepts, and influences associated with the nursing management of women, children, and families.
3. Compare past definitions of health and illness with current definitions, as well as the measurements used to assess health and illness in women and children.
4. Identify the factors that affect maternal, newborn, and child health.
5. Delineate the structures, roles, and functions of the family and how they affect the health of women and children.
6. Identify how society and culture influence the health of women, children, and families.
7. Appraise the health care barriers affecting women, children, and families.
8. Discuss the ethical and legal issues that may arise when caring for women, children, and families.

Sophia Greenly, a 38-year-old woman pregnant with her third child, comes to the prenatal clinic for a routine follow-up visit. Her mother, Betty, accompanies her because Sophia's husband is out of town. Sophia lives with her husband and two children, ages 4 and 9. She works part-time as a lunch aide in the local elementary school. What factors may play a role in influencing the health of Sophia and her family?

Wow

Being pregnant and giving birth is like crossing a narrow bridge: people can accompany you to the bridge, and they can greet you on the other side, but you walk that bridge alone. And the journey doesn't end there: children are the future of a society and special gifts to the world. Due to changes in our society and the world, we must be more vigilant and attentive to our children and their health.

Aperson's ability to lead a fulfilling life and to participate fully in society depends largely on his or her health status. Although the overall health of children has improved and the rates of death and illness in some areas have decreased, the need to focus on the health of women and children remains. Habits and practices established during pregnancy and early childhood can have profound effects on a person's health and wellness throughout life. As a society, creating a population that cares about women, children, and families and promotes solid health care and lifestyle choices is crucial.

Maternal and newborn nursing encompasses a wide scope of practice typically associated with childbearing. It includes care of the woman before pregnancy, care of the woman and her fetus during pregnancy, and care of the woman and her newborn after pregnancy, particularly during the first 6 weeks after birth. The overall goal of maternal and newborn nursing care is to promote and maintain optimal health of the woman and her family. Child health nursing, commonly referred to as pediatric nursing, involves the care of the child from infancy through adolescence. There are approximately 7.83 million children under 18 years of age in Canada, accounting for 23% of the population (Statistics Canada, 2010).

The overall goal of pediatric nursing practice is to promote and assist the child in maintaining optimal levels of health while recognizing the influence of the family on the child's well-being. Achieving this goal involves health promotion and disease and injury prevention as well as assisting with care during illness. The common thread in both of these objectives is the care of the family.

Now more than ever, nurses contribute to nearly every health care experience. Events from birth to death, and every health care emergency in between, will likely involve the presence of a nurse. Involvement of a knowledgeable, supportive, comforting nurse often leads to a positive health care experience. Skilled nursing practice depends on a solid base of knowledge and clinical expertise delivered in a caring, holistic manner. Nurses, using their knowledge and passion, help meet the health care needs of their clients throughout the lifespan, whether the client is a pregnant woman, a fetus, a partner, a child, or the parents or family members of a child. Nurses fill a variety of roles in helping clients to live healthier lives by providing direct care, emotional support, comfort, information, advice, advocacy, and counselling. Nurses are often "in the trenches" advocating for issues, drawing attention to the importance of health care, dealing with the lack of resources and timely access to physician care, and fostering health promotion and illness prevention rather than focusing primarily on acute care needs.

This chapter presents a general overview of the health care of women, children, and families and describes the major factors affecting maternal and child health.

Nurses need to be knowledgeable about these concepts and factors to ensure that they provide professional care.

Historical Development

The health care of children in Canada has changed over the years due to devastating epidemics, social trends in this country and abroad, changes in the health care system, and provincial and federal health care policies that place increasing emphasis on health promotion and early intervention (Public Health Agency of Canada [PHAC], 2009a). By reviewing historical events, nurses can gain a better understanding of the current and future status of maternal and child health nursing.

Evolution of Maternal and Newborn Nursing

Childbirth in the early history of Canada was a difficult and dangerous experience. During the 17th and 18th centuries, women giving birth often died as a result of exhaustion, dehydration, infection, hemorrhage, or seizures (Cassidy, 2006; Historica Dominion Institute, n.d.). During that era, about 50% of all children died before age 5 (Brodsky, 2006; Jolivet, 2006), compared with a child mortality rate of 5% in 2009 (UNICEF, 2010).

Historically, "neighbour midwives" handled the normal birthing process for most women. They learned their skills through an apprenticeship model. Physicians were called only if necessary, and births took place at home (Macdonald & Bourgeault, 2009).

During the early 1900s, an estimated 40% of home births were unattended by any medical personnel, including doctors, nurses, or midwives. In 1691, midwives were one of the three autonomous branches of medicine in Quebec (Herbert, 2011). Midwives underwent compulsory certification in Quebec, Nova Scotia, and New Brunswick between 1872 and 1881. By 1912, midwifery practice was eliminated in most locations with the formation of the Medical Council of Canada. During the war, public health nurses provided midwifery in rural Alberta. In 1946, the Canadian Nurses Association (CNA) approved the practice of RNs as midwives in outlying areas where physicians were not available. With the discovery and utilization of safer anesthesia and antibiotics as well as transfusion for hemorrhage, women started giving birth in hospitals and the high mortality rate associated with the complications of home births decreased dramatically.

In the 1940s and 1950s, as the fear of death during childbirth waned, pain relief became the focus of care. Providing sedation, anesthesia, and twilight sleep (a combination of an amnesic [scopolamine] and an analgesic [morphine] to produce the effect of experiencing some pain with childbirth but having no memory of it) (MedicineNet, 2003) for women during labour and

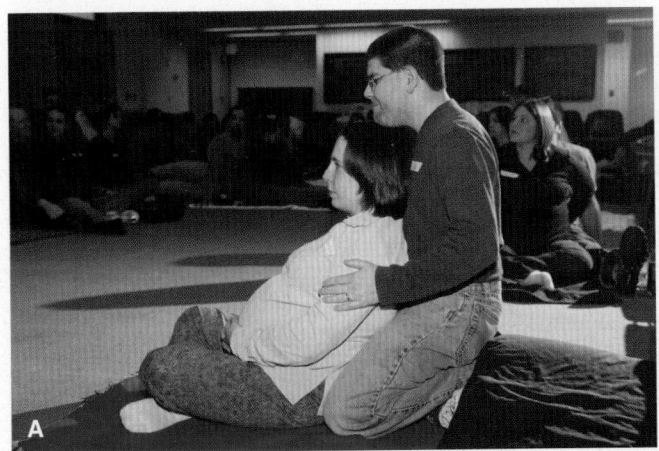
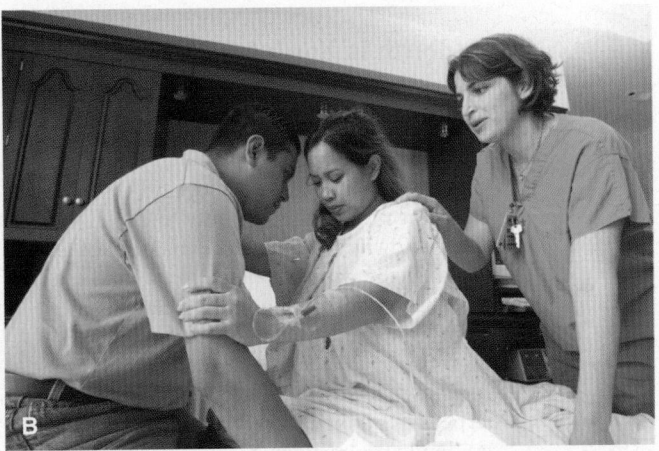

FIGURE 1.1 Today, fathers and partners are welcome to take an active role in the pregnancy and childbirth experience. (**A**) A couple can participate together in childbirth education classes. (Photo by Gus Freedman.) (**B**) Fathers and partners can assist the woman throughout her labour and delivery. (Photo by Joe Mitchell.)

delivery became common practice. As the deleterious consequences of these practices to both mother and baby became known, these practices were rejected.

So-called "natural childbirth," which involves birth without medication and focusing on relaxation techniques, became the preferred way of birthing during the 1960s and 1970s. These techniques opened the door to childbirth education classes and helped bring the father back into the picture. Both partners could participate by taking an active role in pregnancy, childbirth, and parenting (Fig. 1.1). Box 1.1 shows a timeline of childbirth in North America, with an emphasis on Canada.

Today, women have many options for how they want to conduct their labour and delivery, including a variety of what has been practiced in the past. The use of analgesia and anesthesia in the form of nitrous oxide and epidurals is common practice in larger birthing centres. Natural childbirth, using one's own inner resources to labour and birth without any externally administered analgesia, is also practiced.

We have also seen the return of midwives and doulas. The concept of women helping other women during childbirth is not new: women who laboured and gave birth at home were traditionally attended to by relatives and midwives. A **registered midwife** has training in the care of normal pregnancy and delivery and is certified by the Canadian Association of Midwives. A **doula** is a birth assistant who provides emotional, physical, and educational support to the woman and family during childbirth and the postpartum period. Many nurses working in labour and birth areas today are credentialed in their specialty through the CNA certification program. This enhances their knowledge and the level of care provided to the woman and her newborn. Childbirth choices are often based on what works best for the mother, child, and family. See Evidence-based Practice 1.1.

To help ensure that women and babies receive safe, quality care, Health Canada funded the Multidisciplinary Collaborative Primary Maternity Care Project (MCP²) to study and identify ways to reduce barriers to maternity care as well as begin to develop nationwide strategies to enhance the availability and quality of maternity care (MCP², 2006). Based on the work of this initiative, the Society of Obstetricians and Gynaecologists of Canada (SOGC), in conjunction with many of the partners who worked on MCP², called for the implementation of a national birthing initiative (SOGC, 2008). These partners, including the Association of Women's Health, Obstetric and Neonatal Nurses (AWHONN Canada), Canadian Association of Midwives, CNA, the College of Family Physicians of Canada, and the Society of Rural Physicians of Canada, developed strategies to address the issues around a present and growing shortage of qualified health care personnel. The work of the MCP² and the national birthing initiative laid the groundwork for future interdisciplinary collaborations by increasing communication and collaboration between individuals and associations providing the full range of maternal newborn care.

One example of this form of collaborative care is the Managing Obstetrical Risks Efficiently project, developed in partnership by the SOGC and Health Insurance Reciprocal of Canada. This project is presently being used in nine Canadian provinces and one territory and has been adopted in parts of the United States as well (Salus Global Corporation, 2012).

The Aboriginal Birthing Initiative for Canada addresses the needs of First Nations and Inuit women (SOGC, 2007). This initiative was created specifically to address the unique issues and needs of Aboriginal women in Canada and to complement the work of other federal programs, including the First Nations and Inuit Health Branch, the Canada Prenatal Nutrition Program,

BOX 1.1 Childbirth in North America: A Time Line

1700s   Men did not attend births because it was considered indecent.

Women faced birth not with joy and ecstasy but with fear of death.

Female midwives attended the majority of all births at the woman's home.

1800s   There was a shift among middle-class women from using midwives to doctors.

The word *obstetrician* was formed from Latin, meaning "to stand before."

Puerperal (childbed) fever was occurring in epidemic proportions.

Louis Pasteur demonstrated that streptococci were the major cause of puerperal fever that was killing mothers after delivery.

The first cesarean section was performed in Boston in 1894.

The X-ray was developed in 1895 and was used to assess pelvic size for birthing purposes.

1900s   The perinatal mortality rate was 65 per 1,000 births in 1921.

Nurseries were started in hospitals because mothers could not care for their babies for several days after receiving chloroform gas.

Dr. Grantley Dick–Reed (1933) wrote *Childbirth Without Fear,* which reduced the "fear– tension– pain" cycle women experienced during labour and birth.

The perinatal mortality rate dropped to 28 per 1,000 births in 1961; the rate of cesarean section births was less than 5%.

Amniocentesis was first performed to assess fetal growth in 1966.

Dr. Fernand Lamaze (1984) wrote *Painless Childbirth: The Lamaze Method,* which advocated distraction and relaxation to minimize the perception of pain.

In the late 1900s, freestanding birthing centres—labour, delivery, recovery, and postpartum spaces—were designed, and the number of home births began to increase.

The perinatal moratality rate was 6 per 1,000 in 1996.

60% of Canadian women attended childbirth classes.

Almost all hospitals (97%) encouraged the partner to stay with the mother to assist with labour and delivery.

2000s   One in four women undergo a surgical birth (cesarean).

Registered midwives assist couples at home, in hospitals, or in freestanding facilities with natural childbirths. Research shows that midwives are the safest birth attendants for most women, experiencing lower infant and maternal mortality rates and fewer invasive interventions such as episiotomies and cesareans (Hutton, Reitsma, & Kaufman, 2009).

Childbirth in rural and remote areas presents unique challenges. Family physicians are likely to provide the needed care in these areas, although in Canada as a whole 27% of doctors reported delivering babies in 2000 but only 12% of them did so in rural areas; birth centres are not available in some communities.

With the relative scarcity of anesthesiologists and obstetricians in rural areas, the rates of cesarean deliveries and vaginal deliveries with epidurals are lower.

Only a minority of hospitals persist in using the "routine procedures" of perineal shaving, enemas/suppositories, or intravenous fluids. Almost 65% routinely use electronic fetal monitoring upon admission, and 69% separate mom and baby at birth for 1 to 4 hours to observe the baby.

Healthy moms and babies are typically discharged 24 to 48 hours after delivery, and 74% of moms are breastfeeding at time of discharge. Of note, readmission of newborns with jaundice has increased.

94% of hospitals encourage women to walk during labour; 72% have bath and shower facilities available for pain control; 65% use nitrous oxide for pain control; 94% offer narcotics, which 40% of women use; and 55% offer epidurals, which 25% of women use.

The Canadian Association of Midwives, a national regulatory body for midwives, was formed in 2006.

As of 2009, there were 719 Canadian nurses holding CNA certification in perinatal nursing care.

The Canadian Association of Perinatal and Women's Health Nurses (CAPWHN), which represents women's health, obstetric, and newborn nurses from across Canada was formed in 2010.

EVIDENCE-BASED PRACTICE 1.1
How Do Women in Childbirth Respond to Continuous Labour Support?

● **Study**

Throughout history, women have been helping other women in labour by providing emotional support, comfort measures, information, and advocacy. However, in recent years this practice has waned, and facilities frequently adhere to strict specific routines that may leave women feeling "dehumanized." A study was done to assess the effects on mothers and their newborns of continuous, one-to-one intrapartum care in comparison with usual care. The study also evaluated routine practices and policies in the birth environment that might affect a woman's autonomy, freedom of movement, and ability to cope with labour; who the caregiver was (whether the person was a staff member of the facility); and when the support began (early or late in labour).

All published and unpublished randomized clinical trials comparing continuous support during labour with usual care were examined. One author and one research assistant used standard methods for data collection and analysis and extracted the data independently. Clinical trial authors provided additional information. The researchers used relative risk for categorical data and weighted mean difference for continuous data. Sixteen trials from 11 countries involving 13,391 women were examined to provide the data.

▲ **Findings**

Women receiving continuous intrapartum support had a greater chance of a spontaneous vaginal delivery (including without forceps or vacuum extraction). They also had a slight decrease in the length of labour and required less analgesia during this time. These women also reported increased satisfaction with their labour and childbirth experience. Overall, support provided by someone other than a facility staff member and initiated early in labour proved to be more effective.

■ **Nursing Implications**

Based on this research, it is clear that women in labour benefit from one-to-one support. Nurses can use the information gained from this study to educate women about the importance of support persons during labour and delivery. Nurses can also act as client advocates in facilities where they work to foster an environment that encourages the use of support persons during the intrapartum period. The focus of nursing needs to be individualized, supportive, and collaborative with the family during their childbearing experience. In short, nurses should place the needs of the mother and her family first in providing a continuum of care.

Although the study found that support is more effective when provided by someone other than a staff member, support from an individual is key. Assigning the same nurse to provide care to the couple throughout the birthing experience also fosters a one-to-one relationship that helps meet the couple's needs and promote feelings of security. By meeting the couple's needs, the nurse is enhancing their birthing experience.

Source: Hodnett, E. D., Gates, S. Hofmeyr, G. J., & Sakata, C. Continuous support for women during childbirth. *Cochrane Database of Systematic Reviews* 2007. Issue 3. Art No.: CD003766. DOI:10.1002/14651858.CD003766.pub2.

Nursing Services, the Fetal Alcohol Spectrum Disorder Program, and the Aboriginal Head Start Program. The overall goals of Aboriginal Birthing Initiative for Canada include obtaining cultural competency and safety, financial commitment for services, and education.

Evolution of Child Health Nursing

In the 17th and 18th centuries, the overall health of Canadians was poorer than it is today, as demonstrated by high mortality rates and shorter lifespans. Beginning in the early 19th century, a flood of immigrants arrived in Canada, which led to higher rates of infectious diseases as a result of poor public health practices, inadequate and unsanitary living conditions and food (e.g., contaminated milk), harsh working conditions, and lack of experience in coping with the long, cold winters. The devastating epidemics of smallpox, diphtheria, scarlet fever, and measles hit the young the hardest. During this era, health care providers understood that germs caused

disease and parents were discouraged from visiting their children in hospital in an effort to prevent the spread of infections. It was also a time when society viewed children as a commodity to increase the population and share in the work to be done (Canadian Encyclopedia Historica Dominion Institute, 2012; Government of Canada, 2008).

Nursing in Canada and health care for growing families was developing along with the country. The first formal nurse training program began in 1847 at the General and Marine Hospital in St. Catharines, Ontario, and shortly thereafter nursing schools were established in every major hospital in the country. Pediatrics as a nursing specialty was founded later. Toronto's Hospital for Sick Children (known as SickKids) was founded in 1875 by a group of 11 women who rented an 11-bedroom house that could care for sick children. In 1876, the hospital moved to a larger facility, and in 1902, the first nurse graduated from the SickKid's nursing program (SickKids, 2011). Montreal Children's Hospital (2011) opened in 1904, and its training school for nurses was founded in 1905. The timing of pediatric nursing courses in Canada was similar to that in the United States, where the first professional course in pediatric nursing started in the early 1900s at Teachers' College of Columbia University.

These changes in Canada also brought about an increased focus on the health and general well-being of children. Public schools were developed during the 19th century, and the court system began viewing children as minors. In the late 1800s, Lady Ishbel Aberdeen visited Vancouver and learned of the hardship and illness affecting women and children. Around the same time, she also attended the National Council of Women's annual meeting in Halifax and heard similar accounts. This was the impetus she needed to develop a nursing response. After 7 years of Lady Aberdeen's planning and advocacy, Prime Minister Sir Wilfrid Laurier inaugurated the Victorian Order of Nurses Canada as part of the Queen Victoria's diamond jubilee. When the medical community appealed to the government to reverse this decision, Lady Aberdeen appealed to school children across Canada to write letters of support for nurses to care for people in their own homes. This campaign plus other initiatives resulted in the first 12 nurses being admitted to the Victorian Order of Nurses in November 1897 (Victorian Order of Nurses Canada, 2009). In 1903, nurse, midwife, and military nurse Annie A. Bond founded the Margaret Scott Nursing Mission in Winnipeg, Manitoba, the first visiting nurse organization that focused on maternal and child nursing. She is best known as the founder of the Winnipeg Children's Hospital in 1909, which was the culmination of years of tireless work lobbying for sick children whose parents were unable to afford proper medical care (CNA, n.d.).

The turn of the 20th century brought new knowledge about nutrition, sanitation, bacteriology, pharmacology, medication, and psychology. Penicillin, corticosteroids, and vaccines assisted with the fight against communicable diseases. By the end of the 20th century, public health and technological advances significantly affected all aspects of health care. While these advances have led to increased survival rates in children, some of these survivors are left with chronic disabilities. For example, the use of mechanical ventilation and medications to foster lung development in premature infants increases survival but often leads to chronic illnesses such as bronchopulmonary dysplasia, retinopathy of prematurity, cerebral palsy, or developmental delay. These advances have also created new ethical dilemmas as children with hereditary diseases such as cystic fibrosis live long enough to reproduce and have children of their own.

Today, 70% of maternal deaths worldwide are directly related to hemorrhage, infection, unsafe abortion, eclampsia, and obstructed labour. The majority of these deaths occur as a result of unavailable, inaccessible, unaffordable, or poor quality health care (World Health Organization [WHO], 2011b). Health care in Canada is publicly funded, which ensures that finances are not an impediment to accessing health care. The first hospital insurance program in Canada was introduced by Tommy Douglas in Saskatchewan in 1947. Douglas believed if there were enough resources to fund a war, then there were enough resources to provide health care to Canadian citizens. Ten years later, the federal government initiated the national hospital insurance program.

The current Medicare program was created in 1966 under the Canada Health Act. At that time, the federal government paid 50% of the provincial health care costs. Canadian public health care is a provincial responsibility, but the federal government transfer payments are conditional on the provinces upholding the basic principles of Medicare. This ensures that Canadians receive publicly funded, portable, comprehensive, and universal access to necessary physician and hospital services (Canada Health Coalition, 2009). As a result, cost is not a private concern when seeking health care services. However, the covering of costs does not guarantee that quality health care can be provided to all citizens. For example, a study conducted by the PHAC (2009b) found that the shortage of health care professionals negatively impacts the provision of prenatal care. These shortages are most pronounced in isolated and/or rural areas.

Income and social status are closely linked to the health of growing families. Recognizing this, the federal government introduced the Federal Family Allowance in 1944. Initially, families were given monthly payments between $5.00 and $8.00 for every child from birth to age 15. This continued uninterrupted but with minimal increases in payments until 1989, when the universal nature of the family allowance was ended and allocations began to reflect annual income. In 1992, the Canada child tax benefit replaced family allowance. The child tax benefit pays families a maximum of $85 tax free, per child, per month up to the age of 18, but the benefit is based on net family income as filed in the previous year's income tax return. Quebec continues to provide a universal family allowance up to the age of 18 (Guest, 2012).

The 1980s saw the introduction of cost control systems from the federal government as a result of rapid escalation of health care expenditures. The significant changes in the health care system in the 1980s and 1990s have affected pediatric nursing and child health care as outcomes and cost containment were emphasized. Today, more children with chronic illnesses are cared for in the home with the assistance of highly specialized outpatient clinics as well as pediatric home care nurses and government-paid health care aides. These changes also brought more advanced practice nurses, ones who had practiced primarily in specialized areas such as neonatal and pediatric intensive care units, into the field of general pediatrics.

The nurse practitioner role in Canada began in the 1960s in remote northern areas of the country in response to a shortage of doctors willing to service these communities (Nurse Practitioner Association of Ontario, n.d.). Currently modern maternal–child advanced practice nursing, in urban and rural areas, includes nurse practitioners, clinical nurse specialists, and case managers.

Core Concepts of Maternal and Child Health Nursing

Maternal and child health nursing focuses on providing evidence-based, case-managed care to the client within the context of the family. This care involves the implementation of an interdisciplinary plan in a collaborative manner to ensure continuity of care that is cost-effective, quality-oriented, and outcome-focused. In planning for discharge and providing care in the community, pediatric nurses also collaborate with other sectors such as education, social work, and justice. Children should receive atraumatic care to minimize the stress associated with health care procedures or situations.

Family–Centred Care

Family-centred care is the delivery of safe, satisfying, high-quality health care that focuses on and adapts to the physical and psychosocial needs of the family. It is a cooperative effort between the family and their caregivers and recognizes and uses the strengths and integrity of the family. There are three basic principles of family-centred care:

- Childbirth is considered a normal, healthy event in the life of a family.
- Childbirth affects the entire family, and relationships and roles will change.
- Families are capable of making decisions about their own care if given adequate information and professional support (Friedman, Bowden, & Jones, 2003).

The philosophy of family-centred care recognizes the family as the unit of care. The health and functioning of the family affect the health of the client and other members of the family. Family members support one another well beyond the health care provider's brief time with them, such as during the childbearing process or a child's illness. Birth is viewed as a normal life event rather than a medical procedure.

With family-centred care, support and respect for the uniqueness and diversity of families are essential, along with encouragement and enhancement of the family's strengths and competencies. It is important to create opportunities for families to demonstrate their abilities and skills. Families can acquire new abilities and skills to maintain a sense of control and empowerment in meeting their own needs. Family-centred care promotes greater family self-determination, decision-making abilities, control, and self-efficacy, thereby enhancing the client's and family's sense of empowerment. When implementing family-centred care, nurses seek caregiver input. The information, suggestions, and advice are incorporated into the client's plan of care as the nurse counsels and teaches the family about appropriate health care interventions. Today, as nurses partner with various experts to provide high-quality and cost-effective care, one expert partnership that nurses can make is with the client's family.

Unfortunately, some parents feel imposed on by nurses' expectations of what they are to do—a phenomenon that has increased with the recent shortages of nursing staff. Therefore, it is important that nurses negotiate with parents to determine the parent role as well as the preferred types and amounts of communication. This is often the most important factor in the success of interactions during a child's hospital stay (Shields, Pratt, & Hunter, 2006). There are increasing numbers of pediatric day surgeries and children being discharged earlier with the assistance of community health care services. This places a heavy responsibility on families who may have little or no training and often minimal support. There is limited research on family-centred care in this context and a need to quantify the real cost, both emotional and financial, for families who are caring for children with complex health care needs in the home (Shields et al., 2006).

The impact of family-centred care can be seen in the models of care delivery for women. Since the 1980s, childbearing families have been offered increasing options for care, including hospital redesigns (labour, delivery, and recovery rooms; labour, delivery, recovery, and postpartum spaces) aimed at keeping families together during the childbirth experience. This impact also can be seen in the care of children: rooming-in and liberal visiting policies allow parents and other family members to participate in the child's care (Fig. 1.2).

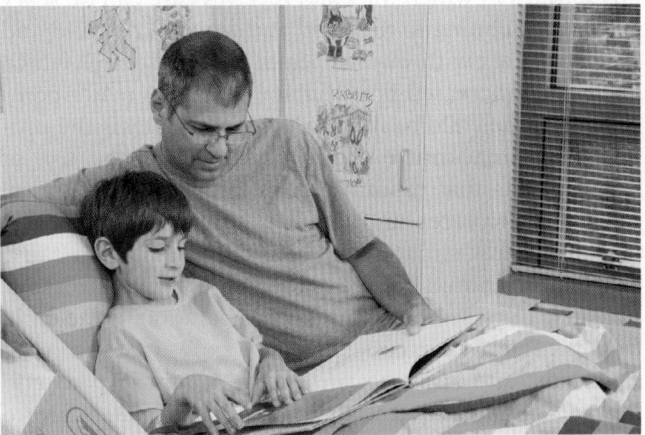

FIGURE 1.2 Providing an opportunity for the parent to interact with the child is an important component of family-centred nursing care.

Evidence-Based, Case-Managed Care

Evidence-based nursing practice involves the use of the best research or evidence in establishing a plan of care and implementing that care. Evidence-based practice is a problem-solving approach to making clinical nursing decisions (Melnyk & Fineout-Overholt, 2005). Widespread use of evidence-based practice may lead to a decrease in variation of care while at the same time increasing the quality of care. Many effective health care innovations at the patient care level are not researched and published in peer-reviewed journals. Some of these are disseminated through presentations at Canadian and international conferences. Health Canada also publishes "best practices" as another means to encourage documentation and circulate local, effective health care innovations.

Modern health care focuses on an interdisciplinary plan of care designed to meet a client's physical, developmental, educational, spiritual, and psychosocial needs. This interdisciplinary type of care is termed **case management**, a collaborative process involving assessment, planning, implementation, coordination, monitoring, and evaluation. It involves the following components:

• Advocacy, communication, and resource management
• Client-focused comprehensive care across a continuum
• Coordinated care with an interdisciplinary approach (Case Management Society of America, 2012)

When the nurse effectively functions in the role of a case manager, client and family satisfaction increases, fragmentation of care decreases, and outcome measurement for a homogenous group of clients becomes possible.

Atraumatic Pediatric Care

Children undergo a wide range of interventions, many of which can be traumatic, stressful, and painful. The various settings in which the child receives care can be scary and overwhelming to the child and family. The child and family interact with various health care personnel, which leads to an increased potential for anxiety. A major component of the child health nursing philosophy is the provision of **atraumatic care**. This involves the use of interventions that minimize physical and psychological distress for children and families. Nurses must be ever-vigilant for any situation that has the potential to cause distress and should be able to identify potential stressors. Pediatric nurses should minimize separation of the child from the family, decrease the child's exposure to stressful situations, and strive to prevent or minimize pain and injury. The importance of providing atraumatic care to children is integrated throughout this text.

A safe sleeping area may assist an anxious child to sleep more soundly. Therefore, nurses are encouraged to perform potentially painful procedures in treatment rooms when possible. This keeps the room the child sleeps in a safe zone in which no traumatic events occur (March & Schub, 2010). Pediatric home care nurses should ask the parents if they can perform assessments, treatments, and interventions in a room other than the child's bedroom.

Think back to Sophia and her mother, Betty, who were described at the beginning of the chapter. Sophia and her husband are planning to use natural childbirth and to have their children present for the birth. While Sophia is waiting to be called for her appointment, Betty says, "Things have changed so much since I was pregnant. It's amazing what happens nowadays." Explain how things have changed in maternal and child health care, focusing on the concept of family-centred care.

Health Status

At one time, health was defined simply as the absence of disease; health was measured by monitoring the mortality and morbidity of a group. These data remain significant for international analysis. For example, WHO (2011a, 2011b) notes that, worldwide, an estimated 8 million children under 5 years of age die every year and 358,000 women die each year as a result of pregnancy and childbirth. Over the past century, however, the focus on health has shifted to disease prevention, health promotion, and wellness. Since 1948, WHO has defined health as "a state of complete physical, mental, and social well-being, and not merely the absence of disease or infirmity" (WHO, 2008).

The definition of health is complex; it is not merely the absence of disease or an analysis of mortality and morbidity statistics. Focusing on the health of the population has resulted in research to determine what factors contribute to making the population healthy and unhealthy. The determinants of health include social and economic conditions that influence health. One significant determinant is healthy child development, which is influenced by family income and social status, parental education, culture, and social supports (Hamilton & Bhatti, 1996; PHAC, n.d). In October 2005, the federal, provincial and territorial Ministers of Health agreed on an overarching goal for every Canadian to be as physically, mentally, emotionally, and spiritually healthy as possible. This broad goal was further divided into more specific objectives, the first of which was that Canadian children reach their full potential and that they grow up to be healthy, confident, secure, and happy (PHAC, 2006).

One significant public health concern is obesity: 26% of Canadian children ages 2 to 17 are overweight and 8% are obese (Shields, 2006). Two major factors contributing to childhood obesity are inactivity and the amount of time a child spends in front of a screen (television, computer, etc). Obesity is a preventable determinant of common chronic health conditions such as cardiovascular disease and diabetes. Among the goals of Canada's Health Living Strategy are that by 2015, there will be a 20% increase in the proportion of Canadians who make healthy food choices, participate in regular physical activity, and are at a "normal" body weight based on body mass index (PHAC, 2009a). Children living in rural areas are at greater risk for obesity than those living in urban settings. Services specializing in pediatric weight management are primarily located in urban settings, however, and lengthy travel times may eliminate rural children from participating in these programs. Pediatric weight management groups in rural settings may not be an option. Although the issue of how to provide this needed service has not been resolved, telehealth and online support are currently being tested (Ambler, Hagedorn, & Ball, 2010).

Measuring health status is not a simple or convenient process. For example, some individuals with chronic illnesses do not see themselves as ill if they can control their condition through self-management. A traditional method used in this country to measure health is to examine mortality and morbidity data. Information is collected and analyzed to provide an objective description of the nation's health. Low birth weight (LBW) is considered a significant indicator of the health of a population. LBW is associated with an infant's survival, growth, and development, and it places an infant at greater risk for developing chronic health problems. The LBW rates in Canada have remained fairly stable over the past 30 years (i.e., 5.5% in 1979 and 6% in 2005), although rates are higher when the mother is under 20 years of age (6.6%), older than 35 years of age (7.1%), or of Aboriginal descent (Human Resources and Skills Development Canada, 2012; Luo, Senecal, Simoniet, et al., 2011; Community Foundations of Canada, 2009). Overall LBW rates increased in 2006 to 7.9% (PHAC, 2009a).

Mortality

Mortality is the incidence or number of individuals who have died over a specific period. This statistic is presented as rates per 100,000 and is calculated from a sample of death certificates. Statistics Canada collects, analyzes, and disseminates the data on Canada's mortality rates (Statistics Canada, 2010).

Maternal Mortality

The **maternal mortality rate** is the number of deaths from any cause during the pregnancy cycle per 100,000 live births. In Canada, the maternal mortality ratio (the number of women dying for every 100,000 live births) was 12 in 2009 (WHO, 2009).

Worldwide, the number of women dying from pregnancy-related causes has dropped more than 35%

over the past 30 years, and the MMR has decreased from 422 deaths in 1980 to 251 deaths in 2008 (Brunner, 2010). However, Canada's MMR has increased from 6 in 1990 to 12 in 2009. The federal government has pledged to improve maternal–child care outcomes and thus reduce mortality rates for women and children. Canada is one of the most medically and technologically advanced nations and has one of the highest per capita rates for health care spending in the world (Kaiser Family Foundation, 2011), but the current mortality rates indicate the need for improvement. For example:

- There has been a rise in the MMR related to atonic postpartum hemorrhage (PPH, 33.8 deaths in 1995 versus 38.7 in 2005).
- There has been a rise in MMR related to PPH with hysterectomy (35.1 deaths in 1995 versus 40.7 in 2005) (PHAC, 2008).

The maternal morbidity and mortality rates among Aboriginal women are dismal (National Aboriginal Health Organization [NAHO], 2008). "Stillbirth and perinatal death rates among [Aboriginals] are about double the Canadian average; among Inuit living in the Northwest Territories, they are about two and a half times the Canadian average" (NAHO, 2008, p. 16). In 1993 (latest information available), the Aboriginal postnatal mortality rate was approximately three and a half times the national rate (NAHO, 2008). In 2003, the breastfeeding rate in the Aboriginal population was 60% compared with 75% in the rest of the population (Stout & Harp, 2009).

In a 2005 roundtable on Aboriginal women's and girls' health hosted by NAHO, the following priority issues for women's reproductive and maternal health were identified:

- Lack of culturally appropriate supports and facilities for pregnancy and birth
- Lack of culturally appropriate education, training, and support for Aboriginal midwives
- Inadequate funding and bursaries to support training
- Long waiting lists to access midwives
- Liability issues for midwives (NAHO, 2008)

Immigrant women may also receive subpar prenatal care, which may be explained by language, cultural, and legal barriers. Further studies are needed to identify and eliminate the disparities in health service provision to this population. Women living in rural settings also have difficulty accessing adequate care.

Fetal Mortality

The **fetal mortality rate** is the number of fetal deaths per 1,000 births (live births and stillbirths) (PHAC, 2008). The definition of a stillbirth in most of Canada includes all deaths at or after 20 weeks' gestation or a birth weight of at least 500 g. Fetal mortality may be attributable to maternal factors (e.g., hypertension, diabetes) or fetal factors (e.g., congenital anomalies, placental abruption, infection, umbilical cord accidents). Over 25% of stillbirths are due to unknown causes. Fetal mortality provides an overall picture of the quality of maternal health and prenatal care.

Neonatal and Infant Mortality

The **neonatal mortality rate** is the number of infant deaths occurring in the first 28 days of life per 1,000 live births. The **infant mortality rate** is the number of deaths occurring in the first 12 months of life per 1,000 live births. The infant mortality rate is used as an index of the general health of a country. Generally, this statistic is one of the most significant measures of children's health. In Canada, the crude neonatal mortality rate was 3.7 per 1,000 in 2004; Nunavut had the highest rate at 9.4 (PHAC, 2008).

In Canada, the infant mortality rate is 5.1 per 1,000 (PHAC, 2008). However, this rate varies among provinces and ethnic groups. Canada ranked 24th in infant mortality out of the 30 most industrialized nations (Government of Canada, 2008).

> ▶ *Take* NOTE!
>
> *The Aboriginal peoples of Canada, including the First Nations, Inuit, and Métis, have consistently had higher infant mortality rates than other ethnic groups (UNICEF Canada, 2009).*

LBW and prematurity are major indicators of infant health and significant predictors of infant mortality (PHAC, 2008). The leading cause of infant death in Canada is prematurity followed by congenital anomalies, asphyxia, and respiratory distress syndrome (PHAC, 2008).

After birth, primary health prevention strategies can significantly improve an infant's health and chances of survival. Breastfeeding has been shown to reduce rates of infection in infants and to improve their long-term health. Emphasizing the importance of placing an infant on his or her back to sleep will reduce the incidence of sudden infant death syndrome (SIDS). Encouraging mothers to join support groups to prevent postpartum depression and learn sound childrearing practices will improve the health of both mothers and their infants.

Childhood Mortality

The **childhood mortality rate** is the number of deaths per 100,000 children 1 to 14 years of age. Canada's childhood mortality rate ranks 12th among the 21 most industrialized countries (Health Canada, 2009). The leading cause of injury-related death in Canadian children is motor vehicle accidents (Pereira, 2011; Safe Kids Canada,

2012). In May 2010, the federal government instituted new regulations that made Canada a world leader in the testing of car seats (Safe Kids Canada, 2011). The changes were made in part because children have become heavier over the past 20 years. With these changes, infants can remain in rear-facing car seats until they reach 20 kg. The maximum allowable weight limit for forward-facing car seats was increased to 30 kg, and there are guidelines for harnesses for special needs children on school buses. Detailed guidelines are available through the Canada Safety Council (visit http://thePoint.lww.com/Chow1e for the direct link). Many motor vehicle–related deaths could be prevented by educating parents about the value of car seat and booster seat use and developing focus group–tested educational materials to educate tweens and teens on the benefits of seat belt use, the dangers of driving under the influence of alcohol and other substances, and the importance of pedestrian safety. Other important causes of childhood mortality in Canada include suicide, homicide, and AIDS.

Morbidity

Morbidity is the measure of the prevalence of a specific illness in a population at a particular time. It is presented in rates per 1,000 population. Morbidity is often difficult to define and record because the types of measurement used vary widely—for example, visits to the physician or diagnosis for hospital admission. Information may be difficult to obtain, such as that gathered by household interviews from research studies. Morbidity statistics are revised less frequently because of this difficulty in defining or obtaining the information.

Women's Health Indicators

Women today face diseases not only of genetic origin but also those that arise from poor personal habits. Even though women represent 51% of the population, only recently have researchers and the medical community focused on their unique health needs. The federal government has initiated a number of programs aimed at identifying and meeting the needs of all Canadian women (Boxes 1.2 and 1.3). Of note, Women and Health Care Reform, a working group of Health Canada, analyzes reforms within the Canadian health care system at the federal, provincial, and territorial levels, as health care is primarily a provincial and territorial responsibility. This group identifies and describes how reforms made will impact women and which women will be impacted (Women and Health Care Reform, 2009).

In 2002, the PHAC funded a study addressing the differences between women's and men's health. Key findings included the following:

• Women had an approximately 20% higher hospitalization rate than men.

BOX 1.2 **Milestones in Support of the Health of Women and Children**

1867 With the British North America Acts, Canada became an independent nation. Health care was addressed only in terms of general guidelines, with management of care left to the provinces.

1900–1970 The federal government set up residential schools, forcing Aboriginal children to be taken from their homes and placed in schools where their language and culture were systematically eliminated from their lives. This created massive mental and physical health issues and social problems for years to come.

1908 The Juvenile Delinquents Act was passed. The group charged with enacting it changed its name to the Canadian Council on Child and Family Welfare in 1930 when it was expanded to include families.

1935 The Canadian Welfare Council replaced the Canadian Council on Child and Family Welfare.

1947 Cooperative Commonwealth Federation leader Tommy Douglas, together with the Government of Saskatchewan, introduced the first publicly funded hospital and medical insurance coverage in portions of Saskatchewan (Wong, 1975).

1957 The Hospital Insurance and Diagnostic Services (HIDS) Act funded 50% of the cost of such programs for any provincial government that adopted them. It outlined five conditions: public administration, comprehensiveness, universality, portability, and accessibility. These remain the pillars of the Canada Health Act.

1960 The Canadian Bill of Rights was passed, making discrimination in the provision of health care based on race, national origin, religion, or colour illegal.

1962 The Government of Saskatchewan introduced the first public health care program with full medical services for permanent residents.

1966 The Canada Assistance Plan was introduced, in which 50% federal funding was provided for designated social programs and new national standards were established for most provincial social assistance programs and services.

1964 A Royal Commission recommended that the Government of Canada implement a universal health care system.

1966 The Canada Assistance Plan provided cost sharing for child welfare and other welfare and pension services formerly solely funded by provinces. The Medical Care Act extended the HIDS Act, enabling cost sharing to allow each province to establish a universal health care plan (i.e., the Medicare system).

1971 The Canadian Council on Social Development replaced the Canadian Welfare Council. Its mission was to develop and promote progressive social policies based on empowerment, social justice, and equity (Canadian Council on Social Development, 2011).

1979 The Children's Aid Foundation was established as a national charity to improve the lives of abused, neglected, and at-risk children (Children's Aid Foundation, 2008). This foundation funded prevention, enrichment, and education programming.

1982 The Canadian Charter of Rights and Freedoms extended the Bill of Rights to include discrimination based on age and physical or mental infirmary.

1984 The Canada Health Act became a vital piece of federal legislation. The act reimburses provinces and territories for health care services delivered and bans extra-billing. The following five principles must be met to receive funding under the Canada Health Act: universally available to permanent residents and citizens, comprehensive in the services it offers, accessible without income barriers, portable within Canada, and publicly funded. The Act also prohibits user fees and extra billing by doctors.

1985 The Canadian Multiculturalism Act stated that cultural pluralism, was to be practiced and honoured within an English–French language base. Therefore, all cultures were to be honoured and individuals of specific cultures were not required to neglect their own cultural practices and take on the Canadian practices.

1988 Criminal Code Section 251 was struck down, which made unrestricted abortions legal in all provinces of Canada.

1995 The Canada Health and Social Transfer Act was introduced, significantly reducing transfer of health and social funding to provinces and territories.

(continued)

BOX 1.2 **Milestones in Support of the Health of Women and Children** (continued)

1996	The Women's Health Contribution Program was created to support community and academic partnerships in development and dissemination of policy research and information on women's health.
1998	Women and Health Care Reform was created as a Working Group from funding by the Women's Health Contribution Program, a Bureau of Women's Health and Gender Analysis at Health Canada.
1999	The Social Union Framework Agreement was signed, recommitting the country to comprehensiveness, universality, portability, public administration, and accessibility to health care services.
2003	The First Minister's Accord on Health Care reaffirmed the five primary principles of the Canada Health Act.
2004	The Multidisciplinary Collaborative Primary Maternity Care Project (MCP²), a nationwide initiative to address the looming shortage of skilled health care professionals in the maternity field, was

completed. Models of care for maternity care as well as models for intercollaborative communication were studied. MCP² includes an amendment addressing specific issues of Aboriginal women.

2005	The National Aboriginal Health Organization is founded with the goal of undertaking knowledge-based activities, including education, research, and dissemination of information to address the health issues of Aboriginal persons.
2006	PHAC was established to assist the Minister of Health in fulfilling responsibilities to help protect the health and safety of all Canadians and to increase the national focus on public health.
2009	The Sex- and Gender-Based Analysis Policy integrated a sex and gender perspective into the development of research, policy and program planning, and decision making, helping to identify and clarify differences between men and women, boys and girls, and their impact on health.

• The most common causes of hospitalization for women were pregnancy and birth, circulatory diseases, digestive diseases, cancer, mental disorders, and musculoskeletal disorders.

BOX 1.3 **Women's Health Issues (in alphabetical order)**

• Aboriginal health
• AIDS
• Breast health (i.e., cancer and breast implants, mammography)
• Cancer, particularly lung, breast, and cervical cancer
• Complications of pregnancy
• Chronic disease, particularly allergies, arthritis, back and limb problems, urethral conditions
• Diabetes
• Family violence and sexual abuse
• Heart disease and stroke
• Lesbian health
• Medication use
• Mental health issues, particularly depression
• Menopause and the use of hormone replacement therapy
• Work–life balance

Source: Public Health Agency of Canada. (2003). *Women's health surveillance report.* Retrieved February 8, 2012 from http://www.phac-aspc.gc.ca/publicat/whsr-rssf/.

• Long-term disability occurred in about 22% of women. Women with disabilities often did not have a partner, had less tangible social support, and had lower income and employment rates than men with disabilities.
• The main causes of death among women included coronary heart disease, cancer, and chronic lung disease.
• Mortality from causes amenable to medical intervention represented 25% of deaths among women.
• Death in women from gender-specific causes (e.g., breast cancer, pregnancy, and its complications) was 40.55 per 100,000, a rate much higher than for male gender-specific causes (29.15 per 100,000).
• The mortality rate for women living in rural areas was significantly higher (at least 20%) than that for women living in urban areas. This was partly due to accidents and chronic diseases (DesMeules, Turner, & Cho, 2003).

Poor health habits can have a negative impact on all women. Smoking, drug abuse, high cholesterol levels, and obesity lead to high mortality and morbidity rates (PHAC, 2009a). Cardiovascular disease is a leading cause of death in Canadian women, regardless of racial or ethnic group (Heart & Stroke Foundation of Alberta, NWT & Nunavut, 2011). Women who have a heart attack are more likely than men to die. Heart attacks in women are often more difficult to diagnose than in men because of their vague and varied symptoms. Heart disease is still thought of as a "man's disease," and thus a heart attack may not be considered in the differential diagnosis when a woman presents to the emergency room. Nurses need to look beyond the obvious "crushing chest pain" textbook symptom that heralds a heart attack in men. Risk factors for heart disease are different between men and women in several ways as well. For example, menopause is associated with a significant rise in coronary events, and women with diabetes are at greater risk than men with diabetes (Framingham.com, n.d.).

Cancer is the second leading cause of death among Canadian women (Canadian Cancer Society [CCS], 2011). Although much attention is focused on cancer of the reproductive system, lung cancer is the leading cause of cancer death in women. This is largely the result of smoking and second-hand smoke. Lung cancer has no early symptoms, making early detection almost impossible. Thus, lung cancer has the lowest survival rate of any cancer: more than 90% of people who get lung cancer die from it (CCS, 2011). Breast cancer occurs in one in every nine women in a lifetime; of the more than 21,000 women diagnosed annually, approximately 5,300 women will die from it (Health Canada, 2006; CCS, 2011). Breast cancer is the most common malignancy in women, second only to lung cancer as a cause of cancer mortality in women (CCS, 2011). A family history of breast cancer, aging, and irregularities in the menstrual cycle at an early age are major risk factors, as are excess weight, not having children, oral contraceptive use, excessive alcohol consumption, a high-fat diet, and long-term use of hormone replacement therapy (Health Canada, 2011c). Breast cancer rates have dropped recently, possibly due to the decreased use of long-term hormone replacement therapy that occurred after the Women's Health Initiative report was released in 2002 (Pace, 2006). Early detection and treatment continue to offer the best chance for a cure, and reducing the risk of cancer by decreasing avoidable risks continues to be the best preventive plan. Colorectral cancer is the third most common cancer diagnosis in women and is the third most common cancer diagnosis to result in death (CCS, 2011).

Women's health is a complex issue, and no single policy is going to change the overall dismal provincial ratings. Although progress in science and technology has helped reduce the incidence of and improve the survival rates for several diseases, women's health issues continue to have an impact on our society. By eliminating or decreasing some of the risk factors and causes for prevalent diseases and illnesses, society and science could minimize certain chronic health problems. Focusing on the causes and effects of particular illnesses could help resolve many of today's women's health issues. Canadian health promotion and prevention efforts include smoking cessation, avoidance of alcohol, folic acid supplementation, exercise, nutrition, and screening for diseases (Health Canada, 2011b).

Childhood Morbidity

With 81.8% of babies born at a healthy weight, Canada ranks 13th out of 21 industrialized countries for health and safety of our children and youth (Health Canada, 2009). The majority of Canadian children are in excellent or very good health (Health Canada, 2009). Factors that may increase morbidity include homelessness, poverty, LBW, chronic health disorders, foreign-born adoption, attending a day care centre, and barriers to health care. Approximately 15% of Canadian children live in poverty, and these children have a higher incidence of disease not only as a result of the inability of parents to provide a healthy diet but also due to inadequate supplemental health care coverage, lack of transportation, and lack of knowledge (UNICEF Innocenti Research Center, 2005). Educating families about how to stay healthy will not be an effective strategy if the family is experiencing food insecurity due to financial concerns. Therefore, nurses also need to advocate for changes in policies and engage in social action strategies that challenge the societal and economic factors that negatively impact health (Williamson & Drummond, 2000).

First Nations, Inuit, and Métis populations have unique health challenges that are critical, complex, and rooted in historical, political, and social factors. Inuit infants in northern Canada die at 3.6 times the average Canadian rate, and 70% of Inuit preschoolers live in homes with food insecurity. Diabetes rates are increasing among Aboriginal youth, and this group is overrepresented in Canada's HIV statistics (Martin, Houston, Yasui, et al., 2011). While the health care challenges are great, there is also the opportunity for change and efforts are being made to close the gap by implementing more holistic approaches to care and addressing the social and economic determinants that are negatively impacting the health of these cultural groups (National Collaborating Centre for Aboriginal Health, n.d.).

The most important aspect of morbidity is the degree of disability it produces, which is measured in children as the number of days missed from school. Missed time at school impacts performance. For example, when children with asthma were compared with children who did not have any chronic condition, the children with asthma scored lower on standardized math and reading tests, and those with the most severe asthma had the poorest outcomes (Kohen, 2010). Asthma affects at least 12% of children in Canada (Asthma Society of Canada, 2005), and 10% of children 0 to 5 years of age live with at least one allergy (Health Canada, 2009). Diseases of the respiratory system are the major cause of hospitalization for children 1 to 9 years of age (Bloom, Dey, & Freeman, 2006). Injury poses a significant threat to the health of children in Canada: every year, one in 230 children is hospitalized with a serious trauma, 20% of which are serious head injuries. In 2008, for every 100,000 children hospitalized, 348 were hospitalized due to unintentional injury, including falls, poisoning, suffocation, and burns (Government of Canada, 2008). Cancer is rare in children but it is the leading cause of disease-related death in Canadian children, with the highest incidence in preschool years (Government of Canada, 2008). Common health problems in children include respiratory disorders, such as asthma and allergies; gastrointestinal disturbances, which lead to malnutrition and dehydration; and injuries. As more immunizations become available, common childhood communicable diseases affect fewer children. Another trend is an increase in the number of children with mental health disorders and other emotional, social, or behavioural problems. The number of Canadian children impacted by mental health disorders is 1.2 million, or 15% of the pediatric population (Canadian Council on Learning, 2009). These conditions can interfere with children's social and academic development and may also increase the risk for significant mental health problems later in life. Adolescents with mental health disorders are more likely to experience injury secondary to reckless driving, promiscuous sexual activity, and substance abuse.

▶ *Take* NOTE!

Environmental and psychosocial factors are now an identified area of concern in the morbidity of children. The "new morbidities" in children include academic difficulties, complex psychiatric disorders, increased incidence of self-harm and harm to others, use of firearms, hostility at school, substance abuse, HIV/AIDS, and adverse media influences (Reasor & Farrell, 2004).

Factors Affecting Maternal and Child Health

From conception, children are shaped by myriad factors, including genetics and the environment. As members of a family, they are also part of a specific population, community, culture, and society. As they learn and grow, children are affected by the multiple, complex, and ever-changing influences around them. For example, dramatic demographic changes in Canada have led to shifts in majority and minority population groups. Globalization has led to an international focus on health. Access to and the types of health care available have changed due to modifications in health care delivery and financing. In addition, Canada is still grappling with issues such as immigration, poverty, homelessness, and violence. Mental health issues that nurses may encounter are impacted by factors such as dramatic demographic changes, which

include increasing numbers of new immigrants and refugees. As a result, nurses must have a more globalized focus on health and mental health as well as an awareness of the types of situations that children may have encountered in refugee camps or war-torn countries.

Across Canada, access to physicians and social supports has changed due to modifications in health care delivery and financing. Nurses are playing an increasingly important role in addressing health needs in situations that were traditionally attended to by physicians. Maternity, pediatric, and community health nurses have assumed a frontline role in:

- Primary prevention, through initiatives to promote health and prevent disease by identifying and addressing modifiable risk factors. Examples are immunization clinics and promotion of breastfeeding.
- Secondary prevention, through early detection and treatment of health concerns. An example is a pediatric nurse assisting a child who has observed domestic violence but who does not show any signs of personal injury (Wolfe & Jaffe, 1999).
- Tertiary prevention, by ensuring that appropriate interventions for illnesses and diseases for high-needs populations are identified and met.

While demographics, genetics, and other health indicators can affect people in a positive way and contribute to healthy growth and development, in some situations they exert a negative influence by increasing a person's health risks. Nurses, especially those working with women and children, need to understand how these influences affect the quality of nursing care and health outcomes. They must examine the impact of these variables to gain the knowledge and skills needed to work with families and populations to develop the best plan for effective care, thereby achieving the best possible outcomes for women, children, and families.

Family

The **family** is considered the basic social unit. Today's families do not fall under a single definition, and the definition of family is changing to reflect today's structural and functional changes. Canada conforms to internationally recognized standards for the definition of family (Statistics Canada, 2009a), which can be summarized as a group of two or more persons related by birth, marriage, or adoption and living together. While earlier definitions of family emphasized the legal ties or genetic relationships of people living in the same household with specific roles, Wright and Leahey (2005), formerly of the Family Nursing Unit at the University of Calgary, define family as whatever the people involved say it is for them.

The family greatly influences the development and health of its members. For example, children learn health

TABLE 1.1 SUMMARY OF MAJOR THEORIES RELATED TO FAMILY

Theory	Description	Key Components
Friedman et al.'s (2003) structural functional theory	Emphasizes the social system of family such as the organization or structure of the family and how the structure relates to the function	Identified five functions of families: • Affective function: meeting the love and belonging needs of each member • Socialization and social placement function: teaching children how to function and assume the adult roles in society • Reproductive role: continuing the family and society in general • Economic function: ensuring the family has necessary resources with appropriate allocation • Health care function: involving the provision of physical needs to keep the family healthy
Duvall's (1977) developmental theory	Emphasizes the developmental stages through which all families evolve, beginning with marriage; the longitudinal career of the family, also known as the family life cycle	Described eight chronological stages with specific predictable tasks that each family completes: • Marriage: beginning of family • Childbearing stage • Family with preschool children • Family with school-age children • Family with adolescents • Family with young adults • Middle-aged parents • Family in later years
Von Bertalanffy's (1968) general systems theory applied to families	Emphasizes the family as a system with interdependent, interacting parts that endure over time to ensure the survival, continuity, and growth of its components; the family is not the total sum of its parts but is characterized by wholeness and unity	Used to define how families interact with and are influenced by the members of their family and society and how to analyze the interrelationships of the members and the impact that change affecting one member will have on the other members
Family stress theory (Boss, 2001)	Addresses the way families respond to stress and how the family copes with the stress as a group and as individuals	Described elements of stress as occurring within the family (such as values, beliefs, structure), which the family can control or change, or from outside the family (such as the culture of the surrounding community, genetics, the family's current time or place), over which the family has no control. Mobilization of family resources results in either a positive response of constructive coping or a negative response of a crisis. Identified the main determinant of adequate coping based on the meaning of the stressful event to the family and its members
Resiliency model of family stress, adjustment, and adaptation	Addresses the way families adapt to stress and can rebound from adversity	Identified the elements of risks and protective factors that aid a family in achieving positive outcomes

care activities, health beliefs, and health values from their family. The family's structure, the roles assumed by family members, and social changes that affect the family's life can influence the child and his or her health status. Families are unique: each one has different views and requires distinct methods for support.

Various theories and models have been generated to explain the concept of family. They have influenced the definition of family, the understanding of the structure and function of the family, and the way family coping and adaptation are assessed. Table 1.1 summarizes some of the major theories related to family.

TABLE 1.2 EXAMPLES OF FAMILY STRUCTURES IN TODAY'S SOCIETY

Theory	Description	Key Components
Nuclear family	Husband, wife, and children living in same household	May include natural or adopted children Once considered the traditional family structure; now less common due to increased divorce rates and child rearing by unmarried persons
Binuclear family	Child who is a member of two families due to joint custody; parenting is considered a "joint venture"	Always works better when the interests of the child are put first and above the parents' needs and desires
Single- or lone-parent family	One parent is solely responsible for care of children	May result from death, desertion, birth outside of marriage, adoption or artificial insemination These families are likely to face challenges because of economic, social, and personal restraints; one person serves as homemaker, caregiver, and financial provider. However, many single-parent families receive financial support from the noncustodial parent
Commuter family	Adults in the family live and work apart for professional or financial reasons, often leaving the daily care of children to one parent.	One parent is responsible for the care of the children and experiences social and personal constraints during the time the other parent is living away for work-related reasons. These families are likely to experience challenges because roles and responsibilities change each time the parent living away leaves and returns to the family unit
Step- or blended family	Adults with children from previous marriages or from the new marriage	May lead to family conflict due to different expectations on the part of the child and adults; they may have different views and practices related to child care and health
Extended family	Nuclear family and grandparents, cousins, aunts, and uncles	Need to identify decision maker and primary caretaker of the children Popular in some cultures, such as Hispanic and Asian cultures
Same-sex family (also called homosexual or gay/lesbian family)	Adults of the same sex living together with or without children	May face negative attitudes about their "different" lifestyle
Communal family	Group of people living together to raise children and manage household; unrelated by blood or marriage	May face negative attitudes about their "different" lifestyle Need to determine the decision-maker and caretaker of the children
Foster family	A temporary family for children who are placed away from their parents to ensure their emotional and physical well-being	May include the foster family's children and other foster children in the home Foster children are more likely to have unmet health needs and chronic health problems because they may have been in a variety of homes
Grandparents-as-parent families	Grandparents raising their grandchildren due to the inability or absence of the parents	May increase the risk for physical, financial, and emotional stress on older adults May lead to confusion and emotional stress for the child if biological parents are in and out of child's life
Adolescent families	Young parents who are still mastering the developmental tasks of their childhood	Are at greater risk for health problems in pregnancy and delivery; more likely to have premature infants, which then leads to risk of subsequent health and developmental problems Probably still need support from their family related to financial, emotional, and school issues

▶ *Take* NOTE!

The lifestyle of the parents basically is the life-style of the children. For instance, parents who are inactive and eat poorly will have children who do the same, and the problems associated with these unhealthy habits, such as diabetes, obesity, and early heart disease, are showing up earlier in children and adolescents. It is important for parents to serve as role models for proper nutrition and physical activity (through sports, hobbies, or other activities).

Family Structure

Family structure is the composition of individuals who interact with one another on a regular, recurring basis in socially sanctioned ways. It involves how the family unit is organized, which often influences the relationships of family members. Family members are gained or lost through events such as divorce, marriage, birth, death, abandonment, and incarceration. All of these events can alter the family structure, leading to roles being redefined or redistributed. Table 1.2 provides examples of the types of family structures found in today's society.

In 2006, 70% of people in Canada lived in family households, with the average household size being 2.5 persons. However, the structure of Canadian families is changing, and the traditional nuclear family is no longer the "norm" (Fig. 1.3). Canada's divorce rate lies around 40% (Hondro, 2010). In 2006, legally married couples with children comprised only 35% of families, down from 55% in 1981. This has created an increase in the number common-law and lone-parent families. In 1981, only 5.6% of families were common-law; and 11.3%, lone-parent families. By 2006, these categories had increased to 15.5% and 15.9%, respectively (Statistics Canada, 2007). Quebec and the territories have the largest numbers of common-law families. There has also been an increase in stepfamilies. In 2001, there were more than a half million stepfamilies in Canada, in about half of which the parents were legally married. The number of women participating in the work force is also increasing, which directly impacts how families care for one another and the way roles are filled. The percentage of women (15 years of age and older) in the work force increased from 45.7% in 1976 to 61.8% in 2005. One interesting trend is the decrease in male participation in the work force (77.7% in 1976 versus 72.8% in 2005) (Human Resources and Skills Development Canada,

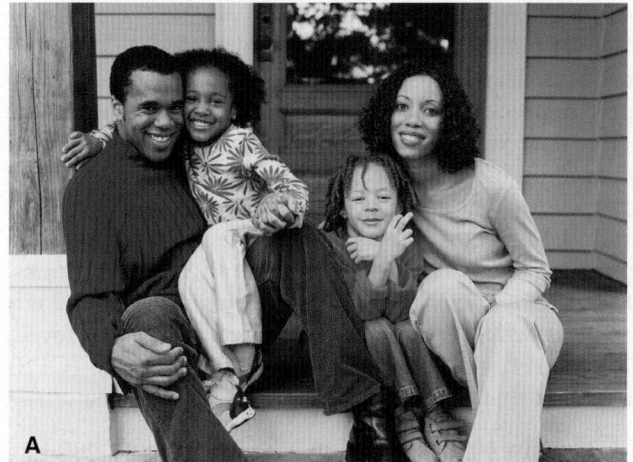

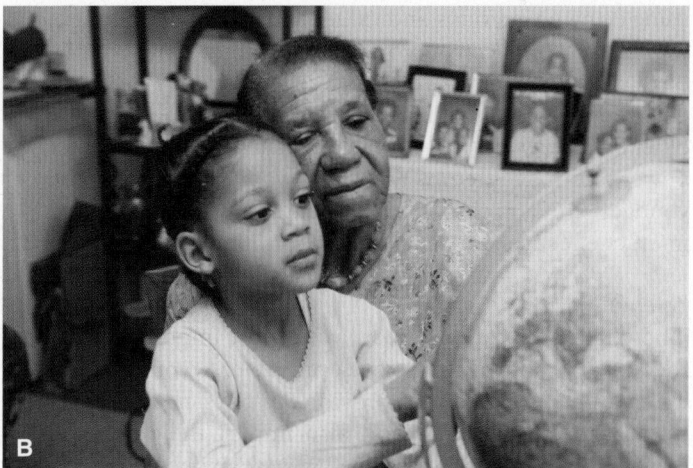

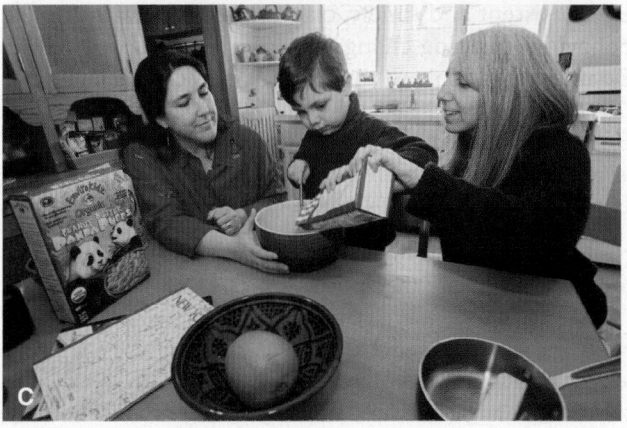

FIGURE 1.3 Nurses must take into account family dynamics when providing health care. There are many different family structures, and they influence the client's needs. (**A**) The traditional nuclear family is composed of two parents and their biological or adopted children. (**B**) The extended family includes the nuclear family plus other family members, such as grandparents, aunts, uncles, and cousins. (**C**) Gay and lesbian families comprise two people of the same sex sharing a committed relationship with or without children.

2006). By understanding clients' family structure and any changes that may occur, nurses can provide them with support to alleviate or prevent less than optimal alterations in family coping and adaptation.

Family Roles and Functions

Each family member has a specific position or status and role when interacting with other members of the family. Typical family roles and their functions include:

- Nurturer: the primary caregiver
- Provider: the person who is primarily responsible for generating the family's income
- Decision maker: the person who is responsible for making choices, especially related to lifestyle and leisure time
- Financial manager: the person who works with the money, such as paying bills and saving
- Problem solver: the person to whom other members go for help in solving problems
- Health manager: the person responsible for maintaining the family members' health, such as scheduling visits and ensuring that immunizations or screenings are up to date
- Gatekeeper: the person who manages information inflow and outflow (Pillitteri, 2007)

Roles and functions are further defined by each family using its own traditions and values and the set of standards for interacting within and outside the family. For example, birth order may affect roles and relationships. First-born children are typically different from those born later. The older child may feel that he or she is in a position of greater power and may attempt to control younger siblings. The youngest child, in response, may learn how to bargain and interact effectively to deal with the situation.

Parental Roles

The parents or caregivers are of utmost importance for the survival and healthy development of a young child. The parents or caregivers provide the physical and emotional care of the child and also impart the rules and expected behaviours of a society. These expected behaviours depend on the culture of the family, the child's developmental stage and physical and cognitive abilities, and the values and beliefs of the family. Parents should nurture their children and provide them with the environmental influences to become competent, productive, self-directed members of society. Young children are particularly dependent on the care they receive; their growth, health, and personhood depend on the capacity of the adults in their lives to understand, perceive, and respond to their bids for assistance and support.

Parenting Styles

The three major parenting styles are authoritarian, authoritative, and permissive. These three styles differ in the amount of control exerted over the child during parenting. Whatever the style, however, sensitive and responsive care is needed for appropriate physical, neurophysiologic, and psychological development.

Authoritarian parents expect unquestioning obedience from the child. The parents' rules and standards are strictly enforced and firm. Parents also expect the children to accept the family's beliefs and values and demand respect for these beliefs. The parents are the ultimate authority on matters and behaviours and allow little if any participation by the child in making decisions. Behaviour that does not adhere to the family rules and standards is forcibly punished.

Authoritative or democratic parents show some respect for the opinions of children. Although parents have the ultimate authority and expect adherence to rules, authoritative parents allow children to be different and believe that each child is an individual. They employ consistent, firm enforcement of the family rules and standards but without the emphasis on punishment of the child.

Permissive or laissez-faire parents exert little control over the behaviour of their children. Rules or standards may be inconsistent, unclear, or nonexistent. Permissive parents allow their children to set their own standards and rules for behaviour. Discipline can be lax, inconsistent, or absent.

Discipline

Much of parenting involves increasing desirable behaviours and decreasing or eliminating undesirable behaviours, a process known as **discipline**. People in our society have various beliefs about the best or most effective method of discipline. Discipline should be based on expectations that are appropriate for the child's age and should be used to set reasonable, consistent limits while permitting choices among acceptable alternatives (Banks, 2002). Discipline is an ongoing learning process, and if it is to be effective, the child needs to feel secure and loved.

In 2011, the Canadian Paediatric Society (CPS) reaffirmed that effective discipline needs to:

- Be given by an adult with an affective or close bond with the child
- Be consistent and timely, or given soon after the behaviour needing change occurs
- Be understandable to the child or perceived as fair by the child
- Be appropriate for the development, age, and temperament of the child
- Ultimately lead to self-discipline (CPS, 2011)

Teaching Guideline 1.1 provides advice about promoting appropriate discipline.

Changes in Parental Roles Over Time

Parental roles have evolved over time due to social and economic changes as well as family changes. Traditionally,

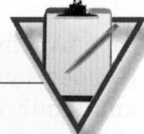

TEACHING GUIDELINE 1.1

Promoting Effective Discipline

- Set clear, consistent, and developmentally appropriate expected behaviours; offer choices whenever possible.
- Maintain consistency in responding to behaviours; provide encouragement and affection.
- Role-model appropriate behaviours.
- Provide an age-appropriate explanation of the consequence if the child demonstrates unacceptable behaviour.
- Always administer the consequence soon after the unacceptable behaviour.
- Keep the consequence appropriate to the age of the child and the situation.
- Stay calm but firm without showing anger when administering the consequence.
- Always praise the child for displaying appropriate behaviour (positive reinforcement).
- Set the environment to assist the child in accomplishing the appropriate behaviour; remove temptations that may lead to inappropriate behaviour.
- Reinforce that the child's behaviour, not the child him- or herself, was "bad."
- Use extinction to reduce or eliminate reinforcement for an inappropriate behaviour (for example, ignore a temper tantrum).
- When using time-out, use 1 minute per year of the child's age (a 3-year-old would have time-out for 3 minutes). Do not exceed 5 minutes.

the role of provider was assigned to the father. However, with increased numbers of women in the workplace and more households with two parents working, today both parents are often the providers as well as the nurturers for the children. Technological expansion has provided parents with opportunities to work at home, allowing some parents to maintain the provider role while simultaneously fulfilling the nurturer and health manager roles. Fathers also are taking on greater responsibilities related to household management and child care. Additionally, the number of single-father parent families and grandparent families are increasing.

Recall Sophia, the pregnant woman described at the beginning of the chapter. Identify the parental roles assumed by Sophia. How might these roles be different from those of her mother when she was Sophia's age?

Changes in Family Structure and Roles

Families today face complex challenges as they attempt to nurture, develop, and socialize their members. Family structure changes such as divorce, blending families, adoption, or foster care can have wide-ranging and life-long effects.

Divorce

As many as 40% of marriages end in divorce (Hondro, 2010). Conflict between the parents and family dysfunction may exert a significant stress on children. Parents need to understand the impact that divorce can have on their children and place the children's interests first. Parents can use the rules given in Teaching Guideline 1.2 to help reduce the tension and conflict associated with divorce.

Single Parenting

Single-parent families may result from divorce or separation, death of a spouse, childbearing by an unmarried woman, or adoption by an unmarried man or woman. For several reasons, any type of single family structure can adversely affect the health of family members. Life in a single-parent household can be stressful for the adult and children. The single parent may feel overwhelmed by the responsibility of juggling child care, maintaining a job, and keeping up with the bills and household chores

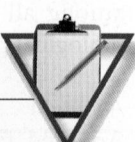

TEACHING GUIDELINE 1.2

Guidelines for Divorcing Parents

- Tell your children about the divorce and the reasons for the divorce in terms they can understand. Be sure that you and your spouse are present together when telling the children; tell all the children at the same time.
- Reassure your children that the divorce is not their fault. Repeat this as often as possible and as necessary.
- Inform the children well in advance before anyone moves out of the house (except when abuse is present or there are concerns for immediate safety).
- Clearly inform the children about the family structure after the divorce, such as who will live with whom and where; also discuss visitation clearly and honestly.
- Do not make your children be or act like adults.
- Do not discuss money or finances with your children.
- Maintain rules and be consistent in this area.
- Never force or allow your children to take sides.
- Avoid belittling your spouse with earshot of the children. However, do not lie to cover up for irresponsible behaviour by the other parent.
- Never put your children between you and your spouse.

Adapted from: Bryner, C. L. (2001). Children of divorce. *Journal of the American Board of Family Practice, 14*(3), 176–183.

(American Psychological Association, 2012). These issues may be compounded by other pressures, such as custody problems, decreased time available to spend with children, continuing conflicts between separated or divorced parents, or changes in relationships with extended family members. Communication and support are essential to the optimal functioning of the single-parent family. The parent and children need to be able to discuss their feelings and work through their problems together.

Blending Families

The creation of a blended family can be a stressful time for the parents and children involved. Although it creates a structure and stability and reduces some of the financial stresses of single parenthood, making the transition to a blended family takes time. Children may feel jealous of the stepparent or feel disloyal to the biological parent. There may be competition or rivalry among the stepchildren. A child may fear that the stepparent is interfering with his or her relationship with the biological parent or taking away his or her source of love, affection, and attention. Mutual respect is necessary to ease the transition to a blended family, as is open, honest communication among all individuals involved—and this includes the biological parent when possible.

Adoption

Adopted families are created in a number of different ways. The parents may contact an agency or intermediary such as an attorney in their own area or country to seek a child. Families may adopt a child from another country (inter-country or international adoption). The child may be of a different culture, race, or ethnicity (Fig. 1.4). Some children may have complex medical, developmental, behavioural, educational, and psychological issues. Children may be adopted after spending time in foster

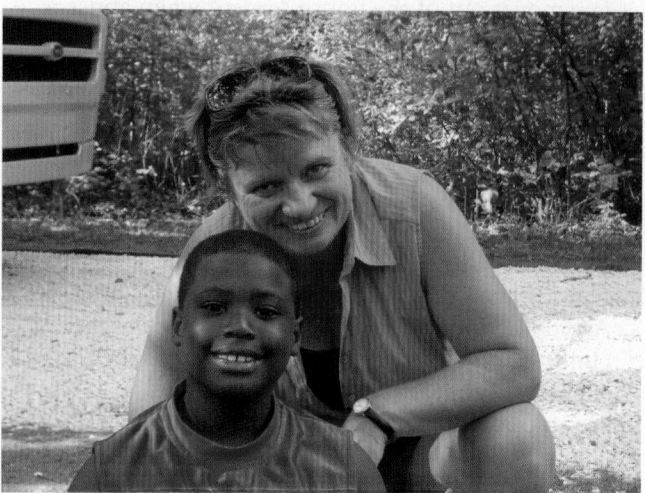

FIGURE 1.4 An adoptive family in which the child is from a different culture.

care. An increasing number of single-parent families, blended families, families with gay or lesbian partners, and families with older parents are providing homes to children through adoption (American Psychological Association, 2005).

The amount of contact between the adoptive parents and the birth mother can vary greatly. There may be no contact at all (closed adoption), or there may be as much direct contact as desired (open adoptions). Regardless of the method used to adopt a child, adoptive families may be faced with unique issues that can affect the health of the family members, such as:

- The adopted child may have been exposed to health risk factors (e.g., poverty, neglect, infectious diseases, and lack of adequate food, clothing, shelter, and consistent caregivers), increasing the child's risk for problems.
- Information about the adopted child's family medical history may be lacking.
- Parents may not know when to tell a child that he or she was adopted.
- The adopted child may be troubled about his or her loss of a "birth family" or the reason for the birth mother's decision for an adoption plan. He or she may have feelings of abandonment, emotional uncertainty, and identity conflict.
- The child and family may experience discrimination or bullying if the child is from a different culture or race.

Foster Care

Foster care refers to the care given to a child who is placed in an alternative living situation apart from his or her parents of origin or legal guardians. The child typically is placed in this living situation due to some difficulty in the family situation, such as abuse, neglect, abandonment, or the parent's inability to meet the child's needs, such as from illness, substance abuse, or death. The living situation may be with relatives (termed kinship care) or foster parents, who are strangers providing protection and shelter in a child welfare–approved foster home. In 2008, more than 76,000 children were living in foster care, with a mean age of 9.5 years. These numbers are increasing yearly (Ponti, 2008).

Child welfare services are under provincial and territorial jurisdictions, each with their own policies and services. The exception to this is children of Aboriginal status. In recognition of the over-representation of Aboriginal children (about 40% of foster children are Aboriginal), a growing number of Métis and First Nations family agencies have been developed to provide culturally based services. Jordan's Principle was unanimously passed in the House of Commons in 2007. This child-first principle ensures that the needs of the child are met by the government of first contact until any jurisdictional dispute can be resolved (Ponti, 2008).

Children in foster care have higher than average medical, emotional, developmental, and educational needs, some of which include:

• Physical health problems
• Self-blame and feelings of guilt
• Feelings of being unwanted
• Feelings of helplessness
• Insecurity and uncertainty about the future
• Ambivalent feelings related to foster parents; feelings of being disloyal to birth parents (American Academy of Child & Adolescent Psychiatry, 2005)

Genetics

Genetics (the study of heredity and its variations) has implications for all stages of life and all types of diseases. The child's biological traits, including gender, race, some behavioural traits, and the presence of certain diseases or illnesses, are directly linked to genetic inheritance. New technologies in molecular biology and biochemistry have led to a better understanding of the mechanisms involved in hereditary transmission, including those associated with genetic disorders. These advances are leading to better diagnostic tests and better management options.

Gender

Gender is established when the sex chromosomes join. A person's gender can influence many aspects, such as physical characteristics and personal attributes, attitudes, and behaviours (Fig. 1.5). Some diseases or illnesses are more common in one gender; for example, scoliosis is more common in females and colour blindness in males.

Race

Race refers to the physical features that distinguish members of a particular group, such as skin colour, bone structure, or blood type. Some physical features that are normal in a particular race may be considered a sign of a

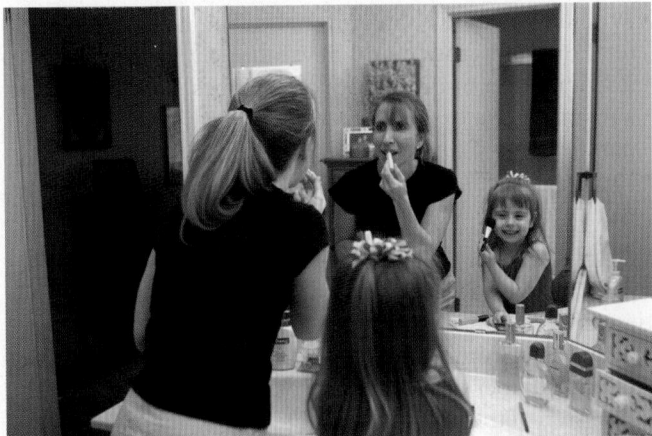

FIGURE 1.5 Interactions with family members and peers as well as activities and societal values affect how children perceive themselves as a certain gender.

disorder in other races. For example, epicanthal folds (the vertical folds of skin that partially or completely cover the inner canthi of the eyes) are normal in Asian children but may occur with Down syndrome or renal agenesis in other races. In addition, certain malformations and diseases are found more commonly in specific races. For example, sickle-cell anemia occurs more often in African and Mediterranean population groups, and cystic fibrosis is seen more often in individuals from the Northwestern European population group.

Society

Society has a major impact on the health of women, children, and families. Major influences include social roles, socioeconomic status, the media, and the expanding global nature of society. Each of these may influence a person's self-concept, where he or she lives, the lifestyle he or she leads—and thus his or her health.

Social Roles

Society often prescribes specific patterns of behaviour, and certain behaviours are permitted while others are prohibited. These social roles are often an important factor in the development of self-concept. Social roles influence a person's ideas about him- or herself. Social roles are generally carried out in groups with which the individual has intimate daily contact, such as the family, school, workplace, or peer groups.

Socioeconomic Status

Another dominant influence is a person's socioeconomic status, his or her relative position in society. This includes the family's economic, occupational, and educational levels. Children are raised differently by parents of different educational levels, occupations, and incomes. Low income levels typically have an adverse influence on individual and family health. The family may not be able to afford sufficient food, health care, and/or housing. Although provincial governments have programs in place to assist families on social assistance or very low income with costs for items such as pediatric medications, dental care, and eyeglasses, these may not cover all health care needs. Housing may be overcrowded or have poor sanitation. These families may not understand the importance of preventive care or may simply not be able to afford it. As a result, they may be exposed to health risks such as lead poisoning, obesity due to poor nutrition, or the negative effects of dental caries.

Poverty

Since 2005, there has been no official government measure of poverty, because Statistics Canada has not identified what is a necessity, which determines the amount of money needed by a family to exist; politicians refuse to provide a consensus definition of poverty (Community Foundations of Canada, 2010).

Poverty is a measurement based on the specific monetary income of a family. The poverty threshold is often measured as a set dollar amount that the government uses to determine whether a family is living in poverty. Poverty in Canada is most commonly measured using the Statistics Canada's low-income cut-off (LICO), which is based on a family spending 20% more of its income on household necessities than the average Canadian family (Human Resources and Skills Development Canada, 2006). LICO is not an absolute number and varies depending on the number of dependents and the population of the community or city. If the individual's or family's income is at or below LICO, then that person or family is said to be living in poverty. Approximately one in six children in Canada, or just over a million, lives in poverty; of those, about 75% live below LICO. The Canadian National Longitudinal Study of Children revealed that the number of children considered to be vulnerable, including vulnerability related to poverty, stands at about 28% (Health Canada, 2007; Statistics Canada, 2007). It is noteworthy that the same children did not necessarily remain vulnerable. With each survey approximately 15% of the formerly vulnerable children no longer met the criteria. However, a new 15% of children had become vulnerable.

Despite the many global economic gains that have been made during the past century, poverty continues to grow and the gap between rich and poor is widening. Major gaps continue between the economic opportunities and status afforded to women and those offered to men. A disproportionate share of the burden of poverty rests on women's shoulders, and this undermines their health. However, poverty, particularly for women, is more than monetary deficiency. Women continue to lag behind men in control of cash, credit, and collateral. Other forms of impoverishment may include deficiencies in literacy, education, skills, employment opportunities, mobility, and political representation, as well as pressures on time and energy linked to their responsibilities. These poverty factors may affect a woman's health (Coll-Back, Bhushan, & Fritsch, 2007).

The effects of poverty on children's health can be wide-ranging. The child may live in substandard housing or housing that poses a threat to his or her health (e.g., unsanitary conditions, exposure to toxins, exposure to violence). Poverty may lead to homelessness for the family. Children living in poverty are more likely than other children to be poorly nourished, to have inadequate health care, to become teen parents, and to have insufficient education. Children living in poverty are also at increased risk for experiencing abuse and violence (Health Canada, 2007).

Homelessness

Homelessness is defined as living in a shelter, on the street, or in other places not intended for human habitation. This includes "couch surfing" (i.e., staying temporarily with family or friends). A person or family is considered to live in vulnerable housing if they have their own place but are at risk for homelessness due to severe financial restrictions (e.g., families who would become homeless if they went one month without a paycheck or persons who have moved at least twice in the past year) (Research Alliance for Canadian Homelessness, Housing, and Health, 2010).

Families with children are the fastest-growing segment of the homeless population. In Calgary, the nonprofit, faith-based organization Inn from the Cold provides shelter to homeless children and their families. In 2010, Inn from the Cold provided emergency shelter to 217 unique families and 319 unique children, which is approximately one of every 1,000 Calgary children. (For a direct link to the organization's website, visit http://thePoint.lww.com/Chow1e). Homeless families commonly are victims of violence and may have mental health challenges. According to the Research Alliance for Canadian Homelessness, Housing, and Health (2010), approximately 200,000 to 300,000 people are homeless on any given night, and for every one person sleeping in a shelter there are 23 more people living with housing vulnerability. There are similar health risks for individuals and families living in unsafe or inadequate housing. Many of these families have the same health and security worries as the absolute homeless. In 2008 in Vancouver, there were 2,660 absolute homeless persons and 9,196 hidden homeless persons who were temporarily staying with another household and who did not have a regular address of their own where they had security of tenure. The hidden homeless included families with children (Eberle, Kraus, & Serge, 2009).

Homelessness has a negative impact on health and well-being in numerous ways, including:

- Increased risk for experiencing hunger
- Increased mental health issues, such as anxiety, depression, or aggressive behaviour
- Higher incidence of chronic health problems and trauma-related injuries
- Problems related to nutritional deficiencies, affecting fetal or child growth and development
- Participation in unhealthy behaviours such as illegal substance use or unprotected sex with multiple partners
- Limited access to health care services, such as preventive care, prenatal care, or dental care

In 2006, the federal government initiated the Homeless Partnering Strategy, which worked with 61 communities experiencing significant homelessness as well as rural and outlying communities and communities where a significant number of people were of Aboriginal descent. The initial step of the program collected data on homelessness, which served as a resource to support the creation of sustainable national and regional collaboration, to enhance community planning processes, and to improve the ability

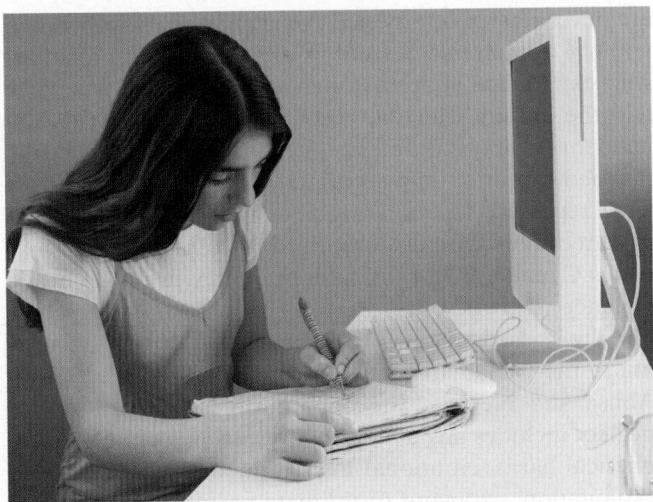

FIGURE 1.6 Computer games can be fun and educational, but the child should be monitored while using the computer and other forms of media to minimize negative effects.

of the Homelessness Partnering Secretariat's ability to measure progress and report results. The final report of this ongoing project has not yet been prepared (Human Resources and Skills Development Canada, 2009).

Media

Today's children are inundated with various forms of media, such as television, the Internet, videos, movies, magazines, books, and newspapers (Fig. 1.6). Some of these present images and information that may not be in the child's best interest. Children may identify with and mimic characters who engage in risky behaviours or lifestyles. They may believe that those lifestyles or behaviours are the acceptable norms. Research has demonstrated that exposure to media violence and risky behaviours is linked to increased risky behaviours in children and adolescents (Fischer, Greitemeyer, Kastenmuller, et al., 2011).

The images that children view every day affect their behaviours and may influence their health. For instance, magazines, movies, and television programs portray thinness as a body type to be emulated, and boys and girls may take up unhealthy dieting or other behaviours to develop that body type. Those whose body type does not fit the ideal may develop depression or self-esteem issues. The most recent content guidelines developed for the telecommunications industry were filed in 1993 by the Canadian Association of Broadcasters and Canadian Radio-Television with Telecommunications Commission (CRTC). They include:

- "Prohibition on airing programs that are gratuitously violent and promote or glamourize violent acts
- A "watershed hour" of 9:00 p.m. before which only violence suitable for children could be aired
- A sensitivity about violence against vulnerable groups such as women and minorities

- A statement that violence would not be shown as a preferred way of solving problems, or as the central theme of children's programming, and that children's programming would not invite dangerous imitation" (Media Awareness Network, 2010).

Entertainment communications are changing quickly. Children have access to wireless handheld technologies, the Internet, video games, and satellite and cable TV airing from a variety of time zones. In 1999, the CRTC, recognizing the challenge in developing and enforcing regulations, announced it would not regulate new media activities under the broadcasting code. In an increasingly globalized, unregulated world, the responsibility for protection of children relies on the vigilance of parents and other adults responsible for children (e.g., teachers and child caregivers) (Media Awareness Network, 2010).

The media's influence relates not only to its content but also to the total viewing time. For example, excessive television viewing has been linked to lack of exercise, weight gain, and obesity. The Internet has fostered closer connections between distant areas of the world. Individuals are no longer limited to their immediate surroundings. The Internet can be a valuable resource for people to access information, learn new things, and communicate, but it also brings threats to health and safety (Iannotti, Kogan, Janssen, et al., 2009; Ogden, Gorber, Dommarco, et al., 2011). Cyberbullying is the use of e-mail, cell phones, or the Internet to physically threaten, harass, or exclude an individual or group. Online exposure to sexual predators, illicit sex, pornography, violence, and racism are a few of the potential threats. Parents, teachers, and nurses need to be alert to these hazards and safeguard their children (Teaching Guideline 1.3) by openly discussing bullying with children in their care and be prepared to act on any problems or situations that arise (Healthy Canadians, 2010).

However, the media may also exert positive influences. Public service messages about the negative effects of substance abuse, smoking, or gang involvement or about teenage pregnancy and birth control are two examples of the media's positive influence. In addition, positive television programs can serve as valuable educational resources. Websites from trustworthy sources provide easily accessed health information. However, it is the responsibility of parents, teachers, nurses, and other caregivers to assist children and youth in assessing the validity of the health information they find online. The Government of Saskatchewan Ministry of Education has created a list of excellent health information websites; visit http://thePoint.lww.com/Chow1e for the direct link.

Violence

Violence can occur in any setting and can involve any individual. Violence against women is a major health concern—it affects thousands of lives and costs the health

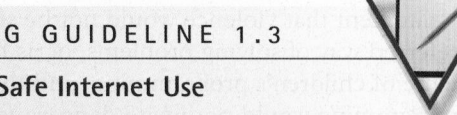

TEACHING GUIDELINE 1.3

Promoting Safe Internet Use

- Determine a specific time limit that your child can spend online each day or week. Be consistent in enforcing this time limit.
- Ensure that Internet use does not replace or interfere with homework, friends, or household or school activities.
- Tell your child NEVER to share personal information with anyone online unless you are sure of the person and the child has your permission to do so.
- Tell your child NEVER to share his or her password with anyone, even friends.
- Review Internet sites with your child, and explain what information and websites are appropriate. Use safety and parental controls offered by your Internet service provider.
- Avoid placing the computer in the child's room. Instead, place the computer in a public area of your home, such as the den or kitchen, so that you can monitor your child's use.
- Discuss with your child the need for maintaining safety while using the Internet. Explain potential hazards in terms the child can understand.
- Advise your child to immediately close any sites or stop any communication that makes him or her confused or uncomfortable. Tell your child NEVER to arrange any face-to-face meeting with persons he or she meets online. Urge your child to seek you out if he or she encounters such a situation.
- Teach the child NEVER to open e-mail from any unknown senders.
- Be aware of computer use policies in your child's school.

care system millions of dollars. Violence affects families, women, and children of all ages, ethnic backgrounds, races, educational levels, and socioeconomic levels. Pregnancy is often a time when physical abuse starts or escalates, resulting in poorer outcomes for the mother and the baby. The nurse is responsible for assessment and follow-up of any abuse or suspected abuse.

Domestic Violence

Violence in the home environment, known as domestic violence, affects many lives in Canada. Violent crime committed by former spouses, boyfriends, or girlfriends is known as intimate partner abuse, family violence, wife beating, battering, marital abuse, or partner abuse. Regardless of the terminology used, the effects of abuse are widespread. It is difficult to obtain an accurate picture of spousal abuse because a large number of cases of abuse

are never reported to police. An estimated 7% of women and 6% of men in a current or previous spousal relationship experience spousal violence (Institute of Marriage and the Family Canada, 2009). In 2007, nearly 40,200 incidents of spousal violence (i.e., violence against legally married, common-law, separated, and divorced partners) were reported, representing about 12% of all reported violent crimes. Women comprised 3% of the victims (Statistics Canada, 2009b). Children often witness domestic violence, and they may be physically, sexually, or emotionally abused themselves (Abell & Ey, 2008). According to the Canadian Incidence Study of Reported Child Abuse and Neglect, the definition of child abuse and neglect includes any action that results in a child's death, physical harm, emotional maltreatment, sexual abuse or exploitation, exposure to intimate partner violence, and multiple other forms of maltreatment that present a risk of harm to a child (PHAC, 2008). In the study of the children identified as being maltreated, 34% were victims of neglect, 20% were victims of physical abuse, 3% were victims of sexual abuse, 9% were victims of emotional or psychological abuse, and 34% were exposed to intimate partner violence. It is notable that 18% of the substantive investigations involved more than one category of substantiated maltreatment. Fortunately, the number of children murdered in Canada for any reason, including child abuse, is very low. Of the 69 children murdered in 2001, 43 were killed by a family member (PHAC, 2008).

On rare occasions, maternal violence to self, her infant, and/or other children can be related to postpartum depression. Because depression places the mother at higher risk for suicide as well as for diminished capacity to adequately and safely care for her infant and other children, nurses working with the growing family need to be aware of the risk and assess for depression (Canadian Children's Rights Council, 2011).

Domestic violence is often accompanied by other major risk factors for children, such as poverty, female-headed households, and low education level of the primary caregiver. Children may feel the need to call for help or to blame themselves for the dispute that led to the abuse. Children who experience domestic violence or child abuse are at risk for problems such as aggressive behaviour, decreased social competencies, withdrawal, developmental regression, fears, anxiety, and learning problems (Children's Defense Fund—Ohio, 2009; Department of Justice Canada, 2011; Royal Canadian Mounted Police, 2007). Additional risks include poor school attendance, inappropriate sexual activity, substance abuse, post-traumatic syndrome, and conducting abuse or sexual assault as an adult (National Coalition Against Domestic Violence, 2007; Royal Canadian Mounted Police, 2007).

Nurses serve their clients best not by trying to rescue them, but by helping them build on their strengths and providing support, thereby empowering them to

> ## BOX 1.4 RADAR
>
> R–Routinely screen every patient for abuse.
> A–Ask direct, supportive, and non-judgmental
>   questions.
> D–Document all findings.
> A–Assess your client's safety.
> R–Review options and provide referrals.

help themselves. All nurses need to include "RADAR" in every client visit (Box 1.4).

Youth Violence

Violence committed by youth, including murder, rape, robbery, and aggravated assault, is an important public health problem. Between 1997 and 2006, violent crime among youth ages 12 to 17 increased 12% in Canada; and between 1991 and 2006, it rose 30%. Assault accounted for 80% of the violent crime committed by youth (Canada.com, 2008). In 2006, 72 males and 12 females under the age of 18 were implicated in homicides, but more than half of the homicides involved more than one perpetrator (Canada.com, 2008). Aboriginals account for 2.8% of the Canadian population but 18% of those who are incarcerated. Historic inequities have resulted in many Aboriginals having fewer protective factors, including social support. It is estimated that up to 80% of Aboriginal children ages 6 years and younger who live in urban areas live in poverty (Canadian Council on Social Development, 2010).

Youth violence affects not only the child and family in terms of injury and death, but also the entire community. Studies have shown that youth violence is associated with a disruption in social services, an increase in health care costs, and a decline in property values.

In recent years, school violence has received much attention, resulting in an increased concern for student safety, which in turn has led to a decline in school violence (Children's Defense Fund, 2005). Students are more likely to be victims of violent crimes away from school, but physical fights, thefts, weapon carrying, teacher victimization, and fear of school environments have increased (National Youth Violence Prevention Resource Center, 2011). There is currently no single resource or directory for school violence in Canada. If violence is to be prevented, families and school personnel must help youth learn to manage conflict in nonviolent ways (Ontario Ministry of Education, 2011). Effective programs to reduce violence in the long term need to involve continued coordination among schools, law enforcement, social services, and mental health systems and the development of effective programs to help to reduce these risk behaviours.

Due to the potential impact of violence on children and families, it is essential to identify and thoroughly assess any violent situation. Assessing and intervening to assist children in dealing with this issue are key, and this includes providing appropriate referrals to children's services, child advocacy centres, law enforcement officials, and shelters.

> ▶ *Take* NOTE!
>
> *Not all children exposed to violence suffer negative consequences. Children are resilient, and preliminary studies indicate that protective factors, such as involvement in social activities, a strong commitment to school and academic performance, and the ability to discuss problems with a supportive adult, can buffer children from the effects of violence, thereby helping to reduce the risk of developing violent behaviours.*

Community

Community encompasses a broad range of concepts, from the country in which a person lives down to a particular neighbourhood or group. The surrounding community affects many aspects of a person's health and general welfare. The quality of life within the community has a great influence on an individual's ability to develop and become a functional member of society. Community influences include the school, which is a community in itself, and peer groups. The support and assistance offered to women, children, and families from other areas of the community, such as school programs and community centres, can improve the individual's overall health and well-being.

Schools

Over the past century, major societal changes have led to children starting school earlier, spending more time in child care settings, and being involved in various community centres and activities. By age 4, many children spend several hours a day in a preschool setting; some children spend more time in school and child care settings than they do at home. In 2002 and 2003, about 54% of Canadian children 6 months to 5 years of age received some type of nonparent child care (Bushnik, 2006) as compared with 42% from 1994 to 1996. As a result, schools and child care services serve as major influences on children.

Although the primary role of schools has always been academic education, today they are performing more health-related functions than in the past. School also serves as a means of socialization, and academic success is linked to healthy behaviours, good mental health, and avoidance of pregnancy and juvenile justice problems, as well as health, jobs, and self-sufficiency in adult life.

School rules about attendance and authority relationships and the system of sanctions and rewards based on achievement transmit to children behavioural expectations that will help them succeed in employment, relationships, and self-sufficiency as adults. Schools can also play a major role in improving health and encouraging healthy behaviours. For example, some Canadian schools offer programs that identify school strengths related to health and health promotion; through groups that include students, parents, school staff, and community health nurses, these programs develop and deliver action plans to address desired next steps to improve the health and well-being of the school population. One such program is the Comprehensive School Health program in Calgary, Alberta (Alberta Health Services, 2011).

Because of social changes in Canada and elsewhere, more children are in child care and after-school programs than ever before. Thus, the socialization process begins earlier and involves a larger percentage of the child's waking hours (Fig. 1.7). Community centres and after-school programs can provide support, empowerment, boundaries and expectations, and constructive use of time (Search Institute, 2011).

Peer Groups

Peer groups can have a great impact on children. Relationships with peers often begin early, and they continue to be a large part of the child's world, particularly in school-age children and adolescents. This influence starts in play groups in early preschool or elementary school. The child comes into contact with a variety of values and belief systems from interactions with peer groups. When these values and beliefs differ from those of the child's family, conflicts can occur, possibly separating children from parents and strengthening the bond with the peer group. When the peer group is involved with school activities, athletics, or other healthy behaviours, the influence

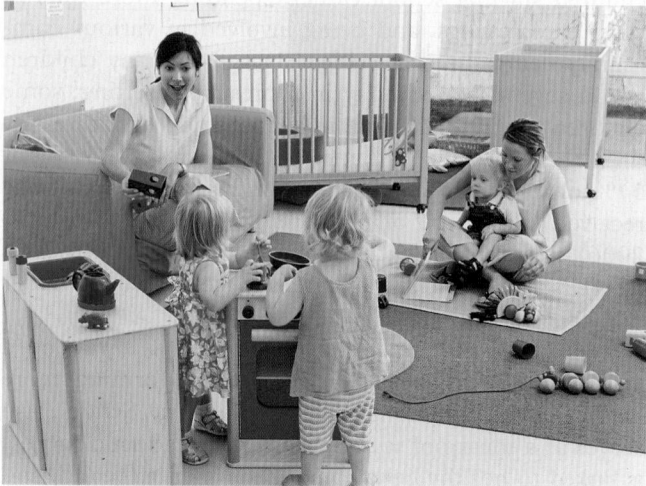

FIGURE 1.7 Day care centres provide socialization and support for young children.

is very positive, but the opposite is also true: peer groups can exert negative influences on the child. Thus, it is vital to identify the important peer groups in a child's life and the positive or negative behaviours associated with these groups.

Community and Neighbourhood Connectedness

Social capital refers to the bonds between individuals that assist social networks in communities to achieve a variety of goals. Basically, social capital is a mechanism by which resources in a community can be mobilized by and from the people, not for them. Such connectedness, relationships, and common interests propel neighbourhoods and communities toward engagement. Connected communities support an environment that makes it easy for people to engage in health-promoting behaviours. Asking a simple question such as, "How is your relationship with your neighbours?" can help give an understanding of a client's social milieu. Three areas to include in nursing assessments and interventions include:

- Bringing families together in communities to set the stage for networking
- Disseminating knowledge about what helps create healthy, supported communities
- Thinking of relationships as investments, with social interactions as the processes by which resources for health are exchanged

Culture

Culture is a view of the world and a set of traditions that are used by a specific social group and are transmitted to the next generation. Culture plays a critical role with women, children, and families. A person's culture influences not only socialization but also his or her experiences related to health and specific health practices. Culture is a complex phenomenon involving many components, such as beliefs, values, language, time, personal space, and view of the world, all of which shape a person's actions and behaviour. Individuals learn these patterns of cultural behaviours from their family and community through a process called enculturation, which involves acquiring knowledge and internalizing values. Culture influences every aspect of development and is reflected in childbearing and childrearing beliefs and practices designed to promote healthy adaptation.

With today's changing demographic patterns, nurses must be able to assimilate cultural knowledge into their interventions so they can care for culturally diverse women, children, and families. Nurses must be aware of the wide range of cultural traditions, values, and ethics. **Cultural safety** is an approach in which nurses are encouraged to recognize that they will never fully understand another person's culture and way of life because cultures and people are complex. People are a blend of many cultures (ethnicity, age, gender, occupation, socioeconomic status, etc), and the relationship between these cultures is fluid, interactive, and dynamic. Therefore, the culturally safe approach is for nurses to acknowledge that they cannot fully predict or standardize a client's cultural needs; however, nurses can create an environment in which the client feels culturally safe. Cultural safety is defined by the person receiving care and not by the nurse; in this way the health care provided can be adapted to meet the client's or patient's needs. Nurses also need to recognize the strengths and capabilities that the patient or client possess that derive from their culture. These need to be acknowledged and incorporated when helping the individual or family develop self- or home management strategies. This approach requires that nurses first examine and reflect on their own culture and biases. For example, nurses should contemplate what they consider to be desirable "universal" moral principles and then think about how they would intervene with a patient whose moral principles are different from their own. In hospitals, patients are already in a position of vulnerability in that they require care they cannot provide for themselves and they are separated from their own cultural contexts. As part of the dominant hospital culture, it is incumbent on nurses to ask the patient or family about cultural preferences. Cultural safety occurs when nurses respond in a way that preserves the patient's identity and that the patient regards as culturally appropriate (Woods, 2010).

▶ **Take** NOTE!

One suggestion to assist in preparing to provide culturally safe care is for nurses to list their desirable "universal" moral principles and then consider how they would intervene with a patient whose moral principles are different from their own.

Cultural Groups

A society typically includes dominant and minority groups. The dominant group, often the largest group, has the greatest authority to control the values and sanctions of the society (Pillitteri, 2007). As a result, the dominant or majority culture may have the largest impact on health care systems. The minority cultural groups may remain in their own communities and maintain some of their traditions and values while mainstreaming into Canadian society. A culture may contain many subcultures, and geographic differences also can occur. Nurses may assume that they understand another's culture, including the Aboriginal culture, but First Nations people from the Algonquin bands in Ontario may be quite different than the Cree in Manitoba, the Blackfoot in Alberta, or the Suquamish in British Columbia. Individuals living in Toronto, Ontario may be quite different from First Nations individuals living in rural Saskatchewan. When providing culturally safe care to a person from an Aboriginal culture,

the culturally safe nurse will not make assumptions but will ask about personal or cultural preferences. Being aware of these differences is essential to providing culturally competent care.

Ethnicity is sometimes used synonymously with culture; the definition basically involves group membership by virtue of common ancestry. The basic groups or divisions are differentiated by customs, characteristics, language, or similar distinguishing factors. Ethnic groups can be identified by their specific family structures, languages, food preferences, religious customs, moral codes, and health care practices. Children learn the group's mode of behaviour by observing and imitating those around them. Most Canadians view themselves as belonging to a specific cultural heritage or ethnic group, though many do not closely identify with their ethnicity. The influences of culture and ethnicity on women, children, and families are highly variable, particularly for new immigrants, and traditional behaviours can change based on new circumstances and a dynamic environment.

Ethnocentrism is a belief that one's own ethnic group is superior to other groups, and thus one's one way of living, ideas, and practices are the best. Some individuals may refuse health care rather than receive it from a cultural group they believe is inferior to their own. Ethnocentrism can lead to a distorted view of the world, and nurses need to evaluate their own biases for any that may hinder their ability to give culturally competent care.

Nurses need to be aware of the health care values and practices that are passed along from one generation to the next. For example, the belief in folk healers relates to how the culture interprets illness and health. Some of these parts of the culture may have major influences on an individual's health. Table 1.3 highlights some major cultural groups and their common health beliefs and practices.

▶ **Take** NOTE!

Nurses can have a lifelong influence on an individual's perceptions of health and use of health services. By providing culturally safe care, nurses can enhance the family's traditional practices, and different cultural practices can become sources of strength rather than areas of conflict.

Spirituality and Religion

Spirituality is a basic human quality involving the belief in something greater than oneself and a faith that affirms life. It is a major influence for many people, providing a meaning or purpose to life and a foundation for and source of love, relationships, and service. Spirituality is considered a universal human phenomenon. During life-changing events and crises, such as a serious illness or the birth of a child with a congenital defect, families often turn to spirituality for hope, comfort, and relief.

TABLE 1.3 BELIEFS AND PRACTICES OF SELECTED CULTURAL GROUPS

Cultural Group	Beliefs and Practices Affecting Maternal and Children's Health
African	Strong extended family relationships; mother as head of household; older family members valued and respected Food as a symbol of health and wealth View of health as harmony with nature; illness as disruption in harmony Use of folk healing and home remedies common View of pregnancy as a state of wellness Emotional support during labour commonly from other women, primarily the woman's own mother Liberal use of oil on newborn's and infant's scalp and skin Belief in illnesses as natural (due to natural forces person hasn't protected self against) and unnatural (due to person or spirit) Illness commonly associated with pain Pain and suffering inevitable; relief achieved through prayers and laying on of hands Individuals vulnerable to external forces
Asian	Strong loyalty to the family Family as the centre, with members expected to care for one another Use of complementary modalities with Western health care practices View of life as a cycle with everything connected to health Pain described by diverse body symptoms Health viewed as a balance between the forces of yang and yin Respect for authority emphasized View of pregnancy as a natural process and happy time for woman Little involvement of the father during labour; quiet, stoic appearance of woman during labour Protection of woman from cold forces for 30 days after birth of newborn
Arab	Women subordinate to men; young individuals subordinate to older persons Family loyalty is primary Good health associated with eating properly, consuming nutritious foods, and fasting to cure disease Illness is due to inadequate diet, shifts in hot and cold, exposure of stomach while sleeping, emotional or spiritual distress, and "evil eye" Little emphasis on preventive care View of pain as unpleasant, requiring immediate control or relief Birthmarks on newborn due to unsatisfied maternal cravings Pain of labour demonstrated via facial expressions, verbalizations, and body movements; reluctant to use breathing and relaxation techniques during labour Wrapping of newborn's stomach at birth to prevent cold or wind from entering baby's body Breastfeeding often delayed for 2 to 3 days after birth Cleanliness important for prayer
Aboriginals (First Nations)	High value on family and tribe; respect for elders Family as an extended network providing care for newborns and children Women as the verbal decision makers View of pregnancy as normal and natural process; entire family may be present at birth Newborn not given colostrum Celebrations to mark the stages of growth and development Use of food to celebrate life events and in healing and religious ceremonies Health as harmony with nature; illness due to disharmony, evil spirits Restoration of physical, mental, and spiritual balance through healing ceremonies View of pain as something to be tolerated
Hispanic	Family important; father as the source of strength, wisdom, and self-confidence Mother as the caretaker and decision maker for health View of children as persons to continue the family and culture Birthmark on baby due to unsatisfied food cravings during pregnancy Mother's legs brought together after birth of newborn to prevent air from entering uterus Possibly boisterous and loud during labour Bed rest for first 3 days postpartum; no bathing for 14 days Newborn protection from the evil eye Use of food for celebrations and socialization Health as God's will, maintainable with a balance of hot and cold food intake Freedom from pain indicative of good health; pain tolerated stoically due to belief that it is God's will Folk medicine practices and prayers, herbal teas and poultices for illness treatment

Though the word "religion" is often used interchangeably with spirituality in our society, the two are distinctly different. Spirituality is considered private and individual. **Religion**, in contrast, is an organized way of sharing beliefs and practicing worship. Less than 75% of Canadians state that they believe in a god (Avery, 2008). This contrasts sharply with the United States, where only 8% do not believe (Avery, 2008). Canadians with spiritual or religious beliefs and views find that they provide strength and support during times of stress and illness. In some religions, illness is seen as a punishment for sin or wrongdoing. Others religions view illness as a test of strength that allows them to strive for faithfulness. Spirituality in Canada cannot be measured or understood solely in terms of organized religion; interest in the afterlife and spiritual references are found in many popular books and movies (Harvey, 1998).

Identifying a client's religious beliefs and customs is important. Families appreciate recognition of and respect for their beliefs. Dietary restrictions, rituals such as baptism or communion, use of amulets or icons, or practices related to birth or newborn care can be incorporated into the plan of care. The best way to meet a family's spiritual needs is to ask them about their preferences and ensure that they are clearly communicated to health care staff interacting with the family.

▶ *Take* NOTE!

Never make assumptions about a family's religious or spiritual affiliation. Although they may belong to a particular religion, they may not adhere to all of its beliefs or participate in all aspects of the religion. Ask the family about their beliefs and preferences, and be alert for clues that provide insight into their specific beliefs.

Diversity of Client Populations

Canada has a history and reputation of being a cultural mosaic, a society where each individual brings a diversity and richness that enriches the country as a whole. Aboriginals and Muslims constitute two of the fastest-growing populations in Canada (Canadian Chamber of Commerce, 2010; Selby, 2007).

According to Statistics Canada (2009a), Asians (including persons from the Middle East) comprise 58.3% of new immigrants and Europeans comprise 16.1%. Between 2001 and 2006, Canada's immigrant population grew by 13.6%; by contrast, the Canadian-born population grew by only 3.3% (Cohen, 2012). In 2010, immigration from all countries reached the highest rate seen in four decades—a 65% increase (Cohen, 2012). Although Canada publicly welcomes new immigrants and maintained its goal of welcoming 240,000 to 265,000 new immigrants in 2010—most other First

World countries are decreasing their immigrant numbers due to economic downturn. Becoming a Canadian citizen is seen to be more difficult. In 2009, the federal government toughened the citizenship testing. As many as one third of immigrants failed the test that year, compared with 4% to 8% in previous years (Guneet, 2010).

Canada is viewed as offering employment and economic opportunities, expanded human rights, educational opportunities, and other types of freedoms and opportunities, thus inspiring many individuals to move to Canada from other countries. Immigration significantly affects the health, educational, and social services offered in this country. It also presents issues related to access to care and the types of care that need to be offered. Canada continually evaluates and amends its immigration policies.

Immigration imposes unique stresses on women, children, and families, including:

• Depression, grief, or anxiety associated with migration and acculturation
• Separation from support systems
• Inadequate language skills in a society that is not tolerant of linguistic differences
• Disparities in social, professional, and economic status between the country of origin and Canada
• Disparities between what the new immigrant anticipated when moving to Canada and reality
• Traumatic events such as war or persecution that may have occurred in the immigrant's native country (American Academy of Pediatrics Committee on Community Health Services, 2005)

Immigrant families may face financial, language, cultural, and other type of barriers that reduce their ability to access health care. For example, they may not seek care if they cannot find health care providers who speak their language or are not confident an interpreter will be available. Stresses experienced by immigrant children and their families, such as those associated with relocation, separation, and traumatic events, can also affect their psychological health. See Evidence-based Practice 1.2.

Health Status and Lifestyle

An individual's chronic health conditions and lifestyle can increase or decrease his or her risk for health problems. Chronic health conditions can begin soon after birth. For example, the incidence of multiple births is on the rise in Canada due to the increased use of in vitro fertilization and other assisted technologies (Behrman & Butler, 2007; PHAC, 2008). Associated complications include intrauterine growth retardation and prematurity (PHAC, 2008), which can lead to chronic health problems that may hinder the child's growth and development. Children with chronic health conditions may

EVIDENCE-BASED PRACTICE 1.2
Perinatal Beliefs and Practices of Immigrant Punjabi Women Living in Canada

● Study

Underutilization of the Canadian health care system by new immigrant Punjabi women has resulted in low birth weight, malnutrition, and genetic anomalies such as neural tube defects in their children. A lack of cultural competence and the provision of culturally safe care were believed to be contributing factors. Previous studies have investigated values and beliefs of various cultures as well as the experiences of immigrant women within the health care systems of various countries and have described cultural norms and guidelines for assessment and care of women from other cultures. Problems associated with those findings included:

- Summaries of norms and values of a cultural group, such as women from India, although helpful in presenting a general understanding, were simplistic and could not address the diversity found within a cultural group.
- Once immigration to Canada had occurred, further differences among individuals, such as economic status, level of English proficiency, and level of integration into the community, were ignored.
- Emphasis was placed on negative stereotypes developed from perceptions of behaviours that do not fit the Western description of "normal" behaviours (e.g., Aboriginal women's belief in the importance of rest in the postnatal period, which runs counter to the Western value of self-care and independence). Positive behaviours such as not smoking were virtually ignored.

To address these and other issues, prenatal classes for new immigrant women have been developed and piloted in Canada with relative success. However, anecdotal reports from British Columbia noted that despite the variety of care options offered, including use of a general practitioner, obstetrician, or midwife, use of translators, and use of CH professionals with the appropriate language skills, uptake of newly immigrated women into these classes was limited.

A naturalistic qualitative study was conducted in a large urban setting in British Columbia to identify and describe the cultural traditions and values of newly immigrated Punjabi women in their perinatal experiences in the Canadian context. All 15 eligible women were first-time mothers who had immigrated to Canada from Punjab, India within the previous 5 years and had given birth to a full-term healthy infant in the previous 3 months. Study findings were confirmed by five South Asian immigrant health professionals who had also given birth in Canada and had provided health care to the Punjabi community for at least 10 years.

▲ Findings

The study showed that Punjabi women have culturally specific beliefs and practices with regard to the prenatal period, dietary practices followed and initiated during the pre- and postnatal period, stress reduction and positive energy practices, familial input, role of the husband, and interactions with health care professionals. Overall, the findings were not homogenous. Adherence to rituals and practices varied widely, based on availability of support and the level of integration into Western culture (i.e., some practices were modified or abandoned).

■ Nursing Implications

Three major recommendations arose from this study. First, ongoing maintenance and updating of professional development opportunities for all health care professionals will address the settlement experience of Punjabi people as well as the intersection of traditional values and beliefs with Western values and beliefs at work in the health care system. Second, inclusion of individuals and leaders within immigrant communities in the development of culturally sensitive and safe health care practices will put their cultural identity in the forefront and will lead to better usage of all levels of health care and more positive postnatal outcomes for both mother and baby. Finally, changing Canada's health care policy and structure will help to better address the individual needs of Punjabi women, such as through policies that better acknowledge the Punjabi value of postpartum rest and the hiring of individuals who speak the Punjabi language.

Source: Grewal, S.K., Bhagat, R., & Balneaves, L.G. (2008). Perinatal beliefs and practices of immigrant women living in Canada. *Journal of Obstetric, Gynecologic and Neonatal Nursing, 37*(3).

experience developmental delays, especially in acquiring skills related to cognition, communication, adaptation, social functioning, and motor functioning. Thus, the beginning health status of a child may affect his or her long-term health and development.

Developmental Level and Disease Distribution

Developmental level has a major impact on an individual's health status. In general, the distribution of diseases or illnesses varies with age. For example, adolescents who become pregnant are at higher risk for certain complications, such as anemia, hypertension, preterm labour, cephalopelvic disproportion, and PPH. Pregnant adolescents also experience higher rates of intimate partner violence and substance abuse. Substance abuse can contribute to LBW, intrauterine growth restriction, preterm births, newborn addiction, and sepsis (Mittendorfer-Rutz & Wasserman, 2008). Women who become pregnant after age 35 are at risk for hypertension, dystocia, and PPH. Older pregnant women are also more likely to have a pre-existing condition that could complicate the pregnancy. Fetuses of older pregnant women are at higher risk for chromosomal abnormalities.

Certain communicable diseases are more commonly associated with certain age groups. Before the use of routine immunizations, conditions such as measles and mumps were commonly seen in younger school-age children. The physiologic immaturity of an infant's body systems increases the risk for infection. Ingestion of toxic substances and poisoning are major health concerns for toddlers as they become more mobile and inquisitive. Adolescents are establishing their identity, which may lead them to distance themselves from their family values and traditions and conform more with their peers for a period of time. This journey may lead to risky behaviours, resulting in injuries or other health problems.

Nutrition

Food provides the body with the calories and nutrients needed to sustain life and promote growth as well as the essentials required to maintain health and prevent illness. Nutritional deficiencies and childhood obesity are frequently a combined problem due to the volume of high-fat food and the low nutritional value of the food consumed. Inadequate food intake, social and cultural food practices or habits that may be nutritionally unsound, the availability of processed and nutritionally inadequate foods, lack of nutrition education in homes and schools, and the presence of illness that interferes with the ingestion, digestion, and absorption of food can all affect an individual's nutrition.

During pregnancy, a woman needs additional calories to support fetal growth and development as well as to support her own needs, and an adequate intake of folic acid is important to prevent neural tube defects (Fig. 1.8). For the child, inadequate nutrition is associated with lowered cognitive ability, poor or altered emotional and mental health, increased susceptibility to childhood illnesses, and stunted physical growth. The "fast food" or "junk food" that is prevalent in today's society is a key factor in the epidemic of childhood obesity and increases in the prevalence of childhood type 2 diabetes. Nutrition and its effects on health status are integrated throughout this text.

Lifestyle Choices

Lifestyle choices that affect an individual's health include patterns of eating, exercise, use of tobacco, drugs, or alcohol, and methods of coping with stress. Most health problems that arise today are due to an individual's lifestyle. For children, the lifestyle of the parents basically is the lifestyle of the child, so parents need to set a good example in terms of nutrition and physical activity. Lifestyle choices are impacted by determinants such as parent income, education, and social support.

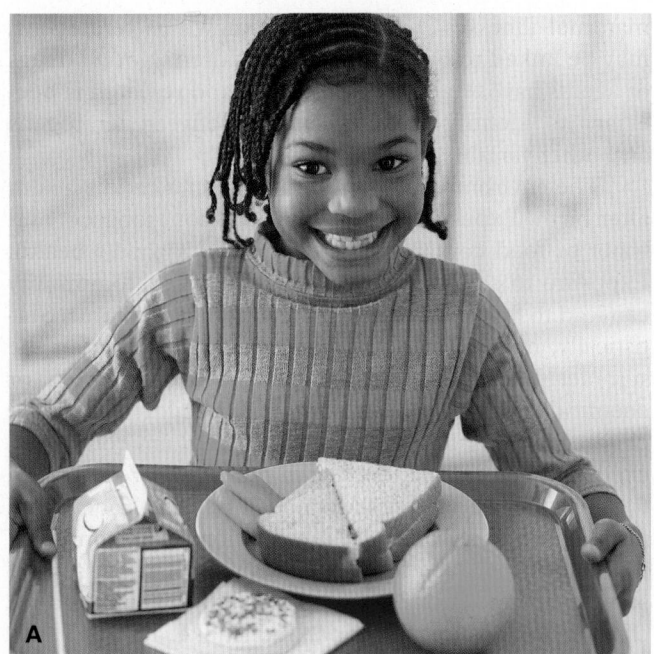

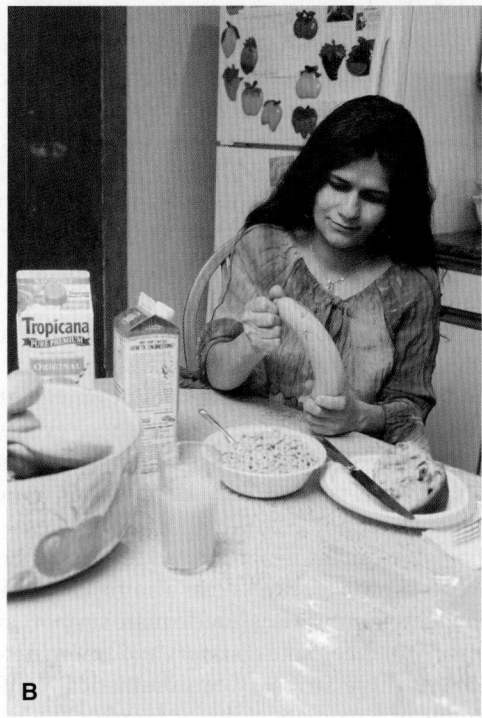

FIGURE 1.8 (**A**) The dietary habits established early in life can have a long-lasting impact on the child's health and quality of life. (**B**) This pregnant client is eating a healthy meal to ensure adequate nutrition.

Environmental Exposure

Some environmental exposures can jeopardize health. In utero, the child can be affected by lack of maternal nutrition, maternal infections, or maternal use of alcohol, tobacco, and drugs. Nurses caring for pregnant women should be aware of the risks to the fetus posed by certain drugs, chemicals, and dietary agents as well as maternal illnesses. These agents, known as teratogens, may be linked to birth defects in children. Not all drugs or agents have fetal effects, however, and research is necessary to identify the correlations between teratogens and other variables.

The environment continues to affect a child's health after birth. Exposure to lead, air pollution, tobacco, and water or food contaminants can impair a child's health. Exposure to safety hazards in the home or community can lead to falls, burns, drowning, or other accidents. Statistically, more drownings occur in children during the summer. Exposure to second-hand smoke, radiation, or chemicals is another health hazard for children. Because children are smaller and still developing, environmental exposures can cause more health problems for them than for adults, both in the short and long term. Therefore, nurses need to advocate for the creation of environments that are supportive of health. Examples of successes are soft playground surfaces and tobacco by-laws that reduce children's exposure to secondhand smoke.

Stress and Coping

Canada is a vast nation, bordered on three sides by ocean. Natural disasters are on the rise worldwide, and Canada is no exception. Forest fires in British Columbia in 2009 and severe rainstorms and tornadoes across Canada in 2005 are just a few examples of natural disasters that had a significant impact on the well-being of women, children, and families. Stressors such as war, terrorism, school violence, and natural disasters may decrease a person's coping ability and lead to alterations in growth and development. Exposure to traumatic events and violence may have long-term effects on an individual's psychosocial development and status. Children who have experienced these events are at risk for the development of post-traumatic stress disorder, behavioural issues, and depression (Andersen, Geary, Portner, et al., 2010).

Exposure to stress is not limited to disasters or traumatic events, however. Stress can also result from inadequate finances, family crises, inadequate support systems, or domestic violence. Like disasters and traumatic events, the effects of these stressors can dramatically affect the health status of a woman, child, or family.

*R*ecall Sophia, the 38-year-old pregnant woman who has come to the prenatal clinic for a visit. While talking with the nurse, Sophia mentions that her children are very involved in activities. She says, "My husband is busy at work, so I do most of the running around. Sometimes I feel like the people at the drive-through know me by name! My husband helps out on the weekends, but during the week, it's all me." What factors may be influencing Sophia's health? How might these factors be influencing the health of her children and the family?

Health Care Cost Containment

The health care system functions within a market setting, offering goods and services that carry a cost to health care consumers and clients. The advent of primary care clinics is part of an attempt to reduce waiting times for health care services, shorten hospital stays, and increase interdisciplinary care in the community setting. The overall challenge is to maintain or improve health outcomes while reducing cost. For example, if a pregnant diabetic woman needs to go to an endocrinologist, the woman will need to go through her primary health care professional to receive a referral to a specialist. However, the primary health care provider may be a nurse practitioner who also refers the woman to a nutritionist.

Canadians have the luxury of a publicly funded health care system that is responsible for meeting the essential health care needs of all Canadians. Care is mostly free at point of use and is provided by private entities (e.g., hospitals, doctors). The Canada Health Act provides guidelines around the quality of care provided and the provinces manage the day to day running of health care delivery. Approximately 70% of payment to providers is made through provincially funded and administered insurance "companies," such as Manitoba Health and the Medical Services Plan of British Columbia, and the remaining 30% is paid through privately funded and administered insurance companies, such as Blue Cross. The majority of funding for health care comes from transfer payments made to each provincial insurance "company" from the federal government, and a lesser amount comes from premiums charged to provincial residents. Not all provinces have chosen to charge residents. Governments provide payment only for what they term "essential services." Each provincial government determines what those "essential services" are. Services provided in hospitals and by most physicians are usually deemed essential. In most cases, pharmaceuticals not administered in the hospital, dental and optometry care, and other services such as privately run physiotherapy are not covered by provincial funding.

Health care systems are continually evolving and costs continually rising—from $39.7 billion in 1975 to $137.3 billion in 2008. Costs were expected to increase by more than 5% in 2009 to $183 billion. The majority of these costs are incurred by hospitals ($51 billion), pharmaceutical companies ($30 billion), and physicians ($26 billion) (Health Canada, 2009).

Although cost containment is important to maintain an affordable publicly funded health care system, such efforts should not reduce the quality or safety of care delivered. Preventive care has been shown to lower costs significantly. Health care professionals are encouraged to promote primary prevention strategies, such as smoking cessation programs, immunizations, and lobbying for equity and social justice, as well as secondary prevention strategies that include increasing public awareness of the importance of mammograms and Pap tests, which yield positive outcomes and reduce overall health care costs. Tertiary prevention, such as using technological advances to diagnose and treat diseases early, also saves both lives and money.

Nurses can be leaders in providing quality care within a limited-resource environment by emphasizing to their clients the importance of making healthy lifestyle choices, seeking early interventions for minor problems before they become major ones, and learning about health-related issues that affect them so they can select the best option for themselves and their families. Prevention services and health education are the cornerstones of delivering quality maternal and child health care. Tobacco addiction and obesity are examples of lifestyle choices that require more than simply education about their harm to health to bring about change. Therefore, nurses also have a role in creating environments that encourage lifestyle changes and make the healthy choice the easy choice.

Health Care System Issues

Canadians enjoy relative freedom of choice with regard to what health care professionals they see, how their care is handled, and where that care is provided. However, this system is not without its issues. One example relates to maternity care. Although over half of the women who were interviewed for the Maternal Experiences Survey stated they were satisfied with their birthing experience, two main issues were neither identified nor addressed (PHAC, 2009b). First, the Aboriginal voice was not heard in this survey. If it had been, the results would have been vastly different. For an Aboriginal woman, the experience of birth is dreaded as it represents a long trip to a hospital where little or no family or social support is present for days to months on end (SOGC, 2007; 2008).

Second, there is a looming shortage of health care professionals who provide maternity care. This shortage has been studied and addressed for a number of years, including at the 2003 First Ministers' Conference and the 2008 SOGC MCP² study, which found that labouring women require 24/7 care provided by skilled attendants, as well as referral and transfer care as needed. Canada's infant mortality, perinatal mortality, and maternal mortality rates are all rising, so the need for trained and skilled health care professionals is imperative.

Currently, family physicians provide the majority of maternity care, although the number of family physicians who attend births has fallen more than 10% in the past decade. The number of practicing obstetricians in Canada was 1,650 in 2008, but the number who actually perform deliveries is declining. Midwifery care is starting to become more widely accepted across Canada, and the demand is rising, but only six provinces (British Columbia, Alberta, Manitoba, Ontario, Quebec, and Nova Scotia) and the Northwest Territories actually recognize midwives. In 2010, there were 850 midwives across Canada, 435 of whom practiced in Ontario. In that province,

10% of births were attended by a midwife, but 40% of mothers who requested to have one could not get one (Hardy, 2011).

As each province is responsible for health care delivery, meeting the needs of women and families has been inconsistent across jurisdictions. As well, changes to the maternity care system may occur at a local level without provincial input (e.g., some hospitals restricting or eliminating care for maternity patients). A national strategy to address fundamental needs across the system is needed to sustain the maternal-child health care services throughout the country.

Access to Health Care

The health care system continues to change as a result of pressures coming from many directions. These changes reflect shifts in social and economic realities and the results of the biomedical and technological progress that has been made over the past several decades. The effects are felt by every individual who seeks health care in any form. The system of providing medical care in a high-tech environment has changed to providing health care in an environment with limited resources and access to services. Ways to allocate our limited health care resources continue to be the focus.

Canadian citizens are entitled to health care coverage, including preventive as well as medical and diagnostic treatment, hospital care, and other services, regardless of their medical history or income. Health care is managed by individual provinces, and provinces also provide publicly funded health care services that are not included in the Canada Health Act. The services offered, restrictions to the services, cost sharing, and whether costs are fixed or variable based on an income-dependent gradient vary from province to province. Examples of provincial health services include home care, physiotherapy, dental care, and prescription medications. In addition to publicly funded health care, private health insurance may be purchased individually, or provided by an employer, to supplement services provided by the province.

Health care services vary among urban, rural, and/or isolated settings. Home intravenous (IV) therapy is not equally accessible across Canada despite research that shows that it is safe and cost-effective and improves the quality of life. In some rural and isolated areas, IV therapy may not be provided if a client's home is too isolated, if there is inadequate home care staffing, or if the health care professionals lack experience in starting and monitoring IV therapy (Moore & Bortolussi, 2011). Rural Canadians have lower survival rates for serious injuries as compared with urban Canadians. Rural ambulance attendants may be volunteers, poorly trained and inadequately equipped, particularly with regard to the care of children. Emergency departments may be staffed with one registered nurse and an on-call physician, neither of whom is likely to be an expert in pediatric care. A child may need to be flown via air ambulance to the nearest acute care referral centre. If the weather is uncooperative, or the air ambulance is busy, it may be many hours before the patient can be transported (Canadian Association of Emergency Physicians, n.d.).

Aboriginal people who live on reservations and Inuit living in the North have direct health services provided and paid for by the federal government and not under the jurisdiction of the provinces. Like all Canadians, they receive health services under the Canada Health Act, but additional services are provided and paid for by Health Canada rather than the province in which a reserve is located. As a result, First Nations people experience different health services and restrictions if they are living on or off the reservation. In the mid-1980s, Health Canada began working with the First Nations and Inuit communities to transition control of health services from the government to the Band councils. The pace of the transition is dependent on each Band council's accountability (Health Canada, 2011a).

Similar models of community intervention have been implemented in First Nations, Inuit, and Aboriginal communities with the addition of a 1-day training program designed to improve the health professional's ability to recognize psychological distress. Evaluation results for this program reveal that suicide rates among youth ages 15 to 19 years were reduced shortly after implementation and sustained for the ensuing 5 years (Health Canada, 2005).

Many attribute Canada's life expectancy (about 80 years) and low infant mortality rate to its universal health care system. Canadian citizens of all income levels and at all stages of life can seek health care for early treatment, maintenance, and preventive interventions without concern about cost (Canadian Health Care, 2007). The most significant issue is the variation in accessibility, which is dependent on factors such as isolation and provincial budgets.

Preventive Care Focus

The emphasis on cost reduction has also led to an emphasis on health promotion, including primary, secondary, and tertiary preventive care services. Assessment of the community includes identifying protective and risk factors as related to determinants of health, such as income, education, and healthy child development. Primary prevention subsequent to the assessment may include lobbying for safe playgrounds or educating families on everything from keeping the home safe to ways to prevent illness, immunizations, and lobbying for school lunches in neighbourhoods where food security is a risk factor. Anticipatory guidance is vital during each health contact with women, children, and families.

The Continuum of Care Emphasis

A "continuum of care" strategy, also called seamless care, is cost-effective and provides more efficient and effective services. This continuum extends from acute care settings such as hospitals to outpatient settings such as ambulatory care clinics, primary care offices, rehabilitative units, community care settings, long-term facilities, homes, and even schools. For example, the hospital stay is now integrated into a continuum that allows the client to complete therapy at home, school, or other community settings, while re-entering the hospital for short periods for specific treatments or illnesses.

Improvements in Diagnosis and Treatments

Because of the tremendous improvements that have been made in technology and biomedicine, disorders and diseases are being diagnosed and treated earlier. The 1990s witnessed remarkable advances in identifying connections between genetics and various pathophysiologic processes. For example, a female fetus with congenital adrenal hyperplasia, a genetic disorder resulting in a steroid enzyme deficiency that can lead to disfiguring anatomic abnormalities, can now receive treatment before birth. In addition, many genetic defects are being identified so counselling and treatment may occur early. With these improved diagnoses and treatments, nurses may now be caring for individuals who have survived situations that once would have been fatal, who are living well beyond their life expectancy for a specific illness, or who are functioning with chronic disabilities. For example, at one time women with congenital heart disease did not live long enough to become pregnant. However, with new surgical techniques to correct the defects, many of these women survive and become pregnant, progressing through their pregnancy and delivery without significant problems.

While positive and exciting, these advances and trends also pose new challenges for the health care community. For example, as health care for premature newborns improves and survival rates increase, the incidence of long-term chronic conditions such as respiratory airway dysfunction or developmental delays has also increased. As a result, nurses are faced with caring for clients at all stages along the health–illness continuum.

Empowerment of Health Care Consumers

Due to the influence of the media as well as the PHAC, the focus on prevention, a more educated population, and technological advances, individuals and families have taken an increased responsibility for their own health. Health consumers are now better informed, and they play a greater role in managing their own health and illness. Families seek information about illnesses, and they participate in making decisions about treatment options. As client advocates valuing family-centred care, nurses are instrumental in promoting this empowerment. To do this effectively, the nurse must respect the family's views and concerns, address all issues and concerns, and always include the family members in decisions.

The Internet provides an abundance of readily accessible health care information. Nurses have a responsibility to direct parents, parents-to-be, and older children to credible sources of information and provide guidance to help them become discerning Internet surfers.

Barriers to Health Care

Women are major consumers of health care services, in many cases arranging not only their own care but also that of family members. Compared with men, women have more health problems, longer life spans, and more significant reproductive health needs. Access to care can be jeopardized by lower incomes and greater responsibilities (juggling work and family). Lack of finances or transportation, language or cultural barriers, inconvenient clinic hours, and poor attitudes of health care workers often discourage clients from seeking health care.

Transportation

Getting to and from appointments can be challenging for clients who do not drive or own a car or cannot use public transportation—if there is public transportation in the area. It can be difficult for these clients to attend all recommended prenatal health care visits or well-child visits, especially if the woman has other small children who must be taken along on the visit. These challenges can reduce the adherence to scheduled appointments and follow-up.

Human Resources

Healthy pregnancy and a healthy delivery can be enhanced when women received pre-conception and prenatal care. On average, a pregnant woman should have between seven and 11 prenatal visits with her family doctor, midwife, or obstetrician (Heaman & O'Brien, 2009). With the shortage of family physicians, obstetricians, and midwives (Haymes, 2007), some pregnant women are finding it challenging to acquire early pregnancy care. In 2006, about 5 million Canadians, or 17% of the population, did not have a family doctor (Canadian Broadcasting Centre, 2006). Moreover, about 70% of family doctors in Canada do not provide prenatal care or attend births; therefore, finding an obstetrician may be even more difficult (Canadian Health Services Research Foundation, 2006). The problem is accentuated in rural areas, and women in these areas are routinely evacuated from their homes, families, and communities to be assured access to appropriate health care.

Language and Culture

Language is how people communicate with each other to increase their understanding or knowledge. If a health care worker cannot speak the same language as the client or does not have a trained interpreter available, a barrier is created. The client's complaints can be misinterpreted or ignored or their significance can be misconstrued. This language barrier might prevent the client from accessing necessary prenatal care or preventive care.

Health determinants such as sociocultural and ethnic factors as well as the age of the mother may pose barriers to health care. Knowledge barriers such as lack of understanding or awareness of the importance of prenatal care or child health promotion and spiritual barriers (e.g., some forms of treatment are proscribed by religions) also cross all ethnic groups and can create barriers to health care.

Health Care Delivery System

The health care delivery system itself can create barriers. Clinic hours must meet the needs of the clients, not the health care providers who work there. Evening or weekend hours might be needed to meet the schedules of working clients. Clinic personnel should evaluate the availability and accessibility of the services they offer. Emergency room visits are often higher than necessary due to the limited number of health care clinics open outside of traditional business hours.

Unfortunately, some health care workers exhibit negative attitudes toward poor or culturally diverse families, and this could deter these clients from seeking health care. Long delays, hurried examinations, and rude comments by staff discourage clients from returning.

▶ *Consider* THIS!

I was a 17-year-old pregnant street worker needing prenatal care. I showed the receptionist the growing bulge on my belly and asked for services. All the receptionist seemed interested in was my Health Care number and whether I had additional health insurance. She proceeded to ask me personal questions concerning who the father was and commented on how young I was. Then I had to step on a scale, which was in an open area where others could see my weight. While she was doing this she talked about how my smoking was hurting my baby. I felt panicky and was glad when she was done. She said I should sit down and wait to be called. It seemed to me like all eyes were on me while I found an empty seat in the waiting room. If I'm anxious I need a smoke but I managed to sit and wait for over an hour without any attention. Then I left.

Critical thinking questions: Why did she leave before receiving any health care service? What must she have been feeling during her wait? Would you come back to this clinic again? Why or why not?

Legal and Ethical Issues in Maternal and Child Health Care

Law and ethics are interrelated and affect all of nursing. Professional nurses must understand their scope of practice, standards of care, institutional or agency policies, and provincial laws. Every nurse is responsible for knowing current information regarding ethics and laws related to their practice (CNA, 2008).

Several areas are of particular importance to the health care of women and children. These include abortion, substance abuse, fetal therapy, informed consent, client rights, and confidentiality.

Abortion

Abortion has always been a volatile legal, social, and political issue. In 1969, the Criminal Code of Canada was amended to decriminalize abortions performed by physicians in hospitals after a "therapeutic abortion committee" determined that the woman's health would be negatively impacted by continuation of the pregnancy. In 1981, Quebec established abortion clinics as part of its community services. In 1988, the Supreme Court deleted abortion from the criminal code, leaving decisions around care of women requesting an abortion to each provincial health care system. In 1991, the Supreme Court ruled that an unborn child is not a "person" and unborn children have no rights unless they are born alive. In 1999, nurses at Markham Stouffville Hospital in Ontario set a Canadian precedent when they were given the right to decline assisting doctors in performing abortions.

Although abortion is a common procedure in Canada today, it remains a hotly debated political issue that separates people into two camps: pro-choice and pro-life. The pro-choice group supports the right of any woman to make decisions about her reproductive functions based on her own moral and ethical beliefs. The pro-life group feels strongly that life starts at conception and abortion is murder, as it deprives the fetus of the basic right to life. In recent years, several parliamentary bills have been introduced, but not passed, that would make it illegal to perform abortions after 20 weeks' gestation and making it a separate crime to kill a fetus in the course of a violent attack on a mother. This very emotional issue will continue to be debated years to come (AbortionInCanada.ca., n.d.; LifeCanada, 2008).

Medical and surgical modalities are available to terminate a pregnancy, depending on how far the pregnancy has developed. A surgical intervention can be performed up to 14 weeks' gestation; a medical intervention can be performed up to 9 weeks' gestation (Gan, Zou, Wu, et al., 2008). All women undergoing abortion need emotional support, a stable environment in which to recover, and non-judgmental care throughout.

Abortion is a complex issue, and the controversy is not only in the public arena: many nurses struggle with the conflict between their personal convictions and their professional duty. Nurses are taught to be supportive client advocates and to interact with a non-judgmental attitude under all circumstances. However, nurses have their own personal and political views, which may be very different from those of their clients. Nurses need to clarify their personal values and beliefs on this issue. The CNA Code of Ethics for Registered Nurses (2008, p. 43) indicates that a "nurse has a right to follow his or her conscience when opposed to certain procedures and practices in health care that others judge to be morally acceptable in its provision for conscientious objection." Ideally, the nurse would be able to anticipate practices and procedures that would not create a conflict with his or her conscience (beliefs and values) in advance. In this case, the nurse should discuss with supervisors, employers or, when the nurse is self-employed, persons receiving care what types of care she or he finds contrary to his or her own beliefs and values (CNA, 2008).

Substance Abuse

Substance abuse for any person is a problem, but when it involves a pregnant woman, substance abuse can cause fetal injury and thus has legal and ethical implications. In some instances, courts have issued jail sentences to pregnant women who caused harm to their fetuses (LifeCanada, 2008). Many provincial laws require nurses to report evidence of prenatal drug exposure, which may lead to charges of negligence and child endangerment against the pregnant woman. This punitive approach to fetal injury raises ethical and legal questions about the degree of governmental control that is appropriate in the interests of child safety (AbortionInCanada.ca., n.d.). Many services are available to assist a pregnant woman to eliminate substance abuse in pregnancy.

Fetal Therapy

Intrauterine fetal surgery is a procedure that involves opening the uterus during pregnancy, performing surgery on the fetus, and placing the fetus back in the uterus. Although the risks to the fetus and the mother are both great, fetal therapy may be used to correct some anatomic lesions (Noble & Rodeck, 2008). Nurses play an important supportive role in caring and advocating for clients and their families. As the use of technology grows, situations will surface more frequently that test a nurse's belief system. Encouraging open discussions to address emotional issues and differences of opinion among staff members is healthy and increases tolerance for differing points of view.

Informed Consent

Informed consent has four key components: disclosure, comprehension, competency, and voluntariness (Taylor, Lillis, & LeMone, 2005). It occurs prior to initiation of the procedure or specific care and addresses the legal and ethical requirement of informing the client about the procedure. The physician or advanced practice nurse is responsible for informing the client about the procedure and obtaining consent by providing a detailed description of the procedure or treatment, its potential risks and benefits, and alternative treatments available. If the client is a child, typically this information is provided to the parents or legal guardians. The nurse's responsibility related to informed consent includes:

- Ensuring that the consent form is completed with signatures from the client (or parents or legal guardians if the client is a child)
- Serving as a witness to the signature process
- Determining whether the client or parents or legal guardians understand what they are signing by asking them pertinent questions

Although laws vary between provinces, certain key elements are associated with informed consent (Box 1.5). Nurses need to be familiar with their specific provincial laws as well as the policies and procedures of the health care agency. Treating clients without obtaining proper consent may result in charges of assault, and the health care provider and/or facility may be held liable for any damages.

Generally, only people over the age of majority (18 years of age) can legally provide consent for health care. Since children are minors, when care is rendered to them, the process involves obtaining written permission from a parent or legal guardian. In cases requiring a signature for consent, usually the parent provides consent for care for children less than 18 years of age, except in certain situations (see further discussion below).

> ▶ *Take* NOTE!
>
> *Allow older children and adolescents to be involved in the decision-making process to the extent possible. However, keep in mind that the parent or guardian is still ultimately responsible for giving consent to treatment.*

Most care rendered in a health care setting is covered by the initial consent for treatment signed when the individual becomes a client at that office or clinic or by the consent to treatment signed upon admission to the hospital or other inpatient facility. Certain procedures, however, require a specific process of informed consent: major and minor surgery; invasive procedures such as amniocentesis, internal fetal monitoring, lumbar puncture, or bone marrow aspiration; treatments placing the client at higher risk, such as chemotherapy or radiation therapy; procedures or treatments involving research; and photography involving the client. Applying restraints to children now requires consent.

If the client cannot provide consent, or in the case of a child, the parent or guardian is not available, then the person closest to the client or in charge of the child (relative, babysitter, or teacher) may give consent for emergency treatment if he or she has a signed form from the parent or legal guardian allowing him or her to do so. During an emergency situation, a verbal consent, via the telephone, may be obtained. Two witnesses must also be listening simultaneously and must sign the consent form, indicating that consent was received via telephone. Health care providers can provide emergency treatment to a child without consent if they have made reasonable attempts to contact the child's parent or legal guardian. Table 1.4 provides additional information about the informed consent process with children.

> ▶ *Take* NOTE!
>
> *Never assume that the adult accompanying the child is the custodial parent or legal guardian. Always clarify the relationship of the accompanying adult.*

Refusal of Medical Treatment

All clients have the right to refuse medical treatment. In Canada, consent is a prerequisite for medical interventions, regardless of whether they are for treatment or diagnosis or performed by a nurse or physician. In the

---

BOX 1.5   Key Elements of Informed Consent

- The decision maker must be of legal age in that province or territory, with full civil rights, and must be competent (have the ability to make the decision).
- Information presented must include all important and relevant aspects required to make an informed decision and must be presented in a manner that is simple, concise, and appropriate to the level of education and language of the individual responsible for making the decision.
- The decision must be voluntary, without coercion or force or under duress.
- There must be a witness to the process of informed consent.
- The witness must sign the consent form.

TABLE 1.4 SPECIAL CONSIDERATIONS RELATED TO INFORMED CONSENT WITH CHILDREN

Issue	Definition	Nursing Considerations
Child not living with biological or adoptive parents	Child is living: • In foster care • With potential adoptive parent • With a relative	– Legally appointed guardian is responsible for providing consent. – Verification of authority of legally appointed guardian – Documentation of the legal guardian in the child's medical record
Parental consent after divorce	Ability to give consent for health care rests with parent who has legal custody by divorce decree	– Determination of joint custody or sole custody by one parent – Parent with only physical custody may give consent for emergency care. Court involvement may be needed if there is joint legal custody but parents disagree on care.
Consent for organ donation	For a minor to donate, the parents must be aware of the risks and benefits and must provide emotional support to child; there should be a close relationship between the donor and recipient.	– Referral of potential donors to local organ procurement organization – Family education about policies related to organ donation – Legal guardian or parental consent to organ donation
Consent for medical experimentation	Requirements include consent of parents, assent of child, and a perceived benefit to the child	Need to comply with all federal regulations if federal funds received (see discussion of assent in text)

case of a child, a custodial parent or legal guardian is authorized to provide consent on the child's behalf, but they do not have the absolute right to refuse treatment on their child's behalf. Refusal of treatment may occur when the treatment conflicts with religious or cultural beliefs. Sometimes common ground may be reached between the family's religious or cultural beliefs and the health care team's recommendations. In some situations, families may decide that treatment to prolong life is not the best decision if it also prolongs their child's pain. In all cases, it is important to educate the client and family about the importance of the recommended treatment without coercing or forcing the client to agree. Communication and education are the keys in this situation.

Intervention by the courts may occur to protect the child. When a child is mature enough to be capable of understanding the nature and consequences of a medical decision, the child is defined as a mature minor and may make his or her own decision. In this situation the legal guardian, parent or caregiver, has no right to consent or refuse treatment. Canadian law is designed to protect the best interest of the child; however, granting guardianship to anyone other than the parent is considered to be a last resort, including in relation to consent for medical intervention. In cases in which the parent's treatment decision for the child is contrary to the preservation of life, health care professionals defer to the courts to make decisions regarding care (Kenny, Downie, & Harrison, 2012). A child's situation may appear before

the courts several times, as they make decisions for each treatment based on the updated health care status of the child. This is referred to as *parens patriae* (the state has a right and a duty to protect children).

Parents may refuse treatment if they perceive that their child's quality of life will be significantly impaired by the medical care that is offered. If the parents refuse treatment but the health care team feels the treatment is reasonable and warranted, the case should be referred to the institution's ethics committee. If the issue remains unresolved, then the judicial system becomes involved (Kon, 2006a, 2006b).

Exceptions to Required Parental Consent for Children

Laws are similar but differ between provinces. In Alberta the mature minor is a person less than 18 years of age who has been "assessed and determined to have the intelligence and maturity to appreciate the nature, risks, benefits, consequences and alternatives of the proposed treatment or procedure including the ethical, emotional and physical aspects" (Alberta Health Services, 2010, p 13). **Emancipated minors** are persons under the age of 18 who are no longer dependent on their parents and may be supporting themselves or living independently. Though provincial and territorial laws vary, emancipated minors are generally treated as mature minors. Provincial and territorial laws also vary in relation to the definition of a mature minor and the types of treatment that may be obtained as a mature minor (without parental consent). According to provincial law, health care may be provided to minors for certain conditions, in a confidential manner, without notifying the parents. These types of care may include pregnancy counselling, prenatal care, contraception, and testing and treatment for sexually transmitted infections. These exceptions provide a confidential environment for children who would avoid care if they were required to inform their parents or legal guardian. Again, the laws vary by province so nurses must be knowledgeable about the laws in the province where they practice.

Additional situations in which persons under the age of 18 are frequently assessed as mature minors include:

• Marriage
• Financial independence and separate living arrangement from parents
• Pregnancy
• Mother of an infant/child less than 18 years of age
• Teen request for birth control (Alberta Health Services, 2010)

Nurses must be familiar with laws of the province in which they work so they can be in compliance when rendering health care and treatment.

Assent

Assent may be defined as agreeing to something. In the care of children, the term refers to the child's participation in the decision-making process about his or her health care (McCullough & Stein, 2007). The age of assent depends on the child's developmental level and maturity. The CPS (2004) recommends the age of primary school for input into decision making. Certainly, the older the child is, the stronger the ethical obligation is to include the child in the decision-making process (Olechnowicz, Eder, Simon, et al., 2002). The CPS (2004) makes the following recommendations related to assent:

• Infants and young children have no significant skill to participate in decision making; therefore, decisions are made by the parent or legal guardian.
• Primary school age children should be given the necessary information at a level they can comprehend and can assent. However, the final legal authority to determine whether a medical treatment or diagnostic test will proceed is the responsibility of the parent or legal guardian.
• Adolescents should be assessed to determine if they qualify as mature minors. However, the parent or legal guardian will make decisions should an adolescent not demonstrate comprehension and appreciation for consequences of the proposed treatment, not reflect fairly stable values or meet all the criteria of a mature minor. An adolescent's consent must be obtained for therapeutic and non-therapeutic research. The assent form

for the involvement of minors in research must be used for all children under the age of 18.

Health Canada (2010a) guidelines for non-therapeutic health research indicates that a primary school-age child must assent to non-therapeutic research; however, parental consent is necessary for participants under 16 years of age (under 18 years of age in Quebec).

Clients' Rights

Canada does not have a patient's bill of rights. One was presented to the federal government in 2002, but it was not passed as the majority of the members of Parliament felt that legal precedent has established that the facility or health care organization providing care has a responsibility to the patient (Government of Canada, 2002). Some established rights of patients in Canada include the right to confidentiality; the right to complete, current information concerning the diagnosis in language that the patient can comprehend; and the right to expect patient safety. The CNA (2008) defines patient safety as not only the "prevention and mitigation of unsafe acts within the health care system," but also "being under the care of a health care provider who, with the person's informed consent, assists the patient to achieve an optimum level of health (p. 1)." The Canadian Institute of Child Health (n.d.) published the "Rights of the Hospitalized Child" in 1980 to raise awareness of the issues faced by hospitalized children. These included the right to be viewed first as a child and then as a patient, the right to be afraid and to cry if hurt, the right to have those dear to them close by when needed, and the right to play and learn even while receiving health care.

Ensuring that clients' rights are upheld is a key aspect in the care of any client. For the pregnant woman, two clients must be considered—the pregnant woman and her fetus. A child, due to his or her age and developmental level, may lack mature decision-making abilities. Many pediatric institutions have adopted a bill of rights for children's health care specific to that institution (Box 1.6).

Parents or legal guardians are ultimately the decision makers for their children. In ethical dilemmas such as babies born with brain damage or extremely preterm birth, parents must be accurately informed about the risks and benefits of treatment before giving consent to treatment or deciding to withdraw or forego treatment (Hurst, 2006; Janvier, Barrington, Aziz, et al., 2008). Some professionals are advocating for prenatal advance directives that would guide care from the time of birth of an extremely premature or otherwise impaired term infant (Catlin, 2005; Janvier et al., 2008).

Confidentiality

The Freedom of Information and Protection of Privacy Act in Alberta, Ontario, and other provinces legislated

BOX 1.6 **Bill of Rights and Responsibilities**

Sincerely, A Child
"I have the right to...
• Be seen as a child first, and then as a patient
• Be called by name
• Know who you are, what you are doing and why
• Have your full attention when you are with me
• Be treated as a unique individual with my own abilities, culture, spirituality and language
• Have my privacy respected
• Be prepared for procedures and how I may feel afterwards
• Have my suggestions heard
• Share my feelings
• Have a support person with me
• Know my choices when my caregiver is not available

I have the responsibility to...
• Be respectful of providers
• Be honest and open with providers
• Ask questions so that I understand
• Learn about my treatment plan
• Be involved in making decisions about my care
• Maintain healthy habits
• Play, learn and be a kid"

Source: Children's Hospital London Health Sciences Centre. (2010). *Bill of rights and responsibilities.* Retrieved February 8, 2012 from http://www.lhsc.on.ca/Patients_Families_Visitors/Childrens_Hospital/CFRC/Rights-Video.htm.

the public's right to access information and established confidentiality of government-held information. The acts vary slightly among provinces and territories but stipulate that information that clearly identifies a client cannot be in public display, including information on a client's chart. In maternal and child health care, information is shared only with the client, legal partner, parents, legal guardians, or individuals as established in writing by the client or the child's parents. This law promotes the security and privacy of health care and health information for all clients. Client information should always be kept confidential in the context of the provincial law as well as the institution's policies.

Exceptions to confidentiality exist. For example, suspicion of physical or sexual abuse and injuries caused by a weapon or criminal act must be reported to the proper authorities. Abuse cases are reported to the appropriate welfare authorities, whereas criminal acts are reported to the police. The health care provider must also follow public health laws related to reporting certain infectious diseases to the local health department (e.g., tuberculosis, hepatitis, HIV, and other sexually transmitted infections). There must be a balance between confidentiality and required disclosure. If health care information must be

disclosed by law, the client must be informed that this will occur (Feldman-Winter & McAbee, 2002).

Implications for Nurses

The health care system is intricately woven into the political and social structure of our society, and nurses must understand social, legal, and ethical health care issues so that they can play an active role in meeting the health care needs of women, children, and families. Nurses need to take a proactive role in advocating for and empowering their clients. For example, nurses can help women in pregnancy and childbirth as well as parents of children and adolescents to increase control over the factors that affect health, thereby improving their health status. They may become empowered by developing skills not only to cope with their environment, but also to change it. Nurses also can assume this mentoring role with children, youth and families, thus helping them to improve their overall health status and health outcomes.

Nurses must have a solid knowledge base about the factors affecting maternal and child health and barriers to health care. They can use this information to provide anticipatory guidance, health counselling, and teaching for women, children, and families. It also is useful in identifying high-risk groups so that interventions can be initiated early on, before problems occur.

When caring for women, children, and families, the nurse operates within the framework of health promotion and disease prevention, which is applicable to all health care settings. Maternal and child health nursing is ever-changing as globalization and the exchange of information expands. Nurses must remain current about new technologies, treatments and approaches; and integrate high-quality, evidence-based interventions into the care they provide.

■■■ Key Concepts

■ Maternal and child health nurses provide care using a philosophy that focuses on the family as the emphasis of care, providing atraumatic care and using evidence-based practice in a case management environment to provide quality, cost-effective care.

■ Health Canada, as well as provinces and territories, have health goals and objectives for adults and children that focus on health promotion and disease prevention.

■ One method to establish the aggregate health status of women, infants, and children is with statistical data, such as mortality, morbidity, and low birth weight rates.

■ The infant mortality rate, although lower in Canada than in many countries in the world, is on the rise. This may be the result of the increase in low-birth-weight infants born in Canada. The low birth weight rate in Canada is low, but there is opportunity for improvement when compared with other industrialized countries.

■ The family is considered the basic social unit. The family greatly influences the development and health of its members. Members learn health care activities, health beliefs, and health values from their family.

■ Social roles are often an important factor in the development of one's self-concept, which can have a very positive influence on health or present various limitations and problems, possibly resulting in a negative influence on health.

■ Culture influences every aspect of development and is reflected in childbearing and childrearing beliefs and practices designed to promote healthy adaptation.

■ Spirituality, a major influence for many individuals, provides a meaning and purpose to life and is a foundation for and a source of love, relationships, and service. Spiritual and religious beliefs and views can provide strength and support to women, children, and their families during times of stress and illness.

■ Other factors impacting the health of women, children, and families include the community and environment in which they live, their level of education, health status and lifestyles, health literacy, access to health care services, and health care consumer empowerment. Family income, transportation, language, culture, and the health care delivery system can create barriers to health care.

■ Advances in science and technology have led to increased ethical dilemmas in health care. Although Canadians have a publicly funded health care system that is responsible for meeting all medically necessary needs, it is not without its problems, which include a looming shortage of trained and skilled health care professionals.

■ All clients have the right to refuse medical treatment. Parents, or legal guardians, have the right to decide for or against medical treatments for children under the age of 18. If the parental decision places the child at risk of harm, the Canadian judicial system is given final determination.

■ In certain provinces, mature minors and emancipated minors may consent to their own health care treatments and certain health care may be provided to adolescents without parental notification, including contraception, pregnancy counselling, prenatal care, testing for and treatment of sexually transmitted infections and communicable diseases (including HIV), substance abuse and mental illness counselling and treatment, and health care required as a result of a crime-related injury.

■ The nurse must be knowledgeable about the laws related to health care of women and children in the specific provinces of nursing practice as well as the specific policies of the health care institution.

REFERENCES

Abell, S., & Ey, J. L. (2008). Domestic violence: Its impact on children. *Clinical Pediatrics, 47*(4), 413–415.

AbortionInCanada.ca. (n.d.). *Abortion in Canada timeline.* Retrieved February 8, 2012 from http://www.abortionincanada.ca/history/Abortion_Canada_Timeline.html

Alberta Health Services. (2010). *Consent to treatment/procedures: Minors/mature minors (Policy PRR-01-03).* Retrieved on February 8, 2012 from http://www.albertahealthservices.ca/ClinicalPolicy/wf-clp-prd-consent-to-treatment-prr-01-03.pdf

Alberta Health Services. (2011). *Comprehensive school health.* Retrieved February 26, 2011 from http://www.healthyalberta.com/Healthy-Places/1026.htm

Ambler, K. A., Hagedorn, D. W. J., & Ball, G. D. C. (2010). Referrals for pediatric weight management: the importance of proximity. *BMC Health Services Research, 10,* 302. Retrieved February 8, 2012 from http://www.biomedcentral.com/content/pdf/1472-6963-10-302.pdf

American Academy of Child & Adolescent Psychiatry. (2005). *Foster care.* Retrieved February 8, 2012 from http://www.aacap.org/cs/root/facts_for_families/foster_care

American Academy of Pediatrics Committee on Community Health Services. (2005). Providing care for immigrant, homeless, and migrant children. *Pediatrics, 115*(4), 1095–1100.

American Psychological Association. (2005). *Lesbian and gay parenting.* Washington, DC: American Psychological Association.

American Psychological Association. (2012). *Single parenting and today's family.* Retrieved February 8, 2012 from http://www.apa.org/helpcenter/single-parent.aspx

Andersen, L., Geary, J., Portner, C., & Verner, D. (2010). Human health. In D. Verner (Ed.), *Reducing poverty, protecting livelihoods, and building assets in a changing climate.* Washington, DC: World Bank.

Asthma Society of Canada. (2005). *Asthma facts and statistics.* Retrieved February 8, 2012 from http://www.asthma.ca/corp/newsroom/pdf/asthmastats.pdf

Avery, T. (2008). *One in four don't believe in God, poll finds.* Retrieved February 8, 2012 from http://www.thestar.com/news/canada/article/434725

Banks, J. B. (2002). Childhood discipline: Challenges for clinicians and parents. *American Family Physician, 66*(8), 1447–1452.

Behrman, R. E., & Butler, A. S. (2007). Medical and pregnancy conditions associated with preterm birth. In *Preterm birth: Causes, consequences, and prevention.* Washington, DC: National Academies Press. Retrieved February 8, 2012 from http://www.ncbi.nlm.nih.gov/books/NBK11363

Bloom, B., Dey, A. N., & Freeman, G. (2006). Summary health statistics for U.S. children: National Health Interview survey, 2005. *Vital Health Statistics, 10*(231), 1–93.

Boss, P. (2001). *Family stress management* (2nd ed.). Thousand Oaks, CA: Sage.

Brodsky, P. L. (2006). Childbirth. A journey through time. *International Journal of Childbirth Education, 21*(3), 10–15.

Brunner, S. (2010). Maternal mortality rises in the USA, Canada and Denmark, and falls in China, Egypt, Ecuador and Bolivia. *Medical News Today.* Retrieved February 8, 2012 from http://www.medical-newstoday.com/articles/185154.php

Bryner, C. L. (2001). Children of divorce. *Journal of the American Board of Family Practice, 14*(3), 176–183.

Bushnik, T. (2006). *Child care in Canada.* Ottawa, ON: Queens Printer.

Canada Health Coalition. (2009). *The history of Medicare.* Retrieved February 8, 2012 from http://medicare.ca/main/the-facts/the-history-of-medicare

Canada.com. (2008). *Youth violence on the rise in Canada.* Retrieved February 8, 2012 from http://www.canada.com/mapleridgetimes/news/story.html?id=6729446e-be1b-49c1-a19a-2650cc741575

Canadian Association of Emergency Physicians. (n.d.). *Rural emergency care.* Retrieved February 8, 2012 from http://caep.ca/advocacy/romanow-commission/rural-emergency-care

Canadian Broadcasting Centre. (2006). *Family doctor shortage major hurdle to health care: study.* Retrieved February 8, 2012 from http://www.cbc.ca/news/canada/montreal/story/2006/11/02/quebec-familydoctors.html

Canadian Cancer Society. (2011). *General cancer statistics at a glance.* Retrieved February 8, 2012 from http://www.cancer.ca/canada-wide/about%20cancer/cancer%20statistics/stats%20at%20a%20glance/general%20cancer%20stats.aspx

Canadian Chamber of Commerce. (2010). *Canada's demographic crunch: Can underrepresented workers save us?* Retrieved February 8, 2012 from http://www.chamber.ca/images/uploads/Reports/2010/Canadas%20Demographic%20Crunch141010.pdf

Canadian Children's Rights Council. (2011). *Child abuse and neglect – Canada statistics.* Retrieved February 8, 2012 from http://www.canadiancrc.com/Child_Abuse/Child_Abuse.aspx

Canadian Council on Learning. (2009). Lessons in learning. A barrier to learning: Mental health disorders among Canadian youth. Retrieved on February 13, 2012 from http://www.ccl-cca.ca/pdfs/LessonsInLearning/04_15_09-E.pdf.

Canadian Council on Social Development. (2010). *Social challenges: The well-being of Aboriginal people.* Retrieved February 8, 2012 from http://www.ccsd.ca/cpsd/ccsd/c_ab.htm

Canadian Council on Social Development. (2011). *Policy initiatives.* Retrieved February 8, 2012 from http://www.ccsd.ca/pi.htm

Canadian Encyclopedia Historica Dominion Institute. (2012). Child labour. Retrieved February 19, 2012 from http://www.thecanadianencyclopedia.com/articles/child-labour

Canadian Health Care. (2007). *Canada Health Act.* Retrieved February 8, 2012 from http://www.canadian-healthcare.org/page2.html

Canadian Health Services Research Foundation. (2006). Allow midwives to participate as full members of the health care team. *Evidence Boost.* Retrieved February 8, 2012 from http://www.alberta-midwives.com/pdfs/EvidenceBoost_June_E.pdf

Canadian Institute of Child Health. (n.d.). *The rights of the child in the health care system* [poster]. Retrieved February 8, 2012 from http://www.cich.ca/PDFFiles/RightHospitalizedPosterENG.pdf

Canadian Nurses Association. (2008). *Code of ethics for registered nurses.* Retrieved February 8, 2012 from http://www.cna-aiic.ca/cna/documents/pdf/publications/Code_of_Ethics_2008_e.pdf

Canadian Nurses Association. (n.d.). *Canadian Nurses Association memorial.* Retrieved February 8, 2012 from http://www.cna-nurses.ca/CNA/documents/pdf/publications/CNA_Memorial_Book_e.pdf

Canadian Paediatric Society. (2004). Treatment decisions regarding infants, children and adolescents. *Paediatrics and Child Health, 9*(2), 99–103. Retrieved February 8, 2012 from http://www.cps.ca/english/statements/B/b04–01.htm

Canadian Paediatric Society. (2011). *Effective discipline for children.* Retrieved February 8, 2012 from http://www.cps.ca/english/statements/CP/pp04–01.htm

Case Management Society of America. (2012). "What is a case manager." Retrieved on February 14, 2012 from http://www.cmsa.org/Home/CMSA/WhatisaCaseManager/tabid/224/Default.aspx

Cassidy, T. (2006). *Birth: The surprising history of how we are born.* Berkeley, CA: Grove/Atlantic, Inc.

Catlin, A. J. (2005). Thinking outside the box: Prenatal care—the call for a prenatal advance directive. *Journal of Perinatal and Neonatal Nursing, 19*(2), 169–176.

Children's Aid Foundation. (2008). *What we do.* Retrieved February 8, 2012 from http://www.cafdn.org/whatwedo.aspx

Children's Defense Fund—Ohio. (2009). *Children who witness domestic violence.* Retrieved February 8, 2012 from http://cdf.childrensdefense.org/site/DocServer/children-who-witness-domestic-violence-ohio.pdf?docID=9961

Children's Defense Fund. (2005). *The state of American's children 2005.* Washington, DC: Author.

Children's Hospital London Health Sciences Centre. (2010). *Bill of rights and responsibilities.* Retrieved February 8, 2012 from http://www.lhsc.on.ca/Patients_Families_Visitors/Childrens_Hospital/CFRC/Rights-Video.htm

Cohen, T. (2012). Immigrants and newcomers drive population growth. National Post. Retrieved Feb. 20, 2012 from http://news.nationalpost.com/2012/02/08/canada-census-2011-immigrants-and-newcomers-drive-population-growth/

Coll-Back, S., Bhushan, A., & Fritsch, K. (2007). Integrating poverty and gender into health programs: A sourcebook for health professionals. *Nursing and Health Sciences, 9*(4), 246–253.

Community Foundations of Canada. (2009). VitalSigns. Retrieved Feb. 21, 2012 from http://www.vitalsignscanada.ca/nr-2009-research-findings-e.html

Community Foundations of Canada. (2010). *Gap between rich & poor.* Retrieved February 8, 2012 from http://vitalsignscanada.ca/research/2010_5gaprichpoor-e.html

Department of Justice Canada. (2011). *Child abuse: A fact sheet from the Department of Justice Canada.* Retrieved February 8, 2012 from http://www.justice.gc.ca/eng/pi/fv-vf/facts-info/child-enf.html#consequences

DesMeules, M., Turner, L., & Cho, R. (2003). *Women's health surveillance report: Mortality, life, and healthy expectancy of Canadian women.* Retrieved February 8, 2012 from http://www.phac-aspc.gc.ca/publicat/whsr-rssf/chap_8-eng.php

Duvall, E. (1977). *Marriage and family development* (5th ed.). Philadelphia: Lippincott.

Eberle, M., Kraus, D., & Serge, L. (2009). *Results of the pilot study to estimate the size of the hidden homeless population in Metro Vancouver.* Retrieved February 8, 2012 from http://www.endhomelessnessnow.ca/homelessness-and-mental-health/ehn-newsletter-issue-9/

Feldman-Winter, L., & McAbee, G. N. (2002). Legal issues in caring for adolescent patients: Physicians can optimize healthcare delivery to teens. *Postgraduate Medicine, 111*(5), 15.

Fischer, P., Greitemeyer, T., Kastenmuller, A., Bogrincic, C., Sauer, A. (2011). The effects of risk-glorifying media exposure on risk-positive cognitions, emotions, and behaviors: A meta-analytic review. *Psychological Bulletin, 137*(3), 367–390. doi: 10.1037/a0022267.

Framingham.com. (n.d.). *Through the looking glass: Women and heart disease.* Retrieved February 8, 2012 from http://www.framingham.com/heart/4stor_04.htm

Friedman, M. M., Bowden, V. R., & Jones, E. G. (2003). *Family nursing: Research, theory, and practice* (5th ed.). Upper Saddle River, NJ: Prentice Hall.

Gan, C., Zou, Y., Wu, S., Li, Y., & Liu, Q. (2008). The influence of medical abortion compared with surgical abortion on subsequent pregnancy outcome. *International Journal of Gynecology and Obstetrics, 101*(3), 231–238.

Government of Canada. (2002). *Patient's bill of rights – A comparative overview.* Depository Services Program PRB 01–31E. Retrieved February 8, 2012 from http://dsp-psd.pwgsc.gc.ca/Collection-R/LoPBdP/BP/prb0131-e.htm

Government of Canada. (2008). *The well-being of Canada's young children – Government of Canada Report 2008.* Retrieved February 2, 2012 from http://publications.gc.ca/collections/collection_2009/rhdcc-hrsdc/HS1-7-2008E.pdf

Grewal, S. K., Bhagat, R., & Balneaves, L. G. (2008). Perinatal beliefs and practices of immigrant Punjabi women living in Canada. *Journal of Obstetric, Gynecologic and Neonatal Nursing, 37*(3), 290–300.

Guest, D. (2012). *Family allowance.* Retrieved February 8, 2012 from http://www.thecanadianencyclopedia.com/index.cfm?PgNm=TCE&Params=A1ARTA0002718

Guneet S. (2010). Increased number of Canadian immigrants failing citizenship test. Canada Updates. Retrieved Feb. 20, 2012 from http://www.canadaupdates.com/content/increased-number-canadian-immigrants-failing-citizenship-test-15906.html

Hamilton, N., & Bhatti, T. (1996) *Population health promotion: An integrated model of population health and health promotion.* Retrieved February 8, 2012 from www.phac-aspc.gc.ca/ph-sp/php-psp/index-eng.php

Hardy, J. (2011). *How Canada's midwife shortage forces healthy mothers into hospitals.* Retrieved February 8, 2012 from http://this.org/magazine/2011/01/07/canada-midwife-shortage

Harvey, B. (1998). *Tips on covering religion in Canada.* Retrieved February 8, 2012 from http://www.faithandmedia.org/articles/show/61

Haymes, M. (2007). *It is time for a national birthing strategy.* Canadian Women's Health Network. Retrieved February 8, 2012 from http://www.cwhn.ca/fr/node/39439

Health Canada. (2005). *Acting on what we know: Preventing youth suicide in First Nations.* Retrieved February 8, 2012 from http://www.hc-sc.gc.ca/fniah-spnia/pubs/promotion/_suicide/prev_youth-jeunes/index-eng.php

Health Canada. (2006). *Healthy living: Breast cancer.* Retrieved February 8, 2012 from http://www.hc-sc.gc.ca/hl-vs/iyh-vsv/diseases-maladies/breast-sein-eng.php

Health Canada. (2007). Reaching for the top: A report by the advisor on healthy children & youth. Healthy Living: Reports and Publications. Retrieved on February 13, 2011 from http://www.hc-sc.gc.ca/hl-vs/pubs/child-enfant/advisor-conseillere/index-eng.php

Health Canada. (2009). *Healthy Canadians: A federal report on comparable health indicators 2008.* Retrieved February 8, 2012 from http://www.

hc-sc.gc.ca/hcs-sss/pubs/system-regime/2008-fed-comp-indicat/index-eng.php

Health Canada. (2010). *Children's assent (consent form for participants under 16 years of age, 18 years of age in Quebec)*. Retrieved February 8, 2012 from http://www.hc-sc.gc.ca/sr-sr/advice-avis/reb-cer/consent/g-eng.php

Health Canada. (2011a). *First Nations, Inuit and Aboriginal health*. Retrieved February 8, 2012 from http://www.hc-sc.gc.ca/fniah-spnia/index-eng.php

Health Canada. (2011b). *Healthy pregnancy*. Retrieved February 8, 2012 from http://www.hc-sc.gc.ca/hl-vs/preg-gros/index-eng.php

Health Canada. (2011c). *Just for you—Women*. Retrieved February 8, 2012 from http://www.hc-sc.gc.ca/hl-vs/jfy-spv/women-femmes-eng.php

Healthy Canadians. (2010). *Bullying*. Retrieved February 8, 2012 from http://healthycanadians.gc.ca/kids/bullying/.

Heaman, M., & O'Brien, B. (2009). Prenatal care provider. In *What Mothers Say: The Canadian Maternity Experience Survey*. Retrieved February 8, 2012 from http://www.phac-aspc.gc.ca/rhs-ssg/pdf/survey-eng.pdf

Heart & Stroke Foundation of Alberta, NWT & Nunavut. (2011). *Women's unique conditions related to heart disease and stroke*. Retrieved February 8, 2012 from http://www.heartandstroke.ab.ca/site/c.lqIRL1PJJtH/b.3650925/k.D932/Heart_Disease__Women_and_heart_disease_and_stroke.htm#wheartattack

Herbert, P. (2011). *A summary of the history of midwifery in Canada*. Retrieved February 2, 2012 from http://www.ucs.mun.ca/~pherbert/Historyofmidincanada.html

Historica Dominion Institute. (n.d.). *Midwife* [video]. Retrieved February 2, 2012 from http://www.histori.ca/minutes/theme.do?id=10185

Hodnett, E. D., Gates, S., Hofmeyr, G. J., & Sakata C. (2007). Continuous support for women during childbirth. *Cochrane Database of Systematic Reviews, 3*(CD003766). DOI: 10.1002/14651858.CD003766.pub2

Hondro, M. (2010). *Divorce rate 40% in Canada as Vanier Inst. releases family report*. Retrieved February 2, 2012 from http://www.suite101.com/content/divorce-rate-40-in-canada-as-vanier-inst-releases-family-report-a293136

Human Resources and Skills Development Canada. (2006). *Canadians in context: Households and families*. Retrieved February 2, 2012 from http://www4.hrsdc.gc.ca/.3ndic.1t.4r@-eng.jsp?iid=37

Human Resources and Skills Development Canada. (2009). *Evaluation of the homelessness partnering strategy - July 2009*. Retrieved February 2, 2012 from http://www.rhdcc-hrsdc.gc.ca/eng/publications_resources/evaluation/2009/ehps/page04.shtml

Human Resources and Skills Development Canada. (2012). *Indicators of well-being in Canada*. Retrieved February 2, 2012 from http://www4.hrsdc.gc.ca/h.4m.2@-eng.jsp

Hurst, I. (2006). The legal landscape at the threshold of viability for extremely premature infants: A nursing perspective, part I. *JONA's Healthcare Law, Ethics, and Regulation, 8*(1), 20–28.

Hutton, E., Reitsma, A., & Kaufman, K. (2009). Outcomes associated with planned home and planned hospital births in low-risk women attended by midwives in Ontario, Canada, 2003–2006: A retrospective cohort study. *Birth, 36*(3), 180–189. DOI: 10.1111/j.1523–536x.209.00322.x

Iannotti, R., Kogan, M., Janssen, I., & Boyce, W. (2009). Patterns of adolescent physical activity, screen-based media use, and positive and negative health indicators in the U.S and Canada. *Journal of Adolescent Health, 44*(5), 493–499. DOI: 10.1016/j.jadohealth.2008.10.142

Institute of Marriage and the Family Canada. (2009). *Canadian spousal abuse statistics*. Retrieved February 2, 2012 from http://www.imf-canada.org/article_files/Canadian%20Spousal%20Abuse%20Statistics.pdf

Janvier, A., Barrington, K., Aziz, K., & Lantos, J. (2008). Ethics ain't easy: do we need simple rules for complicated ethical decisions? *Acta Paediatrica, 94*(4), 402–406.

Jolivet, R. (2006). Nurse-midwives committed to women throughout the lifespan. *The Nurse Practitioner, 9*, 10–13.

Kaiser Family Foundation. (2011). *Health expenditure per capita (PPP; international $) 2008*. Retrieved February 8, 2012 from http://www.globalhealthfacts.org/data/topic/map.aspx?ind=66

Kenny, N, Downie, J., & Harrison, C. (2012). Respectful involvement of children in medical decision making. In F. Baylis, B. Hoffmaster,

S. Sherwin, & K. Borgerson (Eds.), *Health care ethics in Canada* (pp. 233–238) (3rd ed.). Toronto: Nelson Education Ltd.

Kohen, D. E. (2010). *Asthma and school functioning*. Statistics Canada Catalogue no. 82–003-X. Retrieved February 2, 2012 from http://www.statcan.gc.ca/pub/82–003-x/2010004/article/11363-eng.pdf

Kon, A. A. (2006a). Assent in pediatric research. *Pediatrics, 117*(5), 1806–1810.

Kon, A. A. (2006b). When parents refuse treatment for their child. *JONA's Healthcare Law, Ethics, and Regulation, 8*(1), 5–9.

LifeCanada. (2008). *Abortion: Have we gone too far?* Retrieved February 2, 2012 from http://www.lifecanada.org/html/resources/polling/press/Press%20Release_Abortion%20Have%20we%20Gone%20too%20far.pdf

Luo, Z., Senecal, S., Simoniet, S., Guimond, E., Penney, C., & Wilkens, R. (2011). Birth outcomes in the Inuit-inhabited areas of Canada. *Canadian Medical Association Journal, 182*(3), 235–242. DOI: 10.1503/cmaj.082042

Macdonald, M. E., & Bourgeault, I. L. (2009). The Ontario midwifery model of care. In R. Davis-Floyd, L. Barclay, B. Daviss, & J. Tritten (Eds.), *Birth models that work*. Berkley, CA: University of California Press.

March, P. D., & Schub, T. (2010). *Night terrors (sleep disorder) in children. CINAHL Nursing Guide*. Retrieved January 17, 2011 from http://web.ebscohost.com.ezproxy.lib.ucalgary.ca/nrc/detail?hid=122&sid=4f0c593d-bc9c-44a5-a594-0226476c3db3%40sessionmgr115&vid=48&bdata=JnNpdGU9bnJjLWxpdmU%3d#db=nrc&AN=5000003166

Martin, L. J., Houston, S., Yasui, Y., Wild, C., & Saunders, L. D. (2011). All-cause and HIV-related mortality rates among HIV-infected patients after initiating highly active antiretroviral therapy: the impact of Aboriginal ethnicity and injection drug use. *Canadian Journal of Public Health, 102*(2). Retrieved February 8, 2012 from http://journal.cpha.ca/index.php/cjph/article/view/2034

McCullough, L. B., & Stein, F. (2007). *Pediatric assent and confidentiality in clinical practice*. Retrieved February 8, 2012 from http://www.baylorcme.org/assent/presentations/mccullough/mccullough.pdf

MCP². (2006). *Final Report: MCP²*. Retrieved February 8, 2012 from http://webcache.googleusercontent.com/search?q=cache:http://www.mcp2.ca/english/documents/FinalReport-Health Canada.pdf.

Media Awareness Network. (2010). *Government and industry responses to media violence*. Retrieved February 8, 2012 from http://www.media-awareness.ca/english/issues/violence/govt_industry_responses.cfm

MedicineNet. (2003). *Twilight sleep....Childbirth without pain?* Retrieved February 24, 2012 from http://www.medicinenet.com/script/main/art.asp?articlekey=10238

Melnyk, B. M., & Fineout-Overholt, E. (2005). *Evidence-based practice in nursing & healthcare: A guide to best practice*. Philadelphia: Lippincott Williams & Wilkins.

Mittendorfer-Rutz, E., & Wasserman, D. (2008). Pregnancies in high psychosocial risk groups: Research findings and implications for early intervention. *Psychiatric Clinics of North America, 31*(2), 205–212.

Montreal Children's Hospital. (2011). *History*. Retrieved February 8, 2012 from http://thechildren.com/en/about/history.aspx

Moore, D. L., & Bortolussi, R. (2011). Home intravenous therapy: Accessibility for Canadian children and youth. *Paediatrics and Child Health, 16*(2), 105–109.

National Aboriginal Health Organization. (2008). *Celebrating birth: Aboriginal midwifery in Canada*. Retrieved February 8, 2012 from http://www.naho.ca/documents/naho/english/midwifery/celebratingBirth/Midwiferypaper_English.pdf

National Coalition Against Domestic Violence. (2007). *Domestic violence facts*. Retrieved February 8, 2012 from http://www.ncadv.org/files/DomesticViolenceFactSheet(National).pdf

National Collaborating Centre for Aboriginal Health. (n.d.). *Setting the context*. Retrieved April 17, 2012 from http://www.nccah-ccnsa.ca/26/Setting_the_Context.nccah

National Youth Violence Prevention Resource Center. (2011). *About school violence*. Retrieved February 8, 2012 from http://www.cdc.gov/violenceprevention/youthviolence/schoolviolence/

Noble, R., & Rodeck, C. H. (2008). Ethical considerations of fetal therapy. *Bailliere's Best Practice and Research in Clinical Obstetrics and Gynecology, 22*(1), 219–231.

Nurse Practitioner Association of Ontario. (n.d.). *History of NP role development in Ontario.* Retrieved February 8, 2012 from http://npao.org/wp-content/uploads/2011/07/Timeline-of-important-4.pdf

Ogden, C., Gorber, S., Dommarco, J., Carroll, M., Shields, M., & Flegal, K. (2011). The epidemiology of childhood obesity in Canada, Mexico and the United States. *Springer Series in Epidemiology and Public Health, 22*(1), 69–93. DOI: 10.1007/978-1-4419-6039-9_5

Olechnowicz, J. Q., Eder, M., Simon, C., Zyzanski, S., & Kodish, E. (2002). Assent observed: Children's involvement in leukemia treatment and research discussions. *Pediatrics, 109*(5), 806–814.

Ontario Ministry of Education. (2011). *Policy/program memorandum no. 120: Reporting violent incidents to the Ministry of Education.* Retrieved February 8, 2012 from http://www.edu.gov.on.ca/extra/eng/ppm/120.html

Pace, D. T. (2006). Menopause: Studying the research. *Nurse Practitioner, 31*(8), 16–23.

Pereira, J. (2011). *15 accidents that can kill kids.* Retrieved February 8, 2012 from http://www.parentscanada.com/health/15-accidents-that-can-kill-kids.aspx

Ponti, M. (2008). Special considerations for the health supervision of children and youth in foster care. *Paediatrics and Child Health, 13*(2), 129–132. Retrieved February 8, 2012 from http://www.cps.ca/english/statements/CP/cp08–01.htm

Public Health Agency of Canada. (2003). Women's health surveillance report. Retrieved February 8, 2012 from http://www.phac-aspc.gc.ca/publicat/whsr-rssf/

Public Health Agency of Canada. (2006). *Sustainable development in public health: A long term journey begins.* Retrieved February 8, 2012 from http://www.phac-aspc.gc.ca/publicat/sds-sdd/sds-sdd2-a-eng.php

Public Health Agency of Canada. (2008a). *Canadian incidence study of reported child abuse and neglect: Major findings.* Retrieved February 8, 2012 from http://www.phac-aspc.gc.ca/ncfv-cnivf/pdfs/nfnts-cis-2008-rprt-eng.pdf

Public Health Agency of Canada. (2008b). Canadian Perinatal Health Report-2008 edition. Retrieved from http://www.phac-aspc.gc.ca/publicat/2008/cphr-rspc/index-eng.php

Public Health Agency of Canada. (2009a). *The chief public health officer's report on the state of public health in Canada 2009.* Retrieved January 26, 2012 from http://www.phac-aspc.gc.ca/cphorsphc-respcacsp/2009/fr-rc/cphorsphc-respcacsp06-eng.php

Public Health Agency of Canada. (2009b). *What mothers say: The Canadian maternity experiences survey.* Retrieved February 8, 2012 from http://www.phac-aspc.gc.ca/rhs-ssg/pdf/survey-eng.pdf

Public Health Agency of Canada. (n.d). *Healthy child development.* Retrieved January 25, 2012 from http://cbpp-pcpe.phac-aspc.gc.ca/topic/determinants/15/page/1

Reasor, J. E., & Farrell, S. P. (2004). Early childhood mental health: Services that can save a life. *Journal of Pediatric Nursing, 19*(2), 140–144.

Research Alliance for Canadian Homelessness, Housing, and Health. (2010). *Housing vulnerability and health: Canada's hidden emergency.* Retrieved February 8, 2012 from http://www.stmichaelshospital.com/pdf/crich/housing-vulnerability-and-health.pdf

Royal Canadian Mounted Police. (2007). *The effects of domestic violence on children: Where does it hurt?* Retrieved February 8, 2012 from http://www.rcmp-grc.gc.ca/cp-pc/chi-enf-abu-eng.htm

Safe Kids Canada. (2011). *Transport Canada unveils new safety regulations for car seats.* Retrieved February 8, 2012 from http://www.safekidscanada.ca/Professionals/Safety-Information/Child-Passenger-Safety/New-Regulations/New-regulations.aspx

Safe Kids Canada. (2012). *Child passenger safety.* Retrieved February 8, 2012 from http://www.safekidscanada.ca/professionals/safety-information/child-passenger-safety/index.aspx

Salus Global Corporation. (2012). *The MORE^OB program.* Retrieved February 8, 2012 from http://moreob.com/assets/MoreOBBrochure.pdf

Search Institute. (2011). *Developmental assets tools.* Retrieved February 8, 2012 from http://www.search-institute.org/assets

Selby, J. (2007). *Islam in Canada.* Retrieved February 8, 2012 from http://www.euro-islam.info/country-profiles/canada/

Shields, L, Pratt, J., & Hunter, J. (2006). Family centred care: A review of qualitative studies. *Journal of Clinical Nursing, 15,* 1317–1323.

Shields, M. (2006). Overweight and obesity among children and youth. *Health Reports, 17*(3), 27–42.

SickKids. (2011). *About SickKids: History and milestones.* Retrieved February 8, 2012 from http://www.sickkids.ca/AboutSickKids/History-and-Milestones/index.html

Society of Obstetricians and Gynaecologists of Canada. (2007). *An Aboriginal birthing strategy for Canada.* Retrieved February 8, 2012 from http://www.sogc.org/projects/pdf/AboriginalBirthingJune12%2007.pdf

Society of Obstetrics and Gynecologists of Canada. (2008). *A national birthing initiative for Canada.* Retrieved February 8, 2012 from http://www.sogc.org/projects/pdf/BirthingStrategyVersionc-Jan2008.pdf

Statistics Canada. (2007a). National longitudinal survey of children and youth. Survey overview of the 2006/2007 data collection Cycle 7. Government of Canada publications.

Statistics Canada. (2007b). *Census families in private households by family structure and presence of children, by province and territory (2006 Census).* Retrieved February 8, 2012 from http://www40.statcan.gc.ca/l01/cst01/famil54c-eng.htm

Statistics Canada. (2009a). *2006 Census: Immigration in Canada: A portrait of the foreign-born population, 2006 census: Findings.* Retrieved February 8, 2012 from http://www12.statcan.ca/census-recensement/2006/as-sa/97–557/index-eng.cfm

Statistics Canada. (2009b). *Family violence in Canada: A statistical profile* (Cat. No. 85–224-X). Retrieved February 8, 2012 from http://dsp-psd.pwgsc.gc.ca/collection_2009/statcan/85-224-X/85-224-x2009000-eng.pdf

Statistics Canada. (2010). *Population by sex and age groups.* Retrieved February 8, 2012 from http://www40.statcan.gc.ca/l01/cst01/DEMO10A-eng.htm

Stout, R., & Harp, R. (2009). *Aboriginal maternal and infant health in Canada: Review of on-reserve programming.* Retrieved February 8, 2012 from http://pwhce.ca/pdf/AborigMaternal_programmes.pdf

Taylor, C., Lillis, C., & LeMone, P. (2005). *Fundamentals of nursing: The art and science of nursing care* (5th ed.). Philadelphia: Lippincott Williams & Wilkins.

UNICEF. (2010). *At a glance: Canada—Statistics.* Retrieved February 8, 2012 from http://www.unicef.org/infobycountry/canada_statistics.html

UNICEF Canada (2009). *Aboriginal children's health: Leaving no child behind.* Retrieved April 14, 2012 from http://www.nccah-ccnsa.ca/docs/nccah%20partner%20documents/UNICEF%20Report,%20English.pdf

UNICEF Innocenti Research Center. (2005). Report card #6. *Child poverty in rich countries 2005.* Retrieved February 8, 2012 from http://www.unicef-irc.org/publications/pdf/repcard6e.pdf

Victorian Order of Nurses Canada. (2009). *History: A century of caring.* Retrieved February 8, 2012 from http://www.von.ca/en/about/history.aspx

Von Bertalanffy, L. (1968). *General systems theory.* London: Penguin Press.

Williamson, D. L., & Drummond, J. (2000). Enhancing low-income parents' capacities to promote their children's health: education is not enough. *Public Health Nursing, 17*(2), 12–131.

Wolfe, D. A., & Jaffe, G. (1999). Emerging strategies in the prevention of domestic violence. *Domestic Violence and Children, 9*(3), 133–144. Retrieved February 8, 2012 from http://www.princeton.edu/futureofchildren/publications/docs/09_03_9.pdf

Women and Health Care Reform. (2009). *History and future.* Retrieved February 8, 2012 from http://www.womenandhealthcarereform.ca/en/about_history.html

Wong, K. (1975). *Tommy Douglas: A remarkable Canadian.* Retrieved February 8, 2012 from http://www.cupe1975.ca/bursary/burs5.html

Woods, M. (2010). Cultural safety and the socioethical nurse. *Nursing Ethics, 17*(6), 715–725.

World Health Organization. (2000). *Gender, health and poverty fact sheet.* Retrieved February 8, 2012 from https://apps.who.int/inf-fs/en/fact251.html

World Health Organization. (2008). *Frequently asked questions.* Retrieved June 3, 2008 from http://www.who.int/suggestions/faq/en/

World Health Organization. (2009). *Canada: Health profile.* Retrieved February 21, 2012 from http://www.who.int/gho/countries/can.pdf

World Health Organization. (2011a). *Global health advisory*. Retrieved February 8, 2012 from http://www.who.int/gho/en/

World Health Organization. (2011b). *Why do so many women still die in pregnancy or childbirth?* Retrieved February 8, 2012 from http://www.who.int/features/qa/12/en/index.html

Wright, L. M., & Leahey, M. (2005). *Nurses and families: A guide to family assessment and intervention* (5th ed.). Philadelphia: FA Davis.

RECOMMENDED READINGS

American Pregnancy Association. (2011). *Doing it alone*. Retrieved February 8, 2012 from http://www.americanpregnancy.org/unplannedpregnancy/doingitalone.html

Canadian Cancer Society. (2011). *Cancer statistics figures*. Retrieved February 8, 2012 from http://www.cancer.ca/Canada-wide/About%20cancer/Cancer%20statistics/PowerPoint%20slides.aspx?sc_lang=en

Canadian Institute for Health Information. (2009). *Highlights of 2008–2009 selected indicators describing the birthing process in Canada*. Retrieved February 8, 2012 from http://secure.cihi.ca/cihiweb/products/childbirth_highlights_2010_05_18_e.pdf

Canadian Institute for Health Information. (2010a). *Health care in Canada 2010*. Retrieved February 8, 2012 from http://secure.cihi.ca/cihiweb/products/HCIC_2010_Web_e.pdf

Canadian Institute for Health Information. (2010b). *More physicians than ever; greatest percentage increase in physicians in 20 years*. Retrieved February 8, 2012 from http://www.cihi.ca/CIHI-ext-portal/internet/en/Document/spending+health+workforce/workforce/physicians/RELEASE_02DEC10

CIA World Factbook. (2012a). *Country comparison: Infant mortality rate*. Retreived from https://www.cia.gov/library/publications/the-world-factbook/rankorder/2091rank.html?countryName=Canada&countryCode=ca&regionCode=na&rank=187#ca

CIA World Factbook. (2012b). *North America: Canada*. Retrieved February 8, 2012 from https://www.cia.gov/library/publications/the-world-factbook/geos/ca.html

Health Canada. (2010). *The women's health contribution program: Advancing the health of women in Canada*. Retrieved February 8, 2012 from http://www.hc-sc.gc.ca/hl-vs/gender-genre/contribution/index-eng.php

Health Canada. (2011). *Sex and gender-based analysis*. Retrieved February 8, 2012 from http://www.hc-sc.gc.ca/hl-vs/gender-genre/analys/index-eng.php

Mitchinson, W. (2002). *Giving birth in Canada*. Toronto: University of Toronto Press.

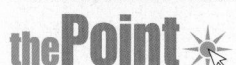

thePoint For additional learning materials, including Internet Resources, visit **http://thePoint.lww.com/Chow1e.**

CHAPTER WORKSHEET

MULTIPLE CHOICE QUESTIONS

1. When preparing a presentation for a local women's group on women's health problems, what would the nurse include as the number-one cause of mortality for women in Canada?

   a. Breast cancer

   b. Childbirth complications

   c. Injury resulting from violence

   d. Heart disease

2. Which factor would most likely be responsible for a pregnant woman's failure to receive adequate prenatal care in Canada?

   a. Age of the pregnant woman

   b. Use of denial to cope with pregnancy

   c. Shortage of health care professionals such as physicians and midwives in their community

   d. Income of the pregnant woman

3. When caring for children, how should the nurse best incorporate the concept of family-centred care?

   a. Encourage the family to allow the physician to make health care decisions for the child.

   b. Use the concepts of respect, family strengths, diversity, and collaboration with family.

   c. Advise the family to choose a pediatric provider who is on the covered child's health care plan.

   d. Recognize that families undergoing stress related to the child's illness cannot make good decisions.

4. When caring for an adolescent, in which instance must the nurse share information with the parents, no matter which province care is provided in?

   a. Delayed cognitive maturity

   b. Depression

   c. Contraception

   d. Tuberculosis

5. The following events were milestones in the health care provided to women and children in Canada. Place the events in the correct sequence, from oldest to most recent.

   ___ a. The first formal nurses training program was instituted in St. Catharines, Ontario.

   ___ b. Medicare was started by Tommy Douglas in Saskatchewan.

   ___ c. Sir Wilfred Laurier inaugurated the Victorian Order of Nurses of Canada.

   ___ d. Annie A. Bond founded the Margaret Scott Nursing Mission in Winnipeg.

   ___ e. The child tax benefit was introduced.

6. Which of the following factors contribute to homelessness? Select all that apply.

   ___ a. Decrease in the number of people living in poverty

   ___ b. Rises in unemployment

   ___ c. Exposure to abuse or neglect

   ___ d. Cutbacks in public welfare programs

   ___ e. Development of community crisis centres

CRITICAL THINKING EXERCISES

1. As a nurse working in a provincially funded low-income clinic offering women's health services primarily to low-income women, you are becoming increasingly frustrated with the number of "no-shows" or appointments missed in your maternity clinic. Some clients come for their initial prenatal intake appointment and never come back. You realize that some just forget their appointments, but most don't even call to notify you. Many of the clients are high risk and thus are jeopardizing their health and the health of their future child.

   a. What assessments might you make prior to deciding on changes needed?

   b. What changes might be helpful to address this situation?

   c. Outline what you might say at your next staff meeting to address the issue of clients making one clinic visit and then never returning.

   d. What strategies might you use to improve attendance and notification?

   e. Describe what cultural and customer service techniques might be needed.

2. A single woman has adopted an 11-month-old infant girl from China and has brought her to the health care facility for a check-up. The mother had no contact with the infant's birth parents. The infant spent 7 months in an orphanage before being adopted. Describe the family structure and the issues that may affect this family.

3. You have been asked by the local school district to speak to a group of middle-school children and their parents about safety. Describe the topics that you should address.

4. A 12-year-old is to undergo research treatment for a serious illness. Explain the concept of assent as it relates to this situation.

STUDY ACTIVITIES

1. Research a current policy, bill, or issue being debated in the community, within your nursing association, or at the provincial or federal government level that pertains to the health and welfare of women or children. Summarize the major facts and supporting and opposing arguments, and prepare an oral report on your findings.

2. Interview a child life specialist about the effects of using the atraumatic approach or the traditional approach for restraining children during procedures. Compare and contrast the effects on children at various developmental stages.

3. Within your clinical group, debate the following statement: Should access to medications and auxiliary health care such as physiotherapy outside a hospital be a right or a privilege?

4. Visit a local community health centre that offers services to women and children from various cultures. Interview the staff about any barriers to health care that they have identified. Investigate what the staff has done to minimize these barriers.

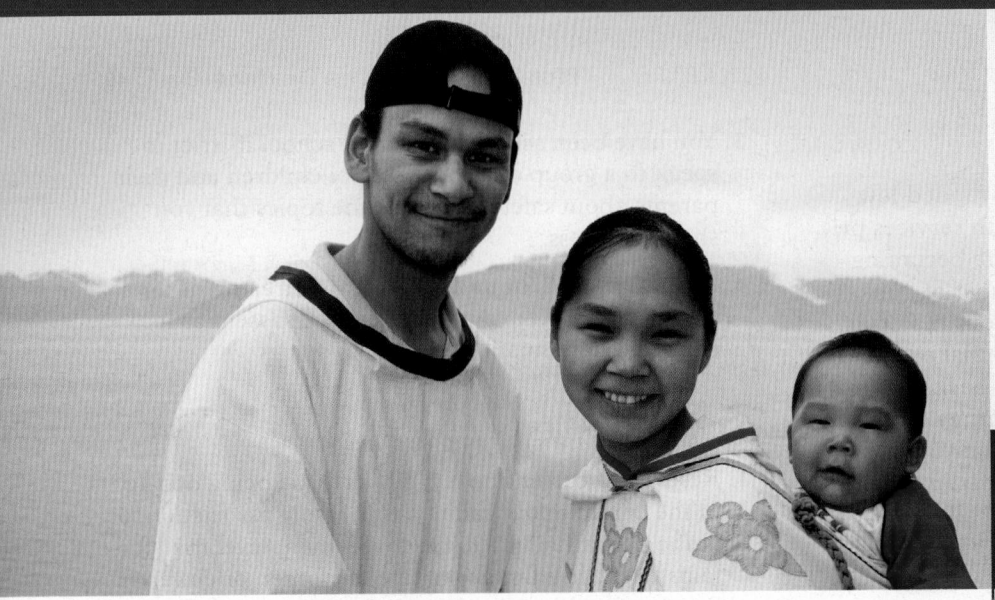

CHAPTER 2

Adapted by Genevieve Currie, Margaret Quance, and Lisa Semple

FAMILY-CENTRED COMMUNITY-BASED CARE

KEY TERMS

community
cultural competence
cultural attunement
cultural safety

epidemiology
family-centred care
family-centred maternity
    care

health literacy
medically fragile
    children
respite care

LEARNING OBJECTIVES

Upon completion of the chapter, the learner will be able to:

1. Examine the major components and key elements of family-centred care.
2. Explain the reasons for the increased emphasis on community health care.
3. Differentiate community health nursing from nursing in acute care settings.
4. Explain the different levels of prevention in community health nursing, providing examples of each.
5. Give examples of cultural issues that may be faced when providing community health nursing.
6. Provide culturally competent care to men, women, children, families, and populations.
7. Identify the variety of settings where community health care can be provided to men, women, children, families, and populations.
8. Outline the various roles and functions assumed by the community health nurse.
9. Demonstrate the ability to use excellent therapeutic communication skills when interacting with men, women, children, and families.
10. Explain the process of health teaching as it relates to men, women, children, and families.
11. Examine the importance of discharge planning and case management in providing community-based care.

Anisha was home 24 hours after giving birth to her first child. She had just changed her newborn son and placed him on his stomach for a nap when the community health nurse arrived for a postpartum visit. Because the nurse didn't speak Punjabi and Anisha didn't speak English, a great deal of gesturing followed. After examining Anisha, the nurse then picked up her son and placed him on his back in the crib. How could the nurse have prepared for this home visit? What message did the nurse convey in changing the newborn's position?

Wow

To recognize diversity in others and respect it, we must first have some awareness of who we are.

Men, women, children, and families receive most of their "health care," both wellness and illness care, in the community setting. During the past several decades, the health care delivery system has placed increasing emphasis on health promotion and disease prevention using primary health care approaches. With a focus on access to health care and reducing the disparities that cause illness, people are living longer and spending more time in the community. Clients often require health care in their homes; many of these clients enter the hospital for shorter stays and then require additional care in the home when they return. The health care system continues to move toward applying the principles of primary health care where essential health care is responsive to the health needs of all Canadians. This is accomplished though the provision of comprehensive health services, considering access to health, intersectoral collaboration and cooperation, use of appropriate technology, increased public participation, and health promotion and illness prevention within the community (World Health Organization, 1978, as cited in Stamler and Yiu, 2012).

Nurses play an important role in the health and wellness of a community. They not only collaborate with individuals to meet their health care needs but also go beyond to assess, plan, and intervene while working with families, communities, and populations. Nurses practice in a variety of settings within a community, such as public health clinics and primary care projects, schools, shelters, churches, community health centres, outreach clinics, outpost nursing stations, and homes. They promote the health of individuals, families, groups, communities, and populations and bolster an environment that supports health.

This chapter describes the concepts of community and community health nursing, addressing the varied settings where such care is provided to men, women, children, and families. The chapter also highlights the major roles and functions of community health nurses, emphasizing their role as facilitators, collaborators, educators in health promotion and disease prevention, and resource brokers (Community Health Nurses of Canada [CHNC], 2008).

Family-Centred Care

Family-centred care (FCC) is such a common phrase that the understanding of this philosophy is often taken for granted in current practice. However, in the history of health care, the concept of FCC is relatively new. It came into being around the mid-1960s in response to consumer activism surrounding the health care experiences of children and women at that time (Jolley & Shields, 2009; Phillips, 2003).

Children's hospital care in the early part of the 20th century was devoid of parental involvement and demonstrations of affection from nursing staff. Parents and families could visit hospitalized children for perhaps 30 minutes per week, if they lived close by, and not at all if they did not (Jolley & Shields, 2009). The primary focus of care for nurses was on preventing the spread of infectious diseases, such as tuberculosis (Jolley & Shields, 2009; McPherson, 1996). During World War II, large numbers of children in Europe were evacuated to the countryside. It was not until after World War II that the psychological effects of the separation of children and parents began to be noticed, principally by psychologist John Bowlby and social worker James Robertson. Bowlby's Theory of Attachment and Robertson's research on the effects of separation of parents from children during hospitalization became the foundation of the pediatric FCC movement (Jolley & Shields, 2009; Shields, 2010).

At the beginning of the 20th century, birth in Canada took place primarily in the home. Formalized prenatal care was rare; women were cared for by unregulated midwives, physicians, and/or sympathetic neighbours with family present. Childbirth was considered part of the life cycle. Pain medication and anaesthesia for birth were not standard protocols. Spurred by technological advances available only in hospitals (such as Twilight Sleep from 1915 to the 1930s), the setting for birth began to move to the hospital (Leavitt, 1986). Another factor influencing the movement of birth to the hospital setting was the view that childbirth was "pathological," a notion promoted by "experts" such as the prominent obstetrician Dr. Joseph De Lee (Phillips, 2003). Women were hospitalized for a week or more with restrictive visiting polices implemented to reduce the possibility of infection. In the late 1940s and into the 1950s, Dr. Grantly Dick-Read developed an educational program for women called "Childbirth Without Fear" and Dr. Ferdinand Lamaze developed the "Lamaze Method for Childbirth Without Pain." Increasing numbers of women began preparing themselves for birth using these methods. The consumer movement of the 1960s as well as the influence of the feminist movement created organizations that continue to influence maternity care to this day, including the International Childbirth Education Association (ICEA) and Childbirth Connections (formerly Maternity Care Association) (Phillips, 2003). Today's **family-centred maternity care** (FCMC) philosophies and programs, found in most birth centres, developed from these historical roots.

Given the history behind each of these movements, models of FCC were developed and implemented differently for hospitalized children and childbearing women. For the care of hospitalized children, visiting hours were loosened followed by 24-hour visiting by parents. Acknowledging the importance of parents in the provision of care to their children, "care-by-parent" models were adopted in which parents "retained responsibility for their child while still being in the care of health professionals" (Jolley & Shields, 2009, p. 168). "Partnership-in-care" models were similar, with the nursing care provided by either nurses or parents with education and support from the nurse. The concept of FCC and the models that developed from it have now spread from acute care sites into community and clinical settings (Rosser, Colwill, Kasperski, & Wilson, 2011).

FCMC has also developed models of care, exemplified by the work of Celeste Phillips (2003). One of the core principles of FCMC is that women should labour and give birth in the same room (unless the woman has a cesarean section), called single room maternity care in labour–delivery–recovery–postpartum (LDRP) rooms.

There are many similarities between FCC and FCMC. No matter which model is used in acute care and community settings, there is similar emphasis on respect and trust between care recipients, their families, and health care providers. There is a requirement for education that promotes the ability of the care recipient to be empowered to make informed choices regarding treatment options. Collaboration between care recipients and health care providers is required, not only in sharing intimate details of one child's or one woman's situation but also from an organizational perspective as well. Often, administrative committees include former care recipients or family members who provide their perspective of the care received. All this is done within the context of the care recipient and his or her family members, including whomever the person defines as "family."

A family-centred approach is associated with positive outcomes that include decreased anxiety, improved pain management, shortened recovery times, and enhanced confidence and problem-solving skills. Communication between the health care team and the family is also improved, leading to greater satisfaction for both health care providers and health care consumers (families). Practicing FCC may empower the family, strengthen family resources, and help the woman or child feel more secure throughout the process.

FCC and FCMC philosophies have influenced many health care organizations, professional bodies, and patient advocacy groups (Table 2.1). These groups and websites meet many of the objectives of FCMC through the provision of information that educates and empowers women to make informed choices about their maternity care:

- The Institute of Family-Centred Care, established in 1992, promotes the FCC philosophy in pediatric, maternity, and newborn intensive care settings. This group's work has now expanded to include adult and geriatric care centres, prompting a name change in 2010 to the Institute for Patient- and Family-Centred Care.
- Planetree is a nonprofit organization that provides education and information within the collaborative community of health care organizations, facilitating efforts to create patient-centred care in healing environments. Part of its mission is to create collaborative relationships and provide information, so patients can make informed decisions concerning their care.
- Childbirth Connection is a well-established American nonprofit advocacy group dedicated to providing women with research-based information on pregnancy and birth.
- BabyCenter is a new Canadian website providing research-based information that has been reviewed by a medical advisory board as well as "moms and dads living the subject first-hand, raising newborns, toddlers, and older children."

The Society of Obstetricians and Gynaecologists of Canada (SOGC) references FCC in its publication *A National Birthing Initiative for Canada* (2008). The Canadian Nurses Association (CNA, 1997) developed a paper on the role of families in care, discussing the differences in care philosophies.

While a number of qualitative studies have demonstrated positive outcomes of FCC (Institute of Patient- and Family-Centred Care, 2010), a *Cochrane* review did not find any randomized controlled trials examining its effectiveness (Shields, Pratt, Davis, & Hunter, 2007). Of more concern are the results of Canadian studies that found the actual practice of FCC and FCMC at the bedside or in the clinic differed from its philosophical beliefs. One study noted that collaboration between parents and nurses concerning the care of their child "changed" to care being delivered by the parents without the required support from the nurses (MacKean, Thurston, & Scott, 2005). Another study suggested that nurses are dependent upon parents' active participation in the organization of the work but that some parents resent being made to do what they perceived to be nurses' work (Coyne, 2007). Another Canadian study found that FCMC was a "mirage" rather than a reality and that the systems of maternity health care did not give priority to women's informed choice (Jimenez, Klein, Hivon, & Mason, 2010). Shields (2010) stated, "In this changing time of short hospital stays, high technology and extremely costly health care, we must question whether or not we should be working to prove the effectiveness of FCC and assuring its continuation as a model of care" (p. 2636). However, in the absence of any other philosophy that has such potential, FCC and FCMC should be maintained. These studies emphasize that it is not only the individual nurse who needs to change and develop but rather a system-wide cultural shift is needed (Phillips, 2003). In order for FCC and FCMC to be effective, the actual workings of the health care system, the environments, the organizational procedures, and all of the participants in care—the woman/child, family, and health care providers—must change.

TABLE 2.1 COMPARISON OF PATIENT– AND FAMILY–CENTRED CARE PRINCIPLES FROM AMERICAN AND CANADIAN ORGANIZATIONS AND PUBLICATIONS

Institute for Patient and Family-Centered Care (United States)	Planetree (United States)	American Academy of Pediatrics (United States)	*Family-Centred Maternity Care* (Canada)	Health Canada (Canada)
Respect and dignity: Health care practitioners listen to and honour patient and family perspectives and choices. Patient and family knowledge, values, beliefs, and cultural backgrounds are incorporated into the planning and delivery of care.	We are human beings, caring for other human beings.	Respecting each child and his or her family	Childbirth is seen as wellness, a normal life event involving dynamic emotional, social, and physical change.	Birth is a celebration, a normal, healthy process.
Information sharing: Health care practitioners communicate and share complete and unbiased information with patients and families in ways that are affirming and useful. Patients and families receive timely, complete, and accurate information in order to effectively participate in care and decision making.	We are all caregivers.	Honouring racial, ethnic, cultural, and socioeconomic diversity and its effect on the family's experience and perception of care	Prenatal care is personalized according to individual needs of each woman and her family.	Pregnancy and birth are unique for each woman.
Participation. Patients and families are encouraged and supported in participating in care and decision making at the level they choose.	Caregiving is best achieved through kindness and compassion.	Recognizing and building on the strengths of each child and family, even in difficult and challenging situations	A comprehensive program of perinatal education prepares families for active participation.	The central objective of care for women, babies, and families is to maximize the probability of a healthy woman giving birth to a healthy baby.
Collaboration. Patients and families are also included on an institution-wide basis. Health care leaders collaborate with patients and families in policy and program development, implementation, and evaluation; in health care facility design; and in professional education, as well as in the delivery of care.	Safe, accessible, high-quality care is fundamental to patient-centred care.	Supporting and facilitating choice for the child and family about approaches to care and support	The hospital team assists the family in making informed choices for care in order to provide them with the experience they desire.	Family-centred maternity and newborn care is based on research evidence.

(continued)

TABLE 2.1 COMPARISON OF PATIENT- AND FAMILY-CENTRED CARE PRINCIPLES FROM AMERICAN AND CANADIAN ORGANIZATIONS AND PUBLICATIONS (continued)

Institute for Patient and Family-Centered Care (United States)	Planetree (United States)	American Academy of Pediatrics (United States)	*Family-Centred Maternity Care* (Canada)	Health Canada (Canada)
	A holistic approach is required in order to meet people's needs of body, mind, and spirit.	Ensuring flexibility in organizational practices, procedures, and provider practices so services can be tailored to the needs, beliefs, and cultural values of each child and family	The father and/or other support persons of the woman's choice are actively involved.	Relationships between women, their families, and health care providers are based on mutual respect and trust.
	Families, friends, and loved ones are vital to the healing process.	Sharing honest and unbiased information with families on an ongoing basis and in ways they find useful and affirming	Whenever the mother wishes, family and friends are encouraged to be present during the entire hospital stay.	Women are cared for within the context of their families.
	Access to understandable health information can empower individuals to participate in their health care.	Providing and/or ensuring formal and informal support for the child and parent(s) and/or guardian(s) during pregnancy, childbirth, infancy, childhood, adolescence, and young adulthood	Each woman's labour and birth are provided in the same location (unless a cesarean is required). When possible, patient and newborn care is given by the same caregivers and in the same location.	In order to make informed choices, women and their families need knowledge about their care.
	The opportunity for individuals to make personal choices related to their care is essential.	Collaborating with families at all levels of health care, in the care of the individual child and in professional education, policy making, and program development	Mothers are the preferred care providers for infants. The nursing role changes from direct care provision to facilitation of care by the mother/family.	Women have autonomy in decision making. Through respect and informed choice, women are empowered to take responsibility.
	Physical environments can enhance healing, health, and well-being.	Empowering each child and family to discover their own strengths, build confidence, and make choices and decisions about their health	When mother-baby care is implemented, the same person cares for the mother and baby, even when they are briefly separated.	Health care providers have a powerful effect on women who are giving birth and their families.

Institute for Patient and Family-Centered Care (United States)	Planetree (United States)	American Academy of Pediatrics (United States)	*Family-Centred Maternity Care* (Canada)	Health Canada (Canada)
	Illness can be a transformational experience for patients, families, and caregivers.		Parents have access to the high-risk newborn at all times and are included in care to the greatest extent possible.	Family-centred care welcomes a variety of health care providers. Technology is used appropriately in family-centred maternity and newborn care. Quality care includes a number of indicators. Language is important.

Sources: American Academy of Pediatrics. (2003). Policy statement: Family centred care and the pediatrician's role. *Pediatrics*, 112(3), 691–696. Retrieved September 13, 2011 from http://aappolicy.aappublications.org/cgi/content/full/pediatrics;112/3/691; Health Canada. (2000). *Family-centred maternity and newborn care: National guidelines.* Retrieved September 12, 2011 from http://www.phac-aspc.gc.ca/hp-ps/dca-dea/publications/fcm-smp/index-eng.php; Institute for Patient- and Family Centered Care. (2010). *What are the core concepts of patient- and family-centered care?* Retrieved September 13, 2011 from http://www.ipfcc.org/faq.html; Phillips, C. R. (2003). *Family-centred maternity care.* Toronto, ON: Jones and Bartlett; Planetree. (2011). *Planetree vision, mission and belief statements.* Retrieved September 13, 2011 from http://www.planetree.org/about.html.

Community Health Care

Community may be defined as a "specific group of people, often living in a defined geographical area, who share a common culture, values, and norms and who are arranged in a social structure according to relationships the community has developed over a period of time" (CHNC, 2008, p. 16). The common features of a community may be common rights and privileges as members of a certain city or common ties of identity, values, norms, culture, language, or social support. Women and increasingly men are caregivers to children, parents, spouses, and neighbours and provide important social support in these roles. The child's community consists of the family, school, neighbourhood, youth organizations, and other peer groups.

A person can be a part of many communities during the course of daily life. Examples might include area of residence (home, apartment, shelter), gender, place of employment (organization or home), language spoken (Tagalog, English, French), educational background or student status, culture (Chinese, South Asian, First Nations, British), career (nurse, businesswoman, housewife), place

of worship (church, temple, mosque, synagogue), and community memberships (community garden, YMCA, support group, school PTA, youth organizations, athletic teams).

In community health care, the community is the unit of service. The providers of care are concerned not only with the clients who present for service but also with the larger population of individuals who have common characteristics and risk factors.

Community Health Nursing

Community health nursing focuses on working with others to improve the health of populations and communities and prevent illness. Population is defined as "a collection of individuals who have one or more personal or environmental characteristics in common" (CHNC, 2008, p. 17). Community health nurses work in geographically and culturally diverse settings to address current and potential health needs of the population or community. They promote and preserve the health of a population but are not limited to particular age groups or diagnoses. Public health nursing is a specialized area of community health nursing focused on epidemiology and the control of disease. In this chapter, public health nurses are referred to using the larger umbrella term of community health nurses (CHNC, 2008).

Epidemiology, defined as the study of the causes, distribution, and control of disease in populations, can determine the health and health needs of a population and assist in planning health services. Community health nurses perform epidemiologic investigations to help analyze trends in the community's health and develop health policy and community health initiatives. Community health initiatives can be focused on the community as a whole or on a specific target population with specific needs. The H1N1 flu vaccine campaign in 2010–2011 is an example of the community as the focus of community health initiatives. An example of a specific population with defined needs would be newly discharged postpartum women and their infants. The focus of health care initiatives is on people and their needs, looking to strengthen their abilities to shape their own lives. The emphasis has shifted away from dependence on health professionals toward personal involvement and personal responsibility. This gives nurses the opportunity to interact with individuals in a variety of self-help roles. Nurses in the community can be the primary force in identifying the challenges and implementing changes in women's and children's health for the future.

Community-Focused Nursing Roles

In the past, the only community-based roles for nurses were community health nurses or public health nurses. CHNC, a national organization for community health nurses providing standards and competencies of practice, defines all community-based nurses under the umbrella term of "community health nurses." This includes home health care nurses who provide illness care within the home. The emphasis on primary health care and illness prevention has increased the demand for community-based and community-focused services. The movement from an illness-oriented "cure" perspective in hospitals to a focus on health promotion and primary health care in community-based settings has dramatically changed employment opportunities for today's nurses. This shift in emphasis to primary health care, primary care networks, and outpatient treatment and management will likely continue. As a result, employment growth in a variety of community-based settings can be expected for nurses possessing the appropriate level of education and/or certification. Statistics from the Canadian Institute for Health Information (CIHI) Nursing Database (2010) show the following trends in registered nurse (RN) employment settings:

• 37.3% of RNs work outside the hospital setting in most Canadian provinces.

• 60% of RNs work outside the hospital setting in the Northern territories and provinces.

It is noteworthy that the delivery of nursing services in the Northern territories differs from that in the provinces (CIHI, 2010).

Community-based nursing encompasses a variety of tasks and care settings, including chronic disease management, ambulatory care, home health care, occupational health, school health, parish nursing, pre- and postnatal care, well child care, communicable disease control, outpost and street clinics, sexual and reproductive health clinics, and hospice settings. Clinical practice within the community may also include case management, research, quality improvement, and discharge planning. Nurses with advanced practice and experience may be employed in areas of research and community development, population health planning and program development, and community education. See Table 2.2 for a list of community-based practice settings.

TABLE 2.2 **COMMUNITY-BASED PRACTICE SETTINGS**

Type of Care	Setting/Description
Ambulatory care	Primary care settings Urgent care centres Family planning clinics Mobile mammography centres Outpost nursing stations Outreach/mobile clinics
Home health care services	High-risk pregnancy/neonate care Maternal/child newborn care Skilled nursing care Respite and hospice care
Public Health Department services	Maternal/child health clinics Family planning clinics School health programs Sexually transmitted infection clinics Immunization clinics Substance abuse/harm reduction programs Jails and prisons Outreach/mobile clinics Outpost nursing stations
Long-term care	Skilled nursing facilities Nursing homes Hospices Assisted living facilities
Other types of care	Parish nursing programs Summer camps Childbirth education programs School health programs Occupational health programs Federal prisons/penitentiaries Street clinics/homeless shelters Disaster shelters

Community Health Nursing Interventions

Nursing interventions involve any treatment the nurse performs to enhance client outcomes. Nursing practice in the community uses the community health nursing process and is similar to that used in the acute care setting. Assessing, planning (including setting goals with the client/family/community), implementing nursing care (including performing procedures, administering medications, coordinating services and equipment, and counselling clients and their families), teaching about care, and evaluating that care are all part of nursing practice for nurses in the community. Table 2.3 highlights the most common nursing interventions used in community health nursing practice.

Community Health Nursing Challenges

Despite the benefits achieved by caring for families in their own homes and communities, challenges also exist. Clients with chronic illnesses are staying in their homes or are being discharged from acute care facilities very early in their recovery and return to the community with more health care needs than in the past. As a result, nursing care and procedures in the home and community are becoming more complex and time-consuming. Consider the example of a woman who is being discharged from the hospital after a cesarean birth who develops a systemic infection, a pelvic abscess, and deep vein thrombosis in her leg. The home health care/community health nurse's primary focus of care in this situation would be to administer heparin and antibiotics intravenously as well as to educate the woman about the care of her infant, including breastfeeding. In the past, this woman would have remained hospitalized for treatment, but infusion therapy delivered in the home is now less costly and allows the client to be discharged sooner.

This demand on the nurse's time may limit the amount of time spent on prevention measures, education, and the family's psychosocial issues. More time may be needed to help families deal with these immediate health issues and concerns. With large client caseloads, nurses may find it difficult to collaborate with families to address the broader influences on health known as the determinants of health (Reutter & Eastlick Kushner, 2010). Nurses working in the community have fewer

TABLE 2.3 COMMUNITY HEALTH NURSING INTERVENTIONS

Intervention	Examples
Health screening—detecting unrecognized or preclinical illness among individuals so they can be referred for definitive diagnosis and treatment	Mammogram or Pap smear, well-child vision and hearing checks
Health education programs—assisting clients in making health-related decisions about self-care, use of health resources, and social health issues such as smoking bylaws and bicycle helmet laws	Childbirth education or breast self-examination, child safety programs, poisoning prevention, youth drug awareness programs
Medication administration—preparing, giving, and evaluating the effectiveness of prescription and over-the-counter drugs	Hormone replacement therapy in menopausal women, childhood immunizations
Telephone consultation—identifying the problem to be addressed; listening and providing support, information, or instruction; documenting advice/instructions given to concerns raised by caller	Consultation for a mother with a newborn with colic, interaction with a parent whose child has a fever or is vomiting
Health system referral—passing along information about the location, services offered, and ways to contact agencies	Referring a woman for a breast prosthesis after a mastectomy, arranging for home tutoring for a child with a long-term illness
Instructional—teaching an individual or group about a medication, disease process, lifestyle changes, community resources, or research findings concerning their environment	Childbirth education class, basic life support classes for parents, child safety education classes
Nutritional counselling—demonstrating the direct relationship between nutrition and illness while focusing on the need for diet modification to promote wellness	Prenatal programs for vulnerable populations; counsellor interviewing a pregnant woman or a child and parents who have anaemia; eating disorders program
Risk identification—recognizing personal or group characteristics that predispose people to develop a specific health problem, and modifying or eliminating them	Genetic counselling of an older pregnant woman at risk for a Down syndrome infant; genetic screening of family members for cystic fibrosis or Huntington's disease

Source: Dochterman, J. M., & Bulechek, G. M. (2008). *Nursing interventions classification (NIC)* (5th ed.). St. Louis: Mosby.

resources available to them compared with nurses in the acute care setting. Decisions often have to be made in isolation. The nurse must possess excellent assessment skills and the ability to communicate effectively and plan appropriate follow-up care with the family in order to be successful in carrying out the appropriate plan of care.

Nurses interested in working in community-based settings must be able to apply the nursing process in an environment that is less structured or controlled than that associated with acute care facilities. Nurses must be able to assimilate information well beyond the immediate physical and psychosocial needs of the client in a controlled acute care setting and reflect upon the broader determinants of health while encountering environmental hazards, diverse lifestyle choices, family issues, different cultural patterns, families experiencing financial burdens, limited access to resources including transportation, employment hazards, communication barriers, limited social supports, and lack of desire to change personal health practices and coping skills.

Although opportunities for employment in community-based settings are available, most positions require a baccalaureate degree and/or specialized certification. Previous medical–surgical experience or experience in particular specialties is an asset (such as perinatal nursing, family newborn or child health nursing) because community health nurses must function fairly independently within the home and community environment.

The nurse must also be familiar with and respectful of many different cultures, socioeconomic levels, and lifestyle choices while remaining objective in managing such diversity. The nurse must also demonstrate an understanding of and appreciation for differences. Interventions must be individualized to address the cultural, social, and economic determinants of health among clients in their own environment (Stamler & Yiu, 2012).

Shift in Responsibilities from Hospital-Based to Community-Based Nursing

Community care, especially home health care, is a rapidly growing need in Canada. The trends contributing to this shift include shorter hospital stays, greater use of outpatient treatment, and a growing population of older Canadians with longer life expectancy. An increasing number of children and adults with chronic and debilitating health conditions have also contributed to the continued shift of health care to the community and home setting. Technology has advanced, allowing for improved monitoring of clients in community settings and at home as well as allowing more complicated procedures, such as intravenous administration of antibiotics, to be performed in the home setting. A major cause for the increase in community care, especially home health care in the pediatric population, is the understanding that an acute care setting is not an appropriate environment for children to grow (Hewitt-Taylor, 2005).

Caring for children at home not only improves their physical health but also allows for adequate growth and development within their family. Children cared for in the home are in a familiar environment with the comfort and support of family, which leads to improved care and quality of life.

Levels of Prevention in Community Health Nursing

Prevention is a key part of community health nursing practice. The emphasis on health care delivery in community-based settings encompasses not only primary preventive health care (e.g., well-child checkups, routine physical examinations, prenatal care, postnatal care, immunizations, treatment of common acute illnesses) but also secondary and tertiary care (Fig. 2.1).

Primary Prevention

The concept of primary prevention concerns preventing a disease or condition before it occurs through health promotion activities, environmental protection, and specific protection against disease or injury. It encompasses a vast array of areas, including nutrition, good hygiene, sanitation, immunization, adequate shelter, smoking cessation, family planning, and the use of seat belts (Stamler & Yiu, 2012).

Prevention of neural tube defects (e.g., anencephaly and spina bifida in children) is an example of primary prevention. The use of folic acid supplementation daily for at least 3 months before and 3 months after conception reduces the risk of first occurrence of neural tube defects (SOGC, 2007). Providing anticipatory guidance to parents about poison prevention and playground safety is another example of primary prevention.

Secondary Prevention

Secondary prevention is the early detection, treatment, and confinement of adverse health conditions, including communicable diseases. Health screenings are the mainstay of secondary prevention. Pregnancy testing, blood pressure evaluations, cholesterol monitoring, fecal occult blood testing, breast examinations, mammography screening, hearing and vision examinations, and Papanicolaou (Pap) smears are examples of secondary-level prevention. Such interventions do not prevent the health problem but are intended for early detection and prompt treatment to prevent complications (Vollman, Anderson, & McFarlane, 2012).

Tertiary Prevention

Tertiary prevention is designed to reduce or limit the progression of a disease or disability. The purpose of tertiary prevention is to restore individuals to their maximum potential (Vollman et al., 2012). Tertiary prevention measures are supportive and restorative. For example,

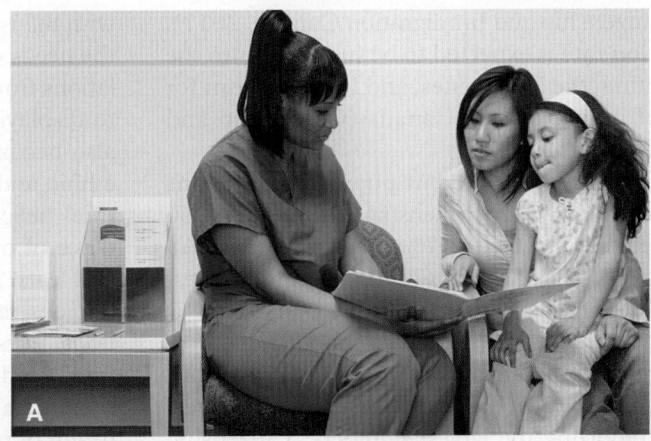

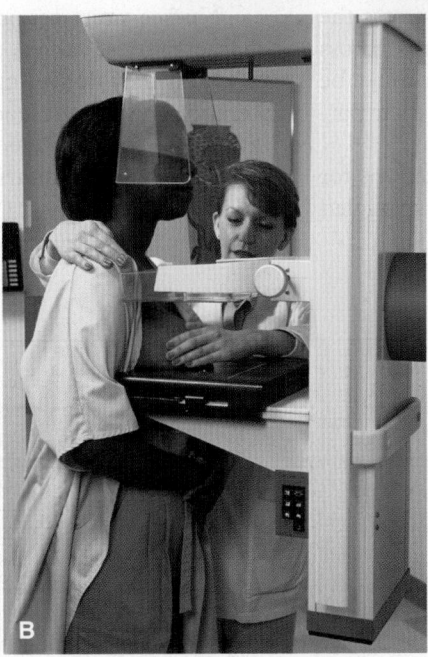

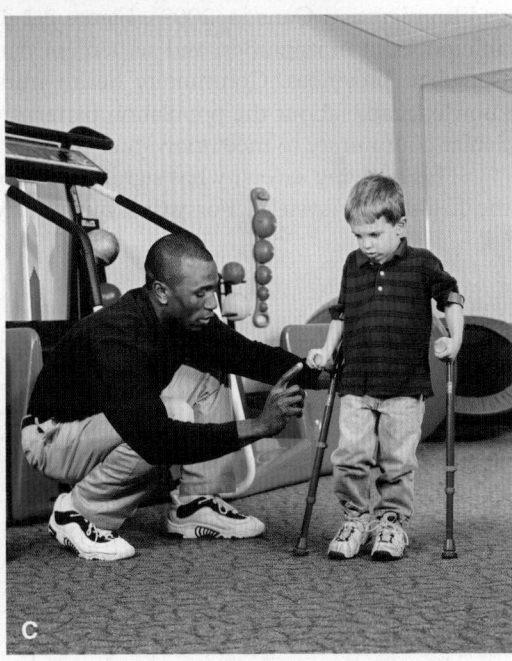

FIGURE 2.1 Levels of prevention in community-based nursing. (**A**) At the primary prevention level, the nurse provides anticipatory guidance and family teaching. (**B**) At the secondary level of prevention, a woman undergoes a mammography screening for early detection of breast problems. (**C**) At the tertiary level of prevention, a child with a developmental disability participates in a rehabilitation program.

tertiary prevention interventions would focus on minimizing and managing the effects of a chronic illness, such as a spinal cord injury or cerebral palsy, or the chronic effects of sexually transmitted infections such as herpes, human immunodeficiency virus (HIV), and untreated chlamydia. Another example would involve working with men and women who have suffered long-term consequences of abuse and violence. The focus of the nurse would be to maximize the person's strengths, help him or her recover from the trauma and loss, build support systems, and refer to appropriate resources.

Organization of Health Care in Canada

Organization of health care in Canada is a provincial responsibility as stipulated by the British North America Act (Petrucka, 2010; Storch, 2010). Each province sets its priorities for funding and services in different ways. The nurse must be familiar with his or her particular provincial organization of health care.

The Nurse's Role in Community Health Preventive Care

All health professionals have a role in health promotion, health protection, and disease prevention. Much of community nursing involves prevention, early identification, and prompt treatment of health problems and monitoring for emerging threats that might lead to health problems. Community health nurses provide health care for men, women, and children at all three levels of prevention. This care often involves advocating for services to meet their needs.

Cultural Context of Community Health Nursing

Canada is described as a multicultural nation. Over the years, attitudes and policies toward immigration have evolved. From 2005 to 2010, the annual rate of immigration to Canada ranged from 236,754 to 280,861 individuals (Citizenship and Immigration Canada, 2011). This immigration rate is expected to be sustained into the near future. China, the Philippines, and India account for the majority of immigrants to Canada (Citizenship and Immigration Canada, 2009).

Each community has different population patterns and demographics. In 2001, Citizenship and Immigration Canada reported that Toronto (43.7%), Vancouver (37.5%), Hamilton (23.6%), and Calgary (20.9%) had the largest percentages of foreign-born citizens. From 1996 to 2001, recent immigrants made up a significant proportion of foreign-born citizens, with Vancouver (23%), Ottawa-Gatineau (20.6%), Toronto (20.4%), and Calgary and Montreal (18.4% each) reporting the largest numbers (Citizenship and Immigration Canada, 2009). Figure 2.2 illustrates the differences in immigration and settlement patterns across Canadian provinces. Community health nurses must be knowledgeable about the population patterns of their particular community to meet individual needs.

This growing diversity has significant implications for the health care system. For years, nurses have struggled with the issues of providing optimal health care that meets the needs of individuals, families, communities, and populations from varied cultures and ethnic groups. In addition to displaying competence in technical skills, nurses must also become competent in caring for clients from varied ethnic and racial backgrounds. Adapting to different cultural beliefs and practices requires flexibility and acceptance of others' viewpoints. Nurses must listen to clients and learn about their beliefs about health and wellness. To demonstrate culturally appropriate care to diverse populations, nurses need to know, understand, and respect culturally influenced health behaviours. Chapter 1 provides a more detailed discussion of culture and its impact on the health of men, women, children, and families.

Nurses must research and understand the cultural characteristics, values, and beliefs of the various people to whom they deliver care so that false assumptions and stereotyping do not lead to insensitive care. Time orientation, personal space, family orientation (patriarchal, matriarchal, or egalitarian), and language are important cultural concepts.

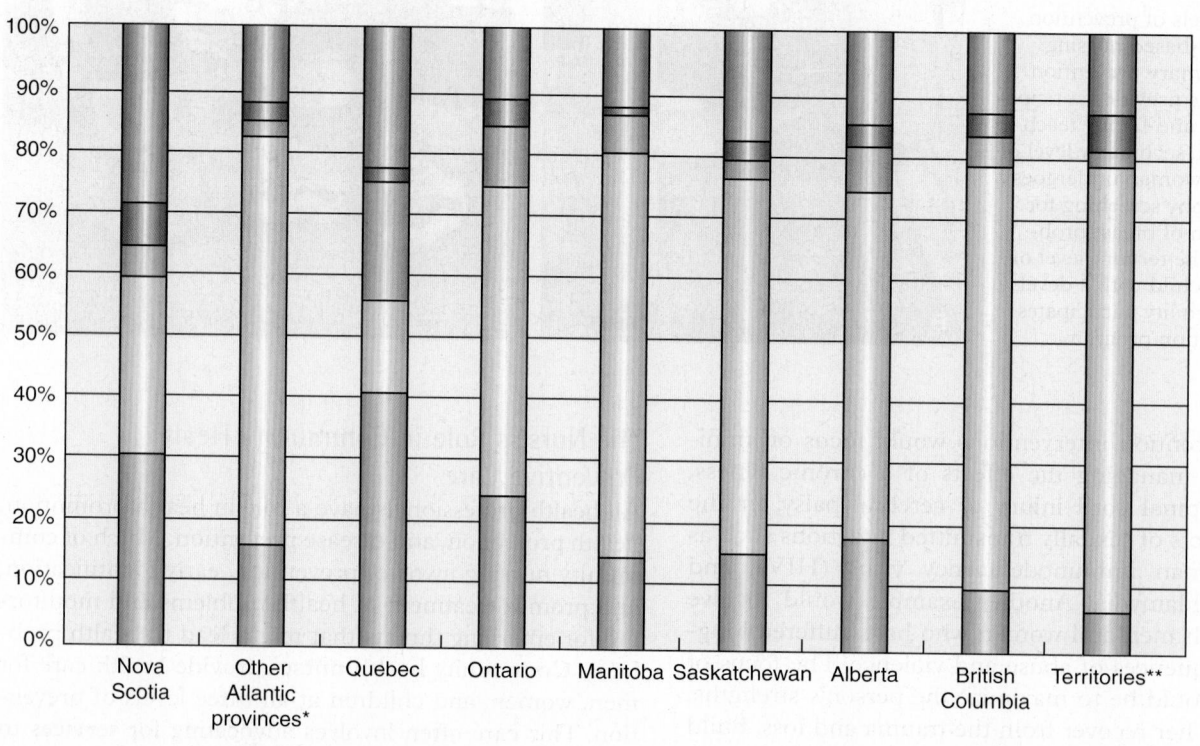

*Newfoundland and Labrador, Prince Edward Island and New Brunswick
** Yokon, Northwest Territories and Nunavut

FIGURE 2.2 Permanent residents of Canada by province or territory and source area, 2010.
Source: *Facts and figures 2010—Immigration overview: Permanent and temporary residents.*
Retrieved January 23, 2012 from http://www.cic.gc.ca/english/resources/statistics/facts2010/
permanent/14.asp. Citizen and Immigration Canada, 2010. Reproduced with the permission of the Minister of Public Works and Government Services Canada, 2011.

Concepts Concerning Culture and Diversity

Canada is a culturally diverse country. Culture forms an important element of the determinants of health that community health nurses consider when working with clients. "Cultural diversity is the variation of cultural factors between people" (CNA, 2010, p. 1). The term *culture* may be interpreted in different ways, depending on the individual's perspective (Aboriginal Nurses Association of Canada, 2009). To ignore or collaborate in only a superficial way with people of varying cultures will negatively impact nursing care and health care outcomes.

There are three particular concepts concerning culture that nurses need to be aware of in order to effectively provide care to clients, families, and/or the community at large: cultural competence, cultural attunement, and cultural safety.

Cultural competence is defined as "a set of congruent behaviour, attitudes, and policies that come together in a system, agency, or among professionals and enables ... [them] to work effectively in cross-cultural situation" (Registered Nurses' Association of Ontario, 2007). Nurses must look at clients through their own eyes as well as through the eyes of clients and family members and develop nonjudgmental acceptance of cultural differences among clients. They must consider diversity as a strength that empowers nurses and clients to achieve mutually acceptable health care goals. Cultural competence must be a goal for health professionals and is considered an ongoing process in a lifelong journey (Vollman et al., 2012) (Box 2.1).

Cultural attunement is a way of being in relation to another. Health care providers need to move beyond the superficial knowledge of a culture to consider the meanings that individuals ascribe to their own ethnicity. This involves carefully listening to understand meaning ascribed to an individual's ethnicity. Cultural attunement requires continuing self-exploration and self-awareness.

Cultural safety is a third concept in providing care and moves health professionals beyond cultural awareness and the mere acknowledgement of "difference." The CNA considers cultural safety "both a process and an outcome whose goal is to promote greater equity. It focuses on root causes of power imbalances and inequitable social relationships in health care" (CNA, 2010, p. 1). Cultural safety is a more inclusive concept that includes cultural awareness, cultural sensitivity, and cultural competence (CNA, 2010). The Aboriginal Nurses Association of Canada (2009) identifies the benefits using a cultural safety lens in order to address health inequities:

- Improve health care access for patients, aggregates, and populations
- Acknowledge that we are all bearers of culture
- Expose the social, political, and historical contexts of care

---

BOX 2.1 **Steps to Developing Cultural Competence**

1. Cultural Self-Awareness
   - Become aware of, appreciative of, and sensitive to the values, beliefs, customs, and behaviours that have shaped one's own culture.
   - Engage in self-exploration beyond one's own culture and "see" clients from different cultures.
   - Examine personal biases and prejudices toward other cultures.
   - Become aware of differences in personal and clients' background.
2. Cultural Knowledge
   - Obtain knowledge about various worldviews of different cultures by reading about different cultures, attending continuing education courses on different cultures, accessing websites, and attending cultural diversity conferences.
   - Become familiar with culturally/ethnically diverse groups, worldviews, beliefs, practices, lifestyles, and problem-solving strategies.
3. Cultural Skills
   - Learn how to perform a competent cultural assessment.
   - Assess each client's unique cultural values, beliefs, and practices without depending solely on written facts about specific cultural groups.
4. Cultural Encounters
   - Engage in cross-cultural interactions with people from culturally diverse backgrounds, such as attending religious services or ceremonies and participating in important family events.
   - Participate in as many cultural encounters as possible to avoid cultural stereotyping.

- Enable practitioners to consider difficult concepts such as racism, discrimination, and prejudice
- Acknowledge that cultural safety is determined by those to whom nurses provide care
- Understand the limitations of "culture" in terms of having people access and safely move through health care systems and encounters with care providers
- Challenge unequal power relations

Barriers to Cultural Competence

Barriers to cultural competence, cultural attunement, and cultural safety have social, political, and historical contexts. Barriers can be grouped into two categories: those related to providers and those related to systems (Godfrey, 2006). When a health care provider lacks knowledge of a client's cultural practices and beliefs or when the provider's beliefs differ from those of the client, the provider may be unprepared to respond when the client makes unexpected health care decisions.

Language differences between the client and provider can also leave the client feeling unsafe and the provider dissatisfied (Vollman et al., 2012). System-related barriers can be found at the unit, programme, policy, or organization level and occur when agencies that have not been designed for cultural diversity require clients to conform to the established rules and regulations, attempting to fit everyone into the same mold. Financial restraints, a system problem, may reduce or eliminate the availability of qualified health translators in assisting with care or teaching, creating feelings of unease and dissatisfaction in the client and the nurse (Vollman et al., 2012).

Community Health Nursing Care Settings for Individuals and Families

Community health nursing takes place in a variety of settings, including primary care networks, public health clinics, health departments, urgent care centres, hospital outpatient centres, family planning clinics, occupational health work settings, schools, camps, churches, outpost stations, shelters, and clients' homes. Nurses provide well care, episodic illness care, and chronic care. They work to promote, preserve, and improve the health of individuals, families, communities, and populations in these settings.

Due to technological advances, cost containment, and shortened hospital stays, the home is a common care setting for men, women, children, and families today. Home health care is geared toward the needs of the client and family. Generally, services are publicly and privately funded. Families may choose to supplement publicly funded services with costs covered either by private insurance plans or the family budget.

Home health care nursing visits may be used for intermittent interventions, such as IV antibiotic administration, follow-up with client teaching, and monitoring. Private-duty nursing care from organizations such as the Victorian Order of Nurses may be used when more extensive care is needed. This care may be delivered hourly (several hours per day) or on a full-time, live-in basis. The cost for private-duty nursing care is borne by the individual and/or family and may be supplemental to publicly funded services. The goals of nursing care in the home setting include promoting, restoring, and maintaining the health of the client. Efforts are directed toward coordinating a network of caregivers.

Home health care focuses on minimizing the effects of the illness or disability along with providing the client with the means to care for the illness or disability at home. Nurses in the home care setting are direct care providers, educators, advocates, and case managers.

Prenatal Care

Early prenatal care with a minimum of four visits is associated with improved pregnancy outcomes (Enkin et al., 2000). Prenatal care is a comprehensive process in which any problems associated with pregnancy are identified and treated. Basic components of prenatal care are early and continuing risk assessment, health promotion, medical and psychosocial interventions, and follow-up. Within the community setting, several services are available to provide health care for pregnant women (Box 2.2).

Not all women are aware of community-based prenatal resources available to them. Perinatal and childbirth education classes are available for a nominal or subsidized fee in most health regions in Canada. Telephone consultation may be available in some jurisdictions such

---

BOX 2.2 **Maternal/Child Community Health Services**

- Public health prenatal clinics provide access to women and their partners depending on the province, health region, and resources available.
- Provincial and territorial community health clinics may be available offering a variety of services, which may include prenatal and postnatal care, well child programs, immunization services, nutritional counselling, perinatal monitoring, telecare services, and dental services.
- Private OB/GYN and family physician offices and clinics are available for women seeking care during their pregnancies. Physician availability will differ depending on the location and resources available in a geographic area.
- Some health regions offer home- and community-based prenatal and postnatal programs for women with limited economic resources (homeless, unemployed, and new immigrant populations). These programs include childbirth education classes, peer support, nutritional resources, and labour support.
- Midwifery services are available in many communities where midwives provide women's health services. In most provinces and territories these services are increasingly covered by provincial health care insurance.
- Childbirth education classes offer pregnant women and their partners a series of educational classes on childbirth and early postpartum preparation. Most classes have fees attached to them but these may be waived for low-income families.
- Local La Leche League groups provide mother-to-mother support for breastfeeding, nutrition, and infant care problem-solving strategies. All women who have an interest in breastfeeding are welcome to participate in the meetings, which are typically held in the home of a La Leche League member.

as Health Link in Alberta, British Columbia, and New Brunswick. Some health regions have written material for the perinatal period available in different languages. An example of such a publication is *From Here to Maternity* (Alberta Health Services, 2010), which is distributed by family physicians' and obstetricians' offices, community health offices, and acute care settings. Postpartum nurses in acute care settings can also be a very helpful link to resources for all parents.

Some technologically advanced care has been shown to improve maternal and child outcomes. For example, fetal monitoring and ultrasound technology traditionally have been used in acute care settings to monitor the progress of many high-risk pregnancies. However, with the increased cost of hospital stays, many services were moved to outpatient facilities and into the home. The intent was to reduce health care costs and to monitor women with complications of pregnancy in the home rather than in the hospital. Examples of services offered in the home setting might include:

- Infusion therapy to treat infections or combat dehydration
- Hypertension monitoring for women with gestational hypertension
- Uterine monitoring for women who are at high risk for preterm labour
- Fetal monitoring to evaluate fetal well-being in high-risk pregnancies
- Portable ultrasound to perform a biophysical profile to assess fetal well-being

As a result, antenatal home care has the potential to produce cost savings compared with admitting women into acute care settings for the duration of their pregnancies.

Labour and Birth Care

The experience of pregnancy and birth involves numerous choices: cloth or disposable diapers, breastfeeding or bottle feeding, doctor or midwife, and where to give birth—at a birthing centre, at home, or at a hospital. Deciding where to give birth depends on the woman's pregnancy risk status. For the pregnant woman who is at high risk as a result of medical or social factors, the hospital is considered the safest place for birth. Potential complications can be addressed because medical technology, skilled professionals, and neonatal services are readily available. For low-risk women, a freestanding birthing centre or a home birth is an option if the personnel and physical resources are available in their geographic location. For example, in Alberta, midwifery services are concentrated in Calgary and Edmonton, so women in rural areas have less access to birthing centres or midwifery care. In contrast, Quebec midwives do not have hospital privileges and are able to provide care only in the home or in birthing centres.

The woman's preferences and expectations about her desired birth experience play a major role in her decisions about birth place and care provider. Some women choose an all-natural birth with no medications and no medical intervention, whereas others feel more comfortable in a setting in which medications and trained staff are available if needed. The nurse's role includes presenting the facts to women and allowing them to choose in collaboration with their health care provider. While safety is paramount, nurses must also protect the woman's right to select birth options and should promote FCC in all maternity settings (see Evidence-Based Practice 2.1).

Birthing Centre

A birthing centre may provide an alternative for women who are uncomfortable with a home birth but who do not want to give birth in a hospital. There may or may not be a cost for families who wish to use a birthing centre. Birthing centres offer a more homelike setting and may have close proximity to a hospital in case of complications (Fig. 2.3). The health care providers in this setting promote a culture of normalcy. Birth is considered a normal physiologic process, and most centres have a non-interventional view of labour and birth. Midwives are often the sole care providers in freestanding birthing centres (such as those in Quebec), but this is dependent upon the organization of health care within the province where the centre is located. Birthing centres usually have fewer restrictions and allow for more freedom in making decisions about labour. American statistics indicate that the rates of cesarean birth and the overall costs associated with giving birth are much lower in birthing centres than in hospitals (Steppe, 2006). However, no Canadian statistics are available. In a birthing centre, the normal discharge time after birth is usually measured in hours (4 to 24 hours) rather than days.

Home Birth

For centuries, women have been giving birth to babies in their homes. Many feel more comfortable and relaxed when giving birth in their own environment. Women who want no medical interventions and a very family-centred birth may choose to have a home birth. Women who opt for home births are usually cared for by midwives. In most provinces, physicians are restricted from attending home births by their professional regulating bodies. Home births may be recommended for pregnant women who are considered to be at low risk for complications during labour and birth. Home birth is advantageous because it:

- Is the least expensive
- Allows the woman to experience labour and birth in the privacy, comfort, and familiarity of home while surrounded by loved ones

EVIDENCE-BASED PRACTICE 2.1
Is an Alternative Institutional Birth Setting Better for Women Than a Conventional Institutional Birth Setting?

● Study

Women have been giving birth to newborns in the home setting since the beginning of time. Births occurring in a facility or institution became the norm during the early 20th century. These institutions continue to be the primary setting for birth. However, with the growing emphasis on the client as a consumer of health care and the desire for family-centred care, greater numbers of facilities and institutions are attempting to incorporate some of the home birth components into their delivery of care. A study was done to compare the effects of care in alternative, more home-like institutional birth settings versus conventional institutional birth settings.

The researchers used standard methods for data collection and analysis to compile information from all randomized and quasi-randomized controlled trials involving a comparison of conventional and alternative institutional birth settings. Alternative birth settings included bedroom-like rooms or Snoezelen rooms, which offer controlled multisensory stimulation. Nine trials involving 10,684 women were included. The researchers were unable to include information related to freestanding birthing centres or Snoezelen rooms because they found no trials on this topic. The researchers reported the results using relative risk and 95% confidence intervals.

▲ Findings

The results showed that women who gave birth in home-like institutional birth settings were less likely to receive or require intrapartum analgesia or anaesthesia, less likely to have an epidural or an episiotomy, and more likely to experience a spontaneous vaginal birth. Other benefits identified included very positive views of intrapartum care and a greater likelihood for initiating breastfeeding with continuation for the next 6 to 8 weeks. There were no apparent effects on perinatal morbidity or mortality, adverse neonatal outcomes, or postpartum hemorrhage.

■ Nursing Implications

The study did identify several important benefits that nurses can integrate into their practice when counselling and teaching pregnant women about available birthing options. Nurses can provide input about incorporating a more "home-like" atmosphere when their facilities are constructing and designing birthing areas. In addition, nurses can advocate for the pregnant woman in labour to ensure that she has freedom to move about the birthing area, allowing her to feel more "at home."

Source: Hodnett, E. D., Downe. S., Walsh, D., & Weston, J. (2010). Alternative versus conventional institutional settings for birth. *Cochrane Database of Systematic Reviews*, 9. Art. No.: CD000012. doi: 10.1002/14651858.CD000012.pub3

- Permits the woman to maintain control over every aspect affecting her labour (e.g., positions, attire, numbers of support people)
- Minimizes interference and unnecessary interventions, allowing labour to progress normally
- Provides continuous one-on-one care by the midwife throughout the birth and early postpartum period

A home birth has some disadvantages, including the limited availability of pain medication as well as safety issues for the mother and baby if an emergency arises (e.g., placental abruption, uterine rupture, cord prolapse, or a distressed fetus). A backup plan for having a health care provider and nearby hospital on standby is usually required by midwifery regulating bodies in each province.

Postpartum and Newborn Care

Recent health care reforms such as postpartum early discharge have reduced hospital stays significantly for women after giving birth. As a result, community health nurses play a major role in extending care beyond the hospital setting. When new mothers are discharged from the hospital, they may feel uncertain about feeding and caring for their newborns. Most are still experiencing perineal discomfort and uterine cramping. They may still have pain from an episiotomy, perineal laceration, or cesarean section incision. They are fatigued and may be constipated. New parents need to be made aware of the resources in their communities such as home visits, telephone consultation by nurses, and postpartum community health clinics.

Postpartum Home Visits

Home visits offer services similar to those offered at a scheduled clinic visit, but they also give the nurse an opportunity to assess the family's adaptation and dynamics in the home environment. During the past decade, hospital stays have averaged 24 to 48 hours or less for vaginal births and 48 to 72 for cesarean births (Public Health Agency of Canada, 2008). These shortened stays have reduced the time available for educating mothers about caring for themselves and their newborns.

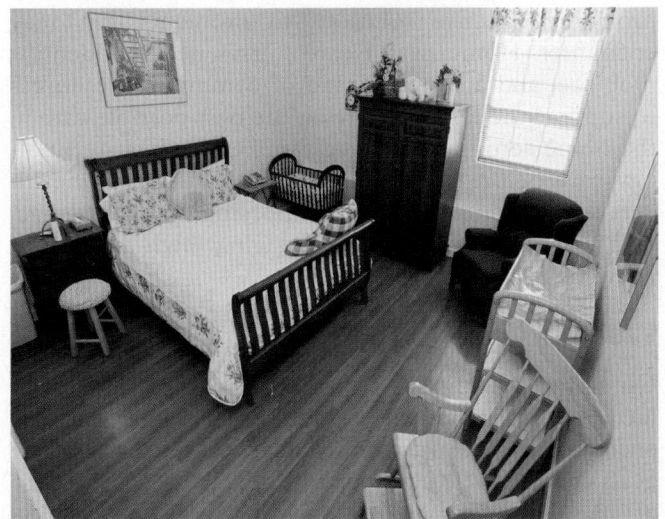

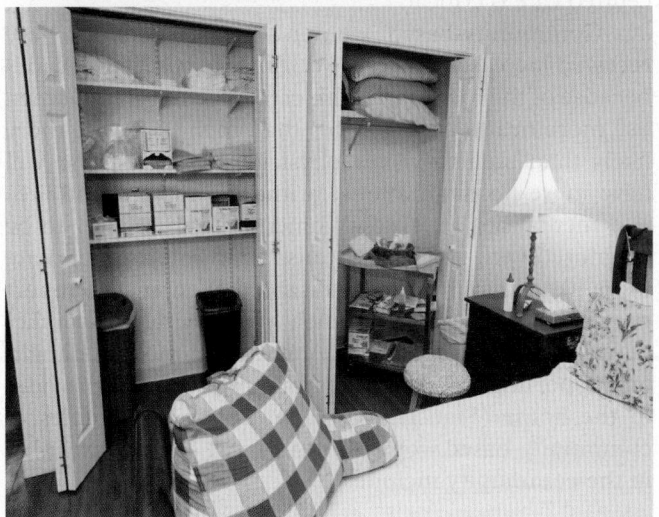

FIGURE 2.3 Birthing centres aim to provide a relaxing home-like environment and promote a culture of normality while offering a full range of health care services to the expectant family. (Photos by Gus Freedman.)

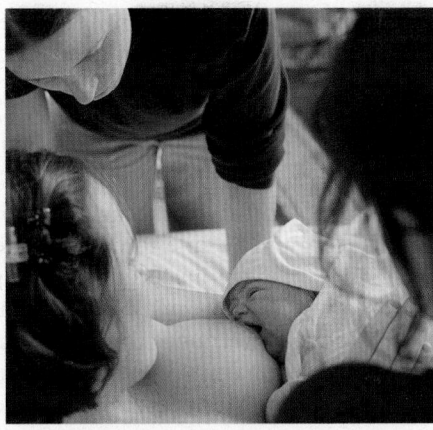

FIGURE 2.4 The nurse makes a postpartum home visit to assess the woman and her newborn. During the visit, the nurse assists the mother with breastfeeding.

Postpartum care in the home environment usually includes:

- Monitoring the physical and emotional well-being of the family members (Fig. 2.4)
- Identifying potential or developing complications for the mother and newborn
- Bridging the gap between discharge and primary care follow-up with the physician and/or other health care providers such as lactation consultants for mothers and their newborns (Public Health Agency of Canada, 2008)

Telephone Consultation

Some health regions may offer a telephone consultation service from family newborn nurses. However, the availability of this service depends on the individual units and facilities as well as the organization of health care within each province. A telephone consultation provides support for parents in addition to home visits and post-partum clinic visits. It may be available in specific regions for extended hours in the evenings and on weekends.

Postpartum Community Clinics

Postpartum community clinics offer another community-based site where the childbearing family can obtain services. These clinics may be in addition to postpartum home visiting services or instead of home-based services. Some health care jurisdictions deem such services to be a more appropriate use of health care resources as the nurse can see multiple postpartum families in a clinical setting. Postpartum community health nurses are willing to answer any questions parents may have about the mother's health or that of her newborn. Appointments usually include an examination of the mother and newborn, education about postpartum and infant care, and nutrition for mother and infant.

High-Risk Newborn Home Care

With the reduced lengths of stay in hospital, high-risk newborns are also being cared for in community settings. High-technology care once was provided only in the hospital. However, the increasing cost of complex care and the influences of managed care have led to the provision of technologically advanced care at home. Families have become "health care systems" by providing physical, emotional, social, and developmental home care for their technology-dependent infants. Suitable candidates for home care may include preterm infants who continue to need oxygen, low-birth-weight infants needing nutritional or hypercaloric formulas or adjunct feeding methods (e.g., tube feedings), or infants with a complex chronic illness. A wide range of equipment may be used, including mechanical ventilation, electronic apnea monitors, home oxygen equipment, intravenous infusions, respiratory nebulizers, phototherapy, and suction equipment. The availability of specialized equipment, in-home health care providers, and funding varies across the provinces and territories.

Family members must work together to provide 24-hour care. They must be able to troubleshoot equipment problems and manage inventories of supplies and equipment. In addition, they must be able to assess the infant for problems; determine the problem; decide when to call the nurse, pharmacist, or physical therapist; and interpret and administer prescriptions. Technology in the home requires nurses to focus on the family "home care system" to provide total care to the infant.

Nurses can play a key role in assisting families in caring for their infants at home by teaching and increasing their confidence. This adaptation begins before discharge from the hospital. Family members are active participants in the transition-to-home plan. Recognition of parental needs and addressing each area in the discharge plan will ease the transition home.

Assessment of the family's preparedness and available resources is essential. The following questions can provide valuable information about this area:

• What do you need to feel well prepared to take care of your infant's physical, emotional, and equipment needs?
• Do you know what resources are available to you in your community/province?
• What in-home support services do you expect to need or hope to access?
• How will you access support for yourself and family to manage the stress of home care?

These simple questions convey the nurse's concern for the infant and family while obtaining a thorough assessment of the family's learning needs.

Once family preparedness has been assessed, the nurse can intervene as necessary. For example, if the caretakers do not think they are prepared to maintain machinery, technology, medication, or developmental therapy, the nurse can provide instructions and hands-on experience within a supportive environment until the family's confidence increases. The nurse can also assist the family to anticipate the common problems that might occur (e.g., advising them to avoid running out of supplies, to have enough medication or special formula mixture to last throughout the weekend, and to keep backup batteries for powering machines or portable oxygen). The outcome of the preparedness assessment and intervention is that the safety of the infant is established and maintained.

Nursing for families who are using complex home care equipment requires caring for the infant and family members' physical and emotional well-being as well as providing effective solutions to problems they may encounter. Home health care nurses need to identify, mobilize, and adapt a myriad of community resources to support the family in giving the best possible care in the home setting. Preparing families for high-technology care before hospital discharge, with home health care nurses continuing and reinforcing that knowledge, will ease the burden of managing high-technology equipment in the home.

Women's Health Care

On average, a woman's reproductive years span half her lifetime. This is not a static period but rather one that encompasses several significant stages. As her reproductive goals change, so do a woman's health care needs. Because of these changing needs, comprehensive community-centred care is critical.

Community-based women's health services have received increased emphasis during the past few decades because of the focus on health care expenditures. Women use more health care services than men. They are more likely than men to visit a physician or dentist and will have more hospitalizations, primarily due to childbirth and mental health issues. Women are more likely to be diagnosed with a sexually transmitted infection and are more likely than men to be disabled. Women also report poorer mental health than men, possibly due to conflict between and within their roles of worker, mother, daughter supporting elderly parents, and primary care provider in the home (Statistics Canada, 2006b). Examples of community-based women's health care services available in the community include:

• Screening centres that offer mammograms, Pap smears, bone density assessments, genetic counselling, ultrasound, breast examinations, laboratory studies (complete blood count, cholesterol testing, thyroid testing, glucose testing for diabetes, follicle-stimulating hormone [FSH] levels), and electrocardiograms. Access to these screening centres is only available after referral from a family physician or midwife.
• Educational centres that provide women's health lectures, instruction on breast self-examinations and Pap smears, and computers for research
• Counselling centres that offer various support groups: genetics, psychotherapy, substance abuse, sexual assault, and domestic violence
• Wellness centres that offer stress reduction techniques, massage therapy, guided imagery, hypnosis, smoking cessation, weight reduction, tai chi, yoga, and women's fitness/exercise classes
• Alternative/wholeness healing centres that provide acupuncture, aromatherapy, biofeedback, therapeutic touch, facials, reflexology, and herbal remedies
• Retail centres that offer specialty equipment, such as breast prostheses, for rental and purchase

Women have multiple choices regarding services, settings, and health care providers. In the past, most women received health care services from physicians such as obstetricians, gynaecologists, and family physicians, but today nurse practitioners are becoming more prevalent in providing well-woman care.

Nurses who work in community health settings need to be familiar with the many health issues commonly encountered by women within their communities. All nurses who work with women of any age in community-based settings, including the workplace, schools, practitioner offices, and clinics, should possess a thorough understanding of the scope of women's health care and should be prepared to intervene appropriately to prevent problems and to promote health.

Child Health Care

The majority of care for a child occurs in community settings that may be broad in focus or highly specialized. One setting may provide well-child care, for example, while a second setting may be limited to diagnostic evaluation, emergency care, or surgical intervention. Other settings may focus on caring for children with a specific condition or diagnosis, such as diabetes or cancer.

Outpatient and Ambulatory Care

Outpatient and ambulatory care is health care provided to individuals who do not require care in an acute setting. Due to advances in medical technology, more medical procedures, such as diagnostic tests and treatments and surgeries, can be performed in outpatient clinics, thereby minimizing the need for the child to be hospitalized overnight. Outpatient and ambulatory care offer convenient and cost-effective access to health care for children and their families, often within their own community. These settings allow for increased independence and permit children to return to their normal routines as quickly as possible. Using a multidisciplinary approach, outpatient programs offer diagnostic, assessment, treatment, and management services for children.

Clinics and Urgent Care Centres

Physician offices, clinics, and urgent care centres are used by children and their families for wellness care, episodic illness care, acute care, and care of chronic conditions. For wellness care and illness or injury, children are often seen by their primary care physician in an office or clinic. For more acute situations or after-hours concerns that cannot wait until clinic operating hours, a child may be seen in an urgent care centre or may be referred to the emergency department. The Canadian Paediatric Society does not encourage the use of urgent care centres or the emergency department for routine care since it is difficult in these settings to provide coordinated, comprehensive FCC that is consistent with a "medical home"

concept (refer to Chapter 30 for more information on medical homes).

The nurse's role in these clinic and urgent care settings includes preparing clients, collecting pertinent health information, performing assessments, assisting the physician with diagnostic testing and procedures, administering injections and medications, changing dressings, assisting with minor surgery, helping to maintain records, and educating the child and family about follow-up care, including when to call the physician or return for follow-up care.

Outpatient Units

Outpatient units are used to keep hospital stays short and therefore decrease the cost of hospitalization. Outpatient units are often part of the hospital. The child and family arrive in the morning; the child has the procedure, test, or surgery and then goes home later in the day. This organization of care is advantageous because there is minimal separation of the child from the family, minimal disruption of the family pattern, lower risk for infection, and decreased cost. However, most outpatient units do not have the equipment or other resources to provide for overnight stays. Thus, if the child develops a complication, he or she will need to be transferred to an acute care, in-patient unit.

Many centres offer pre-surgery health assessment and teaching sessions that allow the parent(s) and child opportunities to voice questions and concerns before the procedure or surgery. On the day of the procedure or surgery, parents usually are allowed to remain with their child until the procedure or surgery begins. Parents may also be allowed to be with their child in the post-anaesthesia care unit as soon as possible. Minimizing separation between the parents and the child provides reassurance, promotes comfort, and meets the physical and emotional needs of the child and family.

Nurses working in the outpatient unit setting are involved with admission and assessment, preoperative teaching and preparation, client assessment and support, postoperative monitoring, case management, discharge planning, and teaching. Before the procedure or surgery, the nurse commonly reviews the routine to be followed and any special instructions, such as nothing by mouth (NPO) orders, and familiarizes the child and family with the setting.

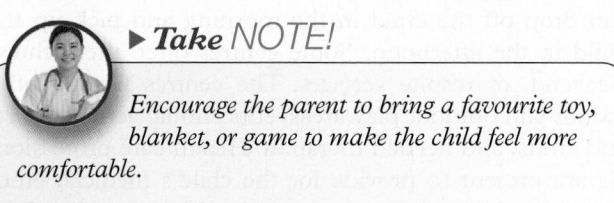

▶ **Take** NOTE!

Encourage the parent to bring a favourite toy, blanket, or game to make the child feel more comfortable.

The nurse performs any surgical preparation and discusses intraoperative procedures as necessary. The nurse also provides provide postprocedural or postoperative care and assessment of the child. Once the child is stable and meets the discharge criteria of the facility, the nurse reviews instructions, including pain management, care of the incision (if appropriate), diet, and activity, including the time frame for returning to school, necessary follow-up, and when to call the physician.

Services for Medically Fragile Children

The number of **medically fragile children**, children who have complex medical needs that require skilled nursing interventions, is growing. In 2006, there were 202,350 children living in Canada who had a physical, mental, or health-related disability (Statistics Canada, 2006a). Historically, these children lived in hospital settings their entire lives. Due to concerns about the high cost of long-term hospitalization and the quality of life for these children, alternative care settings in the community have been developed, facilitated by the increased sophistication of medical and nursing care (Holditch-Davis, Miles, Burchinal, & Goldman, 2011; Mentro, 2003).

The services available for children with complex medical needs vary across Canada and according to the child's needs. Day care, preschool, respite, and hospice services in community settings may be available for families in large urban centres. In the *2006 Participation and Activity Limitation Survey: Disability in Canada* (Statistics Canada, 2006a), 21% of parents stated that child care services or programs had refused to provide care for their child due to the severity of the child's limitations.

With the exception of Hope's Home in Regina, Saskatchewan, examples of day care centres designed to meet the needs of medically fragile children are more often found in the United States. Most of these centres accept children who have complicated medical needs or are technology dependent. Examples include children with multiple congenital anomalies, children who are ventilator dependent, and children with respiratory conditions, cardiac conditions, or cancer. Some centres will accept children with less complicated needs, such as asthma or the need for cardiorespiratory monitoring. In some centres for medically fragile children, children without health care needs are also enrolled in order to promote peer relationships and acceptance.

Day care centres for medically fragile children are similar to typical day care centres. Parents or caregivers can drop off the child in the morning and pick up the child in the afternoon. Some centres offer after-school, weekend, or respite services. The centres usually offer indoor and outdoor play areas, educational activities, arts and crafts, and needed therapies. Health care professionals are present to provide for the child's medical, emotional, and developmental needs. Nurses trained in pediatric and neonatal care, physical therapists, occupational therapists, speech therapists, child life specialists, and social workers work in the day care centres; some centres also have respiratory therapists on site. Children can receive all of their prescribed therapies while at the centre.

Nurses provide direct care such as medication administration and dressing changes, assess and evaluate the child's overall condition, identify potential medical emergencies, determine the need for changes in care or treatment and monitoring, and provide the necessary treatments or interventions to maintain life and health. Most centres are located in the community to help ease transportation issues. Some centres provide transportation to and from home or school. Several jurisdictions in Canada are currently exploring implementation of day care programs for medically fragile children.

Telehealth

Telehealth services use telecommunications technology to improve access to health services and reduce the time, risk, and money spent in travel. Nurses who work in telehealth services may use information and communications technologies such as telephones, audio and video conferencing, smartphones, facsimile machines, and the Internet (CNA, 2007). Telehealth services may be located in many different settings, such as call centres, ambulatory care clinics, physicians' offices, hospital units, and public health units (CNA, 2007). Telehealth is particularly important for rural and remote communities where access to health care providers and travel challenges impede access to universal health care.

Telephone Advice Lines

Telephone advice, a form of telehealth, is available 24 hours a day, 7 days a week in many provinces. Known as "Health Link" in some jurisdictions, families and individuals can call toll free and speak confidentially with an RN regarding community health resources, symptoms, or other concerns. Advice may include referrals and recommendations to visit a physician's office or the local emergency department.

When parents feel comfortable with the providers in their child's medical home office, they often call for advice so they might treat their child's illness at home. This practice saves health care dollars by keeping children with mild illnesses at home rather than seeking care in an emergency department or urgent care centre. If the call is received during office hours and the child's condition warrants evaluation, then the child may be seen in a family physician's office, an outpatient clinic, or the pediatric primary care office.

While telephone triage can be a money-saving and even life-saving intervention, it must be used with caution. Nurses are responsible for ensuring that the services provided are safe, appropriate, and ethical, with careful assessment, planning, implementation, and evaluation of care (CNA, 2007).

Nurses working in telephone advice settings must be able to triage the calls. That is, they determine whether the child needs to be evaluated by a professional and if that evaluation should be made urgently. The nurse must carefully question the parent or caregiver about the specifics of the child's condition to determine whether it fits into a low-risk or high-risk category. When counselling a parent over the phone, the following information is often obtained:

- Signs and symptoms, including their onset and progression and characteristics such as location, severity, and aggravating or relieving factors
- History of the child's present illness, including onset and duration, progression of symptoms, any care given at home, and whether this condition is related to a recent diagnostic procedure, surgery, or hospitalization
- The child's health history, including chronic illnesses and routine medications or alternative treatments
- The child's current status in relation to eating, drinking, elimination, and energy and activity level
- Degree and effectiveness of coping by the child and family to this health alteration (adapted from Simonsen-Anderson, 2002)

After obtaining a thorough assessment, the nurse must use critical thinking skills, experience, and established telephone triage protocols to determine the severity and risk of the child's situation. If the child's situation is determined to be low risk, then home care instruction and advice are appropriate. Children at moderate risk should be seen by their primary care physician or nurse practitioner either that day or within 24 hours. The family is given advice on appropriate care while awaiting the office visit. High-risk children should be evaluated immediately, either in the physician's office or emergency department. Certain high-risk situations warrant activation of the emergency medical system and immediate paramedic evaluation.

> ▶ *Take* NOTE!
>
> *Parents or caregivers often can pick up on subtle problems or cues. Although they may not be able to describe the signs and symptoms accurately, they do know that their child is not acting right. Nurses must listen carefully and act on the parent's or caregiver's concerns.*

Schools

School nursing is a specialized practice of community health nursing that focuses on improving student health and wellness to enhance the achievement and success of students. School nurses are employed by public health departments across Canada and are regulated by the public health system. School nurses are not usually employed by the school system in Canada as they may

be in other parts of the world. School nurses provide this specialty care under the CHNC standards of practice (CHNC, 2008), the public health nursing discipline-specific competencies (CHNC, 2009), and the roles and activities described by the Canadian Public Health Association (CPHA, 2010). School nurses work in partnership with the school community, including students, parents, school personnel, and community agencies, to remove or minimize health barriers to learning, thereby providing students with the best opportunity for academic success. Nurses collaboratively address concerns about school health through direct consultation, school case conferences, referrals to community resources, case management, and community development. School nurses develop, coordinate, and implement health promotion programs and link health service programs such as wellness fairs, immunization services, and injury prevention programs within the school and community. School nurses carry out a variety of roles in providing health care to children (Fig. 2.5, Box 2.3).

School nurses consider the larger socioenvironmental issues of the students and their families within the school population and address the determinants of health that influence long-term health outcomes. These include issues with poverty, diverse cultural backgrounds, lack of social supports, the direct physical environment influencing the school community, and other challenges. Chronic conditions such as obesity, diabetes, asthma, depression, and attention deficit–hyperactivity disorders are more common than in the past. Schools are seeing an increased number of families struggling with social issues such as family violence, addictions, and single parenting with few supports. All of these factors have contributed to an increase in the number of children with diverse and sometimes complex health needs in the school system, changing the responsibilities and expectations of the school nurse. Today's school nurses are

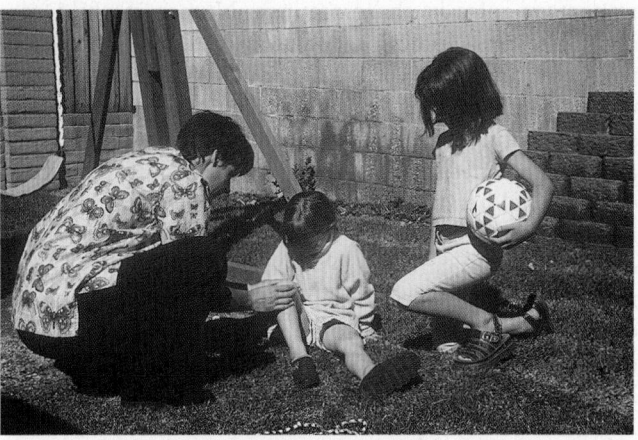

FIGURE 2.5 The school nurse provides nursing assessment as well as health education to students in the school setting.

BOX 2.3 Examples of Activities of the School Nurse

- Assessing, screening, support, care, referrals, and follow-up for identified health issues
- Providing childhood immunizations and communicable disease control
- Providing health promotion and primary and secondary prevention
- Establishing partnerships with community agencies and facilitating community development
- Providing emergency first aid
- Training and educating staff on child health issues
- Educating about health promotion and disease prevention (e.g., immunizations, bike and car safety, and high-risk behaviours such as smoking, drinking, drug use, and sexual activity)
- Advocating for access to resources for individuals, families, and communities within the school community
- Networking with community agencies and making necessary referrals
- Acting as a resource and liaison for health issues and education to students, parents, and school personnel
- Providing case management, consultation, and early referral for children and families who require services

Source: Alberta Health Services. (2003). *Services provided to school communities by public health nurses.* Calgary, AB: Author.

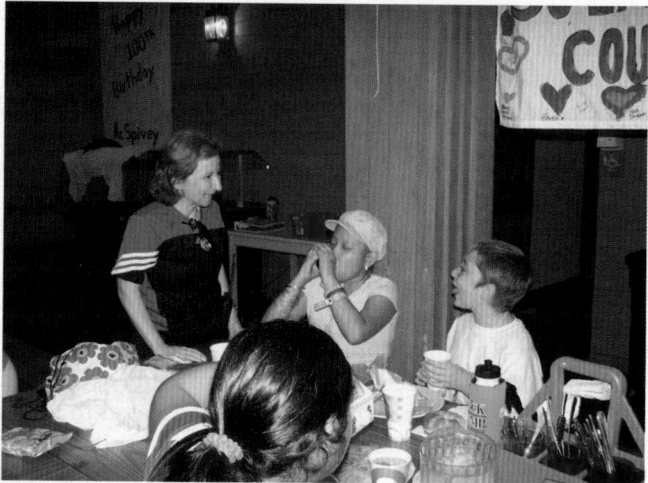

FIGURE 2.6 The camp nurse may care for typical healthy children or may work at a camp for children with special needs or chronic illness.

▶ *Take* NOTE!

Nurses have a unique opportunity to give back to their community by volunteering their services in various settings, such as shelters and clinics in medically underserved areas.

challenged to meet the growing needs of the changing school population while providing comprehensive school health programs.

Child Care Centres, Camps, Public Health Clinics, and Shelters

Other settings in the community, such as child care centres, camps, public health clinics, and shelters, also focus on promoting health, preventing disease and injury, and ensuring a safe environment. Nurses play important roles in these settings. Nurses in child care centres address infection control issues, assess the environment for safety concerns, and provide education and training to staff members. Camp nurses ensure a safe environment for all campers and provide first aid and acute illness care as needed. Camps for children with special health care needs employ specially trained nurses (Fig. 2.6). These camps cater to children with complex health care needs, such as diabetes, head injuries, and physical disabilities, and allow the children the opportunity to experience camp while providing a safe environment and necessary medical care while there. Nurses working in public health clinics and shelters focus on health promotion and disease prevention activities and connecting clients to needed community resources.

Pediatric Health Home Care

Pediatric home health care nurses work under the umbrella of community health nurses to provide short- or long-term services for children and their families at home. Pediatric home health care is also used for medically needy and technology-dependent children, such as children requiring mechanical ventilation. Children with acute illnesses, such as a child with osteomyelitis requiring intravenous antibiotics, or chronic health issues, such as a child with bronchopulmonary dysplasia, who would have traditionally required inpatient care, can often benefit from home care.

Pediatric home health care can be advantageous for the child and family, minimizing the separation of the child from the family and allowing the child to remain in an environment that is familiar and comfortable. However, pediatric home health care does have disadvantages. The presence of health care professionals in the home can be an intrusion on family privacy. Also, caring for children with complex medical needs can be overwhelming for some families. Financial issues may become a burden as well, since families have higher out-of-pocket costs due to lack of reimbursement from a third party for home care. Having one parent or caregiver at home full-time and not earning an income also contributes to increased financial strain, not to mention the social isolation of that person. All of these situations can lead to increased stress on family members. Nurses need to be aware of these potential disadvantages, work in partnership with the family, and provide support and resources as necessary.

Responsibilities of the Pediatric Home Health Care Nurse

As the provider of care, the home health care nurse uses the nursing process. Assessment in the home is similar to that in the acute care setting, but it also involves obtaining assessment data about the family and family functioning. The nurse needs to assess growth and development of the child and thoroughly assess the home environment (refer to Chapter 33 for additional information). The nurse assesses for a safe and nurturing environment for the child by considering the following:

- Availability of resources, such as necessary equipment (e.g., hospital bed, oxygen)
- Suitable physical and emotional surroundings (can the family members deal with the stress of the situation?)
- Ability to contact emergency services
- Power backup if needed
- Ease of evacuation of the child in case of a fire

The nurse also needs to ensure that the home provides electricity, sanitary conditions, heat, possibly air conditioning, and telephone access. If there is no phone in the home, the family needs to plan how they will access a phone in case of emergency. This may include use of a neighbour's phone or relying on a pay phone near the home. The nurse should identify areas of priority and provide appropriate referrals to resources, keeping in mind that some families in rural and remote communities in Canada may not have equal access to services offered in larger urban centres.

During the assessment phase, the nurse identifies the primary caregiver, who must be included in the plan of care. This person may be the mother, father, grandparent, or older sibling. The primary caregiver should be considered the expert about the child and family, providing valuable insights into direct care and the strategies that will be most effective with this child. The primary caregiver can also provide key information about the physical layout of the home, the financial ability of the family, and the family's functioning.

The environment differs greatly between the acute setting and the home setting. In the acute setting the nurse is in control of the environment, while in the home setting the nurse is a guest in the home. It is important for the nurse to establish a trusting relationship with both the child and family (Fig. 2.7), as a trusting therapeutic relationship will enhance all aspects of care.

The pediatric home health care nurse assesses the family's teaching and learning needs. In many situations, some types of care (e.g., frequent dressing changes) must be learned immediately so that the child can be cared for at home. This teaching should begin prior to hospital discharge. However, teaching is ongoing, with teaching

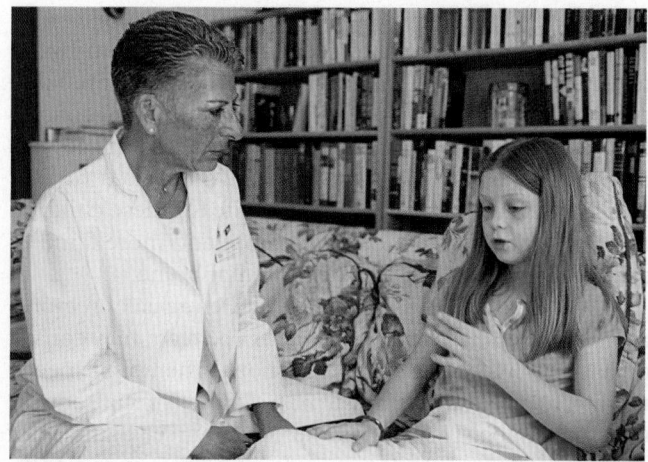

FIGURE 2.7 Listening to the child helps to develop a trusting relationship between the home care nurse and the child and her family.

and learning needs shifting as the child grows and his or her condition changes. The nurse empowers the child and family through education.

After the assessment is complete, the nurse develops and implements a plan of care. This will include the frequency and duration of the home visits. The nurse may provide direct care to the child or may plan and supervise the care given by others, such as unlicensed personnel and family caregivers.

Nursing care in the home requires excellent assessment and critical thinking skills. The nurse has a great deal of independence since there are no other nurses, supervisors, or physicians available in the home as they are in other health care settings. Also, due to the potential complexity of care being provided, the nurse needs to adjust procedures to fit the setting. For example, feeding schedules may be adjusted to fit a child's school schedule, or equipment may be adjusted to allow a child to receive feedings continuously while at school (Fig. 2.8).

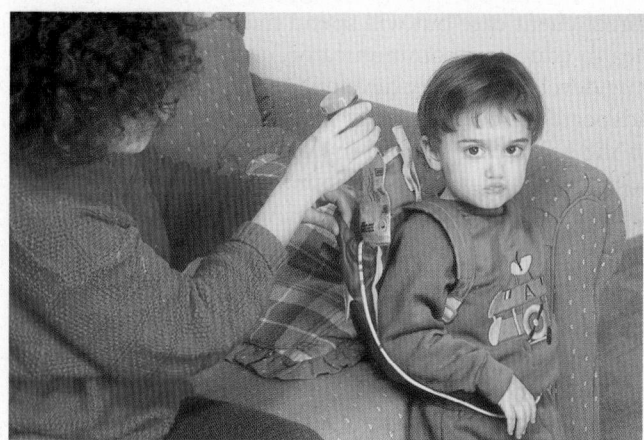

FIGURE 2.8 The home health care nurse may have to adjust procedures and equipment to fit the home setting. Placing a feeding pump in a backpack allows this child to receive feedings continuously while at school.

Home Care of the Technology-Dependent Child

Advances in medicine and technology have contributed to an emerging population of children with chronic diseases and disabilities. Some of these children are considered technology-dependent, meaning they need medical or technical assistance to remain alive or avoid further disability. To improve the quality of life for these children and to reduce health care costs, more and more families are providing care for these children at home.

Meeting the needs of these children usually requires an interdisciplinary team approach. The team may consist of a specialty physician, occupational therapist, speech therapist, physical therapist, nutritionist, special educators, psychologist, social worker, and nurse. Families of children with complex care needs may experience significant emotional, physical, psychological, and financial strain and stigma (Carneval, Alexander, Davis, Rennick, & Troini, 2006; MacDonald & Gibson, 2010). Nurses need to assess the family for these stressors and assist them in finding appropriate resources for assistance.

Due to the intensive, around-the-clock care that many of these children require, physical and emotional exhaustion can occur. Therefore, **respite care**, the provision of support services to temporarily relieve the caregiver from the responsibility of providing care, is crucial. Nurses must assess the need for respite care and assist families in finding appropriate resources. (Refer to Chapter 33 for additional information about respite care.)

Roles and Functions of the Community Health Nurse

Many nurses find the shift from acute care to community settings a challenge. Nurses working in community-based settings share many of the same roles and responsibilities as their colleagues in acute care settings, but there are some differences. For example, in the community or home care setting, the nurse will provide direct client care but will spend more time in the role of health educator, communicator, case manager, community developer, policy developer and implementer, social advocate, resource broker, and manager than the nurse in the acute care setting. In home health care, the nurse will spend a significant amount of time in the supervision or management role (CPHA, 2010).

Communicator

Effective therapeutic communication with men, women, children, and families is critical to the provision of quality nursing care. Client- and family-centred approaches to communication contribute to collaborative interactions and increased satisfaction (McGrath & Hardy, 2008).

Communicating with children can be more difficult than communicating with adults. However, children are able to inform nurses of their experiences reliably and accurately, and nurses need to be able to discern this information when communicating with a child. While communicating with children can be challenging, it is also rewarding, especially if there is good rapport between nurse and child. Treating children as individuals, respecting their views about health, and involving them in their care are essential strategies (Edwards, 2010).

Parents and adults more often require neutral communication—that is, verbal communication that is related to assessing and solving problems. On the other hand, children usually desire affective communication (establishment of rapport and trust, giving comfort). Therefore, nurses need to understand the thought processes from the child's perspective and express honesty, respect, and acceptance of feelings (Boggs, 2011).

Verbal and Nonverbal Communication

Nurses use verbal communication continuously throughout the day when interacting with their clients. Good verbal communication skills are necessary for effective nursing assessment and teaching. Nonverbal communication includes attending to one's own body language as well as others' body language, and active listening. When clients and families feel they are being heard, trust and rapport are established.

*R*ecall Anisha, who recently was discharged from the hospital with her newborn son. How did the nurse communicate with Anisha? Did the nurse's actions during the visit promote the development of trust between Anisha and the nurse? What might have been done differently to foster trust?

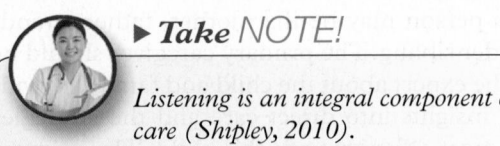

▶ *Take* NOTE!

Listening is an integral component of nursing care (Shipley, 2010).

Active listening is critical to the communication process. Listening may uncover fears or concerns that the nurse may not have discovered through questioning. Critical information may be missed when active listening is not used. The client or family may sense that the nurse is not listening and thus may be reluctant to share further information. During the interaction, determine whether the client's verbal communication is congruent with his or her nonverbal communication.

Communication with Children

To communicate effectively with children, it is necessary to use a variety of age-appropriate methods. Depending on the context and their needs, children prefer to move between the "passive bystander" and "active participant" positions within the communication process (Lambert, Glacken, & McCarron, 2010). If the child is shy, talking to the parents first will to allow the child time to become somewhat comfortable. It is important to engage with each child to determine his or her comfort level and position in the communication process (Lambert et al., 2010). The nurse should use specific, clear phrases in an unhurried, quiet yet confident manner and should place him- or herself at the child's eye level. Instead of direct questioning, the nurse can use dolls, puppets, or stuffed animals to question younger children (Fig. 2.9). Using language that children use themselves and retaining simplicity appropriate to the age of the child will improve communication (Chilman-Blair, 2010).

Older children need privacy. The nurse should provide the child or adolescent with honest answers at a developmentally appropriate level. Allowing children to express their thoughts and feelings and offering choices only when they truly exist facilitates effective communication (Mandleco, 2005). Box 2.4 highlights some guidelines for effective communication with children.

Children will be empowered when they have directly communicated with the nurse. Children may also desire advice about their health care and reassurance about their health status. To be effective when communicating with children of different developmental stages, the nurse must become familiar with how children of different ages communicate and then use age-appropriate techniques. Table 2.4 provides some suggestions for developmentally appropriate communication techniques.

Communication with Families

When communicating with families, the nurse must always be honest. Families want to be valued and should be equal partners in the health care team. This is effective

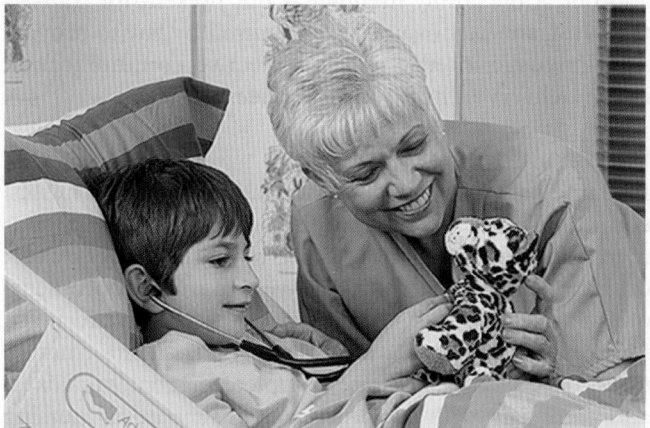

FIGURE 2.9 Sitting at the child's level and allowing the child time for self-expression provide for improved therapeutic communication.

BOX 2.4 Guidelines for Effective Communication with Children

- Introduce yourself and explain your role.
- Position yourself at the child's level.
- Allow the child to remain near the parent if needed, so the child can remain comfortable and relaxed.
- Smile and make eye contact with the child if culturally appropriate.
- Direct your questions and explanations to the child.
- Listen attentively and pause to allow time for the child to formulate his or her thoughts.
- Use the child's or family's terms for body parts and medical care when possible.
- Speak in a calm, quiet, confident, and unhurried voice.
- Use positive rather than negative statements and directions.
- Encourage the child to express his or her feelings and ask questions.
- Observe for nonverbal cues.
- Ask for permission if you need to approach the child to avoid appearing threatening.

---

use of the principles of FCC. The following strategies are effective when working with families:

- Allow family members to verbalize concerns and questions.
- Thoroughly explain the use of equipment and the correct sequence of procedures.
- Help family members understand the long-term as well as short-term effects of the health treatment.
- Teach them what the client will feel like and how he or she will look during a procedure or treatment.
- Remember to ask family members how they are doing and to provide positive reinforcement as well as reassurance (Mandleco, 2005).

When the client is a child, encourage parents to perform as much of the child's care as is reasonable, teaching them how to perform treatments as permitted. Inquire about the parents' perception of the child's progress. Allowing the parents to be involved in the care of their child gives them a sense of control and lets them know that they are valued by the health care team.

Working with an Interpreter

In response to the increasing diversity of the Canadian population, health care systems need to be linguistically competent (Alberta Health Services, 2008). Attempting to communicate with a family who does not speak English can be a difficult, ineffective, and potentially unsafe process. Effective language services can enhance access and

TABLE 2.4 **DEVELOPMENTALLY APPROPRIATE COMMUNICATION TECHNIQUES FOR CHILDREN**

Age	Techniques
Infants	• Respond to crying in a timely fashion. • Allow the infant time to warm up to you. • Use play and playful persuasion. • Use a soothing and calming tone when speaking to the infant. • Talk to the baby directly.
Toddlers	• Approach toddlers carefully, as they often are fearful and quite resistant. • Use the toddler's particular words for objects or actions so that he or she is better able to understand. • Use storytelling, dolls, and books. • Prepare toddlers for procedures just before they are about to occur.
Preschoolers	• Use play, puppetry, or storytelling for a "third-party" approach. • Speak honestly. • Use simple, concrete terms. • Allow the child to have choices as appropriate. • Prepare preschoolers about 1 hour prior to a procedure.
School-age children	• Use diagrams, illustrations, books, and videos. • Allow the child to express feelings honestly. • Use third-party stories to elicit desired information. • Allow the child to ask questions related to care and treatment, and allow adequate time for all of the questions to be answered. • Prepare the child a few days in advance for a procedure.
Adolescents	• Always respect the teenager's need for privacy. • Ensure confidentiality. • Use appropriate medical terminology, defining words as necessary. • Use creativity. • Prepare the teen up to 1 week before a procedure.

the quality of health care for families. Interpreters are an invaluable aid and an essential component of client and family education. Interpreters can be professionals who are certified or accredited, or a family member or a bilingual staff member may be considered an ad hoc interpreter. It should be noted, however, that the medical language and/or the client's symptoms and experiences may not be interpreted accurately when a non-professional interpreter is used (Vollman et al., 2012). For this reason, certified interpreters are preferred in several jurisdictions.

Standards for assessing the qualifications of an interpreter and protocols for requesting and acquiring interpretive services vary across health regions and provinces. Formalized and centrally administered interpretive services are becoming more common. Working with an interpreter, whether in person or over the phone, requires coordination of efforts so that both the family and the interpreter understand the information to be communicated. Working as a team, the nurse questions or informs and the interpreter conveys the information completely and accurately. Box 2.5 presents tips for working with an interpreter to maximize teaching efforts.

Telephone and video interpretation maybe used as a substitute for in-person interpretation. Some health care facilities subscribe to language lines that offer telephone access to interpretation of several different languages. Numerous other interpreters, translators, and language resources are available online.

*R*ecall Anisha, the woman with the newborn who is receiving home care. On the second visit to Anisha's home, the nurse brought a Punjabi-speaking interpreter who explained the reason for the "back to sleep" position and demonstrated to Anisha several other useful positions for feeding and holding. Anisha was smiling when the nurse left and asking when she would be back. What made the difference in their relationship the second visit? What interventions demonstrate culturally competent care?

Communicating With Deaf or Hearing-Impaired Clients and Families

For the hearing-impaired, determine the method of communication used: lip reading, American Sign Language (ASL), another method, or some combination. If the nurse is not proficient in ASL and the client or family uses it, then an ASL interpreter must be available if another adult family member is not present for translation. In Canada, hospitals are required by law to provide sign language interpreters for effective communication in the delivery of health care services.

Documentation of Care

Documentation of care is an essential component of nurses' communication with the multidisciplinary team. Documentation may be done in long hand, in a paper chart or, increasingly, electronically, using narrative, problem-orientation record, or "charting by exception" formats, for example. No matter what the format, the information needs to be factual, accurate, complete, current, organized, and compliant with the provincial and territorial nursing standards (Maxwell & Barry, 2010). Electronic management of records may provide some additional challenges as at each point of electronic transmission, client data must

BOX 2.5   Tips for Working with Interpreters

- **Help the interpreter prepare and understand what needs to be done ahead of time.** A few minutes of preparation may save a lot of time and help communication flow more smoothly in the long run.
- **Remember, the interpreter is the "communication bridge" and not the "content expert."** The nurse's presence at teaching sessions is vital.
- **Be patient. The interpreter's timing may not match that of others involved.** It often takes longer to say in some languages what has already been said in English; therefore, plan for more time than you normally would.
- **Speak slowly and clearly.** Avoid jargon. Use short sentences and be concise. Avoid interrupting the interpreter.
- **Pause every few sentences so the interpreter can translate your information.** After 30 seconds of speaking, stop and let the interpreter express the information. Talk directly to the family, not the interpreter.
- **Give the family and the interpreter a break.** Sessions lasting longer than 20 or 30 minutes are too much for anyone's attention span and concentration.
- **Express the information in two or three different ways if needed.** There may be cultural barriers as well as language and dialect differences that interfere with understanding. Interpreters may often know the correct communication protocols for the family.
- **Use an interpreter to help ensure the family can read and understand translated written materials.** The interpreter can also help answer questions and evaluate learning.
- **Avoid side conversations during sessions.** These can be uncomfortable for the family and jeopardize client–provider relationships and trust.
- **Remember, just because someone speaks another language doesn't mean that he or she will make a good interpreter.** An interpreter who has no medical background may not understand or interpret correctly, no matter how good his or her language skills are.
- **Do not use children as interpreters.** Doing so can affect family relationships, proper understanding, and compliance with health care issues.
- **Remember that interpreters may be hired for a specific period of time** and this may create conflicts if teaching sessions or medical appointments are late.

Adapted from: Weech, W. A. (1999). *Tips for using interpreters.* Foreign Service Institute of the U.S. Department of State.

remain secure and Protection of Privacy and Information Guidelines must be followed.

Direct Care Provider

The community health nurse typically performs less direct physical care than the nurse in the acute care setting. Many times the nurse may observe the client or caregiver performing physical care tasks. Excellent assessment skills are especially important in the community setting. The community health nurse often is functioning in a more autonomous role, and after data collection, he or she will often decide whether to initiate, continue, alter, or end physical nursing care. Assessment extends beyond physical assessment of the client to include the environment and the community.

Management of the Perinatal Client

The nurse provides direct care to the perinatal client, beginning with the woman and/or her partner's first visit to the health care provider and extending through the pregnancy and birth. In addition, the nurse may provide direct care involving the following areas:

- Contraception
- Abortion
- Infertility
- Screening for sexually transmitted infections
- Preconceptual education, risk assessment, and care

- Prenatal education, assessment, and care
- Postpartum education, assessment, and care

Provision of Atraumatic Care for Children

To minimize the stress experienced by children and their families in relation to health care, nurses, child life specialists, and other health care professionals advocate for the provision of atraumatic care. Atraumatic care refers to the delivery of health care in a manner that eliminates or minimizes psychological and physical distress to children and families (Huff et al., 2009; Wong, 2002). The key principles of atraumatic care include:

- Preventing or minimizing physical stressors
- Preventing or minimizing separation of the child from the family
- Promoting a sense of control

Table 2.5 provides suggestions for incorporating the principles of atraumatic care into nursing care for the child and family.

Educator

Due to shortened hospital stays and decreased admissions, providing client and family education is a key role for nurses in the community. Often, teaching begins in the community setting, especially the home, and is frequently focused on assisting the client and family to achieve independence.

TABLE 2.5 SUGGESTIONS FOR PROVIDING ATRAUMATIC CARE

Principle	Suggestions for Nursing Care
Preventing or minimizing physical stressors	• For painful injections, use numbing techniques. • During painful or invasive procedures, avoid traditional restraint or "holding down" of the child. Use alternative positioning such as "therapeutic hugging." • If these positions are not an option, have the parent stand near the child's head to provide comfort. • Insert a saline lock if the child will require multiple doses of parenteral medications. • Advocate for minimal laboratory blood specimen collections. • Avoid use of or minimize intramuscular or subcutaneous injections. • Provide appropriate pain management.
Preventing or minimizing child and family separation	• Promote family-centred care. • Allow the family the choice about whether to stay for invasive procedures, and support them in their decision.
Promoting a sense of control	• Maintain the child's home routine related to activities of daily living. • Encourage the child to have a security item with him or her if desired. • Involve the child and family in planning of care from the first moment of the first encounter. • Empower the family and child by providing knowledge. • Allow the child and family choices when they are available. • Make the environment more inviting, less intimidating.

Nurses are in a unique position to help clients and families manage their own health care needs. Clients and families need to be knowledgeable about areas such as their condition, the health care management plan, and when and how to contact health care providers.

Client education occurs when nurses share information, knowledge, and skills with clients and families, thus empowering them to take responsibility for their health care. Through education, clients and families can overcome feelings of powerlessness and helplessness and gain the confidence and capability to be active members in their plan of care. The goals of client and family education are the following:

• Maintain and promote health and prevent illness
• Restore health
• Optimize quality of life with impaired functioning

Overall, client and family education allows clients and families to make informed decisions, ensures the use of basic health care skills, promotes recognition of problem situations, promotes appropriate responses to problems, and allows for questions to be answered (Edelman & Mandle, 2006).

Steps of Client and Family Education

The steps of client and family education are similar to the steps of the nursing process. The nurse must assess, plan, implement, evaluate and, finally, document education. Once a level of comfort and experience are obtained with each of these steps, they blend together into one harmonious whole that becomes an everyday part of nursing practice. Client education begins with the first client encounter and proceeds through discharge and beyond. Reassessment after each step or change in the process is critical to ensuring success.

Assessing Teaching and Learning Needs

Client education begins with a learning needs assessment that includes the client and family's learning needs, learning styles, and potential barriers to learning. A learning needs assessment also is a good time to establish rapport with the family to demonstrate interest in them and confidence in their ability to learn.

Based on the results of the assessment, an individualized plan can be developed to reduce the time and effort required for nurses to teach while maximizing learning for the client and family. When caring for children, the educational process is targeted at both the child, when developmentally appropriate, and the adult members of the family. Therefore, it is advisable to conduct a learning needs assessment on both the adult caregivers and the child when appropriate.

The completed assessment should be shared with all members of the interdisciplinary team so the entire team can facilitate the learning. Although assessment generally takes place during the first or second meeting with the client and family, it should also occur with each encounter to check for any changes to ensure the success of the education across the continuum of care.

Cultural Impact on Assessment of Learning Needs

Culture can have a significant impact on learning. During the learning needs assessment, the nurse must determine the language(s) spoken in the home and the cultural norms around eye contact and physical touch. The following points should also be considered:

- Who is the person responsible for caring for the client?
- Who is considered the decision maker in the family?
- What is the social support structure?
- Are there special dietary needs and concerns during illness?
- Are there traditional health practices, such as the use of healers, shamans, talismans, folk remedies, and herbs?
- Are special clothes worn or are there other items that help maintain health?
- What are their religious beliefs, ceremonies, and spiritual practices?

▶ *Consider* THIS!

Our medical mission took a team of nurse practitioners into the rural mountains of Guatemala to offer medical services to people who had never had any. One day, a distraught mother brought her 10-year-old daughter to the mission clinic, asking me if there was anything I could do about her daughter's right wrist. She had sustained a fracture a year ago and it had not healed properly. As I looked at the girl's malformed wrist, I asked if it had been splinted to help with alignment, knowing what the answer was going to be. The interpreter enlightened me by saying that this young girl would never marry and have children because of this injury. I appeared puzzled at the interpreter's prediction of this girl's future. It was later explained to me that if the girl couldn't make tortes from corn meal for her husband because of her wrist disability, she would not be worthy of becoming someone's wife and thus would probably live with her parents the rest of her life.

I reminded myself during the week of the medical mission not to impose my cultural values on the women for whom I was caring and to accept their cultural mores without judgment. These silent self-reminders served me well throughout the week, for I was open to learning about their lifestyles and customs.

Thoughts: What must the young girl be feeling at the age of 10, being rejected for a disability that wasn't her fault? What might have happened if I had imposed my value system on this patient? How effective would I have been in helping her if she didn't feel accepted? This incident ripped my heart out, for this young girl will be deprived of a fulfilling family life based on a wrist disability. This is just another example of female suppression that happens all over the world—such a tragedy—and yet a part of their culture, on which nurses should not pass judgment.

Culture influences the interpretation and meaning of illness to a client and family. Questions should be asked about their thoughts or ideas, such as the cause, effects, severity, and hopes for treatment. An individualized teaching plan can then be negotiated with the client and family.

Nurses involved in teaching immigrant or refugee families may encounter specific issues, such as:

- Use of the Imperial versus the metric system for measurement
- Use of measurements such as a "a handful" or "a pinch" rather than specific measurements using a measuring device
- Lack of access to refrigeration for medications requiring cold storage
- Lack of clean water for mixing artificial baby food (formula)
- Breastfeeding practices that differ from Canadian expectations

Literacy Issues

The CPHA established an Expert Panel on Health Literacy to investigate the status of health literacy in Canada. **Health literacy** is defined as the ability to access, understand, evaluate and communicate information as a way to promote, maintain, and improve health in a variety of settings across the life-course (Rootman & Gordon-El-Bihbety, 2008). Health literacy is mediated by education, culture, language, and communication skills; by the nature of materials and messages; and by health care settings. Health literacy is seen as a resource for daily living in settings where people live, learn, and work. Health status and learning are closely linked at all ages and stages of life. Health literacy is essential to managing one's health (Rootman & Gordon-El-Bihbety, 2008).

Using the data from the International Adult Literacy and Skills Survey (Canadian Council on Learning, 2007), the panel concluded that many people in Canada lack the level of literacy needed to respond to the information demands of modern life (Rootman & Gordon-El-Bihbety, 2008). Even more people lack the skills required to respond to the health information demands in different health contexts (Rootman & Gordon-El-Bihbety, 2008). An estimated 55% of adults in Canada have less than adequate health literacy skills. Levels of health literacy vary significantly by province, age, education, language spoken, and gender. There is a notable gap in health literacy between immigrants and non-immigrants. Table 2.6 lists several complex socioeconomic conditions contributing to the individual systemic barriers to health literacy (Rootman & Gordon-El-Bihbety, 2008).

Health and learning are closely related, and studies have shown that the interaction is evident at all

TABLE 2.6 BARRIERS TO HEALTH LITERACY

Individual Barriers	Systemic Barriers
• Increased age • Limited opportunities to gain reading and writing skills • Low levels of formal education • Lack of knowledge and skills about health • Speaking a language other than English or French • Cultural beliefs • Disabilities • Feelings of stigma related to literacy • Exclusion from the benefits available to people with high levels of literacy and education • Exposure to violence • Early childhood experiences	• Provincial, territorial, and regional differences in education and philosophies about health • Changes in curriculum and reduced budgets causing health and physical education to be add-on subjects • Inadequate, inaccessible or non-existent teacher preparation courses and professional development opportunities • A lack of teacher specialists in health and physical education • Insufficient support for public health engagement with schools • Barriers to participating in literacy upgrading: cost, child care, conflict with paid employment • Availability and accessibility of affordable programs for newcomers to Canada • Lack of healthy lifestyle programs in the workplace • Lack of effective access to electronic information and technology and appropriate application • Complex health care, scientific advancements, and new technologies • Increase in chronic or long-term conditions requiring complex medical regimens, lifestyle changes, and self-care • Low levels of awareness and understanding of health literacy among health professionals

Source: Rootman, I., & Gordon-El-Bihbety, R. (2008). *A vision for a literate Canada: Report of the expert panel on health literacy.* Ottawa, ON: Canadian Public Health Association.

ages from early childhood through to the later stages in life (Canadian Council on Learning, 2007). When new and unfamiliar information is disseminated or when emotional distress is present, reading ability and understanding are reduced. In addition, the last grade completed in school does not equate with reading ability. Poor readers often read three to five grade levels below their grade completion. Most health care materials are written at a tenth-grade level (Safeer & Keenan, 2005). Moreover, medical information is becoming increasingly complex, while the amount of time clients have to spend with nurses and other health care providers is decreasing. As a result, many studies have shown that persons with limited literacy skills cannot understand basic medical words and health concepts, whether verbal or written (World Health Communication Associates, 2011). Even persons with adequate literacy skills may have difficulty reading and understanding health care information (Weiss, 2007).

Recognizing poor health literacy skills is difficult. Appearance, verbal ability, employment status, and educational level cannot be used to identify persons who do not read well. People who do not read well often go to great lengths to hide their disability. They may appear to agree with the nurse and suggest that they will read the instructions later (Arnold, 2011).

▶ *Take* NOTE!

Watch for these red flags that may indicate poor literacy skills:

- *Difficulty filling out registration forms, questionnaires, and consent forms*
- *Frequently missed appointments*
- *Noncompliance and lack of follow-up with treatment regimens*
- *Responses such as, "I forgot my glasses" or "I'll read this when I get home"*
- *Inability to answer common questions about their treatment or medicines*
- *Avoidance of asking questions for fear of looking "stupid"*

Planning Education

Once the assessment is completed, mutually agreed-upon achievable learning goals and objectives should be planned with the client and family. It is important that achievement of goals is possible from both the caregiver's and the learner's perspective. Finding common ground and building a bridge between the client's and family's concerns and what the health care team believes they need to know is a critical part of an education plan.

This also is an excellent time to consider client education materials and resources that can be used to maximize learning and retention.

The educational plan should involve input from the entire interdisciplinary team when appropriate. Using good communication and collaboration skills, team members can work together to empower the client and family to become knowledgeable and skilled. Provision of family-centred education requires more thought and skill compared with traditional teacher-centred education.

To achieve maximum success with education, it is beneficial to know how people learn. Dale (1969) suggested that people learn best when actively involved in the learning process. Figure 2.10 provides a summary of his principles, known as the "cone of learning." The implications for client education are clear: the more senses employed and the more actively involved the learner is, the better he or she will remember what was taught.

Interventions to Enhance Learning

Nurses are in an excellent position to foster an environment that is conducive to learning. For example, it is appropriate to say to the client, "Many people have a problem reading and remembering the information on this paper (booklet, manual). Is this ever a problem for you?" Once a problem is acknowledged, the nurse is free to adjust verbal communication techniques and written materials to assist with learning and to communicate this need to the entire interdisciplinary health care team.

Nurses implement individualized teaching techniques based on the assessment information and identified goals. In general, the following techniques can facilitate learning:

- Slow down and repeat information often.
- Speak in conversational style using plain, nonmedical language.
- "Chunk" information and teach it in small bites, using logical steps.
- Prioritize information and teach "survival skills" first.
- Use visuals, such as pictures, videos, and models.
- Teach using an interactive, "hands-on" approach.

If the client or family has poor health literacy skills, learning can be fostered by the use of photos or illustrations, DVDs, CDs or audio tapes, or colour coding (such as medication bottles or steps of a procedure). In addition, teaching can include a "back-up" family member.

Children and adolescents have a great need for information about their illness as they attempt to master feelings of anxiety and restore feelings of competency, self-confidence, and hope for the future. As with adults, they learn best when their input is valued and they are actively included and involved in the learning process. The age and developmental level of the child will determine the amount, format, and timing of the information given. Table 2.7

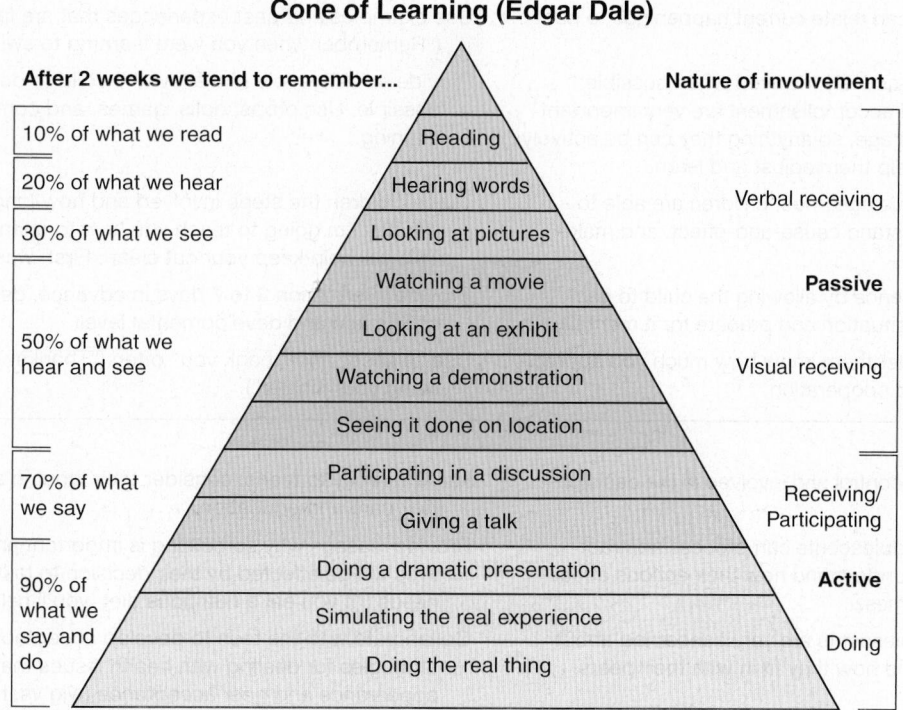

Cone of Learning (Edgar Dale)

After 2 weeks we tend to remember...		Nature of involvement
10% of what we read	Reading	Verbal receiving (Passive)
20% of what we hear	Hearing words	
30% of what we see	Looking at pictures	
50% of what we hear and see	Watching a movie	Visual receiving
	Looking at an exhibit	
	Watching a demonstration	
	Seeing it done on location	
70% of what we say	Participating in a discussion	Receiving/Participating
	Giving a talk	
90% of what we say and do	Doing a dramatic presentation	Active / Doing
	Simulating the real experience	
	Doing the real thing	

FIGURE 2.10 Cone of learning. Adapted from: Dale, E. (1969). *Audio-visual methods in teaching* (3rd ed.). Austin, TX: Holt, Rinehart, and Winston.

TABLE 2.7 GUIDELINES FOR TEACHING CHILDREN

Teaching Tips	Practical Applications
Preschoolers	
Offer simple, concise, concrete explanations based on the assessed needs, questions, and developmental level of the child.	Use a child's senses and relate what a procedure will look, sound, smell, taste, or feel like ("The MRI machine will sound very loud, like a big train").
Be honest, even when the information you need to convey is not positive. This helps the child to form a bond of trust and confidence with caregivers.	Use the family's words that the child understands; use "soft words" ("This will feel warm" instead of "This will burn").
Time explanations to decrease anxiety and excess worry before the event. Avoid telling unpleasant news close to bedtime.	As a general rule, give toddlers information about procedures, medicines, and other interventions immediately beforehand; give 4- to 7-year-olds information 1 or 2 days in advance.
Enlist the aid of the parents because they know their child best. Eliciting information from them about their child's past behaviours and coping skills can often mean the difference between a positive and negative experience for their child.	Teach parents how to coach their child with pain management, visualization, or other methods of distraction when appropriate ("Remember when we went to the beach....").
Provide an active role for the child. This helps to foster a child's sense of self-confidence and control over the situation.	Allow the child to help with simple self-care activities such as holding a dressing or piece of tape. Provide props and dolls to touch and feel as much as possible ("Your job is to keep your hands still").
Respect the child's wishes when he or she verbalizes or demonstrates that he or she does not want more information.	Keep explanations short and simple; know when to stop teaching.
Praise children and let them know how much you appreciate their help and cooperation.	Use "please" and "thank you" often ("Thank you. I like the way you held still for me.").
School-age children	
Allow the child some control and involvement in the decision-making process.	Offer choices whenever possible (taking the medicine with juice or milk), but don't offer choices when there are no alternatives (taking the medicine vs. not taking the medicine).
Know that children can relate current happenings to past experiences.	Use examples and past experiences that are familiar to the child ("Remember when you were learning to swim?").
Allow children to be actively involved when possible; achievement and accomplishment are very important to children at this age, so anything they can be actively involved in will help them adjust and learn.	Provide an active role and allow the child to do as much care as possible. Use props, dolls, games, and computers to enhance learning.
Remember that at this age, most children are able to sequence, understand cause-and-effect, and make sense of time.	Teach children the steps involved and how long they will take ("Today I'm going to teach you how to change your dressing. This will help keep your cut clean. First, wash your hands....").
Enhance self-confidence by allowing the child to gain control over the situation and prepare for it mentally.	Provide information 3 to 7 days in advance, depending on the child's age and developmental level.
Praise children and let them know how much you appreciate their help and cooperation.	Use "please" and "thank you" often ("Thanks! You did a great job using your inhaler").
Adolescents	
Allow teens to be in control and involved in the decision-making process.	Speak directly to teens; consider their input in all decisions about their care and education.
Keep in mind that adolescents can process abstract information and understand how their actions affect long-term outcomes.	Provide reasons why something is important and discuss how their lives will be affected by their decision to take care of their health needs ("If you eat a nutritious diet, you'll help your baby grow").
Remember that adolescents are very concerned about how they look and how they fit in with their peers.	Collaborate with the teen to develop acceptable solutions and strategies for dealing with health issues that affect personal appearance and peer acceptance (wig vs. head scarves for hair loss from chemotherapy).
Know that adolescents strive for independence and have personal values and ideologies that may conflict with those of their parents and the medical community.	Expect some noncompliance with care, despite your best educational efforts. Work together to achieve win–win outcomes of educational goals.

provides some guidelines to keep in mind when teaching children. Before beginning to teach a child, it is important to establish rapport and lay the foundation for good communication.

When teaching preschoolers, the nurse or family assumes part or all of the responsibility for what is learned, how it is learned, and when it is learned. Employing their vivid imaginations, young children often attempt to invent pieces of information, or pick up bits and pieces of misinformation that can lead to false assumptions. Skillfully delivered and timed information as well as proper preparation can help encourage trust, calm, and control for an otherwise apprehensive and uncooperative preschooler.

Unless they are quite ill, school-age children need to cooperate and achieve and usually want to participate in their care. When teaching, speak directly to them and include them in the education plan. Parents can often learn by listening to and observing the care being given to their child (Fig. 2.11).

Adolescents are particularly sensitive about maintaining body image and feelings of control and autonomy. This is especially important with health care processes and decisions that affect them. Education is an essential aspect of care for the adolescent who is pregnant.

Evaluating Learning

Teaching, even when done well, does not necessarily mean learning has occurred. Evaluation of learning is critical to ensure that the client and family have actually learned what the nurse tried to teach. Evaluation should occur with each educational encounter, and goals and interventions should be adjusted accordingly. The nurse, along with the rest of the interdisciplinary team, is responsible for client and family learning. If they have not learned, the health care team must adjust teaching strategies so that the client and family do learn.

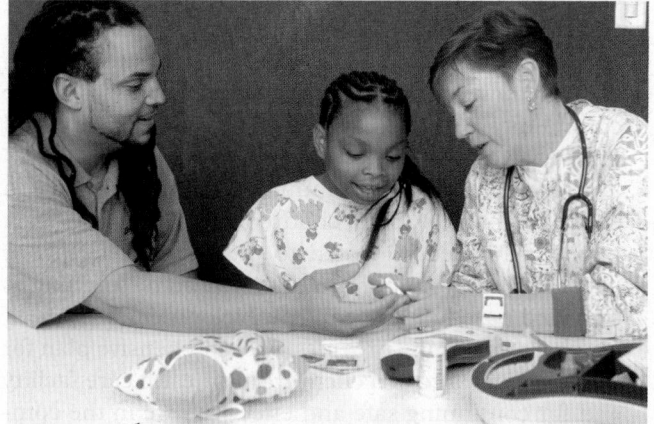

FIGURE 2.11 Nurses need to adapt teaching to the child's developmental level. For the school-age child, teaching the child and parents together fosters the child's need for achievement.

> ▶ *Take* NOTE!
>
> *The ultimate goal of education is a change in behaviour on the part of the client and family; this change can occur in their level of knowledge, skills, or both.*

Evaluation of learning can occur in several different ways, depending on the topic and the method of teaching. The client or family may:

- Demonstrate a skill. Learning can quickly and easily be identified using this method.
- Repeat back or teach back information using their own words.
- Answer open-ended questions. Open-ended questions provide an opportunity to assess for missing or incorrect information. Open-ended questions are those that cannot be answered with a simple "yes" or "no."

Another option to evaluate learning is to provide a "practice" scenario for the client or family, having them verbalize all the steps related to care from the routine measures to those for handling an emergency situation. Information must be conveyed accurately as the client or family walks through the necessary steps.

Documenting Teaching and Learning

Documenting client care and education is part of every nurse's professional practice and serves four main purposes. First and foremost, the client's medical record serves as a communication tool that the interdisciplinary team can use to keep track of what the client and family have learned already and what learning still needs to occur. Next, it serves to testify to the education the family has received if and when legal matters arise. Thirdly, it demonstrates that the nurse is meeting the competencies set for RN practice with respect to teaching and learning (CNA, 2011). Documentation of client and family education is imperative. It is the only means available to ensure that the family's educational plan and objectives have been completed.

Discharge Planner and Case Manager

Due to the short length of stays in acute settings and the shift to community settings for clients with complex health needs, discharge planning and case management have become an important nursing role in the community. Discharge planning involves the development and implementation of a comprehensive plan for the safe discharge of a client from a health care facility and for continuing safe and effective care in the community and at home. Case management focuses on coordinating health care services while balancing quality and cost outcomes. Often clients requiring community-based care, especially home health care, have complex medical needs that require an interdisciplinary team to meet their physical, psychosocial, medical, nursing, developmental, and education needs. Families may experience difficulties receiving consistent coordinated services across the health care continuum. The nurse plays an important role in initiating and maintaining the link between team members and the client to ensure that the client and family are receiving comprehensive, coordinated care.

Advocate and Resource Manager

Client advocate is another important role of the community health nurse to ensure that the client's and family's needs are being met. Advocacy also helps ensure that the client and family have available resources and appropriate health care services. For example, the pregnant woman on bed rest at home may need help in caring for her other children, maintaining the household, or getting to her appointments. Children with complex medical needs may require financial assistance through provincial or federal programs. They may also need assistance in obtaining needed equipment, additional services, and transportation. Community health nurses need a strong understanding of community, provincial, territorial, and federal resources to ensure that clients, families, and populations have access to those required resources for them.

■■■ Key Concepts

■ Family-centred care recognizes the concept of the family as the constant. The health and functioning ability of the family influences and impacts the health of the patient and other members of the family. Family-centred care recognizes and respects family strengths and individuality, encourages referrals for family support, and facilitates collaboration. It ensures flexible, accessible, and responsive health care delivery while incorporating developmental needs and implementing policies to provide emotional and financial support to women, children, and their families.

■ Health care delivery has moved from acute care settings out into the community, with an emphasis on health promotion and illness prevention. Community health nursing focuses on prevention and improvement of the health of populations and communities, addressing current and potential health needs of the population or community, promoting and preserving the health of a population regardless of a particular age group or diagnosis. Community health nurses perform epidemiologic investigations to help analyze and develop health policy and community health initiatives.

■ Community health nurses focus on providing personal care to individuals and families in the community. They centre on promoting and preserving health as well as preventing disease or injury. They help men, women, children, and their families cope with illness and disease. Community health nurses are direct care providers as well as advocators and educators. They focus on minimizing and removing barriers to allow the client, family and populations develop to their full potential.

■ Community health nurses use the nursing process in caring for patients within community settings and apply primary, secondary, and tertiary prevention levels. Nursing interventions in community-based settings include health screening, surveillance, health education, case management, community development, resource consultation and management, social advocacy, health system referral, health and wellness counselling, and risk identification.

■ Nurses working in the community need to develop cultural competence and cultural attunement and practice cultural safety. Steps to gaining cultural competence include cultural self-awareness, cultural knowledge, cultural skills, and cultural encounters.

■ Settings for community health nursing include primary care settings, public health departments, urgent care centres, clients' homes, schools, camps, churches, and shelters such as abuse, homeless, and disaster shelters. Nurses provide both wellness care, episodic illness care, and chronic care to men, women, children, families, and populations.

■ There has been a rise in home health care provision and services due to shorter hospital stays and health care cost containment along with an increase in income and longevity of children with chronic and debilitating health conditions. Technology also has improved, which allows for better monitoring of patients at home and for performing complicated procedures in the home.

■ Roles and functions of the community health nurse include communicator, direct care provider, educator, discharge planner and case manager, and advocate and resource manager.

■ Open, honest lines of communication are essential for community health nurses. The use of an interpreter may be necessary to ensure effective communication with men, women, children, and their families in the community setting. Maintaining confidentiality and privacy are essential skills.

■ Nurses working in the community play a major role in educating men, women, children, and their families. A family's knowledge related to the patient's health or illness is vitally important. For children, teaching is provided based on the child's developmental level.

■ Discharge planning provides a comprehensive plan for the safe discharge of a client from a health care facility and for continuing safe and effective care in the community. Case management focuses on coordinating health care services while balancing quality and cost outcomes. Both contribute to improved transition from the hospital to the community for women, children, their families, and the health care team.

■ Community health nurses act as advocates and resource managers to help ensure that the clients, families, and population groups have the necessary resources and appropriate health care services available to them.

REFERENCES

Aboriginal Nurses Association of Canada. (2009). *Cultural competence and cultural safety in nursing education: A framework for First Nations, Inuit and Métis nursing.* Retrieved January 23, 2012 from http://www.anac.on.ca/Documents/Making%20It%20Happen%20Curriculum%20Project/FINALFRAMEWORK.pdf

Alberta Health Services. (2003). *Services provided to school communities by public health nurses.* Calgary, AB: Author.

Alberta Health Services. (2008). *Best practices in diversity competency: Literature review and environmental scan.* Edmonton, AB: Author.

Alberta Health Services. (2010). *From here to maternity.* Calgary, AB: Author.

American Academy of Pediatrics. (2003). Policy statement: Family centred care and the pediatrician's role. *Pediatrics, 112*(3), 691–696. Retrieved September 13, 2011 from http://aappolicy.aappublications.org/cgi/content/full/pediatrics;112/3/691

Arnold, E. C. (2011). Health promotion and client learning needs. In E. C. Arnold & K. U. Boggs (Eds.), *Interpersonal relationships: Professional communication skills for nurses.* St Louis, MO: Elsevier Saunders.

Boggs, K. U. (2011). Communicating with children. In E. C. Arnold & K. U. Boggs (Eds.), *Interpersonal relationships: Professional communication skills for nurses.* St Louis, MO: Elsevier Saunders.

Canadian Council on Learning. (2007). *Health literacy in Canada: Initial results from the international adult literacy and skills survey 2007.* Retrieved January 23, 2012 from http://www.ccl-cca.ca/pdfs/HealthLiteracy/HealthLiteracyinCanada.pdf

Canadian Institute for Health Information. (2010). *Regulated nurses: Canadian trends, 2005 to 2009.* Retrieved September 12, 2011 from http://secure.cihi.ca/cihiweb/products/nursing_report_2005–2009_en.pdf

Canadian Nurses Association. (1997). The family connection. *Nursing Now, 3,* 1–4. Retrieved September 12, 2011 from http://www.cna-aiic.ca/CNA/documents/pdf/publications/FamilyConnection_Sept1997_e.pdf

Canadian Nurses Association. (2007). *Position statement: Telehealth: The role of the nurse.* Retrieved September 12, 2011 from http://www.cna-nurses.ca/cna/documents/pdf/publications/ps89_telehealth_e.pdf.

Canadian Nurses Association. (2010). *Position statement: Promoting cultural competence in nursing.* Retrieved September 12, 2011 from http://www.cna-aiic.ca/CNA/documents/pdf/publications/PS114_Cultural_Competence_2010_e.pdf

Canadian Nurses Association. (2011). *Canadian Registered Nurse Examination: Competencies.* Retrieved September 12, 2011 from http://www.cna-nurses.ca/CNA/nursing/rnexam/competencies/default_e.aspx

Canadian Public Health Association. (2010). *Public health: Community health nursing practice in Canada: Roles and activities* (4th ed.). Retrieved September 12, 2011 from http://www.chnc.ca/documents/AlexHenteleff-CommunityHealthNursingPracticeinCanad.pdf

Carneval, F. A., Alexander, E., Davis, D., Rennick, J., & Troini, R. (2006). Daily living with distress and enrichment: the moral experience of families with ventilator-assisted children at home. *Pediatrics, 117*(1), 48–60.

Chilman-Blair, K. (2010). Communicating with children about illness. *Practice Nursing, 21*(12), 631–633.

Citizenship and Immigration Canada. (2009). *A description of ethnic segregation/mixing within major Canadian metropolitan areas project.* Retrieved January 23, 2012 from http://www.cic.gc.ca/english/resources/research/ethnic-segregation/city.asp

Citizenship and Immigration Canada. (2011). *Permanent residents of Canada by province or territory and source area, 2010.* Retrieved

January 23, 2012 from http://www.cic.gc.ca/english/resources/statistics/facts2010/permanent/14.asp

Community Health Nurses of Canada. (2008). *Canadian community health nursing standards of practice.* Retrieved January 23, 2012 from http://www.chnc.ca/documents/chn_standards_of_practice_mar08_english.pdf

Community Health Nurses of Canada. (2009). *Public health discipline specific competencies.* Toronto, ON: Author.

Coyne, I. (2007). Disruption of parent participation: Nurses strategies to manage parents on children's wards. *Journal of Clinical Nursing, 17,* 3150–3158. doi: 10.1111/j.1365–2702.2006.01928.x

Dale, E. (1969). *Audio-visual methods in teaching* (3rd ed.). Austin, TX: Holt, Rinehart, and Winston.

Dochterman, J. M., & Bulechek, G. M. (2008). *Nursing interventions classification (NIC)* (5th ed.). St. Louis, MO: Mosby.

Edelman, C. L., & Mandle, C. L. (2006). *Health promotion throughout the lifespan* (6th ed.). St. Louis, MO: Mosby.

Edwards, M. (2010). *Communication skills for nurses: A practical guide on how to achieve successful consultations.* London: Quay Books.

Enkin, M., Keirse, M., Neilson, J., Crowther, C., Duley, L., Hodnett, E., & Hofmeyr, J. (2000). *A guide to effective care in pregnancy and childbirth* (3rd ed.). Toronto, ON: Oxford University Press.

Godfrey, J. R. (2006). Toward optimal health: The need for cultural competence in the healthcare of women. *Journal of Women's Health, 15*(5), 480–484.

Health Canada. (2000). *Family-centred maternity and newborn care: National guidelines.* Retrieved September 12, 2011 from http://www.phac-aspc.gc.ca/hp-ps/dca-dea/publications/fcm-smp/index-eng.php

Hewitt-Taylor, J. (2005). Caring for children with complex and continuing health needs. *Nursing Standard, 19*(42), 41–47.

Hodnett, E. D., Downe S., Walsh D., & Weston, J. (2010). Alternative versus conventional institutional settings for birth. *Cochrane Database of Systematic Reviews, 9.* Art. No.: CD000012. doi: 10.1002/14651858. CD000012.pub3.

Holditch-Davis, D., Miles, M. S., Burchinal, M. R., & Goldman, B. D. (2011). Maternal role attainment with medically fragile infants: part 2. Relationship to quality parenting. *Research in Nursing and Health, 34,* 35–48. doi:10.1002/nur.20418.

Huff, L., Hamlin, A., Wolski, D., McClure, T., Eliades, A., Weaver, L., & Shelestak, D. (2009). Atraumatic care: EMLA cream and application of heat to facilitate peripheral venous cannulation in children. *Issues in Comprehensive Pediatric Nursing, 32*(2), 65–76. doi: 10.1080/01460860902737418.

Institute for Patient- and Family Centered Care. (2010). *What are the core concepts of patient- and family-centered care?* Retrieved January 23, 2012 from http://www.ipfcc.org/faq.html

Jimenez, V., Klein, M., Hivon, M., & Mason, C. (2010). A mirage of change: Family-centred maternity care in practice. *Birth, 37*(2), 160–167.

Jolley, J., & Shields, L. (2009). The evolution of family-centred care. *Journal of Pediatric Nursing, 24*(2), 164–170.

Lambert, V., Glacken, M., & McCarron, M. (2010). Communication between children and health professionals in a child hospital setting: a child transitional communication model. *Journal of Advanced Nursing, 67*(3), 569–582. doi: 10.1111/j.1365–2648.2010.05511.x.

Leavitt, J. W. (1986). *Brought to bed: Childbearing in America. 1750–1950.* New York: Oxford University Press.

MacDonald, H. L., & Gibson, C. H. (2010). Parenting children requiring complex care at home: revisiting normalization and stigma. *Journal of Nursing and Healthcare of Chronic Illness, 2,* 241–251. doi: 10.1111/j.1752–9824.2010.01065.x.

MacKean, G. L., Thurston, W. E., & Scott, C. M. (2005). Bridging the divide between families and health professionals' perspectives on family-centred care. *Health Expectations, 8*(1), 74–85.

Mandleco, B. (2005). *Pediatric nursing skills and procedures.* Clifton Park, NY: Thomson Delmar.

Maxwell, B., & Barry, M. (2010). Documenting and reporting. In P. A. Potter & A. G. Perry (Eds.), *Canadian fundamentals of nursing* (4th ed.). Canadian editors, J. Ross-Kerr & M. Wood. Toronto, ON: Elsevier Canada.

McGrath, J. M., & Hardy, W. (2008). Communication: An essential component to providing quality care. *Newborn and Infant Nursing Reviews, 8*(2), 64–66. doi: 10.1053/j.nainr.2008.03.005.

McPherson, K. (1996). *Bedside matters: The transformation of Canadian nursing, 1900–1990.* Toronto, ON: Oxford University Press.

Mentro, A. (2003). Health care policy for medically fragile children. *Journal of Pediatric Nursing, 18*(4), 225–232.

Petrucka, P. (2010). The Canadian Health Care System. In P. A. Potter & A. G. Perry (Eds.), *Canadian fundamentals of nursing* (4th ed.). Canadian editors, J. Ross-Kerr & M. Wood. Toronto, ON: Elsevier Canada.

Phillips, C. R. (2003). *Family-centred maternity care.* Toronto, ON: Jones and Bartlett Publishers.

Planetree. (2011). *Planetree vision, mission and belief statements.* Retrieved September 13, 2011 from http://www.planetree.org/about.html

Public Health Agency of Canada. (2008). *Canadian perinatal health report, 2008 edition.* Retrieved September 12, 2011 from http://www.phac-aspc.gc.ca/publicat/2008/cphr-rspc/index-eng.php.

Registered Nurses' Association of Ontario. (2007). *Embracing cultural diversity in health care: Developing cultural competence.* Toronto, ON: Author.

Reutter, L & Eastlick Kushner, K. E. Health and Wellness. In P. A. Potter & A. G. Perry (Eds.), *Canadian fundamentals of nursing* (4th ed.). Canadian editors, J. Ross-Kerr & M. Wood. Toronto, ON: Elsevier Canada.

Rootman, I., & Gordon-El-Bihbety, R. (2008). *A vision for a literate Canada: Report of the expert panel on health literacy.* Ottawa, ON: Canadian Public Health Association.

Rosser, W., Colwill, J., Kasperski, J., & Wilson, L. (2011). Progress of Ontario's family health team model: A patient-centered medical home. *Annals of Family Medicine, 9*(2), 165–171.

Safeer, R., & Keenan, J. (2005). Health literacy: The gap between physicians and patients. *American Family Physician, 72*(3), 463–468.

Shields, L. (2010). Questioning family-centred care. *Journal of Clinical Nursing, 19,* 2629–2638.

Shields, L., Pratt, J., Davis, L., & Hunter, J. (2007). Family-centred care for children in hospital. *Cochrane Database of Systematic Reviews, 1,* Art. No.: CD004811. doi: 10.1002/14651858.CD004811.pub2.

Shipley, S. (2010). Listening: A concept analysis. *Nursing Forum, 45*(2), 125–134.

Simonsen-Anderson, S. (2002). Safe and sound: Telephone triage and home recommendations save lives and money. *Nursing Management, 33*(6), 41–43.

Society of Obstetricians and Gynaecologists of Canada. (2007). *Joint SOGC-Motherisk clinical practice guideline: Pre-conceptional vitamin/folic acid supplementation 2007.* Retrieved September 12, 2011 from http://www.sogc.org/media/pdf/advisories/JOGC-dec-07-FOLIC.pdf

Society of Obstetricians and Gynaecologists of Canada. (2008). *A national birthing initiative for Canada.* Ottawa: Author.

Stamler, L. L., & Yiu, L. (2012). *Community health nursing: A Canadian perspective.* Toronto, ON: Pearson Canada.

Statistics Canada. (2006a). *The 2006 participation and activity limitation survey: Disability in Canada.* Retrieved January 23, 2012 from http://www.statcan.gc.ca/bsolc/olc-cel/olc-cel?catno=89–628-X& lang=eng

Statistics Canada. (2006b). *Women in Canada: A gender-based statistical report* (5th ed.). Retrieved January 23, 2012 from http://www.statcan.gc.ca/pub/89–503-x/89–503-x2005001-eng.pdf

Steppe, B. (2006). Experience the experience. *International Journal of Childbirth Education, 21*(3), 33.

Storch, J. L. (2010). Canadian healthcare system. In M. McIntyre & C. McDonald (Eds.), *Realities of Canadian nursing: Professional, practice and power issues.* Toronto, ON: Lippincott Williams & Wilkins.

Vollman, A., Anderson, E. T., & McFarlane, J. (2012). *Canadian community as partner: Theory and practice in nursing* (3rd ed.). Philadelphia: Lippincott Williams & Wilkins.

Weech, W. A. (1999). *Tips for using interpreters.* Foreign Service Institute of the U.S. Department of State.

Weiss, B. (2007). *Health literacy and patient safety: Helping patients understand. A manual for clinicians.* American Medical Association Foundation and the American Medical Association. Retrieved September 27, 2011 from http://www.ama-assn.org/ama1/pub/upload/mm/367/healthlitclinicians.pdf

World Health Communication Associates. (2011). *Health literacy: The "basics" revised edition.* Brussels, Belgium: Author. Retrieved January 23, 2012 from http://www.whcaonline.org/uploads/publications/HL-FINAL-14.7.2011-2.pdf

Wong, D. L. (2002). *Beyond first do no harm: Principles of atraumatic care.* Retrieved June 25, 2006 from http://www3.us.elsevierhealth.com/WOW/op022a.html

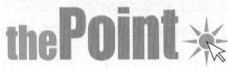

For additional learning materials, including Internet Resources, visit **http://thePoint.lww.com/Chow1e.**

CHAPTER WORKSHEET

MULTIPLE CHOICE QUESTIONS

1. A community health nurse is involved in secondary prevention activities. Which activities might be included? Select all that apply.

   a. Fecal occult blood testing

   b. Hearing screening

   c. Smoking cessation program

   d. Cholesterol testing

   e. Hygiene program

   f. Pregnancy testing

2. A woman is to undergo a colonoscopy at a freestanding outpatient surgery centre. Which would the nurse identify as a major disadvantage associated with this community-based setting?

   a. Increased risk for infection

   b. Increased health care costs

   c. Need to be transferred if overnight stay is required

   d. Increased disruption of family functioning

3. A 2-year-old boy is scheduled to undergo an endoscopic procedure. His parents are asking when they should tell him about it. Based on the nurse's understanding of the child's developmental stage, when would be the most appropriate time to prepare the child for the procedure?

   a. About 1 week before the scheduled date

   b. A few days in advance of the scheduled date

   c. About an hour before the procedure is to occur

   d. Just before the procedure is to be performed

4. When developing a teaching plan for a child and his parents, which action would the nurse do first?

   a. Decide which procedures and medications the child will be discharged on.

   b. Determine the child's and family's learning needs and styles.

   c. Ask the family if they have ever performed this type of procedure.

   d. Tell the child and family what the goals of the teaching session are.

CRITICAL THINKING EXERCISES

1. A 3-year-old girl from Pakistan has become seriously ill while on a visit to Canada. It is projected that she will require a lengthy hospitalization. Describe the steps the nurse should take to communicate with and provide extensive health care teaching to this child's family.

2. A pregnant woman is discharged home from the hospital after admission due to preterm labour. The woman is to be on complete bed rest and will receive home antenatal care through the health region to assist her and her family and to monitor her health status. As the antenatal nurse assigned to this woman, what should your nursing assessment include?

STUDY ACTIVITIES

1. Describe health education topics that would be appropriate in a school setting for elementary students.

2. Shadow a nurse working in a community setting, such as a family planning clinic, school, camp, home health care, or public health department. Identify the role the nurse plays in the health of men, women, children, and families in the setting and the community.

3. Arrange for a visit to a community health centre that offers services to various cultural groups. Interview the staff about the strategies used to overcome communication barriers and different health care practices for the women and children in these groups.

4. Select a website from http://thePoint.lww.com/Chow1e and explore the information provided. How could a community health nurse use this information?

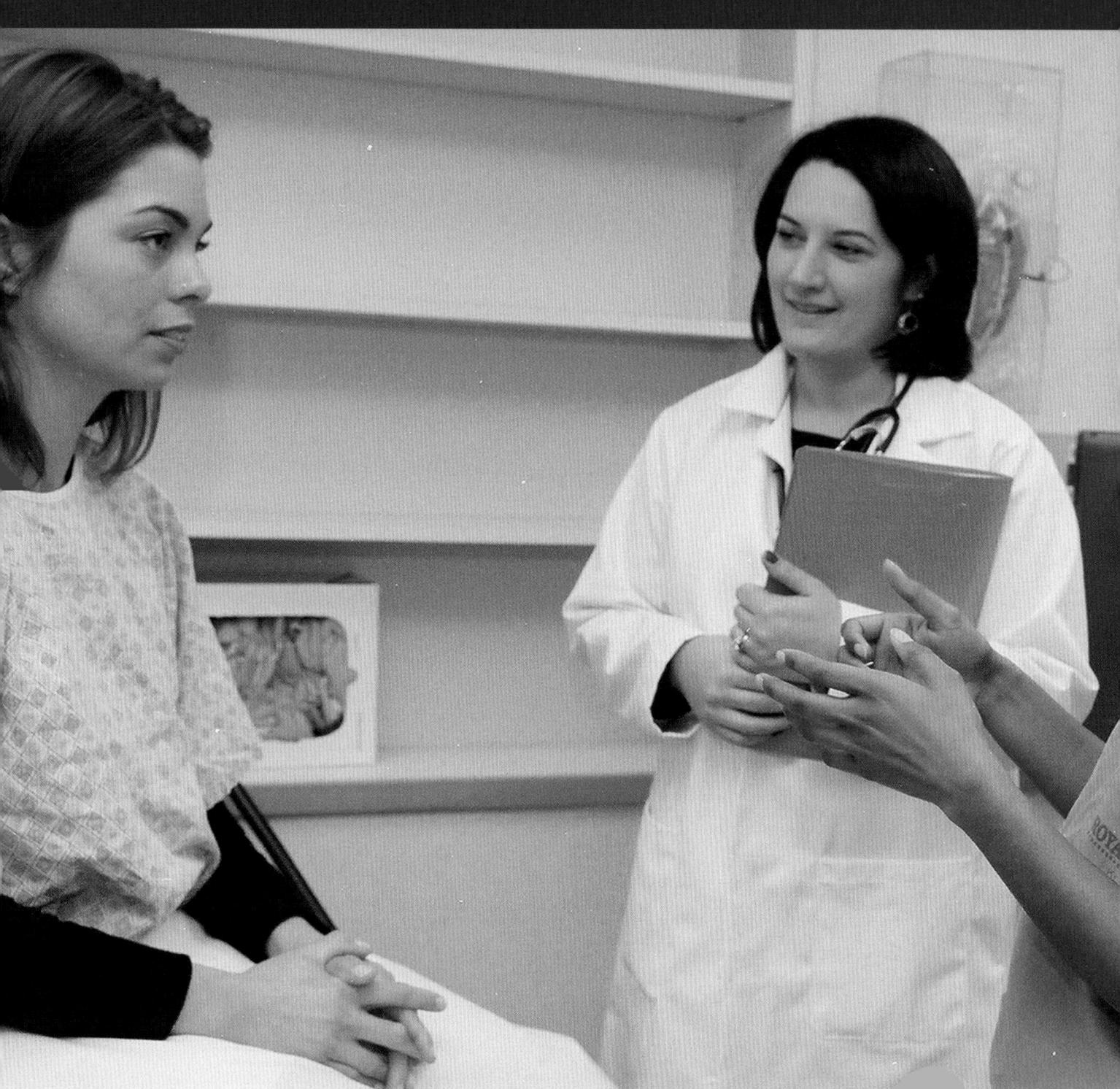

UNIT TWO

WOMEN'S HEALTH THROUGHOUT THE LIFESPAN

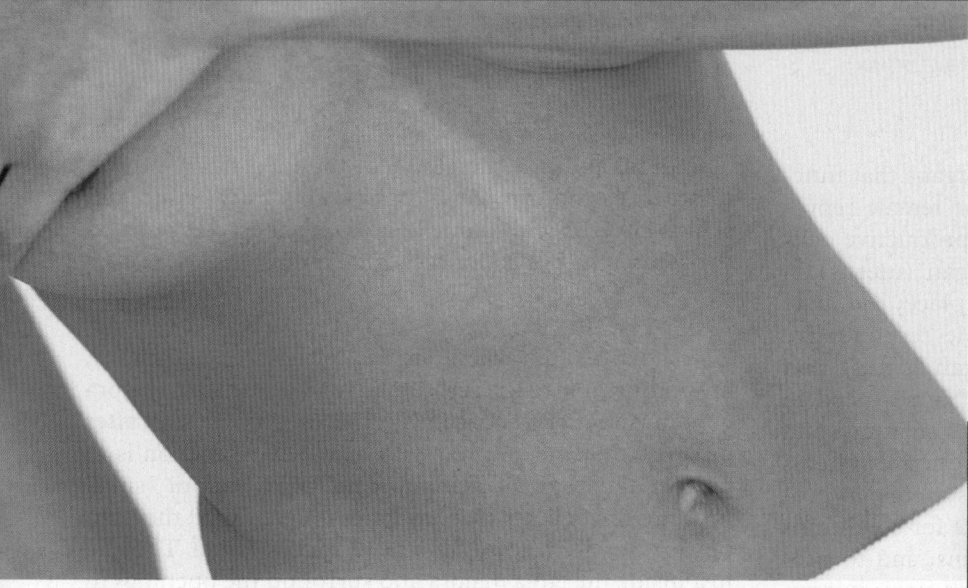

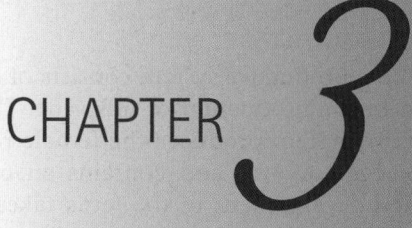

CHAPTER 3

Adapted by Jean Chow

ANATOMY AND PHYSIOLOGY OF THE REPRODUCTIVE SYSTEM

KEY TERMS

breasts
cervix
endometrium
estrogen
fallopian tubes
follicle-stimulating
  hormone (FSH)

luteinizing hormone
  (LH)
menarche
menstruation
ovaries
ovulation
penis

progesterone
testes
uterus
vagina
vulva

LEARNING OBJECTIVES

Upon completion of the chapter, the learner will be able to:

1. Define the key terms used in this chapter.
2. Explain the structure and function of the major external and internal female genital organs.
3. Outline the phases of the menstrual cycle, the dominant hormones involved, and the changes taking place in each phase.
4. Classify external and internal male reproductive structures and the function of each in hormonal regulation.

Linda, 49-year-old, started menstruating when she was 12 years old. Her menstrual periods have always been regular, but now she is experiencing irregular, heavier, and longer ones. She wonders if there is something wrong, or if this is normal.

Wow

All nurses should take care of and respect the human body, for it is a wondrous organism.

The reproductive system consists of organs that function in the production of offspring. The female reproductive system produces the female reproductive cells (the eggs or ova) and contains an organ (uterus) in which development of the fetus takes place; the male reproductive system produces the male reproductive cells (the sperm) and contains an organ (penis) that deposits the sperm within the female. Nurses need to have a thorough understanding of the anatomy and physiology of the male and female reproductive systems to be able to assess the health of these systems, to promote reproductive system health, to care for conditions that might affect the reproductive organs, and to provide client teaching concerning the reproductive system. This chapter will review the female and male reproductive systems and the menstrual cycle as it relates to reproduction.

Female Reproductive Anatomy and Physiology

The female reproductive system is composed of both external and internal reproductive organs.

External Female Reproductive Organs

The external female reproductive organs collectively are called the **vulva** (which means "covering" in Latin). The vulva serves to protect the urethral and vaginal openings and is highly sensitive to touch to increase the female's pleasure during sexual arousal (Alexander, LaRosa, Bader, et al., 2010). The structures that make up the vulva include the mons pubis, the labia majora and minora, the clitoris, the structures within the vestibule, and the perineum (Fig. 3.1).

Mons Pubis

The mons pubis is the elevated, rounded fleshy prominence over the symphysis pubis. This fatty tissue and skin is covered with pubic hair after puberty. It protects the symphysis pubis during sexual intercourse.

Labia

The labia majora, which are relatively large and fleshy, are comparable to the scrotum in males. The labia majora contain sweat and sebaceous (oil-secreting) glands; after puberty, they are covered with hair. Their function is to protect the vaginal opening. The labia minora (small lips) are the delicate hairless inner folds of skin; they can be very small or up to 5.1 cm (2 inches) wide. They lie just inside the labia majora and surround the openings to the vagina and the urethra. The labia minora grow down from the anterior inner part of the labia majora on each side. They are highly vascular and abundant in nerve supply. They lubricate the vulva, swell in response to stimulation, and are highly sensitive.

Clitoris and Prepuce

The clitoris is a small, cylindrical mass of erectile tissue and nerves. It is located at the anterior junction of the labia minora. There are folds above and below the clitoris. The joining of the folds above the clitoris forms the prepuce, a hood-like covering over the clitoris; the junction below the clitoris forms the frenulum.

▶ *Take* NOTE!

The hood-like covering over the clitoris and other parts of the external female genitalia or organs are the sites for female circumcision, which is still practiced in some countries by some cultures (World Health Organization, 2010).

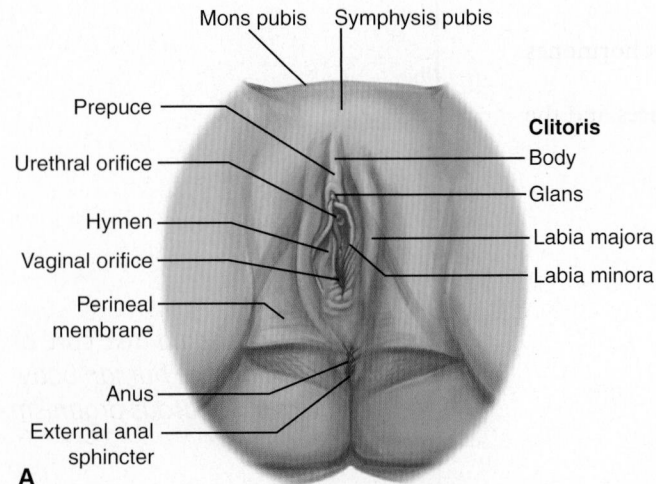

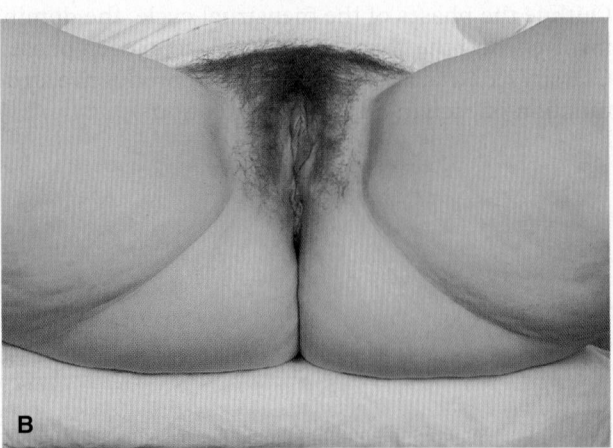

FIGURE 3.1 (**A**) The external female reproductive organs. (**B**) Normal appearance of external structures. (Photo by B. Proud.)

A rich supply of blood vessels gives the clitoris a pink colour. Like the penis, the clitoris is very sensitive to touch, stimulation, and temperature and can become erect. For its small size, it has a generous blood and nerve supply. There are more free nerve endings of sensory reception located on the clitoris than on any other part of the body, and it is, unsurprisingly, the most erotically sensitive part of the genitalia for most females. Its function is sexual stimulation (Ward & Hisley, 2009).

> ▶ **Take** NOTE!
>
> *The word "clitoris" is from the Greek word for key; in ancient times the clitoris was thought to be the key to a woman's sexuality.*

Vestibule

The vestibule is an oval area enclosed by the labia minora laterally. It is inside the labia minora and outside of the hymen and is perforated by six openings. Opening into the vestibule are the urethra from the urinary bladder, the vagina, and two sets of glands. The opening to the vagina is called the introitus, and the half-moon–shaped area behind the opening is called the fourchette. Through tiny ducts beside the introitus, Bartholin's glands, when stimulated, secrete mucus that supplies lubrication for intercourse. Skene's glands are located on either side of the opening to the urethra. They secrete a small amount of mucus to keep the opening moist and lubricate the vagina (Ward & Hisley, 2009).

The vaginal opening is surrounded by the hymen (maidenhead). The hymen is a tough, elastic, perforated, mucosa-covered tissue across the vaginal introitus. In a virgin, the hymen may completely cover the opening, but it usually encircles the opening like a tight ring. Because the degree of tightness varies among women, the hymen may tear at the first attempt at intercourse and cause slight bleeding, or it may be so soft and pliable that no tearing occurs. In a woman who is not a virgin, the hymen usually appears as small tags of tissue surrounding the vaginal opening, but the presence or absence of the hymen can neither confirm nor rule out sexual experience (Ward & Hisley, 2009).

> ▶ **Take** NOTE!
>
> *Heavy physical exertion, use of tampons, or injury to the area can alter the appearance of the hymen in girls and women who have not been sexually active.*

Perineum

The perineum is the most posterior part of the external female reproductive organs. This external region is located between the vulva and the anus. It is made up of skin, muscle, and fascia. The perineum can become lacerated or incised during childbirth and may need to be repaired with sutures. Incising the perineum area to provide more space for the presenting part is called an episiotomy. Although still a common obstetric procedure, the use of episiotomy has decreased over the past 25 years. The procedure should be applied selectively rather than routinely. An episiotomy can add to postpartum discomfort and perineal trauma and can lead to fecal incontinence (Cunningham, Leveno, & Bloom, et al., 2010).

Internal Female Reproductive Organs

The internal female reproductive organs consist of the vagina, uterus, fallopian tubes, and ovaries. These structures develop and function according to the specific hormone influences that affect fertility and childbearing (Fig. 3.2).

Vagina

The **vagina** is a highly distensible musculomembranous canal situated in front of the rectum and behind the bladder. It is a tubular, fibromuscular organ lined with mucous membrane that lies in a series of transverse folds called rugae. The rugae allow for extreme dilation of the canal during labour and birth. The vagina is a canal that connects the external genitals to the uterus. It receives the penis and the sperm ejaculated during sexual intercourse, and it serves as an exit passageway for menstrual blood and for the fetus during childbirth. The front and back walls normally touch each other so that there is no space in the vagina except when it is opened (e.g., during a pelvic examination or intercourse). In the adult, the vaginal cavity is approximately 7.6 to 10.2 cm (3 to 4 inches) long. Muscles that control its diameter surround the lower third of the vagina. The upper two thirds of the vagina lies above these muscles and can be stretched easily. During a woman's reproductive years, the mucosal lining of the vagina has a corrugated appearance and is resistant to bacterial colonization. Before puberty and after menopause (if the woman is not taking estrogen), the mucosa is smooth due to lower levels of estrogen (McBride, Rohoedes, & Shuster, 2010).

The vagina has an acidic environment, which protects it against ascending infections. Antibiotic therapy, douching, perineal hygiene sprays, and deodorants upset the acid balance within the vaginal environment and can predispose women to infections.

Uterus

The **uterus** is a pear-shaped muscular organ at the top of the vagina. It lies behind the bladder and in front of the rectum and is anchored in position by eight ligaments, although it is not firmly attached or adherent to any part of the skeleton. A full bladder tilts the uterus backward; a

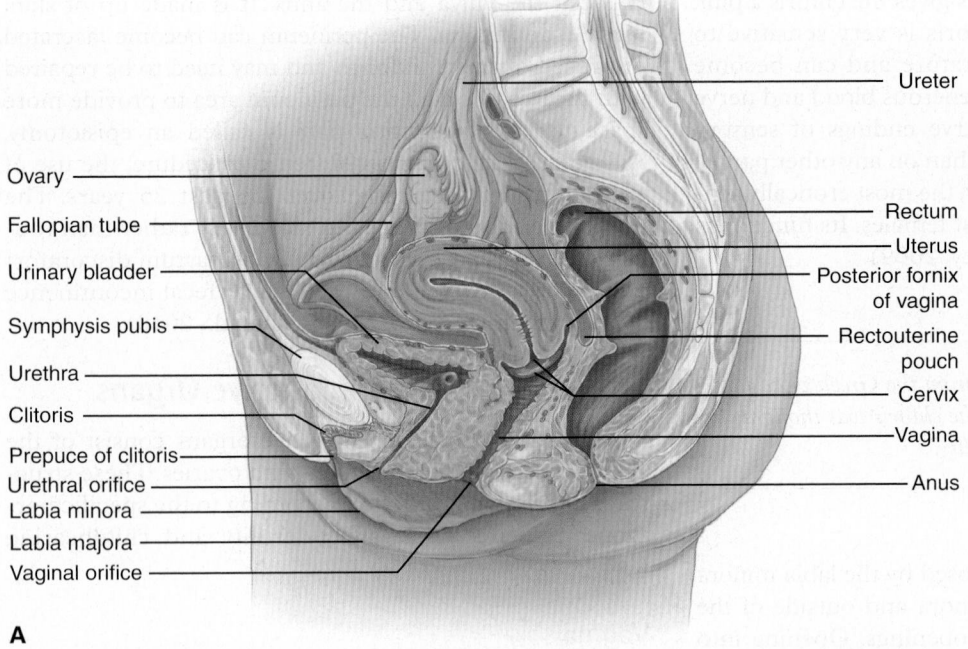

Ureter
Ovary
Fallopian tube
Urinary bladder
Symphysis pubis
Urethra
Clitoris
Prepuce of clitoris
Urethral orifice
Labia minora
Labia majora
Vaginal orifice

Rectum
Uterus
Posterior fornix of vagina
Rectouterine pouch
Cervix
Vagina
Anus

A

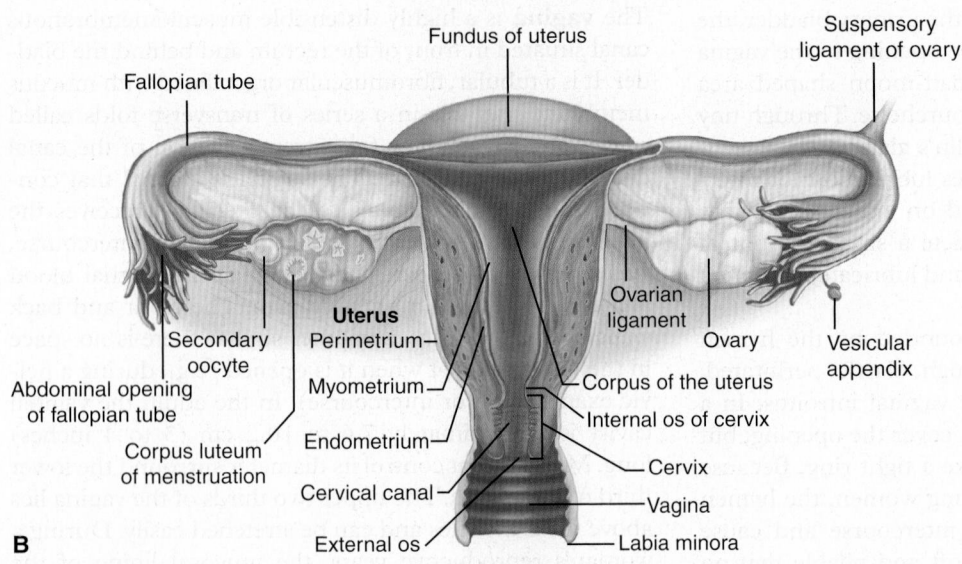

Fundus of uterus
Suspensory ligament of ovary
Fallopian tube
Secondary oocyte
Uterus
Perimetrium
Ovarian ligament
Ovary
Vesicular appendix
Abdominal opening of fallopian tube
Myometrium
Corpus luteum of menstruation
Endometrium
Corpus of the uterus
Internal os of cervix
Cervix
Cervical canal
Vagina
External os
Labia minora

B

FIGURE 3.2 The internal female reproductive organs. (**A**) Lateral view. (**B**) Anterior view. (Source: Anatomical Chart Company [2001]. *Atlas of human anatomy.* Springhouse, PA: Springhouse.)

distended rectum tilts it forward. The uterus alters its position by gravity or with change of posture, and is the size and shape of an inverted pear. It is the site of menstruation, implantation of a fertilized ovum, development of the fetus during pregnancy, and labour. Before the first pregnancy, it measures approximately 7.6 cm (3 inches) long, 5.1 cm (2 inches) wide, and 2.5 cm (1 inch) thick. After a pregnancy, the uterus remains larger than before the pregnancy. After menopause, it becomes smaller and atrophies.

The uterine wall is relatively thick and composed of three layers: the endometrium (innermost layer), the myometrium (muscular middle layer), and the perimetrium (outer serosal layer that covers the body of the uterus). The **endometrium** is the mucosal layer that lines the uterine cavity in non-pregnant women. It varies greatly in thickness from 0.5 to 5 mm and has an abundant supply of

glands and blood vessels (Cunningham et al., 2010). The myometrium makes up the major portion of the uterus and is composed of smooth muscle linked by connective tissue with numerous elastic fibres. During pregnancy, the upper myometrium undergoes marked hypertrophy, but there is limited change in the cervical muscle content.

Anatomic subdivisions of the uterus include the convex portion above the uterine tubes (the fundus); the central portion (the corpus or body) between the fundus and the cervix; and the cervix or neck, which opens into the vagina.

Cervix

The **cervix**, the lower part of the uterus, opens into the vagina and has a channel that allows sperm to enter the uterus and menstrual discharge to exit. It is composed of

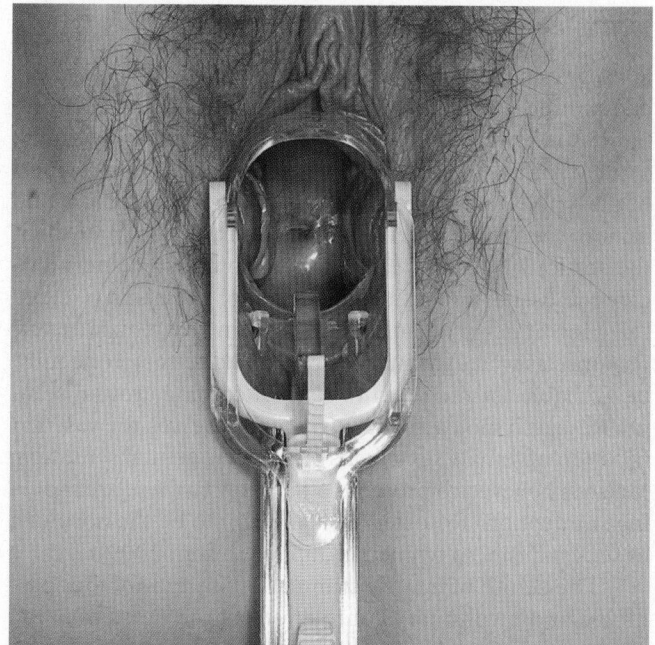

FIGURE 3.3 Appearance of normal cervix. Note: This is the cervix of a multipara female. (Photo by B. Proud.)

fibrous connective tissue. During a pelvic examination, the part of the cervix that protrudes into the upper end of the vagina can be visualized. Like the vagina, this part of the cervix is covered by mucosa, which is smooth, firm, and doughnut-shaped, with a visible central opening called the external os (Fig. 3.3). Before childbirth, the external cervical os is a small, regular, oval opening. After childbirth, the opening is converted into a transverse slit that resembles lips (Fig. 3.4). Except during menstruation or ovulation, the cervix is usually a good barrier against bacteria. The cervix has an alkaline environment, which protects the sperm from the acidic environment in the vagina.

The canal or channel of the cervix is lined with mucus-secreting glands. This mucus is thick and impenetrable to sperm until just before the ovaries release an egg (**ovulation**). At ovulation, the consistency of the mucus changes so that sperm can swim through it, allowing fertilization. At the same time, the mucus-secreting glands of the cervix actually become able to store live sperm for 2 or 3 days. These sperm can later move up through the corpus

and into the fallopian tubes to fertilize the egg; thus, intercourse 1 or 2 days before ovulation can lead to pregnancy. Because some women do not ovulate consistently, pregnancy can occur at varying times after the last menstrual period. The channel in the cervix is too narrow for the fetus to pass through during pregnancy, but during labour it dilates to let the newborn through.

Corpus

The corpus, or the main body of the uterus, is a highly muscular organ that enlarges to hold the fetus during pregnancy. The inner lining of the corpus (endometrium) undergoes cyclical changes as a result of the changing levels of hormones secreted by the ovaries: it is thickest during the part of the menstrual cycle in which a fertilized egg would be expected to enter the uterus and is thinnest just after menstruation. If fertilization does not take place during this cycle, most of the endometrium is shed and bleeding occurs, resulting in the monthly period. If fertilization does take place, the embryo attaches to the wall of the uterus, where it becomes imbedded in the endometrium (about 1 week after fertilization); this process is called implantation (Cunningham et al., 2010). Menstruation then ceases during the 40 weeks (280 days) of pregnancy. During labour, the muscular walls of the corpus contract to push the baby through the cervix and into the vagina.

Fallopian Tubes

The **fallopian tubes** are hollow, cylindrical structures that extend 5.1 to 7.6 cm (2 to 3 inches) from the upper edges of the uterus toward the ovaries. Each tube is about 7 to 10 cm long (4 inches) and approximately 0.7 cm in diameter. The end of each tube flares into a funnel shape, providing a large opening for the egg to fall into when it is released from the ovary. Cilia (beating, hair-like extensions on cells) line the fallopian tube and the muscles in the tube's wall. The fallopian tubes convey the ovum from the ovary to the uterus and sperm from the uterus toward the ovary. This movement is accomplished via ciliary action and peristalsis. If sperm are present in the fallopian tube as a result of sexual intercourse or artificial insemination, fertilization of the ovum can occur in the distal portion of the tube. If the egg is fertilized, it will divide over a period of 4 days while it moves slowly down the fallopian tube and into the uterus.

Ovaries

The **ovaries** are a set of paired glands resembling unshelled almonds set in the pelvic cavity below and to either side of the umbilicus. They are usually pearl-coloured and oblong. They are homologous to the testes. Each ovary is 2.5 to 5 cm long and 0.6 to 1.5 cm thick (Cunningham et al., 2010). The ovaries are not attached to the fallopian tubes but are suspended nearby by several ligaments, which help hold them in position. The development and the release of the ovum and the secretion of the hormones estrogen and progesterone are the two primary

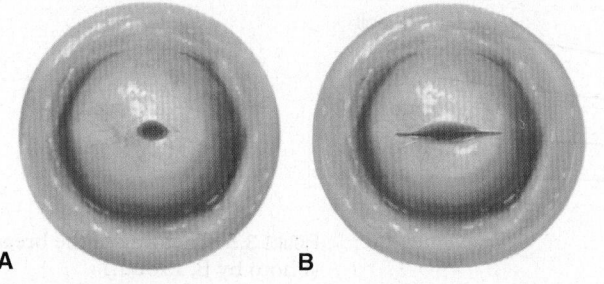

A   **B**

FIGURE 3.4 (**A**) Nulliparous cervical os. (**B**) Parous cervical os.

functions of the ovary. The ovaries link the reproductive system to the body's system of endocrine glands, as they produce the ova (eggs) and secrete, in cyclical fashion, the female sex hormones estrogen and progesterone. After an ovum matures, it passes into the fallopian tubes.

Breasts

The two mammary glands, or **breasts**, are accessory organs of the female reproductive system that are specialized to secrete milk following pregnancy. They overlie the pectoralis major muscles and extend from the second to the sixth ribs and from the sternum to the axilla. Each breast has a nipple located near the tip, which is surrounded by a circular area of pigmented skin called the areola. Each breast is composed of approximately 9 lobes (the number can range between 4 and 18), which contain glands (alveolar) and a duct (lactiferous) that leads to the nipple and opens to the outside (Fig. 3.5). The lobes are separated by dense connective and adipose tissues, which also help support the weight of the breasts (Tarlier & Jarvis, 2009).

During pregnancy, placental estrogen and progesterone stimulate the development of the mammary glands. Because of this hormonal activity, the breasts may double in size during pregnancy. At the same time, glandular tissue replaces the adipose tissue of the breasts.

Following childbirth and the expulsion of the placenta, levels of placental hormones (progesterone and lactogen) fall rapidly, and the action of prolactin (milk-producing hormone) is no longer inhibited. Prolactin stimulates the production of milk within a few days after childbirth, but in the interim, dark yellow fluid called colostrum is secreted. Colostrum contains more minerals and protein, but less sugar and fat, than mature breast milk. Colostrum secretion may continue for approximately a week after childbirth, with gradual conversion to mature milk. Colostrum is rich in maternal antibodies, especially immunoglobulin A (IgA), which offers protection for the newborn against enteric pathogens.

Female Sexual Response

With sexual stimulation, tissues in the clitoris and breasts and around the vaginal orifice fill with blood and the erectile tissues swell. At the same time, the vagina begins to expand and elongate to accommodate the penis. As part of the whole vasocongestive reaction, the labia majora and minora swell and darken. As sexual stimulation intensifies, the vestibular glands secrete mucus to moisten and lubricate the tissues to facilitate insertion of the penis.

Hormones play an integral role in the female sexual response as well. Adequate estrogen and testosterone must be available for the brain to sense incoming arousal stimuli. Research indicates that estrogen preserves the vascular function of female sex organs and affects genital sensation. It also is believed to promote blood flow to these areas during stimulation. Testosterone is thought to be the hormone of sexual desire in women (Krapf & Simon, 2009).

The zenith of intense stimulation is orgasm, the spasmodic and involuntary contractions of the muscles in the region of the vulva, the uterus, and the vagina that produce a pleasurable sensation to the woman. Typically the woman feels warm and relaxed after an orgasm. Within a short time after orgasm, the two physiologic mechanisms that created the sexual response, vasocongestion and muscle contraction, rapidly dissipate.

The Female Reproductive Cycle

The female reproductive cycle is a complex process that encompasses an intricate series of chemical secretions and reactions to produce the ultimate potential for fertility and birth. The female reproductive cycle is a general term encompassing the ovarian cycle, the endometrial cycle, the hormonal changes that regulate them, and the cyclical changes in the breasts. The endometrium, ovaries, pituitary gland, and hypothalamus are all involved in the cyclical changes that help to prepare the body for fertilization. Absence of fertilization results in menstruation, the monthly shedding of the uterine lining. Menstruation

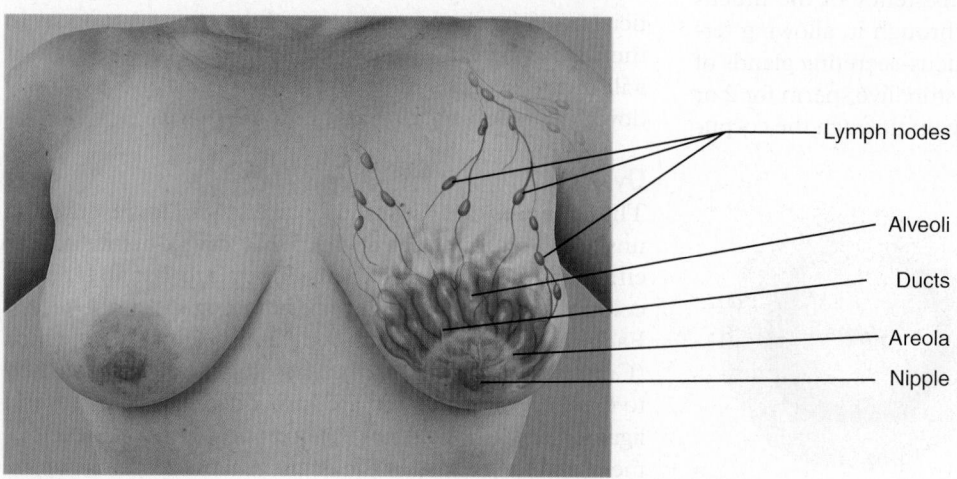

— Lymph nodes

— Alveoli

— Ducts

— Areola

— Nipple

FIGURE 3.5 Anatomy of the breasts. (Photo by B. Proud.)

marks the beginning and end of each menstrual cycle. Menopause is the naturally occurring cessation of regular menstrual cycles.

Menstruation

Menstruation is the normal, predictable physiologic process whereby the inner lining of the uterus (endometrium) is expelled by the body. Typically, this occurs monthly. Menstruation has many effects on girls and women, including emotional and self-image issues. In Canada, the average age at **menarche** (the start of menstruation) has decreased for women born more recently, with the current average age being 12 years (Harris, Prior, & Koehoorn, 2008). The reasons for earlier menarche are not completely understood but may be influenced by nutrition and childhood obesity. Pubertal events preceding the first menses have an orderly progression: thelarche, the development of breast buds; adrenarche, the appearance of pubic and then axillary hair, followed by a growth spurt; and menarche (occurring about 2 years after the start of breast development). In healthy pubertal girls, the menstrual period varies in flow heaviness and may remain irregular in occurrence for up to 2 years following menarche. After that time, the regular menstrual cycle should be established. Most women will experience approximately 400 menstrual cycles within their lifetime (Cunningham et al., 2010). Normal, regular menstrual cycles vary in frequency from 21 to 35 days (with the average cycle lasting 28 days), bleeding lasts 2 to 8 days, and blood loss averages 25 to 60 mL (London, Ladewig, Ball, et al., 2011). Irregular menses can be associated with irregular ovulation, stress, disease, and hormonal imbalances (Cunningham et al., 2010).

Think back to Linda, who was introduced at the beginning of the chapter. What questions might need to be asked to assess her condition? What laboratory work might be anticipated to validate her heavier flow?

Although menstruation is a normal process, various world cultures have taken a wide variety of attitudes toward it, seeing it as everything from a sacred time to an unclean time. In a society where menstruation is viewed negatively, nurses can help women develop a more positive image of this natural physiologic process.

▶ *Take* NOTE!

Knowledge about menstruation has increased significantly and attitudes have changed since early times, when many cultures saw it as "unclean." What was once discussed only behind closed doors is discussed openly today.

Reproductive Cycle

The reproductive cycle, also referred to as the menstrual cycle, results from a functional hypothalamic–pituitary–ovarian axis and a precise sequencing of hormones that lead to ovulation. If conception doesn't occur, menses ensues. The ranges of normal menstrual cycles are as follows:

- Cycle length: 21 to 35 days
- Duration of flow: 2 to 8 days
- Amount of flow: 25 to 60 mL

The female reproductive cycle involves two cycles that occur simultaneously: the ovarian cycle, during which ovulation occurs, and the endometrial cycle, during which menstruation occurs. Ovulation divides these two cycles at midcycle. Ovulation occurs when the ovum is released from its follicle; after leaving the ovary, the ovum enters the fallopian tube and journeys toward the uterus. If sperm fertilizes the ovum during its journey, pregnancy occurs. Figure 3.6 summarizes the menstrual cycle.

Ovarian Cycle

The ovarian cycle is the series of events associated with a developing oocyte (ovum or egg) within the ovaries. While men manufacture sperm daily, often into advanced age, women are born with a single lifetime supply of ova that are released from the ovaries gradually throughout the childbearing years. In the female ovary, 2 million oocytes are present at birth, and about 400,000 follicles are still present at puberty. The excess follicles are depleted during the childbearing years, with only 400 follicles ovulated during the reproductive period (Cunningham et al., 2010). The ovarian cycle begins when the follicular cells (ovum and surrounding cells) swell and the maturation process starts. The maturing follicle at this stage is called a graafian follicle. The ovary raises many follicles monthly, but usually only one follicle matures to reach ovulation. The ovarian cycle consists of three phases: the follicular phase, ovulation, and the luteal phase.

Follicular Phase

This phase is so named because it is when the follicles in the ovary grow and form a mature egg. This phase starts on the first day of the menstrual cycle and continues until ovulation, approximately 10 to 14 days later. The follicular phase is not consistent in duration because of the time variations in follicular development. The hypothalamus is the initiator of this phase. Increasing levels of estrogen secreted from the maturing follicular cells and the continued growth of the dominant follicle cell induce proliferation of the endometrium and myometrium. This thickening of the uterine lining supports an implanted ovum if pregnancy occurs.

Prompted by the hypothalamus, the pituitary gland releases follicle-stimulating hormone (FSH), which

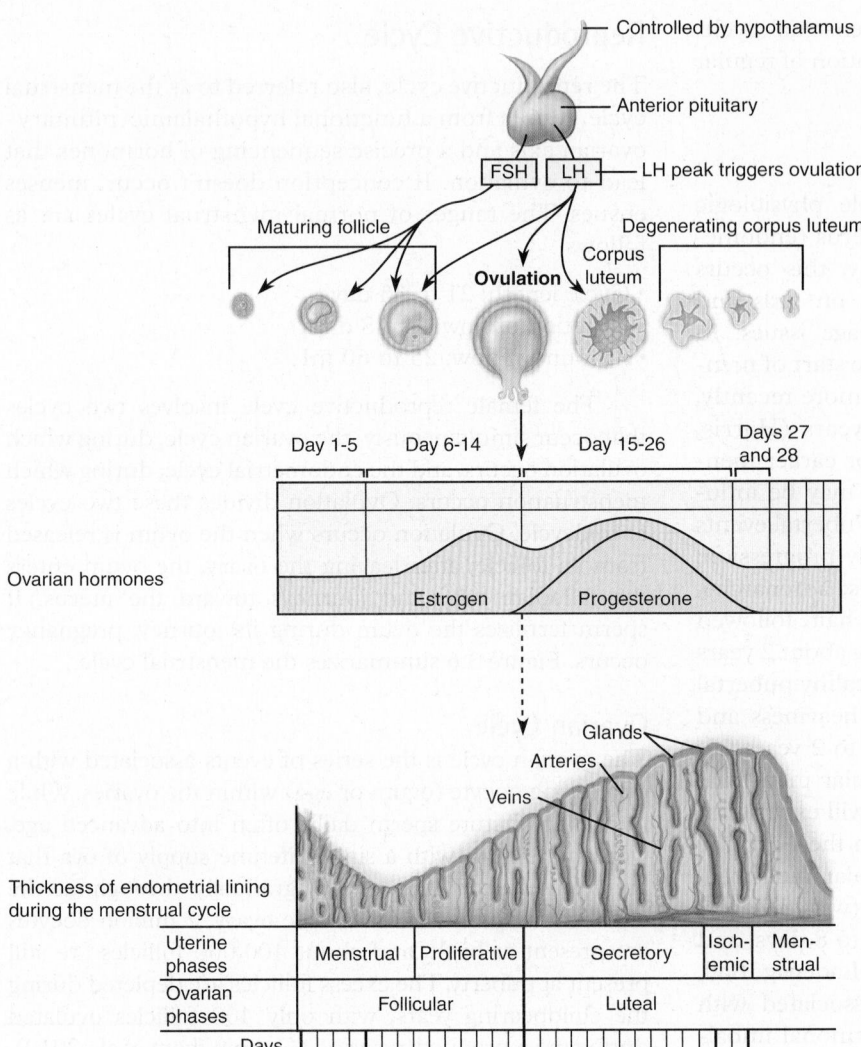

FIGURE 3.6 Menstrual cycle summary based on a 28-day (average) menstrual cycle.

stimulates the ovary to produce 5 to 20 immature follicles. Each follicle houses an immature oocyte or egg. The follicle that is targeted to mature fully will soon rupture and expel a mature oocyte in the process of ovulation. A surge in luteinizing hormone (LH) from the anterior pituitary gland is actually responsible for affecting the final development and subsequent rupture of the mature follicle.

Ovulation

At ovulation, a mature follicle ruptures in response to a surge of LH, releasing a mature oocyte (ovum). This usually occurs on day 14 in a 28-day cycle. When ovulation occurs, there is a drop in estrogen. Typically, ovulation takes place approximately 10 to 12 hours after the LH peak (Cunningham et al., 2010). The distal ends of the fallopian tubes become active near the time of ovulation and create currents that help carry the ovum into the uterus. The lifespan of the ovum is only about 24 hours; unless it meets a sperm on its journey within that time, it will die.

During ovulation, the cervix produces thin, clear, stretchy, slippery mucus that is designed to help the sperm travel up through the cervix to meet the ovum for

fertilization. The one constant, whether a women's cycle is 28 days or 120 days, is that ovulation takes place 14 days before menstruation (Ward & Hisley, 2009).

▶ **Take** *NOTE!*

Some women can feel a pain on one side of the abdomen around the time the egg is released. This midcycle pain is called mittelschmerz and may be experienced as sharp cramps to pain that lasts several hours.

Luteal Phase

The luteal phase begins at ovulation and lasts until the menstrual phase of the next cycle. It typically occurs day 15 through day 28 of a 28-day cycle. After the follicle ruptures, as it releases the egg, it closes and forms a corpus luteum. The corpus luteum secretes increasing amounts of the hormone progesterone, which interacts with the endometrium to prepare it for implantation. At the beginning of the luteal phase, progesterone induces the endometrial glands to secrete glycogen, mucus, and other substances. These glands become tortuous and have large lumens due to increased secretory activity. The progesterone secreted by the corpus luteum causes the temperature of the body to rise slightly until the start of the next period. A slight increase in temperature (approximately 0.5°C) is generally seen just before ovulation occurs (Cunningham et al., 2010); the temperature remains elevated for several days after menstruation begins. This rise in temperature can be plotted on a graph and gives an indication of when ovulation has occurred. In the absence of fertilization, the corpus luteum begins to degenerate and consequently ovarian hormone levels decrease. As estrogen and progesterone levels decrease, the endometrium undergoes involution. In a 28-day cycle, menstruation then begins approximately 14 days after ovulation in the absence of pregnancy. FSH and LH are generally at their lowest levels during the luteal phase and highest during the follicular phase.

▶ *Consider THIS!*

We had been married 2 years when my husband and I decided to start a family. I began thinking back to my high school biology class and tried to remember about ovulation and what to look for. I also used the Internet to find the answers I was seeking. As I was reading, it all started to come into place. During ovulation, a woman's cervical mucus increases and she experiences a wet sensation for several days midcycle. The mucus also becomes stretchable during this time. In addition, body temperature rises slightly and then falls if no conception takes place. Armed with this knowledge, I began to check my temperature daily before arising and began to monitor the consistency of my cervical mucus. I figured that monitoring these two signs of ovulation could help me discover the best time to conceive. After 6 months of trying without results, I wondered what I was doing wrong. Did I really understand my body's reproductive activity?

What additional suggestions might the nurse offer this woman in her journey to conception? What community resources might be available to assist this couple? How does knowledge of the reproductive system help nurses take care of couples who are trying to become pregnant?

Endometrial Cycle

The endometrial cycle occurs in response to cyclical hormonal changes. The four phases of the endometrial cycle are the proliferative phase, secretory phase, ischemic phase, and menstrual phase.

Proliferative Phase

The proliferative phase starts with enlargement of the endometrial glands in response to the increasing amounts

of estrogen. The blood vessels become dilated and the endometrium increases in thickness dramatically in preparation for implantation of the fertilized ovum (Cunningham et al., 2010). Cervical mucus becomes thin, clear, stretchy, and more alkaline, making it more favourable to sperm to enhance the opportunity for fertilization. The proliferative phase starts on about day five of the menstrual cycle and lasts to the time of ovulation. This phase depends on estrogen stimulation resulting from ovarian follicles, and this phase coincides with the follicular phase of the ovarian cycle.

Secretory Phase

The secretory phase begins at ovulation to about 3 days before the next menstrual period. Under the influence of progesterone released by the corpus luteum after ovulation, the endometrium becomes thickened and more vascular (growth of the spiral arteries) and glandular (secreting more glycogen and lipids). These dramatic changes are all in preparation for implantation, if it were to occur. This phase typically lasts from day 15 (after ovulation) to day 28 and coincides with the luteal phase of the ovarian cycle. The secretory phase does not take place if ovulation has not occurred.

Ischemic Phase

If fertilization does not occur, the ischemic phase begins. Estrogen and progesterone levels drop sharply during this phase as the corpus luteum starts to degenerate. Changes in the endometrium occur with spasm of the arterioles, resulting in ischemia of the basal layer. The ischemia leads to shedding of the endometrium down to the basal layer, and menstrual flow begins.

Menstrual Phase

The menstrual phase begins as the spiral arteries rupture secondary to ischemia, releasing blood into the uterus, and the sloughing of the endometrial lining begins. If fertilization does not take place, the corpus luteum degenerates. As a result, both estrogen and progesterone levels fall and the thickened endometrial lining sloughs away from the uterine wall and passes out via the vagina. The beginning of the menstrual flow marks the end of one menstrual cycle and the start of a new one. Most women report bleeding for an average of 3 to 7 days. The amount of menstrual flow varies, but approximately 177 to 237 mm (6 to 8 oz) in volume per cycle is average (Alexander et al., 2010).

Menstrual Cycle Hormones

The menstrual cycle involves a complex interaction of hormones. The predominant hormones include gonadotropin-releasing hormone (GnRH), FSH, LH, estrogen, progesterone, and prostaglandins. Box 3.1 summarizes menstrual cycle hormones.

Gonadotropin–Releasing Hormone

GnRH is secreted from the hypothalamus in a pulsatile manner throughout the reproductive cycle. It pulsates

---

BOX 3.1 **Summary of Menstrual Cycle Hormones**

- LH rises and stimulates the follicle to produce estrogen.
- As estrogen is produced by the follicle, estrogen levels rise, inhibiting the output of LH.
- Ovulation occurs after an LH surge damages the estrogen-producing cells, resulting in a decline in estrogen.
- The LH surge results in establishment of the corpus luteum, which produces estrogen and progesterone.
- Estrogen and progesterone levels rise, suppressing LH output.
- Lack of LH promotes degeneration of the corpus luteum.
- Cessation of the corpus luteum means a decline in estrogen and progesterone output.
- The decline of the ovarian hormones ends their negative effect on the secretion of LH.
- LH is secreted, and the menstrual cycle begins again.

---

slowly during the follicular phase and increases during the luteal phase. GnRH induces the release of FSH and LH to assist with ovulation.

Follicle-Stimulating Hormone

Follicle-stimulating hormone (FSH) is secreted by the anterior pituitary gland and is primarily responsible for the maturation of the ovarian follicle. FSH secretion is highest and most important during the first week of the follicular phase of the reproductive cycle.

Luteinizing Hormone

Luteinizing hormone (LH) is secreted by the anterior pituitary gland and is required for both the final maturation of preovulatory follicles and luteinization of the ruptured follicle. As a result, estrogen production declines and progesterone secretion continues. Thus, estrogen levels fall a day before ovulation, and progesterone levels begin to rise.

Estrogen

Estrogen is secreted by the ovaries and is crucial for the development and maturation of the follicle. Estrogen is predominant at the end of the proliferative phase, directly preceding ovulation. After ovulation, estrogen levels drop sharply as progesterone dominates. In the endometrial cycle, estrogen induces proliferation of the endometrial glands. Estrogen also causes the uterus to increase in size and weight because of increased glycogen, amino acids, electrolytes, and water. Blood supply is expanded as well.

Progesterone

Progesterone is secreted by the corpus luteum. Progesterone levels increase just before ovulation and peak 5 to 7 days after ovulation. During the luteal phase, progesterone induces swelling and increased secretion of the endometrium. This hormone is often called the hormone of pregnancy because of its calming effect (reduces uterine contractions) on the uterus, allowing pregnancy to be maintained.

Prostaglandins

Prostaglandins are a closely related group of oxygenated fatty acids that are produced by the endometrium, with a variety of effects throughout the body. Although they have regulatory effects and are sometimes called hormones, prostaglandins are not classified as hormones; they are found in many parts of the body (Ward & Hisley, 2009). Prostaglandins increase during follicular maturation and play a key role in ovulation by freeing the ovum inside the graafian follicle. Large amounts of prostaglandins are found in menstrual blood.

Menopause

Perimenopause and menopause are biologic markers of the transition from young adulthood to middle age. Neither of these is a symptom or disease, but rather a natural maturing of the reproductive system.

During the perimenopausal years (2 to 8 years prior to menopause), women may experience physical changes associated with decreasing estrogen levels, which may include vasomotor symptoms of hot flashes, irregular menstrual cycles, sleep disruptions, forgetfulness, irritability, mood disturbances, decreased vaginal lubrication, fatigue, vaginal atrophy, palpitations, decreased energy, and depression (Nevin & Ehrenthal, 2008).

Menopause refers to the cessation of regular menstrual cycles. This naturally occurring phase of every woman's life marks the end of menstruation and childbearing capacity. The average age of natural menopause—defined as 1 year without a menstrual period—is 51 years (Alexander et al., 2010). As the average life expectancy for women increases, the number of women reaching and living in menopause has escalated. Most women can expect to spend more than one third of their lives beyond menopause. It is usually marked by atrophy of the breasts, uterus, fallopian tubes, and ovaries (Schorge, Schaffer, Halvorson, et al., 2008).

Many women pass through menopause without untoward symptoms. These women remain active and in good health with little interruption of their daily routines. Other women experience vasomotor symptoms, which give rise to sensations of heat, cold, sweating, headache, insomnia, and irritability (Nevin & Ehrenthal, 2008). Until recently, hormone therapy was the mainstay of menopause pharmacotherapy, but with the recent results of the Women's Health Initiative trial, the use of hormone therapy has become controversial. Many women have turned to nontraditional remedies to manage their menopausal symptoms. Common herbal remedies used include Dong Quai, black cohosh, soy or isoflavone supplementation, ginseng, and St. John's wort. Research to validate their efficacy, safety, and potential harmful effects is lacking at this time, and much of the efficacy is largely anecdotal (Rees, 2008). Nurses can play a major role in assisting menopausal women by educating and counselling them about the multitude of options available for disease prevention, treatment for menopausal symptoms, and health promotion during this time of change in their lives. Menopause should be an opportunity for women to strive for a healthy, long life, and nurses can help to make this opportunity a reality. (See Chapter 4 for more information about menopause.)

Recall Linda, who was experiencing changes in her menstrual patterns. Which hormones might be changing, and which systems might they affect? What approach should the nurse take to enlighten Linda about what is happening to her?

Male Reproductive Anatomy and Physiology

The male reproductive system, like that of the female, consists of those organs that facilitate reproduction. The male organs are specialized to produce and maintain the male sex cells, or sperm; to transport them, along with supporting fluids, to the female reproductive system; and to secrete the male hormone testosterone. The organs of the male reproductive system include the two testes (where sperm cells and testosterone are made), the penis, the scrotum, and the accessory organs (epididymis, vas deferens, seminal vesicles, ejaculatory duct, urethra, bulbourethral glands, and prostate gland).

External Male Reproductive Organs

The penis and the scrotum form the external genitalia in the male (Fig. 3.7).

Penis

The **penis** is the organ for copulation and serves as the outlet for both sperm and urine. The skin of the penis is thin, with no hairs. The prepuce (foreskin) is a circular fold of skin that extends over the glans unless it is removed by circumcision shortly after birth. The urinary meatus, located at the tip of the penis, serves as the external opening to the urethra (Fig. 3.8). The penis is composed mostly of erectile tissue. Most of the body of the penis consists of three cylindrical spaces (sinuses) of erectile tissue. The two larger ones, the corpora cavernosa, are side by side. The third sinus, the corpus spongiosum, surrounds the urethra. Erection results when

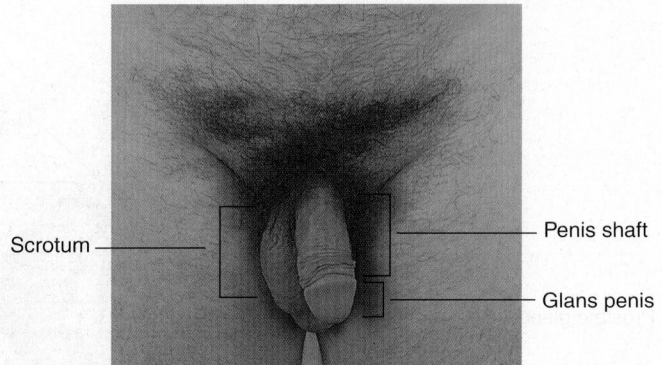

FIGURE 3.7 The external male reproductive organs. (Photo by B. Proud.)

nerve impulses from the autonomic nervous system dilate the arteries of the penis, allowing arterial blood to flow into the erectile tissues of the organ.

Scrotum

The scrotum is the thin-skinned sac that surrounds and protects the testes. The scrotum also acts as a climate-control system for the testes, because they need to be slightly cooler than body temperature to allow normal sperm development. The cremaster muscles in the scrotal wall relax or contract to allow the testes to hang farther from the body to cool or to be pulled closer to the body for warmth or protection (Luctkar-Flude & Jarvis, 2009). A medial septum divides the scrotum into two chambers, each of which encloses a testis.

Internal Male Reproductive Organs

The internal structures include the testes, the ductal system, and accessory glands (Fig. 3.9).

Testes

The **testes** are oval bodies about the size of large olives that lie in the scrotum; usually the left testis hangs a little

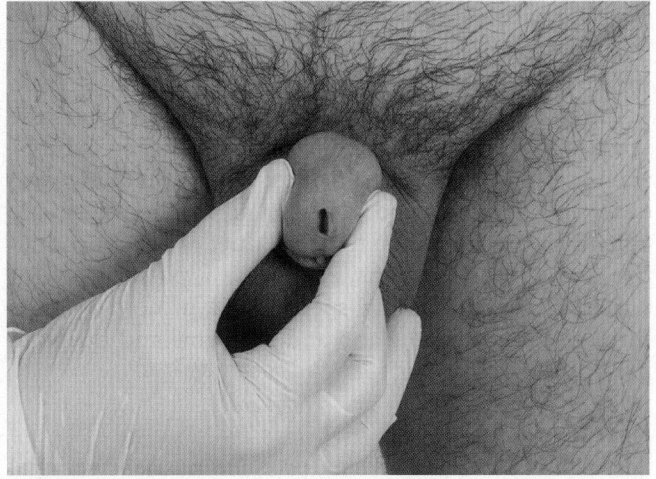

FIGURE 3.8 The urinary meatus. (Photo by B. Proud.)

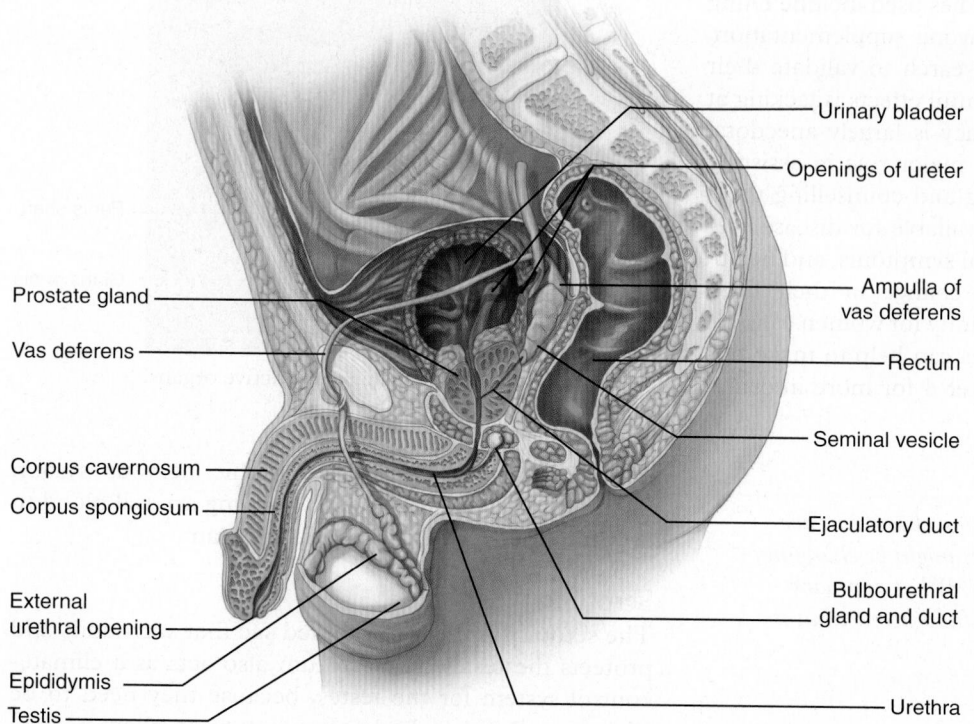

Prostate gland

Vas deferens

Corpus cavernosum

Corpus spongiosum

External
urethral opening

Epididymis

Testis

Urinary bladder

Openings of ureter

Ampulla of
vas deferens

Rectum

Seminal vesicle

Ejaculatory duct

Bulbourethral
gland and duct

Urethra

FIGURE 3.9 Lateral view of the internal male reproductive organs. (Source: Anatomical Chart Company. [2001]. *Atlas of human anatomy*. Springhouse, PA: Springhouse.)

lower than the right one. The testes have two functions: producing sperm and synthesizing testosterone (the primary male sex hormone). Sperm is produced in the seminiferous tubules of the testes. Similar to the female reproductive system, the anterior pituitary releases the gonadotropins, FSH, and LH. These hormones stimulate the testes to produce testosterone, which assists in maintaining spermatogenesis, increases sperm production by the seminiferous tubules, and stimulates production of seminal fluid (Ward & Hisley, 2009). The epididymis, which lies against the testes, is a coiled tube almost 6.1 metres (20 feet) long. It collects sperm from the testes and provides the space and environment for sperm to mature (Fig. 3.10).

The Ductal System

The vas deferens is a cord-like duct that transports sperm from the epididymis. One such duct travels from each testis up to the back of the prostate and enters the urethra to form the ejaculatory ducts. Other structures, such as blood vessels and nerves, also travel along with each vas deferens and together form the spermatic cord. The urethra is the terminal duct of the reproductive and urinary systems, serving as a passageway for semen (fluid containing sperm) and urine. It passes through the prostate gland and the penis and opens to the outside.

Accessory Glands

The seminal vesicles, which produce nutrient seminal fluid, and the prostate gland, which produces alkaline prostatic fluid, are both connected to the ejaculatory

duct leading into the urethra. The paired seminal vesicles are convoluted pouch-like structures lying posterior to, and at the base of, the urinary bladder in front of the rectum. They secrete an alkaline fluid that contains fructose and prostaglandins. The fructose supplies energy to the sperm on its journey to meet the ovum, and the prostaglandins assist in sperm mobility.

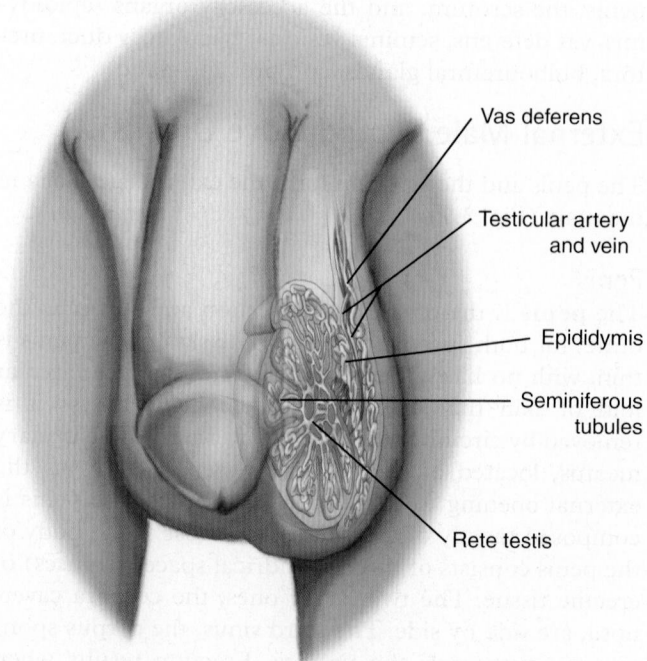

Vas deferens

Testicular artery
and vein

Epididymis

Seminiferous
tubules

Rete testis

FIGURE 3.10 Internal structures of a testis.

The prostate gland lies just under the bladder in the pelvis and surrounds the middle portion of the urethra. Usually the size of a walnut, this gland enlarges with age. The prostate and the seminal vesicles above it produce fluid that nourishes the sperm. This fluid provides most of the volume of semen, the secretion in which the sperm is expelled during ejaculation. Other fluid that makes up the semen comes from the vas deferens and from mucous glands in the head of the penis.

The bulbourethral glands (Cowper's glands) are two small structures about the size of peas, located inferior to the prostate gland. They are composed of several tubes whose epithelial linings secrete a mucus-like fluid. It is released in response to sexual stimulation and lubricates the head of the penis in preparation for sexual intercourse. The bulbourethral glands gradually diminish in size with advancing age.

Male Sexual Response

With sexual stimulation, the arteries leading to the penis dilate and increase blood flow into erectile tissues. At the same time, the erectile tissue compresses the veins of the penis, reducing blood flow away from the penis. Blood accumulates, causing the penis to swell and elongate and producing an erection. As in women, the culmination of sexual stimulation is an orgasm, a pleasurable feeling of physiologic and psychological release.

Orgasm is accompanied by emission (movement of sperm from the testes and fluids from the accessory glands) into the urethra, where it is mixed to form semen. As the urethra fills with semen, the base of the erect penis contracts, which increases pressure and forces the semen through the urethra to the outside (ejaculation). During ejaculation, the ducts of the testes, epididymis, and vas deferens contract, causing expulsion of sperm into the urethra, where the sperm mixes with the seminal and prostatic fluids. These substances, together with mucus secreted by accessory glands, form the semen, which is discharged from the urethra.

■■■ Key Concepts

- The female reproductive system produces the female reproductive cells (the eggs or ova) and contains an organ (uterus) where the fetus develops. The male reproductive system produces the male reproductive cells (the sperm) and contains an organ (penis) that deposits the sperm within the female.
- The internal female reproductive organs consist of the vagina, the uterus, the fallopian tubes, and the ovaries. The external female reproductive organs make up the vulva. These include the mons pubis, the labia majora and minora, the clitoris, structures within the vestibule, and the perineum.
- The breasts are accessory organs of the female reproductive system that are specialized to secrete milk following pregnancy.

- The main function of the reproductive cycle is to stimulate growth of a follicle to release an egg and prepare a site for implantation if fertilization occurs.
- Menstruation, the monthly shedding of the uterine lining, marks the beginning and end of the cycle if fertilization does not occur.
- The ovarian cycle is the series of events associated with a developing oocyte (ovum or egg) within the ovaries.
- At ovulation, a mature follicle ruptures in response to a surge of LH, releasing a mature oocyte (ovum).
- The endometrial cycle is divided into four phases: the follicular or proliferative phase, the luteal or secretory phase, the ischemic phase, and the menstrual phase.
- The menstrual cycle involves a complex interaction of hormones. The predominant hormones are GnRH, FSH, LH, estrogen, progesterone, and prostaglandins.
- The organs of the male reproductive system include the two testes (where sperm cells and testosterone are made), penis, scrotum, and accessory organs (epididymis, vas deferens, seminal vesicles, ejaculatory ducts, urethra, bulbourethral glands, and prostate gland).

REFERENCES

Alexander, L. L., LaRosa, J. H., Bader, H., & Garfield, S. (2010). *New dimensions in women's health* (5th ed.). Boston, MA: Jones and Bartlett.

Cunningham, F. G., Leveno, K. J., Bloom, S. L., et al. (2010). *Williams obstetrics* (23rd ed.). New York: McGraw-Hill.

Harris, M. A., Prior, J. C., & Koehoorn, M. (2008). Age at menarche in the Canadian population: Secular trends and relationship to adulthood BMI. *Journal of Adolescent Health, 43*, 548–554.

Krapf, J. M., & Simon, J. A. (2009). The role of testosterone in the management of hypoactive sexual desire disorder in postmenopausal women, *Maturitus, 63*, 213–219.

London, M. L., Ladewig, P. W., Ball, J. W., Bindler, R. C., & Cowen, K. J. (2011). *Maternal and child nursing care* (3rd ed.). Upper Saddle River, NJ: Pearson.

Luctkar-Flude, M., & Jarvis, C. (2009). Male genitourinary system. In A. J. Browne, J. MacDonald-Jenkins, & M. Luctkar-Flude (Eds.), *Physical examination & health assessment: First Canadian edition.* Toronto, ON: Elsevier.

McBride, M. B., Rohoedes, D. J., & Shuster, L. T. (2010). Vulvovaginal atrophy. *Mayo Clinic Proceedings, 85*(1), 87–94.

Nevin, J. E., & Ehrenthal, D. (2008). Menopause. In A. L. Clouse & K. Sherif (Eds.), *Women's health in clinical practice: A handbook for primary care.* Totowa, NJ: Humana.

Rees, M. (2008). Alternative treatments for the menopause. *Best Practice & Research Clinical Obstetrics and Gynaecology, 23*, 151–161.

Schorge, J. O., Schaffer, J. I., Halvorson, L. M. Hoffman, B. L., Bradshaw, K. D., & Cunningham, F. G. (2008). *Williams gynecology.* New York: McGraw-Hill Medical.

Tarlier, D., & Jarvis, C. (2009). Breasts and regional lymphatics. Physical examination & health assessment. In A. J. Browne, J. MacDonald-Jenkins, & M. Luctkar-Flude (Eds.), *Physical examination & health assessment: First Canadian edition.* Toronto, ON: Elsevier.

Ward, W. L., & Hisley, S. M. (2009). *Maternal-child nursing care.* Philadelphia: FA Davis.

World Health Organization. (2010). *Female genital mutilation.* Retrieved January 13, 2012 from http://www.who.int/mediacentre/factsheets/fs241/en/

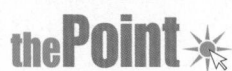

For additional learning materials, including Internet Resources, visit **http://thePoint.lww.com/Chow1e.**

CHAPTER WORKSHEET

MULTIPLE CHOICE QUESTIONS

1. The predominant anterior pituitary hormones that orchestrate the menstrual cycle include:

   a. Thyroid-stimulating hormone (TSH)

   b. Follicle-stimulating hormone (FSH)

   c. Corticotropin-releasing hormone (CRH)

   d. Gonadotropin-releasing hormone (GnRH)

2. Which glands are located on either side of the female urethra and secrete mucus to keep the opening moist and lubricated for urination?

   a. Cowper's

   b. Bartholin's

   c. Skene's

   d. Seminal

3. What event occurs during the proliferative phase of the menstrual cycle?

   a. Menstrual flow starts

   b. Growth hormone is secreted

   c. Ovulation occurs

   d. Progesterone secretion peaks

4. Which hormone is produced in high levels to prepare the endometrium for implantation just after ovulation by the corpus luteum?

   a. Estrogen

   b. Prostaglandins

   c. Prolactin

   d. Progesterone

5. Sperm maturation and storage in the male reproductive system occurs in the:

   a. Testes

   b. Vas deferens

   c. Epididymis

   d. Seminal vesicles

CRITICAL THINKING EXERCISE

1. The school nurse was asked to speak to a 10th-grade biology class about menstruation. The teacher feels that the students do not understand this monthly event and wants to dispel some myths about it. After the nurse explains the factors influencing the menses, one girl asks, "Could someone get pregnant if she had sex during her period?"

   a. How should the nurse respond to this question?

   b. What factor regarding the menstrual cycle was not clarified?

   c. What additional topics might this question lead to that might be discussed?

STUDY ACTIVITIES

1. Go to http://thepoint.lww.com/Chow1e to view a list of Web resources. Select one and visit it to find information concerning a topic of interest regarding women's health. Be prepared to discuss it in class.

2. List the predominant hormones and their function in the menstrual cycle.

3. The ovarian cycle describes the series of events associated with the development of the _____ within the ovaries.

4. Sperm cells and the male hormone testosterone are made in which of the following structures? Select all that apply.

   a. Vas deferens

   b. Penis

   c. Scrotum

   d. Ejaculatory ducts

   e. Prostate gland

   f. Testes

   g. Seminiferous tubules

   h. Bulbourethral glands

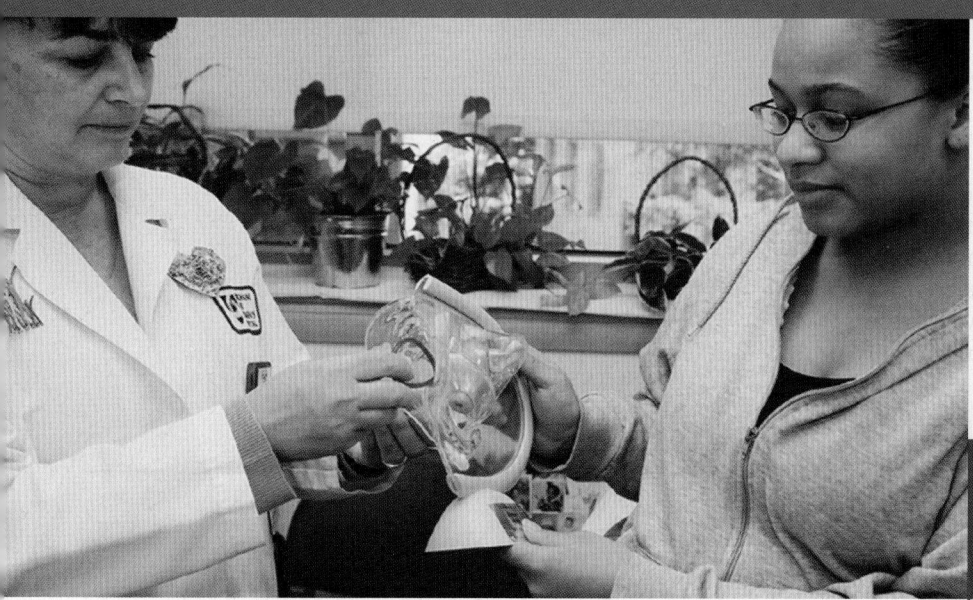

COMMON REPRODUCTIVE ISSUES

KEY TERMS

abortion
abnormal uterine
  bleeding (AUB)
abstinence
amenorrhea
basal body temperature
  (BBT)
cervical cap
cervical mucus ovulation
  method
coitus interruptus
condoms
contraception
contraceptive
  sponge

continuous oral
  contraception (COC)
Depo-Provera
diaphragm
dysfunctional uterine
  bleeding (DUB)
dysmenorrhea
emergency
  contraception
endometriosis
fertility awareness
implant
infertility
intrauterine device
  (IUD)

intrauterine system (IUS)
lactational amenorrhea
  method (LAM)
menopause
oral contraceptives (OCs)
premenstrual syndrome
  (PMS)
standard days method
  (SDM)
sterilization
symptothermal method
transdermal patch
tubal ligation
vaginal ring
vasectomy

LEARNING OBJECTIVES

Upon completion of the chapter, the learner will be able to:

1. Define the key terms used in this chapter.
2. Examine common reproductive concerns in terms of symptoms, diagnostic tests, and appropriate interventions.
3. Identify risk factors and outline appropriate client education needed in common reproductive disorders.
4. Compare and contrast the various contraceptive methods available and their overall effectiveness.
5. Explain the physiologic and psychological aspects of menopause.
6. Delineate the nursing management needed for women experiencing common reproductive disorders.

I zzy, a 27-year-old kindergarten teacher, presents to her health care provider complaining of progressive severe pelvic pain associated with her monthly periods. She has to take off work and "dope up" with pills to endure the pain. In addition, she and her husband Grady have been trying unsuccessfully to conceive for over a year.

Wow

When women bare their souls to us, we must respond without judgment.

Good health throughout the life cycle begins with the individual. Women today can expect to live well into their 80s and need to be proactive in maintaining their own quality of life. Women need to take steps to reduce their risk of disease and become active partners with their health care professional in order to identify problems early, when treatment may be most successful (Teaching Guideline 4.1). Nurses can assist women in maintaining their quality of life by helping them to become more attuned to their body and its clues and can use the assessment period as an opportunity for teaching and counselling.

Common reproductive issues addressed in this chapter that nurses might encounter in caring for women include menstrual disorders, infertility, contraception, abortion, and menopause.

Menstrual Disorders

Many women progress through their monthly menstrual cycle with little or no concern. With few symptoms to worry about, their menses are like clockwork, starting and stopping at nearly the same time every month. For others, the menstrual cycle causes physical and emotional symptoms that initiate visits to their health care provider for consultation. The following menstruation-related conditions will be discussed in this chapter: amenorrhea, dysmenorrhea, dysfunctional uterine bleeding (DUB), premenstrual syndrome (PMS), premenstrual dysphoric disorder (PMDD), and endometriosis. To gain an understanding of menstrual disorders, it is important to know the terms used in describing them (Box 4.1).

TEACHING GUIDELINE 4.1

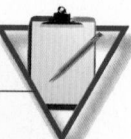

Tips for Being an Active Partner in Managing Your Health

- Become an informed consumer. Read, ask, and search.
- Know your family history, and know the factors that put you at high risk.
- Maintain a healthy lifestyle and let moderation be your guide.
- Schedule regular medical checkups and screenings for early detection.
- Ask your health care professional for a full explanation of any treatment.
- Seek a second medical opinion if you feel you need more information.
- Know when to seek medical care by being aware of disease symptoms.

BOX 4.1 **Menstrual Disorder Vocabulary**

- meno = menstrual-related
- metro = time
- oligo = few
- a = without, none or lack of
- rhagia = excess or abnormal
- dys = not or pain
- rhea = flow

Amenorrhea

Amenorrhea is the absence of menses during the reproductive years. Amenorrhea is normal in prepubertal, pregnant, and postmenopausal females. The most common cause of amenorrhea is pregnancy, but it can also result from disorders of the reproductive organs or conditions associated with the glands that regulate hormone levels (Mayo Clinic Staff, 2011a). Amenorrhea is categorized as primary or secondary. Primary amenorrhea is defined in one of two ways:

- Absence of menses by age 14, with the absence of growth and development of secondary sexual characteristics
- Absence of menses by age 16, with the normal development of secondary sexual characteristics (Bielak & Harris, 2010)

Girls can begin to menstruate around 9 or 10 years of age (Canadian Pediatric Society [CPS], 2012). No wide-ranging Canadian-specific studies have yet been completed that indicate when menstruation occurs in the majority of girls (O'Grady, 2008/2009). Secondary amenorrhea is the absence of menses for three cycles or 6 months in women who have previously menstruated regularly.

Etiology

There are multiple causes of amenorrhea:

- Natural
  - Pregnancy
  - Breastfeeding
- Hormone imbalances
  - Hypothyroid/hyperthyroid conditions
- Lifestyle
  - Extreme or rapid weight gain or loss
  - Emotional stress from a major life event
  - Excessive/vigorous exercise, such as long-distance running
  - Eating disorders (anorexia nervosa or bulimia)/malnutrition
- Medications
  - Tranquilizers/antidepressants

Additional causes of primary amenorrhea may include:

- Birth control medications (oral, injected, implanted, or intrauterine) (Mayo Clinic Staff, 2011a)
- Hormone imbalances, such as Cushing's disease, polycystic ovary syndrome, Turner syndrome, or chronic illness
- Medications, including some street drugs, antipsychotics, or blood pressure medications
- Structural problems, including congenital abnormalities of the reproductive system, imperforate hymen, uterine scarring, or lack of reproductive organs

Other causes of secondary amenorrhea might include:

- Pituitary, ovarian, or adrenal tumours
- Depression
- Hyperprolactinemia
- Chemotherapy or radiation therapy to the pelvic area
- Kidney failure
- Colitis
- Postpartum pituitary necrosis (Sheehan syndrome)

Therapeutic Management

Therapeutic intervention depends on the cause of amenorrhea. The treatment of primary amenorrhea involves correction of any underlying disorders and hormone replacement therapy (HRT) to stimulate the development of secondary sexual characteristics. If a pituitary tumour is the cause, it might be treated with drug therapy, surgical resection, or radiation therapy. Surgery might be needed to correct any structural abnormalities of the genital tract. Therapeutic interventions for amenorrhea may include:

- Cyclic progesterone, when the cause is anovulation, or oral contraceptives (OCs)
- Bromocriptine to treat hyperprolactinemia
- Nutritional counselling to address anorexia, bulimia, or obesity
- Gonadotropin-releasing hormone (GnRH), when the cause is hypothalamic failure
- Thyroid hormone replacement, when the cause is hypothyroidism (Mayo Clinic Staff, 2011a)

Nursing Assessment

Nursing assessment for the young girl or woman experiencing amenorrhea includes a thorough health history and physical examination and several laboratory and diagnostic tests.

Health History and Physical Examination

A thorough history and physical examination are needed to determine the etiology. The history should include questions about the woman's menstrual history; family medical history; past illnesses; hospitalizations and surgeries; obstetric history; use of prescription, over-the-counter, or illicit drugs or natural or homeopathic remedies; recent or past lifestyle changes; and history of present illness, with an assessment of any bodily changes.

The physical examination should begin with an overall assessment of the woman's nutritional status and general health. A sensitive and gentle approach to the pelvic examination is critical in young women. Height and weight should be taken, along with vital signs, with particular attention to blood pressure. Hypothermia, bradycardia, hypotension, and reduced subcutaneous fat may be observed in women with anorexia nervosa. Facial hair and acne might be evidence of androgen excess secondary to a tumour. The presence or absence of axillary and pubic hair may indicate adrenal and ovarian hyposecretion or delayed puberty. A general physical examination (including breasts and genital exam) may uncover unexpected findings that are indirectly related to amenorrhea. For example, hepatosplenomegaly, which may suggest a chronic systemic disease or an enlarged thyroid gland, might point to a thyroid disorder as well as a reason for amenorrhea.

Laboratory and Diagnostic Tests

Common laboratory tests that might be ordered to determine the cause of amenorrhea include:

- Pregnancy test to rule out pregnancy
- Karyotype (might be positive for Turner syndrome)
- Ultrasonography to detect ovarian cysts
- Thyroid function studies to determine thyroid disorder
- Prolactin level (an elevated level might indicate a pituitary tumour)
- Follicle-stimulating hormone (FSH) level (an elevated level might indicate ovarian failure)
- Luteinizing hormone (LH) level (an elevated level might indicate gonadal dysfunction)
- 17-ketosteroid level (an elevated level might indicate an adrenal tumour)
- Laparoscopy to detect polycystic ovary syndrome

Nursing Management

Counselling and education are primary interventions and appropriate nursing roles. Address the diverse causes of amenorrhea, the relationship to sexual identity, possible infertility, and the possibility of a tumour or life-threatening disease. In addition, inform the woman about the purpose of each diagnostic test, how it is performed, and when the results will be available to discuss with her. Sensitive listening, interviewing, and presenting treatment options are paramount to gain the woman's cooperation and understanding.

Nutritional counselling is also vital in managing this disorder, especially if the woman has findings suggestive of an eating disorder. Although not all causes can be addressed by making lifestyle changes, emphasize maintaining a healthy lifestyle (Teaching Guideline 4.2).

TEACHING GUIDELINE 4.2

Tips for Maintaining a Healthy Lifestyle

- Balance energy expenditure with energy intake.
- Modify your diet to maintain ideal weight.
- Avoid excessive use of alcohol and mood-altering or sedative drugs.
- Avoid cigarette smoking.
- Identify areas of emotional stress and seek assistance to resolve them.
- Balance work, recreation, and rest.
- Maintain a positive outlook regarding the diagnosis and prognosis.
- Participate in ongoing care to monitor any medical conditions.
- Maintain bone density through:
  - Calcium intake (1,200 to 1,500 mg daily)
  - Weight-bearing exercise (30 minutes or more daily)
  - Hormone therapy

Source: Popat, V., Sullivan, S. D., Trupin, S. R., et al. (2011). *Amenorrhea*. Retrieved March 4, 2012 from http://www.emedicine.com/med/topic117.htm.

Dysmenorrhea

Dysmenorrhea refers to painful menstruation. The term **dysmenorrhea** is derived from the Greek words "dys," meaning difficult, painful, or abnormal, and "rrhea," meaning flow. Dysmenorrhea is the most common gynecologic symptom reported by women (Lefebvre, Pinsonneault, Antao, et al., 2005). Uterine contractions occur during all periods, but in some women these cramps can be frequent and very intense. Dysmenorrhea is categorized as primary or secondary.

Etiology

Primary dysmenorrhea is caused by increased prostaglandin production by the endometrium in an ovulatory cycle. Prostaglandin causes contraction of the uterus, and levels of this hormone tend to be higher in women with severe menstrual pain than in women who experience mild or no menstrual pain. Increased prostaglandin levels result in increased rhythmic uterine contractions from vasoconstriction of the small vessels of the uterine wall. This condition usually begins after a pre-teen or teen begins menstruation but should become less painful with age or after pregnancy (American College of Obstetricians and Gynecologists [ACOG], 2011b).

Secondary dysmenorrhea is painful menstruation due to pelvic or uterine pathology. It may begin later in life and often lasts longer than normal cramps. It may be caused by endometriosis, adenomyosis, fibroids, pelvic infection, an **intrauterine device (IUD)**, cervical stenosis, or congenital uterine or vaginal abnormalities.

Adenomyosis involves the ingrowth of the endometrium into the uterine musculature. Endometriosis involves ectopic implantation of endometrial tissue in other parts of the pelvis. It occurs most commonly in the third or fourth decade of life and affects 10% of women of reproductive age (Leyland, Casper, Laberge, et al., 2010). Endometriosis is certainly one of the most frequent causes of secondary dysmenorrhea and is a disease that can also affect younger patients (Lefebvre et al., 2005). Fibroids are tumours or growths in the muscles that form outside, inside, or within the walls of the uterus. Some patients with fibroids report both pain and/or heavy menstrual bleeding (ACOG, 2011b). Treatment is directed toward correcting or removing the underlying pathology.

*T*hink back to Izzy from the beginning of chapter. What do you think may be causing her pain? Do you think her pain is a common complaint for women in her age group?

Therapeutic Management

Therapeutic intervention for women with dysmenorrhea is directed toward pain relief and building coping strategies that will promote a productive lifestyle. Treatment measures usually include treating infections if present; suppressing the endometrium if endometriosis is suspected by administering low-dose OCs; administering over-the-counter pain medications, nonsteroidal anti-inflammatory drugs (NSAIDs), or prostaglandin inhibitors to reduce the pain; administering Depo-Provera or inserting an IUD; and initiating lifestyle changes such as exercise, better sleep patterns, and relaxation techniques. Table 4.1 lists selected treatment options for dysmenorrhea.

Nursing Assessment

As with any gynecologic complaint, a thorough, focused history and physical examination are needed to make the diagnosis of primary or secondary dysmenorrhea. In primary dysmenorrhea, the history usually reveals the typical cramping pain with menstruation and the physical examination is completely normal. In secondary dysmenorrhea, the history discloses cramping pain starting after 25 years of age with a pelvic abnormality, a history of infertility, heavy menstrual flow, irregular cycles, and little response to NSAIDs, OCs, or both (Stöppler, 2011).

Health History and Clinical Manifestations

Note past medical history, including any chronic illnesses and family history of gynecologic concerns. Determine medication and substance use, such as prescription medications, contraceptives, anabolic steroids, tobacco, and marijuana, cocaine, or other illegal drugs. A detailed sexual history is essential to assess for inflammation and scarring (adhesions) secondary to pelvic inflammatory disease

TABLE 4.1 **TREATMENT OPTIONS FOR DYSMENORRHEA**

Therapy Options	Dosage	Comments
Nonsteroidal anti-inflammatory drugs (NSAIDs)		
Ibuprofen (Ibuprin, Advil, Motrin)	400–800 mg tid	Take with meals. Don't take with aspirin. Avoid alcohol. Watch for signs of GI bleeding.
Naproxen (Anaprox, Naprelan, Naprosyn, Aleve)	250–500 mg tid	Same as above
Hormonal contraceptives		
Low-dose oral contraceptives	Taken daily (42/7 days, 63/7, or 84/7)	Take active pills for an extended time to reduce number of monthly cycles (Archer, 2006).
Depo-medroxyproges-terone (DMPA) (Depo-Provera)	150 mg IM every 12 weeks	After 12 months of DMPA therapy, 40% to 50% of women will be amenorrheic (Schuiling & Likis, 2013).
Lifestyle changes		
Daily exercise Limit salty foods Weight loss Smoking cessation Relaxation techniques		Gives sense of control over life

(PID). Women with a previous history of PID, sexually transmitted infections (STIs), multiple sexual partners, or unprotected sex are at increased risk.

During the initial interview, the nurse might ask some of the following questions to assess the woman's history of dysmenorrhea:

- At what age did your menstrual cycles begin?
- Have your cycles always been painful, or did the pain start recently?
- When in your cycle do you experience the pain?
- How would you describe the pain you feel?
- Are you sexually active?
- What impact does your cycle have on your physical and social activity?
- When was the first day of your last menstrual cycle?
- Was the flow of your last menstrual cycle a normal amount for you?
- Do your cycles tend to be heavy or last longer than 5 days?
- Are your cycles generally regular and predictable?
- What have you done to relieve your discomfort? Is it effective?
- Has there been a progression of symptom severity?
- Do you have any other symptoms?

Assess for clinical manifestations of dysmenorrhea. Affected women experience sharp, intermittent spasms of pain, usually in the suprapubic area. Pain may radiate to the back of the legs or the lower back. Typically, primary dysmenorrhea is not caused by an underlying medical condition. It is characterized by a crampy suprapubic pain that begins somewhere between several hours before and a few hours after the onset of the menstrual bleeding. Symptoms of dysmenorrhea peak with maximum blood flow and usually last less than 1 day, but the pain may persist up to 2 to 3 days (Lefebvre et al., 2005). Secondary dysmenorrhea usually involves a medical condition that involves a woman's reproductive system. Systemic symptoms of nausea, vomiting, diarrhea, fatigue, fever, headache, or dizziness are fairly common. Explore the history for physical symptoms of bloating, water retention, weight gain, headache, muscle aches, abdominal pain, food cravings, or breast tenderness (Stöppler, 2011).

Physical Examination

When completing a physical examination for concerns related to dysmenorrhea, the health care provider should perform a bimanual pelvic examination. This examination is done during the nonmenstrual phase of the cycle. Explain to the woman how it is to be performed, especially if is her first pelvic examination. Prepare the woman in the examining room by offering her a cover gown to put on and covering her lap with a privacy sheet on the examination table. Remain in the examining room throughout the examination to assist the health care provider with any procedures or specimens and to offer the woman reassurance.

Laboratory and Diagnostic Tests

Common laboratory tests that may be ordered to determine the cause of dysmenorrhea might include:

• Complete blood count to rule out anemia
• Urinalysis to rule out a bladder infection
• Pregnancy test (human chorionic gonadotropin [HCG] level) to rule out pregnancy
• Cervical culture to exclude STI
• Erythrocyte sedimentation rate to detect an inflammatory process
• Stool guaiac to exclude gastrointestinal bleeding or disorders
• Pelvic and/or vaginal ultrasound to detect pelvic masses or cysts
• Diagnostic laparoscopy and/or laparotomy to visualize pathology that may account for the symptoms

What laboratory or diagnostic tests might be ordered to diagnose Izzy's pelvic pain?

Nursing Management

Educating the client about the normal events of the menstrual cycle and the etiology of her pain is paramount in achieving a successful outcome. Explaining the normal menstrual cycle will teach the woman the correct terms so she can communicate her symptoms more accurately and will help dispel myths. Provide the woman with monthly graphs or charts to record menses, the onset of pain, the timing of medication, relief afforded, and coping strategies used. This involves the woman in her care and provides objective information so that therapy can be modified if necessary.

The nurse should explain in detail the dosing regimen and the side effects of the medication selected. According to the Society of Obstetricians and Gynaecologists of Canada (SOGC), commonly prescribed drugs in Canada include NSAIDs such as ibuprofen (Motrin, Advil) and naproxen (Naprosyn) (Lefebvre et al., 2005). They alleviate dysmenorrhea symptoms by decreasing intrauterine pressure and inhibiting prostaglandin synthesis, thus reducing pain (Mannix, 2008). If pain relief is not achieved in two to four cycles, a low-dose combination OC may be initiated. Client teaching and counselling should include information about how to take pills, side effects, and symptoms of adverse reactions.

Encourage the woman to apply a heating pad or warm compress to alleviate menstrual cramps. Additional lifestyle changes that the woman can make to restore some sense of control and active participation in her care are listed in Teaching Guideline 4.3.

Dysfunctional Uterine Bleeding

Dysfunctional uterine bleeding (DUB) is a disorder that occurs most frequently in women at the beginning

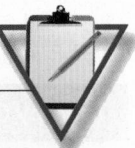

TEACHING GUIDELINE 4.3

Tips to Manage Dysmenorrhea

• Massage
• Acupressure
• Exercise frequently with activities such as walking, jogging, swimming, or biking to produce chemicals that reduce pain
• Use heating pads, hot water bottle or warm baths to increase comfort.
• Take a Vitamin B1 or Magnesium supplement
• Practice relaxation techniques to enhance ability to cope with pain. Yoga or meditation may be helpful

Source: ACOG. (2011b). *Frequently asked questions: Dysmenorrhea.* Retrieved March 4, 2012 from http://www.acog.org/~/media/For%20 Patients/faq046.pdf?dmc=1&ts=20120220T1216121334.

and end of their reproductive years. DUB is also one of the most common reasons that women are referred to a gynecologist (ACOG, 2011a; Telner & Jakubovicz, 2007). One in five women experiences DUB. This problem usually occurs during adolescence and during the 10 years preceding menopause. It is frequently associated with anovulatory cycles, which are common for the first year after menarche and later in life as women approach menopause. A similar condition, called **abnormal uterine bleeding (AUB)**, is defined as changes in the frequency of menses, the duration of flow, or the amount of blood loss (Vilos, Lefebvre, & Graves, 2001).

The pathophysiology of DUB is related to a hormone disturbance. With anovulation, estrogen levels rise as usual in the early phase of the menstrual cycle. In the absence of ovulation, a corpus luteum never forms and progesterone is not produced. The endometrium moves into a hyperproliferative state, ultimately outgrowing its estrogen supply. This leads to irregular sloughing of the endometrium and excessive bleeding (Zieve & Strock, 2011). If the bleeding is heavy enough and frequent enough, anemia can result.

DUB is similar to several other types of uterine bleeding disorders and sometimes overlaps these conditions. They include:

• Menorrhagia (abnormally long, heavy periods)
• Oligomenorrhea (bleeding occurs at intervals of more than 35 days)
• Metrorrhagia (bleeding between periods)
• Menometrorrhagia (bleeding occurs at irregular intervals with heavy flow lasting more than 7 days)
• Polymenorrhea (too frequent periods)

Etiology

The possible causes of DUB may include:

• Adenomyosis
• Pregnancy

- Hormonal imbalance
- Fibroid tumours (see Chapter 7)
- Endometrial polyps or cancer
- Endometriosis
- IUD use
- Polycystic ovary syndrome
- Morbid obesity
- Steroid therapy
- Hypothyroidism
- Blood dyscrasias/clotting disorder

Therapeutic Management

Treatment of DUB depends on the cause of the bleeding and the age of the client. When known, the underlying cause of the disorder is treated. Otherwise, the goal of treatment is to relieve the symptoms so that uterine bleeding does not interfere with a woman's normal activities or cause anemia (Zieve & Strock, 2011).

Management of DUB might include medical care with pharmacotherapy or insertion of an IUD. OCs are used for cycle regulation as well as contraception. They help prevent the risks associated with prolonged unopposed estrogen stimulation of the endometrium. NSAIDs and the levonorgestrel-releasing IUD (Mirena) decrease menstrual blood loss significantly (Lefebvre et al., 2005). The drug categories used in the treatment of DUB are:

- Estrogens: cause vasospasm of the uterine arteries to decrease bleeding
- Progestins: used to stabilize an estrogen-primed endometrium
- OCs: regulate the cycle and suppress the endometrium
- NSAIDs: inhibit prostaglandins
- Levonorgestrel-20 **intrauterine system (IUS)**: suppresses endometrial growth
- Iron salts: replenish iron stores lost during heavy bleeding

If the client does not respond to medical therapy, surgical intervention might include dilation and curettage (D&C), endometrial ablation, or hysterectomy. Endometrial ablation is an alternative to hysterectomy. A thermal balloon or a laser is used to ablate the tissue, producing improvement in 90% of women (McCausland & McCausland, 2010).

Nursing Assessment

A thorough history should be taken to differentiate between DUB and other conditions that might cause vaginal bleeding, such as pregnancy and pregnancy-related conditions (abruptio placentae, ectopic pregnancy, abortion, or placenta previa); systemic conditions such as Cushing syndrome, blood dyscrasias, liver disease, renal disease, or thyroid disease; and genital tract pathology such as infections, tumours, or trauma (Zieve & Strock, 2011).

Assess for clinical manifestations of DUB, which commonly include vaginal bleeding between periods, irregular menstrual cycles (usually less than 28 days between cycles), infertility, mood swings, hot flashes, vaginal tenderness, variable menstrual flow ranging from scanty to profuse, obesity, acne, and diabetes. Signs of polycystic ovary syndrome might be present, since it is associated with unopposed estrogen stimulation, elevated androgen levels, and insulin resistance and is a common cause of anovulation (Collier & Rieder, 2008).

Measure orthostatic blood pressure and orthostatic pulse; a drop in pressure or pulse rate may occur with anemia. The health care provider, with the nurse assisting, performs a pelvic examination to identify any structural abnormalities.

Laboratory and Diagnostic Tests

Common laboratory tests that may be ordered to determine the cause of DUB might include:

- Complete blood count (CBC) to detect anemia
- Prothrombin time (PT) to detect blood dyscrasias
- Pregnancy test (HCG level) to rule out a spontaneous abortion or ectopic pregnancy
- Thyroid-stimulating hormone (TSH) level to screen for hypothyroidism
- Transvaginal ultrasound to measure endometrium
- Pelvic ultrasound to view any structural abnormalities
- Endometrial biopsy to check for intrauterine pathology
- D&C for diagnostic evaluation (Thomas, 2011)

Nursing Management

Educate the client about normal menstrual cycles and the possible reasons for her abnormal pattern. Inform the woman about treatment options, including the contraindications and the risks associated with each treatment. Complications such as infertility can result from lack of ovulation; severe anemia can occur secondary to prolonged or heavy menses; and endometrial cancer can occur in association with prolonged build-up of the endometrial lining without menstrual bleeding. Instruct the woman about any prescribed medications and potential side effects. For example, if high-dose estrogens are prescribed, the woman may experience nausea. Teach her to take antiemetics as prescribed and encourage her to eat small, frequent meals to alleviate nausea. Adequate follow-up and evaluation for women who do not respond to medical management is essential. See Nursing Care Plan 4.1.

Premenstrual Syndrome

Premenstrual syndrome (PMS) describes a wide range of recurrent symptoms that occur during the luteal phase or last half of the menstrual cycle and resolve with the onset

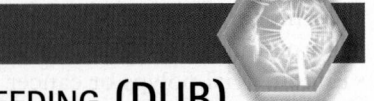

Nursing Care Plan 4.1

OVERVIEW OF A WOMAN WITH DYSFUNCTIONAL UTERINE BLEEDING (DUB)

Stacy, a 52-year-old obese woman, comes to her gynecologist with the complaint of heavy erratic bleeding. Her periods were fairly regular until about 4 months ago, and since that time they have been unpredictable, excessive, and prolonged. Stacy reports she is tired all the time, can't sleep, and feels "out of sorts" and anxious. She is fearful she has cancer.

NURSING DIAGNOSIS: Fear related to current signs and symptoms possibly indicating a life-threatening condition

Outcome Identification and Evaluation
The client will acknowledge her fears as evidenced by statements made that fear and anxiety have been lessened after explanation of diagnosis.

Interventions: Reducing Fear and Anxiety
- Distinguish between anxiety and fear *to determine appropriate interventions.*
- Check complete blood count and assess for possible anemia secondary to excessive bleeding to determine if fatigue is contributing to anxiety and fear. *Fatigue occurs because the oxygen-carrying capacity of the blood is reduced.*
- Reassure client that symptoms can be managed *to help address her current concerns.*
- Provide client with factual information and explain what to expect *to assist client with identifying fears and help in her coping with her condition.*
- Provide symptom management *to reduce concerns associated with the cause of bleeding.*
- Teach client about early manifestations of fear and anxiety *to aid in prompt recognition and to minimize escalation of anxiety.*
- Assess client's use of coping strategies in the past and reinforce use of effective ones *to help control anxiety and fear.*
- Instruct client in relaxation methods, such as deep breathing exercises and imagery, *to provide her with additional methods for controlling anxiety and fear.*

NURSING DIAGNOSIS: Deficient knowledge related to perimenopause and its management

Outcome Identification and Evaluation
The client will demonstrate understanding of her symptoms as evidenced by making health-promoting lifestyle choices, verbalizing appropriate health care practices, and adhering to measures to comply with therapy.

Interventions: Providing Patient Education
- Assess client's understanding of perimenopause and its treatment *to provide a baseline for teaching and developing a plan of care.*
- Review instructions about prescribed procedures and recommendations for self-care, frequently obtaining feedback from the client *to validate adequate understanding of information.*
- Outline link between anovulatory cycles and excessive buildup of uterine lining in perimenopausal women *to assist client in understanding the etiology of her bleeding.*
- Provide written material with pictures *to promote learning and help client visualize what is occurring to her body during perimenopause.*
- Inform client about the availability of community resources and make appropriate referrals as needed *to provide additional education and support.*
- Document details of teaching and learning *to allow for continuity of care and further education, if needed.*

---

of menstruation (Freeman, Halberstadt, Rickels, et al., 2011). More than 80% of Canadian women suffer from some form of PMS symptoms ranging from minor discomfort to significant impairment to normal life. Symptoms usually start 1 to 2 weeks before menstruation but usually go away after menstruation starts (HealthLink Alberta, 2006). Premenstrual symptoms can include mood, behav-

iour, and physical changes that occur prior to a woman's menstrual period.

Premenstrual dysphoric disorder (PMDD) is characterized by severe symptoms that lead to major interference with day-to-day activities and interpersonal relationships; 3% to 8% of women experience PMDD (Komar, 2012; SOGC, 2006c).

Diagnosis and Treatment

The ACOG diagnostic criteria for PMS consist of having at least one of the following affective and somatic symptoms during the 5 days before menses in each of the three successive cycles:

• Mental symptoms: depression, angry outbursts, irritability, anxiety
• Physical symptoms: breast tenderness, abdominal bloating, edema, headache
• Dysfunction in social or economic performance: marriage counselling, parenting difficulties, legal issues

Symptoms must disappear before day 4 of the menstrual cycle and not occur before day 14 to meet the criteria for diagnosis of PMS (ACOG, 2000).

In PMDD, the main symptoms are mood disorders such as depression, anxiety, tension, and persistent anger or irritability. Physical symptoms such as headache, joint and muscle pain, lack of energy, bloating, and breast tenderness are also present. According to the American Psychiatric Association, a woman must have at least five of the typical symptoms to be diagnosed with PMDD (Andoisek & Rapkin, 2007). These must occur during the week before and a few days after the onset of menstruation and must include one or more of the first four of the following symptoms:

1. Affective liability: sadness, tearfulness, irritability
2. Anxiety and tension
3. Persistent or marked anger or irritability
4. Depressed mood, feelings of hopelessness
5. Difficulty concentrating
6. Sleep difficulties
7. Increased or decreased appetite
8. Increased or decreased sexual desire
9. Chronic fatigue
10. Headache
11. Constipation or diarrhea
12. Breast swelling and tenderness

An estimated 20% to 40% of women who experience premenstrual symptoms seek help from their health care provider (Tschudin, Bertea, & Zemp, 2010).

▶ *Take* NOTE!

Because there are no diagnostic tests that can reliably determine the existence of PMS or PMDD, it is the woman herself who must decide that she needs help during this time of the month. The woman must embrace multiple therapies and become an active participant in her treatment plan to find the best level of symptom relief.

Therapeutic Management

Once a diagnosis has been made, several treatment options may be prescribed:

• NSAIDs may be used prior to or at the start of a woman's period to reduce cramps and breast tenderness.
• Certain OCs have been shown to offer relief from symptoms.
• Antidepressants may be used in more severe cases.
• Lifestyle changes such as regular exercise and dietary modifications may relieve mild symptoms (SOGC, 2006c).

Treatment of PMS is often frustrating for both patients and health care providers. Clinical outcomes can be expected to improve as a result of recent consensus on the diagnostic criteria for PMS and PMDD, data from clinical trials, and the availability of evidence-based clinical guidelines.

The management of PMS or PMDD requires a multidimensional approach because these conditions are not likely to have a single cause, and they appear to affect multiple systems within a woman's body; therefore, they are not likely to be amenable to treatment with a single therapy. Education, reassurance, and anticipatory guidance are needed to reduce the negative impact of premenstrual disorders on a woman's life and give her some sense of control over her condition.

Therapeutic interventions for PMS and PMDD address the symptoms because the exact cause of these conditions is still unknown. Treatments may include vitamin supplements, diet changes, exercise, lifestyle changes, and medications (Box 4.2). Medications used in treating PMDD may include antidepressant and anti-anxiety drugs, diuretics, anti-inflammatory medications, analgesics, synthetic androgen agents, OCs, or GnRH (agonists to regulate menses) (Komar, 2012).

Many women use dietary supplements and herbal remedies for their menstrual health and to treat their bleeding disorders, although there has been little research to demonstrate their efficacy. Some of these alternative therapies include calcium, magnesium, vitamin B6, evening primrose oil, vitex, ginkgo biloba, viburnum, dandelion, stinging nettle, burdock, raspberry leaf, skullcap, and St. John's wort (Canning, Waterman, & Dye, 2006).

Although research hasn't validated the efficacy of alternative therapies, it is important for the nurse to be aware of the alternative products that many women choose to use. For example, a recent study suggests that daily treatment with *Hypericum perforatum* (St. John's wort) was more effective than placebo for treating the most common physical and behavioural symptoms associated with PMS (Canning et al., 2006).

Nursing Assessment

Although little consensus exists in the medical literature and among researchers about what constitutes PMS and

BOX 4.2 Treatment Options for PMS and PMDD

- Lifestyle changes:
  Reduce stress.
  Exercise three to five times each week.
  Eat a balanced diet and increase water intake.
  Decrease caffeine intake.
  Stop smoking.
  Limit intake of alcohol.
  Attend a PMS/women's support group.
- Vitamin and mineral supplements:
  Multivitamin daily
  Vitamin E, 400 U/day
  Calcium, 1,200 mg/day
  Magnesium, 200 to 400 mg/day
- Medications:
  NSAIDs taken a week prior to menses
  Oral contraceptives (low dose)
  Antidepressants (SSRIs)
  Anxiolytics (taken during luteal phase)
  Diuretics to remove excess fluid
  Progestins
  Gonadotropin-releasing hormone (GnRH agonists)
  Danazol (androgen hormone that inhibits estrogen production)

PMDD, the physical and psychological symptoms are very real. The extent to which the symptoms debilitate or incapacitate a woman is highly variable.

There are more than 150 symptoms assigned to PMS, but irritability, tension, and dysphoria are the most prominent and consistently described (Freeman et al., 2011). To establish the diagnosis of PMS, elicit a description of cyclic symptoms occurring before the woman's menstrual period. The woman should chart her symptoms daily for two cycles. These data will help demonstrate symptoms clustering around the luteal phase of ovulation, with resolution after bleeding starts. Ask the woman to bring her list of symptoms to the next appointment. Symptoms can be categorized using the following:

- A—anxiety: difficulty sleeping, tenseness, mood swings, clumsiness
- C—craving: headache, cravings for sweets, salty foods, chocolate
- D—depression: feelings of low self-esteem, anger, easily upset
- H—hydration: weight gain, abdominal bloating, breast tenderness
- O—other: hot flashes or cold sweats, nausea, change in bowel habits, aches or pains, dysmenorrhea, acne breakout (Freeman et al., 2011)

Nursing Management

Educate the client about the management of PMS or PMDD. Advise her that lifestyle changes often result in significant symptom improvement without pharmacotherapy. To avoid hypoglycemia and associated mood swings, encourage women to eat a balanced diet by following Canada's Food Guide to Health Eating, which includes nutrient-rich foods. Recommend small, frequent meals with healthy snacks between meals. Administer calcium (1,200 to 1,600 mg/day), magnesium (50 mg/day), and vitamin B6 (50 to 100 mg/day) as prescribed. NSAIDs may be useful for painful physical symptoms, and spironolactone (Aldactone) may help with bloating and water retention. Herbs such as vitex (chaste tree berry) or evening primrose may be recommended; although not harmful, not all herbs have enough clinical or research evidence to document their safety or efficacy (Komar, 2012). Some practitioners may prescribe the OC pill or progesterone to help decrease physical symptoms, but some clients report that these are not always effective (HealthLink Alberta, 2006). A recent research study proposes calcium (1,600 mg/day) and vitamin D (400 IU/day) supplementation in adolescents and women in an effort to prevent PMS (Clayton, 2008).

Encourage clients to participate in aerobic exercise three times a week to promote a sense of well-being, decrease fatigue, and reduce stress. Stress management is also an essential component in decreasing symptoms of PMS. Yoga, Tai Chi, meditation, and deep breathing are activities that can be done throughout the month.

Explain the relationship between cyclic estrogen fluctuation and changes in serotonin levels and how the different management strategies help maintain serotonin levels, thus improving symptoms. It is important to rule out other conditions that might cause erratic or dysphoric behaviour. If the initial treatment regimen does not work, explain to the woman that she should return for further testing. Behavioural counselling and stress management might help women regain control during these stressful periods. Reassuring the woman that support and help are available through many community resources/support groups can be instrumental in her acceptance of this monthly disorder. Nurses can be a very calming force for many women experiencing PMS or PMDD.

▶ **Take** NOTE!

Adolescents and women who experience more extensive emotional symptoms with PMS should be evaluated for PMDD, as they may require antidepressant therapy.

Endometriosis

Endometriosis, one of the most common disease entities confronting gynecologists, is defined as the presence of endometrial glands and stroma tissue outside the uterus. The presence of this ectopic tissue evokes an estrogen-dependent chronic inflammatory process (Leyland et al., 2010). SOGC estimates that 5% to 10% of women are affected by this disease (Leyland et al., 2010). This endometrial tissue is commonly found attached to the ovaries, the fallopian tubes, the outer surface of the uterus, the bowels, the area between the vagina and the rectum (rectovaginal septum), and the pelvic side wall (Fig. 4.1). The places where the tissue attaches are called implants, or lesions. Endometrial tissue found outside the uterus responds to hormones released during the menstrual cycle in the same way as endometrial lining within the uterus.

At the beginning of the menstrual cycle, when the lining of the uterus is shed and menstrual bleeding begins, these abnormally located implants swell and bleed also. In short, the woman with endometriosis experiences several "mini-periods" throughout her abdomen, wherever this endometrial tissue exists.

Think back to Izzy, who visited her health care provider to express her concerns about progressive pelvic pain and infertility. After a thorough health history and pelvic examination, her health care provider suspects she has endometriosis.

Etiology and Risk Factors

It is not currently known why endometrial tissue becomes transplanted and grows in other parts of the body. Several theories exist, but to date none has been scientifically proven. According to the SOCG, there is no consensus on the cellular and molecular origins of the disease but guidelines have been established to improve the care for women who suffer for endometrial symptoms (Leyland et al., 2010). Endometriosis occurs in 25% to 50% of infertile women and in 71% to 87% of women with chronic pelvic pain (Endometriosisinfo.ca, 2011; Kapoor, Alderman, Hiraoka, et al., 2012).

Several factors that increase a woman's risk for developing endometriosis have been identified (Leyland et al., 2010):

- Increasing age
- Family history of endometriosis in a first-degree relative (3 to 10 times the risk)
- Short menstrual cycle (less than 28 days)
- Long menstrual flow (more than 1 week)
- Young age at menarche (younger than 12)
- Few (one or two) or no pregnancies

Therapeutic Management

Endometriosis is a chronic and often progressive inflammatory condition of the pelvis whose predominant symptom is pain. The overall amount of endometriosis is not related to the frequency or severity of symptoms, and the condition's etiology remains unknown. Thus, by necessity, medical therapy is nonspecific and aimed at alleviating symptoms (Leyland et al., 2010). It is theorized that endometriosis may begin in adolescence, and up to 40% of women who experience symptoms do so before the age of 15. Therapeutic management of the client with endometriosis needs to take into consideration the severity of symptoms, the client's desire for

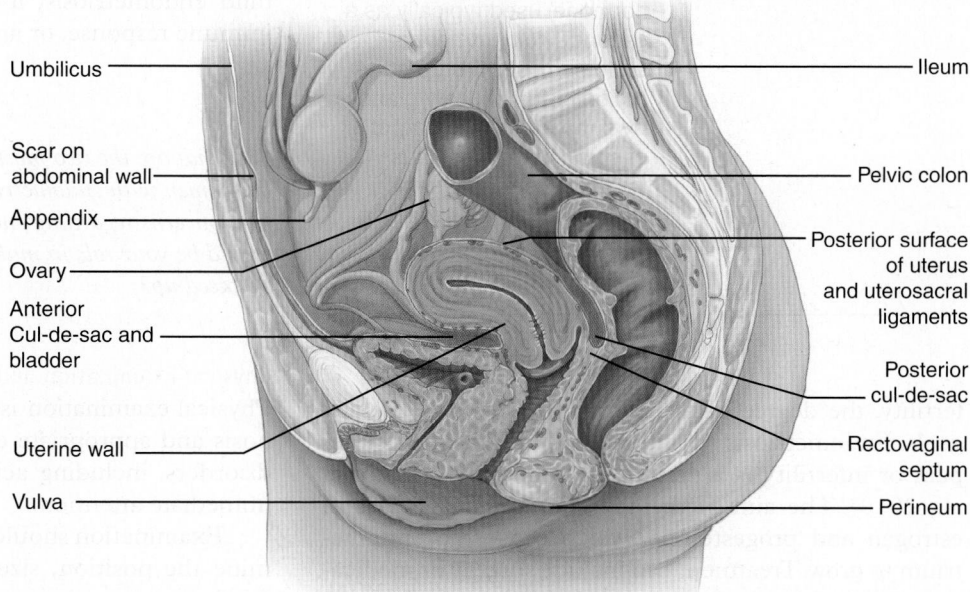

Umbilicus

Scar on abdominal wall

Appendix

Ovary

Anterior Cul-de-sac and bladder

Uterine wall

Vulva

Ileum

Pelvic colon

Posterior surface of uterus and uterosacral ligaments

Posterior cul-de-sac

Rectovaginal septum

Perineum

FIGURE 4.1 Common sites of endometriosis formation.

TABLE 4.2 TREATMENT OPTIONS FOR ENDOMETRIOSIS

Therapy Options	Comment
Surgical intervention	
Conservative surgery	Removal of implants/lesions using laser, cautery, or small surgical instruments. This intervention will reduce pain and allows pregnancy to occur in the future.
Definitive surgery	Abdominal hysterectomy, with or without bilateral salpingo-oophorectomy. This intervention will eliminate pain but will leave a woman unable to become pregnant in the future.
Medication therapy	
NSAIDs	First-line treatment to reduce pain; taken early when premenstrual symptoms are first felt
Oral contraceptives	Suppresses cyclic hormonal response of the endometrial tissue
Progestogens	Used to cast off the endometrial cells and thus destroy them
Antiestrogens	Suppresses a woman's production of estrogen, thus stopping the menstrual cycle and preventing further growth of endometrium
Gonadotropin-releasing hormone analogues (GnRH-a)	Suppresses endometriosis by creating a temporary pseudomenopause
Danazol (Danacrine)	A synthetic androgen (male sex hormone) used typically as a second-line treatment of endometriosis. Disrupts the action of the pituitary gland by suppressing the output of some hormones, thus reducing estrogen, halting menstruation, and resulting in the growth of facial hair and acne.

fertility, the degree of disease, and the client's therapy goals. Endometriosis should only be treated when either pain or infertility is a presenting symptom (Leyland et al., 2010). The aim of therapy is to suppress levels of estrogen and progesterone, which cause the endometrium to grow. Treatment can include surgery or medication (Table 4.2).

Nursing Assessment

Nurses encounter women with endometriosis in a variety of settings, including community health settings, schools, medical clinics, day surgical centres, and hospitals. Health care professionals must take the time to listen to patients who have symptoms of endometriosis and not trivialize or dismiss the concerns of these women, because early recognition is essential to preserve fertility.

Health History

Obtain a health history and elicit a description of signs and symptoms to determine risk factors. Endometriosis is often asymptomatic, but it can be a severe and debilitating condition. It typically is chronic and progressive. Assess the client for clinical manifestations, which include:

• Infertility
• Pain before and during menstrual periods (dysmenorrhea)
• Pain during or after sexual intercourse (dyspareunia)
• Painful urination (dysuria)
• Depression
• Fatigue
• Painful bowel movements (dyschezia)
• Chronic pelvic pain
• Hypermenorrhea (heavy menses)
• Pelvic adhesions
• Irregular and more frequent menses
• Premenstrual vaginal spotting (Endometriosisinfo.ca, 2011)

The two most common symptoms are infertility and pain. While little is known about endometriosis-related infertility, it is possible that the infertility could be caused by scarring, which blocks the fallopian tubes or egg release by the ovaries (Endometriosisinfo.ca, 2011). In mild endometriosis, it is theorized that inflammation, immune response, or angiogenesis could be the cause.

What are the two most common symptoms experienced by women with endometriosis? Do Izzy's symptoms match her concerns regarding endometriosis? As a nurse, what would be your role in making sure Izzy's concerns were followed up?

Physical Examination and Laboratory and Diagnostic Tests

Physical examination is essential to determine the diagnosis and appropriate care, as well as to rule out other disorders, including acute conditions that may require immediate attention.

Examination should include an assessment to determine the position, size, and mobility of the uterus: a fixed, retroverted uterus may suggest severe adhesive disease. A rectovaginal examination may be necessary and appropriate to palpate the uterosacral ligaments and rectovaginal septum, which may reveal tender nodules suggestive of deeply infiltrating endometriosis. Adnexal masses discovered on physical examination may suggest ovarian endometriomas (Leyland et al., 2010).

Usually the first-line investigational tool is ultrasonography, which can determine the presence of ovarian cysts or other pelvic disorders such as fibroids. The gold standard for diagnosis is direct visualization at laparoscopy and histologic study. Laparoscopy will help practitioners determine the severity of endometriotic lesions and the possibility of organ involvement. From this procedure, practitioners usually are able to determine a plan of action to treat the disease (Leyland et al., 2010).

Nurses can play a role by offering a thorough explanation of the condition and explaining why tests are needed to diagnose endometriosis. The nurse can set up appointments for imaging studies and laparoscopy.

Nursing Management

Physical symptoms, whether treated or untreated, can create significant emotional and spiritual distress. It is important to remember each client may experience and perceive their symptoms differently. The nurse should explore how the client is coping with the chronic nature of her disease. In addition to the interventions outlined above, the nurse should encourage the client to adopt healthy lifestyle habits with respect to diet, exercise, sleep, and stress management. Referrals to support groups and Internet resources can help the woman to understand this condition and cope with chronic pain. A number of organizations provide information about the diagnosis and treatment of endometriosis and offer support to women and their families (Box 4.3).

BOX 4.3 Organizations That Can Assist the Client with Endometriosis

- American College of Obstetricians and Gynecologists (ACOG)
- American Society for Reproductive Medicine
- Center for Endometriosis Care
- Endometriosis Association
- Endometriosisinfo.ca
- National Institute of Child Health & Human Development Information Resource Center
- National Women's Health Information Center (U.S. Department of Health and Human Services Office on Women's Health)

Visit http://thePoint.lww.com/Chow1e for direct links to these sites.

After completing several tests, Izzy is diagnosed with endometriosis. She asks you about her chances of becoming pregnant and becoming pain-free. What treatment options would you explain to Izzy? What information can you give about her future childbearing ability?

Infertility

Infertility is defined as the inability to conceive a child after 1 year of regular sexual intercourse unprotected by contraception (Hays, 2009). **Secondary infertility** is the inability to conceive after a previous pregnancy. According to Assisted Human Reproduction Canada (AHRC), 80% of couples who have regular sexual intercourse without contraceptive will get pregnant within 1 year of trying. Of the remaining 20%, the majority will become pregnant within 2 years (AHRC, 2010). An estimated 8.5% of Canadian couples experience problems with infertility.

The condition may be caused by disruptions at various steps of the reproductive process. Management options range from pharmacologic treatment to more advanced techniques referred to as assisted reproductive technologies (AHRC, 2010).

Infertility is a widespread problem that has an emotional, social, and economic impact on couples. Nurses must recognize symptoms of infertility and understand its causes and treatment options so that they can help couples understand the possibilities as well as the limitations of current therapies. Recent studies found that women with infertility wish to be treated with respect and dignity and given appropriate information and support (Greil & McQuillan, 2010). They want their distress to be recognized, to feel cared for, and to have confidence in health care professionals in situations where outcomes are uncertain. The caring aspect of professional nursing is an essential component of meeting the special needs of these couples (Greil & McQuillan, 2010). Prevention of infertility through education should also be incorporated into any client–nurse interaction.

Cultural Considerations

The expectation for couples to reproduce is an accepted norm across cultures, and the inability to conceive may be considered a violation of this cultural norm. In this context, infertility represents a crisis for the couple. The manner in which different cultures, ethnic groups, and religious groups perceive and manage infertility may be very different.

Religion often influences cultural factors and for this reason may also be considered when pursuing treatment for infertility. Nurses must be cognizant of the client's cultural and religious background and how it may dictate which, if any, reproductive treatment options are chosen. Nurses need to include this awareness in their counselling of infertile couples.

Etiology and Risk Factors

Multiple known and unknown factors affect fertility. Female-factor infertility is detected in about 40% of cases, and male-factor infertility is identified in about 30% to 40% of cases. Most cases of male-factor infertility are cause by a low sperm count (oligospermia). Medical conditions, problems with the male anatomy, hormone problems, infections, retrograde ejaculation, genetic disorders, or erectile dysfunction can also affect male fertility.

Female-factor infertility includes the tubal factor (50%), which involves problems with ovulation, and may include (but is less likely) problems with the cervix or with the presence of uterine fibroids or polyps, which is described as the uterine factor. Another cause of female infertility is ovulatory dysfunction. This occurs when a woman has irregular or infrequent menses or does not ovulate at all. Polycystic ovarian syndrome (PCOS) is the most common disorder accounting for 20% of infertility problems. Finally, a very important factor that affects female infertility is age. After the age of 40, the quality of a woman's eggs deteriorates. The remaining 20% of infertility cases fall into a category of combined (both male and female factors) or unexplained infertility (Hays, 2009; Mayo Clinic Staff, 2011c; Regional Fertility Program, 2011).

Risk factors for infertility in women include:

• Age
• Genetics
• Ovulatory problems
• PCOS
• STIs (past or present)
• Uterine factors
• Fallopian tube blockages
• Endometriosis
• Hormone imbalances
• Premature menopause

• Previous cancer treatments
• Weight (overweight or underweight)
• Stress
• Smoking (AHRC, 2010)

Risk factors for infertility in men include:

• Genetics
• Poor sperm quality
• Low sperm count
• Impairment in sexual function
• Reproductive tract blockage (undescended testes, previous surgeries)
• STIs (past or present)
• Hormone imbalances
• Previous cancer treatments
• Weight
• Smoking or excessive alcohol use
• Some prescription medications (AHRC, 2010)

Therapeutic Management

The test results are presented to the couple and different treatment options are suggested. The majority of infertility cases are treated with medications or surgery. Various ovulation-enhancement medications and timed intercourse might be used for the woman with ovulation problems. The woman should understand the medications' benefits and side effects before consenting to take them. Depending on the type of drug used and the dosage, some women may experience multiple births. If the woman's reproductive organs are damaged, surgery may be performed to repair them. Still other couples might opt for the high-tech approaches of intrauterine insemination (IUI) (Fig. 4.2), in vitro fertilization (IVF; Fig. 4.3), and egg donation or contract for a gestational carrier or surrogate (Regional Fertility Program, 2011). Table 4.3 lists selected infertility treatment options.

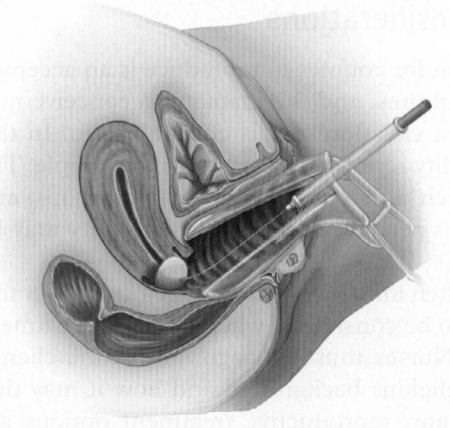
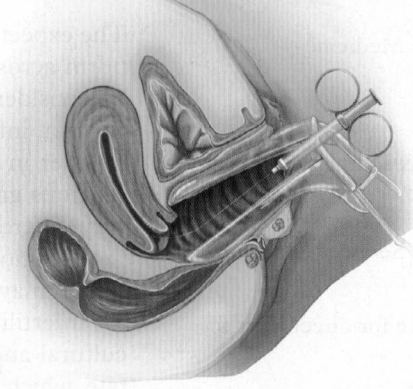

A   **B**

FIGURE 4.2 Intrauterine insemination. Sperm are deposited next to the cervix (**A**) or injected directly into the uterine cavity (**B**).

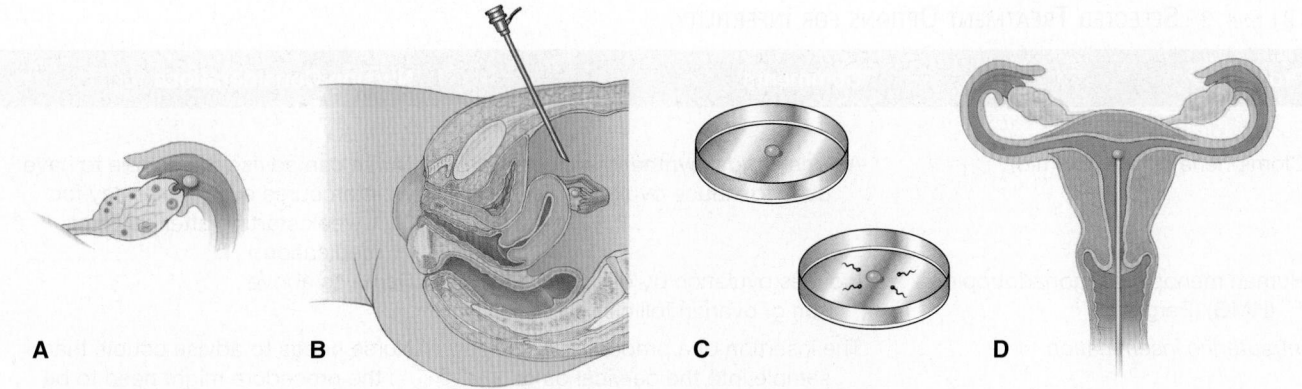

FIGURE 4.3 Steps involved in in vitro fertilization. (**A**) Ovulation. (**B**) Capture of the ova (done here intra-abdominally). (**C**) Fertilization of ova and growth in culture medium. (**D**) Insertion of fertilized ova into uterus.

Nursing Assessment

Infertile couples are under tremendous pressure and may keep their infertility a secret, considering it to be very personal. The couple may experience feelings of inadequacy and guilt, and many are subject to pressures from both family and friends. As their infertility concerns become more chronic, they may begin to blame one another, with consequent marital discord. Seeking help may be a very difficult step for them, and it may take a lot of courage to discuss something about which they feel deeply embarrassed or upset. The nurse working in this specialty setting must be aware of the conflict and concerns couples present with and must be very sensitive to their needs.

A full medical and health history should be taken from both partners, along with a physical examination. The data needed for the infertility evaluation are very sensitive and of a personal nature, so the nurse must use very professional interviewing skills.

There are numerous causes of and contributing factors to infertility, so it is important to use the process of elimination, determining what problems don't exist to better comprehend the problems that do exist. At the first visit, a plan of investigation is outlined and a complete health history is taken. This first visit forces many couples to confront the reality that their desired pregnancy may not occur naturally. Alleviate some of the anxiety associated with diagnostic testing by explaining the timing and reasons for each test.

Assessing Male Factors

The initial screening evaluation for the male partner should include a reproductive history and a semen analysis. From the male perspective, three things must happen for conception to take place: there must be an adequate number of sperm; those sperm must be healthy and mature; and the sperm must be able to penetrate and fertilize the egg. Normal males need to have more than 20 million sperm per millilitre with greater than 50% motility (World Health Organization [WHO], 2007). Semen analysis is the most important indicator of male fertility. The man should abstain from sexual activity or masturbation for 2 to 3 days before giving the sample. For a semen examination, the man is asked to produce a specimen by ejaculating into a specimen container and delivering it to the laboratory for analysis within 1 to 2 hours. When the specimen is brought to the laboratory, it is analyzed for volume, viscosity, number of sperm, sperm viability, motility, and sperm shape. If semen parameters are normal, no further male evaluation is necessary (Regional Fertility Program, 2011). According to Trolice and Witt (2011), 10% to 30% of male infertility is related to scrotal varicocele, 23% is idiopathic, 14% may be caused by an obstruction, and 3% is cryptorchidism (undescended testes).

The physical examination for males experiencing infertility routinely includes:

- Assessment for appropriate male sexual characteristics, such as body hair distribution, development of the Adam's apple, and muscle development
- Examination of the penis, scrotum, testicles, epididymis, and vas deferens for abnormalities (e.g., nodules, irregularities, varicocele)
- Assessment for normal development of external genitalia (small testicles)
- Performance of a digital internal examination of the prostate to check for tenderness or swelling

Assessing Female Factors

The initial assessment of the woman should include a thorough history of factors associated with ovulation and the pelvic organs. Diagnostic tests to determine female infertility may include:

- Assessment of ovarian function
- Menstrual history: regularity of cycles
- Ovulation predictor kits used midcycle
- Urinary LH level
- Clomiphene citrate challenge test
- Endometrial biopsy to document luteal phase
- Assessment of pelvic organs

TABLE 4.3 SELECTED TREATMENT OPTIONS FOR INFERTILITY

Procedure	Comments	Nursing Considerations
Fertility drugs		
Clomiphene citrate (Clomid)	A nonsteroidal synthetic antiestrogen used to induce ovulation	Nurse can advise the couple to have intercourse every other day for 1 week starting after day 5 of medication.
Human menopausal gonadotropin (HMG) (Pergonal)	Induces ovulation by direct stimulation of ovarian follicle	Same as above
Intrauterine insemination	The insertion of a prepared semen sample into the cervical os or intrauterine cavity Enables sperm to be deposited closer to the cervix to improve chances of conception Husband or donor sperm can be used	Nurse needs to advise couple that the procedure might need to be repeated if not successful the first time.
Assisted reproductive technologies*		
In vitro fertilization (IVF)	Oocytes are fertilized in the lab and transferred to the uterus. Usually indicated for tubal obstruction, endometriosis, pelvic adhesions, and low sperm counts	Nurse advises woman to take medication to stimulate ovulation so the mature ovum can be retrieved by needle aspiration.
Gamete intrafallopian transfer (GIFT)	Oocytes and sperm are combined and immediately placed in the fallopian tube so fertilization can occur naturally. Requires laparoscopy and general anesthesia, which increases risk	Nurse needs to inform couple of risks and have consent signed.
Intracytoplasmic sperm injection (ICSI)	One sperm is injected into the cytoplasm of the oocyte to fertilize it. Indicated for male-factor infertility.	Nurse needs to inform the male that sperm will be aspirated by a needle through the skin into the epididymis.
Donor oocytes or sperm	Eggs or sperm are retrieved from a donor and the eggs are inseminated; resulting embryos are transferred via IVF. Recommended for women older than 40 and those with poor-quality eggs.	Nurse needs to support couple in their ethical/religious discussions prior to deciding.
Gestational carrier (surrogacy)	Laboratory fertilization takes place and embryos are transferred to the uterus of another woman, who will carry the pregnancy. Medical-legal issues have resulted over the "true ownership" of the resulting infant.	Nurse should encourage an open discussion regarding implications of this method with the couple.

*When other options have been exhausted, these are considered.

- Papanicolaou (Pap) smear to rule out cervical cancer or inflammation
- Cervical culture to rule out chlamydia infection
- Postcoital testing to evaluate sperm–cervical mucus interaction
- Ultrasound to assess pelvic structures
- Hysterosalpingography to visualize structural defects
- Laparoscopy to visualize pelvic structures and diagnose endometriosis

Laboratory and Diagnostic Testing

The diagnostic procedures that should be done during an infertility workup should be guided by the couple's history. They generally proceed from less to more invasive tests.

Home Ovulation Predictor Kits

Home ovulation predictor kits contain monoclonal antibodies specific for LH and use the enzyme-linked immunosorbent assay (ELISA) test to determine the amount of LH present in the urine. A significant colour change from baseline indicates the LH surge and presumably the most fertile day of the month for the woman.

Clomiphene Citrate Challenge Test

The clomiphene citrate challenge test is used to assess a woman's ovarian reserve (ability of her eggs to become fertilized). FSH levels are drawn on cycle day 3 and again on cycle day 10 after the woman has taken 100 mg clomiphene citrate on cycle days 5 through 9. If the FSH level is greater than 15, the result is considered abnormal and the likelihood of conception with her own eggs is very low (Regional Fertility Program, 2011).

Endometrial Biopsy

Another assessment of ovulation that indicates whether the secretion of progesterone is adequate is an endometrial biopsy. A strip of endometrial tissue is removed just before menstruation. Histologic documentation of secretory endometrial development implies that ovulation has taken place. An endometrium that does not conform to the normal histologic pattern indicates a defect in the luteal phase.

Postcoital Testing

Postcoital testing is done to assess the receptivity of the cervical mucus to sperm. Cervical mucus from the woman is examined 2 to 8 hours after intercourse during the expected time of ovulation, and the number of live, motile sperm present is assessed. Cervical mucus is also evaluated for stretchability (spinnbarkeit) and consistency (Mayo Clinic Staff, 2011b). The results are described in Comparison Chart 4.1.

COMPARISON CHART 4.1 **NORMAL VERSUS ABNORMAL POSTCOITAL TEST RESULTS**

Normal	Abnormal
Normal amounts of sperm are seen in the sample.	No sperm or a large percentage of dead sperm are seen in the sample.
Sperm are moving forward through the cervical mucus.	Sperm are clumped.
The mucus stretches at least 5 cm (2 inches).	Mucus cannot stretch 5 cm (2 inches).
The mucus dries in a fernlike pattern.	Mucus does not dry in a fernlike pattern.

Source: DeSutter, P. (2006). Rational diagnosis and treatment in infertility. *Best Practice & Research: Clinical Obstetrics & Gynecology*, *20*(5), 647–664.

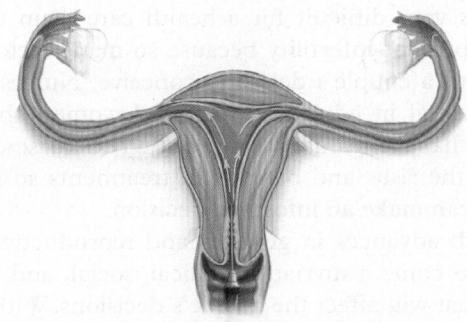

FIGURE **4.4** Insertion of dye for a hysterosalpingogram. The contrast dye outlines the uterus and fallopian tubes on an X-ray to demonstrate patency.

Hysterosalpingogram

In a hysterosalpingogram, 3 to 10 mL of an opaque contrast medium is slowly injected through a catheter into the endocervical canal so that the uterus and tubes can be visualized during fluoroscopy and radiography. If the fallopian tubes are patent, the dye will ascend upward to distend the uterus and the tubes and will spill out into the peritoneal cavity (Fig. 4.4).

Laparoscopy

Laparoscopy is usually performed early in the menstrual cycle. During the procedure, an endoscope is inserted through a small incision in the anterior abdominal wall. Visualization of the peritoneal cavity in an infertile woman may reveal endometriosis, pelvic adhesions, tubal occlusion, fibroids, or polycystic ovaries (Regional Fertility Program, 2011).

Nursing Management

Nurses play an important role in the care of infertile couples. They are pivotal educators about preventive health care. There are a number of potentially modifiable risk factors associated with the development of impaired fertility in women, and women need to be aware of these risks to institute change. For male infertility, modifiable factors must also be identified and corrected. These include poor nutrition, obesity, smoking and excessive alcohol or drug use, or the use of certain prescription medications. The nurse is most effective when he or she offers care and treatment in a professional manner and regards the couple as valued and respected individuals. The nurse's focus must encompass the whole person, not just the results of the various infertility studies. Throughout the entire process, the nurse's role is to provide information, anticipatory guidance, stress management, and counselling. The couple's emotional distress is usually very high, and the nurse must be able to recognize that anxiety and provide emotional support. The nurse may need to refer couples to a reproductive endocrinologist or surgeon, depending on the problem identified.

It is very difficult for a health care team to completely prevent infertility because so many factors contribute to a couple's desire to conceive. Nurses can be instrumental in educating men and women about the factors that contribute to infertility. The nurse can also outline the risks and benefits of treatments so that the couple can make an informed decision.

With advances in genetics and reproductive medicine also come a myriad of ethical, social, and cultural issues that will affect the couple's decisions. With this in mind, provide an opportunity for the couple to make informed decisions in a nondirective, non-judgmental environment. It is important to encourage couples to remain optimistic throughout investigation and treatment. Through the use of advocacy and anticipatory guidance, assist and support couples through the diagnosis and treatment of infertility (Gourounti, Anagnostopoulos, & Vaslamatzis, 2010).

Many infertile couples are not prepared for the emotional roller coaster of grief and loss during infertility treatments. Financial concerns and coping as a couple are two major areas of stress when treatment is undertaken. Universal IVF is usually not publicly funded in Canada. There may be some private benefits that cover the cost of certain portions of fertility treatment. On average, one cycle of IVF costs about $10,000, but the cost can increase to $20,000 for women who require higher doses of medication. Approximately, 15% of couples affected by infertility can afford IVF treatment (Canadian Agency for Drugs and Technologies in Health, 2010).

During the course of what may be months or even years of infertility care, it is essential to develop a holistic approach to nursing care. Stress management and anxiety reduction need to be addressed, and referral to a peer support group such as Resolve might be in order (Box 4.4).

▶ *Consider* THIS!

We had been married for 3 years and wanted to start a family, but much to our dismay nothing happened after a year of trying. I had some irregular periods and was finally diagnosed with endometriosis and put on Clomid. After 3 years of taking Clomid on and off, I went to a fertility expert. The doctor lasered the endometriosis tissue, sent air through my tubes to make sure they were patent, and put me back on Clomid, but still with no luck. Finally, 2 years later, we were put on an IVF waiting list and prayed we would have the money for the procedure when we were chosen. By then I felt a failure as a woman. We then decided that it was more important for us to be parents than it was for me to be pregnant, so we considered adoption. We tried for another year without any results.

We went to the adoption agency to fill out the paperwork for the process to begin. Our blood was taken and we waited for an hour, wondering the whole time why it was taking so long for the results. The nurse finally appeared and handed a piece of paper to me with the word "positive" written on it. I started to cry tears of joy, for a pregnancy had started and our long journey of infertility was finally ending.

Thoughts: for many women the dream of having a child is not easily realized. Infertility can affect self-esteem, disrupt relationships, and result in depression. This couple experienced many years of frustration in trying to have a family. What help can be offered to couples during this time? What can be said to comfort the woman who feels she is a failure?

> ### BOX 4.4 Organizations That Can Assist the Client with Infertility
>
> - American Fertility Association: offers education, referrals, research, support, and advocacy for couples dealing with infertility
> - American Society for Reproductive Medicine (ASRM): provides fact sheets and other resources on infertility, treatments, insurance, and other issues
> - Canadian Fertility and Andrology Society
> - International Consumer Support for Infertility: an international network engaged in advocacy on behalf of infertile couples via fact sheets and information
> - InterNational Counsel on Infertility Information Dissemination (INCIID): provides information about infertility, support forums, and a directory of infertility specialists
> - Infertility Awareness Association of Canada
> - Infertility Network
> - Resolve: a nationwide network of chapters dedicated to providing education, advocacy, and support for men and women facing infertility. They provide a helpline, medical referral services, and a member-to-member contact system.
>
> Visit http://thePoint.lww.com/Chow1e for direct links to these sites.

Contraception

According to the 2002 Canadian Contraception Study, oral contraception, condoms, and sterilization were the contraceptive methods of choice among respondents ages 15 to 44 years. Oral contraception and condoms were the predominant methods reported by unmarried women of ages 15 to 17. Sterilization was the predominant method among married couples of ages 35 to 44, with male sterilization more than twice as common as female sterilization (Fisher & Black, 2007).

BOX 4.5 Outline of Contraceptive Methods

Reversible Methods
Behavioural
• Abstinence
• Fertility awareness
• Withdrawal (coitus interruptus)
• Lactational amenorrhea method (LAM)

Barrier
• Condom (male and female)
• Diaphragm
• Cervical cap
• Sponge

Hormonal
• Oral contraceptives
• Injectable contraceptive
• Transdermal patches
• Vaginal ring
• Implantable contraceptives—Progestin only (available only in the US)
• Intrauterine systems
• Emergency contraceptives

Permanent Methods
• Tubal ligation for women
• Vasectomy for men

Contraception is any method that prevents conception or childbirth. A woman's reproductive life spans almost 40 years, and throughout those years, a variety of contraceptive methods may be used. The barriers to effective use of contraception have been well documented and include personal beliefs and values that can be shaped by both culture and religion (Srikanthan & Reid, 2008).

Couples must decide which contraceptive method is appropriate for them to meet their changing needs throughout their life cycle. In an era when many women wish to delay pregnancy and avoid STIs, choices may be difficult. Box 4.5 outlines the numerous contraceptive methods available today, and Table 4.4 provides a detailed summary of each type, including information on failure rates, advantages, disadvantages, STI protection, and danger signs. Nurses can educate and assist couples during this selection process.

Types of Contraceptive Methods

Contraceptives methods can be divided into three types: behavioural methods, barrier methods, and hormonal methods (SexualityandU.ca, 2006).

Behavioural Methods

Behavioural methods refer to any natural contraceptive method that does not require hormones, pharmaceutical compounds, physical barriers, or surgery to prevent pregnancy. These methods require couples to take an active role in preventing pregnancy through their sexual behaviours.

Abstinence

Abstinence (not having vaginal or anal intercourse) is one of the least expensive forms of contraception and has been used for thousands of years. Basically, pregnancy cannot occur if sperm is kept out of the vagina. It also reduces the risk of contracting human immunodeficiency virus/acquired immunodeficiency syndrome (HIV/AIDS) and other STIs, unless body fluids are exchanged through oral sex; however, some infections, such as herpes and human papillomavirus (HPV), can be passed by skin-to-skin contact. There are many pleasurable options for sex play without intercourse ("outercourse"), such as kissing, masturbation, erotic massage, sexual fantasy, sex toys such as vibrators, and oral sex. Many people have strong feelings about abstinence based on religious, cultural, and moral beliefs. There are many good and personal reasons to choose abstinence. For some it is a way of life, while for others it is a temporary choice. Some people choose abstinence because they want to:

• Wait until they are older
• Wait for a long-term relationship
• Avoid pregnancy or STIs
• Follow religious or cultural expectations

Natural Birth Control

Fertility awareness is a natural method of contraception in which no contraceptive devices are used; instead, certain observations, techniques, and calculations are used to determine the "fertile" and the "safe" periods in a monthly menstrual cycle. There are normal physiologic changes caused by hormonal fluctuations during the menstrual cycle that can be observed and charted. This information can be used to avoid or promote pregnancy. Fertility awareness methods (FAMs) rely upon the following assumptions:

• A single ovum is released from the ovary 14 days before each menstrual period. It lives approximately 24 hours.
• Sperm can live up to 5 days after intercourse. The "unsafe period" during the menstrual cycle is thus approximately 6 days: 3 days before and 3 days after ovulation. Since bodily changes start to occur before ovulation, the woman can become aware of these signs and not have intercourse on these days or use another method to prevent pregnancy.
• The exact time of ovulation cannot be determined, so 2 to 3 days are added to the beginning and end to avoid pregnancy.

The two most common methods of natural birth control are the FAM and natural family planning (NFP)

(text continues on page 126)

TABLE 4.4 **Summary of Contraceptive Methods**

Type	Description	Failure Rate With Typical Use	Pros	Cons	STI Protection	Danger Signs	Comments
Abstinence	Refrain from sexual activity	None	Costs nothing	Difficult to maintain	100%	None	Must be joint couple decision
Fertility awareness	Refrain from sex during fertile period	25%	No side effects; acceptable to most religious groups	High failure rate with incorrect use	None	None	Requires high level of couple commitment
Withdrawal (coitus interruptus)	Man withdraws before ejaculation	27%	Involves no devices and is always available	Requires considerable self-control by the man	None	None	Places woman in trusting and dependent role
Lactational amenorrhea method (LAM)	Uses lactational infertility for protection from pregnancy	1%–2% chance of pregnancy in first 6 months	No cost; not coitus-linked	Temporary method; effective for only 6 months after giving birth	None	None	Mother must breast-feed infant on demand without supplementation for 6 months
Male condom	Thin sheath placed over an erect penis, blocking sperm	15%	Widely available; low cost; physiologically safe	Decreased sensation for man; interferes with sexual spontaneity; breakage risk	Provides protection against STIs	Latex allergy	Couple must be instructed on proper use of condom
Female condom	Polyurethane sheath inserted vaginally to block sperm	21%	Use controlled by woman; eliminates postcoital drainage of semen	Expensive for frequent use; cumbersome; noisy during sex act; for single use only	Provides protection against STIs	Allergy to polyurethane	Couple must be instructed on proper use of condom
Diaphragm with spermicide	Shallow latex cup with spring mechanism in its rim to hold it in place in the vagina	16%	Does not use hormone; considered medically safe; provides some protection against cervical cancer	Requires accurate fitting by health care professional; increase in UTIs	None	Allergy to latex, rubber, polyurethane, or spermicide Report symptoms of toxic shock syndrome. Change size if excessive weight gain or loss.	Woman must be taught to insert and remove diaphragm correctly

Method	Description	Failure rate	Advantages	Disadvantages	STI protection	Side effects	Nursing considerations
Cervical cap with spermicide	Soft cup-shaped latex device that fits over base of cervix	24%	No use of hormones; provides continuous protection while in place	Requires accurate fitting by health care professional; odour may occur if left in too long	None	Irritation, allergic reaction; abnormal Pap test; risk for toxic shock syndrome	Instructions on insertion and removal must be understood by client
Sponge with spermicide	Disk-shaped polyurethane device containing a spermicide that is activated by wetting it with water	25%	Offers immediate and continuous protection for 24 h; OTC	Can fall out of vagina with voiding; is not form-fitting in the vagina	None	Irritation, allergic reactions; toxic shock syndrome can occur if sponge left in too long	Caution woman not to leave sponge in beyond 24 h
Oral contraceptives (combination)	A pill that suppresses ovulation by combined action of estrogen and progestin	8%	Easy to use; high rate of effectiveness; protection against ovarian and endometrial cancer	User must remember to take pill daily; possible undesirable side effects; high cost for some women; prescription needed	None	Dizziness, nausea, mood changes, high blood pressure, blood clots, heart attacks, strokes	Each woman must be assessed thoroughly to make sure she is not a smoker and does not have a history of thromboembolic disease
Oral contraceptives (progestin-only mini-pills)	A pill containing only progestin that thickens cervical mucus to prevent sperm from penetrating	8%	No estrogen-related side effects; may be used by lactating women; may be used by women with history of thrombophlebitis	Must be taken with meticulous accuracy; may cause irregular bleeding	None	Irregular bleeding, weight gain, increased incidence of ectopic pregnancy	Women should be screened for history of functional ovarian cysts, previous ectopic pregnancy, hyperlipidemia prior to giving prescription
Patch (Ortho Evra)	Transdermal patch that releases estrogen and progestin into circulation	8%	Easy system to remember; very effective	May cause skin irritation where it is placed; may fall off and not be noticed and thus provide no protection	None	Less effective in women weighing more than 90.7 kg (200 pounds)	Instruct woman to apply patch every week for 3 weeks and then not to wear one during week 4

(continued)

TABLE 4.4 SUMMARY OF CONTRACEPTIVE METHODS (continued)

Type	Description	Failure Rate With Typical Use	Pros	Cons	STI Protection	Danger Signs	Comments
Ring (Nuva Ring)	Vaginal contraceptive ring about 5.1 cm (2 inches) in diameter that is inserted into the vagina; releases estrogen and progestin	8%	Easy system to remember; very effective	May cause a vaginal discharge; can be expelled without noticing and not offer protection	None	Similar to oral contraceptives	Instruct woman to use a backup method if ring is expelled and remains out for more than 3 h
Depo-Provera injection	An injectable progestin that inhibits ovulation	3%	Long duration of action (3 months); highly effective; estrogen-free; may be used by smokers; can be used by lactating women	Menstrual irregularities; return visit needed every 12 weeks; weight gain, headaches, depression; return to fertility delayed up to 12 months	None	If depression is a problem, this method may increase the depression.	Inform woman that fertility is delayed after stopping the injections
Intrauterine systems	A T-shaped device inserted into the uterus that releases copper, progesterone, or levo- norgestrel	1%	Immediately and highly effective; allows for sexual spontaneity; can be used during lactation; return to fertility not impaired; requires no motivation by the user after insertion	Insertion requires a skilled professional; menstrual irregularities; prolonged amenorrhea; can be unknowingly expelled; may increase the risk of pelvic infection; user must regularly check string for placement; delay of fertility after discontinuing for possibly 6 to 12 months	None	Cramps, bleeding, pelvic inflammatory disease; infertility; perforation of the uterus	Instruct woman how to locate string to check monthly for placement

Postcoital emergency contraceptives (ECs)	Combination of progestin-only pills taken within 72 h after unprotected intercourse	80%	Provides a last chance to prevent a pregnancy	Risk of ectopic pregnancy if EC fails	None	Nausea, vomiting, abdominal pain, fatigue, headache	Inform woman that ECs do not interrupt an established pregnancy, and the sooner they are taken the more effective they are.
Permanent sterilization			One-time decision provides permanent sterility; short recovery time; low long-term risks	Procedures are difficult to reverse; initial cost may be high; chance of regret; some pain/discomfort after procedures	None for both	Postoperative complications: pain, bleeding, infection	Counsel both as to permanence of procedure and urge them to think it through prior to signing consent
Male	Sealing, tying, or cutting the vas deferens	<1%					
Female	Fallopian tubes are blocked to prevent conception	<1%					

Sources: Hatcher, R. A., Trussell, J., Nelson, A. L., Cates, W., Jr., Kowal, D., & Policar, M. (2011). *Contraceptive technology* (20th ed.). New York: Ardent Media, Inc.; Samra-Latif, O. M., & Wood, E. (2011). *Contraception*. Retrieved March 4, 2012 from http://www.emedicine.com/med/topic3211.htm; U.S. Food and Drug Administration. (2006). *FDA approves over-the-counter access for Plan B for women 18 and older; prescription remains required for those 17 and younger.* Retrieved March 4, 2012 from http://www.fda.gov/NewsEvents/Newsroom/PressAnnouncements/2006/ucm108717.htm; and Youngkin, E. Q., & Davis, M. S. (2003). *Women's health: A primary care clinical guide* (3rd ed.). New Jersey: Prentice Hall.

(Leyland et al., 2010). FAMs are moderately effective but are very unforgiving if not carried out as prescribed: not following the guidelines might cause a 4% failure rate with perfect use and 19% failure rate with typical use (Black, Francoeur, Rowe, et al., 2004). Fertility awareness can be used in combination with coital abstinence or barrier methods during fertile days if pregnancy is not desired.

Cervical Mucus Ovulation Method

The **cervical mucus ovulation method** is used to assess the character of the cervical mucus. Cervical mucus changes in consistency during the menstrual cycle and plays a vital role in fertilization of the egg. In the days preceding ovulation, fertile cervical mucus helps draw sperm up and into the fallopian tubes, where fertilization usually takes place. It also helps maintain the survival of sperm. As ovulation approaches, the mucus becomes more abundant, clear, slippery, and smooth; it can be stretched between two fingers without breaking. Under the influence of estrogen, this mucus looks like egg whites. It is called spinnbarkeit mucus (Fig. 4.5). After ovulation, the cervical mucus becomes thick and dry under the influence of progesterone.

The cervical position can also be assessed to confirm changes in the cervical mucus at ovulation. Near ovulation, the cervix feels soft and is high/deep in the vagina, the os is slightly open, and the cervical mucus is copious and slippery (Mayo Clinic Staff, 2012b).

This method works because the woman becomes aware of her body changes that accompany ovulation. When she notices them, she abstains from sexual intercourse or uses another method to prevent pregnancy.

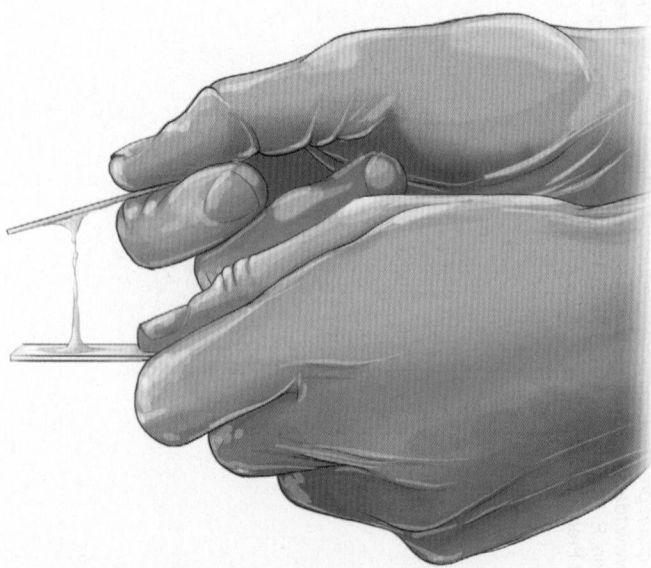

FIGURE 4.5 Spinnbarkeit is the ability of cervical mucus to stretch a distance before breaking.

Each woman is an individual, so each woman's unsafe time of the month is unique and thus must be individually assessed and determined.

Basal Body Temperature

The **basal body temperature** (BBT) refers to the lowest temperature reached upon wakening. The woman takes her temperature orally before rising and records it on a chart. Preovulation temperatures are suppressed by estrogen, whereas postovulation temperatures are increased under the influence of heat-inducing progesterone. Temperatures typically rise within a day or two after ovulation and remain elevated for approximately 2 weeks (at which point bleeding usually begins). If using this method by itself, the woman should avoid unprotected intercourse until the BBT has been elevated for 3 days. Other FAMs should be used along with BBT for better results (Fig. 4.6).

Symptothermal Method

This method uses a combination of BBT change and change in cervical mucus or other cyclic symptoms. A chart of symptoms and BBT is helpful in identifying the fertile days. Some women are aware of ovulation discomfort (Mittelschmerz), which may also be incorporated into the charting. Pain may occur just prior to, during, or just after ovulation. The couple is not protected from STIs, including HIV (SexualityandU.ca, 2006).

Combining all these predictors increases awareness of when ovulation occurs and increases the effectiveness of this method. A home predictor test for ovulation is also available in most pharmacies. It measures LH levels to pinpoint the day before or the day of ovulation. These tests are widely used for fertility and infertility regimens.

The Standard Days Method and the Two-Day Method

The **standard days method (SDM)** and the two-day method are both natural methods of contraception that provide women with simple, clear instructions for identifying fertile days. Women with menstrual cycles between 26 and 32 days long can use the SDM to prevent pregnancy by avoiding unprotected intercourse on days 8 through 19 of their cycles. An international clinical trial of the SDM showed that it is more than 95% effective when used correctly (Black et al., 2004). SDM identifies the 8- to 19-day "fertile window" of a woman's menstrual cycle. These fertile days take into account the lifespan of the women's egg (about 24 hours) and the viability of the sperm (about 5 days) as well as the variation in the actual timing of ovulation from one cycle to another. For the two-day method, women observe the presence or absence of cervical secretions by examining toilet paper or underwear or by monitoring their physical sensations. Every day, the woman asks two simple questions "Did I note any secretions yesterday?" and "Did I note any secretions today?" If the answer to either question is yes, she considers herself fertile and avoids

Basal body temperature

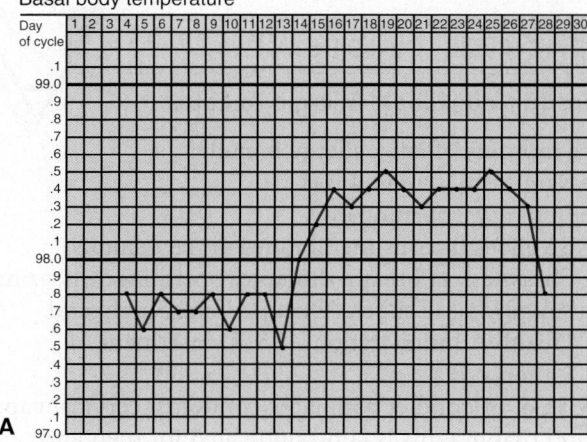

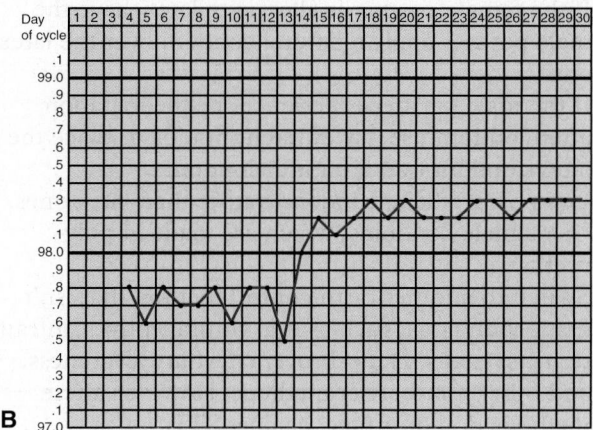

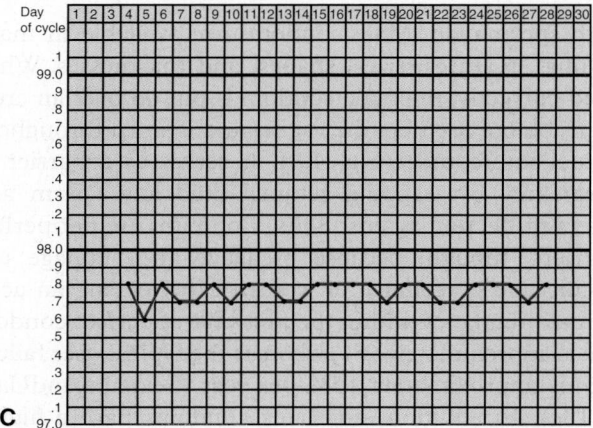

FIGURE **4.6** Basal body temperature graph. (**A**) The woman's temperature dips slightly at midpoint in the menstrual cycle, then rises sharply, an indication of ovulation. Toward the end of the cycle (the 24th day), her temperature begins to decline, indicating that progesterone levels are falling and that she did not conceive. (**B**) The woman's temperature rises at the midpoint in the cycle and remains at that elevated level past the time of her normal menstrual flow, suggesting that pregnancy has occurred. (**C**) There is no preovulatory dip and no rise of temperature anywhere during the cycle. This is the typical pattern of a woman who does not ovulate.

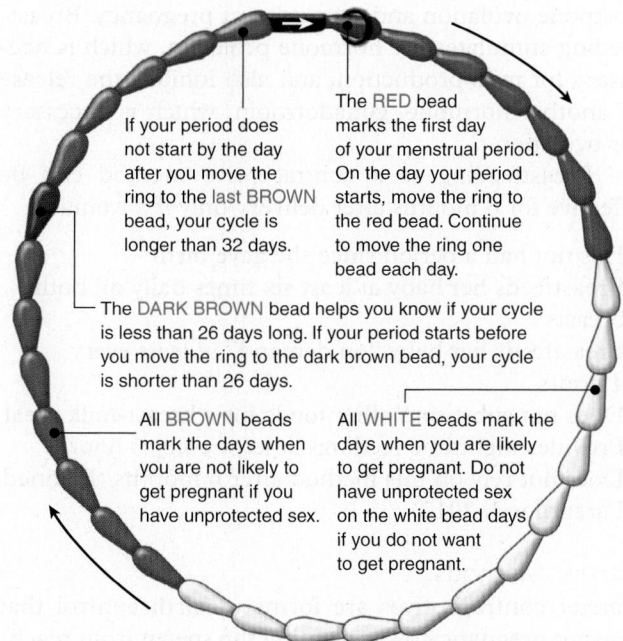

FIGURE **4.7** CycleBeads help women use the standard days method.

unprotected intercourse. If the answers are no, she is unlikely to become pregnant from unprotected intercourse on that day (Sinai, Arevalo, & Jennings, 2006).

To help women keep track of the days on which they should avoid unprotected intercourse, a string of 32 colour-coded beads (CycleBeads) is used, with each bead representing a day of the menstrual cycle. Starting with the red bead, which represents the first day of her menstrual period, the woman moves a small rubber ring one bead each day. The brown beads are the days when pregnancy is unlikely, and the white beads represent her fertile days (Arevalo, 2010). This method has been used in underdeveloped countries for women with limited educational resources (Fig. 4.7).

Withdrawal (Coitus Interruptus)

In **coitus interruptus,** also known as withdrawal, a man controls his ejaculation during sexual intercourse and ejaculates outside the vagina. It is better known colloquially as "pulling out in time" or "being careful." It is one of the oldest and most widely used means of preventing pregnancy in the world (Black et al., 2004). The problem with this method is that the first few drops of the true ejaculate contain the greatest concentration of sperm, and if some pre-ejaculatory fluid escapes from the urethra before orgasm, conception may result. This method requires that the woman rely solely on the cooperation and judgment of the man (Mayo Clinic Staff, 2010).

Lactational Amenorrhea Method

The **lactational amenorrhea method (LAM)** is an effective temporary method of contraception used by breastfeeding mothers. Continuous breastfeeding can postpone ovulation and thus prevent pregnancy. Breast-feeding stimulates the hormone prolactin, which is necessary for milk production, and also inhibits the release of another hormone, gonadotropin, which is necessary for ovulation.

Breastfeeding as a contraceptive method can be effective for 6 months after delivery only if a woman:

• Has not had a period since she gave birth
• Breastfeeds her baby at least six times daily on both breasts
• Breastfeeds her baby "on demand" at least every 4 hours
• Does not substitute other foods for a breast-milk meal
• Provides nighttime feedings at least every 6 hours
• Does not rely on this method after 6 months (Planned Parenthood, 2012)

Barrier Methods

Barrier contraceptives are forms of birth control that prevent pregnancy by preventing the sperm from reaching the ovum. *Mechanical barriers* include condoms, diaphragms, cervical caps, and sponges. These devices are placed over the penis or cervix to physically obstruct the passage of sperm through the cervix. *Chemical barriers* called spermicides, which chemically destroy the sperm in the vagina, may be used along with mechanical barrier devices. They come in creams, jellies, foam, suppositories, and vaginal films. These contraceptives are called barrier methods because they not only provide a physical barrier for sperm but also protect against STIs. Since the HIV/AIDS epidemic started in the early 1980s, these methods have become extremely popular.

Many barrier contraceptives contain latex. Allergy to latex was first recognized in the late 1970s, and since then it has become a major health concern, with increasing numbers of people affected. Natural latex is manufactured from the sap of a rubber tree, and the allergy is to the proteins originating from the rubber tree or the chemicals found in manufactured latex products. The prevalence of latex allergies in Canada is unclear, but the American Academy of Allergy, Asthma, and Immunology (2012) indicates that less than 1% of the general population, 5% to 15% of health care workers, and 24% to 60% of spina bifida patients are sensitive to natural rubber latex. Since the late 1980s, with the establishment of policies dictating barrier requirements resulting from the HIV/AIDS epidemic, there has been an exponential increase in the use of latex gloves and condoms. Teaching Guideline 4.4 provides tips for individuals with latex allergy.

Condoms

Condoms are barrier contraceptives made for both males and females. The male condom is made from latex or polyurethane or natural membrane and may be coated

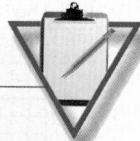

TEACHING GUIDELINE 4.4

Tips for Individuals Allergic to Latex

• Symptoms of latex allergy include:
  • Skin rash, itching, hives
  • Itching or burning eyes
  • Swollen mucous membranes in the genitals
  • Shortness of breath, difficulty breathing, wheezing
  • Anaphylactic shock (Occupational Safety and Health Administration, U.S. Department of Labor, n.d.)
• Use of or contact with latex condoms, cervical caps, and diaphragms is contraindicated for men and women with a latex allergy.
• If the female partner is allergic to latex, have the male partner apply a natural condom over the latex one.
• If the male partner experiences penile irritation after condom use, try different brands or place the latex condom over a natural condom.
• Use polyurethane condoms rather than latex ones.
• Use female condoms, which are made of polyurethane.
• Switch to another birth control method that isn't made with latex, such as oral contraceptives, intrauterine systems, Depo-Provera, fertility awareness, and other non-barrier methods. However, these methods do not protect against STIs.

with spermicide. Male condoms are available in many colours, textures, sizes, shapes, and thicknesses. When used correctly, the male condom is put on over an erect penis before it enters the vagina and is worn throughout sexual intercourse (Fig. 4.8). It serves as a barrier to pregnancy by trapping seminal fluid and sperm and offers protection against STIs. Condoms are not perfect barriers, though, because breakage and slippage can occur. The percentage of women experiencing an accidental pregnancy within the first year of perfect condom use is approximately 2%, whereas the typical user failure rate is approximately 15% per year (SexualityandU.ca, 2010e). In addition, non-latex condoms have a higher risk for pregnancy and STIs than latex condoms (Black et al., 2004).

The female condom (see Fig. 4.8) is a polyurethane pouch inserted into the vagina. It consists of an outer and inner ring that is inserted vaginally and held in place by the pubic bone. Some women complain that the female condom is cumbersome to use and makes noise during intercourse. Female condoms are readily available, are inexpensive, and can be carried inconspicuously by the woman. The female condom was the first woman-controlled method that offered protection

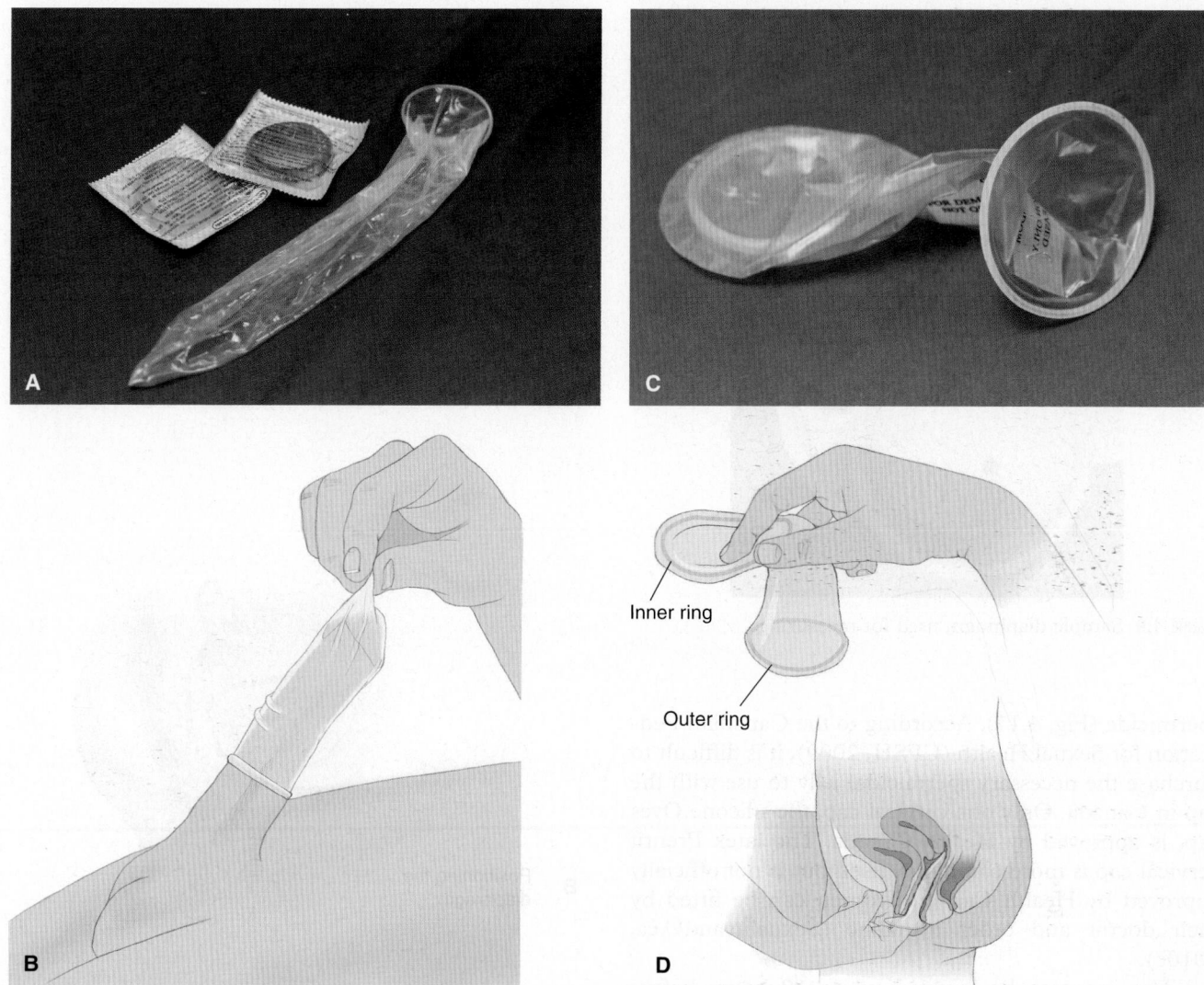

FIGURE 4.8 (**A**) Male condom. (**B**) Applying a male condom. Leaving space at the tip helps to ensure the condom will not break with ejaculation. (**C**) The female condom. (**D**) Insertion technique.

against pregnancy and some STIs. The failure rate of female condoms is around 5% with perfect use and 21% with typical use (SexualityandU.ca, 2010c).

Diaphragm

The **diaphragm** is a soft latex dome surrounded by a metal spring. Used in conjunction with a spermicidal jelly or cream, it is inserted into the vagina to cover the cervix (Fig. 4.9). As of 2009, diaphragms are no longer widely used in Canada and the spermicidal jelly required to eliminate sperm at the cervix is difficult to find (Healthlink BC, 2011). The diaphragm may be inserted up to 4 hours before intercourse but must be left in place for at least 6 hours afterward. Diaphragms are available in a range of sizes and styles. The diaphragm is available only by prescription and must be professionally fitted by

a health care professional. Women may need to be refitted with a different-sized diaphragm after pregnancy, abdominal or pelvic surgery, or weight loss or gain of 4.5 kg or more. As a general rule, diaphragms should be replaced every 1 to 2 years (Female Contraception, 2006). The woman also needs thorough instruction about its use and should practice putting it in and taking it out before she leaves the medical office (Fig. 4.10). Diaphragms are user-controlled, nonhormonal methods that are needed only at the time of intercourse, but they are not effective unless used correctly.

Cervical Cap

The **cervical cap** is smaller than the diaphragm and covers only the cervix; it is held in place by suction. Caps are made from silicone or latex and are used with

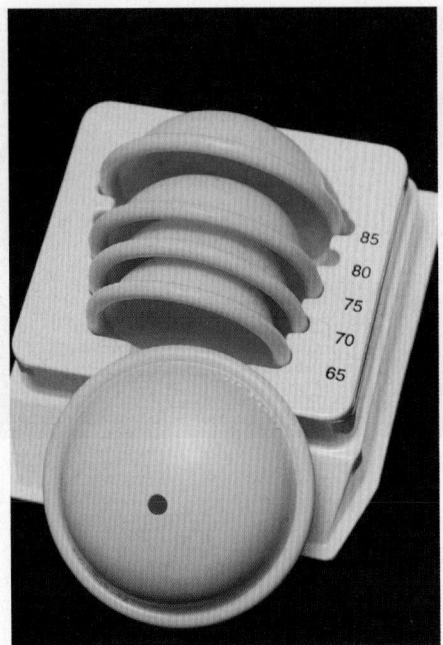

FIGURE 4.9 Sample diaphragm used for measuring.

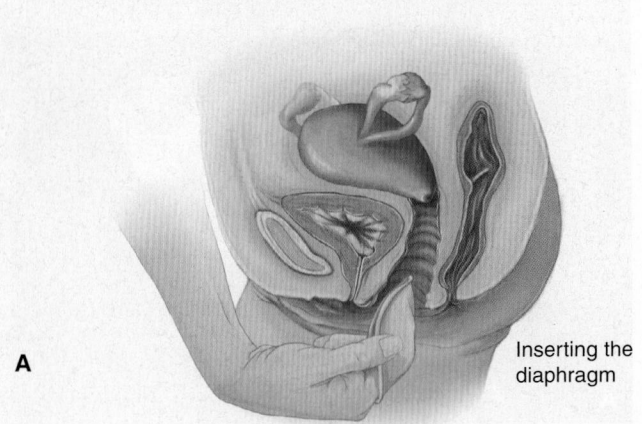

A   Inserting the diaphragm

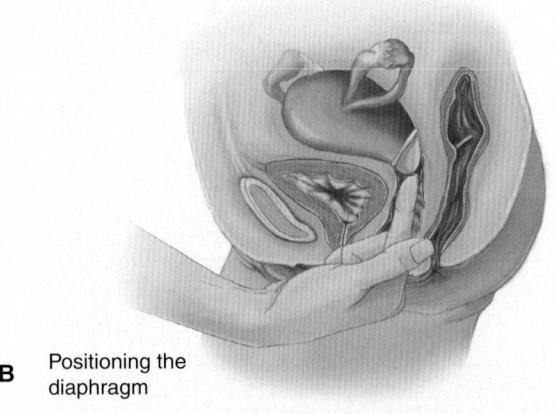

B   Positioning the diaphragm

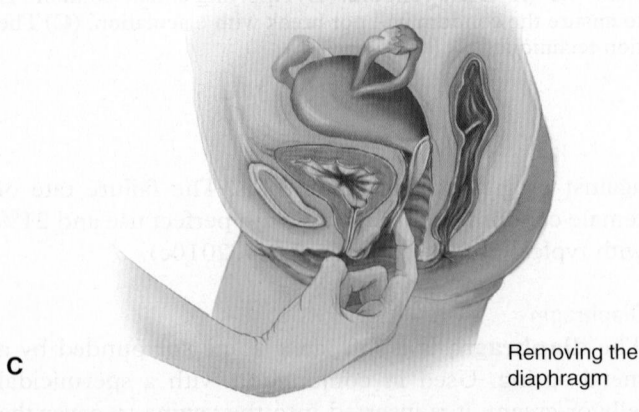

C   Removing the diaphragm

spermicide (Fig. 4.11). According to the Canadian Federation for Sexual Health (CFSH, 2009), it is difficult to purchase the necessary spermicidal jelly to use with the cap in Canada. Only one cervical cap, the silicone Oves cap, is approved by Health Canada. The latex Prentif cervical cap is more commonly used but is not officially approved by Health Canada. Women can be fitted by their doctor and order it online (SexualityandU.ca, 2010c).

The cap may be inserted up to 12 hours before intercourse and provides protection for 48 hours. The cap must be kept in the vagina for 8 hours after the final act of intercourse and should be replaced every 1 to 2 years. A refitting may also be necessary when a women experiences pregnancy, abortion, or weight changes. The dome of the cap is filled about one third full with spermicide. Spermicide should not be applied to the rim because it might interfere with the seal that must form around the cervix. The cap is available only by prescription and must be fitted by a health care professional.

Contraceptive Sponge

The **contraceptive sponge** is a nonhormonal, nonprescription device that includes both a barrier and a spermicide. The sponge provides protection for up to 12 hours (SexualityandU.ca, 2010c). The SOGC states that the contraceptive sponge is not a very effective form of birth control but can be used as a secondary method of contraception (Black et al., 2004). The sponge can be used with the condom. It has been noted that some women have a difficult time removing the sponge or do not remember to take it out (SexualityandU.ca, 2010c).

FIGURE 4.10 Application of a diaphragm. (**A**) To insert, fold the diaphragm in half, separate the labia with one hand, then insert upward and back into the vagina. (**B**) To position, make certain the diaphragm securely covers the cervix. (**C**) To remove, hook a finger over the top of the rim and bring the diaphragm down and out.

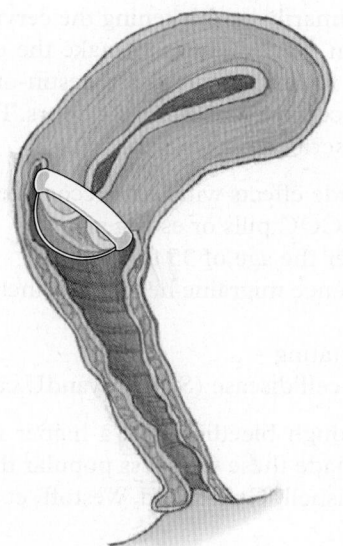

FIGURE 4.11 A cervical cap is placed over the cervix and used with a spermicidal jelly, the same as for a diaphragm.

The contraceptive sponge is a soft polyurethane concave device that prevents pregnancy by covering the cervix and releasing spermicide. While it is less effective than several other methods and does not offer protection against STIs, the sponge achieved a wide following among women who appreciated the spontaneity with which it could be used and its easy availability. To use the sponge, the woman first wets it with water, then inserts it into the vagina with a finger, using a cord loop attachment. It can be inserted up to 24 hours before intercourse and should be left in place for at least 6 hours following intercourse.

Hormonal Methods

Several options are available to women who want long-term but not permanent protection against pregnancy. These methods of contraception work by altering the hormones within a woman's body. They rely on estrogen and progestin or progestin alone to prevent ovulation. When used consistently, these methods are a most reliable way to prevent pregnancy. Hormonal methods include OCs, injectables, implants, vaginal rings, and **transdermal patches**.

Oral Contraceptives

As early as 1937, scientists recognized that the injection of progesterone inhibited ovulation and provided contraception in rabbits. Breakthrough bleeding was reported in early clinical trials in women, and the role of estrogen in cycle control was launched. This established the rationale for modern combination **oral contraceptives (OCs)** that contain both estrogen and progesterone (Fisher & Black, 2007). The OC is the most reliable method for women who seek reversible contraception. In 1960, the FDA approved the first combination OC, Enovid-10 (150 µg estrogen and 9 mg progesterone), for use in the

United States. OCs were approved for use in Canada in 1969. The most notable improvement in OCs in more than 40 years has been the lowering of the estrogen dose to as low as 20 µg and the introduction of new progestins.

OCs are used by millions of women worldwide and are the most common form of birth control chosen by Canadian women (Fig. 4.12). "In Canada, 18% of women of ages 15 to 49 who use birth control use the combined oral contraceptive (COC), and of Canadian women who use contraception, 32% choose COCs as their primary form of birth control" (Blake, Giesbrecht, & Soares, 2009, p. 1). When used perfectly, "The Pill" is 99.7% effective, making it most reliable form of contraception on the market (SexualityandU.ca, 2010b). With typical use, the pill has an effectiveness of 92%. Unlike the original OCs that women took decades ago, the new low-dose forms carry fewer health risks.

While they are most commonly prescribed for contraception, OCs have long been used in the management of a wide range of conditions and have many health benefits such as:

• Reduced incidence of ovarian and endometrial cancer
• Prevention and treatment of endometriosis
• Decreased incidence of acne and hirsutism
• Decreased incidence of ectopic pregnancy
• Decreased incidence of acute PID
• Reduced incidence of fibrocystic breast disease
• Decreased perimenopausal symptoms
• Increased menstrual cycle regularity
• Lower incidence of colorectal cancer
• Reduced iron-deficiency anemia by treating menorrhagia
• Reduced incidence of dysmenorrhea

OCs work primarily by suppressing ovulation by adding estrogen and progesterone to a woman's body, thus mimicking pregnancy. This hormonal level stifles GnRH production, which in turn suppresses FSH and LH and thus inhibits ovulation. Cervical mucus also

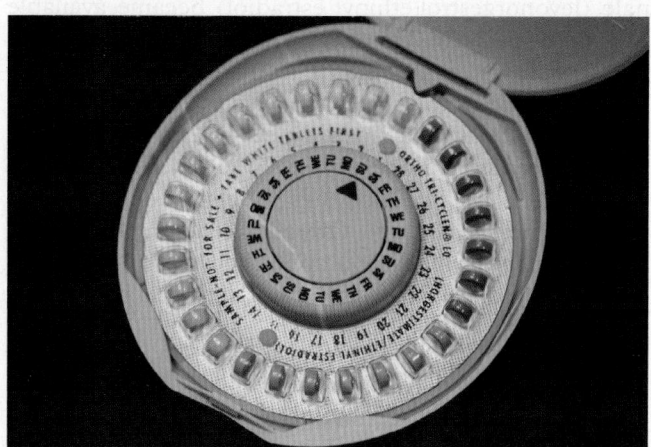

FIGURE 4.12 Oral contraceptive.

thickens, which hinders sperm transport into the uterus. The progestin hormone makes it more difficult for sperm to penetrate the egg because it makes the uterine mucus thicker; it may even prevent ovulation in some women. Implantation is inhibited by suppression of the maturation of the endometrium and alterations of uterine secretions (Leyland et al., 2010).

Two types of OC are available in Canada: combination OCs (which include the extended-cycle preparations) and progestin-only OCs.

Combination Oral Contraceptives

The COCs are available in three forms. *Monophasic pills* deliver fixed dosages of estrogen and progestin each day. *Biphasic pills* deliver the same amount of estrogen for the first 21 days. The progestin:estrogen ratio is lower in the first half of the cycle and this allows the endometrium to become thicker than normal. The progestin and estrogen levels are increased in the second half of the cycle to allow the shedding of the lining of the uterus to occur (Stöppler, 2011). *Triphasic pills* deliver increased doses of estrogen and may have increased doses of progestin concentrations throughout the cycle. A variety of combined OCs may be prescribed:

- Monophasic
  - Levonorgestrel/ethinyl estradiol (Alesse, Min-Ovral)
  - Drospirenone/ethinyl estradiol (Yasmin)
  - Desogestrel/ethinyl estradiol (Linessa/Marvelon)
  - Norethindrone/ethinyl estradiol (Brevicon 0.5/35 or 1/35; Ortho 0.5/35 or 1/35)
  - Norgestimate/ethinyl estradiol (Ortho Cyclen)
- Biphasic
  - Norethindrone/ethinyl estradiol (Synphasic)
- Thriphasic
  - Norgestimate/ethinyl estradiol (Ortho Tri-Cyclen)
  - Desogestrel/ethinyl estradiol (Linessa)

Yaz (drospirenone/ethinyl estradiol), a new combined OC on the market in Canada, provides 24 days of hormone therapy and 4 days of placebo tablets. Seasonale (levonorgestrol/ethinyl estradiol) became available in Canada in 2007. This extended-cycle birth control is a 91-day regimen in which a woman takes a hormone pill for 84 consecutive days followed by 7 days of a placebo pill. The woman can expect to have four withdrawal-bleeding episodes a year (SOCG, 2007).

There is no evidence that women need to have a monthly menstrual cycle. Overall, women report a preference for fewer menstrual cycles because of decreased menstrual complaints and increased quality of life (Mirosh, 2007).

Progestin-Only Oral Contraceptive

OCs that contain progestin only are called mini-pills. In Canada, the mini-pill is available as Micronor. The mini-pill is prescribed for women who cannot take estrogen and works primarily by thickening the cervical mucus to prevent sperm penetration and make the endometrium unfavourable for implantation. Progestin-only pills must be taken at a certain time every 24 hours. These pills are primarily prescribed for women:

- Who have side effects with, or a recognized contraindication to, COC pills or estrogen
- Who are over the age of 35 and smoke
- Who experience migraine headaches, including focal varieties
- Who are lactating
- With sickle-cell disease (SexualityandU.ca, 2010d)

Breakthrough bleeding and a higher risk for pregnancy have made these OCs less popular than combination OCs (Mishell, Guillebaud, Westoff, et al., 2007).

Nursing Management

The balance between the benefits and the risks of OCs must be determined for each woman when she is being assessed for this type of contraceptive. It is a highly effective contraceptive when taken properly but can aggravate many medical conditions, especially in women who smoke. Comparison Chart 4.2 lists advantages and disadvantages of OCs. A thorough history and pelvic examination, including a Pap smear, must be completed before the medication is prescribed and yearly thereafter. Women should also be counselled that the effectiveness of OCs is decreased when the woman is taking antibiotics; thus, the woman will need to use an alternative or secondary method during this period to prevent pregnancy. Women should also be instructed in what to do if they forget to take their pills. Most packages will recommend that if a pill is missed it should be taken as soon as it is forgotten. If more than one day of pills is missed, the woman should refer to the package instructions or to call her pharmacist or physician for further instructions.

Nurses need to provide OC users with a great deal of education before they leave the health care facility. They need to be able to identify early signs and symptoms that might indicate a problem.

▶ *Take* NOTE!

The mnemonic "ACHES" can help women who use OCs remember the early warning signs that necessitate a return to the health care provider (Box 4.6).

Injectable Contraceptives

Depo-Provera is the trade name for an injectable form of a progesterone-only contraceptive given every 12 weeks. Depo-Provera (depot medroxyprogesterone acetate [DMPA]) works by suppressing ovulation and the

COMPARISON CHART 4.2 ADVANTAGES AND DISADVANTAGES OF ORAL CONTRACEPTIVES

Advantages	Disadvantages
Regulate and shorten menstrual cycle	Offer no protection against STIs
Decrease severe cramping and bleeding	Pose a slightly increased risk for breast cancer
Reduce anemia	Modest risk for vein thrombosis and pulmonary emboli
Reduce ovarian and colorectal cancer risk	Increase risk for migraine headaches
Decrease benign breast disease	Increase risk for myocardial infarction, stroke, and hypertension for women who smoke
Reduce risk of endometrial cancer	May increase risk of depression
Improve acne	User must remember to take pill daily
Minimize perimenopausal symptoms	Cost-prohibitive for some women
Decrease incidence of rheumatoid arthritis	
Improve PMS symptoms	
Protect against loss of bone density	

Source: Dirubbo, N. E. (2006). Counsel your patients about contraceptive options. *Nurse Practitioner*, *31*(4), 40–44.

production of FSH and LH by the pituitary gland, by increasing the viscosity of cervical mucus, and by causing endometrial atrophy. A single injection of 150 mg into the buttocks acts like other progestin-only products to prevent pregnancy for 3 months at a time (Fig. 4.13). The SOCG recommends that Depo-Provera be given during the first 5 days of a menstrual cycle to achieve a contraceptive effect in 24 hours (Black et al., 2004). If given after the first 5 days, a backup birth control method should be used for 1 week. Depo-Provera is recommended for women who are not candidates for other forms of birth control. A primary advantage of Depo-Provera is that women only have think about birth control four times a year. It is also safe for women who are breastfeeding. The primary side effect of Depo-Provera is menstrual cycle disturbance (SexualityandU, 2010b).

Research has confirmed that use of DMPA is associated with a decrease in bone mineral density, although this decrease has not been shown to result in adverse outcomes such as osteoporosis or fractures. There is also evidence that the majority of this bone loss is temporary, as bone mineral density is regained once the contraceptive is stopped (SOGC, 2006b). Nevertheless, the SOGC (2006b) recommends that health care professionals counsel their patients on ways to improve their "bone health," such as with calcium and vitamin D supplementation and smoking cessation.

Transdermal Patches

The contraceptive patch (Ortho Evra) has been available in Canada since January 2004. It is a 4 × 4 cm beige patch that sticks to a woman's skin (lower abdomen, upper outer arm, buttocks, or upper torso; avoiding the breasts) and continuously releases estrogen and a progestin into the bloodstream (SexualityandU.ca, 2010b). The patch is applied every 7 days for 3 weeks, followed by a patch-free week during which withdrawal bleeding occurs. Transdermal absorption allows the drug to enter the bloodstream directly, avoiding rapid inactivation in the liver known as first-pass metabolism. Since estrogen

BOX 4.6 **Early Signs of Complications for OC Users**

A:	Abdominal pain may indicate liver or gallbladder problems.
C:	Chest pain or shortness of breath may indicate a pulmonary embolus.
H:	Headaches may indicate hypertension or impending stroke.
E:	Eye problems might indicate hypertension or an attack.
S:	Severe leg pain may indicate a thromboembolic event.

Source: Courtney, K. (2006). The contraceptive patch: Latest developments. *AWHONN Lifelines, 10*(3), 250–253.

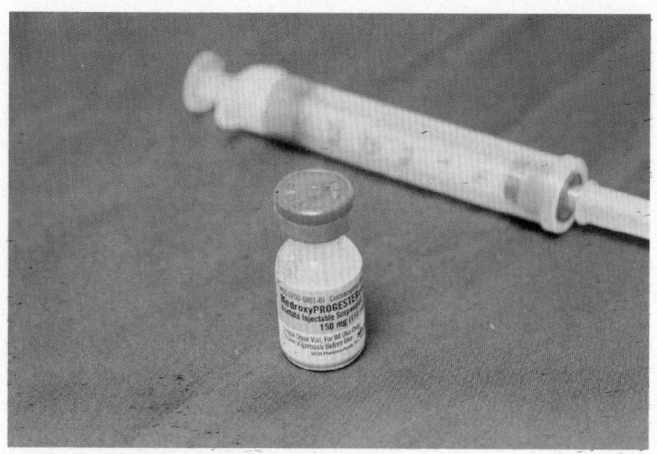

FIGURE 4.13 Injectable contraceptive.

and progesterone are metabolized by liver enzymes, avoiding first-pass metabolism was thought to reduce adverse effects. However, recent evidence suggests that the risk for venous thrombosis and embolism is increased with the patch. The Canadian version of the patch contains less ethinyl estradiol than the version sold in the United States (0.60 mg versus 0.75 mg), and the total estrogen exposure with the Canadian version appears to be closer to that of a 35 μg pill (Fisher & Black, 2007).

Additional studies are under way to understand the clinical significance of these latest findings, but in the interim nurses need to focus on ongoing risk assessment and should be prepared to discuss current research findings with clients.

Compliance with combination contraceptive patch use has been shown to be significantly greater than compliance with OCs (Graziottin, 2006). The patch provides combination hormone therapy with a side effect profile similar to that of OCs. The manufacturer is currently evaluating extended regimens for the patch (Stewart, Kaunitz, LaGuardia, et al., 2006) (Fig. 4.14).

Vaginal Rings

The contraceptive **vaginal ring**, NuvaRing, is a flexible, soft, plastic ring that a woman inserts into her vagina. The ring releases both progestin and estrogen over 3 weeks. The woman removes the ring for a 7-day interval (during which she usually has a period) and then inserts a new ring (Fig. 4.15). The ring does not have to be fitted. To insert the ring, the woman compresses it and places it into the vagina, behind the pubic bone and as far back as possible, but precise placement is not critical. The hormones are absorbed through the vaginal mucosa. Effectiveness and adverse events are similar to those seen with combination OCs. Clients need to be counselled regarding timely insertion of the ring and what to do in case of accidental expulsion. This device is also being tested for extended regimens to reduce menstrual bleeding.

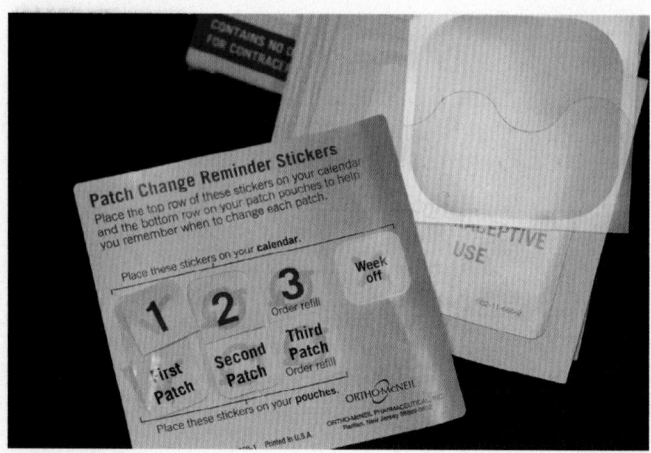

FIGURE **4.14** Transdermal patch.

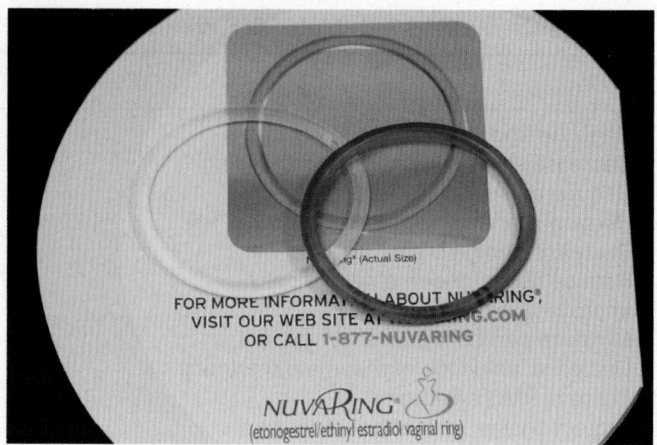

FIGURE **4.15** Vaginal ring.

Implantable Contraceptives

The **implant** is a subdermal time-release contraceptive method that delivers synthetic progestin. Once in place, the implant delivers several years of continuous, highly effective contraception. Like progestin-only pills, implants act by inhibiting ovulation and thickening cervical mucus so sperm cannot penetrate. The side effects are also similar to progestin-only pills: irregular bleeding, headaches, weight gain, breast tenderness, and depression. Fertility is restored quickly after the implant is removed. Placement and removal of contraceptive implants require a minor surgical procedure; therefore, they must be inserted and removed by a health care provider. The implants don't offer any protection against STIs. Contraceptive implants releasing either estrogen and progestin or progestin alone are slow to develop, test, and market, and none are currently available in Canada. Sales of Norplant, the only implant to have been marketed in Canada, were discontinued in September 2002. Second-generation implant systems (Implanon and Jadelle) have been developed to simplify insertion and removal and are effective for 3 years. These new implants contain progestin only (U.S. Food and Drug Administration, 2009).

Intrauterine Systems

Intrauterine systems are small, plastic T-shaped objects that are placed inside the uterus to provide contraception (Fig. 4.16). They prevent pregnancy by making the endometrium of the uterus hostile to implantation of a fertilized ovum by causing a nonspecific inflammatory reaction (Black et al., 2004). Monthly periods become lighter, shorter, and less painful, making this a useful method for women with heavy, painful periods. Some implants may contain copper or progesterone to enhance their effectiveness. One or two attached strings protrude into the vagina so that the user can check for placement.

There are two types of IUDs and systems currently available in Canada: those that do not release hormones

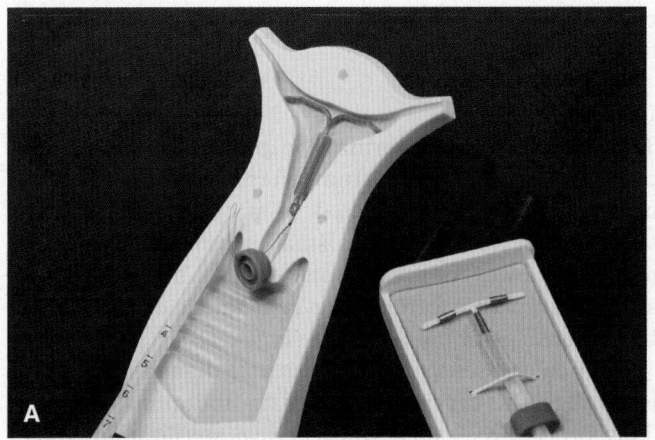
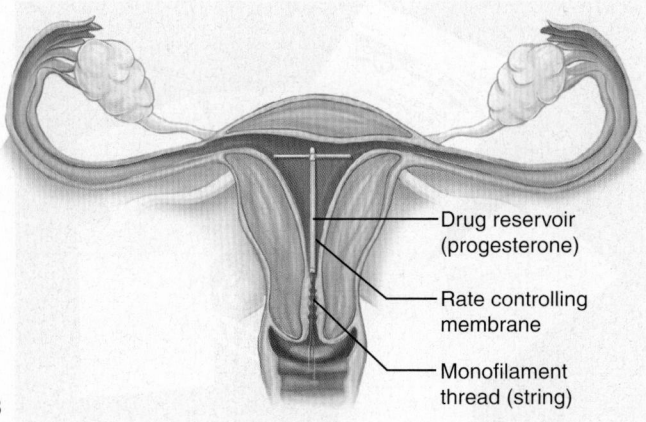

Drug reservoir (progesterone)

Rate controlling membrane

Monofilament thread (string)

FIGURE 4.16 (**A**) Intrauterine system. (**B**) An intrauterine system in place in the uterus.

(Nova-T or Flexi-T 300) and those that release a progestin (levonorgestrel) (Mirena) (SOGC, 2006b). These products do not protect women against STIs. Mirena provides intrauterine contraception for up to 5 years. An advantage of hormonally impregnated intrauterine systems is that they are relatively maintenance-free: users must consciously discontinue using them to become pregnant rather than making a daily decision to avoid conception (French, Vliet, Cowan, et al., 2006). Box 4.7 highlights warning signs of complications.

IUDs and systems are especially suited for women who:

- Desire a reversible, effective, coitally independent method of contraception
- Want a private form of contraception
- Are concerned that they may not remember to use a daily method
- Are considering sterilization
- Desire contraception immediately after delivery or abortion
- Are breastfeeding

> ### BOX 4.7 Warnings for Intrauterine System Users of Potential Complications
>
> P: Period late, pregnancy, abnormal spotting or bleeding
> A: Abdominal pain, pain with intercourse
> I: Infection exposure, abnormal vaginal discharge
> N: Not feeling well, fever, chills
> S: String length shorter or longer or missing
>
> Source: Hatcher, R. A., Trussell, J., Nelson, A. L., Cates, W., Jr., Kowal, D., & Policar, M. (2011). *Contraceptive technology* (20th ed.). New York: Ardent Media, Inc.

- Cannot use a hormonal method of contraception
- Have regular periods and minimal dysmenorrhea
- Want to determine family spacing
- Are considering long-term contraception (SexualityandU.ca, 2010b)

Emergency Contraception

Unplanned pregnancy is a major health, economic, and social issue for women. According to the CFSH (2007, p. 4), "there is no national data on the prevalence of unintended pregnancy in Canada." The CFSH also indicated that national pregnancy rates have declined over the past two decades and induced abortion rates have declined in women under the age of 30. **Emergency contraception** reduces the risk of pregnancy after unprotected intercourse or contraceptive failure such as condom breakage (Lever, 2005). Commonly referred to as the "morning after pill," an emergency contraceptive is used within 72 hours of unprotected intercourse to prevent pregnancy. The sooner emergency contraceptives are taken, the more effective they are. It is believed that emergency contraception works by delaying or inhibiting ovulation. When used properly, emergency contraceptives reduce the risk of pregnancy for a single act of unprotected sex by almost 75% (SexualityandU.ca, 2010a).

Types of emergency contraception include hormonal methods (Yuzpe method and Plan B) and the copper IUD. A copper IUD can be inserted within 7 days of unprotected sex to prevent 99% of pregnancies (SexualityandU.ca, 2010a) Plan B is available in Canada from pharmacists without a prescription (Fig. 4.17) (Fisher & Black, 2007).

Prime points to stress concerning emergency contraceptives are that they:

- Do not offer any protection against STIs or future pregnancies
- Should not be used in place of regular birth control, as they are less effective

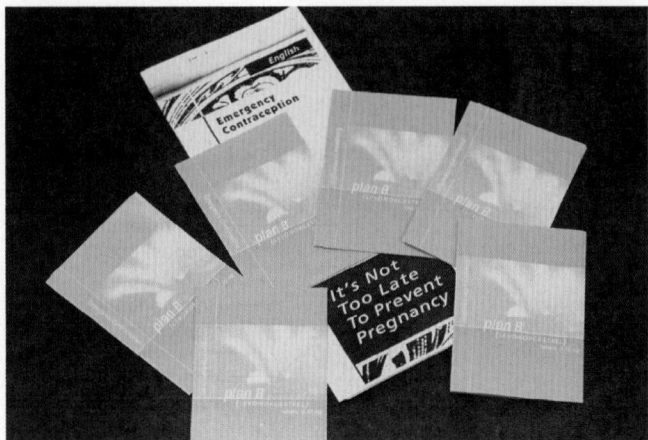

FIGURE 4.17 Emergency contraceptive kit.

- Are regular birth control pills given at higher doses and more frequently
- Are contraindicated during pregnancy because they are considered to be teratogenic

Contrary to popular belief, emergency contraceptives do not induce abortion and are not related to mifepristone (RU-486), the so-called abortion pill. Mifepristone chemically induces abortion by blocking the body's progesterone receptors, which are necessary for pregnancy maintenance. Emergency contraceptives simply prevent embryo creation and uterine implantation from occurring in the first place. There is no evidence that emergency contraceptives have any effect on an already-implanted ovum. The side effects are nausea and vomiting. RU-486 is not available in Canada.

Sterilization

Sterilization is an attractive method of contraception for those who are certain they do not want any, or any more, children. **Sterilization** refers to surgical procedures intended to render a person infertile. Sterilization should be considered a permanent end to fertility because reversal surgery is difficult, expensive, and not highly successful.

Tubal Ligation

Tubal ligation, the sterilization procedure for women, can be performed postpartum, after an abortion, or as an interval procedure unrelated to pregnancy. A laparoscope is inserted through a small subumbilical incision to provide a view of the fallopian tubes. They are grasped and sealed with a cauterizing instrument or with rings, bands, or clips or cut and tied (Fig. 4.18).

A new approach used to visualize the fallopian tubes is through the cervix instead of an abdominal incision. This procedure, called transcervical sterilization, offers several advantages over conventional tubal ligation: general anesthesia and incisions are not needed, thereby increasing safety, lowering costs, and improving access to sterilization. Two methods of transcervical sterilization have been introduced: Essure in 2002 and Adiana in 2009. Only Essure is currently available in Canada. In this procedure, a tiny coil is introduced into the fallopian tubes through the cervix. The coil promotes tissue growth in the fallopian tubes, and over a period of 3 months, this growth blocks the tubes (Mayo Clinic Staff, 2012a). Less invasive than tubal ligation, this technique has become increasingly popular. It can be performed by a trained health care professional in a physician's office or out-patient setting. General anesthesia is not needed, and women usually can go home with minimal post-procedure recovery time (Mayo Clinic Staff, 2012a; Thiel & Carson, 2008).

▶ **Take** NOTE!

According to Thiel and Carson (2008), rates of female sterilization have decreased in Canada. In 1993, 16% of women had permanent contraception versus 7% in 2002. The main method of permanent contraception in Canada remains the vasectomy.

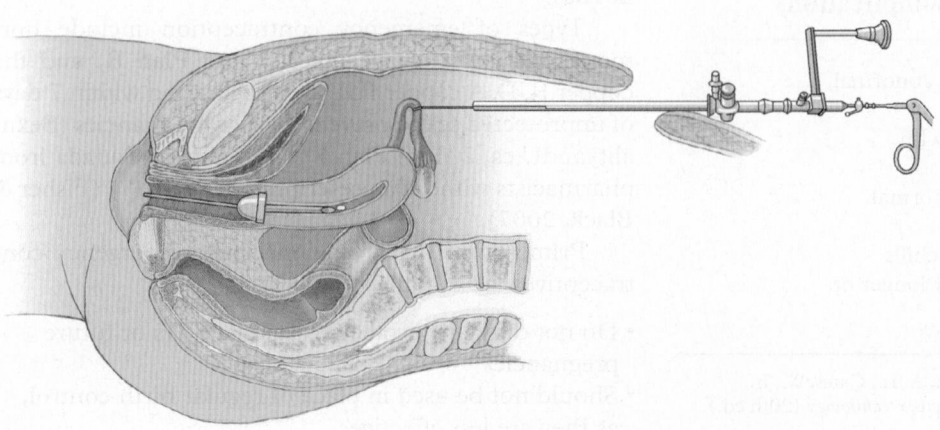

FIGURE 4.18 Laparoscopy for tubal sterilization.

Vasectomy

Male sterilization is accomplished with a surgical procedure known as a **vasectomy**. It is usually performed under local anesthesia in a urologist's office, and most men can return to work and normal activities in a day or two. The procedure involves making a small incision into the scrotum and cutting the vas deferens, which carries sperm from the testes to the penis (Fig. 4.19). After vasectomy, semen no longer contains sperm. This is not immediate, though, and the man must submit semen specimens for analysis until two specimens show that no sperm is present. When the specimen shows azoospermia, the man's sterility is then confirmed (Mammen, Hwang, & Costabile, 2008).

Nursing Management of the Woman Choosing a Contraceptive Method

The choice of a contraceptive method is a very personal one involving many factors. What makes a woman choose one contraceptive method over another? In making contraceptive choices, couples must balance their sexual lives, their reproductive goals, and each partner's health

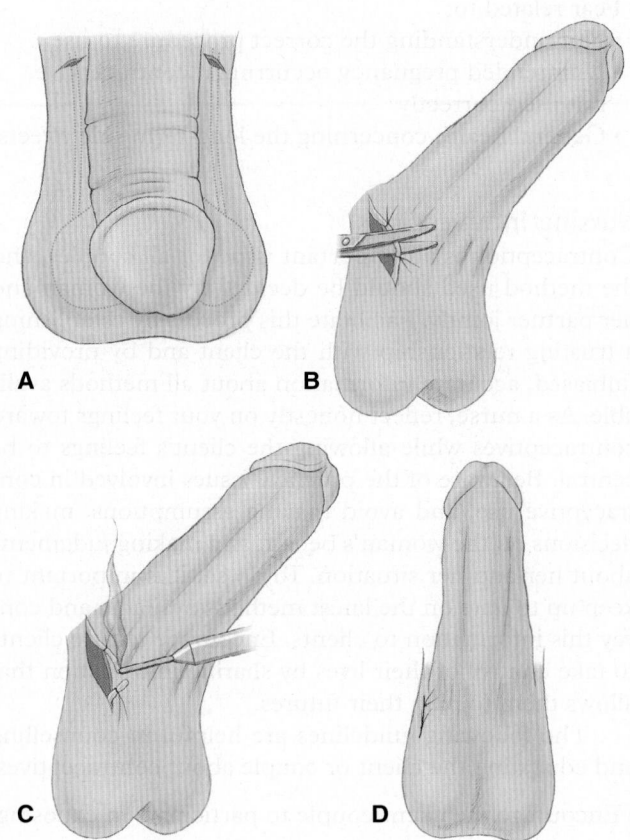

FIGURE 4.19 Vasectomy. (**A**) Site of vasectomy incisions. (**B**) The vas deferens is cut with surgical scissors. (**C**) Cut ends of the vas deferens are cauterized to ensure blockage of the passage of sperm. (**D**) Final skin suture.

BOX 4.8 Selected Religious Choices for Family Planning and Abortion

- Roman Catholic—Abstinence and natural family planning; no abortion
- Judaism—Family planning; abortion accepted in first trimester
- Islam—Family planning accepted; abortion only for serious reasons
- Protestant Christianity—Firmly in favour of family planning; mixed on abortion
- Buddhism—Long experience with family planning and abortion
- Hinduism—Accept both family planning and abortion
- Native American religions—Accept both family planning and abortion
- Chinese religions—Taoism and Confucianism accept both family planning and abortion

---

Source: Srikanthan, A., & Reid, R. (2008). Religious and cultural influences on contraception. *Journal of Obstetrics and Gynecology, February, 30*(2), 129–137. Retrieved March 4, 2012 from http://www.sogc.org/jogc/abstracts/full/200802_WomensHealth_1.pdf.

and safety. The search for a choice that satisfies all three objectives is challenging. A method that works for a sexually active teenage girl may not meet her needs later in life. Several considerations influence a person's choice of contraceptives:

- Motivation
- Cost
- Cultural and religious beliefs (Box 4.8)
- Convenience
- Effectiveness
- Side effects
- Desire for children in the future
- Safety of the method
- Comfort level with sexuality
- Protection from STIs
- Interference with spontaneity

If a contraceptive is to be effective, the woman must understand how it works, must be able to use it correctly and consistently, and must be comfortable and confident with it. If a patient cannot comply with taking a pill daily, consider a method used once a week (transdermal patches), once every 3 weeks (transvaginal ring), or once every 3 months (Depo-Provera injection). Another option may be a progesterone intrauterine system that lasts 3 to 5 years and reduces menstrual flow significantly.

Regardless of which method is chosen, the client's needs should be paramount in the discussion. The nurse can educate clients about which methods are available and their advantages and disadvantages, efficacy, cost, and safety. Counselling can help the woman choose a contraceptive method that is efficacious and fits her preferences and lifestyle.

Nursing Assessment

When assessing which contraceptive method might meet the client's needs, the nurse might ask:

• Do your religious beliefs interfere with any methods?
• Will this method interfere with your sexual pleasure?
• Are you aware of the various methods currently available?
• Is cost a major consideration, or does your insurance cover it?
• Does your partner influence which method you choose?
• Have you heard anything troubling about any of the methods?
• How comfortable are you touching your own body?
• What are your future plans for having children?

Although deciding on a contraceptive is a very personal decision between a woman and her partner, nurses can assist in this process by performing a complete health history and physical examination, and by educating the woman and her partner about necessary laboratory and diagnostic testing. Areas of focus during the nursing assessment are as follows:

• Medical history: smoking status, cancer of the reproductive tract, diabetes mellitus, migraines, hypertension, thromboembolic disorder, allergies, risk factors for cardiovascular disease
• Family history: cancer, cardiovascular disease, hypertension, stroke, diabetes
• Gynecologic history: menstrual disorders, current contraceptive, previous STIs, PID, vaginitis, sexual activity
• Personal history: use of tampons and feminine hygiene products, plans for childbearing, comfort with touching herself, number of sexual partners, involvement of sexual partner in the decision
• Physical examination: height, weight, blood pressure, breast examination, thyroid palpation, pelvic examination
• Diagnostic testing: urinalysis, complete blood count, Pap smear, wet mount to check for STIs, HIV/AIDS tests, lipid profile, glucose level

Figure 4.20 shows an example of a family planning flow record that can be used during the assessment. After collecting the assessment data above, consider the medical factors to help decide if the woman is a candidate for all methods or whether some should be eliminated. For example, if she reports she has multiple sex partners and has a lengthy history of various pelvic infections, she would not be a good candidate for an intrauterine system, based on her infection history. Barrier methods (male or female condoms) of contraception might be recommended to this client to offer protection against STIs.

Nursing Diagnoses

A few nursing diagnoses that might be appropriate based on the nurse's assessment during the decision-making process include:

• Deficient knowledge related to:
 • Methods available
 • Side effects/safety
 • Correct use of method chosen
 • Previous myths believed
• Risk for infection related to:
 • Unprotected sexual intercourse
 • Past history of STIs
 • Methods offering protection

Nursing diagnoses applicable to the contraceptive include:

• Health-seeking behaviours related to:
 • Perceived need for limiting number of children
 • Overall health relative to contraceptives
• Risk for ineffective health maintenance related to:
 • Not being familiar with the various contraceptive methods
 • Being unaware of high-risk sexual behaviour leading to STIs
• Fear related to:
 • Not understanding the correct procedure to use
 • Unintended pregnancy occurring if contraceptive not used correctly
 • General health concerning the long-term side effects

Nursing Interventions

Contraception is an important issue for all couples, and the method used should be decided by the woman and her partner jointly. Facilitate this process by establishing a trusting relationship with the client and by providing unbiased, accurate information about all methods available. As a nurse, reflect honestly on your feelings toward contraceptives while allowing the client's feelings to be central. Be aware of the practical issues involved in contraceptive use, and avoid making assumptions, making decisions on the woman's behalf, and making judgments about her and her situation. To do so, it is important to keep up to date on the latest methods available and convey this information to clients. Encourage female clients to take control of their lives by sharing information that allows them to plan their futures.

The following guidelines are helpful in counselling and educating the client or couple about contraceptives:

• Encourage the client/couple to participate in choosing a method.
• Provide client education. The client/couple must be informed users before the method is agreed upon. Education should be targeted to the client's level so it is understood. Provide step-by-step teaching and an

FAMILY PLANNING FLOW (VISIT) RECORD

Name:_____
ID #:_____
Date of Birth:_____

	Date:			Date:	
Current Method					
Reason for Visit					
LMP					
SUBJECTIVE DATA	**Pt.**	**Comments**	**Pt.**	**Comments**	
Severe headaches					
Depression					
Visual abnormalities					
Dyspnea/chest pain					
Breast changes					
SBE					
Abdominal pain					
Nausea and vomiting					
Dysuria/frequency					
Menstrual irregularities					
Vaginal discharge/infections					
Leg pain					
Surgery, injury, infections, or serious illness since last visit					
Allergic reaction					
Pregnancy plans					
Other					
OBJECTIVE DATA	**Weight**	**B.P.**	**Weight**	**B.P.**	
Other					
Lab					
ASSESSMENT					
Check here if assessment continues on progress notes	O		O		
PLAN					
Type of contraceptive given					
COUNSELING/EDUCATION					
Next appointment					
SIGNATURE/TITLE					
SIGNATURE/TITLE					

O = normal   ✓ = abnormal

FIGURE 4.20 Family planning flow (visit) record.

TEACHING GUIDELINE 4.5

Client Teaching and Counselling for Cervical Caps, Diaphragms, Vaginal Rings, and Condoms

Cervical Cap

• It is important to be involved in the fitting process.
• To insert the cap, pinch the sides together, compress the cap dome, insert into the vagina, and place over the cervix.
• Use one finger to feel around the entire circumference to make sure there are no gaps between the cap rim and the cervix.
• After a minute or two, pinch the dome and tug gently to check for evidence of suction. The cap should resist the tug and not slide off easily.
• To remove the cap, press the index finger against the rim and tip the cap slightly to break the suction, and gently pull out the cap.
• Practice inserting and removing the cervical cap three times to validate your proficiency with this device.
• Fill the dome of the cap up about one third full with spermicide cream or jelly. Do not apply spermicide to the rim, since it may interfere with the seal.
• Wait approximately 30 minutes after insertion before engaging in sexual intercourse to be sure that a seal has formed between the rim and the cervix.
• Leave the cervical cap in place for a minimum of 6 hours after sexual intercourse. It can be left in place for up to 48 hours without additional spermicide being added.
• Do not use during menses due to the potential for toxic shock syndrome. Use an alternative method such as condoms during this time.
• Inspect the cervical cap prior to insertion for cracks, holes, or tears.
• After using the cervical cap, wash it with soap and water, dry thoroughly, and store in its container.

Diaphragm

• Always empty the bladder prior to inserting the diaphragm.
• Inspect diaphragm for holes or tears by holding it up to a light source, or fill it with water and check for a leak.
• Place approximately a tablespoon of spermicidal jelly or cream in the dome and around the rim of the diaphragm.
• The diaphragm can be inserted up to 6 hours prior to intercourse.
• Select the position that is most comfortable for insertion:
  • Squatting
  • Leg up, raising the nondominant leg up on a low stool
  • Reclining position, lying on your back in bed
  • Sitting forward on the edge of a chair

• Hold the diaphragm between the thumb and fingers and compress it to form a "figure-eight" shape.
• Insert the diaphragm into the vagina, directing it downward as far as it will go.
• Tuck the front rim of the diaphragm behind the pubic bone so that the rubber hugs the front wall of the vagina.
• Feel for the cervix through the diaphragm to make sure it is properly placed.
• To remove the diaphragm, insert the finger up and over the top side and move slightly to the side, breaking the suction.
• Pull the diaphragm down and out of the vagina.
• Avoid the use of oil-based products such as baby oil, since this may weaken the rubber.
• Wash the diaphragm with soap and water after use and dry thoroughly.
• Place the diaphragm back into the storage case.
• The diaphragm may need to be refitted after weight loss or gain or childbirth.
• Diaphragms should not be used by women with latex allergies.

Vaginal Ring

• Each ring is used for one menstrual cycle, which consists of 3 weeks of continuous use followed by a ring-free week to allow for menses.
• No fitting is necessary—one size fits all.
• Compress the ring and insert it into the vagina, behind the pubic bone, as far back as possible.
• Precision placement is not essential.
• Backup contraception is needed for 7 days if the ring is expelled for more than 3 hours during the 3-week period of continuous use.
• The vaginal ring is left in place for 3 weeks, then removed and discarded.
• The vaginal ring is not recommended for women with uterine prolapse or lack of vaginal muscle tone (Youngkin & Davis, 2004).

Male Condom

• Always keep the condom in its original package until ready to use.
• Store in a cool, dry place.
• Use spermicidal condoms if available.
• Check expiration date before using.
• Use a new condom for each sexual act.
• Place the condom over the erect penis prior to insertion.
• Place condom on the head of the penis and unroll it down the shaft.

- Leave a half-inch of empty space at the end to collect ejaculate.
- Avoid use of oil-based products because they may cause breakage.
- After intercourse, remove the condom while the penis is still erect.
- Discard condom after use.

Female Condom

- Practice wearing and inserting prior to first use with sexual intercourse.
- Condom can be inserted up to 8 hours before intercourse.

- Condom is intended for one-time use.
- It can be purchased over the counter—one size fits all.
- Avoid wearing rings to prevent tears; long fingernails can also cause tears.
- Spermicidal lubricant can be used if desired.
- Insert the inner ring high in the vagina, against the cervix.
- Place the outer ring on the outside of the vagina.
- Make sure the erect penis is placed inside the female condom.
- Remove the condom after intercourse. Avoid spilling the ejaculate.

opportunity for practice for certain methods (cervical caps, diaphragms, vaginal rings, and condoms). See Teaching Guideline 4.5 and Figure 4.21.

- Obtain written informed consents, which are needed for intrauterine systems, implants, abortion, or sterilization. Informed consent implies that the client is making a knowledgeable, voluntary choice; has received complete information about the method, including the risks; and is free to change her mind before using the method or undergoing the procedure (Fisher & Black, 2007).
- Discuss contraindications for all selected contraceptives.
- Consider the client's cultural and religious beliefs when providing care.
- Address myths and misperceptions about the methods under consideration in your initial discussion of contraceptives.

It is also important to clear up common misconceptions about contraception and pregnancy. Clearing up misconceptions will permit new learning to take hold

and a better client response to whichever methods are explored and ultimately selected. Some common misconceptions include the following:

- Breastfeeding protects against pregnancy.
- Pregnancy can be avoided if the male partner "pulls out" before he ejaculates.
- Pregnancy can't occur during menses.
- Douching after sex will prevent pregnancy.
- Pregnancy won't happen during the first sexual experience.
- Taking birth control pills protects against STIs.
- The woman can be too old to get pregnant.
- Irregular menstruation prevents pregnancy.

When discussing in detail each method of birth control, focus on specific information for each method outlined. Include information such as how this particular method works to prevent pregnancy under normal circumstances of use; the non-contraceptive benefits to overall health; advantages and disadvantages of all methods; the cost involved for each method; danger signs that need to be reported to the health care provider; and the required frequency of office visits needed for each method.

In addition, outline factors that place the client at risk for failure. There are several reasons why contraceptive failures occur. Use Table 4.5 to provide patient education concerning a few of the reasons for contraceptive failure. Help clients who have chosen abstinence or FAMs to define the sexual activities in which they want and don't want to participate. This helps them set sexual limits or boundaries. Help them to develop communication and negotiation skills that will allow them to be successful. Supporting, encouraging, and respecting a couple's choice of abstinence is vital for nurses.

After clients have chosen a method of contraception, it is important to address the following:

- Emphasize that a second method to use as a backup is always needed.

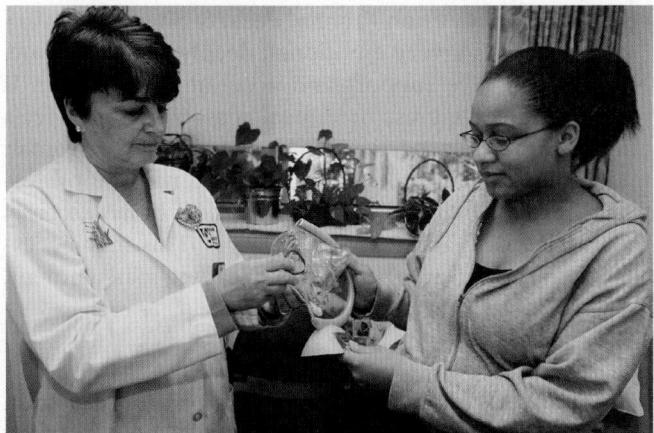
FIGURE 4.21 The nurse demonstrates insertion of a vaginal ring during client teaching.

TABLE 4.5   CONTRACEPTIVE PROBLEMS AND EDUCATIONAL NEEDS

Contraceptive Failure Problem	Client Education Needed
Not following instructions for correct use of contraceptive	Take pill at the same time every day. Use condoms properly and check condition before using. Make sure diaphragm or cervical cap covers cervix completely. Check IUD for placement monthly.
Inconsistent use of contraceptive	Contraceptives must be used regularly to achieve maximum effectiveness. All it takes is one unprotected act of sexual intercourse to become pregnant. 2% to 5% of condoms will break or tear during use.
Condom broke during sex	Check expiration date. Store condoms properly. Use only a water-based lubricant. Watch for tears caused by long fingernails. Use spermicides to decrease possibility of pregnancy if failure occurs.
Use of antibiotics or other herbs taken with OCs	Use alternative methods during the antibiotic therapy, plus 7 additional days. Implement on day 1 of taking antibiotics.
Belief that you can't get pregnant during menses or that it is safe "just this one time"	It may be possible to become pregnant on almost any day of the menstrual cycle.

- Provide both oral and written instructions on the method chosen.
- Discuss the need for STI protection if not using a barrier method.
- Inform the client about the availability of ECs.

Abortion

Abortion is defined as the expulsion of an embryo or fetus before it is viable (Alexander, LaRosa, Bader, et al., 2010). Abortion can be a medical or surgical procedure. The purpose of abortion is to terminate a pregnancy. Canada is one of the very few countries in the world that has no criminal law restricting abortion. Legislation against abortion was liberalized in 1969. In1988, the Supreme Court of Canada struck down Canada's abortion law as unconstitutional. The law was found to violate Section 7 of the Charter of Rights and Freedoms because it infringed upon a woman's right to "life, liberty and security of person" (National Abortion Federation, 2010).

Canadian women obtained fewer induced abortions in 2005 compared with the previous year (Statistics Canada, 2005). A total of 96,815 induced abortions were performed on Canadian women in 2005, down 3.2% from 100,039 in 2004. Specifically, the induced abortion rate decreased from 14.6 abortions for every 1,000 women ages 15 to 44 in 2004 to 14.1 per 1,000 in 2005. Induced abortion rates fell in every age group, except among women ages 35 to 39, where the rate remained the same. Women under 20 experienced the largest decline in abortion rates, from 13.8 for every 1,000 women in 2004 to 13.0 in 2005 (Statistics Canada, 2005).

Surgical Abortion

Surgical abortion is usually carried out by vacuum aspiration or suction curettage. It is an ambulatory procedure done under local anesthesia. The cervix is dilated prior to surgery and then the products of conception are removed by suction evacuation. The uterus may gently be scraped by curettage to make sure that it is empty. The entire procedure lasts about 10 minutes.

Medical Abortion

In a medical abortion, the woman takes certain medications to induce a miscarriage to remove the products of conception. Two methods are currently used to terminate a pregnancy during the first trimester. The first method uses methotrexate (an antineoplastic agent) followed by misoprostol (a prostaglandin agent) given as a vaginal suppository or in oral form 3 to 7 days later. Methotrexate induces abortion because of its toxicity to trophoblastic tissue, the growing embryo. Misoprostol works by causing uterine contractions, which help to expel the products of conception. This method is around 92% successful in completing an abortion (Tanha, Feizi, & Shariat, 2010).

Abortion is a very emotional, deeply personal issue. Nurses must give support and accurate information. If for personal, religious, or ethical reasons a nurse feels unable to actively participate in the care of a woman undergoing an abortion, he or she still has the professional responsibility to ensure that the woman receives the nursing care and help she requires. This may necessitate a transfer to another area or a staffing reassignment.

Menopause

Menopause is defined as the loss of ovarian function (SOGC, 2006d). It "is a retrospective definition made following one year of amenorrhea" (Rees at al., 2009, in Holloway, 2011, p. 47). Menopause marks the end of menstruation and childbearing capacity. In Canada, the average woman reaches menopause at the age of 51, and the SOCG (2006d) estimates that by 2026, 22% of Canadian population will be over 50 years of age.

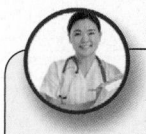

▶ *Take* NOTE!

Humans are virtually the only species to out-live their reproductive capacities.

Menopause signals the end of an era for many women. It concludes their ability to reproduce, and some women find advancing age, altered roles, and these phys-iologic changes to be overwhelming events that may pre-cipitate depression and anxiety (Marnocha, Bergstrom, & Dempsy, 2011). Menopause does not happen in isola-tion. Midlife is often experienced as a time of change and reflection. Change happens in many arenas: children are leaving or returning home, employment pressures intensify as career moves or decisions are required, elderly parents require more care or the death of a parent may have a major impact, and partners are retrenching or undergoing their own midlife crises. Women must negotiate all these changes in addition to menopause. Managing these stressful changes can be very challeng-ing for many women as they make the transition into midlife.

A woman is born with approximately 500,000 ova, but only 300 to 400 ever mature fully to be released dur-ing the menstrual cycle. The absolute number of ova in the ovary is a major determinant of fertility. Over the course of her premenopausal life, there is a steady decline in the number of immature ova. No one understands this depletion, but it does not occur in isolation. Maturing ova are surrounded by follicles that produce two major hormones: estrogen, in the form of estradiol, and proges-terone. The cyclic maturation of the ovum is directed by the hypothalamus. The hypothalamus triggers a cascade of neurohormones, which act through the pituitary and the ovaries as a pulse generator for reproduction.

This hypothalamic–pituitary–ovarian axis begins to break down long before there is any sign that menopause is imminent. Some scientists believe that the pulse gen-erator in the hypothalamus simply degenerates; others speculate that the ovary becomes more resistant to the pituitary hormone FSH and simply shuts down (Brockie, 2008). The final act in this well-orchestrated process is amenorrhea.

As menopause approaches, more and more of the menstrual cycles become anovulatory. This period of time, usually 2 to 8 years before cessation of menstrua-tion, is termed *perimenopause* (Brockie, 2008). In peri-menopause, a woman's body begins to release smaller amounts of estrogen and progesterone (SOCG, 2006d). These fluctuating hormones can cause the ovaries to release an egg in some months but not in others. Some women will also notice that their menstrual cycle may become heavier or mightier in some months and the time frame between periods may be decrease or increase. Perimenopause usually begins around age 39 to 51. When menopause finally appears, viable ova are gone. Estrogen levels plummet by 90%, and estrone, produced in fat cells, replaces estradiol as the body's main form of estrogen. In addition, testosterone levels decrease with menopause.

Menopause, with its dramatic decline in estrogen, affects not only the reproductive organs, but also other body systems:

• Brain: mood and memory, hot flashes, sleep distur-bances
• Cardiovascular: lower levels of high-density lipopro-tein (HDL) and increased risk of cardiovascular dis-ease
• Skeletal: rapid loss of bone density increases the risk of osteoporosis
• Breasts: duct and glandular tissues are replaced by fat
• Genitourinary: vaginal dryness, stress incontinence, cystitis
• Gastrointestinal: less calcium is absorbed from food, increasing the risk for fractures
• Integumentary: skin becomes dry and thin, and colla-gen levels decrease
• Body shape: more abdominal fat; waist size swells rela-tive to hips

Therapeutic Management

Menopause should be managed individually. In the past, despite the wide diversity of symptoms and risks, the tra-ditional reaction was to reach for the one-size-fits-all therapy: HRT. Today the medical community is chang-ing its thinking in light of the Women's Health Initiative (WHI) study and the Heart and Estrogen/Progestin Replacement Study Follow-Up (HERS II), which reported that long-term HRT increased the risks of heart attacks, strokes, and breast cancer; in short, the overall health risks of HRT exceeded the benefits (Writing Group for the Women's Health Initiative Investigators, 2002). In addition, HRT didn't protect against the development of coronary artery disease, nor did it pre-vent the progression of coronary artery disease, as it was previously touted to do (Shelby & O'Hair, 2007). As expected, the fallout from this study and others forced practitioners to re-evaluate their usual therapies and tai-lor treatment to each client's history, needs, and risk fac-tors. The SOGC clinical practice guideline, *Menopause and Osteoporosis Update 2009*, recommends that doctors prescribe HRT in the lowest dose required, and for the duration necessary, to treat troubling menopause symptoms (Reid, Blake, Abramson, et al., 2009). Current research confirms that HRT is both a safe and effective way to treat symptoms of menopause.

There is a universe of treatment options out there, but factors in the client's history and symptoms should be the main consideration when determining therapy. Women need to educate themselves about the latest research findings and collaborate with their health care provider on the right menopause therapy. The following factors should be considered in management:

- HRT is not indicated to treat or prevent cardiovascular disease, according to WHI. Instead, consider lipid-lowering agents and lifestyle changes if risk or disease is present.
- HRT should not be taken for more than 5 years for vasomotor symptoms. Use the lowest dose possible for any HRT.
- HRT is acceptable as long as there is a clear indication for use, the woman is under medical supervision, and she is aware of the risks and benefits (North American Menopause Society, 2004; Palacios, 2008; SOCG, 2006d)
- Consider nonhormonal therapies such as bisphosphonates and selective estrogen receptor modulators (SERMs).
- Consider weight-bearing exercises, calcium, vitamin D, smoking cessation, and avoidance of alcohol to treat or prevent osteoporosis.
- Annual breast examinations and mammograms are essential.
- Local estrogen creams can be used for vaginal atrophy.
- Consider herbal therapies for symptoms (Holloway, 2011; VanDie, 2010).

Although numerous symptoms have been attributed to menopause (Box 4.9), some of them are more closely related to the aging process than to estrogen deficiency. A few of the more common menopausal conditions and their management are discussed here.

Managing Hot Flashes and Night Sweats

Hot flashes and night sweats are classic signs of estrogen deficiency and the predominant complaint of perimenopausal women. A hot flash is a transient and sudden sensation of warmth that spreads over the body, particularly the neck, face, and chest. Hot flashes are caused by vasomotor instability. Nearly 25% of menopausal women experience persistent flushes daily for 5 years or more (Brockie, 2008). Hot flashes are an early and acute sign of estrogen deficiency. These flashes can be mild or extreme and can last from 2 to 30 minutes (Holloway, 2011).

BOX 4.9 **Common Symptoms of Menopause**

- Hot flashes or flushes of the head and neck
- Dryness in the eyes and vagina
- Personality changes
- Anxiety and/or depression
- Loss of libido
- Weight gain and water retention
- Night sweats
- Fatigue
- Irritability
- Insomnia
- Stress incontinence
- Heart palpitations

Source: Chedraui, P., Hidalgo, L., Chavez, D., Morocho, N., Alvarado, M., & Huc, A. (2007). Menopausal symptoms and associated risk factors among postmenopausal women screened for the metabolic syndrome. *Archives of Gynecology & Obstetrics, 275*(3), 161–168.

There are many options for treating hot flashes. Treatment must be based on symptom severity, the client's medical history, and the client's values and concerns. Although the gold standard for the treatment of hot flashes is estrogen, this is not recommended for all women. The following are suggestions for the management of hot flashes:

- Pharmacologic options
  - HRT unless contraindicated
  - Androgen therapy (potentiates estrogen)
  - Estrogen and androgen combinations
  - Progestin therapy (Depo-Provera injection every 3 months)
  - Clonidine (central alpha-adrenergic agonist) weekly patch
  - Propranolol (beta-adrenergic blocker)
  - Gabapentin (Neurontin): antiseizure drug
  - Selective serotonin reuptake inhibitors (SSRIs): venlafaxine (Effexor) and sertraline (Zoloft) have shown promise
  - Vitamin E: 100 mg daily (Rubin, 2007)
- Lifestyle changes
  - Lower room temperature; use fans.
  - Wear clothing in layers for easy removal.
  - Limit caffeine and alcohol intake.
  - Drink 8 to 10 glasses of water daily.
  - Stop smoking or cut back.
  - Avoid hot drinks and spicy food.
  - Take calcium (1,200 to 1,500 mg) and vitamin D (400 to 600 IU).
  - Try relaxation techniques, deep breathing, and meditation.

- Exercise daily, but not just before bedtime.
- Maintain a healthy weight.
- Identify stressors and learn to manage them.
- Keep a diary to identify triggers of hot flashes (Holloway, 2011).
- Alternative therapies (selected non-prescription therapies)
  - Acupuncture reduced frequency of hot flashes
  - Phytoestrogens: isoflavones, ligands, coumenstrols
  - Black cohosh
  - Red clover
  - Vitamin E
  - St. John's wort: reduces depression and fatigue
  - Valerian root: induces sleep and relaxation (Lie, 2006)
  - Chamomile: mild sedative to alleviate insomnia
  - Unopposed transdermal progesterone
  - Compounded bioidentical hormones
    - Estrogen
    - Progesterone
    - Testosterone
  - Dong quai: acts as a form of phytoestrogen

Many women are choosing alternative treatments for managing menopausal symptoms. Because of their natural origin, women perceive that alternative treatments are safer. The interest in phytoestrogens came about because of the low prevalence of hot flashes in Asian women, which was attributed to their diet being rich in phytoestrogens (Manson, 2006). Recent studies have found that black cohosh, multibotanical herbs, and increased soy intake do not reduce the frequency or severity of menopausal hot flashes or night sweats (ACOG, 2004; Huntzinger, 2006; Newton, Reed, LaCroix, et al., 2006; Seppa, 2007). Other remedies for easing menopausal symptoms might include red clover, motherwort, ginseng, sarsaparilla root, valerian root, L-tryptophan, calcium–magnesium, and kelp tablets (Haas, 2007). Again, research thus far has been skeptical about their efficacy, but many women report they ease their symptoms and their use has skyrocketed. While there might be some benefits to their use, evidence of the efficacy of alternative products in menopause is largely anecdotal. Small, preliminary clinical trials might demonstrate the safety of some of the non-pharmacologic products. Nurses should be aware of the purported action of these agents as well as any adverse effects or drug interactions.

Managing Urogenital Changes

Menopause can be a physically and emotionally challenging time for women. In addition to the psychological burden of leaving behind the reproductive phase of life and the stigma of an "aging" body, sexual difficulties due to urogenital changes plague most women but are frequently not addressed. Up to 50% of postmenopausal women experience symptoms of vaginal atrophy (SOCG, 2006a).

Vaginal atrophy occurs during menopause because of declining estrogen levels. These changes include thinning of the vaginal walls, an increase in pH, irritation, increased susceptibility to infection, dyspareunia, loss of lubrication with intercourse, vaginal dryness, and a decrease in sexual desire related to these changes. Decreased estrogen levels can also influence a woman's sexual function. Delayed clitoral reaction, decreased vaginal lubrication, diminished circulatory response during sexual stimulation, and reduced contractions during orgasm have all been linked to low estrogen levels (Holloway, 2011). Women report even that gentle friction can exacerbate symptoms.

Management of these changes might include the use of estrogen vaginal tablets (Vagifem) or cream (Premarin); Estring, an estrogen-releasing vaginal ring that lasts for 3 months; testosterone patches; and over-the-counter moisturizers and lubricants (Astroglide). A positive outlook on sexuality and a supportive partner are also needed to make the sexual experience enjoyable and fulfilling.

▶ *Take* NOTE!

Sexual health is an important aspect of the human experience. By keeping an open mind, listening to women, and providing evidence-based treatment options, the nurse can help improve quality of life for menopausal women.

Preventing and Managing Osteoporosis

Women are greatly affected by osteoporosis after menopause. Osteoporosis is a condition in which bone mass declines to such an extent that fractures occur with minimal trauma. Bone loss begins in the third or fourth decade of a woman's life and accelerates rapidly after menopause. Approximately 2 million Canadian women are living with osteoporosis, and this number is expected to increase as the population ages (MenopauseandU.ca, n.d.). Current research indicates that in the 10 years after menopause a woman can lose up to 30% of her bone mass. According to Papaioannou et al. (2010), osteoporosis is responsible for over 80% of fractures in menopausal women over age 50. The result of these fractures, particularly hip and vertebral fractures, is a possible increased risk for morbidity, institutionalization, and even mortality. Figure 4.22 shows the skeletal changes associated with osteoporosis.

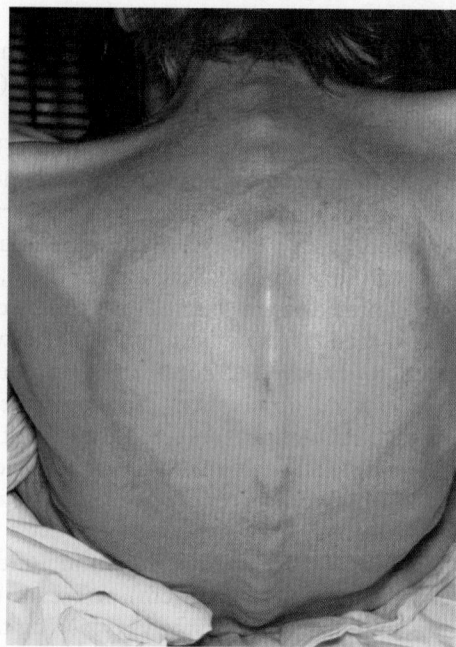

FIGURE 4.22 Skeletal changes associated with osteoporosis. (John Radcliffe Hospital/ Photo Researcher Inc.)

Most women with osteoporosis don't know they have the disease until they sustain a fracture, usually of the wrist or hip. Risk factors include:

- Increasing age
- Postmenopausal status without HRT
- Early menopause (before age 40)
- Small frame, thin-boned
- White or Asian race
- History of irregular periods or eating disorders
- Impaired eyesight
- Rheumatoid arthritis
- Family history of osteoporosis
- Sedentary lifestyle
- History of treatment with:
  - Antacids with aluminum
  - Heparin
  - Corticosteroids
  - Thyroid replacement medication
  - Antiepileptic medications
- Low calcium and vitamin D intake
- Smoking and consuming alcohol
- Excessive amounts of caffeine (MenopauseandU.ca, n.d.)

Screening tests to measure bone density are not good predictors for young women who might be at risk for developing this condition. In Canada, two tools are used to estimate the 10-year risk for a major osteoporotic fracture: the Canadian Association of Radiologists and Osteoporosis Canada (CAROC) tool and the Fracture Risk Assessment Tool (FRAX) developed by the WHO

specifically for Canada (Papaioannou et al., 2010; Osteoporosis Canada, 2011a).

The best management for this painful, crippling, and potentially fatal disease is prevention. Women can modify many risk factors by changing the following nutrition and lifestyle factors:

- Increase calcium and vitamin D intake. Osteoporosis Canada (2011d) recommends 1,000 mg of calcium per day for women 19 to 50 years of age and 1,200 mg for women over age 50. Recommended vitamin D intake is 800 to 2,000 IU for women over 50 (Osteoporosis Canada, 2011b).
- Eat foods that contain calcium that is easily absorbed (milk, cheese, orange juice, salmon, beans, and lentils).
- Avoid excess sodium and caffeine.
- Engage in daily weight-bearing exercise to maintain bone strength. Various exercises also help maintain balance and coordination, which reduces the risk for falls. Women should also consider stretching and toning exercises, such as yoga, to keep muscles toned and limber (MenopauseandU.ca, n.d.).
- Avoid smoking and excessive alcohol.
- Discuss your bone health with your health care provider.

Medications that can help in preventing and managing osteoporosis include:

- HRT (estrogen or estrogen/progesterone)
- SERMs (Evista)
- Calcium and vitamin D supplements (Tums)
- Bisphosphonates (Actonel, Fosamax, Didrocal)
- Denosumab (Prolia)
- Parathyroid hormone (Forteo)
- Calcitonin (Miacalcin) (Osteoporosis Canada, 2011c)

▶ **Take** NOTE!

In 2010, Health Canada approved a new treatment for postmenopausal women with osteoporosis who are at high risk for fracture. Prolia (demosumab) blocks RANK Ligand protein to stop the cells that break down bone while increasing bone mass and bone strength, which reduces the chance of breaking bones at the hip, spine, and non-spine sites. It is administered subcutaneously once every 6 months (Whelan & Raman-Wilms, 2011). See Evidence-Based Practice 4.1.

Preventing and Managing Cardiovascular Disease

According to the Heart and Stroke Foundation of Canada (HSFC, 2011a), women are seven times more likely to die

EVIDENCE-BASED PRACTICE 4.1
Denosumab: A New Injectable Treatment for Postmenopausal Osteoporosis

Osteoporosis, which affects around 1 in 4 women in Canada over the age of 50 years, can result in significant morbidity and mortality, including chronic pain, loss of height, kyphosis, and fractures. It has been reported that individuals with vertebral or hip fracture were more likely to die during the first 5 years of follow-up compared to individuals without fractures. Individuals who have or are at risk for osteoporosis require adequate daily calcium and vitamin D intake. There are also antiresorptive options available for the prophylaxis and/or treatment of osteoporosis; these include bisphosphonates, raloxifene, and calcitonin. However, studies have shown that at least 50% of patients who take oral bisphosphonates quit taking them within a year of receiving the prescription. In 2010, denosumab was approved in Canada to treat postmenopausal women at high risk for fracture. This medication, administered subcutaneously every 6 months, has been shown to increase bone mineral density (BMD). The purpose of this study was to review available data which addressed the mechanism of action, efficacy, and safety of the injectable treatment denosumab for the treatment of osteoporosis.

▲ Findings
Data collected from 3 years of clinical trials suggests that using denosumab for the management of postmenopausal osteoporosis is an effective treatment to maintain or increase BMD. In the phase III randomized, controlled trials, findings included increased BMD at the lumbar spine, hips, femoral neck, and trochanter when compared with placebo. There was also evidence that denosumab was more effective than alendronate in increasing BMD at the hip, trochanter, one third radius, femoral neck, and lumbar spine. The authors recommended more comparison trials with other osteoporosis therapies to provide data regarding denosumab's long-term safety and efficacy.

■ Nursing Implications
According to the results of the study, denosumab is an effective treatment for managing postmenopausal osteoporosis. Nurses should teach women to take the recommended daily dose of calcium and vitamin D either through diet and/or supplements. Women should also be advised to have their serum calcium monitored. As a registered nurse, it is important to teach patients about the adverse effects of the medication. The most common side effects of denosumab reported in the studies included eczema, flatulence, constipation, sore throat, nasopharyngitis, and bronchitis. It is also important for women to report signs and symptoms of serious infections, such as fever, severe abdominal pain, or red or swollen skin.

Source: Whelan, A. M., & Raman-Wilms, L. (2011). Denosumab: A new injectable treatment for postmenopausal osteoporosis. *Canadian Pharmacy Journal, 144*(2), 72–78.

from heart disease than from breast cancer. There is a myth that only women in menopause should be concerned about heart disease, when in fact lifestyle choices in a woman's 20s and 30s have a significant impact on her risk for heart disease (HSFC, 2011b). Half of all postmenopausal women will develop coronary artery disease and one third will die from this disease. A majority of Canadian women (80%) have at least one risk factor for coronary artery disease. In 2008, 29.7% of female deaths in Canada were attributed to cardiovascular disease (HSFC, 2012).

For the first half of a woman's life, estrogen seems to be a protective substance for the cardiovascular system by smoothing, relaxing, and dilating blood vessels. It even helps boost HDL and lower low-density lipoprotein (LDL) levels, helping to keep the arteries clear of plaque accumulation. As a woman reaches menopause, her risk for heart disease increases because of a decrease in estrogen and progesterone. Women may experience increases in total blood cholesterol and blood pressure. Increases in central body fat can contribute to symptoms such as sweating and sleep disturbance (HSFC, 2011b).

Menopause is not the only factor that increases a woman's risk for cardiovascular disease. Lifestyle and medical history factors play a major role. Nine out of ten

Canadians have at least one risk factor that contributes to heart disease:

- Smoking
- Excessive alcohol use
- Obesity
- High-fat diet
- Sedentary lifestyle
- High cholesterol levels
- Family history of cardiovascular disease
- Hypertension
- Apple-shaped body
- Diabetes

Two of the major risk factors for coronary heart disease are hypertension and dyslipidemia. Both are modifiable and can be prevented by lifestyle changes and, if needed, controlled by medication. This is why prevention is essential. Diabetes is another major contributor of heart disease. It has been estimated that 90% of individuals with diabetes have type 2 diabetes (Cremieux, Eapen, Trask, et al., 2011). Among Canadian women of ages 46 to 65, 6% have diabetes, and this percentage increases to 13% after the age of 65

(HSFC, 2012). In addition, women who experience early menopause lose the protection afforded by endogenous estrogen to the cardiac system and are at greater risk for more extensive atherosclerosis. Major preventive strategies include a healthy diet, increased activity, exercise, smoking cessation, decreased alcohol intake, and weight reduction.

Raising awareness of heart disease in women is an essential role for nurses. Lifestyle interventions are effective in preventing cardiovascular disease in all individuals regardless of their underlying risk (HSFC, 2011b). Stressing the importance of lifestyle modifications must begin early in life and should be reinforced from the beginning of a young woman's reproductive years through menopause. Nurses are in an ideal position to teach the importance of good nutrition, healthy weight, and daily exercise before cardiovascular disease becomes clinically evident.

Nursing Assessment

Menopause is a universal and irreversible part of the overall aging process involving a woman's reproductive system. While not a disease state, menopause does place women at greater risk for the development of many conditions of aging. A thorough nursing assessment related to menopause is essential in order to support women and offer appropriate advice for long-term health. Topics to include in a health history are:

- Timing of the last menstrual period
  - Cycle changes
  - Amount of bleeding
- Current use of contraception
- Current use of complementary or herbal supplements
- Personal views on HRT
- Current use of HRT, including type, duration, and side effects or contraindications
- Common menopausal symptoms (Holloway, 2011)

Nurses can help women become aware of their risk for postmenopausal diseases and can promote strategies to prevent them. The nurse can be instrumental in assessing risk factors and planning interventions in collaboration with the client. These might include:

- Screening for osteoporosis, cardiovascular disease, and cancer risk
- Assessment of blood pressure to identify hypertension
- Blood cholesterol to identify hyperlipidemia risk
- Mammogram to find a cancerous lesion
- Pap smear to identify cervical cancer
- Pelvic examination to identify endometrial cancer or masses
- Digital rectal examination to assess for colon cancer

- Bone density testing as a baseline at menopause to identify osteopenia (low bone mass), which might lead to osteoporosis (including calcium and vitamin D consumption)
- Assessing lifestyle to plan strategies to prevent chronic conditions:
  - Dietary intake of fat, cholesterol, and sodium
  - Weight management
  - Calcium intake
  - Use of tobacco, alcohol, and caffeine
  - Performance of breast self-examinations

Nursing Management

Nurses can counsel women about their risks and help them to prevent disease and debilitating conditions with specific health maintenance education. Women should make their own decisions, but the nurse should make sure they are armed with the facts to do so intelligently. Nurses can offer a thorough explanation of the menopausal process, including the latest research findings, to help women understand and make decisions about this inevitable event.

If the woman decides to use HRT to control her menopausal symptoms, she will require a thorough education and frequent reassessment. Women taking HRT should be assessed at least 3 months after starting the medication and should be monitored frequently for breast cancer, deep vein thrombosis, stroke, and coronary heart disease (Holloway, 2011). The nurse can provide realistic expectations of the therapy to reduce the woman's anxiety and concern.

It is also useful to emphasize the value of friends to gain support and share information and resources. Often just talking about emotional difficulties such as the death of a parent or problematic relationships helps solve problems. It also shows the woman that her emotional responses are valid.

Healthy lifestyles and stress management techniques are vital to health and longevity. Evidence-based interventions include lifestyle modifications, risk management therapies, and preventive drug interventions, such as the following:

- Participate actively in maintaining health.
- Control stress.
- Exercise regularly.
- Reduce dietary intake of fat, cholesterol, and sodium to prevent cardiovascular disease.

(Pay particular attention to any trigger foods that may exacerbate hot flashes.)

- Maintain a healthy weight for body frame.
- Reduce caffeine and alcohol intake to prevent osteoporosis and reduce hot flashes, night sweats, and disturbed sleeping.

- Wear lightweight clothing that can be easily removed to health manage hot flashes.
- Take supplemental calcium and eat appropriately to prevent osteoporosis.
- Stop smoking to prevent lung and heart disease.
- Monitor blood pressure, lipids, and diabetes (drug therapy management).
- Use low-dose aspirin.
- Perform breast self-examinations to detect breast lesions.
- Use appropriate moisturizers to prevent vaginal dryness (Holloway, 2011).

These life approaches may seem low-tech, but they can stave off menopause-related complications such as cardiovascular disease, osteoporosis, and depression. These tips for healthy living work well, but the client needs to be motivated to stick with them.

■■■ Key Concepts

■ Establishing good health habits and avoiding risky behaviours early in life will prevent chronic conditions later on.

■ There are more than 200 symptoms of PMS, and at least two different syndromes have been recognized: PMS and PMDD.

■ Endometriosis is a condition in which bits of functioning endometrial tissue are located outside their normal site, the uterine cavity.

■ Infertility is a widespread problem that has an emotional, social, and economic impact on couples.

■ More than half (53%) of all unintended pregnancies occur in women who report using some method of birth control during the month of conception.

■ Hormonal methods include OCs, injectables, vaginal rings, and transdermal patches.

■ Recent studies have shown that the extension of active oral contraceptive pills carries the same safety profile as the conventional 28-day regimens.

■ Menopause, with a dramatic decline in estrogen levels, affects not only the reproductive organs but also other bodily systems.

■ Most women with osteoporosis do not know they have the disease until they sustain a fracture, usually of the wrist or hip.

■ Nurses should aim to have a holistic approach to the sexual health of women from menarche through menopause.

REFERENCES

Alexander, L. L., LaRosa, J. H., Bader, H., & Garfield, S. (2010). *New dimensions in women's health* (5th ed.). Boston, MA: Jones and Bartlett.

American Academy of Allergy, Asthma, and Immunology. (2012). *Latex allergy: Tips to remember*. Retrieved March 4, 2012 from http://www.aaaai.org/patients/publicedmat/tips/latexallergy.stm

American College of Obstetricians and Gynecologists. (2000). Clinical management guidelines for obstetricians–gynecologists, number 15: Premenstrual syndrome. *Obstetrics and Gynecology, 95*, 1–9.

American College of Obstetricians and Gynecologists. (2004). ACOG's task force on hormone therapy. *Obstetrics and Gynecology, 104*(Suppl), S1–S131.

American College of Obstetricians and Gynecologists. (2011a). *Frequently asked questions: Abnormal uterine bleeding*. Retrieved January 31, 2012 from http://www.acog.org/~/media/for%20patients/faq095.ashx

American College of Obstetricians and Gynecologists. (2011b). *Frequently asked questions: Dysmenorrhea*. Retrieved March 4, 2012 from www.acog.org/~/media/For%20Patients/faq046.pdf?dmc=1&ts=20120220T1216121334

Andoisek, K. M., & Rapkin, A. J. (2007). Contraceptive use in women with premenstrual disorders. *USC Dialogues in Contraception, 10*(4), 4–7.

Archer, D. F. (2006). Menstrual-cycle-related symptoms: A review of the rationale for continuous use of oral contraceptives. *Contraception, 74*(5), 359–366.

Arevalo, M. (2010). *CycleBeads*. Retrieved March 4, 2012 from http://www.cyclebeads.com

Assisted Human Reproduction Canada. (2010). *Infertility and AHR*. Retrieved March 4, 2012 from http://www.ahrc-pac.gc.ca/v2/patients/infertility-infertilite-eng.php

Bielak, K. M., & Harris, G. S. (2010). *Amenorrhea*. Retrieved March 4, 2012 from http://www.emedicine.com/ped/topic2779.htm

Black, A. B., Francoeur, D., Rowe, T., et al. (2004). Canadian contraception consensus. No. 143–Part 3 of 3. *Journal of Obstetrics and Gynecology Canada, 26*(4), 347–387. Retrieved March 4, 2012 from http://www.sogc.org/guidelines/public/143E-CPG3-April2004.pdf

Blake, J., Giesbrecht, E., & Soares, C. (2009). Evolving strategies in the dosing of oral contraceptives. *The Canadian Journal of CME, 21*(9), 35–40. Retrieved Retrieved March 4, 2012 from http://www.stacommunications.com/journals/cme/2009/09-Sep-09/WNiCRCME.pdf

Brockie, J. (2008). Physiology and effects of the menopause. *Nurse Prescribing, 6*(5), 202–207.

Canadian Agency for Drugs and Technologies in Health. (2010). *Status of public funding for in vitro fertilization in Canada and internationally*. Retrieved March 4, 2012 from http://www.cadth.ca/media/pdf/Public_Funding_IVF_es-14_e.pdf

Canadian Federation for Sexual Health. (2007). *Sexual health in Canada: Baseline 2007*. Ottawa, ON: Author.

Canadian Federation for Sexual Health. (2009). *Cervical cap*. Retrieved March 4, 2012 from http://www.cfsh.ca/Your_Sexual_Health/Contraception-and-Safer-Sex/Contraception-and-Birth-Control/Cervical-Cap.aspx

Canadian Pediatric Society. (2012). *Growing up: Information for girls about puberty*. Retrieved March 6, 2012 from http://www.caringforkids.cps.ca/handouts/information_for_girls_about_puberty

Canning, S., Waterman, M., & Dye, L. (2006). Dietary supplements and herbal remedies for premenstrual syndrome (PMS): A systematic review of the evidence for their efficacy. *Journal of Reproductive and Infant Psychology, 24*(4), 363–378.

Chedraul, P., Hidalgo, L., Chavez, D., Morocho, N., Alvarado, M., & Huc, A. (2007). Menopausal symptoms and associated risk factors among postmenopausal women screened for the metabolic syndrome. *Archives of Gynecology and Obstetrics, 275*(3), 161–168.

Clayton, A. H. (2008). Symptoms related to the menstrual cycle: Diagnosis, prevalence, and treatment. *Journal of Psychiatric Practice, 14*(1), 13–21.

Collier, M. J., & Rieder, J. (2008). Detecting polycystic ovarian syndrome in teens. *Contemporary OB/GYN, 44*–49. Retrieved March 4, 2012 from http://contemporaryobgyn.modernmedicine.com/obgyn/Endocrinology/Detecting-polycystic-ovarian-syndrome-in-teens/ArticleStandard/Article/detail/548214

Courtney, K. (2006). The contraceptive patch: Latest developments. *AWHONN Lifelines, 10*(3), 250–253.

Cremieux, P. Y., Eapen, S., Trask, S. W., & Ghosh, A. (2011). Weighing the clinical benefits and economic impact of bariatric surgery in morbidly obese patients with diabetes. *Canadian Journal of Diabetes, 35*(2), 89–98.

DeSutter, P. (2006). Rational diagnosis and treatment in infertility. *Best Practice & Research: Clinical Obstetrics & Gynecology, 20*(5), 647–664.

Dirubbo, N. E. (2006). Counsel your patients about contraceptive options. *Nurse Practitioner, 31*(4), 40–44.

Endometriosisinfo.ca. (2011). *Diagnosis and treatment.* Retrieved March 4, 2012 from http://www.endometriosisinfo.ca/treatment_e.aspx

Female Contraception. (2006). *Contraception: Female annual report.* New Canaan, CT: ADAM.

Fisher, W., & Black, A. (2007). Contraception in Canada: A review of method choices, characteristics, adherence and approaches to counseling. *Canadian Medical Association Journal, 176*(7). doi:10.1503/cmaj.060851

Freeman, E. W., Halberstadt, S. M., Rickels, K., et al. (2011). Core symptoms that discriminate premenstrual syndrome. *Journal of Women's Health, 20*(1), 29–35.

French, R., Vliet, H., Cowan, F., et al. (2006). Hormonally impregnated intrauterine systems (IUSs) versus other forms. *Cochrane Database of Systematic Reviews, 3,* CD001776.

Gourounti, K., Anagnostopoulos, F., & Vaslamatzis, G. (2010). Pyschosocial predictors of infertility related stress: A review. *Current Women's Health Reviews, 6,* 318–331.

Graziottin, A. (2006). A review of transdermal hormone contraception: Focus on the ethinyl estradiol/norelgestromin contraceptive patch. *Treatments in Endocrinology, 5*(6), 359–365.

Greil, A. L., & McQuillan, J. M. (2010). "Tying" times: Medicalization, intent and ambiguity in the definition of infertility. *Medical Anthropology Quarterly, 24*(2), 137–156.

Haas, E. (2007). Easing menopause symptoms naturally. *Share Guide, 89,* 29–78.

Hatcher, R. A., Trussell, J., Nelson, A. L., Cates, W., Jr., Kowal, D., & Policar, M. (2011). *Contraceptive technology* (20th ed.). New York: Ardent Media, Inc.

Hays, B. (2009). Infertility: A functional medicine report. *Intergrative Medicine, 8*(6), 20–27.

HealthLink Alberta. (2006). *Premenstrual syndrome: Self-help and other treatments.* Retrieved March 4, 2012 from http://www.healthlinkalberta.ca/Topic.asp?GUID=%7B71910515-78BC-41B7-A751-13AB6C3E35B3%7D

HealthLink BC. (2011). *Diaphragm for birth control: Topic overview.* Retrieved March 4, 2012 from http://www.healthlinkbc.ca/kb//content/special/tw9508.html

Heart and Stroke Foundation of Canada. (2011a). *HeartSmart women: A guide to living with and preventing heart disease and stroke.* Retrieved March 4, 2012 from http://www.heartandstroke.com/site/c.ikIQLcMWJtE/b.4356323/k.89AA/Heart_disease_HeartSmart8482_Women_A_guide_to_living_with_and_preventing_heart_disease_and_stroke.htm

Heart and Stroke Foundation of Canada. (2011b). *Women and heart disease and stroke.* Retrieved March 4, 2012 from http://www.heartandstroke.com/site/c.ikIQLcMWJtE/b.3484041/k.D80A/Heart_disease_Women_and_heart_disease_and_stroke.htm

Heart and Stroke Foundation of Canada. (2012). *Statistics.* Retrieved March 4, 2012 from http://www.heartandstroke.com/site/c.ikIQLcMWJtE/b.3483991/k.34A8/Statistics.htm

Holloway, D. (2011). An overview of the menopause: Assessment and management. *Nursing Standard, 25*(30), 47–57.

Huntzinger, A. (2006). ACOG reports on compounded bioidentical hormones. *American Family Physician, 73*(12), 2242–2245.

Kapoor, D., Alderman, E., Hiraoka, M. K. Y., & Davila, G. W. (2012). *Endometriosis.* Retrieved March 4, 2012 from http://emedicine.medscape.com/article/271899-overview

Komar, B. (2012). Premenstrual syndrome (PMS) and premenstrual dysphoric disorder (PMDD). Retrieved March 4, 2012 from http://www.bcwomens.ca/HealthTopics/SexualHealth/Gynecology/PMSPMDD.htm

Lefebvre, G., Pinsonneault, O., Antao, V., et al. (2005). SOGC clinical practice guideline: Primary dysmenorrhea consensus guideline. *Journal of Obstetrics and Gynaecology, 169,* 1117–1130. Retrieved March 4, 2012 from http://www.sogc.org/guidelines/public/169E-CPG-December2005.pdf

Lever, K. A. (2005) Emergency contraception. *AWHONN Lifelines, 9*(3), 218–225.

Leyland, N., Casper, R., Laberge, P., et al. (2010). Clinical practice guideline: Endometriosis: Diagnosis and management. *Journal of Obstetrics and Gynaecology, 32*(7 Suppl. 2), S1–S36. Retrieved March 4, 2012 from http://www.sogc.org/guidelines/documents/gui244CPG1007E.pdf

Lie, D. (2006). AAFP 2006—Evidence-based complementary and alternative medicine (CAM): What should physicians know? *Medscape News Today.* Retrieved March 4, 2012 from http://www.medscape.com/viewarticle/549067

Mammen, T., Hwang, K., & Costabile, R. A. (2008). Performing vasectomy to ensure future vasovasostomy success: Put the cart before the horse: Four vasectomy considerations that affect future reversal. *Urology Times,* Sept. Retrieved March 4, 2012 from http://goliath.ecnext.com/coms2/gi_0199–9262567/Performing-vasectomy-to-ensure-future.html

Mannix, L. K. (2008). Menstrual-related pain conditions: Dysmenorrhea and migraine. *Journal of Women's Health, 17*(5), 879–891.

Manson, J. E. (2006). Perimenopause, hormones, and midlife health. *Harvard Women's Health Watch, 14*(3), 1–3.

Marnocha, S. K., Bergstrom, M., & Dempsy, L. F. (2011). The lived experience of perimenopause and menopause. *Contemporary Nurse, 37*(2), 229–240.

Mayo Clinic Staff. (2010). *Withdrawal method (ciotus interruptus).* Mayo Clinic Pub No. MY01050. Retrieved March 4, 2012 from http://www.mayoclinic.com/health/withdrawal-method/MY01050

Mayo Clinic Staff. (2011a). *Amenorrhea.* Mayo Clinic Pub No. DS00581. Retrieved March 4, 2012 from http://www.mayoclinic.com/health/amenorrhea/DS00581/DSECTION=tests-and-diagnosis

Mayo Clinic Staff. (2011b). *Cervical mucus method for natural family planning.* Mayo Clinic Pub No. MY01004. Retrieved March 4, 2012 from http://www.mayoclinic.com/health/cervical-mucus-method/MY01004

Mayo Clinic Staff. (2011c). *Infertility.* Mayo Clinic Pub No. DS00310. Retrieved March 4, 2012 from http://www.mayoclinic.com/health/infertility/DS00310

Mayo Clinic Staff. (2012a). *Essure.* Mayo Clinic Pub No. MY00999. Retrieved March 4, 2012 from http://www.mayoclinic.com/health/essure/MY00999

Mayo Clinic Staff. (2012b). *Premenstrual syndrome (PMS).* Mayo Clinic Pub No. DS00134. Retrieved March 4, 2012 from http://www.mayoclinic.com/health/premenstrual-syndrome/DS00134

McCausland, A. M., & McCausland, V. M. (2010). Long-term complications of minimally invasive endometrial ablation devices. *Journal of Gynecologic Surgery, 26*(2), 133–149.

MenopauseandU.ca. (n.d.). *Osteoporosis.* Retrieved February 29, 2012 from http://menopauseandu.ca/health-concerns/osteoporosis_e.aspx

Mirosh, M. (2007). Current usage. In *SOGC clinical practice guideline: Canadian consensus guideline on continuous and extended hormonal contraception, 2007.* Retrieved March 4, 2012 from http://www.sogc.org/guidelines/documents/gui195CPG0707.pdf

Mishell, D. R., Guillebaud, J., Westoff, C., et al. (2007). Combined hormonal contraceptive traits: Variable data collection and bleeding assessment methodologies influence study outcomes and physician perception. *Contraception, 75*(1), 4–10.

National Abortion Federation. (2010). *Legal abortion in Canada.* Retrieved March 4, 2012 from http://www.prochoice.org/canada/legal.html

Newton, K. M., Reed, S. D., LaCroix, A. Z., Grothaus, L. C., Ehrlich, K., & Guiltinan, J. (2006). Treatment of vasomotor symptoms of menopause with black cohosh, multibotanicals, soy, hormone therapy, or placebo. A randomized trial. *Annals of Internal Medicine, 145,* 869–879.

North American Menopause Society. (2004). Recommendations for estrogen and progesterone use in peri-menopausal and post-menopausal women. *Menopause, 11*(6), 589–600.

O'Grady, K. (2008/2009). *Early puberty for girls. The new 'normal' and why we need to be concerned.* Retrieved January 31, 2012 from http://www.cwhn.ca/en/print/en/node/39365

Occupational Safety and Health Administration, U.S. Department of Labor. (n.d.). *Latex allergy.* Retrieved March 4, 2012 from http://www.osha.gov/SLTC/latexallergy

Osteoporosis Canada. (2011a). *Facts and Statistics.* Retrieved March 4, 2012 from http://www.osteoporosis.ca/index.php/ci_id/8867/la_id/1.htm

Osteoporosis Canada. (2011b). *Vitamin D: A key factor in good calcium absorption.* Retrieved March 4, 2012 from http://www.osteoporosis.ca/index.php/ci_id/5536/la_id/1.htm

Osteoporosis Canada. (2011c). *Drug treatments.* Retrieved March 4, 2012 from: http://www.osteoporosis.ca/index.php/ci_id/5514/la_id/1.htm

Osteoporosis Canada. (2011d). *How much calcium do we need?* Retrieved March 4, 2012 from http://www.osteoporosis.ca/index.php/ci_id/5535/la_id/1.htm

Palacios, S. (2008). Advances in hormone replacement therapy: Making the menopause manageable. *BMC Women's Health, 8*(22). Retrieved March 4, 2012 from http://www.biomedcentral.com/1472-6874/8/22

Papaioannou, A., Morin, S., Cheung, A. M., et al. (2010). *2010 clinical practice guidelines for the diagnosis and management of osteoporosis in Canada: Summary.* Retrieved March 4, 2012 from http://www.cmaj.ca/content/early/2010/10/12/cmaj.100771.full.pdf

Planned Parenthood. (2012). *Birth control.* Retrieved March 4, 2012 from http://www.plannedparenthood.org/health-topics/birth-control-4211.htm

Popat, V., Sullivan, S. D., Trupin, S. R., et al. (2011). *Amenorrhea.* Retrieved March 4, 2012 from http://www.emedicine.com/med/topic117.htm

Regional Fertility Program. (2011). *Frequently asked questions.* Retrieved March 4, 2012 from http://www.regionalfertilityprogram. ca/faq.php

Reid, R. L., Blake, J., Abramson, B., et al. (2009). SOGC clinical practice guideline: Menopause and osteoporosis update 2009. *Journal of Obstetrics and Gynaecology, 31*(Suppl. 1), S1–S49. Retrieved March 4, 2012 from http://www.sogc.org/guidelines/documents/Menopause_JOGC-Jan_09.pdf

Rubin, R. (2007). An herbal menopause therapy gets a closer look. *USA Today.* Retrieved March 4, 2012 from http://www.usatoday.com/news/health/2007-01-10-cohosh-usat_x.htm

Samra-Latif, O. M., & Wood, E. (2011). *Contraception.* Retrieved March 4, 2012 from http://www.emedicine.com/med/topic3211.htm

Schuiling, K. D., & Likis, F. E. (2013). *Women's gynecologic health* (2nd ed.). Sudbury, MA: Jones and Bartlett Publishers.

Seppa, N. (2007). Putting the kibosh on black cohosh. *Science News, 171*(2), 29–30.

SexualityandU.ca. (2006). *Choosing a contraceptive that's right for you.* Retrieved March 4, 2012 from http://www.sexualityandu.ca/games-and-apps/contraception-comparison-chart-choosing-a-contraceptive-thats-right-for-you#

SexualityandU.ca. (2010a). *Emergency contraception: How they work: pros and cons.* Retrieved March 4, 2012 from http://www.sexualityandu.ca/health-care-professionals/contraceptive-methods/emergency-contraception

SexualityandU.ca. (2010b). *Hormonal methods.* Retrieved March 4, 2012 from http://www.sexualityandu.ca/birth-control/birth-control-methods-contraception/hormonal-methods

SexualityandU.ca. (2010c). *Non-hormonal methods.* Retrieved March 4, 2012 from http://www.sexualityandu.ca/birth-control/birth-control-methods-contraception/non-hormonal-methods

SexualityandU.ca. (2010d). *Who are good candidates for the progestin only pill?* Retrieved March 4, 2012 from http://www.sexualityandu.ca/faqs/single/who-are-good-candidates-for-the-progestin-only-pill-pop

SexualityandU.ca. (2010e). *Birth Control FAQs* Retrieved March 4, 2012 from http://sexualityandu.ca/faqs/birth-control#

Shelby, K., & O'Hair, K. (2007). *Hormone replacement therapy: What we know now.* Retrieved March 4, 2012 from http://www.nurse.com/ce/course.html?CCID=2325&PageNum= 3&Begin=11545

Sinai, I., Arevalo, M., & Jennings, V. (2006). Fertility awareness-based methods of family planning: Predictors of correct use. *International Family Planning Perspectives, 32*(2), 94–100.

Society of Obstetricians and Gynecologists of Canada. (2006a). Canadian consensus conference on menopause, 2006 update. *Journal of Obstetrics and Gynaecology, 28,* S7–S95.

Society of Obstetricians and Gynecologists of Canada. (2006b). Clinical practice guidelines. Canadian contraceptive consensus—Update on depot medroxyprogesterone acetate (DMPA). *Journal of Obstetrics and Gynaecology, 28*(4), 305–308.

Society of Obstetricians and Gynaecologists of Canada. (2006c). *Premenstrual symptoms being discussed at Society of Obstetricians and Gynaecologists of Canada conference in Mont-Tremblant.* Retrieved March 4, 2012 from http://www.sogc.org/media/advisories-20060928_e.asp

Society of Obstetricians and Gynaecologists of Canada. (2006d). *The menopause handbook: A companion guide to the Society of Obstetricians and Gynecologists of Canada Menopause Consensus Report.* Retrieved March 4, 2012 from http://www.sogc.org/health/pdf/menopause-for-public-e.pdf

Society of Obstetricians and Gynaecologists of Canada. (2007). *New extended-cycle birth control pills safe, effective: Canadian Ob/Gyn Society.* Retrieved March 4, 2012 from http://www.sogc.org/media/advisories-20070712_e.asp

Srikanthan, A., & Reid, R. (2008). Religious and cultural influences on contraception. *Journal of Obstetrics and Gynecology,* February, 30(2), 129–137. Retrieved March 4, 2012 from http://www.sogc.org/jogc/abstracts/full/200802_WomensHealth_1.pdf

Statistics Canada. (2005). *Induced abortion statistics.* Catalogue no. 82–223-X. Retrieved March 4, 2012 from http://publications.gc.ca/collections/collection_2008/statcan/82-223-X/82-223-XIE2008000.pdf

Stewart, F. H., Kaunitz, A. M., LaGuardia, K. D., Karvois, D. L., Fisher, A. C., & Friedman, A. J. (2006). Extended use of transdermal norelgestromin/ethinyl estradiol: A randomized trial. *Obstetrics and Gynecology, 105*(6), 1389–1396.

Stöppler, M. C. (2011). *Menstrual cramps (dysmenorrhea).* Retrieved March 4, 2012 from http://www.medicinenet.com/menstrual_cramps/article.htm

Tanha, F. D., Feizi, M., & Shariat, M. (2010). Sublingual versus vaginal misoprotol for the management of missed abortion. *Journal of Obstetrics and Gynaecology Research, 36*(3), 525–532.

Telner, D. E., & Jakubovicz, D. (2007). Approach to diagnosis and management of abnormal uterine bleeding. *Canadian Family Physician,* 53, 58–64.

Thiel, J. A., & Carson, G. D. (2008). Cost-effectiveness analysis comparing the Essure tubal sterilization procedure and laparoscopic tubal sterilization. *Journal of Obstetrics and Gynaecology Canada, 30*(7), 581–585.

Thomas. (2011). Treatment options for dysfunctional uterine bleeding. *The Nurse Practitioner, 36*(8), 14–20.

Trolice, M., & Witt, M. (2011). Understanding Male Infertility. Retrieved September 26th/2011 from www.theafa.org/article/uinderstanding-maleinfertility

Tschudin, S., Bertea, P. C., & Zemp, E. (2010). Prevalence and predictors of premenstrual syndrome and premenstrual dysphoric disorder in a population-based sample. *Archives of Women's Mental Health,* 13, 485–494. doi:10.1007/s00737-010-0165-3

U.S. Food and Drug Administration. (2006). *FDA approves over-the-counter access for Plan B for women 18 and older; prescription remains required for those 17 and younger.* Retrieved March 4, 2012 from http://www.fda.gov/NewsEvents/Newsroom/PressAnnouncements/2006/ucm108717.htm

U.S. Food and Drug Administration. (2009). *Implanon (etonogestrel implant) 68 mg.* Retrieved March 4, 2012 from http://www.fda.gov/Safety/MedWatch/SafetyInformation/Safety-RelatedDrugLabelingChanges/ucm133061.htm

VanDie, M. D. (2010). Herbal medicine and menopause: An historical perspective. *Australian Journal of Medicinal Herbalism, 22*(4), 121–126.

Vilos, G. A., Lefebvre, G., & Graves, G. R. (2001). SOGC clinical practice guidelines: Guidelines for the management of abnormal uterine bleeding. *Journal of Obstetrics and Gynaecology Canada,* 23(8), 704–709. Retrieved March 4, 2012 from http://www.sogc.org/guidelines/public/106E-CPG-August2001.pdf

Whelan, A. M., & Raman-Wilms, L. (2011). Denosumab: A new injectable treatment for postmenopausal osteoporosis. *Canadian Pharmaceutical Journal, 144*(2), 72–78.

World Health Organization. (2007). Infertility in developing countries. *Reproductive Health.* Retrieved March 4, 2012 from http://www.who.int/ reproductive-health/infertility/index.htm

Writing Group for the Women's Health Initiative Investigators. (2002). Risks and benefits of estrogen plus progestin in healthy postmenopausal women: Principal results from the Women's Health Initiative randomized controlled trial. *Journal of the American Medical Association, 288*(3), 321–333.

Youngkin, E. Q., & Davis, M. S. (2003). *Women's health: A primary care clinical guide* (3rd ed.). New Jersey: Prentice Hall.

Zieve, D., & Strock, S. (2011). *Dysfunctional uterine bleeding (DUB).* Retrieved March 4, 2012 from http://amh.adam.com/content.aspx?productId=117&pid=1&gid=000903

RESOURCES

Amor, C., Rogstad, K. E., Tindall, C., Moore, K. T. H., Giles, D., & Harvey, P. (2008). Men's experiences of vasectomy: A grounded study. *Sexual and Relationship Therapy, 23*(3), 235–345.

Assisted Human Reproduction Canada. (2011). *Your guide to infertility and assisted human preproduction (AHR).* Retrieved March 4, 2012 from http://www.ahrc-pac.gc.ca/v2/pubs/counselling-conseil-eng.php

CaringforKids. (2008). *Growing up: Information for girls about puberty.* Retrieved March 4, 2012 from http://www.caringforkids.cps.ca/handouts/information_for_girls_about_puberty

Storck, S. (2010). *Secondary amenorrhea.* Retrieved February 29, 2012 from http://www.nlm.nih.gov/medlineplus/ency/article/001219.htm

Chapter Worksheet

MULTIPLE CHOICE QUESTIONS

1. A couple is considered infertile after how many months of trying to conceive?

   a. 6 months

   b. 12 months

   c. 18 months

   d. 24 months

2. A couple reports that their condom broke while they were having sexual intercourse last night. What would you advise to prevent pregnancy?

   a. Inject a spermicidal agent into her vagina immediately.

   b. Obtain emergency contraceptives and take them immediately.

   c. Douche with a solution of vinegar and hot water tonight.

   d. Take a strong laxative now and again at bedtime.

3. Which of the following combination OCs has been approved for extended continuous use?

   a. Seasonale

   b. NuvaRing

   c. Ortho Evra

   d. Mirena

4. Which of the following measures helps prevent osteoporosis?

   a. Iron supplementation

   b. Sleeping 8 hours nightly

   c. Eating lean meats only

   d. Walking 4.8 km (3 miles) daily

5. Which of the following activities will increase a woman's risk for cardiovascular disease if she is taking OCs?

   a. Eating a high-fibre diet

   b. Smoking cigarettes

   c. Taking daily multivitamins

   d. Drinking alcohol

6. Hormone therapy taken by menopausal women reduces:

   a. Weight gain

   b. Bone density

   c. Hot flashes

   d. Heart disease

7. Throughout life, a woman's most proactive activity to promote her health would be to engage in:

   a. Consistent exercise

   b. Socialization with friends

   c. Quality quiet time with herself

   d. Consuming water

8. What comment by a woman would indicate that a diaphragm is not the best contraceptive device for her?

   a. "My husband says it is my job to keep from getting pregnant."

   b. "I have a hard time remembering to take my vitamins daily."

   c. "Hormones cause cancer and I don't want to take them."

   d. "I am not comfortable touching myself down there."

CRITICAL THINKING EXERCISE

1. Ms. London, 25, comes to your family planning clinic requesting to have an intrauterine system inserted because "birth control pills give you cancer." In reviewing her history, you note she has been into the STI clinic three times in the past year with vaginal infections and was hospitalized for PID last month. When you question her about her sexual history, she reports having sex with multiple partners and not always using protection.

   a. Is an intrauterine system the most appropriate method for her? Why or why not?

   b. What myths/misperceptions will you address in your counselling session?

   c. Outline the safer sex discussion you plan to have with her.

(question continues on page 154)

STUDY ACTIVITIES

1. Develop a teaching plan for an adolescent with PMS and dysmenorrhea.

2. Arrange to shadow a nurse working in family planning for the morning. What questions does the nurse ask to ascertain the kind of family planning method that is right for each woman? What teaching goes along with each method? What follow-up care is needed? Share your findings with your classmates during a clinical conference.

3. Surf the Internet and locate three Canadian resources for infertile couples to consult that provide support and resources.

4. Male sterilization is the single most prevalent method of permanent contraception used by married couples in Canada. Contact a local urologist and gynecologist to learn about the procedure involved and the cost of male versus female sterilization. Which procedure poses less risk to the person and costs less?

5. Take a field trip to a local drugstore to check out the variety and costs of male and female condoms. How many different brands did you find? What was the range of costs?

6. Noncontraceptive benefits of combined OCs include which of the following? Select all that apply.

    a. Protection against ovarian cancer

    b. Protection against endometrial cancer

    c. Protection against breast cancer

    d. Reduction in incidence of ectopic pregnancy

    e. Prevention of functional ovarian cysts

    f. Reduction in deep venous thrombosis

    g. Reduction in the risk of colorectal cancer

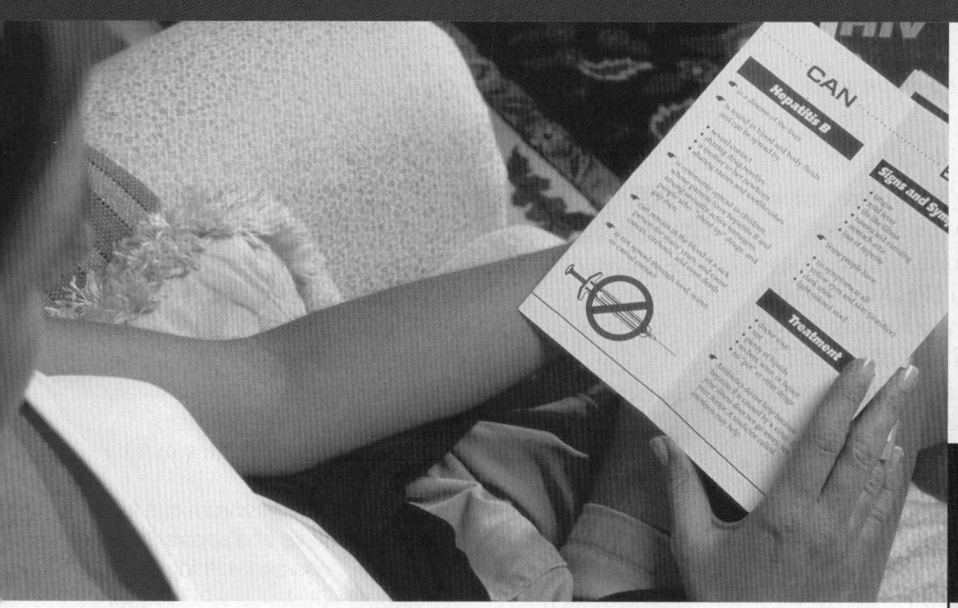

CHAPTER 5

Adapted by Jean Chow and
Pertice Moffitt

SEXUALLY TRANSMITTED INFECTIONS

KEY TERMS

bacterial vaginosis
chlamydia
gonorrhea
herpes
HIV/AIDS

HPV
pelvic inflammatory
   disease (PID)
sexually transmitted
   infection (STI)

syphilis
trichomoniasis
vulvovaginal
   candidiasis

LEARNING OBJECTIVES

Upon completion of the chapter, the learner will be able to:

1. Define the key terms used in this chapter.
2. Discuss the spread and control of sexually transmitted infections.
3. Identify risk factors and outline appropriate client education needed in common sexually transmitted infections.
4. Discuss how contraceptives can play a role in the prevention of sexually transmitted infections.
5. Analyze the physiologic and psychological aspects of sexually transmitted infections.
6. Delineate the nursing management and health promotion needed for women with sexually transmitted infections.

*S*andy, a 19-year-old, couldn't imagine what these "things" were that appeared "down there" in her genital area last week. She was too embarrassed to tell anyone, so she stopped by the college health service today to find out what they were.

Wow

Unconditional self-acceptance in clients is the core to reducing risky behaviour and fostering peace of mind.

Sexually transmitted infections (STIs) are infections of the reproductive tract caused by microorganisms transmitted through vaginal, anal, or oral sexual intercourse (Public Health Agency of Canada [PHAC], 2010). These infections can be transmitted through body fluids such as vaginal secretions, semen, saliva and blood. STIs pose a serious threat not only to women's sexual health but also to the general health and well-being of millions of people worldwide. STIs constitute an epidemic of tremendous magnitude. The incidence of STIs continues to rise in Canada, particularly in certain populations. For example, the rates of gonorrhea and chlamydia in the Northwest Territories are disproportionately higher than in the rest of the country (Government of the Northwest Territories, 2005). However, these findings may be related to the stringent screening and reporting program in this region by registered nurses in advanced practice.

STIs are biologically sexist, presenting greater risk and causing more complications among women than among men. STIs may contribute to cervical cancer, infertility, ectopic pregnancy, chronic pelvic pain, and death. Certain infections can be transmitted in utero to the fetus or during childbirth to the newborn (Table 5.1). STIs know no class, racial, ethnic, or social barriers—all individuals are vulnerable if exposed to the infectious organism. The problem of STIs has still not been tackled adequately on a global scale, and until this is done, numbers worldwide will continue to increase.

A special section on STIs and adolescents is presented below. This is followed by the discussion of specific STIs categorized according to a framework that groups them according to the major symptom manifested (Box 5.1). A section on preventing STIs is included at the end of the chapter.

Sexually Transmitted Infections and Adolescents

The health and well-being of Canadian youth are significantly threatened by STIs (Society of Obstetricians and Gynaecologists of Canada [SOGC], 2004). Teens who are sexually active experience high rates of STIs, and some groups are at higher risk, including sex workers and their clients, men who have sex with men, homeless individuals, travellers, and gay, lesbian, bisexual, and transgendered youth. A subpopulation of these at-risk young Canadians engages in several risky behaviours that include alcohol, drug, tobacco use, and unsafe sex (SOGC, 2004).

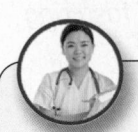

▶ *Take* NOTE!

It is estimated that many adolescents will contract an STI before graduating from high school.

TABLE 5.1 EFFECTS OF STIs ON THE FETUS OR NEWBORN

STI	Effects on Fetus or Newborn
Chlamydia	Can be infected during delivery Eye infections (neonatal conjunctivitis), pneumonia, low birth weight, preterm birth, stillbirth
Gonorrhea	Can be infected during delivery Rhinitis, vaginitis, urethritis, inflammation of sites of fetal monitoring Ophthalmia neonatorum can lead to blindness and sepsis (including arthritis and meningitis).
Herpes type II (genital herpes)	Contamination can occur during birth. Mental retardation, premature birth, low birth weight, death
Syphilis	Can be passed in utero Can result in fetal or infant death Congenital syphilis symptoms include skin ulcers, rashes, fever, weakened or hoarse cry, swollen liver and spleen, jaundice and anemia, various deformations.
Trichomoniasis	Fever, irritability, preterm birth, low birth weight
Venereal warts	May develop warts in throat (laryngeal papillomatosis); uncommon but life-threatening

---

BOX 5.1 **CDC Classification of STIs**

- Infections characterized by vaginal discharge
  - Vulvovaginal candidiasis
  - Trichomoniasis
  - Bacterial vaginosis
- Infections characterized by cervicitis
  - Chlamydia
  - Gonorrhea
- Infections characterized by genital ulcers
  - Genital herpes simplex
  - Syphilis
- Pelvic inflammatory disease (PID)
- Human immunodeficiency virus (HIV)
- Human papillomavirus (HPV) infection
- Vaccine-preventable STI
  - Hepatitis B
- Ectoparasitic infections
- Pediculosis pubis
- Scabies

Biological and behavioural factors place teenagers at high risk. Female adolescents are more susceptible to STIs due to their anatomy. During adolescence and young adulthood, women's columnar epithelial cells are especially sensitive to invasion by sexually transmitted organisms, such as chlamydia and gonococci, because these cells extend out over the vaginal surface of the cervix where they are unprotected by cervical mucus; these cells recede to a more protected location as women age. Behaviourally, adolescents and young adults tend to think they are invincible and deny the risks of their behaviour. This risky behaviour exposes them to STIs and human immunodeficiency virus/acquired immune deficiency syndrome (**HIV/AIDS**). Adolescents frequently have unprotected intercourse, they engage in partnerships of limited duration, and they face many obstacles that prevent them from using the health care system. In the North, Dene elders contend that many influences in modern society, such as rapid cultural transition and loss of cultural practices such as puberty rites, have contributed to risky sexual behaviour (Moffitt, 2008). In an effort to target the increased rates of STIs and develop a community health prevention strategy, researchers in one remote Aboriginal community embarked on community-coordinated research to identify the myriad understandings surrounding sexual attitudes and beliefs (Edwards, Mitchell, Gibson, et al., 2008). Health promotion and prevention strategies are most effective when the community context, along with individual beliefs and practices, is understood.

Nursing Assessment

Many health care providers fail to assess adolescent sexual behaviour and STI risks, to screen for asymptomatic infection during clinic visits, or to counsel adolescents on STI risk reduction. Nurses need to remember that they play a key role in the detection, prevention, and treatment of STIs in adolescents. All provinces and territories allow adolescents to give consent to confidential STI testing and treatment. Table 5.2 discusses clinical manifestations of common STIs in adolescents.

Nursing Management

Encourage the client to complete the antibiotic prescription (specific management for each type of STI is discussed below).

Prevention of STIs among adolescents is critical. The young have the most to lose from acquiring STIs because they will suffer the consequences the longest and might not reach their full reproductive potential. Health care providers have a unique opportunity to provide counselling and education to their clients. Adapt the style, content, and message to the client's developmental level and the community context. Identify risk factors and risk behaviours and guide the client to develop

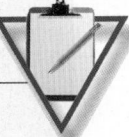

TEACHING GUIDELINE 5.1

Proper Condom Use

- Use latex condoms.
- Use a new condom with each act of sexual intercourse. Never reuse a condom.
- Handle condoms with care to prevent damage from sharp objects such as fingernails and teeth.
- Ensure condom has been stored in a cool, dry place away from direct sunlight. Do not store condoms in wallet or automobile or anywhere they would be exposed to extreme temperatures.
- Do not use a condom if it appears brittle, sticky, or discoloured. These are signs of aging.
- Put condom on before any genital contact.
- Put condom on when penis is erect. Ensure it is placed so it will readily unroll.
- Hold the tip of the condom while unrolling. Ensure there is a space at the tip for semen to collect, but make sure no air is trapped in the tip.
- Ensure adequate lubrication during intercourse. If external lubricants are used, use only water-based lubricants such as K-Y jelly with latex condoms. Oil-based or petroleum-based lubricants, such as body lotion, massage oil, or cooking oil, can weaken latex condoms.
- Withdraw while penis is still erect, and hold condom firmly against base of penis.

Sources: Pickering, L. K. (Ed.) (2006). *Red book: 2006 report of the committee on infectious diseases* (27th ed.). Elk Grove Village, IL: American Academy of Pediatrics; and Public Health Agency of Canada. (2010). *Canadian guidelines on sexually transmitted infections.* Ottawa, ON: Author.

specific individualized actions of prevention. Your interaction with the client needs to be direct, non-judgmental, and culturally appropriate.

Encourage adolescents to postpone initiation of sexual intercourse for as long as possible, but if they choose to have sexual intercourse, explain the necessity of using barrier methods, such as male and female condoms (Teaching Guideline 5.1). For teens who have already had sexual intercourse, the clinician can encourage abstinence at this point. If adolescents are sexually active, they should be directed to teen clinics and contraceptive options should be explained. In areas where specialized teen clinics are not available, nurses should feel comfortable discussing sexuality, safety, and contraception with individual teens and in the community setting. Encourage adolescents to minimize their lifetime number of sexual partners, to use barrier methods consistently and correctly, and to be aware of the connection between drug and alcohol use and the incorrect use of barrier

(text continues on page 162)

TABLE 5.2 **STIs Common in Adolescents**

Disease	Causative Organism	Transmission Mode	Diagnostic Testing	Female Symptoms	Male Symptoms	Treatment
Chlamydia Curable STI Seen frequently among sexually active adolescents and young adults Sexually active adolescents should be screened at least annually.	*Chlamydia trachomatis* (bacteria)	Vaginal, anal, oral sex, and by childbirth	Culture fluid from urethral swabs for males or endocervical swabs for females and conjunctival secretions in neonates	May be asymptomatic Dysuria Vaginal discharge (mucus or pus) Dyspareunia Lower abdominal pain Abnormal vaginal bleeding May lead to pelvic inflammatory disease (PID), ectopic pregnancy, and infertility Can cause inflammation of the rectum and lining of the eye (conjunctivitis) Can infect the throat from oral sexual contact with an infected partner	May be asymptomatic Dysuria Penile discharge (mucus or pus) Urethral itch Urethritis Testicular pain May lead to epididymitis (inflammation of the epididymis, the tubular structure that connects the testicle with the vas deferens) and sterility Can cause inflammation of the rectum and lining of the eye (conjunctivitis) Can infect the throat from oral sexual contact with an infected partner	Azithromycin Doxycycline Erythromycin Ofloxacin Sexual partners need evaluation, testing, and treatment also.
Gonorrhea Curable STI Client is often co-infected with *Chlamydia trachomatis*	*Neisseria gonorrhoeae* (bacteria)	Vaginal, anal, oral sex, and by childbirth	Staining samples directly for the bacterium, detection of bacterial genes or DNA in urine, and growing the bacteria in laboratory cultures More than one test may be used	May be asymptomatic or no recognizable symptoms until serious complications such as PID Urethritis Bartholinitis Urinary frequency Vaginal discharge (yellow, foul) Lower abdominal pain Dyspareunia Endocervicitis Arthritis Abnormal vaginal bleeding	Most produce symptoms but can be asymptomatic Dysuria Penile discharge (pus) Arthritis Epididymitis and may lead to sterility Symptoms of rectal infection include discharge, anal itching, and occasional painful bowel movements with fresh blood.	Usually a single dose of one of the following: Cefixime Ciprofloxacin Ceftriaxone Ofloxacin Spectinomycin Azithromycin Doxycycline Usually will be treated for co-infection with chlamydia, so a combination is given (e.g., ceftriaxone and doxycycline).

Genital Herpes Simplex Virus (HSV) Types 1 and 2						
Genital Herpes Simplex Virus (HSV) Types 1 and 2 Lifelong recurrent viral disease Most people have not been diagnosed. There is no cure.	HSV types I and 2	Having sexual contact (vaginal, oral, or anal) with someone who is shedding the herpes virus either during an outbreak or during a period with no symptoms Can be transmitted through close skin-to-skin contact	Visual inspection and symptoms or culture Presence of IgM indicates primary infection HSV-2 antibody accurate for detection of silent genital HSV-2 but not useful for HSV-1 detection.	May lead to PID, ectopic pregnancy, and infertility Symptoms of rectal infection include discharge, anal itching, and occasional painful bowel movements with fresh blood. Blister-like genital lesions Dysuria Fever, headache, myalgia Tender lymphadenopathy Complications include aseptic meningitis and extragenital lesions	Blister-like genital lesions Dysuria Fever, headache, muscle aches	Sexual partners need evaluation, testing, and treatment also. Acyclovir Famciclovir Valacyclovir Drugs do not cure, just control symptoms Sexual partners benefit from evaluation and counselling. If symptomatic, they need treatment. If asymptomatic, offer testing and education.

(continued)

TABLE 5.2 STIs COMMON IN ADOLESCENTS (continued)

Disease	Causative Organism	Transmission Mode	Diagnostic Testing	Female Symptoms	Male Symptoms	Treatment
Syphilis	*Treponema pallidum* (spirochete bacteria)	Sexual contact with an infected person	Blood tests Venereal Disease Research Laboratory (VDRL), rapid plasma reagin (RPR), and treponemal tests (e.g., fluorescent treponemal antibody absorbed [FTA-ABS]) can lead to a presumptive diagnosis. Darkfield examination and direct fluorescent antibody tests of lesion exudate or tissue provide definitive diagnosis of early syphilis.	Disease is divided into four stages: *Primary infection* • Chancre on place of entrance of bacteria (usually vulva or vagina but can develop in other parts of the body) *Secondary infection* • Maculopapular rash (hands and feet) • Sore throat • Lymphadenopathy • Flu-like symptoms *Latent infection* • No symptoms • No longer contagious • Many people if not treated will suffer no further signs and symptoms. Some people will go on to develop tertiary or late syphilis. *Tertiary infections* • Tumours of skin, bones and liver • Central nervous system symptoms • Cardiovascular symptoms • Usually not reversible at this stage	Disease is divided into four stages: *Primary infection* • Chancre on place of entrance of bacteria (usually on penis but can develop in other parts of the body) *Secondary, latent, and tertiary infections* All similar to female symptoms	Penicillin G injectable (if penicillin allergy, doxycycline or erythromycin) Sexual partners need evaluation and testing.
Trichomoniasis	*Trichomonas vaginalis* (protozoan)	Vaginal intercourse with an infected partner May be picked up from direct genital contact with damp or moist objects, such as towels, wet clothing, or a toilet seat	Microscopic evaluation of vaginal secretions or culture	Many women have symptoms but some may be asymptomatic. Dysuria Urinary frequency Vaginal discharge (yellow, green, or grey and foul odour) Dyspareunia Irritation or itching of genital area	Most infected men are asymptomatic. Dysuria Penile discharge (watery, white)	Metronidazole (Flagyl) Sexual partners need evaluation, testing, and treatment also.

Infection	Pathogen	Transmission	Diagnosis	Symptoms (Female)	Symptoms (Male)	Treatment
Venereal warts (condylomata acuminata) One of the most common STIs Could lead to cancers of the cervix, vulva, vagina, anus, or penis No cure; warts can be removed but virus remains	Human papillomavirus	Vaginal, anal, or oral sex with an infected partner	Visual inspection Abnormal Pap smear may indicate cervical infection of HPV.	Wart-like lesions that are soft, moist, or flesh-coloured and appear on the vulva and cervix and inside and surrounding the vagina and anus Sometimes appear in clusters that resemble cauliflower-like bumps, and are either raised or flat, small or large	Wart-like lesions that are soft, moist, or flesh-coloured and appear on the scrotum or penis Sometimes appear in clusters that resemble cauliflower-like bumps, and are either raised or flat, small or large	May disappear without treatment Treatment is aimed at removing the lesions rather than HPV itself No optimal treatment has been identified, but there are several ways to treat them depending on size and location. Most methods rely on chemical or physical destruction of the lesion: Imiquimod cream 20% Podophyllin antimitotic solution 0.5% Trichloroacetic acid (TCA) Small warts can be removed by: • Freezing (cryosurgery) • Burning (electrocautery) • Laser treatment Large warts that have not responded to treatment may be removed surgically.

161

TABLE 5.3 BARRIERS TO CONDOM USE AND MEANS TO OVERCOME THEM

Perceived Barrier	Intervention Strategy
Decreases sexual pleasure (sensation) Note: often perceived by those who have never used a condom.	• Encourage patient to try the following: • Put a drop of water-based lubricant or saliva inside the tip of the condom or on the glans of the penis before putting on the condom. • Try a thinner latex condom or a different brand or more lubrication.
Decreases spontaneity of sexual activity	• Incorporate condom use into foreplay. • Remind patient that peace of mind may enhance pleasure for self and partner.
Embarrassing, juvenile, "unmanly"	• Remind patient that it is "manly" to protect himself and others.
Poor fit (too small or too big, slips off, uncomfortable)	• Smaller and larger condoms are available.
Requires prompt withdrawal after ejaculation	• Reinforce the protective nature of prompt withdrawal and suggest substituting other postcoital sexual activities.
Fear of breakage may lead to less vigorous sexual activity.	• With prolonged intercourse, lubricant wears off and the condom begins to rub. Have a water-soluble lubricant available to reapply.
Non-penetrative sexual activity	• Condoms have been advocated for use during fellatio; unlubricated condoms may prove best for this purpose due to the taste of the lubricant. • Other barriers, such as dental dams or an unlubricated condom, can be cut down the middle to form a barrier; these have been advocated for use during certain forms of non-penetrative sexual activity (e.g., cunnilingus and anolingual sex).
Allergy to latex	• Polyurethane male and female condoms are available. • A natural skin condom can be used together with a latex condom to protect the man or woman from contact with latex.

From: Public Health Agency of Canada. (2010). *Canadian guidelines on sexually transmitted infections*. Ottawa, ON: Author.

methods. Table 5.3 discusses barriers to condom use and means to overcome them.

Think back to Sandy, who was introduced at the beginning of the chapter. How should the nurse handle Sandy's anxious state? What specific questions should the nurse ask Sandy to determine the source of the possible infection in her genital area?

Infections Characterized by Vaginal Discharge

Vaginitis is a generic term that means inflammation and infection of the vagina. There can be hundreds of causes for vaginitis, but more often than not the cause is infection by one of three organisms:

• *Candida,* a fungus
• *Trichomonas,* a protozoan
• *Gardnerella,* a bacterium

The complex balance of microbiological organisms in the vagina is a key element in the maintenance of health. Subtle shifts in the vaginal environment may allow organisms with pathologic potential to proliferate, causing infectious symptoms.

The nurse's role in managing vaginitis is one of primary prevention and education to limit recurrences of these infections. Primary prevention begins with changing the sexual behaviours that place women at risk for infection. In addition to assessing women for the common signs and symptoms and risk factors, the nurse can help women to avoid vaginitis or to prevent a recurrence by teaching them to take the precautions highlighted in Teaching Guideline 5.2.

Vulvovaginal Candidiasis

Vulvovaginal candidiasis is one of the most common causes of vaginal discharge. It is also referred to as yeast, monilia, and a fungal infection. It is not considered an STI because *Candida* is a normal constituent in the vagina and becomes pathologic only when the vaginal environment becomes altered. An estimated 75% of women will have at least one episode of vulvovaginal candidiasis and 5% to 10% will have more than one episode in their lifetime (PHAC, 2010).

Preventing Vaginitis

- Avoid douching to prevent altering the vaginal environment.
- Use condoms to avoid spreading the organism.
- Avoid tights, nylon underpants, and tight clothes.
- Wipe from front to back after using the toilet.
- Avoid powders, bubble baths, and perfumed vaginal sprays.
- Wear clean cotton underpants.
- Change out of wet bathing suits as soon as possible.
- Become familiar with the signs and symptoms of vaginitis.
- Choose to lead a healthy lifestyle.

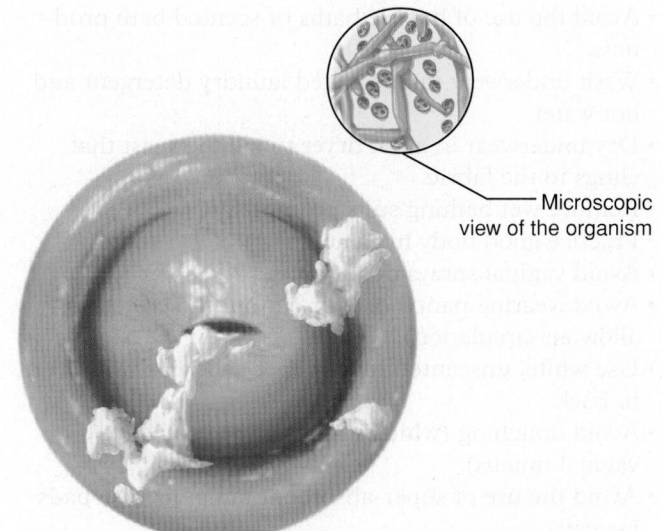

Microscopic view of the organism

FIGURE 5.1 Vulvovaginal candidiasis. (Source: The Anatomical Chart Company. [2002]. *Atlas of pathophysiology.* Springhouse, PA: Springhouse.)

Therapeutic Management

Treatment of uncomplicated vulvovaginal candidiasis includes one of the following medications:

- Miconazole
- Clotrimazole
- Fluconazole (contraindicated in pregnancy) (PHAC, 2010)

Most of the above medications are used intravaginally in the form of a cream, tablet, or suppository used for 3 to 7 days. If fluconazole is prescribed in an uncomplicated case, a 150 mg tablet is taken orally as a single dose (PHAC, 2010).

Recurrent vulvovaginal candidiasis is treated with fluconazole, topical azole, and boric acid (PHAC, 2010). Topical azole preparations are effective in the treatment of vulvovaginal candidiasis, relieving symptoms and producing negative cultures in 2 to 3 days (PHAC, 2010). Topical azoles are the only treatment advised during pregnancy, and treatment for 7 days may be required. Boric acid gelatin capsules are used intravaginally and are contraindicated in pregnancy. If vulvovaginal candidiasis is not treated effectively during pregnancy, the newborn can develop an oral infection known as thrush during the birth process; that infection must be treated with a local azole preparation after birth.

Nursing Assessment

Assess the patient's health history for predisposing factors for vulvovaginal candidiasis, which include:

- Often absent
- Pregnancy
- Sexual activity
- Current or recent antibiotic use
- Poorly controlled diabetes
- Corticosteroid use
- HIV infection

- Immunocompromised state
- Wearing tight, restrictive clothes and nylon underpants
- Trauma to the vaginal mucosa from chemical irritants or douching (PHAC, 2010)

Assess the patient for clinical manifestations of vulvovaginal candidiasis. Although up to 20% of women with this condition are asymptomatic (PHAC, 2010), typical symptoms, which can worsen just before menses, include:

- Pruritus
- Vaginal discharge (thick, white, curd-like)
- Erythema and edema of vagina and vulva
- Superficial dyspareunia
- External dysuria

Figure 5.1 shows the typical appearance of vulvovaginal candidiasis.

Speculum examination will reveal white plaques on the vaginal walls. The vaginal pH is less than 4.5. Definitive diagnosis is made by a wet smear, which reveals the filamentous hyphae and budding yeast characteristic of a fungus when viewed under a microscope (PHAC, 2010).

Nursing Management

Teach preventive measures to women with frequent vulvovaginal candidiasis infections, including:

- Reduce dietary intake of simple sugars and soda.
- Wear white, 100% cotton underpants.
- Avoid wearing tight pants or exercise clothes with spandex.
- Shower rather than taking tub baths.
- Wash with a mild, unscented soap and dry the genitals gently.

- Avoid the use of bubble baths or scented bath products.
- Wash underwear in unscented laundry detergent and hot water.
- Dry underwear in a hot dryer to kill the yeast that clings to the fabric.
- Remove wet bathing suits promptly.
- Practice good body hygiene.
- Avoid vaginal sprays/deodorants.
- Avoid wearing pantyhose (or cut out the crotch to allow air circulation).
- Use white, unscented toilet paper and wipe from front to back.
- Avoid douching (which washes away protective vaginal mucus).
- Avoid the use of super-absorbent tampons (use pads instead).

Trichomoniasis

Trichomoniasis is another common vaginal infection that causes a discharge. *Trichomonas vaginalis* is an ovoid, single-cell protozoa that can be observed under the microscope making a jerky swaying motion. The predisposing factor is multiple sexual partners. In women, it is associated with an increased risk of HIV transmission. The woman may be markedly symptomatic or asymptomatic (10% to 50% of cases). Men are asymptomatic carriers. Although this infection is localized, premature rupture of membranes, preterm birth, and low birth weight may be associated with trichomoniasis (PHAC, 2010).

Therapeutic Management

Recommended treatment for both partners is oral metronidazole (Flagyl) given either as a single 2 g dose or as a 500 mg dose twice daily for 7 days (PHAC, 2010). (See Evidence-based Practice 5.1.) Sex partners of women with trichomoniasis should be treated to avoid recurrence of infection. Men may be asymptomatic or have mild urethritis.

Nursing Assessment

Assess the patient for clinical manifestations of trichomoniasis, which include:

- Off-white or yellow frothy or bubbly discharge
- Vaginal pruritus and vulvar soreness
- Possible cervical bleeding on contact
- Dysuria
- Colpitis macularis ("strawberry" look on cervix)

Figure 5.2 shows the typical appearance of trichomoniasis.

The diagnosis is confirmed when a motile flagellated trichomonad is visualized under the microscope. In addition, a vaginal pH of greater than 4.5 is a typical finding.

Nursing Management

Instruct clients to avoid sex until they and their sex partners are cured (i.e., when therapy has been completed and both partners are symptom-free) and also to avoid consuming alcohol during and for 24 hours after treatment because mixing the medication and alcohol may cause a disulfiram (antabuse) reaction (PHAC, 2010).

EVIDENCE-BASED PRACTICE 5.1
Interventions for Trichomoniasis in Pregnancy

● **Study**

Trichomoniasis is a very common sexually transmitted infection. Trichomoniasis during pregnancy is associated with premature rupture of membranes, preterm birth, and low birth weight. This study examined the association between preterm birth and treatment with metronidazole for maternal trichomoniasis. A retrospective study of live births using billing codes to identify trichomoniasis cases, treatment, and birth outcomes was conducted. Of the 4,274 pregnant women diagnosed with trichomoniasis in this observational study, 3,579 were diagnosed at less than 35 weeks' gestation and undelivered until at least the second day after diagnosis. A comparison was made of the treated and untreated groups of women with respect to preterm birth.

▲ **Findings**

Findings indicate that a woman diagnosed with trichomoniasis during pregnancy is significantly more likely to deliver a preterm infant (less than 37 weeks' gestation). Filling the prescription for metronidazole, a category C drug, varied in women diagnosed with trichomoniasis. Treatment with metronidazole was not associated with an increased risk of preterm births in this study.

■ **Nursing Implications**

The nurse's role concerning this study's results is to counsel women diagnosed with trichomoniasis during pregnancy about the potential risks of treatment. Further research is required to determine whether metronidazole impacts preterm birth risk and the child in the long term. Results of this observational study are not as valid as a randomized trial.

Source: Mann, J. R., McDermott, S., Zhou, L., Barnes, T. L., & Hardin, J. (2009). Treatment of trichomoniasis in pregnancy and preterm birth: An observational study. *Journal of Women's Health, 18*(4), 493–497.

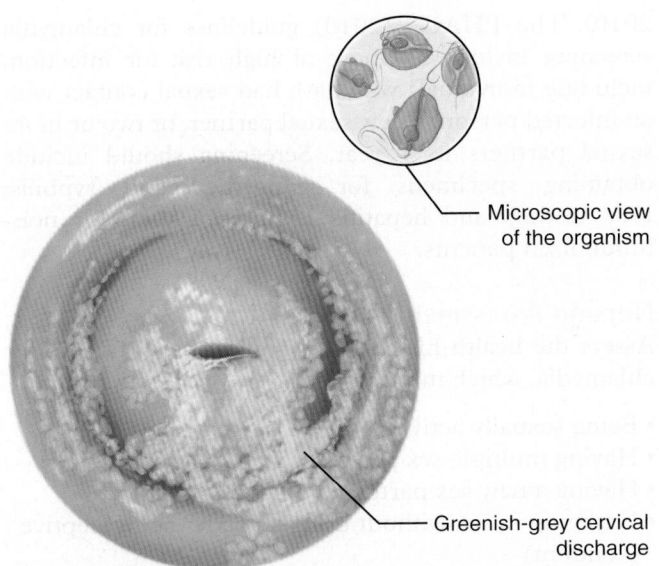

FIGURE 5.2 Trichomoniasis. (Source: The Anatomical Chart Company. [2002]. *Atlas of pathophysiology.* Springhouse, PA: Springhouse.)

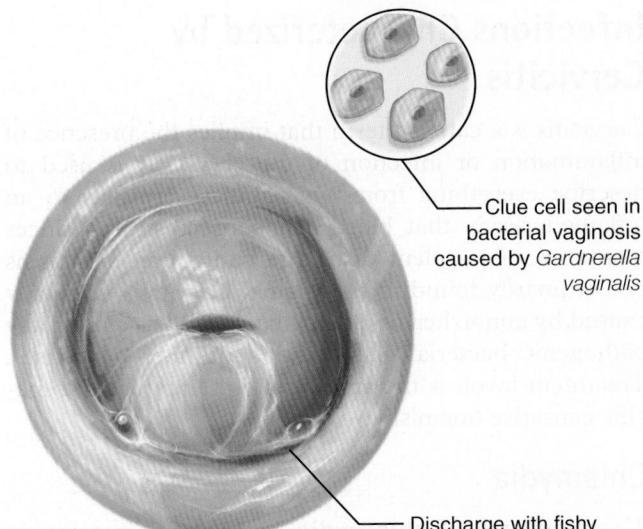

FIGURE 5.3 Bacterial vaginosis. (Source: The Anatomical Chart Company. [2002]. *Atlas of pathophysiology.* Springhouse, PA: Springhouse.)

Bacterial Vaginosis

Bacterial vaginosis, the most common cause of vaginal discharge, is caused by the gram-negative bacilli *Gardnerella, Prevotella,* or *Mobiluncus* spp. and a depletion of lactobacilli (PHAC, 2008). It is prevalent in about 10% to 30% of pregnant women, causes no symptoms in 50% of women, and is associated with increased transmission of HIV. Bacterial vaginosis is not usually considered to be sexually transmitted. It is characterized by alterations in vaginal flora in which lactobacilli in the vagina are replaced with high concentrations of anaerobic bacteria. The cause of the microbial alteration is not fully understood but is associated with being sexually active, having a new sexual partner, intrauterine device (IUD) use, having multiple sex partners, and douching (Centers for Disease Control and Prevention, 2010a; PHAC, 2010). Although routine screening for bacterial vaginosis is not recommended, research suggests that the infection is associated with preterm labour, premature rupture of membranes, chorioamnionitis, preterm birth, and endometritis following a cesarean delivery (PHAC, 2010).

Therapeutic Management

Treatment for symptomatic bacterial vaginosis includes oral metronidazole (Flagyl) 500 mg twice a day for 7 days, metronidazole gel 0.75% once daily intravaginally for 5 days, or clindamycin 2% cream intravaginally once daily for 7 days (PHAC, 2010). Alternative treatments include oral metronidazole 2 g in a single dose or oral clindamycin 300 mg orally twice a day for 7 days. The patient should avoid alcohol during and for 24 hours after oral metronidazole treatment because of a possible disulfiram (Antabuse) reaction (PHAC, 2010). Treatment of asymptomatic bacterial vaginosis is not necessary except for women with a high-risk pregnancy, before IUD insertion, or before undergoing gynecologic surgery/upper tract instrumentation and therapeutic abortion. Treatment of the male partner has not been beneficial in preventing recurrence (PHAC, 2010).

Nursing Assessment

Assess the patient for clinical manifestations of bacterial vaginosis. Primary symptoms are a thin, white homogeneous vaginal discharge and a characteristic "stale fish" odour. Figure 5.3 shows the typical appearance of bacterial vaginosis.

The criteria for diagnosing bacterial vaginosis are:

- Thin, white or grey copious vaginal discharge
- Vaginal pH >4.5
- Positive "whiff test" (secretion is mixed with a drop of 10% potassium hydroxide on a slide, producing a characteristic stale fishy odour)
- The presence of clue cells on wet-mount examination (PHAC, 2010)

Nursing Management

The nurse's role is one of primary prevention and education to limit recurrences of these infections. Primary prevention begins with changing the sexual behaviours that place women at risk for infection. In addition to assessing women for common signs, symptoms, and risk factors, the nurse can help women to avoid vaginitis or to prevent a recurrence by teaching them to take the precautions highlighted in Teaching Guideline 5.2. Recurrence is seen in 15% to 30% of patients 1 to 3 months after treatment (PHAC, 2010).

Infections Characterized by Cervicitis

Cervicitis is a catchall term that implies the presence of inflammation or infection of the cervix. It is used to describe everything from symptomless erosions to an inflamed cervix that bleeds on contact and produces quantities of purulent discharge containing organisms not ordinarily found in the vagina. Cervicitis is usually caused by gonorrhea or chlamydia, as well as almost any pathogenic bacterial agent and a number of viruses. Treatment involves the appropriate therapy for the specific causative organism.

Chlamydia

The incidence of **chlamydia** has been increasing in Canada since 1997 (PHAC, 2010). According to preliminary data, 65,000 Canadians were diagnosed with chlamydia in 2006, with the highest predictor for the infection being age. In 2004, the highest rates of infection were found in those between 15 and 24 years of age, accounting for about two thirds of reported cases (PHAC, 2010). The high rates seen in this age group are due mainly to unplanned sexual relations that sometimes result from pressure or force and the fact that sexual relations in young people typically happen before they have the experience, knowledge, and skills to protect themselves.

Asymptomatic infection is common among both men and women. Men develop urethritis, urethral discharge, and dysuria. In women, chlamydia is linked with cervicitis, dysuria, vaginal discharge, dyspareunia, lower abdominal pain, ectopic pregnancy, pelvic inflammatory disease (PID), and infertility (PHAC, 2010).

Chlamydia trachomatis is the bacterium that causes chlamydia. It is an intracellular parasite that cannot produce its own energy and depends on the host for survival. It is often difficult to detect, and this can pose problems for women due to the long-term consequences of untreated infection. Moreover, lack of treatment provides more opportunity for the infection to be transmitted to sexual partners. Newborns delivered to infected mothers may develop conjunctivitis or pneumonitis and have a 50% chance of acquiring the infection (PHAC, 2010).

Therapeutic Management

Antibiotics are usually used in treating this STI. Treatment options for chlamydia include doxycycline 100 mg orally twice a day for 7 days or azithromycin 1 g orally in a single dose (PHAC, 2010). Alternative treatments include ofloxacin 300 mg orally twice a day for 7 days, or erythromycin given orally, either 2 g per day for 7 days or 1 g per day for 14 days. Because of the common co-infection of chlamydia and gonorrhea, patients treated for gonorrhea should also be treated for chlamydia unless they have already tested negative for chlamydia (PHAC, 2010). The PHAC (2010) guidelines for chlamydia screening include all those at high risk for infection, including individuals who have had sexual contact with an infected person, a new sexual partner, or two or more sexual partners in 1 year. Screening should include obtaining specimens for gonorrhea and syphilis, HIV testing, and hepatitis B immunization for non-immunized patients.

Nursing Assessment

Assess the health history for significant risk factors for chlamydia, which may include:

• Being sexually active under 25 years of age
• Having multiple sex partners
• Having a new sex partner
• Engaging in sex without using a barrier contraceptive (condom)
• Engaging in sexual contact with a person infected with chlamydia
• Being pregnant
• Having a previous STI
• Being part of a vulnerable populations (e.g., sex trade workers, injection drug users, street youth, incarcerated individuals) (PHAC, 2010)

Assess the client for clinical manifestations of chlamydia. Most women are asymptomatic (PHAC, 2010). If the client is symptomatic, clinical manifestations include:

• Mucopurulent vaginal discharge
• Dysuria
• Cervicitis
• Conjunctivitis
• Lower abdominal pain
• Dyspareunia
• Abnormal vaginal bleeding (PHAC, 2010)

The diagnosis can be made by urine testing or by cervical, vaginal, oral, or rectal swab specimens for non-invasive urine-based nucleic acid amplification testing (NAAT) (PHAC, 2010). A conjunctival swab can be obtained for culture, enzyme immunoassay (EIA), and direct fluorescent antibody (DFA) assay.

Gonorrhea

Gonorrhea is a serious bacterial infection. It is highly contagious, potentially very severe, and reportable in all provinces and territories. The incidence of reported gonorrhea in Canada has doubled in recent years, from 4,477 cases in 1997 to 10,808 in 2006 (PHAC, 2010). Gonorrhea increases the risk for PID, infertility, endometritis, systemic neonatal infection, and HIV acquisition and transmission (PHAC, 2010). It is rapidly becoming more and more resistant to cure. Like all other STIs, gonorrhea is an equal-opportunity infection—no one is immune to it regardless of race, creed, gender, age, or sexual preference.

The cause of gonorrhea is the aerobic gram-negative intracellular diplococcus *Neisseria gonorrhoeae*. The site of infection is the columnar epithelium of the endocervix. Gonorrhea is almost exclusively transmitted by sexual activity. In pregnant women, gonorrhea is associated with chorioamnionitis, premature labour, premature rupture of membranes, and postpartum endometritis (Cunningham, Leveno, Bloom, et al., 2010). It can also be transmitted to the newborn in the form of ophthalmia neonatorum during birth by direct contact with gonococcal organisms in the cervix. Ophthalmia neonatorum is highly contagious and if untreated leads to blindness in the newborn.

Therapeutic Management

A rapid increase in quinolone-resistant *N. gonorrhoeae* (ciprofloxacin and ofloxacin) in Canada has resulted in the use of other drugs as preferred treatment for gonorrhea (PHAC, 2010). This has resulted in the use of other drugs as preferred treatment for gonorrhea (PHAC, 2010). The guidelines for the treatment of gonorrhea are being revised. The treatment of choice for those 9 years of age and older consists of a single dose of ceftriaxone 250 mg IM or cefixime 800 mg orally (PHAC, 2011). In situations such as penicillin allergy or known sensitivity to cephalosporin, a single dose of ciprofloxacin 500 mg or ofloxacin 400 mg may be considered only under certain circumstances described by the PHAC. Cefixime is the preferred treatment for pregnant women, but ceftriaxone and spectinomycin are alternative options. Treatment for chlamydial and non-gonococcal infections should follow treatment for each affected population. To prevent gonococcal ophthalmia neonatorum, a prophylactic agent should be instilled into the eyes of all newborns. Erythromycin, tetracycline ophthalmic ointment, or silver nitrate in a single application is recommended (Canadian Paediatric Society, 2010).

Nursing Assessment

Assess the client's health history for risk factors, which may include contact with STI infection, unprotected sex, and sex with multiple partners. Also at risk are travellers to endemic countries who have unprotected sex, sex workers and their partners, individuals under age 25 years, and street-involved youth (PHAC, 2010). Assess the client for clinical manifestations of gonorrhea, keeping in mind that some infected women are totally symptom-free or have symptoms that are not recognized as being due to gonorrhea (PHAC, 2010). Because women are so frequently asymptomatic, they are regarded as a major factor in the spread of gonorrhea. If symptoms are present, they might include (Wong, Lutwick, Heddurshetti, et al., 2009):

• Abnormal vaginal discharge
• Dysuria
• Cervicitis
• Abnormal vaginal bleeding
• Bartholin's abscess
• PID
• Neonatal conjunctivitis in newborns
• Mild sore throat (for pharyngeal gonorrhea)
• Rectal infection (asymptomatic)

Sometimes a local gonorrhea infection is self-limiting (there is no further spread), but usually the organism ascends upward through the endocervical canal to the endometrium of the uterus, further on to the fallopian tubes, and out into the peritoneal cavity. When the peritoneum and the ovaries become involved, the condition is known as PID. The scarring to the fallopian tubes is permanent. This damage is a major cause of infertility and is a possible contributing factor in ectopic pregnancy (Wong et al., 2009).

If gonorrhea remains untreated, it can enter the bloodstream and produce a disseminated gonococcal infection. This severe form of infection can invade the joints (arthritis), the heart (endocarditis), the brain (meningitis), and the liver (toxic hepatitis). Figure 5.4 shows the typical appearance of gonorrhea.

Screening is recommended for all women at risk for gonorrhea. Pregnant women should be screened as early as possible in pregnancy (PHAC, 2010). NAAT can be used for diagnosis, but culture is recommended because antimicrobial susceptibility testing can be performed. However, NAAT may be the only means of diagnosis in some areas in Canada. Any woman suspected of having gonorrhea should be tested for chlamydia also because co-infection is common (PHAC, 2010).

Nursing Management of Chlamydia and Gonorrhea

The prevalence of chlamydia and gonorrhea is increasing dramatically, and these infections can have long-term effects on people's lives. Sexual health is an important

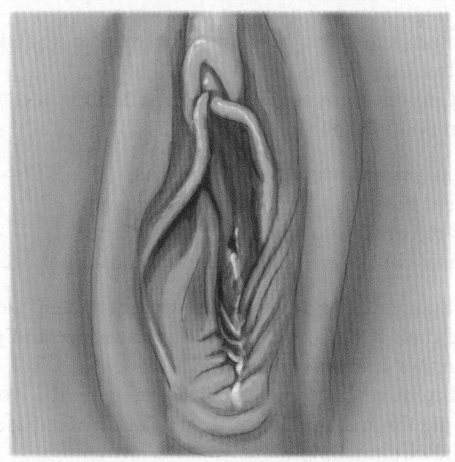

Figure 5.4 Gonorrhea.

part of a person's physical and mental health, and nurses have a professional obligation to address it. Be particularly sensitive when addressing STIs because women are often embarrassed or feel guilty. There is still a social stigma attached to STIs, so women need to be reassured about confidentiality.

The nurse's knowledge about chlamydia and gonorrhea should include treatment strategies, referral sources, and preventive measures. It is important to be skilled at patient education and counselling and to be comfortable talking with, and advising, women diagnosed with these infections.

Provide education about risk factors for these infections. High-risk groups include single women, women younger than 25 years, women with a history of STIs, those with new or multiple sex partners, those who use barrier contraception inconsistently, and women living in communities with high infection rates (PHAC, 2010). Assessment involves taking a health history that includes a comprehensive sexual history. Ask about the number of sex partners and the use of safer sex techniques. Review previous and current symptoms. Emphasize the importance of seeking treatment and informing sex partners. The four-level P-LI-SS-IT model (Box 5.2) can be used to determine interventions for various women because it can be adapted to the nurse's level of knowledge, skill, and experience. Of utmost importance is the willingness to listen and show interest and respect in a non-judgmental manner.

In addition to meeting the health needs of women with chlamydia and gonorrhea, the nurse is responsible for educating the public about the increasing incidence of these infections. This information should include high-risk behaviours associated with these infections, signs and symptoms, and the treatment modalities available. Stress that both of these STIs can lead to infertility

---

BOX 5.2 The P-LI-SS-IT Model

P, Permission—gives the woman permission to talk about her experience

LI, Limited Information—information given to the woman about STIs

• Factual information to dispel myths about STIs
• Specific measures to prevent transmission
• Ways to reveal information to her partner
• Physical consequences, if the infections are untreated

SS, Specific Suggestions—an attempt to help women change their behaviour to prevent recurrence and prevent further transmission of the STI

IT, Intensive Therapy—involves referring the woman or couple for appropriate treatment elsewhere based on their life circumstances

---

and long-term sequelae. Teach safer sex practices to people in non-monogamous relationships. Know the physical and psychosocial responses to these STIs to prevent transmission and the disabling consequences.

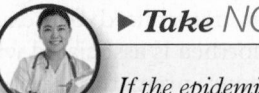

▶ **Take** NOTE!

If the epidemic of chlamydia and gonorrhea is to be halted, nurses must take a major front-line role now.

Infections Characterized by Genital Ulcers

In Canada, the majority of young, sexually active patients who have genital ulcers have genital herpes, syphilis, or chancroid. The frequency of each condition differs by geographic area and patient population; however, genital herpes is the most prevalent of these diseases. More than one of these diseases can be present in a patient who has genital ulcers. All three of these diseases have been associated with an increased risk for HIV infection. Not all genital ulcers are caused by STIs.

Genital Herpes Simplex

Genital **herpes** is a recurrent, lifelong viral infection. The annual incidence of genital herpes in Canada is unknown (PHAC, 2010). Two serotypes of herpes simplex virus (HSV) have been identified: HSV-1 (not sexually transmitted) and HSV-2 (sexually transmitted). HSV-1 causes the familiar fever blisters or cold sores on the lips, eyes, and face. HSV-2 invades the mucous membranes of the genital tract and is known as herpes genitalis. Most persons infected with HSV-2 have not been diagnosed.

HSV is transmitted by contact of mucous membranes or breaks in the skin with visible or nonvisible lesions. Most genital herpes infections are transmitted by individuals who are unaware that they have an infection. Many have mild or unrecognized infections but still shed the herpes virus intermittently. HSV is transmitted primarily by direct contact with an infected individual who is shedding the virus. Kissing, orogenital sex, genital sex, and vaginal delivery are means of transmission.

Having sex with an infected partner places an individual at risk for contracting HSV. After the primary outbreak, the virus remains dormant in the nerve cells for life, resulting in periodic recurrent outbreaks. Recurrent genital herpes outbreaks are triggered by precipitating factors such as emotional stress, menses, and sexual intercourse, but more than half of recurrences occur without a precipitating cause. Immunocompromised women have more frequent and more severe recurrent outbreaks than normal hosts (Salvaggio, Lutwick, Seenivasan, et al., 2012).

Living with genital herpes can be difficult due to the erratic, recurrent nature of the infection, the location of the lesions, the unknown causes of the recurrences, and the lack of a cure. Further, the stigma associated with this infection may affect the individual's feelings about herself and her interaction with her partner(s). Potential psychosocial consequences may include emotional distress, isolation, fear of rejection by a partner, fear of transmission of the disease, loss of confidence, and altered interpersonal relationships (Alexander, LaRosa, Bader, et al., 2010).

Along with the increase in the incidence of genital herpes has been an increase in neonatal HSV infections, which are associated with a high incidence of mortality and morbidity. New maternal HSV-1 or HSV-2 infections cause the greatest risk for the neonate since the mother has not fully developed the immune response by the time of birth (PHAC, 2010). The risk of neonatal infection is up to 50% if the mother has a primary genital HSV infection with lesions present at the time of birth. Approximately 70% of the time, the mother has had no history of genital herpes. If the mother has a recurrent lesion or has asymptomatic genital shedding at the time of birth, the risk is 2% to 8% with a vaginal birth. In most cases, neonatal herpes begins after discharge of an apparently healthy neonate.

Therapeutic Management

No cure for HSV exists, but antiviral drug therapy helps to reduce or suppress symptoms, shedding, and recurrent episodes. For the initial episode, clinically important symptoms require treatment. If the disease is severe, intravenous acyclovir 5 mg/kg every 8 hours is recommended (PHAC, 2010). Other treatments include acyclovir 200 mg orally five times per day for 5 to 10 days, famciclovir 250 mg orally three times per day for 5 days, or valacyclovir 1,000 mg orally twice per day for 10 days (PHAC, 2010). For recurrent episodes of the disease, oral valacyclovir 500 mg twice a day or 1 g every day for 3 days, oral famciclovir 125 mg twice per day for 5 days, or oral acyclovir 200 mg five times daily for 5 days or 800 mg twice per day for 2 days is recommended. Medication is dependent upon the number of outbreaks per year; outbreaks are classified as episodic (less than six per year) and suppressive (more than six per year). Suppressive therapy is recommended for individuals with recurrences at least every 2 months or six times per year (PHAC, 2010).

The management of genital herpes in pregnant women includes antiviral therapy. Acyclovir 200 mg orally five times per day for 5 to 10 days is used for primary infection. For recurrent HSV infection that follows a primary infection within the previous year, prophylactic treatment with oral acyclovir 200 mg four times daily or 400 mg three times daily or oral valacyclovir 500 mg twice daily at 36 weeks of gestation until delivery is recommended. The risk of transmission is present at birth

due to asymptomatic shedding even if there are no lesions; cesarean birth should be considered if the infection occurs late in the third trimester (PHAC, 2010). Therapeutic management also includes counselling regarding the natural history of the disease, the risk of sexual and perinatal transmission, and the use of methods to prevent further spread. Women without a history of HSV should be provided with risk reduction behaviour counselling to avoid contraction of HSV (PHAC, 2010).

Nursing Assessment

Assess the client for clinical manifestations of HSV. Clinical manifestations can be divided into the primary and non-primary episodes and recurrent disease (PHAC, 2010). The first or primary episode is usually the most severe, with a prolonged period of viral shedding. Primary HSV is a systemic disease characterized by extensive painful vesiculoulcerative genital lesions, fever, myalgia, malaise, dysuria, genital irritation, inguinal tenderness, and lymphadenopathy. The lesions in the primary herpes episode are frequently located on the vulva, vagina, and perineal areas. The vesicles will open and weep and finally crust over, dry, and disappear without scar formation (Fig. 5.5). Complications include aseptic meningitis and the development of extragenital lesions. In non-primary infections, a person experiences the first clinically evident episode and testing shows pre-existing antibodies. The manifestation of disease is less severe than in the primary infection. Non-primary infections are characterized by less extensive genital lesions, fewer systemic symptoms, fewer complications, and shorter duration. Asymptomatic shedding is greater in women with HSV-2 and occurs regardless of whether the person is symptomatic (PHAC, 2010).

Recurrent infection episodes are usually much milder and shorter in duration than the primary one. Tingling, itching, pain, localized genital lesions, and a more rapid resolution of lesions are characteristics of recurrent infections. Recurrent herpes is a localized disease characterized by typical HSV lesions at the site of initial viral entry. Recurrent herpes lesions are fewer in number and less painful and resolve more rapidly (Ural, 2010).

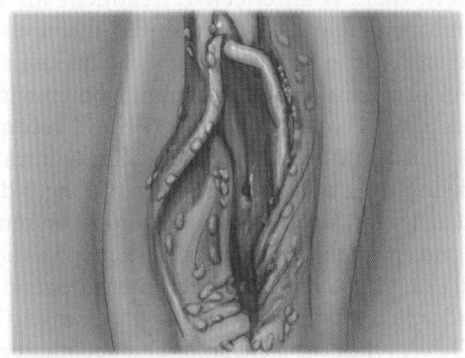

FIGURE 5.5 Genital herpes simplex.

Diagnosis of HSV is often based on clinical signs and symptoms and is confirmed by viral culture of fluid from the vesicle. The absence of HSV antibody in an acute-phase culture demonstrates a primary infection. Testing for type-specific antibodies assists in differentiating between HSV-1 and HSV-2; testing is available in limited laboratories in Canada. The presence of immunoglubulin G antibody indirectly indicates a recent infection (PHAC, 2010).

Syphilis

Syphilis is a complex, curable bacterial infection caused by the spirochete *Treponema pallidum*. It is a serious systemic disease that can lead to disability and death if untreated. Rates of syphilis in Canada are rising, with local outbreaks in several cities across the country (PHAC, 2010). Most of the outbreaks involve men who have sex with men, the sex trade, and locally acquired infection in heterosexual persons. Aboriginal people in British Columbia, Alberta, and the Yukon are disproportionately affected by STIs (PHAC, 2010). Syphilis continues to be one of the most important STIs both because of its biological effect on HIV acquisition and transmission and because of its impact on infant health (PHAC, 2010).

The spirochete rapidly penetrates intact mucous membranes or microscopic lesions in the skin and within hours enters the lymphatic system and bloodstream to produce a systemic infection long before the appearance of a primary lesion. Entry is through microabrasions that may occur in vaginal, rectal, or oral tissues during sexual intercourse (Shah, 2010). The syphilis spirochete can cross the placenta at any time during pregnancy. Congenital syphilis is worrisome, with several cases reported in British Columbia and Ontario in recent years (PHAC, 2010). The consequences of maternal infection include spontaneous abortion, prematurity, stillbirth, and multisystem failure of the heart, lungs, spleen, liver, and pancreas as well as structural bone damage, nervous system involvement, and mental retardation (PHAC, 2010; Waseem & Aslam, 2011).

Therapeutic Management

Fortunately, there is an effective treatment for syphilis. Benzathine penicillin G, administered intramuscularly, is the preferred drug for all stages of the disease (PHAC, 2010). For pregnant or non-pregnant women with syphilis of less than 1 year's duration, PHAC recommends 2.4 million units of benzathine penicillin G intramuscularly in a single dose. If the syphilis is of longer duration (more than 1 year) or unknown duration, the same dose is given once a week for 3 weeks. The preparation used, the dosage, and the length of treatment depend on the stage and clinical manifestations of disease (PHAC, 2010). Doxycycline or ceftriaxone is recommended as an alternative for people who are not pregnant and have

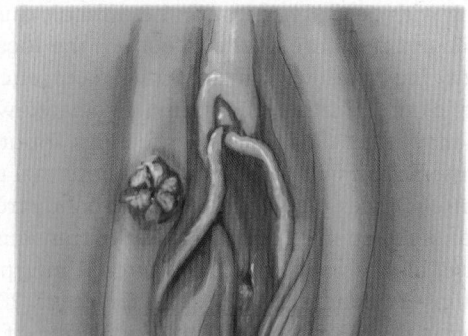

FIGURE 5.6 Chancre of primary syphilis.

penicillin allergies. Pregnant women are treated with penicillin, but there is no alternative treatment available for pregnant women who are allergic to penicillin. In these cases, penicillin desensitization should be considered (PHAC, 2010).

Women should be re-evaluated with additional serologic testing 3, 6, and 12 months after treatment for primary, secondary, and early latent syphilis (PHAC, 2010). Some experts suggest testing at 1 month following treatment to verify the effectiveness of the treatment. Women with late latent and tertiary syphilis should be followed clinically and serologically at 12 and 24 months (PHAC, 2010).

Nursing Assessment

Assess the client for clinical manifestations of syphilis. Syphilis is divided into four stages: primary, secondary, latent, and tertiary. Primary syphilis is characterized by a chancre (painless ulcer) at the site of bacterial entry that will disappear within 1 to 6 weeks without intervention (Fig. 5.6). In addition, painless bilateral adenopathy is present during this highly infectious period. If left untreated, the infection progresses to the secondary stage. Secondary syphilis appears 2 to 6 months after the initial exposure and is manifested by flu-like symptoms and a maculopapular rash of the trunk, palms, and soles. Alopecia and adenopathy are both common during this stage. In addition to rashes, secondary syphilis may present with symptoms of fever, headache, lymphadenopathy, and maculopapular rash on the palms of the hands and soles of the feet (O'Connor, Kleinman, & Goff, 2008). The secondary stage of syphilis lasts about 2 years. Once the secondary stage subsides, the latency period begins. This stage is characterized by the absence of any clinical manifestations of disease, although the serology is positive. This stage can last as long as 20 years. If not treated, tertiary or late syphilis occurs, with life-threatening heart disease and neurologic disease that slowly destroys the heart, eyes, brain, central nervous system, and skin.

Clients with a diagnosis of HIV or another STI should be screened for syphilis, and all pregnant women should be screened at their first prenatal visit. Interpretation of

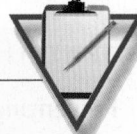

TEACHING GUIDELINE 5.3

Caring for Genital Ulcers

- Abstain from intercourse during the prodromal period and when lesions are present.
- Wash hands with soap and water after touching lesions to avoid autoinoculation.
- Use comfort measures such as wearing cotton underwear and nonconstricting clothes, urinating in water if urination is painful, taking lukewarm sitz baths, and air-drying lesions with a hair dryer on low heat.
- Avoid extremes of temperature such as ice packs or hot pads to the genital area as well as application of steroid creams, sprays, or gels.
- Use condoms with all new or noninfected partners.
- Inform health care professionals of your condition.

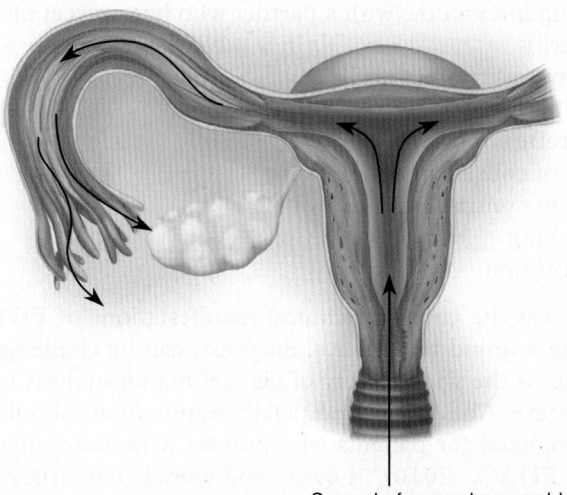

Spread of gonorrhea or chlamydia

FIGURE 5.7 Pelvic inflammatory disease. Chlamydia or gonorrhea spreads up the vagina into the uterus and then to the fallopian tubes and ovaries.

syphilis serology should be made in collaboration with a colleague who has experience in this area (PHAC, 2010). Darkfield microscopic examinations of lesions and DFA/ indirect fluorescent antibody (IFA) tests or NAAT are used to diagnose primary and secondary syphilis.

Nursing Management of Herpes and Syphilis

Genital ulcers from either herpes or syphilis can be devastating to women, and the nurse can be instrumental in helping her through this difficult time. Referral to a support group may be helpful. Address the psychosocial aspects of these STIs with women by discussing appropriate coping skills, acceptance of the lifelong nature of the condition (herpes), and options for treatment and rehabilitation. Teaching Guideline 5.3 highlights appropriate teaching points for the patient with genital ulcers.

Pelvic Inflammatory Disease

Pelvic inflammatory disease refers to an inflammatory state of the upper female genital tract and nearby structures. The fallopian tubes, ovaries, or peritoneum may be involved and endometriosis may also be present. PID results from an ascending polymicrobial infection of the upper female reproductive tract, frequently caused by untreated chlamydia or gonorrhea (Fig. 5.7). An estimated 1 million cases of PID are diagnosed annually in Canada (PHAC, 2010); however, the disease is underreported and up to two thirds of cases go unrecognized. Hospitalizaton rates for PID have decreased because women are being treated as out-patients. However, the number of visits to physician offices has not changed. PID is a serious health problem in Canada. Complications include ectopic pregnancy, tubo-ovarian abscess, infertility, chronic pelvic pain, and Fitz-Hugh–Curtis syndrome (perihepatitis) (PHAC, 2010). Because of the

seriousness of these complications, an accurate diagnosis is critical. To maintain fertility, early diagnosis is imperative (PHAC, 2010).

Therapeutic Management

Treatment of PID must include empiric, broad-spectrum antibiotic coverage of likely pathogens. The client is treated on an out-patient basis with oral antibiotics or is hospitalized and given antibiotics intravenously. The decision to hospitalize a woman is based on clinical judgment and the severity of her symptoms (e.g., severely ill with high fever or with protracted vomiting). Frequently, oral antibiotics are initiated, and if no improvement is seen within 48 to 72 hours, the woman is admitted to the hospital. Treatment then includes intravenous antibiotics, increased oral fluids to improve hydration, bed rest, and pain management. Follow-up is needed to validate that the infectious process is gone to prevent the development of chronic pelvic pain.

Nursing Assessment

Nursing assessment of the woman with PID involves a complete health history and assessment of clinical manifestations, physical examination, and laboratory and diagnostic testing.

Health History and Clinical Manifestations

Explore the client's current and past medical health history for risk factors for PID, which may include:

- Adolescence or young adulthood
- Having multiple sex partners
- Early onset of sexual activity
- History of PID or STI
- Sexual intercourse at an early age
- Alcohol or drug use

- Having intercourse with a partner who has untreated urethritis
- Recent insertion of an IUD
- Nulliparity
- Cigarette smoking
- Lack of consistent condom use
- Lack of contraceptive use
- Douching
- Prostitution

Assess the client for clinical manifestations of PID, keeping in mind that clinical diagnosis can be challenging due to the wide variety of clinical manifestations of the disease. Abdominal and pelvic examinations should be completed for patients who present with abdominal pain (PHAC, 2010). Lower abdominal tenderness, adnexal tenderness, and cervical motion tenderness may be present. Additional supportive criteria that support a diagnosis of PID are:

- Abnormal cervical or vaginal mucopurulent discharge
- Oral temperature above 38.3°C
- Elevated erythrocyte sedimentation rate (inflammatory process)
- Elevated C-reactive protein level (inflammatory process)
- Laboratory documentation of *N. gonorrhoeae* or *C. trachomatis* infection (causative bacterial organism)
- Prolonged or increased menstrual bleeding
- Dysmenorrhea
- Dysuria
- Painful sexual intercourse
- Nausea
- Vomiting

Physical Examination and Laboratory and Diagnostic Tests

Inspect the client for presence of fever (usually over 38 °C) or vaginal discharge. Palpate the abdomen, noting tenderness over the uterus or ovaries. However, the only way to diagnose PID definitively is through an endometrial biopsy, transvaginal ultrasound, or laparoscopic examination. The gold standard is laparoscopy, which can show abnormalities such as fallopian tube erythema and/or purulent exudates (PHAC, 2010).

Nursing Management

If the woman with PID is hospitalized, maintain hydration via intravenous fluids if necessary and administer analgesics as needed for pain. Semi-Fowler's positioning facilitates pelvic drainage. A key element to treatment of PID is education to prevent recurrence. Depending on the clinical setting (hospital or community clinic) where the nurse encounters the woman diagnosed with PID, a risk assessment should be done to ascertain what interventions are appropriate to prevent

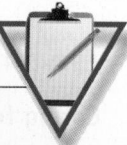

TEACHING GUIDELINE 5.4

Preventing Pelvic Inflammatory Disease

- Advise sexually active girls and women to insist their partners use condoms.
- Discourage routine vaginal douching, as this may lead to bacterial overgrowth.
- Encourage regular sexually transmitted infection screening.
- Emphasize the importance of having each sexual partner receive antibiotic treatment.

a recurrence. Explain the various diagnostic tests needed. Discuss the implications of PID and the risk factors for the infection; her sexual partner should be included if possible. Sexual counselling should include practicing safer sex, limiting the number of sexual partners, using barrier contraceptives consistently, avoiding vaginal douching, considering another contraceptive method if the woman has an IUD and has multiple sexual partners, and completing the course of antibiotics prescribed (Centers for Disease Control and Prevention, 2010b; Womenshealth.gov, 2010a, 2010b). Review the serious sequelae that may occur if the condition is not treated or if the woman does not comply with the treatment plan. Ask the woman to have her partner go for evaluation and treatment to prevent a repeat infection. Provide non-judgmental support while stressing the importance of barrier contraceptive methods and follow-up care. Teaching Guideline 5.4 gives further information related to PID prevention.

Human Papillomavirus

Human papillomavirus (**HPV**) is one of the most common STIs in Canada (PHAC, 2010). Prevalence varies widely among populations, reaching 20% in young women (PHAC, 2010). The SOGC (2009a) estimates that approximately 550,000 Canadians are infected every year and about 75% of Canadians will have at least one HPV infection during their lifetime. Genital warts or condylomata (Greek for warts) are caused by HPV. In addition, infection with certain types of HPV causes cervical cancer, which is the third most common cancer in women during the childbearing years in Canada (SOGC, 2009a).

▶ *Take* NOTE!

The lifetime risk of HPV infection is estimated to be as high as 70% in sexually active individuals.

Nursing Assessment

Nursing assessment of the woman with HPV involves a complete health history and assessment of clinical manifestations, physical examination, and laboratory and diagnostic testing.

Health History and Clinical Manifestations

Skin-to-skin contact is the most common means of transmission of HPV (SOGC, 2009a). Assess the client's health history for risk factors for HPV, which include young age (15 to 25 years) as well as having had multiple sex partners, sex with a male who has had multiple sexual partners, oral sex, or first intercourse at age 15 or younger (SOGC, 2009a). Risk factors contributing to the development of cervical cancer include smoking, few or no screenings for cervical cancer, multiple sex partners, immunosuppressed state, oral contraceptive use, history of STIs, pregnancy (due to increased hormonal level and immunosuppression), nutritional deficiencies, and early onset of sexual activity (Boardman & Matthews, 2011).

Assess the client for clinical manifestations of HPV. Most HPV infections are asymptomatic, unrecognized, or subclinical. Visible genital warts usually are caused by HPV type 6 or 11 (SOGC, 2009a). In addition to the external genitalia, genital warts can occur on the cervix and in the vagina, urethra, anus, and mouth. Depending on the size and location, genital warts can be painful, friable, and pruritic, although most are typically asymptomatic (Fig. 5.8). The strains of HPV associated with genital warts are considered low risk for development of cervical cancer, but other HPV types (16, 18, 31, 33, 35, 39, 45, 51, 52, 56, 58, 59, 68, 73, and 82) have been strongly associated with cervical cancer (PHAC, 2010).

Physical Examination and Laboratory and Diagnostic Tests

Clinically, visible warts are diagnosed by inspection. The warts are fleshy papules with a warty, granular surface. Lesions can grow very large during pregnancy, affecting urination, defecation, mobility, and descent of the fetus (PHAC, 2010). Large lesions, which may resemble cauliflower, exist in coalesced clusters and bleed easily.

Serial Pap smears are performed for low-risk women. These regular Pap smears will detect the cellular changes

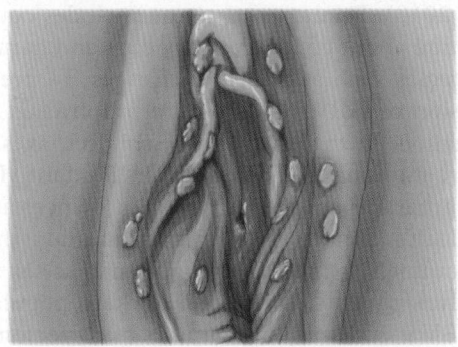

FIGURE 5.8 Genital warts.

associated with HPV. Health Canada has approved Hybrid Capture II, an HPV test used as a follow-up in women who have an ambiguous Pap test. Hybrid Capture II is used to examine the DNA content in cells to determine the specific HPV strain, which is useful in discriminating between low-risk and high-risk HPV types (SOGC, 2009b). The test can has 95% reliability in identifying 13 of the high-risk types of HPV that are associated with the development of cervical cancer and can detect high-risk types of HPV even before there are any conclusive visible changes to the cervical cells. If the test is positive for any of the high-risk types of HPV, the woman should be referred for colposcopy or cervical biopsy (SOGC, 2009b). This test may also be a helpful addition to the Pap test for general screening of women age 30 and over. It is not available everywhere in Canada, however, and patients may have to pay for it.

Upon physical examination, it is determined that Sandy has genital warts. The nurse finds out that Sandy engaged in high-risk behaviour with a stranger she "hooked up" with recently at college. She couldn't imagine that he would give her an STI because "he looked so clean-cut." She wonders how she could possibly have genital warts. What information should be given to Sandy about STIs in general? What specific information about HPV should be stressed?

Therapeutic Management

There is currently no medical treatment or cure for HPV. Instead, therapeutic management focuses heavily on prevention through use of an HPV vaccine and education and on the treatment of lesions and warts caused by HPV.

Two HPV vaccines are used in Canada. In 2006, Gardasil was approved for the prevention of cervical cancer. The vaccine has been recommended for routine administration to males and females between 9 and 26 years of age (SOGC, 2009a). Gardasil is administered intramuscularly in three separate 0.5 mL doses. The deltoid region of the upper arm or anterolateral area of the thigh may be used. The first dose may be given to any individual 9 to 26 years old prior to infection with HPV. The second dose is administered 2 months after the first, and the third dose is given 6 months after the initial dose (MerckVaccines.com, 2011). Gardasil does not protect against all strains of HPV; women must continue to have regular Pap tests (SOGC, 2009a). The real value of the vaccine is in immunizing girls before sexual activity is initiated. In 2010, the Cervarix vaccine was approved for use in females 10 to 25 years of age. Cervarix is used to prevent infection with the HPV strains responsible for 70% of cervical cancers (PHAC, 2010).

If the woman doesn't receive primary prevention with a vaccine, then secondary prevention should focus on education about the importance of receiving regular

Pap smears and, for women over 30, including an HPV test to determine whether the woman has a latent high-risk virus that could lead to precancerous cervical changes. Finally, treatment options for precancerous cervical lesions or genital warts caused by HPV are numerous and may include:

- Topical bichloroacetic or trichloroacetic acid 50% to 80%
- Liquid nitrogen cryotherapy
- Topical imiquimod 5% cream (Aldara) (should not be used in pregnancy)
- Podophyllin/podophyllotoxin 0.5% (applied by patient; should not be used in pregnancy)
- Podophyllin 10% to 25% (applied by health care provider; should not be used in pregnancy)
- CO_2 laser ablation
- Surgical excision
- Electro-fulguration (PHAC, 2010)

The goal of treating genital warts is to remove the warts and induce wart-free periods for the client. Treatment of genital warts should be guided by the preference of the client and available resources. No single treatment has been found to be ideal for all clients, and most treatment modalities appear to have comparable efficacy. Because genital warts can proliferate and become friable during pregnancy, they should be removed using a local agent. A cesarean birth is not indicated solely to prevent transmission of HPV infection to the newborn, unless the pelvic outlet is obstructed by warts (PHAC, 2010).

Nursing Management

An HPV infection has many implications for the woman's health, but most women are unaware of HPV and its role in cervical cancer. The average age of sexual debut is in early adolescence; therefore, it is important to target this population for use of the HPV/cervical cancer vaccine.

Key nursing roles are teaching about prevention of HPV infection and patient education and promotion of vaccines and screening tests in order to reduce the morbidity and mortality associated with cervical cancer caused by HPV infection. Teach all women that the only way to prevent HPV is to refrain from any genital contact with another individual. Although the effect of condoms in preventing HPV infection is unknown, latex condom use has been associated with a lower rate of cervical cancer. Teach women about the link between HPV and cervical cancer. Explain that, in most cases, there are no signs or symptoms of infection with HPV. Strongly encourage all young women between 9 and 26 to consider vaccination. For all women, promote the importance of obtaining regular Pap smears and, for women over 30, suggest an HPV test to rule out the presence of a latent high-risk strain of HPV.

Education and counselling are important aspects of managing genital warts. Teach the woman that:

- Even after genital warts are removed, HPV remains and viral shedding will continue.
- The likelihood of transmission to future partners and the duration of infectivity after treatment for genital warts are unknown.
- The recurrence of genital warts within the first few months after treatment is common and usually indicates recurrence rather than reinfection (SOGC, 2009b).

Sandy is being treated for HPV and is anxious for her "things" to disappear and never return. What education is needed to prevent further transmission from Sandy to any future sexual partners?

Vaccine–Preventable STI: Hepatitis A and B

Hepatitis is an acute, systemic, viral infection that can be transmitted sexually. The viruses associated with hepatitis or inflammation of the liver are hepatitis A, B, C, D, E, and G. Hepatitis A virus (HAV) is spread via the gastrointestinal tract. It can be acquired by drinking polluted water, by eating uncooked shellfish from sewage-contaminated waters or food handled by a hepatitis carrier with poor hygiene, and from oral or anal sexual contact. A person with HAV can easily pass the disease to others within the same household.

Hepatitis B virus (HBV) is transmitted through household contacts, sexual contact (anal, vaginal, or oral), and intravenous drug use as well as from mother to neonate (PHAC, 2010). In Canada, HBV is the most common cause of sexually transmitted hepatitis. The World Health Organization (WHO) estimates the prevalence of HBV worldwide is 350 million chronically infected people (WHO, 2008). Risk factors for infection include having multiple sex partners, using illicit injectable drugs, men having sex with other men, having sex with an HBV-infected person, and having an HBV carrier in the family (PHAC, 2010). Primary prevention includes counselling or education about high-risk behaviours and harm reduction strategies such as needle exchanges. To prevent the transmission of HBV, pre-exposure prophylaxis includes immunization. In the early 1990s, children ages 9 to 13 years were immunized. Today, universal infant HBV vaccination programs are operated in all provinces and territories (Health Canada, 2009). Immunization should be offered routinely to high-risk groups such as sex workers, hemodialysis patients, health care workers, populations in which HBV is endemic, and inmates of correctional facilities. Secondary prevention or post-exposure prophylaxis includes providing hepatitis B immune globulin (HBIG) to people up to 7 days following percutaneous (needlestick) or mucosal exposure and within 14 days to their sexual contacts. Infants born to HBV-infected mothers should be given HBIG immediately after birth and should be vaccinated within 12 hours of birth (PHAC, 2010).

Therapeutic Management

Unlike other STIs, HBV is preventable through immunization. HBV can result in serious, permanent liver damage. Treatment is generally supportive. No specific treatment for acute HBV infection exists.

Nursing Assessment

Assess the client for clinical manifestations of hepatitis. HAV produces flu-like symptoms with malaise, fatigue, anorexia, nausea, pruritus, fever, and upper right quadrant pain. Symptoms of HBV are similar to those of HAV, but with less fever and skin involvement. Although 50% to 70% of adults infected with HBV are asymptomatic (PHAC, 2010), symptoms can include fatigue, nausea, vomiting, rash, arthralgia, and anorexia. Icterus is noted in a small number of cases. The diagnosis of HAV cannot be made based on clinical manifestations alone and requires serologic testing. The presence of IgM antibody to HAV is diagnostic of acute infection. HBV is detected by a blood test that looks for antibodies and proteins produced by the virus and is positively diagnosed by the presence of hepatitis B surface antibody (HBsAg) (PHAC, 2010). Serologic testing should be supplemented by liver function testing and hepatic transaminase levels.

Nursing Management

Nurses should encourage all women to be screened for hepatitis when they have their annual Pap smear, or sooner if high-risk behaviour is identified. Nurses should also encourage women to undergo HBV screening at their first prenatal visit (Perinatology.com, 2010). Nurses can also explain that the HBV vaccine is given to all infants after birth in most hospitals. The vaccination consists of a series of three injections given within 6 months.

A newborn can be infected by the mother through fecal/oral transmission routes (PHAC, 2010). Immunization and/or gammaglobulin can be safely used during pregnancy to provide newborn protection. Household contacts should also be vaccinated against HAV. If a pregnant woman is in contact with an HAV-infected person, gammaglobulin or HAV can be provided to the woman.

Ectoparasitic Infections

Ectoparasites are a common cause of skin rash and pruritus throughout the world, affecting persons of all ages, races, and socioeconomic groups. Overcrowding, delayed diagnosis and treatment, and poor public education contribute to the prevalence of ectoparasites in both industrial and nonindustrial nations. Ectoparasitic infections include infestations of scabies and pubic lice. Since these parasites are easily passed from one person to another during sexual intimacy, clients should be assessed for them when receiving care for other STIs. Scabies is an intensely pruritic dermatitis caused by a mite. The female mite burrows under the skin and deposits eggs, which hatch. The lesions start as a small papule that reddens, erodes, and sometimes crusts. Diagnosis is based on patient history and the appearance of burrows in the webs of the fingers, sides of digits, wrists, axillae, waist, and genitalia (PHAC, 2010). Aggressive infestation can occur in immunodeficient, debilitated, or malnourished people, but healthy people do not usually suffer sequelae.

Clients with pediculosis pubis (pubic lice) usually seek treatment because of the pruritus, because of a rash brought on by skin irritation from scratching, or because they notice lice or nits in their pubic hair, axillary hair, abdominal and thigh hair, and sometimes in the eyebrows, eyelashes, and beard. Infestation is usually asymptomatic until after a week or so, when bites cause pruritus and secondary infections from scratching (Fig. 5.9). Diagnosis is based on history and the presence of nits (small, shiny, yellow, oval, dewdrop-like eggs) affixed to hair shafts or lice (yellowish, oval, wingless insects) (Guenther, Maguiness, & Austin, 2011).

Treatment is directed at the infested area, using 1% permethrin cream, 0.33% pyrethrin–piperonyl butoxide shampoo, or lindane 1% shampoo (PHAC, 2010). Lindane can cause neurotoxicity, which can be minimized by carefully following application instructions. Lindane is contraindicated in children younger than 2 years of age, pregnant women, lactating women, and people with extensive dermatitis.

Bedding, clothing, and fomites should be washed in hot water (50°C) or dry cleaned for decontamination (PHAC, 2010). Alternatively, items (toys and stuffed animals) can be placed in a plastic bag for 1 week. Sexual partner(s) within the previous month should be treated also, as should family members who live in close contact

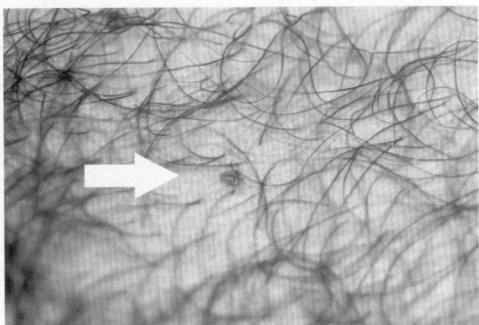

FIGURE 5.9 Pubic lice. A small brown living crab louse is seen at the base of hairs (*arrow*). (Source: Goodheart, H. [2003]. *Goodheart's photoguide of common skin disorders*. Philadelphia: Lippincott Williams & Wilkins.)

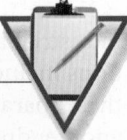

TEACHING GUIDELINE 5.5

Treating and Minimizing the Spread of Scabies and Pubic Lice

- Use the medication according to the manufacturer's instructions.
- Remove nits with a fine-toothed nit comb.
- Do not share any personal items with others or accept items from others.
- Treat objects, clothing, and bedding and wash them in hot water.
- Meticulously vacuum carpets to prevent a recurrence of infestation.

with the infected person. Nursing care of a woman infested with lice or scabies involves a three-tiered approach: eradicating the infestation with medication, removing nits, and preventing spread or recurrence by managing the environment. Over-the-counter products containing pyrethrins (RID, Triple X, Pronto, and Kwell) are safe for use and kill the active lice or mites. Nurses should provide education about these products (Teaching Guideline 5.5). The nurse can follow these same guidelines to prevent the health care facility from becoming infested.

Human Immunodeficiency Virus

The number of Canadians living with HIV is on the rise. According to PHAC surveillance reports, approximately 65,000 were affected at the end of 2008 (PHAC, 2009). From 2000 to 2004, there was a 20% increase in reported HIV-positive tests (PHAC, 2010). To date, there is no cure for this viral infection.

HIV, a retrovirus, is transmitted by intimate sexual contact (oral, anal, or vaginal), by sharing needles for intravenous drug use, or by transfusion of blood or blood products. It can also be passed from mother to fetus during pregnancy. HIV transmission is enhanced by the occurrence of other STIs, such as genital herpes, chlamydia, gonorrhea, trichomoniasis, and bacterial vaginosis (although vaginosis is not generally considered an STI). In 2004, men who had sex with men represented the largest proportion of positive HIV test reports in Canada, followed by men and women infected through heterosexual sex (PHAC, 2010).

The number of women with HIV infection and AIDS has been increasing steadily worldwide; the largest rise in Canada has been in the 15- to 19-year-old age group (PHAC, 2010). Heterosexual contact and intravenous drug use are the two major risk factors for HIV infection in women. Women are particularly vulnerable to heterosexual transmission of HIV due to substantial mucosal exposure to seminal fluids during intercourse.

This biological fact amplifies the risk of HIV transmission in women when coupled with the high prevalence of nonconsensual sex, sex without condoms, and the unknown and/or high-risk behaviours of their partners (National Institute of Allergy and Infectious Diseases, 2009). Therefore, the face of **HIV/AIDS** is becoming the face of young women. This shift will ultimately exacerbate the overall incidence of HIV because women spread it not only through sexual contact but also through nursing and childbirth. Immigrants from HIV-endemic regions represent an increasing number of HIV-positive test reports. In addition to the increased incidence of HIV and AIDS in women, positive HIV test reports and reported AIDS cases are increasing in the Aboriginal population, primarily as a result of injectable drug use (PHAC, 2010). Approximately, 50% of all positive HIV tests in Aboriginal Canadians come from women.

AIDS is a breakdown in the immune function caused by HIV infection. The infected person develops opportunistic infections or malignancies that become fatal. Progression from HIV to AIDS exceeds a median of 10 years after infection (PHAC, 2010). A marked decline in an AIDS diagnoses in Canada has resulted from the use of highly reactive anti-retroviral therapy (HAART). The success of HAART may be creating a relaxed attitude and less caution regarding transmission and acquisition of this infection. HIV has been transformed into a chronic illness, which has increased the burden of care.

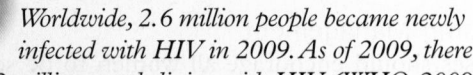

▶ *Take* NOTE!

Worldwide, 2.6 million people became newly infected with HIV in 2009. As of 2009, there were 33.3 million people living with HIV (WHO, 2009).

The fetal and neonatal effects of acquiring HIV through perinatal transmission are devastating and may be fatal. An infected mother can transmit HIV infection to her newborn before or during birth and through breastfeeding. Women infected with HIV in high-income countries are encouraged to avoid breastfeeding because the risk for HIV transmission with breastfeeding is greater than the risk associated with formula feeding (AVERT, 2011). For women in low-income countries where sanitation and access to clean water is problematic, the best option with limited resources and infrastructure is to breastfeed. Women in middle- and low-income countries are advised to take anti-retroviral drugs while the infant is breastfeeding and to breastfeed exclusively for the first 6 months. In areas where anti-retroviral medications are not available, infants should still be breastfed because breastfeeding leads to a higher chance of HIV-free survival (WHO, 2010). Despite the dramatic reduction in perinatal transmission, hundreds of infants worldwide are born infected with HIV each year.

HIV and Adolescents

The effects of HIV and AIDS on adolescents and young adults are of increasing concern, but it is difficult to get accurate data due to the varying ways this population seeks health care services. Some adolescents continue to receive care through pediatricians and adult services, but others have less access due to limited resources related to geography and financial resources. HIV infections are increasing in adolescents and young adults (13 to 24 years).

Most HIV-infected adolescents are exposed to the virus through high-risk sexual behaviours, STIs, and intravenous drug use (PHAC, 2010). Recent data suggest that the majority of HIV-infected adolescent males are infected through sex with men. Because adolescents think they are invincible, they may delay testing, and if they test positive, they may delay or refuse treatment. The inability to trace this population for medical care can lead to increased transmission of HIV.

▶ *Consider* THIS!

> *I was thinking of my carefree college days, when the most important thing was having an active social life and meeting guys. I had been raised by very strict parents and was never allowed to date under their watch. Since I attended an out-of-province college, I figured that my parents' outdated advice and rules no longer applied. Abruptly, my thoughts of the past were interrupted by the HIV counsellor asking about my feelings concerning my positive diagnosis. What was there to say at this point? I had a lot of fun but never dreamed it would haunt me for the rest of my life, which was going to be shortened considerably now. I only wish I could turn back the hands of time and listen to my parents' advice, which somehow doesn't seem so outdated now.*
>
> *Thoughts: all of us have thought back on our lives to better times and wondered how our lives would have changed if we had made better choices or gone down another path. It is a pity that we have only one chance to make good, sound decisions at times. What would you have changed in your life if given a second chance? Can you still make a change for the better now?*

Clinical Manifestations

When a person is initially infected with HIV, he or she goes through an acute primary infection period for about 3 weeks. The HIV viral load drops rapidly because the host's immune system works well to fight this initial infection. The onset of the acute primary infection occurs 2 to 4 weeks after exposure and is often nonspecific or mild (PHAC, 2010). Symptoms may include fever, pharyngitis, rash, headache, lymphadenopathy, sore throat, fatigue, myalgia, oral and/or genital ulcers, weight loss, nausea, vomiting, or diarrhea. Most people do not associate this flu-like condition with HIV infection. After initial exposure, there is a period of 3 to 12 months before seroconversion. The person is considered infectious during this time.

After the acute phase, the infected person becomes asymptomatic, but the HIV virus begins to replicate. The immune system begins a constant battle to fight this viral invasion, but over time it falls behind. A viral reservoir occurs in T cells that can store various stages of the virus. The onset and severity of the disease correlate directly with the viral load: the more HIV virus that is present, the worse the person will feel.

A normal person has a CD4 T-cell count of 450 to 1,200 cells per µL. Because HIV depletes the CD4 cell population over time, infected people become more susceptible to opportunistic infections. At the onset of profound immunosuppression (CD4 T-cell count of 200 or less), an opportunistic infection will occur, qualifying the person for the diagnosis of AIDS. As of now, AIDS will eventually develop in everyone who is HIV-positive. Currently, the AIDS virus and response to treatment are tracked based on CD4 count rather than viral load.

Diagnosis

Serologic testing is used in the diagnosis of HIV (PHAC, 2010). When there is a high index of suspicion (e.g., suspicious clinical symptoms, risky behaviour), serologic testing is recommended.

Approximately, 30% of Canadians with HIV are not aware that they are infected (PHAC, 2010). This means they are not receiving treatment that can prolong their lives, and they may be unknowingly infecting others. In addition, even when people do get tested, one in three fail to return to the testing site to learn their results (PHAC, 2010). Testing for HIV should be offered to anyone seeking evaluation and treatment for STIs. Counselling before and after testing is an integral part of the testing procedure. Informed consent must be obtained before an HIV test is performed. HIV infection is diagnosed by tests for antibodies against HIV-1 and HIV-2 (HIV-1/2). Antibody testing begins with a sensitive screening test (i.e., enzyme-linked immunosorbent immunoassay [ELISA]). This is a specific test for antibodies to HIV that is used to determine whether the person has been exposed to the HIV retrovirus. Reactive screening tests must be confirmed by a more specific test (i.e., the Western blot) on the same specimen. The Western blot is a highly specific test that is used to validate a positive ELISA test finding. A second blood specimen should be used to repeat the initial HIV serologic tests to confirm the diagnosis and rule out laboratory error (PHAC, 2010).

Therapeutic Management

The goals of HIV drug therapy are to:

- Decrease the HIV viral load below the level of detection
- Restore the body's ability to fight off pathogens
- Improve the client's quality of life
- Reduce HIV morbidity and mortality (AVERT, 2011)

Untreated HIV will take years to damage the immune system enough to develop AIDS, but this progression can be delayed by anti-retroviral therapy (AVERT, 2011). HAART, which combines at least three anti-retroviral drugs, has dramatically improved the prognosis of HIV/AIDS. Often treatment begins with combination HAART therapy at the time of the first infection, when the person's immune system is still intact.

There are obvious challenges involved in meeting these goals. The viral load can be reduced much more quickly than the T-cell count can be increased, and this disparity leaves the woman vulnerable to opportunistic infections.

Current therapy to prevent the transmission of HIV from mother to newborn includes a three-part regimen of having the mother take an oral anti-retroviral agent at 14 to 34 weeks of gestation; the medication is continued throughout pregnancy. During labour, an anti-retroviral agent is administered intravenously until delivery. An anti-retroviral syrup is administered to the infant within 12 hours after birth.

Dramatic new treatment advances with anti-retroviral medications have turned a disease that used to be a death sentence into a chronic, manageable condition for individuals who live in countries where anti-retroviral therapy is available. Despite these advances in treatment, however, only a minority of HIV-positive Canadians who take anti-retroviral medications are receiving the full benefits because they are not adhering to the prescribed regimen. Adherence is difficult because of the complexity of the regimen and the lifelong duration of treatment. A typical anti-retroviral regimen may consist of three or more medications taken twice daily. Adherence is made even more difficult because of the unpleasant side effects, such as nausea and diarrhea. Women in early pregnancy already experience these, and the anti-retroviral medication only exacerbates them.

Nursing Management

Nurses can play a major role in caring for the HIV-positive woman by helping her accept the possibility of a shortened lifespan, cope with others' reactions to a stigmatizing illness, and develop strategies to maintain her physical and emotional health. Educate the woman about changes she can make in her behaviour to prevent spreading HIV to others, and refer her to appropriate community resources such as HIV medical care services, substance abuse, mental health services, and social services. See Nursing Care Plan 5.1.

Providing Education About Drug Therapy

The goal of anti-retroviral therapy is to suppress viral replication so that the viral load becomes undetectable. This is done to preserve immune function and delay disease progression but is a challenge because of the side effects of nausea and vomiting, diarrhea, altered taste, anorexia, flatulence, constipation, headaches, anemia, and fatigue. Although not everyone experiences all of the side effects, the majority do have some of them. Current research has not documented the long-term safety of exposure of the fetus to anti-retroviral agents during pregnancy, but collection of data is ongoing.

Help to reduce the development of drug resistance and thus treatment failure by identifying the barriers to adherence; identifying these barriers can help the woman to overcome them. Some of the common barriers exist because the woman:

- Does not understand the link between drug resistance and nonadherence
- Fears revealing her HIV status by being seen taking medication
- Has not adjusted emotionally to the HIV diagnosis
- Does not understand the dosing regimen or schedule
- Experiences unpleasant side effects frequently
- Feels anxious or depressed (AVERT, 2011)

Depending on which barriers are causing nonadherence, work with the woman by educating her about the dosing regimen, helping her find ways to integrate the prescribed regimen into her lifestyle, and making referrals to social service agencies as appropriate. By addressing barriers on an individual level, the nurse can help the woman to overcome them.

Educate the woman about the prescribed drug therapy and stress that it is very important to take the regimen as prescribed. Offer suggestions about how to cope with anorexia, nausea, and vomiting by:

- Separating the intake of food and fluids
- Eating dry crackers upon arising
- Eating six small meals daily
- Using high-protein supplements (Boost, Ensure) to provide quick and easy protein and calories
- Eating "comfort foods," which may appeal when other foods do not

Promoting Drug Adherence

Remaining committed to the recommended drug therapy is a huge challenge for many HIV-infected people. Taking the medication becomes difficult when the same pills that are supposed to thwart the disease are making

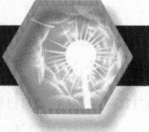

Nursing Care Plan 5.1

OVERVIEW OF THE WOMAN WHO IS HIV-POSITIVE

Annie, a 28-year-old woman, is HIV-positive. She acquired HIV through unprotected sexual contact. She has been inconsistent in taking her anti-retroviral medications and presents today stating she is tired and doesn't feel well.

NURSING DIAGNOSIS: Risk for infection related to positive HIV status and inconsistent compliance with anti-retroviral therapy

Outcome Identification and Evaluation
Client will remain free of opportunistic infections as evidenced by temperature within acceptable parameters and absence of signs and symptoms of opportunistic infections.

Interventions: Minimizing the Risk of Opportunistic Infections
- Assess CD4 count and viral loads *to determine disease progression* (CD4 counts <500/L and viral loads >10,000 copies/L = increased risk for opportunistic infections).
- Assess complete blood count *to identify presence of infection* (>10,000 cells/mm³ may indicate infection).
- Assess oral cavity and mucous membranes for painful white patches in mouth *to evaluate for possible fungal infection.*
- Teach client to monitor for general signs and symptoms of infections, such as fever, weakness, and fatigue, *to ensure early identification.*
- Provide information explaining the importance of avoiding people with infections when possible *to minimize risk of exposure to infections.*
- Teach importance of keeping appointments so her CD4 count and viral load can be monitored *to alert the health care provider about her immune system status.*
- Instruct her to reduce her exposure to infections via:
  - Meticulous handwashing
  - Thorough cooking of meats, eggs, and vegetables
  - Wearing shoes at all times, especially when outdoors
- Encourage a balance of rest with activity throughout the day *to prevent overexertion.*
- Stress importance of maintaining prescribed anti-retroviral drug therapies *to prevent disease progression and resistance.*
- If necessary, refer Annie to a nutritionist to help her understand what constitutes a well-balanced diet with supplements *to promote health and ward off infection.*

NURSING DIAGNOSIS: Knowledge deficit related to HIV infection and possible complications

Outcome Identification and Evaluation
Client will demonstrate increased understanding of HIV infection as evidenced by verbalizing appropriate health care practices and adhering to measures to comply with therapy and reduce her risk of further exposure and reduce risk of disease progression.

Interventions: Providing Patient Education
- Assess her understanding of HIV and its treatment *to provide a baseline for teaching.*
- Establish trust and be honest with Annie; encourage her to talk about her fears and the impact of the disease *to provide an outlet for her concerns.* Encourage her to discuss reasons for her noncompliance.
- Provide a non-judgmental, accessible, confidential, and culturally sensitive approach *to promote Annie's self-esteem and allow her to feel that she is a priority.*
- Explain measures, including safer sex practices and birth control options, to prevent disease transmission; determine her willingness to practice safer sex to protect others *to determine further teaching needs.*
- Discuss the signs and symptoms of disease progression and potential opportunistic infections *to promote early detection for prompt intervention.*
- Outline with the client the availability of community resources and make appropriate referrals as needed *to provide additional education and support.*
- Encourage Annie to keep scheduled appointments *to ensure follow-up and allow early detection of potential problems.*

the person sick. Nausea and diarrhea are just two of the possible side effects. It is often difficult to increase the client's quality of life when so much oral medication is required. The combination medication therapy is challenging for many people, and adhering to the medication regimen over a period of years is extremely difficult. Stress the importance of taking the prescribed anti-retroviral drug therapies by explaining that they help prevent replication of the retrovirus and subsequent progression of the disease, as well as decrease the risk of perinatal transmission of HIV. In addition, provide written materials describing diet, exercise, medications, and signs and symptoms of complications and opportunistic infections. Reinforce this information at each visit. Weight loss is a problem for people with HIV who experience frequent nausea and diarrhea from anti-retroviral therapy (CATIE, 2007). Nutritional guidance from a dietician to consume a high-calorie, high-protein diet along with vitamin and mineral supplements is necessary. For unknown reasons, HIV causes an increased energy expenditure (AVERT, 2011). It is important to maintain weight since weight loss increases morbidity and mortailty in people infected with HIV.

Preventing HIV Infection

The lack of information about HIV infection and AIDS causes great anxiety and fear of the unknown. It is vital to take a leadership role in educating the public about risky behaviours in the fight to control this disease. Prevention of HIV includes sexual abstinence, correct use of barrier methods, risk reduction with intravenous drug users, and reduced number of sexual partners (PHAC, 2010). Individuals who have known risk behaviours should be provided with HIV testing and counselling. This is all good advice for many women, but some simply do not have the economic and social power or choices or control over their lives to put that advice into practice. Barriers to prevention practices should be identified and the means to overcome them should be ascertained (PHAC, 2010). Recognize that fact, and address the factors that will give women more control over their lives by providing anticipatory guidance, giving ample opportunities to practice negotiation techniques and refusal skills in a safe environment, and encouraging the use of female condoms to protect against this deadly virus. Prevention is the key to reversing the current infection trends.

Providing Care During Pregnancy and Childbirth

Voluntary counselling and HIV testing should be offered to all pregnant women as early in the pregnancy as possible to identify HIV-infected women so that treatment can be initiated early. Once a pregnant woman is identified as being HIV-positive, she should be informed about the risk for perinatal infection. Current evidence indicates that in the absence of anti-retroviral medications, 25% of infants born to HIV-infected mothers will become infected with HIV (PHAC, 2010). Use of HAART reduces the transmission rate to 1%. Infants who become infected should be breastfed because breastfeeding leads to a higher chance of HIV-free survival (WHO, 2010).

In addition, the woman needs instructions on ways to enhance her immune system by following these guidelines during pregnancy:

• Getting adequate sleep each night (7 to 9 hours)
• Avoiding infections (e.g., staying out of crowds, handwashing)
• Decreasing stress in her life
• Consulting with a dietician and consuming adequate protein and vitamins
• Increasing her fluid intake to 2 L daily to stay hydrated
• Planning rest periods throughout the day to prevent fatigue

Despite the dramatic reduction in perinatal transmission, Canadian infants continue to be born infected with HIV. The birth of each infected infant is a missed prevention opportunity. To minimize perinatal HIV transmission, identify HIV infection in women, preferably before pregnancy; provide information about disease prevention; and encourage HIV-infected women to follow the prescribed drug therapy.

Providing Appropriate Referrals

The HIV-infected woman may have difficulty coping with the normal activities of daily living because she has less energy and decreased physical endurance. She may be overwhelmed by the financial burdens of medical and drug therapies and the emotional responses to a life-threatening condition, as well as concern about her infant's future, if she is pregnant. A case management approach is needed to deal with the complexity of her needs during this time. Be an empathetic listener and make appropriate referrals for nutritional services, counselling, homemaker services, spiritual care, and local support groups. Many community-based organizations have developed programs to address the numerous issues regarding HIV/AIDS.

Preventing Sexually Transmitted Infections

Education about safer sex practices—and the resulting increase in the use of condoms—can play a vital role in reducing STI rates all over the world. Clearly, knowledge and prevention are the best defenses against STIs. The prevention and control of STIs is based on the following concepts (PHAC, 2010):

1. Education and counselling of persons at risk about safer sexual behaviour
2. Identification of asymptomatic infected individuals and of symptomatic individuals unlikely to seek diagnosis and treatment

3. Effective diagnosis and treatment of infected individuals
4. Evaluation, treatment, and counselling of sex partners of people who are infected with an STI
5. Pre-exposure vaccination of people at risk for vaccine-preventable STIs

Nurses play an integral role in identifying and preventing STIs. They have a unique opportunity to educate the public about this serious public health issue by communicating the methods of transmission and symptoms associated with each condition, tracking the updated PHAC treatment guidelines, and offering clients strategic preventive measures to reduce the spread of STIs.

It is not easy to discuss STI prevention when globally we are failing at it. Knowledge exists on how to prevent every single route of transmission, but the incidence continues to climb. Challenges to prevention of STIs include lack of resources and difficulty in changing the behaviours that contribute to the spread of STIs. Regardless of the challenging factors involved, nurses must continue to educate and to meet the needs of all women to promote their sexual health. Successful treatment and prevention of STIs is impossible without education. Successful teaching approaches include giving clear, accurate messages that are age-appropriate and culturally sensitive.

Primary prevention strategies include education of all women, especially adolescents, regarding the risk of early sexual activity, the number of sexual partners, and STIs. Sexual abstinence is ideal but often not practiced; therefore, the use of barrier contraception (condoms) should be encouraged (see Teaching Guideline 5.1).

Secondary prevention involves the need for annual pelvic examinations with Pap smears for all sexually active women, regardless of age. Many women with STIs are asymptomatic, so regular screening examinations are paramount for early detection. Understanding the relationship between poor socioeconomic conditions and poor patterns of sexual and reproductive self-care is significant in disease-prevention and health-promotion strategies.

Every successful form of prevention requires a change in behaviour. The nursing role in teaching and rendering quality health care is invaluable evidence that the key to reducing the spread of STIs is through behavioural change. Nurses working in these specialty areas have a responsibility to educate themselves, their clients, their families, and the community about STIs and to provide compassionate and supportive care to clients. Some strategies nurses can use to prevent the spread of STIs are detailed in Box 5.3.

Behaviour Modification

Research validates that changing behaviours does result in a decrease in new STI infections, but it must encompass

---

BOX 5.3 Selected Nursing Strategies to Prevent the Spread of STIs

- Provide basic information about STI transmission.
- Outline safer sexual behaviours for people at risk for STIs.
- Refer clients to appropriate community resources to reduce risk.
- Screen asymptomatic persons with STIs.
- Identify barriers to STI testing and remove them.
- Offer pre-exposure immunizations for vaccine-preventable STIs.
- Respond honestly about testing results and options available.
- Counsel and treat sexual partners of persons with STIs.
- Educate school administrators, parents, and teens about STIs.
- Support youth development activities to reduce sexual risk-taking.
- Promote the use of barrier methods (condoms, diaphragms) to prevent the spread of STIs.
- Assist clients to gain skills in negotiating safer sex.
- Discuss reducing the number of sexual partners to reduce risk

---

all levels—governments, community organizations, schools, churches, parents, and individuals. Education must address ways to prevent becoming infected, ways to prevent transmitting infection, symptoms of STIs, and treatment. At this point in the STI epidemic, nurses do not have time to debate the relative merits of prevention versus treatment: both are underused and underfunded, and one leads to the other. But being serious about prevention and focusing on the strategies outlined above will bring about a positive change on everyone's part.

Contraception

The spread of STIs could be prevented by access to safe, efficient, appropriate, modern contraception for everyone who wants it. Nurses can play an important role in helping women to identify their risk of STIs and to adopt preventive measures through the dual protection that contraceptives offer. Traditionally, family planning and STI services have been separate entities in urban centres. Family planning services have addressed a woman's need for contraception without considering her or her partner's risk of STI; meanwhile, STI services have been heavily slanted toward men, ignoring the contraceptive needs of men and their partners.

Many women are at significant risk for unintended pregnancy and STIs, yet with this separation of services, there is limited evaluation of whether they need dual protection—that is, concurrent protection from STIs and unintended pregnancy. This lack of integration of services represents a missed opportunity to identify many at-risk women and to offer them counselling on dual protection.

Nurses can expand their scopes in either setting by discussing dual protection by use of a male or female condom alone or by use of a condom along with a non-barrier contraceptive. Because barrier methods are not the most effective means of fertility control, they have not been typically recommended as a method alone for dual protection. Unfortunately, the most effective pregnancy prevention methods—sterilization, hormonal methods, and IUDs—do not protect against STIs. Dual-method use protects against STIs and pregnancy.

■■■ Key Concepts

- ■ Avoiding risky sexual behaviours may preserve fertility and prevent chronic conditions later in life.
- ■ The most reliable way to avoid transmission of STIs is to abstain from sexual intercourse (i.e., oral, vaginal, or anal sex) or to be in a long-term, mutually monogamous relationship with an uninfected partner.
- ■ Barrier methods of contraception are recommended because they increase protection from contact with urethral discharge, mucosal secretions, and lesions of the cervix or penis.
- ■ The high rate of asymptomatic transmission of STIs calls for teaching high-risk women the nature of transmission and how to recognize infections.
- ■ The SOGC recommends that all women be offered group B streptococcal screening by rectovaginal culture at 35 to 37 weeks of gestation, and that colonized women be treated with intravenous antibiotics at the time of labour or ruptured membranes.
- ■ Nurses should practice good handwashing techniques and follow standard precautions to protect themselves and their patients from STIs.
- ■ Nurses are in an important position to promote the sexual health of all women. Nurses should make their clients and the community aware of the perinatal implications and lifelong sequelae of STIs.

REFERENCES

Alexander, L. L., LaRosa, J. H., Bader, H., Garfield, S., & Alexander, W. J. (2010). *New dimensions in women's health* (5th ed.). Sudbury, MA: Jones and Bartlett Publishers.

AVERT. (2011). *HIV and breastfeeding*. Retrieved January 16, 2012 from http://www.avert.org/hiv-breastfeeding.htm

Boardman, C. H., & Matthews, K. J., Jr. (2011). *Cervical cancer.* Retrieved 16, 2012 from http://emedicine.medscape.com/article/253513-overview

Canadian Paediatric Society. (2010). *Recommendations for the prevention of neonatal ophthalmia. Paediatrics & Child Health,* 7(7), 480–483.

CATIE. (2007). *A practical guide to nutrition for people living with HIV.* Retrieved January 16, 2012 from www.catie.ca/ng_e.nsf?TOC/OEF03E226233AE67852573760070974626?OpenDocument

Centers for Disease Control and Prevention. (2010a). *Bacterial vaginosis—CDC fact sheet.* Retrieved January 16, 2012 from http://www.cdc.gov/std/bv/stdfact-bacterial-vaginosis.htm

Centers for Disease Control and Prevention. (2010b). *Sexually transmitted diseases treatment guidelines: Pelvic inflammatory disease.* Retrieved January 16, 2012 from http://www.cdc.gov/std/treatment/2010/pid.htm

Cunningham, F., Leveno, K., Bloom, S., Hauth, J., Rouse, D., & Spong, C. (2010). *Williams obstetrics* (23rd ed.). New York: McGraw-Hill.

Edwards, K., Mitchell, S., Gibson, N., Martin, J., & Zoe-Martin, C. (2008). Community-coordinated research as HIV/AIDS prevention strategy in Northern Canadian communities. *Pimatisiwan: A Journal of Indigenous and Aboriginal Health,* 6(2), 111–127.

Government of the Northwest Territories. (2005). *NWT health status report.* Yellowknife, NT: Department of Health and Social Services.

Guenther, L., Maguiness, S., & Austin, T. W. (2011). *Pediculosis (lice).* Retrieved January 16, 2012 from http://emedicine.medscape.com/article/1108991-overview

Health Canada. (2009). *It's your health.* Retrieved August 23, 2011 from http://www.hc-sc.gc.ca/hl-vs/iyh-vsv/med/immuniz-eng.php

Mann, J. R., McDermott, S., Zhou, L., Barnes, T. L., & Hardin, J. (2009). Treatment of trichomoniasis in pregnancy and preterm birth: An observational study. *Journal of Women's Health,* 18(4), 493–497.

MerckVaccines.com. (2011). *Homepage for Gardasil.* Retrieved January 16, 2012 from www.merckvaccines.com/vaccines/gardasil/gardasil.html

Moffitt, P. (2008). *"Keep myself well": Perinatal health beliefs and health promotion practices among Tlicho women.* Calgary, AB: Doctoral dissertation, University of Calgary.

National Institute of Allergy and Infectious Diseases. (2009). *HIV/AIDS.* Retrieved January 16, 2012 from www.niaid.nih.gov/topics/HIVAIDS/Understanding?Pages?riskfactors.aspx

O'Connor, M., Kleinman, S., & Goff, M. (2008). Syphilis in pregnancy. *Journal of Midwifery & Women's Health,* 53(3), e17–e21.

Perinatology.com. (2010). *Infections during pregnancy: Hepatitis B virus (HBV).* Retrieved January 16, 2012 from http://www.perinatology.com/exposures/Infection/HepatitisB.htm

Pickering, L. K. (Ed.). (2006). *Red book: 2006 report of the committee on infectious diseases* (27th ed.). Elk Grove Village, IL: American Academy of Pediatrics.

Public Health Agency of Canada. (2009). *Summary: Estimates of HIV prevalence and incidence in Canada, 2008.* Retrieved January 16, 2012 from http://www.phac-aspc.gc.ca/aids-sida/publication/survreport/estimat08-eng.php

Public Health Agency of Canada. (2010). *Guidelines on sexually transmitted infections.* Ottawa, ON: Author.

Public Health Agency of Canada. (2011). *Important notice—Public health information update on the treatment for gonococcal infection.* Retrieved February 14, 2012 from http://www.phac-aspc.gc.ca/std-mts/sti-its/alert/2011/alert-gono-eng.php

Salvaggio, M. R., Lutwick, L. I., Seenivasan, M., & Kumar, S. (2012). *Herpes simplex.* Retrieved January 16, 2012 from http://emedicine.medscape.com/article/218580-overview

Shah, M. (2010). Syphilis. In E. T. Bope, R. E. Rakel, & R. Kellerman (Eds.), *Conn's current therapy 2010.* Philadelphia: Saunders Elsevier.

Society of Obstetricians and Gynaecologists of Canada. (2004). *School-based and school-linked sexual health education and promotion in Canada.* Ottawa, ON: Author.

Society of Obstetricians and Gynaecologists of Canada. (2009a). *HPV info for health-care professionals.* Retrieved January 16, 2012 from http://www.hpvinfo.ca/hpvinfo/professionals/index.aspx

Society of Obstetricians and Gynaecologists of Canada. (2009b). *Signs and symptoms of HPV.* Retrieved January 16, 2012 from http://www.hpvinfo.ca/hpvinfo/adults/signs-testing-diagnosis.aspx

Ural, S. H. (2010). *Genital herpes in pregnancy.* Retrieved January 16, 2012 from http://emedicine.medscape.com/article/274874-overview

Waseem, M., & Aslam, M. (2011). *Pediatric syphilis.* Retrieved January 16, 2012 from http://emedicine.medscape.com/article/969023-overview#a0104

Womenshealth.gov. (2010a). *Douching fact sheet.* Retrieved January 16, 2012 from http://www.womenshealth.gov/publications/our-publications/fact-sheet/douching.cfm

Womenshealth.gov. (2010b). *Pelvic inflammatory disease fact sheet.* Retrieved January 16, 2012 from http://www.womenshealth.gov/publications/our-publications/fact-sheet/pelvic-inflammatory-disease.cfm

Wong, B., Lutwick, L. I., Heddurshetti, R., & Cebular, S. (2009). *Gonococcal infections.* Retrieved January 16, 2012 from http://emedicine.medscape.com/article/218059-overview

World Health Organization. (2008). *Hepatitis B fact sheet.* Retrieved January 16, 2012 from http://www.who.int/mediacentre/factsheets/fs204/en/

World Health Organization. (2009). *Global summary of the AIDS epidemic, 2009.* Retrieved January 16, 2012 from www.who.int/hiv/data/2009_global_summary.png

World Health Organization. (2010). *Guidelines to HIV and infant feeding 2010.* Retrieved January 16, 2012 from http://www.who.int/child_adolescent_health/documents/9789241599535/en/index.html

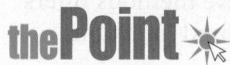

For additional learning materials, including Internet Resources, visit
http://thePoint.lww.com/Chow1e.

CHAPTER WORKSHEET

MULTIPLE CHOICE QUESTIONS

1. Which of the following contraceptive methods offers protection against sexually transmitted infections (STIs)?

   a. Oral contraceptives

   b. Withdrawal

   c. Latex condom

   d. Intrauterine device

2. In teaching about HIV transmission, the nurse explains that the virus cannot be transmitted by:

   a. Shaking hands

   b. Sharing drug needles

   c. Sexual intercourse

   d. Breastfeeding

3. A woman with HPV is likely to present with which nursing assessment finding?

   a. Profuse, pus-filled vaginal discharge

   b. Clusters of genital warts

   c. Single painless ulcer

   d. Multiple vesicles on genitalia

4. The nurse's discharge teaching plan for the woman with PID should reinforce which of the following potentially life-threatening complications?

   a. Involuntary infertility

   b. Chronic pelvic pain

   c. Depression

   d. Ectopic pregnancy

5. To confirm a finding of primary syphilis, the nurse would observe which of the following on the external genitalia?

   a. A highly variable skin rash

   b. A yellow-green vaginal discharge

   c. A nontender, indurated ulcer

   d. A localized gumma formation

CRITICAL THINKING EXERCISE

1. Sally, age 17, comes to the teen clinic saying that she is in pain and has some "crud" between her legs. The nurse takes her into the examining room and questions her about her symptoms. Sally states she had numerous genital bumps that had been filled with fluid, then ruptured and turned into ulcers with crusts. In addition, she has pain on urination and overall body pain. Sally says she had unprotected sex with several men when she was drunk at a party a few weeks back, but she thought they were "clean."

   a. What STI would the nurse suspect?

   b. The nurse should give immediate consideration to which of Sally's complaints?

   c. What should be the goal of the nurse in teaching Sally about STIs?

STUDY ACTIVITIES

1. Select a website from http://thePoint.lww.com/Chow1e to explore. Educate yourself about one specific STI thoroughly and share your expertise with your clinical group.

2. Contact your local health department and request current statistics regarding three STIs. Ask them to compare the current number of cases reported with last year's. Are they less or more? What may be some of the reasons for the change in the number of cases reported?

3. Request permission to attend a local STI clinic to shadow a nurse for a few hours. Describe the nurse's counselling role with patients and what specific information is emphasized to patients.

4. Two common STIs that appear together and commonly are treated together regardless of identification of the secondary one are _____ and _____.

5. Genital warts can be treated with which of the following? Select all that apply.

   a. Penicillin

   b. Podophyllin

   c. Imiquimod

   d. Cryotherapy

   e. Anti-retroviral therapy

   f. Acyclovir

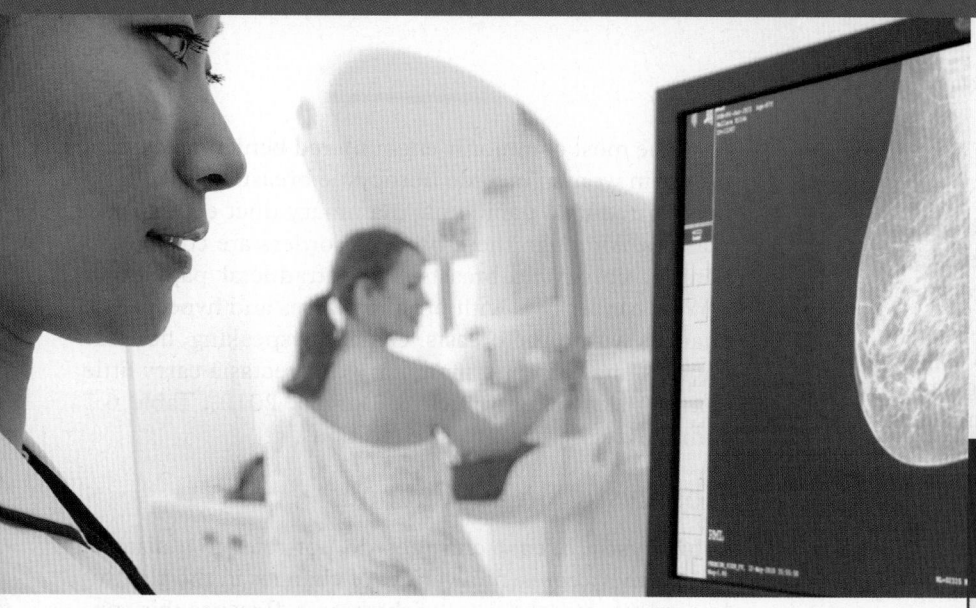

DISORDERS OF THE BREASTS

KEY TERMS

benign breast disorder
breast cancer
breast-conserving
   surgery
breast self-examination
carcinoma

chemotherapy
duct ectasia
endocrine therapy
fibroadenomas
fibrocystic breast
   changes

intraductal papilloma
mammography
mastitis
modified radical
   mastectomy
simple mastectomy

LEARNING OBJECTIVES

Upon completion of the chapter, the learner will be able to:

1. Define the key terms used in this chapter.
2. Identify the incidence, risk factors, screening methods, and treatment modalities for benign breast conditions.
3. Outline preventive strategies for breast cancer through lifestyle changes and health screening.
4. Explain the incidence, risk factors, treatment modalities, and nursing considerations related to breast cancer.
5. Develop an educational plan to teach breast self-examination to a group of young women.

Nancy hasn't been able to sleep well since she felt the lump in her left breast over a month ago, just after her 60th birthday. She knows she is at high risk because her mother died of breast cancer, but she can't bring herself to have it checked out.

Wow

Focus on reducing fear, anxiety, pain, and aloneness in all women diagnosed with a breast disorder.

The female breast is closely linked to womanhood in Canadian culture. Women's breasts act as physical markers for transitions from one stage of life to another, and although the primary function of the breasts is lactation, they are perceived as a symbol of beauty and sexuality.

This chapter discusses assessments, screening procedures, and management of specific benign and malignant breast disorders. Nurses play a key role in helping women maintain breast health by facilitating education and screening. A good working knowledge of early detection techniques, diagnosis, and treatment options is essential.

Benign Breast Disorders

A **benign breast disorder** is any non-cancerous breast abnormality. Though not life-threatening, benign disorders can cause pain and discomfort, and they account for a large number of visits to primary care providers.

Depending on the type of benign breast disorder, treatment might or might not be necessary. Although these disorders are benign, the emotional trauma women experience is phenomenal. Fear, anxiety, disbelief, helplessness, and depression are just a few of the reactions that a woman may have when she discovers a lump in her breast. Many women believe that all lumps are cancerous, but actually more than 90% of the lumps discovered are benign and need no treatment (Alexander, LaRosa, Bader, et al., 2010). Patience, support, and education are the essential components of nursing care.

▶ *Consider THIS!*

> *It was pouring down rain and I was driving alone along dark wet streets to my 8 AM appointment for a breast ultrasound. I recently had my annual mammogram and the radiologist thought he saw something suspicious on my right breast. I was on my way to confirm or refute his suspicions, and I couldn't keep focused on the road ahead. For the past few days I had been a basket case, fearing the worst. I was playing in my mind, what I would do if . . . ? What changes would I make in my life and how would I react when told? I have been through such personal turmoil since that doctor announced he wanted "more tests."*
>
> *Thoughts: this woman is worrying and is emotionally devastated before she even has a conclusive diagnosis. Is this a typical reaction to a breast disorder? Why do women fear the worst? Many women use denial to mask their feelings and hope against hope the doctor made a mistake or misread their mammogram. How would you react if you or your sister, girlfriend, or mother were confronted with a breast disorder?*

The most commonly encountered benign breast disorders in women include fibrocystic breasts, fibroadenomas, intraductal papilloma, mammary duct ectasia, and mastitis. Although these breast disorders are considered benign, fibrocystic breasts and intraductal papillomas carry a cancer risk, with prolific masses and hyperplastic changes within the breasts. Generally speaking, fibroadenomas, mastitis, and mammary duct ectasia carry little cancer risk (Sukumvanich & Borgen, 2010). Table 6.1 summarizes benign breast conditions.

Fibrocystic Breast Changes

Fibrocystic breast changes do not refer to a disease; rather, they represent a variety of changes in the glandular and structural tissues of the breast. Because this condition affects many women at some point, it is more accurately defined as a "change" rather than a "disease." The cause of fibrocystic changes is related to the way breast tissue responds to monthly levels of estrogen and progesterone. During the menstrual cycle, hormonal stimulation of the breast tissue causes the glands and ducts to enlarge and swell. One or both breasts can be involved, and any part of the breast can become tender (Rosolowich, Saettler, & Szuck, 2006). Fibrocystic changes do not increase the risk of breast cancer for most women except when the breast biopsy shows "atypia" or abnormal breast cells. The cause for concern for many women with fibrocystic changes is that breast examinations and mammography become more difficult to interpret, with benign lesions suggesting malignancy, lesions putting the woman at risk for cancer, and lesions co-existing with cancer (Miltenburg & Speights, 2008).

Fibrocystic breast changes are most common in women between the ages of 30 and 50. The condition is rare in postmenopausal women not taking hormone replacement therapy. Fibrocystic breast changes affect at least 50% to 60% of all women at some point in their lives and are the most common breast disorder today (Lee, 2009).

Therapeutic Management

Management of the symptoms of fibrocystic breast changes begins with self-care. In severe cases drugs, including bromocriptine, tamoxifen, or danazol, can be used to reduce the influence of estrogen on breast tissue. However, several undesirable side effects, including masculinization, have been documented. Bromocriptine may cause hepatic impairment and should be used with caution in people with heart disease and mental disorders (Deglin, Vallerand, & Sanoski, 2011). Aspiration or surgical removal of breast lumps will reduce pain and swelling by removing the space-occupying mass.

Nursing Assessment

Nursing assessment consists of a health history, physical examination, and laboratory and diagnostic tests.

TABLE 6.1 SUMMARY OF BENIGN BREAST DISORDERS

Breast Condition	Nipple Discharge	Site	Characteristics/ Age of Client	Tenderness	Diagnosis & Treatment
Fibrocystic breast changes	+ or −	Bilateral; upper outer quadrant	Round, smooth Several lesions Cyclic, palpable 30 to 50 years old	+	Aspiration and biopsy Limit caffeine; ibuprofen; supportive bra
Fibroadenomas	−	Unilateral; nipple area or upper outer quadrant	Round, firm, movable Palpable, rubbery Well delineated Single lesion 15 to 30 years old	−	Mammogram "Watchful waiting" Aspiration and biopsy Surgical excision
Intraductal papilloma	+	Unilateral; near nipple	Small, wart-like Poorly delineated Non-palpable Can become large 40 to 60 years old	+	Culture discharge Mammogram Ultrasound Surgical excision
Duct ectasia	+	Unilateral; behind nipple	Inflammation Pasty, greenish discharge Nonmobile Burning, itching Perimenopausal women	+	Mammogram Ultrasound Culture Antibiotics Surgical excision
Mastitis	−	Unilateral; outer quadrant	Wedge-shaped Warmth, redness Swelling Nipple cracked Breast engorged	+	Antibiotics Warm shower Supportive bra Breastfeeding increase fluids

Sources: Alexander, L. L., LaRosa, J. H., Bader, H., & Garfield, S., Alexander, W. J. (2010). *New dimensions in women's health* (5th ed.). Boston: Jones and Bartlett Publishers; American Cancer Society (2011). *Non-cancerous breast conditions*. Retrieved January 24, 2012 from http://www.cancer.org/docroot/CRI/content/CRI_2_6X_Non_Cancerous_Breast_Conditions_59.asp; and Sukumvanich, P., & Borgen, P. (2010). Diseases of the breast. In R. E. Rakel & E. T. Bope (Eds.), *Conn's current therapy 2007*. Philadelphia: Saunders Elsevier.

Health History

Ask the woman about common clinical manifestations, which include lumpy, tender breasts, particularly during the week before menses. Changes in breast tissue produce pain by nerve irritation from edema in connective tissue and by fibrosis from nerve pinching. The pain is cyclic and frequently dissipates after the onset of menses. The pain is described as a dull, aching feeling of fullness. Masses or nodularities usually appear in both breasts and are often found in the upper outer quadrants. Some women also experience clear to yellow nipple discharge when the breast is squeezed or manipulated.

Physical Examination

It is best to examine a woman's breast a week after menses, when swelling has subsided. Observe the breasts for fibrosis, or thickening of the normal breast tissues, which occurs in the early stages. Cysts form in the later stages and feel like multiple, smooth, well-delineated tiny pebbles or bumpy oatmeal under the skin (Fig. 6.1). On physical examination of the breasts, a few characteristics might be helpful in differentiating a cyst from a cancerous lesion. Cancerous lesions typically are fixed and painless and may cause skin retraction (pulling). Cysts tend to be mobile and tender and do not cause skin retraction in the surrounding tissue.

Laboratory and Diagnostic Tests

Mammography can be helpful in distinguishing fibrocystic changes from breast cancer. Ultrasonography, which produces images of the breasts by sending sound waves through a gel applied to the breasts, is a useful adjunct to mammography for breast evaluation because it helps to differentiate subtle ultrasonic changes that could be associated with malignancy (Fentiman, 2009). Fine-needle aspiration (FNA) biopsy can also be done to differentiate a solid tumour, cyst, or malignancy. FNA biopsy uses a thin needle guided by ultrasound to the

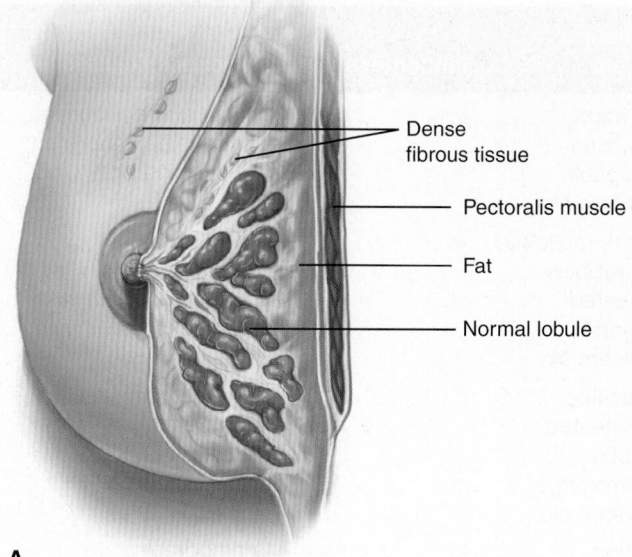

A

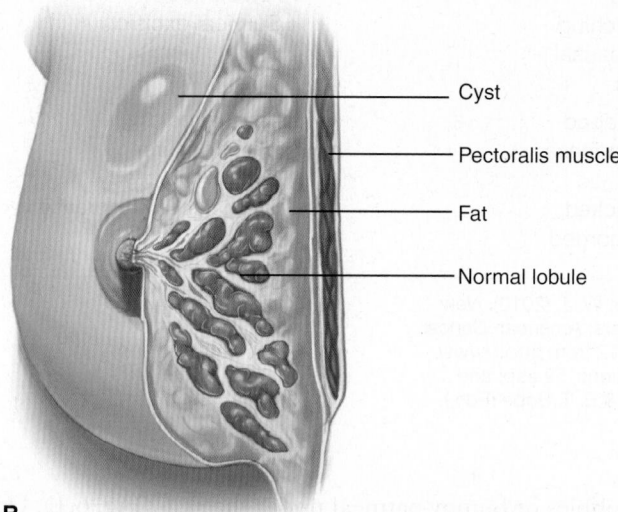

B

FIGURE 6.1 **(A)** Fibrocystic breast changes. **(B)** Cyst. (Source: The Anatomical Chart Company. [2002]. *Atlas of pathophysiology.* Springhouse, PA: Springhouse Corporation.)

mass. In a method called stereotactic needle biopsy, a computer maps the exact location of the mass using mammograms taken from two angles, and the map is used to guide the needle.

Nursing Management

A nurse caring for a woman with fibrocystic breast changes can teach her about the condition, provide tips for self-care (Teaching Guideline 6.1), suggest lifestyle changes, and demonstrate how to perform monthly breast self-examination after her menses to monitor the changes. Nursing Care Plan 6.1 presents a plan of care for a woman with fibrocystic breast changes.

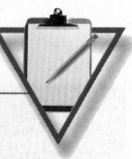

TEACHING GUIDELINE 6.1

Relieving Symptoms of Fibrocystic Breast Changes

- Wear an extra-supportive bra to prevent undue strain on the ligaments of the breasts to reduce discomfort.
- Avoid caffeine, which is a stimulant. This reduces discomfort for some women.
- Take oral contraceptives, as recommended by a health care practitioner, to stabilize the monthly hormonal levels.
- Eat a low-fat diet rich in fruits, vegetables, and grains to maintain a healthy nutritional lifestyle and ideal weight.
- Apply heat to the breasts to help reduce pain via vasodilation of vessels.
- Take diuretics, as recommended by a health care practitioner, to counteract fluid retention and swelling of the breasts.
- Reduce salt intake to reduce fluid retention and swelling in the breasts.
- Take over-the-counter medications, such as aspirin or ibuprofen (Motrin, Advil, Nuprin), to reduce inflammation and discomfort.
- Use thiamine and vitamin E therapy. This has been found helpful for some women, but research has failed to demonstrate a direct benefit from either therapy.
- Take medications as prescribed (e.g., bromocriptine, tamoxifen, or danazol).
- Discuss the possibility of aspiration or surgical removal of breast lumps with a health care practitioner.

Fibroadenomas

Fibroadenomas are common benign solid breast tumours that occur in about 10% of all women and account for up to half of all breast biopsies. They are the most common mass in women (Lee, 2009). They are considered hyperplastic lesions associated with an aberration of normal development and involution rather than a neoplasm. Fibroadenomas can be stimulated by lactation and pregnancy (Sukumvanich & Borgen, 2010). They are composed of both fibrous and glandular tissue and usually occur in women between 20 and 30 years of age (Alexander et al., 2010). Giant fibroadenomas occur most often in pregnant or lactating women. These large lesions may regress in size once hormonal stimulation subsides; lesions that remain large can be excised surgically (Sukumvanich & Borgen, 2010). Fibroadenomas are rarely associated with cancer.

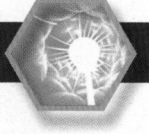

Nursing Care Plan 6.1

Overview of the Woman with Fibrocystic Breast Changes

Sheree Rollins is a 37-year-old woman who comes to the clinic for her routine check-up. During the examination, she says, "Sometimes my breasts feel so heavy and they ache a lot. I noticed a couple of lumpy areas in my breast last week just before I got my period. Is this normal? Now they feel like they're almost gone. Should I be worried?" CBE reveals two small (pea-sized), mobile, slightly tender nodules in each breast bilaterally. No skin retraction noted. Previous mammogram revealed fibrocystic breast changes.

NURSING DIAGNOSIS: Pain related to changes in breast tissue

Outcome Identification and Evaluation
Client will demonstrate a decrease in breast pain as evidenced by a pain rating of 1 or 2 on a pain rating scale of 0 to 10 and statements that pain is lessened.

Interventions: Relieving Pain
- Ask client to rate her pain using a numeric pain rating scale *to establish a baseline.*
- Discuss with client any measures used to relieve pain *to determine effectiveness of the measures.*
- Encourage use of a supportive bra *to aid in reducing discomfort.*
- Instruct client in use of over-the-counter analgesics *to promote pain relief.*
- Advise the client to apply warm compresses or allow warm water from the shower to flow over her breasts *to promote vasodilation and subsequent pain relief.*
- Tell client to reduce her intake of salt to reduce risk of fluid retention and swelling leading *to increased pain.*

NURSING DIAGNOSIS: Deficient knowledge related to fibrocystic breast changes and appropriate care measures

Outcome Identification and Evaluation
Client will verbalize understanding of condition as evidenced by statements about the cause of breast changes and appropriate choices for lifestyle changes, and demonstration of self-care measures.

Interventions: Providing Patient Education
- Assess client's knowledge of fibrocystic breast changes *to establish a baseline for teaching.*
- Explain the role of monthly hormonal level changes and describe the signs and symptoms *to promote understanding of this condition.*
- Teach the client how to perform breast self-examination after her menstrual period *to monitor for changes.*
- Encourage client to report any changes promptly *to ensure early detection of problems.*
- Suggest client speak with her primary care provider about the use of oral contraceptives *to help stabilize monthly hormonal levels.*
- Review lifestyle choices, such as avoiding caffeine, eating a low-fat diet rich in fruits, vegetables, and grains, and adhering to screening recommendations *to promote health.*
- Discuss measures for pain relief *to minimize discomfort associated with breast changes.*

Therapeutic Management
Treatment may include a period of "watchful waiting" because many fibroadenomas stop growing or shrink on their own without any treatment. Other growths may need to be surgically removed if they do not regress or if they remain unchanged. Rapidly enlarging fibroadenomas are surgically excised to rule out a phyllodes tumour, which is difficult to differentiate from fibroadenoma (Sukumvanich & Borgen, 2010). Cryoablation, an alternative to surgery, can also be used to remove a tumour. In this procedure, extremely cold gas is piped into the tumour using ultrasound guidance. The tumour freezes and dies. The current trend is toward a more conservative approach to treatment after careful evaluation and continued monitoring.

Nursing Assessment
Ask the woman about clinical manifestations of fibroadenomas. These lumps are felt as firm, rubbery, well-circumscribed, freely mobile nodules that might or might not be tender when palpated.

Breast fibroadenomas are usually detected incidentally during clinical or self-examinations and are usually located in the upper outer quadrant of the breast; more

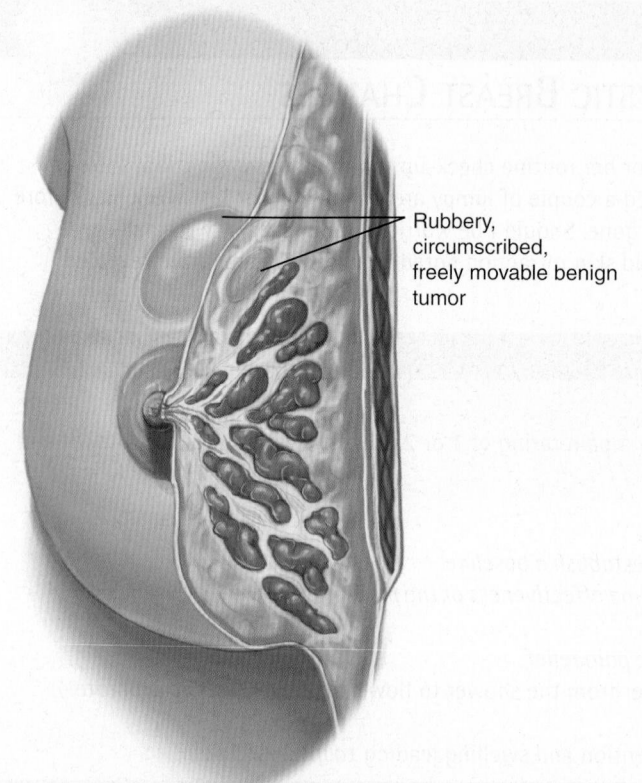

Rubbery, circumscribed, freely movable benign tumor

FIGURE 6.2 Fibroadenoma. (Source: The Anatomical Chart Company. [2002]. *Atlas of pathophysiology.* Springhouse, PA: Springhouse Corporation.)

than one fibroadenoma may be present (Fig. 6.2). Several other breast lesions have similar characteristics, so every woman with a breast mass should be evaluated to exclude cancer. A clinical breast examination (CBE) by a health care professional is critical. In addition, diagnostic studies include imaging studies (mammography, ultrasound, or both) and some form of biopsy, most often FNA, core needle biopsy, or stereotactic needle biopsy. The core needle biopsy removes a small cylinder of tissue from the breast mass, more than the FNA biopsy.

Nursing Management

The nurse should urge the client to return for re-evaluation in 6 months, perform monthly breast self-examinations, and return annually for a CBE.

Intraductal Papilloma

An **intraductal papilloma** is usually a solitary growth found in the mammary ducts, usually near the nipple (Miltenburg & Speights, 2008). This benign growth is thought to be caused by a proliferation and overgrowth of ductal epithelial tissue. An intraductal papilloma is generally less than 1 cm in diameter and might not be palpable. It produces a spontaneous serous, serosanguineous nipple discharge (Miltenburg & Speights,

2008). It mostly affects women between the ages of 40 and 60. A single duct or several ducts may be involved. Women with solitary papilloma without atypia carry a minimally higher risk than the general population for developing breast cancer. These women are not classified as high risk. However, the risk of subsequent breast cancer is increased by four- to fivefold in the presence of atypia (Sukumvanich & Borgen, 2010).

Therapeutic Management

Treatment consists of surgical removal of the papilloma and a part of the duct in which it is found, usually through an incision at the edge of the areola. Excision is usually curative, but some patients may have multiple papillomas that are difficult to remove (Miltenburg & Speights, 2008).

Nursing Assessment

The woman might report a feeling of fullness in the breast and may state that she can manually express a serous, serosanguineous, or watery discharge from the nipple. If the papilloma is large enough, it can be palpated in the nipple area as a soft, nontender, mobile, poorly delineated mass.

Laboratory and diagnostic testing is important to rule out cancer. The nipple discharge is evaluated for the presence of occult blood using a Hemoccult test; a blue colouration on the test card indicates the presence of blood. In addition, a sample of the discharge may be sent for cytologic evaluation to screen for cancer cells. Mammography, ultrasound, or ductography (radiographic dye instilled into a duct outlines the breast ductal system on radiographs) is used to diagnose or differentiate this lesion from a cancerous one. An intraductal papilloma appears as a smooth, lobulated filling defect (Lake, Zapton, Hoda, et al., 2008).

Nursing Management

The nurse should advise the woman to continue monthly breast self-examinations and yearly CBEs.

Duct Ectasia

Duct ectasia is a dilation and inflammation of the ducts behind the nipple. It is most common in perimenopausal women. This benign condition frequently occurs in women who have breastfed their children. The cause is unclear; however, chronic periductal inflammation, fibrosis, and ductal dilation are associated factors. This condition results in noncyclic breast pain, nipple retraction, and discharge (London, Ladewig, Ball, et al., 2011).

Therapeutic Management

This condition frequently improves without any specific treatment, or with warm compresses and antibiotics. If symptoms persist, the abnormal duct is removed through a local incision at the border of the areola. The tissue is sent to the pathology laboratory for evaluation.

Nursing Assessment

Assess the patient for clinical manifestations of duct ectasia. If the ducts have been chronically infected, an erythematous lesion will be present at the edge of the nipple area (American Cancer Society [ACS], 2011). The woman may complain of nipple discharge, which can be green, brown, straw-coloured, reddish, grey, or cream-coloured, with the consistency of toothpaste. In addition, the woman may report a dull nipple pain, subareolar swelling, or a burning sensation accompanied by pruritus around the nipple (Ballestas, Calvry, Cooper, et al., 2008).

Physical examination of the breasts might reveal subareolar redness and swelling, with mild to moderate tenderness on palpation. In addition, palpation will reveal the presence of swellings beneath the areola, along with nipple retraction and dimpling in some postmenopausal women (Ballestas et al., 2008). Diagnostic and laboratory testing includes mammography, ultrasound, and cytology and testing for occult blood on a nipple discharge sample, and ductography may be used to assist in the diagnosis of this lesion.

Nursing Management

The nurse should reassure the woman that this condition is benign and should reinforce the importance of monthly self-examinations as well as annual CBEs by the woman's health care provider. This benign breast condition is typically self-limiting; the only intervention needed is reassurance.

Mastitis

Mastitis is an infection of the connective tissue in the breast that occurs primarily in lactating or engorged women. Mastitis is divided into lactational or nonlactational. The usual causative organisms for lactational mastitis are *Staphylococcus aureus, Haemophilus influenzae,* and *Haemophilus* and *Streptococcus* species, the source of which is the baby's flora. One or more of the ducts drain poorly or become blocked, resulting in bacterial growth in the retained milk (Sukumvanich & Borgen, 2010).

Nonlactational mastitis can be caused by duct ectasia, which occurs when the milk ducts become congested with secretions and debris, resulting in periductal inflammation. These women present with greenish nipple discharge, nipple retraction, and noncyclic pain.

Therapeutic Management

Management of both types of mastitis involves the use of oral antibiotics. Penicillin, dicloxacillin, and cephalosporin are used for staphylococcal and streptococcal organisms (Miltenburg & Speights, 2008). Cephalexin or amoxicillin are used for gram-negative infections. Acetaminophen (Tylenol) is used for pain and fever.

Nursing Assessment

Assess the patient's health history for risk factors for mastitis, which include poor handwashing, ductal abnormalities, nipple cracks and fissures, lowered maternal defenses due to fatigue, tight clothing, poor support of pendulous breasts, failure to empty the breasts properly while breastfeeding, or missing breastfeeding.

Assess the patient for clinical manifestations of mastitis, which include flu-like symptoms of malaise, leukocytosis, fever, and chills. Physical examination of the breasts reveals increased warmth, redness, tenderness, and swelling. The nipple is usually cracked or abraded and the breast is distended with milk (Fig. 6.3). The diagnosis is made based on history and examination.

Nursing Management

Teach the woman about the etiology of mastitis and encourage her to continue to breastfeed, emphasizing that the prescribed medication is safe to take during lactation. Continued emptying of the breast or pumping improves the outcome, decreases the duration of symptoms, and decreases the incidence of breast abscess. Thus, continued breastfeeding is recommended in the presence of mastitis (Miltenburg & Speights, 2008). Instructions for the woman with mastitis are detailed in Teaching Guideline 6.2.

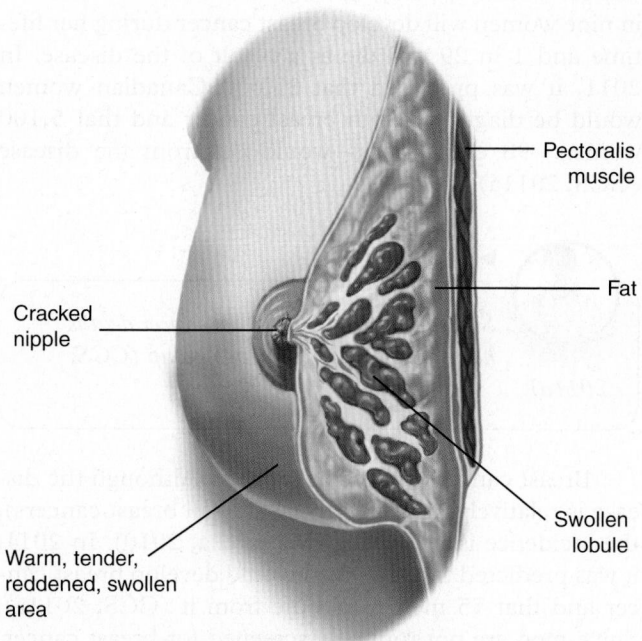

Fat

Pectoralis muscle

Cracked nipple

Swollen lobule

Warm, tender, reddened, swollen area

FIGURE **6.3** Mastitis. (Source: The Anatomical Chart Company. [2002]. *Atlas of pathophysiology.* Springhouse, PA: Springhouse Corporation.)

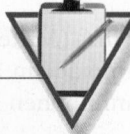

TEACHING GUIDELINE 6.2

Caring for Mastitis

- Take medications as prescribed.
- Continue breastfeeding, as tolerated.
- Wear a supportive bra 24 hours a day to support the breasts.
- Increase fluid intake.
- Make sure infant is positioned correctly on the nipple.
- Practice good handwashing techniques.
- Apply warm compresses to the affected breast or take a warm shower before breastfeeding.
- Frequently change positions while nursing.
- Get adequate rest and nutrition to support or improve the immune system.

Source: Miltenburg, D. M., & Speights, V. O. (2008). Benign breast disease. *Obstetrics and Gynecology Clinics of North America, 35,* 285–300; and Pillitteri, A. (2010). Maternal & child health nursing: Care of the childbearing & childrearing family (6th ed.). Philadelphia: Lippincott Williams & Wilkins.

Malignant Breast Disorders

Breast cancer is a neoplastic disease in which normal body cells are transformed through molecular changes at the cell level accompanied by uncontrolled growth (Swart, Downey, Gohel, et al., 2011). It is the most common cancer in women and the second leading cause of cancer deaths among Canadian women (Canadian Cancer Society [CCS], 2011a). It is estimated that one in nine women will develop breast cancer during her lifetime and 1 in 29 will die as a result of the disease. In 2011, it was predicted that 23,600 Canadian women would be diagnosed with breast cancer and that 5,100 women—98 every week—would die from the disease (CCS, 2011a).

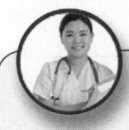

▶**Take** NOTE!

Since the mid-1990s, breast cancer deaths have decreased in every age group (CCS, 2011a).

Breast cancer can also affect men. Although the disease is relatively rare in men (<1% of all breast cancers), the incidence is increasing (Mattarella, 2010). In 2011, it was predicted that 190 men would develop breast cancer and that 55 men would die from it (CCS, 2011a). Since men are not routinely screened for breast cancer, the diagnosis is often delayed. The most common clinical manifestations of male breast cancer is a painless subareolar mass, nipple retraction, bleeding, and

discharge (Onami, Ozaki, Mortimer, et al., 2010). Any male with a suspicious breast mass should undergo diagnostic biopsy. If a malignancy is diagnosed, typical treatment is mastectomy with assessment of the axillary nodes.

The cause of breast cancer, while not well understood, is thought to be a complex interaction between environmental, genetic, and hormonal factors.

Pathophysiology

Cancer is not just one disease, but rather a group of diseases that result from unregulated cell growth. Without regulation, cells divide and grow uncontrollably until they eventually form a tumour. Extensive research has determined that all cancer is the result of changes in DNA or chromosome structure that cause the mutation of specific genes. Cancer development is thought to be clonal in nature, which means that each cell is derived from another cell. If one cell develops a mutation, any daughter cell derived from that cell will have that same mutation, and this process continues until a malignant tumour forms.

Breast cancer starts in the epithelial cells that line the mammary ducts within the breast. The growth rate depends on hormonal influences, mainly estrogen and progesterone. The two major categories of breast cancer are non-invasive and invasive. Non-invasive, or in situ, breast cancers are those that have not extended beyond their duct, lobule, or point of origin into the surrounding breast tissue. Conversely, invasive or infiltrating, breast cancers have extended into the surrounding breast tissue, with the potential to metastasize.

Carcinoma is a malignant tumour that occurs in epithelial tissue; it tends to infiltrate and give rise to metastases. The incidence of this cancer peaks in the seventh decade of life (between 75 and 79 years of age) (Public Health Agency of Canada [PHAC], 2009). Eighty percent of breast cancers occur after the age of 50 (PHAC, 2009). Breast cancer spreads rapidly to axillary and other lymph nodes, even while small. Infiltrating ductal carcinoma may take various histologic forms— well differentiated and slow growing, poorly differentiated and infiltrating, or highly malignant and undifferentiated with numerous metastases. This common type of breast cancer starts in the ducts, breaks through the duct wall, and invades the fatty breast tissue (Jardines, 2008).

Invasive lobular carcinoma, which originates in the terminal lobular units of breast ducts, accounts for 10% of invasive breast cancers (CCS, 2012). Invasive ductal carcinoma accounts for 65% to 89% of invasive cancers. Ductal carcinoma in situ (DCIS), also known as intraductal or non-invasive ductal carcinoma, is the most common type of non-invasive breast cancer, comprising 85% of in situ breast cancers (CCS, 2012). Cancer cells are confined in the breast duct lining. Around 20% of women with newly diagnosed breast cancer will have DCIS. In lobular carcinoma in situ (LCIS), abnormal cells are located in the breast lobules and have not spread outside the glands (CCS, 2012). LCIS makes up 1% to 4% of breast abnormalities and occurs more frequently in premenopausal women. Although LCIS is not breast cancer, women with this condition have a higher incidence of invasive breast cancer. It is worth noting that many women with LCIS do not develop invasive breast cancer. Breast screening and follow-up are important for women with LCIS. Symptoms of inflammatory breast cancer (IBC), which accounts for 1% to 4% of breast cancer cases, can appear suddenly and affect people differently. Symptoms can include breast tenderness or pain, breast swelling, itchiness, nipple discharge or changes, and swollen lymph nodes (CCS, 2012). Paget's disease (2% to 4% of all breast cancers) originates in the nipple and typically occurs in conjunction with invasive ductal carcinoma (Sukumvanich & Borgen, 2010).

Breast cancer is considered to be a highly variable disease. Breast cancer metastasizes widely and to almost all organs of the body, but primarily to the bone, lungs, lymph nodes, liver, and brain. The first sites of metastases are usually local or regional, involving the chest wall or axillary supraclavicular lymph nodes or bone (ACS, 2009).

Breast cancers are classified into three stages based on:

1. Tumour size
2. Extent of lymph node involvement
3. Evidence of metastasis

The purposes of tumour staging are to determine the probability that the tumour has metastasized, to decide on an appropriate course of therapy, and to assess the client's prognosis. Table 6.2 gives details and characteristics of each stage. The overall 10-year survival rate for a woman with stage I breast cancer is 80% to 90%; for a woman with stage II, it is about 50%. The outlook is not as good for women with stage III or stage IV disease (Alexander et al., 2010).

There is no completely accurate way to know whether the cancer has micrometastasized to distant organs, but certain tests can help determine if the cancer has spread. A bone scan can be performed to assess the bones. Magnetic resonance imaging (MRI) can be used to detect metastases to the liver, abdominal cavity, lungs, or brain.

Risk Factors

An estimated 80% of women in whom breast cancer develops have no documented risk factors (Sukumvanich & Borgen, 2010). Breast cancer is thought to develop in response to a number of factors: aging, delayed childbearing or never bearing children, high breast density, family history of cancer, late menopause, and genetic factors (Brower, 2010; CCS, 2011b). Other factors might contribute to breast cancer but have not been scientifically proven. Because rates of breast cancer increase with age, estimates of risk at specific ages are more meaningful than estimates of lifetime risk (Table 6.3).

Being a woman and aging (especially over 50 years) may be the only risk factors for developing breast cancer (CCS, 2011b, 2012). Other risk factors include:

- Previous breast cancer
- Genetic mutations (BRCA-1 and BRCA-2 genes) and family history of breast cancer in a close relative
- Family history of ovarian cancer
- High estrogen levels due to:
  - Dense breast tissue shown by mammogram
  - No pregnancy or first delivery after 30 years of age

TABLE 6.2 **STAGING OF BREAST CANCER**

Stage	Characteristics
0	In situ, early type of breast cancer; ductal carcinoma in situ and lobular carcinoma in situ
I	Localized tumour ≤2 cm in diameter; cancer has not spread beyond the breast
II	Tumour 2–5 cm in diameter, spread to axillary lymph nodes, or both
III	Tumour spread to lymph nodes and nearby tissues (muscles or skin)
IV	Cancer has metastasized to distant parts of body

Source: Canadian Cancer Society. (2012). *Canadian cancer encyclopedia: Breast cancer.* Retrieved January 24, 2012 from info.cancer.ca/cce-ecc/default.aspx?Lang=E&toc=10.

TABLE 6.3 **PROBABILITY OF DEVELOPING BREAST CANCER IN THE NEXT 5 YEARS AT SPECIFIC AGES**

Age (years)	Risk (per 1,000)
30	1.5
35	2.6
40	4.8
45	7.8
50	9.2
55	10.6
60	12.9
65	14.3
70	15.4

Source: Public Health Agency of Canada (PHAC). (2003). *Breast cancer in Canada: Probability of developing breast cancer in the next 5 years.* Retrieved January 24, 2012 from www.phac-aspc.gc.ca/publicat/updates/breast-99-eng.php.

- Early age at menarche
- Menopause later than average
- History of taking hormone replacement therapy (estrogen plus progestin)
- History of one or more breast biopsies indicating abnormal cell changes (atypical hyperplasia)
- Medical radiation to chest area, especially before age 30

The risk of breast cancer can be increased if the woman:

- Drinks alcohol
- Takes oral contraceptives
- Smokes or is exposed to secondhand smoke
- Is obese
- Has a sedentary lifestyle and lacks physical exercise
- Has a high socioeconomic status

The presence of risk factors, especially several of them, calls for careful ongoing monitoring and evaluation to promote early detection. Even though risk factors are important considerations, many women with newly diagnosed breast cancer have no known risk factors. While routine mammography and self-examination are prudent for everyone, these precautions may become lifesavers for at-risk individuals. Mammography screening every 2 years is recommended in Canada for women from 50 to 69 years of age (CCS, 2012). Women ages 40 and 49 should discuss the risk of breast cancer and the risk and benefits of mammography with their doctor. CBE should be performed at least every 2 years by a trained health care professional. While Canadian Cancer Society (CCS) does not advocate any particular routine for breast self-examination, it does advise that women become familiar with their breast tissue with examination of the nipple, tissue up to the collar bone, and under the armpit (CCS, 2012).

Diagnosis

Many studies can be performed to make an accurate diagnosis of a malignant breast lump. Diagnostic tests may include:

- Imaging tests:
  - Mammography
  - Breast ultrasonography
  - Scintimammography
  - Ductography
  - Breast MRI
- Biopsy:
  - FNA biopsy
  - Core needle biopsy
  - Stereotactic core needle biopsy
  - Surgical biopsy
  - Wire localization biopsy
- Laboratory tests:
  - Hormone receptor status
  - Blood tests

- Human epidermal growth factor receptor–2 (HER2) status (CCS, 2010a, 2012)

Mammography

Mammography involves taking low-dose X-ray pictures of the bare breasts while they are compressed between two plastic plates. This procedure is performed to identify and characterize a breast mass and to detect an early malignancy. A screening mammogram typically consists of four views, two per breast (Fig. 6.4). A diagnostic mammogram is performed when the woman has suspicious clinical findings on a breast examination or an abnormality has been found on a screening mammogram. A diagnostic mammogram uses additional views of the affected breast as well as magnification views. Diagnostic mammography provides the radiologist with additional detail to render a more specific diagnosis. A digital mammography machine records electronic images that can be stored on a computer instead of X-ray film. These images can then be enlarged for detailed examination and can be transmitted electronically (CCS, 2012).

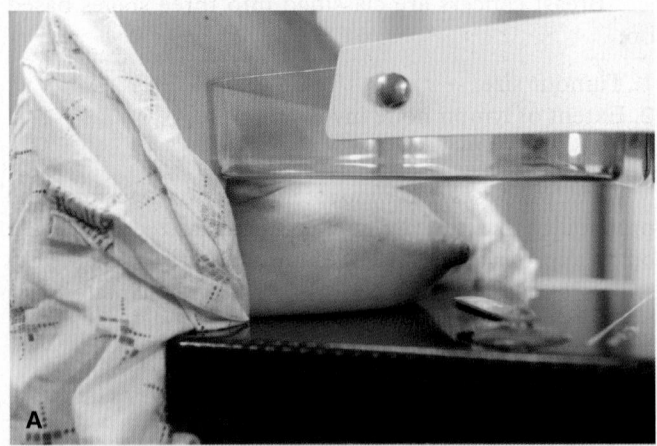

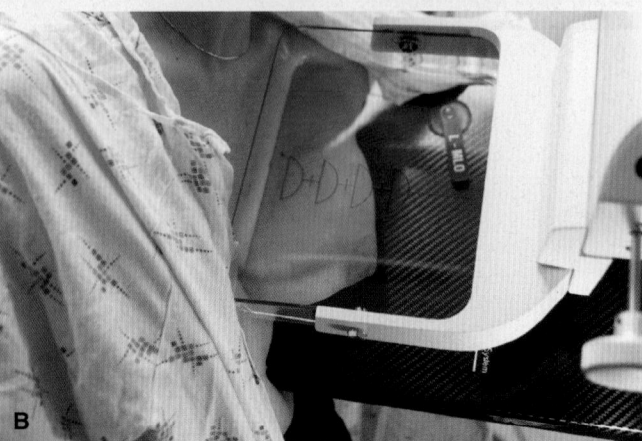

FIGURE 6.4 Mammography. (**A**) A top-to-bottom view of the breast. (**B**) A side view of the breast.

Preparing for a Screening Mammogram

- Schedule the procedure just after menses, when breasts are less tender.
- Avoid caffeinated beverages and food for 5 to 7 days before the procedure.
- Don't use deodorant, powder, antiperspirants, or body lotion on the breasts or under the arms on the day of the procedure because they can appear on the X-ray film as calcium spots.
- Acetaminophen (Tylenol) or aspirin can relieve any discomfort after the procedure.
- Remove all jewellery from around your neck and elsewhere because the metal can cause distortions on the film image.
- Wear clothing that is readily removed above the waist.
- Select a facility listed on the Canadian Association of Radiologists website, or see the CCS website for phone numbers of breast screening centres in each province.

Most women find the 10-minute mammography procedure uncomfortable but not painful. Teaching Guideline 6.3 offers tips for a patient to follow before she undergoes this procedure.

Breast Ultrasound

Ultrasonography uses high-frequency sound waves to make images of the breast structure (CCS, 2012). Ultrasonography can be used to examine a breast lump found during a mammogram, assess whether the lump is a fluid-filled cyst or a solid tumour, and locate an area for biopsy. Gel is placed on the breast and a handheld transducer is used to move across the breast.

Scintimammography (Scintigraphy)

Scintimammography, a second-line diagnostic tool, may be used after mammograms for further breast assessment and is also used to assess axillary lymph nodes (CCS, 2012). Scintimammography involves the use of radioactive isotopes and a specialized camera to take images of breast tissue. This test is done to assess breast lumps that need further examination because of scar tissue, dense breast tissue, and breast implants and when multiple tumours are present. Radiation exposure is considered to be low. Since cancerous cells are more active, they attract more radioactive substances than do benign cells. A radioactive substance such as technetium-99m (Tc-99m) sestamibi is injected via a vein in the arm. Images of the breast are then obtained at different angles and positions (e.g., with the woman lying face up, sitting

with her hands over her head, or lying face down on the imaging table with openings so that the breast can hang down). Scintimammography is not advised for around 2 weeks after FNA or approximately 6 weeks after core needle or excisional biopsy. Detection of small tumours (<1 cm) may be difficult.

Ductography

Ductography, also known as galactography (CCS, 2012), is used in conjunction with mammography to diagnose breast cancer. This X-ray procedure is used to examine breast ducts to determine the cause of nipple discharge. Ductography diagnoses benign intraductal papillomas that are associated with nipple discharge. A thin plastic tube is put into the duct opening on the nipple followed by an injection of contrast medium, which outlines the duct shape when an X-ray is taken. The test takes approximately 20 to 60 minutes and may be uncomfortable.

Breast Magnetic Resonance Imaging

In breast MRI, magnetic forces and radio-frequency waves make cross-sectional breast images (CCS, 2012). A computer changes the images into three-dimensional pictures. MRI is not routinely used as a diagnostic tool but provides a better examination of abnormalities found in mammograms and during clinical exams. It can also differentiate between a benign or malignant abnormality in high-risk women. The test can be used to examine the other breast in newly diagnosed women and assess the condition of breast implants to determine whether a rupture has occurred. The woman lays face down with the breasts hanging into openings with breast coils and the table is moved into an MRI machine. Radio waves are sent and received by the coils to create images. Breast MRI equipment is not available at all hospitals or imaging centres.

Fine-Needle Aspiration

FNA is a biopsy method that uses thin needles to obtain fluid or cells from a lump to assess for malignancy (CCS, 2012). The procedure can be done in a physician's office with or without anesthetic. Ultrasound is used to locate the lump, and then fluid and/or cells from the lump are drawn into a syringe. A cyst will disappear or shrink after the fluid is withdrawn. Although the fluid is usually clear, a green- or yellow-coloured fluid may indicate an infection. Bloody or cloudy fluid may indicate a benign cyst or cancer. Because cysts can redevelop in the same area or other areas of the breast, FNA may need to be repeated. FNA cannot differentiate between early in situ cancer and invasive cancer. A false-negative result may occur if cells were aspirated from an area close to the tumour.

Core Needle Biopsy

The needle used for a core biopsy is thicker than that used for FNA, thus enabling a larger sample (core) of breast tissue for examination (CCS, 2012). The test is performed on solid lumps that are palpable or close to the skin surface. It can be used to differentiate between in situ and invasive cancer. Ultrasound or X-ray imaging can be used to guide the procedure. The results of the core needle biopsy can provide sufficient information about the presence of cancer cells and whether a lumpectomy or mastectomy will be required. If the tissue obtained from a core needle biopsy contains cancer cells but is not sufficient, surgical biopsy may be needed. Core needle biopsies are avoided if vital structures or nerves may be damaged by the procedure. A negative result may be present when, in rare situations, the tumour is missed by the needle.

Stereotactic Core Needle Biopsy

This diagnostic test is also called stereotactic needle biopsy or X-ray guided breast biopsy (CCS, 2012). Mammograms taken at different angles (stereotactic) are used in conjunction with a computer to locate the breast abnormality, and a biopsy needle is placed into it. This type of biopsy is used for non-palpable lumps seen on mammography, to obtain more tissue than can be obtained with FNA, to obtain samples from a new lump in a previous surgery site, or to assess whether a lump is benign without performing surgical biopsy. The woman lays face-down on a special table with openings for the breasts. Breast tissue is compressed and held between two mammography plates. An anesthetic is used before an incision is made into the skin to obtain several tissue samples. Ice and pressure are applied after the biopsy and a bandage is applied to the biopsy site. Slight bleeding, breast tenderness, and bruising may be present after the procedure.

Surgical Biopsy

Parts of a lump or suspicious breast tissue may be removed by excisional or incisional biopsy to detect cancerous tissue (CCS, 2012). Surgical or open biopsy is used by the pathologist to determine the type of cancer cells, tumour grade, hormone receptor status, and HER2 status. The information is used to make treatment decisions.

Surgical biopsy can be done in a physician's office or out-patient clinic. A local anesthetic is used to numb the skin prior to making the incision. In excisional biopsy, both suspicious tissue and normal tissue surrounding it are removed. In very early breast cancer, this type of biopsy may be sufficient to obtain a specimen. In an incisional biopsy, a small part of the abnormal area is removed when it is not possible to remove the entire lump and diagnosis is needed for treatment. Incisional biopsy is not used frequently; wire localization or core needle biopsy is performed instead.

Wire Localization Biopsy

Wire localization biopsy is also called wire localization, fine-wire localization, or needle localization (CCS, 2011b). This type of biopsy is used to locate the exact position of the abnormal tissue before it is removed. It can be used to remove a non-palpable lump, to remove tissue samples in areas where there is more than one abnormality, and to avoid unnecessary breast deformity by removing minimal amounts of normal tissue.

Mammography is used to locate the abnormal tissue, and local anesthetic is used to numb the area (CCS, 2012). A hollow needle is inserted by the radiologist followed by a thin wire with a hook. Once the wire is in place, the needle is removed. Tape is then applied to maintain placement of the wire, and the patient is taken to the operating room where the abnormal tissue is removed.

Sentinel Lymph Node Biopsy

The status of the axillary lymph nodes is an important prognostic indicator in early-stage breast cancer. With a sentinel lymph node biopsy, the clinician can determine whether breast cancer has spread to the axillary lymph nodes without having to perform a traditional axillary lymph node dissection. Experience has shown that the lymph ducts of the breast typically drain to one lymph node first before draining through the rest of the lymph nodes under the arm. The first lymph node is called the sentinel lymph node.

This procedure can be performed under local anesthesia. A radioactive blue dye is injected 1 to 6 hours before the biopsy to identify the afferent sentinel lymph node. The surgeon usually removes one to three nodes and sends them to the pathologist to determine whether cancer cells are present. Sentinel lymph node biopsy is usually performed before a lumpectomy to make sure the cancer has not spread. Removing only the sentinel lymph node can allow women with breast cancer to avoid many of the potential side effects (e.g., lymphedema) (CCS, 2012).

Hormone Receptor Status

Estrogen and progesterone stimulate the growth of some breast cancers (CCS, 2012). Normal breast epithelium has hormone receptors and responds specifically to the stimulatory effects of estrogen and progesterone. The pathologist reports on the amount of estrogen receptor (ER) or progesterone receptor (PR) in the cells (CCS, 2012). The tumour can be ER positive (ER+) or ER negative (ER−). About two thirds of women diagnosed with breast cancer have ER+ cancer, which is more common in postmenopausal than premenopausal women.

Hormone receptor status testing is done to predict how well the cancer will respond to hormone therapy (CCS, 2012). ER+ tumours respond better to hormonal therapy, although PR+ tumours can also be treated with hormonal therapy. A tumour that is both ER+ and PR+ has a better response to endocrine treatment. Hormonal treatment can be used to treat cancer that is sensitive to hormonal manipulation and is used for different stages of breast cancer (CCS, 2012).

HER2 Status

ERBB2, a cancer oncogene more commonly known as HER2 (HER2/Neu), controls HER2 levels (CCS, 2012). This test examines genes (ERBB2) that can help tumours grow. Although healthy breast cells have two copies of the HER2 gene, sometimes too many copies are present, leading to an overabundance of HER2 protein production. Testing can be done on tumour tissues taken by biopsy.

A breast tumour can overexpress HER2 (HER2 positive) or not overexpress HER2 (HER2 negative) (CCS, 2012). HER2-positive breast cancer (15% to 20% of breast cancers) is associated with rapid tumour growth and often has lower estrogen and progesterone receptor levels, making hormone therapy less beneficial. Women with BRCA1 mutations often underexpress HER2.

Therapeutic Management

Women diagnosed with breast cancer have many treatments available to them. The main cancer treatments are surgery, radiation therapy, and chemotherapy (CCS, 2011c). Generally, treatments fall into two categories: local and systemic. Local treatments are surgery and radiation therapy. Effective systemic treatments include chemotherapy, hormonal therapy, and biological therapy (CCS, 2011c).

Treatment plans are based on multiple factors, primarily the type of breast cancer, stage, grade, hormone receptor status (estrogen and progesterone receptors), HER2 status, age, menopausal status, personal health, and personal preferences (CCS, 2012). A combination of surgical treatment and adjunctive therapy is often recommended.

Another consideration in making decisions about a treatment plan is genetic testing for BRCA-1 and BRCA-2. This genetic testing, which became available in 1995, can pinpoint women who have a significantly increased risk for breast and ovarian cancer. Of women with the breast-ovarian cancer syndrome, about 45% have a BRCA-1 gene mutation and 35% have a BRCA-2 mutation (Schorge, Halvorson, Hoffman, et al., 2008).

Testing positive for a BRCA-1 or BRCA-2 mutation can significantly alter health care decisions. Other family members may want to undergo genetic testing. If there is a BRCA gene mutation, early detection is important as well as lifestyle changes to reduce the risk of cancer (CCS, 2012).

Severe psychological distress can occur as a result of genetic testing. Also, many women perceive their breasts as intrinsic to their femininity, self-esteem, and sexuality, and the risk of losing a breast can provoke extreme anxiety (Alexander et al., 2010). Nurses need to address the physical, emotional, and spiritual needs of the women they care for, as well as their families, since this mutation is inherited in an autosomal dominant fashion. Although 20% to 30% of women with breast cancer have a relative

with a breast cancer history, a hereditary predisposition can be identified in only 5% to 10% of breast cancer patients (Swart et al., 2011).

Surgical Options

Generally, the first treatment option for the woman diagnosed with breast cancer is surgery. Neoadjuvant therapy in the form of chemotherapy or radiation is given to shrink a tumour before surgery (CCS, 2012). The surgical options depend on the size and location of the cancer, breast size, extent of the cancer in the same breast, the woman's health, personal preferences, and prior treatment (CCS, 2012). The choices are typically either breast-conserving surgery (lumpectomy with radiation) or mastectomy with or without reconstruction. The overall survival rate with lumpectomy and radiation is about the same as that with modified radical mastectomy (Swart et al., 2011). However, breast-conserving surgery or breast-sparing surgery may not be an option for some women, including those:

- Who have two or more cancer sites that cannot be removed through a single incision
- Whose surgery will not result in a clean margin of tissue
- Who have active connective tissue conditions (lupus or scleroderma) that make body tissues especially sensitive to the side effects of radiation
- Who have had previous radiation to the affected breast
- Whose tumours are larger than 5 cm (2 inches) (National Comprehensive Cancer Network, 2011)
- Who prefer not to undergo daily radiation and do not want to deal with the possible side effects (CCS, 2012)

These decisions are made jointly between the woman and her surgeon. If mastectomy is chosen, either by tumour characteristics or patient preference, then discussion needs to include breast reconstruction and regional lymph node biopsy versus sentinel lymph node biopsy. The mastectomy techniques are a simple mastectomy with sentinel node biopsy or a radical mastectomy with regional node biopsy. Removal of numerous lymph nodes places the patient at high risk for lymphedema.

Breast-Conserving Surgery

Breast-conserving surgery, the least invasive procedure, is the wide local excision (or lumpectomy) of the tumour along with a 1 cm margin of normal tissue. A lumpectomy is often used for early-stage localized tumours. The goal of breast-conserving surgery is to remove the suspicious mass along with tissue free of malignant cells to prevent recurrence. The results are less drastic and emotionally less scarring to the woman. Women undergoing breast-conserving therapy receive radiation after lumpectomy with the goal of eradicating residual microscopic cancer cells to limit locoregional recurrence. In women who do not require adjuvant chemotherapy, radiation therapy typically begins 2 to 4 weeks after surgery to allow healing of the lumpectomy incision site. Radiation is administered to the entire breast at daily doses over a period of several weeks (Swart et al., 2011).

Lymph nodes draining the breast are located primarily in the axilla, and it is recommended that axillary lymph nodes are removed to assess whether they contain cancer (CCS, 2012). Theoretically, if breast cancer is to metastasize to other parts of the body, it will probably do so via the lymphatic system. If malignant cells are found in the nodes, more aggressive systemic treatment may be needed.

Mastectomy

Simple mastectomy or total mastectomy is the removal of all breast tissue, the nipple, areola, and pectoral fascia or chest muscle lining (CCS, 2012). The axillary nodes and pectoral muscles are spared. This procedure is generally used for women with very early non-invasive tumours that have not metastasized to adjacent structures or the lymph nodes and for women who are at high risk for developing breast cancer and wish to reduce their risk (prophylactic mastectomy).

Modified radical mastectomy is another surgical option; survival rates are comparable to those of radical mastectomy, but it is more conducive to breast reconstruction and results in greater mobility and less lymphedema (Alexander et al., 2010). This procedure involves removal of breast tissue, nipple, the axillary nodes, and some chest muscles, but not the pectoralis major, thus avoiding a concave anterior chest (Swart et al., 2011). This type of surgery is seldom performed (CCS, 2009).

In conjunction with mastectomy, lymph node surgery (removal of underarm nodes) may be needed to reduce the risk of distant metastasis and improve a woman's chance of long-term survival. For women with a positive sentinel node biopsy, 10 to 20 underarm lymph nodes may need to be removed. Complications associated with axillary lymph node surgery include nerve damage during surgery, causing temporary numbness down the upper aspect of the arm; seroma formation followed by wound infection; restrictions in arm mobility (some women need physiotherapy); and lymphedema. In many women lymphedema can be avoided by:

- Avoiding the use of affected arm for drawing blood, inserting intravenous lines, or measuring blood pressure (can cause trauma and possible infection)
- Seeking medical care immediately if the affected arm swells
- Wearing gloves when engaging in activities such as gardening that might cause injury
- Wearing a well-fitted compression sleeve to promote drainage return

Women having mastectomies must decide whether to have further surgery to reconstruct the breast. If the woman decides to have reconstructive surgery, it ideally is performed immediately after the mastectomy. The woman must also determine whether she wants the surgeon to use saline implants or natural tissue from her abdomen (transverse rectus abdominis myocutaneous [TRAM] flap method) or back (latissimus dorsi [LAT] flap method).

In the TRAM flap method, the rectus abdominis muscle is transferred from the abdomen via a tunnel under the skin and brought out through a new excision in the breast area. The blood supply is maintained. This tissue is used to reconstruct the breast that has been removed. In the LAT flap method, tissue from the latissimus dorsi muscle in the upper back is tunnelled subcutaneously up to the chest area.

If reconstructive surgery is desired, the ultimate decision regarding the method will be determined by the woman's anatomy (e.g., is there sufficient fat and muscle to permit natural reconstruction) and her overall health status. Both procedures require a prolonged recovery period.

Some women opt for no reconstruction, and many of them choose to wear breast prostheses. Some prostheses are worn in the bra cup and others fit against the skin or into special pockets made into clothing.

Whether to have reconstructive surgery is an individual and very complex decision. Each woman must be presented with all of the options and then allowed to decide. The nurse can play an important role here by presenting the facts to the woman so that she can make an intelligent decision to meet her unique situation.

Adjuvant Therapy

Adjuvant therapy is supportive or additional therapy that is recommended after surgery. This therapy is provided to destroy cancer cells that may have been left behind or transported to other parts of the body (CCS, 2012). Adjunctive therapies include local therapy such as radiation therapy and systemic therapies using chemotherapy, hormonal therapy, and drug therapy. Adjuvant therapy most often begins within 4 to 12 weeks after surgery.

Radiation Therapy

Radiation therapy uses high-energy rays to destroy cancer cells that might have been left behind in the breast, chest wall, or underarm area after the tumour has been removed surgically. Usually serial radiation doses are given 5 days a week to the tumour site for 4 to 6 weeks postoperatively. Each treatment takes only a few minutes, but the dose is cumulative. Women undergoing breast-conserving therapy receive radiation to the entire breast after lumpectomy with the goal of eradicating residual microscopic cancer cells to reduce the chance of recurrence (Swart et al., 2011).

Side effects of traditional radiation therapy include inflammation, local edema, anorexia, swelling, and heaviness in the breast; sunburn-like skin changes in the treated area; and fatigue. This type of therapy can be given several ways: external beam radiation, which delivers a carefully focused dose of radiation from a machine outside the body, or internal radiation, in which tiny pellets that contain radioactive material are placed into the tumour.

Several advances in the field of radiation oncology for the treatment of women with early-stage breast cancer have assisted in reducing the side effects. The treatment position for external radiation has changed from supine to prone, with the arm on the affected side raised above the head, so that the treated breast hangs dependently through the opening of the treatment board.

High-dose brachytherapy is another advance that offers an alternative to traditional radiation treatment. A balloon catheter is used to insert radioactive seeds into the breast after the tumour is removed surgically. The seeds deliver a concentrated dose of radiation directly to the operative site; this is important because most cancer recurrences in the breast (67% to 100%) occur at or near the lumpectomy site. This technique allows a high dose of radiation to be delivered to a small target volume with a minimal dose to the surrounding normal tissue. The procedure takes 4 to 5 days as opposed to the 4 to 6 weeks required for traditional radiation therapy; it also eliminates the need to delay radiation therapy to allow for wound healing. Brachytherapy is occasionally used after breast cancer surgery and is now being examined in clinical trials (CCS, 2012). Side effects include redness or discharge around catheters, fever, and infection. Daily cleansing of the catheter insertion site with a mild soap and application of an antibiotic ointment will minimize the risk for infection.

Chemotherapy

Chemotherapy refers to the use of drugs that are toxic to all cells and interfere with a cell's ability to reproduce. They are particularly effective against malignant cells but affect all rapidly dividing cells, especially those of the skin, the hair follicles, the mouth, the gastrointestinal tract, and the bone marrow. Breast cancer is a systemic disease in which micrometastases are already present in other organs by the time the breast cancer is diagnosed.

Chemotherapy may be indicated (CCS, 2012):

• Prior to surgery to shrink a large tumour
• After surgery to destroy cancer cells left behind or decrease the risk of recurrence
• As an element of combined treatment for locally advanced breast cancer
• For recurring cancer or cancer that has spread after treatment
• To alleviate pain or control metastatic breast cancer symptoms

A combination of chemotherapy drugs is used to treat breast cancer, although sometimes a single drug is used for treatment (e.g., in such recurrent cancer) (CCS, 2012).

Side effects of chemotherapy depend on the type of drug used, the dosage, the dosage schedule, the route, and the client's physical and emotional status (CCS, 2012). Short-term side effects occur during, immediately after, or weeks after treatment and are usually temporary. These include digestive problems (nausea and vomiting, appetite loss), bone marrow suppression (infection, bleeding, and bruising), hair loss, fatigue, skin changes (dryness, rashes, colour changes), changes to fingernails and toenails (lines, cracking, brittleness), bowel problems (diarrhea, constipation), pain, muscle or join pain, weight change (loss or gain), changes to reproductive organ function, organ damage, and allergic reactions. Most people do not experience long-term side effects. However, some people may experience ongoing fatigue, changes in the function of the reproductive organs (fertility or treatment-induced menopause), organ damage (heart, nervous system), and second cancers.

Endocrine or Hormonal Therapy

Hormone levels in the body are altered by endocrine or hormonal therapy, a systemic therapy that affects cancer cells (CCS, 2012). The objective of **endocrine therapy** is to block or counter the effect of estrogen, which plays a central role in the pathogenesis of cancer. In about two thirds of breast cancer cases, estrogen promotes cancer growth as a result of estrogen and/or progesterone receptors (CCS, 2012). Estrogen receptors appear to be the more important receptor. Hormonal therapy treats hormone receptor-positive breast cancers by reducing estrogen production and blocking receptors from binding estrogen. Several different drug classes are used to interfere with or block estrogen receptors. They include selective estrogen receptor modulators (anti-estrogens, SERMs), aromatase inhibitors (used in postmenopausal women to stop tissues from making estrogen), ovarian ablation (ovarian suppression in premenopausal women to stop production of estrogen in the ovaries), progestins, and androgens (CCS, 2012). Treatment depends on whether the woman is premenopausal or postmenopausal, the stage of cancer, other health problems (e.g., osteoporosis or risk of blood clot formation), and the types of hormonal therapies used in the past. Tamoxifen (Nolvadex, Tamofen) is the most commonly used anti-estrogen drug. It is used to prevent breast cancer in women at high risk and in premenopausal or postmenopausal women. It is taken orally on a daily basis.

Fulvestrant (Faslodex) is a newer drug used to reduce estrogen receptors (CCS, 2012). It is used in postmenopausal women with locally advanced or metastatic cancer after hormonal therapy has been used. It can be effective even when tamoxifen does not affect the cancer. Fulvestrant is administered monthly as an intramuscular injection.

Aromatase inhibitors reduce or inhibit estrogen production by blocking aromatase (CCS, 2012). These drugs are not effective in premenopausal women because they do not affect the ovaries. Common aromatase inhibitors taken in pill form include letrozole (Femara), anastrozole (Arimidex), and exemestane (Aromasin). Aromatase inhibitors are taken in early or advanced stages of breast cancer in postmenopausal women. In early-stage breast cancer, aromatase inhibitors may be used after tamoxifen has been taken for 5 years. Women can switch to using aromatase inhibitors after tamoxifen has been taken for 2 to 3 years or if tamoxifen usage results in side effects. In advanced or recurring cancer, aromatase inhibitors can be used instead of tamoxifen. It can be used until there is evidence of cancer progression. Women with hormone-sensitive cancers can live for long periods without any intervention other than hormonal manipulation, but quality-of-life issues need to be addressed in the balance between treatment and side effects.

Ovarian ablation consists of treatments that stop estrogen production by the ovaries (CCS, 2012). Ovarian ablation is performed by surgically removing the ovaries (oophorectomy) to stop estrogen production and may be preferred by women who do not want children. Luteinizing hormone (LH)–releasing hormone (LHRH) antagonists target the pituitary gland and stop the ovaries temporarily from producing estrogen. On occasion, the effect on estrogen production may be permanent. LHRH agonists stimulate the pituitary gland to increase LH production. The pituitary gland eventually stops responding to the stimulus and signals the ovaries to halt estrogen production. Radiation is an uncommon treatment used to destroy ovarian production of estrogen; estrogen levels decrease 3 months after treatment.

Progestins, which are progesterone-like hormonal medications, counteract estrogen effects, stop estrogen production, and compete for receptor sites on breast cancer cells (CCS, 2012). Megestrol (Megace) is a common pill form of progestin drug. Although progestins are infrequently used, women with metastatic breast cancer that is nonresponsive to other hormonal treatments or resistant to tamoxifen can be treated with these drugs.

Androgens, or male hormones, are used to block the pituitary from producing estrogens (CCS, 2012). Although rarely used, androgens are used to treat recurrent cancer or after other hormonal therapies in women with metastatic breast cancer.

Biological or Immunotherapy

Biological or immunotherapy, used as an adjunct to surgery, represents an attempt to stimulate the body's natural defenses to recognize and attack cancer cells or to decrease the side effects of the treatment (CCS, 2012).

Trastuzumab (Herceptin), bevacizumab (Avastin), and colony-stimulating factors (CSFs) are used in breast cancer treatment (CCS, 2012). Some tumours produce excessive amounts of HER2 protein, which regulates cancer cell growth. Trastuzumab is a monoclonal antibody that is designed to block HER2. It interferes with breast cancer cell division and growth and stimulates the immune system to destroy cancer cells. It can be used alone or in combination with other chemotherapy agents to treat clients with metastatic breast disease. Adverse effects of trastuzumab include cardiac toxicity, fever, chills, nausea, vomiting, and allergic reactions.

Bevacizumab targets the vascular endothelial growth factor (VEGF), a protein that builds the blood supply for tumour growth (CCS, 2012). Bevacizumab attaches to VEGF and inhibits the blood supply to a tumour. The delivery of chemotherapy drugs to the tumour is enhanced by bevacizumab. This drug is used for HER2-negative metastatic breast cancer. Because it interferes with healing, bevacizumab is not used for 28 days after surgery.

CSFs lessen the side effects of chemotherapy drugs, especially higher doses (CCS, 2012). CSFs stimulate bone marrow to increase white blood cell production (granulocyte growth factors) and red blood cell production (erythrocyte growth factors).

Nursing Process for the Patient with Breast Cancer

When a woman is diagnosed with breast cancer, she faces treatment that may alter her body shape, may make her feel unwell, and may not carry a certainty of cure. Nurses can support women from the time of diagnosis, through the treatments, and through follow-up after the surgical and adjunctive treatments have been completed. Allowing patients time to ask questions and to discuss any necessary preparations for treatment is critical. As our understanding of breast disorders keeps improving, treatments continue to change. Although the goal of treatment remains improved survival, increasing emphasis is focused on prevention. Nurses can have an impact on early detection of breast disorders, treatment, and symptom management. A nurse who is involved in the woman's treatment plan from the beginning can effectively offer support throughout the whole experience.

Teamwork is important in breast screening and caring for women with breast disorders. Treatment is often fragmented between the hospital and community treatment centres, which can be emotionally traumatic for the woman and her family. The advances being made in the diagnosis and treatment of breast disorders mean that guidelines are constantly changing, requiring all health care professionals to keep up to date. Informed nurses can provide support and information and, most importantly, continuity of care for the woman undergoing treatment for a breast problem.

The nurse plays a particularly important role in providing psychological support and self-care teaching to patients with breast cancer. Nurses can influence both physical and emotional recovery, which are both important aspects of care that help in improving the woman's quality of life and the ability to survive. The nurse's role should extend beyond helping clients; spreading the word in the community about screening and prevention is a big part in the ongoing fight against cancer. The community should see nurses as both educators and valued sources of credible information. This role will help improve clinical outcomes while achieving high levels of client satisfaction.

Remember Nancy from the chapter opener? Is her response typical of many women upon discovering a lump in their breast? Nancy confides her discovery of the lump and her worries to you. What advice would you give her?

Assessment

Early breast cancer has no symptoms. The earliest sign of breast cancer is often an abnormality seen on a screening mammogram before the woman or the health care professional feels it. In the woman presenting with a breast disorder, take a thorough history of the problem and explore the woman's risk factors for breast cancer. Assess the woman for clinical manifestations of breast cancer, such as changes in breast appearance and contour, which become apparent with advancing breast cancer (CCS, 2010b). These changes include:

- Changes in breast shape or size
- A lump or thickening in one breast (a common first sign)
- Persistent nipple or breast irritation
- A lump or swelling in the axilla
- Changes in skin colour or texture
- Nipple retraction, tenderness, or discharge (Fig. 6.5)

Complete a breast examination to validate the clinical manifestations and findings of the health history and risk factor assessment. The CBE involves both inspection and palpation (Nursing Procedure 6.1). Helpful characteristics in evaluating palpable breast masses are described in Box 6.1. If a lump can be palpated, the cancer has been there for quite some time.

Be cognizant of the impact that breast cancer has on a woman's emotional state, coping ability, and quality of life. Women may experience sadness, anger, fear, and guilt as a result of breast cancer. However, despite potential negative outcomes, many women have a positive outlook for their futures and adapt to treatment modalities with a good quality of life. Closely monitor clients for their psychosocial adjustment to diagnosis and treat-

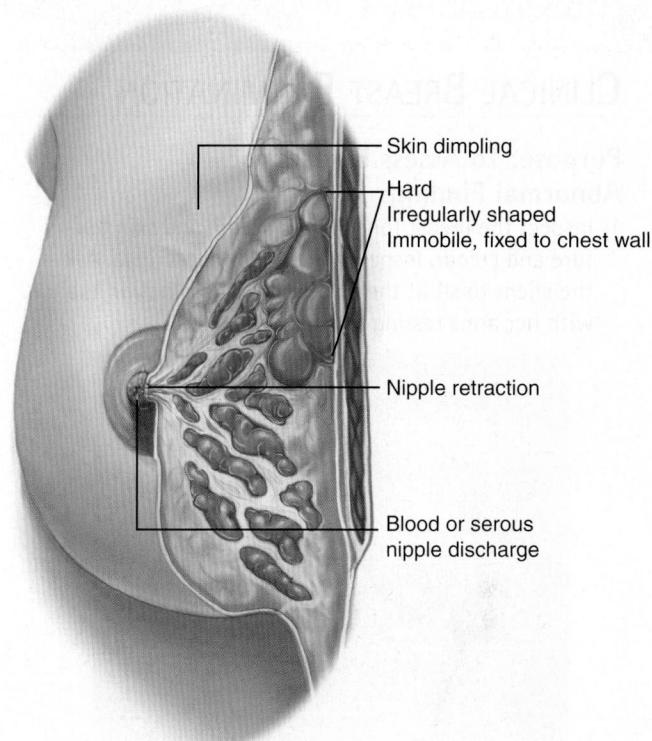

FIGURE 6.5 Malignant breast tumour.

ment and be able to identify those who need further psychological intervention. By giving practical advice, the nurse can help the woman adjust to her altered body image and to accept the changes to her life.

BOX 6.1 Characteristics of Benign Versus Malignant Breast Masses

- **Benign breast masses are described as:**
  - Frequently painful
  - Firm, rubbery mass
  - Bilateral masses
  - Induced nipple discharge
  - Regular margins (clearly delineated)
  - No skin dimpling
  - No nipple retraction
  - Mobile, not affixed to the chest wall
  - No bloody discharge
- **Malignant breast masses are described as:**
  - Hard to palpation
  - Painless
  - Irregularly shaped (poorly delineated)
  - Immobile, fixed to the chest wall
  - Skin dimpling
  - Nipple retraction
  - Unilateral mass
  - Bloody, serosanguineous, or serous nipple discharge
  - Spontaneous nipple discharge

Nursing Procedure 6.1

CLINICAL BREAST EXAMINATION

Purpose: To Assess Breasts for Abnormal Findings

1. Inspect the breast for size, symmetry, and skin texture and colour. Inspect the nipples and areola. Ask the client to sit at the edge of the examination table, with her arms resting at her sides.

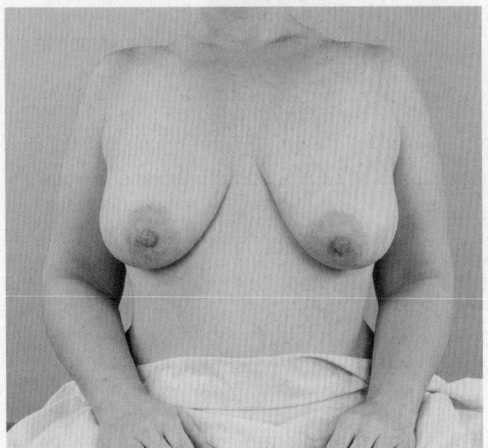

2. Inspect the breast for masses, retraction, dimpling, or ecchymosis.
   - The client places her hands on her hips.

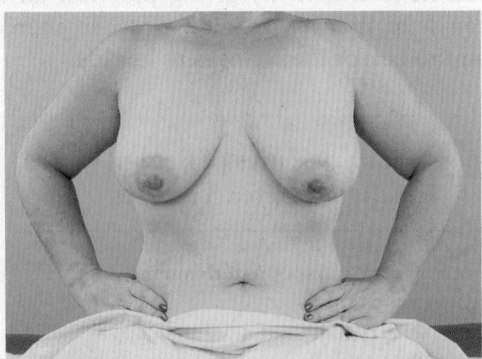

   - She then raises her arms over her head so the axillae can also be inspected.

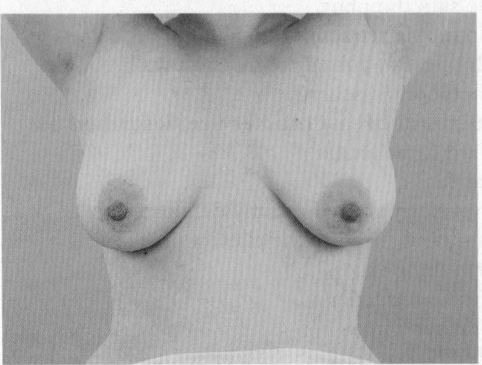

   - The client then stands, places her hands on her hips, and leans forward.

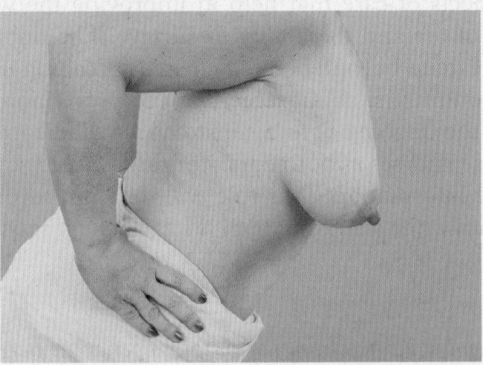

3. Palpate the breasts. Assist the client into a supine position with her arms above her head. Place a pillow or towel under the client's head to help spread the breasts. Three patterns might be used to palpate the breasts:

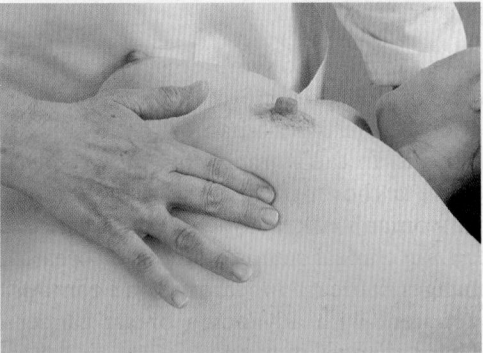

   - Spiral

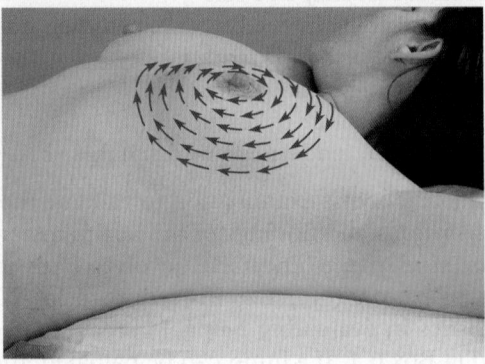

Nursing Procedure 6.1 (continued)

- Pie-shaped wedges

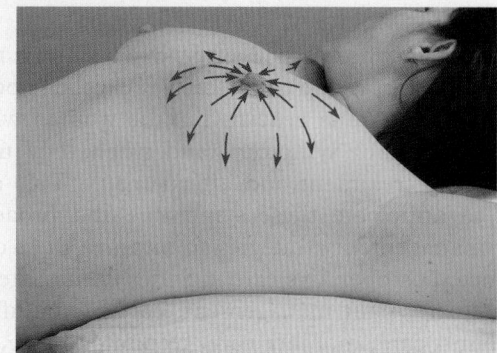

- Vertical strip

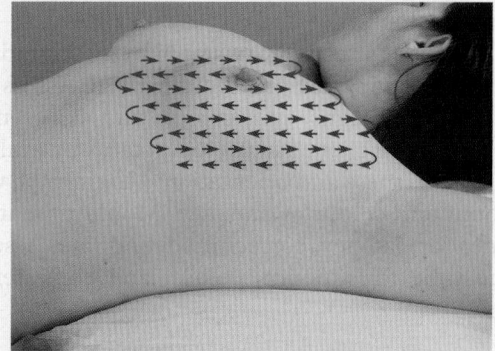

4. Compress the nipple gently between the thumb and index finger to evaluate for masses and squeeze to check for any discharge.

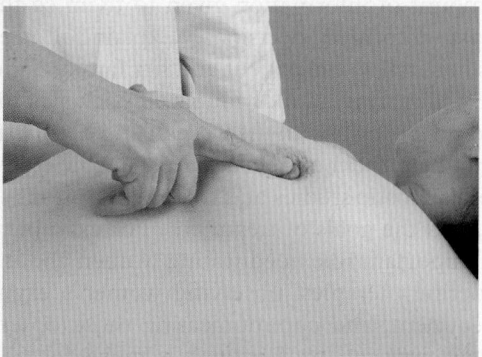

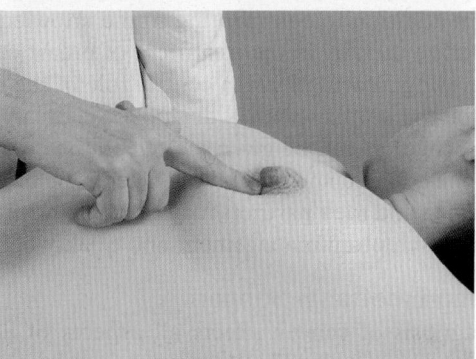

5. Palpate the axillary area for any tenderness or lymph node enlargement. Have the client sit up and move to the edge of the examination table. While supporting the client's arm, palpate downward from the armpit, palpating toward the ribs just below the breast.

Adapted from: Rhoads, J. (2006). *Advanced health assessment and diagnostic reasoning.* Philadelphia: Lippincott Williams & Wilkins.

Because family members play a significant role in supporting women through breast cancer diagnosis and treatment, assess the emotional distress of both partners during the course of treatment and, if needed, make a referral for psychological counselling. By identifying interpersonal strains, negative psychosocial side effects of cancer treatment can be minimized.

Nursing Diagnosis

Appropriate nursing diagnoses for a woman with a diagnosis of breast cancer might include:

- Disturbed body image related to:
  - Loss of body part (breast)
  - Loss of femininity
  - Loss of hair due to chemotherapy
- Fear related to:
  - Diagnosis of cancer
  - Prognosis of disease

- Educational deficit related to:
  - Cancer treatment options
  - Reconstructive surgery decisions
  - Breast self-examination

Nursing Interventions

Offer information, support, and perioperative care to women diagnosed with breast cancer who are undergoing treatment. Implement health-promotion and disease-prevention strategies to minimize the risk for developing breast cancer and to promote optimal outcomes.

Remember Nancy, who discovered a breast lump? You offer to go with her to the doctor. After a full examination and several diagnostic tests, the results come back positive for breast cancer. What treatment options does Nancy have, and what factors need to be considered in selecting those options?

Providing Patient Education

Help the woman and her partner to prioritize the voluminous amount of information given to them so that they can make informed decisions. Explain all treatment options in detail so the patient and her family understand them. By preparing an individualized packet of information and reviewing it with the woman and her partner, the nurse can help them understand her specific type of cancer, the diagnostic studies and treatment options she may choose, and the goals of treatment. For example, nurses play an important role in educating women about the use of endocrine therapies, observing women's experiences with treatment, and communicating those observations to their primary care professionals to make dosage adjustments, in addition to contributing to the knowledge base of endocrine therapy in the treatment of breast cancer.

Providing information is a central role of the nurse in caring for the woman with a diagnosis of breast cancer. This information can be given via telephone counselling, one-to-one contact, and pamphlets. Telephone counselling with women and their partners may be an effective method to improve symptom management and quality of life.

Providing Emotional Support

The diagnosis of cancer affects all aspects of life for a woman and her family. The threatening nature of the disease and feelings of uncertainty about the future can lead to anxiety and stress. Address the woman's needs for:

- Information about diagnosis and treatment
- Physical care while undergoing treatments
- Contact with supportive people
- Education about disease, options, and prevention measures
- Discussion and support by a caring, competent nurse

Reassure the client and her family that the diagnosis of breast cancer does not necessarily mean imminent death, a decrease in attractiveness, or diminished sexuality. Encourage the woman to express her fears and worries. Be available to listen and address the woman's concerns in an open manner to help her toward recovery. All aspects of care must include sensitivity to the patient's personal efforts to cope and heal. Some women will become involved in organizations or charities that support cancer research; they may participate in breast cancer walks to raise awareness or become a CCS volunteer to help others. Each woman copes in her own personal manner, and all of these efforts can be positive motivators for her own healing.

To help women cope with the diagnosis of breast cancer, the CCS launched CancerConnection in 1995. Specially trained breast cancer survivors give women and their family's opportunities to express their feelings, verbalize their fears, and get answers. Most importantly, CancerConnection volunteers offer understanding, support, and hope through face-to-face visits or by telephone; they are proof that people can survive breast cancer and live productive lives. National contact information is 888-939-3333.

Providing Postoperative Care

For the woman who has had surgery to remove a malignant breast lump or an entire breast, excellent postoperative nursing care is crucial. Tell the woman what to expect in terms of symptoms and when they usually occur during treatment and after surgery. This allows women to anticipate these symptoms and proactively employ management strategies to improve their cancer experience. Postoperative care includes immediate postoperative care, pain management, care of the affected arm, wound care, mobility care, respiratory care, emotional care, educational needs, and referrals.

Immediate Postoperative Care

Assess the client's respiratory status by auscultating the lungs and observing the breathing pattern. Assess circulation; note vital signs, skin colour, and skin temperature. Observe the client's neurologic status by evaluating the level of alertness and orientation. Monitor the wound for amount and colour of drainage. Monitor the intravenous lines for patency, correct fluid, and rate. Assess the drainage tube for amount, colour, and consistency of drainage.

Pain Management

Provide analgesics as needed. Reassure the woman that her pain will be controlled. Teach the woman how to communicate her pain intensity on a scale of 0 to 10, with 10 being the worst pain imaginable. Assess the client's pain level frequently and anticipate pain before assisting the woman to ambulate.

Affected Arm Care

Elevate the affected arm on a pillow to promote lymph drainage. Make sure that no treatments are performed on the affected arm, including laboratory draws, intravenous lines, blood pressures, and so on. Place a sign above the bed to warn others not to touch the affected arm.

Wound Care

Observe the wound often and empty drainage reservoirs as needed. Tell the client to report any evidence of infection early, such as fever, chills, or any area of redness or inflammation along the incision line. Also tell the client to report any increase in drainage, foul odour, or separation at the incision site.

Mobility Care

Perform active range-of-motion and arm exercises as ordered. Encourage self-care activities for successful rehabilitation. Perform dressing and drainage care; explain the care during the procedure.

Respiratory Care

Assist with turning, coughing, and deep breathing every 2 hours. Explain that this helps to expand collapsed alveoli in the lungs, promotes faster clearance of inhalation agents from the body, and prevents postoperative pneumonia and atelectasis.

Emotional Care and Referrals

Encourage the client to participate in her care. Assess her coping strategies preoperatively. Explain possible body image concerns after discharge. Promote the CCS websites, which provide the latest cancer therapy news (visit http://thePoint.lww.com/Chow1e for direct links to some of these sites). Encourage the client to attend local support groups for breast cancer survivors, such as CancerConnection, a CCS program in which trained volunteers provide support and up to date information for spouses, children, friends, and other loved ones. Most women younger than 40 years consider the family to be the primary support network, and other women consider friends to be their support network (Snyder & Pearse, 2010). Younger women are less inclined to use support groups. Support may be perceived as emotional, informational, and experiential (support from family and others who have undergone similar experiences).

Educational Needs

Provide follow-up information about adjunctive therapy. Explain that radiation therapy may start within weeks postoperatively. Discuss chemotherapy, its side effects and cycles, home care during treatment, and future monitoring strategies. Explain hormonal therapy, including anti-estrogens or aromatase inhibitors. Teach progressive arm exercises to minimize lymphedema. Explain that ongoing surveillance is needed to detect recurrence of cancer or a new primary site and that the patient will typically see the health care provider every 6 months.

ℕancy underwent a mastectomy with radiation and chemotherapy. What follow-up care is needed? How can the nurse assist Nancy to cope with her uncertain future? What community resources might help her?

Implementing Health-Promotion and Disease-Prevention Strategies

In the past, most women assumed that there was little they could do to reduce their risk of developing breast cancer. However, research has found that the daily choices women make concerning breast cancer screening, diet, exercise, and other health practices have a profound impact on cancer risk. In the fight against cancer, nurses often assume a variety of roles, such as educator, counsellor, advocate, and role model. Nurses can offer education about the following:

• Prevention
• Early detection
• Screening
• Dispelling myths and fears
• Self-examination techniques
• Individual risk status and strategies for risk reduction

It is important to be knowledgeable about the most current evidence-based practices and cognizant of how the media presents this information. Offer prevention strategies within the context of a woman's life. Factors such as lifestyle choices, economic status, and multiple roles need to be taken into consideration when counselling women. Advocate for healthy lifestyles and making sound choices to prevent cancer. Nurses, like all health care professionals, should offer guidance from a comprehensive perspective that acknowledges the unique needs of each individual.

Breast cancer is a frightening experience for women. Like a black cloud hanging over their heads, with little regard for any victim, breast cancer stalks women everywhere they go. Many have a close friend or relative who is battling the disease; many have watched their mothers and sisters die of this dreaded disease. Those with risk factors live with even greater anxiety and fear. No woman wants to hear those chilling words: "The biopsy is positive. You have breast cancer." Provide women with information about detection and risk factors, inform them about the CCS screening guidelines, instruct them on breast self-examination, and outline dietary changes that might reduce their risk of breast cancer.

Awareness is the first step toward a change in habits. Raising the level of awareness about breast cancer is of paramount importance, and nurses can play an important role in health promotion, disease prevention, and education.

Breast Cancer Screening

The three components of early detection are breast self-examination, CBE, and mammography. The CCS (2012) has issued breast cancer screening guidelines that offer specific recommendations for women and greater clarification of the role of breast examinations (Table 6.4).

Women are exposed to multiple sources of cancer prevention information, and much of it may not be sound. Discuss the benefits, risks, and potential limitations of breast self-examination, CBE, and mammography with each woman, and tailor the information to her specific risk factors (CCS, 2012).

Breast self-examination is a technique that enables a woman to detect any changes in her breasts; this could result in early cancer detection. The emphasis is now on awareness of breast changes, not just discovery

TABLE 6.4 CANADIAN CANCER SOCIETY BREAST CANCER SCREENING GUIDELINES

Woman's Age (years)	Screening Activity
40–49	Clinical breast exam by health care professional at least every 2 years
50–69	Clinical breast exam by health care professional at least every 2 years; mammogram every 2 years
≥70	Discuss with health care professional about frequency of testing

Women at increased risk (e.g., family history, genetic tendency, past history of cancer) should discuss with their health care professional the pros and cons of starting mammography screening earlier, undergoing additional diagnostic tests (e.g., ultrasound or MRI), or increasing the frequency of examinations.

Source: Canadian Cancer Society. (2012). *Canadian cancer encyclopedia: Breast cancer.* Retrieved January 24, 2012 from info.cancer.ca/cce-ecc/default.aspx?Lang=E&toc=10.

of cancer. Research has shown that breast self-examination plays a small role in detecting breast cancer compared with self-awareness. However, doing breast self-examination is one way for a woman to know how her breasts normally feel so that she can notice any changes that do occur (CCS, 2012).

There are two steps to conducting a breast self-examination: visual inspection and tactile palpation. The visual part should be done in three separate positions: with the arms up behind the head, with the arms down at the sides, and bending forward. Instruct the woman to look for:

• Changes in shape, size, contour, or symmetry
• Skin discolouration or dimpling, bumps/lumps
• Sores or scaly skin
• Discharge or puckering of the nipple

In the second part, the tactile examination, the woman feels her breasts in one of three specific patterns: spiral, pie-shaped wedges, or up and down. When using any of the three patterns, the woman should use a circular rubbing motion (in dime-sized circles) without lifting the fingers. She checks not only the breasts but also between the breast and the axilla, the axilla itself, and the area above the breast up to the clavicle and across the shoulder. The pads of the three middle fingers on the right hand are used to assess the left breast; the pads of the three middle fingers on the left hand are used to assess the right breast. Instruct the woman to use three different degrees of pressure:

• Light (move the skin without moving the tissue underneath)
• Medium (midway into the tissue)
• Hard (down to the ribs)

Once the tactile examination has been completed while standing in front of a mirror, it should be repeated while lying down. Teaching Guideline 6.4 details breast self-examination.

Nutrition

Nutrition plays a critical role in health promotion and disease prevention (Escott-Stump, 2008). Being overweight or obese is a risk factor for breast cancer in postmenopausal women (CCS, 2012). About 23% of Canadian women are obese, with the lowest obesity rates (12%) noted in women between 18 and 24 years of age (Tjepkema, 2008). A diet high in fruits, vegetables, and high-fibre carbohydrates and low in animal fats seems to offer protection against breast cancer as well as weight control. Women who followed these dietary guidelines decreased their risk of breast cancer (Escott-Stump, 2008).

The American Institute for Cancer Research and the World Cancer Research Fund, which conduct extensive cancer research, made the following recommendations to reduce a woman's risk for developing breast cancer:

1. Be as slim as possible without being underweight.
2. Engage in physical activity for at least 30 minutes per day.
3. Avoid sugar-laden drinks, and eat limited amounts of energy-dense foods.
4. Eat vegetables, fruits, legumes, and whole grains.
5. Eat limited amounts of red meat (beef, pork, lamb), and avoid processed meat.
6. Limit alcohol to one drink per day.
7. Eat less salt and fewer foods processed with sodium.
8. Avoid supplements to prevent cancer.
9. Breastfeed exclusively for up to 6 months after giving birth.
10. Adhere to cancer treatment recommendations (for cancer survivors).

The medical community is also starting to study the role of phytochemicals in health. The unique geographic variability of breast cancer around the world and the low rate of breast cancer in Asian countries compared with Western countries has prompted this interest. This area of research appears hopeful for women seeking to prevent breast cancer as well as those recovering from it. See Evidence-based Practice 6.1. Although the mechanism isn't clear, certain foods demonstrate anticancer properties and boost the immune system. Phytochemical-rich foods include:

• Green tea and herbal teas
• Garlic
• Whole grains and legumes
• Onions and leeks
• Soybeans and soy products

TEACHING GUIDELINE 6.4

How to Perform Breast Self-Examination

Step 1

- Stand before a mirror.
- Check both breasts for anything unusual.
- Look for discharge from the nipple and puckering, dimpling, or scaling of the skin.
   The next two steps are done to check for any changes in the contour of your breasts. As you do them, you should be able to feel your muscles tighten.

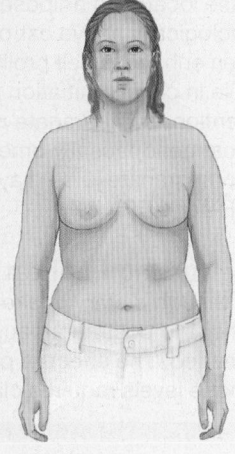

Step 2

- Watch closely in the mirror as you clasp your hands behind your head and press your hands forward.
- Note any change in the contour of your breasts.

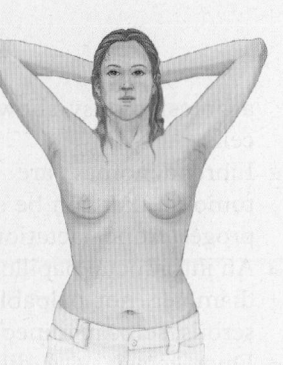

Step 3

- Next, press your hands firmly on your hips and bow slightly toward the mirror as you pull your shoulders and elbows forward.
- Note any change in the contour of your breasts.
   Some women perform the next part of the examination in the shower. Your fingers will glide easily over soapy skin, so you can concentrate on feeling for changes inside the breast.

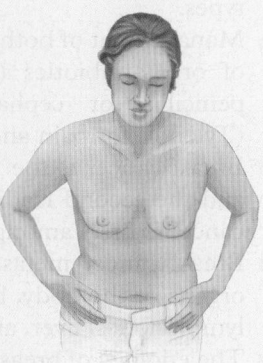

Step 4

- Raise your left arm.
- Use three or four fingers of your right hand to feel your left breast firmly, carefully, and thoroughly.
- Beginning at the outer edge, press the flat part of your fingers in small circles, moving the circles slowly around the breast.
- Gradually work toward the nipple.
- Be sure to cover the whole breast.
- Pay special attention to the area between the breast and the underarm, including the underarm itself.
- Feel for any unusual lumps or masses under the skin.
- If you have any spontaneous discharge during the month—whether or not it is during your self-exam—see your doctor.
- Repeat the examination on your right breast using your left hand.

Step 5

- Lie flat on your back with your left arm over your head and a pillow or folded towel under your left shoulder. (This position flattens your breast and makes it easier to check.)
- Repeat the actions of Step 4 in this position for each breast.

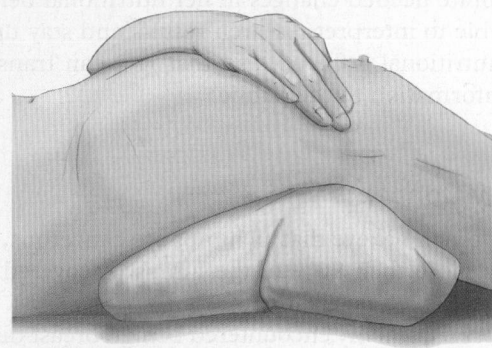

Source: American Cancer Society. (2007). *Breast awareness and self-exam.* Retrieved January 24, 2012 from http://www.cancer.org/Cancer/BreastCancer/DetailedGuide/breast-cancer-detection.

EVIDENCE-BASED PRACTICE 6.1
Can Pomegranate Juice Prevent Breast Cancer?

The hypothesis that pomegranate juice can prevent breast cancer in postmenopausal has been proposed but has not been tested on large population of women.

● Emerging Science

Research examining the effects of diet on breast cancer is ongoing. Recently there has been interest in pomegranates and exploring the benefits of phytochemical properties of the fruit. The pomegranate (*Punica granatum*) has been revered by ancient civilizations and is used in Eastern and Middle Eastern cuisine. Pomegranate juice has recently become popular in North America. The fruit consists of seeds, juice, and the peel. After menopause, most estrogen is converted from adrenal androgens to E1 by aroma-

tase located in adipose tissue. E1 is metabolized to E2, a biologically active estrogen found in breast tissue. Estrogen enhances cell proliferation in the breast and plays a role in cancer initiation and progression. As a dietary intervention, pomegranate may reduce estrogen synthesis in postmenopausal women. In vitro research indicates that pomegranate juice may have an antiproliferative effect on ER+ and ER– cells.

▲ Nursing Implications

Although dietary intake of pomegranate juice may be beneficial to postmenopausal women, more studies are needed. The effect of pomegranate juice on serum hormone levels requires clarification.

Source: Sturgeon, S. R., & Ronnenberg, A. G. (2010). Pomegranate and breast cancer: Possible mechanisms of prevention. *Nutrition Reviews, 68*(2), 122–128.

• Fruits (citrus, apricots, pumpkin, berries)
• Green leafy vegetables (spinach, collards, romaine)
• Colourful vegetables (carrots, squash, tomatoes)
• Cruciferous vegetables (broccoli, cabbage, cauliflower)
• Flax seeds (Escott-Stump, 2008)

Adopt a holistic approach when addressing the nutritional needs of women with breast cancer. Incorporate nutritional assessment into the general overall assessment of all women. Culturally sensitive nutritional assessment tools need to be developed and used to enhance this process. Providing examples of appropriate foods associated with the woman's current dietary habits, relating current health status to nutritional intake, and placing proposed modifications within a realistic personal framework may increase a woman's willingness to incorporate needed changes in her nutritional behaviour. Be able to interpret research results and stay up to date on nutritional influences so that you can transmit this key information to the public.

■■ Key Concepts

■ Many women believe that all lumps are cancerous, but actually more than 90% of the lumps discovered are benign and need no treatment.
■ The most commonly encountered benign breast disorders in women include fibrocystic breasts, fibroadenomas, intraductal papilloma, mammary duct ectasia, and mastitis.
■ Current research suggests that women with fibrocystic breast disease or other benign breast conditions are more likely to develop breast cancer later only if

a breast biopsy shows "atypia" or abnormal breast cells.
■ Fibroadenomas are common benign solid breast tumours that can be stimulated by external estrogen, progesterone, lactation, and pregnancy.
■ An intraductal papilloma is generally less than 1 cm in diameter, not palpable, and produces a spontaneous serous, serosanguineous, or watery nipple discharge.
■ Duct ectasia is a dilation and inflammation of the ducts behind the nipple that results in noncyclic breast pain, nipple retraction, and discharge.
■ Mastitis is an infection of the connective tissue in the breast that occurs primarily in lactating or engorged women; it is divided into lactational or nonlactational types.
■ Management of both types of mastitis involves the use of oral antibiotics (usually a penicillinase-resistant penicillin or cephalosporin) and acetaminophen (Tylenol) for pain and fever.
■ Breast cancer is the most common cancer in women and the second leading cause of cancer deaths (lung cancer is first) among Canadian women.
■ Breast cancer metastasizes widely and to almost all organs of the body, but primarily to the bone, lungs, lymph nodes, liver, and brain.
■ The etiology of breast cancer is unknown, but the disease is thought to develop in response to a number of related factors: aging, delayed childbearing or never bearing children, high breast density, family history of cancer, late menopause, and hormonal factors.
■ Breast cancer treatments fall into two categories: local and systemic. Local treatments are surgery and radiation therapy. Effective systemic treatments include

chemotherapy, hormonal therapy, and biological or immunotherapy.

- Women perceive their breasts as intrinsic to their femininity, self-esteem, and sexuality, and the risk of losing a breast can provoke extreme anxiety.

- Nurses can influence both physical and emotional recovery, which are both important aspects of care that help in improving the woman's quality of life and the ability to survive.

- Providing up to date information and emotional support are central roles of the nurse in caring for the woman with a diagnosis of breast cancer.

REFERENCES

Alexander, L. L., LaRosa, J. H., Bader, H., & Garfield, S., Alexander, W. J. (2010). *New dimensions in women's health* (5th ed.). Boston: Jones and Bartlett Publishers.

American Cancer Society. (2007). *Breast awareness and self-exam.* Retrieved January 24, 2012 from http://www.cancer.org/Cancer/BreastCancer/DetailedGuide/breast-cancer-detection

American Cancer Society. (2009). *How is breast cancer staged?* Retrieved January 24, 2012 from http://www.cancer.org/docroot/CRI/content/CRI_2_4_3X_How_is_breast_cancer_staged_5.asp?sitearea=

American Cancer Society. (2011). *Non-cancerous breast conditions.* Retrieved January 24, 2012 from http://www.cancer.org/docroot/CRI/content/CRI_2_6X_Non_Cancerous_Breast_Conditions_59.asp

Ballestas, H. C., Calvry, J. A., Cooper, K., Gamblian et al. (2008). *Nursing: Interpreting signs and symptoms.* Philadelphia: Lippincott Williams & Wilkins.

Brower, V. (2010). Breast density gains acceptance as breast cancer risk factor. *Journal of the National Cancer Institute, 102*(6), 374–375.

Canadian Cancer Society. (2009). *Mastectomy.* Retrieved January 24, 2012 from http://www.cancer.ca/Canada-wide/About%20cancer/Types%20of%20cancer/Mastectomy.aspx?sc_lang=en

Canadian Cancer Society. (2010a). *Diagnosing breast cancer.* Retrieved January 24, 2012 from http://www.cancer.ca/Canada-wide/About%20cancer/Types%20of%20cancer/Diagnosing%20breast%20cancer.aspx?sc_lang=en

Canadian Cancer Society. (2010b). *Signs and symptoms of breast cancer.* Retrieved January 24, 2012 from http://www.cancer.ca/Canada-wide/About%20cancer/Types%20of%20cancer/Signs%20and%20symptoms%20of%20breast%20cancer.aspx?sc_lang=en

Canadian Cancer Society. (2011a). *Breast cancer statistics at a glance.* Retrieved January 24, 2012 from http://www.cancer.ca/Canada-wide/About%20cancer/Cancer%20statistics/Stats%20at%20a%20glance/Breast%20cancer.aspx?sc_lang=en

Canadian Cancer Society. (2011b). *Causes of breast cancer.* Retrieved January 24, 2012 from http://www.cancer.ca/Canada-wide/About%20cancer/Types%20of%20cancer/Causes%20of%20breast%20cancer.aspx?sc_lang=en

Canadian Cancer Society. (2011c). *Treatment for breast cancer.* Retrieved January 24, 2012 from http://www.cancer.ca/Canada-wide/About%20cancer/Types%20of%20cancer/Treatment%20for%20breast%20cancer.aspx?sc_lan=en

Canadian Cancer Society. (2012). *Canadian cancer encyclopedia: Breast cancer.* Retrieved January 24, 2012 from info.cancer.ca/cce-ecc/default.aspx?Lang=E&toc=10

Deglin, J. H., Vallerand, A. H., & Sanoski, C. A. (2011). *Davis's drug guide for nurses* (12th ed.). Philadelphia: FA Davis.

Escott-Stump, S. (2008). *Nutrition and diagnosis-related care* (6th ed.). Philadelphia: Lippincott Williams & Wilkins.

Fentiman, I. S. (2009). Ultrasound should be intrinsic, not optional, in assessment of breast lesions. *International Journal of Clinical Practice, 63*(11), 1549–1557.

Jardines, L. (2008). Breast disorders. In A. L. Clouse & K. Sherif (Eds.), *Women's health in clinical practice: A handbook for primary care.* Totowa, NJ: Humana Press.

Lake, D., Zapton, D. T., Hoda, R. S., Pope, T. (2008). Radiological case: Intraductal Papilloma with focal atypia. *Applied Radiology, 37*(6), 37–38.

Lee, E. (2009). Evidence-based management of benign breast diseases. *The American Journal for Nurse Practitioners, 13*(7/8), 22–31.

London, M. L., Ladewig, P. W., Ball, J. W., Bindler, R. C., & Cowen, K. J. (2010). *Maternal and child nursing care* (3rd ed.). Upper Saddle River, NJ: Pearson.

Mattarella, A. (2010). Breast cancer in men. *Radiologic Technology, 81*(4), 361–378.

Miltenburg, D. M., & Speights, V. O. (2008). Benign breast disease. *Obstetrics and Gynecology Clinics of North America, 35*, 285–300.

National Comprehensive Cancer Network. (2011). *NCCN guidelines for patients: Breast cancer.* Retrieved January 24, 2012 from http://www.nccn.com/images/patient-guidelines/pdf/breast.pdf

Onami, S., Ozaki, M., Mortimer, J. E., & Pal, S. K. (2010). Male breast cancer: An update in diagnosis, treatment and molecular profiling. *Maturitas, 65*, 308–314.

Pillitteri, A. (2010). *Maternal & child health nursing: Care of the childbearing & childrearing family* (6th ed.). Philadelphia: Lippincott Williams & Wilkins.

Public Health Agency of Canada. (2009). *Breast cancer facts and figures.* Retrieved January 24, 2012 from www.phac-aspc.gc.ca/cd-mc/cancer/breast_cancer_figures-cancer_du_sein_figures-eng.php

Public Health Agency of Canada (PHAC). (2003). *Breast cancer in Canada: Probability of developing breast cancer in the next 5 years.* Retrieved January 24, 2012 from www.phac-aspc.gc.ca/publicat/updates/breast-99-eng.php

Rhoads, J. (2006). *Advanced health assessment and diagnostic reasoning.* Philadelphia: Lippincott Williams & Wilkins.

Rosolowich, V., Saettler, E., & Szuck, B. (2006). Mastalgia. *Journal of Obstetrics and Gynaecology Canada, 170*, 49–57.

Schorge, J. O., Halvorson, L. M., Hoffman, B. L., Bradshaw, K. D., & Cunningham, F. G. (2008). *Williams gynecology.* New York: McGraw-Hill Professional.

Snyder, K. A., & Pearse, W. (2010). Crisis, social support, and the family response: Exploring the narratives of young breast cancer survivors. *Journal of Psychosocial Oncology, 28*(4), 413–431.

Sukumvanich, P., & Borgen, P. (2010). Diseases of the breast. In R. E. Rakel & E. T. Bope (Eds.), *Conn's current therapy 2007.* Philadelphia: Saunders Elsevier.

Swart, R., Downey, L., Gohel, S. G., et al. (2011). *Breast cancer.* Retrieved January 24, 2012 from http://emedicine.medscape.com/article/283561-overview

Tjepkema, M. (2008). *Adult obesity in Canada: Measured height and weight.* Retrieved January 24, 2012 from http://www.statcan.gc.ca/pub/82-620-m/2005001/article/adults-adultes/8060-eng.htm#3

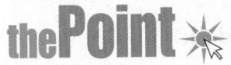 For additional learning materials, including Internet Resources, visit **http://thePoint.lww.com/Chow1e.**

CHAPTER WORKSHEET

MULTIPLE CHOICE QUESTIONS

1. Breast self-examinations involve both touching of breast tissue and:

   a. Palpation of cervical lymph nodes

   b. Firm squeezing of both breast nipples

   c. Visualizing both breasts for any change

   d. A mammogram to evaluate breast tissue

2. Which of the following is the strongest risk factor for breast cancer?

   a. Advancing age and being female

   b. High number of children

   c. Genetic mutations in BRCA-1 and BRCA-2

   d. Family history of colon cancer

3. A biopsy procedure that traces radioisotopes and blue dye from the tumour site through the lymphatic system into the axillary nodes is:

   a. Stereotactic biopsy

   b. Sentinel node biopsy

   c. Axillary dissection biopsy

   d. Advanced breast biopsy

4. The most serious potential adverse reaction from chemotherapy is:

   a. Thrombocytopenia

   b. Deep vein thrombosis

   c. Alopecia

   d. Myelosuppression

5. What suggestion would be helpful for the client experiencing painful fibrocystic breast changes?

   a. Increase her caffeine intake.

   b. Take a mild analgesic when needed.

   c. Reduce her intake of leafy vegetables.

   d. Wear a bra bigger than she needs.

6. A postoperative mastectomy client should be referred to which of the following organizations for assistance?

   a. National Organization for Women

   b. Food and Drug Administration

   c. March of Dimes Foundation

   d. CancerConnection

CRITICAL THINKING EXERCISES

1. Mrs. Gordon, 48 years, presents to the women's community clinic where you work as a nurse. She is very upset and crying. She tells you that she found lumps in her breast: "I know that it's cancer and I will die." When you ask her about her problem, she says she does not check her breasts monthly and hasn't had a mammogram for years because "I don't have time." She also describes the intermittent pain she experiences.

   a. What specific questions would you ask this client to get a clearer picture?

   b. What education is needed for this client regarding breast health?

   c. What community referrals are needed to meet this client's future needs?

2. Ruth Davis, 51 years, stops in at the urgent care facility with an anxious look on her face. She tells the nurse practitioner that she has green discharge coming from her right breast and discomfort intermittently. She can't understand how this would happen since she hasn't previously had any nipple discharge or pain.

   a. What benign breast condition might the nurse practitioner suspect based on her description?

   b. What specific information should the nurse practitioner give Mrs. Davis about duct ectasia?

   c. The typical treatment of this benign breast condition would include what?

STUDY ACTIVITIES

1. Discuss with a group of women what their breasts symbolize to them and to society. Do they symbolize something different to each one?

2. When a woman experiences a breast disorder, what feelings might she be experiencing and how can a nurse help her sort them out?

3. Interview a woman who has fibrocystic breast changes and find out how she manages this condition.

4. An infection of the breast connective tissue that frequently occurs in the lactating woman is

   _____.

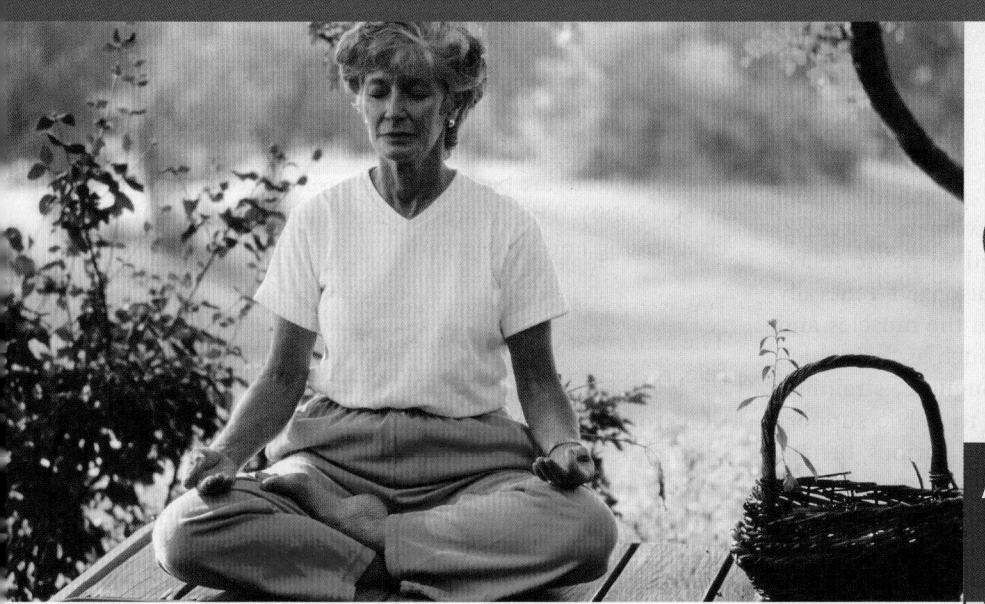

BENIGN DISORDERS OF THE FEMALE REPRODUCTIVE TRACT

KEY TERMS

cystocele
enterocele
Kegel exercises
ovarian cyst

pelvic organ prolapse
pessary
polycystic ovary syndrome
polyps

rectocele
urinary incontinence
uterine fibroids
uterine prolapse

LEARNING OBJECTIVES

Upon completion of the chapter, the learner will be able to:

1. Define the key terms.
2. Identify the major pelvic relaxation disorders in terms of etiology, management, and nursing interventions.
3. Outline the nursing management needed for the most common benign reproductive disorders in women.
4. Discuss urinary incontinence in terms of pathology, clinical manifestations, treatment options, and effect on quality of life.
5. Compare the various benign growths in terms of their symptoms and management.
6. Discuss the emotional impact of polycystic ovarian syndrome and the nurse's role as a counsellor, educator, and advocate.

Liz, a 26-year-old, overweight woman, presented to the clinic with hirsutism and facial acne and told the nurse she was concerned about her irregular menstrual periods. She also said her hair seemed to be falling out on top of her head recently. What diagnostic tests might the nurse anticipate with this patient? How can the nurse prepare Liz for them?

Wow

Women can influence their aging process by making wise lifestyle choices early on.

The incidence of several benign pelvic disorders increases as women age. For instance, women may experience pelvic support disorders related to pelvic relaxation or urinary incontinence. These disorders generally develop after years of wear and tear on the muscles and tissues that support the pelvic floor—such as that which occurs with childbearing, chronic coughing, straining, surgery, or simply aging. In addition to pelvic support disorders, women may also experience various benign neoplasms of the reproductive tract, such as cervical polyps, uterine leiomyomas (fibroids), ovarian cysts, genital fistulas, and Bartholin's cysts. This chapter provides an overview of various pelvic support disorders and benign neoplasms, discussing the assessment, treatment, and prevention strategies for each.

Pelvic Support Disorders

Pelvic support disorders such as pelvic organ prolapse (POP) and urinary and fecal incontinence are common in aging women (Richardson, Hagen, Glazener, et al., 2009). Pelvic support disorders cause significant physical and psychological morbidity and can diminish women's social interactions, emotional well-being, and overall quality of life. Since pelvic support disorders increase with age, the problem will grow worse as the population ages. These disorders occur as a result of weakness of the connective tissue and muscular support of pelvic organs due to a number of factors: vaginal childbirth, intra-abdominal pressure seen in obesity, chronic pulmonary disease, constipation, and smoking (Lazarou & Grigorescu, 2012). The bony pelvis has an exaggerated lumbar spine curve and downward tilt to it. The bladder rests on the symphysis, and the posterior organs rest on the sacrum and coccyx. The pelvis holds the organs, but a woman's erect posture causes a funneling effect and constant downward pressure.

Pelvic Organ Prolapse

Pelvic organ prolapse (from the Latin *prolapsus,* a slipping forth) refers to the abnormal descent or herniation of the pelvic organs from their original attachment sites or their normal position in the pelvis. POP occurs when structures of the pelvis shift and protrude into or outside of the vaginal canal. The Egyptians were the first to describe prolapse of the genital organs. Hippocrates made reference to placing a pomegranate half into the vagina to treat organ prolapse. A disorder exclusive to women, POP rarely results in severe morbidity or mortality but can affect a woman's daily activities and quality of life.

It is difficult to determine the incidence of POP, as the disorder is often asymptomatic and many women do not seek treatment. A primary causative factor for POP is having given birth (Chan, Schultz, Flood, et al., 2010).

With the aging of the population, POP and its associated symptoms are becoming increasingly common (Word et al., 2009). The treatment and diagnosis of POP are challenging and problematic.

Types of Pelvic Organ Prolapse

The four most common types of genital prolapse are cystocele, rectocele, enterocele, and uterine prolapse (Fig. 7.1):

- **Cystocele** occurs when the posterior bladder wall protrudes downward through the anterior vaginal wall.
- **Rectocele** occurs when the rectum sags and pushes against or into the posterior vaginal wall.
- **Enterocele** occurs when the small intestine bulges through the posterior vaginal wall (especially common when straining).
- **Uterine prolapse** occurs when the uterus descends through the pelvic floor and into the vaginal canal. Multiparous women are at particular risk for uterine prolapse.

The extent of uterine prolapse is described in terms of stages:

- First stage: prolapse of the organ into the vaginal canal
- Second stage: cervix descends to the vaginal introitus
- Third stage: cervix is below the vaginal introitus
- Fourth stage: complete vaginal eversion (Lazarou & Grigorescu, 2012)

Etiology

Anatomic support of the pelvic organs is mainly provided by the levator ani muscle complex and the connective tissue attachments of the pelvic organ fascia. Dysfunction of one or both of these components can lead to loss of support and eventually POP. Weakened pelvic floor muscles also prevent complete closure of the urethra, resulting in urine leakage during physical stress. This problem is not limited to older women: urinary incontinence has been documented in women of varying ages, including young women (Rahn, 2009).

Many risk factors for POP have been suggested, but the true cause is likely to be multifactorial. Causes might include:

- Constant downward gravity because of erect human posture
- Atrophy of supporting tissues with aging and decline of estrogen levels
- Weakening of pelvic support related to childbirth trauma
- Reproductive surgery
- Family history of POP
- Young age at first birth
- Connective tissue disorders
- Introital lacerations at childbirth
- Pelvic radiation

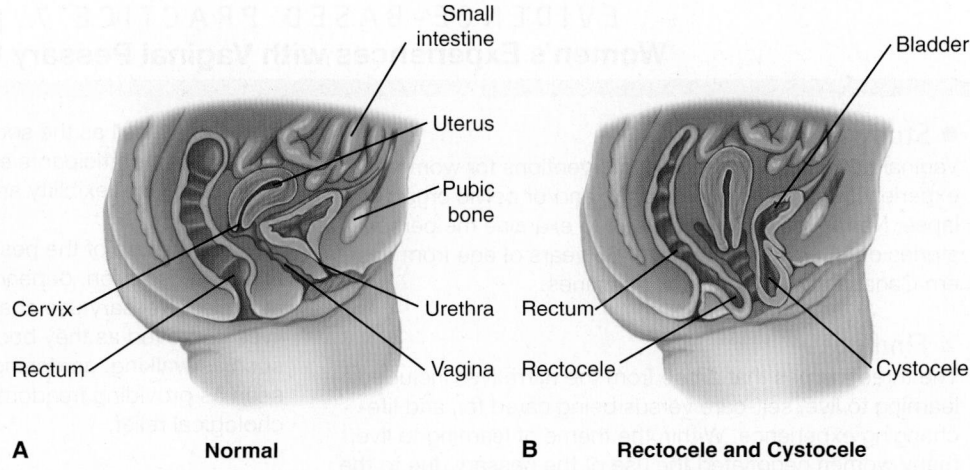

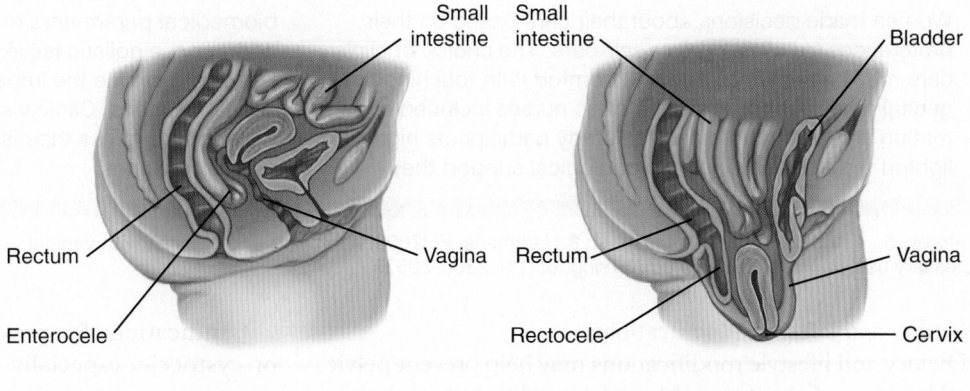

FIGURE 7.1 Types of pelvic prolapse. (**A**) Normal. (**B**) Rectocele and cystocele. (**C**) Enterocele. (**D**) Uterine prolapse.

- Increased abdominal pressure secondary to:
  - Lifting of children or heavy objects
  - Straining due to chronic constipation
  - Respiratory problems or chronic coughing
  - Obesity (O'Dell & Morse, 2008; Word et al., 2009)

Therapeutic Management

Treatment options for POP depend on the symptoms and their effect on the woman's quality of life. Important considerations when deciding on nonsurgical or surgical options include the severity of symptoms; the woman's preferences; the woman's health status, age, and suitability for surgery; and the presence of other pelvic conditions (urinary or fecal incontinence). When surgery is being considered, the nature of the procedure and the likely outcome must be fully explained and discussed with the woman and her partner. Treatment options for POP include Kegel exercises, estrogen replacement therapy, dietary and lifestyle modifications, and the use of pessaries and surgery (see Evidence-based Practice 7.1).

Kegel Exercises

Kegel exercises strengthen the pelvic floor muscles to support the inner organs and prevent further prolapse.

The purpose of pelvic floor exercises is to increase the muscle volume, which will result in a stronger muscular contraction. Kegel exercises might limit the progression of mild prolapse and alleviate mild prolapse symptoms, including low back pain and pelvic pressure. They will not, however, help severe uterine prolapse.

Hormone Replacement Therapy

Hormone replacement therapy (orally, transdermally, or vaginally) may improve the tone and vascularity of the supporting tissue in perimenopausal and menopausal women by increasing blood perfusion and the elasticity of the vaginal wall.

▶ *Take* NOTE!

Before hormone therapy is considered, a thorough medical history must be taken to assess the patient's risk for complications (e.g., endometrial cancer, myocardial infarction, stroke, breast cancer, pulmonary emboli, and deep vein thrombosis). Hormonal therapy in the treatment of POP is unclear (Society of Obstetricians and Gynaecologists Canada, 2006).

EVIDENCE-BASED PRACTICE 7.1
Women's Experiences with Vaginal Pessary Use

● Study

Vaginal pessaries are used as interventions for women experiencing urinary incontinence and/or pelvic organ prolapse. Narrative inquiry was used to examine the personal stories of 11 white women over 65 years of age from eastern Canada about the use of pessaries.

▲ Findings

The three themes that arose from the narratives included learning to live, self-care versus being cared for, and life-changing experience. Within the theme of learning to live, many women negotiated the use of the pessary due to the fear of surgery and surgical complications.

Women made decisions about their care based on their preferences for clinic care or self-care. The choice of clinic care may be related to age and comfort with touching the genital area. Support from the clinic nurses included information and instruction, and the study participants highlighted the emotional and psychological support they

received as well as the social aspect of the clinic visits. Some of the participants engaged in self-care based on their desire for flexibility and confidence.

Without the use of the pessary, the women suffered confinement, isolation, dependence, and sacrificed social activities. Pessary use changed their lives. The women's lives improved as they became more engaged in activities such as walking, gardening, and dancing. The pessary was seen as providing freedom, including emotional and psychological relief.

■ Nursing Implications

The use of pessaries impacts women's lives beyond the biomedical parameters of symptom relief. Nurses need to address the holistic issues surrounding the use of pessaries and examine the impact of the pessary on lifestyle and sexual relations. Clinic visits need to include time for women to express their issues and concerns about the use of pessaries.

Storey, S., Aston, M., Price, S., Irving, L., & Hemmens, E. (2009). Women's experiences with vaginal pessary use. *Journal of Advanced Nursing*, *65*(11), 2350–2357.

Dietary and Lifestyle Modifications

Dietary and lifestyle modifications may help prevent pelvic relaxation and chronic problems later in life. Dietary habits can exacerbate the prolapse by causing constipation and consequently chronic straining. The stools of a constipated person are hard and dry, and typically one must strain while bearing down to defecate. This straining to pass a hard stool increases intra-abdominal pressure, which over time causes the pelvic organs to prolapse. Dietary modifications can help to establish regular bowel movements without discomfort and eliminate flatus and bloating.

Pessaries

A **pessary** is a silicone or plastic device that is placed into the vagina to support the uterus, bladder, and rectum as a space-filling device, replacing normal pressure on the vaginal walls when levator ani support is unreliable (Fig. 7.2). Although there are many types and shapes, the most commonly used pessary is a firm ring that presses against the wall of the vagina and urethra to help decrease leakage and support a prolapsed vagina or uterus. Pessaries are of two main types:

- Support pessaries, which rest under the symphysis and sacrum and elevate the vagina (e.g., Ring, Gehrung, and Hodge pessaries)
- Space-occupying pessaries, which are designed to manage severe prolapse by supporting the uterus even with a lack of vaginal tone (e.g., cube, doughnut, and inflatable Gellhorn pessaries)

Indications for pessary use include uterine prolapse or cystocele, especially among elderly clients for whom surgery is contraindicated; younger women with prolapse who plan to have additional children; and women with marked prolapse who prefer to use a pessary rather than undergo surgery (Atnip, 2009). Many women use pessaries for only a short period of time and then become free of symptoms. Long-term use can lead to pressure necrosis in some women; in this situation other methods of support should be explored.

Pessaries are fitted by trial and error; the woman often needs to try several sizes or styles. The largest pessary that the woman can wear comfortably is generally the most effective. The woman should be instructed to report any discomfort or difficulty with urination or defecation while wearing the pessary.

Surgical Interventions

Surgical interventions for genital organ prolapse are designed to correct specific defects, with the goals being to restore normal anatomy and preserve function (Maher, Feiner, Baessler, et al., 2010). Surgery is not an option for all women. Since there is a high rate of failure for surgical intervention (Richardson et al., 2009), noninvasive treatment strategies should be discussed.

Surgical interventions might include anterior or posterior colporrhaphy (to repair a cystocele or rectocele, respectively) and vaginal hysterectomy (for uterine prolapse). An anterior or posterior colporrhaphy may be

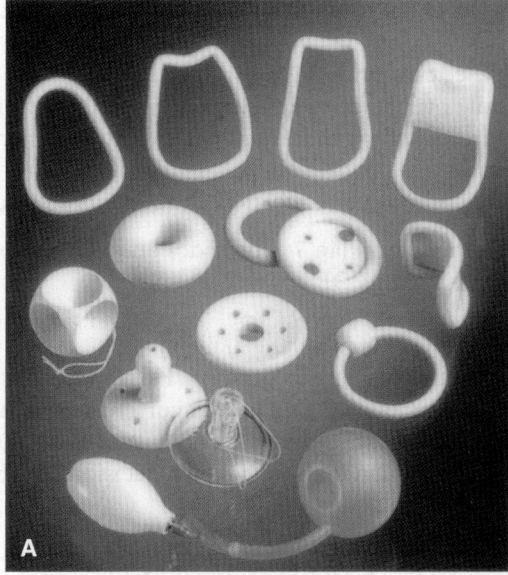

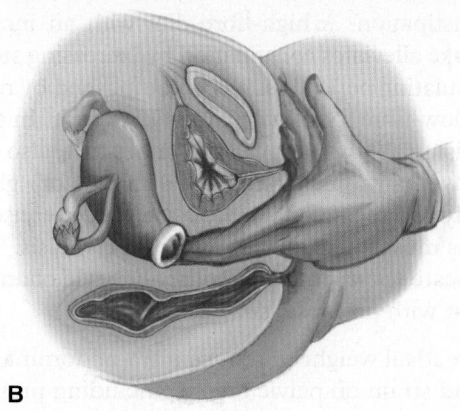

FIGURE 7.2 Examples of pessaries. (**A**) Various shapes and sizes of pessaries available. (**B**) Insertion of one type of pessary.

effective for a first-degree prolapse. This surgical procedure tightens the anterior or posterior vaginal wall, thus repairing the cystocele or rectocele. The pubocervical fascia (supportive tissue between the vagina and bladder) is folded and sutured to bring the bladder and urethra in proper position (Lazarou & Grigorescu, 2012).

A vaginal hysterectomy is the treatment of choice for uterine prolapse because it removes the prolapsed organ that is bringing down the bladder and rectum with it. It can be combined with an anterior or posterior repair if a cystocele or rectocele is present.

Nursing Assessment

Nursing assessment for women with POP includes a thorough health history and physical examination as well as several laboratory and diagnostic tests.

Health History and Clinical Manifestations

The cause of prolapse is multifactorial, with vaginal childbirth, advancing age, and increasing body mass index the

most consistent risk factors (O'Dell & Morse, 2008). Assessment of risk factors (chronic straining, hysterectomy, normal aging, and abnormalities of connective tissue) in the woman's history will assist the health care provider in the diagnosis and treatment of POP. The history should include questions about:

- The woman's obstetric history (number of pregnancies, weight of newborns, pregnancy spacing)
- Chronic respiratory condition (chronic coughing)
- Menopausal status
- Weight history (loss or gain)
- Constipation (frequency and chronicity)
- Age
- Family history (family member with POP)
- Urinary incontinence
- Previous pelvic surgeries

Assess for clinical manifestations of POP. POP is often asymptomatic, but when symptoms do occur, they are often related to the site and type of prolapse. Symptoms common to all types of prolapses are a feeling of dragging, a lump in the vagina, or something "coming down." Women with POP can present either with one symptom, such as vaginal bulging or pelvic pressure, or with several complaints, including many bladder, bowel, and pelvic symptoms. Symptoms associated with POP are summarized in Box 7.1.

Women present with varying degrees of descent. Uterine prolapse is the most troubling type of pelvic relaxation because it is often associated with concomitant defects of the vagina in the anterior, posterior, and lateral compartments (Lazarou & Grigorescu, 2012).

Physical Examination

The pelvic examination performed by the health care provider includes an external genital inspection to visualize any obvious protrusion of the uterus, bladder, urethra, or vaginal wall occurring at the vaginal opening. Usually the woman is asked to perform the Valsalva maneuver (bearing down) while the examiner notes which organ prolapses first and the degree to which it occurs. Any urine leakage during the examination is important to note. The woman is asked to contract the pubococcygeal muscles (Kegel exercise); the health care provider inserts two fingers into the vagina to assess the strength and symmetry of the contraction. Since genital organ prolapse can cause urinary symptoms such as incontinence, bladder function should be assessed by determining postvoid residual with a catheter. If the woman has more than 100 mL of retained urine, she should be referred for further urodynamic evaluation and testing.

Laboratory and Diagnostic Tests

Common laboratory tests that may be ordered to determine the cause of POP might include a urinalysis to rule out a bacterial infection, urine culture to identify the

BOX 7.1 Symptoms Associated with Pelvic Organ Prolapse

- Urinary symptoms
  - Stress incontinence
  - Frequency (diurnal and nocturnal)
  - Urgency and urge incontinence
  - Hesitancy
  - Poor or prolonged stream
  - Feeling of incomplete emptying
- Bowel symptoms
  - Difficulty in defecation
  - Incontinence of flatus or liquid or solid stool
  - Urgency of defecation
  - Feeling of incomplete evacuation
  - Rectal protrusion or prolapse after defecation
- Sexual symptoms
  - Inability to have frequent intercourse
  - Dyspareunia
  - Lack of satisfaction or orgasm
  - Incontinence during sexual activity
- Other local symptoms
  - Pressure or heaviness in the vagina
  - Pain in the vagina or perineum
  - Low back pain after long periods of standing
  - Palpable bulge in the vaginal vault
  - Difficulty walking due to a protrusion from the vagina
  - Difficulty inserting or keeping a tampon in place
  - Vaginal-cervical mucosa hypertrophy, excoriation, ulceration, and bleeding
  - Abdominal pressure or pain

Sources: Feiner, Baessler, & Glazener, 2010; O'Dell, K. K., & Morse, A. N. (2008). It's not all about birth: Biomechnics applied to pelvic organ prolapsed prevention. *Journal of Midwifery and Women's Health*, 53(1), 28–36; Strohbehn, K., & Richter, H. E. (2008). Operative management of pelvic organ prolapsed. In R. S. Gibbs, B. Y. Karlan, A. F. Haney, I. E. Nygaard (Eds.). *Danforth's obstetrics and gynecology* (pp. 839–865). Philadelphia: Wolters Kluwer; & Word, A., Pathi, S, & Schaffer, J. I. (2009). Pathophysiology of pelvic organ prolapsed. *Obstetrics and Gynecology Clinics of North America*, 36(3), 521–530.

specific organism if present, visualization of urine loss during the pelvic examination, and measurement of postvoid urine volume.

Nursing Management

Help the woman understand the nature of the condition, the treatment options, and the likely outcomes. Nursing considerations might include the following:

- Describe normal anatomy and causes of pelvic prolapse.
- Assess how this condition has affected the woman's life.
- Outline the options, with the advantages and disadvantages of each.

- Allow the client to make the decision that is right for her.
- Provide education.
- Schedule preoperative activities needed for surgery.
- Reassure the client that there is a solution for her symptoms.
- Provide community education about genital prolapse.

Nursing Care Plan 7.1 provides an overview of care for a woman with POP.

Encourage Pelvic Floor Muscle Training

Encourage the woman to perform Kegel exercises daily (Teaching Guideline 7.1). Discuss current research findings and educate the woman about hormone therapy, allowing the woman to make her own decision on whether to use hormones.

Encourage Dietary and Lifestyle Modifications

Instruct clients to increase dietary fibre and fluids to prevent constipation. A high-fibre diet with an increase in fluid intake alleviates constipation by increasing stool bulk and stimulating peristalsis. It is accomplished by replacing refined, low-fibre foods with high-fibre foods. In addition to increasing the amount of fibre in her diet, also encourage the woman to drink eight 250 mL (8 oz) glasses of fluid daily and to engage in regular aerobic exercise, which promotes muscle tone and stimulates peristalsis.

Educate the client about other lifestyle changes that will assist with prolapse, such as:

- Achieve ideal weight to reduce intra-abdominal pressure and strain on pelvic organs, including pressure on the bladder.
- Wear a girdle or abdominal support to support the muscles surrounding the pelvic organs.
- Avoid lifting heavy objects to reduce the risk of increasing intra-abdominal pressure, which can push the pelvic organs downward.

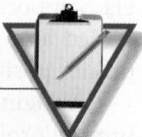

TEACHING GUIDELINE 7.1

Performing Kegel Exercises

- Squeeze the muscles in your rectum as if you are trying to prevent passing flatus.
- Stop and start urinary flow to help identify the pubococcygeus muscle.
- Tighten the pubococcygeus muscle for a count of three, and then relax it.
- Contract and relax the pubococcygeus muscle rapidly 10 times.
- Try to bring up the entire pelvic floor and bear down 10 times.
- Repeat Kegel exercises at least five times daily.

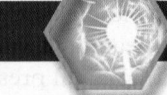

Nursing Care Plan 7.1

OVERVIEW OF A WOMAN WITH PELVIC ORGAN PROLAPSE (POP)

Katherine, a 62-year-old multiparous woman, came to her gynecologist with complaints of a chronic dragging or heavy painful feeling in her pelvis, lower backache, constipation, and urine leakage. Her symptoms increase when she stands for long periods. She hasn't had menstrual cycles for at least a decade. She tells you, "I'm not taking any of those menopausal hormones."

NURSING DIAGNOSIS: Pain related to relaxation of pelvic support and elimination difficulties

Outcome Identification and Evaluation
Client will report an acceptable level of discomfort within 1 to 2 hours of intervention as evidenced by a rating of less than 4 on a 0-to-10 pain scale.

Interventions: Providing Pain Management
* Obtain a thorough pain history, including ongoing pain experiences, methods of pain control used, what worked, what didn't, any allergies to pain medications, and the effect of pain on her activities of daily living *to provide a baseline and enable a systematic approach to pain management.*
* Assess the location, frequency, severity, duration, precipitating factors, and aggravating/alleviating factors *to identify characteristics of the client's pain to plan appropriate interventions.*
* Educate client about any medications prescribed (correct dosage, route, side effects, and precautions) *to increase the client's understanding of the therapy and promote compliance.*
* Assess problematic elimination patterns *to identify underlying factors from which to plan appropriate prevention strategies.*
* Encourage client to increase fluids and fibre in diet and increase physical activity daily *to promote peristalsis.*
* Assist client with establishing regular toileting patterns by setting aside time daily for bowel elimination *to promote regular bowel function and evacuation.*
* Urge client to avoid the routine use of laxatives *to reduce risk of compounding constipation.*

NURSING DIAGNOSIS: Knowledge deficit related to causes of structural disorders and treatment options

Outcome Identification and Evaluation
Client will demonstrate understanding of current condition and treatments as evidenced by identifying treatment options, making health-promoting lifestyle choices, verbalizing appropriate health care practices, and adhering to treatment plan.

Interventions: Provide Client Education
* Assess client's understanding of pelvic organ prolapse and its treatment options *to provide a baseline for teaching.*
* Review information provided about surgical procedures and recommendations for healthy lifestyle, obtaining feedback frequently, *to validate client's understanding of instructions.*
* Discuss association between uterine, bladder, and rectal prolapse and symptoms *to help client understand the etiology of her symptoms and pain.*
* Have client verbalize and discuss information related to diagnosis, surgical procedure, preoperative routine, and postoperative regimen *to ensure adequate understanding and provide time for correcting or clarifying any misinformation or misconceptions.*
* Provide written material with pictures *to promote learning and help client visualize what has occurred to her body secondary to aging, weight gain, childbirth, and gravity.*
* Discuss pros and cons of hormone replacement therapy, osteoporosis prevention, and cardiovascular events common in postmenopausal women *to promote informed decision making by the client about available menopausal therapies.*
* Inform client about the availability of community resources and make appropriate referrals as needed *to provide additional education and support.*
* Document details of teaching and learning *to allow for continuity of care and further education, if needed.*

• Avoid high-impact aerobics, jogging, or jumping repeatedly to minimize the risk of increasing intra-abdominal pressure, which places downward pressure on the organs.
• Give up smoking to minimize the risk for a chronic "smoker's cough," which increases intra-abdominal pressure and forces the pelvic organs downward.

Provide Teaching for Pessary Use

Educate the woman about pessary use. Discuss complications as part of the instruction. Although the pessary is a safe device, it is still a foreign body in the vagina. Because of this, the most common side effects of pessary use are increased vaginal discharge, urinary tract infections, vaginitis, and odour. These effects can be reduced by douching with dilute vinegar or hydrogen peroxide. Postmenopausal women with thin vaginal mucosa are susceptible to vaginal ulceration with the use of a pessary. Advise the woman to use estrogen cream to make the vaginal mucosa more resistant to erosion and to strengthen the vaginal walls.

The woman must be capable of managing the use of the pessary, either alone or with the help of a caretaker. The most common recommendations for pessary care include removing the pessary twice weekly and cleaning it with soap and water; using a lubricant for insertion; and having regular follow-up examinations every 6 to 12 months after an initial period of adjustment. Educate the woman in the care of her pessary so she feels comfortable with all aspects of care before leaving the health care facility.

Provide Perioperative Care

Prepare the woman for surgery by reinforcing the risks and benefits of surgery and describing the postoperative course. Explain that a Foley catheter will be in place for up to 1 week, and that she might not be able to urinate due to the swelling after the catheter has been removed. Provide home care instructions for the Foley catheter. She should cleanse the perineal area daily with mild soap and water, especially around where the catheter enters the urinary meatus. If the woman is provided with a leg bag to be worn during waking hours, instruct her to empty it frequently and keep it below the level of the bladder to prevent backflow. The same principles are applied to the primary Foley bag when emptying.

During the recovery period, instruct the client to avoid for several weeks activities that cause an increase in abdominal pressure, such as straining, sneezing, and coughing. In addition, advise her to avoid lifting anything heavy or straining to push anything. Explain to the woman that stool softeners and gentle laxatives might be prescribed to prevent constipation and straining with bowel movements. Pelvic rest will be prescribed until the operative area is healed in 6 weeks.

Promote Prevention Strategies

Limited data are available on ways to prevent POP. Approaches include lifestyle changes that reduce modifiable risk factors, such as losing weight, avoiding heavy lifting, and relieving constipation. Explore with the woman what factors in her lifestyle might be modified to reduce her risk of developing POP (primary prevention) or improve her quality of life after receiving treatment (secondary prevention).

Urinary Incontinence

Urinary incontinence is the involuntary loss of urine sufficient enough to be a social or hygiene problem (Vasavada, Carmel, & Rackley, 2012). It has been estimated that 10% to 40% of women experience urinary incontinence at some time in their lives, varying in severity from mild to severe (Dannecker, Friese, Stief, et al., 2010). It is more common than diabetes and Alzheimer's disease, both of which receive a great deal of press attention. About half the women with incontinence have never discussed the problem with their health care provider because they feel ashamed or embarrassed (Howard & Steggall, 2010).

> ▶ **Take** NOTE!
>
> *Incontinence is preventable, treatable, and often curable. However, many women believe that loss of bladder function is a normal and expected part of aging.*

Incontinence can have far-reaching effects. Some women experience anxiety, depression, social isolation, and disruptions in their self-esteem and dignity. It can cause the woman to stop working, travelling, socializing, and enjoying sexual relationships. In addition, incontinence can create a tremendous burden for caretakers and is a common reason for admission to a long-term care facility (Vasavada, Carmel, & Rackley., 2012).

The three most common types of incontinence are urge incontinence (overactive bladder caused by detrusor muscle contractions), stress incontinence (inadequate urinary sphincter function), and mixed incontinence (involves both stress and urge incontinence) (Vasavada et al., 2012). Comparison Chart 7.1 details the differences between stress and urge incontinence.

Pathophysiology and Etiology

Urinary continence requires several factors, including effective functioning of the bladder, adequate pelvic floor muscles, neural control from the brain, and integrity of the neural connections that facilitate voluntary control. The bladder neck and proximal urethra function as a sphincter. During urination the sphincter relaxes and the bladder empties. The ability to control urination requires

COMPARISON CHART 7.1 URGE INCONTINENCE VERSUS STRESS INCONTINENCE

	Urge Incontinence	Stress Incontinence
Description	Precipitous loss of urine, preceded by a strong urge to void, with increased bladder pressure and detrusor contraction	Accidental leakage of urine that occurs with increased pressure on the bladder from coughing, sneezing, laughing, or physical exertion
Etiology	Causes might be neurologic, idiopathic, or infectious	Develops commonly in women in their 40s and 50s, usually as the result of weakened muscles and ligaments in the pelvis following childbirth
Signs and Symptoms	Urgency, frequency, nocturia, and a large amount of urine loss	Involuntary loss of a small amount of urine in response to physical activity that raises intra-abdominal pressure

the integrated function of numerous components of the lower urinary tract, which must be structurally sound and function normally. Incontinence can develop if the bladder muscles become overactive due to weakened sphincter muscles, if the bladder muscles become too weak to contract properly, or if signals from the nervous system to the urinary structures are interrupted. A major factor in women that contributes to urinary continence is the estrogen level, because this hormone helps maintain bladder sphincter tone. In perimenopausal or menopausal women, incontinence can be a problem as estrogen levels begin to decline and genitourinary changes occur. In simple terms, the bladder is the reservoir, the urethra is the seal, and the levator ani muscle is the gate that holds pressure against the outflow of urine by supporting the urethra and bladder from below. When there is a dysfunction of any of the three structures, incontinence occurs.

Contributing factors in urinary incontinence include:

- Fluid intake, particularly caffeinated beverages: adequate fluid intake is necessary, but caffeinated beverages can provoke urgency.
- Constipation: alters the position of the pelvic organs and puts pressure on the bladder
- Habitual "preventive" emptying: may result in training the bladder to hold only small amounts of urine
- Advancing age: age-related anatomic changes provide less pelvic support
- Pregnancy and childbirth: damage to pelvic structures during childbirth
- Smoking: risk of damage to urinary sphincter from chronic coughing and bladder irritation from tobacco by-products
- Obesity: increases abdominal pressure (Amir & Bent, 2008; Goode, Burgio, Richter, et al., 2010)

Therapeutic Management

Treatment options depend on the type of urinary incontinence. In general, the least invasive procedure with the fewest risks is the first choice for treatment. Surgery is used only if other methods have failed. There is a widespread belief that urinary incontinence is an inevitable problem of getting older and that little or nothing can be done to relieve symptoms or reverse it. Nothing is further from the truth, and attitudes must change so that women feel comfortable seeking help for this embarrassing condition.

For many women with urge incontinence, simple reassurance and lifestyle interventions might help. However, if more than simple lifestyle measures are needed, effective treatments might include:

- Bladder training to establish normal voiding intervals (every 3 to 5 hours)
- Kegel exercises to strengthen the pelvic floor musculature
- Pessary ring to support pelvic structures that have weakened
- Pharmacotherapy to reduce the urge to void. Anticholinergic agents such as oxybutynin or tolterodine might be prescribed. The most common side effects of anticholinergic agents include dry mouth and confusion, so consideration for use in the elderly must be taken (Johnston, 2006). Imipramine, an antidepressant with anticholinergic and alpha-adrenergic effects, may enhance urethral sphincter tone and be useful for mixed urinary incontinence.

For women with stress incontinence, treatment is not always a cure, but it can minimize the impact of this condition on the woman's quality of life. Some treatment options for stress incontinence might include:

- Weight loss if needed
- Avoidance of constipation
- Smoking cessation
- Kegel exercises to strengthen the pelvic floor
- Pessaries
- Weighted vaginal cones to improve the tone of pelvic floor muscles

- Periurethral injection (injecting a bulking agent [collagen] to form a bulge that brings the urethral walls closer together to achieve a better closure)
- Alpha-adrenergic agonists. These drugs have had variable results in enhancing intrinsic urethral sphincter tone and have serious side effects of hypertension and cardiac arrhythmias (Johnston, 2006).
- Surgery to correct genital prolapse and improve urethral and bladder tone

Nursing Assessment

The assessment of the incontinent woman includes a history, physical examination, laboratory tests, and possibly urodynamic testing. The onset, frequency, severity, and pattern of incontinence should be determined, as well as any associated symptoms such as frequency, dysuria, urgency, and nocturia. Incontinence may be quantified by asking the woman if she wears a pad and how often the pad is changed. A review of the woman's current medications, including over-the-counter medications, should be included in the history.

A complete physical examination should be carried out by the health care provider; it should include a neurologic assessment and pelvic and rectal examinations. The presence of associated POP should be noted because it can contribute to the woman's voiding problems and may have an impact on diagnosis and treatment. A rectal examination is done to evaluate sphincter tone and perineal sensation.

A urinalysis is performed to look for hematuria, pyuria, glucosuria, or proteinuria. A urine culture is done if there is pyuria or bacteriuria. Postvoid residual should be measured either with pelvic ultrasound or directly with a catheter. If the residual exceeds the limit set, urodynamic testing is then used to diagnose the incontinence.

Nursing Management

Incontinence can be devastating and can cause psychosocial concerns and isolation. Nurses can encourage women with troublesome symptoms to seek help. Discuss the treatment options with the client, including benefits and potential outcomes, and encourage her to select the continence treatment best for her lifestyle. Provide education about good bladder habits and strategies to reduce the incidence or severity of incontinence (Teaching Guideline 7.2). Provide support and encouragement to ensure compliance. Remember that aging can increase the risk of incontinence, but incontinence is not an inevitable part of aging. Review the anatomy and physiology of the urinary system and offer simple explanations to help the woman cope with urinary alterations. Therapeutic listening is important. Be aware of the courage it takes for a woman to disclose an embarrassing condition.

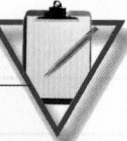

TEACHING GUIDELINE 7.2

Managing Urinary Incontinence

- Avoid drinking too much fluid (i.e., 1.5 L total daily limit), but do not decrease your intake of fluids.
- Reduce intake of fluids and foods that are bladder irritants and precipitate urgency, such as chocolate, caffeine, carbonated beverages, alcohol, artificial sweetener, hot spicy foods, orange juice, and tomatoes (Women's Health Matters, 2012).
- Increase fibre and fluids in your diet to reduce constipation.
- Control blood glucose levels to prevent polyuria.
- Treat chronic cough.
- Remove any barriers that delay you from reaching the toilet.
- Practice good perineal hygiene by using mild soap and water. Wipe from front to back to prevent urinary tract infections.
- Become aware of adverse drug effects.
- Take your medications as prescribed.
- Continue to do pelvic floor (Kegel) exercises.

▶ *Consider* THIS!

Life can be complicated and embarrassing at times when we least expect it. I met a man in church who seemed interested in me, and he asked me out for coffee after Sunday services. I have been alone for 10 years and this prospect seemed exciting to me. We talked for hours over coffee and seemed to have a great deal in common, especially since both of us had lost our spouses to cancer. He asked me to go square dancing with him, since that was an activity we both had enjoyed in the past with our spouses. I hadn't been out or physically active for ages and didn't realize how my body had changed with age.

It was during the first dance that I noticed a wet sensation between my legs, which I was unable to control. I managed to continue on and pretend that all was fine, but then realized what many of my friends were talking about—stress incontinence. Not being able to control one's urine is very embarrassing and it complicates your life, but I made up my mind that it wasn't going to control me!

Thoughts: Gravity and childbirth take a toll on women's reproductive organs by bringing them downward. This woman is not going to let stress incontinence curtail her outside activity, which demonstrates a good attitude. What can be done about her embarrassing accidents? Were there any preventive strategies she could have used at an earlier age?

Benign Growths

The most common benign growths of the reproductive tract include cervical, endocervical, and endometrial polyps; uterine fibroids (leiomyomas); ovarian cysts; genital fistulas; and Bartholin's cysts.

Polyps

Polyps are small benign growths. The cause of polyp growth is not well understood, but they are frequently the result of infection. Polyps might be associated with chronic inflammation, an abnormal local response to increased levels of estrogen, or local congestion of the cervical vasculature (Schnatz, Ricci, & O'Sullivan, 2009). Single or multiple polyps might occur. They are most common in multiparous women. Polyps can appear anywhere but are most common on the cervix and in the uterus (Fig. 7.3).

Cervical polyps often appear after menarche. Endocervical polyps are commonly found in multiparous women between 40 and 60 years of age. Endocervical polyps are more common than cervical polyps, with a stalk of varied width and length. Endometrial polyps are benign tumours or localized overgrowths of the endometrium. Most endometrial polyps are solitary, and they

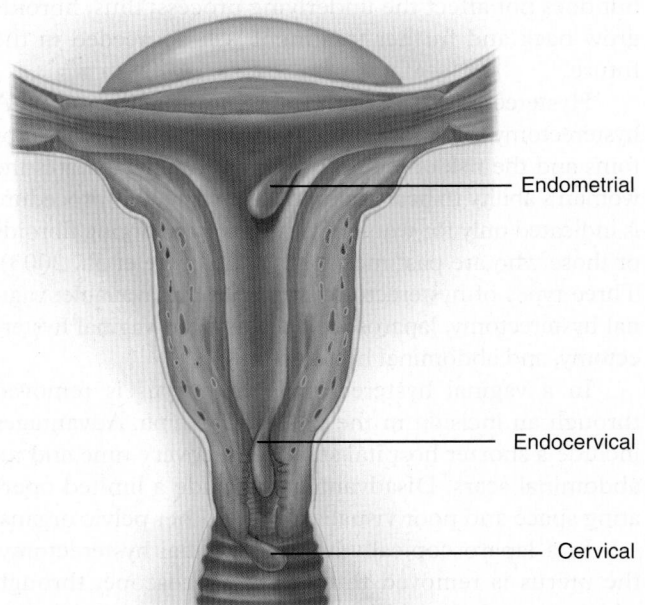

FIGURE 7.3 Cervical, endocervical, and endometrial polyps.

rarely occur in women younger than 20 years of age. The incidence of these polyps rises steadily with increasing age, peaks in the fifth decade of life, and gradually declines after menopause. They often present with abnormal bleeding (Schnatz et al., 2009).

Therapeutic Management

Treatment of polyps usually consists of simple removal with small forceps done on an outpatient basis, removal during hysteroscopy, or dilation and curettage (D&C). The polyp base can be removed by laser vaporization. Because many polyps are infected, an antibiotic may be ordered after removal as a preventive measure or to treat early signs of infection.

Although polyps are rarely cancerous, a specimen should be sent after surgery to a pathology laboratory to exclude malignancy. A cervical biopsy typically reveals mildly atypical cells and signs of infection. Polyps rarely return after they are removed. Regularly scheduled Pap smears are suggested for women with cervical polyps to detect any future abnormal growths that may be malignant.

Nursing Assessment

Nursing assessment for a woman with polyps includes assisting with the physical examination and preparing the collected specimen to be sent to the cytologist.

Clinical Manifestations

Assess for clinical manifestations of polyps, which arise from the endocervical canal and sometimes from the ectocervix. These fleshy growths are often pedunculated and range in colour from red to purplish red (Schnatz et al., 2009). Cervical and endocervical polyps are often asymptomatic, but they can produce mild symptoms such as abnormal vaginal bleeding (after intercourse or douching, between menses) or discharge. The most common clinical manifestation of endometrial polyps is metrorrhagia (irregular, acyclic uterine bleeding).

Physical Examination and Laboratory and Diagnostic Studies

Typically, cervical polyps are diagnosed when the cervix is visualized through a speculum during the woman's annual gynecologic examination. Endometrial polyps are not detected on physical examination but rather with ultrasound or hysteroscopy (introduction of a small camera through the cervix to visualize the uterine cavity).

Nursing Management

Nursing management of polyps involves explaining the condition and the rationale for removal and giving follow-up care instructions. The nurse also assists the health care provider with the removal procedure.

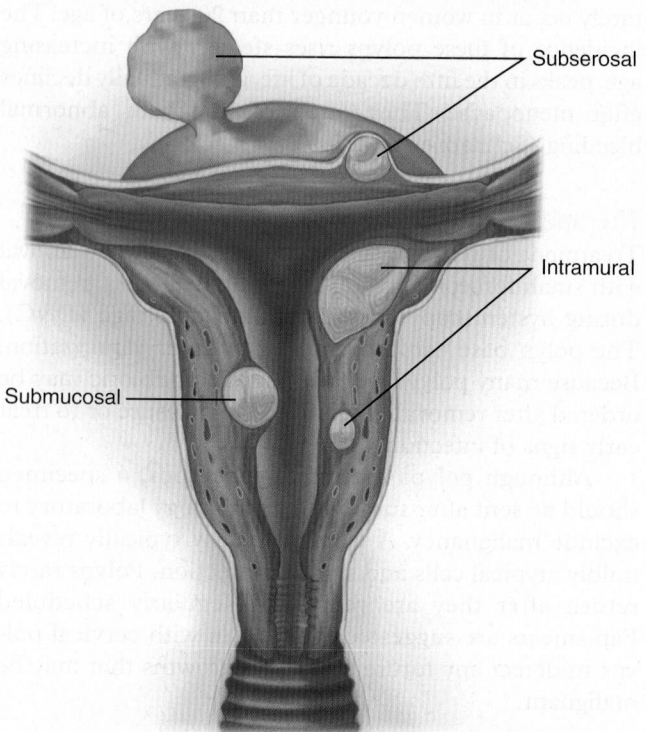

FIGURE 7.4 Submucosal, intramural, and subserosal fibroids.

Uterine Fibroids

Uterine fibroids, or leiomyomas, are benign proliferations composed of smooth muscle and fibrous connective tissue in the uterus. Fibroids can occur in the submucous layer, the intramural layer, or the subserous layer of the uterus (Fig. 7.4). They are estrogen-dependent and thus grow rapidly during the childbearing years, when estrogen is plentiful, but they shrink during menopause, when estrogen levels decline. It is believed that these benign tumours develop in up to 20% of women older than age 35 and 40% of women older than 50 (Aeby & Dantas, 2010). Fibroids are the most common indication for hysterectomy in Canada.

Etiology

Although the cause of fibroids is unknown, several predisposing factors have been identified, including:

• Age (late reproductive years)
• Genetic predisposition
• African ethnicity
• Nulliparity
• Steroid hormone concentrations (Gupta, Holloway, & Kubba, 2010)

Therapeutic Management

Treatment depends on the size of the fibroids and the woman's symptoms. There are several options, from watchful waiting to surgery.

Medical Management

Medical therapy should be tailored to the woman's needs and geared toward alleviating the symptoms (Lefebvre, Vilos, Allaire, et al., 2003). Gonadotropin-releasing hormone (GnRH) agonists, available as a nasal spray, slow release injection, and subcutaneous injection, can shrink the fibroids within 3 months by up to 50% of the original volume. Tranexamic acid may decrease the menorrhagia that is associated with fibroids. Danazol has been shown to reduce fibroid volume by 20% to 25%. The cost and side effects of medical treatments may limit their long-term use (Lefebvre et al., 2003). Once therapy is stopped, the fibroids typically recur.

Uterine artery embolization (UAE) is an option in which polyvinyl alcohol pellets, trisacryl gelatin microspheres, and gelatin sponge are injected into selected blood vessels via a catheter to block circulation to the fibroid, causing it to shrink and producing symptom resolution (Goodwin & Spies, 2009). After treatment, the fibroids shrink over the course of months to years, but they may recur. The effect of UAE on future pregnancy is unknown because ovarian function may be impaired by the procedure.

Surgical Management

For women with large fibroids or severe menorrhagia, surgery is preferred over medical treatment. Surgical management might involve myomectomy, laser surgery, or hysterectomy.

Myomectomy involves removing the fibroid alone. Myomectomy is performed via laparoscopy, either through either abdominal incision or via a vaginal approach. The advantage is that only the fibroid is removed; fertility is not jeopardized because this procedure leaves the uterine muscle walls intact. Myomectomy relieves symptoms but does not affect the underlying process; thus, fibroids grow back and further treatment will be needed in the future.

Hysterectomy is the surgical removal of the uterus. A hysterectomy to remove fibroids eliminates both the symptoms and the risk of recurrence, but it also terminates the woman's ability to bear children. Therefore, this procedure is indicated only for women with rapidly enlarging fibroids or those who are past menopause (Lefebvre et al., 2003). Three types of hysterectomy surgeries are available: vaginal hysterectomy, laparoscopically assisted vaginal hysterectomy, and abdominal hysterectomy.

In a vaginal hysterectomy, the uterus is removed through an incision in the posterior vagina. Advantages include a shorter hospital stay and recovery time and no abdominal scars. Disadvantages include a limited operating space and poor visualization of other pelvic organs.

In a laparoscopically assisted vaginal hysterectomy, the uterus is removed through a laparoscope, through which structures within the abdomen and pelvis are visualized. Small incisions are made in the abdominal wall to permit the laparoscope to enter the surgical site. Advantages include a better surgical field, less pain, lower health care costs, and a shorter recovery time. Disadvantages include potential injury to the bladder and the inability to remove enlarged uteruses and scar tissue.

In abdominal hysterectomy, the uterus and other pelvic organs are removed through an incision in the abdomen. This procedure allows the surgeon to visualize all pelvic organs and is typically used when a malignancy is suspected or a very large uterus is present. Disadvantages include the need for general anesthesia, a longer hospital stay and recovery period, more pain, higher health care costs, and a visible scar on the abdomen.

Nursing Assessment

Nursing assessment for the woman with uterine fibroids includes a thorough health history and physical examination.

Health History and Clinical Manifestations

The history should include questions about the woman's menstrual cycle, including alterations in the menstrual pattern (e.g., pain or pressure, aggravating and alleviating factors), history of infertility, and any history of spontaneous abortion, which might indicate a space-occupying uterine lesion. Ask if any female relatives have had fibroids, as there is a familial predisposition. Assess for clinical manifestations of uterine fibroids. Symptoms of fibroids depend on their size and location and may include:

- Chronic pelvic pain
- Low back pain
- Iron deficiency anemia secondary to bleeding
- Bloating
- Infertility (with large tumours)
- Dysmenorrhea
- Dyspareunia
- Urinary frequency, urgency, or incontinence
- Irregular vaginal bleeding (menorrhagia)
- Feeling of heaviness in the pelvic region

Physical Examination and Laboratory and Diagnostic Studies

The bimanual examination performed by the health care provider typically shows an enlarged, irregular uterus. The uterus may be palpable abdominally if the fibroid is very large. Ultrasound may be used to confirm the diagnosis.

Nursing Management

Provide information about surgery so the woman can make an informed decision. Offer a thorough explanation of the procedure and aftercare (Box 7.2). A woman undergoing a hysterectomy for the treatment of fibroids often needs special care.

Genital Fistulas

Genital fistulas are abnormal openings between a genital tract organ and another organ, such as the urinary tract or the gastrointestinal tract. A fistula can result from a congenital anomaly, surgical complications, Bartholin's gland abscesses, radiation, or malignancy, but the majority of fistulas that occur worldwide are related to obstetric trauma (Schorge, Schaffer, Halvorson, et al., 2008). During normal labour, the bladder is displaced upward into the abdomen and the anterior vaginal wall, the base of the bladder, and the urethra are compressed between the fetal head and the posterior pubis. When labour is obstructed or prolonged, this unrelieved compression causes ischemia, which causes pressure necrosis and subsequent fistula formation.

Common types of fistulas include:

- Vesicovaginal: communication between the bladder and the genital tract
- Urethrovaginal: communication between the urethra and the vagina
- Rectovaginal: communication between the rectum or sigmoid colon and the vagina

The direct consequences of this damage include urinary incontinence and fecal incontinence if the rectum is involved. This tragic condition has plagued women since the beginning of history (Spurlock, 2012).

Therapeutic Management

Many small fistulas will heal without treatment, but large fistulas often require surgical repair; surgery may be postponed until the edema or inflammation in the surrounding tissues has dissipated. Surgical repair of fistulas is associated with a high success rate if it is done in a timely manner, but individualized intervention should be attempted, taking into account quality of life (Schorge et al., 2008).

Nursing Assessment

The history should include questions about any changes in the woman's urinary and bowel patterns. Assess for common signs and symptoms of fistulas, which are related to the type of fistula. If the opening involves the rectum, feces and flatus will leak through the vagina. If it involves the bladder, urine will leak from the vagina. Depending on the location and size of the fistula, the woman may or may not experience discomfort. The health care provider can detect these abnormal openings through inspection and palpation during the pelvic examination. Diagnostic or laboratory tests are generally not ordered once this condition is found.

Nursing Management

Provide guidance and support. Offer information to help the woman learn about her condition and, with

---

BOX 7.2 **Nursing Interventions for a Woman Undergoing a Hysterectomy**

Preoperative Care
- Instruct the patient and her family about the procedure and aftercare.
- Provide interventions to reduce anxiety (due to perceived threats to the woman's self-concept and role functioning) and fear of alteration in body image, complications, and pain. Prepare the woman so she knows what to expect throughout her perioperative experience. Explain postoperative pain management procedures that will be used. Identify the high-risk woman early to reduce her stress.
- Teach turning, deep breathing, and coughing before surgery to prevent postoperative atelectasis and respiratory complications such as pneumonia.
- Encourage the woman to discuss her feelings. Some women equate their femaleness with their reproductive capability, and loss of the uterus could evoke grieving.
- Complete all preoperative orders in a timely manner to allow for rest.

Postoperative Care
- Provide comfort measures.
- Administer analgesics promptly or use a patient-controlled analgesia pump.
- Administer antiemetics to control nausea and vomiting per order.
- Change the client's linens and gown frequently to promote hygiene.
- Change the client's position frequently and use pillows for support to promote comfort and pain management.
- Assess the incision, the dressing, and vaginal bleeding and report if bleeding is excessive (soaking perineal pad within an hour).

- Monitor elimination and provide increased fluids and fibre to prevent constipation and straining.
- Encourage ambulation and active range-of-motion exercises when in bed to prevent thrombophlebitis and venous stasis.
- Monitor vital signs to detect early complications.
- Be comfortable discussing sexual concerns with the client.

Discharge Planning
- Advise the client to reduce her activity level to avoid fatigue, which might inhibit healing.
- Advise the client to rest when she is tired and to increase her activity level slowly.
- Educate the client on the need for pelvic rest (nothing in the vagina) for 6 weeks.
- Instruct the client to avoid heavy lifting or straining for about 6 weeks to prevent an increase in intra-abdominal pressure, which could weaken her sutures.
- Teach the client the signs and symptoms of infection.
- Advise the woman to take showers instead of tub baths to reduce the risk for infection.
- Encourage the client to eat a healthy diet with increased intake of fluids to prevent dehydration and fluid and electrolyte imbalance.
- Instruct the client to change her perineal pad frequently to prevent infection.
- Explain and schedule follow-up care appointments as needed.
- Provide information about community resources for support/help.

---

appropriate intervention, to improve her quality of life. Begin by making sure the woman understands her anatomy and why she is having such symptoms. Provide a thorough explanation of the treatment options so that she can make an informed decision. Be sensitive to the woman's feeling of shame and fear about her incontinence; these feelings may be why she delayed seeking treatment. Address all of the woman's needs, both physical and emotional.

Bartholin's Cysts

A Bartholin's cyst is a swollen, fluid-filled, sac-like structure that results when one of the ducts of the Bartholin's gland becomes blocked. The cyst may become infected and an abscess may develop in the gland. The Bartholin's glands are two mucus-secreting glandular structures with duct openings bilaterally at the base of the labia minora near the opening of the vagina that provide lubrication during sexual arousal. Bartholin's cysts are common cystic growths in the vulva (Boardman, 2008).

Therapeutic Management

Treatment can be conservative or surgical depending on the symptoms, the size of the cyst, and whether it is infected or not. Small, asymptomatic cysts do not require treatment. For cysts that do require treatment, there are many nonsurgical options. Sitz baths along with analgesics are used to reduce discomfort. Antibiotics are prescribed if the gland is infected.

Treatment options include placement of a Word catheter for drainage, excision using carbon dioxide laser, needle aspiration, silver nitrate gland ablation, marsupialization, gland excision, and incision and drainage (Wechter, Wu, Marzano, et al., 2009). A review of the literature did not reveal a best treatment approach. Cysts or abscesses tend to recur. Treatment for a pregnant woman with a Bartholin's cyst depends on the severity of the symptoms and whether an infection is present. Surgery may be delayed until after the woman gives birth if there are no symptoms.

Nursing Assessment

Nursing assessment for the woman with a Bartholin's cyst includes a thorough health history and physical examination and laboratory and diagnostic tests.

Health History

The history should include questions about the woman's sexual practices and protective measures used. Assess for common signs and symptoms of Bartholin's cysts. The woman may be asymptomatic if the cyst is small (less than 5 cm) and not infected. If infection is present, symptoms include varying degrees of pain, especially when walking or sitting; unilateral edema; redness around the gland; and dyspareunia. Extensive inflammation may cause systemic symptoms. Abscess formation occurs when the cystic fluid becomes infected. An abscess usually develops rapidly over a 2- to 3-day period and may rupture spontaneously.

Physical Examination and Laboratory and Diagnostic Studies

The diagnosis of Bartholin's cysts or abscesses is primarily made during a physical examination when a protruding tender labial mass is located. Cultures of the purulent abscess fluid and of the cervix should be obtained for *Neisseria gonorrhoeae* and *Chlamydia trachomatis* to rule out a sexually transmitted infection.

Nursing Management

Nurses must be aware of and knowledgeable about vulvar cysts and treatment options. The woman may be aware of a vulvar cyst secondary to the pain or may be unaware if the cyst is asymptomatic. A Bartholin's cyst may be an incidental finding during a routine pelvic examination. Explain the cause of the cyst and assist with cultures if needed. Provide reassurance and support.

Ovarian Cysts

An **ovarian cyst** is a fluid-filled sac that forms on the ovary (Fig. 7.5). These very common growths are usually benign and are asymptomatic in many women (Gupta et al., 2010). When the cysts grow large and exert pressure on surrounding structures, women often seek medical help.

Types of Ovarian Cysts

The most common benign ovarian cysts are follicular cysts, corpus luteum (lutein) cysts, theca-lutein cysts, and polycystic ovarian syndrome (PCOS).

Follicular Cysts

Follicular cysts are caused by the failure of the ovarian follicle to rupture at the time of ovulation. Follicular cysts seldom grow larger than 5 cm in diameter; most regress and require no treatment. They can occur at any age but are more common in reproductive-aged women

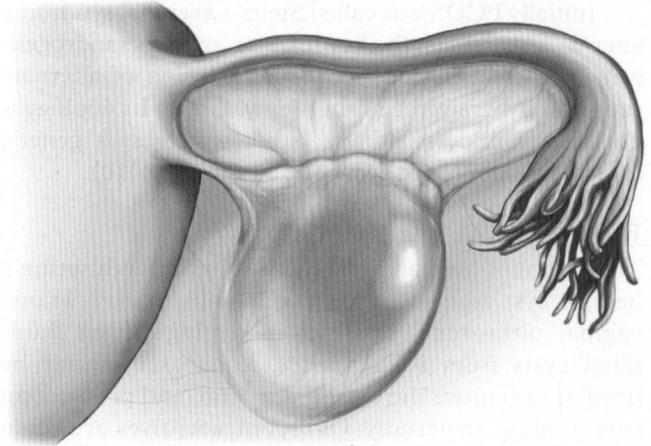

FIGURE 7.5 Ovarian cyst.

and are rare after menopause. They are detected by vaginal ultrasound.

Corpus Luteum (Lutein) Cysts

A corpus luteum cyst forms when the corpus luteum becomes cystic or hemorrhagic and fails to degenerate after 14 days. These cysts might cause pain and delay the next menstrual period. A pelvic ultrasound helps to make this diagnosis. Typically these cysts appear after ovulation and resolve without intervention.

Theca-Lutein Cysts

Prolonged abnormally high levels of human chorionic gonadotropin (hCG) stimulate the development of theca-lutein cysts. Although rare, these cysts are associated with hydatidiform mole, choriocarcinoma, PCOS, and Clomid therapy.

Polycystic Ovarian Syndrome

Polycystic ovary syndrome involves the presence of multiple inactive follicle cysts within the ovary that interfere with ovarian function. It is associated with obesity, hyperinsulinemia, elevated luteinizing hormone levels (linked to ovulation), elevated androgen levels (virilization), hirsutism (male-pattern hair growth), follicular atresia (ovarian growth failure), ovarian growth and cyst formation, anovulation (failure to ovulate), and amenorrhea (absence of menstruation or irregular periods). PCOS is the most common cause of androgen excess, affecting approximately 5% to 10% of women in the childbearing age group (Vause & Cheung, 2010).

▶ *Take* NOTE!

Careful attention should be given to PCOS because affected women are at increased risk for long-term health problems such as cardiovascular disease, type 2 diabetes, infertility, and cancer (Ferry, 2010).

Initially PCOS was called Stein–Leventhal syndrome after its researchers; the key features are hyperandrogenism, menstrual dysfunction, and exclusion of alternate causes of hyperandrogenism (Ferry, 2010). Its etiology is not clearly understood, but studies suggest a genetic (autosomal-dominant) component (Ferry, 2010).

Therapeutic Management

Treatment of ovarian cysts focuses on differentiating a benign cyst from a solid ovarian malignancy. Transvaginal ultrasound is useful in distinguishing fluid-filled cysts from solid masses. Laparoscopy may be needed to remove the cyst, if it is large and pressing on surrounding structures. Oral contraceptives are often prescribed to suppress gonadotropin levels, which may help resolve the cysts. Pain medication is also prescribed if needed.

Management of PCOS includes both drug and non-drug therapy, along with lifestyle modifications. Goals of therapy focus on reducing the production and circulating levels of androgens, protecting the endometrium against the effects of unopposed estrogens, supporting lifestyle changes to achieve ideal body weight, lowering the risk of cardiovascular disease, avoiding the effects of hyperinsulinemia on the risk of cardiovascular disease and diabetes, and inducing ovulation to achieve pregnancy if desired. Treatment modalities for PCOS are highlighted in Box 7.3.

BOX 7.3 Treatment Modalities for PCOS

- Oral contraceptives to treat menstrual irregularities and acne
- Mechanical hair removal (shaving, waxing, plucking, or electrolysis) to treat hirsutism
- Glucophage (metformin), which improves insulin uptake by fat and muscle cells, to treat hyperinsulinemia
- Ovulation induction agents (clomiphene citrate) as the first-line therapy
- Lifestyle changes (e.g., weight loss; exercise; balanced, low-fat, low glycemic index diets)
- Referral to support groups to help improve emotional state and build self-esteem

---

Sources: Barron, A. M., & Falsetti, D. (2008). Polycystic ovary syndrome in adolescents. *Advance for Nurse Practitioners, 16*(3), 49–54; Lindsey, A. B., & Mercurio, M.G. (2010). Hirsutism: Diagnosis and management. *Gender Medicine, 7*(2), 79–87; Marsh, K. A., Steinbeck, K. S., Atkinson, F. S., Petocz, P., & Brand-Miller, J. C. (2010). Effect of a low glycemic index compared with a conventional healthy diet on polycystic ovary syndrome. *American Journal of Clinical Nutrition, 92*(1), 83–92; & Vause, T. D. R., & Cheung, A. P. (2010). Ovulation induction in polycystic ovary syndrome. *SOGC Clinical Practice Guideline, 5*, 495–502.

Nursing Assessment

Nursing assessment for the woman with PCOS includes a thorough health history and physical examination as well as laboratory and diagnostic tests.

Health History

The history should include questions about the woman's symptoms, including onset, location, frequency, quality, intensity, and aggravating and alleviating factors of her discomfort. Note the last menstrual period and whether or not her cycles are regular. Ask about her overall general health and any changes recently noticed, such as a change in abdominal girth without a concomitant weight gain.

Assess for common signs and symptoms of ovarian cysts. Findings might include:

- Hirsutism (face and chin, upper lip, areola, lower abdomen, and perineum)
- Alopecia (frontal region and crown of head)
- Virilization (clitoral hypertrophy, deepening of voice, increased muscle mass, breast atrophy, male-pattern baldness)
- Menstrual irregularity and infertility (oligomenorrhea, amenorrhea, irregular menses, anovulation)
- Polycystic ovaries (numerous follicles on ovaries)
- Obesity (occurs in more than 50% of women with PCOS; occurs in abdominal region, with an increase in the waist–hip ratio)
- Insulin resistance (hyperinsulinemia, glucose intolerance)
- Dyslipidemia (reduced high-density lipoprotein, elevated serum triglycerides)
- Cardiovascular disease and hypertension
- Increased risk for endometrial cancer, ovarian cancer, breast cancer
- Psychological impact (depression, frustration, anxiety, eating disorders)
- Acne (face and shoulders) (Gupta et al., 2010)

Physical Examination and Laboratory and Diagnostic Studies

The physical examination includes inspection, auscultation, and palpation of the abdomen because large ovarian masses may cause visible changes in the abdomen. A complete pelvic examination is performed to assess the location, size, shape, texture, mobility, and tenderness of any palpable mass.

Diagnostic tests include a pregnancy test to rule out an ectopic pregnancy. Gonorrhea and chlamydia testing is warranted if an ovarian abscess is suspected. An ultrasound may be ordered to differentiate between functional or simple ovarian cysts and a solid tumour. Additional tests may be performed depending on the findings.

Remember Liz, the client with irregular menses, facial hair, and acne? Her glucose level is elevated, multiple cysts were felt on her ovaries during the pelvic examination, and laboratory tests found elevated lipid and lipoprotein levels. What education should the nurse provide Liz regarding her PCOS diagnosis? What medications might be prescribed to address her abnormal laboratory values?

Nursing Management

Nursing care should include education about the condition, treatment options, diagnostic test arrangements, and referral for surgery if needed. Provide support and reassurance during the diagnostic period to allay anxiety in the client and her family. Reassure the woman that the majority of ovarian cysts are benign, but regardless stress the importance of follow-up care. Listen to the woman's concerns about her appearance, infertility, and facial hair growth. Offer suggestions to help the woman feel better about herself and her health.

Nurses can have a positive impact on women with PCOS through counselling and education. Provide support for women dealing with negative self-image secondary to the physical manifestations of PCOS. Through education, help the woman understand the syndrome and its associated risk factors to prevent long-term health problems. Encourage the woman to make positive lifestyle changes. Make community referrals to local support groups to help the woman build her coping skills.

Liz returns to the clinic a month later for re-evaluation of her PCOS. She has been taking metformin to reduce her insulin resistance and has followed her exercise regimen and reduced her caloric intake to lose weight, but she still complains about her facial hair and acne. What interventions might be helpful to address this problem? What medication might also be prescribed to regularize her menses and relieve the hirsutism?

■■■ Key Concepts

- Pelvic support disorders such as pelvic organ prolapse and urinary and fecal incontinence are prevalent conditions in aging women. They cause significant physical and psychological morbidity, with obvious detriment to women's social interactions, emotional well-being, and overall quality of life.
- The four most common types of genital prolapse are cystocele, rectocele, enterocele, and uterine prolapse.
- The purpose of pelvic-floor exercises is to increase the muscle volume, which will result in a stronger muscular contraction. Kegel exercises might limit the progression

of mild prolapse and alleviate mild prolapse symptoms, including low back pain and pelvic pressure.

- Urinary incontinence is the involuntary loss of urine sufficient enough to be a social or hygiene problem.
- The three most common types of incontinence are urge incontinence (overactive bladder caused by detrusor muscle contractions), stress incontinence (inadequate urinary sphincter function), and mixed incontinence (involves both stress and urge incontinence).
- The most common benign growths of the reproductive tract include cervical, endocervical, and endometrial polyps; uterine fibroids (leiomyomas); and ovarian cysts.
- PCOS involves the presence of multiple inactive follicle cysts within the ovary that interfere with ovarian function. Hyperandrogenism, insulin resistance, and chronic anovulation characterize PCOS. Careful attention should be given to this condition because women with it are at increased risk for long-term health problems such as cardiovascular disease, hypertension, dyslipidemia, type 2 diabetes, and cancer (endometrial, breast, and ovarian).

REFERENCES

Aeby, T. C., & Dantas, S. (2010). Uterine leiomyomas. In E. T. Bope, R. E. Rakel, & R. D. Kellerman (Eds.), *Conn's current therapy 2010*. Philadelphia: Saunders.

Amir, B., & Bent, A. E. (2008). Nonsurgical management of urinary incontinence and overactive bladder. In R. S. Gibbs, B. Y. Karlan, A. F. Haney, I. E. Nygaard (Eds.), *Danforth's obstetrics and gynecology*. Philadelphia: Wolters Kluwer.

Atnip, S. D. (2009). Pessary use and management for pelvic organ prolapse. *Obstetrics and Gynecology Clinics of North America, 36*(3), 541–563.

Barron, A. M., & Falsetti, D. (2008). Polycystic ovary syndrome in adolescents. *Advance for Nurse Practitioners, 16*(3), 49–54.

Boardman, L.A. (2008). Benign vulvovaginal disorders. In R. S. Gibbs, B. Y. Karlan, A. F. Haney, & I. E. Nygaard (Eds.), *Danforth's obstetrics and gynecology*. Philadelphia: Wolters Kluwer.

Chan, M. C., Schultz, J. A., Flood, C. G., & Rosychuk, R. J. (2010). A retrospective review of patients seen in a multidisciplinary pelvic floor clinic. *Journal of Obstetrics and Gynaecology Canada, 32*(1), 35–40.

Dannecker, C., Friese, K., Stief, C., & Bauer, R.,(2010). Urinary incontinence in women. *Deutsches Arzteblatt International, 107*(24), 420–426.

Ferry, R. J. (2010). Polycystic ovarian syndrome: Follow-up. Retrieved February 1, 2012 from http://emedicine.medscape.com/article/924698-overview

Goode, P. S., Burgio, K. L., Richter, H. E., & Markland, A. D. (2010). Incontinence in older women. *Journal of the American Medical Association, 303*(21), 2172–2181.

Goodwin, S. C., & Spies, J. B. (2009). Uterine fibroid embolization. *New England Journal of Medicine, 361*(7), 690–697.

Gupta, S., Holloway, D., & Kubba, A. (2010). *Oxford handbook of women's health nursing*. New York: Oxford University Press.

Howard, F., & Steggall, M. (2010). Urinary incontinence in women: Quality of life and help-seeking. *British Journal of Nursing, 19*(12), 742–749.

Johnston, S. (2006). Urogenital concerns. *Journal of Obstetrics and Gynaecology Canada, 28*(2), S33–S42.

Lazarou, B., & Grigorescu, B. A. (2012). Pelvic organ prolapse. Retrieved February 2, 2012 from http://emedicine.medscape.com/article/276259-overview

Lefebvre, G., Vilos, G., Allaire, C., & Jeffrey, J. (2003). The management of uterine leiomyomas. *Journal of Obstetrics and Gynaecology Canada, 5,* 1–10.

Lindsey, A. B., & Mercurio, M. G. (2010). Hirsutism: Diagnosis and management. *Gender Medicine, 7*(2), 79–87.

Maher, C., Feiner, B., Baessler, K., & Glazener, K. (2010). Surgical management of pelvic organ prolapse in women. *Cochrane Database of Systematic Reviews, 4,* 1–202.

Marsh, K. A., Steinbeck, K. S., Atkinson, F. S., Petocz, P., & Brand-Miller, J. C. (2010). Effect of a low glycemic index compared with a conventional healthy diet on polycystic ovary syndrome. *American Journal of Clinical Nutrition, 92*(1), 83–92.

O'Dell, K. K., & Morse, A. N. (2008). It's not all about birth: Biomechanics applied to pelvic organ prolapsed prevention. *Journal of Midwifery and Women's Health, 53*(1), 28–36.

Rahn, D. D. (2009). Pathophysiology of urinary incontinence, voiding dysfunction, and overactive bladder. *Obstetrics and Gynecology Clinics of North America, 36*(3), 464–474.

Richardson, K., Hagen, S., Glazener, C., & Stark, D. (2009). The role of nurses in the management of women with pelvic organ prolapse. *British Journal of Nursing, 18*(5), 294–300.

Schorge, J. O., Schaffer, J. I., Halvorson, L. M., Hoffman, B. L., Bradshaw, K. D., & Cunningham, F. G. (2008). Genitourinary fistula and urethral diverticulum. In J. O. Schorge, J. I. Schaffer, L. M. Halvorson, B. L. Hoffman, K. D. Bradshaw, & F. G. Cunningham (Eds.), *Williams Gynecology.* Columbus, OH: McGraw-Hill Professional.

Schnatz, P. F., Ricci, S., & O'Sullivan, D. M. (2009). Cervical polyps in postmenopausal women: Is there a difference in risk? *Menopause, 16*(3), 524–528.

Society of Obstetricians and Gynaecologists Canada. (2006). Canadian consensus conference on menopause, 2006 uddate. *Journal of Obstetrics and Gynaecology Canada, 29*(Suppl), S7–S94. Retrieved February 5, 2012 from www.sogc.org/guidelines/public/171e-cons-february2006.pdf

Spurlock, J. (2012). Vesicovaginal fistula. Retrieved February 2, 2012 from http://emedicine.medscape.com/article/267943-overview

Strohbehn, K., & Richter, H. E. (2008). Operative management of pelvic organ prolapsed. In R. S. Gibbs, B. Y. Karlan, A. F. Haney, I. E. Nygaard (Eds.). *Danforth's obstetrics and gynecology.* Philadelphia: Wolters Kluwer.

Vasavada, S. P., Carmel, M. E., & Rackley, R. (2012). Urinary incontinence. Retrieved February 1, 2012 from http://emedicine.medscape.com/article/452289-overview

Vause, T. D. R., & Cheung, A. P. (2010). SOGC clinical practice guideline: Ovulation induction in polycystic ovary syndrome. *Journal of Obstetrics and Gynaecology Canada, 32*(5), 495–502. Retrieved February 2, 2012 from http://sogc.org/guidelines/documents/gui242CPG1005E.pdf

Wechter, M. E., Wu, J. M., Marzano, D., & Haefner, H. (2009). Management of Bartholin duct cysts and abscesses: A systematic review. *Obstetrical and Gynecological Survey, 64*(6), 395–404.

Women's Health Matters. (2012). *Coping.* Retrieved August 30, 2010 from http://www.womenshealthmatters.ca/health-resources/pelvic-health/urinary-incontinence/coping/

Word, A., Pathi, S, & Schaffer, J. I. (2009). Pathophysiology of pelvic organ prolapsed. *Obstetrics and Gynecology Clinics of North America, 36*(3), 521–530.

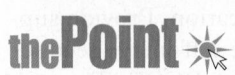

For additional learning materials, including Internet Resources, visit **http://thePoint.lww.com/Chow1e.**

CHAPTER WORKSHEET

MULTIPLE CHOICE QUESTIONS

1. When you are interviewing a patient with uterine fibroids, what subjective data would you expect to find in her history?

   a. Cyclic migraine headaches

   b. Urinary urgency

   c. Chronic pelvic pain

   d. Chronic constipation

2. Treatment options available for women with pelvic organ prolapse are:

   a. Pessaries and Kegel exercises

   b. External pelvic fixation devices

   c. Weight gain and yoga

   d. Firm panty-and-girdle garments

3. Which of the following dietary and lifestyle modifications might the nurse recommend to help prevent pelvic relaxation as women age?

   a. Eat a high-fibre diet to avoid constipation and straining.

   b. Avoid sitting for long periods; get up and walk around frequently.

   c. Limit the amount of exercise to prevent overdeveloping muscles.

   d. Space children a year apart to reduce wear and tear on the uterus.

4. Women with PCOS are at increased risk for developing which of the following long-term health problems?

   a. Osteoporosis

   b. Lupus

   c. Type 2 diabetes

   d. Migraine headaches

5. Side effects experienced by women taking GnRH agonists for the treatment of fibroids closely resemble those of:

   a. Osteoporosis

   b. Osteoarthritis

   c. Depression

   d. Menopause

CRITICAL THINKING EXERCISE

1. Faith, a 42-year-old multiparous woman, presents to the women's health clinic complaining of pelvic pain, menorrhagia, and vaginal discharge. She says she has been having these problems for several months. On examination, her uterus is enlarged and irregular in shape. Her blood studies reveal anemia.

   a. What condition might Faith have, based on her symptoms?

   b. What treatment options are available to address this condition?

   c. What educational interventions should the nurse discuss with Faith?

STUDY ACTIVITIES

1. Prepare an educational session to teach women how to do Kegel exercises to prevent stress incontinence and pelvic floor relaxation.

2. In a small group, discuss the personal, social, and sexual issues that might affect a woman with pelvic organ prolapse. How might these issues affect her socialization? How might a support group help?

3. List the symptoms that a woman with uterine fibroids might have. Discuss how these symptoms might mimic a more frightening condition and why the woman might delay seeking treatment.

4. A bladder that herniates into the vagina is a _____.

5. A rectum that herniates into the vagina is a _____.

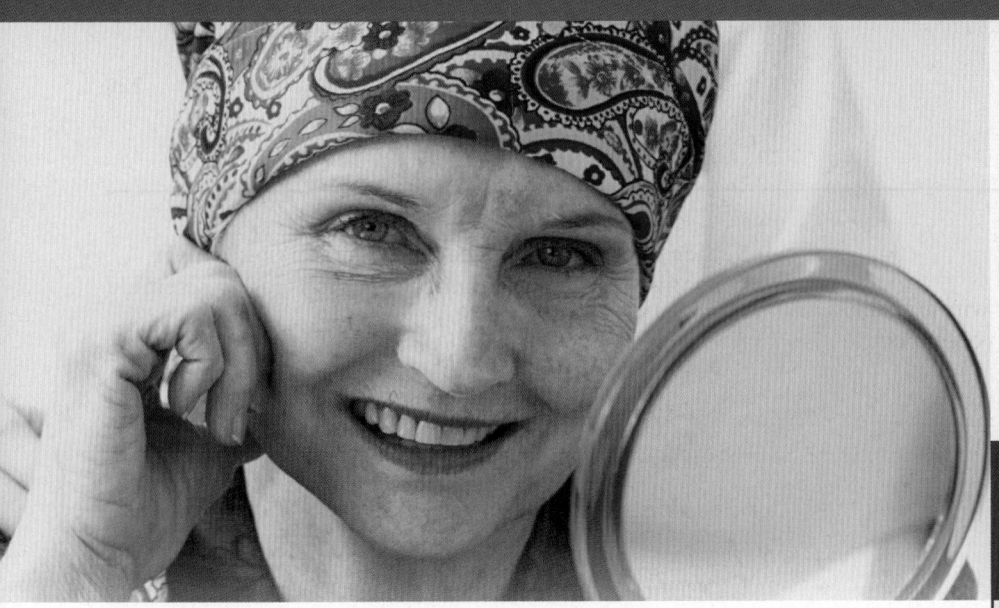

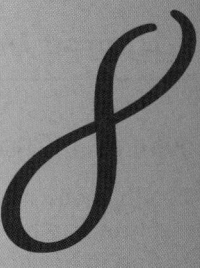

CHAPTER 8

Adapted by Shelley Cobbett

CANCERS OF THE FEMALE REPRODUCTIVE TRACT

KEY TERMS

cervical cancer
cervical dysplasia
colposcopy
cone biopsy

cryotherapy
endometrial cancer
human papillomavirus
ovarian cancer

Papanicolaou (Pap) test
vaginal cancer
vulvar cancer

LEARNING OBJECTIVES

Upon completion of the chapter, the learner will be able to:

1. Define the key terms in the chapter.
2. Identify the major modifiable risk factors for reproductive tract cancers.
3. Discuss the risk factors, screening methods, and treatment modalities for cancers of the female reproductive tract.
4. Outline the nursing management needed for the most common malignant reproductive tract cancers in women.
5. Discuss lifestyle changes and health screenings that can reduce the risk of or prevent reproductive tract cancers.
6. List the community resources available for a woman undergoing surgery for cancer of the reproductive tract.
7. Explain the psychological distress felt by women diagnosed with cancer, and outline information that can help them to cope.

*C*armella is an obese, 55-year-old woman who presents to her health care provider with vaginal bleeding. She has been through menopause and wonders why she is having a period again. Her medical history includes infertility and hypertension. Three years ago she had a mastectomy for breast cancer, and she has been taking tamoxifen (Nolvadex-D) to prevent recurrent breast cancer since her surgery. What risk factors in Carmella's history might predispose her to a reproductive tract cancer? What additional information is needed to make a diagnosis?

WoW

The word "cancer" can strike fear into anyone who hears it. But when it involves a reproductive organ, this fear is often magnified.

Cancer is the leading cause of death among women in Canada, surpassing cardiovascular disease in 2003 (Statistics Canada, 2009). Women have a one-in-three lifetime risk of developing cancer, and one out of every four deaths is due to cancer (Canadian Cancer Society [CCS], 2009b). Approximately 81,700 new cases of cancer are diagnosed in women each year, with more than 23,000 cancer-related deaths annually in women ages 40 to 79 (CCS, 2009b). Cancer incidence is rising in young women ages 20 to 39 years. According to the CCS (2009b), an estimated 4,400 new cases of uterine cancer (5.4% of all cancers) and 2,500 cases of ovarian cancer (3% of all cancers) were diagnosed in 2009, with the estimated number of related deaths exceeding 800 and 1,750 respectively.

Breast, lung, and colorectal cancer account for over half of all female cancers, with breast cancer having the highest incidence (22,700 new cases) and lung cancer being the leading cause of death (9,400 deaths) (CCS, 2009b). Nurses need to focus their energies on screening, education, and early detection to reduce these numbers. Because cancer risk is strongly associated with lifestyle and behaviour, screening programs are of particular importance for early detection. Overall cancer incidence rates for women show modest increases, but mortality rates are declining, suggesting better survival for some cancers (CCS, 2009b).

This chapter begins with a nursing process overview of the care of women with reproductive cancer. It then describes selected cancers of the reproductive system—ovarian, endometrial, cervical, vaginal, and vulvar cancer. The chapter discusses the nurse's role through diagnosis, intervention, and follow-up care. Cancer management requires a multidisciplinary approach, including specialists in surgical, medical, and radiation oncology. The nurse can provide guidance and support to the client as she finds her way through the health care maze.

NURSING PROCESS OVERVIEW FOR THE WOMAN WITH CANCER OF THE REPRODUCTIVE TRACT

The word "cancer" is laden with fear and dread. These feelings may be worsened when the cancer involves a woman's reproductive tract. The diagnosis of a reproductive tract cancer can have a profound impact on a woman's sexuality because it affects the very core of her identity as a female. The loss of the reproductive body part as well as the possible loss of childbearing ability can have a significant effect on women and their partners. Nurses need to remember this impact when counselling women and their partners about cancer treatment and side effects and changes in gender roles and sexuality.

When a woman is first diagnosed with a reproductive tract cancer, two primary needs arise: information and emotional support. When the diagnosis is made, the woman typically has many questions, such as "What is going to happen to me?," "How will this change my life?," and "Will I survive?" Nurses can play a major role in helping women find the answers to their questions and directing them to the resources they need. Two reliable sources of general cancer information are the National Cancer Institute (NCI) of the United States and the CCS.

The nurse also plays a key role in offering emotional support, determining appropriate sources of support, and helping the woman use effective coping strategies. Schroevers, Schroevers, Helgeson, et al., (2010) found that the more emotional support received after a cancer diagnosis, the greater the positive consequences of the illness will be for the woman. Women without a social support network may need a social work referral or may need to be guided toward support groups to receive the emotional support they need.

In addition, cancer clients have a strong need for hope. Strategies for inspiring hope may include active listening, touch, presence, and helping clients overcome communication barriers. Often it is not what nurses say or do but just their presence that counts.

Assessment

Assessment of a woman with cancer of the reproductive tract involves a thorough history and physical examination. In addition, various laboratory and diagnostic tests may be done to evaluate for a malignancy.

Health History and Physical Examination

Interview the woman carefully to determine any current or past factors that might increase her risk for cancer, such as early menarche, late menopause, sexually transmitted infections (STIs), use of hormonal agents, or infertility. Find out if the woman has a family history of cancer. Be thorough in obtaining the woman's past medical history, especially her reproductive, obstetric, and gynecologic history. Ask about her lifestyle and behaviours, including risky behaviours such as engaging in unprotected sexual intercourse or sexual intercourse with multiple partners. Find out if she has had routine or recommended screening procedures.

Ask if the woman has had any symptoms, such as abnormal vaginal bleeding or discharge or vaginal discomfort. Often the symptoms of cancer are vague and nonspecific and the woman may attribute them to another problem, such as aging, stress, or improper diet.

Perform a complete physical examination, including a review of body systems and a pelvic examination.

COMMON LABORATORY AND DIAGNOSTIC TESTS 8.1

Test	Explanation	Indications	Nursing Implications
Clinical breast examination	Assessment of the breast for abnormal findings; patient may discover lump herself; high-risk history for breast cancer	Identifies palpable mass, skin change, inverted nipple, or unresolved rash	• Educate client to perform breast self-examination and report any abnormalities. • Reinforce need for frequent clinical breast examinations if risk factors are present.
Mammography	Screening modality for breast cancer or any distortion in breast tissue architecture	Detects calcifications, densities, and nonpalpable cancer lesions	Stress importance of annual mammograms for all women after the age of 40 or 50, depending on their risk history.
Pap smear	Cervical cytology screening to diagnose cervical cancers	Aids in detecting abnormal cells of the cervix (from squamocolumnar junction of the cervix; most cervical cancers arise here)	Encourage all sexually active women to receive an annual pelvic examination, including a Pap smear, to promote early detection of cervical cancer.
Transvaginal ultrasound	Screening for pelvic pathology to assist in diagnosing endometrial cancers	Allows measurement of endometrial thickness to determine if endometrial biopsy is needed for postmenopausal bleeding	• Review the risk factors for the development of endometrial cancer and reason for this screening test. • Assist in preparing the patient for this examination.
CA-125	Nonspecific blood test used as a tumour marker	Elevation of marker suggests malignancy but is not specific to ovarian cancer.	• Review risk factors for ovarian cancer and explain that a series of diagnostic tests may be performed (transvaginal ultrasound, CT scan, CA-125) to assist in the diagnosis and treatment plan. • Elevated marker levels are not specific to ovarian cancer; they can be elevated in other types of cancer.

Observe for lesions or masses in the perineal area. Note any masses when palpating the abdomen or when performing the pelvic examination.

Laboratory and Diagnostic Testing

Some of the laboratory and diagnostic tests used to help diagnose cancer of the reproductive tract are discussed in Common Laboratory and Diagnostic Tests 8.1.

Nursing Diagnoses and Related Interventions

Upon completion of a thorough assessment, the nurse might identify several nursing diagnoses, including:

• Deficient knowledge
• Disturbed body image
• Anxiety
• Fear
• Pain

Nursing goals, interventions, and evaluation for the woman with a reproductive cancer are based on the

nursing diagnoses. Nursing Care Plan 8.1 may be used as a guide in planning nursing care for the woman with a reproductive cancer. It should be individualized based on the woman's symptoms and needs.

Nurses have traditionally served as advocates in the health care arena and should continue to be on the forefront of health education and diagnosis, acting as leaders in the fight against cancer. It was predicted that 81,000 women would be diagnosed with cancer in 2009 and more than 35,000 would die as a result of the disease (CCS, 2009b). The public needs to know that not only are these deaths preventable but also many of the cancers themselves are preventable. Nurses need to work to improve the availability and quality of cancer-screening services, making them accessible to underserved and socioeconomically disadvantaged clients. Through a unified effort by health care professionals, health policy experts, government agencies, health insurance companies, the media, educational institutions, and women themselves, along with consistency and continuity, nurses can offer quality care to all women with cancer.

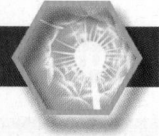

Nursing Care Plan 8.1

OVERVIEW OF A WOMAN WITH A REPRODUCTIVE TRACT CANCER

Molly, a thin 28-year-old Aboriginal woman, comes to the free health clinic complaining of a thin, watery vaginal discharge and spotting after sex. She says she is homeless and has lived "on the streets" for years. Molly says she has had multiple sex partners to pay for her food and cigarettes. She had an abnormal Pap smear "a while back" but didn't return to the clinic for follow-up. She hopes nothing "bad" is wrong with her because she just found a job that will allow her to get off the streets. "I'm worried that I won't be the same if there is something wrong. I don't know what I'd do if there is a problem," she tells you. Cervical cancer is suspected.

NURSING DIAGNOSIS: Anxiety related to uncertainty of diagnosis, possible diagnosis of cancer, and eventual outcome as evidenced by client's report of signs and symptoms, statements of being worried and not knowing what she would do

Outcome Identification and Evaluation
Client will demonstrate measures to cope with anxiety *as evidenced by statements acknowledging anxiety, use of positive coping strategies, and verbalization that anxiety has decreased.*

Interventions: Reducing Anxiety
- Encourage client to express her feelings and concerns *to reduce her anxiety and to determine appropriate interventions.*
- Assess the meaning of the diagnosis to the client, clarify misconceptions, and provide reliable, realistic information *to enhance her understanding of her condition, subsequently reducing her anxiety.*
- Assess client's psychological status *to determine degree of emotional distress related to diagnosis and treatment options.*
- Identify and address verbalized concerns, providing information about what to expect *to decrease uncertainty about the unknown.*
- Assess the client's use of coping mechanisms in the past and their effectiveness *to foster use of positive strategies.*
- Teach client about early signs of anxiety and help her recognize them (e.g., fast heartbeat, sweating, or feeling flushed) *to minimize escalation of anxiety.*
- Provide positive reinforcement that the client's condition can be managed *to relieve her anxiety.*

NURSING DIAGNOSIS: Deficient knowledge related to diagnosis, prevention strategies, disease course, and treatment as evidenced by client's statements about hoping nothing bad is wrong, lack of follow-up for previous abnormal Pap test, and high-risk behaviours

Outcome Identification and Evaluation
Client will demonstrate understanding of diagnosis, *as evidenced by making health-promoting lifestyle choices, verbalizing appropriate health care practices, describing condition once diagnosed, and adhering to measures to comply with therapy.*

Interventions: Providing Client Teaching
- Assess client's current knowledge about her diagnosis and proposed therapeutic regimen *to establish a baseline from which to develop a teaching plan.*
- Review contributing factors associated with development of reproductive tract cancer, including lifestyle behaviours, *to foster an understanding of the etiology of cervical cancer.*
- Review information about treatments and procedures and recommendations for healthy lifestyle, obtaining feedback frequently *to validate adequate understanding of instructions.*
- Discuss strategies, including using condoms and limiting the number of sexual partners, *to reduce the risk of transmission of STIs,* including human papillomavirus (HPV), which is associated with cervical cancer.
- Encourage client to obtain prompt treatment of any vaginal or cervical infections *to minimize the risk for cervical cancer.*
- Urge the client to have an annual Pap smear *to allow screening and early detection.*
- Describe the treatment measures used *to provide client with knowledge of what may be necessary.*
- Provide written material with pictures *to allow for client review and help her visualize what is occurring in her body.*
- Inform client about available community resources and make appropriate referrals as needed *to provide additional education and support.*
- Document details of teaching and learning *to allow for continuity of care and further education, if needed.*

(continued)

Nursing Care Plan 8.1 (continued)

NURSING DIAGNOSIS: Disturbed body image related to suspected reproductive tract cancer and impact on client's sexuality and sense of self as evidenced by statement of being worried about not being the same

Outcome Identification and Evaluation

Client will verbalize or demonstrate a positive self-esteem in relation to body image as evidenced by positive statements about self, sexuality, and participation in activities with others.

Interventions: Promoting Healthy Body Image

- Assess client's use of self-criticism *to determine client's current state of coping and adjustment.*
- Determine if the client's change in body image has contributed to social isolation *to provide a direction for care.*
- Provide opportunities for client to explore her feelings related to issues of sexuality, including past behaviours that may have placed her at risk, *to minimize feelings of guilt about her condition.*
- Acknowledge the client's feelings about possible changes in her body and sexuality and her illness *to foster trust and allow client to ventilate feelings and concerns.*
- Facilitate contact with other clients with the same type of cancer *to promote sharing of feelings and decrease feelings of isolation.*
- Initiate referrals for counselling and community support groups as necessary *to assist client in gaining a positive image of herself.*

These are examples of the nursing diagnoses that may fit this scenario. You may be able to identify others for your practice.

Educating to Prevent Cancer

Nurses need to provide clients with information to help prevent disease and enhance quality of life. Educate women about the importance of consistent and timely screenings to identify cancer early. Emphasize the importance of having an annual pelvic examination. Also stress the need for follow-up screenings as recommended. Provide clients with information if further diagnostic testing is required.

Nurses also play a key role in promoting cancer awareness, prevention, and control. Advocate to improve the availability of cancer screening services and work to provide public education about risk factors for cancer.

Nurses can be instrumental in helping women to identify and change behaviours that put them at risk for various reproductive tract cancers (Teaching Guideline 8.1). Do not limit your interventions to providing preventive education only: inform women about the consequences of doing nothing about their conditions and what the long-range outcomes might be without treatment. For example, stress the importance of visiting a health care professional if certain signs and symptoms appear:

- Blood in a bowel movement
- Unusual vaginal discharge or chronic vulvar itching
- Persistent abdominal bloating or constipation
- Irregular vaginal bleeding
- Persistent low backache not related to standing

TEACHING GUIDELINE 8.1

Reducing Your Risk for Cancer

- Don't smoke.
- Drink alcohol only in moderation (no more than one drink daily).
- Be physically active daily.
- Eat a healthy diet.
- Stay current with immunizations.
- Reach and maintain a healthy weight.
- Take preventive medicines if needed.
- Get recommended screening tests:
- Body mass index (BMI) to identify obesity
- Mammogram every 1 to 2 years starting at age 40
- Pap smear every 1 to 3 years, if sexually active, between the ages of 21 and 70
- Cholesterol checked annually starting at age 45
- Blood pressure checked at least every 2 years
- Diabetes test if hypertensive or hypercholesterolemic
- Check for sexually transmitted infections (STIs) if sexually active

Sources: Mayo Clinic. (2010). *Cancer prevention: 7 steps to reduce your risk.* Retrieved February 6, 2012 from http://www.mayoclinic.com/health/cancer-prevention/CA00024; World Health Organization. (2012). *Cancer prevention.* Retrieved February 6, 2012 from http://www.who.int/cancer/prevention/en/.

- Elevated or discoloured vulvar lesions
- Bleeding after menopause
- Pain or bleeding after sexual intercourse

Teaching the Client About Her Diagnosis

Provide information about tests that may be required to confirm or rule out the diagnosis. Review with the woman what she has been told about her diagnosis and her understanding of her condition. It is not unusual for the woman to hear the diagnosis and then become overwhelmed by the thought of cancer, blocking out whatever is said after that. Answer any questions she may have. Go slowly and repeat the information as necessary. Use written materials to explain and reinforce the teaching. Provide information about her condition and recommended therapies. For example, if a client is undergoing surgery, discuss postoperative issues such as incision care, pain, and activity level. Instruct the client on health maintenance activities after treatment, and inform her and her family about available support resources.

Providing Emotional Support

Once the diagnosis is made, provide the woman and her family with emotional support. Validate the client's feelings and provide realistic hope, using a nonjudgmental approach and therapeutic communication skills during all interactions. Individualize the care based on the client's cultural traditions and beliefs.

Ensuring Culturally Competent Cancer Care

Cultural diversity in Canada is increasing, and as diverse cultures interact, conflicts inevitably ensue. These conflicts can affect health care outcomes. Providing culturally competent cancer care can improve outcomes and decrease disparities in care. Work to develop cultural competence by learning about and showing respect for all cultures. Culture plays a critical role in the differing perceptions of a cancer diagnosis by patients, their families, and health care providers. Because behaviours and world views are influenced by an individual's cultural background, culture can influence beliefs about experiences of health and illness and client health-seeking behaviours (Huang, Yates, & Prior, 2009).

In some cultures, sharing news of a serious illness such as cancer is considered disrespectful and impolite. Culturally competent communication is the key! For example, with an Aboriginal family, it is very important to find out who is considered the decision maker. Someone nominated in the family—usually the oldest male— will make the health care decisions; it is very important to find out who that person is and communicate effectively with him or her (Huang et al., 2009). Integrate this knowledge into your care to ensure a culturally competent approach.

▶ *Take NOTE!*

When a diagnosis of cancer is made, assessing an individual's strengths and weaknesses from a cultural perspective will help the nurse to provide culturally competent care.

As life becomes increasingly multilingual, multicultural, and multi-faith, learning about clients' values and cultural beliefs becomes challenging. Be willing to learn about client preferences; doing so promotes caring and nurturing.

Supporting the Pregnant Woman with Cancer

Theoretically, changes in the mother's immune system during pregnancy can increase the risk of malignancy because cell-mediated immunity, which is suppressed in pregnant women, normally protects against cancerous tumours (Blackburn, 2007). Some research has hinted at an increased rate of progression and decreased survival times in women who develop breast and cervical cancer and then become pregnant, but this generally has not been validated by research studies.

Ovarian cancer during pregnancy is rare because the disease typically occurs in older women. Because most pregnant women receive frequent medical care, including pelvic examinations, most ovarian cancers in pregnant women are found at early stages. According to the Society of Obstetricians and Gynaecologists of Canada (SOGC), oral contraceptives have been shown to reduce the risk of future ovarian cancer by 10% to 12% after 1 year of use, by 50% after 5 years, and by 80% after 10 years. Since routine screening for endometrial cancer is currently not recommended in the general population (Rahaman & Cohen, 2010), few cases would be detected in the relatively young pregnant population. The low incidence of ovarian neoplasia detected during pregnancy appears to reflect the low prevalence of ovarian cancer in young women (Palmer, Vatish, & Tidy, 2008). Cervical cancer is more common in the pregnant population than other reproductive malignancies, and it can affect the woman's health status and the pregnancy.

Physical examination and ultrasound investigation during pregnancy may lead to early diagnosis of an ovarian tumour, and tumours may be detected incidentally during caesarean delivery (Stensheim, Moller, Dijk, et al., 2009). The wishes of the pregnant woman and her family are of paramount importance when making decisions about continuing the pregnancy and undergoing cancer treatment. Some women will decide to terminate the pregnancy for the sake of their own health; others will undergo treatment during the pregnancy to preserve the life of the unborn child. Regardless of the woman's decision, provide support and education during treatment, birth, and beyond.

Ovarian Cancer

Ovarian cancer is malignant neoplastic growth of the ovary (Fig. 8.1). It is the seventh most common cancer among women and the fourth most common cause of cancer deaths among women in Canada (CCS, 2009b). The CCS estimates that about 2,500 new cases of ovarian cancer are diagnosed in Canada each year and 1,750 deaths result from the disease. A woman's risk for getting ovarian cancer during her lifetime is 1 in 71, and the lifetime probability of dying from ovarian cancer is 1 in 87. Women who are older than 69 years of age at the time of diagnosis have a less favourable prognosis than women who are younger at diagnosis.

The most important variable influencing the prognosis is the extent of the disease. Survival depends on the stage of the tumour, grade of differentiation, gross findings at surgery, amount of residual tumour after surgery, and effectiveness of any adjunct treatment postoperatively. Many women with ovarian cancer will experience recurrence despite the best efforts of eradicating the cancer through surgery, radiation, or chemotherapy to eliminate residual tumour cells. The prognosis for women with a recurrence of ovarian cancer is poor (Green, Ahmed, Al Husaini, et al., 2011). The 5-year survival rates (the percentage of women who live at least 5 years after their diagnosis) are shown in Table 8.1 according to stage. The overall 5-year survival rate for women with ovarian cancer is 42% (Green et al., 2011).

TABLE 8.1 SURVIVAL RATES FOR OVARIAN CANCER

Stage	Five-Year Relative Survival Rate
I	80% to 90%
II	65% to 75%
III & IV	20% to 22%
All stages	*<40%*

Source: Duarte-Franco, E., & Franco, E. (2003). Other gynecologic cancers. In *Women's health surveillance report: A multi-dimensional look at the health of Canadian women.* Ottawa, ON: Canadian Institute for Health Information. Retrieved February 6, 2012 from http://secure.cihi.ca/cihiweb/products/CPHI_WomensHealth_e.pdf.

Pathophysiology

Ovarian cancer, the cause of which is unknown, can originate from different cell types. Most ovarian cancers originate in the ovarian epithelium. They usually present as solid masses that have spread beyond the ovary and seeded into the peritoneum prior to diagnosis. An inherited genetic mutation is the causative factor in 5% to 10% of cases of epithelial ovarian cancer.

Screening and Diagnosis

Seventy-five percent of ovarian cancers are not diagnosed until the cancer has advanced to stage III or IV, primarily because there is still no adequate screening test. Two genes, BRCA-1 and BRCA-2, are linked with hereditary breast and ovarian cancers. Blood tests can be performed to assess DNA in white blood cells to detect

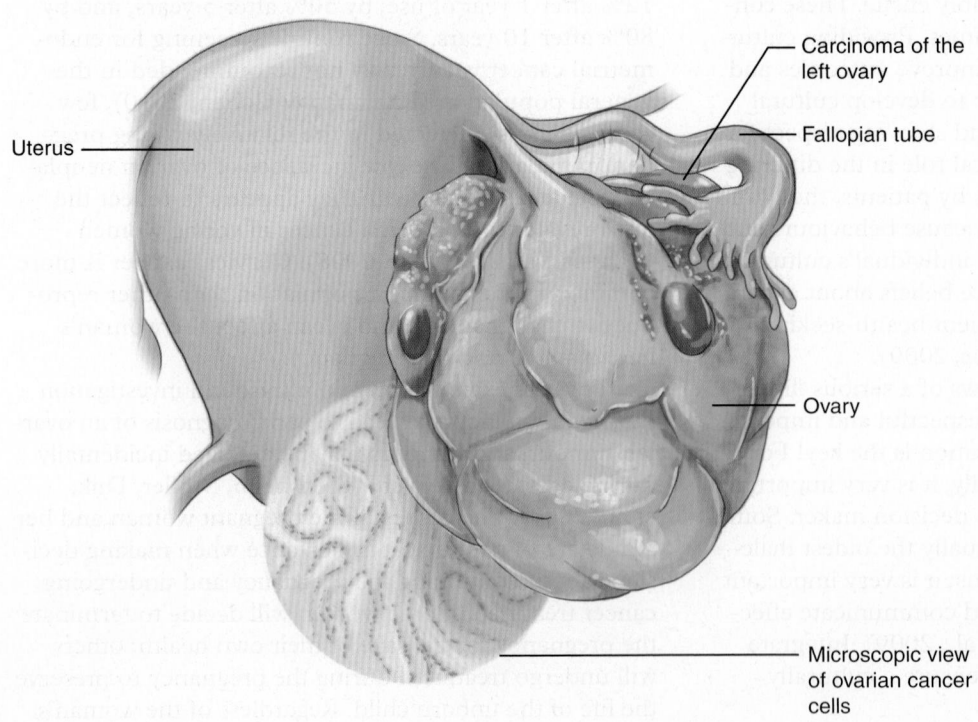

Uterus

Carcinoma of the left ovary

Fallopian tube

Ovary

Microscopic view of ovarian cancer cells

FIGURE 8.1 Ovarian cancer. (The Anatomical Chart Company. [2005]. *Atlas of pathophysiology* [2nd ed.]. Philadelphia: Lippincott Williams & Wilkins.)

mutations in the BRCA genes. The inherited genetic abnormalities carried in these genes have been shown to be a factor in 5% to 10% of breast cancers. Women who carry one of these genes are much more likely to have breast cancer and to be diagnosed at a younger age; these mutations also increase the woman's probability of developing ovarian cancer (CCS, 2009a).

To assist in screening, researchers have been developing an ovarian cancer symptom index that includes pelvic and abdominal pain, urinary frequency and urgency, increased abdominal size (bloating), and difficulty eating (feeling full) (Nelson, 2008). The symptom index is considered positive if any of these symptoms occur more than 12 times a month and persist for more than 1 year. The utility of this symptom index as a general screening tool remains to be assessed.

Specific clinical guidelines for ovarian cancer screening have not been developed, so the disease is often not diagnosed until after it has metastasized. Cancer antigen 125 (CA-125) is a biologic tumour marker associated with ovarian cancer. Although levels are elevated in many women with ovarian cancer, CA-125 is not specific for this cancer and levels may be elevated with other malignancies as well (pancreatic, liver, colon, breast, and lung cancers). CA-125 is not higher than normal in 50% of women with early-stage ovarian cancer, so it does not detect ovarian cancer early in half of women (CCS, 2009d).

Therapeutic Management

Treatment options for ovarian cancer vary depending on the stage and severity of the disease. Usually a laparoscopy (abdominal exploration with an endoscope) is performed for diagnosis and staging, as well as evaluation for therapy. In stage 1 the cancer is limited to the ovaries. In stage 2 the growth involves one or both ovaries, with pelvic extension. Stage 3 cancer has spread to the lymph nodes and other organs or structures inside the abdominal cavity. In stage 4, the cancer has metastasized to distant sites (Green et al., 2011). Figure 8.2 shows the likely metastatic sites for ovarian cancer.

Surgical intervention remains the mainstay of management of ovarian cancer. Surgery generally includes a total abdominal hysterectomy, bilateral salpingo-oophorectomy, peritoneal biopsies, omentectomy, and pelvic para-aortic lymph node sampling to evaluate cancer extension (Green et al., 2011). Because most women are diagnosed with advanced-stage ovarian cancer, aggressive management involving debulking or cytoreductive surgery is commonly performed. This surgery involves resecting all visible tumours from the peritoneum, taking peritoneal biopsies, sampling lymph nodes, and removing all reproductive organs and the omentum. This aggressive surgery has been shown to improve long-term survival rates.

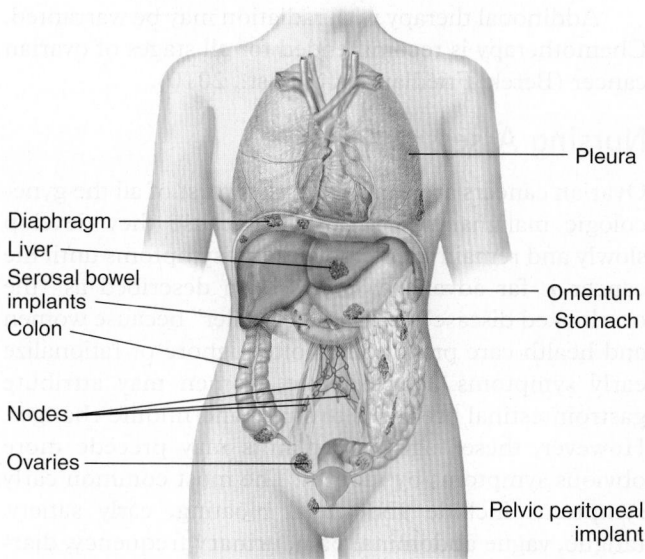

FIGURE 8.2 Common metastatic sites for ovarian cancer. (The Anatomical Chart Company. [2005]. *Atlas of pathophysiology* [2nd ed.]. Philadelphia: Lippincott Williams & Wilkins.)

▶ *Consider* THIS!

I felt I was a lucky woman because I had been in remission from breast cancer for 12 years, and I had been given the gift of life to share with my beloved family. Recently I became ill with stomach problems: pain, indigestion, bloating, and nausea. My doctor treated me for GERD (acid reflux disease), but the symptoms persisted. I then was referred to a gastroenterologist, an urologist, and then a gynecologist, who did an ultrasound, which was negative. I received reassurance from all three that there was nothing wrong with me. As time went by, I experienced more pain, more symptoms, and increased frustration. Six months after seeing all three specialists, a repeat ultrasound revealed I had ovarian cancer, and I needed surgery as soon as possible. I underwent a complete hysterectomy and my surgeon found I was in stage 3. Since then, I have undergone chemotherapy and participated in a clinical cancer study that wasn't successful for me, and now I am facing the fact that I am going to die soon.

Thoughts: This woman has tried everything to save her life, but, alas, time has run out for her with advanced ovarian cancer. Women diagnosed with breast cancer are at a significant risk for developing ovarian cancer later in life. Of the string of doctors she saw, one has to ponder why none ordered a CA-125 blood test with her history of breast cancer. The question remains: if they had and it was elevated, would she be in stage 3 now? I guess we will never know.

Additional therapy with radiation may be warranted. Chemotherapy is recommended for all stages of ovarian cancer (Berek, Friedlander, & Bast., 2010).

Nursing Assessment

Ovarian cancers are considered the worst of all the gynecologic malignancies, primarily because they develop slowly and remain silent and without symptoms until the cancer is far advanced. It has been described as "the overlooked disease" or "the silent killer" because women and health care practitioners often ignore or rationalize early symptoms. For example, women may attribute gastrointestinal problems to stress and midlife changes. However, these vague complaints may precede more obvious symptoms by months. The most common early symptoms include abdominal bloating, early satiety, fatigue, vague abdominal pain, urinary frequency, diarrhea or constipation, and unexplained weight loss or gain. The later symptoms include anorexia, dyspepsia, ascites, a palpable abdominal mass, pelvic pain, and back pain (CCS, 2009d).

Obtain a thorough history of the woman's symptoms, including their onset, duration, and frequency. Review the woman's history for risk factors such as:

- Nulliparity
- Early menarche (before 12 years old)
- Late menopause (after 55 years old)
- Increasing age (over 50 years of age)
- High-fat diet
- Obesity
- Persistent ovulation over time
- First-degree relative with ovarian cancer
- Use of perineal talcum powder or hygiene sprays
- Older than 30 years at first pregnancy
- Positive BRCA-1 and BRCA-2 mutations
- Personal history of breast, bladder, or colon cancer
- Hormone replacement therapy for more than 10 years
- Ashkenazi Jewish ancestry
- Infertility (CCS, 2009d)

Perform a complete physical examination. Inspect the abdomen, noting any distention or bloating. Palpate the abdomen. Be alert for a mass or pain on palpation. Anticipate further testing to confirm the diagnosis.

Nursing Management

The complexities of ovarian cancer make a multidisciplinary approach necessary for optimal management. With the subtle nature and high risk of recurrence and mortality of this condition, most women find it an emotionally exhausting and devastating experience. Nursing management focuses on measures to promote early detection, educate the woman about the disease and its treatments, and provide emotional support. Nurses should show a positive attitude that communicates understanding and reassurance.

Promoting Early Detection

Nurses need to ensure that women are aware of the risk factors for ovarian cancer. Urge women not to dismiss seemingly innocuous symptoms as "just a part of aging." Encourage women to describe such nonspecific complaints at health visits.

Assess the woman's family and personal history for risk factors and encourage genetic testing for women with affected family members. Outline screening guidelines for women with hereditary cancer syndrome and inform women at high risk about the appropriate screening strategies.

Urge women to have yearly bimanual pelvic examinations and a transvaginal ultrasound to allow identification of ovarian masses in their early stages. After menopause, a mass on an ovary is not a cyst: physiologic cysts can arise only from a follicle that has not ruptured or from the cystic degeneration of the corpus luteum.

▶ **Take** NOTE!

A small ovarian "cyst" found on ultrasound in an asymptomatic postmenopausal woman should arouse suspicion. Women with simple ovarian "cysts" or masses, a common incidental finding among women over 55 years of age, do not appear to be at increased risk for the development of invasive ovarian cancer. However, these women need follow-up management (Greenlee, Kessel, Williams, et al., 2010).

Educating the Client

Education is a major focus of nursing care. This teaching involves risk reduction and health promotion. Teach the woman about risk-reduction strategies; for instance, pregnancy, use of oral contraceptives, and breastfeeding reduce the risk of ovarian cancer. Instruct women to avoid using talc and hygiene sprays on their genitals. Review the lifetime risks related to BRCA-1 and BRCA-2 genes and options available should the woman test positive for these genes. Help to promote community awareness of ovarian cancer by educating the public about risk-reducing behaviours.

Instruct the woman about the importance of healthy lifestyles. Stress the importance of maintaining a healthy weight to reduce risk. Encourage women to eat a low-fat diet.

For the woman who is diagnosed with ovarian cancer, describe in simple terms the tests, treatment modalities, and follow-up needed. For example, if the woman will be having surgery, provide thorough teaching about what to expect before, during, and after surgery. Outline treatment options and the implications of choices. Assist the woman and her family to decipher the myriad of information related to staging, tests, and treatments. Teach the woman about additional treatment measures, such as radiation therapy or chemotherapy, including how to handle the common adverse effects of treatment.

Supporting the Client and Family

The diagnosis of ovarian cancer, like any cancer, can be overwhelming. In addition, the treatments and their effects can be highly stressful, both physically and emotionally. Provide one-to-one support for women facing treatment for ovarian cancer. Ovarian cancer involves the reproductive system, which has a direct impact on the woman's view of herself. Encourage open discussion of sexuality and the impact of cancer. Listen to and support the woman and her family as they try to cope with this disease. Encourage the use of appropriate coping strategies to allow for the best quality of life. Try to restore hope to women with ovarian cancer, and stress treatment compliance. If appropriate, encourage participation in clinical trials to offer hope for all women. Continue to offer support to the woman and her family members as they experience sadness and grief.

Endometrial Cancer

Endometrial cancer (also known as uterine cancer) is malignant neoplastic growth of the uterine lining. Currently, endometrial cancer is the fourth most commonly diagnosed cancer in women in Canada. The CCS estimates about 4,400 new cases of endometrial cancer are diagnosed annually in Canada, and 800 deaths result from the disease (CCS, 2009e). The lifetime probability of a woman developing endometrial cancer is 1 in 42. The most common presentation of endometrial cancer is postmenopausal bleeding (Buchanan, Weinstein, & Hillson, 2009).

Pathophysiology

Two mechanisms are believed to be involved in the development of endometrial cancer. A history of exposure to unopposed estrogen is the cause in 75% of women. Those that are spontaneous and are unrelated to estrogen or endometrial hyperplasia represent the other 25% of endometrial cancers.

Endometrial cancer may originate in a polyp or in a diffuse multifocal pattern. The pattern of spread partially depends on the degree of cellular differentiation. Well-differentiated tumours tend to limit their spread to the surface of the endometrium. Metastatic spread occurs in a characteristic pattern and most commonly involves the lungs, inguinal and supraclavicular nodes, liver, bones, brain, and vagina (CCS, 2009e). Early tumour growth is characterized by friable and spontaneous bleeding. Later tumour growth is characterized by myometrial invasion and growth toward the cervix (Fig. 8.3).

Adenocarcinoma of the endometrium is typically preceded by hyperplasia. Carcinoma in situ is found only on the endometrial surface. In stage I, it has spread to the muscle wall of the uterus. In stage II, it has spread to the cervix. In stage III, it has spread to the bowel or vagina, with metastases to pelvic lymph nodes. In stage IV, it has invaded the bladder or bowel mucosa, with distant metastases to the lungs, liver, and bone (CCS, 2009e).

Type I carcinomas, the most common, begin as endometrial hyperplasia and progress to carcinomas. Giving estrogen preparations without progestin for hormone replacement therapy leads to an increased risk for endometrial cancer. Type I is generally found at an earlier stage and treatment results are more favourable.

Unlike type I endometrial carcinoma, type II carcinomas appear spontaneously, are associated with a poorly differentiated cell type, and have a poor prognosis (Buchanan et al., 2009). They account for less than 10% of all endometrial cancers but contribute to the majority of all endometrial cancer deaths.

Screening and Diagnosis

Remember Carmella, the woman with postmenopausal bleeding? In postmenopausal women, any bleeding is abnormal and warrants further assessment. What testing would the nurse anticipate as being ordered to confirm the diagnosis? What would be the nurse's role during this testing?

Screening for endometrial cancer is not routinely done because it is not practical or cost-effective. The CCS recommends that women should be informed about the risks and symptoms of endometrial cancer at the onset of menopause and strongly encouraged to report any unexpected bleeding or spotting to their health care provider. A pelvic examination is frequently normal in the early stages of the disease. Changes in the size, shape, or consistency of the uterus or its surrounding support structures may exist when the disease is more advanced.

An endometrial biopsy is the diagnostic procedure of choice. It can be done in the health care provider's office without anesthesia. A slender suction catheter is used to obtain a small sample of tissue for pathology. The development of newer office-based sampling tools and techniques, such as the Pipelle device, has simplified this evaluation. This device consists of a disposable plastic core and a drinking-straw-like sheath that obtains endometrial biopsies through gentle suctioning. The sensitivity of the Pipelle in detecting endometrial cancer has been calculated to be as high as 99% in postmenopausal women and 91% in premenopausal women (Buchanan et al., 2009). The

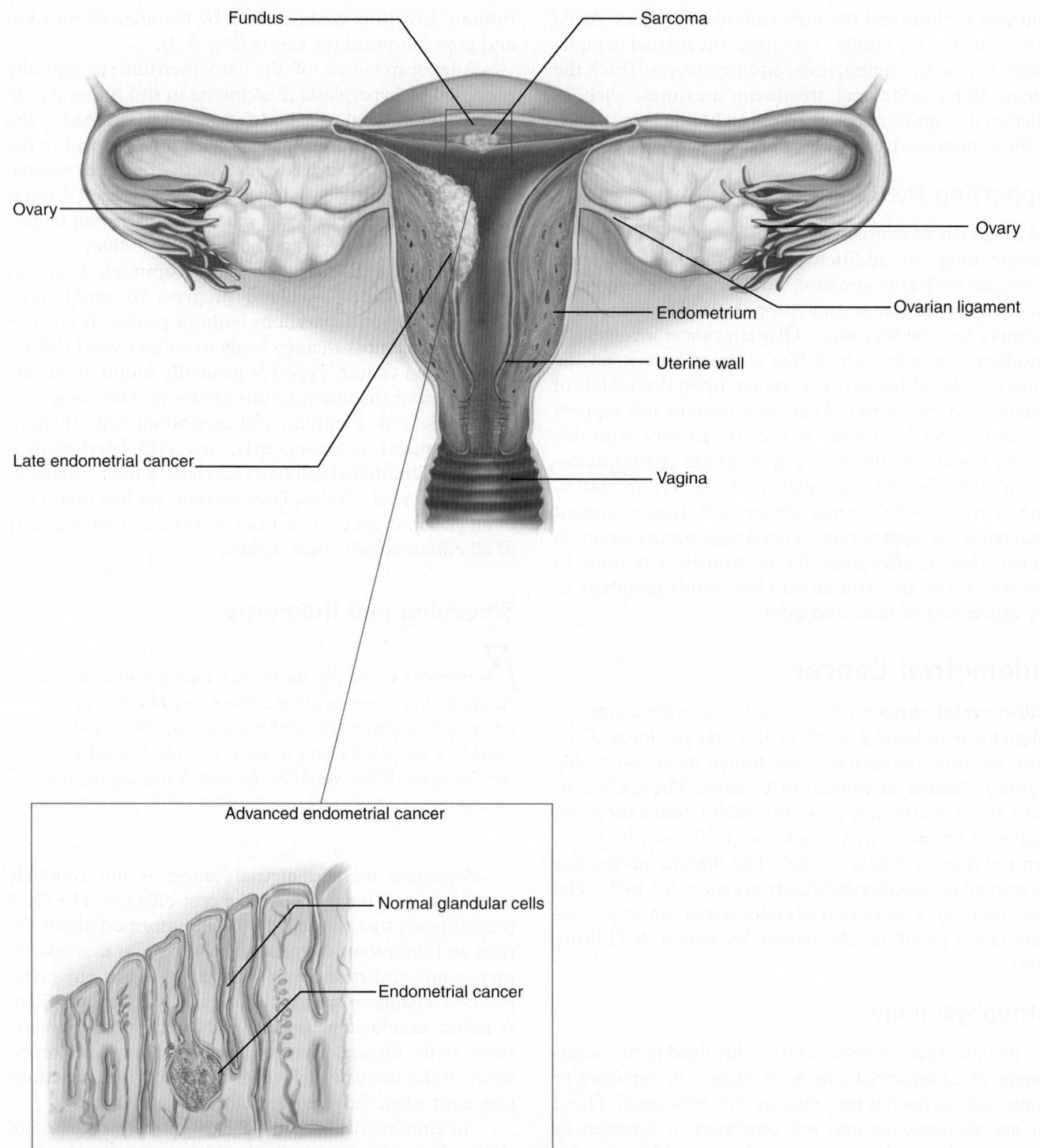

FIGURE 8.3 Progression of endometrial cancer. (The Anatomical Chart Company. [2005]. *Atlas of pathophysiology* [2nd ed.]. Philadelphia: Lippincott Williams & Wilkins.)

woman may experience mild cramping and bleeding after the procedure for about 24 hours, but mild pain medication typically will reduce this discomfort.

Transvaginal ultrasound can be used to evaluate the endometrial cavity and measure the thickness of the endometrial lining. It can be used to detect endometrial hyperplasia. In one recent study, endometrial thickness

of less than 4 mm had a negative predictive value of 100% for endometrial cancer (Goldstein, 2009).

Therapeutic Management

Typically, the stage of the disease directs treatment. It usually involves surgery with adjunct therapy based on pathologic findings. Surgery most often involves removal of the uterus (hysterectomy) and the fallopian tubes and ovaries (salpingo-oophorectomy). Removal of the tubes and ovaries is recommended because tumour cells spread early to the ovaries, and any dormant cancer cells could be stimulated to grow by ovarian estrogen. In more advanced cancers, radiation and chemotherapy are used as adjuncts to surgery. Routine surveillance intervals for follow-up care are typically every 3 months then every 6 months for the 3 years following treatment; thereafter, annual examination is appropriate (Whitcomb, 2008).

Nursing Assessment

Obtain a thorough history from the woman, ascertaining her primary complaint. Most commonly, the major initial symptom of endometrial cancer is abnormal and painless vaginal bleeding.

▶ **Take** NOTE!

Any episode of bright-red bleeding that occurs after menopause should be investigated. Abnormal uterine bleeding is rarely the result of uterine malignancy in a young woman, but in the postmenopausal woman it should be regarded with suspicion.

Also review the woman's history for any risk factors, including:

- Nulliparity
- Obesity (more than 23 kg overweight)
- Liver disease
- Infertility
- Diabetes mellitus
- Hypertension
- History of pelvic radiation
- Polycystic ovary syndrome
- Infertility
- Early menarche (before 12 years old)
- High-fat diet
- Use of prolonged exogenous unopposed estrogen with an intact uterus
- Endometrial hyperplasia
- Family history of endometrial cancer
- Personal history of hereditary nonpolyposis colon cancer
- Personal history of breast or ovarian cancer
- Late onset of menopause (after age 52 years)
- Tamoxifen use
- Chronic anovulation (CCS, 2009e)

Assess the woman for additional manifestations, such as dyspareunia, low back pain, purulent genital discharge, dysuria, pelvic pain, weight loss, and a change in bladder and bowel habits. These may suggest advanced disease.

Perform a physical examination and assist with or perform, as appropriate, a pelvic examination. Observe for vaginal discharge. Note any changes in the size, shape, or consistency of the uterus or surrounding structures or client reports of pain during examination. Anticipate the need for transvaginal ultrasound to identify endometrial hyperplasia (usually >4 mm) and endometrial biopsy to identify malignant cells.

Nursing Management

Ensure that the woman understands all the treatment options. Address any concerns the woman expresses, including those of a sexual nature. Ensure that follow-up appointments are scheduled appropriately. Refer the client to a support group. Offer the woman and family explanations and emotional support throughout.

Educate the client about preventive measures or follow-up care if she has been treated for cancer. Education may be the most important tool currently available for the early detection of endometrial cancer. Many risk factors for endometrial cancer are modifiable, including obesity, hypertension, and diabetes. Educating women about risk factors and ways to decrease the risks is essential so that women can learn about their own risk and can become partners in the fight against the number-one gynecologic cancer (Teaching Guideline 8.2).

*C*armella's endometrial biopsy indicates endometrial adenocarcinoma. Her health care provider recommends surgery and adjuvant radiation therapy. How long will Carmella need to follow up after surgery? What lifestyle changes will the nurse need to stress with Carmella?

Cervical Cancer

Cervical cancer is cancer of the uterine cervix. The CCS (2009c) estimates that approximately 1,300 cases of invasive cervical cancer will be diagnosed annually in Canada and that approximately 380 will die as a result of the disease. Some researchers estimate that noninvasive cervical cancer (carcinoma in situ) is about four times more common than invasive cervical cancer. Cervical cancer with a low grade has a more favourable prognosis. Grade as a prognostic factor appears to be more important for adenocarcinoma of the cervix because grade 3 tumours have a greater risk for metastasis and a less favourable prognosis than grade 1 or 2 tumours. The odds of a woman in Canada developing cervical cancer is approximately 1 in 148 (CCS, 2009c).

The incidence and mortality rates of cervical cancer have decreased noticeably in the past several decades, with most of the reduction attributed to the **Papanicolaou (Pap) test**, which detects cervical cancer and

TEACHING GUIDELINE 8.2

Preventive and Follow-Up Measures for Endometrial Cancer

- Schedule regular pelvic examinations after the age of 21.
- Visit health care practitioner for early evaluation of any abnormal bleeding after menopause.
- Maintain a low-fat diet throughout life.
- Exercise daily.
- Manage weight to discourage hyperestrogenic states, which predispose to endometrial hyperplasia.
- Pregnancy serves as a protective factor by reducing estrogen.
- Ask your doctor about the use of combination estrogen and progestin pills.
- When combination oral contraceptives are taken to facilitate the regular shedding of the uterine lining, take risk-reduction measures.
- Be aware of risk factors for endometrial cancer and make modifications as needed.
- Report any of the following symptoms immediately:
- Bleeding or spotting after sexual intercourse
- Bleeding that lasts longer than a week
- Reappearance of bleeding after 6 months or more of no menses
- After cancer therapy, schedule follow-up appointments for the next few years.
- After cancer therapy, frequently communicate with your health care provider concerning your status.
- After surgery, maintain a healthy weight.

precancerous lesions. Cervical cancer is one of the most treatable cancers when detected at an early stage (CCS, 2009c).

Pathophysiology

Cervical cancer starts with abnormal changes in the cellular lining or surface of the cervix. Typically these changes occur in the squamous–columnar junction of the cervix. Here, cylindrical secretory epithelial cells (columnar) meet the protective flat epithelial cells (squamous) from the outer cervix and vagina in what is termed the transformation zone. The continuous replacement of columnar epithelial cells by squamous epithelial cells in this area makes these cells vulnerable to take up foreign or abnormal genetic material (Jhingran, 2010). Figure 8.4 shows the pathophysiology of cervical cancer.

The development of cervical cancer has been linked to the **human papillomavirus (HPV)**, which is acquired through sexual activity (CCS, 2009c). More than 90% of squamous cervical cancers contain HPV DNA, and the virus is now accepted as a major causative factor in the development of cervical cancer and its precursor, **cervical dysplasia** (disordered growth of abnormal cells).

Screening and Diagnosis

Screening for cervical cancer is very effective because the presence of a precursor lesion, cervical intraepithelial neoplasia (CIN), helps determine whether further tests are needed. Lesions start as dysplasia and progress in a predictable fashion over a long period, allowing ample opportunity for intervention at a precancerous stage.

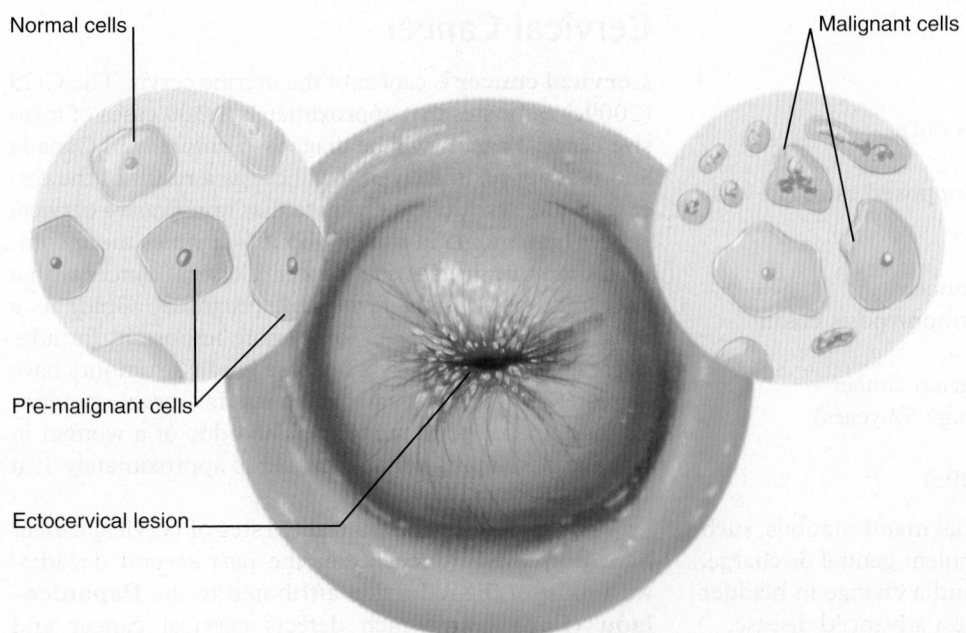

Carcinoma in situ

Squamous cell carcinoma

Normal cells

Malignant cells

Pre-malignant cells

Ectocervical lesion

FIGURE 8.4 Cervical cancer. (The Anatomical Chart Company. [2005]. *Atlas of pathophysiology* [2nd ed.]. Philadelphia: Lippincott Williams & Wilkins)

Progression from low-grade to high-grade dysplasia takes an average of 9 years, and progression from high-grade dysplasia to invasive cancer takes up to 2 years (Porth, 2009).

Widespread use of the Pap test (also known as a Pap smear), a procedure used to obtain cells from the cervix for cytology screening, is credited with saving tens of thousands of women's lives. From 1996 to 2005, the incidence of cervical cancer in Canada decreased 2.3% (CCS, 2009b). Despite its outstanding record of success as a screening tool for cervical cancer (it detects approximately 90% of early cancer changes), the conventional Pap test has a 20% false-negative rate. False-negative Pap test results are more common than false-positive Pap test results (CCS, 2009c). Many technologies have been developed to improve the sensitivity and specificity of Pap testing, including:

- Thin-Prep: in this liquid-based technique, the cervical specimen is placed into a vial of preservative solution rather than on a glass slide.
- Computer-assisted automated Pap test rescreening (AutoPap; PAPNET): an algorithm-based decision-making technology identifies slides that should be rescreened by cytopathologists by selecting samples that exceed a certain threshold for the likelihood of abnormal cells.
- HPV-DNA typing (Hybrid Capture): this system uses the association between certain types of HPV (16, 18, 31, 33, 35, 45, 51, 52, and 56) and the development of cervical cancer. This system can identify high-risk HPV types and improves detection and management.
- Computer-assisted technology (CDS-1000, AutoCyte, AcCell): these computerized instruments can detect abnormal cells that are sometimes missed by technologists (Ricci & Kyle, 2009).

The high rate of false-negative results may also be due to other factors, including errors in sampling the cervix, in preparing the slide, and in client preparation.

According to the SOGC, women should have their first Pap test within 3 years of any sexual contact or by age 21. They should then have regular Pap tests as often as their health care provider recommends. According to the Public Health Agency of Canada (PHAC, 2003), 15% of women have never been screened and 30% have not been screened in the past 3 years. If the results of annual Pap smears are normal for 3 consecutive years, screening can be spaced out to once every 3 years. Women at risk for cervical cancer, including immunosuppressed women and women with a history of cervical cancer or high-grade abnormalities, still need annual Pap smears (Table 8.2).

Pap smear results are classified using the Bethesda System (Box 8.1), which provides a uniform diagnostic terminology that allows clear communication between the laboratory and the health care provider. The information provided by the laboratory is divided into three categories:

TABLE 8.2 PAP SMEAR GUIDELINES

First Pap	Age 21 or within 3 years of first sexual intercourse
Age 21–29	Every 2 years using glass slide or liquid-based method
Age 30–70	Every 3 years if last 3 Pap tests were normal
After age 70	May discontinue if: —Past 3 Pap tests were normal and —No Pap tests in the past 10 years were abnormal

Source: American College of Obstetricians and Gynecologists. (2009). Practice bulletin: cervical cytology screening. *Obstetrics and Gynecology, 114*(6), 1409–1420.

specimen adequacy, general categorization of cytologic findings, and interpretation/result (CCS, 2009c).

Therapeutic Management

Treatment for abnormal Pap smears depends on the severity of the results and the health history of the woman. Therapeutic choices all involve destroying as many affected cells as possible. Box 8.2 describes treatment options.

Using the Bethesda system, the following management guidelines for abnormal Pap results were developed by the U.S. National Cancer Institute and are used in Canada to provide direction to health care providers and clients:

- Atypical squamous cells—unknown significance (ASC-US): repeat the Pap smear in 4 to 6 months or refer for colposcopy.
- Atypical squamous cells—high grade changes (ASC-H): refer for colposcopy without HPV testing.
- Atypical glandular cells (AGC) and adenocarcinoma in situ (AIS): immediate colposcopy; follow-up is based on the findings.

Colposcopy is a microscopic examination of the lower genital tract using a magnifying instrument called a colposcope. Specific patterns of cells that correlate well with certain histologic findings can be visualized.

Nursing Assessment

Obtain a thorough history and physical examination of the woman. Investigate her history for risk factors such as:

- Early age at first intercourse (within 1 year of menarche)
- Lower socioeconomic status
- Promiscuous male partners
- Unprotected sexual intercourse
- Family history of cervical cancer (mother or sisters)
- Sexual intercourse with uncircumcised men

BOX 8.1 The Bethesda System for Classifying Pap Smears

Specimen Type: conventional Pap smear vs. liquid-based

Specimen Adequacy: satisfactory or unsatisfactory for evaluation

General Categorization: (optional)

• Negative for intraepithelial lesion or malignancy
• Epithelial cell abnormality. See interpretation/result.

Automated Review: if case was examined by automated device or not

Ancillary Testing: provides a brief description of the test methods and report results so health care provider understands

Interpretation/Result:

• Negative for intraepithelial lesion or malignancy
• Organisms: *trichomonas vaginalis,* fungus, bacterial vaginosis, herpes simplex
• Other non-neoplastic findings: reactive cellular changes associated with inflammation, radiation, IUDs, atrophy
• Other: Endometrial cells in a woman >40 years of age
• Epithelial cell abnormalities:

• *Squamous cell*
  • Atypical squamous cells
  • Of undetermined significance (ASC-US)
  • Cannot exclude HSIL (ASC-H)
  • Low-grade squamous intraepithelial lesion (LSIL)
  • Encompassing HPV/mild dysplasia/CIN-1
  • High-grade squamous intraepithelial lesion (HSIL)
  • Encompassing moderate and severe dysplasia CIS/CIN-2 and CIN-3
  • With features suspicious for invasion
  • Squamous cell carcinoma
• *Glandular Cell:* atypical
  • Endocervical, endometrial, or glandular cells
  • Endocervical cells—favour neoplastic
  • Glandular cells—favour neoplastic
  • Endocervical adenocarcinoma in situ
  • Adenocarcinoma
  • Endocervical, endometrial, extrauterine
• Other malignant neoplasms (specify)

Educational Notes and Suggestions: (optional)

Source: National Institutes of Health. (2007). *Cervical cancer prevention.* Retrieved February 6, 2012 from http://www.cancer.gov/cancertopics/pdq/prevention/cervical/HealthProfessional

• Female offspring of mothers who took diethylstilbestrol (DES)
• Infections with genital herpes or chronic chlamydia
• Multiple sex partners
• Cigarette smoking

• Immunocompromised state
• Human immunodeficiency virus (HIV) infection
• Oral contraceptive use
• Moderate dysplasia on Pap smear within past 5 years
• HPV infection (CCS, 2009c)

BOX 8.2 Treatment Options for Cervical Cancer

• *Cryotherapy*—destroys abnormal cervical tissue by freezing with liquid nitrogen, Freon, or nitrous oxide. Studies show a 90% cure rate (Jhingran, 2010). Healing takes up to 6 weeks, and the client may experience a profuse, watery vaginal discharge for 3 to 4 weeks.
• *Cone biopsy* or *conization*—removes a cone-shaped section of cervical tissue. The base of the cone is formed by the ectocervix (outer part of the cervix) and the point or apex of the cone is from the endocervical canal. The transformation zone is contained within the cone sample. The cone biopsy can be used to completely remove any precancers and very early cancers. There are two methods commonly used for cone biopsies:
  • LEEP (loop electrosurgical excision procedure) or LLETZ (large loop excision of the transformation zone)—the abnormal cervical tissue is removed with a wire that is heated by an electrical current. For this procedure, a local anesthetic is used. It is performed in the health care provider's office in approximately 10 minutes.

Mild cramping and bleeding may persist for several weeks after the procedure.
• Cold knife cone biopsy—a surgical scalpel or a laser is used instead of a heated wire to remove tissue. This procedure requires general anesthesia and is done in a hospital setting. After the procedure, cramping and bleeding may persist for a few weeks.
• *Laser therapy*—destroys diseased cervical tissue by using a focused beam of high-energy light to vaporize it (burn it off). After the procedure, the woman may experience a watery brown discharge for a few weeks. Very effective in destroying precancers and preventing them from developing into cancers.
• *Hysterectomy*—removes the uterus and cervix surgically
• *Radiation therapy*—delivered by internal radium applications to the cervix or external radiation therapy that includes lymphatics of the pelvis
• *Chemoradiation*—weekly cisplatin therapy concurrent with radiation. Investigation of this therapy is ongoing.

Nursing Procedure 8.1

ASSISTING WITH COLLECTION OF A PAP SMEAR

Purpose: To Obtain Cells from the Cervix for Cervical Cytology Screening

1. Explain procedure to the client (Fig. A).
2. Instruct client to empty her bladder.
3. Wash hands thoroughly.
4. Assemble equipment, maintaining sterility of equipment (Fig. B).
5. Position client on stirrups or foot pedals so that her knees fall outward.
6. Drape client with a sheet for privacy, covering the abdomen but leaving the perineal area exposed.
7. Open packages as needed.
8. Encourage client to relax.

9. Provide support to client as the practitioner obtains a sample by spreading the labia; inserting the speculum; inserting the cytobrush and swabbing the endocervix; and inserting the plastic spatula and swabbing the cervix (Fig. C–H).
10. Transfer specimen to container (Fig. I) or slide. If a slide is used, spray the fixative on the slide.
11. Place sterile lubricant on the practitioner's fingertip when indicated for the bimanual examination.
12. Wash hands thoroughly.
13. Label specimen according to facility policy.
14. Rinse reusable instruments prior to sterilization, and dispose of waste appropriately (Fig. J).
15. Wash hands thoroughly.

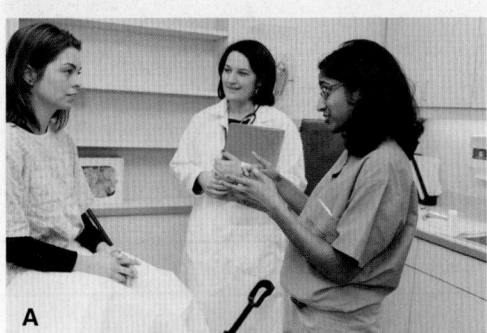

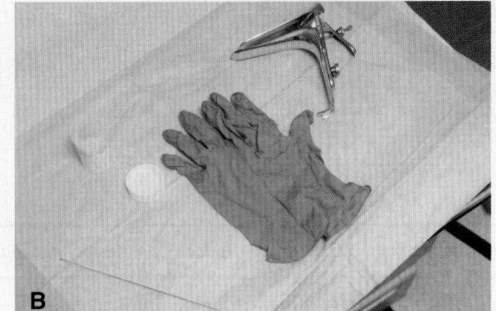

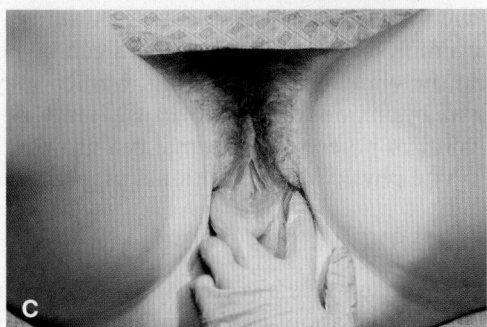

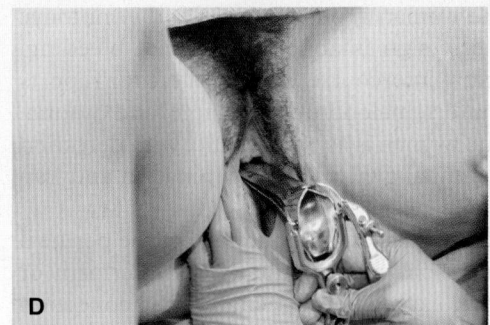

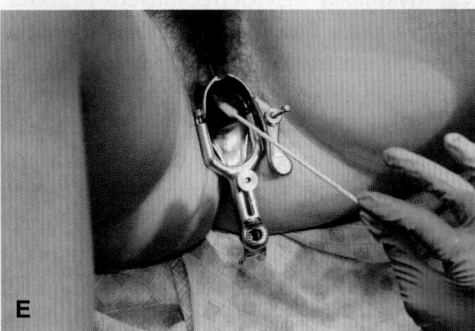

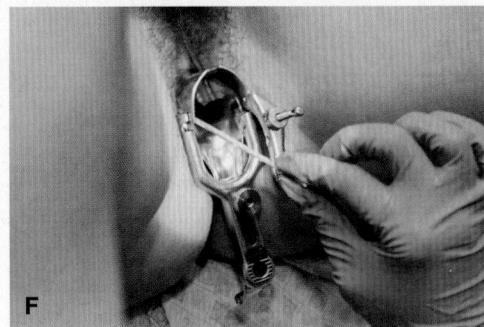

(continued)

Nursing Procedure 8.1 (continued)

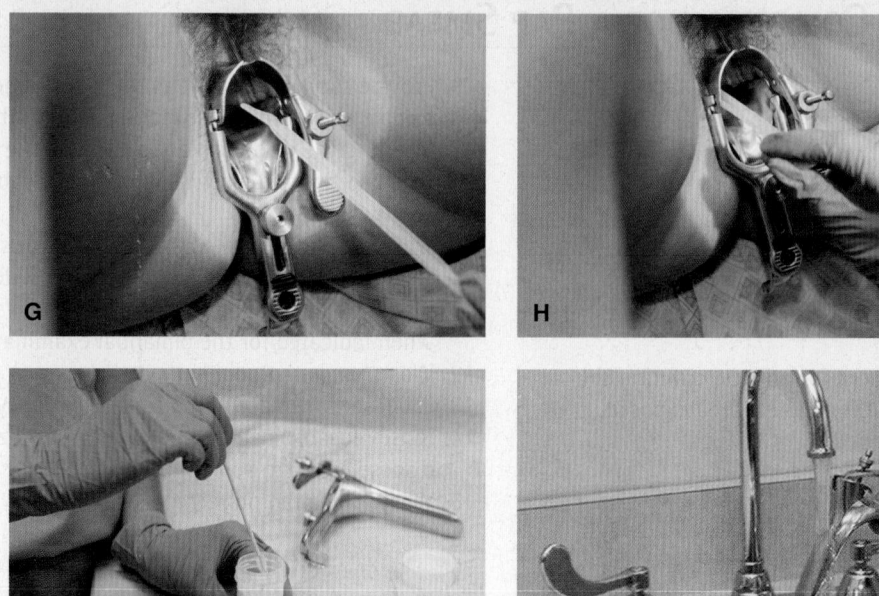

Used with permission from Klossner, N. J. (2006). *Introductory maternity nursing*. Philadelphia: Lippincott Williams & Wilkins.

Question the woman about any signs and symptoms. Clinically, the first sign is abnormal vaginal bleeding, usually after sexual intercourse. Also be alert for reports of vaginal discomfort, malodorous discharge, and dysuria. In some cases the woman is asymptomatic, with detection occurring at an annual gynecologic examination and Pap test.

Perform a physical examination. Inspect the perineal area for vaginal discharge or genital warts. Perform or assist with a pelvic examination, including the collection of a Pap smear as indicated (Nursing Procedure 8.1).

▶ **Take** NOTE!

Suspect advanced cervical cancer in women with pelvic, back, or leg pain, weight loss, anorexia, weakness and fatigue, and fractures.

Prepare the woman for further diagnostic testing if indicated, such as a colposcopy. In a colposcopy, the woman is placed in the lithotomy position and her cervix is cleansed with acetic acid solution. Acetic acid makes abnormal cells appear white, which is referred to as acetowhite. These white areas are then biopsied and sent to the pathologist for assessment. Although this test is not painful, has no side effects, and can be performed safely in the clinic or office setting, women may be apprehensive or anxious about it because it is done to identify and confirm potential abnormal cell growth. Provide appropriate physical and emotional preparation for this test.

Nursing Management

The nurse's role involves primary prevention by educating women about risk factors and ways to prevent cervical dysplasia (Evidence-based Practice 8.1). Cervical cancer rates have decreased in Canada because of the widespread use of Pap testing, which can detect precancerous lesions of the cervix before they develop into cancer. Nevertheless, during 2009, an estimated 1,300 new cases were diagnosed and approximately 380 women were estimated to die from cervical cancer (CCS, 2009c).

Gardasil, the first vaccine developed to protect girls and women from HPV, is now available. The vaccine prevents infection from four HPV types: HPV 6, 11, 16, and 18. These types are responsible for 70% of cervical cancers and 90% of genital warts (Merck Frosst Canada, 2010). Clinical trials indicate that the vaccine has high efficacy in preventing persistent HPV infection, cervical cancer precursor lesions, vaginal and vulvar cancer precursor lesions,

EVIDENCE-BASED PRACTICE 8.1
Smoking and Cervical Cancer Risk, Independent of Infection with High-Risk HPV Types

● Background

Because cervical cancer is common, prevention is paramount. Prevention can be either primary or secondary. Primary prevention is characterized by health education to promote lifestyles and behaviours that minimize the risk for cervical cancer. With the recent availability of the HPV vaccine, we may have developed a false sense of security with regard to cervical cancer. However, it is important to remember that HPV is not the only risk factor for cervical cancer. Smoking increases a woman's risk for cervical cancer. Interventions to promote the cessation of smoking continue to be of major importance. This nested case-control prospective study considered whether smoking is an independent risk factor for cervical cancer after controlling for infection with high-risk types of HPV. The sample included more than 1 million women, most of whom were pregnant. Smoking status was assessed objectively by serum cotinine concentration.

▲ Findings

After controlling for infection with high-risk HPV types, the risk for invasive cervical cancer overall and for squamous cell carcinoma (but not adenocarcinoma) was increased in both light and heavy smokers compared with nonsmokers. Smoking increased a woman's risk for invasive cervical cancer approximately twofold, independent of infection with high-risk types of HPV.

■ Nursing Implications

Nurses can use the information from this research to design appropriate strategies for client teaching and can encourage women who smoke to practice health promotion by means of smoking cessation. It is important to inform women that smoking cessation will minimize their risk for the development of cervical cancer. Educational interventions and smoking cessation programs targeting socially and economically disadvantaged women who smoke are positive health promotion practices that have the potential to reduce the incidence of cervical carcinoma. Increased knowledge will strengthen women's desire to protect themselves from the many hazards of smoking, including cervical cancer.

Kapeu, A.S., Luostarinen, T., Jellum, E., Dillner, J., Hakama, M., Koskela, P., et al. (2009). Is smoking an independent risk factor for invasive cervical cancer? A nested case–control study within Nordic biobanks. *American Journal of Epidemiology, 169*(4), 480–488.

and genital warts. The vaccine is administered by intramuscular injection, and the recommended schedule is a three-dose series with the second and third doses administered 2 and 6 months after the first dose. The recommended age for vaccination of females is 11 to 12 years old, but the vaccine can be administered to girls as young as 9 years old (Merck Frosst Canada, 2010). The long-term efficacy of HPV vaccines remains to be determined. Sustained efficacy up to 4.5 years has been documented, but it could be that boosters will be needed (Centers for Disease Control and Prevention, 2007). However, the vaccine is not a substitute for routine cervical cancer screening, and vaccinated women should have Pap smears as recommended.

Focus primary prevention education on the following:

- Identify high-risk behaviours in clients and teach them how to reduce them:
  - Take steps to prevent STIs.
  - Avoid early sexual activity.
  - Faithfully use barrier methods of contraception.
  - Avoid smoking and drinking.
  - Receive the HPV vaccine.
- Instruct women on the importance of screening for cervical cancer by annual Pap smears. Outline the

proper preparation before having a Pap smear (Teaching Guideline 8.3). Reinforce specific guidelines for screening.

Nurses also can advocate for clients by making sure that the Pap smear is sent to an accredited laboratory for interpretation. Doing so reduces the risk of false-negative results.

Secondary prevention focuses on reducing or limiting the area of cervical dysplasia. Tertiary prevention focuses on minimizing disability or spread of cervical cancer. Explain in detail all procedures that might be needed. Encourage the client who has undergone any cervical treatment to allow the pelvic area to rest for approximately 1 month. Discuss this rest period with the client and her partner to gain his cooperation. Outline alternatives to vaginal intercourse, such as cuddling, holding hands, and kissing. Remind the woman about any follow-up procedures that are needed and assist her with scheduling if necessary.

Throughout the process, provide emotional support to the woman and her family. During the decision-making process, the woman may be overwhelmed by the diagnosis and all the information being presented. Refer the woman and her family to appropriate community resources and support groups as indicated.

Vaginal Cancer

Vaginal cancer is malignant tissue growth arising in the vagina. It is rare, representing less than 3% of all genital cancers. According to the PHAC, the reported annual age-standardized incidence rate (ASIR) for vaginal cancer is fewer than 1 in 100,000 women in all countries with the exceptions of Argentina (1.5/100,000) and Colombia (1.2/100,000). Nova Scotia is the Canadian province with the highest ASIR for vaginal cancers; at 0.8 per 100,000, it is ranked fourth highest in the world. Survival in patients with vaginal cancers is generally poor: stage I disease has a 5-year survival rate of 64% to 90%, stage II 29% to 66%, and stages III and IV 0% to 40%. Vaginal cancer can be effectively treated, and when found early it is often curable.

Pathophysiology

The etiology of vaginal cancer has not been identified. Malignant diseases of the vagina are either primary vaginal cancers or metastatic forms from adjacent or distant organs. About 80% of vaginal cancers are metastatic, primarily from the cervix and endometrium. These cancers invade the vagina directly. Cancers from distant sites that metastasize to the vagina through the blood or lymphatic system are typically from the colon, kidneys, skin (melanoma), or breast. Tumours in the vagina commonly occur on the posterior wall and spread to the cervix or vulva (Rotmensh, 2010).

Squamous cell carcinomas that begin in the epithelial lining of the vagina account for about 90% of vaginal cancers (Rotmensh, 2010). This type of cancer usually occurs in women over age 50. They develop slowly over a period of years, commonly in the upper third of the vagina. They tend to spread early by directly invading the bladder and rectal walls. They also metastasize through blood and lymphatics. The remaining 10% are adenocarcinomas, which differ from squamous cell carcinoma by an increase in pulmonary metastases and supraclavicular and pelvic node involvement (Rotmensh, 2010).

Therapeutic Management

Treatment of vaginal cancer depends on the type of cells involved and the stage of the disease. If the cancer is localized, radiation, laser surgery, or both may be used. If the cancer has spread, radical surgery might be needed, such as a hysterectomy or removal of the upper vagina with dissection of the pelvic nodes in addition to radiation therapy.

Nursing Assessment

Begin the history and physical examination by reviewing for risk factors. Although direct risk factors for the initial development of vaginal cancer have not been identified, associated risk factors include advancing age (over 60 years old), previous pelvic radiation, exposure to diethylstilbestrol (DES) in utero, vaginal trauma, history of genital warts (HPV infection), HIV infection, cervical cancer, chronic vaginal discharge, smoking, obesity, hypertension, diabetes, and low socioeconomic level (Rotmensh, 2010).

Question the woman about any complaints. Most women with vaginal cancer are asymptomatic. Those with symptoms have painless vaginal bleeding (often after sexual intercourse), abnormal vaginal discharge, dyspareunia, dysuria, urinary frequency, constipation, and pelvic pain (Rotmensh, 2010). During the physical examination, observe for any obvious vaginal discharge or genital warts, or changes in the appearance of the vaginal mucosa. Anticipate colposcopy with biopsy of suspicious lesions to confirm the diagnosis.

Nursing Management

Nursing management for this cancer is similar to that for other reproductive cancers, with emphasis on sexuality counselling and referral to local support groups. Women undergoing radical surgery need intensive counselling about the nature of the surgery, risks, potential complications, changes in physical appearance and physiologic function, and sexuality alterations.

Vulvar Cancer

Vulvar cancer is an abnormal neoplastic growth on the external female genitalia (Fig. 8.5). The SOGC (2006) indicates that vulvar cancer is responsible for 5% of all

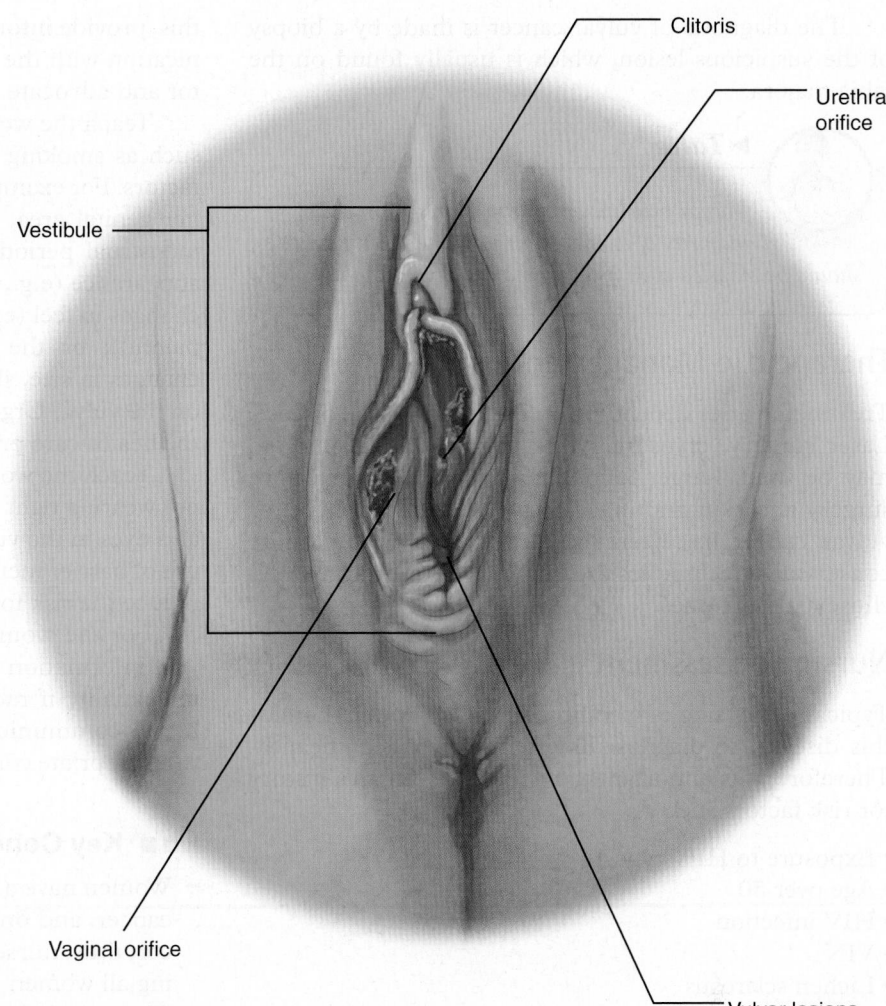

FIGURE 8.5 Vulvar cancer. (The Anatomical Chart Company. [2005]. *Atlas of pathophysiology* [2nd ed.]. Philadelphia: Lippincott Williams & Wilkins)

female genital cancers. All provinces have rates above 1 in 100,000 women and these are among the highest reported worldwide; the highest incidence rate of vulvar cancer is found in Prince Edward Island (2.6/100,000 women; Duarte-France & Franco, 2003). When detected early, vulvar cancer is highly curable.

Vulvar cancer is found most commonly in older women between 65 and 75 years of age, but the incidence in women younger than 35 years old has increased over the past few decades (SOGC, 2006). Health Canada's Women's Health Surveillance Report states that the overall 5-year survival rate of vulvar cancer is 46%.

Pathophysiology

Approximately 90% of vulvar tumours are squamous cell carcinomas. This type of cancer forms slowly over several years and is usually preceded by precancerous changes, termed vulvar intraepithelial neoplasia (VIN). The two major types of VIN are classic (undifferentiated) and simplex (differentiated). Currently, HPV types 6 and 11 are most frequently found in benign vulvar warts, and HPV types 16, 18, 31, 33, and 45 are more

frequently associated with intraepithelial neoplasia or invasive carcinoma. Most vulvar carcinomas occur in older women, with more than 50% of cases diagnosed in women between 60 and 79 years of age (Rotmensh, 2010). Invasive vulvar carcinomas are being seen with increasing frequency in younger patients, however, with 15% of vulvar cancers arising in women under the age of 40 years. This increased frequency in younger patients may be attributed to an increase in the number of sexual partners or to venereal viral infections within the population (Rotmensh, 2010).

Screening and Diagnosis

Annual vulvar examination is the most effective way to prevent vulvar cancer. Careful inspection of the vulva during routine annual gynecologic examinations remains the most productive diagnostic technique. Liberal use of biopsies of any suspicious vulvar lesion is usually necessary to make the diagnosis and to guide treatment. However, many women do not seek health care evaluation for months or years after noticing an abnormal lump or lesion.

The diagnosis of vulvar cancer is made by a biopsy of the suspicious lesion, which is usually found on the labia majora.

> ▶ *Take* NOTE!
>
> *Vulvar pruritus or a lump is present in the majority of women with vulvar cancer. Lumps should be biopsied even if the woman is asymptomatic.*

Therapeutic Management

Treatment varies depending on the extent of the disease. Laser surgery, cryosurgery, or electrosurgical incision may be used. Larger lesions may need more extensive surgery and skin grafting. The traditional treatment for vulvar cancer has been radical vulvectomy, but more conservative techniques are being used to improve psychosexual outcomes.

Nursing Assessment

Typically, no single specific clinical symptom heralds this disease, so diagnosis is often delayed significantly. Therefore, it is important to review the woman's history for risk factors such as:

- Exposure to HPV type 16
- Age over 50
- HIV infection
- VIN
- Lichen sclerosus
- Melanoma or atypical moles
- Exposure to herpes simplex virus (HSV) type II
- Multiple sex partners
- Smoking
- History of breast cancer
- Immune suppression
- Hypertension
- Diabetes mellitus
- Obesity (Rotmensh, 2010)

Vulvar atypias can present with a variety of symptoms. In most cases, the woman reports persistent vulvar itching that does not improve with the use of creams or ointments; however, 20% of patients are asymptomatic. During the physical examination, observe for any masses or thickening of the vulvar area. A vulvar lump or mass most often is noted. Lesions can be flat, raised (maculopapular), or verrucous; they may be brown (hyperpigmented), red (erythroplastic), white, or discoloured (Rotmensh, 2010). Less commonly, the woman may present with vulvar bleeding, discharge, dysuria, and pain.

Nursing Management

Women with vulvar cancer must clearly understand their disease, treatment options, and prognosis. To accomplish this, provide information and establish effective communication with the client and her family. Act as an educator and advocate.

Teach the woman about healthy lifestyle behaviours, such as smoking cessation and measures to reduce risk factors. For example, instruct the woman how to examine her genital area, urging her to do so monthly between menstrual periods. Tell her to look for any changes in appearance (e.g., whitened or reddened patches of skin); changes in feel (e.g., areas of the vulva becoming itchy or painful); or the development of lumps, moles (e.g., changes in size, shape, or colour), freckles, cuts, or sores on the vulva. Urge the woman to report these changes to the health care provider (Cancer.net, 2010).

Teach the woman about preventive measures such as not wearing tight undergarments and not using perfumes and dyes in the vulvar region. Also educate her about the use of barrier methods of birth control (e.g., condoms) to reduce the risk for contracting HIV, HSV, and HPV.

For the woman diagnosed with vulvar cancer, provide information and support. Discuss potential changes in sexuality if radical surgery is performed. Encourage her to communicate openly with her partner. Refer her to appropriate community resources and support groups.

■■■ Key Concepts

- Women have a one-in-three lifetime risk of developing cancer, and one out of every four deaths is from cancer; thus, nurses must focus on screening and educating all women regardless of risk factors.
- The nurse plays a key role in offering emotional support, determining appropriate sources of support, and helping the woman use effective coping strategies when facing a diagnosis of cancer of the reproductive tract. Although reproductive tract cancer is rare during pregnancy, the woman's vigilance and routine screenings should continue throughout.
- A woman's sexuality and culture are inextricably interwoven, and it is essential that nurses working with women of various cultures recognize this and remain sensitive to the vast changes that will take place when the diagnosis of cancer is made.
- Ovarian cancer is the seventh most common cancer among women and the fourth most common cause of cancer deaths for women in Canada, accounting for more deaths than any other cancer of the reproductive system.
- Ovarian cancer has been described as "the overlooked disease" or "silent killer," because women and/or health care practitioners often ignore or rationalize early symptoms. It is typically diagnosed in advanced stages.
- Unopposed endogenous and exogenous estrogens, obesity, nulliparity, menopause after the age of 52 years, and diabetes are the major etiologic risk factors associated with the development of endometrial cancer.

- The CCS recommends that women should be informed about risks and symptoms of endometrial cancer at the onset of menopause and strongly encouraged to report any unexpected bleeding or spotting to their health care providers.
- Malignant diseases of the vagina are either primary vaginal cancers or metastatic forms from adjacent or distant organs. Vaginal cancer tumours can be effectively treated and, when found early, are often curable.
- Cervical cancer incidence and mortality rates have decreased noticeably in the past several decades, with most of the reduction attributed to the Pap test, which detects cervical cancer and precancerous lesions.
- The nurse's role involves primary prevention of cervical cancer through education of women regarding risk factors and preventive techniques to avoid cervical dysplasia.
- Diagnosis of vulvar cancer is often delayed significantly because there is no single specific clinical symptom that heralds it. The most common presentation is persistent vulvar itching that does not improve with the application of creams or ointments.

REFERENCES

American College of Obstetricians and Gynecologists. (2009). ACOG practice bulletin: cervical cytology screening. *Obstetrics and Gynecology, 114*(6), 1409–1420.

Berek, J. S., Friedlander, M. L., & Bast, R. C. (2010). Ovarian cancer. In W. K. Hong, R. C. Bast, W. N. Hait, et al. (Eds.), *Holland-Frei cancer medicine* (8th ed.). Shelton, CT: Peoples Medical Publishing House.

Blackburn, S. T. (2007). *Maternal, fetal and neonatal physiology: A clinical perspective* (3rd ed.). St. Louis, MO: Saunders Elsevier.

Buchanan, E., Weinstein, L., & Hillson, C. (2009). Endometrial cancer. *American Family Physician, 80*(10), 1075–1080.

Canadian Cancer Society. (2009a). *Background on the patenting of BRCA1 and 2 genes.* Toronto, ON: Author.

Canadian Cancer Society. (2009b). *Canadian cancer statistics 2009.* Toronto, ON: Author.

Canadian Cancer Society. (2009c). *Cervical cancer.* Toronto, ON: Author.

Canadian Cancer Society. (2009d). *Ovarian cancer.* Toronto, ON: Author.

Canadian Cancer Society. (2009e). *Uterine cancer.* Toronto, ON: Author.

Cancer.net. (2010). *Vulvar cancer: Risk factors and prevention.* Retrieved February 6, 2012 from http://www.cancer.net/patient/Cancer+Types/Vulvar+Cancer?sectionTitle = Risk%20Factors%20and%20Prevention

Centers for Disease Control and Prevention. (2007). Quadrivalent human papillomavirus vaccine: Recommendations of the Advisory Committee on Immunization Practices (ACIP). *Morbidity and Mortality Weekly Report, 56*(RR-2), 1–24.

Duarte-Franco, E., & Franco, E. (2003). Other gynecologic cancers. In *Women's health surveillance report: A multi-dimensional look at the health of Canadian women.* Ottawa, ON: Canadian Institute for Health Information. Retrieved February 6, 2012 from http://secure.cihi.ca/cihiweb/products/CPHI_WomensHealth_e.pdf

Goldstein, S. R. (2009). The role of transvaginal ultrasound or endometrial biopsy in the evaluation of the menopausal endometrium. *American Journal of Obstetrics and Gynecology, 201*(1), 5–11.

Green, A. E., Ahmed, S., Al Husaini, H. H., et al. (2011). Ovarian cancer. Retrieved February 6, 2012 from http://emedicine.medscape.com/article/265651.

Greenlee, R., Kessel, B., Williams, C., et al. (2010). Prevalence, incidence and natural history of simple ovarian cysts among women >55 years old in a large cancer screening trial. *The American Journal of Obstetrics and Gynecology, 202*(4), 373.e1–e9.

Huang, Y., Yates, P., & Prior, D. (2009). Accommodating the diverse cultural needs of cancer patients and their families in palliative care. *Cancer Nursing, 32*(1), E12–E21.

Jhingran, A. (2010). Neoplasms of the cervix. In W. K. Hong, R. C., Bast, W. N. Hait, et al. (Eds.), *Holland-Frei cancer medicine.* (8th ed.). Shelton, CT: Peoples Medical Publishing House.

Mayo Clinic. (2010). *Cancer prevention: 7 steps to reduce your risk.* Retrieved February 6, 2012 from http://www.mayoclinic.com/health/cancer-prevention/CA00024.

Merck Frosst Canada. (2010). *Product monograph: Gardasil.* Kirkland, QC: Author. Retrieved February 6, 2012 from http://www.merckfrosst.ca/mfcl/en/corporate/products/gardasil.html

National Institutes of Health. (2007). *Cervical cancer prevention.* Retrieved February 6, 2012 from http://www.cancer.gov/cancertopics/pdq/prevention/cervical/HealthProfessional

Nelson, R. (2008). Combining symptom index with CA125 improves detection of ovarian cancer. *Cancer, 12*(13), 2424–2456.

Palmer, J., Vatish, M., & Tidy, J. (2008). Epithelial ovarian cancer in pregnancy: A review of the literature. *International Journal of Obstetrics and Gynaecology, 116*(4), 480–491.

Porth, C. (2009). *Pathopyhsiology* (8th ed.). Philadephia: Lippincott Williams & Wilkins.

Public Health Agency of Canada. (2003). *Cervical cancer in Canada.* Ottawa, ON: Author. Retrieved February 6, 2012 from http://www.phac-aspc.gc.ca/publicat/updates/cervix-98-eng.php.

Rahaman, J., & Cohen, C. (2010). Endometrial cancer. In W. K. Hong, R. C., Bast, W. N. Hait, et al. (Eds.), *Holland-Frei cancer medicine* (8th ed.). Shelton, CT: Peoples Medical Publishing House.

Ricci, S. S., & Kyle, T. (2009). *Maternity and pediatric nursing.* Philadephia: Lippincott Williams & Wilkins.

Rotmensh, J. H. (2010). Neoplasms of the vulva and vagina. In W. K. Hong, R. C., Bast, W. N. Hait, et al. (Eds.), *Holland-Frei cancer medicine.* (8th ed.). Shelton, CT: Peoples Medical Publishing House.

Schroevers, M. J., Schroevers, M. J., Helgeson, V. S., Sanderman, R., & Ranchor A. V. (2010). Type of social support matters for prediction of posttraumatic growth among cancer survivors. *Psycho-Oncology, 19*(1), 46–53.

Society of Obstetricians and Gynaecologists of Canada. (2006). *Clinical practice guidelines: Management of squamous cell cancer of the vagina.* *JOGC, 180*, 640–645. Retrieved May 8, 2012 from http://www.sogc.org/guidelines/documents/180E-CPG-July2006.pdf

Statistics Canada. (2009). *Mortality, summary list of causes. Catalogue no. 84F0209X.* Ottawa, ON: Author.

Stensheim, H., Moller, B., Dijk, T., & Fossa, S. (2009). Cause-specific survival for women diagnosed with cancer during pregnancy or lactation: A registry-based cohort study. *Journal of Clinical Oncology, 27*(1), 45–51.

Whitcomb, B. (2008). Gynecologic malignancies. *Surgical Clinics of North America, 88*(2), 301–317.

World Health Organization. (2012). *Cancer prevention.* Retrieved February 6, 2012 from http://www.who.int/cancer/prevention/en/

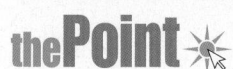 For additional learning materials, including Internet Resources, visit **http://thePoint.lww.com/Chow1e.**

CHAPTER WORKSHEET

MULTIPLE CHOICE QUESTIONS

1. When describing ovarian cancer to a local women's group, the nurse states that ovarian cancer often is not diagnosed early because:

   a. The disease progresses very slowly.

   b. The early stages produce very vague symptoms.

   c. The disease usually is diagnosed only at autopsy.

   d. Clients don't follow up on acute pelvic pain.

2. A postmenopausal woman reports that she has started spotting again. Which of the following would the nurse do?

   a. Instruct the client to keep a menstrual diary for the next few months.

   b. Tell her not to worry, since this a common but not serious event.

   c. Have her start warm-water douches to promote healing.

   d. Anticipate that the doctor will do an endometrial biopsy.

3. Which of the following would the nurse identify as the priority psychosocial need for a women diagnosed with reproductive cancer?

   a. Clear information

   b. Hand-holding

   c. Cheerfulness

   d. Offering of hope

4. When teaching a group of women about screening and early detection of cervical cancer, the nurse would include which of the following as most effective?

   a. Fecal occult blood test

   b. Urine test for culture and sensitivity

   c. CA-125 blood test

   d. Pap smear

5. After teaching a group of students about reproductive tract cancers, the nursing instructor determines that the teaching was successful when the students identify which of the following as the most lethal type of female reproductive cancer?

   a. Vulvar

   b. Ovarian

   c. Endometrial

   d. Cervical

CRITICAL THINKING EXERCISES

1. Tammy Scott, a 27-year-old sexually active white woman, visits the Public Health Department family planning clinic and requests information about the various contraceptive methods available. In taking her history, the nurse learns that she started having sex at age 15 and has had multiple sex partners since then. She smokes two packs of cigarettes daily. She has never previously obtained any gynecologic care.

   a. Based on her history, which risk factors for cervical cancer are present?

   b. What recommendations would you make for her, and why?

   c. What are this client's educational needs concerning health maintenance?

2. Jennifer Nappo, a 60-year-old nulliparous woman, presents to the gynecologic oncology clinic after her health care provider palpated an adnexal mass on her right ovary. In taking her history, the nurse learns that she has experienced mild abdominal bloating and weight loss for the past several months but felt fine otherwise. She was diagnosed with breast cancer 15 years ago and was treated with a lumpectomy and radiation. She has occasionally used talcum powder in her perineal area over the past 20 years.

   A transvaginal ultrasound reveals a complex mass in the right adnexa. She undergoes a total abdominal hysterectomy and bilateral salpingo-oophorectomy and lymph node biopsy. Pathology confirms a diagnosis of stage III ovarian cancer with abdominal metastasis and positive lymph nodes.

   a. Is this client's profile typical for a woman with this diagnosis?

   b. What in her history might increase her risk for ovarian cancer?

   c. What can the nurse do to increase awareness of this cancer for all women?

STUDY ACTIVITIES

1. During your surgical clinical rotation, interview a female client undergoing surgery for cancer of her reproductive organs. Ask her to recall the symptoms that brought her to the health care provider. Ask her what thoughts, feelings, and emotions went through her mind before and after her diagnosis. Finally, ask her how this experience will change her life in the future.

2. Visit an oncology and radiology treatment centre to find out about the various treatment modalities available for reproductive cancers. Contrast the various treatment methods and report your findings to your class.

3. Visit one of the websites listed online for Chapter 8 at http://thePoint.lww.com/Chow1e to explore a topic of interest concerning reproductive cancers. How correct and current is the content? What is its level? Share your assessment with your classmates.

4. Taking oral contraceptives provides protection against _____ cancer.

5. Two genes, BRCA-1 and BRCA-2, are linked with hereditary _____ and _____ cancers.

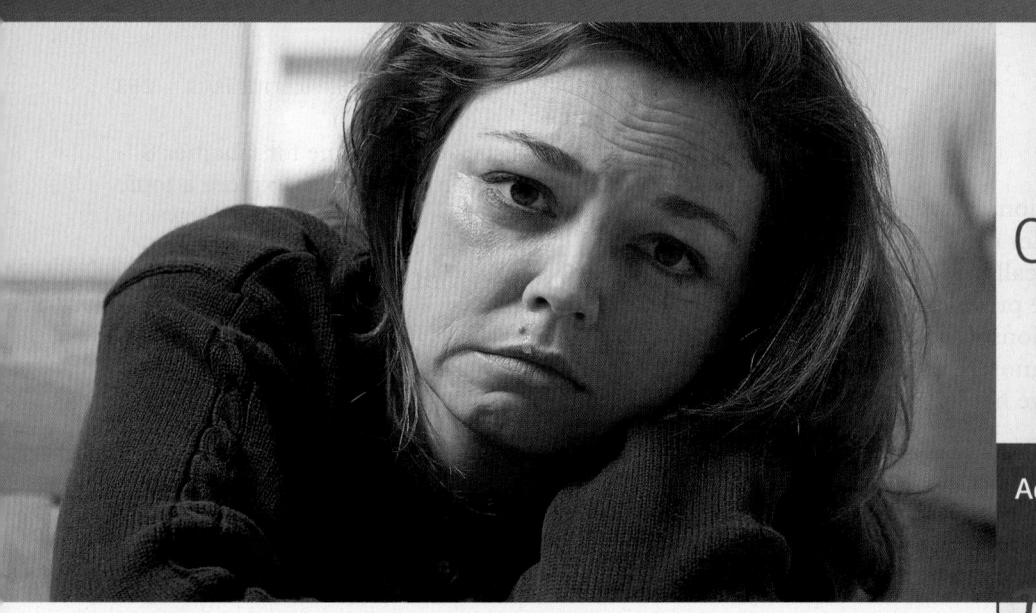

CHAPTER 9

Adapted by Jean Chow

VIOLENCE AND ABUSE

KEY TERMS

acquaintance rape
age of consent
battered woman
  syndrome
cycle of violence

date rape
female genital mutilation
honour crime
human trafficking
incest

intimate partner violence
post-traumatic stress
  disorder
rape
sexual abuse

LEARNING OBJECTIVES

After completion of the chapter, the student should be able to:

1. Define the key terms.
2. Discuss the incidence of violence in women.
3. Outline the cycle of violence and appropriate interventions.
4. Discuss the myths and facts about violence.
5. Analyze the dynamics of rape and sexual abuse.
6. Describe the resources available to women experiencing abuse.
7. Discuss the role of the nurse who cares for abused women.

*D*orothy came to the prenatal clinic with a complaint of recurring headaches. She had been in twice this week already, but insisted she be seen today and started to cry. When the nurse called her into the examination room, Dorothy's cell phone rang. She hurried to answer it and told the person on the other end that she was at the store. When the nurse asked if she was afraid at home, Dorothy answered "at times." What cues did the nurse pick up on to ask that question? How common is this problem in women?

Wow

After being traumatized, women can decide not to accept help or to seek help.

Violence against women and children is a significant health and social problem affecting virtually all societies, but often it goes unrecognized and unreported. In fact, in many countries violence against women is still accepted as part of normal behaviour. Family violence occurs in interpersonal relationships that are characterized by intimacy, kinship, and dependency (National Clearinghouse on Family Violence, 2010) and can include physical, financial, verbal, and emotional abuse (Statistics Canada, 2011).

For all the strides Canadian women have made in the past 100 years, obliterating violence against themselves is not one of them. Although violence against women in Canada is costly in terms of health and social ramifications, it remains under-recognized and shrouded in secrecy. Violence against women is a growing problem and in many countries it is still accepted as part of normal behaviour. The 13th annual *Family Violence in Canada* report, based on results from the 2009 General Social Survey on Victimization (Statistics Canada, 2011), focused on self-reported incidents of spousal abuse and provided the following statistics:

- Females were twice as likely as males to report an injury resulting from spousal violence (42% versus 18%). Of those women who did report an injury, 13% were hospitalized as a result of the injury.
- Younger Canadians (25 to 34 years of age) were three times more likely than older Canadians (age 45 and older) to report being victims of spousal violence (i.e., physical or sexual assault).
- Common-law couples had a higher incidence of spousal violence than legally married couples.
- Women were about three times more likely to be victims of spousal homicide than men.

Children are also affected by family violence. In 2009, 55,000 children and youth encountered physical abuse or sexual abuse (Statistics Canada, 2011). Three in 10 of these offences were perpetrated by a family member. Girls were more than four times more likely than boys to be victims of sexual abuse; physical assault rates for girls and boys were similar (Statistics Canada, 2011).

In Canada, many abused women seek shelter in transition homes and emergency facilities (Sauvé & Burns, 2009). Over half of these women are admitted with their children (Sauvé & Burns, 2009). Between April 1, 2007 and March 31, 2008, approximately 101,000 women and children were admitted to such facilities (Sauvé & Burns, 2009). Emergency housing is provided for 1 day to 11 weeks in transition houses (Sauvé & Burns, 2009). Long-term or second-stage housing (3 to 12 months) includes support to assist women to find permanent accommodations. Safe homes are private settings that provide emergency housing. Some housing provides bilingual services as well as services for mobility, hearing, and vision deficits. The National Clearinghouse on Family Violence provides a comprehensive list of all transition houses and shelters in Canada, including the services each provides; visit http://thePoint.lww.com/Chow1e for a direct link.

According to results of the 2008 Transition Home Survey, which profiles Canadian shelter residents on a specific day of the year, 4,273 women and 3,361 children were living in shelters across Canada on April 16, 2008 (Sauvé & Burns, 2009). Of these women, 3,222 were there to escape an abusive situation and they were accompanied by 2,900 children. The women reported that they wanted to escape psychological, physical, sexual, and financial abuse as well as harassment and threats.

In many cases, a victim escapes her abuser only to be turned away from a local shelter because it is full. Between April 2009 and March 2010, 6,169 women and 5,601 children were accommodated in shelters in Alberta (Alberta Council of Women's Shelters, 2010). During the same period, 9,934 women and 6,342 children could not be accommodated (Alberta Council of Women's Shelters, 2011).

Nurses play a major role in assessing women who have suffered some type of violence. Often, after a woman is victimized, she will complain about physical ailments that give her the opportunity to visit a health care setting. A visit to a health care agency is an ideal time for women to be assessed for violence. Nurses are often viewed as trustworthy and sensitive about very personal subjects, and many women feel comfortable in confiding in or discussing these issues with them. It is important to discuss this issue with clients.

▶ *Take* NOTE!

Nurses will come in contact with violence and sexual abuse no matter what health care setting they work in. Nurses must be ready to ask the right questions and to act on the answers, because such action could be life-saving.

This chapter addresses two types of violence against women: intimate partner violence and sexual abuse. Both types of violence against women have devastating and costly consequences for all of society.

Intimate Partner Violence

The Public Health Agency of Canada (PHAC, 2009a) indicates that intimate partner abuse happens in male, female, and same-sex relationships. **Intimate partner violence** is actual or threatened physical or sexual violence or psychological/emotional abuse. It includes threats of physical or sexual violence when the threat is used to control a person's actions (Cherniak, Grant,

Mason, et al., 2005). It can include psychological abuse, financial abuse, physical abuse, forced intercourse and other means of sexual coercion, and controlling behaviours such as isolating victims from family or friends or preventing the person from obtaining assistance. Intimate partners include individuals who are currently in dating, cohabitating, or marital relationships, or those who have been in such relationships in the past. Men and women can both be victims of abuse, but in most cases men are the abusers. Most of the offenders are current and former partners. Some of the common terms used to describe intimate partner violence are domestic abuse, spouse abuse, wife abuse, domestic violence, family violence, assault, battering, and rape. Intimate partner violence occurs regardless of education, economic status, ethnicity, race, or religion.

There are common warning signs for intimate partner violence (PHAC, 2009a). The partner has to be right, makes decisions about daily activities, controls the financial resources, and demands to know the whereabouts of the partner and who is with the partner. Intimate partner violence affects a distressingly high percentage of the population and has physical, psychological, social, and economic consequences (Fig. 9.1).

A nurse may be the first health care professional to assess and identify the signs of intimate partner violence and can have a profound impact on a woman's decision to seek help. Thus, it is important for nurses to be able to identify abuse and aid the victim. Intimate partner violence can leave significant psychological scars, and a well-trained nurse can have a positive impact on the victim's mental and emotional health.

Incidence

Data from the 2009 General Social Survey on Victimization indicate that the 5-year rate of intimate partner violence has remained stable at 6% since 2004 (Statistics

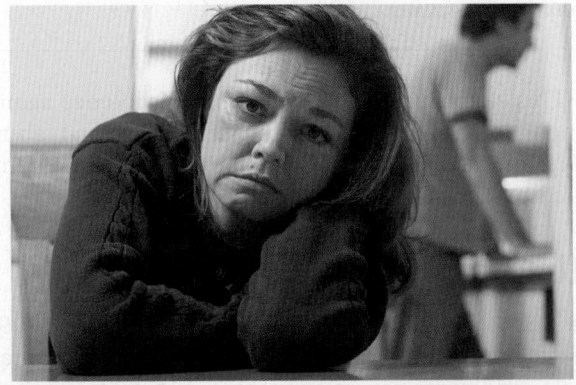

FIGURE 9.1 Intimate partner violence has significant physical, psychological, social, and economic consequences. An important role of the health care provider is to identify abusive or potentially abusive situations as soon as possible and provide support for the victim.

Canada, 2011). The proportion of reported spousal abuse was similar across the country. Only Newfoundland, Labrador, and Quebec reported spousal violence rates below the national average. In 2009, the highest rates of spousal homicide were in Manitoba, Saskatchewan, British Columbia, Nunavut, and Northwest Territories. Women are more likely to be murdered by a legally married spouse, while men are more likely to be murdered by a common-law partner (Beattie & Cotter, 2010; Statistics Canada, 2011).

Women are at risk for violence at nearly every stage of their lives. Old, young, beautiful, unattractive, married, single—no woman is completely safe from the risk of intimate partner violence. Approximately 1 billion dollars was spent in 2002 on direct medical costs related to abuse against women (Women, Information and Advocacy, 2009). Annual costs for related short- and long-term psychiatric care are estimated to be $506 million (SexualityandU.ca, 2010b).

Abuse among certain groups requires particular attention. Violence within gay and lesbian relationships may go unreported for fear of harassment or ridicule. These people may already be stigmatized by society and find it difficult to seek help and support (Department of Justice Canada, 2009). Disabled and dependent people may be vulnerable to abuse as well. Disability is regarded as difficulty with the activities with daily living, physical or cognitive difficulty, or a health issue (PHAC, 2009c). Abuse may be perpetrated by an intimate partner, family member or care provider. Disabled women who are dependent on others for care are vulnerable to abuse. When abuse is present, the incidents are rarely isolated and occur on an ongoing basis. Women with disabilities are abused at a much greater rate than women without disabilities. Challenges to disabled women include decreased financial resources, dependency on care providers, decreased availability of support services, decreased accessibility to settings where assistance can be provided, barriers to contacting police, and control issues that accompany dependency.

Most Aboriginal women have experienced physical domestic abuse, and child sexual abuse is prevalent (Smylie, 2001). Aboriginal communities have a higher incidence of intimate partner abuse than the rest of Canada (National Clearinghouse on Family Violence, 2008). In 2009, nearly 67,000 Aboriginal women 15 years of age or older reported being victims of violence (Brennan, 2011). The reported incidence of sexual assault among Aboriginals in 2009 was 70 per 1,000 versus 23 per 1,000 in the non-Aboriginal population (Perreault, 2011). Of nonspousal violent events involving Aboriginal women, 76% were not reported to police—a rate similar to that among non-Aboriginal women (70%) (Brennan, 2011). When violence occurs, Aboriginal women reported that it must be very severe before it is reported to police or before the woman leaves home (National Clearinghouse on Family Violence, 2008). Due to the

EVIDENCE-BASED PRACTICE 9.1
An Exploratory Study of Help-Seeking Behaviours in South Asian Immigrant Women Experiencing Partner Abuse

The goal of this qualitative study using critical emancipatory and feminist perspectives was to examine help-seeking in South Asian immigrant women experiencing partner abuse.

● **Study**

Twenty-two South Asian women who immigrated from India, Pakistan, and Bangladesh were recruited to participate in three focus groups located at three community centres in Toronto. Each focus group meeting lasted 1.5 to 2 hours. Only two of the meetings were audiotaped because the third group expressed discomfort with recording; detailed notes were made during this meeting. Participants received reimbursement to cover travel costs and time. The discussions were held in Hindi, and a bilingual assistant took notes. The discussion covered sources of help-seeking, timing of help-seeking, and reasons for delaying help-seeking. After data interpretation, the participations were debriefed about the findings.

▲ **Findings**

The themes of reasons for delaying help-seeking, turning points, and professional support arose from the findings. All the women sought professional help only after a lengthy time period during which their health suffered. The women delayed help-seeking because of stigma, culturally defined gender roles, concern about their children's well-being, loss of social support, and lack of knowledge about available resources. The turning point for seeking professional help came after the women's coping resources were depleted. Interactions with health professionals were facilitated by trust, non-judgmental attitude, cultural understanding, and having a female physician. The availability of social services was appreciated. The women indicated that physicians should ask about abuse in patient visits.

■ **Nursing Implications**

As immigrants arrive in Canada, it is important for nurses to assess for possible abuse issues. Prevention is needed in addressing partner abuse, and community education and grass-roots organizations, religious centres, social services, and media may be utilized to address the issue. Nurses need to be aware that South Asian immigrant women experiencing intimate partner abuse may delay help-seeking. Nurses should learn about culturally competent interventions and know how to utilize them.

Ahmed, F., Driver, N., McNally, M. J., & Stewart, D. E. (2009). "Why doesn't she seek help for partner abuse?" An exploratory study with South Asian immigrant women. *Social Science & Medicine, 69,* 613–622.

ethnocentric nature of the Canadian judicial system, Aboriginal women perceive police to be unresponsive and indifferent to their safety (Dylan, Regehr, & Alaggia, et al., 2008). See Evidence-based Practice 9.1.

Background

Until recently, Canadian society tended to legitimize a man's power and control over a woman. The Canadian legal and judicial systems considered intervention into family disputes wrong and a violation of the family's right to privacy. Intimate partner violence was often tolerated and even socially acceptable. Fortunately, attitudes and laws have changed to protect women and punish abusers.

Characteristics of Intimate Partner Violence

Intimate partner violence is a complex issue, and both men and women can be victims or perpetrate violence (Caetano, Vaeth, & Ramisetty-Mikler, 2008). Multiple factors can lead to either victimization or perpetration of violence:

• Use and abuse of substances such as alcohol (increases the risk of victimization for men)

• Powerlessness
• History of victimization
• Member of an ethnic minority group
• Impulsivity
• Age (less violent relationships exist with older age)
• Prior criminal charges (Caetano et al., 2008; Eke, Hilton, Harris, et al., 2011)

Generation-to-Generation Continuum of Violence

Violence is a learned behaviour that, without intervention, is self-perpetuating. It is a cyclical health problem. The long-term effects of violence on victims and children can be profound. Children who witness one parent abuse another are more likely to become delinquents or batterers themselves because they see abuse as an integral part of a close relationship. Thus, an abusive relationship between father and mother can perpetuate future abusive relationships. Children who witness family violence are at risk for emotional disorders, post-traumatic stress disorder (PTSD), anxiety, depression, developmental problems, irregular school attendance, and violence against others (PHAC, 2009b).

Childhood maltreatment is a major health problem that is associated with a wide range of physical conditions and leads to high rates of psychiatric morbidity and social problems in adulthood. In 2008, 235,842 investigations of child maltreatment were conducted in Canada, similar to the 235,315 investigations conducted in 2003 (PHAC, 2010). Of these investigations, 85,440 were substantiated (14.19 per 1,000 children), with 18,510 (22%) involving children of Aboriginal heritage. Exposure to intimate partner violence and neglect were the two most frequently occurring groupings.

In a telephone survey conducted in Quebec, 22.1% of female respondents and 9.7% of male respondents indicated that they had experienced childhood sexual abuse (Hebert, Tourigny, Cyr, et al., 2009). Few had ever previously disclosed the abuse (about one in five), and men were less likely than women to have disclosed. Women who were physically or sexually abused as children are at increased risk for victimization and experience adverse physical and mental health conditions such as depression, anxiety, lack of trust in the community, higher body mass index, joint pain, and nausea and vomiting (Bonomi, Cannon, Anderson, et al., 2008; Cannon, Anderson, Rivara, et al., 2010).

When a parent is abused, the children are abused as well (Society of Obstetricians and Gynaecologists of Canada [SOGC], 2011). Exposure to violence has a negative impact on children's physical, emotional, and cognitive well-being. The cycle continues into another generation through learned responses and violent acting out. While there are always exceptions, most children deprived of their basic physical, psychological, and spiritual needs do not develop healthy personalities. They struggle with depression, self-blame, life dissatisfaction, relationship difficulties, low self-esteem, and trust issues (PHAC, 2009b). The health effects of domestic violence on children depend on the age of the child and may include failure to thrive, PTSD, anxiety, cruelty to animals, aggression, bullying, property destruction, suicide, somatic concerns, running away from home, and problems with school attendance and performance (SexualityandU.ca, 2010c). Men who assault their partners will assault their children; in turn, women who are assaulted will assault their children (Chambliss, 2008).

The Cycle of Violence

In an abusive relationship, the **cycle of violence** comprises three distinct phases: the tension-building phase, the acute battering phase, and the honeymoon phase (Dutton, 2006). The cyclical behaviour begins with a time of tension-building arguments, progresses to violence, and settles into a making-up or calm period. This cycle of violence increases in frequency and severity as it is repeated over and over again. The cycle can cover a long or short period of time. The honeymoon phase gradually shortens and eventually disappears altogether.

Abuse in relationships typically becomes accelerated and thus more dangerous over time. The abuser no longer feels the need to apologize and indulge in a honeymoon phase as the woman becomes increasingly disempowered in the relationship.

Phase 1: Tension-Building

During the first—and usually the longest—phase of the cycle, tension escalates between the couple. Excessive drinking, jealousy, or other factors might lead to name-calling, hostility, and friction. The woman might sense that her partner is reacting to her more negatively, that he is on edge and reacts heatedly to any trivial frustration. A woman often will accept her partner's building anger as legitimately directed toward her. She internalizes what she perceives as her responsibility to keep the situation from exploding. In her mind, if she does her job well, he remains calm. But if she fails, the resulting violence is her fault.

Phase 2: Acute Battering

The second phase of the cycle is the explosion of violence. The batterer loses control both physically and emotionally. This is when the victim may be assaulted or murdered. After a battering episode, most victims consider themselves lucky that the abuse was not worse, no matter how severe their injuries. They often deny the seriousness of their injuries and refuse to seek medical treatment.

Phase 3: Honeymoon

The third phase of the cycle is a period of calm, loving, contrite behaviour on the part of the batterer. He may be genuinely sorry for the pain he caused his partner. He attempts to make up for his brutal behaviour and believes he can control himself and never again hurt the woman he loves. The victim wants to believe that her partner really can change. She feels responsible, at least in part, for causing the incident, and she feels responsible for her partner's well-being (Box 9.1).

Types of Abuse

Abusers may use whatever it takes to control a situation—from emotional abuse and humiliation to physical assault. Victims often tolerate emotional, physical, financial, and sexual abuse. Many remain in abusive relationships because they believe they deserve the abuse.

Emotional Abuse

Emotional abuse includes:

• Promising, swearing, or threatening to hit the victim
• Forcing the victim to perform degrading or humiliating acts
• Threatening to harm children, pets, or close friends
• Humiliating the woman by name-calling and insults
• Threatening to leave her and the children

- Destroying valued possessions
- Controlling the victim's every move

Physical Abuse

Physical abuse includes:

- Hitting or grabbing the victim so hard that it leaves marks
- Throwing things at the victim
- Slapping, spitting at, biting, burning, pushing, choking, or shoving the victim
- Kicking or punching the victim, or slamming her against things
- Attacking the victim with a knife, gun, rope, or electrical cord
- Controlling access to health care for injury

Financial Abuse

Financial abuse includes:

- Preventing the woman from getting a job
- Sabotaging a current job
- Controlling how all money is spent
- Failing to contribute financially

Sexual Abuse

Sexual abuse includes:

- Forcing the woman to have vaginal, oral, or anal intercourse against her will
- Biting the victim's breasts or genitals
- Shoving objects into the victim's vagina or anus
- Forcing the victim to perform sexual acts on other people or animals

Myths and Facts About Intimate Partner Violence

There are many myths about intimate partner violence (Table 9.1). Health care providers should take steps to dispel these myths.

Abuse Profiles

Victims

Ironically, victims rarely describe themselves as abused. In **battered woman syndrome**, the woman has experienced deliberate and repeated physical or sexual assault by an intimate partner. She is terrified and feels trapped, helpless, and alone. She reacts to any expression of anger or threat by avoidance and withdrawal behaviour.

Some women believe that the abuse is caused by a personality flaw or inadequacy in themselves (e.g., inability to keep the man happy). These feelings of failure are reinforced and exploited by their partners. After being told repeatedly that they are "bad," some women begin to believe it. Many victims were abused as children and may have mental and physical health issues as a result (Cannon et al., 2010).

Abusers

Abusers come from all walks of life and often feel insecure, powerless, and helpless, feelings that are not in line with the image they would like to project. The abusers can be family members, ex-partners, friends, acquaintances, or strangers (Statistics Canada, 2011).

Violence typically occurs at home and is usually directed toward the woman's or man's intimate partner or the children who live there. Abusers may fail to accept responsibility or blame others for their own problems. They may tend to express negative feelings and meet their needs through controlling behaviours (SexualityandU.ca, 2010a). They may have stereotypical perceptions about male and female roles and relationships. Abusers may be jealous and dependent on their partners. They may minimize and blame their partners for the abuse. They may be pleasant outside of the home but show the reverse behaviours at home.

Violence Against Pregnant Women

Many think of pregnancy as a time of celebration and planning for the unborn child's future, but in a troubled relationship it can be a time of escalating violence. For women who have been abused before, beatings and violence during pregnancy are "business as usual" for them.

Women are at a higher risk for violence during pregnancy. Pregnant women are vulnerable during this time,

TABLE 9.1 COMMON MYTHS AND FACTS ABOUT VIOLENCE

Myths	Facts
Battering of women occurs only in lower socioeconomic classes.	Violence occurs in all socioeconomic classes.
Violence occurs to only a small percentage of women.	One in five Canadian men admits to being violent toward a partner; 10% of Canadian women live with an abusive partner.
Substance abuse causes the violence.	Drugs and alcohol can be used as an excuse for violence, but abuse occurs even when the person is sober and not under the influence of drugs.
Women can easily choose to leave the abusive relationship.	Women stay in the abusive relationship because they feel they have no options.
Survivors/men who abuse have mental health problems.	Survivors and abusers often seem normal and don't appear to suffer from personality disorders or other forms of mental illness.
Pregnant women are protected from abuse by their partners.	Women are physically abused during pregnancy. The effects of violence on infant outcomes can include preterm delivery, fetal distress, low birth weight, and child abuse.
Women provoke their partners to abuse them.	Women may be willing to blame themselves for someone else's bad behaviour, but nobody deserves to be beaten.
The woman is to blame for abuse.	A woman is prevented from moving away from the abuser by being blamed.
Abuse only occurs once.	Abuse occurs multiple times before it is disclosed.
Injuries related to abuse are typically not serious.	Twenty percent of homicides in Canada are related to family violence. One quarter of the women who are abused attempt suicide.

Sources: Canadian Divorce Laws. (2011). *Domestic violence.* Retrieved February 7, 2012 from www.canadiandivorcelaws.com/domestic-violence/; Manitoba Association of Women's Shelters. (2008). *What is abuse?* Retrieved February 7, 2012 from www.maws.mb.ca/domestic_violence. htm; SexualityandU.ca. (2010a). *Characteristics of abusers.* Retrieved February 7, 2012 from http://www.sexualityandu.ca/health-care-professionals/domestic-violence/characteristics-of-abuse; SexualityandU.ca (2010b). *Domestic violence.* Retrieved February 7, 2012 from www.sexuality-andu.ca/en/health-care-professionals/domestic-violence; SexualtyandU.ca (2010c). *Health effects of abuse.* Retrieved February 7, 2012 from http://www.sexualityandu.ca/health-care- professionals/domestic_violence/health_effects_of_abuse; & Westbrook, L. (2009). Information myths and intimate partner violence: Sources, contexts, and consequences. *Journal of the American Society for Information Science and Technology, 60*(4), 826–836.

and abusers can take advantage of it. Abuse during pregnancy poses special risks and dynamics. Women with planned pregnancies may choose to have abortions if they have been victims of physical or sexual abuse within the past year (Bourassa & Berube, 2007; Chambliss, 2008).

Various factors may lead to battering during pregnancy, including:

• Inability of the couple to cope with the stressors of pregnancy
• Resentment toward the interference of the growing fetus and change in the woman's shape
• Doubts about paternity or the expectant mother's fidelity during pregnancy
• Perception that the baby will be a competitor
• Outside attention the pregnancy brings to the woman
• Unwanted pregnancy
• The woman's new interest in herself and her unborn baby

• Insecurity and jealousy about the pregnancy and the responsibilities it brings
• Financial burden related to the expense of pregnancy and loss of income
• Stress of the role transition from adult man to becoming the father of a child
• Physical and emotional changes of pregnancy that make the woman vulnerable
• Previous isolation from family and friends that limit the couple's support system

Abuse during pregnancy and postpartum threatens the well-being of the mother and fetus. Physical violence may involve injuries to the breasts, genitals, and abdomen (Cherniak et al., 2005). The mental health consequences are also significant. Several studies have confirmed the relationship between abuse and poor mental health, especially depression (Antoniou, Vivilaki, & Daglas, 2008; Beydoun, Al-Sahab, Beydoun, et al., 2010). For the pregnant woman, this most often manifests itself as postpartum depression.

▶ *Take* NOTE!

Frequently, the fear of harm to her unborn child will motivate a woman to escape an abusive relationship.

Women assaulted during pregnancy are at risk for:

- Injuries to themselves and the fetus
- Maternal depression
- Maternal stress
- Miscarriage
- Fetal injury, fetal death
- Maternal infections (e.g., vaginal, cervical, uterine)
- Exacerbation of chronic illness
- Placental abruption
- Premature rupture of membranes
- Insufficient weight gain
- Abdominal trauma
- Delayed or no prenatal care
- Preterm labour and low birth weight
- Risk of infectious complications in pregnancy due to the effect of stress on the immune system (Chambliss, 2008; Cherniak et al., 2005; Shah & Shah, 2010)

Signs of abuse can emerge during pregnancy and may include poor attendance at prenatal visits, unrealistic fears, weight fluctuations, difficulty with pelvic examinations, and noncompliance with treatment.

Intimate partner violence during pregnancy is as common or more so than routinely tested conditions such as pre-eclampsia, diabetes, aneuploidy in advanced age, HIV, abnormal Pap smear, or abnormal serum screen (Chambliss, 2008). Uncovering abuse in pregnant women requires a consistent and direct approach to every client by the nurse. Multiple assessments may enhance reporting by enabling the nurse to establish trust and rapport with the woman and identify changes in her behaviour. Once abuse is discovered in a pregnant woman, interventions should include development of a safety plan, emotional support, counselling, referral to community services, ongoing prenatal care, and interventions related to children and adolescents (SOGC, 2005).

Violence Against Older Women

Intimate partner violence affects women of all ages, but often the literature focuses on women in the childbearing years, ignoring the problems of aging women experiencing abuse. Abuse is covered by the Criminal Code of Canada (Canadian Network for the Prevention of Elder Abuse, 2010). Reporting of abuse falls under provincial and territorial jurisdiction.

Although an injury may bring the older woman into the health care system, the physical and emotional sequelae of intimate partner violence may be more subtle and can include psychological problems (e.g., panic attacks, acute anxiety), depression, detrimental effect on family relationships, insomnia, loss of self-esteem, chronic pain, frustration, hopelessness, and shame (McGarry, Simpson, & Mansour, 2010). There is little research about older women and domestic violence. Accurate detection and assessment of abuse in elderly women are essential duties of all nurses.

Nursing Management

Nurses encounter thousands of abuse victims each year in their practice settings, but many victims slip through the cracks. There are many things that nurses can do to help victims. Early recognition and intervention can significantly reduce the morbidity and mortality associated with intimate partner violence. To stop the cycle of violence, nurses need to know how to assess for and identify violence and implement appropriate actions. The key is astute assessment and identification.

Assessment

Routine screening for intimate partner violence is the first way to detect abuse. In its best practice guideline for woman abuse, the Registered Nurses' Association of Ontario (RNAO, 2005) provides the following universal screening recommendations for females 12 years of age and older:

- Screening should take place when the woman's condition is stable.
- Questions should be asked face-to-face in a private area.
- Screening should take place when the woman is alone and not in the presence of a partner, family members, or children over the age of 3.
- Nurses need to be mindful of the woman's safety.
- If language barriers are present, trained cultural interpreters should be utilized.

Despite the importance of assisting women, nurses need maintain awareness that there are risks in screening women (Cory & Dechief, 2007). The health and safety of the woman may not be improved when she is identified as experiencing abuse. The nurse should build rapport by showing an interest in the woman's concerns, listening, and creating an atmosphere of openness. Communicating support through a non-judgmental attitude, or telling her that no one deserves to be abused, is the first step toward establishing trust and rapport. Rather than overlooking abused women as "chronic complainers," astute nurses need to be vigilant for subtle clues of abuse. When a woman denies abuse, information and education about abuse should be provided and her response should be documented (RNAO, 2005). Nurses in screening and responding to abuse need to pay attention to race, ethnicity, economic status, spiritual beliefs, age, sexual orientation, and language ability.

Learning how to assess for abuse is critical. Some basic assessment guidelines follow.

Screen for Abuse During Every Health Care Visit

Screening for violence takes only a few minutes and can have an enormously positive effect on the outcome for the abused woman. Any woman could be a victim; no single sign marks a woman as an abuse victim, but the following clues may be helpful:

- Injuries: bruises, scars from blunt trauma, or weapon wounds on the face, head, and neck
- Injury sequelae: headaches, hearing loss, joint pain, sinus infections, teeth marks, clumps of hair missing, dental trauma, pelvic pain, breast or genital injuries
- Reported history of injury that is not consistent with the actual presenting problem
- Mental health problems: depression, anxiety, substance abuse, eating disorders, suicidal ideation or suicide attempts
- Frequent health care visits for chronic, stress-related disorders such as chest pain, headaches, back or pelvic pain, insomnia, and gastrointestinal disturbances
- Partner's behaviour at the health care visit: appears overly solicitous or overprotective, is unwilling to leave her alone with the health care provider (although in cross-cultural settings, this may not be applicable [SOGC, 2005]).

Look for the following indicators of abuse:

- Previous history of assault
- Previous injuries inflicted by weapons
- Multiple medical visits for injuries or anxiety symptoms
- History of depression, substance use, or suicide attempts
- Tranquilizer or sedative use
- Sexually transmitted infections (STIs) or pelvic inflammatory disease
- Bruises to the upper arm, neck and face, abdomen, or breasts
- Comments about emotional or physical abuse of "a friend"
- Hovering behaviour of male partner during visit (may not be applicable in some cultural settings) (SOGC, 2005)

Dorothy, whom you met at the beginning of the chapter, has been frequenting the clinic with vague somatic complaints in recent weeks and admits she is sometimes afraid at home. She tells the nurse her partner doesn't want her to work, even though he was only sporadically employed at low-paying jobs. What cues in her assessment might indicate abuse? What physical signs might the nurse observe?

Isolate Patient Immediately From Family

If abuse is detected, immediately isolate the woman to provide privacy and to prevent potential retaliation from the abuser. Asking about abuse in front of the perpetrator may trigger an abusive episode during the interview or at home. Ways to ensure the woman's safety would be to take the victim to an area away from the abuser to ask questions. The assessment can take place anywhere—x-ray area, ultrasound room, elevator, ladies' room, laboratory—that is private and away from the abuser.

If abuse is detected, the nurse can do the following to enhance the nurse–client relationship:

- Educate the woman about the connection between the violence and her symptoms.
- Help the woman acknowledge what has happened to her and begin to deal with the situation.
- Offer her referrals so she can get the help that will allow her to begin to heal.

Dorothy returns to the prenatal clinic a month later with anemia, inadequate weight gain, bruises on her face and neck, and second-trimester bleeding. This time she is accompanied by her partner, who stays close to Dorothy. What questions should the nurse ask to assess the situation? Where is the appropriate location to ask these questions? What legal responsibilities does the nurse have concerning her observations?

Ask Direct or Indirect Questions About Abuse

Questions to screen for abuse should be routine and handled just like any other question. Many nurses feel uncomfortable asking questions of this nature, but broaching the subject is important even if the answer comes later. Just knowing that someone else knows about the abuse offers a victim some relief.

Ask difficult questions in an empathetic and non-threatening manner and remain non-judgmental in all responses and interactions. Choose the type of question that makes you most comfortable. Direct and indirect questions produce the same results. "Does your partner hit you?" or "Have you ever been or are you now in an abusive relationship?" are direct questions. If that approach feels uncomfortable, try indirect questions: "We see many women with injuries or complaints like yours and often they are being abused. Is that what is happening to you?" or "Many women in our community experience abuse from their partners. Is anything like that happening in your life?" With either approach, nurses need to maintain a non-judgmental acceptance of whatever answer the woman offers.

The SAVE Model is a screening protocol that nurses can use when assessing women for violence (Box 9.2).

BOX 9.2 **Save Model**

Screen All of Your Patients for Violence by Asking:
- Do you feel safe in your home?
- Do you feel you are in control of your life?
- Have you ever been sexually or physically abused?
- Can you talk about your abuse with me now?

Ask Direct Questions in a Non-Judgmental Way:
- Begin by normalizing the topic to the woman.
- Make continuous eye contact with the woman.
- Stay calm; avoid emotional reactions to what she tells you.
- Never blame the woman, even if she blames herself.
- Don't dismiss or minimize what she tells you, even if she does.
- Wait for each answer patiently. Don't rush to the next question.
- Do not use formal, technical, or medical language.
- Use a nonthreatening, accepting approach.

Validate the Patient by Telling Her:
- You believe her story.
- You do not blame her for what happened.
- It is brave of her to tell you this.
- Help is available for her.
- Talking with you is a hopeful sign and a first big step.

Evaluate, Educate, and Refer This Patient by Asking Her:
- What type of violence was it?
- Is she now in any danger?
- How is she feeling now?
- Does she know that there are consequences to violence?
- Is she aware of community resources available to help her?

Sources: Dutton, D. G. (2006). Rethinking domestic violence. Vancouver, BC: University of British Columbia Press; Du Plat-Jones, J. (2006). Domestic violence: The role of health professionals. *Nursing Standard, 21*(14), 44–48; & Thackeray J., Stelzner, S., Downs, S. M., & Miller, C. (2007). Screening for intimate partner violence. *Journal of Interpersonal Violence, 22*(6), 659–670.

Assess Immediate Safety

The Danger Assessment Tool helps women and health care providers assess the potential for homicidal behaviour in an ongoing abusive relationship. It is based on research that showed several risk factors for abuse-related murders:

- Increased frequency or severity of abuse
- Presence of firearms
- Sexual abuse
- Substance abuse
- Generally violent behaviour outside of the home
- Control issues (e.g., daily chores, friends, job, money)
- Physical abuse during pregnancy
- Suicide threats or attempts (victim or abuser)
- Child abuse (Kelly, 2007)

Document and Report Your Findings

If the interview reveals a history of abuse, accurate documentation is critical because this evidence may support the woman's case in court. Documentation must include details about the frequency and severity of abuse; the location, extent, and outcome of injuries; and any treatments or interventions. When documenting, use direct quotes and be very specific: "He choked me." Describe any visible injuries, and use a body map (outline of a woman's body) to show where the injuries are. Obtain photos (with informed consent) or document her refusal if the woman declines photos. Pictures or diagrams can be worth a thousand words. Figure 9.2 shows a sample documentation form for intimate partner violence.

Mandatory reporting to police of any injuries that involve knives, firearms, or other deadly weapons or that present life-threatening emergencies remains controversial in Canada. Ontario passed a bill in 2004 requiring mandatory reporting of weapon-related injuries.

Nursing Diagnosis

When violence is suspected or validated, the nurse needs to formulate nursing diagnoses based on the completed assessment. Possible nursing diagnoses related to violence against women might include the following:

- Deficient knowledge related to understanding the cycle of violence and availability of resources
- Fear related to the possibility of severe injury to self or children during cycle of violence
- Low self-esteem related to feelings of worthlessness
- Hopelessness related to prolonged exposure to violence
- Compromised individual and family coping related to persistence of victim–abuser relationship

Interventions

If abuse is identified, nurses can undertake interventions that can increase the woman's safety and improve her health. The goal of intervention is to enable the victim to gain control of her life. Provide sensitive, predictable care in an accepting setting. Offer step-by-step explanations of procedures. Provide educational materials about violence. Allow the victim to actively participate in her care and have control over all health care decisions. Pace your nursing interventions and allow the woman to take the lead. Communicate support through a non-judgmental attitude. Carefully document assessment findings and nursing interventions.

Depending on when in the cycle of violence the nurse encounters the abused woman, goals may fall into three groups:

- Primary prevention: aimed at breaking the abuse cycle through community educational initiatives by nurses, physicians, law enforcement, teachers, and clergy

Woman Abuse: Screening, Identification and Initial Response

Appendix C: Assessment Tools for the Nurse

ABUSE ASSESSMENT SCREEN[1] (AAS)

1. **WITHIN THE LAST YEAR**, have you been hit, slapped, kicked, or otherwise physically hurt by someone?　　　　YES　　NO

   If YES, by whom?_____
   Total number of times_____

2. **SINCE YOU'VE BEEN PREGNANT**, have you been hit, slapped, kicked, or otherwise physically hurt by someone?　　YES　　NO

   If YES, by whom?_____
   Total number of times_____

MARK THE AREA OF INJURY ON THE BODY MAP.
SCORE EACH INCIDENT ACCORDING TO THE FOLLOWING SCALE:　　SCORE

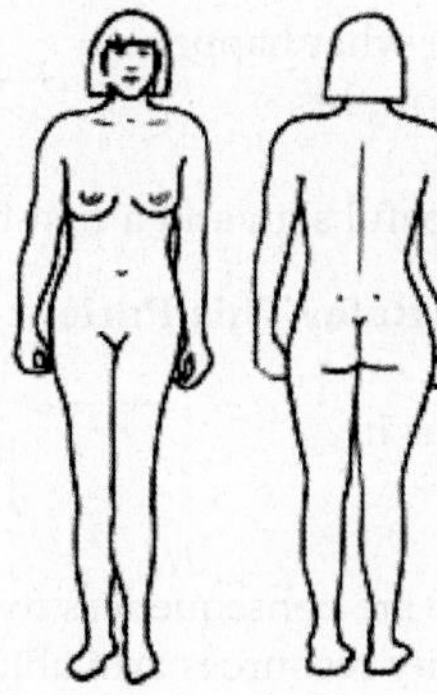

1 = Threats of abuse including use of a weapon
2 = Slapping, pushing; no injuries and/or lasting pain
3 = Punching, kicking, bruises, cuts and/or continuing pain
4 = Beating up, severe contusions, burns, broken bones
5 = Head injury, internal injury, permanent injury
6 = Use of weapon; wound from weapon

If any of the descriptions for the higher number apply, use the higher number.

3. **WITHIN THE LAST YEAR**, has anyone forced you to have sexual activities?　　　　YES　　NO

   If YES, by whom?_____
   Total number of times_____

Source: McFarlane & Parker, (1994). In Fishwick, N. (1998). Assessment of women for partner abuse. *Journal of Obstetric, Gynecologic, & Neonatal Nursing, 27,* 661–670. Reproduced with permission.

[1] Note: this tool is validated

FIGURE 9.2 Intimate partner violence documentation form.

• Secondary prevention: focuses on dealing with victims and abusers in early stages, with the goal of preventing progression of abuse
• Tertiary prevention: activities are geared toward helping severely abused women and children recover and become productive members of society and rehabilitating abusers to stop the cycle of violence. These activities are typically long term and expensive.

A tool developed by Holtz and Furniss (1993)—the ABCDES—provides a framework for providing sensitive nursing interventions to abused women (Box 9.3).

Specific nursing interventions for the abused woman include educating her about community services, providing emotional support, and offering a safety plan.

BOX 9.3 The ABCDES of Caring for Abused Women

- **A** is reassuring the woman that she is not alone. The isolation by her abuser keeps her from knowing that others are in the same situation and that health care providers can help her.
- **B** is expressing the belief that violence against women is not acceptable in any situation and that it is not her fault.
- **C** is confidentiality, since the woman might believe that if the abuse is reported, the abuser will retaliate.
- **D** is documentation, which includes the following:
  1. A clear quoted statement about the abuse
  2. Accurate descriptions of injuries and the history of them
  3. Photos of the injuries (with the woman's consent)
- **E** is education about the cycle of violence and that it will escalate.
- **S** is safety, the most important aspect of the intervention, to ensure that the woman has resources and a plan of action to carry out when she decides to leave.

Educate the Woman About Community Services

A wide range of support services are available to meet the needs of victims of violence. Nurses should be prepared to help the woman take advantage of these opportunities. Services will vary by community but might include psychological counselling, legal advice, social services, crisis services, support groups, hotlines, housing, vocational training, and other community-based referrals.

Give the woman information about shelters or services even if she initially rejects it. She may be able to use this information at a later point. Give the woman the National Domestic Violence hotline number: 800-363-9010.

Provide Emotional Support

Providing reassurance and support to a victim of abuse is key if the violence is to end. Nurses in all clinical settings can help victims to feel a sense of personal power and provide them with a safe and supportive environment. Appropriate action can help victims to express their thoughts and feelings in constructive ways, manage stress, and move on with their lives. Appropriate interventions are:

Strengthen the woman's sense of control over her life by:

- Teaching coping strategies to manage her stress
- Assisting with activities of daily living to improve her lifestyle
- Allowing her to make as many decisions as she can
- Educating her about the symptoms of PTSD and their basis

Encourage the woman to establish realistic goals for herself by:

- Teaching problem-solving skills
- Encouraging social activities to connect with other people

Provide support and allow the woman to grieve for her losses by:

- Listening to and clarifying her reactions to the traumatic event
- Discussing shock, disbelief, anger, depression, and acceptance

Explain to the woman that:

- Abuse is never OK. She didn't ask for it and she doesn't deserve it.
- She is not alone and help is available.
- Abuse is a crime and she is a victim.
- Alcohol, drugs, money problems, depression, or jealousy does not cause violence, but these things can give the abuser an excuse for losing control and abusing her.
- The actions of the abuser are not her fault.
- Her history of abuse is believed.
- Making a decision to leave an abusive relationship can be very hard and takes time.

Offer a Safety Plan

The choice to leave must rest with the victim. Nurses cannot choose a life for the victim; they can only offer choices. Leaving is a process, not an event. Victims may try to leave their abusers as many as seven or eight times before succeeding (SOGC, 2005). Women planning to leave an abusive relationship should have a safety plan, if possible (Teaching Guideline 9.1).

Sexual Violence

Sexual violence is both a public health problem and a human rights violation. Over the course of their lives, women may experience more than one type of violence.

Sexual violence can have a variety of devastating short- and long-term effects. Women can experience psychological, physical, and cognitive symptoms that affect them daily. These can include chronic pain (headaches, backache, arthritis), STIs, pregnancy, sleep disturbances, chronic fatigue, neurologic disorders (numbness, tingling, seizures), eating and gastrointestinal disorders, alcohol and substance abuse, depression, anxiety disorders, suicide or suicidal ideation, sexual dysfunction, and PTSD (Cherniak et al., 2005). A traumatic experience not only damages a woman's sense of safety in the world, but it can also reduce her self-esteem and her abilities to function in the world.

Assailants, like their victims, come from all walks of life and all ethnic backgrounds; there is no typical profile. Why do men rape? No theory provides a satisfactory explanation. So few assailants are caught and convicted

TEACHING GUIDELINE 9.1

Safety Plan for Leaving an Abusive Relationship

- When leaving an abusive relationship, take the following items:
  - Driver's license or photo ID, passport, immigration papers
  - Social insurance number or identification cards, health cards
  - Birth certificates for you and your children
  - School and immunization records
  - The deed or lease to your home or apartment
  - Any court papers or orders
  - Cheque book, bank cards, credit cards, and cash
  - Divorce papers, custody papers, marriage document
  - Keys for house, car, safety deposit box
  - Insurance cards, address or telephone book
  - Photo of spouse or partner (SOGC, 2005)
  - If you need to leave a domestic violence situation immediately, turn to authorities for assistance in gathering this material.
- Develop a "game plan" for leaving and rehearse it.
- Don't use phone cards—they leave a trail to follow.

that a clear profile remains elusive. What is known is that many assailants have trouble dealing with the stresses of daily life. Such men become angry and experience feelings of powerlessness. Sexual violence is a broad term that can be used to describe sexual abuse, incest, rape, female genital mutilation, and human trafficking.

Sexual Abuse

Sexual abuse occurs when a female is forced to have sexual contact of any kind (vaginal, oral, or anal) without her consent. Marriage does not constitute a tacit agreement for a spouse to inflict one's demands on the other without permission. The Canadian Incidence Study of Reported Child Abuse and Neglect (Trocmé, Fallon, MacLaurin, et al., 2003) examined aspects of sexual abuse, including attempted penetration, genital fondling, oral sex, exposure of adult genitals, sex talk, voyeurism, and sexual exploitation (child prostitution and pornography).

Childhood sexual abuse has a lifelong impact on its survivors. Women who experience childhood sexual abuse are more likely to be re-victimized sexually as adults (Lemieux & Byers, 2008). This is because the early abuse lowers their self-esteem and their ability to protect themselves and set firm boundaries. Childhood sexual abuse is a trauma that influences the way victims form relationships, deal with adversity, cope with daily problems, relate to their children and peers, protect their

health, and live. Girls and boys raised in violent homes are more likely to become adolescent parents and to repeat violent behaviour as adults (Chambliss, 2008).

Incest

Childhood sexual abuse involves any kind of sexual experience between a child and another person that violates the social taboos of family roles; examples include fondling, intercourse, exhibitionism, pornography, sodomy, and incest (Canadian Resource Centre for Victims of Crime, 2006). **Incest** is any type of sexual exploitation between blood relatives or surrogate relatives. Sibling incest may be motivated by the older sibling's need for comfort and acceptance rather than sexual gratification (Thompson, 2009). Such sexual abuse is not only a crime but also a symptom of acute and irreversible family dysfunction. Survivors of incest are often tricked, coerced, or manipulated. All adults appear to be powerful to children. Perpetrators might threaten victims so that they are afraid to disclose the abuse or might tell them the abuse is their fault. Often these threats serve to silence victims.

Incestual relationships in the home endanger not only the child's intellectual and moral development, but also the health of the child. Many children do not ask for help because they do not want to expose their "secret." For this reason, just the tip of the iceberg is statistically visible—serious injuries, internal damage, STIs, or pregnancy. Incest can have serious long-term effects on its victims, including eating disorders, sexual problems in their adult life, PTSD, guilt and shame, low self-esteem, self-loathing, self-directed disgust, depression, and self-destructive behaviour (Kluft, 2010; National Center for Victims of Crime, 2008).

Whether an incest victim endured an isolated incident of abuse or ongoing assaults over an extended period, recovery can be painful and difficult. The recovery process begins with admission of abuse and the recognition that help and services are needed. Resources for incest victims include books, self-help groups, workshops, therapy programs, and possibly legal remedies. In addition to listening to and believing incest victims, nurses need to search for ways to prevent future generations from enduring such abuse and from continuing the cycle of abuse in their own family and relationships.

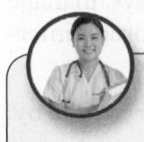

▶ **Take** NOTE!

Childhood sexual abuse is a trauma that can affect every aspect of the victim's life.

Rape

Rape is an expression of violence, not a sexual act. It is not an act of lust or an overzealous release of passion: it is a

▶ *Consider* THIS!

> At 53 years old, I stood and looked at myself in the mirror. The image staring back at me was one of a frightened, middle-aged, cowardly woman hiding her past. I had been sexually abused by my father for many years as a child and never told anyone. My mother knew of the abuse but felt helpless to make it stop. I married right out of high school to escape and felt I lived a "happy normal life" with my husband and three children. My children have left home and live away, and my husband recently died of a sudden heart attack. I am now experiencing dreams and thoughts about my past abuse and feeling afraid again.
>
> Thoughts: This woman suppressed her abusive past for most of her life and now her painful experience has surfaced. What can be done to reach out to her at this point? Did her health care providers miss the "red flags" that are common to women with a history of childhood sexual abuse all those years?

violent, aggressive assault on the victim's body and integrity. Rape is a legal rather than a medical term. It denotes penile penetration of the vagina, mouth, or rectum of a female or male without consent. It may or may not involve the use of a weapon. The **age of consent** in Canada is 16 years (Department of Justice Canada, 2010). When sexual exploitation is involved, however, as in the case of prostitution, pornography, or a relationship of trust, authority, or dependency (e.g., teacher, coach), the age of consent is 18 years. A "close-in-age" exception exists for 12- and 13-year-olds when the person is less than 2 years older and there is no exploitation of the young person. As long as the partner is less than 5 years older, a 14- or 15-year-old can consent to sexual activity as long there is no exploitation or relationship of trust, authority, or dependency involved. Enforcement of laws, education, and community empowerment are all needed to prevent rape.

Many people believe that rape usually occurs on a dark night when a stranger assaults a provocatively dressed, promiscuous woman. They believe that rapists are sex-starved people seeking sexual gratification. Such myths and the facts are presented in Table 9.2.

Acquaintance Rape

In **acquaintance rape**, someone is forced to have sex by a person he or she knows. Rape by a coworker, a teacher, a husband's friend, or a boss is considered acquaintance rape. **Date rape**, an assault that occurs within a dating relationship or marriage without consent of one of the participants, is a form of acquaintance rape. Acquaintance and date rapes commonly occur on university and college campuses. In the United States, one in four college women

has been raped—that is, has been forced, physically or verbally, actively or implicitly, to engage in sexual activity (Elliott, 2008).

These forms of rape are physically and emotionally devastating for the victims. Research has indicated that the survivors of acquaintance rape report similar levels of depression, anxiety, complications in subsequent relationships, and difficulty attaining pre-rape levels of sexual satisfaction to what survivors of stranger rape report. Although acquaintance rape and date rape do not always involve drugs, a rapist might use alcohol or other drugs to sedate his victim. The Canadian government has legislation that provides tougher penalties for trafficking date rape drugs.

Date rape drugs are also known as "club drugs" because they are often used at dance clubs, fraternity parties, and all-night raves. The most common is Rohypnol (also known as roofies, forget pills, and the drop drug). It comes in the form of a liquid or pill that quickly dissolves in liquid with no odor, taste, or colour. This drug is 10 times as strong as diazepam (Valium) and produces memory loss for up to 8 hours. Gamma hydroxybutyrate (GHB; called liquid ecstasy or easy lay) produces euphoria, an out-of-body high, sleepiness, increased sex drive, and memory loss. It comes in a white powder or liquid and may cause unconsciousness, depression, and coma. The third date rape drug, ketamine (known as Special K, vitamin K, or super acid), acts on the central nervous system to separate perception and sensation. Combining ketamine with other drugs can be fatal.

Date rape drugs can be very dangerous, and there are a variety of ways that women can protect themselves (Teaching Guideline 9.2).

Rape Recovery

Rape survivors take a long time to heal from their traumatic experience. Some women never heal and never get professional counselling, but most can cope. Rape is viewed as a situational crisis that the survivor is unprepared to handle because it is an unforeseen event. Survivors typically go through four phases of recovery following rape (Table 9.3).

TEACHING GUIDELINE 9.2

Protecting Yourself Against Date Rape Drugs

- Avoid parties where alcohol is being served.
- Never leave a drink of any kind unattended.
- Don't accept a drink from someone else. Accept drinks from a bartender or in a closed container only.
- Don't drink from a punch bowl or a keg.
- If you think someone drugged you, call 911.

TABLE 9.2 COMMON MYTHS AND FACTS ABOUT RAPE

Myths	Facts
Women who are raped get over it quickly.	It can take several years to recover emotionally and physically from rape.
Most rape victims tell someone about it. Victims report the violence to their friends, family, and police.	The majority of women never tell anyone about their experience. In fact, almost two thirds of victims never report it to the police.
Once the rape is over, a survivor can again feel safe in her life.	The victim feels vulnerable, betrayed, and insecure afterward.
If a woman does not want to be raped, it cannot happen.	A woman can be forced and overpowered by most men.
Women fabricate stories about being raped.	It is unlikely that a woman will make up a story about being raped. It is very traumatizing to be a victim.
Women who feel guilty after having sex then say they were raped.	Victims perceive that they lack credibility and that police will not help.
Women blame themselves for the rape, believing they did something to provoke it.	Women should never blame themselves for being the victim of someone else's violence.
Women who wear tight, short clothes are "asking for it."	No victim invites sexual assault, and what she wears is irrelevant.
Women have rape fantasies and want to be raped.	Reality and fantasy are different. Dreams have nothing to do with the brutal violation of rape.
Medication can help women forget about the rape.	Initially medication can help, but counselling is needed.
A man cannot rape his wife.	The law recognizes that rape against a spouse is a crime.
In dating relationships, sexual urges cannot be controlled.	Sexual urges can be controlled. When a partner says "no," the person has the right to control her body.
Rapists are mentally ill.	Rapists can be found anywhere in society.

Sources: Baugher, S. N., Elhai, J. D., Monroe, J. R., & Gray, M. J. (2010). Rape myth acceptance, sexual trauma history, and posttraumatic stress disorder. *Journal of Interpersonal Violence, 25*(11), 2036–2053; Centers for Disease Control and Prevention. (2012). *Understanding intimate partner violence fact sheet.* Retrieved February 7, 2012 from http://www.cdc.gov/violenceprevention/pdf/ ipv_factsheet-a.pdf; Dutton, D. G. (2006). *Rethinking domestic violence.* Vancouver, BC: University of British Columbia Press; Medicine Net. (2012). *Rape (sexual assault).* Retrieved February 7, 2012 from http://www.medicinenet.com/rape_sexual_assault/article.htm; National Clearinghouse on Family Violence. (2006). *Violence in dating relationships.* Ottawa, ON: Government of Canada. Retrieved February 7, 2012 from http://www.phac-aspc.gc.ca/ncfv-cnivf/pdfs/fem-2006-dat_e.pdf; & Westbrook, L. (2009). Information myths and intimate partner violence: Sources, contexts, and consequences. *Journal of the American Society for Information Science and Technology, 60*(4), 826–836.

A significant proportion of women who are raped also experience symptoms of **post-traumatic stress disorder**. PTSD develops when an event outside the range of normal human experience occurs that produces marked distress in the person. Symptoms of PTSD are divided into three groups:

- Intrusion (re-experiencing the trauma, including nightmares, flashbacks, recurrent thoughts)
- Avoidance (avoiding trauma-related stimuli, social withdrawal, emotional numbing)
- Hyperarousal (increased emotional arousal, exaggerated startle response, irritability)

TABLE 9.3 FOUR PHASES OF RAPE RECOVERY

Phase	Survivor's Response
Acute phase (disorganization)	Shock, fear, disbelief, anger, shame, guilt, feelings of uncleanliness, insomnia, nightmares, and sobbing
Outward adjustment phase (denial)	Appears outwardly composed and returns to work or school; refuses to discuss the assault and denies need for counselling
Reorganization	Denial and suppression don't work, and the survivor attempts to make life adjustments by moving or changing jobs and uses emotional distancing to cope.
Integration and recovery	Survivor begins to feel safe and starts to trust others. She may become an advocate for other rape victims.

Nursing Management

Research has found that rape survivors undergo a profound and complex trauma. Immediate treatment needs to address legal, medical, and psychosocial dimensions (Luce & Schrager, 2010). The survivor should be provided with a safe and comfortable environment for a forensic examination. Nursing care of the rape survivor should focus on providing supporting care, collecting and documenting evidence, assessing for STIs, preventing pregnancy, and assessing for PTSD. Once initial treatment and evidence collection are completed, follow-up care should include counselling, medical treatment, and crisis intervention. There is mounting evidence that early intervention and immediate counselling speed a rape survivor's recovery. Nursing Care Plan 9.1 highlights a sample plan of care for a victim of rape.

▶ *Take* NOTE!

Many rape survivors seek treatment in the hospital emergency room if there are no rape crisis centres available. Unfortunately, many emergency room doctors and nurses have little training in how to treat rape survivors or in collecting evidence. To make matters worse, if they have to wait for hours in public waiting rooms, survivors may leave the hospital, never to receive treatment or supply the evidence needed to arrest and convict their assailants.

Providing Supporting Care

Establishing a therapeutic and trusting relationship will help the survivor describe her experience. Take the woman

Nursing Care Plan 9.1

OVERVIEW OF THE WOMAN WHO IS A VICTIM OF RAPE

Lucia, a 20-year-old college student, was admitted to the emergency room after police found her when a passerby called 911 to report an assault. She stated, "I think I was raped a few hours ago while I was walking home through the park." Assessment reveals the following: numerous cuts and bruises of varying sizes on her face, arms, and legs; lip swollen and cut; right eye swollen and bruised; jacket and shirt ripped and bloodied; hair matted with grass and debris; vital signs within acceptable parameters; client tearful, clutching her clothing, and trembling; perineal bruising and tearing.

NURSING DIAGNOSIS: Rape-trauma syndrome related to report of recent sexual assault

Outcome Identification and Evaluation

Client will demonstrate adequate coping skills related to effects of rape as evidenced by her ability to discuss the event, verbalize her feelings and fears, and exhibit appropriate actions to return to her pre-crisis level of functioning.

Interventions: Promoting Adequate Coping Skills

- Stay with the client *to promote feelings of safety.*
- Explain the procedures to be completed based on facility's policy *to help alleviate client's fear of the unknown.*
- Assist with physical examination for specimen collection *to obtain evidence for legal proceedings.*
- Administer prophylactic medication as ordered *to prevent pregnancy and sexually transmitted infections.*
- Provide care to wounds as ordered *to prevent infection.*
- Assist client with hygiene measures as necessary *to promote self-esteem.*
- Allow client to describe the events as much as possible *to encourage ventilation of feelings about the incident;* engage in active listening and offer non-judgmental support *to facilitate coping and demonstrate understanding of the client's situation and feelings.*
- Help the client identify positive coping skills and personal strengths used in the past *to aid in effective decision making.*
- Assist client in developing additional coping strategies and teach client relaxation techniques *to help deal with the current crisis and anxiety.*
- Contact the rape counsellor in the facility *to help the client deal with the crisis.*
- Arrange for follow-up visit with rape counsellor *to provide continued care and to promote continuity of care.*
- Encourage the client to contact a close friend, partner, or family member to accompany her home *to provide support.*
- Provide the client with the telephone number of a counselling service or community support groups *to help her cope and obtain ongoing support.*
- Provide written instructions related to follow-up appointments, care, and testing *to ensure adequate understanding.*

to a secure, isolated area away from family, friends, and other patients and staff so she can be open and honest when asked about the assault. Provide a change of clothes, access to a shower and toiletries, and a private waiting area for family and friends.

Collecting and Documenting Evidence

The victim should be instructed to bring all clothing, especially undergarments, worn at the time of the assault to the medical facility. The victim should not shower or bathe before presenting for care. Typically a specially trained nurse will collect the evidence from the victim.

Assessing for Sexually Transmitted Infections

As part of the assessment, a pelvic examination will be done to collect vaginal secretions to rule out any STIs. This examination is very emotionally stressful for most women and should be carried out very gently and sensitively.

Preventing Pregnancy

An essential element in the care of rape survivors involves offering them pregnancy prevention. After unprotected intercourse, including rape, pregnancy can be prevented by using emergency contraceptive pills, sometimes called postcoital contraception. Emergency contraceptive pills (Plan B or levonorgestrel) involve high doses of the same oral contraceptives that millions of women take every day. The emergency regimen consists of two doses: the first dose is taken within 72 hours of the unprotected intercourse and the second dose is taken 12 hours after the first dose or sooner. Emergency contraception works by preventing ovulation, fertilization, or implantation. It does not disrupt an established pregnancy and should not be confused with mifepristone (RU-486), a drug that has not been approved by Health Canada for abortion (Pancham & Dunn, 2007).

Assessing for PTSD

Nurses can begin to assess the extent to which a survivor is suffering from PTSD by asking the following questions:

To assess the presence of intrusive thoughts:

• Do upsetting thoughts and nightmares of the trauma bother you?
• Do you feel as though you are actually reliving the trauma?
• Does it upset you to be exposed to anything that reminds you of that event?

To assess the presence of avoidance reactions:

• Do you find yourself trying to avoid thinking about the trauma?
• Do you stay away from situations that remind you of the event?
• Do you have trouble recalling exactly what happened?
• Do you feel numb emotionally?

To assess the presence of physical symptoms:

• Are you having trouble sleeping?
• Have you felt irritable or experienced outbursts of anger?
• Do you have heart palpitations and sweating?
• Do you have muscle aches and pains all over?

Female Genital Mutilation

Female genital mutilation, also known as female circumcision, is a cultural practice carried out predominantly in countries of Africa and in some areas of the Middle East and Asia. Due to immigration, genital mutilation practices have spread to Latin America, North America, Europe, and Australia (Kontoyannis & Katsetos, 2010). The World Health Organization (WHO) defines female genital mutilation as all procedures involving the partial or total removal or other injury to the female genital organs, whether for cultural or other nontherapeutic purposes (WHO, 2010). An estimated 100 to 140 million girls have undergone female genital mutilation (WHO, 2010).

This issue has drawn increasing global attention over the past several years. Nongovernmental organizations such as Amnesty International are conducting research and campaign work on the practice. Female genital mutilation in Canada is viewed as child assault and is considered under sections of the Criminal Code. WHO is fighting tirelessly to eradicate this practice through advocacy, policy development, research, and training for health care providers (WHO, 2010). In fact, WHO, the United Nations Population Fund, and the United Nations Children's Fund have issued a joint plea for the eradication of the practice, saying it would be a major step forward in the promotion of human rights worldwide (WHO, 2010).

▶ *Take* NOTE!

Female genital mutilation results from an intersection of cultural, religious, and social factors on family and community levels. Social pressure to conform perpetuates the practice (WHO, 2010).

Background

Reasons for performing the ritual reflect the ideology and cultural values of each community that practices it. Some consider it a rite of passage into womanhood; others use it as a means of preserving virginity until marriage. In cultures where it is practiced, it is an important part of culturally defined gender identity. In any case, all the reasons are cultural and traditional and may have existed for at least 5,000 years (Kontoyannis & Katsetos, 2010). Female genital mutilation causes injury to women and does not benefit them.

Female genital mutilation is usually performed when the girl is between infancy and 15 years old, an age when

> ### BOX 9.4 Four Major Types of Female Genital Mutilation Procedures
>
> Type I: Excision of the prepuce with or without excision of part or all of the clitoris
>
> Type II: Excision of the clitoris and part or all of the labia minora
>
> Type III (infibulation): Excision of all or part of the external genitalia and stitching/narrowing of the vaginal opening
>
> Type IV: Pricking, piercing, or incision of the clitoris or labia
>
> Stretching of the clitoris and/or labia
>
> Cauterizing by burning the clitoris and surrounding tissues
>
> Scraping or cutting the vaginal orifice
>
> Introduction of a corrosive substance into the vagina
>
> Placing herbs into the vagina to narrow it

Sources: Keleher, H., & Franklin, L. (2008). Changing gendered norms about women and girls at the level of household and community: A review of the evidence. *Global Public Health, Suppl. 1*(3), 42–57; & World Health Organization (WHO). (2010). *Female genital mutilation.* Retrieved February 7, 2012 from http://www.who.int/mediacentre/factsheets/fs241/en/.

she cannot give informed consent for a procedure with lifetime health consequences (WHO, 2010). It is performed occasionally on adult women. In its mildest form, the clitoris is partially or totally removed. In the most extreme form, called infibulation, the clitoris, labia minora, labia majora, and the urethral and vaginal openings are cut away. The vagina is then stitched or held together, leaving a small opening for menstruation and urination. Cutting and restitching may be necessary to permit the woman to have sexual intercourse and bear children. Box 9.4 lists types of female genital mutilation procedures.

Untrained village practitioners, using no form of anesthesia, generally perform the operation. Cutting instruments may include broken glass, knives, tin lids, scissors, unspecialized razors, or other crude instruments. In addition to causing intense pain, the procedure carries with it a number of health risks. Immediate complications include:

- Hemorrhage
- Shock
- Pain
- Tetanus or sepsis
- Urinary retention
- Open lesions and injury to genital tissue (WHO, 2010)

Long-term consequences include:

- Recurrent urinary tract and bladder infections
- Cysts
- Infertility
- Risk of childbirth complications and newborn death
- Need for future surgeries (WHO, 2010)

Nursing Management

Because of increasing migration, more nurses throughout the world are exposed to women who have suffered these procedures and thus need to know about its impact on women's reproductive health. Helping women who have had one of these procedures requires good communication skills and often an interpreter, since many may not speak English or French. Nurses have the opportunity to educate patients by providing accurate information and positive health care experiences. Make sure that you are comfortable with your own feelings about this practice before dealing with patients. Some guidelines are as follows:

- Let the client know you are concerned and interested and want to help.
- Speak clearly and slowly, using simple, accurate terms.
- Use the term or name for this practice the recipient uses, not "female genital mutilation."
- Use pictures and diagrams to help the woman understand what you are saying.
- Be patient in allowing the client to answer questions.
- Repeat back your understanding of the client's statements.
- Always look and talk directly to the client, not the interpreter.
- Place no judgment on the cultural practice.
- Encourage the client to express herself freely.
- Maintain strict confidentiality.
- Provide culturally competent care to all women.

Human Trafficking

A girl who was just 16 years old was held captive in a residence in Toronto, where she was forced to have sex with dozens of men daily. On her night stand was a teddy bear that reminded her of her childhood.

This scenario describes **human trafficking**, the enslavement of persons for exploitation. Human trafficking is both a global and a domestic problem, a modern form of slavery that may affect 4 million women and girls worldwide (Stewart & Gajic-Veljanoski, 2005). Canada is a receiver of trafficked persons, and the country's open immigration policy and support for refugees facilitates the practice. Human trafficking claimants in Canada in recent years have been from Romania, the Philippines, Moldova, and China (Perrin, 2009). Canadian statistics on human trafficking have been collected only since 2006 (Perrin, 2010), and Canada needs to focus more attention on this issue. The Palermo Protocol was adopted by the United Nations in 2000 to prevent human trafficking, protect its victims, and prosecute offenders (the "3P paradigm"; Perrin, 2010).

Women and children are the primary victims of human trafficking, many in the sex trade as described above and others through forced-labour domestic servitude. In Canada, trafficked women forced into prostitution, slavery, or marriage are discovered through police raids or when victims seek asylum (Perrin, 2009). Victims often are unable or afraid to seek legal help due to abusive situations, fear of retaliation, language barriers, deportation expectations, and fear of criminal charges. Canada is more focused on criminal and educational approaches rather than human rights approaches that would provide assistance to victims, protection, and right to health.

- Victims are primarily women and children who lack education, employment, and economic opportunities in their own countries.
- Traffickers promise victims employment as nannies, maids, dancers, factory workers, sales clerks, or models in Canada.
- Traffickers transport the victims from their countries to unfamiliar destinations away from their support systems.
- Once they are here, traffickers coerce them, using rape, torture, starvation, imprisonment, threats, or physical force, into prostitution, pornography, sex trade, forced labour, or involuntary servitude.

Victims of human trafficking are exposed to many serious physical and psychological health risks, such as repeated rape, food and sleep deprivation, emotional manipulation, forced or unsafe abortions, torture, HIV/AIDS, STIs, anxiety, depression, somaticized symptoms such as headaches and body aches, persistent sexual exploitation, social marginalization, and suicidality (Stewart & Gajic-Veljanoski, 2005). Health care is one of the most pressing needs of these victims, yet limited care is available for undocumented individuals. As a nurse it is important to be alert for trafficking victims in any setting and to recognize cues (Box 9.5).

Trafficking persons is hugely profitable: one estimate places global profits at approximately $5 to $7 billion US annually (Stewart & Gajic-Veljanoski, 2005). Among illegal enterprises, trafficking is second only to drug dealing and is tied with the illegal arms industry in its ability to generate dollars. As a destination country and transit point for traffickers, profits gained from Canadian operations contribute to organized criminal enterprises worldwide (Royal Canadian Mounted Police, 2010). Human trafficking suspects may be linked to other criminal activities, such as credit card fraud, mortgage fraud, and organized prostitution in Canada or internationally.

Human trafficking is a violation of human rights. If you suspect a trafficking situation, notify local law enforcement and a regional social service organization that has experience in dealing with trafficking victims. It is imperative to reach out to these victims and stop the cycle of abuse by following through on your suspicions.

Honour Violence

The Government of Canada has been encouraged to condemn honour killings (Canada Newswire, 2010). **Honour crime** is violence that is considered to be culturally acceptable. The Canadian government offers a guide called

---

BOX 9.5 **Identifying Victims of Human Trafficking**

Cues
Look beneath the surface and ask yourself: Is this person....
- A female or a child in poor health?
- Foreign-born and doesn't speak English or French?
- Lacking immigration documents?
- Giving an inconsistent explanation of injury?
- Reluctant to give any information about self, injury, home, or work?
- Fearful of authority figure or "sponsor" if present? ("Sponsor" might not leave victim alone with health care provider.)
- Living with the employer?

Sample questions to ask the potential victim of human trafficking:
- Can you leave your job or situation if you wish?
- Can you come and go as you please?
- Have you been threatened if you try to leave?
- Has anyone threatened your family with harm if you leave?
- What are your working and living conditions?
- Do you have to ask permission to go to the bathroom, eat, or sleep?
- Is there a lock on your door so you cannot get out?
- What brought you to Canada? Are your plans the same now?
- Are you free to leave your current work or home situation?
- Who has your immigration papers? Why don't you have them?
- Are you paid for the work you do?
- Are there times you feel afraid?
- How can your situation be changed?

Sources: humantrafficking.org; Jones, L., Engstrom, D. W., Hilliard, T, & Diaz, M. (2007). *The Joint Commission accreditation manual for hospitals.* Chicago, IL: JCAHO.

Discover Canada: The Rights and Responsibilities of Citizenship, which explains that Canada does not tolerate cultural practices of gender-based violence such as honour killings, spousal abuse, or female genital mutilation (Citizenship and Immigration Canada, 2011). Unlike violence perpetrated by an intimate partner, honour violence occurs in the family context and can be perpetrated by several family members (Papp, 2010). Honour violence may be condoned and facilitated by the family and community. Honour crimes are meant to restore family honour and have a cleansing effect on the family name.

Summary

The causes of violence against women are complex. Many women will experience some type of violence in their lives, and it can have a debilitating effect on their health and future relationships. Violence frequently leaves a "legacy of pain" to future generations. Nurses can empower women and encourage them to move forward and take control of their lives. When women live in peace and security and free from violence, they have an enormous potential to contribute to their own communities and to the national and global society. Violence against women is not normal, legal, or acceptable and it should never be tolerated or justified. It can and must be stopped by the entire world community.

■■■ Key Concepts

■ Violence against women is a major public health and social problem because it violates a woman's very being and causes numerous mental and physical health sequelae.

■ Every woman has the potential to become a victim of violence.

■ Abuse may be mental, physical, or sexual in nature or a combination.

■ The cycle of violence includes three phases: tension-building, acute battering, and honeymoon.

■ Many women experience post-traumatic stress disorder (PTSD) after being sexually assaulted. PTSD can inhibit a survivor from adapting or coping in a healthy manner.

■ Pregnancy can precipitate or escalate violence toward the woman.

■ The nurse's role in dealing with survivors of violence is to establish rapport; open up lines of communication; apply the nursing process to assess and screen all patients in all settings; and implement and intervene as appropriate.

REFERENCES

Aggeles, T. B. (2012). *Domestic violence advocacy, Florida, update.* Retrieved February 7, 2012 from http://ce.nurse.com/60133/domestic-violence-advocacy-florida-update-2007/

Alberta Council of Women's Shelters. (2010). *New shelter statistics highlight children* [press release]. Retrieved February 7, 2012 from http://www.acws.ca/documents/MEDIARELEASENOV1ShelterStats.pdf

Alberta Council of Women's Shelters. (2011). *Position paper on the Victims of Crime Fund Alberta Council of Women's Shelters February, 2011.* Retrieved February 7, 2012 from http://www.acws.ca/documents/POSITIONPAPERontheVictimsofCrimeFund.pdf

Antoniou, E., Vivilaki, V., & Daglas, M. (2008). Correlation of domestic violence during pregnancy with postnatal depression: Systematic review of bibliography. *Health Science Journal, 2*(1), 15–19.

Baugher, S. N., Elhai, J. D., Monroe, J. R., & Gray, M. J. (2010). Rape myth acceptance, sexual trauma history, and posttraumatic stress disorder. *Journal of Interpersonal Violence, 25*(11), 2036–2053.

Beattie, S., & Cotter, A. (2010). Homicide in Canada, 2009. *Juristat, 30*(3). Statistics Canada catalogue no.85–002-X; retrieved February 7, 2012 from http://www.statcan.gc.ca/pub/85-002-x/2010003/article/11352-eng.htm

Beydoun, H. A., Al-Sahab, B., Beydoun, M. A., & Tamim, H. (2010). Intimate partner violence as a risk factor for postpartum depression among Canadian women in the maternity experience survey. *Annals of Epidemiology, 20*(8), 575–583.

Bonomi, A. E., Cannon, E. A., Anderson, M. L., Rivara, F. P., & Thompson, R. S. (2008). Association between self-reported health and physical and/or sexual abuse experienced before age 18. *Child Abuse & Neglect, 32*(7), 693–701.

Bourassa, D., & Berube, J. (2007). The prevalence of intimate partner violence among women and teenagers seeking abortion compared with those continuing pregnancy. *Journal of Obstetrics and Gynaecology Canada, 29*(5), 415–423.

Brennan, S. (2011). Violent victimization of Aboriginal women in the Canadian provinces, 2009. *Juristat.* Statistics Canada catalogue no.85–002-X; retrieved February 7, 2012 from http://www.statcan.gc.ca/pub/85-002-x/2011001/article/11439-eng.pdf

Burgess, A. W. (2007). How many red flags does it take? *American Journal of Nursing, 107*(1), 28–31.

Caetano, R., Vaeth, P.A., & Ramisetty-Mikler, S. (2008). Intimate partner violence victim and perpetrator characteristics among couples in the United States. *Journal of Family Violence, 23*, 507–518.

Campbell, J. C., & Furniss, K. K. (2002). *Violence against women: Identification, screening and management of intimate partner violence.* Washington, DC: The Association of Women's Health, Obstetric and Neonatal Nurses.

Canadian Divorce Laws. (2011). *Domestic violence.* Retrieved February 7, 2012 from www.canadiandivorcelaws.com/domestic-violence/

Canadian Network for the Prevention of Elder Abuse. (2010). *Canadian laws on abuse and neglect.* Retrieved February 7, 2012 from http://www.cnpea.ca/canadian_laws_on_abuse_and_negle.htm

Canada Newswire. (2010). *Minister Ambrose calls for community action to help end "honour crimes"* [news release]. Retrieved February 7, 2012 from http://www.newswire.ca/en/story/711243/minister-ambrose-calls-for-community-action-to-help-end-honour-crimes

Canadian Resource Centre for Victims of Crime. (2006). *The devastation of sexual assault.* Retrieved February 7, 2012 from http://crcvc.ca/docs/sexual_assault.pdf

Cannon, E. A., Anderson, M. L., Rivara, F. P., & Thompson, R. S. (2010). Adult health and relationship outcomes among women with abuse experiences during childhood. *Violence and Victims, 25*(3), 291–305.

Centers for Disease Control and Prevention. (2012). *Understanding intimate partner violence fact sheet.* Retrieved February 7, 2012 from http://www.cdc.gov/violenceprevention/pdf/ipv_factsheet-a.pdf

Chambliss, L. R. (2008). Intimate partner violence and its implication for pregnancy. *Clinical Obstetrics and Gynecology, 51*(2), 385–387.

Cherniak, D., Grant, L., Mason, R., Moore, B., & Pellizari, R. (2005) Intimate partner violence consensus statement. *Journal of Obstetrics and Gynaecology Canada, 4*, 365–388.

Citizenship and Immigration Canada. (2011). *Discover Canada: The rights and responsibilities of citizenship.* Retrieved February 7, 2012 from http://www.cic.gc.ca/english/pdf/pub/discover.pdf

Cory, J., & Dechief, L. (2007). *SHE framework: Safety and health enhancement for women experiencing abuse.* Vancouver, BC: Institute Against Family Violence.

Department of Justice Canada. (2009). *Family violence: Department of Justice: Overview paper.* Retrieved February 7, 2012 from http://www.justice.gc.ca/eng/pi/fv-vf/facts-info/fv-vf/fv-vf.pdf

Department of Justice Canada. (2010). *Age of consent to sexual activity.* Retrieved February 7, 2012 from www.justice.gc.ca/eng/dept-min/clp/faq.html

Du Plat-Jones, J. (2006). Domestic violence: The role of health professionals. *Nursing Standard, 21*(14), 44–48.

Dutton, D. G. (2006). *Rethinking domestic violence.* Vancouver, BC: University of British Columbia Press.

Dylan, A., Regehr, C., & Alaggia, R. (2008). And justice for all? Aboriginal victims of sexual violence. *Violence Against Women, 14*(6), 678–696.

Eke, A.W., Hilton, N. Z., Harris, G. T., Rice, M. E., & Houghton, R. E. (2011). Intimate partner homicide: Risk assessment and prospects for prediction. *Journal of Family Violence, 26*, 211–216.

Elliott, S. M. (2008). Drug-facilitated sexual assault: Educating women about the risks. *Nursing for Women's Health, 12*(1), 30–37.

Hebert, M., Tourigny, M., Cyr, M., McDuff, P., & Joly, J. (2009). Prevalence of childhood sexual abuse and timing of disclosure in a representative sample of adults from Quebec. *Canadian Journal of Psychiatry, 54*(9), 631–636.

Holtz, H., & Furniss, K. K. (1993). The health care provider's role in domestic violence. *Trends in Health Care Law and Ethics, 15,* 519–522.

Keleher, H., & Franklin, L. (2008). Changing gendered norms about women and girls at the level of household and community: A review of the evidence. *Global Public Health, Suppl 1*(3), 42–57.

Kelly, P. J. (2007). Integrating intimate partner violence prevention into daily practice. *Journal of Psychosocial Nursing, 45*(4), 8–10.

Kluft, R.P. (2010). Ramifications of incest. *Psychiatric Times, 27*(12), 48–55.

Kontoyannis, M., & Katsetos, C. (2010). Female genital mutilation. *Health Science Journal, 4*(1), 31–36.

Lemieux, S., & Byers, E.S. (2008). The sexual well-being of women who have experienced child sexual abuse. *Psychology of Women Quarterly, 32,* 126–144.

Luce, H., & Schrager, S. (2010). Sexual assault of women. *American Family Physician, 81*(4), 489–495.

Manitoba Association of Women's Shelters. (2008). *What is abuse?* Retrieved February 7, 2012 from www.maws.mb.ca/domestic_violence.htm

McGarry, J., Simpson, C., & Mansour, M. (2010). How domestic abuse affects the wellbeing of older women. *Nursing Older People, 22*(5), 33–37.

Medicine Net. (2012). *Rape (sexual assault).* Retrieved February 7, 2012 from http://www.medicinenet.com/rape_sexual_assault/article.htm

National Center for Victims of Crime. (2008). *Incest.* Retrieved February 7, 2012 from http://www.ncvc.org/ncvc/AGP.Net/Components/documentViewer/Download.aspxnz?DocumentID=45715

National Clearinghouse on Family Violence. (2006). *Violence in dating relationships.* Ottawa, ON: Government of Canada. Retrieved February 7, 2012 from http://www.phac-aspc.gc.ca/ncfv-cnivf/pdfs/fem-2006-dat_e.pdf

National Clearinghouse on Family Violence. (2008). *Aboriginal women and family violence.* Ottawa, ON: Government of Canada. Retrieved February 7, 2012 from http://www.phac-aspc.gc.ca/ncfv-cnivf/pdfs/fem-abor_e.pdf

National Clearinghouse on Family Violence. (2010). *Family violence initiative: Performance report for April 2004 to March 2008.* Retrieved February 7, 2012 from http://webapps01.un.org/vawdatabase/uploads/Canada%20FVI%20Performance%20Report%202008.pdf

Pancham, A., & Dunn, S. (2007). Emergency contraception in Canada: An overview and recent developments. *The Canadian Journal of Human Sexuality, 16*(3–4), 129–133.

Papp, A. (2010). *Culturally driven violence against women: A growing problem in Canada's immigrant communities.* Winnipeg, MB: Frontier Centre for Public Policy. Retrieved February 7, 2012 from http://www.fcpp.org/files/1/Culturally-Driven%20Violence%20Against%20Women.pdf

Perreault, S. (2011). Violent victimization of Aboriginal people in the Canadian provinces, 2009. *Juristat.* Statistics Canada catalogue no. 85–002-X; retrieved February 7, 2012 from http://www.statcan.gc.ca/pub/85-002-x/2011001/article/11415-eng.pdf

Perrin, B. (2009). Confronting human trafficking in Canada. *The Lawyers Weekly;* retrieved September 7, 2011 from http://www.lawyersweekly.ca/index.php?section=article&articleid=849

Perrin, B. (2010). *Canada's underground world of human trafficking: Invisible chains.* Toronto, ON: Penguin Group.

Public Health Agency of Canada. (2009a). *Spousal and partner abuse— It can be stopped.* Retrieved February 7, 2012 from http://www.phac-aspc.gc.ca/ncfv-cnivf/publications/rcmp-grc/fem-partnrabus-eng.php

Public Health Agency of Canada. (2009b). *The effects of domestic violence on children—Where does it hurt?* Retrieved February 7, 2012 from http://www.phac-aspc.gc.ca/ncfv-cnivf/publications/rcmp-grc/fem-vioeffects-eng.php

Public Health Agency of Canada. (2009c). *Violence against women with disabilities.* Retrieved February 7, 2012 from http://www.phac-aspc.gc.ca/ncfv-cnivf/publications/femdisabus-eng.php

Public Health Agency of Canada. (2010). *Canadian incidence study of reported child abuse and neglect—2008: Major findings.* Retrieved February 7, 2012 from http://www.phac-aspc.gc.ca/ncfv-cnivf/pdfs/nfnts-cis-2008-rprt-eng.pdf

Registered Nurses' Assocation of Ontario. (2005). *Nursing best practice guidelines—Woman abuse: Screening, identification and initial response.* Toronto, ON: Author.

Royal Canadian Mounted Police. (2010). *Human trafficking in Canada: A threat assessment.* Retrieved February 7, 2012 from www.rcmp-grc.gc.ca/pubs/ht-tp/htta-tpem-eng.htm

Sauvé, J., & Burns, M.,(2009). Residents of Canada's shelters for abused women 2008. *Juristat, 29*(2), 1–21. Statistics Canada catalogue no. 85–002-X; retrieved February 7, 2012 from http://www.phac-aspc.gc.ca/ncfv-cnivf/pdfs/fem-residents-eng.pdf

SexualityandU.ca. (2010a). *Characteristics of abusers.* Retrieved February 7, 2012 from http://www.sexualityandu.ca/health-care-professionals/domestic-violence/characteristics_of_abuse

SexualityandU.ca. (2010b). *Domestic violence.* Retrieved February 7, 2012 from http://www.sexualityandu.ca/health-care-professionals/domestic_violence

SexualtyandU.ca. (2010c). *Health effects of abuse.* Retrieved February 7, 2012 from http://www.sexualityandu.ca/health-care- professionals/domestic_violence/health_effects_of_abuse

Shah, P. S., & Shah, J. (2010). Maternal exposure to domestic violence and pregnancy and birth outcomes: A systematic review and meta-analyses. *Journal of Women's Health, 19*(11), 2017–2031.

Smylie, J. (2001). A guide for health professionals working with aboriginal peoples: SOGC policy guide. *Journal of Obstetrics and Gynaecology Canada, 100,* 1–15.

Society of Obstetricians and Gynecologists of Canada. (2005). *Intimate partner violence consensus statement.* Retrieved May 14, 2012 from http://www.sogc.org/guidelines/public/157E-CPG-April2005.pdf

Society of Obstetricians and Gynaecologists of Canada. (2011). *General health: Intimate partner violence.* Retrieved February 7, 2012 from www.sogc.org/health/health-ipv_e.asp

Statistics Canada. (2011). *Family violence in Canada: A statistical profile.* Ottawa, ON: Author.

Stewart, D. E., & Gajic-Veljanoski, O. (2005). Trafficking in women: the Canadian perspective. *Canadian Medical Association Journal, 173*(1), 25–26.

Thackeray J., Stelzner, S., Downs, S. M., & Miller, C. (2007). Screening for intimate partner violence. *Journal of Interpersonal Violence, 22*(6), 659–670.

Thompson, K. M. (2009). Sibling incest: A model for group practice with adult female victims of brother-sister incest. *Journal of Family Violence, 24,* 531–537.

Trocmé, N., Fallon, B., MacLaurin, B., Daciuk, J. Felstiner, C., et al. (2003). *Canadian incidence study of reported child abuse and neglect— 2003: Major findings.* Retrieved February 7, 2012 from http://www.phac-aspc.gc.ca/cm-vee/csca-ecve/index-eng.php

Westbrook, L. (2009). Information myths and intimate partner violence: Sources, contexts, and consequences. *Journal of the American Society for Information Science and Technology, 60*(4), 826–836.

Women, Information and Advocacy. (2009). *Statistics on family violence in Canada.* Retrieved September 7, 2011 from http://www.domesticabusemuststop.org/resources.php?subaction=showfull&id=1248128300&archive=&start_from=&ucat=2&

World Health Organization (WHO). (2010). *Female genital mutilation.* Retrieved February 7, 2012 from http://www.who.int/mediacentre/factsheets/fs241/en/

RECOMMENDED READING

Peter, T. (2009). Exploring taboos: Comparing male- and female- perpetrated child sexual abuse. *Journal of Interpersonal Violence, 24*(7), 1111–1128.

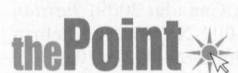

For additional learning materials, including Internet Resources, visit **http://thePoint.lww.com/Chow1e.**

CHAPTER WORKSHEET

MULTIPLE CHOICE QUESTIONS

1. The primary goal of intervention in working with abused women is to:

   a. Set up an appointment for the woman with a mental health counsellor

   b. Convince the woman to set up a safety plan to use when she leaves

   c. Help the woman to develop courage and financial support to leave the abuser

   d. Empower the woman and improve her self-esteem to regain control of her life

2. The first phase of the abuse cycle is characterized by:

   a. The woman provoking the abuser to bring about battering

   b. Tension-building and verbal or minor battery

   c. A honeymoon period that lulls the victim into forgetting

   d. An acute episode of physical battering

3. Women recovering from abusive relationships need to learn ways to improve their:

   a. Cooking skills and provide more nutritious meals for their children

   b. Creativity so as to improve their decorating skills within the home

   c. Communication and negotiation skills to increase their assertiveness

   d. Personal appearance by losing weight and exercising more

4. Which of the following statements might empower abuse victims to take action?

   a. "You deserve better than this."

   b. "Your children deserve to grow up in a two-parent family."

   c. "Try to figure out what you do to trigger his abuse and stop it."

   d. "Give your partner more time to come to his senses about this."

CRITICAL THINKING EXERCISE

1. Mrs. Boggs has three children under the age of 5 and is 6 months pregnant with her fourth child. She has made repeated unscheduled visits to your clinic with vague somatic complaints regarding the children as well as herself but has missed several scheduled prenatal appointments. On occasion she has worn sunglasses to cover bruises around her eyes. As a nurse you sense there is something else bothering her, but she doesn't seem to want to discuss it with you. She appears sad and the children cling to her.

   a. Outline your conversation when you broach the subject of abuse with Mrs. Boggs.

   b. What is your role as a nurse in caring for a family in which you suspect abuse?

   c. What ethical/legal considerations are important in planning care for this family?

STUDY ACTIVITIES

1. Visit the Canadian Women's Foundation website for information about violence (see http://thePoint.lww.com/Chow1e for the direct link). Discuss what you discovered on this site and your reactions to it.

2. Research the statistics about violence against women in your province. Are law enforcement and community interventions reducing the incidence of sexual assault and intimate partner violence?

3. Attend a residence orientation at a local university to hear about measures in place to protect women on campus. Find out the number of sexual assaults reported and what strategies the university uses to reduce this number.

4. Identify three community resources that could be useful to a victim of violence. Identify their sources of funding and the services they provide.

UNIT THREE

PREGNANCY

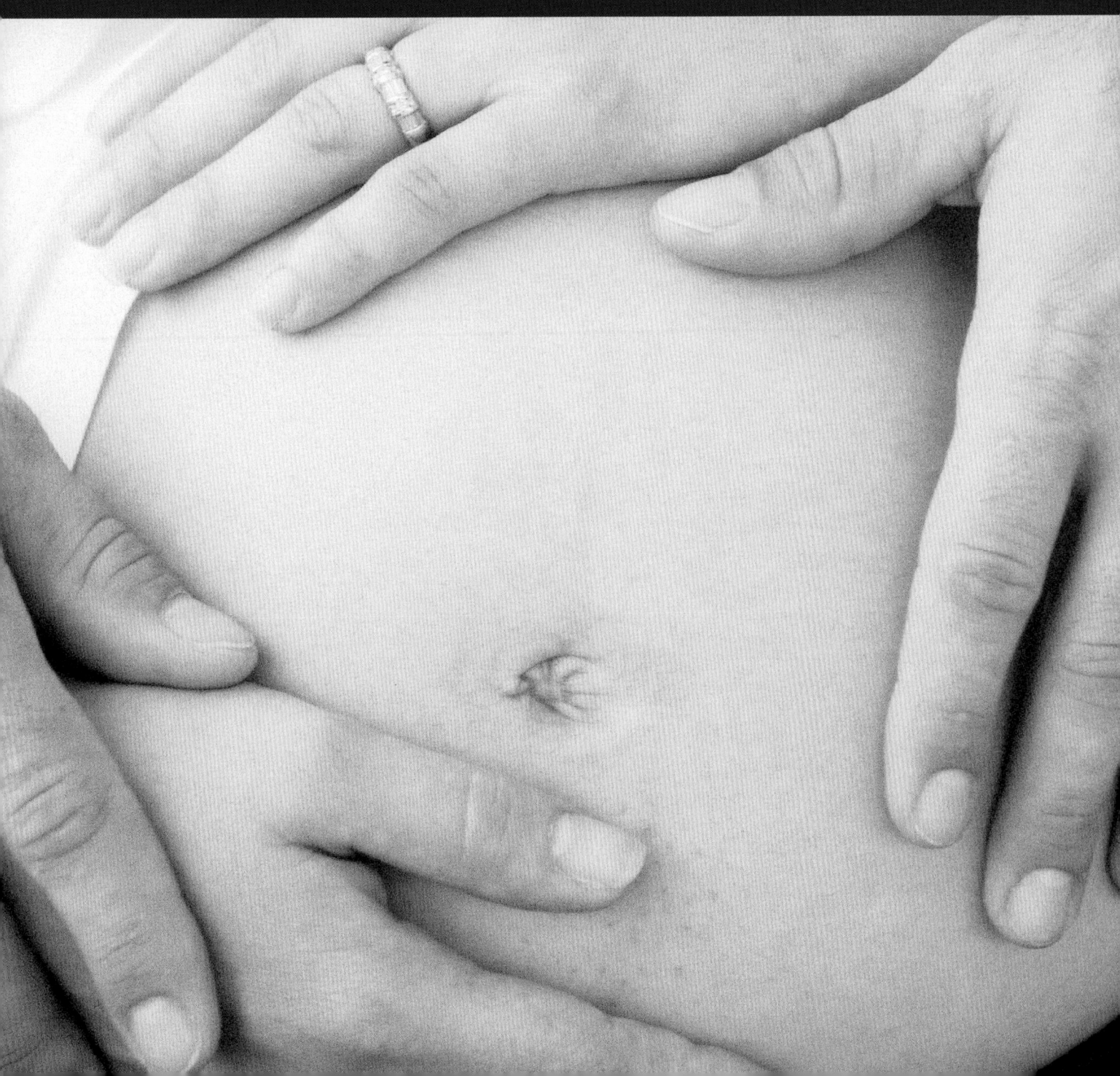

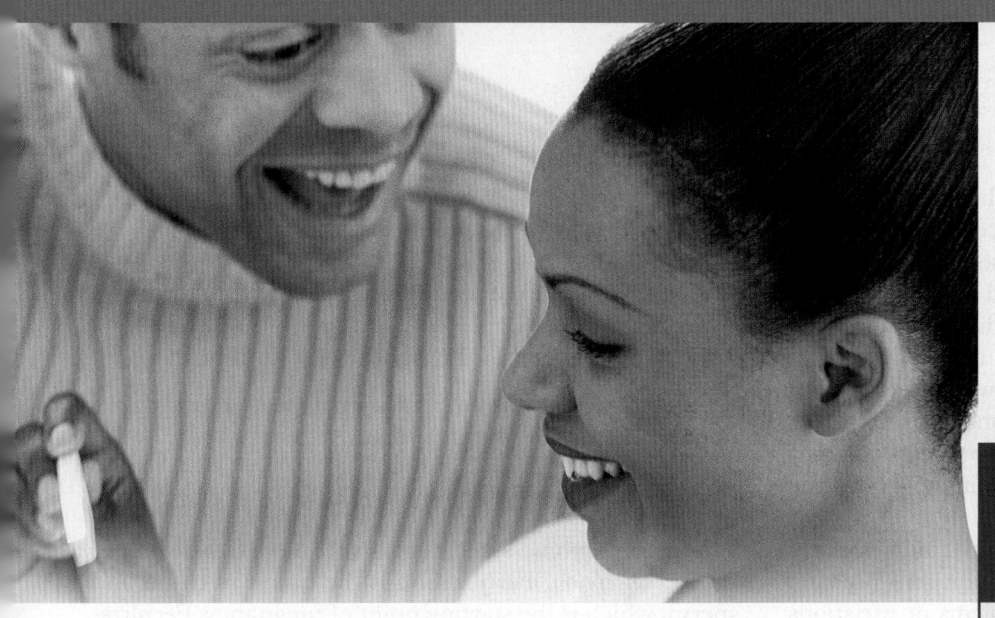

FETAL DEVELOPMENT AND GENETICS

KEY TERMS

allele
blastocyst
chromosome
conceptus
dominant
embryonic stage
epigenetics
fertilization
fetal stage
genes
genetic counselling
genetics

genome
genotype
heterozygous
homozygous
karyotype
mosaicism
monosomies
morula
multifactorial inheritance
mutation
organogenesis
phenotype

placenta
polyploidy
preembryonic stage
recessive
teratogen
trisomies
trophoblast
umbilical cord
zona pellucida
zygote

LEARNING OBJECTIVES

Upon completion of the chapter, the learner will be able to:

1. Describe the process of fertilization, implantation, and cell differentiation.
2. Explain the functions of the placenta, umbilical cord, and amniotic fluid.
3. Outline typical fetal development from conception through birth.
4. Compare the various inheritance patterns, including nontraditional patterns of inheritance.
5. Give examples of ethical and legal issues surrounding genetic testing.
6. Explain the role of the nurse in genetic counselling and genetic-related activities.
7. Discuss advances in the science of human genetics and our understanding of multifactorial influences on genetics and fetal development.
8. Describe recent advances in the field of epigenetics.

*R*obert and Kate Shafer have just received the good news that Kate's pregnancy test was positive. It had been a long and anxious 3 years of trying to start a family. Although both were elated about the prospect of becoming parents, they were concerned about the possibility of a genetic problem because Kate was 38 years old. What might be their first step in looking into their genetic concern? As a nurse, what might raise concerns for you?

Wow

Witnessing the miracle of life can be awe-inspiring for nurses.

Human reproduction is one of the most intimate spheres of an individual's life. For conception to occur, a healthy ovum from the woman is released from the ovary, passes into an open fallopian tube, and starts its journey downward. Sperm from the male is deposited into the vagina and swims to meet the ovum at the outermost portion of the fallopian tube, the area where fertilization takes place (Gilbert, 2010). When one spermatozoon penetrates the ovum's thick outer membrane, pregnancy begins. All this activity takes place within a 5-hour time span.

Nurses caring for the childbearing family need to have a basic understanding of conception and prenatal development so they can identify problems or variations and can initiate appropriate interventions should any problems occur. This chapter presents an overview of fetal development, beginning with conception. It also discusses hereditary and socio-environmental influences on fetal development and the nurse's role in genetic counselling.

Fetal Development

Fetal development during pregnancy is measured in number of weeks after fertilization. The duration of pregnancy is about 40 weeks from the time of fertilization. This equates to 9 calendar months or approximately 266 to 280 calendar days. The three stages of fetal development during pregnancy are:

1. **Preembryonic stage:** fertilization through the second week
2. **Embryonic stage:** end of the second week through the eighth week
3. **Fetal stage:** end of the eighth week until birth

Fetal circulation is a significant aspect of fetal development that spans all three stages.

Preembryonic Stage

The preembryonic stage begins with **fertilization**, also called *conception*. Fertilization is the union of ovum and sperm, which is the starting point of pregnancy. Fertilization typically occurs around 2 weeks after the last normal menstrual period in a 28-day cycle (Cunningham, Leveno, Bloom, et al., 2010). Fertilization requires a timely interaction between the release of the mature ovum at ovulation and the ejaculation of enough healthy, mobile sperm to survive the vaginal environment through which they must travel to meet the ovum. Sperm last up to only 48 hours in the female genital tract, and the ovum usually dies within 24 hours if not fused with a sperm (Blackburn, 2007). All things considered, the act of conception is difficult at best. To say merely that it occurs when the sperm fertilizes the ovum is overly simple

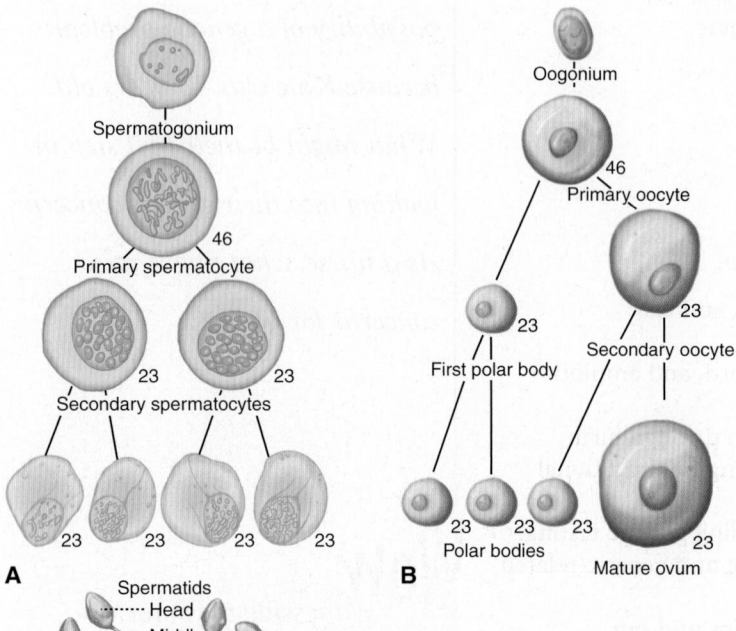

FIGURE 10.1 The formation of gametes by the process of meiosis is known as gametogenesis. (**A**) Spermatogenesis. One spermatogonium gives rise to four spermatozoa. (**B**) Oogenesis. From each oogonium, one mature ovum and three abortive cells are produced. The chromosomes are reduced to one half the number characteristic for the general body cells of the species. In humans, the number in the body cells is 46, and that in the mature spermatozoon and secondary oocyte is 23.

because this union requires an intricate interplay of hormonal preparation and overcoming an overwhelming number of natural barriers. Conception is truly an amazing outcome of this elaborate process.

Prior to fertilization, the ovum and the spermatozoon undergo the process of meiosis. The primary oocyte completes its first meiotic division before ovulation. The secondary oocyte begins its second meiotic division just before ovulation. Primary and secondary spermatocytes undergo meiotic division while still in the testes (Fig. 10.1).

Although more than 200 million sperm/mL are contained in the ejaculated semen, only one is able to enter the ovum to fertilize it. All others are blocked by the clear protein layer called the **zona pellucida**. The zona pellucida disappears in about 5 days. Once the sperm reaches the plasma membrane, the ovum resumes meiosis and forms a nucleus with half the number of **chromosomes** (23). When the nucleus from the ovum and the nucleus from the sperm make contact, they lose their respective nuclear membranes and combine their maternal and paternal chromosomes. Because each nucleus contains a haploid number of chromosomes (23), this union restores the diploid number (46). The resulting **zygote** (fertilized oocyte) begins the process of embryonic and fetal development. The genetic information from both ovum and sperm establishes the unique physical characteristics of the individual. Sex determination is also determined at fertilization and depends on whether the ovum is fertilized by a Y-bearing sperm or an X-bearing sperm. An XX zygote will become a female and an XY zygote will become a male (Fig. 10.2).

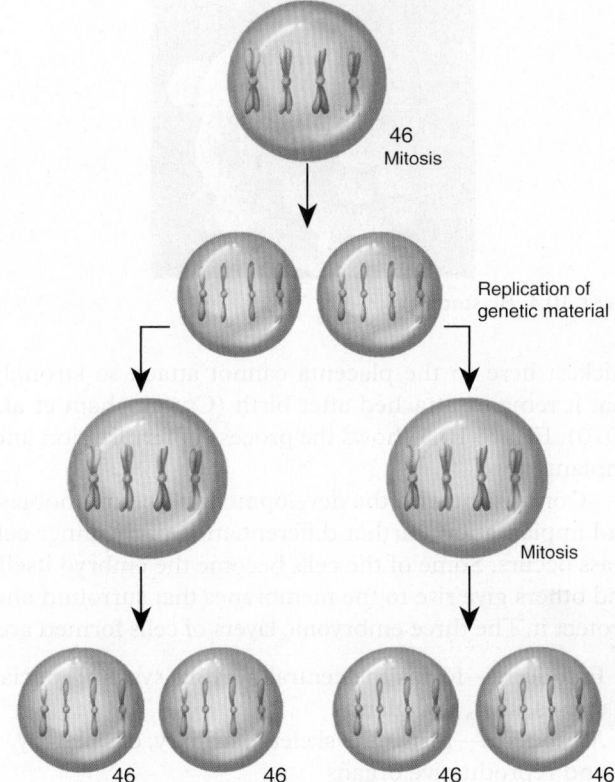

FIGURE 10.3 Mitosis of the stoma cells.

Fertilization takes place in the outer third of the ampulla of the fallopian tube. When the ovum is fertilized by the sperm (now called a zygote), a great deal of activity immediately takes place. Mitosis, or *cleavage,* occurs as the zygote is slowly transported into the uterine cavity by tubal muscular movements (Fig. 10.3). After a series of four cleavages, the 16 cells appear as a solid ball of cells or **morula**, meaning "little mulberry." The morula reaches the uterine cavity about 72 hours after fertilization (Johnson, 2007).

With additional cell division, the morula divides into specialized cells that will later form fetal structures. Within the morula, an off-centre, fluid-filled space appears, transforming it into a hollow ball of cells called a **blastocyst** (Fig. 10.4). The inner surface of the blastocyst will form the embryo and amnion. The outer layer of cells surrounding the blastocyst cavity is called a **trophoblast**. Eventually, the trophoblast develops into one of the embryonic membranes, the chorion, and helps to form the placenta.

At this time, the developing blastocyst needs more nutrients to keep growing. The trophoblast attaches itself to the surface of the endometrium for further nourishment. Normally, implantation occurs in the upper uterus (fundus), where a rich blood supply is available. This area also contains strong muscular fibres, which clamp down on blood vessels after the placenta separates from the inner wall of the uterus. Additionally, the lining is

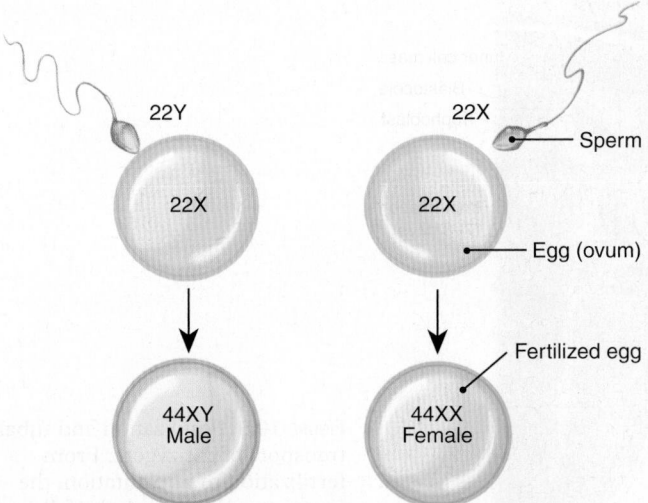

FIGURE 10.2 Inheritance of gender. Each ovum contains 22 autosomes and an X chromosome. Each spermatozoon (sperm) contains 22 autosomes and either an X chromosome or a Y chromosome. The gender of the zygote is determined at the time of fertilization by the combination of the sex chromosomes of the sperm (either X or Y) and the ovum (X).

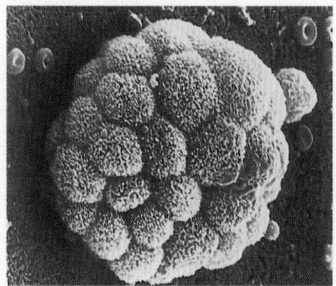

FIGURE 10.4 Blastocyst.

thickest here so the placenta cannot attach so strongly that it remains attached after birth (Cunningham et al., 2010). Figure 10.5 shows the process of fertilization and implantation.

Concurrent with the development of the trophoblast and implantation, further differentiation of the inner cell mass occurs. Some of the cells become the embryo itself, and others give rise to the membranes that surround and protect it. The three embryonic layers of cells formed are:

1. Ectoderm—forms the central nervous system, special senses, skin, and glands
2. Mesoderm—forms the skeletal, urinary, circulatory, and reproductive organs
3. Endoderm—forms the respiratory system, liver, pancreas, and digestive system

BOX 10.1 Summary of Preembryonic Development

- Fertilization takes place in ampulla of the fallopian tube.
- Union of sperm and ovum forms a *zygote* (46 chromosomes).
- Cleavage cell division continues to form a *morula* (mass of 16 cells).
- The inner cell mass is called *blastocyst*, which forms the embryo and amnion.
- The outer cell mass is called *trophoblast*, which forms the placenta and chorion.
- Implantation occurs 7 to 10 days after conception in the endometrium.

These three layers are formed at the same time as the embryonic membranes, and all tissues, organs, and organ systems develop from these three primary germ cell layers (Dillon, 2007). Box 10.1 summarizes preembryonic development.

Despite the intense and dramatic activities going on internally during this period of preembryonic development, many women are unaware that pregnancy has

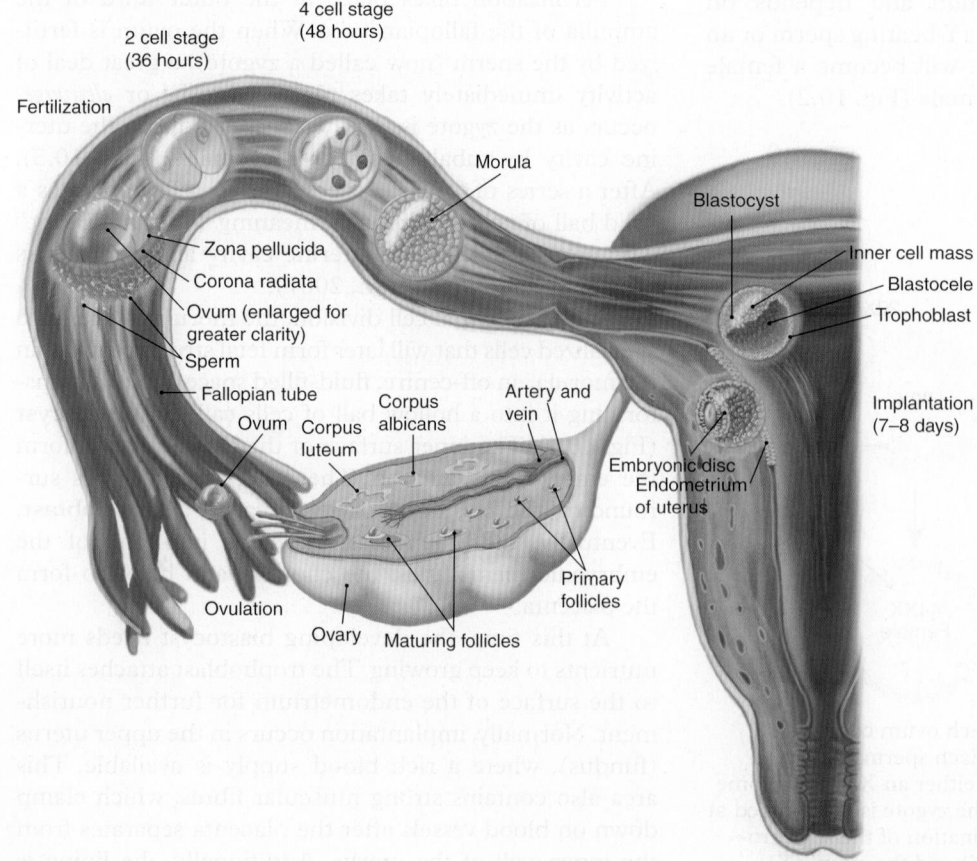

FIGURE 10.5 Fertilization and tubal transport of the zygote. From fertilization to implantation, the zygote travels through the fallopian tube, experiencing rapid mitotic division (cleavage). During the journey toward the uterus the zygote evolves through several stages, including morula and blastocyst.

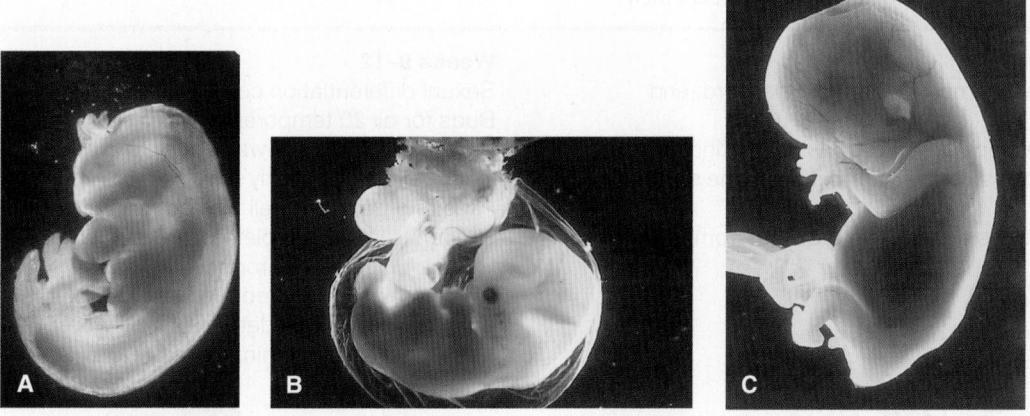

FIGURE 10.6 Embryonic development. (**A**) 4-week embryo. (**B**) 5-week embryo. (**C**) 6-week embryo.

begun. Several weeks will pass before even one of the presumptive signs of pregnancy—missing the first menstrual period—will take place.

Embryonic Stage

The embryonic stage of development begins at day 15 after conception and continues through week 8. Basic structures of all major body organs and the main external features are completed during this time period. Table 10.1 and Figure 10.6 summarize embryonic development.

The embryonic membranes (Fig. 10.7) begin to form around the time of implantation. The chorion consists of trophoblast cells and a mesodermal lining. It has finger-like projections called *chorionic villi* on its surface. The amnion originates from the ectoderm germ layer during the early stages of embryonic development. It is a thin protective membrane that contains amniotic fluid. As the embryo grows, the amnion expands until it touches the chorion. These two fetal membranes form the fluid-filled amniotic sac, or bag of waters, that protects the floating embryo (Blackburn, 2007; Creatsas, Chrousos, & Mastorakos, 2007; Moore, 2007).

Amniotic fluid surrounds the embryo and increases in volume as the pregnancy progresses, reaching approximately a litre at term. Amniotic fluid is derived from two sources: fluid transported from the maternal blood across the amnion and fetal urine. Its volume changes constantly as the fetus swallows and voids. Sufficient amounts of amniotic fluid help maintain a constant body temperature for the fetus, permit symmetric growth and development, cushion the fetus from trauma, allow the **umbilical cord** to be relatively free from compression, and promote fetal movement to enhance musculoskeletal development. Amniotic fluid is composed of 98% water and 2% organic matter. It is slightly alkaline and contains albumin, urea, uric acid, creatinine, bilirubin, lecithin, sphingomyelin, epithelial cells, vernix, and fine hair called lanugo (Cunningham et al., 2010).

The volume of amniotic fluid is important in determining fetal well-being. It gradually fluctuates throughout the pregnancy. Alterations in amniotic fluid volume can be associated with problems in the fetus. Too little amniotic fluid (<500 mL at term), termed *oligohydramnios,* is associated with uteroplacental insufficiency and fetal renal abnormalities. Too much amniotic fluid (>2,000 mL at term), termed *hydramnios,* is associated with maternal diabetes, neural tube defects, chromosomal deviations, and malformations of the central nervous system and/or gastrointestinal tract

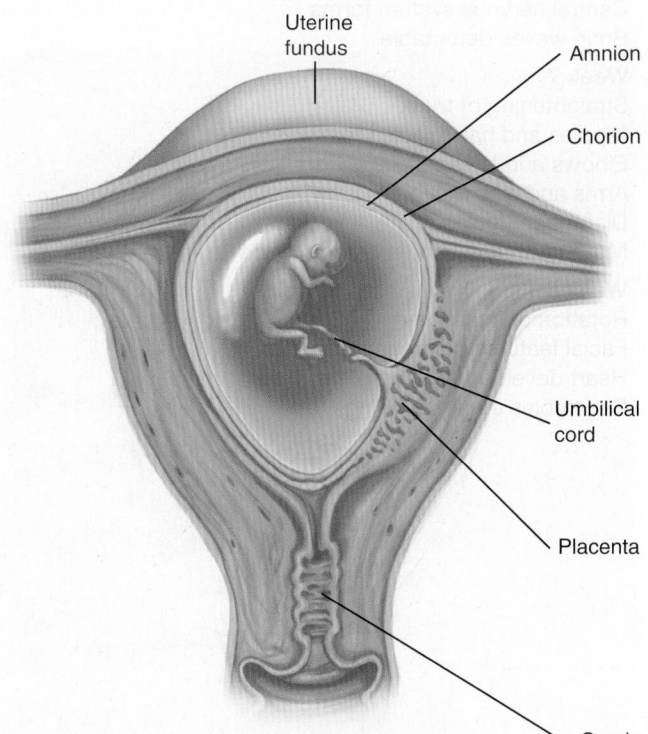

FIGURE 10.7 The embryo is floating in amniotic fluid, surrounded by the protective fetal membranes (amnion and chorion).

TABLE 10.1 EMBRYONIC AND FETAL DEVELOPMENT

Week 3
Beginning development of brain, spinal cord, and
  heart
Beginning development of the gastrointestinal tract
Neural tube forms, which later becomes the spinal
  cord
Leg and arm buds appear and grow out from body

Week 4
Brain differentiates
Limb buds grow and develop more

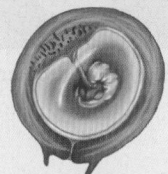
4 weeks

Week 5
Heart now beats at a regular rhythm
Beginning structures of eyes and ears
Some cranial nerves are visible
Muscles innervated

Week 6
Beginning formation of lungs
Fetal circulation established
Liver produces red blood cells
Further development of the brain
Primitive skeleton forms
Central nervous system forms
Brain waves detectable

Week 7
Straightening of trunk
Nipples and hair follicles form
Elbows and toes visible
Arms and legs move
Diaphragm formed
Mouth with lips and early tooth buds

Week 8
Rotation of intestines
Facial features continue to develop
Heart development complete
Resembles a human being

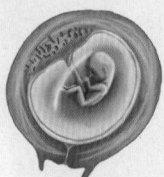
8 weeks

Weeks 9–12
Sexual differentiation continues
Buds for all 20 temporary teeth laid down
Digestive system shows activity
Head comprises nearly half the fetus size
Face and neck are well formed
Urogenital tract completes development
Red blood cells are produced in the liver
Urine begins to be produced and excreted
Fetal gender can be determined by week 12
Limbs are long and thin; digits are well formed

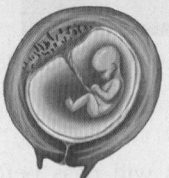
12 weeks

Weeks 13–16
A fine hair called lanugo develops on the head
Fetal skin is almost transparent
Bones become harder
Fetus makes active movement
Sucking motions are made with the mouth
Amniotic fluid is swallowed
Fingernails and toenails present
Weight quadruples
Fetal movement (also know as quickening) detected by
  mother

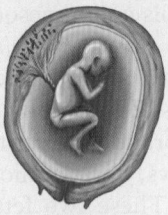
16 weeks

Weeks 17–20
Rapid brain growth occurs
Fetal heart tones can be heard with stethoscope
Kidneys continue to secret urine into amniotic fluid
Vernix caseosa, a white greasy film, covers the fetus
Eyebrows and head hair appear
Brown fat deposited to help maintain temperature
Nails are present on both fingers and toes
Muscles are well developed

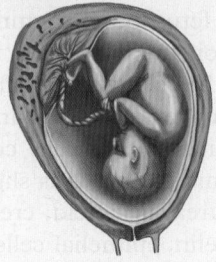
20 weeks

Weeks 21–24
Eyebrows and eyelashes are well formed
Fetus has a hand grasp and startle reflex
Alveoli forming in lungs
Skin is translucent and red
Lungs begin to produce surfactant

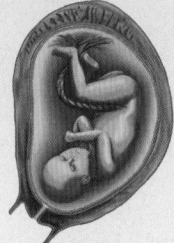

25 weeks

Weeks 25–28
Fetus reaches a length of 38.1 cm (15 inches)
Rapid brain development
Eyelids open and close
Nervous system controls some functions
Fingerprints are set
Blood formation shifts from spleen to bone marrow
Fetus usually assumes head-down position

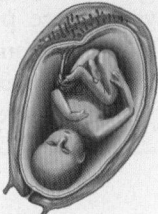

28 weeks

Weeks 29–32
Rapid increase in the amount of body fat
Increased central nervous system control over body
    functions
Rhythmic breathing movements occur
Lungs are not fully mature
Fetus stores iron, calcium, and phosphorus

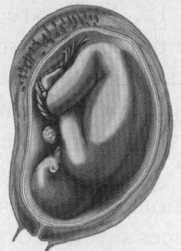

32 weeks

Weeks 33–38
Testes are in scrotum of male fetus
Lanugo begins to disappear
Increase in body fat
Fingernails reach the end of fingertips
Small breast buds are present on both sexes
Mother supplies fetus with antibodies against disease
Fetus is considered full term at 38 weeks
Fetus fills uterus

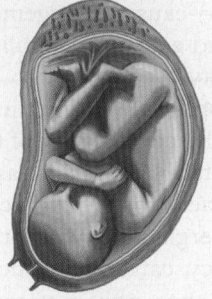

37 weeks

that prevent normal swallowing of amniotic fluid by the fetus (Gilbert, 2010).

While the placenta is developing (end of the second week), the umbilical cord is also formed from the amnion. It is the lifeline from the mother to the growing embryo. It contains one large vein and two small arteries. Wharton's jelly (a specialized connective tissue) surrounds these three blood vessels in the umbilical cord to prevent compression, which would cut off fetal blood and nutrient supply. At term, the average umbilical cord is 55.9 cm (22 inches) long and about 2.54 cm (1 inch) wide (Cunningham et al., 2010).

The precursor cells of the placenta—the trophoblasts—first appear 4 days after fertilization as the outer layer of cells of the blastocyst. These early blastocyst trophoblasts differentiate into all the cells that form the **placenta.** When fully developed, the placenta serves as

the interface between the mother and the developing fetus. As early as 3 days after conception, the trophoblasts make human chorionic gonadotropin (hCG), a hormone that ensures that the endometrium will be receptive to the implanting embryo. During the next few weeks the placenta begins to make hormones that control the basic physiology of the mother in such a way that the fetus is supplied with the nutrients and oxygen needed for growth. The placenta also protects the fetus from immune attack by the mother, removes waste products from the fetus, induces the mother to bring more food to the placenta and, near the time of delivery, produces hormones that ready fetal organs for life outside the uterus (Cunningham et al., 2010).

Normally during pregnancy the mother's blood does not mix with fetal blood because there is no direct contact between their bloods; layers of fetal tissue always separate the maternal blood and the fetal blood. These fetal tissues are called the *placental barrier.* Materials can be interchanged only through diffusion. The maternal uterine arteries deliver nutrients to the placenta, which in turn provides nutrients to the developing fetus; the mother's uterine veins carry fetal waste products away. The structure of the placenta is usually completed by week 12. There are some rare circumstances in which the potential exists for fetal-maternal blood mixing, including some placental abnormalities, tubal pregnancy, significant antenatal bleeding, and invasive procedures such as amniocentesis (Blackburn, 2007).

The placenta is not only a transfer organ but a factory as well. It produces several hormones necessary for normal pregnancy:

- hCG—preserves the corpus luteum and its progesterone production so that the endometrial lining of the uterus is maintained; this is the basis for pregnancy tests
- Human placental lactogen (hPL)—modulates fetal and maternal metabolism, participates in the development of maternal breasts for lactation, and decreases maternal insulin sensitivity to increase its availability for fetal nutrition
- Estrogen (estriol)—causes enlargement of a woman's breasts, uterus, and external genitalia; stimulates myometrial contractility
- Progesterone (progestin)—maintains the endometrium, decreases the contractility of the uterus, stimulates maternal metabolism and breast development, provides nourishment for the early **conceptus**
- Relaxin—acts synergistically with progesterone to maintain pregnancy, causes relaxation of the pelvic ligaments, softens the cervix in preparation for birth (Cunningham et al., 2010)

The placenta acts as a pass-through between the mother and fetus, not a barrier. Almost everything the mother ingests (food, alcohol, drugs, and medications) passes through to the developing conceptus. This is why it is so important to counsel and support pregnant women about the use of drugs, alcohol, and tobacco, because these substances can be harmful to the conceptus. In particular, counselling and support are important for women (even before pregnancy) about alcohol use as it can cause fetal alcohol spectrum disorder (Society of Obstetricians and Gynaecologists of Canada [SOGC], 2005). Care also needs to be taken with over-the-counter, herbal, and prescription medications during pregnancy.

During the embryonic stage, the conceptus grows rapidly as all organs and structures are forming. During this critical period of differentiation the growing embryo is most susceptible to damage from external sources, including **teratogens** (substances that cause birth defects, such as alcohol as well as some drugs and

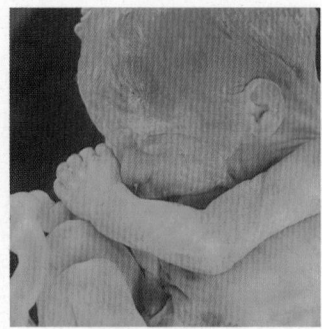

FIGURE 10.8 Fetal development: 12- to 15-week fetus.

medications), infections (such as rubella or cytomegalovirus), radiation, and nutritional deficiencies.

Fetal Stage

The average pregnancy lasts 280 days from the first day of the last menstrual period. The fetal stage is the time from the end of the eighth week until birth. It is the longest period of prenatal development. During this stage, the conceptus is mature enough to be called a fetus. Although all major systems are present in their basic form, dramatic growth and refinement of all organ systems take place during the fetal period (see Table 10.1). Figure 10.8 depicts a 12- to 15-week-old fetus.

Fetal Circulation

The circulation through the fetus during uterine life differs from that of a child or an adult. Fetal circulation involves the circulation of blood from the placenta to and through the fetus, and back to the placenta. A properly functioning fetal circulation system is essential to sustain the fetus. Before it develops, nutrients and oxygen diffuse through the extraembryonic coelom and the yolk sac from the placenta. As the embryo grows, its nutrient needs increase and the amount of tissue easily reached by diffusion increases. Thus, the circulation must develop quickly and accurately (Blackburn, 2007).

The circulatory system of the fetus functions much differently from that of a newborn. The most significant difference is that oxygen is received from the placenta during fetal life and via the lungs after birth. In addition, the fetal liver does not perform the metabolic functions that it will after birth because the mother's body performs these functions. Three shunts also are present during fetal life:

1. Ductus venosus—connects the umbilical vein to the inferior vena cava
2. Ductus arteriosus—connects the main pulmonary artery to the aorta
3. Foramen ovale—anatomic opening between the right and left atria

The oxygenated blood is carried from the placenta to the fetus via the umbilical vein. About half of this blood passes through the hepatic capillaries and the rest flows through the ductus venosus into the inferior vena cava. Blood from the vena cava is mostly deflected through the foramen ovale into the left atrium, then to the left ventricle, into the ascending aorta, and on to the head and upper body. This allows the fetal coronary circulation and the brain to receive the blood with the highest level of oxygenation.

Deoxygenated blood from the superior vena cava flows into the right atrium, the right ventricle, and then the pulmonary artery. Because of high pulmonary vascular resistance, only a small percentage (5% to 10%) of the blood in the pulmonary artery flows to the lungs; the majority is shunted through the patent ductus arteriosus and then to the descending aorta (Blackburn, 2007). The fetal lungs are essentially non-functional because they are filled with fluid, making them resistant to incoming blood flow. They receive only enough blood for proper nourishment. Finally, two umbilical arteries carry the unoxygenated blood from the descending aorta back to the placenta.

At birth, a dramatic change in the fetal circulatory pattern occurs. The foramen ovale, ductus arteriosus, ductus venosus, and umbilical vessels are no longer needed. With the newborn's first breath, the lungs inflate, which leads to an increase in blood flow to the lungs from the right ventricle. This increase raises the pressure in the left atrium, causing a one-way flap on the left side of the foramen ovale, called the septum primum, to press against the opening, creating a functional separation between the two atria. Blood flow to the lungs increases because blood entering the right atrium can no longer bypass the right ventricle. As a result, the right ventricle pumps blood into the pulmonary artery and on to the lungs. The ductus venosus closes with the clamping of the umbilical cord and inhibition of blood flow through the umbilical vein. The ductus arteriosus constricts partly in response to the higher arterial oxygen levels that occur after the first few breaths. This closure prevents blood from the aorta from entering the pulmonary artery (Blackburn, 2007). All of these changes leave the newborn with the typical adult pattern of circulation. Figure 10.9 shows fetal circulation.

Genetics

Genetics is the study of heredity and its variation (Slee, Slee, & Schmidt, 2008). According to the Public Health Agency of Canada (PHAC, 2002), serious birth defects and genetic disorders occur in about 2% to 3% of all infants born in Canada. Traditionally, genetics has been associated with making decisions about childbearing and caring for children with genetic disorders. Recently, genetic and technologic advances are expanding our understanding of how genetic changes affect human diseases such as diabetes, cancer, Alzheimer's disease, and other multifactorial diseases that are prevalent in adults (Beery & Smith, 2011; Solomon, Jack, & Feero, 2008). Our ability to diagnose genetic conditions is more advanced than our ability to cure or treat the disorders. However, accurate diagnosis has led to improved treatment and outcomes for those affected with these disorders.

Today, nurses are required to have basic skills and knowledge in genetics, genetic testing, and genetic counselling so they can assume new roles and provide information and support to women, children, and families (American Nurses Association [ANA], 2009; Bottorff, McCullum, Balneaves, et al., 2005; Canadian Nurses Association, 2002).

Advances in Genetics

Recent advances in genetic knowledge and technology have affected all areas of health. These advances have increased the number of health interventions that can be undertaken with regard to genetic disorders. For example, genetic diagnosis is now possible before conception and very early in pregnancy (see Evidence-based Practice 10.1). Genetic testing can now identify presymptomatic conditions in children and adults. Gene therapy can be used to replace or repair defective or missing genes with normal ones. Gene therapy has been used for a variety of disorders, including cystic fibrosis, melanoma, diabetes, human immunodeficiency virus (HIV), and hepatitis (Beery & Smith, 2011; Giacca, 2010). Genetic agents may replace drugs, general surgery may be replaced by gene surgery, and genetic intervention may replace radiation (Beery & Smith, 2011; Giacca, 2010). Gene therapy may also be used to treat many chronic illnesses.

The Human Genome Project (HGP) was an international 13-year effort to produce a comprehensive

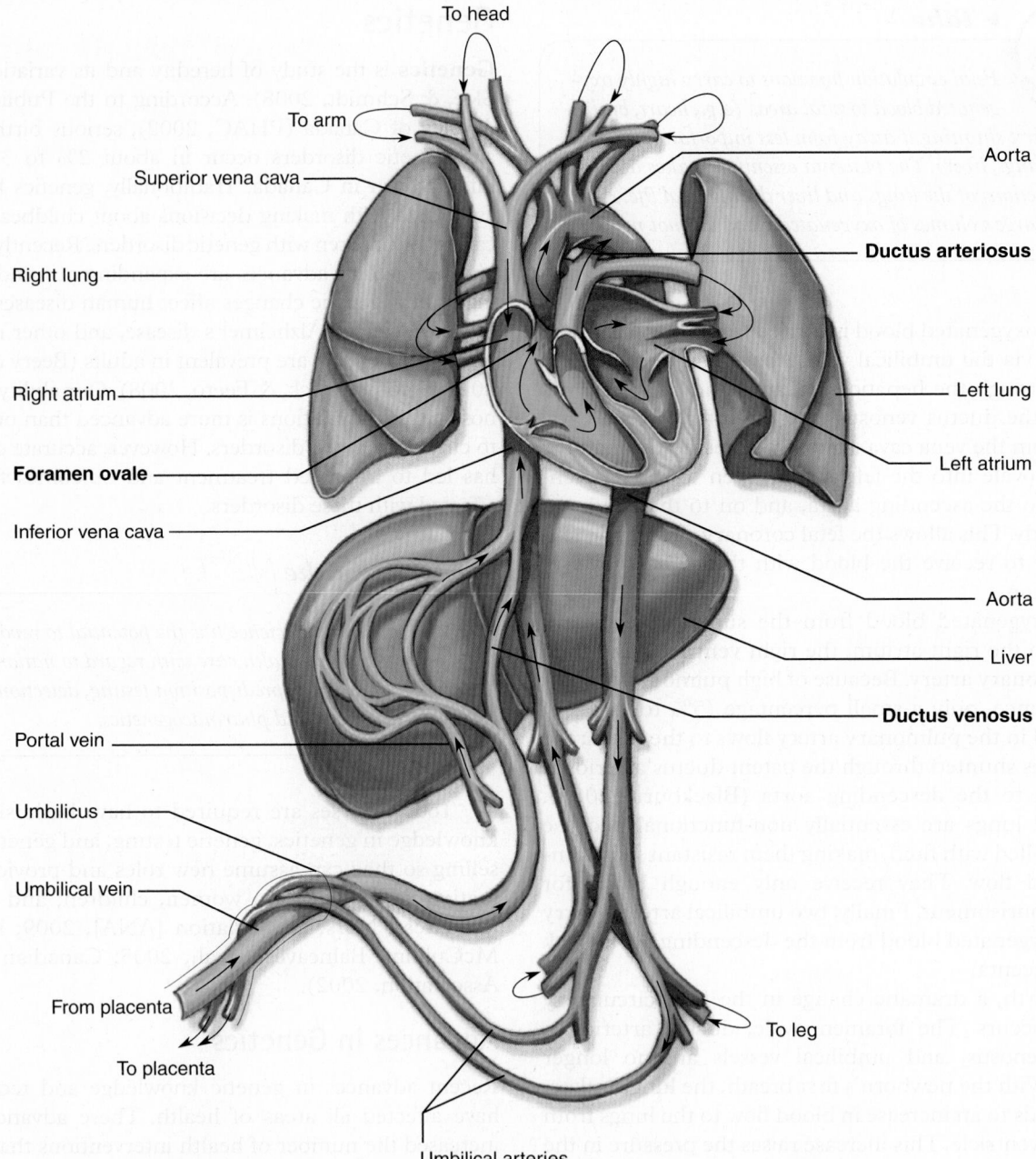

To head

To arm

Superior vena cava

Right lung

Right atrium

Foramen ovale

Inferior vena cava

Portal vein

Umbilicus

Umbilical vein

From placenta

To placenta

Aorta

Ductus arteriosus

Left lung

Left atrium

Aorta

Liver

Ductus venosus

To leg

Umbilical arteries

FIGURE 10.9 Fetal circulation. Arrows indicate the path of blood. The umbilical vein carries oxygen-rich blood from the placenta to the liver and through the ductus venosus. From there it is carried to the inferior vena cava to the right atrium of the heart. Some of the blood is shunted through the foramen ovale to the left side of the heart, where it is routed to the brain and upper extremities. The rest of the blood travels down to the right ventricle and through the pulmonary artery. A small portion of the blood travels to the non-functioning lungs, while the remaining blood is shunted through the ductus arteriosus into the aorta to supply the rest of the body.

sequence of the human genome. It was started in 1990 by the U.S. Department of Energy and the National Institutes of Health and was completed in May 2003. It has brought advances to the field of genetics and genetic testing (ANA, 2009). An individual's **genome** represents his or her genetic blueprint, which determines **genotype** (the gene pairs inherited from parents; the

specific genetic makeup) and **phenotype** (observed outward characteristics of an individual) (Giacca, 2010).

A primary goal of the HGP was to translate the findings into new strategies for the prevention, diagnosis, and treatment of genetic diseases and disorders. Two key findings from the project were that all human beings are 99.9% identical at the DNA level, and approximately

EVIDENCE-BASED PRACTICE 10.1
Preimplantation Genetic Screening and Promoting Pregnancy with Assisted Reproductive Technologies

● Study

Assisted reproductive technologies such as in vitro fertilization (IVF) and intracytoplasmic sperm injection (ICSI) involve the transfer of an embryo to the mother to achieve pregnancy. The physician selects the embryos for transfer based on specific criteria related to their structure and form. These "good-quality" embryos are then implanted in the mother in the hopes of achieving a pregnancy. Unfortunately, many women do not experience a pregnancy. The reasons for these failures are not known. One belief is that the embryos being transferred, although they meet the criteria for structure and form, may have an abnormal number of chromosomes, which affects implantation and the development of a pregnancy. Preimplantation genetic screening (PGS) is a tool being used to identify embryos of good quality with the normal number of chromosomes. Based on the screening, only these embryos are implanted; in theory, this would increase the rate of pregnancy. However, there are questions as to how effective PGS is in improving the rates of pregnancy and live birth.

In this updated review two independent authors used predetermined quality criteria to collect and analyze data from numerous databases, registers, and reference lists of articles. The researchers also gathered additional data from other authors as necessary. The researchers selected all relevant randomized controlled trials dealing with IVF or ICSI with and without PGS. The researchers measured the outcome based primarily on the live birth rate.

In the initial review in 2006 the researchers reviewed two randomized controlled trials. Both trials involved IVF or ICSI with and without the use of PGS. The group without PGS was considered the control group. The trials also involved women of advanced maternal age (over age 35). In this update, the researchers reviewed nine randomized controlled trials.

▲ Findings

Compared with the control group, the PGS group showed significant decreases in the live birth rates in women of advanced maternal age and those with repeated IVF failure. However, the researchers noted that PGS technique development is still ongoing in an effort to increase its efficacy. They recommend that these new developments should still be properly evaluated before their routine clinical application and that it is not yet appropriate to offer PGS as routine patient care.

■ Nursing Implications

Although the study showed some increasing effectiveness of PGS in the past six years, nurses need to be aware of the continually emerging technology and techniques associated with genetics so that they can provide women and their families with the most appropriate information about available options and therapies. Nurses can incorporate information from this study in their teaching, anticipatory guidance, and counselling activities related to options so that couples can make the best-informed decision possible.

Twisk, M., Mastenbroek, S., van Wely, M., Heineman, M. J., Van der Veen, F., Repping, S. (2006). Preimplantation genetic screening for abnormal number of chromosomes (aneuploidies) in in vitro fertilisation or intracytoplasmic sperm injection. *Cochrane Database of Systematic Reviews,* (1). Art. No.: CD005291. doi:10.1002/14651858.CD005291.pub2

30,000 genes make up the human genome (International Human Genome Sequencing Consortium, 2004). For a direct link to more information about the HGP, visit http://thePoint.lww.com/Chow1e.

Current and potential applications for the HGP to health care include rapid and more specific diagnosis of disease, with hundreds of genetic tests available in research or clinical practice; earlier detection of genetic predisposition to disease; less emphasis on treating the symptoms of a disease and more emphasis on looking at the fundamental causes of the disease; new classes of drugs; avoidance of environmental conditions that may trigger disease; and possible augmentation or replacement of defective genes through gene therapy. This new genetic knowledge and technology, along with the commercialization of this knowledge, will change both professional and parental understanding of genetic disorders.

The potential benefits of these discoveries are vast, but so is the potential for misuse. These advances challenge all health care professionals to consider the many ethical, legal, and social ramifications of genetics in human lives. In the near future, individual risk profiling based on an individual's unique genetic makeup will be used to tailor prevention, treatment, and ongoing management of health conditions. This profiling will raise issues associated with patient privacy and confidentiality related to workplace discrimination and access to health insurance. Issues of autonomy are equally problematic as society considers how to address the injustices that will inevitably surface when disease risk can be determined years in advance of its occurrence. Nurses will play an important role in developing policies and providing direction and support in this arena, and to do so they will need a basic understanding of genetics, including inheritance and inheritance patterns. (For a direct link to more information on the ethical, social, and legal issues sur-rounding human genetic research and advances, visit http://thePoint.lww.com/Chow1e.)

A newer field of study is **epigenetics**, which examines factors other than the DNA sequence that influence the development of an organism, including the environment, inheritance, nutrition, behaviour, and stress. The U.S. National Institutes of Health has heavily funded this area of research and notes that epigenetics has the potential to explain the mechanisms of aging and human development as well as the origins of cancer, heart disease, mental illness, and other conditions. Many important epigenetic interactions between the genome and the environment occur during embryonic development. Maternal nutrition is a current focus of research in this field. There is much still to learn, but epigenetics will most likely have a significant impact on public health in the future.

Inheritance

The nucleus within the cell is the controlling factor in all cellular activities because it contains chromosomes, long continuous strands of deoxyribonucleic acid (DNA) that carry genetic information. Each chromosome is made up of **genes**. Genes are individual units of heredity of all traits and are organized into long segments of DNA that occupy a specific location on a chromosome and determine a particular characteristic in an organism.

DNA stores genetic information and encodes the instructions for synthesizing specific proteins needed to maintain life. DNA is double-stranded and takes the form of a double helix. The side pieces of the double helix are made up of a sugar, deoxyribose, and a phosphate, occurring in alternating groups. The cross-connections or rungs of the ladder are attached to the sides and are made up of four nitrogenous bases: adenine, cytosine, thymine, and guanine. The sequence of the base pairs as they form each rung of the ladder is referred to as the genetic code (Fig. 10.10; Wright & Hastie, 2007).

Each gene has a segment of DNA with a specific set of instructions for making proteins needed by body cells for proper functioning. Genes control the types of proteins made and the rate at which they are produced (Solomon et al., 2008). Any change in gene structure or location leads to a **mutation**, which may alter the type and amount of protein produced (Fig. 10.11). Genes never act in isolation; they always interact with other genes and the environment. They are arranged in a specific linear formation along a chromosome.

The genotype, the specific genetic makeup of an individual, usually in the form of DNA, is the internally coded inheritable information. It refers to the particular **allele**, which is one of two or more alternative versions of gene at a given position or locus on a chromosome that imparts the same characteristic of that gene. For instance, each human has a gene that controls height, but there are

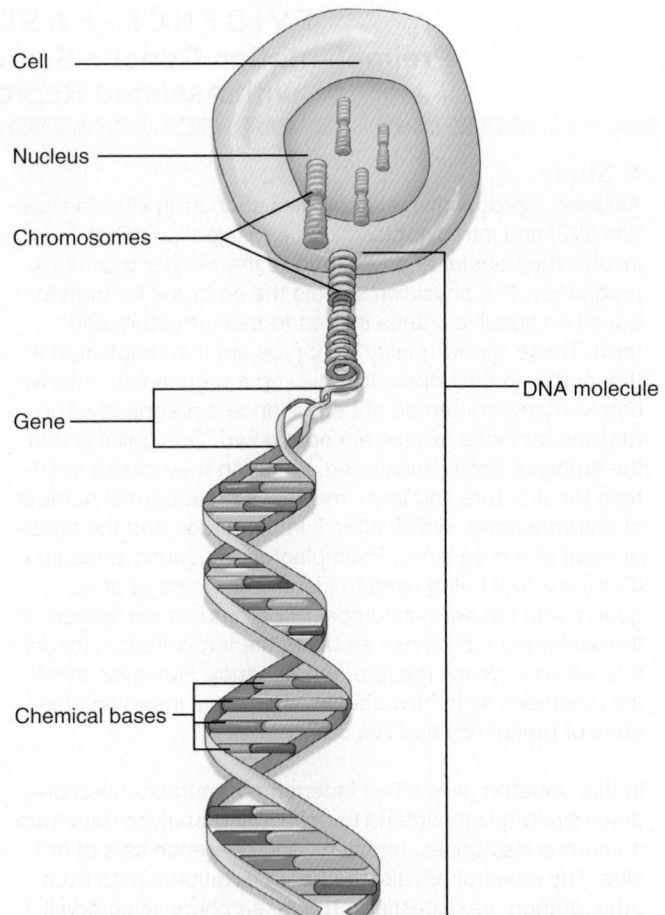

FIGURE 10.10 DNA is made up of four chemical bases. Tightly coiled strands of DNA are packaged in units called chromosomes, housed in the cell's nucleus. Working subunits of DNA are known as genes. (From the National Institutes of Health and National Cancer Institute [1995]. *Understanding gene testing* [NIH Pub. No. 96–3905]. Washington, DC: U.S. Department of Human Services.)

variations of these genes, which are alleles, in accordance with the specific height for which the gene codes. A gene that controls eye colour may have an allele that produces blue eyes or an allele that produces brown eyes. The genotype, together with environmental variation that influences the individual, determines the phenotype, or the observed, outward characteristics of an individual. A human inherits two genes, one from each parent. Therefore, one allele comes from the mother and one from the father. These alleles may be the same for the characteristic (**homozygous**) or different (**heterozygous**). For example, WW stands for homozygous **dominant**; ww stands for homozygous **recessive**. Heterozygous would be indicated as Ww. If the two alleles differ, such as Ww, the dominant one will usually be expressed in the phenotype of the individual.

Human beings typically have 46 chromosomes. This includes 22 pairs of non-sex chromosomes or autosomes

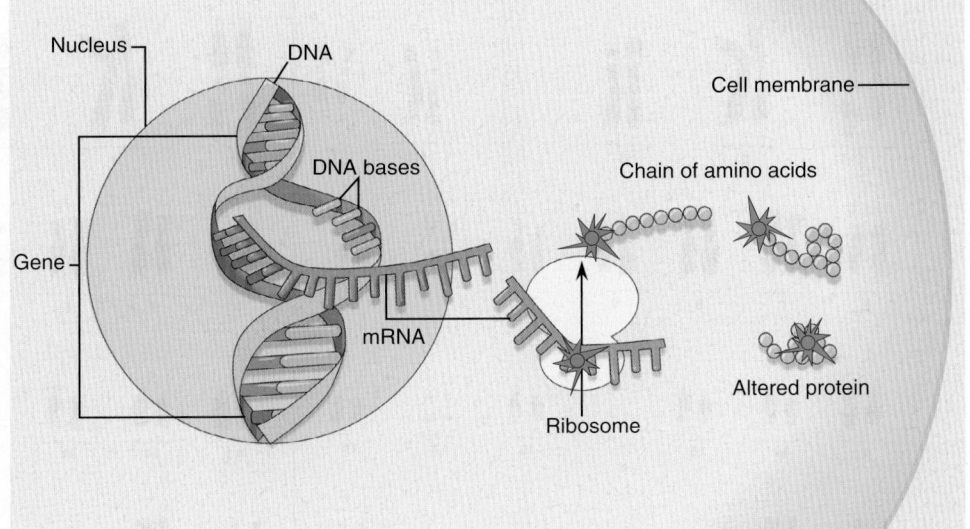

FIGURE 10.11 When a gene contains a mutation, the protein encoded by that gene will be abnormal. Some protein changes are insignificant, while others are disabling. (From the National Institutes of Health and National Cancer Institute. [1995]. *Understanding gene testing* [NIH Pub. No. 96–3905]. Washington, DC: U.S. Department of Human Services.)

and one pair of sex chromosomes (two X chromosomes in females, and an X chromosome and a Y chromosome in males). Offspring receive one chromosome of each of the 23 pairs from each parent.

Regulation and expression of the thousands of human genes is very complex and is the result of many intricate interactions within each cell. Alterations in gene structure, function, transcription, translation, and protein synthesis can influence an individual's health (Wright & Hastie, 2007). Gene mutations are a permanent change in the sequence of DNA. Some mutations have no significant effect, whereas others can have a tremendous impact on the health of the individual. Several genetic disorders can result from these mutations, such as cystic fibrosis, sickle-cell disease, phenylketonuria, or hemophilia.

The pictorial analysis of the number, form, and size of an individual's chromosomes is termed the **karyotype**. This analysis commonly uses white blood cells and fetal cells in amniotic fluid. The chromosomes are numbered from the largest to the smallest, 1 to 22, and the sex chromosomes are designated by the letter X or Y. A female karyotype is designated as 46,XX and a male karyotype is designated as 46,XY. Figure 10.12 illustrates an example of a karyotyping pattern.

Patterns of Inheritance

A genetic disorder is a disease caused by an abnormality in an individual's genetic material or genome. Diagnosis of a genetic disorder is usually based on clinical signs and symptoms or on laboratory confirmation of an altered gene associated with the disorder. Accurate diagnosis can be aided by the recognition of the pattern of inheritance within a family. The pattern of inheritance is also vital to understand when teaching and counselling families about the risks in future pregnancies. Some genetic disorders occur in multiple family members, while others may

occur in only a single family member. A genetic disorder is caused by completely or partially altered genetic material, while a familial disorder is more common in relatives of the affected individual but may be caused by environmental influences and not genetic alterations. For a more detailed discussion of specific types of genetic disorders, see Chapter 50.

Monogenic Disorders

Patterns of inheritance demonstrate how a genetic disorder can be passed on to offspring. Principles of genetic disease inheritance of single gene disorders are the same principles that govern the inheritance of other traits, such as eye and hair colour. These are known as Mendel's laws of inheritance, named for the genetic work of Gregor Mendel, an Austrian naturalist. These patterns occur due to a single gene being defective and are referred to as monogenic or sometimes Mendelian disorders. If the defect occurs on the autosome, the genetic disorder is termed autosomal; if the defect is on the X chromosome, the genetic disorder is termed X-linked. The defect also can be classified as dominant or recessive. Monogenic disorders include autosomal dominant, autosomal recessive, X-linked dominant, and X-linked recessive patterns.

Autosomal Dominant Inheritance Disorders

Autosomal dominant inherited disorders occur when a single gene in the heterozygous state is capable of producing the phenotype. In other words, the abnormal or mutant gene overshadows the normal gene and the individual will demonstrate signs and symptoms of the disorder. The affected person generally has an affected parent, and an affected person has a 50% chance of passing the abnormal gene to each of his or her children (Fig. 10.13). Affected individuals are present in every generation. Males and family members who are phenotypically

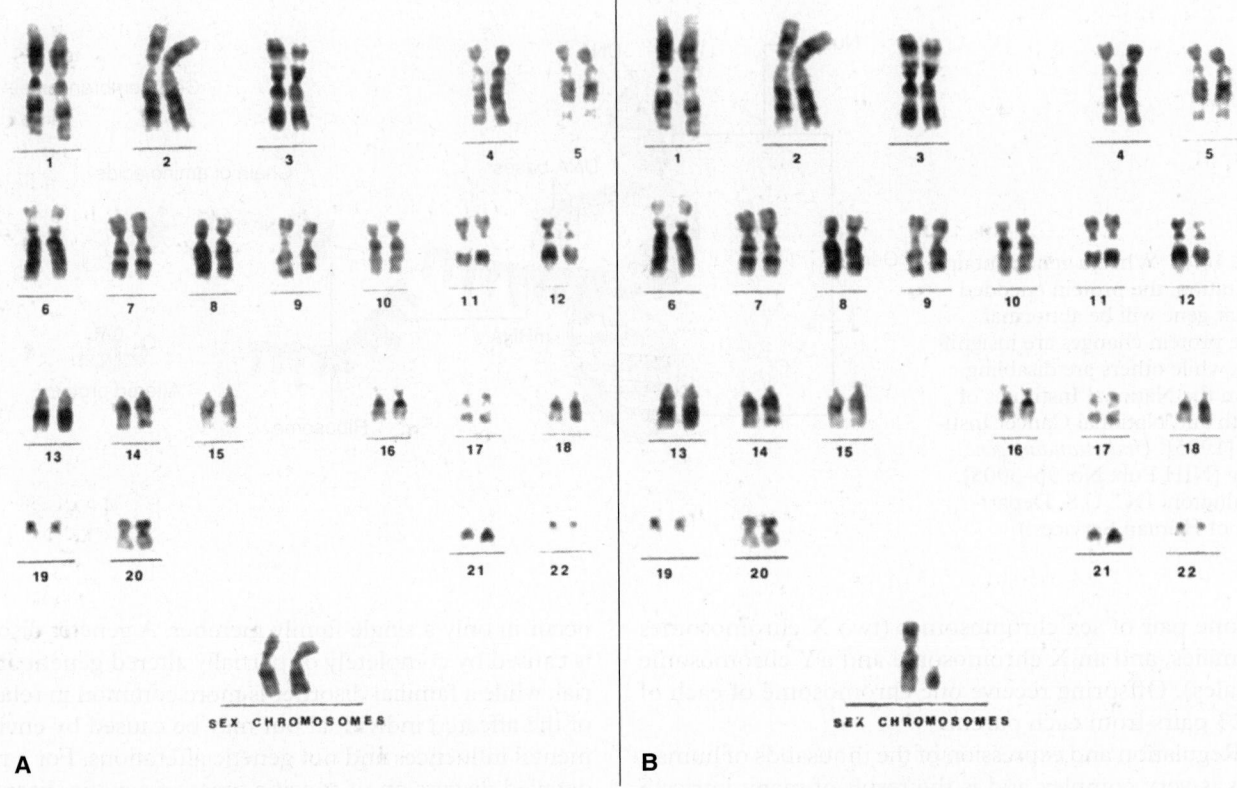

FIGURE 10.12 Karyotype pattern. (**A**) Normal female karyotype. (**B**) Normal male karyotype.

normal (do not show signs or symptoms of the disorder) do not transmit the condition to their offspring. Females and males are equally affected and a male can pass the disorder on to his son. This male-to-male transmission is important in distinguishing autosomal dominant inheritance from X-linked inheritance. There are varying degrees of presentation among individuals in a family. Therefore, a parent with a mild form could have a child with a more severe form. Common types of genetic disorders that follow the autosomal dominant pattern of inheritance include neurofibromatosis, Huntington's disease, achondroplasia, and polycystic kidney disease.

Autosomal Recessive Inheritance Disorders

Autosomal recessive inherited disorders occur when two copies of the mutant or abnormal gene in the homozygous state are necessary to produce the phenotype. In other words, two abnormal genes are needed for the individual to demonstrate signs and symptoms of the disorder. These disorders are generally less common than autosomal dominant disorders (Kliegman et al., 2011). Both parents of the affected person must be heterozygous carriers of the gene (clinically normal but carry the gene), and their offspring have a 25% chance of being homozygous (a 50% chance of getting the mutant gene from each parent and therefore a 25% chance of inheriting two mutant genes). If the child is clinically normal, there is a 50% chance that the child is a carrier (Fig. 10.14).

Affected individuals are usually present in only one generation of the family. Females and males are equally affected and a male can pass the disorder on to his son. The chance that any two parents will both be carriers of

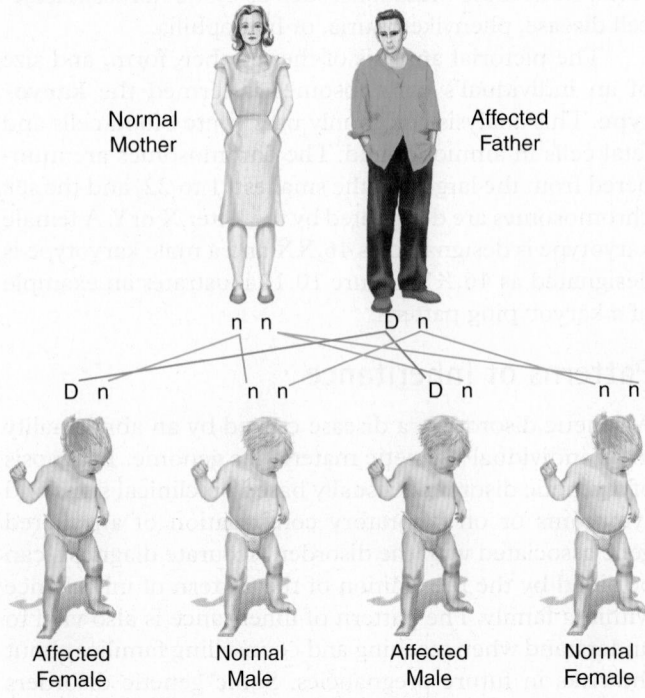

FIGURE 10.13 Autosomal dominant inheritance.

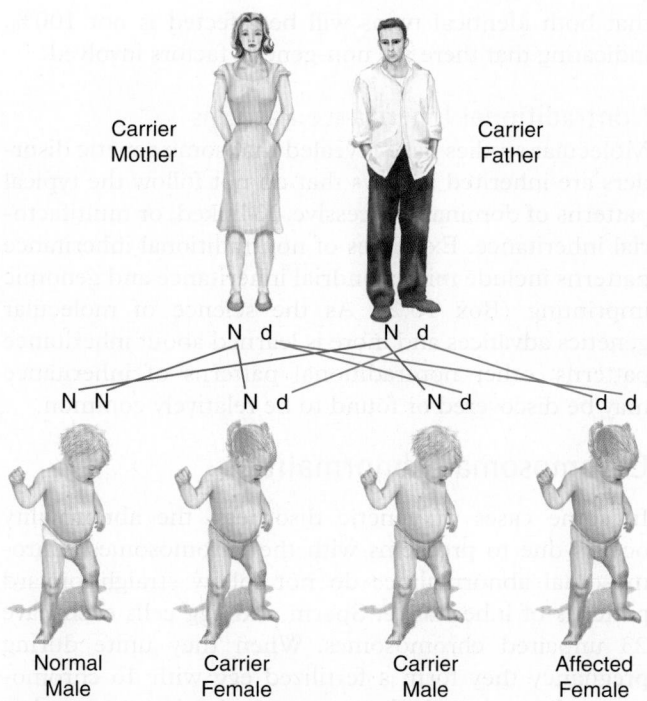

FIGURE 10.14 Autosomal recessive inheritance.

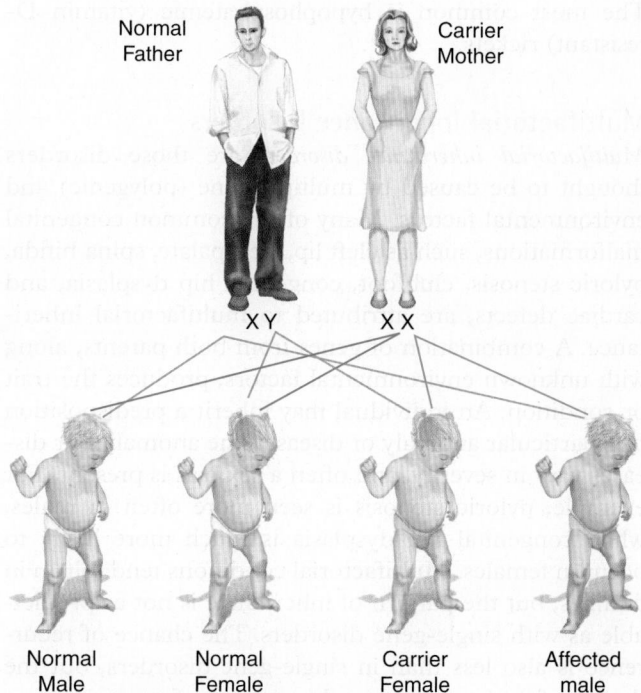

FIGURE 10.15 X-linked recessive inheritance.

the mutant gene is increased if the couple is consanguineous (having a common ancestor). Common types of genetic disorders that follow the autosomal recessive inheritance pattern include cystic fibrosis, phenylketonuria, Tay–Sachs disease, and sickle-cell disease.

X-linked Inheritance Disorders

X-linked inherited disorders are those associated with altered genes present on the X chromosome. They differ in characteristic from autosomal disorders. If a male inherits an X-linked altered gene, he will express the condition. Since a male has only one X chromosome, all the genes on his X chromosome will be expressed (the Y chromosome carries no normal allele to compensate for the altered gene). Since females inherit two X chromosomes, they can be either heterozygous or homozygous for any allele. Therefore, X-linked disorders in females are expressed similarly to autosomal disorders.

Most X-linked disorders demonstrate a recessive pattern of inheritance. Males are more affected than females. A male has only one X chromosome and all the genes on his X chromosome will be expressed, whereas a female will usually need both X chromosomes to carry the disease. There is no male-to-male transmission (since no X chromosome from the male is transmitted to male offspring), but any man who is affected will have carrier daughters. If a woman is a carrier, there is a 50% chance that her sons will be affected and a 50% chance that her daughters will be carriers (Fig. 10.15). Common types of genetic disorders that follow X-linked recessive inheritance patterns include hemophilia, colour blindness, and Duchenne muscular dystrophy.

X-linked dominant inheritance is present if heterozygous female carriers demonstrate signs and symptoms of the disorder. All of the daughters and none of the sons of an affected male have the condition, while both male and female offspring of an affected woman have a 50% chance of inheriting and presenting with the condition (Fig. 10.16). X-linked dominant disorders are rare.

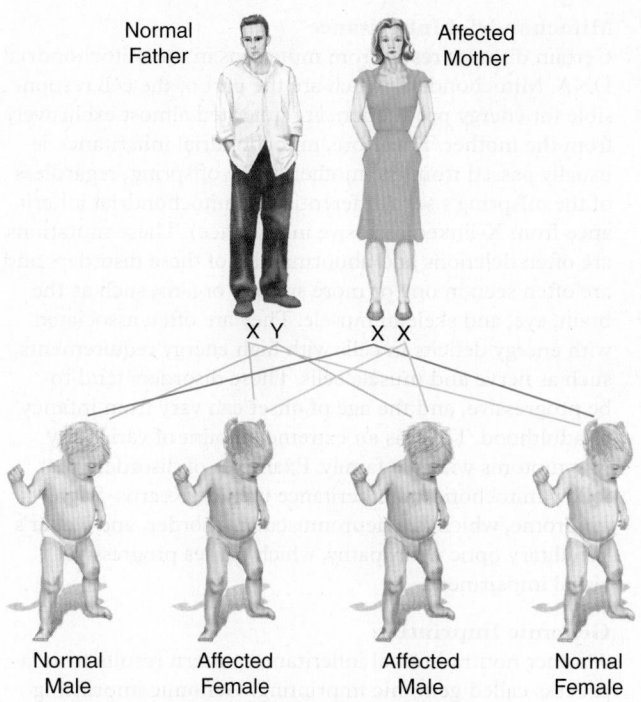

FIGURE 10.16 X-linked dominant inheritance.

The most common is hypophosphatemic (vitamin D-resistant) rickets.

Multifactorial Inheritance Disorders

Multifactorial inheritance disorders are those disorders thought to be caused by multiple gene (polygenic) and environmental factors. Many of the common congenital malformations, such as cleft lip, cleft palate, spina bifida, pyloric stenosis, clubfoot, congenital hip dysplasia, and cardiac defects, are attributed to multifactorial inheritance. A combination of genes from both parents, along with unknown environmental factors, produces the trait or condition. An individual may inherit a predisposition to a particular anomaly or disease. The anomalies or diseases vary in severity, and often a sex bias is present. For example, pyloric stenosis is seen more often in males, while congenital hip dysplasia is much more likely to occur in females. Multifactorial conditions tend to run in families, but the pattern of inheritance is not as predictable as with single-gene disorders. The chance of recurrence is also less than in single-gene disorders, but the degree of risk is related to the number of genes in common with the affected individual. The closer the degree of relationship, the more genes an individual has in common with the affected family member, resulting in a higher chance the individual's offspring will have a similar defect. In **multifactorial inheritance**, the likelihood

that both identical twins will be affected is not 100%, indicating that there are non-genetic factors involved.

Nontraditional Inheritance Patterns

Molecular studies have revealed that some genetic disorders are inherited in ways that do not follow the typical patterns of dominant, recessive, X-linked, or multifactorial inheritance. Examples of nontraditional inheritance patterns include mitochondrial inheritance and genomic imprinting (Box 10.2). As the science of molecular genetics advances and more is learned about inheritance patterns, other nontraditional patterns of inheritance may be discovered or found to be relatively common.

Chromosomal Abnormalities

In some cases of genetic disorders, the abnormality occurs due to problems with the chromosomes. Chromosomal abnormalities do not follow straightforward patterns of inheritance. Sperm and egg cells each have 23 unpaired chromosomes. When they unite during pregnancy they form a fertilized egg with 46 chromosomes. Sometimes before pregnancy begins, an error has occurred during the process of cell division, leaving an egg or sperm with too many or too few chromosomes. If this egg or sperm cell joins with a normal egg or sperm cell, the resulting embryo has a chromosomal abnormality. Chromosomal abnormalities can also occur due to

---

BOX 10.2 **Nontraditional Inheritance Patterns**

Mitochondrial Inheritance
Certain diseases result from mutations in the mitochondrial DNA. Mitochondria, which are the part of the cell responsible for energy production, are inherited almost exclusively from the mother. Therefore, mitochondrial inheritance is usually passed from the mother to the offspring, regardless of the offspring's sex (differentiating mitochondrial inheritance from X-linked recessive inheritance). These mutations are often deletions and abnormalities of these disorders and are often seen in one or more specific organs, such as the brain, eye, and skeletal muscle. They are often associated with energy deficits in cells with high energy requirements, such as nerve and muscle cells. These disorders tend to be progressive, and the age of onset can vary from infancy to adulthood. There is an extreme amount of variability in symptoms within a family. Examples of disorders that follow mitochondrial inheritance include Kearns–Sayre syndrome, which is a neuromuscular disorder, and Leber's hereditary optic neuropathy, which causes progressive visual impairment.

Genomic Imprinting
Another nontraditional inheritance pattern results from a process called genomic imprinting. Genomic imprinting

plays a critical role in fetal growth and development and placental functioning. In genomic imprinting, the expression of a gene is determined by its parental origin. In genomic imprinting both the maternal and paternal alleles are present, but only one is expressed; the other is inactive. Genomic imprinting does not alter the genetic sequence itself but affects the phenotype observed. In these cases the altered genes in a certain region of the genome have very different expressions depending on whether they were inherited from the mother or the father. Several human syndromes are known to be associated with defects in gene imprinting. Disorders that result from a disruption of imprinting usually involve a growth phenotype and include varying degrees of developmental problems. Common examples include Prader–Willi syndrome (a condition resulting in severe hypotonia and hyperphagia leading to obesity and mental retardation), Angelman syndrome (a neurodevelopmental disorder associated with mental retardation, jerky movements, and seizures), and Beckwith–Wiedemann syndrome (characterized by somatic overgrowth, congenital malformations, and a predisposition to embryonic neoplasia).

an error in the structure of the chromosome. Small pieces of the chromosome may be deleted, duplicated, inverted, misplaced, or exchanged with part of another chromosome. Most chromosomal abnormalities occur due to an error in the egg or sperm. Therefore, the abnormality is present in every cell of the body. However, some abnormalities can happen after fertilization during mitotic cell division and result in **mosaicism**. Mosaicism or mosaic form refers to when the chromosomal abnormalities do not show up in every cell and only some cells or tissues carry the abnormality. In mosaic forms of the disorder, the symptoms are usually less severe than if all the cells were abnormal.

About one in 150 live-born infants is born with a chromosomal abnormality (March of Dimes, 2009). These often cause major defects because they involve added or missing genes. Congenital anomalies and mental retardation are often associated with chromosomal abnormalities. These abnormalities occur on autosomal as well as sex chromosomes and can result from changes in the number of chromosomes or changes in the structure of the chromosomes.

Numerical Abnormalities

Chromosomal abnormalities of number often result from nondisjunction, or failure of the chromosome pair to separate during cell division, meiosis, or mitosis. Few chromosomal numerical abnormalities are compatible with full-term development and most result in spontaneous abortion. There are some numerical abnormalities that do support development to term because the chromosome on which the abnormality is present carries relatively few genes (such as chromosome 13, 18, 21, or X). Two common abnormalities of chromosome number are monosomies or trisomies. In **monosomies**, there is only one copy of a particular chromosome instead of the usual pair (an entire single chromosome is missing). In these cases, all fetuses spontaneously abort in early pregnancy. Survival is seen only in mosaic forms of these disorders. In **trisomies**, there are three of a particular chromosome instead of the usual two (an entire single chromosome is added). The most common trisomies include trisomy 21 (Down syndrome), trisomy 18, and trisomy 13. Figure 10.17 shows the karyotype of a child with Down syndrome. (See Chapter 50 for a detailed discussion of these disorders.) Trisomies may be present in every cell or may present in the mosaic form.

Another type of abnormal chromosome number is **polyploidy**. Polyploidy causes an increase in the number of haploid sets (23) of chromosomes in a cell. Triploidy refers to three whole sets of chromosomes in a single cell (in humans, a total of 69 chromosomes per cell); tetraploidy refers to four whole sets of chromosomes in a single cell (in humans, a total of 92 chromosomes per cell). Polyploidy usually results in an early spontaneous abortion and is incompatible with life.

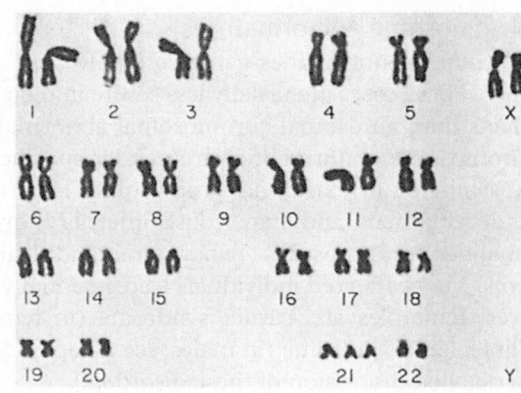

FIGURE 10.17 Karyotype of a child with Down syndrome.

Structural Abnormalities

Chromosome abnormalities of structure usually occur when there is a breakage and loss of a portion of one or more chromosomes and during the repair process the broken ends are rejoined incorrectly. Structural abnormalities usually lead to having too much or too little genetic material. Altered chromosome structure can take on several forms. Deletions occur when a portion of the chromosome is missing or deleted, resulting in a loss of that portion of the chromosome. Duplications are seen when a portion of the chromosome is duplicated and an extra chromosomal segment is present. Clinical findings vary depending on how much chromosomal material is involved. Inversions occur when a portion of the chromosome breaks off at two points and is turned upside down and reattached; therefore, the genetic material is inverted. With inversion, there is no loss or gain of chromosomal material and carriers are phenotypically normal, but they do have an increased risk for miscarriage and chromosomally abnormal offspring. Ring chromosomes are seen when a portion of a chromosome has broken off in two places and formed a circle or ring.

The most clinically significant structural abnormality is a translocation. This occurs when a portion of one chromosome is transferred to another chromosome and an abnormal rearrangement is present.

Structural abnormalities can be balanced or unbalanced. Balanced abnormalities involve the rearrangement of genetic material with neither an overall gain nor loss. Individuals who inherit a balanced structural abnormality are usually phenotypically normal but are at a higher risk for miscarriages and having chromosomally abnormal offspring. Examples of structural rearrangements that can be balanced include inversions, translocation, and ring chromosomes. Unbalanced structural abnormalities are similar to numerical abnormalities because genetic material is either gained or lost. Unbalanced structural abnormalities can encompass several genes and result in severe clinical consequences.

Sex Chromosome Abnormalities

Chromosomal abnormalities can also involve sex chromosomes. These cases are usually less severe in their clinical effects than autosomal chromosomal abnormalities. Sex chromosome abnormalities are gender-specific and involve a missing or extra sex chromosome. They affect sexual development and may cause infertility, growth abnormalities, and possibly behavioural and learning problems. Many affected individuals lead essentially normal lives. Examples are Turner syndrome (in females) and Klinefelter's syndrome (in males; see Chapter 50 for a more detailed discussion of these disorders).

Genetic Evaluation and Counselling

The Canadian Association of Genetic Counsellors (CAGC, 2006) defines **genetic counselling** as providing information about genetic conditions with counselling support so that individuals can make personal decisions about the management of their health, their children's health, or their pregnancies. There are a variety of reasons an individual should be referred for genetic counselling. Box 10.3 lists situations in which families may benefit from genetic counselling. In many cases, geneticists and genetic counsellors provide information to families regarding genetic diseases. However, an experienced family physician, pediatrician, or nurse who has received special training in genetics may also provide the information.

A genetic consultation involves evaluation of an individual or a family. Its purposes are to confirm, diagnose, or rule out genetic conditions; to identify medical management issues; to calculate and communicate genetic risks to a family; to discuss ethical and legal issues; and to provide and arrange psychosocial support. Genetic counsellors serve as educators and resource persons for other health care providers and the general public.

The ideal time for genetic counselling is before conception. Preconception counselling gives people the chance to identify and reduce potential pregnancy risks, plan for known risks, and establish early prenatal care. Unfortunately, many women delay seeking prenatal care until their second or third trimester, after the crucial time of **organogenesis**. Therefore, it is important that preconception counselling is offered to all women and men as they seek health care throughout their childbearing years, especially if they are contemplating having children. This requires health care providers to take an active role.

Preconception screening and counselling can raise serious ethical and moral issues. The results of prenatal genetic testing can lead to the decision to terminate a pregnancy, even if the results are not conclusive but indicate a strong possibility that the child will have an abnormality. The severity of the abnormality may not be known, and some may find the decision to terminate unethical. Another difficult situation that provides an example of the

---

> **BOX 10.3** **Situations in Which Genetic Counselling may be Beneficial**
>
> - Maternal age 35 years or older when the baby is born (note, however, that maternal age alone is a relatively poor predictor of fetal chromosomal abnormalities) (Best Start, 2007; SOGC, 2001)
> - Although there is no clear accepted definition of advanced paternal age, sources recommend counselling for paternal age 45 to 50 years or older (American College of Medical Genetics, 2007)
> - Previous child, parent, or close relative with an inherited disease, congenital anomaly, metabolic disorder, developmental disorder, or chromosomal abnormality
> - Consanguinity or incest
> - Pregnancy screening abnormality, including alpha-fetoprotein, quad screen, integrated prenatal screen, serum integrated prenatal screen, amniocentesis, ultrasound, and nuchal translucency
> - Stillborn with congenital anomalies
> - Two or more pregnancy losses
> - Teratogen exposure or risk
> - Concerns about genetic defects that occur frequently in their ethnic or racial group (for instance, those of African descent are most at risk for having a child with sickle-cell anemia)
> - Abnormal newborn screening
> - Child born with one or more major malformations in a major organ system
> - Child with abnormalities of growth
> - Child with developmental delay, mental retardation, blindness, or deafness

---

ethical and moral issues surrounding genetic screening and counselling involves disorders that affect only one gender of offspring. A father or mother may find that he or she is a carrier of a gene for a disorder for which there is no prenatal screening test available. In these cases, the decision may be made to terminate any pregnancy in which the fetus is the affected sex, even though there is a 50% chance that the child will not inherit the disorder. In these situations, information and support must be provided in a manner that "recognizes and respects the ability of individuals and families to balance the risks and benefits of services offered and then to make the appropriate decisions for themselves" (CAGC, 2006, page 2).

Genetic counselling is particularly important if a congenital anomaly or genetic disease has been diagnosed prenatally or if a child is born with a life-threatening congenital anomaly or genetic disease. In these cases, families need information urgently so they can make immediate decisions. If a diagnosis with genetic implications is made later in life, if a couple with a family history of a genetic disorder or a previous child with a genetic disorder is planning a family, or if there is suspected

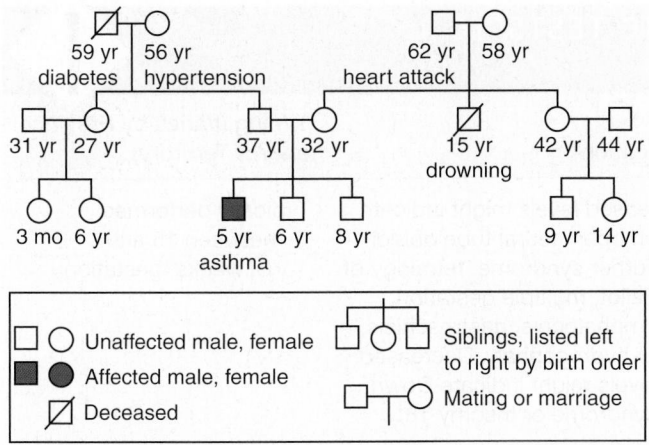

FIGURE 10.18 A genogram or pedigree is a diagram made using symbols that demonstrates the links between family members and focuses on medical and health information for each relative.

teratogen exposure, urgency of information is not such an issue. In these situations, the family needs time to ponder all of its options. This may involve several meetings over a longer period of time.

Genetic counselling involves gathering information regarding birth history, past medical history, and current health status as well as a family history of congenital anomalies, mental retardation, genetic diseases, reproductive history, general health, and causes of death. A detailed family history is imperative and in most cases will include the development of a genogram, or pedigree, which is like a family tree (Fig. 10.18). Information is ideally gathered on three generations, but if the family history is complicated, information from more distant relatives may be needed. Families receiving genetic counselling may benefit from being told in advance that this information will be necessary; they may need to discuss these sensitive, private issues with family members to obtain the needed facts. When necessary, medical records may be requested for family members, especially those who have a genetic disorder, to help ensure accuracy of the information. Sometimes a pedigree may reveal confidential information not known by all family members, such as an adoption, a child conceived through in vitro fertilization, or a husband not being the father of a baby. Therefore, maintaining confidentiality is extremely important. After careful analysis of the data obtained, referral to a genetic counsellor when indicated is appropriate.

Medical genetic knowledge has increased dramatically over the past few decades. Not only is it possible to detect specific diseases with genetic mutations, but it is also possible to test for a genetic predisposition to various diseases or conditions and certain physical characteristics. This leads to complex ethical, moral, and social issues. Maintaining client privacy and confidentiality and administering care in a nondiscriminatory manner

are essential while maintaining sensitivity to cultural differences. It is essential to respect client autonomy and present information in a nondirective, non-judgmental, and ethical manner.

Nursing Roles and Responsibilities

The nurse is likely to interact with the client in a variety of ways related to genetics—taking a family history, scheduling genetic testing, explaining the purposes of all screening and diagnostic tests, answering questions, and addressing concerns raised by family members. Nurses are often the first health care providers to encounter women with preconception and prenatal issues. Nurses play an important role in beginning the preconception counselling process and referring women and their partners for further genetic testing when indicated.

An accurate and thorough family history is an essential part of preconception counselling. Nurses in any practice setting can obtain a family history during the initial encounter. The purpose is to gather patient and family information that may provide clues as to whether the patient has a genetic trait, inherited condition, or inherited predisposition (ANA, 2009). At a basic level, all nurses should be able to take a family medical history to help identify those at risk for genetic conditions and then initiate a referral when appropriate. Box 10.4

BOX 10.4 **Taking a Preconception History for Assessment and Counselling**

"A thorough preconception history identifies couples who are genetically at risk. When women and their partners are informed of the risks of having a baby with birth defects or a genetic disorder prior to pregnancy, they are then able to determine their options regarding a pregnancy (including contraception, artificial insemination, adoption, prenatal invasive testing, or chance) (SOGC, 2011, page 59).

The SOGC has recently released a new guideline on genetic considerations for a women's preconception evaluation. The guideline presents questions and strategies for exploring the genetic and health history of individuals in the following areas. This history outline is adapted from the PHAC. *Family-centred Maternity and Newborn Care: National Guidelines* (2000).
- Family history
- Ethnic history
- Age
- Chronic conditions
- Infectious conditions
- Reproductive history
- Lifestyle assessment

Source: SOGC, 2011

COMMON LABORATORY AND DIAGNOSTIC TESTS 10.1
PRENATAL TESTS TO ASSESS RISK FOR GENETIC DISORDERS

Test	Description	Indication	Timing (Varies by Province and/or Territory)
Alpha-fetoprotein (AFP)	A sample of the woman's blood is drawn to evaluate plasma protein that is produced by the fetal liver, yolk sac, and GI tract and crosses from the amniotic fluid into the maternal blood.	Increased levels might indicate an open neural tube defect, Turner syndrome, tetralogy of Fallot, multiple gestation, omphalocele, gastroschisis, or hydrocephaly. Decreased levels might indicate Down syndrome or trisomy 18.	Typically performed between 15 and 17 weeks' gestation
Amniocentesis	Amniotic fluid aspirated from the amniotic sac; safety concerns include infection, pregnancy loss, and fetal needle injuries	To perform chromosome analysis, alpha-fetoprotein, DNA markers, viral studies, and karyotyping; and to identify inborn errors of metabolism	Usually performed between 15 and 20 weeks' gestation to allow for adequate amniotic fluid volume to accumulate; results take 2 to 3 weeks
Chorionic villus sampling	Removal of small tissue specimen from the fetal portion of the placenta, which reflects the fetal genetic makeup; main complications include severe transverse limb defects and spontaneous pregnancy loss	To detect fetal karyotype, sickle-cell anemia, phenylketonuria, Down syndrome, Duchenne muscular dystrophy, and numerous other genetic disorders	Typically performed between 15 and 16 weeks' gestation, with results available in 2 to 3 weeks
Percutaneous umbilical blood sampling (PUBS) or cordocentesis	Insertion of a needle directly into a fetal umbilical vessel under ultrasound guidance; two potential complications: fetal hemorrhage and infection	Used for prenatal diagnosis of inherited blood disorders such as hemophilia A, karyotyping, detection of fetal infection, determination of acid–base status, and assessment and treatment of isoimmunization. Procedure can also be used for fetal therapy.	Generally performed after 16 weeks' gestation
Nuchal translucency (NT)	An intravaginal ultrasound that measures fluid collection in the subcutaneous space between the skin and the cervical spine of the fetus	To identify fetal anomalies; abnormal fluid collection can be associated with genetic disorders (trisomies 13, 18, and 21), Turner syndrome, cardiac deformities, and/or physical anomalies. When the NT is greater than 3.0 or 3.5 mm (depending on the testing facility), the measurement is considered abnormal.	Performed between 10 and 14 weeks' gestation
Ultrasound/fetal scan—level 1 (basic anatomy) and level II (targeted examination)	Use of high-frequency sound waves to visualize the fetus. Level I ultrasound of fetal anatomy is regarded as standard practice. Level II is done when there are more risk factors for congenital and/or growth abnormalities.	Enables early identification of structural changes	Level I typically performed between 18 and 20 weeks' gestation Level II typically performed after 18 weeks' gestation

Test	Description	Indication	Timing (Varies by Province and/or Territory)
Serum quad marker screen	Measurement of second-trimester serum quad markers (AFP, unconjugated estriol [uE3], hCG, and inhibin A)	To identify risk for Down syndrome, open neural tube defects, and other chromosomal disorders. Elevated hCG combined with lower than normal estriol and maternal serum AFP levels indicate increased risk for Down syndrome or other trisomy condition.	Performed between 16 and 18 weeks' gestation
Integrated prenatal screen (IPS)	A screening process that combines first- and second-trimester screening tests. Includes serum screening tests using the levels of first trimester maternal serum markers (pregnancy-associated plasma protein A [PAPP-A]), second trimester quad markers (see quad screening), and NT—in combination with consideration of other variables, including maternal age, to calculate risk.	Tests for Down syndrome, trisomy 18, and open neural tube defects	First trimester measurements usually carried out between 11 and 14 weeks' gestation
Serum integrated prenatal screen (SIPS)	The same combined screening process as IPS but with no NT (serum testing only).	Tests for Down syndrome, trisomy 18, and open neural tube defects	Two blood tests Part 1: 10–13 + 6 weeks Part 2: 15–20 + 6 weeks (ideally at 11 and 16 weeks)

Note: Provinces and territories across Canada vary in their prenatal genetic screening protocols. As new developments in maternal serum and ultrasound screening emerge, it is anticipated that there will be a decreased need for invasive testing (amniocentesis and chorionic villus sampling) (Summers, Langlois, Wyatt, et al., 2007).

Sources: Perinatal Services BC. (2010). *PSBC obstetric guideline 17: Prenatal screening for Down Syndrome, Trisomy 18 and open neural tube defects.* Retrieved February 3, 2011 from http://www.bcprenatalscreening.ca/sites/prenatal2/files/Prenatal_Screening_Guideline.pdf; and Summers, A. M., Langlois, S., Wyatt, P., Wilson, R. D., et al. (2007). SOGC Clinical practice guideline: Prenatal screening for fetal aneuploidy. *Journal of Obstetrics and Gynaecology Canada, 29*(2), 146–161. Retrieved February 3, 2011 from http://www.sogc.org/media/pdf/advisories/JOGC-feb_07-CPG.pdf.

presents examples of focused assessment questions that can be used. Based on the information gathered during the history, the nurse must decide whether a referral to a genetic specialist is necessary or further evaluation is needed. Prenatal screening to assess for genetic risks and defects might be used to identify genetic disorders. These tests are described in Common Laboratory and Diagnostic Tests 10.1. There have been significant advances in the field of genetic screening, and programs vary across Canada. In addition to guidelines from the SOGC, each province or territory may offer specific guidelines.

*R*emember Robert and Kate Shafer? Based on the information gathered from their genetic history, they were referred to a genetic specialist. What prenatal tests might be ordered to assess their risk for genetic disorders? What would be the nurse's role related to genetic counselling?

Nurses working with families involved with genetic counselling typically have certain responsibilities. The American Nurses Association (ANA) has developed essential competencies for genetic and genomic nursing within five areas (professional responsibilities, nursing assessment, identification, referral activities and provision of education, care and support). Specific competencies include:

- Using interviewing and active listening skills to identify genetic concerns
- Knowing basic genetic terminology and inheritance patterns
- Explaining basic concepts of probability and disorder susceptibility
- Safeguarding the privacy and confidentiality of patients' genetic information
- Providing complete informed consent to facilitate decisions about genetic testing
- Discussing costs of genetic services and the benefits and risks of using health insurance to pay for genetic services, including potential risks of discrimination
- Recognizing and defining ethical, legal, and social issues, including knowing one's own attitudes and values related to this science
- Providing accurate information about the risks and benefits of genetic testing
- Providing culturally appropriate methods to convey genetic information
- Monitoring the emotional reactions of individuals and families after receiving genetic analysis
- Providing information on appropriate local or online support groups and facilitating referrals
- Knowing their own limitations and making appropriate referrals (ANA, 2009)

Talking with families who have recently been diagnosed with a genetic disorder or who have had a child born with congenital anomalies is very difficult. Many times the nurse may be the one who has first contact with these parents and will be the one to provide follow-up care.

Genetic disorders are significant, life-changing, and possibly life-threatening situations. The information is highly technical and the field is undergoing significant technologic advances. Nurses need an understanding of who will benefit from genetic counselling and must be able to discuss the role of the genetic counsellor with families. The nurse wants to ensure that families at risk are aware that genetic counselling is available before they attempt to have another baby.

*B*ased on the results of their genetic tests, Robert and Kate are placed at moderate risk for having an infant with an autosomal recessive genetic disorder. The couple asks the nurse what all of this means. What information should the nurse provide about concepts of probability and disorder susceptibility for this couple? How can the nurse help this couple to make knowledgeable decisions concerning their reproductive future?

Nurses play an essential role in providing emotional support to the family through this challenging time. This is especially important with follow-up counselling after the couple or family has been to the genetic specialist.

▶ *Take* NOTE!

Nurses need to be actively engaged with patients and their families and help them consider the facts, values, and context in which they are making decisions. Nurses need to be open and honest with families as they discuss these sensitive and emotionally laden choices.

The nurse is in an ideal position to help families review what has been discussed during the genetic counselling sessions and to answer any additional questions they might have. Referral to appropriate agencies, support groups, and resources, such as a social worker, a chaplain, or an ethicist, is another key role when caring for families with suspected or diagnosed genetic disorders.

▶ *Consider* THIS!

As I waited for the genetic counsellor to come into the room, my mind was filled with numerous fears and questions. What does an inconclusive amniocentesis really mean? What if this pregnancy produced an abnormal baby? How would I cope with a special child in my life? If only I had gone to the midwife sooner when I thought I was pregnant, but still in denial. Why did I wait so long to admit this pregnancy and get prenatal care? If only I had started to take my folic acid pills when prescribed. Why didn't I research my family's history to know of any hidden genetic conditions? What about my sister with a Down syndrome child? What must I have been thinking? I guess I could play the "what-if" game forever and never come up with answers. It was too late to do anything about this pregnancy because I was in my last trimester. I started to pray silently when the counsellor opened the door. . . .

Thoughts: this woman is reviewing the last several months, looking for answers to her greatest fears. Inconclusive screenings can introduce emotional torment for many women as they wait for validating results. Are these common thoughts and fears for many women facing potential genetic disorders? What supportive interventions might the nurse offer?

■■■ Key Concepts

- Fertilization, which takes place in the outer third of the ampulla of the fallopian tube, leads to the formation of a zygote. The zygote undergoes cleavage, eventually implanting in the endometrium about 7 to 10 days after conception.

■ Three embryonic layers of cells are formed and include the ectoderm, which forms the central nervous system, special senses, skin, and glands; the mesoderm, which forms the skeletal, urinary, circulatory, and reproductive systems; and the endoderm, which forms the respiratory system, liver, pancreas, and digestive system.

■ Amniotic fluid surrounds the embryo and increases in volume as the pregnancy progresses, reaching approximately a litre in volume by term.

■ At no time during pregnancy is there any direct connection between the blood of the fetus and the blood of the mother, so there is no mixing of blood.

■ A specialized connective tissue known as Wharton's jelly surrounds the three blood vessels in the umbilical cord to prevent compression, which would choke off the supply of blood and nutrients to the growing life inside.

■ The placenta protects the fetus from immune attack by the mother, removes waste products from the fetus, induces the mother to bring more food to the placenta, and, near the time of delivery, produces hormones that mature fetal organs in preparation for life outside the uterus.

■ The purpose of fetal circulation is to carry highly oxygenated blood to vital areas (heart and brain) while first shunting it away from less vital ones (lungs and liver).

■ Humans have 46 paired chromosomes that are found in all cells of the body, except the ovum and sperm cells, which have just 23 chromosomes. Each person has a unique genetic constitution, or genotype.

■ Research from the HGP has provided a better understanding of the genetic contribution to disease.

■ Genetic disorders can result from abnormalities in patterns of inheritance or chromosomal abnormalities involving chromosomal number or structure.

■ Autosomal dominant inheritance occurs when a single gene in the heterozygous state is capable of producing the phenotype. Autosomal recessive inheritance occurs when two copies of the mutant or abnormal gene in the homozygous state are necessary to produce the phenotype. X-linked inheritance disorders are those associated with altered genes present on the X chromosome. They can be dominant or recessive. Multifactorial inheritance is thought to be caused by multiple genetic and environmental factors.

■ In some cases of genetic disorders, a chromosomal abnormality occurs. Chromosomal abnormalities do not follow straightforward patterns of inheritance. These abnormalities occur on autosomal as well as sex chromosomes and can result from changes in the number or structure of the chromosomes.

■ Genetic counselling involves evaluation of an individual or a family. Its purpose is to confirm, diagnose, or rule out genetic conditions; identify medical management issues; calculate and communicate genetic risks to a family; discuss ethical and legal issues; and assist in providing and arranging psychosocial support.

■ Legal, ethical, and social issues can arise related to genetic testing and may include the privacy and confidentiality of genetic information, who should have access to personal genetic information, psychological impact and stigmatization due to individual genetic differences, use of genetic information in reproductive decision making and reproductive rights, and whether testing should be performed if no cure is available.

■ Preconception screening and counselling can raise serious ethical and moral issues for individuals and families. Prenatal genetic screening and testing can lead to the decision to terminate a pregnancy based on the results.

■ Nurses play an important role in beginning the preconception counselling process and referring women and their partners for further genetic information when indicated. Many times the nurse is the one who has first contact with these women and will be the one to provide follow-up care.

■ Nurses need to have a solid understanding of who will benefit from genetic counselling and be able to discuss the role of the genetic counsellor with families, ensuring that families at risk are aware that genetic counselling is available before they attempt to have another baby.

■ Nurses play an essential role in providing emotional support and referrals to appropriate agencies, support groups, and resources when caring for families with suspected or diagnosed genetic disorders. Nurses can assist patients with their decision making by referring them to a social worker, a chaplain, or an ethicist.

REFERENCES

American College of Medical Genetics. (2007). *Statement on guidance for genetic counseling in advanced paternal age.* Retrieved February 3, 2011 from http://www.acmg.net/StaticContent/StaticPages/Paternal_Age.pdf

American Nurses Association. (2009). *Essentials of genetic and genomic nursing: Competencies, curricula guidelines and outcome indicators* (2nd ed.). Bethesda, MD: Author.

Beery, T., & Smith, C. (2011). Genetics/genomics advances to influence care for patients with chronic disease. *Rehabilitation Nursing, 36*(2), 54–60.

Best Start. (2007). *Reflecting on the trend: Pregnancy after age 35.* Toronto, ON: Author. Retrieved February 3, 2011 from http://www.beststart.org/resources/rep_health/pdf/bs_pregnancy_age35.pdf.

Blackburn, S. T. (2007). *Maternal, fetal and neonatal physiology* (3rd ed.). Philadelphia: Saunders.

Bottorff, J., McCullum, M., Balneaves, L., et al. (2005). Canadian nursing in the genomic era: A call for leadership. *Nursing Leadership, 18*(2), 56–72.

Canadian Association of Genetic Counsellors. (2006). *Code of ethics for Canadian genetic counsellors.* Oakville, ON: Author. Retrieved February 3, 2011 from http://cagc-accg.ca/images/docs/Professional_Issues/code%20of%20ethics%20e-070628.pdf

Canadian Nurses Association. (2002). *Position statement: The role of the nurse in reproductive and genetic technologies.* Ottawa, ON: Author.

Creatsas, G., Chrousos, G. P., & Mastorakos, G. (2007). *Women's health and disease: Gynecologic and reproductive issues.* Malden, MA: Blackwell Publishers.

Cunningham, F., Leveno, K., Bloom, S., Hauth, J., Rouse, D., & Spong, C. (2010). *Williams obstetrics* (23rd ed.). New York: McGraw-Hill.

Dillon, P. M. (2007). *Nursing health assessment: A critical thinking, case studies approach* (2nd ed.). Philadelphia: FA Davis.

Giacca, M. (2010). *Gene therapy.* Milan: Springer.

Gilbert, E. S. (2010). *Manual of high-risk pregnancy and delivery* (5th ed.). St. Louis, MO: Mosby Inc.

International Human Genome Sequencing Consortium. (2004). Finishing the euchromatic sequence of the human genome. *Nature, 431,* 931–945.

Johnson, M. H. (2007). *Essential reproduction* (6th ed.). Malden, MA: Blackwell Publishers.

Kliegman, R., Stanton, B., St. Geme, J., Schor, N., & Behrman, R. (2011). *Nelson's textbook of pediatrics* (19th ed.). Philadelphia: WB Saunders.

March of Dimes. (2009). *Birth defects: Chromosomal abnormalities.* Retrieved February 7, 2012 from http://www.marchofdimes.com/baby/birthdefects_chromosomal.html

Moore, K. (2007). *The developing human: Clinically oriented embryology* (5th ed.). Philadelphia: WB Saunders.

Perinatal Services BC. (2010). *PSBC obstetric guideline 17: Prenatal screening for Down Syndrome, Trisomy 18 and open neural tube defects.* Retrieved February 3, 2011 from http://www.bcprenatalscreening.ca/sites/prenatal2/files/Prenatal_Screening_Guideline.pdf

Public Health Agency of Canada. (2000). *Family-centered maternity and newborn care: National guidelines.* Retrieved May 14, 2012 from http://www.phac-aspc.gc.ca/hp-ps/dca-dea/publications/fcm-smp/index-eng.php

Public Health Agency of Canada. (2002). *Congenital anomalies in Canada: A perinatal health report, 2002.* Ottawa, ON: Author. Retrieved February 3, 2011 from http://www.phac-aspc.gc.ca/publicat/cac-acc02/index-eng.php

Slee, D., Slee, V., & Schmidt, H. (2008). *Slee's health care terms* (5th ed.). Mississauga, ON: Jones & Bartlett.

Society of Obstetricians and Gynaecologists of Canada. (2001). *Canadian guidelines for prenatal diagnosis: Genetic indications for prenatal diagnosis.* Retrieved May 14, 2012 from http://www.sogc.org/guidelines/public/105e-cpg1-june2001.pdf

Society of Obstetricians and Gynaecologists of Canada. (2005). *Alcohol use and pregnancy consensus clinical guidelines.* Retrieved May 14, 2012 from http://www.sogc.org/guidelines/documents/gui245CPG1008E.pdf

Society of Obstetricians and Gynaecologists of Canada. (2011). *Genetic considerations for a woman's pre-conception evaluation.* Retrieved May 21, 2012 from http://www.sogc.org/guidelines/documents/gui253CO1101E.pdf

Solomon, B., Jack, B., & Feero, G. (2008). The clinical content of preconception care: Genetics and genomics. *American Journal of Obstetrics and Gynecology, 199*(6B), S340–S344.

Summers, A. M., Langlois, S., Wyatt, P., Wilson, R. D., et al. (2007). SOGC Clinical practice guideline: Prenatal screening for fetal aneuploidy. *Journal of Obstetrics and Gynaecology Canada, 29*(2), 146–161. Retrieved February 3, 2011 from http://www.sogc.org/media/pdf/advisories/JOGC-feb_07-CPG.pdf

Wright, A., & Hastie, N. (2007). *Genes and common diseases.* New York: Cambridge University Press.

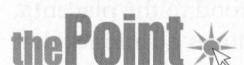

the Point For additional learning materials, including Internet Resources, visit **http://thePoint.lww.com/Chow1e.**

CHAPTER WORKSHEET

MULTIPLE CHOICE QUESTIONS

1. After teaching a group of students about fertilization, the instructor determines that the teaching was successful when the group identifies which as the usual site of fertilization?

   a. Fundus of the uterus

   b. Endometrium of the uterus

   c. Upper portion of the fallopian tube

   d. Follicular tissue of the ovary

2. A client comes to the clinic for pregnancy testing. The nurse explains that the test detects the presence of which hormone?

   a. hPL

   b. hCG

   c. FSH

   d. TSH

3. The nurse is counselling a couple, one of whom is affected by an autosomal dominant disorder. They express concerns about the risk of transmitting the disorder. What is the best response by the nurse regarding the risk that their baby may have for the disease?

   a. "You have a one in four (25%) chance."

   b. "The risk is 12.5%, or a one in eight chance."

   c. "The chance is 100%."

   d. "Your risk is 50%, or a one in two chance."

4. What is the first step in determining a couple's risk for a genetic disorder?

   a. Observing the patient and family over time

   b. Conducting extensive psychological testing

   c. Obtaining a thorough family health history

   d. Completing an extensive exclusionary list

5. A nurse is working in a women's health clinic. Genetic counselling would be most appropriate for the woman who:

   a. Just had her first miscarriage at 10 weeks

   b. Is 30 years old and planning to conceive

   c. Has a history that reveals a close relative with Down syndrome

   d. Is 18 weeks pregnant with a normal triple screen result

CRITICAL THINKING EXERCISE

1. Sue and David wish to start a family, but they can't agree on something important. David wants Sue to be tested for cystic fibrosis (CF) to see if she is a carrier. David had a brother with CF and watched his parents struggle with the hardship and the expense of caring for him for years, and he doesn't want to experience it in his own life. David has found out he is a CF carrier. Sue doesn't want to have the test because she figures that once a baby is in their arms, they will be glad, no matter what.

   a. What information/education should this couple consider before deciding whether to have the test?

   b. How can you assist this couple in their decision-making process?

   c. What is your role in this situation if you don't agree with their decision?

STUDY ACTIVITIES

1. Select one of the websites on http://thePoint.lww.com/Chow1e to explore the topic of genetics. Critique the information presented. Was it understandable to a layperson? What specifically did you learn? Share your findings with your classmates during a discussion group.

2. Draw your own family pedigree, identifying inheritance patterns. Share it with your family to validate its accuracy. What did you discover about your family's past health?

3. Select one of the various prenatal genetic screening tests (alpha-fetoprotein, amniocentesis, chorionic villus sampling, integrated prenatal screen, percutaneous umbilical blood screening, quad marker screen, serum integrated prenatal screen, ultrasound, or nuchal translucency) and research it in depth. Role-play with another nursing student how you would explain its purpose, the procedure, and potential findings to an expectant parent who is at risk for a fetal abnormality.

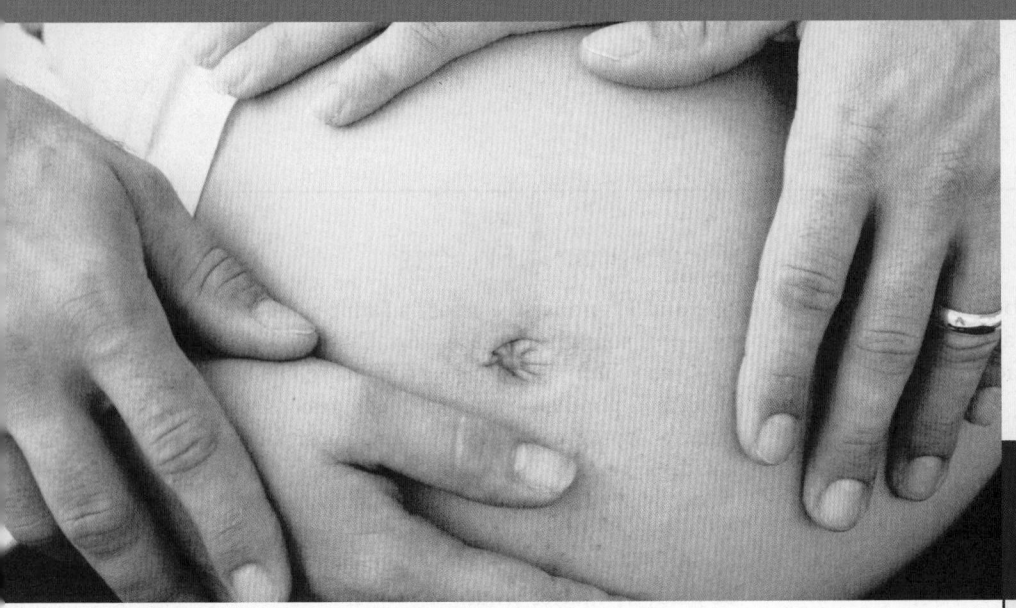

MATERNAL ADAPTATION DURING PREGNANCY

KEY TERMS

ballottement
Braxton Hicks
  contractions
Chadwick's
  sign

dietary reference
  intakes (DRIs)
Goodell's sign
Hegar's sign
linea nigra

physiologic anemia of
  pregnancy
pica
quickening
trimester

LEARNING OBJECTIVES

Upon completion of the chapter, the learner will be able to:

1. Define the key terms used in this chapter.
2. Differentiate between subjective (presumptive), objective (probable), and diagnostic (positive) signs of pregnancy.
3. Explain maternal physiologic changes that occur during pregnancy.
4. Summarize the nutritional needs of the pregnant woman and her fetus.
5. Identify the emotional and psychological changes that occur during pregnancy.

*M*arva, age 17, appeared at the walk-in clinic complaining that she had a stomach virus and needed to be seen today. When the nurse asked her additional questions about her illness, Marva reported that she had been sick to her stomach and "beat tired" for days. She had stopped eating to avoid any more nausea and vomiting.

Wow

When a woman discovers that she is pregnant, she must remember to protect and nourish the fetus by making wise choices.

Pregnancy is a normal life event that involves considerable physical and psychological adjustments for the mother. A pregnancy is divided into three **trimesters** of 13 weeks each (Ricci, 2009). Within each trimester, numerous adaptations take place that facilitate the growth of the fetus. The most obvious are physical changes to accommodate the growing fetus. However, pregnant women also undergo psychological changes as they prepare for parenthood.

Signs and Symptoms of Pregnancy

Traditionally, signs and symptoms of pregnancy have been grouped into the following categories: presumptive, probable, and positive (Box 11.1). The only signs that can determine a pregnancy with 100% accuracy are positive signs.

What additional information is necessary to complete the assessment of Marva, the 17-year-old with nausea and vomiting? What diagnostic tests might be done to confirm the nurse's suspicion that she is pregnant?

Subjective (Presumptive) Signs

Presumptive signs are those signs experienced by the woman herself. The most obvious presumptive sign of pregnancy is the absence of menstruation. Skipping a period is not a reliable sign of pregnancy by itself, but if

▶ ***Consider*** *THIS!*

Jim and I decided to start our family, so I stopped taking the Pill 3 months ago. One morning when I got out of bed to take the dog out, I felt queasy and lightheaded. I sure hoped I wasn't coming down with the flu. By the end of the week, I was feeling really tired and started taking naps in the afternoon. In addition, I seemed to be going to the bathroom frequently, despite not drinking much fluid. When my breasts started to tingle and ache, I decided to make an appointment with my doctor to see what "illness" I had contracted.

After listening to my list of physical complaints, the office nurse asked me if I might be pregnant. My eyes opened wide: I had somehow missed the link between my symptoms and pregnancy. I started to think about when my last period was, and it had been 2 months ago. The office ran a pregnancy test and much to my surprise it was positive!

Thoughts: many women stop contraceptives in an attempt to achieve pregnancy but miss the early signs of pregnancy. This woman was experiencing several signs of early pregnancy—urinary frequency, fatigue, morning nausea, and breast tenderness. What advice can the nurse give this woman to ease these symptoms? What additional education related to her pregnancy would be appropriate at this time?

it is accompanied by consistent nausea, fatigue, breast tenderness, and urinary frequency, pregnancy would seem very likely.

Presumptive changes are the least reliable indicators of pregnancy because any one of them can be caused by

---

BOX 11.1 Signs and Symptoms of Pregnancy

Presumptive (Time of Occurrence)	Probable (Time of Occurrence)	Positive (Time of Occurrence)
Fatigue (12 weeks)	Braxton Hicks contractions (16–28 weeks)	Ultrasound verification of embryo or fetus (4–6 weeks)
Breast tenderness (3–4 weeks)	Positive pregnancy test (4–12 weeks)	Fetal movement felt by experienced clinician (20 weeks)
Nausea and vomiting (4–14 weeks)	Abdominal enlargement (14 weeks)	Auscultation of fetal heart tones via Doppler (10–12 weeks)
Amenorrhea (4 weeks)	Ballottement (16–28 weeks)	
Urinary frequency (6–12 weeks)	Goodell's sign (5 weeks)	
Hyperpigmentation of the skin (16 weeks)	Chadwick's sign (6–8 weeks)	
Fetal movements (**quickening**; 16–20 weeks)	Hegar's sign (6–12 weeks)	
Uterine enlargement (7–12 weeks)		
Breast enlargement (6 weeks)		

Sources: Cunningham, F. G., Leveno, K. J., Bloom, S. L., Hauth, J. C., Rouse, D. J., & Spong, C. Y. (2010). *Williams's obstetrics* (23rd ed.). New York: McGraw-Hill Companies, Inc.: and Simpson, K. R., & Creehan, P. A. (Eds.). (2008). *AWHONN perinatal nursing* (3rd ed.). Philadelphia: Lippincott Williams & Wilkins.

conditions other than pregnancy (Fraser & Cooper, 2009). For example, amenorrhea can be caused by early menopause, endocrine dysfunction, malnutrition, anemia, diabetes mellitus, long-distance running, cancer, or stress. Nausea and vomiting can be caused by gastrointestinal (GI) disorders, food poisoning, acute infections, or eating disorders. Fatigue could be caused by anemia, stress, or viral infections. Breast tenderness may result from chronic cystic mastitis, premenstrual changes, or the use of oral contraceptives. Urinary frequency could have a variety of causes other than pregnancy, such as infection, cystocele, structural disorders, pelvic tumours, or emotional tension (Fraser & Cooper, 2009).

Objective (Probable) Signs

Probable signs of pregnancy are those that are apparent on physical examination by a health care professional. Common probable signs of pregnancy include softening of the lower uterine segment or isthmus (Hegar's sign), softening of the cervix (Goodell's sign), and a bluish-purple colouration of the vaginal mucosa and cervix (Chadwick's sign). Other probable signs include changes in the shape and size of the uterus, abdominal enlargement, Braxton Hicks contractions, and **ballottement** (the examiner pushes against the woman's cervix during a pelvic examination and feels a rebound from the floating fetus).

Along with these physical signs, pregnancy tests are also considered a probable sign of pregnancy. Several pregnancy tests are available (Table 11.1). The tests vary in sensitivity, specificity, and accuracy and are influenced by the length of gestation, specimen concentration, presence of blood, and the presence of some drugs (Shields, 2012).

Human chorionic gonadotropin (hCG) is the earliest biochemical marker for pregnancy, and many pregnancy tests are based on the recognition of hCG or a beta subunit of hCG. hCG levels in normal pregnancy usually double every 48 to 72 hours until they peak approximately 60 to 70 days after fertilization; levels then decrease to a plateau at 100 to 130 days of pregnancy (Shields, 2012).

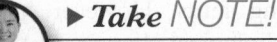

▶ *Take* NOTE!

This elevation of hCG corresponds to the morning sickness period of approximately 6 to 12 weeks during early pregnancy.

Home pregnancy tests are available over the counter and have become quite popular since their introduction in 1975. These tests are very sensitive, cost-effective, and faster than traditional laboratory pregnancy tests. Enzyme-linked immunosorbent assay (ELISA) technology is the basis for most home pregnancy tests.

Although probable signs suggest pregnancy and are more reliable than presumptive signs, they still are not 100% reliable in confirming a pregnancy. For example, uterine tumours, polyps, infection, and pelvic congestion can cause changes in uterine shape, size, and consistency. And although pregnancy tests are used to establish the diagnosis of pregnancy when the physical signs are still inconclusive, they are not completely reliable because conditions other than pregnancy (e.g., ovarian cancer, choriocarcinoma, hydatidiform mole) can also elevate hCG levels.

Positive Signs

Usually within 2 weeks after a missed period, enough subjective symptoms are present so that a woman can be

TABLE 11.1 SELECTED PREGNANCY TESTS

Type	Specimen	Example	Remarks
Agglutination inhibition test	Urine	Pregnosticon, Gravindex	If hCG is present in urine, agglutination does not occur, which is positive for pregnancy; reliable 14–21 days after conception; 95% accurate in diagnosing pregnancy
Immunoradiometric assay	Blood serum	Neocept, Pregnosis	Measures ability of blood sample to inhibit the binding of radiolabelled hCG to receptors; reliable 6–8 days after conception; 99% accurate in diagnosing pregnancy
Enzyme-linked immunosorbent assay (ELISA)	Blood serum or urine	Over-the-counter home/office pregnancy tests	Uses an enzyme to bond with hCG in the urine if present; reliable 4 days after implantation; 99% accurate if hCG specific

Source: Gibbs, R. S., Karlan, B. Y., Haney, A. F., &., Nygaard, I. E. (2008). *Danforth's obstetrics and gynecology* (10th ed.). Philadelphia: Lippincott Williams & Wilkins.

reasonably sure she is pregnant. However, an experienced health care professional can confirm her suspicions by identifying positive signs of pregnancy. The positive signs of pregnancy confirm that a fetus is growing in the uterus. Visualizing the fetus by ultrasound, palpating for fetal movements, and hearing a fetal heartbeat are all signs that make the pregnancy a certainty.

Once pregnancy is confirmed, the health care professional will set up a schedule of prenatal visits to assess the woman and her fetus throughout the entire pregnancy. Assessment and education begin at the first visit and continue throughout the pregnancy (see Chapter 12).

*R*emember Marva, who thought she had a stomach virus? Her pregnancy test was positive. On questioning by the nurse, she acknowledged missing two menstrual periods and being sexually active with her boyfriend without using protection. What is the nurse's role at this point with Marva? What instructions might be given to her while she waits for her first prenatal visit?

Physiologic Adaptations During Pregnancy

Every system of a woman's body changes during pregnancy to accommodate the needs of the growing fetus, and with startling rapidity. The physical changes of pregnancy can be uncomfortable, although every woman reacts uniquely.

Reproductive System Adaptations

Significant changes occur throughout the woman's body during pregnancy to accommodate the growing human being within her. Many have a protective role for maternal homeostasis and are essential to meet the demands of both the mother and the fetus. Many adaptations are reversible after the woman gives birth, but some persist for life.

Uterus

During the first few months of pregnancy, estrogen stimulates uterine growth, and the uterus undergoes a tremendous increase in size, weight, length, width, depth, volume, and overall capacity throughout pregnancy. The weight of the uterus increases from 70 g to about 1,100 g at term; its capacity increases from 10 to 5,000 mL or more at term (Cunningham, Leveno, Bloom, et al., 2010). The uterine walls thin to 1.5 cm or less; from a solid globe, the uterus becomes a hollow vessel.

Uterine growth occurs as a result of both hyperplasia and hypertrophy of the myometrial cells, which do not increase much in number but do increase in size. Blood vessels elongate, enlarge, dilate, and sprout new

branches to support and nourish the growing muscle tissue, and the increase in uterine weight is accompanied by a large increase in uterine blood flow necessary to perfuse the uterine muscle and accommodate the growing fetus (Simpson & Creehan, 2008).

Uterine contractility is enhanced as well. Spontaneous, irregular, and painless contractions, called **Braxton Hicks contractions**, begin at about 12 weeks' gestation (Evans, Evans, Brown, et al., 2010). These contractions continue throughout pregnancy, becoming especially noticeable during the last month, when they function to thin out or efface the cervix before birth (see Chapter 12 for more information).

Changes in the uterus occurring during the first 6 to 8 weeks of gestation produce some of the typical findings, including a positive **Hegar's sign**. This softening and compressibility of the lower uterine segment results in exaggerated uterine anteflexion during the early months of pregnancy, which adds to urinary frequency (Fraser & Cooper, 2009).

The uterus remains in the pelvic cavity for the first 3 months of pregnancy, after which it progressively ascends into the abdomen (Fig. 11.1). As the uterus grows, it presses on the urinary bladder and causes the increased frequency of urination experienced during early pregnancy. In addition, the heavy gravid uterus in

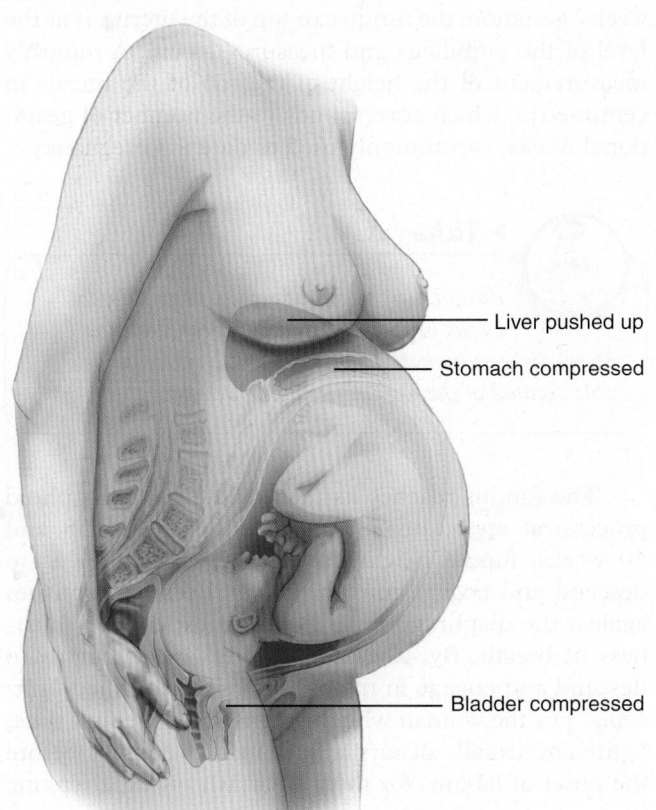

— Liver pushed up

— Stomach compressed

— Bladder compressed

FIGURE 11.1 The growing uterus in the abdomen.

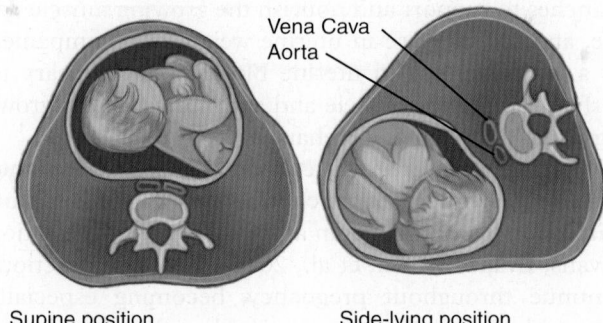

Vena Cava
Aorta

Supine position   Side-lying position

FIGURE 11.2 Supine hypotensive syndrome.

the last trimester can fall back against the inferior vena cava in the supine position, resulting in vena cava compression, which reduces venous return and decreases cardiac output and blood pressure, with increasing orthostatic stress. This occurs when the woman changes her position from recumbent to sitting to standing. This acute hemodynamic change, termed supine hypotensive syndrome, causes the woman to experience symptoms of weakness, lightheadedness, nausea, dizziness, or syncope (Fig. 11.2). These changes are reversed when the woman is in the left lateral position, which displaces the uterus to the left and off the vena cava.

The uterus, which starts as a pear-shaped organ, becomes ovoid as length increases over width. By 20 weeks' gestation, the fundus, or top of the uterus, is at the level of the umbilicus and measures 20 cm. A monthly measurement of the height of the top of the uterus in centimetres, which corresponds to the number of gestational weeks, is commonly used to date the pregnancy.

> ▶ **Take** NOTE!
>
> *Fundal height can be typical of gestational weeks between 18 and 32 weeks, but after 36 weeks' gestation, this measurement is no longer reliable because of the beginning of fetal descent.*

The fundus reaches its highest level, at the xiphoid process, at approximately 36 weeks. Between 38 and 40 weeks, fundal height drops as the fetus begins to descend and engage into the pelvis. Because it pushes against the diaphragm, many women experience shortness of breath. By 40 weeks, the fetal head begins to descend and engage in the pelvis, which is termed *lightening*. For the woman who is pregnant for the first time, lightening usually occurs approximately 2 weeks before the onset of labour; for the woman who is experiencing her second or subsequent pregnancy, it usually occurs at the onset of labour. Although breathing becomes easier because of this descent, the pressure on the urinary

bladder now increases and women experience urinary frequency again.

Cervix

Between 6 and 8 weeks of pregnancy, the cervix begins to soften (**Goodell's sign**) due to vasocongestion. Along with the softening, the endocervical glands increase in size and number and produce more cervical mucus. Under the influence of progesterone, a thick mucus plug is formed that blocks the cervical os and protects the opening from bacterial invasion. At about the same time, increased vascularization of the cervix causes **Chadwick's sign**. Cervical ripening (softening, effacement, and increased distensibility) begins about 4 weeks before birth. Ripening is an inflammatory process and is not dependent on uterine contractions (Timmons, Akins, & Mahendroo, 2010).

Vagina

During pregnancy, there is increased vascularity because of the influences of estrogen, resulting in pelvic congestion and hypertrophy of the vagina in preparation for the distention needed for birth. The vaginal mucosa thickens, the connective tissue begins to loosen, the smooth muscle begins to hypertrophy, and the vaginal vault begins to lengthen (Fraser & Cooper, 2009).

Vaginal secretions become more acidic, white, and thick. Most women experience an increase in a whitish vaginal discharge, called leukorrhea, during pregnancy. This is normal except when it is accompanied by itching and irritation, possibly suggesting *Candida albicans*, a monilial vaginitis, which is a very common occurrence in this glycogen-rich environment (Akinbiyi, Watson, & Feyi-Waboso, 2008). Monilial vaginitis is a benign fungal condition that is uncomfortable for the woman, but it can be transmitted from an infected mother to her newborn at birth. Neonates develop an oral infection known as thrush, which presents as white patches on the mucous membranes of the mouth. It is self-limiting and is treated with local antifungal agents.

Ovaries

The increased blood supply to the ovaries causes them to enlarge until approximately the 12th to 14th week of gestation. The ovaries are not palpable after that time because the uterus fills the pelvic cavity. Ovulation ceases during pregnancy because of the elevated levels of estrogen and progesterone, which block secretion of follicle-stimulating hormone (FSH) and luteinizing hormone (LH) from the anterior pituitary. The ovaries are very active in hormone production to support the pregnancy until about weeks 6 to 7, when the corpus luteum regresses and the placenta takes over the major production of progesterone.

Breasts

The breasts increase in fullness, become tender, and grow larger throughout pregnancy under the influence of estrogen and progesterone. The breasts become highly vascular, and veins become visible under the skin. The nipples become larger and more erect. Both the nipples and the areola become deeply pigmented, and tubercles of Montgomery (sebaceous glands) become prominent. These sebaceous glands keep the nipples lubricated for breastfeeding.

Changes that occur in the connective tissue of the breasts, along with the tremendous growth, lead to striae (stretch marks). Initially striae appear as pink to purple lines on the skin, but they eventually fade to a silver colour. Although they become less conspicuous in time, they never completely disappear.

Creamy, yellowish breast fluid called colostrum can be expressed by the third trimester. This fluid provides nourishment for the breastfeeding newborn during the first few days of life (see Chapters 15 and 16 for more information).

Table 11.2 summarizes reproductive system adaptations.

General Body System Adaptations

In addition to changes in the reproductive system, the pregnant woman also experiences changes in virtually every other body system in response to the growing fetus.

Gastrointestinal System

The GI system begins in the oral cavity and ends at the rectum. During pregnancy, the gums become hyperemic, swollen, and friable and tend to bleed easily. This change is influenced by estrogen and increased proliferation of blood vessels and circulation to the mouth. In addition, the saliva produced in the mouth becomes more acidic. Some women complain about excessive salivation, termed ptyalism, which may be caused by the decrease in unconscious swallowing by the woman when nauseated (Cunningham et al., 2010). Dental plaque, calculus, and debris deposits increase during pregnancy and are all associated with gingivitis. It had been suggested that there was a link between periodontal disease and preterm birth, but a recent study indicates this may not be so (Macones, Parry, Nelson, et al., 2010).

Smooth muscle relaxation and decreased peristalsis occur as a result of the influence of progesterone. Elevated progesterone levels cause smooth muscle relaxation, which results in delayed gastric emptying and decreased peristalsis. Transition time of food throughout the GI tract may be so much slower that more water than normal is reabsorbed, leading to bloating and constipation. Constipation can also result from low-fibre food choices, reduced fluid intake, use of iron supplements, decreased activity level, and intestinal displacement secondary to a growing uterus. Constipation, increased venous pressure, and the pressure of the gravid uterus contribute to the formation of hemorrhoids.

The slowed gastric emptying combined with relaxation of the cardiac sphincter allows reflux, which causes heartburn. Acid indigestion or heartburn (pyrosis) seems to be a universal problem for pregnant women.

TABLE 11.2 SUMMARY OF REPRODUCTIVE SYSTEM ADAPTATIONS

Reproductive Organ	Adaptations
Uterus	Size increases to 20 times non-pregnant size. Capacity increases by 2,000 times to accommodate the developing fetus. Weight increases from 70 g to approximately 1,100 g at term. Uterine growth occurs as a result of both hyperplasia and hypertrophy of the myometrial cells. Increased strength and elasticity allow uterus to contract and expel fetus during birth.
Cervix	Increases in mass, water content, and vascularization. Changes from a relatively rigid to a soft, distensible structure that allows the fetus to be expelled. Under the influence of progesterone, a thick mucus plug is formed, which blocks the cervical os and protects the developing fetus from bacterial invasion.
Vagina	Increased vascularity because of estrogen influences, resulting in pelvic congestion and hypertrophy. Increased thickness of mucosa, along with an increase in vaginal secretions to prevent bacterial infections.
Ovaries	Increased blood supply to the ovaries causes them to enlarge until approximately the 12th to 14th week of gestation, when the placenta takes over their function. Ovulation ceases during pregnancy because of the elevated levels of estrogen and progesterone.
Breasts	Breast changes begin soon after conception; they increase in size and areolar pigmentation. The tubercles of Montgomery enlarge and become more prominent, and the nipples become more erect. The blood vessels become more prominent, and blood flow to the breast doubles.

It is caused by regurgitation of the stomach contents into the upper esophagus and may be associated with the generalized relaxation of the entire digestive system. Over-the-counter antacids will usually relieve the symptoms, but they should be taken with the health care provider's knowledge and only as directed.

The emptying time of the gallbladder is prolonged secondary to the smooth muscle relaxation from progesterone. Hypercholesterolemia can follow, increasing the risk for gallstone formation. Other risk factors for gallbladder disease include obesity, Hispanic ethnicity, and increasing maternal age (Hurt, Guile, Bienstock, et al., 2011). Nausea and vomiting, better known as morning sickness, plagues about 50% to 80% of pregnant women (Sanu & Lamont, 2011). Although it occurs most often in the morning, the nauseated feeling can last all day in some women. The highest incidence of morning sickness is between 6 and 12 weeks. The physiologic basis for morning sickness is still debatable. It has been linked to the high levels of hCG, high levels of circulating estrogens, reduced stomach acidity, and the lowered tone and motility of the digestive tract (Sanu & Lamont, 2011).

Cardiovascular System

Cardiovascular changes occur early during pregnancy to meet the demands of the enlarging uterus and the placenta for more blood and more oxygen. Perhaps the most striking cardiac alteration occurring during pregnancy is the increase in blood volume.

Blood Volume

During pregnancy, blood volume increases by approximately 1,500 mL, or 50% above non-pregnant levels (Evans et al., 2010). The increase is made up of 1,000 mL plasma plus 450 mL red blood cells (RBCs). It begins at weeks 10 to 12, peaks at weeks 32 to 34, and decreases slightly at week 40.

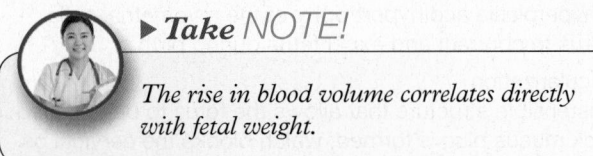

▶ **Take** NOTE!

The rise in blood volume correlates directly with fetal weight.

This increase in blood volume is needed to provide adequate hydration of fetal and maternal tissues, to supply blood flow to perfuse the enlarging uterus, and to provide a reserve to compensate for blood loss at birth and during the postpartum period (Cunningham et al., 2010; Preeti, Shiozawa, Haut, et al., 2011). This increase is also necessary to meet the increased metabolic needs of the mother and the need for increased perfusion of other organs, especially the woman's kidneys, because she is excreting waste products for herself and the fetus.

Cardiac Output and Heart Rate

Cardiac output is the product of stroke volume and heart rate. It increases from 30% to 50% over the non-pregnant rate by the 32nd week of pregnancy and declines to about a 20% increase at 40 weeks' gestation. The increase in cardiac output is associated with an increase in venous return and greater right ventricular output, especially in the left lateral position (Crawford, 2009). Heart rate increases by 10 to 15 beats/minute between 14 and 20 weeks of gestation, and this persists to term. There is slight hypertrophy or enlargement of the heart during pregnancy. This is probably to accommodate the increase in blood volume and cardiac output. The heart works harder and pumps more blood to supply the oxygen needs of the fetus as well as those of the mother. Both heart rate and venous return are increased in pregnancy, contributing to the increase in cardiac output seen throughout gestation. A woman with preexisting heart disease may become symptomatic and begin to decompensate during the time the blood volume peaks. Close monitoring is warranted from 28 to 35 weeks' gestation.

Blood Pressure

Blood pressure, especially the diastolic pressure, declines slightly during pregnancy as a result of peripheral vasodilation caused by progesterone. It reaches a low point at mid-pregnancy and thereafter increases to pre-pregnant levels until term (Crawford, 2009). During the first trimester, blood pressure typically remains at the pre-pregnancy level. During the second trimester, the blood pressure decreases 5 to 10 mm Hg and thereafter returns to first-trimester levels (Crawford, 2009). Any significant rise in blood pressure during pregnancy should be investigated to rule out gestational hypertension.

Blood Components

The number of RBCs also increases throughout pregnancy to a level 25% to 33% higher than non-pregnant values, depending on the amount of iron available. This increase is necessary to transport the additional oxygen required during pregnancy. Although there is an increase in RBCs, there is a greater increase in the plasma volume as a result of hormonal factors and sodium and water retention. Because the plasma increase exceeds the increase of RBC production, normal hemoglobin, and hematocrit values decrease. This state of hemodilution is referred to as **physiologic anemia of pregnancy**. Changes in RBC volume are due to increased circulating erythropoietin and accelerated RBC production. The rise in erythropoietin in the last two trimesters is stimulated by progesterone, prolactin, and human placental lactogen (Evans et al., 2010).

Iron requirements during pregnancy increase because of the demands of the growing fetus and the increase in maternal blood volume. The fetal tissues take predominance over the mother's tissues with respect to the use of iron stores. With the accelerated production of RBCs, iron is necessary for hemoglobin formation, the oxygen-carrying component of RBCs.

> ▶ *Take* NOTE!
>
> *Many women enter pregnancy with insufficient iron stores and thus need supplementation to meet the extra demands of pregnancy.*

Both fibrin and plasma fibrinogen levels increase, along with various blood-clotting factors. These factors make pregnancy a hypercoagulable state. These changes, coupled with venous stasis secondary to venous pooling, which occurs during late pregnancy after long periods of standing in the upright position with the pressure exerted by the uterus on the large pelvic veins, contribute to slowed venous return, pooling, and dependent edema. These factors also increase the woman's risk for venous thrombosis (Chan, 2010).

Respiratory System

The growing uterus and the increased production of the hormone progesterone cause the lungs to function differently during pregnancy. During the pregnancy, the amount of space available to house the lungs decreases as the uterus puts pressure on the diaphragm and causes it to shift upward by 4 cm above its usual position. The growing uterus does change the size and shape of the thoracic cavity, but diaphragmatic excursion increases, chest circumference increases by 5 to 7.5 cm, and the transverse diameter increases by 2.5 cm, allowing a larger tidal volume as evidenced by deeper breathing (Cunningham et al., 2010). Tidal volume, or the volume of air inhaled, increases gradually by 30% to 40% (from 500 to 700 mL) as the pregnancy progresses. As a result of these changes, the women's breathing becomes more diaphragmatic than abdominal (Luks, 2011).

A pregnant woman breathes faster and more deeply because she and the fetus need more oxygen. Oxygen consumption increases during pregnancy as airway resistance and lung compliance remain unchanged. Changes in the structures of the respiratory system take place to prepare the body for the enlarging uterus and increased lung volume (Hegewald & Crapo, 2011). As muscles and cartilage in the thoracic region relax, the chest broadens, with a conversion from abdominal breathing to thoracic breathing. This leads to a 50% increase in air volume per minute. All these structural alterations are temporary and revert back to their pre-pregnant state at the end of the pregnancy.

Increased vascularity of the respiratory tract is influenced by increased estrogen levels, leading to congestion. This congestion gives rise to nasal and sinus stuffiness, epistaxis (nosebleed), and changes in the tone and quality of the woman's voice (Luks, 2011).

Renal/Urinary System

The renal system must handle the effects of increased maternal intravascular and extracellular volume and metabolic waste products as well as excretion of fetal wastes. The predominant structural change in the renal system during pregnancy is dilation of the renal pelvis and uterus. Changes in renal structure occur from hormonal influences of estrogen and progesterone, pressure from an enlarging uterus, and an increase in maternal blood volume. Like the heart, the kidneys work harder throughout the pregnancy. Changes in kidney function occur to accommodate a heavier workload while maintaining a stable electrolyte balance and blood pressure. As more blood flows to the kidneys, the glomerular filtration rate (GFR) increases, leading to an increase in urine flow and volume, substances delivered to the kidneys, and filtration and excretion of water and solutes (Norwitz & Robinson, 2010).

Anatomically, the kidneys enlarge during pregnancy. Each kidney increases in length and weight as a result of hormonal effects that cause increased tone and decreased motility of the smooth muscle. The renal pelvis becomes dilated. The ureters (especially the right ureter) elongate, widen, and become more curved above the pelvic rim as early as the 10th gestational week (Cornelis, Odutayo, Keunen, et al., 2011). Progesterone is thought to cause both these changes because of its relaxing influence on smooth muscle.

Blood flow to the kidneys increases by 50% to 80% as a result of the increase in cardiac output. This in turn leads to an increase in the GFR by as much as 40% to 60% starting during the second trimester. This elevation continues until birth (Cunningham et al., 2010).

The activity of the kidneys normally increases when a person lies down and decreases on standing. This difference is amplified during pregnancy, which is one reason that a pregnant woman feels the need to urinate frequently while trying to sleep. Late in the pregnancy, the increase in kidney activity is even greater when the woman lies on her side rather than her back. Lying on the side relieves the pressure that the enlarged uterus puts on the vena cava carrying blood from the legs. Subsequently, venous return to the heart increases, leading to increased cardiac output. Increased cardiac output results in increased renal perfusion and glomerular filtration (Blackburn, 2008).

Musculoskeletal System

Changes in the musculoskeletal system are progressive, resulting from the influence of hormones, fetal growth, and maternal weight gain. Pregnancy is characterized by changes in posture and gait. By the 10th to 12th week of pregnancy, the ligaments that hold the sacroiliac joints and the pubic symphysis in place begin to soften and stretch, and the articulations between the joints widen and become more movable (Ricci, 2009). The relaxation of the joints peaks by the beginning of the third trimester. The purpose of these changes is to increase the size of the pelvic cavity and to make delivery easier.

The postural changes of pregnancy—an increased swayback and an upper spine extension to compensate for the enlarging abdomen—coupled with the loosening of the sacroiliac joints may result in lower back pain. The woman's centre of gravity shifts forward, requiring a realignment of the spinal curvatures. An increase in the normal lumbosacral curve (lordosis) occurs and a compensatory curvature in the cervicodorsal area develops to assist her in maintaining her balance (Fig. 11.3). In addition, relaxation and increased mobility of joints occur because of the hormones, progesterone and relaxin, which lead to the characteristic "waddle gait" that pregnant women demonstrate toward term. Increased weight gain can add to this discomfort by accentuating the lumbar and dorsal curves.

Integumentary System

The skin of pregnant women undergoes hyperpigmentation primarily as a result of estrogen, progesterone, and melanocyte-stimulating hormone (MSH) levels. These changes are mainly seen on the nipples, areola, umbilicus, perineum, and axilla. Although many integumentary changes disappear after giving birth, some only fade. Many pregnant women express concern about stretch marks, skin colour changes, and hair loss. Unfortunately, little is known about how to avoid these changes.

Complexion changes are not unusual. The increased pigmentation that occurs on the breasts and genitalia also develops on the face to form the "mask of pregnancy," or facial melasma that occurs in up to 70% of pregnant women. There is a genetic predisposition toward melasma, which is exacerbated by the sun; it tends to recur in subsequent pregnancies. This blotchy, brownish pigment covers the forehead and cheeks in dark-haired women. Most fade as the hormones subside at the end of the pregnancy, but some may linger. The skin in the middle of the abdomen may develop a pigmented line called **linea nigra**, which extends from the umbilicus to the pubic area (Fig. 11.4).

Striae gravidarum, or stretch marks, are irregular reddish streaks that appear on the abdomen, breasts, and buttocks in about half of pregnant women. Striae are most prominent by 6 to 7 months. They result from reduced connective tissue strength resulting from the elevated adrenal steroid levels and stretching of the structures secondary to growth (Soutou, Régnier, Nassar, et al., 2009). They are more common in younger women, women with larger infants, and women with higher body mass indices. Nonwhites and women with a history of breast or thigh striae or a family history of striae gravidarum also are at higher risk (Cunningham et al., 2010).

Vascular changes during pregnancy manifested in the integumentary system include varicosities of the legs, vulva, and perineum. Varicose veins commonly are the result of distention, instability, and poor circulation secondary to prolonged standing or sitting and the heavy gravid uterus placing pressure on the pelvic veins,

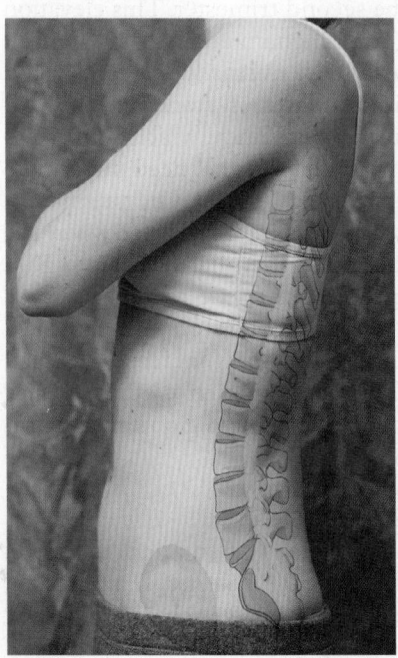
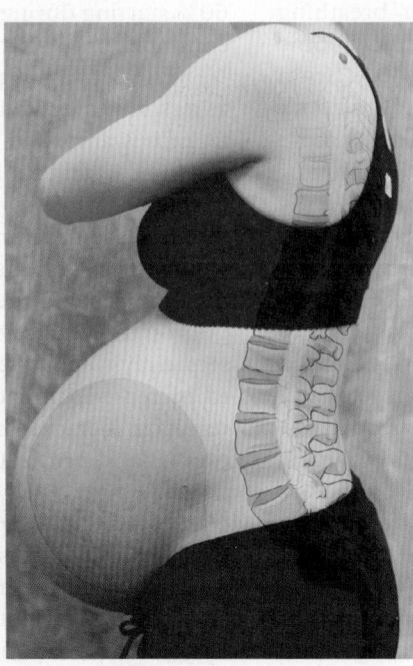

A. Early pregnancy   **B.** Late pregnancy

FIGURE 11.3 Postural changes during (**A**) the first trimester and (**B**) the third trimester.

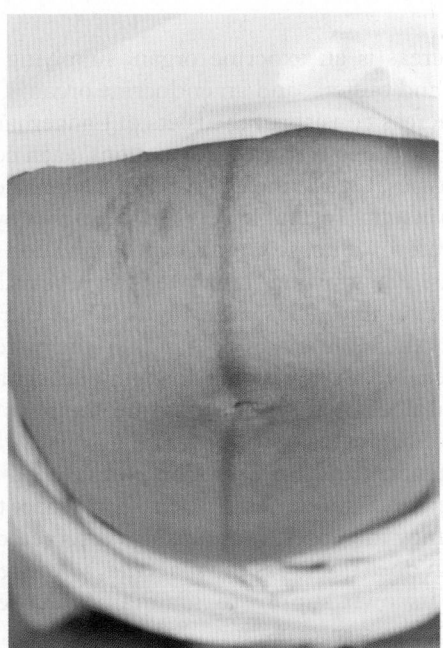

FIGURE 11.4 Linea nigra.

preventing complete venous return. Interventions to reduce the risk of developing varicosities include:

- Elevating both legs when sitting or lying down
- Avoiding prolonged standing or sitting; changing position frequently
- Resting in the left lateral position
- Walking daily for exercise
- Avoiding tight clothing or knee-high hosiery
- Wearing support hose if varicosities are a preexisting condition to pregnancy

Another skin manifestation, believed to be secondary to vascular changes and high estrogen levels, is the appearance of small blood vessels called vascular spiders. They may appear on the neck, thorax, face, and arms. They are especially obvious in white women and typically disappear after childbirth (Geraghty & Pomeranz, 2011). Palmar erythema is a well-delineated pinkish area on the palmar surface of the hands. This integumentary change is also related to elevated estrogen levels (Geraghty & Pomeranz, 2011).

Some women also notice a decline in hair growth during pregnancy. The hair follicles normally undergo a growing and resting phase. The resting phase is followed by a loss of hair; the hairs are then replaced by new ones. During pregnancy, fewer hair follicles go into the resting phase. After delivery, the body catches up with subsequent hair loss for several months. Nails typically grow faster during pregnancy. Pregnant women may experience increased brittleness and transverse grooves on the nails, but most of these conditions resolve in the postpartum period (Geraghty & Pomeranz, 2011).

Endocrine System

The endocrine system undergoes many changes during pregnancy because hormonal changes are essential in meeting the needs of the growing fetus. Hormonal changes play a major role in controlling the supplies of maternal glucose, amino acids, and lipids to the fetus. Although estrogen and progesterone are the main hormones involved in pregnancy changes, other endocrine glands and hormones also change during pregnancy.

Thyroid Gland

The thyroid gland enlarges slightly and becomes more active during pregnancy as a result of increased vascularity and hyperplasia. Increased gland activity results in an increase in thyroid hormone secretion starting during the first trimester; levels taper off within a few weeks after birth and return to normal limits (Cunningham et al., 2010). With an increase in the secretion of thyroid hormones, the basal metabolic rate (BMR, the amount of oxygen consumed by the body over a unit of time in millilitres per minute) progressively increases by 25%, along with heart rate and cardiac output (Cunningham et al., 2010).

Pituitary Gland

The pituitary gland, also known as the hypophysis, is a small, oval gland about the size of a pea that is connected to the hypothalamus by a stalk called the infundibulum. During pregnancy, the pituitary gland enlarges; it returns to normal size after birth.

The anterior lobe of the pituitary is glandular tissue and produces multiple hormones. The release of these hormones is regulated by releasing and inhibiting hormones produced by the hypothalamus. Some of these anterior pituitary hormones induce other glands to secrete their hormones. The increase in blood levels of the hormones produced by the final target glands (e.g., the ovary or thyroid) inhibits the release of anterior pituitary hormones. Changes in levels of pituitary hormones are discussed in the following paragraphs.

FSH and LH secretion are inhibited during pregnancy, probably as a result of hCG produced by the placenta and corpus luteum and the increased secretion of prolactin by the anterior pituitary gland. Levels remain decreased until after delivery.

Thyroid-stimulating hormone (TSH) is reduced during the first trimester but usually returns to normal for the remainder of the pregnancy. Decreased TSH is thought to be one of the factors, along with elevated hCG levels, associated with morning sickness, nausea, and vomiting during the first trimester.

Growth hormone (GH) is an anabolic hormone that promotes protein synthesis. It stimulates most body cells to grow in size and divide, facilitating the use of fats for fuel and conserving glucose. During pregnancy, there is a decrease in the number of GH-producing cells and a corresponding decrease in GH blood levels. The action of human placental lactogen (hPL) is thought to decrease the need for and use of GH.

During pregnancy, the secretion of prolactin increases 10-fold to promote breast development and the lactation process. High levels of progesterone secreted by the placenta inhibit the direct influence of prolactin on the breast during pregnancy, thus suppressing lactation. At birth, as soon as the placenta is expelled and there is a drop in progesterone, lactogenesis can begin (Blackburn, 2008).

MSH, another anterior pituitary hormone, increases during pregnancy. For many years, its increase was thought to be responsible for many of the skin changes of pregnancy, particularly changes in skin pigmentation (e.g., darkening of the areola, melasma, and linea nigra). However, currently it is thought that the skin changes are due to estrogen (and possibly progesterone) as well as the increase in MSH.

The two hormones oxytocin and antidiuretic hormone (ADH) released by the posterior pituitary are actually synthesized in the hypothalamus. They migrate along nerve fibres to the posterior pituitary and are stored until stimulated to be released into the general circulation.

Oxytocin is released by the posterior pituitary gland, and its production gradually increases as the fetus matures (Ward & Hisley, 2009). Oxytocin is responsible for uterine contractions, both before and after delivery. The muscle layers of the uterus (myometrium) become more sensitive to oxytocin near term. Toward the end of a term pregnancy, levels of progesterone decline and contractions that were previously suppressed by progesterone begin to occur more frequently and with stronger intensity. This change in the hormonal levels is believed to be one of the initiators of labour.

Oxytocin is responsible for stimulating the uterine contractions that bring about delivery. Contractions lead to cervical thinning and dilation. They also exert pressure, helping the fetus to descend in the pelvis for eventual delivery. After delivery, oxytocin secretion continues, causing the myometrium to contract and helping to constrict the uterine blood vessels, decreasing the amount of vaginal bleeding after delivery.

Oxytocin is also responsible for milk ejection during breastfeeding. Stimulation of the breasts through sucking or touching stimulates the secretion of oxytocin from the posterior pituitary gland. Oxytocin causes contraction of the myoepithelial cells in the lactating mammary gland. With breastfeeding, "afterpains" often occur, signalling that oxytocin is being released.

Vasopressin (ADH) functions to inhibit or prevent the formation of urine via vasoconstriction, which results in increased blood pressure. Vasopressin also exhibits an antidiuretic effect and plays an important role in the regulation of water balance (Blackburn, 2008).

Pancreas

The pancreas is an exocrine organ, supplying digestive enzymes and buffers, and an endocrine organ. The endocrine pancreas consists of the islets of Langerhans, which are groups of cells scattered throughout, each containing four cell types. One of the cell types is the beta cell, which produces insulin. Insulin lowers blood glucose by increasing the rate of glucose uptake and utilization by most body cells. The growing fetus needs significant amounts of glucose, amino acids, and lipids. Even during early pregnancy the fetus makes demands on the maternal glucose stores. Ideally, hormonal changes of pregnancy help meet fetal needs without putting the mother's metabolism out of balance.

A woman's insulin secretion works on a "supply-versus-demand" mode. As the demand to meet the needs of pregnancy increases, more insulin is secreted. Maternal insulin does not cross the placenta, so the fetus must produce its own supply to maintain glucose control (Box 11.2 gives information about pregnancy, glucose, and insulin).

During the first half of pregnancy, much of the maternal glucose is diverted to the growing fetus, and thus the mother's glucose levels are low. hPL and other hormonal antagonists increase during the second half of

---

BOX 11.2 **Pregnancy, Insulin, and Glucose**

- During early pregnancy, there is a decrease in maternal glucose levels because of the heavy fetal demand for glucose. The fetus is also drawing amino acids and lipids from the mother, decreasing the mother's ability to synthesize glucose. Maternal glucose is diverted across the placenta to assist the growing embryo/fetus during early pregnancy. As a result, maternal glucose concentrations decline to a level that would be considered "hypoglycemic" in a non-pregnant woman. During early pregnancy there is also a decrease in maternal insulin production and insulin levels.
- The pancreas is responsible for the production of insulin, which facilitates entry of glucose into cells. Although glucose and other nutrients easily cross the placenta to the fetus, insulin does not. Therefore, the fetus must produce its own insulin to facilitate the entry of glucose into its own cells.
- After the first trimester, hPL from the placenta and steroids (cortisol) from the adrenal cortex act against insulin. hPL acts as an antagonist against maternal insulin, and thus more insulin must be secreted to counteract the increasing levels of hPL and cortisol during the last half of pregnancy.
- Prolactin, estrogen, and progesterone are also thought to oppose insulin. As a result, glucose is less likely to enter the mother's cells and is more likely to cross over the placenta to the fetus (Cunningham et al., 2010).

pregnancy. Therefore, the mother must produce more insulin to overcome the resistance by these hormones.

If the mother has normal beta cells of the islets of Langerhans, there is usually no problem meeting the demands for extra insulin. However, if the woman has inadequate numbers of beta cells, she may be unable to produce enough insulin and will develop glucose intolerance during pregnancy. If the woman has glucose intolerance, she is not able to meet the increasing demands and her blood glucose level increases.

Adrenal Glands

Pregnancy does not cause much change in the size of the adrenal glands themselves, but there are changes in some secretions and activity. One of the key changes is the marked increase in the secretion of cortisol, which regulates carbohydrate and protein metabolism and is helpful in times of stress (Ward & Hisley, 2009). Although pregnancy is considered a normal condition, it is a time of stress for a woman's body. Cortisol increases in response to increased estrogen levels throughout pregnancy and returns to normal levels within 6 weeks postpartum (Cunningham et al., 2010).

During the stress of pregnancy, cortisol:

- Helps keep up the level of glucose in the plasma by breaking down noncarbohydrate sources, such as amino and fatty acids, to make glycogen. Glycogen, stored in the liver, is easily broken down to glucose when needed so that glucose is available in times of stress.
- Breaks down proteins to repair tissues and manufacture enzymes
- Has anti-insulin, anti-inflammatory, and antiallergic actions
- Is needed to make the precursors of adrenaline, which the adrenal medulla produces and secretes

Aldosterone, also secreted by the adrenal glands, is increased during pregnancy. It normally regulates absorption of sodium from the distal tubules of the kidney. During pregnancy, progesterone allows salt to be "wasted" (or lost) in the urine. Aldosterone is produced in increased amounts by the adrenal glands as early as 15 weeks of pregnancy (Taylor, Badell, & Martina, 2011).

Prostaglandin Secretion During Pregnancy

Prostaglandins are not protein or steroid hormones; they are chemical mediators, or "local" hormones. Although hormones circulate in the blood to influence distant tissues, prostaglandins act locally on adjacent cells. The fetal membranes of the amniotic sac—the amnion and chorion—are both believed to be involved in the production of prostaglandins. Various maternal and fetal tissues, as well as the amniotic fluid itself, are considered to be sources of prostaglandins, but details about their composition and sources are limited. It is widely believed that prostaglandins play a part in softening the cervix and

initiating and/or maintaining labour, but the exact mechanism is unclear.

Placental Secretion

The placenta has a feature possessed by no other endocrine organ—the ability to form protein and steroid hormones. Very early during pregnancy, the placenta begins to produce the following hormones:

- hCG
- hPL
- Relaxin
- Progesterone
- Estrogen

Table 11.3 summarizes the roles of these hormones.

Immune System

The immune system is made up of organs and specialized cells whose primary purpose is to defend the body from foreign substances (antigens) that may cause tissue injury or disease. The mechanisms of innate and adaptive immunity work cooperatively to prevent, control, and eradicate foreign antigens in the body.

A general enhancement of innate immunity (inflammatory response and phagocytosis) and suppression of adaptive immunity (protective response to a specific foreign antigen) takes place during pregnancy. These immunologic alterations help prevent the mother's immune system from rejecting the fetus (foreign body), increase her risk of developing certain infections such as urinary tract infections, and influence the course of chronic disorders such as autoimmune diseases. Some chronic conditions worsen (diabetes) while others seem to stabilize (asthma) during pregnancy, but this is individualized and not predictable. In general, immune function in pregnant women is similar to immune function in non-pregnant women (Witkin, Linhares, Bongiovanni, et al., 2011).

*M*arva returns for her first prenatal appointment and tells the nurse that her whole body is "out of sorts." Outline the bodily changes Marva can expect each trimester to help her understand the adaptations taking place. What guidance can the nurse give Marva to help her understand the changes of pregnancy?

Table 11.4 summarizes the general body systems adaptations to pregnancy.

Changing Nutritional Needs of Pregnancy

Healthy eating during pregnancy enables optimal gestational weight gain and reduces complications, both

TABLE 11.3 PLACENTAL HORMONES

Hormone	Description
hCG	• Responsible for maintaining the maternal corpus luteum, which secretes progesterone and estrogens, with synthesis occurring before implantation • Produced by fetal trophoblast cells until the placenta is developed sufficiently to take over that function • Basis for early pregnancy tests because it appears in the maternal bloodstream soon after implantation • Production peaks at 8 weeks and then gradually declines
hPL (also known as human chorionic somatomam-motropin [hCS])	• Prepares mammary glands for lactation and is involved in the process of making glucose available for fetal growth by altering maternal carbohydrate, fat, and protein metabolism • Antagonist of insulin because it decreases tissue sensitivity or alters the ability to use insulin • Increases the amount of circulating free fatty acids for maternal metabolic needs and decreases maternal metabolism of glucose to facilitate fetal growth
Relaxin	• Secreted by the placenta as well as the corpus luteum during pregnancy • Thought to act synergistically with progesterone to maintain pregnancy • Increases flexibility of the pubic symphysis, permitting the pelvis to expand during delivery • Dilates the cervix, making it easier for the fetus to enter the vaginal canal; thought to suppress the release of oxytocin by the hypothalamus, thus delaying the onset of labour contractions (Cunningham et al., 2010)
Progesterone	• Often called the "hormone of pregnancy" because of the critical role it plays in supporting the endometrium of the uterus • Supports the endometrium to provide an environment conducive to fetal survival • Produced by the corpus luteum during the first few weeks of pregnancy and then by the placenta until term • Initially, causes thickening of the uterine lining in anticipation of implantation of the fertilized ovum. From then on, it maintains the endometrium, inhibits uterine contractility, and assists in the development of the breasts for lactation (Simpson & Creehan, 2008).
Estrogen	• Promotes enlargement of the genitals, uterus, and breasts, and increases vascularity, causing vasodilation. • Relaxes pelvic ligaments and joints (Cunningham et al., 2010) • Associated with hyperpigmentation, vascular changes in the skin, increased activity of the salivary glands, and hyperemia of the gums and nasal mucous membranes (Geraghty & Pomeranz, 2011) • Aids in developing the ductal system of the breasts in preparation for lactation (Simpson & Creehan, 2008)

of which are associated with positive birth outcomes. During pregnancy, maternal nutritional needs change to meet the demands of the pregnancy. Healthy eating can help ensure that adequate nutrients are available for both mother and fetus.

Nutritional intake during pregnancy has a direct effect on fetal well-being and birth outcome (Scholl, 2008). Inadequate nutritional intake, for example, is associated with preterm birth, low birth weight, and congenital anomalies. Excessive nutritional intake is connected with fetal macrosomia (>4,000 g), leading to a difficult birth, neonatal hypoglycemia, and continued obesity in the mother (Davis & Olson, 2009).

Since the requirements for so many nutrients increase during pregnancy, pregnant women should take a vitamin and mineral supplement daily. Prenatal vitamins are prescribed routinely as a safeguard against a less-than-optimal diet. In particular, iron and folic acid need to be supplemented because their increased requirements during pregnancy are usually too great to be met through diet alone (Health Canada, 2009d, 2011; Widen & Siega-Riz, 2010). Iron and folic acid are needed to form new blood cells for the expanded maternal blood volume and to prevent anemia. Folic acid is essential before pregnancy and in the early weeks of pregnancy to prevent neural tube defects in the fetus (Health Canada, 2011; Public Health Agency of Canada, 2008). For most pregnant women, Health Canada recommends supplements of 16 to 20 mg of iron and 0.4 mg (400 µg) of folic acid per day (Cockell, Miller, & Lowell, 2009). Women

TABLE 11.4 SUMMARY OF GENERAL BODY SYSTEM ADAPTATIONS

System	Adaptation
GI system	*Mouth and pharynx:* gums become hyperemic, swollen, and friable and tend to bleed easily. Saliva production increases. *Esophagus:* decreased lower esophageal sphincter pressure and tone, which increases the risk of developing heartburn *Stomach:* decreased tone and mobility with delayed gastric emptying time, which increases the risk of gastro-esophageal reflux and vomiting. Decreased gastric acidity and histamine output, which improves symptoms of peptic ulcer disease. *Intestines:* decreased intestinal tone motility with increased transit time, which increases risk of constipation and flatulence *Gallbladder:* decreased tone and motility, which may increase risk of gallstone formation
Cardiovascular system	*Blood volume:* marked increase in plasma (50%) and RBCs (25% to 33%) compared with non-pregnant values. Causes hemodilution, which is reflected in a lower hematocrit and hemoglobin. *Cardiac output (CO) and heart rate:* CO increases from 30% to 50% over the non-pregnant rate by the 32nd week of pregnancy. The increase in CO is associated with an increase in venous return and greater right ventricular output, especially in the left lateral position. Heart rate increases by 10–15 beats/min between 14 and 20 weeks of gestation, and this increase persists to term. *Blood pressure:* diastolic pressure decreases typically 10–15 mm Hg to reach its lowest point by mid-pregnancy; it then gradually returns to non-pregnant baseline values by term. *Blood components:* the number of RBCs increases throughout pregnancy to a level 25% to 33% higher than non-pregnant values. Both fibrin and plasma fibrinogen levels increase, along with various blood-clotting factors. These factors make pregnancy a hypercoagulable state.
Respiratory system	Enlargement of the uterus shifts the diaphragm up to 4 cm above its usual position. As muscles and cartilage in the thoracic region relax, the chest broadens, with conversion from abdominal breathing to thoracic breathing. This leads to a 50% increase in air volume per minute. Tidal volume, or the volume of air inhaled, increases gradually by 30% to 40% (from 500–700 mL) as the pregnancy progresses.
Renal/urinary system	The renal pelvis becomes dilated. The ureters (especially the right ureter) elongate, widen, and become more curved above the pelvic rim. Bladder tone decreases and bladder capacity doubles by term. GFR increases 40% to 60% during pregnancy. Blood flow to the kidneys increases by 50% to 80% as a result of the increase in cardiac output.
Musculoskeletal system	Distention of the abdomen with growth of the fetus tilts the pelvis forward, shifting the centre of gravity. The woman compensates by developing an increased curvature (lordosis) of the spine. Relaxation and increased mobility of joints occur because of the hormones progesterone and relaxin, which lead to the characteristic "waddle gait" that pregnant women demonstrate toward term.
Integumentary system	Hyperpigmentation of the skin is the most common alteration during pregnancy. The most common areas include the areola, genital skin, axilla, inner aspects of the thighs, and linea nigra. Striae gravidarum, or stretch marks, are irregular reddish streaks that may appear on the abdomen, breasts, and buttocks in about half of pregnant women. The skin in the middle of the abdomen may develop a pigmented line called linea nigra, which extends from the umbilicus to the pubic area. Melasma ("mask of pregnancy") occurs in 45% to 70% of pregnant women. It is characterized by irregular, blotchy areas of pigmentation on the face, most commonly on the cheeks, chin, and nose.
Endocrine system	Controls the integrity and duration of gestation by maintaining the corpus luteum via hCG secretion; production of estrogen, progesterone, hPL, and other hormones and growth factors via the placenta; release of oxytocin (by the posterior pituitary gland), prolactin (by the anterior pituitary), and relaxin (by the ovary, uterus, and placenta)
Immune system	A general enhancement of innate immunity (inflammatory response and phagocytosis) and suppression of adaptive immunity (protective response to a specific foreign antigen) takes place during pregnancy. These immunologic alterations help prevent the mother's immune system from rejecting the fetus (foreign body), increase her risk of developing certain infections, and influence the course of chronic disorders such as autoimmune diseases.

with a previous history of a fetus with a neural tube defect are often prescribed a higher dose (Health Canada, 2009c, 2010d).

There is an abundance of conflicting advice about nutrition during pregnancy and what is good or bad to eat. Overall, the following guidelines are helpful:

• Increase your consumption of fruits and vegetables, especially brightly coloured ones.
• Include a small amount of unsaturated fat daily.
• Include grain products each day, especially whole grains.
• Use reduced-fat dairy products instead of full-fat ones.
• Eat fish weekly, choosing types and amounts of fish that are low in mercury (Health Canada, 2011).
• Include an extra two to three servings each day from any of the four food groups listed in Canada's Food Guide (Health Canada, 2010a).

In the months before conception, food choices are key. The foods and vitamins consumed can ensure that the woman and her fetus will have the nutrients that are essential for the very start of pregnancy (Health Canada, 2010b).

Nutritional Requirements During Pregnancy

Pregnancy is one of the most nutritionally demanding periods of a woman's life. Gestation involves rapid cell division and organ development, and an adequate supply of nutrients is essential to support this tremendous fetal growth (Widen & Siega-Riz, 2010).

Most women are usually motivated to eat properly during pregnancy for the sake of the fetus. The general recommendations for nutrient intake made by Health Canada (2009a) are not limited to preventing deficiency diseases; rather, the **dietary reference intakes (DRIs)** incorporate current concepts about the role of nutrients and food components in reducing the risk for chronic disease, developmental disorders, and other related problems. The DRIs can be used to plan and assess diets for healthy people (Health Canada, 2009a).

These dietary recommendations also include information for women who are pregnant or lactating, because growing fetal and maternal tissues require increased quantities of essential dietary components. For example, the current DRIs suggest an increase in the pregnant woman's intake of protein from 46 to 71 g/day, iron from

TABLE 11.5 DAILY DIETARY RECOMMENDATIONS FOR PREGNANT AND LACTATING WOMEN

Nutrient	Non-Pregnant Women	Pregnant Women	Lactating Women
Calories	2,200	2,500	2,700
Protein	60 g	80 g	80 g
Water/fluids	6–8 glasses	8 glasses	8 glasses
Vitamin A	700 µg	770 µg	1,300 µg
Vitamin C	75 mg	85 mg	120 mg
Vitamin D	5 µg	5 µg	5 µg
Vitamin E	15 µg	15 µg	19 µg
Vitamin B1 (thiamine)	1.1 mg	1.5 mg	1.5 mg
Vitamin B2 (riboflavin)	1.1 mg	1.4 mg	1.6 mg
Vitamin B3 (niacin)	14 mg	18 mg	17 mg
Vitamin B6 (pyridoxine)	1.3 mg	1.9 mg	2 mg
Vitamin B12 (cobalamin)	2.4 µg	2.6 µg	2.8 µg
Folate	400 µg	600 µg	500 µg
Calcium	1,000 mg	1,000 mg	1,000 mg
Phosphorus	700 mg	700 mg	700 mg
Iodine	150 µg	220 µg	290 µg
Iron	18 mg	27 mg	9 mg
Magnesium	310 mg	350 mg	310 mg
Zinc	8 mg	11 mg	12 mg

Source: Health Canada. (2009a). *Prenatal nutrition guidelines for health professionals: Background on Canada's Food Guide.* Retrieved February 20, 2012 from http://www.hc-sc.gc.ca/fn-an/pubs/nutrition/guide-prenatal-eng.php.

18 to 27 g/day, and folate from 400 to 600 μ/day, along with an increase of 300 calories per day over the recommended caloric intake of 1,800 to 2,200 for non-pregnant women (Table 11.5) (HealthLink BC, 2011).

For a pregnant woman to meet recommended DRIs, it is important for her to eat according to Canada's Food Guide (Fig. 11.5). Health Canada developed the Food Guide based on nutrient standards from DRIs, current evidence linking diet and chronic disease, food supply, and food choices available to Canadians (Katamay, Esslinger, Vigneault, et al., 2007). During development of Canada's Food Guide, attention was paid to include food choices and cultural eating patterns of First Nations and Inuit Canadians. These adaptations are further explained in the Health Canada publication, *Eating Well with Canada's Food Guide: First Nations, Inuit and Métis* (2010c), which is available in English as well as numerous First Nations languages. Overall, the Food Guide provides a pattern to help implement these guidelines rather than a prescriptive daily diet and should provide sufficient nutrients for a healthy pregnancy. Except for iron, folic acid, vitamin D (Barrett & McElduff, 2010; Ginde, Sullivan, Mansbach, et al., 2010), and calcium, most of the nutrients a woman needs during pregnancy can be obtained by making healthy food choices. However, a vitamin and mineral supplement is generally prescribed.

> ▶ *Take* NOTE!
>
> *Good food sources of folic acid include dark green vegetables, such as broccoli, romaine lettuce, and spinach; baked beans; black-eyed peas; citrus fruits; peanuts; and liver.*

Fish and shellfish are an important part of a healthy diet because they contain high-quality protein, are low in saturated fat, and contain omega-3 fatty acids. Some types of fish and shellfish contain traces of mercury and

---

▌▌	Health Canada	Santé Canada	*Your health and safety... our priority.*	*Votre santé et votre sécurité... notre priorité.*

My Food Guide Servings Tracker

NAME: _____   DATE: _____

	Food Guide Servings per day	
	7–8	**PREGNANT FEMALE AGED 19–50**

Vegetables and Fruit

1 Food Guide Serving =
125 mL (½ cup) fresh, frozen or canned vegetable or fruit or 100% juice or
250 mL (1 cup) leafy raw vegetables or salad or
1 piece of fruit

6–7 Grain Products

1 Food Guide Serving =
1 slice (35 g) of bread or ½ pita or tortilla (35 g) or
125 mL (½ cup) cooked rice, pasta or couscous or
30 g cold cereal or 175 mL (¾ cup) hot cereal

2 Milk and Alternatives

1 Food Guide Serving =
250 ml (1 cup) milk or fortified soy beverage or
175 g (¾ cup) yogurt or
50 g (1 ½ oz) cheese

2 Meat and Alternatives

1 Food Guide Serving =
75 g (2 ½ oz)/125 mL (½ cup) cooked fish, shellfish, poultry or lean meat or
175 mL (¾ cup) cooked legumes or tofu or
60 mL (¼ cup) shelled nuts and seeds

2–3 Include an extra 2 to 3 Food Guide Servings from any of the four food groups each day.

30 to 45 mL (2 to 3 Tbsp) each day Oils and Fats
Include a small amount of unsaturated fat each day. This includes oil used for cooking, salad dressings, margarine and mayonnaise.

Checklist:
- Include a multivitamin containing folic acid and iron every day.
- Eat at least one dark green and one orange vegetable each day.
- Choose vegetables and fruit prepared with little or no added fat, sugar or salt.
- Have vegetables and fruit more often than juice.
- Make at least half of your grain products whole grain each day.
- Choose grain products that are lower in fat, sugar or salt.
- Drink skim, 1% or 2% milk each day.
- Select lower fat milk alternatives.
- Have meat alternatives such as beans, lentils and tofu often.
- Eat at least two Food Guide Servings of fish each week.
- Select lean meat and alternatives prepared with little or no added fat or salt.
- Satisfy your thirst with water.
- Limit foods and beverages high in calories, fat, sugar or salt.
- Be active regularly as part of a healthy pregnancy. See your doctor before increasing your activity level.

For more information and to order copies of Canada's Food Guide visit Canada's Food Guide on line.

www.healthcanada.gc.ca/foodguide

Canada

FIGURE 11.5 Canada's Food Guide for Pregnant Females.

other contaminants that may harm a developing fetus if ingested by pregnant women in large amounts, but the benefits of eating fish outweigh the potential risks (Institute of Medicine [IOM], 2006). With this in mind, Health Canada (2009b) advises women who may become pregnant, pregnant women, and nursing mothers to do the following:

- Limit their intake of tuna (fresh or frozen), shark, swordfish, orange roughy, and escolar to no more than 150 g (5 ounces) per month
- Have at least 150 g (5 ounces) of cooked fish each week, choosing from a variety of non-predatory fish, such as:
  - Salmon, trout, lake whitefish, Atlantic mackerel
  - Canned light tuna, pollock, herring, and haddock
- Check with local health units about the safety of fish caught by family and friends in local lakes, rivers, and coastal areas (Health Canada, 2009c)

Maternal Weight Gain

All pregnant women should aim for a steady rate of weight gain throughout pregnancy. During the first trimester, for women whose pre-pregnant weight is within the normal range, the weight gain overall should be about 2 kg. Much of the weight gained during the first trimester is caused by growth of the uterus and expansion of the blood volume. During the second and third trimesters, a weight gain of about 0.5 kg per week is expected (HealthLink BC, 2011). (Table 11.6). The Society of Obstetricians and Gynaecologists of Canada (SOGC) (Davies, Maxwell, McLeod, et al., 2010) and Health Canada (2010e) recommend that optimal weight gains during pregnancy be based on pre-pregnancy body mass index (BMI) (Box 11.3, Teaching

TABLE 11.6 NORMAL DISTRIBUTION OF WEIGHT GAIN DURING PREGNANCY

Component	Weight
Fetus	3,294 g (7.3 pounds)
Blood	1,442 g (3.2 pounds)
Uterus	970 g (2 pounds)
Breasts	397 g (14 ounces)
Placenta and umbilical cord	644 g (1.4 pounds)
Fat and protein stores	3,345 g (7.4 pounds)
Tissue fluids	1,496 g (3.3 pounds)
Amniotic fluid	795 g (1.8 pounds)
Approximate total weight gain	12.4 kg (27.3 pounds)

Source: Cunningham, F. G., Leveno, K. J., Bloom, S. L., Hauth, J. C., Rouse, D. J., & Spong, C. Y. (2010). *Williams's obstetrics* (23rd ed.). New York: McGraw-Hill Companies, Inc.

BOX 11.3 Body Mass Index

Body mass index (BMI) provides an accurate estimate of total body fat and is considered a good method to assess overweight and obesity in people. BMI is a weight-to-height ratio calculation that can be determined by dividing a woman's weight in kilograms by her height in metres squared. BMI can also be calculated by weight in pounds divided by the height in inches squared, multiplied by 704.5. Health Canada (2008) categorizes BMI as follows:
- Underweight: <18.5
- Healthy weight: 18.5–24.9
- Overweight: 25–29.9
- Obese: ≥30

Use this example to calculate BMI:
Mary is 5 feet 5 inches tall and weighs 150 pounds.
1. Convert weight into kilograms: 150 lb/2.2 lb/kg = 68.18 kg
2. Convert height into metres:
   a. 5-foot-5 = 65 inches × 2.54 cm/inch = 165.1 cm
   b. 165.1 cm/100 cm = 1.65 m
3. Then square the height in metres: 1.65 × 1.65 = 2.72 m²
4. Calculate BMI: 68.18 kg/2.72 m² = 25

Guideline 11.1). Weight gain tracking charts based on pre-pregnancy BMI have been developed for all categories of recommended weight gain (Health Canada, 2010e). These charts, which are available online, provide

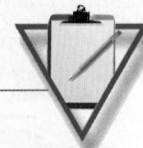

TEACHING GUIDELINE 11.1

Teaching to Promote Optimal Nutrition During Pregnancy

- Follow Canada's Food Guide, selecting a variety of foods from each group.
- Gain weight in a gradual and steady manner as follows:
  - Normal-weight woman: 11.5–16 kg (25–35 pounds)
  - Underweight woman: 12.5–18 kg (28–40 pounds)
  - Overweight woman: 7–11.5 kg (15–25 pounds)
  - Obese woman: 5–9 kg (11–15 pounds)
- Take your prenatal vitamin/mineral supplementation daily.
- Avoid weight-reduction diets.
- Do not skip meals; eat three meals with one or two snacks daily.
- Limit your intake of sodas and caffeine-rich drinks.
- Avoid the use of diuretics.
- Do not restrict the use of salt unless instructed to do so by your health care provider.
- Engage in reasonable physical activity daily.

visual cues to evaluate the overall pattern of weight gain during pregnancy. (Visit http://thePoint.lww.com/Chow1e for a direct link.)

Gaining either too much or too little weight during pregnancy can have undesirable effects on both the mother and the fetus (Rasmussen & Yaktine, 2009). There is evidence that babies born to mothers who gain either too much or too little weight during pregnancy are less likely to be breastfed, which has implications for the infant's future health and wellness (Viswanathan, Siega-Riz, Moos, et al., 2008). Health Canada (2010e) and the SOGC (Davies et al., 2010) both recommend that the ideal time to evaluate and counsel women on gestational weight gain is prior to conception and to continue throughout the pregnancy. See Evidence-based Practice 11.1.

Excess maternal weight gain during pregnancy is associated with large-for-gestational-age infants. With larger infants, there is a higher risk for prolonged labour and birth, cesarean delivery, birth trauma, birth asphyxia, and perinatal mortality (Crane, White, Murphy, et al., 2009; Viswanathan et al., 2008; Zhang, Decker, Platt, et al., 2008). As well, infants born to obese mothers have been shown to be at higher risk for congenital anomalies (Davies et al., 2010), childhood obesity, and

type 2 diabetes later in life (Margerison Zilko, Rehkopf, & Abrams, 2010; Oken, Rifas-Shiman, Field, et al., 2008; Schack-Nielson, Michaelsen, Gamborg, et al., 2010). Mothers with a pre-pregnancy BMI higher than 25 are at increased risk for development of gestational diabetes (Hedderson, Gunderson, & Ferrara, 2010). If they fail to lose this weight 6 months after giving birth, they are at much higher risk for developing cardiovascular and other chronic health problems (Rasmussen & Yaktine, 2009). Therefore, SOGC recommends that women who are overweight when beginning a pregnancy should gain no more than 7 to 11.5 kg during the pregnancy, depending on their nutritional status and degree of obesity (Crane et al., 2009; Davies et al., 2010; Hinkle, Sharma, & Dietz, 2010).

Although not gaining enough weight during pregnancy or having a pre-pregnancy BMI below 18.5 is less common, it is also a concern. Being underweight or not gaining adequate amounts during pregnancy increases the risk for having a preterm birth, a small-for-gestational-age baby, or a low birth weight baby (Viswanathan et al., 2008) and also increases the risk of neonatal mortality, cognitive and physical disabilities, and chronic health problems in later life (Health Canada, 2010a). Studies

EVIDENCE-BASED PRACTICE 11.1
Weight Gain Measures in Women with Gestational Diabetes Mellitus

● Study

The incidences of gestational diabetes mellitus (GDM) and excessive gestational weight gain have increased in recent years among pregnant women in Canada. GDM is associated with potential adverse consequences for both mother and infant, such as hypertensive disorders and type 2 diabetes in the mother and neonatal hypoglycemia, macrosomia and, in the future, type 2 diabetes, obesity, and glucose intolerance in the child. The incidence of operative births also increases with the increased size of the fetus. In 2009, the Institute of Medicine (IOM) recommended that gestational weight gains for all pregnant women be based on the woman's pre-pregnancy BMI. The total weight gain recommended varies depending on the BMI category— underweight, normal, overweight, or obese. In all categories, the recommended weight gain for the first trimester is 0.5 to 2 kg. In this study, the charts of 1,181 women who gave birth in a Quebec hospital were reviewed to examine whether a relationship existed between weight gain in the first trimester and GDM.

▲ Findings

Weight gain patterns and amounts were studied, and the resulting statistical analysis revealed that there was no difference in total weight gain between patients with GDM, but first trimester weight gain was higher in women with GDM compared with controls. In contrast, patients with GDM had a lower third trimester weight gain. The study found that even in a model including traditional risk factors for GDM, such as maternal age and obesity, first trimester weight gain remained an independent predictor of GDM. The study also revealed that women diagnosed with GDM and followed by an interdisciplinary team were able to maintain their total gestational weight gain to close to the IOM recommendations.

■ Nursing Implications

Excessive first trimester weight gain has been shown to be a risk factor for GDM that is independent of other traditional predictors. Management of GDM through medical and nutritional intervention in the third trimester seems to be effective in managing appropriate weight gain in line with IOM recommendations. Therefore, it is suggested that nurses focus especially on education and attention to informing and monitoring first trimester weight gain in pregnant women to reduce their risk for development of GDM.

Morisset, A. D., Tchernof, A., Dubé, M. C., Veillette, J., Weisnagel, J., & Robitaille, J. (2011). Weight gain measures in women with gestational diabetes mellitus. *Journal of Women's Health, 20*(3), 375–380. doi:10.1089 = jwh.2010.2252

suggest this is more common in women who are multiparous, have a lower household income, or were born outside Canada (Lowell & Miller, 2010). Any woman who has a pre-pregnancy BMI of less than 18.5 is considered to be high risk and should be referred to a nutritionist. Their activity, exercise patterns, and the food intake patterns should be assessed, and they should be encouraged to gain 12.5 to 18 kg during the pregnancy (Davies et al., 2010).

Nutrition Promotion

Through education, nurses can play an important role in ensuring adequate nutrition for pregnant women. During the initial prenatal visit, health care providers conduct a thorough assessment of a woman's typical dietary practices and address any conditions that may cause inadequate nutrition, such as nausea and vomiting or lack of access to adequate food. Assess and reinforce dietary information at every prenatal visit to promote good nutrition. A normal well-balanced diet generally provides most of the recommended nutrients except iron and folate, both of which must be supplemented in the form of prenatal vitamins. It is also important to assess and advise women on exercise habits. The SOGC and the Canadian Society for Exercise Physiology (CSEP) advise that regular exercise is important for all pregnant women who have no contraindication against it. A form developed by CSEP (PARmed-X for Pregnancy: Physical Activity Readiness Medical Examination) can be used by the health care provider as a screening tool and to initiate discussion relating to the benefits of appropriate exercise during pregnancy. Visit http://thePoint.lww.com/Chow1e for a link to this form, which can be downloaded for free.

Canada's Food Guide is the typical tool used for nutritional education and is recognized by the general population as the gold standard for healthy eating patterns. In pregnancy, women should continue to follow the pre-pregnancy guideline but add an additional two to three serving from any of the four food groups. Health Canada offers many online resources that are helpful when providing nutritional information for pregnant women (see Teaching Guideline 11.1).

Special Nutritional Considerations

Many factors play an important role in shaping a person's eating habits, and these factors must be taken into account if nutritional counselling is to be realistic and appropriate. Nurses need to be aware of these factors to ensure individualized teaching and care. To accommodate Canada's diverse population, the Food Guide has been translated into 10 languages in addition to English and French. An adaptation of the guide, *Eating Well with Canada's Food Guide: First Nation, Inuit, and Métis,* is also available (Health Canada, 2010c). In addition, interactive resources are available free of charge on the Health Canada website.

Cultural Variations and Restrictions

Food is important to every cultural group. It is often part of celebrations and rituals. The nurse needs to adapt Canadian nutritional guidelines when working with women from various cultures in order to meet nutritional needs within their cultural framework. Food choices and variations for different cultures might include the following:

- Grain products:
  - Bolillo
  - Couscous
  - Hua juan
  - Flaxseed
  - Bannock
- Vegetables and fruits:
  - Agave
  - Bok choy
  - Jicama
  - Okra
  - Water chestnuts
  - Catabopy
  - Kumquats
  - Plantain
  - Yucca fruit
  - Zapate
- Meat and alternatives:
  - Traditional wild meats and game
  - Bean paste
  - Blood sausage
  - Legumes
  - Shellfish
- Milk alternatives:
  - Buttermilk
  - Buffalo milk
  - Soybean milk

Traditional fats that are liquid at room temperature, such as seal and whale oil, or ooligan grease contain unsaturated fats and can be used as all or part of the 2 to 3 tablespoons of unsaturated fats recommended per day.

Lactose Intolerance

The best source of calcium is milk and dairy products, but for women with lactose intolerance, adaptations are necessary. Women with lactose intolerance lack an enzyme (lactase) needed for the breakdown of lactose into its component simple sugars, glucose, and galactose. Without adequate lactase, lactose passes through the small intestine undigested and causes abdominal discomfort, gas, and diarrhea. Lactose intolerance is especially common among women of African, Asian, and Middle Eastern descent (Sabella & Cunningham, 2010).

Additional or substitute sources of calcium may be necessary. These may include peanuts, almonds, sunflower seeds, broccoli, salmon, kale, soy, and molasses (Amit, 2010). In addition, encourage the woman to drink lactose-free dairy products or calcium-enriched orange juice or soy milk.

Vegetarians

Vegetarian diets are becoming increasingly prevalent in Canada. People choose a vegetarian diet for various reasons, including environmental, animal rights, philosophical, religious, and health beliefs (Amit, 2010). Vegetarians choose not to eat meat, chicken, and fish. Their diets consist mostly of plant-based foods, such as legumes, vegetables, whole grains, nuts, and seeds. Vegetarians fall into groups defined by the types of foods they eat. Lacto-ovo-vegetarians omit red meat, fish, and poultry but eat eggs, milk, and dairy products in addition to plant-based foods. Lacto-vegetarians consume milk and dairy products along with plant-based foods; they omit eggs, meat, fish, and poultry. Vegans eliminate all foods from animals, including milk, eggs, and cheese, and eat only plant-based foods (Dieticians of Canada, 2010).

The concern with any form of vegetarianism, especially during pregnancy, is that the diet may be inadequate in nutrients. This may lead to low gestational weight gain, iron-deficiency anemia, compromised protein utilization, and decreased mineral absorption. A diet can become so restrictive that a woman is not gaining weight or is consistently not eating enough from one or more of the food groups. Generally, the more restrictive the diet, the greater the chance there is for nutrient deficiencies.

Well-balanced vegetarian diets that include dairy products provide adequate caloric and nutrient intake and do not require special supplementation; however, vegan diets do not include any meat, eggs, or dairy products. In addition to taking a prenatal multivitamin supplement that includes, iron, folate and vitamin B12, pregnant vegetarians must pay special attention to their intake of protein, iron, calcium, and vitamin B12 (Dieticians of Canada, 2010). Suggestions include:

- For protein: substitute soy foods, beans, lentils, nuts, grains, and seeds.
- For iron: eat a variety of meat alternatives, along with vitamin C–rich foods.
- For calcium: substitute soy, calcium-fortified orange juice, and tofu.
- For vitamin B12: eat fortified soy foods, fortified meat alternatives, and a B12 supplement.

Pica

Many women experience unusual food cravings during their pregnancy. Having cravings during pregnancy is perfectly normal. Sometimes, however, women crave substances that have no nutritional value and can even be dangerous to themselves and their fetus. **Pica** is the compulsive ingestion of non-food substances. Pica is derived from the Latin term for magpie, a bird that is known to consume a variety of non-food substances. Unlike the bird, however, pregnant women who develop a pica habit typically have one or two specific cravings.

The exact cause of pica is not known. Many theories have been advanced to explain it, but none has been proven scientifically. The incidence of pica is difficult to determine, since it is under-reported. The practice of pica is not limited to any one geographic area, race, creed, or culture (Young, 2010). The three main substances consumed by women with pica are soil or clay (geophagia), ice (pagophagia), and laundry starch (amylophagia). Nutritional implications include:

- Soil: replaces nutritive sources and causes iron-deficiency anemia
- Clay: produces constipation; can contain toxic substances and cause parasitic infection
- Ice: can cause iron-deficiency anemia, tooth fractures, freezer burn injuries
- Laundry starch: replaces iron-rich foods, leads to iron deficiencies, and replaces protein metabolism, thus depriving the fetus of amino acids needed for proper development (Young, 2010)

Clinical manifestations of anemia often precede the identification of pica because it is rarely addressed by the health care provider and the woman does not usually volunteer such information (Cunningham et al., 2010). Secrecy surrounding this habit makes research and diagnosis difficult because some women fail to view their behaviour as anything unusual, harmful, or worth reporting. Because of the clinical implications, pica should be discussed with all pregnant women as a preventive measure. The topic can be part of a general discussion of cravings, and the nurse should stress the harmful effects outlined above.

Suspect pica when the woman exhibits anemia even though her dietary intake is appropriate. Ask about her usual dietary intake, and include questions about the ingestion of non-food substances. Consider the potential negative outcomes for the pregnant woman and her fetus, and take appropriate action.

Psychosocial Adaptations During Pregnancy

WATCH&LEARN

Pregnancy is a unique time in a woman's life. It is a time of dramatic alterations in her body and her appearance, as well as a time of change in her social status. All these changes occur simultaneously. Concurrent with the physiologic changes within her body systems are psychosocial changes within the mother and family members as they face significant role and lifestyle changes.

Maternal Emotional Responses

Motherhood, perhaps more than any role in society, has acquired a special significance for women. Women are taught that they should find fulfillment and satisfaction in the role of the "ever-bountiful, ever-giving, self-sacrificing mother" (Ricci, 2009). With such high expectations, many pregnant women experience various emotions throughout their pregnancy. The woman's approach to these emotions is influenced by her emotional makeup, her sociologic and cultural background, her acceptance or rejection of the pregnancy, whether the pregnancy was planned, whether the father is known, and her support network (Simpson & Creehan, 2008).

Despite the wide-ranging emotions associated with the pregnancy, many women experience similar responses. These responses commonly include ambivalence, introversion, acceptance, mood swings, and changes in body image.

Ambivalence

The realization of a pregnancy can lead to fluctuating responses, possibly at the opposite ends of the spectrum. For example, regardless of whether the pregnancy was planned, the woman may feel proud and excited at her achievement while at the same time fearful and anxious of the implications. The reactions are influenced by several factors, including the way the woman was raised, her current family situation, the quality of the relationship with the expectant father, and her hopes for the future. Some women express concern over the timing of the pregnancy, wishing that goals and life objectives had been met before becoming pregnant. Other women may question how a newborn or infant will affect their career or their relationships with friends and family. These feelings can cause conflict and confusion about the pregnancy (Borisoff, 2011).

Ambivalence, or having conflicting feelings at the same time, is a universal feeling and is considered normal when preparing for a lifestyle change and new role. Pregnant women commonly experience ambivalence during the first trimester. Usually ambivalence evolves into acceptance by the second trimester, when fetal movement is felt. The woman's personality, her ability to adapt to changing circumstances, and the reactions of her partner will affect her adjustment to being pregnant and her acceptance of impending motherhood.

Introversion

Introversion, or focusing on oneself, is common during the early part of pregnancy. The woman may withdraw and become increasingly preoccupied with herself and her fetus. As a result, her participation with the outside world may be less, and she will appear passive to her family and friends.

This introspective behaviour is a normal psychological adaptation to motherhood for most women. Introversion seems to heighten during the first and third trimesters, when the woman's focus is on behaviours that will ensure a safe and health pregnancy outcome. Couples need to be aware of this behaviour and should be informed about measures to maintain and support the focus on the family.

Acceptance

During the second trimester, the physical changes of the growing fetus with an enlarging abdomen and fetal movement bring reality and validity to the pregnancy. There are many tangible signs that someone separate from herself is present. The pregnant woman feels fetal movement and may hear the heartbeat. She may see the fetal image on an ultrasound screen and feel distinct parts, recognizing independent sleep and wake patterns. She becomes able to identify the fetus as a separate individual and accepts this.

Many women will verbalize positive feelings about the pregnancy and will conceptualize the fetus. The woman may accept her new body image and talk about the new life within. Generating a discussion about the woman's feelings and offering support and validation at prenatal visits are important.

Mood Swings

Emotional lability is characteristic throughout most pregnancies. One moment a woman can feel great joy, and within a short time she can feel shock and disbelief. Frequently, pregnant women will start to cry without any apparent cause. Some women feel as though they are riding an "emotional roller-coaster." These extremes in emotion can make it difficult for partners and family members to communicate with the pregnant woman without placing blame on themselves for their mood changes. Clear explanations about how common mood swings are during pregnancy are essential.

Change in Body Image

The way in which pregnancy affects a woman's body image varies greatly from person to person. Some women feel as if they have never been more beautiful, whereas others spend their pregnancy feeling overweight and uncomfortable. For some women pregnancy is a relief from worrying about weight, whereas for others it only exacerbates their fears of weight gain. Changes in body image are normal but can be very stressful for the pregnant woman. Offering a thorough explanation and initiating discussion of the expected bodily changes may help the family to cope with them.

Maternal Role Tasks

Many nursing theorists, including Reva Rubin and Ramona Mercer, have identified maternal tasks that a woman must accomplish to incorporate the maternal role into her personality. Mercer (2004) suggested that the term "maternal role attainment" be replaced with "becoming a mother" as the maternal role is an ongoing process that continues throughout the lifespan. Accomplishing these tasks helps the expectant mother to develop her self-concept as a mother and to form a mutually gratifying relationship with her infant. These tasks are listed in Box 11.4.

Pregnancy and Sexuality

The way a pregnant woman feels and experiences her body during pregnancy can affect her sexuality. The woman's changing shape, emotional status, fetal activity,

BOX 11.4 Maternal Role Tasks

- **Ensuring safe passage throughout pregnancy and birth**
  - Primary focus of the woman's attention
  - First trimester: woman focuses on herself, not on the fetus
  - Second trimester: woman develops attachment of great value to her fetus
  - Third trimester: woman has concern for herself and her fetus as a unit
  - Participation in positive self-care activities related to diet, exercise, and overall well-being
- **Seeking acceptance of infant by others**
  - First trimester: acceptance of pregnancy by herself and others
  - Second trimester: family needs to relate to the fetus as member
  - Third trimester: unconditional acceptance without rejection
- **Seeking acceptance of self in maternal role to infant ("binding in")**
  - First trimester: mother accepts idea of pregnancy, but not of infant
  - Second trimester: with sensation of fetal movement (quickening), mother acknowledges fetus as a separate entity within her
  - Third trimester: mother longs to hold infant and becomes tired of being pregnant
- **Learning to give of oneself**
  - First trimester: identifies what must be given up to assume new role
  - Second trimester: identifies with infant, learns how to delay own desires
  - Third trimester: questions her ability to become a good mother to infant (Rubin, 1984)

changes in breast size, pressure on the bladder, and other discomforts of pregnancy result in increased physical and emotional demands. These can produce stress on the sexual relationship between the pregnant woman and her partner. As the changes of pregnancy ensue, many partners become confused, anxious, and fearful of how the relationship may be affected.

Sexual desire of pregnant women may change throughout the pregnancy. During the first trimester, the woman may be less interested in sex because of fatigue, nausea, and fear of disturbing the early embryonic development. During the second trimester, her interest may increase because of the stability of the pregnancy. During the third trimester, her enlarging size may produce discomfort during sexual activity (Jones, Chan, & Farine, 2011).

A woman's sexual health is intimately linked to her own self-image. Sexual positions to increase comfort as the pregnancy progresses as well as alternative noncoital modes of sexual expression, such as cuddling, caressing, and holding, should be discussed. Giving permission to talk about and then normalizing sexuality can help enhance the sexual experience during pregnancy and, ultimately, the couple's relationship. If avenues of communication are open regarding sexuality during pregnancy, any fears and myths the couple may have can be dispelled.

Pregnancy and the Partner

Nursing care related to childbirth has expanded from a narrow emphasis on the physical health needs of the mother and infant to a broader focus on family-related, social, and emotional needs. One prominent feature of this family-centred approach is the recent movement toward promoting the mother–infant bond. To achieve a truly family-centred practice, nurses must make a comparable commitment to understanding and meeting the needs of the partner in the emerging family. Recent studies suggest that the partner's potential contribution to the infant's overall development has been misperceived or devalued and that the partner's ability and willingness to assume a more active role in the infant's care may have been underestimated (Hohmann-Marriott, 2009).

Reactions to pregnancy and to the psychological and physical changes by the woman's partner vary greatly. Some enjoy the role of being the nurturer, whereas others experience alienation and may seek comfort or companionship elsewhere. Some expectant fathers may view pregnancy as proof of their masculinity and assume the dominant role, whereas others see their role as minimal, leaving the pregnancy up to the woman entirely. Each expectant partner reacts uniquely.

Emotionally and psychologically, expectant partners may undergo less visible changes than women, but most of these changes remain unexpressed and unappreciated

(Newman & Newman, 2012). Expectant partners also experience a multitude of adjustments and concerns. Physically, they may gain weight around the middle and experience nausea and other GI disturbances—what is termed couvade syndrome, a sympathetic response to their partner's pregnancy. They also experience ambivalence during early pregnancy, with extremes of emotions (e.g., pride and joy versus an overwhelming sense of impending responsibility).

During the second trimester of pregnancy, partners go through acceptance of their role of breadwinner, caretaker, and support person. They come to accept the reality of the fetus when movement is felt, and they experience confusion when dealing with the woman's mood swings and introspection. During the third trimester, the expectant partner prepares for the reality of this new role and negotiates what the role will be during the labour and birthing process. Many express concern about being the primary support person during labour and birth and worry about how they will react when faced with their loved one in pain. Expectant partners share many of the same anxieties as their pregnant partners. However, it is uncommon for them to reveal these anxieties to the pregnant partner or health care professionals. Often, how the expectant partner responds during the third trimester depends on the state of the marriage or partnership. When the marriage or partnership is struggling, the impending increase in responsibility toward the end of pregnancy acts to drive the expectant partner further away. Often it manifests as working late, staying out late with friends, or beginning new or superficial relationships. In the stable marriage or partnership, the expectant partner who may have been struggling to find his or her place in the pregnancy now finds concrete tasks to do—for example, painting the nursery, assembling the car seat, attending Lamaze classes, and so on.

Pregnancy and Siblings

A sibling's reaction to pregnancy is age-dependent. Some children might express excitement and anticipation, whereas others might have negative reactions. A young toddler might regress in toilet training or ask to drink from a bottle again. An older school-aged child may ignore the new addition to the family and engage in outside activities to avoid the new member. The introduction of an infant into the family is often the beginning of sibling rivalry, which results from the child's fear of change in the security of the relationship with his or her parents (Veltri, 2010). Preparation of the siblings for the anticipated birth is imperative and must be designed according to the age and life experiences of the sibling at home. Constant reinforcement of love and caring will help to reduce the older child's fear of change and worry about being replaced by the new family member.

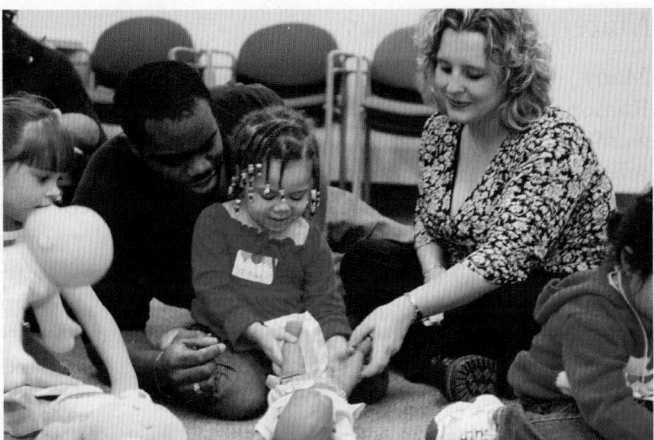

FIGURE 11.6 Parents preparing sibling for the birth of a new baby.

If possible, parents should include siblings in preparation for the birth of the new baby to help them feel as if they have an important role to play (Fig. 11.6). Parents must also continue to focus on the older sibling after the birth to reduce regressive or aggressive behaviour toward the newborn.

■■■ Key Concepts

■ Pregnancy is a normal life event that involves considerable physical, psychosocial, emotional, and relationship adjustments.

■ The signs and symptoms of pregnancy have been grouped into those that are subjective (presumptive) and experienced by the woman herself, those that are objective (probable) and observed by the health care professional, and those that are the definite, positive signs.

■ Physiologically, almost every system of a woman's body changes during pregnancy with startling rapidity to accommodate the needs of the growing fetus. A majority of the changes are influenced by hormonal changes.

■ The placenta is a unique kind of endocrine gland; it has a feature possessed by no other endocrine organ—the ability to form protein and steroid hormones.

■ Occurring in conjunction with the physiologic changes in the woman's body systems are psychosocial changes occurring within the mother and family members as they face significant role and lifestyle changes.

■ Commonly experienced emotional responses to pregnancy in the woman include ambivalence, introversion, acceptance, mood swings, and changes in body image.

■ Reactions of expectant partners to pregnancy and to the physical and psychological changes in the woman vary greatly.

■ A sibling's reaction to pregnancy is age dependent. The introduction of a new infant to the family is often the beginning of sibling rivalry, which results from the established child's fear of change in security of their relationships with their parents. Therefore, preparation of the siblings for the anticipated birth is imperative.

REFERENCES

Akinbiyi, A. A., Watson, R., & Feyi-Waboso, P. (2008). Prevalence of *Candida albicans* and bacterial vaginosis in asymptomatic pregnant women in South Yorkshire, United Kingdom: Outcome of a prospective study. *Archives of Gynecology and Obstetrics, 278,* 463–466. doi:10.1007/s00404–008-0593–8

Amit, M. (2010). Vegetarian diets in children and adolescents. *Paediatrics & Child Health, 15*(5), 303–314.

Barrett, H., & McElduff, A. (2010). Vitamin D and pregnancy: An old problem revisited. *Best Practice & Research: Clinical Endocrinology & Metabolism, 24,* 527.

Blackburn, S. T. (2008). Physiologic changes of pregnancy. In K. R. Simpson & P. A. Creehan (Eds.), *AWHONN perinatal nursing* (3rd ed.). Philadelphia: Lippincott Williams & Wilkins.

Borisoff, D. (2011). Transforming motherhood: "We've come a long way," maybe. *Review of Communication, 5*(1), 1–11.

Chan, W. S. (2010). Venous thromboembolism in pregnancy. *Expert Review of Cardiovascular Therapy, 8*(12), 1731–1740.

Cockell, K. A., Miller, D. C., & Lowell, H. (2009). Application of the dietary reference intakes in developing a recommendation for pregnancy iron supplements in Canada. *American Journal of Clinical Nutrition, 90,* 1023–1028.

Cornelis, T., Odutayo, A., Keunen, J., & Hladunewich, M. (2011). The kidney in normal pregnancy and preeclampsia. *Seminars in Nephrology, 31*(1), 4–14.

Crane, J. M. G., White, J., Murphy, P., Burrage, L., Hutchens, D. (2009). The effect of gestational weight gain by body mass index on maternal and neonatal outcomes. *Journal of Obstetrics and Gynaecology Canada, 31*(1):28–35.

Crawford, M. H. (2009). *Current diagnosis & treatment: Cardiology* (3rd ed.). Columbus, OH: The McGraw-Hill Companies, Inc.

Cunningham, F. G., Leveno, K. J., Bloom, S. L., Hauth, J. C., Rouse, D. J., & Spong, C. Y. (2010). *Williams's obstetrics* (23rd ed.). New York: McGraw-Hill Companies, Inc.

Davies, G. A., Maxwell, C., McLeod, L., et al. (2010). SOGC clinical practice guideline: Obesity in pregnancy. *Journal of Obstetrics and Gynaecology Canada, 32*(2), 165–173. Retrieved February 20, 2012 from http://www.sogc.org/guidelines/documents/gui239ECPG1002.pdf

Davis, E., & Olson, C. (2009). Obesity in pregnancy. *Primary Care: Clinics in Office Practice, 36*(2), 341–356. doi:10.1016/i.pop 2009. 01.005

Dieticians of Canada. (2010). *Eating guidelines for vegans.* Retrieved February 20, 2012 from http://www.dietitians.ca/getattachment/c8c30477-aad8-4283-9164-079855fabb6d/FactSheet-Eating-Guidelines-for-Vegans.pdf.aspx

Evans, R., Evans, M., Brown, Y., & Orshan, S. (2010). *Canadian maternity, newborn and women's health nursing: Comprehensive care across the lifespan.* Philadelphia: Lippincott Williams & Wilkins.

Fraser, D. M., & Cooper, M. A. (Eds.). (2009). *Myles textbook for midwives.* Philadelphia: Elsiever.

Geraghty, L. N., & Pomeranz, M. K. (2011). Physiologic changes and dermatoses of pregnancy. *International Journal of Dermatology, 50,* 771–782. doi:10.1111/j.1365–4632.2010.04869.x

Gibbs, R. S., Karlan, B. Y., Haney, A. F., & Nygaard, I. E. (2008). *Danforth's obstetrics and gynecology* (10th ed.). Philadelphia: Lippincott Williams & Wilkins.

Ginde, A. A., Sullivan, A. F., Mansbach, J. M., & Camargo, C. A., Jr. (2010). Vitamin D insufficiency in pregnant and non-pregnant women of childbearing age in the United States. *American Journal of Obstetrics & Gynecology, 202*(5), 436e1–436e8.

HealthLink BC. (2011). *Nutrition and weight gain during pregnancy.* Retrieved February 20, 2012 from http://www.healthlinkbc.ca/kb/content/special/hw194870.html#hw194870-Credits

Health Canada. (2008). *Canadian guidelines for body weight classification in adults—Quick reference tool for professionals.* Retrieved February 20, 2012 from http://www.hc-sc.gc.ca/fn-an/nutrition/weights-poids/guide-ld-adult/cg_quick_ref-ldc_rapide_ref-eng.php

Health Canada. (2009a). *Prenatal nutrition guidelines for health professionals: Background on Canada's Food Guide.* Retrieved February 20, 2012 from http://www.hc-sc.gc.ca/fn-an/pubs/nutrition/guide-prenatal-eng.php

Health Canada. (2009b). *Prenatal nutrition guidelines for health professionals: Fish and omega-3 fatty acids.* Retrieved February 20, 2012 from http://www.hc-sc.gc.ca/fn-an/pubs/nutrition/omega3-eng.php

Health Canada. (2009c). *Prenatal nutrition guidelines for health professionals: Folate contributes to a healthy pregnancy.* Retrieved February 20, 2012 from http://www.hc-sc.gc.ca/fn-an/pubs/nutrition/folate-eng.php

Health Canada. (2009d). *Prenatal nutrition guidelines for health professionals: Iron contributes to a healthy pregnancy.* Retrieved February 20, 2012 from http://www.hc-sc.gc.ca/fn-an/pubs/nutrition/iron-fer-eng.php

Health Canada. (2010a). *Canada's Food Guide: Servings tracker for pregnant females.* Retrieved February 20, 2012 from http://www.hc-sc.gc.ca/fn-an/alt_formats/hpfb-dgpsa/pdf/food-guide-aliment/table_female-femme_preg-ence_age19–50-eng.pdf

Health Canada. (2010b). *Dietary reference intakes tables.* Retrieved February 20, 2012 from http://www.hc-sc.gc.ca/fn-an/nutrition/reference/table/index-eng.php

Health Canada. (2010c). *Eating well with Canada's Food Guide: First Nations, Inuit and Métis.* Retrieved February 20, 2012 from http://www.hc-sc.gc.ca/fn-an/food-guide-aliment/fnim-pnim/index-eng.php

Health Canada. (2010d). *High-dose folic acid supplementation: Questions and answers for health professionals.* Retrieved February 20, 2012 from http://www.hc-sc.gc.ca/fn-an/nutrition/prenatal/fol-qa-qr-eng.php

Health Canada. (2010e). *Prenatal nutrition guidelines for health professionals: Gestational weight gain.* Retrieved February 20, 2012 from http://www.hc-sc.gc.ca/fn-an/nutrition/prenatal/ewba-mbsa-eng.php#t3

Health Canada. (2011). *Prenatal nutrition.* Retrieved February 20, 2012 from http://www.hc-sc.gc.ca/fn-an/nutrition/prenatal/index-eng.php

Hedderson, M. M., Gunderson, E. P., & Ferrara, A. (2010). Gestational weight gain and risk of gestational diabetes mellitus. *Obstetrics and Gynecology, 115*(3), 597–604.

Hegewald, M. J., & Crapo R. O. (2011). Respiratory physiology in pregnancy. *Clinics in Chest Medicine, 32*(1), 1–13.

Hinkle, S. N., Sharma, A. J., & Dietz, P. M. (2010). Gestational weight gain in obese mothers and associations with fetal growth. *American Journal of Clinical Nutrition, 92*(3), 644–651.

Hohmann-Marriott, B. (2009). The couple context of pregnancy and its effects on prenatal care and birth outcomes. *Maternal & Child Health Journal, 13*(6), 745–754. doi:10.1007/s10995–009-0467–0

Hurt, K. J., Guile, M. W., Bienstock, J. L., Fox, H. E., & Wallach, E. E. (2011). *Johns Hopkins manual of gynecology and obstetrics* (4th ed.). Philadelphia: Lippincott Williams & Wilkins.

Institute of Medicine. (2006). *Seafood choices: Balancing benefits and risks.* Washington, DC: National Academies Press. Retrieved February 20, 2012 from http://www.iom.edu/Reports/2006/Seafood-Choices-Balancing-Benefits-and-Risks.aspx

Jones, C., Chan, C., & Farine, D. (2011). Sex in pregnancy. *Canadian Medical Association Journal, 183*(7), 815–818.

Katamay, S. W., Esslinger, S. K., Vigneault, M., et al. (2007). *Eating well with Canada's Food Guide (2007). Development of the food intake pattern.* Retrieved September 5, 2011 from http://www.hc-sc.gc.ca/fn-an/pubs/fd_int_pat-ela_mod_alim-eng.php

Lowell, H., & Miller, D. C. (2010). Weight gain during pregnancy: Adherence to Health Canada's Guidelines. *Health Reports, 21*(2):31–36.

Luks, A. M. (2011). Pregnancy and critical care medicine, part 1: Normal physiologic changes in pregnancy. *Critical Care Alert, 18*(12), 89–94.

Macones, G. A., Parry, S., & Nelson D. B., et al. (2010). Treatment of localized periodontal disease in pregnancy does not reduce the occurrence of preterm birth: Results from the Periodontal Infections and Prematurity Study (PIPS). *American Journal of Obstetrics and Gynecology, 202,* 147.e1–147.e8.

Margerison Zilko, C. E., Rehkopf, D., & Abrams, B. (2010). Association of maternal gestational weight gain with short- and long-term maternal and child health outcomes. *American Journal of Obstetrics & Gynecology, 202*(6), 574.e1–574.e8.

Mercer, R. T. (2004). Becoming a mother versus maternal role attainment. *Journal of Nursing Scholarship, 36*(3), 226–232.

Newman, B. M., & Newman, P. R. (2012). *Development through life: A psychosocial approach* (11th ed.). Toronto, ON: Nelson.

Norwitz, E. R., & Robinson, J. N. (2010). Pregnancy-induced physiologic alterations. In M. A. Belfort, G. Saade, M. R. Foley, J. P. Phelan, & G. A. Dildy (Eds.), *Critical care obstetrics* (5th ed.). Oxford, UK: Wiley-Blackwell.

Oken, E., Rifas-Shiman, S. L., Field, A. E, Frazier, A. L., & Gillman, M. W. (2008). Maternal gestational weight gain and offspring weight in adolescence. *Obstetrics & Gynecology, 112*(5), 999–1006.

Preeti, R. J., Shiozawa, A., Haut, E., et al. (2011). An assessment of the impact of pregnancy on trauma. *Surgery, 149*(1), 94–98.

Public Health Agency of Canada. (2008). *Folic acid: Why all women who could become pregnant should be taking folic acid.* Retrieved February 20, 2012 from http://www.phac-aspc.gc.ca/fa-af/index-eng.php

Rasmussen, K. M., & Yaktine, K. L. (Eds.). (2009). *Weight gain during pregnancy: Reexamining the guidelines.* Retrieved February 20, 2012 from http://www.nap.edu/catalog.php?record_id=12584

Ricci, S. (2009). *Essentials of maternity, newborn and women's health nursing.* Philadelphia: Lippincott Williams & Wilkins.

Rubin, R. (1984). *Maternal identity and the maternal experience.* New York: Springer.

Sabella, C., & Cunningham, R. J., III. (Eds.). (2010). *The Cleveland Clinic intensive review of pediatrics* (3rd ed.). Philadelphia: Lippincott Williams & Wilkins.

Sanu, O., & Lamont, R. (2011). Hyperemesis gravidarum: Pathogenesis and the use of antiemetic agents. *Expert Opinion on Pharmacotherapy, 12*(5), 737–748.

Schack-Nielson, L., Michaelsen, K. F., Gamborg, M., Mortensen, E. L., & Sørensen, T. I. (2010). Gestational weight gain in relation to offspring body mass index and obesity from infancy through adulthood. *International Journal of Obesity, 34*(1), 67–74.

Scholl, T. (2008). Maternal nutrition and pregnancy outcome. In C. Duggan, J. Watkins, & W. Walker (Eds.), *Nutrition in pediatrics: Basic science & clinical applications.* Hamilton, ON: BC Decker Inc.

Shields, A. (2012). *Pregnancy diagnosis.* Retrieved February 20, 2012 from http://emedicine.medscape.com/article/262591-overview#aw2aab6b4

Simpson, K. R., & Creehan, P. A. (Eds.). (2008). *AWHONN perinatal nursing* (3rd ed.). Philadelphia: Lippincott Williams & Wilkins.

Soutou, B., Régnier, S., Nassar, D. Parant, O., Khosroterhrani, K., & Aractingi, S. (2009). Dermatological manifestations associated with pregnancy. *Expert Review of Dermatology, 4*(4), 329–340.

Taylor, R., Badell, N., & Martina, L. (2011). The endocrinology of pregnancy. In D. G. Gardner & D. Shoback (Eds.), *Greenspan's Basic & Clinical Endocrinology* (9th ed.). New York: McGraw-Hill Medical.

Timmons, B., Akins, M., & Mahendroo, M. (2010). Cervical remodeling during pregnancy and parturition. *Trends in Endocrinology & Metabolism, 21*(6), 353–361.

Veltri, L. (2010). Family nursing with childbearing families. In J. Kaakinen, V. Gedaly-Duff, D. Padgett Coehlo, & S. Harmon Hanson (Eds.), *Family health care nursing: Theory, practice and research* (4th ed.). Philadelphia: FA Davis.

Viswanathan, M., Siega-Riz, A. M., Moos, M. K., et al. (2008). *Outcomes of maternal weight gain: Evidence report/technology assessment no. 168. AHRQ Publication No. 08-E009.* Rockville, MD: Agency for Healthcare Research and Quality.

Ward, S. L., & Hisley, S. M. (2009). *Maternal-child nursing care: Optimizing outcomes for mothers, children & families.* Philadelphia: FA Davis.

Widen, E., & Siega-Riz, A. (2010). Prenatal nutrition: A practical guide for assessment and counselling. *Journal of Midwifery & Women's Health, 55*(6), 540–549. doi:10.1016/j.jmwh.2010.06.017

Witkin, S., Linhares, I., Bongiovanni, A., Herway, C., & Skupski, D. (2011). Unique alterations in infection-induced immune activation during pregnancy. *BJOG: An International Journal of Obstetrics & Gynaecology, 118*(2), 145–153.

Young, S. L. (2010). Pica in pregnancy: New ideas about an old condition. *Annual Review of Nutrition, 30,* 403–422. doi:10.1146/annurev.nutr.012809.104713

Zhang, X., Decker, A., Platt, R. W., & Kramer, M. S. (2008). How big is too big? The perinatal consequences of fetal macrosomia. *American Journal of Obstetrics and Gynecology, 198*(5):517.e1–517.e6.

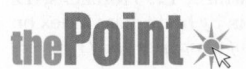

CHAPTER WORKSHEET

MULTIPLE CHOICE QUESTIONS

1. What factors would change during a pregnancy if the hormone progesterone were reduced or withdrawn?

    a. The woman's gums would become red and swollen and would bleed easily.

    b. The uterus would contract more and peristalsis would increase.

    c. Morning sickness would increase and would be prolonged.

    d. It would inhibit the secretion of prolactin by the pituitary gland.

2. Which of the following is a presumptive sign or symptom of pregnancy?

    a. Restlessness

    b. Elevated mood

    c. Urinary frequency

    d. Low backache

3. When obtaining a blood test for pregnancy, which hormone would the nurse expect the test to measure?

    a. hCG

    b. hPL

    c. FSH

    d. LH

4. During pregnancy, which of the following should the expectant mother reduce or avoid?

    a. Raw meat or uncooked shellfish

    b. Fresh, washed fruits and vegetables

    c. Whole grains

    d. Protein and iron from meat sources

5. A feeling expressed by most women upon learning they are pregnant is:

    a. Acceptance

    b. Depression

    c. Jealousy

    d. Ambivalence

6. Reva Rubin identified four major tasks that the pregnant woman undertakes to form a mutually gratifying relationship with her infant. What is "binding in"?

    a. Ensuring safe passage through pregnancy, labour, and birth

    b. Seeking acceptance of this infant by others

    c. Seeking acceptance of self as mother to the infant

    d. Learning to give of oneself on behalf of the infant

CRITICAL THINKING EXERCISES

1. When interviewing a woman at her first prenatal visit, the nurse asks about her feelings. The woman replies, "I'm frightened and confused. I don't know whether I want to be pregnant or not. Being pregnant means changing our whole life, and now having somebody to care for all the time. I'm not sure I will be a good mother. Plus I'm a bit afraid of all the changes that will happen to my body. Is this normal? Am I okay?"

    a. How should the nurse answer these questions?

    b. What specific information is needed to support the client during this pregnancy?

2. Sally, age 23, is 9 weeks pregnant. At her clinic visit she says, "I'm so tired I can barely make it home from work. Then once I'm home, I don't have the energy to make dinner." She says she is so sick in the morning that she is frequently late to work and spends much of the day in the bathroom. Sally's current lab work is within normal limits.

    a. What explanation can the nurse offer Sally about her discomforts?

    b. What interventions can the nurse offer to Sally?

3. Bringing a new infant into the family affects the siblings. What strategies can a nurse discuss when a mother asks how to deal with this?

(question continues on page 330)

STUDY ACTIVITIES

1. Go to your local health department's maternity clinic and interview several women regarding their feelings and the bodily changes that have taken place since they became pregnant. Based on your findings, place them into appropriate trimesters of their pregnancy.

2. Search the Internet for information about the psychological changes that occur during pregnancy. Share your websites with your clinical group.

3. During pregnancy, the plasma volume increases by 50% but the RBC volume increases by only 25% to 33%. This disproportion is manifested as

   _____.

4. When a pregnant woman in her third trimester lies on her back and experiences dizziness and lightheadedness, the underlying cause of this is

   _____.

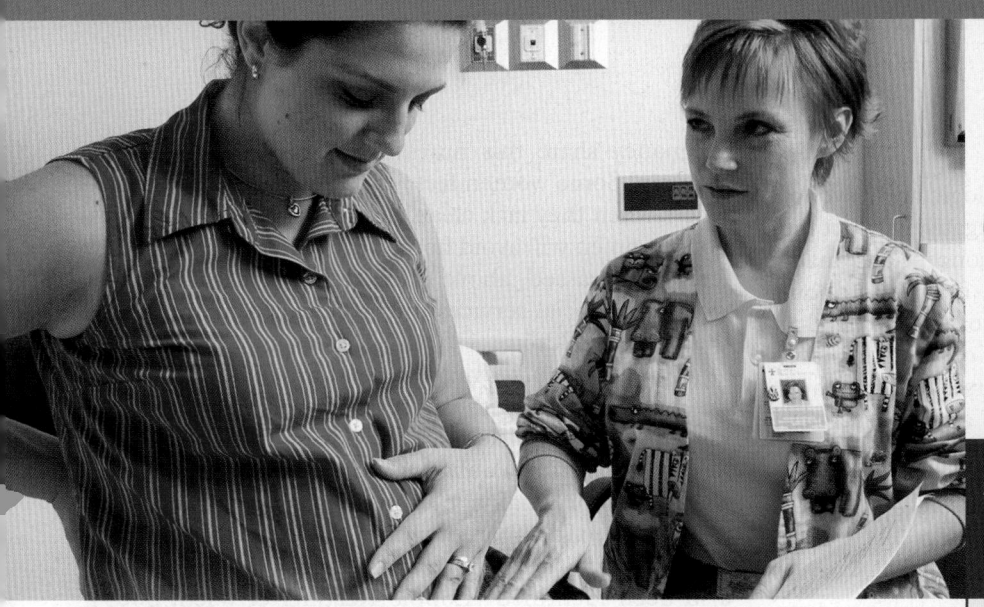

NURSING MANAGEMENT DURING PREGNANCY

KEY TERMS

alpha-fetoprotein
amniocentesis
biophysical profile
chorionic villus sampling
  (CVS)

gravida
high-risk pregnancy
nuchal translucency
para
perinatal education

preconception care
risk factors
teratogen

LEARNING OBJECTIVES

Upon completion of the chapter, the learner will be able to:

1. Define the key terms used in this chapter.
2. Discuss the opportunities for health promotion from preconception throughout pregnancy and the contributions nurses make working in partnership with pregnant women and their families.
3. Identify risk factors that affect pregnancy outcomes (the health of mothers and babies) and substances that may have teratogenic effects on the fetus.
4. Describe the components of health assessment for the woman before and during pregnancy (includes appropriate history taking, physical examination, and laboratory evaluation).
5. Describe the components of fetal health assessment.
6. Discuss strategies that promote health and comfort during pregnancy.
7. Describe the range of approaches to perinatal education in Canada.

Linda and her partner, Rob, are eager to start a family within the next year. They decide to check out a new midwifery practice located in their community, and they go for a preconception appointment. They leave their appointment overwhelmed with all the information they were given about having a healthy pregnancy.

Wow

Pregnancy has been called the "teachable moment" in the lives of women and families as pregnancy provides many opportunities for health teaching. However, "teaching is more than telling" (Tiedje, 2004) and requires skilled nurses who can build relationships with childbearing women and help them to make sense of the health information in the context of their lives.

Pregnancy is a time of many physiologic and psychological changes that can positively or negatively affect the woman, her fetus, and her family. Misconceptions, inadequate information, and unanswered questions about pregnancy, birth, and parenthood are common. The ultimate goal of any pregnancy is the birth of a healthy newborn within a healthy family, and nurses play a major role in helping the pregnant woman and her partner achieve this goal. Ongoing assessment and health education are essential.

This chapter describes nursing management for health promotion during pregnancy. It begins with a brief discussion of preconception care and then describes the assessment of the woman at the first prenatal visit and on follow-up visits. The chapter discusses tests commonly used to assess maternal and fetal well-being, including specific nursing management related to each test. The chapter also identifies important strategies to minimize the common discomforts of pregnancy and promote self-care. Lastly, the chapter discusses perinatal education, including childbirth education, birthing options, care provider options, preparation for breastfeeding or bottle-feeding, and final preparation for labour and birth.

Registered nurses (RNs) in Canada work with childbearing women in a variety of settings with a primary focus on promoting health and preventing pregnancy risks or adverse outcomes. For example, an RN might work in a rural, remote, or Aboriginal community providing comprehensive primary health care services. In other settings the RN may provide prenatal education or care in collaboration with a physician, midwife, or nurse practitioner (NP). In large urban settings, the RN may provide nursing care in a highly specialized out-patient clinic or for women hospitalized with pregnancy complications. Some women experiencing pregnancy complications are cared for by nurses working in small community hospitals or in the community. Some RNs provide perinatal health education classes for women and their partners as they prepare for childbirth, newborn care, and/or parenting (Wallace, Dodd, McNeil, et al., 2009).

The purpose of preconception and prenatal care is to promote the health of the woman, baby, and family and to identify and modify **risk factors** that are known to influence pregnancy outcomes. Some of these known pregnancy risks reflect broad social determinants of health, such as poverty. Poverty influences health in pregnancy and may interact with other social factors such as age, race, ethnicity, and sexual orientation. Poverty limits resources such as safe housing and food security and may also be linked to lower educational levels, decreased health literacy, and under- or unemployment. The lack of money may also limit access to prenatal care since women may lack reliable child care and transportation. Some women who receive food supplements in pregnancy share this nutritious food with their other children. Some women feel judged by prenatal care providers when they lack clean clothing or shower facilities. Some women will avoid home visits by nurses when they feel embarrassed about their home environment or worry that social services might be called to apprehend their other children.

Canadian nurses need to be aware of how the social determinants of health can result in health inequities or institutionalized differences in access to the resources needed for health (Pauly, MacKinnon, & Varcoe, 2009). Because Aboriginal women have poor pregnancy outcomes when compared with Canadian women as a whole, social determinants of Aboriginal health have also been identified (Loppie Reading & Wien, 2009). Addressing these broad social factors requires a comprehensive, intersectoral community development approach. In Canada, many such teams have been led by public health nurses working in collaboration with groups and communities. Nurses can act as advocates and educators, creating healthy, supportive communities for women and their partners in the childbearing phases of their lives.

Preconception Care

Preconception care is the promotion of the health and well-being of a woman and her partner before pregnancy. The goal of preconception care is to identify health problems, lifestyle habits, or social concerns that might unfavourably affect pregnancy and to promote health for the childbearing woman and her family (Centers for Disease Control and Prevention [CDC], 2012; Society of Obstetricians and Gynaecologists of Canada [SOGC], 2011a).

A lifespan approach to preconception care has been proposed as a strategy to decrease poor birth outcomes (Malnory & Johnson, 2011). "A lifecourse model suggests a complex interplay of biological, behavioural, psychological, and social protective and risk factors that contribute to health outcomes" (p. 110). The goal of the lifespan approach is to decrease prematurity and unintended pregnancy. Primary health care for women focuses on optimizing women's health to decrease health risks prior to conception. When providing nursing care during the preconception or interconception intervals, RNs work in collaborative partnerships with women and family members and frequently with other maternity care providers. Nursing management focuses on health promotion and risk prevention.

Health Promotion

Women's health promotion needs to be grounded in the principles of woman and family-centred care and provided in culturally safe ways that acknowledge the woman's culture and life ways. The principles for woman-centred perinatal care include:

- Recognition that pregnancy and childbirth are normal life events for most women
- The need to support women to participate fully in their care
- Provision of woman-centred services that are grounded in understanding women's values and needs
- Engaging women and their family members as partners in maternity care services (Perinatal Services BC, 2010a)

These principles reflect a philosophical approach to care that is congruent with cultural competence and cultural safety.

Cultural safety is a complex concept that recognizes many cultural differences, including age, gender, race, ethnicity, and social class, as well the culture of health care professions and health systems (Browne, Varcoe, Smye, et al., 2009). Cultural safety is congruent with the concept of cultural competence (Leininger & McFarland, 2002) but goes beyond cultural awareness and sensitivity toward acknowledgement of power differentials that exist in nursing encounters. As such, cultural safety builds on transcultural nursing (Maier-Lorentz, 2008) to help nurses develop the skills needed for truly collaborative partnerships between nurses and their "patients" (women and family members). Rather than providing the same care to everyone regardless of culture, cultural safety is mindful of cultural differences (Richardson & MacGibbon, 2010). For example, women who are not accustomed to the prevalent culture of potential risk in childbearing may be frightened or overwhelmed by some Canadian maternity care practices (Lewallen, 2011).

Preventing Adverse Pregnancy Outcomes

Preconception care is just as important as prenatal care to reduce adverse pregnancy outcomes such as maternal and infant mortality, preterm births, and low birth weight infants. Adverse pregnancy outcomes constitute a major public health challenge. In 2004, for example, 8.2% of infants born in Canada were premature, 7.8% were born at less than the 10th percentile of weight for gestational age (small for gestational age [SGA]), 11.6% were born above the 90th percentile of weight for gestational age (large for gestational age [LGA]), and 4.8% had major congenital anomalies (Public Health Agency of Canada [PHAC], 2008a). One recent success story is that the prevalence of neural tube defects (NTDs) in Canada decreased by more than 50% between 1995 and 2004; this was largely attributed to the addition of folic acid to enriched flour and other cereals and the inclusion of folic acid in women's vitamin supplements. Although rates of

maternal mortality are low, maternal morbidity remains a significant health issue (PHAC, 2008a). It remains troubling, however, that for almost every indicator measured, young women, women who have less than a high school education, women who live in households below the low-income cut-off, and women who live in the Northern territories have relatively poorer pregnancy outcomes (PHAC, 2009).

Additional risk factors for adverse pregnancy outcomes are prevalent among women of reproductive age, as demonstrated by the following statistics from PHAC (2008a, 2009):

- 22% of Canadian women report smoking in the 3 months preceding pregnancy, and 23.4% are exposed to secondhand smoke in the home environment during pregnancy.
- Maternal alcohol consumption in pregnancy in known to be under-reported, with 10% to 20% of Canadian women stating that they consume alcohol during pregnancy.
- 42% of women do not take folic acid supplements before pregnancy, increasing the risk of NTDs in the newborn.
- 13.6% of Canadian women starting a pregnancy are obese (body mass index [BMI] of 30 kg/m² or greater), which may increase their risk of developing hypertension, diabetes, and thromboembolic disease and may increase the need for cesarean birth.
- Some women take prescription or over-the-counter drugs that are known **teratogens** (substances harmful to the developing fetus).
- About 5% of women have preexisting medical conditions that can negatively affect pregnancy if unmanaged.

All of these factors pose risks to pregnancy, and many of them should be addressed during every interaction with a health provider. Specific recognized risk factors for adverse pregnancy outcomes and some interventions to prevent them are listed in Table 12.1.

The PHAC (2005) has identified three effective preconception interventions to improve the health of women and newborns:

- Smoking cessation programs before and during pregnancy
- Screening and counselling women who drink alcohol in pregnancy to reduce consumption
- Folic acid supplementation before pregnancy.

RNs can take an active role in reducing pregnancy risks by learning how to provide smoking cessation interventions (Registered Nurses' Association of Ontario [RNAO], 2007), by counselling women about the use of alcohol and other harmful substances during pregnancy, and by ensuring that all women of childbearing age have

TABLE 12.1 RISK FACTORS FOR ADVERSE PREGNANCY OUTCOMES AND AVAILABLE INTERVENTIONS

Risk Factor or Condition of Vulnerability	Available Interventions	Demonstrated Health Effects
Retinoic acid (Accutane) for cystic acne	Pregnancy prevention	Eliminates teratogenic effects on fetus
Alcohol use	Eliminating alcohol use (effects are related to timing and dose, so no safe level of alcohol use in pregnancy has been identified) (SOGC, 2010a).	Controlling alcohol binge drinking and/or frequent drinking prevents fetal alcohol spectrum disorders and other known teratogenic effects
Anti-epileptic drugs	Changing to a less teratogenic regimen before pregnancy	Decreases teratogenic effects
Anti-coagulants (oral)	Switching women off teratogenic anticoagulants (Warfarin) before pregnancy	Decreases teratogenic effects
Not breastfeeding	Promoting breastfeeding for the majority of women and babies. Exclusive breastfeeding for the first 6 months of the baby's life is currently recommended (CPS, 2009).	Protects against respiratory and gastrointestinal illness in the newborn; also results in fewer allergies, lower rates of sudden infant death syndrome (SIDS), and may prevent childhood obesity; improves weight loss in the mother
Diabetes (preconception)	Diabetes management (SOGC, 2007f)	Substantially reduces the risk of birth defects among infants of diabetic mothers
Folic acid deficiency	Folic acid supplementation (SOGC, 2007d)	Reduces occurrence of neural tube defects (NTDs) by two thirds
Hepatitis B	Hepatitis B vaccination for women of reproductive age (SOGC, 2009b)	Prevents transmission of infection to infants in utero and eliminates the risks of hepatic failure, liver carcinoma, cirrhosis, and death in the mother
Hypothyroidism	Adjusting levothyroxine dosage early in pregnancy	Protects fetal neurologic development
HIV/AIDS	HIV screening and treatment (SOGC, 2006a)	Allows for timely treatment for women (couples) and the administration of anti-retroviral drugs during pregnancy to prevent transmission to the fetus
Maternal phenylketonuria (PKU)	Maternal PKU management before pregnancy	Prevents babies from being born with PKU-related mental retardation
Mental health challenges or mood disorders (including depression and anxiety)	Identification and treatment of depression before, during, or after pregnancy; mobilization of maternal support systems	Helps prevent negative health effects in the mother, infant, and other family members
Rubella seronegativity	Rubella vaccination before pregnancy (or postpartum) (SOGC, 2007c)	Provides protection against congenital rubella syndrome
Obesity	Reaching a healthy weight before pregnancy and achieving a healthy weight gain during pregnancy based on pre-pregnancy BMI (SOGC, 2010b)	Helps reduce the risk of NTDs, preterm birth, and diabetes in the newborn; decreases risk of cesarean birth; and helps reduce the risk of hypertensive disorders and thromboembolic disease in the mother
Poor oral hygiene	Oral hygiene and dental care before and during pregnancy	Decreases preterm birth rates, improves maternal health
Sexually transmitted infections (STIs)	STI screening and treatment (Perinatal Services BC, 2010a)	Reduces the risk of ectopic pregnancy, infertility, and chronic pelvic pain (*Chlamydia trachomatis* and *Neisseria gonorrhoeae*) and also reduces the possible risk to a fetus of death or disability (including mental retardation and blindness)

Risk Factor or Condition of Vulnerability	Available Interventions	Demonstrated Health Effects
Smoking	Smoking cessation programs and counselling; programs that include partners and family members to promote health and decrease environmental exposure (secondhand smoke) (RNAO, 2007)	Prevents preterm birth, low birth weight, and other adverse outcomes (e.g., SIDS) associated with smoking during pregnancy
Street drug use (may be an indirect indicator as it is also associated with smoking, alcohol use, and poor nutrition); poly-drug use is common	Early prenatal care with referral to addiction counselling services as needed; housing support may be required	Can help prevent low birth weight, preterm birth, and development/behavioural problems in childhood; some drugs (e.g., cocaine) can cause placental abruption and fetal death
Underweight and poor nutrition	Nutrition counselling and taking food and vitamin supplements as needed	Preterm birth, low birth weight
Violence or physical abuse	Screening for abuse (physical, emotional, domination, or sexual) when the partner is not in the room; discussing a safety plan; valuing the woman and promoting self-esteem (SOGC, 2005c)	Helps to prevent adverse effects in the mother and infant
Working conditions (heavy lifting, strenuous work, prolonged standing, shift work or highly stressful working conditions)	Job re-assignments or early maternity leave as indicated	May help prevent preterm birth and adverse maternal health effects

Adapted from: Public Health Agency of Canada. (2008a). *The Canadian Perinatal Health Report, 2008 edition.* Retrieved February 21, 2012 from http://www.phac-aspc.gc.ca/publicat/2008/cphr-rspc/index-eng.php; and Public Health Agency of Canada. (2009). *What mothers say: The Canadian Maternity Experiences Survey.* Retrieved February 21, 2012 from http://www.phac-aspc.gc.ca/rhs-ssg/pdf/survey-eng.pdf.

folic acid supplementation. For women with pre-existing health challenges or familial genetic risk factors, RNs can encourage women and their partners to have a pre-conception health assessment with their primary care provider. All women need to be encouraged and supported to be as healthy as possible both prior to and during pregnancy (SOGC, 2011a).

Preconception Health Assessment

Ideally, couples thinking about having a child schedule a visit with their health care provider for preconception counselling to ensure that they are in the best possible state of health before pregnancy. The period of greatest environmental sensitivity and consequent risk for the developing embryo is between days 17 and 56 after conception (Coad & Dunstall, 2011). The first prenatal visit, which is usually a month or more after a missed menstrual period, may occur too late to affect reproductive outcomes associated with abnormal organogenesis. In some cases, such as with unintended pregnancies, women may delay seeking health care, denying that they are pregnant. Thus, commonly used prevention practices

may begin too late to avert the morbidity and mortality associated with congenital anomalies and low birth weight (PHAC, 2005; SOGC, 2011a). Therefore, before conception (and between pregnancies) is considered an optimal time for health promotion and prevention of adverse pregnancy outcomes.

What is the purpose of couples like Linda and Rob going for preconception counselling? What are the goals of preconception care for this couple? Consider the resources available for this English-speaking couple. What difference would it make if they spoke limited or no English? Where could you find appropriate prenatal resources in other languages spoken in Canada?

Nursing Management

Preconception care involves obtaining a complete health history and physical examination of the woman and her partner. The health history helps identify the impact and implications of chronic medical conditions and past obstetric/gynecologic history on future fertility and pregnancies. Women with chronic medical conditions may be referred to the appropriate specialist. Key areas to consider in preconception health assessment for women and their partners include:

- Underlying medical conditions, such as cardiovascular and respiratory problems or genetic disorders
- Communicable disease history, including rubella susceptibility, varicella, human immunodeficiency virus (HIV), and herpes
- Immunization status of the woman to ensure that her immunizations are up to date
- Reproductive health data, such as pelvic examinations, use of contraceptives, and other sexually transmitted infections (STIs)
- Sexuality (gender) and sexual practices, such as safer-sex practices and body image issues
- Nutrition history, present nutrition status (e.g., folic acid intake), and BMI
- Lifestyle and health practices, including occupation, exercise, and recreational activities
- Psychosocial issues, such as levels of stress and exposure to abuse and violence
- Medication and drug use, including use of tobacco, alcohol, over-the-counter and prescription medications, and illicit drugs
- Family history to identify any medical or genetic conditions (e.g., Bloom syndrome, cystic fibrosis, familial dysautonomia, Tay–Sachs disease, thalassemia, sickle-cell anemia) that require treatment or a referral to specialists
- Support systems, including family, friends, and community (SOGC, 2006a, 2006c, 2008a, 2008b, 2008e, 2011a; PHAC, 2005, 2006)

The information obtained during the history and physical examination also provides a foundation for tailored health education. Nurses play an important role in the provision of appropriate and understandable health information. It is important to enter into a collaborative partnership with the woman and her partner, enabling them to examine their own health and its influence on the health of their future baby. Provide information to allow the woman and her partner to make an informed decision about having a baby (see Box 12.1), but keep in mind that this decision rests solely with the couple.

▶ **Take** NOTE!

Health promotion activities, such as preconception care, should be integrated into women's primary health care.

BOX 12.1 Preconception Health Information

The following topics have been identified as appropriate for discussion with all women of reproductive age:
- Benefits of a planned pregnancy and good health prior to conception
- Contraceptive choices that meet the timing of desired pregnancy
- Importance of taking folic acid before conception to prevent neural tube defects
- Vitamin supplementation (including vitamin D) and a healthy diet (may include a diet history and referral to nutritionist as needed)
- Food safety and how to reduce the risk of a food-acquired infection
- Weight management, including healthy pre-pregnancy weight (BMI of 19 to 27) and risks associated with underweight, overweight, and obesity.
- Physical fitness and activity
- Genetic testing and counselling as appropriate
- Safe use of medications, herbs, and supplements
- Substance use issues, including smoking, alcohol, and drugs.
- Smoking cessation counselling and prevention of fetal alcohol spectrum disorders
- Referrals for substance use as appropriate
- Stressors in the work environment and any needed changes to promote health
- Environmental hazards, including metals and other contaminants
- Accident prevention, including seat belt use
- Healthy sexuality and safer sex
- Healthy relationship and parenting information
- Building a social support network to promote self-esteem and prevent anxiety and depression
- Housing options and social services available (as needed)
- Developing a safety plan and getting help for victims of violence
- Self-management of chronic conditions such as diabetes and asthma

Adapted from: Perinatal Services BC. (2010a). *BCPHP Obstetric Guide 19: Maternity care pathway.* Retrieved February 21, 2012 from http://www.perinatalservicesbc.ca//sites/bcrcp/files/Guidelines/Obstetrics/Guideline_19.pdf.

Linda and Rob decide to change several aspects of their lifestyle and nutritional habits before conceiving a baby, based on advice from the midwife. They both want to lose weight, stop smoking, and increase their intake of fruits and vegetables. How will these alterations in health practices benefit Linda's future pregnancy and promote health for the family? How could you help this couple with smoking cessation?

Prenatal Care

Women and their families are important partners in prenatal care and health promotion. Prenatal care in Canada is publicly funded and provided as part of primary health care services. Physicians, midwives, and NPs are responsible for the care of pregnant women and may work in multidisciplinary teams with other nurses, nutritionists, social workers, physiotherapists, and childbirth educators. Given Canada's vast and varied geography and the difficulties providing comprehensive maternity services in rural, remote, and Aboriginal communities, multidisciplinary collaborative maternity care has been proposed as the way to ensure appropriate access to prenatal care and health education and to address health inequities. The Multidisciplinary Collaborative Primary Maternity Care Project explored ways to address the impact of the human resource shortage in maternity care by maximizing the collaboration of all professional groups. Although representatives of national professional associations supported multidisciplinary collaborative maternity care, they also identified educational, structural, and relational barriers to collaborative practice (Peterson, Medves, Davies, et al., 2007).

The new models of prenatal care that are being implemented across Canada are more congruent with woman- and family-centred collaborative maternity care principles and cultural safety. Examples include programs that share health information, promote informed decision making, and incorporate health promotion strategies as early in pregnancy as possible (Wallace et al., 2009). Some creative programs utilize online technologies to promote prenatal education and collaborative maternity care (Alberta Health Services, 2009).

Group prenatal care or centering pregnancy programs integrate health education with maternity care visits from a multidisciplinary team that includes nurses (BC Women's Hospital, 2010). Many of these programs include counselling for smoking cessation and other identified health concerns (Bottorff, Lalaw, Johnson, et al., 2005; Okoli, Greaves, Bottorff, et al., 2010). Some programs, such as the Canada Prenatal Nutrition Program, are designed to address the social determinants of health and provide multidisciplinary care along with food supplements (PHAC, 2010d). The Canada Prenatal Nutrition Program also provides services in Inuit communities and on many First Nations reserves. Special programs are also available for new immigrants to Canada (Best Start Resource Centre, 2009).

Because nurses provide perinatal care to women and families from diverse cultural backgrounds, they need to remain open to learning about the woman's values, beliefs, and health practices that affect childbearing. Providing culturally competent nursing care also requires learning how to advocate for women and families, assess health literacy, and use interpreter services (Lewallen, 2011). As discussed earlier, Canadian RNs are also learning to provide culturally safe nursing care (Browne et al., 2009).

Specialized services, such as perinatal mental health programs, may also be available in larger urban centres. For women who may have experienced violence, racism, street involvement or homelessness, or substance use, women-centred care principles can also include harm reduction and trauma-informed "one-stop" coordinated prenatal care (BC Centre of Excellence for Women's Health, 2010; Garm, 1999).

The First Prenatal Visit

Once a pregnancy is suspected and, in many cases, tentatively confirmed by a home pregnancy test, women seek prenatal care to promote a healthy outcome. The assessment process begins at this initial prenatal visit and continues throughout the pregnancy. The initial visit is an ideal time to screen for factors that might place the woman and her fetus at risk for problems such as preterm delivery. The initial visit also is an optimal time to begin working in partnership with the woman to provide health information about changes that will affect her life. Pregnant women and their partners frequently have questions, misinformation, or misconceptions about what to eat, weight gain, physical discomforts, drug and alcohol use, sexuality, and the birthing process. The nurse needs to allow time during all prenatal visits to answer questions and provide anticipatory guidance and to make appropriate community referrals to meet the needs of these women.

Comprehensive Health History

During the initial visit, a comprehensive health history is obtained, including age, menstrual history, prior obstetric history, past medical and surgical history, family health history, genetic screening, medication or drug use, and history of exposure to infections (including STIs) (Perinatal Services BC, 2010a). Prenatal forms vary from province to province but have many similarities. The Antenatal Psychosocial Health Assessment (Reid, Biringer, Carroll, et al., 1998) has been incorporated into many provincial assessment forms and includes family factors, maternal factors, substance abuse, and family violence. Nurses need to be aware that many pregnant women experience intimate partner violence and be prepared when women disclose abuse in pregnancy (SOGC, 2005c). To encourage more collaborative relationships between women and their maternity care providers, Perinatal Services BC (2012) released a Pregnancy Passport that women can carry with them throughout the childbearing year.

The initial health history typically includes questions about three major areas: the reason for seeking care; the woman's past medical, surgical, and personal health history, including that of her family and her partner; and the woman's reproductive history. During the history-taking process, the nurse and woman establish the foundation for a trusting relationship and jointly develop a plan of care for the pregnancy. Tailor this plan to the woman's lifestyle as much as possible and focus primarily on education for overall wellness during pregnancy. The ultimate goal is health promotion and early detection and prevention of any problems that occur during pregnancy (SOGC, 2011a).

Reason for Seeking Care

The woman commonly comes for prenatal care based on the suspicion that she is pregnant. She may report that she has missed her menstrual period or has had a positive result on a home pregnancy test. Ask the woman for the date of her last menstrual period (LMP). Also ask about any presumptive or probable signs of pregnancy that she might be experiencing. Typically, a urine or blood test to check for evidence of human chorionic gonadotropin (hCG) is done to confirm the pregnancy.

Health History

Ask about the woman's health history, including medical conditions and surgery. This information is important because health conditions that the woman experienced in the past (e.g., urinary tract infections) may recur or be exacerbated during pregnancy. Also, chronic illnesses, such as diabetes or heart disease, can increase the risk for complications during pregnancy for the woman and her fetus. Ask about any history of allergies to medications, foods, or environmental substances. Ask about any mental health problems, such as depression or anxiety. Gather similar information about the woman's family and her partner.

The woman's social and environmental health history also are important. Ask about her occupation, possible exposure to teratogens (substances with the potential to alter the fetus permanently in form or function), exercise and activity level, recreational patterns, use of substances such as alcohol, tobacco, and drugs, use of alternative and complementary therapies, sleep patterns, nutritional habits, and general lifestyle. Each of the social determinants of health may have an impact on the woman's health and the outcome of her pregnancy (PHAC, 2010o). For example, if the woman smokes during pregnancy, nicotine in cigarettes causes vasoconstriction in the mother, leading to reduced placental perfusion. As a result, the newborn may be SGA and at increased risk for sudden infant death syndrome (SIDS) (SIDS Canada, 2010). In addition, no safe level of alcohol consumption in pregnancy has been determined (PHAC, 2010a). Many fetuses exposed to heavy alcohol levels during pregnancy develop fetal alcohol spectrum disorders (FASD), a collection of deformities and disabilities believed to result from maternal alcohol use during pregnancy (SOGC, 2010a).

Reproductive History

The woman's reproductive history includes a menstrual, obstetric, and gynecologic history. Typically, this history begins with a description of the woman's menstrual cycle, including her age at menarche, number of days in her cycle, typical flow characteristics, and any discomfort experienced. The use of contraception also is important, including when the woman last used any contraception.

The average age of childbearing for women in Canada is on the rise, and more women are turning to assisted reproductive technologies, such as in vitro fertilization (IVF), to become pregnant (SOGC, 2006b). The nurse should tactfully inquire about the woman's experiences with these complex programs and procedures.

Ask the woman the date of her LMP to determine the estimated or expected date of birth (EDB). Several methods may be used to estimate this date. Using Nagele's rule, subtract 3 months and then add 7 days to the first day of the LMP. Then correct the year by adding 1. This date has a margin of error of plus or minus 2 weeks. For instance, if a woman reports that her LMP started on October 14, 2011, you would subtract 3 months (July) and add 7 days (21), then add 1 year (2012). This woman's EDB is July 21, 2012. A gestational or birth calculator or wheel can also be used to calculate the due date (Fig. 12.1). Web tools are also available to assist women with this calculation (PHAC, 2010h).

Because of the normal variations in women's menstrual cycles, differences in the normal length of gestation between ethnic groups, and errors in dating methods, there is no such thing as an exact "due date." In general, a birth 2 weeks before or 2 weeks after the EDB is considered normal. Nagele's rule is less accurate if the woman's menstrual cycles are irregular, if the woman conceives while breastfeeding or before her regular menstrual cycle is established, if she is ovulating even though she is amenorrheic, or if she conceives soon after discontinuing oral contraceptives (Cunningham, Leveno, Bloom, et al., 2010). Some practitioners use ultrasound to more accurately determine the gestational age and date the pregnancy; this is increasingly becoming the norm in Canada, where most women have two or more ultrasounds during pregnancy (PHAC, 2009).

Typically, an obstetric history provides information about the woman's past pregnancies, including any problems encountered during the pregnancy, labour, delivery, and afterward. Such information can provide clues to problems that might develop in the current pregnancy. Some common terms used to describe and document an obstetric history include:

- **Gravid:** the state of being pregnant
- **Gravida:** a pregnant woman; gravida I (primigravida) during the first pregnancy, gravida II (secundigravida) during the second pregnancy, and so on

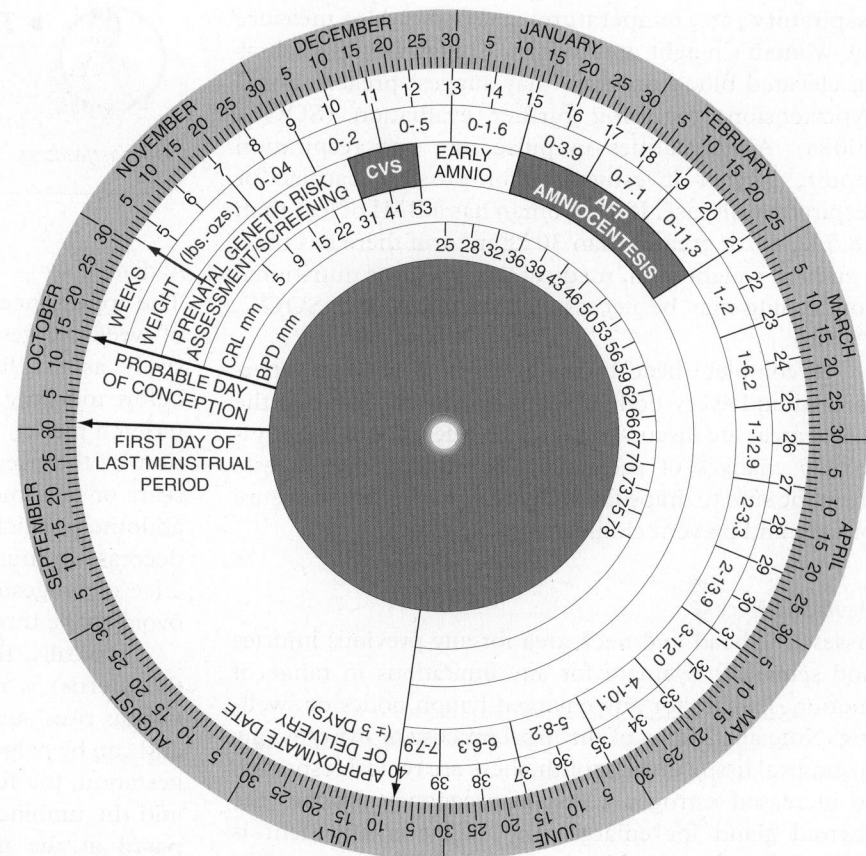

FIGURE 12.1 Estimating the date of birth using a birth wheel. The first day of the woman's last normal menstrual period was October 1. Using the birth wheel, her EDB would be approximately July 8 of the following year. (Used with permission. © 2007, March of Dimes.)

- **Para:** Parity refers to the number of times a woman has given birth to a child (live or stillborn) after 20 weeks' gestation. (Para means "having given birth" [Fraser & Cooper, 2009]). Babies born before 20 weeks are counted as an abortion (therapeutic or spontaneous).
  - Nullipara (para 0) is a woman who has not yet given birth after 20 weeks' gestation.
  - Primipara (para 1) is a woman who has given birth once after 20 weeks' gestation.
  - Multipara (para 2 or more) is a woman who has given birth more than once.

Other systems may be used to document a woman's obstetric history. These systems often break down the category of para more specifically and may include abortions (Box 12.2).

Information about the woman's gynecologic history is important. Ask about any reproductive tract surgeries the woman has undergone. For example, surgery on the uterus may affect its ability to contract effectively during labour. A history of tubal pregnancy increases the woman's risk for another tubal pregnancy. Also ask about safe-sex practices and any history of STIs.

Physical Examination

The next step in the assessment process is the physical examination, which detects any physical problems that may affect the pregnancy outcome. The initial physical examination provides the baseline for evaluating changes during future visits.

Begin the physical examination by obtaining a urine sample and vital signs, including blood pressure,

---

BOX 12.2 Obstetric History Terms

GTPAL or TPAL

G = gravida, T = term births, P = preterm births, A = abortions, L = living children

G—the current pregnancy

T—the number of term births at >37 weeks' gestation

P—the number of preterm births (between 20 and before completion of 37 weeks' gestation)

A—the number of births before 20 weeks' gestation

L—the number of children currently living

Consider this example:

Mary Johnson is pregnant for the fourth time. She had one abortion at 8 weeks' gestation. She has a daughter who was born at 40 weeks' gestation and a son born at 34 weeks. Mary's obstetric history would be documented as follows:

Using the gravida/para method: gravida 4, para 2

Using the TPAL method: 1112 (T = 1 [daughter born at 40 weeks]; P = 1 [son born at 34 weeks], A = 1 [abortion at 8 weeks]; L = 2 [two living children])

respiratory rate, temperature, and pulse. Also measure the woman's height and weight. Abnormalities such as an elevated blood pressure may suggest pregestational hypertension, requiring further evaluation (SOGC, 2008a). Abnormalities in pulse rate and respiration require further investigation for possible cardiac or respiratory disease. If the woman has a BMI of less than 18.5 kg/m^2 or greater than 30 kg/m^2 or if there has been a sudden weight gain, medical treatment or nutritional counselling may be necessary (PHAC, 2008b; SOGC, 2010b).

A complete head-to-toe assessment is usually performed and every body system is assessed. Some of the major areas are discussed here with reference to the physiologic changes of pregnancy. Throughout the assessment, be sure to drape the woman appropriately to ensure privacy and prevent chilling.

Head and Neck

Assess the head and neck area for any previous injuries and sequelae. Evaluate for any limitations in range of motion. Palpate for any enlarged lymph nodes or swelling. Note any edema of the nasal mucosa or hypertrophy of gingival tissue in the mouth; these are typical responses to increased estrogen levels in pregnancy. Palpate the thyroid gland for enlargement. Slight enlargement is normal, but marked enlargement may indicate hyperthyroidism, requiring further investigation.

Chest

Auscultate heart sounds, noting any abnormalities. A soft systolic murmur caused by the increase in blood volume may be noted. Anticipate an increase in heart rate by 10 to 15 beats/minute (starting between 14 and 20 weeks of pregnancy) secondary to increases in cardiac output and blood volume. The body adapts to the increase in blood volume with peripheral dilation to maintain blood pressure. Progesterone causes peripheral dilation (Coad & Dunstall, 2011).

Auscultate the chest for breath sounds, which should be clear. Also note symmetry of chest movement and thoracic breathing patterns. Estrogen promotes relaxation of the ligaments and joints of the ribs, with a resulting increase in the anteroposterior chest diameter. Expect a slight increase in respiratory rate to accommodate the increase in tidal volume and oxygen consumption.

Inspect and palpate the breasts. Increases in estrogen and progesterone and blood supply make the breasts feel full and more nodular, with increased sensitivity to touch. Blood vessels become more visible and there is an increase in breast size. Striae gravidarum (stretch marks) may be visible in some women. Darker pigmentation of the nipple and areola is present, along with enlargement of Montgomery's glands.

▶ **Take** NOTE!

Use this opportunity to teach breast self-examination and begin a discussion about breastfeeding.

Abdomen

The appearance of the abdomen depends on the number of weeks of gestation. The abdomen enlarges progressively as the fetus grows. Inspect the abdomen first before touching. Inspection may reveal striae gravidarum (stretch marks) and linea nigra, depending on the duration of the pregnancy. Look also for previous surgical scars or fetal movement. With warm hands, palpate the abdomen, which should be rounded and nontender. A decrease in muscle tone may be noted due to the influence of progesterone. The uterus maintains a globular/ovoid shape throughout pregnancy.

Typically, the height of the uterine fundus (top of the uterus) is measured to evaluate fetal growth. The fundus rises out of the pelvis at 12 to 14 weeks' gestation and can be palpated at the symphysis pubis. At 16 weeks' gestation, the fundus is midway between the symphysis and the umbilicus. At 20 weeks, the fundus can be palpated at the umbilicus and measures approximately 20 cm from the symphysis pubis. By 36 weeks the fundus is just below the ensiform cartilage and measures approximately 36 cm. This measurement is referred to as the symphysis–fundal height, which is measured from the symphysis pubis (pubic bone) to the uterine fundus (Coad & Dunstall, 2011).

Extremities

Inspect and palpate both legs for dependent edema, pulses, and varicose veins. If edema is present in early pregnancy, further evaluation may be needed to rule out pregestational hypertension. Ask the woman if she has any pain in her calf that increases when she ambulates. This might indicate a deep vein thrombosis (DVT). High levels of estrogen during pregnancy place women at higher risk for DVT (Coad & Dunstall, 2011).

Pelvic Examination

The pelvic examination provides information about the internal and external reproductive organs. In addition, it aids in assessing some of the early signs of pregnancy and allows for determination of pelvic adequacy. During the pelvic examination, remain in the examining room to assist the primary maternity care provider with any specimen collection, fixation, and labelling. Also provide comfort and emotional support for the woman, who might be anxious. Throughout the examination, explain what is happening and why, and answer questions.

External Genitalia

After the woman is placed in the lithotomy position and draped appropriately, the external genitalia are inspected visually. They should be free from lesions, discharge, hematomas, varicosities, and inflammation upon inspection. A culture for STIs may be collected at this time.

Internal Genitalia

Next, the internal genitalia are examined via a speculum. The cervix should be smooth, long, thick, and closed. Because of increased pelvic congestion, the cervix will be softened (Goodell's sign), the uterine isthmus will be softened (Hegar's sign), and there will be a bluish colouration of the cervix and vaginal mucosa (Chadwick's sign).

The uterus typically is pear-shaped and mobile, with a smooth surface. It will undergo cell hypertrophy and hyperplasia so that it enlarges throughout the pregnancy to accommodate the growing fetus.

During the pelvic examination, a Papanicolaou (Pap) smear is obtained. Additional cultures, such as for gonorrhea and chlamydia screening and group B streptococcus (GBS) screening, also may be obtained. Ensure that all specimens obtained are labelled correctly and sent to the laboratory for evaluation. A rectal examination is done last to assess for lesions, masses, prolapse, or hemorrhoids.

Once the examination of the internal genitalia is completed and the speculum is removed, a bimanual examination is performed to estimate the size of the uterus to confirm dates and to palpate the ovaries. The ovaries should be small and nontender, without masses.

Pelvic Size, Shape, and Measurements

The size and shape of the woman's pelvis can affect her ability to deliver vaginally. Pelvic shape is typically classified as one of four types: gynecoid, android, anthropoid, and platypelloid. Refer to Chapter 13 for an in-depth discussion of pelvic size and shape. The maternity care provider may also take internal pelvic measurements to determine the actual diameters of the inlet and outlet through which the fetus will pass. This can be important if the woman has never given birth vaginally. Three measurements are assessed: diagonal conjugate, true conjugate, and ischial tuberosity diameter (Fig. 12.2). Taking pelvic measurements is unnecessary for the woman who has given birth vaginally before (unless she has experienced some type of trauma to the area) because vaginal delivery demonstrates that the pelvis is adequate for the passage of the fetus.

Laboratory Tests

A series of tests is generally ordered during the initial visit so that baseline data can be obtained, allowing for early detection and prompt intervention if any problems occur. Tests that are generally conducted for all pregnant women include urinalysis and blood studies. The urine is analyzed for albumin, glucose, ketones, and bacteria. Blood studies usually include a complete blood count, blood typing, red cell antibodies and Rh factor, a rubella titer, hepatitis B surface antigen, HIV, and thyroid-stimulating hormone (TSH). STI testing (for syphilis, chlamydia, and gonorrhea) and a Pap test are also conducted (Perinatal Services BC, 2010a). (For more detailed information, see Table 12.2.)

The need for additional laboratory studies is determined by a woman's history, physical examination

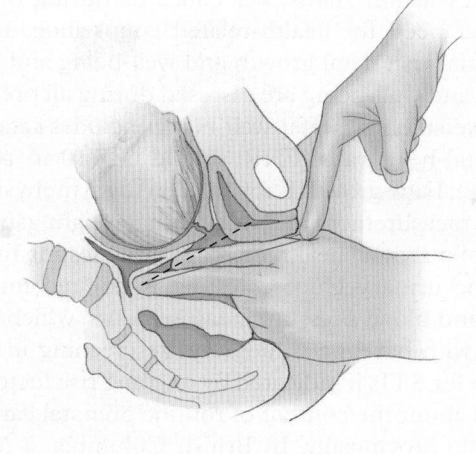

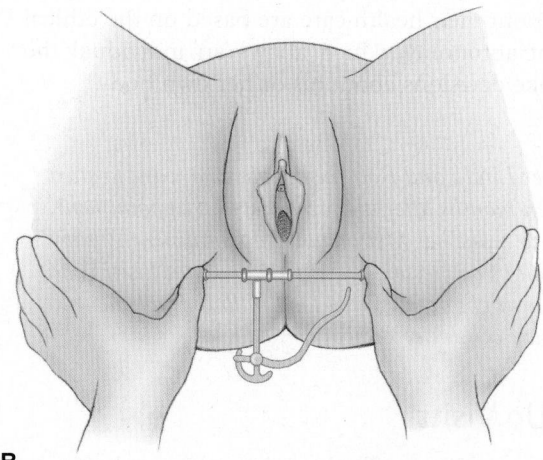

A   **B**

FIGURE 12.2 Pelvic measurements. (**A**) Diagonal conjugate (solid line) and true conjugate (dotted line). (**B**) Ischial tuberosity diameter.

TABLE 12.2 COMMON LABORATORY AND DIAGNOSTIC TESTS FOR PREGNANT WOMEN

Test	Explanation
Complete blood cell count	Evaluates hemoglobin and mean corpuscular volume levels and red blood cell count (4.2–5.4 million/mm^3) to detect presence of anemia; determines white blood cell count (5,000–10,000/mm^3), which if elevated may indicate an infection; determines platelet count (150,000–450,000/mm^3) to assess clotting ability
Blood typing	Determines woman's blood type and Rh status to rule out any blood incompatibility issues early; Rh-negative mother would likely receive RhoGAM (at 28 weeks) if she is Rh sensitive via indirect Coombs' test
Rubella titer	Detects antibodies for the virus that causes German measles; if titer is 1:8 or less, the woman is not immune, requires immunization after birth, and is advised to avoid people with undiagnosed rashes
Hepatitis B	Determines if mother has hepatitis B by detecting presence of hepatitis B surface antigen (HBsAg) in her blood
HIV testing	Detects HIV antibodies and, if positive, requires more specific testing, counselling, and treatment during pregnancy with anti-retroviral medications to prevent transmission to fetus
STI screening: Venereal Disease Research Laboratory (VDRL) or rapid plasma reagin (RPR) serologic tests	Detects STIs (such as syphilis, herpes, human papillomavirus, and gonorrhea) so that treatment can be initiated early to prevent transmission to fetus
Cervical smear	Detects abnormalities such as cervical cancer (Pap test) or infections such as gonorrhea, chlamydia, or group B streptococcus so that treatment can be initiated if positive

Source: Perinatal Services BC. (2010a). *BCPHP Obstetric Guide 19: Maternity care pathway.* Retrieved February 21, 2012 from http://www.perinatalservicesbc.ca//sites/bcrcp/files/Guidelines/Obstetrics/Guideline_19.pdf.

findings, current health status, and risk factors identified in the initial interview. Additional tests can be offered, but ultimately the woman and her partner make the decision about undergoing them. Educate the woman and her partner about the tests, including the rationale for each. In addition, support the woman and her partner in their decision-making process, regardless of whether or not you agree with the couple's decision. The couple's decisions about their health care are based on the ethical principle of autonomy, which allows an individual the right to make decisions about his or her own body.

Remember Linda and Rob, the couple who want to start a family? Ten months after the preconception appointment, Linda calls to make her first prenatal appointment. What key areas will be addressed at this first prenatal visit? What interventions might be suggested for Linda to implement in order to ensure a healthy newborn?

Follow-Up Visits

Prenatal care is more effective when women begin to receive care in the first trimester and continue at regular intervals throughout pregnancy (PHAC, 2009). PHAC (2000) recommends the following schedule for visits with a primary maternity care provider:

• Early pregnancy: every 4 to 6 weeks
• After 30 weeks' gestation: every 2 to 3 weeks
• After 36 weeks' gestation: every 1 to 2 weeks

The frequency of prenatal visits depends on the woman's health status, her concerns during pregnancy, and her need for health-related counselling. Following the initial visit, fetal growth and well-being and maternal health and well-being are assessed during all prenatal visits. Assessment of fetal well-being includes fetal activity and fetal heart rate (FHR; should be 110 to 160 beats/minute). Fetal growth is reflected in the symphysis–fundal height measurement and in maternal weight gain. Assessment of maternal health includes urine testing for protein (routine urinary glucose testing is not recommended), pulse and blood pressure measurements, which are compared with baseline values, and rescreening in each trimester for STIs if indicated by ongoing risk factors. More details about the content of routine prenatal care may be available provincially. In British Columbia, a Maternity Care Pathway has been developed to ensure that all women receive the same standard of care (Perinatal Services BC, 2010a).

At each follow-up visit, the nurse can answer questions, provide anticipatory guidance and health education, and review nutritional guidelines and practices (including prenatal vitamin therapy). Throughout the pregnancy, encourage the woman's partner to participate as desired and when possible.

Assessment of Fetal Growth and Wellbeing
Fetal Movement Patterns
Fetal movement is usually perceived by the woman between 16 and 20 weeks' gestation. Perceived fetal movement is most often related to trunk and limb motion and rollovers or flips and is a gross indicator of fetal well-being. Decreased fetal movement may indicate poor placental perfusion and possible fetal compromise as the fetus attempts to compensate, decreasing oxygen requirements by decreasing activity (SOGC, 2007a). A decrease in fetal movement may also be related to other factors, such as fetal sleep cycles, maternal use of central nervous system depressants, and fetal anomalies, such as hydrocephalus or anencephaly (SOGC, 2007a).

Being aware of and counting fetal movements is a non-invasive method of screening and can be taught easily to all pregnant women. The healthy pregnant woman without risk factors needs to be aware of her baby's usual movement patterns and be able to perform a fetal movement count in the third trimester if she perceives a decrease in movement (SOGC, 2007a). SOGC recommends that women count distinctive movements until they reach a count of six. If the woman does not feel six fetal movements in a 2-hour period she should notify her maternity care provider. Further investigation with a fetal non-stress test (NST) and/or biophysical profile is warranted (SOGC, 2007a).

Instruct the woman about how to count fetal movements, the reasons for doing so, and the significance of decreased fetal movements. Suggest that she pay attention to her baby's movements periodically through the day. Counting movements in a relaxed environment and a comfortable position is an important way to get to know her baby's usual activity pattern.

Fetal Heart Rate Assessment
FHR measurement is integral to fetal surveillance throughout pregnancy, and hearing the fetal heartbeat is reassuring for the woman and her partner. Auscultating the FHR with a handheld Doppler at each prenatal visit helps confirm that the intrauterine environment is still supportive to the growing fetus. The purpose of assessing FHR is to determine rate and rhythm. Nursing Procedure 12.1 lists the steps in assessing the FHR.

Symphysis–Fundal Height Measurement
Symphysis–fundal height is the distance (in centimetres) from the top of the pubic bone (symphysis) to the top of

Nursing Procedure 12.1
MEASURING FETAL HEART RATE

Purpose: To Assess Fetal Well-Being
1. Assist the woman onto the examining table and have her lie down with her head slightly elevated.
2. Cover her with a sheet to ensure privacy, and then expose her abdomen.
3. Visually inspect the abdomen before touching. Observe for skin changes (such as linea nigra, straie gravidarum), scars from previous surgery, and fetal movement.
4. With warm hands, palpate the abdomen to determine the fetal lie, position, and presentation.
5. When auscultating the fetal heart **before** fetal parts are identifiable, palpate the fundus and measure the symphysis–fundal height first. Then apply gel and move the Doppler around until the fetal heart is located.
6. When auscultating the fetal heart **after** fetal parts are identifiable (third trimester), locate the back of the fetus (the ideal position to hear the heartbeat). Apply lubricant gel to the abdomen in the area where the back has been located. Turn on the hand-held Doppler device and place it on the spot over the fetal back. Listen for the sound of the amplified heartbeat, moving the device slightly from side to side as necessary to obtain the loudest sound.
7. Assess the woman's pulse rate and compare it with the amplified sound. If the rates appear the same, reposition the Doppler device.
8. Once the fetal heartbeat has been identified, count the number of beats in 1 minute and record the results.
9. Remove the Doppler device and wipe off any remaining gel from the woman's abdomen and the device.
10. Record the heart rate in the woman's medical record.
11. Provide information to the woman regarding fetal well-being based on findings.

the uterus (fundus); it is measured using a tape measure with the woman lying on her back with her knees slightly flexed (Fig. 12.3). Symphysis–fundal height typically increases as the pregnancy progresses; it reflects fetal growth and provides a gross estimate of the duration of the pregnancy. Symphysis–fundal height should approximately equal the number of weeks of gestation until week 36. For example, a fundal height of 24 cm suggests a fetus at 24 weeks' gestation. After 36 weeks, the fundal height drops due to lightening and may no longer correspond with the week of gestation.

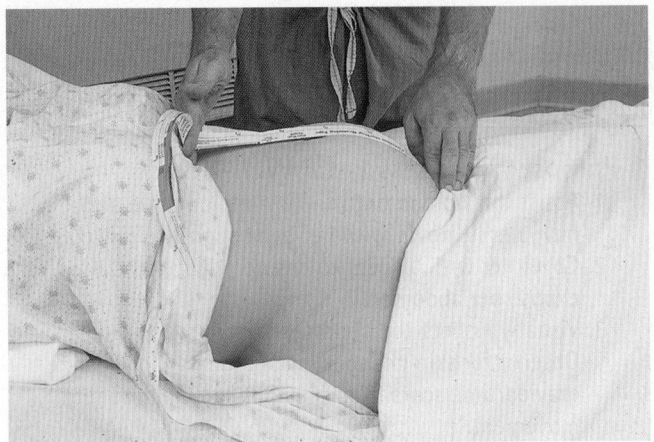

FIGURE 12.3 Symphysis–fundal height measurement.

Fundal height is expected to increase progressively throughout the pregnancy, reflecting fetal growth. A growth curve that flattens or remains stable may be a short-term normal variation or it may indicate a problem with fetal growth such as intrauterine growth restriction (IUGR). If the fundal height measurement differs from the estimated gestational age by more than 4 cm, further evaluation is warranted if a multifetal gestation has not been diagnosed or hydramnios has not been ruled out (D'Amico, Barbarito, Twomey, et al., 2011).

Assessment of Maternal Health and Well-Being

First Trimester (0 to 14 Weeks)

In the first trimester, the focus of prenatal visits is on assisting the woman to quit smoking and avoid alcohol and other harmful substances and ensuring that her folic acid intake is adequate. Many women experience taste changes in the first trimester and may find smoking or drinking distasteful. This provides an opportunity for the nurse to assist with smoking cessation and for referral to substance use rehabilitation programs.

The nurse should follow the five A's in an attempt to help the woman quit smoking. **Ask** about smoking, **advise** or strongly urge pregnant women to quit, **assess** her willingness to make a quit attempt, **assist** the woman with quitting, and **arrange** follow-up as needed. Guidelines to help nurses learn motivational interviewing techniques and brief interventions are available (RNAO, 2007). Information for women is readily available (PHAC, 2010m). See Evidence-based Practice 12.1.

The first trimester may also provide an opportunity for nutritional assessment and dietary change. Women

---

EVIDENCE-BASED PRACTICE 12.1
Health Care Providers' Engagement in Smoking Cessation with Pregnant Smokers

● **Study**

Several studies have shown that health care provider advice is critical for smoking cessation. The Registered Nurses' Association of Ontario (RNAO) has developed best practice guidelines to help nurses have the knowledge needed to take a more informed and active role in brief smoking cessation interventions. This study reviews how health care providers (HCPs) engage in smoking cessation (SC) with pregnant smokers.

This study reviewed literature from a variety of databases and identified 28 publications that met their inclusion criteria. Selected studies had clearly defined behavioural outcomes for HCP's delivery of smoking cessation interventions to pregnant women.

▲ **The Findings**

Although more than 50% of HCPs *asked* women about their smoking status and *advised* pregnant smokers to quit, few *assessed* readiness for change, *assisted* in smoking cessation interventions (brief or intensive), or *arranged* follow-up appointments or referrals. The five A's in italics are considered best practice for nurses in Canada (RNAO, 2007). Barriers to providing brief interventions included a lack of knowledge and confidence, perceptions that women lacked interest in smoking cessation, and a lack of time to engage in SC interventions.

■ **Nursing Implications**

In addition to assessing motivation for smoking cessation, nurses need to assess the role that tobacco plays in the woman's life (not just during pregnancy). When assisting by providing brief interventions, nurses need to de-emphasize smoking cessation solely for pregnancy-related reasons and focus on motivations for women's health in general. Intensive interventions may need to be tailored to the needs of particular groups, such as adolescents and women living in poverty. Nurses may need to adopt a woman-centred harm reduction approach, address the stigma associated with smoking, and include both relapse prevention and strategies to integrate partners and social support networks.

Source: Okoli, C., Greaves, L. Bottorff, J., & Marcellus, L. (2010). Health care providers' engagement in smoking cessation with pregnant smokers. *Journal of Obstetric, Gynecologic, and Neonatal Nursing, 39*(1), 64–77.

can also be counselled to limit their caffeine intake (PHAC, 2010c). Early prenatal genetic testing may also be completed during the first trimester (discussed later in the chapter). Women should also receive anticipatory guidance about relevant pregnancy discomforts and be given the opportunity to discuss their particular concerns. A discussion about culturally relevant prenatal care practices may assist the nurse to provide culturally safe care.

Second Trimester (14 to 27 Weeks)

In addition to assessing fetal growth and well-being, prenatal visits should focus on maternal health concerns. Follow-up visits usually involve assessment of the woman's blood pressure and weight, urine testing for protein, and other diagnostic tests as per protocol. Genetic screening and a detailed obstetric ultrasound are usually recommended between 15 and 20 weeks' gestation (SOGC, 2005a, 2005b, 2011b).

Between weeks 24 and 28, a blood glucose screening test is usually conducted using a 50 g glucose load followed by a 1-hour plasma glucose determination. If the result is positive, further diagnostic testing, such as a 3-hour 100 g glucose tolerance test, is warranted to determine whether gestational diabetes is present (SOGC, 2002b). For unsensitized Rh-negative women, Rh immunoglobulin is usually administered at 28 weeks (SOGC, 2003c).

The woman also is evaluated to determine her risk of preterm labour. At each visit, ask if she is experiencing any common signs or symptoms of preterm labour, such as uterine contractions, dull backache, a feeling of pressure in the pelvic area or thighs, increased vaginal discharge, menstrual-like cramps, or vaginal bleeding (MacKinnon, 2006). If the woman is experiencing any of these symptoms, a sterile speculum examination may be performed for fetal fibronectin testing (BC Perinatal Health Program, 2005). If the woman has had a previous preterm birth, she is at increased risk for another and close monitoring is warranted (SOGC, 2010c).

During this time, review the common discomforts of pregnancy, discuss any of the woman's concerns, and answer questions. Reinforce the importance of good nutrition and daily exercise, and commend the woman for the good work she is doing in caring for herself and her baby. The decision about infant feeding is usually made during pregnancy, so the second trimester is a good time to provide balanced information about the advantages and disadvantages of breastfeeding. Women need accurate information to participate in making informed decisions.

Third Trimester (28 Weeks Until Delivery)

During the third trimester assessments for prenatal depression/anxiety and for pre-eclampsia are performed in addition to all the assessments of previous visits. Pregnant women commonly experience dependent edema of the lower extremities from constriction of blood vessels secondary to the heavy gravid uterus. However, periorbital edema, edema of the hands, and pretibial edema are abnormal and could be signs of gestational hypertension. Inspecting and palpating both extremities, listening for complaints of tight rings on fingers, and observing for swelling around the eyes are important assessments. Abnormal findings in any of these areas need to be reported (SOGC, 2008b).

Nurses also need to assess the woman's emotional adjustment to pregnancy and identify mood disorders, such as prenatal depression or anxiety. These pregnancy health challenges are more common than previously thought and women may need to be referred for counselling or treatment, including medications and psychotherapy (McKillop, Martin, Bowen, et al., 2011).

If the baby is in the breech position, an ultrasound may be performed at about 34 weeks' gestation and a referral made for external cephalic version if available or desired. Re-evaluate hemoglobin level and mean corpuscular volume (MCV) to assess for anemia.

Reinforce the importance of fetal activity monitoring as an indicator of fetal well-being in the last weeks of pregnancy. The woman can also use this opportunity to get to know her unborn baby's usual patterns of activity. Between 35 and 37 weeks, a rectovaginal swab may be obtained to check for GBS (SOGC, 2004). If the woman has had a previous baby affected by GBS or has had GBS bacteriuria during her current pregnancy, she is considered GBS positive and further screening is not indicated (Perinatal Services BC, 2010a).

The third trimester is also the time to review the signs and symptoms of labour and discuss when the woman should come to the hospital for assessment. Discuss the woman's plans and preferences for labour and birth. Also review the woman's decision about infant feeding and provide information on breastfeeding or formula preparation and bottle-feeding as appropriate. This is also a good time to discuss sexual health and review her desire for family planning after birth. Assess the woman's knowledge and decisions about infant care and remind her that an infant car seat is required by law and must be used to drive the newborn home from the hospital or birthing centre.

Beginning at 41 weeks, the woman needs to be aware that increased fetal assessment with NSTs, amniotic fluid measurement, and fetal movement counting are required (SOGC, 2008c). Induction may be offered between 41 and 42 weeks of pregnancy (Perinatal Services BC, 2010a).

Teaching About the Danger Signs of Pregnancy

It is important to educate the woman about danger signs during pregnancy that require further evaluation. Explain that she should contact her health care provider **immediately** if she experiences any of the following:

- During the first trimester: spotting or bleeding (miscarriage); painful urination (infection); severe, persistent vomiting (hyperemesis gravidarum); fever higher than 38°C (infection); and lower abdominal pain with dizziness and accompanied by shoulder pain (ruptured ectopic pregnancy)
- During the second trimester: menstrual-like cramps or uterine contractions (preterm labour); pain in the calf, often increased with foot flexion (blood clot in deep vein); sudden gush or leakage of fluid from the vagina (premature rupture of membranes); and sudden change in fetal movement patterns or fewer than six movements in a 2-hour counting period (possible fetal distress or demise)
- During the third trimester: sudden weight gain; periorbital or facial edema, severe upper abdominal pain, or headache with visual changes (pregnancy-induced hypertension); and sudden decrease in daily fetal movements (possible demise). Any of the previous warning signs and symptoms can also be present in this last trimester.

Preterm Birth Prevention

One of the warning signs that should be emphasized during prenatal visits is early contractions, which can lead to preterm birth. All pregnant women need to be able to recognize early signs of contractions to prevent preterm labour, which is a major public health problem. In Canada, approximately 8% of all live births occur before 37 weeks' gestation (PHAC, 2008a). Preterm infants can suffer lifelong health consequences such as mental retardation, chronic lung disease, cerebral palsy, seizure disorders, and blindness, among other problems (March of Dimes, 2011). Preterm labour can occur in any pregnant woman and is not an indication that the woman was not taking good care of herself and her unborn baby.

If the woman experiences menstrual-like cramps occurring every 10 minutes accompanied by a low, dull backache, she should stop what she is doing and lie down on her left side for 1 hour and drink two or three glasses of water (dehydration increases uterine contractions). If the symptoms worsen or don't subside after 1 hour, she should contact her health care provider. Although there is little good evidence for the efficacy of tocolytic medications or drugs that decrease contractions, it is recommended that the corticosteroid betamethasone be administered to women experiencing preterm labour to hasten fetal lung maturity (SOGC, 2003a).

Screening and Diagnostic Tests

During the antepartum period, additional screening tests are performed routinely to monitor fetal well-being and to detect possible problems. When screening tests detect a possible health problem, diagnostic tests are used to confirm the problem and as a guide for appropriate interventions. In addition, some women experience high-risk pregnancy and require additional health surveillance. Tests discussed in this section include ultrasonography, tests used to identify the fetus at risk for congenital anomalies, and technologies used for closer monitoring of high-risk pregnancies.

Ultrasonography

Since its introduction in the late 1950s, ultrasonography has become a very useful diagnostic tool in obstetrics. Real-time scanners can produce a continuous picture of the fetus that is transmitted on a monitor. A transducer that emits high-frequency sound waves is placed on the mother's abdomen and moved to visualize the fetus (Fig. 12.4). The fetal heartbeat and any malformations in the fetus can be assessed, and measurements can be made accurately from the picture on the monitor.

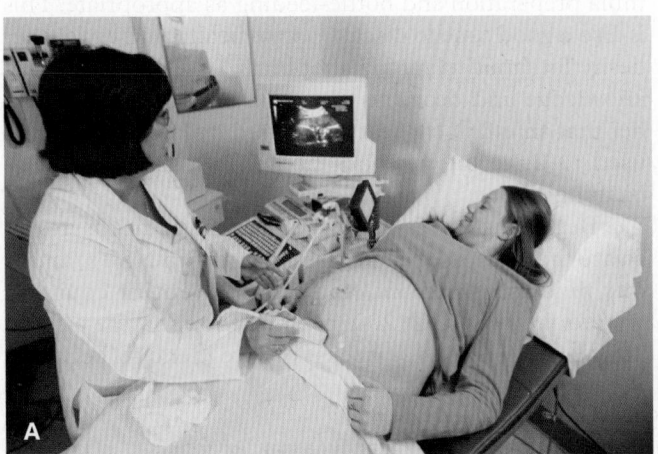
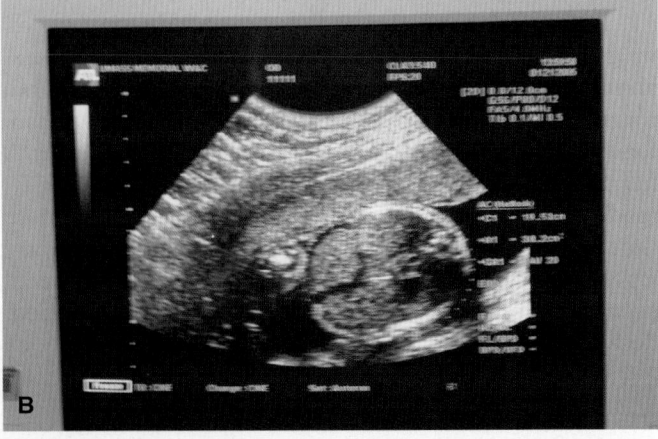

FIGURE 12.4 Ultrasound. (**A**) Ultrasound device being applied to a woman's abdomen. (**B**) View of the monitor.

Ultrasound is considered a safe, accurate, and cost-effective tool. It provides important information about fetal activity, growth, and gestational age; assesses fetal well-being; and determines the need for more invasive intrauterine tests (Coad & Dunstall, 2011).

There are no hard-and-fast rules as to the number of ultrasounds a pregnant woman should have, but most Canadian women today undergo two or three ultrasound tests during their pregnancy (PHAC, 2009). An ultrasound may be performed in the first trimester to confirm pregnancy and to exclude ectopic or molar pregnancies. A second scan is usually performed at about 18 to 20 weeks to look for congenital malformations, exclude multi-fetal pregnancies, and verify dates and growth. An ultrasound scan may also be done at around 34 weeks to evaluate fetal size, assess fetal growth, and verify fetal/placental position (SOGC, 2010d). An ultrasound is used to confirm placental location during amniocentesis and to provide visualization during chorionic villus sampling (CVS). An ultrasound is also ordered whenever an abnormality is suspected (SOGC, 2009a, 2010d).

Nursing management during the ultrasound focuses on educating the woman about the test and reassuring her that there is no evidence that the sound waves used during the test will harm the baby. However, nonmedical uses of ultrasound, such as determining the sex of the fetus, are not recommended (SOGC, 2007c). No special preparation is needed before performing an ultrasound, although in early pregnancy the woman may need to have a full bladder. Inform her that she may experience some discomfort from the pressure on the full bladder during the scan, but it will last only a short time. Tell the woman that the conducting gel used on the abdomen during the scan may feel cold initially.

Tests Used to Identify the Fetus at Risk for Congenital Anomalies

Both screening and diagnostic tests are used to identify the fetus at risk for congenital anomalies. RNs play an important role in providing information to childbearing women and their families about routine pregnancy screening tests and discussing the differences between screening and diagnostic testing. For example, genetic screening tests will have a higher false-positive rate but will usually be less invasive than diagnostic testing (SOGC, 2011b). Women and their families need to understand what a positive screening test means as well as receive support when they are referred for genetic counselling and further diagnostic testing.

Genetic Screening Tests

Screening is the process of testing a population using specific biomarkers and predefined screening cut-off levels to identify individuals at greater risk for a particular disorder (SOGC, 2011b). Screening should only be offered to women when an accurate diagnostic test and, ideally, effective intervention are available. Women and their family members need accurate information and support to make an informed decision about participating in screening programs. Nurses play an important role ensuring that women who undergo genetic testing understand that: (1) it is their choice to undergo screening for genetic diseases, (2) there are differences between screening and diagnostic testing, and (3) false-positive screening test results are relatively common.

Pregnancy screening protocols are organized into comprehensive programs and vary by province and territory, so each province has slightly different procedures and processes for genetic screening, diagnosis, and counselling. For example, Perinatal Services BC (2011) recently revised its guideline for prenatal screening as a result of improvements in serologic screening and additional information that can be obtained from detailed ultrasound scans (including nuchal translucency testing). Current information and recommendations can be found on many of the provincial reproductive or perinatal health services websites. (For direct links to some of these websites, visit http://thePoint.lww.com/Chow1e.)

Serum markers commonly tested include alpha-fetoprotein (AFP), pregnancy-associated plasma protein A (PAPP-A), unconjugated estriol, hCG, and inhibin A. Ultrasound testing includes nuchal translucency testing in the first trimester and detailed ultrasound examinations looking for physical changes between 18 and 20 weeks' gestation (Perinatal Services BC, 2011).

Maternal Serum Biomarkers

Maternal blood or serum screening tests may be used to determine the risk of open NTDs, Down syndrome, trisomy 18, and other inherited conditions. The risk (or probability) of these disorders is calculated from a combination of factors, including maternal age, ethnicity, weight, diabetes status, smoking status and, when available, ultrasound measurements of nuchal translucency. The screening tests offered commonly vary according to the gestational age of the fetus at the time the woman begins prenatal care as well as the woman's age at her baby's EDB.

Correct information about gestational dating as well as maternal weight, race, number of fetuses, and insulin dependency is necessary to ensure the accuracy of these screening tests. If incorrect maternal information is submitted or the blood specimen is not drawn during the appropriate time frame, false-positive results may occur, increasing the woman's anxiety. Further testing might then be ordered based on an inaccurate interpretation, resulting in additional financial and emotional costs.

Alpha-Fetoprotein Analysis

Alpha-fetoprotein is a substance produced by the fetal liver between weeks 13 and 20 of gestation. Elevated levels of maternal serum AFP or amniotic fluid AFP were first linked to the occurrence of fetal NTDs about 30 years ago. AFP is present in amniotic fluid in low concentrations between 10 and 14 weeks of gestation and can be detected in maternal serum beginning approximately at 12 to 14 weeks of gestation (Gilbert, 2011). If a developmental defect is present, such as failure of the neural tube to close, more AFP escapes into amniotic fluid from the fetus. AFP then enters the maternal circulation by crossing the placenta, and the level in maternal serum can be measured.

A variety of situations can lead to elevation of maternal serum AFP, including an open NTD, underestimation of gestational age, the presence of multiple fetuses, gastrointestinal defects, slow fetal growth, oligohydramnios, and decreased maternal weight (Gilbert, 2011). Lower-than-expected maternal serum AFP levels are seen when fetal gestational age is overestimated or in cases of fetal death, hydatidiform mole, increased maternal weight, maternal type 1 diabetes, and fetal trisomy 21 (Down syndrome) or trisomy 18 (Edward's syndrome) (Gilbert, 2011). Measurement of maternal serum AFP detects approximately 80% of all open NTDs and open abdominal wall defects in early pregnancy (SOGC, 2011b). AFP has now been combined with other biomarker screening tests and with detailed ultrasound testing to more accurately determine the risk for NTDs and Down syndrome.

Other Serum Biomarkers Used for Genetic Screening Tests

Additional serum markers include PAPP-A, unconjugated estriol, hCG, and inhibin A. These additional markers were added to AFP testing to enhance detection (improve the sensitivity of the test) and help decrease the frequency of false-positive results (improve the specificity of the test). For example, inhibin A is used to increase the accuracy of screening for Down syndrome in women younger than 35 years of age; low inhibin A levels indicate the possibility of Down syndrome (Gilbert, 2011). Again, the timing of testing influences the number of specific biomarkers included in the genetic serum screen. These biomarkers are merely screening tests and identify women who require further definitive procedures (ie, amniocentesis or ultrasound) to make a diagnosis of NTDs (anencephaly, spina bifida, and encephalocele), Down syndrome, or trisomy 18 in the fetus. Most screening tests are performed between 15 and 22 weeks of gestation (Perinatal Services BC, 2011).

Nursing management related to genetic screening tests consists primarily of providing education about the tests. Prenatal screening has become standard in prenatal care in Canada. However, for many couples it remains confusing, emotionally charged, and filled with uncertain risks. Offer a thorough explanation of the screening tests, including a description of the risks and benefits of each, and emphasize that these tests are for screening

purposes only. Remind the couple that a definitive diagnosis is not made without further diagnostic tests, such as an amniocentesis. Answer any questions about prenatal screening tests and respect the couple's decision if they choose not to have them done. Couples need to be aware that deciding to undergo genetic screening does not mean that they would necessarily have an abortion if a test result were positive (Perinatal Services BC, 2011).

Nursing management for the woman who chooses maternal serum screening testing also consists of preparing her for the screening test by gathering accurate information about the date of her LMP, weight, race, and gestational dating. The nurse would explain that genetic testing involves obtaining one or two blood specimens and at least one ultrasound examination and may make arrangements for this testing to be completed.

Nuchal Translucency Screening and Detailed Ultrasound Examinations

Nuchal translucency screening (ultrasound) is done in the first trimester of pregnancy between 11 and 14 weeks. This test allows for earlier detection and diagnosis of some fetal chromosomal and structural abnormalities. Ultrasound is used to identify an increase in nuchal translucency, which is due to the subcutaneous accumulation of fluid behind the fetal neck. Increased nuchal translucency is associated with chromosomal abnormalities such as trisomies 21, 18, and 13. Infants with trisomies tend to have more collagen and elastic connective tissue, allowing for fluid accumulation (SOGC, 2005b).

In the second trimester, the presence or absence of "soft markers" (physical signs of genetic disorders) on an ultrasound examination may identify structural anomalies (such as diaphragmatic hernias) or may be used to modify the calculated risk established by maternal age or prior screening (SOCG, 2011b).

Genetic Counselling and Diagnostic Tests

Women with positive screening test results should have rapid access to appropriate follow-up (diagnostic testing with amniocentesis or CVS) and genetic counselling. Some diagnostic tests may only be available in large urban perinatal centres, and expectant parents are understandably anxious during this time. RNs may be employed in settings where they assist during genetic testing, so limited information about nursing management during some of these tests will be provided.

Health professionals with advanced training in human genetics provide genetic counselling, diagnosis, and sometimes therapy (Jones & Ciofani, 2010). The goal of genetic counselling is to provide accurate information so that the woman and family can make an informed decision about the options available to them. The birth of a child with significant health challenges affects the whole family, so time for reflection and discussion are as important as the information provided.

Amniocentesis

Amniocentesis involves a transabdominal puncture of the amniotic sac to obtain a sample of amniotic fluid for analysis. The fluid contains fetal cells that are examined to detect chromosomal abnormalities and several hereditary metabolic defects in the fetus before birth. In addition, amniocentesis is used to confirm a fetal abnormality when other screening tests detect a possible problem. More than 40 different chromosomal abnormalities, inborn errors of metabolism, and NTDs can be diagnosed with amniocentesis. Amniocentesis can replace a genetic probability with a diagnostic certainty, allowing the woman and her partner to make an informed decision about the option of therapeutic abortion.

Amniocentesis is usually performed to diagnose chromosomal abnormalities, evaluate the fetal condition when the woman is sensitized to the Rh-positive blood, diagnose intrauterine infections, and investigate amniotic fluid AFP when the maternal serum AFP level is elevated (Gilbert, 2011). The second trimester is the most common time to have an amniocentesis for any prenatal diagnosis because the risk to the fetus is greater the earlier amniocentesis is performed (SOGC, 2007b). By 14 to 16 weeks of gestation, there is sufficient amniotic fluid for sampling yet enough time for a safe abortion, if desired. Amniocentesis may be offered to women who are 40 years of age or older, women who have a child with an NTD, and women with elevated maternal serum AFP levels or a positive genetic screen. It also may be used to detect chromosomal aberrations when a parent has a chromosomal abnormality or is a carrier for a metabolic disease (Cunningham et al., 2010).

In the third trimester, amniocentesis is most commonly indicated to determine fetal lung maturity after the 35th week of gestation via analysis of lecithin-to-sphingomyelin ratios and to evaluate the fetal condition with Rh isoimmunization. Table 12.3 lists amniotic fluid analysis findings and their implications.

Procedure

Amniocentesis is performed after an ultrasound examination identifies an adequate pocket of amniotic fluid

TABLE 12.3 AMNIOTIC FLUID ANALYSIS AND IMPLICATIONS

Test Component	Normal Findings	Fetal Implications of Abnormal Findings
Colour	Clear with white flecks of vernix caseosa in a mature fetus	Blood of maternal origin is usually harmless. "Port wine" fluid may indicate abruptio placentae. Fetal blood may indicate damage to the fetal, placental, or umbilical cord vessels.
Bilirubin	Absent at term	High levels indicate hemolytic disease of the neonate in isoimmunized pregnancy.
Meconium	Absent (except in breech presentation)	Presence indicates fetal hypotension or distress.
Creatinine	More than 2 mg/dL in a mature fetus	Decrease may indicate immature fetus (less than 37 weeks).
Lecithin–sphingomyelin ratio (L–S ratio)	More than 2 generally indicates fetal pulmonary maturity.	A ratio of less than 2 indicates pulmonary immaturity and subsequent respiratory distress syndrome.
Phosphatidylglycerol	Present	Absence indicates pulmonary immaturity.
Glucose	Less than 45 mg/dL	Excessive increases at term or near term indicate hypertrophied fetal pancreas and subsequent neonatal hypoglycemia.
Alpha-fetoprotein	Variable, depending on gestational age and laboratory technique; highest concentration (about 18.5 µg/mL) occurs at 13 to 14 weeks	Inappropriate increases indicate neural tube defects such as spina bifida or anencephaly, impending fetal death, congenital nephrosis, or contamination of fetal blood.
Bacteria	Absent	Presence indicates chorioamnionitis.
Chromosomes	Normal karyotype	Abnormal karyotype may indicate fetal sex and chromosome disorders.
Acetylcholinesterase	Absent	Presence may indicate neural tube defects, exomphalos, or other serious malformations.

Sources: Blackburn, S. T. (2007). *Maternal, fetal, and neonatal physiology: A clinical perspective* (3rd ed.). St. Louis, MO: Saunders Elsevier; and D'Amico, D., Barbarito, C., Twomey, C. & Harder, N. (2011). *Health and physical assessment in nursing: Canadian Edition.* Toronto: Pearson Education Canada.

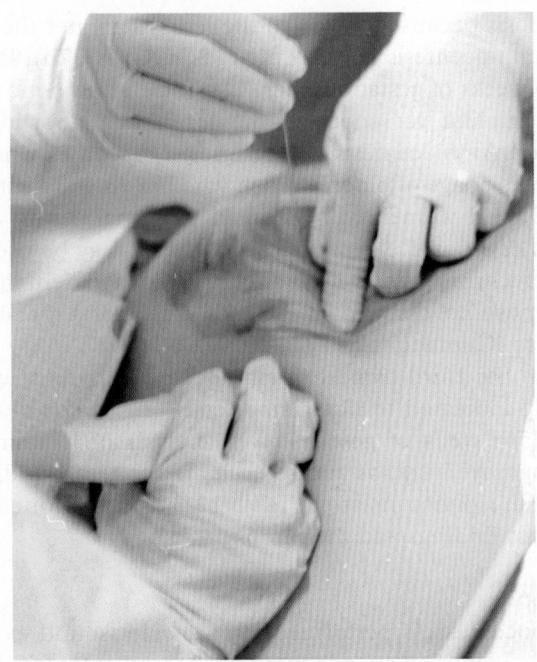

FIGURE 12.5 Technique for amniocentesis: inserting needle.

free of fetal parts, the umbilical cord, or the placenta (Fig. 12.5). The health care provider inserts a long pudendal or spinal needle, a 22-gauge, 12.7 cm (5 inches) needle, into the amniotic cavity and aspirates amniotic fluid, which is placed in an amber or foil-covered test tube to protect it from light. When the desired amount of fluid has been withdrawn, the needle is removed and slight pressure is applied to the site. If there is no evidence of bleeding, a sterile bandage is applied to the needle site. The specimens are then sent to the laboratory immediately for cytologic evaluation.

Examining a sample of fetal cells directly produces a definitive diagnosis rather than a "best guess" diagnosis based on indirect screening tests. Amniocentesis is an invaluable diagnostic tool, but the risks include spontaneous abortion (1 in 200), maternal or fetal infection, fetalmaternal hemorrhage, leakage of amniotic fluid, and maternal discomfort after the procedure. The test results may take up to 3 weeks (SOGC, 2005a).

Nursing Management

When preparing the woman for an amniocentesis, explain the procedure and encourage her to empty her bladder just before the procedure to avoid the risk of bladder puncture. Inform her that a 20-minute electronic fetal monitoring strip usually is obtained to evaluate fetal wellbeing and obtain a baseline to compare after the procedure is completed. Obtain and record maternal vital signs.

After the procedure, assist the woman to a position of comfort and administer RhoGAM intramuscularly if the woman is Rh negative to prevent potential sensitization to fetal blood. Assess maternal vital signs and fetal heart rate every 15 minutes for an hour after the procedure. Observe

the puncture site for bleeding or drainage. Instruct the woman to rest after returning home and remind her to report fever, leaking amniotic fluid, vaginal bleeding, or uterine contractions or any changes in fetal activity (increased or decreased) to the health care provider.

When the test results come back, be available to offer support, especially if a fetal abnormality is found. Also prepare the woman and her partner for the need for genetic counselling. Trained genetic counsellors can provide accurate medical information and help couples to interpret the results of the amniocentesis so they can make the decisions that are right for them as a family.

Chorionic Villus Sampling

There has been an impetus to develop earlier prenatal diagnostic procedures so that couples can make an early decision to terminate the pregnancy if an anomaly is confirmed. Early prenatal diagnosis by CVS was proposed as an alternative to amniocentesis. **Chorionic villus sampling** is a procedure for obtaining a sample of the chorionic villi for prenatal evaluation of chromosomal disorders, enzyme deficiencies, and fetal gender determination and to identify sex-linked disorders such as hemophilia, sickle-cell anemia, and Tay–Sachs disease (Blackburn, 2007; Jones & Ciofani, 2010). Chorionic villi are finger-like projections that cover the embryo and anchor it to the uterine lining before the placenta is developed. Because they are of embryonic origin, sampling provides information about the developing fetus. CVS can be used to detect numerous genetic disorders, with the exception of NTDs (Coad & Dunstall, 2011; Jones & Ciofani, 2010). Results of CVS testing are available more quickly than those of amniocentesis, usually within 48 hours (SOGC, 2005a).

Procedure

CVS is generally performed 10 to 13 weeks after the LMP. Earlier, chorionic villi may not be sufficiently developed for adequate tissue sampling and the risk for limb defects is increased (Cunningham et al., 2010). First, an ultrasound is done to confirm gestational age and viability. Then, under continuous ultrasound guidance, CVS is performed using either a transcervical or transabdominal approach. With the transcervical approach, a sterile catheter is introduced through the cervix and inserted into the placenta, where a sample of chorionic villi is aspirated. This approach requires the woman to have a full bladder to push the uterus and placenta into a position that is more accessible to the catheter. With the transabdominal approach, an 18-gauge spinal needle is inserted through the abdominal wall into the placental tissue and a sample of chorionic villi is aspirated. Regardless of the approach used, the sample is sent to the cytogenetics laboratory for analysis.

Potential complications of CVS include mild vaginal bleeding and cramping, spontaneous abortion, limb abnormalities, rupture of membranes, infection, chorioamnionitis, and fetal-maternal hemorrhage (Blackburn, 2007). The pregnancy loss rate is approximately 1.3%, which is somewhat higher than with traditional amniocentesis (SOGC, 2007b). In addition, women who are Rh negative should receive immune globulin (RhoGAM) to avoid isoimmunization (Gilbert, 2011).

Nursing Management

Explain to the woman that the procedure will last about 15 minutes. An ultrasound will be done first to locate the embryo, and a baseline set of vital signs will be taken before starting. Make sure she is informed of the risks related to the procedure and what to expect during the procedure.

After either procedure instruct the woman about signs to watch for and report, such as fever, cramping, and vaginal bleeding. Urge her not to engage in any strenuous activity for the next 48 hours. Assess the fetal heart rate for changes, and administer RhoGAM to an unsensitized Rh-negative woman after the procedure.

Percutaneous Umbilical Blood Sampling

Percutaneous umbilical blood sampling (PUBS) permits the collection of a blood specimen directly from the fetal circulation (Fig. 12.6). This test also allows for rapid chromosomal analysis to achieve a timely diagnosis. It is also done when the fetus is at risk for genetic anomalies or blood disorders, such as blood incompatibility or hemoglobinopathies.

Procedure

Under continuous ultrasound guidance, a fine needle is inserted through the mother's abdomen and uterine wall into an umbilical cord vessel. Specimens can be evaluated for coagulation studies, blood group typing, complete blood count, karyotyping, and blood gas analysis (Singh, Singh, & Vanita, 2012). Fetal infection, Rh incompatibility, and fetal acid–base status can be determined. The blood sample is usually drawn late in the second trimester to assist in medical management, but PUBS can be done any time after 16 weeks of gestation.

Although the information gained from this procedure is valuable and can be life-saving for many fetuses, PUBS is not without risks. Potential complications include leakage of blood from the puncture site, cord laceration, cord hematomas, transient fetal bradycardia, infection, thromboembolism in the umbilical cord, preterm labour, infection, and premature rupture of membranes (Blackburn, 2007; Cunningham et al., 2010).

Nursing Management

Explain the procedure to the woman and her partner. Position her on the examination table and monitor vital signs and FHR throughout the procedure. Assess FHR continuously and perform external fetal monitoring for up to 2 hours before the woman is discharged from the out-patient area. A repeat ultrasound is usually done within an hour after the procedure to rule out bleeding or hematoma formation. Prior to discharge, instruct the woman to report signs of infection, an increase in contractions, or a change in fetal activity level. Reinforce the need to count fetal movements, and review the technique so she can assess complete a fetal activity record when she is discharged home.

Additional Health Surveillance Used for High-Risk Pregnancies

When a high-risk pregnancy is identified, additional antepartum testing can be initiated to promote positive maternal, fetal, and neonatal outcomes. **High-risk pregnancies** include those that are complicated by maternal or fetal health challenges (coincidental with or unique to pregnancy) that jeopardize the health status of the mother and put the fetus at risk for uteroplacental insufficiency, hypoxia, and death. However, additional antepartum fetal testing should take place only when the results obtained will guide future care, whether it is reassurance, more frequent testing, admission to the hospital, or the need for immediate delivery (Gilbert, 2011).

Fetal Activity Monitoring

Fetal health surveillance includes fetal movement or activity monitoring, which becomes increasingly important in the third trimester or when the woman experiences pregnancy complications. Women experiencing health challenges in pregnancy are commonly asked to diligently monitor changes in their baby's activity and to complete a fetal activity record. Provide the woman with detailed information concerning fetal movement counts and stress the need for consistency in monitoring (at approximately the same time each day) and the importance of informing the health care provider promptly of

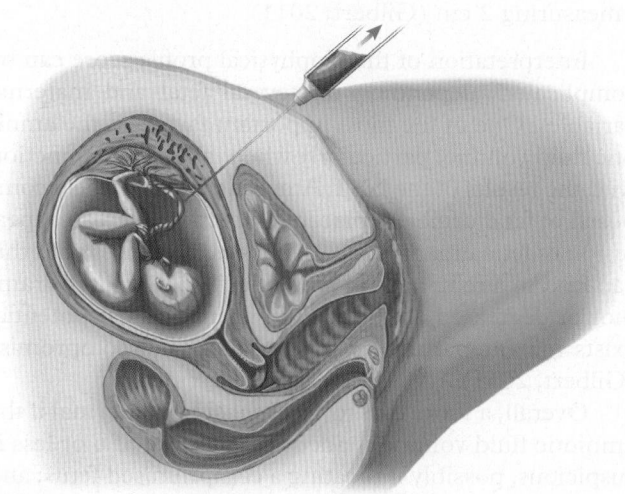

FIGURE 12.6 Collecting blood sample for PUBS.

any reduced movements. Providing "fetal kick count" charts to record movement helps promote participation. When changes are identified, further investigation with an NST and/or biophysical profile or early delivery may be warranted (SOGC, 2007a).

Non-Stress Test

The NST is an indirect measurement of uteroplacental function. Unlike the fetal movement counting done by the mother alone, this procedure requires specialized equipment and trained personnel. The basis for the NST is that the normal fetus produces characteristic FHR patterns in response to fetal movements. In the healthy fetus the FHR accelerates with fetal movement. Currently, an NST is recommended once or twice weekly (after 28 weeks of gestation) for women with diabetes and other high-risk conditions, such as IUGR, pre-eclampsia, post-term pregnancy, and renal disease (Cunningham et al., 2010; SOGC, 2007a). An NST is a non-invasive test that requires no initiation of contractions. It is quick to perform and has no known side effects. However, it is associated with a high false-positive rate due to fetal sleep periods, so additional testing may be required (Gilbert, 2011).

Procedure

Before the procedure the woman eats food to stimulate fetal activity. An external electronic fetal monitoring device is applied to her abdomen. The device consists of two belts, each with a sensor. One of the sensors records uterine activity; the second sensor records fetal heart rate. The woman is handed an "event marker" with a button that she pushes every time she perceives fetal movement. When the button is pushed, the fetal monitor strip is marked to identify that fetal movement has occurred. The procedure usually lasts 20 to 30 minutes.

Nursing Management

Prior to the NST, explain the testing procedure and have the woman empty her bladder. Position her in a semi-Fowler's position and apply the two external monitor belts. Document the date and time the test is started, patient information, the reason for the test, and the maternal vital signs. Obtain a baseline fetal monitor strip over 15 to 30 minutes.

During the test, observe for signs of fetal activity with a concurrent acceleration of the fetal heart rate. Interpret the NST as normal, atypical, or abnormal, as per current SOGC guidelines (2007a). A normal NST includes at least two FHR accelerations from the baseline of at least 15 beats/minute for at least 15 seconds within the 20-minute recording period. The baseline rate should also be normal, with variability and without significant decelerations. An atypical NST requires further assessment, and an abnormal NST requires urgent action. After the NST is completed, the nurse or maternity care

provider will discuss the results and their implications with the woman and her partner.

Biophysical Profile

A **biophysical profile** uses a real-time ultrasound to assess fetal behaviour (fetal tone, breathing, and movements) and/or amniotic fluid volume. These four parameters, together with the NST, constitute the biophysical profile. Each parameter is controlled by a different structure in the fetal brain: fetal tone by the cortex, fetal movements by the cortex and motor nuclei, fetal breathing by the centres close to the fourth ventricle, and the NST by the posterior hypothalamus and medulla. The amniotic fluid is the result of fetal urine volume. Not all facilities perform an NST unless other parameters of the profile are abnormal (Gilbert, 2011). The biophysical profile is based on the concept that a fetus that experiences hypoxia loses certain behavioural parameters in the reverse order in which they were acquired during fetal development (normal order of development: tone at 8 weeks; movement at 9 weeks; breathing at 20 weeks; and FHR reactivity at 24 weeks).

Scoring and Interpretation

The biophysical profile is a scored test with four or five components, each worth 2 points if present. A total score of 10 is possible if the NST is used. Thirty minutes are allotted for testing, although fewer than 10 minutes are usually needed. The following criteria must be met to obtain a score of 2 (normal); anything less is scored as 0 (abnormal):

- Body movements: three or more discrete limb or trunk movements
- Fetal tone: one or more instances of full extension and flexion of a limb or trunk
- Fetal breathing: one or more fetal breathing movements of more than 30 seconds
- Amniotic fluid volume: one or more pockets of fluid measuring 2 cm (Gilbert, 2011)

Interpretation of the biophysical profile score can be complicated, depending on several fetal and maternal variables. One of the most important factors is the amniotic fluid volume, particularly when taken in conjunction with the results of the NST. Amniotic fluid is largely composed of fetal urine. As placental function decreases, perfusion of fetal organs, such as kidneys, decreases, and this can lead to a reduction of amniotic fluid. If oligohydramnios or decreased amniotic fluid is present, the potential exists for antepartum or intrapartum fetal compromise (Gilbert, 2011).

Overall, a score of 8 to 10 is considered normal if the amniotic fluid volume is adequate. A score of 6 or less is suspicious, possibly indicating a compromised fetus; and further investigation of fetal well-being is needed. A score of 4 or less is associated with a high probability of fetal asphyxia and requires prompt intervention (SOGC, 2007a).

Because the biophysical profile is an ultrasonographic assessment of fetal behaviour, it requires more extensive equipment and more highly trained personnel than other testing modalities. Although the cost is greater than with less sophisticated tests, the biophysical profile permits conservative therapy and prevents premature or unnecessary intervention. There are also fewer false-positive results with the biophysical profile than with the NST alone (Cunningham et al., 2010).

Nursing Management

Nursing management focuses primarily on offering the woman support and answering her questions. The nurse might be asked to complete the NST before scheduling the biophysical profile. Explain why further testing might be needed and tell the woman that the ultrasound will be done in the diagnostic imaging department.

Doppler Flow Studies

Doppler flow studies of the uterine or umbilical artery can be used to measure the velocity of blood flow via ultrasound. Doppler flow studies can detect fetal compromise in high-risk pregnancies. The test is non-invasive and has no contraindications. The colour images produced help to identify abnormalities in diastolic flow within the umbilical vessels. The velocity of the fetal red blood cells can be determined by measuring the change in the frequency of the sound wave reflected off the cells. Thus, Doppler flow studies can detect the movement of red blood cells in vessels (Gilbert, 2011).

In pregnancies that are complicated by hypertension or IUGR, diastolic blood flow may be absent or even reversed (Gilbert, 2011). Doppler flow studies also can be used to evaluate the blood flow through other fetal blood vessels, such as the aorta and those in the brain. Research continues to determine the indications for Doppler flow studies to improve pregnancy outcomes. Nursing management of the woman undergoing Doppler flow studies is similar to that described for an ultrasound.

Nursing Management for the Common Discomforts of Pregnancy

Most women experience common discomforts during pregnancy and ask a nurse's advice about ways to minimize them. However, other women will not bring up their concerns unless asked. A collaborative partnership approach to care is highly recommended (Gottlieb & Feeley, 2006). The nurse needs to address the common discomforts that occur in each trimester and provide suggestions to help the woman deal with them (Teaching Guideline 12.1). Nursing Care Plan 12.1 applies the nursing process to the care of a woman experiencing some discomforts of pregnancy.

First-Trimester Discomforts

During the first 3 months of pregnancy, the woman's body is undergoing numerous changes. Some women experience many discomforts, but others have few. These discomforts are caused by the changes taking place within the body and may pass as the pregnancy progresses.

Urinary Frequency or Incontinence

Urinary frequency or incontinence is common in the first trimester because the growing uterus compresses the bladder. This also is a common complaint during the third trimester, especially when the fetal head settles into the pelvis. However, the discomfort tends to improve in the second trimester, when the uterus becomes an abdominal organ and moves away from the bladder region.

After infection and gestational diabetes have been ruled out as causative factors of increased urinary frequency, suggest that the woman decrease her fluid intake 2 to 3 hours before bedtime and limit her intake of caffeinated beverages. Increased voiding is normal, but encourage the woman to report any pain or burning during urination. Also explain that increased urinary frequency may subside as she enters her second trimester, only to recur in the third trimester. Teach the woman to perform Kegel or pelvic floor exercises throughout the day to help strengthen perineal muscle tone, thereby enhancing urinary control and decreasing the possibility of incontinence.

Fatigue

Fatigue plagues all pregnant women, primarily in the first and third trimesters (the highest energy levels typically occur during the second trimester), even if they get their normal amount of sleep at night. First-trimester fatigue most often is related to the many physical changes (e.g., increased oxygen consumption, increased levels of progesterone and relaxin, increased metabolic demands) and psychosocial changes (e.g., mood swings, multiple role demands) of pregnancy. Third-trimester fatigue can be caused by sleep disturbances from increased weight (many women cannot find a comfortable sleeping position due to the enlarging abdomen), physical discomforts such as heartburn, anxiety and/or insomnia, and a decrease in exercise (Coad & Dunstall, 2011; Schuurmans, Senikas, & Lalonde, 2010).

Once anemia, infection, and blood dyscrasias have been ruled out as contributing to the woman's fatigue, advise her to arrange work, child care, and other responsibilities to permit additional rest periods. Work with the woman to devise a realistic schedule for rest and activity. Using pillows for support in the side-lying position relieves pressure on major blood vessels that supply

TEACHING GUIDELINE 12.1

Teaching to Manage the Discomforts of Pregnancy

Urinary Frequency or Incontinence

- Try Kegel exercises to increase control over leakage.
- Empty your bladder when you first feel a full sensation.
- Avoid caffeinated drinks, which stimulate voiding.
- Reduce your fluid intake after dinner to reduce nighttime urination.

Fatigue

- Attempt to get a full night's sleep, without interruptions.
- Eat a healthy balanced diet.
- Schedule a nap in the early afternoon daily.
- When you are feeling tired, rest.

Nausea and Vomiting

- Eat whenever and whatever you like. Avoid an empty stomach.
- Munch on dry crackers/toast in bed before arising.
- Eat several small meals throughout the day.
- Drink fluids between meals rather than with meals.
- Avoid greasy, fried foods or ones with a strong odour.
- Try ginger supplements or acupressure (Sea Bands).
- If symptoms persist, discuss taking a doxylamine/pyridoxine supplement (Diclectin).

Backache

- Avoid standing or sitting in one position for long periods.
- Apply a heating pad (low setting) to the small of your back.
- Support your lower back with pillows when sitting.
- Stand with your shoulders back to maintain correct posture.

Leg Cramps

- Elevate legs above heart level frequently throughout the day.
- If you get a cramp, straighten both legs and flex your feet toward your body.
- Ask your health care provider about taking calcium supplements, which may reduce leg spasms.

Varicosities

- Walk daily to improve circulation to the extremities.
- Elevate both legs above the heart level while resting.
- Avoid standing in one position for long periods of time.
- Don't wear constrictive stockings and socks.
- Don't cross the legs when sitting for long periods.
- Wear support stockings to promote better circulation.

Constipation

- Increase your intake of foods high in fibre and drink at least eight 8-ounce glasses of fluid daily.
- Exercise each day (brisk walking) to promote movement through the intestine.
- Reduce the amount of cheese consumed.

Hemorrhoids

- Establish a regular time for daily bowel elimination.
- Prevent straining by drinking plenty of fluids and eating fibre-rich foods and exercising daily.
- Use warm sitz baths and cool witch hazel compresses for comfort.

Heartburn/Indigestion

- Avoid spicy or greasy foods and eat small, frequent meals.
- Sleep on several pillows so that your head is elevated.
- Stop smoking and avoid caffeinated drinks to reduce stimulation.
- Avoid lying down for at least 2 hours after meals.
- Try drinking sips of water to reduce the burning sensation.
- Take antacids sparingly if the burning sensation is severe (Tums are a good choice).

Braxton Hicks or Prelabour Contractions

- Before 37 weeks it is important to identify preterm labour and seek early treatment
- Try changing your position or engaging in mild exercise to help reduce the sensation.
- Drink more fluids if possible.

oxygen and nutrients to the fetus when resting (Fig. 12.7). Also recommend the use of relaxation techniques, providing instructions as necessary, and suggest she increase her daily exercise level.

Nausea and Vomiting

Nausea and vomiting are common discomforts during the first trimester: up to 90% of women experience nausea during pregnancy (Lane, 2007). The physiologic changes that cause nausea and vomiting are unknown, but research suggests that unusually high levels of estrogen, progesterone, and hCG and a vitamin B6 deficiency may be contributing factors. Nausea and vomiting of pregnancy may be an adaptation rather than a disease as the symptoms lead women to avoid alcohol and smoking (known teratogens). Symptoms usually last until the

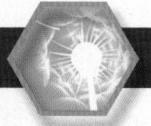

Nursing Care Plan 12.1

OVERVIEW OF THE WOMAN EXPERIENCING COMMON DISCOMFORTS OF PREGNANCY

Alicia, a 32-year-old, G1 P0, at 10 weeks' gestation, comes to the clinic for a visit. During the interview she tells you, "I'm running to the bathroom to urinate it seems like all the time, and I'm so nauseated that I'm having trouble eating." She denies any burning or pain on urination. Vital signs are within acceptable limits.

NURSING DIAGNOSIS: Impaired urinary elimination related to frequency secondary to physiologic changes of pregnancy

Outcome Identification and Evaluation
Woman will report a decrease in urinary complaints, as evidenced by a decrease in the number of times she uses the bathroom to void, reports that she feels her bladder is empty after voiding, and use of Kegel exercises.

Interventions: Promoting Normal Urinary Elimination Patterns
- Assess woman's usual bladder elimination patterns *to establish a baseline for comparison.*
- Obtain a urine specimen for analysis *to rule out infection or glucosuria.*
- Review with woman the physiologic basis for the increased frequency during pregnancy; inform woman that frequency should abate during the second trimester and that it most likely will return during her third trimester. *This will promote understanding of the problem.*
- Encourage the woman to empty her bladder when first feeling a sensation of fullness *to minimize risk of urinary retention.*
- Suggest woman avoid caffeinated drinks, *which can stimulate the need to void.*
- Encourage woman to drink adequate amounts of fluid throughout the day; however, have woman reduce her fluid intake before bedtime to reduce nighttime urination.
- Urge woman to keep the perineal area clean and dry *to prevent irritation and excoriation from any leakage.*
- Instruct woman in Kegel exercises *to increase perineal muscle tone and control over leakage.*
- Teach woman about the signs and symptoms of urinary tract infection and urge her to report them should they occur *to ensure early detection and prompt intervention.*

NURSING DIAGNOSIS: Imbalanced nutrition, less than body requirements, related to nausea and vomiting

Outcome Identification and Evaluation
Woman will ingest adequate amounts of nutrients for maternal and fetal well-being as evidenced by acceptable weight gain pattern and statements indicating an increase in food intake with a decrease in the number of episodes of nausea and vomiting.

Interventions: Promoting Adequate Nutrition
- Obtain weight and compare with baseline *to determine effects of nausea and vomiting on nutritional intake.*
- Review woman's typical dietary intake over 24 hours *to determine nutritional intake and patterns so that suggestions can be individualized.*
- Encourage woman to eat five or six small, frequent meals throughout the day *to prevent her stomach from becoming empty.*
- Suggest that she munch on dry crackers, toast, cereal, or cheese or drink a small amount of lemonade before arising *to minimize nausea.*
- Encourage woman to arise slowly from bed in the morning and avoid sudden movements *to reduce stimulation of the vomiting centre.*
- Advise woman to drink fluids between meals rather than with meals *to avoid overdistention of the abdomen and subsequent increase in abdominal pressure.*
- Encourage woman to increase her intake of foods high in vitamin B6, such as meat, poultry, bananas, fish, green leafy vegetables, peanuts, raisins, walnuts, and whole grains, as tolerated, *to ensure adequate nutrient intake.*
- Advise the woman to avoid greasy, fried, or highly spiced foods and to avoid strong odours, including foods such as cabbage, *to minimize gastrointestinal upset.*
- Encourage the woman to avoid wearing tight or restricting clothes *to minimize pressure on the expanding abdomen.*
- Arrange for consultation with nutritionist as necessary *to assist with diet planning.*
- Discuss taking a doxylamine/pyridoxine supplement (Diclectin) *to help ease nausea.*
- Provide appropriate online resources. (For links to some relevant websites, visit http://thePoint.lww.com/Chow1e.)

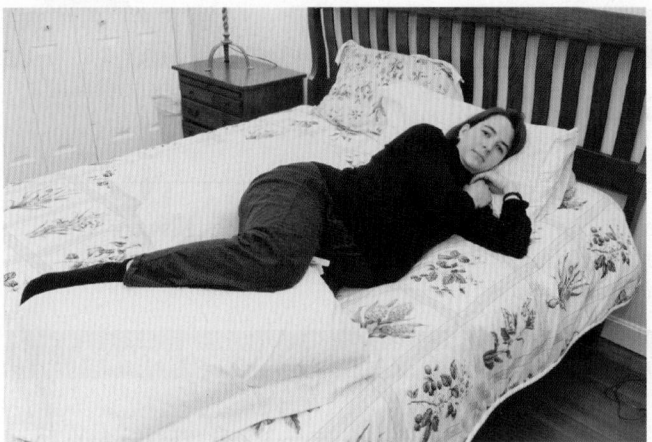

FIGURE 12.7 Using pillows for support in the side-lying position.

second trimester and are generally associated with a positive pregnancy outcome. Some women also experience ptyalism (excessive salivation), which requires frequent mouth care and sucking on hard candy to relieve symptoms (PHAC, 2010j).

To help alleviate nausea and vomiting, advise the woman to eat small, frequent meals (five or six a day) to prevent her stomach from becoming completely empty. Other helpful suggestions include eating dry crackers, Cheerios, lemonade, or cheese before getting out of bed in the morning and increasing her intake of foods high in vitamin B6 (such as meat, poultry, bananas, fish, green leafy vegetables, peanuts, raisins, walnuts, and whole grains), or making sure she is receiving enough vitamin B6 by taking her prescribed prenatal vitamins. Other helpful tips to deal with nausea and vomiting include the following:

- Get out of bed in the morning very slowly, and avoid sudden movements.
- Open a window to remove odours of food being cooked and avoid strong smells.
- Have someone else prepare meals if possible.
- Trust your body. Eat whatever you feel like and whenever you want.
- Limit intake of fluids or soups during meals (drink them between meals).
- Avoid fried foods and foods cooked with grease, oils, or fatty meats.
- Avoid highly seasoned foods (garlic, onions, peppers, and chili).
- Drink a small amount of a caffeine-free carbonated beverage (ginger ale) if nauseated.
- Avoid wearing tight or restricting clothes, which might place increased pressure on the expanding abdomen.
- Try alternative therapies, such as ginger supplements, acupressure (Sea Bands), or acupuncture (PHAC, 2010j; SOGC, 2002a).

For some women, nausea and vomiting of pregnancy is a serious health concern and additional treatment is recommended. Diclectin (a doxylamine/pyridoxine combination) is the treatment of choice since it has the best evidence to support its safety and effectiveness (SOGC, 2002a). Motherisk, an organization of The Hospital for Sick Children that aims to promote wellness in pregnant women and their unborn children, has developed a treatment algorithm for moderate to severe nausea and vomiting of pregnancy (Einarson, Maltepe, Boskovic, et al., 2007). (For a direct link to the Motherisk website, visit http://thePoint.lww.com/Chow1e.)

Breast Tenderness

Due to increased estrogen and progesterone levels, which cause the breast tissues to thicken and the number of milk ducts and glands to increase during the first trimester, many women experience breast tenderness (Coad & Dunstall, 2011). Offering a thorough explanation to the woman about the reasons for the breast discomfort is important. Wearing a larger bra with good support can help alleviate this discomfort. Some women need to wear a supportive bra, even while sleeping. As her breasts increase in size, advise her to change her bra size to ensure adequate support (Schuurmans et al., 2010).

Constipation

Increasing levels of progesterone during pregnancy lead to decreased contractility of the gastrointestinal tract, slowed movement of substances through the colon, and a resulting increase in water absorption (Coad & Dunstall, 2011). All of these factors lead to constipation. Lack of exercise or too little fibre or fluids in the diet can also promote constipation. In addition, the large bowel is mechanically compressed by the enlarging uterus, adding to this discomfort. The iron and calcium in prenatal vitamins can also contribute to constipation during the first and third trimesters.

Explain how pregnancy exacerbates the symptoms of constipation and offer the following suggestions:

- Eat fresh or dried fruit daily.
- Eat more raw fruits and vegetables, including their skins.
- Eat whole-grain cereals and breads such as raisin bran or bran flakes.
- Participate in physical activity every day.
- Eat meals at regular intervals.
- Establish a time of day to defecate, and elevate your feet on a stool to avoid straining.
- Drink six to eight glasses of water daily.
- Decrease your intake of refined carbohydrates.
- Drink warm fluids on arising to stimulate bowel motility.
- Decrease your consumption of sugary sodas.
- Avoid eating large amounts of cheese (PHAC, 2010e; Schuurmans et al., 2010).

If the suggestions above are ineffective, suggest that the woman use a bulk-forming laxative such as Metamucil.

Nasal Stuffiness, Epistaxis, Bleeding Gums

Increased levels of estrogen cause edema of the mucous membranes of the nasal and oral cavities (Coad & Dunstall, 2011). Advise the woman to drink extra water for hydration of the mucous membranes or to use a cool mist humidifier in her bedroom at night. Local application of petroleum jelly may also be helpful. If she needs to blow her nose to relieve nasal stuffiness, advise her to blow gently, one nostril at a time. Advise her to avoid the use of nasal decongestants and sprays.

If a nosebleed occurs, advise the woman to loosen the clothing around her neck, sit with her head tilted slightly forward, and pinch the bridge of her nose with her thumb and forefinger for 10 to 15 minutes.

If the woman has bleeding gums, encourage her to practice good oral hygiene by using a soft toothbrush and flossing daily. Warm saline mouthwashes can relieve discomfort. If the gum problem persists, instruct her to see her dentist (PHAC, 2010k).

▶ *Take* NOTE!

Poor oral hygiene is associated with preterm labour and birth. Some women will need assistance accessing inexpensive dental health services.

Cravings

Desires for certain foods and beverages are likely to begin during the first trimester but do not appear to reflect any physiologic need. Foods with a high sodium or sugar content often are the ones craved. At times, some women crave non-food substances such as clay, cornstarch, laundry detergent, baking soda, soap, paint chips, dirt, ice, or wax. This craving for non-food substances, termed pica, may indicate a severe dietary deficiency of minerals or vitamins, or it may have cultural roots (Coad & Dunstall, 2011). Pica is also discussed in Chapter 11.

Leukorrhea

Increased vaginal discharge begins during the first trimester and continues throughout pregnancy. The physiologic changes behind leukorrhea arise from the high levels of estrogen, which cause increased vascularity and hypertrophy of cervical glands and vaginal cells (Cunningham et al., 2010). The result is increased vaginal secretions throughout pregnancy.

Advise the woman to keep the perineal area clean and dry, washing the area with mild soap and water during her daily shower. Also recommend that she avoid wearing pantyhose and other tight-fitting nylon clothes that prevent air from circulating to the genital area. Encourage the use of cotton underwear and suggest wearing a nightgown rather than pajamas to allow for increased airflow. Also instruct the woman to avoid douching and tampon use (Schuurmans et al., 2010).

Second-Trimester Discomforts

A sense of well-being typically characterizes the second trimester for most women. By this time, the fatigue, nausea, and vomiting have subsided and the uncomfortable changes of the third trimester are a few months away. Not every woman experiences the same discomforts during this time, so nursing assessments and interventions must be individualized.

Backache

Backache, experienced by many women during the second trimester, is due to a shift in the centre of gravity caused by the enlarging uterus that results in muscle strain. In addition, a high level of circulating progesterone softens cartilage and loosens joints, thus increasing discomfort. Upper back pain also can be caused by increased breast size (SOGC, 2003b).

After exploring other reasons that might cause backache, such as uterine contractions, urinary tract infection, ulcers, or musculoskeletal back disorders, the following instructions may be helpful:

- Maintain correct posture, with head up and shoulders back.
- Wear low-heeled shoes with good arch support.
- When standing for long periods, place one foot on a stool or box.
- Use good body mechanics when lifting objects.
- When sitting, use foot supports and pillows behind the back.
- Try pelvic tilt or rocking exercises to strengthen the back (Schuurmans et al., 2010).

The pelvic tilt or pelvic rock is used to alleviate pressure on the lower back during pregnancy by stretching the lower back muscles. It can be done sitting, standing, or on all fours. To do it on all fours, the hands are positioned directly under the shoulders and the knees under the hips. The back should be in a neutral position with the head and neck aligned with the straight back. The woman then presses up with the lower back and holds this position for a few seconds, then relaxes to a neutral position. This action of pressing upward is repeated frequently throughout the day to prevent a sore back (SOGC, 2003b).

Leg Cramps

Leg cramps occur primarily in the second and third trimesters and could be related to the pressure of the gravid uterus on pelvic nerves and blood vessels (Coad & Dunstall, 2011). Diet can also be a contributing factor if the woman is not consuming enough of certain minerals, such as calcium and magnesium. The sudden stretching of leg muscles may also play a role in causing leg cramps (Schuurmans et al., 2010).

Encourage the woman to gently stretch the muscle by dorsiflexing the foot up toward the body. Wrapping a warm, moist towel around the leg muscle can also help the muscle to relax. Advise the woman to avoid stretching her legs and pointing her toes. Stress the importance of wearing low-heeled shoes and arising slowly from a sitting position. If the leg cramps result from deficiencies in minerals (such as calcium), eating more foods that are rich in these nutrients may relieve the condition. Also instruct the woman on calf-stretching exercises: have her stand .91 metres (3 feet) from the wall and lean toward it, resting her lower arms against it while keeping her heels on the floor. This may help reduce cramping if it is done before going to bed.

Elevating the legs throughout the day will help relieve pressure and minimize strain. Wearing support hose and avoiding curling the toes may help to relieve leg discomfort. Also instruct the woman to avoid standing in one spot for a prolonged period or crossing her legs. If she must stand for prolonged periods, suggest that she change her position at least every 2 hours by walking or sitting to reduce the risk of leg cramps. Encourage her to drink eight 236.6 millilitres (8 ounces) glasses of fluid throughout the day to ensure adequate hydration (Schuurmans et al., 2010).

Varicosities of the Vulva and Legs

Varicosities of the vulva and legs are associated with increased venous stasis caused by the pressure of the gravid uterus on pelvic vessels and the vasodilation resulting from increased progesterone levels. Progesterone relaxes the vein walls, making it difficult for blood to return to the heart from the extremities; pooling can result. Genetic predisposition, inactivity, obesity, and poor muscle tone are contributing factors (Coad & Dunstall, 2011).

Encourage the woman to wear support hose and teach her how to apply them properly. Advise her to elevate her legs above her heart while lying on her back for 10 minutes before she gets out of bed in the morning, thus promoting venous return before she applies the hose. Instruct the woman to avoid crossing her legs and wearing knee-high stockings because these actions cause constriction of leg vessels and muscles and contribute to venous stasis. Also encourage the woman to elevate both legs above the level of the heart for 5 to 10 minutes at least twice a day (Fig. 12.8), to wear low-heeled shoes, and to avoid long periods of standing or sitting, frequently changing her position. If the woman has vulvar varicosities, suggest she apply ice packs to the area when she is lying down.

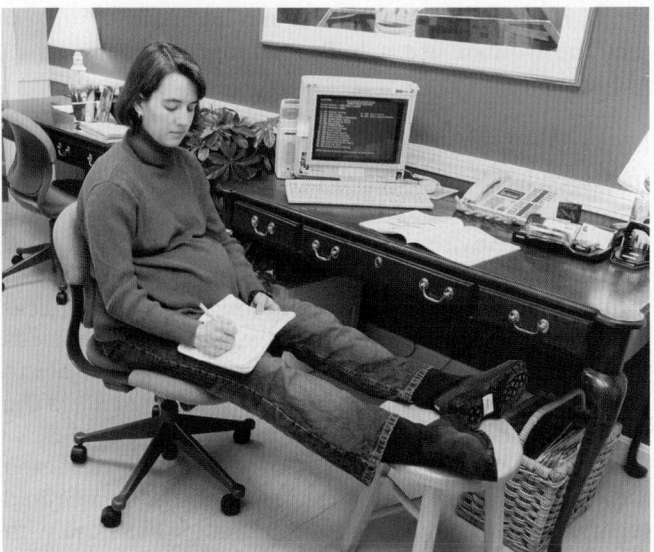

FIGURE 12.8 Woman elevating her legs while working.

Hemorrhoids

Hemorrhoids are varicosities of the rectum and may be external (outside the anal sphincter) or internal (above the sphincter). They occur as a result of progesterone-induced vasodilation and from pressure of the enlarged uterus on the lower intestine and rectum (Coad & Dunstall, 2011). Hemorrhoids are more common in women with constipation, poor fluid intake or poor dietary habits, smokers, or those with a previous history of hemorrhoids (Cunningham et al., 2010).

Instruct the woman in measures to prevent constipation, including increasing fibre intake and drinking at least 2 L of fluid per day. Recommend the use of topical anesthetics (e.g., Preparation H, Anusol) to reduce pain, itching, and swelling. Teach the woman about local comfort measures such as warm sitz baths, witch hazel compresses, or cold compresses. To minimize her risk of straining while defecating, suggest that she elevate her feet on a stool. Also encourage her to avoid prolonged sitting or standing (Schuurmans et al., 2010).

Flatulence with Bloating

The physiologic changes that result in constipation (reduced gastrointestinal motility and dilation secondary to progesterone's influence) may also result in increased flatulence. As the enlarging uterus compresses the bowel, it delays the passage of food through the intestines, thus allowing more time for gas to be formed by bacteria in the colon (Coad & Dunstall, 2011). The woman usually reports increased passage of rectal gas, abdominal bloating, or belching. Instruct the woman to avoid gas-forming foods, such as beans, cabbage, and onions, as well as foods that have a high content of white sugar. Adding more fibre to the diet, increasing fluid intake, and increasing physical exercise are also helpful in reducing flatus. In addition, reducing the swallowing of air when chewing gum or smoking will reduce gas build-up. Reducing the intake of carbonated beverages and cheese and eating mints can also help reduce flatulence during pregnancy (Schuurmans et al., 2010).

Third-Trimester Discomforts

As women enter their third trimester, many experience a return of the first-trimester discomforts of fatigue, urinary frequency, leukorrhea, and constipation. These discomforts are secondary to the ever-enlarging uterus compressing adjacent structures, increasing hormone levels, and the metabolic demands of the fetus. In addition to these discomforts, many women experience shortness of breath, heartburn and indigestion, swelling, and Braxton Hicks contractions.

Shortness of Breath

The increasing growth of the uterus prevents complete lung expansion late in pregnancy. As the uterus enlarges upward, the expansion of the diaphragm is limited. Shortness of breath can occur when the woman lies on her back and the pressure of the gravid uterus against the vena cava reduces venous return to the heart (Coad & Dunstall, 2011).

Explain to the woman that shortness of breath is normal and will improve when the fetus drops into the pelvis (lightening). Instruct her to adjust her body position to allow for maximum expansion of the chest and to avoid large meals, which increase abdominal pressure. Raising the head of the bed on blocks or placing pillows behind her back is helpful too. In addition, stress that lying on her side will displace the uterus off the vena cava, avoid supine hypotension syndrome, and improve her breathing. Advise the woman to avoid exercise that precipitates dyspnea, to rest after exercise, and to avoid overheating in warm climates. If she still smokes, encourage her to stop and/or refer her to a smoking cessation program (RNAO, 2007).

Heartburn and Indigestion

Heartburn and indigestion result when high progesterone levels cause relaxation of the cardiac sphincter, allowing food and digestive juices to flow backward from the stomach into the esophagus. Irritation of the esophageal lining occurs, causing the burning sensation known as heartburn. In addition, the stomach is displaced upward and compressed by the large uterus in the third trimester, thus limiting the stomach's capacity to empty quickly. Food sits, causing heartburn and indigestion (Coad & Dunstall, 2011). It occurs in up to 70% of women at some point during pregnancy, with an increased frequency seen in the third trimester (Blackburn, 2007).

Heartburn pain may radiate to the neck and throat. It worsens when the woman lies down, bends over after eating, or wears tight clothes. Indigestion (vague abdominal discomfort after meals) results from eating too much or too fast; from eating when tense, tired, or emotionally upset; from eating food that is too fatty or spicy; and from eating heavy food or food that has been badly cooked or processed (Schuurmans et al., 2010).

Review the woman's usual dietary intake and suggest that she limit or avoid gas-producing or fatty foods and large meals. Encourage the woman to maintain proper posture and remain in the sitting position for 1 to 3 hours after eating to prevent reflux of gastric acids into the esophagus by gravity. Urge the woman to eat slowly, chewing her food thoroughly to prevent excessive swallowing of air, which can lead to increased gastric pressure. Instruct the woman to avoid highly spiced foods, chocolate, coffee, alcohol, sodas, and spearmint or peppermint. These items stimulate the release of gastric digestive acids, which may cause reflux into the esophagus. Avoid late-night or large meals and gum chewing (PHAC, 2010i).

Dependent Edema

Swelling is the result of increased capillary permeability caused by elevated hormone levels and increased blood volume. Sodium and water are retained and thirst increases. Edema occurs most often in dependent areas such as the legs and feet throughout the day due to gravity; it improves after a night's sleep. Warm weather or prolonged standing or sitting may increase edema. Generalized edema, appearing in the face, hands, and feet, can signal pre-eclampsia if accompanied by dizziness, blurred vision, headaches, upper quadrant pain, or nausea (Gilbert, 2011). Generalized edema should be reported to the health care provider.

Appropriate suggestions to minimize dependent edema include the following:

- Elevate your feet and legs above the level of the heart.
- Wear support hose when standing or sitting for long periods.
- Change position frequently throughout the day.
- Walk at a sensible pace to help contract leg muscles to promote venous return.
- When taking a long car ride, stop to walk around every 2 hours.
- When standing, rock from the ball of the foot to the toes to stimulate circulation.
- Lie on your left side to keep the gravid uterus off the vena cava to return blood to the heart.
- Avoid foods high in sodium, such as lunch meats, potato chips, and bacon.
- Avoid wearing knee-high stockings.
- Drink six to eight glasses of water daily to replace fluids lost through perspiration.
- Avoid high intake of sugar and fats, which cause water retention.

Carpal Tunnel Syndrome

Pregnant women may experience tingling, numbness, and/or burning in the fingers and hands due to the physiologic changes of pregnancy (edema), which compress the median nerve (Cunningham et al., 2010). The nurse can suggest gentle range-of-motion exercises and/or elevation of the affected hand. Women should avoid repetitive wrist motion and take frequent breaks from work activities. Some women may require referral to a physiotherapist for a soft wrist splint.

Round Ligament Pain

Some women experience pain under the ribs from tension placed on the round ligament due to uterine enlargement. Slow position changes may help prevent this pain, and bringing the knees up to the abdomen may decrease it. For unremitting round ligament pain, assuming a hands-and-knees position with the head down and buttocks elevated may be helpful.

Braxton Hicks or Prelabour Contractions

Braxton Hicks contractions are irregular, painless contractions that occur without cervical dilation. Typically they intensify in the third trimester in preparation for labour. In reality, they have been present since early in the pregnancy but may have gone unnoticed. They are thought to increase the tone of uterine muscles for labour purposes.

Reassure the woman that these contractions are normal. Instruct the woman in how to differentiate between Braxton Hicks and labour contractions. Explain that in labour contractions grow longer, stronger, and closer together and occur at regular intervals. Walking usually strengthens true labour contractions, whereas Braxton Hicks contractions tend to decrease in intensity and taper off. Advise the woman to keep herself well hydrated and to rest in a side-lying position to help relieve the discomfort. Suggest that she use relaxation and breathing techniques to ease the discomfort.

Nursing Management to Promote Health in Pregnancy

RNs work in collaboration with childbearing women and their families to promote health and positive childbearing experiences. Pregnancy is considered a time of health, not illness. Health promotion and maintenance activities are important for promoting an optimal outcome for the woman and her fetus. Pregnant women commonly have many questions about the changes occurring during pregnancy; how these changes affect their usual routine, such as working, travelling, exercising, or engaging in sexual activity; how the changes influence their typical self-care activities, such as bathing, perineal care, or dental care; and whether these changes are signs of a problem. A number of resources are available to guide pregnant women. Many of these, such as PHAC's "The Sensible Guide to a Healthy Pregnancy," are available online (PHAC, 2008b).

> ▶ *Take* NOTE!
>
> *Women may have heard stories about or been told by others what to do and what not to do during pregnancy, leading to many misconceptions and much misinformation. However, nurses also need to respect traditional knowledge in order to provide culturally safe care.*

Nurses can play a major role in providing anticipatory guidance and teaching to promote the woman's health, helping to clarify misconceptions and correct any misinformation. Educating the woman to identify health risks posed by her health practices, lifestyle, or environment situations and proposing ways to modify them to avoid a negative outcome are important health promotion strategies. Counselling should include instructions for healthy ways to prepare food, advice to avoid medications unless they are prescribed for her, and discussion about identifying teratogens within her environment or at work and how to reduce her risk from exposure. The pregnant woman can better care for herself and the fetus if her concerns are anticipated. Nurses also have an advocacy role in lobbying for health policies, programs,

> ▶ *Consider* THIS!
>
> *One has to wonder sometimes why women go through what they do. During my first pregnancy I was sick for the first 2 months. I would experience waves of nausea from the moment I got out of bed until midmorning. Needless to say, I wasn't the happiest camper around. After the third month, my life seemed to settle down and I was beginning to think that being pregnant wasn't too bad after all. For the moment, I was fooled. Then, during my last 2 months, another wave of discomfort struck—heartburn and constipation—a double whammy! I now feared eating anything that might trigger acid indigestion and also might remain in my body too long. I literally had to become the "fibre queen" to combat these two challenges. Needless to say, my "suffering" was well worth our bright-eyed baby girl in the end.*
>
> *Thoughts: despite the various discomforts associated with pregnancy, most women wouldn't change their end result. Do most women experience these discomforts? What suggestions could be made to reduce them?*

and appropriate services, particularly for Canadian women living in rural, remote, or Aboriginal communities (MacKinnon, 2008).

Personal Hygiene

Counsel women to wash their hands frequently throughout the day to lower the bacterial count on their hands and under their fingernails. During pregnancy a woman's sebaceous (sweat) glands become more active under the influence of hormones, and sweating is more profuse. The cervical and vaginal glands also produce more secretions during pregnancy. Frequent showering helps to promote better hygiene. Encourage the use of cotton underwear to allow greater air circulation. Taking a tub bath in pregnancy is permitted as long as the fetal membranes are intact. In the third trimester, the woman's centre of gravity shifts so extra precautions are needed to prevent the risk of slipping.

Hot Tubs and Saunas

Caution pregnant women to avoid using hot tubs, saunas, whirlpools, and tanning beds during pregnancy. The heat may cause fetal tachycardia as well as raise the maternal temperature. Exposure to bacteria in hot tubs that have not been cleaned sufficiently is another reason to avoid them during pregnancy (PHAC, 2010l).

Perineal Care

The glands in the cervical and vaginal areas become more active during pregnancy secondary to hormonal influences. This increase in activity will produce more vaginal secretions, especially in the last trimester. Advise pregnant women to shower frequently and wear all-cotton underwear to minimize the effects of these secretions. Caution pregnant women not to douche, because douching can increase the risk of infection, and not to wear panty liners, which block air circulation and retain moisture. Explain that they should also avoid perfumed soaps, lotions, perineal sprays, and harsh laundry detergents to help prevent irritation and potential infection.

Dental Care

Research has established that the elevated levels of estrogen and progesterone during pregnancy cause women to be more sensitive to the effects of bacterial dental plaque, which can cause gingivitis, an oral infection characterized by swollen and bleeding gums (Schuurmans et al., 2010). Brushing and flossing teeth twice daily will help reduce bacteria in the mouth. Advise the woman to visit her dentist early in the pregnancy to address any dental caries and have a thorough cleaning to prevent possible infection later in the pregnancy. Advise her to avoid exposure to X-rays by informing the hygienist of the pregnancy (PHAC, 2010k).

Researchers are exploring a link between prematurity and periodontitis (SOGC, 2010c), an oral infection that spreads beyond the gum tissues to invade the supporting structures of the teeth. Periodontitis is characterized by bleeding gums, loss of tooth attachment, loss of supporting bone, and bad breath due to pus formation. Unfortunately, because this infection is chronic and often painless, women frequently don't realize they have it. Additional guidelines that the nurse should stress regarding maintaining dental health include the following:

- Seek professional dental care during the first trimester for assessment and care.
- Obtain treatment for dental pain and infection promptly during pregnancy.
- Brush twice daily for 2 minutes with fluoridated toothpaste, especially before bed, and rinse well. Use a soft-bristled toothbrush and be sure to brush at the gum line to remove food debris and plaque to keep gums healthy.
- Eat healthy foods, especially those high in vitamins A, C, and D and calcium.
- Avoid sugary snacks. Chew sugar-free gum for 10 minutes after a meal if brushing isn't possible.
- Prevent tooth decay that results from morning sickness. After vomiting, rinse your mouth immediately with water as soon as possible (PHAC, 2010j).

Breast Care

Since the breasts enlarge significantly and become heavier throughout pregnancy, stress the need to wear a firm, supportive bra with wide straps to balance the weight of the breasts. Instruct the woman to anticipate buying a larger-sized bra about halfway through her pregnancy because of the increasing size of the breasts. Advise her to avoid using soap on the nipple area because it can be very drying. Encourage her to rinse the nipple area with plain water while bathing to keep it clean. The Montgomery glands secrete a lubricating substance that keeps the nipples moist and discourages growth of bacteria, so there is no need to use soap or antiseptics on the nipples. Colostrum secretion begins at around 16 weeks' gestation, at which time the woman may notice as moisture in her bra. Advise the woman to place cotton breast pads in her bra and change them frequently to prevent build-up, which may lead to excoriation.

If the mother has chosen to breastfeed, nipple preparation is unnecessary unless her nipples are inverted and do not become erect when stimulated. Consider referring the woman with inverted nipples or other breastfeeding concerns to a lactation consultant (Johnson & Strube, 2011).

Clothing

Many contemporary clothes are loose-fitting and layered, so the woman may not need to buy an entirely new wardrobe to accommodate her pregnancy. While some pregnant women continue to wear tight clothes, loose clothing may be more comfortable for the woman and her expanding waistline. Advise pregnant women to avoid wearing constricting clothes and girdles that compress the growing abdomen. Urge the woman to avoid knee-high hose, which might impede lower-extremity circulation and increase the risk of developing DVT. Low-heeled shoes will minimize falls and prevent backache. Wearing layered clothing may be more comfortable, especially toward term, when the woman may feel overheated.

Exercise

Exercise is well tolerated by a healthy woman during pregnancy. It promotes a feeling of well-being, improves circulation, helps reduce constipation, bloating, and swelling, increases energy level, improves posture, helps sleep, promotes relaxation and rest, and relieves the lower back discomfort that often arises as the pregnancy progresses. However, the duration and difficulty of exercise should be modified throughout pregnancy because of a decrease in performance efficiency with gestational age. Some women continue to push themselves to maintain their prior level of exercise, but most find that as their shape changes and their abdominal area enlarges, they must modify their exercise routines. Modification also helps to reduce the risk of injury caused by laxity of the joints and connective tissue, which results from hormonal effects (SOGC, 2003b).

Exercise during pregnancy is contraindicated in women with preterm labour, ruptured membranes, hypertensive disorders of pregnancy, an incompetent cervix, a growth-restricted fetus, higher-order multiple gestation, persistent antepartum bleeding, placenta previa, or serious systemic diseases such as cardiac disease. Table 12.4 provides a list of absolute and relative contraindications that have been approved by both the SOGC and the Canadian Society for Exercise Physiology.

It is believed that pregnancy is a unique time for behaviour change and that healthy behaviours maintained or adopted during pregnancy may improve the woman's health for the rest of her life. The excess weight gained in pregnancy, which some women never lose, is a major public health problem (PHAC, 2008a). Obese women should be advised that they are at risk for medical complications such as cardiac disease, pulmonary disease, gestational hypertension, gestational diabetes, and obstructive sleep apnea (SOGC, 2010b). Regular exercise during pregnancy may help to reduce some of these risks.

Exercise during pregnancy helps return a woman's body to good health after the baby is born. The long-term benefits of exercise include improved posture, weight control, and improved muscle tone; exercise also aids in the prevention of osteoporosis after menopause

TABLE 12.4 CONTRAINDICATIONS TO EXERCISE IN PREGNANCY

Absolute Contraindications	Relative Contraindications
Ruptured membranes	Previous spontaneous abortion
Preterm labour	Previous preterm birth
Hypertensive disorders of pregnancy	Mild/moderate cardiovascular disorder
Incompetent cervix	Mild/moderate respiratory disorder
Growth-restricted fetus	Anemia (hemoglobin <100 g/L)
Higher-order multiple gestation (triplets)	Twin pregnancy after 28 weeks
Placenta previa after 28th week	Malnutrition or eating disorder
Persistent second or third trimester bleeding	Other significant medical conditions
Uncontrolled type 1 diabetes, thyroid disease, or other serious medical disorder	

Adapted from: Society of Obstetricians and Gynaecologists of Canada. (2003b). SOGC Clinical Practice Guideline No. 129: Exercise in pregnancy and the postpartum period. *Journal of Obstetrics and Gynaecology Canada, 25*(6), 516–522. Retrieved February 21, 2012 from http://www.sogc.org/guidelines/public/129E-JCPG-June2003.pdf.

and assists in keeping the birth weight of the fetus within the normal range (PHAC, 2010l). Teaching Guideline 12.2 highlight recommendations for exercise during pregnancy.

Sleep and Rest

Getting enough sleep helps a person feel better and promotes optimal performance levels during the day. The body releases its greatest concentration of growth hormone during sleep, helping the body to repair damaged tissue and grow. Also, with the increased metabolic demands during pregnancy, fatigue is a constant challenge to many pregnant women, especially during the first and third trimesters. A recent nursing study demonstrated that 25% of women have high childbirth fears and more than 20% reported sleeping fewer than 6 hours per night (Hall, Hauch, Carty, et al., 2009). Providing an opportunity for women to express their fear of childbirth may be an effective nursing intervention.

The following tips can help promote adequate sleep:

• Stay on a regular schedule by going to bed and waking up at the same times.

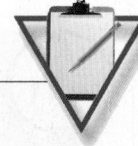

TEACHING GUIDELINE 12.2

Teaching to Promote Exercise During Pregnancy

- Consume liquids before, during, and after exercising.
- Exercise three or four times each week, not sporadically.
- Engage in brisk walking, swimming, biking, or low-impact aerobics; these are considered ideal activities.
- Avoid getting overheated during exercise.
- Reduce the intensity of workouts in late pregnancy.
- Avoid jerky, bouncy, or high-impact movements.
- Avoid lying flat (supine) after the fourth month because of supine hypotension.
- Use pelvic tilt and pelvic rocking to relieve backache.
- Start with 5 to 10 minutes of stretching exercises.
- Rise slowly following an exercise session to avoid dizziness.
- Avoid activities such as skiing, surfing, scuba diving, and ice hockey.
- Never exercise to the point of exhaustion.

Sources: Public Health Agency of Canada. (2008b). *The sensible guide to a healthy pregnancy.* Retrieved February 21, 2012 from http://www.phac-aspc.gc.ca/hp-gs/guide-eng.php; and Society of Obstetricians and Gynaecologists of Canada. (2003b). SOGC Clinical Practice Guideline No. 129: Exercise in pregnancy and the postpartum period. *Journal of Obstetrics and Gynaecology Canada, 25*(6), 516–522. Retrieved February 21, 2012 from http://www.sogc.org/guidelines/public/129E-JCPG-June2003.pdf.

- Eat meals at regular times to keep external body cues consistent.
- Take time to unwind and relax before bedtime.
- Establish a bedtime routine or pattern and follow it.
- Create a restful sleep environment by reducing the light and lowering the room temperature.
- Go to bed when you feel tired; if sleep doesn't occur, read a book until you are sleepy.
- Reduce caffeine intake later in the day.
- Limit fluid intake after dinner to minimize trips to the bathroom.
- Exercise daily to improve circulation and well-being.
- Avoid lying flat on your back after the fourth month, which may compromise circulation to the uterus and result in supine hypotension syndrome.
- Keep anxieties and worries out of the bedroom. Set aside a specific area in the home or time of day for them (PHAC, 2010c).

See Evidence-based Practice 12.2.

Emotional Health

One in ten women suffers from depression during pregnancy (PHAC, 2010g), so women and family members need to be aware of the signs and symptoms of depression as well as the availability of treatment when needed. Women who have experienced postpartum depression with a previous pregnancy may need additional nursing

---

EVIDENCE-BASED PRACTICE 12.2
Childbirth Fear, Anxiety, Fatigue, and Sleep Deprivation in Pregnant Women

● **Study**

This study explored relationships between women's levels of childbirth fear, sleep deprivation, anxiety, and fatigue during the third trimester of pregnancy. The study is important because these variable cause women distress and have been associated with increased childbirth interventions, such as caesarean birth.

This cross-sectional survey included 650 women living in one Canadian province and planning to give birth in the next few weeks at a hospital with a minimum of 150 births/year. Women who responded to the survey were an average of 31.5 years old, predominantly well educated, and Canadian citizens. Sixty percent of respondents were nulliparous; 40% were multiparous. Respondents were cared for during pregnancy by a family physician (39%), an obstetrician (36%), or a midwife (25%).

▲ **The Findings**

Twenty-five percent of women reported high levels of childbirth fear, 54% reported moderate levels, and 21% reported low levels. Childbirth fear, fatigue, sleep deprivation, and anxiety were positively correlated. Women's fear of childbirth appears to be part of a complex picture of women's emotional experiences during late pregnancy.

■ **Nursing Implications**

Women who have high childbirth fear are more likely to have significantly less help available, more daily stressors, and more fatigue and anxiety. Women cared for by midwives have lower anxiety and fear levels, so perhaps nurses could recommend supportive midwifery care and help women mobilize their support networks. Nursing interventions to reduce fatigue and childbirth fear require further study.

Source: Hall, W., Hauch, Y., Carty, E., Hutton, E., Fenwick, J., & Stoll, K. (2009). Childbirth fear, anxiety, fatigue, and sleep deprivation in pregnant women. *Journal of Obstetric, Gynecologic, & Neonatal Nursing, 38,* 567–576. doi:10.1111/j.1552–6909.2009.01054.x

BOX 12.3 Symptoms of Depression

Women should check with their health care provider if they experience four or more of the following symptoms for a 2-week period or if any of the symptoms causes undue concern.
- Anxiety or inability to concentrate
- Frequent mood swings or extreme irritability
- Sleep problems or extreme fatigue
- Persistent sadness or a feeling that nothing is fun anymore
- Lack of interest in things you usually care about
- A dramatic change in appetite (increased or decreased)

Adapted from: Public Health Agency of Canada. (2008b). *The sensible guide to a healthy pregnancy.* Retrieved February 21, 2012 from http://www.phac-aspc.gc.ca/hp-gs/guide-eng.php.

support and should be encouraged to mobilize their support network. The following activities promote emotional health and may help prevent depression in pregnancy or following birth:

- Maintain a healthy balance of activity and rest. Exercise and eat well to help limit mood swings.
- Get adequate sleep and rest. Accept offers of help from family and friends.
- Share your thoughts and feelings with others when you are worried, anxious, sad, or upset.
- Avoid stress as much as possible and build your social support network.
- Know the symptoms of depression (Box 12.3), and contact your health care provider if you experience four or more of these symptoms for at least 2 weeks or if any of them is a particular concern.
- Screen women for intimate partner violence at every opportunity, when their partner is not present (SOGC, 2005c), and know how to respond if the answer is "yes."

Sexual Activity and Sexuality

Pregnancy is characterized by intense biological, psychological, and social changes. These changes have direct and indirect, conscious and unconscious effects on a woman's sexuality. The woman experiences dramatic alterations in her physiology, her appearance, and her body, as well as her relationships. A woman's sexual responses during pregnancy vary widely. Common symptoms such as fatigue, nausea, vomiting, breast soreness, and urinary frequency may reduce her desire for sexual intimacy. However, many women report enhanced sexual desire due to increasing levels of estrogen and pelvic congestion (Kitzinger, 2005).

▶ *Take* NOTE!

Fluctuations in sexual desire are normal and a highly individualized response throughout pregnancy.

The physical and emotional adjustments of pregnancy can cause changes in body image, fatigue, mood swings, and sexual activity. The woman's changing shape, emotional status, fetal activity, changes in breast size, pressure on the bladder, and other common discomforts of pregnancy result in increased physical and emotional demands. These can produce stress on the sexual relationship of the pregnant woman and her partner. However, most women adjust well to the alterations and experience a satisfying sexual relationship.

Often pregnant women ask whether sexual intercourse is allowed during pregnancy or whether there are specific times when they should refrain from having sex. This is a good opportunity to educate women about sexual activity during pregnancy and also to ask about their expectations and experiences related to sexuality and pregnancy changes. It is also a good time for nurses to address the impact of the changes associated with pregnancy on sexual desire and behaviour. Some women experience increased sexual desire while others experience less. Couples may enjoy sexual activity more because there is no fear of pregnancy and no need to disrupt spontaneity by using birth control. An increase in pelvic congestion and lubrication secondary to estrogen influence may heighten orgasm for many women. Some women have a decrease in desire because of a negative body image, fear of harming the fetus by engaging in intercourse, and fatigue, nausea, and vomiting A couple may need assistance to adjust to the various changes brought about by pregnancy. Reassure the woman and her partner that sexual activity is permissible during pregnancy unless there is a history of any of the following:

- Vaginal bleeding
- Placenta previa
- Risk of preterm labour
- Incompetent cervix
- Premature rupture of membranes
- Presence of infection (SexualityandU, 2010)

Inform the couple that the fetus will not be injured by intercourse. Suggest that alternative positions may be more comfortable (e.g., woman on top, side-lying), especially during the later stages of pregnancy (Kitzinger, 2005). Many women feel a particular need for closeness during pregnancy, and the woman should communicate this need to her partner. Emphasize to the couple that closeness and cuddling need not culminate in intercourse and that other forms of sexual expression, such as mutual masturbation, foot massage, holding hands, kissing, and hugging can be very satisfying (SexualityandU, 2010). Women will experience a myriad of symptoms, feelings, and physical sensations during their pregnancy. Having a satisfying sexual relationship during pregnancy is certainly possible, but it requires honest communication between partners to determine what works best for them and a good relationship with their health care provider to ensure safety (SexualityandU, 2010).

You may also encounter childbearing women who identify as a lesbian couple. Nurses need to first reflect on their own values and assumptions about lesbian motherhood and refer to current literature (Larsson & Dykes, 2009).

Employment

For the most part, women can continue working until delivery if they have no complications during their pregnancy and the workplace does not present any special hazards. Hazardous occupations include health care workers, day care providers, laboratory technicians, chemists, painters, hairstylists, veterinary workers, and carpenters. Jobs that require strenuous work, such as heavy lifting, climbing, carrying heavy objects, and standing for prolonged periods, place a pregnant woman at risk for falls and for preterm labour if modifications are not instituted (Schuurmans et al., 2010).

Assess for environmental and occupational factors that place a pregnant women and her fetus at risk for injury. Interview the woman about her employment environment. Ask about possible exposure to teratogens and the physical demands of employment: is she exposed to temperature extremes? Does she need to stand for prolonged periods in a fixed position? A description of the work environment is important in providing anticipatory guidance to the woman. Stress the importance of taking rest periods throughout the day, because constant physically intensive workloads increase the likelihood of low birth weight and preterm labour and birth (Cunningham et al., 2010).

Due to the numerous physiologic and psychosocial changes that women experience during pregnancy, the employer may need to make special accommodations to reduce the pregnant woman's risk of hazardous exposures and heavy workloads. The employer may need to provide adequate coverage so that the woman can take rest breaks; remove the woman from any areas where she might be exposed to toxic substances; and avoid work assignments that require heavy lifting, hard physical labour, continuous standing, or constant moving (Schuurmans et al., 2010). Women who are employed may be eligible for maternity and parental leave benefits. Service Canada provides information about these benefits. Some recommendations for working while pregnant are given in Teaching Guideline 12.3.

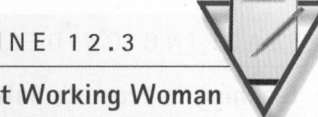

TEACHING GUIDELINE 12.3

Teaching for the Pregnant Working Woman

- Plan to take two 10- to 15-minute breaks within an 8-hour workday.
- Be sure there is a place available for you to rest, preferably in the side-lying position, with a restroom readily available.
- Avoid jobs that require strenuous workloads; if this is not possible, request a modification of work duties (lighter tasks) to reduce your workload.
- Change your position from standing to sitting or vice versa at least every 2 hours.
- Ensure that you are allowed time off without penalty, if necessary, to ensure a healthy outcome for you and your baby.
- Make sure the work environment is free of toxic substances.
- Ensure the work environment is smoke-free so passive smoking isn't a concern.
- Minimize heavy lifting if associated with bending.

Sources: Public Health Agency of Canada. (2008b). *The sensible guide to a healthy pregnancy*. Retrieved February 21, 2012 from http://www.phac-aspc.gc.ca/hp-gs/guide-eng.php; and Schuurmans, N., Senikas, V., & Lalonde, A. (2010). *Healthy beginnings* (4th ed.). Ottawa: Society of Obstetricians and Gynaecologists of Canada.

Travel

Pregnancy does not curtail a woman's ability to travel in a car or in a plane. However, women should follow a few safety guidelines to minimize risk to themselves and their fetuses. Pregnant women can travel safely throughout their pregnancy, although the second trimester is perhaps the best time to travel because there is the least chance of complications (Schuurmans et al., 2010). Pregnant women planning international travel should consider the problems that could occur during the journey as well as the quality of medical care available at the destination. In addition, pregnant women have an increased risk of blood clots during prolonged travel so having an aisle seat and walking during long flights is recommended (Foreign Affairs and International Trade Canada, 2011; PHAC, 2010f).

▶ *Take* NOTE!

It is often difficult to find pasteurized milk in developing countries. When travelling to developing countries, pregnant women are encouraged to take powdered milk to mix into other foods to help ensure that they get enough calcium (Foreign Affairs and International Trade Canada, 2011).

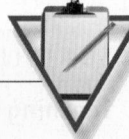

TEACHING GUIDELINE 12.4

Teaching to Promote Safe Travel on Planes and in Foreign Countries

- Bring along a copy of the prenatal record if your travel will be prolonged in case there is a medical emergency away from home.
- When travelling abroad, carry a foreign dictionary that includes words or phrases for the most common pregnancy emergencies.
- Travel with at least one companion at all times for personal safety.
- Check with your health care provider before receiving any immunizations necessary for foreign travel; some may be harmful to the fetus.
- When in some foreign countries, avoid fresh fruit, vegetables, and local water.
- Avoid any milk that is not pasteurized.
- Eat only meat that is well cooked to avoid toxoplasmosis.
- Request an aisle seat and walk about the airplane every 2 hours.
- While sitting on long flights, practice ankle-circling exercises to improve circulation to the lower extremities.
- Be aware of typical problems encountered by pregnant travellers, such as fatigue, heartburn, indigestion, constipation, vaginal discharge, leg cramps, urinary frequency, and hemorrhoids.
- Always wear support hose while flying to prevent the development of blood clots.
- Drink plenty of water to keep well hydrated throughout the flight.

Source: Foreign Affairs and International Trade Canada. (2011). *Her own way: A woman's guide to safe and successful travel.* Retrieved February 21, 2012 from http://www.voyage.gc.ca/publications/pdf/her_own_way-en.pdf.

Advise pregnant women to be aware of the potential for injuries and trauma related to travel, and teach women ways to prevent these from occurring. Teaching Guideline 12.4 offers tips for safe travel on planes and to foreign areas.

When travelling by car, the major risk is a car accident. The impact and momentum can lead to traumatic separation of the placenta from the wall of the uterus. Shock and massive hemorrhage might result. Transport Canada recommends that pregnant women take extra care when adjusting their seat belt. "Sit as upright as you can, and wear the lap belt under your abdomen and as low over the hips as possible. The shoulder strap should go between your breasts and off to the side above your belly" (Transport Canada, 2007).

Tips that nurses can offer to promote safety during ground travel include the following:

- Always wear a three-point seat belt, no matter how short the trip, to prevent ejection or serious injury from collision.
- Apply a nonpadded shoulder strap properly; it should cross between the breasts and over the upper abdomen, above the uterus (Fig. 12.9).
- If no seat belts are available (buses or vans), ride in the back seat of the vehicle.
- Use a lap belt that crosses over the pelvis below the uterus.
- Avoid cell phone use while driving to prevent distraction.
- Avoid driving when very fatigued, especially in the first and third trimesters.
- Avoid late-night driving, when visibility might be compromised.
- Direct a tilting steering wheel away from the abdomen (Schuurmans et al., 2010; Transport Canada, 2007)

Pets

Pets can be great stress reducers, providing companionship to pregnant women and their family members. After the baby is born, some pets respond with jealousy, not unlike sibling rivalry. Many books and online resources offer suggestions for dealing with these concerns. Nurses need to be aware of current resources.

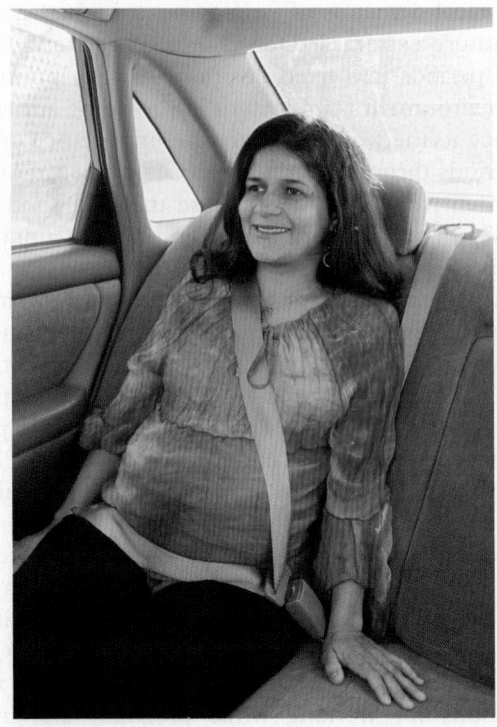

FIGURE 12.9 Proper application of a seat belt during pregnancy.

Toxoplasmosis is an illness that is caused by a protozoan and may result in harm to the developing baby if the mother gets the disease in pregnancy. Cats infected with the organism can spread the disease through their feces. Women should be counselled to avoid emptying the cat litter box or working in gardens frequented by cats. Eating undercooked meat and drinking unpasteurized milk are also not recommended (PHAC, 2010n).

Immunizations and Medications

Ideally, women should receive all childhood immunizations before conception to protect the fetus from any risk of congenital anomalies. If the woman comes for a preconception visit, discuss immunizations such as measles, mumps, and rubella (MMR), hepatitis B, and diphtheria/tetanus (every 10 years); administer them at this time if needed (SOGC, 2009b).

The risk to a developing fetus from vaccination of the mother during pregnancy is primarily theoretical. Routine immunizations are not usually indicated during pregnancy. However, no evidence exists of risk from vaccinating pregnant women with inactivated virus or bacterial vaccines or toxoids. A number of other vaccines have not been studied adequately, and thus the theoretical risks of vaccination must be weighed against the potential risks of the disease to mother and fetus (SOGC, 2009b). Guidelines for immunization during pregnancy are highlighted in Box 12.4 (SOGC, 2009b).

► *Take* NOTE!

Advise pregnant women to avoid live virus vaccines (MMR and varicella) and to avoid becoming pregnant within 1 month of having received one of these vaccines because of the theoretical risk of transmission to the fetus (Bozzo, Narducci, & Einararson, 2011).

It is best for pregnant women not to take any unnecessary medications. Encourage women to discuss with the health care provider their current medications and any herbal remedies they take so that they can learn about any potential risks should they continue to take the medications during pregnancy. Generally, if the woman is taking medicine for seizures, high blood pressure, asthma, or depression, the benefits of continuing the medicine during pregnancy outweigh the risks to the fetus. The safety profile of some medications may change according to the gestational age of the fetus (Schuurmans et al., 2010).

The U.S. Food and Drug Administration (FDA) has developed a system of ranking drugs that appears on the labels and in the package inserts in Canada. These risk categories are summarized in Box 12.5. About one in five Canadian women uses FDA category C, D, and X drugs at least once in pregnancy (Wen, Yang, Krewski, et al., 2008). The most common prescription drugs taken in pregnancy are antiasthmatics, antibiotics, nonsteroidal anti-inflammatory drugs, antianxiety or antidepressant medications, and oral contraceptives. Nurses play an important role in discussing medication use (including herbal medications and vitamin therapy) with childbearing women and should have access to reference books on drugs in pregnancy and lactation.

A common concern of many pregnant women involves the use of over-the-counter medications and herbal agents. Many women consider these products benign simply because they are available without a prescription. While herbal medications are commonly thought of as "natural" alternatives to other medicines, they can be just as potent as some prescription medications. A major concern about herbal medicine is the lack of consistent potency in the active ingredients in any given batch of product, making it difficult to know the exact strength by reading the label. Also, many herbs contain chemicals that cross the placenta and may cause harm to the fetus (Schuurmans et al., 2010).

Nurses are often asked about the safety of over-the-counter medicines and herbal agents. Unfortunately, many drugs have not been evaluated in controlled studies, and it is difficult to make general recommendations

---

BOX 12.4 Guidelines for Immunization in Pregnancy

Vaccines That Should be Considered if Otherwise Indicated
- Hepatitis A or B
- Influenza (recommend inactivated vaccine)
- Tetanus/diphtheria
- Meningococcal
- Rabies

Vaccines Contraindicated During Pregnancy
- Influenza (live, live-attenuated vaccine)
- Measles
- Mumps
- Rubella
- Varicella
- Yellow fever (no data on safety)
- Poliomyelitis (oral polio vaccine)

Adapted from: Society of Obstetricians and Gynaecologists of Canada. (2009b). SOGC Clinical Practice Guideline No. 236: Immunization in pregnancy. *Journal of Obstetrics and Gynaecology Canada, 31*(11), 1085–1092. Retrieved February 21, 2012 from http://www.sogc.org/guidelines/documents/gui236CPG0911.pdf.

FDA Pregnancy Risk Classification of Drugs

- Category A: these drugs have been tested and found safe during pregnancy. Examples: folic acid, vitamin B_6, and thyroid medicine.
- Category B: These drugs have been used frequently during pregnancy and do not appear to cause major birth defects or other fetal problems. Examples: antibiotics, acetaminophen (Tylenol), aspartame (artificial sweetener), famotidine (Pepcid), prednisone (cortisone), insulin, and ibuprofen.
- Category C: these drugs are more likely to cause problems, and safety studies have not been completed. Examples: prochlorperazine (Compazine), fluconazole (Diflucan), ciprofloxacin (Cipro), and some antidepressants.
- Category D: these drugs have clear health risks for the fetus. Examples: alcohol, lithium (treats bipolar disorders), phenytoin (Dilantin); all chemotherapeutic agents used to treat cancer.
- Category X: these drugs have been shown to cause birth defects and should never be taken during pregnancy. Examples: Accutane (treats cystic acne), androgens (treat endometriosis), Coumadin (prevents blood clots), antithyroid medications for overactive thyroid; radiation therapy (cancer treatment), Tegison or Soriatane (treats psoriasis), streptomycin (treats tuberculosis); thalidomide (treats insomnia), diethylstilbestrol (DES) (treats menstrual disorders), and organic mercury from contaminated food.

Source: Wen, S., Yang, T., Krewski, D., et al. (2008). Patterns of exposure to prescription FDA C, D and X drugs in a Canadian population. *Journal of Perinatology, 28,* 324–329.

for these products. Therefore, encourage pregnant women to check with their health care provider before taking anything. SOGC (2007e) offers a helpful review of drug, chemical, and infectious exposures for maternity care providers. (For additional online resources about over-the-counter drugs and herbal remedies in pregnancy, visit http://thePoint.lww.com/Chow1e.)

Alcohol and substance use are serious concerns in pregnancy, and the nurse needs to be prepared to assess their use in a nonthreatening manner (SOGC, 2010a). FASD includes a variety of harms resulting from prenatal exposure to alcohol. Although malnutrition and binge drinking increase the risk of FASD, evidence is insufficient to identify a threshold for low-level drinking in pregnancy; therefore, abstinence is recommended. Women who continue to use alcohol or other illicit substances during pregnancy benefit from a harm reduction approach (SOGC, 2011c).

Nursing Management to Prepare the Woman and Her Partner for Labour, Birth, and Parenthood

Childbirth today is a very different experience from childbirth in previous generations. In the first half of the 20th century, women were literally "put to sleep" with anesthetics, and they woke up with a baby. Most women never remembered the details and had a passive role in childbirth as the physician delivered the newborn in an antiseptic hospital setting. With the second wave of feminism in the 1960s, women began to insist on taking a more active role in their health care, including childbirth. Couples wanted to be together during the extraordinary event of childbirth, and partners were prepared as labour "coaches." Beginning in the 1970s, family-centred maternity care was introduced and many obstetric practices (such as shave preps and enemas) were questioned. The significance of childbirth in the life of the woman was recognized (Simkin, 1991), as were the needs of other family members (MacKinnon, Churchill, & Hotelling, 2010).

Childbirth education began because women demanded to become more involved in their birthing experience rather than simply turning control over to a health care provider. Traditional childbirth education classes focused on developing and practicing techniques for use in managing pain and facilitating the progress of labour. Recently, the focus of this education has broadened: it now encompasses not only preparation for childbirth but also preparation for pregnancy, breastfeeding, infant care, transition to new parenting roles, relationship skills, family health promotion, and sexuality (Wallace et al., 2009). The term used to describe this broad range of topics is **perinatal education**.

Perinatal Education

Perinatal education classes teach pregnant women and their support person about pregnancy, birth, and parenting. The goals of perinatal education include health promotion for pregnancy, informed decision making, childbirth preparation, and preparation for the postpartum period and parenting (MacKinnon et al., 2010). The classes are offered in local communities or online and are usually taught by certified childbirth educators. In Calgary, for example, Birth and Babies offers a comprehensive array of classes and has recently launched an online program designed for women and families who live in rural and remote locations and may not have access to group classes (Alberta Health Services, 2009). In addition, many nurses provide brief educational encounters such as bench-style teaching in physicians' offices or "baby care fairs," a form of interactive learning exhibits found in shopping malls. In addition to community colleges, both Lamaze International and the International Childbirth Education Association (ICEA) offer certification programs for perinatal educators.

Childbirth Preparation

In the past, most childbirth classes focused on preparing women for natural childbirth (a birth without pain-relieving medications) so that the woman could be in control as much as possible throughout the experience. The classes differ in their approach to specific comfort techniques and breathing patterns. The four most common childbirth methods in Canada are the Lamaze (psychoprophylactic) method, the Bradley (partner-coached childbirth) method, HypnoBirthing, and Birthing From Within.

Lamaze Method

Lamaze is a psychoprophylactic ("mind prevention") method of preparing for labour and birth that promotes the use of body awareness, relaxation, and specific breathing techniques. Dr. Fernand Lamaze, a French obstetrician, popularized this method of childbirth preparation in the 1960s. Lamaze believed in conquering fear through knowledge and that women needed to alter their perception of suffering during childbirth by learning conditioned reflexes that, instead of signalling pain, would signal the work of producing a child (labour) and thus would carry the woman through labour awake, aware, and in control of her own body (Leonard, 2007). Lamaze felt strongly that all women have the right to deliver their babies with minimal or no medication while maintaining their dignity, minimizing their pain, maximizing their self-esteem, and enjoying the miracle of birth.

Lamaze classes include information on toning exercises, relaxation, and breathing techniques for labour. The breathing techniques are used during labour to enhance relaxation and reduce the woman's perception of pain. The goal is for women to work with their body during childbirth to maintain relaxation, decrease pain, and ensure adequate oxygenation of the fetus. Paced breathing techniques are taught as an effective attention-focusing strategy to reduce pain.

Paced breathing begins with the woman signalling her partner by taking a cleansing breath at the onset and end of each contraction. This cleansing breath is a cue to the woman to let go of tension while enhancing oxygenation for the work of labour. Three types of paced breathing are usually taught: slow-paced, modified-paced, and pattern-paced breathing. All of these breathing techniques build on body awareness and relaxation.

Slow-paced breathing is associated with relaxation and should be about half the normal breathing rate (six to nine breaths per minute). This type of breathing is the most relaxed pattern and is recommended throughout labour. Abdominal or chest breathing may be used. It is generally best to breathe in through the nose and breathe out either through the nose or mouth, whichever is more comfortable for the woman.

Modified-paced breathing can be used for increased work or stress during labour to increase alertness or focus attention or when slow-paced breathing is no longer effective in keeping the woman relaxed. The woman's respiratory rate increases, but it does not exceed twice her normal rate. Modified-paced breathing is a quiet upper chest breath that is increased or decreased according to the intensity of the contraction. The inhalation and the exhalation are equal. This breathing technique should be practiced during pregnancy for optimal use during labour.

Patterned-paced breathing is similar to modified-paced breathing but takes on a rhythmic pattern. Patterned-paced breathing uses a variety of patterns, with an emphasis on the exhalation breath at regular intervals. Different patterns can be used, such as 4/1, 6/1, 4/1. A 4/1 rhythm is four upper chest breaths followed by an exhalation (a sighing out of air, like blowing out a candle). Random patterns can be chosen for use as long as the basic principles of rate and relaxation are met.

Couples practice these breathing patterns typically during the last few months of pregnancy until they feel comfortable using them. Focal points (visual fixation on a designated object), effleurage (light abdominal massage), massage, and imagery (journey of the mind to a relaxing place) are also added to aid in relaxation.

Bradley Method (Partner-Coached)

Dr. Robert Bradley, a US-based obstetrician, advocated a completely unmedicated labour and natural birth experience. In 1965, he wrote *Husband-Coached Childbirth*, which enlisted the active participation of the husband as labour coach. The Bradley method proposes that having a baby is an experience that should be rooted in love, supported by a strong husband and a sustaining wife who flowers beautifully in childbirth. The Bradley method emphasizes the pleasurable sensations of childbirth, teaching women to concentrate on these sensations while "turning on" to their own bodies (Leonard, 2007).

The Bradley method stresses that childbirth is a joyful, natural process and emphasizes the partner's involvement during pregnancy, labour, birth, and the early newborn period. Thus, the training techniques are directed toward the coach, not the mother. The coach is educated in massage/comfort techniques to use on the mother throughout the labour and birth process. Health care providers encourage the family to give birth together.

HypnoBirthing

In HypnoBirthing, therapeutic suggestions, visualization, and relaxation breathing are used to induce a trance-like state in the woman, thereby decreasing her need for medications and minimizing her stress during childbirth. It builds on the work of Grantly Dick-Read, a British obstetrician, who in 1944 wrote *Childbirth Without Fear.* He believed that fear is the primary pain-producing agent in an otherwise normal labour and that fear builds a state of tension, creating an antagonistic effect on the labouring muscles of the uterus, which results in pain. Pain causes more fear, which further increases the tension, and the vicious cycle of "fear–tension–pain" is established (Leonard, 2007). Dick-Read sought to interrupt the circular pattern of fear, tension, and pain during the labour and birthing process by promoting his belief that the degree of fear could be diminished with increased understanding of the normal physiologic response to labour (Alexander, LaRosa, Bader, et al., 2009). Dick-Read believed that prenatal instruction was essential for pain relief and that emotional factors during labour interfered with the normal labour progression.

In HypnoBirthing (also called the Mongan method), the woman is conditioned to work in harmony with her body during labour by using breath control and deep abdominopelvic breathing to promote general body relaxation. The woman learns how the birthing muscles work in perfect harmony—as they were designed to—when her body is sufficiently relaxed. The woman also learns to use her natural birthing instincts for a calm, serene, and comfortable birth. When the woman has her baby she is not in a deep trance but rather experiences sensations similar to the focusing that occurs when you are engrossed in a good movie or book (Fritsch, 2011).

Birthing from Within

The Birthing From Within approach stresses self-discovery as the essence of childbirth preparation. Rather than learning about obstetric procedures, this approach stresses that childbirth is a profound rite of passage and not a medical event. The goal of this approach is to help women give birth-in-awareness—not to achieve a specific birth outcome (e.g., an unmedicated birth) (England & Horowitz,

1998). Fathers and/or partners provide assistance simply by their presence, not as coaches, and their needs during the birth process are acknowledged. This approach has recently gained in popularity because it allows women and their partners to receive support from biomedical technologies (such as epidurals) rather than focusing on one right way to give birth.

Nursing Support and Childbirth Preparation

Regardless of the childbirth preparation approach chosen, it is the nurse's role to recognize and work with the patterns of the woman's breathing and movements. The nurse can offer support by commending the woman's/couple's efforts, by suggesting position changes or other comfort measures, and by reinforcing breathing patterns that allow the woman to cope with contractions (Simkin, 2008). It is important to take cues from the woman and to remain quiet during the woman's periods of imagery and focal point visualization to avoid breaking her concentration.

The overall aim of any of the approaches to childbirth education is to enable each woman to work with her own body and yield to the powerful process of birth. As the woman gains success and tangible benefits from the exercises she is taught, she begins to believe in her own strength to give birth to her baby (Fig. 12.10). Nurses play a key role in supporting and encouraging each couple's use of the techniques taught in childbirth education classes.

Every woman's labour is unique, and it is important for nurses not to generalize or stereotype women. The most effective support a nurse can offer couples using prepared childbirth methods is encouragement and presence (MacKinnon, McIntyre, & Quance, 2005). These nursing measures must be adapted to each individual throughout the labour process. Offering encouraging with phrases such as "great job" or "you can do it" helps to reinforce their efforts and at the same time empowers them to continue. Using eye-to-eye contact to

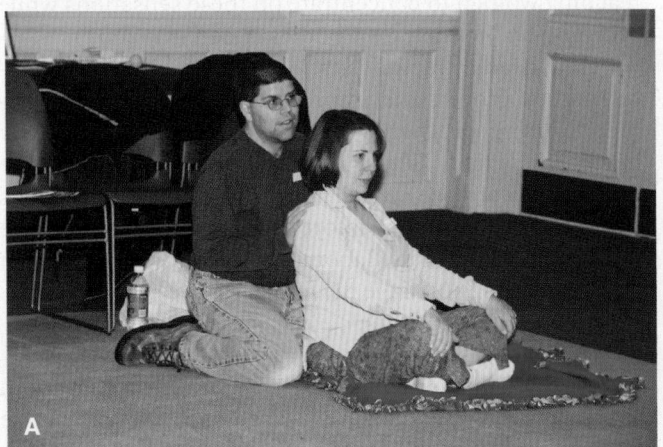
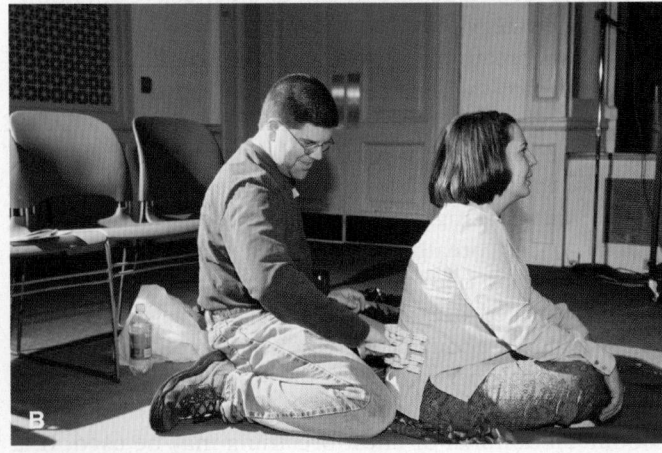

FIGURE 12.10 A couple practicing the techniques taught in a childbirth education class.

engage the woman's total attention is important if she seems overwhelmed or appears to lose control during the transition phase of labour. This strategy has been named the "taking charge routine" (Simkin, 2008).

Nurses play a significant role in enhancing the couple's relationship by respecting the involvement of the partner and demonstrating concern for his or her needs throughout labour. Offering to stay with the woman facilitates the partner's needs for periodic breaks while at the same time supporting active participation. The nurse can offer anticipatory guidance to the couple and suggest additional comfort measures and/or demonstrate coping techniques to the partner and praise their successful use, which increases self-esteem. Focus on the couple's strengths and the positive elements of the labour experience. Congratulating the couple for a job well done is paramount. Throughout the labour experience, the nurse can demonstrate personal warmth and project a friendly attitude. Frequently, a nurse's touch may help to prevent a crisis by reassuring the mother that she is doing fine.

Options for Birth Settings and Care Providers

From the moment a woman discovers she is pregnant, numerous decisions await her—where the infant will be born, what birth setting is best, and who will assist with the birth. The great majority of women are healthy and can consider the full range of birth settings—hospital, birth centre, or home—and care providers. They should be given information about each to ensure the most informed decision.

Birth Settings

Hospitals

Hospitals are the most common site for birth in Canada. If the woman has a serious medical condition or is at high risk for developing one, she will probably need to plan to give birth in a hospital setting under the care of

an obstetrician. Giving birth in a hospital is advantageous for several reasons. Hospitals are best equipped to diagnose and treat women and newborns with complications; trained personnel are available if necessary; and no transportation is needed if a complication should arise during labour or birth. Disadvantages include the high-tech atmosphere, strict policies and restrictions that might limit who can be with the woman, and the medical model of care, which can result in more cesarean and operative deliveries (SOGC, 2008d).

Within the hospital setting, birth environments have become more family friendly. In the past, the conventional delivery room resembled an operating room, where the health care professional delivered the newborn from the woman, who was positioned in stirrups. The woman was then transferred to the recovery area on a stretcher and then again to the postpartum unit. Today the birthing suite or labour/delivery/recovery (LDR) room is the most common option available. With LDR rooms, the woman and her partner remain in the same place for labour, birth, and recovery. The LDR is a private room decorated to look as home-like as possible. For example, the bed converts to allow for various birthing positions, and there may be a rocking chair or an easy chair for the woman's partner. Despite the homey atmosphere, the room is still equipped with emergency resuscitative equipment and electronic fetal monitors in case they are needed quickly (Fig. 12.11A). Such settings provide a more personal childbirth experience in a less formal and intimidating atmosphere compared with the traditional delivery room.

Birth Centres

A birth centre (Fig. 12.11B) can be a good choice for a woman who wants more personalized care than in a hospital but does not feel comfortable with a home birth. In contrast to the institutional environment of a hospital, most birth centres have a home-like atmosphere, and many are, in fact, located in converted homes. Some are

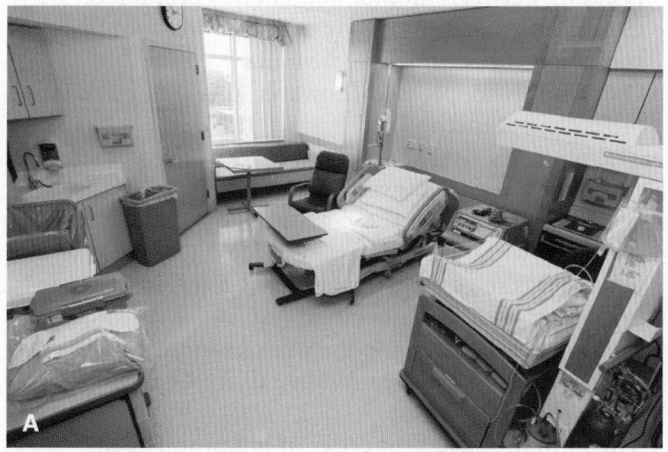
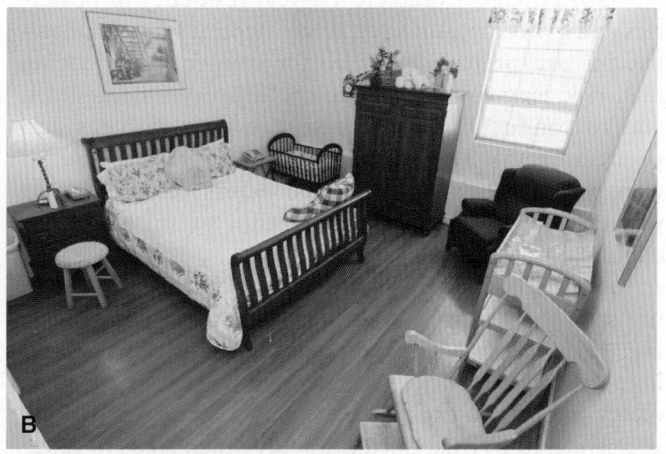

FIGURE 12.11 (**A**) Birthing suite. (**B**) Birthing centre.

located on hospital property and affiliated with the hospital. Birth centres are designed to provide maternity care to women who are judged to be at low risk for obstetric complications. Women are encouraged to give birth in the position that is most comfortable for them. Care in birth centres is often provided by midwives and is more relaxed, without routine intravenous lines, fetal monitoring, and restrictive protocols. A disadvantage of the birth centre is the need to transport the woman to a hospital quickly should an emergency arise because some equipment (such as an operating room) is not readily available. Birth centres are only available in some Canadian cities, such as Calgary, Winnipeg, and Montreal. The province of Quebec has the most extensive experience with birth centres in Canada.

Home

Most women who choose a home birth believe that birth is a natural process that requires little medical intervention. Home births can be safe if there are qualified, experienced attendants and an emergency transfer system in place in case of serious complications. Many women choose the home setting out of a strong desire to actively participate in their child's birth and to give birth surrounded by family members. Most home birth caregivers are midwives who have provided continuous care to the woman throughout the pregnancy. Disadvantages of home births include the need to transport the woman to the hospital during or after labour if a problem arises as well as the limited pain management available in the home setting.

Care Providers

While most women in Canada still receive pregnancy care from a physician (an obstetrician or family doctor), an increasing number are choosing a midwife for their care. In some settings, NPs provide care during pregnancy and the postpartum period. RNs remain the most frequent maternity care providers during labour and birth in the hospital setting.

Obstetricians complete a 4-year residency in obstetrics and gynecology in addition to medical school. Obstetricians are prepared to care for women experiencing high-risk pregnancies, to manage delivery emergencies, and to conduct most operative deliveries (forceps and cesarean birth). Some family physicians provide care for women during childbirth, while others refer pregnant women to colleagues who specialize in working with childbearing women.

Registered midwives (RMs) complete a 4-year degree program that focuses on women's health and childbearing. Midwives work in hospitals, birthing centres, and home settings to deliver care. They believe in the normalcy of birth and may tolerate wider variations of what is considered normal during labour, which leads to fewer interventions applied during the childbirth process. "The midwifery model of care promotes, normal birth, enables women to make informed choices, and provides continuity of care and support throughout the childbearing experience" (Canadian Association of Midwives, 2011). Midwives are able to handle most birth emergencies but refer women experiencing a high-risk pregnancy or birth to an obstetric team for management.

In addition to the woman's primary health care professional, some women hire a doula to be with them during the childbearing process. *Doula* is a Greek word that means "woman's servant." A doula is a laywoman trained to provide women and their families with encouragement, emotional and physical support, and information throughout pregnancy, labour, birth, and/or postpartum. Doulas provide the woman with continuous support throughout labour but do not perform any clinical procedures.

Preparation for Breastfeeding or Bottle-Feeding

A pregnant woman is faced with a decision about which method of infant feeding will work best for her particular situation. The woman and her partner need to explore the advantages and disadvantages of breastfeeding first, as breastfeeding for 1 year remains the recommended feeding option for most newborns (Canadian Paediatric Society, 2009; PHAC, 2010b). Providing the woman and her partner with information and resources to support their decision will increase the likelihood of a successful experience.

Breastfeeding

Substantial scientific evidence exists documenting the health benefits of breastfeeding for newborns. Human milk provides an ideal balance of nutrients for newborns (Breastfeeding Committee of Canada, 2002). Breastfeeding is advantageous for the following reasons:

- Human milk is digestible, economical, and requires no preparation.
- Bonding between mother and child is promoted.
- Cost is less than purchasing artificial breast milk substitutes or commercial formula.
- Ovulation is suppressed (however, this is not a reliable birth control method).
- The mother's risks for ovarian cancer and premenopausal breast cancer are reduced.
- Extra calories are used, which promotes weight loss gradually without dieting.
- Oxytocin is released to promote more rapid uterine involution with less bleeding.
- Sucking helps to develop the muscles in the infant's jaw.
- Absorption of lactose and minerals in the newborn is improved.
- The immunologic properties of breast milk help prevent infections in the baby.

- The composition of breast milk adapts to meet the infant's changing needs.
- Constipation in the baby is not a problem with adequate intake.
- Food allergies are less likely to develop in the breastfed baby.
- The incidence of otitis media and upper respiratory infections in the infant is reduced.
- Breastfed babies are less likely to be overfed, thus reducing the risk of adult obesity.
- Breastfed newborns are less prone to vomiting (Feldman & Frati, 2008; PHAC, 2010b).

One could say that lactation and breastfeeding are so natural that they should just happen on their own accord, but this is not the case. Learning to breastfeed takes practice, requires support from the partner, and demands dedication and patience on the part of the mother and baby. Learning to breastfeed has been compared with learning to dance. All nurses who work with breastfeeding dyads need to know how to help women get started with breastfeeding and be familiar with proper techniques for positioning and latch (RNAO, 2003). More information on breastfeeding is provided in Chapter 16. In some situations, a referral to a lactation consultant may be helpful or needed.

Breastfeeding also has potential disadvantages for the mother. These include breast discomfort, sore nipples, mastitis, engorgement, milk stasis, vaginal dryness, and decreased libido (Blackburn, 2007). Some mothers feel that breastfeeding is inconvenient or embarrassing, limits other activities, limits partner involvement, and restricts their use of alcohol or drugs. Nurses can help mothers to address their fears by making practical suggestions to minimize discomfort and embarrassment.

Nipple preparation is not necessary during the prenatal period unless the nipples are inverted and do not become erect when stimulated. Assess for this by placing the forefinger and thumb above and below the areola and compressing behind the nipple. If the nipple flattens or inverts, some lactation consultants advise the woman to wear breast shields during the last 2 months of pregnancy, although there is no current evidence that this treatment is effective (Johnson & Strube, 2011).

Encourage the woman to attend a breastfeeding support group (e.g., La Leche League), provide her with sources of information about infant feeding, and suggest that she read a good reference book about lactation. All of these activities will help in her decision-making process and will be invaluable to her should she choose to breastfeed her newborn.

It is important for nurses to remember that while breastfeeding may be the best choice for most newborns, it may not be the best choice for all women. Some women simply feel that breastfeeding is not right for them and their decision should be supported. Other women may have medical reasons for not breastfeeding or may have experienced sexual abuse in the past. Some women with mental health disorders may require medications that are not recommended for the baby (Humphries, 2010). Nurses need to support all women regardless of the choices that they make.

Bottle-Feeding

Women may choose to bottle-fed their newborns with expressed breast milk or commercially prepared breast milk substitutes commonly referred to as "infant formulas." Women who desire to continue breastfeeding are usually advised not to introduce bottles until breastfeeding is well established (usually after about 6 to 8 weeks). Some women are unable to breastfeed their baby in the early weeks (e.g., if the baby is ill or very premature) but are encouraged to pump their breasts to stimulate milk production and may feed their baby expressed breast milk using a variety of methods, sometimes including bottle-feeding.

Bottle-feeding an infant isn't simply a matter of "open, pour, and feed." Parents need information on types of formulas, preparation and storage of formula, equipment, and feeding positions. It is recommended that normal full-term infants receive conventional cow's milk-based formula. If the infant has a reaction to the first formula (diarrhea, vomiting, abdominal pain, excessive gas), another formula should be tried. Sometimes a soy-based formula is substituted. In terms of preparation and use of formula, the following guidelines should be stressed:

- Obtain adequate equipment (six 120 mL and eight 240 mL bottles, plus nipples).
- Consistency is important. Stay with a nipple that is comfortable to the infant.
- Assess nipples frequently for any loose pieces of rubber at the opening.
- Correct formula preparation is critical to the health and development of the infant. Formula is available in three forms: ready-to-feed, concentrate, and powder.
- Correct formula dilution is important to avoid fluid imbalances. Read the formula label thoroughly before mixing. Use ready-to-use formula as is, without dilution. Dilute concentrated formula with equal parts water. Mix one scoop of powdered formula with 60 mL (2 ounces) of water.
- If the water supply is safe, sterilization is not necessary; if the water supply is questionable, water should be boiled for 5 minutes before use.
- Bottles and nipples should be washed in hot, sudsy water using a bottle brush.
- Formula should be served at room temperature. It should not be heated in a microwave oven because it will be heated unevenly.
- Formula can be prepared 24 hours in advance and stored in the refrigerator (BC Ministry of Health, 2010)

Teach the woman and other caregivers to feed the infant in a semi-upright position using the cradle hold. This position allows for face-to-face contact between the infant and caretaker. Advise the caretaker to hold the bottle so that the nipple is kept full of formula to prevent excessive air swallowing. Instruct the caretaker to feed the infant every 3 to 4 hours and adapt the feeding times to the infant's needs. Frequent burping of the infant helps prevent gas from building up in the stomach. Caution the caretaker not to prop the bottle as this can cause choking (Health Link BC, 2010).

Bottle-feeding should mirror breastfeeding as closely as possible. While nutrition is important, so are the emotional and interactive components of feeding. Encourage the caretaker to cuddle the infant closely and position the infant so that his or her head is in a comfortable position. Also encourage communication with the infant during feedings.

> ▶ **Take** NOTE!
>
> *Warn the caretaker about the danger of putting the infant to bed with a bottle; this can lead to "baby bottle tooth decay" because sugars in the formula stay in contact with the infant's developing teeth for prolonged periods.*

Final Preparations for Labour and Birth

In addition to providing support and education throughout pregnancy, the nurse can help to prepare couples for their "big day" by reviewing the following topics (as appropriate):

• Touring the birthing facility
• Packing a suitcase to take to the birthing facility when labour starts
• Making arrangements to have siblings and/or pets taken care of during labour
• Understanding the signs and symptoms of labour
• Knowing how and when to contact their care provider
• Knowing what to do if membranes rupture prior to going into labour
• Discussing comfort measures for early labour and pain relief options
• Knowing what to expect during labour and birth
• Knowing how to communicate their needs and desires for labour and birth
• Anticipating the possibility of a cesarean birth if complications occur
• Exploring possible names for the newborn and knowing about the birth registration process
• Communicating their choices related to infant feeding and preparing for getting started

• Making a decision regarding circumcision should they have a boy
• Purchasing an approved infant car seat and reading the instructions carefully
• Having items needed for the mother's and newborn's homecoming, including:
  • Infant clothes in several sizes, soft blankets, and towels
  • Infant crib made after 1986 with a tight-fitting mattress (Health Canada, 2008)
  • Diapers (cloth or disposable)
  • Nursing bras, breast pads, and a breast pump, if desired (if breastfeeding)
  • Sanitary supplies for lochia
  • Infant thermometer and a small bath or back rest for bathing
  • Bottles and formula (if bottle-feeding)
• Considering a family planning method to use after birth, and discussing when to resume sexual activity

Nurses have many opportunities to help women and their partners prepare for the birth of their baby and early parenting. Although it may be difficult for independent women to accept help, the postpartum period is an ideal time to learn to say "yes" to offers of assistance from friends and family members. Each woman and family is unique and may have cultural practices that need to be considered during pregnancy, childbirth, and the postpartum period. The nurse can ask about cultural practices, anticipate the need for additional health services (such as an interpreter during labour and birth), advocate for women and families, and remain available to provide support and answer questions. There is so much information available on the Internet today that many parents need assistance from the nurse to make sense of it all. The nurse can then support the couple's ability to make informed decisions needed for their particular situation.

Pregnancy, childbirth, and early parenting are important transitions for families. To provide culturally safe nursing care, the nurse needs to remain open to learning about many cultural beliefs, values, and practices and to advocate for woman- and family-centred, evidence-informed maternity care.

■■■ Key Concepts

■ Preconception care is the promotion of the health and well-being of a woman and her partner before pregnancy. The goal of preconception care is to identify health problems, lifestyle practices, or social concerns that might unfavourably affect pregnancy.

■ A primary aspect of nursing management during the antepartum period is educating and counselling the pregnant woman and her partner to promote healthy outcomes for all involved.

- The nurse needs to maximize opportunities for health promotion during pregnancy. The nurse can help women and family members make sense of the information that is currently available.
- Women who have prenatal care, do not live in poverty, and are more educated are more likely to have successful pregnancy outcomes. For women who experience health inequities, the nurse's role may be that of an advocate for needed programs and services
- A thorough history and physical examination are performed on the initial prenatal visit.
- Symphysis–fundal height is measured when the uterus arises out of the pelvis to evaluate fetal growth; the fundus reaches the level of the umbilicus at approximately 20 weeks.
- Symphysis–fundal height should approximately equal the number of weeks of gestation until week 36.
- Prenatal screening has become standard in prenatal care to detect NTDs and genetic abnormalities.
- All pregnant women need to be able to recognize warning signs in pregnancy so that they can take appropriate action and contact their maternity care provider.
- At each visit the woman is asked whether she is having any symptoms of preterm labour, which include uterine contractions, dull backache, pressure in the pelvic area or thighs, increased vaginal discharge, menstrual-like cramps, and vaginal bleeding.
- The nurse should address common discomforts that occur in each trimester and provide realistic suggestions to promote comfort for the woman.
- The pregnant woman can better care for herself and the fetus if she has the opportunity to ask questions and if anticipatory guidance is incorporated into each prenatal visit.
- Since pregnancy is an opportunity for health promotion, nutritional assessment, nutritional information (such as Canada's Food Guide), and sometimes referral to a nutritionist are recommended.
- The recommended weight gain during pregnancy depends on the woman's pregnant BMI.
- Iron and folic acid supplementation is needed during pregnancy because the increased requirements at this time are usually too great to be met through diet alone.
- Pregnancy may be an opportunity for smoking cessation, and the nurse should **ask** about smoking, **advise** or strongly urge pregnant women to quit, **assess** their willingness to make a quit attempt, **assist** women with quitting, and **arrange** follow-up as needed (the five A's).
- The focus of perinatal education has broadened to include preparation for pregnancy and family adaptation to parenting.
- Childbirth education began because of increasing pressure from consumers who wanted to become more involved in their birthing experience. The four

childbirth education approaches currently available in Canada are Lamaze (psychoprophylactic), Bradley (partner-coached childbirth), HypnoBirthing, and Birthing From Within.
- The great majority of women in Canada are healthy and can consider the full range of birth settings: hospital, birth centre, or home setting.
- Pregnancy, childbirth, and early parenting are important transitions for families. To provide culturally competent nursing care the nurse needs to remain open to learning about many cultural beliefs, values, and practices and advocate for woman- and family-centred, culturally safe maternity care.

REFERENCES

Alberta Health Services. (2009). *Birth and babies program.* Retrieved February 21, 2012 from www.online.birthandbabies.com

Alexander, L. L., LaRosa, J. H., Bader, H., & Garfield, S. (2009). *New dimensions in women's health* (5th ed.). Sudbury, MA: Jones and Bartlett Publishers.

BC Centre of Excellence for Women's Health. (2010). *Woman centred harm reduction approaches.* Retrieved February 21, 2012 from http://www.coalescing-vc.org/virtualLearning/section4/default.htm

BC Ministry of Health. (2010). *Baby's best chance: Parents' handbook of pregnancy and baby care* (6th ed., 2nd Rev.). Retrieved February 21, 2012 from http://www.health.gov.bc.ca/library/publications/year/2010/bbc.pdf

BC Perinatal Health Program. (2005). *Obstetric guideline 2A: Preterm labour.* Retrieved February 21, 2012 from http://www.perinatalservicesbc.ca/NR/rdonlyres/F9BCBC50-5C68-467F-A756-042689313FBD/0/OBGuidelinesPretermLabour2A.pdf

BC Women's Hospital. (2010). *Connecting pregnancy group prenatal care.* Retrieved February 21, 2012 from http://www.bcwomens.ca/HealthTopics/HavingBaby/GettingReady/TypesofCareOffered/prenatalgroup.htm

Best Start Resource Centre. (2009). *Giving birth in a new land: Strategies for service providers working with newcomers.* Toronto, ON: Author. Retrieved February 21, 2012 from http://www.beststart.org/resources/rep_health/Newcomer_%20Guide_Final.pdf

Blackburn, S. T. (2007). *Maternal, fetal, and neonatal physiology: A clinical perspective* (3rd ed.). St. Louis, MO: Saunders Elsevier.

Bottorff, J., Lalaw, C., Johnson, J., et al. (2005). Unraveling smoking ties: How tobacco use is embedded in couple interactions. *Research in Nursing and Health, 28*(4), 316–328.

Bozzo, P., Narducci, A., & Einararson, A. (2011). Vaccination during pregnancy. *Canadian Family Physician, 57*(5), 555–557.

Breastfeeding Committee of Canada. (2002). *Breastfeeding statement of the Breastfeeding Committee for Canada.* Retrieved February 21, 2012 from http://breastfeedingcanada.ca/documents/webdoc5.pdf

Browne, A., Varcoe, C., Smye, V., et al. (2009). Cultural safety and the challenges of translating critically oriented knowledge in practice. *Nursing Philosophy, 10,* 167–179.

Canadian Association of Midwives. (2011). What is a Canadian registered midwife? Retrieved February 21, 2012 from http://www.canadianmidwives.org/what-is-a-midwife.html

Canadian Paediatric Society. (2009). Exclusive breastfeeding should continue to six months. *Paediatrics and Child Health, 10*(3), 148. Retrieved February 21, 2012 from http://www.cps.ca/english/statements/n/breastfeedingmar05.htm

Centers for Disease Control and Prevention. (2012). *What is preconception care?* Retrieved February 21, 2012 from http://www.cdc.gov/ncbddd/preconception/default.htm

Coad, J., & Dunstall, M. (2011). *Anatomy and physiology for midwives* (3rd ed.). Edinburgh: Elsevier Churchill Livingstone.

Cunningham, F., Leveno, K. J., Bloom, S. L., et al. (Eds.). (2010). *William's obstetrics* (23rd ed.). New York: McGraw-Hill.

D'Amico, D., Barbarito, C., Twomey, C., & Harder, N. (2011). *Health and physical assessment in nursing: Canadian Edition.* Toronto: Pearson Education Canada.

Einarson, A., Maltepe, C., Boskovic, R., & Korean, G. (2007). Treatment of nausea and vomiting in pregnancy: An updated algorithm. *Canadian Family Physician, 53*(12), 2109–2111.

England, P., & Horowitz, R. (1998). *Birthing from within.* Albuquerque, NM: Partera Press.

Feldman, P., & Frati, F. (2008). *Evidence-based benefits of breastfeeding for the Breastfeeding Committee for Canada: An annotated bibliography.* Retrieved February 21, 2012 from http://breastfeedingcanada.ca/documents/BCC%20Annotated%20Bibliography_Revised%20Aug%202007_corrected%2010%20March%202008.pdf

Foreign Affairs and International Trade Canada. (2011). *Her own way: A woman's guide to safe and successful travel.* Retrieved February 21, 2012 from http://www.voyage.gc.ca/publications/pdf/her_own_way-en.pdf

Fraser, D., & Cooper, M. (2009). *Myles textbook for midwives* (15th ed.) Edinburgh: Churchill Livingstone.

Fritsch, I. (2011). *About HypnoBirthing.* Retrieved February 21, 2012 from http://www.hypnobirthingcanada.com/hypnobirthing/?page_id=2

Garm, A. (1999). The Sheway Project. *Canadian Nurse, 95*(10), 22–25.

Gilbert, E. S. (2011). *Manual of high-risk pregnancy and delivery* (5th ed.). St. Louis, MO: Mosby Elsevier.

Gottlieb, L., & Feeley, N. (2006). *The collaborative partnership approach to care—A delicate balance.* Toronto, ON: Mosby Elsevier.

Hall, W., Hauch, Y., Carty, E., Hutton, E., Fenwick, J., & Stoll, K. (2009). Childbirth fear, anxiety, fatigue, and sleep deprivation in pregnant women. *Journal of Obstetric, Gynecologic, and Neonatal Nursing, 38,* 567–576. doi:10.1111/j.1552–6909.2009.01054.x

Health Canada. (2008). *Crib safety.* Retrieved February 21, 2012 from http://www.hc-sc.gc.ca/cps-spc/alt_formats/hecs-sesc/pdf/pubs/cons/cribs-lits_enfants-eng.pdf

Health Link BC. (2010). *Formula feeding your baby: Safely preparing and storing formula.* Retrieved February 21, 2012 from http://www.healthlinkbc.ca/healthfiles/hfile69b.stm

Humphries, J. (2010). *Are we hurting when we try to help? Exploring the experiences of infant feeding for women with mental health challenges.* VIHA Research Newsletter. Retrieved February 21, 2012 from http://www.viha.ca/NR/rdonlyres/30F39EA4–50AA-4FB6–8360-DCD574BC2CBB/0/Researchnewsletterspring2010.pdf

Johnson, T., & Strube, K. (2011). Breast care during pregnancy. *Journal of Obstetric, Gynecologic, and Neonatal Nursing, 40*(2), 144–148.

Jones, S., & Ciofani, L. (2010). Genetics, embryology, and preconceptual/prenatal assessment and screening. In R. Evans, M. Evans, Y. Brown & S. Orshan (Eds.). *Canadian maternity, newborn and women's health nursing: Comprehensive care across the life span.* Philadelphia: Lippincott Williams & Wilkins.

Kitzinger, S. (2005). *The complete book of pregnancy and childbirth* (4th ed.). New York: Alfred A Knopf.

Lane, C. A. (2007). Nausea and vomiting in pregnancy: A tailored approach treatment. *Clinical Obstetrics and Gynecology, 50*(1), 100–111.

Larsson, A., & Dykes, A. (2009). Care during pregnancy and childbirth in Sweden: Perspectives of lesbian women. *Midwifery, 25,* 682–690.

Leininger, M., & McFarland, M. R. (2002). *Transcultural nursing concepts, theories, research & practice.* New York: McGraw Hill.

Leonard, P. (2007). *Childbirth education: A handbook for nurses.* Retrieved February 21, 2012 from http://ce.nurse.com/60057/childbirth-education-a-handbook-for-nurses/

Lewallen, L. (2011). The importance of culture in childbearing. *Journal of Obstetric, Gynecologic, and Neonatal Nursing, 40*(1), 4–8.

Loppie Reading, C., & Wien, F. (2009). *Health inequalities and social determinants of Aboriginal peoples' health.* Prince George, BC: The National Collaborating Centre for Aboriginal Health. Retrieved February 21, 2012 from http://www.nccah-ccnsa.ca/docs/social%20determinates/NCCAH-Loppie-Wien_Report.pdf

MacKinnon, K. (2006). Living with the threat of preterm labor: Women's work of keeping the baby in. *Journal of Obstetric, Gynecologic, and Neonatal Nursing, 35*(6), 700–708.

MacKinnon, K. (2008). Labouring to nurse: The work of rural nurses who provide maternity care. *Rural and Remote Health (Online), 8,* 1047.

MacKinnon, K., Churchill, J., & Hotelling, B. (2010). Educational preparation for pregnancy, childbirth and parenthood. In R. Evans, M. Evans, Y. Brown, & S. Orchan (Eds.), *Maternity, newborn & women's health nursing.* Philadelphia: Lippincott Williams & Wilkins.

MacKinnon, K., McIntyre, M., & Quance, M. (2005). The meaning of the nurse's presence during childbirth. *Journal of Obstetrical Gynecologic and Neonatal Nursing, 34*(1), 28–36.

Maier-Lorentz, M. (2008). Transcultural nursing: Its importance in nursing practice. *Journal of Cultural Diversity, 15*(1), 37–43.

Malnory, M., & Johnson, T. (2011). The reproductive life plan as a strategy to decrease poor birth outcomes. *Journal of Obstetric, Gynecologic, and Neonatal Nursing, 40*(1), 109–121.

March of Dimes. (2011). *Prematurity research.* Retrieved February 21, 2012 http://www.marchofdimes.com/research/prematurityresearch.html

McKillop, E., Martin, S., Bowen, A., & Muhajarine, N. (2011). The best and worst time of my life: The lived experience and meaning of pregnancy in women with mild to moderate depression. *Journal of Prenatal and Perinatal Psychology and Health, 24*(3), 174–195.

Okoli, C., Greaves, L., Bottorff, J., & Marcellus, L. (2010). Health care providers' engagement in smoking cessation with pregnant smokers. *Journal of Obstetric, Gynecologic, and Neonatal Nursing, 39*(1), 64–77.

Pauly, B., MacKinnon, K., & Varcoe, C. (2009). Revisiting "Who Gets Care?" Health equity as an arena for nursing action. *Advances in Nursing Science, 32*(2), 118–127.

Perinatal Services BC. (2010a). *BCPHP Obstetric Guide 19: Maternity care pathway.* Retrieved February 21, 2012 from http://www.perinatalservicesbc.ca//sites/bcrcp/files/Guidelines/Obstetrics/Guideline_19.pdf

Perinatal Services BC. (2012). *Pregnancy passport.* Retrieved February 21, 2012 from http://www.perinatalservicesbc.ca/FamilyResources/PregnancyPassport/default.htm

Perinatal Services BC. (2011). *BC Prenatal Genetic Screening Program update.* Retrieved February 21, 2012 from http://bcprenatalscreening.ca/sites/prenatal2/files/PGSP_Mar11_Update.pdf

Peterson, W., Medves, J., Davies, B., & Graham, I. (2007). Multidisciplinary Collaborative Maternity Care in Canada: Easier Said Than Done. *Journal of Obstetrics and Gynaecology Canada, 29*(11): 880–886.

Public Health Agency of Canada. (2000). *Family centred maternity and newborn care: National guidelines.* Retrieved February 21, 2012 from http://www.phac-aspc.gc.ca/hp-ps/dca-dea/publications/fcm-smp/index-eng.php

Public Health Agency of Canada. (2005). *Make every mother and child count: Report on Maternal and Child Health in Canada.* Retrieved February 21, 2012 from http://www.phac-aspc.gc.ca/rhs-ssg/pdf/whd_05epi_e.pdf

Public Health Agency of Canada. (2006). *Canadian Immunization Guide: Part 3. Recommended immunizations* (7th ed.). Retrieved February 21, 2012 from http://www.phac-aspc.gc.ca/publicat/cig-gci/pdf/cig-gci-2006-part-3_e.pdf

Public Health Agency of Canada. (2008a). *The Canadian Perinatal Health Report, 2008 edition.* Retrieved February 21, 2012 from http://www.phac-aspc.gc.ca/publicat/2008/cphr-rspc/index-eng.php

Public Health Agency of Canada. (2008b). *The sensible guide to a healthy pregnancy.* Retrieved February 21, 2012 from http://www.phac-aspc.gc.ca/hp-gs/guide-eng.php

Public Health Agency of Canada. (2009). *What mothers say: The Canadian Maternity Experiences Survey.* Retrieved February 21, 2012 from http://www.phac-aspc.gc.ca/rhs-ssg/pdf/survey-eng.pdf

Public Health Agency of Canada. (2010a). *Alcohol and pregnancy.* Retrieved February 21, 2012 from http://www.phac-aspc.gc.ca/hp-gs/know-savoir/alc-eng.php

Public Health Agency of Canada. (2010b). *Breastfeeding.* Retrieved February 21, 2012 from http://www.phac-aspc.gc.ca/dca-dea/prenatal/nutrition-eng.php

Public Health Agency of Canada. (2010c). *Caffeine and pregnancy.* Retrieved February 21, 2012 from http://www.phac-aspc.gc.ca/hp-gs/know-savoir/caffeine-eng.php

Public Health Agency of Canada. (2010d). *Canada Prenatal Nutrition Program (CPNP).* Retrieved February 21, 2012 from http://www.phac-aspc.gc.ca/dca-dea/programs-mes/cpnp_main-eng.php

Public Health Agency of Canada. (2010e). *Constipation.* Retrieved February 21, 2012 from http://www.phac-aspc.gc.ca/hp-gs/know-savoir/constipation-eng.php

Public Health Agency of Canada. (2010f). *Don't drink the water.* Retrieved February 21, 2012 from http://www.phac-aspc.gc.ca/tmp-pmv/ddtw/index-eng.php

Public Health Agency of Canada. (2010g). *Emotional health.* Retrieved February 21, 2012 from http://www.phac-aspc.gc.ca/hp-gs/know-savoir/ment-eng.php

Public Health Agency of Canada. (2010h). *Your healthy pregnancy calendar.* Retrieved February 21, 2012 from http://www.phac-aspc.gc.ca/hp-gs/calendar/calendar-eng.php

Public Health Agency of Canada. (2010i). *Heartburn.* Retrieved February 21, 2012 from http://www.phac-aspc.gc.ca/hp-gs/know-savoir/heartburn-eng.php

Public Health Agency of Canada. (2010j). *Nausea and vomiting.* Retrieved February 21, 2012 from http://www.phac-aspc.gc.ca/hp-gs/know-savoir/sick-eng.php

Public Health Agency of Canada. (2010k). *Oral health.* Retrieved February 21, 2012 from http://www.phac-aspc.gc.ca/hp-gs/know-savoir/ora-dent-eng.php

Public Health Agency of Canada. (2010l). *Physical activity and pregnancy.* Retrieved February 21, 2012 from http://www.phac-aspc.gc.ca/hp-gs/know-savoir/phys-eng.php

Public Health Agency of Canada. (2010m). *Smoking and pregnancy.* Retrieved February 21, 2012 from http://www.phac-aspc.gc.ca/hp-gs/know-savoir/smoke-fumer-eng.php

Public Health Agency of Canada. (2010n). *Toxoplasmosis.* Retrieved February 21, 2012 from http://www.inspection.gc.ca/english/fssa/concen/cause/toxoplasmae.shtml

Public Health Agency of Canada. (2010o). *What determines health?* Retrieved February 21, 2012 from http://www.phac-aspc.gc.ca/ph-sp/determinants/index-eng.php

Registered Nurses' Association of Ontario. (2003). *Nursing best practice guideline: Breastfeeding best practice guidelines for nurses.* Retrieved February 21, 2012 from http://www.rnao.org/Storage/11/564_BPG_Breastfeeding.pdf

Registered Nurses' Association of Ontario. (2007). *Nursing best practice guideline: Integrating smoking cessation into daily nursing practice.* Retrieved February 21, 2012 from http://www.rnao.org/Storage/29/2338_Final_-_revised_smoking.pdf

Reid, A., Biringer, A., Carroll, J., Midmer, D., Wilson, L., et al. (1998). Using the ALPHA form in practice to assess antenatal psychosocial health. *Canadian Medical Association Journal, 159*(6), 677–684.

Richardson, F., & MacGibbon, L. (2010). Cultural safety: Nurses' accounts of negotiating the order of things. *Women's Studies Journal, 24*(2), 54–65.

Schuurmans, N., Senikas, V., & Lalonde, A. (2010). *Healthy beginnings* (4th ed.). Ottawa, ON: Society of Obstetricians and Gynaecologists of Canada.

SexualityandU. (2010). *Sex during pregnancy.* Retrieved February 21, 2012 from http://www.sexualityandu.ca/sexual-health/pregnancy/sex-during-pregnancy

SIDS Canada. (2010). *Smoking & SIDS.* Retrieved February 21, 2012 from http://www.sidscanada.org/smoking.html

Simkin, P. (1991). Just another day in a woman's life? Women's long-term perceptions of their first birth experience. *Birth, 18*(4), 203–210.

Simkin, P. (2008). *The birth partner: A complete guide to childbirth for dads, doulas, and all other labor companions.* Boston, MA: The Harvard Common Press.

Singh, D., Singh, J. R., & Vanita, V. (2012). *Prenatal diagnosis for congenital malformations and genetic disorders.* Retrieved February 21, 2012 from http://www.emedicine.com/oph/topic485.htm

Society of Obstetricians and Gynaecologists of Canada. (2002a). SOGC Clinical Practice Guideline No. 120: The management of nausea and vomiting of pregnancy. *Journal of Obstetrics and Gynaecology Canada, 24*(10), 817–823. Retrieved February 21, 2012 from http://www.sogc.org/guidelines/public/120E-CPG-October2002.pdf

Society of Obstetricians and Gynaecologists of Canada. (2002b). SOGC Clinical Practice Guideline No. 121: Screening for gestational diabetes mellitus. *Journal of Obstetrics and Gynaecology Canada, 24*(11), 894–903. Retrieved February 21, 2012 from http://www.sogc.org/guidelines/public/121E-CPG-November2002.pdf

Society of Obstetricians and Gynaecologists of Canada. (2003a). SOGC Clinical Practice Guideline No. 122: Antenatal corticosteroid therapy for fetal maturation. *Journal of Obstetrics and Gynaecology Canada, 25*(1), 45–48. Retrieved February 21, 2012 from http://www.sogc.org/guidelines/public/122E-CO-Janvier2003.pdf

Society of Obstetricians and Gynaecologists of Canada. (2003b). SOGC Clinical Practice Guideline No. 129: Exercise in pregnancy and the postpartum period. *Journal of Obstetrics and Gynaecology Canada, 25*(6), 516–522. Retrieved February 21, 2012 from http://www.sogc.org/guidelines/public/129E-JCPG-June2003.pdf

Society of Obstetricians and Gynaecologists of Canada. (2003c). SOGC Clinical Practice Guideline No. 133: Prevention of Rh alloimmunization. *Journal of Obstetrics and Gynaecology Canada, 25*(9), 765–773. Retrieved February 21, 2012 from http://www.sogc.org/guidelines/documents/133E-CPG-September2003.pdf

Society of Obstetricians and Gynaecologists of Canada. (2004). SOGC Clinical Practice Guideline No. 149: The prevention of early-onset neonatal group B streptococcal disease. *Journal of Obstetrics and Gynaecology Canada, 26*(9), 826–832. Retrieved February 21, 2012 from http://www.sogc.org/guidelines/public/149E-CPG-September2004.pdf

Society of Obstetricians and Gynaecologists of Canada. (2005a). SOGC Clinical Practice Guideline No. 168: Amended Canadian Guideline for Prenatal Diagnosis Change to 2005-Techniques for Prenatal Diagnosis. *Journal of Obstetrics and Gynaecology Canada, 25*(1), 45–48. Retrieved February 21, 2012 from http://www.sogc.org/guidelines/public/122E-CO-Janvier2003.pdf

Society of Obstetricians and Gynaecologists of Canada. (2005b). SOGC Clinical Practice Guideline No. 199: Fetal soft markers in obstetric ultrasound. *Journal of Obstetrics and Gynaecology Canada, 27*(6), 592–612. Retrieved February 21, 2012 from http://www.sogc.org/guidelines/public/162E-CPG-June2005.pdf

Society of Obstetricians and Gynaecologists of Canada. (2005c). SOGC Clinical Practice Guideline No. 157: Intimate partner violence consensus statement. *Journal of Obstetrics and Gynaecology Canada, 27*(4), 365–388. Retrieved February 21, 2012 from http://www.sogc.org/guidelines/public/157E-CPG-April2005.pdf

Society of Obstetricians and Gynaecologists of Canada. (2006a). SOGC Clinical Practice Guideline No. 185: HIV screening in pregnancy. *Journal of Obstetrics and Gynaecology Canada, 28*(12), 1103–1107. Retrieved February 21, 2012 from http://www.sogc.org/guidelines/documents/185E-CPG-December2006.pdf

Society of Obstetricians and Gynaecologists of Canada. (2006b). SOGC Clinical Practice Guideline No. 173: Pregnancy outcomes after assisted reproductive technology. *Journal of Obstetrics and Gynaecology Canada, 28*(3), 220–233. Retrieved February 21, 2012 from http://www.sogc.org/guidelines/public/173E-JCPG-March2006.pdf

Society of Obstetricians and Gynaecologists of Canada. (2007a). SOGC Clinical Practice Guideline No. 197: Fetal health surveillance: Antepartum and intrapartum consensus guideline. *Journal of Obstetrics and Gynaecology Canada, 29*(9 Suppl. 4), S1–S56. Retrieved February 21, 2012 from http://www.sogc.org/guidelines/documents/gui197CPG0709r.pdf

Society of Obstetricians and Gynaecologists of Canada. (2007b). SOGC Clinical Practice Guideline No. 162: Mid-trimester amniocentesis fetal loss rate. *Journal of Obstetrics and Gynaecology Canada, 29*(7), 586–590. Retrieved February 21, 2012 from http://www.sogc.org/guidelines/documents/gui194CPG0707.pdf

Society of Obstetricians and Gynaecologists of Canada. (2007c). SOGC Policy Statement No. 191: Non-medical use of fetal ultrasound. *Journal of Obstetrics and Gynaecology Canada, 29*(4), 364–365. Retrieved February 21, 2012 from http://www.sogc.org/guidelines/documents/191E-PS-April2007.pdf

Society of Obstetricians and Gynaecologists of Canada. (2007d). SOGC Clinical Practice Guideline No. 201: Pre-conceptional vitamin/folic acid supplementation. *Journal of Obstetrics and Gynaecology Canada, 29*(12), 1003–1013. Retrieved February 21, 2012 from http://www.sogc.org/guidelines/documents/guiJOGC201JCPG0712.pdf

Society of Obstetricians and Gynaecologists of Canada. (2007e). SOGC Clinical Practice Guideline No. 199: Principles of human teratology: Drug, chemical, and infectious exposure. *Journal of Obstetrics and Gynaecology Canada, 29*(11), 911–917. Retrieved February 21, 2012 from http://www.sogc.org/guidelines/documents/guiJOGC199CPG0711.pdf

Society of Obstetricians and Gynaecologists of Canada. (2007f). SOGC Clinical Practice Guideline No. 200: Teratogenicity associated with pre-existing and gestational diabetes. *Journal of Obstetrics and*

Gynaecology Canada, 29(11), 927–934. Retrieved February 21, 2012 from http://sogc.org/guidelines/documents/guiJOGC200CPG0711.pdf

Society of Obstetricians and Gynaecologists of Canada. (2008a). SOGC Clinical Practice Guideline No. 206: Diagnosis, evaluation, and management of the hypertensive disorders of pregnancy. *Journal of Obstetrics and Gynaecology Canada, 30*(3 Suppl. 1), S1–S52. Retrieved February 21, 2012 from http://www.sogc.org/guidelines/documents/gui206CPG0803hypertensioncorrection.pdf

Society of Obstetricians and Gynaecologists of Canada. (2008b). SOGC Clinical Practice Guideline No. 208: Guidelines for the management of herpes simplex virus in pregnancy. *Journal of Obstetrics and Gynaecology Canada, 30*(6), 514–519. Retrieved February 21, 2012 from http://www.sogc.org/guidelines/documents/gui208CPG0806.pdf

Society of Obstetricians and Gynaecologists of Canada. (2008c). SOGC Clinical Practice Guideline No. 214: Guidelines for the management of pregnancy at 41 + 0 to 42 + 0 weeks. *Journal of Obstetrics and Gynaecology Canada, 30*(9), 800–810. Retrieved February 21, 2012 from http://www.sogc.org/guidelines/documents/gui214CPG0809.pdf

Society of Obstetricians and Gynaecologists of Canada. (2008d). SOGC Joint Policy Statement No. 221: Joint policy statement on normal childbirth. *Journal of Obstetrics and Gynaecology Canada, 30*(12), 1163–1165. Retrieved February 21, 2012 from http://www.sogc.org/guidelines/documents/gui221PS0812.pdf

Society of Obstetricians and Gynaecologists of Canada. (2008e). SOGC Clinical Practice Guideline No. 203: Rubella in pregnancy. *Journal of Obstetrics and Gynaecology Canada, 30*(2), 152–158. Retrieved February 21, 2012 from http://www.sogc.org/guidelines/documents/guiJOGC203CPG0802.pdf

Society of Obstetricians and Gynaecologists of Canada. (2009a). SOGC Clinical Practice Guideline No. 234: Evaluation of prenatally diagnosed structural congenital anomalies. *Journal of Obstetrics and Gynaecology Canada, 31*(9), 875–881. Retrieved February 21, 2012 from http://www.sogc.org/guidelines/documents/gui234CO0909.pdf

Society of Obstetricians and Gynaecologists of Canada. (2009b). SOGC Clinical Practice Guideline No. 236: Immunization in pregnancy. *Journal of Obstetrics and Gynaecology Canada, 31*(11), 1085–1092. Retrieved February 21, 2012 from http://www.sogc.org/guidelines/documents/gui236CPG0911.pdf

Society of Obstetricians and Gynaecologists of Canada. (2010a). SOGC Clinical Practice Guideline No. 245: Alcohol use and pregnancy consensus clinical guidelines. *Journal of Obstetrics and Gynaecology Canada, 32*(8 Suppl. 3), S1–S36. Retrieved February 21, 2012 from http://www.sogc.org/guidelines/documents/gui245CPG1008E.pdf

Society of Obstetricians and Gynaecologists of Canada. (2010b). SOGC Clinical Practice Guideline No. 239: Obesity in pregnancy. *Journal of Obstetrics and Gynaecology Canada, 32*(2), 165–173. Retrieved February 21, 2012 from http://www.sogc.org/guidelines/documents/gui239ECPG1002.pdf

Society of Obstetricians and Gynaecologists of Canada. (2010c). *Women's Health Information: Preterm labour.* Retrieved February 21, 2012 from http://www.sogc.org/health/pregnancy-preterm_e.asp

Society of Obstetricians and Gynaecologists of Canada. (2010d). *Women's health information: Ultrasound in pregnancy.* Retrieved February 21, 2012 from http://www.sogc.org/health/pregnancy-ultrasound_e.asp

Society of Obstetricians and Gynaecologists of Canada. (2011a). Genetic considerations for a woman's pre-conception evaluation. *Journal of Obstetrics and Gynaecology Canada, 33*(1), 57–64.

Society of Obstetricians and Gynaecologists of Canada. (2011b). Prenatal screening for fetal aneuploidy in singleton pregnancies. *Journal of Obstetrics and Gynaecology Canada, 33*(7), 736–750.

Society of Obstetricians and Gynaecologists of Canada. (2011c). Substance use in pregnancy. *Journal of Obstetrics and Gynaecology Canada, 33*(4), 367–372.

Tiedje, L. (2004). Teaching is more than telling: Education about prematurity in a prenatal clinic waiting room. *MCN, The American Journal of Maternal/Child Nursing, 29*(6), 373–378.

Transport Canada. (2007). *Seat belt sense—The case for restraints: What you need to know about seat belts, air bags and child restraints.* Retrieved February 21, 2012 from http://www.tc.gc.ca/eng/roadsafety/tp-tp14646-menu-191.htm

Wallace, D., Dodd, M., McNeil, D., et al. (2009). A pregnancy wellness guide to enhance care through self-assessment, personal reflection, and self-referral. *Journal of Obstetric, Gynaecologic, and Neonatal Nursing, 38*(2), 134–147.

Wen, S., Yang, T., Krewski, D., et al. (2008). Patterns of exposure to prescription FDA C, D and X drugs in a Canadian population. *Journal of Perinatology, 28*, 324–329.

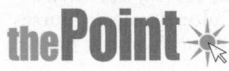

CHAPTER WORKSHEET REVIEW

MULTIPLE CHOICE QUESTIONS

1. Which of the following biophysical profile findings indicate poor oxygenation to the fetus?

   a. Two pockets of amniotic fluid

   b. Well-flexed arms and legs

   c. Nonreactive fetal heart rate

   d. Fetal breathing movements noted

2. The nurse teaches the pregnant woman how to perform Kegel exercises as a way to accomplish which of the following?

   a. Prevent perineal lacerations

   b. Stimulate postdates labour

   c. Increase pelvic muscle tone

   d. Lose pregnancy weight quickly

3. During a clinic visit, a pregnant woman at 30 weeks' gestation tells the nurse, "I've had some mild cramps and some backache. What does this mean?" The nurse should:

   a. Prepare the woman as she is in the very early stages of labour

   b. Assess for other symptoms of preterm labour

   c. Suggest that her symptoms are related to overhydration

   d. Discuss Braxton Hicks contractions, which occur throughout pregnancy

4. The nurse teaches a pregnant woman about exercise and activity, including activities not recommended during pregnancy. The nurse determines that the teaching was effective when the pregnant woman states that which of the following activities is not recommended during pregnancy?

   a. Swimming

   b. Walking

   c. Scuba diving

   d. Bike riding

5. A pregnant woman's last normal menstrual period was on August 10. Using Nagele's rule, the nurse calculates that her EDB will be which of the following?

   a. May 3

   b. June 10

   c. June 17

   d. May 17

CRITICAL THINKING EXERCISES

1. Dominique Doucette comes to the women's health centre where you work as a nurse. She is in her first trimester of pregnancy and tells you her main complaints are nausea and fatigue, to the point that she wants to sleep most of the time and eats only one meal daily. She appears pale and tired. Her mucous membranes are pale. She reports that she gets 8 to 9 hours of sleep each night but still can't seem to stay awake and alert at work. She tells you she knows that she is not eating as she should, but she isn't hungry. Her hemoglobin level and hematocrit are low.

   a. What subjective and objective data do you have to make your assessment?

   b. What is your impression of this woman?

   c. What nursing interventions would be appropriate for this woman?

   d. How will you evaluate the effectiveness of your interventions?

2. Monica Adamson, a 16-year-old high school student, is here for her first prenatal visit. Her last normal menstrual period was 2 months ago, and she states that she has been "sick ever since." She is 1.7 m tall and weighs 50 kg. In completing her dietary assessment, the nurse asks Monica about her intake of milk and other dairy products. Monica reports that she doesn't like "that stuff" and doesn't want to put on too much weight because it "might ruin my figure."

   a. In addition to the routine obstetric assessments, which additional assessments might be warranted for this teenager?

   b. What dietary instruction should be provided to this teenager based on her history?

   c. What follow-up monitoring should be included in subsequent prenatal visits?

(question continues on page 380)

3. Maria Mendes, a 27-year-old Hispanic woman in her last trimester of pregnancy (34 weeks), complains to the clinic nurse that she is constipated and feels miserable most of the time. She reports that she has started taking laxatives, but mostly they don't help her. When questioned about her dietary habits, she replies that she eats beans and rice and drinks tea with most meals. She says she has tried to limit her fluid intake so she doesn't have to go to the bathroom so much because she doesn't want to miss any of her daytime soap operas on television.

a. What additional information would the nurse need to assess her complaint?

b. What interventions would be appropriate for Maria?

c. What adaptations will Maria need to make to alleviate her constipation?

STUDY ACTIVITIES

1. Visit a birth centre and compare it with a traditional hospital setting in terms of restrictions, type of pain management available, and costs.

2. Arrange to shadow a midwife for a day to learn about her role in working with the childbearing family.

3. Select two of the websites listed on http://thePoint. lww.com/Chow1e, note their target audience, the validity of information offered, and their appeal to expectant couples. Present your findings.

4. Request permission to attend a childbirth education class in your local area and help a woman without a partner practice the paced breathing exercises. Present the information you learned and think about how you can apply it while taking care of a woman during labour.

5. A laywoman with specialized education and experience in assisting women during labour is a _____.

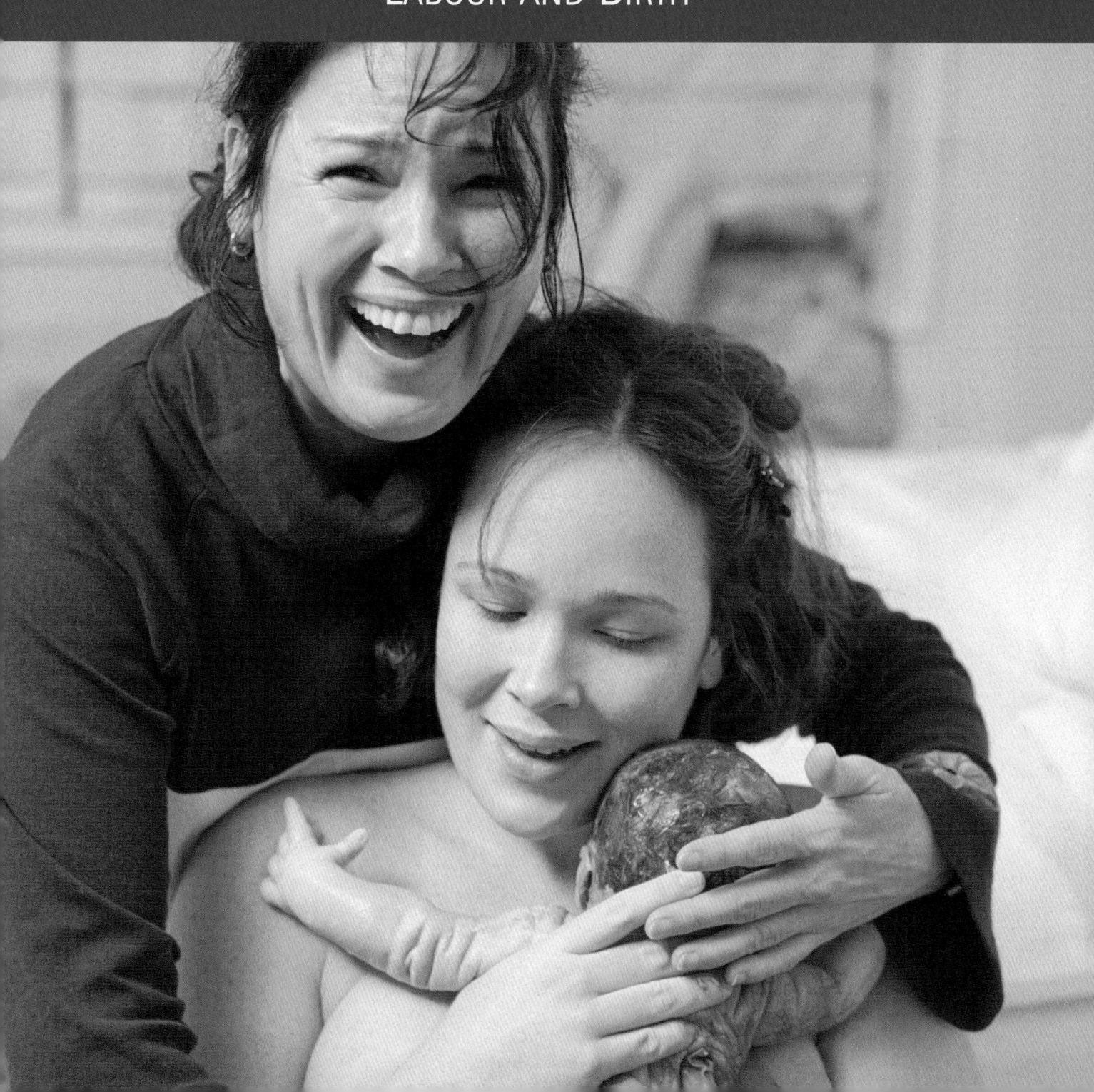

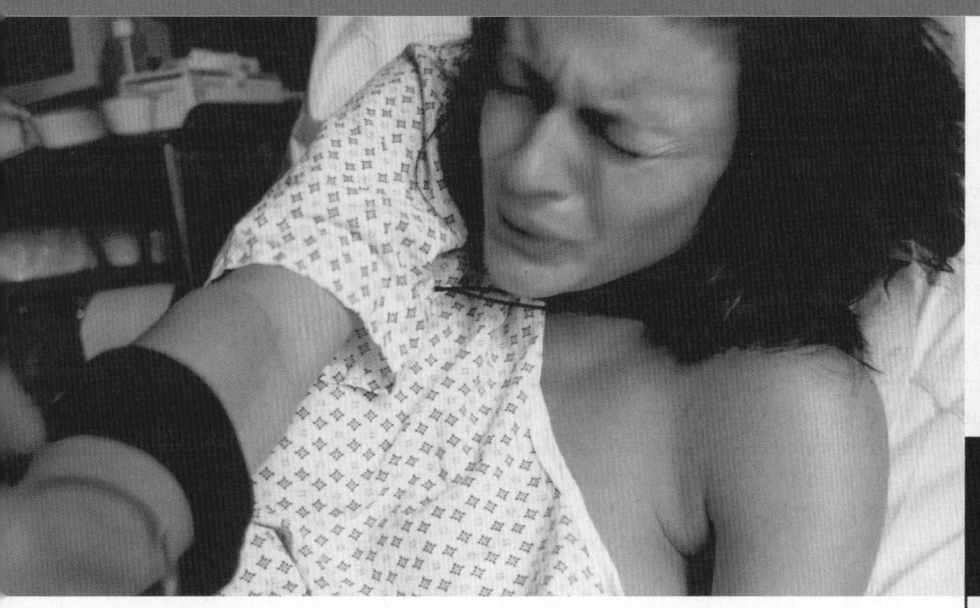

LABOUR AND BIRTH PROCESS

KEY TERMS

attitude
dilation
doula
duration
effacement

engagement
frequency
intensity
lie
lightening

moulding
position
presentation
station

LEARNING OBJECTIVES

Upon completion of the chapter, the learner will be able to:

1. Outline premonitory signs of labour.
2. Compare and contrast true versus false labour.
3. Categorize the critical factors affecting labour and birth.
4. Analyze the cardinal movements of labour.
5. Identify the maternal and fetal responses to labour and birth.
6. Classify the stages of labour and the critical events in each stage.
7. Explain the normal physiologic/psychological changes occurring during all four stages of labour.
8. Formulate the concept of pain as it relates to the woman in labour.

*K*athy and Chuck have been eagerly awaiting the birth of their first child for what seems to them an eternity. When Kathy finally feels contractions in her abdomen, she and Chuck rush to the hospital. After the OB nurse obtains a complete history and physical assessment, she informs Kathy and her husband that Kathy must have experienced "false labour" and that they should return home until she starts true labour.

Wow

Intense physical and emotional support promotes a positive and memorable birthing experience.

The process of labour and birth involves more than the birth of a newborn. Numerous physiologic and psychological events occur that ultimately result in the birth of a newborn and the creation or expansion of the family.

This chapter describes labour and birth as a process. It addresses initiation of labour, the premonitory signs of labour, including true and false labour, critical factors affecting labour and birth, maternal and fetal response to the labouring process, and the four stages of labour. The chapter also identifies critical factors related to each stage of labour: the "10 P's" of labour.

Initiation of Labour

Labour is a complex, multifaceted interaction between the mother and the fetus. It is a series of processes by which the fetus is expelled from the uterus. It is difficult to determine exactly why labour begins and what initiates it. Although several theories have been proposed to explain the onset and maintenance of labour, none of these have been proved scientifically. It is widely believed that labour is influenced by a combination of factors, including uterine stretch, progesterone withdrawal, increased oxytocin sensitivity, and increased release of prostaglandins.

One theory suggests that labour is initiated by a change in the estrogen-to-progesterone ratio. During the last trimester of pregnancy, estrogen levels increase and progesterone levels decrease. This change leads to an increase in the number of myometrium gap junctions. Gap junctions are proteins that connect cell membranes and facilitate coordination of uterine contractions and myometrial stretching (Cunningham et al., 2010).

Although physiologic evidence for the role of oxytocin in the initiation of labour is inconclusive, the number of oxytocin receptors in the uterus increases at the end of pregnancy. This creates an increased sensitivity to oxytocin. Estrogen, the levels of which are also rising, increases myometrial sensitivity to oxytocin. With the increasing levels of oxytocin in the maternal blood in conjunction with fetal production, initiation of uterine contractions can occur. Oxytocin also aids in stimulating prostaglandin synthesis through receptors in the decidua. Prostaglandins lead to additional contractions, cervical softening, gap junction induction, and myometrial sensitization, thereby leading to a progressive cervical **dilation** (the opening or enlargement of the external cervical os) (Martin & Kennedy, 2009b).

Prostaglandins are produced in the decidua and fetal membranes and have a central role in the initiation of labour. Prostaglandin levels increase late during pregnancy secondary to elevated estrogen levels. Prostaglandins stimulate smooth muscle contraction of the uterus.

An increase in prostaglandins leads to myometrial contractions and a reduction in cervical resistance. Subsequently, the cervix softens, thins out, and dilates during labour.

Premonitory Signs of Labour

Before the onset of labour, a pregnant woman's body undergoes several changes in preparation for the birth of the newborn. The changes that occur often lead to characteristic signs and symptoms that suggest that labour is near. These premonitory signs and symptoms can vary, and not every woman experiences every one of them.

Cervical Changes

Before labour begins, cervical softening and possible cervical dilation with descent of the presenting part into the pelvis occur. These changes can occur 1 month to 1 hour before actual labour begins.

As labour approaches, the cervix changes from an elongated structure to a shortened, thinned segment. Cervical collagen fibres undergo enzymatic rearrangement into smaller, more flexible fibres that facilitate water absorption, leading to a softer, more stretchable cervix. These changes occur secondary to the effects of prostaglandins and pressure from Braxton Hicks contractions (Murray & Huelsmann, 2009).

Lightening

Lightening occurs when the fetal presenting part begins to descend into the maternal pelvis. The uterus lowers and moves into a more anterior position. The shape of the abdomen changes as a result of the change in the uterus. With this descent, the woman usually notes that her breathing is much easier. However, she may complain of increased pelvic pressure, cramping, and low back pain. She may notice an increase in vaginal discharge and more frequent urination. Also, edema of the lower extremities may occur as a result of the increased stasis of pooling blood. In primigravidas, lightening can occur 2 weeks or more before labour begins; among multigravidas, it may not occur until labour (Ward & Hisley, 2009).

Increased Energy Level

Some women report a sudden increase in energy before labour. This is sometimes referred to as nesting, because many women will focus this energy toward childbirth preparation by cleaning, cooking, preparing the nursery, and spending extra time with other children in the household. The increased energy level usually occurs 24 to 48 hours before the onset of labour.

Bloody Show

At the onset of labour, the mucous plug that fills the cervical canal during pregnancy is expelled as a result of cervical softening and increased pressure of the presenting part. These ruptured cervical capillaries release a small amount of blood that mixes with mucus, resulting in the pink-tinged secretions known as bloody show.

Braxton Hicks Contractions

Braxton Hicks contractions, which the woman may have been experiencing throughout the pregnancy, may become stronger and more frequent. Braxton Hicks contractions are typically felt as a tightening or pulling sensation of the top of the uterus. They occur primarily in the abdomen and groin and gradually spread downward before relaxing. In contrast, true labour contractions are more commonly felt in the lower back. These contractions aid in moving the cervix from a posterior position to an anterior position. They also help in ripening and softening the cervix. However, the contractions are irregular and can be decreased by walking, voiding, eating, increasing fluid intake, or changing position.

Braxton Hicks contractions usually last about 30 seconds but can persist for as long as 2 minutes. As birth draws near and the uterus becomes more sensitive to oxytocin, the frequency and intensity of these contractions increase. However, if the contractions last longer than 30 seconds and occur more often than four to six times an hour, advise the woman to contact her health care provider so that she can be evaluated for possible preterm labour, especially if she is less than 38 weeks pregnant.

> ▶ *Take* NOTE!
>
> *An infant born between 34 and 36 completed weeks of gestation is identified as "late preterm" and experiences many of the same health issues as other preterm birth infants (Association of Women's Health, Obstetric and Neonatal Nurses [AWHONN], 2007).*

Spontaneous Rupture of Membranes

Spontaneous rupture of membranes precedes contractions in 10% of term pregnancies and in 40% of preterm pregnancies (Murray & Huelsmann, 2009). The rupture of membranes can result in either a sudden gush or a steady leakage of amniotic fluid. Although much of the amniotic fluid is lost when the rupture occurs, a continuous supply is produced to ensure protection of the fetus until birth.

After the amniotic sac has ruptured, the barrier to infection is gone and an ascending infection is possible. In addition, there is a danger of cord prolapse if engagement has not occurred with the sudden release of fluid and pressure with rupture. Due to the possibility of these complications, advise women to notify their health care provider and go in for an evaluation.

> ▶ *Consider* THIS!
>
> *I always pictured myself a dignified woman and behaved in ways to demonstrate that, for that was the way I was raised. My mother and grandmother always stressed that you should look good, dress well, and do nothing to embarrass yourself in public. I did a fairly good job of living up to their expectations until I become pregnant. I recall I was overdue according to my dates and was miserable in the summer heat. I decided to go to the store for some ice cream. As I waddled down the grocery aisles, all of a sudden my water broke and came pouring down my legs all over the floor. Not wanting to make a spectacle of myself and remembering what my mother always said about being dignified at all times in public, I quickly reached up onto the grocery shelf and "accidentally" knocked off a large jar of pickles right where my puddle was. As I walked hurriedly away from that mess without my ice cream, I heard on the store loudspeaker, "Clean-up on aisle 13!"*
>
> *Thoughts: we tend to live by what we are taught, and in this case, this woman needed to save face from her ruptured membranes. Many women experience ruptured membranes before the onset of labour, so it is not out of the ordinary for this to happen in public. What risks can occur when membranes do rupture? What action should this woman take now to minimize these risks? How will the nurse validate this woman's ruptured membranes?*

True Versus False Labour

False labour is a condition occurring during the latter weeks of some pregnancies in which irregular uterine contractions are felt, but the cervix is not affected. In contrast, true labour is characterized by contractions occurring at regular intervals that increase in frequency, duration, and intensity. True labour contractions bring about progressive cervical dilation and effacement. Table 13.1 summarizes the differences between true and false labour. False labour, prodromal labour, and Braxton Hicks contractions are all names for contractions that do not contribute in a measurable way toward the goal of birth.

Many women fear being sent home from the hospital with "false labour." All women feel anxious when they feel contractions, but they should be informed that labour could be a long process, especially if it is their first pregnancy. Encourage the woman to think of false labour or "pre-labour signs" as positive, as they are part of the

TABLE 13.1   DIFFERENCES BETWEEN TRUE AND FALSE LABOUR

Parameters	True Labour	False Labour
Contraction timing	Regular, becoming closer together, usually 4–6 min apart, lasting 30–60 s	Irregular, not occurring close together
Contraction strength	Become stronger with time, vaginal pressure is usually felt	Frequently weak, not getting stronger with time or alternating (a strong one followed by weaker ones)
Contraction discomfort	Starts in the back and radiates around toward the front of the abdomen	Usually felt in the front of the abdomen
Any change in activity	Contractions continue no matter what positional change is made	Contractions may stop or slow down with walking or making a position change
Stay or go?	Stay home until contractions are 5 min apart, last 45–60 s, and are strong enough so that a conversation during one is not possible—then go to the hospital or birthing centre.	Drink fluids and walk around to see if there is any change in the intensity of the contractions; if the contractions diminish in intensity after either or both—stay home.

Source: Cunningham et al. (2010). *Williams obstetrics* (23rd ed.). New York: McGraw-Hill.

entire labour continuum. With first pregnancies, the cervix can take up to 20 hours to dilate completely (Cunningham et al., 2010). In clinical care, it is difficult to differentiate between prolonged latent phase and false labour (McDonald, 2010). There is no consensus on how long latent labour should last and it is important to watch and wait for labour.

Remember Kathy and Chuck, the anxious couple who came to the hospital too early? Kathy felt sure she was in labour and is now confused. What explanations and anticipatory guidance should be offered to this couple? What term would describe her earlier contractions?

Factors Affecting the Labour Process

In many references, the critical factors that affect the process of labour and birth are outlined as the "five P's":

1. Passageway (birth canal)
2. Passenger (fetus and placenta)
3. Powers (contractions)
4. Position (maternal)
5. Psychological response

These critical factors are commonly accepted and discussed by health care professionals. However, five additional "P's" can also affect the labour process:

1. Philosophy (low tech, high touch)
2. Partners (support caregivers)
3. Patience (natural timing)
4. Patient preparation (childbirth knowledge base)
5. Pain control (comfort measures)

These five additional "P's" are helpful in planning care for the labouring family. These patient-focused factors are an attempt to foster labour that can be managed through the use of high touch, patience, support, knowledge, and pain management.

Passageway

The birth passageway is the route through which the fetus must travel to be born vaginally. The passageway consists of the maternal pelvis and soft tissues. Of the two, however, the maternal bony pelvis is more important because it is relatively unyielding (except for the coccyx). Typically the pelvis is assessed and measured during the first trimester, often at the first visit to the health care provider, to identify any abnormalities that might hinder a successful vaginal birth. As the pregnancy progresses, the hormones relaxin and estrogen cause the connective tissues to become more relaxed and elastic and cause the joints to become more flexible to prepare the mother's pelvis for birth. Additionally, the soft tissues usually yield to the forces of labour.

Bony Pelvis

The maternal bony pelvis can be divided into the true and false portions. The false (or greater) pelvis is composed of the upper flared parts of the two iliac bones with their concavities and the wings of the base of the sacrum. The false pelvis is divided from the true pelvis by an imaginary line drawn from the sacral prominence at the back to the superior aspect of the symphysis pubis at the front of the pelvis. This imaginary line is called

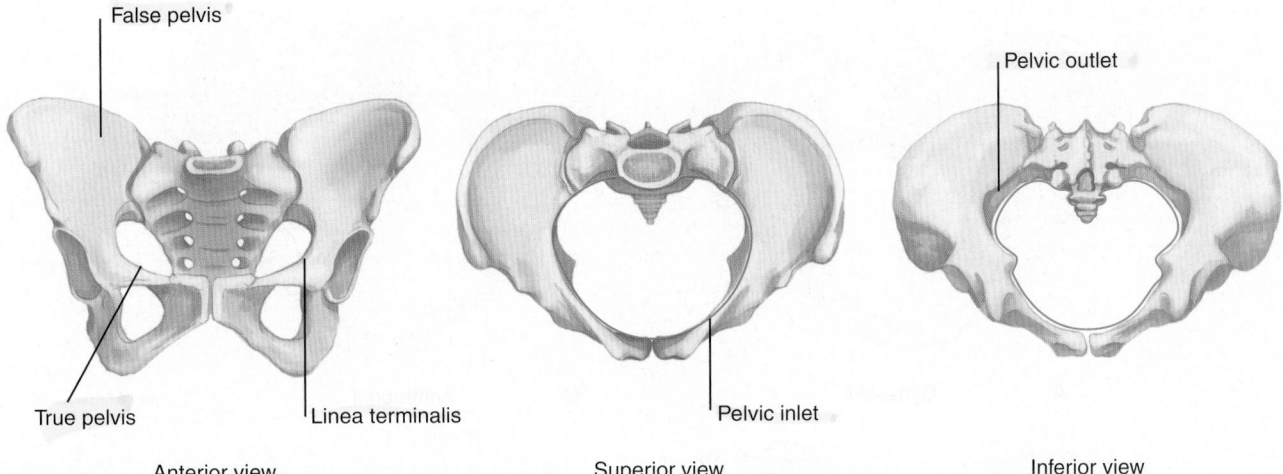

FIGURE 13.1 The bony pelvis.

linea terminalis. The false pelvis lies above this imaginary line; the true pelvis lies below it (Fig. 13.1). The true pelvis is the bony passageway through which the fetus must travel. It is made up of three planes: the inlet, the midpelvis (cavity), and the outlet.

Pelvic Inlet

The pelvic inlet allows entrance to the true pelvis. It is bounded by the sacral prominence in the back, laterally by the lineal terminalis, and by the superior aspect of the symphysis pubis in the front (Cunningham et al., 2010). The pelvic inlet is wider in the transverse aspect (sideways) than it is from front to back.

Midpelvis

The midpelvis (cavity) occupies the space between the inlet and the outlet. It is through this snug, curved space that the fetus must travel to reach the outside. As the fetus passes through this small area, its chest is compressed, causing lung fluid and mucus to be expelled. This expulsion removes the space-occupying fluid so that air can enter the lungs with the newborn's first breath.

Pelvic Outlet

The pelvic outlet is bound by the ischial tuberosities, the lower rim of the symphysis pubis, and the tip of the coccyx. In comparison with the pelvic inlet, the outlet is wider from front to back. For the fetus to pass through the pelvis, the outlet must be large enough.

To ensure the adequacy of the pelvic outlet for vaginal birth, the following pelvic measurements are assessed:

- Diagonal conjugate of the inlet (distance between the anterior surface of the sacral prominence and the anterior surface of the inferior margin of the symphysis pubis)
- Transverse or ischial tuberosity diameter of the outlet (distance at the medial and lowest aspect of the ischial

tuberosities, at the level of the anus; a known hand span or clenched-fist measurement is generally used to obtain this measurement)
- True or obstetric conjugate (distance estimated from the measurement of the diagonal conjugate; 1.5 cm is subtracted from the diagonal conjugate measurement)

For more information about pelvic measurements, see Chapter 12.

If the diagonal conjugate measures at least 11.5 cm and the true or obstetric conjugate measures 10 cm or more (1.5 cm less than the diagonal conjugate, or about 10 cm), then the pelvis is large enough for a vaginal birth of what would be considered a normal-size newborn.

Pelvic Shape

In addition to size, the shape of a woman's pelvis is a determining factor for a vaginal birth. The pelvis is divided into four main shapes: gynecoid, anthropoid, android, and platypelloid (Fig. 13.2).

The gynecoid pelvis is considered the true female pelvis, occurring in about 50% of all women (Martin & Kennedy, 2009a). Vaginal birth is most favourable with this type of pelvis because the inlet is round and the outlet is roomy. This shape offers the optimal diameters in all three planes of the pelvis. This type of pelvis allows early and complete fetal internal rotation during labour.

The anthropoid pelvis is common in men and occurs in 25% of women (Martin & Kennedy, 2009a). The pelvic inlet is oval and the sacrum is long, producing a deep pelvis (wider front to back [anterior to posterior] than side to side [transverse]). Vaginal birth is more favourable with this pelvic shape compared with the android or platypelloid shape (Ward & Hisley, 2009).

The android pelvis is considered the male-shaped pelvis and is characterized by a funnel shape. It occurs in approximately 20% of women (Martin & Kennedy, 2009a). The pelvic inlet is heart-shaped and the posterior

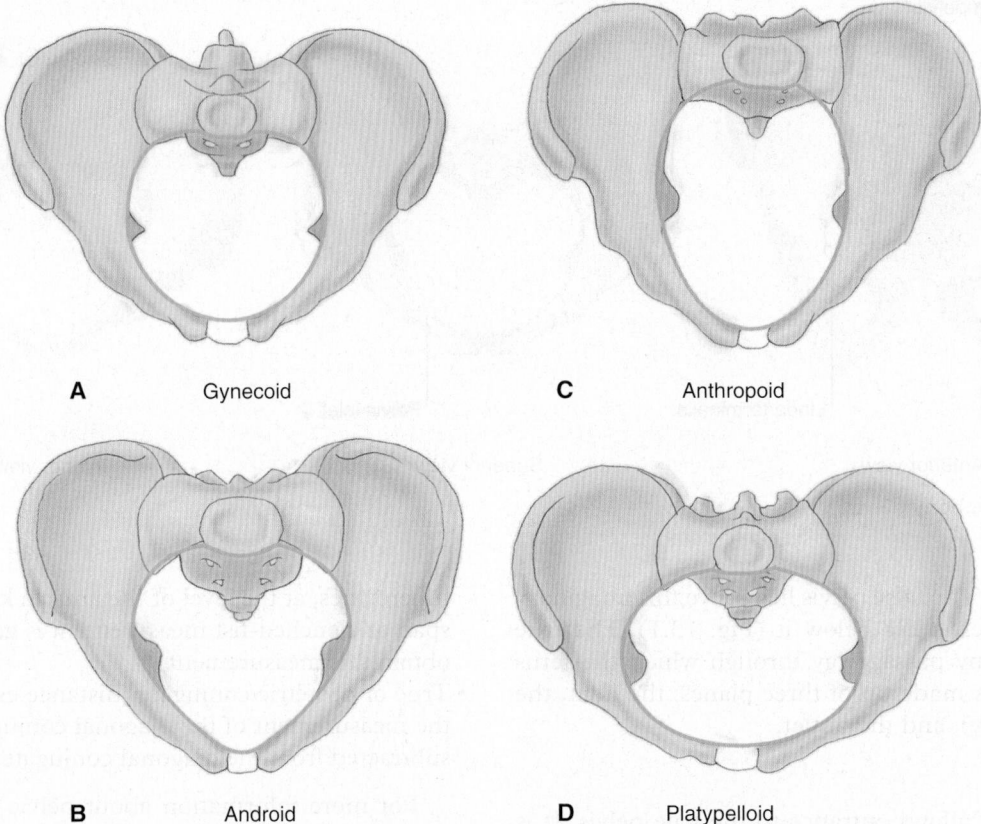

A   Gynecoid   C   Anthropoid

B   Android   D   Platypelloid

FIGURE 13.2 Pelvic shapes. (**A**) Gynecoid. (**B**) Android. (**C**) Anthropoid. (**D**) Platypelloid.

segments are reduced in all pelvic planes. Descent of the fetal head into the pelvis is slow, and failure of the fetus to rotate is common. The prognosis for labour is poor, subsequently leading to cesarean birth.

The platypelloid or flat pelvis is the least common type of pelvic structure among men and women, with an approximate incidence of 5% (Martin & Kennedy, 2009a). The pelvic cavity is shallow but widens at the pelvic outlet, making it difficult for the fetus to descend through the midpelvis. It is not favourable for a vaginal birth unless the fetal head can pass through the inlet. Women with this type of pelvis usually require cesarean birth.

An important principle is that most pelves are not purely defined but occur in nature as mixed types. Many women have a combination of these four basic pelvis types, with no two pelves being exactly the same. Regardless of the shape, the newborn will be born if size and positioning remain compatible. The narrowest part of the fetus attempts to align itself with the narrowest pelvic dimension (e.g., biparietal to interspinous diameters, which means the fetus generally tends to rotate to the most ample portion of the pelvis).

Soft Tissues

The soft tissues of the passageway consist of the cervix, the pelvic floor muscles, and the vagina. Through **effacement**,

the cervix effaces (thins) and dilates (opens) to allow the presenting fetal part to descend into the vagina.

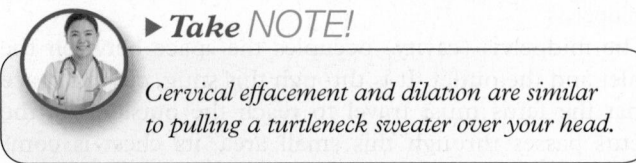

▶ **Take** NOTE!

Cervical effacement and dilation are similar to pulling a turtleneck sweater over your head.

The pelvic floor muscles help the fetus to rotate anteriorly as it passes through the birth canal. The soft tissues of the vagina expand to accommodate the fetus during birth.

Passenger

The fetus (with placenta) is the passenger. The fetal head (size and presence of moulding), fetal attitude (degree of body flexion), fetal lie (relationship of body parts), fetal presentation (first body part), fetal position (relationship to maternal pelvis), fetal station, and fetal engagement are all important factors that have an impact on the ultimate outcome in the birthing process.

Fetal Head

The fetal head is the largest and least compressible fetal structure, making it an important factor in relation to labour and birth. Considerable variation in the size and diameter of the fetal skull is often seen.

Compared with an adult, the fetal head is large in proportion to the rest of the body (Ward & Hisley, 2009). The bones that make up the face and cranial base are fused and essentially fixed. However, the bones that make up the rest of the cranium (two frontal bones, two parietal bones, and the occipital bone) are not fused; rather, they are soft and pliable, with gaps between the plates of bone. These gaps, which are membranous spaces between the cranial bones, are called sutures, and the intersections of these sutures are called fontanels. Sutures are important because they allow the cranial bones to overlap in order for the head to adjust in shape (elongate) when pressure is exerted on it by uterine contractions or the maternal bony pelvis. Some diameters shorten whereas others lengthen as the head is moulded during the labour and birthing process. This malleability of the fetal skull may decrease fetal skull dimensions (Cunningham et al., 2010). After birth, the sutures close as the bones grow and the brain reaches its full growth.

The changed (elongated) shape of the fetal skull at birth as a result of overlapping of the cranial bones is known as **moulding**. Along with moulding, fluid can also collect in the scalp (caput succedaneum) or blood can collect beneath the scalp (cephalohematoma), further distorting the shape and appearance of the fetal head. Caput succedaneum can be described as edema of the scalp at the presenting part. This swelling crosses suture lines and disappears within 3 to 4 days. Cephalohematoma is a collection of blood between the periosteum and the bone. It does not cross suture lines and is generally reabsorbed over weeks or months (Cunningham et al., 2010).

▶ *Take* NOTE!

Parents may become concerned about the distortion of their newborn's head. However, reassurance that the oblong shape is only temporary is usually all that is needed to reduce their anxiety.

Sutures also play a role in helping to identify the position of the fetal head during a vaginal examination. Figure 13.3 shows a fetal skull. The coronal sutures are located between the frontal and parietal bones and extend transversely on both sides of the anterior fontanels. The frontal suture is located between the two frontal bones. The lambdoidal sutures are located between the occipital bone and the two parietals, extending transversely on either side of the posterior fontanels. The sagittal suture is located between the parietal bones and divides the skull into the right and left halves. During a pelvic examination, palpation of these sutures by the examiner reveals the position of the fetal head and the degree of rotation that has occurred.

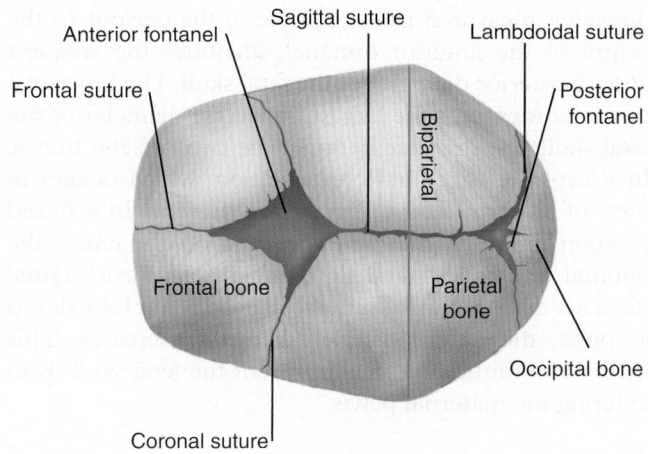

FIGURE 13.3 Fetal skull.

The anterior and posterior fontanels are also useful in helping to identify the position of the fetal head, and they allow for moulding. In addition, the fontanels are important when evaluating the newborn. The anterior fontanel is the famous "soft spot" of the newborn's head. It is diamond-shaped and measures about 2 to 3 cm. It remains open up to 18 months after birth to allow for growth of the brain (Davidson, London, & Ladewig, 2008). The posterior fontanel corresponds to the anterior one but is located at the back of the fetal head; it is triangular. This one closes within 8 to 12 weeks after birth and measures, on average, 0.5 to 1 cm at its widest diameter (Kenner & Lott, 2007).

The diameter of the fetal skull is an important consideration during the labour and birth process. Fetal skull diameters are measured between the various landmarks of the skull. Diameters include occipitofrontal, occipitomental, suboccipitobregmatic, and biparietal (Fig. 13.4). The two most important diameters that can affect the birth process are the suboccipitobregmatic (approximately 9.5 cm at term) and the biparietal (approximately 9.25 cm at term) diameters. The suboccipitobregmatic

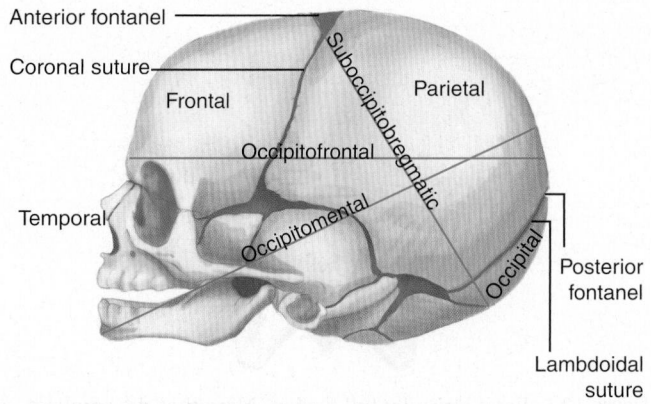

FIGURE 13.4 Fetal skull diameters.

diameter, measured from the base of the occiput to the centre of the anterior fontanel, identifies the smallest anteroposterior diameter of the fetal skull. The biparietal diameter measures the largest transverse diameter of the fetal skull: the distance between the two parietal bones. In a cephalic (headfirst) presentation, which occurs in 95% of all term births, if the fetus presents in a flexed position in which the chin is resting on the chest, the optimal or smallest fetal skull dimensions for a vaginal birth are demonstrated. If the fetal head is not fully flexed at birth, the anteroposterior diameter increases. This increase in dimension might prevent the fetal skull from entering the maternal pelvis.

Fetal Attitude

Fetal attitude is another important consideration related to the passenger. Fetal **attitude** refers to the posturing (flexion or extension) of the joints and the relationship of fetal parts to one another. The most common fetal attitude when labour begins is with all joints flexed—the fetal back is rounded, the chin is on the chest, the thighs are flexed on the abdomen, and the legs are flexed at the knees (Fig. 13.5). This normal fetal position is most favourable for vaginal birth, presenting the smallest fetal skull diameters to the pelvis.

When the fetus presents to the pelvis with abnormal attitudes (no flexion or extension), the diameter can increase the diameter of the presenting part as it passes through the pelvis, increasing the difficulty of birth. An attitude of extension tends to present larger fetal skull diameters, which may make birth difficult.

Fetal Lie

Fetal **lie** refers to the relationship of the long axis (spine) of the fetus to the long axis (spine) of the mother. There are two primary lies: longitudinal (which is the most common) and transverse (Fig. 13.6).

A longitudinal lie occurs when the long axis of the fetus is parallel to that of the mother (fetal spine to maternal spine side-by-side). A transverse lie occurs when the long axis of the fetus is perpendicular to the long axis of

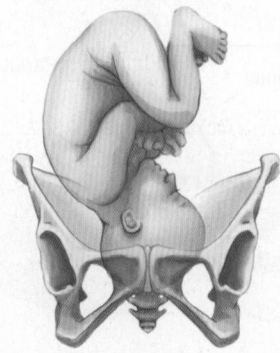

FIGURE 13.5 Fetal attitude: full flexion. Note that the smallest diameter presents to the pelvis.

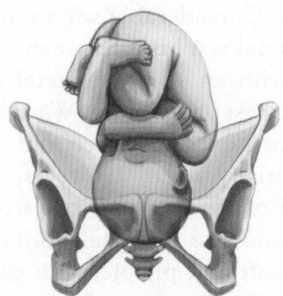

A. Longitudinal lie

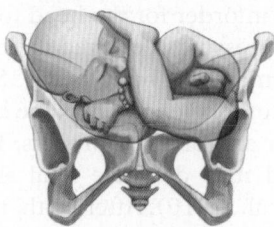

B. Transverse lie

FIGURE 13.6 Fetal lie.

the mother (fetus spine lies across the maternal abdomen and crosses her spine). A fetus in a transverse lie position cannot be delivered vaginally (Cunningham et al., 2010).

Fetal Presentation

Fetal **presentation** refers to the body part of the fetus that enters the pelvic inlet first (the "presenting part"). This is the fetal part that lies over the inlet of the pelvis or the cervical os. Knowing which fetal part is coming first at birth is critical for planning and initiating appropriate interventions.

The three main fetal presentations are cephalic (head first), breech (pelvis first), and shoulder (scapula first). The majority of term newborns enter this world in a cephalic presentation; breech and shoulder presentations are uncommon. In a cephalic presentation, the presenting part is usually the occiput portion of the fetal head (Fig. 13.7). This presentation is also referred to as a vertex presentation. Variations in a vertex presentation include the military, brow, and face presentations.

Breech presentation occurs when the fetal buttocks or feet enter the maternal pelvis first and the fetal skull enters last. This abnormal presentation poses several challenges at birth. Primarily, the largest part of the fetus (skull) is born last and may become "hung up" or stuck in the pelvis. In addition, the umbilical cord can become compressed between the fetal skull and the maternal pelvis after the fetal chest is born because the head is the last to exit. Moreover, unlike the hard fetal skull, the buttocks are soft and are not as effective as a cervical dilator during labour compared with a cephalic presentation.

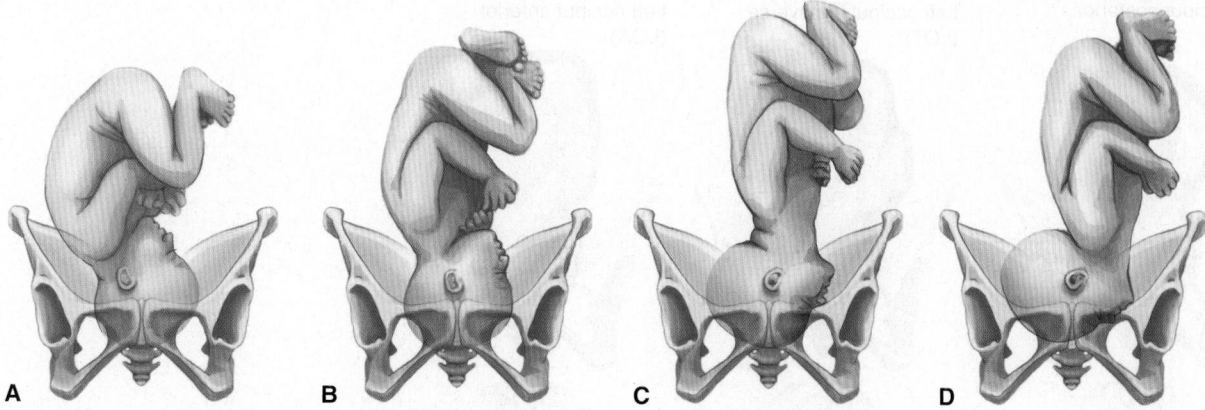

FIGURE 13.7 Fetal presentation: cephalic presentations. (**A**) Vertex. (**B**) Military. (**C**) Brow. (**D**) Face.

Finally, there is the possibility of trauma to the head as a result of the lack of opportunity for moulding.

The types of breech presentations are determined by the positioning of the fetal legs (Fig. 13.8). In a frank breech (50% to 70%), the buttocks present first with both legs extended up toward the face. In a full or complete breech (5% to 10%), the fetus sits cross-legged above the cervix. In a footling or incomplete breech (10% to 30%), one or both legs are presenting. Breech presentations are associated with hydramnios, oligohydramnios, prematurity, placenta previa, multiparity, previous breech delivery, uterine abnormalities (fibroids), multiple fetuses, and some congenital anomalies such as hydrocephaly (Cunningham et al., 2010). A frank breech can result in a vaginal birth, but complete and footling (incomplete) breech presentations generally necessitate a cesarean birth.

A shoulder presentation occurs when the fetal shoulders present first, with the head tucked inside. The fetus is in a transverse lie with the shoulder as the presenting part. Conditions associated with shoulder presentation include placenta previa, multiple gestation, or fetal anomalies. A cesarean birth is typically necessary (Cunningham et al., 2010).

Fetal Position

Fetal **position** describes the relationship of a given point on the presenting part of the fetus to a designated point of the maternal pelvis (Cunningham et al., 2010). The landmark fetal presenting parts include the occipital bone (O), which designates a vertex presentation; the chin (mentum [M]), which designates a face presentation; the buttocks (sacrum [S]), which designate a breech presentation; and the scapula (acromion process [A]), which designates a shoulder presentation.

In addition, the maternal pelvis is divided into four quadrants: right anterior, left anterior, right posterior, and left posterior. These quadrants designate whether the presenting part is directed toward the front, back, left, or right side of the pelvis. Fetal position is determined first by identifying the presenting part and then

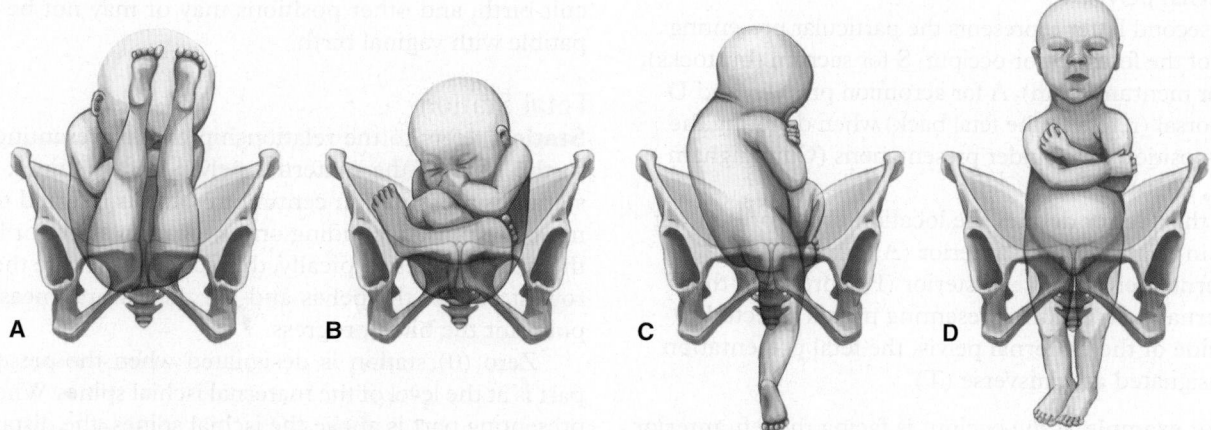

FIGURE 13.8 Breech presentations. (**A**) Frank breech. (**B**) Complete breech. (**C**) Single footling breech. (**D**) Double footling breech.

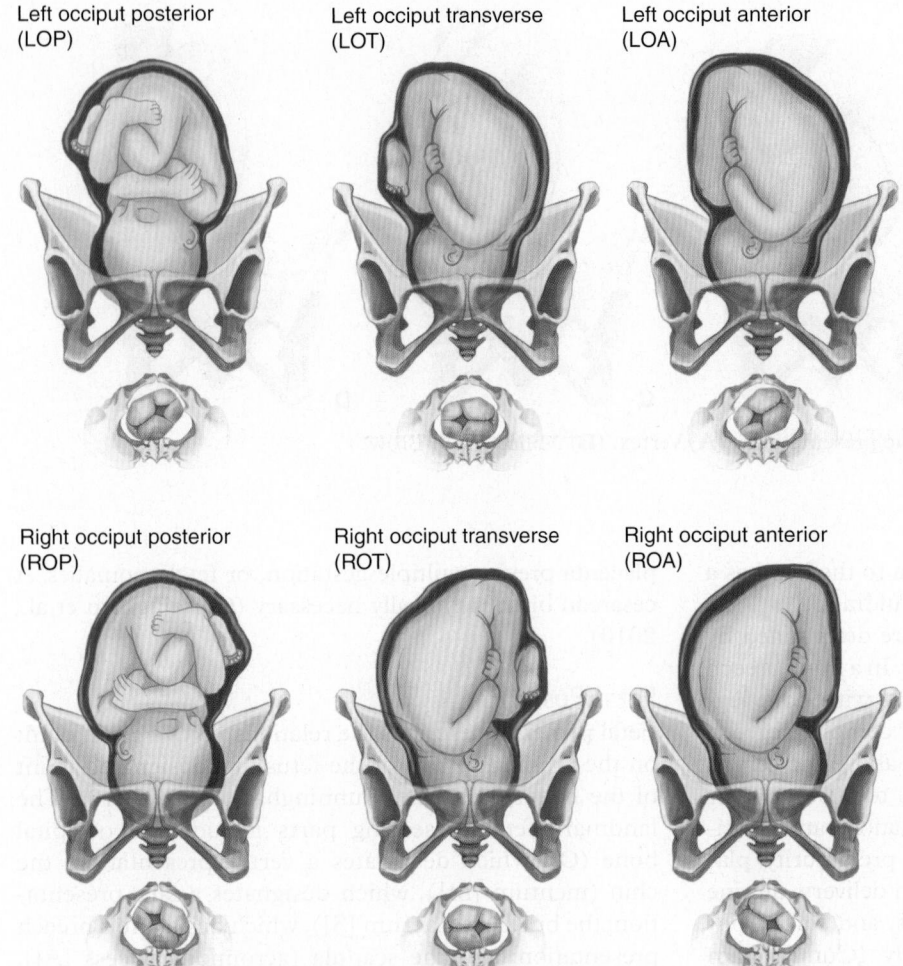

Left occiput posterior
(LOP)

Left occiput transverse
(LOT)

Left occiput anterior
(LOA)

Right occiput posterior
(ROP)

Right occiput transverse
(ROT)

Right occiput anterior
(ROA)

FIGURE 13.9 Examples of fetal positions in a vertex presentation. The lie is longitudinal for each illustration. The attitude is one of flexion. Notice that the view of the top illustration is seen when facing the pregnant woman. The bottom view is that seen with the woman in a dorsal recumbent position.

the maternal quadrant the presenting part is facing (Fig. 13.9). Position is indicated by a three-letter abbreviation as follows:

- The first letter defines whether the presenting part is tilted toward the left (L) or the right (R) side of the maternal pelvis.
- The second letter represents the particular presenting part of the fetus: O for occiput, S for sacrum (buttocks), M for mentum (chin), A for acromion process, and D for dorsal (refers to the fetal back) when denoting the fetal position in shoulder presentations (Cunningham et al., 2010).
- The third letter defines the location of the presenting part in relation to the anterior (A) portion of the maternal pelvis or the posterior (P) portion of the maternal pelvis. If the presenting part is directed to the side of the maternal pelvis, the fetal presentation is designated as transverse (T).

For example, if the occiput is facing the left anterior quadrant of the pelvis, then the position is termed left occipitoanterior and is recorded as LOA. LOA is the

most common (and most favourable) fetal position for birthing today, followed by right occipitoanterior (ROA).

The positioning of the fetus allows the fetal head to contour to the diameters of the maternal pelvis. LOA and ROA are optimal positions for vaginal birth. An occiput posterior position may lead to a long and difficult birth, and other positions may or may not be compatible with vaginal birth.

Fetal Station

Station refers to the relationship of the presenting part to the level of the maternal pelvic ischial spines. Fetal station is measured in centimetres and is referred to as a minus or plus, depending on its location above or below the ischial spines. Typically, the ischial spines are the narrowest part of the pelvis and are the natural measuring point for the birth progress.

Zero (0) station is designated when the presenting part is at the level of the maternal ischial spines. When the presenting part is above the ischial spines, the distance is recorded as minus stations. When the presenting part is below the ischial spines, the distance is recorded as plus stations. For instance, if the presenting part is above the ischial spines by 1 cm, it is documented as being a –1 station; if the presenting part is below the ischial spines by 1 cm, it is documented as being a +1 station. An easy way to understand this concept is to think in terms of meeting the goal, which is the birth. If the fetus is descending downward (past the ischial spines) and moving toward meeting the goal of birth, then the station is positive and the centimetre numbers grow bigger from +1 to +4. If the fetus is not descending past the ischial spines, then the station is negative and the centimetre numbers grow bigger from –1 to –4. The farther away the presenting part from the outside, the larger the negative number (–4 cm). The closer the presenting part of the fetus is to the outside, the larger the positive number (+4 cm). Figure 13.10 shows stations of presenting part.

Fetal Engagement

Engagement signifies the entrance of the largest diameter of the fetal presenting part (usually the fetal head) into the smallest diameter of the maternal pelvis (Cunningham et al., 2010). The fetus is said to be "engaged" in the pelvis when the presenting part reaches 0 station. Engagement is determined by pelvic examination.

The largest diameter of the fetal head is the biparietal diameter. It extends from one parietal prominence to the other. It is an important factor in the navigation through the maternal pelvis. Engagement typically occurs in primigravidas 2 weeks before term, whereas multigravidas may experience engagement several weeks before the onset of labour or not until labour begins.

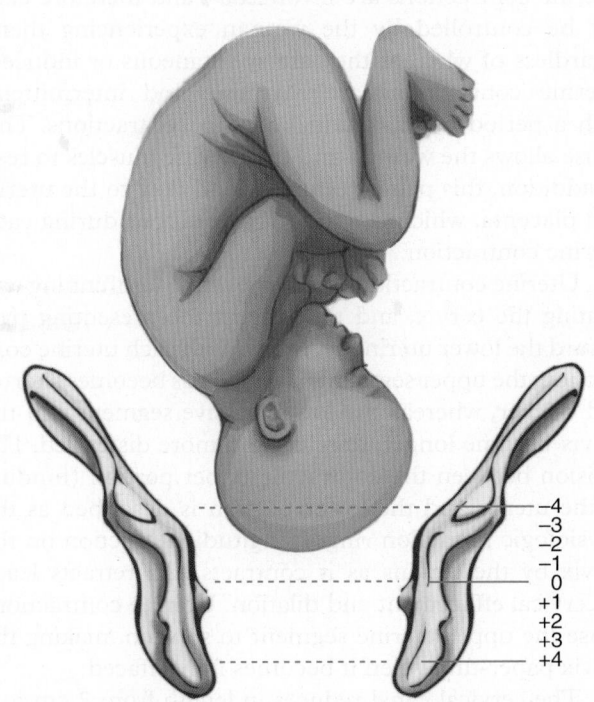

FIGURE 13.10 Fetal stations.

> ▶ **Take** NOTE!
>
> *The term floating is used when engagement has not occurred, because the presenting part is freely movable above the pelvic inlet.*

Cardinal Movements of Labour

The fetus goes through many positional changes as it travels through the passageway. These positional changes are known as the cardinal movements of labour. They are deliberate, specific, and very precise movements that allow the smallest diameter of the fetal head to pass through a corresponding diameter of the mother's pelvic structure. Although cardinal movements are conceptualized as separate and sequential, the movements are typically concurrent (Fig. 13.11).

Engagement

Engagement occurs when the greatest transverse diameter of the head in vertex (biparietal diameter) passes through the pelvic inlet (usually 0 station). The head usually enters the pelvis with the sagittal suture aligned in the transverse diameter.

Descent

Descent is the downward movement of the fetal head until it is within the pelvic inlet. Descent occurs intermittently with contractions and is brought about by one or more of the following forces:

- Pressure of the amniotic fluid
- Direct pressure of the fundus on the fetus' buttocks or head (depending on which part is located in the top of the uterus)
- Contractions of the abdominal muscles (second stage)
- Extension and straightening of the fetal body

Descent occurs throughout labour, ending with birth. During this time, the mother experiences discomfort, but she is unable to isolate this particular fetal movement from her overall discomfort.

Flexion

Flexion occurs as the vertex meets resistance from the cervix, the walls of the pelvis, or the pelvic floor. As a result, the chin is brought into contact with the fetal thorax and the presenting diameter is changed from occipitofrontal to suboccipitobregmatic (9.5 cm), which achieves the smallest fetal skull diameter presenting to the maternal pelvic dimensions.

Internal Rotation

After engagement, as the head descends, the lower portion of the head (usually the occiput) meets resistance from one side of the pelvic floor. As a result, the head

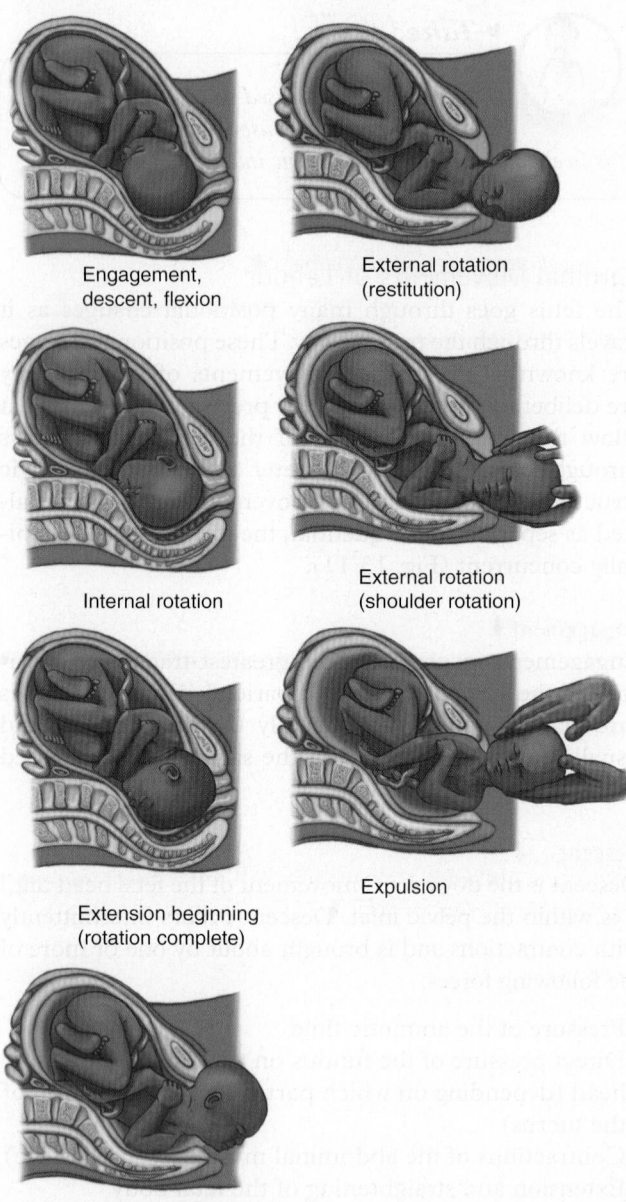

Engagement, descent, flexion

External rotation (restitution)

Internal rotation

External rotation (shoulder rotation)

Extension beginning (rotation complete)

Expulsion

Extension complete

FIGURE 13.11 Cardinal movements of labour.

rotates about 45 degrees anteriorly to the midline under the symphysis. This movement is known as internal rotation. Internal rotation brings the anteroposterior diameter of the head in line with the anteroposterior diameter of the pelvic outlet. It aligns the long axis of the fetal head with the long axis of the maternal pelvis. The widest portion of the maternal pelvis is the anteroposterior diameter, and thus the fetus must rotate to accommodate the pelvis.

Extension

With further descent and full flexion of the head, the nucha (the base of the occiput) becomes impinged under the symphysis. Resistance from the pelvic floor causes the fetal head to extend so that it can pass under the pubic arch. Extension occurs after internal rotation is complete. The head emerges through extension under the symphysis pubis along with the shoulders. The anterior fontanel, brow, nose, mouth, and chin are born successively.

External Rotation (Restitution)

After the head is born and is free of resistance, it untwists, causing the occiput to move about 45 degrees back to its original left or right position (restitution). The sagittal suture has now resumed its normal right-angle relationship to the transverse (bisacromial) diameter of the shoulders (i.e., the head realigns with the position of the back in the birth canal). External rotation of the fetal head allows the shoulders to rotate internally to fit the maternal pelvis.

Expulsion

Expulsion of the rest of the body occurs more smoothly after the birth of the head and the anterior and posterior shoulders (Cunningham et al., 2010).

Powers

The primary stimulus powering labour is uterine contractions. Contractions cause complete dilation and effacement of the cervix during the first stage of labour. The secondary powers in labour involve the use of intra-abdominal pressure (voluntary muscle contractions) exerted by the woman as she pushes and bears down during the second stage of labour.

Uterine Contractions

Uterine contractions are involuntary and therefore cannot be controlled by the woman experiencing them, regardless of whether they are spontaneous or induced. Uterine contractions are rhythmic and intermittent, with a period of relaxation between contractions. This pause allows the woman and the uterine muscles to rest. In addition, this pause restores blood flow to the uterus and placenta, which is temporarily reduced during each uterine contraction.

Uterine contractions are responsible for thinning and dilating the cervix, and they thrust the presenting part toward the lower uterine segment. With each uterine contraction, the upper segment of the uterus becomes shorter and thicker, whereas the lower passive segment and the cervix become longer, thinner, and more distended. The division between the contractile upper portion (fundus) of the uterus and the lower portion is described as the physiologic retraction ring. Longitudinal traction on the cervix by the fundus as it contracts and retracts leads to cervical effacement and dilation. Uterine contractions cause the upper uterine segment to shorten, making the cervix paper-thin when it becomes fully effaced.

The cervical canal reduces in length from 2 cm to a paper-thin entity and is described in terms of percentages from 0% to 100%. In primigravidas, effacement typically starts before the onset of labour and usually begins before dilation; in multigravidas, however, neither effacement nor dilation may start until labour ensues (Nettina, 2010). On clinical examination, the following may be assessed:

• Cervical canal 2 cm in length would be described as 0% effaced.
• Cervical canal 1 cm in length would be described as 50% effaced.
• Cervical canal 0 cm in length would be described as 100% effaced.

Dilation is dependent on the pressure of the presenting part and the contraction and retraction of the uterus. The diameter of the cervical os increases from less than 1 cm to approximately 10 cm to allow for birth. When the cervix is fully dilated, it is no longer palpable on vaginal examination. Descriptions may include the following:

• External cervical os closed: 0 cm dilated
• External cervical os half open: 5 cm dilated
• External cervical os fully open: 10 cm dilated

During early labour, uterine contractions are described as mild, they last about 30 seconds, and they occur about every 5 to 7 minutes. As labour progresses, contractions last longer (60 seconds), occur more frequently (2 to 3 minutes apart), and are described as being moderate to high in intensity.

Each contraction has three phases: increment (build-up of the contraction), acme (peak or highest intensity), and decrement (descent or relaxation of the uterine muscle fibres; Fig. 13.12).

Uterine contractions are monitored and assessed according to three parameters: frequency, duration, and intensity.

1. **Frequency** refers to how often the contractions occur and is measured from the increment of one contraction to the increment of the next contraction.

2. **Duration** refers to how long a contraction lasts and is measured from the beginning of the increment to the end of the decrement for the same contraction.

3. **Intensity** refers to the strength of the contraction determined by manual palpation or measured by an internal intrauterine pressure catheter (IUPC). The catheter is positioned in the uterine cavity through the cervix after the membranes have ruptured. It reports intensity by measuring the pressure of the amniotic fluid inside the uterus in millimetres of mercury (Murray & Huelsmann, 2009).

Intra–Abdominal Pressure

Increased intra-abdominal pressure (voluntary muscle contractions) compresses the uterus and adds to the power of the expulsion forces of the uterine contractions (Murray & Huelsmann, 2009). Coordination of these forces in unison promotes birth of the fetus and expulsion of the fetal membranes and placenta from the uterus. Interference with these forces (such as when a woman is highly sedated or extremely anxious) can compromise the effectiveness of these powers.

Psychological Response

Childbearing can be one of the most life-altering experiences for a woman. The experience of childbirth goes beyond the physiologic aspects: it influences her self-confidence, self-esteem, and view of life, relationships, and children. Her state of mind (psyche) throughout the entire process is critical to bring about a positive outcome for her and her family. Factors promoting a positive birth experience include:

• Clear information about procedures
• Support; not being alone
• Sense of mastery, self-confidence
• Trust in staff caring for her
• Positive reaction to the pregnancy

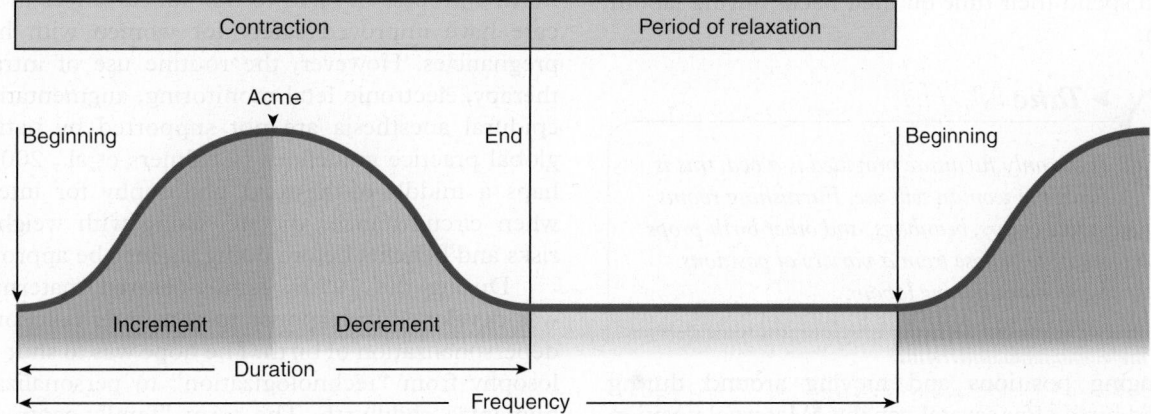

FIGURE 13.12 The three phases of a uterine contraction.

• Personal control over breathing
• Preparation for the childbirth experience

Having a strong sense of self and meaningful support from others can often help women manage labour well. Feeling safe and secure typically promotes a sense of control and ability to withstand the challenges of the childbearing experience. Anxiety and fear, however, decrease a woman's ability to cope with the discomfort of labour. Maternal catecholamines secreted in response to anxiety and fear can inhibit uterine blood flow and placental perfusion. In contrast, relaxation can augment the natural process of labour (Murray & Huelsmann, 2009). Preparing mentally for childbirth is important so that the woman can work with, rather than against, the natural forces of labour.

Position (Maternal)

Maternal positioning during labour has only recently been the subject of well-controlled research. Scientific evidence has shown that nonmoving, back-lying positions during labour are not healthy (Zwelling, 2010). However, despite this evidence to the contrary, most women continue to lie flat on their backs during labour. Some of the reasons why this practice continues include the following:

• Belief that labouring women need to conserve their energy and not tire themselves
• Belief that nurses cannot keep track of the whereabouts of ambulating women
• Belief that the supine position facilitates vaginal examinations and external belt adjustment
• Belief that a bed is "where one is supposed to be" in a hospital setting
• Belief that the position is more convenient for the delivering health professional
• Belief that labouring women are "connected to things" that impede movement (Zwelling, 2010)

Although many labour and birthing facilities claim that all women are allowed to adopt any position of comfort during their labouring experience, the great majority of women spend their time on their backs during labour and birth.

▶ *Take* NOTE!

If the only furniture provided is a bed, this is what the woman will use. Furnishing rooms with comfortable chairs, beanbags, and other birth props allows a woman to choose from a variety of positions and to be free to move during labour.

Changing positions and moving around during labour and birth offer several benefits. Maternal position can influence pelvic size and contours. Changing position

and walking affect the pelvic joints, which may facilitate fetal descent and rotation. Squatting enlarges the pelvic outlet by approximately 25%, whereas a kneeling position removes pressure on the maternal vena cava and helps to rotate the fetus in the posterior position (Zwelling, 2010). The use of any upright or lateral position, compared with supine or lithotomy positions, may:

• Reduce the length of the first stage of labour
• Reduce the duration of the second stage of labour
• Reduce the number of assisted deliveries (vacuum and forceps)
• Reduce episiotomies and perineal tears
• Contribute to fewer abnormal fetal heart rate patterns
• Increase comfort/reduce requests for pain medication
• Enhance a sense of control by the mother
• Alter the shape and size of the pelvis, which assists in descent
• Assist gravity to move the fetus downward (Zwelling, 2010)

Using the research available can bring better outcomes, heightened professionalism, and evidence-based practice to childbearing practices.

Philosophy

Not everyone views childbirth in the same way. A philosophical continuum exists that extends from viewing labour as a disease process to a normal process. One philosophy assumes that women cannot manage the birth experience adequately and therefore need constant expert monitoring and management. The other philosophy assumes that women are capable, reasoning individuals who can actively participate in their birth experience.

The health care system in Canada today appears to be leaning toward the former philosophy, applying technological interventions to most mothers who enter the hospital system. For many women in the 21st century, giving birth in a hospital has become "intervention intensive"—designed to start, continue, and end labour through medical management rather than allowing the normal process of birth to unfold. Advances in medical care have improved safety for women with high-risk pregnancies. However, the routine use of intravenous therapy, electronic fetal monitoring, augmentation, and epidural anesthesia are not supported by national or global practice guidelines (Chalmers et al., 2009). Perhaps a middle-of-the-road philosophy for intervening when circumstances dictate, along with weighing the risks and benefits before doing so, may be appropriate.

During the 1970s, family-centred maternity care was developed in response to consumer reaction to the depersonalization of birth. The hope was to shift the philosophy from "technologization" to personalization to humanize childbirth. The term "family-centred birthing" is more appropriate today to denote the low-tech, high-touch approach requested by many childbearing women, who view childbirth as a normal process. In Canada, there have been positive improvements to family-centred maternity care but more change is needed to assist women and families to achieve positive birthing experiences (Jimenez, Klein, Hivon, & Mason, 2010).

Registered midwives are champions of family-centred birthing, and their participation in the childbirth process is associated with fewer unnecessary interventions when compared with participation by obstetricians. Registered midwives subscribe to a normal birth process in which the woman uses her own instincts and bodily signs during labour. In short, midwives empower women within the birthing environment (Leap, Sandall, Buckland, & Huber, 2010).

No matter what philosophy is held, it is ideal if everyone involved in the particular birth process—from the health care provider to the mother—shares the same philosophy toward the birth process.

Partners

Women desire attentive care during labour and birth from partners who can convey emotional support by offering their continued presence and words of encouragement. Partners can play an important role in providing this comfort (Hanson, Hunter, Bormann, & Sobo, 2009), although they may experience fear related to their role at birth. Although the presence of the baby's father at the birth provides special emotional support, a partner can be anyone who is present to support the woman throughout the experience. See Evidence-based Practice 13.1.

Worldwide, women usually support other women in childbirth. Hodnett, Gates, Hofmeyr, & Sakala (2011) reported that the continuous presence of a trained female support person (**doula**) reduced the need for medication for pain relief, the use of vacuum or forceps delivery, and the need for cesarean births. Continuous support was also associated with a slight reduction in the length of labour. The doula, who is an experienced labour companion, provides the woman and her partner with emotional and physical support and information throughout the entire labour and birth experience.

Given the many benefits of intrapartum support, labouring women should always have the option to receive partner support, whether from nurses, doulas, significant others, or family. Whoever the support partner is, he or she should provide the mother with continuous presence and hands-on comfort and encouragement.

Patience

The birth process takes time. If more time were allowed for women to labour naturally without intervention, the cesarean birth rate would most likely be reduced (Chalmers et al., 2010; Romano & Lothian, 2008; Wilson, Effkren, & Butler, 2010). The literature suggests that delaying interventions can give a woman enough time to

EVIDENCE–BASED PRACTICE 13.1
Continuous Support for Women During Childbirth

● **Study**

Historically, women have been attended and supported by other women during labour. However, in recent decades in hospitals worldwide, continuous support during labour has become the exception rather than the rule. Concerns about the consequent dehumanization of the birth experience have led to calls for a return to continuous support by women for women during labour.

This review of studies included 16 trials from 11 countries, involving more than 13,000 women in a wide range of settings and circumstances. The primary goal of the review was to assess the effects, on mothers and their babies, of continuous, one-to-one intrapartum support compared with usual care. The secondary goal was to determine whether the effects of continuous support are influenced by (1) routine practices and policies in the birth environment that may affect a woman's autonomy, freedom of movement, and ability to cope with labour; (2) whether the caregiver is a member of the staff of the institution; and (3) whether the continuous support begins early or later in labour.

▲ **Findings**

Women who received continuous labour support were more likely to give birth "spontaneously" (vaginally, without vacuum or forceps). They were less likely to use pain medications, were more likely to be satisfied with their experience, and had slightly shorter labours. In general, labour support appeared to be more effective when it was provided by women who were not part of the hospital staff. It also appeared to be more effective when started early in labour. No adverse effects were identified.

■ **Nursing Implications**

Knowing the results of this evidence-based study, all nurses should strive to be a real "presence" for all of their labouring couples. Based on the findings, continuous nursing support promotes positive birthing outcomes and fewer technical/surgical interventions. Both maternal and fetal well-being is preserved when nurses are present and involved during the childbirth experience.

Hodnett, E. D., Gates, S., Hofmeyr, G. J., & Sakala, C. (2011). Continuous support for women during childbirth. *Cochrane Database of Systematic Reviews, 2*, CD003766. doi: 10.1002/14651858. CD003766.pub3

progress in labour and reduce the need for surgical inter-vention (Romano & Lothian, 2008).

The current cesarean birth rate in Canada was reported to be 25.6 per 100 hospital deliveries in 2004 and 2005, yet the World Health Organization (WHO) rec-ommends a rate of 10% to 15% (Chalmers et al., 2010; Public Health Agency of Canada [PHAC], 2008). Cesar-ean birth is associated with increased morbidity and mor-tality for both mother and infant as well as increased in-patient length of stay and health care costs (Society of Obstetricians and Gynaecologists of Canada [SOGC], 2008). The elective/other category of cesarean births rep-resented 6.7 per 100 hospital births (PHAC, 2008).

It is difficult to predict how any given labour will progress and therefore equally difficult to determine how long a woman's labour will last. There is no way to estimate the likely strength and frequency of uterine contractions, the extent to which the cervix will soften and dilate, and how much the fetal head will mould to fit the birth canal. We cannot know beforehand whether the complex fetal rotations needed for an efficient labour will take place properly. All of these factors are unknowns when a woman starts labour.

There is a trend in health care, however, to attempt to manipulate the process of labour through medical means such as artificial rupture of membranes and augmentation of labour with oxytocin (Chalmers et al., 2010). In Canada, the labour induction rate ranges from 21.6% to 52.5% and the labour augmentation rate ranges from 16.1% to 40.6% (Chalmers et al., 2009). An amniotomy (artificial rupture of the fetal membranes) may be performed to aug-ment or induce labour when the membranes have not ruptured spontaneously. Doing so allows the fetal head to have more direct contact with the cervix in order to dilate it. This procedure is performed with the fetal head at −2 station or lower, with the cervix dilated to at least 3 cm. Synthetic oxytocin (Syntocinon) is also used to induce or augment labour by stimulating uterine contractions. It is administered piggybacked into the primary intravenous line with an infusion pump titrated to uterine activity.

There is compelling evidence that elective induction of labour significantly increases the risk of cesarean birth, especially for nulliparous women (Murray & Huelsmann, 2009). The belief is that many cesarean births could be avoided if women were allowed to labour longer and if the natural labour process were allowed to complete the job. The longer wait (using the intervention of patience) usually results in less intervention.

The Society of Obstetricians and Gynaecologists of Canada (SOGC) suggests that induction should be offered at 41 to 42 weeks' gestation based on evidence that sug-gests decreased perinatal mortality without an increased rate of cesarean section (Delaney & Roggensack, 2008). Determination of gestational age should be based on ultra-sound in the first trimester. Sweeping of the membranes should be offered between 38 and 41 weeks based on a discussion of the risks and benefits. There are medical indi-cations for inducing labour, such as premature rupture of membranes and when labour does not start; a pregnancy more than 41 weeks' gestation; maternal hypertension, diabetes, or a uterine infection; or fetal demise (Dunne, Da Silva, Schmidt, & Natale, 2009). However, more women today are requesting induction for reasons of convenience.

When the labouring woman feels the urge to bear down, pushing begins. Most women respond extremely well to messages from their body without being directed by the nurse. A more natural, undirected approach allows the woman to wait and bear down when she feels the urge to push. Having patience and letting nature take its course will reduce the incidence of physiologic stress in the mother, resulting in less trauma to her perineal tissue.

Patient Preparation

Basic prenatal education can help women manage their labour process and feel in control of their birthing expe-rience. The literature indicates that if a woman is pre-pared before the labour and birth experience, the labour is more likely to remain normal or natural (without the need for medical intervention) (Leap et al., 2010). An increasing body of evidence also indicates that the well-prepared woman, with good labour support, is less likely to need analgesia or anesthesia and is unlikely to require cesarean birth (Barrett & Stark, 2010).

Prenatal education teaches the woman about the childbirth experience and increases her sense of control. She is then able to work as an active participant during the labour and birth experience (International Childbirth Education Association, n.d.). Research also suggests that prenatal preparation may affect intrapartum and postpar-tum psychosocial outcomes. For example, prenatal edu-cation covering parenting communication classes had a significant effect on postpartum anxiety and adjustment. Prenatal education should be viewed as an opportunity to strengthen families by providing anticipatory guidance and improving their life skills. In short, prenatal educa-tion helps to promote healthy families during the transi-tion to parenthood and beyond (International Childbirth Education Association, n.d.).

> ▶ *Take* NOTE!
>
> *Learning about labour and birth allows women and couples to express their needs and preferences, enhances their confidence, and improves communication between themselves and the staff.*

Pain Management

Labour and birth, although a normal physiologic pro-cess, can produce significant pain. Pain during labour is a nearly universal experience. Controlling the pain without harm to the fetus or labour process is the major focus of pain management during childbirth.

Pain is a subjective experience involving a complex interaction of physiologic, spiritual, sensory, behavioural, cognitive, psychosocial, and cultural influences (Murray & Huelsmann, 2009). Cultural values and learned behaviours influence perception and response to pain, as do anxiety and fear, both of which tend to heighten the sense of pain (Murray & Huelsmann, 2009). The challenge for health care providers is to find the right combination of pain management methods to keep the pain manageable while being mindful of the maternal and fetal outcomes. Chapter 14 presents a full discussion of pain management during labour and birth.

Physiologic Responses to Labour

Labour is the physiologic process by which the uterus expels the fetus and placenta from the body. During pregnancy, progesterone secreted from the placenta suppresses the spontaneous contractions of a typical uterus, keeping the fetus within the uterus. In addition, the cervix remains firm and noncompliant. At term, however, changes that occur in the cervix make it softer. In addition, uterine contractions become more frequent and regular, signalling the onset of labour.

The labour process involves a series of rhythmic, involuntary, usually quite uncomfortable uterine muscle contractions. They bring about a shortening of muscle fibres that causes effacement and dilation of the cervix and a bursting of the fetal membranes. Then, accompanied by both reflex and voluntary contractions of the abdominal muscles (pushing), the uterine contractions result in the birth of the baby (Murray & Huelsmann, 2009). During labour, the mother and fetus make several physiologic adaptations.

Maternal Responses

The labour process stresses several of the woman's body systems, which react through numerous compensatory mechanisms. As the woman progresses through childbirth, numerous physiologic responses occur that help her adapt to the labouring process:

- Heart rate increases by 10 to 20 bpm.
- Cardiac output increases by 10% to 15% during the first stage of labour and by 30% to 50% during the second stage of labour.
- Blood pressure increases by 10 to 30 mm Hg during uterine contractions in all labour stages.
- White blood cell count increases by 25,000 to 30,000 cells/mm³, perhaps as a result of tissue trauma.
- Respiratory rate increases and more oxygen is consumed related to the increase in metabolism.

- Gastric motility and food absorption decrease, which may increase the risk of nausea and vomiting during the transition stage of labour.
- Gastric emptying and gastric pH decrease, increasing the risk for vomiting with aspiration.
- Temperature rises slightly, possibly due to an increase in muscle activity.
- Muscular aches/cramps occur as a result of the stressed musculoskeletal system.

A woman's ability to adapt to the stress of labour is influenced by her psychological and physical state. Among the many factors that affect her coping ability are:

- Previous birth experiences and their outcomes
- Current pregnancy experience (planned versus unplanned, discomforts experienced, age, risk status of pregnancy, chronic illness, weight gain)
- Cultural considerations (values and beliefs about health status)
- Support system (presence and support of a valued partner during labour)
- Childbirth preparation (attended childbirth classes and has practiced paced breathing techniques)
- Exercise during pregnancy
- Expectations of the birthing experience
- Anxiety level
- Fear of labour and loss of control
- Fatigue and weariness (Murray & Huelsmann, 2009)

Fetal Responses

Although the focus during labour may be on assessing the mother's adaptations, several physiologic adaptations occur in the fetus as well. The fetus is experiencing labour along with the mother. If the fetus is healthy, the stress of labour usually has no adverse effects. The nurse needs to be alert to any abnormalities in the fetus' adaptation to labour. Fetal responses to labour include:

- Periodic fetal heart rate accelerations and slight decelerations related to fetal movement, fundal pressure, and uterine contractions
- Decrease in circulation and perfusion to the fetus secondary to uterine contractions (a healthy fetus is able to compensate for this drop)
- Increase in arterial carbon dioxide pressure (PCO_2)
- Decrease in fetal breathing movements throughout labour

▶ *Take* NOTE!

Respiratory changes during labour help to prepare the fetus for extrauterine respiration immediately after birth.

Stages of Labour

Labour is typically divided into four stages: dilation, expulsive, placental, and restorative. Table 13.2 summarizes the major events of each stage.

The first stage is the longest: it begins with the first true contraction and ends with full dilation (opening) of the cervix. Because this stage lasts so long, it is divided into three phases, each corresponding to the progressive dilation of the cervix.

Stage two of labour, or the expulsive stage, begins when the cervix is completely dilated and ends with the birth of the newborn. The expulsive stage can last from minutes to hours.

The third stage, or the placental stage, starts after the newborn is born and ends with the separation and birth of the placenta. Continued uterine contractions typically cause the placenta to be expelled within 5 to 30 minutes.

The fourth stage, or the restorative stage, lasts from 1 to 4 hours after birth. This period is when the mother's

TABLE 13.2 STAGES AND PHASES OF LABOUR

	First Stage	Second Stage	Third Stage	Fourth Stage
Description	From 0 to 10 cm dilation; consists of three phases	From complete dilation (10 cm) to birth of the newborn; lasts up to 1 h	Separation and delivery of the placenta	1–4 h after the birth of the newborn; time of maternal physiologic adjustment
Phases	**Latent phase** (0–3 cm dilation) • Cervical dilation from 0 to 3 cm • Cervical effacement from 0% to 40% • Nullipara, lasts up to 6 h; multigravida, lasts up to 4.5 h • Contraction frequency every 5–10 min • Contraction duration 30–45 s • Contraction intensity mild to palpation **Active phase** (4–7 cm dilation) • Cervical dilation from 4 to 7 cm • Cervical effacement from 40% to 80% • Nullipara, averages 9 h; multigravida averages 6.5 h • Contraction frequency every 2–5 min • Contraction duration 45–60 s • Contraction intensity moderate to palpation **Transition phase** (8–10 cm dilation) • Cervical dilation from 8 to 10 cm • Cervical effacement from 80% to 100% • Nullipara lasts up to 3 h; multigravida, lasts up to 1 h • Contraction frequency every 1–2 min • Contraction duration 60–90 s • Contraction intensity strong by palpation	**Pelvic phase** (period of fetal descent) **Perineal phase** (period of active pushing) • Nullipara, lasts up to 1 h; multigravida, lasts up to 30 min • Contraction frequency every 2–3 min or less • Contraction duration 60–90 s • Contraction intensity strong by palpation • Strong urge to push during the later perineal phase	**Placental separation:** detaching from uterine wall **Placental expulsion:** coming outside the vaginal opening	

body begins to stabilize after the hard work of labour and the loss of the products of conception.

First Stage

During the first stage of labour, the fundamental change underlying the process is progressive dilation of the cervix. Cervical dilation is gauged subjectively by vaginal examination and is expressed in centimetres. The first stage ends when the cervix is dilated to 10 cm in diameter and is large enough to permit the passage of a fetal head of average size. The fetal membranes, or bag of waters, usually rupture during the first stage, but they may have burst earlier or may even remain intact until birth. For the primigravida, the first stage of labour lasts about 12 hours. However, this time can vary widely: for the multiparous woman, it is usually only half that.

During the first stage of labour, women usually perceive the visceral pain of diffuse abdominal cramping and uterine contractions. Pain during the first stage of labour is primarily a result of the dilation of the cervix and lower uterine segment and the distention (stretching) of these structures during contractions. The first stage is divided into three phases: latent or early phase, active phase, and transition phase.

Latent or Early Phase

The latent or early phase gives rise to the familiar signs and symptoms of labour. This phase begins with the start of regular contractions and ends when rapid cervical dilation begins. Cervical effacement occurs during this phase, and the cervix dilates from 0 to 3 cm.

Contractions usually occur every 5 to 10 minutes, last 30 to 45 seconds, and are described as mild by palpation. Effacement of the cervix is from 0% to 40%. Most women are very talkative during this period, perceiving their contractions to be similar to menstrual cramps. Women may remain at home during this phase, contacting their health care professional about the onset of labour.

For the nulliparous woman, the latent phase typically lasts about 6 hours; in the multiparous woman, it lasts about 4.5 hours (Pillitteri, 2010). During this phase, women are apprehensive but excited about the start of labour after their long gestational period.

*T*hink back to the couple who were sent home from the hospital birthing centre. Three days later Kathy awoke with a wet sensation and intense discomfort in her back, spreading around to her abdomen. She decided to go for a walk, but her contractions didn't diminish; instead, they continued to occur every few minutes and grew stronger in intensity. She and Chuck decided to go back to the hospital birthing centre. Was there a difference in the location of Kathy's discomfort this time? What changes will the admission nurse find in Kathy if this is true labour?

Active Phase

Cervical dilation begins to occur more rapidly during the active phase. The cervix usually dilates from 4 to 7 cm, with 40% to 80% effacement taking place. This phase can last about 9 hours for the nulliparous woman and 6.5 hours for the multiparous woman (Varney, Kriebs, & Gegor, 2004). The fetus descends farther in the pelvis. Contractions become more frequent (every 2 to 5 minutes) and increase in duration (45 to 60 seconds). The woman's discomfort intensifies (moderate to strong by palpation). She becomes more intense and inwardly focused, absorbed in the serious work of her labour. She limits interactions with those in the room. If she and her partner have attended childbirth education classes, she will begin to use the relaxation and paced breathing techniques that they learned to cope with the contractions. The typical dilation rate for the nulliparous woman is 1.2 cm/hour; for the multiparous woman, it is 1.5 cm/hour (Cunningham et al., 2010).

Transition Phase

The transition phase is the last phase of the first stage of labour. During this phase, dilation slows, progressing from 8 to 10 cm, with effacement from 80% to 100%. The transition phase is the most difficult and, fortunately, the shortest phase for the woman. During transition, the contractions are stronger (hard by palpation), more painful, and more frequent (every 1 to 2 minutes), and they last longer (60 to 90 seconds). The average rate of fetal descent is 1 cm/hour in nulliparous women and 2 cm/hour in multiparous women. Pressure on the rectum is great and there is a strong desire to contract the abdominal muscles and push.

Other maternal features during the transitional phase include nausea and vomiting, trembling extremities, backache, increased apprehension and irritability, restless movement, increased bloody show from the vagina, inability to relax, diaphoresis, feelings of loss of control, and being overwhelmed (the woman may say, "I can't take it anymore"). This phase should not last longer than 3 hours for nulliparas and 1 hour for multigravidas (Cunningham et al., 2010).

*I*n assessing Kathy, the nurse finds she is 4 cm dilated and 50% effaced with ruptured membranes. In what stage and phase of labour would this assessment finding place Kathy?

Second Stage

The second stage of labour begins with complete cervical dilation (10 cm) and effacement and ends with the birth of the newborn. Although the previous stage of labour primarily involved the thinning and opening of the cervix, this stage involves moving the fetus through

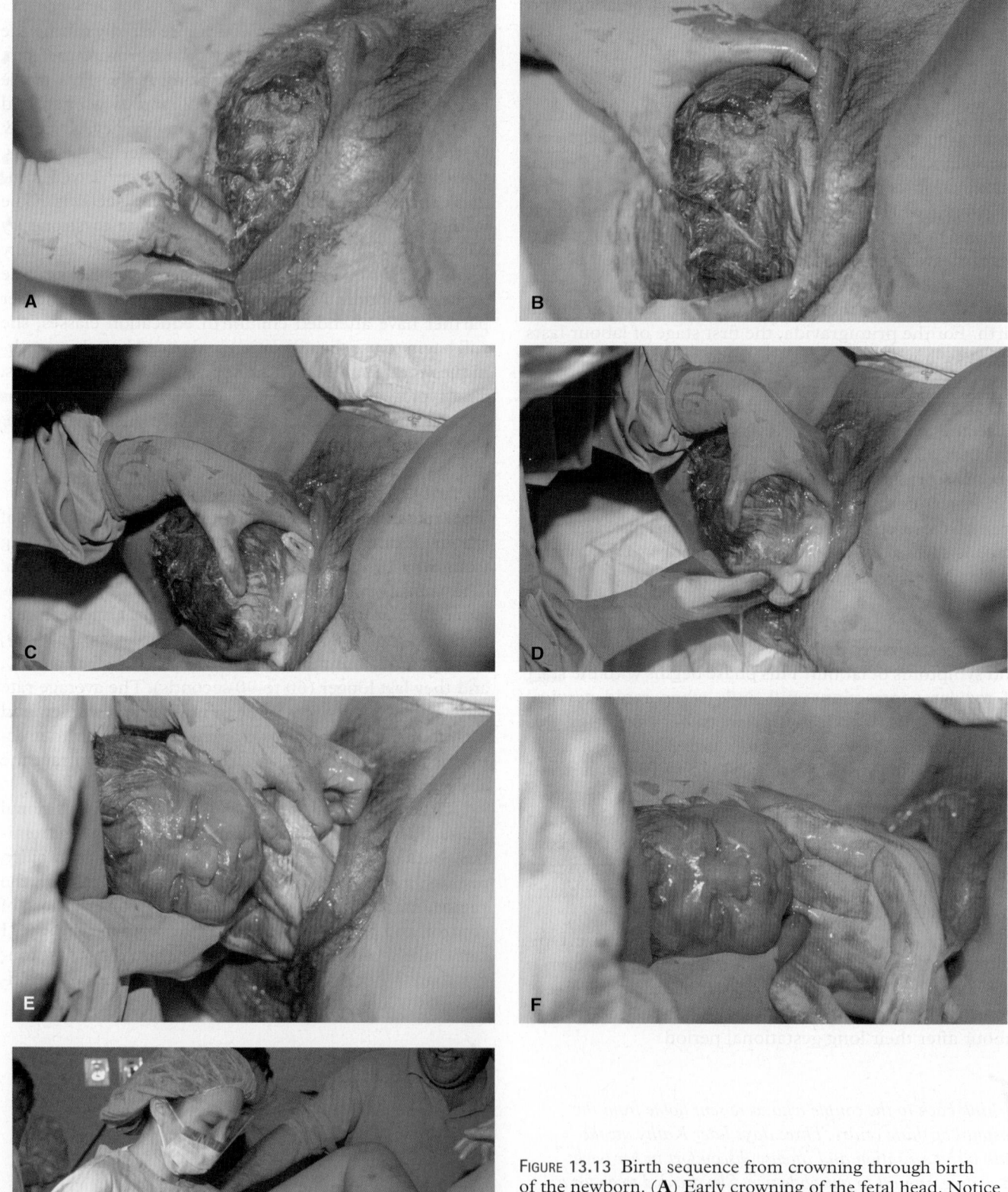

FIGURE 13.13 Birth sequence from crowning through birth of the newborn. (**A**) Early crowning of the fetal head. Notice the bulging of the perineum. (**B**) Late crowning. Notice that the fetal head is appearing face down. This is the normal OA position. (**C**) As the head extends, you can see that the occiput is to the mother's right side—ROA position. (**D**) The cardinal movement of extension. (**E**) The shoulders are born. Notice how the head has turned to line up with the shoulders—the cardinal movement of external rotation. (**F**) The body easily follows the shoulders. (**G**) The newborn is held for the first time! (© B. Proud.)

the birth canal and out of the body. The cardinal movements of labour occur during the early phase of passive descent in the second stage of labour.

Contractions occur every 2 to 3 minutes, last 60 to 90 seconds, and are described as strong by palpation. The average length of the second stage of labour in a nullipara is approximately 1 hour and less than half that time for the multigravida (Fig. 13.13). During this expulsive stage, the mother usually feels more in control and less irritable and agitated. She is focused on the work of pushing. Traditionally, women have been taught to hold their breath to the count of 10, inhale again, push again, and repeat the process several times during a contraction. This sustained, strenuous style of pushing has been shown to lead to hemodynamic changes in the mother and interfere with oxygen exchange between the mother and the fetus. In addition, it is associated with pelvic floor damage: the longer the push, the more damage to the pelvic floor (Cooke, 2010). The newest protocol from Association of Women's Health, Obstetric and Neonatal Nurses (AWHONN) recommends an open-glottis method in which air is released during pushing to prevent the build-up of intrathoracic pressure. Doing so also supports mother's involuntary bearing-down efforts (Roberts, Gonzalez, & Sampselle, 2007).

During the second stage of labour, pushing can either follow the mother's spontaneous urge or be directed by the caregiver. Much debate still exists between spontaneous and directed pushing during the second stage of labour. Although directed pushing is common practice in hospitals, there is evidence to suggest that directed pushing should be avoided. Research seems to support spontaneous pushing—when the woman is allowed to follow her own instincts (Hanson, 2009). Evidence is mounting that the management of the second stage, particularly pushing, is a modifiable risk factor in long-term perinatal outcomes. Valsalva (holding breath) bearing down and supine maternal position are linked to negative maternal–fetal hemodynamics and outcomes. The adoption of a physiologic, woman-directed approach to bearing down is advocated (Cooke, 2010).

Evidence-based practice focuses on a physiologic approach to the second stage of labour. Behaviours demonstrated by labouring women during this time include pushing at the onset of the urge to bear down, using their own pattern and technique of bearing down in response to sensations they experience, using open-glottis bearing down with contractions, pushing with variations in strength and duration, pushing down with progressive intensity, and using multiple positions to increase progress and comfort. This approach is in stark contrast to management by arbitrary time limits and the directed bearing-down efforts seen in practice today (Martin, 2009).

Labouring down (promotion of passive descent) is an alternative strategy for second-stage management in women with epidurals. Using this approach, the fetus descends and is born without coached maternal pushing.

The second stage of labour has two phases (pelvic and perineal) related to the existence and quality of the maternal urge to push and to obstetric conditions related to fetal descent. The early phase of the second stage is called pelvic phase because it is during this phase that the fetal head is negotiating the pelvis, rotating, and advancing in descent. The later phase is called perineal phase because at this point the fetal head is lower in the pelvis and is distending the perineum. The occurrence of a strong urge to push characterizes the later phase of the second stage and has also been called phase of active pushing (Hanson, 2009).

The later perineal phase occurs when the mother feels a tremendous urge to push as the fetal head is lowered and is distending the perineum. The perineum bulges and there is an increase in bloody show. The fetal head becomes apparent at the vaginal opening but disappears between contractions. When the top of the head no longer regresses between contractions, it is said to have crowned. The fetus rotates as it manoeuvres out (Fig. 13.13).

Third Stage

The third stage of labour begins with the birth of the newborn and ends with the separation and birth of the placenta. It consists of two phases: placental separation and placental expulsion.

Placental Separation

After the infant is born, the uterus continues to contract strongly and can now retract, decreasing markedly in size. These contractions cause the placenta to pull away from the uterine wall. The following signs of separation indicate that the placenta is ready to deliver:

- The uterus rises upward.
- The umbilical cord lengthens.
- A sudden trickle of blood is released from the vaginal opening.
- The uterus changes its shape to globular.

Spontaneous birth of the placenta occurs in one of two ways: the fetal side (shiny grey side) presenting first (called Schultz's mechanism or, more commonly, "shiny Schultz's") or the maternal side (red raw side) presenting first (termed Duncan's mechanism or "dirty Duncan").

Placental Expulsion

After separation of the placenta from the uterine wall, continued uterine contractions cause the placenta to be expelled within 2 to 30 minutes unless there is gentle external traction to assist. After the placenta is expelled, the uterus is massaged briefly by the attending physician or midwife until it is firm so that uterine blood vessels constrict, minimizing the possibility of hemorrhage. Normal blood loss is approximately 500 to 600 mL for a vaginal birth and 1,000 mL for a cesarean birth (Cunningham et al., 2010).

If the placenta does not spontaneously deliver, the health care professional assists with its removal by manual extraction. On expulsion, the placenta is inspected for its intactness by the health care professional and the nurse to make sure that all sections are present. If any piece is still attached to the uterine wall, it places the woman at risk for postpartum hemorrhage because it becomes a space-occupying object that interferes with the ability of the uterus to contract fully and effectively.

Fourth Stage

The fourth stage begins with completion of the expulsion of the placenta and membranes and ends with the initial physiologic adjustment and stabilization of the mother (1 to 4 hours after birth). This stage initiates the postpartum period. The mother usually feels a sense of peace and excitement, is wide awake, and is very talkative initially. The attachment process begins with her inspecting her newborn and desiring to cuddle and breastfeed him or her. The mother's fundus should be firm and well contracted. Typically it is located at the midline between the umbilicus and the symphysis, but it then slowly rises to the level of the umbilicus during the first hour after birth (Ward & Hisley, 2009). If the uterus becomes boggy, it is massaged to keep it firm. The lochia (vaginal discharge) is red, mixed with small clots, and of moderate flow. If the woman has had an episiotomy during the second stage of labour, it should be intact, with the edges approximated and clean and no redness or edema present.

The focus during this stage is to monitor the mother closely to prevent hemorrhage, bladder distention, and venous thrombosis. Usually the mother is thirsty and hungry during this time and may request food and drink. Her bladder is hypotonic and thus she has limited sensation to acknowledge a full bladder or to void. Vital signs, the amount and consistency of the vaginal discharge (lochia), and the uterine fundus are usually monitored every 15 minutes for at least 1 hour. The woman will be feeling cramp-like discomfort during this time due to the contracting uterus.

■■■ Key Concepts

- Labour is a complex, multifaceted interaction between the mother and the fetus. Thus, it is difficult to determine exactly why labour begins and what initiates it.
- Before the onset of labour, a pregnant woman's body undergoes several changes in preparation for the birth of the newborn, often leading to characteristic signs and symptoms that suggest that labour is near. These changes include cervical changes, lightening, increased energy level, bloody show, Braxton Hicks contractions, and spontaneous rupture of membranes.
- False labour is a condition seen during the latter weeks of some pregnancies in which irregular uterine contractions are felt, but the cervix is not affected.
- The critical factors in labour and birth are designated as the 10 P's: passageway (birth canal), passenger (fetus and placenta), powers (contractions), psychological response, maternal position, philosophy (low tech, high touch), partners (support caregivers), patience (natural timing), patient preparation (childbirth knowledge base), and pain control (comfort measures).
- The size and shape of a woman's pelvis are determining factors for a vaginal birth. The female pelvis is classified according to four main groups: anthropoid, android, gynecoid, and platypelloid.
- The labour process comprises of a series of rhythmic, involuntary, usually quite uncomfortable uterine muscle contractions that bring about a shortening (effacement) and opening (dilation) of the cervix and a bursting of the fetal membranes. Important parameters of uterine contractions are frequency, duration, and intensity.
- The diameters of the fetal skull vary considerably, with some diameters shortening and others lengthening as the head is moulded during the labour and birth process.
- Pain during labour is a nearly universal experience for childbearing women. Having a strong sense of self and meaningful support from others can often help women manage labour well and reduce their sensation of pain.
- Preparing mentally for childbirth is important for women to enable them to work with the natural forces of labour and not against them.
- As the woman experiences and progresses through childbirth, numerous physiologic responses occur that assist her adaptation to the labouring process.
- Labour is typically divided into four stages that are unequal in length.
- During the first stage of labour, the fundamental change underlying the process is progressive dilation of the cervix. It is further divided into three phases: latent phase, active phase, and transition.
- The second stage of labour begins with complete cervical dilation (10 cm) and effacement and ends with the birth of the infant.
- The third stage of labour is that of separation and birth of the placenta. It consists of two phases: placental separation and placental expulsion.
- The fourth stage of labour begins after the birth of the placenta and membranes and ends with the initial physiologic adjustment and stabilization of the mother (1 to 4 hours).

REFERENCES

Association of Women's Health, Obstetric and Neonatal Nurses. (2007). *AWHONN late preterm infant initiative: What parents of late preterm (near-term) infants need to know.* Retrieved February 10, 2012 from http://www.awhonn.org/awhonn/content.do?name=02_PracticeResources/2C3_Focus_NearTermInfant.htm

Barrett, S. J., & Stark, M. A. (2010). Factors associated with labour support behaviors of nurses. *Journal of Perinatal Education, 19*(1), 12–18.

Chalmers, B., Kaczorowski, J., Darling, E., Heaman, M., Fell, D. B., O'Brien, B., & Lee, L. (2010). Cesarean and vaginal birth in Canadian women: A comparison of experiences. *Birth, 37*(1), 44–49.

Chalmers, B., Kaczorowski, J., Levitt, C., Dzakpasu, S., O'Brien, B., Lee, L., Boscoe, M., & Young, D. (2009). Use of routine interventions in vaginal labour and birth: Findings from the Maternity Experiences Survey. *Birth, 36*(1), 13–25.

Cooke, A. (2010). When will we change practice and stop directing pushing in labour? *British Journal of Midwifery, 18*(2), 76–81.

Cunningham, F. G., Leveno, K. J., Bloom, S. L., Hauth, J. C., Rouse, D. J., & Spong, C. Y. (2010). *Williams obstetrics* (23rd ed.). New York: McGraw-Hill.

Davidson, M. R., London, M. L., Ladewig, P. A. W. (2008). *Olds' maternal–newborn nursing and women's health across the lifespan.* Upper Saddle River, NJ: Pearson/Prentice Hall.

Delaney, M., & Roggensack, A. (2008). Guidelines for the management of pregnancy at 41 + 0 to 42 + 0 weeks. *Journal of Obstetrics and Gynaecology Canada, 214*, 800–810.

Dunne, C., Da Silva, O., Schmidt, G., & Natale, R. (2009). outcomes of elective labour induction and elective caesarean section in low-risk pregnancies between 37 and 41 weeks' gestation. *Journal of Obstetrics and Gynaecology Canada, 31*(12), 1124–1130.

Hanson, L. (2009). Second-stage labour care: Challenges in spontaneous bearing down. *Journal of Perinatal and Neonatal Nursing, 23*(1), 31–39.

Hanson, S., Hunter, L. P., Bormann, J. R., & Sobo, E. J. (2009). Paternal fears of childbirth: A literature review. *Journal of Perinatal Education, 18*(4), 12–20.

Hodnett, E. D., Gates, S., Hofmeyr, G. J., & Sakala, C. (2011). Continuous support for women during childbirth. *Cochrane Database of Systematic Reviews, 2*, CD003766. doi: 10.1002/14651858. CD003766.pub3

International Childbirth Education Association. (n.d.). *Mission and philosophy.* Retrieved February 10, 2012 from www.icea.org/content/mission

Jimenez, V., Klein, M., Hivon, M., & Mason, C. (2010). A mirage of change: Family-centered maternity care in practice. *Birth, 37*(2), 160–167.

Kenner, C., & Lott, J. W. (2007). *Comprehensive neonatal care: An interdisciplinary approach* (4th ed.). St. Louis, MO: Saunders Elsevier.

Leap, N., Sandall, J., Buckland, S., & Huber, U. (2010). Journey to confidence: Women's experiences of pain in labour and relational continuity of care. *Journal of Midwifery and Women's Health, 55*(3), 234–242.

Martin, C. J. H. (2009). Effects of Valsalva manoeuvre on maternal and fetal wellbeing. *British Journal of Midwifery, 17*(5), 279–285.

Martin, E. J., & Kennedy, B. B. (2009a). Maternal and fetal response to labor. In B. B. Kennedy, D. J. Ruth, & E. J. Martin (Eds.), *Intrapartum management modules* (pp. 17–45). Philadelphia: Wolters Kluwer.

Martin, E. J., & Kennedy, B. B. (2009b). Overview of labour. In B. B. Kennedy, D. J. Ruth, & E. J. Martin (Eds.), *Intrapartum management modules.* Philadelphia: Wolters Kluwer.

McDonald, G. (2010). Diagnosing the latent phase of labour: Use of the partogram. *British Journal of Midwifery, 18*(10), 630–637.

Murray, M. L., & Huelsmann, G. M. (2009). *Labor and delivery nursing: A guide to evidence-based practice.* New York: Springer.

Nettina, S. M. (2010). *Lippincott manual of nursing practice.* Philadelphia: Lippincott.

Pillitteri, A. (2010). *Maternal & child health nursing: Care of the childbearing & childrearing family* (6th ed.). Philadelphia: Wolters Kluwer.

Public Health Agency of Canada. (2008). *Canadian perinatal health report, 2008 edition.* Retrieved February 10, 2012 from www.publichealth.gc.ca/cphr/

Roberts, J. M., Gonzalez, C. B., & Sampselle, C. (2007). Why do supportive birth attendants become directive of maternal bearing-down efforts in second-stage labor? *Journal of Midwifery and Women's Health, 52*(2), 134–141.

Romano, A. M., & Lothian, J. A. (2008). Promoting, protecting, and supporting normal birth: A look at the evidence. *Journal of Obstetric, Gynecologic, & Neonatal Nursing, 37*(1), 94–105.

Society of Obstetricians and Gynaecologists of Canada. (2008). *Rising C-section rates add risks during childbirth and place excess strain on the healthcare system, warn Canadian obstetricians.* Retrieved February 10, 2012 from www.sogc.org/media/pdf/advisories/ACM_June2008_C-Sections_e.pdf

Varney, H., Kriebs, J. M., & Gegor, C. L. (2004). *Varney's midwifery* (4th. ed.). Boston: Jones and Bartlett.

Ward, S., & Hisley, S. (2009). *Maternal-child nursing care.* Philadelphia: F.A. Davis.

Wilson, B. L., Effkren, J., & Butler, R. J. (2010). Relationship between cesarean section and labor induction. *Journal of Nursing Scholarship, 42*(2), 130–138.

Zwelling, E. (2010). Overcoming the challenges: Maternal movement. *The American Journal of Maternal/Child Nursing, 35*(2), 72–78.

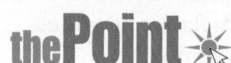

the Point ✷ For additional learning materials, including Internet Resources, visit
http://thePoint.lww.com/Chow1e.

CHAPTER WORKSHEET

MULTIPLE CHOICE QUESTIONS

1. When determining the frequency of contractions, the nurse would measure which of the following?

    a. Start of one contraction to the start of the next contraction

    b. Beginning of one contraction to the end of the same contraction

    c. Peak of one contraction to the peak of the next contraction

    d. End of one contraction to the beginning of the next contraction

2. Which fetal lie is most conducive to a spontaneous vaginal birth?

    a. Transverse

    b. Longitudinal

    c. Perpendicular

    d. Oblique

3. Which of the following observations would suggest that placental separation is occurring?

    a. Uterus stops contracting altogether.

    b. Umbilical cord pulsations stop.

    c. Uterine shape changes to globular.

    d. Maternal blood pressure drops.

4. As the nurse is explaining the difference between true versus false labour to her childbirth class, she states that the major difference between them is:

    a. Discomfort level is greater with false labour.

    b. Progressive cervical changes occur in true labour.

    c. There is a feeling of nausea with false labour.

    d. There is more fetal movement with true labour.

5. The shortest but most intense phase of labour is the:

    a. Latent phase

    b. Active phase

    c. Transition phase

    d. Placental expulsion phase

6. A labouring woman is admitted to the labour and birth suite at 6 cm dilation. She would be in which phase of the first stage of labour?

    a. Latent

    b. Active

    c. Transition

    d. Early

7. Which assessment would indicate that a women is in true labour?

    a. Membranes are ruptured and fluid is clear

    b. Presenting part is engaged and not floating

    c. Cervix is 4 cm dilated, 90% effaced

    d. Contractions last 30 seconds, every 5 to 10 minutes

CRITICAL THINKING EXERCISES

1. Cindy, a 20-year-old primigravida, calls the birthing centre where you work as a nurse and reports she thinks she is in labour because she feels labour pains. Her due date is this week. The midwives have been giving her prenatal care throughout this pregnancy.

    a. What additional information do you need to respond appropriately?

    b. What suggestions/recommendations would you make to her?

    c. What instructions need to be given to guide her decision making?

    d. What other premonitory signs of labour might the nurse ask about?

    e. What manifestations would be found if Cindy is experiencing true labour?

2. You are assigned to lead a community education class for women in their third trimester of pregnancy to prepare them for their upcoming birth. Prepare an outline of topics that should be addressed.

STUDY ACTIVITIES

1. During clinical postconference, share with the other nursing students how the critical forces of labour influenced the length of labour and the birthing process for a labouring woman assigned to you.

2. The cardinal movements of labour include which of the following? Select all that apply.

   a. Extension and rotation

   b. Descent and engagement

   c. Presentation and position

   d. Attitude and lie

   e. Flexion and expulsion

3. Interview a woman on the mother–baby unit who has given birth within the past few hours. Ask her to describe her experience and examine psychological factors that may have influenced her labouring process.

4. On the following illustration, identify the parameters of uterine contractions by marking an "X" where the nurse would measure the duration of the contraction.

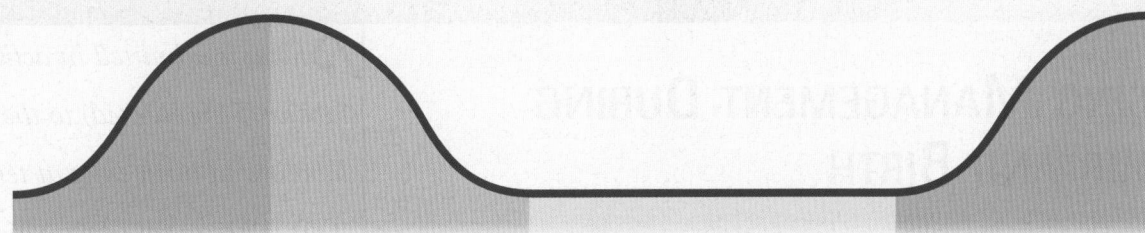

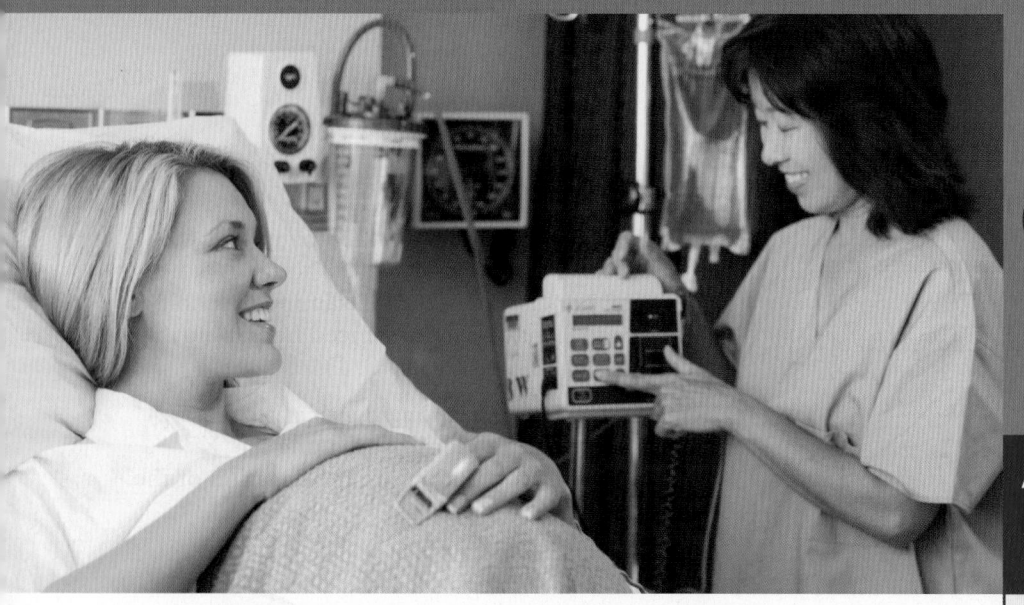

CHAPTER14

Adapted by Cyndee L. MacPhee

NURSING MANAGEMENT DURING LABOUR AND BIRTH

KEY TERMS

accelerations
artefact
baseline fetal heart rate
baseline variability
crowning

deceleration
electronic fetal monitoring
episiotomy
Leopold's manoeuvres

neuraxial analgesia/
  anesthesia
periodic baseline changes

LEARNING OBJECTIVES

Upon completion of the chapter, the learner will be able to:

1. Define the key terms related to the labour and birth process.
2. Discuss the measures used to evaluate maternal status during labour and birth.
3. Explain the advantages and disadvantages of external and internal fetal monitoring, including the appropriate use for each.
4. Choose appropriate nursing interventions to address abnormal fetal heart rate patterns.
5. Outline the nurse's role in fetal assessment.
6. Explain the various comfort-promotion and pain-relief strategies used during labour and birth.
7. Summarize the assessment data collected on admission to the perinatal unit.
8. Discuss the ongoing assessments involved in each stage of labour and birth.
9. Explain the nurse's role throughout the labour and birth process.

Sheila is admitted in active labour (5 cm dilated) to the labour and birth suite at term. This is her second pregnancy and she is prepared to avoid pain medications this time so she can be more involved with the birthing process. She has been using modified-paced breathing with success thus far.

Wow

Wise nurses are not always silent, but they know when to be during the miracle of birth.

The labouring and birthing process is a life-changing event for many women. Nurses need to be respectful, available, encouraging, supportive, and professional in dealing with all women. A recent study by Bryanton, Gagnon, Johnston, et al. (2008) demonstrated that nurses can promote a positive birth experience by responding to the needs of the labouring woman through appropriate nursing interventions.

The health of mothers and their infants is of critical importance, both as a reflection of the current health status of a large segment of our population and as a predictor of the health of the next generation. The Society of Obstetricians and Gynaecologists of Canada (SOGC) established a National Birthing Initiative in 2008 with the overall goal of ensuring that all Canadian women have access to quality maternity care that is centred around women and family. The framework for this initiative arose from the Multidisciplinary Collaborative Primary Maternity Care Project (MCP²), which produced national guidelines in 2006 for collaborative models of care in Canada (SOGC, 2008a).

This chapter provides information about nursing management during labour and birth. First, the essentials for in-depth assessment of maternal and fetal status during labour and birth are discussed. This is followed by a thorough description of the major methods of promoting comfort and providing pain management. The chapter concludes by putting all the information together with a discussion of the nursing care specific to each stage of labour, including the necessary data to be obtained with the admission assessment, methods to evaluate labour progress during the first stage of labour, and key nursing measures that focus on maternal and fetal assessments and pain relief for all stages of labour.

Maternal Assessment During Labour and Birth

During labour and birth, various techniques are used to assess maternal status. These techniques provide an ongoing source of data to determine the woman's response and her progress in labour. Assess maternal vital signs, including temperature, blood pressure, pulse, respiration, and pain, which are primary components of the physical examination and ongoing assessment. Also review the prenatal record to identify risk factors that may contribute to a decrease in uteroplacental circulation during labour. If there is no vaginal bleeding on admission, a vaginal examination is performed to assess cervical dilation, after which it is monitored periodically as necessary to identify progress. Evaluate maternal pain and the effectiveness of pain-management strategies at regular intervals during labour and birth.

Vaginal Examination

Although not all nurses perform vaginal examinations on labouring women in all practice settings, most nurses working in community hospitals do so because physicians are not routinely present in labour and birth suites. Nurses care for women and attend almost every birth in Canada. It is not uncommon for the nurse to be the only health care provider present, in the absence of a physician or midwife. Thus appropriate educational preparation for nurses in these settings is imperative as new models of interprofessional collaborative care come into play (SOGC, 2008a).

> ▶ **Take** NOTE!
>
> *A vaginal examination is an assessment skill that takes time and experience to develop; only by doing it frequently in clinical practice can the practitioner's skill level improve.*

The purpose of performing a vaginal examination is to assess the amount of cervical dilation, the percentage of cervical effacement, and the fetal membrane status and to gather information on presentation, position, station, degree of fetal head flexion, and presence of fetal skull swelling or molding (Fig. 14.1). Prepare the woman by informing her about the procedure, what information will be obtained from it, how she can assist with the procedure, how it will be performed, and who will be performing it.

The woman is typically on her back during the vaginal examination. The vaginal examination is performed gently, with concern for the woman's comfort. If it is the

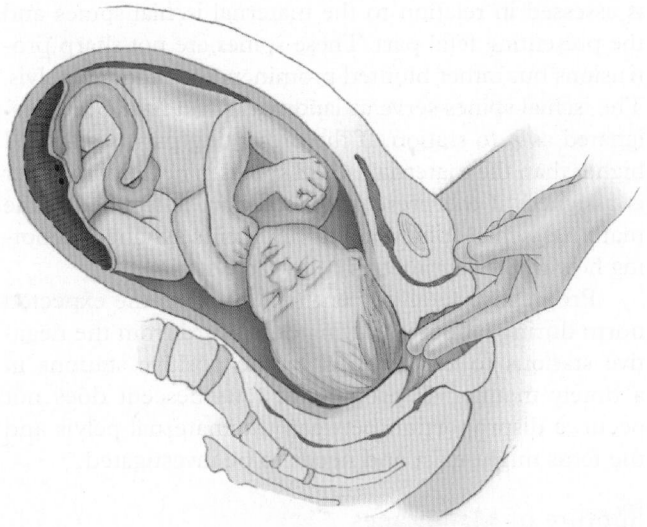

FIGURE 14.1 Vaginal examination to determine cervical dilation and effacement.

initial vaginal examination to check for membrane status, water is used as a lubricant. If the membranes have already ruptured, an antiseptic solution is used to prevent an ascending infection. After donning sterile gloves, the examiner inserts his or her index and middle fingers into the vaginal introitus. Next, the cervix is palpated to assess dilation, effacement, and position (e.g., posterior or anterior). If the cervix is open to any degree, the presenting fetal part, fetal position, station, and presence of molding can be assessed. In addition, the membranes can be evaluated and described as intact, bulging, or ruptured.

At the conclusion of the vaginal examination, the findings are discussed with the woman and her partner to bring them up to date about labour progress. In addition, the findings are documented either electronically or in writing and reported to the primary health care professional in charge of the case.

Cervical Dilation and Effacement

The amount of cervical dilation and the degree of cervical effacement are key areas assessed during the vaginal examination as the cervix is palpated with the gloved index finger. Although this finding is somewhat subjective, experienced examiners typically come up with similar findings. The width of the cervical opening determines dilation, and the length of the cervix assesses effacement. The information yielded by this examination serves as a basis for determining which stage of labour the woman is in and what her ongoing care should be.

Fetal Descent and Presenting Part

In addition to cervical dilation and effacement findings, the vaginal examination can also determine fetal descent (station) and presenting part. During the vaginal examination, the gloved index finger is used to palpate the fetal skull (if vertex presentation) through the opened cervix or the buttocks in the case of a breech presentation. Station is assessed in relation to the maternal ischial spines and the presenting fetal part. These spines are not sharp protrusions but rather blunted prominences at the midpelvis. The ischial spines serve as landmarks and have been designated as zero station. If the presenting part is palpated higher than the maternal ischial spines, a negative number is assigned; if the presenting fetal part is felt below the maternal ischial spines, a plus number is assigned, denoting how many centimetres below zero station.

Progressive fetal descent (−5 to +4) is the expected norm during labour—moving downward from the negative stations to zero station to the positive stations in a timely manner. If progressive fetal descent does not occur, a disproportion between the maternal pelvis and the fetus might exist and needs to be investigated.

Rupture of Membranes

The integrity of the membranes can be determined during the vaginal examination. Typically, if intact, the membranes will be felt as a soft bulge that is more prominent during a contraction. If the membranes have ruptured, the woman may have reported a sudden gush of fluid. Membrane rupture also may occur as a slow trickle of fluid. When membranes rupture, the priority focus should be on assessing fetal heart rate (FHR) first to identify a deceleration, which might indicate cord compression secondary to cord prolapse. If the membranes are ruptured when the woman comes to the hospital, it is important to ascertain when it occurred. Prolonged ruptured membranes increase the risk of infection as a result of ascending vaginal organisms for both mother and fetus. Signs of intrauterine infection to be alert for include maternal fever, fetal and maternal tachycardia, foul odour of vaginal discharge, and an increase in white blood cell count.

To confirm that membranes have ruptured, a sample of fluid is taken from the vagina and tested with nitrazine paper to determine the fluid's pH. Vaginal fluid is acidic, whereas amniotic fluid is alkaline and turns nitrazine paper blue. Sometimes, however, false-positive results may occur, especially in women experiencing a large amount of bloody show, because blood is alkaline. The membranes are most likely intact if the nitrazine test tape remains yellow to olive green, suggesting an acidic pH from 5 to 6. The membranes are probably ruptured if the nitrazine test tape turns a blue-green to deep blue, suggesting an alkaline pH from 6.5 to 7.5 (Evans, Evans, Brown, et al., 2010; Ladewig, London, & Davidson, 2009; Moldenhauer, 2008).

If the nitrazine test is inconclusive, an additional test, called the fern test, can be used to confirm rupture of membranes. With this test, a sample of fluid is obtained, applied to a microscope slide, and allowed to dry. Using a microscope, the slide is examined for a characteristic fern pattern that indicates the presence of amniotic fluid.

Assessing Uterine Contractions

The primary power of labour is uterine contractions, which are involuntary. Uterine contractions increase intrauterine pressure, causing tension on the cervix. This tension leads to cervical dilation and thinning, which in turn eventually forces the fetus through the birth canal. Normal uterine contractions have a contraction (systole) and a relaxation (diastole) phase. The contraction resembles a wave, moving downward to the cervix and upward to the fundus of the uterus. Each contraction starts with a building up (increment), gradually reaching an acme (peak intensity), and then a letting down (decrement). Each contraction is followed by an interval of rest, which ends when the next contraction begins. At the acme (peak) of the contraction, the entire uterus is contracting, with the greatest intensity in the fundal area. The relaxation phase follows and occurs simultaneously throughout the uterus.

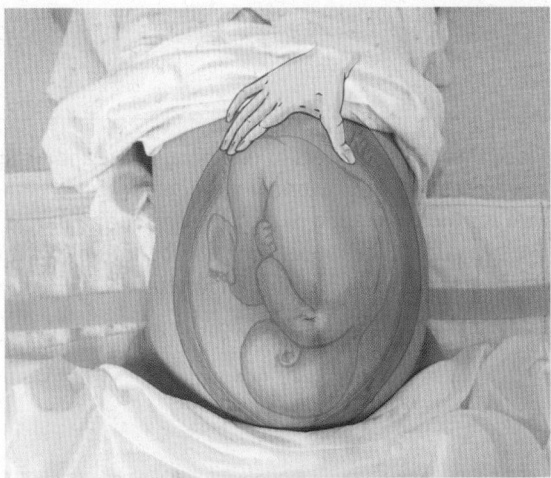

FIGURE 14.2 Nurse palpating the woman's fundus during a contraction.

Uterine contractions during labour are monitored by palpation, external fetal monitoring (tocodynamometer), or internal monitoring (intrauterine pressure catheter [IUPC]). Assessment of the contractions includes frequency, duration, intensity, and uterine resting tone. The type of information obtained is determined by the method selected (Kennedy, Ruth, & Martin, 2009). (See Chapter 13 for a more detailed discussion.) To palpate the fundus for contraction intensity, place the pads of your fingers on the fundus and describe how it feels: like the tip of the nose (mild), like the chin (moderate), or like the forehead (strong). Palpation of intensity is a subjective judgment of the indentability of the uterine wall; a descriptive term is assigned (mild, moderate, or strong) (Fig. 14.2).

▶ **Take** NOTE!

Frequent clinical experience is needed to gain accuracy in assessing the intensity of uterine contractions.

The second method used to assess the intensity of uterine contractions is electronic fetal monitoring (EFM). EFM can be done either externally or internally, although internal monitoring provides a more accurate measurement of intensity than external monitoring (Matsuo, Scanlon, Atlas, et al., 2008). When using the tocodynamometer, contraction intensity must also be assessed by palpation (Kennedy et al., 2009).

For women at risk for preterm birth, home uterine activity monitoring can be used to screen for prelabour uterine contractility so that escalating contractility can be identified, allowing earlier intervention to prevent preterm birth. The home uterine activity monitor consists of a pressure sensor attached to a belt that is held against the abdomen and a recording/storage device that is carried on a belt or hung from the shoulder. Uterine activity is typically recorded by the woman for 1 hour twice daily, while she is performing routine activities. The stored data are transmitted via telephone to a perinatal nurse, and a receiving device prints out the data. The woman is contacted if there are any problems.

There is no consensus in the literature to show that home monitoring improves outcomes for high-risk mothers and fetuses (Currell, Urquhart, Harlow, et al., 2009). Iams, Romero, Culhane, et al. (2008) reviewed the literature to identify what primary, secondary, or tertiary approaches work best to reduce the morbidity and mortality associated with preterm birth from early contractions. They found that even when high-risk women met daily with health care professionals, their rates of preterm birth did not change. The most successful efforts identified thus far have been from active tertiary treatment to stop contractions with, for example, the use of tocolytics. The SOGC (2007) recommends that the frequency of antenatal fetal testing should be individualized to reflect the risk factor(s) present.

Performing Leopold's Manoeuvres

Leopold's manoeuvres are a method for determining the presentation, position, and lie of the fetus through the use of four specific steps (Pillitteri, 2010). This method involves inspection and palpation of the maternal abdomen as a screening assessment for malpresentation. A longitudinal lie is expected, and the presentation can be cephalic, breech, or shoulder. Each manoeuvre answers a question:

- What fetal part (head or buttocks) is located in the fundus (top of the uterus)?
- On which maternal side is the fetal back located? (Fetal heart tones are best auscultated through the back of the fetus.)
- What is the presenting part?
- Is the fetal head flexed and engaged in the pelvis?

Leopold's manoeuvres are described in Nursing Procedure 14.1.

Fetal Assessment During Labour and Birth

A fetal assessment identifies well-being or signs that indicate compromise. The character of the amniotic fluid is assessed, but the fetal assessment focuses primarily on determining the FHR pattern. Fetal scalp sampling, fetal pulse oximetry (FPO), and fetal stimulation are additional assessments performed as necessary in the case of questionable FHR patterns.

Nursing Procedure 14.1

PERFORMING LEOPOLD'S MANOEUVRES

Purpose: To Determine Fetal Presentation, Position, and Lie

1. Place the woman in the supine position and stand beside her.
2. Perform the first manoeuvre to determine presentation.
   a. Facing the woman's head, place both hands on the abdomen to determine fetal position in the uterine fundus.
   b. Feel for the buttocks, which will feel soft and irregular (indicates vertex presentation); feel for the head, which will feel hard, smooth, and round (indicates a breech presentation).

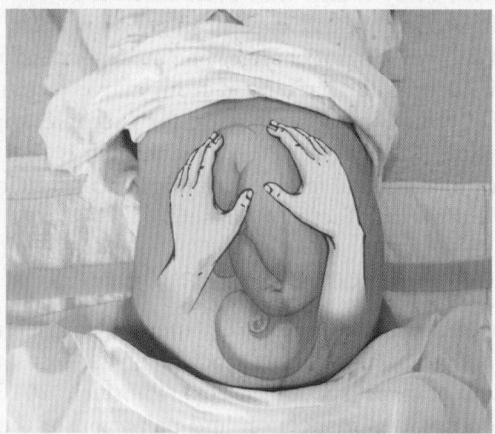

3. Complete the second manoeuvre to determine position.
   a. While still facing the woman, move hands down the lateral sides of the abdomen to palpate on which side the back is located (feels hard and smooth).
   b. Continue to palpate to determine on which side the limbs are located (irregular nodules with kicking and movement).

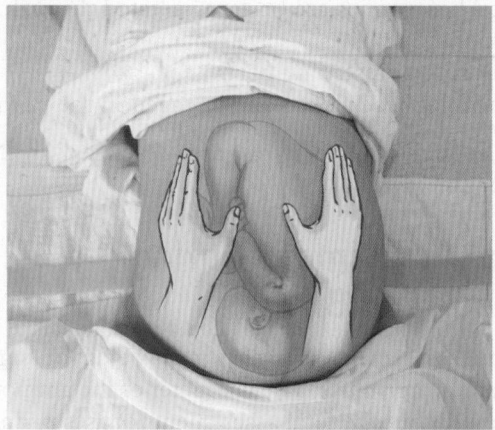

4. Perform the third manoeuvre to confirm presentation.
   a. Move hands down the sides of the abdomen to grasp the lower uterine segment and palpate the area just above the symphysis pubis.

   b. Place thumb and fingers of one hand apart and grasp the presenting part by bringing fingers together.
   c. Feel for the presenting part. If the presenting part is the head, it will be round, firm, and ballottable; if it is the buttocks, it will feel soft and irregular.

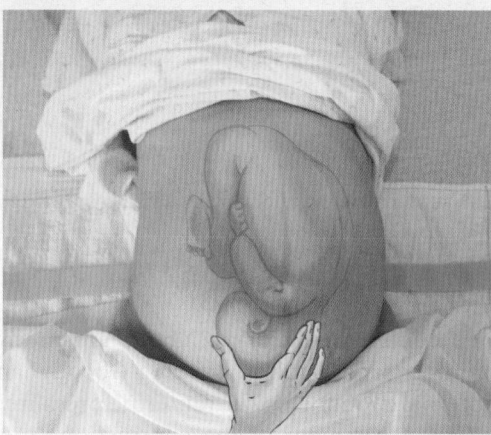

5. Perform the fourth manoeuvre to determine attitude.
   a. Turn to face the client's feet and use the tips of the first three fingers of each hand to palpate the abdomen.
   b. Move fingers toward each other while applying downward pressure in the direction of the symphysis pubis. If you palpate a hard area on the side opposite the fetal back, the fetus is in flexion, because you have palpated the chin. If the hard area is on the same side as the back, the fetus is in extension, because the area palpated is the occiput.

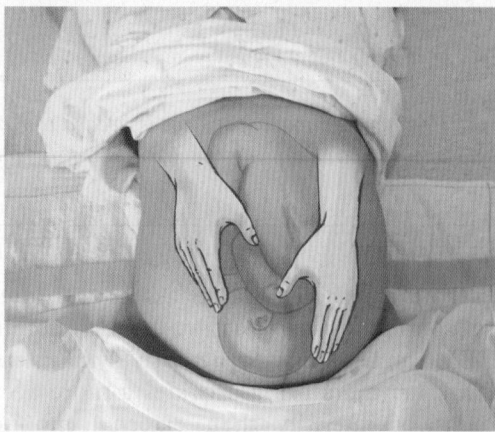

   Also, note how your hands move. If the hands move together easily, the fetal head is not descended into the woman's pelvic inlet. If the hands do not move together and stop because of resistance, the fetal head is engaged into the woman's pelvic inlet (Lowdermilk et al., 2010).

Analysis of Amniotic Fluid

Amniotic fluid should be clear when the membranes rupture, either spontaneously or artificially through an amniotomy (a disposable plastic hook [Amnihook] is used to perforate the amniotic sac). Cloudy or foul-smelling amniotic fluid indicates infection. Green fluid may indicate that the fetus has passed meconium secondary to transient hypoxia; however, it is considered a normal occurrence if the fetus is in a breech presentation. If it is determined that meconium-stained amniotic fluid is due to fetal hypoxia, the maternity and pediatric teams work together to prevent meconium aspiration syndrome. This would necessitate suctioning after the head is born before the infant takes a breath and perhaps direct tracheal suctioning after birth if the Apgar score is low. In some cases, an amnioinfusion (introduction of warmed, sterile normal saline or Ringer's lactate solution into the uterus) is used to dilute moderate to heavy meconium released in utero to assist in preventing meconium aspiration syndrome.

Analysis of the FHR

Analysis of the FHR is one of the primary evaluation tools used to determine fetal oxygen status indirectly. FHR assessment can be done intermittently using a fetoscope (a modified stethoscope attached to a headpiece) or a Doppler (ultrasound) device, or continuously with an electronic fetal monitor applied externally or internally.

Intermittent FHR Monitoring

FHR monitoring through intermittent auscultation involves the use of a fetoscope or a hand-held Doppler device that uses ultrasound waves that bounce off the fetal heart, producing echoes or clicks that reflect the rate of the fetal heart (Fig. 14.3). The SOGC (2007) recommends the use of intermittent auscultation as the preferred method of intrapartum fetal surveillance in low-risk women in the active phase of labour.

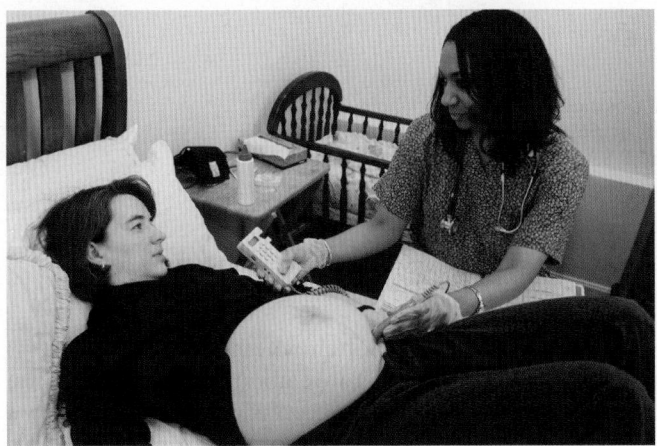

FIGURE 14.3 Auscultating fetal heart rate.

> ▶ **Take** NOTE!
>
> *Intermittent auscultation is less invasive, inexpensive, easy to use, and does not restrict movement (Lowdermilk, Perry, & Cashion, 2010; SOGC, 2007), whether in hospital or community-based settings. Studies show little difference in fetal or neonatal outcomes when intermittent auscultation is used as an alternative to EFM (Lavender, Hart, & Smyth, 2008; Steer, 2008.)*

Intermittent FHR monitoring allows the woman to be mobile in the first stage of labour. She is free to move around and change position at will since she is not attached to a stationary electronic fetal monitor. However, intermittent monitoring does not provide a continuous FHR recording and does not document how the fetus responds to the stress of labour (unless listening is done during the contraction). The best way to assess fetal well-being would be to start listening to the FHR at the end of the contraction (not after one) so that late decelerations can be detected. However, the pressure of the device during a contraction is uncomfortable and can distract the woman from using her paced-breathing patterns.

Intermittent FHR auscultation can be used to detect FHR baseline and rhythm and changes from baseline. However, it cannot be used to assess variability and transient changes as no visual record is available to assess FHR patterns (Tucker, Miller, & Miller, 2009). During intermittent auscultation to establish a baseline, the FHR is assessed for a full minute after a contraction. From then on, unless there is a problem, listening for 30 seconds and multiplying the value by two is sufficient. The FHR should be assessed regularly to ensure that it is in the same range after the contraction as it was in the previous assessments. If not, assess possible causes for the change (SOGC, 2007). If the woman experiences a change in condition during labour, auscultation assessments should be more frequent. The SOGC (2007) also recommends checking the FHR after any invasive procedure, rupture of membranes, vaginal examinations, and administration of medications. The FHR is heard most clearly at the fetal back. In a cephalic presentation, the FHR is best heard in the lower quadrant of the maternal abdomen. In a breech presentation, it is heard at or above the level of the maternal umbilicus (Fig. 14.4). As labour progresses, the FHR location will change accordingly as the fetus descends into the maternal pelvis for the birthing process. To ensure that the maternal heart rate is not confused with the FHR, palpate the client's radial pulse simultaneously while the FHR is being auscultated through the abdomen.

The procedure for using a fetoscope or Doppler device to assess FHR is similar (see Nursing Procedure 12.1

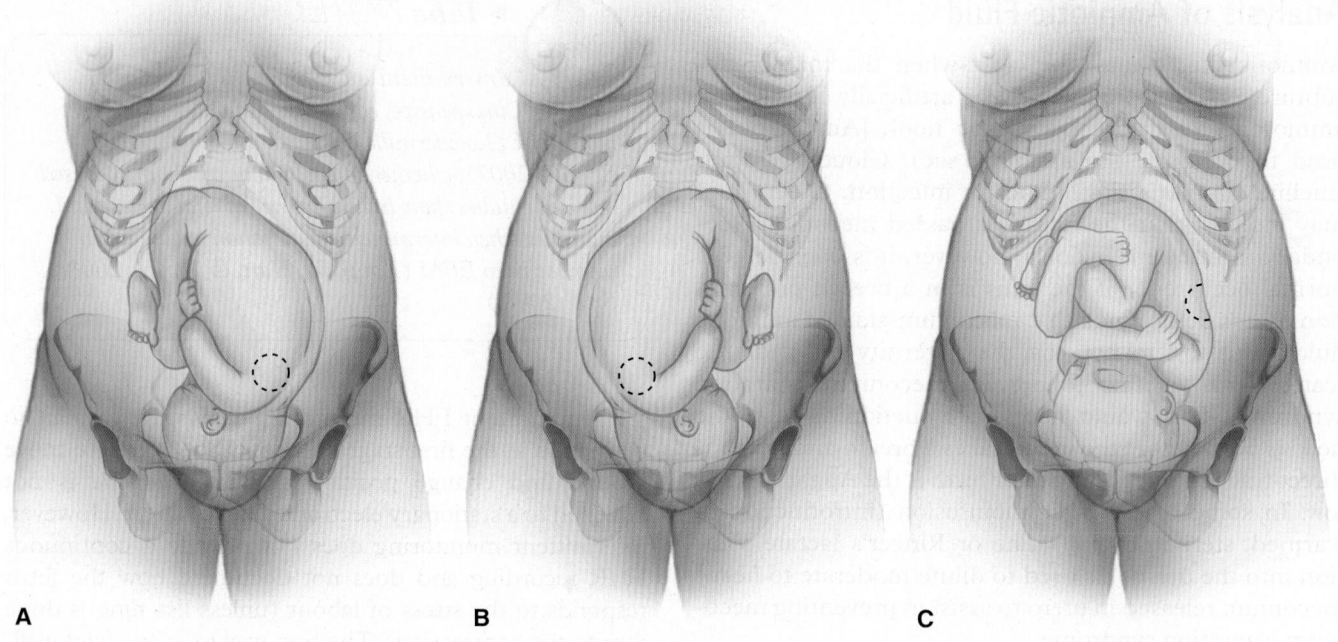

A   B   C

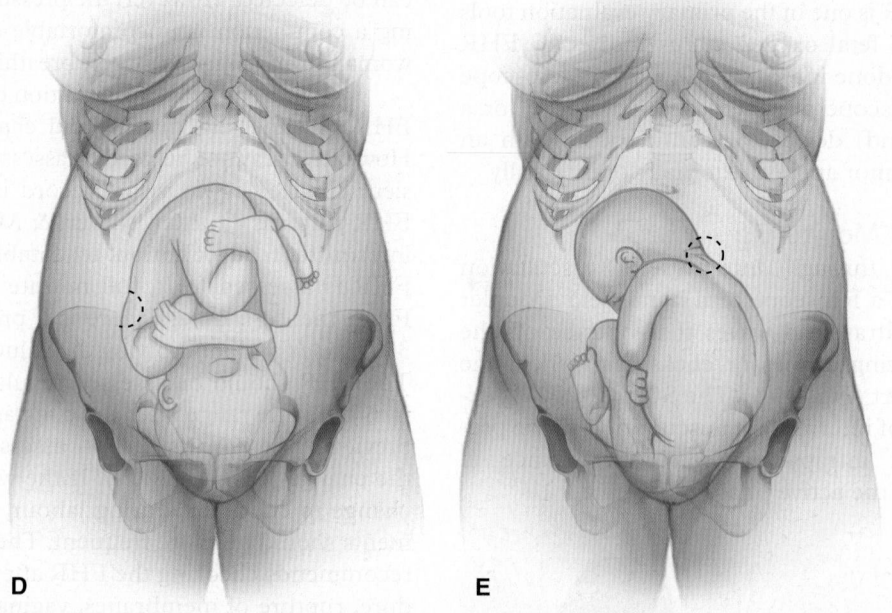

D   E

FIGURE 14.4 Locations for auscultating fetal heart rate based on fetal position. (**A**) Left occiput anterior (LOA). (**B**) Right occiput anterior (ROA). (**C**) Left occiput posterior (LOP). (**D**) Right occiput posterior (ROP). (**E**) Left sacral anterior (LSA).

in Chapter 12). The main difference is that a small amount of water-soluble gel is applied to the woman's abdomen or ultrasound device before auscultation with the Doppler device to promote sound wave transmission. This gel is not needed when a fetoscope is used. Usually the FHR is best heard in the woman's lower abdominal quadrants; if it is not found quickly, it may help to locate the fetal back by performing Leopold's manoeuvres.

Although the intermittent method of FHR assessment allows the client to move about during labour, the information obtained fails to provide a complete picture of the well-being of the fetus moment to moment. This leads to the question of what the fetal status is during the times that are not assessed. For women who are considered at low risk for complications, this period of non-assessment is not a problem. However, for the undiagnosed high-risk woman, it might prove ominous.

The SOGC is the leading national obstetric professional organization in Canada and provides guidelines for evidence-based obstetric care, including guidelines for assessment during labour and delivery. Comprising gynaecologists, obstetricians, family physicians, nurses, midwives, and allied health professionals, the SOGC works collaboratively with several other national maternity health care providers: the College of Family Physicians of Canada (CFP), the Canadian Association of Midwives (CAM), the Canadian Association of Perinatal and Women's Health Nurses (CAPWHN), and the Society of Rural Physicians of Canada (SRPC), all of whom help inform the clinical practice guidelines and support the initiatives of the SOGC. The SOGC cautions that the information it provides should not dictate an exclusive course of treatment/procedure and should not substitute for the advice of a physician.

Intermittent auscultation is the recommended fetal surveillance method during labour for healthy women without identified risk factors for adverse perinatal outcome (SOGC, 2007, 2008b). The following guidelines are recommended for assessing FHR by intermittent auscultation:

- Admission fetal heart tracings are not recommended for healthy women at term in labour in the absence of risk factors for adverse perinatal outcome, as there is no evident benefit.
- Intensive fetal surveillance by intermittent auscultation or EFM requires the continuous presence of nursing or midwifery staff.
  - Assess FHR on admission and every hour in the latent phase of the first stage of labour.
  - Assess FHR every 15 to 30 minutes during the active phase of the first stage of labour.
  - Assess FHR every 5 minutes during the active second stage of labour.

The SOGC recommendation of having the continuous presence of a nurse or nurse midwife suggests that adequate staffing is essential with intermittent FHR monitoring to ensure optimal outcomes for mother and fetus. The overall goal of these guidelines is to contribute to the best possible fetal outcomes while maintaining the lowest possible rates of intervention (SOGC, 2007).

Continuous Electronic Fetal Monitoring (Cardiotocography)

Electronic fetal monitoring is a term used interchangeably with **cardiotocography (CTG)**, which uses an external monitor to record changes in the FHR with an aim to identify babies who may be short of oxygen

(hypoxic) (Alfirevic, Devane, & Gyte, 2008; SOGC, 2007). The monitor produces a sound with each heartbeat and provides a visual graphic record of the FHR pattern. CTG is considered by some to be a more precise term than EFM because it also monitors the mother's contractions. In addition, other forms of fetal monitoring are also considered electronic, such as electrocardiography and FPO (Alfirevic et al., 2008). The purpose of FHR monitoring is to identify fetal hypoxemia and acidemia in order to allow early intervention in an effort to prevent fetal morbidity and mortality (ICSI, 2011).

In a recent review of randomized controlled trials, Alfirevic et al. (2008) found insufficient evidence to identify specific situations in which continuous EFM might result in better outcomes when compared with intermittent auscultation. However, continuous EFM is associated with an increase in cesarean section and instrumental vaginal births. Nevertheless, SOGC guidelines (2007) state that women with risk factors for adverse perinatal outcomes should receive EFM. However, with an identified normal tracing, maternal stability, and no increase in the rate of oxytocin infusions, mothers can be allowed up to ambulate for periods of up to 30 minutes.

Current methods of continuous EFM were introduced in Canada and the United States during the 1960s specifically for use in clients whose babies were considered to be at high risk for hypoxia. However, the use of these methods gradually increased and they eventually came to be used in non–high risk cases as well. This increased use is now the centre of controversy as continuous EFM is known to be associated with the steadily increasing rates of cesarean births in Canada and abroad (Low, 2009; Menacker & Martin, 2009; Public Health Agency of Canada [PHAC], 2008; SOGC, 2008c). Additional studies also suggest that the use of intrapartum EFM increases the number of preterm and surgical births with no significant effect on reducing the incidence of intrapartum death or long-term neurologic injury (Alfirevic et al., 2008; ICSI, 2011). With EFM, there is a continuous record of the FHR: no gaps exist, as they do with intermittent auscultation. The concept of hearing and evaluating every beat of the fetus's heart to allow for early intervention seems logical. On the downside, however, continuous monitoring can limit maternal movement and encourages the woman to lie in the supine position, which reduces placental perfusion and potentially contributes to problems. Despite the criticisms, EFM remains an accurate method for determining fetal health status by providing moment-to-moment information about FHR status. However, FHR readings are dynamic and transient and require frequent reassessment and interpretation (Macones, Hankins, Spong, et al., 2008).

Various groups within the medical community have criticized the use of continuous fetal monitoring for all pregnant clients, whether high risk or low risk. Concerns about the efficiency and safety of routine EFM in labour have led expert panels in Canada to recommend that such monitoring be limited to high-risk pregnancies (SOGC, 2008d). Continuous EFM can be performed externally (indirectly), with the equipment attached to the maternal abdominal wall, or internally (directly), with the equipment attached to the fetus. Both methods provide a continuous printout of the FHR, but they differ in their specificity. The efficacy of EFM depends on the accurate interpretation of the tracings, not necessarily which method (external versus internal) is used.

Continuous External Monitoring

In external or indirect monitoring, two ultrasound transducers, each of which is attached to a belt, are applied around the woman's abdomen. They are similar to the hand-held Doppler device. One transducer, which is pressure sensitive, is called a tocodynamometer. It is placed over the uterine fundus in the area of greatest contractility to monitor and record uterine contractions (Evans et al., 2010). The other ultrasound transducer records the baseline FHR, long-term variability, accelerations, and decelerations. It is positioned on the maternal abdomen in the midline between the umbilicus and the symphysis pubis. The diaphragm of the ultrasound transducer is moved to either side of the abdomen to obtain a stronger sound and is then attached to the second elastic belt. This transducer converts the fetal heart movements into beeping sounds and records them on graph paper (Fig. 14.5).

Good continuous data are provided on the FHR. External monitoring can be used while the membranes are still intact and the cervix is not yet dilated. It is non-invasive and can detect relative changes in abdominal pressure between uterine resting tone and contractions. External monitoring also measures the approximate duration and frequency of contractions, providing a permanent record of FHR (Tucker et al., 2009).

However, external monitoring can restrict the mother's movements. It also cannot detect short-term

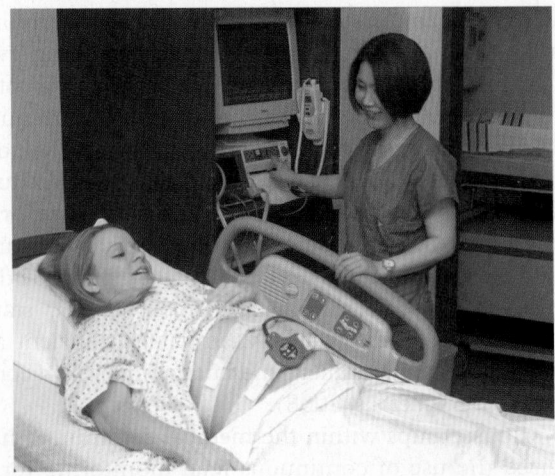

FIGURE 14.5 Continuous external electronic fetal monitoring device applied to the woman in labour.

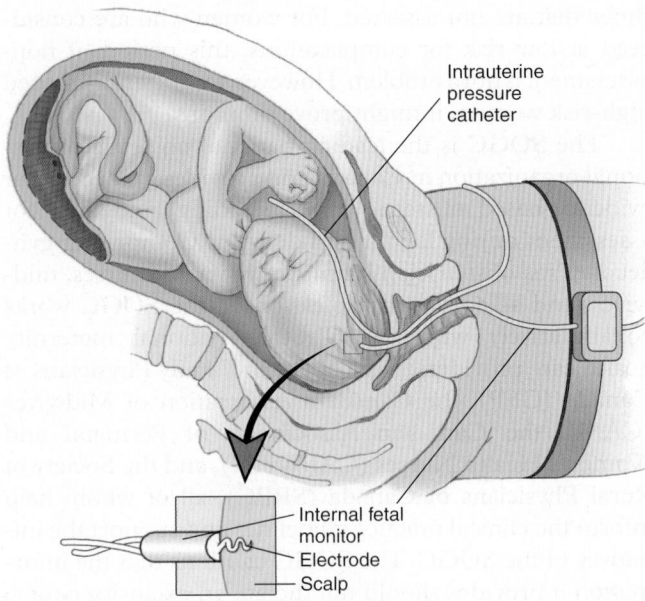

FIGURE 14.6 Continuous internal electronic fetal monitoring.

variability. Signal disruptions can occur due to maternal obesity, fetal malpresentation, and fetal movement, as well as by artefact. **Artefact** describes irregular variations or the absence of FHR on the fetal monitor record that result from mechanical limitations of the monitor or electrical interference. For instance, the monitor may pick up transmissions from CB radios used by truck drivers on nearby roads and translate them into a signal. Additionally, gaps in the monitor strip can occur periodically without explanation.

Continuous Internal Monitoring

Continuous internal monitoring is usually indicated for women or fetuses considered to be at high risk. Possible conditions might include multiple gestation, decreased fetal movement, abnormal FHR on auscultation, intrauterine growth restriction (IUGR), maternal fever, preeclampsia, dysfunctional labour, preterm birth, or medical conditions such as diabetes or hypertension. It involves the placement of a spiral electrode on the fetal presenting part, usually the head, to assess FHR and a pressure transducer placed internally within the uterus to record uterine contractions (Fig. 14.6). The fetal spiral electrode is considered the most accurate method of detecting fetal heart characteristics and patterns because it involves receiving a signal directly from the fetus (Menihan & Kopel, 2008). Trained labour and birth nurses can place the spiral electrode on the fetal head when the membranes rupture in some health care facilities, but they do not place the IUPC in the uterus. Internal monitoring does not have to include both an IUPC and a scalp electrode. A fetal scalp electrode can be used to monitor the fetal heartbeat without monitoring the maternal intrauterine pressure.

Both the FHR and the duration and interval of uterine contractions are recorded on the graph paper. This method permits evaluation of baseline heart rate and changes in rate and pattern.

Four specific criteria must be met for this type of monitoring to be used:

- Ruptured membranes
- Cervical dilation of at least 2 cm
- Presenting fetal part low enough to identify correctly and allow placement of the scalp electrode
- Skilled practitioner available to insert spiral electrode (Ladewig et al., 2009)

Compared with external monitoring, continuous internal monitoring can accurately detect both short-term (moment-to-moment) changes and long-term variability (fluctuations within the baseline) as well as FHR dysrhythmias. In addition, maternal position changes and movement do not interfere with the quality of the tracing.

Determining FHR Patterns

It is imperative for all obstetric nurses, midwives, and physicians who deliver newborns to achieve competence in FHR monitoring and analysis (Macones et al., 2008; SOGC, 2007). FHR patterns provide information on the current acid–base status of the fetus and, although they may fluctuate from time to time, require prompt ongoing evaluation (Macones et al., 2008; SOGC, 2007). Assessment parameters of the FHR are classified as baseline rate, baseline variability, and periodic changes in the rate (accelerations and decelerations). To effectively care for women during labour and birth, the nurse must accurately interpret FHR tracings to determine if the pattern is normal (indicating fetal well-being), atypical or indeterminate (necessitating continued surveillance and re-evaluation), or abnormal (indicating the need for immediate intervention) (Macones et al., 2008; SOGC, 2007). The National Institute of Child Health & Human Development (NICHD) and the Institute for Clinical Systems Improvement (ICSI), both United States-based organizations, recently recommended a three-tier system for the categorization of FHR patterns that is very similar to the Canadian guidelines (ICSI, 2011; Macones et al., 2008).

Table 14.1 summarizes these patterns.

Baseline FHR

Baseline fetal heart rate refers to the average FHR that occurs during a 10-minute segment that excludes periodic or episodic rate changes (such as tachycardia or bradycardia) and periods of marked variability. It is assessed when the woman has no contractions. The normal baseline FHR ranges between 110 and 160 beats/minute (Alfirevic et al., 2008) and can be obtained by auscultation, ultrasound, Doppler, or an internal fetal spiral electrode.

TABLE 14.1 INTERPRETING FHR PATTERNS

Normal FHR signs	• Normal baseline (110–160 beats/min) • Moderate bradycardia (100–110 beats/min); good variability • Good beat-to-beat variability and fetal accelerations
Atypical signs	• Fetal tachycardia (>160 beats/min) • Moderate bradycardia (100–110 beats/min); lost variability • Absent beat-to-beat variability • Marked bradycardia (90–100 beats/min) • Moderate variable decelerations
Abnormal signs	• Fetal tachycardia with loss of variability • Prolonged marked bradycardia (<90 beats/min) • Severe variable decelerations (<70 beats/min) • Persistent late decelerations

Sources: Institute for Clinical Systems Improvement. (2011). *Health care guideline: Management of labor* (4th ed.). Retrieved February 22, 2012 from http://www.icsi.org/labor/labor__management_of__full_version__2.html; Macones, G. A., Hankins, G. D. V., Spong, C. Y., Hauth, J., & Moore, T. (2008). The 2008 National Institute of Child Health and Human Development workshop report on electronic fetal monitoring: Update on definitions, interpretation, and research guidelines. *Journal of Obstetric, Gynecologic, & Neonatal Nursing, 37*(5), 510–515; & Society of Obstetricians and Gynecologists of Canada. (2007). *SOGC clinical practice guidelines: Fetal health surveillance: Antepartum and intrapartum consensus guideline. Journal of Obstetrics and Gynecology in Canada, 29*(9), S3–S56. Retrieved February 22, 2012 from http://www.sogc.org/guidelines/documents/gui197CPG0709.pdf.

Fetal bradycardia occurs when the FHR is below 110 beats/minute and lasts 10 minutes or longer (Tucker et al., 2009). It can be the initial response of a healthy fetus to asphyxia. Causes of fetal bradycardia might include fetal hypoxia, prolonged maternal hypoglycemia, fetal acidosis, viral infections, administration of drugs to the mother, maternal hypothermia, maternal hypotension, prolonged umbilical cord compression, and fetal congenital heart block (SOGC, 2007; Tucker et al., 2009). Bradycardia may be benign if it is an isolated event, but it is considered an ominous sign when accompanied by a decrease in long-term variability and late decelerations.

Fetal tachycardia is a baseline FHR greater than 160 beats/minute that lasts for 10 minutes or longer (SOGC, 2007; Tucker et al., 2009). It can represent an early fetal compensatory response to asphyxia and can be maternal or fetal in nature (Tucker et al., 2009). Maternal causes such as fever, medication, and dehydration are amenable to interventions. Other causes include fetal hypoxia/acidosis, maternal anxiety, thyroid disease, fetal heart failure, and fetal arrhythmias (Tucker et al., 2009). Fetal tachycardia is considered an ominous sign if it is accompanied by a decrease in variability and late decelerations (Lowdermilk et al., 2010).

Baseline Variability

Baseline variability is defined as normal physiologic variations in the time intervals that elapse between each fetal heartbeat observed along the baseline in the absence of contractions, decelerations, and accelerations (Menihan & Kopel, 2008). It represents the interplay between the parasympathetic and sympathetic nervous systems producing moment-to-moment changes in the FHR. Because variability is in essence the combined result of autonomic nervous system branch function, its presence implies that both branches are working and receiving adequate oxygen (Tucker et al., 2009). Thus, variability is one of the most important characteristics of the FHR.

Variability is described in three ways: minimal or absent, moderate, and marked. Minimal or absent variability typically is caused by uteroplacental insufficiency, cord compression, maternal hypotension, uterine hyperstimulation (tachysystole), abruptio placentae, or a fetal dysrhythmia. Interventions to improve uteroplacental blood flow and perfusion through the umbilical cord include lateral positioning of the mother, increasing the IV fluid rate to improve maternal circulation, administering oxygen at 8 to 10 L/min by mask, considering internal fetal monitoring, documenting findings, and reporting to the health care provider. Preparation for a surgical birth may be necessary if no changes occur after attempting the interventions.

Moderate variability indicates that the autonomic and central nervous systems of the fetus are well developed and well oxygenated. It is considered a good sign of fetal well-being and correlates with the absence of significant metabolic acidosis (Fig. 14.7).

Marked variability occurs when there are more than 25 beats of fluctuation in the FHR baseline. Causes of this include cord prolapse or compression, maternal hypotension, uterine hyperstimulation (tachysystole), and abruptio placentae. Interventions include determining the cause, if possible, lateral positioning, increasing the IV fluid rate, administering oxygen at 8 to 10 L/min by mask, discontinuing oxytocin infusion, observing for changes in tracing, considering internal fetal monitoring,

communicating an abnormal pattern to the health care provider, and preparing for a surgical birth if no change in pattern is noted (Menihan & Kopel, 2008).

FHR variability is an important clinical indicator that is predictive of fetal acid–base balance and cerebral tissue perfusion (Tucker et al., 2009). As the central nervous system is desensitized by hypoxia and acidosis, FHR decreases until a smooth baseline pattern appears. Loss of variability may be associated with a poor outcome. Some causes of decreased variability include fetal hypoxia/acidosis, drugs that depress the central nervous system, congenital abnormalities, fetal sleep, prematurity, and fetal tachycardia (Tucker et al., 2009).

> ▶ *Take* NOTE!
>
> *External EFM cannot assess short-term variability. Therefore, if external monitoring shows a baseline that is smoothing out, use of an internal spiral electrode should be considered to gain a more accurate picture of the fetal health status.*

Periodic Baseline Changes

Periodic baseline changes are temporary, recurrent changes made in response to a stimulus such as a contraction. The FHR can demonstrate patterns of acceleration or deceleration in response to most stimuli. Fetal **accelerations** are transitory increases in the FHR above the baseline associated with sympathetic nervous stimulation. They are visually apparent, with elevations of FHR of more than 15 beats/minute above the baseline, and their duration is less than 2 minutes (Macones et al., 2008). They are generally considered transient and require no interventions. Accelerations denote fetal movement and fetal well-being and are the basis for non-stress testing.

A **deceleration** is a transient fall in FHR caused by stimulation of the parasympathetic nervous system. Decelerations are described by their shape and association with a uterine contraction. They are classified as early, late, variable, and prolonged (Fig. 14.8).

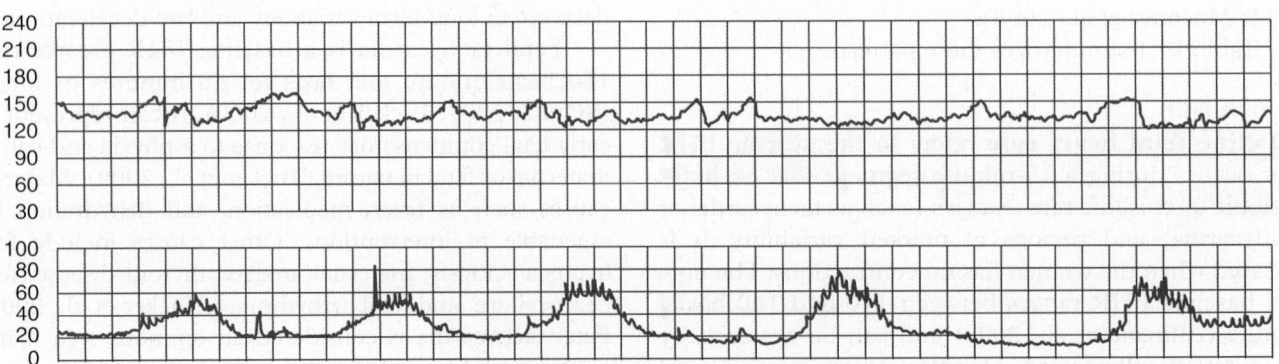

FIGURE 14.7 Long-term variability (average or moderate).

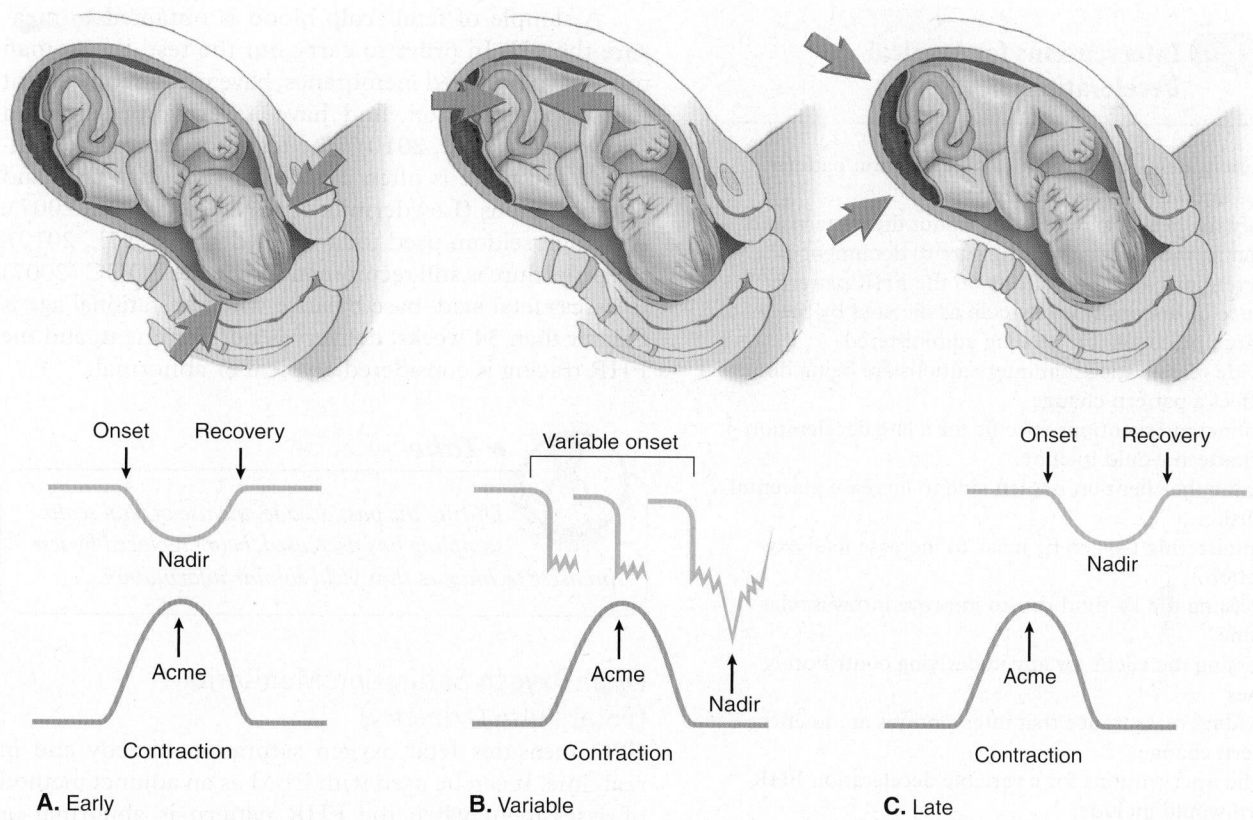

FIGURE 14.8 Decelerations. (**A**) Early. (**B**) Variable. (**C**) Late.

Early decelerations are characterized by a gradual decrease in the FHR in which the nadir (lowest point) occurs at the peak of the contraction. They rarely decrease more than 30 to 40 beats/minute below the baseline. Typically, the onset, nadir, and recovery of the deceleration occur at the same time as the onset, peak, and recovery of the contraction. They are most often seen during the active stage of any normal labour, during pushing, crowning, or vacuum extraction. They are thought to be a result of fetal head compression that results in a reflex vagal response with a resultant slowing of the FHR during uterine contractions. Early decelerations are not indicative of fetal distress and do not require intervention.

Late decelerations are transitory decreases in FHR that occur after a contraction begins. The FHR does not return to baseline levels until well after the contraction has ended. In most cases, the onset, nadir, and recovery of the deceleration occur after the beginning, peak, and ending of the contraction, respectively (Macones et al., 2008). Late decelerations are associated with uteroplacental insufficiency, causing hypoxemia from inadequate placental perfusion during contractions. Conditions that may decrease uteroplacental perfusion with resultant decelerations include maternal hypotension, gestational hypertension, placental aging secondary to diabetes and postmaturity, uterine hyperstimulation (tachysystole) via

oxytocin infusion, maternal smoking, anemia, and cardiac disease. Repetitive late decelerations and late decelerations with decreasing baseline variability are ominous signs (Tucker et al., 2009). Box 14.1 highlights interventions for decelerations. When decelerations are repetitive, the fetal scalp pH should be obtained if clinically appropriate and prepare for delivery (SOGC, 2007).

Variable decelerations present as visually apparent abrupt decreases in FHR below baseline and have an unpredictable shape on the FHR baseline, possibly demonstrating no consistent relationship with uterine contractions. Variable decelerations are usually associated with cord compression. These are usually uncomplicated variable decelerations. However, they can also be complicated and abnormal when the FHR decreases to less than 70 beats/minute, persists at that level for at least 60 seconds, and is repetitive (SOGC, 2007). The pattern of variable deceleration consistently related to the contractions with a slow return to FHR baseline may also be indicative of hypoxemia.

Prolonged decelerations are gradual or abrupt FHR declines of at least 15 beats/minute that last longer than 2 minutes but less than 10 minutes (Macones et al., 2008). The rate usually drops to less than 90 beats/minute. These decelerations are caused by some disruption to the oxygen supply. Many factors are associated with this pattern, including prolonged cord compression,

BOX 14.1 Interventions for Atypical Decelerations

If a patient develops an atypical deceleration pattern such as late or variable decelerations:
- Notify the health care provider about the pattern and obtain further orders, making sure to document all interventions and their effects on the FHR pattern.
- Reduce or discontinue oxytocin as dictated by the facility's protocol, if it is being administered.
- Provide reassurance that interventions are being done to effect a pattern change.

Additional interventions specific for a late deceleration FHR pattern would include:
- Turning the client on her left side to increase placental perfusion
- Administering oxygen by mask to increase fetal oxygenation
- Increasing the IV fluid rate to improve intravascular volume
- Assessing the client for any underlying contributing causes
- Providing reassurance that interventions are to effect pattern change

Specific interventions for a variable deceleration FHR pattern would include:
- Changing the client's position to relieve compression on the cord
- Providing reassurance that interventions are to effect pattern change
- Giving oxygen and IV fluids as ordered

abruptio placentae, cord prolapse, and supine maternal position (Lowdermilk et al., 2010). Prolonged decelerations can be remedied by identifying the underlying cause and correcting it.

Other Fetal Assessment Methods

In situations suggesting the possibility of fetal compromise, such as inconclusive or atypical FHR patterns, further ancillary testing such as fetal scalp sampling, FPO, and fetal stimulation may be used to validate the FHR findings and assist in planning interventions.

Fetal Scalp Blood Sampling

Fetal scalp blood sampling was developed as a means of measuring fetal distress in conjunction with EFM to make critical decisions about the management of labour and to prevent unnecessary operative interventions resulting from the use of EFM alone. Abnormal FHR patterns may not necessarily indicate fetal hypoxia or acidosis. Therefore, assessing fetal acid–base status through fetal scalp blood sampling may help to prevent unnecessary surgical intervention.

A sample of fetal scalp blood is obtained to measure the pH. In order to carry out the test, the woman must have ruptured membranes, have met a requirement for cervical dilation, and have a vertex presentation (Lowdermik et al., 2010). The test procedure is complicated, and there is often a need for repetitive tests and interpretations (Lowdermilk et al., 2010; SOGC, 2007). Although seldom used today (Lowdermilk et al., 2010), the procedure is still recommended by the SOGC (2007) to assess fetal acid–base balance when gestational age is greater than 34 weeks, delivery is not imminent, and the FHR tracing is considered atypical or abnormal.

> ▶ *Take* NOTE!
>
> *During the past decade, the use of fetal scalp sampling has decreased, being replaced by less invasive techniques that yield similar information.*

Fetal Oxygen Saturation Monitoring (Fetal Pulse Oximetry)

FPO measures fetal oxygen saturation directly and in real time. It can be used with EFM as an adjunct method of assessment when the FHR pattern is abnormal or atypical. A soft sensor is introduced through the dilated cervix and placed on the cheek, forehead, or temple of the fetus. It is held in place by the uterine wall. The sensor then is attached to a special adapter on the fetal monitor that provides a real-time recording that is displayed on the uterine activity panel of the tracing. FPO is a noninvasive and safe method for assessing fetal oxygenation. However, recent research shows that FPO has not proven to be clinically useful in determining fetal status (American College of Obstetricians and Gynecologists [ACOG], 2009; East, Chan, Colditz, et al., 2007) or reducing overall cesarean section rates. Based on earlier evidence, the SOGC (2007) does not recommend routine use of FPO during intrapartum care.

Fetal Stimulation

An indirect method used to evaluate fetal oxygenation and acid–base balance to identify fetal hypoxia is fetal scalp stimulation and vibroacoustic stimulation. If the fetus does not have adequate oxygen reserves, carbon dioxide builds up, leading to acidemia and hypoxemia. These metabolic states are reflected in abnormal FHR patterns as well as fetal inactivity. Fetal stimulation is performed to promote fetal movement with the hope that FHR accelerations will accompany the movement.

Fetal movement can be stimulated with a vibroacoustic stimulator (artificial larynx) applied to the woman's lower abdomen and turned on for a few seconds to produce sound and vibration or by tactile stimulation via pelvic examination and stimulation of the fetal scalp with the gloved fingers. A well-oxygenated fetus will respond when stimulated (tactile or by noise) by moving in conjunction with an acceleration of 15 beats/minute above the baseline heart rate that lasts at least 15 seconds. This FHR acceleration reflects a pH of more than 7 and a fetus with an intact central nervous system. However, the absence of a response does not necessarily indicate fetal compromise (SOGC, 2007; Tucker et al., 2009). The SOGC recommends the use of digital fetal scalp stimulation in response to atypical electronic fetal heart tracings.

Promoting Comfort and Pain Management During Labour

Pain during labour is a universal experience, although the intensity of the pain may vary. Although labour and childbirth are viewed as natural processes, both can produce significant pain and discomfort. The acute pain of labour is primarily physical in nature, has a fixed duration, and can often be relieved by non-pharmacologic methods (Evans et al., 2010).

Pain is uniquely personal, and the pain of labour can be influenced by personality traits, cultural expectations, anxiety, access to social and emotional support, social status, environment, and past experiences (Wolf, 2009). Therefore, techniques used to manage labour pain vary according to geography and culture. At the beginning of regular-onset uterine contractions, the appearance of bloody show, or membrane rupture, for example, Orthodox Jewish women observe the law of *niddah*. At this point, the husband will no longer touch his wife but may remain in the room providing spiritual support. He may or may not look at his wife during the birth (Berkowitz, 2008). Korean women do not express pain outwardly for fear of shaming the family, and silence is valued by the Chinese (Ladewig et al., (2009). Canada has a substantial Aboriginal population for whom childbirth is a sacred event that traditionally involved the family and community as a whole (National Aboriginal Health Organization, 2008). Many Aboriginals today not only need to leave their communities to experience the birth alone but also they are limited in the number of support people who are allowed to attend the birth. This can create anxiety for the mother, potentially increasing pain, lengthening the labour, and contributing to complications.

Culturally diverse childbearing families present to the labour and birth suites with the same needs and desires of all families. Regardless of the expression of pain, it is imperative for nurses to explore with labouring mothers their perception of the pain and how best to support them. Give them and their families the same respect and sense of welcome shown to all families. Make sure they have a high-quality birth experience by upholding their religious, ethnic, and cultural values and integrating them into care. Today, women have many safe non-pharmacologic and pharmacologic choices for the management of pain during labour and birth, which may be used separately or in combination with one another.

Nurses are in an ideal position to provide childbearing women with balanced, clear, concise information about effective non-pharmacologic and pharmacologic measures to relieve pain. It is important for nurses to be knowledgeable about the most recent scientific research on labour pain-relief modalities, to make sure that accurate and unbiased information about effective pain-relief measures is available to labouring women, to be sure that the woman determines what is an acceptable labour pain level for her, and to allow the woman the choice of pain-relief method.

Non-pharmacologic Measures

Non-pharmacologic measures may include continuous labour support, hydrotherapy, ambulation and position changes, acupuncture and acupressure, attention focusing and imagery, therapeutic touch and massage, breathing techniques, and effleurage. Most of these methods are based on the "gate control" theory of pain, which proposes that local physical stimulation can interfere with pain stimuli by closing a hypothetical gate in the spinal cord, thus blocking pain signals from reaching the brain (Lowdermilk et al., 2010). It has long been a standard of care for labour nurses to first provide or encourage a variety of non-pharmacologic measures before moving to the pharmacologic interventions.

Reynolds (2010) reviewed the role of pain, stress, and loss of maternal control on the development of progressive fetal metabolic acidosis. Unmanaged increased stress leads to the release of cortisol and catecholamines, prolonging labour and impairing fetal blood flow. In addition, maternal hyperventilation can lead to fetal respiratory alkalosis and metabolic acidosis. This supports the need for the labouring mother to gain control through one or a combination of non-pharmacologic measures that are usually simple, safe, and inexpensive. Many of these measures are taught in childbirth classes and should be practiced for best results with the partner/coach before the onset of labour. The nurse's role is to provide support and encouragement for the woman and her partner during this time. Although women can't consciously direct the labour contractions, they can control how they respond to the contractions, thereby enhancing their feelings of control.

Continuous Labour Support

Continuous labour support involves offering a sustained presence to the labouring woman by providing emotional support, comfort measures, advocacy, information and advice, and support for the partner. A woman's family, a midwife, a nurse, a doula, or anyone else close to the woman can provide this continuous presence (Adams & Bianchi, 2008; Leap, Sandall, Buckland, et al., 2010;

Simkin, 2008). A support person can assist the woman to ambulate, reposition herself, and use breathing techniques. A support person can also aid with the use of acupressure, massage, music therapy, or therapeutic touch. During the natural course of childbirth, a labouring woman's functional ability is limited secondary to pain, and she often has trouble making decisions. The support person can help her make decisions based on his or her knowledge of the woman's birth plan and personal wishes.

A recent *Cochrane* review concluded that women who received continuous labour support were more likely to give birth spontaneously (vaginally), had shorter labours, were less likely to use pain medications, and expressed more satisfaction with the birth experience (Hodnett, Gates, Hofmeyr, et al., 2009a). The SOGC (2007) and Association of Women's Health, Obstetric, and Neonatal Nurses (2011) both stress the importance of having continuous labour support from a registered nurse or other trained personnel for the labouring woman and her family.

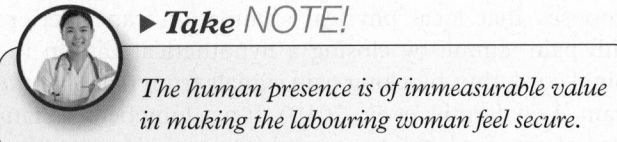

▶ *Take* NOTE!

The human presence is of immeasurable value in making the labouring woman feel secure.

Hydrotherapy

Hydrotherapy is a non-pharmacologic measure in which the woman immerses herself in warm water for relaxation and relief of discomfort. The warm water releases endorphins and provides better circulation and oxygenation (Lowdermilk et al., 2010). Contractions are usually less painful in warm water because the warmth and buoyancy of the water have a relaxing effect.

Hydrotherapy may shorten the length of labour and enhance coping by encouraging an upright position and increased movements (Stark, Rudell, & Haus, 2008).

Evidence indicates that water immersion in the first stage of labour reduces pain and the use of epidural/spinal analgesia (Cluett & Burns, 2009). There is no evidence of increased adverse outcomes for the fetus, neonate, or woman from labouring in water. Immersion during the second stage of labour needs further investigation (Cluett & Burns, 2009), but at present, there is no clear evidence to support or not support a woman's decision to give birth in water. The Royal Australian and New Zealand College of Obstetricians and Gynaecologists (2008) cautions against the consequences of unintended water birth, while the SOGC has not issued any position statement to date on hydrotherapy.

A wide range of hydrotherapy options is available, from ordinary bathtubs to whirlpool baths and showers, combined with low lighting and music. Many hospitals provide showers and whirlpool baths for labouring women for pain relief. However, hydrotherapy is more commonly practiced in birthing centres managed by midwives.

Hydrotherapy is an effective pain-management option for many women. Women who are experiencing a healthy pregnancy can be offered this option.

Ambulation and Position Changes

Ambulation and position changes during labour are another extremely useful comfort measure. The medical profession traditionally has influenced women to assume a recumbent position throughout labour but without evidence to demonstrate its appropriateness (Lawrence, Lewis, Hofmeyr, et al., 2009). Changing position frequently (every 30 minutes or so)—sitting, walking, kneeling, standing, lying down, getting on hands and knees, and using a birthing ball—helps relieve pain (Fig. 14.9). Walking, moving around, and changing positions throughout labour make use of gravity to facilitate movement of the baby downward, helping to increase pelvic diameter and promote fetal rotation, thereby shortening the length of the first stage of labour (Lawrence et al., 2009). Supine and sitting positions for prolonged time should be avoided because they may interfere with the progress of labour and can cause compression of the vena cava and decreased blood return to the heart.

A recent pilot study in Canada demonstrated favourable outcomes for women who laboured in an "ambient room," where the hospital bed was removed and additional equipment was added to promote relaxation, mobility, and a calm atmosphere. Sixty-two participants were allocated to either a standard birthing room or the "ambient room." The women in the ambient group spent 50% or less time labouring in bed, and the need for artificial oxytocin infusions was reduced (Hodnett, Stremler, Weston, et al., 2009b).

Swaying from side to side, rocking, or other rhythmic movements may also be comforting. If labour is progressing slowly, ambulating may speed it up again. Upright positions such as walking, kneeling forward, or doing the lunge on the birthing ball give most women a greater sense of control and active movement than just lying down. Table 14.2 highlights some of the more common positions that can be used during labour and birth.

Acupuncture and Acupressure

Acupuncture and acupressure can be used to relieve pain during labour. Acupuncture involves stimulating key trigger points with needles. This form of Chinese medicine has been practiced for approximately 3,000 years. Classic Chinese teaching holds that throughout the body there are meridians or channels of energy (*qi*) that when in balance regulate body functions. Pain

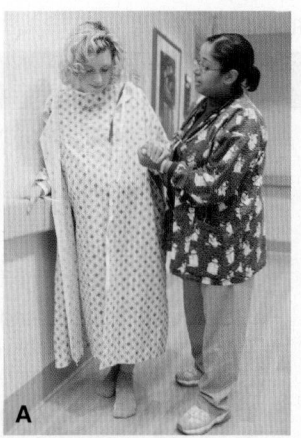
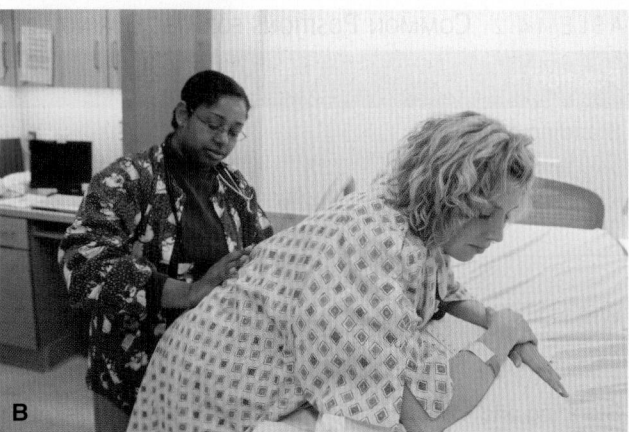
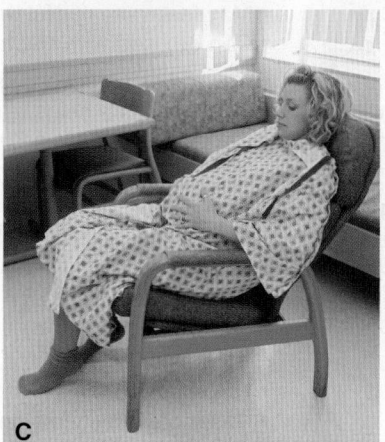
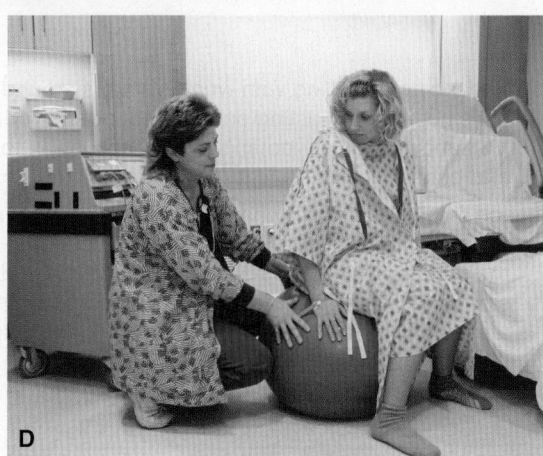

FIGURE 14.9 Various positions for use during labour. (**A**) Ambulation. (**B**) Leaning forward. (**C**) Sitting in a chair. (**D**) Using a birthing ball.

reflects an imbalance or obstruction of the flow of energy. Stimulating the trigger points causes the release of endorphins, reducing the perception of pain. Although controlled research studies are limited, Smith et al. (2006) found that acupuncture may be helpful for pain management during labour. In addition, a recent large randomized controlled trial of more than 600 Danish women demonstrated that acupuncture reduced the need for pharmacologic and invasive methods during delivery and was a good supplement to existing pain relief methods (Borup, Wurlitzer, Hedegaard, et al., 2009).

Acupressure involves the application of a firm finger or massage at the same trigger points to reduce the pain sensation. The amount of pressure is important. The intensity of the pressure is determined by the needs of the woman. Holding and squeezing the hand of a woman in labour may trigger the point most commonly used for both techniques. Acupressure points are found along the spine, neck, shoulder, toes, wrists, lower back (including sacral points), hips, below kneecaps, ankles, and along the toenails (Lowdermilk et al., 2010). A recent *Cochrane* review found that while acupressure does significantly shorten the length of labour, evidence regarding its

effectiveness in pain management is insufficient and further research is required (Smith et al., 2009).

Attention Focusing and Imagery

Attention focusing or distraction and imagery use many of the senses and the mind to focus on stimuli. Distraction entails the use of specific activities such as the use of a visual focal point, guided imagery, visualization, hypnosis, or rituals (Adams & Bianchi, 2008). The woman can focus on tactile stimuli such as touch, massage, or stroking. She may focus on auditory stimuli such as music, humming, or verbal encouragement. Guided imagery supports distraction by visually allowing the mind to create a pleasant image and enhance relaxation in early labour, such as by imagining a beach scene (Adams & Bianchi, 2008) or revisiting a happy memory. Breathing, relaxation, positive thinking, and positive visualization work well for mothers in labour and are examples of labour support behaviours (Adams & Bianchi, 2008). Practicing these behaviours with maternal clients in labour will positively affect birth experiences. Adams & Bianchi (2008) states that a call to action is necessary to design and implement a certification program that would lend importance and credibility to these concepts.

TABLE 14.2 COMMON POSITIONS FOR USE DURING LABOUR AND BIRTH

Position	Potential Advantages
Standing	• Takes advantage of gravity during and between contractions • Makes contractions feel less painful and be more productive • Helps fetus line up with angle of maternal pelvis • Helps to increase urge to push in second stage of labour
Walking	• Has the same advantages as standing • Causes changes in the pelvic joints, helping the fetus move through the birth canal
Standing and leaning forward on partner, bed, birthing ball	• Has the same advantages as standing • Is a good position for a backrub • May feel more restful than standing • Can be used with electronic fetal monitor
Slow dancing (standing with woman's arms around partner's neck, head resting on his chest or shoulder, with his hands rubbing woman's lower back; sway to music and breathe in rhythm if it helps)	• Has the same advantages as walking • Back pressure helps relieve back pain • Rhythm and music help woman relax and provide comfort
Lunge (having a straight chair to side of the labouring woman with one foot on the seat with knee and foot to the side; woman bends raised knee and hip and lunges sideways repeatedly during a contraction, holding each lunge for 5 seconds; partner holds chair and helps with balance)	• Widens one side of the pelvis (the side toward lunge) • Encourages rotation of baby • Can also be done in a kneeling position
Sitting upright	• Helps promote rest • Has more gravity advantage than lying down • Can be used with electronic fetal monitor
Semi-sitting (setting the head of the bed at a 45-degree angle with pillows used for support)	• Has the same advantages as sitting upright • Is an easy position if on a bed
Sitting on toilet or commode	• Has the same advantages as sitting upright • May help relax the perineum for effective bearing down
Rocking in a chair	• Has the same advantages as sitting upright • May help speed labour (rocking movement)
Sitting, leaning forward with support	• Has the same advantages as sitting upright • Is a good position for a backrub
On all fours, on hands and knees	• Helps relieve backache • Assists rotation of baby in posterior position • Allows for pelvic rocking and body movement • Relieves pressure on hemorrhoids • Allows for vaginal examinations • Is sometimes preferred as a pushing position by women with back labour
Kneeling, leaning forward with support on a chair seat, the raised head of the bed, or on a birthing ball	• Has the same advantages as all-fours position • Puts less strain on wrists and hands
Side-lying	• Is a very good position for resting and convenient for many kinds of medical interventions • Helps lower elevated blood pressure • May promote progress of labour when alternated with walking • Is useful to slow a very rapid second stage • Takes pressure off hemorrhoids • Facilitates relaxation between contractions

Position	Potential Advantages
Squatting	• May relieve backache • Takes advantage of gravity • Requires less bearing-down effort • Widens pelvic outlet • May help fetus turn and move down in a difficult birth • Helps if the woman feels no urge to push • Allows freedom to shift weight for comfort • Offers an advantage when pushing, since upper trunk presses on the top of the uterus
Supported squat (leaning back against partner, who supports woman under the arms and takes the entire woman's weight; standing up between contractions)	• Requires great strength in partner • Lengthens trunk, allowing more room for fetus to manoeuvres into position • Lets gravity help
Dangle (partner sitting high on bed or counter with feet supported on chairs or footrests and thighs spread; woman leaning back between partner's legs, placing flexed arms over partner's thighs; partner gripping sides with his thighs; woman lowering herself and allowing partner to support her full weight; standing up between contractions)	• Has the same advantages of a supported squat • Requires less physical strength from the partner than with supported squat position

Sources: Adams, E. D., & Bianchi, A. L. (2008). A practical approach to labor support. *Journal of Obstetric, Gynecologic, & Neonatal Nursing, 37,* 106–115; Lowdermilk, D. L., Perry, S. E., & Cashion, K. (2010). *Maternity nursing* (8th ed.). Maryland Heights, MO: Mosby Elsevier; & Rice Simpson, K., & Creehan, P. A. (2008). *Perinatal nursing.* Philadelphia: AWHONN & Lippincott Williams & Wilkins.

Therapeutic Touch and Massage

Touch is an integral part of human nature and is used in many ways in health and illness, including assessment, diagnosis, and healing (Rose, 2009). Both therapeutic touch and massage can serve to relax patients and distract them from discomfort (Evidence-based Practice 14.1).

Therapeutic touch is an intentionally directed process of energy exchange that uses the hands to promote relaxation and reduce pain and anxiety without actually

EVIDENCE-BASED PRACTICE 14.1
The Effects of Complementary and Alternative Therapies for Pain Management in Labour on Maternal and Perinatal Morbidity

● Study

The pain of labour can be intense, with tension, anxiety, and fear making it worse. Many women would like to labour without using drugs and turn to alternatives to manage pain. These alternative methods include acupuncture, mind–body techniques, massage, reflexology, herbal medicines or homeopathy, hypnosis, and music. This review examined currently available evidence supporting the use of alternative and complementary therapies for pain management during labour. Fourteen trials were reviewed, with data reporting on 1,537 women using different modalities of pain management; 1,448 women were included in the meta-analysis.

▲ Findings

There is insufficient evidence regarding the benefits of music, massage, relaxation, white noise, acupressure, and aromatherapy and no evidence about the effectiveness of massage or other complementary therapies. Acupuncture and hypnosis may be beneficial for the management of pain during labour; however, the number of women studied has been small. Few other complementary therapies have been subjected to proper scientific study.

■ Nursing Implications

Although this study didn't offer conclusive evidence that alternative therapies for pain management work better than pharmacologic or invasive methods, they should not be discounted. Many women wish to avoid artificial means to control the discomfort of labour. The nurse should be supportive and open-minded about a woman's efforts to meet her pain management goals.

Source: Smith, C. A., Collins, C. T., Cyna, A. M., & Crowther, C. A. (2006). Complementary and alternative therapies for pain management in labour. *Cochrane Database of Systematic Reviews, 4,* CD003521.

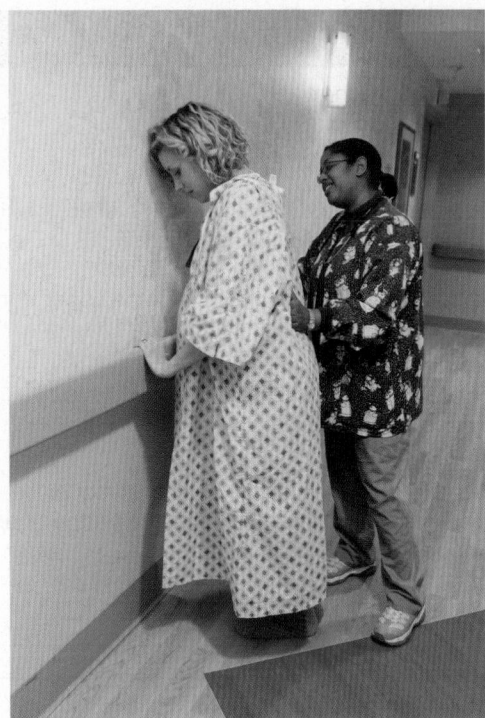

FIGURE 14.10 Nurse massaging the client's back during a contraction while she ambulates during labour.

touching the physical body of the patient (Monroe, 2009; Therapeutic Touch International Association [TTIA], 2010). In order to perform therapeutic touch correctly, the technique must be learned and practiced (TTIA, 2010). Therapeutic touch is often used in conjunction with massage for women during labour.

During massage, some women prefer a light touch while others find a firmer touch more soothing. Massage of the neck, shoulders, back, thighs, feet, and hands can be very comforting. The use of firm counterpressure in the lower back or sacrum is especially helpful for back pain during contractions (Fig. 14.10). Problems with the skin, such as skin rashes, varicose veins, bruises, or infections, are contraindications for massage. In a study of 93 labouring women in Taiwan, most considered massage for low back pain to provide effective pain relief but a few thought massage made the labour even worse (Tzeng & Su, 2008). Thus an individualized approach to massage during labour is recommended. While performing this intervention, nurses should assess the reaction of the woman in order to provide individualized nursing care.

Effleurage is a form of massage that uses light, stroking, superficial touch of the abdomen in rhythm with breathing during contractions. Like traditional massage and therapeutic touch, effleurage is used as a relaxation technique and a distraction from discomfort. However, external fetal monitor belts may interfere with the ability to perform effleurage properly.

Breathing Techniques

Breathing techniques are effective in producing relaxation and pain relief through the use of distraction. If the woman is concentrating on slow-paced rhythmic breathing, she isn't likely to fully focus on contraction pain. Breathing techniques are often taught in childbirth education classes (see Chapter 12 for additional information).

Breathing techniques use controlled breathing to reduce the pain experienced through a stimulus-response conditioning. The woman selects a focal point within her environment to stare at during the first sign of a contraction. This focus creates a visual stimulus that goes directly to her brain. The woman takes a deep cleansing breath, which is followed by rhythmic breathing. Verbal commands from her partner supply an ongoing auditory stimulus to her brain. Effleurage can be combined with the breathing to provide a tactile stimulus, all blocking pain sensations to her brain. There are many benefits to breathing exercises during labour:

- Increased confidence
- Enhanced sense of control
- Distraction from pain
- Enhanced relaxation
- An even flow of oxygen and carbon dioxide
- Prevention of breath holding during contractions
- Relief of labour pain (Adams & Bianchi, 2008; Simkin, 2010)

In their childbirth education classes, many couples learn some form of rhythmic breathing for use during labour. Various patterns may be taught, but each begins and ends with a cleansing breath that involves inhaling through the nose with the shoulders relaxed and exhaling through the mouth and releasing all tension.

In the first pattern, also known as slow-paced breathing, the breathing rate is half the number of breaths normally taken per minute. Following the cleansing breath, the woman inhales through the nose to a count of four and then exhales through the mouth to a count of four, repeating until the end of the contraction when another cleansing breath is taken. In the second pattern, modified-paced breathing, the breathing rate is slightly faster than normal but not more than twice the resting rate. Following the cleansing breath, inhalation and exhalation are done to the count of two following the procedure for slow-paced breathing. The third pattern, pant blow breathing, uses the same rate as with modified-paced breathing except that the breathing is punctuated every few breaths by blowing softly through pursed lips. The pant is an in-breath and an out-breath (touching the tip of the tongue to the roof of the mouth to keep the mouth moist). Patterns may vary: pant-2–3–4-blow or pant-2–3-blow (Perinatal Education Associates, Inc., 2010).

Many childbirth educators do not recommend specific breathing techniques or trying to teach parents the "right" way to breathe during labour and birth. Couples are encouraged to find breathing styles that enhance their relaxation and use them. There are numerous benefits to controlled and rhythmic breathing in childbirth, and many women choose these techniques to manage their discomfort during labour.

Pharmacologic Measures

With varying degrees of success, generations of women have sought ways to relieve the pain of childbirth. Pharmacologic pain relief during labour includes systemic analgesia and regional or local anesthesia. Women have seen dramatic changes in pharmacologic pain management options over the years. Methods have evolved from biting down on a stick to a more complex pharmacologic approach such as epidural/intrathecal analgesia. Systemic analgesia and regional analgesia/anesthesia have become less common, while newer neuraxial analgesia/anesthesia techniques involving minimal motor blockade have become more popular. **Neuraxial analgesia/anesthesia** is the administration of analgesic (opioids) or anesthetic (medication capable of producing a loss of sensation in an area of the body) agents, either continuously or intermittently, into the epidural or intrathecal space to relieve pain. Low-dose and ultra-low-dose epidural analgesia, spinal analgesia, and combined spinal-epidural (CSE) analgesia have replaced the traditional epidural for labour (Simmons, Cyna, Dennis, et al., 2009). This shift in pain management allows a woman to be an active participant in labour.

▶ *Take* NOTE!

Regardless of which approach is used during labour, the woman has the right to choose the methods of pain control that will best suit her and meet her needs.

▶ *Consider* THIS!

When I was expecting my first child, I was determined to put my best foot forward and do everything right. I was an experienced OB nurse, and in my mind doing everything right was expected behaviour. I was already 2 weeks past my calculated due date and I was becoming increasingly worried. That particular day I went to work with a backache but felt no contractions.

I managed to finish my shift but felt completely wiped out. As I walked to my car outside the hospital, my water broke and I felt the warm fluid run down my legs. I went back inside to be admitted for this much-awaited event.

Although I had helped thousands of women go through their childbirth experience, I was now the one in the bed and not standing alongside it. My husband and I had practiced our breathing techniques to cope with the discomfort of labour, but this "discomfort" in my mind was more than I could tolerate. So despite my best intentions of doing everything right, within an hour I begged for a painkiller to ease the pain. While the medication took the edge off my pain, I still felt every contraction and truly now appreciate the meaning of the word "labour." Although I wanted to use natural childbirth without any medication, I know that I was a full participant in my son's birthing experience, and that is what "doing everything right" was for me!

Thoughts: doing what is right varies for each individual, and as nurses we need to support whatever that is. Having a positive outcome from the childbirth experience is the goal; the means it takes to achieve it is less important. How can nurses support women in making their personal choices to achieve a healthy outcome? Are any women "failures" if they ask for pain medication to tolerate labour? How can nurses help women overcome this stigma of being a "wimp"?

Systemic Analgesia

Systemic analgesia involves the use of one or more drugs administered orally, intramuscularly, or intravenously (IV); they become distributed throughout the body via the circulatory system. Depending on which administration method is used, the therapeutic effect of pain relief can occur within minutes and last for several hours. The most important complication associated with the use of this class of drugs is respiratory depression. Therefore, women given these drugs require careful monitoring. Opioids given close to the time of birth can cause central nervous system depression in the newborn, necessitating the administration of naloxone (Narcan) to reverse the depressant effects of the opioids.

Several drug categories may be used for systemic analgesia:

- Opioids, such as butorphanol (Stadol), nalbuphine (Nubain), meperidine (Demerol), or fentanyl (Sublimaze)
- Ataractics, such as hydroxyzine (Vistaril) or promethazine (Phenergan)
- Benzodiazepines, such as diazepam (Valium) or midazolam (Versed)
- Barbiturates, such as secobarbital (Seconal) or pentobarbital (Nembutal)

Drug Guide 14.1 highlights some of the major drugs used for systemic analgesia.

DRUG GUIDE 14.1 Common Agents Used for Systemic Analgesia

Type	Drug	Comments
Opioids	Morphine 2–5 mg IV	May be given IV, intrathecally, or epidurally
		Rapidly crosses the placenta
		Can cause maternal and neonatal CNS depression
		Decreases uterine contractions
		May be given IV or epidurally with maximal fetal uptake 2–3 hours after administration
		Can cause fetal CNS depression
	Meperidine (Demerol) 25–50 mg IV[a]	Decreases fetal variability
		Naloxone does not reverse and may even worsen fetal neurotoxicity
		Is given IV
		Is rapidly transferred across the placenta
		Causes neonatal respiratory depression
		Is given IV
	Butorphanol (Stadol) 1 mg IV q3–4h	Causes less maternal nausea and vomiting
		Causes decreased FHR variability, fetal bradycardia, and respiratory depression
		Is given IV or epidurally
	Nalbuphine (Nubain) 10 mg IV	Can cause maternal hypotension, maternal and fetal respiratory depression
		Rapidly crosses placenta
		Rapid action and short duration of 1–2 hours
	Fentanyl (Sublimaze) 25–50 mcg IV	
Ataractics	Hydroxyzine (Vistaril) 50 mg IM	Does not relieve pain but reduces anxiety and potentiates opioid analgesic effects
		Is used to decrease nausea and vomiting
		Is used for antiemetic effect when combined with opioids
	Promethazine (Phenergan) 25 mg IV	Causes sedation and reduces apprehension
		May contribute to maternal hypotension and neonatal depression
Benzodiazepines	Diazepam (Valium) 2–5 mg IV	Is given to enhance pain relief of opioid and cause sedation
		May be used to stop eclamptic seizures
		Decreases nausea and vomiting
		Can cause newborn depression; therefore, lowest possible dose should be used
		Is not used for analgesic but amnesia effect
		Is used as adjunct for anesthesia
		Is excreted in breast milk
	Midazolam (Versed) 1–5 mg IV	
Barbiturates	Secobarbital (Seconal) 100 mg PO/IM	Causes sedation
		Is used in very early labour to alter a dysfunctional pattern
		Is not used for pain relief in active labour
	Pentobarbital (Nembutal) 100 mg PO/IM	Crosses placenta and is secreted in breast milk

[a]Not recommended.

Sources: British Columbia Perinatal Health Program. (2009). *Core competencies: Management of labour in an institutional setting if the primary maternal care provider is absent. Guidelines for registered nurses.* Vancouver, BC: BC Perinatal Health Program. Retrieved February 22, 2012 from http://www.perinatalservicesbc.ca/sites/bcrcp/files/FHS/Linked_Core_Competencies_with_DST.pdf; Datta, S., Kodali, B. S., & Segal, S. (2009). *Obstetric anesthesia handbook* (5th ed.). New York: Springer; deglin, J. H., Vallerand, A. H., & Sanoski, C. A. (2011). *Davis's drug guide for nurses* (12th ed.). Philadelphia: FA Davis Company; & The Merck Manual. (2007). *Management of normal labor.* Retrieved February 22, 2012 from http://www.merck.com/mmpe/sec18/ch260/ch260d.html#sec18-ch260-ch260d-1073.

Systemic analgesics are typically administered parenterally, usually through an existing IV line. Maternal analgesia during labour often directly affects the baby because of placental transfer of drugs administered to the mother; the baby is also affected indirectly by the secondary physiologic or biochemical changes experienced by the mother (Evans et al., 2010; Reynolds, 2010). Historically, opioids have been administered by nurses, but in the past decade there has been increasing use of client-controlled IV analgesia (patient-controlled analgesia [PCA]). With this system, the woman is given a button connected to a computerized pump on the IV line. When the woman desires analgesia, she presses the button and the pump delivers a preset amount of medication. This system provides the woman with a sense of control over her own pain management and active participation in the childbirth process.

Opioids

Opioids are morphine-like medications that are most effective for the relief of moderate to severe pain. Opioids typically are administered IV. Meperidine [Demerol] was once the most commonly used of all the synthetic opioids (others include butorphanol [Stadol], nalbuphine [Nubain], fentanyl [Sublimaze]) for the management of pain during labour. However, many hospitals are now reconsidering this standard because meperidine metabolizes to normeperidine, leading to neurobehavioural depression in many women lasting for several days (British Columbia Perinatal Health Program, 2009; Rice Simpson & Creehan, 2008; The Merck Manual, 2007). Opioids can impact early breastfeeding (Reynolds, 2010) and are associated with newborn respiratory depression, yet they do not achieve adequate maternal analgesia (Akerman & Dresner, 2009; Reynolds, 2010).

All opioids are considered good analgesics. However, respiratory depression can occur in both mother and fetus depending on the dose given. They may also cause a decrease in FHR variability identified on the fetal monitor strip. This FHR pattern change is usually transient. Other systemic side effects include nausea, vomiting, pruritus, delayed gastric emptying, drowsiness, hypoventilation, and newborn respiratory depression. To reduce the incidence of newborn respiratory depression, birth should occur within 1 hour or after 4 hours of administration to prevent the fetus from receiving the peak concentration (Deglin, Vallerand, & Sanoski, 2011). Opioid antagonists such as naloxone (Narcan) are given to reverse the effects of the central nervous system depression, including respiratory depression, caused by opioids. Nurses need to be aware of the fact that the duration of naloxone's effect is very short, and they should therefore be alert for a potential return of respiratory depression and the need for repeated doses (Evans et. al., 2010). Opioid antagonists also are used to reverse the side effects of neuraxial opioids, such as pruritus (Deglin et al., 2011).

Ataractics

The ataractic group of medications is used in combination with an opioid to decrease nausea and vomiting and lessen anxiety. These adjunct drugs potentiate the effectiveness of the opioid so that a lesser dose can be given. They may also be used to increase sedation.

Benzodiazepines

Benzodiazepines are used for minor tranquilizing and sedative effects. Diazepam (Valium) is given IV to stop seizures due to pregnancy-induced hypertension. However, it is not used during labour itself. It can be administered to calm a woman who is out of control, thereby enabling her to relax enough so that she can participate effectively during her labour process rather than fighting against it. Lorazepam (Ativan) can also be used for its tranquilizing effect, but increased sedation is experienced with this medication (Deglin et al., 2011). Midazolam (Versed), also given IV, produces amnesia but no analgesia. It is most commonly used as an adjunct for anesthesia but is given in small doses and should be used cautiously due to its amnesic effect (Datta, Kodali, & Segal, 2009). Diazepam and midazolam cause central nervous system depression in both the woman and the newborn (Deglin et al., 2011).

Barbiturates

Barbiturates are used only in early labour to promote sleep when birth is unlikely for 12 to 24 hours. The goal is to promote therapeutic rest for a few hours to enhance the woman's ability to cope with active labour. These drugs cross the placenta and cause central nervous system depression in the newborn (Rice Simpson & Creehan, 2008).

Regional Analgesia/Anesthesia

Regional techniques, also referred to as neuraxial analgesia/anesthesia, provide unrivaled pain relief in labour with minimal side effects. The drugs are administered into a specific region, the lower neuraxis. Only small doses are needed as this technique provides a local effect in blocking pain pathways.

The routes for regional pain relief include epidural block, CSE block, local infiltration, pudendal block, and intrathecal (spinal) analgesia/anesthesia (Grant, 2010). Local and pudendal routes are used during birth for episiotomies; epidural and intrathecal routes are used for pain relief during active labour and birth. The major advantage of regional pain-management techniques is that the woman can participate in the birthing process and still have good pain control.

Epidural Block

While the rates of epidural use during labour vary among provinces and territories in Canada, nationally there has been a significant overall increase. Approximately two-thirds of all vaginal deliveries in Quebec (69%) and

Ontario (60%), were preceded by an epidural. Rates have continued to climb in six of the remaining eight provinces and in two of the three territories (Canadian Institute for Health Information, 2010). Over just a 2-year period, from 2006–2007 to 2008–2009, the largest increases noted were in Nova Scotia (increasing by 6.2% for a total of 54.6%) and Prince Edward Island (increasing by 9.3% for a total of 39.5%). The Canadian Anesthesiologists' Society [CAS], (2010) has developed consensus-based guidelines for acute pain management using neuraxial analgesia (intrathecal or epidural administration of opioids and/or local anesthetics). Among these are the availability of an anesthesiologist at all times and appropriate education of nurses involved in the care of patients in receipt of this treatment (CAS, 2010). Despite the rising rates of epidural use, many rural Canadian communities are unable to offer this service to their clients during labour based on these guidelines.

An epidural block involves the injection of a drug into the epidural space, which is located outside the dura mater between the dura and the spinal canal. The epidural space is typically entered through the third and fourth lumbar vertebrae with a needle, and a catheter is threaded into the epidural space. The needle is removed and the catheter is left in place to allow for continuous infusion or intermittent injections of medicine (Fig. 14.11). An epidural block provides analgesia and anesthesia and can be used for both vaginal and cesarean births. It has evolved from a regional block producing total loss of sensation to analgesia with minimal blockade. The effectiveness of epidural analgesia depends on the technique and medications used. It is usually started after labour is well established, typically when cervical dilation is greater than 5 cm.

Theoretically, epidural local anesthetics could block all labour pain if used in large volumes and high concentrations. However, pain relief is balanced against other goals such as walking during the first stage of labour, pushing effectively in the second stage, and minimizing maternal and fetal side effects.

An epidural is contraindicated for women with a previous history of spinal surgery or spinal abnormalities, coagulation defects, infections, and hypovolemia. It also is contraindicated for the woman who is receiving anticoagulation therapy.

Complications may include nausea and vomiting, hypotension, fever, pruritus, intravascular injection, and respiratory depression (*Childbirth: An epidural*, 2011). Effects on the fetus during labour include fetal distress secondary to maternal hypotension (British Columbia Perinatal Health Program, 2009). Ensuring that the woman avoids a supine position after an epidural catheter has been placed will help to minimize hypotension.

Changes in epidural drugs and techniques have been made to optimize pain control while minimizing side effects. Today many women receive a continuous lumbar epidural infusion of a local anesthetic as well as an opioid (Rice Simpson & Creehan, 2008). The addition of

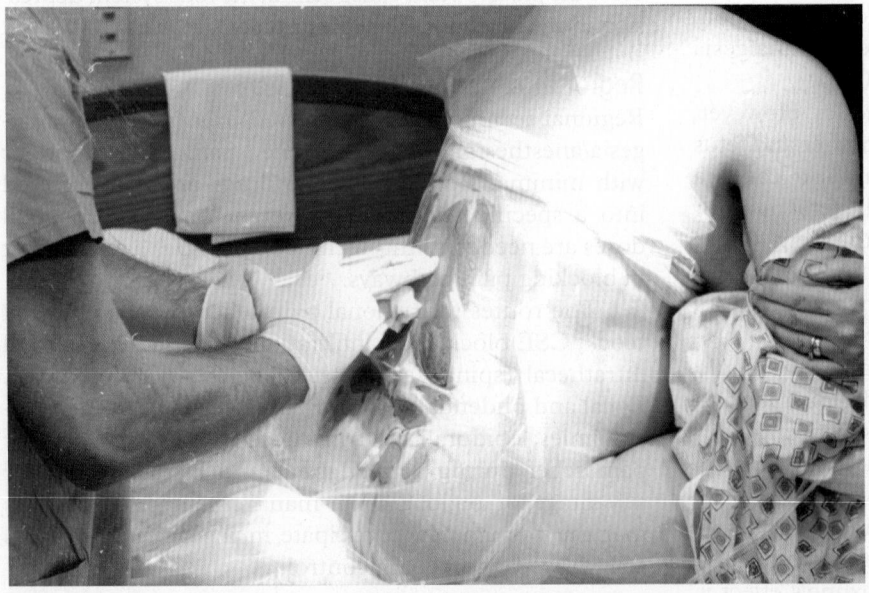

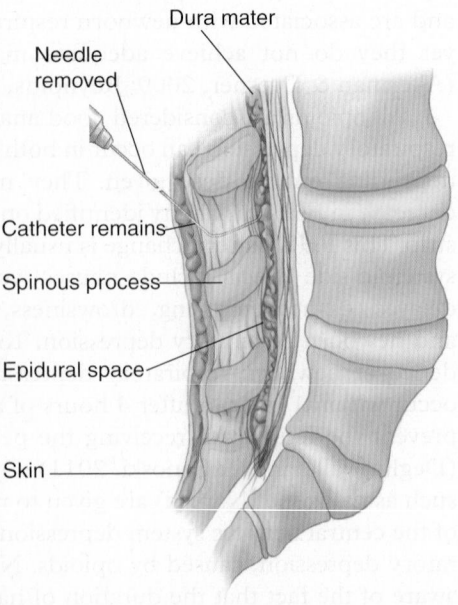

A

B

FIGURE 14.11 Epidural catheter insertion. (**A**) A needle is inserted into the epidural space. (**B**) A catheter is threaded through the needle into the epidural space; the needle is then removed. The catheter allows medication to be administered intermittently or continuously to relieve pain during labour and childbirth.

opioids, such as fentanyl or morphine, to the local anesthetic helps decrease the amount of motor block obtained (Reynolds, 2010). Continuous infusion pumps are often used to administer the epidural analgesia, allowing the woman to be in control and administer a bolus dose on demand (Akerman & Dresner, 2009).

Spinal (Intrathecal) Analgesia/Anesthesia

The spinal (intrathecal) pain-management involves the injection of an anesthetic "caine" agent, with or without opioids, into the subarachnoid space to provide pain relief during labour or cesarean birth. The contraindications are similar to those for the epidural block. Potential adverse reactions for the woman include hypotension and spinal headache.

Combined Spinal–Epidural Analgesia

Another epidural technique is CSE analgesia. This technique involves inserting the epidural needle into the epidural space and subsequently inserting a small-gauge spinal needle through the epidural needle into the subarachnoid space. An opioid, without a local anesthetic, is injected into this space. The spinal needle is then removed and an epidural catheter is inserted for later use.

CSE is advantageous because of its rapid onset of pain relief (within 3 to 5 minutes) that can last up to 3 hours. In a recent review of CSE analgesia studies, Cheng & Caughey (2012) found this method to offer superior pain control. In their review of 19 randomized, controlled trials involving close to 3,000 women, Simmons and colleagues (2009) concluded that CSE had a faster onset of action and was associated with less pruritus than with epidurals; however, there was no difference in the woman's ability to mobilize or in the obstetric or neonatal outcomes. Although women can theoretically walk with CSE, they often choose not to because of poor mobility and leg weakness (Simmons et al., 2009).

Ambulating during labour provides several benefits: it may help control pain better, shorten the first stage of labour, increase the intensity of the contractions, and decrease the possibility of an operative vaginal or cesarean birth. However, nurses need to be cognizant of the potential for injury in patients using CSE analgesia if the client is verbalizing or demonstrating poor mobility or weakness.

Other complications include maternal hypotension, which can lead to fetal distress; postdural puncture headache (Alam, Raheen, Iqbal, et al., 2011); inadequate or failed block (Evans et al., 2010); pruritus; and urinary retention (Akerman & Dresner, 2009). In addition, the procedure is known to slow down the first stage or labour and/or extend the second stage (Evans et al., 2010; Klein, Kaczorowski, Hall, et al., 2009). Hypotension and associated FHR changes are managed with maternal positioning (semi-Fowler's, left lateral tilt), intravenous

hydration, and supplemental oxygen (Evans et al., 2010). The patient may need a urinary catheter to either prevent (inserted during labour) or relieve urinary retention postpartum (Akerman & Dresner, 2009; Evans et al., 2010). Itching and rash may occur secondary to the anesthetic and is often easily managed with diphenhydramine hydrochloride (Benadryl).

Patient-Controlled Epidural Analgesia

Epidural PCA involves the use of an indwelling epidural catheter with an infusion of medication and a programmed pump that allows the woman to control the dosing. This method allows the woman to have a sense of control over her pain and reach her own individually acceptable analgesia level. Studies have shown that women report high levels of satisfaction with both CSE and epidural PCA, but they appear to prefer controlling their pain with the push of a button (Landau, 2009).

With epidural PCA, the woman uses a hand-held device connected to an analgesic agent that is attached to an epidural catheter. When she pushes the button, a bolus dose of agent is administered via the catheter to reduce her pain. This method allows the woman to manage her pain at will without having to ask a staff member to provide pain relief.

Local Infiltration

Local infiltration involves the injection of a local anesthetic, such as lidocaine, into the superficial perineal nerves to numb the perineal area. This technique is done by the physician or midwife just before performing an episiotomy (surgical incision into the perineum to facilitate birth) or before suturing a laceration. Local infiltration does not alter the pain of uterine contractions, but it does numb the immediate area of the episiotomy or laceration. Local infiltration does not cause side effects for the woman or her newborn.

Pudendal Nerve Block

A pudendal nerve block refers to the injection of a local anesthetic agent (e.g., bupivacaine, ropivacaine) into the pudendal nerves near each ischial spine. It provides pain relief in the lower vagina, vulva, and perineum (Fig. 14.12).

A pudendal block is used for the second stage of labour, an episiotomy, or an operative vaginal birth with outlet forceps or vacuum extractor. It must be administered about 15 minutes before it is needed to ensure its full effect. A transvaginal approach is generally used to inject an anesthetic agent at or near the pudendal nerve branch. Neither maternal nor fetal complications are common.

General Anesthesia

General anesthesia is typically reserved for emergency cesarean births when there is not enough time to provide

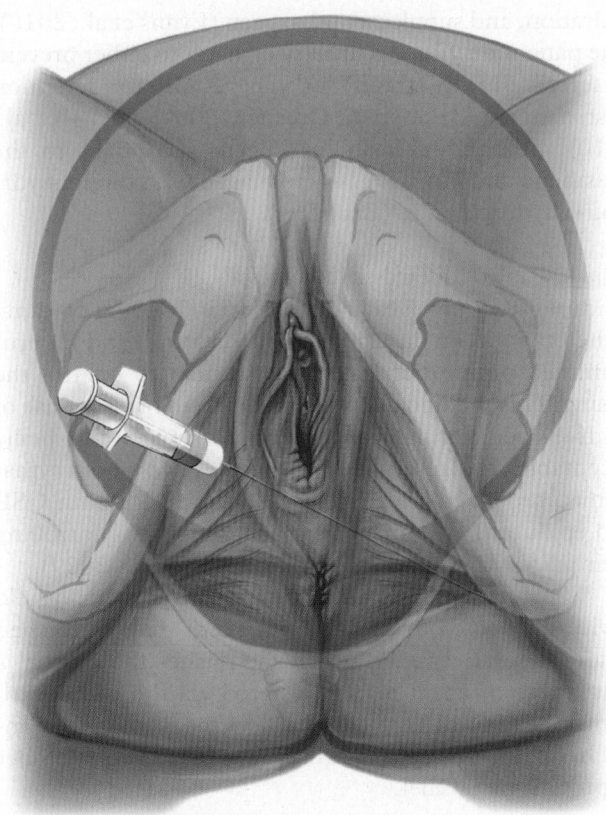

FIGURE 14.12 Pudendal nerve block.

spinal or epidural anesthesia or if the woman has a contraindication to the use of regional anesthesia. It can be started quickly and causes a rapid loss of consciousness. General anesthesia can be administered by IV injection, inhalation of anesthetic agents, or both. Commonly, thiopental, a short-acting barbiturate, is given IV to produce unconsciousness. This is followed by administration of a muscle relaxant. After the woman is intubated, nitrous oxide and oxygen are administered.

All anesthetic agents cross the placenta and affect the fetus. The primary complication with general anesthesia is fetal depression, along with uterine relaxation and potential maternal vomiting and aspiration.

Although the anesthesiologist or nurse anesthetist administers the various general anesthesia agents, the nurse needs to be knowledgeable about the pharmacologic aspects of the drugs used and must be aware of airway management. Ensure that the woman is NPO and has a patent IV. In addition, administer a nonparticulate (clear) oral antacid (e.g., Bicitra or sodium citrate) or a proton pump inhibitor (Protonix) as ordered to reduce gastric acidity. Assist with placement of a wedge under the woman's right hip to displace the gravid uterus and prevent vena cava compression in the supine position. Once the newborn has been removed

from the uterus, assist the perinatal team in providing supportive care.

Nursing Care During Labour and Birth

WATCH & LEARN

Childbirth, a physiologic process that is fundamental to all human existence, is one of the most significant cultural, psychological, spiritual, and behavioural events in a woman's life. Although the act of giving birth is a universal phenomenon, it is a unique experience for each woman. Continuous evaluation and appropriate intervention for women during labour are the keys to promoting a positive outcome for the family.

The nurse's role in childbirth is to ensure a safe environment for the mother and her newborn. Nurses begin evaluating the mother and fetus during the admission procedures at the health care agency and continue to do so throughout labour. It is critical to provide anticipatory guidance and explain each procedure (fetal monitoring, IV therapy, medications given, and expected reactions) and what will happen next. This will prepare the woman for the upcoming physical and emotional challenges, thereby helping to reduce her anxiety. Acknowledging her support systems (family or partner) helps allay their fears and concerns, thereby assisting them in carrying out their supportive role. Knowing how and when to evaluate a woman during the various stages of labour is essential for all labour and birth nurses to ensure a positive maternal experience and a healthy newborn.

A major focus of care for the woman during labour and birth is assisting her with maintaining control over her pain, emotions, and actions while being an active participant. Nurses can help and support women to be actively involved in their childbirth experience by allowing time for discussion, offering companionship, listening to worries and concerns, paying attention to the woman's emotional needs, and offering information to help her understand what is happening in each stage of labour.

Nursing Care During the First Stage of Labour

Depending on how far advanced the woman's labour is when she arrives at the facility, the nurse will determine assessment parameters of maternal–fetal status and plan care accordingly. The nurse will provide high-touch, low-tech supportive nursing care during the first stage of labour when admitting the woman and orienting her to the labour and birth suite. Nursing care during this stage will include taking an admission history (reviewing the prenatal record); checking the results of routine laboratory tests and any special tests such as chorionic villi sampling, amniocentesis, genetic studies, and biophysical profile done during pregnancy; asking the woman about her childbirth preparation (birth plan, classes taken, coping skills); and completing a physical assessment of the woman to establish a baseline of values for future comparison.

Key nursing interventions include:

- Identifying the estimated date of birth from the client and the prenatal chart
- Validating the client's prenatal history to determine fetal risk status
- Determining fundal height to validate dates and fetal growth
- Performing Leopold's manoeuvres to determine fetal position, lie, and presentation
- Checking FHR
- Performing a vaginal examination (as appropriate) to evaluate effacement and dilation progress
- Instructing the client and her partner about monitoring techniques and equipment
- Assessing fetal response and FHR against contractions and recovery time
- Interpreting fetal monitoring strips
- Checking FHR baseline for accelerations, variability, and decelerations
- Repositioning the client to obtain an optimal FHR pattern
- Recognizing FHR problems and initiating corrective measures
- Checking amniotic fluid for meconium staining, odour, and amount
- Comforting the client throughout the testing period and labour
- Supporting the client's decisions regarding intervention or avoidance of intervention
- Assessing the client's support system and coping status frequently

In addition to these interventions to promote optimal outcomes for the mother and fetus, the nurse must document care accurately and in a timely fashion. The purpose of the health record is to communicate the health status of the mother to other members of the team. In addition, accurate and timely documentation of the care provided and the responses shown will be critical in potential cases of litigation (Rice Simpson & Creehan, 2008), which is prevalent in the childbirth arena. In addition to following provincial and agency policies, guidelines for recording care include the following:

- Ensure that only factual and objective information on care provided is recorded
- Include all communication with other health care team members (direct or indirect)
- Document only clinically relevant information
- Include comprehensive data about maternal–fetal status
- Record nursing interventions and patient response

The SOGC (2007) stresses the importance of good, clear, effective communication and accurate documentation pertaining to fetal health assessments. In particular, specific required documentation inclusions are listed as they pertain to intermittent auscultation and EFM.

Assessing the Woman Upon Admission

The nurse usually first comes in contact with the woman either by phone or in person. It is important to ascertain whether the woman is in true or false labour and whether she should be admitted or sent home. Upon admission to the labour and birth suite, the highest priorities include assessing FHR, assessing cervical dilation/effacement, and determining whether membranes have ruptured or are intact. These assessment data will guide the critical thinking in planning care for the patient.

If the initial contact is by phone, establish a therapeutic relationship with the woman. Speaking in a calm, caring tone facilitates this. When completing a phone assessment, include questions about the following:

- Estimated date of birth, to determine if term or preterm
- Fetal movement (frequency in the past few days)
- Other premonitory signs of labour experienced
- Parity, gravida, and previous childbirth experiences
- Time from start of labour to birth in previous labours
- Characteristics of contractions, including frequency, duration, and intensity
- Appearance of any vaginal bloody show
- Membrane status (ruptured or intact)
- Presence of supportive adult in household or if she is alone

When speaking with the woman over the telephone, review the signs and symptoms that denote true versus false labour, and suggest various positions she can assume to provide comfort and increase placental perfusion. Also suggest walking, massage, and taking a warm shower to promote relaxation. Outline what foods and fluids are appropriate for oral intake in early labour. Throughout the phone call, listen to the woman's concerns and answer any questions clearly.

Rice Simpson and Creehan (2008) advise against telephone triage; they advise nurses simply to instruct women to call their primary health care provider or come to the hospital to be evaluated. Ruling out true labour and possible maternal–fetal complications cannot be done accurately over the phone.

Additional nursing responsibilities associated with a phone assessment include:

- Consulting the woman's prenatal record for parity status, estimated date of birth, and untoward events
- Calling the health care provider to inform him or her of the woman's status
- Preparing for admission to the perinatal unit to ensure adequate staff assignment
- Notifying the admissions office of a pending admission

If the nurse's first encounter with the woman is in person, an assessment is completed to determine whether she should be admitted to the perinatal unit or sent home until her labour advances. Entering a facility is often an intimidating and stressful event for women since it is an unfamiliar environment. Giving birth for the first time is a pivotal event in the lives of most women. Therefore, demonstrate respect when addressing the client; listen carefully and express interest and concern. As part of the National Birthing Initiative for Canada, the SOGC (2008a) recognizes the importance of ensuring that maternity care is patient centred and empowering for women and identifies listening to women's voices as the highest priority. Inviting the labouring woman to share her birth plan and making her a part of the decisions that affect her care demonstrates respect and will enhance her sense of self-control.

An admission assessment includes maternal health history, physical assessment, fetal assessment, laboratory studies, and assessment of psychological status. Usually the facility has a form that can be used throughout labour and birth to document assessment findings (Fig. 14.13).

Maternal Health History

A maternal health history should include typical biographical data such as the woman's name and age and the name of the delivering health care provider. Other information that is collected includes the prenatal record data, including the estimated date of birth, a history of the current pregnancy, and the results of any laboratory and diagnostic tests, such as blood type, Rh status, and group B streptococcal status; past pregnancy and obstetric history; past health history and family history; prenatal education; list of medications; risk factors such as diabetes, hypertension, and use of tobacco, alcohol, or illicit drugs; reason for admission, such as labour, cesarean birth, or observation for a complication; history of potential domestic violence; history of previous preterm births; allergies; time of last food ingestion; method chosen for infant feeding; name of birth attendant and pediatrician; and pain management plan.

Ascertaining this information is important so that an individualized plan of care can be developed for the woman. If, for example, the woman's due date is still 2 months away, it is important to establish this information so interventions can be initiated to arrest the labour immediately or notify the intensive perinatal team to be available. In addition, if the woman is a diabetic, it is critical to monitor her glucose levels during labour, to prepare for a surgical birth if dystocia of labour occurs, and to alert the newborn nursery of potential hypoglycemia in the newborn after birth. By collecting important information about each woman they care for, nurses can help improve the outcomes for all concerned.

Be sure to observe the woman's emotions, support system, verbal interaction, body language and posture, perceptual acuity, and energy level. Also note her cultural background and language spoken. This psychosocial information provides cues about the woman's emotional state, culture, and communication systems. For example, if the woman arrives at the labour and birth suite extremely anxious, alone, and unable to communicate in English, how can the nurse meet her needs and plan her care appropriately? It is only by assessing each woman physically and psychosocially that the nurse can make astute decisions regarding proper care. In this case, an interpreter would be needed to assist in the communication process between the staff and the woman to initiate proper care.

It is important to acknowledge and try to understand the cultural differences in women with cultural backgrounds different from that of the nurse. Attitudes toward childbirth are heavily influenced by the culture in which the woman has been raised. As a result, within every society, specific attitudes and values shape the woman's childbearing behaviours. Be aware of what these are. When carrying out a cultural assessment during the admission process, ask questions (Box 14.2) to help plan culturally competent care during labour and birth.

Physical Examination

The physical examination typically includes a generalized assessment of the woman's body systems, including hydration status, vital signs, auscultation of heart and lung sounds, and measurement of height and weight.

BOX 14.2 Questions for Providing Culturally Competent Care During Labour and Birth

- Where were you born? How long have you lived in Canada?
- What languages do you speak and read?
- Who are your major support people?
- What are your religious practices?
- How do you view childbearing?
- Are there any special precautions or restrictions that are important?
- Is birth considered a private or a social experience?
- Are there any practices in your culture related to the birth of your child that are important?
- Are there any practices in your culture related to your newborn that are important, such as a naming ceremony?
- How would you like to manage your labour discomfort?
- Who will provide your labour support?

Source: D'Avanzo, C. E. (2008). *Cultural health assessment* (4th ed.). St. Louis, MO: Mosby Elsevier.

ADMISSION ASSESSMENT OBSTETRICS

▲ PATIENT IDENTIFICATION ▲

ADMISSION DATA

Date		Time		Via
				☐ Ambulatory ☐ Wheelchair ☐ Stretcher

Grav.	Term	Pre-term	Ab.	Living	EDC	LMP	GA

Prev. adm. date _____ Reason _____

Obstetrician _____ Pediatrician _____

Ht. _____ Wt. _____ Wt. gain _____

Allergies (meds/food) ☐ None _____ ☐ Hx latex sensitivity

BP _____ T _____ P _____ R _____

FHR _____ Vag exam _____

Reason for Admission

☐ Labor / SROM   ☐ Induction _____

☐ Primary C/S _____ ☐ Repeat C/S

☐ Observation _____

☐ OB / Medical complication _____

Onset of labor: ☐ Not in labor

Date _____ Time _____

Membranes: ☐ Intact

☐ Ruptured / Date _____ Time _____

☐ Clear   ☐ Meconium   ☐ Bloody   ☐ Foul

Vaginal bleeding: ☐ None

☐ Normal show   ☐ _____

Current Pregnancy Labs   ☐ NPC

☐ POL	☐ PPROM	☐ Cerclage
☐ PIH	☐ Chr. HTN	☐ Other _____

☐ Diabetes _____ Diet _____

☐ Insulin _____

☐ Amniocentesis _____ Results _____

Bld type / RH ____ Date Rhogam ____

Antibody screen ☐Neg ☐Pos

Rubella ☐ Non-immune ☐ Immune

Diabetic screen ☐ Normal ☐ Abnormal

Recent exposure to chick pox ☐

Current meds: _____

_____

	Pos	Neg	Tested
Hepatitis B	☐	☐	☐ No
HIV	☐	☐	☐ No
Group B strep	☐	☐	☐ No
GC	☐	☐	☐ No
Chlamydia	☐	☐	☐ No
RPR	☐	☐	☐ No

Previous OB History

☐ POL   ☐ Multiple gestation

☐ Prev C/S type _____ Reason _____

☐ PIH   ☐ Chronic HTN   ☐ Diabetes _____

☐ Stillbirth/demise   ☐ Neodeath   ☐ Anomalies

☐ Precipitous labor (<3 H) ☐ Macrosomia

☐ PP Hemorrhage

☐ Hx Transfusion reaction ☐Yes ☐ No

☐ Other _____

Latest risk assessment   ☐ None

1. _____ 3. _____

2. _____ 4. _____

Signature _____   Date _____

    Time _____

NEUROLOGICAL

☐ WNL

Variance: ☐ HA

☐ Scotoma / visual changes

Reflexes   ☐ < 2 +   ☐ > 2 +

    ☐ Clonus ____ bts

☐ Numbness   ☐ Tingling

☐ Hx Seizures

☐ _____

RESPIRATORY

☐ WNL

Variance: ☐ Hx Asthma ☐ URI

Respirations: ☐< 12 ☐ > 24

Effort: ☐ SOB

☐ Shallow ☐ Labored

Auscultation:

☐ Diminished ☐ Crackles

☐ Wheezes ☐ Rhonchi   No Yes

	No	Yes
Cough for greater than 2 weeks?	☐	☐
Is the cough productive?	☐	☐
Blood in the sputum?	☐	☐
Experiencing any fever or night sweats?	☐	☐
Ever had TB in the past?	☐	☐
Recent exposure to TB?	☐	☐
Weight loss in last 3 weeks?	☐	☐

If the patient answers yes to any three of the above questions implement policy and procedure # 5725-0704.

GASTROINTESTINAL

☐ WNL

Variance: ☐ Heartburn

☐ Epigastric pain   Nausea

☐ Vomiting ☐ Diarrhea

☐ Constipation ☐ Pain

☐ Wt. Gain < 2lbs / month**

☐ Recent change in appetite of
< 50% of usual intake for > 5 days

☐ _____

INTEGUMENTARY

☐ WNL

Variance: ☐ Rash ☐ Lacerations

☐ Abrasion ☐ Swelling

☐ Uticaria ☐ Bruising

☐ Diaphoretic/hot

☐ Clammy/cold

☐ Scars

☐ _____

FETAL ASSESSMENT

☐ WNL

Variance:

☐ NRFS

FHR ☐ < 110   ☐ > 160

LTV ☐ Absent ☐ Minimal

    ☐ Increased

STV Absent

Decelerations: _____

    ☐ Decreased fetal movement

    ☐ IUGR

☐ _____

CARDIOVASCULAR

☐ WNL

Variance:

☐ MVP

Heart rate: ☐ < 60 ☐ > 100

B/P: Systolic: ☐ < 90 ☐ > 140

    Diastolic: ☐ < 50 ☐ > 90

☐ Edema _____

☐ Chest pain / palpitations

☐ _____

MUSCULOSKELETAL

☐ WNL

Variance:

☐ Numbness   ☐ Tingling

☐ Paralysis   ☐ Deformity

☐ Scoliosis

☐ _____

GENITOURINARY

☐ WNL

Variance: ☐ Albumin _____

Output: ☐ < 30 cc/Hr.

☐ UTI   ☐ Rx   ☐ Frequency

☐ Dysuria   ☐ Hematuria

☐ CVA Tenderness

☐ Hx STD _____

☐ Vag. discharge _____

☐ Rash   ☐ Blisters

☐ Warts   ☐ Lesions

☐ _____

EARS, NOSE, THROAT, AND EYES

☐ WNL

Variance:

☐ Sore throat   ☐ Eyeglasses

☐ Runny nose ☐ Contact lenses

☐ Nasal congestion

PSYCHOSOCIAL

☐ WNL

Variance: ☐ Hx depression

    ☐ Yes ☐ No

☐ Emotional behavioral care

Affect: ☐ Flat ☐ Anxious

☐ Uncooperative ☐ Combative

Living will ☐ Yes ☐ No

    ☐ On chart

Healthcare surrogate ☐ Yes ☐No

    ☐ On chart

Are you being hurt, hit, frightened by anyone
at home or in your life? ☐ Yes ☐ No

Religious preference _____

	Denies	Yes	
Tobacco use	☐ Denies	☐ Yes	Amt _____
Alcohol use	☐ Denies	☐ Yes	Amt _____
Drug use	☐ Denies	☐ Yes	Amt type _____
Primary language	☐ English	☐ Spanish	☐ _____

PAIN ASSESSMENT

1. Do you have any ongoing pain problems?   ☐ No ☐ Yes
2. Do you have any pain now?   ☐ No ☐ Yes
3. If any of the above questions are answered yes, the patient has a positive pain screening.
4. Patient to be given pain management education material.
   Complete pain / symptom assessment on flowsheet.
5. *Please proceed to complete pain assessment.*

FIGURE 14.13 Sample documentation form used for admission to the perinatal unit. (Used with permission. Briggs Corporation, 2001.)

The physical examination also includes the following assessments:

- Fundal height measurement
- Uterine activity, including contraction frequency, duration, and intensity
- Status of membranes (intact or ruptured)
- Cervical dilation and degree of effacement
- Fetal status, including heart rate, position, and station
- Pain level

These assessment parameters form a baseline against which the nurse can compare all future values throughout labour. The findings should be similar to those of the woman's prepregnancy and pregnancy findings, with the exception of her pulse rate, which might be elevated secondary to her anxious state with beginning labour.

Laboratory Studies

On admission, laboratory studies typically are done to establish a baseline. Although the exact tests may vary among facilities, they usually include a urinalysis via clean-catch urine specimen and complete blood count (CBC). Blood typing and Rh factor analysis may be necessary if the results of these are unknown or unavailable. In addition, if the following test results are not included in the maternal prenatal history, it may be necessary to perform them at this time. They include syphilis screening, hepatitis B surface antigen (HBsAg) screening, group B streptococcus (GBS) testing, human immunodeficiency virus (HIV) testing (if the woman gives consent), and possible drug screening if the history is positive.

GBS is a gram-positive organism that is present in the vaginal and gastrointestinal tract of 15% to 45% of women (Woods & Levy, 2011). These women are asymptomatic carriers but can cause GBS disease of the newborn through vertical transmission. The mortality rate of infected newborns varies according to time of onset (early or late). Risk factors for GBS include maternal intrapartum fever, prolonged ruptured membranes, previous birth of an infected newborn, and GBS bacteriuria in the present pregnancy.

In 2004, the SOGC issued guidelines that advised universal screening of pregnant women at 35 to 37 weeks' gestation for GBS and intrapartum antibiotic therapy for GBS carriers. In addition, women at term whose membranes ruptured more than 18 hours previously should receive treatment (SOGC, 2004a). Maternal infections associated with GBS include acute chorioamnionitis, endometritis, and urinary tract infection. Neonatal clinical manifestations include pneumonia and sepsis. Identified GBS carriers receive IV antibiotic prophylaxis (penicillin G or ampicillin) at the onset of labour or when membranes rupture.

The SOGC (2001) recommends elective cesarean section at 38 weeks for HIV-positive women who meet one of the following criteria: women who have not received any anti-retroviral therapy, women receiving anti-retroviral monotherapy regardless of the viral load, women with detectable viral load regardless of the amount of therapy received, women with unknown viral load status, and women who have received no prenatal care. Read and Newell's (2009) findings in a *Cochrane* review support elective cesarean section for women not taking anti-retrovirals or for those only in receipt of zidovudine. However, they say the relationship between mother to child transmission is less clear when HIV-positive women have low viral loads and recommend further study in this area. Additional interventions to reduce the transmission risk include avoiding use of a scalp electrode for fetal monitoring or doing a scalp blood sampling for fetal pH, delaying amniotomy, and avoiding invasive procedures such as forceps or vacuum-assisted delivery. The nurse stresses the importance of all interventions and the goal to reduce transmission of HIV to the newborn.

Continuing Assessment During the First Stage of Labour

After the admission assessment is complete, assessment continues for changes that would indicate that labour is progressing as expected. Assess the woman's knowledge, experience, and expectations of labour. Typically, blood pressure, pulse, and respirations are assessed every hour during the latent phase of labour unless the clinical situation dictates that vital signs be taken more frequently. During the active and transition phases, they are assessed every 30 minutes. The temperature is taken every 4 hours throughout the first stage of labour unless the clinical situation dictates more frequent measurement (maternal fever).

Vaginal examinations are performed periodically to track labour progress. This assessment information is shared with the woman to reinforce that she is making progress toward the goal of birth. Uterine contractions are monitored for frequency, duration, and intensity every 30 to 60 minutes during the latent phase, every 15 to 30 minutes during the active phase, and every 15 minutes during transition. Note the changes in the character of the contractions as labour progresses, and inform the woman of her progress. Continually determine the woman's level of pain and her ability to cope and use relaxation techniques effectively.

When the fetal membranes rupture, spontaneously or artificially, assess the FHR and check the amniotic fluid for colour, odour, and amount. Assess the FHR intermittently or continuously via electronic monitoring. During the latent phase of labour, assess the FHR every 30 to 60 minutes; in the active phase, assess FHR at least every 15 to 30 minutes. Also, be sure to assess the FHR before ambulation, prior to any procedure, and before administering analgesia or anesthesia to the mother. Table 14.3 summarizes assessments for the first stage of labour.

TABLE 14.3 SUMMARY OF ASSESSMENTS DURING THE FIRST STAGE OF LABOUR

Assessments[a]	Latent Phase (0–3 cm)	Active Phase (4–7 cm)	Transition (8–10 cm)
Vital signs (blood pressure, pulse, respirations)	Every 30–60 min	Every 30 min	Every 15–30 min
Temperature	Every 4 hours	Every 4 hours	Every 4 hours
Contractions (frequency, duration, intensity)	Every 30–60 min by palpation or continuously by electronic fetal monitoring (EFM)	Every 15–30 min by palpation or continuously by EFM	Every 15 min by palpation or continuously by EFM
Fetal heart rate	Every hour by Doppler or continuously by EFM	Every 30 min by Doppler or continuously by EFM	Every 15–30 min by Doppler or continuously by EFM
Vaginal examination	Initially on admission to determine phase and as needed based on maternal cues to document labour progression	As needed to monitor labour progression	As needed to monitor labour progression
Behaviour/psychosocial	With every client encounter: talkative, excited, anxious	With every client encounter: self-absorbed in labour; intense and quiet now	With every client encounter: discouraged, irritable, feels out of control, declining coping ability

[a]The frequency of assessments is dictated by the health status of the woman and fetus and can be altered if either one of their conditions changes.

*R*emember Sheila from the chapter-opening scenario? What is the nurse's role with Sheila in active labour? What additional comfort measures can the labour nurse offer Sheila?

Nursing Interventions

Nursing interventions during the admission process should include:

- Asking about the client's expectations of the birthing process
- Providing information about labour, birth, pain-management options, and relaxation techniques
- Presenting information about fetal monitoring equipment and the procedures needed
- Monitoring FHR and identifying patterns that need further intervention
- Monitoring the mother's vital signs to obtain a baseline for later comparison
- Reassuring the client that her labour progress will be monitored closely and nursing care will focus on ensuring fetal and maternal well-being throughout

As the woman progresses through the first stage of labour, nursing interventions include:

- Encouraging the woman's partner to participate
- Keeping the woman and her partner up to date on the progress of the labour
- Orienting the woman and her partner to the labour and birth unit and explaining all of the birthing procedures
- Providing clear fluids (e.g., ice chips) as needed or requested
- Maintaining the woman's parenteral fluid intake at the prescribed rate if she has an IV
- Initiating or encouraging comfort measures, such as backrubs, cool cloths to the forehead, frequent position changes, ambulation, showers, slow dancing, leaning over a birth ball, side-lying, or counterpressure on lower back (Teaching Guideline 14.1)
- Encouraging the partner's involvement with breathing techniques
- Assisting the woman and her partner to focus on breathing techniques
- Informing the woman that the discomfort will be intermittent and of limited duration; urging her to rest between contractions to preserve her strength; and encouraging her to use distracting activities to lessen the focus on contractions
- Changing bed linens and gown as needed
- Keeping the perineal area clean and dry

TEACHING GUIDELINE 14.1

Positioning During the First Stage of Labour

- Walking with support from your partner (adds the force of gravity to contractions to promote fetal descent)
- Slow-dancing position with your partner holding you (adds the force of gravity to contractions and promotes support from and active participation of your partner)
- Side-lying with pillows between the knees for comfort (offers a restful position and improves oxygen flow to the uterus)
- Semi-sitting in bed or on a couch leaning against the partner (reduces back pain because fetus falls forward, away from the sacrum)
- Sitting in a chair with one foot on the floor and one on the chair (changes pelvic shape)
- Leaning forward by straddling a chair, a table, or a bed or kneeling over a birth ball (reduces back pain, adds the force of gravity to promote descent; possible pain relief if partner can apply sacral pressure)
- Sitting in a rocking chair or on a birth ball and shifting weight back and forth (provides comfort because rocking motion is soothing; uses the force of gravity to help fetal descent)
- Lunge by rocking weight back and forth with foot up on chair during contraction (uses force of gravity by being upright; enhances rotation of fetus through rocking)

Sources: Adams, E. D., & Bianchi, A. L. (2008). A practical approach to labor support. *Journal of Obstetric, Gynecologic, & Neonatal Nursing, 37,* 106–115; Evans, R. J., Evans, M. K., Brown, Y. M. R., & Orshan, S. A. (2010). *Canadian maternity, newborn, & women's health nursing.* Philadelphia: Lippincott Williams & Wilkins; Lawrence, A., Lewis, L., Hofmeyr, G. J., Dowswell, T., & Styles, C. (2009). Maternal positions and mobility during first stage labour. *Cochrane Database of Systematic Reviews, 2,* CD003934; Lowdermilk, D. L., Perry, S. E., & Cashion, K. (2010). *Maternity nursing* (8th ed.). Maryland Heights, MO: Mosby Elsevier; & Schilling, T. (2009). *Healthy birth practices from Lamaze International: #2 Walk, move around, and change positions throughout labor.* Retrieved February 22, 2012 from http://www.lamaze.org/Portals/0/carepractices/CarePractice2.pdf.

- Supporting the woman's decisions about pain management
- Monitoring maternal vital signs frequently and reporting any abnormal values
- Ensuring that the woman takes deep cleansing breaths before and after each contraction to enhance gas exchange and oxygen to the fetus
- Educating the woman and her partner about the need for rest and helping them plan strategies to conserve strength
- Monitoring FHR for baseline, accelerations, variability, and decelerations

- Checking on bladder status and encouraging voiding at least every 2 hours to make room for birth
- Repositioning the woman as needed to obtain optimal heart rate pattern
- Communicating requests from the woman to appropriate personnel
- Respecting the woman's sense of privacy by covering her when appropriate
- Offering human presence by being present with the woman, not leaving her alone for long periods
- Being patient with the natural labour pattern to allow time for change
- Reporting any deviations from normal to the health care professional so that interventions can be initiated early to be effective (SOGC, 2007).

See Nursing Care Plan 14.1.

Remember Sheila, who was admitted in active labour? She has progressed to the transition phase (8 cm dilated) and is becoming increasingly more uncomfortable. She is using a patterned-paced breathing pattern now but thrashing around in the hospital bed.

Nursing Management During the Second Stage of Labour

Nursing care during the second stage of labour focuses on supporting the woman and her partner with interventions such as assisting with positioning and breathing techniques and providing instruction and assistance as needed. Research suggests that delaying pushing in the second stage of labour reduces the time spent in this stage, decreases the need for instrument-assisted delivery, and lessens postpartum fatigue, which ultimately affect both mother and newborn (Man-Lung, Kuan-Chia, Hsin Yang, et al., 2009). Shortening the phase of active pushing and lengthening the early phase of passive descent can be achieved by encouraging the woman not to push until she has a strong desire to do so and until the descent and rotation of the fetal head are well advanced. Berghella, Baxter, & Chauhan. (2008), in a review of evidence-based interventions, found upright positions such as sitting, semi-recumbency, kneeling, and squatting to be associated with shorter birth intervals, less pain and perineal damage, and fewer operative births.

Perineal lacerations or tears can occur during the second stage when the fetal head emerges through the vaginal introitus. The extent of the laceration is defined by depth: a first-degree laceration extends through the skin; a second-degree laceration extends through the muscles of the perineal body; a third-degree laceration continues through the anal sphincter muscle; and a

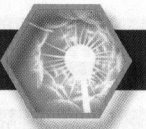

Nursing Care Plan 14.1

OVERVIEW OF THE WOMAN IN THE ACTIVE PHASE OF THE FIRST STAGE OF LABOUR

Candice, a 23-year-old gravida 1, para 0 (G1,P0) is admitted to the labour and birth suite at 39 weeks' gestation having contractions of moderate intensity every 5 to 6 minutes. A vaginal examination reveals her cervix is 80% effaced and 5 cm dilated. The presenting part (vertex) is at 0 station and her membranes ruptured spontaneously 4 hours ago at home. She is admitted and an IV is started for hydration and vascular access. An external fetal monitor is applied. FHR is 140 beats/minute and regular. Her partner is present at her bedside. Candice is now in the active phase of the first stage of labour, and her assessment findings are as follows: cervix dilated 7 cm, 80% effaced; moderate to strong contractions occurring regularly, every 3 to 5 minutes, lasting 45 to 60 seconds; at 0 station on pelvic examination; FHR auscultated loudest below umbilicus at 140 beats/minute; vaginal show—pink or bloody vaginal mucus; currently apprehensive, inwardly focused, with increased dependency; voicing concern about ability to cope with pain; limited ability to follow directions.

NURSING DIAGNOSIS: Anxiety related to labour and birth process and fear of the unknown related to client's first experience

Outcome Identification and Evaluation
Client will remain calm and in control as evidenced by ability to make decisions and use positive coping strategies.

Interventions: Promoting Positive Coping Strategies
• Provide instruction regarding the labour process *to allay anxiety.*
• Reorient the woman to the physical environment and equipment as necessary *to keep her informed of events.*
• Encourage verbalization of feelings and concerns *to reduce anxiety.*
• Listen attentively to woman and partner *to demonstrate interest and concern.*
• Inform woman and partner of standard procedures/processes *to ensure adequate understanding of events and procedures.*
• Frequently update woman of progress and labour status *to provide positive reinforcement for actions.*
• Reinforce relaxation techniques and provide instruction if needed *to aid in coping.*
• Encourage participation of the partner in the coaching role; role-model to facilitate partner participation in labour process *to provide support and encouragement to the client.*
• Provide a presence and remain with woman as much as possible *to provide comfort and support.*

NURSING DIAGNOSIS: Pain related to effects of contractions and cervical dilation and events of labour

Outcome Identification and Evaluation
Client will maintain a tolerable level of pain and discomfort as evidenced by statements of pain relief, pain rating of 2 or less on pain rating scale, and absence of adverse effects in client and fetus from analgesia or anesthesia.

Interventions: Providing Pain Relief
• Monitor vital signs, observe for signs of pain, and have client rate pain on a scale of 0 to 10 *to provide baseline for comparison.*
• Encourage client to void every 1 to 2 hours *to decrease pressure from a full bladder.*
• Assist woman to change positions frequently *to increase comfort and promote labour progress.*
• Encourage use of distraction *to reduce focus on contraction pain.*
• Suggest pelvic rocking, massage, or back counterpressure *to reduce pain.*
• Assist with use of relaxation and breathing techniques *to promote relaxation.*
• Use touch appropriately (backrub) when desired by the woman *to promote comfort.*
• Integrate use of non-pharmacologic measures for pain relief, such as warm water, birthing ball, or other techniques *to facilitate pain relief.*
• Administer pharmacologic agents as ordered when requested *to control pain.*
• Provide reassurance and encouragement between contractions *to foster self-esteem and continued participation in labour process.*

(continued)

Nursing Care Plan 14.1 (continued)

NURSING DIAGNOSIS: Risk of infection related to vaginal examinations following rupture of membranes

Outcome Identification and Evaluation
Client will remain free of infection as evidenced by absence of signs and symptoms of infection, vital signs and FHR within acceptable parameters, lab test results within normal limits, and clear amniotic fluid without odour.

Interventions: Preventing Infection
• Monitor vital signs (every 1 to 2 hours after rupture of membranes) and FHR frequently as per protocol *to allow for early detection of problems;* report fetal tachycardia (early sign of maternal infection) *to ensure prompt treatment.*
• Provide frequent perineal care and pad changes *to maintain good perineal hygiene.*
• Change linens and woman's gown as needed *to maintain cleanliness.*
• Ensure that vaginal examinations are performed only when needed *to prevent introducing pathogens into the vaginal vault.*
• Monitor lab test results such as white blood cell count *to assess for elevations indicating infection.*
• Use aseptic technique for all invasive procedures *to prevent infection transmission.*
• Carry out good handwashing techniques before and after procedures and use standard precautions as appropriate *to minimize risk of infection transmission.*
• Document amniotic fluid characteristics—colour, odour—*to establish baseline for comparison.*

fourth-degree laceration also involves the anterior rectal wall. Third- and fourth-degree lacerations need to be repaired carefully to retain fecal continence (Lowdermilk et al., 2010). The primary care provider should repair any lacerations during the third stage of labour.

An **episiotomy** is an incision made in the perineum to enlarge the vaginal outlet and theoretically to shorten the second stage of labour. An episiotomy can be either midline or mediolateral. There is insufficient evidence to determine which type of incision is better (Carroli & Mignini, 2009). Figure 14.14 shows episiotomy locations.

Registered midwives can perform and repair episiotomies, but they frequently use alternative measures if possible. Alternative measures such as warm compresses

and continual massage with oil have been successful in stretching the perineal area to prevent cutting it. The routine use of episiotomies as compared with a needed (restrictive) approach has been studied for several years; conclusions support use of a restrictive approach, which yields many benefits for the recipients (Carroli & Mignini, 2009). The use of restrictive episiotomy results in less pain postpartum, better sexual function later, and less relaxation of pelvic musculature (Schuurmans, Senikas, & Lalonde, 2009).

Despite the lack of evidence supporting the routine use of episiotomies (PHAC, 2000; SOGC, 2004b, 2010), the Canadian Maternity Experiences Survey reported that one in five women has undergone one. Women who

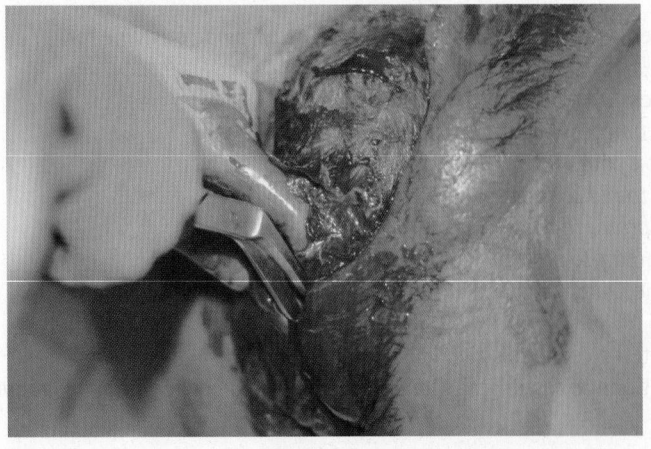

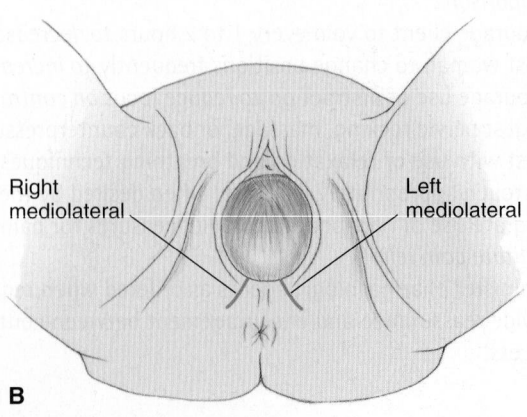

A

B

FIGURE 14.14 Location of an episiotomy. (**A**) Midline episiotomy. (**B**) Right and left mediolateral episiotomies.

TABLE 14.4 SUMMARY OF ASSESSMENTS DURING THE SECOND, THIRD, AND FOURTH STAGES OF LABOUR

Assessments[a]	Second Stage of Labour (Birth of Neonate)	Third Stage of Labour (Placenta Expulsion)	Fourth Stage of Labour (Recovery)
Vital signs (blood pressure, pulse, respirations)	Every 5–15 min	Every 15 min	Every 15 min
Fetal heart rate	Every 5–15 min by Doppler or continuously by electroinc fetal monitoring (EFM)	Apgar scoring at 1 and 5 min	Newborn—complete head-to-toe assessment; vital signs every 15 min until stable
Contractions/ uterus	Palpate every one	Observe for placental separation	Palpate for firmness and position every 15 min for first hour
Bearing down/ pushing	Assist with every effort	None	None
Vaginal discharge	Observe for signs of descent—bulging of perineum, crowning	Assess bleeding after expulsion	Assess every 15 min with fundus firmness check
Behaviour/ psychosocial	Observe every 15 min: cooperative, focus is on work of pushing newborn out	Observe every 15 min: often feelings of relief after hearing newborn crying; calmer	Observe every 15 min: usually excited, talkative, awake; needs to hold newborn, be close, and inspect body

[a]The frequency of assessments is dictated by the health status of the woman and fetus and can be altered if either one of their conditions changes.

have episiotomies are more likely than women who do not have episiotomies to experience more severe perineal trauma, more suturing, more pain, and more healing complications (Carroli & Mignini, 2009).

Assessment

Assessment is continuous during the second stage of labour. Hospital policies dictate the specific type and timing of assessments, as well as the way in which they are documented. Assessment involves identifying the signs typical of the second stage of labour, including:

- Increase in apprehension or irritability
- Spontaneous rupture of membranes
- Sudden appearance of sweat on upper lip
- Increase in blood-tinged show
- Low grunting sounds from the woman
- Complaints of rectal and perineal pressure
- Beginning of involuntary bearing-down efforts

Other ongoing assessments include the contraction frequency, duration, and intensity; maternal vital signs every 5 to 15 minutes; fetal response to labour as indicated by FHR monitor strips; amniotic fluid for colour, odour, and amount when membranes are ruptured; and the coping status of the woman and her partner (Table 14.4).

Assessment also focuses on determining the progress of labour. Associated signs include bulging of the perineum, labial separation, advancing and retreating of the newborn's head during and between bearing-down efforts, and **crowning** (fetal head is visible at vaginal opening; Fig. 14.15).

A vaginal examination is completed to determine if it is appropriate for the woman to push. Pushing is appropriate if the cervix has fully dilated to 10 cm and the woman feels the urge to do so.

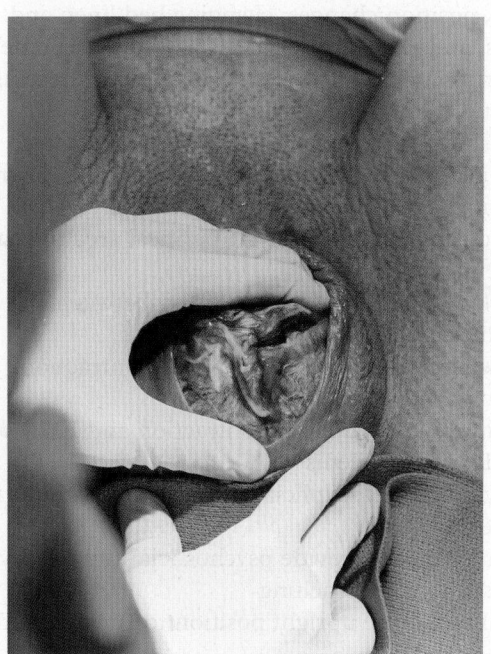

FIGURE 14.15 Crowning.

Nursing Interventions

Nursing interventions during this stage focus on motivating the woman, encouraging her to put all her efforts to pushing this newborn to the outside world, and giving her feedback on her progress. If the woman is pushing and not making progress, suggest that she keep her eyes open during the contractions and look toward where the infant is coming out. Changing positions every 20 to 30 minutes will also help in making progress. Positioning a mirror so the woman can visualize the birthing process and how successful her pushing efforts are can help motivate her.

The benefits of upright positioning during the second stage of labour are related to gravity with less aortovagal compression, improved fetal alignment, and larger anterior–posterior and transverse pelvic outlets (Berghella et al., 2008). Some suggestions for positions in the second stage include:

- Lithotomy with feet up in stirrups: most convenient position for caregivers
- Semi-sitting with pillows underneath knees, arms, and back
- Lateral/side-lying with curved back and upper leg supported by partner
- Sitting on birthing stool: opens pelvis, enhances the pull of gravity, and helps with pushing
- Squatting/supported squatting: gives the woman a sense of control
- Kneeling with hands on bed and knees comfortably apart

Other important nursing interventions during the second stage include:

- Providing continuous comfort measures such as mouth care, position changes, changing bed linen and underpads, and providing a quiet, focused environment
- Instructing the woman on the following bearing-down positions and techniques:
  - Pushing only when she feels an urge to do so
  - Using abdominal muscles when bearing down
  - Using short pushes of 6 to 7 seconds
  - Focusing attention on the perineal area to visualize the newborn
  - Relaxing and conserving energy between contractions
  - Pushing several times with each contraction (Lowdermilk et al., 2010)
- Continuing to monitor contraction and FHR patterns to identify problems
- Providing brief, explicit directions throughout this stage
- Continuing to provide psychosocial support by reassuring and coaching
- Facilitating the upright position to encourage the fetus to descend

- Continuing to assess blood pressure, pulse, respirations, uterine contractions, bearing-down efforts, FHR, coping status of the client and her partner
- Providing pain management if needed
- Providing a continuous nursing presence
- Offering praise for the client's efforts
- Preparing for and assisting with delivery by:
  - Notifying the health care provider of the estimated time frame for birth
  - Preparing the delivery bed and positioning the client
  - Preparing the perineal area according to the facility's protocol
  - Offering a mirror and adjusting it so the woman can watch the birth
  - Explaining all procedures and equipment to the client and her partner
  - Setting up delivery instruments needed while maintaining sterility
  - Receiving newborn and transporting him or her to a warming environment, or covering the newborn with a warmed blanket on the woman's abdomen
  - Providing initial care and assessment of the newborn (see the Birth section that follows)

Sheila is completely dilated now and experiencing the urge to push. How can the nurse help Sheila with her pushing efforts? What additional interventions can the labour nurse offer Sheila now?

Birth

The second stage of labour ends with the birth of the newborn. The maternal position for birth varies from the standard lithotomy position to side-lying to squatting to standing or kneeling, depending on the birthing location, the woman's preference, and standard protocols. Once the woman is positioned for birth, cleanse the vulva and perineal areas. The primary health care provider then takes charge after donning protective eyewear, mask, gown, and gloves and performing hand hygiene.

Once the fetal head has emerged, the primary care provider explores the fetal neck to see if the umbilical cord is wrapped around it. If it is, the cord is slipped over the head to facilitate delivery. As soon as the head emerges, the health care provider suctions the newborn's mouth first (because the newborn is an obligate nose breather) and then the nares with a bulb syringe to prevent aspiration of mucus, amniotic fluid, or meconium (Fig. 14.16). The umbilical cord is double-clamped and cut between the clamps. With the first cries of the newborn, the second stage of labour ends.

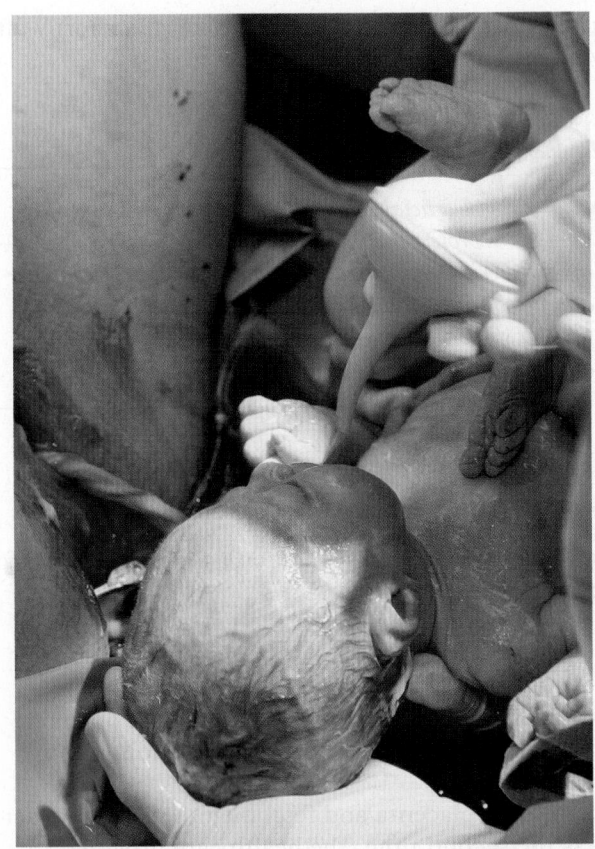

FIGURE 14.16 Suctioning the newborn immediately after birth.

In addition to encouraging Sheila to rest between pushing and offering praise for her efforts, what is the nurse's role during the birthing process?

Immediate Care of the Newborn

Once the infant is born, place him or her under the radiant warmer, dry him or her, assess him or her, wrap him or her in warmed blankets, and place him or her on the woman's abdomen for warmth and closeness. In some health care facilities, the newborn is placed on the woman's abdomen immediately after birth and covered with a warmed blanket. In either scenario, the stability of the newborn dictates the location of aftercare. The nurse can also assist the mother with breastfeeding her newborn for the first time.

Assessment of the newborn begins at the moment of birth and continues until the newborn is discharged. Drying the newborn and providing warmth to prevent heat loss by evaporation is essential to help support thermoregulation and provide stimulation. Placing the newborn under a radiant heat source and putting on a stockinet cap will further reduce heat loss after drying.

Assess the newborn by assigning an Apgar score at 1 and 5 minutes. The Apgar score assesses five parameters—heart rate (absent, slow, or fast), respiratory effort (absent,

weak cry, or good strong yell), muscle tone (limp, or lively and active), response to irritation stimulus, and colour—that evaluate a newborn's cardiorespiratory adaptation after birth. The parameters are arranged from the most important (heart rate) to the least important (colour). The newborn is assigned a score of 0 to 2 in each of the five parameters. The purpose of the Apgar assessment is to evaluate the physiologic status of the newborn; see Chapter 18 for additional information on Apgar scoring.

To verify his or her identity, secure two identification bands on the newborn, one on the wrist and one on the ankle, that match the band on the mother's wrist. This identification process is completed in the birthing suite before anyone leaves the room. Some facilities provide an additional identical band for the father as well (Lowdermilk et al., 2010). The bands should fit snugly to prevent loss.

Other types of newborn security systems can also be used to prevent abduction. Some systems have sensors that are attached to the newborn's identification bracelet or cord clamp. An alarm is set off if the bracelet or clamp activates receivers near exits. Others have an alarm that is activated when the sensor is removed from the newborn (Fig. 14.17). Although newborn abduction is not common in hospitals, additional security measures in maternity wards are now common across Canada and are supported by policies. Visitors are often screened in some way before they are allowed access to the newborn (Evans et al., 2010). Examples include controlled unit access with videos and alarms, family and support people wearing identification bracelets to match baby's, all newborns transported in cribs and those carrying a newborn in their arms are questioned. Parents are educated in the basics of hospital security (Evans et al., 2010).

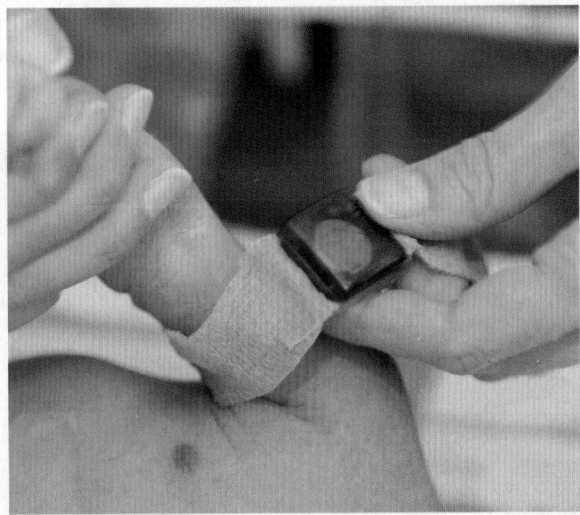

FIGURE 14.17 An example of a security sensor applied to a newborn's arm.

Sheila gave birth to a healthy 7-pound, 7-ounce baby girl (3,500 g). She is eager to hold and nurse her newborn. What is the initial care of the newborn? How can the nurse meet the needs of both the newborn and Sheila, who is exhausted but eager to bond with her newborn?

Nursing Management During the Third Stage of Labour

During the third stage of labour, strong uterine contractions continue at regular intervals under the continuing influence of oxytocin. The uterine muscle fibres shorten, or retract, with each contraction, leading to a gradual decrease in the size of the uterus, which helps shear the placenta away from its attachment site. The third stage is complete when the placenta is delivered. Nursing care during the third stage of labour focuses primarily on immediate newborn care and assessment and being available to assist with the delivery of the placenta and inspecting it for intactness.

Three hormones play important roles in the third stage. During this stage the woman experiences peak levels of oxytocin and endorphins, while the high adrenaline levels that occurred during the second stage of labour to aid with pushing begin falling. The hormone oxytocin causes uterine contractions and helps the woman to enact instinctive mothering behaviours such as holding the newborn close to her body and cuddling the baby.

Skin-to-skin contact immediately after birth and the newborn's first attempt at breastfeeding further augment maternal oxytocin levels, strengthening the uterine contractions that will help the placenta to separate and the uterus to contract to prevent hemorrhage. Endorphins, the body's natural opiates, produce an altered state of consciousness and aid in blocking out pain. In addition, the drop in adrenaline level from the second stage, which had kept the mother and baby alert at first contact, causes most women to shiver and feel cold shortly after giving birth.

> ▶ **Take** NOTE!
>
> *A crucial role for nurses during this time is to protect the natural hormonal process by ensuring unhurried and uninterrupted contact between mother and newborn after birth, providing warmed blankets to prevent shivering, and allowing skin-to-skin contact and breastfeeding.*

Assessment

Assessment during the third stage of labour includes:

- Monitoring placental separation by looking for the following signs:
  - Firmly contracting uterus
  - Change in uterine shape from discoid to globular ovoid
  - Sudden gush of dark blood from vaginal opening
  - Lengthening of umbilical cord protruding from vagina
- Examining placenta and fetal membranes for intactness the second time (the health care provider assesses the placenta for intactness the first time) (Fig. 14.18)
- Assessing for any perineal trauma, such as the following, before allowing the birth attendant to leave:
  - Firm fundus with bright-red blood trickling: laceration
  - Boggy fundus with red blood flowing: uterine atony
  - Boggy fundus with dark blood and clots: retained placenta
- Inspecting the perineum for condition of episiotomy, if performed
- Assessing for perineal lacerations and ensuring repair by birth attendant

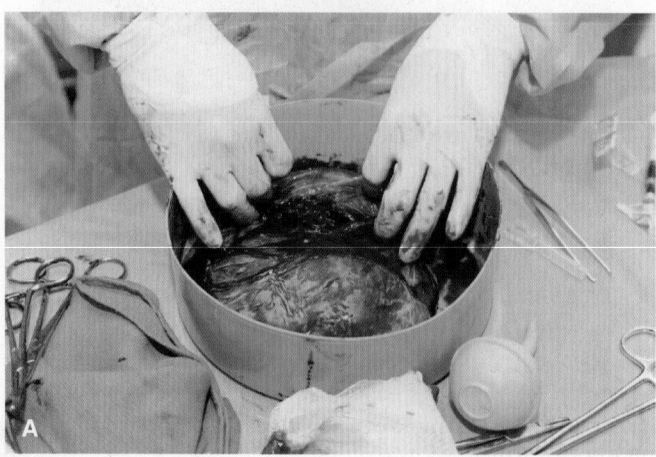 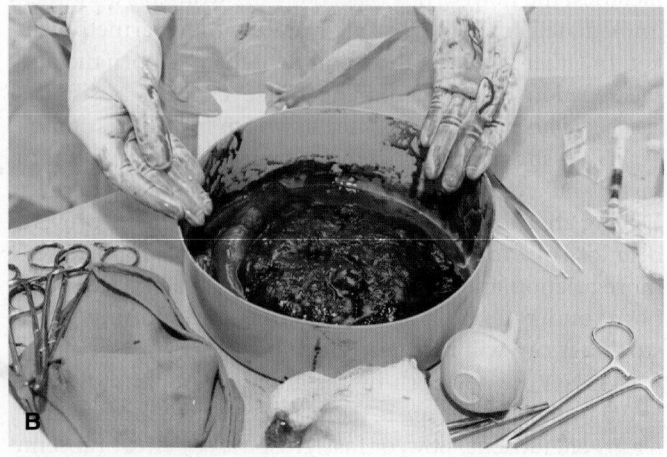

FIGURE 14.18 Placenta. (**A**) Fetal side. (**B**) Maternal side.

Nursing Interventions

Interventions during the third stage of labour include:

- Describing the process of placental separation to the couple
- Instructing the woman to push when signs of separation are apparent
- Administering oxytocin if ordered and indicated after placental expulsion
- Providing support and information about episiotomy and/or laceration
- Cleaning and assisting the client into a comfortable position after birth, making sure to lift both legs out of stirrups (if used) simultaneously to prevent strain
- Repositioning the birthing bed to serve as a recovery bed if applicable
- Assisting with transfer to the recovery area if applicable
- Providing warmth by replacing warmed blankets over the woman
- Applying an ice pack to the perineal area to provide comfort to episiotomy if indicated
- Explaining what assessments will be carried out over the next hour and offering positive reinforcement for actions
- Ascertaining any needs
- Monitoring maternal physical status by assessing:
  - Vaginal bleeding: amount, consistency, and colour
  - Vital signs: blood pressure, pulse, and respirations taken every 15 minutes
  - Uterine fundus, which should be firm, in the midline, and at the level of the umbilicus
- Recording all birthing statistics and securing the primary caregiver's signature
- Documenting birthing event in the birth book (official record of the facility that outlines every birth event), detailing any deviations

Nursing Management During the Fourth Stage of Labour

The fourth stage of labour begins after the placenta is expelled and lasts up to 4 hours after birth, during which time recovery takes place. This recovery period may take place in the same room where the woman gave birth, in a separate recovery area, or in her postpartum room. During this stage, the woman's body is beginning to undergo the many physiologic and psychological changes that occur after birth. The focus of nursing management during the fourth stage of labour involves frequent close observation for hemorrhage, provision of comfort measures, and promotion of family attachment.

Assessment

Assessments during the fourth stage centre on the woman's vital signs, status of the uterine fundus and perineal area, comfort level, lochia amount, and bladder status. During the first hour after birth, vital signs are taken every 15 minutes, then every 30 minutes for the next hour if needed. The woman's blood pressure should remain stable and within normal range after giving birth. A decrease may indicate uterine hemorrhage; an elevation might suggest pre-eclampsia.

The pulse usually is typically slower (60 to 70 beats/minute) than during labour. This may be associated with a decrease in blood volume following placental separation. An elevated pulse rate may be an early sign of blood loss. The blood pressure usually returns to its pre-pregnancy level and therefore is not a reliable early indicator of shock. Fever is indicative of dehydration (<100.4°F or 38°C) or infection (>101°F or 38.3°C), which may involve the genitourinary tract. Respiratory rate is usually between 16 and 24 breaths/minute and regular. Respirations should be unlaboured unless there is an underlying preexisting respiratory condition.

Assess fundal height, position, and firmness every 15 minutes during the first hour following birth. The fundus needs to remain firm to prevent excessive postpartum bleeding. The fundus should be firm (feels like the size and consistency of a grapefruit), located in the midline and below the umbilicus. If it is not firm (boggy), gently massage it until it is firm (see Nursing Procedure 22.1 in Chapter 22 for more information). Once firmness is obtained, stop massaging.

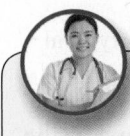

> ▶ *Take* NOTE!
>
> *If the fundus is displaced to the right of the midline, suspect a full bladder as the cause.*

The vagina and perineal areas are quite stretched and edematous following a vaginal birth. Assess the perineum, including the episiotomy if present, for possible hematoma formation. Suspect a hematoma if the woman reports excruciating pain or cannot void or if a mass is noted in the perineal area. Also assess for hemorrhoids, which can cause discomfort.

Assess the woman's comfort level frequently to determine the need for analgesia. Ask the woman to rate her pain on a scale of 1 to 10; it should be less than 3. If it is higher, further evaluation is needed to make sure there aren't any deviations contributing to her discomfort.

Assess vaginal discharge (lochia) every 15 minutes for the first hour and every 30 minutes for the next hour. Palpate the fundus at the same time to ascertain its firmness and help to estimate the amount of vaginal discharge. In addition, palpate the bladder for fullness, since many women receiving an epidural block experience limited sensation in the bladder region. Voiding should produce large amounts of urine (diuresis) each time. Palpation of the woman's bladder after each voiding helps to ensure complete emptying. A full bladder will displace the uterus to either side of the midline and potentiate uterine hemorrhage secondary to bogginess.

Nursing Interventions

Nursing interventions during the fourth stage might include:

- Providing support and information to the woman regarding episiotomy repair and related pain-relief and self-care measures
- Applying an ice pack to the perineum to promote comfort and reduce swelling
- Assisting with hygiene and perineal care; teaching the woman how to use the perineal bottle after each pad change and voiding; helping the woman into a new gown
- Monitoring for return of sensation and ability to void (if regional anesthesia was used)
- Encouraging the woman to void by ambulating to bathroom, listening to running water, or pouring warm water over the perineal area with the peri bottle
- Monitoring vital signs and fundal and lochia status every 15 minutes and documenting them
- Promoting comfort by offering analgesia for afterpains and warm blankets to reduce chilling
- Offering fluids and nourishment if desired
- Encouraging parent–infant attachment by providing privacy for the family
- Being knowledgeable about and sensitive to typical cultural practices after birth
- Assisting the mother to nurse, if she chooses, during the recovery period to promote uterine firmness (the release of oxytocin from the posterior pituitary gland stimulates uterine contractions)
- Teaching the woman how to assess her fundus for firmness periodically and to massage it if it is boggy
- Describing the lochia flow and normal parameters to observe for postpartum
- Teaching safety techniques to prevent newborn abduction
- Demonstrating the use of the portable sitz bath as a comfort measure for her perineum if she had a laceration or an episiotomy repair
- Explain comfort/hygiene measures and when to use them
- Assisting with ambulation when getting out of bed for the first time
- Providing information about the routine on the mother–baby unit or nursery for her stay
- Assessing for signs of early parent–infant attachment: provides touch at times other than during feedings, meets all of baby's physical needs (Rice Simpson & Creehan, 2010)

▪▪▪ Key Concepts

- A nurse provides physical and emotional support during the labour and birth process to assist a woman to achieve her goals.
- When a woman is admitted to the labour and birth area, the admitting nurse must assess and evaluate the risk status of the pregnancy and initiate appropriate interventions to provide optimal care for the client.
- Completing an admission assessment includes taking a maternal health history; performing physical assessment on the woman and fetus, including her emotional and psychosocial status; and obtaining the necessary laboratory studies.
- The nurse's role in fetal assessment for labour and birth includes determining fetal well-being and interpreting signs and symptoms of possible compromise. Determining the FHR pattern and assessing amniotic fluid characteristics are key.
- FHR can be assessed intermittently or continuously. Although the intermittent method allows the client to move about during labour, the information obtained intermittently does not provide a complete picture of fetal well-being from moment to moment.
- Assessment parameters of the FHR are classified as baseline rate, baseline variability (long-term and short-term), and periodic changes in the rate (accelerations and decelerations).
- The nurse monitoring the labouring client needs to be knowledgeable about which parameters are normal, atypical, and abnormal so that appropriate interventions can be instituted.
- For an atypical FHR pattern, the nurse should notify the health care provider about the pattern and obtain further orders, making sure to document all interventions and their effects on the FHR pattern.
- In addition to interpreting assessment findings and initiating appropriate inventions for the labouring client, accurate and timely documentation must be carried out continuously.
- Today's women have many safe non-pharmacologic and pharmacologic choices for the management of pain during childbirth. They may be used individually or in combination to complement one another.
- Nursing management for the woman during labour and birth includes comfort measures, emotional support, information and instruction, advocacy, and support for the partner.
- Nursing care during the first stage of labour includes taking an admission history (reviewing the prenatal record), checking the results of routine laboratory work and special tests done during pregnancy, asking the woman about her childbirth preparation (birth plan, classes taken, coping skills), and completing a physical assessment of the woman to establish a baseline of values for future comparison.

- Nursing care during the second stage of labour focuses on supporting the woman and her partner in making decisions about her care and labour management, implementing strategies to prolong the early passive phase of fetal descent, supporting involuntary bearing-down efforts, providing instruction and assistance, and encouraging the use of maternal positions that can enhance descent and reduce the pain.

- Nursing care during the third stage of labour primarily focuses on immediate newborn care and assessment and being available to assist with the delivery of the placenta and inspecting it for intactness.

- The focus of nursing management during the fourth stage of labour involves frequently observing the mother for hemorrhage, providing comfort measures, and promoting family attachment.

REFERENCES

Adams, E. D., & Bianchi, A. L. (2008). A practical approach to labor support. *Journal of Obstetric, Gynecologic, and Neonatal Nursing, 37,* 106–115.

Akerman, N., & Dresner, M. (2009). The management of breakthrough pain during labour. *CNS Drugs, 23*(8), 669–679.

Alam, R., Raheen, M. R., Iqbal, K. M., & Chowdhury, R. A. (2011). Headache following spinal anaesthesia: A review on recent update. *Journal of Bangladesh College of Physicians and Surgeons, 29*(1), 32–40.

Alfirevic, Z., Devane, D., & Gyte, G. M. L. (2008). Continuous cardiotocography (CTG) as a form of electronic fetal monitoring (EFM) for fetal assessment during labour. *Cochrane Database of Systematic Reviews, 3,* CD006066.

American College of Obstetricians and Gynecologists. (2009). *Intrapartum fetal heart rate monitoring: Nomenclature, interpretation, and general management principles. ACOG Practice Bulletin No. 106.* Washington, DC: Author.

Association of Women's Health, Obstetric, and Neonatal Nurses. (2011). *Nursing support of laboring women [Clinical Position Statement].* Washington, DC: Author. Retrieved from http://www.awhonn.org/awhonn/content.do?name=05_HealthPolicyLegislation/5H_PositionStatements.htm

Berghella, V., Baxter, J. K., & Chauhan, S. K. (2008). Evidence-based labor and delivery management. *American Journal of Obstetrics and Gynecology, 100*(5), 445–454.

Berkowitz, B. (2008). Cultural aspects in the care of the orthodox Jewish woman. *Journal of Midwifery and Women's Health, 53*(1), 62–67.

Borup, L., Wurlitzer, W., Hedegaard, M., Kesmodel, U., & Hvidman, L. (2009). Acupuncture as pain relief during delivery: a randomized controlled trial. *Birth: Issues in Perinatal Care, 36*(1), 5–12.

British Columbia Perinatal Health Program. (2009). *Core competencies: Management of labour in an institutional setting if the primary maternal care provider is absent. Guidelines for registered nurses.* Vancouver, BC: BC Perinatal Health Program. Retrieved February 22, 2012 from http://www.viha.ca/NR/rdonlyres/A20CC622-1C76-4ADA-9CE5-06A464AD99F3/0/mol_linked_core_competencies_with_dst_june_2010.pdf

Bryanton, J., Gagnon, A., Johnston, C., & Hatem, M. (2008). Predictor of women's perceptions of the childbirth experience. *Journal of Obstetric, Gynecologic, and Neonatal Nursing, 37*(1), 24–34.

Canadian Anesthesiologists' Society. (2010). *Guidelines for acute pain management using neuraxial analgesia.* Retrieved September 4, 2010 from http://www.cas.ca/members/

Canadian Institute for Health Information. (2010). *Highlights of 2008–2009 selected indicators describing the birthing process in Canada.* Retrieved February 22, 2012 from http://secure.cihi.ca/cihiweb/products/childbirth_highlights_2010_05_18_e.pdf

Carroli, G., & Mignini, L. (2009). Episiotomy for vaginal birth. *Cochrane Database of Systematic Reviews, 1,* CD000081.

Cheng, Y., & Caughey, A. B. (2012). *Normal labor and delivery.* Retrieved February 20, 2012 from http://emedicine.medscape.com/article/260036-print

Childbirth: An epidural. (2011). Retrieved September 4, 2010 from http://womenshealthmatters.info/centres/pregnancy/childbirth/epidural.html

Cluett, E. R., & Burns, E. (2009). Immersion in water in labour and birth. *Cochrane Database of Systematic Reviews, 2,* CD000111.

Currell, R., Urquhart, C., Harlow, F., & Callow, L. (2009). Home uterine monitoring for detecting preterm labour. *Cochrane Database of Systematic Reviews, 1,* CD006172.

D'Avanzo, C. E. (2008). *Cultural health assessment* (4th ed.). St. Louis, MO: Mosby Elsevier.

Datta, S., Kodali, B. S., & Segal, S. (2009). *Obstetric anesthesia handbook* (5th ed.). New York: Springer.

Deglin, J. H., Vallerand, A. H., & Sanoski, C. A. (2011). *Davis's drug guide for nurses* (12th ed.). Philadelphia: FA Davis Company.

East, C. E., Chan, F. Y., Colditz, P. B., & Begg, L. (2007). Fetal pulse oximetry for fetal assessment in labour. *Cochrane Database of Systematic Reviews, 2,* CD004075.

Evans, R. J., Evans, M. K., Brown, Y. M. R., & Orshan, S. A. (2010). *Canadian maternity, newborn, & women's health nursing.* Philadelphia: Lippincott Williams & Wilkins.

Grant, G. J. (2010). Neuraxial analgesia and anesthesia for labor and delivery: Drugs. Retrieved February 22, 2012 from http://www.uptodate.com/patients/content/topic.do?topicKey=~.vo.0WZNfzauWD

Hodnett, E. D., Gates, S., Hofmeyr, G. J., & Sakala, C. (2009a). Continuous support for women during childbirth. *Cochrane Database of Systematic Reviews, 3,* CD003766.

Hodnett, E. D., Stremler, R., Weston, J. A., & McKeever, P. (2009b). Re-conceptualizing the hospital labor room: The PLACE (Pregnant and Laboring in an Ambient Clinical Environment) pilot trial. *Birth, 36*(2), 159–166 DOI: 10.1111/j.1523-536X.2009.00311.x

Iams, J. D., Romero, R., Culhane, J. F., & Goldenberg, R. L. (2008). Primary, secondary, and tertiary interventions to reduce the morbidity and mortality of preterm birth. *Lancet, 37*(9607), 164–175.

Institute for Clinical Systems Improvement. (2011). *Health care guideline: Management of labor* (4th ed.). Retrieved February 22, 2012 from http://www.icsi.org/labor/labor__management_of_full_version__2.html

Kennedy, B. B., Ruth, D. J., & Martin, E. J. (2009). *Intrapartum management modules: A perinatal education program* (4th ed.). Philadelphia: Lippincott Williams & Wilkins.

Klein, M. C., Kaczorowski, J., Hall, W. A., et al. (2009). The attitudes of Canadian maternity care practitioners towards labour and birth: Many differences but important similarities. *Journal of Obstetrics and Gynaecology Canada, 31*(9), 827–840.

Ladewig, P. A., London, M. L., & Davidson, M. R. (2009). *Contemporary maternal-newborn nursing care* (7th ed.). Upper Saddle River, NJ: Pearson.

Landau, R. (2009). What's new in obstetric anesthesia. *International Journal of Obstetric Analgesia, 18,* 368–372.

Lavender, T., Hart, A., & Smyth, R. M. D. (2008). Effect of partogram use on outcomes for women in spontaneous labour at term. *Cochrane Database of Systematic Reviews, 4,* CD005461.

Lawrence, A., Lewis, L., Hofmeyr, G. J., Dowswell, T., & Styles, C. (2009). Maternal positions and mobility during first stage labour. *Cochrane Database of Systematic Reviews, 2,* CD003934.

Leap, N., Sandall, J., Buckland, S., & Huber, U. (2010). Journey to confidence: Women's experiences of pain in labour and relational continuity of care. *Journal of Midwifery and Women's Health, 55*(3), 234–242.

Low, J. (2009). Operative delivery: Yesterday and today. *Journal of Obstetrics and Gynaecology Canada, 29*(2), 132–141.

Lowdermilk, D. L., Perry, S. E., & Cashion, K. (2010). *Maternity nursing* (8th ed.). Maryland Heights, MO: Mosby Elsevier.

Macones, G. A., Hankins, G. D. V., Spong, C. Y., Hauth, J., & Moore, T. (2008). The 2008 National Institute of Child Health and Human Development workshop report on electronic fetal monitoring: Update on definitions, interpretation, and research guidelines. *Journal of Obstetric, Gynecologic, and Neonatal Nursing, 37*(5), 510–515.

Man-Lung, L., Kuan-Chia, L., Hsin Yang, L., Kuang-Shing, S., & Meei-Ling, G. (2009). Effects of delayed pushing during the second stage of labor on postpartum fatigue and birth outcomes in nulliparous women. *Journal of Nursing Research, 17*(1), 62–72.

Matsuo, K., Scanlon, J. T., Atlas, R. O., & Kopelman, J. N. (2008). Staircase sign: A newly described uterine contraction pattern seen in rupture of unscarred gravid uterus. *Journal of Obstetrics and Gynaecological Research, 34*(1), 100–104.

Menacker, F., & Martin, J. (2009). BirthStats: rates of cesarean delivery, and unassisted and assisted vaginal delivery, United States, 1996, 2000, and 2006. *Birth: Issues in Perinatal Care, 36*(2), 167.

Menihan, C. A., & Kopel, E. (2008). *Fetal monitoring: Concepts and applications.* Philadelphia: Lippincott Williams & Wilkins.

Moldenhauer, J. S. (2008). Premature rupture of membranes (PROM). *The Merck Manual for Healthcare Professionals.* Retrieved February 20, 2012 from http://www.merck.com/mmpe/sec18/ch264/ch264j.html

Monroe, C. M. (2009). The effects of therapeutic touch on pain. *Journal of Holistic Nursing, 27*(2), 84–92.

National Aboriginal Health Organization. (2008). *Celebrating birth: Aboriginal midwifery in Canada.* Ottawa, ON: Author. Retrieved February 20, 2012 from http://www.naho.ca/documents/naho/english/midwifery/celebratingBirth/Midwiferypaper_English.pdf

Perinatal Education Associates, Inc. (2010). *Breathing.* Retrieved February 20, 2012 from http://www.birthsource.com/scripts/article.asp?articleid=211

Pillitteri, A. (2010). *Maternal & child health nursing: Care of the childbearing & childrearing family.* Philadelphia: Wolters Kluwer.

Public Health Agency of Canada. (2000). *Family-centred maternity and newborn care: National Guidelines.* Retrieved February 20, 2012 from http://www.phac-aspc.gc.ca/hp-ps/dca-dea/publications/fcm-smp/index-eng.php

Public Health Agency of Canada. (2008). *Canadian perinatal health report, 2008 edition.* Retrieved February 20, 2012 from http://www.publichealth.gc.ca/cphr/

Read, J. S., & Newell, M. L. (2009). Efficacy and safety of cesarean delivery for prevention of mother-to-child transmission of HIV-1. *Cochrane Database of Systematic Reviews, 1*, 1–15.

Reynolds, F. (2010). The effects of maternal labour analgesia on the fetus. *Best Practice and Research: Clinical Obstetrics and Gynaecology, 24*(3), 289–302.

Rice Simpson, K., & Creehan, P. A. (2008). *Perinatal nursing.* Philadelphia: AWHONN & Lippincott Williams & Wilkins.

Rose, M. K. (2009). *Comfort touch: Massage for the elderly and the ill.* Philadelphia: Lippincott Williams & Wilkins.

Royal Australian and New Zealand College of Obstetricians and Gynaecologists. (2008). *Warm water immersion during labour and birth: College statement C-Obs 24.* Retrieved February 22, 2012 from http://www.ranzcog.edu.au/womens-health/statements-a-guidelines/college-statements/424-warm-water-immersion-in-labour-and-birth-c-obs-24.html

Schilling, T. (2009). *Healthy birth practices from Lamaze International: #2 Walk, move around, and change positions throughout labor.* Retrieved February 22, 2012 from http://www.lamaze.org/Portals/0/carepractices/CarePractice2.pdf

Schuurmans, N., Senikas, V., & Lalonde, A. B. (2009). *Healthy beginnings* (4th ed.). Mississauga: Wiley.

Simkin, P. (2008). *The birth partner: A complete guide to childbirth for dads, doulas, and all other labor companions* (3rd ed.). Boston, MA: The Harvard Common Press.

Simkin, P. (2010). Ten ways to relieve labor pain. *Pregnancy Birth and Beyond: Lamaze International.* Retrieved February 22, 2012 from http://magazine.lamaze.org/Birth/ComfortZone/tabid/195/Default.aspx

Simmons, S. W., Cyna, A. M., Dennis, A. T., & Hughes, D. (2009). Combined spinal-epidural versus epidural analgesia in labour. *Cochrane Database of Systematic Reviews, 1*, CD003401.

Smith, C. A., Collins, C. T., Cyna, A. M., & Crowther, C. A. (2006). Complementary and alternative therapies for pain management in labour. *Cochrane Database of Systematic Reviews, 4*, CD003521.

Society of Obstetricians and Gynaecologists of Canada. (2008a). *A National Birthing Initiative for Canada.* Retrieved February 22, 2012 from http://www.sogc.org/projects/birthing-strategy_e.asp

Society of Obstetricians and Gynaecologists of Canada. (2008b). Joint policy statement on normal childbirth. *Journal of Obstetrics and Gynecology in Canada, 30*(12), 1163–1165. Retrieved February 22, 2012 from http://www.sogc.org/guidelines/documents/gui221PS0812.pdf

Society of Obstetricians and Gynaecologists of Canada. (2008c). *Media advisories: Rising C-section rates add risks during childbirth and place excess strain on the healthcare system, warn Canadian obstetricians.* Retrieved February 22, 2012 from http://www.sogc.org/media/advisories-20080625_e.asp

Society of Obstetricians and Gynaecologists of Canada. (2008d). Joint policy statement on normal childbirth. *Journal of Obstetrics and Gynaecology Canada, 30*(12), 1163–1165.

Society of Obstetricians and Gynecologists of Canada. (2001). SOGC clinical practice guidelines: Mode of delivery for pregnant women infected by the human immunodeficiency virus. *Journal of Obstetrics and Gynaecology Canada, 23*(4), 348–350. Retrieved February 22, 2012 from http://www.sogc.org/guidelines/public/101E-CPG-April2001.pdf

Society of Obstetricians and Gynecologists of Canada. (2004a). SOGC clinical practice guidelines: The prevention of early-onset neonatal group B streptococcal disease. *Journal of Obstetrics and Gynaecology Canada, 26*(9), 826–832. Retrieved February 22, 2012 from http://www.sogc.org/guidelines/public/149E-CPG-September2004.pdf

Society of Obstetricians and Gynecologists of Canada. (2004b). SOGC clinical practice guidelines: Guidelines for operative vaginal birth. *Journal of Obstetrics and Gynaecology Canada, 26*(8), 747–753. Retrieved February 22, 2012 from http://www.sogc.org/guidelines/public/148E-CPG-August2004.pdf

Society of Obstetricians and Gynecologists of Canada. (2007). SOGC clinical practice guidelines: Fetal health surveillance: Antepartum and intrapartum consensus guideline. *Journal of Obstetrics and Gynecology in Canada, 29*(9), S3–S56. Retrieved February 22, 2012 from http://www.sogc.org/guidelines/documents/gui197CPG0709.pdf

Stark, M. A., Rudell, B., & Haus, G. (2008). Observing position and movements in hydrotherapy: A pilot study. *Journal of Obstetric, Gynecologic, and Neonatal Nursing, 37*(1), 116–122.

Steer, P. J. (2008). Has electronic fetal heart rate monitoring made a difference. *Seminars in Fetal and Neonatal Medicine, 13*(1), 2–3.

The Merck Manual. (2007). *Management of normal labor.* Retrieved February 22, 2012 from http://www.merck.com/mmpe/sec18/ch260/ch260d.html#sec18-ch260-ch260d-1073

Therapeutic Touch International Association. (2010). *Therapeutic touch policy and procedure for health care professionals.* Retrieved February 22, 2012 from http://www.therapeutic-touch.org/newsarticle.php?newsID=6

Tucker, S. M., Miller, L. A., & Miller, D. A. (2009). *Mosby's pocket guide to fetal monitoring: A multidisciplinary approach* (6th ed.). St. Louis, MO: Mosby.

Tzeng, Y., & Su, T. (2008). Low back pain during labor and related factors. *Journal of Nursing Research, 16*(3), 231–240.

Wolf, J. H. (2009). *Deliver me from pain: Anesthesia and Birth in America.* Baltimore, MD: The Johns Hopkins University Press.

Woods, C. J., & Levy, C. S. (2011). *Streptococcus group B infections.* Retrieved September 4, 2010 from http://emedicine.medscape.com/article/229091-overview

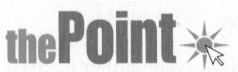

For additional learning materials, including Internet Resources, go to http://thePoint.lww.com/Chow1e.

CHAPTER WORKSHEET

MULTIPLE CHOICE QUESTIONS

1. When a client in labour is fully dilated, which instruction would be most effective to assist her in encouraging effective pushing?

   a. Hold your breath and push through entire contraction.

   b. Use chest-breathing with the contraction.

   c. Pant and blow during each contraction.

   d. Push for 6 to 7 seconds several times during each contraction.

2. During the fourth stage of labour, the nurse palpates the uterus on the right side and sees a saturated perineal pad. What is the nurse's first action?

   a. Massage the uterus vigorously.

   b. Have the client void and reassess her.

   c. Notify the primary care provider.

   d. Document as a normal finding.

3. When managing a client's pain during labour, nurses should:

   a. Make sure the agents given don't prolong labour.

   b. Know that all pain-relief measures are similar.

   c. Support the client's decisions and requests.

   d. Not recommend non-pharmacologic methods.

4. When caring for a client during the active phase of labour without continuous EFM, the nurse would intermittently assess FHR every:

   a. 15 minutes

   b. 5 minutes

   c. 30 minutes

   d. 60 minutes

5. The nurse notes the presence of transient fetal accelerations on the fetal monitoring strip. Which intervention would be most appropriate?

   a. Reposition the client on the left side.

   b. Begin 100% oxygen via face mask.

   c. Document this reassuring pattern.

   d. Call the health care provider immediately.

CRITICAL THINKING EXERCISES

1. Carrie, a 20-year-old primigravida at term, comes to the birthing centre in active labour (dilation 5 cm and 80% effaced, -1 station) with ruptured membranes. She states she wants an "all-natural" birth without medication. Her partner is with her and appears anxious but supportive. On the admission assessment, Carrie's prenatal history is unremarkable; vital signs are within normal limits; FHR via Doppler ranges between 140 and 144 beats/minute and is regular.

   a. Based on your assessment data and the woman's request not to have medication, what non-pharmacologic interventions could you offer her?

   b. What positions might be suggested to facilitate fetal descent?

2. Several hours later, Carrie complains of nausea and turns to her partner and angrily tells him to not touch her and to go away.

   a. What assessment needs to be done to determine what is happening?

   b. What explanation can you offer Carrie's partner regarding her change in behaviour?

STUDY ACTIVITIES

1. Share experiences within a postclinical conference group regarding the pain management interventions of the patients to which you were assigned. Compare and evaluate the effectiveness of different methods used, maternal behaviour observed, and neonatal outcome in terms of Apgar scores.

2. On the fetal heart monitor, the nurse notices an elevation of the fetal baseline with the onset of contractions. This elevation would describe _____.

3. Compare and contrast a local birthing centre to a community hospital's birthing suite in terms of the pain-management techniques and fetal monitoring used.

4. Select a childbirth website for expectant parents and critique the information provided in terms of its educational level and amount of advertising.

UNIT FIVE

POSTPARTUM PERIOD

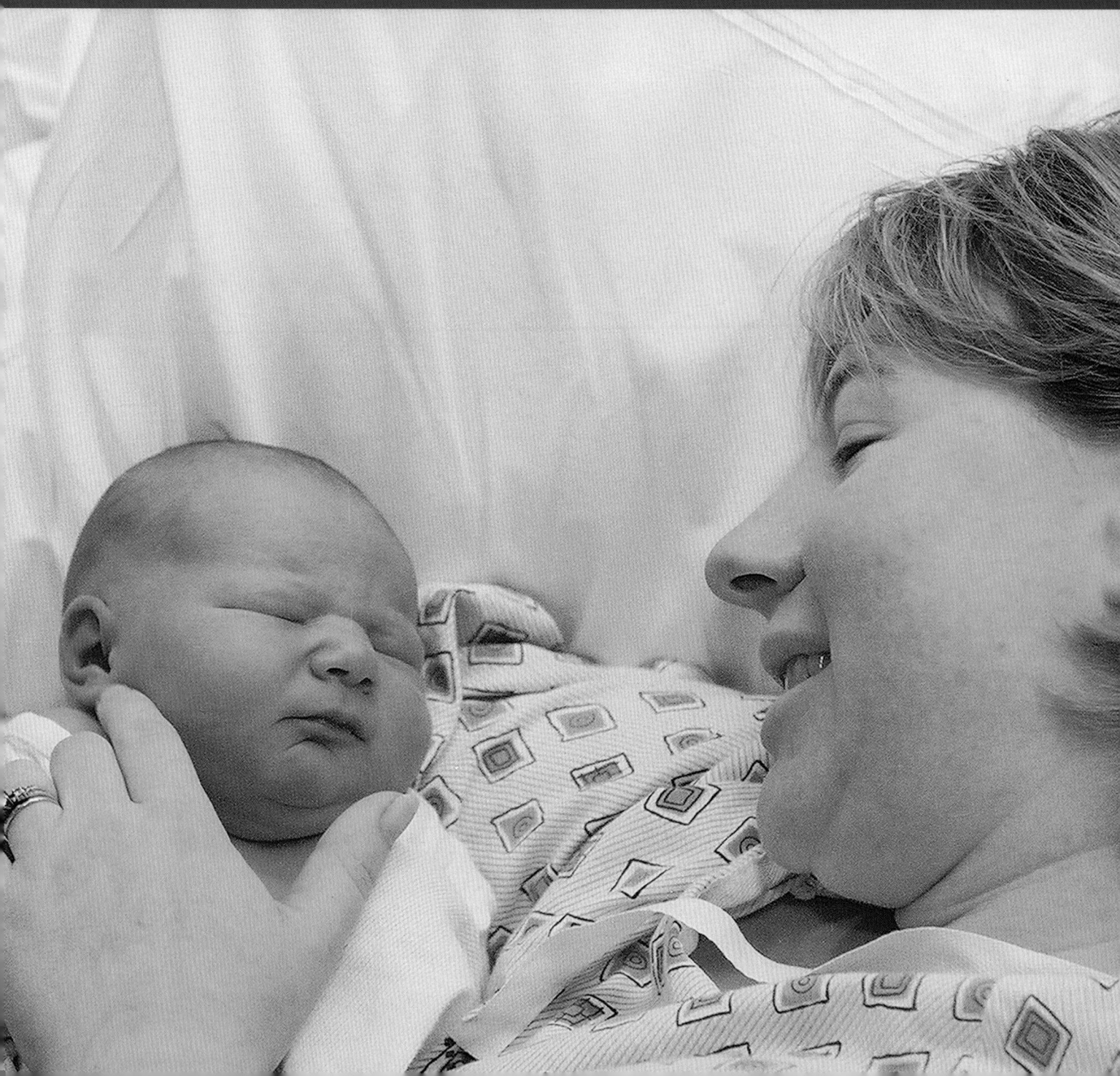

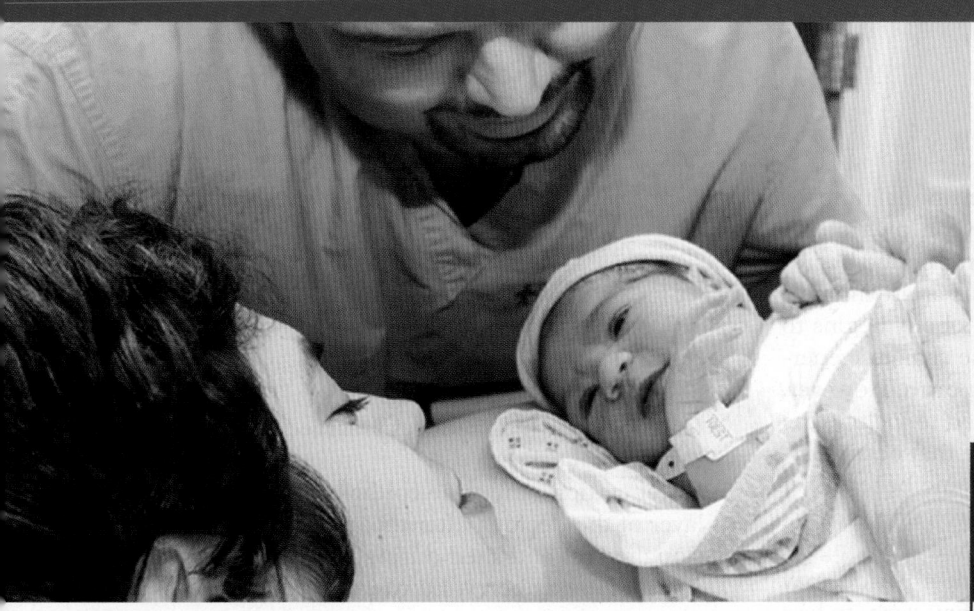

POSTPARTUM ADAPTATIONS

KEY TERMS

engorgement
engrossment
involution
lactation

letting-go phase
lochia
puerperium
taking-hold phase

taking-in phase
uterine atony

LEARNING OBJECTIVES

Upon completion of the chapter, the learner will be able to:

1. Define the key terms used in this chapter.
2. Explain the systemic physiologic changes occurring in the woman after childbirth.
3. Identify the phases of maternal role adjustment as described by Reva Rubin.
4. Analyze the psychological adaptations occurring in the mother's partner after childbirth.

Betsy had been home only 3 days when she called the OB unit where she had given birth and asked to speak to the lactation consultant. She reported pain in both breasts. Her nipples were tender due to frequent breastfeeding and she described her breasts as heavy, hard, and swollen.

Wow

A new mother's expectations are seen through rose-coloured glasses, and at times her fantasy is better than the reality.

The postpartum period is a critical transitional time for a woman, her newborn, and her family on physiologic and psychological levels. The **puerperium** period begins after the delivery of the placenta and lasts approximately 8 weeks. During this period the woman's body begins to return to its pre-pregnant state, and these changes generally resolve by the sixth week after giving birth. However, the postpartum period can also be defined to include the changes in all aspects of the mother's life that occur during the first year after a child is born. Some believe that the postpartum adjustment period lasts well into the first year, making the fourth phase of labour the longest. Keeping this in mind, the true postpartum period may last between 9 and 12 months as the mother works to lose the weight she gained while pregnant, adjusts psychologically to the changes in her life, and takes on the new role of mother.

This chapter describes the major physiologic and psychological changes that occur in a woman after childbirth. Various systemic adaptations take place throughout the woman's body. In addition, the mother and the family adjust to the new addition psychologically. The birth of a child changes the family structure and the roles of the family members. The adaptations are dynamic and continue to evolve as physical changes occur and new roles emerge.

Maternal Physiologic Adaptations

During pregnancy, the woman's entire body changed to accommodate the needs of the growing fetus. After birth, the woman's body once again undergoes significant changes in all body systems to return her body to its pre-pregnant state.

Reproductive System Adaptations

The reproductive system goes through tremendous adaptations to return to the pre-pregnancy state. All organs and tissues of the reproductive system are involved. The female reproductive system is unique in its capacity to remodel throughout the woman's reproductive life. The events after birth, with the shedding of the placenta and subsequent uterine involution, involve substantial tissue destruction and subsequent repair and remodelling. For example, the woman's menstrual cycle, interrupted during pregnancy, will begin to return several weeks after childbirth. The uterus, which has undergone tremendous expansion during pregnancy to accommodate progressive fetal growth, will return to its pre-pregnancy size typically over 6 weeks (American College of Nurse Midwives, n.d.). The mother's breasts have grown to prepare for lactation and do not return to their pre-pregnancy size as the uterus does.

Uterus

The uterus returns to its normal size through a gradual process of **involution**, which involves retrogressive changes that return it to its pre-pregnant size and condition (Borgelt et al., 2010). Involution involves three retrogressive processes:

1. Contraction of muscle fibres to reduce those previously stretched during pregnancy
2. Catabolism, which reduces enlarged, individual myometrial cells
3. Regeneration of uterine epithelium from the lower layer of the decidua after the upper layers have been sloughed off and shed during lochial discharge (Perry, Hockenberry, Lowdermilk, et al., 2010).

The uterus, which weighs approximately 1,000 g (2.2 lb) soon after birth, undergoes physiologic involution as it returns to its non-pregnant state. Approximately 1 week after birth, the uterus shrinks in size by 50% and weighs about 500 g (1 lb); at the end of 6 weeks, it weighs approximately 60 g (2 oz), about the weight before the pregnancy (Evans, Evans, Brown, et al., 2010; Perry et al., 2010; Fig. 15.1). During the first few days after birth, the uterus typically descends from the level of the umbilicus at a rate of 1 cm (1 fingerbreadth) per day. By 3 days, the fundus lays 2 to 3 fingerbreadths below the umbilicus (or slightly higher in multiparous women). By the end of 10 days, the fundus usually cannot be palpated because it has descended into the true pelvis.

If these retrogressive changes do not occur as a result of retained placental fragments or infection, subinvolution results. Subinvolution is generally responsive to early diagnosis and treatment. Factors that facilitate uterine involution include complete expulsion of amniotic

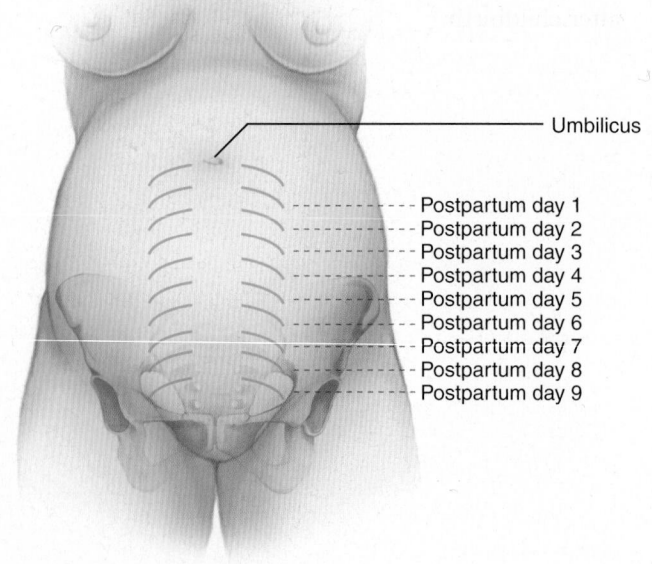

Umbilicus

Postpartum day 1
Postpartum day 2
Postpartum day 3
Postpartum day 4
Postpartum day 5
Postpartum day 6
Postpartum day 7
Postpartum day 8
Postpartum day 9

FIGURE 15.1 Uterine involution.

membranes and placenta at birth, a complication-free labour and birth process, breastfeeding, and early ambulation. Factors that inhibit involution include a prolonged labour and difficult birth, incomplete expulsion of amniotic membranes and placenta, uterine infection, overdistention of uterine muscles (such as by multiple gestation, hydramnios, or a large singleton fetus), a full bladder (which displaces the uterus and interferes with contractions), anesthesia (which relaxes uterine muscles), and close childbirth spacing (frequent and repeated distention decreases tone and causes muscular relaxation).

Lochia

Lochia is the vaginal discharge that occurs after birth. It results from involution, during which the superficial layer of the decidua basalis becomes necrotic and is sloughed off. Immediately after childbirth, lochia is bright red and consists mainly of blood (red and white blood cells), fibrinous products, and decidual cells. The lochia from the uterus is alkaline but becomes acidic as it passes through the vagina. It is roughly equal to the amount occurring during a heavy menstrual period. The average amount of lochial discharge in the first week is typically 240 to 270 mL (8 to 9 oz) (Perry et al., 2010).

Women who have had cesarean births tend to have less flow because the uterine debris is removed manually along with delivery of the placenta. Lochia is present in most women for at least 3 weeks after childbirth, but it persists in some women for as long as 6 weeks.

Lochia passes through three stages: lochia rubra, lochia serosa, and lochia alba:

- Lochia rubra is a deep-red mixture of mucus, tissue debris, and blood that occurs for the first 3 to 4 days after birth. As uterine bleeding subsides, it becomes paler and more serous.
- Lochia serosa is the second stage. It is pinkish brown and is expelled 3 to 10 days postpartum. Lochia serosa primarily contains leukocytes, decidual tissue, red blood cells, and serous fluid.
- Lochia alba is the final stage. The discharge is creamy white or light brown and consists of leukocytes, decidual tissue, and reduced fluid content. It occurs from days 10 to 14 but can last 3 to 6 weeks postpartum in some women and still be considered normal.

Lochia at any stage should have a fleshy smell; an offensive odour usually indicates an infection, such as endometritis.

> ▶ *Take* NOTE!
>
> *A danger sign is the reappearance of bright-red blood after lochia rubra has stopped. Re-evaluation by the health care professional is essential if this occurs.*

Afterpains

Part of the involution process involves uterine contractions, and many women are bothered by painful uterine contractions termed afterpains. All women may experience afterpains, but they may be more acutely painful in multiparous women secondary to repeated stretching of the uterine muscles. This repeated stretching reduces muscle tone, allowing for alternate uterine contraction and relaxation. The uterus of a primiparous woman tends to remain contracted after giving birth unless she has had a prolonged, difficult labour and birth or an overdistended uterus secondary to multiple gestation, hydramnios, or retained blood clots or placental fragments.

> ▶ *Take* NOTE!
>
> *Afterpains are usually stronger during breast-feeding because oxytocin released by the sucking reflex strengthens the contractions. Mild analgesics can reduce this discomfort.*

Cervix

The cervix typically returns to its pre-pregnancy state by week 6 of the postpartum period. The cervix gradually closes but never regains its pre-pregnancy appearance. Immediately after childbirth, the cervix is shapeless and edematous and is easily distensible for several days. The cervical os gradually closes and returns to normal by 2 weeks, whereas the external os widens and never appears the same after childbirth. The external cervical os is no longer shaped like a circle but instead appears as a jagged slit-like opening, often described as a "fish mouth" (Fig. 15.2).

Vagina

Shortly after birth, the vaginal mucosa is edematous and thin, with few rugae. As ovarian function returns and estrogen production resumes, the mucosa thickens and rugae return in approximately 3 to 4 weeks. The vagina gapes at the opening and is generally lax. The vagina returns to its approximate pre-pregnancy size by

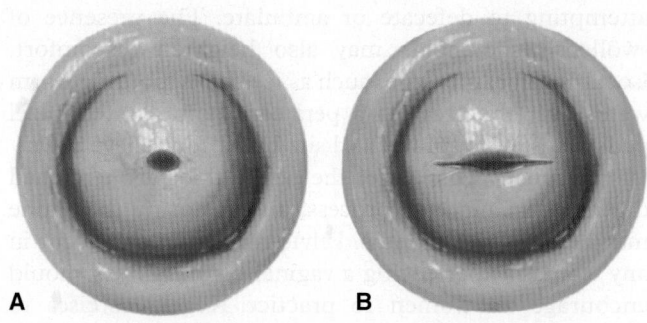

FIGURE 15.2 Appearance of the cervical os. (**A**) Before the first pregnancy. (**B**) After pregnancy.

6 to 8 weeks postpartum but will always remain a bit larger than it had been before pregnancy.

The breastfeeding woman may note that her vaginal mucosa is pale and without rugae; this is related to being in a hypoestrogenic state (Ladewig, London, & Davidson, 2010). Ovulation can return as early as a month after childbirth in women who are not breastfeeding, with a mean time frame of 3 months. The mean time to ovulation in breastfeeding women is approximately 4 to 6 months, but this can vary greatly depending on breastfeeding patterns (Ladewig et al., 2010). Localized dryness and coital discomfort (dyspareunia) usually plague most women until menstruation returns. Water-soluble lubricants can reduce discomfort during intercourse. Box 15.1 lists some commonly available water-soluble lubricants.

Perineum

The perineum is often edematous and bruised for the first day or two after birth. If the birth involved an episiotomy or laceration, complete healing may take as long as 4 to 6 months in the absence of complications at the site, such as hematoma or infection (Perry et al., 2010). Perineal lacerations may extend into the anus and cause considerable discomfort for the mother when she is attempting to defecate or ambulate. The presence of swollen hemorrhoids may also heighten discomfort. Local comfort measures such as ice packs, pouring warm water over the area via a peri care bottle, witch hazel pads, anesthetic sprays, and sitz baths can relieve pain.

Supportive tissues of the pelvic floor are stretched during the childbirth process, and restoring their tone may take up to 6 months. Pelvic relaxation can occur in any woman experiencing a vaginal birth. Nurses should encourage all women to practice Kegel exercises to improve pelvic floor tone, strengthen the perineal muscles, and promote healing.

▶ **Take** NOTE!

Failure to maintain and restore perineal muscular tone may lead to urinary incontinence later in life for many women (Menezes, Pereira, & Hextall, 2010).

Cardiovascular System Adaptations

The cardiovascular system undergoes dramatic changes after birth. During pregnancy, the heart is displaced slightly upward and to the left. This reverses as the uterus undergoes involution. Cardiac output remains high for the first few days postpartum and then gradually declines to non-pregnancy values within 3 months of birth.

Blood volume, which increased substantially during pregnancy, drops rapidly after birth and returns to normal within 4 weeks postpartum (Evans et al., 2010). The decrease in both cardiac output and blood volume reflects the birth-related blood loss (an average of 500 mL with a vaginal birth and 1,000 mL with a cesarean birth). Blood plasma volume is further reduced through diuresis, which occurs during the early postpartum period (Perry et al., 2010). Despite the decrease in blood volume, the hematocrit level remains relatively stable and may even increase, reflecting the predominant loss of plasma. Thus, an acute decrease in hematocrit is not an expected finding and may indicate hemorrhage.

Pulse and Blood Pressure

The increase in cardiac output during pregnancy begins to diminish after birth. This decrease in cardiac output is reflected in bradycardia (heart rate 50 to 70 bpm) for the first 2 weeks postpartum. This slowing of the heart rate is related to the increased blood that flows back to the heart and to the central circulation after it is no longer perfusing the placenta. This increase in central circulation brings about an increased stroke volume and allows a slower heart rate to provide ample maternal circulation. Gradually, cardiac output returns to pre-pregnancy levels by 3 months after childbirth (Perry et al., 2010).

Tachycardia (heart rate above 100 bpm) in the postpartum woman warrants further investigation. It may indicate hypovolemia, dehydration, or hemorrhage. However, because of the increased blood volume during pregnancy, a considerable loss may be well tolerated and not cause a compensatory cardiovascular response such as tachycardia. In most instances of postpartum hemorrhage, blood pressure and cardiac output remain increased because of the compensatory increase in heart rate. Thus, a decrease in blood pressure and cardiac output are not expected changes during the postpartum period. Early identification is essential to ensure prompt intervention.

Blood pressure values should be similar to those obtained during the labour process. In some women there may be a slight transient increase lasting for about a week after childbirth (Ladewig et al., 2010). A significant increase accompanied by headache might indicate pre-eclampsia and requires further investigation. A decreased blood pressure may suggest orthostatic hypotension or uterine hemorrhage.

Coagulation

Clotting factors that increased during pregnancy tend to remain elevated during the early postpartum period. Giving birth stimulates this hypercoagulability state further. As a result, these coagulation factors remain elevated for 2 to 3 weeks postpartum (Hackley, Kriebs, & Rousseau, 2007). This hypercoagulable state, combined with vessel damage during birth and immobility, places the woman at risk for thromboembolism (blood clots) in the lower extremities and the lungs.

Blood Cellular Components

Red blood cell production ceases early in the puerperium, causing mean hemoglobin and hematocrit levels to decrease slightly in the first 24 hours. Over the next 2 weeks, both levels rise slowly. The white blood count, which increases for unknown reasons during labour, remains elevated for the first 4 to 6 days after birth but then falls to 6,000 to $10,000/mm^3$. This white blood cell elevation can create the impression that there is a postpartum infection occurring or can complicate a diagnosis of an actual postpartum infection in the immediate postpartum period.

Urinary System Adaptations

Pregnancy and birth can have profound effects on the urinary system. During pregnancy, the glomerular filtration rate and renal plasma flow increase significantly. Both usually return to normal by 6 weeks after birth.

Many women have difficulty feeling the sensation to void after giving birth if they received an anesthetic block during labour (which inhibits neural functioning of the bladder) or if they received oxytocin to induce or augment their labour (antidiuretic effect). These women will be at risk for incomplete emptying, bladder distention, difficulty voiding, and urinary retention. In addition, urination may be impeded by:

• Perineal lacerations
• Generalized swelling and bruising of the perineum and tissues surrounding the urinary meatus
• Hematomas
• Decreased bladder tone as a result of regional anesthesia
• Diminished sensation of bladder pressure as a result of swelling, poor bladder tone, and numbing effects of regional anesthesia used during labour (Kennedy, Ruth, & Martin, 2009)

Difficulty voiding can lead to urinary retention, bladder distention, and ultimately urinary tract infection. Urinary retention and bladder distention can cause displacement of the uterus from the midline to the right and can inhibit the uterus from contracting properly, which increases the risk of postpartum hemorrhage. Urinary retention is a major cause of **uterine atony**, which can cause excessive bleeding in the immediate postpartum period. Frequent voiding of small amounts (less than 150 mL) suggests urinary retention with overflow, and catheterization may be necessary to empty the bladder to restore tone.

Postpartum diuresis occurs as a result of several mechanisms: the large amounts of intravenous fluids given during labour, a decreasing antidiuretic effect of oxytocin as its level declines, the buildup and retention of extra fluids during pregnancy, and a decreasing production of aldosterone—the hormone that decreases sodium retention and increases urine production (Perry et al., 2010). All these factors contribute to rapid filling of the bladder within 12 hours of birth. Diuresis begins within 12 hours after childbirth and continues throughout the first week postpartum. Normal function returns within a month after birth (Ladewig et al., 2010).

▶ **Consider** *THIS!*

Have you ever felt like a real idiot by not being able to complete a simple task in life? I had a beautiful baby boy after only 6 hours of labour. My epidural worked well and I actually felt very little discomfort throughout my labour. Because it was the middle of the night when they brought me to my postpartum room, I felt a few hours of sleep would be all I needed to be back to normal. During an assessment early the next morning, the nurse found my uterus had shifted to the right from my midline, and I was instructed to empty my bladder. I didn't understand why the nurse was concerned about where my uterus was located and, besides, I didn't feel any sensation of a full bladder. But I did get up anyway and tried to comply. Despite all the nurse's tricks of running the faucet for sound effects, in addition to having warm water poured over my thighs via the peri bottle, I was unable to urinate. How could I not accomplish one of life's simplest tasks?

Thoughts: women who receive regional anesthesia frequently experience reduced sensation to their perineal area and do not feel a full bladder. The nursing assessment revealed a displaced uterus secondary to a full bladder. What additional "tricks" can be used to assist this woman to void? What explanation should be offered to her regarding why she is having difficulty urinating?

Gastrointestinal System Adaptations

The gastrointestinal system quickly returns to normal after childbirth because the gravid uterus is no longer filling the abdominal cavity and producing pressure on the abdominal organs. Progesterone levels, which caused relaxation of smooth muscle during pregnancy and diminished bowel tone, also are declining.

Regardless of the type of delivery, most women experience decreased bowel tone and sluggish bowels for several days after birth. Decreased peristalsis occurs in response to analgesics, surgery, diminished intra-abdominal pressure, low-fibre diet and insufficient fluid intake, and diminished muscle tone. In addition, women with an episiotomy, perineal laceration, or hemorrhoids may fear pain or damage to the perineum with their first bowel movement and may attempt to delay it. Subsequently, constipation is a common problem during the postpartum period. A stool softener is often prescribed for this reason.

Most women are hungry and thirsty after childbirth, commonly related to NPO restrictions and the energy expended during labour. Their appetite returns to normal immediately after giving birth.

▶ **Take** NOTE!

Anticipate the woman's need to replenish her body with food and fluids, and provide both soon after she gives birth.

Musculoskeletal System Adaptations

The effects of pregnancy on the muscles and joints vary widely. During pregnancy, the hormones relaxin, estrogen, and progesterone relax the joints. After birth, levels of these hormones decline, resulting in a return of all joints to their pre-pregnancy state. Some women may experience an increase in shoe size after the delivery of their baby due to the ligaments in the feet relaxing, which has been influenced by the hormone relaxin during pregnancy. The ligaments in the feet may or may not return to their original pre-pregnant size. Women's shoe size may also increase due to the extra weight being carried during the pregnancy, which may result in the flattening of a woman's arches therefore potentially increasing her shoe size—particularly in width (Weber & Kelley, 2010).

Women commonly experience fatigue and activity intolerance and have a distorted body image for weeks after birth secondary to declining relaxin and progesterone levels, which cause hip and joint pain that interferes with ambulation and exercise. Good body mechanics and correct position are important during this time to prevent low back pain and injury to the joints. Within 6 to 8 weeks after delivery, joints are completely stabilized and return to normal.

During pregnancy, stretching of the abdominal wall muscles occurs to accommodate the enlarging uterus. This stretching leads to a loss in muscle tone and possibly separation of the longitudinal muscles (rectus abdominis muscles) of the abdomen. Separation of the rectus abdominis muscles, called diastasis recti, may be more common in women who have poor abdominal muscle tone before pregnancy (Ricci, 2010). After birth, muscle tone is diminished and the abdominal muscles are soft and flabby. Specific exercises are necessary to help the woman regain muscle tone. Fortunately, diastasis responds well to exercise, and abdominal muscle tone can be improved (see Chapter 16 for more information about exercises to improve muscle tone).

▶ **Take** NOTE!

If rectus muscle tone is not regained through exercise, abdominal wall support may not be adequate during future pregnancies, which may lead to abdominal discomfort or pain as the pregnancy progresses. Multiple births or repeated pregnancies increase the risk.

Integumentary System Adaptations

Another system that experiences lasting effects of pregnancy is the integumentary system. As estrogen and progesterone levels decrease, the darkened pigmentation on the abdomen (linea nigra), face (melasma), and nipples gradually fades. Some women experience hair loss during pregnancy and the postpartum periods. Approximately 90% of hairs are growing at any one time, with the other 10% entering a resting phase. Because of the high estrogen levels present during pregnancy, an increased number of hairs go into the resting phase, which is part of the normal hair loss cycle. The most common period for hair loss is within 3 months after birth, when estrogen returns to normal levels and more hairs are allowed to fall out. This hair loss is temporary, and re-growth generally returns to normal levels in 6 to 12 months.

Striae gravidarum (stretch marks) that developed during pregnancy on the breasts, abdomen, and hips gradually fade to silvery lines. However, these lines do not disappear completely. Although many products on the market claim to make stretch marks disappear, their effectiveness is highly questionable.

The profuse diaphoresis (sweating) that is common during the early postpartum period is one of the most noticeable adaptations in the integumentary system. Many women will wake up drenched with perspiration during the puerperium. This postpartal diaphoresis is a mechanism to reduce the amount of fluids retained during pregnancy and restore fluid level to a pre-pregnancy state. It can be profuse at times and is common, especially at night during the first week after birth. Reassure the client that this is normal and encourage her to change her gown to prevent chilling.

Respiratory System Adaptations

Respirations usually remain within the normal adult range of 16 to 24 breaths/minute. As the abdominal organs resume their non-pregnancy position, the diaphragm returns to its usual position. Anatomic changes in the thoracic cavity and rib cage caused by increasing uterine growth resolve quickly. As a result, discomforts such as shortness of breath and rib aches are relieved. Tidal volume, minute volume, vital capacity, and functional residual capacity return to pre-pregnancy values, typically within 1 to 3 weeks after birth (Perry et al., 2010).

Endocrine System Adaptations

The endocrine system undergoes several changes rapidly after birth. Levels of circulating estrogen and progesterone drop quickly with delivery of the placenta. Decreased estrogen levels are associated with breast engorgement and with the diuresis of excess extracellular fluid accumulated during pregnancy (Ladewig et al., 2010). Estrogen is at its lowest level a week after birth. For the woman who is not breastfeeding, estrogen levels begin to increase by 2 weeks after birth. For the breastfeeding woman, estrogen levels remain low until breastfeeding frequency decreases.

Other placental hormones (human chorionic gonadotropin [hCG], human placenta lactogen [hPL], progesterone) decline rapidly after birth. hCG levels are nonexistent at the end of the first postpartum week, and hPL is undetectable within 1 day after birth (Perry et al., 2010). Progesterone levels are undetectable by 3 days after childbirth, and production is reestablished with the first menses. Prolactin levels decline within 2 weeks for the woman who is not breastfeeding and remain elevated for the lactating woman (Perry et al., 2010).

Think back to Betsy, the woman experiencing painful changes in her breasts. What is Betsy describing to the lactation consultant? Why has the condition of her breasts changed compared with when she was in the hospital?

Lactation

Lactation is the secretion of milk by the breasts. It is thought to be triggered by the interaction of progesterone, estrogen, prolactin, and oxytocin. Breast milk typically appears 3 days after childbirth.

During pregnancy, the breasts increase in size and functional ability in preparation for breastfeeding. Within the first month of gestation, the ducts of the mammary glands grow branches, forming more lobules and alveoli. These structural changes make the breasts larger, more tender, and heavy. Each breast gains nearly 454 g (1 lb) in weight by term, the glandular cells fill with secretions, blood vessels increase in number, and there are increased amounts of connective tissue and fat cells (Perry et al., 2010).

Prolactin from the anterior pituitary gland, secreted in increasing levels throughout pregnancy, triggers the synthesis and secretion of milk after the woman gives birth. During pregnancy, prolactin, estrogen, and progesterone cause synthesis and secretion of colostrum, which contains protein and carbohydrate but no milk fat. It is only after birth takes place, when the high levels of estrogen and progesterone are abruptly withdrawn, that prolactin is able to stimulate the glandular cells to secrete milk instead of colostrum. This takes place within 2 to 3 days after giving birth. Oxytocin acts with in the breasts by triggering the milk ejection reflex so that milk can be ejected from the alveoli to the nipple. Therefore, sucking by the newborn will release milk. Prolactin levels increase in response to nipple stimulation during feedings. Prolactin and oxytocin result in milk production if stimulated by sucking (Ladewig et al., 2010) (Fig. 15.3). If the stimulus (sucking) is not present, as with a woman who is not breastfeeding, breast engorgement and milk production will begin to subside within 2 to 3 days postpartum.

Typically, during the first 2 days after birth, the breasts are soft and nontender. The woman also may report a tingling sensation in both breasts. After this time, breast changes depend on whether the mother is breastfeeding or taking measures to prevent lactation.

Engorgement is the process of swelling of the breast tissue as a result of an increase in blood and lymph supply as a precursor to lactation (Helms & Darbishire, 2009). Breasts increase in vascularity and swell in response to prolactin 2 to 4 days after birth. If engorged, the breasts will be hard and tender to touch. They are temporarily full, tender, and very uncomfortable until the milk supply is ready. Frequent feedings (every 2 to 3 hours) help to minimize discomfort and resolve engorgement. Standing in a warm shower or applying warm compresses immediately before feedings will help to soften the breasts and nipples in order to allow the newborn to latch on easier. These measures will also enhance the letdown reflex. Applying cold compresses to the breasts between feedings helps to reduce swelling, and women should be instructed to wear a comfortable bra that is not too tight (Scott Ricci, 2010) (see Chapter 18). To maintain milk supply, the breasts need to be stimulated by a nursing infant, a breast pump, or manual expression of the milk (Fig. 15.4). Ensuring that the infant has a correct latch will help to lessen the discomfort. Some women may experience

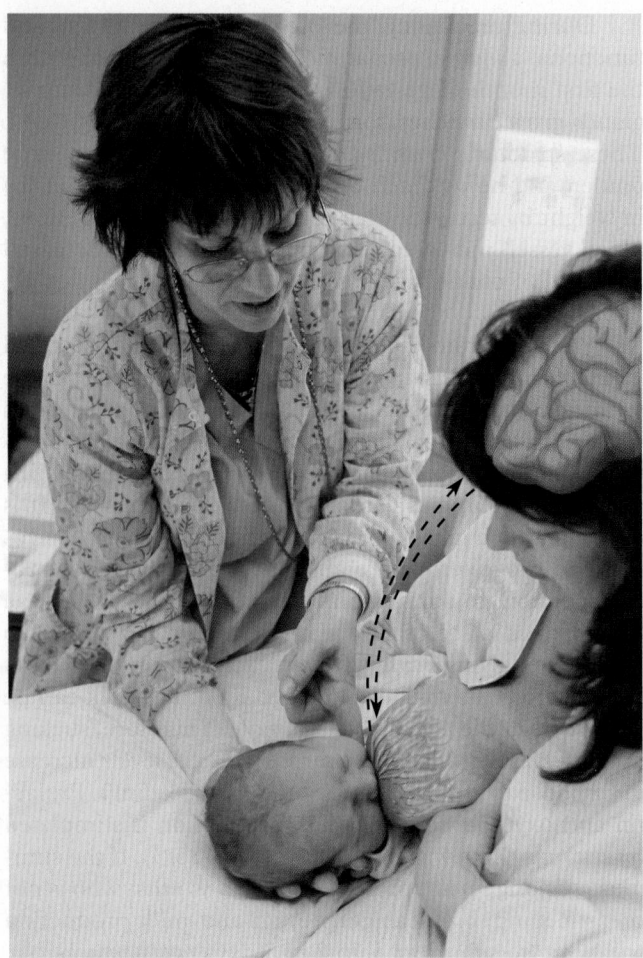

FIGURE 15.3 Physiology of lactation.

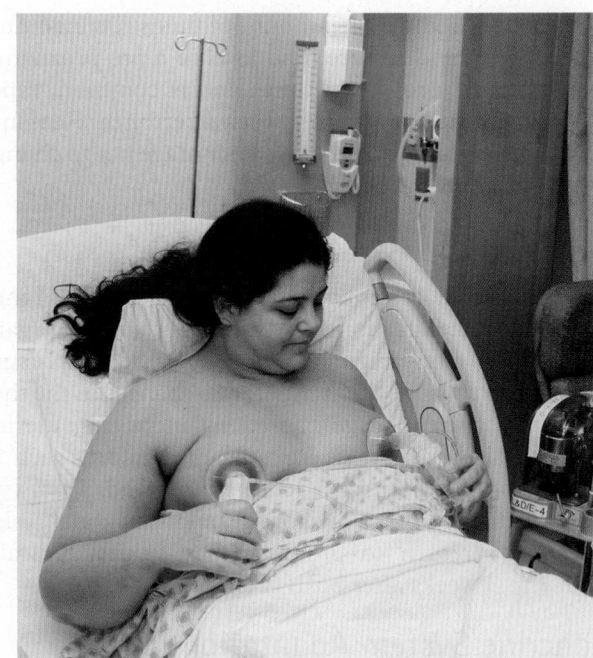

FIGURE 15.4 Mother using breast pumps to stimulate milk production.

engorgement that causes the areola to become extremely full and may make it difficult for a baby to correctly latch. Mothers should be taught to gently express breast milk manually from the areola before breastfeeding to soften the area, thereby allowing the baby to achieve a correct deep latch.

*R*emember Betsy, with the breast discomfort? The lactation consultant explained that she was experiencing normal breast engorgement and offered several suggestions to help her. What relief measures might they be? What reassurance can be given to Betsy at this time?

If the woman is not breastfeeding, relief measures include wearing a comfortable, supportive bra 24 hours daily, applying ice to her breasts for approximately 15 to 20 minutes every other hour, and not stimulating the breasts by squeezing or manually expressing milk from the nipples or encouraging the baby to nuzzle at the breast. In addition, avoiding exposure of the breasts to warmth and stimulation (e.g., by avoiding hot showers

and not letting the infant nuzzle at the breast) will help relieve breast engorgement. In women who are not breast-feeding, engorgement typically subsides within 2 to 3 days with these measures. See Evidence-based Practice 15.1.

*B*etsy tries several of the measures the lactation consultant suggested to relieve her breast discomfort but is still having heaviness and pain. She feels discouraged and tells the nurse she is thinking of reducing her breastfeeding and using formula to feed her newborn. Is that a good choice? Why or why not? What interventions will help Betsy get through this difficult time?

Ovulation and Return of Menstruation

Changing hormone levels constantly interact with one another to produce bodily changes. Four major hormones are influential during the postpartum period: estrogen, progesterone, prolactin, and oxytocin. Estrogen is the major female hormone during pregnancy, but levels drop profoundly at birth and reach their lowest level a week into the postpartum period. Progesterone quiets the uterus to prevent a preterm birth during pregnancy, and its increasing levels during pregnancy prevent lactation from starting before birth takes place. As with estrogen, progesterone levels decrease dramatically after birth and are undetectable 72 hours after birth. Progesterone levels are reestablished with the first menstrual cycle (Perry et al., 2010).

EVIDENCE-BASED PRACTICE 15.1
Effects of Cigarette Smoking Cessation on Breastfeeding Duration

● Study

Breastfeeding provides improved maternal and infant health and is recommended by the World Health Organization as the exclusive means of infant feeding for the first 6 months of life. While initiation rates of breastfeeding have continued to rise, inadequate duration of breastfeeding remains a challenge for health care practitioners in both developed and developing countries. Many factors influence the duration of breastfeeding, including age, marital status, and education level.

Maternal cigarette smoking has been identified as a predictor of early breastfeeding cessation. The authors of this controlled trial placed women who were smokers at the start of their prenatal care into two groups. The women were assigned to either an incentive-based smoking cessation intervention, in which those who abstained from smoking received vouchers that could be exchanged for retail items, or to the control group, in which women received the vouchers independent of their smoking status.

▲ Findings

At the 2-week and 4-week postpartum time points, the researchers found no significant difference in the percentage of women reporting to be breastfeeding. However, at the 8-week time point, 41% of the women in the incentive group were still breastfeeding versus 26% in the control group. Differences in breastfeeding rates were observed again 12 weeks postpartum, with the incentives group reporting a 35% rate of breastfeeding versus 17% in the control group. At the end of 24 weeks, there continued to be a discernable difference in breastfeeding rates between the groups (incentives = 20%, control group = 13%).

■ Nursing Implications

According to the authors, while there is a need for continued research and improved observation of the outcomes, offering a smoking cessation intervention appeared to have increased the length of breastfeeding for a number of women. Nurses can offer this information to women who are smoking and wanting to breastfeed and explain the evidence-based practice behind the research. Nurses can also become advocates for easily accessible and affordable smoking cessation programs for postpartum mothers.

Source: Higgins, T., Higgins, S., Heil, S., Badger, G., Skelly, J. Bernstein, I., Solomon, L., Washido, Y., & Preston, A. (2010). Effects of cigarette smoking cessation on breastfeeding duration. *Nicotine & Tobacco Research, 12*(5), 483–488.

During the postpartum period, oxytocin stimulates the uterus to contract during the breastfeeding session and for as long as 20 minutes after each feeding. Oxytocin also acts on the breast by eliciting the milk letdown reflex during breastfeeding. Prolactin is also associated with the breastfeeding process by stimulating milk production. In women who breastfeed, prolactin levels remain elevated into the sixth week after birth (Kennedy et al., 2009). The levels of the hormone increase and decrease in proportion to nipple stimulation. Prolactin levels decrease in nonlactating women, reaching prepregnancy levels by the third postpartum week (Ladewig et al., 2010). High levels of prolactin have been found to delay ovulation by inhibiting ovarian response to follicle-stimulating hormone (Ladewig et al., 2010).

The timing of first menses and ovulation after birth differs between women who are and are not breastfeeding. For nonlactating women, menstruation usually resumes 7 to 9 weeks after giving birth, with the first cycle being anovulatory (Ladewig et al., 2010). The return of menses in the lactating woman depends on breastfeeding frequency and duration. It can return any time from 2 to 18 months after childbirth, depending on whether the woman is exclusively breastfeeding or supplementing with formula. The first postpartum menstrual period may be heavier than pre-pregnancy ones and is frequently anovulatory (Hackley et al., 2007).

▶ *Take* NOTE!

Ovulation may occur before menstruation (as early as 28 days); therefore, breastfeeding may not a reliable method of contraception. Other methods of family planning should be discussed with families of newborns to ensure child spacing that the family/mother desires (Royal College of Obstetricians and Gynecologists Faculty of Sexual & Reproductive Healthcare, 2009).

Psychological Adaptations

Mothers' and fathers' experiences of pregnancy are necessarily different, and this difference continues after childbirth as they both adjust to their new parenting roles. Parenting involves caring for infants physically and emotionally to foster the growth and development into responsible, caring adults. During the early months of parenthood, mothers experience more life changes and get more satisfaction from their new roles than fathers do. However, fathers interact with their newborns much like mothers do (Premberg, Hellstrom, & Berg, 2008). Early parent–infant contact after birth improves attachment behaviours. Other members of the newborn's family, such as siblings and grandparents, also experience changes related to the birth of the newborn. Chapter 16 describes these changes.

Maternal Psychological Adaptations

Postpartum depression affects the transition to the maternal role for many mothers. Between 50% and 80% of new mothers suffer from the short-lived postpartum mood disorder termed "baby blues." In addition, up to 16% of new mothers in Canada, or more than 335,202 women, suffer debilitating postpartum depression each year, a prevalence that continues unabated (Centre for Addiction and Mental Health, 2011). Postpartum depression can lead to alienation from loved ones, daily dysfunction secondary to overwhelming sorrow and disorientation, and, at its most extreme, personal terror resulting in dangerous thoughts and violent actions. For additional information, see Chapter 22.

The woman experiences a variety of responses as she adjusts to a new family member, postpartum discomforts, changes in her body image, and the reality of change in her life. In the early 1960s, Reva Rubin identified three phases that a mother goes through to adjust to her new maternal role. Rubin's maternal role framework can be used to monitor the client's progress as she "tries on" her new role as a mother. Absence of these processes or inability to progress through the phases satisfactorily may impede the appropriate development of the maternal role (Rubin, 1984). Although Rubin's maternal role development theories are of value, some of her observations regarding the length of each phase may not be completely relevant for the contemporary woman of the 21st century. Today, many women know their infant's gender, have "seen" their fetus in utero through four-dimensional ultrasound, and have a working knowledge of childbirth and child care. They are less passive than in years past and progress through the phases of attaining the maternal role at a much faster pace than Rubin would have imagined. Still, Rubin's framework is timeless for assessing and monitoring expected role behaviours when planning care and appropriate interventions.

Taking–In Phase
The **taking-in phase** is the time immediately after birth when the new mother needs sleep, depends on others to meet her needs, and relives the events surrounding the birth process. This phase is characterized by dependent behaviour. During the first 24 to 48 hours after giving

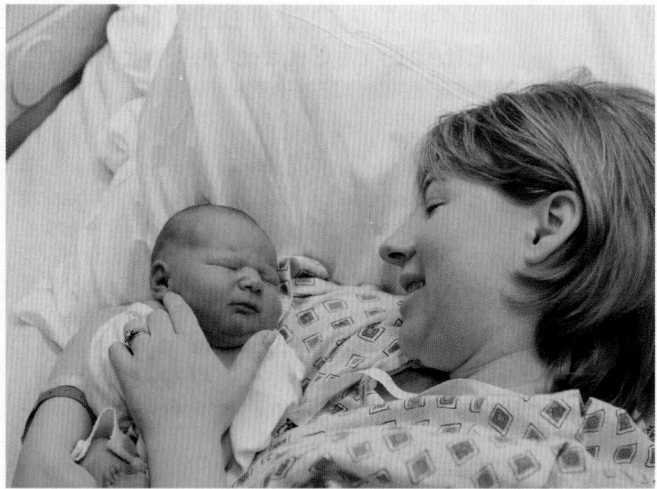

FIGURE 15.5 Mother bonding with newborn during the taking-in phase.

birth, mothers often assume a very passive role in meeting their own basic needs for food, fluids, and rest, allowing the nurse to make decisions for them concerning activities and care. They spend time recounting their labour experience to anyone who will listen. Such actions help the mother integrate the birth experience into reality—that is, the pregnancy is over and the newborn is now a unique individual, separate from herself. When interacting with the newborn, new mothers spend time claiming the newborn and touching him or her, commonly identifying specific features in the newborn, such as "he has my nose" or "his fingers are long like his father's" (Fig. 15.5).

▶ **Take** *NOTE!*

The taking-in phase typically lasts 1 to 2 days and may be the only phase observed by nurses in the hospital setting because of the shortened postpartum stays that are the norm today.

Taking–Hold Phase
The **taking-hold phase**, the second phase of maternal adaptation, is characterized by dependent and independent maternal behaviour. This phase typically starts on the second to third day postpartum and may last several weeks.

As the client regains control over her bodily functions during the next few days, she will be taking hold and becoming preoccupied with the present. She will be particularly concerned about her health, the infant's condition, and her ability to care for him or her. She demonstrates increased autonomy and mastery of her own body's functioning and a desire to take charge with support and help from others. She will show independence by caring for herself and learning to care for her newborn, but she still requires assurance that she is doing well as a mother. She expresses a strong interest in caring for the infant by herself.

Letting-Go Phase

In the **letting-go phase**, the third phase of maternal adaptation, the woman reestablishes relationships with other people. She adapts to parenthood through her new role as a mother. She assumes the responsibility and care for the newborn with a bit more confidence now (Evans et al., 2010). The focus of this phase is to move forward by assuming the parental role and to separate herself from the symbiotic relationship that she and her newborn had during pregnancy. She establishes a lifestyle that includes the infant. The mother relinquishes the fantasy infant and accepts the real one.

Partner Psychological Adaptations

For partners, whether they are husbands, significant others, boyfriends, same-sex life partners, or just friends, becoming a parent or just sharing the childbirth experience can be a perplexing time as well as a time of great change. This transition is influenced by many factors, including participation in childbirth, relationships with significant others, competence in child care, the family role organization, the individual's cultural background, and the method of infant feeding.

> ▶ *Take* NOTE!
>
> *Most research findings stress the importance of early contact between the father or significant other and the newborn, as well as participation in infant care activities, to foster the relationship (Premberg et al., 2008).*

Infants have a powerful effect on their fathers and others, who become intensely involved with them (Fig. 15.6). The father's or significant other's developing bond with the newborn—a time of intense absorption, preoccupation, and interest—is called engrossment.

Engrossment

Engrossment is characterized by seven behaviours:

1. Visual awareness of the newborn—the father or partner perceives the newborn as attractive, pretty, or beautiful.
2. Tactile awareness of the newborn—the father or partner has a desire to touch or hold the newborn and considers this activity to be pleasurable.
3. Perception of the newborn as perfect—the father or partner does not "see" any imperfections.

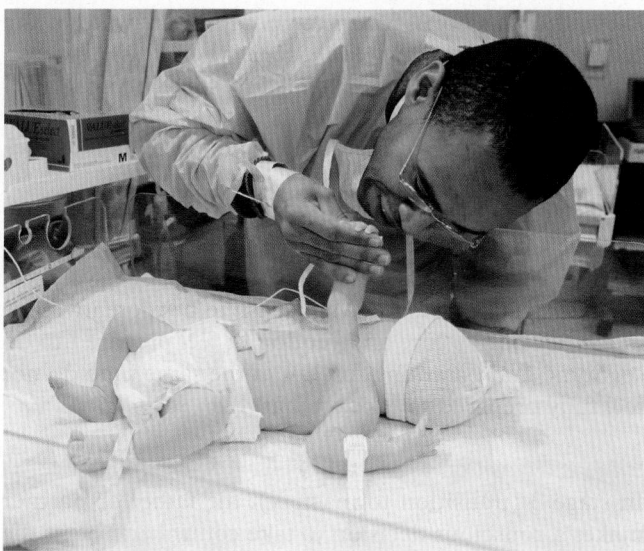

FIGURE 15.6 Engrossment of the father and his newborn.

4. Strong attraction to the newborn—the father or partner focuses all attention on the newborn when he or she is in the room.
5. Awareness of distinct features of the newborn—the father or partner can distinguish his or her newborn from others in the nursery.
6. Extreme elation—the father or partner feels a "high" after the birth of the child.
7. Increased sense of self-esteem—the father or partner feels proud, "bigger," more mature, and older after the birth of the child (Sears & Sears, 2006).

Frequently, fathers or partners are portrayed as well-meaning but bumbling when caring for newborns. However, they have their own unique way of relating to their newborns and can become as nurturing as mothers. A father's or partner's nurturing responses may be less automatic and slower to unfold than a mother's, but they are capable of a strong bonding attachment to their newborns (Sears & Sears, 2006). Encouraging fathers or partners to express their feelings by seeing, touching, and holding their son or daughter and by cuddling, talking to, and feeding him or her will help to cement this new relationship. Reinforcement of this engrossing behaviour helps fathers or partners to make a positive attachment during this critical period.

Three-Stage Role Development Process

Similar to mothers, fathers or partners also go through a predictable three-stage process during the first 3 weeks as they too "try on" their roles as parents. The three stages are expectations, reality, and transition to mastery (Sears & Sears, 2006).

Stage 1: Expectations

New fathers or partners pass through stage 1 (expectations) with preconceptions about what home life will be like with a newborn. Many men may be unaware of the dramatic changes that can occur when this newborn comes home to live with them. For some, it is an eye-opening experience.

Stage 2: Reality

Stage 2 (reality) occurs when fathers or partners realize that their expectations in stage 1 are not realistic. Their feelings change from elation to sadness, ambivalence, jealousy, and frustration. Many wish to be more involved in the newborn's care and yet do not feel prepared to do so. Some find parenting fun but at the same time do not feel fully prepared to take on that role.

Stage 3: Transition to Mastery

In stage 3 (transition to mastery), the father or partner makes a conscious decision to take control and be at the centre of his newborn's life regardless of his preparedness. This adjustment period is similar to that of the mother's letting-go phase, when she incorporates the newest member into the family.

■■■ Key Concepts

- The puerperium refers to the first 6 weeks after delivery. During this period, the mother experiences many physiologic and psychological adaptations to return her to the pre-pregnant state.

- Involution involves three processes: contraction of muscle fibres to reduce stretched ones, catabolism (which reduces enlarged, individual cells), and regeneration of uterine epithelium from the lower layer of the decidua after the upper layers have been sloughed off and shed in lochia.

- Lochia passes through three stages during the postpartum period: lochia rubra, lochia serosa, and lochia alba.

- Maternal blood plasma volume decreases rapidly after birth and returns to normal within 4 weeks postpartum.

- Reva Rubin (1984) identified three phases the mother goes through to adjust to her new maternal role. The phases of maternal postpartum adjustment are taking in, taking hold, and letting go.

- The transition to fatherhood is influenced by many factors, including participation in childbirth, relationships with significant others, competence in child care, the family role organization, the father's cultural background, and the method of infant feeding.

- Like mothers, fathers and partners go through a predictable three-stage process during the first 3 weeks as they too "try on" their role as fathers or partners. The three stages include expectations, reality, and transition to mastery.

References

American College of Nurse Midwives. (n.d.) *Recovering from pregnancy.* Retrieved May 21, 2012 from http://www.mymidwife.org/index.asp?bid=151

Borgelt, L., O'Connell, M. B., Smith, J., & Calis, K. A. (2010). *Women's health across the lifespan.* Bethesda, MD: American Society of Health-System Pharmacists.

Centre for Addiction and Mental Health. (2011). *Postpartum depression.* Retrieved February 12, 2012 from http://www.camh.net/About_Addiction_Mental_Health/Mental_Health_Information/Postpartum_Depression/ppd_ci_ppd.html

Evans, R., Evans, M., Brown, Y., & Orshan, S. (2010). *Canadian maternity, newborn, & women's health nursing.* Philadelphia: Lippincott Williams & Wilkins.

Hackley, B., Kriebs, J. M., & Rousseau, M. E. (2007). *Primary care of women: A guide for midwives and women's health providers.* Sudbury, MA: Jones & Bartlett Publishers.

Helms, S., & Darbishire, P. (2009). *Understanding breastfeeding: Beyond medication.* Retrieved February 12, 2012 from http://www.uspharmacist.com/content/d/feature/c/15751/

Higgins, T., Higgins, A., Heil, S., Badger, G., Skelly, J. Bernstein, I., Solomon, L., Washido, Y., & Preston, A. (2010). Effects of cigarette smoking cessation on breastfeeding duration. *Nicotine & Tobacco Research, 12*(5), 483–488.

Kennedy, B., Ruth, D. J., & Martin, E. J. (2009). *Intrapartum management modules: A perinatal education program* (4th ed.). Philadelphia: Lippincott Williams & Wilkins.

Ladewig, P., London, M., & Davidson, M. (2010). *Contemporary maternal-newborn nursing care.* New York: Pearson.

Menezes, M., Pereira, M., & Hextall, A. (2010). Predictors of urinary incontinence at midlife and beyond. *Maturitas, 65*(2), 167–171. doi:10.1016/jmarturitas.2009.10.004

Perry, S., Hockenberry, M., Lowdermilk, D., & Wilson, D. (2010). *Maternal child nursing care* (4th ed.). St. Louis, MO: Mosby Elsevier.

Premberg, A., Hellstrom, A. L., & Berg, M. (2008). Experiences of the first year of the father. *Nordic College of Caring Science, 22*(1), 56–63.

Ricci, S. S. (2010). *Essentials of maternity, newborn, and women's health nursing.* Philadelphia: Lippincott Williams & Wilkins.

Royal College of Obstetricians and Gynecologists Faculty of Sexual & Reproductive Healthcare. (2009). *Clinical guidance: Postnatal sexual and reproductive health.* Retrieved February 12, 2012 from http://www.fsrh.org/pdfs/CEUGuidancePostnatal09.pdf

Rubin, R. (1984). *Maternal identity and the maternal experience.* New York: Springer.

Sears, R. W., & Sears, J. M. (2006). *Fathers' first steps: 25 things every dad should know.* Boston, MA: Harvard Common Press.

Weber, J., & Kelley, J. (2010). *Health assessment in nursing* (4th ed.). Lippincott, Williams, & Wilkins: Philadelphia.

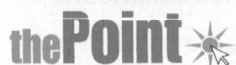

For additional learning materials, including Internet Resources, visit http://thePoint.lww.com/Chow1e.

CHAPTER WORKSHEET

MULTIPLE CHOICE QUESTIONS

1. Postpartal breast engorgement occurs 48 to 72 hours after giving birth. What physiologic change influences breast engorgement?

   a. An increase in blood and lymph supply to the breasts

   b. A decrease in estrogen and progesterone levels

   c. Dramatically increased colostrum production

   d. Fluid retention in the breasts due to the intravenous fluids given during labour

2. In the taking-in maternal role phase described by Rubin (1984), the nurse would expect the woman's behaviour to be characterized as which of the following?

   a. Gaining self-confidence

   b. Adjusting to her new relationships

   c. Being passive and dependent

   d. Resuming control over her life

3. The nurse is explaining to a postpartal woman that the afterpains she is experiencing can be the result of which of the following?

   a. Manipulation of the uterus during labour

   b. An infant weighing more than 3,629 g (8 lb)

   c. Pregnancies that were too closely spaced

   d. Contractions of the uterus after birth

4. The nurse would expect a postpartal woman to demonstrate lochia in which sequence?

   a. Rubra, alba, serosa

   b. Rubra, serosa, alba

   c. Serosa, alba, rubra

   d. Alba, rubra, serosa

5. The nurse is assessing Ms. Smith, who gave birth to her first child 5 days ago. What findings by the nurse would be expected?

   a. Cream-coloured lochia; uterus above the umbilicus

   b. Bright-red lochia with clots; uterus two finger-breadths below umbilicus

   c. Light pink or brown lochia; uterus four to five fingerbreadths below umbilicus

   d. Yellow, mucous-filled lochia; uterus at the level of the umbilicus

6. Prioritize the postpartum mother's needs 4 hours after giving birth by placing a number 1, 2, 3, or 4 in the blank before each need.

   _____ Learn how to hold and cuddle the infant

   _____ Watch a baby bath demonstration given by the nurse

   _____ Sleep and rest without being disturbed for a few hours

   _____ Interaction time with the infant to facilitate bonding

CRITICAL THINKING EXERCISES

1. A new nurse assigned to the postpartum mother–baby unit makes a comment to the oncoming shift that Ms. Griffin, a 25-year-old primipara, seems lazy and shows no initiative in taking care of herself or her baby. The nurse reported that Ms. Griffin talks excessively about her labour and birth experience and seems preoccupied with herself and her needs, not her newborn's care. She wonders if something is wrong with this mother because she seems so self-centred and has to be directed to do everything.

   a. Is there something "wrong" with Ms. Griffin's behaviour? Why or why not?

   b. What maternal role phase is being described by the new nurse?

   c. What role can the nurse play to support the mother through this phase?

(question continues on page 466)

2. Mrs. Lenhart, a primipara, gave birth to a healthy baby boy yesterday. Her husband John seemed elated at the birth, calling his friends and family on his cell phone minutes after the birth. He passed out cigars and praised his wife for her efforts. Today, when the nurse walked into their room, Mr. Lenhart seemed very anxious around his new son and called for the nurse whenever the baby cried or needed a diaper change. He seemed standoffish when asked to hold his son, and he spent time talking to other fathers in the waiting room, leaving his wife alone in the room.

a. Would you consider Mr. Lenhart's paternal behaviour to be normal at this time?

b. What might Mr. Lenhart be feeling at this time?

c. How can the nurse help this new father adjust to his new role?

STUDY ACTIVITIES

1. Find an Internet resource that discusses general postpartum care for new mothers who might have questions after discharge. Evaluate the website's information as to how credible, accurate, and current it is.

2. Prepare a teaching plan for new mothers, outlining the various physiologic changes that will take place after discharge.

3. The term that describes the return of the uterus to its pre-pregnancy state is _____.

4. A deviated fundus to the right side of the abdomen would indicate a _____.

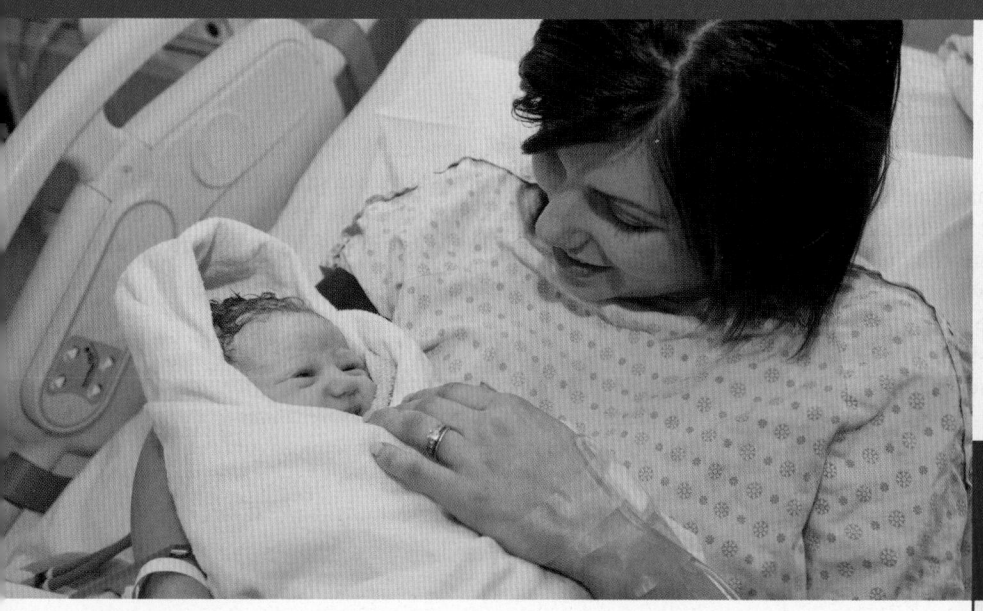

NURSING MANAGEMENT DURING THE POSTPARTUM PERIOD

KEY TERMS

attachment
bonding
en face position

Kegel exercises
mastitis
peri bottle

postpartum blues
sitz bath

LEARNING OBJECTIVES

Upon completion of the chapter, the learner will be able to:

1. Define the key terms.
2. List the parameters that need to be assessed during the postpartum period.
3. Compare the bonding and attachment processes.
4. Identify behaviours that enhance or inhibit the attachment process.
5. Outline nursing management for the woman and her family during the postpartum period.
6. Discuss the role of the nurse in promoting successful breastfeeding.
7. List areas of health education needed for discharge planning, home care, and follow-up.

Raina is a 24-year-old Muslim primipara who has just been admitted to the postpartum unit. Her husband sits at the bedside but doesn't seem to give her any physical or emotional support after her lengthy labour and difficult birth.

WOW

Parenting is an intimate, interactive, continuous, lifelong process.

The postpartum period is a time of major adjustments and adaptations not just for the mother but for all members of the family. It is during this time that parenting starts and a relationship with the newborn begins. A positive, loving relationship between parents and their newborn promotes the emotional well-being of all. This relationship endures and has profound effects on the child's growth and development.

▶ **Take** NOTE!

Parenting is a skill that is often learned by trial and error, with varying degrees of success. Successful parenting, a continuous and complex interactive process, requires the parents to learn new skills and to integrate the new member into the family.

Once the infant is born, each system in the mother's body takes several weeks to return to its non-pregnant state. The physiologic changes in women during the postpartum period are dramatic. Nurses should be aware of these changes and should be able to make observations and assessments to validate normal occurrences and detect any deviations.

In addition to physical assessment and care of the woman in the postpartum period, strong social support is vital to help her integrate the baby into the family. In today's mobile society, extended families may live far away and may be unable to help care for the new family. As a result, many new parents turn to health care professionals for information as well as physical and emotional support during this adjustment period. Nurses can be an invaluable resource by serving as mentors, teaching about self-care measures and baby care basics, and providing emotional support. Nurses can "mother" the new mother by offering physical care, emotional support, and information and practical help. The nurse's support and care through this critical time can increase the new parents' confidence, giving them a sense of accomplishment in their parenting skills.

One important intervention during the postpartum period is the promotion of breastfeeding. All women require individualized assessment and support around infant feeding decisions. Women also require attention and support for breastfeeding challenges (Breastfeeding Committee for Canada [BCC], 2011).

As in all nursing care, nurses should provide culturally competent care during the postpartum period. The nurse should engage in ongoing cultural self-assessment to ensure that appropriate understanding exists around the concepts of race, ethnicity, and the need to avoid stereotyping (London, Ladewig, Ball, et al., 2011). Providing culturally competent nursing care during the postpartum

period requires time, open-mindedness, and patience. To promote positive outcomes, the nurse should be sensitive to the woman's and family's culture, religion, and ethnic influences (see Providing Optimal Cultural Care in the Nursing Interventions section).

Remember the couple introduced at the beginning of the chapter? When the postpartum nurse comes to examine Raina, her husband quickly leaves the room and returns a short time later after the examination is complete. How do you interpret his behaviour toward his wife? What might you communicate to this couple?

This chapter describes the nursing management of the woman and her family during the postpartum period. It outlines physical assessment parameters for new mothers and newborns. It also focuses on bonding and attachment behaviours; nurses need to be aware of these behaviours so they can perform appropriate interventions. Steps to address physiologic needs such as comfort, self-care, nutrition, and contraception are described. Ways to help the woman and her family adapt to the birth of the newborn are also discussed (Fig. 16.1).

Nursing management during the postpartum period focuses on assessing the woman's ability to adapt to the physiologic and psychological changes occurring at this time (see Chapter 15 for a detailed discussion of these adaptations). Family members are also assessed to determine how well they are making the transition to this new stage. Based on the assessment findings, the nurse plans and implements care to address the family's needs. Because of today's shortened lengths of hospital stay, the nurse may be able to focus only on priority needs and may need to arrange for follow-up in the home to ensure that all the family's needs are met.

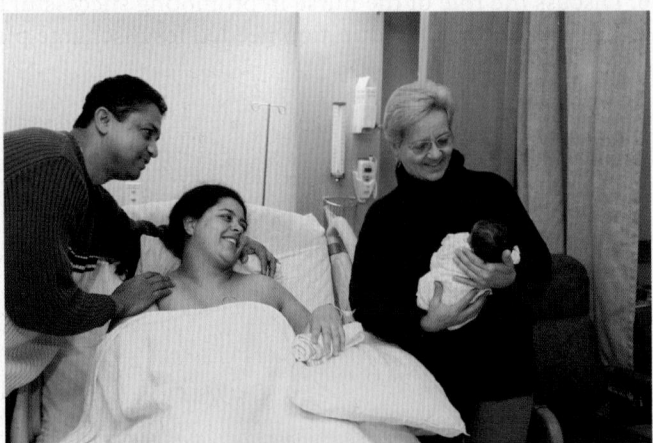

FIGURE 16.1 Parents and grandmother interacting with the newborn.

Assessment

Comprehensive nursing assessment begins within an hour after the woman gives birth and continues through discharge.

▶ *Take* NOTE!

Nurses need a firm grasp of normal findings so that they can recognize abnormal findings and intervene appropriately.

This assessment includes vital signs and physical and psychosocial assessments. Although the exact protocol may vary among facilities, postpartum assessment typically is performed at 5- to 15-minute intervals during the initial recovery period as needed. After that, vital signs should be taken:

• Every 30 minutes for 1 hour
• Every hour for 2 hours
• Every 4 to 8 hours (London et al., 2011)

During each assessment, keep in mind risk factors that may lead to complications, such as infection or hemorrhage, during the recovery period (Box 16.1). Early identification is critical to ensure prompt intervention.

As with any assessment, always review the woman's medical record for information about her pregnancy, labour, and birth. Note any preexisting conditions; any complications that occurred during pregnancy, labour, birth, and immediately afterward; and any treatments provided. This information is usually recorded on the labour record and any documents that were completed on admission as well as on the antenatal record that is provided by the physician. Postpartum assessment of the mother typically includes vital signs, pain level, and a systematic head-to-toe review of body systems. The acronym BUBBLE-EE—breasts, uterus, bladder, bowels, lochia, episiotomy/perineum, extremities, and emotional status—can be used as a guide for this head-to-toe review (Evans, Evans, Brown, et al., 2010). While assessing the woman and her family during the postpartum period, be alert for danger signs (Box 16.2). Notify the primary health care provider immediately if any are noted.

Postpartum assessment also includes assessing the parents and other family members, such as siblings and grandparents, for attachment and bonding with the newborn.

Vital Signs

Obtain vital signs and compare them with the previous values, noting and reporting any deviations. Vital sign changes can be an early indicator of complications.

BOX 16.1   Factors Increasing the Woman's Risk for Postpartum Complications

Risk Factors for Postpartum Infection
• Operative procedure (forceps, cesarean birth, vacuum extraction)
• History of diabetes, including gestational-onset diabetes
• Prolonged labour (more than 24 hours)
• Use of indwelling urinary catheter
• Anemia (hemoglobin <120 g/L)
• Multiple vaginal examinations during labour
• Prolonged rupture of membranes (more than 24 hours)
• Manual extraction of placenta
• Compromised immune system (HIV positive)

Risk Factors for Postpartum Hemorrhage
• Precipitous labour (less than 3 hours)
• Uterine atony
• Placenta previa or abruptio placentae
• Labour induction or augmentation
• Operative procedures (vacuum extraction, forceps, cesarean birth)
• Retained placental fragments
• Prolonged third stage of labour (more than 30 minutes)
• Multiparity, more than three births closely spaced
• Uterine overdistention (large infant, twins, hydramnios)

Temperature

Use a consistent measurement technique (oral, axillary, or tympanic) to get the most accurate readings. Typically, the new mother's temperature during the first 24 hours postpartum is within the normal range. Some women experience a slight fever, up to 38°C (100.4°C), during the first 24 hours as a result of the exertion of labour and the possibility of dehydration that subsequently occurs. Temperature should be normal after 24 hours with replacement of fluids lost during labour

---

BOX 16.2   Postpartum Danger Signs

• Fever higher than 38°C (100.4 °F)
• Foul-smelling lochia or an unexpected change in colour or amount
• Visual changes, such as blurred vision or spots, or headaches
• Calf pain with dorsiflexion of the foot
• Swelling, redness, or discharge at the episiotomy site
• Dysuria, burning, or incomplete emptying of the bladder
• Shortness of breath or difficulty breathing
• Depression or extreme mood swings

and birth (London et al., 2011). A temperature above 38°C (100.4°C) at any time or an abnormal temperature after the first 24 hours may indicate infection and must be reported. Abnormal temperature readings warrant continued monitoring until an infection can be ruled out through cultures or blood studies.

Pulse

Because of the changes in blood volume and cardiac output after delivery, relative bradycardia may be noted. The woman's pulse rate may range from 50 to 70 beats/minute as a decreased cardiac output takes hold following the expulsion of the placenta and the body adjusts to decreased circulating blood volume and a subsequent increased stroke volume. Pulse usually stabilizes to pre-pregnancy levels within 10 days (London et al., 2011).

Tachycardia in the postpartum woman can suggest anxiety, excitement, fatigue, pain, excessive blood loss, infection, or underlying cardiac problems. Further investigation is warranted to rule out complications.

Respirations

Respiratory rates in the postpartum woman should be within the normal range of 16 to 20 breaths/minute. Any change in respiratory rate out of the normal range might indicate respiratory infection, pulmonary edema, atelectasis, or pulmonary embolism and must be reported. Lungs should be clear on auscultation.

Blood Pressure

Assess the woman's blood pressure and compare it with her usual range. Report any deviation from this range. Elevations in blood pressure from baseline might suggest pregnancy-induced hypertension; decreases may suggest dehydration or excessive blood loss. A diastolic blood pressure reading of 90 to 95 mm Hg is suggestive of pregnancy-induced hypertension and needs to be reported.

Blood pressure also may vary based on the woman's position, so assess blood pressure with the woman in the same position every time. Be alert for orthostatic hypotension, which can occur when the woman moves rapidly from a lying or sitting position to a standing one. This potential is especially significant after childbirth, since there has been a significant change in body fluid volume and blood loss (London et al., 2011). Consider mobilizing the woman initially with the assistance of another nurse in case of fainting.

Pain

Pain, the fifth vital sign, is assessed along with the other four parameters. Question the woman about the type of pain and its location and severity. Have the woman rate the pain using a numeric scale from 0 to 10 points.

Many postpartum orders will have the nurse pre-medicate the woman routinely for afterbirth pains rather than wait for her to experience them first. The goal of pain management is to have the woman's pain scale rating maintained between 0 and 2 points at all times, especially after breastfeeding. This can be accomplished by assessing the woman's pain level frequently and preventing pain by administering analgesics. Comfort measures such as warm showers, deep breathing, reassurance, and a calm environment can also be helpful in preventing and alleviating postpartum discomfort. If the woman has severe pain in the perineal region despite use of physical comfort measures, check for a hematoma by inspecting and palpating the area. If one is found, notify the health care provider immediately.

Breasts

Inspect the breasts for size, contour, asymmetry, engorgement, or erythema. Check the nipples for cracks, redness, fissures, or bleeding, and note whether they are erect, flat, or inverted. Flat or inverted nipples can make breastfeeding challenging for both mother and infant. Cracked, blistered, fissured, bruised, or bleeding nipples in the breastfeeding woman are generally indications that the baby is improperly positioned on the breast. Palpate the breasts lightly to ascertain if they are soft, filling, or engorged, and document your findings. For women who are not breastfeeding, use a gentle, light touch to avoid breast stimulation, which will exacerbate engorgement. As milk is starting to come in, the breasts become firmer; this is charted as "filling." Engorged breasts are hard, tender, and taut. Ask the woman if she is having any nipple discomfort. Palpate the breasts for any nodules, masses, or areas of warmth, which may indicate a plugged duct that may progress to **mastitis** if not treated promptly. Any discharge from the nipple should be described and documented if it is not colostrum (creamy yellow) or foremilk (bluish white).

Uterus

Assess the fundus (top portion of the uterus) to determine the degree of uterine involution. If possible, have the woman empty her bladder before assessing the fundus. If the patient has had a cesarean birth and has a patient-controlled anesthesia pump, instruct her to self-medicate prior to fundal assessment to decrease her discomfort. Using a two-handed approach with the woman in the supine position and the bed in a flat position or as low as possible, palpate the abdomen gently, feeling for the top of the uterus while the other hand is placed on the lower segment of the uterus to stabilize it (Fig. 16.2).

The fundus should be midline and should feel firm. A boggy or relaxed uterus is a sign of uterine atony. This can be the result of bladder distention, which displaces the uterus upward and to the right, or retained placental fragments. Either situation predisposes the woman to

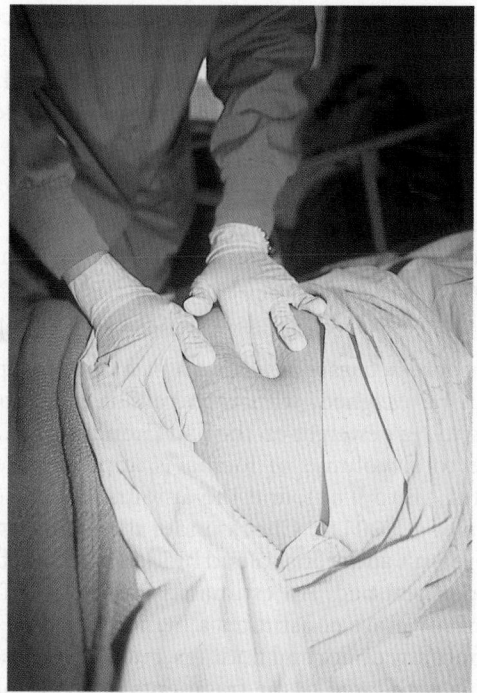

FIGURE 16.2 Palpating the fundus.

hemorrhage. Once the fundus is located, place your index finger on the fundus and count the number of fingerbreadths between the fundus and the umbilicus (one fingerbreadth is approximately equal to 1 cm). One to two hours after birth, the fundus typically is between the umbilicus and the symphysis pubis. Approximately 6 to 12 hours after birth, the fundus usually is at the level of the umbilicus (U/U).

Normally, the fundus progresses downward at a rate of one fingerbreadth (or 1 cm) per day after childbirth (London et al., 2011). On the first postpartum day, the top of the fundus is located 1 cm below the umbilicus and is recorded as U-1. Similarly, on the second postpartum day, the fundus would be 2 cm below the umbilicus and should be recorded as U-2, and so on. If the fundus is not firm, gently massage the uterus using a circular motion until it becomes firm.

Bladder

Considerable diuresis (called "puerperal diuresis")—as much as 3,000 mL—may follow for several days after childbirth as the woman's body adjusts its fluid balance to its pre-pregnant state. This heightened state of diuresis begins during the first 12 to 24 hours after delivery (London et al., 2011). However, many postpartum women do not sense the need to void even if their bladder is full. Women who received regional anesthesia during labour are at risk for bladder distention and for difficulty voiding until sensation returns within several hours after birth. Impediments to normal voiding could also be attributed to the tissue trauma that may have

occurred during the birthing process (especially in the case of a large baby, use of forceps during delivery, or a prolonged second stage of labour). It is important to consider the possibility of urethral edema, which has the potential to make the passage of urine difficult.

Assess for voiding problems by asking the woman the following questions:

• Have you (passed your water, urinated, gone to the bathroom) yet?
• Have you noticed any burning or discomfort with urination?
• Do you have any difficulty passing your urine?
• Do you feel that your bladder is empty when you finish urinating?
• Do you have any signs of infection such as urgency, frequency, or pain?
• Are you able to control the flow of urine by squeezing your muscles?
• Have you noticed any leakage of urine when you cough, laugh, or sneeze?

Assess the bladder for distention and adequate emptying after efforts to void. Palpate the area over the symphysis pubis. If empty, the bladder is not palpable. Palpation of a rounded mass suggests bladder distention. Also percuss the area: a full bladder is dull to percussion. If the bladder is full, lochia drainage will be more than normal because the uterus cannot contract to suppress the bleeding. The nurse must review the fluid intake and output (including blood loss) measurements during labour and into the postpartum period in order to evaluate for dehydration as a possible reason for low urine output.

▶ **Take** NOTE!

Note the location and condition of the fundus; a full bladder tends to displace the uterus up and to the right.

After the woman voids, palpate and percuss the area again to determine adequate emptying of the bladder. If the bladder remains distended, the woman may be retaining urine in her bladder, and measures such as urinary catheterization should be instituted in order to ensure that the bladder has been emptied. Be alert for signs of infection, including infrequent or insufficient voiding, fever, chills, nausea, discomfort, burning, urgency, or foul-smelling urine (Potter & Perry, 2010). Document urine output.

Bowels

Spontaneous bowel movements may not occur for 2 to 3 days after giving birth because of a decrease in muscle tone in the intestines during labour or because of bowel evacuation during delivery. Women with lacerations or an episiotomy or those who have undergone a cesarean birth may be reluctant to bear down to achieve a bowel movement; these women may benefit from stool softeners (London et al., 2011).

Inspect the woman's abdomen for distention, auscultate for bowel sounds in all four quadrants, and palpate for tenderness. The abdomen typically is soft, nontender, and nondistended. Bowel sounds are present in all four quadrants. Ask the woman if she has had a bowel movement or has passed gas since giving birth because constipation is a common problem during the postpartum period (especially following cesarean birth) and most women do not offer this information unless asked about it. Normal assessment findings are active bowel sounds, passing gas, and a nondistended abdomen.

Lochia

Assess lochia in terms of amount, colour, odour, and change with activity and time. To assess how much a woman is bleeding, ask her how many perineal pads she has used in the past 1 to 2 hours and how much drainage was on each pad. For example, did she saturate the pad completely, or was only half of the pad covered with drainage? Ask about the colour and odour of the drainage as well as the presence of any clots. Lochia has a definite musky scent, with an odour similar to that of menstrual flow without any large clots. Foul-smelling lochia suggests an infection, and large clots suggest poor uterine involution, necessitating additional intervention.

To determine the amount of lochia, observe the amount of lochia saturation on the perineal pad and relate it to time (Fig. 16.3). Lochia flow will increase when the woman gets out of bed (lochia pools in the vagina and the uterus while she is lying down) and when

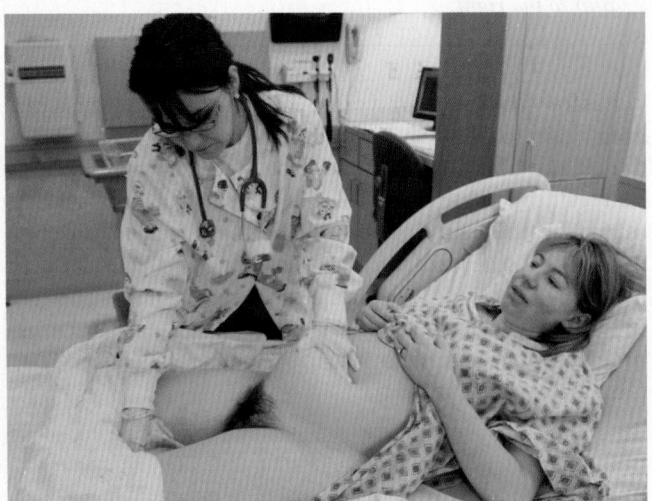

FIGURE 16.3 Assessing lochia.

she breastfeeds (oxytocin release causes uterine contractions). A woman who saturates a perineal pad within 30 to 60 minutes is bleeding much more than one who saturates a pad in 2 hours. Typically, the amount of lochia is described as follows:

• Scant: a 2.5 to 5 cm (1- to 2-inch) lochia stain on the perineal pad
• Light or small: an approximately 10 cm (4-inch) stain
• Moderate: a 10 to 15 cm (4- to 6-inch) stain
• Large or heavy: the pad is saturated within 1 hour

For more accurate assessment of blood loss, perineal pads can be weighed, with each millilitre of blood loss equating to 1 g of weight on the pad (London et al., 2011).

The total volume of lochia is approximately 240 to 270 mL (8 to 9 oz), and the amount decreases daily (London et al., 2011). Check under the woman to make sure there isn't additional blood hidden and not absorbed on her perineal pad. An estimated blood loss of 500 to 1,000 mL or more constitutes a hemorrhage.

Report any abnormal findings, such as heavy, bright-red lochia with large tissue fragments or a foul odour. If excessive bleeding occurs, the first step would be to massage the boggy fundus until it is firm to reduce the flow of blood. Document all findings.

Women who had a cesarean birth will usually have less lochia discharge than those who had a vaginal birth, but stages and colour changes remain the same. There is also a risk for postpartum hemorrhage among women who give birth by cesarean section, and it is important to assess for excessive bleeding according to the same guidelines used following a vaginal birth. Although the woman's abdomen will be tender after surgery, the nurse must palpate the fundus and assess the lochia to make sure they are within the normal range and that there is no excessive bleeding. Administering analgesic prior to the assessment is helpful when possible.

Anticipatory guidance to give the woman at discharge should include information about lochia and the expected changes. Urge the woman to notify her health care provider if lochia rubra returns after the serosa and alba transitions have taken place. This is abnormal and may indicate subinvolution or that the woman is too active and needs to rest more. Lochia is an excellent medium for bacterial growth. Explain to the woman that frequent changing of perineal pads, continued use of her peri bottle for rinsing the perineal area, and handwashing before and after pad changes are important infection control measures.

Episiotomy and Perineum

To assess the episiotomy and perineal area, position the woman on her side with her top leg flexed upward at the knee and drawn up toward her waist. If necessary, use a penlight to provide adequate lighting during the

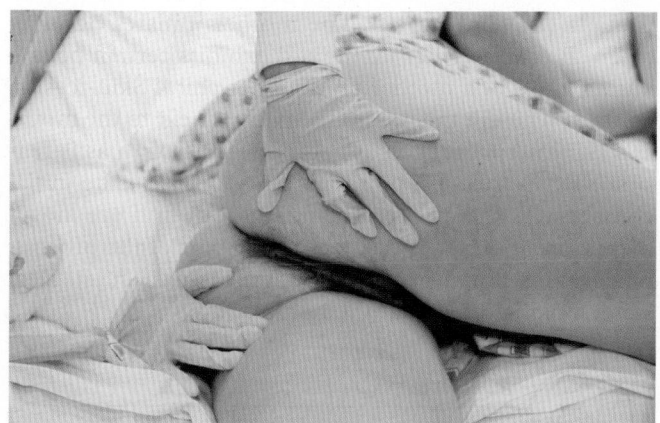

FIGURE 16.4 Inspecting the perineum.

assessment. Wearing gloves and standing at the woman's side with her back to you, gently lift the upper buttock to expose the perineum and anus (Fig. 16.4). Inspect the episiotomy for irritation, ecchymosis, tenderness, or hematomas. Assess for hemorrhoids and their condition.

During the early postpartum period, the perineal tissue surrounding the episiotomy is typically edematous and slightly bruised. The normal episiotomy site should not have redness, discharge, or edema. The majority of healing takes place within the first 2 weeks, but it may take 4 to 6 months for the episiotomy to heal completely (London et al., 2011). Lacerations to the perineal area sustained during the birthing process that were identified and repaired also need to be assessed to determine their healing status. Lacerations are classified based on their severity and tissue involvement:

• First-degree laceration—involves only skin and superficial structures above muscle
• Second-degree laceration—extends through perineal muscles
• Third-degree laceration—extends through the anal sphincter muscle
• Fourth-degree laceration—continues through anterior rectal wall

Assess the episiotomy and any lacerations at least every 8 hours to detect hematomas or signs of infection. Large areas of swollen, bluish skin with complaints of severe pain in the perineal area indicate pelvic or vulvar hematomas. Redness, swelling, increasing discomfort, or purulent drainage may indicate infection. Both findings need to be reported immediately.

A white line the length of the episiotomy is a sign of infection, as is swelling or discharge. Severe, intractable pain, perineal discolouration, and ecchymosis indicate a perineal hematoma, a potentially dangerous condition. Report any unusual findings. Ice can be applied to relieve discomfort and reduce edema; sitz baths also can promote comfort and perineal healing (see Promoting Comfort in the Nursing Interventions section).

Extremities

During pregnancy, the state of hypercoagulability protects the mother against excessive blood loss during childbirth and placental separation. However, this hypercoagulable state can increase the risk of thromboembolic disorders during pregnancy and postpartum. Three factors predispose women to thromboembolic disorders during pregnancy: stasis (compression of the large veins because of the gravid uterus), altered coagulation (state of pregnancy), and localized vascular damage (may occur during birthing process). All of these increase the risk of clot formation.

> ▶ *Take* NOTE!
>
> *Changes in coagulation during pregnancy, in combination with compression of the common iliac vein because of the pregnant uterus, increase the risk for thromboembolic disease in pregnant and postpartum women. Approximately 1 in 500 to 700 women experience superficial vein thrombosis.*

Pulmonary embolus is a potentially life-threatening event that occurs when thrombi originating from the extremities travel to the pulmonary artery and obstruct the flow of blood to the lungs. Risk factors associated with thromboembolic conditions include:

• Anemia
• Diabetes mellitus
• Cigarette smoking
• Obesity
• Pre-eclampsia secondary to exaggeration of hypercoagulable state
• Hypertension
• Varicose veins
• Pregnancy
• Oral contraceptive use or hormone replacement therapy
• Cesarean birth
• Previous thromboembolic disease
• Multiparity
• Inactivity
• Advanced maternal age (London et al., 2011)

Because of the subtle presentation of thromboembolic disorders, the physical examination may not be enough to detect them. The woman may report lower extremity tightness or aching when ambulating that is relieved with rest and elevation of the leg. Edema in the affected leg (typically the left), along with warmth and tenderness, may also be noted. Diagnosis is dependent on a variety of factors and tests, including client history, physical examination, and venous ultrasonography or occlusive impedance plethysmography. Women at increased risk for this condition during the postpartum period should wear antiembolism stockings or use sequential compression devices to reduce their risk for thrombophlebitis. Encouraging the client to ambulate after childbirth reduces the incidence of thrombophlebitis. Heparin therapy is used for deep vein thrombosis (London et al., 2011).

Emotional Status

Assess the woman's emotional status by observing how she interacts with her family, her level of independence, energy levels, eye contact with her infant (within a cultural context), posture and comfort level while holding the newborn, and sleep and rest patterns. Be alert for mood swings, irritability, or crying episodes.

Remember Raina and her "quiet" husband, the Muslim couple? The postpartum nurse informs Raina that her doctor, Nancy Schultz, has been called away for emergency surgery and won't be available the rest of the day. The nurse explains that Dr. Robert Nappo will be making rounds for her. Raina and her husband become upset. Why? Is culturally competent care being provided to this couple?

Bonding and Attachment

Nurses can be instrumental in promoting attachment by assessing attachment behaviours (positive and negative) and intervening appropriately if needed. Nurses must be able to identify any family discord that might interfere with the attachment process. Remember, however, that mothers from different cultures may behave differently from what is expected in your own culture. Use of herbal remedies after childbirth, for example, may be common among women of Aboriginal or Chinese descent (London et al., 2011). Don't assume that different behaviour is wrong. Engaging in conversation with the woman regarding different practices can be helpful for both the nurse and the patient in order to deepen cultural awareness.

Meeting their newborn for the first time after birth can be an exhilarating experience for parents. Although the mother has spent many hours dreaming of her unborn child and how he or she will look, it is not until after birth that they meet face to face. They both need to get to know one another and to develop feelings for one another.

Bonding is the close emotional attraction to a newborn by the parents that optimally develops during the first 30 to 60 minutes after birth. It is unidirectional, from parent to infant. It is thought that optimal bonding of the parents to a newborn requires a period of close contact within the first few minutes to a few hours after birth (Society of Obstetricians and Gynaecologists of Canada [SOGC], 2010). The mother initiates bonding when she caresses her infant and exhibits certain behaviours typical of a mother tending her child. Skin-to-skin contact, wherein the unclothed baby is next to the mother's skin, is encouraged as soon after the birth as is feasible (BCC, 2011). The infant's responses to the initial contact with the mother, including body and eye movements, are thought to be a necessary part of the process. During this initial period, the infant is in a quiet, alert state, looking directly at the holder.

▶ ***Take* NOTE!**

The length of time necessary for bonding depends on the health of the infant and mother as well as the circumstances surrounding the labour and birth (London et al., 2011).

Attachment is the development of strong affection between an infant and a significant other (mother, father, sibling, or caretaker) (McKinney, James, Murray, et al., 2009). The process of attachment follows a progressive or developmental course that changes over time. Attachment is an individualized and multifactorial process that differs based on the health of the infant, the mother, and environmental circumstances such as the need to care for other children (McKinney et al., 2009). It occurs through mutually satisfying experiences. Maternal attachment begins during pregnancy as the result of fetal movement and maternal fantasies about the infant and continues through the birth and postpartum periods. Attachment behaviours include seeking, staying close to, and exchanging gratifying experiences with the infant. In a high-risk pregnancy, the attachment process may be complicated by premature birth (lack of time to develop a relationship with the unborn baby) and by parental stress due to the fetal and/or maternal vulnerability (McKinney et al., 2009).

Bonding is a vital component of the attachment process and is necessary in establishing parent–infant attachment and a healthy, loving relationship. During this early period of acquaintance, mothers touch their infants in a very characteristic manner. Mothers visually and physically "explore" their infants, initially using their fingertips on the infant's face and extremities and progressing to massaging and stroking the infant with their fingers. This is followed by palm contact on the trunk. Eventually, mothers draw their infant toward them and hold the infant. Mothers also interact with their infants through eye-to-eye contact in the ***en face* position** (Fig. 16.5) (McKinney et al., 2009).

Generally, research on attachment has found that the process is similar for fathers as for mothers. Fathers develop an emotional tie with their infants in a variety of ways. They seek and maintain closeness with the infant

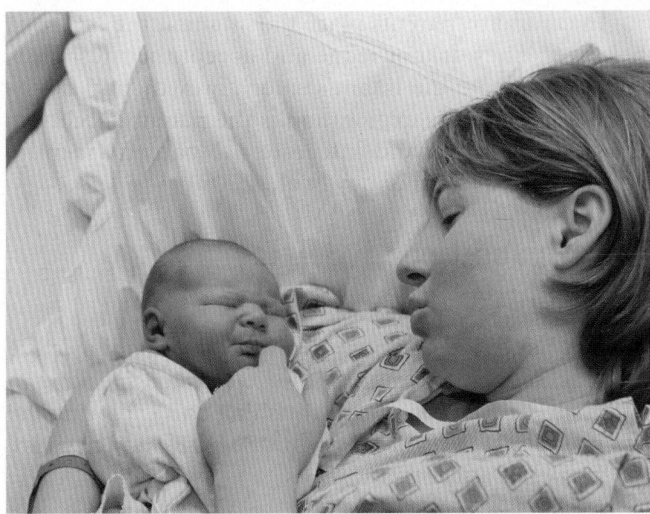

FIGURE 16.5 *En face* position.

and can recognize characteristics of the infant. Initially, the father (like the mother) will spend time inspecting the new infant and experience the euphoria that can be a part of the birth experience. For the father, attachment increases as the baby responds to him. It is important for the father to be included in the teaching and care of the infant so that his involvement will be as complete as possible (McKinney et al., 2009). Attachment is a process; it does not occur instantaneously, even though many parents believe in a romanticized version of attachment, which happens right after birth. A delay in the attachment process can occur if a mother's physical and emotional states are adversely affected by exhaustion, pain, the absence of a support system, anesthesia, or an unwanted outcome (London et al., 2011).

> ▶ *Take* NOTE!
>
> *Many midwives teach fathers to massage their partners, which has been proven to have a positive effect on the pregnancy, labour, bonding and attachment, and perhaps on family dynamics (Whitehouse, 2006).*

The developmental task for the infant is learning to differentiate between trust and mistrust. If the mother or caretaker is consistently responsive to the infant's care, meeting the baby's physical and psychological needs, the infant will likely learn to trust the caretaker, view the world as a safe place, and grow up to be secure, self-reliant, trusting, cooperative, and helpful. However, if the infant's needs are not met, the child is more likely to face developmental delays, neglect, and child abuse (Logsdon, Wisner, Pinto-Foltz, 2006).

"Becoming" a parent may take 4 to 6 months. The transition to parenthood involves four stages:

1. Commitment, attachment, and preparation for an infant during pregnancy, including the choice of care provider for the birth, acquiring prenatal instruction, and seeking out mentors and role models to learn about mothering behaviours.
2. Acquaintance with, and increasing attachment to, the infant, learning how to care for the infant, and physical restoration during the first weeks after birth. This phase often requires many supports from family, friends, and care providers. Women are intent on learning how to interpret their baby's cues.
3. Moving toward a new normal routine in the first 4 months after birth. Mothers gain confidence about their abilities to mother the infant based on their individual situation, as opposed to relying on textbooks or following other's instructions without question.
4. Achievement of a parenthood role around 4 months, wherein mothers have integrated the role of parent into their lives.

The stages overlap, and the timing of each is affected by variables such as the environment, family dynamics, and the partners (McKinney et al., 2009).

Factors Affecting Attachment

Attachment behaviours are influenced by three major factors:

1. Parents' background (includes the care that the parents received when growing up, cultural practices, relationship within the family, experience with previous pregnancies and planning and course of events during pregnancy, postpartum depression)
2. Infant (includes the infant's temperament and health at birth)
3. Care practices (the behaviours of physicians, midwives, nurses, and hospital personnel; care and support during labour; first day of life in separation of mother and infant; and rules of the hospital or birthing centre) (Grossman, Grossman, Waters, 2006)

Attachment occurs more readily with the infant whose temperament, health, appearance, and gender fit the parent's expectations. If the infant does not meet these expectations, parents may grieve the loss of the fantasy that they held about the infant during the pregnancy (McKinney et al., 2009).

Factors associated with the health care facility or birthing unit can also hinder attachment. These include:

- Separation of infant and parents immediately after birth and for long periods during the day
- Policies that discourage unwrapping and exploring the infant

- Intensive care environment, restrictive visiting policies
- Staff indifference or lack of support for parent's care-taking attempts and abilities

Critical Attributes of Attachment

The terms "bonding" and "attachment" are often used interchangeably, even though they involve different time frames and interactions. Bonding refers to the initial connection toward the infant that is felt by the parents during pregnancy and the initial contact 30 to 60 minutes following the birth. Attachment is a reciprocal process that continues to develop as mutually satisfying interactions occur between the parents and the child. Parents who are sensitive and responsive to their infant's cues will promote the infant's development and growth. Parents who become skilled at recognizing the ways their infant communicates will respond appropriately by smiling, vocalizing, and touching.

Maternal behaviours that facilitate attachment include:

- "Fingertipping," in which the mother explores the baby's face, fingers, and toes with her fingertips only
- Stroking the baby's chest with her palm, beginning to enfold the child, and engaging in consoling behaviours
- Beginning to identify specific features of the infant, including resemblance to family members
- Speaking to the infant in a high-pitched and soothing voice, and referring to the infant according to the child's gender rather than as "it" (McKinney et al., 2009)

In centrality, parents place the infant at the centre of their lives. They acknowledge and accept their responsibility to promote the infant's safety, growth, and development. Parent role exploration is the parents' ability to find their own way and integrate the parental identity into themselves (McKinney et al., 2009).

Positive and Negative Attachment Behaviours

Positive bonding behaviours include maintaining close physical contact, making eye-to-eye contact, speaking in soft, high-pitched tones, and touching and exploring the infant. Table 16.1 highlights typical positive and negative behaviours of attachment.

Nursing Interventions

In terms of postpartum hospital stays today, "less is more." If the woman had a vaginal delivery, she may be discharged in 24 hours or less, depending on her condition and her preferences. If she had a cesarean birth, she may remain hospitalized for 72 hours. This shortened stay leaves little time for nurses to prepare the woman and her family for the many changes that will occur when she returns home. Nurses need to use this limited time to address the following topics: pain and discomfort, immunizations, nutrition, activity and exercise, lactation, discharge teaching, sexuality and contraception, and follow-up (Nursing Care Plan 16.1).

TABLE 16.1 POSITIVE AND NEGATIVE ATTACHMENT BEHAVIOURS

	Positive Behaviours	Negative Behaviours
Infant	Smiles; is alert; demonstrates strong grasp reflex to hold parent's finger; sucks well, feeds easily; enjoys being held close; makes eye-to-eye contact; follows parent's face; appears facially appealing; is consolable when crying	Feeds poorly, regurgitates often; cries for long periods, colicky and inconsolable; shows flat affect, rarely smiles even when prompted; resists holding and closeness; sleeps with eyes closed most of the time; stiffens body when held; is unresponsive to parents; doesn't pay attention to parents' faces
Parent	Makes direct eye contact; assumes *en face* position when holding infant; claims infant as family member, pointing out common features; expresses pride in infant; assigns meaning to infant's actions; smiles and gazes at infant; touches infant, progressing from fingertips to holding; names infant; requests to be close to infant as much as allowed; speaks positively about infant	Expresses disappointment or displeasure in infant; fails to "explore" infant visually or physically; fails to claim infant as part of family; avoids caring for infant; finds excuses not to hold infant close; has negative self-concept; appears uninterested in having infant in room; frequently asks to have infant taken back to nursery to be cared for; assigns negative attributes to infant and calls infant inappropriate, negative names (e.g., frog, monkey, tadpole)

Sources: Grossman, K. E., Grossman, K., & Waters, E. (2006). *Attachment from infancy to adulthood.* New York: Guilford Publications, Inc; Nash, L. R. (2007). Postpartum care. In R. E. Rakel & E. T. Bope (Eds.), *Conn's current therapy 2007.* Philadelphia: Saunders Elsevier; & Oppenheim, D., & Goldsmith, D. F. (2007). *Attachment theory in clinical work with children: Bridging the gap between research and practice.* New York: Guilford Publications, Inc.

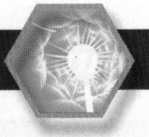

Nursing Care Plan 16.1

OVERVIEW OF THE POSTPARTUM WOMAN

Belinda, a 26-year-old G2P2, is a patient on the mother–baby unit after giving birth to a term 3.7 kg (8 lb, 2 oz) baby boy yesterday. The night nurse reports that she has an episiotomy, complains of a pain rating of 7 points on a scale of 1 to 10, is having difficulty breastfeeding, and had heavy lochia most of the night. The nurse also reports that the patient seems focused on her own needs and not on her infant. Assessment this morning reveals the following:

B: Breasts are soft with colostrum leaking; nipples cracked
U: Uterus is one fingerbreadth below the umbilicus; deviated to right
B: Bladder is palpable; patient states she hasn't been up to void yet
B: Bowels have not moved; bowel sounds present; passing flatus
L: Lochia is moderate; perineal pad soaked from night accumulation
E: Episiotomy site intact; swollen, bruised; hemorrhoids present
—
E: Extremities; no edema over tibia, no warmth or tenderness in calf
E: Emotional status is "distressed" as a result of discomfort and fatigue

NURSING DIAGNOSIS: Impaired tissue integrity related to episiotomy

Outcome Identification and Evaluation
The woman remains free of infection, without any signs and symptoms of infection, and exhibits evidence of progressive healing as demonstrated by a clean, dry, intact episiotomy site.

Interventions: Promoting Tissue Integrity
- Monitor episiotomy site *to check for redness, edema, and signs of infection.*
- Assess vital signs at least every 4 hours *to identify changes suggesting infection.*
- Apply ice pack to episiotomy site *to reduce swelling.*
- Instruct patient on use of sitz bath *to promote healing, hygiene, and comfort.*
- Encourage frequent perineal care and perineal pad changes *to prevent infection.*
- Recommend ambulation *to improve circulation and promote healing.*
- Instruct patient on positioning *to relieve pressure on perineal area.*
- Demonstrate use of anesthetic sprays *to numb perineal area.*

NURSING DIAGNOSIS: Pain related to episiotomy, sore nipples, and hemorrhoids

Outcome Identification and Evaluation
The woman experiences a decrease in pain, reporting that her pain has diminished to a tolerable level, rating it as 2 points or less.

Interventions: Providing Pain Relief
- Thoroughly inspect perineum *to rule out hematoma as cause of pain.*
- Administer analgesic medication as ordered *to promote comfort.*
- Carry out comfort measures to episiotomy as outlined earlier *to reduce pain.*
- Explain discomforts and reassure the client that they are time-limited to assist in coping with pain.
- Apply Tucks pads to swollen hemorrhoids *to induce shrinkage and reduce pain.*
- Suggest frequent use of sitz bath *to reduce hemorrhoid pain.*
- Administer stool softener and laxative *to prevent straining with first bowel movement.*
- Observe positioning and latching-on technique during breastfeeding. Offer suggestions based on observations to correct positioning/latching-on *to minimize trauma to the breast.*
- Suggest air-drying of nipples after breastfeeding and use of plain water *to prevent nipple cracking.*
- Teach relaxation techniques when breastfeeding *to reduce anxiety and discomfort.*

(continued)

Nursing Care Plan 16.1 (continued)

NURSING DIAGNOSIS: Risk for ineffective coping related to mood alteration and pain

Outcome Identification and Evaluation
The woman copes with mood alterations, as evidenced by positive statements about newborn and participation in newborn care.

Interventions: Promoting Effective Coping
- Provide a supportive, nurturing environment and encourage the mother to vent her feelings and frustrations to relieve anxiety.
- Provide opportunities for the mother to rest and sleep *to combat fatigue.*
- Encourage the mother to eat a well-balanced diet *to increase her energy level.*
- Provide reassurance and explanations that mood alterations are common after birth secondary to waning hormones after pregnancy *to increase the mother's knowledge.*
- Allow the mother relief from newborn care *to afford opportunity for self-care.*
- Discuss with partner expected behaviour from mother and how additional support and help are needed during this stressful time *to promote partner's participation in care.*
- Make appropriate community referrals for mother–infant support *to ensure continuity of care.*
- Encourage frequent skin-to-skin contact and closeness between mother and infant *to facilitate bonding and attachment behaviours.*
- Encourage client to participate in infant care and provide instructions as needed *to foster a sense of independence and self-esteem.*
- Offer praise and reinforcement of positive mother–infant interactions *to enhance self-confidence in care.*

▶ *Take* NOTE!

Always adhere to standard precautions when providing direct care to reduce the risk of disease transmission.

Providing Optimal Cultural Care

As Canadian culture becomes more diverse, nurses must be prepared to care for childbearing families from various cultures. In many cultures, women and their families are cared for and nurtured by their community for weeks and even months after the birth of a new family member. Box 16.3 highlights some of the major cultural variants during the postpartum period.

Many Aboriginal women from remote areas are encouraged to relocate to major centres to await the birth of a child, since their home communities are not seen as having the appropriate resources to deliver babies. These women may experience a sense of social and cultural isolation from family and loved ones and may be separated from their other children or partners. The SOGC (2010) recommends a new model of care for women whose pregnancies are considered low risk so that they can stay in their home communities and be attended by local health care providers such as midwives or physicians. Resource development in remote communities (in the form of trained care providers) would be necessary before the current model of care could be

changed (SOGC, 2010). Nurses need to remember that childbearing practices and beliefs vary across cultures. To provide appropriate nursing care, the nurse should determine the patient's preferences before intervening. Cultural practices may include dietary restrictions, certain clothes, taboos, activities for maintaining mental health, and the use of silence, prayer, or meditation.

*R*aina and her husband are upset at the thought of having a male doctor care for her because Muslim women are very modest and prefer having a same-sex care provider. What should the nurse do in this situation?

Promoting Comfort

The postpartum woman may have discomfort and pain from a variety of sources, such as an episiotomy, perineal lacerations, an edematous perineum, inflamed hemorrhoids, engorged breasts, afterbirth pains secondary to uterine contractions in breastfeeding and multiparous mothers, and sore nipples if breastfeeding. Non-pharmacologic and pharmacologic measures can be used to decrease pain and discomfort. See Evidence-based Practice 16.1.

Applications of Cold and Heat
Commonly, an ice pack is the first measure used after a vaginal birth to relieve perineal discomfort from edema,

BOX 16.3 **Cultural Influences During the Postpartum Period**

French Canadian

Traditional French Canadian culture is comprised of people of European and Aboriginal heritage. Historically, contraceptive practices in French Canada were closely tied with the Roman Catholic religion. However, that is no longer the case and women today exercise conscious health and lifestyle decision making. In recent years, "francophones" of other origins who are French speaking (such as people from French-speaking African countries) also comprise French Canadian culture. If the nurse has the ability, speaking French with the family is a helpful way to include the extended family and connect with community resources (Evans et al., 2010).

- The practice of "la culbute" is when a parent holds the baby above the crib and rotates him or her in hopes that the infant will sleep during the night and be awake during the day.

First Nations

Aboriginal women comprise a diverse population in which unique cultural practices may be passed down using the oral tradition. Cultural practices may therefore be communicated among specific groups and may differ from one another. Because these cultural practices are communicated orally, it is important for the nurse to gain understanding by direct communication with the mother and her family (L. Barney, personal communication, January 20, 2011).

The importance of extended family is deeply embedded in the traditions and beliefs of Aboriginal people. Therefore, the nurse should consider individual accommodations such as encouraging the elder woman to be present when needed. The person who will be the infant's primary caregiver (which may not be the mother) should be included in all teaching. Health care services, in general, attempt to accommodate traditional native healing practices whenever possible, as those practices attempt to foster harmony with the environment and with the family (Evans et al., 2010).

Asian

The term "Asian" refers to people from Korea, China, Japan, the Philippines, and Southeast Asia. The importance of family is a core value, as are honour and harmony. In general, mothers of Asian descent tend to exhibit more protective behaviour of their children compared with Western approaches. The authority of the elders is unquestioned (Evans et al., 2010).

Japanese

- Cleanliness and protection from cold are essential components of newborn care. Nurses should give the daily bath to the infant.
- Newborns routinely are not taken outside the home because it is believed that they should not be exposed to outside or cold air. Infants should be kept in a quiet, clean, warm place for the first month of life.
- Breastfeeding is the primary method of feeding.
- Many women stay in their parents' home for 1 to 2 months after birth.
- Bathing the infant can be the centre of family activity at home (Bowers, 2007).

Filipino

- Grandparents often assist in the care of their grandchildren.
- Breastfeeding is encouraged, and some mothers breastfeed their children for up to 2 years.
- Women have difficulty discussing birth control and sexual matters.
- Strong religious beliefs prevail, and bedside prayer is common.
- Families are very close-knit, and numerous visitors can be expected at the hospital after childbirth (Srivastava, 2007).

Hispanic

People from Latin America, Central America, and South America are represented by the term "Hispanic." The Hispanic culture is primarily patriarchal, but in matters of health the woman usually makes the decisions, as her role is to care for the women and children. Often the extended family members are consulted before the medical community in case of illness. Home remedies and folk remedies may be valued (Evans et al., 2010).

Mexican

- The newborn's grandmother lives with the mother for several weeks after birth to help with housekeeping and child care.
- Most women will breastfeed more than 1 year. The infant is carried in a *rebozo* (shawl) that allows easy access for breastfeeding.
- Women may avoid eye contact and may not feel comfortable being touched by a stranger. Nurses need to respect this feeling.
- Some women may bring religious icons to the hospital and may want to display them in their room (Srivastava, 2007).

Muslim

Muslim families are patriarchal, but within the marriage the woman may have considerable influence over decision making. Culturally, the birth of a child is welcomed, as it promotes family status. Because Muslim women are concerned with modesty, they may have a preference for female birth attendants only (Evans et al., 2010).

- Modesty is a primary concern; nurses need to protect the client's modesty.
- Muslims are not permitted to eat pork; check all food items before serving.
- Male–female touching is prohibited except in an emergency situation.
- A Muslim woman stays in the house for 40 days after birth, being cared for by the female members of her family.
- Most Muslim women will breastfeed, but religious events call for periods of fasting, which may increase the risk of dehydration or malnutrition.
- Women are exempt from obligatory five-times-daily prayers as long as lochia is present.
- Extended family is likely to be present throughout much of the woman's hospital stay. They will need an empty room to perform their prayers without having to leave the hospital (Cassar, 2006).

EVIDENCE-BASED PRACTICE 16.1
Administration of Paracetamol (Acetaminophen) to Relieve Postpartum Perineal Pain

The perineum often incurs trauma following a vaginal delivery because of the stretching and/or tearing of tissue that occurs during the birth, especially if forceps or vacuum extraction is used or an episiotomy has been performed. Perineal pain and swelling can interfere with mobilization, breastfeeding positioning, and general well-being of new mothers.

● **Study**

Because the discomfort in the sensitive perineal area has the potential to diminish the quality of experience in the important first few days of the postpartum period, a meta-analysis of studies was conducted to ascertain whether administration of acetaminophen (at a dose of 500 to 1,000 mg) would alleviate discomfort in the perineal region.

It is important to note that this medication is generally assumed to be safe with breastfeeding.

▲ **Findings**

The use of acetaminophen was more effective than the placebo for treating perineal pain.

■ **Nursing Implications**

This study concluded that women should be offered pain relief for perineal pain, even though some women may choose to decline it. It appears that a dose of either 500 or 1,000 mg of acetaminophen is effective, and there does not appear to be any rise in adverse effects if the medication is used according to instructions. Women can also be reassured that the medication does not pose a heightened risk to their breastfeeding newborn.

Source: Chou, D., Abalos, E., Gyte, G. M. L., Gülmezoglu, A. M. (2010). Paracetamol/acetaminophen (single administration) for perineal pain in the early postpartum period [review]. *The Cochrane Library*, 3:CD008407

an episiotomy, or laceration. It is applied during the fourth stage of labour and can be used for the first 24 hours to reduce perineal edema and prevent hematoma formation, thus reducing pain and promoting healing. Ice packs are wrapped in a disposable covering or clean washcloth and are applied to the perineal area. Usually the ice pack is applied for 20 minutes and removed for 10 minutes. Many commercially prepared ice packs are available, but a latex glove filled with crushed ice and covered can also be used if the mother is not allergic to latex. Ensure that the ice pack is changed frequently to promote good hygiene and to allow for periodic assessments.

The **peri bottle** is a plastic squeeze bottle filled with warm tap water that is sprayed over the perineal area after each voiding and before applying a new perineal pad. Usually the peri bottle is introduced to the woman when she is assisted to the bathroom to freshen up and void for the first time—in most instances, once vital signs are stable after the first hour. Provide the woman with instructions on how and when to use the peri bottle. Reinforce this practice each time she changes her pad, voids, or defecates, making sure that she understands to direct the flow of water from front to back. The woman can take the peri bottle home and use it over the next several weeks until her lochia discharge stops. The peri bottle can be used by women who had either vaginal or cesarean births to provide comfort and hygiene to the perineal area.

After the first 24 hours, a **sitz bath** with warm water may be prescribed and substituted for the ice pack to reduce local swelling and promote comfort for

an episiotomy, perineal trauma, or inflamed hemorrhoids. The change from cold to warm therapy enhances vascular circulation and healing (London et al., 2011). Before using a sitz bath, the woman should cleanse the perineum with a peri bottle or take a shower using mild soap.

Most health care agencies use plastic disposable sitz baths that women can take home. The plastic sitz bath

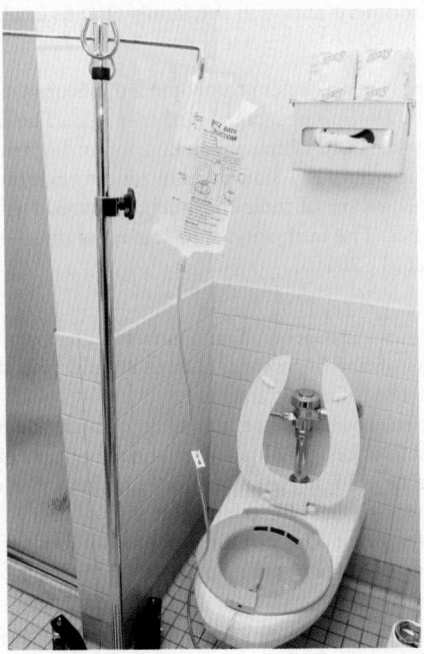

FIGURE 16.6 Sitz bath setup.

consists of a basin that fits on the commode; a bag filled with warm water is hung on a hook and connected via a tube onto the front of the basin (Fig. 16.6). Teaching Guideline 16.1 highlights the steps in using a sitz bath.

Advise the woman to use the sitz bath several times daily to provide hygiene and comfort to the perineal area. Encourage her to continue this measure after discharge.

Keep in mind that tremendous hemodynamic changes are taking place within the mother during this early postpartum period, and her safety must be a priority. Fatigue, blood loss, the effects of medications, and lack of food may cause her to feel weak when she stands up. Assisting the woman to the bathroom to instruct her on how to use the peri bottle and sitz bath is necessary to ensure her safety. Many women become lightheaded or dizzy when they get out of bed and need direct physical assistance. Staying in the woman's room, ensuring that the emergency call light is readily available, and being available if needed during this early period will ensure safety and prevent accidents and falls.

Topical Preparations

Several treatments may be applied topically for temporary relief of pain and discomfort. One such treatment is a local anesthetic spray such as Dermoplast or Americaine. These agents numb the perineal area and are used after cleansing the area with water via the peri bottle and/or a sitz bath.

For hemorrhoid discomfort, cool witch hazel pads, such as Tucks Medicated Pads, can be used. The pads are placed at the rectal area, between the hemorrhoids and the perineal pad. These pads cool the area, help relieve swelling, and minimize itching.

Analgesics

Analgesics such as acetaminophen (Tylenol) and oral nonsteroidal anti-inflammatory drugs (NSAIDs) such as ibuprofen (Motrin) are prescribed to relieve mild postpartum discomfort. For moderate to severe pain, a narcotic analgesic such as codeine or oxycodone in conjunction with aspirin or acetaminophen may be prescribed. Instruct the woman about the possible adverse effects of any medication prescribed. Common adverse effects of oral opioid analgesics include dizziness, lightheadedness, nausea and vomiting, constipation, urinary retention, myoclonus, and sedation (Potter & Perry, 2010).

Also inform the woman that the drugs are secreted in breast milk. Nearly all medications that the mother takes are passed into her breast milk; however, mild analgesics (e.g., acetaminophen or ibuprofen) are considered relatively safe for breastfeeding mothers (Moretti, Lee, Ito, 2000). Administering a mild analgesic approximately an hour before breastfeeding will usually relieve afterpains and/or perineal discomfort.

Assisting with Elimination

The bladder is edematous, hypotonic, and congested immediately postpartum. Consequently, bladder distention, incomplete emptying, and inability to void are common. A full bladder interferes with uterine contraction and may lead to hemorrhage because it will displace the uterus out of the midline. Encourage the woman to void. Often, assisting her to assume the normal voiding position on the commode facilitates this. If the woman has difficulty voiding, pouring warm water over the perineal area, listening to the sound of running tap water, blowing bubbles through a straw, taking a warm shower, drinking fluids, or placing her hand in a basin of warm water may stimulate the urge to void. If these actions do not stimulate urination within 4 to 6 hours after giving birth, catheterization may be needed. Palpate the bladder for distention and ask the woman if she is voiding in small amounts (less than 100 mL) frequently (retention with overflow). If catheterization is necessary, use sterile technique to reduce the risk of infection.

Decreased bowel motility during labour, high iron content in prenatal vitamins, postpartum fluid loss, and the adverse effects of pain medications and/or anesthesia may predispose the postpartum woman to constipation.

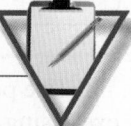

TEACHING GUIDELINE 16.1

Using a Sitz Bath

1. Close clamp on tubing before filling bag with water to prevent leakage.
2. Fill sitz bath basin and plastic bag with warm water (comfortable to touch).
3. Place the filled basin on the toilet with the seat raised and the overflow opening facing toward the back of the toilet.
4. Hang the filled plastic bag on a hook close to the toilet or on an IV pole.
5. Attach the tubing to the opening on the basin.
6. Position the basin on the toilet seat and release the clamp to allow warm water to irrigate the perineum.
7. Remain seated on the basin for approximately 15 to 20 minutes.
8. Stand up and pat the perineum area dry. Apply a clean perineal pad.
9. Tip the basin to remove any remaining water and flush the toilet.
10. Wash the basin with warm water and soap and dry it in the sink.
11. Store basin and tubing in a clean, dry area until the next use.
12. Wash hands with soap and water.

In addition, the woman may fear that bowel movements will cause pain or injury, especially if she had an episiotomy or a laceration that was repaired with sutures.

Usually a stool softener, such as docusate (Colace), with or without a laxative might be helpful if the client has difficulty with bowel elimination. Other measures, such as ambulating and increasing fluid and fibre intake, may also help. Nutritional instruction might include increasing fruits and vegetables in the diet; drinking plenty of fluids (8 to 12 cups daily) to keep the stool soft; drinking small amounts of prune juice and/or hot liquids to stimulate peristalsis; eating high-fibre foods such as bran cereals, whole grains, dried fruits, fresh fruits, and raw vegetables; and walking daily.

Promoting Activity, Rest, and Exercise

The postpartum period is an ideal time for nurses to promote the importance of physical fitness, help women incorporate exercise into their lifestyle, and encourage them to overcome barriers to exercise. The lifestyle changes that occur postpartum may affect a woman's health for decades. Early ambulation is encouraged to reduce the risk of thromboembolism and to improve strength.

Many changes occur postpartum, and caring for a newborn alters the woman's eating and sleeping habits, work schedules, and time allocation. Postpartum fatigue is common during the early days after childbirth, and it may continue for weeks or months. Fatigue should be assessed as a symptom of postpartum depression or a thyroid condition (London et al., 2011). Fatigue affects the mother's relationships with significant others and her ability to fulfill household and child care responsibilities. Be sure that the mother recognizes her need for rest and sleep and is realistic about her expectations. Some suggestions for new mothers include the following:

- Nap when the infant is sleeping, because getting uninterrupted sleep at night is difficult.
- Reduce participation in outside activities and limit the number of visitors.
- Determine the infant's sleep–wake cycles and attempt to increase wakeful periods during the day so the baby sleeps for longer periods at night.
- Eat a balanced diet to promote healing and to increase energy levels.
- Share household tasks to conserve your energy.
- Ask the father or other family members to provide infant care during the night periodically so that you can get an uninterrupted night of sleep.
- Review your family's daily routine and see if you can "cluster" activities to conserve energy and promote rest.

The demands of parenthood may reduce or prevent exercise in even the most committed person, but walking at a brisk pace or pushing the baby in a stroller are excellent ways for new mothers to maintain healthy exercise. In some communities, fitness classes for postnatal women can provide exercise and an important supportive social outlet. Women are encouraged to take a few months to lose the pregnancy weight while ensuring they are attending to important nutritional needs (SOGC, 2009). Emphasize the following benefits of a regular exercise program:

- Helps the woman to lose pregnancy weight
- Increases energy level so the woman can cope with her new responsibilities
- Speeds the return to pre-pregnant size and shape
- Provides an outlet for stress

Breastfeeding and exercise may help to control weight in the long term (SOGC, 2009).

> ▶ **Take** NOTE!
>
> *Women with a body mass index greater than 29 have both the least weight gain during pregnancy and the least weight loss after birth. From 6 to 18 months after giving birth, women weigh an average of 3.6 kg more than their pre-pregnancy weight (Evans et al., 2010).*

The postpartum woman may face some obstacles to exercising, including physical changes (ligament laxity), competing demands (newborn care), lack of information about weight retention (inactivity equates to weight gain), and stress incontinence (leaking of urine during activity).

A healthy woman with an uncomplicated vaginal birth can resume exercise in the immediate postpartum period. Women who experience cesarean birth should follow the advice of their physician about when to safely resume exercise. Encourage the woman to start slowly and increase the level of exercise over a period of several weeks as tolerated. Jogging strollers may be an option for some women, allowing them to exercise with their newborns. Also, exercise videos and DVDs, television programs, and home exercise equipment allow mothers to work out while the newborn naps.

Exercising after giving birth promotes feelings of well-being and restores muscle tone lost during pregnancy. Routine exercise should be resumed gradually, beginning with Kegel exercises on the first postpartum day and progressing as appropriate for the type of delivery. Walking is an excellent form of early exercise as long as the woman avoids jarring and bouncing movements, because joints do not stabilize until 6 to 8 weeks postpartum. Exercising too much too soon can cause the woman to bleed more, and her lochia may return to bright red.

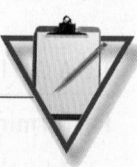

Exercising During the Postpartum Period

Abdominal Breathing

1. While lying on a flat surface (floor or bed), take a deep breath through your nose and expand your abdominal muscles (they will rise up from your midsection).
2. Slowly exhale and tighten your abdominal muscles for 3 to 5 seconds.
3. Repeat this several times.

Head Lift

1. Lie on a flat surface with the knees flexed and feet flat on the surface.
2. Lift your head off the flat surface, tuck it onto your chest, and hold for 3 to 5 seconds.
3. Relax your head and return to the starting position.
4. Repeat this several times.

Modified Sit-Ups

1. Lie on a flat surface and raise your head and shoulders 14 to 18 cm (6 to 8 inches) so that your outstretched hands reach your knees.
2. Keep your waist on the flat surface.

3. Slowly return to the starting position.
4. Repeat, increasing in frequency as your comfort level allows.

Double Knee Roll

1. Lie on a flat surface with your knees bent.
2. While keeping your shoulders flat, slowly roll your knees to your right side to touch the flat surface (floor or bed).
3. Roll your knees back over your body to the left side until they touch the opposite side of the flat surface.
4. Return to the starting position on your back and rest.
5. Repeat this exercise several times.

Pelvic Tilt

1. Lie on your back on a flat surface with your knees bent and your arms at your side.
2. Slowly contract your abdominal muscles while lifting your pelvis up toward the ceiling.
3. Hold for 3 to 5 seconds and slowly return to your starting position.
4. Repeat several times.

Should that occur, women can take it as a sign that they need to decrease their activity level (London et al., 2011).

Recommended exercises for the first few weeks postpartum include abdominal breathing, head lifts, modified sit-ups, double knee roll, and pelvic tilt (Teaching Guideline 16.2). The number of exercises and their duration are gradually increased as the woman gains strength.

Remember that cultures may have different attitudes toward exercise. Some cultures expect new mothers to observe a specific period of bed rest or activity restriction. It would be inappropriate to recommend active exercise during the early postpartum period, since that recommendation may indicate a lapse in attention to cultural competence in nursing, which is of the utmost importance in the maternal/child setting (Evans et al., 2010).

Preventing Stress Incontinence

Stress incontinence refers to urine loss associated with coughing, sneezing, laughing, or lifting. Weak pelvic floor muscles and supportive tissue often account for the condition (Potter & Perry, 2010). Therefore, the more vaginal deliveries a woman has had, the more likely she is to have stress incontinence, as each pregnancy and delivery challenges the tone of the pelvic

floor. Postpartum women might consider low-impact activities such as walking, biking, swimming, or low-impact aerobics so they can resume physical activity while strengthening the pelvic floor.

Suggestions to prevent stress incontinence include:

- Start a regular program of Kegel exercises after childbirth.
- Lose weight if necessary; obesity is associated with stress incontinence.
- Avoid smoking; limit intake of alcohol and caffeinated beverages, which irritate the bladder.

Kegel exercises help to strengthen the pelvic floor muscles if done properly and regularly, since they facilitate structural support and maintain the bladder neck in position so as not to leak during increases in intra-abdominal pressure (Potter & Perry, 2010). Kegel exercises were originally developed by Dr. Arnold Kegel as a method of controlling incontinence in women after childbirth. While providing postpartum care, instruct women on primary prevention of stress incontinence by discussing the value and purpose of Kegel exercises. Approach the subject sensitively, avoiding the term "incontinent." The terms "leakage," "loss of urine," or "bladder control issues" are more acceptable to most women.

Women can perform Kegel exercises, doing ten 5-second contractions, whenever they change diapers,

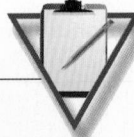

TEACHING GUIDELINE 16.3

Performing Kegel Exercises

1. Identify the correct pelvic floor muscles by contracting them to stop the flow of urine while sitting on the toilet.
2. Repeat this contraction several times to become familiar with it.
3. Start the exercises by emptying the bladder.
4. Tighten the pelvic floor muscles and hold for 10 seconds.
5. Relax the muscle completely for 10 seconds.
6. Perform 10 exercises at least three times daily. Progressively increase the number that you perform.
7. Perform the exercises in different positions, such as standing, lying, and sitting.
8. Keep breathing during the exercises.
9. Don't contract your abdominal, thigh, leg, or buttocks muscles during these exercises.
10. Relax while doing Kegel exercises and concentrate on isolating the right muscles.
11. Attempt to tighten your pelvic muscles before sneezing, jumping, or laughing.
12. Remember that you can perform Kegel exercises anywhere without anyone noticing.

talk on the phone, or watch TV. Teach the woman to perform Kegel exercises properly; help her to identify the correct muscles by trying to stop and start the flow of urine when sitting on the toilet (Teaching Guideline 16.3). Kegel exercises can be done without anyone knowing.

Assisting with Self-Care Measures

Demonstrate and discuss with the woman ways to prevent infection during the postpartum period. Because she may experience lochia drainage for as long as a month after childbirth, describe practices to promote well-being and healing. These measures include:

- Frequently change perineal pads (at least four times daily) by applying and removing them from front to back to prevent spreading contamination from the rectal area to the genital area.
- Avoid using tampons after giving birth to decrease the risk of infection.
- Shower once or twice daily using a mild soap. Avoid using soap on the nipples.
- Use a sitz bath after every bowel movement to cleanse the rectal area and relieve enlarged hemorrhoids.

- Use the peri bottle filled with warm water after urinating and before applying a new perineal pad
- Wash your hands before changing perineal pads, after disposing of soiled pads, and after voiding (London et al., 2011).

To reduce the risk for infection at the episiotomy site, reinforce proper perineal care with the client, showing her how to rinse her perineum with the peri bottle after she voids or defecates. Stress the importance of always patting gently from front to back and washing her hands thoroughly before and after perineal care. For hemorrhoids, have the client apply witch hazel-soaked pads (Tucks Medicated Pads), ice packs to relieve swelling, or hemorrhoidal cream or ointment if ordered.

Ensuring Safety

One of the safety concerns during the postpartum period is orthostatic hypotension. When the woman moves rapidly from a lying or sitting position to a standing one, her blood pressure can drop suddenly, causing her pulse rate to increase. She may become dizzy and faint. Be aware of this problem and initiate the following safeguards:

- Check blood pressure first before ambulating the client.
- Elevate the head of the bed for a few minutes before ambulating the client.
- Have the client sit on the side of the bed for a few moments before getting up.
- Help the client to stand up, and stay with her.
- Ambulate alongside the client and provide support if needed.
- Frequently ask the client how her head feels.
- Stay close by to assist if she feels lightheaded.

Additional topics to address concern infant safety. Instruct the woman to place the newborn back in the crib on his or her back if she is feeling sleepy. If the woman falls asleep while holding the infant, she might drop him or her. Also, instruct mothers to keep the door to their room closed when their infant is in their room with them. They should check the identification of anyone who enters their room or who wants to take the infant out of the room. Many hospitals emphasize safety strategies to parents and have added security measures to protect families from infant abduction.

Counselling About Sexuality and Contraception

Sexuality is an important part of every woman's life. Women want to get back to "normal" as soon as possible after giving birth, but the couple's sexual relationship cannot be isolated from the psychological and psychosocial adjustments that both partners are going through.

Most couples wait to have sexual intercourse for about 4 to 6 weeks after the delivery (SOGC, 2009). Fatigue, the physical demands made by the infant, and the stress of new roles and responsibilities may stress the emotional reserves of couples. To promote comfort, the body needs time to recover from the delivery and for the organs to return to their pre-pregnant state. Body image issues may also be a factor for women whose bodies are still changed. New parents may not get much privacy or rest, both of which are necessary for sexual pleasure (SOGC, 2009).

Men may feel they now have a secondary role within the family, and they may not understand their partner's daily routine. These issues, combined with the woman's increased investment in the mothering role, can strain the couple's sexual relationship.

Although couples are reluctant to ask, they often want to know when they can safely resume sexual intercourse after childbirth. Typically, sexual intercourse can be resumed once bright-red bleeding has stopped and the perineum is healed from an episiotomy or lacerations. This is usually by the third to the sixth week postpartum. However, there is not a set, prescribed time to resume sexual intercourse after childbirth. Each couple must set their own time frame when they feel it is appropriate to resume sexual intercourse (SOGC, 2009).

When counselling the couple about sexuality, determine what knowledge and concerns the couple have about their sexual relationship. Inform them that fluctuations in sexual interest are normal. Also inform the couple about what to expect when resuming sexual intercourse and how to prevent discomfort. Precoital vaginal lubrication may be impaired during the postpartum period, especially in women who are breastfeeding. Use of water-based gel lubricants (K-Y jelly, Astroglide) can help, as can position changes during intercourse (SOGC, 2009). Pelvic floor exercises, in addition to preventing stress incontinence, can also enhance sensation.

Contraceptive options should be included in the discussions with the couple so that they can make an informed decision before resuming sexual activity. Many couples are overwhelmed with the amount of new information given to them during their brief hospitalization, so many are not ready for a lengthy discussion about contraceptives. Presenting a brief overview of the options, along with literature, may be appropriate. It may be suitable to ask them to think about contraceptive needs and preferences and advise them to use a barrier method (condom with spermicidal gel or foam) until they choose another form of contraceptive. This advice is especially important if the follow-up appointment will not occur for 4 to 6 weeks after childbirth, as many couples will resume sexual activity before this time. Some postpartum women ovulate before their menstrual period returns and thus need contraceptive protection to prevent another pregnancy. It is important to emphasize that there is a chance to become pregnant, even if women are breastfeeding and experiencing amenorrhea. Contraception is therefore an important consideration.

Open and effective communication is necessary for effective contraceptive counselling so that information is clearly understood. Provide clear, consistent information appropriate to the woman and her partner's language, culture, and educational level. Recommending resources such as *Healthy Beginnings* (SOGC, 2009) or other pamphlets about contraception that have been developed in the local community could also be helpful.

Promoting Nutrition

The postpartum period can be a stressful one for myriad reasons, such as fatigue, the physical stress of pregnancy and birth, and the nonstop work required to take care of the newborn and to meet the needs of other family members. As a result, the new mother may ignore her own nutrition needs. Whether she is breastfeeding or bottle-feeding, encourage the new mother to take good care of herself and eat a healthy diet so that the nutrients lost during pregnancy can be replaced and she can return to a healthy weight. In general, nutrition recommendations for the postpartum woman include the following:

- Eat a wide variety of foods with high nutrient density.
- Eat meals that require little or no preparation.
- Avoid high-fat fast foods.
- Drink plenty of fluids daily—at least 2,500 mL (approximately 84 oz).
- Avoid fad weight-reduction diets and harmful substances such as alcohol, tobacco, and drugs.
- Avoid excessive intake of fat, salt, sugar, and caffeine.
- Eat the recommended daily servings from each food group.

The following summary outlines Canada's Food Guide daily nutrition requirements for postpartum women (Health Canada, 2011):

- Seven to eight servings of vegetables and fruits
- Six or seven servings of grain products
- Two servings of milk or milk alternatives
- Two servings of meat or meat alternatives
- 30 to 45 mL (2 to 3 tbsp) of unsaturated oils and fats

The breastfeeding mother's nutritional needs are higher than they were during pregnancy. The mother's diet and nutritional status influence the quantity and quality of breast milk. To meet the needs for milk production, breastfeeding women require an extra two or three Food Guide servings per day. These servings can be included as additions to regular meals or as extra snacks.

Following are some examples of dietary additions to achieve these additional requirements:

- One piece of fruit and 175 g (¾ cup) of yogurt
- An extra piece of toast at breakfast and an extra 250 mL (1 cup) of milk at supper
- Half a bagel (45 g) with 50 g (1½ oz) of cheese
- 30 g of cereal with 250 mL (1 cup) of milk
- Spinach salad made with 250 mL (1 cup) of spinach, one hard-boiled egg, and 30 mL (2 tbsp) of walnuts (Health Canada, 2011)

According to Food Guide recommendations (Health Canada, 2011), breastfeeding mothers should take a daily multivitamin that contains 400 µg (0.4 mg) of folic acid. When combined with foods rich in folic acid, daily requirements will be met.

Certain foods (usually gaseous or strong-flavoured ones) eaten by the mother may affect the flavour of the breast milk or cause gastrointestinal problems for the infant. Not all infants are affected by the same foods. If the particular food item seems to cause a problem, urge the mother to eliminate that food for a few days to see if the problem disappears.

> ▶ **Take** NOTE!
>
> *During the woman's brief stay in the health care facility, she may demonstrate a healthy appetite and eat well. Nutritional problems usually start at home when the mother needs to make her own food selections and prepare her own meals. This is a crucial area to address during follow-up.*

Supporting the Woman's Choice of Feeding Method

While there is considerable evidence that breastfeeding has numerous health benefits, many mothers choose to feed their infants formula for the first year of life. Nurses must be able to deliver sound, evidence-based information to help the new mother choose the best way to feed her infant and must support her in her decision (London et al., 2011).

Many factors affect a woman's choice of feeding method, such as culture, employment demands, support from significant others and family, and knowledge base. Although breastfeeding is encouraged, be sure that couples have the information they need to make an informed decision. Whether a couple chooses to breast-feed or bottle-feed their newborn, support and respect their choice.

Certain women should not breastfeed. Drugs such as antithyroid drugs, antineoplastic drugs, alcohol, or street drugs (amphetamines, cocaine, PCP, marijuana) enter the breast milk and will harm the infant, so women taking these substances should not breastfeed. Women with mental health challenges face decision making concerning the safety of breastfeeding while taking antidepressant or antipsychotic medication. Many medications are considered safe in the context of breastfeeding, but not all, so women will need information about the safety of their particular medication in the context of breastfeeding. Despite reassurances about the safety of a given medication, some women may choose not to breastfeed because they are uncomfortable with the knowledge that the medications will be transferred to the infant through the breast milk. To prevent HIV transmission to the newborn, women who are HIV positive should not breastfeed. Other contraindications to breastfeeding include a newborn with an inborn error of metabolism such as galactosemia or phenylketonuria, a current pregnancy, or a serious mental health disorder that would prevent the mother from remembering to feed the infant consistently.

Providing Assistance with Breastfeeding and Bottle-Feeding

First-time mothers often have many questions about feeding, and even women who have had experience with feeding a newborn may have questions. Regardless of whether the postpartum woman is breastfeeding or bottle-feeding her newborn, she can benefit from instruction.

Providing Assistance with Breastfeeding

WATCH & LEARN

The World Health Organization (WHO) and UNICEF (2009) and the Breastfeeding Committee for Canada (BCC, 2011) recommend breastfeeding for all full-term newborns. Exclusive breastfeeding is sufficient to support optimal growth and development for approximately the first 6 months of life. Breastfeeding for the first 6 months of life and up to 2 years of age or older is optimal (SOGC, 2009). Education and support for a mother regarding breastfeeding choice will increase the likelihood of a successful breastfeeding experience.

At birth, all newborns should be quickly dried, assessed and, if stable, placed immediately in uninterrupted skin-to-skin contact with their mother. This is good practice whether the mother is going to breastfeed or bottle-feed her infant. Skin-to-skin care provides the newborn with optimal physiologic stability, warmth, and opportunities for the first feed (BCC, 2011; WHO, UNICEF, 2009). The benefits of breastfeeding are clear (see Chapter 18). To promote breastfeeding, the Baby-Friendly Hospital Initiative, an international program of the World Health Organization and the United Nations Children's Fund, was started in 1991 (UNICEF, n.d.). As part of this program, the hospital or birth centre should take the following 10 steps to provide "an optimal environment for the promotion, protection, and support of breastfeeding":

1. Have a written breastfeeding policy that is communicated to all staff.
2. Educate all staff to implement this written policy.
3. Inform all women about the benefits and management of breastfeeding.
4. Show all mothers how to initiate breastfeeding within 30 minutes of birth.
5. Give no food or drink other than breast milk to all newborns.
6. Demonstrate to all mothers how to initiate and maintain breastfeeding.
7. Encourage breastfeeding on demand.
8. Allow no pacifiers to be given to breastfeeding infants.
9. Establish breastfeeding support groups and refer mothers to them.
10. Practice rooming-in 24 hours daily (BCC, 2011; WHO, UNICEF, 2009)

The nurse is responsible for encouraging breastfeeding when appropriate. For the woman who chooses to breastfeed her infant, the nurse or lactation consultant will need to spend time instructing her how to do so successfully. Many women have the impression that breastfeeding is simple. Although it is a natural process, women may experience some difficulty in breastfeeding their newborns. Nurses can assist mothers with this transition. Assist and provide one-to-one support for breastfeeding mothers, especially first-time breastfeeding mothers, to encourage appropriate technique. Suggestions are highlighted in Teaching Guideline 16.4.

▶ *Take NOTE!*

Some newborns "latch on and catch on" right away, while others take more time and patience. Inform new mothers about this to reduce their frustration and uncertainty about their ability to breastfeed.

Encourage mothers to believe in themselves and their ability to accomplish successful breastfeeding. They should not panic if breastfeeding does not go smoothly at first; it takes time and practice. Additional suggestions to help mothers relax and feel more comfortable while breastfeeding, especially when they return home, include the following:

• Select a quiet corner or room where you won't be disturbed.
• Use a rocking chair to soothe both you and your infant.

• Take long, slow deep breaths to relax before nursing.
• Drink while breastfeeding to replenish body fluids.
• Listen to soothing music while breastfeeding.
• Cuddle and caress the infant while feeding.
• Set out extra cloth diapers within reach to use as burping cloths.
• Allow sufficient time to enjoy each other in an unhurried atmosphere.
• Involve other family members in all aspects of the infant's care from the start.

Providing Assistance with Bottle-Feeding

If the mother or couple has chosen to bottle-feed their newborn, the nurse should respect and support their decision. Some women experience feelings of guilt and stigmatization as a result of the decision to feed their infant with formula. That potential needs to be understood and addressed by nurses. Discuss with the parents what type of formula they will use. Commercial formulas are classified as cow's milk-based (Enfamil, Similac), soy protein-based (Isomil, Prosobee, Nursoy), or specialized or therapeutic formulas for infants with protein allergies (Nutramigen, Pregestimil, Alimentum). The Canadian Pediatric Society (2009) advises caution regarding the use of soy formula in cases in which there is neither a cultural reason to avoid cow's milk nor an allergy to cow's milk. Some studies indicate that there can be short- or long-term consequences for the infant (such as hormonal disturbances or thyroid malfunction) as a result of exposure to soy products.

Because of the emphasis on breastfeeding promotion in maternal/child care settings, nurses can overlook the need for education around formula preparation. There are many considerations for new parents around formula use, including the methods of maintaining asepsis, sterility, the importance of the concentration of formula, and other issues associated with safe feeding practice, and these should be addressed with the new parents (London et al., 2011).

Commercial formulas can be purchased in various forms: powdered (must be mixed with water), condensed liquid (must be diluted with equal amounts of water), ready to use (poured directly into bottles), and prepackaged (ready to use in disposable bottles). One way to calculate the amount of formula an infant will require per day is to give 150 to 200 mL (5 to 6 oz) of formula milk per kilogram of body weight each day. The amount required also depends on the baby's age, however, and guidelines change as the baby ages. For example, a newborn only needs 30 to 60 mL per feed for the first week of life. This amount will increase to 90 to 120 mL per feed by 1 month of age and 120 to 180 mL per feed from 2 to 6 months. After that, the infant will take 180 to 220 mL at

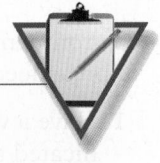

TEACHING GUIDELINE 16.4

Breastfeeding Suggestions

• Explain that breastfeeding is a learned skill for both parties.
• Offer a thorough explanation about the procedure.
• Instruct the mother to wash her hands before starting.
• Inform the mother that her afterpains will increase during breastfeeding.
• Make sure the mother is comfortable (pain-free) and not hungry.
• Tell the mother to start the feeding with an awake and alert infant showing hunger signs.
• Assist the mother to position herself correctly for comfort.
• Urge the mother to relax to encourage the let-down reflex.
• Guide the mother's hand to form a "C" to access the nipple.
• Have the mother lightly tickle the infant's upper lip with her nipple to stimulate the infant to open the mouth wide.
• Help her to latch on by bringing the infant rapidly to the breast with a wide-open mouth.
• Show her how to check that the newborn's mouth position is correct, and tell her to listen for a sucking noise.
• Demonstrate correct removal from the breast, using her finger to break the suction.
• Instruct the mother on how to burp the infant between breasts.
• Show her different positions, such as cradle and football holds and side-lying positions (see Chapter 18).
• Reinforce and praise the mother for her efforts.
• Allow ample time to answer questions and address concerns.
• Refer the mother to support groups and community resources.

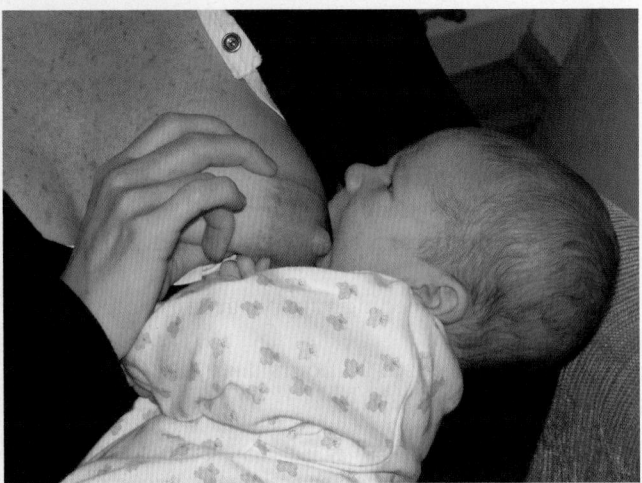

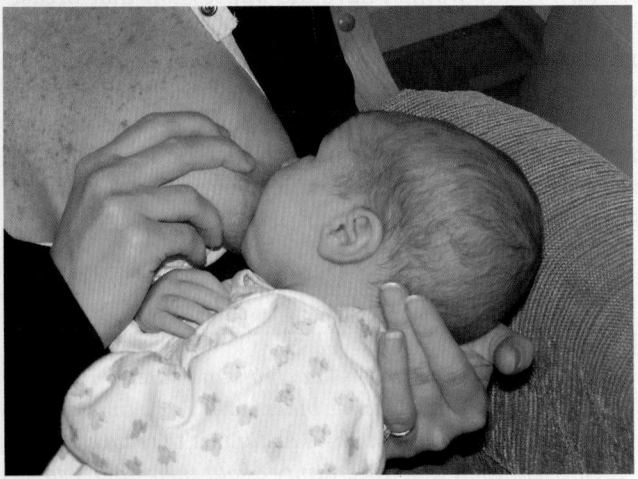

each feeding. The baby's cues will be the guide for how much to feed (rooting, crying) and when to discontinue the feeding (Babycenter, 2011). After 6 months of age, the number of feedings declines to accommodate other foods in the baby's diet, such as fruits, cereals, and vegetables (Babycenter, 2012). For more information on newborn nutrition and bottle-feeding, see Chapter 18.

When teaching parents and other caretakers about bottle-feeding, provide the following guidelines:

• Make feeding a relaxing time, a time to provide both food and comfort to your newborn.

• Use the feeding period to promote bonding by smiling, singing, making eye contact, and talking to the infant.
• Always hold the newborn when feeding. Never prop the bottle as this can cause choking and/or dental carries. Cuddle the baby close and ensure that the baby's head is higher than his or her body. Support the head to make swallowing easier.
• Use a comfortable position when feeding the newborn. Place the newborn in your dominant arm, which is supported by a pillow. Alternatively, have the newborn in a semi-upright position supported in the

crook of your arm (this position reduces choking and the flow of milk into the middle ear).

- Tilt the bottle so that the nipple and the neck of the bottle are always filled with formula. This prevents the infant from taking in too much air. Let the baby set the pace.
- Stimulate the sucking reflex by touching the nipple to the infant's lips.
- Observe expiry dates on formula containers. When purchasing formula, avoid cans with bumps or indents.
- Refrigerate any powdered formula that has been combined with tap water after constitution.
- Discard any formula not taken; do not save it for future feedings.
- Follow the baby's cues for hunger before feeding, and stop feeding when the baby shows signs of feeling full (such as turning away).
- Burp the infant frequently, and place the baby on his or her back for sleeping.
- Do not let the baby hold the bottle until after 1 year of age.
- Use only iron-fortified infant formula for first year (HealthLink, 2010).

Teaching About Breast Care

Regardless of whether or not the mother is breastfeeding her newborn, urge her to wear a very supportive, snug bra 24 hours a day to support enlarged breasts and promote comfort. A woman who is breastfeeding should wear a supportive bra throughout the lactation period. A woman who is not nursing should wear a supportive bra until engorgement ceases and then should wear a less restrictive one. The bra should fit snugly while still allowing the mother to breathe without restriction. All new mothers should use plain water to clean their breasts, especially the nipple area; soap is drying and should be avoided.

Assessing the Breasts

Instruct the mother how on to examine her breasts daily. Daily assessment includes the milk supply (breasts will feel full as they are filling), the condition of the nipples (red, bruised, fissured, or bleeding), and the success of breastfeeding. The fullness of the breasts may progress to engorgement in the breastfeeding mother if feedings are delayed or breastfeeding is ineffective. Palpating both breasts will help identify whether the breasts are soft, filling, or engorged. A similar assessment of the breasts should be completed on the nonlactating mother to identify any problems, such as engorgement or mastitis.

Alleviating Breast Engorgement

Breast engorgement usually occurs during the first week postpartum. It is a common response of the breasts to the sudden change in hormones and the presence of an increased amount of milk. Reassure the woman that this condition is temporary and usually resolves within 72 hours.

Alleviating Breast Engorgement in the Breastfeeding Woman

If the mother is breastfeeding, encourage frequent feedings, at least every 2 to 3 hours, using manual expression just before feeding to soften the breast so the newborn can latch on more effectively. Advise the mother to allow the newborn to feed on the first breast until it softens before switching to the other side. See Chapter 18 for more information on alleviating breast engorgement and other common breastfeeding concerns.

Alleviating Breast Engorgement and Suppressing Lactation in the Bottle-Feeding Woman

If the woman is bottle-feeding, explain that breast engorgement is a self-limiting phenomenon that disappears as increasing estrogen levels suppress milk formation (i.e., lactation suppression). Encourage the woman to use ice packs, to wear a snug, supportive bra 24 hours a day, and to take mild analgesics such as acetaminophen. Encourage her to avoid any stimulation to the breasts that might foster milk production, such as warm showers or pumping or massaging the breasts. Medication is no longer given to hasten lactation suppression. Teaching Guideline 16.5 provides tips on lactation suppression.

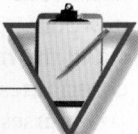

TEACHING GUIDELINE 16.5

Suppressing Lactation

1. Wear a supportive, snugly fitting bra starting at approximately 6 hours post-delivery. Remove the bra only when taking showers.
2. Milk suppression may take 5 to 7 days to accomplish.
3. Take mild analgesics to reduce breast discomfort.
4. Let shower water flow over your back rather than your breasts so that the heat of the water does not stimulate milk production and delay the suppression process.
5. Avoid any breast stimulation in the form of sucking or massage.
6. Ice packs may be applied over axillary area of each breast for 20 minutes at a time four times daily.
7. Medications to suppress lactation are no longer recommended. (London et al., 2011).

Promoting Family Adjustment and Well-Being

The postpartum period involves extraordinary physiologic, psychological, and sociocultural changes in the life of a woman and her family. Adapting to the role of a parent is not an easy process. The postpartum period is a "getting-to-know-you" time when parents begin to integrate the newborn into their lives as they reconcile the fantasy child with the real one. This can be a very challenging period for families. Nurses play a major role in assisting families to adapt to the changes, promoting a smooth transition into parenthood. Appropriate and timely interventions can help parents adjust to the role changes and promote attachment to the newborn.

For couples who already have children, the addition of a new member may bring role conflict and challenges. The nurse should provide anticipatory guidance about siblings' responses to the new baby, increased emotional tension, child development, and meeting the multiple needs of the expanding family. Although the multiparous woman has had experience with newborns, do not assume that her knowledge is current and accurate, especially if some time has elapsed since her previous child was born. Reinforcing information is important for all families.

Promoting Parental Roles

Parents' roles develop and grow when they interact with their newborn (see Chapter 15 for information on maternal and paternal adaptation). The pleasure they derive from this interaction stimulates and reinforces this behaviour. With repeated, continued contact with the newborn, parents learn to recognize cues and understand the newborn's behaviour. This positive interaction contributes to family harmony.

Nurses need to know the stages parents go through as they make their new parenting roles fit into their life experience. Assess the parents for attachment behaviours (normal and deviant), adjustment to the new parental role, family member adjustment, social support system, and educational needs. To promote parental role adaptation and parent–newborn attachment, include the following nursing interventions:

- Provide as much opportunity as possible for parents to interact with their newborn. Encourage exploration, holding, and providing care.
- Model behaviours by holding the newborn close and speaking positively.
- Always refer to the newborn by name in front of the parents.
- Speak directly to the newborn in a calm voice.
- Encourage both parents to pick up and hold the newborn.

- Point out the newborn's response to parental stimulation.
- Point out the positive physical features of the newborn.
- Involve both parents in the newborn's care and praise them for their efforts.
- Evaluate the family's strengths and weaknesses and readiness for parenting.
- Assess for risk factors such as lack of social support and the presence of stressors.
- Observe the effect of culture on the family interaction to determine whether it is appropriate.
- Monitor parental attachment behaviours to determine whether alterations require referral. Positive behaviours include holding the newborn closely or in an *en face* position, talking to or admiring the newborn, or demonstrating closeness. Negative behaviours include avoiding contact with the newborn, calling the baby derogatory names, or showing a lack of interest in caring for the newborn (see Table 16.1).
- Monitor the parents' coping behaviours to determine alterations that need intervention. Positive coping behaviours include positive conversations between the partners, both parents wanting to be involved with newborn care, and lack of arguments between the parents. Negative behaviours include not visiting, limited conversations or periods of silence, and heated arguments or conflict.
- Identify the support systems available to the new family and encourage them to ask for help. Ask direct questions about home or community support. Make referrals to community resources to meet the family's needs.
- Arrange for community home visits in high-risk families to provide positive reinforcement of parenting skills and nurturing behaviours with the newborn.
- To reduce the new parents' frustration, provide anticipatory guidance about the following before discharge:
  - Newborn sleep–wake cycles (they may be reversed)
  - Variations in newborn appearance
  - Infant developmental milestones (growth spurts)
  - How to interpret crying cues (hunger, wet, discomfort)
  - Techniques to quiet a crying infant (e.g., car ride)
  - Sensory enrichment/stimulation (e.g., colourful mobile)
  - Signs and symptoms of illness and how to assess for fever
  - Important phone numbers, follow-up care, and needed immunizations
  - Physical and emotional changes associated with the postpartum period

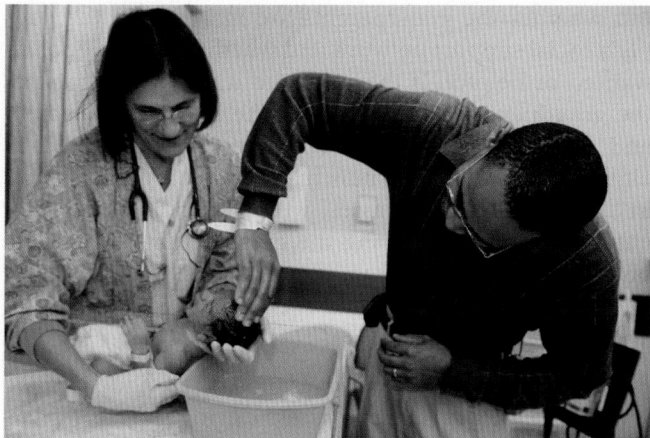
Figure 16.7 Father participating in newborn care.

Katie and Molly have been excited about having a new baby sister since they were told about their mother's pregnancy. The 6-year-old twins are eagerly looking out the front window, waiting for their parents to bring their new sister, Jessica, home. The girls are big enough to help their mother care for their new sibling, and for the past few months they have been fixing up the new nursery and selecting baby clothes. They practiced diapering their dolls—their mother was specific about not using any powder or lotion on Jessica's bottom—and holding them correctly to feed them bottles. Finally, their mother arrives home from the hospital with Jessica in her arms!

The girls notice that their mother is very protective of Jessica and watches them carefully when they care for her. They fight over the opportunity to hold her or feed her. What is special to both of them is the time they spend alone with their parents. Although a new family member has been added, the twins still feel special and loved by their parents.

Thoughts: Bringing a new baby into an established family can cause conflict and jealousy. What preparation did the older siblings have before Jessica arrived? Why is it important for parents to spend time with each sibling separately?

In addition, nurses can help fathers to feel more competent in assuming their parental role by teaching and providing information (Fig. 16.7). Education can dispel any unrealistic expectations they may have, helping them to cope more successfully with the demands of fatherhood and thereby fostering a nurturing family relationship.

Explaining Sibling Roles

It can be overwhelming to a young child to have another family member introduced into his or her small, stable world. Although most parents try to prepare siblings for the arrival of their new little brother or sister, many young children experience stress. They may view the new infant as competition or fear that they will be replaced in the parents' affection. All siblings need extra attention from their parents and reassurance that they are loved and important.

Many parents need reassurance that sibling rivalry is normal. Suggest the following to help parents minimize sibling rivalry:

- Expect and tolerate some regression (thumb-sucking, bedwetting).
- Explain childbirth in an appropriate way for the child's age.
- Encourage discussion about the new infant during relaxed family times.
- Encourage the sibling(s) to participate in decisions, such as the baby's name and toys to buy.
- Take the sibling on the tour of the maternity suite.

- Need to integrate siblings into care of the newborn; stress that sibling rivalry is normal and offer ways to reduce it
- Ways for the couple to make time together
- Appropriate community referral resources

- Buy a T-shirt that says "I'm the [big brother or big sister]."
- Spend "special time" with the child.
- Read with the child. Some suggested title include *Things to Do with A New Baby* (Ormerod, 1984); *Betsy's Baby Brother* (Wolde, 1975); *The Berenstain Bears' New Baby* (Berenstain, 1974); and *Mommy's Lap* (Horowitz & Sorensen, 1993).
- Plan time for each child throughout the day.
- Role-play safe handling of a newborn, using a doll. Give the preschooler or school-age child a doll to care for.
- Encourage older children to verbalize emotions about the newborn.
- Purchase a gift that the child can give to the newborn.
- Purchase a gift that can be given to the child by the newborn.
- Arrange for the child to come to the hospital to see the newborn (Fig. 16.8).
- Move the sibling from his or her crib to a youth bed months in advance of the birth of the newborn.
- Encourage grandparents to pay attention to the older child when visiting (Rector, 2007).

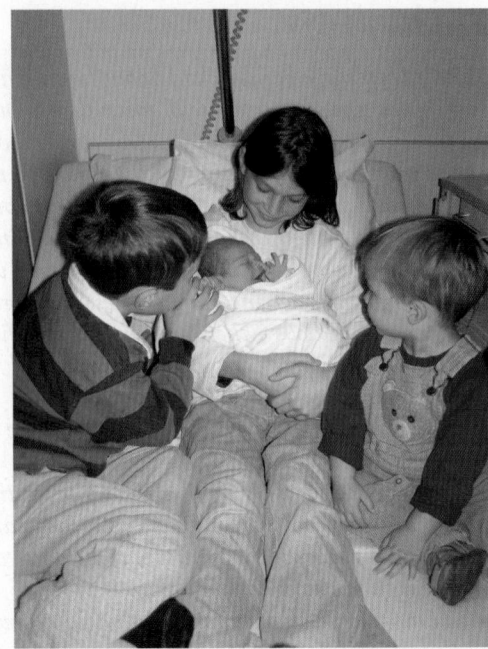

FIGURE 16.8 Sibling visitation.

Discussing Grandparents' Role

Grandparents can be a source of support and comfort to the postpartum family if effective communication skills are used and roles are defined. The grandparents' role and involvement will depend on how close they live to the family, their willingness to become involved, and cultural expectations of their role. Just as parents and siblings go through developmental changes, so too do grandparents. These changes can have a positive or negative effect on the relationship.

Newborn care, feeding, and childrearing practices have changed since the grandparents raised the parents. New parents may lack parenting skills but nonetheless want their parents' support without criticism. A grandparent's "take-charge approach" may not be welcome by new parents who are testing their own parenting roles, and family conflict may ensue. However, many grandparents respect their adult children's wishes for autonomy and remain "resource people" for them when requested.

> ▶ *Take* NOTE!
>
> *Grandparents' involvement can enrich the lives of the entire family if accepted in the right context and dose by the family.*

Nurses can assist in the grandparents' role transition by assessing their communication skills, role expectations, and support skills during the prenatal period. Find out whether the grandparents are included in the couple's social support network and whether their support is wanted or helpful. If they are, and it is, then encourage the grandparents to learn about the parenting, feeding, and childrearing skills their children have learned in childbirth classes. This information is commonly found in "grandparenting" classes, which introduce new parenting concepts and bring the grandparents up to date on current childbirth practices.

Teaching About Postpartum Blues

Issues such as sleep deprivation and exhaustion are important for the nurse to assess during the early postpartum period. Not only is a woman adjusting to the needs of her infant over a 24-hour period but she may also be coping with interruptions and visitors while in the hospital. In general, it is difficult for women to achieve the societal expectations of motherhood, which include high levels of coping and capability (Evans et al., 2010). The postpartum period is typically a happy yet stressful time because the birth of an infant is accompanied by enormous physical, social, and emotional changes.

The postpartum woman may report feelings of emotional lability, such as crying one minute and laughing the next. **Postpartum blues** are transient emotional disturbances beginning in the first week after childbirth and are characterized by a wide range of labile emotions such as uneven energy capacities, insomnia, difficulty with decision making, emotional insecurity, and grieving for a former sense of self and body image. These symptoms typically begin 3 to 4 days after childbirth and resolve by day 10 (SOGC, 2009). These mood swings may be confusing to new mothers but are usually self-limiting.

Postpartum blues are thought to affect up to 70% of all new mothers (Evans et al., 2010). In mothers who maintain contact with reality and enjoy a firm support system, the symptoms tend to resolve spontaneously without therapy within 1 to 2 weeks.

> ▶ *Take* NOTE!
>
> *If the baby blues do not resolve but become more severe and last longer than 2 weeks, it is possible that postpartum depression is developing. Typical manifestations of postpartum depression include feelings of hopelessness, isolation, and despair. Thoughts of harming oneself or one's baby may persist. Immediate medical attention is warranted (SOGC, 2009)*

Postpartum blues requires no formal treatment other than support and reassurance because it does not usually interfere with the woman's ability to function and care for her infant. Further evaluation is necessary, however, if symptoms persist more than 2 weeks (SOGC, 2009). Nurses can ease a mother's distress by encouraging her to vent her feelings and by demonstrating patience and understanding with her and her family. Suggest that getting outside help with housework and infant care might help her to feel less overwhelmed until the blues ease. Provide telephone numbers she can call when she feels down during the day. Making women aware of postpartum blues while they are pregnant will increase their knowledge about this mood disturbance, which may lessen their embarrassment and increase their willingness to ask for and accept help if it does occur.

The postpartum woman also is at risk for postpartum depression and postpartum psychosis; these conditions are discussed in Chapter 22.

Preparing for Discharge

The length of stay in the health care facility should be individualized for each mother and baby, but in Canada the average hospital stay is 2.1 days following a vaginal birth and 3.8 days following a cesarean birth (Public Health Agency of Canada [PHAC], 2009). A shortened hospital stay may be indicated if the following criteria are met:

- Mother is afebrile and vital signs are within normal range.
- Lochia is appropriate in amount and colour for stage of recovery.
- Hemoglobin and hematocrit values are within normal range.
- Uterine fundus is firm; urinary output is adequate.
- ABO blood groups and RhD status are known and, if indicated, anti-D immunoglobulin has been administered.
- Surgical wounds are healing and no signs of infection are present.
- Mother is able to ambulate without difficulty.
- Food and fluids are taken without difficulty.
- Self-care and infant care are understood and demonstrated.
- Family or other support system is available to care for both mother and baby.
- Mother is aware of possible complications

Teaching About Safe Sleeping

PHAC (2011a) recently issued the following recommendations about infant safe sleeping:

1. Provide a smoke-free environment before and after birth.
2. Always place the baby on his or her back to sleep.
3. Place the baby to sleep in a crib next to the adult's bed for the first 6 months.

4. Use a safe crib environment that has no toys or loose bedding.

Bed-sharing (referring to adults sharing any sleep surface with infants) is not recommended as it is associated with a higher risk of sudden infant death syndrome (SIDS) and suffocation.

Providing Immunizations

Prior to discharge, check the immunity status for rubella for all mothers and give a subcutaneous injection of rubella vaccine if the mother is not serologically immune (titer less than 1:10). Be sure that the client signs a consent form to receive the vaccine. Nursing mothers can be vaccinated because the live, attenuated rubella virus is not communicable. Inform all mothers receiving immunization about adverse effects (rash, joint symptoms, and a low-grade fever 5 to 21 days later) and the need to avoid pregnancy for at least 3 months after being vaccinated because of the risk of teratogenic effects (PHAC, 2011b).

If the client is Rh negative, check the Rh status of the newborn. Verify that the woman is Rh negative and has not been sensitized, that the Coombs' test is negative, and that the newborn is Rh positive. Mothers who are Rh negative and have given birth to an infant who is Rh positive should receive an injection of Rh immunoglobulin within 72 hours after birth to prevent a sensitization reaction in the Rh-negative woman who received Rh-positive blood cells during the birthing process. The usual protocol for the Rh-negative woman is to receive two doses of Rh immunoglobulin (RhoGAM), one dose at 28 weeks' gestation and the second within 72 hours after childbirth. A signed consent form is needed after a thorough explanation about the procedure is provided, including its purpose, possible adverse effects, and effect on future pregnancies.

Ensuring Follow-Up Care

New mothers and their families need to be attended to over an extended period of time by nurses knowledgeable about mother care, infant feeding (breastfeeding and bottle-feeding), infant care, and nutrition. Although continuous nursing care stops on discharge from the hospital or birthing centre, extended episodic nursing care needs to be provided at home. Some of the challenges faced by families after discharge are described in Box 16.4.

Many new mothers are reluctant to "cut the cord" after their brief stay in the health care facility and need expanded community services. Women who are discharged too early from the hospital run the risk of uterine subinvolution, discomfort at an episiotomy or cesarean site, infection, fatigue, and maladjustment to their new role. Postpartum nursing care should include a range of family-focused care, including telephone calls, out-patient

BOX 16.4 **Challenges Facing Families After Discharge**

- Lack of role models for breastfeeding and infant care
- Lack of support from the new mother's own mother if she did not breastfeed
- Increased mobility of society, which means that extended family may live far away and cannot help care for the newborn and support the new family
- Feelings of isolation and limited community ties for women who work full-time
- Shortened hospital stays: parents may be overwhelmed by all the information they are given during the brief hospital stay
- Prenatal classes usually focus on the birth itself rather than on skills parents need to care for themselves and the newborn during the postpartum period
- Limited access to education and support systems for families from diverse cultures

Source: Nash, L. R. (2007). Postpartum care. In R. E. Rakel & E. T. Bope (Eds.), *Conn's current therapy 2007*. Philadelphia: Saunders Elsevier.

clinics, and home visits. Typically, public health nurses or community nurses will provide postpartum care after hospital discharge. Ideally, a postpartum home visit or a telephone call from a public health nurse will occur within a week of discharge (PHAC, 2009). It is important for the postpartum nurse to document any concerns that may require follow-up in the community.

Providing Telephone Follow-Up

Telephone follow-up typically occurs during the first week after discharge to check on how things are going at home. Calls can be made by perinatal nurses within the agency as part of follow-up care or by the local public health nurses. A disadvantage to a phone call assessment is that the nurse cannot see the client and thus must rely on the mother's or family's observations. The experienced nurse needs to be able to recognize distress and give appropriate advice and referral information if needed.

Providing Out-Patient Follow-Up

For mothers with established health care providers, such as midwives, family physicians, pediatricians, and obstetricians, visits to the office are arranged soon after discharge. For the woman with an uncomplicated vaginal birth, an office visit is usually scheduled for 4 to 6 weeks after childbirth. A woman who has had a cesarean birth frequently is seen within 2 weeks after hospital discharge. Hospital discharge orders will specify when these visits

should be made. Newborn examinations and further diagnostic laboratory studies are scheduled within the first week.

▶ *Take NOTE!*

In Canada, women may deliver at home under the care of a registered midwife. Women may also choose midwifery care but deliver in hospital and leave within hours of delivery. In both cases, women and babies are followed at home daily for several days by the midwife. Guidelines for follow-up with mothers and infants vary according to the nature of the professional providing maternal/child care.

Out-patient clinics are available in many communities. If family members run into a problem, the local clinic is available to provide assessment and treatment. Clinic visits can replace or supplement home visits. Although these clinics are open during daytime hours only and the staff members are unfamiliar with the family, they can be a valuable resource for the new family with a problem or concern.

Providing Home Visit Follow-Up

Depending on the part of the country, home visits are usually made within the first week after discharge to assess the mother and newborn. During the home visit, the nurse assesses for and manages common physical and psychosocial problems. In addition, the home nurse can help the new parents adjust to the change in their lives. The postpartum home visit usually includes the following:

- Maternal assessment: general well-being, vital signs, breast health and care, abdominal and musculoskeletal status, voiding status, fundus and lochia status, psychological and coping status, family relationships, proper feeding technique, environmental safety check, newborn care knowledge and health teaching needed (Fig. 16.9 shows sample assessment forms)
- Infant assessment: physical examination, general appearance, vital signs, home safety check, child development status, any education needed to improve parents' skills
- The homecare nurse must be prepared to support and educate the woman and her family in the following areas:
- Breastfeeding or bottle-feeding technique and procedures
- Appropriate parenting behaviour and problem solving
- Maternal/newborn physical, psychosocial, and culture-environmental needs

(text continues on page 498)

Maternal Assessment
Maternal/Newborn Record System

Page 1 of 2

Date _MO_ / _DAY_ / _YR_ Time begin: _____
Time end: _____   Date of delivery _MO_ / _DAY_ / _YR_

Medication allergy   ☐ None Identify_____
Significant health history   ☐ None Identify_____

PHYSICAL

TEMP.	PULSE	RESP.	BP	/

Breasts   ☐ Nursing   ☐ Non-nursing
Color   ☐ Normal   ☐ Reddened
Condition   ☐ Soft   ☐ Firm   ☐ Engorged   ☐ Blocked ducts
Secretion   ☐ Colostrum   ☐ Milk   ☐ Other _____
Support bra   ☐ No   ☐ Yes, fit   ☐ Appropriate
                                                 ☐ Inappropriate

Nipples (If nursing) ☐ Erect ☐ Flat   ☐ Inverted
Condition   ☐ Intact   ☐ Bruised   ☐ Blistered
            ☐ Fissured ☐ Bleeding ☐ Scabbed
Care   ☐ Water only ☐ Soap   ☐ Air dry
            ☐ Topical agent (type/frequency) _____

            ☐ Other _____
Self-exam   ☐ Accurate   ☐ Inaccurate/instructed

Abdomen

Diastasis recti   ☐ Absent   ☐ Present_____cm
                  ☐ Exercise taught
Incision   ☐ None
Type   ☐ Transverse ☐ Vertical ☐ Umbilical
Closure   ☐ Staples   ☐ Sutures   ☐ Steri-strips
Condition   ☐ Approximated   ☐ Open_____ cm
                  ☐ Redness _____
                  ☐ Swelling _____
                  ☐ Discharge _____
                  ☐ Other_____

Reproductive Tract

Uterus   ☐ Firm ☐ Firm with massage ☐ Boggy
         Height_____ ☐ Midline ☐ Displaced L R
         ☐ Non tender ☐ Tender ☐ With touch ☐ Constant
Lochia   ☐ Rubra ☐ Serosa ☐ Alba
         ☐ Clots (describe)_____
         ☐ Fleshy odor ☐ Foul odor
         Pads Type_____ Number/day_____

         Saturation %├───┼───┼───┼───┤
                     0   25 50 75 100

Perineum   ☐ Intact ☐ Laceration
           ☐ Episiotomy Type_____ Extension_____
Condition ☐ Redness_____
           ☐ Edema_____
           ☐ Ecchymoses_____
           ☐ Discharge_____
           ☐ Approximation_____
Care   ☐ Front-to-back cleansing ☐ Peri-bottle
           ☐ Soap/water
           ☐ Ice ☐ Sitz bath ☐ Warm ☐ Cool
           ☐ Topical agent (type/frequency) _____

           ☐ Other _____

Elimination

Urinary tract
  Voiding pattern   ☐ Normal ☐ Incontinence
                    ☐ Bladder distention ☐ Catheter (type)
  Signs of infection ☐ None/reviewed ☐ Urgency ☐ Frequency
                    ☐ Dysuria ☐ CVA tenderness L R
Gastrointestinal tract
  Bowel pattern   ☐ Normal ☐ No BM
                  ☐ Constipation ☐ Diarrhea
                  ☐ Meds/treatments (type, frequency, effect) _____

  Hemorrhoids   ☐ No ☐ Yes (describe) _____
                ☐ Meds/treatments (type, frequency, effect) _____

Lower Extremities

Edema   ☐ None ☐ Pedal ☐ Ankle ☐ Pretibial ☐ Thigh
        ☐ Pitting (describe)_____
Signs of thrombophlebitis   ☐ None

	L	R		L	R
Homan's sign	☐	☐	Redness	☐	☐
Pain	☐	☐	Warmth	☐	☐
Swelling	☐	☐			

Pain	**No**	**Yes**	
		Managed	Problematic
Abdominal incision	☐	☐	☐
Back	☐	☐	☐
Breasts	☐	☐	☐
Headache	☐	☐	☐
Hemorrhoid	☐	☐	☐
Nipple	☐	☐	☐
Perineum	☐	☐	☐
Uterine cramping	☐	☐	☐
Other _____	☐	☐	☐

Analgesic   ☐ No
            ☐ Yes (type/dose/frequency) _____

Reportable danger signs ☐ Aware ☐ Unaware/instructed

TESTS   ☐ None
            ☐ Urinalysis
            ☐ CBC
            ☐ _____

IDENTIFIED NEEDS

_____
_____
_____
_____
_____
_____
_____
_____

Signature _____

A

FIGURE 16.9 Sample postpartum home visit assessment form. (**A**) Maternal assessment. (*continued*)

Maternal Assessment
Maternal/Newborn Record System

Page 2 of 2

PATIENT IDENTIFICATION

Record No. _____

Name _____

Home address _____

STREET

CITY   STATE   ZIP

ACTIVITIES OF DAILY LIVING - 24 HOUR HISTORY

Date MO / DAY / YR

Nutrition

Appetite	☐ Good	☐ Fair	☐ Poor
Usual pattern	☐ Yes	☐ No	
Special diet	☐ No	☐ Yes	
Food intolerance/allergy	☐ No	☐ Yes	
Vitamin/mineral supplement	☐ No	☐ Yes	

Fluid intake (type/amount) _____

BREAKFAST	LUNCH	DINNER	SNACKS

General Hygiene   ☐ Adequate   ☐ Inadequate (describe)

Sleep/Activity

Amount of Activity	**Activities**	**Exercise**
Night, uninterrupted _____ hrs	Limitations ☐ None Identify _____	☐ None

Amount of Activity

Night, uninterrupted _____ hrs

Naps ☐ No ☐ Yes _____ hrs

Fatigue ☐ None ☐ Minimal ☐ Moderate ☐ Exhausted

Activities

Limitations ☐ None Identify _____

☐ Self-care   ☐ Infant care

	Appropriate	Inappropriate/instructed
Stair climbing	☐	☐
Lifting	☐	☐
Household tasks	☐	☐
Outside home	☐	☐

Other _____

Exercise

☐ None

	Accurate	Inaccurate/instructed
Kegel	☐	☐
Postpartum	☐	☐

Other _____

PSYCHOLOGICAL

Review of Labor and Birth

Missing pieces	☐ No	☐ Yes
Unmet expectations	☐ No	☐ Yes
Unresolved feelings	☐ No	☐ Yes

Pertinent data _____

Postpartum Timetable   (Key on reverse side)

☐ Taking in   ☐ Taking hold   ☐ Letting go

Emotional Status   ☐ Happy ☐ Ambivalent ☐ Anxious
☐ Sad ☐ Other _____

Postpartum-depression (Key on reverse side)

☐ 0 ☐ 1 ☐ 2 ☐ 3 ☐ 4

☐ Signs/Symptoms Reviewed

General Comments   (body image, role changes, concerns) _____

SEXUALITY

	Aware	Unaware/instructed
Relationship with partner		
Adjustment	☐	☐
Expressions of affection	☐	☐
Resuming Intercourse		
Timing (lack of lochia, comfort)	☐	☐
Vaginal dryness	☐	☐
Milk ejection (if lactating)	☐	☐
Position variation	☐	☐
Libidinal changes	☐	☐
Return of Menses	☐	☐

Contraceptive Method

☐ None   ☐ Undecided/aware of options
☐ Natural family planning
☐ Cervical cap
☐ Condom
☐ Diaphragm
☐ Hormones ☐ Pill ☐ Injection ☐ Implant
☐ IUD
☐ Spermicide
☐ Sterilization ☐ Female ☐ Male
☐ Other _____

Accurate use ☐ Yes ☐ No/instructed

IDENTIFIED NEEDS

_____

Signature _____

FIGURE 16.9 (continued)

Newborn Assessment
Maternal/Newborn Record System

Date MO / DAY / YR   Time begin: _____   Date of Birth MO / DAY / YR
                     Time end: _____

Significant history ☐ None   Identify_____

PHYSICAL

Temp _____   Pulse (rate/rhythm) _____   Resp _____
Weight _____   Birth weight _____   % Change _____
Length_____   Head _____   Chest _____

HEAD/NECK

	Level	Bulging	Depressed
1. Fontanels			
Anterior	☐	☐	☐
Posterior	☐	☐	☐

Sutures   ☐ Open   ☐ Closed   ☐ Overriding
2. Variations   ☐ Molding   ☐ Caput   ☐ Cephalhematoma

	NORMAL	ABNORMAL	DETAIL VARIATIONS/ ABNORMAL FINDINGS
3. Face (symmetry)	☐	☐	
4. Eyes (symmetry, conjunctiva, sciera, eyelids, PERL)	☐	☐	
5. Ears (shape, position, auditory response)	☐	☐	
6. Nose (patency)	☐	☐	
7. Mouth (lip, mucous membranes, tongue, palate)	☐	☐	
8. Neck (ROM, symmetry)	☐	☐	
Chest			
9. Appearance (shape, breasts, nipples)	☐	☐	
10. Breath sounds	☐	☐	
11. Clavicles	☐	☐	
Cardiovascular			
12. Heart sounds	☐	☐	
13. Brachial/femoral pulses (compare strength, equality)	☐	☐	
Abdomen			
14. Appearance (shape, size)	☐	☐	
15. Cord (condition)	☐	☐	
16. Liver (less than or equal to 3 cm ↓ ®costal margin)	☐	☐	
Genitalia			
17. Female (labia, introitus, discharge)	☐	☐	
18. Male (meatus, scrotum, testes)	☐	☐	

19. Circumcision ☐ No   ☐ Yes

Musculoskeletal			
20. Muscle tone	☐	☐	
21. Extremities (symmetry, digits, ROM)	☐	☐	
22. Hips (symmetry, ROM)	☐	☐	
23. Spine (alignment, integrity)	☐	☐	
Neurologic			
24. Reflexes (presence, symmetry)			
Moro	☐	☐	
Grasp	☐	☐	
Babinski	☐	☐	
25. Cry (presence, quality)	☐	☐	

PHYSICAL (CONT'D)
Skin

Turgor   ☐ Good   ☐ Poor
Condition ☐ Smooth   ☐ Dry, cracked   ☐ Peeling
Color   ☐ Pink   ☐ Ruddy   ☐ Cyanotic   ☐ Pale
☐ Jaundice (note levels)
   ☐ Head (3 mg/dl)
   ☐ Head and upper chest (6 mg/dl)
   ☐ Head and entire chest (9 mg/dl)
   ☐ Head, chest and abdomen to umbilicus (12 mg/dl)
   ☐ Head, chest and entire abdomen (15 mg/dl)
   ☐ Head, chest, abdomen, legs and feet (18 mg/dl)
Variations (Rashes, lesions, birthmarks). _____

NUTRITION
Feeding

Reflexes ☐ Root   ☐ Suck   ☐ Swallow
Hunger cues identified ☐ Yes   ☐ No/instructed

BREAST	FORMULA
Frequency____times in _____ hours	Type _____
Time per breast_____ min _____ min	Amount _____ oz.
Positioning ☐ Correct	Frequency _____
☐ Incorrect_____	Preparation ☐ Correct
Latch ☐ Correct	☐ Incorrect _____
☐ Incorrect_____	
Appropriate audible swallows	☐ Correct
☐ Yes ☐ No_____	☐ _____

Satiation demonstrated   ☐ Yes
☐ No (describe) _____
Regurgitation ☐ No   ☐ Yes (describe) _____
Pacifier use ☐ No   ☐ Yes (type/pattern)_____

Stool (number/day, color, consistency)_____
Urine (number/day, color)_____

BEHAVIOR
Sleep/Activity Pattern (24 hours)

Sleep (16–20 hrs)   ☐ Yes ☐ No (describe)_____

Awake-alert (2–3 hrs)   ☐ Yes ☐ No (describe)_____

Awake-crying (2–4 hrs)   ☐ Yes ☐ No (describe)_____

Consolability (Key on reverse)   ☐ 0 ☐ 1 ☐ 2 ☐ 3 ☐ 4

TESTS   ☐ None   Time
☐ Metabolic screen kit no. _____   _____
☐ Bilirubin   _____
☐ Hematocrit   _____
☐ _____   _____
☐ _____   _____

IDENTIFIED NEEDS _____
_____
_____
_____
_____
Signature _____

B

FIGURE 16.9 (continued) (**B**) Newborn assessment. (Used with permission: Copyright Briggs Corporation. Professional Nurse Associates.)

• Emotional needs of the new family
• Warning signs of problems and how to prevent or eliminate them
• Sexuality issues, including contraceptive use
• Immunization needs for both mother and infant
• Family dynamics for smooth transition
• Links to health care providers and community resources

■■■ Key Concepts

■ The transitional adjustment period between birth and parenthood includes education about baby care basics, the role of the new family, emotional support, breastfeeding or bottle-feeding support, and maternal mentoring.

■ Sensitivity to how childbearing practices and beliefs vary for multicultural families and knowledge about how best to provide appropriate nursing care to meet their needs are important during the postpartum period.

■ A thorough postpartum assessment is the key to preventing complications, as is frequent handwashing by the nurse, especially between handling mothers and infants.

■ The postpartum assessment using the acronym BUBBLE-EE (breasts, uterus, bowel, bladder, lochia, episiotomy/perineum, extremities, and emotions) is a helpful guide in performing a systematic head-to-toe postpartum assessment.

■ Lochia is assessed according to its amount, colour, and change with activity and time. It proceeds from lochia rubra to serosa to alba.

■ Because of shortened agency stays, nurses must use this brief time with the client to address areas of comfort, elimination, activity, rest and exercise, self-care, sexuality and contraception, nutrition, family adaptation, discharge, and follow-up.

■ The BCC (2011) and the SOGC (2009) advocate breastfeeding for all full-term newborns, maintaining that, ideally, breast milk should be the sole nutrient for infants for the first 6 months, followed by breastfeeding along with foods until 12 months of age or longer.

■ Successful parenting is a continuous and complex interactive process that requires the acquisition of new skills and the integration of the new member into the existing family unit.

■ Bonding is a vital component of the attachment process and is necessary in establishing parent–infant attachment and a healthy, loving relationship; attachment behaviours include seeking and maintaining close proximity to, and exchanging gratifying experiences with, the infant.

■ Nurses can be instrumental in facilitating attachment by first understanding attachment behaviours

(positive and negative) of newborns and parents, and intervening appropriately to promote and enhance attachment.

■ New mothers and their families need to be attended to over an extended period of time by nurses knowledgeable about mother care, newborn feeding (breastfeeding and bottle-feeding), newborn care, and nutrition.

REFERENCES

Babycenter. (2011). *How do I know if my baby is getting enough formula?* Retrieved February 28, 2012 from http://www.babycenter.ca/baby/formula/gettingenoughexpert/

Babycenter. (2012). *How much formula milk does my baby need?* Retrieved February 28, 2012 from http://www.babycenter.ca/baby/formula/howmuchmilk/

Bowers, P. (2007). *Cultural perspectives in childbearing.* Retrieved February 28, 2012 from http://www.nurse.com/ce/course.html?CCID=3245

Breastfeeding Committee for Canada. (2011). *Summary 1: Integrated 10 steps practice indicators for hospitals and community health services.* Retrieved March 10, 2012 from http://breastfeedingcanada.ca/documents/2011–03-30_BCC_BFI_Integrated_10_Steps_summary.pdf

Canadian Paediatric Society. (2009). Concerns for the use of soy-based formulas in infant nutrition. *Paediatrics and Child Health, 14*(3):109–113.

Cassar, L. (2006). Cultural expectations of Muslims and Orthodox Jews in regard to pregnancy and the postpartum period: A study in comparison and contrast. *International Journal of Childbirth Education, 21*(2), 27–30.

Evans, R. J., Evans, M. K., Brown, Y. M. R., & Orshan, S. A. (2010). *Canadian maternity, newborn & women's health nursing.* Philadelphia: Lippincott Williams & Wilkins.

Grossman, K. E., Grossman, K., & Waters, E. (2006). *Attachment from infancy to adulthood.* New York: Guilford Publications, Inc.

Health Canada. (2011). *Canada's Food Guide: Pregnancy and breastfeeding.* Retrieved August 30, 2011 from http://hc-sc.gc.ca/fn-an/food-guide-aliment/choose-choix/advice-conseil/women-femmes-eng.php

HealthLink, B. C. (2010). *Formula feeding your baby; getting started.* Retrieved February 28, 2012 from http://www.hc-sc.gc.ca/fn-an/food-guide-aliment/choose-choix/advice-conseil/women-femmes-eng.php

Logsdon, M. C., Wisner, K. L., & Pinto-Foltz, M. D. (2006). The impact of postpartum depression on mothering. *Journal of Obstetric, Gynecologic, and Neonatal Nursing, 35*(5), 652–658.

London, M. L., Ladewig, P. W., Ball, J. W., Bindler, R. C., & Cowen, K. J. (2011). In M. Connor (Ed.), *Maternal and child nursing care* (3rd ed.). Upper Saddle River, NJ: Pearson.

McKinney, E. S., James, S. R., Murray, S. S., & Ashwill, J. W. (Eds.). (2009). *Maternal-child nursing* (3rd ed.). Canada: Saunders Elsevier.

Moretti, M. E., Lee, A., Ito, S. (2000). *Cancer in pregnancy: Which drugs are contraindicated during breastfeeding?* Retrieved February 28, 2012 from http://www.motherisk.org/prof/commonDetail.jsp?content_id=232

Nash, L. R. (2007). Postpartum care. In R. E. Rakel & E. T. Bope (Eds.), *Conn's current therapy 2007.* Philadelphia: Saunders Elsevier.

Oppenheim, D., & Goldsmith, D. F. (2007). *Attachment theory in clinical work with children: Bridging the gap between research and practice.* New York: Guilford Publications, Inc.

Potter, P. A., & Perry, A. G. (2010). Urinary elimination. In P. A. Potter, A. G. Perry, M. J. Wood & J. C. Ross-Kerr (Eds.), *Canadian fundamentals of nursing* (4th ed.). Toronto, ON: Mosby Elsevier.

Public Health Agency of Canada. (2009). *What mothers say: The Canadian maternity experiences survey.* Retrieved February 28, 2012 from http://www.phac-aspc.gc.ca/rhs-ssg/pdf/survey-eng.pdf

Public Health Agency of Canada. (2011a). *Sleep safe for your baby.* Retrieved February 28, 2012 from http://www.phac-aspc.gc.ca/hp-ps/dca-dea/stages-etapes/childhood-enfance_0–2/sids/index-eng.php

Public Health Agency of Canada. (2011b). *Vaccine preventable diseases: Rubella*. Retrieved February 28, 2012 from http://www.phac-aspc.gc.ca/im/vpd-mev/rubella-eng.php

Rector, L. (2007). *Supporting siblings and their families during intensive baby care*. Baltimore: Paul H. Brookes Publishing.

Society of Obstetricians and Gynaecologists of Canada (SOGC). (2009). *Healthy Beginnings: Giving your baby the best start, from preconception to birth* (4th ed.). In N. Schuurmans, V. Senikas & A. Lalonde (Eds.), Mississauga, Ontario: John Wiley & Sons Canada Ltd.

Society of Obstetricians and Gynaecologists of Canada (SOGC). (2010). Returning birth to Aboriginal, rural, and remote communities. *Journal of Obstetrics and Gynaecology Canada, 32*(12), 1186–1118. Retrieved February 28, 2012 from http://www.sogc.org/guidelines/documents/gui251PS1012E.pdf

Srivastava, R. (2007). *The healthcare professional's guide to clinical cultural competence*. Philadelphia: Elsevier Health Sciences.

UNICEF. (n.d.) *The baby-friendly hospital initiative*. Retrieved February 28, 2012 from http://www.unicef.org/programme/breastfeeding/baby.htm

Whitehouse, K. (2006). That loving touch. *Practicing Midwife, 9*(3), 22–25.

WHO, UNICEF. (2009). *Baby Friendly Initiative*. Retrieved March 10, 2012 from http://www.who.int/nutrition/publications/infantfeeding/bfhi_trainingcourse/en/

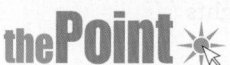

the Point For additional learning materials, including Internet Resources, visit **http://thePoint.lww.com/Chow1e.**

CHAPTER WORKSHEET

MULTIPLE CHOICE QUESTIONS

1. When assessing a postpartum woman, which of the following would lead the nurse to suspect postpartum blues?

   a. Panic attacks and suicidal thoughts

   b. Anger toward self and infant

   c. Periodic crying and insomnia

   d. Obsessive thoughts and hallucinations

2. Which of these activities would best help the postpartum nurse to provide culturally sensitive care for the childbearing family?

   a. Taking a transcultural course

   b. Caring for only families of his or her cultural origin

   c. Teaching Western beliefs to culturally diverse families

   d. Educating him- or herself about diverse cultural practices

3. Which of the following suggestions would be most appropriate to include in the teaching plan for a postpartum woman who needs to lose weight?

   a. Increase fluid intake and acid-producing foods in her diet.

   b. Avoid empty-calorie foods and increase exercise.

   c. Start a high-protein diet and restrict fluids.

   d. Eat no snacks or carbohydrates.

4. After teaching a group of breastfeeding women about nutritional needs, the nurse determines that the teaching was successful when the women state that they need to increase their intake of which nutrients?

   a. Carbohydrates and fibre

   b. Fats and vitamins

   c. Calories and protein

   d. Iron-rich foods and minerals

5. Which of the following would lead the nurse to suspect that a postpartum woman was developing a complication?

   a. Fatigue and irritability

   b. Perineal discomfort and pink discharge

   c. Pulse rate of 60 beats/minute

   d. Swollen, tender, hot area on breast

6. Which of the following would the nurse assess as indicating positive bonding between the parents and their newborn?

   a. Holding the infant close to the body

   b. Having visitors hold the infant

   c. Buying expensive infant clothes

   d. Requesting that the nurses care for the infant

7. Which activity would the nurse include in the teaching plan for parents with a newborn and an older child to reduce sibling rivalry when the newborn is brought home?

   a. Punishing the older child for bedwetting behaviour

   b. Sending the sibling to the grandparents' house

   c. Planning a special time daily for the older sibling

   d. Allowing the sibling to share a room with the infant

8. The major purpose of the first postpartum home care visit is to:

   a. Identify complications that require interventions

   b. Obtain a blood specimen for phenylketonuria testing

   c. Complete the official birth certificate

   d. Support the new parents in their parenting roles

CRITICAL THINKING EXERCISES

1. As a nurse working on a postpartum unit, you enter the room of Ms. Jones, a 22-year-old primipara, and find her chatting on the phone while her newborn is crying loudly in the bassinette, which has been pushed into the bathroom. You pick up and comfort the newborn. While holding the baby, you ask the client if she was aware her newborn was crying. She replies, "That's about all that monkey does since she was born!" You hand the newborn to her and she places the newborn on the bed away from her and continues her phone conversation.

   a. What is your nursing assessment of this encounter?

   b. What nursing interventions would be appropriate?

   c. What specific discharge interventions may be needed?

2. Jennifer Adamson, a 34-year-old single primipara, left the hospital after a 36-hour stay with her newborn son. She lives alone in a one-bedroom walk-up apartment. As the postpartum home health nurse visiting her 2 days later, you find the following:

   - Tearful client pacing the floor holding her crying son
   - Home cluttered and in disarray
   - Fundus firm and displaced to right of midline
   - Moderate lochia rubra; episiotomy site clean, dry, and intact
   - Vital signs within normal range; pain rating less than 3 points on scale of 1 to 10
   - Breasts engorged slightly; supportive bra on
   - Newborn assessment within normal limits
   - Distended bladder upon palpation; reporting urinary frequency

   a. Which of these assessment findings warrants further investigation?

   b. What interventions are appropriate at this time, and why?

   c. What health teaching is needed before you leave this home?

3. The nurse walks into the room of Lisa Drew, a 24-year-old primigravida. She asks the nurse to hand her the bottle sitting on the bedside table, stating, "I'm going to finish it off because my baby only ate half of it 3 hours ago when I fed him."

   a. What response by the nurse would be appropriate at this time?

   b. What action should the nurse take?

   c. What health teaching is needed for Lisa prior to discharge?

STUDY ACTIVITIES

1. Identify three questions that a nurse would ask a postpartum woman to assess for postpartum blues.

2. Find a website that offers advice to new parents about breastfeeding. Critique the site, the author's credentials, and the accuracy of the content.

3. Outline instructions you would give to a new mother on how to use her peri bottle.

4. Breast tissue swelling secondary to vascular congestion after childbirth and preceding lactation describes _____.

5. Listen to the postpartum story of one of your assigned patients and share it with your peers in class or as part of an online discussion.

UNIT SIX

THE NEWBORN

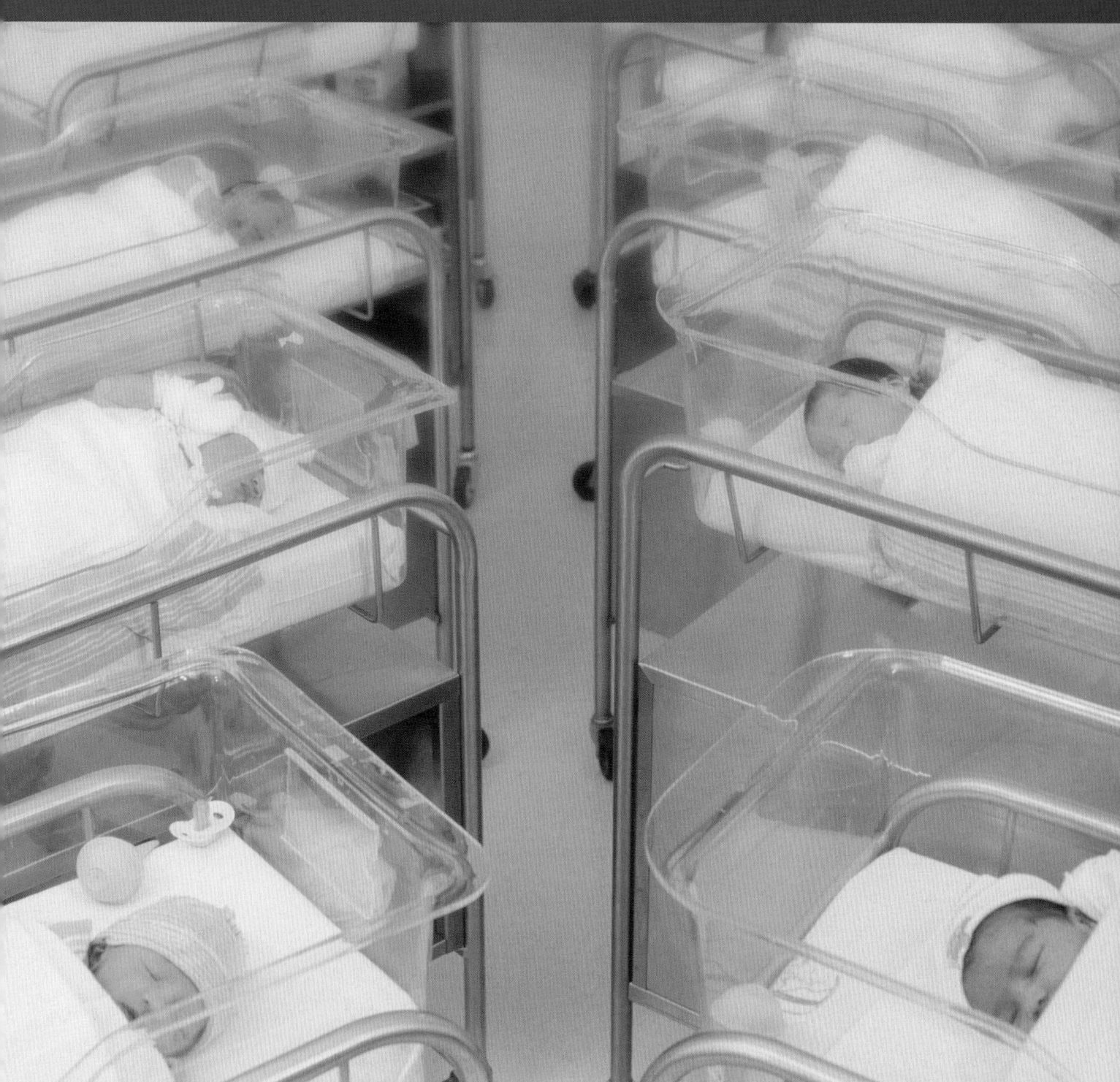

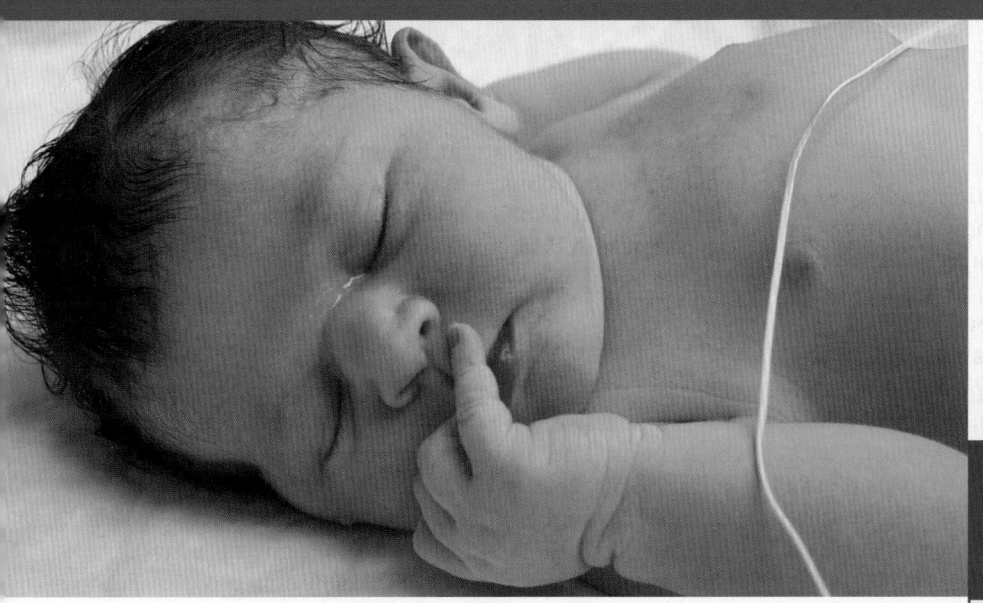

CHAPTER 17

Adapted by Andrea Brandt

NEWBORN ADAPTATION

KEY TERMS

cold stress
jaundice
meconium
neonatal period

neurobehavioural
response
neutral thermal
environment (NTE)

periodic breathing
reflex
thermoregulation

LEARNING OBJECTIVES

Upon completion of the chapter, the learner will be able to:

1. Define the key terms used in this chapter.
2. Identify the major changes in body systems that occur as the newborn adapts to extrauterine life.
3. List the primary challenges faced by the newborn during the adaptation to extrauterine life.
4. Explain the three behavioural patterns of newborn behavioural adaptation.
5. Discuss the five typical behavioural responses of the newborn.

The postpartum unit nurse reviewed the patient's file prior to entering the room: 18-year-old primipara, 1 day postpartum with a term newborn girl weighing 3.2 kg (7 lb). The new mother, Maria, greeted the nurse when she entered the room. After performing a postpartum assessment on Maria and an assessment of her newborn daughter, the nurse asked Maria if she had any questions or concerns. Maria's eyes welled up with tears: she is worried that her daughter can't see.

Wow

Newborns can't always be judged by their outer wrapping; rather, we should focus on the awesome gift inside.

When a child is born, the exhaustion and stress of labour are over for the parents, but now the newborn must begin the work of physiologically and behaviourally adapting to the new environment. The first 24 hours of life can be the most precarious (Blackburn, 2007).

The **neonatal period** is defined as the first 28 days of life. After birth, the newborn is exposed to a whole new world of sounds, colours, smells, and sensations. The newborn, previously confined to the warm, dark, wet intrauterine environment, is now thrust into an environment that is much brighter and cooler. As the newborn adapts to life after birth, numerous physiologic changes occur (Table 17.1).

Awareness of the adaptations that are occurring forms the foundation for providing support to the newborn during this crucial time. Physiologic and behavioural changes occur quickly during this transition period. Being aware of any deviations from the norm is crucial to ensure early identification and prompt intervention.

This chapter describes the physiologic changes of the newborn's major body systems. It also discusses the behavioural adaptations, including behavioural patterns and the newborn's behavioural responses that occur during this transition period.

Physiologic Adaptations

The mechanics of birth require a change in the newborn for survival outside the uterus. Immediately, respiratory gas exchange, along with circulatory modifications, must occur to sustain extrauterine life. During this time, as newborns strive to attain homeostasis, they also experience complex changes in major organ systems. Although the transition usually takes place within the first 6 to 10 hours of life, many adaptations take weeks to attain full maturity.

Cardiovascular System Adaptations

During fetal life, the heart relies on certain unique structures that assist it in providing adequate perfusion of vital body parts. The umbilical vein carries oxygenated blood from the placenta to the fetus. The ductus venosus allows the majority of the umbilical vein blood to bypass the liver and merge with blood moving through the vena cava, bringing it to the heart sooner. The foramen ovale allows more than half the blood entering the right atrium to cross immediately to the left atrium, thereby passing the pulmonary circulation. The ductus arteriosus connects the pulmonary artery to the aorta, which allows bypassing of the pulmonary circuit. Only a small portion of blood passes through the pulmonary circuit for the main purpose of perfusion of the structure, rather than for oxygenation. The fetus depends on the placenta to provide oxygen and nutrients and to remove waste products.

At birth, the circulatory system must switch from fetal to newborn circulation and from placental to pulmonary gas exchange. The physical forces of the contractions of labour and birth, mild asphyxia, increased intracranial pressure as a result of cord compression and uterine contractions, as well as cold stress immediately experienced after birth lead to an increased release of catecholamines, which are critical for the changes involved in the transition to extrauterine life. The increased catecholamine level

TABLE 17.1 ANATOMIC AND PHYSIOLOGIC COMPARISON OF THE FETUS AND NEWBORN

Comparison	Fetus	Newborn
Respiratory system	Fluid-filled, high-pressure system causes blood to be shunted from the lungs through the ductus arteriosus to the rest of the body.	Air-filled, low-pressure system encourages blood flow through the lungs for gas exchange; increased oxygen content of blood in the lungs contributes to the closing of the ductus arteriosus (becomes a ligament).
Site of gas exchange	Placenta	Lungs
Circulation through the heart	Pressures in the right atrium are greater than in the left, encouraging blood flow through the foreman ovale.	Pressures in the left atrium are greater than in the right, causing the foreman ovale to close.
Hepatic portal circulation	Ductus venosus bypasses; maternal liver performs filtering functions	Ductus venosus closes (becomes a ligament); hepatic portal circulation begins.
Thermoregulation	Body temperature is maintained by maternal body temperature and the warmth of the intrauterine environment.	Body temperature is maintained through a flexed posture, muscle activity, and metabolism.

Source: Klossner, N. J., & Hatfield, N. T. (2010). *Introductory maternity and pediatric nursing.* Philadelphia: Lippincott Williams & Wilkins.

(epinephrine) assists with promotion of pulmonary fluid clearance (Evans, Evans, Brown, et al., 2010; Meeks, Hallsworth, & Yeo, 2010).

Fetal Structures

Changes in circulation occur immediately at birth as the fetus separates from the placenta (Fig. 17.1). As the fetus emerges from the vaginal canal, the chest is compressed. Upon exiting the canal the chest recoils, allowing air to be sucked into the lung fields (Evans et al., 2010). At this point, the umbilical cord is clamped. This affects "chemoreceptors sensitive to changes in arterial oxygen and carbon dioxide content," which contributes to the onset of the first breath and continued lung functioning (Askin, 2009a; Evans et al., 2010, p. 775). As a result, systemic vascular resistance increases, and with this change comes a rapid decrease in pulmonary vascular resistance and an increase in pulmonary blood flow (Askin, 2009a; Evans et al., 2010; Meeks et al., 2010). The foramen ovale functionally closes with a decrease in pulmonary vascular resistance, which leads to a decrease in right-sided heart pressures. An increase in systemic pressure, after clamping of the cord, leads to an increase in left-sided heart pressures. The ductus arteriosus, ductus venosus, and umbilical vessels that were vital during fetal life are no longer needed. Over a period of months, these fetal vessels form non-functional ligaments.

Before birth, the foramen ovale allowed most of the oxygenated blood entering the right atrium from the inferior vena cava to pass into the left atrium of the heart. With the newborn's first breath, air pushes into the lungs, triggering an increase in pulmonary blood flow and pulmonary venous return to the left side of the heart. As a result, the pressure in the left atrium becomes higher than in the right atrium. The increased left atrial pressure causes the foramen ovale to close, thus allowing the output from the right ventricle to flow entirely to the lungs. With closure of this fetal shunt, oxygenated blood is now separated from nonoxygenated blood. The subsequent increase in tissue oxygenation further promotes the increase in systemic blood pressure and continuing blood flow to the lungs. The foramen ovale normally closes functionally at birth when left atrial pressure increases and right atrial pressure decreases. Permanent anatomic closure, though, really occurs throughout the next several weeks.

During fetal life, the ductus arteriosus, located between the aorta and the pulmonary artery, protected the lungs against circulatory overload by shunting blood (right to left) into the descending aorta, bypassing the pulmonary circulation. Its patency during fetal life is promoted by continual production of prostaglandin E2 (PGE2) by the placenta (Askin, 2009a; Ladewig, London, & Davidson, 2010). The ductus arteriosus becomes

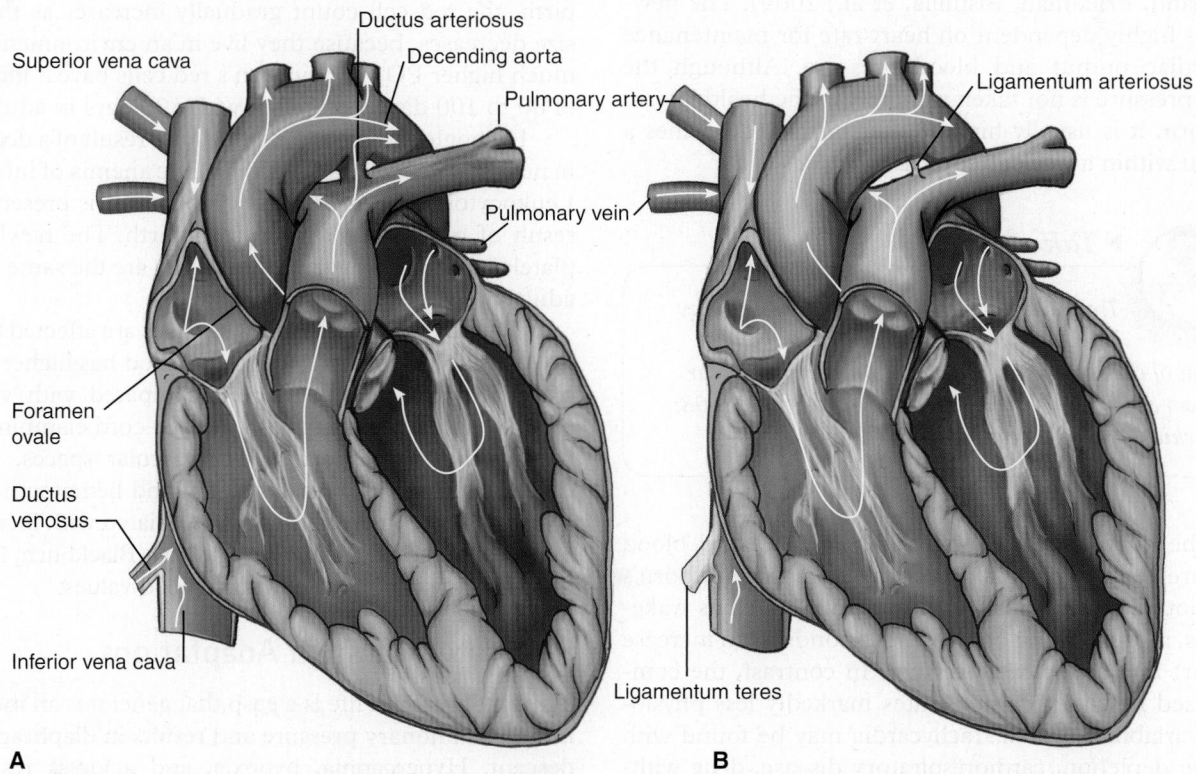

A

Superior vena cava

Ductus arteriosus

Decending aorta

Pulmonary artery

Pulmonary vein

Foramen ovale

Ductus venosus

Inferior vena cava

B

Ligamentum arteriosus

Ligamentum teres

FIGURE 17.1 Cardiovascular adaptations of the newborn. Note the changes in oxygenation between (**A**) prenatal circulation and (**B**) postnatal (pulmonary) circulation.

functionally closed within the first few hours after birth. Oxygen is the most important factor in controlling its closure. Closure depends on the high oxygen content of the aortic blood resulting from aeration of the lungs at birth. At birth, pulmonary vascular resistance decreases, allowing pulmonary blood flow to increase and oxygen exchange to occur in the lungs. It occurs secondary to an increase in the partial pressure of oxygen (PO_2) coincident with the first breath and umbilical cord occlusion when it is clamped.

The ductus venosus shunted blood from the left umbilical vein to the inferior vena cava during intrauterine life. It closes within a few days after birth, because this shunting is no longer needed as a result of activation of the liver. The activated liver now takes over the functions of the placenta (which was expelled at birth). The ductus venosus becomes a ligament in extrauterine life.

The two umbilical arteries and one umbilical vein begin to constrict at birth, because with placental expulsion, blood flow ceases. In addition, peripheral circulation increases. Thus, the vessels are no longer needed and they too become ligaments.

Heart Rate

During the first few minutes after birth, the newborn's heart rate is approximately 120 to 180 beats/min. Thereafter, it begins to decrease to an average of 110 to 160 beats/min but can vary depending on the newborn's sleep or wake level (Davidson, London, & Ladewig 2012; Dipchand, Friedman, Bismilla, et al., 2009). The newborn is highly dependent on heart rate for maintenance of cardiac output and blood pressure. Although the blood pressure is not taken routinely in the healthy term newborn, it is usually highest after birth and reaches a plateau within a week after birth.

> ▶ **Take** NOTE!
>
> *Transient functional cardiac murmurs may be heard during the neonatal period as a result of the changing dynamics of the cardiovascular system at birth (Askin, 2009b; Cochran & Lee, 2008; Mackie, Jutras, Dancea, et al., 2009).*

The fluctuations in both the heart rate and blood pressure tend to follow the changes in the newborn's behavioural state. An increase in activity, such as wakefulness, movement, or crying, corresponds to an increase in heart rate and blood pressure. In contrast, the compromised newborn demonstrates markedly less physiologic variability overall. Tachycardia may be found with volume depletion, cardiorespiratory disease, drug withdrawal, and hyperthyroidism. Bradycardia is often associated with apnea and is often seen with hypoxia.

Blood Volume

The blood volume of the newborn depends on the amount of blood transferred from the placenta at birth. It is usually estimated to be 80 to 85 mL/kg of body weight in the term infant (Blackburn, 2007). However, the volume may vary by as much as 25% to 40%, depending on when clamping of the umbilical cord occurs. Early (before 30 to 40 seconds) or late (after 3 minutes) clamping of the umbilical cord changes circulatory dynamics during transition. It is important to note that the definition of what constitutes early and late cord clamping is still a point of discussion and controversy (Hutton & Hassan, 2007; McDonald & Middleton, 2009). Recent studies show the benefits of delayed cord clamping as improving the newborn's cardiopulmonary adaptation, preventing childhood anemia without increasing hypervolemia-related risks, increasing blood pressure, improving oxygen transport, and increasing red blood cell flow (McDonald & Middleton, 2009). Although a tailored approach is required in the case of cord clamping, the balance of available data suggests that delayed cord clamping should be the method of choice (Gutierrez, Velasquez, & Iriarte, 2010). Further research is needed to explain the relationship among oxygen transport, red blood cell volume, and initiation of breathing, thereby indicating whether early or delayed cord clamping is beneficial.

Blood Components

Fetal red blood cells are large but few in number. After birth, the red cell count gradually increases as the cell size decreases, because they live in an environment with much higher PO_2. A newborn's red cells have a life span of 80 to 100 days, compared with 120 days in adults.

Hemoglobin initially declines as a result of a decrease in neonatal red cell mass (physiologic anemia of infancy). Leukocytosis (elevated white blood cells) is present as a result of birth trauma soon after birth. The newborn's platelet count and aggregation ability are the same as the adult's.

The newborn's hematologic values are affected by the site of the blood sample (capillary blood has higher levels of hemoglobin and hematocrit compared with venous blood), placental transfusion (delayed cord clamping and normal shift of plasma to extravascular spaces, which causes higher levels of hemoglobin and hematocrit), and gestational age (increased age is associated with increased numbers of red cells and hemoglobin) (Blackburn, 2007). Table 17.2 lists normal newborn blood values.

Respiratory System Adaptations

The first breath of life is a gasp that generates an increase in transpulmonary pressure and results in diaphragmatic descent. Hypercapnia, hypoxia, and acidosis resulting from normal labour become stimuli for initiating respirations. Inspiration of air and expansion of the lungs allow

TABLE 17.2   NORMAL NEWBORN BLOOD VALUES

Lab Data	Age	Normal Range
Hemoglobin	<6 days	150–220 g/L
	7–30 days	140–220 g/L
Hematocrit	≤6 days	0.460–0.700
	7–30 days	0.400–0.650
Platelets		$150–400 \times 10^9$/L
Red blood cells	≤30 days	$3.50–6.00 \times 10^{12}$/L
White blood cells	≤6 days	$9.0–30.0 \times 10^9$/L
	7–13 days	$5.0–21.0 \times 10^9$/L
	14 days–2 months	$5.0–20.0 \times 10^9$/L

Source: Dipchand, A. I., Friedman, J. N., Bismilla, Z., Gupta, S., & Lam, C. (Eds.). (2009). *The hospital for sick children handbook of pediatrics* (11th ed.). Toronto: Saunders Elsevier.

for an increase in tidal volume (amount of air brought into the lungs). Surfactant is a surface tension-reducing lipoprotein found in the newborn's lungs that prevents alveolar collapse at the end of expiration and loss of lung volume. It lines the alveoli to enhance aeration of gas-free lungs, thus reducing surface tension and lowering the pressure required to open the alveoli. Normal lung function is dependent upon surfactant, which permits a decrease in surface tension at end-expiration (to prevent atelectasis) and an increase in surface tension during lung expansion (to facilitate elastic recoil on inspiration). Surfactant provides the lung stability needed for gas exchange. The newborn's first breath, in conjunction with surfactant, overcomes the surface forces to permit aeration of the lungs. The chest wall of the newborn is floppy because of the high cartilage content and poorly developed musculature. Thus, accessory muscles to help in breathing are ineffective.

One of the most crucial adaptations that the newborn makes at birth is adjusting from a fluid-filled intrauterine environment to a gaseous extrauterine environment. During fetal life, the lungs are expanded with an ultrafiltrate of the amniotic fluid. During and after birth, this fluid must be removed and replaced with air. Passage through the birth canal allows intermittent compression of the thorax, which helps eliminate the fluid in the lungs. Pulmonary capillaries and the lymphatics remove the remaining fluid.

If fluid is removed too slowly or incompletely (e.g., with decreased thoracic squeezing during birth or diminished respiratory effort), transient tachypnea (respiratory rate above 60 beats/min) of the newborn occurs. Examples of situations involving decreased thoracic compression and diminished respiratory effort include cesarean birth and sedation in newborns (Askin, 2009a; Evans et al., 2010; Ladewig et al., 2010).

> ▶ *Take* NOTE!
>
> *A baby born by cesarean delivery does not have the same benefit of the birth canal squeeze as does the newborn born by vaginal delivery. Closely observe the respirations of the newborn after cesarean delivery.*

Lungs

Before the newborn's lungs can maintain respiratory function, the following events must occur:

- Initiation of respiratory movement
- Lung expansion
- Establishment of functional residual capacity (air remaining in the lungs at the end of expiration)
- Decreased pulmonary vascular resistance (Askin, 2009a; Ladewig et al., 2010)

Initial breathing is probably the result of a reflex triggered by pressure changes, noise, light, chilling, compression of the fetal chest during delivery, and high carbon dioxide and low oxygen concentrations in the newborn's blood. Several factors stimulate respiration, but the exact science of this transition still requires further investigation to identify the precise nature of this process (Askin, 2009a; Evans et al., 2010).

Respirations

After respirations are established in the newborn, they are shallow and irregular, ranging from 30 to 60 breaths/min, with short periods of apnea (less than 15 seconds). The newborn's respiratory rate varies according to his or her activity; the more active the newborn, the higher the respiratory rate, on average. Signs of respiratory distress to observe for include cyanosis, tachypnea, expiratory grunting, sternal retractions, and nasal flaring. Respirations should not be laboured, and the chest movements should be symmetric. In some cases, **periodic breathing** may occur, which is the cessation of breathing that lasts 5 to 15 seconds without changes in colour or heart rate (Ladewig et al., 2010). Periodic breathing may be observed in newborns within the first few days of life and requires close monitoring.

> ▶ *Take* NOTE!
>
> *Apneic periods lasting more than 20 seconds with cyanosis and heart rate changes are not periodic breathing episodes but are considered true apneic spells that require further evaluation (Ladewig et al., 2010).*

Body Temperature Regulation

Newborns are dependent on their environment for the maintenance of body temperature, much more so immediately after birth than later in life. One of the most important elements in a newborn's survival is obtaining a stable body temperature to promote an optimal transition to extrauterine life. On average, a newborn's rectal temperature ranges from 36.6° to 38.0 °C (97.9° to 100.4 °F) (Canadian Pediatric Society [CPS], 2011b; Evans et al., 2010). Although there has been discussion surrounding rectal perforation (which occurs in less than 1 in 2 million cases) and the need to avoid rectal temperatures in the newborn population, it is still the definitive recommended standard in Canada, followed by the axilla (CPS, 2011b).

Thermoregulation is the process of maintaining the balance between heat loss and heat production. It is a critical physiologic function that is closely related to the transition and survival of the newborn. An appropriate thermal environment is essential for maintaining a normal body temperature. Compared with adults, newborns tolerate a narrower range of environmental temperatures and are extremely vulnerable to both under- and overheating. Nurses play a key role in providing an appropriate environment to help newborns maintain thermal stability.

▶ *Consider THIS!*

When I look down at my little miracle of life in my arms, I can't help but beam with pride at this great accomplishment. She seems so vulnerable and defenseless and yet is equipped with everything she needs to survive at birth. When the nurse brought my daughter in for the first time after birth, I wanted to see and feel every part of her. Much to my dismay, she was wrapped up like a mummy in a blanket and she had a pink knit cap on her head. I asked the nurse why all the babies had to look like they were bound for the North Pole with all these layers on. Wasn't she aware it was summertime and probably at least 27 degrees outside?

The nurse explained that newborns lose body heat easily and need to be kept warm until their temperature stabilizes. Even though I wanted to get up close and personal with my baby, I decided to keep the pink polar bear outfit on her.

Thoughts: newborns may be born with "everything they need to survive" on the outside, but they still experience temperature instability and lose heat through radiation, evaporation, convection, and conduction. Because the newborn's head is the largest body part, a great deal of heat can be lost if a cap is not kept on the head. What guidance can be given to this mother before discharge to stabilize her daughter's temperature while at home? What simple examples can be used to demonstrate your point?

Heat Loss

Newborns have several characteristics that predispose them to heat loss:

- Thin skin with blood vessels close to the surface
- Lack of shivering ability to produce heat involuntarily
- Limited stores of metabolic substrates (glucose, glycogen, fat)
- Limited use of voluntary muscle activity or movement to produce heat
- Large body surface area relative to body weight
- Lack of subcutaneous fat, which provides insulation
- Little ability to conserve heat by changing posture (fetal position)
- No ability to adjust their own clothing or blankets to achieve warmth
- Inability to communicate that they are too cold or too warm

Every newborn struggles to maintain body temperature from the moment of birth, when the newborn's wet body is exposed to the much cooler environment of the birthing room. The amniotic fluid covering the newborn cools as it evaporates rapidly in the low humidity and air-conditioning of the room. The newborn's temperature can drop 0.25° to 1° per minute after leaving the warmth of the mother's uterus due to evaporation (Baumgart, 2008; Evans et al., 2010).

The transfer of heat depends on the temperature of the environment, air speed, and water vapour pressure or humidity. Heat exchange between the environment and the newborn involves the same mechanisms as those with any physical object and its environment. These mechanisms are conduction, convection, evaporation, and radiation (Fig. 17.2). Prevention of heat loss is a key nursing intervention.

Conduction

Conduction involves the transfer of heat from one object to another when the two objects are in direct contact with each other. Conduction refers to heat fluctuation between the newborn's body surface when in contact with other solid surfaces, such as a circumcision restraining board. Heat loss by conduction can also occur when touching a newborn with cold hands or when the newborn has direct contact with a colder object such as a metal scale. Using a warmed cloth diaper or blanket to cover any cold surface touching a newborn directly helps to prevent heat loss through conduction.

Convection

Convection involves the flow of heat from the body surface to cooler surrounding air or to air circulating over a body surface. An example of convection-related heat loss would be a cool breeze that flows over the newborn. To prevent heat loss by this mechanism, keep the newborn out of direct cool drafts (open doors, windows, fans, air

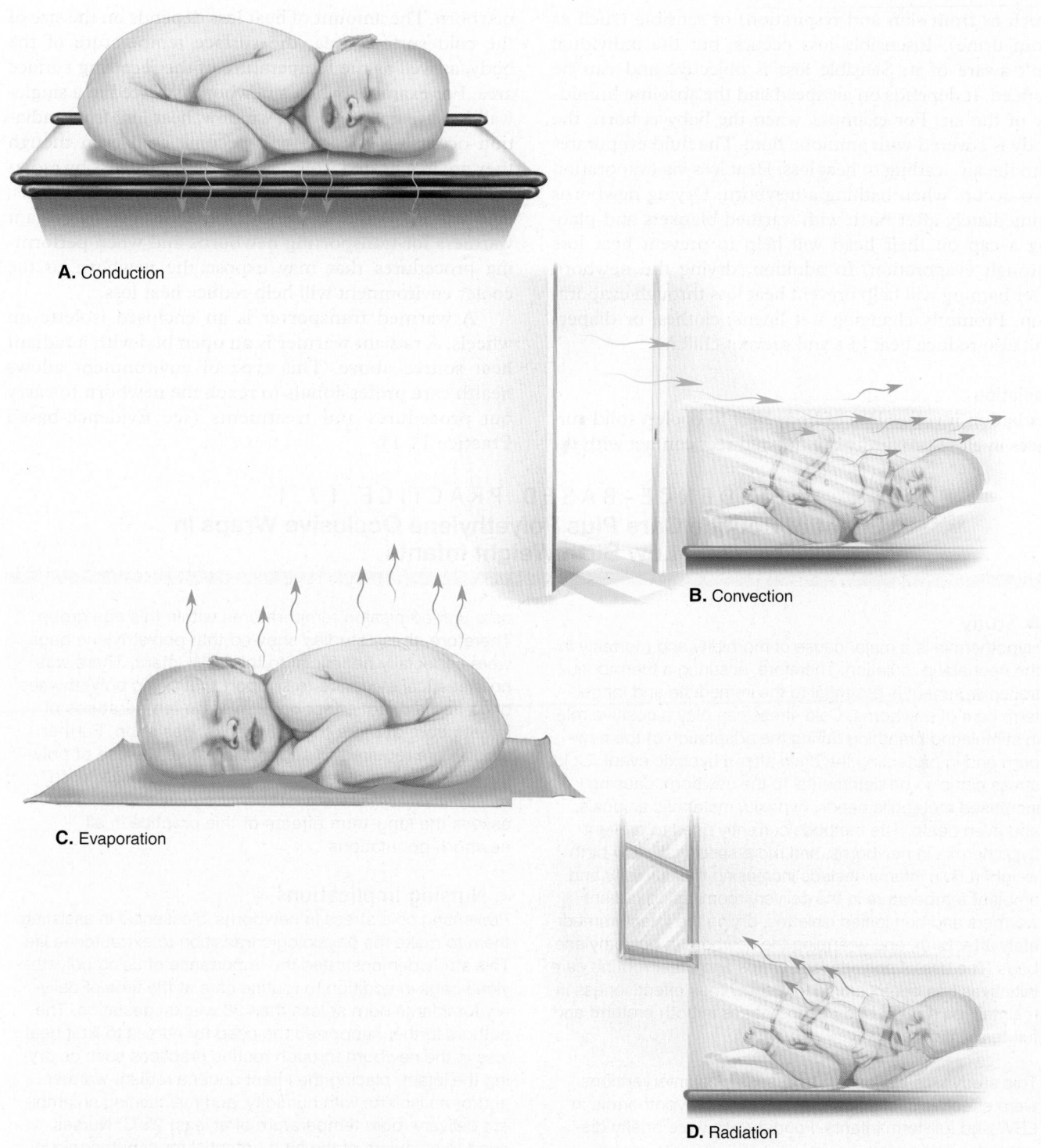

FIGURE 17.2 The four mechanisms of heat loss in the newborn. (**A**) Conduction.
(**B**) Convection. (**C**) Evaporation. (**D**) Radiation.

conditioners) in the environment, work inside an isolette as much as possible and minimize opening portholes that allow cold air to flow inside, and warm any oxygen or humidified air that comes in contact with the newborn. Using clothing and blankets in isolettes is an effective means of reducing the newborn's exposed surface area and providing external insulation. Also, transporting the

newborn to the nursery in a warmed isolette, rather than carrying him or her, helps to maintain warmth and reduce exposure to the cool air.

Evaporation

Evaporation involves the loss of heat when a liquid is converted to a vapour. Evaporative loss may be insensible (such as from skin and respiration) or sensible (such as from urine). Insensible loss occurs, but the individual isn't aware of it. Sensible loss is objective and can be noticed. It depends on air speed and the absolute humidity of the air. For example, when the baby is born, the body is covered with amniotic fluid. The fluid evaporates into the air, leading to heat loss. Heat loss via evaporation also occurs when bathing a newborn. Drying newborns immediately after birth with warmed blankets and placing a cap on their head will help to prevent heat loss through evaporation. In addition, drying the newborn after bathing will help prevent heat loss through evaporation. Promptly changing wet linens, clothes, or diapers will also reduce heat loss and prevent chilling.

Radiation

Radiation involves loss of body heat to cooler, solid surfaces in close proximity but not in direct contact with the newborn. The amount of heat loss depends on the size of the cold surface area, the surface temperature of the body, as well as the temperature of the receiving surface area. For example, when a newborn is placed in a single-wall isolette next to a cold window, heat loss from radiation occurs. Newborns will become cold even though they are in a heated isolette. To reduce heat loss by radiation, keep cribs and isolettes away from outside walls, cold windows, and air conditioners. Also, using radiant warmers for transporting newborns and when performing procedures that may expose the newborn to the cooler environment will help reduce heat loss.

A warmed transporter is an enclosed isolette on wheels. A radiant warmer is an open bed with a radiant heat source above. This type of environment allows health care professionals to reach the newborn to carry out procedures and treatments (see Evidence-based Practice 17.1).

EVIDENCE-BASED PRACTICE 17.1
Effect of Routine Care Plus Polyethylene Occlusive Wraps in Low Birth Weight Infants

● Study

Hypothermia is a major cause of morbidity and mortality in the neonatal population. Therefore, ensuring a thermoneutral environment is essential to the immediate and longer-term care of newborns. Cold stress can play a positive role in stimulating breathing during the adaptation of the newborn and in protecting the brain after a hypoxic event. Cold stress can also be detrimental to the newborn, causing increased metabolic needs, hypoxia, metabolic acidosis, and even death. The methods currently used to prevent hypothermia in newborns, and more specifically low birth weight (LBW) infants, include increasing the humidity and ambient temperature in the delivery room, using radiant warmers and humidified isolettes, drying the infant immediately after birth, and wrapping the newborn in polyethylene bags. The use of polyethylene wraps and other routine care initiatives has been studied to identify their effectiveness in maintaining normal body temperatures in both preterm and full-term infants.

This study was performed to assess what interventions were effective in alleviating or preventing hypothermia in LBW and full-term infants. Four studies were briefly discussed in this review.

▲ Findings

Results from this study demonstrated that the use of polyethylene bags assists in decreasing the chance of a hypothermic episode at delivery for infants born at less than 28 weeks' gestation. Of the four studies reviewed, each found a significant increase in neonatal intensive care unit admission temperatures within this age group. Therefore, these studies showed that polyethylene bags were especially beneficial to the LBW infant. There was no statistical evidence to support that using polyethylene bags had a direct effect on admission temperatures of infants born at more than 28 weeks' gestation. Further studies are required to support or refute the use of polyethylene bags in other critical newborn settings, such as extremely small for gestational age infants, and to assess the long-term effects of this practice in all newborn populations.

■ Nursing Implications

Preventing cold stress in newborns is essential in assisting them to make the physiologic transition to extrauterine life. This study demonstrated the importance of using polyethylene bags in addition to routine care at the time of delivery for infants born at less than 28 weeks' gestation. The authors further supported the need for nurses to limit heat loss in the newborn through routine practices such as drying the infant, placing the infant under a radiant warmer and/or an isolette with humidity, and maintaining an ambient delivery room temperature of at least 25°C. Nurses need to be aware of the high potential for hypothermia in the newborn and provide interventions that will assist in preventing the various mechanisms of heat loss, such as drafts or contact with cold surfaces, in addition to the use of humidity and warmers. Furthermore, nurses can assist in future research about heat sources that support thermoregulation in the newborn and the effects of these sources on the various gestational ages.

Mance, M. J. (2008). Keeping infants warm: Challenges of hypothermia. *Advances in Neonatal Care, 8*(1), 6–12.

Overheating

The newborn is also prone to overheating. Limited insulation and limited sweating ability can predispose any newborn to overheating. Control of body temperature is achieved via a complex negative feedback system that creates a balance between heat production, heat gain, and heat loss. The primary heat regulator is located in the hypothalamus and the central nervous system. The immaturity of the newborn's central nervous system makes it difficult to create and maintain this balance. Therefore, the newborn can become overheated easily. For example, an isolette that is too warm or one that is left too close to a sunny window may lead to hyperthermia. Although heat production can substantially increase in response to a cool environment, basal metabolic rate and the resultant heat produced cannot be reduced. Overheating increases fluid loss, the respiratory rate, and the metabolic rate considerably.

Thermoregulation

Thermoregulation, the balance between heat loss and heat production, is related to the newborn's rate of metabolism and oxygen consumption. The newborn attempts to conserve heat and increase heat production in the following ways: increasing the metabolic rate, increasing muscular activity through movement, increasing peripheral vasoconstriction, and assuming a fetal position to hold in heat and minimize exposed body surface area.

An environment in which body temperature is maintained without an increase in metabolic rate or oxygen use is called a **neutral thermal environment (NTE)**. Within an NTE, the rates of oxygen consumption and metabolism are minimal, and internal body temperature is maintained because of thermal balance. It promotes growth and stability and minimizes heat (energy) and water loss (McLenan, 2010). Since newborns have difficulty maintaining their body heat through shivering or other mechanisms, they need a higher environmental temperature to maintain an NTE. If the environmental temperature decreases, the newborn responds by consuming more oxygen. The respiratory rate increases (tachypnea) in response to the increased need for oxygen. As a result, the newborn's metabolic rate increases.

The newborn's primary method of heat production is through nonshivering thermogenesis, a process in which brown fat (adipose tissue) is oxidized in response to cold exposure. Brown fat is a special kind of highly vascular fat found only in newborns. The brown colouring is derived from the fat's rich supply of blood vessels and nerve endings. These fat deposits, which are capable of intense metabolic activity—and thus generate a great deal of heat—are found between the scapulae, at the nape of the neck, in the mediastinum, and in areas surrounding the kidneys and adrenal glands. Brown fat makes up about 2% to 6% of body weight in the full-term newborn

(Blackburn, 2007). When the newborn experiences a cold environment, the release of norepinephrine increases, which in turn stimulates brown fat metabolism by the breakdown of triglycerides. Cardiac output increases, increasing blood flow through the brown fat tissue. Subsequently, this blood becomes warmed as a result of the increased metabolic activity of the brown fat.

Newborns can experience heat loss through all four mechanisms, ultimately resulting in cold stress. **Cold stress** is excessive heat loss that requires a newborn to use compensatory mechanisms (such as nonshivering thermogenesis, brown fat stores, and tachypnea) to maintain core body temperature (Askin, 2009a; Ladewig et al., 2010). The consequences of cold stress can be quite severe. As the body temperature decreases, the newborn becomes less active, lethargic, hypotonic, and weaker. All newborns are at risk for cold stress, particularly within the first 12 hours of life. However, preterm newborns are at the greatest risk for cold stress and experience more profound effects than full-term newborns because they have fewer fat stores, poorer vasomotor responses, and less insulation to cope with a hypothermic event.

Cold stress in the newborn can lead to the following problems if not reversed: depleted brown fat stores, increased oxygen needs, respiratory distress, increased glucose consumption leading to hypoglycemia, metabolic acidosis, jaundice, hypoxia, and decreased surfactant production (Baumgart, 2008; Evans et al., 2010).

> ▶ *Take* NOTE!
>
> *Nurses must be aware of the thermoregulatory needs of the newborn and must ensure that these needs are met to provide the newborn with the best start possible.*

To minimize the effects of cold stress and maintain an NTE, the following interventions are helpful:

- Prewarming blankets and hats to reduce heat loss through conduction
- Keeping the infant transporter (warmed isolette) fully charged and heated at all times
- Drying the newborn completely after birth to prevent heat loss from evaporation
- Encouraging skin-to-skin contact (kangaroo care) with the mother if the newborn is stable and has been dried and a hat applied (Baumgart, 2008; Mance, 2008)
- Promoting early breastfeeding to provide fuels for nonshivering thermogenesis
- Using heated and humidified oxygen
- Always using radiant warmers and double-wall isolettes to prevent heat loss from radiation
- Defer bathing until the newborn is medically stable, and using a radiant heat source while bathing (Fig. 17.3)

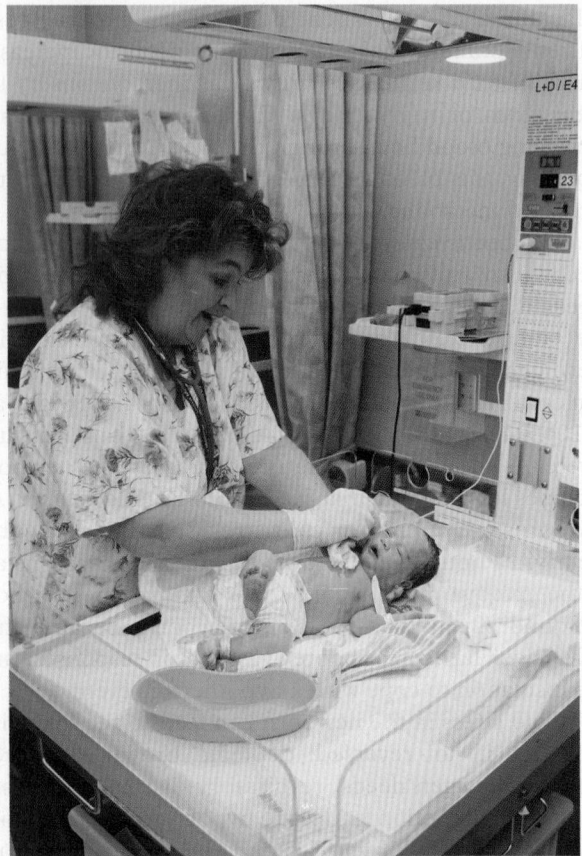

FIGURE 17.3 Bathing a newborn under a radiant warmer to prevent heat loss.

• Avoiding the placement of a skin temperature probe over a bony area or one with brown fat, because it does not give an accurate assessment of the whole body temperature (most temperature probes are placed over the liver when the newborn is supine or side-lying)

Hepatic System Function

At birth, the newborn's liver assumes the functions that the placenta handled during fetal life. These functions include iron storage, carbohydrate metabolism, blood coagulation, and conjugation of bilirubin.

Iron Storage

As red blood cells are destroyed after birth, the iron is released and is stored by the liver until new red cells need to be produced. Newborn iron stores are determined by total body hemoglobin content and length of gestation. At birth, the term newborn has iron stores sufficient to last approximately 4 to 6 months (Perry, Hockenberry, Lowdermilk, et al., 2010).

Carbohydrate Metabolism

When the placenta is lost at birth, the maternal glucose supply is cut off. Initially, the newborn's serum glucose levels decline. Usually, the term newborn's blood glucose level is lower than the maternal blood glucose level (Ladewig et al., 2010).

Glucose is the main source of energy for the first several hours after birth. With the newborn's increased energy needs after birth, the liver releases glucose from glycogen stores for the first 24 hours. Initiating feedings helps to stabilize the newborn's blood glucose levels. The CPS does not recommend routine glucose checks for all newborns (CPS, 2011a). Typically, blood glucose levels are assessed using a heel stick sample of blood only if the newborn is considered at risk for hypoglycemia (<2.6 mmol/L). At-risk newborns include those who are large or small for gestational age, premature, or unwell as well as infants who have suffered asphyxia or whose mothers have diabetes (CPS, 2011a).

Bilirubin Conjugation

The liver is also responsible for the conjugation of bilirubin—a yellow to orange bile pigment produced by the breakdown of red blood cells. In utero, elimination of bilirubin in the blood is handled by the placenta and the mother's liver. However, once the cord is cut, the newborn must now assume this function.

Bilirubin normally circulates in plasma, is taken up by liver cells, and is changed to a water-soluble pigment that is excreted in the bile. This conjugated form of bilirubin is excreted from liver cells as a constituent of bile.

The principal source of bilirubin in the newborn is the hemolysis of erythrocytes. This is a normal occurrence after birth, when fewer red blood cells are needed to maintain extrauterine life.

When red blood cells die after approximately 80 days of life, the heme in their hemoglobin is converted to bilirubin. Bilirubin is released in an unconjugated form called indirect bilirubin, which is fat-soluble. Enzymes, proteins, and different cells in the reticuloendothelial system and liver process the unconjugated bilirubin into conjugated bilirubin or direct bilirubin. This form is water-soluble and now enters the gastrointestinal system via the bile and is eventually excreted through feces. The kidneys also excrete a small amount.

Newborns produce bilirubin at a rate of approximately 6 to 8 mg/kg/day. This is more than twice the production rate in adults, primarily because of relative polycythemia and increased red blood cell turnover. Bilirubin production typically declines to the adult level shortly after birth (Ladewig et al., 2010). In addition, the metabolic pathways of the liver are relatively immature and thus cannot conjugate bilirubin as quickly as needed.

Failure of the liver cells to break down and excrete bilirubin can cause an increased amount of bilirubin in the bloodstream, leading to jaundice (Maisels & McDonagh, 2008). Bilirubin is toxic to the body and must be excreted. Blood tests ordered to determine bilirubin levels measure bilirubin in the serum. Total bilirubin is a combination of indirect (unconjugated) and direct (conjugated) bilirubin.

When unconjugated bilirubin pigment is deposited in the skin and mucous membranes, jaundice typically results. **Jaundice**, also known as icterus, refers to the yellowing of the skin, sclera, and mucous membranes that results from increased bilirubin blood levels. Visible jaundice as a result of increased blood bilirubin levels occurs in more than half of all healthy newborns. Even in healthy term newborns, extremely elevated blood levels of bilirubin during the first week of life can cause kernicterus, a permanent and devastating form of brain damage (Hansen, 2012; Simmons, 2011).

Common risk factors for the development of jaundice include fetal–maternal blood group incompatibility; prematurity; breastfeeding; drugs; maternal diabetes; infrequent feedings; male gender; trauma during birth that results in cephalhematoma; cutaneous bruising; polycythemia; previous sibling with hyperbilirubinemia; infections such as toxoplasmosis, cytomegalovirus, and other viruses; and ethnicity such as Asian or Aboriginal (Hansen, 2012).

The causes of newborn jaundice can be classified into three groups based on the mechanism of accumulation:

1. Bilirubin overproduction, such as from blood incompatibility (Rh or ABO), glucose-6-phosphate dehydrogenase (G6PD) deficiency, drugs, trauma at birth (such as forceps or vacuum delivery), polycythemia, delayed cord clamping, and breast milk jaundice
2. Decreased secretion or undersecretion of bilirubin, as seen in physiologic jaundice (physiologic jaundice appears after 24 hours of life, whereas pathologic jaundice occurs within first 24 hours of life), hypothyroidism, and breastfeeding
3. Impaired bilirubin excretion, as seen in biliary obstruction (biliary atresia, neoplasm), sepsis, cystic fibrosis, and drugs (aspirin, acetaminophen, sulfonamides, alcohol, steroids, antibiotics) (Davidson, London & Ladewig, 2012; Martin & Cloherty, 2008; Stokowski, 2011)

Jaundice in the newborn is discussed in more detail in Chapter 24.

Gastrointestinal System Adaptations

The full-term newborn has the capacity to swallow, digest, metabolize, and absorb food taken in soon after birth. At birth, the pH of the stomach contents is mildly acidic, reflecting the pH of the amniotic fluid. The once-sterile gut changes rapidly, depending on what feeding is received.

Mucosal Barrier Protection

An important adaptation of the gastrointestinal system is the development of a mucosal barrier to prevent the penetration of harmful substances (bacteria, toxins, and antigens) present within the intestinal lumen. At birth, the newborn must be prepared to deal with bacterial colonization of the gut. Colonization is dependent on oral intake. It usually occurs within 24 hours of age and is required for the production of vitamin K (Pillitteri, 2010). If harmful substances are allowed to penetrate the mucosal epithelial barrier under pathologic conditions, they can cause inflammatory and allergic reactions (Blackburn, 2007).

▶ *Take* NOTE!

Human breast milk provides a passive mechanism to protect the newborn against the dangers of a deficient intestinal defense system. It contains antibodies, viable leukocytes, and many other substances that can interfere with bacterial colonization and prevent harmful penetration (Riordan & Wambach, 2009).

Stomach and Digestion

The stomach of the newborn has a capacity ranging from 30 to 90 mL, with a variable emptying time of 2 to 4 hours. The cardiac sphincter and nervous control of the stomach are immature, which may lead to uncoordinated peristaltic activity and frequent regurgitation. Immaturity of the pharyngoesophageal sphincter and absence of lower esophageal peristaltic waves also contribute to the reflux of gastric contents. Avoid overfeeding and stimulating frequent burping may minimize regurgitation. Most digestive enzymes are available at birth, allowing newborns to digest simple carbohydrates and protein. However, they have limited ability to digest complex carbohydrates and fats because amylase and lipase levels are low at birth. As a result, newborns excrete a fair amount of lipids, resulting in fatty stools.

Adequate digestion and absorption are essential for newborn growth and development. Normally, term newborns lose 5% to 10% of their birth weight as a result of insufficient caloric intake within the first week after birth, shifting of intracellular water to extracellular space, and insensible water loss. To gain weight, the term newborn requires an intake of 120 kcal/kg/day (Ladewig et al., 2010).

Bowel Elimination

The frequency, consistency, and type of stool passed by newborns vary widely. The evolution of a stool pattern begins with a newborn's first stool, which is meconium. **Meconium** is composed of amniotic fluid, shed mucosal cells, intestinal secretions, and blood. It is greenish black, has a tarry consistency, and is usually passed within 12 to 24 hours of birth. The first meconium stool passed is sterile, but this changes rapidly with ingestion of bacteria through feedings. After feedings are initiated, a transitional stool develops, which is greenish brown to yellowish brown, thinner in consistency, and seedy in appearance.

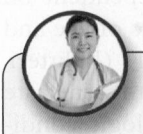

▶ *Take* NOTE!

Newborns who are fed early pass stools sooner, which helps to reduce bilirubin buildup.

The last development in the stool pattern is the milk stool. The characteristics differ in breastfed and formula-fed newborns. The stools of the breastfed newborn are yellow-gold, loose and stringy to pasty in consistency, and typically sour-smelling. The stools of the formula-fed newborn vary depending on the type of formula ingested. They may be yellow, yellow-green, or greenish and loose, pasty, or formed in consistency, and they have an unpleasant odour.

Renal System Changes

The majority of term newborns void immediately after birth, indicating adequate renal function. Although the newborn's kidneys can produce urine, they are limited in their ability to concentrate it until about 3 months of age, when the kidneys begin to mature. Full kidney maturation does not occur until approximately 2 years of age (Evans et al., 2010). Until that time, a newborn voids frequently and the urine has a low specific gravity (1.001 to 1.020). About six to eight voidings daily is average for most newborns; this indicates adequate fluid intake, although in the first 2 days the newborn may void as few as two times (Davidson, London & Ladewig, 2012; Perry et al., 2010).

The renal cortex is relatively underdeveloped at birth and does not reach maturity until 12 to 18 months of age. At birth, the glomerular filtration rate (GFR) is approximately 30% of normal adult values, reaching approximately 50% of normal adult values by the 10th day of life and full adult values by the first year of life (Blackburn, 2007). The low GFR and the limited excretion and conservation capability of the kidney affect the newborn's ability to excrete salt, water loads, and drugs.

▶ *Take* NOTE!

The possibility of fluid overload is increased in newborns; keep this in mind when administering intravenous therapy to a newborn.

Immune System Adaptations

Essential to the newborn's survival is the ability to respond effectively to hostile environmental forces. The newborn's immune system begins working early in gestation, but many of the responses do not function adequately during the early neonatal period. The intrauterine environment usually protects the fetus from harmful microorganisms and the need for defensive immunologic responses. With exposure to a wide variety of microorganisms at birth, the newborn must develop a balance between its host defenses and the hostile environmental organisms to ensure a safe transition to the outside world.

Responses of the immune system serve three purposes: defense (protection from invading organisms), homeostasis (elimination of worn-out host cells), and surveillance (recognition and removal of enemy cells). The newborn's immune system response involves recognition of the pathogen or other foreign material, followed by activation of mechanisms to react against and eliminate it. All immune responses primarily involve leukocytes (white blood cells).

The immune system's responses can be divided into two categories: natural and acquired immunity. These mechanisms are interrelated and interdependent; both are required for immunocompetency.

Natural Immunity

Natural immunity includes responses or mechanisms that do not require previous exposure to the microorganism or antigen to operate efficiently. Physical barriers (such as intact skin and mucous membranes), chemical barriers (such as gastric acids and digestive enzymes), and resident non-pathologic organisms make up the newborn's natural immune system. Natural immunity involves the most basic host defense responses: ingestion and killing of microorganisms by phagocytic cells.

Acquired Immunity

Acquired immunity involves two primary processes: (1) the development of circulating antibodies or immuno-globulins capable of targeting specific invading agents (antigens) for destruction, and (2) formation of activated lymphocytes designed to destroy foreign invaders. Acquired immunity is absent until after the first invasion by a foreign organism or toxin.

Immunoglobulins are subdivided into five classes: IgA, IgD, IgE, IgG, and IgM. The newborn depends largely on three immunoglobulins for defense mechanisms: IgG, IgA, and IgM. IgG is the major immunoglobulin and the most abundant, making up about 80% of all circulating antibodies (Blackburn, 2007). It is found in serum and interstitial fluid. It is the only class able to cross the placenta, with active placental transfer beginning at approximately 20 to 22 weeks' gestation. IgG produces antibodies against bacteria, bacterial toxins, and viral agents.

IgA is the second most abundant immunoglobulin in the serum. IgA, also known as secretory IgA (sIgA), is the major immunoglobulin that provides "the initial bolus that supplements immunoglobulins transferred earlier across the placenta to the fetus" and has "immense immunological value to the neonate" (Riordan & Wambach, 2009, p. 142). This immunoglobulin is found initially in higher levels while the newborn receives colostrum but then decreases as the mature milk comes in (Riordan & Wambach, 2009). Furthermore, this immunoglobulin provides passive immunity to protect the newborns gastrointestinal tract since at birth the infant is deficient in IgA (Riordan & Wambach, 2009).

IgA does not cross the placenta, and maximum levels are reached during childhood. This immunoglobulin is believed to protect mucous membranes from viruses and bacteria. IgA is predominantly found in the gastrointestinal and respiratory tracts, tears, saliva, colostrum, and breast milk.

> ▶ *Take* NOTE!
>
> *A major source of IgA is human breast milk and more specifically colostrum, so breastfeeding is believed to have significant immunologic advantages over formula feeding (Davidson, London & Ladewig, 2012; Wagner, 2010)*

IgM is found in blood and lymph fluid and is the first immunoglobulin to respond to infection. It does not cross the placenta, and levels are generally low at birth unless there is a congenital intrauterine infection. IgM offers a major source of protection from blood-borne infections. The predominant antibodies formed during neonatal or intrauterine infection are of this class.

Integumentary System Adaptations

The most important function of the skin is to provide a protective barrier between the body and the environment. It limits the loss of water, prevents absorption of harmful agents, protects thermoregulation and fat storage, and protects against physical trauma. The epidermal barrier begins to develop during mid-gestation and is fully formed by about 32 weeks' gestation. Although the neonatal epidermis is similar to the adult epidermis in thickness and lipid composition, skin development is not complete at birth (Douma, 2008; Meeks et al., 2010). Although the basic structure is the same as that of an adult, the less mature the newborn, the less mature the skin functions. Fewer fibrils connect the dermis and epidermis in the newborn compared with the adult. Also, the risk for breaking the skin from tape, monitors, and handling is greater in newborns than in adults. In addition, sweat glands are present at birth, but some newborns cannot perspire initially (especially if born at less than 36 weeks' gestation) and full adult functioning of these glands is not present until later in life (Davidson, London & Ladewig, 2012; Meeks et al., 2010).

Newborns vary greatly in appearance. Many of the variations are temporary and reflect the physiologic adaptations that the newborn is experiencing. Skin colouring varies, depending on the newborn's age, race or ethnic group, temperature, and whether he or she is crying. Skin colour changes with both the environment and health status. At birth, the newborn's skin is dark red to purple. As the newborn begins to breathe air, the skin colour changes to red. This redness normally begins to fade the first day.

Neurologic System Adaptations

The nervous system consists of the brain, spinal cord, 12 cranial nerves, and a variety of spinal nerves that come from the spinal cord. Neurologic development follows cephalocaudal (head to toe) and proximal–distal (centre to outside) patterns. Myelin develops early on in sensory impulse transmitters. Thus, the newborn has an acute sense of hearing, smell, and taste. The newborn's sensory capabilities include:

- Hearing—responds to noise by turning to sound; newborns hear best in low and midrange frequencies
- Taste—ability to distinguish between different tastes; term newborn has full complement of taste receptors
- Smell—ability to distinguish between mother's breast milk and breast milk from others
- Touch—well developed at birth; responds to tactile stimuli
- Vision—ability to focus on objects only in close proximity (5 cm away) but prefer objects such as faces and colours 20 to 30 cm away; tracks objects to midline or beyond; the least mature sense at birth (Davidson, London & Ladewig, 2012; Evans et al., 2010)

Remember Maria, the new mother who is worried that her daughter can't see? What might the new mother notice about her daughter's behaviour? What might be the new mother's expectations?

Successful adaptations demonstrated by the respiratory, circulatory, thermoregulatory, and musculoskeletal systems indirectly indicate the central nervous system's successful transition from fetal to extrauterine life, because the central nervous system plays a major role in all these adaptations. In the newborn, congenital reflexes are the hallmarks of maturity of the central nervous system, viability, and adaptation to extrauterine life.

The presence and strength of a reflex is an important indication of neurologic development and function. A **reflex** is an involuntary muscular response to a sensory stimulus. It is built into the nervous system and does not need the intervention/involvement of conscious thought or will to take effect (Mosby, 2009). Many neonatal reflexes disappear with maturation, although some remain throughout adulthood.

The arcs of these reflexes end at different levels of the spine and brain stem, reflecting the function of the cranial nerves and motor systems. The way newborns blink, move their limbs, focus on a caretaker's face, turn toward sound, suck, swallow, and respond to the environment are all indications of their neurologic abilities.

Assessment of newborn reflexes assists in identifying neurologic integrity. Through these assessments, the health care provider may be able to identify abnormalities in tone, posture, or behaviour that would increase the index of suspicion for neurologic dysfunction (Davidson, London & Ladewig, 2012; White, Duncan, & Baumle, 2011). Damage to the nervous system during the birthing process (birth trauma, perinatal hypoxia) can cause delays in the normal growth, development, and functioning of the newborn. Early identification may help to identify the cause and to start early intervention to decrease long-term complications or permanent sequelae.

Newborn reflexes are assessed to evaluate neurologic function and development. Absent or abnormal reflexes in a newborn, persistence of a reflex past the age when it is normally lost, or re-development of an infantile reflex in an older child or adult may indicate neurologic pathology (see Chapter 18 for a description of newborn reflex assessment).

The public health nurse explained to Maria that all newborns are born with some degree of myopia (can't see distances) and that 20/20 vision isn't generally achieved until 2 years of age. What developmental information should the nurse discuss with Maria?

Behavioural Adaptations

In addition to adapting physiologically, the newborn also adapts behaviourally. All newborns progress through a specific pattern of events after birth, regardless of their gestational age or the type of birth they experienced.

Behavioural Patterns

The newborn usually demonstrates a predictable pattern of behaviour during the first several hours after birth, characterized by two periods of reactivity separated by a sleep phase. Behavioural adaptation is a defined progression of events triggered by stimuli from the extrauterine environment after birth.

First Period of Reactivity

The first period of reactivity begins at birth and lasts for 30 minutes. The newborn is alert and moving and may appear hungry. This period is characterized by uncoordinated bilateral extremity movements, myoclonic movements of the eyes, spontaneous Moro reflexes, sucking motions, rooting, and fine tremors of the extremities (Ladewig et al., 2010). Respiration and heart rate are elevated but gradually begin to slow as the next period begins.

This period of alertness allows parents to interact with their newborn and to enjoy close contact with their new baby (Fig. 17.4). The appearance of sucking and rooting behaviours provides a good opportunity for

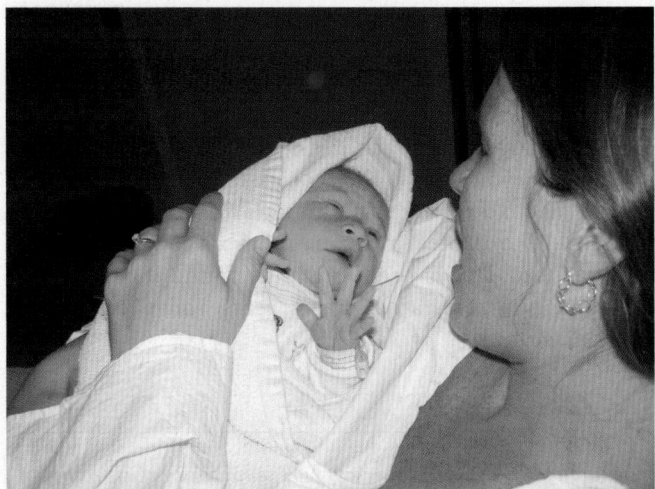

FIGURE 17.4 The first period of reactivity is an optimal time for interaction.

initiating breastfeeding. Many newborns latch onto the nipple and suck well during this first experience.

Period of Deceased Responsiveness

At 30 to 120 minutes of age, the newborn enters the second stage of transition—that of sleep or a decrease in activity. This phase is referred to as a period of decreased responsiveness. Movements are less jerky and less frequent. Heart and respiratory rates decline as the newborn enters the sleep phase. The muscles become relaxed, and responsiveness to outside stimuli diminishes. During this phase, it is difficult to arouse or interact with the newborn. No interest in sucking is shown. This quiet time can be used for both mother and newborn to remain close and rest together after labour and the birthing experience.

Second Period of Reactivity

The second period of reactivity begins as the newborn awakens and shows an interest in environmental stimuli. This period lasts 4 to 6 hours in the normal newborn (Ladewig et al., 2010). Heart and respiratory rates increase. Peristalsis also increases. Thus, it is not uncommon for the newborn to pass meconium during this period. In addition, motor activity and muscle tone increase in conjunction with an increase in muscular coordination (Fig. 17.5).

Interaction between the mother and the newborn during this second period of reactivity is encouraged if the mother has rested and desires it. This period also provides a good opportunity for the parents to examine their newborn and ask questions.

▶ *Take* NOTE!

Teaching about feeding, positioning for feeding, and diaper-changing techniques can be reinforced during this time.

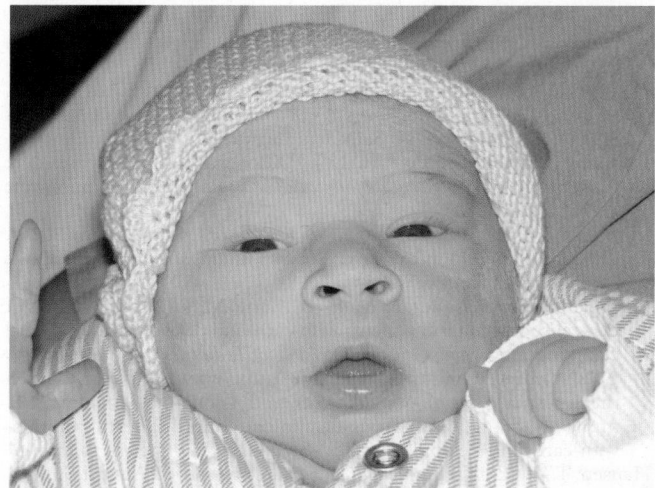

FIGURE 17.5 Newborn during the second period of reactivity. Note the newborn's wide-eyed interest.

Newborn Behavioural Responses

Newborns demonstrate several predictable responses when interacting with their environment. How they react to the world around them is termed a **neurobehavioural response**. It comprises predictable periods that are probably triggered by external stimuli.

Expected newborn behaviours include orientation, habituation, motor maturity, self-quieting ability, and social behaviours. Any deviation in behavioural responses requires further assessment, because it may indicate a complex neurobehavioural problem.

Orientation

The response of newborns to stimuli is called orientation. They become more alert when they sense a new stimulus in their environment. Orientation reflects newborns' response to auditory and visual stimuli, demonstrated by their movement of head and eyes to focus on that stimulus. Newborns prefer the human face and bright, shiny objects. As the face or object comes into their line of vision, newborns respond by staring at the object intently. Newborns use this sensory capacity to become familiar with people and objects in their surroundings.

Remember Maria, who was concerned about her newborn daughter's vision? She told the nurse that her daughter didn't show any interest in her pastel-coloured homemade mobile she had hung near the window in her hospital room across from the isolette. What suggestions can the nurse make to Maria regarding the placement of the mobile and the types and colours of objects used to promote orientation in her newborn daughter?

Habituation

Habituation is the newborn's ability to process and respond to visual and auditory stimuli—that is, how well and appropriately he or she responds to the environment. Habituation is the ability to block out external stimuli after the newborn has become accustomed to the activity. During the first 24 hours after birth, newborns should increase their ability to habituate to environmental stimuli and sleep. Habituation provides a useful indicator of their neurobehavioural intactness.

Motor Maturity

Motor maturity depends on gestational age and involves evaluation of posture, tone, coordination, and movements. These activities enable newborns to control and coordinate movement. When stimulated, newborns with good motor organization demonstrate movements that are rhythmic and spontaneous. Bringing the hand up to the mouth is an example of good motor organization. As newborns adapt to their new environment, smoother movements should be observed. Such motor behaviour is a good indicator of the newborn's ability to respond and adapt accordingly—that is, process stimuli appropriately by the central nervous system.

Self-Quieting Ability

Self-quieting ability refers to newborns' ability to quiet and comfort themselves. Newborns vary in their ability to console themselves or to be consoled. "Consolability" is how newborns are able to change from the crying state to an active alert, quiet alert, drowsy, or sleep state. They console themselves by hand-to-mouth movements and sucking, alerting to external stimuli and motor activity (Ladewig et al., 2010). Assisting parents to identify consoling behaviours to quiet their newborn if the newborn is not able to self-quiet is important. These behaviours include rocking, holding, gently patting, and softly singing to them.

Social Behaviours

Social behaviours include cuddling and snuggling into the arms of the parent when the newborn is held. Usually newborns are very sensitive to being touched, cuddled, and held. Cuddliness is very important to parents, because they frequently gauge their ability to care for their newborn by the newborn's acceptance or positive response to their actions. This can be assessed by the degree to which the newborn nestles into the contours of the holder's arms. Most newborns cuddle, but some will resist. Assisting parents to assume comforting behaviours (e.g., by cooing while holding their newborn) and praising them for their efforts can help foster cuddling behaviours.

■■■ Key Concepts

- The neonatal period is defined as the first 28 days of life. As the newborn adapts to life after birth, numerous physiologic changes occur.

- At birth, the cardiopulmonary system must switch from fetal to neonatal circulation and from placental to pulmonary gas exchange.

- One of the most crucial adaptations that the newborn makes at birth is the adjustment of a fluid medium exchange from the placenta to the lungs and that of a gaseous environment.

- Neonatal red blood cells have a life span of 80 to 100 days in comparison with the adult red blood cell life span of 120 days, which causes several adjustment problems.

- Thermoregulation is the maintenance of balance between heat loss and heat production. It is a critical physiologic function that is closely related to the transition and survival of the newborn.

- The newborn's primary method of heat production is through nonshivering thermogenesis, a process in which brown fat (adipose tissue) is oxidized in response to cold exposure. Brown fat is a special kind of highly vascular fat found only in newborns.

- Heat loss in the newborn is the result of four mechanisms: conduction, convection, evaporation, and radiation.

- Responses of the immune system serve three purposes: defense (protection from invading organisms), homeostasis (elimination of worn-out host cells), and surveillance (recognition and removal of enemy cells).

- In the newborn, congenital reflexes are the hallmarks of maturity of the central nervous system, viability, and adaptation to extrauterine life.

- The newborn usually demonstrates a predictable pattern of behaviour during the first several hours after birth, characterized by two periods of reactivity separated by a sleep phase.

REFERENCES

Askin, D. F. (2009a). Fetal-to-neonatal transition—What is normal and what is not? Part 1: The physiology of transition. *Neonatal Network, 28*(3), e33–e36.

Askin, D. F. (2009b). Fetal-to-neonatal transition—What is normal and what is not? Part 2: Red flags. *Neonatal Network, 28*(3), e37–e40.

Baumgart, S. (2008). Iatrogenic hyperthermia and hypothermia in the neonate. *Clinics in Perinatology, 35*, 183–197.

Blackburn, S. T. (2007). *Maternal fetal and neonatal physiology: A clinical perspective.* (3rd ed.). Philadelphia: Saunders Elsevier.

Canadian Pediatric Society. (2011a). *Screening guidelines for newborns at risk for low blood glucose* [Position Statement FN2004–01]. *Paediatrics & Child Health, 9*(10), 723–729. Retrieved August 3, 2011 from http://www.cps.ca/english/statements/FN/fn04-01.htm

Canadian Pediatric Society (2011b). *Temperature measurement in pediatrics.* Retrieved May 29, 2012 from http://www.cps.ca/english/statements/cp/cp00-01.htm

Cochran, W. D., & Lee, K. G. (2008). Assessment of the newborn history and physical examination of the newborn. In J. P. Cloherty, E. C. Eichenwald, & A. R. Stark (Eds.), *Manual of neonatal care.* Philadelphia: Lippincott Williams & Wilkins.

Davidson, M. R., London, M. L., & Ladewig, P. A. W. (2012). *Olds' maternal-newborn nursing & women's health across the lifespan* (9th ed.). Upper Saddle River, NJ: Pearson.

Dipchand, A. I., Friedman, J. N., Bismilla, Z., Gupta, S., & Lam, C. (Eds.). (2009). *The hospital for sick children handbook of pediatrics* (11th ed.). Toronto, ON: Saunders Elsevier.

Douma, C. E. (2008). Skin care. In J. P. Cloherty, E. C. Eichenwald, & A. R. Stark (Eds.), *Manual of neonatal care.* Philadelphia: Lippincott Williams & Wilkins.

Evans, R. J., Evans, M. K., Brown, Y. R. M., & Orshan, S. A. (2010). *Canadian maternity, newborn, & women's health nursing.* Philadelphia: Lippincott Williams & Wilkins.

Gutierrez, A. O., Velasquez, R. M. E., & Iriarte, M. T. (2010). Analysis of clinical course in term patients with early and delayed umbilical cord clamping after birth. *Internet Journal of Pediatrics and Neonatology, 11*(2). Retrieved August 3, 2011 from http://www.ispub.com/journal/the_internet_journal_of_pediatrics_and_neonatology/volume_12_number_1_8/article/analysis-of-clinical-course-in-term-patients-with-early-and-delayed-umbilical-cord-clamping-after-birth.html

Hansen, T. W. R. (2012). *Neonatal jaundice.* Retrieved August 3, 2011 from http://emedicine.medscape.com/article/974786-overview

Hutton, E. K., & Hassan, E. S. (2007). Late vs early clamping of the umbilical cord in full-term neonates: Systematic review and meta-analysis of controlled trials. *Journal of the American Medical Association, 297*(11), 1241–1252.

Klossner, N. J., & Hatfield, N. T. (2010). *Introductory maternity and pediatric nursing.* Philadelphia: Lippincott Williams & Wilkins.

Ladewig, P. A. W., London, M. L., & Davidson, M. R. (2010). *Contemporary maternal-newborn nursing care* (7th ed.). New York: Pearson.

Mackie, A. S., Jutras, L. C., Dancea, A. B., Rohlicek, C. V., Platt, R., & Beland, M. J. (2009). Can cardiologists distinguish innocent from pathologic murmurs in neonates? *The Journal of Pediatrics, 154*(1), 50–54.

Maisels, M. J., & McDonagh, A. F. (2008). Phototherapy for neonatal jaundice. *The New England Journal of Medicine, 358*(9), 920–928.

Mance, M. J. (2008). Keeping infants warm: Challenges of hypothermia. *Advances in Neonatal Care, 8*(1), 6–12.

Martin, C. R., & Cloherty, J. P. (2008). Neonatal hyperbilirubinemia. In J. P. Cloherty, E. C. Eichenwald, & A. R. Stark (Eds.), *Manual of neonatal care.* Philadelphia: Lippincott Williams & Wilkins.

McDonald, S. J., & Middleton, P. (2009). Effect of timing on umbilical clamping of term infants on maternal and neonatal outcomes. *The Cochrane Database of Systematic Reviews, (2)*, CD004074. doi:10.1002/14651858.CD004074.pub2

McLenan, D. (2010). Care of the high-risk neonate. In E. T. Bope, R. E. Rakel, & R. Kellerman (Eds.), *Conn's current therapy 2010.* Philadelphia: Saunders Elsevier.

Meeks, M., Hallsworth, M., & Yeo, H. (2010). *Nursing the neonate* (2nd ed.). United Kingdom: Wiley—Blackwell.

Mosby. (2009). In *Mosby's dictionary of medicine, nursing & health professions.* (8th ed.). St. Louis: Mosby Elsevier.

Perry, S. E., Hockenberry, M. J., Lowdermilk, D. L., & Wilson, D. (2010). *Maternal child nursing care* (4th ed.). St. Louis, MO: Mosby Elsevier.

Pillitteri, A. (2010). *Maternal & child health nursing: Care of the childbearing & childrearing family* (6th ed.). Philadelphia: Lippincott Williams & Wilkins.

Riordan, J., & Wambach, K. (2009). *Breastfeeding and human lactation* (4th ed.). Sudbury: Jones and Bartlett Publishers.

Simmons, S. (2011). Hyperbilirubinemia in neonates: Prevention, early identification, and treatment. *Advances in Neonatal Care, 11*(5s), s22–s27.

Stokowski, L. (2011). Reviewing the needs of jaundice management. *Advances in Neonatal Care, 11*(5s), s1–s2.

Wagner, C. L. (2010). *Human milk and lactation.* Retrieved May 21, 2012 from http://emedicine.medscape.com/article/1835675-overview

White, L., Duncan, G., & Baumle, W. (2011). *Foundations of maternal & pediatric nursing* (3rd ed.). South Melbourne, Australia: CENGAGE Learning.

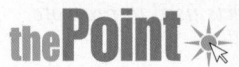
For additional learning materials, including Internet Resources, visit http://thePoint.lww.com/Chow1e.

CHAPTER WORKSHEET

MULTIPLE CHOICE QUESTIONS

1. When assessing the term newborn, the following are observed: newborn is alert, heart and respiratory rates have stabilized, and meconium has been passed. The nurse determines that the newborn is exhibiting behaviours indicating:

   a. Initial period of reactivity

   b. Second period of reactivity

   c. Decreased responsiveness period

   d. Period of sleep

2. When caring for a newborn, the nurse ensures that the doors of the nursery are closed and minimizes opening of the isolette portholes to prevent heat loss via which mechanism?

   a. Conduction

   b. Evaporation

   c. Convection

   d. Radiation

3. After teaching a group of nursing students about thermoregulation and appropriate measures to prevent heat loss by evaporation, which of the following student behaviours would indicate successful teaching?

   a. Transporting the newborn in an isolette

   b. Maintaining a warm room temperature

   c. Placing the newborn on a warmed surface

   d. Drying the newborn immediately after birth

4. After birth, the nurse would expect which fetal structure to close as a result of increases in the pressure gradients on the left side of the heart?

   a. Foramen ovale

   b. Ductus arteriosus

   c. Ductus venosus

   d. Umbilical vein

5. Which of the following newborns could be described as breathing normally?

   a. Newborn A is breathing deeply, with a regular rhythm, at a rate of 20 beats/min

   b. Newborn B is breathing diaphragmatically with sternal retractions, at a rate of 70 beats/min

   c. Newborn C is breathing shallowly, with 40-second periods of apnea and cyanosis

   d. Newborn D is breathing shallowly, at a rate of 36 beats/min, with short periods of apnea

6. When assessing a term newborn (6 hours old), the nurse auscultates bowel sounds and documents recent passing of meconium. These findings would indicate:

   a. Abnormal gastrointestinal newborn transition and need to be reported

   b. An intestinal anomaly that needs immediate surgery

   c. A patent anus with no bowel obstruction and normal peristalsis

   d. A malabsorption syndrome resulting in fatty stools

CRITICAL THINKING EXERCISES

1. As the nurse manager, you have been orienting a new nurse in the nursery for the past few weeks. Although she has been demonstrating adequacy with most procedures, today you observe her bathing several newborns without covering them, weighing them on the scale without a cover, leaving the storage door open with the transporter nearby, and leaving the newborns' head covers and blankets off after showing them to family members through the nursery observation window.

   a. What is your impression of this behaviour?

   b. What principles concerning thermoregulation need to be reinforced?

   c. How will you evaluate whether your instructions have been effective?

(question continues on page 522)

2. The most important adaptations for the newborn to make after birth are to establish respirations, make cardiovascular adjustments, and establish thermoregulation. Nursing care focuses on monitoring and supporting adjustments to extrauterine adaptation. Write an appropriate nursing intervention to help achieve the following newborn adaptations:

   a. Respiratory adaptation

   b. Safety, including prevention of infection

   c. Thermoregulation

STUDY ACTIVITIES

1. While in the nursery clinical setting, identify the period of behavioural reactivity (first, inactivity, or second period) for two newborns born at different times. Share your findings in postconference that clinical day.

2. Obtain a set of vital signs (temperature, pulse, respiration) for a newborn on admission to the nursery. Repeat this procedure and compare changes in the values several hours later. Discuss what changes in the vital signs you would expect during this transitional period.

3. Find two websites about transition to extrauterine life that can be shared with other nursing students as well as nursery nurses. Critique the information presented in terms of how accurate and current it is.

4. The most common mechanism of heat loss in the newborn is _____.

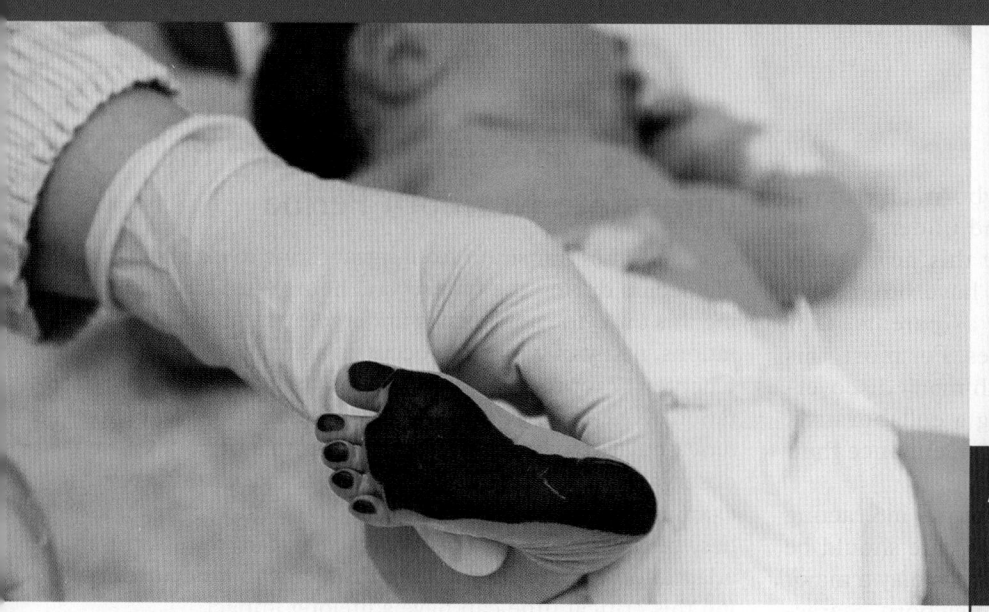

CHAPTER 18

Adapted by Tara Loutit and
Lenora Marcellus

NURSING MANAGEMENT OF THE NEWBORN

KEY TERMS

acrocyanosis	grunting	nevus vasculosus
Apgar score	harlequin sign	ophthalmia neonatorum
apnea	hypoglycemia	phototherapy
bed sharing	infant abduction	pseudomenstruation
bradycardia	immunizations	retractions
caput succedaneum	jaundice	room sharing
cephalhematoma	lanugo	stork bites
circumcision	meconium	suture line
co-sleeping	milia	tachycardia
erythema toxicum	molding	tachypnea
fontanel	Mongolian spots	vernix caseosa
gestational age	nevus flammeus	

LEARNING OBJECTIVES

Upon completion of the chapter, the learner will be able to:

1. Define the key terms.
2. Discuss the assessments performed during the immediate newborn period.
3. Select interventions that meet the immediate needs of the term newborn.
4. List the components of a typical physical examination of a newborn.
5. Identify common variations that can be noted during a newborn's physical examination.
6. List common concerns in the newborn and appropriate interventions.
7. Describe the importance of the newborn screening tests.
8. Explain common interventions that are appropriate during the early newborn period.
9. Discuss the nurse's role in meeting the newborn's nutritional needs.
10. Outline collaborative discharge planning and education needed for the family with a newborn.

*K*elly, a 16-year-old first-time mother, calls the hospital maternity unit 3 days after being discharged home. She tells the nurse that her newborn son "looks like a canary" and "isn't nursing well." She wonders what is wrong.

Wow

You can send a more powerful message with your actions and behaviour than with words alone.

Immediately after the birth of a newborn, all parents are faced with the task of learning and understanding as much as possible about caring for this new family member, even if the parents already have other children. In their new or expanded role as parents, they will face many demands and challenges. For most, this is a wonderful, exciting time filled with many discoveries and much information. Promoting a collaborative, enabling relationship with the family can enhance their experience.

Parents learn as they watch the nurse interacting with and caring for their newborn. This care should be individualized and family-centred as nurses play a major role in teaching parents about typical newborn characteristics and about ways to foster optimal growth and development. This role is even more important today because of limited hospital stays.

The newborn has come from a dark, small, enclosed space in the mother's uterus into the bright, cold extrauterine environment. Nurses can easily forget that they are caring for a small human being who is experiencing his or her first taste of human interaction outside the uterus. The newborn period is an extremely important and vulnerable one, and health goals and guidelines have been developed to address this critical period (Health Canada, 2000).

It is also easy to overlook the intensity with which parents, family members, and other visitors observe the actions of nurses as they care for their new family member. Nurses need to serve as a model for giving nurturing care to newborns and play a profound role at the time of birth in facilitating attachment between mothers and newborns as well as family closeness. Therefore, the mother and her newborn, within the context of their family or personal support, should be viewed as a unit.

This chapter provides information about assessment and interventions in the period immediately following the birth of a newborn and during the early newborn period. For the purposes of this chapter, information is presented within the context of hospital birth, but it is important to note that an increasing number of births in Canada occur at home or in a birth centre setting. The information in this chapter is also general in nature. Most provinces and territories, as well as Health Canada, have developed a number of guidelines related to the care of newborns. It is important to be aware of the recommendations that are followed in each practice setting. Finally, although the term *parents* is used frequently throughout the chapter, it is important to note that there is great diversity in our population in family structures and cultural practices related to birth and the many roles that mothers, fathers, aunts, uncles, other relatives, foster families, adoptive families, and friends play in raising children in our society.

Nursing Management During the Immediate Newborn Period

The period of transition from intrauterine to extrauterine life occurs during the first several hours after birth. During this time, the newborn is undergoing numerous adaptations, many of which are occurring simultaneously (see Chapter 17 for more information on the newborn's adaptation). The neonate's temperature, respiration, and cardiovascular dynamics stabilize during this period. Close observation of the newborn's status is essential. Careful examination of the newborn at birth can detect anomalies, birth injuries, and disorders that can compromise adaptation to extrauterine life. Problems that occur during this critical time can have a lifelong impact.

Assessment

The initial newborn assessment is completed in the birthing area, with the uncompromised baby placed directly on the mother's chest to remain warm and to complete transition. A more thorough assessment can be done within the first 2 to 4 hours, once the parents have had time to bond with their newborn. In addition to ongoing vital sign and physical assessment, a third and more thorough assessment is completed before discharge. The purpose of these assessments is to determine whether the baby is transitioning effectively into the extrauterine environment, to identify apparent physical abnormalities, and to provide parents with information and health teaching (Fraser & Cooper, 2009).

During the initial newborn assessment, look for signs that might indicate a problem, including:

- Nasal flaring
- Chest retractions
- **Grunting** on exhalation
- Laboured breathing
- Generalized cyanosis
- Abnormal breath sounds: rhonchi, crackles (rales), wheezing, stridor
- Abnormal respiratory rate (**tachypnea**, more than 60 breaths/minute; bradypnea, less than 25 breaths/minute)
- Flaccid body posture
- Abnormal heart rate (**tachycardia**, more than 160 beats/minute; bradycardia, less than 100 beats/minute)
- Abnormal newborn size: small or large for gestational age

If any of these findings are noted, medical intervention may be necessary. The US-based Neonatal Resuscitation Program (NRP) provides recommendations for nurses and physicians to manage complications that arise at or shortly after birth. A subcommittee of the Canadian NRP Program Steering Committee was convened to review the textbook as they may apply within the health care system and culture of care in Canada (Canadian Pediatric Society [CPS], n.d.).

Apgar Scoring

The **Apgar score**, introduced in 1952 by Dr. Virginia Apgar, is used to evaluate newborns at 1 minute and 5 minutes after birth. An additional Apgar assessment is done at 10 minutes if the 5-minute score is less than 7 points or if resuscitation is prolonged (Kattwinkel, 2011; Kliegman, Behrman, Jenson, et al., 2011). Assessment of the newborn at 1 minute provides data about the newborn's initial adaptation to extrauterine life. Assessment at 5 minutes provides a clearer indication of the newborn's overall central nervous system status.

Five parameters are assessed with Apgar scoring. A quick way to remember the parameters of Apgar scoring is as follows:

- A = appearance (colour)
- P = pulse (heart rate)
- G = grimace (reflex irritability)
- A = activity (muscle tone)
- R = respiratory (respiratory effort)

Each parameter is assigned a score ranging from 0 to 2 points. A score of 0 indicates an absent or poor response; a score of 2 indicates a normal response (Table 18.1). A normal newborn's score should be 8 to 10 points. It is rare for an infant to receive a score of 10 on the Apgar because pink hands and feet are usually not seen (acrocyanosis) in the newborn in the first few minutes of life. The higher the score, the better the condition of the newborn. If the Apgar score is 8 or higher, no intervention is needed other than supporting normal respiratory efforts and maintaining thermoregulation. Scores of 4 to 7 signify moderate difficulty, and scores of 0 to 3 represent severe distress in adjusting to extrauterine life. The Apgar score is influenced by a variety of factors, including the presence of maternal medications, infection, and fetal malformations (Cunningham, Leveno, Bloom, et al., 2010).

When the newborn experiences physiologic depression, the Apgar score characteristics disappear in a predictable manner: first the pink colouration is lost, next the respiratory effort, and then the tone, followed by reflex irritability and, finally, heart rate (Cunningham et al., 2010).

> ▶ **Take** NOTE!
>
> Although Apgar scoring is done at 1 and 5 minutes, it also can be used as a guide during the immediate newborn period to evaluate the newborn's status for any changes because it focuses on critical parameters that must be assessed throughout the early transition period.

Length and Weight

Parents are eager to know their newborn's length and weight. Accurate measurements of these characteristics are important as they will provide a foundation for assessment of growth and development and will be needed if the infant requires fluids or medications during his or her

TABLE 18.1 **APGAR SCORING FOR NEWBORNS**

Parameter (Assessment Technique)	0 Point	1 Point	2 Points
Heart rate (auscultation of apical heart rate for 1 full min)	Absent	Slow (<100 beats/min)	>100 beats/min
Respiratory effort (observation of the volume and vigour of the newborn's cry; auscultation of depth and rate of respirations)	Apneic	Slow, irregular, shallow	Regular respirations (usually 30–60 breaths/min), strong, good cry
Muscle tone (observation of extent of flexion in the newborn's extremities and newborn's resistance when the extremities are pulled away from the body)	Limp, flaccid	Some flexion, limited resistance to extension	Tight flexion, good resistance to extension with quick return to flexed position after extension
Reflex irritability (flicking of the soles of the feet or suctioning of the nose with a bulb syringe)	No response	Grimace or frown when irritated	Sneeze, cough, or vigorous cry
Skin colour (inspection of trunk and extremities with the appropriate colour for ethnicity appearing within minutes after birth)	Cyanotic or pale	Appropriate body colour; blue extremities (acrocyanosis)	Completely appropriate colour (pink on both trunk and extremities)

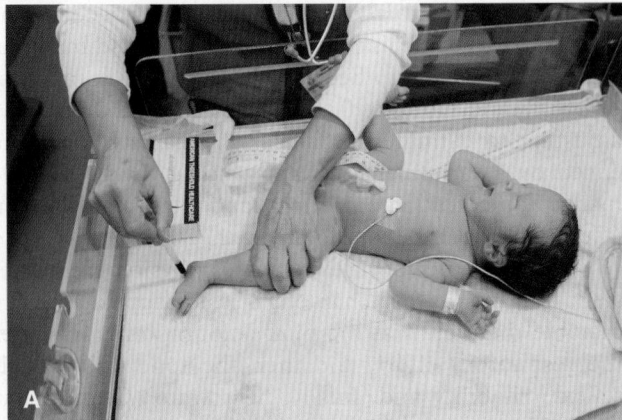 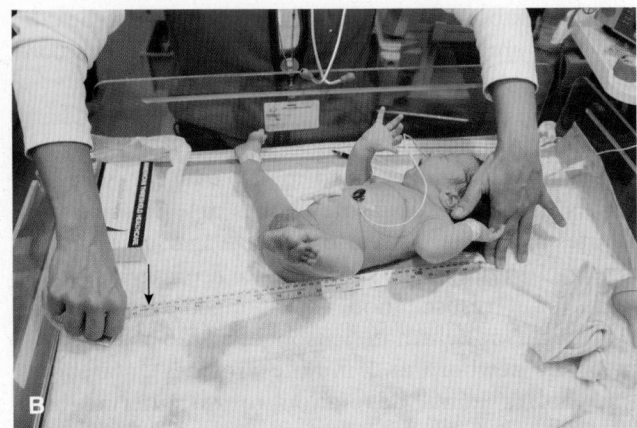

FIGURE 18.1 Measuring a newborn's length. (**A**) The nurse extends the newborn's leg and marks the pad at the heel. (**B**) The nurse measures from the newborn's head to the heel mark.

stay in the hospital. These measurements are taken within the first 1 to 2 hours after birth. A disposable tape measure or a built-in measurement board located on the side of the scale can be used. Obtaining an accurate length measurement is challenging with a moving infant; research has shown that measuring with calibrated equipment such as a board is more accurate (Fraser & Cooper, 2009). Length is measured from the head of the newborn to the heel with the newborn unclothed (Fig. 18.1). Because of the flexed position of the newborn after birth, place the newborn in a supine position and extend the leg completely when measuring the length. The expected length of a full-term newborn is usually 48 to 53 cm (19 to 21 inches). Molding can affect measurement (Kliegman et al., 2011; Tappero & Honeyfield, 2009).

Most often, newborns are weighed using a digital scale that reads the weight in grams. First, balance the scale if it is not balanced. Place a warmed protective cloth or paper as a barrier on the scale to prevent heat loss by conduction; recalibrate the scale to zero after applying the barrier. Next, place the unclothed newborn in the centre of the scale. Keep a hand above the newborn for safety (Fig. 18.2).

Typically, the term newborn weighs 2,500 to 4,000 g (5.5 to 8.5 lb). In 2006, the World Health Organization developed updated child growth standards based on breastfed infants and appropriately fed infants of different ethnic origins. Birth weights less than 10% or more than 90% on a growth chart are outside the normal range and need further investigation. Weights taken at later times are compared with previous weights and are documented with regard to gain or loss on a nursing flow sheet. Newborns typically lose approximately 10% of their initial birth weight by 3 to 4 days of age secondary to loss of meconium and extracellular fluid as well as limited food intake. This weight is usually regained by the 10th day of life (Kliegman et al., 2011). Weight loss may also be influenced by the method of feeding; infants who are breastfed normally lose weight over a longer period of time and take

longer to regain initial weight loss. It is important to keep this in mind when assessing the adequacy of feeding.

Newborns can be classified by their birth weight regardless of their gestational age (Canadian Perinatal Surveillance System, 2008) as follows:

- Low birth weight: <2,500 g (<5.5 lb)
- Very low birth weight: <1,500 g (<3.5 lb)
- Extremely low birth weight: <1,000 g (<2.5 lb)

Vital Signs

Heart rate and respiratory rate are assessed immediately after birth with Apgar scoring. Heart rate, obtained by

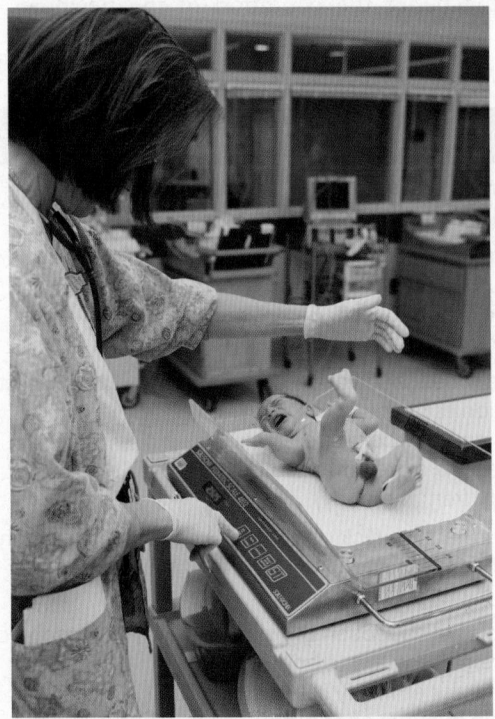

FIGURE 18.2 Weighing a newborn. Note how the nurse guards the newborn from above to prevent injury.

taking an apical pulse for 1 full minute, typically is 120 to 160 beats/minute. Some term newborns may have a resting heart rate as low as 80 beats/minute depending on their level of arousal (Acute Care of at-Risk Newborns [ACoRN] Neonatal Society, 2010). Newborns' respirations are assessed when they are quiet or sleeping. Place a stethoscope on the right side of the chest and count the breaths for 1 full minute to identify any irregularities. The normal newborn respiratory rate is 40 to 60 breaths/minute with symmetric chest movement.

All babies are at risk for temperature instability because their ability to regulate body temperature has not yet fully developed. Maintaining a neutral thermal environment is one of the key physiologic challenges a newborn faces after delivery; the risk for hypothermia is real and potentially dangerous (Soll, 2008). Maintaining temperature within the normal range by providing warmth and minimizing heat loss is an important component of newborn care (ACoRN Neonatal Society, 2010). When there are no contraindications, skin-to-skin thermal management should be encouraged. This has been shown to improve axillary temperature 90 minutes after birth and improved abdominal temperature within the first 21 minutes after birth (Soll, 2008). The normal axillary temperature for a term newborn is 36.5° to 37.5°C (97.9° to 99.7°F). Although mild variations from normal are common, wider variations can be detrimental. If the baby's temperature falls outside this normal range, readings should be done more frequently (every 15 to 30 minutes) until the temperature is normalized. Rectal temperatures are no longer taken because of the risk for perforation (Blackburn, 2007). The thermometer or temperature probe is held in the midaxillary space according to manufacturer's directions and hospital protocol.

Blood pressure is not usually assessed as part of a newborn examination unless there is a clinical indication or low Apgar scores. If assessed, an oscillometer (electronic blood pressure monitor) is used. The typical range is 50 to 75 mm Hg (systolic) and 30 to 45 mm Hg (diastolic). Crying, moving, and late clamping of the umbilical cord will increase systolic pressure (Tappero & Honeyfield, 2009). The proper-size cuff must be used when measuring blood pressure; the most common cause of a hypertensive measurement is a cuff that is too small. It is recommended that the cuff width should be 40% to 50% of the circumference of the extremity or 25% to 55% wider than the diameter of the extremity being measured, and that the bladder should entirely circle the extremity without overlapping (Tappero & Honeyfield, 2009). Typical values for newborn vital signs are provided in Table 18.2.

Gestational Age Assessment

To determine a newborn's **gestational age** (the stage of maturity), physical signs and neurologic characteristics are assessed. Typically, gestational age is determined by

TABLE 18.2   NEWBORN VITAL SIGNS

Newborn Vital Signs	Ranges of values
Temperature	36.5°–37.5°C (97.9°–99.7°F)
Heart rate (pulse)	120–160 beats/min; can increase to 180 during crying
Respirations	30–60 breaths/min at rest; will increase with crying
Blood pressure	50–75 mm Hg systolic, 30–45 mm Hg diastolic

using a tool such as the Dubowitz/Ballard or New Ballard Score system (Fig. 18.3). This scoring system provides an objective estimate of gestational age by scoring the specific parameters of physical and neuromuscular maturity. Points are given for each assessment parameter, with a low score of –1 or –2 points for extreme immaturity to 4 or 5 points for postmaturity. The scores from each section are added together to correspond to a specific gestational age in weeks.

The physical maturity section of the examination is done during the first 2 hours after birth. The physical maturity assessment section of the Ballard examination evaluates physical characteristics that appear different at different stages depending on a newborn's gestational maturity. Newborns who are physically mature have higher scores than those who are not. The areas assessed on the physical maturity examination include:

- Skin texture—typically ranges from sticky and transparent to smooth, with varying degrees of peeling and cracking, to parchment-like or leathery with significant cracking and wrinkling
- **Lanugo**—soft downy hair on the newborn's body, which is absent in preterm newborns, appears with maturity, and then disappears again with postmaturity
- Plantar creases—creases on the soles of the feet, which range from absent to covering the entire foot, depending on maturity (the greater the number of creases, the greater the newborn's maturity)
- Breast tissue—the thickness and size of breast tissue and areola (the darkened ring around each nipple), which range from being imperceptible to full and budding
- Eyes and ears—eyelids can be fused or open and ear cartilage and stiffness determine the degree of maturity (the greater the amount of ear cartilage with stiffness, the greater the newborn's maturity)
- Genitals—in males, evidence of testicular descent and appearance of scrotum (which can range from smooth to covered with rugae) determine maturity; in females, appearance and size of clitoris and labia determine maturity (a prominent clitoris with flat labia suggests

NEUROMUSCULAR MATURITY

NEUROMUSCULAR MATURITY SIGN	SCORE							RECORD SCORE HERE
	−1	0	1	2	3	4	5	
POSTURE								
SQUARE WINDOW (Wrist)	>90°	90°	60°	45°	30°	0°		
ARM RECOIL		180°	140°–180°	110°–140°	90°–110°	<90°		
POPLITEAL ANGLE	180°	160°	140°	120°	100°	90°	<90°	
SCARF SIGN								
HEEL TO EAR								
						TOTAL NEUROMUSCULAR MATURITY SCORE		

SCORE

Neuromuscular ____
Physical ____
Total ____

MATURITY RATING

Score	Weeks
−10	20
−5	22
0	24
5	26
10	28
15	30
20	32
25	34
30	36
35	38
40	40
45	42
50	44

PHYSICAL MATURITY

PHYSICAL MATURITY SIGN	SCORE							RECORD SCORE HERE
	−1	0	1	2	3	4	5	
SKIN	sticky, friable, transparent	gelatinous, red, translucent	smooth, pink, visible veins	superficial peeling and/or rash, few veins	cracking pale areas, rare veins	parchment, deep cracking, no vessels	leathery, cracked, wrinkled	
LANUGO	none	sparse	abundant	thinning	bald areas	mostly bald		
PLANTAR SURFACE	heel-toe 40–50 mm:−1 <40 mm:−2	>50 mm no crease	faint red marks	anterior transverse crease only	creases ant. 2/3	creases over entire sole		
BREAST	impercep-tible	barely perceptible	flat areola no bud	stippled areola 1–2 mm bud	raised areola 3–4 mm bud	full areola 5–10 mm bud		
EYE-EAR	lids fused loosely: −1 tightly: −2	lids open pinna flat stays folded	sl. curved pinna; soft; slow recoil	well-curved pinna; soft but ready recoil	formed and firm instant recoil	thick cartilage, ear stiff		
GENITALS (Male)	scrotum flat, smooth	scrotum empty, faint rugae	testes in upper canal, rare rugae	testes descending, few rugae	testes down, good rugae	testes pendulous, deep rugae		
GENITALS (Female)	clitoris prominent and labia flat	prominent clitoris and small labia minora	prominent clitoris and enlarging minora	majora and minora equally prominent	majora large, minora small	majora cover clitoris and minora		
						TOTAL PHYSICAL MATURITY SCORE		

Figure 18.3 Gestational age assessment tool. (Source: Ballard, J. L., Khoury, J. C., Wedig, K., et al. [1991]. New Ballard Score, expanded to include extremely premature infants. *Journal of Pediatrics*, 119[3], 417–423.)

prematurity, whereas a clitoris covered by labia suggests greater maturity)

The neuromuscular maturity section typically is completed within 24 hours after birth. Six activities or manoeuvres that the newborn performs with various body parts are evaluated to determine the newborn's degree of maturity:

1. Posture—how does the newborn hold his or her extremities in relation to the trunk? The greater the degree of flexion, the greater the maturity. For example, extension of arms and legs is scored as 0 point and full flexion of arms and legs is scored as 4 points.
2. Square window—how far can the newborn's hands be flexed toward the wrist? The angle is measured

and scored from more than 90 degrees to 0 degree to determine the maturity rating. As the angle decreases, the newborn's maturity increases. For example, an angle of more than 90 degrees is scored as −1 point and an angle of 0 degree is scored as 4 points.

3. Arm recoil—how far do the newborn's arms "spring back" to a flexed position? This measure evaluates the degree of arm flexion and the strength of recoil. The reaction of the arm is then scored from 0 to 4 points based on the degree of flexion as the arms are returned to their normal flexed position. The higher the points assigned, the greater the neuromuscular maturity (for example, recoil less than a 90-degree angle is scored as 4 points).

4. Popliteal angle—how far will the newborn's knees extend? The angle created when the knee is extended is measured. An angle less than 90 degrees indicates greater maturity. For example, an angle of 180 degrees is scored as −1 point and an angle of less than 90 degrees is scored as 5 points.

5. Scarf sign—how far can the elbows be moved across the newborn's chest? An elbow that does not reach midline indicates greater maturity. For example, if the elbow reaches or nears the level of the opposite shoulder, this is scored as −1 point; if the elbow does not cross the proximate axillary line, it is scored as 4 points.

6. Heel to ear—how close can the newborn's feet be moved to the ears? This manoeuvre assesses hip flexibility: the lesser the flexibility, the greater the newborn's maturity. The heel-to-ear assessment is scored in the same manner as the scarf sign.

After the scoring is completed, the 12 scores are totalled and then compared with standardized values to determine the appropriate gestational age in weeks. Scores range from very low in preterm newborns to very high for mature and postmature newborns.

Typically newborns are also classified according to gestational age as:

- Preterm or premature—born before 37 weeks' gestation, regardless of birth weight
- Term—born between 38 and 42 weeks' gestation
- Postterm or postdates—born after completion of week 42 of gestation
- Postmature—born after 42 weeks and demonstrating signs of placental aging

Using the information about gestational age and then considering birth weight, newborns can also be classified as follows:

- Small for gestational age (SGA)—weight less than the 10th percentile on standard growth charts (usually <5.5 lb)

- Appropriate for gestational age (AGA)—weight between 10th and 90th percentiles on standard growth charts
- Large for gestational age (LGA)—weight more than the 90th percentile on standard growth charts (usually >9 lb)

Chapter 23 describes these variations in birth weight and gestational age in greater detail.

▶ **Take** NOTE!

Gestational age assessment is important because it allows the nurse to plot growth parameters and to anticipate problems related to prematurity, postmaturity, and growth abnormalities. Most provincial and territorial birth forms have reference charts to document gestational age assessment as well as growth parameters.

Nursing Interventions

During the immediate newborn period, care focuses on helping the newborn to make the transition to extrauterine life. Nursing interventions include maintaining airway patency, promoting skin-to-skin contact, ensuring proper identification, administering prescribed medications, and maintaining thermoregulation.

Maintaining Airway Patency

Once the baby has been delivered and placed on the mother's chest, the nurse can continue to assess the need for resuscitation by noting respiratory effort, heart rate, and skin colour. If excessive secretions are noted that the newborn is unable to clear on his or her own, consider oral and nasal suctioning and turn the baby's head to the side. Turning the newborn's head "will allow secretions to collect in the cheek where they can be removed more easily" (Kattwinkel, 2011, p. 46). Typically, the newborn's mouth is suctioned gently first with a bulb syringe to remove debris and then the nose is suctioned. Suctioning in this manner helps to prevent aspiration of fluid into the lungs by an unexpected gasp. Routine suctioning of the newborn's oral and nasal passages is no longer recommended in the vigorous infant (Kattwinkel, 2011).

When suctioning a newborn with a bulb syringe, compress the bulb before placing it into the oral or nasal cavity. Release the bulb slowly, making sure the tip is placed away from the mucous membranes to draw up the excess secretions. Remove the bulb syringe from the mouth or nose and then, while holding the bulb syringe tip over an emesis basin lined with paper towel or tissue, compress the bulb to expel the secretions. Repeat the procedure gently as needed until all secretions are removed.

▶ *Take* NOTE!

Always keep a bulb syringe near the newborn in case he or she develops sudden choking or a blockage in the nose.

▶ *Take* NOTE!

It make take several minutes for the newborn to transition and for his or her colour to improve. Continued assessment can take place while the baby is on his or her mother's chest.

Skin-to-Skin Contact

Early skin-to-skin contact ideally begins immediately after birth and involves placing the naked newborn, covered with a warm blanket, on the mother's bare chest. This practice between mother and baby has been shown to reduce maternal bleeding, improve oxygenation, stabilize the baby's glucose, reduce crying, improve mother–baby interaction, maintain thermoregulation, and assist with successful breastfeeding (Caruana, 2008). If the newborn is healthy and stable, wipe the newborn from head to toe with a dry cloth and place him or her skin-to-skin on the mother's abdomen. Then cover the newborn and mother with another warmed blanket to hold in the warmth. Immediate mother–newborn contact takes advantage of the newborn's natural alertness after a vaginal birth and fosters bonding. Skin-to-skin care can also be modified for those parents who are not comfortable with immediate full skin-to-skin care, and can also be done with the father or other caregivers.

Initiating Breastfeeding

Helping mother breastfeed immediately after birth is gradually becoming the norm instead of attending immediately to what have become routine delivery room interventions. Since infants are the most alert within the first 60 to 90 minutes following birth, it is an ideal time to initiate breastfeeding. Helping mothers initiate breastfeeding within half an hour of birth is one of the World Health Organization's 10 Steps to Successful Breastfeeding (La Leche League International, 2010).

Left alone on the mother's abdomen, a healthy newborn moves upward, pushing with the feet, pulling with the arms, and bobbing the head until finding and latching on to the mother's nipple. A newborn's sense of smell is highly developed, which also helps in finding the nipple. As the newborn moves to the nipple, the mother produces high levels of oxytocin, which contracts the uterus, thereby minimizing bleeding. Oxytocin also causes the breasts to release colostrum when the newborn sucks on the nipple. Colostrum is rich in antibodies and thus provides the newborn with his or her "first immunization" against infection.

Ensuring Proper Identification

Starting at birth and throughout the hospital stay, attention to the safety and security of the newborn is important. The newborn commonly receives two ID bracelets, one on a wrist and one on an ankle. The mother receives a matching one, usually on her wrist. Four-band systems are also available. The ID bands usually state the infant's name, sex, date and time of birth, and identification number. The same identification number is on the bracelets of all the family members. If there are twins, each baby will have his or her own set of bracelets that will also identify birth order (Twin A for the first born and Twin B for the second born).

These ID bracelets provide for the safety of the newborn and must be secured before the mother and newborn leave the birthing area. The ID bracelets are checked by all nurses to validate that the correct newborn is brought to the right mother if they are separated for any period of time (Fig. 18.4). They also serve as the official newborn identification and are checked before initiating any procedure on that newborn and on discharge from the unit. Taking the newborn's picture within 2 hours after birth with a colour camera or colour video/digital image also helps prevent mix-ups and abduction. Some facilities use electronic devices that sound an alarm if the newborn is removed from the area. Parents are also key partners in safety and are encouraged to ask to see the photo identification of staff before giving their baby to someone (Association of Women's Health, Obstetric and Neonatal Nurses [AWHONN], 2007; Colling & York, 2010).

Although abductions from Canadian hospitals are rare, hospital security staff must always be well prepared to handle such incidents. Local law enforcement officials can be helpful in these situations too, especially if an Amber Alert search and recovery plan is activated. Many

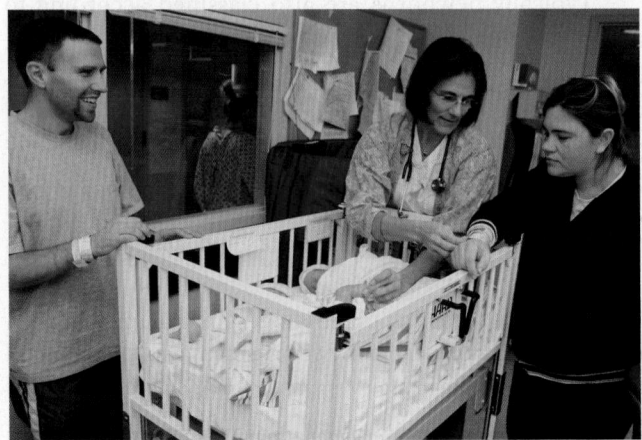

FIGURE 18.4 The nurse checks the newborn's identification band against the mother's.

DRUG GUIDE 18.1	DRUGS FOR THE NEWBORN	
Drug	**Action/Indication**	**Nursing Implications**
Phytonadione (vitamin K [Aqua-MEPHYTON, Konakion, Mephyton])	Provides the newborn with vitamin K (necessary for production of adequate clotting factors II, VII, IX, and X by the liver) during the first week of birth until newborn can manufacture it Prevents vitamin K deficiency bleeding	• Administer within 1 to 2 h after birth. • Give as an IM injection at a 90-degree angle into the middle third of the vastus lateralis muscle. • Use a 25 gauge, 5/8 in needle for injection. • Hold the leg firmly and inject medication slowly after aspirating. • Adhere to standard precautions. • Assess for bleeding at injection site after administration.
Erythromycin ophthalmic ointment 0.5% or tetracycline ophthalmic ointment 1%	Provides bactericidal and bacteriostatic actions to prevent *Neisseria gonorrhoeae* and *Chlamydia trachomatis* conjunctivitis Prevents ophthalmia neonatorum	• Be alert for chemical conjunctivitis for 1–2 days. • Wear gloves, and open eyes by placing thumb and finger above and below the eye. • Gently squeeze the tube or ampoule to apply medication into the conjunctival sac from the inner canthus to the outer canthus of each eye. • Do not touch the tip to the eye. • Close the eye to make sure the medication permeates. • Wipe off excess ointment after 1 min.

facilities now have protocols and procedures in place for this situation.

Administering Prescribed Medications

During the immediate newborn period, two medications are commonly ordered: vitamin K and eye prophylaxis with either erythromycin or tetracycline ophthalmic ointment (Drug Guide 18.1).

Vitamin K

Vitamin K, a fat-soluble vitamin, promotes blood clotting by increasing the synthesis of prothrombin by the liver. A deficiency of this vitamin would delay clotting and might lead to unexpected bleeding.

Generally, the bacteria of the intestine produce vitamin K in adequate quantities. However, the newborn's bowel is sterile, so vitamin K is not produced in the intestine until after microorganisms are introduced, such as with the first feeding.

The administration of vitamin K to prevent early vitamin K deficiency bleeding has been the standard of care since the early 1960s. CPS recommends that vitamin K be given as a single intramuscular dose of 0.5 mg (birth weight 1,500 g or less) or 1.0 mg (birth weight greater than 1,500 g) to all newborns within the first 6 hours after birth following initial stabilization and an appropriate opportunity for maternal and family interaction (Fig. 18.5) (CPS,

2011b). If parents are not comfortable with intramuscular administration, oral vitamin K is available. Oral administration requires three doses, however, and parents need to be informed that there is an increased risk for late hemorrhagic disease.

Eye Prophylaxis

The CPS (2002) recommends that all newborns, whether delivered vaginally or by cesarean section, receive an instillation of a prophylactic agent in their eyes as soon as

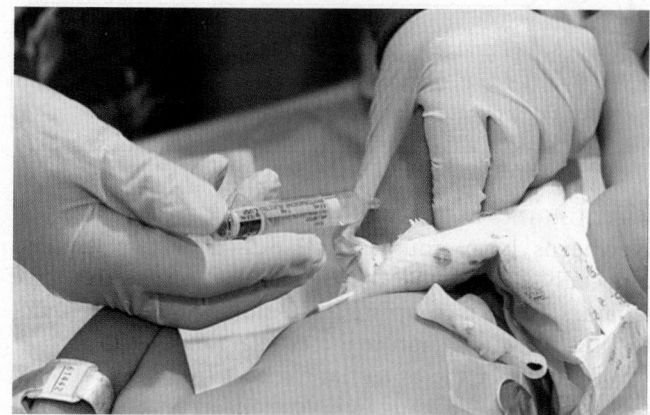

FIGURE 18.5 The nurse administers vitamin K intramuscularly to the newborn.

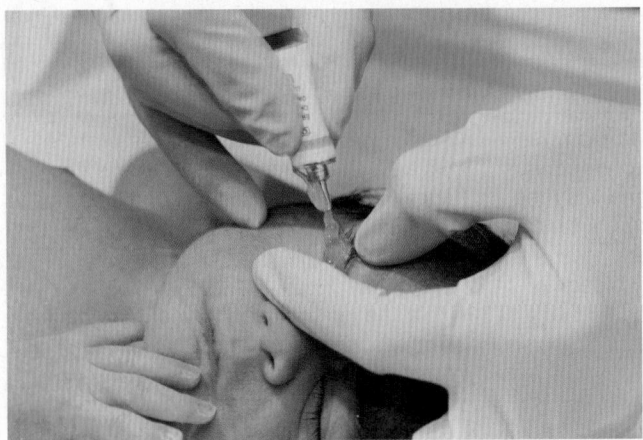

FIGURE 18.6 The nurse administers eye prophylaxis.

possible after birth. This is to prevent **ophthalmia neo-natorum** (chlamydia trachomatis is the most common organism) and **gonoccocal ophthalmia**, which can cause neonatal blindness (CDC, 2010). Ophthalmia neonatorum is a hyperacute purulent conjunctivitis occurring during the first 10 days of life. It is usually contracted during birth when the baby comes in contact with infected vaginal discharge of the mother (CDC, 2010). Most often both eyelids become swollen and red with purulent discharge.

Prophylactic agents that are currently recommended include erythromycin 0.5% ophthalmic ointment or tetracycline 1% ophthalmic ointment in a single application; 1% silver nitrate solution was formerly used but has little efficacy in preventing chlamydial eye disease (CDC, 2010). Regardless of which agent is used, the medication should be instilled within 1 hour after birth (Fig. 18.6). (Health Canada, 2000).

Inform all parents about the eye treatment, including why it is recommended, what problems may arise if the treatment is not given, and possible adverse effects of the treatment.

▶ **Take** NOTE!

Parents have the right to refuse this treatment. Ensure this is an informed decision based on accurate information and teaching.

Maintaining Thermoregulation

Newborns have trouble regulating their temperature, especially during the first few hours after birth (see Chapter 17 for a complete discussion). Therefore, maintaining body temperature is a crucial nursing role.

Remember the potential for heat loss in newborns, and perform all nursing interventions in a way that minimizes heat loss and prevents hypothermia. Thoroughly drying the infant, placing a cap on his or her head, and

ensuring skin-to-skin contact with the mother while the infant is covered with a warm blanket all minimize heat loss. Ongoing care to prevent hypothermia involves making sure the newborn is not exposed to cold surfaces or cool drafts and wrapping the newborn in warm blankets when skin-to-skin contact is not possible. If the newborn is to be placed under a heat warmer, unwrap the infant and put a sensor in place to monitor temperature and avoid hyperthermia.

A wide variety of devices are available to measure temperature in newborns; most birthing facilities are now using electronic thermometers. Axillary temperatures are recommended to assess the newborn's body temperature. At one time, rectal thermometers were routinely used to monitor body temperature, but their use is no longer recommended because of the risk for traumatizing the rectal lining (Blackburn, 2007). Axillary temperature should be maintained between 36.3° and 37.0°C (inclusive) and skin temperature between 36.5° and 37.0°C (ACoRN Neonatal Society, 2010). Nursing interventions to help maintain body temperature include:

- Promote skin-to-skin contact with the newborn's mother or another caregiver immediately after birth.
- Dry the newborn immediately after birth to prevent heat loss through evaporation.
- Cover or wrap the baby in warmed blankets to reduce heat loss via convection.
- Use a warmed cover on the scale to weigh the unclothed newborn to prevent heat loss through conduction.
- Warm stethoscopes and hands before examining the baby or providing care.
- Avoid placing newborns in drafts or near air vents to prevent heat loss through convection.
- Delay the initial bath until the baby's temperature has stabilized to prevent heat loss through evaporation.
- Avoid placing cribs near cold outer walls to prevent heat loss through radiation.
- Put a cap on the newborn's head after it is thoroughly dried after birth.
- Place the newborn in an incubator or under a temperature-controlled radiant warmer if other interventions are not effective at improving the temperature (Fig. 18.7).

Nursing Management During the Early Newborn Period

The early newborn period is a time of great adjustment for both the mother and the newborn, both of whom are adapting to many physiologic and psychological changes. In the past, mothers and newborns remained in a health care facility while these dramatic changes were taking place, with nurses and doctors readily available. Today, however, shorter hospital stays as well as delivery in birth centres and at home are increasingly the norm, and new

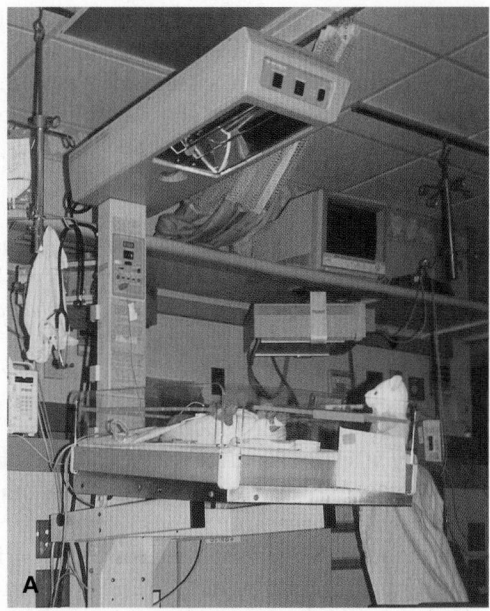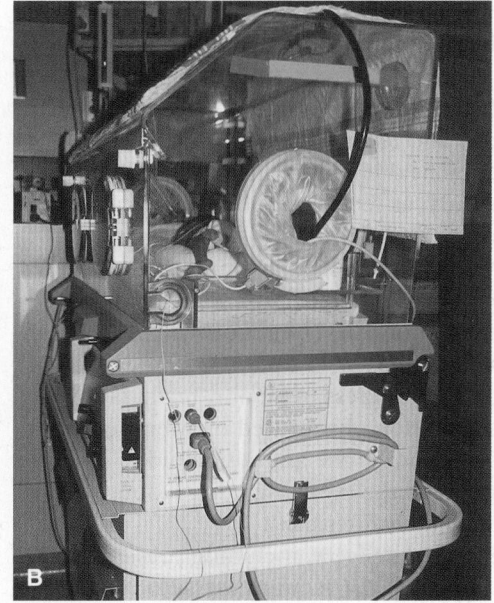

FIGURE 18.7 Maintaining thermoregulation. (**A**) Radiant warmer. (**B**) Isolette.

mothers can easily be overwhelmed by having to go through all of these changes in such a short time: the woman gives birth, experiences marked physiologic and psychological changes, and must adapt to her newborn and learn the skills needed to care for herself and the baby, all within 24 to 48 hours.

The nurse's role is to promote parent–infant attachment by encouraging the family to spend time "getting to know" their infant and assist them through this transition period. The parent–infant bond is formative to a child's sense of security and has long-lasting effects; therefore, keeping babies and parents together should be a high priority. The newborn needs continued health assessment, and the family's needs should be assessed as they learn to care for their new baby. Nurses can support and strengthen the mother's knowledge within her particular family and cultural situation and enhance her confidence in her and in her baby's health by maintaining open lines of communication, sharing information, and teaching about newborn care.

Assessment

The newborn requires ongoing assessment to ensure that his or her transition to extrauterine life is progressing without problems. The nurse uses the data gathered during the initial assessment as a baseline for comparison. The baby should be assessed and cared for while he or she is with the parents, thus providing an opportunity for parental education and attachment.

Perinatal History

Pertinent maternal and fetal data are vital to formulate a plan of care for the mother and her newborn. Historical

information is obtained from the medical record and from interviewing the mother. Review the maternal history because it provides pertinent information, such as the presence of certain risk factors that could affect the newborn. Keep in mind that a comprehensive maternal history may not be available, especially if the mother has had limited or no prenatal care. Many birthing facilities in Canada have been shifting to a single-room model of care versus separate birthing and postpartum units, so you may already be familiar with the maternal history by the time of the infant's birth.

Historical information usually includes the following:

- Mother's name, medical record number, blood type, serology result, and rubella and hepatitis status
- Other maternal tests that are relevant to the newborn and care, such as HIV and group B streptococcus status
- Intrapartum maternal antibiotic therapy (type, dose, and duration)
- Maternal illness that can affect the pregnancy, evidence of chorioamnionitis, maternal use of medications such as steroids
- Gestational diabetes
- Prenatal care, including timing of first visit and subsequent visits
- Risk for blood group incompatibility, including Rh status and blood type
- Fetal distress or any nonreassuring fetal heart rate patterns during labour
- Known inherited conditions such as sickle cell anemia and phenylketonuria (PKU)
- Birth weights of previous live-born children, along with identification of any newborn problems

- Any social determinants of health that impact the family's well-being, such as social support and safe and adequate housing
- History of substance use, including tobacco, alcohol, and prescription and recreational drug use
- History of mental health conditions (including cognitive challenges such as fetal alcohol spectrum disorder [FASD]), trauma, or violence
- Cultural factors, including primary language
- Pregnancy complications associated with abnormal fetal growth, fetal anomalies, or abnormal results from tests of fetal well-being
- Information on the progress of labour, birth, labour complications, duration of ruptured membranes, and presence of meconium in the amniotic fluid
- Medications given to the mother during labour, at birth, and immediately after birth
- Time and method of delivery, including presentation and the use of forceps or a vacuum extractor
- Status of the newborn at birth, including Apgar scores at 1 and 5 minutes, the need for suctioning, weight, gestational age, vital signs, and umbilical cord status
- Medications administered to the newborn
- Postbirth maternal information, including placental findings, positive cultures, and presence of fever

Newborn Physical Examination

The initial newborn physical examination, which may demonstrate subtle differences related to the newborn's age, is carried out within the first 24 hours after birth. For example, a newborn who is 30 minutes old has not yet completed the normal transition from intrauterine to extrauterine life, and thus variability may exist in vital signs and in respiratory, neurologic, gastrointestinal, skin, and cardiovascular systems. Therefore, a comprehensive examination should be delayed until after the newborn has completed the transition. The assessment process also provides an opportunity to share information with parents about their infant, help them begin to appreciate the capacities that their infant already is demonstrating, and model safe practices such as handwashing and proper positioning. Techniques of physical assessment of the newborn include observation, auscultation, palpation, percussion, and transillumination (Tappero & Honeyfield, 2009).

In a quiet newborn, begin with the least invasive and noxious elements of the examination (such as observation and auscultation) and then progress to the areas most likely to irritate the newborn (e.g., examining the hips and eliciting the Moro reflex). A general visual assessment provides a significant amount of information about the well-being of a newborn. Initial observation gives an impression of a healthy (stable) versus an ill newborn and a term versus a preterm newborn.

A typical physical examination of a newborn includes a general survey of skin colour, posture, state of alertness, head size, overall behavioural state, respiratory status,

sex, and any obvious congenital anomalies. Check the overall appearance for anything unusual. Then complete the examination in a systematic fashion. An important point to consider and to share with parents is that there is a wide range of "typical" for newborns.

Remember Kelly, who called the home health nurse and said her newborn son "looks like a canary"? What additional information is needed about the baby? What might be causing his yellow colour?

Anthropometric Measurements

Shortly after birth, after the sex of the child is revealed, most parents want to know the "vital statistics" of their newborn—length and weight—to report to their family and friends. Additional measurements, including head and chest circumference, are also taken and recorded. Abdominal measurements are not routinely obtained unless there is a suspicion of pathology that causes abdominal distention. The newborn's progress from that point on will be validated based on these early measurements. These measurements will be compared with future serial measurements to determine growth patterns, which are plotted on growth charts to evaluate normalcy. Therefore, accuracy is key.

Weight is affected by racial origin, maternal age, size of the parents, maternal nutrition, and placental perfusion (Tappero & Honeyfield, 2009). Weight should be correlated with gestational age. A newborn who weighs more than normal might be LGA or an infant of a diabetic mother (IDM); a newborn who weighs less than normal might be SGA or preterm or might have a genetic syndrome. It is important to identify the cause for the deviation in size and to monitor the newborn for complications common to that etiology.

Head Circumference

The average newborn head circumference is 32 to 38 cm (13 to 15 in). Measure the circumference at the head's widest diameter (the occipitofrontal circumference). Wrap a flexible, non-stretchable or paper measuring tape snugly around the newborn's head and record the measurement (Fig. 18.8A).

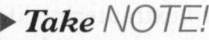

▶ *Take* NOTE!

Head circumference may need to be remeasured at a later time if the shape of the head is altered from birth.

The head circumference should be approximately one fourth of the newborn's length (Tappero & Honeyfield, 2009). A small head might indicate microcephaly caused

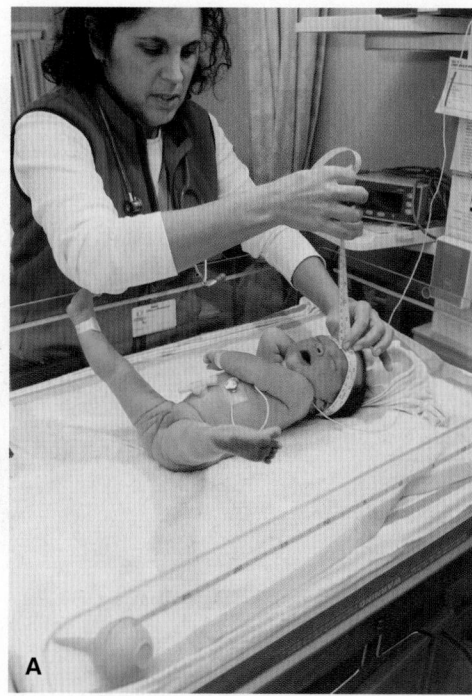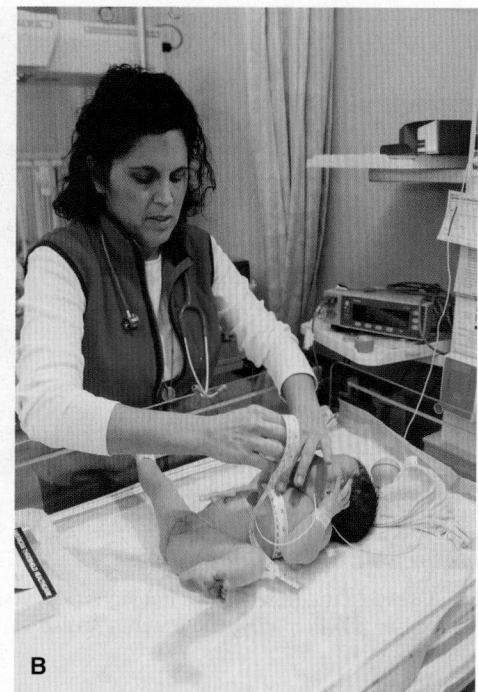

FIGURE 18.8 (**A**) Measuring head circumference. (**B**) Measuring chest circumference.

by rubella, toxoplasmosis, prenatal cocaine or alcohol exposure, or SGA status; an enlarged head might indicate hydrocephalus or increased intracranial pressure. Both need to be documented and reported for further investigation. The head circumference measurement may need to be repeated at a later date if the shape of the head was significantly altered during the birth process and if the delivery was instrument-assisted.

Chest Circumference

The average chest circumference in a newborn is 30 to 36 cm (12 to 14 in). It is generally equal to or about 2 to 3 cm less than the head circumference (Burns, Dunn, Brady, et al., 2009). Place a flexible, non-stretchable or paper tape measure around the unclothed newborn's chest at the nipple line during expiration without pulling it taut (see Fig. 18.8B).

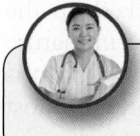 ▶ *Take* NOTE!

The head and chest circumferences are usually equal by about 1 year of age.

Vital Signs

In the newborn, temperature, pulse, and respirations are monitored frequently and compared with baseline data obtained immediately after birth. Temperature, pulse, and respirations are reassessed at 1 and 2 hours following the first vital signs, at hour 6, and once per shift until

discharge (Perinatal Services BC, 2011b). If the newborn has been cool and is being warmed, check the temperature every 15 to 30 minutes until within normal range. Blood pressure is not routinely assessed in a normal newborn unless the baby's clinical condition warrants it. This schedule can change depending on the baby's health status.

Obtain an apical pulse by placing the stethoscope over the fourth intercostal space on the chest. Listen for a full minute, noting rate, rhythm, and abnormal sounds such as murmurs. In the typical newborn, the heart rate is 120 to 160 beats/minute, with wide fluctuations with activity and sleep. Sinus arrhythmia is a normal finding. Murmurs detected during the newborn period do not necessarily indicate congenital heart disease, but they need to be assessed frequently over the next several months to see if they persist.

Also palpate the apical, femoral, and brachial pulses for presence and equality (Fig. 18.9). Report any abnormalities to the primary health care provider for evaluation.

Assess respirations by observing the rise and fall of the chest for 1 full minute. Respirations should be symmetric, slightly irregular, shallow, and unlaboured at a rate of 30 to 60 breaths/minute. The newborn's respirations are predominantly diaphragmatic, but they are synchronous with abdominal movements. Also auscultate breath sounds. Note any abnormalities, such as tachypnea, bradypnea, grunting, gasping, periods of **apnea** lasting longer than 20 seconds, asymmetry or decreased chest expansion, abnormal breath sounds (rhonchi,

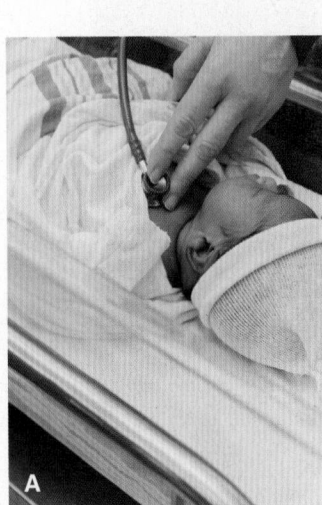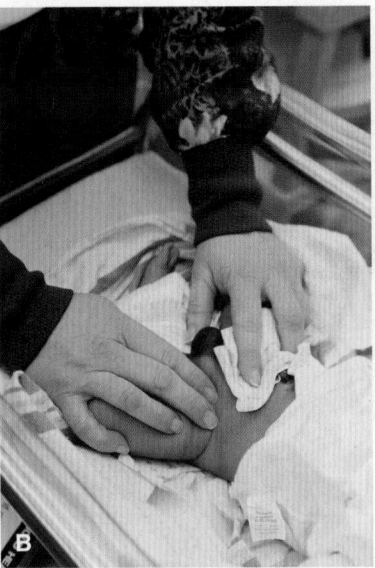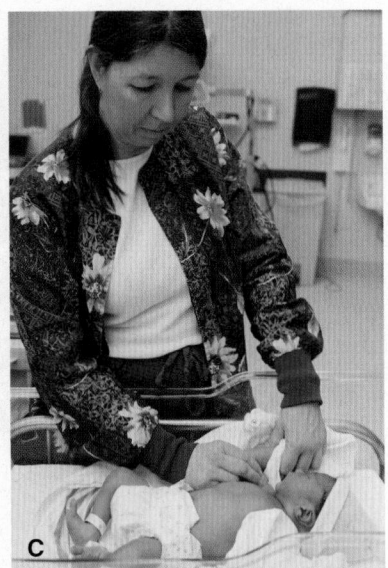

FIGURE 18.9 Assessing the newborn's vital signs. (**A**) Assessing the apical pulse. (**B**) Palpating the femoral pulse. (**C**) Palpating the brachial pulse.

crackles), or sternal retractions. Some variations might exist early after birth, but if the abnormal pattern persists, notify the primary health care provider.

Skin

Observe the overall appearance of the skin, including colour, texture, turgor, and integrity. The newborn's skin should be smooth and flexible, and the colour should be consistent with genetic background.

Skin Condition and Colour

Check skin turgor by gently pinching a small area of skin over the chest or abdomen and note how quickly it returns to its original position. In a well-hydrated newborn, the skin should return to its normal position immediately. Skin that remains "tented" after being pinched indicates dehydration. A small amount of lanugo (fine downy hair) may be observed over the shoulders and on the sides of the face and upper back. There may be some cracking and peeling of the skin. The skin should be warm to the touch and intact.

The newborn's skin often appears blotchy or mottled, especially in the extremities. Persistent cyanosis of fingers, hands, toes, and feet with mottled blue or red discolouration and coldness is called **acrocyanosis**. It may be seen in newborns during the first few weeks of life in response to exposure to cold. Acrocyanosis is normal and intermittent.

Newborn Skin Variations

While assessing the skin, note any rashes, ecchymoses or petechiae, nevi, or dark pigmentation. Skin lesions can be congenital or transient; they may be a result of infection or may result from the mode of birth. If any are present, observe the anatomic location, arrangement, type, and colour. Bruising may result from the use of devices such as a vacuum extractor during delivery. Petechiae may be the result of pressure on the skin during the birth process. Forceps marks may be observed over the cheeks and ears. A small puncture mark may be seen if internal fetal scalp electrode monitoring was used during labour.

Common skin variations include vernix caseosa, stork bites or salmon patches, milia, Mongolian spots, erythema toxicum, harlequin sign, nevus flammeus, and nevus vasculosus (Fig. 18.10).

Vernix caseosa is a thick white substance that protects the skin of the fetus. It is formed by secretions from the fetus's oil glands and is found during the first 2 or 3 days after birth in body creases and the hair. It does not need to be removed because it will be absorbed into the skin.

Stork bites or salmon patches are superficial vascular areas found on the nape of the neck, on the eyelids, and between the eyes and upper lip (see Fig. 18.10A). The name comes from the marks on the back of the neck where, as myth goes, a stork may have picked up the baby. They are caused by a concentration of immature blood vessels and are most visible when the newborn is crying. They are considered a normal variant, and most fade and disappear completely within the first year.

Milia are unopened sebaceous glands frequently found on a newborn's nose. They may also appear on the chin and forehead (see Fig. 18.10B). They form from oil glands and disappear on their own within 2 to 4 weeks. When they occur in a newborn's mouth and gums, they are termed **Epstein's pearls**.

Mongolian spots are blue or purple splotches that appear on the lower back and buttocks of newborns (see

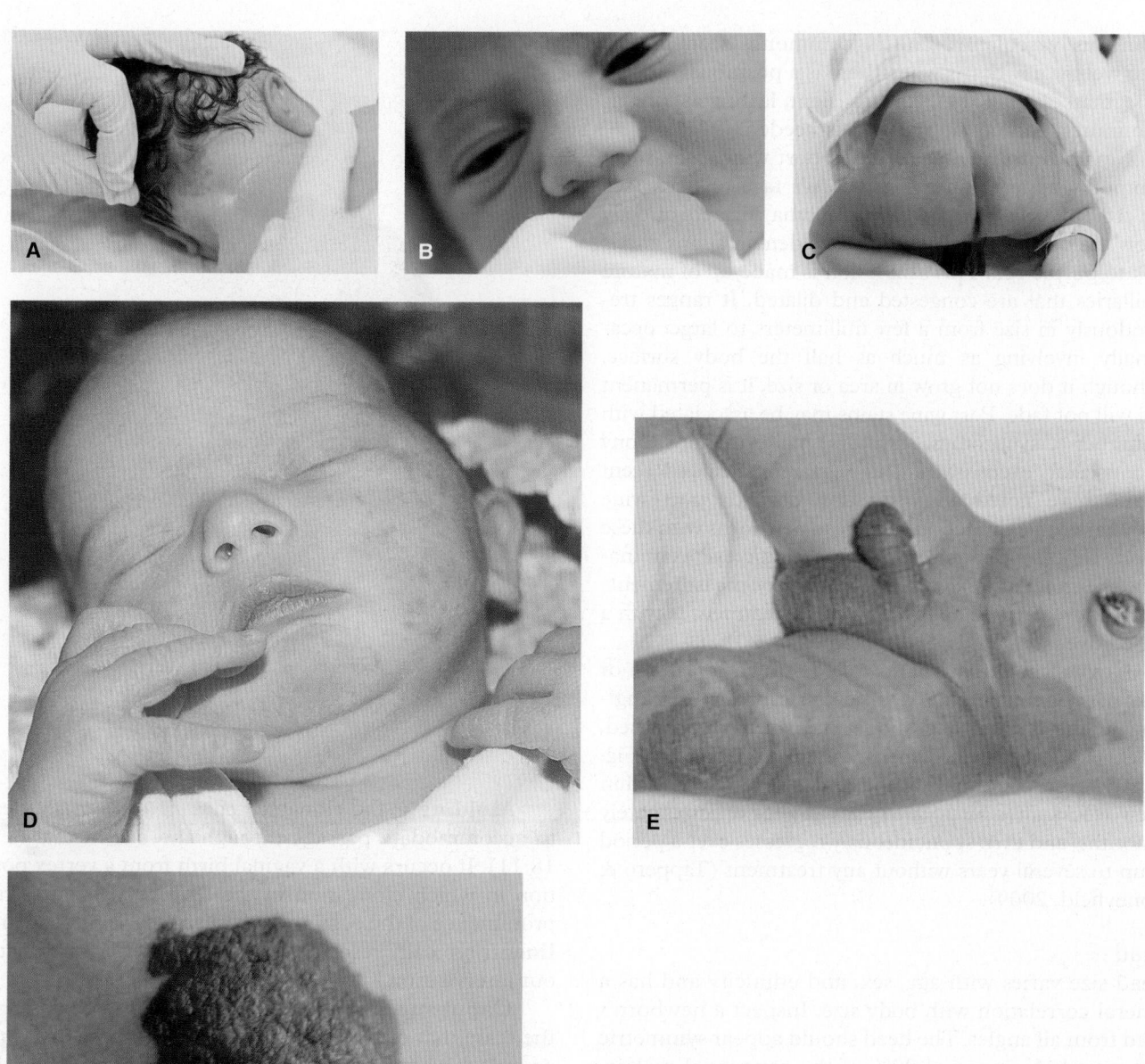

FIGURE 18.10 Common skin variations. (**A**) Stork bite. (**B**) Milia. (**C**) Mongolian spots. (**D**) Erythema toxicum. (**E**) Nevus flammeus (port-wine stain). (**F**) Strawberry hemangioma.

Fig. 18.10C). They tend to occur in black, Asian, and Indian newborns but can occur in dark-skinned newborns of all races. The spots are caused by a concentration of pigmented cells and usually disappear within the first 4 years of life (Kliegman et al., 2011.

Erythema toxicum (newborn rash) is a benign, idiopathic, generalized, transient rash that occurs in up to 70% of all newborns during the first week of life. It consists of small white or yellow papules or vesicles on the skin. The rash is common on the face, chest, back, and extremities (see Fig. 18.10D). One of the chief characteristics of this rash is its lack of pattern. It is caused by the newborn's eosinophils reacting to the environment as the immune system matures (It does not require any treatment and disappears in a few days (Tappero & Honeyfield, 2009).

Harlequin sign refers to the dilation of blood vessels on only one side of the body, giving the newborn the appearance of wearing a clown suit. It gives a distinct midline demarcation, which is described as pale on the nondependent side and red on the opposite, dependent side. It is caused by a temporary autonomic imbalance of cutaneous vasculature and is commonly seen in low birth weight newborns when there is a positional change (Kliegman et al., 2011). It is transient, lasting as long as 30 minutes, and no intervention is needed.

Nevus flammeus, also called port wine stain, most commonly appears on the newborn's face or neck (see Fig. 18.10E). It is a capillary angioma located directly below the dermis. It is flat with sharp demarcations and is pink to purple-red. This skin lesion is made up of mature capillaries that are congested and dilated. It ranges tremendously in size from a few millimeters to large, occasionally involving as much as half the body surface. Although it does not grow in area or size, it is permanent and will not fade. Port wine stains may be associated with a number of syndromes, structural malformations, bony or muscular overgrowth, and certain cancers. Recent studies have noted an association between port wine birthmarks and childhood cancer, so newborns with these lesions should be monitored with periodic eye examinations, neurologic imaging, and extremity measurements (McHoney, 2010). The most effective treatment is with a pulsed dye laser (PDL) (Kliegman et al., 2011).

Nevus vasculosus, also called strawberry mark or strawberry hemangioma, is a benign capillary hemangioma in the dermal and subdermal layers. It is raised, rough, dark red, and sharply demarcated (see Fig. 18.10F). It is commonly found in the head region within a few weeks after birth, grows rapidly for approximately 6 months, and then spontaneously regresses over a period of up to several years without any treatment (Tappero & Honeyfield, 2009).

Head

Head size varies with age, sex, and ethnicity and has a general correlation with body size. Inspect a newborn's head from all angles. The head should appear symmetric and round. As many as 90% of the congenital malformations present at birth are visible on the head and neck, so careful assessment is very important (Tappero & Honeyfield, 2009).

The newborn has two **fontanels** at the juncture of the cranial bones. The anterior fontanel is diamond-shaped and closes by 18 to 24 months. Typically it measures 4 to 6 cm at the largest diameter (bone to bone). The posterior one is triangular, smaller than the anterior fontanel (usually fingertip size or 0.5 to 1 cm), and closes by 6 to 12 weeks. Palpate both fontanels, which should be soft, flat, and open. Then palpate the skull. It should feel smooth and fused, except at the area of the fontanels. Also assess the size of the head and the anterior and posterior fontanels, and compare them with appropriate standards.

Variations in Head Size and Appearance

During inspection and palpation, be alert for common variations that may cause asymmetry. These include caput succedaneum, cephalhematoma, and molding.

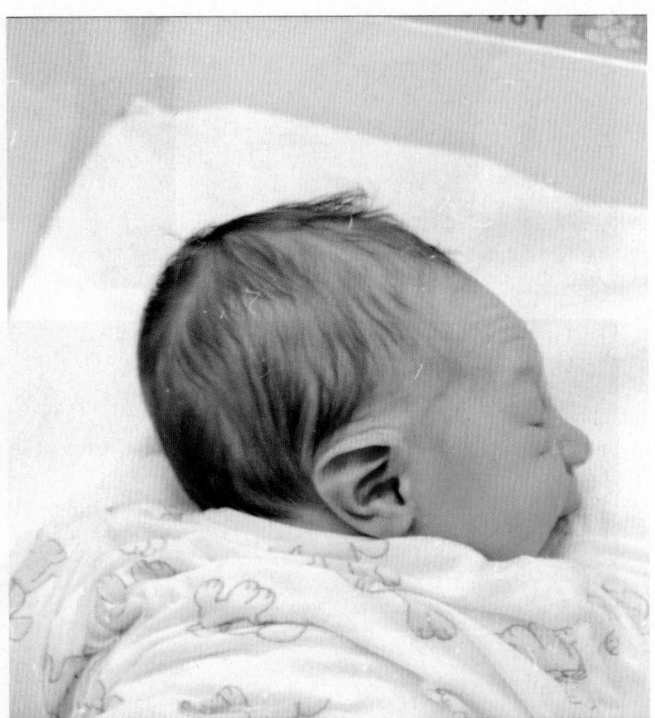

FIGURE 18.11 Molding in a newborn's head.

Molding is the elongated shaping of the fetal head to accommodate passage through the birth canal (Fig. 18.11). It occurs with a vaginal birth from a vertex position in which elongation of the fetal head occurs with prominence of the occiput and overriding sagittal **suture line**. It typically resolves within a week after birth without intervention.

Caput succedaneum describes localized edema on the scalp that occurs from the pressure of the birth process. It is commonly observed after prolonged labour. Clinically, it appears as a poorly demarcated soft tissue swelling that crosses suture lines. Pitting edema and overlying petechiae and ecchymosis are noted (Fig. 18.12A). The swelling will gradually dissipate in about 3 days without any treatment. Newborns who were delivered via vacuum extraction usually have a caput in the area where the cup was used.

Cephalhematoma is a localized effusion of blood beneath the periosteum of the skull. This condition is due to disruption of the vessels during birth. It occurs after prolonged labour and use of obstetric interventions such as low forceps or vacuum extraction. The clinical features include a well-demarcated, often fluctuant swelling with no overlying skin discolouration. The swelling does not cross suture lines and is firmer to the touch than an edematous area (see Fig. 18.12B). Cephalhematoma usually appears on the second or third day after birth and disappears within weeks or months (Tappero & Honeyfield, 2009).

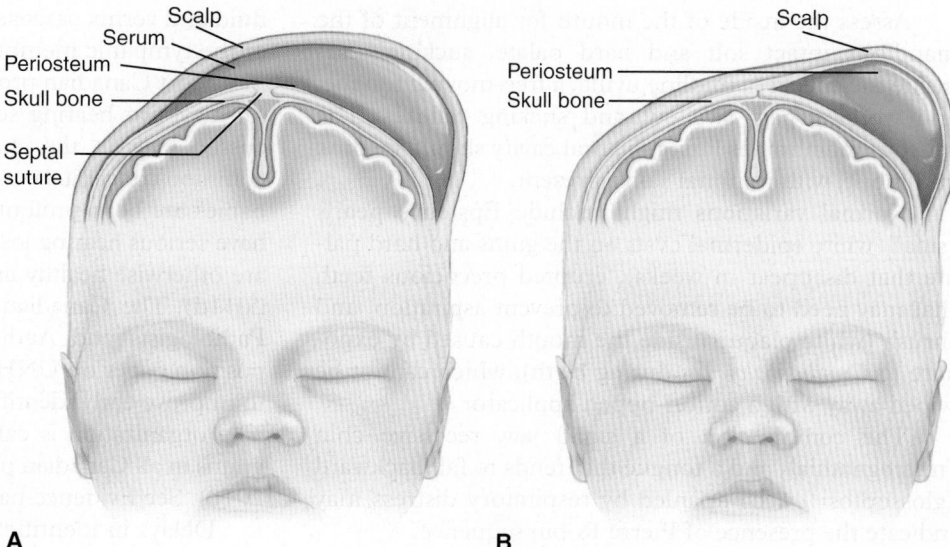

FIGURE 18.12 (**A**) Caput succedaneum involves the collection of
serous fluid and often crosses the
suture line. (**B**) Cephalhematoma
involves the collection of blood
and does not cross the suture
line.

A   **B**

Common Abnormalities in Head or Fontanel Size

Common abnormalities in head or fontanel size that
may indicate a problem include:

- Microcephaly—a head circumference more than
  2 standard deviations below average or less than 10%
  of normal parameters for gestational age, caused by
  failure of brain development. It can be familial, with
  autosomal dominant or recessive inheritance, and it
  may be associated with infections (cytomegalovirus),
  syndromes such as trisomies 13 and 18, and FASD
  (Kliegman et al., 2011).
- Macrocephaly—a head circumference more than 90%
  of normal, typically related to hydrocephalus. It is
  often familial (with autosomal dominant inheritance)
  and can be either an isolated anomaly or a manifestation of other anomalies, including hydrocephalus and
  skeletal disorders (achondroplasia) (Kliegman et al.,
  2011).
- Large fontanels—more than 6 cm in the anterior
  diameter bone to bone or more than a 1 cm diameter
  in the posterior fontanel. This condition is possibly
  associated with malnutrition, hydrocephaly, congenital
  hypothyroidism, trisomies 13, 18, and 21, and various
  bone disorders such as osteogenesis imperfecta.
- Small or closed fontanels—smaller-than-normal anterior and posterior diameters or fontanels that are
  closed at birth. This condition is associated with
  microcephaly or premature synostosis (union of two
  bones by osseous material) (Blackburn, 2007).

Face

Observe the newborn's face for fullness and symmetry.
The face should have full cheeks and should be symmetric when the baby is resting and crying. If forceps were
used during birth, the newborn may have bruising and
reddened areas over both cheeks and parietal bones

secondary to the pressure of the forceps blades. Reassure
the parents that this resolves without treatment, and
point out improvement each day.

Problems with the face can also involve facial nerve
paralysis caused by trauma from the use of forceps.
Paralysis is usually apparent on the first or second day of
life. Typically, the newborn will demonstrate asymmetry
of the face with the inability to close the eye and move
the lips on the affected side. Newborns with facial nerve
paralysis have difficulty making a seal around the nipple,
and consequently milk or formula drools from the paralyzed side of the mouth. Most facial nerve palsies resolve
spontaneously within days, although full recovery may
require weeks to months.

Nose

Inspect the nose for size, symmetry, position, and lesions.
The newborn's nose is small and narrow. The nose
should have a midline placement, patent nares, and an
intact septum. The nostrils should be of equal size and
should be patent. A slight mucus discharge may be present, but there should be no actual drainage. The newborn is a preferential nose breather and will use sneezing
to clear the nose if needed. The newborn can smell after
the nasal passages are cleared of amniotic fluid and
mucus (Tappero & Honeyfield, 2009).

Mouth

Inspect the newborn's mouth, lips, and interior structures. The lips should be intact with symmetric movement and positioned in the midline; there should not be
any lesions. Inspect the lips for pink colour, moisture,
and cracking. The lips should encircle the examiner's finger to form a vacuum. Variations involving the lip might
include cleft upper lip (separation extending up to the
nose) or thin upper lip associated with FASD.

Assess the inside of the mouth for alignment of the mandible, intact soft and hard palate, sucking pads inside the cheeks, a midline uvula, a free-moving tongue, and working gag, swallow, and sucking reflexes. The mucous membranes lining the oral cavity should be pink and moist, with minimal saliva present.

Normal variations might include Epstein's pearls (small, white epidermal cysts on the gums and hard palate that disappear in weeks), erupted precocious teeth that may need to be removed to prevent aspiration, and thrush (white plaque inside the mouth caused by exposure to *Candida albicans* during birth), which cannot be wiped away with a cotton-tipped applicator.

The combination of a small jaw, recessive chin (micrognathia), and a tongue that tends to fall backward (glossoptosis) accompanied by respiratory distress may indicate the presence of Pierre Robin sequence.

Eyes

Inspect the external eye structures, including the eye colour, eyelids, lashes, conjunctiva, sclera, iris, and pupils, for position, colour, size, and movement. There may be marked edema of the eyelids and subconjunctival hemorrhages due to pressure during birth. The eyes should be clear and symmetrically placed. Test the blink reflex by bringing an object close to the eye; the newborn should respond quickly by blinking. Also test the newborn's pupillary reflex: pupils should be equal, round, and reactive to light bilaterally. Assess the newborn's gaze: he or she should be able to track objects to the midline. Movement may be uncoordinated during the first few weeks of life. Many newborns have transient strabismus (deviation or wandering of eyes independently) and searching nystagmus (involuntary repetitive eye movement), which is caused by immature muscular control. These are normal for the first 3 to 6 months of life.

Examine the internal eye structures. A red reflex (luminous red appearance seen on the retina) should be seen bilaterally on retinoscopy. The red reflex normally shows no dullness or irregularities.

Chemical conjunctivitis commonly occurs within 24 hours of instillation of eye prophylaxis after birth. There is lid edema with sterile discharge from both eyes. Usually it resolves within 48 hours without treatment.

Ears

Inspect the ears for size, shape, skin condition, placement, amount of cartilage, and patency of the auditory canal. The ears should be soft and pliable and should recoil quickly and easily when folded and released. Ears should be aligned with the outer canthi of the eyes. Low-set ears are characteristic of many syndromes and genetic abnormalities, such as trisomies 13 and 18, and internal organ abnormalities involving the renal system.

An otoscopic examination is not typically done because the newborn's ear canals are filled with amniotic fluid and vernix caseosa, which would make visualization of the tympanic membrane difficult.

Most Canadian provinces and territories have universal newborn hearing screening (UNHS) programs (discussed later in the chapter). Hearing loss is the most common congenital condition in Canada: about 3 in 1,000 babies are born profoundly deaf, and another 3 in 1,000 have serious hearing loss. Most hearing-impaired children are otherwise healthy and born to hearing parents (CPS, 2011d). The Canadian Association of Speech-Language Pathologists and Audiologists (CASLPA) submitted a position paper on UNHS as part of its national campaign to improve early identification of hearing loss in children. The organization is calling for adoption of UNHS programs in all Canadian provinces and territories (CASLPA, 2010). See Evidence-based Practice 18.1.

Delays in identification and intervention may affect the child's cognitive, verbal, behavioural, and emotional development. Screening at birth has reduced the age at which newborns with hearing loss are identified and has improved early intervention rates dramatically. Prior to universal newborn screening, children were usually older than 2 years before significant congenital hearing loss was detected; by this time it had already affected their speech and language skills (CASLPA, 2010).

Causes of hearing loss can be conductive, sensorineural, or central. Risk factors for congenital hearing loss include cytomegalovirus infection and preterm birth necessitating a stay in the neonatal intensive care unit.

To assess for hearing ability generally, observe the newborn's response to noises and conversations. The newborn typically turns toward these noises and startles with loud ones.

Neck

Inspect the newborn's neck for movement and ability to support the head. The newborn's neck will appear almost nonexistent because it is so short. Creases are usually noted. Webbing (lateral folds of skin) indicates the presence of Turner's syndrome, a genetic condition seen in girls that is caused by the absence of an X chromosome. The neck should move freely in all directions and should be capable of holding the head in a midline position. The newborn should have enough head control to be able to hold the head up briefly without support. Report any deviations such as restricted neck movement or absence of head control.

Also inspect and palpate the clavicles, which should be straight and intact. The clavicle is the most frequently injured bone during labour and delivery and accounts for 90% of all obstetric fractures. The primary cause of fractured clavicles is mechanical compression seen during difficult deliveries, such as with shoulder dystocia. In most cases, the fractured clavicle is asymptomatic, but decreased or absent movement, crepitus (grating that can be felt or heard with movement), and pain or tenderness

EVIDENCE-BASED PRACTICE 18.1
Universal Neonatal Hearing Screening Versus Selective Screening as Part of the Management of Childhood Deafness

● Study
The principal factors that determine how deafness affects a child's development are the degree of hearing impairment and the age at which it is diagnosed. A number of factors are thought to increase the risk for hearing impairment, such as low birth weight, prematurity, and perinatal hypoxia and jaundice. The high incidence of deafness in children without risk factors and the introduction of simple new screening tests with high sensitivity and specificity have led many prestigious bodies to recommend universal early detection programs for deafness rather than screening that targets high-risk groups. A study was performed to compare the long-term effectiveness of a universal neonatal screening and early treatment program for hearing impairment versus screening and treatment of high-risk neonates only.

▲ Findings
This updated review was withdrawn as the researchers still did not find any randomized trials that compared the long-term results of these screening programs. Controlled trials and before-and-after studies continue to be needed to address this issue.

■ Nursing Implications
Although additional research is needed, nurses should encourage all parents to have their newborns screened. The CPS (2011d) recommends hearing screening for all newborns so that early interventions can be provided to prevent speech, language, and cognitive development impairments. This information should be stressed during discharge planning activities and follow-up tests if warranted.

Source: Puig, T., Municio, A., & Medà, C. (2009). WITHDRAWN: Universal neonatal hearing screening versus selective screening as part of the management of childhood deafness. *Cochrane Database of Systematic Reviews* 2009, Issue 2. Art. No.: CD003731. doi:10.1002/14651858.CD003731.pub2.

on movement of the arm on the affected side may be noted (Tappero & Honeyfield, 2009). Treatment involves immobilization and minimizing pain.

Chest
Inspect the newborn's chest for size, shape, and symmetry. The newborn's chest should be round and symmetric, with a circumference 2 to 3 cm smaller than the head circumference. The xiphoid process may be prominent at birth, but it usually becomes less apparent when adipose tissue accumulates. Nipples may be engorged and may secrete a white discharge. This discharge, which occurs in both boys and girls, is a result of exposure to high levels of maternal estrogen while in utero. This enlargement and milky discharge usually dissipates within a few weeks. Some newborns may have extra nipples, called supernumerary nipples. They are typically small, raised, pigmented areas vertical to the main nipple line, 5 to 6 cm below the normal nipple. They tend to be familial and do not contain glandular tissue. Reassure parents that these extra small nipples are harmless.

The newborn chest is usually barrel-shaped, with equal anteroposterior and lateral diameters, and symmetric. Auscultate the lungs bilaterally for equal breath sounds. Normal breath sounds should be heard, with little difference between inspiration and expiration. Fine crackles can be heard on inspiration soon after birth as a result of clearing amniotic fluid from the lungs. Diminished breath sounds might indicate atelectasis, effusion, or poor respiratory effort. Respiratory issues are the most

frequent cause of admission for neonatal intensive care (Kliegman et al., 2011).

Listen to the heart when the newborn is quiet or sleeping. S1 and S2 heart sounds are accentuated at birth. The point of maximal impulse (PMI) is a lateral to midclavicular line located at the fourth intercostal space. A displaced PMI may indicate tension pneumothorax or cardiomegaly. Murmurs are often heard and are usually benign, but if present after the first 12 hours of life should be evaluated to rule out a cardiac disorder (Kliegman et al., 2011).

Abdomen
Inspect the abdomen for shape and movement. Typically the newborn's abdomen is protuberant but not distended. This contour is a result of the immaturity of the abdominal muscles. Abdominal movements are synchronous with respirations because newborns are, at times, abdominal breathers.

Auscultate bowel sounds in all four quadrants and then palpate the abdomen for consistency, masses, and tenderness. Perform auscultation and palpation systematically in a clockwise fashion until all four quadrants have been assessed. Palpate gently to feel the liver, the kidneys, and any masses. The liver is normally palpable 1 to 3 cm below the costal margin in the midclavicular line. The kidneys are 1 to 2 cm above and to both sides of the umbilicus. Normal findings would include bowel sounds in all four quadrants and no masses or tenderness on palpation. Absent or hyperactive bowel sounds might indicate an intestinal obstruction. Abdominal distention might indicate air swallowing, ascites, obstruction or perforation of the gastrointestinal tract, infection, masses, or an enlarged abdominal organ. A sunken (or scaphoid) abdomen may indicate a diaphragmatic hernia (Kliegman et al., 2011).

Inspect the umbilical cord area for the correct amount of blood vessels (two arteries and one vein). The umbilical vein is larger than the two umbilical arteries. Evidence of only a single umbilical artery is associated with cardiovascular, renal, and gastrointestinal anomalies. Also inspect the umbilical area for signs of bleeding, infection, granuloma, or abnormal or persistent communication with the intra-abdominal organs (Tappero & Honeyfield, 2009).

Genitalia

Inspect the penis and scrotum in the male. In the uncircumcised male, the foreskin should cover the glans. In the circumcised male newborn, the glans should be smooth, with the meatus centred at the tip of the penis. It will appear reddened until it heals. Check the position of the urinary meatus: it should be in the midline at the glans tip. If it is on the ventral surface of the penis, hypospadias is present; if it is on the dorsal surface of the penis, it is termed epispadias. In either case, circumcision should be avoided until further evaluation.

Inspect the scrotum for size, symmetry, colour, presence of rugae, and location of testes. The scrotum usually appears relatively large and should be pink in white neonates and dark brown in neonates of colour. Rugae should be well formed and should cover the scrotal sac. There should not be bulging, excessive edema, or discolouration (Fig. 18.13A). The presence of some edema is common, often due to a hydrocele (a collection of fluid in the scrotum) that usually disappears during the first 3 to 6 months.

Palpate the scrotum for evidence of the testes, which should be in the scrotal sac. The testes should feel firm and smooth and should be of equal size on both sides of the scrotal sac in the term newborn. Undescended testes (cryptorchidism) might be palpated in the inguinal canal in preterm infants; they can be unilateral or bilateral. If the testes are not palpable within the scrotal sac, further investigation is needed.

In the female newborn, inspect the external genitalia. The urethral meatus is located below the clitoris in the midline (Kliegman et al., 2011). In contrast to the male genitalia, the female genitalia will be engorged: the labia majora and minora may both be edematous. The labia majora are large and cover the labia minora. The clitoris is large and the hymen is thick. These findings are due to the maternal hormones estrogen and progesterone (see Fig. 18.13B). A vaginal discharge composed of mucus mixed with blood may also be present during the first few weeks of life. This discharge, called **pseudomenstruation**,

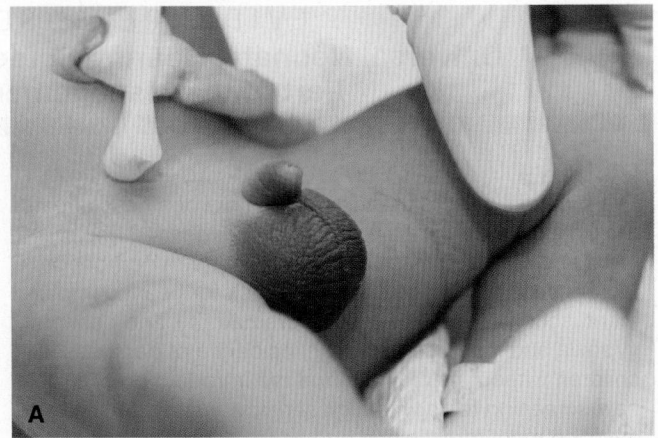

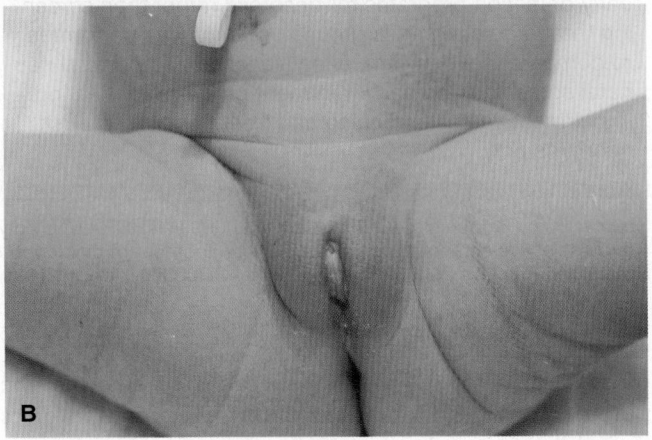

FIGURE 18.13 Newborn genitalia. (**A**) Male genitalia. Note the darkened colour of the scrotum. (**B**) Female genitalia.

requires no treatment. Explain this phenomenon to the parents.

Variations in female newborns may include a labial bulge, which might indicate an inguinal hernia; ambiguous genitalia; a rectovaginal fistula with feces present in the vagina; and an imperforate hymen.

Inspect the anus in both male and female newborns for position and patency. An imperforate anus should be obvious with examination, but may not become apparent until meconium is not passed by 24 hours of age.

Extremities and Back

Inspect the newborn's upper extremities for appearance and movement. Inspect the hands for shape, number, and position of fingers and presence of palmar creases. The newborn's arms and hands should be symmetric and should move through range of motion without hesitation. Observe for spontaneous movement of the extremities. Each hand should have five digits. Note any extra digits (polydactyly) or fusing of two or more digits (syndactyly). Most newborns have three palmar creases on the hand. A single palmar crease, called simian line, is frequently associated with Down syndrome.

A brachial plexus injury can occur in macrosomic infants and during a difficult birth involving shoulder dystocia. Erb's palsy is an injury resulting from damage to the upper plexus during labour and birth. The affected arm hangs limp alongside the body, and the affected shoulder and arm are adducted, extended, and internally rotated with a pronated wrist. The Moro reflex is absent on the affected side in brachial palsy. Complete recovery occurs for most infants, but may take a few months (Kliegman et al., 2011).

Assess the lower extremities in the same manner. They should be of equal length, with symmetric skin folds. Inspect the feet for clubfoot (a turning-inward position), which is secondary to intrauterine positioning. This may be positional or structural. Perform the Ortolani and Barlow manoeuvres to identify congenital hip dislocation, commonly termed developmental dysplasia of the hip (DDH). Nursing Procedure 18.1 highlights the steps for performing these manoeuvres.

Inspect the back. The spine should appear straight and flat and should be easily flexed when the baby is held in a prone position. Observe for the presence of a skin disruption, tuft of hair, a pilonidal dimple in the midline, a cyst, sinus tract, or a mass along the spine. These abnormal findings may be signs of a congenital spinal or neurologic anomaly and should be documented and reported to the primary health care provider (Tappero & Honeyfield, 2009).

Table 18.3 summarizes the newborn assessment.

Neurologic Status

Assess the newborn's state of alertness, posture, muscle tone, and reflexes.

Newborn Alertness, Posture, and Muscle Tone

The newborn should be alert and not persistently lethargic. The normal posture is hips abducted and partially flexed, with knees flexed. Arms are adducted and flexed at the elbow. Fists are often clenched, with fingers covering the thumb.

To assess for muscle tone, support the newborn with one hand under the chest. Observe how the neck muscles

---

Nursing Procedure 18.1

PERFORMING ORTOLANI AND BARLOW MANOEUVRES

Purpose: To Detect Congenital Developmental Dysplasia of the Hip

Ortolani Manoeuvre

1. Place the newborn in the supine position and flex the hips and knees to 90 degrees at the hip.
2. Grasp the inner aspect of the thighs and abduct the hips (usually to approximately 180 degrees) while applying upward pressure.

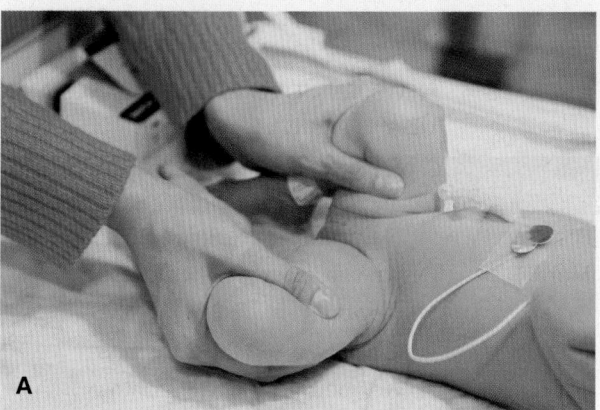

A

3. Listen for any sounds during the manoeuvre. There should be no "cluck" or "click" heard when the legs are abducted. Such a sound indicates the femoral head hitting the acetabulum as the head re-enters the area. This suggests developmental hip dysplasia.

Barlow Manoeuvre

1. With the newborn still lying supine and grasping the inner aspect of the thighs (as just mentioned), adduct the thighs while applying outward and downward pressure to the thighs.

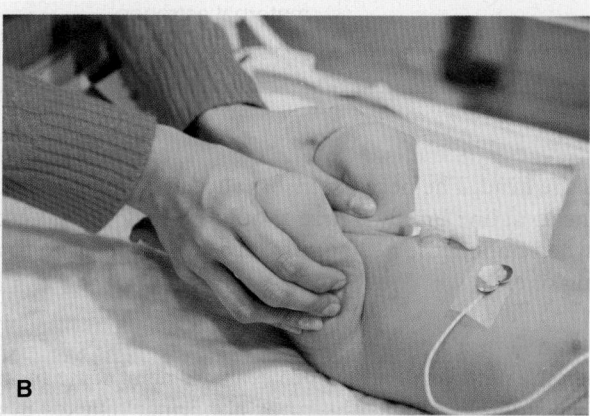

B

2. Feel for the femoral head slipping out of the acetabulum; also listen for a click (Dillon, 2007).

TABLE 18.3   NEWBORN ASSESSMENT SUMMARY

Assessment	Usual Findings	Variations and Common Problems
Anthropometric measurements	Head circumference: 33–37 cm (13–14 in) Chest circumference: 30–33 cm (12–13 in) Weight: 2,500–4,000 g (5.5–8.5 lb) Length: 48–53 cm (19–21 in)	SGA, LGA, preterm, postterm
Vital signs	Temperature: 36.5°–37.5°C (97.9°–99.7°F) Apical pulse: 120–160 beats/min Respirations: 30–60 breaths/min	
Skin	Smooth, flexible, good skin turgor, warm	Jaundice, acrocyanosis, milia, Mongolian spots, stork bites
Head	Varies with age, sex, ethnicity	Microcephaly, macrocephaly, enlarged fontanels
Face	Full cheeks, facial features symmetric	Facial nerve paralysis, nevus flammeus, nevus vasculosus
Nose	Small, placement in the midline and narrow, ability to smell	Malformation or blockage
Mouth	Aligned in midline, symmetric, intact soft and hard palate	Epstein's pearls, erupted precocious teeth, thrush
Neck	Short, creased, moves freely, baby holds head in midline	Restricted movement, clavicular fractures
Eyes	Clear and symmetrically placed on face	Chemical conjunctivitis, subconjunctival hemorrhages
Ears	Soft and pliable with quick recoil when folded and released	Low-set ears, hearing loss
Chest	Round, symmetric, smaller than head	Nipple engorgement, whitish discharge
Abdomen	Protuberant contour, soft, three vessels in umbilical cord	Distended, only two vessels in umbilical cord
Genitals	Male: smooth glans, meatus centred at tip of penis Female: swollen genitals as a result of maternal estrogen	Edematous scrotum in males, vaginal discharge in females
Extremities and spine	Extremities symmetric with free movement	Congenital hip dislocation, tuft or dimple on spine

hold the head. The neck extensors should be able to hold the head in line briefly. There should be only slight head lag when pulling the newborn from a supine position to a sitting one.

Newborn Reflexes

Assess the newborn's reflexes to evaluate neurologic function and development. Absent or abnormal reflexes in a newborn, persistence of a reflex past the age when the reflex is normally lost, or return of an infantile reflex in an older child or adult may indicate neurologic pathology (Table 18.4). Reflexes commonly assessed in the newborn include sucking, Moro, stepping, tonic neck, rooting, Babinski, and palmar grasp reflex. Spinal reflexes tested include truncal incurvation (Galant reflex) and anocutaneous reflex (anal wink).

The sucking reflex is elicited by gently stimulating the newborn's lips by touching them. The newborn will

TABLE 18.4   NEWBORN REFLEXES: APPEARANCE AND DISAPPEARANCE

Reflex	Appearance	Disappearance
Blinking	Newborn	Persists into adulthood
Moro	Newborn	3–6 months
Grasp	Newborn	3–4 months
Stepping	Birth	1–2 months
Tonic neck	Newborn	3–4 months
Sneeze	Newborn	Persists into adulthood
Rooting	Birth	4–6 months
Gag reflex	Newborn	Persists into adulthood
Cough reflex	Newborn	Persists into adulthood
Babinski sign	Newborn	12 months

typically open the mouth and begin a sucking motion. Placing a gloved finger in the newborn's mouth will also elicit a sucking motion (Fig. 18.14A).

The Moro reflex, also called embrace reflex, occurs when the neonate is startled. To elicit this reflex, place the newborn on his or her back. Support the upper body weight of the supine newborn by the arms, using a lifting motion, without lifting the newborn off the surface. Then release the arms suddenly. The newborn will throw the arms outward and flex the knees; the arms then return to the chest. The thumbs and the forefingers also spread to form a C. The newborn initially appears startled and then relaxes to a normal resting position (see Fig. 18.14B).

Assess the stepping reflex by holding the newborn upright and inclined forward with the soles of the feet touching a flat surface. The baby should make a stepping or walking motion, alternating flexion and extension with the soles of the feet (see Fig. 18.14C).

The tonic neck reflex resembles the stance of a fencer and is often called fencing reflex. Test this reflex by having the newborn lie on the back. Turn the baby's head to one side. The arm toward which the baby is facing should extend straight away from the body with the hand partially open, whereas the arm on the side away from the face is flexed and the fist is clenched tightly. Reversing the direction to which the face is turned reverses the position (see Fig. 18.14D).

Elicit the rooting reflex by stroking the newborn's cheek. The newborn should turn toward the side that was stroked and should begin to make sucking movements (see Fig. 18.14E).

The Babinski reflex should be present at birth and disappears at approximately 1 year of age. It is elicited by stroking the lateral sole of the newborn's foot from the heel toward and across the ball of the foot. The toes should fan out. A diminished response indicates a neurologic problem and needs follow-up (see Fig. 18.14F).

The newborn exhibits two grasp reflexes: palmar grasp and plantar grasp. Elicit the palmar grasp reflex by placing a finger on the newborn's open palm. The baby's hand will close around the finger. Attempting to remove the finger causes the grip to tighten. Newborns have strong grasps and can almost be lifted from a flat surface if both hands are used. The grasp should be equal bilaterally (see Fig. 18.14G).

The plantar grasp is similar to the palmar grasp. Place a finger just below the newborn's toes. The toes typically curl over the finger (see Fig. 18.14H).

Blinking, sneezing, gagging, and coughing are all protective reflexes and are elicited when an object or light is brought close to the eye (blinking), something irritating is swallowed or a bulb syringe is used for suctioning (gagging and coughing), or an irritant is brought close to the nose (sneezing).

The truncal incurvation reflex (Galant reflex) is present at birth and disappears in a few days to 4 weeks.

With the newborn in a prone position or held in ventral suspension, apply firm pressure and run a finger down either side of the spine. This stroking will cause the pelvis to flex toward the stimulated side. This indicates T2–S1 innervation. Lack of response indicates a neurologic or spinal cord problem.

The anocutaneous reflex (anal wink) is elicited by stimulating the perianal skin close to the anus. The external sphincter will constrict (wink) immediately with stimulation. This indicates S4–5 innervation. Absence of this reflex indicates that there may be an abnormality of the central nervous system (Tappero & Honeyfield, 2009).

Nursing Interventions

Developing confidence to care for their newborn is challenging for most parents. It takes time and patience, and nurses should individualize care according to the needs and uniqueness of each family—as identified by the family. Educating and empowering parents about their newborn and all the procedures (e.g., feeding, bathing, changing, handling) involved in daily care are key nursing interventions. The nurse functions as a resource for the family, providing guidance, suggestions, and assistance as needed.

Providing General Newborn Care

Generally, newborn care involves bathing and hygiene, diaper care, cord care, circumcision care, use of appropriate clothing, environmental safety measures, and prevention of infection. Nurses should teach these skills to parents and should serve as role models for appropriate and consistent interaction with newborns. Demonstrating respect for the newborn and family helps foster a positive atmosphere to promote the newborn's growth and development.

Bathing and Hygiene

Immediately after birth, drying the newborn and removing blood may minimize the risk for infection caused by hepatitis B, herpes virus, and HIV, but the specific benefits of this practice remain unclear. Until the newborn has been thoroughly bathed, universal precautions should be used when handling the newborn, including wearing gloves. Residual vernix can be left on the skin and allowed to wear off with normal care and handling (AWHONN, 2007).

Newborns are bathed primarily for aesthetic reasons, and bathing is postponed until thermal and cardiorespiratory stability are ensured. Traditional reasons why nurses bathe the newborn are so they can conduct a physical assessment, reduce the effect of hypothermia, and allow the mother to rest (Cohen, 2007). However, research suggests that nurses do not need to give the newborn an initial bath to reduce heat loss; rather, the parents should be given this opportunity, supported by nurses (Medves &

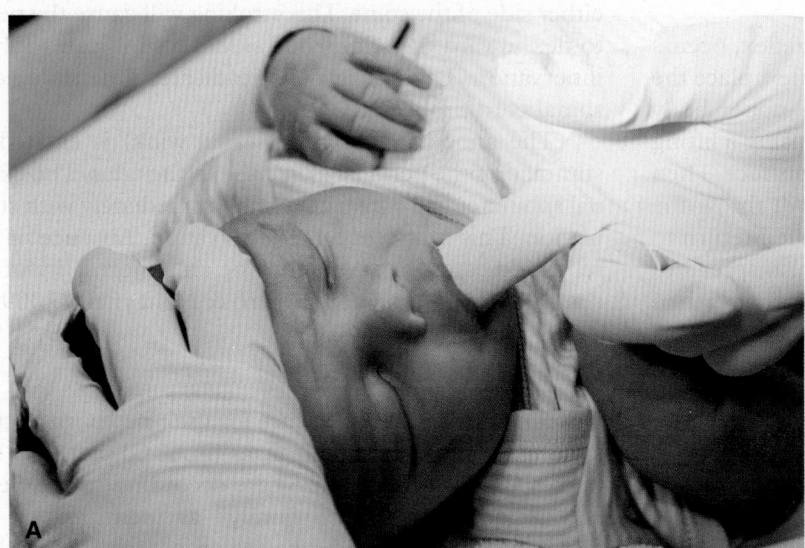

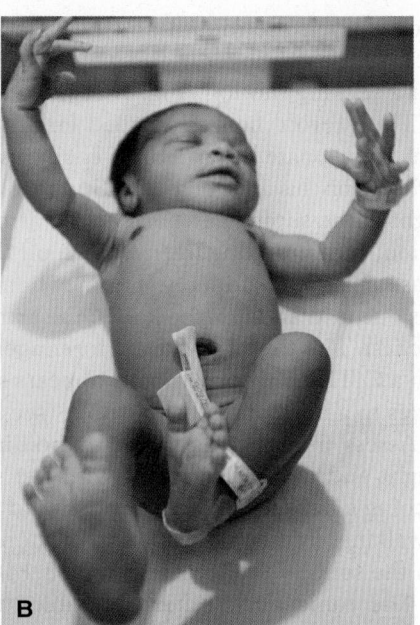

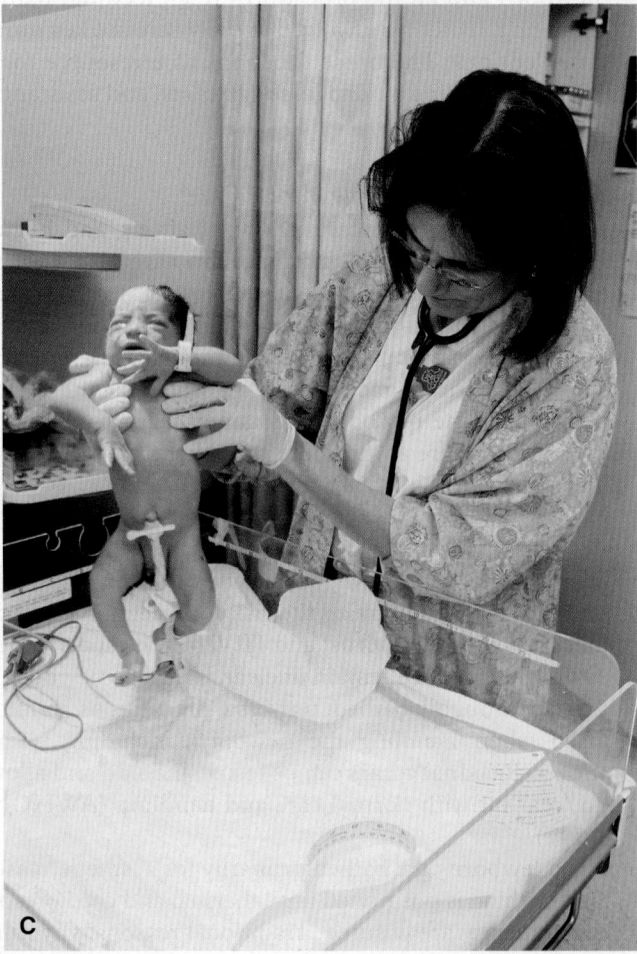

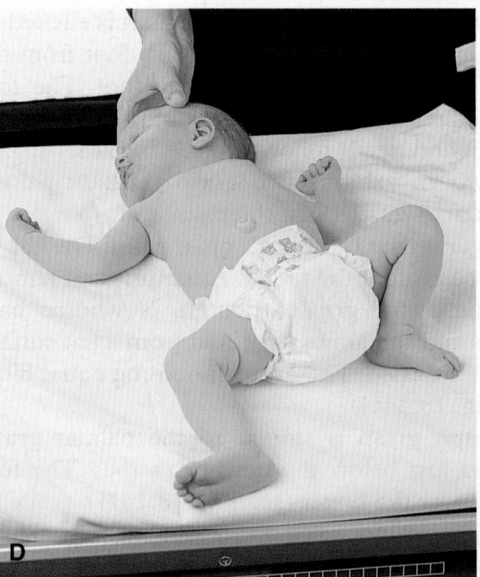

FIGURE 18.14 Newborn reflexes. (**A**) Sucking reflex. (**B**) Moro reflex. (**C**) Stepping reflex.
(**D**) Tonic neck reflex. (*continued*)

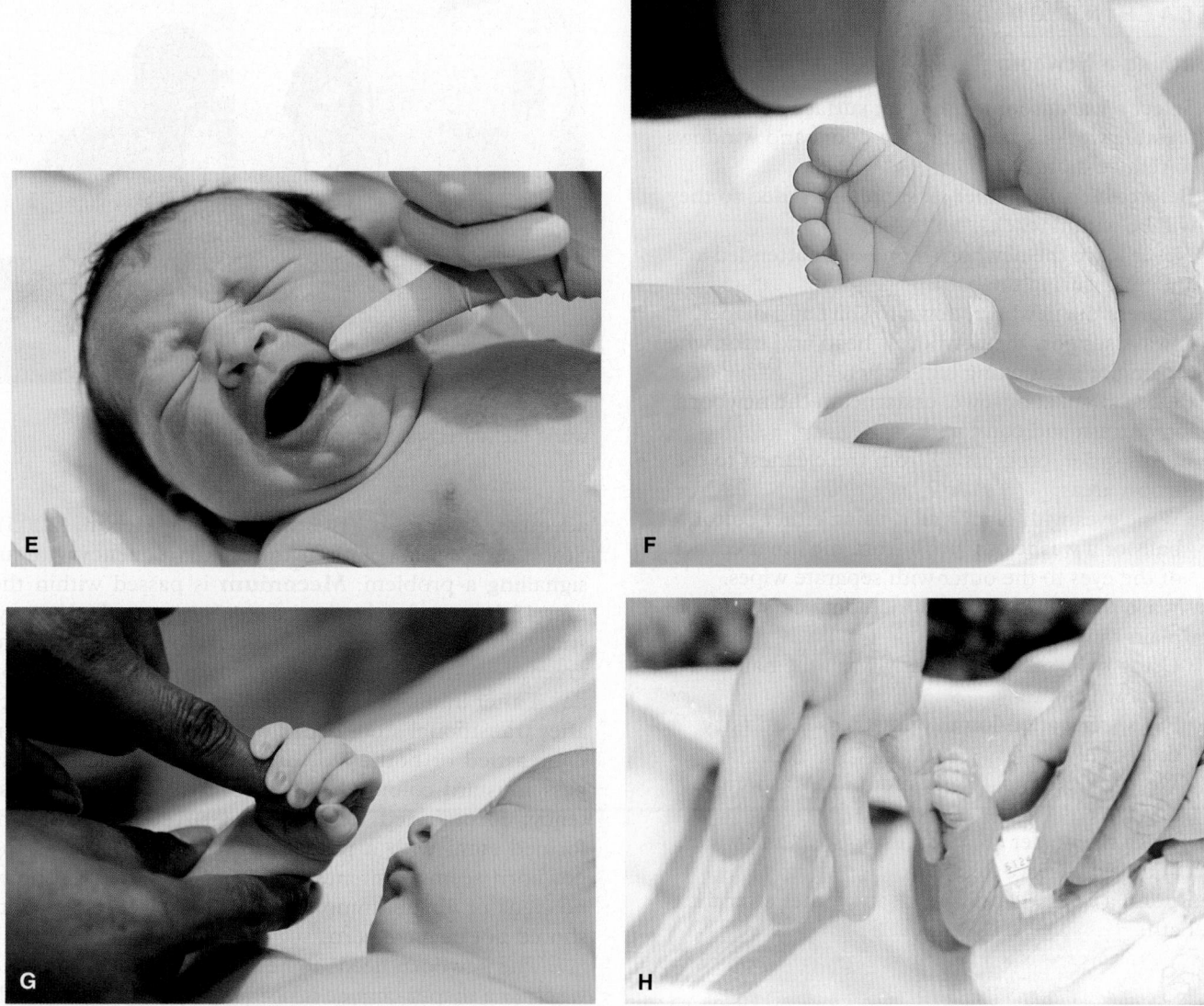

FIGURE 18.14 (continued) (**E**) Rooting reflex. (**F**) Babinski reflex. (**G**) Palmar grasp.
(**H**) Plantar grasp.

O'Brien, 2004). The benefits of daily bathing have not been clearly justified (AWHONN, 2007).

The literature suggests that tub bathing for the first bath, as opposed to sponge bathing, can be done without significantly lowering the newborn's temperature or increasing rates of cord infection in healthy term newborns. The bath should be kept as short as possible and take place in a warm room with the door closed to minimize air currents. The 2007 AWHONN skin care guideline provides detailed evidence-based practice recommendations for maintaining neonatal skin integrity, including bathing strategies. Encourage the parents to gather all items needed before starting the bath: a soft, clean washcloth; two cotton balls to clean the eyes; mild, unscented soap and shampoo; towels or blankets; a tub or basin with warm water; a clean diaper; and a change

of clothes. Other guidelines for bathing newborns are given in Teaching Guideline 18.1.

Move from the "cleanest" area (the eyes) to the most soiled area (the diaper area) to prevent cross-contamination. Use plain warm water on the face and eyes, adding a mild soap to cleanse the remainder of the body. Guide the parents to wash the face and neck gently after each feeding to prevent rashes and to prevent the odour that can develop when milk accumulates in the neck creases. Teach the parents to wrap a finger with a soft, clean, damp cloth and wipe the gums daily prior to eruption of the first teeth (Canadian Dental Association, 2012).

Wash the hair using running water so that the scalp can be thoroughly rinsed. A mild shampoo or soap can be used. Wash both fontanel areas. Parents often avoid these "soft spots" because they fear that they will "hurt

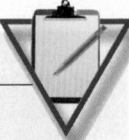

TEACHING GUIDELINE 18.1

Bathing a Newborn

- Select a warm room with a flat surface at a comfortable working height. Close doors and windows to reduce drafts.
- Before the bath, gather all supplies needed so they will be within reach.
- Never leave the newborn alone or unattended at any time during the bath.
- Undress the newborn down to shirt and diaper.
- Always support the newborn's head and neck when moving or positioning him or her.
- Place a blanket or towel underneath the newborn for warmth and comfort.
- In this order, progressing from the cleanest to the dirtiest areas:
  - Wipe eyes with plain water, using either cotton balls or a washcloth. Wipe from the inner corner of the eyes to the outer with separate wipes.
  - Wash the rest of the face, including ears, with plain water.
  - Using baby shampoo, gently wash the hair and rinse with water.
  - Pay special attention to body creases, and dry thoroughly.
  - Wash extremities, trunk, and back. Wash, rinse, dry, cover.
  - Wash the diaper area last, using soap and water, and dry; observe for rash.
- Put on a clean diaper and clean clothes after the bath.

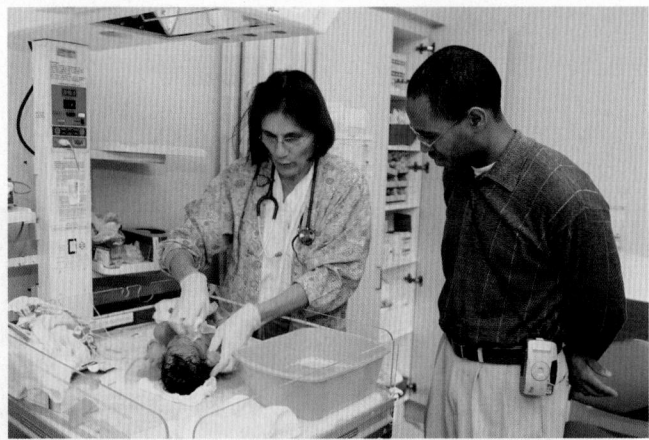

FIGURE 18.15 The nurse demonstrates bathing a newborn while the father watches.

adequate hydration (BC Ministry of Health, 2005). Stools can vary in colour, texture, and frequency without signalling a problem. **Meconium** is passed within the first 48 hours after birth; the stools appear thick, tarry, sticky, and dark green. Transitional stools (thin, brown to green, less sticky than meconium) typically appear by day 3 after initiation of feeding. The stool characteristics after transitional stool depend on whether the newborn is breastfed or bottle-fed. Breastfed newborns typically pass mustard-coloured, soft stool with a seedy consistency; formula-fed newborns pass yellow to brown, formed stool with a pasty consistency. As long as the newborn seems content, is eating normally, and shows no signs of illness, minor changes in bowel movements should not be a concern.

The newborn needs to be checked frequently to see whether a diaper change is needed, especially after feeding. Adhere to universal precautions when providing diaper area care. Teach parents to keep the top edge of the diaper below the umbilical cord area to prevent irritation and to allow air to help dry the cord. The diaper area will be cleansed at each diaper change, and any milk spilled will be cleaned. Clear water and a mild soap (neutral pH, 5.5 to 7.0) are appropriate to cleanse the diaper area. The use of lotions, fragranced items, and baby oil is not encouraged because these can lead to skin irritation and can cause rashes. Powders should not be used because they can be inhaled, causing respiratory distress. If the parents want to use oils and lotions, have them apply a small amount onto their hand first, away from the newborn; this warms the lotion. Then the parents should apply the lotion or oil sparingly.

Meconium can be difficult to remove from the skin. Use plain water or special cleansing wipes if necessary to clean the area. Teach parents how to clean the diaper area properly and how to prevent skin irritation. One of the decisions parents are immediately faced with is whether to use cloth or disposable diapers. Discuss the

the baby's brain" if they rub too hard. Reassure parents that there is a strong membrane providing protection. In Figure 18.15, the nurse is showing the father how to bathe his newborn.

To prevent chilling after bathing, dry the infant immediately, diaper, use a hat, and double wrap in warm blankets. Check the baby's temperature within an hour to make sure it is within normal limits. If it is low, consider skin-to-skin contact and refreshing the warm blankets. Teach parents that a bath approximately every other day is sufficient for the first year; more frequent bathing may dry the skin (BC Ministry of Health, 2005).

Elimination and Diaper Area Care

Newborn elimination patterns are highly individualized. All newborns should have voided by 24 hours of age. When the infant is hydrated, the urine is light amber in colour. Once urination is established after the first 4 to 6 days of life, wetting five or more diapers a day indicates pros and cons of using cloth diapers versus disposable diapers so that the parents can make informed decisions. Regardless of the type of diapers used, up to 10 diapers a day, or about 70 a week, will be needed.

Additional information about diapering might include:

- Before diapering, make sure all supplies are within reach, including clean diaper, cleaning agent or wipes, and ointment.
- Lay the newborn on a changing table and remove the dirty diaper.
- Use water and mild soap or wipes to gently wipe the genital area clean; wipe from front to back for girls to avoid urinary tract infections.
- Wash your hands thoroughly before and after changing diapers.

While performing diaper area care, parents should observe the area closely for irritation or rash. Tips for preventing or healing a diaper rash include:

- Change diapers frequently, especially after bowel movements.
- Apply a "barrier" cream after cleaning with mild soap and water.
- Use dye- and fragrance-free detergents to wash cloth diapers.
- Avoid the use of plastic pants because they tend to hold in moisture.
- Expose the newborn's bottom to air several times a day.

> ▶ *Take* NOTE!
>
> *Advise parents that a rash that persists for more than 3 days may be fungal in origin and may require additional treatment. Encourage the parents to notify the health care provider.*

Cord Care

The umbilical cord begins drying within hours after birth and is shrivelled and blackened by the second or third day. Within 7 to 10 days, it sloughs off and the umbilicus heals. During this transition, frequent assessments of the area are necessary to detect any bleeding or signs of infection. Cord bleeding is abnormal and may occur if the cord clamp is loosened. Any cord drainage is also abnormal and is generally caused by infection, which requires immediate treatment.

Inspect the cord area during each diaper change to ensure that it is clean and dry. For initial cord care, water alone is sufficient for cleaning. Dry thoroughly with an absorbent gauze to remove excess moisture, and then discard gauze. On an ongoing basis use natural drying (keeping the cord area clean and dry without the routine application of topical agents). Keep the baby's diaper folded down to avoid irritation and rubbing and to reduce contamination by urine or stool (AWHONN, 2007).

Expect to remove the cord clamp approximately 24 hours after birth by using a cord-cutting clamp. However, if the cord is still moist, keep the clamp in place and provide a referral to a community health care centre so that a nurse can remove the cord clamp after discharge. Always adhere to agency policies regarding cord care; changes in policy may be necessary based on new research findings.

Many parents avoid contact with the cord site to make sure they don't "bother" it. Teach them how to care for the cord site when they go home to prevent complications (Teaching Guideline 18.2). Advise parents not to pull on the stump even when it starts to come off. It will fall off on its own. Parents should continue to clean the belly button for a few days after the cord falls off.

Circumcision Care

Circumcision is the surgical removal of all or part of the foreskin (prepuce) of the penis. This has been traditionally done for hygiene and medical reasons and is the oldest known religious rite. In the Jewish faith, circumcision is a ritual that is performed by a *mohel* (ordained circumciser) on the eighth day after birth if possible. The circumcision is followed by a religious ceremony during which the newborn is named.

The debate over routine newborn circumcision continues in Canada. For many years, the purported benefits and harms of circumcision have been debated in the medical literature and society at large, with no clear consensus to date.

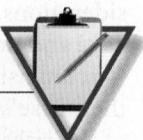

TEACHING GUIDELINE 18.2

Umbilical Cord Care

- Observe for bleeding, redness, drainage, or foul odour from the cord stump and report any of these findings to your newborn's primary care provider immediately.
- Water is used for cleaning. Continue to clean the belly button for a few days after the cord falls off.
- Expose the cord stump to the air as much as possible throughout the day.
- Fold diapers below the level of the cord to prevent contamination of the site and to promote air-drying of the cord.
- Observe the cord stump, which will change colour from yellow to brown to black. This is normal.
- Never pull the cord stump or attempt to loosen it, even when it starts to come off on its own; it will fall off naturally.

A policy statement by the CPS (1996) indicates that newborn circumcision has potential disadvantages and risks as well as medical benefits and advantages. Risks to the newborn include infection, hemorrhage, skin dehiscence, adhesions, urethral fistula, and pain. Benefits to the newborn include lower rates of urinary tract infections, sexually transmitted infections (including HIV), and penile cancer. Although some studies have shown a reduction in HIV rates with circumcision, there is currently international controversy about the benefits (Doctors Opposing, 2008).

The CPS guidelines state that if parents decide to circumcise their newborn, pain relief must be provided. Research has found that newborns circumcised without analgesia experience pain and stress, as indicated by changes in heart rate, blood pressure, oxygen saturation, and cortisol levels (Ridings & Amaya, 2007). Analgesic measures may include EMLA cream (a topical mixture of local anesthetics), a dorsal penile nerve block with buffered lidocaine, acetaminophen, a sucrose pacifier, and swaddling (Cunningham et al., 2010).

The CPS recommends that parents be given accurate and unbiased information about the risks and benefits of circumcision and that routine circumcision not be performed (CPS, 1996). As with other newborn procedures, research continues. New position statements by both the CPS and American Academy of Pediatrics are expected in the near future. Nurses must remain knowledgeable about current medical research to allow parents to make informed decisions. The absence of compelling medical evidence in favour of or against newborn circumcision makes informed consent of parents of paramount importance. The circumcision discussion involves cultural, religious, medical, and emotional considerations. Nurses may have difficulty remaining unbiased and unemotional as they present the facts to parents. Circumcision is a very personal decision for parents, and the nurse's major responsibility is to inform the parents of the risks and benefits of the procedure and to address

concerns so that the parents can reach a fully informed decision.

> ▶ **Take** NOTE!
>
> *The decision to circumcise the male newborn is often a social one, with the strongest factor being whether the newborn's father is himself circumcised (CPS, 1996).*

There are three commonly used methods of circumcision: the Gomco clamp, the Plastibell device, and the Mogen clamp (Cunningham et al., 2010). During the circumcision procedure, part of the foreskin is removed by clamping and cutting with a scalpel (Gomco or Mogen clamp) or by using a Plastibell. The Plastibell is fitted over the glans, and the excess foreskin is pulled over the plastic ring. A suture is tied around the rim to apply pressure to the blood vessels, creating hemostasis. The excess foreskin is cut away. The plastic rim remains in place until healing occurs. The plastic ring typically loosens and falls off in approximately 1 week (Kenner & Lott, 2007) (Fig. 18.16).

Immediately after circumcision, the tip of the penis is usually covered with petroleum jelly–coated gauze to keep the wound from sticking to the diaper. Continued care of this site includes:

- Assess for bleeding every 30 minutes for at least 2 hours.
- Document the first voiding to evaluate for urinary obstruction or edema.
- Squeeze water over the area daily and then rinse with warm water. Pat dry. Use water only for the first 3 to 4 days after the procedure.
- Apply a small amount of petroleum jelly with every diaper change if the Plastibell was used; clean with water if other techniques were used.

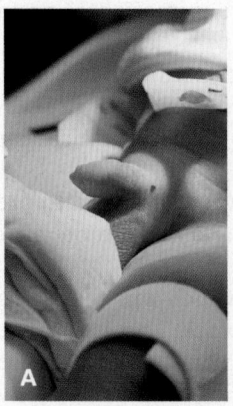 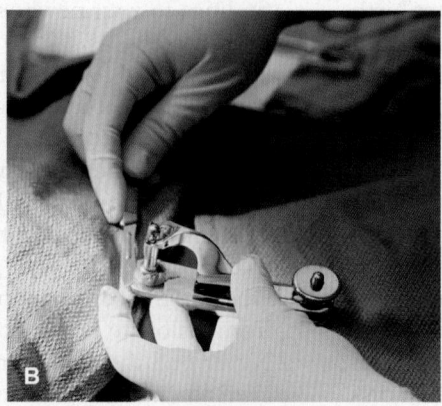 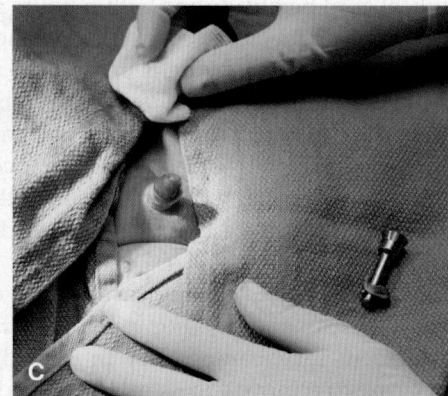

FIGURE 18.16 Circumcision. (**A**) Before the procedure. (**B**) Clamp applied and foreskin removed. (**C**) Appearance after circumcision.

- Fasten the diaper loosely over the penis to prevent friction.

If a Plastibell has been used, it will fall off by itself in about a week. Inform parents of this and advise them not to pull it off sooner. Also instruct the parents to check daily for any foul-smelling drainage, bleeding, or unusual swelling.

If the newborn is uncircumcised, wash the penis with water after each diaper change and do not force the foreskin back; it will retract normally over time.

Safety

Newborns are completely dependent on those around them to ensure their safety. Their safety must be ensured while in the health care facility and after they are discharged. Parental education is key, especially as the newborn grows and develops and begins to respond to and explore his or her surroundings (Teaching Guideline 18.3).

Environmental Safety

People who enter a health care facility for treatment expect to be safe there until they return home, but ensuring a safe environment can be a daunting challenge to a health care facility.

Consider this scenario: a woman dressed in nurse's clothing entered the hospital room of a new mother soon after she had given birth. This "nurse" told the mother she needed to take her newborn to the nursery to have him weighed. Sometime later, a staff nurse making her routine rounds realized something was wrong when she saw that the newborn's bassinet in the mother's room was empty and the mother was sound asleep in her bed. The staff nurse called security immediately because she suspected that a newborn abduction had taken place.

This is a typical (albeit extremely rare) abduction scenario that has occurred in Canada. In **infant abduction**, someone who is not a family member takes a child less than 1 year old (AWHONN, 2007). Infant abductions are traumatic for the parents, the community, and the health care facility. The facility may also face huge financial liability if a lawsuit is filed by the parents.

Abductions typically occur during the day and are usually carried out by women who are not criminally sophisticated. Many of these women experienced a pregnancy loss in the past; they are often emotionally immature and compulsive, with low self-esteem. Most female

TEACHING GUIDELINE 18.3

General Newborn Safety

- Have emergency telephone numbers readily available, such as those for emergency medical assistance and the poison control centre.
- Keep small or sharp objects out of reach to prevent them from being aspirated.
- Put safety plugs in wall sockets within the child's reach to prevent electrocution.
- Always supervise the newborn in the tub: a newborn can drown in 2 inches of water.
- Make sure the crib or changing table is sturdy, without any loose hardware, and is painted with lead-free paint.
- Avoid placing the crib or changing table near blinds or curtain cords.
- Ensure that toys are soft, nontoxic, and washable.
- Provide a smoke-free environment for all infants.
- Place all infants on their backs to sleep to reduce the risk for sudden infant death syndrome.
- To prevent falls, do not leave the newborn alone on any elevated surface. Keep one hand on your baby at all times.

- Use sun shields on strollers and hats to avoid overexposing the newborn to the sun.
- To prevent infection, thoroughly wash your hands before feeding your baby and after using the bathroom, handling diapers, handling pets, or sneezing and coughing.
- Know how to help a choking baby. Courses on basic first aid and baby and home safety may be available in your community.
- Thoroughly investigate any infant care facility before using it.
- Never hold your baby while drinking a hot beverage, cooking, or smoking.
- Check the temperature of bottles by squirting a small amount of the formula or milk on the inside of your wrist.
- Check bath water temperature with your elbow before bathing your infant.
- Keep the temperature in your hot water heater below 49°C.

Sources: British Columbia Ministry of Health. (2005). *Baby's best chance: Parent's handbook of pregnancy and baby care* (revised 6th ed.). Retrieved March 7, 2012 from http://www.health.gov.bc.ca/library/publications/year/2005/babybestchance.pdf; and Public Health Agency of Canada. (2011). *Joint statement on safe sleep: Preventing sudden infant death syndrome.* Retrieved September from http://www.phac-aspc.gc.ca/hp-ps/dca-dea/stages-etapes/childhood-enfance_0–2/sids/jsss-ecss-eng.php.

abductors can play the role of a hospital employee convincingly (Colling & York, 2010).

Health care agencies are challenged to prevent infant abduction by instituting sound security practices and systems (AWHONN, 2007). Such measures include the following:

- All newborns must be transported in cribs and not carried.
- Nurses must respond immediately to any security alarm that sounds on the unit.
- Newborns must never be unattended at any time, especially in hallways.
- All staff must wear appropriate identification at all times.
- Scrubs should not be worn by nursing staff on the postpartum unit.
- Personnel should be wary of visitors who do not seem to be visiting a specific mother.
- The electronic security system should be checked to make sure it works.
- Proper functioning and placement of any electronic sensors used on newborns should be ensured.
- Parents should be taught what infant abduction is; why infant security is important; the schedule of nursery, feeding, and visiting hours; rules about visitor access; the facility's security policies and procedures; what parents can do to protect their infant in the hospital; which staff members are allowed to handle the newborn; and what a proper ID looks like.

Providing a safe and secure environment is a shared responsibility of the facility, staff, and parents. Preventing abductions requires everyone to learn and follow the protocols and procedures.

Car Safety

All provinces and territories require the use of car seats for infants and children (Transport Canada, 2009). Health Canada (2007) reports that motor vehicle passenger injuries are a leading cause of death in children and youth. In more than half of these deaths, the child is unrestrained.

All infant and child car seats and booster cushions now sold in Canada have an expiration date on them. People using these devices past their expiry, or useful life date, do so at their own risk. Transport Canada (2009) strongly advises parents and caregivers to follow all of the manufacturer's instructions and respect the expiration dates on the products.

Despite evidence that the use of car seats can reduce morbidity and mortality related to motor vehicle crashes, parents who lack knowledge about them may underuse or misuse them. It is estimated that car seat restraint systems are used correctly only 64% of the time (Snowdon, Hussein, & Ahmed, 2010). Hospitals and community health agencies vary in their approach to education and

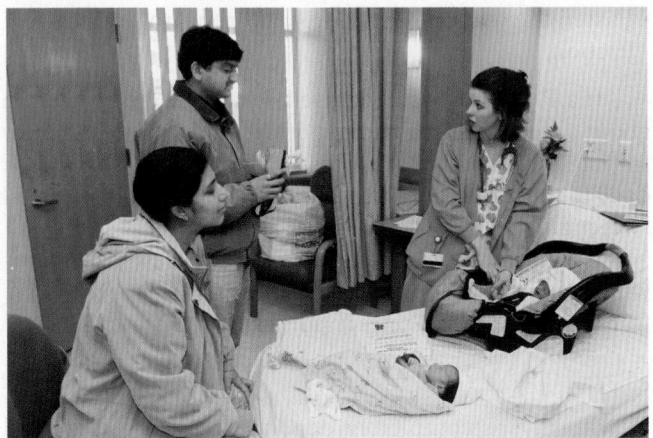

FIGURE 18.17 Newborn in a properly secured car seat.

support on car seat safety. Be sure to familiarize yourself with the policies in your facility and the guidelines for your province. Make sure that parents understand the importance of correct restraint and safely transporting their newborn in an approved car safety seat every time the infant rides in a car (Fig. 18.17). If they cannot afford one, many community organizations will provide one for them. According to Health Canada, no one car seat is considered to be the "safest" or the "best"; instead, consistent and proper use of the seat is the key to preventing injuries and deaths. Instruct parents in the following:

- Select a car seat that is appropriate for the child's size and weight.
- Use the car seat correctly, every time the child is in the car.
- Make sure the harness (most seats have a 3- to 5-point harness) is in the slots at or below the shoulders.

Infection Prevention

The nurse plays a major role in preventing infection in the newborn environment. Ways to control infection are as follows:

- Minimize exposure of newborns to organisms.
- Wash your hands before and after providing care, and insist that all personnel wash their hands before handling any newborn.
- Do not allow ill staff or visitors to visit or handle newborns.
- Monitoring the umbilical cord stump and circumcision site for signs of infection.
- Providing eye prophylaxis by instilling prescribed medication soon after birth.
- Educate parents about appropriate home measures that will prevent infections, such as practicing good handwashing before and after diaper changes, keeping the newborn well hydrated, avoiding bringing the infant into crowds (which may expose him or her to cold and flu viruses), observing for early signs of

infection (fever, vomiting, loss of appetite, lethargy, laboured breathing, green watery stools, drainage from umbilical cord site or eyes), and keeping appointments for routine immunizations.

Promoting Sleep and Safe Sleep

Although many parents feel their newborns need them every minute of the day, babies actually need to sleep much of the day initially. Usually newborns sleep up to 15 hours daily. They sleep for 2 to 4 hours at a time but do not sleep through the night because their stomach capacity is too small to go long periods without nourishment.

> ▶ *Take* NOTE!
>
> *All newborns develop their own sleep patterns and cycles, but it may take several months before the newborn sleeps through the night.*

Parents should place the newborn on his or her back to sleep (Perinatal Services BC, 2011a). To prevent suffocation, all fluffy bedding, quilts, sheepskins, stuffed animals, and pillows should be removed from the crib.

It is important to distinguish between the terms co-sleeping, bed sharing, and room sharing as they are often used inconsistently (Trifunov, 2009). **Co-sleeping** is a term used to refer to both the broad range of infant sleeping practices (including room sharing and bed sharing) and also as a distinct term for bed sharing. **Bed sharing** is when the infant shares the same sleeping surface with another person; this is a controversial issue in Canada but at present there is limited evidence regarding its prevalence. **Room sharing** is when the infant does not share the same sleeping surface but sleeps in the same room as the parents. Parents should be informed that the practice of bed sharing is not recommended because it has been associated with a higher incidence of sudden infant death syndrome (SIDS) (Rourke, Leduc, Constantin, et al., 2010). Suffocation can occur when the infant gets entangled in bedding or caught under pillows or when the infant slips between the bed and the wall or the head-board and mattress. Also, the parent may accidentally roll against or on top of the baby.

The safest place for an infant to sleep for the first 6 months of life is in a crib, cradle, or bassinet that meets current Canadian regulations, near the parent or caregiver's bed (Public Health Agency of Canada [PHAC], 2011). All leading child safety organizations recommend the following for safe sleep for infants:

- Place the infant in the "back to sleep" position.
- Maintain a smoke-free environment.
- Do not place the infant to sleep on chairs, sofas, waterbeds, or cushions, either alone or with another person (Trifunov, 2009).

Teach parents to avoid other unsafe sleeping conditions, such as placing the newborn in the prone position, using a crib that does not meet federal safety guidelines, using extra soft bedding items, allowing window cords to hang loose and in close proximity to the crib, or setting the room temperature too high (can cause overheating) (PHAC, 2011).

Enhancing Bonding

Encourage and enhance parent–newborn interaction and the development of early relationships by involving both parents with the baby and demonstrating appropriate nurturing behaviours:

- Say "hello" and introduce yourself to the newborn.
- Ask the parents' permission to care for and hold their newborn. This helps parents to realize that they are responsible for their child and reminds nurses of their role.
- Show parents the power of a soothing voice to calm the newborn.
- Provide care to the newborn in the least stressful way.
- Demonstrate ways to wake the newborn up gently to feed better.
- Tell parents what you are doing, why you are doing it, and how they can duplicate what you are doing at home.
- Offer the opportunity for parents to perform care while you observe them. Support their efforts to soothe the newborn throughout the care process.
- Help parents to interpret the communication cues the newborn uses.
- Point out the efforts the newborn is making to connect with the parents (e.g., alerting to the familiar voice, following the parents while they are speaking, quieting when held securely).

One of the most pleasurable aspects of newborn care is being close to them. Bonding begins before birth and continues afterward when parents cradle their newborn and gently stroke him or her with their fingers. Provide parents with opportunities for "skin-to-skin" contact with the newborn, holding the baby against their own skin when feeding or cradling. Many newborns respond very positively to gentle massage. If necessary, recommend books and videos that cover the subject.

Soothing the Baby

For newborns, crying is their only way to communicate that something is wrong. Try to find out the reason why: is the diaper wet? Is the room too hot or too cold? Is the baby uncomfortable (e.g., diaper rash or tight clothing)? Suggest the following ways in which parents can soothe an upset newborn:

- Try feeding or burping to relieve air or stomach gas.
- Lightly rub the newborn's back and speak softly to him or her.

TABLE 18.5 SELECTED CONDITIONS SCREENED FOR IN THE NEWBORN[a]

Condition	Description	Clinical Picture/Effect if not Treated	Treatment	Timing of Screening
PKU	Autosomal recessive inherited deficiency in one of the enzymes necessary for the metabolism of phenylalanine to tyrosine—essential amino acids found in most foods	Irritability, vomiting of protein feedings, and a musty odour to the skin or body secretions of the newborn; if not treated, mental and motor retardation, seizures, microcephaly, and poor growth and development	Lifetime diet of foods low in phenylalanine (low protein) and monitoring of blood levels (Lawson, 2007); special newborn formulas available	Universally screened for in Canada; testing is done 24–48 h after protein feeding
Congenital hypothyroidism	Deficiency of thyroid hormone necessary for normal brain growth, calorie metabolism, and development; may result from maternal hypothyroidism	Increased risk in newborns with birth weight <2,000 g or >4,500 g, and those from Hispanic and Asian ethnic groups; feeding problems, growth and breathing problems; if not treated, irreversible brain damage and mental retardation	Lifelong thyroid replacement therapy (Dudek, 2006)	Testing (measures thyroxine [T_4] and thyroid-stimulating hormone [TSH]) is done between days 4 and 6 of life.
Medium-chain Acyl CoA dehydrogenase deficiency (MCAD)	The inheritance is autosomal recessive. MCAD is an enzyme responsible for the metabolism of medium-chain fatty acids. Deficiency results from the mutations in the MCAD gene resulting in absent or decreased activity.	At risk for a combination for hypoglycemia, vomiting, lethargy, encephalopathy, respiratory arrest, hepatomegaly, seizures, apnea, cardiac arrest, coma, and sudden death. Long-term outcomes may include developmental and behavioural disability, chronic muscle weakness, failure to thrive, cerebral palsy, and attention deficit disorder.	Lifetime special diet involving additional supplements and avoiding fasting.	Universally screened in most provinces. Tandem mass spectrometry (MS/MS) is the screening technology used to diagnose MCAD using newborn blood samples.
Galactosemia	Absence of the enzyme needed for the conversion of the milk sugar galactose to glucose	Poor weight gain, vomiting, jaundice, mood changes, loss of eyesight, seizures, and mental retardation; if untreated, galactose build-up causing permanent damage to the brain, eyes, and liver, and eventually death	Eliminate milk from diet; substitute soy milk	First test done on discharge from the hospital with a follow-up test within 1 month

[a]Note: Screening criteria vary among provinces and territories.

- Gently sway side to side, or rock back and forth in a rocking chair.
- Talk with the newborn while making eye contact.
- Take the newborn for a walk in a stroller or carriage to get fresh air.
- Change the baby's position from back to side or vice versa.
- Try singing, reciting poetry and nursery rhymes, or reading to the baby.
- Turn on a musical mobile above the newborn's head.
- Give more physical contact by walking, rocking, or patting the newborn.
- Swaddle the newborn to provide a sense of security and comfort. To do this:
  - Spread out a receiving blanket, with one corner folded slightly.
  - Lay the newborn face up with head at the folded corner. Position the baby's hands close to his or her mouth for self-soothing.
  - Wrap the left corner over the baby's body and tuck it beneath the baby.
  - Bring the bottom corner over the baby's feet.
  - Wrap the right corner around the baby, leaving only the head exposed.

It is important for parents to realize that for some of the crying times, they will not be able to soothe their baby—no matter what strategy they use. There may be periods of increased crying, and this is part of the normal early behavioural development of their baby. Prolonged, unsoothable crying is heart-wrenching and frustrating to most parents. It is important to discuss strategies for coping with crying and inconsolability with every parent and caregiver. The Period of PURPLE Crying is one example of a program that offers information on coping with infant crying. Visit http://thePoint.lww.com/Chow1e for a direct link to this program and other information about coping strategies.

Assisting with Screening Tests

Screening newborns for problems is important because some potentially life-threatening metabolic diseases may not be obvious at birth. Throughout Canada, newborn screening tests are required before discharge to check for certain genetic and inborn errors of metabolism and hearing. Early identification and initiation of treatment can prevent significant complications and can minimize the negative effects of untreated disease.

Genetic and Inborn Errors of Metabolism Screening

There is no one specific Canadian guideline for newborn screening, so panels vary across the country. Although each province and territory mandate which conditions must be tested, the most common screening tests are for PKU, hypothyroidism, and medium-chain acyl CoA dehydrogenase deficiency (Table 18.5). More recently,

some provinces have been expanding the number of tests that are routinely conducted following birth.

The trend toward early discharge of newborns can affect the timing of screening and the accuracy of some test results. For example, the newborn needs to ingest enough breast milk or formula to elevate phenylalanine levels for the screening test to identify PKU accurately, so newborn screening for PKU testing should not be performed before 24 hours of age.

Screening tests for genetic and inborn errors of metabolism require a few drops of blood taken from the newborn's heel (Fig. 18.18). These tests are usually performed shortly before discharge. Newborns who are discharged before 24 hours of age need to have repeat tests done within a week in an outpatient facility or by a community health nurse.

Be aware of which conditions your province or territory regularly screens for at birth to ensure that the parents are taught about the tests and the importance of early treatment. Also be familiar with the optimal time frame for screening and conditions that could affect the results. Ensure that a satisfactory specimen has been obtained at the appropriate time and that circumstances

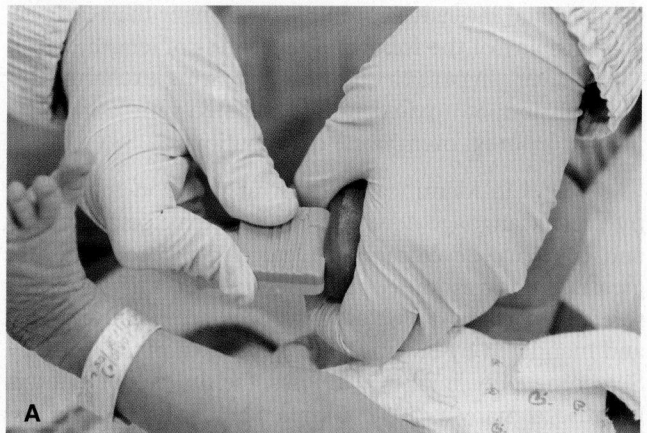

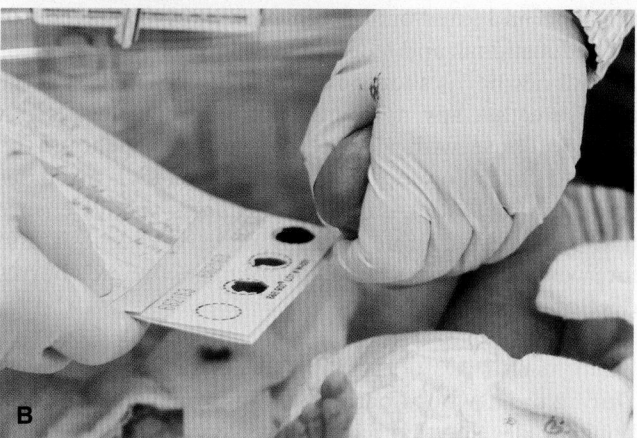

FIGURE 18.18 Screening for PKU. (**A**) Performing a heel stick. (**B**) Applying the blood specimen to the card for screening.

that could cause false results have been minimized. Send out specimens and completed forms within 24 hours of collection to the appropriate laboratory (Merenstein & Gardner, 2011).

Hearing Screening

Hearing loss is one of the most common congenital conditions in Canada: approximately one to three newborns out of every 1,000 have some degree of hearing loss (CASLPA, 2010; CPS, 2011d). Unlike a physical deformity, hearing loss is not clinically detectable at birth and thus remains difficult to assess. For infants with risk factors the prevalence can be as high as 10 per 1,000 live births. Factors associated with an increased risk for hearing loss include:

- Family history of childhood sensory hearing loss
- Congenital infections such as cytomegalovirus, rubella, toxoplasmosis, herpes, or bacterial meningitis
- Congenital craniofacial defects involving the external ear

Physical findings consistent with an underlying syndrome associated with hearing loss include:

- Low birth weight (<1,500 g) or prematurity (<37 weeks)
- A neonatal intensive care unit stay longer than 2 days or with any of the following regardless of length of stay: severe hyperbilirubinemia requiring exchange transfusion, ototoxic drug use, assisted ventilation, extracorporeal membrane oxygenation

Delays in identification and intervention may affect the child's language development, academic performance, and cognitive development. Detection before 3 months greatly improves outcomes. Because of this, auditory screening programs for all newborns are recommended and mandated by law in throughout most of the country. Screening only infants with risk factors is not enough because as many as 50% of infants born with hearing loss have no known risk factors (CASLPA, 2010). Early identification and intervention can prevent severe psychosocial, educational, and language development delays.

All newborns should be screened prior to discharge to ensure that any newborn with a hearing loss is not missed. Those with suspected hearing loss should be referred for follow-up assessment (Box 18.1 discusses screening methods). In addition, nurses should ensure that testing is accurate to facilitate early diagnosis and intervention services and to optimize the newborn's developmental potential.

Dealing with Common Health Concerns

During the newborn period of transition, certain conditions can develop that require intervention. These conditions, although not typically life-threatening, can be a source of anxiety for the parents. Common concerns

---

> ### BOX 18.1 Newborn Hearing Screening Methods
>
> A newborn's hearing can be screened in one of two ways: otoacoustic emission (OAE) or automated auditory brain stem response (ABR) (CPS, 2011d). In OAE, a tiny flexible plug is placed in the infant's ear canal and the sounds produced by the newborn's inner ear are measured in response to certain tones or clicks presented through the earphone. Preset parameters in the equipment decide whether the OAEs are sufficient for the newborn to pass or whether a referral is necessary for further evaluation.
>
> In ABR, small disk-shaped sensors are placed behind each ear and on the infant's forehead. Sounds are then presented to the ears using miniature earphones. In the hospital the test is done while the baby is in natural sleep. Electrodes placed around the newborn's head, neck, and shoulders record neural activity from the infant's brain stem in response to the tapping noises. The ABR tests how well the ear and the nerves leading to the brain work. Like OAEs, automated ABR screening is sensitive to more than mild degrees of hearing loss, but a "pass" does not guarantee normal hearing.
>
> A two-step screening procedure has been used in most UNHS programs, using the OAE as the first test in newborns with no risk factors, followed by ABR in newborns who do not pass the test (CPS, 2011d). The ABR is also recommended in infants with risk factors.

---

include transient tachypnea of the newborn, physiologic jaundice, and hypoglycemia.

Transient Tachypnea of the Newborn

Transient tachypnea of the newborn appears soon after birth. It is accompanied by retractions, expiratory grunting, or cyanosis and can be relieved by low-dose oxygen therapy. Mild or moderate respiratory distress typically is present at birth or within 6 hours of birth. This condition usually resolves within 72 hours.

Transient tachypnea of the newborn occurs most frequently in full-term infants born by cesarean section or having experienced a perinatal hypoxic event. This can be due to the lack of thoracic squeezing that occurs during a cesarean birth, altered permeability of pulmonary capillary vessels, aspiration of amniotic fluid, or diminished respiratory effort if the mother received central nervous system depressant medication. Prolonged labour, fetal macrosomia, and maternal asthma also have been associated with this condition (Blackburn, 2007).

Nursing interventions include providing supportive care (giving oxygen, ensuring warmth, observing respiratory status frequently, and allowing time for the pulmonary capillaries and the lymphatics to remove the remaining fluid). The clinical course is relatively benign, but any newborn respiratory issue can be very frightening to the parents. Provide a thorough explanation and reassure them that the condition will resolve over time.

Physiologic Jaundice

Physiologic **jaundice** is very common in newborns, with approximately 60% of newborns demonstrating yellowish skin, mucous membranes, and sclera within the first 3 days of life (CPS, 2011a). Jaundice is the visible manifestation of hyperbilirubinemia. It typically results from the deposition of unconjugated bilirubin pigment in the skin and mucous membranes.

Factors that contribute to the development of physiologic jaundice in the newborn include an increased bilirubin load because of relative polycythemia, a shortened erythrocyte life span (80 days compared with the adult 120 days), and immature hepatic uptake and conjugation processes (Blackburn, 2007). Normally the liver removes bilirubin from the blood and changes it to a form in which it can be excreted. As the red blood cell breakdown continues at a fast pace, the newborn's liver cannot keep up with bilirubin removal. Thus, bilirubin accumulates in the blood, causing a yellowish discolouration of the skin. The CPS (2011a) recommends the following for recognizing and treating hyperbilirubinemia:

• Universal screening for jaundice among newborns should be implemented in Canada.
• Adequate follow-up should be ensured for all infants who are jaundiced.
• A program for breastfeeding support should be instituted in every facility where babies are delivered.

Assess for jaundice in all newborns by pressing gently with a fingertip on the bridge of the nose, sternum, or forehead. If jaundice is present, the blanched area will appear yellow before the capillary refill (Merenstein & Gardner, 2011).

Measures that parents can take to reduce the risk of jaundice include exposing the newborn to natural sunlight for short periods of time throughout the day to help oxidize the bilirubin deposits on the skin, provide breastfeeding on demand to promote elimination of bilirubin through urine and stooling, and avoiding glucose water supplementation, which hinders elimination.

If or when the levels of unconjugated serum bilirubin increase and do not return to normal levels with increased hydration, phototherapy is used. The serum level of bilirubin at which phototherapy is initiated is a matter of clinical judgment by the physician, midwife, or nurse practitioner, and is based on factors such as gestational age, feeding and hydration status, and bruising (CPS, 2011a). **Phototherapy** involves exposing the newborn to ultraviolet light, which converts unconjugated bilirubin into products that can be excreted through feces and urine.

▶ **Take** NOTE!

Exposure of newborns to sunlight represents the first documented use of phototherapy in the medical literature. Sister J. Ward, a charge nurse in Essex, England, in 1956 recognized that when jaundiced newborns were exposed to the sun they became less yellow. This observation changed the entire treatment of jaundice in newborns (Maisels, 2006).

Phototherapy reduces bilirubin levels in the blood by breaking down unconjugated bilirubin into colourless compounds. These compounds can then be excreted in the bile. Phototherapy aims to curtail the increase in bilirubin blood levels, thereby preventing kernicterus, a condition in which unconjugated bilirubin enters the brain. If not treated, kernicterus can lead to brain damage and death.

During the past several decades, phototherapy has generally been administered with either banks of fluorescent lights or spotlights. Factors that determine the dose of phototherapy include spectrum of light emitted, irradiance of light source, design of light unit, surface area of newborn exposed to the light, and distance of the newborn from the light source (Vreman, 2008). For phototherapy to be effective, the rays must penetrate as much of the skin as possible. Thus, the newborn must be naked and turned frequently to ensure maximum exposure of the skin. Several side effects of standard phototherapy have been identified: frequent loose stools, increased insensible water loss, transient rash, and potential retinal damage if the newborn's eyes are not covered sufficiently.

Fibreoptic pads have been developed that can be wrapped around the newborn or on which the newborn can lie. The light is delivered from a tungsten–halogen bulb through a fibreoptic cable and is emitted from the sides and ends of the fibres inside a plastic pad (Vreman, 2008). These products work on the premise that phototherapy can be improved by delivering higher-intensity therapeutic light to decrease bilirubin levels. The pads do not produce appreciable heat like the banks of lights or spotlights do, so insensible water loss is not increased. Eye patches also are not needed; thus, parents can feed and hold their newborns continuously to promote bonding.

When caring for newborns receiving phototherapy for jaundice, nurses must do the following:

• Closely monitor body temperature and fluid and electrolyte balance.
• Observe skin integrity (as a result of exposure to diarrhea and phototherapy lights).
• Provide eye protection to prevent corneal injury related to phototherapy exposure.
• Encourage parents to participate in their newborn's care to reduce parent–infant separation.

See Chapter 24 for a more detailed discussion of hyperbilirubinemia.

The home health nurse made a postpartum visit to Kelly to assess the situation. Kelly's son was slightly jaundiced when the home health nurse pressed gently over his sternum, but Kelly said he was nursing better compared with the previous 2 days. What home suggestions can the nurse make to Kelly to reduce the jaundice? What specific education about physiologic jaundice is needed?

Hypoglycemia

Healthy, term babies do not require blood glucose screening. Blood glucose levels may be as low as 1.8 to 2.0 mmol/L (32 to 36 mg/dL) at 1 hour of age, increasing to up to 2.6 mmol/L (≤47 mg/dL) by 2 hours of age and to normal adult levels (≥3.3 mol/L or >60 mg/dL) in the next 2 days (ACoRN Neonatal Society, 2010). In newborns, blood glucose levels fall to a low point during the first few hours of life because the source of maternal glucose is removed when the placenta is expelled. This period of transition is usually smooth, but certain newborns are at greater risk for **hypoglycemia**: infants of diabetic mothers, preterm newborns, and newborns with intrauterine growth restriction, inadequate caloric intake, sepsis, asphyxia, hypothermia, polycythemia, glycogen storage disorders, and endocrine deficiencies (Kliegman et al., 2011).

Most newborns experience transient hypoglycemia and are asymptomatic. The symptoms, when present, are nonspecific and include jitteriness, lethargy, cyanosis, apnea, seizures, high-pitched or weak cry, and poor feeding. If hypoglycemia is prolonged or is left untreated, serious, long-term adverse neurologic sequelae such as learning disabilities and mental retardation can occur (Hoe, 2008). Therefore, at-risk newborns should be identified, assessed, and monitored as needed.

Nursing care of the hypoglycemic newborn includes monitoring for signs of hypoglycemia or identifying high-risk newborns prone to this disorder based on their perinatal history, physical examination, body measurements, and gestational age. Recommendations for blood glucose monitoring are available through several sources, including the CPS (2011c) and the ACoRN Neonatal Society (2010). More frequent monitoring and early feeding may be necessary for newborns considered to be at high risk. Prevent hypoglycemia in at-risk newborns by initiating early feedings with breast milk or formula. If hypoglycemia persists despite feeding, notify the primary health care provider for orders such as intravenous therapy with dextrose solutions. Anticipate hypoglycemia in certain high-risk newborns and begin assessments immediately on nursery admission.

Promoting Nutrition

Several physiologic changes dictate the type and method of feeding throughout the newborn's first year. Some of these changes include the following:

• Stomach capacity is limited to about 20 mL at birth for an infant of average weight (Blackburn, 2007). The emptying time is short (2 to 3 hours), and peristalsis is rapid. Therefore, small, frequent feedings are needed at first, with amounts progressively increasing with maturity.
• The immune system is immature at birth, so the baby is at a high risk for food allergies during the first 4 to 6 months of life. Introducing solid foods prior to this time increases the risk of developing food allergies.
• Pancreatic enzymes and bile to assist in digestion of fat and starch are in limited supply until about 3 to 6 months of age. Infants cannot digest cereal prior to this time.
• The kidneys are immature and unable to concentrate urine until about 4 to 6 weeks of age. Excess protein and mineral intake can place a strain on kidney function and can lead to dehydration. Infants need to consume more water per unit of body weight than adults do as a result of their high body weight from water.
• Immature muscular control at birth changes over time to assist in the feeding process by improving head and neck control, hand–eye coordination, swallowing, and ability to sit, grasp, and chew.

Newborn Nutritional Needs

As newborns grow, their energy and nutrient requirements change to meet their body's changing needs. During infancy, energy, protein, vitamin, and mineral requirements per pound of body weight are higher than at any other time of life. These high levels are needed to fuel the rapid growth and development during this stage of life. Generally, an infant's birth weight doubles in the first 4 to 6 months of life and triples within the first year (Kliegman et al., 2011).

A newborn's caloric needs range from 80 to 120 cal/kg body weight. For the first 3 months, the infant needs 110 cal/kg/day; this decreases to 100 cal/kg/day from 3 to 6 months (Begany & Mascarenhas, 2007; Health Canada, 2005). Breast milk and formulas contain approximately 20 cal/oz, so the caloric needs of young infants can be met if several feedings are given throughout the day.

Fluid requirements for the newborn and infant range from 100 to 150 mL/kg/day. This requirement can be met through breast- or bottle-feedings. Additional water supplementation is not necessary. Adequate carbohydrates, fats, protein, and vitamins are achieved through consumption of breast milk or formula. The breastfed infant draws on iron reserves for the first 6 months and then needs iron-rich foods or supplementation added at 6 months of age. Health Canada (2005) recommends that bottle-fed infants be given iron-fortified formula from birth and that all infants (breast- and bottle-fed) receive a daily supplement of 400 IU of vitamin D starting at birth to prevent rickets and vitamin D deficiency. Vitamin D deficiency is common in Canada, especially among northern native communities where lack of light and dressing for intense cold decreases the opportunity for vitamin D production in the skin. Furthermore, dependence on traditional vitamin D–rich foods has diminished (CPS, 2010. The use of fluoride-supplemented toothpaste in infants is determined by their level of risk (water not fluoridated, visible tooth defect, or special health care needs) and families should consult a health professional (Canadian Dental Association, 2008).

Supporting the Choice of Feeding Method

Women typically decide about the method of feeding well before the infant is born. Prenatal and childbirth classes present information about breastfeeding versus bottle-feeding and allow the parents to make up their minds about which method is best for them. Various factors can influence their decision, including socioeconomic status; culture; employment; social support available; level of education; the media; the range of care interventions provided during pregnancy, childbirth, and the early postpartum period; and especially partner and family support (Pryor & Huggins, 2007). Nurses can provide evidence-based information to assist the woman and her family in making their decision. Regardless of which method is chosen, the nurse needs to respect and support the decision.

Feeding the Newborn

Extensive resources are available related to newborn nutrition to support both professionals and parents. Sources of information include Health Canada, PHAC, provincial health organizations (including public health), breastfeeding organizations (e.g., La Leche League), and health professional organizations. Nurses need to be familiar with the resources and guidelines that are used in their practice settings.

The newborn can be fed at any time during the transition period if assessments are stable. During feeding observe his or her ability to suck and swallow. Most newborns are on demand feeding schedules and are fed when they awaken. When they go home, mothers are encouraged to feed their newborns every 2 to 4 hours during the day and when the newborn awakens during the night.

Parents often have many questions about feeding. Generally, newborns should be fed on demand whenever they seem hungry. Most newborns will give cues about their hunger status by crying, placing their fingers or fist in their mouth, rooting around, and sucking.

Newborns differ in their feeding needs and preferences, but most breastfed infants need to be fed every 2 to 3 hours. There is no set time for how long babies

should breastfeed, although most references suggest between 10 to 30 minutes on the first breast followed by offering the second breast. The length of feedings is up to the mother and newborn. Encourage the mother to respond to cues from her infant and not feed according to a standard or preset schedule.

Formula-fed newborns usually feed every 3 to 4 hours, finishing a bottle in 30 minutes or less. Most babies drink about 60 to 120 mL each feeding during the first month. Babies gradually have more until they are drinking about 180 to 240 mL at a time and double their intake within a few weeks of age (HealthLink BC, 2010). If the newborn seems satisfied, wets six to 10 diapers daily, produces several stools a day, sleeps well, and is gaining weight regularly, then he or she is probably receiving sufficient breast milk or formula.

Newborns may swallow air during feedings, which causes discomfort and fussiness. Parents can prevent this by burping them frequently throughout the feeding. Tips about burping include:

- Hold the newborn upright with his or her head on the parent's shoulder (Fig. 18.19A).
- Support the head and neck while the parent gently pats or rubs the newborn's back (Fig. 18.19B).
- Have the newborn sit on the parent's lap, while supporting the baby's chest and head. Gently rub the newborn's back with the other hand.
- Lay the newborn on the parent's lap with the baby's back facing up.
- Support the newborn's head in the crook of the parent's arm and gently pat or rub the back.

▶ **Take** NOTE!

It is the upright position, not the strength of the patting or rubbing, that allows the newborn to release air accumulated in the stomach.

Stress to parents that feeding time is more than an opportunity to get nutrients into their newborn; it is also a time for closeness and sharing. Feedings are as much for the baby's emotional pleasure as his or her physical well-being. Encourage parents to maintain eye contact with the newborn during the feeding, hold him or her comfortably close to them, and talk softly during the feeding to promote closeness and security.

Breastfeeding

There is consensus in the medical community that breastfeeding is optimal for all newborns. The CPS and the Breastfeeding Committee of Canada (BCC) recommend breastfeeding exclusively for the first 6 months of life, continuing it in conjunction with other food for up to

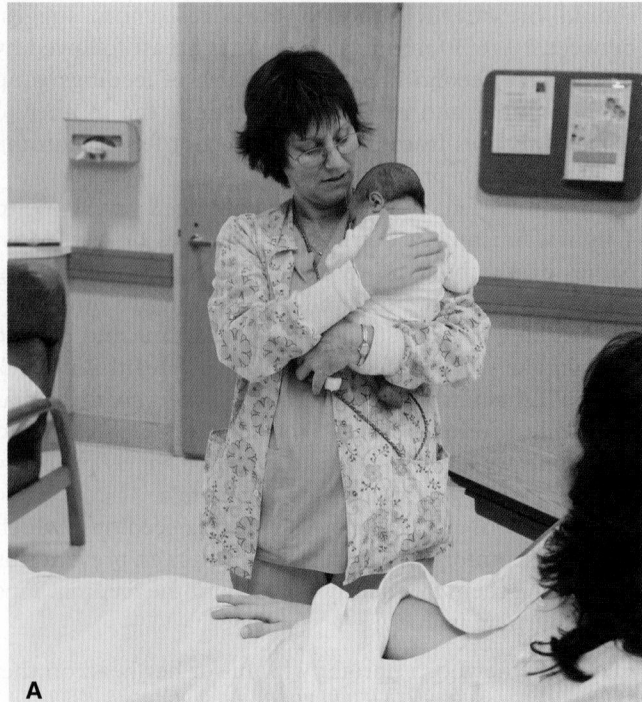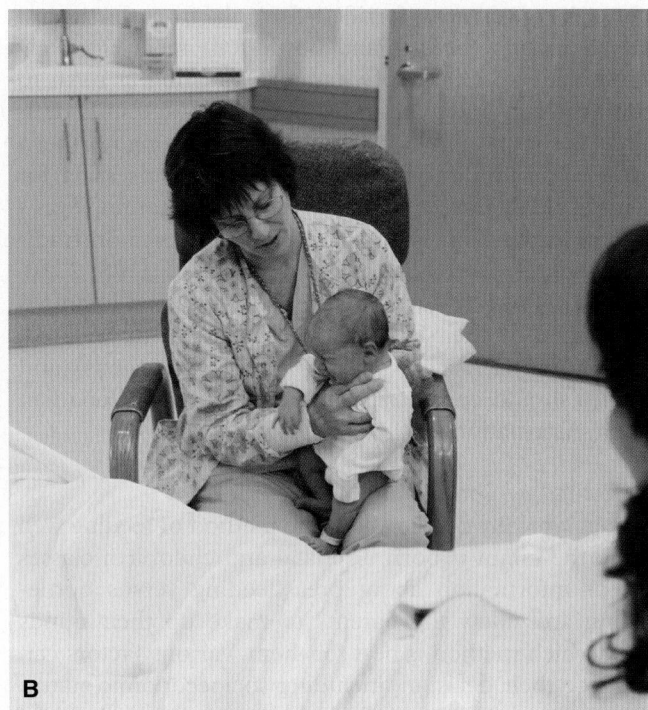

A **B**

FIGURE 18.19 The nurse demonstrates holding the newborn upright over the shoulder (**A**) and sitting the newborn upright, supporting the neck and chin (**B**), to elicit burps during feeding.

2 years and beyond (BCC, 2002; CPS, 2009). Box 18.2 highlights the advantages of breastfeeding for the mother and newborn.

Mothers should continue to breastfeed during mild illnesses such as colds or the flu. However, there are some situations in which women are advised not to breastfeed, including being HIV positive, using certain prescription medications and illicit substances, and having active herpes simplex lesions on the breast.

The composition of breast milk changes over time from colostrum to transitional milk and finally to mature milk. Colostrum is a thick, yellowish substance secreted during the first few days after birth. It is high in protein, minerals, and fat-soluble vitamins. It is rich in immunoglobulins (IgA), which help protect the newborn's gastrointestinal tract against infections. It is a natural laxative that helps rid the intestinal tract of meconium quickly (Pryor & Huggins, 2007).

Transitional milk occurs between colostrum and mature milk and contains all the nutrients in colostrum, but it is thinner and less yellow than colostrum. This transitional milk is replaced by true or mature milk around day 10 after birth. Mature milk appears bluish and is not as thick as colostrum. It provides 20 cal/oz and contains:

- Protein—although the content is lower than in formula, it is ideal to support growth and development for the newborn. The majority of protein is whey, which is easy to digest.

- Fat—approximately 58% of total calories are fat, but they are easy to digest. Essential fatty acid content is high, as is the level of cholesterol, which helps develop enzyme systems capable of handling cholesterol later in life.
- Carbohydrate—approximately 35% to 40% of total calories are in the form of lactose, which stimulates the growth of natural defense bacteria in the gastrointestinal system and promotes calcium absorption.
- Water—water, the major nutrient in breast milk, makes up 85% to 95% of the total volume. Total milk volume varies with the age of the infant and demand.
- Minerals—breast milk contains calcium, phosphorus, chlorine, potassium, and sodium, with trace amounts of iron, copper, and manganese. Iron absorption is about 50%, compared with about 4% for iron-fortified formulas.
- Vitamins—if a mother is well nourished, vitamin supplementation is not necessary, with the exception of vitamin D.
- Enzymes—lipase and amylase are found in breast milk to assist with digestion (Dudek, 2006).

Breastfeeding Assistance

Keys to successful breastfeeding include:

- Initiating breastfeeding within the first hour of life if the newborn is stable
- Following the newborn's feeding schedule—8 to 12 times in 24 hours

---

BOX 18.2 **Advantages of Breastfeeding for the Newborn**

- Contributes to the development of a strong immune system
- Stimulates growth of positive bacteria in digestive tract
- Strong protective effect for infant gastrointestinal infection
- Reduces incidence of stomach upset, diarrhea, and colic
- Begins the immunization process at birth by providing passive immunity
- Promotes optimal mother–infant bonding
- Reduces risk of newborn constipation
- Promotes greater developmental gains in preterm infants
- Provides easily tolerated and digestible formula that is sterile, at proper temperature, and readily available with no artificial colourings, flavourings, or preservatives
- Is less likely to result in overfeeding, leading to obesity

- Promotes better tooth and jaw development as a result of sucking hard
- Provides protection against food allergies
- Is associated with avoidance of type 1 diabetes and heart disease
- Offers possible protective effect against SIDS

Advantages for the Mother
- Can facilitate postpartum weight loss
- Stimulates uterine contractions to control bleeding
- Promotes uterine involution as a result of release of oxytocin
- Offers protection for some women against breast cancer, ovarian cancer, endometrial cancer, osteoporosis, and anemia
- Increases spacing between pregnancies; prolongs lactational amenorrhea

---

Sources: Breastfeeding Committee of Canada. (2002). *Breastfeeding statement of the Breastfeeding Committee of Canada.* Retrieved March 7, 2012 from http://breastfeedingcanada.ca/documents/webdoc5.pdf; Canadian Pediatric Society (reaffirmed 2009). Exclusive breastfeeding should continue to six months. *Paediatrics & Child Health, 10*(3), 148. Retrieved February 21, 2011 from http://www.cps.ca/english/statements/n/breastfeedingmar05.htm; and La Leche League International. (2010). *The womanly art of breastfeeding* (8th ed.). New York: Ballantyne.

- Providing unrestricted periods of breastfeeding
- Offering no supplement unless medically indicated
- Having a nurse with breastfeeding expertise or a lactation consultant observe a feeding session
- Avoiding artificial nipples and pacifiers except during a painful procedure
- Feeding from both breasts over each 24-hour period
- Watching for indicators of sufficient intake from infant:
  - 6 to 10 wet diapers daily
  - Waking up hungry 8 to 12 times in 24 hours
  - Acting content and falling asleep after feeding
- Keeping the newborn with the mother throughout the hospital stay

Help position the newborn so that latching-on is effective and is not painful for the mother. Placing pillows or a folded blanket under the mother's head may help, or rolling her to one side and tucking the newborn next to her. Assess both the mother and newborn during this initial session to determine needs for assistance and education. One tool used frequently in this assessment is the LATCH scoring tool (Table 18.6). The higher the score, the less nursing intervention is needed by the mother and baby.

Breastfeeding Positioning

The mother and infant must be in comfortable positions to ensure breastfeeding success. The four most common positions for breastfeeding are the football, cradle, cross-cradle, and side-lying holds. Each mother, on experimentation, can decide which positions feel most comfortable for her (Fig. 18.20).

In the football hold, the mother holds the infant's back and shoulders in her palm and tucks the infant under her arm. Remind the mother to keep the infant's ear, shoulder, and hip in a straight line. The mother supports the breast with her hand and brings it to the infant's lips to latch on. She continues to support the breast until the infant begins to nurse. This position allows the mother to see the infant's mouth as she guides her infant to the nipple. This is a good choice for mothers who have had a cesarean birth because it avoids pressure on the incision.

The cradling position is the one most commonly used. The mother holds the baby in the crook of her arm, with the infant facing the mother. The mother supports the breast with her opposite hand.

In the cross-cradle position, the mother places a pillow across her lap, with the infant facing the mother. The mother supports the infant's back and shoulders with her palm and supports her breast from underneath. After the infant is in position, the infant is pulled forward to latch on.

In the side-lying position, the mother lies on her side with a pillow supporting her back and another pillow supporting the newborn in the front. To start, the mother props herself up on an elbow and supports the newborn with that arm, while holding her breast with the opposite hand. Once nursing is started, the mother lies down in a comfortable position.

TABLE 18.6 THE LATCH SCORING TOOL

Parameters	0 Point	1 Point	2 Points
L: Latch	Sleepy infant, no sustained latch achieved	Must hold nipple in infant's mouth to sustain latch and suck; must stimulate infant to continue to suck	Grasps nipple; tongue down; rhythmic sucking
A: Audible swallowing	None	A few observed with stimulation	Spontaneous and intermittent both <24 h old and afterward
T: Type of nipple	Inverted (drawn inward into breast tissue)	Flat (not protruding)	Everted or protruding out after stimulation
C: Comfort of nipple	Engorged, cracked bleeding; severe discomfort	Filling; reddened, small blisters or bruises; mild to moderate discomfort	Soft, nontender
H: Hold (positioning)	Nurse must hold infant to breast	Minimal assistance; help with positioning, then mother takes over	No assistance needed by nurse

Sources: Centers for Disease Control and Prevention. (2010). *2010 STD treatment guidelines.* Retrieved February 21, 2011 from http://www.cdc.gov/STD/treatment/2010/default.htm; Canadian Pediatric Society. (2002). Recommendations for the prevention of neonatal ophthalmia. *Paediatrics & Child Health, 7*(7), 480–483. Retrieved September 28, 2011 from http://www.cps.ca/english/statements/ID/Id02–03.htm; and Canadian Pediatric Society (2011d). Universal newborn hearing screening. *Paediatrics & Child Health, 16*(5), 301–305. Retrieved February 21, 2011 from http://www.cps.ca/english/statements/CP/cp11–02.htm.

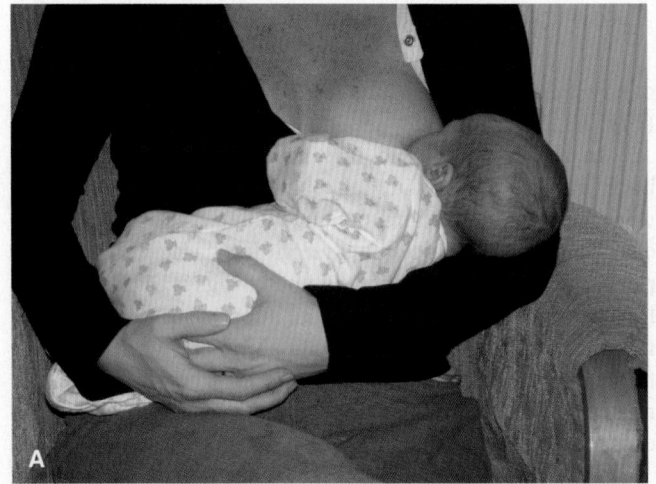

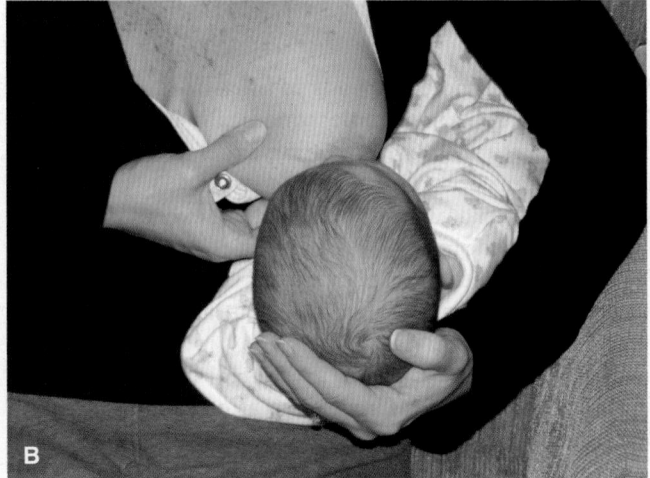

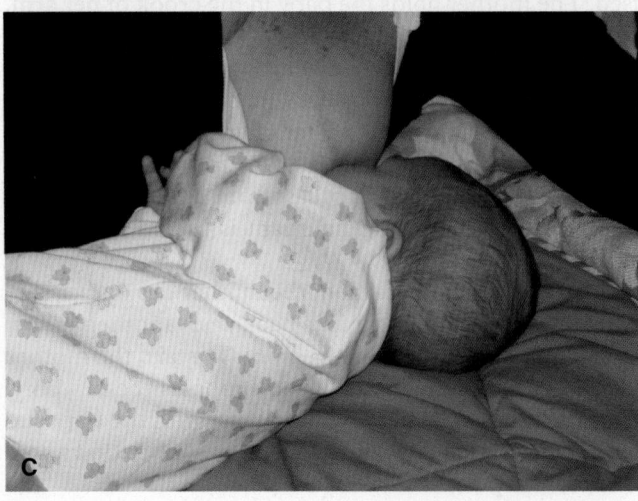

FIGURE 18.20 Breastfeeding positions. (**A**) Cradle hold. (**B**) Football hold. (**C**) Side-lying position.

To promote latching-on, instruct the mother to make a C or a V with her fingers. In the C hold, the mother places her thumb well above the areola and the other four fingers below the areola and under the breast. In the V hold, the mother places her index finger above the areola and her other three fingers below the areola and under the breast. Either method can be used as long as the mother's hand is well away from the nipple so the infant can latch on.

Breastfeeding Education

Breastfeeding is not an innate skill in human mothers. Almost all women have the potential to breastfeed successfully, but many fail because of inadequate knowledge or support. Nursing Care Plan 18.1 gives typical nursing diagnoses, outcomes, and interventions. For many mothers and newborns, breastfeeding goes smoothly from the start, but for others it is a struggle. Nurses can help throughout the experience by demonstrating techniques and offering encouragement and praise for success. Nurses should emphasize that the key to successful breastfeeding is correct positioning and latching-on.

Breastfeeding support and teaching by nurses has been shown to have a significant effect on both the ability to breastfeed successfully and the duration of lactation (Spatz, 2010). During the first few breastfeeding sessions, mothers want to know how often they should be nursing, whether breastfeeding is going well, if the newborn is getting enough nourishment, and what problems may ensue and how to cope with them. Education for the breastfeeding mother is highlighted in Teaching Guideline 18.4.

TEACHING GUIDELINE 18.4

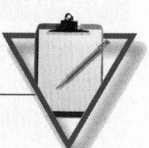

Breastfeeding

- Set aside a quiet place where you can be relaxed and won't be disturbed. Relaxation promotes milk letdown.
- Sit in a comfortable chair or rocking chair or lie on a bed. Be sure you are in a comfortable position to nurse. Try to make each feeding calm, quiet, and leisurely. Avoid distractions.
- Listen to soothing music and sip a nutritious drink during feedings.
- Initially, nurse the newborn every few hours to stimulate milk production. Remember that the supply of milk is equal to the demand—the more sucking, the more milk.
- Watch for cues from the infant to indicate that he or she is hungry, such as:
  - Nuzzling against the breasts
  - Demonstrating the rooting reflex by making sucking motions
  - Placing fist or hands in mouth to suck on
  - Crying and squirming
  - Smacking of the lips
- Stimulate the rooting reflex by touching the newborn's cheek to initiate sucking.
- Look for signs indicating that the newborn has latched on correctly: wide-open mouth with the nipple and much of the areola in the mouth, lips rolled outward, and tongue over lower gum; visible jaw movement drawing milk out; rhythmic sucking with an audible swallowing (soft "ka" or "ah" sound indicates the infant is swallowing milk).
- Hold the newborn closely, facing the breast, with the newborn's ear, shoulder, and hip in direct alignment.
- Nurse the infant on demand, not on a rigid schedule. Feed every 2 to 3 hours within a 24-hour period for a total of 8 to 12 feedings.
- Alternate the breast you offer first; identify with a safety pin on bra.
- Vary your position for each feeding to empty breasts and reduce soreness.
- Look for signs that the newborn is getting enough milk:
  - At least six wet diapers and two to five loose yellow stools daily after approximately the first week
  - Steady weight gain after the first week of age
  - Pale-yellow urine, not deep yellow or orange
  - Sleeping well, yet looks alert and healthy when awake (La Leche League International, 2010)
- Wake up the newborn if he or she has nursed less than 5 minutes by unwrapping him or her.
- Before removing the baby from the breast, break the infant's suction by inserting a finger.
- Burp the infant to release air when changing breasts and at the end of the breastfeeding session.
- Avoid supplemental formula feedings to prevent "nipple confusion" (Pryor & Huggins, 2007).
- Do not take drugs or medications unless approved by the health care provider. This includes being careful with herbal products. Medications with codeine (such as Tylenol #3) may not be safe during breastfeeding. If you need pain medication after birth, talk with your health care provider.
- Avoid drinking alcohol or caffeinated drinks because they pass through milk.
- Do not smoke while breastfeeding; it increases the risk of SIDS.
- Always wash your hands before expressing or handling milk to store.
- Wear nursing bras and clothes that are easy to undo.

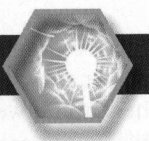

Nursing Care Plan 18.1

OVERVIEW OF THE MOTHER AND NEWBORN HAVING DIFFICULTY WITH BREASTFEEDING

Baby boy James, weight 7 lb 4 oz, was born a few hours ago. His mother, Jane, is a 19-year-old gravida 1, para 1. His Apgar scores were 9 points at both 1 and 5 minutes. Labour and birth were unremarkable, and James was placed on Jane's chest for skin-to-skin contact. James began to show readiness to feed and the nurse assisted Jane with positioning and latching-on and left the room for a few minutes. On returning, Jane was upset, James was crying, and Jane stated she wanted a bottle of formula to feed him since she didn't have milk and her nipples hurt.

    Assessment reveals a young, inexperienced mother placed in an uncomfortable situation with limited knowledge of breastfeeding. Anxiety from the mother transferred to James, resulting in crying. The mother, apprehensive about breastfeeding, needs additional help.

NURSING DIAGNOSIS: Knowledge deficit related to breastfeeding skills

Outcome Identification and Evaluation
Mother will demonstrate understanding of breastfeeding skills as evidenced by use of correct positioning and technique, and verbalization of appropriate information related to breastfeeding.

Interventions: Providing Education
- Instruct mother on proper positioning for breastfeeding; suggest use of football hold, side-lying position, modified cradle, and across-the-lap position *to ensure comfort and to promote ease in breastfeeding.*
- Review breast anatomy and milk letdown reflex *to enhance mother's understanding of lactation.*
- Observe newborn's ability to suck and latch on to the nipple *to assess whether newborn has adequate ability.*
- Monitor sucking and newborn swallowing for several minutes *to ensure adequate latching on and to assess intake.*
- Reinforce nipple care with water and exposure to air *to maintain nipple integrity.*

NURSING DIAGNOSIS: Anxiety related to breastfeeding ability and irritable, crying newborn

Outcome Identification and Evaluation
Mother will verbalize increased comfort with breastfeeding as evidenced by positive statements related to breastfeeding and verbalization of desire to continue to breastfeed newborn.

Interventions: Reducing Anxiety
- Ensure that the environment is calm and soothing without distractions *to promote maternal and newborn relaxation.*
- Show mother correct latching-on technique *to promote breastfeeding.*
- Assist in calming newborn by holding and talking *to ensure that the newborn is relaxed prior to latching on.*
- Reassure mother she can be successful at breastfeeding *to enhance her self-esteem and confidence.*
- Encourage frequent trials and attempts *to enhance confidence.*
- Encourage the mother to verbalize her anxiety/fears *to reduce anxiety.*

NURSING DIAGNOSIS: Pain related to breastfeeding and incorrect latching-on technique

Outcome Identification and Evaluation
Mother will experience a decrease in pain during breastfeeding as evidenced by statements of less nipple pain.

Interventions: Reducing Pain
- Suggest several alternate positions for breastfeeding *to increase comfort.*
- Demonstrate how to break suction before removing infant from breast *to minimize trauma to nipple.*
- Inspect nipple area *to promote early identification of trauma.*
- Reinforce correct latching-on technique *to prevent nipple trauma.*
- Administer pain medication if indicated *to relieve pain.*
- Instruct about nipple care between feedings *to maintain nipple integrity.*

Remember Kelly, who was concerned about jaundice in her newborn son? At her son's 2-week well-baby checkup at the clinic, his bilirubin level came back within normal limits. Kelly still felt he was not getting enough to eat and stated that she might switch to formula-feeding her son. What information can the nurse present to promote and reinforce breastfeeding? Should the nurse make a referral to a breastfeeding clinic or lactation consultant?

Breast Milk Storage and Expression

If the breastfeeding mother becomes separated from the newborn for any reason (e.g., work, travel, illness), she needs instruction on how to express and store milk safely. Expressing milk can be done manually (hand compression of breast) or by using a breast pump. Manual or hand pumps are inexpensive and can be used by mothers who occasionally need an extra bottle if they are going out (Fig. 18.21). Electric breast pumps are used for mothers who experience a lengthy separation from their infants and need to pump their breasts regularly.

To ensure the safety of expressed breast milk, instruct the mother in the following:

- Wash your hands before expressing milk or handling breast milk.
- Use clean containers to store expressed milk.
- Discard any milk that has been refrigerated more than 72 hours.
- Use any frozen expressed milk within 1 month after storage in the freezer compartment of a refrigerator, or within 6 months after storage in a deep freezer.

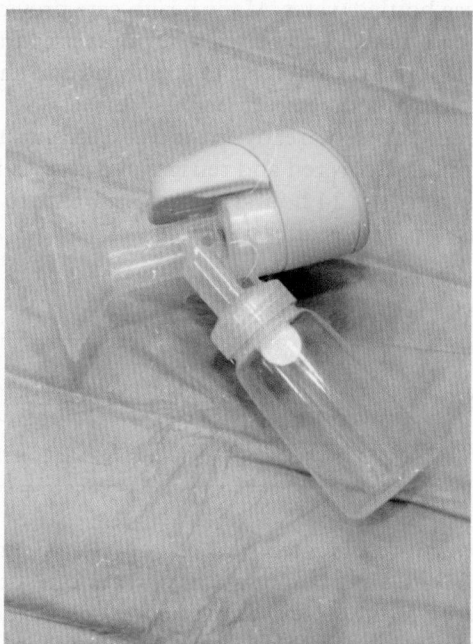

FIGURE 18.21 Hand-held breast pump.

- Do not use microwave ovens to warm chilled milk. Do not heat breast milk on the stove. Excessive heat can destroy important proteins and nutrients in the milk.
- Discard any used milk; never refreeze it.
- Store milk in quantities to be used for each feeding (2 to 4 oz).
- Thaw milk in warm water before using (BC Ministry of Health, 2005). Once milk has been thawed, it may be refrigerated up to 24 hours.
- You may want to warm up the milk again by placing the bottle of expressed milk into a container of warm water before the actual feeding.

Common Breastfeeding Concerns

Breastfeeding women may experience problems such as cracked nipples, engorgement, or mastitis. Breastfeeding should not be painful for the mother. If she has sore, cracked nipples, the first step is to find the cause. Incorrect positioning or latching-on, removing the infant from the breast without first breaking the suction, or wearing a bra that is too tight can cause cracked or sore nipples. Cracked nipples can increase the risk of mastitis because a break in the skin may allow *Staphylococcus aureus* or other organisms to enter the body.

Sore nipples usually are caused by improper infant attachment, which traumatizes the tissue. The nurse should review techniques for proper positioning and latching-on. Recommend the following to the mother:

- Use only water, not soap, to clean the nipples to prevent dryness.
- Express some milk before feeding to stimulate the milk ejection reflex.
- Avoid using breast pads with plastic liners, and change pads when they are wet.
- Wear a comfortable bra that is not too tight.
- Apply a few drops of breast milk to the nipples after feeding.
- Rotate positions when feeding the infant to promote complete breast emptying.
- Leave the nursing bra flaps down after feeding to allow nipples to air-dry.
- Inspect the nipples daily for redness or cracks (BC Ministry of Health, 2005).

To ease nipple pain and trauma, reinforce appropriate latching-on and remind the woman about the need to break the suction at the breast before removing the newborn from the breast. Additional measures may include applying cold compresses over the area and massaging breast milk onto the nipple after feeding.

Engorgement may occur as the milk comes in around day 3 or 4 after birth of the newborn. Explain to the mother that engorgement, though uncomfortable, is self-limited and will resolve as the newborn continues to nurse. The mother should continue to nurse during engorgement to avoid a plugged milk duct, which could lead to mastitis. Provide the following tips for relieving engorgement:

• Take warm to hot showers to encourage milk release.
• Express some milk manually before breastfeeding.
• Wear a supportive nursing bra 24 hours a day to provide support.
• Feed the newborn in a variety of positions—sitting up and then lying down.
• Massage the breasts from under the axillary area down toward the nipple.
• Increase the frequency of feedings.
• Apply warm compresses to the breasts prior to nursing.
• Stay relaxed while breastfeeding.
• Use a breast pump if nursing or manual expression is not effective.
• Remember that this condition is temporary and resolves quickly.

Mastitis, or inflammation of the breast, causes flu-like symptoms, chills, fever, and malaise. These symptoms may occur before the development of soreness, aching, swelling, and redness in the breast (usually the upper outer quadrant). This condition usually occurs in just one breast when a milk duct becomes blocked, causing inflammation, or through a cracked or damaged nipple, allowing bacteria to infect a portion of the breast. Treatment consists of rest, warm compresses, antibiotics, breast support, and continued breastfeeding (the infection will not pass into the breast milk). Explain to the mother that it is important to keep the milk flowing in the infected breast, whether it is through nursing or manual expression or with a breast pump.

Formula Feeding

Despite the general acknowledgment that breastfeeding is the most desirable means of feeding infants, some mothers choose formula feeding and need education about this procedure.

Formula feeding requires more than just opening, pouring, and feeding. Parents need information about the types of formula available, preparation and storage of formula, equipment, feeding positions, and the amount to feed their newborn. The mother also needs to know how to prevent lactation (see Chapter 16 for more information).

Commercially prepared formulas are regulated by the Canadian Food Inspection Agency and Health Canada. Healthy full-term infants usually receive conventional cow's milk–based formula, but this decision is made by the health care provider. If the infant shows signs of a reaction or lactose intolerance, a switch to another formula type is recommended. The general recommendation is for all infants to receive iron-fortified formula until the age of 1 year. The latest generation of infant formulas includes some fortification with docosahexaenoic acid (DHA) and arachidonic acid (ARA), two natural components of breast milk. Researchers have found that formulas with DHA and ARA can enhance visual and cognitive development in children (Lawson, 2007).

Commercial formulas come in three forms: powder, concentrate, and easy to feed or ready to use. All are similar in terms of nutritional content but differ in expense. Powdered formula is the least expensive, with concentrated formula the next most expensive. Both must be mixed with water before using. Ready-to-feed formula is the most expensive; it can be opened and poured into a bottle and fed directly to the infant.

Parents need information about the equipment needed for formula feeding. Basic supplies are four to six 4 oz (118 mL) bottles, eight to ten 8 oz (237 mL) bottles, 8 to 10 nipple units, a bottle brush, and a nipple brush. A key area of instruction is assessing for flow of formula through the nipple and checking for any nipple damage. When the bottle is filled and turned upside down, the flow from the nipple should be approximately one drop per second. If the parents are using bottles with disposable bags, instruct them to make sure they have a tight-fitting nipple to prevent leaks. Frequent observation of the flow rate from the nipple and the condition of the nipple will prevent choking and aspiration associated with too fast a rate of delivery. Ask the parents to fill a bottle with formula and then turn it upside down and observe the rate at which the formula drips from the bottle. If it is too fast (more than one drop/ second), then the nipple should be replaced.

Correct formula preparation is critical to the newborn's health and development. Mistakes in dilution may result if the parents do not understand how to prepare the formula or make measurement errors. The safety of the water supply should be considered. If well water is used, parents should sterilize the water by boiling it or should use bottled water. Many health care providers still recommend that all water used in formula preparation be brought to a rolling boil for 1 to 2 minutes and should be cooled to room temperature before use.

Opened cans of ready-made or concentrated formula should be covered and refrigerated after being prepared for the day (24 hours). Instruct parents to discard any unused portions after 48 hours.

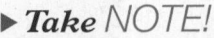

▶ *Take* NOTE!

Any formula left in the bottle after feeding should also be discarded, because the infant's saliva has been mixed with it.

To warm refrigerated formula, advise the parents to place the bottle in a pan of warm water and test the temperature by letting a few drops fall on the inside of the wrist. If it is comfortably warm to the mother, it is the correct temperature.

Formula-Feeding Assistance

The process of feeding a newborn formula from a bottle should mirror breastfeeding as closely as possible. Although nutrition is important, so are the emotional and interactive components of feeding. Encourage parents to cuddle their newborn closely and position him or her so that the head is in a comfortable position, not too far back or turned, which makes swallowing difficult. Also urge parents to communicate with their newborn during the feedings by talking and singing to him or her.

Although it may seem that bottle-feeding is not a difficult task, many new parents find it awkward. At first glance, holding an infant and a bottle appears simple enough, but both the position of the baby and the angle of the bottle must be correct.

Formula-Feeding Positions

Advise mothers, fathers, and caregivers to feed the newborn in a relaxed and quiet setting to create a sense of calm for themselves and the baby. Make sure that comfort is a priority for both mother and newborn. The mother can sit in a comfortable chair, using a pillow to support the arm in which she is holding the baby. The mother can cradle the newborn in a semi-upright position, supporting the newborn's head in the crook of her arm. Holding the newborn close during feeding provides stimulation and helps prevent choking. Holding the newborn's head raised slightly will help prevent formula from washing backward into the eustachian tubes in the ears, which can lead to an ear infection.

Formula-Feeding Education

Parents require teaching about the correct preparation and storage of formula as well as the techniques for feeding (HealthLink BC, 2010). See Teaching Guideline 18.5.

Proper positioning makes bottle-feeding easier and more enjoyable for both mother and newborn. As in breastfeeding, frequent burping is key. Advise the parents to hold the bottle so that formula fills the nipple, thus allowing less air to enter. Infants get fussy when they swallow air during feedings and need to be relieved of it every 60 to 80 mL (2 to 3 ounces).

Emphasize to parents that an electrolyte imbalance can occur in infants who are fed formula that has been incorrectly mixed. Hypernatremia can result from formula that is mixed too thickly; the high concentration of sodium is too much for the baby's immature kidneys to handle. As a result, sodium is excreted along with water, leading to dehydration. Mixing the formula with too much water in an effort to save money can lead to failure to thrive and lack of weight gain.

Weaning and Introduction of Solid Foods

Eventually, breastfeeding or formula feeding ends. Weaning involves the transition from breast to bottle, from breast or bottle to cup, or from liquids to solids. Weaning

---

TEACHING GUIDELINE 18.5

Formula Feeding

- Wash your hands with soap and water before preparing formula.
- Mix the formula and water amounts exactly as the label specifies. Check the expiration date. Make sure you use powdered formula within 1 month after opening.
- Always hold the newborn and bottle during feedings; never prop the bottle.
- Never freeze formula or warm it in the microwave.
- Heat formula by holding the bottle under warm tap water or by placing the bottle in a bowl of warm water or bottle warmer for no more than 15 minutes.
- Test the temperature of the formula by shaking a few drops on the wrist.
- Hold the bottle like a pencil, keeping it tipped to prevent air from entering. Position the bottle so that the nipple remains filled with milk.
- Burp the infant after every few millilitres to allow air swallowed to escape.

- Move the nipple around in the infant's mouth to stimulate sucking.
- Always keep a bulb syringe close by to use if choking occurs.
- Avoid putting the infant to bed with a bottle to prevent "baby bottle tooth decay."
- Feed the newborn approximately every 3 to 4 hours.
- Use an iron-fortified formula for the first year.
- It is safest to prepare powdered infant formula one bottle at a time and to feed your baby right after you have prepared the bottle. If you do prepare bottles ahead of time, they must be prepared using water that is at least 70° C, cooled quickly under running water or in ice water, and stored in the refrigerator.
- Check nipples regularly and discard any that are sticky, cracked, or leaking.
- Store unmixed, open liquid formula in the refrigerator for up to 48 hours.
- Throw away any formula left in the bottle after each feeding.

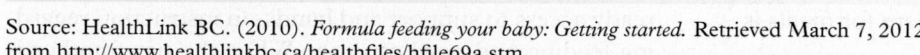

Source: HealthLink BC. (2010). *Formula feeding your baby: Getting started.* Retrieved March 7, 2012 from http://www.healthlinkbc.ca/healthfiles/hfile69a.stm.

from breastfeeding to cup has several advantages over weaning to a bottle because it eliminates the step of weaning first to a bottle and then to a cup. Another advantage is that the bottle does not become a security object for the infant.

Weaning may be done because the mother is returning to work and cannot keep breastfeeding or because the infant is losing interest in breastfeeding and showing signs of independence. There is no "right" time to wean; it depends on the desires of the mother and infant. Weaning represents a significant change in the way the mother and infant interact, and each mother must decide for herself when she and her infant are ready to take that step. Either one can start the weaning process, but usually it occurs between 6 months and 1 year of age.

To begin weaning from the breast, instruct mothers to substitute breastfeeding with a cup or bottle. Often the midday feeding is the easiest feeding to replace. A trainer cup with two handles and a snap-on lid with a spout is appropriate and minimizes spilling. Since weaning is a gradual process, it may take months. Instruct parents to proceed slowly and let the infant's willingness and interest guide them.

Weaning from the bottle to the cup also needs to be timed appropriately for mother and infant. Typically, the night bottle is the last to be given up, with cup drinking substituted throughout the day. Slowly diluting the formula with water over a week can help in this process; the final result is an all-water bottle. Solids can be offered to infants starting at 6 months of age, when they show signs of readiness cues, including:

- Consumption of 1,000 mL (32 oz) of formula or breast milk daily (estimated)
- Ability to sit up with minimal support and turn head away to indicate fullness
- Reduction of protrusion reflex so cereal can be propelled to back of throat
- Demonstration of interest in food others around them are eating
- Ability to open mouth automatically when food approaches it

When introducing solid foods, certain principles apply:

- Only one new single-ingredient food should be introduced at a time to watch for allergies.
- Infants should be allowed to set the pace regarding how much they wish to eat.
- New foods should not be introduced more frequently than every 3 to 5 days.
- Fruits are added after cereals; then vegetables and meats are introduced; eggs are introduced last. Iron-rich first foods are important to offer.
- A relaxed, unhurried, calm atmosphere for meals is important.

- A variety of foods are provided to ensure a balanced diet.
- Infants should never be force-fed (Lawson, 2007).

Nurses can promote good feeding practices by actively listening to new mothers, helping them clarify their feelings and discussing solutions. A warm, sincere manner and tone of voice will put an anxious mother at ease. Giving accurate information, making suggestions, and presenting options will enable the mother to decide what is best for her and her infant. Nurses should be sensitive to the individual, family, and economic and cultural differences among mothers before offering suggestions for feeding practices that may not be appropriate.

Preparing for Discharge

Preparing the parents and their families for discharge is an essential task for the nurse. Because of today's shorter hospital stays, the nurse must identify the major teaching topics that need to be covered. Nurses should assess the parents' baseline knowledge and learning needs and plan how to meet them. Using the following principles fosters a learner-centred approach:

- Make the environment conducive to learning. Encourage the parents to feel comfortable during this intense time by using support and praise.
- Allow the parents to provide input about the content and the process of learning. What do they want and need to learn?
- Build the parents' self-esteem by confirming that their responses to the entire birthing process and aftercare are legitimate, and others have felt the same way.
- Ensure that what the parents learn is relevant to their day-to-day home situation.
- Encourage responsibility by reinforcing that their emotional and physical responses are within the normal range.
- Respect cultural, ethnic, and religious beliefs and practices that are important to the family by taking into account their particular health and social beliefs regarding newborn and postpartum care. The Aboriginal population is the fastest-growing group in Canada, with a birth rate 1.5 times higher than that in the non-Aboriginal population. In addition, Canada's immigration policy is reflected in the diversity of our population; in 2006 the top five source countries were China, India, the Philippines, Pakistan, and the United States. When caring for people within these broad populations, it is important to acknowledge the diversity within groups, communities, and even families (Gagnon, Zimbeck, Zeitlin, et al., 2009; Smith, Edwards, Varcoe, et al., 2006).

While in the hospital, women and their families have ready access to support and hands-on instruction regarding feeding and newborn care. When the new mother is discharged, this close supervision and support by nurses should not end abruptly. It is important to inform parents of the supports that are available to them in the community, including community health nurses, breastfeeding and parenting support groups, and primary health care providers.

▶ *Consider THIS!*

I have always prided myself on being very organized and in control in most situations, but survival at home after childbirth wasn't one of them. I left the hospital 24 hours after giving birth to my son because my doctor said I could. The postpartum nurse encouraged me to stay longer, but wanting to be in control and sleeping in my own bed again won out. I thought my baby would be sleeping while I sent out birth announcements to my friends and family—wrong! What happened instead was my son didn't sleep as I imagined and my nipples became sore after breastfeeding every few hours. I was weary and tired and wanted to sleep, but I couldn't. Somehow I thought I would be getting a full night's sleep because I was up throughout the day, but that was a fantasy too. At 2 o'clock in the morning when you are up feeding your baby, you feel you are the only one in the world up at that time and feel very much alone. My feelings of being organized and in control all the time have changed dramatically since I left the hospital. I have learned to yield to the important needs of my son and derive satisfaction from being able to bring comfort to him and to let go of my control.

Thoughts: it is interesting to see how a newborn changed this woman's need to organize and control her environment. What "survival tips" could the nurse offer this woman to help in her transition to home with her newborn? How can friends and family help when women arrive home from the hospital with their newborns?

Ensuring Follow-Up Care

Most newborns are scheduled for a health follow-up appointment with their physician or midwife within the first week after discharge so that additional laboratory testing can be done as part of the newborn screening series, especially if they were discharged within 48 hours. After this first visit, the typical schedule of assessment and immunization visits is as follows: 2, 4, 6, 12, and 18 months (PHAC, 2006). These appointments provide an opportunity for parents to ask questions and receive anticipatory guidance as their newborn grows and develops. In many communities this series of visits is provided by community health nurses; in other areas they are provided by physicians or nurse practitioners.

In addition to encouraging parents to keep follow-up appointments, advise parents to call their health care provider if they notice signs of illness in their newborn. They should know which over-the-counter medicines should be kept on hand. Review the following warning signs of illness with parents:

- Temperature of 38.3°C (101°F) or higher
- Forceful, persistent vomiting (not just spitting up)
- Refusal to take feedings
- Two or more green, watery, diarrheal stools
- Infrequent wet diapers and change in bowel movements from normal pattern
- Lethargy or excessive sleepiness
- Inconsolable crying and extreme fussiness
- Abdominal distention
- Difficult or laboured breathing

Providing Immunization Information

Parents also need instructions about immunizations for their newborn. **Immunization** is the process of rendering an individual immune or of becoming immune to certain communicable diseases (PHAC, 2006). The purpose of the immune system is to identify unknown (non-self) substances in the body and develop a defense against these invaders. Disease prevention by immunization is a public health priority, and immunization is one of the leading health indicators for PHAC and provincial and territorial public health authorities. Nurses can help to support the health of the public by educating new parents about the importance of disease prevention through immunizations.

Immunity can be provided either passively or actively. Passive immunity is protection transferred via already formed antibodies from one person to another. Passive immunity includes transplacental passage of antibodies from a mother to her newborn, immunity passed through breast milk, and immunity from immunoglobulins. Passive immunity provides limited protection and decreases over a period of weeks or months (Blackburn, 2007). Active immunity is protection produced by an individual's own immune system. It can be obtained by having the actual disease or by receiving a vaccine that produces an immunologic response by that person's body. Active immunity may be lifelong either way.

Young infants and children are susceptible to various illnesses because their immune systems are not yet mature. Many of these illnesses can be prevented by following the recommended schedule of childhood immunizations (PHAC, 2006) (Fig. 18.22). There may also be some provincial schedule differences, and it will be important to identify those. The schedule for immunizations should be reviewed with parents, stressing the importance of continued follow-up health care to preserve their infant's health.

In some provinces the newborn's first immunization (hepatitis B) is received in the hospital soon after birth.

Timing	DTaP-IPV	Hib	MMR	Var	HB	Pneu- C-7	Men-C	Tdap	Inf
Infants and Children									
Birth					Infancy 3 doses ★ or Pre-teen/ teen 2–3 doses				
2 months	⊖	✦				■	⊙		
4 months	⊖	✦				■	(⊙)		
6 months	⊖	✦				■	⊙ or		6–23 months ⊠ 1–2 doses
12 months			■	●		■ 12–15 months	⊙ if not yet given		
18 months	⊖	✦	■ or						
4–6 years	⊖		■						
14–16 years							⊙ if not yet given	▲	

()	Symbols with brackets around them imply that these doses may not be required, depending on the age of the child or adult.
⊖	**Diphtheria, tetanus, acellular pertussis and inactivated polio virus vaccine (DTaP-IPV):** DTaP-IPV(± Hib) vaccine is the preferred vaccine for all doses in the vaccination series, including completion of the series in children who have received one or more doses of DPT (whole cell) vaccine (e.g., recent immigrants). The 4- to 6-year dose can be omitted if the fourth dose was given after the child's fourth birthday.
✦	*Haemophilus influenzae* **type b conjugate vaccine (Hib):** The Hib schedule shown is for the *Haemophilus* b capsular polysaccharide–polyribosylribitol phosphate (PRP) conjugated to tetanus toxoid (PRP-T). For catch-up, the number of doses depends on the age at which the schedule is begun. Not usually required past age 5 years.
■	**Measles, mumps, and rubella vaccine (MMR):** A second dose of MMR is recommended for children at least 1 month after the first dose for the purpose of better measles protection. For convenience, options include giving it with the next scheduled vaccination at 18 months of age or at school entry (age 4–6 years) (depending on the provincial/territorial policy) or at any intervening age that is practical. In the catch-up schedule (i.e., children <7 years of age not immunized in early infancy), the first dose should not be given until the child is ≥12 months old. MMR should be given to all susceptible adolescents and adults.
●	**Varicella vaccine (Var):** Children aged 12 months to 12 years should receive one dose of varicella vaccine. Susceptible individuals ≥13 years of age should receive two doses at least 28 days apart.
★	**Hepatitis B vaccine (HB):** Hepatitis B vaccine can be routinely given to infants or pre-adolescents, depending on the provincial/territorial policy. For infants born to chronic carrier mothers, the first dose should be given at birth (with hepatitis B immunoglobulin); otherwise the first dose can be given at 2 months of age to fit more conveniently with other routine infant immunization visits. The second dose should be administered at least 1 month after the first dose, and the third at least 2 months after the second dose, but these may fit more conveniently into the 4- and 6-month immunization visits. A two-dose schedule for adolescents is an option.
■	**Pneumococcal conjugate vaccine-7-valent (Pneu-C-7):** Recommended for all children under 2 years of age. The recommended schedule depends on the age of the child when vaccination is begun.
⊙	**Meningococcal C conjugate vaccine (Men-C):** Recommended for children <5 years of age, adolescents, and young adults. The recommended schedule depends on the age of the individual and the conjugate vaccine used. At least one dose in the primary infant series should be given after 5 months of age. If the provincial/territorial policy is to give Men-C to persons ≥12 months of age, one dose is sufficient.

FIGURE **18.22** Recommended childhood immunization schedule. (Source: Canadian Immunization Guide (7th ed.). Public Health Agency of Canada, 2006. Reproduced with the permission of the Minister of Health, 2011.) (*continued*)

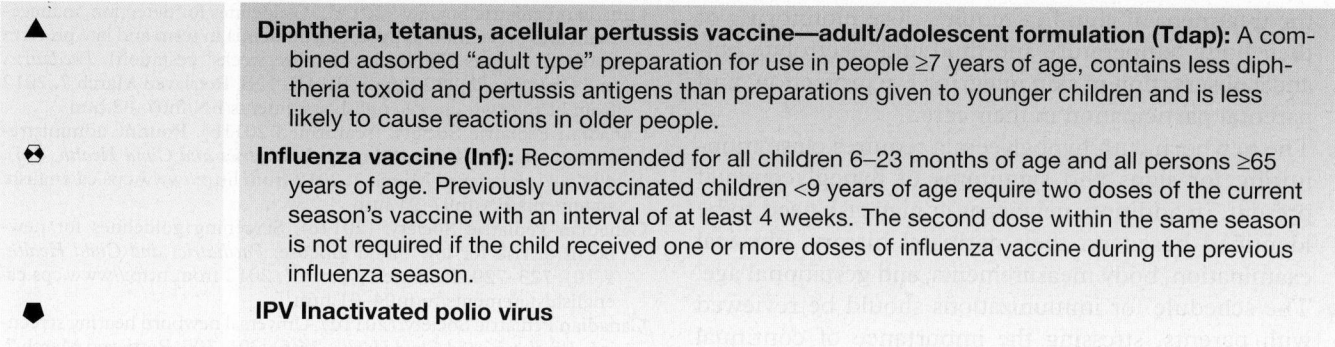

Diphtheria, tetanus, acellular pertussis vaccine—adult/adolescent formulation (Tdap): A combined adsorbed "adult type" preparation for use in people ≥7 years of age, contains less diphtheria toxoid and pertussis antigens than preparations given to younger children and is less likely to cause reactions in older people.

Influenza vaccine (Inf): Recommended for all children 6–23 months of age and all persons ≥65 years of age. Previously unvaccinated children <9 years of age require two doses of the current season's vaccine with an interval of at least 4 weeks. The second dose within the same season is not required if the child received one or more doses of influenza vaccine during the previous influenza season.

IPV Inactivated polio virus

FIGURE 18.22 (continued)

The first dose can also be given by age 2 months if the mother is hepatitis B surface antigen (HBsAg) negative. If the mother is HBsAg positive, then the newborn should receive hepatitis B vaccine and hepatitis B immunoglobulin within 12 hours of birth (PHAC, 2006).

Education for the parents should include the risks and benefits for each vaccine and possible adverse effects. Federal law requires a consent form to be signed before administering a vaccine. Parents have the right to refuse immunizations based on their religious or personal beliefs and can sign a waiver noting their decision. The nurse administering the vaccine must document the date and time it was given; the name and manufacturer, lot number, and expiration date of the vaccine given; site and route of administration; and the name and title of the nurse who administered the vaccine.

■■■ Key Concepts

- The period of transition from intrauterine to extra-uterine life occurs during the first several hours after birth. It is a time of stabilization for the newborn's temperature, respiration, and cardiovascular dynamics.
- The newborn's bowel is sterile at birth. It usually takes about a week for the newborn to produce vitamin K in sufficient quantities to prevent vitamin K deficiency bleeding.
- It is recommended that all newborns in Canada receive an instillation of a prophylactic agent (usually erythromycin or tetracycline ophthalmic ointment) in their eyes within 1 hour of birth.
- Nursing measures to maintain newborns' body temperature include drying them immediately after birth to prevent heat loss through evaporation, placing them in skin-to-skin contact with their mother, covering them in prewarmed blankets, and putting a hat on their head.
- The specific components of a typical newborn examination include a general survey of skin colour, posture, state of alertness, head size, overall behavioural

state, respiratory status, sex, and any obvious congenital anomalies.

- Gestational age assessment is pertinent because it allows the nurse to plot growth parameters and to anticipate potential problems related to prematurity/postmaturity and growth abnormalities such as SGA/LGA.
- After the newborn has passed the transitional period and stabilized, the nurse needs to complete ongoing assessments, vital signs, weight and measurements, cord care, hygiene measures, newborn screening tests, and various other tasks until the newborn is discharged home from the birthing unit.
- Important topics about which to educate parents include environmental safety, newborn characteristics, feeding and bathing, circumcision and cord care, sleep and elimination patterns of newborns, safe infant car seats, holding/positioning, and follow-up care.
- Newborn screening is conducted to test for hearing ability and for certain genetic and inborn errors of metabolism; requirements for such screening prior to discharge from the hospital vary across Canada.
- The CPS and the BCC recommend that women breastfeed their children exclusively for the first 6 months of life and that it continue along with other food for up to 2 years and beyond.
- Parents who choose not to breastfeed need to know what types of formula are available, preparation and storage of formula, equipment, feeding positions, and how much to feed their infant.
- Common problems associated with the newborn include transient tachypnea, physiologic jaundice, and hypoglycemia.
- Transient tachypnea of the newborn appears soon after birth; is accompanied by retractions, expiratory grunting, or cyanosis; and is relieved by low-dose oxygen.
- Physiologic jaundice is a very common condition in newborns, with the majority demonstrating yellowish skin, mucous membranes, and sclera within the first 3 days of life. Newborns undergoing phototherapy in

the treatment of jaundice require close monitoring of their body temperature and fluid and electrolyte balance; observation of skin integrity; eye protection; and parental participation in their care.

■ The newborn with hypoglycemia requires close monitoring for signs and symptoms of hypoglycemia if present. In addition, newborns at high risk need to be identified based on their perinatal history, physical examination, body measurements, and gestational age.

■ The schedule for immunizations should be reviewed with parents, stressing the importance of continual follow-up health care to preserve their infant's health.

REFERENCES

Acute Care of at-Risk Newborns (ACoRN) Neonatal Society. (2010). *A resource and learning tool for health professionals* (2nd ed.). Vancouver, BC: Author.

Association of Women's Health, Obstetric and Neonatal Nurses (AWHONN). (2007). *Neonatal skin care* (2nd ed.). Evidence-based clinical practice guideline. Washington (DC): Association of Women's Health, Obstetric and Neonatal Nurses (AWHONN).

Association of Women's Health, Obstetric and Neonatal Nurses. (2007). Preventing infant abduction: A parent's guide. *AWHONN Lifelines, 10*(6), 521–522.

BC Ministry of Health. (2005). *Baby's best chance: Parent's handbook of pregnancy and baby care* (revised 6th ed.). Retrieved March 7, 2012 from http://www.health.gov.bc.ca/library/publications/year/2005/babybestchance.pdf

Begany, M., & Mascarenhas, M. (2007). Normal infant feeding. In R. E. Rakel & E. T. Bope (Eds.), *Conn's current therapy 2007.* Philadelphia: Saunders Elsevier.

Blackburn, S. T. (2007). *Maternal, fetal, and neonatal physiology: A clinical perspective* (3rd ed.). St. Louis, MO: Saunders Elsevier.

Breastfeeding Committee of Canada. (2002). *Breastfeeding statement of the Breastfeeding Committee of Canada.* Retrieved March 7, 2012 from http://breastfeedingcanada.ca/documents/webdoc5.pdf

Burns, C. E., Dunn, A. M., Brady, M. A., Starr, N. B., & Blosser, C. G. (2009). *Pediatric primary care* (4th ed.). St. Louis, MO: Saunders Elsevier.

Canadian Association of Speech-Language Pathologists and Audiologists. (2010). *CASLPA position paper on universal newborn hearing screening.* Retrieved March 7, 2012 from http://www.caslpa.ca/PDF/position%20papers/Universal_Newborn_Hearing_Screening_Position_Paper_2010.pdf

Canadian Dental Association. (2008). *CDA position on use of fluorides in caries prevention.* Retrieved March 7, 2012 from http://www.cda-adc.ca/_files/position_statements/fluorides.pdf

Canadian Dental Association. (2012). *Dental care for children.* Retrieved March 7, 2012 from http://www.cda-adc.ca/en/oral_health/cyft/dental_care_children/

Canadian Pediatric Society. (1996). Neonatal circumcision revisited. *Canadian Medical Association Journal, 154*(6), 769–780. Retrieved March 7, 2012 from http://www.cps.ca/english/statements/fn/fn96–01.htm

Canadian Pediatric Society. (2002). Recommendations for the prevention of neonatal ophthalmia. *Paediatrics and Child Health, 7*(7), 480–483. Retrieved March 7, 2012 from http://www.cps.ca/english/statements/ID/Id02–03.htm

Canadian Pediatric Society. (reaffirmed 2009). Exclusive breastfeeding should continue to six months. *Paediatrics and Child Health, 10*(3), 148. Retrieved March 7, 2012 from http://www.cps.ca/english/statements/n/breastfeedingmar05.htm

Canadian Pediatric Society. (reaffirmed 2010). Vitamin D supplementation: Recommendations for Canadian mothers and infants. *Paediatrics and Child Health, 12*(7), 583–589. Retrieved March 7, 2012 from http://www.cps.ca/english/statements/ii/fnim07–01.htm

Canadian Pediatric Society. (2011a). Guidelines for detection, management and prevention of hyperbilirubinemia in term and late preterm newborn infants (35 weeks or more weeks' gestation). *Paediatrics and Child Health,* (12 Suppl. B), 1B–12B. Retrieved March 7, 2012 from http://www.cps.ca/english/statements/FN/fn07–02.htm

Canadian Pediatric Society. (reaffirmed 2011b). Routine administration of vitamin K to newborns. *Paediatrics and Child Health, 2*(6), 429–431. Retrieved March 7, 2012 from http://www.cps.ca/english/statements/FN/fn97–01.htm

Canadian Pediatric Society. (2011c). Screening guidelines for newborns at risk for low blood glucose. *Paediatrics and Child Health, 9*(10), 723–729. Retrieved March 7, 2012 from http://www.cps.ca/english/statements/fn/fn04–01.htm

Canadian Pediatric Society. (2011d). Universal newborn hearing screening. *Paediatrics and Child Health, 16*(5), 301–305. Retrieved March 7, 2012 from http://www.cps.ca/english/statements/CP/cp11–02.htm

Canadian Pediatric Society. (n.d.). *Addendum to the NRP provider textbook 6th edition: Recommendations for specific modifications in the Canadian context.* Retrieved March 14, 2012 from http://www.cps.ca/nrp/addendum.pdf

Canadian Perinatal Surveillance System. (2008). *Canadian Perinatal Health Report 2008.* Retrieved March 7, 2012 from http://www.phac-aspc.gc.ca/publicat/2008/cphr-rspc/index-eng.php

Caruana, E. (2008). Early skin-to-skin contact for mothers and their healthy newborn infants. *Journal of Advanced Nursing, 62*(4), 439–440.

Centers for Disease Control and Prevention. (2010). *2010 STD treatment guidelines.* Retrieved March 7, 2012 from http://www.cdc.gov/STD/treatment/2010/default.htm

Cohen, S. (2007). *Critical thinking in the pediatric unit Skills to assess, analyze, and act.* Marblehead, MA: HCPro, Inc.

Colling, R., & York, T. (2010). *Hospital and health care security* (5th ed.). Burlington, MA: Elsevier.

Cunningham, F. G., Leveno, K. J., Bloom, S. L., Hauth, J. C., Gilstrap, L. C., & Wenstrom, K. D. (2010). *Williams obstetrics* (23rd ed.). New York: McGraw-Hill.

Doctors Opposing Circumcision. (2008). *Doctors Opposing Circumcision: HIV statement.* Seattle, WA. Retrieved March 14, 2012 from http://www.doctorsopposingcircumcision.org/info/HIVStatement.html

Dudek, S. G. (2006). *Nutrition essentials for nursing practice* (5th ed.). Philadelphia: Lippincott Williams & Wilkins.

Fraser, D., & Cooper, M. (2009). *Myles textbook for midwives* (15th ed.). London: Elsevier.

Gagnon, A., Zimbeck, M., Zeitlin, J., & the ROAM Collaboration. (2009). Migration to Western industrialized countries and perinatal health: A systematic review. *Social Science and Medicine, 69*(6), 934–946. doi:10.1016/j.socoscimed.209.06.027

Health Canada. (2000). *Family-centered maternity and newborn care: National guidelines.* Retrieved March 7, 2012 from http://www.phac-aspc.gc.ca/hp-ps/dca-dea/publications/fcm-smp/index-eng.php

Health Canada. (2005). *Nutrition for healthy term infants—Statement of the joint working group: Canadian Pediatric Society, Dieticians of Canada, and Health Canada.* Retrieved March 7, 2012 from http://www.hc-sc.gc.ca/fn-an/pubs/infant-nourrisson/nut_infant_nourrisson_term-eng.php

Health Canada. (2007). *Reaching for the top: A report by the advisor on healthy children & youth: Injury prevention and safety.* Retrieved March 7, 2012 from http://www.hc-sc.gc.ca/hl-vs/pubs/child-enfant/advisor-conseillere/prevention-eng.php

HealthLink BC. (2010). *Formula feeding your baby: Getting started.* Retrieved March 7, 2012 from http://www.healthlinkbc.ca/healthfiles/hfile69a.stm

Hoe, F. M. (2008). Hypoglycemia in infants and children. *Advances in Pediatrics, 55,* 367–384. doi:10.1016/j.yapd.2008.07.008

Kattwinkel, J. (Ed.). (2011). *Neonatal resuscitation textbook* (6th ed.), American Heart Association, American Academy of Pediatrics.

Kenner, C., & Lott, J. W. (2007). *Comprehensive neonatal care: An interdisciplinary approach* (4th ed.). St. Louis, MO: Saunders Elsevier.

Kliegman, R. M., Behrman, R. E., Jenson, H. B., & Stanton, B. F. (2011). *Nelson's textbook of pediatrics* (19th ed.). St. Louis, MO: Saunders Elsevier.

La Leche League International. (2010). *The womanly art of breastfeeding* (8th ed.). New York: Ballantyne.

Lawson, M. (2007). Contemporary aspects of infant feeding. *Pediatric Nursing, 19*(2), 39–45.

Maisels, M. J. (2006). What's in a name? Physiologic and pathologic jaundice: The conundrum of defining normal bilirubin levels in the newborn. *Pediatrics, 118*(2), 805–807.

McHoney, M. (2010). Early human development: Neonatal tumors, vascular tumors. *Early Human Development, 86*(10), 613–618.

Medves, J., & O'Brien, B. (2004). The effect of bather and location of first bath on maintaining thermal stability in newborns. *Journal of Obstetrics, Gynecologic and Neonatal Nursing, 33*(2), 175–182.

Merenstein, G. B., & Gardner, S. L. (2011). *Handbook of neonatal intensive care.* St. Louis, MO: Mosby.

Perinatal Services BC. (2011a). *Health promotion guidelines 1: Safe sleep environment guideline for infants 0 to 12 months of age.* Retrieved March 7, 2012 from http://perinatalservicesbc.ca/sites/bcrcp/files/Guidelines/Health_Promotion_and_Prevention/Infant_Sleep_Environment.pdf

Perinatal Services BC. (2011b). *Newborn guideline 13: Newborn nursing care pathway.* Retrieved March 7, 2012 from http://perinatalservicesbc.ca/sites/bcrcp/files/Guidelines/Newborn/NB13NursingCarePathway.pdf

Pryor, G., & Huggins, K. (2007). *Nursing mother, working mother: The essential guide to breastfeeding your baby before and after you return to work* (2nd ed.). Harvard, MA: The Harvard Common Press.

Public Health Agency of Canada. (2006). *Canadian immunization guide* (7th ed.). Retrieved March 7, 2012 from http://www.phac-aspc.gc.ca/publicat/cig-gci/

Public Health Agency of Canada. (2011). *Joint statement on safe sleep: Preventing sudden infant death syndrome.* Retrieved March 7, 2012 from http://www.phac-aspc.gc.ca/hp-ps/dca-dea/stages-etapes/childhood-enfance_0–2/sids/jsss-ecss-eng.php

Ridings, H., & Amaya, M. (2007). Male neonatal circumcision: An evidence-based review. *Journal of the American Academy of Physician Assistants, 20*(2), 32–36.

Rourke, L., Leduc, D., Constantin, E., Carsley, S., & Rourke, J. (2010). Update on well-baby and well-child care from 1 to 5 years. *Canadian Family Physician, 56*, 1285–1290.

Smith, D., Edwards, N., Varcoe, C., Martens, P., & Davies, B. (2006). Bringing safety and responsiveness into the forefront of care for pregnant and parenting Aboriginal people. *Advances in Nursing Science, 29*(2), E27–E44.

Snowdon, A., Hussein, A., & Ahmed, E. (2010). *Canadian National Survey on Child Restraint use 2010.* Retrieved March 7, 2012 from http://www.tc.gc.ca/eng/roadsafety/resources-researchstats-child-restraint-survey-2010–1207.htm

Soll, R. F. (2008). Heat loss prevention in neonates. *Journal of Perinatology, 28,* S57–S59. doi:10.1038/jp.2008.51

Spatz, D. L. (2010). The critical role of nurses in lactation support. *Journal of Obstetric, Gynecologic, and Neonatal Nursing, 39*(5), 499–500.

Tappero, E., & Honeyfield, M. (2009). *Physical assessment of the newborn: A comprehensive approach to the art of physical examination* (4th ed.). Santa Rosa, CA: NICU Ink Book Publishers.

Transport Canada. (2009). *Consumer information notice—Children's car seats and booster cushions: How long are they safe?* Retrieved March 7, 2012 from http://www.tc.gc.ca/eng/roadsafety/safedrivers-childsafety-notices-2007c10-menu-355.htm

Trifunov, W. (2009). *The practice of bedsharing: A systematic literature and policy review.* Ottawa, ON: Public Health Agency of Canada. Retrieved March 7, 2012 from http://www.phac-aspc.gc.ca/hp-ps/dca-dea/stages-etapes/childhood-enfance_0–2/sids/pbs-ppl-eng.php

Vreman, H. J. (2008). Standardized bench method for evaluating the efficacy of phototherapy devices. *Acta Pædiatrica, 97,* 308–316. doi:10.1111/j.1651-2227.2007.00631.x

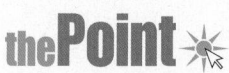

For additional learning materials, including Internet Resources, visit http://thePoint.lww.com/Chow1e.

CHAPTER WORKSHEET

MULTIPLE CHOICE QUESTIONS

1. At birth, a newborn's assessment reveals the following: heart rate of 140 beats/minute, loud crying, some flexion of extremities, crying when bulb syringe is introduced into the nares, and a pink body with blue extremities. The nurse would document the newborn's Apgar score as:

   a. 5 points

   b. 6 points

   c. 7 points

   d. 8 points

2. The nurse is explaining phototherapy to the parents of a newborn. The nurse would include which of the following as the purpose?

   a. Increase surfactant levels

   b. Stabilize the newborn's temperature

   c. Destroy Rh-negative antibodies

   d. Oxidize bilirubin on the skin

3. The nurse administers a single dose of vitamin K intramuscularly to a newborn after birth to promote:

   a. Conjugation of bilirubin

   b. Blood clotting

   c. Foramen ovale closure

   d. Digestion of complex proteins

4. A prophylactic agent is instilled in both eyes of all newborns to prevent which of the following conditions?

   a. Gonorrhea and chlamydia

   b. Thrush and *Enterobacter* infection

   c. *Staphylococcus* infection and syphilis

   d. Hepatitis B and herpes

5. The CPS recommends that all newborns be placed on their backs to sleep to reduce the risk of:

   a. Respiratory distress syndrome

   b. Bottle mouth syndrome

   c. Sudden infant death syndrome

   d. GI regurgitation syndrome

6. Which of the following immunizations is received by newborns before hospital discharge?

   a. Pneumococcus

   b. Varicella

   c. Hepatitis A

   d. Hepatitis B

7. Which condition would be missed if newborns are screened before they have tolerated protein feedings for at least 48 hours?

   a. Hypothyroidism

   b. Cystic fibrosis

   c. Phenylketonuria

   d. Sickle cell disease

CRITICAL THINKING EXERCISES

1. Linda Scott, a mother who delivered her first baby, calls the nurse into her room and expresses concern about how her daughter looks. Ms. Scott tells the nurse that her baby's head looks like a "banana" and is mushy to the touch, and she has "white spots" all over her nose. In addition, there appear to be red marks on the back of her baby's neck. She wants to know what is wrong with her baby and whether these problems will go away.

   a. How should the nurse respond to Ms. Scott's questions?

   b. What additional newborn instruction might be appropriate at this time?

   c. What reassurance can be given to Ms. Scott regarding her daughter's appearance?

2. At approximately 12:30 a.m. on a Friday, a woman enters a hospital through a busy emergency room. She is wearing a white uniform and a lab coat with a stethoscope around her neck. She identifies herself as a new nurse coming back to check on something she had left on the unit on an earlier shift. She enters a client's room containing the mother's newborn, pushes the open crib down a hallway, and escapes through an exit. The security cameras aren't working. The infant isn't discovered missing until the 2 a.m. check by the nurse.

a. What impact does an infant abduction have on the family and the hospital?

b. What security measure was the weak link in the chain of security?

c. What can hospitals do to prevent infant abduction?

STUDY ACTIVITIES

1. Interview a new mother on her second day after birth about the changes she has noticed in her newborn's appearance and behaviour within the past 24 hours. Discuss your interview findings at post-conference.

2. Teach newborn bathing to new parents in their room, using the principle of bathing from the cleanest to the dirtiest body part. Discuss the questions asked by the parents and their reaction to the experience in post-conference.

3. Go to the La Leche League website (visit http://thePoint.lww.com/Chow1e for the direct link). Review the information it provides on breastfeeding. How helpful would it be to a new mother?

4. Debate the risks and benefits of neonatal circumcision within your nursing group at post-conference. Did either side present a stronger position? What is your opinion, and why?

CHILDBEARING AT RISK

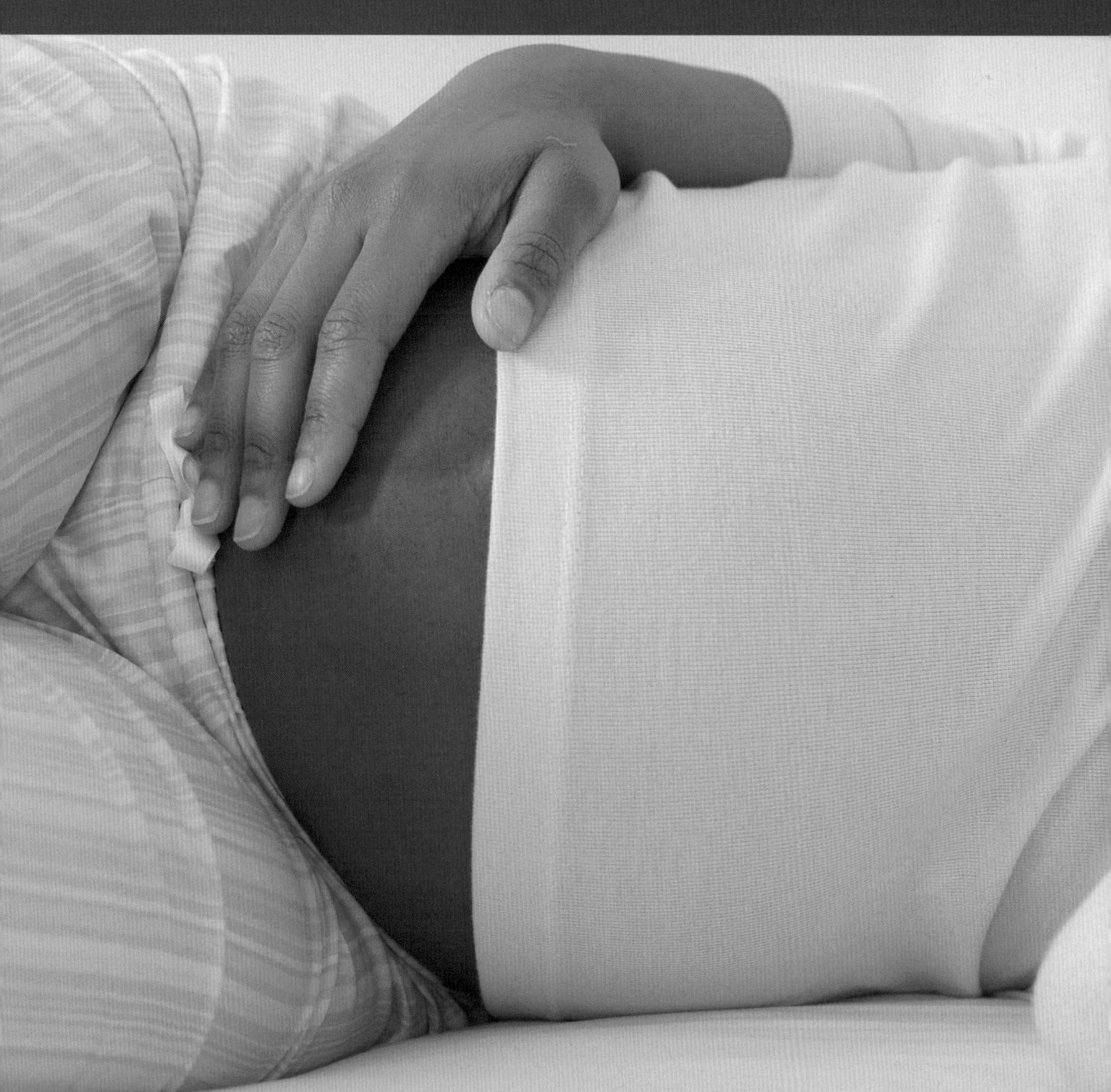

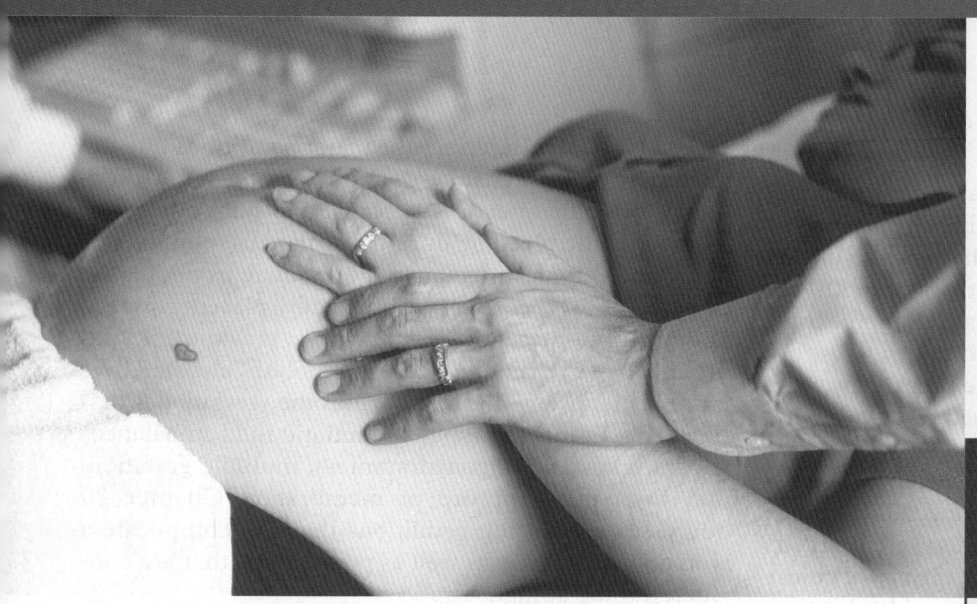

NURSING MANAGEMENT OF PREGNANCY AT RISK: PREGNANCY–RELATED COMPLICATIONS

KEY TERMS

abortion
abruptio placentae
ectopic pregnancy
gestational hypertension
gestational trophoblastic
   disease (GTD)

high–risk pregnancy
hyperemesis gravidarum
multiple gestation
oligohydramnios
polyhydramnios
placenta previa

premature rupture of
   membranes (PROM)
preterm premature
   rupture of membranes
   (PPROM)

LEARNING OBJECTIVES

Upon completion of the chapter, the learner will be able to:

1. Define the term "high-risk pregnancy."
2. Explain common factors that might place a pregnancy at high risk.
3. Identify the causes of vaginal bleeding during early and late pregnancy.
4. Outline nursing assessment and management for the pregnant woman experiencing vaginal bleeding.
5. Develop a plan of care for the woman experiencing pre-eclampsia, eclampsia, and HELLP syndrome.
6. Explain the pathophysiology of polyhydramnios and subsequent management.
7. Select factors in a woman's prenatal history that place her at risk for premature rupture of membranes (PROM).
8. Formulate a teaching plan for maintaining the health of pregnant women experiencing a high-risk pregnancy.

*H*elen, a 35-year-old G5 P4, presented to the labour and birth suite with severe abdominal pain. She reports that the pain began suddenly about an hour ago while she was resting. She has had two prior cesarean births and thus far has had an uneventful 32 weeks of pregnancy. Helen appears distressed and is moaning. What additional assessments do you need to care for Helen? What might be your immediate nursing action?

Wow

Detours and bumps along the road of life can be managed, but many cannot be entirely cured.

Most people view pregnancy as a natural process with a positive outcome—the birth of a healthy newborn. Unfortunately, conditions can occur that may result in negative outcomes for the fetus, mother, or both. A **high-risk pregnancy** is one in which a condition exists that jeopardizes the health of the mother, her fetus, or both. The condition may result from the pregnancy, or it may be a condition that was present before the woman became pregnant.

In Canada, approximately 10% of all pregnancies are considered high risk. According to the Canadian Institute for Health Information (2004), "Pregnancies are deemed high-risk if there is a higher-than-average chance of complications developing. For example, women with a history of medical conditions such as gestational diabetes, heart disease, or those carrying more than one child, may be considered high-risk." The risk status of a woman and her fetus can change during the pregnancy, with a number of problems occurring during labour, birth, or afterward, even in women without any known previous antepartal risk. Examples of high-risk conditions include gestational diabetes and ectopic pregnancy. Early identification of the woman at risk is essential to ensure that appropriate interventions are instituted promptly, increasing the opportunity to change the course of events and provide a positive outcome.

The term "risk" may mean different things to different groups. For example, health care professionals may focus on the disease processes and treatments to prevent complications. Nurses may focus on nursing care and on the psychosocial impact on the woman and her family. The woman's attention may be focused on her own needs and those of her family. Together, working as a collaborative team, the ultimate goal of care is to ensure the best possible outcome for the woman, her fetus, and her family.

Risk assessment begins at the first antepartal visit and continues with each subsequent visit because factors may be identified in later visits that were not apparent during earlier visits. For example, as the nurse and client develop a trusting relationship, previously unidentified or unsuspected factors (such as drug abuse or intimate partner violence) may be revealed. Through education and support, the nurse can encourage the client to inform her health care provider of these concerns, and necessary interventions or referrals can be made.

A comprehensive approach to high-risk pregnancy is needed. For example, prenatal stress and distress have been shown to have significant consequences for the mother, child, and family (Reid, Power, & Cheshire, 2009). Risks are grouped into broad categories based on threats to health and pregnancy outcome. Current categories of risk are biophysical, psychosocial, sociodemographic, and environmental (Gilbert, 2010) (Box 19.1).

This chapter describes the major conditions directly related to the pregnancy that can complicate a pregnancy, possibly affecting maternal and fetal outcomes. These include bleeding during pregnancy (spontaneous abortion, ectopic pregnancy, gestational trophoblastic disease (GTD), cervical insufficiency, placenta previa, and abruptio placentae), hyperemesis gravidarum, gestational hypertension, HELLP (hemolysis, elevated liver enzymes, and low platelets) syndrome, gestational diabetes, blood incompatibility, amniotic fluid imbalances (hydramnios and oligohydramnios), multiple gestation, and premature rupture of membranes. Chapter 20 addresses preexisting conditions that can complicate a woman's pregnancy as well as populations that are considered to be at high risk.

Bleeding During Pregnancy

Bleeding at any time during pregnancy is potentially life-threatening. Bleeding can occur early or late in the pregnancy and may result from numerous conditions. Conditions commonly associated with early bleeding (first half of pregnancy) include spontaneous abortion, ectopic pregnancy, GTD, and conditions associated with midtrimester bleeding, such as cervical insufficiency. Conditions associated with late bleeding include placenta previa and abruptio placentae, which usually occur after the 20th week of gestation.

Spontaneous Abortion

An **abortion** is the loss of an early pregnancy, usually before week 20 of gestation. Abortion can be spontaneous or induced. A spontaneous abortion refers to the loss of a fetus resulting from natural causes—that is, not elective or therapeutically induced by a procedure. The term *miscarriage* is often used by nonmedical people to denote an abortion that has occurred spontaneously. A miscarriage can occur during early pregnancy, and many women who miscarry may not even be aware that they are pregnant. About 80% of spontaneous abortions occur within the first trimester.

The overall rate of spontaneous abortion in Canada is reported to be 8% of recognized pregnancies (Einarson, Choi, Einarson, et al., 2009). However, with the development of highly sensitive assays for human chorionic gonadotropin (hCG) levels that detect pregnancies prior to the expected next menses, the incidence of pregnancy loss increases significantly—from 22% to 57% (Stephenson, 2008).

Pathophysiology

The causes of spontaneous abortion are varied and often unknown. The most common cause for first-trimester abortions is fetal genetic abnormalities, usually unrelated to the mother. The major non-genetic causes, at any time

BOX 19.1 Factors Placing a Woman at Risk During Pregnancy

Biophysical Factors
- Genetic conditions
- Chromosomal abnormalities
- Multiple pregnancy
- Defective genes
- Inherited disorders
- ABO incompatibility
- Large fetal size
- Medical and obstetric conditions
- Preterm labour and birth
- Cardiovascular disease
- Chronic hypertension
- Incompetent cervix
- Placental abnormalities
- Infection
- Diabetes
- Maternal collagen diseases
- Pregnancy-induced hypertension
- Asthma
- Postterm pregnancy
- Hemoglobinopathies
- Nutritional status
- Inadequate dietary intake
- Food fads
- Excessive food intake
- Under- or overweight status
- Hematocrit value less than 33%
- Eating disorder

Psychosocial Factors
- Smoking
- Caffeine
- Alcohol
- Drugs
- Inadequate support system
- Situational crisis
- History of violence
- Emotional distress
- Unsafe cultural practices

Sociodemographic Factors
- Poverty status
- Lack of prenatal care
- Age younger than 15 years or older than 35 years
- Parity—all first pregnancies and more than five pregnancies
- Marital status—increased risk for unmarried
- Accessibility to health care
- Ethnicity—increased risk in nonwhite women

Environmental Factors
- Infections
- Radiation
- Pesticides
- Illicit drugs
- Industrial pollutants
- Secondhand cigarette smoke
- Personal stress

Source: Gilbert, E. (2010). *Manual of high-risk pregnancy and delivery* (5th ed.). St. Louis, MO: Mosby.

in the pregnancy, include maternal–fetal infection, including rubella virus, cytomegalovirus, herpes simplex virus, bacterial vaginosis, and toxoplasmosis; obstetric complications, including placental abruption and hemorrhage; and maternal medical conditions, including diabetes, hypertension, hypothyroidism, and chronic nephritis. (Silver, 2009).

Nursing Assessment

When a pregnant woman calls to report vaginal bleeding, she must be seen as soon as possible by a health care professional to ascertain the etiology. Varying degrees of vaginal bleeding, low back pain, abdominal cramping, and passage of products of conception tissue may be reported. Ask the woman about the colour of the vaginal bleeding (bright red is significant) and the amount—for example, question her about the frequency with which she is changing her peripads (saturation of one peripad hourly is significant) and the passage of any clots or tissue. Instruct her to save any tissue or clots passed and bring them with her to the health care facility. Also obtain a description of any other signs and symptoms the

woman may be experiencing, along with a description of their severity and duration. It is important to remain calm and listen to the woman's description.

When the woman arrives at the health care facility, assess her vital signs and observe the amount, colour, and characteristics of the bleeding. Ask her to rate her current pain level, using an appropriate pain assessment tool. Also evaluate the amount and intensity of the woman's abdominal cramping or contractions, and assess the woman's level of understanding about what is happening to her. A thorough assessment helps in determining the type of spontaneous abortion, such as threatened abortion, inevitable abortion, incomplete abortion, complete abortion, missed abortion, and habitual abortion, that the woman may be experiencing (Table 19.1).

Nursing Management

Nursing management of the woman with a spontaneous abortion focuses on providing continued monitoring and psychological support, for the family is experiencing acute loss and grief. An important component of this support is reassuring the woman that spontaneous abortions usually

TABLE 19.1 CATEGORIES OF SPONTANEOUS ABORTION

Category	Assessment Findings	Diagnosis	Therapeutic Management
Threatened abortion	Vaginal bleeding (often slight) early in a pregnancy No cervical dilation or change in cervical consistency Mild abdominal cramping Closed cervical os No passage of fetal tissue	Vaginal ultrasound to confirm whether sac is empty Declining maternal serum hCG and progesterone levels to provide additional information about viability of pregnancy	Conservative supportive treatment Possible reduction in activity in conjunction with nutritious diet and adequate hydration
Inevitable abortion	Vaginal bleeding (greater than that associated with threatened abortion) Rupture of membranes Cervical dilation Strong abdominal cramping Possible passage of products of conception	Ultrasound and hCG levels to indicate pregnancy loss	Vacuum curettage if products of conception are not passed, to reduce risk for excessive bleeding and infection Prostaglandin analogues such as misoprostol to empty uterus of retained tissue (only used if fragments are not completely passed)
Incomplete abortion (passage of some of the products of conception)	Intense abdominal cramping Heavy vaginal bleeding Cervical dilation	Ultrasound confirmation that products of conception are still in uterus	Client stabilization Evacuation of uterus via dilation and curettage (D&C) or prostaglandin analogue
Complete abortion (passage of all products of conception)	History of vaginal bleeding and abdominal pain Passage of tissue with subsequent decrease in pain and significant decrease in vaginal bleeding	Ultrasound demonstrating an empty uterus	No medical or surgical intervention necessary Follow-up appointment to discuss family planning
Missed abortion (nonviable embryo retained in utero for at least 6 weeks)	Absent uterine contractions Irregular spotting Possible progression to inevitable abortion	Ultrasound to identify products of conception in uterus	Evacuation of uterus (if inevitable abortion does not occur): suction curettage during first trimester, dilation and evacuation during second trimester Induction of labour with intravaginal PGE2 suppository to empty uterus without surgical intervention
Habitual abortion	History of three or more consecutive spontaneous abortions Not carrying the pregnancy to viability or term	Validation via client's history	Identification and treatment of underlying cause (possible causes such as genetic or chromosomal abnormalities, reproductive tract abnormalities, chronic diseases or immunologic problems) Cervical cerclage in second trimester if incompetent cervix is the cause

result from an abnormality and that her actions did not cause the abortion.

Providing Continued Monitoring

Continued monitoring and ongoing assessments are essential for the woman experiencing a spontaneous abortion. Monitor the amount of vaginal bleeding through pad counts and observe for passage of products of conception tissue. Assess the woman's pain and provide appropriate pain management to address the cramping discomfort.

Assist in preparing the woman for procedures and treatments such as surgery to evacuate the uterus or medications such as misoprostol or prostaglandin E2 (PGE2). If the woman is Rh negative and not sensitized, expect to administer Rh immune globulin (WinRho) within 72 hours after the abortion is complete. Drug Guide 19.1 gives more information about these medications.

Providing Support

A woman's emotional reaction may vary depending on her desire for this pregnancy and her available support network. Provide both physical and emotional support. In addition, prepare the woman and her family for the assessment process, and answer their questions about what is happening.

Explaining some of the causes of spontaneous abortions can help the woman to understand what is happening and may allay her fears and guilt that she did something to cause this pregnancy loss. Most women experience an acute sense of loss and go through a grieving process with a spontaneous abortion. Providing sensitive listening, counselling, and anticipatory guidance to the woman and her family will allow them to verbalize their feelings and ask questions about future pregnancies.

The grieving period may last as long as 2 years after a pregnancy loss, with each person grieving in his or her own way. Encourage friends and family to be supportive but give the couple space and time to work through their loss. Referral to a community support group for parents who have experienced a miscarriage can be very helpful during this grief process.

DRUG GUIDE 19.1 MEDICATIONS USED FOR SPONTANEOUS ABORTIONS

Medication	Action/Indications	Nursing Implications
Misoprostol (Cytotec)	Stimulates uterine contractions to terminate a pregnancy Evacuates the uterus after abortion to ensure passage of all the products of conception	Monitor for side effects such as diarrhea, abdominal pain, nausea, vomiting, dyspepsia. Assess vaginal bleeding and report any increased bleeding, pain, or fever. Monitor for signs and symptoms of shock, such as tachycardia, hypotension, and anxiety.
Mifepristone (RU-486)	Acts as progesterone antagonist, allowing prostaglandins to stimulate uterine contractions; causes the endometrium to slough May be followed by administration of misoprostol within 48 h	Monitor for headache, vomiting, diarrhea, and heavy bleeding. Anticipate administration of antiemetic prior to use to reduce nausea and vomiting. Encourage client to use acetaminophen to reduce discomfort from cramping.
PGE2, dinoprostone (Cervidil, Prepidil Gel, Prostin E2)	Stimulates uterine contractions, causing expulsion of uterine contents Expels uterine contents in fetal death or missed abortion during second trimester Effaces and dilates the cervix in pregnancy at term	Bring gel to room temperature before administering. Avoid contact with skin. Administer using sterile technique. Keep client supine 30 min after administering. Document time of insertion and dosing intervals. Remove insert with retrieval system after 12 h or at the onset of labour. Explain purpose and expected response to client.
Rh(D) immunoglobulin (WinRho, Gamulin, HydroRho-D, RhoGAM)	Suppresses immune response of non-sensitized Rh-negative patients who are exposed to Rh-positive blood Prevents isoimmunization in Rh-negative women exposed to Rh-positive blood after abortions, miscarriages, and pregnancies	Administer intramuscularly in deltoid area. Give only WinRho for abortions and miscarriages <12 weeks unless fetus or father is Rh negative (unless patient is Rh positive, Rh antibodies are present). Educate woman that she will need this after subsequent deliveries if newborns are Rh positive; also check lab study results prior to administering the drug.

Ectopic Pregnancy

An **ectopic pregnancy** is any pregnancy in which the fertilized ovum implants outside the uterine cavity. In Canada, ectopic and molar pregnancies account for a maternal mortality ratio of 2 per 1,000,000, live births (Public Health Agency of Canada [PHAC], 2008). Between 2004 and 2005, the ectopic pregnancy rate was 11.9 per 1,000 reported pregnancies, with varying incidences across provinces and territories. In Prince Edward Island, there were 6.4 per 1,000 reported pregnancies, while in the Northwest Territories, the rate was 31.8 per 1,000 reported pregnancies. The rates increase from east to west as well as with increasing maternal age and the presence of sexually transmitted infections (STIs). Canadian data on ectopic pregnancy are limited by the data collection process: in-patient data were gathered, but data were not collected from day surgery and out-patient settings. More sensitive serum hCG testing and the use of transvaginal ultrasound have resulted in the earlier detection of ectopic pregnancies (Peel, 2009).

With an ectopic pregnancy, rupture and hemorrhage may occur due to the growth of the embryo. A ruptured ectopic pregnancy is a medical emergency. It is a potentially life-threatening condition and involves pregnancy loss. According to Murray, Baakdah, Bardell, et al. (2005), "Ectopic pregnancy remains an important cause of maternal death, accounting for about 4% of the approximately 20 annual pregnancy-related deaths in Canada" (p. 905).

Pathophysiology

Normally, the fertilized ovum implants in the uterus. With an ectopic pregnancy, the ovum implants outside the uterus. The most common site for implantation is the fallopian tubes, but some ova may implant in the ovary, the cervix, or the abdominal cavity (Fig. 19.1) (Varma & Gupta, 2009). None of these anatomic sites can accommodate placental attachment or a growing embryo.

Ectopic pregnancies usually result from conditions that obstruct or slow the passage of the fertilized ovum through the fallopian tube to the uterus. This may be a physical blockage in the tube or failure of the tubal epithelium to move the zygote (the cell formed after the egg is fertilized) down the tube into the uterus. In the general population, most cases are the result of tubal scarring secondary to pelvic inflammatory disease (PID). Organisms such as *Neisseria gonorrhoeae* and *Chlamydia trachomatis* may cause tubal pathology. Gibbs, Danforth, Karlan, et al. (2008) reported a two- to fourfold increased risk of ectopic pregnancy in women with a history of a chlamydia, gonorrhea, and/or nonspecific PID. Even with early treatment, tubal damage can occur.

Therapeutic Management

The therapeutic management of ectopic pregnancy depends on whether the tube is intact or has ruptured.

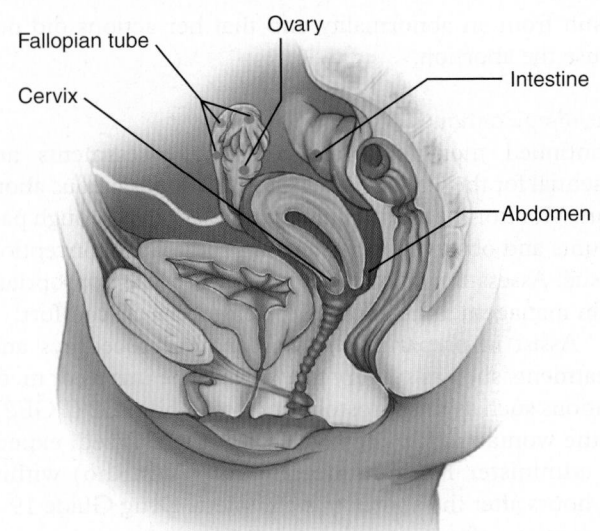

FIGURE 19.1 Possible sites for implantation with an ectopic pregnancy.

Historically, the treatment of ectopic pregnancy was limited to surgery, but medical therapy is currently available.

If the fallopian tube is still intact, medical management becomes an option. To be eligible for medical therapy, the client must be hemodynamically stable with a mass measuring less than 3.5 cm, have no signs of tubal rupture, show no fetal cardiac activity, and agree to frequent out-patient follow-up (Varma & Gupta, 2009). The potential advantages of medical management include avoidance of surgery, the preservation of tubal patency and function, and lower cost. Methotrexate is the most commonly used agent in the medical (nonsurgical) management of ectopic pregnancy (Lipscomb, 2011; Sepilian, 2011). Surgery is used for the treatment of hemodynamic unstable patients, patients who want no further pregnancies, or patients who are unsuitable or do not want to risk medical treatment with methotrexate (Lipscomb, 2011).

Methotrexate is a folic acid antagonist that inhibits cell division in the developing embryo. It typically has been used as a chemotherapeutic agent in the treatment of leukemias, lymphomas, and carcinomas. It has been shown to be very effective without the potential for fallopian tube damage, infertility complications, and other risks associated with surgical interventions (Lavanya, Deepika, & Patil, 2009). Adverse effects associated with methotrexate include nausea, vomiting, stomatitis, diarrhea, gastric upset, increased abdominal pain, and dizziness. Prior to receiving the single-dose intramuscular injection to treat unruptured pregnancies, the woman needs to be counselled on the risks, benefits, adverse effects, and possibility of failure of medical therapy, which would result in tubal rupture, necessitating surgery (Stucki & Buss, 2008). The woman is then instructed to return weekly for follow-up laboratory studies for the next several weeks until beta-hCG titers decrease.

Surgical management for the unruptured fallopian tube might involve a linear salpingostomy to preserve the tube—an important consideration for the woman wanting to preserve her future fertility.

With a ruptured ectopic pregnancy, surgery is necessary as a result of possible uncontrolled hemorrhage. A laparotomy with removal of the tube (salpingectomy) may be necessary. With earlier diagnosis and medical management, the focus has changed from preventing maternal death to facilitating rapid recovery and preserving fertility.

Regardless of the treatment approach (medical or surgical), the woman's beta-hCG level is monitored until it is undetectable to ensure that any residual trophoblastic tissue that forms the placenta is gone. Also, all Rh-negative unsensitized clients are given WinRho to prevent isoimmunization in future pregnancies. See Evidence-based Practice 19.1.

Nursing Assessment

Nursing assessment focuses on determining the existence of an ectopic pregnancy and whether or not it has ruptured.

Health History and Physical Examination

Assess the client thoroughly for signs and symptoms that may suggest an ectopic pregnancy. The onset of signs and symptoms varies, but they usually begin at about the seventh or eighth week of gestation. A missed menstrual period, adnexal fullness, and tenderness may indicate an unruptured tubal pregnancy. As the tube stretches, the pain increases. Pain may be unilateral, bilateral, or diffuse over the abdomen.

▶ **Take** NOTE!

The hallmark of ectopic pregnancy is abdominal pain with spotting within 6 to 8 weeks after a missed menstrual period. Although this is the classic triad, all three of these signs and symptoms occur in only about 50% of cases. Many women have symptoms typical of early pregnancy, such as breast tenderness, nausea, fatigue, shoulder pain, and low back pain.

In addition, review the client's history for possible contributing factors. These may include:

- PID
- Previous treatment of gonorrhea and/or chlamydia
- Prior ectopic pregnancy
- Prior tubal surgery and conception after tubal ligation
- Use of an intrauterine device

EVIDENCE-BASED PRACTICE 19.1
Ectopic Pregnancy: Selecting the Best Intervention

● **Study**

The incidence of ectopic pregnancy, which involves implantation of the fertilized ovum outside the uterine cavity, has increased over the past several decades due to advances in diagnostic methods. The most common site for implantation is in the fallopian tube (thus the name tubal pregnancy). If left untreated, tubal rupture and hemorrhage can occur. At one time, surgery was the only available treatment option. However, treatment today may involve expectant care, medication therapy, or surgery (laparoscopic or open approach). Questions have arisen as to the effectiveness and safety of these treatments.

A study was conducted to evaluate the effectiveness of major types of treatment for ectopic pregnancy. Data were collected from 35 randomized controlled trials that compared the treatments for ectopic pregnancies.

▲ **Findings**

The open approach to surgery was significantly more effective in removing the ectopic pregnancy than the laparoscopic approach, but the laparoscopic approach was more cost-effective. Medication therapy involving fixed multiple doses of methotrexate was effective in women who had low pregnancy hormone levels without any evidence of bleeding. Expectant management was less successful than drug therapy, but the information on this treatment option was inadequate.

■ **Nursing Implications**

This study identified three important treatment options available to a woman with an ectopic pregnancy. Nurses can use this information in their practice as a basis for formulating a teaching plan about treatment options and when reviewing the health care provider's recommendations for treatment. As a result, women can make a more informed decision. Nurses also can advocate for medication therapy for women who have low pregnancy hormone levels and no bleeding.

Source: Hajenius, P. J., Mol, F., Mol, B. W. J., Bossuyt, P. M. M., Ankum, W. M., & van der Veen, F. (2009). Interventions for tubal ectopic pregnancy. *Cochrane Database of Systematic Reviews, 1,* CD000324. Retrieved March 9, 2012 from http://onlinelibrary.wiley.com/doi/10.1002/14651858. CD000324.pub2/abstract.

- Cigarette smoking
- Use of fertility drugs or assisted reproductive technology
- Age between 35 and 44
- Prior diethylstilbestrol (DES) exposure
- Salpingitis isthmica nodosa
- A T-shaped uterus
- Prior abdominal surgery
- Pregnancy due to a failure with progestin-only contraception
- Prior ruptured appendix (Sepilian & Wood, 2011)

If rupture or hemorrhage occurs before treatment begins, symptoms may worsen and include severe, sharp, and sudden pain in the lower abdomen as the tube tears open and the embryo is expelled into the pelvic cavity; feelings of faintness; referred pain to the shoulder area, indicating bleeding into the abdomen, caused by phrenic nerve irritation; hypotension; marked abdominal tenderness with distention; and hypovolemic shock.

Laboratory and Diagnostic Testing

The use of transvaginal ultrasound to visualize the misplaced pregnancy and low levels of serum beta-hCG assist in diagnosing an ectopic pregnancy. The ultrasound determines whether the pregnancy is intrauterine, assesses the size of the uterus, and provides evidence of fetal viability. The visualization of an adnexal mass and the absence of an intrauterine gestational sac are diagnostic for ectopic pregnancy (Madani, 2008). In a normal intrauterine pregnancy, beta-hCG levels typically double every 2 to 4 days until peak values are reached 60 to 90 days after conception. Concentrations of hCG peak at week 10, then decline steadily until reaching a low-level plateau by week 14 to 18 (Cole, 2010). Therefore, low beta-hCG levels are suggestive of an ectopic pregnancy or impending abortion. Additional tests may be done to rule out other conditions such as spontaneous abortion, ruptured ovarian cyst, appendicitis, and salpingitis.

Nursing Management

Nursing management for the woman with an ectopic pregnancy focuses on preparing the woman for treatment, providing support, and providing education about preventive measures.

Preparing the Woman for Treatment

Administer analgesics as ordered to relieve discomfort from abdominal pain. Although the intensity of the pain can vary, women often report a great deal of pain. If the woman is treated medically, explain the medication that will be used and what she can expect. Also review signs and symptoms of possible adverse effects. If treatment will occur on an out-patient basis, outline the signs and symptoms of ectopic rupture (severe, sharp, stabbing, unilateral abdominal pain; vertigo/fainting; hypotension;

and increased pulse) and advise the woman to seek medical help immediately if any of these symptoms occur.

If surgery is needed, close assessment and monitoring of the client's vital signs, bleeding (peritoneal or vaginal), and pain status are critical to identify hypovolemic shock, which may occur with tubal rupture. Prepare the client physiologically and psychologically for surgery or any procedure. Provide a clear explanation of the expected outcome. Astute vigilance and early referral will help reduce short- and long-term morbidity.

Providing Emotional Support

The woman with an ectopic pregnancy requires support throughout diagnosis, treatment, and aftercare. A woman's psychological reaction to an ectopic pregnancy is unpredictable. However, it is important to recognize she has experienced a pregnancy loss in addition to undergoing treatment for a potentially life-threatening condition. The woman may find it difficult to comprehend what has happened to her because events occur so quickly. In the woman's mind, she had just started a pregnancy and now it has ended abruptly. Help her to make this experience "more real" by encouraging her and her family to express their feelings and concerns openly, and validating that this is a loss of pregnancy and it is okay to grieve over the loss.

Provide emotional support, spiritual care, client education, and information about community support groups available (a variety of programs exist across Canada) as the client grieves for the loss of her unborn child and comes to terms with the medical complications of the situation. Acknowledge the client's pregnancy and allow her to discuss her feelings about what the pregnancy means. Also, stress the need for follow-up blood testing for several weeks to monitor hCG titers until they return to zero, indicating resolution of the ectopic pregnancy. Ask about her feelings and concerns about her future fertility, and provide teaching about the need to use contraceptives for at least three menstrual cycles to allow her reproductive tract to heal and the tissue to be repaired. Include the woman's partner in this discussion to make sure both parties understand what has happened, what intervention is needed, and what the future holds regarding childbearing.

Educating the Client

Preventing ectopic pregnancies through screening and client education is essential. Many can be prevented by avoiding conditions that might cause scarring of the fallopian tubes. In addition, a contributing factor to the development of ectopic pregnancy is a previous ectopic pregnancy. Therefore, educating the woman is crucial.

Prevention education may include the following:

- Reduce risk factors such as sexual intercourse with multiple partners or intercourse without a condom.

- Avoid contracting STIs that lead to PID.
- Obtain early diagnosis and adequate treatment of STIs.
- Avoid the use of intrauterine contraceptive methods to reduce the risk for repeat ascending infections, which can be responsible for tubal scarring.
- Use condoms to decrease the risk for infections that cause tubal scarring.
- Seek prenatal care early to confirm the location of pregnancy.

Gestational Trophoblastic Disease

Gestational trophoblastic disease (GTD) comprises a spectrum of neoplastic disorders that originate in the placenta. Gestational tissue is present, but the pregnancy is not viable. The incidence is about 0.6 to 1.1 in 1,000 pregnancies in North America (Gerulath, 2002). The two most common types of GTD are hydatidiform mole (partial and complete) and choriocarcinoma.

Pathophysiology

Hydatidiform mole is a benign neoplasm of the chorion in which the chorionic villi degenerate and become transparent vesicles containing clear, viscid fluid. Hydatidiform mole is classified as complete or partial. The complete mole contains no fetal tissue and develops from an "empty egg," which is fertilized by a normal sperm (the paternal chromosomes replicate, resulting in 46 all-paternal chromosomes). The embryo is not viable and dies. No circulation is established, and no embryonic tissue is found. The complete mole is associated with the development of choriocarcinoma. The partial mole has a triploid karyotype (69 chromosomes) because two sperm have provided a double contribution by fertilizing the ovum (Fig. 19.2).

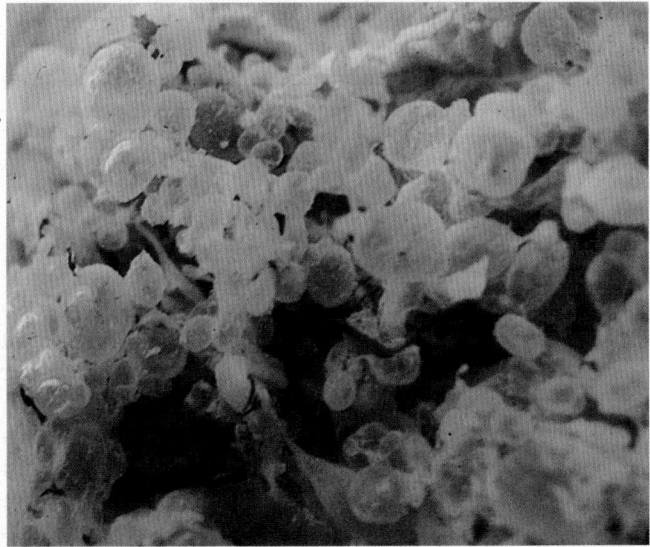

FIGURE 19.2 Complete hydatidiform mole. The chorionic villi degenerate and become filled with a viscid fluid, forming transparent vesicles.

> ▶ *Consider* THIS!
>
> *We had lived across the dorm hall from each other during nursing school but really didn't get to know each other except for a casual hello in passing. When we graduated, Rose went to work in the emergency room and I in OB. We saw each other occasionally in the employee cafeteria, but a quick hello was all that we usually exchanged. I heard she married one of the paramedics who worked in the ER and was soon pregnant. I finally got to say more than hello when she was admitted to the OB unit bleeding during her fourth month of pregnancy. What was discovered was gestational trophoblastic disease and not a normal pregnancy. I remember holding her in my arms as she wept. After surgery, she was told she had a complete molar pregnancy and would need extensive follow-up for the next year. I lost track of her that summer as my life became busier. Around Thanksgiving time, I heard she had died from choriocarcinoma. I attended her funeral, finally, to get the time to say a final hello and good-bye, but this time with sadness and tears.*
>
> *Thoughts: Rose was only 26 years old when she succumbed to this very virulent cancer. I think back and realize I missed knowing this brave young woman and wished that I had taken the time to say more than hello. Could her outcome have been different? Why wasn't it recognized earlier? Did she not follow up after her diagnosis? I can only speculate regarding the whom, what, and where. She lived a short but purposeful life, and hopefully continued research will change other women's outcomes in the future.*

The exact cause of molar pregnancy is unknown, but researchers are looking into a genetic basis. Studies have revealed some remarkable features about molar pregnancies, including:

- Ability to invade into the wall of the uterus
- Tendency to recur in subsequent pregnancies
- Possible development into choriocarcinoma, a virulent cancer with metastasis to other organs
- Influence of nutritional factors, such as protein deficiency
- Tendency to affect older women more often than younger women

Having a molar pregnancy (partial or complete) results in the loss of the pregnancy and the possibility of developing choriocarcinoma, a chorionic malignancy from the trophoblastic tissue. The most frequent sites of metastases are the lungs, lower genital tract, brain, liver, and kidney (Sierra-Bergua, Sánchez-Marteles, Cabrerizo-García, 2008).

Therapeutic Management

Treatment consists of immediate evacuation of the uterine contents as soon as the diagnosis is made and long-term follow-up of the client to detect any remaining trophoblastic tissue that might become malignant. Dilation and suction curettage (D&C) is used to empty the uterus. The tissue obtained is sent to the laboratory for analysis to evaluate for choriocarcinoma. Serial levels of hCG are used to detect residual trophoblastic tissue for 1 year. If any tissue remains, hCG levels will not regress. In 80% of women with a benign hydatidiform mole, serum hCG titers steadily drop to normal within 8 to 12 weeks after evacuation of the molar pregnancy. In the other 20% of women with a malignant hydatidiform mole, serum hCG levels begin to rise (Hernandez, 2012).

Due to the increased risk for cancer, the client is advised to receive extensive follow-up therapy for the next 12 months. The follow-up protocol may include:

- Baseline hCG level, chest radiograph, and pelvic ultrasound
- Weekly serum hCG level until it drops to zero and remains at that level for 3 consecutive weeks, then monthly for 6 months, then every 2 months for the remainder of the year
- Chest radiograph every 6 months to detect pulmonary metastasis
- Regular pelvic examinations to assess uterine and ovarian regression
- Systemic assessments for symptoms indicative of lung, brain, liver, or vaginal metastasis
- Strong recommendation to avoid pregnancy for 1 year because the pregnancy can interfere with the monitoring of hCG levels
- Use of a reliable contraceptive for at least 1 year (Gilbert, 2010)

Nursing Assessment

The nurse plays a crucial role in identifying and bringing this condition to the attention of the health care provider based on sound knowledge of the typical clinical manifestations and through astute antepartal assessments.

Clinical manifestations of GTD are very similar to those of spontaneous abortion at about 12 weeks of pregnancy. Assess the woman for potential clinical manifestations at each antepartal visit. Be alert for the following:

- Early signs of pregnancy, such as amenorrhea, breast tenderness, fatigue
- Brownish vaginal bleeding/spotting
- Anemia
- Severe morning sickness (due to high hCG levels)
- Fluid retention and swelling
- Uterine size larger than expected for pregnancy dates
- Extremely high hCG levels present; no single value considered diagnostic

- Early development of pre-eclampsia (usually not present until after 24 weeks)
- Absence of fetal heart rate or fetal activity
- Expulsion of grape-like vesicles (possible in some women)

The diagnosis is made by high hCG levels and the characteristic appearance of the vesicular molar pattern in the uterus via transvaginal ultrasound.

Nursing Management

Nursing management of the woman with GTD focuses on preparing her for a D&C, providing emotional support to deal with the loss and potential risks, and educating her about the risk that cancer may develop after a molar pregnancy and the strict adherence needed with the follow-up program. The woman must understand the need for the continued follow-up care regimen to improve her chances of becoming pregnant in the future and to ensure her continued quality of life.

Preparing the Client

Upon diagnosis, the client will need an immediate evacuation of the uterus. Perform preoperative care, preparing the client physically and psychologically for the procedure.

Providing Emotional Support

To aid the client and her family in coping with the loss of the pregnancy and the possibility of a cancer diagnosis, use the following interventions:

- Listen to their concerns and fears.
- Allow them time to grieve for the pregnancy loss.
- Acknowledge their loss and sad feelings (say you are sorry for their loss).
- Encourage them to express their grief; allow them to cry.
- Provide them with as much factual information as possible to help them make sense of what is happening.
- Enlist support from additional family and friends as appropriate and with the client's permission.

Educating the Client

After GTD is diagnosed, teach the client about the condition and appropriate interventions that may be necessary to save her life. Explain each phase of treatment accurately and provide support for the woman and her family as they go through the grieving process.

As with any facet of health care, be aware of the latest research and new therapies. Inform the client about her follow-up care, which will probably involve close clinical surveillance for approximately 1 year, and reinforce its importance in monitoring the client's condition. Tell the client that serial serum beta-hCG levels are used to detect residual trophoblastic tissue. Continued high or increasing hCG titers are abnormal and need further evaluation.

Inform the client about the possible use of chemotherapy, such as methotrexate, which may be started as prophylaxis. Strongly urge the client to use a reliable contraceptive to prevent pregnancy for 1 year, as a pregnancy would interfere with tracking the serial beta-hCG levels used to identify a potential malignancy. Stress the need for the client to cooperate and adhere to the plan of therapy throughout this year-long follow-up.

Cervical Insufficiency

Cervical insufficiency, also called premature dilation of the cervix, describes a weak, structurally defective cervix that spontaneously dilates in the absence of contractions in the second trimester, resulting in the loss of the pregnancy. The incidence of cervical insufficiency is less than 1%; estimates range from 1 in 500 to 1 in 2,000 pregnancies, accounting for approximately 20% to 25% of midtrimester losses (Fox & Chervenak, 2008).

Pathophysiology

The exact mechanism contributing to cervical insufficiency is not known. Some studies have linked the incompetent cervix with having less collagen and more smooth muscle than the normal cervix, while others have disproven this link (Oxlund, Ørtoft, Brüel, et al., 2010). Several theories have been proposed that focus on damage to the cervix as a key component.

Cervical insufficiency is likely to be the clinical end point of many pathologic processes, such as congenital cervical disorders, deep cervical laceration secondary to prior vaginal or cesarean birth, infection/inflammation, trauma to the cervix (conization, amputation, obstetric laceration, or forced cervical dilation, which may occur during elective pregnancy termination). However, the exact etiology of cervical insufficiency is not known.

Cervical length also has been associated with cervical insufficiency and subsequently preterm birth. Recent studies have examined the association between a short cervical length and the risk for preterm birth. Some have demonstrated a continuum of risk between a shorter cervix on ultrasound and a higher risk for preterm birth, leading to the hypothetical argument that women with a short cervix on ultrasound might benefit from cervical cerclage, but there have been conflicting results (Mancuso & Owen, 2009).

Therapeutic Management

Cervical insufficiency may be treated in a variety of ways: bed rest, pelvic rest, avoidance of heavy lifting, or surgically, via a procedure of cervical cerclage in the second trimester. Cervical cerclage involves using a heavy purse-string suture to secure and reinforce the internal os of the cervix (Fig. 19.3).

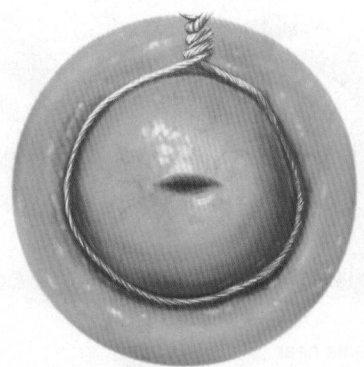

FIGURE 19.3 Cervical cerclage.

According to the Society of Obstetricians and Gynaecologists of Canada (SOGC), to reduce the risk for preterm labour, cervical cerclage should be considered for asymptomatic pregnant women with a history of preterm birth and a cervical measurement of less than 25 mm prior to 24 weeks' gestation (Lim, Butt, & Crane, 2011). Asymptomatic women are defined as those with no signs of infections, are not in labour, and who's membranes are intact.

Nursing Assessment

Nursing assessment focuses on obtaining a thorough history to determine any risk factors that might have a bearing on this pregnancy—previous cervical trauma, preterm labour, fetal loss in the second trimester, or previous surgeries or procedures involving the cervix. History may reveal a previous loss of pregnancy around 20 weeks.

Also be alert for complaints of vaginal discharge or pelvic pressure. Commonly with cervical insufficiency the woman will report a pink-tinged vaginal discharge or an increase in pelvic pressure. Cervical dilation also occurs. If this continues, rupture of the membranes, release of amniotic fluid, and uterine contractions occur, subsequently resulting in delivery of the fetus, often before it is viable.

▶ *Take* NOTE!

The diagnosis of cervical insufficiency remains difficult in many circumstances. The cornerstone of diagnosis is a history of midtrimester pregnancy loss associated with painless cervical dilation without evidence of uterine activity.

Transvaginal ultrasound typically is done around 20 weeks' gestation to determine cervical length and evaluate for shortening. Cervical shortening occurs from the internal os outward and can be viewed on ultrasound as funnelling. The amount of funnelling can be determined by dividing funnel length by cervical length. The most

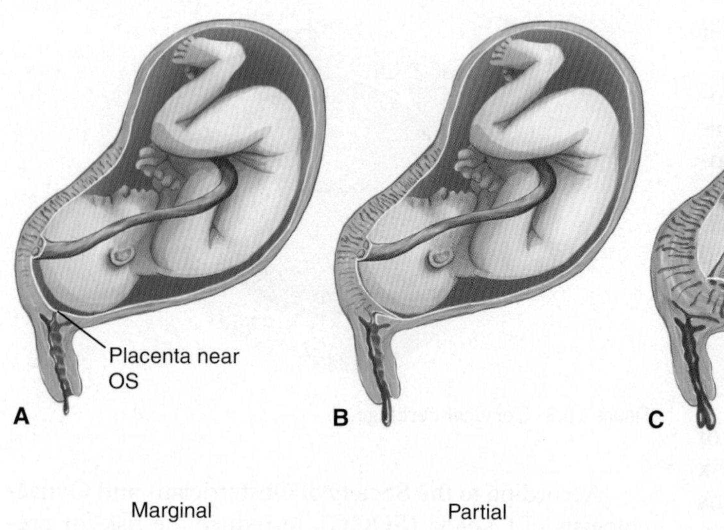

FIGURE 19.4 Classification of placenta previa. (**A**) Marginal. (**B**) Partial. (**C**) Complete.

common time at which a short cervix or funnelling develops is 18 to 22 weeks, so ultrasound screening should be performed during this interval (Fox & Chervenak, 2008). A cervical length less than 25 mm is abnormal between 14 and 24 weeks and may increase the risk for preterm labour.

Nursing Management

Nursing management focuses on monitoring the woman very closely for signs of preterm labour: backache, increased vaginal discharge, rupture of membranes, and uterine contractions. Provide emotional support and education to allay the couple's anxiety about the well-being of their fetus. Provide preoperative care and teaching as indicated if the woman will be undergoing cerclage. Teach the client and her family about the signs and symptoms of preterm labour and the need to report any changes immediately. Also reinforce the need for activity restrictions (if appropriate) and continued regular follow-up. Continuing surveillance throughout the pregnancy is important to promote a positive outcome for the family.

Placenta Previa

Placenta previa is a bleeding condition that occurs during the last two trimesters of pregnancy. In placenta previa (literally, "afterbirth first"), the placenta implants over the cervical os. This condition may cause serious morbidity and mortality to the fetus and the mother. It complicates approximately 3.5 to 6 of every 1,000 births and is associated with potentially serious consequences from hemorrhage, abruption (separation) of the placenta, preterm birth, or emergency cesarean birth (Bahar, Abusham, Eskandar, et al., 2009; Joy, Lyon, & Stone, 2010).

Pathophysiology

The exact cause of placenta previa is unknown. It is initiated by implantation of the embryo in the lower uterus.

With placental attachment and growth, the cervical os may become covered by the developing placenta. Placental vascularization is defective, allowing the placenta to attach directly to the myometrium (accreta), invade the myometrium (increta), or penetrate the myometrium (percreta).

Placenta previa is generally classified according to the degree of coverage or proximity to the internal os, as follows (Fig. 19.4):

- Complete placenta previa: the internal cervical os is completely covered by the placenta
- Partial placenta previa: the internal os is partially covered by the placenta
- Marginal placenta previa: the placenta is at the margin or edge of the internal os
- Low-lying placenta previa: the placenta is implanted in the lower uterine segment and is near the internal os but does not reach it

Therapeutic Management

Therapeutic management depends on the extent of bleeding, the amount of placenta over the cervical os, whether the fetus is developed enough to survive outside the uterus, the position of the fetus, the mother's parity, and the presence or absence of labour (Zeltzer, 2011).

If the mother and fetus are both stable, therapeutic management may involve expectant ("wait-and-see") care. This care can be carried out at home or on an antepartal unit in the health care facility. If there is no active bleeding and the client has readily available access to reliable transportation, can maintain bed rest at home, and can comprehend instructions, expectant care at home is appropriate. However, if the client requires continuous care and monitoring and cannot meet the home care requirements, the antepartal unit is the best environment.

Nursing Assessment

Nursing assessment involves a thorough history, including possible risk factors, and physical examination. Evaluate the client closely for these risk factors:

- Advancing maternal age (more than 35 years)
- Previous cesarean birth
- Multiparity
- Uterine insult or injury
- Prior placenta previa
- Multiple gestations
- Previous induced surgical abortion
- Smoking (Ko & Yoon, 2011)

Health History and Physical Examination

Ask the client if she has had any problems associated with bleeding, now or in the recent past. The classic clinical presentation is painless, bright-red vaginal bleeding occurring during the second or third trimester. The initial bleeding usually is not profuse and it ceases spontaneously, only to recur. The first episode of bleeding occurs (on average) at 27 to 32 weeks' gestation. The bleeding is thought to arise secondary to the thinning of the lower uterine segment in preparation for the onset of labour. When the bleeding occurs at the implantation site in the lower uterus, the uterus cannot contract adequately and stop the flow of blood from the open vessels. Typically with normal placental implantation in the upper uterus, minor disruptive placental attachment is not a problem because there is a larger volume of myometrial tissue able to contract and constrict bleeding vessels.

Assess the client for uterine contractions, which may or may not occur with the bleeding. Palpate the uterus; typically it is soft and nontender on examination. Auscultate the fetal heart rate; it commonly is within normal parameters. Fetal distress is usually absent but may occur when cord problems arise, such as umbilical cord prolapse or cord compression, or when the client has experienced blood loss to the extent that maternal shock or placental abruption has occurred (Liston, Sawchuk, & Young, 2007).

Laboratory and Diagnostic Testing

To validate the position of the placenta, a transvaginal ultrasound is done. In addition, magnetic resonance imaging may be ordered when preparing for delivery because it allows identification of placenta accreta (placenta abnormally adherent to the myometrium), increta (placenta accreta with penetration of the myometrium), or percreta (placenta accreta with invasion of the myometrium to the peritoneal covering, causing rupture of the uterus) in addition to placenta previa. These placental abnormalities, although rare, carry a very high morbidity and mortality rate, possibly necessitating a hysterectomy at delivery.

Nursing Management

Whether the care setting is in the client's home or in the health care facility, the nurse focuses on monitoring the maternal–fetal status, including assessing for signs and symptoms of vaginal bleeding and fetal distress, and providing support and education to the client and her family, including what events and diagnostic studies are being performed. For the majority of women, a cesarean birth will be planned. Nursing Care Plan 19.1 discusses the nursing process for the woman with placenta previa.

Monitoring Maternal–Fetal Status

Assess the degree of vaginal bleeding; inspect the perineal area for blood that may be pooled underneath the woman. Estimate and document the amount of bleeding. Perform a peripad count on an ongoing basis, making sure to report any changes in amount or frequency to the health care provider. If the woman is experiencing active bleeding, prepare for blood typing and cross-matching in the event a blood transfusion is needed.

▶ *Take* NOTE!

Avoid performing vaginal examinations in the woman with placenta previa. They may disrupt the placenta and cause hemorrhage.

Monitor maternal vital signs and uterine contractility frequently for changes. Have the client rate her level of pain using an appropriate pain rating scale.

Assess fetal heart rates via Doppler or electronic monitoring to detect fetal distress. Monitor the woman's cardiopulmonary status, reporting any difficulties in respirations, changes in skin colour, or complaints of difficulty breathing. Have oxygen equipment readily available should fetal or maternal distress develop. Encourage the client to lie on her side to enhance placental perfusion.

If the woman has an intravenous (IV) line inserted, inspect the IV site frequently. Alternately, anticipate the insertion of an intermittent IV access device such as a saline lock, which can be used if quick access is needed for fluid restoration and infusion of blood products. Obtain laboratory tests as ordered, including complete blood count (CBC), coagulation studies, and Rh status if appropriate.

Administer pharmacologic agents as necessary. Give WinRho if the client is Rh negative at 28 weeks' gestation. Monitor tocolytic medication if prevention of preterm labour is needed.

Providing Support and Education

Determine the woman's level of understanding about placenta previa and the associated procedures and treatment plan. Doing so is important to prevent confusion

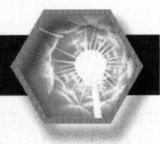

Nursing Care Plan 19.1

OVERVIEW OF THE WOMAN WITH PLACENTA PREVIA

Sandy, a 39-year-old G5, P4, multigravida client at 32 weeks' gestation, was admitted to the labour and birth suite with sudden vaginal bleeding. Sandy had no further active bleeding and did not complain of any abdominal discomfort or tenderness. She did complain of occasional "tightening" in her stomach. Her abdomen palpated soft. Fetal heart rates were in the 140s with accelerations with movement. Sandy was placed on bed rest with bathroom privileges. Ultrasound identified a low-lying placenta with a viable, normal-growth fetus. She was diagnosed with placenta previa and admitted for observation and surveillance of fetal well-being. Her history revealed two previous cesarean births, smoking half a pack of cigarettes per day, and endometritis infection after the birth of her last child. Additional assessment findings included painless, bright-red vaginal bleeding with initial bleeding ceasing spontaneously; irregular, mild, and sporadic uterine contractions; fetal heart rate and maternal vital signs within normal range; fetus in transverse lie; anxiety related to the outcome of pregnancy; and expression of feelings of helplessness.

NURSING DIAGNOSIS: Ineffective tissue perfusion (fetal and maternal) related to blood loss

Outcome Identification and Evaluation
Client will maintain adequate tissue perfusion as evidenced by stable vital signs, decreased blood loss, few or no uterine contractions, normal fetal heart rate patterns and variability, and positive fetal movement

Interventions: Maintaining Adequate Tissue Perfusion
- Establish IV access *to allow for administration of fluids, blood, and medications as necessary.*
- Obtain type and cross-match for at least 2 U of blood products *to ensure availability should bleeding continue.*
- Obtain specimens as ordered for blood studies, such as CBC and clotting studies, *to establish a baseline and use for future comparison.*
- Monitor output *to evaluate adequacy of renal perfusion.*
- Administer IV fluid replacement therapy as ordered *to maintain blood pressure and blood volume.*
- Palpate for abdominal tenderness and rigidity *to determine bleeding and evidence of uterine contractions.*
- Institute bed rest *to reduce oxygen demands.*
- Assess for rupture of membranes *to evaluate for possible onset of labour.*
- Avoid vaginal examinations *to prevent further bleeding episodes.*
- Complete an Rh titer *to identify need for WinRho.*
- Avoid nipple stimulation *to prevent uterine contractions.*
- Continuously monitor for contractions or PROM *to allow for prompt intervention.*
- Administer tocolytic agents as ordered *to stall preterm labour.*
- Monitor vital signs frequently *to identify possible hypovolemia and infection.*
- Assess frequently for active vaginal bleeding *to minimize risk for hemorrhage.*
- Continuously monitor fetal heart rate with electronic fetal monitor *to evaluate fetal status.*
- Assist with fetal surveillance tests as ordered *to aid in determining fetal well-being.*
- Observe for abnormal fetal heart rate patterns, such as loss of variability, decelerations, tachycardia, *to identify fetal distress.*
- Position patient in side-lying position with wedge for support *to maximize placental perfusion.*
- Assess fetal movement *to evaluate for possible fetal hypoxia.*
- Teach woman to monitor fetal movement *to evaluate well-being.*
- Administer oxygen as ordered *to increase oxygenation to mother and fetus.*

NURSING DIAGNOSIS: Anxiety related to threats to self and fetus

Outcome Identification and Evaluation
Client will experience a decrease in anxiety as evidenced by verbal reports of less anxiety, use of effective coping measures, and calm demeanor

Nursing Care Plan 19.1 (continued)

Interventions: Minimizing Anxiety

- Provide factual information about the diagnosis and treatment, and explain interventions and the rationale behind them *to provide client with a clear understanding of her condition.*
- Answer questions about health status honestly *to establish a trusting relationship.*
- Speak calmly to patient and family members *to minimize environmental stress.*
- Encourage the use of past effective techniques for coping *to promote relaxation and feelings of control.*
- Acknowledge and facilitate the woman's spiritual needs *to promote effective coping.*
- Involve the woman and family in the decision-making process *to foster self-confidence and control over situation.*
- Maintain a presence during stressful periods *to allay anxiety.*
- Use the sense of touch if appropriate *to convey caring and concern.*
- Encourage talking as a means *to release tension.*

---

and gain her cooperation. Provide information about the condition and make sure that all information related is consistent with information from the primary care provider. Explain all assessments and treatment measures as needed. Act as a client advocate in obtaining information for the family.

Teach the woman how to perform and record daily fetal movement. This action serves two purposes. One, it provides valuable information about the fetus. Two, it is an activity that the client can participate in, thereby fostering some feeling of control over the situation.

If the woman will require prolonged hospitalization or home bed rest, assess the physical and emotional impact that this may have on her. Evaluate her coping mechanisms to help determine how well she will be able to adjust to and cooperate with the treatment plan. Allow the client to verbalize her feelings and fears and provide emotional support. Also, provide opportunities for distraction—educational videos or DVDs, arts and crafts, computer games, reading books—and evaluate the client's response.

In addition to the emotional impact of prolonged bed rest, thoroughly assess the woman's skin to prevent skin breakdown and to help alleviate her discomfort secondary to limited physical activity. Instruct the woman in appropriate skin care measures. Encourage her to eat a balanced diet with adequate fluid intake to ensure that adequate nutrition and hydration and prevent complications associated with urinary and bowel elimination secondary to bed rest.

Teach the client and family about any signs and symptoms that should be reported immediately. In addition, prepare the woman for the possibility of a cesarean birth. The woman must notify her health care provider about any bleeding episodes or backaches (may indicate preterm labour contractions) and must adhere to the prescribed bed rest regimen. To ensure compliance and a positive outcome, she needs to be aware of the purpose of all of the observations that need to be made.

Abruptio Placentae

Abruptio placentae is the separation of a normally located placenta after the 20th week of gestation and prior to birth that leads to hemorrhage. It is a significant cause of third-trimester bleeding and carries a high mortality rate. It occurs in about 1% of all pregnancies throughout the world (Deering, 2011), or 1 in 120 pregnancies. The overall fetal mortality rate for placental abruption is 20% to 40%, depending on the extent of the abruption. Maternal mortality is approximately 6% in abruptio placentae and is related to cesarean birth and/or hemorrhage/coagulopathy (Deering, 2011).

Pathophysiology

The etiology of this condition is unknown; however, it has been proposed that abruption starts with degenerative changes in the small maternal arterioles, resulting in thrombosis, degeneration of the decidua, and possible rupture of a vessel. Bleeding from the vessel forms a retroplacental clot. The bleeding causes increased pressure behind the placenta and results in separation (Deering, 2011).

Fetal blood supply is compromised and fetal distress develops in proportion to the degree of placental separation. This is caused by the insult of the abruption itself and by issues related to prematurity when early birth is required to alleviate maternal or fetal distress.

Abruptio placentae is classified according to the extent of separation and the amount of blood loss from the maternal circulation. Classifications include:

- Mild (grade 1): minimal bleeding (less than 500 mL), marginal separation (10% to 20%), tender uterus, no coagulopathy, no signs of shock, no fetal distress
- Moderate (grade 2): moderate bleeding (1,000 to 1,500 mL), moderate separation (20% to 50%), continuous abdominal pain, mild shock
- Severe (grade 3): absent to moderate bleeding (more than 1,500 mL), severe separation (more than 50%),

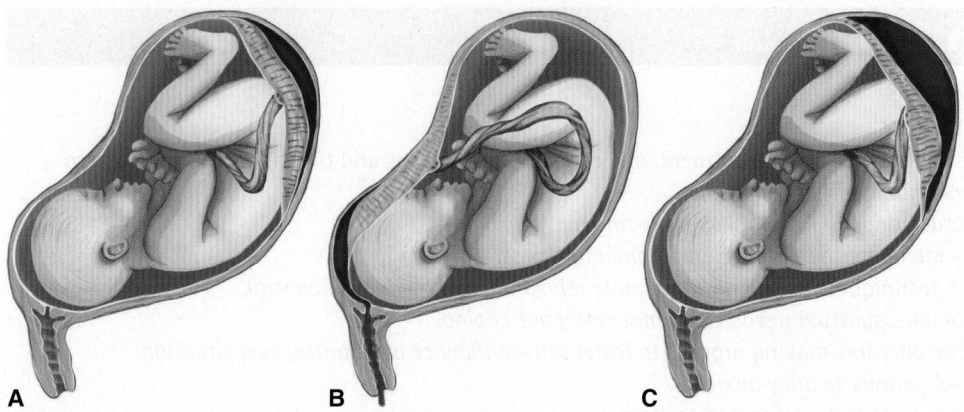

A Partial abruption, concealed hemorrhage

B Partial abruption, apparent hemorrhage

C Complete abruption, concealed hemorrhage

FIGURE 19.5 Classification of abruptio placentae. (**A**) Partial abruption with concealed hemorrhage. (**B**) Partial abruption with apparent hemorrhage. (**C**) Complete abruption with concealed hemorrhage.

profound shock, agonizing abdominal pain, and development of disseminated intravascular coagulopathy (DIC) (Gilbert, 2010)

Abruptio placentae also may be classified as partial or complete, depending on the degree of separation. Alternately, it can be classified as concealed or apparent, by the type of bleeding (Fig. 19.5).

*R*emember Helen, the pregnant woman with severe abdominal pain? Electronic fetal monitoring revealed uterine hypertonicity with absent fetal heart sounds. Palpation of her abdomen revealed rigidity and extreme tenderness in all four quadrants. Her vital signs were as follows—temperature, afebrile; pulse, 94; respirations, 22; blood pressure, 130/90 mm Hg. What might you suspect as the cause of Helen's abdominal pain? What course of action would you anticipate for Helen?

Therapeutic Management

Treatment of abruptio placentae is designed to assess, control, and restore the amount of blood lost; to provide a positive outcome for both mother and newborn; and to prevent coagulation disorders, such as DIC (Box 19.2). Emergency measures include starting two large-bore IV lines with normal saline or lactated Ringer's solution to combat hypovolemia, obtaining blood specimens for evaluating hemodynamic status values and for typing and cross-matching, and frequently monitoring fetal and maternal well-being. After the severity of abruption is determined and appropriate blood and fluid replacement is given, cesarean birth is done immediately if fetal distress is evident. If the fetus is not in distress, close monitoring continues, with delivery planned at the earliest signs of fetal distress. Because of the possibility of fetal blood loss through the placenta, a neonatal intensive care team should be available during the birth process to

assess and treat the newborn immediately for shock, blood loss, and hypoxia.

If the woman develops DIC, treatment focuses on determining and correcting the underlying cause. Replacement therapy of the coagulation factors is achieved by

---

BOX 19.2 **Disseminated Intravascular Coagulation (DIC)**

DIC is a bleeding disorder characterized by an abnormal reduction in the elements involved in blood clotting resulting from their widespread intravascular clotting (Day, Paul, Williams, et al., 2010). This disorder can occur secondary to abruptio placentae.

Simply put, the clinical and pathologic manifestations of DIC can be described as a loss of balance between the clot-forming activity of thrombin and the clot-lysing activity of plasmin. Therefore, too much thrombin tips the balance toward the prothrombic state and the client develops clots. Alternately, too much clot lysis (fibrinolysis) results from plasmin formation and the client hemorrhages. Small clots form throughout the body, and eventually the blood-clotting factors are used up, rendering them unavailable to form clots at sites of tissue injury. Clot-dissolving mechanisms are also increased, which results in bleeding (possibly severe).

DIC can be stimulated by many factors, including sepsis, malignancy, and obstetric conditions such as placental abruption, missed abortion or retained dead fetus, amniotic fluid embolism, and eclampsia.

Laboratory studies that assist in the diagnosis include:
- Decreased fibrinogen and platelets
- Prolonged PT and aPTT
- Positive D-dimer tests and fibrin (split) degradation products (objective evidence of the simultaneous formation of thrombin and plasmin) (Levi & Schmaier, 2011)

transfusion of fresh-frozen plasma along with cryoprecipitate to maintain the circulating volume and provide oxygen to the cells of the body. Anticoagulant therapy (low-molecular-weight heparin), packed red cells, platelet concentrates, antithrombin concentrates, and nonclotting protein-containing volume expanders are also used to combat this serious condition (Levi & Schmaier, 2011). Prompt identification and early intervention are essential for a woman with acute DIC associated with abruptio placentae to treat DIC and possibly save her life.

Nursing Assessment

Abruptio placentae is a medical emergency. The nurse plays a critical role in assessing the pregnant woman presenting with abdominal pain and/or experiencing vaginal bleeding, especially in a concealed hemorrhage, in which the extent of bleeding is not recognized. Rapid assessment is essential to ensure prompt, effective interventions to prevent maternal and fetal morbidity and mortality. Comparison Chart 19.1 compares placenta previa with abruptio placentae.

Health History and Physical Examination

Begin the health history by assessing the woman for risk factors that may predispose her to abruptio placentae, such as maternal smoking, advanced maternal age (over 35 years old), poor nutrition, multiple gestation, excessive intrauterine pressure caused by hydramnios, hypertension, severe trauma (e.g., auto accident, intimate partner violence), cocaine use, alcohol ingestion, and multiparity (Norwitz & Schorge, 2010; Zeltzer, 2011). Ask the woman about her previous pregnancies to determine whether she has experienced a prior abruption. In addition, be alert for other notable risk factors, such as male fetal gender, chorioamnionitis, prolonged ruptured membranes (more than 24 hours), pre-eclampsia, and low socioeconomic status (Deering, 2011).

Assess the woman for bleeding. As the placenta separates from the uterus, hemorrhage ensues. It can be apparent, appearing as vaginal bleeding, or it can be concealed. Vaginal bleeding is present in 80% of women diagnosed with abruptio placentae and may be significant enough to jeopardize both maternal and fetal health within a short time frame. The remaining 20% of abruptions are associated with a concealed hemorrhage and the absence of vaginal bleeding. Monitor the woman's level of consciousness, noting any signs or symptoms that may suggest shock.

> ▶ **Take** NOTE!
>
> Vital signs can be within normal range, even with significant blood loss, because a pregnant woman can lose up to 40% of her total blood volume without showing signs of shock (Gilbert, 2010).

Assess the woman for complaints of pain, including the type, onset, and location. Ask if she has had any contractions. Palpate the abdomen, noting any contractions, uterine tenderness, tenseness, or rigidity. Ask if she has noticed any changes in fetal movement and activity. Decreased fetal movement may be the presenting complaint, resulting from fetal jeopardy or fetal death (Deering, 2011). Assess fetal heart rate and continue to monitor it electronically.

> ▶ **Take** NOTE!
>
> Classic manifestations of abruptio placentae include painful, dark-red vaginal bleeding (port wine colour) because the bleeding comes from the clot that was formed behind the placenta; "knife-like" abdominal pain; uterine tenderness; contractions; and decreased fetal movement. Rapid assessment is essential to ensure prompt, effective interventions to prevent maternal and fetal morbidity and mortality.

COMPARISON CHART 19.1 **PLACENTA PREVIA VERSUS ABRUPTIO PLACENTAE**

Manifestation	Placenta Previa	Abruptio Placentae
Onset	Insidious	Sudden
Type of bleeding	Always visible; slight, then more profuse	Can be concealed or visible
Blood description	Bright red	Dark
Discomfort/pain	None (painless)	Constant; uterine tenderness on palpation
Uterine tone	Soft and relaxed	Firm to rigid
Fetal heart rate	Usually in normal range	Fetal distress or absent
Fetal presentation	May be breech or transverse lie; engagement is absent	No relationship

Laboratory and Diagnostic Testing

Laboratory and diagnostic tests may be helpful in diagnosing the condition and guiding management. These studies may include:

- CBC: determines the current hemodynamic status; however, it is not reliable for estimating acute blood loss
- Fibrinogen levels: typically are increased in pregnancy (hyperfibrinogenemia); thus, a moderate dip in fibrinogen levels might suggest coagulopathy (DIC) and, if profuse bleeding occurs, the clotting cascade might be compromised
- Prothrombin time (PT)/activated partial thromboplastin time (aPTT): determines the client's coagulation status, especially if surgery is planned
- Type and cross-match: determines blood type if a transfusion is needed
- Kleihauer–Betke test: detects fetal red blood cells in the maternal circulation, determines the degree of fetal–maternal hemorrhage, and helps calculate the appropriate dosage of WinRho to give to Rh-negative clients
- Nonstress test: demonstrates findings of fetal jeopardy manifested by late decelerations or bradycardia
- Biophysical profile: aids in evaluating clients with chronic abruption; a low score (less than 6 points) suggests possible fetal compromise (Deering, 2011)

Ultrasound is not useful for making a definitive diagnosis because the clot is sonographically visible in less than 50% of the cases (Zeltzer, 2011).

Nursing Management

Nursing management of the woman with abruptio placentae warrants immediate care to provide the best outcome for both mother and fetus.

Ensuring Adequate Tissue Perfusion

Upon arrival to the facility, place the woman on strict bed rest and in a left lateral position to prevent pressure on the vena cava. This position provides uninterrupted perfusion to the fetus. Expect to administer oxygen therapy via nasal cannula to ensure adequate tissue perfusion. Monitor oxygen saturation levels via pulse oximetry to evaluate the effectiveness of interventions.

Obtain maternal vital signs frequently, as often as every 15 minutes as indicated, depending on the woman's status and amount of blood loss. Observe for changes in vital signs suggesting hypovolemic shock and report them immediately. Also expect to insert an indwelling urinary (Foley) catheter to assess hourly urine output and initiate an IV infusion for fluid replacement using a large-bore catheter.

Assess fundal height for changes. An increase in size would indicate bleeding. Monitor the amount and characteristics of any vaginal bleeding as frequently as every 15 to 30 minutes. Be alert for signs and symptoms of DIC, such as bleeding gums, tachycardia, oozing from the IV insertion site, and petechiae, and administer blood products as ordered if DIC occurs.

Institute continuous electronic fetal monitoring. Assess uterine contractions and report any increased uterine tenseness or rigidity. Also observe the tracing for tetanic uterine contractions or changes in fetal heart rate patterns suggesting fetal compromise.

Providing Support and Education

A woman diagnosed with abruptio placentae may be filled with a sense of heightened anxiety and apprehension, for her own health as well as that of her fetus. Communicate empathy and understanding of the client's experience, and provide emotional support throughout this frightening time. Remain with the couple, acknowledge their emotions and fears, and address their spiritual and cultural needs. Answer their questions about the status of their fetus openly and honestly, being sure to explain indicators of fetal well-being. Provide information about the various diagnostic tests, treatments, and procedures that may be done, including the possible need for a cesarean birth.

Depending on the client's status, extent of bleeding, and length of gestation, the fetus may not survive. If the fetus does survive, he or she most likely will require neonatal intensive care. Assist the client and family to deal with the loss or with the birth of a newborn in the neonatal intensive care unit.

Although abruptio placentae is not a preventable condition, client education is important to help reduce the risk for a recurrence of this condition. Encourage the woman to avoid drinking, smoking, or using drugs during pregnancy. Urge her to seek early and continuous prenatal care and to receive prompt health care if any signs and symptoms occur in future pregnancies.

Think back to Helen, the pregnant woman described at the beginning of the chapter. She was diagnosed with abruptio placentae and was prepared for an emergency cesarean birth. On exploration, there was almost a 75% abruption, with approximately 800 mL of concealed blood between the uterus and the placenta. In addition, she lost an additional 500 mL during surgery. What in Helen's history may have placed her at increased risk for abruption? What assessments and interventions would be essential during her postpartum recovery secondary to her large blood loss? What psychosocial interventions would be necessary due to her fetal loss?

Hyperemesis Gravidarum

More than half of pregnant women experience nausea and vomiting during their pregnancy (Society of Obstetricians and Gynaecologists of Canada [SOGC], 2010).

The terms *nausea and vomiting of pregnancy* and *morning sickness* are often used to describe this condition when symptoms are relatively mild. Such symptoms usually disappear after the first trimester. This mild form of nausea and vomiting mostly affects the quality of life of the woman and her family, whereas the severe form—hyperemesis gravidarum—results in dehydration, electrolyte imbalance, and the need for hospitalization (Wilcox, 2010).

Unlike morning sickness, **hyperemesis gravidarum** is a complication of pregnancy characterized by persistent, uncontrollable nausea and vomiting causing weight loss of more than 5% of pre-pregnancy body weight, electrolyte imbalance, and ketonuria (Arsenault & Lane, 2002).

Hyperemesis is estimated to occur in approximately 5 in every 1,000 pregnancies. The prevalence increases in molar pregnancies and multiple gestations. Its peak incidence occurs between 8 and 12 weeks of pregnancy, and it usually resolves by week 14 (Ogunyemi, Fong, & Chen Herrero, 2011).

> ▶ *Take* NOTE!
>
> *Every pregnant woman needs to be instructed to report any episodes of severe nausea and vomiting or episodes that extend beyond the first trimester.*

Pathophysiology

Although the exact cause of nausea and vomiting is unknown, its effects—decreased placental blood flow, decreased maternal blood flow, and acidosis—can threaten the health of the mother and fetus. Dehydration can also lead to preterm labour (Stan, Boulvian, Pfister, et al., 2009). Numerous theories abound, but few studies have produced scientific evidence to identify the etiology of this condition. It is likely that multiple factors contribute to it.

Elevated levels of hCG are present in all pregnant women during early pregnancy, usually declining after 12 weeks. This corresponds to the usual duration of morning sickness. In hyperemesis gravidarum, the hCG levels are often higher and extend beyond the first trimester. Symptoms exacerbate the disease. Decreased fluid intake and prolonged vomiting cause dehydration; dehydration increases the serum concentration of hCG, which in turn exacerbates the nausea and vomiting—a vicious cycle. A few other theories that have been proposed to explain its etiology include:

- Endocrine theory: high levels of hCG and estrogen during pregnancy
- Metabolic theory: vitamin B6 deficiency
- Psychological theory: psychological stress increases the symptoms

Therapeutic Management

Conservative management in the home is the first line of treatment for the woman with hyperemesis gravidarum. This usually focuses on dietary and lifestyle changes.

If conservative management fails to alleviate the client's symptoms and nausea and vomiting continue, medications are available (Drug Guide 19.2). Motherisk has developed an algorithm to assist in the management of nausea and vomiting in pregnancy (Einarson, Maltepe, Boskovic, et al., 2007). In the event dehydration occurs, hospitalization is necessary to reverse the effects of severe nausea and vomiting.

On admission to the hospital, blood tests are ordered to assess the severity of the client's dehydration, electrolyte imbalance, ketosis, and malnutrition. Parenteral fluids and drugs are ordered to rehydrate the woman and reduce the symptoms. Rehydration includes IV fluids as per hospital policy with vitamins (pyridoxine [B6]) and electrolytes added (Einarson et al., 2007). Antiemetics may be administered rectally or intravenously to control the nausea and vomiting. Once her condition stabilizes and she is able to tolerate fluids, medications may be administered orally.

If the client does not improve after several days of bed rest, "gut rest," IV fluids, and antiemetics, total parenteral nutrition or feeding through a percutaneous endoscopic gastrostomy tube is instituted to prevent malnutrition.

Finding a drug that works for any given client is largely a matter of trial and error. If one drug is ineffective, another class of drugs with a different mechanism of action may help. The SOGC recommends doxylamine–pyridoxine (Diclectin) as the first drug of choice for the treatment of nausea and vomiting in pregnancy. Metoclopramide or ondansetron (Zofran) may be used if treatment with Diclectin is unsuccessful (see Drug Guide 19.2).

Few women receive complete relief of symptoms from any one therapy. Complementary and alternative medicine therapies appeal to many to help supplement traditional ones. Some popular therapies include acupressure, massage, therapeutic touch, ginger, and the wearing of Sea-bands to prevent nausea and vomiting. Research has reported a positive effect of using acupressure over the Neiguan point on the wrist, via wrist bands, to control nausea and vomiting associated with pregnancy (SOGC, 2010).

Nursing Assessment

Nursing assessment of the woman with hyperemesis gravidarum requires a thorough history and physical examination to identify signs and symptoms associated with this disorder. The client is extremely uncomfortable. She may experience many hours of lost work productivity and sleep, and hyperemesis may damage family

DRUG GUIDE 19.2   MEDICATIONS USED FOR HYPEREMESIS GRAVIDARUM

Medication	Action/Indications	Nursing Implications
Doxylamine and pyridoxine (Diclectin)	Antinausea, antihistamine, vitamin Prevents nausea and vomiting in pregnancy	May cause drowsiness, vertigo, nervousness, disorientation Counsel patient to avoid driving or operating machinery until effects of the drug are known. Do not combine with alcohol or other CNS depressants. Not for use in patients with epilepsy
Prochlorperazine (Compazine)	Acts centrally to inhibit dopamine receptors in the CTZ and peripherally to block vagus nerve stimulation in the GI tract Controls severe nausea and vomiting	Be alert for abnormal movements and for neuroleptic malignant syndrome such as seizures, hyper-/hypotension, tachycardia, and dyspnea. Assess mental status, intake/output Caution patient not to drive as a result of drowsiness or dizziness Advise to change position slowly to minimize effects of orthostatic hypotension.
Promethazine (Phenergan)	Diminishes vestibular stimulation and acts on the chemoreceptor trigger zone (CTZ) Symptomatic relief of nausea and vomiting, and motion sickness	Be alert for urinary retention, dizziness, hypotension, and involuntary movements. Institute safety measures to prevent injury secondary to sedative effects Offer hard candy and frequent rinsing of mouth for dryness.
Metoclopromide	Antiemetic, peristaltic stimulant	Do not use in patients with gastrointestinal bleeding. May increase risk for bronchospasms in asthmatic patients May increase the incidence of seizures in patients with epilepsy
Ondansetron (Zofran)	Blocks serotonin peripherally, centrally, and in the small intestine Prevents nausea and vomiting	Monitor for possible side effects, such as diarrhea, constipation, abdominal pain, headache, dizziness, drowsiness, and fatigue. Monitor liver function studies as ordered.

Sources: Brophy, K., Scarlett-Fergusen, H., & Webber, K. (2008). *Clinical drug therapy for Canadian practice* (1st Canadian ed.). Philadelphia: Lippincott Williams & Wilkins; Karch, A. M. (2011). *2011 Lippincott's nursing drug guide.* Philadelphia: Lippincott Williams & Wilkins; King, T. L., & Brucker, M. C. (2011) *Pharmacology for women's health.* Sudbury, MA: Jones and Bartlett Publishers; Society of Obstetrics and Gynaecologists of Canada. (2002). *Clinical practice guidelines: The management of nausea and vomiting of pregnancy.* Retrieved April 4, 2012 from http://www.sogc.org/guidelines/public/120E-CPG-October2002.pdf; and Wilcox, S. R. (2012). Pregnancy, hyperemesis gravidarum. *eMedicine.* Retrieved April 4, 2012 from http://emedicine.medscape.com/article/796564-overview.

relationships. If hyperemesis progresses untreated, it may cause neurologic disturbances, renal or liver damage, or death (McParlin, Graham, & Robson, 2008). Laboratory and diagnostic tests aid in determining the severity of the disorder.

Health History and Physical Examination

Begin the history by asking the client about the onset, duration, and course of her nausea and vomiting. Ask her about any medications or treatments she used and how effective they were in relieving her nausea and vomiting. Obtain a diet history from the client, including a dietary recall for the past week. Note the client's knowledge of

nutrition and need for appropriate nutritional intake. Be alert for patterns that may contribute to or trigger her distress. Also ask about any complaints of ptyalism (excessive salivation), anorexia, indigestion, and abdominal pain or distention. Ask if she has noticed any blood or mucus in her stool.

Review the client's history for possible risk factors, such as young age, nausea and vomiting with previous pregnancy, history of intolerance of oral contraceptives, nulliparity, trophoblastic disease, multiple gestation, emotional or psychological stress, gastro-esophageal reflux disease, primigravida status, obesity, hyperthyroidism, and *Helicobacter pylori* seropositivity (Ogunyemi et al., 2011). Weigh the client and compare this weight with her weight before she began experiencing symptoms as well as with her pre-pregnancy weight to estimate the degree of loss. With hyperemesis, weight loss usually exceeds 5% of body mass.

Inspect the mucous membranes for dryness and check skin turgor for evidence of fluid loss and dehydration. Assess blood pressure for changes, such as hypotension, that may suggest a fluid volume deficit. Also note any complaints of weakness, fatigue, activity intolerance, dizziness, or sleep disturbances.

Assess the client's perception of the situation. Note any evidence of depression or anxiety, which can add to her emotional distress (McParlin et al., 2008). Determine the woman's support systems that are available for help.

Laboratory and Diagnostic Testing

The results of laboratory and diagnostic tests may provide clues to the severity or etiology of the disorder. These may include:

- Liver enzymes: aspartate aminotransferase (AST) and alanine aminotransferase (ALT) levels are usually elevated
- CBC: elevated levels of red blood cells and hematocrit, indicating dehydration
- Urine ketones: positive when the body breaks down fat to provide energy in the absence of inadequate intake
- Blood urea nitrogen (BUN): increased in the presence of salt and water depletion
- Urine specific gravity: greater than 1.025, possibly indicating concentrated urine linked to inadequate fluid intake or excessive fluid loss
- Serum electrolytes: decreased levels of potassium, sodium, and chloride resulting from excessive vomiting and loss of hydrochloric acid in the stomach
- Ultrasound: evaluation for molar pregnancy or multiple gestation (Wilcox, 2010)

Nursing Management

Nursing management for the client with hyperemesis gravidarum focuses on promoting comfort by controlling the client's nausea and vomiting and promoting adequate nutrition. In addition, the nurse plays a major role in supporting and educating the client and her family.

Promoting Comfort and Nutrition

During the initial period, expect to withhold all oral food and fluids, maintaining NPO status to allow the GI tract to rest. In addition, administer prescribed antiemetics to relieve the nausea and vomiting and IV fluids to replace fluid losses. Monitor the rate of infusion to prevent overload and assess the IV insertion site to prevent infiltration or infection. Also administer electrolyte replacement

therapy as ordered to correct any imbalances, and periodically check serum electrolyte levels to evaluate the effectiveness of therapy.

Provide physical comfort measures such as hygiene measures and oral care. Pay special attention to the environment, making sure to keep the area free of pungent odours. As the client's nausea and vomiting subside, gradually introduce oral fluids and foods in small amounts. Monitor intake and output and assess the client's tolerance to the increase in intake.

Providing Support and Education

Women with hyperemesis gravidarum commonly are fatigued physically and emotionally. Many are exhausted, frustrated, and anxious. Offer reassurance that all interventions are directed toward promoting positive pregnancy outcomes for both the woman and her fetus. Providing information about the expected plan of care may help to alleviate the client's anxiety. Listen to her concerns and feelings, answering all questions honestly. Educate the woman and her family about the condition and its treatment options (Teaching Guideline 19.1). Teach the client about therapeutic lifestyle changes, such as avoiding stressors and fatigue that may trigger nausea and vomiting. Offer ongoing support and encouragement

TEACHING GUIDELINE 19.1

Teaching to Minimize Nausea and Vomiting

- Avoid noxious stimuli—such as strong flavours, perfumes, or strong odours such as frying bacon—that might trigger nausea and vomiting.
- Avoid tight waistbands to minimize pressure on the abdomen.
- Eat small, frequent meals throughout the day—six small meals.
- Separate fluids from solids by consuming fluids between meals.
- Avoid lying down or reclining for at least 2 hours after eating.
- Use high-protein supplement drinks.
- Avoid foods high in fat.
- Increase your intake of carbonated beverages.
- Increase your exposure to fresh air to improve symptoms.
- Eat when you are hungry, regardless of normal mealtimes.
- Drink herbal teas containing peppermint or ginger.
- Avoid fatigue and learn how to manage stress in life.
- Schedule daily rest periods to avoid becoming overtired.
- Eat foods that settle the stomach, such as dry crackers, toast, or soda.

and promote active participation in care decisions, thereby empowering the client and her family. Attempting to provide the client with a sense of control may help her overcome the feeling that she has lost control. If necessary, refer the client to a spiritual advisor or counsellor. Also suggest local or national support groups that the client may contact for additional information.

Arrange for possible home care follow-up for the client and reinforce discharge instructions to promote understanding. Collaborate with community resources to ensure continuity of care.

Gestational Hypertension

Gestational hypertension is characterized by hypertension without proteinuria after 20 weeks of gestation and a return of the blood pressure to normal postpartum. Previously, gestational hypertension was known as pregnancy-induced hypertension or toxemia of pregnancy, but these terms are no longer used. Gestational hypertension is clinically characterized by a blood pressure of 140/90 mm Hg or more on two occasions at least 6 hours apart (Magee, Helewa, Moutquin, et al., 2008). Gestational hypertension can be differentiated from chronic hypertension, which appears before the 20th week of gestation or before the current pregnancy and continues after the woman gives birth. Regardless of its onset, hypertension jeopardizes the well-being of the mother as well as the fetus.

Gestational hypertension with edema and proteinuria is one of the causes of maternal death in Canada (Statistics Canada, 2011). Hypertension complicates 2% to 3% of pregnancies (Carson & Gibson, 2012). The highest rates are in women younger than 20 or older than 40 years of age (Magee et al., 2008). "The classification of the hypertensive disorders of pregnancy is based on the two most common manifestations of pre-eclampsia: hypertension and proteinuria" (Magee et al., 2008, p. 9). The recommended classification of hypertensive disorders in pregnancy is based on guidelines from the SOGC (Magee et al., 2008) (Box 19.3).

Gestational hypertension can be classified as pre-eclampsia or eclampsia, each of which is associated with specific criteria. Pre-eclampsia is further categorized as mild or severe.

Pathophysiology

Gestational hypertension remains an enigma. The condition can be devastating to both the mother and fetus, and yet the etiology remains a mystery to medical science despite decades of research. Many theories exist, but none have truly explained the widespread pathologic changes that result in pulmonary edema, oliguria, seizures, thrombocytopenia, coagulation, abnormal liver function, and abnormal liver enzymes (Lindheimer, Taler,

---

BOX 19.3 SOGC Hypertension Classifications

1. Hypertensive disorders of pregnancy should be classified as pre-existing hypertension or gestational hypertension on the basis of different diagnostic and therapeutic factors.
2. The presence or absence of pre-eclampsia must be ascertained, given its clear association with more adverse maternal and perinatal outcomes.
3. In women with pre-existing hypertension, pre-eclampsia should be defined as resistant hypertension, new *or* worsening proteinuria, *or* one or more of the other adverse conditions.*
4. In women with gestational hypertension (blood pressure elevation to 140/90 mm Hg identified after mid-pregnancy without proteinuria), pre-eclampsia should be defined as new-onset proteinuria *or* one or more of the other adverse conditions.*
5. Severe pre-eclampsia should be defined as pre-eclampsia with onset before 34 weeks' gestation, with heavy proteinuria *or* one or more of the other adverse conditions.*
6. The term pregnancy-induced hypertension should be abandoned, as its meaning in clinical practice is unclear.

*Other adverse conditions consist of maternal symptoms (persistent or new/unusual headache, visual disturbances, persistent abdominal or right upper quadrant pain, severe nausea or vomiting, chest pain or dyspnea), maternal signs of end-organ dysfunction, abnormal maternal laboratory testing (elevated serum creatinine [according to local laboratory criteria]; elevated AST, ALT or LDH with symptoms; platelet count <100 × 10⁹/L; or serum albumin <20 g/L), or fetal morbidity (oligohydramnios, IUGR, absent or reversed end-diastolic flow in the umbilical artery by Doppler velocimetry, or intrauterine fetal death).

Source: Magee, L. A., Helewa, M., Moutquin, J.-M., & von Dadelszen, P. (2008). SOGC clinical practice guidelines: Diagnosis, evaluation and management of the hypertensive disorders of pregnancy. *Journal of Obstetrics and Gynaecology Canada, 30*(3 Suppl. 1), S1–S52. Retrieved March 9, 2012 from http://www.sogc.org/guidelines/documents/gui206CPG0803_001.pdf.

& Cunningham, 2008). Despite the results of several research studies, low-dose aspirin; supplementation with calcium, magnesium, zinc, or antioxidant therapy (vitamin C and E); salt restriction; diuretic therapy; and fish oils have not proven to prevent this destructive condition (Carson & Gibson, 2012; Lindheimer et al., 2008). Only low-dose aspirin and calcium have shown minimal protective effects (Lindheimer et al., 2008). Vitamin C and E supplementation have been shown to have no effect and may be harmful in some high-risk populations.

The underlying mechanisms involved with this disorder are vasospasm and hypoperfusion. In addition, endothelial injury occurs, leading to platelet adherence, fibrin deposition, and the presence of schistocytes (fragment of an erythrocyte).

Generalized vasospasm results in elevation of blood pressure and reduced blood flow to the brain, liver, kidneys, placenta, and lungs. Decreased liver perfusion leads to impaired liver function and subcapsular hemorrhage. This is demonstrated by epigastric pain and elevated liver enzymes in the maternal serum. Decreased brain perfusion leads to small cerebral hemorrhages and symptoms of arterial vasospasm such as headaches, visual disturbances, blurred vision, and hyperactive deep tendon reflexes (DTRs). A thromboxane/prostacyclin imbalance leads to increased thromboxane (potent vasoconstrictor and stimulator of platelet aggregation) and decreased prostacyclin (potent vasodilator and inhibitor of platelet aggregation), which contribute to the hypertensive state. Decreased kidney perfusion reduces the glomerular filtration rate (GFR), resulting in decreased urine output and increased serum levels of sodium, BUN, uric acid, and creatinine, further increasing extracellular fluid and edema. Increased capillary permeability in the kidneys allows albumin to escape, which reduces plasma colloid osmotic pressure and moves more fluid into extracellular spaces; this leads to pulmonary edema and generalized edema. Poor placental perfusion resulting from prolonged vasoconstriction helps to contribute to intrauterine growth restriction (IUGR), premature separation of the placenta (abruptio placentae), persistent fetal hypoxia, and acidosis. In addition, hemoconcentration (resulting from decreased intravascular volume) causes increased blood viscosity and elevated hematocrit (Ross, 2011; Stokes, 2011).

Therapeutic Management

The SOGC recently revised its guidelines for the treatment of hypertension in the pregnant woman (Magee et al., 2008). Management of the woman with gestational hypertension varies depending on the severity of her condition and its effects on the fetus. Typically the woman is managed conservatively if she is experiencing mild symptoms. However, if the condition progresses, management becomes more aggressive.

Management for Mild Pre-Eclampsia

Conservative strategies for mild pre-eclampsia are used if the woman exhibits no signs of renal or hepatic dysfunction or coagulopathy. A woman with mild elevations in blood pressure may be placed on bed rest at home. She is encouraged to rest as much as possible in the lateral recumbent position to improve uteroplacental blood flow, reduce her blood pressure, and promote diuresis. In addition, antepartal visits and diagnostic testing—such as CBC, clotting studies, liver enzymes, and platelet levels—increase in frequency. The woman will be asked to monitor her blood pressure daily (every 4 to 6 hours while awake) and report any increased readings; she will also measure the amount of protein found in her urine using a dipstick and will weigh herself to detect any weight gain. Daily fetal movement counts also are implemented. If there is any decrease in movement, the woman needs to be evaluated by her health care provider that day. A balanced, nutritional diet with no sodium restriction is advised. In addition, she is encouraged to drink six to eight 8-oz glasses of water daily.

If home management fails to reduce the blood pressure, admission to the hospital is warranted and the treatment strategy is individualized based on the severity of the condition and the gestational age at the time of diagnosis. During the hospitalization, the woman with mild pre-eclampsia is monitored closely for signs and symptoms of severe pre-eclampsia or impending eclampsia (e.g., persistent headache, hyperreflexia). Blood pressure measurements are frequently recorded along with daily weights to detect excessive weight gain resulting from edema. Fetal surveillance is instituted in the form of daily fetal movement counts, nonstress testing, and serial ultrasounds to evaluate fetal growth and amniotic fluid volume to confirm fetal well-being. Expectant management usually continues until the pregnancy reaches term, fetal lung maturity is documented, or complications develop that warrant immediate birth (Han & Norwitz, 2011).

Prevention of disease progression is the focus of treatment during labour. Blood pressure is monitored frequently, and a quiet environment is important to minimize the risk for stimulation and to promote rest. IV magnesium sulphate is infused to prevent any seizure activity, along with antihypertensives if blood pressure values begin to rise. Calcium gluconate is kept at the bedside in case the magnesium level becomes toxic. Continued close monitoring of neurologic status is warranted to detect any signs or symptoms of hypoxemia, impending seizure activity, or increased intracranial pressure. An indwelling urinary (Foley) catheter usually is inserted to allow for accurate measurement of urine output.

Management for Severe Pre-Eclampsia

Severe pre-eclampsia may develop suddenly and bring with it high blood pressure of more than 160/110 mm Hg, proteinuria of more than 5 g in 24 hours, oliguria of less than 400 mL in 24 hours, cerebral and visual symptoms, and rapid weight gain. This clinical picture signals severe pre-eclampsia, and immediate hospitalization is needed.

Treatment is highly individualized and based on disease severity and fetal age. Birth of the infant is the only cure because pre-eclampsia depends on the presence of trophoblastic tissue. Therefore, the exact age of the fetus is assessed to determine viability.

Severe pre-eclampsia is treated aggressively because hypertension poses a serious threat to mother and fetus. The goal of care is to stabilize the mother–fetus dyad and prepare for birth. Therapy focuses on controlling hypertension, preventing seizures, preventing long-term morbidity, and preventing maternal, fetal, or newborn death (Magee et al., 2008). Intense maternal and fetal surveillance starts when the mother enters the hospital and continues throughout her stay.

The woman in labour with severe pre-eclampsia typically receives oxytocin to stimulate uterine contractions and magnesium sulphate to prevent seizure activity. Oxytocin and magnesium sulphate can be given simultaneously via infusion pumps to ensure both are administered at the prescribed rate. The client is evaluated closely for magnesium toxicity. If at all possible, a vaginal delivery is preferable to a cesarean birth. PGE2 gel may be used to ripen the cervix. A cesarean birth may be performed if the client is seriously ill. A pediatrician/neonatologist must be available in the birthing room to care for the newborn. A newborn whose mother received magnesium sulphate needs to be monitored for respiratory depression, hypotension, and hypotonia (Deglin, Vallerand, & Sanoski, 2011).

Management of Eclampsia

In the woman who develops an eclamptic seizure, the convulsive activity begins with facial twitching, followed by generalized muscle rigidity. Respirations cease for the duration of the seizure, resulting from muscle spasms, thus compromising fetal oxygenation. Coma usually follows the seizure activity, with respiration resuming. Eclamptic seizures are life-threatening emergencies and require immediate treatment to decrease maternal morbidity and mortality.

As with any seizure, the initial management is to clear the airway and administer adequate oxygen. Positioning the woman on her left side and protecting her from injury during the seizure are key. Suction equipment must be readily available to remove secretions from her mouth after the seizure is over. IV fluids are administered after the seizure at a rate to replace urine output and additional insensible losses. Fetal heart rate is monitored closely. Magnesium sulphate is administered IV to prevent further seizures. Hypertension is controlled with antihypertensive medications. After the seizures are controlled, the woman's stability is assessed and birth commences via induction or cesarean delivery (Magee et al., 2008).

If the woman's condition remains stable, she will be transferred to the postpartum unit for care. If she becomes unstable after giving birth, she may be transferred to the critical care unit for closer observation.

Nursing Assessment

Preventing complications related to hypertension during pregnancy requires the use of assessment, advocacy, and counselling skills. Assessment begins with the accurate measurement of the client's blood pressure at each encounter. In addition, nurses need to assess for subjective complaints that may indicate progression of the disease—visual changes, severe headaches, unusual bleeding or bruising, right upper quadrant pain, sudden weight gain, or nausea and vomiting (Mistovich, Krost, & Limmer, 2008). The significant signs of gestational hypertension—proteinuria and hypertension—occur without the woman's awareness. Unfortunately, by the time symptoms are noticed, gestational hypertension can be severe.

> ▶ **Take** NOTE!
>
> *The absolute blood pressure (value that validates elevation) of 140/90 mm Hg should be obtained on two occasions 6 hours apart to be diagnostic of gestational hypertension. Proteinuria is defined as 0.3 g or more of urinary protein per 24 hours or more than 1+ protein by chemical reagent strip or dipstick of at least two random urine samples collected at least 6 hours apart with no evidence of urinary tract infection (Magee et al., 2008).*

Health History and Physical Examination

Take a thorough history during the first antepartal visit to identify whether the woman is at risk for pre-eclampsia. Risk factors include:

- Primigravida status
- Multifetal pregnancy
- History of pre-eclampsia in a previous pregnancy
- Family history of pre-eclampsia (mother or sister)
- Lower socioeconomic group
- History of diabetes, hypertension, or renal disease
- Black race
- Age extremes (younger than 20 or older than 35)
- Obesity (Magee et al., 2008; Mistovich et al., 2008)

In addition, complete a nutritional assessment that includes the woman's usual intake of protein, calcium, daily calories, and fluids.

Women at risk for pre-eclampsia require more frequent prenatal visits throughout their pregnancy, and they require teaching about problems so that they can report them promptly.

Blood pressure must be measured carefully and consistently. Obtain all measurements with the woman in the same position (blood pressure is highest in the sitting position and lowest in the side-lying position) and by using the same technique (automated versus manual). This standardization in position and technique will yield the most accurate readings (Magee et al., 2008).

Obtain the client's weight (noting gain since last visit), and assess for amount and location of edema. Asking questions such as "Do your rings still fit on your fingers?" or "Is your face puffy when you get up in the morning?"

will help to determine whether fluid retention is present or if the woman's status has changed since her last visit.

> ▶ *Take* NOTE!
>
> *Although edema is not a cardinal sign of pre-eclampsia, weight should be monitored frequently to identify sudden gains in a short time span. Current research relies less on the classic triad of symptoms (hypertension, proteinuria, and edema or weight gain) and more on decreased organ perfusion, endothelial dysfunction (capillary leaking and proteinuria), and elevated blood pressure as key indicators (Carson & Gibson, 2012).*

If edema is present, assess the distribution, degree, and pitting. Document your findings and identify whether the edema is dependent or pitting. Dependent edema is present on the lower half of the body if the client is ambulatory, where hydrostatic pressure is greatest. It is usually observed in the feet and ankles or in the sacral area if the client is on bed rest.

Pitting edema is edema that leaves a small depression or pit after finger pressure is applied to a swollen area (Brodovicz, McNaughton, Uemura, et al., 2009). Record the depth of pitting demonstrated when pressure is applied. Although subjective, the following is used to record relative degrees:

- 1+ pitting edema = 2-mm depression into skin; disappears rapidly
- 2+ pitting edema = 4-mm skin depression; disappears in 10 to 15 seconds
- 3+ pitting edema = 6-mm depression into skin; lasts more than 1 minute
- 4+ pitting edema = 8-mm depression into skin; lasts 2 to 3 minutes

At every antepartal visit, assess the fetal heart rate with a Doppler device. Also check a clean-catch urine specimen for protein using a dipstick.

Laboratory and Diagnostic Testing

Various laboratory tests may be performed to evaluate the woman's status. Typically these include a CBC, serum electrolytes, BUN, creatinine, and hepatic enzyme levels. Urine specimens are checked for protein; if levels are 1+ to 2+ or greater, a 24-hour urine collection is completed.

Nursing Management

Nursing management of the woman with gestational hypertension focuses on close monitoring of blood pressure and ongoing assessment for evidence of disease progression. Throughout the client's pregnancy, fetal surveillance is key.

Intervening with Pre-Eclampsia

The woman with mild pre-eclampsia requires frequent monitoring to detect changes because pre-eclampsia can progress rapidly. Instruct all women about the signs and symptoms of pre-eclampsia and urge them to contact their health care professional for immediate evaluation should any occur.

Typically women with mild pre-eclampsia can be managed at home if they have a good understanding of the disease process, are stable, have no abnormal laboratory test results, and demonstrate good fetal movement (Teaching Guideline 19.2). The home care nurse makes frequent visits and follow-up phone calls to assess the woman's condition, to assist with scheduling periodic

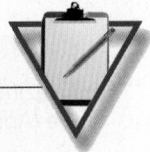

TEACHING GUIDELINE 19.2

Teaching for the Woman with Mild Pre-Eclampsia

- Rest in a quiet environment to prevent cerebral disturbances.
- Drink 8 to 10 glasses of water daily.
- Consume a balanced, high-protein diet including high-fibre foods.
- Obtain intermittent bed rest to improve circulation to the heart and uterus.
- Limit your physical activity to promote urination and subsequent decrease in blood pressure.
- Enlist the aid of your family so that you can obtain appropriate rest time.
- Perform self-monitoring as instructed, including:
  - Taking your own blood pressure twice daily
  - Checking and recording weight daily
  - Performing urine dipstick twice daily
  - Recording the number of fetal kicks daily
- Contact the home health nurse if any of the following occurs:
  - Increase in blood pressure
  - Protein present in urine
  - Gain of more than 450 g (1 lb) in 1 week
  - Burning or frequency when urinating
  - Decrease in fetal activity or movement
  - Headache (forehead or posterior neck region)
  - Dizziness or visual disturbances
  - Increase in swelling in hands, feet, legs, and face
  - Stomach pain, excessive heartburn, or epigastric pain
  - Decreased or infrequent urination
  - Contractions or low back pain
  - Easy or excessive bruising
  - Sudden onset of abdominal pain
  - Nausea and vomiting

DRUG GUIDE 19.3 MEDICATIONS USED WITH PRE-ECLAMPSIA AND ECLAMPSIA

Medication	Action/Indications	Nursing Implications
Magnesium sulphate	Blocks neuromuscular transmission, vasodilation Prevents and treats eclamptic seizures	Administer IV loading dose of 4–6 g over 30 min, continue maintenance infusion of 2–4 g/h as ordered. Monitor serum magnesium levels closely. Assess DTRs and check for ankle clonus. Have calcium gluconate readily available in case of toxicity. Monitor for signs and symptoms of toxicity, such as flushing, sweating, hypotension, and cardiac and central nervous system depression.
Methyldopa (Aldomet)	Antihypertensive Stimulates alpha-adrenergic receptor sites, decreasing sympathetic stimulation to heart and blood vessels	250–500 mg PO bid-qid (max 2 g/day) Sedation is common; caution patient about driving or other hazardous activities until effect is known Monitor for possible adverse effects such as jaundice and hepatitis
Hydralazine hydrochloride (Apresoline)	Vascular smooth muscle relaxant, thus improving perfusion to renal, uterine, and cerebral areas Reduction in blood pressure	Administer 5–10 mg by slow IV bolus every 20 min as needed Use parenteral form immediately after opening ampule. Withdraw drug slowly to prevent possible rebound hypertension. Monitor for adverse effects such as palpitations, headache, tachycardia, anorexia, nausea, vomiting, and diarrhea.
Labetalol hydrochloride (Normodyne)	Alpha-1 and beta blocker Reduces blood pressure	Be aware that drug lowers blood pressure without decreasing maternal heart rate or cardiac output. Administer IV bolus dose of 10–20 mg and then administer IV infusion of 2 mg/min until desired blood pressure value is achieved. Monitor for possible adverse effects such as gastric pain, flatulence, constipation, dizziness, vertigo, and fatigue.
Nifedipine (Procardia)	Calcium-channel blocker Dilates coronary arteries, arterioles, and peripheral arterioles Reduces blood pressure Stops preterm labour	Administer 10 mg orally for three doses and then every 4–8 h. Monitor for possible adverse effects such as dizziness, peripheral edema, angina, diarrhea, nasal congestions, cough.
Sodium nitroprusside	Causes rapid vasodilation (arterial and venous) Used for severe hypertension requiring rapid reduction in blood pressure	Administer via continuous IV infusion with dose titrated according to blood pressure levels. Wrap IV infusion solution in foil or opaque material to protect from light. Monitor for possible adverse effects, such as apprehension, restlessness, retrosternal pressure, palpitations, diaphoresis, abdominal pain.

Medication	Action/Indications	Nursing Implications
Furosemide (Lasix)	Diuretic action, inhibiting the reabsorption of sodium and chloride from the ascending loop of Henle Pulmonary edema (used only if condition is present)	Administer via slow IV bolus at a dose of 10–40 mg over 1–2 min. Monitor urine output hourly. Assess for possible adverse effects such as dizziness, vertigo, orthostatic hypotension, anorexia, vomiting, electrolyte imbalances, muscle cramps, and muscle spasms.

Sources: Brophy, K., Scarlett-Fergusen, H., & Webber, K. (2008). *Clinical drug therapy for Canadian practice* (1st Canadian ed.). Philadelphia: Lippincott Williams & Wilkins; Gilbert, E. S. (2011). *Manual of high-risk pregnancy and delivery* (5th ed.). St. Louis, MO: Mosby Elsevier; Karch, A. M. (2011). *2011 Lippincott's nursing drug guide*. Philadelphia: Lippincott Williams & Wilkins; King, T. L., & Brucker, M. C. (2011) *Pharmacology for women's health*. Sudbury, MA: Jones and Bartlett Publishers; and Magee, L. A., Helewa, M., Moutquin, J.-M., & von Dadelszen, P. (2008). SOGC clinical practice guidelines: Diagnosis, evaluation and management of the hypertensive disorders of pregnancy. *Journal of Obstetrics and Gynaecology Canada, 30*(3 Suppl. 1), S1–S52. Retrieved March 9, 2012 from http://www.sogc.org/guidelines/documents/gui206CPG0803_001.pdf.

evaluations of the fetus (such as nonstress tests), and to evaluate any changes that might suggest a worsening of the woman's condition.

Early detection and management of mild pre-eclampsia is associated with the greatest success in reducing progression of this condition. As long as the client carries out the guidelines of care as outlined by the health care provider and she remains stable, home care can continue to maintain the pregnancy until the fetus is mature. If disease progression occurs, hospitalization is required.

Intervening with Severe Pre-Eclampsia

The woman with severe pre-eclampsia requires hospitalization. Maintain the client on complete bed rest in the left lateral lying position. Ensure that the room is dark and quiet to reduce stimulation. Give sedatives as ordered to encourage quiet bed rest. The client is at risk for seizures if the condition progresses. Therefore, institute and maintain seizure precautions, such as padding the side rails and having oxygen, suction equipment, and call light readily available to protect the client from injury.

▶ *Take* NOTE!

Pre-eclampsia increases the risk for placental abruption, preterm birth, IUGR, and fetal distress during childbirth. Be prepared!

Closely monitor the client's blood pressure. Administer antihypertensives as ordered to reduce blood pressure (Drug Guide 19.3). Assess the client's vision and level of consciousness. Report any changes and any complaints of headache or visual disturbances. Offer a high-protein diet with eight to 10 glasses of water daily. Monitor the client's intake and output every hour and administer fluid and

electrolyte replacements as ordered. Assess the woman for signs and symptoms of pulmonary edema, such as crackles and wheezing heard on auscultation, dyspnea, decreased oxygen saturation levels, cough, anxiety, confusion, and restlessness (Sovari, Kocheril, & Bass, 2012).

To achieve a safe outcome for the fetus, prepare the woman for possible testing to evaluate fetal status as pre-eclampsia progresses. These may include the nonstress test, serial ultrasounds to track fetal growth, amniocentesis to determine fetal lung maturity, Doppler velocimetry to screen for fetal compromise, and biophysical profile to evaluate ongoing fetal well-being (Carson & Gibson, 2012).

Other laboratory tests may be performed to monitor the disease process and to determine whether it is progressing into HELLP syndrome. These include liver enzymes such as lactic dehydrogenase (LDH), ALT, and AST; chemistry panel, such as creatinine, BUN, uric acid, and glucose; CBC, including platelet count; coagulation studies, such as PT, PTT, fibrinogen, and bleeding time; and a 24-hour urine collection for protein and creatinine clearance.

Administer parenteral magnesium sulphate as ordered to prevent seizures. Assess DTRs to evaluate the effectiveness of therapy. Clients with pre-eclampsia commonly present with hyperreflexia. Severe pre-eclampsia causes changes in the cortex, which disrupts the equilibrium of impulses between the cerebral cortex and the spinal cord. Brisk reflexes (hyperreflexia) are the result of an irritable cortex and indicate central nervous system involvement (Lim, Sayah, Steinberg, et al., 2011).

Diminished or absent reflexes occur when the client develops magnesium toxicity. Because magnesium is a potent neuromuscular blocker, the afferent and efferent nerve pathways do not relay messages properly and hyporeflexia develops. Common sites used to assess DTRs are the biceps, triceps, patella, Achilles, and heel.

Nursing Procedure 19.1

ASSESSING THE PATELLAR REFLEX

Purpose: To Evaluate for Nervous System Irritability Related to Pre-Eclampsia

1. Place the woman in the supine position (or sitting upright with the legs dangling freely over the side of the bed or examination table).
2. If lying supine, have the woman flex her knee slightly.
3. Place a hand under the knee to support the leg and locate the patellar tendon. It should be midline just below the knee cap.
4. Using a reflex hammer or the side of your hand, strike the area of the patellar tendon firmly and quickly.
5. Note the movement of the leg and foot. A patellar reflex occurs when the leg and foot move (documented as 2+).
6. Repeat the procedure on the opposite leg.

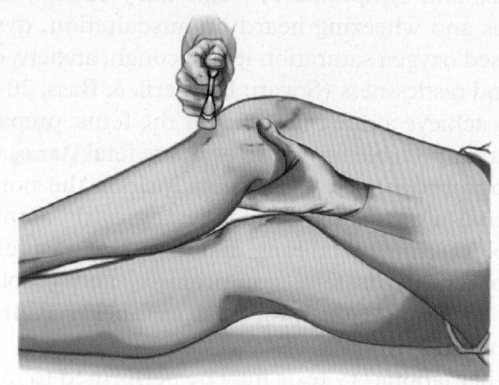

Nursing Procedure 19.1 highlights the steps for assessing the patellar reflex.

The National Institute of Neurological Disorders and Stroke (NINDS), a division of the US National Institutes of Health, published a scale in the early 1990s that, although subjective, remains widely in use today. It grades reflexes from 0 to 4+. Grades 2+ and 3+ are considered normal, whereas grades 0 and 4 may indicate pathology (Table 19.2). Because these are subjective assessments, to improve communication of reflex results, condensed descriptor categories such as absent, average, brisk, or clonus should be used rather than numeric codes (Gilbert, 2010).

Clonus is the presence of rhythmic involuntary contractions, most often at the foot or ankle. Sustained clonus confirms central nervous system involvement. Nursing Procedure 19.2 highlights the steps used to test for ankle clonus.

With magnesium sulphate administration, the client is at risk for magnesium toxicity. Closely assess the client

TABLE 19.2 GRADING DEEP TENDON REFLEXES

Description of Finding	Grade
Reflex absent, no response detected	0
Diminished, low normal	1
Average, normal	2
Brisker than average, may indicate disease	3
Hyperactive, brisk, clonus present	4

Source: Jarvis, C. (2009). *Physical examination & health assessment* (1st Canadian ed.). Toronto, Ontario: Saunders Elsevier.

for signs of toxicity, which include a respiratory rate of less than 12 breaths/minute, absence of DTRs, and a decrease in urinary output, below 30 mL per hour. Also monitor serum magnesium levels. Although exact levels may vary among agencies, serum magnesium levels ranging from 4 to 7 mEq/L are considered therapeutic, whereas levels higher than 8 mEq/dL are generally considered toxic. As levels increase, the woman is at risk for adverse effects:

- Respiratory paralysis
- Hypothermia

Nursing Procedure 19.2

TESTING FOR ANKLE CLONUS

Purpose: To Evaluate for Nervous System Irritability Related to Pre-Eclampsia

1. Place the woman in the supine position.
2. Have the client slightly bend her knee and place a hand under the knee to support it.
3. Dorsiflex the foot briskly and then quickly release it.
4. Watch for the foot to rebound smoothly against your hand. If the movement is smooth without any rapid contractions of the ankle or calf muscle, then clonus is not present; if the movement is jerky and rapid, clonus is present.
5. Repeat on the opposite side.

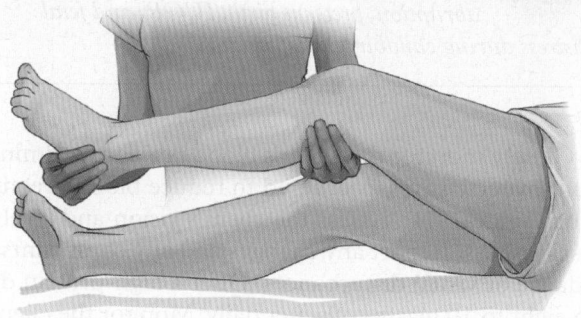

- Pulmonary edema
- Depressed reflexes
- Hypotension
- Flushing
- Drowsiness
- Depressed cardiac function
- Diaphoresis
- Hypocalcemia
- Hypophosphatemia
- Hyperkalemia
- Visual changes (Medscape Reference, 2011)

If signs and symptoms of magnesium toxicity develop, expect to administer calcium gluconate as the antidote.

Throughout the client's stay, closely monitor her for signs and symptoms of labour. Perform continuous electronic fetal monitoring to assess fetal well-being. Note trends in baseline rate and presence or absence of accelerations or decelerations. Also observe for signs of fetal distress and report them immediately. Administer glucocorticoid treatment as ordered to enhance fetal lung maturity and prepare for labour induction if the mother's condition warrants.

Keep the client and family informed of the woman's condition and educate them about the course of treatment. Provide emotional support for the client and family. Severe pre-eclampsia is very frightening for the client and her family, and most expectant mothers are very anxious about their own health as well as that of the fetus. To allay anxiety, use light touch to comfort and reassure her that the necessary actions are being taken. Actively listening to her concerns and fears and communicating them to the health care provider is important in keeping lines of communication open. Offering praise for small accomplishments can provide positive reinforcement for behaviours that should be continued.

Intervening with Eclampsia

The onset of seizure activity identifies eclampsia. Typically, eclamptic seizures are generalized and start with facial twitching. The body then becomes rigid, in a state of tonic muscular contraction. The clonic phase of the seizure involves alternating contraction and relaxation of all body muscles. Respirations stop during seizure activity and resume shortly after it ends. Client safety is the primary concern during eclamptic seizures. If possible, turn the client to her side and remain with her. Make sure that the side rails are up and padded. Dim the lights and keep the room quiet.

Document the time and sequence of events as soon as possible. After the seizure activity has ceased, suction the nasopharynx as necessary and administer oxygen. Continue the magnesium sulphate infusion to prevent further seizures. Ensure continuous electronic fetal monitoring, evaluating fetal status for changes. Also assess the client for uterine contractions. After the client is stabilized, prepare her for the birthing process as soon as possible to reduce the risk for perinatal mortality.

Providing Follow-Up Care

After delivery of the newborn, continue to monitor the client for signs and symptoms of pre-eclampsia/eclampsia for at least 48 hours. Expect to continue to administer magnesium sulphate infusion for 24 hours to prevent seizure activity, and monitor serum magnesium levels for toxicity.

Assess vital signs at least every 4 hours, along with routine postpartum assessments—fundus, lochia, breasts, bladder, bowels, and emotional state attention when performing the fundal assessment and assessing lochia. Monitor urine output closely. Diuresis is a positive sign that, along with a decrease in proteinuria, signals resolution of the disease.

HELLP

HELLP is an acronym for hemolysis, elevated liver enzymes, and low platelets. HELLP syndrome occurs in about 20% of pregnant women diagnosed with severe pre-eclampsia. Typically, HELLP develops in the third trimester, though it can develop either earlier in the pregnancy or up to 48 hours postpartum (Hagel-Fenton, 2008). HELLP syndrome leads to an increased maternal risk for liver hematoma or rupture, placental abruption, DIC, stroke, pulmonary edema, cerebral edema, renal damage, sepsis, and death as well as an increased fetal risk for respiratory distress, IUGR, and death (Haram, Svendsen, & Abildgaard, 2009).

Pathophysiology

The hemolysis that occurs is termed microangiopathic hemolytic anemia. It is thought to happen when red blood cells become fragmented as they pass through small, damaged blood vessels. Elevated liver enzymes are the result of reduced blood flow to the liver secondary to obstruction from fibrin deposits. Hyperbilirubinemia and jaundice result from liver impairment. Low platelet levels are caused by vascular damage, which results from vasospasm, and platelets aggregate at sites of damage, resulting in thrombocytopenia (Haram et al., 2009).

Therapeutic Management

The treatment for HELLP syndrome is based on the severity of the disease, the gestational age of the fetus, and the condition of the mother and the fetus. The client should be admitted or transferred to a tertiary centre with a neonatal intensive care unit. Additional treatments include magnesium sulphate, antihypertensives, and correction of the coagulopathies that accompany HELLP syndrome. After this syndrome is diagnosed and the woman's condition is stable, birth of the infant is indicated.

Magnesium sulphate is used prophylactically to prevent seizures. Antihypertensives such as hydralazine or labetalol are given to control blood pressure. Blood component therapy—such as fresh-frozen plasma, packed red cells, or platelets—is transfused to address the microangiopathic hemolytic anemia. Birth may be delayed up to 96 hours so that betamethasone or dexamethasone can be given to stimulate lung maturation in the preterm fetus.

Nursing Assessment

Nursing assessment of the woman with HELLP is similar to that for the woman with severe pre-eclampsia. Be alert for complaints of nausea (with or without vomiting), malaise, epigastric or right upper quadrant pain, and demonstrable edema. Perform systematic assessments frequently, as indicated by the woman's condition and response to therapy.

A diagnosis of HELLP syndrome is made based on laboratory test results, including:

- Low hematocrit that is not explained by any blood loss
- Elevated LDH (liver impairment)
- Elevated AST (liver impairment)
- Elevated ALT (liver impairment)
- Elevated BUN
- Elevated bilirubin level
- Elevated uric acid and creatinine levels (renal involvement)
- Low platelet count (less than $100,000 \times 10^9/L$)

Nursing Management

Nursing management of the woman diagnosed with HELLP syndrome is the same as that for the woman with severe pre-eclampsia. Closely monitor the client for changes and provide ongoing support throughout this experience.

Gestational Diabetes

Gestational diabetes is a condition involving glucose intolerance that occurs during pregnancy. It is discussed in greater detail in Chapter 20.

Blood Incompatibility

Blood incompatibility most commonly involves blood type or the Rh factor. Blood type incompatibility, also known as ABO incompatibility, is not as severe a condition as Rh incompatibility. ABO incompatibility rarely causes significant hemolysis, and antepartum treatment is not warranted. Rh sensitization occurs in approximately 0.4 in 1,000 births (Fung & Eason, 2003).

Dr. D. B. Chown, a Canadian physician living in Winnipeg, worked with Connaught Laboratories to manufacture the Rh immune serum, which was licensed in 1968. Approximately, 15% of white Canadian women are Rh negative (Beaulieu, 1993). About 35,000 Rh-negative women become pregnant every year and carry 24,500 Rh-positive fetuses who are at risk for Rh disease. Maternal alloimmunization occurs in 1% to 2% of Rh-negative women in Canada (Fung & Eason, 2003).

Pathophysiology

Hemolysis associated with ABO incompatibility is limited to mothers with type O blood whose fetuses have type A or B blood. In mothers with type A and B blood, naturally occurring antibodies are of the IgM class, which do not cross the placenta, whereas in type O mothers the antibodies are predominantly IgG in nature. Because A and B antigens are widely expressed in a variety of tissues besides red blood cells, only a small portion of antibodies crossing the placenta are available to bind to fetal red cells. In addition, fetal red cells appear to have less surface expression of A or B antigen, resulting in few reactive sites—hence the low incidence of significant hemolysis in affected neonates.

With ABO incompatibility, usually the mother is blood type O, with anti-A and anti-B antibodies in her serum; the infant is blood type A, B, or AB. The incompatibility arises as a result of the interaction of antibodies present in maternal serum and the antigen sites on the fetal red cells.

Rh incompatibility is a condition that develops when a woman with Rh-negative blood is exposed to Rh-positive blood cells and subsequently develops circulating titers of Rh antibodies. Individuals with an Rh-positive blood type have the D antigen present on their red cells, whereas individuals with an Rh-negative blood type do not. The presence or absence of the Rh antigen on the red blood cell membrane is genetically controlled. Fifteen percent to twenty percent of whites have Rh-negative blood (Salem, 2012).

Rh incompatibility most commonly arises with exposure of an Rh-negative mother to Rh-positive fetal blood during pregnancy or birth, during which time erythrocytes from the fetal circulation leak into the maternal circulation. After a significant exposure, alloimmunization or sensitization occurs. As a result, maternal antibodies are produced against the foreign Rh antigen.

Theoretically, fetal and maternal blood do not mix during pregnancy. In reality, however, small placental accidents (transplacental bleeds secondary to minor separation), abortions, ectopic pregnancy, abdominal trauma, trophoblastic disease, amniocentesis, placenta previa, and abruptio placentae allow fetal blood to enter the maternal circulation and initiate the production of antibodies to destroy Rh-positive blood. The amount of fetal blood necessary to produce Rh incompatibility varies. In one study, less than 1 mL of Rh-positive blood was shown to result in sensitization of women who are Rh negative (Salem, 2012).

Once sensitized, it takes approximately a month for Rh antibodies in the maternal circulation to cross over into the fetal circulation. In most cases, sensitization occurs during delivery (Salem, 2012). Thus, most firstborn infants with Rh-positive blood are not affected because the short period from first exposure of Rh-positive fetal erythrocytes to the birth of the infant is insufficient to produce a significant maternal IgG antibody response.

The risk and severity of alloimmune response increase with each subsequent pregnancy involving a fetus with Rh-positive blood. A second pregnancy with an Rh-positive fetus often produces a mildly anemic infant, whereas succeeding pregnancies produce infants with more serious hemolytic anemia.

Nursing Assessment

At the first prenatal visit, determine the woman's blood type and Rh status. Also obtain a thorough health history, noting any reports of previous events involving hemorrhage to delineate the risk for prior sensitization. When the client's history reveals an Rh-negative mother who may be pregnant with an Rh-positive fetus, prepare the client for an antibody screen (indirect Coombs test) to determine whether she has developed isoimmunity to the Rh antigen. This test detects unexpected circulating antibodies in a woman's serum that could be harmful to the fetus (Gilbert, 2010).

Nursing Management

If the indirect Coombs test is negative (meaning no antibodies are present), then the woman is a candidate for WinRho. If the test is positive, WinRho is of no value because isoimmunization has occurred. In this case, the fetus is monitored carefully for hemolytic disease.

The incidence of isoimmunization has declined dramatically as a result of prenatal and postnatal WinRho administration after any event in which blood transfer may occur. The standard dose is 300 μg, which is effective for 30 mL of fetal blood. Rh immunoglobulin helps to destroy any fetal cells in the maternal circulation before sensitization occurs, thus inhibiting maternal antibody production. This provides temporary passive immunity, thereby preventing maternal sensitization.

The current recommendation is that every Rh-negative nonimmunized woman receives WinRho at 28 weeks' gestation and again within 72 hours after giving birth. Other indications for WinRho include:

- Ectopic pregnancy
- Chorionic villus sampling
- Amniocentesis

- Prenatal hemorrhage
- Molar pregnancy
- Maternal trauma
- Percutaneous umbilical sampling
- Therapeutic or spontaneous abortion
- Fetal surgery (Fung & Eason, 2003; Koelewijn, de Haas, Vrijkotte, et al., 2009)

Despite the availability of WinRho and laboratory tests to identify women and newborns at risk, isoimmunization remains a serious clinical reality that continues to contribute to perinatal and neonatal mortality. Nurses, as client advocates, are in a unique position to make sure test results are brought to the health care provider's attention so appropriate interventions can be initiated. In addition, nurses must stay abreast of current literature and research regarding isoimmunization and its management. Stress to all women that early prenatal care can help identify and prevent this condition. Since Rh incompatibility is preventable with the use of WinRho, prevention remains the best treatment. Nurses can make a tremendous impact to ensure positive outcomes for the greatest possible number of pregnancies through education.

Amniotic Fluid Imbalances

Amniotic fluid develops from several maternal and fetal structures, including the amnion, chorion, maternal blood, fetal lungs, GI tract, kidneys, and skin. Any alteration in one or more of the various sources will alter the amount of amniotic fluid. Polyhydramnios and oligohydramnios are two imbalances associated with amniotic fluid.

Polyhydramnios

Polyhydramnios, also called hydramnios, is a condition in which there is too much amniotic fluid (more than 2,000 mL) surrounding the fetus between 32 and 36 weeks. It occurs in approximately 3% of all pregnancies and is associated with fetal anomalies of development (Rajiah, 2011). It is associated with poor fetal outcomes because of the increased incidence of preterm births, fetal malpresentation, and cord prolapse.

There are several causes of polyhydramnios. Generally, too much fluid is being produced, there is a problem with the fluid being taken up, or both. It can be associated with maternal disease and fetal anomalies, but it can also be idiopathic in nature.

Therapeutic Management

Treatment may include close monitoring and frequent follow-up visits with the health care provider if the hydramnios is mild to moderate. In severe cases in which the woman is in pain and experiencing shortness of breath, an amniocentesis or artificial rupture of the membranes is done to reduce the fluid and the pressure. Removal of fluid by amniocentesis is only transiently effective. A non-invasive treatment may involve the use of a prostaglandin synthesis inhibitor (indomethacin) to decrease amniotic fluid volume by decreasing fetal urinary output, but this may cause premature closure of the fetal ductus arteriosus (Carter & Boyd, 2012).

Nursing Assessment

Begin the assessment with a thorough history, being alert to risk factors such as maternal diabetes or multiple gestation. Review the maternal history for information about possible fetal anomalies, including fetal esophageal or intestinal atresia, neural tube defects, chromosomal deviations, fetal hydrops, central nervous system or cardiovascular anomalies, and hydrocephaly.

Determine the gestational age of the fetus and measure the woman's fundal height. With hydramnios, there is a discrepancy between fundal height and gestational age, or a rapid growth of the uterus is noted. Assess the woman for complaints of discomfort in her abdomen, such as being severely stretched and tight. Also note any reports of uterine contractions, which may result from overstretching of the uterus. Assess for shortness of breath resulting from pressure on her diaphragm and inspect her lower extremities for edema, which results from increased pressure on the vena cava.

Palpate the abdomen and obtain fetal heart rate. Often the fetal parts and heart rate are difficult to obtain because of the excess fluid present.

Prepare the woman for possible diagnostic testing to evaluate for the presence of possible fetal anomalies. An ultrasound usually is done to measure the pockets of amniotic fluid to estimate the total volume. In some cases, ultrasound also is helpful in finding the etiology of polyhydramnios, such as multiple pregnancy or a fetal structural anomaly.

Nursing Management

Nursing management of the woman with polyhydramnios focuses on ongoing assessment and monitoring for symptoms of abdominal pain, dyspnea, uterine contractions, and edema of the lower extremities. Explain to the woman and her family that this condition can cause her uterus to become overdistended and may lead to preterm labour and preterm rupture of membranes. Outline the signs and symptoms of both conditions and instruct the woman to contact her health care provider if they do occur. If a therapeutic amniocentesis is performed, assist the health care provider and monitor maternal and fetal status throughout for any changes.

Oligohydramnios

Oligohydramnios is a decreased amount of amniotic fluid (less than 500 mL) between 32 weeks and 36 weeks' gestation. It occurs in 5% to 8% of all pregnancies. Oligohydramnios may result from any condition that prevents the fetus from making urine or blocks it from going into the amniotic sac.

This condition puts the fetus at an increased risk for perinatal morbidity and mortality (Carter & Boyd, 2012). Reduction in amniotic fluid reduces the ability of the fetus to move freely without risk for cord compression, which increases the risk for fetal death and intrapartal hypoxia.

Therapeutic Management

The woman with oligohydramnios can be managed on an out-patient basis with serial ultrasounds and fetal surveillance through nonstress testing and biophysical profiles. As long as fetal well-being is demonstrated with frequent testing, no intervention is necessary. If fetal well-being is compromised, however, birth is planned along with amnioinfusion (the transvaginal infusion of crystalloid fluid to compensate for the lost amniotic fluid). The fluid is introduced into the uterus through an intrauterine pressure catheter. The infusion is administered in a controlled fashion to prevent overdistention of the uterus. Amnioinfusion is thought to improve abnormal fetal heart rate patterns, decrease cesarean births, and possibly minimize the risk for neonatal meconium aspiration syndrome (Norwitz & Schorge, 2010).

Nursing Assessment

Review the maternal history for factors associated with oligohydramnios, including:

- Uteroplacental insufficiency
- Premature rupture of membranes prior to labour onset
- Hypertension of pregnancy
- Maternal diabetes
- IUGR
- Postterm pregnancy
- Fetal renal agenesis
- Polycystic kidneys
- Urinary tract obstructions

Assess the client for complaints of fluid leaking from the vagina. Leaking of amniotic fluid from the vagina occurs with rupture of the amniotic sac. Leaking in conjunction with a uterus that is small for expected dates of gestation also suggests oligohydramnios. Unfortunately, the woman may not present with any symptoms. Typically, the reduced volume of amniotic fluid is identified on ultrasound.

Nursing Management

Nursing management of the woman with oligohydramnios involves continuous monitoring of fetal well-being during nonstress testing or during labour and birth by identifying nonreassuring patterns on the fetal monitor. Variable decelerations indicating cord compression are common. Changing the woman's position might be therapeutic in altering this fetal heart rate pattern. After the birth, evaluate the newborn for signs of postmaturity, congenital anomalies, and respiratory difficulty.

Assist with amnioinfusion as indicated and continue to assess the woman's vital signs, contraction status, and fetal heart rate throughout the procedure. Provide comfort measures such as changing the bed linens and the woman's bed clothes frequently because of the constant leakage of fluid from the vagina. Also provide frequent perineal care during the infusion.

Multiple Gestation

Multiple gestation is defined as more than one fetus being born to a pregnant woman. This includes twins, triplets, and higher-order multiples such as quadruplets on up. In the past three decades, the number of multiple gestations in Canada has exploded dramatically because of the widespread use of fertility drugs, older women having babies, and assisted reproductive technologies to treat infertility. The overall prevalence of multiple births in Canada is approximately 3 in 100 (Statistics Canada, 2008). The increasing number of multiple gestations is a concern because women who are expecting more than one infant are at high risk for preterm labour, hydramnios, hyperemesis gravidarum, anemia, pre-eclampsia, and antepartum hemorrhage. Fetal/newborn risks or complications include prematurity, respiratory distress syndrome, birth asphyxia, congenital anomalies (central nervous system), twin-to-twin transfusion syndrome (transfusion of blood from one twin [i.e., donor] to the other twin [i.e., recipient]), IUGR, and becoming conjoined twins (Fletcher, Zach, Pramanik, et al., 2009).

The two types of twins are monozygotic and dizygotic (Fig. 19.6). Monozygotic twins develop when a single, fertilized ovum splits during the first 2 weeks after conception. Monozygotic twins also are called identical twins. Two sperm fertilizing two ova produce dizygotic twins, which are called fraternal twins. Separate amnions, chorions, and placentas are formed in dizygotic twins. Triplets can be monozygotic, dizygotic, or trizygotic.

Therapeutic Management

When a multiple gestation is confirmed, the woman is followed with serial ultrasounds to assess fetal growth patterns and development. Biophysical profiles along with nonstress tests are ordered to determine fetal well-being. Many women are hospitalized in late pregnancy to prevent preterm labour and receive closer surveillance. During the intrapartum period the woman is monitored closely, with a perinatal team available to assist after birth. Operative delivery is frequently needed due to fetal malpresentation.

Nursing Assessment

Obtain a health history and physical examination. Be alert for complaints of fatigue and severe nausea and vomiting. Assess the woman's abdomen and fundal height. Typically with a multiple gestation the uterus is larger than expected based on the estimated date of birth. Laboratory test results may reveal anemia. Prepare the woman for ultrasound, which typically confirms the diagnosis of a multiple gestation.

Nursing Management

During the prenatal period, care focuses on providing education and support for the woman in areas of nutrition, increased rest periods, and close observation for pregnancy complications—anemia, excessive weight gain, proteinuria, edema, vaginal bleeding, and hypertension. Instruct the woman to be alert for and report immediately any signs and symptoms of preterm labour—contractions, uterine cramping, low backache, increased vaginal discharge, loss of mucus plug, pelvic pain, and pressure.

With the onset of labour, expect to monitor fetal heart rates continuously. Prepare the woman for an ultrasound to assess the presentation of each fetus to

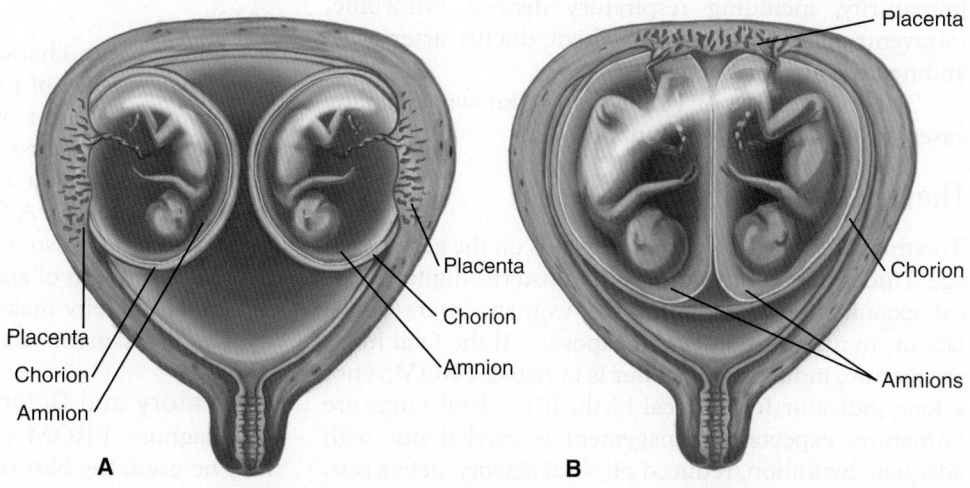

FIGURE 19.6 Multiple gestation with twins. (**A**) Dizygotic twins, where each fetus has its own placenta, amnion, and chorion. (**B**) Monozygotic twins, where the fetuses share one placenta, two amnions, and one chorion.

determine the best delivery approach. Ensure that extra nursing staff and the perinatal team are available for any birth or newborn complications.

After the babies are born, closely assess the woman for hemorrhage by frequently assessing uterine involution. Palpate the uterine fundus and monitor the amount and characteristics of lochia.

Throughout the entire pregnancy, birth, and hospital stay, inform and support the woman and her family. Encourage them to ask questions and verbalize any fears and concerns.

Premature Rupture of Membranes

Premature rupture of membranes (PROM) is the rupture of the bag of waters before the onset of true labour. There are a number of associated conditions and complications, such as infection, prolapsed cord, abruptio placentae, and preterm labour. This is the single most common diagnosis associated with preterm births (Gilbert, 2010).

PROM occurs in approximately 6% to 19% of all births (Crane, 2001). If prolonged (greater than 24 hours), the woman's risk for infection (chorioamnionitis, endometritis, sepsis, and neonatal infections) increases, and this risk continues to increase as the duration of rupture time increases. The time interval from rupture of membranes to the onset of regular contractions is termed the latent period.

The terminology pertaining to PROM can be confusing. PROM is rupture of the membranes prior to the onset of labour and is used appropriately when referring to a woman who is beyond 37 weeks' gestation, has presented with spontaneous rupture of the membranes, and is not in labour. Related terms include **preterm premature rupture of membranes (PPROM)**, which is defined as rupture of membranes prior to the onset of labour in a woman who is *less* than 37 weeks of gestation. Perinatal risks associated with PPROM may stem from immaturity, including respiratory distress syndrome, intraventricular hemorrhage, patent ductus arteriosus, and necrotizing enterocolitis.

The exact cause of PROM is not known. In many cases, PROM occurs spontaneously.

Therapeutic Management

Treatment of PROM typically depends on the gestational age. Under no circumstances is an unsterile digital cervical examination done until the woman enters active labour, to minimize infection exposure. If the fetal lungs are mature, induction of labour is initiated. PROM is not a lone indicator for surgical birth. If the fetal lungs are immature, expectant management is carried out with adequate hydration, reduced physical activity, pelvic rest,

and close observation for possible infection, such as with frequent monitoring of vital signs and laboratory test results (e.g., the white blood cell count). Corticosteroids may be given to enhance fetal lung maturity if lungs are immature, although this remains controversial. Recent studies have shown clear benefits of antibiotics to decrease neonatal morbidity associated with PPROM (Yudin, van Schalkwyk, & Van Eyk, 2009).

Nursing Assessment

Nursing assessment focuses on obtaining a complete health history and performing a physical examination to determine maternal and fetal status. An accurate assessment of the gestational age and knowledge of the maternal, fetal, and neonatal risks are essential to appropriate evaluation, counselling, and management of women with PROM and PPROM.

Health History and Physical Examination

Review the maternal history for risk factors such as infection, increased uterine size (hydramnios, macrosomia, multifetal gestation), uterine and fetal anomalies, lower socioeconomic status, STIs, cervical insufficiency, vaginal bleeding, and cigarette smoking during pregnancy. Ask about any history or current symptoms of urinary tract infection (frequency, urgency, dysuria, or flank pain) or pelvic or vaginal infection (pain or vaginal discharge).

Assess for signs and symptoms of labour, such as cramping, pelvic pressure, or back pain. Also assess her vital signs, noting any signs indicative of infection such as fever and tachycardia (Jazayeri, 2011).

Institute continuous electronic fetal heart rate monitoring to evaluate fetal well-being. Conduct a vaginal examination to ascertain the cervical status in PROM. If PPROM exists, a sterile speculum examination (where the examiner inspects the cervix but does not palpate it) is done rather than a digital cervical examination because digital examination may diminish latency (period of time from rupture of membranes to birth) and increase newborn morbidity (Cunningham, Leveno, Bloom, et al., 2010).

Observe the characteristics of the amniotic fluid. Note any evidence of meconium, or a foul odour. When meconium is present in the amniotic fluid, it typically indicates fetal distress related to hypoxia. Meconium stains the fluid yellow to greenish brown, depending on the amount present. A foul odour of amniotic fluid indicates infection. Also observe the amount of fluid. A decreased amount of amniotic fluid reduces the cushioning effect, thereby making cord compression a possibility. Key assessments are summarized in Box 19.4.

Laboratory and Diagnostic Testing

To diagnose PROM or PPROM, several procedures may be used: the Nitrazine test, fern test, or ultrasound.

Key Assessments with Premature Rupture of Membranes

For the woman with PROM, the following assessments are essential:

- Determine the date, time, and duration of membrane rupture by client interview.
- Ascertain the gestational age of the fetus based on date of mother's last menstrual period, fundal height, and ultrasound dating.
- Question the woman about possible history of or recent urinary tract infection or vaginal infection that might have contributed to PROM.
- Assess for any associated labour symptoms, such as back pain or pelvic pressure.
- Assist with or perform diagnostic tests to validate leakage of fluid, such as Nitrazine test, "ferning" on slide, and ultrasound.
- Continually assess for signs of infection, including:
  - Elevation of maternal temperature and pulse rate
  - Abdominal/uterine tenderness
  - Fetal tachycardia more than 160 bpm
  - Elevated white blood cell count and C-reactive protein
  - Cloudy, foul-smelling amniotic fluid

After the insertion of a sterile speculum, a sample of the fluid in the vaginal area is obtained. With a Nitrazine test, the pH of the fluid is tested; amniotic fluid is more basic (7.0) than normal vaginal secretions (4.5). Nitrazine paper turns blue in the presence of amniotic fluid. However, false-positive results can occur if blood, urine, semen, or antiseptic chemicals are also present; all will increase the pH.

For the fern test, a sample of vaginal fluid is place on a slide to be viewed directly under a microscope. Amniotic fluid will develop a fern-like pattern when it dries because of sodium chloride crystallization.

Other laboratory and diagnostic tests that may be used include:

- Urinalysis and urine culture for urinary tract infection or asymptomatic bacteriuria
- Cervical test or culture for chlamydia or gonorrhea
- Vaginal culture for bacterial vaginosis and trichomoniasis
- Vaginal introital/rectal culture for group B streptococcus

Nursing Management

Nursing management for the woman with PROM or PPROM focuses on preventing infection and identifying uterine contractions. The risk for infection is great because of the break in the amniotic fluid membrane and its close proximity to vaginal bacteria. Therefore, monitor

maternal vital signs closely. Be alert for a temperature elevation or an increase in pulse, which could indicate infection. Also monitor the fetal heart rate continuously, reporting any fetal tachycardia (which could indicate a maternal infection) or variable decelerations (suggesting cord compression). If variable decelerations are present, anticipate amnioinfusion based on agency policy. Evaluate the results of laboratory tests such as a CBC. An elevation in white blood cells would suggest infection. Administer antibiotics if ordered.

Encourage the woman and her partner to verbalize their feelings and concerns. Educate them about the purpose of the protective membranes and the implications of early rupture. Keep them informed about planned interventions, including potential complications and required therapy. As appropriate, prepare the woman for induction or augmentation of labour as appropriate if she is near term.

If labour doesn't start within 48 hours, the woman with PPROM may be discharged home on expectant management, which may include:

- Antibiotics if cervicovaginal cultures are positive
- Activity restrictions
- Education about signs and symptoms of infection and when to call with problems or concerns (Teaching Guideline 19.3)

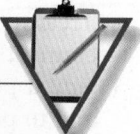

TEACHING GUIDELINE 19.3

Teaching for the Woman with PPROM

- Monitor your baby's activity by performing fetal kick counts daily.
- Check your temperature daily and report any temperature increases to your health care provider.
- Watch for signs related to the beginning of labour. Report any tightening of the abdomen or contractions.
- Avoid any touching or manipulating of your breasts, which could stimulate labour.
- Do not insert anything into your vagina or vaginal area.
- Maintain any specific activity restrictions as recommended.
- Wash your hands thoroughly after using the bathroom and make sure to wipe from front to back each time.
- Keep your perineal area clean and dry.
- Take your antibiotics as directed if your health care provider has prescribed them.
- Call your health care provider with changes in your condition, including fever, uterine tenderness, feeling like your heart is racing, and foul-smelling vaginal discharge.

- Frequent fetal testing for well-being
- Ultrasound every 3 to 4 weeks to assess amniotic fluid levels
- Possible corticosteroid treatment depending on gestational age
- Daily kick counts to assess fetal well-being

■■■ Key Concepts

■ Identifying risk factors early on and throughout the pregnancy is important to ensure the best outcome for every pregnancy. Risk assessment should start with the first prenatal visit and continue with subsequent visits.

■ The three most common causes of hemorrhage early in pregnancy (first half of pregnancy) are spontaneous abortion, ectopic pregnancy, and GTD.

■ Ectopic pregnancies occur in about 1 in 50 pregnancies and have increased dramatically during the past few decades.

■ Having a molar pregnancy results in the loss of the pregnancy and the possibility of developing choriocarcinoma, a chronic malignancy from the trophoblastic tissue.

■ The classic clinical presentation for placenta previa is painless, bright-red vaginal bleeding occurring during the third trimester.

■ Treatment of abruptio placentae is designed to assess, control, and restore the amount of blood lost; to provide a positive outcome for both mother and infant; and to prevent coagulation disorders.

■ DIC can be described in simplest terms as a loss of balance between the clot-forming activity of thrombin and the clot-lysing activity of plasmin.

■ Hyperemesis gravidarum is a complication of pregnancy characterized by persistent, uncontrollable nausea and vomiting before the 20th week of gestation.

■ Gestational hypertension is the most common complication reported during pregnancy (Carson & Gibson, 2012).

■ HELLP is an acronym for hemolysis, elevated liver enzymes, and low platelets.

■ Rh incompatibility is a condition that develops when a woman of Rh-negative blood type is exposed to Rh-positive fetal blood cells and subsequently develops circulating titers of Rh antibodies.

■ Hydramnios occurs in approximately 3% to 4% of all pregnancies and is associated with fetal anomalies of development.

■ Nursing care related to the woman with oligohydramnios involves continuous monitoring of fetal well-being during nonstress testing or during labour and birth by identifying nonreassuring patterns on the fetal monitor.

■ The increasing number of multiple gestations is a concern because women who are expecting more than one infant are at high risk for preterm labour, hydramnios, hyperemesis gravidarum, anemia, pre-eclampsia, and antepartum hemorrhage.

■ Nursing care related to PROM centres on infection prevention and identification of preterm labour contractions.

■ Early identification of preterm labour would allow for appropriate interventions that may prolong the pregnancy, such as transferring the woman to a facility with a neonatal intensive care unit for prenatal care, administering glucocorticoids to the mother to promote fetal lung maturity, and giving appropriate antibiotics to treat infections to arrest the labour process.

■ It is essential that nurses teach all pregnant women how to detect the early symptoms of preterm labour and what to do if they experience contractions or cramping that does not go away.

REFERENCES

Arsenault, M. Y., & Lane, C. (2002). SOGC clinical practice guidelines: The management of nausea and vomiting in pregnancy. *Journal of Obstetrics and Gynaecology Canada, 24*(10), 817–823.

Bahar, A., Abusham, A., Eskandar, M., Sobande, A., & Alsunaidi, M. (2009). Risk factors and pregnancy outcome in different types of placenta previa. *Journal of Obstetrics and Gynaecology Canada, 31*(2), 126–131.

Beaulieu, M. D. (1993). *Screening for D (Rh) sensitization in pregnancy.* Retrieved March 9, 2012 from http://www.phac-aspc.gc.ca/publicat/clinic-clinique/pdf/s1c11e.pdf

Brodovicz, K. G., McNaughton, K., Uemura, N., Meininger, G., Girman, C. J., & Yale, S. H. (2009). Reliability and feasibility of methods to quantitatively assess peripheral edema. *Clinical Medicine and Research, 7*(1–2), 21–31.

Brophy, K., Scarlett-Fergusen, H., & Webber, K. (2008). *Clinical drug therapy for Canadian practice* (1st Canadian ed.). Philadelphia: Lippincott Williams & Wilkins.

Canadian Institute for Health Information. (2004). *Giving birth in Canada: Providers of maternity and infant care.* Retrieved March 9, 2012 from http://dsp-psd.pwgsc.gc.ca/Collection/H118-25-2004E.pdf

Carson, M. P., & Gibson, P. (2012). *Hypertension and pregnancy.* Retrieved March 9, 2012 from http://emedicine.medscape.com/article/261435-overview#showall

Carter, B. S., & Boyd, R. L. (2012). *Pediatric polyhydramnios and oligohydramnios medication.* Retrieved March 9, 2012 from http://emedicine.medscape.com/article/975821-medication#showall

Cole, L. (2010). Biological functions of hCG and hCG-related molecules. *Reproductive Biology and Endocrinology, 8,* 102. doi:10.1186/1477-7827-8-102

Crane, J. (2001). SOGC clinical practice guideline: Induction of labour at term. *Journal of Obstetrics and Gynaecology Canada, 23*(8), 717–728. Retrieved March 9, 2012 from http://www.sogc.org/guidelines/public/107E-CPG-August2001.pdf

Cunningham, F. G. N. F., Leveno, K. J., Bloom, S., Hauth, J. C., Rouse, D., & Sponc, C. (2010). *Williams' obstetrics* (23rd ed.). New York: McGraw-Hill.

Day, R., Paul, P., Williams, B., Smeltzer, S., & Bare, B. (2010). *Brunner & Suddarth's textbook of medical-surgical nursing* (2nd Canadian ed.). Philadelphia: Lippincott Williams & Wilkins.

Deering, S. (2011). *Abruptio placentae.* Retrieved March 9, 2012 from http://emedicine.medscape.com/article/252810-overview#showall

Deglin, J., Vallerand, A., Sanoski, C. (2011). *Davis's drug guide for nurses* (12th ed.). Philadelphia: FA Davis Company.

Einarson, A., Choi, J., Einarson, T. R., & Koren, G. (2009). Rates of spontaneous and therapeutic abortions following use of antidepressants in pregnancy: Results from a large prospective database. *Journal of Obstetrics and Gynaecology Canada, 31*(5), 452–456.

Einarson, A., Maltepe, C., Boskovic, R., & Koren, G. (2007). *Treatment of nausea and vomiting in pregnancy.* Retrieved March 9, 2012 from http://www.motherisk.org/women/updatesDetail.jsp?content_id=875

Fletcher, G., Zach, T., Pramanik, A. K., & Ford, S. P. (2009). *Multiple births.* Retrieved March 9, 2012 from http://emedicine.medscape.com/article/977234-overview#showall

Fox, N. S., & Chervenak, F. A. (2008). Cervical cerclage: A review of the evidence. *Obstetrical and Gynecological Survey, 63*(1), 58–65.

Fung, K., & Eason, E. (2003). SOGC clinical practice guidelines: Prevention of RH alloimmunization. *Journal of Obstetrics and Gynaecology Canada, 25*(9), 765–773. Retrieved March 9, 2012 from http://www.sogc.org/guidelines/public/133e-cpg-september2003.pdf

Gerulath, A. H. (2002). SOGC clinical practice guidelines: Gestational trophoblastic disease. *Journal of Obstetrics and Gynaecology Canada, 24*(5), 434–439. Retrieved March 9, 2012 from http://www.sogc.org/guidelines/public/114E-CPG-May2002.pdf

Gibbs, R. S., Danforth, D. N., Karlan, B. Y., & Haney, A. F. (2008). *Danforth's obstetrics and gynecology* (10th ed.). Philadelphia: Lippincott Williams & Wilkins.

Gilbert, E. (2010). *Manual of high-risk pregnancy and delivery* (5th ed.). St. Louis, MO: Mosby.

Hagel-Fenton, D. J. (2008). Beyond preeclampsia: HELLP syndrome. *RN, 71*(3), 22–26.

Hajenius, P. J., Mol, F., Mol, B. W. J., Bossuyt, P. M. M., Ankum, W. M., & van der Veen, F. (2009). Interventions for tubal ectopic pregnancy. *Cochrane Database of Systematic Reviews, 1*, CD000324. doi:10.1002/14651858.CD000324.pub2

Han, C., & Norwitz, E. R. (2011). Expectant management of severe preeclampsia remote from term: Not for everyone. *Contemporary OB/GYN, 56*(2), 50–55.

Haram, K., Svendsen, E., & Abildgaard, U. (2009). The HELLP syndrome: Clinical issues and management. A review. *BMC Pregnancy and Childbirth, 9,* 8. Retrieved March 9, 2012 from http://www.ncbi.nlm.nih.gov/pmc/articles/PMC2654858/?tool=pubmed. doi:10.1186/1471-2393-9-8

Hernandez, E. (2012). Gestational trophoblastic neoplasia. Retrieved March 9, 2012 from http://emedicine.medscape.com/article/279116-overview#showall

Jarvis, C. (2009). *Physical examination & health assessment* (1st Canadian ed.). Toronto, Ontario: Saunders Elsevier.

Jazayeri, A. (2011). *Premature rupture of membranes.* Retrieved April 28, 2011 from http://emedicine.medscape.com/article/261137-overview#

Joy, S., Lyon, D., & Stone, R. A. (2010). *Placenta previa.* Retrieved March 9, 2012 from http://emedicine.medscape.com/article/262063-overview

Karch, A. M. (2011). *2011 Lippincott's nursing drug guide.* Philadelphia: Lippincott Williams & Wilkins.

Ko, P., & Yoon, Y. (2011). *Placenta previa in emergency medicine clinical presentation. eMedicine.* Retrieved March 9, 2012 from http://emedicine.medscape.com/article/796182-clinical#showall

Koelewijn, J. M., de Haas, M., Vrijkotte, T. G. M., van der Schoot, C. E., & Bonsel, G. E. (2009). Risk factors for RhD immunisation despite antenatal and postnatal anti-D prophylaxis. *British Journal of Obstetrics and Gynaecology, 116*(10), 1304–1314.

Lavanya, R., Deepika, K., & Patil, M. (2009). Successful pregnancy following medical management of heterotopic pregnancy. *Journal of Human Reproductive Science, 2*(1), 35–40.

Levi, M., & Schmaier, A. H. (2011). *Disseminated intravascular coagulation treatment & management.* Retrieved March 9, 2012 from http://emedicine.medscape.com/article/199627-treatment#a1127

Lim, K., Butt, K., & Crane, J. M. (2011). SOGC clinical practice guidelines: Ultrasonographic cervical length assessment in predicting preterm birth in singleton pregnancies. *Journal of Obstetrics and Gynaecology Canada, 25*(9), 765–773. Retrieved March 9, 2012 from http://www.sogc.org/guidelines/documents/gui257CPG1106E.pdf

Lim, K. H., Sayah, A. J., Steinberg, G., Semenovskaya, Z., Erogul, M., & Zwanger, M. (2011). *Preeclampsia.* Retrieved March 9, 2012 from http://www.emedicine.com/med/topic1905.htm

Lindheimer, M. D., Taler, S. J., & Cunningham, F. G. (2008). Hypertension in pregnancy. *Journal of the American Society of Hypertension, 2*(6), 484–494.

Lipscomb, G. H. (2011). Ectopic pregnancy. In E. T. Bope, R. Kellerman, & R. E. Rakel (Eds.), *Conn's current therapy 2011.* Philadelphia: Saunders Elsevier.

Liston, R., Sawchuk, D., & Young, D. (2007). Fetal health surveillance: Antepartum and intrapartum consensus guideline. *Journal of Obstetrics and Gynaecology Canada, 29*(9 Suppl. 4), S3–S56. Retrieved March 9, 2012 from http://www.sogc.org/guidelines/documents/gui197CPG0709.pdf

Madani, Y. (2008). The use of ultrasonography in the diagnosis of ectopic pregnancy: A case report and review of the literature. *The Medscape Journal of Medicine, 10*(2), 35.

Magee, L. A., Helewa, M., Moutquin, J.-M., & von Dadelszen, P. (2008). SOGC clinical practice guidelines: Diagnosis, evaluation and management of the hypertensive disorders of pregnancy. *Journal of Obstetrics and Gynaecology Canada, 30*(3 Suppl. 1), S1–S52. Retrieved March 9, 2012 from http://www.sogc.org/guidelines/documents/gui206CPG0803_001.pdf

Mancuso, M., & Owen, J. (2009). Prevention of preterm birth based on a short cervix: Cerclage. *Seminars in Perinatology, 33*(5), 325–333. doi:10.1053/j.semperi.2009.06.005

McParlin, C., Graham, R. H., & Robson, S. C. (2008). Caring for women with nausea and vomiting in pregnancy: New approaches. *British Journal of Midwifery, 16*(5), 280–285.

Medscape Reference. (2011). *Magnesium sulfate (Rx).* Retrieved March 9, 2012 from http://reference.medscape.com/drug/mgso4-magnesium-sulfate-344444#0

Mistovich, J. J., Krost, W. S., & Limmer, D. D. (2008). Beyond the basics: Preeclampsia and eclampsia. *EMS Magazine, 37*(11), 51–55.

Murray, H., Baakdah, H., Bardell, T., & Tulandi, T. (2005). Diagnosis and treatment of ectopic pregnancy. *Canadian Medical Association Journal, 173*(8), 905–912.

Norwitz, E. R., & Schorge, J. O. (2010). *Obstetrics and gynecology at a glance* (3rd ed.). Malden, MA: Blackwell Publishing Ltd.

Ogunyemi, D. A., Fong, A., & Chen Herrero, T. (2011). *Hyperemesis gravidarum.* Retrieved March 9, 2012 from http://emedicine.medscape.com/article/254751-overview

Oxlund, B., Ørtoft, G., Brüel, A., Danielsen, C., Oxlund, H., & Uldbjerg, N. (2010). Cervical collagen and biomechanical strength in non-pregnant women with a history of cervical insufficiency. *Reproductive Biology and Endocrinology, 8,* 92. doi:10.1186/1477-7827-8-92

Peel, A. (2009). Diagnosis of an interstitial ectopic pregnancy with two-dimensional transvaginal sonography. *Ultrasound, 17*(2), 93–95.

Public Health Agency of Canada. (2008). *Canadian perinatal health report, 2008 edition.* Retrieved March 9, 2012 from http://www.phac-aspc.gc.ca/publicat/2008/cphr-rspc/pdf/cphr-rspc08-eng.pdf

Rajiah, P. (2011). *Polyhydramnios.* Retrieved March 9, 2012 from http://emedicine.medscape.com/article/404856-overview

Reid, H., Power, M., & Cheshire, K. (2009). Factors influencing antenatal depression, anxiety and stress. *British Journal of Midwifery, 17*(8), 501–508.

Ross, M. (2011). *Eclampisa.* Retrieved March 9, 2012 from http://emedicine.medscape.com/article/253960-overview#aw2aab6c10

Salem, L. (2012). *Rh incompatibility.* Retrieved April 28, 2011 from http://emedicine.medscape.com/article/797150-overview#showall

Sepilian, V. (2011). *Ectopic pregnancy treatment and management.* Retrieved March 9, 2012 from http://emedicine.medscape.com/article/258768-treatment

Sepilian, V., & Wood, E. (2011). *Ectopic pregnancy.* Retrieved March 9, 2012 from http://emedicine.medscape.com/article/258768-overview#showall

Sierra-Bergua, B., Sánchez-Marteles, M., Cabrerizo-García, J. L., & Sanjoaquin-Conde, I. (2008). Choriocarcinoma with pulmonary and cerebral metastases. *Singapore Medical Journal, 49*(10), 286–288.

Silver, R. M. (2009). Evaluation of fetal death from nongenetic causes. *Contemporary OB/GYN, 54*(12), 35–43.

Society of Obstetrics and Gynaecologists of Canada. (2010). *Women's health information: Nausea and vomiting in pregnancy.* Retrieved March 9, 2012 from http://www.sogc.org/health/pregnancy-nausea_e.asp

Sovari, A. A., Kocheril, A. G., & Bass, A. S. (2012). *Cardiogenic pulmonary edema clinical presentation.* Retrieved March 9, 2012 from http://emedicine.medscape.com/article/157452-clinical#showall

Stan, C. M., Boulvian, M., Pfister, R., & Hirsbrunner-Almagbaly, P. (2009). Hydration for treatment of preterm labour. *Cochrane Database of Systematic Reviews, 2,* CD003096.

Statistics Canada. (2008). Live births and fetal deaths (stillbirths), by geography—Type of birth (single or multiple). Retrieved March 9, 2012 from http://www.statcan.gc.ca/pub/84f0210x/2008000/t025-eng.pdf

Statistics Canada. (2011). *Deaths, by cause—Chapter XV: Pregnancy, childbirth and the puerperium (O00 to O99), age group and sex, Canada.* Retrieved March 9, 2012 from http://www5.statcan.gc.ca/cansim/a05?lang=eng&id=1020535

Stephenson, M. (2008). Recurrent early pregnancy less: Is miscarriage evaluation the missing link? *Contemporary OB/GYN, 53*(10), 50–55.

Stokes, B. (2011). Hypertensive disease of pregnancy. In E. T. Bope, R. Kellerman, & R. E. Rakel (Eds.), *Conn's current therapy 2011.* Philadelphia: Saunders Elsevier.

Stucki, D., & Buss, J. (2008). The ectopic pregnancy, a diagnostic and therapeutic challenge. *Journal of Medicine and Life, 1*(1), 40–48.

Varma, R., & Gupta, J. (2009). Tubal ectopic pregnancy. *Clinical Evidence, 1406,* 1–15.

Wilcox, S. R. (2010). *Pregnancy, hyperemesis gravidarum.* Retrieved March 9, 2012 from http://emedicine.medscape.com/article/796564-overview

Yudin, M. H., van Schalkwyk, J., & Van Eyk, N. (2009). SOGC clinical practice guideline: Antibiotic therapy in preterm premature rupture of the membranes. *Journal of Obstetrics and Gynaecology Canada, 31*(9), 863–867. Retrieved March 9, 2012 from http://www.sogc.org/guidelines/documents/gui233CPG0909.pdf

Zeltzer, J. S. (2011). Vaginal bleeding in late pregnancy. In R. D. Kellerman & E. T. Bope (Eds.), *Conn's current therapy 2011.* Philadelphia: Saunders Elsevier.

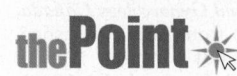

For additional learning materials, including Internet Resources, visit http://thePoint.lww.com/Chow1e.

CHAPTER WORKSHEET

MULTIPLE CHOICE QUESTIONS

1. A woman diagnosed with pre-eclampsia is to receive magnesium sulphate. The rationale for this drug is to:

   a. Reduce CNS irritability to prevent seizures

   b. Provide supplementation of an important mineral she needs

   c. Prevent constipation during and after the birthing process

   d. Decrease musculoskeletal tone to augment labour

2. A woman is suspected of having abruptio placentae. Which of the following would the nurse expect to assess as a classic symptom?

   a. Painless, bright-red bleeding

   b. "Knife-like" abdominal pain

   c. Excessive nausea and vomiting

   d. Hypertension and headache

3. WinRho is given to Rh-negative women to prevent maternal sensitization. In addition to pregnancy, Rh-negative women would also receive this medication after which of the following?

   a. Therapeutic or spontaneous abortion

   b. Head injury from a car accident

   c. Blood transfusion after a hemorrhage

   d. Unsuccessful artificial insemination procedure

4. After teaching a woman about hyperemesis gravidarum and how it differs from the typical nausea and vomiting of pregnancy, which statement by the woman indicates that the teaching was successful?

   a. "I can expect the nausea to last through my second trimester."

   b. "I should drink fluids with my meals instead of in between them."

   c. "I need to avoid strong odours, perfumes, or flavours."

   d. "I should lie down after I eat for about 2 hours."

5. A pregnant woman, approximately 12 weeks' gestation, comes to the emergency department after calling her health care provider's office and reporting moderate vaginal bleeding. Assessment reveals cervical dilation and moderately strong abdominal cramps. She reports that she has passed some tissue with the bleeding. The nurse interprets these findings to suggest which of the following?

   a. Threatened abortion

   b. Inevitable abortion

   c. Incomplete abortion

   d. Missed abortion

CRITICAL THINKING EXERCISES

1. Suzanne, a 16-year-old primigravida, presents to the maternity clinic complaining of continual nausea and vomiting for the past 3 days. She states she is approximately 15 weeks pregnant and has been unable to hold anything down or take any fluids in without throwing up for the past 3 days. She reports she is dizzy and weak. On examination, Suzanne appears pale and anxious. Her mucous membranes are dry, skin turgor is poor, and her lips are dry and cracked.

   a. What is your impression of this condition?

   b. What risk factors does Suzanne have?

   c. What intervention is appropriate for this woman?

2. Gloria is an obese 9-year-old primigravida of African descent who is diagnosed with gestational hypertension. Her history reveals that her sister developed pre-eclampsia during her pregnancy. When describing her diet to the nurse, Gloria mentions that she tends to eat a lot of fast food.

   a. What risk factors does Gloria have that increase her risk for gestational hypertension?

   b. When assessing Gloria, what assessment findings would lead the nurse to suspect that Gloria has developed severe pre-eclampsia?

(question continues on page 618)

STUDY ACTIVITIES

1. Ask a community health maternity nurse how the signs and symptoms of gestational hypertension (including pre-eclampsia and eclampsia) are taught, and how effective efforts have been to reduce the incidence in the area.

2. Find a website designed to help parents who have suffered a pregnancy loss secondary to a spontaneous abortion. What is its audience level? Is the information up to date?

3. A pregnancy in which the blastocyst implants outside the uterus is an _____ pregnancy.

4. The most serious complication of hydatidiform mole is the development of _____ afterward.

5. Discuss various activities a woman with a multiple gestation could engage in to help pass the time when ordered to be on bed rest at home for 2 months.

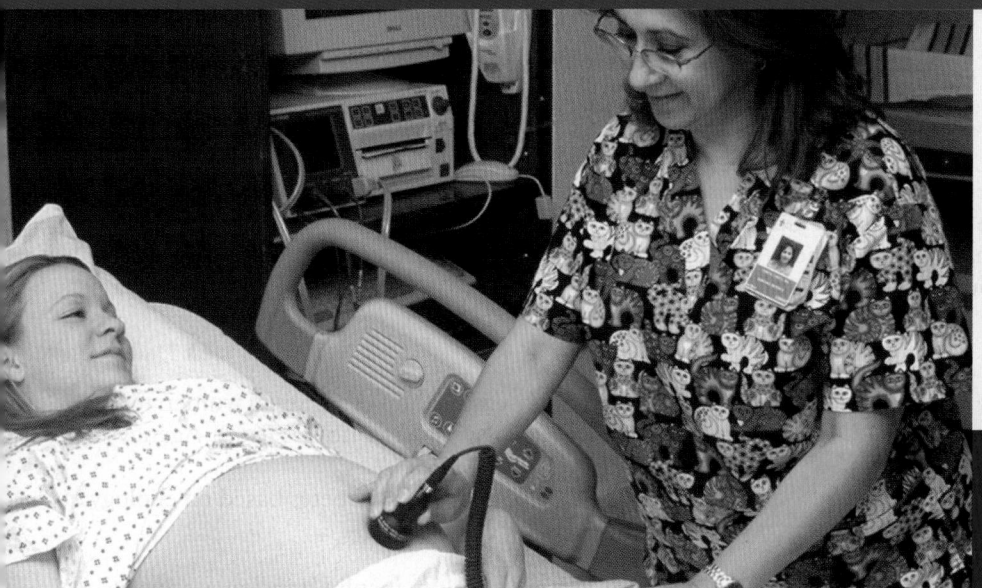

NURSING MANAGEMENT OF THE PREGNANCY AT RISK: SELECTED HEALTH CONDITIONS AND VULNERABLE POPULATIONS

KEY TERMS

acquired
   immunodeficiency
   syndrome (AIDS)
adolescence
anemia
fetal alcohol spectrum
   disorder (FASD)
gestational diabetes
   mellitus (GDM)

glycated hemoglobin
   (A1C) level
human immunodeficiency
   virus (HIV)
impaired fasting glucose
impaired glucose
   tolerance
neonatal abstinence
   syndrome

perinatal drug abuse
pica
pregestational diabetes
pregnancy after 35 years
   of age
teratogen
type 1 diabetes
type 2 diabetes

LEARNING OBJECTIVES

Upon completion of the chapter, the learner will be able to:

1. Identify at least two conditions present before pregnancy that can have a negative effect on a pregnancy.
2. Explain how a condition present before pregnancy can affect the woman physiologically and psychologically when she becomes pregnant.
3. Differentiate the nursing assessment and management for a pregnant woman with diabetes from that of a pregnant woman without diabetes.
4. Explore how congenital and acquired heart conditions can affect a woman's pregnancy.
5. Describe the nursing assessment and management of a pregnant woman with cardiovascular disorders and respiratory conditions.
6. Differentiate among the types of anemia affecting pregnant women in terms of prevention and management.
7. Describe the most common infections that can jeopardize a pregnancy, and propose possible preventive strategies.

*R*ose, a thin 16-year-old appearing very pregnant, came into the clinic wheezing and having difficulty catching her breath. She had missed several previous prenatal visits but arrived at the clinic today in distress. Rose has a history of asthma since she was 5 years old. How might Rose's current condition affect her pregnancy? Is this picture typical of the pregnant asthmatic?

Wow

As the sun sets each day, nurses should make sure they have done something for others, and should try to be understanding even under the most difficult of conditions.

LEARNING OBJECTIVES (continued)

8. Explain the nurse's role in the prevention and management of adolescent pregnancy.
9. Identify the impact of pregnancy on a woman over the age of 35.
10. Develop a plan of care for the pregnant woman who is HIV positive.
11. Examine the effects of substance abuse during pregnancy.

Pregnancy and childbirth are exciting yet complex facets within the continuum of women's health. Ideally the pregnant woman is free of any conditions that can affect a pregnancy, but in reality many women enter pregnancy with a multitude of health-related or psychosocial issues that can have a negative impact on the outcome.

Many pregnant women express the wish, "I hope my baby is born healthy." Nurses can play a major role in helping this become a reality by educating women before they become pregnant. Conditions such as diabetes, cardiac and respiratory disorders, anemias, and specific infections frequently can be controlled through close prenatal management so that their impact on pregnancy is minimized. Nurses can provide pregnancy-prevention strategies when counselling teenagers. Meeting the developmental needs of pregnant adolescents is a challenge. Finally, lifestyle choices, such as the use of alcohol, nicotine, and illicit substances, can place many women at risk during pregnancy, and nurses need to remain non-judgmental in working with these special populations.

Chapter 19 described pregnancy-related conditions that place the woman at risk. This chapter addresses common conditions that can have a negative impact on the pregnancy and special populations at risk, outlining appropriate nursing assessment and management for each condition or situation. The unique skills of nurses, in conjunction with the other members of the health care team, can increase the potential for a positive outcome in many high-risk pregnancies.

Diabetes Mellitus

Diabetes mellitus is a common chronic disease characterized by a relative lack of insulin or absence of the hormone, which is necessary for glucose metabolism. The chronic hyperglycemia of diabetes is associated with long-term damage, dysfunction, and failure of the eyes, kidneys, nerves, heart, and blood vessels. The incidence of diabetes is increasing at an alarming rate in Canada, already reaching epidemic proportions. According to the Canadian Diabetes Cost Model, the number of Canadians living with diabetes will grow from 2.5 million in 2010 to 3.7 million by 2020. A contributing factor to these increasing rates is the incidence of obesity (Canadian Diabetes Association [CDA], 2009). In pregnancy, the prevalence of diabetes is population specific, ranging from 3.7% in multi-ethnic, non-Aboriginal women to 8% to 18% in Aboriginal women (Public Health Agency of Canada [PHAC], 2009a).

The CDA (2008) classifies diabetes based on etiology. These groups include:

- **Type 1 diabetes:** absolute insulin deficiency (due to an autoimmune process); usually appears in childhood or adolescence; approximately 10% of those diagnosed have type 1 diabetes
- **Type 2 diabetes:** insulin resistance or deficiency (related to obesity, sedentary lifestyle); diagnosed primarily in adults older than 40 years of age but is now being seen in children; accounts for 90% of all diagnosed cases
- **Gestational diabetes mellitus (GDM):** glucose intolerance with its onset during pregnancy or first detected in pregnancy; affects approximately 4% of all pregnancies and increases the mother's risk for developing type 2 diabetes
- **Other specific types:** includes a wide variety of relatively uncommon conditions; primarily specific genetically defined forms of diabetes or diabetes associated with other diseases or drug use.

During pregnancy, diabetes typically is categorized into two groups: **pregestational diabetes** is the alteration in carbohydrate metabolism identified before conception that can occur in women with type 1 or type 2 disease; and, **gestational diabetes**, which develops during pregnancy. In Canada, pregestational diabetes complicates 0.7% to 1.8% of all pregnancies and affects more than 11,000 women annually. GDM occurs in approximately 3.7% of all pregnant women, and those rates are higher among Aboriginal women (CDA, 2008; PHAC, 2009a). GDM is associated with either neonatal complications, such as macrosomia, hypoglycemia, and birth trauma, or maternal complications, such as pre-eclampsia and cesarean birth (Hod & Simeoni, 2009; Langer, 2008).

Before the discovery of insulin in 1922 by Canadian scientist Dr. Fredrick Banting, most women with diabetes were infertile or experienced spontaneous abortion (Hod et al., 2008). Over the past several decades, great strides have been made in improving the outcomes of pregnancy in women with diabetes, but this chronic metabolic disorder remains a high-risk condition during pregnancy. A favourable outcome requires commitment on the woman's part to comply with frequent prenatal visits, dietary restrictions, self-monitoring of blood glucose levels, frequent laboratory tests, intensive fetal surveillance, and perhaps hospitalization (Boinpally & Jovanovic, 2009; CDA, 2008; Kitzmiller, Block, Brown, et al., 2008).

Pathophysiology

With diabetes, there is a deficiency of or resistance to insulin. This alteration interferes with the body's ability to obtain essential nutrients for fuel and storage. If a pregnant woman has pregestational diabetes or develops GDM, the profound metabolic alterations that occur during pregnancy and that are necessary to support the growth and development of fetus can be affected.

▶ **Consider** THIS!

Scott and I had been busy all day setting up the new crib and nursery, and we finally sat down to rest. I was due any day, and we had been putting this off until we had a long weekend to complete the task. I was excited to think about all the frilly pinks that decorated her room. I was sure that my new daughter would love it as much as I loved her already. A few days later I barely noticed any fetal movement, but I thought that she must be as tired as I was by this point.

That night I went into labour and kept looking at the worried faces of the nurses and the midwife in attendance. I had been diagnosed with gestational diabetes a few months ago and had tried to follow the instructions regarding diet and exercise, but old habits are hard to change when you are 38 years old. I was finally told after a short time in the labour unit that they couldn't pick up a fetal heartbeat and an ultrasound was to be done—still no heartbeat was detected. Scott and I were finally told that our daughter was a stillborn. All I could think about was that she would never get to see all the pink colours in the nursery. . . .

Maternal metabolism is directed toward supplying adequate nutrition for the fetus. In pregnancy, placental hormones cause insulin resistance at a level that tends to parallel the growth of the fetoplacental unit. As the placenta grows, more placental hormones are secreted. Human placental lactogen (hPL) and growth hormone (somatotropin) increase in direct correlation with the growth of placental tissue, rising throughout the last 20 weeks of pregnancy and causing insulin resistance. Subsequently, insulin secretion increases to overcome the resistance of these two hormones. In the nondiabetic pregnant woman, the pancreas can respond to the demands for increased insulin production to maintain normal glucose levels throughout the pregnancy (Klieger, Pollex, & Koren, 2008). However, the woman with

glucose intolerance or diabetes during pregnancy cannot cope with changes in metabolism resulting from insufficient insulin to meet the needs during gestation (Devlieger, Casteels, & Van Assche, 2008).

Over the course of pregnancy, insulin resistance changes. It peaks in the last trimester to provide more nutrients to the fetus. The insulin resistance typically results in postprandial hyperglycemia, although some women also have an elevated fasting blood glucose level (Kaaja & Rönnemaa, 2008). With this increased demand on the pancreas in late pregnancy, women with diabetes or glucose intolerance cannot accommodate the increased insulin demand; glucose levels rise as a result of insulin deficiency, leading to hyperglycemia. Consequently, the mother and her fetus can experience major problems (Table 20.1).

Therapeutic Management

Preconception care is key for the woman with pregestational diabetes (the alteration in carbohydrate metabolism is identified before conception) to ensure that her disease state is stable. The goals of preconception care are to:

- Integrate the woman into the management of her diabetes
- Achieve the lowest glycated hemoglobin A1C test results without excessive hypoglycemia
- Ensure effective contraception until stable glycemia is achieved
- Supplement the diet with multivitamins containing 5 mg folic acid starting at least 3 months preconception and continuing until 12 weeks postconception
- Identify and evaluate long-term diabetic complications such as retinopathy, nephropathy, neuropathy, cardiovascular disease, and hypertension (CDA, 2008)

Excellent control of blood glucose, as evidenced by normal fasting blood glucose levels and a **glycated hemoglobin (A1C) level** (a measurement of the average glucose levels over the past 100 to 120 days), is crucial to achieve the best pregnancy outcome. An A1C level of less than 7% indicates good control; a value of more than 8% indicates poor control and warrants intervention (CDA, 2008).

Preconception counselling also is important in helping to reduce the risk for congenital malformation. The most common malformations associated with diabetes occur in the renal, cardiac, skeletal, and central nervous systems (CNS). Since these defects occur by the eighth week of gestation, preconception counselling is critical. The rate of congenital anomalies in women with pregestational diabetes can be reduced if excellent glycemic control is achieved at the time of conception (Cheng & Caughey, 2008). This information needs to be stressed with all diabetic women contemplating a pregnancy.

TABLE 20.1   DIABETES AND PREGNANCY: EFFECTS ON THE MOTHER AND FETUS

Effects on the Mother	Effects on the Fetus/Neonate
• Polyhydramnios due to fetal diuresis caused by hyperglycemia • Gestational hypertension of unknown etiology • Ketoacidosis due to uncontrolled hyperglycemia • Preterm labour secondary to premature membrane rupture • Stillbirth in pregnancies complicated by ketoacidosis and poor glucose control • Hypoglycemia as glucose is diverted to the fetus (occurring in first trimester) • Urinary tract infections resulting from excess glucose in the urine (glucosuria), which promotes bacterial growth • Chronic monilial vaginitis due to glucosuria, which promotes growth of yeast • Difficult labour, cesarean birth, postpartum hemorrhage secondary to an overdistended uterus to accommodate a macrosomic infant	• Cord prolapse secondary to polyhydramnios and abnormal fetal presentation • Congenital anomaly due to hyperglycemia in the first trimester (cardiac problems, neural tube defects, skeletal deformities, and genitourinary problems) • Macrosomia resulting from hyperinsulinemia stimulated by fetal hyperglycemia • Birth trauma due to increased size of fetus, which complicates the birthing process (shoulder dystocia) • Preterm birth secondary to hydramnios and an aging placenta, which places the fetus in jeopardy if the pregnancy continues • Fetal asphyxia secondary to fetal hyperglycemia and hyperinsulinemia • Intrauterine growth restriction (IUGR) secondary to maternal vascular impairment and decreased placental perfusion, which restricts growth • Perinatal death due to poor placental perfusion and hypoxia • Respiratory distress syndrome resulting from poor surfactant production secondary to hyperinsulinemia inhibiting the production of phospholipids, which make up surfactant • Polycythemia due to excessive red blood cell (RBC) production in response to hypoxia • Hyperbilirubinemia due to excessive RBC breakdown from hypoxia and an immature liver unable to break down bilirubin • Neonatal hypoglycemia resulting from ongoing hyperinsulinemia after the placenta is removed • Subsequent childhood obesity and carbohydrate intolerance

Sources: Gilbert, E. S. (2011). *Manual of high risk pregnancy & delivery* (5th ed.). St. Louis, MO: Mosby Elsevier; & Nodine, P. M., Arruda, J., & Hastings-Tolsma, M. (2011). Prenatal environment: Effect on neonatal outcome. In S. L. Gardner, B. S. Carter, M. Enzman-Hines, & J. A. Hernandez (Eds.), *Merenstein & Gardner's handbook of neonatal intensive care* (7th ed.). St. Louis, MO: Mosby Elsevier.

In addition, the woman with pregestational diabetes needs to be evaluated for complications of diabetes. This evaluation should be part of baseline screening and continuing assessment during pregnancy (Retnakaran & Shah, 2009).

Normal maternal blood glucose and A1C levels during pregnancy are considerably lower than in nonpregnant women (CDA, 2008). Therapeutic management for the woman with GDM (defined as glucose intolerance with its onset during pregnancy or first detected during pregnancy) focuses on tight plasma glucose (PG) control. The CDA (2008) recommends maintaining a fasting and preprandial PG level between 3.8 and 5.2 mmol/L, with 1- and 2-hour postprandial PG levels between 5.5 and 7.7 and between 5.0 and 6.6 mmol/L, respectively. In comparison, for pregnant women without diabetes, near-normal fasting and PG levels (mean ± SD) include a fasting value of 4.3 (± 0.7) mmol/L, a 1-hour postprandial PG value of 6.1 (± 0.9) mmol/L, and a 2-hour postprandial value of 5.4 (± 0.6). Values are higher in obese women. Such tight control has been advocated

because it is associated with a reduction in macrosomia (Cheung, 2009).

Women with diabetes need comprehensive prenatal care. The primary goals of care are to maintain glycemic control and minimize the risks of the disease on the fetus. Key aspects of treatment include nutritional management, insulin regimens, and close maternal and fetal surveillance.

Nutritional management focuses on maintaining balanced glucose levels, providing sufficient energy and nutrients for the pregnant woman while avoiding ketosis, and minimizing the risk for hypoglycemia in women treated with insulin (Lapolla, Dalfra, Mello, et al., 2008). Women who receive dietary instruction and follow it have been shown to have a better pregnancy outcome than those who don't receive dietary advice (CDA, 2008; Cheung, 2009). For the woman with GDM, nutritional management may be all that is necessary.

Insulin, which doesn't cross the placenta, historically has been the medication of choice for treating hyperglycemia in pregnancy. Recent studies have examined the use of oral hypoglycemic medications in pregnancy. Several studies have used glyburide (Diabeta) with promising results (Balani, Hyer, Rodin, et al., 2009; Nicholson, Bolen, Witkop, et al., 2009). When oral agents are prescribed, additional treatment with insulin may be necessary as the pregnancy advances (Nicholson et al., 2009). More research is indicated to establish the drug's safety and efficacy in managing diabetes in pregnancy before it can be considered an evidence-based practice (Klieger et al., 2008).

The CDA (2008) recommends that women diagnosed with GDM receive nutritional counselling from a registered dietitian. The CDA also recommends insulin therapy if diet is unsuccessful in achieving a fasting glucose level below 5.2 mmol/L, a 1-hour postprandial level below 7.7 mmol/L, or 2-hour postprandial level below 5.2 mmol/L.

The use of diet or insulin to achieve a 1-hour postprandial blood glucose level of 7.7 mmol/L is recommended (CDA, 2008). Further studies are needed to establish the safety of oral antidiabetic agents (Klieger et al., 2008).

Glycemic control—regardless of whether it involves diet, insulin, or oral agents—leads to fewer cases of shoulder dystocia, hyperbilirubinemia requiring phototherapy, nerve palsy, bone fracture, large-for-gestational-age status, and fetal macrosomia (CDA, 2008; Nodine, Arruda, & Hastings-Tolsma, 2011).

Insulin remains the medication of choice for glycemic control in pregnant and lactating women with any type of diabetes (CDA, 2008). Generally, insulin doses are reduced in the first trimester to prevent hypoglycemia resulting from increased insulin sensitivity as well as from nausea and vomiting. Newer short-acting insulins such as lispo (Humalog) and aspart (Novolog), which do not cross the placenta, may help reduce postprandial hyperglycemia and episodes of hypoglycemia between meals (CDA, 2008; Cheung, 2009). Changes in diet and activity level add to the need for changes in insulin dosages throughout pregnancy.

Insulin regimens vary, and controversy remains over the best strategy for insulin delivery in pregnancy. Many health care providers use a split-dose therapy (two thirds of the daily dose in the morning and the remaining one third in the evening). Others advocate the use of an insulin pump to deliver a continuous subcutaneous insulin infusion. Regardless of which protocol is used, frequent blood glucose measurements are necessary, and the insulin dosage is adjusted on the basis of daily glucose levels. See Evidence-based Practice 20.1.

Close maternal and fetal surveillance is also essential. Frequent laboratory tests are done during pregnancy to monitor the woman's status and glucose control. Fetal surveillance via diagnostic testing aids in evaluating fetal well-being and assisting in determining the best time for birth.

For the labouring woman with diabetes, intravenous saline is given and blood glucose levels are monitored every 1 to 2 hours. Glucose levels are monitored throughout labour to reduce the likelihood of neonatal hypoglycemia. If necessary, an infusion of regular insulin may be given to maintain this level (CDA, 2008). If the woman was receiving insulin during her pregnancy, adjustments in dosage may be necessary after birth since glucose diversion across the placenta to supply the growing fetus is no longer present and insulin resistance is now removed. Frequently, the woman with GDM can remain controlled through diet and weight management; the woman with type 1 diabetes usually returns to pre-pregnancy levels of insulin administration (Modder, 2008).

Nursing Assessment

Nursing assessment begins at the first prenatal visit. A thorough history and physical examination in conjunction with specific laboratory and diagnostic testing aids in developing an individualized plan of care for the woman with diabetes.

Health History and Physical Examination

For the woman with pregestational diabetes, obtain a thorough history of the preexisting diabetic condition. Ask about her duration of disease, management of glucose levels (insulin injections, insulin pump, or oral hypoglycemic agents), dietary adjustments, presence of vascular complications and current vascular status, current insulin regimen, and technique used for glucose testing. Review any information that she may have received as part of her preconception counselling and measures that were implemented at that time.

Be knowledgeable about the woman's nutritional requirements, and assess the adequacy and pattern of her dietary intake. Assess her blood glucose self-monitoring in terms of technique, frequency, and her ability to adjust the insulin dose based on the changing patterns. Ask about the frequency of episodes of hypoglycemia or hyperglycemia to ascertain the woman's ability to recognize and treat them. Continue to assess her for signs and symptoms of hypo- and hyperglycemia.

During antepartum visits, assess the client's knowledge about her disease, including the signs and symptoms of hypoglycemia, hyperglycemia, and diabetic ketoacidosis; insulin administration techniques; and the impact of pregnancy on her chronic condition. If possible, have the woman demonstrate her technique for blood glucose monitoring and insulin administration if appropriate. Although the client may have had diabetes for some time, do not assume that she has a firm knowledge base about her disease process or management of it.

Assess the woman's risk for GDM at the first prenatal visit. The CDA (2008) recommends assessing all women for risk factors and then determining the need

EVIDENCE-BASED PRACTICE 20.1
Selecting Methods of Insulin Administration for Pregnant Women with Diabetes

● Study

A woman who has diabetes and becomes pregnant is at risk for various problems, both for herself and her fetus. The goal during pregnancy is to maintain optimal glucose control. For these women, insulin is the mainstay of treatment. Unfortunately, blood glucose levels are not static and insulin requirements change throughout pregnancy.

Insulin typically is administered subcutaneously, commonly in multiple doses throughout the day. However, it also may be administered via a continuous subcutaneous infusion. The question arises as to which method of insulin administration affords the best control of blood glucose levels for pregnant women. The belief is that the continuous infusions would provide better blood glucose control and thus reduce the risks for problems for the mother and fetus.

Two studies, one prospective nonrandomized and one retrospective, were conducted comparing the effects of continuous subcutaneous insulin infusions with multiple daily doses of insulin therapy and their effect on neonatal birth weight, perinatal mortality, fetal anomalies, and maternal hypoglycemia and hyperglycemia. The two studies, including 84 women in all, were reviewed and an analysis was performed.

▲ Findings

The researchers found no significant differences in birth weight, perinatal mortality, fetal anomalies, fetal morbidity, or maternal hypoglycemia and hyperglycemia between the two groups. The researchers attributed this to the methods and limited sample size of participants in the study. They concluded that there was insufficient evidence to support one method being better than the other. The researchers recommended additional research using a more vigorous approach and larger samples of women.

■ Nursing Implications

These studies, although inconclusive, do underscore the need for glucose control in women with pregestational diabetes. Nurses need to be aware of these findings so that they can integrate knowledge of adequate blood glucose control when teaching pregnant women with diabetes about its potential effects, regardless of the method of insulin administration. Nurses also need to be cognizant of the various methods available for insulin administration so that they can incorporate the information from these studies to provide individualized care to the pregnant woman with diabetes, thereby promoting the best possible outcomes for the mother and her fetus.

Sources: Kernaghan, D., Farrell, T., Hammond, P., & Owen, P. (2008). Fetal growth in women managed with insulin pump therapy compared to conventional insulin. *European Journal of Obstetrics, Gynecology, and Reproductive Biology, 137*(1), 47–49.

Volpe, L., Pancani, F., Aragona, M., et al. (2010). Continuous subcutaneous insulin infusion and multiple dose insulin injections in type 1 diabetic pregnant women: a case-control study. *Gynecological Endocrinology, 26*(3), 193–196.

for additional testing in the high-risk group only. Factors that place a woman at high risk include:

- History of gestational diabetes in a previous pregnancy
- Family history of diabetes
- Previous infant weighing more 4,000 g (9 lb)
- Previous unexplained fetal demise or neonatal death
- Maternal obesity (body mass index [BMI] >30 kg/m²)
- Member of high-risk ethnic group (Aboriginal, Hispanic, African, South Asian, Asian)
- Acanthosis nigricans
- Corticosteroid use
- Vascular disease
- Polycystic ovary disease
- Glycosuria or proteinuria (CDA, 2008)

Women with clinical characteristics consistent with a high risk for GDM should undergo glucose testing as soon as feasible.

Provide close ongoing assessment throughout the antepartal period. Women with GDM are at increased risk for pre-eclampsia and glucose control-related complications such as hypoglycemia, hyperglycemia, and ketoacidosis. GDM of any severity increases the risk for fetal macrosomia. It is also associated with an increased frequency of maternal hypertensive disorders and operative births. This may be the result of fetal growth disorders (CDA, 2008). Even though GDM is diagnosed during pregnancy, the woman may have had glucose intolerance before the pregnancy. Therefore, monitor the woman closely for signs and symptoms of possible complications.

Also assess the woman's psychosocial adaptation to her condition. This assessment is critical to gain her cooperation for a change in regimen or the addition of a new regimen throughout pregnancy. Identify her support systems and note any financial constraints, as she will need more intense monitoring and frequent fetal surveillance.

Laboratory and Diagnostic Testing

The results of laboratory and diagnostic tests provide valuable information about maternal and fetal well-being.

Women with pregestational diabetes and those discovered to have GDM require ongoing maternal and fetal surveillance to promote the best outcome.

Screening

The CDA currently recommends a risk analysis of all pregnant women at their first prenatal visit and additional screening of all high-risk pregnant women again at 24 to 28 weeks, or earlier if risk factors are present. If the initial screening risk assessment is low, additional screening may not be necessary. Pregnant women who fulfill all of the following criteria need not be screened:

- No previous history of GDM or glucose intolerance
- Maternal age less than 25 years
- Pregnant BMI less than 27
- No family history (first-degree relative) of diabetes
- No history of GDM or poor obstetric outcome
- Not from an ethnic/racial group with a high prevalence of diabetes (CDA, 2008)

If the initial risk assessment is high, re-screening should take place between 24 and 28 weeks. A woman with abnormal early results may have had diabetes before the pregnancy, and her fetus is at great risk for congenital anomalies. An elevated A1C level supports the likelihood of GDM (Cheung & Caughey, 2008).

There is little universal consensus regarding the appropriate screening method. Typically, screening is based on a 50 g 1-hour glucose challenge test, usually performed between weeks 24 and 28 of gestation (CDA, 2008). A 50 g oral glucose load is given, without regard to the timing or content of the last meal. Blood glucose is measured 1 hour later; a level above 10.2 mmol/L is abnormal. If the result is abnormal, a 75 g oral glucose tolerance test is conducted to test normal blood glucose levels. Normal values are:

- Fasting blood glucose level: less than 5.3 mmol/L
- At 1 hour: less than 10.6 mmol/L
- At 2 hours: less than 8.9 mmol/L (CDA, 2008)

A diagnosis of GDM can be made only after an abnormal result is obtained on the 75 g oral glucose tolerance test. Two or more abnormal values confirm the diagnosis (CDA, 2008).

Surveillance

Maternal surveillance may include the following:

- Urine check for protein (may indicate the need for further evaluation for pre-eclampsia) and for nitrates and leukocyte esterase (may indicate a urinary tract infection)
- Urine check for ketones (may indicate the need for evaluation of eating habits)
- Kidney function evaluation every trimester for creatinine clearance and protein levels

- Eye examination in the first trimester to evaluate the retina for vascular changes
- Measurement of A1C level every 4 to 6 weeks to monitor glucose trends (CDA, 2008; Cheung, 2009)

Fetal surveillance may include ultrasound to provide information about fetal growth, activity, and amniotic fluid volume and to validate gestational age. Alpha-fetoprotein levels may be obtained to detect congenital anomalies such as an open neural tube or ventral wall defects of omphalocele or gastroschisis, and a fetal echocardiogram may be necessary to rule out cardiac anomalies. A biophysical profile helps to monitor fetal well-being and uteroplacental profusion, and nonstress tests commonly are performed weekly after 28 weeks' gestation to evaluate fetal well-being. As the pregnancy progresses, an amniocentesis may be done to determine the lecithin/sphingomyelin (L/S) ratio and the presence of phosphatidyl glycerol to evaluate whether the fetal lung is mature enough for birth (Nodine et al., 2011).

Nursing Management

The ideal outcome of every pregnancy is a healthy newborn and mother. Nurses can be pivotal in realizing this positive outcome for women with pregestational diabetes or GDM by implementing measures to minimize risks and complications. Since the woman with diabetes is considered to be at high risk for complications, antepartal visits occur more frequently (every 2 weeks up to 28 weeks and then twice a week until birth), providing the nurse with numerous opportunities for ongoing assessment, education, and counselling (Nursing Care Plan 20.1).

Promoting Optimal Glucose Control

At each visit, review the mother's blood glucose levels, including any laboratory tests and self-monitoring results. Reinforce with the woman the need to perform blood glucose monitoring (usually four times a day, before meals and at bedtime) and to keep a record of the results. If appropriate, obtain a fingerstick blood glucose level to evaluate the accuracy of self-monitoring results. Also assess the woman's techniques for self-monitoring blood glucose levels and for administering insulin if ordered, and offer support and guidance (Fig. 20.1). If the woman is receiving insulin therapy, assist with any changes needed if glucose levels are not controlled.

Obtain a urine specimen and check for glucose, protein, and ketones. Ask the woman if she has had any episodes of hypoglycemia and what she did to alleviate them.

Discuss dietary measures related to blood glucose control (Fig. 20.2). In addition, recommend the following:

- Avoid weight loss and dieting during pregnancy.
- Ensure that food intake is adequate to prevent ketone formation and promote weight gain.

Nursing Care Plan 20.1

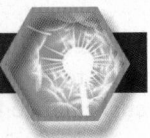

OVERVIEW OF THE PREGNANT WOMAN WITH TYPE 1 DIABETES

Donna, a 30-year-old woman with type 1 diabetes, presents to the maternity clinic for preconception care. She has been a diabetic for 8 years and takes insulin twice daily by injection. She does blood glucose self-monitoring four times daily. She reports that her disease is fairly well controlled, but "I'm worried about how my diabetes will affect a pregnancy and my baby. Will I need to make changes in my routine? Will my baby be normal?" She reports that she recently had a foot infection and needed to go to the emergency room because it led to an episode of ketoacidosis. She states that her last A1c test results were abnormal.

NURSING DIAGNOSIS: Deficient knowledge related to type 1 diabetes, blood glucose control, and effects of condition on pregnancy as evidenced by questions about effect on pregnancy, possible changes in regimen, and pregnancy outcome

Outcome Identification and Evaluation
Client will demonstrate increased knowledge of type 1 diabetes and effects on pregnancy *as evidenced by proper techniques for blood glucose monitoring and insulin administration, ability to modify insulin doses and dietary intake to achieve control, and verbalization of need for glycemic control prior to pregnancy, with blood glucose levels remaining within normal range.*

Interventions: Providing Client Teaching
- Assess client's knowledge of diabetes and pregnancy *to establish a baseline from which to develop an individualized teaching plan.*
- Review the underlying problems associated with diabetes and how pregnancy affects glucose control *to provide client with a firm knowledge base for decision making.*
- Review signs and symptoms of hypoglycemia and hyperglycemia and prevention and management measures *to ensure client can deal with them should they occur.*
- Provide written materials describing diabetes and care needed for control *to provide opportunity for client's review and promote retention of learning.*
- Observe client administering insulin and self-glucose testing for technique and offer suggestions for improvement if needed *to ensure adequate self-care ability.*
- Discuss proper foot care *to prevent future infections.*
- Teach home treatment for symptomatic hypoglycemia *to minimize risk to client and fetus.*
- Outline acute and chronic diabetic complications *to reinforce the importance of glucose control.*
- Discuss use of contraceptives until blood glucose levels can be optimized before conception occurs *to promote best possible health status before conception.*
- Explain the rationale for good glucose control and the importance of achieving excellent glycemic control before pregnancy *to promote a positive pregnancy outcome.*
- Review self-care practices (blood glucose monitoring and frequency of testing; insulin administration; adjustment of insulin dosages based on blood glucose levels) *to foster independence in self-care and feelings of control over the situation.*
- Refer client for dietary counselling *to ensure optimal diet for glycemic control.*
- Outline obstetric management and fetal surveillance needed for pregnancy *to provide client with information on what to expect.*
- Discuss strategies for maintaining optimal glycemic control during pregnancy *to minimize risks to client and fetus.*

NURSING DIAGNOSIS: Anxiety related to future pregnancy and its outcome secondary to underlying diabetes as evidenced by questions about her condition's effect on the baby and baby being normal

Outcome Identification and Evaluation
Client will openly express her feelings related to her diabetes and pregnancy *as evidenced by statements of feeling better about her pre-existing condition and pregnancy outlook, and statements of understanding related to future childbearing by linking good glucose control with positive outcomes for both herself and offspring.*

Nursing Care Plan 20.1 (continued)

Interventions: Minimizing Anxiety

- Review the need for a physical examination *to evaluate for any effects of diabetes on the client's health status.*
- Explain the rationale for assessing client's blood pressure, vision, and peripheral pulses at each visit *to provide information related to possible effects of diabetes on health status.*
- Identify any alterations in present diabetic condition that need intervention *to aid in minimizing risks that may increase client's anxiety level.*
- Review potential effects of diabetes on pregnancy *to promote client understanding of risks and ways to control or minimize them.*
- Encourage active participation in decision making and planning pregnancy *to promote feelings of control over the situation and foster self-confidence.*
- Discuss feelings about future childbearing and managing pregnancy *to help reduce anxiety related to uncertainties.*
- Encourage client to ask questions or voice concerns *to help decrease anxiety related to the unknown.*
- Emphasize the use of frequent and continued surveillance of client and fetal status during pregnancy *to reduce the risk for complications and aid in alleviating anxieties related to the unknown.*
- Provide positive reinforcement for healthy behaviours and actions *to foster continued use and enhancement of self-esteem.*

- Eat three meals a day plus three snacks to promote glycemic control:
  - 40% of calories from good-quality complex carbohydrates
  - 35% of calories from protein sources
  - 25% of calories from unsaturated fats (CDA, 2008)

▶ *Take* NOTE!

Nutrient requirements and recommendations for weight gain for the pregnant woman with diabetes are the same as those for the pregnant nondiabetic woman.

If necessary, arrange for consultation with a dietitian or nutritionist to individualize the dietary plan. Also encourage the woman to participate in an exercise program that includes at least three sessions lasting longer than 15 minutes per week. Exercise may lessen the need for insulin or dosage adjustments.

When caring for the labouring woman with pregestational diabetes or GDM, adjust the intravenous flow rate and the rate of supplemental regular insulin based on the blood glucose levels as ordered. Monitor blood glucose levels every 1 to 2 hours or more frequently if necessary. Keep a syringe with 50% dextrose solution available at the bedside to treat profound hypoglycemia. Monitor fetal heart rate patterns throughout labour to detect nonreassuring patterns. Assess maternal vital signs every hour, in addition to assessing the woman's urinary output

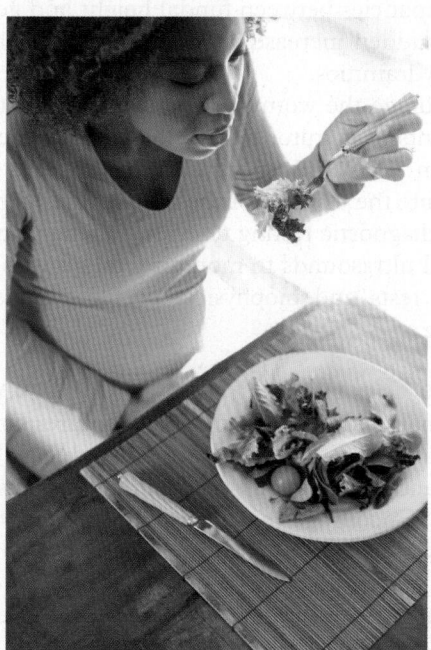

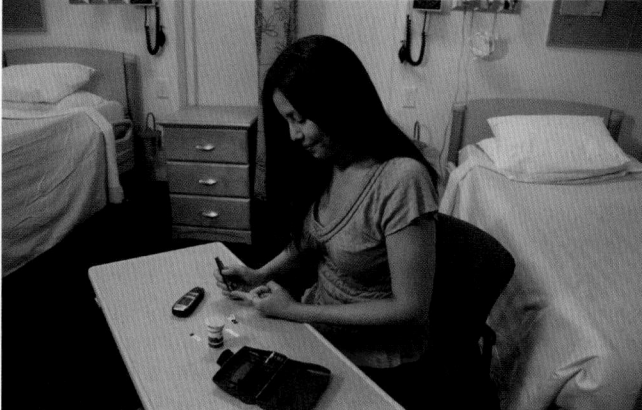

FIGURE 20.1 The client is demonstrating the technique for self-blood glucose monitoring.

FIGURE 20.2 The pregnant client eating a nutritious meal to ensure adequate glucose control.

with an indwelling catheter. If a cesarean birth is scheduled, monitor the woman's blood glucose levels hourly and administer short-acting insulin or glucose based on the blood glucose levels as ordered.

After birth, monitor blood glucose levels every 2 to 4 hours and continue intravenous fluid administration as ordered. Encourage breastfeeding to assist in maintaining good glucose control. For the woman with pregestational diabetes and type 1 or 2 diabetes, expect insulin needs to decrease rapidly after birth: they may be reduced by half of the antepartum dose as meals are started (Cheung, 2009). Some women may return to their pre-pregnancy insulin dosage.

The therapy plan after childbirth is individualized for each woman. If recommended dietary modifications are carried out along with weight loss, the woman with GDM may return to her normal glucose levels. This is also true for the woman with pregestational diabetes, except that she will return to her pre-pregnancy insulin administration levels. This provides the nurse with a wonderful opportunity to reinforce healthy lifestyle interventions on the postpartum unit. Nurses can also become involved with community-based education to continue to offer their expertise.

Preventing Complications

Assess the woman closely at each visit for signs and symptoms of complications. Anticipate possible complications and plan appropriate interventions or referrals. Check the woman's blood pressure for changes and evaluate for proteinuria when obtaining a urine specimen. These might suggest the development of pre-eclampsia. Measure fundal height and review gestational age. Note any discrepancies between fundal height and gestational age or a sudden increase in uterine growth. These may suggest hydramnios.

Encourage the woman to perform daily fetal movement counts to monitor fetal well-being. Tell her specifically when she should notify her health care provider. Also prepare the woman for the need for frequent laboratory and diagnostic testing to evaluate fetal status. Assist with serial ultrasounds to monitor fetal growth and with nonstress tests and biophysical profiles to assess fetal well-being.

Providing Client Education and Counselling

The pregnant woman with diabetes requires counselling and education about the need for strict glucose monitoring, diet and exercise, and signs and symptoms of complications. Encourage the client and her family to make any lifestyle changes needed to optimize the pregnancy outcome. Providing dietary education and lifestyle advice that extends beyond pregnancy may lower the risk that the woman will have GDM in subsequent pregnancies as well as type 2 diabetes (CDA, 2008; Kapustin, 2008). At each visit, stress the importance of performing blood glucose screening and documenting the results. With proper instruction, the client and her family will be able to cope with all the changes in her body during pregnancy (Teaching Guideline 20.1).

Review discussions about the timing of birth and the rationale. Counsel the client about the possibility of cesarean birth for large-for-gestational-age infant, or inform the woman who will be giving birth vaginally about the possible need for augmentation with oxytocin (Pitocin).

▶ *Take* NOTE!

In the woman with well-controlled diabetes, birth is typically not induced before term unless there are complications, such as pre-eclampsia or fetal compromise. An early delivery date might be set for the woman with poorly controlled diabetes who is having complications.

Instruct the client about the benefits of breastfeeding related to blood glucose control. Breastfeeding helps to normalize blood glucose levels. Therefore, encourage the woman to breastfeed her newborn. Also teach the woman receiving insulin for her diabetes that her insulin needs after birth will drastically decrease. Inform her that she will need a repeat glucose challenge test at a postpartum visit (CDA, 2008; Cheng & Caughey, 2008).

For the woman with GDM, the focus is on lifestyle education. Women with GDM have a greater than 50% increased risk for developing type 2 diabetes (CDA, 2008; Feig, Zinman, Wang, et al., 2008). Inform the woman that screening most likely will be done at the postpartum follow-up appointment in 6 weeks. Women with normal results at that visit typically are screened every 3 years thereafter (CDA, 2008). Teach her how to maintain an optimal weight to reduce her risk for developing diabetes. If necessary, refer the woman to a dietitian to help outline a balanced nutritious diet.

Cardiovascular Disorders

In 2006, a Canadian woman died of cardiovascular disease every 7 minutes (Heart and Stroke Foundation, 2012). Cardiovascular disease is the leading cause of death for women in Canada, killing nearly 40,000 women each year. Despite the prominent reduction in cardiovascular mortality among men, the rate has not declined for women. Cardiovascular disease has killed more women than men since the early 1980s (Heart and Stroke Foundation, 2012). In addition to being the number one killer of women, at the time of diagnosis women have both a poorer overall prognosis and a higher risk for death than men diagnosed with heart disease. More women die of heart disease, stroke, and other cardiovascular diseases

TEACHING GUIDELINE 20.1

Teaching for the Pregnant Woman with Diabetes

- Be sure to keep your appointments for frequent prenatal visits and tests for fetal well-being.
- Perform blood glucose self-monitoring as directed, usually before each meal and at bedtime. Keep a record of your results and call your health care provider with any levels outside the established range. Bring your results to each prenatal visit.
- Perform daily "fetal kick counts." Document them and report any decrease in activity.
- Drink eight to ten 8-ounce glasses of water each day to prevent bladder infections and maintain hydration.
- Wear proper, well-fitted footwear when walking to prevent injury.
- Engage in a regular exercise program such as walking to aid in glucose control, but avoid exercising in temperature extremes.
- Consider breastfeeding your infant to lower your blood glucose levels.
- If you are taking insulin:
  - Administer the correct dose of insulin at the correct time every day.
  - Eat breakfast within 30 minutes after injecting regular insulin to prevent a reaction.
  - Plan meals at a fixed time and snacks to prevent extremes in glucose levels.

- Avoid simple sugars (cake, candy, cookies), which raise blood glucose levels.
- Know the signs and symptoms of hypoglycemia and treatment needed:
- Sweating; tremors; cold, clammy skin; headache
- Feeling hungry, blurred vision, disorientation, irritability
- Treatment: Drink 8 ounces of milk and eat two crackers or glucose tablets
- Carry "glucose boosters" (such as Life Savers) to prevent hypoglycemia.
- Know the signs and symptoms of hyperglycemia and treatment needed:
  - Dry mouth, frequent urination, excessive thirst, rapid breathing
  - Feeling tired, flushed, hot skin, headache, drowsiness
  - Treatment: Notify health care provider, since hospitalization may be needed
- Wear a diabetic identification bracelet at all times.
- Wash your hands frequently to prevent infections.
- Report any signs and symptoms of illness, infection, and dehydration to your health care provider, because these can affect blood glucose control.

than men, yet many women do not realize they are at risk (PHAC, 2009b).

Approximately 1% to 3% of pregnant women in Western countries have cardiac disease, which is responsible for 10% to 25% of maternal deaths (Stangl Schad, Gossing, et al., 2008). The prevalence of cardiac disease is increasing as a result of lifestyle patterns, including cigarette smoking, diabetes, and stress (PHAC, 2010b). As women are delaying childbearing, the incidence of cardiac disease in pregnancy will continue to increase. Rheumatic heart disease used to represent the majority of cardiac conditions during pregnancy, but congenital heart disease now constitutes nearly half of all cases of heart disease encountered during pregnancy. Classic symptoms of heart disease mimic common symptoms of late pregnancy, such as palpitations, shortness of breath with exertion, and occasional chest pain. Few women with heart disease die during pregnancy, but they are at risk for other complications, such as heart failure, arrhythmias, and stroke (Moghbeli, Pare, & Webb, 2008). Their offsprings are also at risk for complications, such as premature birth, low birth weight for gestational age, respiratory distress syndrome, intraventricular hemorrhage, and death (Nodine et al., 2011).

Congenital and Acquired Heart Disease

Congenital heart disease often involves structural defects that are present at birth but may not be discovered at that time (Table 20.2). Until recently, women with congenital heart disease didn't live long enough to bear children. Today, due to new surgical techniques to correct these defects, many of these women can complete a successful pregnancy at relatively low risk when appropriate counselling and optimal care are provided. Increasing numbers of women with complex congenital heart disease are reaching childbearing age. Complications such as growth restriction and preterm and premature birth and fetal and neonatal mortality are more common among children of women with congenital heart disease. The risk for complications is determined by the severity of the cardiac lesion, the presence of cyanosis, the maternal functional class, and the use of anticoagulation (Moghbeli et al., 2008).

Women with certain congenital conditions should avoid pregnancy. These include uncorrected tetralogy of Fallot, transposition of the great arteries, and Eisenmenger's syndrome, a defect with both cyanosis and pulmonary hypertension (Blanchard & Shabetai, 2009).

TABLE 20.2 SELECTED HEART CONDITIONS AFFECTING PREGNANCY

Condition	Description	Management
Tetralogy of Fallot	Congenital defect involving four structural anomalies: obstruction to pulmonary flow; ventricular septal defect (abnormal opening between the right and left ventricles); dextroposition of the aorta (aortic opening overriding the septum and receiving blood from both ventricles); and right ventricular hypertrophy (increase in volume of the myocardium of the right ventricle) (Gilbert, 2011)	Hospitalization and bed rest possible after the 20th week with hemodynamic monitoring via a pulmonary artery catheter to monitor volume status Oxygen therapy may be necessary during labour and birth.
Atrial septal defect (ASD)	Congenital heart defect involving a communication or opening between the atria with left-to-right shunting due to greater left-sided pressure Arrhythmias present in some women	Treatment with atrioventricular nodal blocking agents and, at times, with electrical cardioversion (Gilbert, 2011)
Ventricular septal defect (VSD)	Congenital heart defect involving an opening in the ventricular septum, permitting blood flow from the left to the right ventricle. Complications include arrhythmias, heart failure, and pulmonary hypertension (Gilbert, 2011).	Rest with limited activity if symptomatic
Patent ductus arteriosus	Abnormal persistence of an open lumen in the ductus arteriosus between the aorta and the pulmonary artery after birth; results in increased pulmonary blood flow and redistribution of flow to other organs (Gilbert, 2011)	Surgical ligation of the open ductus during infancy; subsequent problems minimal after surgical correction
Mitral valve prolapse	Very common in the general population, occurring most often in younger women Leaflets of the mitral valve prolapse into the left atrium during ventricular contraction. The most common cause of mitral valve regurgitation if present during pregnancy (Gilbert, 2011). Usually improvement in mitral valve function due to increased blood volume and decreased systemic vascular resistance of pregnancy; most women are able to tolerate pregnancy well.	Most women are asymptomatic; diagnosis is made incidentally. Occasional palpations, chest pain, or arrhythmias in some women, possibly requiring beta-blockers Usually no special precautions are necessary during pregnancy.
Mitral valve stenosis	Most common chronic rheumatic valvular lesion in pregnancy Causes obstruction of blood flow from the atria to the ventricle, thereby decreasing ventricular filling and causing a fixed cardiac output Resultant pulmonary edema, pulmonary hypertension, and right ventricular failure (Gilbert, 2011) Most pregnant women with this condition can be managed medically.	General symptomatic improvement with medical management involving diuretics, beta-blockers, and anticoagulant therapy Activity restriction, reduction in sodium, and potentially bed rest if condition severe
Aortic stenosis	Narrowing of the opening of the aortic valve, leading to an obstruction to left ventricular ejection (Xiushui et al., 2012) Women with mild disease can tolerate hypervolemia of pregnancy; with progressive narrowing of the opening, cardiac output becomes fixed.	Diagnosis confirmed with echocardiography Pharmacologic treatment with beta-blockers and/or antiarrhythmic agents to reduce risk for heart failure and/or dysrhythmias Bed rest/limited activity and close monitoring

Condition	Description	Management
Peripartum cardio-myopathy	Rare congestive cardiomyopathy that may arise during pregnancy. Multiparity, age, multiple fetuses, hypertension, an infectious agent, autoimmune disease, or cocaine use may contribute to its presence (Gilbert, 2011). Development of heart failure in the last month of pregnancy or within 5 months of giving birth without any preexisting heart disease or any identifiable cause	Preload reduction with diuretic therapy Afterload reduction with vasodilators Improvement in contractility with inotropic agents Non-pharmacologic approaches include salt restriction and daily exercise such as walking or biking. The question of whether another pregnancy should be attempted is controversial due to the high risk for repeat complications.
Myocardial infarction (MI)	Rare during pregnancy but incidence is expected to increase as older women are becoming pregnant and the risk factors for coronary artery disease become more prevalent Factors contributing to MI include family history, stress, smoking, age, obesity, multiple fetuses, hypercholesterolemia, and cocaine use (Burt & Durbridge, 2009). Increased plasma volume and cardiac output during pregnancy increase the cardiac workload as well as the myocardial oxygen demands; imbalance in supply and demand may contribute to myocardial ischemia.	Usual treatment modalities for any acute MI along with consideration for the fetus Anticoagulant therapy, rest, and lifestyle changes to preserve the health of both parties

Sources: Gilbert, E. S. (2011). *Manual of high risk pregnancy & delivery* (5th ed.). St. Louis, MO: Mosby Elsevier, & Xiushui, R., Aggarwal, K., Balentine, J., et al. (2012). *Aortic stenosis.* Retrieved February 13, 2012 from http://www.emedicine.com/EMERG/topic40.htm.

Acquired heart disease is typically rheumatic in origin (see Table 20.2). The incidence of rheumatic heart disease has declined dramatically in the past several decades because of prompt identification of streptococcal throat infections and treatment with antibiotics. When the heart is involved, valvular lesions such as mitral stenosis, prolapse, or aortic stenosis are common.

Many women are postponing childbearing until the fourth or fifth decade of life. With advancing maternal age, underlying medical conditions such as hypertension, diabetes, and hypercholesterolemia contributing to ischemic heart disease become more common and increase the incidence of acquired heart disease complicating pregnancy. Coronary artery disease and myocardial infarction may result.

A woman's ability to function during the pregnancy is often more important than the actual diagnosis of the cardiac condition. The following functional classification system, based on disability and physical signs, was developed by the Canadian Cardiovascular Society (1976):

- Class I: asymptomatic with no limitation of ordinary physical activity
- Class II: symptomatic (dyspnea, chest pain) with slight limitation of ordinary activity
- Class III: symptomatic (fatigue, palpitations) with marked limitation of activity
- Class IV: symptomatic at rest or with any physical activity

The classification may change as the pregnancy progresses and the woman's body must cope with the increasing stress on the cardiovascular system resulting from the numerous physiologic changes taking place. Typically, a woman with class I or II cardiac disease can go through a pregnancy without major complications. A woman with class III disease usually has to maintain bed rest during pregnancy. A woman with class IV disease should avoid pregnancy (Moghbeli et al., 2008). Women with cardiac disease may benefit from preconception counselling so that they know the risks before deciding to become pregnant.

Maternal mortality varies directly with the functional class at pregnancy onset. The American College of Obstetrics and Gynecology has adopted a three-tiered classification according to the risk for death during pregnancy (Box 20.1).

Pathophysiology

Numerous hemodynamic changes occur in all pregnant women. These normal physiologic changes can overstress

---

BOX 20.1 **Classification of Maternal Mortality Risk**

Group I (minimal risk) has a mortality rate of 1% and comprises women with:
- Patent ductus arteriosus
- Tetralogy of Fallot, corrected
- Atrial septal defect
- Ventricular septal defect
- Mitral stenosis, class I and II

Group II (moderate risk) has a mortality rate of 5% to 15% and comprises women with:
- Tetralogy of Fallot, uncorrected
- Mitral stenosis with atrial fibrillation
- Aortic stenosis, class III and IV
- Aortic coarctation without valvular involvement
- Artificial valve replacement

Group III (major risk) has a 25% to 50% mortality rate and comprises women with:
- Pulmonary hypertension
- Complicated aortic coarctation
- Previous myocardial infarction

Source: Gilbert, E. S. (2011). *Manual of high risk pregnancy & delivery* (5th ed.). St. Louis, MO: Mosby Elsevier.

---

the woman's cardiovascular system, increasing her risk for problems. Increased cardiac workload and greater myocardial oxygen demand during pregnancy place the woman's cardiovascular system at high risk for morbidity and mortality.

▶ *Take NOTE!*

Uterine blood flow increases by at least 1 L per minute during pregnancy, requiring the body to produce more blood. This results in a 25% increase in red blood cells, a 50% expansion of plasma volume, and an overall hemodilution. In addition, the increase in total red blood cellular volume includes an increase in clotting factors and platelets, defining the hypercoagulable state of pregnancy (Burt & Durbridge, 2009). These changes start as early as the second month of gestation.

Similarly, cardiac output increases steadily during pregnancy by 30% to 50% over pre-pregnancy levels: stroke volume increases 20% to 30% from pre-pregnant levels, and the maternal heart rate increases by 10 to 20 beats per minute. The increase is due to both the expansion in blood volume and the augmentation of stroke volume and heart rate. Other hemodynamic changes associated with pregnancy include a decrease in both the systemic vascular resistance and pulmonary vascular resistance, thereby lowering the systolic and diastolic blood pressure. In addition, the hypercoagulability associated with pregnancy might increase the risk for arterial thrombosis and embolization. These normal physiologic changes are important for a successful adaptation to pregnancy but create unique physiologic challenges for the woman with cardiac disease (Blanchard & Shabetai, 2009) (Comparison Chart 20.1).

Therapeutic Management

Ideally, a woman with a history of congenital or acquired heart disease should consult her health care provider before becoming pregnant and should undergo a risk assessment. This risk assessment must consider the woman's functional capacity, exercise tolerance, degree of cyanosis, medication needs, and history of arrhythmias. Data needed for risk assessment can be acquired from a thorough cardiovascular history and examination, a 12-lead electrocardiogram (EKG), and evaluation of oxygen saturation levels by pulse oximetry. The impact of heart disease on a woman's childbearing potential needs to be clearly explained, and information on how pregnancy may affect her and the fetus is important. This allows women to make an informed decision about whether they wish to accept the risks associated with pregnancy. When possible, any surgical procedures, such as valve replacement, should be done before pregnancy to improve fetal and maternal outcomes (Patel, Asopa, Tang, et al., 2008).

If the woman presents for care after she has become pregnant, prenatal counselling focuses on the impact of the hemodynamic changes of pregnancy, the signs and symptoms of cardiac compromise, and dietary and lifestyle changes needed. More frequent prenatal visits (every 2 weeks until the last month and then weekly) are usually needed to ensure the health and safety of the mother and fetus.

Nursing Assessment

Frequent and thorough assessments are crucial during the antepartum period to ensure early detection of and prompt intervention for problems. Assess the woman's vital signs, noting any changes. Auscultate the apical heart rate and heart sounds, being especially alert for abnormalities, including irregularities in rhythm or murmurs. Check the client's weight and compare with baseline and weights obtained on previous visits. Report any weight gain outside recommended parameters. Inspect the extremities for edema and note any pitting.

Question the woman about fetal activity, and ask if she has noticed any changes. Report any changes such as a decrease in fetal movements. Ask the woman about any symptoms of preterm labour, such as low back pain, uterine contractions, and increased pelvic pressure and vaginal discharge, and report them immediately. Assess

COMPARISON CHART 20.1 CARDIOVASCULAR CHANGES: PREPREGNANCY VS PREGNANCY

Measurement	Prepregnancy	Pregnancy
Heart rate	72 (±10) bpm	+10%–20%
Cardiac output	4.3 (±0.9) L/min	+30% to 50%
Blood volume	5 L	+20% to 50%
Stroke volume	73.3 (±9) mL	+30%
Systemic vascular resistance	1,530 (±520) dyne/cm/sec	–20%
Oxygen consumption	250 mL/min	+20%–30%

Source: Gilbert, E. S. (2011). *Manual of high risk pregnancy & delivery* (5th ed.). St. Louis, MO: Mosby Elsevier.

the fetal heart rate and review serial ultrasound results to monitor fetal growth.

Assess the client's lifestyle and her ability to cope with the changes of pregnancy and its effect on her cardiac status and ability to function. Evaluate the client's understanding of her condition and what restrictions and lifestyle changes may be needed to provide the best outcome for her and her fetus. A healthy infant and mother at the end of pregnancy is the ultimate goal. As the client's pregnancy advances, expect her functional class to be revised based on her level of disability. Suggest realistic modifications.

The nurse plays a major role in recognizing the signs and symptoms of cardiac decompensation. Decompensation refers to the heart's inability to maintain adequate circulation. As a result, tissue perfusion in the mother and the fetus is impaired. The pregnant woman is most vulnerable for this complication from 28 to 32 weeks of gestation and in the first 48 hours postpartum (Moghbeli et al., 2008). Assess the woman for the following signs and symptoms:

- Shortness of breath on exertion, dyspnea
- Cyanosis of lips and nail beds
- Swelling of face, hands, and feet
- Jugular vein engorgement
- Rapid respirations
- Abnormal heartbeats, reports of heart racing or palpitations
- Chest pain with effort or emotion
- Syncope with exertion
- Increasing fatigue
- Moist, frequent cough

▶ *Take* NOTE!

Assessing the pregnant woman with heart disease for cardiac decompensation is vital because the mother's hemodynamic status determines the health of the fetus.

Nursing Management

Nursing management of the pregnant woman with heart disease focuses on assisting with measures to stabilize the mother's hemodynamic status, because a decrease in maternal blood pressure or volume will cause blood to be shunted away from the uterus, thus reducing placental perfusion. Pregnant women with cardiac disease also need assistance in reducing risks that would lead to complications or further cardiac compromise. Therefore, education and counselling are critical. Collaboration between the cardiologist, obstetrician, perinatologist, and nurse is needed to promote the best possible outcome.

Encourage the woman to continue taking her cardiac medications as prescribed. Review the indications, actions, and potential side effects of the medications. Reinforce the importance of frequent antepartal visits and close medical supervision throughout the pregnancy.

Discuss the need to conserve energy. Help the client to prioritize household chores and child care to allow rest periods. Encourage the client to rest in the side-lying position, which enhances placental perfusion.

Encourage the client to eat nutritious foods and consume a high-fibre diet to prevent straining and constipation. Discuss limiting sodium intake if indicated to reduce fluid retention. Contact a dietitian to assist the woman in planning nutritionally appropriate meals.

Assist the woman in preparing for diagnostic tests to evaluate fetal well-being. Describe the tests that may be done, such as EKG and echocardiogram, and explain the need for serial nonstress testing, usually beginning at approximately 32 weeks.

Instruct the woman how to monitor fetal activity and movements. Urge her to do this daily and report any changes in activity immediately.

Although the morbidity and mortality rates of pregnant women with cardiac disease have decreased greatly, congestive heart failure, cardiac arrhythmia, thromboembolism, angina, hypoxemia, and infective endocarditis can occur (Gilbert, 2011). Explain the signs and symptoms of these complications and review the sign and symptoms of cardiac decompensation, encouraging the woman to notify her health care provider if any occur.

Provide support and encouragement throughout the antepartal period. Assess the support systems available to the client and her family, and encourage her to use them. If necessary, assist with referrals to community services for additional support.

During labour, anticipate the need for invasive hemodynamic monitoring, and make sure the woman has been prepared for this beforehand. Monitor her fluid volume carefully to prevent overload. Anticipate the use of epidural anesthesia if a vaginal birth is planned. After birth, assess the client for fluid overload as peripheral fluids mobilize. This fluid shift from the periphery to the central circulation taxes the heart, and signs of heart failure such as cough, progressive dyspnea, edema, palpitations, and crackles in the lung bases may ensue before postpartum diuresis begins. Because hemodynamics do not return to baseline for several days after childbirth, women at intermediate or high risk require monitoring for at least 48 hours postpartum (Burt & Durbridge, 2009).

Chronic Hypertension

Chronic hypertension exists when the woman has high blood pressure before pregnancy or before the 20th week of gestation, or when hypertension persists for more than 12 weeks postpartum. The Society of Obstetricians and Gynaecologists of Canada (SOGC) has classified blood pressure as follows:

- Normal: systolic less than 120 mm Hg, diastolic less than 80 mm Hg
- Prehypertension: systolic 120 to 139 mm Hg, diastolic 80 to 89 mm Hg
- Mild hypertension: systolic 140 to 159 mm Hg, diastolic 90 to 99 mm Hg
- Severe hypertension: systolic 160 mm Hg or higher, diastolic 100 mm Hg or higher (Magee, Helewa, Moutquin, et al., 2008)

Chronic hypertension in pregnancy is defined as diastolic blood pressure exceeding 90 mm Hg based on the average of at least two measurements taken using the same arm. Women with systolic blood pressure higher than 140 mm Hg should be followed closely for the development of diastolic hypertension. Severe hypertension is defined as systolic blood pressure exceeding 160 mm Hg or diastolic blood pressure higher than 110 mm Hg (Magee et al., 2008).

Hypertension affects 10% of pregnant women, with the prevalence varying according to age, race, and BMI (Moreira, Gus, Nunes, et al., 2009). One in four hypertensive women develops pre-eclampsia during pregnancy. Chronic hypertension is typically seen in older, obese women with glucose intolerance. The most common complication of hypertension in pregnancy is pre-eclampsia, which is seen in approximately 25% of women who enter the pregnancy with hypertension (Magee et al., 2008). (See Chapter 19 for more information about pre-eclampsia.)

Therapeutic Management

Preconception counselling is important in fostering positive outcomes. Typically, it involves lifestyle changes such as diet, exercise, weight loss, and smoking cessation.

Treatment for women with chronic hypertension focuses on maintaining normal blood pressure, preventing superimposed pre-eclampsia/eclampsia, and ensuring normal fetal development. Once the woman is pregnant, antihypertensive agents are typically reserved for those with severe hypertension (150 to 160/100 to 110 mm Hg). Methyldopa (Aldomet) is commonly prescribed because of its safety record during pregnancy. This slow-acting antihypertensive agent helps to improve uterine perfusion. Other antihypertensive agents that can be used include labetalol (Transdate), atenolol (Tenorium), and nifedipine (Procardia) (Caton, Bell, Druschel, et al., 2009; Gilbert, 2011).

Lifestyle changes are needed and should continue throughout the pregnancy. The woman with chronic hypertension will be seen more frequently (every 2 weeks until 28 weeks and then weekly until birth) to monitor her blood pressure and to assess for any signs of pre-eclampsia. At approximately 24 weeks' gestation, the woman will be instructed to document fetal movement. At this same time, serial ultrasounds will be ordered to monitor fetal growth and amniotic fluid volume. Additional tests will be included if the client's status changes.

Nursing Assessment

Nursing assessment of the woman with chronic hypertension involves a thorough history and physical examination. Review the woman's history closely for risk factors. The pathogenesis of hypertension is multifactorial and includes many modifiable risk factors such as smoking, obesity, caffeine intake, excessive alcohol intake, excessive salt intake, and use of nonsteroidal anti-inflammatory drugs. Also be alert for nonmodifiable risk factors such as increasing age and black race (Gilbert, 2011; Magee et al., 2008). Ask if the woman has received any preconception counselling and what measures have been used to prevent or control hypertension.

Assess the woman's vital signs, in particular her blood pressure. Evaluate her blood pressure in all three positions (sitting, lying, and standing), and note any major differences in the readings. Assess her for orthostatic hypertension when she changes her position from sitting to standing. Document your findings.

Ask the woman if she monitors her blood pressure at home; if so, inquire about the typical readings. Ask the woman if she uses any medications for blood pressure control, including the drug, dosage, and frequency of administration, as well as any side effects. Ask the woman about lifestyle modifications that she has used to address any modifiable risk factors, and their effectiveness.

Hypertension during pregnancy decreases uteroplacental perfusion. Therefore, fetal well-being must be assessed and closely monitored. Anticipate serial ultrasounds to assess fetal growth and amniotic fluid volume. Question the woman about fetal movement and evaluate her report of daily "kick counts." Assess fetal heart rate at every visit.

Nursing Management

Preconception counselling is the ideal time to discuss lifestyle changes to prevent or control hypertension. One area to cover during this visit would be a diet that contains an adequate amount of potassium, magnesium, and calcium. Sodium is usually limited to 2.4 g. Suggest aerobic exercise, although the woman should cease exercising once the pregnancy is confirmed. Encourage smoking cessation and avoidance of alcohol. If the woman is overweight, encourage her to lose weight before becoming pregnant, not during the pregnancy (Magee et al., 2008). Stressing the positive benefits of a healthy lifestyle might help motivate the woman to make the modifications and change unhealthy habits.

Assist the woman in scheduling appointments for antepartum visits every 2 weeks until 28 weeks' gestation and then weekly. Prepare the woman for frequent fetal assessments. Explaining the rationale for the need to monitor fetal growth is important to gain the woman's cooperation. Carefully monitor the woman for signs and symptoms of abruptio placentae (abdominal pain, rigid abdomen, vaginal bleeding) as well as superimposed pre-eclampsia (elevation in blood pressure, weight gain, edema, proteinuria). Alerting the woman to these risks allows early identification and prompt intervention.

Stress the importance of daily periods of rest (1 hour) in the left lateral recumbent position to maximize placental perfusion. Encourage women with chronic hypertension to use home blood pressure monitoring devices. Urge the woman to report any elevations. As necessary, instruct the woman and her family how to measure and record a daily blood pressure, and reinforce the need for her to take her medications as prescribed to control her blood pressure and to ensure the well-being of her unborn child. Praising her for her efforts at each prenatal visit may motivate her to continue the regimen throughout her pregnancy.

Close monitoring of the woman with chronic hypertension continues during labour and birth and during the postpartum period to prevent or identify the onset of pre-eclampsia. Accurate and frequent blood pressure readings and careful administration of antihypertensive medications, if prescribed, are essential components of care. Stressing the need for continued medical supervision after childbirth is vital to motivate the woman to maintain or initiate lifestyle changes and dietary habits and stay compliant with her medication regimen.

Respiratory Conditions

During pregnancy, the respiratory system is affected by hormonal changes, mechanical changes, and prior respiratory conditions. These changes can cause a woman with a history of compromised respiration to decompensate during pregnancy. While upper respiratory infections are typically self-limiting, chronic respiratory conditions, such as asthma or tuberculosis (TB), can have a negative effect on the growing fetus when alterations in oxygenation occur in the mother. The outcome of pregnancy in a woman with a respiratory condition depends on the severity of the oxygen alteration as well as the degree and duration of hypoxia on the fetus.

Asthma

Asthma affects approximately 3.4% to 8.4% of pregnancies worldwide (Davel, Irusen, & Hall, et al., 2009). It affects 2.4 million Canadians and is one of the most common and potentially serious medical conditions to complicate pregnancy (Canadian Lung Association [CLA], 2011a; Kennedy, 2009). Maternal asthma is associated with an increased risk forinfant death, pre-eclampsia, intrauterine growth restriction (IUGR), preterm birth, and low birth weight (Nodine et al., 2011). These risks are linked to the severity of asthma: more severe asthma increases the risk (Chapman, 2008).

*R*emember Rose, the pregnant teenager with asthma in acute distress described at the beginning of the chapter? What therapies might be offered to control her symptoms? Should she be treated differently than someone who is not pregnant? Why or why not?

Pathophysiology

Asthma, an allergic-type inflammatory response of the respiratory tract to various stimuli, is also known as reactive airway disease because the bronchioles constrict in response to allergens, irritants, and infections. In addition to bronchoconstriction, inflammation of the airways produces thick mucus that further limits the movement of air and makes breathing difficult.

The normal physiologic changes of pregnancy affect the respiratory system. While the respiratory rate does not change, hyperventilation increases at term by 48% due to high progesterone levels. Diaphragmatic elevation and a decrease in functional lung residual capacity occur late in pregnancy, which may reduce the woman's ability to inspire deeply to take in more oxygen. Oxygen consumption and the metabolic rate both increase, placing additional stress on the woman's respiratory system (Hardy-Fairbanks & Baker, 2010).

Both the woman and her fetus are at risk if asthma is not well managed during pregnancy. When a pregnant woman has trouble breathing, her fetus also has trouble getting the oxygen it needs for adequate growth and development. Severe persistent asthma has been linked to the development of maternal hypertension, pre-eclampsia, placenta previa, uterine hemorrhage, and oligohydramnios. Women whose asthma is poorly controlled during pregnancy are at increased risk for pre-eclampsia, preterm birth, low birth weight, and stillbirth (Gilbert, 2011).

The severity of the condition improves in one third of pregnant women, remains unchanged in one third, and worsens in one third (CLA, 2011a). However, the effect of pregnancy on asthma is unpredictable. The greatest increase in asthma attacks usually occurs between 24 and 36 weeks' gestation; flare-ups are rare during the last 4 weeks of pregnancy and during labour (Davel et al., 2009).

Therapeutic Management

Asthma should be treated as aggressively in pregnant women as in non-pregnant women because the benefits of averting an asthma attack outweigh the risks of medications. The goals of treatment are to prevent hospitalization, emergency room visits, work loss, and chronic disability. Three specific drugs to control asthma are recommended for use during pregnancy:

- Budesonide (inhaled-corticosteroid)
- Albuterol (short-acting beta$_2$ agonist)
- Salmeterol (long-acting beta$_2$ agonist) (Davel et al., 2009)

Oral corticosteroids are not recommended for the treatment of asthma during pregnancy, but they can be used to treat severe asthma attacks during pregnancy (Barclay, 2009).

Nursing Assessment

Obtain a thorough history of the disease, including the woman's usual therapy and control measures. Question the woman about asthma triggers and strategies used to reduce exposure to them (Box 20.2). Review the client's medication therapy regimen.

Auscultate the lungs and assess respiratory and heart rates. Include the rate, rhythm, and depth of respirations; skin colour; blood pressure and pulse rate; and signs of fatigue. Patients with an acute asthma attack often present with wheezing, chest tightness, tachypnea, nonproductive coughing, shortness of breath, and dyspnea. Lung auscultation findings might include diffuse wheezes and rhonchi, bronchovesicular sounds, and a more prominent expiratory phase of respiration compared with the inspiratory phase (Benninger & McCallister, 2010). If the

---

| BOX 20.2 | **Common Asthma Triggers** |

- Smoke and chemical irritants
- Air pollution
- Dust mites
- Animal dander
- Seasonal changes with pollen, molds, and spores
- Upper respiratory infections
- Esophageal reflux
- Medications, such as aspirin and nonsteroidal anti-inflammatory drugs (NSAIDs)
- Exercise
- Cold air
- Emotional stress

Sources: Canadian Lung Association. (2011a). *Pregnancy & asthma.* Retrieved February 13, 2012 from http://www.lung.ca/diseases-maladies/asthma-asthme/pregnancy-grossesse/index_e.php; & Little, M., & Sinert, R. (2011). *Asthma in pregnancy.* Retrieved February 13, 2012 from http://www.emedicine.com/emerg/TOPIC476.HTM.

---

pregnancy is far enough along, the fetal heart rate is measured and routine prenatal assessments (weight, blood pressure, fundal height, urine for protein) are completed.

Laboratory studies usually include a complete blood count with differential (to assess the degree of nonspecific inflammation and identify anemia) and pulmonary function tests (to assess the severity of an attack and to provide a baseline to evaluate the client's response to treatment).

Nursing Management

Nursing management focuses on client education about the condition and the skills necessary to manage it: self-monitoring, correct use of inhalers, identifying and limiting exposure to asthma triggers, and following a long-term plan for managing asthma and for promptly handling signs and symptoms of worsening asthma. Client education fosters adherence to the treatment regimen, thereby promoting an optimal environment for fetal growth and development.

Ensure that the woman understands drug actions and interactions, the uses and potential abuses of asthma medications, and the signs and symptoms that require medical evaluation. Reviewing potential perinatal complications with the woman is helpful in motivating her to adhere to the prescribed regimen. At each antepartum visit, reassess the efficacy of the treatment plan to determine whether adjustments are needed.

Taking control of asthma in pregnancy is the responsibility of the client along with her health care team. Providing the client with the knowledge and tools to monitor her condition, control triggers and her environment (Teaching Guideline 20.2), and use medications to prevent acute exacerbations assist the client in taking

TEACHING GUIDELINE 20.2

Teaching to Control Environmental Asthma Triggers

- Remove any carpeting in the house, especially the bedroom, to reduce dust mites.
- Use an allergen-proof casing on the mattress, box spring, and pillows.
- Wash all bedding in hot water.
- Remove dust collectors in house, such as stuffed animals, books, and knick-knacks.
- Avoid pets in the house to reduce exposure to pet dander.
- Use a high-efficiency particulate air-filtering system in the bedroom.
- Do not smoke, and avoid places where you can be exposed to passive cigarette smoke from others.
- Stay indoors and use air conditioning when the pollen or mold count is high or air quality is poor.
- Wear a covering over your nose and mouth when going outside in the cold weather.
- Avoid exposure to persons with colds, flu, or viruses.

control. Facilitating a partnership with the woman will improve perinatal outcomes.

When teaching the pregnant woman with asthma, cover the following topics:

- Signs and symptoms of asthma progression and exacerbation
- Importance and safety of medication to the fetus and to herself
- Warning signs that indicate the need to contact the health care provider
- Potential harm to the fetus and to herself by undertreatment or delay in seeking help
- Prevention and avoidance of known triggers
- Home use of metred-dose inhalers
- Adverse effects of medications

During labour, monitor the client's oxygenation saturation by pulse oximetry and provide pain management through epidural analgesia to reduce stress, which may trigger an acute attack. Continuously monitor the fetus for distress during labour and assess fetal heart rate patterns for hypoxia. Assess the newborn for signs and symptoms of hypoxia.

▶ *Take NOTE!*

Successful asthma management can reduce adverse perinatal outcomes: pre-eclampsia, preterm birth, and low birth weight.

Rose, the pregnant teenager described earlier, is concerned about passing her asthma on to her baby. What should the nurse discuss with her? What questions should the nurse ask to help in identifying triggers in Rose's environment to prevent future asthma attacks?

Tuberculosis

TB is a disease that has been around for years but never seems to go away completely. Globally, TB is second only to HIV/AIDS as a cause of illness and death in adults, accounting for over 9.2 million cases of active disease and 2 million deaths each year (World Health Organization [WHO], 2010a). Someone in the world is newly infected with TB every second. Overall, one third of the world's population is currently infected with TB. Left undiagnosed and untreated, each person with active TB will infect on average of 10 to 15 people every year (WHO, 2010a).

Although it is not prevalent in Canada, a resurgence of TB was noted starting in the mid-1980s secondary to the AIDS epidemic, immigration, and the emergence of drug-resistant strains. The majority of TB cases in Canada (70%) originate from outside the country, with 1,669 cases reported in 2007 (CLA, 2011b). With the large numbers of immigrants coming to Canada, all nurses must be skilled in screening for and managing this condition.

A person becomes infected by inhaling the infectious organism, *Mycobacterium tuberculosis*, which is carried on a droplet nuclei and spread by airborne transmission. The lung is the major site of involvement, but the lymph glands, meninges, bones, joints, and kidneys can become infected. Women can remain asymptomatic for long periods of time as the organism may lie dormant. Pregnant women with untreated TB are more likely to have pre-eclampsia, miscarriage, preterm labour, a low birth weight infant, IUGR, an infant with a low Apgar score, and perinatal death (Whittaker & Kampmann, 2008). The newborn is at risk for acquiring TB postnatally if the mother still has active TB at the time of birth. Therefore, prenatal diagnosis and effective treatment of the mother are essential.

Therapeutic Management

Therapeutic management of TB during pregnancy is essentially the same as that for the general population. Medications are the cornerstone of treatment to prevent infection from progressing. The medical therapy for pregnant women is a combination of medications such as isoniazid, rifampin, and ethambutol, taken daily for up to 9 months. These anti-TB agents appear to have minimal teratogenic risks and may be started as soon as the diagnosis of TB is made. However, extensive research has not been done to determine the definitive safety of these drugs (Maddineni & Panda, 2008).

Nursing Assessment

Review the woman's history for risk factors such as immunocompromised status, recent immigration status, homelessness or overcrowded living conditions, and injectable drug use. Women emigrating from developing countries such as Latin America, Asia, the Indian subcontinent, Eastern Europe, Russia, China, Mexico, Haiti, and Africa with high rates of TB also are at risk.

At antepartum visits, be alert for clinical manifestations of TB, including fatigue, fever or night sweats, nonproductive cough, slow weight loss, anemia, hemoptysis, and anorexia (Whittaker & Kampmann, 2008). If TB is suspected or the woman is at risk for developing TB, anticipate screening with purified protein derivative (PPD) administered by intradermal injection. If the client has been exposed to TB, a reddened induration will appear within 72 hours. If the test is positive, anticipate a follow-up chest x-ray with lead shielding over the abdomen and sputum cultures to confirm the diagnosis.

Nursing Management

Compliance with the multidrug therapy is critical to protect the woman and her fetus from progression of TB. Provide education about the disease process, the mode of transmission, prevention, potential complications, and the importance of adhering to the treatment regimen.

Stressing the importance of health-promotion activities throughout the pregnancy is important. Some suggestions might include avoiding crowded living conditions, avoiding sick people, maintaining adequate hydration, eating a nutritious, well-balanced diet, keeping all prenatal appointments to evaluate fetal growth and well-being, and getting plenty of fresh air by going outside frequently. Determining the woman's understanding of her condition and treatment plan is important for compliance. A language interpreter may be needed to validate and reinforce her understanding if she does not speak English.

Breastfeeding is not contraindicated during the medication regimen and should in fact be encouraged. Management of the newborn of a mother with TB involves preventing transmission by teaching the parents not to cough, sneeze, or talk directly into the newborn's face. Nurses need to stay current about new therapies and screening techniques to treat this centuries-old disease.

Hematologic Conditions

Anemia, a reduction in red blood cell volume, is measured by hematocrit (Hct) or a decrease in the concentration of hemoglobin (Hgb) in the peripheral blood. This results in reduced capacity of the blood to carry oxygen to the vital organs of the mother and fetus. Anemia is a sign of an underlying problem but does not indicate its origin.

Iron-Deficiency Anemia

Iron-deficiency anemia affects one in four pregnancies and is usually related to an inadequate dietary intake of iron (Milman, 2008). It is a very common state in pregnant women. Anemia during the early part of pregnancy can increase the likelihood of preterm birth, low birth weight, and perinatal mortality (Gautam, Saha, Sekhri, et al., 2008; Shah & Ohlsson, 2009). With significant maternal iron depletion, the fetus will attempt to store iron, but at the cost to the mother. Anemia at term increases the perinatal risk for both the mother and newborn. The risks of hemorrhage (impaired platelet function) and infection during and after birth also are increased.

Therapeutic Management

The goals of treatment for iron-deficiency anemia in pregnancy are to eliminate symptoms, correct the deficiency, and replenish iron stores. The SOGC–Canadian College of Medical Geneticists (CCMG) (Langlois, Ford, Chitayat, et al., 2008) and WHO (2001) recommend routine iron supplementation for all pregnant women at a low dose of 30 mg/day beginning at the first prenatal visit. Attempting to meet maternal iron requirements solely through diet in the face of diminished iron stores is difficult.

Nursing Assessment

Review the mother's history for factors that may contribute to the development of iron-deficiency anemia, including poor nutrition, hemolysis, **pica** (consuming non-food substances), multiple gestation, limited intervals between pregnancies, and blood loss. Assess the woman's dietary intake as well as the quantity and timing of ingestion of substances that interfere with iron absorption, such as tea, coffee, chocolate, and high-fibre foods. Ask the woman if she has fatigue, weakness, malaise, anorexia, or increased susceptibility to infection, such as frequent colds. Inspect the skin and mucous membranes, noting any pallor. Obtain vital signs and report any tachycardia.

Prepare the woman for laboratory testing. Laboratory tests usually reveal low Hgb (<6.8 mmol/L), low Hct (<35%), low serum iron (<30 µg/dL), microcytic and hypochromic cells, and low serum ferritin (<30 µg/L) (Milman, 2008; WHO, 2001).

▶ **Take** NOTE!

Hgb and Hct decrease normally during pregnancy in response to an increase in blood plasma in comparison with red blood cells. This hemodilution can lead to physiologic anemia of pregnancy, which is expected in the second trimester of pregnancy. This hemodilution phenomenon should not be confused with an iron-deficiency anemia, in which the Hgb would be below 6.8 mmol/L and Hct would be below 35%.

Nursing Management

Nursing management of the woman with iron-deficiency anemia focuses on encouraging compliance with drug therapy and providing dietary instruction about the intake of foods high in iron. Although iron constitutes a minimal percentage of the body's total weight, it has several major roles: it assists in the transport of oxygen and carbon dioxide throughout the body, it aids in the production of red blood cells, and it plays a role in the body's immune response.

Stress the importance of taking the prenatal vitamin and iron supplement consistently. Encourage the woman to take the iron supplement with vitamin C-containing fluids such as orange juice, which will promote absorption, rather than milk, which can inhibit iron absorption. Taking iron on an empty stomach improves its absorption, but many women cannot tolerate the gastrointestinal discomfort it causes. In such cases, advise the woman to take it with meals. Instruct the woman about adverse effects, which are predominantly gastrointestinal and include gastric discomfort, nausea, vomiting, anorexia, diarrhea, metallic taste, and constipation. Suggest that the woman take the iron supplement with meals and increase her intake of fibre and fluids to help overcome the most common side effects.

Provide dietary counselling. Recommend foods high in iron, such as dried fruits, whole grains, green leafy vegetables, meats, peanut butter, and iron-fortified cereals (Health Canada, 2011). Anticipate the need for a referral to a dietitian. Teaching Guideline 20.3 highlights instructions for the pregnant woman with iron-deficiency anemia.

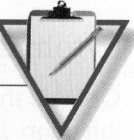

TEACHING GUIDELINE 20.3

Teaching for the Woman with Iron-Deficiency Anemia

- Take your prenatal vitamin daily; if you miss a dose, take it as soon as you remember.
- For best absorption, take iron supplement between meals.
- Avoid taking iron supplement with coffee, tea, chocolate, and high-fibre food.
- Eat foods rich in iron, such as:
  - Meats, green leafy vegetables, legumes, dried fruits, whole grains
  - Peanut butter, bean dip, whole-wheat–fortified breads and cereals
- For best iron absorption from foods, consume the food along with a food high in vitamin C.
- Increase your exercise, fluids, and high-fibre foods to reduce constipation.
- Plan frequent rest periods during the day.

Thalassemia

Thalassemia is a group of hereditary anemias in which synthesis of one or both chains of the hemoglobin molecule (alpha and beta) is defective. A low Hgb and a microcytic, hypochromic anemia result. The prevalence and severity of thalassemia depend on the woman's racial background: persons of Mediterranean, Southeast Asian, Middle Eastern, Western Pacific, Caribbean, South American, and African heritage are most frequently affected. Over 3.7 million Canadians, 12.5% of the population, identify their ethnic origin as one known to be at increased risk for thalassemia (Langlois et al., 2008).

Thalassemia occurs in two forms: alpha-thalassemia and beta-thalassemia. Alpha-thalassemia (minor), the heterozygous form, results from the inheritance of one abnormal gene from either parent, placing the offspring in a carrier trait state. These women have little or no hematologic disease and are clinically asymptomatic (silent carrier state). Beta-thalassemia (major) is the form involving inheritance of the gene from both parents. Beta-thalassemia major can be very severe. Genetic counselling might be necessary when decisions about childbearing are being made.

Thalassemia minor has little effect on the pregnancy, although the woman will have mild, persistent anemia. This anemia does not respond to iron therapy, and iron supplements should not be prescribed. Women with thalassemia major do not usually become pregnant because of lifelong severe hemolysis, anemia, and premature death (Bajoria & Chatterjee, 2009).

Management of thalassemia during pregnancy depends on the severity of the disease. Identification and screening are important to plan care. The woman's ethnic background, medical history, and blood studies are analyzed. If the woman is determined to be a carrier, screening of the father of the child is indicated. Knowledge of the carrier state of each parent provides the genetic counsellor with knowledge about the risk that the fetus will be a carrier or will have the disease (Langlois et al., 2008).

Mild anemia may be present, and instructions to rest and avoid infections are helpful. Nurses should provide supportive care and expectant management throughout the pregnancy.

Sickle-Cell Anemia

Sickle-cell anemia is an autosomal recessive inherited condition that results from a defective Hgb molecule, hemoglobin S (Hb S). It is found most commonly in people whose families are from Africa, Southeast Asia, and the Middle East (Mann-Jiles & Morris, 2009). About 1 in 20 people from these risk groups are carriers of the trait, while approximately 1 in 500 are affected with the disease (Sickle Cell Association of Ontario, n.d.; Yu, Stasiowska, Stephens, et al., 2009). People with only one gene for the trait (heterozygous) will have sickle-cell trait without obvious symptoms of the disease and with little effect on the pregnancy.

Pathophysiology

In the human body, the Hgb molecule serves as the oxygen-carrying component of the red blood cells. Most people have several types of circulating hemoglobin (Hb A and Hb A2) that make up the majority of their circulatory system. In sickle-cell disease, the abnormal Hb S replaces Hb A and Hb A2. Hb S becomes sickle-shaped as a result of any stress or trauma such as infection, fever, acidosis, dehydration, physical exertion, excessive cold exposure, or hypoxia (Inati, Koussa, Taher, et al., 2008). Significant anemia results. (See Chapter 46 for more information about sickle-cell disease.)

Sickle-cell anemia during pregnancy is associated with more severe anemia and frequent vaso-occlusive crises, with increased maternal and perinatal morbidity and mortality. In pregnant women with sickle-cell anemia, complications can occur at any time during gestation, labour and birth, or postpartum (Langlois et al., 2008). This is believed to be secondary to hormonal modifications, hypercoagulable state, and increased susceptibility to infection. Microvascular sickling in the placental circulation is associated with miscarriages, placental abruption, pre-eclampsia, preterm labour, IUGR, and low birth weight (Villers, Jamison, De Castro, et al., 2008).

Therapeutic Management

Ideally, women with hemoglobinopathies are screened before conception and are made aware of the risks of sickle-cell anemia to themselves and to the fetus. A blood hemoglobin electrophoresis is done for all women from high-risk ancestry at their first prenatal visit to determine the types and percentages of hemoglobin present. This information should help them in making reproductive decisions.

Treatment depends on the health status of the woman. During pregnancy, only supportive therapy is used: blood transfusions for severe anemia, analgesics for pain, and antibiotics for infection.

Nursing Assessment

Assess the woman for signs and symptoms of sickle-cell anemia. Ask the woman if she has anorexia, dyspnea, or malaise. Inspect the colour of the skin and mucous membranes, noting any pallor. Be alert for indicators of sickle-cell crisis, including severe abdominal pain, muscle spasms, leg pains, joint pain, fever, stiff neck, nausea and vomiting, and seizures (Villers et al., 2008).

Nursing Management

Clients require emotional support, education, and follow-up care to deal with this chronic condition, which can have a great impact on the woman and her family. Moni-

tor vital signs, fetal heart rate, weight gain, and fetal growth. Assess hydration status at each visit and urge the client to drink eight to 10 glasses of fluid daily to prevent dehydration. Teach the client about the need to avoid infections (including meticulous handwashing), cigarette smoking, alcohol consumption, and temperature extremes (Inati, Chabtini, Mounayar, et al., 2009).

Assist the woman in scheduling frequent fetal well-being assessments, such as biophysical profiles, nonstress tests, and contraction stress tests, and monitor laboratory test results for changes. Throughout the antepartal period, be alert for early signs and symptoms of crisis.

During labour, encourage rest and provide pain management. Oxygen supplementation is typically used throughout labour, along with intravenous fluids to maintain hydration. The fetal heart rate is monitored closely. After giving birth, the woman is fitted with antiembolism stockings to prevent blood clot formation. Before discharge from the facility after birth of the newborn, discuss family planning options.

Infections

A wide variety of infections can affect the progression of pregnancy, possibly having a negative impact on the outcome. The effect of the infection depends on the timing and severity of the infection and the body systems involved. Common viral infections include cytomegalovirus (CMV), rubella, herpes simplex, hepatitis B, varicella, parvovirus B19, and several sexually transmitted infections (STIs) (Table 20.3). Toxoplasmosis and group B streptococcus are common nonviral infections. Only the most common infections are discussed here.

Cytomegalovirus

CMV is the most common congenital and perinatal viral infection in the world. Infection is more prevalent in underdeveloped countries and among lower socioeconomic groups in developed countries where crowding is more common. (Nigro, 2009). CMV occurs in 1% to 2% of all live births in North America (Harvey & Dennis, 2008). Pregnant women acquire active disease primarily from sexual contact, blood transfusions, kissing, and contact with children in day care centres. The virus can be found in virtually all body fluids. Prevalence is influenced by many factors, including age, geographic distribution, socioeconomic status, and childbearing practices (Nigro, 2009). CMV infection during pregnancy may result in abortion, stillbirth, low birth weight, IUGR, microcephaly, deafness, blindness, mental retardation, jaundice, or congenital or neonatal infection. The first or primary infection, if it occurs during pregnancy, is the most dangerous to the fetus: the fetus has a 30% to 40% chance of being infected (Blaho, 2010; Yinon, Farine, Yudin, et al., 2010).

TABLE 20.3 SEXUALLY TRANSMITTED INFECTIONS AFFECTING PREGNANCY

Infection (Organism)	Effect on Pregnancy and Fetus/Newborn	Implications
Syphilis (*Treponema pallidum*)	Maternal infection increases risk for premature labour and birth. Newborn may be born with congenital syphilis—jaundice, rhinitis, anemia, IUGR, and CNS involvement.	All pregnant women should be screened for this STI and treated with benzathine penicillin G 2.4 million units IM to prevent placental transmission.
Gonorrhea (*Neisseria gonorrhoeae*)	Majority of women are asymptomatic. It causes ophthalmia neonatorum in the newborn from birth through infected birth canal.	All pregnant women should be screened at first prenatal visit, with repeat screening in the third trimester. All newborns receive mandatory eye prophylaxis with tetracycline or erythromycin within the first hour of life. Mother is treated with ceftriaxone (Rocephin) 125 mg IM in single dose before going home.
Chlamydia (*Chlamydia trachomatis*)	Majority of women are asymptomatic. Infection is associated with infertility and ectopic pregnancy, spontaneous abortions, preterm labour, premature rupture of membranes, low birth weight, stillbirth, and neonatal mortality. Infection is transmitted to newborn through vaginal birth. Neonate may develop conjunctivitis or pneumonia.	All pregnant women should be screened at first prenatal visit and treated with erythromycin.
Human papillomavirus (HPV)	Infection causes warts in the anogenital area, known as condylomata acuminata. These warts may grow large enough to block a vaginal birth. Fetal exposure to HPV during birth is associated with laryngeal papillomas.	Warts are treated with trichlorocetic acid, liquid nitrogen, or laser therapy under colposcopy. A quadrivalent HPV vaccine (Gardasil) against the viral types most likely to cause cervical cancer (types 16 and 18) and genital warts (types 6 and 11) has been licensed in Canada for girls and women 9 to 26 years old. The vaccine is 95% to 100% effective (Association of Women's Health, Obstetric and Neonatal Nurses, 2008). It is hoped that this vaccine will reduce the number of HPV-positive pregnant women in the future.
Trichomonas (*Trichomonas vaginalis*)	Infection produces itching and burning, dysuria, strawberry patches on cervix, and vaginal discharge. Infection is associated with premature rupture of membranes and preterm birth.	Treatment is with a single 2 g dose of metronidazole (Flagyl).

Sources: Public Health Agency of Canada. (2008a). *Genital herpes simplex virus (HSV) infections.* Retrieved February 13, 2012 from http://www.phac-aspc.gc.ca/std-mts/sti-its/pdf/504genherp-vhs-eng.pdf; Public Health Agency of Canada. (2008b). *Genital human papilloma virus (HPV) infections.* Retrieved February 13, 2012 from http://www.phac-aspc.gc.ca/std-mts/sti-its/pdf/505hpv-vph-eng.pdf; Public Health Agency of Canada. (2008c). *Hepatitis B virus (HBV) infections.* Retrieved February 13, 2012 from http://www.phac-aspc.gc.ca/std-mts/sti-its/pdf/507hepb-eng.pdf; Public Health Agency of Canada. (2008d). *Human immunodeficiency virus (HIV) infections.* Retrieved February 13, 2012 from http://www.phac-aspc.gc.ca/std-mts/sti-its/pdf/508hiv-vih-eng.pdf; & Public Health Agency of Canada. (2010a). *Hepatitis B—get the facts.* Retrieved February 13, 2012 from http://www.phac-aspc.gc.ca/hcai-iamss/bbp-pts/hepatitis/hep_b-eng.php.

Most women are asymptomatic and don't know they have been exposed to CMV. Symptoms of CMV in the fetus and newborn, known as cytomegalovirus inclusion disease, include hepatosplenomegaly, thrombocytopenia, IUGR, jaundice, purpura, microcephaly, hearing loss, chorioretinitis, and mental retardation (Venkatesh, Adams, & Weisman., 2011; Yinon et al., 2010). Since there is no therapy that prevents or treats CMV infections, nurses are responsible for educating and supporting women of childbearing age who are at risk for CMV infection. Stressing the importance of good handwashing and use of sound hygiene practices can help to reduce transmission of the virus (Harvey & Dennis, 2008).

Rubella

Rubella, commonly called German measles, is spread by droplets or through direct contact with a contaminated object. Large rubella outbreaks occurred in Canada in the 1990s, a reflection of Canadian immigration policies in the 1970s and 1980s as well as international immunization policies. The incidence of rubella in Canada is approximately 1,000 reported cases per year (Canadian Paediatric Society, 2007).

The risk for a pregnant woman transmitting this virus through the placenta to her fetus increases with earlier exposure to the virus. When infection occurs within the first trimester, fetal infection rates are near 80%; rates drop to 25% in the late second trimester and increase again in the third trimester, from 35% at 30 weeks' gestation to nearly 100% beyond 36 weeks' gestation (Yinon et al., 2010).

Education for primary prevention is key. Ideally, all women have been vaccinated and have adequate immunity against rubella. However, all women are still screened at their first prenatal visit to determine their status. A rubella antibody titre of 1:8 or greater proves immunity. Women who are not immune should be vaccinated during the immediate postpartum period so they will be immune before becoming pregnant again (SOGC, 2008). Nurses need to check the rubella immune status of all new mothers and should make sure all mothers with a titre of less than 1:8 are immunized prior to discharge after birth of the newborn.

Herpes Simplex Virus

The prevalence of herpes simplex virus (HSV) genital infection has been rising worldwide (PHAC, 2008a). The annual incidence of genital herpes due to HSV infection in Canada is not known due to inconsistent provincial reporting methods. In the United States, it is estimated that HSV occurs in approximately 8.4 per 1,000 persons. Females are at a higher risk for acquiring genital herpes from a male partner than males are from a female partner (PHAC, 2008a). Despite strategies designed to prevent perinatal transmission, the number of cases of newborn HSV infection continues to rise, mirroring the rising prevalence of genital herpes infection in women of childbearing age (Money, Seben, Wong, et al., 2008).

HSV is a DNA virus with two subtypes: HSV-1 and HSV-2. HSV-1 infections were traditionally associated with oral lesions (fever blisters), whereas HSV-2 infections occurred in the genital region. Currently, either type can be found in either location (Anzivino, Fioriti, Mischitelli, et al., 2009).

In Canada, the rate of HSV-2 seropositivity in pregnant women is 17%, with a range of 7.1% to 28.1%. Neonatal HSV continues to be a dire medical consequence of genital herpes. Canadian neonatal HSV surveillance data show a rate of 1 in 17,000 live births (Money et al., 2008).

Infection occurs by direct contact of the skin or mucous membranes with an active lesion through such activities as kissing, sexual (vaginal, oral, anal) contact, or routine skin-to-skin contact. HSV is associated with infections of the genital tract that, when acquired during pregnancy, can result in severe systemic symptoms in the mother and significant morbidity and mortality in the newborn (Ural, 2011). Once the virus enters the body, it never leaves.

Infants born to mothers with a primary HSV infection have a 30% to 50% risk for acquiring the infection via perinatal transmission near or during birth. Recurrent genital HSV infections carry a 2% risk for neonatal infection if the recurrence occurs around the time of vaginal birth (PHAC, 2008a).

The greatest risk for transmission is when the mother develops a primary infection near term and it is not recognized. Most neonatal infections are acquired at or around the time of birth through either ascending infection after ruptured membranes or contact with the virus at the time of birth. The method and timing of birth in a woman with genital herpes are controversial. It is recommended that in the absence of active lesions, a vaginal birth is acceptable, but if the woman has active herpetic lesions near or at term, a cesarean birth should be planned (Money et al., 2008; PHAC, 2008a).

Management for the woman with genital herpes during pregnancy involves caring for her as well as reducing the risk for newborn herpes. Since the majority of newborn herpes cases result from perinatal transmission of the virus during vaginal birth, and because transmission can result in severe neurologic impairment or death, treatment of the mother with an antiviral agent such as acyclovir must be started as soon as the culture comes back positive. Universal screening for herpes is not economically sound, so nurses need to remain knowledgeable about current practice to provide accurate and sensitive care to all women.

Hepatitis B Virus

Hepatitis B virus (HBV) is one of the most prevalent chronic diseases in the world. HBV can be transmitted through contaminated blood, illicit drug use, and sexual contact. The virus is 100 times more infectious than HIV and, unlike HIV, can live outside the body in dried blood for more than a week (Parry, 2010).

It is estimated that between 0.7% and 0.9% of Canada's population is chronically infected by HBV. In 2008, the overall reported rate of acute HBV infection in Canada was 0.74 (individuals infected) per 100,000 people living in Canada (PHAC, 2008c). Sexual transmission accounts for most adult HBV infections in the Canada. Acutely infected women develop hepatitis with anorexia, nausea, vomiting, fever, abdominal pain, and jaundice. In women with acute HBV, vertical transmission occurs in approximately 10% of newborns when infection occurs in the first trimester and in 80% to 90% of newborns when acute infection occurs in the third trimester. Without intervention, 70% to 90% of infants born to women who are positive for HBV will have chronic HBV by 6 months of age (Jonas, 2009).

In addition, HBV infection during pregnancy is associated with an increased risk for preterm birth, low birth weight, and neonatal death. Newborns infected with HBV are likely to become chronic carriers of the virus, becoming reservoirs for continued infection in the population (PHAC, 2008c; Venkatesh et al., 2011). The fetus is at particular risk during birth because of the possible contact with contaminated blood at this time.

Nursing Assessment

Review the woman's history for factors placing her at high risk:

- History of STIs
- Household contact with HBV-infected persons
- Employment as a health care worker
- Abuse of intravenous drugs
- Sex worker (prostitute)
- Foreign born
- Multiple sexual partners
- Chinese, Southeast Asian, or African heritage
- Sexual partners who are HBV infected (PHAC, 2008c)

At the first prenatal visit, all pregnant women should be screened for hepatitis B surface antigen (HBsAg) via blood studies. Expect to repeat this screening later in pregnancy for women in high-risk groups (Jonas, 2009).

Nursing Management

If a woman tests positive for HBV, expect to administer HBV immune globulin (HBIG, Hep-B-Gammagee). The newborn receives HBV vaccine (Recombivax-HB, Engerix-B) within 12 hours of birth. The second and third doses of the vaccine are given at 1 and 6 months of age. Routine HBV vaccination is recommended for all newborns, regardless of the infection status of the mother (PHAC, 2008c).

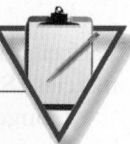

TEACHING GUIDELINE 20.4

Teaching to Prevent Hepatitis B Virus Infection

- Abstain from alcohol.
- Avoid intravenous drug exposure or sharing of needles.
- Encourage all household contacts and sexual partners to be vaccinated.
- Receive immediate treatment for any sexually transmitted infection.
- Know that your newborn will receive the hepatitis B vaccine soon after birth.
- Use good handwashing techniques at all times.
- Avoid contact with blood or body fluids.
- Use barrier methods such as condoms during sexual intercourse.
- Avoid sharing any personal items, such as razors, toothbrushes, or eating utensils.

Women who are HBsAg-negative may be vaccinated safely during pregnancy. No current research supports the use of surgical births to reduce vertical transmission of HBV. Breastfeeding by mothers with chronic HBV infection does not increase the risk for viral transmission to their newborns (Venkatesh et al., 2011; PHAC, 2008c).

Client education related to prevention of HBV infection is essential. Teach the woman about safer sex practices, good handwashing techniques, and the use of standard precautions (Teaching Guideline 20.4). Protection can be afforded with the highly effective HBV vaccine.

Permanent remission of the disease rarely occurs, even with treatment. Therefore, therapy is directed at long-term suppression of viral replication and prevention of end-stage liver disease. Urge the woman to consume a high-protein diet and avoid fatigue. A healthy lifestyle can help delay disease progression. Initiate an open discussion about the modes of transmission and use of condoms to prevent spread.

Varicella Zoster Virus

Varicella zoster virus (VZV), a member of the herpes virus family, is the virus that causes both varicella (chickenpox) and herpes zoster (shingles). Pregnant women are at risk for developing varicella when they come in close contact with children who have active infection. Maternal varicella can be transmitted to the fetus through the placenta, leading to congenital varicella syndrome, if the mother is infected during the first half of pregnancy; via an ascending infection during birth; or by direct contact with infectious lesions, leading to infection after birth.

Varicella occurs in approximately 1 to 7 of 10,000 pregnancies (Sauerbrei, 2010).

Congenital varicella syndrome can occur in newborns of mothers infected during early pregnancy. It is characterized by low birth weight, skin lesions in a dermatomal distribution, spontaneous abortion, chorioretinitis, cataracts, cutaneous scarring, limb hypoplasia, microcephaly, ocular abnormalities, mental retardation, and early death (Daley, Thorpe, & Garland, 2008).

Preconception counselling is important for preventing this condition. A major component of counselling involves determining the woman's varicella immunity. The vaccine is administered if needed. Provide education to women who work in occupations that increase the risk for exposure to the virus, such as day care workers, teachers of young children, and staff caring for children in institutional settings.

Varicella during pregnancy can be associated with severe illnesses for both the mother and her newborn. If contracted in the first half of pregnancy, some pregnant women are at risk for developing varicella pneumonia, which may put them at risk for life-threatening ventilatory compromise and death. If the mother develops varicella rashes close to her due date, generalized neonatal varicella leading to death in about 20% of cases can be expected (Sauerbrei, 2010). Maternal infection is preventable by preconception vaccination.

Parvovirus B19

Parvovirus B19 infection occurs worldwide. The incidence of acute B19 infection in pregnancy is about 3% (Crane, Armson, de la Ronde, et al., 2002). Parvovirus B19 is a common, self-limiting benign childhood virus that causes erythema infectiosum, also known as fifth disease (referring to its "fifth place" in a list of common childhood infections). Approximately 50% to 65% of women of reproductive age have developed immunity to parvovirus B19 (Beigi, Wiesenfeld, Landers, et al., 2008).

Pathophysiology

The infection is spread transplacentally, by the oropharyngeal route in casual contact, and through infected blood. Infection of the fetus occurs through transplacental passage of the virus. Acute infection in pregnancy can cause B19 infection in the fetus, leading to non-immune fetal hydrops secondary to severe anemia or fetal loss, depending on the gestational age at the time of infection. The risk to the fetus is greatest when the woman is exposed and infected within the first 20 weeks of gestation. In addition to hydrops, other fetal effects of parvovirus include spontaneous abortion, congenital anomalies (CNS, craniofacial, and eye), and long-term effects such as hepatic insufficiency, myocarditis, and learning disabilities (Beigi et al., 2008; Crane et al., 2002).

Therapeutic Management

Generally, diagnosis of parvovirus is based on clinical symptoms and serologic antibody testing for parvovirus immunoglobulin G (IgG) and parvovirus immunoglobulin M (IgM). Parvovirus B19 infection is followed by life-long immunity, which is shown by positive serum B19 IgG. Pregnant women who have been exposed to or who develop symptoms of parvovirus B19 require assessment to determine whether they are susceptible to infection (non-immune). If the woman is immune, she can be reassured that she will not develop infection and that the virus will not adversely affect her pregnancy. If she is non-immune, then referral to a perinatologist is recommended and counselling regarding the risks of fetal transmission, fetal loss, and hydrops is necessary. Knowledge of how best to manage it during pregnancy lags behind our understanding of the potential adverse consequences.

Intrauterine B19 infection is a cause of fetal anemia, hydrops, and demise, and perhaps also of congenital anomalies. The best strategy for surveillance of the infected pregnant woman is serial ultrasounds for detection of hydropic changes and fetal anemia, and treatment for severe fetal anemia. Serial ultrasounds are advocated because the rates of fetal death and complications peak 4 to 6 weeks after exposure, but they can occur as late as 3 months following onset of symptoms (Rawlinson, Hall, Jones, et al., 2008).

The infected newborn is assessed for any anomaly and followed for up to 6 years to identify any sequelae (Beigi et al., 2008).

Nursing Assessment

Review the mother's history for any risk factors. Schoolteachers, day care workers, and women living with school-age children are at highest risk for being seropositive for parvovirus B19, especially if a recent outbreak has occurred in those settings. Also assess the woman for specific signs and symptoms. The characteristic rash starts on the face with a "slapped-cheeks" appearance and is followed by a generalized maculopapular rash. Fever, arthralgia, and generalized malaise are usually present in the mother. Prepare the mother for antibody testing.

Nursing Management

Prevention is the best strategy. Stress the need for handwashing after handling children, cleaning toys and surfaces with which children have been in contact, and avoiding the sharing of food and drinks. Screening for parvovirus B19 during early pregnancy may help in early diagnosis, but the cost-effectiveness of a national screening program has not been accepted to date. The nurse can provide information regarding risk factors and potential complications if exposed and support the parent's decision.

Group B Streptococcus

Group B streptococcus (GBS) is a naturally occurring bacterium found in 10% to 35% of healthy adults. Women who test positive for the GBS bacteria are considered carriers. Carrier status is transient and doesn't indicate illness. Approximately 25% of pregnant women carry GBS in the rectum or vagina, thus introducing the risk for colonization of the fetus during birth. The incidence of neonatal disease in Canada and the United States is 0.5 to 1 per 1,000 live births (El Aila, Tency, Claeys, et al., 2009; SOGC, 2011a). Approximately 1 in every 100 to 200 newborns born to mothers who carry GBS will develop signs and symptoms of GBS disease. Although GBS is rarely serious in adults, it can be life-threatening to newborns. GBS is the most common cause of sepsis and meningitis in newborns and is a frequent cause of newborn pneumonia (Dechen, Sumit, & Ranabir, 2010). Newborns with early-onset (within a week after birth) GBS infections may have pneumonia or sepsis, whereas late-onset (after the first week) infections often manifest with meningitis (Venkatesh et al., 2011).

Genital tract colonization poses the most threat to the newborn because of exposure during birth and to the mother because of ascending infection after the membranes rupture. GBS colonization in the mother is thought to cause chorioamnionitis, endometritis, and postpartum wound infection.

Therapeutic Management

Antibiotic therapy usually is effective in treating women with GBS infections of the urinary tract or uterus, or chorioamnionitis without any sequelae. According to the SOGC guidelines (Money et al., 2004), all pregnant women should be screened for GBS at 35 to 37 weeks' gestation. Vaginal and rectal specimens are cultured for the presence of the bacterium. If positive, the woman should be treated with intravenous antibiotics during labour.

Penicillin G is the treatment of choice for GBS infection because of its narrow spectrum. Alternative antibiotics can be prescribed for clients with a penicillin allergy. The drug is usually administered intravenously at least 4 hours before birth so that it can reach adequate levels in the serum and amniotic fluid to reduce the risk for newborn colonization. Close monitoring is required during the administration of intravenous antibiotics because severe allergic reactions can occur rapidly.

Nursing Assessment

Review the woman's prenatal history, asking about any previous infection. Determine whether the woman's membranes have ruptured and the time of rupture. The risk for infection is increased if the infant is not born within 18 hours after rupture of amniotic membranes.

Monitor the mother's vital signs, reporting any maternal fever greater than 38°C. Assess the woman for other risk factors for perinatal transmission of GBS, including previous colonization with GBS, low socioeconomic status, black race, age less than 20 years, positive colonization at 35 to 37 weeks' gestation, GBS in urine sample, previous birth of GBS-positive newborn, preterm birth, and use of invasive obstetric procedures (El Aila et al., 2009; Money et al., 2004). Document this information to help prevent vertical transmission to the newborn.

Many women with GBS infection are asymptomatic, but they may have urinary tract infections, uterine infections, and chorioamnionitis.

Nursing Management

Nurses play major roles as educators and advocates for all women and newborns to reduce the incidence of GBS infections. Ensure that pregnant women between 35 and 37 weeks' gestation are screened for GBS infection during a prenatal visit. Record the results and notify the birth attendant if the woman has tested positive for GBS. During labour, be prepared to administer intravenous antibiotics to all women who are GBS positive.

Toxoplasmosis

Toxoplasmosis is a relatively widespread parasitic infection caused by a one-celled organism, *Toxoplasma gondii* (Tridapalli, Capretti, Farneti, et al., 2008). Estimates suggest that one third of Canadians have been infected (Canadian Centre for Occupational Health and Safety [CCOHS], 2011). When a pregnant woman is exposed to this protozoan, the infection can pose serious risks to her fetus (Habib, 2008). Approximately 1,400 newborns are born infected with toxoplasmosis in Canada every year (CCOHS, 2011). It is transferred hand to mouth after touching cat feces while changing the cat litter box or through gardening in contaminated soil. Consuming undercooked meat, such as pork, lamb, or venison, can also transmit this organism.

Although the woman typically remains asymptomatic, transmission of toxoplasmosis to her fetus can occur throughout pregnancy. A pregnant woman who contracts toxoplasmosis for the first time in the first trimester has a 15% chance of passing the infection to her fetus; miscarriage is common (CCOHS, 2011). The risk for transmission to the fetus increases to 30% in the second trimester and 60% in the third trimester. A fetus that contracts congenital toxoplasmosis typically is premature and small for gestational age. Other manifestations may include seizures, enlarged liver and spleen, thrombocytopenia, chorioretinitis, jaundice, hydrocephalus, cerebral calcification, lymphedema, and a rash (Venkatesh et al., 2011).

Treatment of the woman during pregnancy to reduce the risk for congenital infection is with a combination of pyrimethamine and sulfadiazine. Treatment

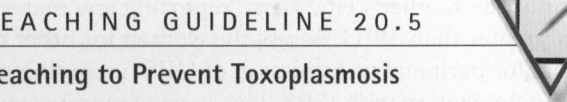

TEACHING GUIDELINE 20.5

Teaching to Prevent Toxoplasmosis

- Avoid eating raw or undercooked meat, especially lamb or pork. Cook all meat to an internal temperature of 160°F throughout.
- Clean cutting boards, work surfaces, and utensils with hot soapy water after contact with raw meat or unwashed fruits and vegetables.
- Peel or thoroughly wash all raw fruits and vegetables before eating them.
- Wash hands thoroughly with warm water and soap after handling raw meat.
- Avoid feeding the cat raw or undercooked meats.
- Avoid emptying or cleaning the cat's litterbox. Have someone else do it daily.
- Keep the cat indoors to prevent it from hunting and eating birds or rodents.
- Avoid uncooked eggs and unpasteurized milk.
- Wear gardening gloves when in contact with outdoor soil.
- Avoid contact with children's sandboxes, because cats can use them as litterboxes.

with sulfonamides during pregnancy has been shown to reduce the risk for congenital infection.

Prevention is the key to managing this infection. Nurses play a key role in educating the woman about measures to prevent toxoplasmosis (Teaching Guideline 20.5).

Vulnerable Populations

In 2008 there were an estimated 220 million pregnancies worldwide, with about 500,000 of them in Canada (Luong, 2008). Each pregnancy runs the risk for an adverse outcome for the mother and the baby, but risks are dramatically increased for certain vulnerable populations: adolescents, women over the age of 35, women who are HIV positive, and women who abuse substances. While risks cannot be totally eliminated once pregnancy has begun, they can be reduced through appropriate and timely interventions.

Every woman's experience with pregnancy is unique and personal. The circumstances each one faces and what pregnancy means to her involve emotions and experiences that belong solely to her. Many women in these special population groups go through this experience in confusion and isolation, feeling desperately in need of help but not knowing where to go. Although all pregnant women experience these emotions to a certain extent, they are heightened in women who have numerous psychosocial issues. Pregnancy is a stressful time. Pregnant women face wide-ranging changes in their lives, relationships, and bodies as they move toward parenthood. These changes can be challenging for a woman without any additional stresses but are even more so in the face of age extremes, illness, or substance abuse.

Skilled nursing interventions are essential to promote the best outcome for the client and her baby. Timely support and appropriate interventions during the perinatal period can have longstanding implications for the mother and her newborn, with the ultimate goal of stability and integration of the family as a unit.

Pregnant Adolescent

Adolescence lasts from the onset of puberty to the cessation of physical growth, roughly from 11 to 19 years of age. Adolescents vacillate between being children and being adults. They need to adjust to the physiologic changes their bodies are undergoing and establish a sexual identity during this time. They search for personal identity and desire freedom and independence of thought and action. However, they continue to have a strong dependence on their parents (McKay & Barrett, 2010).

Each year in Canada, approximately 31,000 adolescents between the ages of 15 and 19 years become pregnant (Luong, 2008). These pregnancies, which account for 6% of all births, are typically unintended and occur outside of marriage. In addition, about half of all teen pregnancies occur within 6 months of first having sexual intercourse. Of girls who become pregnant, one in six will have a repeat pregnancy within 1 year (Aruda, Waddicor, Frese, et al., 2010; Briggs, Hopman, & Jamieson, 2007; DeVito, 2010). Most of these girls are unmarried, and many are not ready for the emotional, psychological, and financial responsibilities of parenthood. Adolescent pregnancy is further complicated by the teen's lack of financial resources: the income of teen mothers is half that of women who give birth in their 20s (DeVito, 2010).

In Canada, the incidence of teenage pregnancy decreased by 36.7% between 1996 and 2006, and it continues to be lower than in the United Kingdom, United States, and other developed countries (McKay & Barrett, 2010). However, even this reduced incidence represents what is considered an unacceptably high level of pregnancy in an age group that is likely to suffer the social consequences of early pregnancy most. Consequently, adolescent pregnancy is considered a major health problem.

Impact of Pregnancy in Adolescence

Adolescents are a unique group with special needs related to their stage of development. Adolescent pregnancy can be an emotionally charged situation, laden with ethical dilemmas and decisions. Topics such as abstinence, safer sex, abortion, and the decision to have a child are sensitive issues (Kramer & Lancaster, 2010).

Adolescent pregnancy is an area in which a nurse's moral convictions may influence the care that he or she provides to clients. Nurses need to examine their own beliefs about teen sexuality to identify personal assumptions. Putting aside one's moral convictions may be difficult, but it is necessary when working with pregnant adolescents. To be effective, health care providers must be able to communicate with adolescents in a manner they can understand and respect them as individuals.

Developmental Issues

An adolescent must accomplish certain developmental tasks to advance to the next stage of maturity. These developmental tasks include:

- Seeking economic and social stability
- Developing a personal value system
- Building meaningful relationships with others (Fig. 20.3)
- Becoming comfortable with their changing bodies
- Working to become independent from their parents
- Learning to verbalize conceptually (Duncan, Harris, Reedy, et al., 2008; Strunk, 2008).

Adolescents have special needs when working to accomplish their developmental tasks and making a smooth transition to young adulthood. One of the biggest areas of need is sexual health. Adolescents commonly lack the information, skills, and services necessary to make informed choices related to their sexual and reproductive health. Developmentally, adolescents are trying to figure out who they are and how they fit into society. As adolescents mature, their parents become less influential and peers become more influential. Peer pressure can lead adolescents to participate in sexual activity, as can the typical adolescent's belief that "it won't happen to me" (Box 20.3).

As a result, unplanned pregnancies occur. Work on the developmental tasks of adolescence, especially identity, can be interrupted as the adolescent attempts to

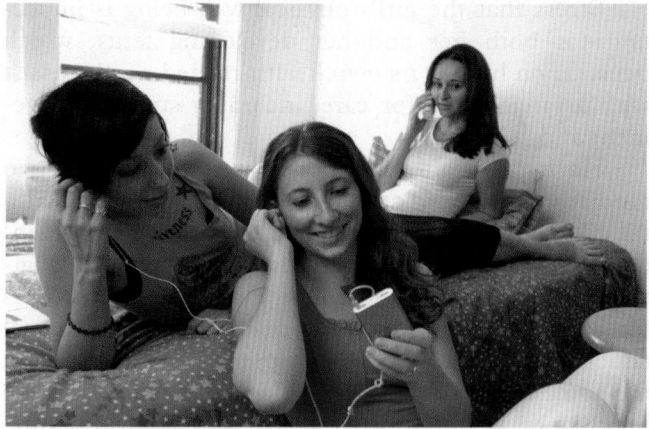

FIGURE 20.3 Adolescent girls sharing time together.

BOX 20.3 Possible Factors Contributing to Adolescent Pregnancy

- Early menarche
- Peer pressure to become sexually active
- Sexual or other abuse as a child
- Lack of accurate contraceptive information
- Fear of telling parents about sexual activity
- Feelings of invulnerability
- Poverty (majority of births occur in poor families)
- Culture or ethnicity (high incidence in Hispanic and black girls)
- Unprotected sex
- Low self-esteem and inability to negotiate
- Lack of appropriate role models
- Strong need for someone to love
- Drug use, truancy, or other behavioural problems
- Wish to escape a bad home situation
- Early dating without supervision

Sources: March of Dimes. (2009). *Teenage pregnancy.* Retrieved February 13, 2012 from http://www.marchofdimes.com/professionals/medicalresources_teenpregnancy.html; & McKay, A., & Barrett, M. (2010). Trends in teen pregnancy rates from 1996–2006: A comparison of Canada, Sweden, U.S.A., and England/Wales. *Canadian Journal of Human Sexuality, 19*(1–2), 43–52.

---

integrate the tasks of pregnancy, bonding, and preparing to care for another with the tasks of developing self-identity and independence. A pregnant adolescent must try to meet her own needs along with those of her fetus. The process of learning how to separate from the parents while learning how to bond and attach to a newborn brings conflict and stress. A pregnancy can exacerbate an adolescent's feeling of loss of control (Kramer & Lancaster, 2010).

Health and Social Issues

Adolescent pregnancy has a negative impact in terms of both health and social consequences. For example, most pregnant teens will drop out of school. More than half will receive public assistance within a few years of having their first child. In addition, children of adolescent mothers are at greater risk for preterm birth, low birth weight, child abuse, neglect, poverty, and death (Chedraui, 2008). The younger the adolescent is at the time of the first pregnancy, the more likely it is that she will have another pregnancy during her teens (Dehlendorf, Marchi, Vittinghoff, et al., 2010).

The psychosocial risks associated with early childbearing often have an even greater impact on mothers, families, and society than the obstetric or medical risks (Kramer & Lancaster, 2010). Pregnant adolescents experience higher rates of domestic violence and substance abuse. Those experiencing abuse are more likely to abuse substances, receive inadequate prenatal care, and have lower pregnancy weight compared with those who are not abused (Heavey, 2010). Moreover, substance abuse (cigarettes, alcohol, or illicit drugs) can contribute to low birth weight, IUGR, preterm birth, newborn addiction, and sepsis (Baker, Wheeler, Sanders, et al., 2009).

Although early childbearing (12 to 19 years of age) occurs in all socioeconomic groups, it is more prevalent among poor women and those from minority backgrounds, who face more obstetric and newborn risks than their more affluent counterparts (Dehlendorf et al., 2010). Poverty often contributes to delayed prenatal care and medical complications related to poor nutrition, such as anemia.

The financial burden of adolescent pregnancy is high (Rosenthal et al., 2009). Much of the expense stems from cash assistance, prenatal care, supplemental nutrition, and health care at delivery (Adams, Gavin, Femi Ayadi, et al., 2009). However, this amount does not address the costs to society in terms of the loss of human resources and the far-reaching intergenerational effects of adolescent parenting.

For some adolescents, pregnancy may be seen as a hopeless situation: a grim story of poverty and lost dreams, of being trapped in a life that was never wanted. Health-related behaviours, such as smoking, diet, sexual behaviour, and help-seeking behaviours, that are developed during adolescence often endure into later life (Heavey, 2010; Milne & Glasier, 2008). The consequences associated with an adolescent's less-than-optimal health status at this age as a result of pregnancy can ultimately affect her long-term health and that of her children.

However, some adolescents can create a happy, stable life for themselves and their children by facing their challenges and working hard to beat the odds.

*R**ecall Rose, the pregnant teenager with asthma. What issues would be important for the nurse to discuss with her related to her pregnancy, her asthma, and her age?*

Nursing Assessment

Assessment of the pregnant adolescent is the same as that for any pregnant woman. However, when dealing with pregnant teens, the nurse also needs to ask:

- How does the girl see herself in the future?
- Are realistic role models available to her?
- How much does she know about child development?
- What financial resources are available to her?
- Does she work? Does she go to school?
- What emotional support is available to her?
- Can she resolve conflicts and manage anger?
- What does she know about health and nutrition for herself and her child?

- Will she need help dealing with the challenges of the new parenting role?
- Does she need information about community resources?

Having an honest regard for adolescents requires getting to know them and being able to appreciate the important aspects of their life. Doing so forms a basis for the nurse's clinical judgment and promotes care that takes into account the concerns and practical circumstances of the teen and her family. Skillful practice includes knowing how and when to advise a teen and when to listen and refrain from giving advice. Giving advice can be misinterpreted as "preaching," and the adolescent will probably ignore the information. The nurse must be perceptive, flexible, and sensitive and must work to establish a therapeutic relationship.

Nursing Management

For adolescents, as for all women, pregnancy can be a physically, emotionally, and socially stressful time. The pregnancy is often both the result and cause of social problems and stressors that can be overwhelming to them. Nurses must support adolescents during the transition from childhood into adulthood, which is complicated by their emergence into motherhood. Assist the adolescent in identifying family and friends who want to be involved and provide support throughout the pregnancy.

Help the adolescent identify the options for this pregnancy, such as abortion, self-parenting of the child, temporary foster care for the baby or herself, or placement of the child for adoption. Explore with the adolescent why she became pregnant. Becoming aware of why she decided to have a child is necessary to help with the development of the adolescent and her ability to parent. Identify barriers to seeking prenatal care, such as lack of transportation, too many problems at home, financial concerns, the long wait for an appointment, and lack of sensitivity on the part of the health care system. Encourage the girl to set goals and work toward them. Assist her in returning to school and furthering her education. As appropriate, initiate a referral for career or job counselling.

Stress that the girl's physical well-being is important for both her and her developing fetus, which depends on her for its own health-related needs. Assist with arrangements for care, including stress management and self-care.

Having a healthy newborn eases the transition to motherhood somewhat, rather than having to deal with the added stress of caring for an unhealthy baby (Dehlendorf et al., 2010). Monitor weight gain, sleep and rest patterns, and nutritional status to promote positive outcomes for both. Stress the importance of attending prenatal education classes. Provide appropriate teaching based on the adolescent's developmental level and emphasize the importance of continued prenatal and follow-up care. Monitor maternal and fetal well-being throughout pregnancy and labour (Fig. 20.4).

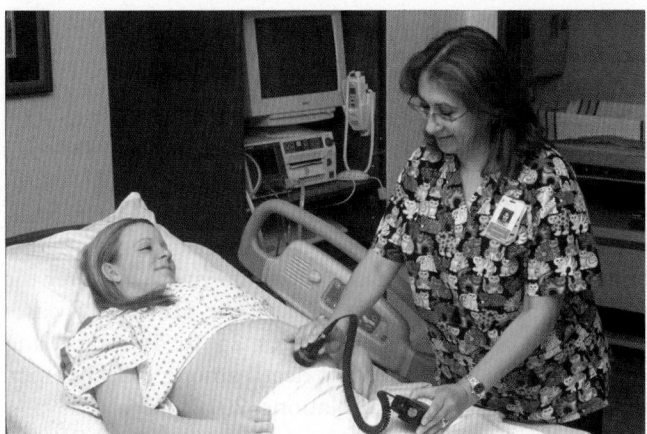

FIGURE 20.4 A pregnant adolescent receiving care during labour.

Nurses can also play a major role in preventing adolescent pregnancies, perhaps by volunteering to talk to teen groups. Box 20.4 highlights the key areas for teaching adolescents about pregnancy prevention.

Tackling the many issues surrounding adolescent pregnancy is difficult. Making connections with clients is crucial regardless of how complex their situation is. The future challenges nurses to find solutions to teenage pregnancy. Nurses must take proactive positions while working with adolescents, parents, schools, and communities to reduce the problems associated with early childbearing.

BOX 20.4 **Topics for Teaching Adolescents to Prevent Pregnancy**

- High-risk behaviours that lead to pregnancy
- Involvement in programs such as Free Teens, Teen Advisors, or Postponing Sexual Involvement
- Planning and goal setting to visualize their futures in terms of career, college, travel, and education
- Choice of abstinence or taking a step back to become a "second-time virgin"
- Discussions about sexuality with a wiser adult—someone they respect can help put things in perspective
- Protection against sexually transmitted infections and pregnancy if they choose to remain sexually active
- Critical observation and review of peers and friends to make sure they are creating the right atmosphere for friendship
- Empowerment to make choices that will shape their life for years to come, including getting control of their own lives now
- Appropriate use of recreational time, such as sports, drama, volunteer work, music, jobs, church activities, and school clubs

---

Sources: King-Jones, T. C. (2008). Caring for pregnant adolescents: Perils and pearls of communication. *Nursing for Women's Health, 12*(2), 114–119; & March of Dimes. (2009). *Teenage pregnancy.* Retrieved February 13, 2012 from http://www.marchofdimes.com/professionals/medicalresources_teenpregnancy.html.

The Pregnant Woman Over Age 35

The term "elderly primip" is used to describe a woman age 35 or older who is pregnant for the first time. A few decades ago, a woman having a baby after the age of 35 probably was giving birth to the last of several children, but today she may be having her first. With advances in technology and the tendency of women to seek career advancement prior to childbearing, the dramatic increase in women having first pregnancies after the age of 35 will likely continue.

Impact of Pregnancy on the Older Woman

Whether childbearing is delayed by choice or by chance, starting a family at age 35 is different and not without risks. Women in this age group may already have chronic health conditions that may put the pregnancy at risk. In addition, numerous studies have shown that increasing maternal age is a risk factor for infertility and spontaneous abortions, gestational diabetes, chronic hypertension, preeclampsia, preterm labour and birth, multiple pregnancy, genetic disorders and chromosomal abnormalities, placenta previa, IUGR, low Apgar scores, and surgical births (Al Shami, Kadasne, Khalfan, et al., 2011). However, even though increased age implies increased complications, most women today who become pregnant after age 35 have healthy pregnancies and healthy newborns (Clift-Matthews, 2010; Lisonkova, Sheps, Janssen, et al., 2011).

Nursing Assessment

Nursing assessment of the pregnant woman over age 35 is the same as that for any pregnant woman. For a woman of this age, a preconception visit is important to identify chronic health problems that might affect the pregnancy and also to address lifestyle issues that may take time to modify. Encourage the older woman to plan for the pregnancy by seeing her health care provider before getting pregnant to discuss preexisting medical conditions, medications, and lifestyle choices. Assess the woman for risk factors such as cigarette smoking, poor nutrition, overweight or underweight, alcohol use, or illicit drug use.

A preconception visit also provides the opportunity to educate the woman about risk factors and provide information on how to modify her lifestyle habits to improve the pregnancy outcome. Assist the woman with lifestyle changes so that she can begin pregnancy in an optimal state of health. For example, if the woman is overweight, educate her about weight loss so that she can start the pregnancy at a healthy weight. If the woman smokes, encourage smoking cessation to reduce the effects of nicotine on herself and her fetus.

Prepare the woman for laboratory and diagnostic testing to establish a baseline for future comparisons. The risk for having a baby with Down syndrome increases with age, especially over age 35. Amniocentesis is routinely offered to all older women to allow the early detection of numerous chromosomal abnormalities, including Down syndrome. Additionally, a quadruple blood screen (alpha-fetoprotein, human chorionic gonadotropin, unconjugated estriol, and inhibin A [placental hormone]) drawn between 15 and 20 weeks of pregnancy can be helpful in screening for Down syndrome and neural tube defects.

Nursing Management

During routine prenatal visits, the nurse can play a key role in promoting a healthy pregnancy. Consider social, genetic, and environmental factors that are unique to the older pregnant women and prepare to address these factors when providing care. Although research has shown increases in preterm labour and births, low birth weight newborns, and operative interventions for older women, many carry their pregnancies to term without incident (Mahavarkar, Madhu, & Mule., 2008).

Assess the woman's knowledge about risk factors and measures to reduce them. Educate her about measures to promote a positive outcome. Encourage her to get early and regular prenatal care. Advise her to eat a variety of nutritious foods, especially fortified cereals, enriched grain products, and fresh fruits and vegetables and to drink at least six to eight glasses of water daily and take the prescribed vitamin containing 4 g of folic acid daily. Also stress the need for her to avoid alcohol intake during pregnancy, avoid exposure to secondhand smoke, and take no drugs unless they are prescribed. Provide continued surveillance of the mother and fetus throughout the pregnancy.

Women Who Are HIV Positive

Human immunodeficiency virus (HIV) is a retrovirus that is transmitted by blood and body fluids. The Joint United Nations Programme on HIV/AIDS (United Nations, 2010) estimates the number of people living with HIV infection worldwide is nearly 33.3 million, including approximately 16 million women of childbearing age and 2.5 million children, most of whom acquired HIV as a result of mother-to-child transmission. In Canada, the number of people living with HIV infection is estimated to be between 43,000 and 110,000 (Merson, O'Malley, Serwadda, et al., 2008).

Despite the revolutionary strides that have been made in treatment and detection and recent clinical advances and cautious optimism associated with combination therapies and vaccines, the number of individuals who are HIV positive continues to climb worldwide. Intensive efforts notwithstanding, there remains no real "cure" on the horizon (United Nations, 2010).

Historically, HIV/AIDS was associated with the male homosexual community and intravenous drug users, but the prevalence of HIV/AIDS is now increasing more rapidly among women than men. Women are the fastest-growing segment of persons becoming infected with HIV;

transmission in women occurs most frequently from sexual contact (75%) and from intravenous drug use (25%) (United Nations, 2010). Most women, a large number of whom are mothers, have acquired the disease through heterosexual contact. The risk for acquiring HIV through heterosexual contact is greater for women due to exposure to the higher viral concentration in semen. In addition, sexual intercourse may cause breaks in the vaginal lining, increasing the chances that the virus will enter the woman's body. Fifty percent of all the HIV/AIDS cases worldwide occur in women ages 25 to 44 years, and AIDS is the leading cause of death among black women in this age group (United Nations, 2010).

Pathophysiology

The three recognized modes of HIV transmission are unprotected sexual intercourse with an infected partner, contact with infected blood or blood products, and perinatal transmission.

> ▶ **Take** NOTE!
>
> *HIV is not transmitted by doorknobs, faucets, toilets, dirty dishes, mosquitoes, wet towels, coughing or sneezing, shaking hands, or being hugged or by any other indirect method.*

The virus attacks the T4 cells, decreases the CD4 cell count, and disables the immune system. The HIV condition can progress to a severe immunosuppressed state termed **acquired immunodeficiency syndrome (AIDS)**. AIDS is a progressive, debilitating disease that suppresses cellular immunity, predisposing the infected person to opportunistic infections and malignancies. The defining conditions of AIDS include opportunistic infections, primary neurologic disease, or malignancy (PHAC, 2008d). Eventually, death occurs. The time from infection with HIV to development of AIDS is a median of 11 years but varies depending on whether the patient is taking current anti-retroviral therapy (Mahy, Stover, Kiragu, et al., 2010). Research indicates that pregnancy does not accelerate the progression of HIV to AIDS or death (Kilmarx, 2009).

Once infected with HIV, the woman develops antibodies that can be detected with the enzyme-linked immunosorbent assay (ELISA) and confirmed with the Western blot test. Antibodies develop within 6 to 12 weeks after exposure, although this latent period is much longer in some women. Table 20.4 highlights the four stages of HIV infection.

Impact of HIV on Pregnancy

When a woman who is infected with HIV becomes pregnant, the risks to herself, her fetus, and the newborn are

TABLE 20.4 **STAGES OF HIV INFECTION**

Stages	Description	Clinical Picture
I	Acute infection	Early stage with pervasive viral production Flu-like symptoms 2–4 weeks after exposure Signs and symptoms: weight loss, low-grade fever, fatigue, sore throat, night sweats, and myalgia
II	Asymptomatic infection	Viral replication continues within lymphatics Usually free of symptoms; lymphadenopathy
III	Persistent generalized lymphadenopathy	Possibly remaining in this stage for years; AIDS develops in most within 7–10 years Opportunistic infections occur
IV	End-stage disease (AIDS)	Severe immune deficiency High viral load and low CD4 counts Signs and symptoms: bacterial, viral, or fungal opportunistic infections; fever; wasting syndrome; fatigue; neoplasms; and cognitive changes

Source: (PHAC, 2011a).

great. The risks are compounded by problems such as drug abuse, lack of access to prenatal care, poverty, poor nutrition, and high-risk behaviours such as unsafe sex practices and multiple sex partners, which can predispose the woman to additional STIs such as herpes, syphilis, or human papillomavirus (HPV). Additional risk factors to assess for include women who exchange sex for money or drugs or have sex partners who do, women whose past or present sex partners are or were HIV infected, and women who had a blood transfusion before 1985 (Do & Meekers, 2009). Pregnant women who are HIV positive are at risk for preterm delivery, premature rupture of membranes, intrapartum or postpartum hemorrhage, postpartum infection, poor wound healing, and genitourinary tract infections (United Nations, 2010).

Perinatal transmission of HIV (from the mother to the fetus or child) also can occur. However, the incidence of such cases has decreased in the past several years in developed countries, primarily due to the use of zidovudine therapy in pregnant women infected with HIV. This has not been the case in poor countries without similar resources. UNAIDS estimates that more than 370,000 new infections resulting from mother-to-child transmission occurred in 2009. This number is expected to increase rapidly as the prevalence of HIV rises in Southeast Asia (United Nations, 2010). Perinatal transmission rates are as high as 35% when there is no intervention (anti-retroviral therapy) and less than 5% when anti-retroviral treatment and appropriate care are available.

With perinatal transmission, approximately 25% to 50% of children manifest AIDS within the first year of life, and about 80% have clinical symptoms of the disease within 3 to 5 years (Williams, Keane-Tarchichi, Bettica, et al., 2009). Breastfeeding is a major contributing factor for mother-to-child transmission, and the infected mother must be informed about this. Infant feeding guidelines

recommend that HIV-positive mothers in high-income countries should avoid breastfeeding as the risk for HIV transmission to the child markedly outweighs the risks associated with replacement feeding (feeding of commercial infant formula or modified animal milk rather than breast milk) (WHO, 2010b). In low- and middle-income countries, recommendations on infant feeding differ from those in high-income countries as a result of limited resources (i.e., little access to health services, clean water and sanitation). The WHO recommends that in low- and middle-income countries, HIV-positive mothers should continue to breastfeed until the age of 12 months provided the HIV-positive mother or baby continues to receive anti-retroviral therapy (Slater et al., 2010; WHO, 2010b). Given the devastating effects of HIV infection on children, preventing its transmission is critical (Unicef, 2009).

In addition to perinatal transmission, the fetus and newborn also are at risk for prematurity, IUGR, low birth weight, and infection. Prompt treatment with anti-retroviral medications for the HIV-infected infant may slow the progression of the disease (Mirpuri & Jain, 2010).

Therapeutic Management

Women who are seropositive for HIV require counselling about the risk for perinatal transmission and the potential for obstetric complications. The risk for perinatal transmission directly correlates with the viral load (Betancourt, Abrams, McBain, et al., 2010). A discussion of the options on continuing the pregnancy, medication therapy, risks, perinatal outcomes, and treatment is warranted. Women who elect to continue with the pregnancy should be treated with anti-retroviral therapy regardless of their CD4 count or viral load.

Drug therapy is the mainstay of treatment for pregnant women infected with HIV. The standard treatment is oral anti-retroviral drugs given twice daily from 14 weeks' gestation until giving birth, intravenous administration during labour, and oral syrup for the newborn in the first 6 weeks of life (Mnyani & McIntyre, 2009). The goal of therapy is to reduce the viral load as much as possible, thereby reducing the risk for transmission to the fetus.

Decisions about the birthing method to be used are made on an individual basis based on several factors involving the woman's health. Some reports suggest that cesarean birth may reduce the risk for HIV infection (Buchanan & Cunningham, 2009). Efforts to reduce instrumentation, such as avoiding the use of an episiotomy, fetal scalp electrodes, and fetal scalp sampling, will reduce the newborn's exposure to bodily fluids.

With appropriate therapies, the prognosis for pregnant women with HIV infection has improved significantly. In addition, the newborns of women with HIV infection who have received treatment usually do not become infected. Unfortunately, therapy is complicated and medications are expensive. Moreover, the medications are associated with numerous adverse effects and possible toxic reactions. These therapies offer a dual purpose: reduce the likelihood of mother-to-infant transmission and provide optimal suppression of the viral load in the mother. The core goal of all medical therapy is to bring the client's viral load to an undetectable level, thus minimizing the risk for transmission to the fetus and newborn.

Nursing Assessment

Nursing assessment begins with a thorough history and physical examination. In addition, the woman is offered screening for HIV antibodies.

Health History and Physical Examination

Review the woman's history for risk factors, such as unsafe sex practices, multiple sex partners, and injectable drug use. Also have the woman complete a risk assessment survey. In addition, question the woman about any flu-like symptoms such as a low-grade fever, fatigue, sore throat, night sweats, diarrhea, cough, skin lesions, or muscle pain.

Perform a complete physical examination. Obtain the woman's weight and determine whether she has lost weight recently. Assess for signs and symptoms of STIs, such as vulvovaginal candidiasis, bacterial vaginosis, HSV, chancroid, CMV, or chlamydia because of the increased risk for STIs.

▶ *Take* NOTE!

Women who request an HIV test despite reporting no individual risk factors should be considered at risk, since many are not likely to disclose their high-risk behaviours.

Laboratory and Diagnostic Testing

The SOGC (2011b) recommends that all pregnant women be offered HIV antibody testing, regardless of their risk for infection, and that testing be done during the initial prenatal evaluation. Testing is essential because treatments are available that can reduce the likelihood of perinatal transmission and maintain the health of the woman (Giles, 2009).

▶ *Take* NOTE!

Screening only women who are identified as high risk based on their histories is inadequate due to the prolonged latency period that can exist after exposure. Also, research indicating that treatment with anti-retroviral agents could reduce vertical transmission from the infected mother to the newborn has dramatically increased the importance of HIV antibody screening in pregnancy.

Offer all women who are pregnant or planning a pregnancy HIV testing using ELISA. Prepare the woman with a reactive screening test for an additional test, such as the Western blot or an immunofluorescence assay. The Western blot is the confirmatory diagnostic test. A positive antibody test confirmed by a supplemental test indicates that the woman has been infected with HIV and can pass it on to others. HIV antibodies are detectable in at least 95% of women within 3 months after infection (Clark, Lampe, & Jamieson, 2008).

In addition to the usual screening tests done in normal pregnancy, additional testing for STIs may be necessary. Women infected with HIV have high rates of STIs, especially HPV, vulvovaginal candidiasis, bacterial vaginosis, syphilis, HSV, chancroid, CMV, gonorrhea, chlamydia, and hepatitis B (Gilbert, 2011).

Nursing Management

Women infected with HIV should receive comprehensive prenatal care, which starts with pretest and posttest counselling. In pretest counselling, the client completes a risk assessment survey and the nurse explains the meaning of positive versus negative test results, obtains informed consent for HIV testing, and educates the woman on how to prevent HIV infection by changing lifestyle behaviours if needed. Posttest counselling includes informing the client of the test results, reviewing the meaning of the results again, and reinforcing safer sex guidelines. All pretest and posttest counselling should be documented in the client's chart.

Educating the Client

Pregnant clients are dealing with many issues at their first prenatal visit. The confirmation of pregnancy may be accompanied by feelings of joy, anxiety, depression, or other emotions. Simultaneously, the client is given many pamphlets and receives advice and counselling about many important health issues (e.g., nutrition, prenatal development, appointment schedules). This health teaching may be done while the woman feels excited, tired, and anxious. To expect women to understand detailed explanations of a complex disease entity such as HIV/AIDS at this time may be unrealistic. Determine the client's readiness for this discussion.

Identify the client's individual needs for teaching, emotional support, and physical care. Approach education and counselling of HIV-positive pregnant women in a caring, sensitive manner. Address the following information:

- Infection control issues at home
- Safer sex precautions
- Stages of the HIV disease process and treatment for each stage
- Symptoms of opportunistic infections
- Preventive drug therapies for her unborn infant
- Avoidance of breastfeeding
- Referrals to community support, counselling, and financial aid
- Client's support system and potential caretaker
- Importance of continual prenatal care
- Need for a well-balanced diet
- Measures to reduce exposure to infections

Be knowledgeable about HIV infection and how HIV is transmitted and share this knowledge with all women. Nurses also can work to influence legislators, public health officials, and the entire health establishment toward policies to address the HIV epidemic. Research toward treatment and cure is tremendously important, but the major key to prevention of the spread of the virus is education. Nurses play a major role in this education.

Supporting the Client

Be aware of the psychosocial sequelae of HIV/AIDS. A diagnosis of HIV can put a woman into an emotional tailspin, where she is worried about her own health and that of her unborn infant. She may experience grief, fear, or anxiety about the future of her children. Along with the medications that are so important to her health maintenance, address the woman's mental health needs, family dynamics, capacity to work, and social concerns and provide appropriate support and guidance.

Be aware of your personal beliefs and attitudes toward women who are HIV positive or have AIDS. Incorporate this awareness in your actions as you help the woman face the reality of the diagnosis and treatment options. Empathy, understanding, caring, and assistance are key to helping the client and her family.

Preparing for Labour, Birth, and Afterward

Current evidence suggests that cesarean birth performed before the onset of labour and before the rupture of membranes significantly reduces the rate of perinatal transmission. The SOCG and UNAIDS recommend that HIV-positive women be offered elective cesarean birth to reduce the rate of transmission beyond that which may be achieved through anti-retroviral therapy (SOGC, 2011b; United Nations, 2010). They further suggest that operative births be performed at 38 weeks' gestation and that amniocentesis be avoided to prevent contamination of the amniotic fluid with maternal blood. Decisions concerning the method of delivery should be based on the woman's viral load, the duration of ruptured membranes, the progress of labour, and other pertinent clinical factors (Giles, 2009).

Prepare the woman physically and emotionally for the possibility of cesarean birth and assist as necessary. Ensure that she understands the rationale for the surgical birth.

After the birth of the newborn, the motivation for taking anti-retroviral medications may be lower, thus affecting the woman's compliance with therapy. Encourage the woman to continue therapy for her own sake as well as that of the newborn. Nurses can make a difference in helping women to adhere to their complex drug regimens.

Reinforce family planning methods during this time, incorporating a realistic view of the woman's disease status. The use of oral contraceptives with concurrent use of condoms is recommended. Advise the woman that breastfeeding is not recommended unless she is on anti-retroviral medications (United Nations, 2010). Instruct the HIV-positive woman in self-care measures, including the proper method for disposing of perineal pads to reduce the risk for exposing others to infected body fluids. Finally, teach the HIV-positive woman the signs and symptoms of infection in newborns and infants, encouraging her to report any to the health care provider.

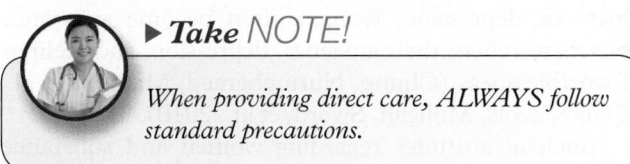

▶ *Take* NOTE!

When providing direct care, ALWAYS follow standard precautions.

The Pregnant Woman with Substance Abuse

Perinatal drug abuse is the use of alcohol and other drugs by pregnant women. The incidence of substance abuse during pregnancy is highly variable because most pregnant women are reluctant to reveal the extent of their use. Illicit drugs include alcohol, cigarettes, cocaine, marijuana, heroin, and psychotherapeutic drugs that were not prescribed by a health care professional (Scott & Lust, 2010).

Impact of Substance Abuse on Pregnancy

The use of drugs, legal or not, increases the risk for medical complications in the mother and poor birth outcomes in the newborn. The placenta acts as an active transport mechanism, not as a barrier, and substances pass from a mother to her fetus through the placenta. Thus, both the fetus and the mother experience substance use, abuse, and addiction. Additionally, fetal vulnerability to drugs is much greater because the fetus has not developed the enzymatic system needed to metabolize drugs (Gareri, Brieni, Reynolds, et al., 2009).

A woman who claims to have taken no drugs while pregnant may be unaware that substances such as hair dye, diet cola, paint, or over-the-counter (OTC) medications for colds or headaches are considered drugs. Thus, it is very difficult to get a true picture of the real use of drugs by pregnant women.

Many drugs are considered to have a teratogenic effect on growing fetuses. A **teratogen** is any environmental substance that can cause physical defects in the developing embryo and fetus. Pregnant women with substance abuse commonly present with polysubstance abuse, which is likely to be more damaging than the use of any single substance. Thus, it is inherently difficult to ascribe a specific perinatal effect to any one substance (Rubio et al., 2008).

Effects of Addiction

Addiction is a multifaceted process that is affected by environmental, psychological, family, and physical factors. Women who use drugs, alcohol, or tobacco come from all socioeconomic backgrounds, cultures, and lifestyles. Factors associated with substance abuse during a pregnancy may include low self-esteem, inadequate support systems, low self-expectations, high levels of anxiety, socioeconomic barriers, involvement in abusive relationships, chaotic familial and social systems, and a history of psychiatric illness or depression. Women often become substance abusers to relieve their anxieties, depression, and feelings of worthlessness (Chung, Nurmohamed, Mathew, et al., 2010; Niccols, Milligan, Sword, et al., 2010).

Societal attitudes regarding women and substance abuse may prohibit them from admitting the problem and seeking treatment. Society sanctions women for failing to live up to expectations of how a pregnant woman "should" behave, thereby possibly driving them further away from the treatment they so desperately need. For many reasons, pregnant women who abuse substances feel unwelcome in prenatal clinics or medical settings. Often they seek prenatal care late or not at all. They may fear being shamed or reported to legal or child protection authorities. A non-judgmental atmosphere and unbiased teaching to all pregnant women regardless of their life-style is crucial. A caring, concerned manner is critical to help these women feel safe and respond honestly to assessment questions.

Pregnancy can be a motivator for some who want to try treatment. The goal of therapy is to help the client deal with pregnancy by developing a trusting relationship. Providing a full spectrum of medical, social, and emotional care is needed.

Effects of Commonly Abused Substances

Substance abuse during pregnancy, particularly in the first trimester, has a negative effect on the health of the mother and the growth and development of the fetus. The fetus experiences the same systemic effects as the mother, but often more severely. The fetus cannot metabolize drugs as efficiently as the expectant mother and will experience the effects long after the drugs have left the women's system. Substance abuse during pregnancy is associated with preterm labour, abortion, IUGR, abruptio placentae, low birth weight, neurobehavioural abnormalities, and long-term childhood developmental consequences (Thompson, Levitt, & Stanwood, 2009; Walton-Moss, McIntosh, Conrad, et al., 2009). Table 20.5 summarizes the effects of selected drugs during pregnancy.

Alcohol

Alcohol abuse is a major public health issue in Canada. Alcohol is a teratogen, a substance known to be toxic to human development. Approximately 10.5% of pregnant women report alcohol consumption (Carson, Vitale Cox, Crane, et al., 2010). Theoretically, no mother would give a glass of wine, beer, or hard liquor to her newborn, but when she drinks, her embryo or fetus is exposed to the same blood alcohol concentration as she is. The teratogenic effects of heavy maternal drinking have been recognized since 1973, when fetal alcohol syndrome was first described. Fetal alcohol syndrome is now classified under the broader term of **fetal alcohol spectrum disorder (FASD)**; this disorder includes the full range of birth defects, such as structural anomalies and behavioural and neurocognitive disabilities caused by prenatal exposure to alcohol (Carson et al., 2010). With an average incidence in Canada of 10 cases per 1,000 live births, FASD is estimated to affect approximately 1% of the population. Some communities report incidence rates of 190 per 1,000 live births (Carson et al., 2010). More than 3,000 Canadian babies each year are born with FASD, and approximately 300,000 people are currently living with it. The occurrence of FASD is significantly greater in Aboriginal populations and in rural, remote, and northern communities (Health Canada, 2006). FASD is the leading cause of mental retardation (Carson et al., 2010).

Not every woman who drinks during pregnancy will give birth to an affected child. Based on the best research

TABLE 20.5 EFFECTS OF SELECTED DRUGS ON PREGNANCY

Substance	Effect on Pregnancy
Alcohol	Spontaneous abortion, inadequate weight gain, IUGR, fetal alcohol spectrum disorder; the leading cause of mental retardation
Caffeine	Vasoconstriction and mild diuresis in mother, fetal stimulation; but teratogenic effects not documented via research
Nicotine	Vasoconstriction, reduced uteroplacental blood flow, decreased birth weight, abortion, prematurity, abruptio placentae, fetal demise
Cocaine	Vasoconstriction, gestational hypertension, abruptio placentae, abortion, "snow baby syndrome," CNS defects, IUGR
Marijuana	Anemia, inadequate weight gain, "amotivational syndrome," hyperactive startle reflex, newborn tremors, prematurity, IUGR
Narcotics	Maternal and fetal withdrawal, abruptio placentae, preterm labour, premature rupture of membranes, perinatal asphyxia, newborn sepsis and death, intellectual impairment, malnutrition
Sedatives	CNS depression, newborn withdrawal, maternal seizures in labour, newborn abstinence syndrome, delayed lung maturity

Source: Gilbert, E. S. (2011). *Manual of high risk pregnancy & delivery* (5th ed.). St. Louis, MO: Mosby Elsevier.

available, the following is known about alcohol consumption during pregnancy:

- Intake increases the risk for alcohol-related birth defects, including growth deficiencies, facial abnormalities, CNS impairment, behavioural disorders, and intellectual development.
- No amount of alcohol consumption is considered safe during pregnancy.
- Damage to the fetus can occur at any stage of pregnancy, even before a woman knows she is pregnant.
- Cognitive defects and behavioural problems resulting from prenatal exposure are lifelong.
- Alcohol-related birth defects are completely preventable (Carson et al., 2010).

Risk factors for giving birth to an alcohol-affected newborn include maternal age, socioeconomic status, ethnicity, genetic factors, poor nutrition, depression, family disorganization, unplanned pregnancy, and late

BOX 20.5 **Common Cognitive and Behavioural Problems Associated with FASD**

- Attention-deficit/hyperactivity disorder (ADHD)
- Inability to foresee consequences
- Inability to learn from previous experience
- Lack of organization
- Learning difficulties
- Poor abstract thinking
- Poor impulse control
- Speech and language problems
- Poor judgment

prenatal care (Carson et al., 2010). Identification of risk factors strongly associated with alcohol-related birth outcomes could help identify high-risk pregnancies requiring intervention.

Characteristics of FASD include craniofacial dysmorphia (thin upper lip, small head circumference, and small eyes), IUGR, microcephaly, and congenital anomalies such as skeletal abnormalities and cardiac defects. Long-term sequelae include postnatal growth restriction, attention deficits, delayed reaction time, and poor scholastic performance (Nodine et al., 2011). The complex neurobehavioural problems typically manifest themselves insidiously. Children with prenatal alcohol exposure struggle with cognitive, academic, social, emotional, and behavioural challenges. These challenges reduce the child's ability to learn and function successfully in many structured environments (Greenbaum, Stevens, Nash, et al., 2009). Common cognitive and behavioural problems are listed in Box 20.5, and Figure 20.5 illustrates the characteristic facial features. See Chapter 24 for a more detailed discussion of the newborn with FASD.

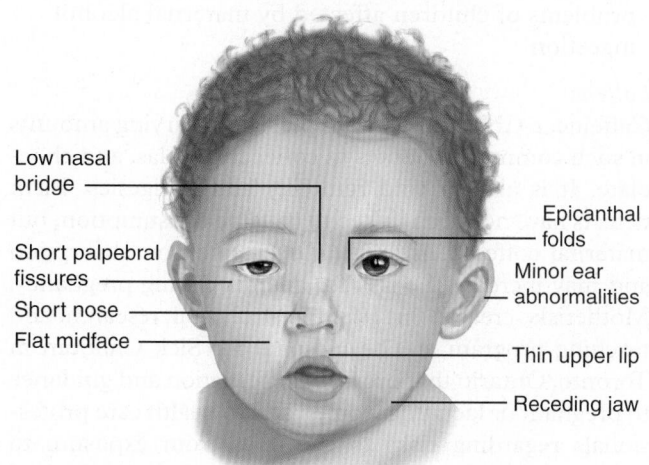

FIGURE 20.5 Typical facial characteristics of a newborn with FASD.

One of the biggest challenges in determining the true prevalence of FASD is how to recognize the syndrome, which depends in part on the age and physical features of the person being assessed. Difficulty in identifying alcohol abuse is due to the client's denial of alcohol use, unwillingness to report alcohol consumption, under-reporting, and limited ability to recollect the frequency, quantity, and type of alcohol consumed. This makes it difficult to identify women who are drinking during pregnancy, institute preventive measures, or refer them for treatment.

Women who drink excessively while pregnant are at high risk for giving birth to children with birth defects. To prevent these defects, women should stop drinking during all phases of a pregnancy. Unfortunately, many women continue to drink during their pregnancy despite warnings from professionals.

Currently, it is not known whether there is a minimum amount of alcohol that is safe to drink during pregnancy; an occasional glass of wine might be harmless or might not be. Therefore, eliminating alcohol consumption during pregnancy is the ultimate goal to prevent FASD. Most women know they shouldn't drink during pregnancy, but the "window of vulnerability"—the time lag between conception and the discovery of pregnancy—may put substantial numbers of children at risk. Additionally, traditional alcohol-screening questionnaires, such as the Michigan Alcoholism Screening Test (MAST) and the CAGE Questionnaire, are not sensitive enough to detect low levels of alcohol consumption among women.

Several challenges remain in preventing birth defects due to alcohol consumption:

- Ways to improve clinical recognition of high-risk women who drink alcohol
- Ways to intervene more effectively to modify drinking behaviours
- In utero approaches to prevent or minimize fetal injury
- Strategies to address the neurodevelopmental problems of children affected by maternal alcohol ingestion

Caffeine

Caffeine, a CNS stimulant, is present in varying amounts in such common products as coffee, tea, colas, and chocolate. It is also in cold remedies and analgesics. Birth defects have not been linked to caffeine consumption, but maternal coffee consumption decreases iron absorption and may increase the risk for anemia during pregnancy. Motherisk, created in 1985, is a clinical research and teaching program at The Hospital for Sick Children in Toronto, Ontario that provides information and guidance to pregnant or lactating women and to health care professionals regarding risks to the fetus from exposure to drugs, chemicals, diseases, radiation and environmental agents. Motherisk recommends that pregnant women eliminate or limit their consumption of caffeine to less than 150 mg/day, or the equivalent of 1½ cups of coffee or cola (Anderson, Juliano, & Schulkin, 2009).

Nicotine

Nicotine, found in cigarettes, is another substance that is harmful to the pregnant woman and her fetus. Nicotine, which causes vasoconstriction, transfers across the placenta and reduces blood flow to the fetus, contributing to fetal hypoxia. When compared with alcohol, marijuana, and other illicit drug use, tobacco use is less likely to decline as the pregnancy progresses (Crawford, Tolosa, & Goldenberg, 2008; Varvarigou, Fouzas, & Beratis, 2010). Smoking is associated with adverse pregnancy outcomes. However, these adverse outcomes can be avoided if the woman stops smoking before becoming pregnant.

Smoking increases the risk for spontaneous abortion, preterm labour and birth, maternal hypertension, placenta previa, and abruptio placentae. The perinatal death rate among infants of smoking mothers is 20% to 35% higher than among infants of nonsmoking mothers (Aliyu, Lynch, Saidu, et al, 2010).

Smoking has also been considered an important risk factor for low birth weight, sudden infant death syndrome (SIDS), and cognitive deficits, especially in language, reading, and vocabulary, as well as poorer performances on tests of reasoning and memory. Researchers have also reported behaviour problems, such as increased activity, inattention, impulsivity, opposition, and aggression (Blood-Siegfried & Rende, 2010).

Women who smoke during the pregnancy also continue to smoke after giving birth, and thus the infant will be exposed to nicotine after birth. This environmental or passive exposure affects the child's development and increases the risk for childhood respiratory disorders.

Cocaine

Cocaine use is second only to marijuana use in women who abuse illicit drugs during pregnancy. The incidence of cocaine exposure in utero is reported to be 0.3% to 9.5% (Bhuvaneswar, Chang, Epstein, et al., 2008).

Cocaine is a psychoactive drug derived from the leaves of the coca plant, which grows in the Andes Mountains of Peru, Ecuador, and Bolivia. The freebase form, called "crack" because of the cracking or popping noise made in its preparation, is less expensive, easily made, and smokable. Cocaine is a powerful vasoconstrictor. When sniffed into the mucous membranes of the nose, it produces an intense "rush" that some have compared to an orgasmic experience. Smoked crack is absorbed rapidly by the pulmonary vasculature and reaches the brain's circulation in 6 to 8 seconds (Canadian Centre on Substance Abuse [CCSA], 2012).

Cocaine use produces vasoconstriction, tachycardia, and hypertension in both the mother and the fetus (Hull, May, Farrell-Moore, et al., 2010). Uteroplacental insufficiency may result from reduced blood flow and placental perfusion. Chronic use can result in low birth weight, the most common effect of cocaine use in pregnancy (Malek, Obrist, Wenzinger, et al., 2009).

Studies suggest that perinatal cocaine use increases the risk for preterm labour, abortion, abruptio placentae, IUGR, intrauterine fetal distress and demise, seizures, withdrawal, and cerebral infarcts. Cocaine may increase the risk for uterine rupture and congenital anomalies (Weiner & Finnegan, 2011). Fetal anomalies associated with cocaine use in early pregnancy involve neurologic problems such as neural tube defects and microcephaly; cardiovascular anomalies such as congenital heart defects; genitourinary conditions such as prune belly syndrome, hydronephrosis, and ambiguous genitalia; and gastrointestinal system problems such as necrotizing enterocolitis (Weiner & Finnegan, 2011). Some infants exposed to cocaine in utero show increased irritability and are difficult to calm and soothe to sleep (Schuetze, Eiden, & Edwards, 2009).

Marijuana

Marijuana is the most commonly used illicit drug in Canada. According to the 2008 Canadian Alcohol and Drug Use Monitoring Study (CADUMS), 11.4% of Canadians 15 years of age and older reported using cannabis (CCSA, 2012). It is often called pot, reefer, herb, widow, hash, grass, weed, Mary Jane, or MJ (Leslie, 2008). Marijuana is a preparation of the leaves and flowering tops of *Cannabis sativa*, the hemp plant, which contains a number of pharmacologically active agents. Tetrahydrocannabinol (THC) is the most active ingredient of marijuana. With heavy smoking, THC narrows the bronchi and bronchioles and produces inflammation of the mucous membranes. Smoking marijuana causes tachycardia and a reduction in blood pressure, resulting in orthostatic hypotension.

The effects of marijuana smoking on pregnancy are not yet fully understood because there are very few studies on its long-term effects on child development. One can speculate that the effects of marijuana on the immature nervous system may be subtle and not detected until more complex functions are required, usually in a formal educational setting. There is some evidence that marijuana increases the risk for spontaneous abortion and preterm delivery (Weiner & Finnegan, 2011). Although marijuana is not considered teratogenic, many newborns display altered responses to visual stimuli, increased tremulousness, and a high-pitched cry, which might indicate CNS insults (van Gelder, Reefhuis, Caton, et al., 2010). A strong correlation exists between the use of marijuana and the use of alcohol and cigarettes.

Opiates and Narcotics

Opiates and narcotics include opium, heroin (known as horse, junk, smack, downtown), morphine, codeine, hydromorphone (Dilaudid, little D), oxycodone (Percodan, perkies), meperidine (Demerol, demise), and methadone (meth, dollies). These drugs are CNS depressants that soothe and lull. They may be used medically for pain, but all have a high potential for abuse. Most cause an intense addiction in both mother and newborn.

Narcotic dependence is particularly problematic in pregnant women. It leads to medical, nutritional, and social neglect by the woman due to the long-term risks of physical dependence, malnutrition, compromised immunity, hepatitis, and fatal overdose (Kumar, 2009). Taking opiates or narcotics during pregnancy places the woman at increased risk for preterm labour, IUGR, and preeclampsia (Malek et al., 2009).

Heroin is the most common illicitly used opioid. It is derived from the seeds of the poppy plant and can be sniffed, smoked, or injected. It crosses the placenta via simple diffusion within 1 hour of maternal consumption (CCSA, 2012). Use of heroin during pregnancy is believed to affect the developing brain of the fetus and may cause behavioural abnormalities in childhood (Weiner & Finnegan, 2011).

The most common harmful effect of heroin and other narcotics on newborns is withdrawal, or **neonatal abstinence syndrome** (see Chapter 24). This collection of symptoms may include irritability, hypertonicity, a high-pitched cry, vomiting, diarrhea, respiratory distress, disturbed sleeping, sneezing, diaphoresis, fever, poor sucking, tremors, and seizures (Lall, 2008; Murphy-Oikonen, Montelpare, Southon, et al., 2010).

Withdrawal from opiates during pregnancy is extremely dangerous for the fetus, so a prescribed oral methadone maintenance program combined with psychotherapy is recommended for the pregnant woman. This closely supervised treatment program reduces withdrawal symptoms in the newborn, reduces drug cravings, and blocks the euphoric effects of narcotic drugs in order to reduce illicit drug use. Methadone maintenance provides a steady state of opiate levels, thus reducing the risk for withdrawal to the fetus and exposure to HIV and other STIs because the mother is no longer injecting drugs. However, methadone has the same withdrawal consequences for women and newborns as heroin does (Keegan, Parva, Finnegan, et al., 2010).

Sedatives

Sedatives relax the CNS and are used medically for inducing relaxation and sleep, relieving tension, and treating seizures. Sedatives easily cross the placenta and can cause birth defects and behavioural problems. Infants born to mothers who abuse sedatives during pregnancy may be physically dependent on the drugs themselves and are more prone to respiratory problems, feeding difficulties, disturbed sleep, sweating, irritability, and fever (Howland, 2009; Wang, 2012).

Methamphetamines

Methamphetamine use among pregnant women has increased rapidly in North America (Wang, 2012). This highly addictive stimulant is commonly known as speed, meth, crystal, jib, crank, ice, or chalk. In its smoked form, it is often referred to as ice, crystal, crank, and glass. It is a white, odourless, bitter-tasting powder that was developed from its parent drug, amphetamine, and was used originally in nasal decongestants and bronchial inhalers. The maternal effects include increased energy and alertness, an intense rush, decreased appetite, tachycardia, and tachypnea. Chronic use can lead to psychosis, including paranoia, hallucinations, memory loss, and aggressive or violent behaviour (Buxton & Dove, 2008). Few studies have been done on the effects of methamphetamine abuse during pregnancy, but the few done indicate an increased risk for preterm births, placental abruption, IUGR, and congenital anomalies (Wang, 2012; Weiner & Finnegan, 2011). These findings are hard to interpret, however, due to small sample size and polydrug use of the participants.

Nursing Assessment

Complete a thorough history and physical examination to evaluate a client for substance use and abuse. Substance abuse screening in pregnancy is done to detect the use of any substance known or suspected to exert a deleterious effect on the client or her fetus. Routinely ask about substance abuse with all women of childbearing age, inform them of the risks involved, and advise them against continuing. Screening questionnaires are helpful in identifying potential users, may reduce the stigma of asking clients about substance abuse, and result in a more accurate and consistent evaluation. The questions in Box 20.6 may be helpful in assessing a client who is at risk for substance abuse during pregnancy. Using "accepting" terminology may encourage the woman to give honest answers without fear of reproach.

A urine toxicology screen may also be helpful in determining drug use, although a urine screen identifies only recent or heavy use of drugs. The length of time a drug is present in urine is as follows:

- Cocaine: 24 to 48 hours in an adult, 72 to 96 hours in an infant
- Heroin: 24 hours in an adult, 24 to 48 hours in an infant
- Marijuana: 1 week to 1 month in an adult, up to a month or longer in an infant
- Methadone: up to 10 days in an adult and an infant (Wang, 2012)

Nursing Management

If the woman's drug screen is positive, use this as an opportunity to discuss prenatal exposure to substances that may be harmful. The discussion may lead the nurse to refer the client for a diagnostic assessment or identify an intervention such as counselling that may be helpful. Being non-judgmental is a key to success; a client is more apt to trust and reveal patterns of abuse if the nurse does not judge her and her lifestyle choices.

> ### BOX 20.6 Sample Questions for Assessing Substance Use
>
> - Have you ever used recreational drugs? If so, when and what?
> - Have you ever taken a prescription drug other than as intended?
> - What are your feelings about drug use during pregnancy?
> - How often do you smoke cigarettes? How many per day?
> - How often do you drink alcohol?
>
> If the assessment reveals substance use, obtain additional information by using the RAFFT questions, which are a sensitive screening instrument for identifying substance abuse (Weekes & Lee, 2006):
>
> **R:** Do you drink or take drugs to **R**elax, improve your self-image, or fit in?
> **A:** Do you ever drink or take drugs while **A**lone?
> **F:** Do you have any close **F**riends who drink or take drugs?
> **F:** Does a close **F**amily member have a problem with alcohol or drugs?
> **T:** Have you ever gotten in **T**rouble from drinking or taking drugs?

A positive drug screen in a newborn warrants an investigation by the provincial child protection agency. In the interim, institute measures to reduce stress and stimuli to promote the newborn's comfort (see Chapter 24 for a more in-depth discussion).

Be proactive, supportive, and accepting when caring for the client. Assure women with substance abuse problems that sharing information of a confidential nature with health care providers will not render them liable to criminal prosecution. Provide counselling and education, emphasizing the following:

- Effects of substance exposure on the fetus
- Interventions to improve mother–child attachment and improve parenting
- Psychosocial support if treatment is needed to reduce substance abuse
- Referral to outreach programs to improve access to treatment facilities
- Hazardous legal substances to avoid during pregnancy
- Follow-up of children born to substance-dependent mothers
- Dietary counselling to improve the pregnancy outcome for both mother and child
- Drug screening to identify all drugs a client is using
- More frequent prenatal visits to monitor fetal well-being
- Maternal and fetal benefits of remaining drug-free

• Cultural sensitivity
• Coping skills, support systems, and vocational assistance

Substance abuse is a complex problem that requires sensitivity to each woman's unique situation and contributing factors. Be sure to address individual psychological and sociocultural factors to help the woman to regain control of her life. Treatment must combine different approaches and provide ongoing support for women learning to live drug-free. Developing personal strengths, such as communication skills and assertiveness, and self-confidence will help the woman in resisting the drug use. Encourage the use of appropriate coping skills. Enhancing self-esteem also helps provides a foundation to avoid drugs.

■■■ Key Concepts

■ Preconception counselling for the woman with diabetes is helpful in promoting blood glucose control to prevent congenital anomalies.

■ The classification system for diabetes commonly used is based on disease etiology and not pharmacologic management; the classification includes type 1 diabetes, type 2 diabetes, gestational diabetes, and **impaired fasting glucose** and **impaired glucose tolerance**.

■ A functional classification for heart disease during pregnancy is based on past and present disability: class I, asymptomatic with no limitation of physical activity; class II, symptomatic (dyspnea, chest pain) with increased activity; class III, symptomatic (fatigue, palpitation) with normal activity; and class IV, symptomatic at rest or with any physical activity.

■ Chronic hypertension exists when the woman has a blood pressure of 140/90 mm Hg or higher before pregnancy or before the 20th week of gestation or when hypertension persists for more than 12 weeks postpartum.

■ Successful management of asthma in pregnancy involves elimination of environmental triggers, drug therapy, and client education.

■ Ideally, women with hematologic conditions are screened before conception and are made aware of the risks to themselves and to a pregnancy.

■ A wide variety of infections, such as rubella, herpes simplex, hepatitis B, varicella, parvovirus B19, and many STIs can affect the pregnancy, having a negative impact on its outcome.

■ The younger the adolescent is at the time of the first pregnancy, the more likely it is that she will have another pregnancy during her teens. About 1 million teenagers between the ages of 15 and 19 become pregnant each year; about half give birth and keep their infants.

■ The nurse's role in caring for the pregnant adolescent is to assist her in identifying the options for this pregnancy, including abortion, self-parenting of the child, temporary foster care for the baby or herself, or placement for adoption.

■ The prevalence of HIV/AIDS is increasing more rapidly among women than men: half of all HIV/AIDS cases worldwide now occur in women. There are only three recognized modes of HIV transmission: unprotected sexual intercourse with an infected partner, contact with infected blood or blood products, and perinatal transmission. Breastfeeding is a major contributing factor in mother-to-child transmission of HIV.

■ Cases of perinatal AIDS have decreased in the past several years in Canada, primarily because of the use of zidovudine therapy in pregnant women with HIV. SOGC and UNAIDS recommend that all pregnant women should be offered HIV antibody testing regardless of their risk for infection, and that testing should be done during the initial prenatal evaluation.

■ Pregnant women with substance abuse problems commonly abuse several substances, making it difficult to ascribe a specific perinatal effect to any one substance. Societal attitudes regarding pregnant women and substance abuse may prohibit them from admitting the problem and seeking treatment.

■ Substance abuse during pregnancy is associated with preterm labour, abortion, low birth weight, CNS and fetal anomalies, and long-term childhood developmental consequences.

■ Fetal alcohol spectrum disorder is a lifelong yet completely preventable set of physical, mental, and neurobehavioural birth defects; it is the leading cause of mental retardation in Canada.

■ Nursing management for the woman with substance abuse focuses on screening and preventing substance abuse to reduce the high incidence of obstetric and medical complications as well as the morbidity and mortality among passively addicted newborns.

REFERENCES

Adams, E. K., Gavin, N. I., Femi Ayadi, M., Santelli, J., & Raskind-Hood, C. (2009). The costs of public services for teenage mothers post-welfare reform: A ten-state study. *Journal of Health Care Finance, 35*(3), 44–58.

Al Shami, H., Kadasne, A., Khalfan, M., Iqbal, S., & Mirghani, H. (2011). Pregnancy outcome in late maternal age in a high-income developing country. *Archives of Gynecology and Obstetrics, 284,* 1113–1116.

Aliyu, M. H., Lynch, O., Saidu, R., Alio, A. P., Marty, P. J., & Salihu, H. M. (2010). Intrauterine exposure to tobacco and risk of medically indicated and spontaneous preterm birth. *American Journal of Perinatology, 27*(5), 405–410. doi:10.1055/s-0029-1243316

Anderson, B. L., Juliano, L. M., & Schulkin, J. (2009). Caffeine's implications for women's health and survey of obstetrician-gynecologists' caffeine knowledge and assessment practices. *Journal of Women's Health, 18*(9), 1457–1466.

Anzivino, E., Fioriti, D., Mischitelli, M., et al. (2009). Herpes simplex virus infection in pregnancy and in neonate: Status of art of epidemiology, diagnosis, therapy and prevention. *Virology Journal, 6,* 1–11. doi:10.1186/1743-422X-6-40

Aruda, M. M., Waddicor, K., Frese, L., Cole, J., & Burke, P. (2010). Early pregnancy in adolescents: Diagnosis, assessment, options counseling, and referral. *Journal of Pediatric Healthcare, 24*(1), 4–13. doi:10.1016/j.pedhc.2008.11.003

Association of Women's Health, Obstetric and Neonatal Nurses. (2008). *HPV counseling: A clinician resource.* Washington, DC: Author.

Bajoria, R., & Chatterjee, R. (2009). Current perspectives of fertility and pregnancy in thalassemia. *Hemoglobin, 33,* S131–S135. doi:10.3109/03630260903365023

Baker, P. N., Wheeler, S. J., Sanders, T. A., et al. (2009). A prospective study of micronutrient status in adolescent pregnancy. *The American Journal of Clinical Nutrition, 89*(4), 1114–1124.

Balani, J., Hyer, S. L., Rodin, D. A., & Shehata, H. (2009). Pregnancy outcomes in women with gestational diabetes treated with metformin or insulin: A case-control study. *Diabetic Medicine, 26*(8), 798–802.

Barclay, L. (2009). New guidelines for asthma management. *American Journal of Respiratory Critical Care Medicine, 180,* 59–99.

Beigi, R. H., Wiesenfeld, H. C., Landers, D. V., & Simhan, H. N. (2008). High rate of severe fetal outcomes associated with maternal parvovirus B19 infection in pregnancy. *Infectious Diseases in Obstetrics & Gynecology, 2008,* 1–4. doi:10.1155/2008/524601

Benninger, C., & McCallister, J. (2010). Asthma in pregnancy: Reading between the lines. *The Nurse Practitioner, 35*(4), 10–19.

Betancourt, T. S., Abrams, E. J., McBain, R., & Fawzi, M. C. S. (2010). Family-centred approaches to the prevention of mother to child transmission of HIV. *Journal of the International AIDS Society, 13*(Suppl 2), S2–S2.

Bhuvaneswar, M. D., Chang, G., Epstein, L. A., & Stern, T. A. (2008). *Cocaine and opioid use during pregnancy: Prevalence and management.* Retrieved May 29, 2012 from http://www.ncbi.nlm.nih.gov/pmc/articles/PMC2249829/

Blaho, J. A. (2010). Human cytomegalovirus infection in pregnant women and neonates: A new risk factor for cardiovascular disease? *Archives of Clinical Microbiology, 1*(1), 1–3.

Blanchard, D., & Shabetai, R. (2009). Cardiac diseases. In R. Creasy, R. Resnik, J. Iams, C. Lockwood, & T. Moore (Eds.), *Creasy and Resnik's maternal-fetal medicine: principles and practices* (6th ed.). Philadelphia: Saunders.

Blood-Siegfried, J., & Rende, E. K. (2010). The long-term effects of prenatal nicotine exposure on neurologic development. *Journal of Midwifery & Women's Health, 55*(2), 143–152. doi:10.1016/j.jmwh.2009.05.006

Briggs, M. M., Hopman, W. M., & Jamieson, M. A. (2007). Comparing pregnancy in adolescents and adults: Obstetric outcomes and prevalence of anemia. *Journal of Obstetrics & Gynecology Canada, 29*(7), 546–555.

Boinpally, T., & Jovanovic, L. (2009). Management of type 2 diabetes and gestational diabetes in pregnancy. *The Mount Sinai Journal of Medicine, New York, 76*(3), 269–280.

Buchanan, A. M., & Cunningham, C. K. (2009). Advances and failures in preventing perinatal human immunodeficiency virus infection. *Clinical Microbiology Reviews, 22*(3), 493–507.

Burt, C. C., & Durbridge, J. (2009). Management of cardiac disease in pregnancy. *Continuing Education in Anaesthesia, Critical Care & Pain, 9*(2), 44–47.

Buxton, J. A., & Dove, N. A. (2008). The burden and management of crystal meth use. *Canadian Medical Association Journal, 178*(12), 1537–1539.

Canadian Cardiovascular Society. (1976). *Functional classification of angina pectoris.* Retrieved February 13, 2012 from http://www.ccs.ca/position_statements/index_e.aspx

Canadian Centre for Occupational Health and Safety. (2011). *Toxoplasmosis.* Retrieved February 13, 2012 from http://www.ccohs.ca/oshanswers/diseases/toxoplasmosis.html

Canadian Centre on Substance Abuse. (2012). *General health and addiction statistics.* Retrieved February 13, 2012 from http://www.ccsa.ca/Eng/Statistics/Canada/GHAS/Pages/default.aspx

Canadian Diabetes Association. (2008). Canadian Diabetes Association 2008 clinical practice guidelines for the prevention and management of diabetes in Canada. *Canadian Journal of Diabetes, 32*(Suppl 1), S1–S201.

Canadian Diabetes Association. (2009). *An economic tsunami: The cost of diabetes in Canada.* Retrieved February 13, 2012 from http://www.diabetes.ca/documents/get-involved/FINAL_Economic_Report.pdf

Canadian Lung Association. (2011a). *Pregnancy & asthma.* Retrieved February 13, 2012 from http://www.lung.ca/diseases-maladies/asthma-asthme/pregnancy-grossesse/index_e.php

Canadian Lung Association. (2011b). *Tuberculosis.* Retrieved February 13, 2012 from http://www.lung.ca/diseases-maladies/tuberculosis-tuberculose_e.php

Canadian Paediatric Society. (2007). Rubella (German measles) in pregnancy. *Paediatrics & Child Health, 12*(9), 798. Retrieved February 13, 2012 from http://www.ncbi.nlm.nih.gov/pmc/articles/PMC2532864/

Carson, G., Vitale Cox, L., Crane, J., et al. (2010). SOGC clinical practice guideline: Alcohol use and pregnancy consensus clinical guidelines. *Journal of Obstetrics and Gynaecology Canada, 32*(8 Suppl 3), S1–S31. Retrieved February 13, 2012 from http://www.sogc.org/guidelines/documents/gui245CPG1008E.pdf

Caton, A. R., Bell, E. M., Druschel, C. M., et al. (2009). Antihypertensive medication use during pregnancy and the risk of cardiovascular malformations. *Hypertension, 54*(1), 63–70.

Chapman, K. R. (2008). Asthma in Canada: Missing the treatment targets. *Canadian Medical Association Journal, 178*(8), 1027–1028.

Chedraui, P. (2008). Pregnancy among young adolescents: Trends, risk factors and maternal-perinatal outcome. *Journal of Perinatal Medicine, 36*(3), 256–259. doi:10.1515/JPM.2008.047

Cheng, Y. W., & Caughey, A. B. (2008). Gestational diabetes: Diagnosis and management. *Journal of Perinatology 28*(10), 657–664.

Cheung, N. W. (2009). The management of gestational diabetes. *Vascular Health and Risk Management, 5,* 153–164. Retrieved February 13, 2012 from http://www.ncbi.nlm.nih.gov/pmc/articles/PMC2672462/

Chung, E. K., Nurmohamed, L., Mathew, L., Elo, I. T., Coyne, J. C., & Culhane, J. F. (2010). Risky health behaviors among mothers-to-be: The impact of adverse childhood experiences. *Academic Pediatrics, 10*(4), 245–251.

Clark, J., Lampe, M. A., & Jamieson, D. J. (2008). Testing women for human immunodeficiency virus infection: Who, when, and how? *Clinical Obstetrics and Gynecology, 51*(3), 507–517.

Clift-Matthews, V. (2010). Flexible care for pregnant teenagers. *British Journal of Midwifery, 18*(10), 616–616.

Crane, J., Armson, A., de la Ronde, S., et al. (2002). SOGC clinical practice guideline: Parvovirus B19 infection in pregnancy. *Journal of Obstetrics and Gynaecology Canada, 119,* 1–8. Retrieved February 12, 2012 from http://www.sogc.org/guidelines/public/119e-cpg-september2002.pdf

Crawford, J. T., Tolosa, J. E., & Goldenberg, R. L. (2008). Smoking cessation in pregnancy: Why, how, and what next? *Clinical Obstetrics and Gynecology, 51*(2), 419–435.

Daley, A. J., Thorpe, S., & Garland, S. M. (2008). Varicella and the pregnant woman: Prevention and management. *Australian & New Zealand Journal of Obstetrics & Gynaecology, 48*(1), 26–33. doi:10.1111/j.1479-828X.2007.00797.x

Davel, S., Irusen, E. M., & Hall, D. (2009). Asthma in pregnancy—don't lose control. *Current Allergy & Clinical Immunology, 22*(1), 4–9. Retrieved February 13, 2012 from http://www.pntonline.co.za/index.php/PNT/article/view/440/441

Dechen, T. C., Sumit, K., & Ranabir, P. (2010). Correlates of vaginal colonization with group B streptococci among pregnant women. *Journal of Global Infectious Diseases, 2*(3), 236–241. doi:10.4103/0974-777X.68536

Dehlendorf, C., Marchi, K., Vittinghoff, E., & Braveman, P. (2010). Sociocultural determinants of teenage childbearing among Latinas in California. *Maternal & Child Health Journal, 14*(2), 194–201. doi:10.1007/s10995-009-0443-8

DeVito, J. (2010). How adolescent mothers feel about becoming a parent. *Journal of Perinatal Education, 19*(2), 25–34. doi:10.1624/105812410×495523

Devlieger, R., Casteels, K., & Van Assche, F. A. (2008). Reduced adaptation of the pancreatic B cells during pregnancy is the major causal factor for gestational diabetes: Current knowledge and metabolic effects on the offspring. *Acta Obstetricia Et Gynecologica Scandinavica, 87*(12), 1266–1270.

Do, M., & Meekers, D. (2009). Multiple sex partners and perceived risk of HIV infection in zambia: Attitudinal determinants and gender differences. *AIDS Care, 21*(10), 1211–1221. doi:10.1080/09540120902730047

Duncan, B., Harris, G., Reedy, J., Krahe, S., Gillis, R., & Laguna, M. (2008). Common/unity: An innovative program to address 3 root causes of many of the social ills seen in adolescents. *Clinical Pediatrics, 47*(3), 280–288.

El Aila, N. A., Tency, I., Claeys, G., et al. (2009). Genotyping of *Streptococcus agalactiae* (group B streptococci) isolated from vaginal and rectal swabs of women at 35–37 weeks of pregnancy. *BMC Infectious Diseases, 9*, 153–153.

Feig, D. S., Zinman, B., Wang, X., & Hux, J. E. (2008). Risk of development of diabetes mellitus after diagnosis of gestational diabetes. *Canadian Medical Association Journal, 179*(3), 229–234.

Gareri, J., Brieni, J., Reynolds, J., & Koren, G. (2009). Potential role of the placenta in fetal alcohol spectrum disorder. *Pediatric Drugs, 11*(1), 26–29.

Gautam, C. S., Saha, L., Sekhri, K., & Saha, P. K. (2008). Iron deficiency in pregnancy and the rationality of iron supplements prescribed during pregnancy. *Medscape Journal of Medicine, 10*(12), 283–283.

Gilbert, E. S. (2011). *Manual of high risk pregnancy & delivery* (5th ed.). St. Louis, MO: Mosby Elsevier.

Giles, M. (2009). HIV and pregnancy: Screening and management update. *Current Opinion in Obstetrics & Gynecology, 21*(2), 131–135.

Greenbaum, R. L., Stevens, S. A., Nash, K., Koren, G., & Rovet, J. (2009). Social cognitive and emotion processing abilities of children with fetal alcohol spectrum disorders: A comparison with attention deficit hyperactivity disorder. *Alcoholism: Clinical & Experimental Research, 33*(10), 1656–1670. doi:10.1111/j.1530–0277.2009.01003.x

Habib, F. A. (2008). Post-treatment assessment of acute *Toxoplasma* infection during pregnancy. *Journal of Obstetrics & Gynaecology, 28*(6), 593–595. doi:10.1080/01443610802344332.

Hardy-Fairbanks, A., & Baker, E. R. (2010). Asthma in pregnancy: Pathophysiology, diagnosis and management. *Obstetrics and Gynecology Clinics of North America, 37*(2), 159–172.

Harvey, J., & Dennis, C. (2008). Hygiene interventions for prevention of cytomegalovirus infection among childbearing women: Systematic review. *Journal of Advanced Nursing, 63*(5), 440–450.

Health Canada. (2006). *Fetal alcohol spectrum disorder.* Retrieved February 13, 2012 from http://www.hc-sc.gc.ca/hl-vs/alt_formats/pacrb-dgapcr/pdf/iyh-vsv/diseases-maladies/fasd-etcaf-eng.pdf

Health Canada. (2011). *Prenatal nutrition.* Retrieved February 13, 2012 from http://www.hc-sc.gc.ca/fn-an/nutrition/prenatal/index-eng.php

Heart and Stroke Foundation. (2012). *Statistics.* Retrieved February 13, 2012 from http://www.heartandstroke.com/site/c.ikIQLcMWJtE/b.3483991/k.34A8/Statistics.htm

Heavey, E. (2010). Don't miss preconception opportunities for adolescents. *American Journal of Maternal Child Nursing, 35*(4), 213–219. doi:10.1097/NMC.0b013e3181dd9d5a

Hod, M., Jovanovic, L., Di Renzo, G. C., De Leiva, S., & Langer, O. (2008). *Textbook of diabetes and pregnancy* (2nd ed.). New York: Informa.

Hod, M., & Simeoni, U. (2009). Maternal, fetal and neonatal complications of diabetic pregnancy-delivering optimal care while awaiting for cure. *Seminars in Fetal & Neonatal Medicine, 14*(2), 63–65. doi:10.1016/j.siny.2008.09.003.

Howland, R. H. (2009). Prescribing psychotropic medications during pregnancy and lactation: Principles and guidelines. *Journal of Psychosocial Nursing & Mental Health Services, 47*(5), 19–23.

Hull, L., May, J., Farrell-Moore, D., & Svikis, D. S. (2010). Treatment of cocaine abuse during pregnancy: Translating research to clinical practice. *Current Psychiatry Reports, 12*(5), 454–461.

Inati, A., Chabtini, L., Mounayar, M., & Taher, A. (2009). Current understanding in the management of sickle cell disease. *Hemoglobin, 33*, S107–S115. doi:10.3109/03630260903347682.

Inati, A., Koussa, S., Taher, A., & Perrine, S. (2008). Sickle cell disease: New insights into pathophysiology and treatment. *Pediatric Annals, 37*(5), 311–321.

Jonas, M. M. (2009). Hepatitis B and pregnancy: An underestimated issue. *Liver International, 29*, 133–139. doi:10.1111/j.1478–3231.2008.01933.x

Kaaja, R., & Rönnemaa, T. (2008). Gestational diabetes: Pathogenesis and consequences to mother and offspring. *The Review of Diabetic Studies, 5*(4), 194–202.

Kapustin, J. F. (2008). Postpartum management for gestational diabetes mellitus: Policy and practice implications. *Journal of the American Academy of Nurse Practitioners, 20*(11), 547–554.

Keegan, J., Parva, M., Finnegan, M., Gerson, A., & Belden, M. (2010). Addiction in pregnancy. *Journal of Addictive Diseases, 29*(2), 175–191. doi:10.1080/10550881003684723.

Kennedy, S. (2009). Providing specialist care for pregnant women with asthma. *Nursing Standard, 23*(20), 43–48.

Kilmarx, P. H. (2009). Global epidemiology of HIV. *Current Opinion in HIV and AIDS, 4*(4), 240–246.

King-Jones, T. C. (2008). Caring for pregnant adolescents: Perils and pearls of communication. *Nursing for Women's Health, 12*(2), 114–119.

Kitzmiller, J. L., Block, J. M., Brown, F. M., et al. (2008). Managing preexisting diabetes for pregnancy: Summary of evidence and consensus recommendations for care. *Diabetes Care, 31*(5), 1060–1079.

Klieger, C., Pollex, E., & Koren, G. (2008). Treating the mother—protecting the unborn: The safety of hypoglycemic drugs in pregnancy. *Journal of Maternal-Fetal & Neonatal Medicine, 21*(3), 191–196.

Kramer, K. L., & Lancaster, J. B. (2010). Teen motherhood in crosscultural perspective. *Annals of Human Biology, 37*(5), 613–628. doi:10.3109/03014460903563434.

Kumar, M. T. (2009). S64–04 epidemiology of substance use in pregnancy. *European Psychiatry, 24*, S308–S308. doi:10.1016/S0924–9338(09)70541–3.

Lall, A. (2008). Neonatal abstinence syndrome. *British Journal of Midwifery, 16*(4), 220–223.

Langer, O. (2008). Type 2 diabetes in pregnancy: Exposing deceptive appearances. *Journal of Maternal-Fetal & Neonatal Medicine, 21*(3), 181–189.

Langlois, S., Ford, J. C., Chitayat, D., et al. (2008). Joint SOGC-CCMG clinical practice guideline: Carrier screening for thalassemia and hemoglobinopathies in Canada. *Journal of Obstetrics and Gynaecology Canada, 218*(10), 950–960. Retrieved February 13, 2012 from http://www.sogc.org/guidelines/documents/gui218CPG0810.pdf.

Lapolla, A., Dalfra, M. G., Mello, G., et al. (2008). Early detection of insulin sensitivity and beta cell function with simple tests indicates future derangements in late pregnancy. *The Journal of Clinical Endocrinology & Metabolism, 93*(3), 976–980. doi:10.1210/jc.2007–1363.

Leslie, K. (2008). Alcohol and drug use among teenagers. *Canadian Medical Association Journal, 178*(2), 149. doi:10.1503/cmaj.071622.

Lisonkova, S., Sheps, S. B., Janssen, J. A., Lee, S. K., & Dahlgren, L. (2011). Effect of older maternal age on birth outcomes in twin pregnancies: A population-based study. *Journal of Perinatology, 31*, 85–91. doi:10.1038/jp.2010.114.

Little, M., & Sinert, R. (2011). *Asthma in pregnancy.* Retrieved February 13, 2012 from http://www.emedicine.com/emerg/TOPIC476.HTM.

Luong, M. (2008). Life after teenage motherhood. *Statistics Canada (No. 75–001-X).* Retrieved February 13, 2012 from http://www.statcan.gc.ca/pub/75–001-x/2008105/pdf/10577-eng.pdf.

Maddineni, M., & Panda, M. (2008). Pulmonary tuberculosis in a young pregnant female: Challenges in diagnosis and management. *Infectious Diseases in Obstetrics and Gynecology, 2008*, 628985.doi:10.1155/2008/628985.

Magee, L. A., Helewa, M., Moutquin, J.-M., et al. (2008). SOGC clinical practice guidelines: Diagnosis, evaluation, and management of the hypertensive disorders of pregnancy. *Journal of Obstetrics and Gynaecology Canada, 30*(3 Suppl 1), S1–S38. Retrieved February 13, 2012 from http://www.sogc.org/guidelines/documents/gui206CPG0803_001.pdf.

Mahavarkar, S. H., Madhu, C. K., & Mule, V. D. (2008). A comparative study of teenage pregnancy. *Journal of Obstetrics & Gynaecology, 28*(6), 604–607. doi:10.1080/01443610802281831.

Mahy, M., Stover, J., Kiragu, K., et al. (2010). What will it take to achieve virtual elimination of mother-to-child transmission of HIV? an assessment of current progress and future needs. *Sexually Transmitted Infections, 86*(Suppl 2), ii48–ii55.

Malek, A., Obrist, C., Wenzinger, S., & von Mandach, U. (2009). The impact of cocaine and heroin on the placental transfer of methadone. *Reproductive Biology and Endocrinology, 7*, 61. doi:10.1186/1477–7827-7-61.

Mann-Jiles, V., & Morris, D. L. (2009). Quality of life of adult patients with sickle cell disease. *Journal of the American Academy of Nurse Practitioners, 21*(6), 340–349.

March of Dimes. (2009). *Teenage pregnancy.* Retrieved February 13, 2012 from http://www.marchofdimes.com/professionals/medicalresources_teenpregnancy.html.

McKay, A., & Barrett, M. (2010). Trends in teen pregnancy rates from 1996–2006: A comparison of Canada, Sweden, U.S.A., and England/Wales. *Canadian Journal of Human Sexuality, 19*(1–2), 43–52.

Merson, M. H., O'Malley, J., Serwadda, D., & Apisuk, C. (2008). The history and challenge of HIV prevention. *The Lancet, 372,* 475–478. doi:10.1016/S0140–6736(08)60884–3

Milman, N. (2008). Prepartum anaemia: Prevention and treatment. *Annals of Hematology, 87*(12), 949–959.

Milne, D., & Glasier, A. (2008). Preventing repeat pregnancy in adolescents. *Current Opinion in Obstetrics & Gynecology, 20*(5), 442–446.

Mirpuri, J., & Jain, L. (2010). Issues of prematurity and HIV infection. *Clinics in Perinatology, 37*(4), 887.

Mnyani, C. N., & McIntyre, J. A. (2009). Preventing mother-to-child transmission of HIV. *BJOG: An International Journal of Obstetrics and Gynaecology, 116*(Suppl 1), 71–76.

Modder, J. (2008). Diabetes in pregnancy: Can we make a difference? *BJOG: An International Journal of Obstetrics and Gynaecology, 115*(4), 419–420.

Moghbeli, N., Pare, E., & Webb, G. (2008). Practical assessment of maternal cardiovascular risk in pregnancy. *Congenital Heart Disease, 3*(5), 308–316.

Money, D. M., Dobson, S., Boucher, M., et al. (2004). SOGC clinical practice guidelines: The prevention of early-onset neonatal group B streptococcal disease. *Journal of Obstetrics and Gynaecology Canada, 149,* 826–832. Retrieved February 13, 2012 from http://www.sogc.org/guidelines/public/149E-CPG-September2004.pdf.

Money, D., Seben, M., Wong, T., et al. (2008). SOGC clinical practice guidelines: Guidelines for the management of herpes simplex virus in pregnancy. *Journal of Obstetrics and Gynaecology Canada, 208,* 514–519. Retrieved February 13, 2012 from http://www.sogc.org/guidelines/documents/gui208CPg0806.pdf.

Moreira, L. B., Gus, M., Nunes, G., et al. (2009). Association between pregnancy-related hypertension and severity of hypertension. *Journal of Human Hypertension, 23*(6), 415–419.

Murphy-Oikonen, J., Montelpare, W. J., Southon, S., Bertoldo, L., & Persichino, N. (2010). Identifying infants at risk for neonatal abstinence syndrome: A retrospective cohort comparison study of 3 screening approaches. *Journal of Perinatal & Neonatal Nursing, 24*(4), 366–372. doi:10.1097/JPN.0b013e3181fa13ea.

Niccols, A., Milligan, K., Sword, W., et al. (2010). Maternal mental health and integrated programs for mothers with substance abuse issues. *Psychology of Addictive Behaviors, 24*(3), 466–474.

Nicholson, W., Bolen, S., Witkop, C. T., Neale, D., Wilson, L., & Bass, E. (2009). Benefits and risks of oral diabetes agents compared with insulin in women with gestational diabetes: A systematic review. *Obstetrics and Gynecology, 113*(1), 193–205.

Nigro, G. (2009). Maternal-fetal cytomegalovirus infection: From diagnosis to therapy. *Journal of Maternal-Fetal & Neonatal Medicine, 22*(2), 169–174.

Nodine, P. M., Arruda, J., & Hastings-Tolsma, M. (2011). Prenatal environment: Effect on neonatal outcome. In S. L. Gardner, B. S. Carter, M. Enzman-Hines, & J. A. Hernandez (Eds.), *Merenstein & Gardner's handbook of neonatal intensive care* (7th ed.). St. Louis, MO: Mosby Elsevier.

Parry, J. (2010). At last a global response to viral hepatitis. *Bulletin of the World Health Organization, 88*(11), 801–802. doi:10.2471/BLT.10.011110.

Patel, A., Asopa, S., Tang, A. T. M., & Ohri, S. K. (2008). Cardiac surgery during pregnancy. *Texas Heart Institute Journal, 35*(3), 307–312.

Public Health Agency of Canada. (2008a). *Genital herpes simplex virus (HSV) infections.* Retrieved February 13, 2012 from http://www.phac-aspc.gc.ca/std-mts/sti-its/pdf/504genherp-vhs-eng.pdf.

Public Health Agency of Canada. (2008b). *Genital human papilloma virus (HPV) infections.* Retrieved February 13, 2012 from http://www.phac-aspc.gc.ca/std-mts/sti-its/pdf/505hpv-vph-eng.pdf.

Public Health Agency of Canada. (2008c). *Hepatitis B virus (HBV) infections.* Retrieved February 13, 2012 from http://www.phac-aspc.gc.ca/std-mts/sti-its/pdf/507hepb-eng.pdf.

Public Health Agency of Canada. (2008d). *Human immunodeficiency virus (HIV) infections.* Retrieved February 13, 2012 from http://www.phac-aspc.gc.ca/std-mts/sti-its/pdf/508hiv-vih-eng.pdf.

Public Health Agency of Canada. (2009a). *Report from the National Diabetes Surveillance System: Diabetes in Canada, 2009.* Retrieved February 13, 2012 from http://www.phac-aspc.gc.ca/publicat/2009/ndssdic-snsddac-09/pdf/report-2009-eng.pdf.

Public Health Agency of Canada. (2009b). *Tracking heart disease & stroke in Canada.* Her Retrieved February 13, 2012 from http://www.phac-aspc.gc.ca/publicat/2009/cvd-avc/pdf/cvd-avs-2009-eng.pdf.

Public Health Agency of Canada. (2010a). *Hepatitis B—get the facts.* Retrieved February 13, 2012 from http://www.phac-aspc.gc.ca/hcai-iamss/bbp-pts/hepatitis/hep_b-eng.php.

Public Health Agency of Canada. (2010b). *Report from the Canadian Chronic Disease Surveillance System: Hypertension in Canada, 2010.* Retrieved February 13, 2012 from http://www.phac-aspc.gc.ca/cd-mc/cvd-mcv/ccdss-snsmc-2010/pdf/CCDSS_HTN_Report_FINAL_EN_20100513.pdf.

Rawlinson, W. D., Hall, B., Jones, C. A., et al. (2008). Viruses and other infections in stillbirth: What is the evidence and what should we be doing? *Pathology, 40*(2), 149–160. doi:10.1080/00313020701813792.

Retnakaran, R., & Shah, B. R. (2009). Abnormal screening glucose challenge test in pregnancy and future risk of diabetes in young women. *Diabetic Medicine, 26*(5), 474–477.

Rosenthal, M. S., Ross, J. S., Bilodeau, R., Richter, R. S., Palley, J. E., & Bradley, E. H. (2009). Economic evaluation of a comprehensive teenage pregnancy prevention program: Pilot program. *American Journal of Preventive Medicine, 37*(6), S280–S287. doi:10.1016/j.amepre.2009.08.014.

Rubio, D. M., Kraemer, K. L., Farrell, M. H., & Day, N. L. (2008). Factors associated with alcohol use, depression, and their co-occurrence during pregnancy. *Alcoholism, Clinical and Experimental Research, 32*(9), 1543–1551.

Sauerbrei, A. (2010). Review of varicella-zoster virus infections in pregnant women and neonates. *Health, 2*(2), 143–152. doi:10.4236/health.2010.22022.

Schuetze, P., Eiden, R. D., & Edwards, E. P. (2009). A longitudinal examination of physiological regulation in cocaine-exposed infants across the first 7 months of life. *Infancy, 14*(1), 19–43. doi:10.1080/15250000802569660.

Scott, K., & Lust, K. (2010). Illicit substance use in pregnancy—a review. *Obstetric Medicine (1753–495X), 3*(3), 94–100. doi:10.1258/om.2010.100014.

Shah, P. S., & Ohlsson, A. (2009). Effects of prenatal multimicronutrient supplementation on pregnancy outcomes: A meta-analysis. *Canadian Medical Association Journal, 180*(12), E99–E108.

Sickle Cell Association of Ontario. (n.d.). *About sickle cell.* Retrieved February 13, 2012 from http://www.sicklecellontario.org/sickle-cell-101.

Slater, M., Stringer, E. M., & Stringer, J. S. A. (2010). Breastfeeding in HIV-positive women: What can be recommended? *Paediatric Drugs, 12*(1), 1–9.

Society of Obstetricians and Gynaecologists of Canada. (2008). *Rubella in pregnancy.* Retrieved May 29, 2012 from http://www.sogc.org/guidelines/documents/guiJOGC203CPG0802.pdf

Society of Obstetricians and Gynaecologists of Canada. (2011a). *Group B streptococcus infection in pregnancy.* Retrieved February 13, 2012 from http://www.sogc.org/health/pregnancy-groupb_e.asp.

Society of Obstetricians and Gynaecologists of Canada. (2011b). *HIV testing in pregnancy.* Retrieved February 13, 2012 from http://www.sogc.org/health/pregnancy-hiv_e.asp.

Stangl, V., Schad, J., Gossing, G., Borges, A., Baumann, G., & Stangl, A. (2008). Maternal heart disease and pregnancy outcome: A single centre experience. *European Journal of Heart Failure, 10,* 855–860. doi:10.1016/j.ejheart.2008.07.017.

Strunk, J. A. (2008). The effect of school-based health clinics on teenage pregnancy and parenting outcomes: An integrated literature review. *The Journal of School Nursing, 24*(1), 13–20.

Thompson, B. L., Levitt, P., & Stanwood, G. D. (2009). Prenatal exposure to drugs: Effects on brain development and implications for policy and education. *Nature Reviews Neuroscience, 10*(4), 303–312.

Tridapalli, E., Capretti, M. G., Farneti, G., Marangoni, A., Cevenini, R., & Faldella, G. (2008). Congenital toxoplasmosis: The importance of the western blot method to avoid unnecessary therapy in potentially infected newborns. *Acta Paediatrica, 97*(9), 1298–1300, doi: 10.1111/j.1651–2227.2008.00905.x.

Unicef. (2009). *Children and HIV and AIDS.* Retrieved February 13, 2012 from http://www.unicef.org/aids/index_statistics.html.

United Nations (Joint United Nations Programme on HIV/AIDS). (2010). *UNAIDS report on the global aids epidemic 2010.* Geneva: Switzerland: WHO. Retrieved February 13, 2012 from http://www.unaids.org/globalreport/Global_report.htm.

Ural, S. H. (2011). *Genital herpes in pregnancy.* Retrieved February 13, 2012 from http://emedicine.medscape.com/article/274874-print.

van Gelder, M. M. H. J., Reefhuis, J., Caton, A. R., Werler, M. M., Druschel, C. M., & Roeleveld, N. (2010). Characteristics of pregnant illicit drug users and associations between cannabis use and perinatal outcome in a population-based study. *Drug and Alcohol Dependence, 109*(1–3), 243–247.

Varvarigou, A. A., Fouzas, S., & Beratis, N. G. (2010). Effect of prenatal tobacco smoke exposure on fetal growth potential. *Journal of Perinatal Medicine, 38*(6), 683–687. doi:10.1515/JPM.2010.101.

Venkatesh, M. P., Adams, K. M., & Weisman, L. E. (2011). Infection in the neonate. In S. L. Gardner, B. S. Carter, M. Enzman-Hines & J. A. Hernandez (Eds.), *Merenstein & Gardner's handbook of neonatal intensive care* (7th ed.). St. Louis, MO: Mosby Elsevier.

Villers, M. S., Jamison, M. G., De Castro, L., & James, A. H. (2008). Morbidity associated with sickle cell disease in pregnancy. *American Journal of Obstetrics & Gynecology, 199*(2), 125.e1–e5.

Volpe, L., Pancani, F., Aragona, M., et al. (2010). Continuous subcutaneous insulin infusion and multiple dose insulin injections in type 1 diabetic pregnant women: A case-control study. *Gynecological Endocrinology, 26*(3), 193–196.

Walton-Moss, B., McIntosh, L. C., Conrad, J., & Kiefer, E. (2009). Health status and birth outcomes among pregnant women in substance abuse treatment. *Women's Health Issues, 19*(3), 167–175.

Wang, M. (2012). *Perinatal drug abuse and neonatal drug withdrawal.* Retrieved February 12, 2012 from http://emedicine.medscape.com/article/978492-overview.

Weiner, S. M., & Finnegan, L. P. (2011). Drug withdrawal in the neonate. In S. L. Gardner, B. S. Carter, M. Enzman-Hines & J. A. Hernandez (Eds.), *Merenstein & Gardner's handbook of neonatal intensive care* (7th ed.). St. Louis, MO: Mosby Elsevier.

Whittaker, E. & Kampmann, B. (2008). Perinatal tuberculosis: New challenges in the diagnosis and treatment of tuberculosis in infants and the newborn. *Early Human Development, 84*(12), 795–799.

Williams, S. F., Keane-Tarchichi, M., Bettica, L., Dieudonne, A., & Bardeguez, A. D. (2009). Pregnancy outcomes in young women with perinatally acquired human immunodeficiency virus-1. *American Journal of Obstetrics & Gynecology, 200*(2), 149.e1–e5.

World Health Organization. (2001). *Iron deficiency anemia: Assessment, prevention and control: A guide for programme managers.* Retrieved February 13, 2012 from http://www.who.int/nutrition/publications/micronutrients/anaemia_iron_deficiency/WHO_NHD_01.3/en/index.html.

World Health Organization. (2010a). *Tuberculosis.* Retrieved February 13, 2012 from www.who.int/mediacentre/factsheets/fs104/en/.

World Health Organization. (2010b). *WHO HIV & AIDS guidelines for PMTCT & breastfeeding.* Retrieved February 12, 2012 from http://www.avert.org/pmtct-guidelines.htm.

Xiushui, R., Aggarwal, K., Balentine, J., et al. (2012). *Aortic stenosis.* Retrieved February 13, 2012 from http://www.emedicine.com/EMERG/topic40.htm.

Yinon, Y., Farine, D., Yudin, M. H., et al. (2010). SOGC clinical practice guidelines: Cytomegalovirus in pregnancy. *Journal of Obstetrics and Gynaecology Canada, 32*(4), 348–354. Retrieved February 13, 2012 from http://www.sogc.org/guidelines/documents/gui240CPG1004E.pdf.

Yu, C. K. H., Stasiowska, E., Stephens, A., Awogbade, M., & Davies, A. (2009). Outcome of pregnancy in sickle cell disease patients attending a combined obstetric and haematology clinic. *Journal of Obstetrics and Gynaecology, 29*(6), 512–516.

RECOMMENDED READINGS

Agrawal, A., Scherrer, J. F., Grant, J. D., Sartor, C. E., Pergadia, M. L., Duncan, A. E., et al. (2010). The effects of maternal smoking during pregnancy on offspring outcomes. *Preventive Medicine, 50*(1–2), 13–18. doi:10.1016/j.ypmed.2009.12.009.

Albright, B. B., & Rayburn, W. F. (2009). Substance abuse among reproductive age women. *Obstetrics and Gynecology Clinics of North America, 36*(4), 891.

Asthma Society of Canada. (2011). *Resources & support: Your healthcare team.* Retrieved June 30, 2011 from http://www.asthma.ca/adults/community/askExpert3.php.

Balen, A., Creighton, S., & Martin-Hirsch, P. (2010). Adolescent reproductive health [editorial: special issue]'s choice. *BJOG: An International Journal of Obstetrics & Gynaecology, 117*(2), i–i.

Hellwig, J. P. (2009). Hypertension in women: More evidence for the role of lifestyle. *Nursing for Women's Health, 13*(5), 367–372.

Barrett, H. L., Morris, J., & McElduff, A. (2009). Watchful waiting: A management protocol for maternal glycaemia in the peripartum period. *Australian & New Zealand Journal of Obstetrics & Gynaecology, 49*(2), 162–167.

Dontigny, L., Arsenault, M.-Y., Martel, M.-J., et al. (2008). SOGC clinical practice guidelines: Rubella in pregnancy. *Journal of Obstetrics and Gynaecology Canada, 203*, 152–158. Retrieved February 13, 2012 from http://www.sogc.org/guidelines/documents/guiJOGC-203CPG0802.pdf.

Herrman, J. W. (2010). Assessing the teen parent family: The role for nurses. *Nursing for Women's Health, 14*(3), 212–221. doi:10.1111/j.1751–486X.2010.01542.x.

Kumar, V., Das, S., & Jameel, S. (2010). The biology and pathogenesis of hepatitis viruses. *Current Science, 98*(3), 312–325.

Radesky, J. S., Oken, E., Rifas-Shiman, S., Kleinman, K. P., Rich-Edwards, J., & Gillman, M. W. (2008). Diet during early pregnancy and development of gestational diabetes. *Paediatric & Perinatal Epidemiology, 22*(1), 47–59. doi:10.1111/j.1365–3016.2007.00899.x.

Sarris, I., Litos, M., Bewley, S., Okpala, I., Seed, P., & Oteng-Ntim, E. (2008). Platelet count as a predictor of the severity of sickle cell disease during pregnancy. *Journal of Obstetrics & Gynaecology, 28*(7), 688–691. doi:10.1080/01443610802462977.

Weekes, A. J., & Lee, D. S. (2006). Substance abuse: Cocaine. eMedicine. Retrieved June 2, 2012 from http://www.emedicine.com/ped/topic2666.htm.

Winklbaur, B., Baewert, A., Jagsch, R., Rohrmeister, K., Metz, V., Aeschbach Jachmann, C., et al. (2009). Association between prenatal tobacco exposure and outcome of neonates born to opioid-maintained mothers. implications for treatment. *European Addiction Research, 15*(3), 150–156.

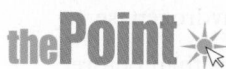

thePoint For additional learning materials, including Internet Resources, visit **http://thePoint.lww.com/Chow1e.**

CHAPTER WORKSHEET

MULTIPLE CHOICE QUESTIONS

1. Which of the following would the nurse include when teaching a pregnant woman about the pathophysiologic mechanisms associated with gestational diabetes?

    a. Pregnancy fosters the development of carbohydrate cravings.

    b. There is progressive resistance to the effects of insulin.

    c. Hypoinsulinemia develops early in the first trimester.

    d. Glucose levels decrease to accommodate fetal growth.

2. When providing prenatal education to a pregnant woman with asthma, which of the following would be important for the nurse to do?

    a. Explain that she should avoid steroids during her pregnancy.

    b. Demonstrate how to assess her blood glucose levels.

    c. Teach correct administration of subcutaneous bronchodilators.

    d. Ensure she seeks treatment for any acute exacerbation.

3. Which of the following conditions would most likely cause a pregnant woman with type 1 diabetes the greatest difficulty during her pregnancy?

    a. Placenta previa

    b. Hyperemesis gravidarum

    c. Abruptio placentae

    d. Rh incompatibility

4. Women who drink alcohol during pregnancy:

    a. Often produce more alcohol dehydrogenase

    b. Usually become intoxicated faster than before

    c. Can give birth to an infant with fetal alcohol spectrum disorder

    d. Gain fewer pounds throughout the gestation

5. When explaining to a pregnant woman about HIV infection and transmission, which of the following would the nurse include?

    a. It primarily occurs when there is a large viral load in the blood.

    b. HIV is most commonly transmitted via sexual contact.

    c. It affects the majority of infants of mothers with HIV infection.

    d. Nurses are most frequently affected due to needle sticks.

CRITICAL THINKING EXERCISES

1. A client at 26 weeks' gestation came to the clinic to follow up on her previous 1-hour glucose screening. Her results had come back outside the accepted screening range, and a 3-hour glucose tolerance test had been ordered. It resulted in three abnormal values, confirming a diagnosis of gestational diabetes. As the nurse in the prenatal clinic you are seeing her for the first time.

    a. What additional information will you need to provide care for her?

    b. What education will she need to address this new diagnosis?

    c. How will you evaluate the effectiveness of your interventions?

2. A 14-year-old girl comes to the public health clinic with her mother. The mother tells you that her daughter has been "out messing around and has gotten herself pregnant." The girl is crying quietly in the corner and avoids eye contact with you. The mother reports that her daughter "must be following in my footsteps" because she became pregnant when she was only 15 years old. The client's mother goes back out into the waiting room and leaves the client with you.

    a. What is your first approach with the client to gain her trust?

    b. List the client's educational needs during this pregnancy.

    c. What prevention strategies are needed to prevent a second pregnancy?

3. Linda, a 27-year-old G3P2, is admitted to the labour and birth suite because of preterm rupture of membranes at an estimated 35 weeks' gestation. She has received no prenatal care and reports this was an unplanned pregnancy. Linda appears distracted and very thin. She reports that her two previous children have been in foster care since birth because the child welfare authorities "didn't think I was an adequate mother." She denies any recent use of alcohol or drugs, but you smell alcohol on her breath. She has a spontaneous vaginal birth a few hours later, producing a 4-lb baby boy with Apgar scores of 8 at 1 minute and 9 at 5 minutes.

   a. What aspects of this woman's history may lead the nurse to suspect that this infant may be at risk for fetal alcohol spectrum disorder?

   b. What additional screening or laboratory tests might validate your suspicion?

   c. What physical and neurodevelopmental deficits might present later in life if the infant has fetal alcohol spectrum disorder?

STUDY ACTIVITIES

1. In the maternity clinic or hospital setting, interview a pregnant woman with a preexisting medical condition (e.g., diabetes, asthma, sickle-cell anemia) and find out how this condition affects her life and this pregnancy, especially her lifestyle choices.

2. You have a close friend who has a problem with alcohol but denies it. She now admits to you that she thinks she is pregnant because she missed her period. What specific information and advice should you give her concerning alcohol use during pregnancy?

3. Should marijuana be legalized in Canada? What impact might your view (pro or con) have on pregnant women and their offspring?

4. Outline a discussion you might have with an HIV-positive pregnant woman who doesn't see the need to take anti-retroviral agents to prevent perinatal transmission.

5. The nurse is preparing a teaching session about breastfeeding for a group of pregnant women who have various infections listed below. The nurse would include women with which of the following conditions? Select all that apply.

   a. Hepatitis B

   b. Parvovirus B19

   c. Herpes virus type 2

   d. HIV-positive status

   e. Cytomegalovirus

   f. Varicella zoster virus

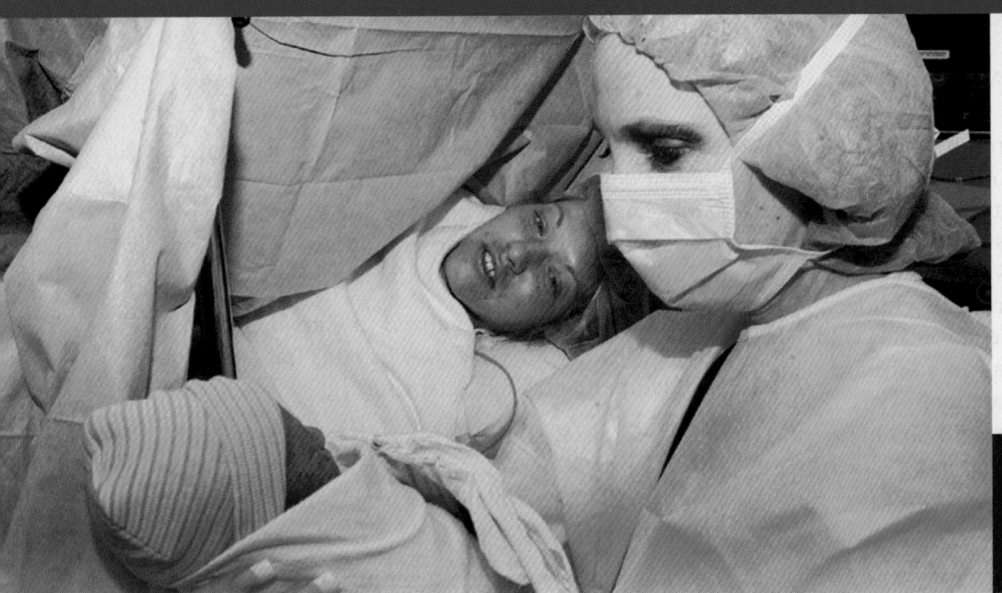

Adapted by Kala Streibel

NURSING MANAGEMENT OF LABOUR AND BIRTH AT RISK

Jennifer, a 29-year-old G1P0, is at 41 weeks' gestation. Her health care provider has recommended that she come in for induction. She is very anxious about doing this since she has heard "horror stories" about the "hard, painful contractions" that can result. What can the nurse do to calm her fears?

KEY TERMS

amnioinfusion
cesarean birth
dystocia
forceps
hypertonic uterine
   dysfunction

hypotonic uterine
   dysfunction
labour induction
macrosomia
postterm pregnancy
precipitous labour
preterm labour

shoulder dystocia
tocolytic
umbilical cord prolapse
vacuum extractor
vaginal birth after
   cesarean (VBAC)

LEARNING OBJECTIVES

Upon completion of the chapter, the learner will be able to:

1. Define dystocia.
2. Identify the four major abnormalities or problems associated with dysfunctional labour patterns, giving examples of each problem.
3. Describe the nursing management for the woman with dysfunctional labour experiencing a problem with the powers, passenger, passageway, and psyche.
4. Develop a plan of care for the woman experiencing preterm labour.
5. Discuss the nursing assessment and management of the woman experiencing a postterm pregnancy.
6. Explain four obstetric emergencies that can complicate labour and birth, including appropriate management for each.
7. Compare and contrast the nursing management for the woman undergoing labour induction or augmentation, forceps- and vacuum-assisted birth.
8. Summarize the plan of care for a woman who is to undergo a cesarean birth.
9. Discuss the key areas to be addressed when caring for a woman who is to undergo vaginal birth after cesarean (VBAC).

Wow

In face of a crisis or a potentially bad outcome, add a mixture of warmth and serenity to your technical abilities.

Most women describe pregnancy as an exciting time in their life, but the development of an unexpected problem can suddenly change this description dramatically. Consider the woman who has had a problem-free pregnancy and then suddenly develops a condition during labour, changing a routine situation into a possible crisis. Many complications occur with little or no warning and present challenges for the perinatal health care team as well as the family. The nurse plays a major role in identifying the problem quickly and coordinating immediate intervention, ultimately achieving a positive outcome.

This chapter addresses several conditions occurring during labour and birth that may increase the risk for an adverse outcome for the mother and the fetus. It also describes birth-related procedures that may be necessary for the woman who develops a condition that increases her risk or that may be needed to reduce the woman's risk for developing a condition, thus promoting optimal maternal and fetal outcomes. Nursing management of the woman and her family focuses on professional support and compassionate care.

Dystocia

Dystocia, defined as abnormal or difficult labour, can be influenced by a vast number of maternal and fetal factors. Dystocia is said to exist when the progress of active labour deviates from normal; it is characterized by a slow and abnormal progression of labour (Joy et al., 2011) and has been identified in approximately 10% of hospital deliveries in Canada. Dystocia is the leading indicator for cesarean section (Public Health Agency of Canada [PHAC], 2008).

To characterize a labour as abnormal, a basic understanding of normal labour is essential. Normal labour starts with regular uterine contractions that are strong enough to result in cervical effacement and dilation. Early in labour, uterine contractions are irregular and cervical effacement and dilation occur gradually. When cervical dilation reaches 4 cm and uterine contractions become more powerful, the active phase of labour begins. Because dystocia cannot be predicted or diagnosed with certainty, the term "failure to progress" is often used. This term includes lack of progressive cervical dilation (>4 hours with <0.5 cm per hour) and lack of descent of the fetal head (>1 hour of effective pushing with no descent of the head) (Cheng & Caughey, 2012). An adequate trial of labour is needed to declare with confidence that dystocia or "failure to progress" exists. Understanding normal labour patterns and early identification of factors associated with dystocia are essential to reducing the prevalence and risk related to dystocia.

According to the Society of Obstetricians and Gynaecologists of Canada (SOGC, 2008), dystocia can be prevented through prenatal education, allowing for spontaneous onset of labour, and providing continuous labour support, free movement in labour, no routine interventions, and appropriate non-pharmacologic and pharmacologic pain relief measures.

Early identification of and prompt interventions for dystocia are essential to minimize the risk to the woman and the fetus. Factors associated with an increased risk for dystocia include epidural analgesia, excessive analgesia, multiple gestation, hydramnios, maternal exhaustion, ineffective maternal pushing technique, occiput posterior position, unripe cervix with induction, longer first stage of labour, nulliparity, contracted pelvis, short maternal stature, fetal macrosomia, maternal obesity, fetal malpresentation, fetal anomalies (hydrocephalus), maternal age older than 35 years, gestational age more than 41 weeks, chorioamnionitis, ineffective uterine contractions, and high fetal station at complete cervical dilation (Joy et al., 2011).

Dystocia can result from problems or abnormalities involving the expulsive forces (known as the "powers"); presentation, position, and fetal development (the "passenger"); the maternal bony pelvis or birth canal (the "passageway"); and maternal stress (the "psyche"). Table 21.1 summarizes the diagnosis, therapeutic management, and nursing management of the common problems associated with dystocia (Joy et al., 2011).

Problems with the Powers

When the expulsive forces of the uterus become dysfunctional, the uterus may either never fully relax (hypertonic contractions), placing the fetus in jeopardy, or relax too much (hypotonic contractions), causing ineffective contractions. Still another dysfunction can occur when the uterus contracts so frequently and with such intensity that a very rapid birth will take place (precipitous labour).

Hypertonic uterine dysfunction occurs when the uterus never fully relaxes between contractions. Subsequently, contractions are erratic and poorly coordinated because more than one uterine pacemaker is sending signals for contraction. Placental perfusion becomes compromised, thereby reducing oxygen to the fetus. These hypertonic contractions exhaust the mother, who is experiencing frequent, intense, and painful contractions with little progression (Watts, 2010).

Hypotonic uterine dysfunction occurs during active labour (dilation more than 4 cm) when contractions become poor in quality and lack sufficient intensity to dilate and efface the cervix. Contributing factors to hypotonic uterine function are overdistention, malposition of the fetus, and excessive analgesia (Watts, 2010). The major risk with this complication is hemorrhage after giving birth because the uterus cannot contract effectively to compress blood vessels.

Precipitous labour is one that is completed in less than 3 hours. Women experiencing precipitous labour

(text continues on page 676)

TABLE 21.1 DIAGNOSIS AND MANAGEMENT OF COMMON PROBLEMS ASSOCIATED WITH DYSTOCIA

Problem	Description	Diagnosis	Therapeutic Management	Nursing Management
Problems with the powers				
Hypertonic uterine dysfunction	Occurs in the latent phase of the first stage of labour (cervical dilation <4 cm); uncoordinated Force of contraction typically in the midsection of the uterus at the junction of the active upper and passive lower segments of the uterus rather than in the fundus Loss of downward pressure to push the presenting part against the cervix (Watts, 2010) Woman commonly becomes discouraged due to lack of progress; also has increased pain secondary to uterine anoxia	Characteristic hypertonicity of the contractions and the lack of labour progress	Therapeutic rest with the use of sedatives to promote relaxation and stop the abnormal activity of the uterus Hydration to promote fluid and electrolyte balance Identification of and intervention for any contributing factors Ruling out placental abruption (also associated with high resting tone and persistent pain) Onset of a normal labour pattern occurs in many women after a 4–6 h rest period (Watts, 2010).	Institute bed rest and sedation to promote relaxation and reduce pain. Assist with measures to rule out fetopelvic disproportion and fetal malpresentation. Evaluate fetal tolerance to labour pattern, such as monitoring of FHR patterns. Assess for signs of maternal infection. Promote adequate hydration through IV therapy. Provide pain management via epidural or IV analgesics. Assist with amniotomy to augment labour. Explain to woman and family about dysfunctional pattern. Plan for operative birth if normal labour pattern is not achieved.
Hypotonic uterine dysfunction	Often termed secondary uterine inertia because the labour begins normally and then the frequency and intensity of contractions decrease Possible contributing factors: overdistended uterus (i.e., multifetal pregnancy, macrosomia, polyhydramnios), too much pain medicine given too early in labour, fetal malposition, and regional anesthesia (Watts, 2010)	Evaluation of the woman's labour to confirm that she is having hypotonic active labour rather than a long latent phase Evaluation of maternal pelvis and fetal presentation and position to ensure that they are not contributing to the prolonged labour without noticeable progress	Identification of possible cause of inefficient uterine action (a malpositioned fetus, a too small maternal pelvis, overdistention of the uterus with fluid or a macrosomic fetus) Rupture of amniotic sac (amniotomy) if all causes ruled out Possible augmentation with oxytocin (Syntocin) to stimulate effective uterine contractions Cesarean birth if amniotomy and augmentation ineffective	Administer oxytocin as ordered once fetopelvic disproportion is ruled out. Assist with amniotomy if membranes are intact. Provide fetal surveillance as appropriate. Monitor vital signs, contractions, and cervix continually. Assess for signs of maternal and fetal infection. Explain to woman and family about dysfunctional pattern. Plan for surgical birth if normal labour pattern is not achieved or fetal distress occurs.

Precipitous labour	Abrupt onset of higher-intensity contractions occurring in a shorter period of time instead of the more gradual increase in frequency, duration, and intensity that typifies most spontaneous labours	Identification based on the rapidity of progress through the stages of labour	Vaginal delivery if maternal pelvis is adequate	Closely monitor woman with previous history. Anticipate use of scheduled induction to control labour rate. Stay in constant attendance to monitor progress. Be prepared for delivery in the absence of the primary care provider. Anticipate postpartum hemorrhage.
Problems with the passenger				
Persistent occiput posterior position	Engagement of fetal head in the left or right occipito-transverse position with the occiput rotating posteriorly rather than into the more favourable occiput anterior position (fetus born facing upward instead of the normal downward position) Labour usually much longer and more uncomfortable (causing increased back pain during labour) if fetus remains in this position Possible extensive caput succedaneum and moulding from the sustained occiput posterior position	Leopold manoeuvres and vaginal examination to determine position of fetal head in conjunction with the mother's complaints of severe back pain (back of fetal head pressing on mother's sacrum and coccyx)	Labour to proceed, preparing the woman for a long labour (spontaneous resolution possible) Comfort measures and maternal positioning to help promote fetal head rotation	Assess for complaints of back pain in first stage of labour. Perform fetal surveillance as appropriate. Encourage maternal position changes to promote fetal head rotation: hands and knees and rocking pelvis back and forth; side-lying position; side lunges during contractions; sitting, kneeling, or standing while leaning forward; squatting position to give birth and enlarge pelvic outlet (Simkin, 2010). Apply low back counter-pressure during contractions to ease the discomfort. Use other helpful measures to attempt to rotate the fetal head, including lateral abdominal stroking in the direction that the fetal head should rotate; assisting the client into a hands-and-knees position (all fours); and squatting, pelvic rocking, stair climbing, assuming a side-lying position toward the side that the fetus should rotate, and side lunges.

(continued)

TABLE 21.1 DIAGNOSIS AND MANAGEMENT OF COMMON PROBLEMS ASSOCIATED WITH DYSTOCIA (continued)

Problem	Description	Diagnosis	Therapeutic Management	Nursing Management
				Provide measures to reduce anxiety, including continuous support.
				Continuously reinforce the woman's progress.
				Teach the woman and support person(s) about measures to facilitate fetal head rotation.
				Administer agents as ordered for pain relief (effective pain relief is crucial to help the woman to tolerate the back discomfort).
				Assess for prolonged second stage of labour with arrest of descent (common with this malposition).
				Anticipate possible use of forceps to rotate to anterior position at birth or manual rotation to anterior position at end of second stage.
				Prepare for possible cesarean birth if rotation is not achieved.
Face and brow presentation	Face presentation with complete extension of the fetal head	Diagnosis via vaginal examination only once labour is well established; palpation of facial features as the presenting part rather than the fetal head	Vaginal birth possible with face presentation with an adequate maternal pelvis and fetal head rotation; cesarean birth if head rotates backward	Assist with evaluating for feto-pelvic disproportion. Anticipate cesarean birth if vertex position is not achieved.
	Brow presentation: fetal head between full extension and full flexion so that the largest fetal skull diameter presents to the pelvis		Cesarean birth for brow presentation unless head flexes	Explain fetal malposition to the woman and her partner. Provide close observation for any signs of fetal hypoxia, as evidenced by late decelerations on the fetal monitor.

| Breech presentation | Fetal buttocks, or breech, presenting first rather than the head
1. Frank breech: buttock as the presenting part, with hips flexed and legs and knees extended upward
2. Complete breech (or full breech): buttock as presenting part, with hips flexed and knees flexed in a "cannonball" position
3. Footling or incomplete breech: One or two feet as the presenting part, with one or both hips extended | Vaginal examination to determine breech presentation. Ideally, ultrasound to confirm a clinically suspected presentation and to identify any fetal anomalies | The optimal method of birth is controversial and depends on a variety of factors: anticipated size of fetus, maternal pelvis, cord position, availability of early labour ultrasound assessment, comfort of care provider with breech delivery, and availability of cesarean birth

Regardless of the birth method selected, the risk for trauma is high. Breech vaginal births are recommended by SOGC only when early labour ultrasound is available, no contraindications to vaginal breech delivery exist, and the estimated fetal weight is between 2,500 and 4,000 g (Kotaska et al., 2009).
Vaginal delivery: fetus allowed to spontaneously deliver up to the umbilicus; then manoeuvres to assist in the delivery of the remainder of the body, arms, and head; fetal membranes left intact as long as possible to act as a dilating wedge and to prevent cord prolapse; anesthesiologist and pediatrician present
Caesarean birth: use of external cephalic version to reduce the chance of breech presentation at birth; attempted after the 36th week of gestation but before the start of labour (some fetuses spontaneously turn to a cephalic | Assess for associated conditions such as placenta previa, hydramnios, fetal anomalies, and multiple gestation.
Arrange for ultrasound to confirm fetal presentation.
Assist with external cephalic version possible after 36 weeks, and administer tocolytics to assist with external cephalic version.
Anticipate trial labour for 4–6 h to evaluate progress if version is unsuccessful.
Plan for cesarean birth if no progress is seen or fetal distress occurs.
After external cephalic version, administer RhoGAM to the Rh-negative woman to prevent a sensitization reaction if trauma has occurred and the potential for mixing of blood exists (Hofmeyr & Kulier, 2010). |

(continued)

TABLE 21.1 DIAGNOSIS AND MANAGEMENT OF COMMON PROBLEMS ASSOCIATED WITH DYSTOCIA (continued)

Problem	Description	Diagnosis	Therapeutic Management	Nursing Management
			presentation on their own toward term, and some will return to the breech presentation if external cephalic version is attempted too early) (Hofmeyr & Kulier, 2010); variable success rates, with risk for fractured bones, ruptured viscera, abruptio placentae, fetomaternal hemorrhage, and umbilical cord entanglement; tocolytic drugs to relax the uterus, as well as other methods to facilitate external cephalic version at term; individual evaluation of each woman for all factors before any interventions are initiated (Fischer, 2011)	
Shoulder dystocia	Delivery of fetal head with neck not appearing; retraction of chin against the perineum; shoulders remaining wedged behind the mother's pubic bone, causing a difficult birth with potential for injury to both mother and baby If shoulders still above the brim at this stage, no advancement. Newborn's chest trapped within the vaginal vault; chest unable to expand with respiration (although nose and mouth are outside)	Emergency, often unexpected complication. Diagnosis made when newborn's head delivers without delivery of neck and remaining body structures; "turtle sign" Primary risk factors, including suspected infant macrosomia, maternal diabetes mellitus, excessive maternal weight gain, abnormal maternal pelvic anatomy, maternal obesity,	If anticipated, preparatory tasks instituted: alerting of key personnel; education of woman and family regarding steps to be taken in the event of a difficult birth; emptying of woman's bladder to allow additional room for possible manoeuvres needed for the birth McRobert's maneuvre or suprapubic pressure (not fundal) (see Fig. 21.1). Combination of manoeuvres effective in more than 100% of cases of shoulder dystocia (Allen & Gurewitsch, 2010)	Intervene immediately due to cord compression. Perform McRobert's manoeuvre (application of suprapubic pressure) and be prepared to assist in other manoeuvres. Assist with positioning the woman in squatting position, hands-and-knees position, or lateral recumbent position for birth to free shoulder. Clear room of unnecessary clutter to make room for additional personnel and equipment.

	Risk for umbilical cord compression between the fetal body and the maternal pelvis	post-dates pregnancy, short stature, a history of previous shoulder dystocia, precipitous second stage, multiple pregnancy, induction of labour, prolonged labour, operative vaginal delivery, and use of epidural analgesia (Allen & Gurewitsch, 2010; Davies, Maxwell, & McLeod, 2010)	Newborn resuscitation team readily available	After the birth, assess newborn for crepitus, deformity, Erb's palsy, or bruising, which might suggest neurologic damage or a fracture of clavicle or humorous (Allen & Gurewitsch, 2010).
Multiple gestation	More than one fetus, leading to uterine overdistention and possibly resulting in hypotonic contractions and abnormal presentations of the fetuses. Fetal hypoxia during labour a significant threat due to placenta providing oxygen and nutrients to more than one fetus	Nearly all multiples are now diagnosed early by ultrasound. Most women go into labour before 37 weeks.	Admission to facility with specialized care unit if woman goes into labour. Spontaneous progression of labour if woman has no complicating factors and first fetus is in longitudinal lie. Separate monitoring of each FHR during labour and birth. After birth of first fetus, clamping of cord and lie of the second twin assessed. Possible external cephalic version necessary to assist in providing a longitudinal lie. Second and subsequent fetuses at greater risk for birth-related complications, such as umbilical cord prolapse, malpresentation, and placental abruption regardless of the method of delivery (Schmitz, Carnavalet, Azria, et al., 2008). Cesarean birth if risk factors high.	Assess for hypotonic labour pattern due to overdistention. Evaluate for fetal presentation, maternal pelvic size, and gestational age to determine mode of delivery. Ensure presence of neonatal team for birth of multiples. Anticipate need for cesarean birth.

(continued)

TABLE 21.1 DIAGNOSIS AND MANAGEMENT OF COMMON PROBLEMS ASSOCIATED WITH DYSTOCIA (continued)

Problem	Description	Diagnosis	Therapeutic Management	Nursing Management
Excessive fetal size and abnormalities	Macrosomia leading to fetopelvic disproportion (fetus unable to fit through the maternal pelvis to be born vaginally) Reduced contraction strength due to overdistention by large fetus leading to a prolonged labour and the potential for birth injury and trauma Fetal abnormalities possibly interfering with fetal descent, leading to prolonged labour and difficult birth	A diagnosis of fetal macrosomia can be confirmed by measuring the birth weight after birth. Suspicion of macrosomia based on increased fundal height measurements or ultrasound examination before onset of labour (if suspected due to conditions such as maternal diabetes or obesity, estimation of fetal weight via ultrasound). Leopold's manoeuvres to estimate fetal weight and position on admission to labour and birth unit	Possible trial of labour to evaluate progress Possible planned cesarean section	Assess for inability of fetus to descend. Plan for cesarean birth if maternal parameters are inadequate to give birth to large fetus.
Problems with the passageway	Contraction of one or more of the three planes of the pelvis Poorer prognosis for vaginal birth in women with android and platypelloid types of pelvis Contracted pelvis involving reduction in one or more of the pelvic diameters interfering with progress of labour: inlet, midpelvis, and outlet contracture Obstruction in the birth canal, such as placenta previa that partially or completely obstructs the internal os of the cervix, fibroids in the	Shortest AP diameter <10 cm or greatest transverse diameter <12 cm (approximation of AP diameter via measurement of diagonal conjugate, which in the contracted pelvis is <11.5 cm) Interischial tuberous diameter of <8 cm possibly compromising outlet contracture (outlet and midpelvic contractures frequently occur together)	Focus on allowing natural forces of labour contractions to push the largest diameter (biparietal) of the fetal head beyond the obstruction or narrow passage	Assess for poor contractions, slow dilation, and prolonged labour. Evaluate bowel and bladder status to reduce soft tissue obstruction and allow increased pelvic space. Anticipate trial of labour; if no labour progression after an adequate trial, plan for cesarean birth.

| Problems with the psyche | lower uterine segment, a full bladder or rectum, an edematous cervix caused by premature bearing-down efforts, and human papillomavirus (HPV) warts | Release of stress-related hormones (catecholamines, cortisol, epinephrine, beta-endorphin), which act on smooth muscle (uterus) and reduce uterine contractility (Romano & Lothian, 2008). Excessive release of catecholamines and other stress-related hormones not therapeutic. Release also results in decreased uteroplacental perfusion and increased risk for poor newborn adjustment (Romano & Lothian, 2008). | Ruling out of other possible causes of dystocia | Treatment dependent on woman's responses, such as anxiety, fear, anger, frustration, or denial (highly variable due to woman's understanding of the condition itself, past experiences, previous coping mechanisms, and the amount of family and nursing support received) Appropriate medical or surgical interventions depending on the underlying condition | Provide comfortable environment—dim lighting, music. Encourage partner to participate. Provide pain management to reduce anxiety and stress. Ensure continuous presence of staff to allay anxiety. Provide frequent updates concerning fetal status and progress. Provide ongoing encouragement to minimize the woman's stress and help her to cope with labour and to promote a positive, timely outcome (Romano & Lothian, 2008). Assist in relaxation and comfort measures to help her body work more effectively with the forces of labour. Engage the woman in conversation about her emotional well-being; offer anticipatory guidance and reassurance to increase her self-esteem and ability to cope, decrease frustration, and encourage cooperation. |

typically have soft perineal tissues that stretch readily, permitting the fetus to pass through the pelvis quickly and easily. Maternal complications are rare if the maternal pelvis is adequate and the soft tissues yield to a fast fetal descent, although perineal lacerations and postpartum hemorrhage are possible. Potential fetal complications may include head trauma, such as intracranial hemorrhage or nerve damage, and hypoxia due to the rapid progression of labour (Cunningham, Leveno, Bloom, et al., 2010).

Problems with the Passenger

Any presentation other than occiput anterior or a slight variation of the fetal position or size increases the probability of dystocia. These variations can affect the contractions or fetal descent through the maternal pelvis. Common problems involving the fetus include occiput posterior position, breech presentation, multifetal pregnancy, excessive size (macrosomia) as it relates to cephalopelvic disproportion, and structural anomalies.

Persistent occiput posterior is one of the most common malpositions. The reasons for this malposition are often unclear. This position presents slightly larger diameters to the maternal pelvis, thus slowing fetal descent. A fetal head that is poorly flexed may be responsible. In addition, poor uterine contractions may not push the fetal head down into the pelvic floor to the extent that the fetal occiput sinks into it rather than being pushed to rotate in an anterior direction. Persistent occiput posterior may be associated with a more painful labour, prolonged labour, and dystocia (Hunter, Hofmeyr, & Kulier, 2007).

Face and brow presentations are rare and are associated with fetal malformations and polyhydramnios (Bashiri, Burstein, Bar-David, et al., 2008).

Breech presentation, which occurs in 3% to 4% of labours, is frequently associated with high parity with uterine relaxation, previous breech delivery, uterine anomalies, multifetal pregnancies, placenta previa, oligohydramnios, polyhydramnios, preterm births, and fetal anomalies such as hydrocephaly and anencephaly (Cunningham et al., 2010). Perinatal mortality is increased with a breech presentation, regardless of the mode of delivery (Hofmeyr & Hannah, 2010). Women with breech presentation at term may be offered external cephalic version, which is an attempt to turn the fetus to cephalic presentation and is performed under carefully controlled clinical conditions (Hofmeyr & Kulier, 2010).

Shoulder dystocia is defined as the obstruction of fetal descent and birth by the axis of the fetal shoulders after the fetal head has been delivered. It is one of the most anxiety-provoking emergencies encountered in labour. Failure of the shoulders to deliver spontaneously places both the woman and the fetus at risk for injury. Postpartum hemorrhage, secondary to uterine atony or vaginal lacerations, is the major complication to the mother. Transient Erb's or Duchenne's brachial plexus palsies and clavicular or humeral fractures are the most common fetal injuries encountered with shoulder dystocia. Failure to deliver the whole body within 6 minutes has been shown to increase the incidence of acidosis, asphyxia, permanent central nervous system impairment, and death (Allen & Gurewitsch, 2010). Risks for shoulder dystocia include a history of shoulder dystocia, macrosomia, maternal diabetes, excessive weight gain, maternal obesity, postterm pregnancy, precipitous second stage, operative delivery (forceps or vacuum), and prolonged second stage. Prompt recognition and appropriate management, such as with McRobert's manoeuvre or suprapubic pressure, can reduce the severity of injuries to the mother and the newborn (Fig. 21.1).

> ▶ *Take* NOTE!
>
> *Prompt recognition and appropriate management of shoulder dystocia can reduce the severity of injuries to the mother and the infant. Immediately assess the infant for signs of trauma such as a fractured clavicle, Erb's palsy, or neonatal asphyxia. Assess the mother for excessive vaginal bleeding and blood in the urine from bladder trauma.*

Multiple gestation refers to twins, triplets, or more infants within a single pregnancy (Box 21.1). The incidence of multiple gestation is increasing, primarily as a result of infertility treatment (medical and surgical) and an increased number of women giving birth at older ages. The incidence of multiple births in Canada is 3 in 100 births (PHAC, 2008). The most common maternal complication is postpartum hemorrhage resulting from uterine atony.

Excessive fetal size and abnormalities can also contribute to labour and birth dysfunctions. **Macrosomia**, in which a newborn weighs more than 4,000 g (8 pounds 13 oz) at birth, complicates approximately 10% of all pregnancies but has a higher incidence in Aboriginal women (PHAC, 2008). Fetal abnormalities may include hydrocephalus, ascites, or a large mass on the neck or head. Complications associated with dystocia related to excessive fetal size and anomalies include an increased risk for postpartum hemorrhage, dysfunctional labour, increased incidence of instrumental delivery and cesarean section, increased length of hospital stay, fetopelvic disproportion, soft tissue laceration during vaginal birth, fetal injuries or fractures, asphyxia, lower Apgar scores, and increased incidence of neonatal intensive care unit admission (Pundir & Sinha, 2009).

Problems with the Passageway

Problems with the passageway (pelvis and birth canal) are related to a contraction of one or more of the three

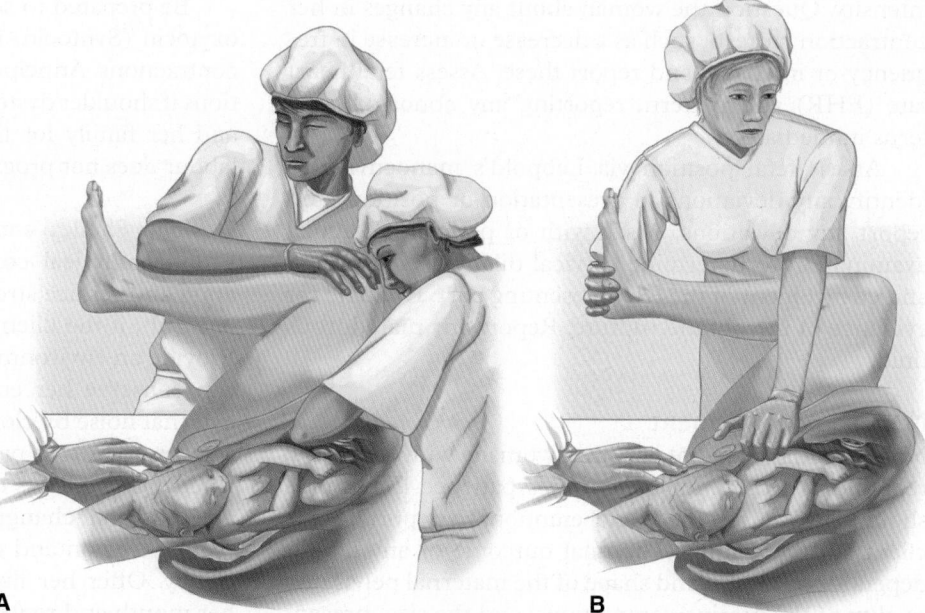

FIGURE 21.1 Manoeuvres to relieve shoulder dystocia. (**A**) McRobert's manoeuvre. The mother's thighs are flexed and abducted as much as possible to straighten the pelvic curve. (**B**) Suprapubic pressure. Pressure is applied just above the pubic bone, pushing the fetal anterior shoulder downward to displace it from above the mother's symphysis pubis. The newborn's head is depressed toward the mother's anus while suprapubic pressure is applied.

A   **B**

BOX 21.1   **Multiple Gestation**

As the name implies, multiple gestation involves more than one fetus. These fetuses can result from fertilization of a single ovum or multiple ova. Twin pregnancies that are single-ovum conceptions (monozygotic twins) share one chorion (membrane closest to the uterus), and each twin has his or her own amnion (membrane surrounding the amniotic fluid). One fertilized ovum splits into two separate individuals who are said to be natural clones. They have separate amniotic sacs and placentas, are identical in appearance, and are always the same gender. Twin pregnancies that are multiple-ova conceptions (dizygotic twins) result from two ova fertilized by two sperm. Genetically, dizygotic twins are as alike (or unlike) as any other pair or siblings (Fletcher, 2009).

The fetuses of a twin gestation, whether monozygotic or dizygotic, are slightly "squashed" because two fetuses develop in a space usually occupied by one. This compression is reflected in the slowing of weight gain in both twins compared with that for singletons.

Multiple births other than twins can be of the identical type, the fraternal type, or combinations of the two. Triplets can occur from the division of one zygote into two, with one dividing again, producing identical triplets, or they can come from two zygotes, one dividing into a set of identical twins, and the second zygote developing as a single fraternal sibling, or from three separate zygotes (Fletcher, 2009). In recent years, fertility drugs used to induce ovulation have resulted in a greater frequency of quadruplets, quintuplets, sextuplets, and even octuplets.

---

planes of the maternal pelvis: inlet, midpelvis, and outlet. The female pelvis can be classified into four types based on the shape of the pelvic inlet, which is bounded anteriorly by the posterior border of the symphysis pubis, posteriorly by the sacral promontory, and laterally by the linea terminalis. The four basic types are gynecoid, anthropoid, android, and platypelloid (see Chapter 12 for additional information). Contraction of the midpelvis is more common than inlet contraction and typically causes an arrest of fetal descent. Obstructions in the maternal birth canal, such as swelling of the soft maternal tissue and cervix, termed soft tissue dystocia, also can hamper fetal descent and impede labour progression outside the maternal bony pelvis.

Problems with the Psyche

Many women experience an array of emotions during labour, which may include fear, anxiety, helplessness, being alone, and weariness. These emotions can lead to psychological stress, which indirectly can cause dystocia.

Nursing Assessment

Begin the assessment by reviewing the client's history to look for risk factors for dystocia. Include in the assessment the mother's frame of mind to identify fear, anxiety, stress, lack of support, and pain, which can interfere with uterine contractions and impede labour progress. Helping the woman to relax will promote normal labour progress.

Assess the woman's vital signs. Note any elevation in temperature (might suggest an infection) or changes in heart rate or blood pressure (might signal hypovolemia). Evaluate the uterine contractions for frequency and intensity. Question the woman about any changes in her contraction pattern, such as a decrease or increase in frequency or intensity, and report these. Assess fetal heart rate (FHR) and pattern, reporting any abnormal patterns immediately.

Assess fetal position via Leopold's manoeuvres to identify any deviations in presentation or position, and report any deviations. Assist with or perform a vaginal examination to determine cervical dilation, effacement, and engagement of the fetal presenting part. Evaluate for evidence of membrane rupture. Report any malodorous fluid.

Nursing Management

Nursing management of the woman with dystocia, regardless of the etiology, requires patience. The nurse should provide physical and emotional support to the client and her family. The final outcome of any labour depends on the size and shape of the maternal pelvis, the quality of the uterine contractions, and the size, presentation, and position of the fetus. Thus, dystocia is diagnosed not at the start of labour but rather after labour has progressed for a time.

Promoting the Progress of Labour

The nurse plays a major role in determining the progress of labour. Continue to assess the woman, frequently monitoring cervical dilation and effacement, uterine contractions, and fetal descent, and document that all assessed parameters are progressing. Evaluate progress in active labour by using a partogram. When the woman's membranes rupture, if they have not already ruptured, observe for colour, odour, and visible cord prolapse. Continue to assess fetal well-being and document the FHR on the partogram.

> ▶ *Take* NOTE!
>
> *If a dysfunctional labour occurs, contractions will slow or fail to advance in frequency, duration, or intensity; the cervix will fail to respond to uterine contractions by dilating and effacing; and the fetus will fail to descend.*

Throughout labour, assess the woman's fluid balance status. Check skin turgor and mucous membranes. Monitor intake and output. Also monitor the client's bladder for distention at least every 2 hours and encourage her to empty her bladder often. In addition, monitor her bowel status. A full bladder or rectum can impede descent.

Continue to monitor fetal well-being. If the presenting part is high or the fetus is in the breech position, be especially observant for visible cord prolapse and note any variable decelerations in heart rate. If either occurs, report it immediately.

Be prepared to administer a labour stimulant such as oxytocin (Syntocin) if ordered to treat hypotonic labour contractions. Anticipate the need to assist with manipulations if shoulder dystocia is diagnosed. Prepare the woman and her family for the possibility of a cesarean birth if labour does not progress.

Providing Physical and Emotional Comfort

Employ physical comfort measures to promote relaxation and reduce stress. Offer blankets for warmth and a backrub, if the client wishes, to reduce muscle tension. Provide an environment conducive to rest so the woman can conserve her energy. Lower the lights and reduce external noise by closing the hallway door. Offer a warm shower or bath to promote relaxation (if not contraindicated). Use pillows to support the woman in a comfortable position, changing her position every 30 minutes to reduce tension and to enhance uterine activity and efficiency. Offer her fluids/food as appropriate to moisten her mouth and replenish her energy (Fig. 21.2).

Assist with providing counter-pressure along with backrubs if the fetus is in the occiput posterior position. Encourage the woman to ambulate or assume different positions to promote fetal rotation. Upright positions are helpful in facilitating fetal rotation and descent. Also encourage the woman to visualize the descent and birth of the fetus.

Assess the woman's level of pain and degree of distress. Administer analgesics as ordered or according to the facility's protocol.

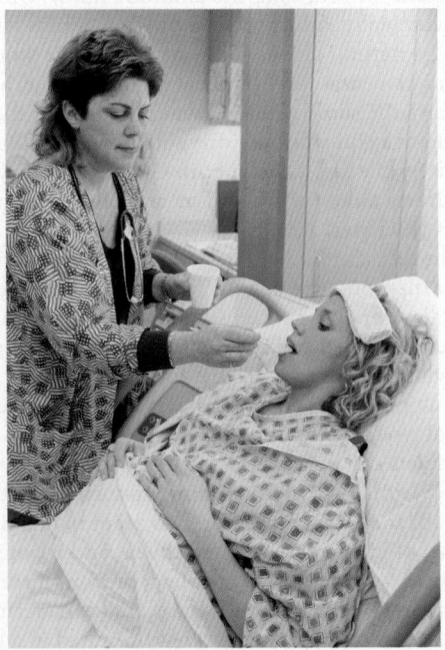

FIGURE 21.2 The nurse applies a cool, moist washcloth to the forehead and offers ice chips to combat thirst and provide comfort for the woman experiencing dystocia.

Evaluate the mother's level of fatigue throughout labour, such as verbal expressions of feeling exhausted, inability to cope in early labour, or inability to rest or calm down between contractions. Praise the woman and her partner for their efforts. Provide empathetic listening to increase the client's coping ability, and remain with the client to demonstrate caring (Romano & Lothian, 2008).

Promoting Empowerment

Educate the client and family about dysfunctional labour and its causes and therapies. Explain therapeutic interventions that may be needed to assist with the labour process. Encourage the client and her partner to participate in decision making about interventions.

Assist the woman and partner in expressing their fears and anxieties. Provide encouragement to help them to maintain control. Support the client and her partner in their coping efforts. Keep the woman and her partner informed of progress and advocate for them.

Preterm Labour

Preterm labour is defined as the occurrence of regular uterine contractions accompanied by cervical effacement and dilation before the end of the 37th week of gestation. If not halted, it leads to preterm birth. Contributing factors include infection, prior preterm birth, periodontal disease, genetic influence, working during pregnancy, lifestyle (e.g., cigarette smoking, illicit drug use, inadequate weight gain, psychological factors such as anxiety or chronic stress), and ethnicity (e.g., Aboriginal women and in the African background in the United States) (Cunningham et al., 2010; Women's Health Data Directory, 2011). The exact cause of preterm labour is not known. Currently, prevention is the goal.

Preterm births remain one of the biggest contributors to perinatal morbidity and mortality in the world. According to PHAC (2008), about 8.2% of births in Canada are preterm. One percent to 2% of deliveries occur before 34 weeks. Late preterm deliveries (between 34 and 37 weeks) occurring in a level III centre have a 99% to 100% survival rate, with the infant often appearing to be the "same" as a term baby; however, these infants require observation and interventions to maintain thermoregulation and glycemic control (Ishiguro, Namai, & Yoichi, 2009).

Preterm birth is one of the most common obstetric complications, and its sequelae have a profound effect on the survival and health of the newborn. The rate of preterm births in Canada has increased over the past 25 years. Preterm births prior to 32 weeks' gestation account for 50% of neurologic morbidity and 60% of perinatal mortality (PHAC, 2008). Infants born prematurely also are at risk for serious sequelae such as respiratory distress syndrome, respiratory failure, central nervous system hemorrhage, infections, thermoregulation problems that can lead to acidosis and weight loss, gastrointestinal complications including necrotizing enterocolitis and feeding difficulties, and long-term cognitive, visual, motor, hearing, growth, and behavioural problems (PHAC, 2008; Ross & Eden, 2011). Although great strides have been made in neonatal intensive care, prematurity remains the leading cause of infant death in Canada (PHAC, 2008).

Therapeutic Management

Predicting the risk for preterm labour is valuable only if there is an available intervention that is likely to improve the situation. Many factors influence the decision to intervene when women present with symptoms of preterm labour, including the probability of progressive labour, gestational age, and the risks of treatment. Accurate dating of the fetus is essential (Ross & Eden, 2011).

The treatment for preterm labour often includes tocolysis and varying degrees of activity restriction (Fig. 21.3). Antibiotics may be prescribed to treat presumed or confirmed infections. Steroids may be given to enhance fetal lung maturity between 24 weeks and 34 weeks' gestation.

Tocolytic Therapy

The decision to stop preterm labour is individualized based on risk factors, extent of cervical dilation, membrane status, fetal gestational age, and presence or absence of infection. **Tocolytic** therapy is most likely ordered if preterm labour occurs before the 34th week of gestation in an attempt to delay birth and thereby to reduce the severity of respiratory distress syndrome and other complications associated with prematurity. Tocolytic therapy does not typically prevent preterm birth, but it may delay it for 24 to 48 hours, allowing corticosteroid treatment to promote fetal lung maturity (Ross & Eden, 2011). It is contraindicated for abruptio placentae, acute fetal distress or death, eclampsia or severe preeclampsia, lethal fetal anomalies, significant antepartum

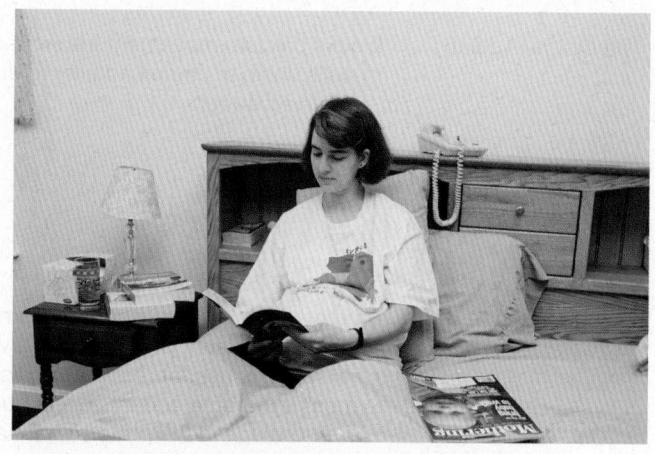

FIGURE 21.3 The mother with preterm labour resting in bed at home.

hemorrhage, imminent delivery, chorioamnionitis, other maternal indication for delivery, and maternal cardiac or renal disease (Ross & Eden, 2011).

Medications most commonly used for tocolysis include indomethacin (Indocid, a prostaglandin synthetase inhibitor) and nifedipine (Adalat, a calcium-channel blocker). These drugs are used "off label": this means while they may be effective for this purpose, they have not been officially tested, developed, and approved for this purpose by Health Canada under the Food and Drugs Act (Health Canada, 2011). These medications have serious side effects, and the woman needs close supervision when they are being administered (Drug Guide 21.1). Oxytocin antagonists (e.g., atosiban) and beta-adrenergic agonists (e.g., terbutaline) are not approved for use in Canada.

Corticosteroids

Corticosteroids given to the mother in preterm labour can help prevent or reduce the frequency and severity of respiratory distress syndrome in premature infants

delivered between 24 weeks and 34 weeks' gestation. The beneficial effects of corticosteroids on fetal lung maturation have been reported within 48 hours of initial administration (Brownfoot, Crowther, & Middleton, 2008). These drugs require at least 24 hours to become effective, so timely administration is crucial.

Nursing Assessment

The preterm birth rate cannot be reduced until there are ways to predict the risk for preterm birth. Because the etiology is often multifactorial, an individualized approach is needed.

Health History and Physical Examination

The signs of preterm labour are subtle and may be overlooked by the client as well as the health care professional. Obtain a thorough health history and be alert for risk factors associated with preterm labour and birth (Box 21.2).

Frequently, women are unaware that uterine contractions, effacement, and dilation are occurring, thus

---

DRUG GUIDE 21.1   MEDICATIONS USED WITH PRETERM LABOUR

Drug	Action/Indications	Nursing Implications
Indomethacin (Indocid)	Inhibits prostaglandins, which stimulate contractions; inhibits uterine activity to arrest preterm labour	Continuously assess vital signs, uterine activity, and FHR. Administer oral form with food to reduce GI irritation. Do not give to women with peptic ulcer disease. Schedule ultrasound to assess amniotic fluid volume and function of ductus arteriosus before initiating therapy; monitor for signs of maternal hemorrhage. Be alert for maternal adverse effects such as nausea, vomiting, heartburn, rash, prolonged bleeding time, oligohydramnios, and hypertension. Monitor for neonatal adverse effects, including constriction of ductus arteriosus, premature ductus closure, necrotizing enterocolitis, oligohydramnios, and pulmonary hypertension.
Nifedipine (Adalat)	Blocks calcium movement into muscle cells, inhibits uterine activity to arrest preterm labour	Use caution if giving this drug with magnesium sulfate because of increased risk for hypotension. Monitor for fetal effects such as decreased uteroplacental blood flow manifested by fetal bradycardia, which can lead to fetal hypoxia. Monitor for adverse effects, such as flushing of the skin, headache, transient tachycardia, palpitations, postural hypertension, peripheral edema, and transient fetal tachycardia.
Betamethasone (Celestone)	Promotes fetal lung maturity by stimulating surfactant production, prevents or reduces risk for respiratory distress syndrome and intraventricular hemorrhage in the preterm neonate less than 34 weeks' gestation	Administer two doses intramuscularly 24 h apart. Monitor for maternal infection or pulmonary edema. Educate parents about potential benefits of drug to preterm infant. Assess maternal lung sounds and monitor for signs of infection.

BOX 21.2 Risk Factors Associated with Preterm Labour and Birth

- African-American race (more than double the risk)
- Maternal age extremes: less than 16 years and more than 40 years old
- Low socioeconomic status
- Alcohol or other drug use, especially cocaine
- Poor maternal nutrition
- Maternal periodontal disease
- Cigarette smoking
- History of prior preterm birth (triples the risk)
- Uterine abnormalities
- Preexisting diabetes or hypertension
- Multiple gestation
- Premature rupture of membranes
- Late or no prenatal care
- Short cervical length
- Sexually transmitted infections: gonorrhea, *Chlamydia*, trichomoniasis
- Bacterial vaginosis (50% increased risk)
- Chorioamnionitis
- Hydramnios
- Hypertensive disorders of pregnancy
- Cervical insufficiency
- Short interpregnancy interval: less than 1 year between births
- Placental problems, such as placenta previa and placental abruption
- Maternal anemia
- Urinary tract infection
- Intimate partner violence
- Stress, acute and chronic

Source: Menon, R. (2008). Spontaneous preterm birth, a clinical dilemma: Etiologic, pathophysiologic and genetic heterogeneities and racial disparity. *Acta Obstetricia et Gynecologica Scandinavica, 87*(6), 590–600. doi:10.1080/0001634080205126.

making early intervention ineffective in arresting preterm labour and preventing the birth of a premature newborn. Ask the woman about any complaints, being alert for the subtle symptoms of preterm labour, which may include:

- Change or increase in vaginal discharge
- Pelvic pressure (pushing-down sensation)
- Low, dull backache
- Menstrual-like cramps
- Heaviness or aching in the thighs
- Regular uterine contractions, with or without pain

Assess the pattern of the contractions: the contractions must be persistent, such that six contractions occur in 1 hour, resulting in cervical change. Evaluate cervical dilation and effacement. On examination, engagement of the fetal presenting part will be noted.

Laboratory and Diagnostic Testing

Commonly used diagnostic testing for preterm labour risk assessment includes a complete blood count to detect infection, which may be a contributing factor to preterm labour; urinalysis to detect bacteria and nitrites, which are indicative of a urinary tract infection; endocervical cultures, which may indicate infections (e.g., bacterial vaginosis); a sterile speculum assessment for rupture of membranes; and a biophysical profile to evaluate fetal age and status, including amniotic fluid volume.

Other tests that may be used for preterm labour prediction include fetal fibronectin testing and cervical length evaluation by transvaginal ultrasound. However, these tests have a high negative predictive value and are thus better at predicting which pregnant women are unlikely to have a preterm birth as opposed to predicting those who will (Kiefer & Vintzileous, 2008).

Fetal Fibronectin

Fetal fibronectin, a glycoprotein produced by the chorion, is found at the junction of the chorion and decidua (fetal membranes and uterus). It is present in cervicovaginal fluid prior to delivery, regardless of gestational age. It is not found in vaginal secretions unless there has been a disruption between the chorion and decidua. The test is a useful marker for impending membrane rupture within 7 to 14 days if the level increases to greater than 0.05 µg/mL. Conversely, if fetal fibronectin is not present, there is a 99.5% chance that the woman will not go into preterm labour (Kiefer & Vintzileous, 2008).

A sterile applicator is used to collect a cervicovaginal sample during a speculum examination. The result is either positive (fetal fibronectin is present) or negative (fetal fibronectin is not present). Interpretation of fetal fibronectin results must always be viewed in conjunction with the clinical findings; it is not used as a lone indicator for predicting preterm labour.

Transvaginal Ultrasound

Transvaginal ultrasound of the cervix has been used as a tool to predict preterm labour in high-risk pregnancies and to differentiate between true and false preterm labour. Three parameters are evaluated during the transvaginal ultrasound: cervical length and width, funnel width and length, and percentage of funnelling. Measurement of the closed portion of the cervix visualized during the transvaginal ultrasound is the single most reliable parameter for prediction of preterm delivery in high-risk women (Ross & Eden, 2011).

Cervical length varies during pregnancy and can be measured fairly reliably after 16 weeks' gestation using an ultrasound probe inserted in the vagina. A cervical length of 3 cm or more indicates that delivery within 14 days is unlikely. Women with a short cervical length of 2.5 cm during the mid-trimester have a substantially greater risk for preterm birth prior to 35 weeks' gestation. As with fetal fibronectin testing, negative results can be reassuring and prevent unnecessary interventions (Kiefer & Vintzileous, 2008).

Nursing Management

Nurses play a key role in reducing preterm labour and births to improve pregnancy outcomes for both mothers and their infants. Early detection of preterm labour is currently the best strategy to improve outcomes. It is challenging to identify and address all of factors associated with preterm labour, especially when women experiencing contractions are frequently falsely reassured and not assessed thoroughly to determine the cause. This delay impedes initiation of interventions to reduce infant death and morbidity.

Preterm birth prevention programs for women at high risk have used self-monitoring of symptoms and patterns, weekly cervical examinations, telephone monitoring, home visiting, and home uterine activity monitoring, alone or in combination, with mixed results (Currell, Urquhart, Harlow, et al., 2009).

Nursing management of the woman with preterm labour involves administering tocolytic therapy if indicated, thoroughly educating the client, and providing psychological support during the process.

Administering Tocolytic Therapy

A firm diagnosis of preterm labour is necessary before treatment is considered. Diagnosis requires the presence of both uterine contractions and cervical change. A cause for preterm labour should always be sought. Absolute contraindications to tocolytic agents include intrauterine infection, fetal distress, vaginal bleeding, prolonged premature rupture of the membranes, and intrauterine demise. Bed rest and hydration are commonly recommended, but without proven efficacy.

Short-term pharmacologic therapy remains the cornerstone of management. However, there are no studies to suggest that any tocolytic agent can delay birth for longer than 48 hours (Ross & Eden, 2011). No single agent has a clear therapeutic advantage. Administer tocolytics as ordered and monitor both mother and fetus carefully for side effects.

Supportive nursing care is needed for the woman in preterm labour regardless of whether the contractions are stopped with tocolytic therapy. Nursing tasks include monitoring vital signs, measuring intake and output, encouraging bed rest on the woman's left side to enhance placental perfusion, continuously monitoring the FHR via an external monitor, limiting vaginal examinations to prevent an ascending infection, and monitoring the mother and fetus closely for any adverse effects from the tocolytic agents. Offering the couple ongoing explanations will help prepare them for the birth.

Educating the Client

Ensure that every pregnant woman receives basic education about preterm labour, including information about harmful lifestyles, the signs of genitourinary infections and preterm labour, and the appropriate response to these symptoms. Teach the client how to palpate for and time uterine contractions. Provide written materials to support this education at a level and in a language appropriate for the client. Also educate clients about the importance of prenatal care, risk reduction, and recognizing the signs and symptoms of preterm labour. Teaching Guideline 21.1 highlights important instructions related to preventing preterm labour.

Explaining to the couple what is happening in terms of labour progress, the treatment regimen, and the status of the fetus is important to reduce the anxiety associated with the risk for giving birth to a preterm infant. Educate them about the importance of promoting fetal lung maturity with corticosteroids. Include supportive family members in all education. Allow time for the woman and her family to express their concerns about the possible outcome for the infant and the possible side effects of the tocolytic therapy. Encourage them to vent any feelings, fears, and anger they may experience. Provide the woman and her family with an honest appraisal of the situation and plan of treatment throughout her care.

Providing Psychological Support

Preterm labour and birth present multifactorial challenges for everyone involved. If the woman's activities are restricted, additional stresses may be placed on the family, contributing to the crisis. Assess the stress levels of the client and family, and make appropriate referrals. Emphasize the need for more frequent supervision and office visits, and encourage clients to talk to their health care provider for reassurance.

Every case of spontaneous preterm labour is unique. Care must take into account the clinical circumstances, and the full and informed consent of the woman and her partner is needed. Half of all women who ultimately give birth prematurely have no identifiable risk factors. Nurses should be sensitive to any complaint and should provide appropriate assessment, information, and follow-up. Sensitivity to the subtle differences between normal pregnancy sensations and the prodromal symptoms of preterm labour is a key factor in ensuring timely care. Offer clarification and validation of the woman's symptoms.

If tocolytic therapy isn't successful in stopping uterine contractions, support the couple through this stressful period to prepare them for the birth. Keep them informed of all progress and changes; for example, continuously monitor maternal and fetal vital signs, especially the maternal temperature to detect signs of early infection. Offer one-on-one contact and be available throughout this difficult and anxiety-producing period.

TEACHING GUIDELINE 21.1

Teaching to Prevent Preterm Labour

- Take a daily prenatal vitamin during the pregnancy.
- Seek early prenatal care from a qualified provider and attend all prenatal appointments.
- Visit a dentist in early pregnancy to evaluate and treat periodontal disease.
- Enrol in a smoking cessation program if you are unable to quit on your own.
- Curtail sexual activity until after 37 weeks if experiencing preterm labour symptoms.
- Consume a well-balanced diet to gain appropriate weight.
- Avoid the use of substances such as marijuana, cocaine, and heroin.
- Identify factors and areas of stress in your life, and use stress management techniques to reduce them.
- If you are experiencing intimate partner violence, seek resources to modify the situation.

Recognize the signs and symptoms of preterm labour and notify your birth attendant if any occur:
- Uterine contractions, cramping, or low back pain
- Feeling of pelvic pressure or fullness
- Increase in vaginal discharge
- Nausea, vomiting, and diarrhea
- Leaking of fluid from vagina (SOGC, 2006)

If you are experiencing any of these signs or symptoms, do the following:
- Stop what you are doing and rest for 1 hour.
- Empty your bladder.
- Lie down on your side.
- Drink two to three glasses of water.
- Feel your abdomen and make note of the hardness of the contraction. Call your health care provider and describe the contraction as:
  - Mild if it feels like the tip of the nose
  - Moderate if it feels like the tip of the chin
  - Strong if it feels like your forehead

Postterm Labour

A term pregnancy usually lasts 38 to 42 weeks. A **postterm pregnancy** is one that continues past the end of the 42nd week of gestation, or 294 days from the first day of the last menstrual period. Postterm pregnancies account for about 4% to 14% of births in Canada (PHAC, 2008). Incorrect dates account for the majority of these cases because many women have irregular menses and thus cannot identify the date of their last menstrual period accurately.

*R*ecall *Jennifer, described at the beginning of the chapter, who was at 41 weeks' gestation. What information would be most important to determine on admission to the facility? What interventions might the nurse anticipate when she arrives?*

The exact etiology of a postterm pregnancy is unknown because the mechanism for the initiation of labour is not completely understood. Theories suggest there may be a deficiency of estrogen and continued secretion of progesterone that prohibits the uterus from contracting, but no evidence has validated this. A woman who has one postterm pregnancy is at greater risk for another in subsequent pregnancies.

Postterm pregnancies may adversely affect both the mother and fetus or newborn. Maternal risk is related to the large size of the fetus at birth, which increases the

chances that a cesarean birth will be needed. Other issues might include dystocia, birth trauma, postpartum hemorrhage, and infection. Mechanical or artificial interventions such as forceps- or vacuum-assisted birth and labour induction with oxytocin may be necessary. In addition, maternal exhaustion and feelings of despair over this prolonged gestation can add to the woman's anxiety level and reduce her coping ability.

Fetal risks associated with a postterm pregnancy include meconium aspiration, macrosomia, shoulder dystocia, brachial plexus injuries, and cephalopelvic disproportion. All of these conditions predispose the fetus to birth trauma or a surgical birth. The perinatal mortality rate at more than 42 weeks' gestation is twice that at term and increases fourfold and higher at 43 weeks' gestation and beyond (Delaney & Roggensack, 2008). Uteroplacental insufficiency, meconium aspiration, and intrauterine infection contribute to the increased rate of perinatal deaths (Caughey & Butler, 2011). As the placenta ages, its perfusion decreases and it becomes less efficient at delivering oxygen and nutrients to the fetus. Amniotic fluid volume also begins to decline by 40 weeks of gestation, possibly leading to oligohydramnios, subsequently resulting in fetal hypoxia and an increased risk for cord compression because the cushioning effect offered by adequate fluid is no longer present. Placental insufficiency, maternal hypertensive disorders, maternal infection, maternal substance use (especially smoking and cocaine), hypoxia, and oligohydramnios predispose the fetus to aspiration of meconium, which is released by the fetus in response to a hypoxic insult (Clark & Clark, 2010). All of these issues can compromise fetal well-being and lead to fetal distress.

Nursing Assessment

Obtain a thorough history to determine the estimated date of birth. Many women are unsure of the date of their last menstrual period, so the date given may be unreliable. Despite numerous methods used to date pregnancies, many are still misdated. Accurate gestational dating via ultrasound is essential.

Antepartum assessment for a postterm pregnancy typically includes daily fetal movement counts done by the woman, nonstress tests done twice weekly, amniotic fluid assessments as part of the biophysical profile, and weekly cervical examinations to evaluate for ripening. In addition, assess the following:

- Client's understanding of the various fetal well-being tests
- Client's stress and anxiety concerning her lateness
- Client's coping ability and support network

Nursing Management

Once the dates are established and postdate status is confirmed, monitoring fetal well-being becomes critical. When determining the plan of care for a woman with a postterm pregnancy, the first decision is whether to deliver the baby or wait. If the decision is to wait, then fetal surveillance is the key. If the decision is to have the woman deliver, labour induction is initiated. Both decisions remain controversial, and there is no clear answer about which option is more appropriate. Therefore, the plan must be individualized.

Think back to Jennifer, who is scheduled for labour induction. What ongoing nursing assessments would be important when providing care for her?

Providing Support
The intense surveillance is time-consuming and intrusive, adding to the anxiety and worry already being experienced by the woman about her overdue status. Be alert to the woman's anxiety and allow her to discuss her feelings. Provide reassurance about the expected time range for birth and the well-being of the fetus based on the assessment tests. Validating the woman's stressful state due to the prolonged pregnancy provides an opportunity for her to verbalize her feelings openly.

Educating the Woman and Her Partner
Teach the woman and her partner about the testing required and the reasons for each test. Also describe the methods that may be used for cervical ripening if indicated.

Explain about the possibility of induction if the woman's labour isn't spontaneous or if a dysfunctional labour pattern occurs. Also prepare the woman for the possibility of a surgical delivery if fetal distress occurs.

Providing Care During the Intrapartum Period
During the intrapartum period, continuously assess and monitor FHR to identify potential fetal compromise early (e.g., atypical or abnormal FHR) so that interventions can be initiated. Also monitor the woman's hydration status to ensure maximal placental perfusion. When the membranes rupture, assess amniotic fluid characteristics (colour, amount, and odour) to identify previous fetal hypoxia and prepare for prevention of meconium aspiration. Report meconium-stained amniotic fluid immediately when the membranes rupture. Anticipate the need for amnioinfusion to minimize the risk for meconium aspiration by diluting the meconium in the amniotic fluid expelled by the hypoxic fetus. In addition, monitor the woman's labour pattern closely because dysfunctional patterns are common.

Encourage the woman to verbalize her feelings and concerns, and answer all her questions. Provide support, presence, information, and encouragement throughout this time.

Women Requiring Labour Induction and Augmentation

Ideally, all pregnancies go to term, with labour beginning spontaneously. However, many women need help to initiate or sustain the labour process. **Labour induction** involves the stimulation of uterine contractions by medical or surgical means to produce delivery before the onset of spontaneous labour. The labour induction rate in Canada is approximately 20% (PHAC, 2008). Evidence is compelling that medical induction of labour increases the risk for cesarean birth (Wilson, Effken, & Butler, 2010).

Labour induction is not an isolated event: it brings about a cascade of other interventions that may or may not produce a favourable outcome. Labour induction also involves intravenous therapy, continuous electronic fetal monitoring, and significant discomfort from stimulating uterine contractions. It may also involve increased use of epidural analgesia/anesthesia and a prolonged stay on the labour unit.

Labour augmentation enhances ineffective contractions after labour has begun. Continuous electronic FHR monitoring is necessary.

There are multiple medical and obstetric reasons for inducing labour, the most common being postterm gestation. Other indications for inductions include prelabour rupture of membranes, hypertensive disorders, renal disease, chorioamnionitis, intrauterine fetal demise, and preexisting diabetes (PHAC, 2008). According to the SOGC, contraindications to labour induction are the same as contraindications to labour and vaginal delivery and may include complete placenta previa, transverse fetal lie, prolapsed umbilical cord, a prior classic uterine incision that entered the uterine cavity, previous myomectomy, previous uterine rupture, vasa previa, invasive cervical cancer, active genital herpes infection, and abnormal FHR patterns (Crane, 2001). In general, labour induction is indicated when the benefits of birth outweigh the risks to the mother or the fetus for continuing the pregnancy. However, the balance between risk and benefit remains controversial. See Evidence-based Practice 21.1.

▶ **Take** NOTE!

Before labour induction is started, fetal maturity (dating, ultrasound, amniotic fluid studies) and cervical readiness (vaginal examination, Bishop scoring) must be assessed. Both need to be favourable for a successful induction.

Therapeutic Management

The decision to induce labour is based on a thorough evaluation of maternal and fetal status. Typically, this includes an assessment to evaluate fetal size, position, and gestational age; nonstress test to evaluate fetal well-being; Nitrazine paper and/or fern test to confirm ruptured membranes; complete blood count; and vaginal examination to evaluate the cervix for inducibility. Accurate dating of the pregnancy is also essential before cervical ripening and induction are initiated to prevent a preterm birth.

Cervical Ripening

There has been increasing awareness that if the cervix is unfavourable or unripe, a successful vaginal birth is less likely. Cervical ripeness is an important variable when labour induction is being considered. A ripe cervix is shortened, centred (anterior), softened, and partially dilated. An unripe cervix is long, closed, posterior, and firm. Cervical ripening usually begins prior to the onset of labour contractions and is necessary for cervical dilation and the passage of the fetus.

Various scoring systems to assess cervical ripeness have been introduced, but the Bishop score is most

EVIDENCE-BASED PRACTICE 21.1
Labour Induction and Outcomes for Women Beyond Term

● **Study**

Postterm pregnancies may adversely affect both the mother and the fetus or newborn. Placental perfusion decreases as the placenta ages and becomes less efficient at delivering oxygen and nutrients to the fetus. Amniotic fluid volume also begins to decline by 40 weeks of gestation, increasing the fetus's risk for oligohydramnios, meconium aspiration, and cord compression. However, questions arise: what is the best time for inducing labour in a postterm pregnancy? Does labour induction improve maternal and fetal outcomes, or would it be better to wait for spontaneous labour to begin?

A study was conducted to compare the effects of inducing labour in women between 41 and 42 weeks of gestation or waiting for spontaneous labour to begin. A search was conducted for randomized, controlled trials that compared labour induction with expectant management in women who were greater than 41 + 0 weeks of gestation. Two review authors collected the data and analyzed the trials. A total of 19 trials were evaluated.

▲ **Findings**

Based on the trials analyzed, fewer perinatal deaths occurred in women who were offered labour induction at 41 + 0 weeks of gestation. There was a statistically significant rate of cesarean sections performed in the group that was not induced. There were fewer instances of fetal distress and fewer newborns experienced meconium aspiration syndrome with induction at 41 weeks or more. Statistical analysis; however, showed that these differences were not significant.

■ **Nursing Implications**

Nurses need to be aware of the potential benefits and limitations associated with labour induction so that they can provide women and their families with the most appropriate information about options for a postterm pregnancy. Nurses can integrate information from this study in their teaching about the risks associated with postterm pregnancy. They can also use this information to help answer the couple's questions about induction and its effectiveness as well as provide anticipatory guidance about the procedure. Doing so fosters empowerment of the woman and her family, promoting optimal informed decision making.

Source: Delaney, M., & Roggensack, A. (2008). SOGC clinical practice guideline: Guidelines for management of pregnancy at 41 + 0 to 42 + 0 weeks. *Journal of Obstetrics and Gynaecology Canada*, *30*(9), 800–1810. Retrieved February 28, 2012 from http://www.sogc.org/guidelines/documents/gui214CPG0809.pdf.

TABLE 21.2 BISHOP SCORING SYSTEM

Score	Dilation (cm)	Effacement (%)	Station	Cervical Consistency	Position of Cervix
0	Closed	0%–30%	−3	Firm	Posterior
1	1–2	40%–50%	−2	Medium	Midposition
2	3–4	60%–70%	−1 or 0	Soft	Anterior
3	5–6	80%	+1 or +2	Very soft	Anterior

Modified from: Bishop, E. H. (1964). Pelvic scoring for elective induction. *Obstetrics & Gynecology*, 24(2), 267.

commonly used today. The Bishop score helps identify women who would be most likely to achieve a successful induction (Table 21.2). The duration of labour is inversely correlated with the Bishop score: a score over 8 indicates a successful vaginal birth. Bishop scores of less than 6 usually indicate that a cervical ripening method should be used prior to induction (Blickstein, 2009).

Non-Pharmacologic Methods

Non-pharmacologic methods for cervical ripening are less frequently used today, but nurses need to be aware of them and question clients about their use. Methods may include herbal agents such as evening primrose oil, black haw, black and blue cohosh, and red raspberry leaves. In addition, castor oil, hot baths, and enemas are used for cervical ripening and labour induction. The risks and benefits of these agents have not been adequately studied.

Other non-pharmacologic methods suggested for labour induction are sexual intercourse and breast stimulation. Both actions promote the release of oxytocin, which stimulates uterine contractions. In addition, human semen is a biological source of prostaglandins used for cervical ripening. Sexual intercourse with breast stimulation may be beneficial, but its effectiveness has not been fully compared with other induction methods; therefore, this method for labour induction is not validated by research (Blickstein, 2009).

Mechanical Methods

Mechanical methods are used to open the cervix and stimulate the progression of labour. All share a similar mechanism of action—application of local pressure stimulates the release of prostaglandins to ripen the cervix. Potential advantages of mechanical methods, compared with pharmacologic methods, may include simplicity or preservation of the cervical tissue or structure, lower cost, and fewer side effects. The risks associated with these methods include infection, bleeding, membrane rupture, and placental disruption (Delaney & Roggensack, 2008).

For example, an indwelling (Foley) catheter (e.g., 26 French) can be inserted into the endocervical canal to ripen and dilate the cervix. This direct pressure stimulates the release of prostaglandins (Caughey & Butler, 2011).

Hygroscopic dilators such as laminaria (a type of dried seaweed) absorb endocervical and local tissue fluids. As they enlarge, they expand the endocervix and provide controlled mechanical pressure. Absorption of water leads to expansion of the dilators and opening of the cervix (Caughey & Butler, 2011).

Surgical Methods

Surgical methods used to ripen the cervix and induce labour include stripping of the membranes and performing an amniotomy. Stripping of the membranes is accomplished by inserting a finger through the internal cervical os and moving it in a circular direction. This motion causes the membranes to detach. Manual separation of the amniotic membranes from the cervix is thought to induce cervical ripening and the onset of labour (Boulvain, Stan, & Irion, 2005).

An amniotomy involves inserting a cervical hook (Amniohook) through the cervical os to deliberately rupture the membranes. This promotes pressure of the presenting part on the cervix and stimulates an increase in the activity of prostaglandins locally. Risks associated with these procedures include umbilical cord prolapse or compression, maternal or neonatal infection, FHR deceleration, bleeding, and client discomfort (Joy et al., 2011).

When either of these techniques is used, amniotic fluid characteristics (such as whether it is clear, bloody, or meconium is present) and the FHR pattern must be monitored closely.

Pharmacologic Agents

The use of pharmacologic agents has revolutionized cervical ripening. The use of prostaglandins to attain cervical ripening has been found to be highly effective in producing cervical changes independent of uterine contractions (Blickstein, 2009). In some cases, women will go into labour, requiring no additional stimulants for induction. Induction of labour with prostaglandins offers the advantage of promoting both cervical ripening and uterine contractility. A drawback of prostaglandins is their ability to induce excessive uterine contractions, which can increase maternal and perinatal morbidity (Crane, 2001; Kho, Sadler, & McCowan, 2008). Prostaglandin analogues commonly used for cervical ripening include dinoprostone gel (Prepidil), dinoprostone inserts (Cervidil), and misoprostol (Cytotec). Misoprostol, a synthetic PGE1 analogue, is a gastric cytoprotective agent used in the treatment and prevention of peptic ulcers. It can be administered intravaginally or orally to ripen the cervix or induce labour. Since the best route and dose of misoprostal have not been established, it is not used in Canada for induction of labour with a live fetus (Crane, 2001) (Drug Guide 21.2). Furthermore, it is contraindicated for women with prior uterine scars and therefore should not be used for cervical ripening in women attempting a **vaginal birth after cesarean (VBAC)**.

Oxytocin

Oxytocin is a potent endogenous uterotonic agent used for both artificial **induction** and **augmentation** of labour and is the most common induction agent used worldwide (Blickstein, 2009). It is produced naturally by the posterior pituitary gland and stimulates contractions of the uterus. For women with low Bishop scores, cervical ripening is typically initiated before oxytocin is administered. Once the cervix is ripe, oxytocin is the most popular pharmacologic agent used for inducing or augmenting labour. A woman with an unfavourable cervix may be admitted the evening before induction to ripen her cervix with one of the prostaglandin agents. Then induction begins with oxytocin the next morning if she has not already gone into labour. Doing so markedly enhances the success of induction.

Response to oxytocin varies widely: some women are very sensitive to even small amounts. The most common adverse effect of oxytocin is uterine hyperstimulation, leading to fetal compromise and impaired oxygenation (Hayes & Weinstein, 2008). The response of the uterus to

DRUG GUIDE 21.2	DRUGS USED FOR CERVICAL RIPENING AND LABOUR INDUCTION	
Drug	**Action/Indications**	**Nursing Implications**
Dinoprostone (Cervidil insert; Prepidil gel)	Directly softens and dilates the cervix/to ripen cervix and induce labour	Provide emotional support. Administer pain medications as needed. Frequently assess degree of effacement and dilation. Monitor uterine contractions for frequency, duration, and strength. Assess maternal vital signs and FHR pattern frequently. Monitor woman for possible adverse effects such as headache, nausea and vomiting, and diarrhea.
Misoprostol (Cytotec)	Ripens cervix/to induce labour with intrauterine fetal demise. Misoprostol is not recommended for use with induction for live births.	Instruct client about purpose and possible adverse effects of medication. Ensure informed consent is signed per hospital policy. Assess vital signs frequently. Monitor client's reaction to drug. Initiate oxytocin for labour induction at least 4 h after last dose was administered. Monitor for possible adverse effects such as nausea and vomiting, diarrhea, and uterine hyperstimulation.
Oxytocin (Syntocin)	Acts on uterine myofibrils to contract/to initiate or reinforce labour	Administer as an IV infusion via pump, increasing dose based on protocol until adequate labour progress is achieved. Assess baseline vital signs and FHR and then frequently after initiating oxytocin infusion. Determine frequency, duration, and strength of contractions frequently. Notify health care provider of any uterine hypertonicity or abnormal FHR patterns. Maintain careful intake and output, being alert for water intoxication. Keep client informed of labour progress. Monitor for possible adverse effects such as hyperstimulation of the uterus, impaired uterine blood flow leading to fetal hypoxia, rapid labour leading to cervical lacerations or uterine rupture, water intoxication (if oxytocin is given in electrolyte-free solution or at a rate exceeding 20 mU/min), and hypotension.

the drug is closely monitored throughout labour so that the oxytocin infusion can be titrated appropriately. In addition, oxytocin has an antidiuretic effect, resulting in decreased urine flow that may lead to water intoxication. Symptoms to watch for include headache and vomiting.

Oxytocin is administered via an intravenous infusion pump piggybacked into the main intravenous line at the port most proximal to the insertion site. Usually 10 units of oxytocin is added to 1 L of isotonic solution to achieve an infusion rate of 0.5 to 20 mU/minute (6 to 120 mL/ hour) with consistent assessment (Crane, 2001). The dose is titrated according to protocol to achieve stable contractions every 2 to 3 minutes lasting 40 to 60 seconds (Hayes & Weinstein, 2008; Joy et al., 2011). The uterus should relax between contractions. If the resting uterine tone remains above 20 mm Hg, uteroplacental insufficiency and fetal hypoxia can result. This underscores the importance of continuous FHR monitoring.

Oxytocin has many advantages: it is potent and easy to titrate, it has a short half-life (3 to 10 minutes), and it is generally well tolerated. Induction using oxytocin has side effects (water intoxication, hypotension, and uterine hypertonicity), but because the drug does not cross the placental barrier, no direct fetal problems have been observed (Hayes & Weinstien, 2008) (Fig. 21.4).

Remember Jennifer, the young woman described at the beginning of the chapter? After her cervix is ripened, an oxytocin infusion is started and her progress is slow. What encouragement can the nurse offer? After a few hours, her contractions begin to increase in intensity and frequency. What typical pain management measures can the nurse implement, and how would the nurse evaluate the effectiveness of these measures?

Nursing Assessment

Nursing assessment of the woman who is undergoing labour induction or augmentation involves a thorough history and physical examination. Review the woman's history for relative indications for induction or augmentation, such as diabetes, hypertension, postterm status, dysfunctional labour pattern, prolonged ruptured membranes, and maternal or fetal infection, and for contraindications such as placenta previa, overdistended uterus, active genital herpes, fetopelvic disproportion, fetal malposition, or severe fetal distress.

Assist with determining the gestational age of the fetus to prevent a preterm birth. Assess fetal well-being to validate the client's and fetus's ability to withstand labour contractions. Evaluate the woman's cervical status, including cervical dilation and effacement, and station via vaginal examination as appropriate before cervical ripening or induction is started. Determine the Bishop score to determine the probable success of induction.

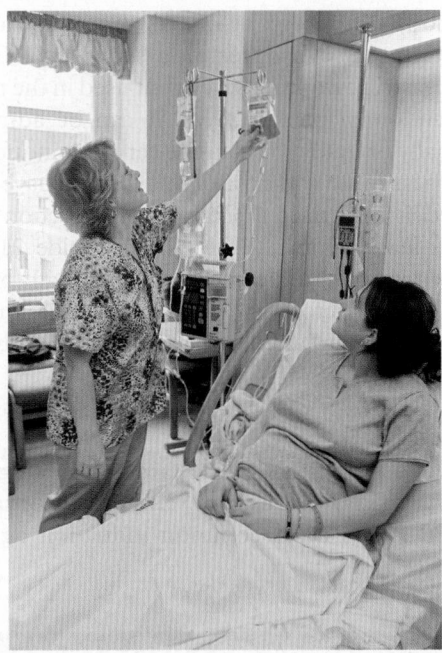

FIGURE 21.4 The nurse monitors an intravenous infusion of oxytocin being administered to a woman in labour.

▶ **Take** NOTE!

Nurses working with women in labour play an important role acting as the "eyes" and "ears" for the birth attendant because they remain at the client's bedside throughout the entire experience. Close, frequent assessment and follow-up interventions are essential to ensure the safety of the mother and her unborn child during cervical ripening and labour induction or augmentation.

Nursing Management

Explain to the woman and her partner about the induction or augmentation procedure clearly, using simple terms (Teaching Guideline 21.2). Ensure that an informed consent has been signed after the client and her partner have received complete information about the procedure, including its advantages, disadvantages, and potential risks. Ensure that the Bishop score has been determined before proceeding. Nursing Care Plan 21.1 presents an overview of the nursing care for a woman undergoing labour induction.

Administering Oxytocin

If not already done, prepare the oxytocin infusion by diluting 10 units of oxytocin in 1,000 mL of lactated Ringer's solution. Use an infusion pump on a secondary line connected to the primary infusion. Start the oxytocin infusion in mU/minute or mL/hour as ordered. Typically,

TEACHING GUIDELINE 21.2

TEACHING GUIDELINE 21.2

Teaching in Preparation for Labour Induction

- Your health care provider may recommend that you have your labour induced. This may be necessary for a variety of reasons, such as elevated blood pressure, a medical condition, prolonged pregnancy over 41 weeks, or problems with FHR patterns or fetal growth.
- Your health care provider may use one or more methods to induce labour, such as stripping the membranes, breaking the amniotic sac to release the fluid, administering medication close to or in the cervix to soften it, or administering a medication called oxytocin (Syntocin) to stimulate contractions.
- Labour induction is associated with some risks and disadvantages, such as overactivity of the uterus; nausea, vomiting, or diarrhea; and changes in FHR.
- Prior to inducing your labour, your health care provider may perform a procedure to ripen your cervix to help ensure a successful induction.
- Medication may be placed around your cervix the day before you are scheduled to be induced.
- During the induction, your contractions may feel stronger than normal. However, the length of your labour may be reduced with induction.
- Medications for pain relief and comfort measures will be readily available.
- Health care staff will be present throughout labour.

the initial dose is 1 to 2 mU/minute; anticipate increasing the rate in increments of 1 to 2 mU/minute every 30 minutes to a maximum of 20 mU/minute. Maintain the rate once the desired contraction frequency has been reached. To ensure adequate maternal and fetal surveillance during induction or augmentation, the SOGC recommends a nurse-to-client ratio that does not exceed 1:1 (Rowe, 2007).

During induction or augmentation, monitoring of the maternal and fetal status is essential. Apply an external electronic fetal monitor or assist with placement of an internal device. Obtain the mother's vital signs and the FHR every 15 minutes during the first stage. Evaluate and document the contractions (frequency, duration, and intensity) and resting tone, and adjust the oxytocin infusion rate accordingly. Monitor and document the FHR, including baseline rate, baseline variability, and decelerations, to determine whether the oxytocin rate needs adjustment. Discontinue the oxytocin and notify the birth attendant if uterine hyperstimulation or an abnormal FHR pattern occurs. Perform or assist with periodic vaginal examinations to determine cervical dilation and fetal descent, and document labour progress on the partogram.

Continue to monitor the FHR continuously and document it every 15 minutes during the active phase of labour and every 5 minutes during the second stage. Assist with pushing efforts during the second stage.

Measure and record intake and output to prevent excess fluid volume. Encourage the client to empty her bladder every 2 hours to prevent soft tissue obstruction.

Providing Pain Relief and Support

Assess the woman's level of pain. Ask her frequently to rate her pain and provide pain management as needed. Offer position changes and other non-pharmacologic measures. Note her reaction to any medication given, and document its effect. Monitor her need for comfort measures as contractions increase.

Throughout induction and augmentation, frequently reassure the woman and her partner about the fetal status and labour progress. Provide them with frequent updates on the condition of the woman and the fetus. Assess the woman's ability to cope with stronger contractions. Provide support and encouragement as indicated.

After a very long day, Jennifer gives birth to a healthy baby boy with Apgar scores of 9 at 1 minute and 10 at 5 minutes. When transferring her to the postpartum unit, what information is essential to include for the accepting nurse? What specific nursing information should be given to the nursery nurse regarding the labouring experience? With such a lengthy labour, what assessments might the postpartum nurse be especially focused on for the first few hours after birth?

Intrauterine Fetal Demise

When an unborn life suddenly ends with fetal loss, the family members are profoundly affected. The sudden loss of an expected child is tragic and the family's grief can be very intense: it can leave families struggling with a variety of mental health challenges (Bennett, Litz, Maguen, et al., 2008).

Fetal death can be due to numerous conditions, such as infection, hypertension, advanced maternal age, maternal obesity, multiple pregnancy, diabetes, congenital anomalies, umbilical cord accident, placental abruption, hemorrhage, or coagulopathies; or it may go unexplained (PHAC, 2008). Early pregnancy loss (less than 20 weeks' gestation) may be through a spontaneous abortion (miscarriage), an induced abortion (therapeutic abortion), or a ruptured ectopic pregnancy. A wide spectrum of feelings

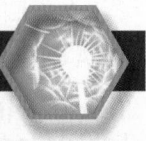

Nursing Care Plan 21.1

OVERVIEW OF THE WOMAN UNDERGOING LABOUR INDUCTION

Rose, a 29-year-old primipara, is admitted to the labour and birth suite at 40 weeks' gestation for induction of labour. Assessment reveals that her cervix is ripe and 80% effaced, and dilated to 2 cm. Rose says, "I'm a bit nervous about being induced. I've never been through labour before and I'm afraid that I'll have a lot of pain from the medicine used to start the contractions." She consents to being induced but wants reassurance that this procedure won't harm the baby. Upon examination, the fetus is engaged and in a cephalic presentation, with the vertex as the presenting part. Her partner is at her side. Induction is initiated with oxytocin. Rose reports that contractions have started and are beginning to get stronger.

NURSING DIAGNOSIS: Anxiety related to induction of labour and lack of experience with labour *as evidenced by statements about being nervous, not having gone through labour before, and fear of pain*

Outcome Identification and Evaluation

Client will experience decrease in anxiety as evidenced by ability to verbalize understanding of procedures involved and use of positive coping skills to reduce anxious state.

Interventions: Minimizing Anxiety

- Provide a clear explanation of the labour induction process *to provide client and partner with a knowledge base.*
- Maintain continuous physical presence *to provide physical and emotional support and demonstrate concern for maternal and fetal well-being.*
- Explain each procedure before carrying it out and answer questions *to promote understanding of procedure and rationale for use and decrease fears of the unknown.*
- Review with client measures used in the past to deal with stressful situations *to determine effectiveness;* encourage use of past effective coping strategies *to aid in controlling anxiety.*
- Instruct client's partner in helpful measures to assist client in coping and encourage their use *to foster joint participation in the process and feelings of being in control and to provide support to the client.*
- Offer frequent reassurance of fetal status and labour progress *to help alleviate client's concerns and foster continued participation in the labour process.*

NURSING DIAGNOSIS: Risk for injury (maternal or fetal) related to induction procedure *as evidenced by client's concerns about fetal well-being and possible adverse effects of oxytocin administration*

Outcome Identification and Evaluation

Client will remain free of complications associated with induction *as evidenced by progression of labour as expected, delivery of healthy newborn, and absence of signs and symptoms of maternal and fetal adverse effects.*

Interventions: Promoting Maternal and Fetal Safety

- Follow agency's protocol for medication use and infusion rate *to ensure accurate, safe drug administration.*
- Set up oxytocin IV infusion to piggyback into the primary IV infusion line *to allow for prompt discontinuation should adverse effects occur.*
- Use an infusion pump *to deliver accurate dose as ordered.*
- Gradually increase oxytocin dose in increments of 1 to 2 mU/minute every 30 to 60 minutes based on assessment findings and protocol *to promote effective uterine contractions.*
- Maintain oxytocin rate once desired frequency of contractions has been reached *to ensure continued progress in labour.*
- Accurately monitor contractions for frequency, duration, and intensity and resting tone *to prevent development of hypertonic contractions.*
- Monitor FHR via continuous electronic fetal monitoring to observe the FHR response to titrated medication rate *to ensure fetal well-being and identify adverse effects immediately.*
- Obtain maternal vital signs every 1 to 2 hours or as indicated by agency's protocol, reporting any deviations, *to promote maternal well-being and allow for prompt detection of problems.*
- Communicate with birth attendant frequently concerning progress *to ensure continuity of care.*
- Discontinue oxytocin infusion if tetanic contractions (>90 seconds), uterine hyperstimulation (<2 minutes apart), elevated uterine resting tone, or an atypical or abnormal FHR pattern occurs *to minimize the risk for adverse drug effects.*
- Provide client with frequent reassurance of maternal and fetal status *to minimize anxiety.*

Nursing Care Plan 21.1 (continued)

NURSING DIAGNOSIS: Pain related to uterine contractions *as evidenced by client's statements about contractions increasing in intensity and expected effect of oxytocin administration*

Outcome Identification and Evaluation
Client will report a decrease in pain as evidenced by statements of increased comfort and pain rating of 3 or less on numeric pain rating scale.

Interventions: Promoting Comfort and Pain Relief
- Explain to the client that she will experience discomfort sooner than with naturally occurring labour *to promote client's awareness of events and prepare client for the experience.*
- Frequently assess client's pain using a pain rating scale *to quantify client's level of pain and evaluate effectiveness of pain-relief measures.*
- Provide comfort measures, such as hygiene, backrubs, music, and distraction, and encourage the use of breathing and relaxation techniques *to help promote relaxation.*
- Provide support for her partner *to aid in alleviating stress and concerns.*
- Employ non-pharmacologic methods, such as position changes, birthing ball, hydrotherapy, visual imagery, and effleurage, *to help manage pain and foster feelings of control over situation.*
- Administer pharmacologic agents such as analgesia or anesthesia as appropriate and as ordered *to control pain.*
- Continuously reassess client's pain level *to evaluate effectiveness of pain management techniques used.*

---

may be expressed, from relief to sadness and despair. A stillbirth can occur at any gestational age (after 20 weeks' gestation), and typically there is little or no warning other than reduced fetal movement.

The period following a fetal death is extremely difficult for the family. For many women, emotional healing takes much longer than physical healing. The feelings of loss can be intense. The grief response in some women may be so great that their relationships become strained, and healing can become hampered unless appropriate interventions and support are provided.

Fetal death also affects the health care staff. Despite the trauma that the loss of a fetus causes, some staff members avoid dealing with the bereaved family, never talking about or acknowledging their grief. This seems to imply that not discussing the problem will allow the grief to dissolve and vanish. As a result, the family's needs go unrecognized. Failing to keep the lines of communication open with a bereaved client and her family closes off some of the channels to recovery and healing that may be desperately needed. Subsequently, the bereaved family members may feel isolated.

Nursing Assessment

History and physical examination are of limited value in the diagnosis of fetal death, since the only history tends to be recent absence of fetal movement. An inability to obtain fetal heart sounds on examination suggests fetal demise, but an ultrasound is necessary to confirm the absence of fetal cardiac activity. Once fetal demise is confirmed, induction of labour is indicated.

Nursing Management

The nurse can play a major role in assisting the grieving family. With skillful intervention, the bereaved family may be better prepared to resolve their grief and move forward. To assist families in the grieving process, include the following measures:

- Provide accurate, understandable information to the family.
- Encourage discussion of the loss and venting of feelings of grief and guilt.
- Provide the family with baby mementos and pictures to validate the reality of death.
- Allow unlimited time with the stillborn infant after birth to validate the death; provide time for the family members to be together and grieve; offer the family the opportunity to see, touch, and hold the infant.
- Use appropriate touch, such as holding a hand or touching a shoulder.
- Inform the chaplain or the religious leader of the family's denomination about the death and request his or her presence.
- Assist the parents with the funeral arrangements or disposition of the body.
- Provide the parents with brochures offering advice about how to talk to other siblings about the loss.
- Refer the family to a local support group designed for those who have lost an infant through abortion, miscarriage, fetal death, stillbirth, or other tragic circumstances.
- Make community referrals to promote a continuum of care after discharge.

Women Experiencing an Obstetric Emergency

Obstetric emergencies are challenging to all labour and birth personnel because of the increased risk for adverse outcomes for the mother and fetus. Quick clinical judgment and good critical decision making will increase the odds of a positive outcome for both mother and fetus. This chapter discusses a few of these emergencies: umbilical cord prolapse, placental abruption, uterine rupture, and amniotic fluid embolism.

Umbilical Cord Prolapse

An **umbilical cord prolapse** is the protrusion of the umbilical cord alongside (occult) or ahead of the presenting part of the fetus (Fig. 21.5). This condition occurs in 0.6% of deliveries and requires prompt recognition and intervention for a positive outcome (Beall & Ross, 2012). The risk is increased further when the presenting part does not fill the lower uterine segment, as is the case with incomplete breech presentations (5% to 10%), premature infants, and multiparous women (Beall & Ross, 2012). With a 50% perinatal mortality rate, cord prolapse is one of the most catastrophic events in the intrapartum period (Rodgers & Schiavone, 2008).

Pathophysiology

Prolapse usually leads to total or partial occlusion of the cord. Since this is the fetus's only lifeline, fetal perfusion deteriorates rapidly. Complete occlusion renders the fetus helpless and oxygen-deprived. The fetus will die if the cord compression is not relieved.

Nursing Assessment

Prevention is the key to managing cord prolapse by identifying clients at risk for this condition. Carefully assess each client to help predict her risk status. Be aware that cord prolapse is more common in pregnancies involving malpresentation, prematurity, ruptured membranes with a fetus at a high station, polyhydramnios, grand multiparity, and multifetal gestation (Beall & Ross, 2012). Continuously assess the client and fetus to detect changes and to evaluate the effectiveness of any interventions performed.

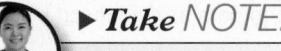

▶ **Take** NOTE!

When the presenting part does not fully occupy the pelvic inlet, prolapse is more likely to occur.

Nursing Management

Prompt recognition of a prolapsed cord is essential to reduce the risk for fetal hypoxia resulting from prolonged cord compression. When membranes are artificially ruptured, assist with verifying that the presenting part is well applied to the cervix and engaged into the pelvis. If pressure or compression of the cord occurs, assist with measures to relieve the compression. Typically, the examiner places a sterile gloved hand into the vagina and holds the presenting part of the umbilical cord until delivery. Changing the woman's position to a modified Sims, Trendelenburg, or knee–chest position also helps relieve cord pressure. Monitor FHR, maintain bed rest, and administer oxygen if ordered. Provide emotional support and explanations as to what is going on to allay the woman's fears and anxiety. If the mother's cervix is not fully dilated, prepare the woman for an emergency cesarean birth to save the fetus's life.

Placental Abruption

Placental abruption refers to premature separation of a normally implanted placenta from the maternal myometrium. Placental abruption occurs in about 1% of all

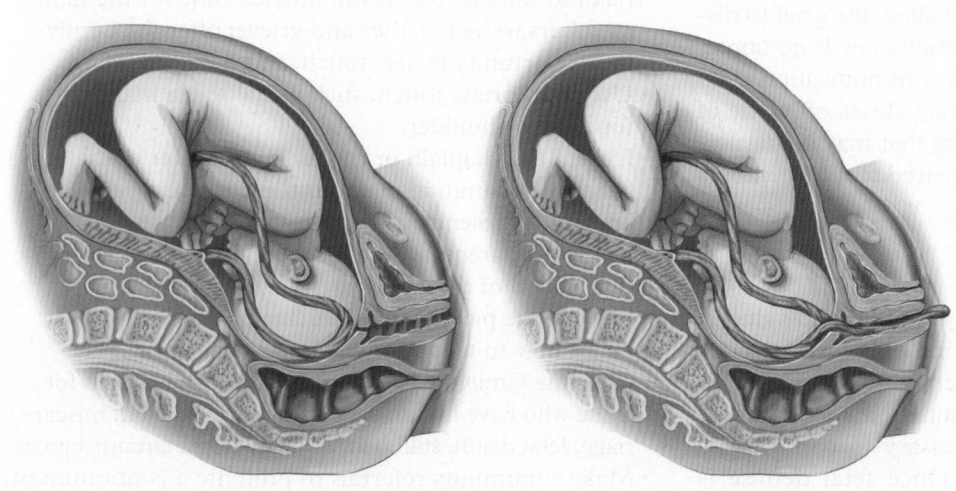

FIGURE 21.5 Prolapsed cord. (**A**) Prolapse within the uterus. (**B**) Prolapse with the cord visible at the vulva.

pregnancies throughout the world. Risk factors include hypertensive disorders, intrauterine growth restriction, prolonged rupture of membranes, chorioamnionitis, advanced maternal age, seizure activity, uterine rupture, trauma, smoking, cocaine use, coagulation defects, previous history of abruption, trauma (including domestic violence), and placental pathology. These conditions may force blood into the underlayer of the placenta and cause it to detach (Neilson, 2003).

Management of placental abruption depends on the gestational age, the extent of the hemorrhage, and maternal–fetal oxygenation perfusion/reserve status (see Chapter 19 for additional information on abruptio placenta). Treatment is based on the circumstances. Typically once the diagnosis is established, the focus is on maintaining the cardiovascular status of the mother and developing a plan to deliver the fetus quickly. A cesarean birth takes place if the fetus is still alive. A vaginal birth may take place if there is fetal demise.

Uterine Rupture

Uterine rupture is a catastrophic tearing of the uterine wall into the abdominal cavity. Its onset is often marked only by sudden fetal bradycardia, and treatment requires rapid surgery for good outcomes. From the time of diagnosis to delivery, only 10 to 37 minutes are available before clinically significant fetal morbidity occurs. Fetal morbidity occurs secondary to catastrophic hemorrhage, fetal anoxia, or both (Nahum & Pham, 2010).

Nursing Assessment

Review the mother's history for risk conditions such as previous uterine surgery (including cesarean section), prior rupture, trauma, prior invasive molar pregnancy, history of placenta percreta or increta, malpresentation, labour induction with excessive uterine stimulation, dystocia, overdistended uterus (multiple gestation or polyhydramnios), and crack cocaine use (Nahum & Pham, 2010). Reviewing a client's history for risk factors might prove to be life-saving for both mother and fetus.

Generally, the first and most reliable symptom of uterine rupture is sudden fetal distress. Other signs may include decreased baseline uterine pressure, loss of uterine contractility, abdominal pain with or without an epidural, hemorrhage, irregular abdominal wall contour, loss of station in the fetal presenting part, and hypovolemic shock in the woman, fetus, or both (Nahum & Pham, 2010).

Timely management of uterine rupture depends on prompt detection. Because many women desire a trial of labour after a previous cesarean birth, the nurse must be familiar with the signs and symptoms of uterine rupture. It is difficult to prevent uterine rupture or to predict which women will experience rupture, so constant preparedness is necessary.

Screening all women with previous uterine surgical scars is important, and continuous electronic fetal monitoring should be used during labour because this may provide the only indication of an impending rupture.

Nursing Management

Because the presenting signs may be nonspecific, the initial management will be the same as that for any other cause of acute fetal distress. Urgent delivery by cesarean birth is usually indicated. Monitor maternal vital signs and observe for hypotension and tachycardia, which might indicate hypovolemic shock. Assist in preparing for an emergency cesarean birth by alerting the operating room staff, anesthesia provider, and neonatal team. Insert an indwelling urinary (Foley) catheter if one is not in place already. Inform the woman of the seriousness of this event and remind her that the health care staff will be working quickly to ensure her health and that of her fetus. Remain calm and provide reassurance that everything is being done to ensure a safe outcome for both.

The life-threatening nature of uterine rupture is underscored by the fact that the maternal circulatory system delivers approximately 500 mL of blood to the term uterus every minute. Maternal death is a real possibility without rapid intervention. Newborn outcome after rupture depends largely on the speed with which surgical rescue is carried out.

> ▶ *Take* NOTE!
>
> *When excessive bleeding occurs during the childbirth process and it persists or signs such as bruising or petechiae appear, disseminated intravascular coagulation (DIC) should be suspected.*

Amniotic Fluid Embolism

Amniotic fluid embolism is a rare and often fatal event characterized by the sudden onset of hypotension, hypoxia, and coagulopathy. Amniotic fluid containing particles of debris (e.g., hair, skin, vernix, or meconium) enters the maternal circulation and obstructs the pulmonary vessels, causing respiratory distress and circulatory collapse (Spiliopoulos, Puri, Neetu, et al., 2009). The incidence is approximately 1 case per 8,000 to 80,000 pregnancies. Due to improvements in early recognition and treatment, the maternal mortality rate has decreased to 61% (Toy, 2009).

Pathophysiology

Normally, amniotic fluid does not enter the maternal circulation because it is contained within the uterus, sealed off by the amniotic sac. An embolus occurs when the barrier between the maternal circulation and the amniotic fluid is broken and amniotic fluid enters the maternal venous system via the endocervical veins, the placental site (if the placenta is separated), or a site of uterine trauma. This condition has a high mortality rate: as many as 50% of women die within the first hour after the onset of symptoms, and most survivors have permanent neurologic impairment (Moore, 2012).

Although medical science has supplied many answers to questions about this condition, health care providers remain largely unable to predict or prevent an amniotic fluid embolism or to significantly decrease its mortality rate.

Nursing Assessment

No test can diagnose an amniotic fluid embolism. Therefore, the nurse's assessment skills are critical. Immediate recognition and diagnosis of this condition are essential to improve maternal and fetal outcomes. Until recently, the diagnosis could be made only after an autopsy of the mother revealed squamous cells, lanugo, or other fetal and amniotic material in the pulmonary arterial vasculature (Moore, 2012).

The clinical appearance is varied, but most women experience difficulty breathing and hypotension. Other symptoms may include cyanosis, seizures, tachycardia, coagulation failure, DIC, pulmonary edema, uterine atony with subsequent hemorrhage, acute respiratory distress syndrome, and cardiac arrest (Moore, 2012).

> ▶ **Take** NOTE!
>
> *Amniotic fluid embolism should be suspected in any pregnant women with an acute onset of dyspnea, hypotension, and DIC. By knowing how to intervene, the nurse can promote a better chance of survival for both the mother and her newborn.*

Nursing Management

Upon recognizing the signs and symptoms, institute supportive measures: oxygenation (resuscitation and 100% oxygen), circulation (intravenous fluids, inotropic agents to maintain cardiac output and blood pressure), control of hemorrhage and coagulopathy (oxytocic agents to control uterine atony and bleeding), seizure precautions, and administration of steroids to control the inflammatory response (Moore, 2012).

Care is largely supportive and aimed at maintaining oxygenation and hemodynamic function and correcting coagulopathy. There is no specific therapy that is lifesaving once this condition starts. Adequate oxygenation is necessary, with endotracheal intubation and mechanical ventilation for most women. Vasopressors are used to maintain hemodynamic stability. Management of DIC may involve replacement with packed red blood cells or fresh-frozen plasma as necessary. Oxytocin infusions and prostaglandin analogues can be used to address uterine atony.

Explain to the client and family what is happening and what therapies are being instituted. The woman is usually transferred to a critical care unit for intensive observation and care. Assist the family to express their feelings and provide support as needed.

Women Requiring Birth-Related Procedures

Most women can give birth without the need for operative obstetric interventions. Most will expect to have a "natural" birth experience and don't anticipate the need for medical intervention. However, in some situations interventions are necessary to safeguard the health of the mother and the fetus. The most common birth-related procedures are amnioinfusion, episiotomy (see Chapter 14), forceps-assisted or vacuum-assisted birth, cesarean birth, and vaginal birth following a previous cesarean birth. Nurses play a major role in helping the couple to cope with any unanticipated procedures by offering a thorough explanation of the procedure, its anticipated benefits and risks, and any other options available.

Amnioinfusion

Amnioinfusion is a technique in which a volume of warmed, sterile, normal saline or Ringer's lactate solution is introduced into the uterus through an intrauterine pressure catheter to increase the volume of fluid when oligohydramnios is present (Carter & Boyd, 2012). It is used to change the relationship of the uterus, placenta, cord, and fetus to improve placental and fetal oxygenation. Instilling an isotonic glucose-free solution into the uterus helps to cushion the umbilical cord or dilute thick meconium (Prieto, Badillo, Galán, et al., 2008).

This procedure is commonly indicated for severe variable decelerations due to cord compression, oligohydramnios due to placental insufficiency, postmaturity or rupture of membranes, preterm labour with premature rupture of membranes, and thick meconium fluid. However, it does not prevent meconium aspiration syndrome (Hofmeyr & Xu, 2010). Contraindications to amnioinfusion include vaginal bleeding of unknown origin, umbilical cord prolapse, amnionitis, uterine hypertonicity, and severe fetal distress.

There is no standard protocol for amnioinfusion. After obtaining informed consent, a vaginal examination is performed to evaluate for cord prolapse, establish dilation, and confirm presentation. Next, 250 to 500 mL of warmed normal saline or lactated Ringer's solution is administered using an infusion pump over 20 to 30 minutes. Overdistention of the uterus is a risk, so the amount of fluid infused must be monitored closely (Carter & Boyd, 2012).

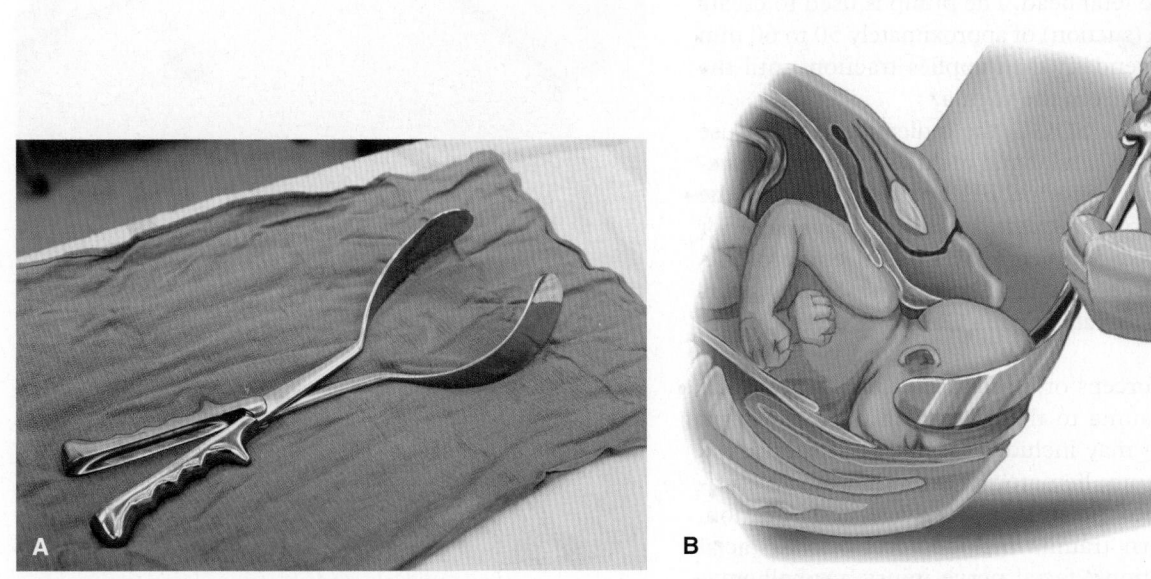

FIGURE 21.6 Forceps delivery. (**A**) Example of forceps. (**B**) Forceps being applied to the fetus.

When caring for the woman who is receiving an amnioinfusion, include the following:

- Explain the need for the procedure, what it involves, and how it may solve the problem.
- Inform the mother that she will need to remain on bed rest during the procedure.
- Assess the mother's vital signs and associated discomfort level.
- Maintain intake and output records.
- Assess the duration and intensity of uterine contractions frequently to identify overdistention or increased uterine tone.
- Monitor the FHR pattern to determine whether the amnioinfusion is improving the fetal status.
- Prepare the mother for a possible cesarean birth if the FHR does not improve after the amnioinfusion.

Forceps- or Vacuum–Assisted Birth

Forceps or a vacuum extractor may be used to apply traction to the fetal head or to provide a method of rotating the fetal head during birth. **Forceps** are stainless-steel instruments, similar to tongs, with rounded edges that fit around the fetus's head. Some forceps have open blades and some have solid blades. Outlet forceps are used when the fetal head is crowning and low forceps are used when the fetal head is at a +2 station or lower but not yet crowning. The forceps are applied to the sides of the fetal head. The type of forceps used is determined by the birth attendant. All forceps have a locking mechanism that prevents the blades from compressing the fetal skull (Fig. 21.6).

A **vacuum extractor** is a cup-shaped instrument attached to a suction pump used for extraction of the fetal head (Fig. 21.7). The suction cup is placed against

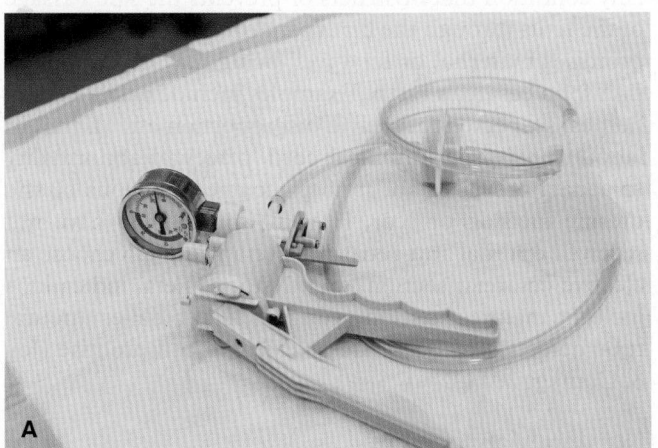

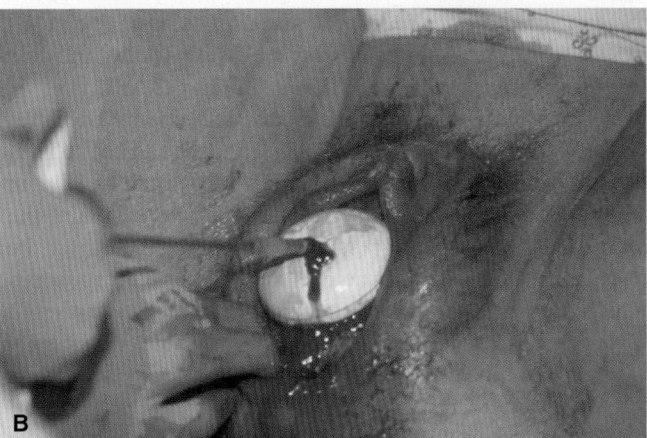

FIGURE 21.7 Vacuum extractor for delivery. (**A**) Example of a vacuum extractor. (**B**) Vacuum extractor applied to the fetal head to assist in delivery.

the occiput of the fetal head. The pump is used to create negative pressure (suction) of approximately 50 to 60 mm Hg. The birth attendant then applies traction until the fetal head emerges from the vagina.

According to the SOGC, the indications for the use of either method are similar and include a prolonged second stage of labour, abnormal FHR pattern, failure of the presenting part to fully rotate to the occiput anterior position, presumed fetal jeopardy or fetal compromise, maternal heart disease, maternal cerebrovascular malformations, and maternal fatigue (Cargill & MacKinnon, 2004).

The use of forceps or a vacuum extractor poses the risk for tissue trauma to the mother and the newborn. Maternal trauma may include lacerations of the cervix, vagina, or perineum; hematoma; extension of the episiotomy incision into the anus; hemorrhage; and infection. Potential newborn trauma includes ecchymosis, facial and scalp lacerations, facial nerve injury, cephalhematoma, intracranial hemorrhage, and caput succedaneum (Cargill & MacKinnon, 2004).

Prevention is the key to reducing the use of these techniques. Preventive measures include frequently changing the client's position, encouraging upright posture and ambulation if permitted, frequently reminding the client to empty her bladder to allow maximum space for birth, and providing adequate hydration throughout labour. Additional measures include assessing maternal vital signs, the contraction pattern, the fetal status, and the maternal response to the procedure. Provide a thorough explanation of the procedure and the rationale for its use. Reassure the mother that any marks or swelling on the newborn's head or face will disappear without treatment within 2 to 3 days. Alert the postpartum nursing staff about the use of the technique so that they can observe for any bleeding or infection related to genital lacerations.

Cesarean Birth

A **cesarean birth** is the delivery of the fetus through an incision in the abdomen and uterus. A classic (vertical) or low transverse incision may be used; today, the low transverse incision is more common (Fig. 21.8).

The number of cesarean births has risen steadily in Canada; approximately 26% of infants are delivered via this method today compared with approximately 17% in 1996 (PHAC, 2008). Several factors may explain the increased incidence of cesarean deliveries, including the widespread use of continuous electronic fetal monitoring, which identifies fetal distress early; the reduced number of forceps-assisted births; maternal obesity; older maternal age and reduced parity, with more nulliparous women having infants; convenience to the client and doctor; elective repeat cesarean sections; elective cesarean section for breech presentation as a result of the Term Breech Trial; and attitudes of clients, nurses, and physicians about birth

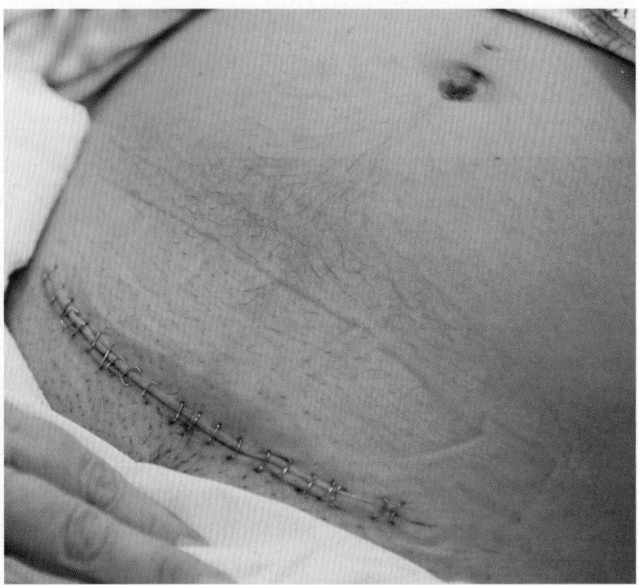

FIGURE 21.8 Low transverse incision for cesarean birth.

(Hewer, Boschma, & Hall, 2009; Kotaska, Menticoglou, & Gagnon, 2009; PHAC, 2008).

High cesarean birth rates are an international concern. Cesarean birth is a major surgical procedure with a fourfold increase in mortality compared with a vaginal birth. The client is at risk for complications such as infection, hemorrhage, aspiration, venous thromboembolus, and bowel and urinary tract trauma. Fetal injury and respiratory difficulty for the newborn also may occur (Cargill & MacKinnon, 2004).

Spinal, epidural, or general anesthesia is used for cesarean births. Epidural anesthesia is most commonly used today because it is associated with less risk and most women wish to be awake and aware of the birth experience.

Nursing Assessment

Review the woman's history for indications associated with cesarean birth and complete a physical examination. Any condition that obstructs or prevents the safe passage of the fetus through the birth canal or that seriously compromises maternal or fetal well-being may be an indication for a cesarean birth. Examples include active genital herpes, suspected fetopelvic disproportion after a trial of labour, prolapsed umbilical cord, placental abnormality (placenta previa or abruptio placentae), previous classic uterine incision or scar, HIV in women who have not received optimal anti-retroviral therapy or who choose an elective cesarean section, and dystocia. Fetal indications include malpresentation, congenital anomalies (neural tube defects, hydrocephalus), and fetal compromise (Joy & Contag, 2011).

Nursing Management

Once the decision has been made to proceed with a cesarean birth, assess the woman's knowledge of the procedure and necessary preparation. Assist with obtaining diagnostic tests as ordered. These tests are usually ordered to ensure the well-being of both parties and may include a complete blood count; blood type and cross-match so that blood is available for transfusion if needed; and an ultrasound to determine fetal position and placental location.

Although the nurse's role in a cesarean birth can be very technical and skill-oriented at times, the focus must remain on the woman, not the equipment surrounding the bed. Care should be centred on the family, not the surgery. Provide education and minimize separation of the mother, father, and newborn. Remember that the client is anxious and concerned about her welfare as well as that of her child. Use touch, eye contact, therapeutic communication, and genuine caring to provide couples with a positive birth experience, regardless of the type of delivery.

Providing Preoperative Care

Client preparation varies depending on whether the cesarean birth is planned or unplanned. The major difference is the time allotted for preparation and teaching. In an unplanned cesarean birth, institute measures quickly to ensure the best outcomes for the mother and the fetus. Ensure that the woman has signed an informed consent, and allow for discussion of fears and expectations. Provide essential teaching and explanations to reduce the woman's fears and anxieties.

Ascertain the client's and family's understanding of the surgical procedure. Reinforce the reasons for surgery given by the surgeon. Outline the procedure and expectations of the surgical experience. Ensure that all diagnostic tests ordered have been completed, and evaluate the results. Explain to the woman and her family about what to expect postoperatively. Reassure the woman that pain management will be provided throughout the procedure and afterward. Encourage the woman to report any pain.

Ask the woman about the time she last had anything to eat or drink. Document the time and what was consumed. Throughout the preparations, assess maternal and fetal status frequently.

Provide preoperative teaching to reduce the risk for postoperative complications. Demonstrate the use of the incentive spirometer and deep-breathing and leg exercises. Instruct the woman on how to splint her incision.

Complete the preoperative procedures, which may include:

• Preparing the surgical site as ordered
• Starting an intravenous infusion for fluid replacement therapy as ordered
• Inserting an indwelling (Foley) catheter and informing the client about how long it will remain in place (usually 24 hours)
• Administering any preoperative medications as ordered; documenting the time administered and the client's reaction

Maintain a calm, confident manner in all interactions with the client and the family. Help transport the client and her partner to the operative area.

Providing Postoperative Care

Postoperative care for the mother who has had a cesarean delivery is similar to that for one who has had a vaginal birth, with a few additional measures. Assess vital signs and lochia flow every 15 minutes for the first hour, then every 30 minutes for the next hour, and then every 4 hours if stable. Assist with perineal care and instruct the client in the same. Inspect the abdominal dressing and document the description, including any evidence of drainage. Assess uterine tone to determine fundal firmness. Check the patency of the intravenous line, making sure the infusion is flowing at the correct rate. Inspect the infusion site frequently for redness.

Assess the woman's level of consciousness if sedative drugs were administered. Institute safety precautions until the woman is fully alert and responsive. If a regional anesthetic was used, monitor for the return of sensation to the legs.

Assess for evidence of abdominal distention and auscultate bowel sounds. Assist with early ambulation to prevent respiratory and cardiovascular problems and to promote peristalsis. Monitor intake and output at least every 4 hours initially and then every 8 hours as indicated.

Encourage the woman to cough, perform deep-breathing exercises, and use the incentive spirometer every 2 hours. Administer analgesics as ordered and provide comfort measures, such as splinting the incision and pillows for positioning. Assist the client to move in bed and turn side to side to improve circulation. Also encourage the woman to ambulate to promote venous return from the extremities.

Encourage early touching and holding of the newborn to promote bonding. Assist with breastfeeding initiation and offer continued support. Suggest alternate positioning techniques to reduce incisional discomfort while breastfeeding.

Review with the couple their perception of the surgical birth experience. Allow them to verbalize their feelings and assist them in positive coping measures. Prior to discharge, teach the woman about the need for adequate rest, activity restrictions such as lifting, and signs and symptoms of infection.

Vaginal Birth After Cesarean

Vaginal birth after cesarean describes a woman who gives birth vaginally after having at least one previous cesarean birth. SOGC guidelines suggest that most women who have had a cesarean birth are candidates for vaginal birth and should be offered a trial of labour for subsequent pregnancies (Martel & MacKinnon, 2005).

The choice of a vaginal or a repeat cesarean birth can be offered to women who had a lower abdominal incision. However, controversy remains. The argument against VBAC focuses on the risk for uterine rupture and hemorrhage. Although the risk for uterine rupture is relatively low, 1 in 200, the rate of fetal mortality in the event of a uterine rupture is extremely high (Nahum & Pham, 2010).

Contraindications to VBAC include a prior classic uterine incision, prior hysterotomy or myomectomy, previous uterine rupture, or the presence of a contraindication to labour (Martel & MacKinnon, 2005). Most women go through a trial of labour to see how they progress, but this must be performed in an environment capable of providing continuous electronic fetal monitoring and cesarean section if needed. The use of prostaglandin E2 and misoprostol (Cytotec) increases the risk for uterine rupture and thus is not recommended in VBAC clients. The woman considering induction of labour after a previous cesarean birth needs to be informed of the increased risk for uterine scar dehiscence with an induction than with spontaneous labour (Martel & MacKinnon, 2005).

Women are the primary decision makers about the choice of birth method, but they need education about VBAC during their prenatal course. Management is similar for any women experiencing labour, but certain areas require special focus:

- Consent: fully informed consent is essential for the woman who wants to have a trial of labour after cesarean birth. The client must be advised about the risks as well as the benefits. She must understand the ramifications of uterine rupture, even though the risk is small.
- Documentation: recordkeeping is an important component of safe client care. If an emergency occurs, it is imperative not only to take care of the client but also to keep track of the plan of care, interventions and their timing, and the client's response. Events and activities can be written right on the fetal monitoring tracing to correlate with the change in fetal status.
- Surveillance: an abnormal fetal monitor tracing in a woman undergoing a trial of labour after a cesarean birth should alert the nurse to the possibility of uterine rupture. Terminal bradycardia must be considered an emergency situation, and the nurse should prepare the team for an emergency delivery.
- Readiness for emergency: according to SOGC criteria for a safe trial of labour for a woman who has had a previous cesarean birth, the physician, anesthesia provider, and operating room team must be available. Anything less would place the women and fetus at risk (Martel & MacKinnon, 2005).

Nurses must act as advocates, giving input on the appropriate selection of women who wish to undergo VBAC. Nurses also need to become experts at reading fetal monitoring tracings to identify an atypical or abnormal pattern and set in motion an emergency delivery. Including all these nursing strategies will make VBAC safer for all.

■■■ Key Concepts

- Risk factors for dystocia include epidural analgesia, excessive analgesia, multiple gestation, maternal exhaustion, hydramnios, ineffective pushing, unripe cervix with induction, maternal obesity, malpresentation, fetal anomalies, occiput posterior position, longer first stage of labour, nulliparity, short maternal stature, maternal age older than 35 years, gestational age more than 41 weeks, chorioamnionitis, pelvic contractions, macrosomia, and high station at complete cervical dilation.

- Dystocia may result from problems in the powers, passenger, passageway, or psyche.

- Problems involving the powers that lead to dystocia include hypertonic uterine dysfunction, hypotonic uterine dysfunction, and precipitous labour.

- Management of hypertonic labour pattern involves therapeutic rest with the use of sedatives to promote relaxation and stop the abnormal activity of the uterus.

- Any presentation other than occiput or a slight variation of the fetal position or size increases the probability of dystocia.

- Multiple gestation may result in dysfunctional labour due to uterine overdistention, which may lead to hypotonic dystocia, and abnormal presentations of the fetuses.

- During labour, evaluation of fetal descent, cervical effacement and dilation, and characteristics of uterine contractions are paramount to determine progress or lack thereof.

- Antepartum assessment for a postterm pregnancy typically includes daily fetal movement counts done by the woman, nonstress tests done twice weekly, amniotic fluid assessments as part of the biophysical profile, and weekly cervical examinations to check for ripening for induction.

- Once the cervix is ripe, oxytocin is the most popular pharmacologic agent used for inducing or augmenting labour.

- Generally, the first and most reliable symptom of uterine rupture is fetal distress.

- Amniotic fluid embolism is a rare but often fatal event characterized by the sudden onset of hypotension, hypoxia, and coagulopathy.

- Cesarean births have steadily risen in Canada; today, approximately one in four births occurs this way. Cesarean birth is a major surgical procedure and has increased risks over vaginal birth.

REFERENCES

Allen, R. H., & Gurewitsch, E. D. (2010). *Shoulder dystocia.* Retrieved February 28, 2012 from http://emedicine.medscape.com/article/1602970-overview

Bashiri, A., Burstein, E., Bar-David, J., Levy, A., & Mazor, M. (2008). Face and brow presentation: Independent risk factors. *The Journal of Maternal-Fetal and Neonatal Medicine, 21*(6), 357–360. doi:10.1080/14767050802037647

Beall, M. H., & Ross, M. G. (2012). *Umbilical cord complications.* Retrieved February 28, 2012 from http://emedicine.medscape.com/article/262470-overview

Bennett, S. M., Litz, B. T., Maguen, S., & Ehrenreich, J. T. (2008). An exploratory study of the psychological impact and clinical care of perinatal loss. *Journal of Loss and Trauma, 13*(6), 485–510. doi:10.1080/15325028021712668

Bishop, E. H. (1964). Pelvic scoring for elective induction. *Obstetrics and Gynecology, 24*(2), 267.

Blickstein, I. (2009). Induction of labour. *Journal of Maternal-Fetal and Neonatal Medicine, 22*(S2), 31–37.

Boulvain, M., Stan, C. M., & Irion, O. (2005). Membrane sweeping for induction of labour. *Cochrane Database of Systematic Reviews, 1,* CD000451. doi:10.1002/14651858.CD000451.pub2

Brownfoot, F. C., Crowther, C. A., & Middleton, P. (2008). Different corticosteroids and regimens for accelerating fetal lung maturity for women at risk for preterm birth. *Cochrane Database of Systematic Reviews, 4.* doi:10.1002/14651858.CD0006764.pub2

Cargill, Y. M., & MacKinnon, C. J. (2004). Guidelines for operative vaginal birth. *Journal of Obstetrics and Gynaecology Canada, 26*(8), 747–753.

Carter, B. S., & Boyd, R. L. (2012). *Pediatric polyhydramnios and oligohydramnios.* Retrieved February 28, 2012 from http://www.emedicine.com/ped/topic1854.htm

Caughey, A. B., & Butler, J. R. (2011). *Postterm pregnancy.* Retrieved February 28, 2012 from http://www.emedicine.medscape.com/article/261369-overview

Cheng, Y., & Caughey, A. B. (2012). *Normal labor and delivery.* Retrieved February 28, 2012 from http://emedicine.medscape.com/article/260036-overview

Clark, M. B., & Clark, D. A. (2010). *Meconium aspiration syndrome.* Retrieved February 28, 2012 from http://emedicine.medscape.com/article/974110-overview

Crane, J. M. (2001). SOGC clinical practice guideline: Induction of labour at term. *Journal of Obstetrics and Gynaecology Canada, 23*(8), 717–728. Retrieved February 28, 2012 from http://www.sogc.org/guidelines/public/107E-CPG-August2001.pdf

Cunningham, F., Leveno, K., Bloom, S., Hauth, J., Rouse, D., & Spong, C. (2010). *Williams obstetrics.* New York: McGraw-Hill.

Currell, R., Urquhart, C, Harlow, F., & Callow, L. (2009). Home uterine monitoring for detecting preterm labour. *Cochrane Database of Systematic Reviews, 4,* CD006172. doi:10.1002/14651858.CD006172

Davies, G. A. L., Maxwell, C., & McLeod, L. (2010). SOGC clinical practice guideline: Obesity in pregnancy. *Journal of Obstetrics and Gynaecology Canada, 32*(2), 165–173. Retrieved February 28, 2012 from http://www.sogc.org/guidelines/documents/gui239ECPG1002.pdf

Delaney, M., & Roggensack, A. (2008). SOGC clinical practice guideline: Guidelines for management of pregnancy at 41 + 0 to 42 + 0 weeks. *Journal of Obstetrics and Gynaecology Canada, 30*(9), 800–1810. Retrieved February 28, 2012 from http://www.sogc.org/guidelines/documents/gui214CPG0809.pdf

Fischer, R. (2011). *Breech presentation.* Retrieved February 28, 2012 from http://emedicine.medscape.com/article/262159-overview

Fletcher, G. E. (2009). *Multiple birth.* Retrieved February 28, 2012 from http://emedicine.medscape.com/article/977234-overview

Hayes, E. J., & Weinstein, L. (2008). Improving patient safety and uniformity of care by a standardized regimen for the use of oxytocin. *American Journal of Obstetrics and Gynecology, 198,* 622.e1–622.e7.

Health Canada. (2011). *Drugs and health products.* Retrieved September 1, 2011 from http://www.hc-sc.gc.ca/dhp-mps/prodpharma/index-eng.php

Hewer, N., Boschma, G., & Hall, W. A. (2009). Elective cesarean section as a transformative technological process: Players, power, and context. *Journal of Advanced Nursing, 65*(8), 1762–1771. doi:10.1111/j.1365–2648.2009.05021.x

Hofmeyr, G. J., & Hannah, M. (2010). Planned cesarean section for term breech delivery. *Cochrane Database of Systematic Reviews, 8,* CD 000166. doi:10.1002.14651858.CD000166

Hofmeyr, G. J., & Kulier, R. (2010). External cephalic version for breech presentation at term. *Cochrane Database of Systematic Reviews, 1,* CD000083. doi:10.1002/14651858.Cd000083

Hofmeyr, G. J., & Xu, H. (2010). Amnioinfusion for meconium-stained liquor in labour. *Cochrane Database of Systematic Reviews, 1,* CD000014. doi:10.1002/14651888.CD000014.pub3

Hunter, S., Hofmeyr, G. J., & Kulier, R. (2007). Hands and knees posture in late pregnancy or labour for fetal malposition (lateral or posterior). *Cochrane Database of Systematic Reviews, 4,* CD 001063. doi:10.1002/14651858.CD001063.pub3

Ishiguro, A., Namai, Y., & Yoichi, M. I. (2009). Managing "healthy" late preterm infants. *Pediatrics International, 51*(5), 720–725. doi:10.1111/j.1442–200X.2009.02837.x

Joy, S., & Contag, S. A. (2011). *Cesarean delivery.* Retrieved February 28, 2012 from http://emedicine.medscape.com/article/263424-overview#Indications

Joy, S., Scott, P. L., & Lyon, D. (2011). *Abnormal labour.* Retrieved February 28, 2012 from http://www.emedicine.medscape.com/article/273053-overview

Kho, E. M., Sadler, L., & McCowan, L. (2008). Induction of labour: A comparison between controlled-release dinoprostone vaginal pessary (Cervadil®) and dinoprostone intravaginal gel (Prostin E2®). *Australian and New Zealand Journal of Obstetrics and Gynecology, 48,* 473–477. doi:10.1111/j.1479–828X.2008.00901.x

Kiefer, D. G., & Vintzileous, A. M. (2008). The utility of fetal fibronectin in the prediction and prevention of spontaneous preterm birth. *Reviews in Obstetrics and Gynecology, 1*(3), 106–112.

Kotaska, A., Menticoglou, S., & Gagnon, G. (2009). SOGC clinical practice guideline: Vaginal delivery of breech presentation. *Journal of Obstetrics and Gynaecology Canada, 31*(6), 557–566. Retrieved February 28, 2012 from http://www.sogc.org/guidelines/documents/gui226CPG0906.pdf

Martel, M., & MacKinnon, C. J. (2005). SOGC clinical practice guideline: Guidelines for a vaginal birth after previous Caesarean birth. *Journal of Obstetrics and Gynaecology Canada, 27*(2), 164–174. Retrieved February 28, 2012 from http://www.sogc.org/guidelines/public/155E-CPG-February2005.pdf

Menon, R. (2008). Spontaneous preterm birth, a clinical dilemma: Etiologic, pathophysiologic and genetic heterogeneities and racial disparity. *Acta Obstetricia et Gynecologica Scandinavica, 87*(6), 590–600. doi:10.1080/00016340802055126

Moore, L. E. (2012). *Amniotic fluid embolism.* Retrieved February 28, 2012 from http://emedicine.medscape.com/article/253068-zoverview

Nahum, G. G., & Pham, K. Q. (2010). Uterine rupture in pregnancy. Retrieved February 28, 2012 from http://emedicine.medscape.com/article/275854-overview

Neilson, J. P. (2003). Interventions for treating placental abruption. *Cochrane Database of Systematic Reviews, 1,* CD003247. doi:10.1002/14651858.CD003247

Prieto, A. P., Badillo, M. P. C., Galán, S. M., & Ventoso, F. M. (2008). Prophylactic intrapartum transcervical amnioinfusion. *Current Women's Health Reviews, 4*(2), 133–140.

Public Health Agency of Canada. (2008). *Canadian perinatal health report, 2008 edition.* Retrieved February 28, 2012 from http://www.phac-aspc.gc.ca/publicat/2008/cphr-rspc/index-eng.php

Pundir, J., & Sinha, P. (2009). Non-diabetic macrosomia: An obstetrical dilemma. *Journal of Obstetrics and Gynecology, 29*(3), 200–205. doi:10.1080/01443610902735140

Rodgers, C., & Schiavone, N. (2008). Cord prolapse audit: Recognition, management and outcome. *British Journal of Midwifery, 16*(5), 315–318.

Romano, A. M., & Lothian, J. A. (2008). Promoting, protecting, and supporting normal birth: A look at the evidence. *Journal of Obstetric, Gynecologic, & Neonatal Nursing, 37*(1), 94–105. doi:10.1111/j.1552–6909.2007.00210.x

Ross, M. G., & Eden, R. D. (2011). *Preterm labour.* Retrieved February 28, 2012 from http://emedicine.medscape.com/article/260998-overview

Rowe, T. (2007). Fetal health surveillance: Antepartum and intrapartum consensus guideline. *Journal of Obstetrics and Gynaecology Canada, 29*(9 Suppl. 4), S1–S56.

Schmitz, T., Carnavalet, C. C., Azria, E., Lopez, E., Carbrol, D., & Goffinet, F. (2008). Neonatal outcomes of twin pregnancy according to the planned mode of delivery. *Obstetrics and Gynecology, 111*(3), 695–703. doi:10.1097/AOG.0b013e318163c435

Simkin, P. (2010). The fetal occiput posterior position: State of science and a new perspective. *BIRTH, 37*(1), 61–71.

Society of Obstetricians and Gynaecologists of Canada. (2006). *Preterm labour.* Retrieved February 28, 2012 from http://www.sogc.org/health/pdf/preterme.pdf

Society of Obstetricians and Gynaecologists of Canada. (2008). Joint policy statement on normal childbirth. *Journal of Obstetrics and Gynaecology Canada, 30*(12), 1163–1165.

Spiliopoulos, M., Puri, I., Neetu, J., Kruse, L., Mastrogiannis, D., & Dandolu, V. (2009). Amniotic fluid embolism-risk factors, maternal and neonatal outcomes. *Journal of Maternal-Fetal and Neonatal Medicine, 22*(5), 439–444. doi:10.1080/14767050902787216

Toy, H. (2009). Amniotic fluid embolism. *European Journal of General Medicine, 6*(2), 108–115.

Watts, N. (2010). High-risk labour and childbirth. In R. J. Evans, M. K. Evans, Y. M. Brown, & S. Orshan (Eds.), *Canadian maternity, newborn, & women's health.* Philadelphia: Lippincott Williams & Wilkins.

Wilson, B. L., Effken, J., & Butler, R. J. (2010). The relationship between cesarean section and labour induction. *Journal of Nursing Scholarship, 64*(4), 371–377.

Women's Health Data Directory. (2011). Premature/preterm birth. Retrieved March 6, 2012 from http://www.womenshealthdata.ca/category.aspx?catid=95&rt=1

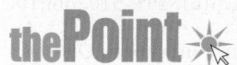

the Point For additional learning materials, including Internet Resources, visit
http://thePoint.lww.com/Chow1e.

CHAPTER WORKSHEET

MULTIPLE CHOICE QUESTIONS

1. When reviewing the medical record of a client, the nurse notes that the woman has a condition in which the fetus cannot physically pass through the maternal pelvis. The nurse interprets this as:

   a. Cervical insufficiency

   b. Contracted pelvis

   c. Maternal disproportion

   d. Fetopelvic disproportion

2. The nurse would anticipate a cesarean birth for a client who has which active infection present at the onset of labour?

   a. Hepatitis

   b. Herpes simplex virus

   c. Toxoplasmosis

   d. Human papillomavirus

3. After a vaginal examination, the nurse determines that the client's fetus is in an occiput posterior position. The nurse would anticipate that the client will have:

   a. Intense back pain

   b. Frequent leg cramps

   c. Nausea and vomiting

   d. A precipitous birth

4. When assessing the following women, which would the nurse identify as being at the greatest risk for preterm labour?

   a. Woman who had twins in a previous pregnancy

   b. Client living in a large city

   c. Woman working full-time as a computer programmer

   d. Client with a history of a previous preterm birth

5. The rationale for using a prostaglandin gel for a client prior to the induction of labour is to:

   a. Stimulate uterine contractions

   b. Numb cervical pain receptors

   c. Prevent cervical lacerations

   d. Soften and efface the cervix

6. A client who was in active labour and whose cervix had dilated to 4 cm experiences a weakening in the intensity and frequency of her contractions and exhibits no further progress in labour. The nurse interprets this as a sign of:

   a. Hypertonic labour

   b. Precipitous labour

   c. Hypotonic labour

   d. Dysfunctional labour

CRITICAL THINKING EXERCISES

1. Marsha, a 26-year-old multipara, is admitted to the labour and birth suite in active labour. After a few hours, the nurse notices a change in her contraction pattern—poor contraction intensity and no progression of cervical dilation beyond 5 cm. Marsha keeps asking about her labour progress and appears anxious about "how long this labour is taking."

   a. Based on the nurse's findings, what might you suspect is going on?

   b. How can the nurse address Marsha's anxiety?

   c. What are the appropriate interventions to change this labour pattern?

2. Marsha activates her call light and states, "I feel increased wetness down below."

   a. What might be occurring?

   b. How will the nurse confirm the suspicions?

   c. What interventions are appropriate for this finding?

STUDY ACTIVITIES

1. Visit a local pregnancy and infant loss support website (visit http://thePoint.lww.com/Chow1e for a link) and assess its helpfulness to parents.

2. Outline the fetal and maternal risks associated with a postterm pregnancy.

3. An abnormal or difficult labour describes

   _____.

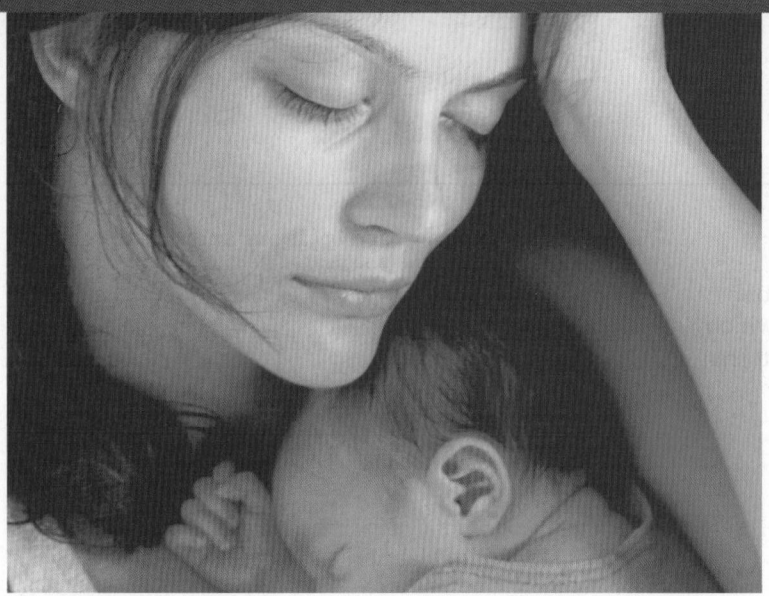

CHAPTER 22

Adapted by Susan Ruth Beischel

NURSING MANAGEMENT OF THE POSTPARTUM WOMAN AT RISK

KEY TERMS

mastitis	postpartum hemorrhage	uterine atony
metritis	(PPH)	uterine inversion
postpartum depression	subinvolution	
(PPD)	thrombophlebitis	

LEARNING OBJECTIVES

After studying the chapter, the student should be able to:

1. Define the key terms.
2. Discuss the risk factors, clinical manifestations, preventive measures, and management of common postpartum complications.
3. Describe at least two affective disorders that can occur in women after birth and specific therapeutic management to address them.
4. Differentiate the causes of postpartum hemorrhage and list appropriate assessments and interventions.
5. Outline the role of the nurse in assessing and managing care of women with selected postpartum complications.

Joan gave birth about an hour ago to her fifth baby boy, who weighed 4.55 kg (10 lb), and she is resting in bed when the nurse comes in to assess her. She tells the nurse that she feels like there is "something really wet" between her legs. She also feels a bit lightheaded. What would the nurse suspect is happening? What findings would support the nurse's suspicion? What should the nurse do first?

Wow

After holding their breath during the childbirth experience, nurses shouldn't let it out fully and relax until discharge.

Typically, recovery from childbirth proceeds normally in both physiologic and psychological aspects. It is a time filled with many changes and wide-ranging emotions, and the new mother commonly experiences a great sense of accomplishment. However, the woman can experience deviations from the norm, developing a postpartum condition that places her at risk. The development of a high-risk condition or complication can become a life-threatening event. This chapter addresses the nursing management of the most common conditions that place the postpartum woman at risk: hemorrhage, infection, thromboembolic disease, and postpartum emotional disorders.

Postpartum Hemorrhage

Postpartum hemorrhage (PPH) is a potentially life-threatening complication of both vaginal and cesarean births. It occurs in 5% of deliveries and is the leading cause of maternal death worldwide, with an estimated mortality rate of 140,000 per year or one maternal death every 4 minutes (Leduc, Senikas, & Lalonde, 2009). In Canada, the incidence of direct maternal mortality from hemorrhage is 2.5 per 1,000,000 live births (Public Health Agency of Canada [PHAC], 2008).

Primary or early PPH is defined as excessive bleeding that occurs in the first 24 hours after delivery (Leduc et al., 2009). Blood loss that occurs 24 hours to 6 weeks after birth is termed secondary or late PPH. Traditionally, the definition of PPH has been blood loss greater than 500 mL after vaginal birth and more than 1,000 mL after abdominal birth (Leduc et al., 2009). However, this definition is arbitrary because estimates of blood loss at birth are subjective and generally inaccurate. Studies have suggested that health care providers consistently underestimate actual blood loss (Leduc et al., 2009; Maslovitz, Barkai, Lessing, et al., 2008; Tebruegge, Misra, Pantazidou, et al., 2009). A more objective definition of PPH would be any amount of bleeding that places the mother in hemodynamic instability (Leduc et al., 2009).

Factors that place a woman at risk for PPH are listed in Box 22.1.

Etiology

Excessive bleeding can occur at any time between the separation of the placenta and its expulsion or removal. The most common cause of PPH is **uterine atony,** failure of the uterus to contract and retract after birth. The uterus must remain contracted after birth to control bleeding from the placental site. Any factor that causes the uterus to relax after birth will cause bleeding—even a full bladder that displaces the uterus.

Over the course of a pregnancy, maternal blood volume increases by approximately 50% (4 to 6 L). The

---

BOX 22.1 Factors Placing A Woman at Risk for Postpartum Hemorrhage

- Prolonged first, second, or third stage of labour
- Previous history of postpartum hemorrhage
- Multiple gestation
- Uterine infection
- Manual extraction of placenta
- Arrest of descent
- Maternal exhaustion, malnutrition, or anemia
- Mediolateral episiotomy
- Pre-eclampsia
- Precipitous birth
- Maternal hypotension
- Previous placenta previa
- Coagulation abnormalities
- Birth canal lacerations
- Operative birth (forceps or vacuum)
- Augmented labour with medication
- Coagulation abnormalities
- Grand multiparity
- Hydramnios

Sources: Gilbert, E. S. (2011). *Manual of high risk pregnancy & delivery* (5th ed.). St. Louis: MO: Mosby Elsevier; & Leduc, D., Senikas, V., & Lalonde, A. B. (2009). SOGC clinical practice guideline: Active management of the third stage of labour: Prevention and treatment of postpartum hemorrhage. *Journal of Obstetrics and Gynaecology Canada, 31*(10), 980–993. Retrieved March 12, 2012 from http://www.sogc.org/guidelines/documents/gui235CPG0910.pdf.

---

plasma volume increases somewhat more than the total red blood cell volume, leading to a fall in the hemoglobin and hematocrit levels. The increase in blood volume meets the perfusion demands of the low-resistance uteroplacental unit and provides a reserve for the blood loss that occurs at delivery (Blackburn, 2008). Given this increase, the typical signs of hemorrhage (i.e., falling blood pressure, increasing pulse rate, and decreasing urinary output) do not appear until as much as 1,800 to 2,100 mL has been lost (Gilbert, 2011). In addition, accurate determination of actual blood loss is difficult because of pooling inside the uterus and on peripads, mattresses, and the floor. Because no universal clinical standard exists, nurses must be vigilant of risk factors, checking clients carefully before letting the primary care provider leave.

Other causes of PPH include lacerations of the genital tract, episiotomy, retained placental fragments, uterine inversion, coagulation disorders, and hematomas of the vulva, vagina, or subperitoneal areas (Cabero Roura & Keith, 2009). A helpful way to remember the causes of PPH is the "4T's": tone, tissue, trauma, and thrombosis (Leduc et al., 2009).

Tone

Altered uterine muscle tone most commonly results from overdistention of the uterus. Overdistention can be caused by multifetal gestation, fetal macrosomia, hydramnios, fetal abnormality, or placental fragments. Other causes might include prolonged or rapid, forceful labour, especially if stimulated; bacterial toxins (e.g., chorioamnionitis, endomyometritis, septicemia); use of anesthesia, especially halothane; and magnesium sulfate used in the treatment of pre-eclampsia (Leduc et al., 2009). Overdistention of the uterus is a major risk factor for uterine atony, the most common cause of early PPH, which can lead to hypovolemic shock.

Tissue

Uterine contraction and retraction lead to detachment and expulsion of the placenta after birth. Complete detachment and expulsion of the placenta permit continued contraction and optimal occlusion of blood vessels. Failure of complete separation of the placenta and expulsion does not allow the uterus to contract fully, since retained fragments occupy space and prevent the uterus from contracting fully to clamp down on blood vessels; this can lead to hemorrhage. After the placenta is expelled, a thorough inspection is necessary to confirm its intactness; tears or fragments left inside may indicate an accessory lobe or placenta accreta. Placenta accreta is an uncommon condition in which the chorionic villi adhere to the myometrium. This causes the placenta to adhere abnormally to the uterus and not separate and deliver spontaneously. Profuse hemorrhage results because the uterus cannot contract fully.

A prolapse of the uterine fundus to or through the cervix so that the uterus is turned inside out after birth is called **uterine inversion**. This condition is associated with abnormal adherence of the placenta, excessive traction on the umbilical cord, vigorous fundal pressure, precipitous labour, or vigorous manual removal of the placenta. Acute postpartum uterine inversion is rare, with an estimated incidence of 1 per 2,500 births (Mirza & Gaddipati, 2009). Prompt recognition and rapid treatment to replace the inverted uterus will avoid morbidity and mortality for this serious complication (Majd, Nawaz, Ismail, et al., 2009).

Subinvolution refers to the incomplete involution of the uterus or failure to return to its normal size and condition after birth (Al-Mehaisen, Al-Kuran, Amarin, et al., 2008). Complications of subinvolution include hemorrhage, pelvic peritonitis, salpingitis, and abscess formation (Leduc et al., 2009). Causes of subinvolution include retained placental fragments, distended bladder, uterine myoma, and infection. The clinical picture includes a postpartum fundal height that is higher than expected, with a boggy uterus; the lochia fails to change colour from red to serosa to alba within a few weeks. This condition is usually identified at the woman's postpartum examination 4 to 6 weeks after birth via a bimanual vaginal examination or ultrasound. Treatment is directed toward stimulating the uterus to expel fragments with a uterine stimulant, and antibiotics are given to prevent infection.

Trauma

Damage to the genital tract may occur spontaneously or through the manipulations used during birth. For example, a cesarean birth results in more blood loss than a vaginal birth. The amount of blood loss depends on suturing, vasospasm, and clotting for hemostasis. Uterine rupture is more common in women with previous cesarean scars or those who have undergone any procedure resulting in disruption of the uterine wall, including myomectomy, uteroplasty for a congenital anomaly, perforation of the uterus during a dilation and curettage (D&C), biopsy, or intrauterine device (IUD) insertion (Cabero Roura & Keith, 2009).

Trauma can also occur after prolonged or vigorous labour, especially if the uterus has been stimulated with oxytocin or prostaglandins. Trauma can also occur after extrauterine or intrauterine manipulation of the fetus.

Cervical lacerations commonly occur during a forceps delivery or in mothers who have not been able to resist bearing down before the cervix is fully dilated. Vaginal sidewall lacerations are associated with operative vaginal births but may occur spontaneously, especially if the fetal hand presents with the head. Lacerations can arise during manipulations to resolve shoulder dystocia. Lacerations should always be suspected in the face of a contracted uterus with bright-red blood continuing to trickle out of the vagina.

Thrombosis

Thrombosis (blood clots) helps to prevent PPH immediately after birth by providing a homeostasis in the woman's circulatory system. As long as there is a normal clotting mechanism that is activated, postpartum bleeding will not be exacerbated. Disorders of the coagulation system do not always appear in the immediate postpartum period due to the efficiency of stimulating uterine contractions through medications to prevent hemorrhage. Fibrin deposits and clots in supplying vessels play a significant role in the hours and days after birth. Coagulopathies should be suspected when postpartum bleeding persists without any identifiable cause (Peyvandi, Menegatti, & Siboni, 2011).

Ideally, the client's coagulation status is determined during pregnancy. However, if she received no prenatal care, coagulation studies should be ordered immediately to determine her status. Abnormal results typically include decreased platelet and fibrinogen levels; increased prothrombin time, partial thromboplastin time, and fibrin degradation products; and a prolonged bleeding time (Kadir, Chi, & Bolton-Maggs, 2009). Conditions associated with coagulopathies in the postpartum client include idiopathic thrombocytopenic purpura (ITP), von

Willebrand disease (vWD), and disseminated intravascular coagulation (DIC).

Idiopathic Thrombocytopenia Purpura

ITP is a disorder of increased platelet destruction caused by the development of autoantibodies to platelet-membrane antigens. The incidence of ITP in young women is approximately 1 to 2 per 1,000 pregnancies (Belkin, Levy, & Sheiner,. 2009). Thrombocytopenia, capillary fragility, and increased bleeding time define the disorder. Clinical manifestations include easy bruising, bleeding from mucous membranes, menorrhagia, epistaxis, bleeding gums, hematomas, and severe hemorrhage after a cesarean birth or lacerations (Fujita, Sakai, Matsuura, et al., 2010). Glucocorticoids and immune globulin are the mainstays of medical therapy.

von Willebrand Disease

vWD is a congenital bleeding disorder, inherited as an autosomal dominant trait, that is characterized by a prolonged bleeding time, a deficiency of von Willebrand factor, and impairment of platelet adhesion (Peyvandi et al., 2011). It is estimated to affect 1 in 1,000 or 30,000 Canadians (Canadian Hemophilia Society, 2007). Most cases remain undiagnosed from lack of awareness, difficulty in diagnosis, a tendency to attribute bleeding to other causes, and variable symptoms (Castaman, Tosetto, & Rodeghiero, 2010). Symptoms include excessive bruising, prolonged nosebleeds, and prolonged oozing from wounds after surgery and after childbirth. The goal of therapy is to correct the defect in platelet adhesiveness by raising the level of von Willebrand factor with medications (Castaman et al., 2010).

Disseminated Intravascular Coagulation

DIC is a life-threatening, acquired pathologic process in which the clotting system is abnormally activated, resulting in widespread clot formation in the small vessels throughout the body (Peyvandi et al., 2011). It can cause PPH by altering the blood clotting mechanism. DIC is always a secondary diagnosis that occurs as a complication of abruptio placentae, amniotic fluid embolism, intrauterine fetal death with prolonged retention of the fetus, severe pre-eclampsia, septicemia, and hemorrhage. Clinical features include petechiae, ecchymoses, bleeding gums, tachycardia, uncontrolled bleeding during birth, and acute renal failure (Thachil & Toh, 2009). The treatment goal is to maintain tissue perfusion through aggressive administration of fluid therapy, oxygen, and blood products.

Nursing Management

Pregnancy and childbirth involve significant health risks, even for women with no preexisting health problems. There are approximately 50 cases of pregnancy-related hemorrhage per 1,000 pregnancies every year in Canada, with some of these women bleeding to death (PHAC, 2008). Most of these deaths occur within 4 hours of giving birth and are a result of problems during the third stage of labour (Leduc et al., 2009). The period after the birth and the first hours of postpartum are crucial times for the prevention, assessment, and management of bleeding. Compared with other maternal risks such as infection, bleeding can rapidly become life-threatening, and nurses, along with other health care providers, need to identify this condition quickly and intervene appropriately.

Nursing Assessment

Since the most common cause of immediate severe PPH is uterine atony (failure of the uterus to properly contract after birth), assessing uterine tone after birth by palpating the fundus for firmness and location is essential. A soft, boggy fundus indicates uterine atony.

> ▶ **Take** NOTE!
>
> *A soft, boggy uterus that deviates from the midline suggests a full bladder interfering with uterine involution. If the uterus is not in correct position (midline), it will not be able to contract to control bleeding.*

Assess the amount of bleeding. If bleeding continues even though there are no lacerations, suspect retained placental fragments. The uterus remains large with painless dark-red blood mixed with clots. This cause of hemorrhage can be prevented by carefully inspecting the placenta for intactness.

If trauma is suspected, attempt to identify the source and document it. Typically, the uterus will be firm with a steady stream or trickle of unclotted bright-red blood noted in the perineum. Most deaths from PPH are not due to gross bleeding, but rather to inadequate management of slow, steady blood loss (Cabero Roura & Keith, 2009).

Assessment for a suspected hematoma would reveal a firm uterus with bright-red bleeding. Observe for a localized bluish bulging area just under the skin surface in the perineal area (Fig. 22.1). Often, the woman will report severe perineal or pelvic pain and will have difficulty voiding. In addition, she will have hypotension, tachycardia, and anemia (Gilbert, 2011).

Assessment for coagulopathies as a cause of PPH would reveal prolonged bleeding from the gums and venipuncture sites, petechiae on the skin, and ecchymotic areas. The amount of lochia would be much greater also. Urinary output would be diminished, with signs of acute renal failure. Vital signs would show an increase in pulse rate and a decrease in level of consciousness. Signs of

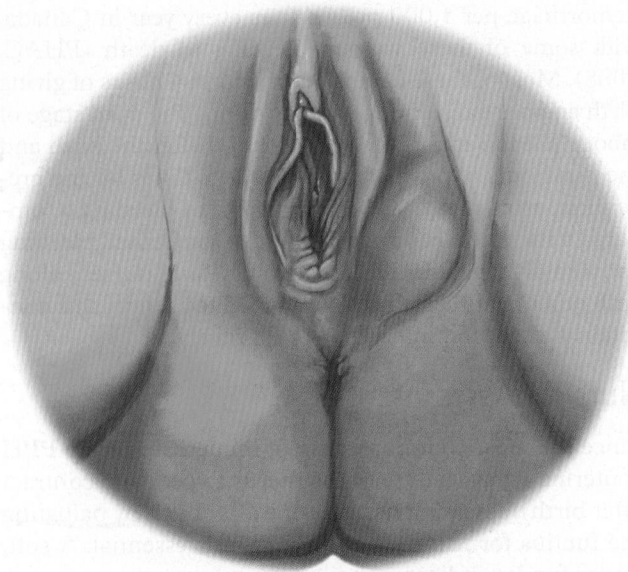

FIGURE 22.1 Perineal hematoma. Note the bulging, swollen mass.

shock do not appear until hemorrhage is far advanced due to the increased fluid and blood volume of pregnancy.

Nursing Management

Massage the uterus if uterine atony is noted. The uterine muscles are sensitive to touch; massage aids in stimulating the muscle fibers to contract. Massage the boggy uterus while supporting the lower uterine segment to stimulate contractions and expression of any accumulated blood clots. As blood pools in the vagina, stasis of blood causes clots to form; they need to be expelled as pressure is placed on the fundus. Overly forceful massage can tire the uterine muscles, resulting in further uterine atony and increased pain. See Nursing Procedure 22.1 for the steps in massaging the fundus.

If repeated fundal massage and expression of clots fail, medication is probably needed to contract the uterus to control bleeding from the placental site. The injection of a uterotonic drug immediately after birth is an important intervention used to prevent PPH. Oxytocin (Pitocin, Syntocinon); methylergonovine maleate (Methergine); ergonovine maleate (Ergotrate); a synthetic analogue of prostaglandin E1 misoprostol (Cytotec); and prostaglandin F2-alpha (PGF2-alpha, carboprost [Hemabate]) are drugs used to manage PPH (Drug Guide 22.1). The choice of which uterotonic drug to use for management of bleeding depends on the clinical judgment of the health care provider, the availability of drugs, and the risks and benefits of the drug.

Remember Joan, the woman described at the beginning of the chapter? The nurse assesses her and finds that her uterus is boggy. What would the nurse do next? What additional nursing measures might be used if Joan's fundus remains boggy? When should the health care provider be notified?

Nursing Procedure 22.1

MASSAGING THE FUNDUS

Purpose: To Promote Uterine Contraction

1. After explaining the procedure to the woman, place one gloved hand (usually the dominant hand) on the fundus.
2. Place the other gloved hand on the area above the symphysis pubis (this helps to support the lower uterine segment).
3. With the hand on the fundus, gently massage the fundus in a circular manner. Be careful not to over massage the fundus, which could lead to muscle fatigue and uterine relaxation.
4. Assess for uterine firmness (uterine tissue responds quickly to touch).
5. If firm, apply gentle yet firm pressure in a downward motion toward the vagina to express any clots that may have accumulated.
6. Do not attempt to express clots until the fundus is firm because the application of firm pressure on an uncontracted uterus could cause uterine inversion, leading to massive hemorrhage.

7. Assist the woman with perineal care and applying a new perineal pad.
8. Remove gloves and wash hands.

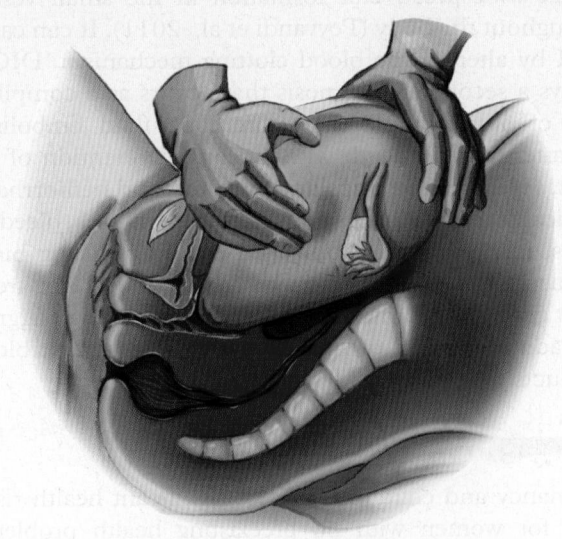

DRUG GUIDE 22.1   DRUGS USED TO CONTROL POSTPARTUM HEMORRHAGE

Drug	Action/Indication	Nursing Implications
Oxytocin (Pitocin, Syntocinon)	Stimulates the uterus to contract to control bleeding from the placental site	Assess fundus for evidence of contraction and compare amount of bleeding every 15 minutes or according to orders. Monitor vital signs every 15 minutes. Monitor uterine tone to prevent hyperstimulation. Reassure client about the need for uterine contraction and administer analgesics for comfort. Offer explanation to client and family about what is happening and the purpose of the medication. Provide non-pharmacologic comfort measures to assist with pain management. Set up the IV infusion to be piggybacked into a primary IV line. This ensures that the medication can be discontinued readily if hyperstimulation or adverse effects occur while maintaining the IV site and primary infusion.
Misoprostol (Cytotec)	Stimulates the uterus to contract to reduce bleeding; a prostaglandin analogue	As above. Very effective drug therapy for acute postpartum hemorrhage. Contraindications: allergy, active CVD, pulmonary or hepatic disease; use with caution in women with asthma
Ergonovine maleate (Ergotrate)	Stimulates the uterus/to prevent and treat postpartum hemorrhage due to atony or subinvolution	Assess baseline bleeding, uterine tone, and vital signs every 15 minutes or according to protocol. Offer explanation to client and family about what is happening and the purpose of the medication. Monitor for possible adverse effects, such as nausea, vomiting, weakness, muscular pain, headache, or dizziness.
Prostaglandin (PGF2-alpha, carboprost [Hemabate])	Stimulates uterine contractions/to treat postpartum hemorrhage due to uterine atony when not controlled by other methods	Assess vital signs, uterine contractions, client's comfort level, and bleeding status as per protocol. Offer explanation to client and family about what is happening and the purpose of the medication. Monitor for possible adverse effects, such as fever, chills, headache, nausea, vomiting, diarrhea, flushing, and bronchospasm.

Sources: King, T.L., and Brucker, M.C. (2011). *Pharmacology for women's health*. Sudbury, MA: Jones and Bartlett Publishers; Lilley, L., Collins, S.R., Harrington, S., and Snyder, J. (2011). *Pharmacology and the nursing process*. St. Louis, MO: Mosby Elsevier; Skidmore-Roth, L. (2012). *Mosby's 2012 nursing drug reference*. (25th edition), St. Louis, MO: Mosby Elsevier; and Society of Obstetrics and Gynaecologists of Canada. (2009). Active management of the third stage of labour: Prevention and treatment of postpartum hemorrhage. *Clinical practice guideline*. Retrieved April 4, 2012 from http://www.sogc.org/guidelines/documents/gui235CPG0910.pdf.

Maintain the primary IV infusion and be prepared to start a second infusion at another site in case blood transfusions are necessary. Draw blood for type and cross-match and send it to the laboratory. Administer oxytocics as ordered, correlating and titrating the IV medication infusion rate to assessment findings of uterine firmness and lochia. Assess for visible vaginal bleeding, and count or weigh perineal pads.

▶ *Take NOTE!*

When weighing perineal pads to determine blood loss, remember that 1 g of pad weight is equivalent to 1 mL of blood loss (Gilbert, 2011; Leduc et al., 2009).

Check vital signs every 15 to 30 minutes, depending on the acuity of the mother's health status. Monitor her complete blood count to identify any deficit or assess the adequacy of replacement. In addition, assess the woman's level of consciousness to determine changes that may result from inadequate cerebral perfusion.

If a full bladder is present, assist the woman to empty her bladder to reduce displacement of the uterus. If the woman cannot void, anticipate the need to catheterize her to relieve bladder distention.

Retained placental fragments usually are manually separated and removed by the birth attendant. Be sure that the birth attendant remains long enough after birth to assess the bleeding status of the woman and determine the etiology. Assist the birth attendant with suturing any lacerations immediately to control hemorrhage and repair the tissue.

For the woman who develops ITP, glucocorticoids, intravenous immunoglobulin, intravenous anti-Rho D, and platelet transfusions may be administered. A splenectomy may be needed if the bleeding tissues do not respond to medical management.

In vWD, there is a decrease in von Willebrand factor, which is necessary for platelet adhesion and aggregation. It binds to and stabilizes factor VIII of the coagulation cascade (Peyvandi et al., 2011). Desmopressin, a synthetic form of vasopressin (antidiuretic hormone), may be used to treat vWD. This drug stimulates the release of stored factor VIII and von Willebrand factor from the lining of blood vessels, which increases platelet adhesiveness and shortens bleeding time. Other treatments that may be ordered include clotting factor concentrates, replacement of von Willebrand factor and factor VIII (Alphanate, Humate-P), antifibrinolytics (Amicar), and nonsteroidal anti-inflammatory drugs (NSAIDs) that do not cause platelet dysfunction (Bextra) (Castaman et al., 2010).

Be alert for women with abnormal bleeding tendencies, ensuring that they receive proper diagnosis and treatment. Teach them how to prevent severe hemorrhage by learning how to feel for and massage their fundus when boggy, assisting the nurse to keep track of the number of and amount of bleeding on perineal pads, and avoiding any medications with antiplatelet activity such as aspirin, antihistamines, or NSAIDS.

If the woman develops DIC, institute emergency measures to control bleeding and impending shock and prepare to transfer her to the intensive care unit. Identification of the underlying condition and elimination of the causative factor are essential to correct the coagulation problem. Be ready to replace fluid volume, administer blood component therapy, and optimize the mother's oxygenation and perfusion status to ensure adequate cardiac output and end-organ perfusion. Continually reassess the woman's coagulation status via laboratory studies.

Monitor vital signs closely, being alert for changes that signal an increase in bleeding or impending shock.

Observe for signs of bleeding, including spontaneous bleeding from gums or nose, petechiae, excessive bleeding from the cesarean incision site, hematuria, and blood in the stool. These findings correlate with decreased blood volume, decreased organ and peripheral tissue perfusion, and clots in the microcirculation (Pacheco, Costantine, Saade, et al., 2010).

> ▶ **Take** NOTE!
>
> *Always remember the four causes of PPH and the appropriate intervention for each: 1. Uterine atony—massage and oxytocics; 2. Retained placental tissue—evacuation and oxytocics; 3. Lacerations or hematoma—surgical repair; 4. Thrombosis (bleeding disorders)—blood products.*

Institute measures to avoid tissue trauma or injury, such as giving injections and drawing blood. Also provide emotional support to the client and her family throughout this critical time by being readily available and providing explanations and reassurance.

An IV oxytocin infusion is started for Joan. What assessments will need to be done frequently to make sure Joan is not losing too much blood? What discharge instructions need to be reinforced with Joan?

Thromboembolic Conditions

A thrombosis (blood clot within a blood vessel) can cause an inflammation of the blood vessel lining (**thrombophlebitis**), which in turn can lead to a possible thromboembolism (obstruction of a blood vessel by a blood clot carried by the circulation from the site of origin). Thrombi can involve the superficial or deep veins in the legs or pelvis. Superficial venous thrombosis usually involves the saphenous venous system and is confined to the lower leg. In some women, superficial thrombophlebitis may be caused by the use of the lithotomy position during birth. Deep venous thrombosis can involve deep veins from the foot to the calf, thighs, or pelvis. In both locations, thrombi can dislodge and migrate to the lungs, causing a pulmonary embolism (PE) (James, 2009).

PE is a potentially fatal thromboembolic condition that occurs when the pulmonary artery is obstructed by a blood clot that has travelled from another vein into the lungs, causing an obstruction and infarction. When the clot is large enough to block one or more of the pulmonary vessels that supply the lungs, it can result in sudden death. PE is one of the leading causes of pregnancy-related deaths worldwide (Liu, Rouleau, Joseph, et al., 2009).

The incidence of PE in Canada is 5 in 1,000,000 live births (PHAC, 2008).

Pathophysiology

The major causes of a thrombus formation (blood clot) are venous stasis, injury to the innermost layer of the blood vessel, and hypercoagulation. Venous stasis and hypercoagulation are both common in the postpartum period. Other factors that place women at risk for thrombosis include prolonged bed rest, diabetes, obesity, cesarean birth, smoking, progesterone-induced distensibility of the veins of the lower legs during pregnancy, severe anemia, history of previous thrombosis, varicose veins, diabetes mellitus, advanced maternal age (older than 35 years), multiparity, and use of oral contraceptives before pregnancy (Jacobsen, Skjeldestad, & Sandset, 2008; Liu et al., 2009).

Nursing Assessment

Assess the woman closely for risk factors and signs and symptoms of thrombophlebitis. Look for risk factors in the woman's history such as use of oral contraceptives before the pregnancy, employment that necessitates prolonged standing, history of thrombophlebitis or endometritis, or evidence of current varicosities. Suspect superficial venous thrombosis in a woman with varicose veins who reports tenderness and discomfort over the site of the thrombosis, most commonly in the calf area. The area appears reddened along the vein and is warm to the touch. The woman will report increased pain in the affected leg when she ambulates and bears weight.

Manifestations of deep venous thrombosis are often absent and diffuse. If they are present, they are caused by an inflammatory process and obstruction of venous return. Calf swelling, erythema, warmth, tenderness, and pedal edema may be noted. A positive Homans sign (pain in the calf upon dorsiflexion) is not a definitive diagnostic sign because pain can also be caused by a strained muscle or contusion (Lindqvist, Torsson, Almqvist, et al., 2008; Liu et al., 2009).

Assess for signs and symptoms of PE, including unexplained sudden onset of shortness of breath, tachypnea, sudden chest pain, tachycardia, cardiac arrhythmias, apprehension, profuse sweating, hemoptysis, and sudden change in mental status as a result of hypoxemia (Liu et al., 2009). Expect a lung scan to be done to confirm the diagnosis.

Nursing Management

The three most common thromboembolic conditions occurring during the postpartum period are superficial venous thrombosis, deep venous thrombosis, and PE.

Preventing Thrombotic Conditions

Prevention of thrombotic conditions is an essential aspect of nursing management. Many deaths related to these conditions can be prevented by the routine use of simple measures:

- Developing public awareness about risk factors, symptoms, and preventive measures
- Preventing venous stasis by encouraging activity that causes leg muscles to contract and promotes venous return (leg exercises and walking)
- Using intermittent sequential compression devices to produce passive leg muscle contractions until the woman is ambulatory
- Elevating the woman's legs above her heart level to promote venous return
- Stopping smoking to reduce or prevent vascular vasoconstriction
- Applying compression stockings and removing them daily for inspection of legs
- Performing passive range-of-motion exercises while in bed
- Using postoperative deep-breathing exercises to improve venous return by relieving the negative thoracic pressure on leg veins
- Reducing hypercoagulability with the use of warfarin, aspirin, and heparin
- Preventing venous pooling by avoiding pillows under the knees, not crossing the legs for long periods, and not leaving the legs up in stirrups for long periods
- Padding stirrups to reduce pressure against the popliteal angle
- Avoiding sitting or standing in one position for prolonged periods
- Using a bed cradle to keep linens and blankets off extremities
- Avoiding trauma to legs to prevent injury to the vein wall
- Increasing fluid intake to prevent dehydration
- Avoiding the use of oral contraceptives

In women at risk, early ambulation is the easiest and most cost-effective method of prevention. Use of elastic compression stockings (TED hose or Jobst stockings) decreases distal calf vein thrombosis by decreasing venous stasis and augmenting venous return (Liu et al., 2009). Women who are at a high risk for thromboembolic disease based on risk factors or previous history of deep vein thrombosis or PE may be placed on prophylactic heparin therapy during pregnancy. Standard heparin or a low-molecular-weight heparin such as enoxaparin (Lovenox) can be given, since neither of these crosses the placenta. It is typically discontinued during labour and birth and then restarted during the postpartum period.

Treating Thromboembolic Disorders

Although thromboembolic disorders occur in less than 1% of all postpartum women, pulmonary embolus can be fatal if a clot obstructs the lung circulation; thus, early identification and treatment are paramount. For the woman with superficial venous thrombosis, care includes administering NSAIDs for analgesia, providing for rest and elevation of the affected leg, applying warm compresses to the affected area to promote healing, and using antiembolism stockings to promote circulation to the extremities.

Nursing interventions for a woman with deep vein thrombosis include bed rest and elevation of the affected extremity to decrease interstitial swelling and promote venous return from that leg. Apply antiembolism stockings to both extremities as ordered. Fit the stockings correctly and urge the woman to wear them at all times. Sequential compression devices can also be used for women with varicose veins, a history of thrombophlebitis, or a surgical birth. Anticoagulant therapy using a continuous IV infusion of heparin is started to prolong clotting time and prevent extension of the thrombosis. Monitor the woman's coagulation studies closely; these might include activated partial thromboplastin time (APTT), whole blood partial thromboplastin time, and platelet levels. Therapeutic APTT values typically range from 35 to 45 seconds, depending on which standard values are used (Liu et al., 2009). Also apply warm, moist compresses to the affected leg and administer analgesics as ordered to decrease the discomfort.

After several days of IV heparin therapy, expect to begin oral anticoagulant therapy with warfarin (Coumadin) as ordered. In most cases, the woman will continue to take this medication for several months after discharge.

For the woman who develops a PE, institute emergency measures immediately. The objectives of treatment are to prevent further growth or multiplication of thrombi in the lower extremities, prevent further thrombi from travelling to the pulmonary vascular system, and provide cardiopulmonary support if needed. Interventions include administering oxygen via mask or cannula and continuous IV heparin titrated according to the laboratory results, maintaining the client on bed rest, and administering analgesics for pain relief. Thrombolytic agents, such as tissue plasminogen activator (t-PA), might be used to dissolve pulmonary emboli and the source of the thrombus in the pelvis or deep leg veins, thus reducing the potential for a recurrence.

Educating the Client

Provide teaching about the use of anticoagulant therapy and possible danger signs (Teaching Guideline 22.1). Additional interventions include providing anticipatory guidance, support, and education about anticoagulants and associated signs of complications and risks. Focus discharge teaching on the importance of the following:

- Eliminating modifiable risk factors for deep vein thrombosis (smoking, use of oral contraceptives, a sedentary lifestyle, and obesity)
- Using compression stockings

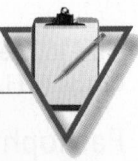

TEACHING GUIDELINE 22.1

Teaching to Prevent Bleeding Related to Anticoagulant Therapy

- Watch for possible signs of bleeding and notify your health care provider if any occur:
  - Nosebleeds
  - Bleeding from the gums or mouth
  - Black, tarry stools
  - Brown "coffee ground" vomitus
  - Red to brown speckled mucus from a cough
  - Oozing at incision, episiotomy site, cut, or scrape
  - Pink-, red-, or brown-tinged urine
  - Bruises, "black and blue marks"
  - Increased lochia discharge (from present level)
- Practice measures to reduce your risk for bleeding:
  - Brush your teeth gently using a soft toothbrush.
  - Use an electric razor for shaving.
  - Avoid activities that could lead to injury, scrapes, bruising, or cuts.
  - Do not use any over-the-counter products containing aspirin or aspirin-like derivatives.
  - Avoid consuming alcohol.
  - Inform other health care providers about the use of anticoagulants, especially dentists.
  - If you accidentally cut or scrape yourself, apply firm direct pressure to the site for 5 to 10 minutes. Do the same after receiving any injections or having blood specimens drawn.
  - Avoid constrictive clothing and prolonged standing or sitting in a motionless, leg-dependent position.

- Making sure to comply with follow-up laboratory testing as scheduled
- Wearing an identification bracelet or band that indicates that you are taking an anticoagulant
- Knowing the danger signs and symptoms (sudden onset of chest pain, dyspnea, and tachypnea) to report to the health care provider

Postpartum Infection

Infection during the postpartum period is a common cause of maternal morbidity and mortality. Overall, postpartum infection is estimated to occur in up to 8% of all births. There is a higher occurrence in cesarean births than in vaginal births (Belfort, Clark, Saade, et al., 2010; Clark, Belfort, Dildy, et al., 2008). The incidence of postpartum infections is expected to increase because of the earlier discharge of postpartum women from the hospital (Wong & Rosh, 2010).

Postpartum infection is defined as a fever of 38°C or higher after the first 24 hours after childbirth, occurring on at least 2 of the first 10 days after birth, exclusive of the first 24 hours (Gilbert, 2011; Wong & Rosh, 2010). Infections can easily enter the female genital tract externally and ascend through the internal genital structures. In addition, the normal physiologic changes of childbirth increase the risk for infection by decreasing the vaginal acidity due to the presence of amniotic fluid, blood, and lochia, all of which are alkaline. An alkaline environment encourages the growth of bacteria. Because today women are commonly discharged 24 to 48 hours after giving birth, nurses must assess new mothers for risk factors and identify early subtle signs and symptoms of an infectious process.

The common bacterial etiology of postpartum infections involves organisms that constitute the normal vaginal flora, typically a mix of aerobic and anaerobic species. Postpartum infections generally are polymicrobial and involve the following microorganisms: *Staphylococcus aureus, Escherichia coli, Klebsiella, Gardnerella vaginalis,* gonococci, coliform bacteria, group A or B hemolytic streptococci, *Chlamydia trachomatis,* and the anaerobes that are common to bacterial vaginosis (Arianpour, Safari, & Hatami, 2009; Paruk, 2008). Common postpartum infections include metritis, wound infections, urinary tract infections, and mastitis. Signs and symptoms of these postpartum infections are listed in Table 22.1.

Metritis

Although usually referred to clinically as endometritis, postpartum uterine infections typically involve more than just the endometrial lining. Metritis is an infectious condition that involves the endometrium, decidua, and adjacent myometrium of the uterus. Extension of metritis can result in parametritis, which involves the broad ligament and possibly the ovaries and fallopian tubes, or septic pelvic thrombophlebitis, which results when the infection spreads along venous routes into the pelvis (Wong & Rosh, 2010).

The uterine cavity is sterile until rupture of the amniotic sac. As a consequence of labour, birth, and associated manipulations, anaerobic and aerobic bacteria can contaminate the uterus. In most cases, the bacteria responsible for pelvic infections are those that normally reside in the bowel, vagina, perineum, and cervix, such as *E. coli, Klebsiella pneumoniae,* or *G. vaginalis.*

The risk for metritis increases dramatically after a cesarean birth; it complicates 10% to 20% of cesarean births. This is typically an extension of chorioamnionitis that was present before birth (indeed, that may have been why the cesarean birth was performed). In addition, trauma to the tissues and a break in the skin (incision) provide portals for bacteria to enter the body and multiply (Belfort et al., 2010).

Primary prevention of metritis is key and focuses on reducing the risk factors and incidence of cesarean

TABLE 22.1 SIGNS AND SYMPTOMS OF POSTPARTUM INFECTIONS

Postpartum Infection	Signs and Symptoms
Metritis	Lower abdominal tenderness or pain on one or both sides Temperature elevation (>38°C) Foul-smelling lochia Anorexia Nausea Fatigue and lethargy Leukocytosis and elevated sedimentation rate
Wound infection	Weeping serosanguineous or purulent drainage Separation of or unapproximated wound edges Edema Erythema Tenderness Discomfort at the site Maternal fever Elevated white blood cell count
Urinary tract infection	Urgency Frequency Dysuria Flank pain Low-grade fever Urinary retention Hematuria Urine positive for nitrates Cloudy urine with strong odour
Mastitis	Flu-like symptoms, including malaise, fever, and chills Tender, hot, red, painful area on one breast Inflammation of breast area Breast tenderness Cracking of skin or around nipple or areola Breast distention with milk

births. When metritis occurs, broad-spectrum antibiotics are used to treat the infection. Management also includes measures to restore and promote fluid and electrolyte balance, provide analgesia, and offer emotional support. In most treated women, reduction of fever and elimination of symptoms will occur within 48 to 72 hours after the start of antibiotic therapy.

Wound Infections

Any break in the skin or mucous membranes provides a portal for bacteria. In the postpartum woman, sites of wound infection include cesarean surgical incisions, the

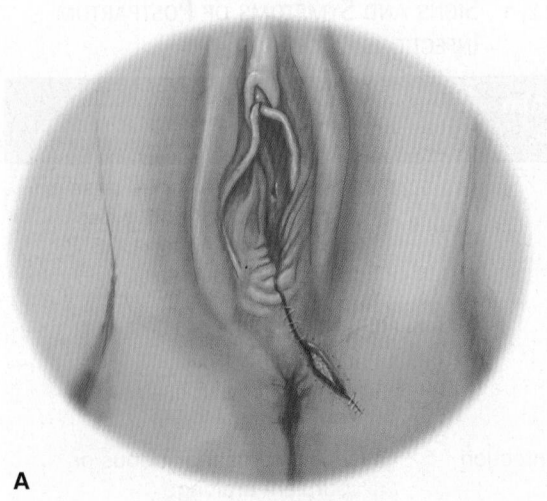

A

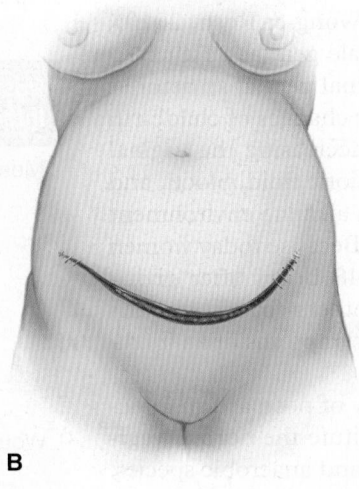

B

FIGURE 22.2 Postpartum wound infections. (**A**) Infected episiotomy site. (**B**) Infected cesarean birth incision.

episiotomy site in the perineum, and the genital tract as a result of laceration (Fig. 22.2). Wound infections are usually not identified until the woman has been discharged from the hospital because symptoms may not manifest until 24 to 48 hours after birth. Therefore, instructions about signs and symptoms to look for should be included in all discharge teaching. When a low-grade fever (<38°C), poor appetite, and a low energy level persist for a few days, a wound infection should be suspected.

Management of wound infections involves recognition of the infection followed by opening of the wound to allow drainage. Aseptic wound management with sterile gloves and frequent dressing changes if applicable, good handwashing, frequent perineal pad changes, hydration, and ambulation to prevent venous stasis and improve circulation are initiated to prevent development of a more serious infection or spread of the infection to adjacent structures. Parenteral antibiotics are the mainstay of treatment. Analgesics are also important because women often experience discomfort at the wound site.

Urinary Tract Infections

Urinary tract infections are most commonly caused by bacteria often found in bowel flora, including *E. coli, Klebsiella, Proteus,* and *Enterobacter* species. Any form of invasive manipulation of the urethra, such as urinary catheterization, frequent vaginal examinations, and genital trauma increase the likelihood of a urinary tract infection. Treatment consists of administering fluids if dehydration exists and antibiotics if appropriate.

Mastitis

Mastitis is an inflammation of the breast tissue caused by milk stasis and bacterial invasion that can develop in the first several postpartum weeks (Lowdermilk, Perry, Cashion, et al., 2011; Wilson-Clay & Hoover, 2008). Signs and symptoms of mastitis are the appearance of a

painful, hot and reddened area on the breast, fatigue, fever, flu-like symptoms, tachycardia, and headache (see Table 22.1). The infection is usually unilateral and located in the outer breast quadrants (Fig. 22.3) (Riordan & Wambach, 2010).

A number of risk factors predispose a woman to mastitis, including stress and fatigue, cracked nipples, plugged or blocked ducts, ample milk supply and/or decrease in number of feedings, and engorgement and stasis (Riordan & Wambach, 2010). Mastitis can be caused by a missed infant feeding, constriction from a bra that is too tight, breast trauma, poor drainage of duct and alveolus, poor maternal nutrition, vigorous exercise, or an infection.

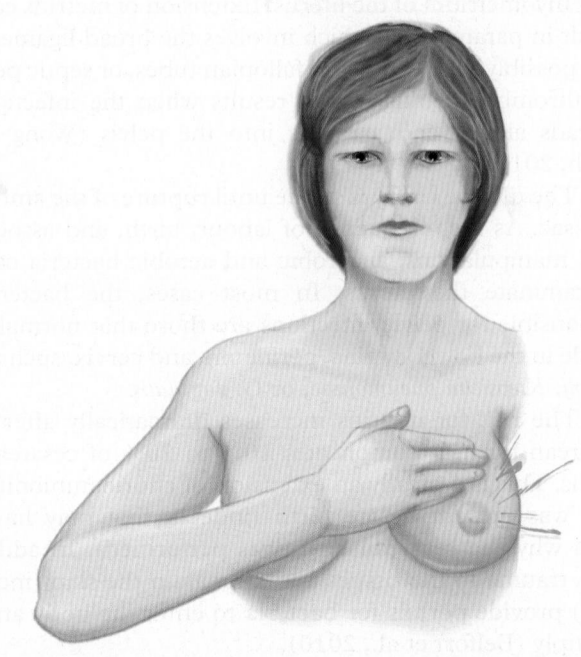

FIGURE 22.3 With mastitis, an area on one breast is tender, hot, red, and painful.

BOX 22.2 **Factors Placing A Woman at Risk for Postpartum Infection**

- Prolonged (>6 hours) premature rupture of membranes (removes the protective barrier to fetus and amniotic fluid so bacteria can ascend)
- Insertion of fetal scalp electrode or intrauterine pressure catheter for internal fetal monitoring during labour (provides entry into uterine cavity)
- Cesarean birth (allows bacterial entry due to break in protective skin barrier)
- Instrument-assisted childbirth, such as forceps or vacuum extraction (increases risk for trauma to genital tract, which provides bacteria access to grow)
- Urinary catheterization (could allow entry of bacteria into bladder due to break in aseptic technique)
- Regional anesthesia that decreases perception to void (causes urinary stasis and increases risk for urinary tract infection)
- Unwell staff attending to woman (promotes droplet infection from personnel)
- Compromised health status, such as anemia, obesity, smoking, drug abuse (reduces the body's immune system and decreases ability to fight infection)

- Preexisting colonization of lower genital tract with bacterial vaginosis, *C. trachomatis*, group B streptococci, *S. aureus*, and *E. coli* (allows microbes to ascend)
- Retained placental fragments (provides medium for bacterial growth)
- Manual removal of a retained placenta (causes trauma to the lining of the uterus and thus opens up sites for bacterial invasion)
- Trauma to the genital tract, such as episiotomy or lacerations (provides a portal of entry for bacteria)
- Prolonged labour with frequent vaginal examinations to check progress (allows time for bacteria to multiply and increases potential exposure to microorganisms or trauma)
- Poor nutritional status (reduces body's ability to repair tissue)
- Gestational diabetes (decreases body's healing ability and provides higher glucose levels on skin and in urine, which encourages bacterial growth)
- Break in aseptic technique during surgery or birthing process by the birth attendant or nurses (allows entry of bacteria)

The most common infecting organism is *S. aureus,* which comes from the breastfeeding infant's mouth or throat (Wong & Rosh, 2010). Infection can be transmitted from the lactiferous ducts to a secreting lobule, from a nipple fissure to periductal lymphatics, or by circulation (Riordan & Wambach, 2010).

The diagnosis is usually made without a culture being taken. Unless mastitis is treated adequately, it may progress to a breast abscess. Treatment of mastitis focuses on two areas: emptying the breasts and controlling the infection. The breast can be emptied either by the infant sucking or by manual expression. Increasing the frequency of nursing is advised. Lactation need not be suppressed. Control of infection is achieved with antibiotics. In addition, ice or warm packs and analgesics may be needed.

▶ **Take** NOTE!

Regardless of the etiology of mastitis, the focus is on reversing milk stasis, maintaining milk supply, and continuing breastfeeding, along with providing maternal comfort and preventing recurrence.

Nursing Assessment

Perinatal nurses are primary caregivers for postpartum women and have the unique opportunity to identify subtle changes that place women at risk for infection. Because women today are commonly discharged 24 to 48 hours after giving birth, nurses must assess new mothers for

risk factors (Box 22.2) and identify early signs and symptoms of an infectious process, which may be subtle or specific depending on the type and location of the infection (see Table 22.1).

Review the client's history and physical examination and labour and birth record for factors that might increase her risk for developing an infection. Then complete the assessment (using the "BUBBLE-EE" parameters discussed in Chapter 16), paying particular attention to areas such as the abdomen and fundus, breasts, urinary tract, episiotomy, lacerations, or incisions, being alert for signs and symptoms of infection (see Table 22.1).

▶ **Take** NOTE!

A postpartum infection is commonly associated with an elevated temperature. Other generalized signs and symptoms may include chills, foul-smelling vaginal discharge, headache, malaise, restlessness, anxiety, and tachycardia. In addition, the woman may have specific signs and symptoms based on the type and location of the infection.

When assessing the episiotomy site, use the acronym "REEDA" (redness, erythema or ecchymosis, edema, drainage or discharge, and approximation of wound edges) to ensure complete evaluation of the site (Gilbert, 2011; Wong & Rosh, 2010). Monitor the woman's vital signs, especially her temperature, for changes that may signal an infection.

Nursing Management

Nursing care focuses on preventing postpartum infections. Use the following guidelines to help reduce the incidence of postpartum infections:

- Maintain aseptic technique when performing invasive procedures such as urinary catheterization, when changing dressings, and during all surgical procedures.
- Use good handwashing technique before, after, and in between each patient care activity.
- Reinforce measures for maintaining good perineal hygiene.
- Use adequate lighting and turn the client to a side-lying position to assess the episiotomy site.
- Screen all visitors for any signs of active infections to reduce the client's risk for exposure.
- Review the client's history for preexisting infections or chronic conditions.
- Monitor vital signs and laboratory results for any abnormal values.
- Monitor the frequency of vaginal examinations and length of labour.
- Assess frequently for early signs of infection, especially fever and the appearance of lochia.
- Inspect wounds frequently for inflammation and drainage.
- Encourage rest, adequate hydration, and healthy eating habits.
- Reinforce preventive measures during any interaction with the client.

Client teaching is essential. Review the signs and symptoms of infection, emphasizing the danger signs and symptoms that need to be reported to the health care provider. Most importantly, stress proper handwashing, especially after perineal care and before and after breastfeeding. Also reinforce measures to promote breastfeeding, including proper breast care (see Chapter 16).

If the woman develops an infection, also review treatment measures, such as antibiotic therapy if ordered, and any special care measures, such as dressing changes (Nursing Care Plan 22.1). Teaching Guideline 22.2 highlights the major teaching points for a woman with a postpartum infection.

Postpartum Emotional Disorders

The postpartum period involves extraordinary physiologic, psychological, and social and cultural changes in the life of a woman and her family. Women have varied reactions to their childbearing experiences, exhibiting a wide range of emotions. The norm of some cultures is that birth is a happy time for all new mothers and is associated with positive feelings such as joy and gratitude for a healthy infant. But for others, it may not be a happy event. New mothers may also feel weepy, overwhelmed,

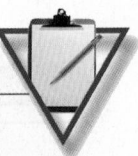

TEACHING GUIDELINE 22.2

Teaching for the Woman with a Postpartum Infection

- Continue your antibiotic therapy as prescribed:
  - Take the medication exactly as ordered and continue with the medication until it is finished.
- Do not stop taking the medication even when you are feeling better.
- Check your temperature every day and call your health care provider if it is above 38°C.
- Watch for other signs and symptoms of infection, such as chills, increased abdominal pain, change in the colour or odour of your lochia, or increased redness, warmth, swelling, or drainage from a wound site such as your cesarean incision or episiotomy. Report any of these to your health care provider immediately
- Practice good infection prevention:
  - Always wash your hands thoroughly before and after eating, using the bathroom, touching your perineal area, or providing care for your newborn.
  - Wipe from front to back after using the bathroom.
  - Remove your perineal pad using a front-to-back motion. Fold the pad in half so that the inner sides of the pad that were touching your body are against each other. Wrap in toilet tissue or place in a plastic bag and discard.
  - Wash your hands before applying a new pad.
  - Apply a new perineal pad using a front-to-back motion. Handle the pad by the edges (top and bottom or sides) and avoid touching the inner aspect of the pad that will be against your body.
  - When performing perineal care with the peri bottle, angle the spray of water to that it flows from front to back.
  - Drink plenty of fluids each day and eat a variety of foods that are high in vitamins, iron, and protein.
  - Be sure to get adequate rest at night and periodically throughout the day.

or unsure of what is happening to them. They may experience fear about loss of control; they may feel scared, alone, or guilty, or as if they have somehow failed. Although the exact cause is unknown, a lower incidence of postpartum emotional disorders occurs in cultures that promote open expression of emotions and woman-centred care (Lowdermilk et al., 2011).

Postpartum emotional disorders have been documented for years, but only recently have they received medical attention. Plummeting levels of estrogen and progesterone immediately after birth can contribute to postpartum mood disorders. It is believed that the greater the change in these hormone levels between pregnancy and

Nursing Care Plan 22.1

OVERVIEW OF THE WOMAN WITH A POSTPARTUM COMPLICATION

Jennifer, a 16-year-old G1P1, gave birth to a boy by cesarean 3 days ago due to cephalopelvic disproportion following 25 hours of labour with ruptured membranes. Her temperature is 39.2°C. She is complaining of chills and malaise and severe pain at the incision site. The site is red and warm to the touch with purulent drainage. Jennifer's lochia is scant and dark red, with a strong odour. She tells the nurse to take her baby back to the nursery because she doesn't feel well enough to care for him.

NURSING DIAGNOSIS: Ineffective thermoregulation related to bacterial invasion *as evidenced by fever, complaints of chills and malaise, and statement of not feeling well.*

Outcome Identification and Evaluation
Jennifer will exhibit a return to normothermia *as evidenced by a body temperature being maintained around 37°C, reports of a decrease in chills and malaise, and statements of feeling better.*

Interventions: Promoting Fever Reduction
- Assess vital signs every 2 to 4 hours and record results *to monitor progress of infection.*
- Offer cool bed bath or shower *to reduce temperature.*
- Place cool cloth on forehead and/or back of neck *for comfort.*
- Change bed linen and gown when damp from diaphoresis *to provide comfort and hygiene.*
- Administer antipyretics as ordered *to reduce temperature.*
- Administer antibiotic therapy and wound care as ordered *to treat infection.*
- Use aseptic technique *to prevent spread of infection.*
- Force fluids to 2,000 mL per shift to hydrate patient; document intake and output *to assess hydration status.*

NURSING DIAGNOSIS: Impaired skin integrity related to wound infection as *evidenced by purulent drainage, redness, swelling, and separation of wound edges*

Outcome Identification and Evaluation
Jennifer will experience a resolution of wound infection as *evidenced by a reduction in redness, swelling, and drainage from wound, absence of purulent drainage, and beginning signs and symptoms of wound healing.*

Interventions: Promoting Wound Healing
- Administer antibiotic therapy as ordered *to treat infection.*
- Perform frequent dressing changes and wound care as ordered *to promote wound healing;* monitor dressing for drainage, including amount, colour, and characteristics, *to evaluate for resolution of infection.*
- Use aseptic technique *to prevent spread of infection.*
- Encourage fluid intake *to maintain fluid balance;* encourage adequate dietary intake, including protein, *to promote healing.*

NURSING DIAGNOSIS: Acute pain related to infectious process

Outcome Identification and Evaluation
Patient reports decreased pain *as evidenced by a rating of 0 or 1 on pain scale, verbalization of relief with pain management, and statements of feeling better and ability to rest comfortably.*

Interventions: Relieving Pain
- Place client in semi-Fowler's position to facilitate drainage and relieve pressure.
- Assess pain level on pain scale of 0 to 10 to quantify pain; reassess pain level after intervening to determine effectiveness of intervention.
- Assess fundus gently to ensure appropriate involution.
- Administer analgesics as needed and on time as ordered to maintain pain relief.
- Provide for rest periods to allow for the healing process.
- Encourage good dietary intake to promote healing.
- Assist with positioning in bed with pillows to promote comfort. Offer a backrub or other non-pharmacologic pain relief measure to ease aches and discomfort if desired.

(continued)

Nursing Care Plan 22.1 (continued)

NURSING DIAGNOSIS: Risk for impaired parental/infant attachment related to effects of postpartum infection *as evidenced by mother's request to take baby back to the nursery*

Outcome Identification and Evaluation

Client begins to bond with newborn appropriately with each exposure *as evidenced by desire to spend time with newborn, expression of positive feelings toward newborn when holding him or her, increasing participation in care of newborn as client's condition improves, and statements about help and support at home to care for self and newborn.*

Interventions: Promoting Mother–Newborn Interaction

- Promote adequate rest and sleep *to promote healing.*
- Bring newborn to mother after she is rested and had an analgesic *to allow mother to focus her energies on the child.*
- Progressively allow the client to care for or comfort her infant as her energy level and pain level improve *to promote self-confidence in caring for the newborn.*
- Offer praise and positive reinforcement for caretaking tasks; stress positive attributes of newborn to mother while caring for him or her *to facilitate bonding and attachment.*
- Contact family members to participate in care of the newborn *to allow mother to rest and recover from infection.*
- Encourage mother to care for herself first and then the newborn *to ensure adequate energy for newborn's care.*
- Arrange for assistance and support after discharge from hospital *to aid in providing necessary backup.*
- Refer to community health nurse for follow-up care of mother and newborn at home *to foster continued development of maternal–infant relationship.*

---

postpartum, the greater the chance is for developing a mood disorder (Joy, Contag, & Templeton, et al., 2012).

Many types of emotional disorders occur in the postpartum period. Although their description and classification may be controversial, the disorders are commonly classified on the basis of their severity as postpartum or baby blues, postpartum depression, and postpartum psychosis.

Postpartum or Baby Blues

Many postpartum women (approximately 50% to 85%) experience the "baby blues." The woman exhibits mild depressive symptoms of anxiety, irritability, mood swings, tearfulness, increased sensitivity, and fatigue (Joy et al., 2012). The "blues" typically peak on postpartum days 4 and 5 and usually resolve by postpartum day 10. Although the woman's symptoms may be distressing, they do not reflect psychopathology and usually do not affect the mother's ability to function and care for her infant. Baby blues are usually self-limiting and require no formal treatment other than reassurance and validation of the woman's experience, as well as assistance in caring for herself and the newborn. However, follow-up of women with postpartum blues is important, as up to 20% go on to develop postpartum depression (Doucet, Dennis, Letourneau, et al., 2009).

Postpartum Depression

Depression is more prevalent in women than in men, which may be related to biological, hormonal, and psy-

chosocial factors. If the symptoms of postpartum blues last beyond 6 weeks and seem to get worse, the mother may be experiencing **postpartum depression**, a major depressive episode associated with childbirth (Joy et al., 2012). In Canada, as many as 8% to 23% of mothers develop postpartum depression in the first year following childbirth (Sharma & Penava, 2010). Unlike the postpartum blues, women with postpartum depression feel worse over time, and changes in mood and behaviour do not go away on their own.

The exact etiology is unknown but it appears to be a multi-factorial disorder and several factors can increase a mother's risk for developing postpartum depression:

- History of previous depression
- History of postpartum depression
- Evidence of depressive symptoms during pregnancy
- Family history of depression
- Life stress
- Childcare stress
- Prenatal anxiety
- Lack of social support
- Relationship stress
- Difficult or complicated pregnancy
- Traumatic birth experience
- Birth of a high-risk or special-needs infant (Doucet et al., 2009; Sharma & Penava, 2010)

Postpartum depression affects not only the woman but also the entire family. Identifying depression early can substantially improve the client and family outcomes. Postpartum depression usually has a more gradual onset

▶ *Consider THIS!*

As an assertive practicing attorney in her thirties, my first pregnancy was filled with nagging feelings of doubt about this upcoming event in my life. Throughout my pregnancy I was so busy with trial work that I never had time to really evaluate my feelings. I was always reading about the bodily changes that were taking place, and on one level I was feeling excited, but on another level I was emotionally drained. Shortly after the birth of my daughter, those suppressed nagging feelings of doubt surfaced big time and practically immobilized me. I felt exhausted all the time and was only too glad to have someone else care for my daughter. I didn't breastfeed because I thought it would tie me down too much. Although at the time I thought this "low mood" was normal for all new mothers, I have since found out it was postpartum depression. How could any woman be depressed about this wondrous event?

Thoughts: Now that postpartum depression has been recognized as a real emotional disorder, it can be treated. This woman showed tendencies during her pregnancy but was able to suppress the feelings and go forward. Her description of her depression is very typical of many women who suffer in silence, hoping to get over these feelings in time. What can nurses do to promote awareness of this disorder? Can it be prevented?

and becomes evident within the first 6 weeks postpartum. Some of the common manifestations are listed in Box 22.3.

Postpartum depression lends itself to prophylactic intervention because its onset is predictable, the risk

---

BOX 22.3) **Common Manifestations of Postpartum Depression**

- Loss of pleasure or interest in life
- Low mood, sadness, tearfulness
- Exhaustion that is not relieved by sleep
- Feelings of guilt
- Irritability
- Inability to concentrate
- Anxiety
- Despair
- Compulsive thoughts
- Loss of libido
- Loss of confidence
- Sleep difficulties (insomnia)
- Loss of appetite
- Feelings of failure as a mother (Gilbert, 2011)

---

period for illness is well defined, and women at high risk can be identified using a screening tool. Prophylaxis starts with a prenatal risk assessment and education. Based on the woman's history of prior depression, prophylactic antidepressant therapy may be needed during the third trimester or immediately after giving birth. See Evidence-based Practice 22.1.

Management of postpartum depression mirrors that of any major depression—a combination of antidepressant medication, antianxiety medication, and psychotherapy in an out-patient or in-patient setting (Gilbert, 2011). Marital counselling may be necessary when marital problems may be contributing to the woman's depressive symptoms.

Postpartum Psychosis

At the severe end of the continuum of postpartum emotional disorders is postpartum psychosis, which occurs in 1 woman per 1,000 births (Sharma & Penava, 2010). It generally surfaces within 3 weeks of giving birth. Symptoms of postpartum psychosis include sleep disturbances, fatigue, depression, and hypomania. The mother will be tearful, confused, and preoccupied with feelings of guilt and worthlessness. Early symptoms resemble those of depression, but they may escalate to delirium, hallucinations, anger toward herself and her infant, bizarre behaviour, manifestations of mania, and thoughts of hurting herself and the infant. The mother frequently loses touch with reality and experiences a severe regressive breakdown, associated with a high risk for suicide or infanticide (Doucet et al., 2009).

Most women with postpartum psychosis are hospitalized for up to several months. Psychotropic drugs are almost always part of treatment, along with individual psychotherapy and support group therapy.

▶ *Take NOTE!*

The greatest hazard of postpartum psychosis is suicide. Infanticide and child abuse are also risks if the woman is left alone with her infant. Early recognition and prompt treatment of this disorder is imperative (Pacagnella, Cecatti, Camargo, et al., 2010).

Nursing Assessment

Postpartum emotional disorders are often overlooked and go unrecognized despite the large percentage of women who experience them (Pacagnella et al., 2010). The postpartum period is a time of increased vulnerability, but few women receive education about the possibility of depression after birth. In addition, many women

EVIDENCE-BASED PRACTICE 22.1
Psychosocial and Psychological Interventions to Prevent Postpartum Depression

● Study

Postpartum depression is a devastating condition that affects approximately 13% of new mothers. The negative maternal and newborn outcomes associated with postpartum depression are well documented in the literature. There is a lack of knowledge about its cause and mortality, and it often remains undetected, as women are reluctant to disclose symptoms of depression or seek treatment. The two clinical questions guided the study toward preventing postpartum depression: how can nurses confirm depressive symptoms in postpartum women, and what effective prevention interventions can nurses implement in practice?

Reviewers searched multiple databases to identify 106 peer-reviewed research articles and two guidelines published in English. A panel of experts and 46 stakeholders representing diverse perspectives, including women who experienced postpartum depression, reviewed the articles and guidelines. In total, 10 specific recommendations were developed, including two prevention recommendations.

▲ Findings

Women who received preventive psychosocial or psychological interventions for reducing the risk for developing postpartum depression suggest that intensive, professionally based support may prevent women from developing postpartum depression. The first practice recommendation is for individualized and flexible nursing preventive interventions based on the self-identification or diagnosis of depressive symptoms of at-risk families. Preventive interventions included antenatal and postnatal education, lay home visits, and early postpartum follow-up. The second recommendation is for nurses to initiate prevention strategies in the early postpartum period.

■ Nursing Implications

The study provided some useful information for nurses to incorporate when providing care to pregnant women throughout the perinatal period. Nurses need to remain alert for risk factors associated with postpartum depression so they can initiate appropriate interventions for these vulnerable women and their families. Nurses can implement flexible and individually based psychosocial and psychological interventions during the prenatal period, keeping in mind that these interventions need to be continued throughout the postpartum period. They can also advocate for their clients upon discharge to ensure appropriate follow-up and support in the community and minimize impact on the family.

Source: McQueen, K., Montgomery, P., Lappan-Gracon, S., Evans, M., & Hunter, J. (2008). Evidence-based recommendations for depressive symptoms in postpartum women. *Journal of Obstetric, Gynecologic and Neonatal Nursing, 37,* 127–136. doi:10.1111/j.1552-6909.2008.00215.x

may feel ashamed of having negative emotions at a time when they "should" be happy; thus, they don't seek professional help. Nurses can play a major role in providing guidance about postpartum emotional disorders, detecting manifestations, and assisting women to obtain appropriate care.

Assessment should begin by reviewing the woman's history to identify risk factors that could predispose her to depression:

- Poor coping skills
- Low self-esteem
- Numerous life stressors
- Mood swings and emotional stress
- Previous psychological problems or a family history of psychiatric disorders
- Substance abuse
- Limited social support networks

Be alert for possible physical findings. Assess the woman's activity level, including her level of fatigue. Ask about her sleeping habits, noting any problems with insomnia. When interacting with the woman, observe for verbal and nonverbal indicators of anxiety as well as her ability to concentrate during the interaction. Difficulty concentrating and anxious behaviours suggest a problem. Also assess her nutritional intake: weight loss due to poor food intake may be seen. Assessment can identify women with a high-risk profile for depression, and the nurse can educate them and make referrals for individual or family counselling if needed.

Nursing Management

Nursing interventions that are appropriate to assist any postpartum woman to cope with the changes of this period include the following:

- Encourage the client to verbalize her feelings of what she is going through.
- Recommend that the woman seek help for household chores and child care.
- Stress the importance of good nutrition and adequate exercise and sleep.
- Encourage the client to develop a support system with other mothers.

- Assist the woman to structure her day to regain a sense of control.
- Emphasize the importance of keeping her expectations realistic.
- Discuss postponing major life changes, such as moving or changing jobs.
- Provide information about bodily changes (Canadian Mental Health Association, 2011).

The nurse can play an important role in assisting women and their partners with postpartum adjustment. Providing facts about the enormous changes that can occur during the postpartum period is critical. Review the signs and symptoms of all three emotional disorders. This information is typically included as part of prenatal visits and childbirth education classes. Know the risk factors associated with these disorders and review the history of clients and their families. Use specific, non-threatening questions to aid in early detection.

Discuss factors that may increase a woman's vulnerability to stress during the postpartum period, such as sleep deprivation and unrealistic expectations, so couples can understand and respond to those problems if they occur. Stress that many women need help after childbirth and that help is available from many sources, including people they already know. Assisting women to learn how to ask for help is important so they can gain the support they need. Also provide educational materials about postpartum emotional disorders. Have available referral sources for psychotherapy and support groups appropriate for women experiencing postpartum adjustment difficulties.

■■■ Key Concepts

- PPH is a potentially life-threatening complication of both vaginal and cesarean births. It is the leading cause of maternal mortality in Canada.
- A good way to remember the causes of PPH is the "4 T's": tone, tissue, trauma, and thrombosis.
- Uterine atony is the most common cause of early PPH, which can lead to hypovolemic shock.
- Oxytocin (Pitocin, Syntocinon), methylergonovine maleate (Methergine), ergonovine maleate (Ergotrate), and prostaglandin (PGF2-alpha, carboprost [Hemabate]) are drugs used to manage PPH.
- Failure of the placenta to separate completely and be expelled interferes with the ability of the uterus to contract fully, thereby leading to hemorrhage.
- Causes of subinvolution are retained placental fragments, distended bladder, uterine myoma, and infection.
- Lacerations should always be suspected when the uterus is contracted and bright-red blood continues to trickle out of the vagina.
- Conditions that cause coagulopathies may include ITP, vWD, and DIC.

- Pulmonary embolism is a potentially fatal condition that occurs when the pulmonary artery is obstructed by a blood clot that has travelled from another vein into the lungs, causing obstruction and infarction.
- The major causes of a thrombus formation (blood clot) are venous stasis and hypercoagulation, both of which are common in the postpartum period.
- Postpartum infection is defined as a fever of 38°C or higher after the first 24 hours after childbirth, occurring on at least 2 of the first 10 days exclusive of the first 24 hours.
- Common postpartum infections include metritis, wound infections, urinary tract infections, and mastitis.
- Postpartum emotional disorders are commonly classified on the basis of their severity: "baby blues," postpartum depression, and postpartum psychosis.
- Management of postpartum depression mirrors the treatment of any major depression—a combination of antidepressant medication, antianxiety medication, and psychotherapy in an out-patient or in-patient setting.

REFERENCES

Al-Mehaisen, L., Al-Kuran, O., Amarin, Z. O., Matalka, I., Beitawi, S., & Muhtaseb, A. (2008). Secondary postpartum hemorrhage following placental site vessel subinvolution: A case report. *Archives of Gynecology and Obstetrics, 278*(6), 585–587.

Arianpour, N., Safari, A., & Hatami, F. (2009). Bacteria isolated from post-partum infections. *Journal of Family & Reproductive Health, 3*(2), 63–66.

Belfort, M. A., Clark, S. L., Saade, G. R., et al. (2010). Hospital readmission after delivery: Evidence for an increased incidence of non-urogenital infection in the immediate postpartum period. *American Journal of Obstetrics and Gynecology, 202*(1), 35.e1–35.e7.

Belkin, A., Levy, A., & Sheiner, E. (2009). Perinatal outcomes and complications of pregnancy in women with immune thrombocytopenic purpura. *Journal of Maternal-Fetal & Neonatal Medicine, 22*(11), 1081–1085. doi:10.3109/14767050903029592

Blackburn, S. T. (2008). Physiologic changes in pregnancy. In K. R. Simpson, & P. A. Creehan (Eds.), *AWHONN's perinatal nursing* (3rd ed.). Philadelphia: Lippincott Williams & Wilkins.

Cabero, Roura, L., & Keith, L. G. (2009). Post-partum haemorrhage: Diagnosis, prevention and management. *Journal of Maternal-Fetal & Neonatal Medicine, 22*, 38–45.

Canadian Hemophilia Society. (2007). *Von Willebrand disease.* Retrieved March 12, 2012 from http://www.hemophilia.ca/en/bleeding-disorders/von-willebrand-disease/

Canadian Mental Health Association. (2011). *Post partum depression.* Retrieved March 12, 2012 from http://www.cmha.ca/bins/content_page.asp?cid=3-86-87-88&lang=1

Castaman, G., Tosetto, A., & Rodeghiero, F. (2010). Pregnancy and delivery in women with von Willebrand's disease and different von Willebrand factor mutations. *Haematologica, 95*(6), 963–969.

Clark, S.L., Belfort, M.A., Dildy, G.A., Herbst, M.A., Meyers, J.A., & Hankins, G.D. (2008). Maternal death in the 21st century: Causes, prevention, and relationship to cesarean delivery. *American Journal of Obstetrics and Gynecology, 199*(1), 36.e1–36.e5; discussion 91-2. e7–91-2.e11.

Doucet, S., Dennis, C., Letourneau, N., & Blackmore, E. R. (2009). Differentiation and clinical implications of postpartum depression and postpartum psychosis. *Journal of Obstetric, Gynecologic, and Neonatal Nursing, 38*(3), 269–279.

Fujita, A., Sakai, R., Matsuura, S., et al. (2010). A retrospective analysis of obstetric patients with idiopathic thrombocytopenic purpura:

A single center study. *International Journal of Hematology, 92*(3), 463–467.

Gilbert, E. S. (2011). *Manual of high risk pregnancy & delivery* (5th ed.). St. Louis: MO: Mosby Elsevier.

Jacobsen, A. F., Skjeldestad, F. E., & Sandset, P. M. (2008). Ante- and postnatal risk factors of venous thrombosis: A hospital-based case-control study. *Journal of Thrombosis and Haemostasis, 6*(6), 905–912.

James, A. H. (2009). Venous thromboembolism in pregnancy. *Arteriosclerosis, Thrombosis, and Vascular Biology, 29*(3), 326–331.

Joy, S., Contag, S. A., & Templeton, H. B. (2012). Postpartum depression. Retrieved March 12, 2012 from http://emedicine.medscape.com/article/271662-overview

Kadir, R., Chi, C., & Bolton-Maggs, P. (2009). Pregnancy and rare bleeding disorders. *Haemophilia, 15*(5), 990–1005. doi:10.1111/j.1365-2516.2009.01984.x

Leduc, D., Senikas, V., & Lalonde, A. B. (2009). SOGC clinical practice guideline: Active management of the third stage of labour: Prevention and treatment of postpartum hemorrhage. *Journal of Obstetrics and Gynaecology Canada, 31*(10), 980–993. Retrieved March 12, 2012 from http://www.sogc.org/guidelines/documents/gui235CPG0910.pdf

Lindqvist, P. G., Torsson, J., Almqvist, A., & Björgell, O. (2008). Postpartum thromboembolism: Severe events might be preventable using a new risk score model. *Vascular Health and Risk Management, 4*(5), 1081–1087.

Liu, S., Rouleau, J., Joseph, K. S., et al. (2009). Epidemiology of pregnancy-associated venous thromboembolism: A population-based study in Canada. *Journal of Obstetrics and Gynaecology Canada, 31*(7), 611–620. Retrieved March 12, 2012 from http://www.sogc.org/jogc/abstracts/full/200907_Obstetrics_2.pdf

Lowdermilk, D. L., Perry, S. E., Cashion, K., & Alden, K. R. (2011). *Maternity and women's health care* (10th ed.). Philadelphia: Mosby Elsevier.

Majd, H. S., Nawaz, T., Ismail, L., Luker, R., & Kalla, S. (2009). Acute uterine inversion as a cause of major post-partum haemorrhage: A case report and review of the literature. *Internet Journal of Gynecology & Obstetrics, 12*(1). Retrieved March 12, 2012 from http://www.ispub.com/journal/the_internet_journal_of_gynecology_and_obstetrics/volume_12_number_1_4/article/acute-uterine-inversion-as-a-cause-of-major-post-partum-haemorrhage-a-case-report-and-review-of-the-literature.html

Maslovitz, S., Barkai, G., Lessing, J. B., Ziv, A., & Many, A. (2008). Improved accuracy of postpartum blood loss estimation as assessed by simulation. *Acta Obstetrica & Gynecologica Scandinavica, 87*(9), 929–934. doi:10.1080/00016340802317794

Mirza, F. G., & Gaddipati, S. (2009). Obstetric emergencies. *Seminars in Perinatology, 33*(2), 97–103.

Pacagnella, R. C., Cecatti, J. G., Camargo, R. P., et al. (2010). Rationale for a long-term evaluation of the consequences of potentially life-threatening maternal conditions and maternal "near-miss" incidents using a multidimensional approach. *Journal of Obstetrics and Gynaecology Canada, 32*(8), 730–738. Retrieved March 12, 2012 from http://www.sogc.org/jogc/abstracts/full/201008_Obstetrics_1.pdf

Pacheco, L. D., Costantine, M. M., Saade, G. R., Mucowski, S., Hankins, G. D. V., & Sciscione, A. C. (2010). Von Willebrand disease and pregnancy: A practical approach for the diagnosis and treatment. *American Journal of Obstetrics and Gynecology, 203*(3), 194–200.

Paruk, F. (2008). Infection in obstetric critical care. *Best Practice & Research: Clinical Obstetrics & Gynaecology, 22*(5), 865–883.

Peyvandi, F., Menegatti, M., & Siboni, S.M. (2011). Post-partum hemorrhage in women with rare bleeding disorders. *Thrombosis Research, 127*, S116–S119. doi:10.1016/S0049-3848(11)70031-7

Public Health Agency of Canada. (2008). *Canadian perinatal health report*, 2008 edition. Ottawa: ON. Retrieved March 12, 2012 from http://www.phac-aspc.gc.ca/publicat/2008/cphr-rspc/pdf/cphr-rspc08-eng.pdf

Riordan, J., & Wambach, K. (2010). Breast-related problems. In J. Riordan, & K. Wambach (Eds.), *Breastfeeding and human lactation* (4th ed.). Toronto: ON: Jones & Bartlett.

Sharma, V., & Penava, D. (2010). Screening for bipolar disorder during pregnancy and the postpartum period [comment]. *Journal of Obstetrics and Gynaecology Canada, 32*(3), 278–281. Retrieved March 12, 2012 from http://www.sogc.org/jogc/abstracts/full/201003_Commentary_1.pdf

Tebruegge, M., Misra, I., Pantazidou, A., et al. (2009). Estimating blood loss: Comparative study of the accuracy of parents and health care professionals. *Pediatrics, 124*(4), e729–e736.

Thachil, J., & Toh, C. (2009). Disseminated intravascular coagulation in obstetric disorders and its acute haematological management. *Blood Reviews, 23*(4), 167–176.

Wilson-Clay, B., & Hoover, K. L. (2008). *The breastfeeding atlas*. (4th ed.). Manchaca, Texas: LactNews Press.

Wong, A. W., & Rosh, A. J. (2010). *Postpartum infections*. Retrieved March 12, 2012 from http://emedicine.medscape.com/article/796892-overview

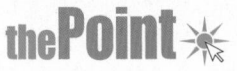

For additional learning materials, including Internet Resources, visit
http://thePoint.lww.com/Chow1e.

CHAPTER WORKSHEET

MULTIPLE CHOICE QUESTIONS

1. A postpartum mother appears very pale and states she is bleeding heavily. The nurse should first:

   a. Call the client's health care provider immediately.

   b. Immediately set up an intravenous infusion of magnesium sulfate.

   c. Assess the fundus and ask her about her voiding status.

   d. Reassure the mother that this is a normal finding after childbirth.

2. Hallucinations and expressions of suicide or infanticide are indicative of:

   a. Postpartum psychosis

   b. Postpartum anxiety disorder

   c. Postpartum depression

   d. Postpartum blues

3. The nurse assesses a woman closely in the first few hours after giving birth because which of the following could occur?

   a. Thrombophlebitis

   b. Breast engorgement

   c. Uterine infection

   d. PPH

4. Which of the following would the nurse expect to include in the plan of care for a woman with mastitis who is receiving antibiotic therapy?

   a. Stop breastfeeding and apply lanolin.

   b. Administer analgesics and bind both breasts.

   c. Apply warm or cold compresses and give analgesics.

   d. Remove the nursing bra and expose the breast to fresh air.

CRITICAL THINKING EXERCISES

1. Mrs. Griffin had a 12-hour labour before a cesarean birth. Her membranes ruptured 6 hours before she came to the hospital. Her fetus showed signs of distress, so internal electronic fetal monitoring was used. Her most recent test results indicate she is anemic.

   a. What postpartum complication is this new mother at highest risk for? Why?

   b. What assessments need to be done to detect this potential complication?

   c. What nursing measures will the nurse use to prevent this complication?

2. Tammy, a 32-year-old G9P9, had a spontaneous vaginal birth 2 hours ago. Tammy has been having a baby each year for the past 9 years. Tammy's lochia has been heavy, with some clots. She hasn't been up to void since she had epidural anesthesia and has decreased sensation to her legs.

   a. What factors place Tammy at risk for PPH?

   b. What assessments are needed before planning interventions?

   c. What nursing actions are needed to prevent a PPH?

3. Lucy, a 25-year-old G2P2, gave birth 2 days ago and is expected to be discharged today. She has a history of severe postpartum depression 2 years ago with her first child. Lucy has not been out of bed for the past 24 hours, is not eating, and provides no care for herself or her newborn. Lucy states she already has a boy at home and not having a girl this time is disappointing.

   a. What factors/behaviours place Lucy at risk for an emotional disorder?

   b. Which interventions might be appropriate at this time?

   c. What education does the family need prior to discharge?

STUDY ACTIVITIES

1. Compare and contrast postpartum blues, postpartum depression, and postpartum psychosis in terms of their unique features and medical management.

2. Select a website from the ones on http://thePoint. lww.com/Chow1e. Critique it regarding its helpfulness to parents, the correctness of the information supplied, and when was it last updated.

3. Interview a woman who has given birth and ask about any complications she may have had and what was most helpful to her during the experience.

4. The number-one cause of PPH is

   _____.

5. When giving report to the nurse who will be caring for a woman and her newborn in the postpartum period, what information should the labour nurse convey?

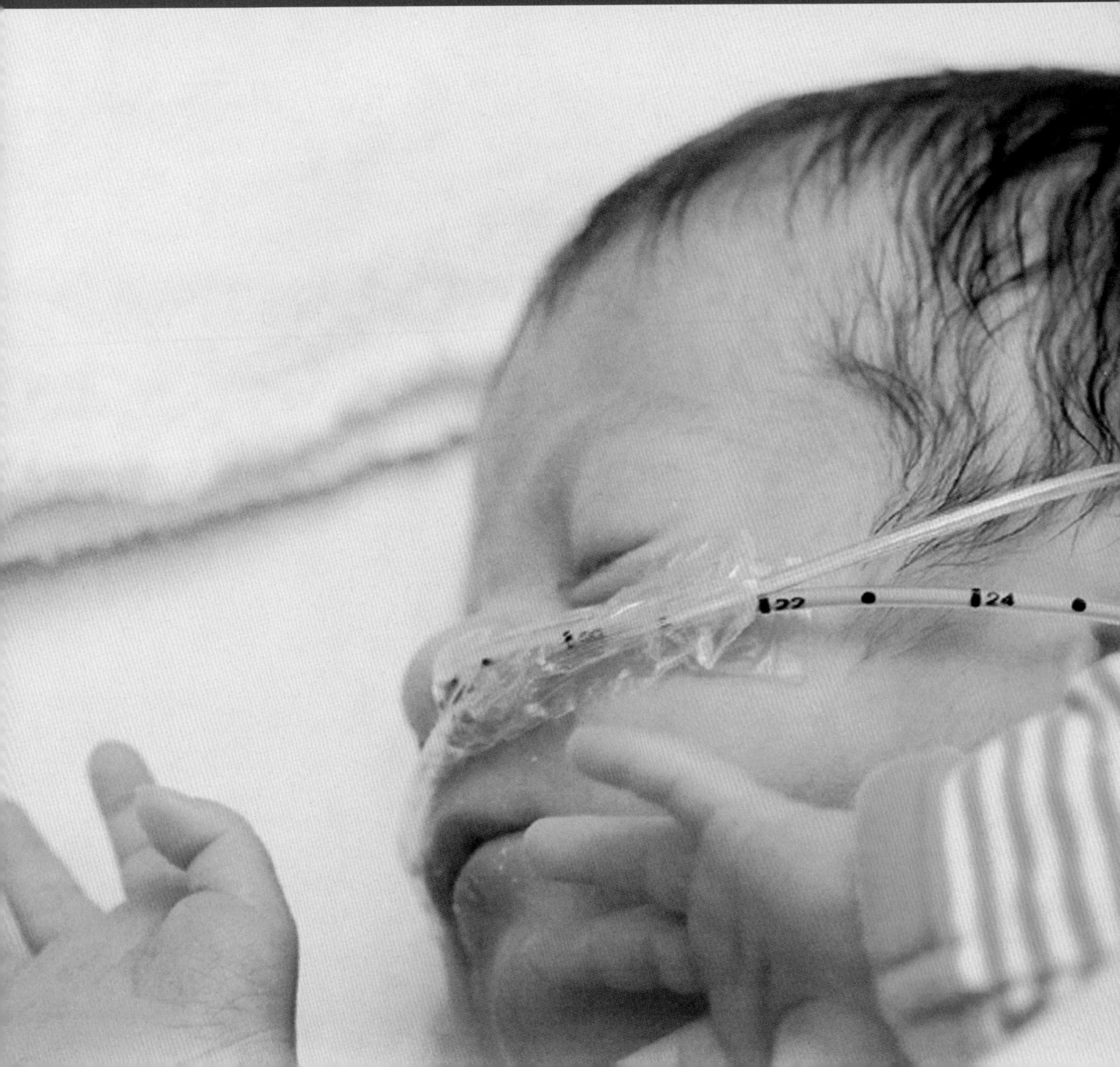

UNIT EIGHT

THE NEWBORN AT RISK

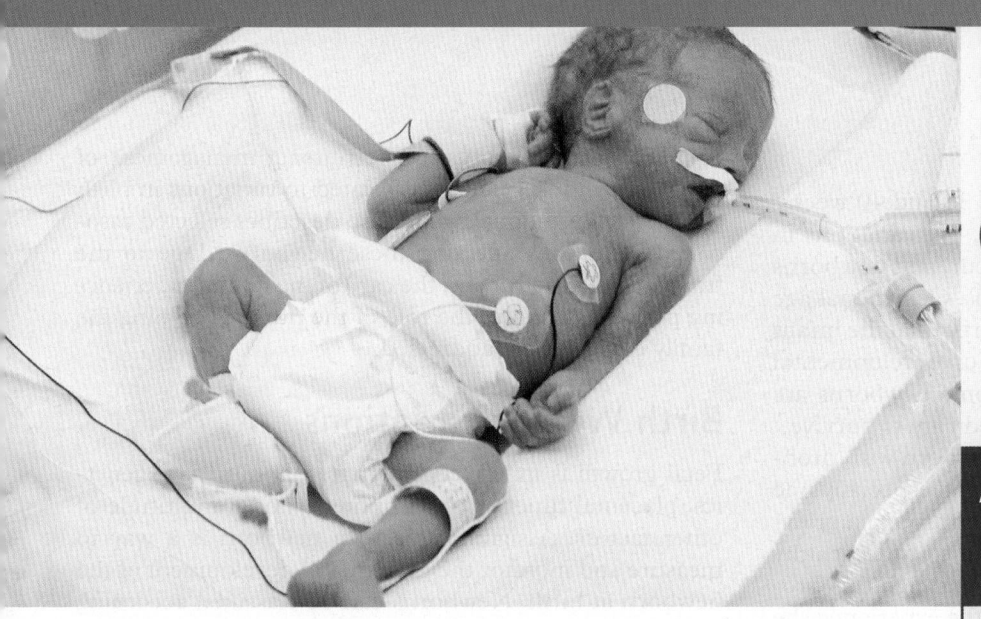

Adapted by Lynne Harwood–Lunn

NURSING CARE OF THE NEWBORN WITH SPECIAL NEEDS

KEY TERMS

appropriate for
   gestational age
asphyxia
extremely low birth
   weight

large for gestational age
late preterm newborn
low birth weight
postterm newborn
preterm newborn

retinopathy of
   prematurity
small for gestational age
term newborn
very low birth weight

LEARNING OBJECTIVES

Upon completion of the chapter, the learner will be able to:

1. Explain factors that assist in identifying a newborn at risk due to variations in birth weight and gestational age.
2. Select contributing factors and common complications associated with dysmature infants and their management.
3. Compare and contrast a small-for-gestational-age newborn and a large-for-gestational-age newborn; a postterm and preterm newborn.
4. Discuss associated conditions that affect the newborn with variations in birth weight and gestational age, including appropriate management.
5. Outline the nurse's role in helping parents experiencing perinatal grief or loss.
6. Integrate knowledge of the risks associated with late preterm births into nursing interventions, discharge planning, and parent education.

Anna and her husband were stunned when she went into labour at 7 months' gestation. They couldn't understand what would cause her to give birth early, but it happened. When they approached the NICU, Anna took a deep breath and looked down at her tiny baby with tubes coming from everywhere. What feelings might they be experiencing at this moment? Do you think that guilt would be one of those feelings? If so, why?

Wow

Guiding a parent's hand to touch a frail or ill newborn demonstrates courage and compassion under very difficult circumstances and is a powerful tool in helping to deal with the newborn's special needs.

ost newborns are born between 38 and 40 weeks' gestation and weigh 2,700 to 4,000 g, but variations in birth weight or gestational age can occur, and newborns with these variations have special needs. Gestational age at birth is inversely correlated with the risk that the infant will experience physical, neurologic, or developmental sequelae (March of Dimes, 2011). Some newborns are born very ill and need special advanced care to survive.

When a woman gives birth to a newborn with problems involving immaturity or birth weight, especially one who is considered high risk, she may go through a grieving process in which she mourns the loss of the healthy full-term newborn she had expected. Through this process, she learns to come to terms with the experience she now faces.

The development of new technologies and regionalized care centres for the care of newborns with special needs has resulted in significant improvements. Nurses need to have a sound knowledge base to identify the newborn with special needs and to provide coordinated care.

The key to identifying a newborn with special needs related to birth weight or gestational age variation is an awareness of the factors that could place a newborn at risk. These factors are similar to those that would suggest a high-risk pregnancy and include:

- Maternal nutrition (malnutrition or overweight)
- Substandard living conditions
- Low socioeconomic status
- Maternal age of less than 20 or more than 35 years old
- Substance abuse
- Failure to seek prenatal care
- Smoking or exposure to passive smoke
- Periodontal disease
- Multiple gestation
- Extreme maternal stress
- Abuse and violence
- Placental complications (placenta previa or abruptio placentae)
- History of previous preterm birth
- Maternal disease (e.g., hypertension or diabetes)
- Maternal infection (e.g., urinary tract infection or chorioamnionitis)
- Exposure to occupational hazards (Joseph, 2008)
- Recent immigration to Canada (Urquia, Frank, Glazier, et al., 2007)
- Use of assisted reproductive technologies (Gundby, Bissonnette, Librach, et al., 2008)

Being able to anticipate the birth of a newborn at risk allows the birth to take place at a health care facility equipped with the necessary resources to meet the mother's and newborn's needs. This is important in reducing mortality and morbidity.

This chapter discusses the nursing management of newborns with special needs related to variations in birth weight and gestational age. It also describes selected associated conditions affecting these newborns. Due to the frailty of these newborns, the care of the family experiencing perinatal loss and the role of the nurse in helping the family cope also are addressed.

Birth Weight Variations

Fetal growth is influenced by maternal nutrition, genetics, placental function, environment, and a multitude of other factors. Assigning size to a newborn is a way to measure and monitor the growth and development of the newborn at birth. Newborns can be classified according to their weight and weeks of gestation, and knowing the group into which a newborn fits is important.

Appropriate for gestational age (AGA) characterizes approximately 80% of newborns and describes a newborn with a normal height, weight, head circumference, and body mass index (BMI) (Dorland, 2007). Being in the AGA group confers the lowest risk for any problems. These infants have lower morbidity and mortality than other groups.

Small-for-gestational-age (SGA) newborns typically weigh less than 2,500 g (5 lb 8 oz) at term due to less growth in utero than expected. A newborn is also classified as SGA if his or her birth weight is at or below the 10th percentile as correlated with the number of weeks of gestation on a growth chart.

Large for gestational age (LGA) describes newborns whose birth weight is above the 90th percentile on a growth chart regardless of gestational age; infants who weigh more than 4,000 g are considered to have high birth weight (Luo, Senecal, Simonet, et al., 2010).

The following terms describe other newborns with marginal weights at birth and of any gestational age:

- **Low birth weight:** less than 2,500 g (5.5 lb) (Fig. 23.1)
- **Very low birth weight:** less than 1,500 g (3 lb 5 oz)
- **Extremely low birth weight:** less than 1,000 g (2 lb 3 oz)

Small-for-Gestational-Age Newborns

Newborns are considered SGA when they weigh less than two standard deviations for gestational age or fall below the 10th percentile on a growth chart for gestational age. In Canada, 8.3% of infants are born SGA, with the highest rates in Ontario and Alberta (Canadian Institute for Health Information, 2009). These infants can be preterm, term, or postterm.

In some SGA newborns, the rate of growth does not meet the expected growth pattern. Termed intrauterine growth restriction (IUGR), these newborns also are considered at risk, with the perinatal morbidity and mortality

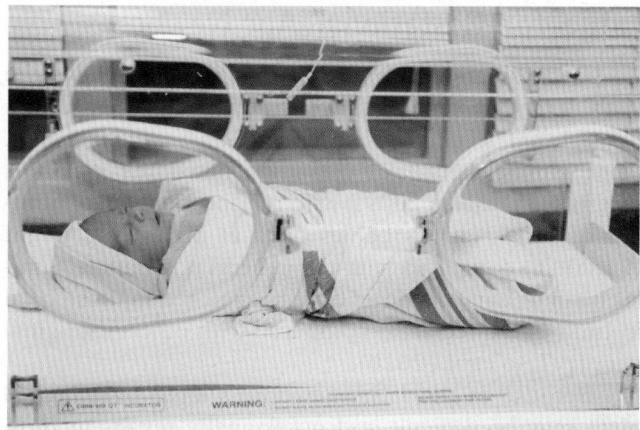

FIGURE 23.1 A low birth weight newborn in an isolette.

rate increased substantially compared with that of the AGA newborn (Zhong, Tuuli, & Odido, 2010). IUGR is the pathologic counterpart of SGA. However, an important distinction to make between SGA newborns and IUGR is that not all newborns who are SGA have IUGR. The converse also is true: not all newborns who have IUGR are SGA. Some SGA newborns are constitutionally small: they are statistically small but otherwise healthy.

Conditions altering fetal growth produce insults that affect all organ systems and are known to produce two patterns of growth that depend on the timing of the insult to the developing embryo or fetus. An early insult (typically occurring before 28 weeks) results in overall growth restriction, with all organs being small. These SGA infants never catch up in size when compared with normal children. An insult later in gestation (after 28 weeks) results in intrauterine malnutrition, but optimal postnatal nutrition generally restores normal growth potential and carries a better prognosis than earlier insults (Ricci & Kyle, 2009).

Historically, IUGR has been categorized as symmetric or asymmetric. Symmetric IUGR is characterized by equal delay of growth of all organs and reflects very early growth failure or reduced growth potential. In asymmetric IUGR, brain growth is preserved in comparison with growth of other organs such as the liver. Asymmetric IUGR classically develops in the third trimester as a result of fetal malnutrition (Rodek & Whittle, 2009).

Fetal growth is dependent on genetic, placental, and maternal factors. Cognitive and motor development during infancy forms the basis for children's subsequent development. Newborns who experience nutritional deficiencies in utero and are born SGA are at risk for cognitive deficits that can undermine their academic performance throughout their lives (Beckmann, Ling, Barzansky, et al., 2010).

The fetus is thought to have an inherent growth potential that, under normal circumstances, yields a healthy newborn of appropriate size. The maternal–placental–fetal units act in harmony to meet the needs of the fetus during gestation. However, growth potential in the fetus can be limited, and this is analogous to failure to thrive in the infant. The causes of both can be intrinsic or environmental. Factors that can contribute to the birth of an SGA newborn are highlighted in Box 23.1.

Nursing Assessment

Assessment of the SGA infant begins with a review of the maternal history to identify risk factors such as smoking, drug abuse, chronic maternal illness, hypertension, multiple gestation, or genetic disorders. This information allows the nurse to anticipate a possible problem and to be prepared to intervene quickly should one occur. At birth, perform a thorough physical examination, closely observing the newborn for typical characteristics, including:

- Head disproportionately large compared with rest of body
- Wasted appearance of extremities
- Reduced subcutaneous fat stores
- Decreased amount of breast tissue
- Scaphoid abdomen (sunken appearance)

BOX 23.1 Factors Contributing to the Birth of SGA Newborns

- Preconceptional or preexisting risk factors
- Chronic hypertension/renal disease
- Diabetes with vasculopathy
- Autoimmune syndromes—antiphospholipid syndrome, lupus
- Thrombophilia
- Maternal hypoxemia—cyanotic heart disease, severe chronic anemia, chronic pulmonary disease
- Uterine anomalies—large submucous myomas, septate uterus, synechia
- Low maternal age (teenagers)
- Smoking
- Substance abuse—alcohol, heroin, methadone, cocaine, therapeutic agents
- Malnutrition
- Environmental pollution (e.g., sulfur dioxide, nitrogen dioxide, carbon monoxide)
- Family history of IUGR
- Pregnancy-related risk factors in the first trimester
- Fetal chromosomal abnormality—trisomy 13, 18, and 21; triploidy; uniparental disomy
- Fetal malformations—gastroschisis, omphalocele, diaphragmatic hernia, congenital heart defect
- Maternal infection—malaria, rubella, cytomegalovirus, herpes, toxoplasmosis
- Multiple gestation

Source: Zhong, Y., Tuuli, M., & Odido, A. O. (2010). First-trimester assessment of placenta function and the prediction of preeclampsia and intrauterine growth restriction. *Prenatal Diagnoses, 30,* 293–308.

- Wide skull sutures secondary to inadequate bone growth
- Poor muscle tone over buttocks and cheeks
- Loose and dry skin that appears oversized
- Thin umbilical cord

Also assess the SGA newborn for any congenital malformations, neurologic insults, or indications of infection. SGA newborns commonly face problems after birth because of the decrease in placental function during gestation. Table 23.1 highlights some of the common problems associated with SGA newborns and others experiencing a variation in birth weight or gestational age. Anticipate the need for and provide resuscitation as indicated by the newborn's condition.

Nursing Management

Interventions for the SGA infant may include obtaining weight, length, and head circumference, comparing them with standards, and documenting the findings. Perform frequent serial blood glucose measurements as ordered and monitor vital signs, being particularly alert for changes in respiratory status that might indicate respiratory distress. Institute measures to maintain a neutral thermal environment to prevent cold stress and acidosis.

Initiate early and frequent oral feedings unless contraindicated. Any newborn who is stressed at birth depletes available glucose stores with resulting hypoglycemia. The Canadian Paediatric Society (CPS, 2011) recognizes that neonatal hypoglycemia cannot be defined by a single value but proposes that intervention should be implemented when repeated blood glucose values are less than 2.6 mmol/L. With the loss of the placenta at birth, the newborn now must assume control of glucose homeostasis through intermittent oral feedings. If oral feedings are not accepted or blood glucose remains below 2.6 mmol/L despite feeds, an intravenous infusion with 10% dextrose at a rate of 80 mL/kg/day may be needed to maintain the glucose level above 2.6 mmol/L (CPS, 2011). Weigh the newborn daily and ensure that he or she has adequate rest periods to decrease metabolic requirements.

Observe for clinical signs of polycythemia and monitor blood results. Asymptomatic newborns with a hematocrit between 60% and 70% may simply be supported with fluids, close observation, and a repeat hematocrit level in 4 to 6 hours (Sankar, Agarwal, Deorari, et al., 2010). If the newborn is symptomatic, partial exchange transfusion may be used, but this treatment is considered controversial.

Provide anticipatory guidance to parents about any treatments and procedures that are being done. Emphasize the need for close follow-up and careful monitoring of the infant's growth in length, weight, and head circumference and feeding patterns throughout the first year of life to confirm any "catch-up" growth taking place.

Large-for-Gestational-Age Newborns

To be considered LGA, newborns must be above the 90th percentile on a birth weight chart and weigh more than 4,000 g (Luo, Kierans, Wilkins, et al., 2004). Approximately 1.9% of Canadian newborns are LGA (Statistics Canada, 2009), with a disproportionate number of First Nations babies born at high birth weight (>4,000 g) compared with the general population. Similar birth weight outcomes have been noted in those born in Inuit-inhabited areas compared with other Aboriginal people (Luo et al., 2010).

Because of the LGA newborn's large size, vaginal birth may be difficult and occasionally results in birth injury. Shoulder dystocia, clavicular fractures, and facial palsies are common. The incidence of cesarean births is very high among LGA newborns to avoid arrested labour and birth trauma.

▶ *Take* NOTE!

Diabetes is commonly associated with LGA newborns. However, due to poor placental perfusion, the newborn may experience IUGR and be SGA.

Nursing Assessment

Assessment of the LGA newborn begins with a review of the maternal history, which can provide clues as to whether the woman has an increased risk for giving birth to an LGA newborn. Maternal factors that increase the chance of bearing an LGA newborn include diabetes mellitus or glucose intolerance, multiparity, prior history of a macrosomic infant, postdates gestation, obesity, and age over 35 years (Kierans, Luo, Wilkins, et al., n.d).

At birth, assess the newborn for common characteristics. The typical LGA newborn has a large body and appears plump and full-faced. The increase in body size is proportional. However, the head circumference and body length are in the upper limits of intrauterine growth. These newborns have poor motor skills and have difficulty in regulating behavioural states. LGA newborns are more difficult to arouse to a quiet alert state (Neonatal Handbook, 2011).

Thoroughly assess the LGA newborn at birth to identify traumatic birth injuries such as fractured clavicles, brachial palsy, facial paralysis, phrenic nerve palsy, skull fractures, or hematomas. Perform a neurologic examination to identify any nerve palsies, looking for abnormalities such as immobility of the upper arm. Observe and document any injuries discovered to allow for early intervention and improved outcomes.

Glucose screening guidelines dictate that asymptomatic infants at risk for hypoglycemia should receive one effective feed before a blood glucose check at 2 hours of

(text continues on page 732)

TABLE 23.1 COMMON PROBLEMS ASSOCIATED WITH NEWBORNS EXPERIENCING A VARIATION IN BIRTH WEIGHT OR GESTATIONAL AGE

Problem	Occurrence	Etiology/Pathophysiology	Assessment Findings	Nursing Implications
Perinatal asphyxia	SGA newborns (common) Postterm newborns Preterm newborns (common)	Poor tolerance to stress of labour, frequently leading to acidosis and hypoxia Living in hypoxic environment prior to birth, leaving little to no oxygen reserves available to withstand stress of labour: • Uterine contractions increase hypoxic stress • Possible depletion of glycogen stores due to chronic hypoxic state, leading to fetal distress • Impaired uteroplacental circulation due to maternal and uterine conditions predisposing to perinatal depression Compromised newborn at birth experiencing difficulty adjusting to extra-uterine environment Placental deprivation or oligohydramnios, leading to cord compression and subsequent reduction in perfusion to fetus Surfactant deficiency Unstable chest wall Immaturity of respiratory control centres in the CNS Small respiratory passages, increasing risk for obstruction Inability to clear mucus from airways	Fetal distress (bradycardia, decelerations) during labour Low Apgar scores (Kiess, Chernausek, & Hokken-Koelega, 2009)	Anticipate possible problem; assess for maternal risk factors. Initiate resuscitation measures immediately at birth.
Difficulty with thermoregulation	SGA newborns (common) Postterm newborns Preterm newborns (common) Late preterm infant (common)	Less muscle mass, less brown fat, less heat-preserving subcutaneous fat, and limited ability to control skin capillaries (Bissinger & Annibale, 2010) Associated with depleted glycogen stores, poor subcutaneous fat stores, and disturbances in CNS thermoregulation due to hypoxia (Darcy, 2009)	Temperature <36.4°C; temperature instability; skin cool to touch; cyanosis of hands and feet Bradypnea (<25 beats/min) and tachypnea (>60 breaths/minute) Tremors, irritability Wheezing, crackles, retractions Restlessness, lethargy Hypotonia Weak or high-pitched cry	Maintain a neutral thermal environment to promote stabilization of newborn's temperature. Assess skin temperature and respiration characteristics. Monitor arterial blood gases and blood glucose levels.

(continued)

TABLE 23.1 Common Problems Associated with Newborns Experiencing a Variation in Birth Weight or Gestational Age (continued)

Problem	Occurrence	Etiology/Pathophysiology	Assessment Findings	Nursing Implications
		Increased risk for acidosis and hypoglycemia secondary to metabolic stress (Neonatal Handbook, 2007) Loss of subcutaneous fat second to placental insufficiency Use of stored nutrients for nutrition due to lost ability of placenta to nourish fetus Subsequent wasting of subcutaneous fat, muscle, or both (Darcy, 2009) Loss of natural insulation (subcutaneous fat) important in temperature regulation Immaturity of CNS (temperature-regulating centre) interferes with ability to regulate body temperature Inadequate amounts of subcutaneous fat Lack of muscle tone and flexion to conserve heat Inadequate brown fat to generate heat Limited muscle mass activity, reducing ability to produce own heat Inability to shiver to generate heat	Seizures Poor feeding Grunting (Chen et al., 2010) Acidosis	Eliminate sources of heat loss: • Dry newborn thoroughly. • Wrap in warmed blanket with stockinette cap on head. • Use radiant heat source.
Hypoglycemia	SGA newborns (common) LGA newborns (common) Postterm newborns Preterm newborns Late preterm infants	Increased metabolic rate and lack of adequate glycogen stores to meet newborn's metabolic needs Commonly associated with infants of diabetic mothers Abrupt cessation of high-glucose maternal blood supply with birth and continued insulin production by the newborn Limited ability to release glucagons and catecholamines, which normally stimulate glucagon breakdown and glucose release	Often subtle Lethargy, tachycardia Respiratory distress Jitteriness Drowsiness Poor feeding, feeble sucking Hypothermia, temperature instability Diaphoresis Weak cry Seizures Hypotonia Blood glucose levels <40 mg/dL for term newborns, <20 mg/dL for preterm newborns (CPS, 2011)	Monitor blood glucose levels, initially on arrival to nursery and hourly thereafter. Maintain fluid and electrolyte balance. Watch for subtle changes. Initiate early oral feedings if possible; if not, administer IV infusion with 10% dextrose in water.

Problem	Occurrence	Etiology/Pathophysiology	Assessment Findings	Nursing Implications
		Hypoxia secondary to depleted glycogen reserves Placental insufficiency secondary to placental aging contributing to chronic fetal nutritional deficiency further depleting glycogen stores Immature sucking and swallowing leading to insufficient intake Perinatal hypoxia Increased energy expenditure Decreased subcutaneous and brown fat with little to no glycogen stores		
Polycythemia	SGA newborns LGA newborns Postterm newborns	Chronic mild hypoxia secondary to placental insufficiency Stimulation of erythropoietin release, leading to increased RBC production Secondary to fetal hypoxia, trauma with bleeding, increased erythropoietin production, or delayed cord clamping (Sankar et al., 2010) Intrauterine hypoxia triggers increased RBC cell production to compensate for lower oxygen levels.	Venous hematocrit >65% Plethora (ruddy appearance) Weak sucking reflex Tachypnea Jaundice Lethargy Jitteriness Hypotonia Irritability Feeding difficulties Difficulty in arousing Seizures	Ensure adequate hydration (orally or IV). Monitor hematocrit levels (goal is ~60%). Administer partial exchange transfusion, albumin or normal saline IV to reduce RBC volume and increase fluid volume (controversial).
Meconium aspiration	SGA newborns Postterm newborns	Release of meconium into amniotic fluid prior to birth Inhalation of meconium-containing amniotic fluid by the newborn, leading to aspiration Commonly associated with chronic intrauterine hypoxia Struggling by fetus making respiratory efforts and bearing down with abdominal muscles, leading to expulsion of meconium into amniotic fluid Normal sucking and swallowing by fetus leads to meconium filling airways.	Green amniotic fluid with rupture of membranes during labour Green staining of the umbilical cord or fingernails Difficulty initiating respirations	Initiate resuscitation measures as necessary. Suction airways and support ventilation (see Chapter 24 for more information).

(continued)

TABLE 23.1   COMMON PROBLEMS ASSOCIATED WITH NEWBORNS EXPERIENCING A VARIATION IN
BIRTH WEIGHT OR GESTATIONAL AGE (continued)

Problem	Occurrence	Etiology/Pathophysiology	Assessment Findings	Nursing Implications
Hyperbilirubi-nemia	LGA newborns (common) Preterm newborns Late preterm infants	Associated with polycythe-mia and RBC breakdown Inability to tolerate feedings in the first few days of life, leading to increased enterohepatic circulation of bilirubin Excessive bruising second-ary to birth trauma, lead-ing to higher-than-normal bilirubin levels Increased breakdown of RBCs and immature liver function to handle excess load	Elevated serum biliru-bin levels Jaundice Tea-coloured urine Clay-coloured stools	Ensure adequate hydration. Institute early feed-ings if possible. Administer photo-therapy (see Chapter 24 for more information).
Birth trauma	LGA newborns	Large size requiring use of operative birth procedure	Obvious deformities Bruising Edema Asymmetric movement	Perform complete physical and neu-rologic assess-ment of the newborn. Note symmetry of structure and function. Assist parents in understanding situation (see Chapter 24 for more information).

age (CPS, 2011). Screening should continue every 3 to 6 hours thereafter (before feeds) until feeding is established and the glucose level remains at 2.6 mmol/L or higher (CPS, 2011). The clinical signs of hypoglycemia are often subtle and include lethargy, apathy, drowsiness, irritability, tachypnea, weak cry, temperature instability, jitteriness, seizures, apnea, bradycardia, cyanosis or pallor, feeble suck and poor feeding, hypotonia, and coma. Other disorders, including septicemia, severe respiratory distress, and con-genital heart disease, may present with similar findings. In addition, be alert for other common problems, such as polycythemia and hyperbilirubinemia (see Table 23.1).

Nursing Management

Assist in stabilizing the LGA newborn. Because studies have indicated that hypoglycemia in LGA infants occurs on average 2.9 hours after birth, it is recommended that screening be initiated in at-risk babies at 2 hours of age (after an initial feed) and continued until the period of risk is considered over. However, symptomatic infants should have a blood glucose assessment without delay as part of the workup for diagnostic and therapeutic pur-poses (CPS, 2011).

If an infant's blood glucose level is below 1.8 mmol/L at 2 hours of age or below 2.0 mmol/L at subsequent checks, initiate an intravenous infusion of 10% dextrose at a rate of 5.5 mg/kg/minute (CPS, 2011). Monitor and record intake and output and obtain daily weights to aid in evaluating nutritional intake.

Observe for signs of polycythemia and hyperbiliru-binemia and report any immediately to the health care provider so that early interventions can be taken to pre-vent poor long-term neurologic development outcomes. Polycythemia and hyperviscosity are associated with fine and gross motor delays, speech delays, and neuro-logic sequelae (Neonatal Handbook, n.d.). Increasing fluid volume aids in decreasing blood viscosity. Partial exchange transfusion with plasma or normal saline may be used to lower hematocrit and decrease blood viscos-ity, but this treatment remains controversial. Hydra-tion, early feedings, and phototherapy are used to treat hyperbilirubinemia (see Chapter 24 for more informa-tion about hyperbilirubinemia). Provide parental guid-ance about the treatments and procedures being done and about the need for follow-up care for any abnor-malities identified.

Gestational Age Variations

The mean duration of pregnancy, calculated from the first day of the last normal menstrual period, is approximately 280 days, or 40 weeks. Gestational age is typically measured in weeks: a newborn born before completion of 37 weeks is classified as a **preterm newborn** and one born after completion of 42 weeks is classified as a **postterm newborn**. An infant born from the first day of 38th week through 42 weeks is classified as a **term newborn**. As of 2006, a new classification has been added, the **late preterm newborn**—one who is born between 34 weeks and 36 weeks, 6 days of gestation.

Precise knowledge of a newborn's gestational age is imperative for effective postnatal management. Determination of gestational age by the nurse assists in planning appropriate care for the newborn and provides important information regarding potential problems that need interventions. See Chapter 18 for more information on assessing gestational age.

▶ **Take** NOTE!

Although preterm and postterm newborns may appear to be at opposite ends of the gestational age spectrum and are very different in size and appearance, both are at high risk and need special care.

Postterm Newborn

A pregnancy that extends beyond 42 weeks' gestation produces a postterm newborn. Other terms used to describe these late births include postmature, prolonged pregnancy, or postdates pregnancy. Postterm newborns may be LGA, SGA, or dysmature (newborn weighs less than established normal parameters for estimated gestational age [IUGR]), depending on placental function. Perinatal mortality (intrauterine fetal demise plus neonatal deaths), meconium aspiration, infectious morbidity, birth trauma, low umbilical artery pH levels, and low Apgar scores are identified complications associated with the postterm newborn (Cheng, Nicholson, Nakagawa, et al., 2008).

The reason why some pregnancies last longer than others is not completely understood. What is known is that women who experience one postterm pregnancy are at increased risk in subsequent pregnancies. The incidence of prolonged pregnancy in Canada is approximately 5.8 births per 1,000 (Statistics Canada, 2009).

The ability of the placenta to provide adequate oxygen and nutrients to the fetus after 42 weeks' gestation is thought to be compromised, leading to perinatal mortality and morbidity. As the placenta loses its ability to nourish the fetus, the fetus uses stored nutrients to stay alive, and wasting occurs. This wasted appearance at birth is secondary to the loss of muscle mass and subcutaneous fat.

▶ *Consider* THIS!

I had been waiting for this baby my whole married life and now I was told to wait even longer. I was into my third week past my due date and was just told that if I didn't go into labour on my own, the doctor would induce me on Monday. As I waddled out of his office into the hot summer sun, I thought about all the comments that would await me at the office: "You're not still pregnant, are you?" "Weren't you due last month?" "You look as big as a house." "Are you sure you aren't expecting triplets?" I started to get into my car when I felt warm fluid slide down my legs. Although I was embarrassed at my wetness, I was thrilled I wouldn't have to go back to the office and drove myself to the hospital. Within hours my wait was finally over with the birth of my son, a postterm infant with peeling skin and a thick head of hair. He was certainly worth the wait!

Thoughts: although most due dates are within plus or minus 2 weeks, we can't "go to the bank with it" because so many factors influence the start of labour. This woman was anxious about her overdue status, but nature prevailed. The old adage "when the fruit is ripe, it will fall" doesn't always bring a good outcome: many women need a little push to bring a healthy newborn forth. What happens when the fetus stays inside the uterus too long? What other features are typical of postterm infants?

Nursing Assessment

A thorough assessment of the postterm newborn upon admission to the nursery provides a baseline from which to identify changes in clinical status. Review the maternal history for any risk factors associated with postterm birth. Also be aware of the common physical characteristics and be able to identify any deviation from the expected. Postterm newborns typically exhibit the following characteristics:

- Dry, cracked, wrinkled skin
- Long, thin extremities
- Creases that cover the entire soles of the feet
- Wide-eyed, alert expression
- Abundant hair on scalp
- Thin umbilical cord
- Limited vernix and lanugo
- Meconium-stained skin
- Long nails (Hatfield, 2008)

Assess the newborn's gestational age and complete a physical examination to identify any abnormalities. Review the medical record to determine the colour of the amniotic fluid when membranes ruptured and observe for a meconium-stained umbilical cord and fingernails to assess for possible meconium aspiration. Careful suctioning at the time of birth and afterward, if the condition dictates it, reduces the incidence of meconium aspiration. Also be alert for other typical complications associated with a postterm newborn, such as perinatal asphyxia, hypoglycemia, hypothermia, and polycythemia, and be prepared to initiate early interventions (see Table 23.1).

Nursing Management

The birth of a postterm newborn creates a crisis for the mother and her family. In most situations, birth of a newborn requiring special care was not anticipated. Postterm newborns are susceptible to several birth challenges secondary to placental dysfunction that place them at risk for asphyxia, hypoglycemia, and respiratory distress. The nurse must be vigilant for complications when managing these newborns.

The postterm newborn is at high risk for perinatal asphyxia, which is usually attributed to placental deprivation or oligohydramnios that leads to cord compression, thereby reducing perfusion to the fetus. Anticipating the need for newborn resuscitation is a priority. The newborn resuscitation team needs to be available in the birthing suite for immediate backup. The newborn may require transport to the neonatal intensive care unit (NICU) for continuous assessment, monitoring, and treatment, depending on his or her status after resuscitation.

Monitor and maintain the postterm newborn's blood glucose levels once stabilized. Intravenous dextrose 10% and/or early initiation of feedings will help stabilize the blood glucose levels to prevent central nervous system (CNS) sequelae.

Also monitor the postterm newborn's skin temperature, respiration characteristics, results of blood studies such as arterial blood gases (ABGs) and serum bilirubin levels, and neurologic status. Institute measures to prevent or reduce the risk of hypothermia by eliminating sources of heat loss: thoroughly dry the newborn at birth, wrap him or her in a warmed blanket, and place a stockinet cap on the newborn's head. Providing environmental warmth via a radiant heat source will help stabilize the newborn's temperature.

Closely assess all postterm newborns for polycythemia. Providing adequate hydration helps to reduce the viscosity of the newborn's blood to prevent thrombosis. Be alert to the early, often subtle signs to promote early identification and prompt treatment to prevent any neurodevelopmental delays.

Preterm Newborn

A preterm newborn is one who is born before the completion of 37 weeks of gestation. Recent national birth rates indicate an upward trend in Canada that began in 2002. Approximately 8% of Canadian births are preterm infants (Statistics Canada, 2009).

Despite the recognition that preterm birth is the most important perinatal challenge facing industrialized countries, two decades of clinical and community efforts at preterm birth prevention have failed to reduce rates of preterm birth. Several factors are associated with the rise in preterm rates, including increased medical intervention, older maternal age, and increases in multiple births (Joseph, 2008).

Changes in perinatal care practices, including regional care, have reduced newborn mortality rates. Transporting high-risk pregnant women to a tertiary centre for birth rather than transferring the neonate after birth is associated with a reduction in neonatal mortality and morbidity (Vargo & Trotter, 2007). Despite increasing survival rates, preterm infants continue to be at high risk for neurodevelopmental disorders such as cerebral palsy or mental retardation, intraventricular hemorrhage, congenital anomalies, neurosensory impairment, behavioural problems, and chronic lung disease (Pillitteri, 2009). Making sure that all pregnant women receive quality prenatal care throughout pregnancy is a major method for preventing preterm births.

Effects of Prematurity on Body Systems

Since the preterm newborn did not remain in utero long enough, every body system may be immature, affecting the newborn's transition from intrauterine to extrauterine life and placing him or her at risk for complications. Prematurity results in incomplete brain development: therefore, many higher-order functions regulated by the cerebellum and cerebral cortex are not fully developed, predisposing the infant to short-term and long-term morbidities (March of Dimes, 2011).

*R*ecall Anna, who was described at the beginning of the chapter; she gave birth to a newborn at 7 months' gestation. What problems would you anticipate that her newborn might have?

Respiratory System

The respiratory system is one of the last body systems to mature. Therefore, the preterm newborn is at great risk for respiratory complications. A few of the problems that affect the preterm newborn's breathing ability and adjustment to extrauterine life include:

- Surfactant deficiency, leading to the development of respiratory distress syndrome
- Unstable chest wall, leading to atelectasis
- Immature respiratory control centres, leading to apnea
- Smaller respiratory passages, leading to an increased risk for obstruction
- Inability to clear fluid from passages, leading to transient tachypnea

Cardiovascular System

The preterm newborn has great difficulty in making the transition from intrauterine to extrauterine life in terms of changing from a fetal to a newborn circulation pattern. Higher oxygen levels in the circulation once air breathing begins spur this transition. If the oxygen levels remain low secondary to perinatal asphyxia, the fetal pattern of circulation may persist, causing blood flow to bypass the lungs. Another problem affecting the cardiovascular system is the increased incidence of congenital anomalies associated with continued fetal circulation—patent ductus arteriosus and an open foramen ovale. In addition, impaired regulation of blood pressure in preterm newborns may cause fluctuations throughout the circulatory system. There is a significant association between the prevalence of hypotension and hemorrhagic or ischemic brain injuries (du Plessis, 2009).

Gastrointestinal System

Preterm newborns usually lack the neuromuscular coordination required to maintain the suck, swallow, and breathing regimen necessary for sufficient calorie and fluid intake to support growth. Perinatal hypoxia causes shunting of blood from the gut to more important organs such as the heart and brain. Subsequently, ischemia and damage to the intestinal wall can occur. This combination of shunting, ischemia, damage to the intestinal wall, and poor sucking ability places the preterm infant at risk for malnutrition and weight loss.

In addition, preterm newborns have a small stomach capacity, weak abdominal muscles, compromised metabolic function, limited ability to digest proteins and absorb nutrients, and weak or absent suck and gag reflexes. All of these limitations place the preterm newborn at risk for nutritional deficiency and subsequent growth and development delays (Shah & Shah, 2009).

Currently, minimal enteral feeding is used to prepare the preterm newborn's gut to overcome the many feeding difficulties associated with gastrointestinal immaturity. It involves the introduction of small amounts, usually 0.5 to 1 mL/kg/hour, of enteral feeding to induce surges in gut hormones that enhance maturation of the intestine. This minute amount of breast milk or formula given via gavage feeding prepares the gut to absorb future introduction of nutrients. It builds mucosal bulk, stimulates development of enzymes, enhances pancreatic function, stimulates maturation of gastrointestinal hormones, reduces gastrointestinal distention and malabsorption, and enhances transition to oral feedings (Blackburn, 2007).

Renal System

The renal system of the preterm newborn is immature, reducing the baby's ability to concentrate urine and slowing the glomerular filtration rate. As a result, the risk for fluid retention, with subsequent fluid and electrolyte disturbances, increases. In addition, preterm newborns have limited ability to clear drugs from their systems, thereby increasing the risk of drug toxicity. Close monitoring of the preterm newborn's acid–base and electrolyte balance is critical to identify metabolic inconsistencies. Prescribed medications require strict evaluation to prevent overwhelming the preterm baby's immature renal system.

Immune System

The preterm newborn's immune system is very immature, increasing his or her susceptibility to infections. A deficiency of IgG may occur because transplacental transfer does not occur until after 34 weeks' gestation. This protection is lacking if the baby was born before this time. In addition, preterm newborns have an impaired ability to manufacture antibodies to fight infection if they were exposed to pathogens during the birth process. Moreover, the preterm newborn's thin skin and fragile blood vessels provide a limited protective barrier, adding to the increased risk for infection. Thus, anticipating and preventing infections is the goal; preventing infections has a better outcome than treating them.

Central Nervous System

The preterm newborn is susceptible to injury and insult to the CNS, increasing the potential for long-term disability into adulthood. Like all newborns, preterm newborns have difficulty in temperature regulation and maintaining stability. However, their risk for heat loss is compounded by inadequate amounts of insulating subcutaneous fat; lack of muscle tone and flexion to conserve heat; inadequate brown fat to generate heat; limited muscle mass activity, reducing the possibility of producing their own heat; inability to shiver to generate heat; and an immature temperature-regulating centre in the brain (Blackburn, 2007). Preventing cold stress is critical, as cold stress can hinder a successful transition to the extrauterine environment or precipitate persistence of the fetal circulation or pulmonary hypertension. Recognition of cold stress and rapid interventions to prevent deleterious effects are key (Mally, Bailey, & Hendricks-Munoz, 2010).

In addition, the preterm newborn is especially susceptible to hypoglycemia due to immature glucose control mechanisms, decreased glucose stores, and a reduced availability of alternative fuels such as ketone bodies.

> ▶ **Take** NOTE!
>
> *Glucose is needed by the brain and CNS to maintain and support numerous body system functions.*

Nursing Assessment

Preterm newborns are at high risk for numerous problems and require special care. When preterm labour develops and cannot be stopped by medical interventions, plans for appropriate management of the mother and the preterm newborn are necessary, such as transporting them to a regional centre with facilities to care for preterm newborns or notifying the facility's NICU.

EVIDENCE-BASED PRACTICE 23.1
Improving the Quality of Care of Infants in Neonatal Intensive Care Areas

● Study

The Canadian Neonatal Network consists of 30 tertiary-level regional NICUs across Canada and maintains a prospective national database for all infants admitted to neonatal intensive care unit (NICU). Approaches for continuous quality improvement have been used to improve outcomes; however, the National Institutes of Child Health and Human Development Quality Collaborative indicate little or no effect has been seen in NICU. Quality improvement methods have been critiqued since they are based on intuition and anecdotes rather than on evidence.

Researchers developed a new method called the Evidence-based Practice for Improving Quality for continuous quality improvement. The method is based on the use of published literature, data from participating hospitals to gather information about hospital specific practices, and the employment of the national network to communicate expertise. The goal of the study was to evaluate the Evidence-based Practice for Improving Quality method by conducting a prospective cluster randomized controlled trial to reduce nosocomial infection and bronchopulmonary dysplasia in newborns at 32 or fewer weeks' gestation and admitted to one of 12 Canadian Neonatal Network hospitals during a 36-month period. The hypothesis was that nosociomial infections would be reduced in infants in NICUs randomized to reduce infection but reduction in infection would not be seen in NICUs randomized to reduced bronchopulmonary dysplasia. Another hypothesis was that bronchopulmonary dysplasia would be reduced in NICUs randomized for this outcome but not in the NICUs randomized to reduce infection.

Negative blood culture or cerebrospinal fluid culture and no culture taken defined the absence of nosocomial infection. Growth of one or more organisms in blood or cerebrospinal cultures taken after 48 hours of admission indicated the presence of a nosocomial infection. Nosocomial infection was differentiated from maternal isolates according to study criteria. Oxygen dependency at 36 weeks' corrected gestational age and infants discharged from NICU on oxygen before 36 weeks' corrected age defined brochopulmonary dysplasia.

Twelve NICU units from across Canada participated in the study, Six NICUs were randomized to the nosocomial infection reduction group and six NICUs were randomized to the bronchopulmonary dysplasia reduction group. Each group served as the control for the other group and each group was blinded to the inventions and discussions related to the other group. During phase 1 of the study, information was gathered on the baseline population characteristics of all infants born at 32 weeks or earlier including outcomes and practices. Site investigators attended a 3-day critical appraisal workshop to learn about systematic reviews, principles of continuous quality improvement, neonatal infections, bronchopulmonary dysplasia, data interpretation, and research methods. Parents and staff were interviewed to identify change barriers. During phase 2, single or multiple practice changes were implemented in rapid cycles (1–3 months). Monitoring for compliance was a component of the study.

Participant groups developed potentially useful practices and priorities as well as potential strategies for implementing practice change. Each hospital used group consensus in conjunction with hospital-specific data and culture to develop its own unique recommendations for practice change.

▲ Findings

Prior to the initiation of evidenced-based strategies, 40% of nosocomial infections in NICUs were associated with central lines, with percutaneously inserted central catheters carrying the highest risk. Following the trial, there was a significant decrease in the incidence of nosocomial infections in the infection group compared to incidence prior to commencement of the study. Infection rates could be compared between hospitals, and strategies that yielded the best results could be adopted by other institutions. In the pulmonary group, there no significant alteration in the incidence of bronchopulmonary dysplasia. However, there was a significant decrease in the incidence of nosocomial infection.

In the Evidence-based Practice for Improving Quality method in this study allowed NICUs to choose practice changes pertinent to them. The decreased incidence of nosocomial infections in the pulmonary group may be related to improved lung status and a reduced need for assisted respirations and invasive interventions, and better feeding and growth. The change in NICU practices had a spill-over effect in affecting other outcomes. This explains the decrease in nosocomial infections in both the infection and pulmonary groups.

■ Nursing Implications

The Evidence-based Practice for Improving Quality method focuses on changing organizational culture and supports behavioural modifications. This multidimensional research method may be used by nurses as a means to changing NICU practices.

Source: Lee, S. K., et al. (2009). Improving the quality of care for infants: a cluster randomized controlled trial. *Canadian Association Medical Journal*, 181(8), 469–476.

Depending on the degree of prematurity, the preterm newborn may be kept in the NICU for months, and evidence-based nursing practice is essential to providing appropriate care. (See Evidenced-based Practice 23.1.)

A thorough assessment of the preterm newborn upon admission to the nursery provides a baseline from which to identify changes in clinical status. Be aware of the common physical characteristics and be able to identify any deviation from the expected (Fig. 23.2). Common physical characteristics of preterm infants may include:

- Birth weight of less than 2,500 g
- Scrawny appearance

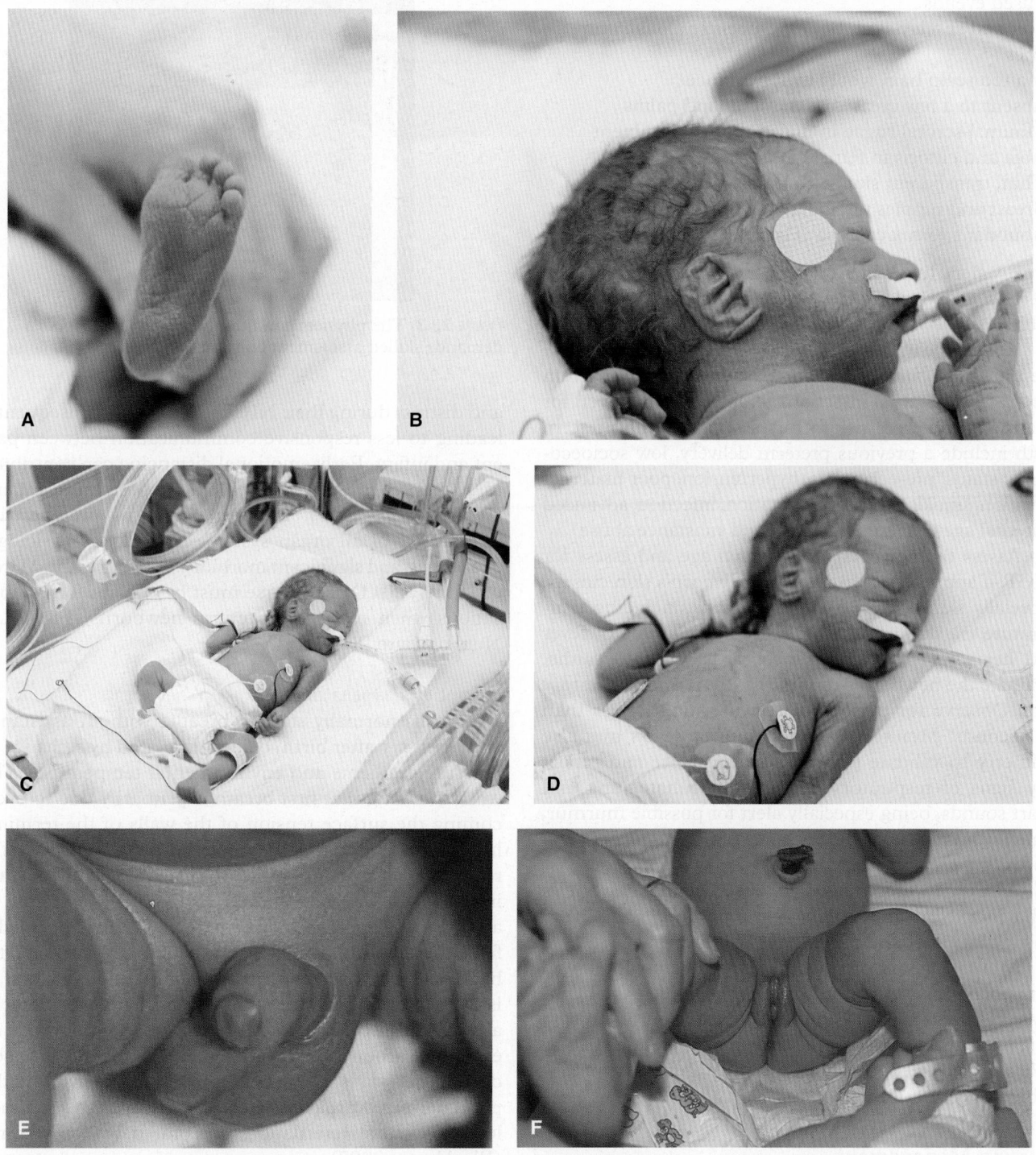

FIGURE 23.2 Characteristics of a preterm newborn. (**A**) Few plantar creases. (**B**) Soft, pliable ear cartilage, matted hair, and fused eyelids. (**C**) Lax posture with poor muscle tone. (**D**) Breast and nipple area barely visible. (**E**) Male genitalia with minimal rugae on scrotum. (**F**) Female genitalia with prominent labia and clitoris.

- Head circumference disproportionately larger than chest circumference
- Poor muscle tone
- Minimal subcutaneous fat
- Undescended testes
- Plentiful lanugo (soft, downy hair), especially over the face and back
- Poorly formed pinnae, with soft, pliable cartilage
- Fused eyelids
- Soft and spongy skull bones, especially along suture lines
- Matted scalp hair, wooly in appearance
- Absent to a few creases in the soles and palms
- Minimal scrotal rugae in male infants; prominent labia and clitoris in female infants
- Thin, transparent skin with visible veins
- Breast and nipples not clearly delineated
- Abundant vernix caseosa (Hatfield, 2008)

Be alert for evidence that might suggest that the preterm newborn is developing a complication (see Table 23.1).

Review the maternal history to identify risk factors for preterm birth and check antepartum and intrapartum records for maternal infections to anticipate the need for treatment. Maternal risk factors associated with preterm birth include a previous preterm delivery, low socioeconomic status, pre-eclampsia, hypertension, poor maternal nutrition, smoking, multiple gestation, infection, advanced maternal age or teen pregnancy, and substance abuse.

Assess the newborn's gestational age and assess for IUGR if appropriate. Inspect the newborn's skin closely, especially skin colour. Assess vital signs, including temperature via skin probe to identify hypothermia or fever and heart rate to identify tachycardia or bradycardia. Evaluate the newborn's respiratory effort and respiratory rate. Observe for periods of apnea lasting longer than 20 seconds. Monitor oxygen saturation levels by pulse oximetry to validate perfusion status. Note and report any signs of respiratory distress. Auscultate lung and heart sounds, being especially alert for possible murmur, which would indicate the presence of patent ductus arteriosus in a preterm newborn.

Assess neurologic status by observing the newborn's behaviour. Note any restlessness, hypotonia, or weak cry or sucking effort and report unusual findings.

Monitor laboratory studies such as hemoglobin and hematocrit for signs of polycythemia. Screen for hypoglycemia upon admission and then hourly, always observing for nonspecific signs of hypoglycemia such as lethargy, poor feeding, and seizures. Evaluate serum bilirubin concentrations.

Nursing Management

The birth of a preterm newborn creates a crisis for the mother and family. Many parents experience depression

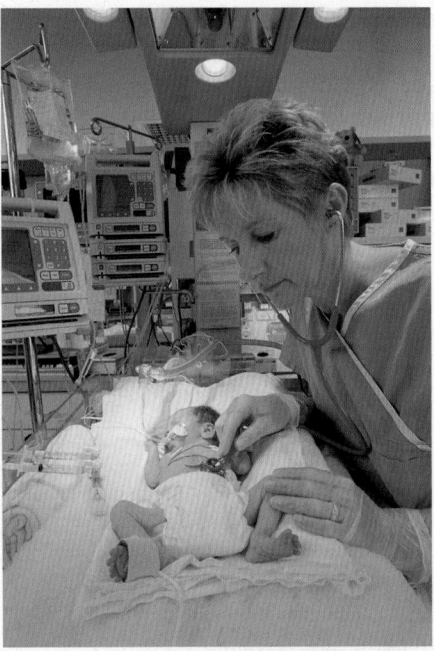

FIGURE 23.3 The physical condition of a preterm newborn demands skilled assessment and nursing care.

and distress during their NICU experience, consequently leading to less responsive communication between parent and infant. Early emotional distancing can contribute to poorer cognitive development of premature infants (Whittington, 2010). Preterm newborns present with immaturity of all organ systems, abundant physiologic challenges, and significant morbidity and mortality (March of Dimes, 2011). The nurse must be vigilant for complications when managing preterm newborns (Fig. 23.3, Nursing Care Plan 23.1).

Promoting Oxygenation

Newborns normally start to breathe without assistance and often cry after birth, being stimulated by a change in pressure gradients and environmental temperature. The work of taking that first breath is primarily due to overcoming the surface tension of the walls of the terminal lung units at the gas–tissue interface. Subsequent breaths require less inspiratory pressure since there is an increase in functional capacity and air retained. By 1 minute of age, most newborns are breathing well. A newborn who fails to establish adequate, sustained respiration after birth is said to have **asphyxia**. On a physiologic level, it is defined as an impairment in gas exchange resulting in a decrease in oxygen in the blood (hypoxemia) and an excess of carbon dioxide or hypercapnia that leads to acidosis. Asphyxia is the most common clinical insult in the perinatal period that results in brain injury, which may lead to mental retardation, cerebral palsy, or seizures (Blackburn, 2007).

The preterm infant lacks surfactant. Surfactant lowers surface tension in the alveoli and stabilizes them to

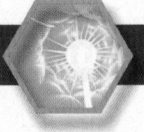

Nursing Care Plan 23.1

OVERVIEW OF THE CARE OF A PRETERM NEWBORN

Alice, an 18-year-old, felt she had done everything right during her first pregnancy and certainly didn't anticipate giving birth to a preterm newborn at 32 weeks' gestation. When Mary Kaye was born, she had respiratory distress and hypoglycemia and couldn't stabilize her temperature. Assessment revealed the following: newborn described as scrawny in appearance; skin thin and transparent with prominent veins over abdomen; hypotonia with lax, extended positioning; weak sucking reflex when nipple offered; respiratory distress with tachypnea (70 breaths/minute), nasal flaring, and sternal retractions; low blood glucose level suggested by lethargy, tachycardia, jitteriness; axillary temperature of 36°C (96.8°F) despite warmed blanket; weight 2,146 g (4.73 lb); length 45 cm (17.72 inches).

NURSING DIAGNOSIS: Ineffective breathing pattern related to immature respiratory system and respiratory distress as evidenced by tachypnea, nasal flaring, and sternal retractions

Outcome Identification and Evaluation
Newborn's respiratory status returns to adequate level of functioning as evidenced by rate remaining within 30 to 60 breaths/minute, maintenance of acceptable oxygen saturation levels, and minimal to absent signs of respiratory distress.

Interventions: Promoting Optimal Breathing Pattern
- Assess gestational age and risk factors for respiratory distress *to allow early detection.*
- Anticipate need for bag and mask setup and wall suction *to allow for prompt intervention should respiratory status continue to worsen.*
- Assess respiratory effort (rate, character, effort) *to identify changes.*
- Assess heart rate for tachycardia and auscultate heart sounds *to determine worsening of condition.*
- Observe for cues (grunting, shallow respirations, tachypnea, apnea, tachycardia, central cyanosis, hypotonia, increased effort) *to identify need for additional oxygen.*
- Maintain slight head elevation *to prevent upper airway obstruction.*
- Assess skin colour *to evaluate tissue perfusion.*
- Monitor oxygen saturation level via pulse oximetry *to provide objective indication of perfusion status.*
- Provide supplemental oxygen as indicated and ordered *to ensure adequate tissue oxygenation.*
- Assist with any ordered diagnostic tests, such as chest X-ray and arterial blood gases, *to determine effectiveness of treatments.*
- Cluster nursing activities *to reduce oxygen consumption.*
- Maintain a neutral thermal environment *to reduce oxygen consumption.*
- Monitor hydration status *to prevent fluid volume deficit or overload.*
- Explain all events and procedures to the parents *to help alleviate anxiety and promote understanding of the newborn's condition.*

NURSING DIAGNOSIS: Ineffective thermoregulation related to lack of fat stores and hypotonia as evidenced by extended positioning, low axillary temperature despite warmed blanket, respiratory distress, and lethargy

Outcome Identification and Evaluation
Newborn will demonstrate ability to regulate temperature as evidenced by temperature remaining in normal range (36.5°C to 37.5°C) and absent signs of cold stress.

Interventions: Promoting Thermoregulation
- Assess the axillary temperature every hour or use a thermistor probe *to monitor for changes.*
- Review maternal history *to identify risk factors contributing to problem.*
- Monitor vital signs, including heart rate and respiratory rate, every hour *to identify deviations.*
- Check radiant heat source or isolette *to ensure maintenance of appropriate temperature of the environment.*
- Assess environment for sources of heat loss or gain through evaporation, conduction, convection, or radiation *to minimize risk of heat loss.*
- Avoid bathing and exposing newborn *to prevent cold stress.*
- Warm all blankets and equipment that come in contact with newborn; place warmed cap on the newborn's head and keep it on *to minimize heat loss.*

(continued)

Nursing Care Plan 23.1 (continued)

- Encourage kangaroo care (mother or father holds preterm infant underneath clothing skin-to-skin and upright between breasts) *to provide warmth.*
- Educate parents on how to maintain a neutral thermal environment, including importance of keeping the newborn warm with a cap and double-wrapping with blankets and changing them frequently to keep dry *to promote newborn's adjustment.*
- Demonstrate ways to safeguard warmth and prevent heat loss.

NURSING DIAGNOSIS: Risk for imbalanced nutrition: less than body requirements related to poor sucking and lack of glycogen stores necessary to meet the newborn's increased metabolic demands as evidenced by weak sucking reflex, low birth weight, and signs and symptoms of hypoglycemia, including lethargy, tachycardia, and jitteriness

Outcome Identification and Evaluation
Newborn will demonstrate adequate nutritional intake, remaining free of signs of hypoglycemia as evidenced by blood glucose levels being maintained above 45 mg/dL, enhanced sucking ability, and appropriate weight gain.

Interventions: Promoting Optimal Nutrition
- Identify newborn at risk based on behavioural characteristics, body measurements, and gestational age *to establish a baseline and allow for early detection.*
- Assess blood glucose levels as ordered *to determine status and establish a baseline for interventions.*
- Obtain blood glucose measurements upon admission to nursery and every 1 to 2 hours as indicated *to evaluate for changes.*
- Observe behaviour for signs of low blood glucose *to allow early identification.*
- Initiate early oral feedings or gavage feedings *to maintain blood glucose levels.*
- If oral or gavage feedings aren't tolerated, initiate an IV glucose infusion *to aid in stabilizing blood glucose levels.*
- Assess skin for pallor and sweating *to identify signs of hypoglycemia.*
- Assess neurologic status for tremors, seizures, jitteriness, and lethargy *to identify further drops in blood glucose levels.*
- Monitor weight daily for changes *to determine effectiveness of feedings.*
- Maintain temperature using warmed blankets, radiant warmer, or warmed isolette *to prevent heat loss and possible cold stress and reduce energy demands.*
- Monitor temperature *to prevent cold stress resulting in decreased blood glucose levels.*
- Offer opportunities for non-nutritive sucking on premature-size pacifier *to satisfy sucking needs.*
- Monitor for tolerance of oral feedings, including intake and output, *to determine effectiveness.*
- Administer IV dextrose if newborn is symptomatic *to raise blood glucose levels quickly.*
- Decrease energy requirements, including clustering care activities and providing rest periods, *to conserve glucose and glycogen stores.*
- Inform parents about procedures and treatments, including rationale for frequent blood glucose levels, *to help reduce their anxiety.*

prevent their collapse. Even if preterm newborns can initiate respirations, they have a limited ability to retain air due to insufficient surfactant. Therefore, preterm newborns develop atelectasis quickly without alveoli stabilization. The inability to initiate and establish respirations leads to hypoxemia and ultimately hypoxia (decreased oxygen), acidosis (decreased pH), and hypercarbia (increased carbon dioxide). This change in the newborn's biochemical environment may inhibit the transition to extrauterine circulation, thus allowing fetal circulation patterns to persist.

Failure to initiate extrauterine breathing or failure to breathe well after birth leads to hypoxia (too little oxygen in the cells of the body). As a result, the heart rate falls, cyanosis develops, and the newborn becomes hypotonic and unresponsive. Although this can happen with any newborn, the risk is higher in preterm newborns.

Prevention and early identification of newborns at risk are key. Prenatal risk factors that can help identify the newborn who may need resuscitation at birth secondary to asphyxia include:

- History of substance abuse
- Gestational hypertension
- Fetal distress due to hypoxia before birth
- Chronic maternal diseases such as diabetes or a heart or renal condition
- Maternal or perinatal infection
- Placental problems (placenta previa or abruptio placentae)
- Umbilical cord problems (nuchal or prolapsed)
- Difficult or traumatic birth
- Multiple births

• Congenital heart disease
• Maternal anesthesia or recent analgesia
• Preterm or postterm birth (Cloherty, Eichenwald, & Stark, 2008)

Note the newborn's Apgar score at 1 and 5 minutes. If the score is below 7 at either time, resuscitation efforts are needed. Rarely, infants do not respond to initial resuscitative efforts. If an infant fails to respond to properly executed resuscitation, investigation is necessary to determine possible causes. Some contributing factors may include mechanical blockage, impaired lung function, congenital heart disease, heart block, brain injury, congenital neuromuscular disorder, or respiratory depression from maternally administered opioids (Fernandes, 2012). Monitor vital signs continuously, check blood glucose levels for hypoglycemia secondary to stress, and maintain a neutral thermal environment to promote energy conservation and minimize oxygen consumption.

Resuscitating the Newborn

Any newborn can be born with asphyxia without warning. Approximately 10% of newborns require some assistance to begin breathing at birth. Anticipation, adequate preparation, accurate evaluation, and prompt initiation of support are critical for successful newborn resuscitation. Have all basic equipment immediately available and in working order. Ensure that the equipment is evaluated daily, and document its condition and any needed repairs. Box 23.2 lists the equipment needed for basic newborn resuscitation.

BOX 23.2 **Basic Equipment for Newborn Resuscitation**

• A wall vacuum suction apparatus
• A wall source or tank source of 100% oxygen with a flow meter
• Exhaled CO_2 detector or capnograph
• T-piece resuscitator
• A neonatal self-inflating or flow-inflating ventilation bag with correct-size facemasks
• A selection of endotracheal tubes (2.5, 3.0, or 3.5 mm) with introducers
• A laryngoscope with a small, straight blade and spare batteries and bulbs
• Epinephrine 1:10,000 ampules; 1 and 3 mL syringes
• Ampules of naloxone (Narcan) with syringes and needles
• A wall clock to document timing of activities and events
• A supply of disposable gloves in a variety of sizes for staff to use

---

Determine the need for resuscitation by performing a rapid assessment using the following four questions:

• What is the gestational age of this newborn?
• Was the amniotic fluid clear of meconium or cloudy (infection present)?
• Is the newborn breathing or crying now?
• Does the newborn have good muscle tone?

If the answers are "yes" to all questions, then routine care is initiated: provide warmth, clear the airway, dry the newborn, and assess colour. If the answer to any of these questions is "no," the newborn should receive one or more of the following actions, according to this sequence:

1. Stabilization—Dry the newborn thoroughly with a warm towel; provide warmth by placing him or her under a radiant heater to prevent rapid heat loss through evaporation; position the head in a neutral position to open the airway; clear the airway with a bulb syringe or suction catheter; stimulate breathing. At times, handling and rubbing the newborn with a dry towel may be all that is needed to stimulate respirations.
2. Ventilation
3. Chest compressions
4. Administration of epinephrine and/or volume expansion (Kattwinkel, Perlman, Aziz, et al., 2010).

The decision to progress beyond the initial steps is determined by simultaneous assessment of two vital characteristics: respirations (apnea, gasping, or laboured or unlaboured breathing) and heart rate (whether greater than or less than 100 beats/minute) (Kattwinkel et al., 2010).

When performing newborn resuscitation, use the mnemonic "ABCDs" (airway, breathing, circulation, and drugs) to remember the sequence of steps (Box 23.3). Coordinated chest compressions and ventilations should continue until the spontaneous heart rate exceeds 60 beats/minute (Kattwinkel et al., 2010).

Throughout the resuscitation period, keep the parents informed of what is happening to their newborn and what is being done and why. Provide support through this initial crisis. Once the newborn is stabilized, encourage bonding by having the parents stroke, touch and, when appropriate, hold the newborn.

Administering Oxygen

Oxygen administration is a common therapy in newborn nurseries. Although it has been used in newborns for over 75 years, there is no universal agreement on the most appropriate range at which oxygen levels should be maintained for newborns experiencing hypoxia, nor is there a standard time frame for oxygen to be administered (Walsh, Brooks, & Grenier, 2009). While this uncertainty continues, nurses will experience a wide variation in practice in terms of modes of administration, monitoring,

BOX 23.3 ABCDs of Newborn Resuscitation

- **Airway**
  - Place infant's head in "sniffing" position.
  - Suction mouth, then nose.
  - Suction trachea if meconium-stained and newborn is NOT vigorous (strong respiratory effort, good muscle tone, and heart rate >100 beats/minute).
- **Breathing**
  - Use positive-pressure ventilation (PPV) for apnea, grasping, or pulse <100 beats/minute.
  - Ventilate at rate of 40 to 60 breaths/minute.
  - Listen for rising heart rate, audible breath sounds.
  - Look for slight chest movement with each breath.
  - Use carbon dioxide detector after intubation.
- **Circulation**
  - Start compressions if heart rate is <60 beats/minute after 30 seconds of effective PPV.
  - Give 3 compressions: 1 breath = 1 event, or 120 events per minute or 1 event per ½ second.
  - Compress one third of the anterior–posterior diameter of the chest.
- **Drugs**
  - Give epinephrine if heart rate is <60 beats/minute after 30 seconds of compressions and ventilation.
  - *Caution:* Epinephrine dosage is different for endotracheal and IV routes!
    - Epinephrine: 1:10,000 concentration
      - Endotracheal route: 1 mL/kg of 1:10,000 solution to a maximum dose of 3 mL
      - Intravenous route: 0.1 mL/kg of 1:10,000 solution (Kattwinkel et al., 2010)

blood levels, and target ranges for both short- and long-term oxygen therapy.

A guiding principle, though, is that oxygen therapy should be targeted to levels appropriate to the condition, gestational age, and postnatal age of the newborn. Oxygen therapy must be used judiciously to prevent **retinopathy of prematurity (ROP)**, a major cause of blindness in preterm newborns in the past. ROP is a potentially blinding eye disorder that occurs when abnormal blood vessels grow and spread through the retina, eventually leading to retinal detachment. The incidence of ROP is inversely proportional to the preterm baby's birth weight.

Although the role of oxygen in the pathogenesis of ROP is unclear, current evidence suggests that it is linked to the duration of oxygen use rather than the concentration. Currently, there is no published evidence to indicate that high oxygen saturations increase ROP risk; however, duration of oxygen supplementation has been suggested to be related to ROP severity (Chen, Guo, Smith, et al., 2010). An ophthalmologic consult for follow-up after discharge is essential for preterm infants who have received extensive oxygen therapy. See Chapter 38 for a more in-depth discussion of this condition.

Respiratory distress in preterm infants is commonly caused by a deficiency of surfactant, retained fluid in the lungs (wet lung syndrome), meconium aspiration, pneumonia, hypothermia, or anemia. The principles of care are the same regardless of the cause of respiratory distress. First, keep the newborn warm, preferably in a warmed isolette or with an overhead radiant warmer, to conserve the baby's energy and prevent cold stress. Handle the newborn as little as possible, because stimulation often increases the oxygen requirement. Provide energy through calories via intravenous dextrose or gavage or continuous tube feedings to prevent hypoglycemia. Treat cyanosis with an oxygen hood or blow-by oxygen placed near the newborn's face if respiratory distress is mild and short-term therapy is needed. Record the following important observations every hour or more frequently if indicated, and document any deterioration or changes in respiratory status:

- Respiratory rate, quality of respirations, and respiratory effort
- Airway patency, including removal of secretions per facility policy
- Skin colour, including any changes to duskiness, blueness, or pallor
- Lung sounds on auscultation to differentiate breath sounds in upper and lower fields
- Equipment required for oxygen delivery, such as:
  - Blow-by oxygen delivered via mask or tube for short-term therapy
  - Oxygen hood (oxygen is delivered via a plastic hood placed over the newborn's head)
  - Nasal cannula (oxygen is delivered directly through the nares) (Fig. 23.4A)
  - Continuous positive airway pressure (CPAP), which prevents collapse of unstable alveoli and delivers high levels of inspired oxygen into the lungs
  - Mechanical ventilation, which delivers consistent assisted ventilation and oxygen therapy, reducing the work of breathing for the fatigued infant (see Fig. 23.4B)
- Correct placement of endotracheal tube (if present)
- Heart rate, including any changes
- Oxygen saturation levels via pulse oximetry to evaluate need for therapy modifications based on hemoglobin
- Maintenance of oxygen saturation level of 85% to 93% (Finer & Leone, 2009)
- Nutritional intake, including calories provided, to prevent hypoglycemia and method of feeding, such as gavage, intravenous, or continuous enteral feedings
- Hydration status, including any signs and symptoms of fluid overload
- Laboratory tests, including ABGs, to determine effectiveness of oxygen therapy
- Administration of medication, such as exogenous surfactant

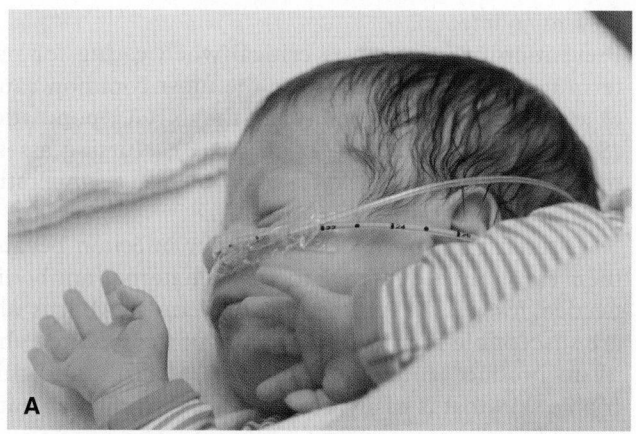
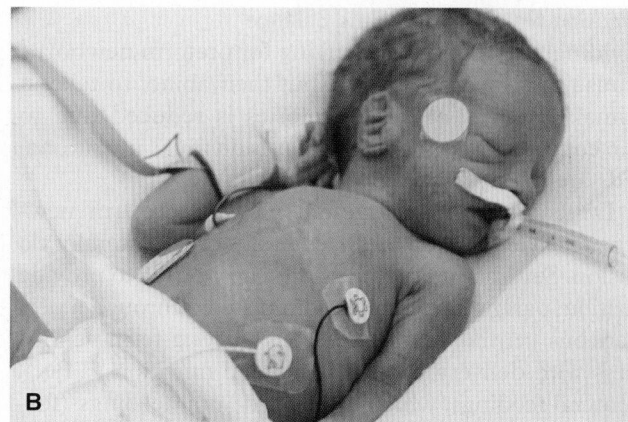

FIGURE 23.4 (**A**) A preterm newborn receiving oxygen therapy via a nasal cannula. The newborn also has an enteral feeding tube inserted for nutrition. (**B**) A preterm newborn receiving mechanical ventilation.

If the newborn shows worsening cyanosis or if oxygen saturation levels fall below 85%, prepare to give additional oxygen as ordered. Throughout the care, strict asepsis, including handwashing, is vital to reduce the risk of infection.

Maintaining Thermal Regulation

Immediately after birth, dry the newborn with a warmed towel and then place him or her in a second warm, dry towel before performing the assessment. This drying prevents rapid heat loss secondary to evaporation. Newborns who are active, breathing well, and crying are stable and can be placed on their mother's chest ("kangaroo care") to promote warmth and prevent hypothermia. Preterm newborns who are not considered stable may be placed under a radiant warmer or in a warmed isolette after they are dried with a warmed towel.

Typically newborns use nonshivering thermogenesis for heat production by metabolizing their own brown adipose tissue. However, the preterm newborn has an inadequate supply of brown fat because he or she left the uterus before it was adequate. The preterm newborn also has decreased muscle tone and thus cannot assume the flexed fetal position, which reduces the amount of skin exposed to a cooler environment. In addition, preterm newborns have large body surface areas compared with weight. This allows an increased transfer of heat from their bodies to the environment.

Typically, a preterm newborn who is having problems with thermal regulation is cool to cold to the touch. The hands, feet, and tongue may appear cyanotic. Respirations are shallow or slow, or signs of respiratory distress are present. The newborn is lethargic and hypotonic, feeds poorly, and has a feeble cry. Blood glucose levels are probably low, leading to hypoglycemia due to the energy expended to keep warm.

When promoting thermal regulation for the preterm newborn:

- Remember the four mechanisms for heat transfer and ways to prevent loss:
  - Convection: heat loss through air currents (avoid drafts near the newborn)
  - Conduction: heat loss through direct contact (warm everything the newborn comes in contact with, such as blankets, mattress, stethoscope)
  - Radiation: heat loss without direct contact (keep isolettes away from cold sources and provide insulation to prevent heat transfer)
  - Evaporation: heat loss by conversion of liquid into vapour (keep the newborn dry and delay the first bath until the baby's temperature is stable)
- Frequently assess the temperature of the isolette or radiant warmer, adjusting the temperature as necessary to prevent hypo- or hyperthermia.
- Assess the newborn's temperature every hour until stable.
- Observe for clinical signs of cold stress, such as respiratory distress, central cyanosis, hypoglycemia, lethargy, weak cry, abdominal distention, apnea, bradycardia, and acidosis.
- Remember the complications of hypothermia and frequently assess the newborn for signs:
  - Metabolic acidosis secondary to anaerobic metabolism used for heat production, which results in the production of lactic acid
  - Hypoglycemia due to depleted glycogen stores
  - Pulmonary hypertension secondary to pulmonary vasoconstriction
- Monitor the newborn for signs of hyperthermia such as tachycardia, tachypnea, apnea, warm to touch, flushed skin, lethargy, weak or absent cry, and CNS depression; adjust the environmental temperature appropriately.
- Explain to the parents the need to maintain the newborn's temperature, including the measures used; demonstrate ways to safeguard warmth and prevent heat loss.

Promoting Nutrition and Fluid Balance

Providing nutrition is challenging for preterm newborns because their needs are great but their ability to take in optimal amounts of energy/calories is reduced due to their compromised health status. Individual nutritional needs are highly variable.

Depending on their gestational age, preterm newborns receive nutrition orally, enterally, or parenterally via infusion. Several different methods can be used to provide nutrition: parenteral feedings administered through a percutaneous central venous catheter for long-term venous access with delivery of total parenteral nutrition (TPN), or enteral feedings, which can include oral feedings (formula or breast milk), continuous nasogastric tube feedings, or intermittent gavage tube feedings. Gavage feedings are commonly used for compromised newborns to allow them to rest during the feeding process. Many have a weak suck and become fatigued and thus cannot consume enough calories to meet their needs.

Most newborns born after 34 weeks' gestation without significant complications can feed orally. Those born before 34 weeks' gestation typically start with parenteral nutrition within the first 24 hours of life. Then enteral nutrition is introduced and advanced based on the degree of maturity and clinical condition. Ultimately, enteral nutrition methods replace parenteral nutrition.

To promote nutrition and fluid balance in the preterm newborn:

- Measure daily weight and plot it on a growth curve.
- Monitor intake; calculate fluid and caloric intake daily.
- Assess fluid status by monitoring weight; urinary output; urine specific gravity; laboratory test results such as serum electrolyte levels, blood urea nitrogen, creatinine, and hematocrit; skin turgor; and fontanels (Ambalavanan, 2010). Be alert for signs of dehydration, such as a decrease in urinary output, sunken fontanels, temperature elevation, lethargy, and tachypnea.
- Continually assess for enteral feeding intolerance; measure abdominal girth, auscultate bowel sounds, and measure gastric residuals before the next tube feeding.
- Encourage and support breastfeeding by facilitating maternal breast pumping.
- Encourage nuzzling at the breast in conjunction with kangaroo care if the newborn is stable.

▶ *Take NOTE!*

When assessing the fluid status of a preterm newborn, palpate the fontanels. Sunken fontanels suggest dehydration; bulging fontanels suggest overhydration.

Preventing Infection

Prevention of infection is critical when caring for preterm newborns. Infections are the most common cause of morbidity and mortality in the NICU population (Simpson, Ye, Hellmann, et al., 2010). Nursing assessment and early identification of problems are imperative to improve outcomes.

Preterm newborns are at risk for infection because their early birth deprived them of maternal antibodies needed for passive protection. Preterm newborns also are susceptible to infection because of their limited ability to produce antibodies, asphyxia at birth, and thin, friable skin that is easily traumatized, providing an entry portal for microorganisms.

Early detection is crucial. The clinical manifestations can be nonspecific and subtle: apnea, diminished activity, poor feeding, temperature instability, respiratory distress, seizures, tachycardia, hypotonia, irritability, pallor, jaundice, and hypoglycemia. Report any of these to the primary care provider immediately so that treatment can be instituted.

Include the following interventions when caring for a preterm or postterm newborn to prevent infection:

- Assess for risk factors in maternal history that place the newborn at increased risk.
- Monitor for changes in vital signs such as temperature instability, tachycardia, or tachypnea.
- Assess oxygen saturation levels and initiate oxygen therapy as ordered if oxygen saturation levels fall below acceptable parameters.
- Assess feeding tolerance, typically an early sign of infection.
- Monitor laboratory test results for changes.
- Avoid using tape on the newborn's skin to prevent tearing.
- Use equipment that can be thrown away after use.
- Adhere to standard precautions; use clean gloves to handle dirty diapers and dispose of them properly.
- Use sterile gloves when assisting with any invasive procedure; attempt to minimize the use of invasive procedures.
- Remove all jewelry on your hands before washing hands; wash hands upon entering the nursery and in between caring for newborns.
- Avoid coming to work when ill, and screen all visitors for contagious infections.

Preventing Complications

Preterm newborns face a myriad of possible complications as a result of their fragile health status or the procedures and treatments used. Some of the more common complications in preterm newborns include respiratory distress syndrome, periventricular–intraventricular hemorrhage, bronchopulmonary dysplasia, ROP, hyperbilirubinemia, anemia, necrotizing enterocolitis, hypoglycemia, infection or septicemia, delayed growth and development, and mental or motor delays (March of Dimes, 2011). Several of these complications are described in Chapter 24.

Remember Anna, who was in a state of shock when she entered the NICU to see her preterm baby for the first time? How could the nurse have prepared her for this event? What information needs to be given at the isolette to reduce her anxiety and fear now?

Providing Appropriate Stimulation

Newborn stimulation involves a series of activities to encourage normal development. Research on developmental interventions shows that tactile–kinesthetic stimulation, such as rocking, skin-to-skin contact with parents, containment (swaddling and surrounded by blanket rolls), music, non-nutritive sucking, breastfeeding, massage, holding, and sleeping on waterbeds, is linked to gains in weight, growth, head circumference, activity level, general health status, and cognitive and motor development in newborns, particularly preterm newborns (Teti, Black, Viscardi, et al., 2009).

Conversely, overstimulation may have negative effects by reducing oxygenation and causing stress. A newborn reacts to stress by flaying the hands or bringing an arm up to cover the face. When overstimulated (such as by noise, lights, excessive handling, alarms, and procedures) and stressed, heart and respiratory rates decrease and periods of apnea or bradycardia may follow (Blackburn, 2007).

Appropriate developmental stimulation that would not overtax the compromised newborn might include kangaroo (skin-to-skin) holding, rocking, soft singing or music, cuddling, gentle stroking of the infant's skin, colourful mobiles, gentle massage, waterbed mattresses, and non-nutritive sucking opportunities (Fig. 23.5) or providing sucrose if tolerated.

The NICU environment can be altered to provide periods of calm and rest for the newborn by dimming the lights, lowering the volume and tone of conversations, closing doors gently, setting the telephone ringer to the lowest volume possible, clustering nursing activities, and covering the isolette with a blanket to act as a light shield to promote rest at night.

Encourage parents to hold and interact with their newborn. Doing so helps to acquaint the parents with their newborn, promotes self-confidence, and fosters parent–newborn attachment (Fig. 23.6).

Think back to Anna, the woman who gave birth to a preterm newborn at 7 months' gestation. Anna will be discharged, but her newborn will be staying in the NICU for a while. What interventions would be appropriate to facilitate bonding despite their separation? What support can be provided specifically to her family?

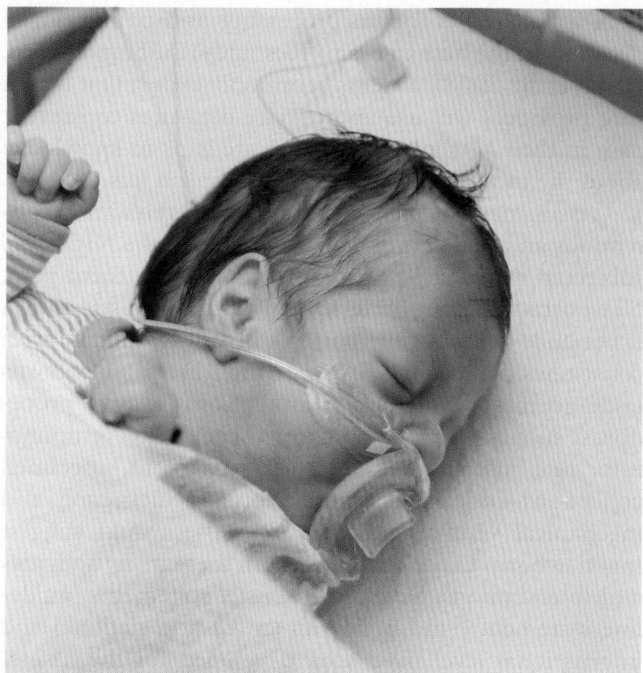

FIGURE 23.5 A preterm newborn receiving non-nutritive sucking.

Managing Pain

Pain is an unpleasant sensory and emotional experience felt by all humans. Newborns feel pain and require the same level of pain assessment and management as adults. Common indicators of pain in the newborn who is unable to vocalize include crying, facial expressions, body movements, and physiologic changes. Painful procedures in the early stages of development lead to long-term changes

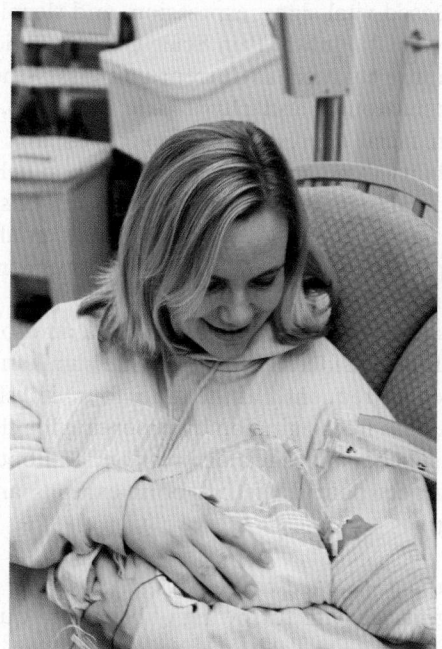

FIGURE 23.6 A mother bonding with her preterm newborn.

such as higher-level pain processing and pain-induced plasticity in the human brain (Kostandy, Ludington-Hoe, Cong, et al., 2008). Parents commonly expect that health care providers will use appropriate measures to prevent pain in their newborns, but there are gaps in knowledge about the most effective way to accomplish this.

Assessment of pain in the newborn remains a contentious and vexing problem. Newborns in the NICU are subjected to repeated procedures that cause them pain. Newborns, whether preterm, full term, or postterm, do experience pain, but the pain is difficult to validate with consistent behaviours. Considering that ill newborns undergo multiple noxious stimuli from invasive procedures, such as lumbar punctures, heelsticks, venipuncture, line insertions, chest tube placement, specimen collections, endotracheal intubation and suctioning, and mechanical ventilation, common sense would suggest that newborns experience pain from these many activities and interventions. Several consensus statements, guideline statements, and policy directives at a national and international level have been developed for the assessment and management of newborn pain. However, despite the volume of evidence, there remains a wide practice gap between what is known and what occurs in practice (Spence, Henderson-Smart, New, et al., 2010). An international consortium established principles of newborn pain prevention and management that all nurses must be familiar with and apply (Box 23.4).

Several psychometric tools are available to assess pain in the newborn. Examples include the Pain Assessment Tool (PAT), which evaluates respirations, heart rate, oxygen saturation, and blood pressure; the Premature Infant Pain Profile (PIPP), which assesses heart rate and oxygen saturation; the CRIES tool (cry, requires oxygen, increased vital signs, expression, and sleeplessness); and the Neonatal Infant Pain Scale (NIPS), which evaluates respiratory patterns. Current pain assessment tools rely on behavioural and physiologic measures, such as change in facial expression; however, research suggests the possibility that pain assessment based on behavioural tools alone may underestimate the pain response in premature infants (Slater, Cantarella, Franck, et al., 2008). See Chapter 35 for a more in-depth discussion of pain assessment and management.

Nurses play a key role in assessing a newborn's pain level. Pain is considered the "fifth vital sign" and should be assessed as frequently as the other four vital signs. Differentiate pain from agitation by observing for changes in vital signs, behaviour, facial expression, and body movement. Suspect pain if the newborn exhibits any of the following:

- Sudden high-pitched cry
- Facial grimace with furrowing of brow and quivering chin
- Increased muscle tone

BOX 23.4 Newborn Pain Prevention and Management Guidelines

- Newborn pain frequently goes unrecognized and undertreated.
- Pain assessment is an essential activity prior to pain management.
- Newborns experience pain, and analgesics should be given.
- A procedure considered painful for an adult should also be considered painful for a newborn.
- Developmental maturity and health status must be considered when assessing for pain in newborns.
- Newborns may be more sensitive to pain than adults.
- Pain behaviour is frequently mistaken for irritability and agitation.
- Newborns are more susceptible to the long-term effects of pain.
- Adequate pain management may reduce complications and mortality.
- Non-pharmacologic measures can prevent, reduce, or eliminate newborn pain.
- Sedation does not provide pain relief and may mask pain responses.
- A newborn's response to both pharmacologic and non-pharmacologic pain therapy should be assessed within 30 minutes of administration or intervention.
- Health care professionals are responsible for pain assessment and treatment.
- Written guidelines are needed on each newborn unit.

Source: Spence, K., Henderson-Smart, D., New, K., et al. (2010). Evidence-based clinical practice guideline for management of newborn pain. *Journal of Paediatrics and Child Health, 46*(4), 184–192.

- Oxygen desaturation
- Body posturing, such as squirming, kicking, or arching
- Limb withdrawal and thrashing movements
- Increase in heart rate and respirations, shallow breathing, increased or decreased blood pressure; additionally neonates may demonstrate bradycardia or apnea (Ballweg, 2008)
- Fussiness and irritability (Ballantyne, Fishman, & Rathmell, 2009; Ballweg, 2008)

The goals of pain management are to minimize the amount, duration, and severity of pain and to assist the newborn in coping. Effective pain management strategies for newborns include preventing, limiting, or avoiding noxious stimuli; using non-pharmacologic techniques to reduce pain; and administering pharmacologic agents when appropriate. Box 23.5 lists some of the more commonly used non-pharmacologic pain management techniques for the preterm newborn.

The number of analgesics available for use with preterm newborns is limited. Morphine and fentanyl,

---

BOX 23.5 Non-pharmacologic Techniques to Reduce Pain in the Preterm Newborn

- Gentle handling, rocking, caressing, cuddling, and massaging
- Rest periods before and after painful procedures
- Kangaroo care (skin-to-skin contact) during procedures
- Breastfeeding, if able, to reduce pain from minor procedures
- Use of a facilitated tuck (holding arms and legs in a flexed position)
- Application of topical anesthetics prior to venipuncture or lumbar puncture
- Swaddling and positioning to establish physical boundaries
- Non-nutritive sucking (pacifier dipped in sucrose) prior to procedure
- Minimal use of tape, with gentle removal to avoid skin tears
- Warm blankets for wrapping to facilitate relaxation
- Reduction of noxious environmental stimuli by removing or turning down noise from alarms, beepers, loud conversations, and bright lights
- Distraction, such as with coloured objects or mobiles

Sources: Spence et al., 2010; Kostandy, R., Ludington-Hoe, S., Cong, X., et al. (2008). Kangaroo care (skin contact) reduces crying response to pain in preterm neonates: Pilot results. *Pain Management Nursing, 9*(2), 55–65.

---

usually administered intravenously, are the most commonly used opioids for moderate to severe pain. Acetaminophen is effective for mild pain. Benzodiazepines are used as sedatives during painful procedures and can be combined with opioids for more effectiveness. Local or topical anesthetics (e.g., EMLA cream) also may be used before procedures such as venipuncture, lumbar puncture, and intravenous catheter insertion (Ballweg, 2008).

Be vigilant in assessing for adverse effects (respiratory depression or hypotension) when administering pharmacologic agents for pain management, especially in preterm newborns with neurologic impairment. These negative effects are usually dose- and route-related, so be knowledgeable about the pharmacokinetics and therapeutic dosing of any drug administered.

Promoting Growth and Development

In the late 1970s, researchers evaluated the NICU environment in terms of light and sound levels, caregiving activities, and handling of newborns. As a result of this research, many environmental modifications were made to reduce the stress and overstimulation of the NICU, and the concept of developmentally supportive care was introduced. Developmentally supportive care is defined as care of a newborn or infant to support positive growth and development. Developmental care focuses on what

newborns or infants can do at that stage of development; it uses therapeutic interventions only to the point that they are beneficial; and it provides for the development of the newborn–family unit (Neonatal Handbook, 2010).

- Developmental care is a philosophy of care that requires rethinking the relationships between newborns, families, and health care providers. It includes a variety of activities designed to manage the environment and individualize the care of the preterm or high-risk ill newborn based on behavioural observations. The aim of developmental care is to reduce stress and agitation, preserve energy and promote growth, enhance recovery, facilitate self-regulatory capabilities, and promote central nervous system organization (Neonatal Handbook, 2010).

Developmental care includes these strategies:

- Clustering care to promote rest and conserve the infant's energy
- Flexed positioning to simulate in utero positioning
- Environmental management to reduce noise and visual stimulation
- Kangaroo care to promote skin-to-skin sensation
- Placement of twins in the same isolette or open crib to reduce stress
- Activities to promote self-regulation and state regulation:
  - Surrounding the newborn with nesting rolls/devices
  - Swaddling with a blanket to maintain the flexed position
  - Providing sheepskin or a waterbed to simulate the uterine environment
  - Providing non-nutritive sucking (calms the infant)
  - Providing objects to grasp (comforts the newborn)
- Promotion of parent–infant bonding by making parents feel welcome in the NICU
- Open, honest communication between parents and staff
- Collaboration with the parents in planning the infant's care (Gooding, Cooper, Blaine, et al., 2011)

Developmental care can be fostered by clustering the lights in one area so that no lights are shining directly on newborns, installing visual alarm systems and limiting overhead pages to minimize noise, and monitoring continuous and peak noise levels. Nurses can play an active role by serving on committees that address these issues. In addition, nurses can provide direct developmentally supportive care. Doing so involves careful planning of nursing activities to provide the ideal environment for the newborn's development. For example:

- Dim the lights and cover isolettes at night to simulate nighttime.
- Support early extubation from mechanical ventilation.
- Encourage early and consistent feedings with breast milk.

- Administer prescribed antibiotics judiciously.
- Position the newborn as if he or she were still in utero (a nesting fetal position).
- Promote kangaroo care by encouraging parents to hold the newborn against the chest for extended periods each day.
- Coordinate care to respect sleep and awake states.

Throughout the newborn's stay, work with the parents, developing a collaborative partnership so they feel comfortable caring for their newborn. Be prepared to make referrals to community support groups to enhance coping (Kearvell & Grant, 2010).

Promoting Parental Coping

Generally, pregnancy and the birth of a newborn are exciting times, but when the newborn has serious, perhaps life-threatening problems, the exciting experience suddenly changes to one of anxiety, fear, guilt, loss, and grief.

Parents are typically unprepared for the birth of a preterm newborn and commonly experience an array of emotions, including disappointment, fear for the survival of the newborn, and anxiety due to the separation from their newborn immediately after birth (Kearvell & Grant, 2010). Early interruptions in the bonding process and concern about the newborn's survival can create extreme anxiety and interfere with attachment (Kearvell & Grant, 2010).

Nursing interventions aimed at reducing parental anxiety include:

- Reviewing with them the events that have occurred since birth
- Providing simple relaxation and calming techniques (visual imagery, breathing)
- Exploring their perception of the newborn's condition and offering explanations
- Validating their anxiety and behaviours as normal reactions to stress and trauma
- Providing a physical presence and support during emotional outbursts
- Exploring the coping strategies they used successfully in the past and encouraging their use now
- Encouraging frequent visits to the NICU
- Addressing their reactions to the NICU environment and explaining all equipment used
- Identifying family and community resources available to them (Roland & Goodnight, 2009)

Preparing for Discharge

Discharge planning typically begins with evidence that recovery of the newborn is certain. However, the exact date of discharge may not be predictable. The goal of the discharge plan is to make a successful transition to home care. Essential elements for discharge are a physiologically stable infant, a family who can provide the neces-

---

> ### BOX 23.6 Critical Components of Discharge Planning
>
> - Parental education—involvement and support in newborn care during NICU stay will ensure their readiness to care for the infant at home
> - Evaluation of unresolved medical problems—review of the active problem list and determination of what home care and follow-up are needed
> - Implementation of primary care—completion of newborn screening tests, immunizations, examinations such as funduscopic exam for ROP, and hematologic status evaluation
> - Development of home care plan, including assessment of:
>   - Equipment and supplies needed for care
>   - In-home caregiver's preparation and ability to care for infant
>   - Adequacy of the physical facilities in the home
>   - An emergency care and transport plan if needed
>   - Financial resources for homecare costs
>   - Family needs and coping skills
>   - Community resources, including how they can be accessed

sary care with appropriate support services in place in the community, and a primary care physician available for ongoing care.

The care of each high-risk newborn after discharge requires careful coordination to provide ongoing multidisciplinary support for the family. The discharge planning team typically includes the parents, primary care physician, neonatologists, neonatal nurses, and a social worker. Other professionals, such as surgical specialists and pediatric subspecialists, occupational, physical, speech, and respiratory therapists, nutritionists, home health care nurses, and a case manager, may be included as needed. Critical components of discharge planning are summarized in Box 23.6.

Nurses involved in the discharge process are instrumental in bridging the gap between the hospital and home. Interventions typically include:

- Assessing the physical status of the mother and the newborn
- Discussing the early signs of complications and what to do if they occur
- Reinforcing instructions for infant care and safety
- Stressing the importance of proper car seat use
- Providing instructions for medication administration
- Reinforcing instructions for equipment operation, maintenance, and troubleshooting
- Teaching infant cardiopulmonary resuscitation and emergency care

- Demonstrating techniques for special care procedures such as dressings, ostomy care, artificial airway maintenance, chest physiotherapy, suctioning, and infant stimulation
- Providing breastfeeding support or instruction on gavage feedings
- Assisting with defining roles in the adjustment period at home
- Assessing the parents' emotional stability and coping status
- Providing support and reassurance to the family
- Reporting abnormal findings to the health care team for intervention
- Following up with parents to assure them that they have a "lifeline"

Dealing with Perinatal Loss

Perinatal loss is a profound experience for the family. It engenders a unique kind of mourning since the infant is so much a part of the parents' identity. Instead of celebrating a new life as they expected, parents are mourning the loss of dreams and hopes and the loss of an extension of themselves. NICU nurses face a difficult situation when caring for newborns who may not survive. Newborn death is incomprehensible to most parents. This makes the grieving process more difficult because what is happening "can't be real." Deciding whether to see, touch, or hold the dying newborn is extremely difficult for many parents. Nurses play a major role in assisting parents to make their dying newborn "real" to them by providing them with as many memories as possible and encouraging them to see, hold, touch, dress, and take care of the infant and take photographs. These actions help to validate the parents' sense of loss, relive the experience, and attach significance to the meaning of loss. A lock of hair, a name card, or an identification bracelet may serve as important mementoes that can ease the grieving process. The memories created by these interventions can be useful allies in the grieving process and in resolving grief (Harvey, Snowdon, & Elbourne, 2008; National Association of Neonatal Nurses, 2010).

Parent–newborn interaction is vital to the normal processes of attachment and bonding. The detachment process involved in a newborn's death is equally important for parents. Nurses can aid in this process by helping parents to see their newborn through the maze of equipment, explaining the various procedures and equipment, encouraging them to express their feelings about the newborn's status, and providing time for them to be with their dying newborn (Kearvell & Grant, 2010).

A common reaction by many people when learning that a newborn is not going to survive is one of avoidance. Nurses are no exception. It is difficult to initiate a conversation about such a sensitive issue without knowing how the parents are going to react and cope with the impending loss. One way to begin a conversation with the parents is to convey concern and acknowledge their loss. Active listening can give parents a safe place to begin the healing process. The relationship that the nurse establishes with the parents is a unique one, providing an opportunity for both the nurse and the parents to share their feelings.

Be aware of personal feelings about loss and how these feelings are part of one's own life and personal belief system. Actively listen to the parents when they are talking about their experiences. Communicate empathy (understanding and feeling what another person is feeling), respect their feelings, and respond to them in helpful and supportive ways (Roland & Goodnight, 2009). Table 23.2 highlights appropriate interventions for a family experiencing a perinatal loss before and after a newborn dies.

In a time of crisis or loss, individuals are often more sensitive to other people's reactions. For example, the parents may be extremely aware of the nurse's facial expressions, choice of words, and tone of voice. Talking quickly, in a businesslike fashion, or ignoring the loss may inhibit parents from discussing their pain or how they are coping with it. Parents may need to vent their frustrations and anger, and the nurse may become the target. Validate their feelings and attempt to reframe or re-focus the anger toward the real issue of loss. An example would be to say, "I understand your frustration and anger about this situation. You have experienced a tremendous loss and it must be difficult not to have an explanation for it at this time." Doing so helps to defuse the anger while allowing them to express their feelings.

When assisting bereaved parents, start where the parents are in the grief process to avoid imposing your own agenda on them. Remember that while the parents are struggling over the loss of the same child, they may not be synchronized in the grieving process. You may feel uncomfortable at not being able to change the situation or take the pain away. The nurse's role is to provide immediate emotional support and facilitate the grieving process. Supporting and strengthening the family bond in the face of perinatal loss is essential. Follow-up phone calls within 1 to 2 weeks, after the parents have had time to process the birth and loss experience, help to evaluate the parent's well-being and provide an opportunity for them to ask questions. Providing the family with community support groups and contacts is essential (Roland & Goodnight, 2009).

Late Preterm Newborn

A late preterm newborn is an infant born between 34 weeks, 0 days and 36 weeks, 6 days of gestation. Approximately 5.7% of Canadian births are late preterm; however, this group represents approximately 74% of all preterm births (Statistics Canada, 2009). High morbidity and mortality have been documented in recent

TABLE 23.2 ASSISTING PARENTS TO COPE WITH PERINATAL LOSS

Before the newborn's death	Respect variations in the family's spiritual needs and readiness. Assess cultural beliefs and practices that may bring comfort; respect culturally appropriate requests for truth telling and informed refusal. Initiate spiritual comfort by calling the hospital clergy if appropriate; offer to pray with the family if appropriate. Encourage the parents to take photographs, make memory boxes, and record their thoughts in a journal. Explore with family members how they dealt with previous losses. Discuss techniques to reduce stress, such as meditation and relaxation. Recommend that family members maintain a healthy diet and get adequate rest and exercise to preserve their health. Participate in early and repeated care conferencing to reduce family stress. Allow the family to be present at both medical rounds and resuscitation; provide explanations of all procedures, treatments, and findings; answer questions honestly and as completely as possible. Provide opportunities for the family to hold the newborn if they choose to. Assess the family's support network. Provide suggestions as to how friends can be helpful to the family.
After the newborn's death	Help the family to accept the reality of death by using the word "died." Acknowledge their grief and the fact that their newborn has died. Help the family to work through their grief by validating and listening. Provide the family with realistic information about the causes of death. Offer condolences to the family in a sincere manner. Encourage the father to cry and grieve with his partner. Provide opportunities for the family to hold the newborn if they desire.
At the time of the release of the newborn's body	Reassure the family that their feelings and grieving responses are normal. Encourage the parents to have a funeral or memorial service to bring closure. Suggest that the parents plant a tree or flowers to remember the infant. Address attachment issues concerning subsequent pregnancies. Provide information about local support groups. Provide anticipatory guidance regarding the grieving process. Present information about any impact on future childbearing, and refer the parents to appropriate specialists or genetic resources.

Sources: Branchett, K., & Sretton, J. (2012). Neonatal palliative and end of life care: What parents want from professionals. *Journal of Neonatal Nursing, 18*, 40–44; and National Association of Neonatal Nurses. (2010). Palliative care for newborns and infants: Position statement for the advances in neonatal care. *Advances in Neonatal Care, 10*(6), 287–293.

years in this population (Kitsommart, Janes, Mahajan, et al., 2009).

Perinatal nurses need to understand the risks of late preterm births and the unique needs of this population to facilitate timely assessment and intervention to improve outcomes. In a recent Canadian tertiary-care centre study, the need for respiratory support and the incidence of intensive care admission, pneumothorax, and mortality in late preterm infants was significantly higher (12-fold) than in infants born at term (Kitsommart et al., 2009).

Some of the challenges facing the late preterm newborn include respiratory distress (secondary to cesarean births, maternal gestational diabetes, chorioamnionitis, premature rupture of membranes, and fetal distress); thermoregulation issues related to limited ability to flex the trunk and extremities to decrease exposed surface area; hypoglycemia related to the first two challenges (respiratory distress and cold stress); jaundice and hyperbilirubinemia related to a gestational age of 36 weeks or less; and feeding challenges related to immature suck and swallowing reflexes (Darcy, 2009). These challenges are similar to those facing the preterm newborn and require similar management. Nurses and parents must be aware of the risks associated with late preterm births to optimize care and outcomes for this group of newborns.

■■■ Key Concepts

■ Variations in birth weight and gestational age can place a newborn at risk for problems that require special care.

■ Variations in birth weight include the following categories: small for gestational age, AGA, and large for gestational age. Newborns who are small or large for gestational age have special needs.

■ The SGA newborn faces problems related to a decrease in placental function in utero; these problems may include perinatal asphyxia, hypothermia, hypoglycemia, polycythemia, and meconium aspiration.

■ Risk factors for the birth of an LGA infant include maternal diabetes mellitus or glucose intolerance, multiparity, prior history of a macrosomic infant, postdates gestation, maternal obesity, male fetus, and genetics. LGA newborns face problems such as birth trauma due to cephalopelvic disproportion, hypoglycemia, and jaundice secondary to hyperbilirubinemia.

■ Variations in gestational age include postterm and preterm newborns. Postterm newborns may be large or small for gestational age or dysmature, depending on placental function.

■ The postterm newborn may develop several complications after birth, including fetal hypoxia, hypoglycemia, hypothermia, polycythemia, and meconium aspiration.

■ Preterm birth is the leading cause of death in the neonatal period, and congenital anomalies are the leading cause of death in the postneonatal period (Public Health Agency of Canada, 2008).

■ The preterm newborn is at risk for complications because his or her organ systems are immature, thereby impeding the transition from intrauterine life to extrauterine life.

■ Newborns can experience pain, but their pain is difficult to validate with consistent behaviours.

■ Strategies for pain prevention and management using both pharmacologic and non-pharmacologic therapies are essential.

■ Newborns with gestational age variations, primarily preterm newborns, benefit from developmental care, which includes a variety of activities designed to manage the environment and individualize the care based on behavioural observations.

■ Nurses play a key role in assisting the parents and family of a newborn with special needs to cope with this crisis situation, including dealing with the possibility that the newborn may not survive. Nurses working with parents experiencing a perinatal loss can help by actively listening, understanding the parents' experiences, and communicating empathy.

■ The goal of discharge planning is to make a successful transition to home care.

REFERENCES

Ambalavanan, N. (2010). *Fluid, electrolyte and nutrition management of the newborn*. Retrieved March 13, 2012 from http://emedicine.medscape.com/article/976386-overview#aw2aab6b3

Ballantyne, J. C., Fishman, S. M., & Rathmell, J. P. (2009). *Bonica's management of pain* (4th ed.). Philadelphia: Lippincott Williams & Wilkins.

Ballweg, D. (2008). Neonatal and pediatric pain management: standards and application. *Paediatrics & Child Health, 17*(Suppl), S61–S66.

Beckmann, C., Ling, F., Barzansky, B., Herbert, W., Laube, D.W., & Smith, R. (2010). *Obstetrics and Gynecology* (6th ed.). Philadelphia: Lippincott Williams & Wilkins.

Bissinger, R. & Annibale, D. (2010). Thermoregulation in low-birth-weight infants during the golden hour: Results and implications. *Advances in Neonatal Care, 10*(5), 230–238.

Blackburn, S. (2007). *Maternal, fetal and neonatal physiology: A clinical perspective* (3rd ed.). Philadelphia: Saunders Elsevier.

Branchett, K. & Sretton, J. (2012). Neonatal palliative and end of life care: What parents want from professionals. *Journal of Neonatal Nursing, 18*, 40–44.

Canadian Institute for Health Information. (2009). *Too early, too small: A profile of small babies across Canada*. Retrieved March 13, 2012 from http://secure.cihi.ca/cihiweb/products/too_early_too_small_en.pdf

Canadian Paediatric Society. (2011). *Screening guidelines for newborns at risk for low blood glucose*. Retrieved March 13, 2012 from http://www.cps.ca/english/statements/FN/fn04-01.htm

Chen, M. L., Guo, L., Smith, L. E., Dammann, C. E., & Dolmman, O. (2010). High or low oxygen saturation and severe retinopathy or prematurity: A meta-analysis. *Pediatrics, 125*(6), 1483–1492.

Cheng, Y. W., Nicholson, J. M., Nakagawa, S. Bruckner, T. A., Washington, A. E., & Caughey, A. B. (2008). Perinatal outcomes in low-risk term pregnancies: do they differ by week of gestation?. *American Journal of Obstetrics and Gynecology, 199*(4), 370e1–370e7.

Cloherty, J., Eichenwald, E., & Stark, A. (2008). *Manual of neonatal care*. Philadelphia: Lippincott Williams & Wilkins.

Darcy, A. E. (2009). Complications of the late preterm infant. *Journal of Perinatal and Neonatal Nursing, 23*(1), 78–86.

Dorland, W. A. N. (2007). *Dorland's illustrated medical dictionary* (30th ed.). St. Louis: Saunders Elsevier.

du Plessis, A. J. (2009). The role of systematic hemodynamic disturbances in prematurity-related brain injury. *Journal of Child Neurology, 24*(9), 1127–1140.

Ferndandes, C. (2012). *Neonatal resuscitation in the delivery room*. Retrieved March 13, 2012 from http://www.uptodate.com/contents/neonatal-resuscitation-in-the-delivery-room

Finer, N., & Leone, T. (2009). Oxygen saturation monitoring for the preterm infant: The evidence basis for current practice. *Pediatric Research, 65*(4), 375–380.

Gooding, J., Cooper, L., Blaine, A., Franck, L., Howse, J. & Berns, S. (2011). Family support and family-centered care in the neonatal intensive care unit: Origins, advances, impact. *Seminars in Perinatology, 35*(1), 20–28.

Gundby, J., Bissonnette, F., Librach, C., & Cowan, L. (2008). Assisted reproductive technologies (ART) in Canada. *Fertility and Sterility, 89*(5), 1123–1132.

Harvey, S., Snowdon, C., & Elbourne, D. (2008). Effectiveness of bereavement interventions in neonatal intensive care: A review of the evidence. *Seminars in Fetal and Neonatal Medicine, 13*, 341–356.

Hatfield, N. (2008). *Broadribb's introductory pediatric nursing*. Philadelphia: Lippincott Williams & Wilkins.

Joseph, K. S. (2008). An overview of perinatal health in Canada. *Canadian Perinatal Health Report, 2008 edition*. Retrieved March 13, 2012 from http://www.phac-aspc.gc.ca/publicat/2008/cphr-rspc/pdf/overview-apercu-eng.pdf

Kattwinkel, J., Perlman, J., Aziz, K., et al. (2010). Neonatal resuscitation: 2010 American Heart Association guidelines for cardiopulmonary resuscitation and emergency cardiovascular care. *Pediatrics, 126*(5), e1400–e1413. Retrieved March 13, 2012 from http://pediatrics.aappublications.org/cgi/content/full/126/5/e1400

Kearvell, H., & Grant, J. (2010). Getting connected: How nurses can support mother/infant attachment in the neonatal intensive care unit. *Australian Journal of Advanced Nursing, 27*(3), 75–82.

Kierans, W., Luo, Z., Wilkins, R., Taylor-Clapp, S., & Foster, L. (n.d.). *Infant macrosomia among First Nations in British Columbia—Prevalence, trends and characteristics*. Retrieved March 13, 2012 from http://www.vs.gov.bc.ca/stats/indian/REPORT_Only_Macros.pdf

Kiess, W., Chernausek, S. D. & Hokken-Koelega, A.C.S. (Eds.). (2009). *Small for gestational age: causes and consequences*. Basel, NY: Karger.

Kitsommart, R., Janes, M., Mahajan, V., et al. (2009). Outcomes of late-preterm infants: A retrospective, single-center, Canadian study. *Clinical Pediatrics, 48*(8), 844–850.

Kostandy, R., Ludington-Hoe, S., Cong, X., et al. (2008). Kangaroo care (skin contact) reduces crying response to pain in preterm neonates: Pilot results. *Pain Management Nursing, 9*(2), 55–65.

Lee, S.K., Aziz, K., Singhal, N., et al. (2009). Improving the quality of care for infants: a cluster randomized controlled trial. *Canadian Association Medical Journal, 181*(8), 469–476.

Luo, Z., Kierans, W. J., Wilkins, R., Liston, R. M., Uh, S., & Kramer, M. S. (2004). Infant mortality among First Nations versus non-First Nations in British Columbia: temporal trends in rural versus urban areas, 1981–2000. *International Journal of Epidemiology, 33,* 1252–1259.

Luo, Z., Senecal, S., Simonet, F., Guimond, E., Penney, C., & Wilkins, R. (2010). Birth outcomes in the Inuit-inhabited areas of Canada. *Canadian Medical Association Journal, 182*(3), 235–242.

Mally, P., Bailey, S., & Hendricks-Munoz, K. (2010). Clinical issues in the management of late preterm infants. *Current Problems in Pediatric and Adolescent Health Care, 40*(9), 218–233.

March of Dimes. (2011). *Healthy babies are worth the wait—Preventing preterm babies through community-based interventions: An implementation manual.* Retrieved March 13, 2012 from http://www.marchofdimes.com/HBWW_manual_12-21-10.pdf

National Association of Neonatal Nurses. (2010). Palliative care for newborns and infants: Position statement for the advances in neonatal care. *Advances in Neonatal Care, 10*(6), 287–293.

Neonatal Handbook. (2007). *Metabolic diseases.* Retrieved March 13, 2012 from http://www.rch.org.au/nets/handbook/index.cfm?doc_id=895

Neonatal Handbook. (2010). *Developmental care.* Retrieved March 13, 2012 from http://www.netsvic.org.au/nets/handbook/?doc_id=719

Neonatal Handbook. (2011). Infant of a diabetic mother. Retrieved March 13, 2012 from http://www.rch.org.au/nets/handbook/index.cfm?doc_id=889

Neonatal Handbook. (n.d.). *Polycythaemia.* Retrieved March 13, 2012 from http://www.netsvic.org.au/nets/handbook/?doc_id=636

Pillitteri, A. (2009). *Maternal and child health nursing: Care of the childbearing and childrearing family.* Philadelphia: Lippincott Williams & Wilkins.

Public Health Agency of Canada. (2008). *Canadian perinatal health report, 2008 edition.* Retrieved March 13, 2012 from http://www.phac-aspc.gc.ca/publicat/2008/cphr-rspc/pdf/cphr-rspc08-eng.pdf

Ricci, S., & Kyle, T. (2009). *Maternity and pediatric nursing.* Philadelphia: Lippincott Williams & Wilkins.

Rodek, C., & Whittle, M. (2009). *Fetal medicine: Basic science and clinical practice* (2nd ed.). Philadelphia: Elsevier.

Roland, A., & Goodnight, W. H. (2009). Fetal loss: Addressing the evaluation and supporting the emotional needs of parents. *Journal of Midwifery & Women's Health, 54*(3), 241–248.

Sankar, M. J., Agarwal, R., Deorari, A., & Paul, V. (2010). *Management of polycythemia in neonates.* Retrieved March 13, 2012 from http://www.newbornwhocc.org/pdf/Polycythemia_2010_200810.pdf

Shah, M. D., & Shah, S. R. (2009). Nutritional deficiencies in the premature infant. *Pediatric Clinics of North America, 56*(5), 1069–1083.

Simpson, C., Ye., X., Hellmann, J., & Tomlinson, C. (2010). Trends in cause-specific mortality at a Canadian outborn NICU. *Pediatrics, 126*(6), e1538–e1544.

Slater, R., Cantarella, A., Franck, L., Meek, J., & Fitzgerald, M. (2008). *How well do clinical pain assessment tools reflect pain in infants?* Retrieved March 13, 2012 from http://www.plosmedicine.org/article/info%3Adoi%2F10.1371%2Fjournal.pmed.0050129

Spence, K., Henderson-Smart, D., New, K., et.al. (2010). Evidence-based clinical practice guideline for management of newborn pain. *Journal of Paediatrics and Child Health, 46*(4), 184–192.

Statistics Canada. (2009). *Births 2007.* (Catalogue no. 84F0210X). Retrieved March 13, 2012 from http://www.statcan.gc.ca/pub/84f0210x/2007000/userinfo-usagerinfo-eng.htm

Teti, D., Black, M., Viscardi, R., et al. (2009). Interventions with African American premature infants: Four-month results of an early intervention program. *Journal of Early Intervention, 31*(2), 146–166.

Urquia, M. L., Frank, J. W., Glazier, R. H., & Moineddin, R. (2007). *Birth outcomes by neighbourhood income and recent immigration in Toronto.* Retrieved March 13, 2012 from http://www.statcan.gc.ca/pub/82-003-x/2006010/article/birth-naissance/10356-eng.pdf

Vargo, L. E., & Trotter, C. W. (2007). The premature infant: Nursing assessment and management. *March of Dimes Nursing Modules* (2nd ed.). #33-1995-05.

Walsh, B., Brooks, T., & Grenier, B. (2009). Oxygen therapy in the neonatal care environment. *Respiratory Care, 54*(9), 1193–1202.

Whittington, C. (2010). *Parental perceptions of touch between parents and infants in the neonatal intensive unit [Doctoral dissertation].* Available from Dissertation Express database. (UMI No. 3438747).

Zhong, Y., Tuuli, M., & Odido, A. O. (2010). First-trimester assessment of placenta function and the prediction of preeclampsia and intrauterine growth restriction. *Prenatal Diagnoses, 30,* 293–308.

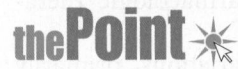 **For additional learning materials, including Internet Resources, visit http://thePoint.lww.com/Chow1e.**

CHAPTER WORKSHEET

MULTIPLE CHOICE QUESTIONS

1. The nurse documents that a newborn is postterm based on the understanding that he or she was born after:

   a. 38 weeks' gestation

   b. 40 weeks' gestation

   c. 42 weeks' gestation

   d. 44 weeks' gestation

2. SGA and LGA newborns have an excessive number of red blood cells because of:

   a. Hypoxia

   b. Hypoglycemia

   c. Hypocalcemia

   d. Hypothermia

3. Because subcutaneous and brown fat stores were used for survival in utero, the nurse would assess an SGA newborn for which of the following?

   a. Hyperbilirubinemia

   b. Hypothermia

   c. Polycythemia

   d. Hypoglycemia

4. In assessing a preterm newborn, which of the following findings would be of greatest concern?

   a. Milia over the bridge of the nose

   b. Thin, transparent skin

   c. Poor muscle tone

   d. Heart murmur

5. In dealing with parents experiencing a perinatal loss, which of the following nursing interventions would be most appropriate?

   a. Sheltering the parents from the bad news

   b. Making all the decisions regarding care

   c. Encouraging them to participate in the newborn's care

   d. Leaving them by themselves to allow time to grieve

6. The nurse is providing care to several newborns with variations in gestational age and birth weight. When developing the plan of care for these newborns, the nurse focuses on energy conservation to promote growth and development. Which measures would the nurse include in the nursing plan of care? Select all that apply.

   a. Keeping the handling of the newborn to a minimum

   b. Maintaining a neutral thermal environment

   c. Decreasing environmental stimuli

   d. Initiating early oral feedings

   e. Using thermal warmers in all cribs

7. Which of the following concepts would the nurse incorporate into the plan of care when assessing pain in a newborn with special needs?

   a. Newborns experience pain primarily with surgical procedures.

   b. Preterm newborns in the NICU are at least risk for pain.

   c. Pain assessment needs to be comprehensive and frequent.

   d. A newborn's facial expression is the primary indicator of pain.

CRITICAL THINKING EXERCISES

1. After fetal distress was noted on the monitor, a postterm newborn was delivered via a difficult vacuum extraction. The newborn had low Apgar scores and had to be resuscitated before being transferred to the nursery. Once admitted, the nurse observed the following behaviours: jitteriness, tremors, hypotonia, lethargy, and rapid respirations.

   a. What might these behaviours indicate?

   b. For what other conditions might this newborn be at high risk?

   c. What intervention is needed to address this newborn's condition?

(question continues on page 754)

2. A preterm newborn was born at 35 weeks following an abruptio placentae due to a car accident. He was transported to the NICU at a nearby regional medical centre. After being stabilized, he was placed in an isolette close to the door and placed on a cardiac monitor. A short time later, the nurse notices that he is cool to the touch and lethargic, has a weak cry, and has an axillary temperature of 36°C.

   a. What might have contributed to this newborn's hypothermic condition?

   b. What transfer mechanism may have been a factor?

   c. What intervention would be appropriate for the nurse to initiate?

3. A term SGA newborn weighing 1,800 g was brought to the nursery for admission a short time after birth. The labour and birth nurse reports the mother was a heavy smoker and a cocaine addict and experienced physical abuse throughout her pregnancy. After stabilizing the newborn and correcting the hypoglycemia with oral feedings, the nurse observes the following: acrocyanosis, ruddy colour, poor circulation to the extremities, tachypnea, and irritability.

   a. What complication might this SGA newborn be manifesting?

   b. What factors may have contributed to this complication?

   c. What would be an appropriate intervention to manage this condition?

STUDY ACTIVITIES

1. At a community health department maternity clinic, secure permission to interview the parents of a special needs child. Ask about their feelings throughout the experience. How are they managing and coping now?

2. Visit the March of Dimes website and review this group's national campaign to reduce the incidence of prematurity. Are their strategies workable or not? Explain your reasoning.

3. A common metabolic disorder present in both SGA and LGA newborns after birth is

   _____.

4. A 4.5 kg LGA newborn is brought to the nursery after a difficult vaginal birth. The nursery nurse should focus on detecting birth injuries such as

   _____.

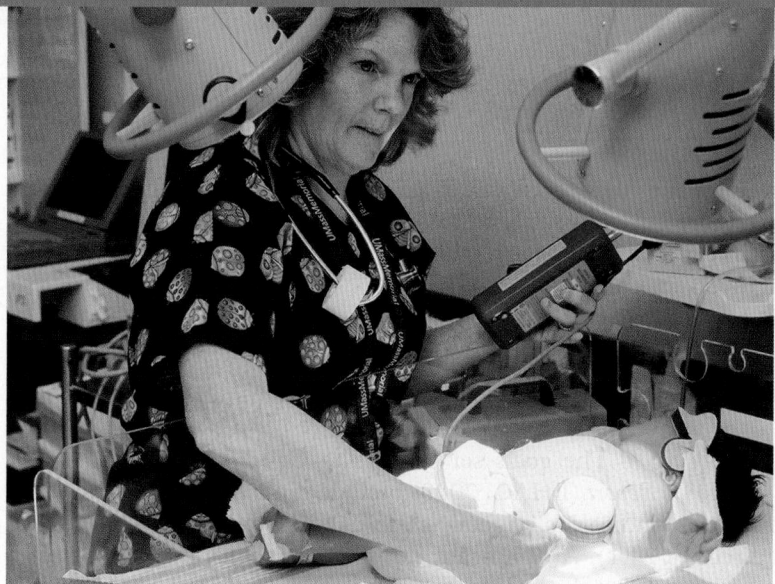

NURSING MANAGEMENT OF THE NEWBORN AT RISK: ACQUIRED AND CONGENITAL NEWBORN CONDITIONS

Adapted By Cathy Ringham

KEY TERMS

alcohol–related birth defects

asphyxia

caput succedaneum

cephalhematoma

fetal alcohol spectrum disorder

fetal alcohol syndrome

gastroschisis

hyperbilirubinemia

infant of a diabetic mother

kernicterus

meconium aspiration syndrome

neonatal abstinence syndrome

neonatal sepsis

omphalocele

respiratory distress syndrome

Kelly, a 27-year-old G2P1, comes to the labour and birth area in active labour. She tells you she is overdue and relieved to finally be giving birth. Her membranes rupture on admission, revealing meconium-stained fluid. What additional nursing assessments need to be carried out now? What risk factors need to be considered when developing Kelly's plan of care?

LEARNING OBJECTIVES

After completion of the chapter, the learner will be able to:

1. Identify the most common acquired conditions affecting the newborn.
2. Describe the nursing management of a newborn experiencing respiratory distress syndrome.
3. Outline the birthing room preparation and procedures necessary to prevent meconium aspiration syndrome in the newborn at birth.
4. Differentiate risk factors for the development of necrotizing enterocolitis.
5. Explain the impact of maternal diabetes on the newborn and the care needed.
6. Describe the assessment and intervention for a newborn experiencing substance withdrawal after birth.
7. Identify assessment and nursing management for newborns sustaining trauma and birth injuries.
8. Outline the assessment, interventions, prevention, and management of hyperbilirubinemia in newborns.
9. Summarize the interventions appropriate for a newborn with neonatal sepsis.

WoW *Nurses are uniquely capable of creating a calm environment that empowers pregnant women to persevere through a potentially complicated labour.*

LEARNING OBJECTIVES (continued)

10. Describe four gastrointestinal system congenital anomalies that can occur in a newborn.
11. Formulate a plan of care for a newborn with an acquired or congenital condition.
12. Discuss the importance of parental participation in care of the newborn with a congenital or acquired condition, including the nurse's role in facilitating parental involvement.

Advances in prenatal and neonatal medical and nursing care throughout the industrialized world have led to a marked increase in the number of newborns who have survived a high-risk pregnancy but experience acquired or congenital conditions. These newborns are considered at risk; that is, they are susceptible to morbidity and mortality because of the acquired or congenital disorder.

The Public Health Agency of Canada's (PHAC) vision is to promote and protect the health of Canadians. As part of this mandate, the agency publishes numerous reports addressing the health challenges of women and children, including at-risk newborns. The *Canadian Perinatal Health Report* highlights goals for improving outcomes for newborns with acquired and congenital conditions (PHAC, 2008).

The goals set out in the *Canadian Perinatal Health Report* (PHAC, 2008) include reporting on 42 significant indicators of fetal, maternal, and newborn health (Box 24.1). A significant number of these indicators directly affect the health and well-being of vulnerable newborns.

Technological and pharmacologic advances over the past several decades, in conjunction with standardized policies and procedures, have significantly improved survival rates for at-risk newborns. However, morbidity remains an important sequela. For example, some of these newborns are at risk for continuing health problems that require long-term technological support. Other newborns remain at risk for physical and developmental

---

BOX 24.1 Indicators of Fetal, Maternal, and Newborn Health

The *Canadian Perinatal Health Report* provides data on the following "significant indicators" of fetal, maternal, and newborn health (ranked from most to least important):

- Infant mortality rate
- Small-for-gestational-age rate
- Large-for-gestational-age rate
- Preterm birth rate
- Postterm birth rate
- Maternal mortality ratio
- Rate of live births to teenage mothers
- Severe maternal morbidity rate
- Rate of cesarean delivery
- Rate of breastfeeding
- Rate of maternal alcohol consumption during pregnancy
- Multiple birth rate
- Rate of neonatal hospital readmission after discharge
- Birth rate of ectopic pregnancy
- Severe neonatal morbidity rate
- Use of antenatal steroids in <34 weeks of gestation
- Induced abortion ratio
- Rate of labour induction
- Rate of maternal readmission after discharge following childbirth
- Proportion of mothers with low weight gain rate
- Rate of operative vaginal delivery
- Rate of early neonatal discharge from hospital after birth
- Spontaneous abortion rate

- Proportion of births in women with no first trimester prenatal visit
- Rate of mother/infant separation
- Proportion of mothers with a low pre-pregnancy body mass index (BMI)
- Rate of early maternal discharge from hospital after childbirth
- Rate of low maternal education
- Prevalence of exposure to environmental tobacco smoke during pregnancy
- Proportion of pregnant women living without a partner
- Proportion of pregnant women with no social support
- Rate of general anesthesia use in cesarean deliveries
- Rate of regional anesthesia use in deliveries
- Use of surfactant in pregnancies of <34 weeks of gestation
- Resuscitation rate in low birth weight neonates
- Rate of trauma to the perineum
- Proportion of low birth weight neonates with low 5-minute Apgar score
- Proportion of pregnant women reporting physical abuse
- Proportion of pregnant women reporting high psychosocial stress
- Proportion of low birth weight neonates with low cord blood pH
- Proportion of low birth weight neonates with abnormal cord blood base deficit
- Circumcision rate

Source: Public Health Agency of Canada. (2008). *Canadian perinatal health report, 2008 edition.* Retrieved March 14, 2012 from http://www.phac-aspc.gc.ca/publicat/2008/cphr-rspc/pdf/cphr-rspc08-eng.pdf.

problems into the school years and beyond. Providing the complex care needed to maintain the child's health and well-being will have a tremendous emotional and economic impact on the family. Nurses are challenged to provide support to mothers and their families when neonatal well-being is threatened.

Acquired disorders typically occur at or soon after birth. They may result from problems or conditions experienced by the woman during her pregnancy or at birth, such as diabetes, maternal infection, or substance abuse, or conditions associated with labour and birth, such as prolonged rupture of membranes or fetal distress. However, there may be no identifiable cause for the disorder.

Congenital disorders are disorders present at birth, usually due to some type of malformation that occurred during the antepartum period. Congenital disorders, which typically involve a problem with inheritance, include structural anomalies (commonly referred to as birth defects), chromosomal disorders, and inborn errors of metabolism. Most congenital disorders have a complex etiology, involving many interacting genes, gene products, and social and environmental factors during organogenesis. Some alterations can be prevented or compensated for with pharmacologic, nutritional, or other types of interventions, while others cannot be changed. Only through a better understanding of the complex interplay of genetic, environmental, social, and cultural factors can these devastating and life-changing outcomes be prevented (PHAC, 2008).

This chapter addresses selected acquired and congenital newborn conditions. In addition, it describes the nurse's role in assessment and management, emphasizing parental education and support. Nurses play a key role in helping the parents cope with the stress of having an ill newborn.

Acquired Disorders

Neonatal Asphyxia

As the newborn makes the transition to life outside the fluid-filled intrauterine environment, dramatic changes must occur to facilitate newborn respirations. Newborns normally start to breathe on their own as they are placed on their mother's abdomen and stimulated with the process of drying them off. Most newborns make this transition such that by 1 minute of age, they are breathing well on their own. A newborn who fails to establish adequate, sustained respiration after birth is said to have **asphyxia**. Physiologically, asphyxia can be defined as impairment in gas exchange resulting in a decrease in blood oxygen levels (hypoxemia) and an excess of carbon dioxide (hypercapnia) that leads to acidosis.

Asphyxia is the most common clinical insult in the perinatal period. As many as 10% of newborns require some degree of active resuscitation to stimulate breathing and less than 1% require significant intervention (Kattwinkel, Perlman, Aziz, et al., 2010). Each year 4 million infants die during the neonatal period, nearly a quarter of whom succumb to the effects of perinatal asphyxia (Saugstad, 2010). A significant number of the newborns who survive develop long-term problems such as cerebral palsy, mental retardation, and speaking, hearing, visual, and learning disabilities (Cooper, 2011).

Pathophysiology

Asphyxia occurs when oxygen delivery is insufficient to meet metabolic demands, resulting in hypoxia, hypercarbia, and metabolic acidosis. Any condition that reduces oxygen delivery to the fetus can result in asphyxia. These conditions may include maternal hypoxia, such as from cardiac or respiratory disease, anemia, or postural hypotension; maternal vascular disease that leads to placental insufficiency, such as diabetes or hypertension; cord problems such as compression or prolapse; and postterm pregnancies, which may trigger meconium release into the amniotic fluid.

Initially, the newborn uses compensatory mechanisms including tachycardia and vasoconstriction to help bring oxygen to the vital organs for a time. However, without intervention, these mechanisms fail, leading to hypotension, bradycardia, and eventually cardiopulmonary arrest. With failure to breathe effectively after birth, the newborn will develop hypoxia (too little oxygen in the cells of the body). As a result, the heart rate falls, cyanosis develops, and the newborn becomes hypotonic and unresponsive.

Think back to Kelly, described at the beginning of the chapter. She gives birth to a son weighing approximately 2,500 g; he is born postterm and small for gestational age. His skin is stained yellow-green and he is limp, cyanotic, and apneic at birth. The initial assessment once the newborn is under the radiant warmer indicates that resuscitation and tracheal suctioning are needed. What is the nurse's role during resuscitation? What assessments will be needed during this procedure?

Nursing Assessment

The key to successful treatment of newborn asphyxia is early identification and recognition of newborns who may be at risk. Review the perinatal history for risk factors, including:

• Trauma: injury to the central or peripheral nervous system secondary to a long or difficult labour, a precipitous birth, multiple gestation, abnormal presentation, cephalopelvic disproportion, shoulder dystocia, or extraction by forceps or vacuum

- Intrauterine asphyxia: for example, fetal hypoxia secondary to maternal hypoxia, diabetes, hypertension, anemia, cord compression, or meconium aspiration
- Sepsis: acquired bacterial or viral organisms from infected amniotic fluid, maternal infection, or direct contact while passing through the birth canal
- Malformation: congenital anomalies including facial or upper airway deformities, renal anomalies, pulmonary hypoplasia, neuromuscular disorders, esophageal atresia, or neural tube defects
- Hypovolemic shock: secondary to abruptio placentae, placenta previa, or cord rupture resulting in blood loss to the fetus
- Medication: drugs taken during pregnancy or given to mother during labour that can affect the fetus by causing hypotension and placental hypoperfusion; these drugs may include hypnotics, analgesics, anesthetics, narcotics, oxytocin, and street drugs

The Canadian Paediatric Society (CPS) mandates use of Neonatal Resuscitation Program (NRP) principles at every delivery, including having at least one health care provider dedicated to caring for the newborn. This may include one or more of the following: nurse, respiratory technologist, pediatrician, or physician who is trained in neonatal resuscitation (Kattwinkel et al., 2010).

NRP guidelines suggest asking three questions regarding the newborn's status at the time of delivery:

- Is the infant of term gestation?
- Is the infant crying or breathing?
- Is there good muscle tone? (Finan, Aylward, Aziz, et al., 2011)

In addition, at the time of birth all infants are expected to be provided with warmth, positioned to ensure their airway is clear, dried, and stimulated as needed. These initial steps can occur on the mother's abdomen if the newborn is vigorous; that is, crying or breathing and with good muscle tone. Infants who have no respiratory effort and poor or no muscle tone must be taken to the overhead warmer for immediate assessment and intervention. A newborn with marked pallor and flaccid tone has likely experienced significant hypoxia in utero or during the delivery process (Kattwinkel et al., 2010).

Assess the work of breathing. Be alert for apnea, tachypnea, gasping respirations, grunting, nasal flaring, or retractions. Evaluate heart rate and note bradycardia. Assess the newborn's temperature, noting hypothermia or hyperthermia. Determine the Apgar score at 1 and 5 minutes. Although the Apgar score is useful in identifying infants who might have experienced asphyxia, resuscitation measures must not be delayed in order to measure the Apgar score; this could result in unnecessary hypoxia (Kattwinkel et al., 2010).

Anticipate diagnostic testing to identify etiologies for the newborn's asphyxia. For example, a chest X-ray may identify structural abnormalities that might interfere with respiration. A blood culture may identify an infectious process. A blood toxicology screen may detect any maternal drugs in the newborn.

Nursing Management

Management of the newborn experiencing asphyxia includes immediate resuscitation. Ensure that the equipment needed for resuscitation is readily available and in working order and appropriate staff trained in neonatal resuscitation have been called to attend the delivery. Essential equipment includes a radiant warmer or area with radiant heat, a wall suction apparatus, medical air and oxygen sources, an infant T-piece resuscitator (preferred for practitioners with limited experience in resuscitation) or a flow-inflating (anesthetic) ventilation bag with a mask for experienced providers, endotracheal tubes (2.5 to 4.0 mm), a laryngoscope, and ampules of naloxone (Narcan) with syringes and needles for administration (see Chapter 23 for a more detailed discussion of resuscitation).

In the event of a flaccid newborn without spontaneous respirations, take the infant to the radiant warmer as quickly as possible. Dry the newborn with a warm towel to prevent rapid heat loss through evaporation, and remove the wet linen. Handling and rubbing the newborn with a dry towel may be all that is needed to stimulate the onset of breathing. If the newborn fails to respond to stimulation, then active resuscitation is needed. At this point the steps outlined in the NRP (Kattwinkel et al., 2010) program should be followed.

The procedure for newborn resuscitation is easily remembered by the "ABCs"—airway, breathing, and circulation. (see Chapter 23, Box 23.3). Continue resuscitation until the newborn has a pulse above 100 beats/minute, a good cry or good breathing efforts, and good tone. Newborns who have received interventions such as positive pressure ventilation, supplemental oxygen, and cardiac compressions will require close observation by a registered nurse and physician experienced with post-resuscitation care (Kattwinkel et al., 2010). Initial assessment and care can take place at the mother's bedside when there is no nursery facility. Newborns who have been significantly compromised will need to be transported to a facility capable of caring for newborns with more complex needs.

▶ **Take** NOTE!

Resuscitation guidelines taught in the NRP and endorsed by the CPS suggest resuscitation efforts may be stopped if the newborn exhibits no detectable heartbeat after 10 minutes of adequate resuscitation (Kattwinkel et al., 2010).

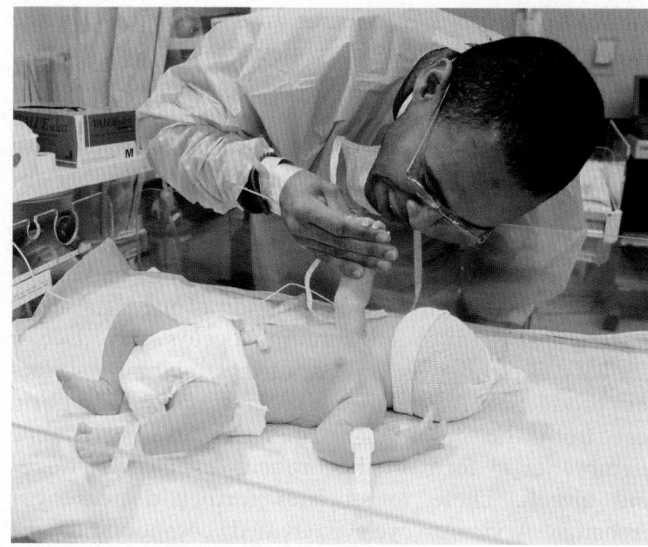

FIGURE 24.1 A father interacting with his newborn once the newborn's condition has stabilized.

Provide continued observation and assessment of the newborn who has been successfully resuscitated. Monitor the newborn's vital signs and oxygen saturation levels closely for changes. Maintain a neutral thermal environment to prevent hypothermia, which would increase the newborn's metabolic and oxygen demands. Check the blood glucose level and observe for signs of hypoglycemia; if this develops, it can further stress the newborn.

The need for resuscitative measures can be extremely upsetting for the parents. Explain to them the initial resuscitation activities being performed and offer ongoing explanations about any procedures being done, equipment being used, or medications given. Provide physical and emotional support to the parents through the initial crisis and throughout the newborn's stay. Give frequent updates on their infant's status. When the newborn is stable, encourage the parents to hold their newborn to promote bonding (Fig. 24.1). Supporting the parents to hold and care for their newborn helps to decrease the parents' anxiety and promote family-focused care.

*R*emember Kelly, the young woman described at the beginning of the chapter? Because her son has poor tone and no respiratory effort, he is intubated and tracheal suctioning is performed in order to clear the airway of meconium. Positive-pressure ventilation is also started using room air initially; oxygen may be introduced gradually as needed (Kattwinkel et al., 2010). Ventilation is continued for 1 minute and then gradually discontinued. The heart rate is now 120 beats/minute, and spontaneous respirations are noted. Oxygen is gradually withdrawn as the newborn begins to cry and turn pink. What continued care is needed in the special care nursery? What explanation should be offered to Kelly regarding her son?

Transient Tachypnea of the Newborn

Transient tachypnea of the newborn (TTN) is a condition involving a mild degree of respiratory distress. It is described as the retention of lung fluid or transient pulmonary edema (Gardner, Enzman-Hines, & Dickey, 2011). It usually occurs within a few hours of birth and resolves by 72 hours of age. TTN occurs in approximately 11 per 1,000 live births (Asenjo, 2011).

Pathophysiology

Most newborns make the transition from fetal to newborn life without incident. During fetal life, the lungs are filled with a serous fluid because the placenta, not the lungs, is used for nutrient and gas exchange. During and after birth, this fluid must be removed and replaced with air. Passage through the birth canal during a vaginal birth compresses the thorax, which helps remove some of this fluid. Pulmonary circulation and the lymphatic drainage remove the remaining fluid shortly after birth. TTN occurs when the liquid in the lung is removed slowly or incompletely.

Nursing Assessment

Astutely observe the newborn with respiratory distress because TTN is a diagnosis of exclusion. Initially it might be difficult to distinguish this condition from respiratory distress syndrome (RDS) or group B streptococcal pneumonia, since the clinical picture is similar. However, the symptoms of transient tachypnea rarely last more than 72 hours (Gardner et al., 2011; Louis, 2008).

History and Physical Examination

Review the perinatal history for contributing factors. TTN is commonly seen in newborns who are sedated or have been born via cesarean birth. Also check the history for evidence of a prolonged labour, fetal macrosomia, and maternal asthma and smoking. These factors are associated with a higher incidence of TTN (Louis, 2008).

Closely assess the newborn for signs of TTN. Within the first few hours of birth, observe for tachypnea, expiratory grunting, retractions, laboured breathing, nasal flaring, and mild cyanosis (Gardner et al., 2011). Mild to moderate respiratory distress is present by 6 hours of age, with respiratory rates as high as 100 to 140 breaths/minute (Louis, 2008). Also inspect the newborn's chest for hyperextension or a barrel shape. Auscultate breath sounds, which may be slightly diminished secondary to reduced air entry.

Laboratory and Diagnostic Testing

To aid in the diagnosis, a chest X-ray may be obtained. It usually reveals mild symmetric lung overaeration and prominent perihilar interstitial markings and streaking. These findings correlate with lymphatic engorgement of retained fetal fluid (Asenjo, 2011).

Nursing Management

Nursing management focuses on providing adequate oxygenation and determining whether the newborn's respiratory manifestations appear to be resolving or persisting. Provide supportive care while the retained lung fluid is reabsorbed. Administer intravenous (IV) fluids and/or gavage feedings until the respiratory rate decreases enough to allow safe oral feeding. Provide supplemental oxygen via a nasal cannula or oxygen hood to maintain adequate oxygen saturation. Maintain a neutral thermal environment with minimal stimulation to minimize oxygen demand.

Provide ongoing assessment of the newborn's respiratory status. As TTN resolves, the newborn's respiratory rate declines to 60 breaths/minute or less, the oxygen requirement decreases, and the chest X-ray shows resolution of the perihilar streaking. Provide reassurance and progress reports to the parents to help them cope with this crisis.

Respiratory Distress Syndrome

Despite improved survival rates and advances in perinatal care, many high-risk newborns are at risk for respiratory problems, particularly **respiratory distress syndrome**, a breathing disorder resulting from lung immaturity and lack of alveolar surfactant. Since the link between RDS and surfactant deficiency was discovered more than 30 years ago, tremendous strides have been made in understanding the pathophysiology and treatment of this disorder. The introduction of prenatal steroids to accelerate lung maturity and the development of synthetic surfactant can be credited with the dramatic improvements in the outcome of newborns with RDS (Bhakti, 2008; PHAC, 2007).

Although 66% of infants born preterm, before 35 weeks' gestation, receive antenatal steroids, there remain a significant number of infants who require intervention for RDS. There were an estimated 380,000 births in Canada in 2009 (Statistics Canada, 2011), and nearly 10% of these newborns were preterm. Furthermore, the rate of preterm births is rising due to increasing maternal age, assisted conception, and an increase in the number of women with complex health issues who are choosing to get pregnant (Whyte, 2010). With this increase in preterm births, more infants are at risk for RDS and other complications associated with prematurity. RDS represents significant morbidity in the preterm population in spite of new treatments and technologies (Consortium on Safe Labour, 2010; PHAC, 2007). Intensive respiratory care, usually with mechanical ventilation, is necessary.

Pathophysiology

Lung immaturity and surfactant deficiency contribute to the development of RDS. Surfactant is a complex mixture of phospholipids and proteins that adheres to the alveolar surface of the lungs. Surfactant forms a coating over the inner surface of the alveoli, reducing the surface tension and preventing alveolar collapse at the end of expiration. In the affected newborn, surfactant is deficient or lacking, and this deficit results in stiff lungs and alveoli that tend to collapse, leading to diffuse atelectasis. The work of breathing is increased because increased pressure similar to that required to initiate the first breath is needed to inflate the lungs with each successive breath. Hypoxemia and acidemia result, leading to vasoconstriction of the pulmonary vasculature. Right-to-left shunting occurs and alveolar capillary circulation is limited, further inhibiting surfactant production. As the disease progresses, fluid and fibrin leak from the pulmonary capillaries, causing hyaline membranes to form in the bronchioles, alveolar ducts, and alveoli. These membranes further decrease gas exchange. A vicious cycle is created, compounding the problem (Gardner et al., 2011).

Nursing Assessment

Nursing assessment focuses on keen observation to identify the signs and symptoms of respiratory distress. In addition, assessment aids in differentiating RDS from other respiratory conditions, such as TTN or group B streptococcal pneumonia.

History and Physical Examination

Review the history for risk factors associated with RDS; these include perinatal asphyxia regardless of gestational age, cesarean birth in the absence of preceding labour (related to the lack of thoracic squeezing), male gender, and maternal diabetes. It is believed that each of these conditions has an impact on surfactant production, thus resulting in RDS in the term infant (Bhakti, 2008).

▶ *Take NOTE!*

Prolonged rupture of membranes, intrauterine growth restriction (IUGR), gestational hypertension, maternal heroin addiction, and use of prenatal corticosteroids may reduce the newborn's risk for RDS because of the physiologic stress imposed on the fetus. Chronic stress experienced by the fetus in utero is believed to accelerate the production of surfactant before the 35th week of gestation and thus reduces the incidence of RDS at birth. However, it is important to be aware that every preterm and newborn exposed to intrauterine stress will not necessarily have benefitted from increased surfactant production.

The newborn with RDS usually demonstrates signs at birth or within a few hours of birth. Observe the infant for expiratory grunting, nasal flaring, chest wall retractions, see-saw respirations, and generalized cyanosis. Auscultate the heart and lungs, noting tachycardia (rates above 150 to 180), fine inspiratory crackles, and tachypnea (rates above 60 breaths/minute). Use the Silverman–Anderson index assessment tool to determine the degree of respiratory distress. The index involves observation of five features, each of which is scored as 0, 1, or 2 (Fig. 24.2). The higher the score, the greater the respiratory distress is. A score over 7 suggests severe respiratory distress.

Laboratory and Diagnostic Testing

The diagnosis of RDS is based on the clinical picture and X-ray findings. A chest X-ray reveals hypoaeration, underexpansion, and a "ground glass" pattern (Bhakti, 2008; Gardner et al., 2011).

Nursing Management

If untreated, RDS will worsen. However, it appears to be a self-limiting disease, with respiratory symptoms declining after 72 hours. This decline parallels the production of surfactant in the alveoli (Gardner et al., 2011). The newborn needs supportive care until surfactant is produced. Effective therapies for established RDS include conventional mechanical ventilation, continuous positive airway pressure (CPAP) or positive end-expiratory pressure (PEEP) to prevent volume loss during expiration, and surfactant therapy. The use of exogenous surfactant replacement therapy to stabilize the newborn's lungs until postnatal surfactant synthesis matures has become a life-saver.

Score

Feature observed	0	1	2
Chest movement	Synchronized respirations	Lag on respirations	Seesaw respirations
Intercostal retraction	None	Just visible	Marked
Xiphoid retraction	None	Just visible	Marked
Nares dilation	None	Minimal	Marked
Expiratory grunt	None	Audible by stethoscope	Audible by unaided ear

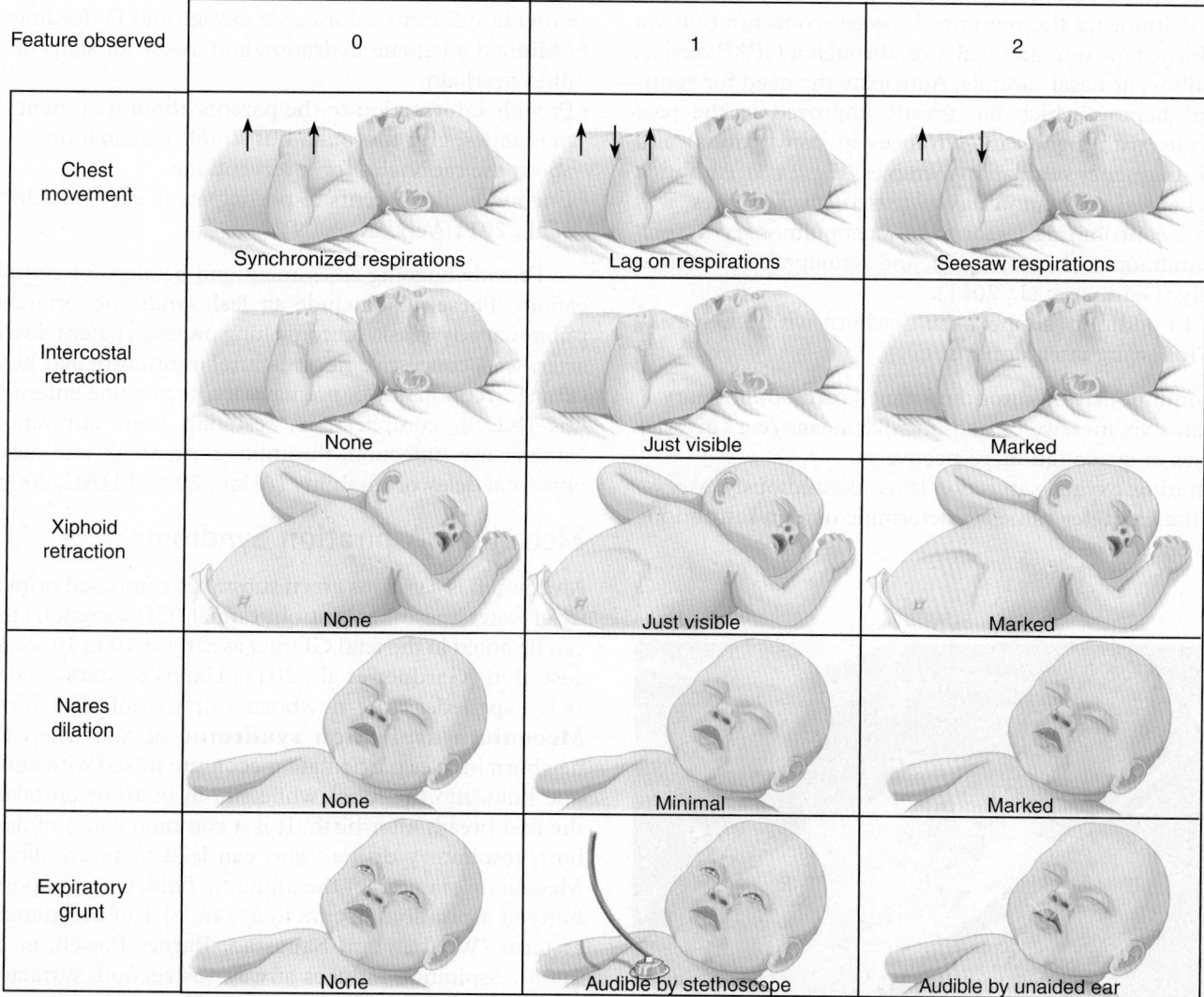

FIGURE 24.2 Assessing the degree of respiratory distress. (Used with permission from: Silverman, W. A., & Anderson, D. H. [1956]. A controlled clinical trial of effects of water mist on obstructive respiratory signs, death rate, and necroscopy findings among premature infants. *Pediatrics, 17*[4], 1–9.)

Care of the newborn with RDS is primarily supportive and requires a multidisciplinary approach to obtain the best outcomes. Therapy focuses on improving oxygenation and maintaining optimal lung volumes. Expect to transfer the newborn to the neonatal intensive care unit (NICU) soon after birth. Apply the basic principles of newborn care, such as thermoregulation, cardiovascular and nutritional support, normal glucose level maintenance, and infection prevention, to achieve the therapeutic goals of reducing mortality and minimizing lung trauma.

Anticipate the administration of surfactant replacement therapy, prophylactically or as a rescue approach. With prophylactic administration, surfactant is given within minutes after birth, thus providing replacement surfactant before severe RDS develops. Rescue treatment is indicated for newborns with established RDS who require mechanical ventilation and supplemental oxygen. The earlier the surfactant is administered, the better the effect on gas exchange (Soll & Ozek, 2010).

Administer the prescribed oxygen concentration via ambient flow into an incubator, through a CPAP device, headbox, or nasal cannula. Anticipate the need for ventilator therapy, which has greatly improved in the past decade, with significant advances in conventional and high-frequency ventilation therapies (Fig. 24.3). Although mechanical ventilation has increased survival rates, it is also a contributing factor to bronchopulmonary dysplasia, pulmonary hypertension, and retinopathy of prematurity (Gardner et al., 2011).

In addition, support the newborn with RDS using the following interventions:

- Continuously monitor the infant's cardiopulmonary status via invasive or non-invasive means (e.g., arterial lines or auscultation, respectively).
- Monitor oxygen saturation levels continuously; assess pulse oximeter values to determine oxygen saturation levels.
- Closely monitor vital signs, acid–base status, and arterial blood gases.
- Administer broad-spectrum antibiotics if blood cultures are positive.
- Administer sodium bicarbonate or acetate as ordered to correct metabolic acidosis.
- Provide fluids and vasopressor agents as needed to prevent or treat hypotension.
- Test blood glucose levels and administer dextrose as ordered for prevention or treatment of hypoglycemia.
- Cluster caretaking activities to avoid overtaxing and compromising the newborn.
- Place the newborn in the prone position (only when on continuous cardiorespiratory monitoring) to optimize respiratory status and reduce stress.
- Perform gentle suctioning to remove secretions and maintain a patent airway.
- Assess level of consciousness to identify intraventricular hemorrhage.
- Provide sufficient calories via gavage and IV feedings.
- Maintain adequate hydration and assess for signs of fluid overload.
- Provide information to the parents about treatment modalities; give thorough but simple explanations about the rationales for interventions.
- Encourage the parents to participate in care (Gardner et al., 2011; Verklan, 2009).

Provide ongoing assessment and be alert for complications. These may include air leak syndrome, bronchopulmonary dysplasia (chronic lung disease), patent ductus arteriosus, congestive heart failure, intraventricular hemorrhage, retinopathy of prematurity, necrotizing enterocolitis (NEC), complications resulting from intravenous catheter use (infection, thrombus formation), and developmental delay or disability (Askin, 2009; PHAC, 2008).

Meconium Aspiration Syndrome

Meconium is a viscous green substance composed primarily of water and other gastrointestinal (GI) secretions that can be noted in the fetal GI tract as early as 10 to 16 weeks' gestation (Gardner et al., 2011; Harris & Stark, 2008). It is expelled as the newborn's first stool after birth. **Meconium aspiration syndrome** occurs when the newborn inhales particulate meconium mixed with amniotic fluid into the lungs while still in utero or on taking the first breath after birth. It is a common cause of newborn respiratory distress and can lead to severe illness. Meconium staining of the amniotic fluid, with the possibility of aspiration, occurs in 8% to 20% of pregnancies at term (Wiedemann, Saugstad, Barnes-Powell, et al., 2008). Aspiration induces airway obstruction, surfactant dysfunction, hypoxia, and chemical pneumonitis with inflammation of pulmonary tissues. In severe cases, it progresses to persistent pulmonary hypertension and death (Wiedemann et al., 2008). About 5% of infants

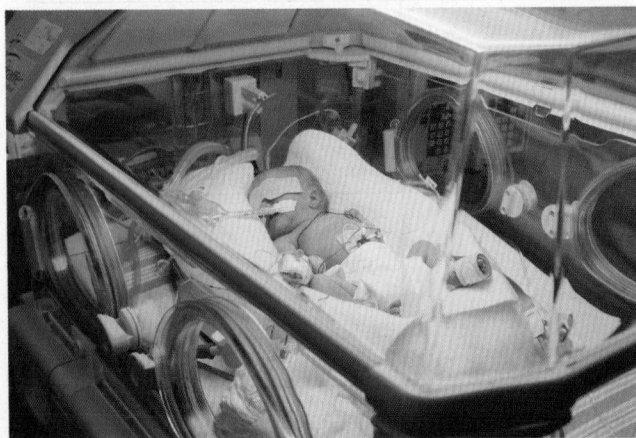

FIGURE 24.3 A newborn with RDS receiving mechanical ventilation.

who aspirate meconium-stained fluid develop meconium aspiration syndrome (Harris & Stark, 2008).

Pathophysiology

Meconium may be passed in utero secondary to hypoxic stress. Hypoxia induces the fetus to gasp or attempt to breathe. The fetus may bear down and pass meconium into the amniotic fluid or he or she may experience a vagal reflex that causes relaxation of the anal sphincter, allowing meconium to be passed into the amniotic fluid. The fetus then sucks or swallows this amniotic fluid in utero, or the infant may aspirate meconium with the first breath after birth as air rushes into the lungs.

Although the etiology is not well understood, the effects of meconium can be harmful to the fetus. Meconium alters the amniotic fluid by reducing antibacterial activity and subsequently increasing the risk for perinatal bacterial infection. Additionally, meconium is very irritating because it contains enzymes from the fetal pancreas.

When aspirated into the lungs, meconium blocks the bronchioles, causing an inflammatory reaction as well as a decrease in surfactant production. Gas exchange is impaired and atelectasis occurs. A ball–valve effect occurs when air is inspired into the alveoli but cannot be fully expired secondary to reduced airway diameter. Significant respiratory distress is followed by persistent pulmonary hypertension, right-to-left shunting of blood, and patent ductus arteriosus. Conventional mechanical ventilation, extracorporeal membrane oxygenation (ECMO), nitric oxide, high-frequency ventilation, or liquid ventilation may be necessary.

Nursing Assessment

Review prenatal and birth records to identify newborns who may be at high risk for meconium aspiration. Predisposing factors for meconium aspiration syndrome include postterm pregnancy; breech, forceps, or vacuum extraction births; prolonged or difficult labour associated with fetal distress in a term or postterm newborn; maternal hypertension or diabetes; oligohydramnios; IUGR; prolapsed cord; or acute or chronic placental insufficiency (Gardner et al., 2011).

Assess the amniotic fluid for meconium staining when the maternal membranes rupture. Green-stained amniotic fluid suggests the presence of meconium in the amniotic fluid and should be reported immediately. After birth, note any yellowish-green staining of the umbilical cord and nails and skin. This staining indicates that meconium has been present for some time.

*C*onsider Kelly, the 27-year-old woman who gave birth to a son who required resuscitation. What findings would lead the nurse to suspect that her son aspirated meconium? What risk factors in Kelly's history would support the diagnosis of meconium aspiration syndrome?

▶ *Take* NOTE!

Recent evidence suggests that newborns with meconium staining do not routinely require intrapartum suctioning (before the birth of the shoulders) or following delivery. Tracheal suctioning is only warranted if the newborn is flaccid and has no respiratory effort, and a heart rate less than 60 beats/minutes (Kattwinkel et al., 2010).

Observe the newborn for a barrel-shaped chest with an increased anterior–posterior chest diameter (similar to that found in a patient with chronic obstructive pulmonary disease), prolonged tachypnea, progression from mild to severe respiratory distress, intercostal retractions, end-expiratory grunting, and cyanosis (Gardner et al., 2011). Auscultate the lungs, noting coarse crackles and rhonchi.

Chest X-rays show patchy, fluffy infiltrates unevenly distributed throughout the lungs and marked hyperaeration mixed with areas of atelectasis. Arterial blood gas analysis will indicate metabolic acidosis with a low blood pH, decreased arterial oxygen pressure (PaO_2), and increased partial pressure of arterial carbon dioxide ($PaCO_2$) (Acute Care of at-Risk Newborns (ACoRN) Neonatal Society, 2009). Direct visualization of the vocal cords for meconium staining using a laryngoscope can confirm the presence of meconium below the larynx.

Nursing Management

Nursing management focuses on ensuring adequate tissue perfusion and minimizing oxygen demand and energy expenditure. Caring for the newborn with meconium aspiration begins in the birthing unit when the birth attendant identifies meconium-stained amniotic fluid with membrane rupture during labour. Note that NRP guidelines no longer recommend suctioning the nose or pharynx upon delivery of the head, prior to the first breath. If the newborn has poor tone and has significant respiratory depression at birth, direct tracheal suctioning with a meconium aspirator may be necessary prior to beginning resuscitative efforts (Kattwinkel et al., 2010). Repeated suctioning and stimulation are limited to infants with significant respiratory depression (Gardner et al., 2011; Harris & Stark, 2008). Following resuscitation the newborn is usually transferred to the NICU for close monitoring.

Maintain a neutral thermal environment, including placing the newborn under a radiant warmer or in a warmed isolette, to prevent hypothermia. In addition, minimize handling to reduce energy expenditure and oxygen consumption that could lead to further hypoxemia and acidosis.

Administer oxygen therapy as ordered via positive-pressure ventilation, CPAP device, or ambient oxygen delivered into an incubator. Monitor oxygen saturation levels via pulse oximetry to evaluate the newborn's response to treatment and to detect changes. Increased pulmonary pressures associated with meconium aspiration may cause blood to be shunted away from the lungs. The newborn may exhibit uneven pulmonary ventilation, with hyperinflation in some areas and atelectasis in others. This leads to poor perfusion and subsequent hypoxemia, which in turn may increase pulmonary vasoconstriction, resulting in a worsening of hypoxemia and acidosis.

Hyperoxygenation is seldom recommended to dilate the pulmonary vasculature and close the ductus arteriosus; rather, oxygen is delivered to maintain saturations within strictly prescribed levels. Nitric oxide inhalation may be used to decrease pulmonary vascular resistance, or high-frequency oscillatory ventilation may be used to increase the chance of air trapping (Wiedemann et al., 2008). In addition, administer vasopressors and pulmonary vasodilators as prescribed and administer surfactant as ordered to counteract inactivation by meconium. Monitor arterial blood gas results for changes and assist with measures to correct acid–base imbalances to facilitate perfusion of tissues and prevent pulmonary hypertension (Harris & Stark, 2008). If these measures are ineffective, be prepared to assist with the use of ECMO, a modified type of heart–lung machine.

In addition, perform the following interventions:

- Cluster newborn care to minimize oxygen demand.
- Administer broad-spectrum antibiotics to treat bacterial pneumonia.
- Administer sedation to reduce oxygen consumption and energy expenditure.
- Continuously monitor the newborn's condition.
- Reassure and support the parents throughout the experience (Cleveland, 2009; Siegel, Gardner, & Dickey, 2011).

Persistent Pulmonary Hypertension of the Newborn

Persistent pulmonary hypertension of the newborn, previously referred to as persistent fetal circulation, is a cardiopulmonary disorder characterized by marked pulmonary hypertension that causes right-to-left extrapulmonary shunting of blood and hypoxemia. Persistent pulmonary hypertension can occur idiopathically or as a complication of perinatal asphyxia, meconium aspiration syndrome, pneumonia, congenital heart defects, metabolic disorders such as hypoglycemia, hypothermia, hypovolemia, hyperviscosity, acute hypoxia with delayed resuscitation, sepsis, and RDS. Persistent pulmonary hypertension occurs in 2 to 6 per 1,000 live infants born at term, near term, or postterm (Spillers, 2010).

Pathophysiology

Normally, pulmonary artery pressure decreases when the newborn takes the first breath. However, interference with this ability to breathe allows pulmonary pressures to remain increased. Hypoxemia and acidosis also occur, leading to vasoconstriction of the pulmonary artery. These events cause an elevation in pulmonary vascular resistance. Normally, the decrease in pulmonary artery pressure and pulmonary vascular resistance with breathing leads to the closure of the ductus arteriosus and foramen ovale. However, with persistent pulmonary hypertension, pulmonary vascular resistance is elevated to the point that venous blood is diverted to some degree through fetal structures, such as the ductus arteriosus or foramen ovale, causing them to remain open, leading to a right-to-left shunting of blood into the systemic circulation. This diversion of blood bypasses the lungs, resulting in systemic arterial hypoxemia.

Nursing Assessment

Assess the newborn's status closely. A newborn with persistent pulmonary hypertension demonstrates tachypnea within 12 hours after birth. Observe for marked cyanosis, grunting, and retractions. Auscultate the heart, noting a systolic ejection murmur, and measure blood pressure for hypotension resulting from both heart failure and persistent hypoxemia (Gardner et al., 2011). Measure oxygen saturation via pulse oximetry, and report low values. Prepare the newborn for an echocardiogram, which will reveal right-to-left shunting of blood that confirms the diagnosis.

Nursing Management

When caring for the newborn with persistent pulmonary hypertension, pay meticulous attention to detail, with continuous monitoring of the newborn's oxygenation and perfusion status and blood pressure. The goals of therapy include improving alveolar oxygenation, inducing metabolic alkalosis by administering sodium bicarbonate, correcting hypovolemia and hypotension with the administration of volume replacement and vasopressors, and anticipating use of ECMO when support has failed to maintain acceptable oxygenation (Spillers, 2010).

Provide immediate resuscitation after birth and administer oxygen therapy as ordered. Early and effective resuscitation and correction of acidosis and hypoxia are helpful in preventing persistent pulmonary hypertension. Monitor arterial blood gases frequently to evaluate the effectiveness of oxygen therapy. Provide respiratory support, which frequently necessitates the use of mechanical ventilation. Administer prescribed medications, monitor cardiopulmonary status, cluster care to reduce stimulation, and provide support and education to the parents.

▶ *Take* NOTE!

Almost any procedure, such as suctioning, weighing, changing diapers, or positioning, can precipitate severe hypoxemia due to the instability of the pulmonary vasculature. Therefore, minimize the newborn's exposure to stimulation as much as possible.

Periventricular–Intraventricular Hemorrhage

Periventricular–intraventricular hemorrhage is defined as bleeding that usually originates in the subependymal germinal matrix region of the brain, with extension into the ventricular system (Martin, 2011). It is a common problem in preterm infants, especially in those born before 32 weeks' gestation. A significant number of these newborns will incur brain injury, leading to complications that may include hydrocephalus, seizure disorders, periventricular leukomalacia (an ischemic injury resulting from inadequate perfusion of the white matter adjacent to the ventricles), cerebral palsy, learning disabilities, vision or hearing deficits, and mental retardation. Identifying preventive strategies to reduce the incidence of these brain insults is a national public health priority (PHAC, 2008).

The incidence of ventricular hemorrhage depends on the gestational age at birth. Up to 50% of newborns weighing 1,500 g or less or born at 30 weeks' gestation or less will have evidence of hemorrhage. Only about 4% of term newborns show evidence of ventricular hemorrhage. Very low birth weight infants have the earliest onset of hemorrhage and the highest mortality rate (Verklan & Lopez, 2011).

Pathophysiology

The preterm newborn is at greatest risk for periventricular–intraventricular hemorrhage because cerebral vascular development is immature, making the brain tissue more vulnerable to injury. The shorter the gestation period, the greater the risk of brain damage in the infant (Vassilyadi, Tataryn, Shamji, et al., 2009). While all areas of the brain can be injured, the periventricular area is the most vulnerable.

Each ventricular area contains a rich network of capillaries that are very thin and fragile and can rupture easily. The causes of rupture vary and include fluctuations in systemic and cerebral blood flow, increases in cerebral blood flow from hypertension, IV infusions, seizure activity, increases in cerebral venous pressure due to vaginal delivery, hypoxia, and respiratory distress. With a preterm birth, the fetus is suddenly transported from a well-controlled uterine environment into a highly stimulating one. This tremendous physiologic stress and shock may contribute to the rupture of periventricular capillaries and subsequent hemorrhage. Most hemorrhages occur in the first 72 hours after birth (Verklan & Lopez, 2011).

Periventricular–intraventricular hemorrhage is classified on a grading system of I (least severe) to V (most severe) (Vassilyadi et al., 2009). The prognosis is guarded, depending on the grade and severity of the hemorrhage. Generally, newborns with mild hemorrhage (grades I and II) have a much better developmental outcome than those with severe hemorrhage (grades III to V). However, some newborns diagnosed with severe bleeds early in the neonatal period present with grade I or grade II during subsequent investigations and show no evidence of neurologic compromise in the long term (Gardner et al., 2011).

Nursing Assessment

The signs of periventricular–intraventricular hemorrhage vary significantly; no clinical signs may be evident. Closely monitor newborns who are at an increased risk, such as those who are preterm or of low birth weight. Also assess for risk factors such as acidosis, asphyxia, unstable blood pressure, meningitis, seizures, acute blood loss, hypovolemia, respiratory distress with mechanical ventilation, intubation, apnea, hypoxia, suctioning, use of hyperosmolar solutions, rapid volume expansion, and activities that involve handling (Martin, 2011).

Evaluate the newborn for an unexplained drop in hematocrit, pallor, and poor perfusion as evidenced by respiratory distress and oxygen desaturation. Note seizures, lethargy or other changes in level of consciousness, weak suck, high-pitched cry, or hypotonia. Palpate the anterior fontanel for tenseness. Assess vital signs, noting bradycardia and hypotension. Evaluate laboratory data for changes indicating metabolic acidosis or glucose instability. Frequently a bleed can progress rapidly and result in shock and death. Prepare the newborn for cranial ultrasonography, the diagnostic tool of choice to detect hemorrhage.

Nursing Management

Prevention of preterm birth is essential in preventing periventricular–intraventricular hemorrhage. Promote community awareness of factors that may contribute to periventricular–intraventricular hemorrhage, such as a lack of prenatal care, maternal infection, alcohol consumption, and smoking (Martin, 2011). Identify risk factors that can lead to hemorrhage, and focus care on interventions to decrease the risk for hemorrhage. For example, institute measures to prevent perinatal asphyxia and birth trauma and provide developmental care in the NICU. If a preterm birth is expected, having the mother deliver at a tertiary care facility with a NICU would be most appropriate.

Care of the newborn with periventricular–intraventricular hemorrhage is primarily supportive. Correct anemia, acidosis, and hypotension with fluids and medications. Administer fluids slowly to prevent fluctuations in blood pressure. Avoid rapid volume expansion to minimize changes in cerebral blood flow. Keep the newborn in a flexed, contained position with the head elevated to prevent or minimize fluctuations in intracranial pressure. Continuously monitor the newborn for signs of hemorrhage, such as changes in the level of consciousness, bulging fontanel, seizures, apnea, and reduced activity level. Also, measure head circumference daily.

Minimize handling of the newborn by clustering nursing care, and limit stimulation in the newborn's environment to reduce stress. Also reduce the newborn's exposure to noxious stimuli to avoid a fluctuation in blood pressure and energy expenditure. Provide adequate oxygenation to promote tissue perfusion but controlled ventilation to decrease the risk for pneumothorax.

The long-term neurodevelopmental outcome is unpredictable. Researchers have observed that while more very low birth weight infants are surviving, there are fewer complications related to intraventricular hemorrhage due to improved diagnosis and treatment during the infant's hospitalization (Vassilyadi et al., 2009). Support for the parents to cope with the diagnosis and potential long-term sequelae is essential. Provide education and emotional support for the parents throughout the newborn's stay. Discuss expectations for short-term and long-term care needs with the parents and assist them in obtaining the necessary support from appropriate community resources.

Necrotizing Enterocolitis

NEC is a serious GI disease occurring in newborns. It is the most common and most serious acquired GI disorder among hospitalized preterm neonates and is associated with significant acute and chronic morbidity and mortality (Bradshaw, 2009; Gregory, 2008). NEC occurs in 1 to 3 of every 1,000 live births, affecting 1% to 5% of all newborns in NICUs (Gregory, 2008). Attempts to improve GI function and reduce the risk for NEC include enteral antibiotics, judicious administration of parenteral fluids, human milk feedings, antenatal corticosteroids, enteral probiotics (*Lactobacillus acidophilus*), and slow continuous drip feedings (Bradshaw, 2009).

Pathophysiology

The pathophysiology of NEC is not clearly understood and is thought to be multifactorial in nature. Current research points to three major pathologic mechanisms that lead to NEC: bowel ischemia, bacterial flora, and the effect of feeding (Bradshaw, 2009).

During perinatal or postnatal stress, oxygen is shunted away from the gut to more important organs such as the heart and the brain. Ischemia and intestinal wall damage occur, allowing bacteria to invade. High-solute feedings allow bacteria to flourish. Mucosal or transmucosal necrosis of part of the intestine occurs (Gregory, 2008). Although any region of the bowel can be affected, the distal ileum and proximal colon are the regions most commonly involved. NEC usually occurs between 3 and 12 days of life, but it can occur weeks later in some newborns.

Nursing Assessment

NEC can be devastating, and astute assessment is crucial. Assessing the newborn for the development of NEC includes the health history and physical examination as well as laboratory and diagnostic testing.

Health History and Physical Examination

Assess the newborn's history for risk factors associated with NEC. In addition to preterm birth, prenatal and postnatal predisposing risk factors are highlighted in Box 24.2.

Also observe the newborn for common signs and symptoms, which may include:

- Abdominal distention and tenderness
- Bloody stools
- Feeding intolerance, characterized by bilious vomiting
- Signs of sepsis
- Lethargy
- Apnea
- Shock

BOX 24.2 Predisposing Factors for the Development of Necrotizing Enterocolitis

Prenatal Factors
- Preterm labour
- Prolonged rupture of membranes
- Pre-eclampsia
- Maternal sepsis
- Amnionitis
- Uterine hypoxia

Postnatal Factors
- Respiratory distress syndrome
- Patent ductus arteriosus
- Congenital heart disease
- Exchange transfusion
- Low birth weight
- Low Apgar scores
- Umbilical catheterization
- Hypothermia
- Gastrointestinal infection
- Hypoglycemia
- Asphyxia

Always keep the possibility of NEC in mind when dealing with preterm newborns, especially when enteral feedings are being administered. Note respiratory distress, cyanosis, lethargy, decreased activity level, temperature instability, feeding intolerance, diarrhea, bile-stained emesis, or grossly bloody stools. Assess blood pressure, noting hypotension. Evaluate the neonate's abdomen for distention, tenderness, and visible loops of bowel (Bradshaw, 2009). Measure the abdominal circumference, noting an increase. Determine residual gastric volume prior to feeding; when it is elevated, be suspicious for NEC.

Laboratory and Diagnostic Testing

Common laboratory and diagnostic tests ordered for assessment of NEC include:

- Kidney, ureter, and bladder (KUB) abdominal X-ray: confirms the presence of pneumatosis intestinalis (air in the bowel wall) and persistently dilated loops of bowel (Bradshaw, 2009; Gregory, 2008)
- Blood values: may demonstrate metabolic acidosis, increased white blood cells, thrombocytopenia, neutropenia, electrolyte imbalance, or disseminated intravascular coagulation (DIC)

Nursing Management

Nursing management of the newborn with NEC focuses on maintaining fluid and nutritional status, providing supportive care, and teaching the family about the condition and prognosis. Therapeutic management initially consists of bowel rest and antibiotic therapy. Serial KUB X-rays are used to assess the resolution or progression of NEC. If medical treatment fails to stabilize the newborn or if free air is present on a left lateral decubitus film, surgical intervention will be necessary to resect the portion of necrotic bowel. Surgery for NEC usually requires the placement of a proximal enterostomy until the anastomosis site is ready for reconnection.

Maintaining Fluid and Nutritional Status

If NEC is suspected, immediately stop enteral feedings until a diagnosis is made. Administer IV fluids initially to restore proper fluid balance. If ordered, administer total parenteral nutrition (TPN) to keep the newborn supported nutritionally. Give prescribed IV antibiotics to prevent sepsis from the necrotic bowel (if surgery is required, antibiotics may be needed for an extended period of time). Institute gastric decompression as ordered with an orogastric tube attached to low intermittent suction. Carefully monitor intake and output. Restart enteral feedings once the disease has resolved (normal abdominal examination and KUB negative for pneumatosis) or as determined postoperatively by the surgeon.

Providing Supportive Care

Manage pain by administering analgesics as ordered. Infection control is important, with an emphasis on careful handwashing. In addition, implement these interventions in an ongoing manner:

- Check stools for evidence of blood and report any positive findings.
- Measure the abdominal girth.
- Palpate the abdomen for tenderness and rigidity.
- Auscultate for normal bowel sounds.
- Observe the abdomen for redness or shininess, which indicates peritonitis.

Teaching the Family

The diagnosis of NEC may cause significant anxiety. Listen to the family's worries and fears. Answer their questions honestly. Inform the family that medically treated NEC is usually limited to a short period and resolves within 48 hours of stopping oral feedings. Explain that surgical treatment of NEC, however, can be a much lengthier process. When a large amount of bowel has become necrosed, as determined during the bowel resection, the likelihood of long-term medical problems increases significantly. Short bowel syndrome may result from a large resection (short bowel syndrome is discussed in Chapter 41). Reassure the family that although some infants have more involved cases of NEC, the improved parenteral nutrition formulations have improved the outcomes for these infants. Provide education about ostomy care if surgery is required (refer to page xxx for a discussion of ostomy care). Promote interaction with their newborn.

Infants of Diabetic Mothers

An **infant of a diabetic mother** is one born to a woman with pregestational or gestational diabetes (see Chapter 20 for additional information). The newborn of a diabetic woman is at high risk for numerous health-related complications, especially hypoglycemia. In light of the increasing incidence of type 2 diabetes among women of childbearing age as a result of obesity, it is important to educate women about the potential impact of poor glycemic control on their offspring.

Impact of Diabetes on the Newborn

For more than a century, it has been known that diabetes during pregnancy can have severe adverse effects on fetal and newborn outcomes. Infants of diabetic mothers have increased morbidity and mortality in the perinatal period. The incidence of major congenital anomalies is much greater for these newborns than for other newborns. Poor glycemic control in the first trimester, during organogenesis, is thought to be a major reason for congenital malformations. The most common types of malformations in infants of diabetic mothers involve the cardiovascular, skeletal, central nervous, GI, and genitourinary systems. Cardiac anomalies are the most common (Gardner et al., 2011).

Infants of diabetic mothers are longer and weigh more than newborns of similar gestational age born to non-diabetic mothers. They also have increased organ weights (organomegaly) and excessive fat deposits on the shoulders and trunk, contributing to the increased overall body weight and predisposing them to shoulder dystocia. These newborns are macrosomic (an infant whose birth weight exceeds 4,500 g). These oversized newborns frequently require cesarean delivery for cephalopelvic disproportion and are often hypoglycemic in the first few hours after birth.

Despite their increased size and weight, they may be remarkably frail, showing behaviours similar to those of a preterm newborn. Thus, birth weight may not be a reliable criterion of maturity. Newborns of women with diabetes but without vascular complications often tend to be large for gestational age (LGA), whereas those of women with diabetes and vascular disease are usually small for gestational age (SGA) (Hatfield, Shwoebel, & Lynyak, 2011).

Pathophysiology

The large size of the infant born to a diabetic mother is due to secondary to exposure to high levels of maternal glucose crossing the placenta into the fetal circulation. Maternal hyperglycemia acts as a fuel to stimulate increased production of fetal insulin, which in turn promotes somatic growth within the fetus. The fetus responds to these high levels by producing more insulin, which acts as a growth factor in the fetus. How the fetus will be affected and the problems that the newborn experiences depend on the severity, duration, and control of the diabetes in the mother. Table 24.1 summarizes the common problems that may occur in infants of diabetic mothers.

Nursing Assessment

Assessment begins in the prenatal period by identifying women with diabetes and taking measures to control maternal glucose levels (see Chapter 20 for information on management of the pregnant woman with diabetes).

Physical Examination

At birth, inspect the newborn for these characteristic features:

- Full rosy cheeks with a ruddy skin colour
- Short neck (some describe "no-neck" appearance)
- Buffalo hump over the nape of the neck
- Massive shoulders with a full intrascapular area
- Distended upper abdomen due to organ overgrowth
- Excessive subcutaneous fat tissue, producing fat extremities (Fig. 24.4)

Be alert for hypoglycemia, which may occur immediately after birth or within an hour. Assess blood glucose levels, which should remain above 2.6 mmol/L (Rozance & Hay, 2010). Closely assess the newborn for signs of

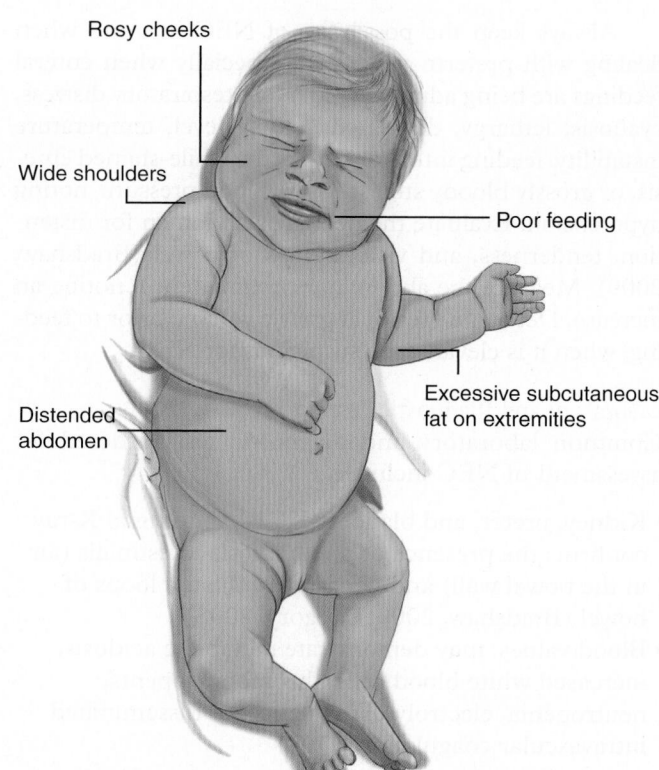

Rosy cheeks

Wide shoulders

Poor feeding

Distended abdomen

Excessive subcutaneous fat on extremities

FIGURE 24.4 Characteristics of an infant of a diabetic mother.

hypoglycemia, including listlessness, hypotonia, apathy, poor feeding, apneic episodes with a drop in oxygen saturation, cyanosis, temperature instability, pallor and sweating, tremors, irritability, and seizures.

Assess the newborn for signs of birth trauma involving the head (tense, bulging fontanels, cephalhematoma, skull fractures, and facial nerve paralysis), shoulders and extremities (posturing, paralysis), and skin (bruising). Inspect the newborn for compromised oxygenation by examining the skin for cyanosis, pallor, mottling, and sluggish capillary refill. Take the newborn's temperature frequently and provide a neutral thermal environment to prevent cold stress, which would increase the glucose utilization and contribute to the hypoglycemic state.

Laboratory and Diagnostic Testing

Determine baseline serum calcium, magnesium, and bilirubin levels and monitor them frequently for changes (Table 24.2). Hypocalcemia is typically manifested in the first 2 to 3 days of life as a result of birth injury or a prolonged delay in parathyroid hormone production. Hypomagnesemia parallels calcium levels and is suspected only when hypocalcemia does not respond to calcium replacement therapy. Red blood cell breakdown leads to increased hematocrit and polycythemia. In addition, hyperbilirubinemia may be caused by slightly decreased extracellular fluid volume, hepatic immaturity, and birth trauma forming enclosed hemorrhages. It can appear

TABLE 24.1   COMMON PROBLEMS OF INFANTS OF DIABETIC MOTHERS

Condition	Description	Effects
Macrosomia	Newborn with an excessive birth weight; arbitrarily defined as a birth weight >4,000 g (8 lb 13 oz) or >90% for gestational age Complication in 10% of all pregnancies in Canada	Increased risk for shoulder dystocia, traumatic birth injury, birth asphyxia Risks for newborn hypoglycemia and hypomagnesemia, polycythemia, and electrolyte disturbances Increased maternal risk for surgical birth, post-partum hemorrhage and infection, and birth canal lacerations Increased risk for developing type 2 diabetes later in life for both Higher weight and accumulation of fat in childhood and a higher rate of obesity in adults
Respiratory distress syndrome (RDS)	Cortisol-induced stimulation of lecithin/sphingomyelin (phospholipids) necessary for lung maturation is antagonized due to the high insulin environment within the fetus due to mother's hyperglycemia. Less mature lung development than expected for gestational age Decrease in the phospholipid phosphatidylglycerol (PG), which stabilizes surfactant, compounding risk	Most commonly, breathing normally at birth but developing laboured, grunting respiration with cough and a hoarse complaining cry within a few hours with chest retractions and varying degrees of cyanosis Infants of diabetic mothers with vascular disease seldom develop RDS because the chronic stress of poor intrauterine perfusion leads to increased production of steroids, which accelerates lung maturation.
Hypoglycemia	Glucose is the major source of energy for organ function. Typical characteristics: • Poor feedings • Jitteriness • Lethargy • High-pitched or weak cry • Apnea • Cyanosis and seizures Some newborns asymptomatic.	Low blood glucose levels are problematic during early post-birth period due to abrupt cessation of high-glucose maternal blood supply and the continuation of insulin production by the newborn. Limited ability to release glucagon and catecholamines, which normally stimulate glucagon breakdown and glucose release Prolonged and untreated hypoglycemia leads to serious, long-term adverse neurologic sequelae such as learning disabilities and mental retardation.
Hypocalcemia and hypomagnesemia	Hypocalcemia (drop in calcium levels) manifested by tremors, hypotonia, apnea, high-pitched cry, and seizures due to abrupt cessation of maternal transfer of calcium to fetus primarily in third trimester and experiencing birth asphyxia Associated hypomagnesemia directly related to the maternal level before birth About half of infants of diabetic mothers affected	Newborn is at risk for a prolonged delay in parathyroid hormone production and cardiac dysrhythmias.
Polycythemia	Venous hematocrit of >65% in the newborn Increased oxygen consumption by infants of diabetic mothers secondary to fetal hyperglycemia and hyperinsulinemia Increased fetal erythropoiesis secondary to intrauterine hypoxia due to placental insufficiency from maternal diabetes Hypoxic stimulation of increased red blood cell (RBC) production as compensatory mechanism	Increased viscosity, resulting in poor blood flow predisposing newborn to decreased tissue oxygenation and development of microthrombi

(continued)

TABLE 24.1 COMMON PROBLEMS OF INFANTS OF DIABETIC MOTHERS (continued)

Condition	Description	Effects
Hyperbilirubinemia	Usually seen within the first few days after birth, manifested by a yellow appearance of the sclera and skin Excessive red cell hemolysis necessary to break down increased RBCs in circulation due to polycythemia Resultant elevated bilirubin levels Excessive bruising secondary to birth trauma of macrosomic infants, further adding to high bilirubin levels	If untreated, high levels of unconjugated bilirubin may lead to kernicterus (neurologic syndrome that results in irreversible damage) with long-term sequelae that include cerebral palsy, sensorineural hearing loss, and mental retardation.
Congenital anomalies	Occur in up to 10% of infants of diabetic mothers, accounting for 30% to 50% of perinatal deaths. Incidence is greatest among SGA newborns. Overall, approximately three times the usual incidence of congenital anomalies compared with newborns from the non-diabetic general population.	Most common anomalies: • Coarctation of the aorta • Atrial and ventricular septal defects • Transposition of the great vessels • Sacral agenesis • Hip and joint malformations • Anencephaly • Spina bifida • Caudal dysplasia • Hydrocephalus

Sources: Gardner, S. L., Enzman-Hines, M., & Dickey, L. (2011). Respiratory diseases. In S. Gardner, B. Carter, M. Enzman-Hines, & J. Hernandez (Eds.), *Merenstein & Gardner's handbook of neonatal intensive care.* St. Louis, MO: Mosby Elsevier; and Hatfield, L. Shwoebel, A., & Lynyak, C. (2011). Caring for the infant of the diabetic mother. *Maternal/Child Nursing, 36*(1), 10–16.

within the first 24 hours of life (pathologic) or after 24 hours of life (physiologic).

Nursing Management

The focus of care for these infants is early detection and initiation of therapy to address potential problems (Nursing Care Plan 24.1). Perform a head-to-toe physical assessment to identify congenital anomalies. Institute measures to correct hypoglycemia, hypocalcemia, hypomagnesemia, dehydration, and jaundice. Provide oxygenation and ventilatory support as necessary.

Preventing Hypoglycemia

Prevent hypoglycemia by promoting breastfeeding within 30 minutes of delivery. Breast milk facilitates glycemic stability better than formula. However, formula may need to be given when the mother is unable to breastfeed or chooses to formula feed (Chertok, Raz, Shoham, et al., 2009). Feedings must be at frequent intervals (every 2 to 3 hours) to help to control glucose levels, reduce hematocrit, and promote bilirubin excretion. Maintain a neutral thermal environment to avoid cold stress, which may stimulate the metabolic rate, thereby increasing the demand for glucose. Provide rest periods to decrease energy demand and expenditure.

Monitor blood glucose levels via heel stick at 1 hour of age then every 3 hours as long as the infant remains well and the glucose level is 2.6 mmol/L or higher (Rozance & Hay, 2010). Consider discontinuing monitoring once three readings of 2.6 mmol/L or higher have been achieved and the infant is asymptomatic (Rozance & Hay, 2010). Document the results. Report unstable glucose values if oral feedings do not maintain and stabilize the newborn's blood glucose levels. If glucose levels are not stabilized, initiate IV glucose infusions as ordered and monitor to ensure that the infusions are flowing at the prescribed rate.

Maintaining Fluid and Electrolyte Balance

Monitor serum calcium levels for changes indicating the need for supplementation, such as with oral or IV calcium gluconate. Assess the newborn for signs of hypocalcemia, such as tremors, jitteriness, twitching, seizures, and high-pitched cry.

TABLE 24.2 CRITICAL LABORATORY VALUES FOR INFANTS OF DIABETIC MOTHERS

Hypoglycemia	<2.6 mmol/L
Hypocalcemia	<7 mg/dL
Hypomagnesemia	<1.5 mg/dL
Hyperbilirubinemia	>425 mmol/L (term infant)
Polycythemia	>65% (venous hematocrit)

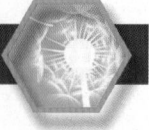

Nursing Care Plan 24.1

OVERVIEW OF AN INFANT OF A DIABETIC MOTHER

Jamie, a 38-year-old woman, gave birth to a term large-for-gestational-age newborn weighing 4,500 g (10 lb). She had a history of gestational diabetes but had not received any prenatal care. She arrived at the hospital in active labour. Despite macrosomia, the newborn's Apgar scores were 8 and 9 at 1 and 5 minutes, respectively. No resuscitative measures were needed.

One hour after birth, assessment revealed a pale, irritable newborn with sweating and several episodes of apnea. A glucose level obtained at this time via a heel stick was 2.2 mmol/L. Two hours later, the newborn begins exhibiting signs of respiratory distress—grunting, nasal flaring, retractions, tachypnea (respiratory rate 88 breaths/minute), and tachycardia (heart rate 176 beats/minute).

NURSING DIAGNOSIS: Risk for unstable glucose level related to hypoglycemia secondary to intrauterine hyperinsulin state resulting from maternal gestational diabetes as indicated by low blood glucose level, irritability, pallor, sweating, and apnea

Outcome Identification and Evaluation
The newborn will exhibit adequate glucose control *demonstrated by maintaining blood glucose levels above 2.6 mmol/L and an absence of clinical signs of hypoglycemia.*

Interventions: Promoting Glucose Control
- Monitor blood glucose levels via heel stick 1 hour after initial low reading and subsequent intervention, then every 3 hours until three consecutive point-of-care glucometer readings are >2.6 mmol/L. *Glucose levels less than 1.8 require immediate intervention: IV glucose and dedicated care by a nurse who can observe and monitor glucose levels closely to minimize the risk for complications associated with hypoglycemia.*
- Continue to observe for manifestations of hypoglycemia, such as pallor, tremors, jitteriness, lethargy, and poor feeding, *to allow for early detection and prompt intervention, thereby minimizing the risk for complications associated with hypoglycemia.*
- Monitor temperature frequently and institute measures to maintain a neutral thermal environment *to prevent cold stress, which would increase metabolic demands and further deplete glycogen stores.*
- Initiate early feedings every 2 to 3 hours or as appropriate or administer glucose supplements as ordered *to prevent hypoglycemia caused by the newborn's hyperinsulin state. Administer IV glucose infusions as ordered to correct hypoglycemia if glucose levels do not stabilize with feeding.*
- Cluster infant care activities and provide for rest periods *to conserve the newborn's energy and reduce use of glucose and glycogen stores.*
- Reduce environmental stimuli by dimming lights and speaking softly *to reduce energy demands and further utilization of glucose.*
- Explain all events and procedures to the mother *to help alleviate anxiety and promote understanding of the newborn's condition.*

NURSING DIAGNOSIS: Impaired gas exchange related to respiratory distress secondary to delayed lung maturity resulting from inhibition of pulmonary surfactant production due to fetal hyperinsulinemia as evidenced by grunting, nasal flaring, retractions, tachypnea, and tachycardia

Outcome Identification and Evaluation
Newborn will demonstrate signs of adequate oxygenation without respiratory distress *as demonstrated by respiratory rate and vital signs within acceptable parameters, absence of nasal flaring, retractions, and grunting, and oxygen saturation and arterial blood gas levels within acceptable parameters.*

Interventions: Promoting Oxygenation
- Monitor newborn's vital signs *to establish a baseline and evaluate for changes.*
- Assess airway patency and perform gentle suctioning as ordered *to ensure patency and allow for adequate oxygen intake.*
- Position the newborn prone *to optimize respiratory status and reduce stress.*
- Assess lung sounds for changes *to allow early detection of change in status.*

(continued)

Nursing Care Plan 24.1 (continued)

- Continuously monitor oxygen saturation levels via pulse oximetry *to determine adequacy of tissue perfusion.*
- Assess arterial or venous blood gas results *to detect changes indicating acidosis, hypoxemia, or hypercarbia, which would suggest hypoxia.* Administer treatment as ordered *to correct acidosis.*
- Administer oxygen as ordered *to promote adequate tissue perfusion.*
- Assess newborn's skin to identify cyanosis, pallor, and mottling *to detect changes indicating compromised oxygenation.*
- Administer surfactant replacement therapy as ordered *to aid in stabilizing the newborn's lungs until postnatal surfactant synthesis improves.*
- Institute measures to maintain normal blood glucose levels and a neutral thermal environment, cluster care activities, and reduce excessive stimuli *to reduce oxygen demand and consumption.*

Sources: Asenjo, M. (2011). *Imaging in transient tachypnea of the newborn.* Retrieved March 14, 2012 from http://www.emedicine.com/radio/topic710.htm; Gardner, S. L., Enzman-Hines, M., & Dickey, L. (2011). Respiratory diseases. In S. Gardner, B. Carter, M. Enzman-Hines, & J. Hernandez (Eds.), *Merenstein & Gardner's handbook of neonatal intensive care.* St. Louis, MO: Mosby Elsevier; and Verklan, T. (2009). So, he's a little premature... What's the big deal? *Critical Care Clinics of North America, 21,* 149–161.

Also administer fluid therapy as ordered to maintain adequate hydration. Monitor serum bilirubin levels and institute phototherapy if the newborn is over 24 hours old.

Providing Parental Support

Assist the parents and family in understanding the newborn's condition and need for frequent monitoring. Offer support and information to the parents and family. They may erroneously interpret the newborn's large size as an indication that the newborn is free of problems. Encourage open communication and listen with empathy to the family's fears and concerns. Provide frequent opportunities for the parents to interact with their newborn. Make appropriate referrals to social services and community resources as necessary to help the family cope.

Birth Trauma

Injuries to the newborn from the forces of labour and birth are categorized as birth trauma. In the past, numerous injuries were associated with difficult births requiring external or internal version or mid- or high forceps deliveries. Today, however, cesarean births have contributed to the decline in birth trauma. Improved prenatal diagnosis, monitoring of risk factors, and close monitoring during labour have also helped to reduce the incidence of birth injuries (Verklan & Lopez, 2011).

Pathophysiology

The process of birth is a blend of compression, contractions, torques, and traction. Birth traumas are injuries sustained by the newborn during the birthing process. When fetal size, presentation, or unusual progression of labour complicates this process, the forces of labour and birth may lead to tissue damage, edema, hemorrhage, or fracture in the newborn. For example, birth trauma may result from the pressure of birth, especially in a prolonged or abrupt labour, abnormal or difficult presentation, or mechanical forces, such as forceps or vacuum used during delivery. Table 24.3 summarizes the most common types of birth trauma.

Nursing Assessment

Recognition of trauma and birth injuries is imperative so that early treatment can be initiated. Review the labour and birth history for risk factors including prolonged or precipitous labour, breech presentation, and use of forceps or vacuum to assist delivery (Verklan & Lopez, 2011). Also review the history for multiple fetus deliveries, large-for-date infants, extreme prematurity, large fetal head, or newborns with congenital anomalies.

Complete a careful physical and neurologic assessment of every newborn admitted to the nursery to establish whether injuries exist. Inspect the head for lumps, bumps, or bruises. Note whether swelling or bruising crosses the suture line. Assess the eyes and face for facial paralysis, observing for asymmetry of the face with crying or appearance of the mouth being drawn to the unaffected side. Ensure that the newborn spontaneously moves all extremities. Note any absence of or decrease in deep tendon reflexes or abnormal positioning of extremities.

Assess and document symmetry of structure and function. Be prepared to assist with scheduling diagnostic studies to confirm trauma or injuries, which will be important in determining treatment modalities.

Nursing Management

Nursing management is primarily supportive and focuses on assessing for resolution of the trauma or any associated complications along with providing support and education to the parents. Provide the parents with explanations and reassurance that these injuries usually resolve with minimal or no treatment. Parents are alarmed when

TABLE 24.3   COMMON TYPES OF BIRTH TRAUMA

Type	Description	Findings	Treatment
Fractures	Most often occur during breech births or shoulder dystocia in newborns with macrosomia Mid-clavicular fractures are the most common type of fracture, secondary to shoulder dystocia. Long bone fractures of humorous or femur, usually mid-shaft, also can occur.	Mid-clavicular fractures: the newborn presents with irritability and does not move the arm on the affected side either spontaneously or when the Moro reflex is elicited. Femoral or humeral long bone fractures: the newborn shows loss of spontaneous leg or arm motion, respectively; usually swelling and pain accompany the limited movement. X-rays confirm the fracture.	Mid-clavicular fractures typically heal rapidly and uneventfully; arm motion may be limited by pinning the newborn's sleeve to the shirt. Femoral and humeral shaft fractures are treated with splinting. Healing and complete recovery are expected within 2 to 4 weeks without incident. Explanation to the parents and reassurance are needed.
Brachial plexus injury	Primarily in large babies, babies with shoulder dystocia, or breech delivery Results from stretching, hemorrhage within a nerve, or tearing of the nerve or the roots associated with cervical cord injury. Associated traumatic injuries include fracture of the clavicle or humorous or subluxations of the shoulder or cervical spine. Erb's palsy is an upper brachial plexus injury. Klumpke's palsy is an injury to the lower brachial plexus (lower brachial injuries are less common).	In Erb's palsy, the involved extremity usually presents adducted, prone, and internally rotated; shoulder movement is absent; Moro, bicep, and radial reflexes are absent, but the grasp reflex is usually present. Klumpke's palsy is manifested by weakness in the hand and wrist; grasp reflex is absent.	Erb's palsy usually involves immobilization of the upper arm across the upper abdomen/chest to protect the shoulder from excessive motion for the first week; then gentle passive range-of-motion exercises are performed daily to prevent contractures. There is usually no associated sensory loss, and this condition usually improves rapidly. Treatment for Klumpke's palsy involves placing the hand in a neutral position and using passive range-of-motion exercises. In some cases deficits may persist, requiring continuing observation.
Cranial nerve trauma	Most common is facial nerve palsy. Frequently attributed to pressure resulting from forceps. May also result from pressure on the nerve in utero, related to fetal positioning such as the head lying against the shoulder.	Physical findings include asymmetry of the face when crying; mouth may be drawn toward the unaffected side; wrinkles are deeper on the unaffected side. The paralyzed side may be smooth, with a swollen appearance. Eye is persistently open on the affected side.	Most infants begin to recover in the first week, but full resolution may take up to several months; parents need reassurance about this. In most cases, treatment is not necessary, only observation. If the eye is affected and unable to close, protection with patches and synthetic tears may be necessary. Parents need instruction about how to feed the newborn, since he or she cannot close the lips around the nipple without having milk seep out.

(continued)

TABLE 24.3 COMMON TYPES OF BIRTH TRAUMA (continued)

Type	Description	Findings	Treatment
Head trauma	Mild trauma can cause soft tissue injuries such as cephalhematoma and caput succedaneum; greater trauma can cause depressed skull fractures. **Cephalhematoma** (subperiosteal collection of blood secondary to the rupture of blood vessels between the skull and periosteum) occurs in 2.5% of all births and typically appears within hours after birth (Nicholson, 2007). **Caput succedaneum** (soft tissue swelling) is caused by edema of the head against the dilating cervix during the birth process. Subarachnoid hemorrhage (one of the most common types of intracranial trauma) may be due to hypoxia/ischemia, variations in blood pressure, and the pressure exerted on the head during labour. Bleeding is of venous origin, and underlying contusions also may occur (Laroia, 2010). Subdural hemorrhage (hematomas) occurs less often today because of improved obstetric techniques. Typically, tears of the major veins or venous sinuses overlying the cerebral hemispheres or cerebellum (most common in newborns of primiparas and large newborns, or after an instrumented birth) are the cause. Increased pressure on the blood vessels inside the skull leads to tears. Depressed skull fractures (rare) may result from the pressure of a forceps delivery; can also occur during spontaneous or cesarean births and may be associated with other head trauma causing subdural bleeding, subarachnoid hemorrhage, or brain trauma (Laroia, 2010).	In cephalhematoma, suture lines delineate its extent; usually located on one side, over the parietal bone. In caput succedaneum, swelling is not limited by suture lines: it extends across the midline and is associated with head moulding. It does not usually cause complications other than a misshapen head. Swelling is maximal at birth and then rapidly decreases in size. In subarachnoid hemorrhage, some RBCs may appear in the cerebrospinal fluid of full-term newborns. Newborns may present with apnea, seizures, lethargy, or abnormal findings on a neurologic examination. Subdural hemorrhage can be asymptomatic, or the neonate can exhibit seizures, enlarging head size, decreased level of consciousness, or abnormal findings on a neurologic examination, with hypotonia, a poor Moro reflex, or extensive retinal hemorrhages. Depressed skull fractures can be observed and palpated as depressions. Confirmation by X-ray is necessary.	Cephalhematoma resolves gradually over 2 to 3 weeks without treatment (see Chapter 18). Caput succedaneum usually resolves over the first few days without treatment (see Chapter 18). Subarachnoid hemorrhage requires minimal handling to reduce stress. Subdural hematoma requires aspiration; can be life-threatening if it is in an inaccessible location and cannot be aspirated. Depressed skull fractures typically require a neurosurgical consultation.

Source: Verklan, T., & Lopez, S. M. (2011). Neurologic disorders. In S. Gardner, B. Carter, M. Enzman-Hines, & J. Hernandez (Eds.), *Merenstein & Gardner's handbook of neonatal intensive care*. St. Louis, MO: Mosby Elsevier.

their newborn is unable to move an extremity or demonstrates asymmetric facial movements. Provide parents with a realistic picture of the situation to gain their understanding and trust. Be readily available to answer questions and teach them how to care for the newborn, including any modifications that might be necessary. Allow parents adequate time to understand the implications of the birth trauma or injury and what treatment modalities are needed, if any. Provide them with information about the length of time until the injury will resolve and when and if they need to seek further medical attention for the condition. Spending time with the parents and providing them with support, information, and teaching are important to allow them to make decisions and care for their newborn. Anticipate the need for community referral for ongoing follow-up and care, if necessary.

Newborns of Substance–Abusing Mothers

It is generally assumed that all pregnant women want to provide a healthy environment for their unborn child and know how to avoid harm. However, for women who use substances such as drugs or alcohol, this may not be the case. Substance use during pregnancy exposes the fetus to the possibility of IUGR, prematurity, neurobehavioural and neurophysiologic dysfunction, birth defects, infections, and long-term developmental sequelae (Schechner, 2008; Weiner & Finnegan, 2011).

It is difficult to establish the true prevalence of substance use in pregnant women; many women deny taking any nonprescribed substance because of the associated social stigma and legal implications (Wong, Ordean, & Kahan, 2011). The extent of licit and illicit drug use in pregnancy is thought to be significantly under-reported (Schechner, 2008). Drug exposure may go unrecognized in newborns whose mothers do not self-report, and these infants may be discharged home at increased risk for medical and social problems, including abuse and neglect.

Tobacco, alcohol, and marijuana are the substances most commonly abused during pregnancy. Other substances may include opioids such as morphine, codeine, methadone, meperidine, and heroin; central nervous system (CNS) stimulants such as amphetamines and cocaine; CNS depressants such as barbiturates, diazepam (Valium), and sedative–hypnotics; and hallucinogens, such as LSD, inhalants, glue, paint thinner, nail polish remover, and nitrous oxide (Weiner & Finnegan, 2011). Table 24.4 highlights commonly used substances and their effects on the fetus and newborn.

Substance abuse during pregnancy is the subject of much controversy. The timing of drug ingestion usually determines the type and severity of damage to the fetus. Frequently, the woman uses more than one substance, which compounds the problem. Nurses must be knowledgeable about the issues of substance abuse and must be

▶ *Consider THIS!*

I admit, I was pretty reckless as a teen. I was rebellious, hated my mother's authority, and started smoking and doing drugs just to "check out" of my painful world. It was one big blast after another with crazy highs and lows. I didn't think about my behaviour and never thought it would hurt anyone. Then I got pregnant. When I was about 4 months I convinced myself that if I cut back, everything would be fine for my baby and me.

Now I see my tiny son fight for air and shake all over, I am not so sure that I didn't hurt anyone except myself. My son is fighting against MY nicotine and drug addiction, and I feel so guilty. Sooner or later my addiction would hurt someone I cared about, but I didn't care at the time. I had no idea what the impact would be on my mother and my baby. How could I do this to them?

Thoughts: this woman honestly regrets what her addiction has done to her son as she stands watching him go through withdrawal. Her lifestyle choices do affect others, despite her previous denial. One problem with addiction is the difficulty in getting help after deciding to finally quit. There aren't enough rehab centres to deal with the large numbers needing their services, and it can be difficult to get into one. What can be offered to pregnant women who abuse substances? How can nurses increase community awareness about the impact of this problem, especially during pregnancy?

alert for opportunities to identify, prevent, manage, and educate women and families about this key public health issue.

Fetal Alcohol Syndrome

The adverse effects of alcohol consumption have been recognized for centuries, but the associated pattern of fetal anomalies was not labelled until the early 1970s. The distinctive pattern identified three specific findings: growth restriction (prenatal and postnatal), craniofacial structural anomalies, and CNS dysfunction. These distinctive findings were called **fetal alcohol syndrome**, characterized by physical and mental disorders that appear at birth and remain problematic throughout the child's life. However, there are also circumstances in which the effects of prenatal alcohol exposure are apparent but the newborn does not meet all of the criteria. In an attempt to include those who do not meet the strict criteria, the terms "fetal alcohol effects," "alcohol-related birth defects," and "alcohol-related neurologic defects" are used to describe children with a variety of problems thought to be related to alcohol consumption during

(text continues on page 779)

TABLE 24.4 SUBSTANCES AND THEIR EFFECTS ON THE FETUS AND NEWBORN

Substance	Description	Effects on Fetus and Newborn	Nursing Implications
Alcohol	Consumption is pervasive and widely accepted with use, abuse, and addiction affecting all levels of society. It is a common misconception that a substance sold to the public without restriction is safe.	Fetal alcohol syndrome (one of the most common known causes of mental retardation) Fetal alcohol spectrum disorders Alcohol-related birth defects	Provide education that decreasing or eliminating alcohol consumption during pregnancy is the only way to prevent fetal alcohol syndrome and fetal alcohol effects. Assist pregnant woman in finding a treatment program if possible. Inform all women who are pregnant or planning to become pregnant about the detrimental effects of alcohol during pregnancy. Educate women using a non-judgmental, culturally connected approach. Warn women that there is no safe time to drink or amount of alcohol they can consume while pregnant.
Tobacco/ nicotine	Nicotine is an addictive substance. It causes epinephrine release from adrenal cortex, leading to initial stimulation followed by depression and fatigue, causing the user to seek more nicotine. Increased numbers of women are smoking. Over 2,500 chemicals are found in cigarette smoke, including nicotine, tar, carbon monoxide, and cyanide. It is unknown which are harmful, but nicotine and carbon monoxide are believed to play a role in causing adverse pregnancy outcomes.	Impaired oxygenation of mother and fetus due to nicotine crossing placenta and carbon monoxide combining with hemoglobin Increased risk for low birth weight (risk almost doubled), small for gestational age, and preterm birth. Increased risk for sudden infant death syndrome (SIDS) and chronic respiratory illness.	Provide teaching to women about healthy behaviours. Provide support for smoking cessation. Individualize counselling based on factors associated with the woman's smoking and challenges faced (why woman smokes, stressors in life, and social support network). Suggest options such as group smoking cessation programs, relaxation techniques, individual counselling, hypnosis, and partner-support counselling.
Marijuana	Most widely used illicit psychoactive substance in Western world. Derived from *Cannabis sativa* plant.	Not shown to have teratogenic effects on fetus; no consistent types of malformations identified. Intrauterine growth restriction (IUGR) is common due to delivery of carbon monoxide to fetus. Increased risk for small for gestational age.	

Substance	Description	Effects on Fetus and Newborn	Nursing Implications
		Altered responses to visual stimuli, sleep-pattern abnormalities, photophobia, lack of motor control, hyper-irritability, increased tremulousness, and high-pitched cry noted in infants of mothers who smoked marijuana. Research related to long-term effects is continuing. Provide teaching to women about healthy behaviours. Provide support for cessation of marijuana use.	
Methamphetamine	Addictive stimulant; use releases high levels of dopamine, which stimulates brain cells, enhancing mood and body movement. High potential for abuse and addiction; can be inhaled, injected, smoked, or taken orally. Many street names, such as speed, meth, ice, and chalk. Primary effects include accelerated heart and respiratory rate, elevated blood pressure, pupillary dilation; secondary effects include loss of appetite. Used medically as treatment for obesity and narcolepsy in adults and hyperactivity in children.	Little research on use during pregnancy because its use is less common than cocaine or narcotics Fetal effects similar to cocaine (suggesting vasoconstriction as possible underlying mechanism). Possible maternal malnutrition, leading to problems with fetal growth and development. Increased risk for preterm birth and low birth weight. Infants may have withdrawal symptoms, including dysphoria, agitation, jitteriness, poor weight gain, abnormal sleep patterns, poor feeding, frantic fist sucking, high-pitched cry, respiratory distress soon after birth, frequent infections, and significant lassitude (Arenson & Drake, 2007). Long-term effects are not known.	Provide teaching to women about healthy behaviours. Provide support for cessation of methamphetamine use. Monitor the woman for weight changes; emphasize the need for adequate nutritional intake to support fetal growth and development.
Cocaine	Strong CNS stimulant that interferes with reabsorption of dopamine. Physical effects: vasoconstriction; pupillary dilation; increased temperature, heart rate, and blood pressure. Taken orally, sublingually, intranasally, intravenously, or via inhalation. Estimated that 30% to 40% of cocaine addicts are female.	Preterm birth and lower birth weight. Unclear impact on later development. Speculation that cocaine interferes with infant's cognitive development, leading to learning and memory difficulties later in life. Associated congenital anomalies: genitourinary, cardiac, and CNS defects, and prune belly syndrome	Educate the woman about the effects of cocaine use on the fetus and newborn. Assess for use of other substances. Provide teaching to women about healthy behaviours. Provide support and guidance for cessation of cocaine and other substance use.

(continued)

TABLE 24.4 SUBSTANCES AND THEIR EFFECTS ON THE FETUS AND NEWBORN (continued)

Substance	Description	Effects on Fetus and Newborn	Nursing Implications
	Maternal cocaine use during pregnancy is a significant health problem (CPS, 2007). Increased potential for use of multiple drugs if mother using cocaine (Marcellus, 2007).	Other typical newborn characteristics: smaller head circumference, piercing cry, limb defects, ambiguous genitalia, poor feeding, poor visual and auditory responses, poor sleep patterns, decreased impulse control, stiff, hyperextended positioning, irritability and hypersensitivity, inability to respond to caretaker (Blackburn, 2007)	
Heroin	Illegal, highly addictive opiate derived from morphine that can be sniffed, smoked, or injected. Possible consequences include HIV infection, tuberculosis, crime, violence, and family disruption. Severe physical addiction; CNS depressant producing mental dullness and drowsiness.	Newborns of heroin-addicted mothers are born dependent on heroin. Increased risk for transmission of hepatitis B and C and HIV to newborns when mothers share needles. Significantly increased rates of stillbirth, IUGR, preterm birth, and newborn mortality. Small-for-gestational age newborns, meconium aspiration, high incidence of SIDS, and delayed effects from subacute withdrawal (restlessness, continual crying, agitation, sneezing, vomiting, fever, diarrhea, seizures, irritability, and poor socialization [possibly persisting for 4 to 6 months]; March of Dimes, 2007) Intrauterine death or preterm birth is possible with abrupt cessation of heroin use.	Educate the woman about the effects of heroin use on the fetus and newborn. Assess for use of other substances. Provide teaching to women about healthy behaviours. Warn the woman not to abruptly stop heroin use. Encourage her to enrol in a methadone maintenance program.
Methadone	Synthetic opiate narcotic used primarily as maintenance therapy for heroin addiction.	Improvement in many of the detrimental fetal effects associated with heroin use. Withdrawal symptoms are common in newborns. Possible low birth weight due to symmetric fetal growth restriction. Increased severity and longer period of withdrawal (due to methadone's longer half-life). Seizures (commonly severe) do not usually occur until 2 to 3 weeks of age, when the newborn is at home.	

Substance	Description	Effects on Fetus and Newborn	Nursing Implications
		Increased rate of SIDS. Methadone maintenance programs are the standard of care for women with narcotic addiction. Inform the woman about the benefits and risks of methadone use vs. heroin use. Advantages include improved fetal and newborn growth, reduced risk for fetal death, and reduced risk for HIV infection. Advise the woman that she will need to return consistently to receive the prescribed methadone dose. Reinforce the need for continued prenatal care. Inform the woman that she can breastfeed her newborn while receiving methadone. Teach mother and caregivers about signs and symptoms of methadone withdrawal.	

Sources: Steiker, L. K. H. (2009). A dialogue on fetal alcohol spectrum disorder (FASD) and the prenatal impact of substances on children: An interview with Elizabeth C. Pomeroy. *Journal of Social Work Practice in the Addictions*, 9(4), 417–422; Jansson, L. M., Choo, R., Velez, M. L., et al. (2008). Methadone maintenance and breastfeeding in the neonatal period. *Pediatrics*, 121, 106–114; Marcellus, L. (2007). Neonatal abstinence syndrome: Reconstructing the evidence. *Neonatal Network*, 26(1), 33–40; Centers for Disease Control and Prevention. (2007). *Surgeon general's report: Women and smoking fact sheet: Tobacco use and reproductive outcomes.* Retrieved XXXX, 2012 from http://www.cdc.gov/tobacco/sgr/sgr_forwomen/factsheet_outcomes.htm; National Center on Birth Defects and Developmental Disabilities, Centers for Disease Control and Prevention, & Department of Health and Human Services. (2004). *Fetal alcohol syndrome: Guidelines for referral and diagnosis.* Retrieved March 14, 2012 from http://www.cdc.gov/ncbddd/fasd/documents/fas_guidelines_accessible.pdf; Public Health Agency of Canada. (2008). *Canadian perinatal health report, 2008 edition.* Retrieved March 14, 2012 from http://www.phac-aspc.gc.ca/publicat/2008/cphr-rspc/pdf/cphr-rspc08-eng.pdf; and Wong, S., Ordean, A., Kahan, M. (2011). SOGC clinical practice guideline: Substance use in pregnancy. *Journal of Obstetrics & Gynaecology Canada, 33*(4), 367–384. Retrieved March 14, 2012 from http://www.sogc.org/guidelines/documents/gui256CPG1104E.pdf.

pregnancy. The US Institute of Medicine coined the term **fetal alcohol spectrum disorder** as a way of describing the broader effects of prenatal alcohol exposure. Children with fetal alcohol syndrome are at the severe end of the spectrum (Premji & Semenic, 2009). Newborns with some but not all of the symptoms of fetal alcohol syndrome are described as having **alcohol-related birth defects**. Fetal alcohol effects may include such problems as low birth weight, developmental delays, and hyperactivity. Box 24.3 summarizes the manifestations of fetal alcohol syndrome.

Approximately 3,000 infants born in Canada each year are affected by fetal alcohol syndrome (FAS) (Thanh & Jonsson, 2010). Higher rates of FAS have also been suggested in infants born to women with chronic alcoholism, a condition reported to be significantly higher in remote Aboriginal populations across Canada (Premji & Semenic, 2009).

Fetal alcohol syndrome is one of the most common known causes of cognitive delays and the only cause that is entirely preventable. The effects last a lifetime. Children with this syndrome have varying degrees of psychological and behavioural problems and often find it difficult to hold a job and live independently (Premji & Semenic, 2009; Thanh & Jonsson, 2010).

Decreasing or eliminating alcohol consumption during pregnancy is the only way to prevent fetal alcohol syndrome and fetal alcohol effects. Unfortunately, few treatment programs address the needs of pregnant women, so many newborns are exposed to alcohol in utero.

Neonatal Abstinence Syndrome

Newborns of women who abuse tobacco, illicit substances, caffeine, and alcohol can exhibit withdrawal behaviour. Withdrawal symptoms occur in 60% to 90% of

BOX 24.3 Clinical Picture of Fetal Alcohol Syndrome

- Microcephaly (head circumference <10th percentile)*
- Small palpebral (eyelid) fissures*
- Abnormally small eyes
- Intrauterine growth restriction
- Maxillary hypoplasia (flattened or absent)
- Epicanthal folds (folds of skin of the upper eyelid over the eye)
- Thin upper lip*
- Missing vertical groove in median portion of upper lip*
- Short upturned nose
- Short birth length and low birth weight
- Joint and limb defects
- Altered palmar crease pattern
- Prenatal or postnatal growth ≤10th percentile*
- Congenital cardiac defects (septal defects)
- Delayed fine and gross motor development
- Poor eye–hand coordination
- Clinically significant brain abnormalities*
- Mental retardation
- Narrow forehead
- Performance substantially below expected level in cognitive or developmental functioning, executive or motor functioning, and attention or hyperactivity; social or language skills*
- Inadequate sucking reflex and poor appetite

---

*Diagnosis of fetal alcohol syndrome requires the presence of three findings:

1. Documentation of all three facial abnormalities
2. Documentation of growth deficits (height, weight, or both below 10th percentile)
3. Documentation of CNS abnormalities (structural, neurologic, or functional)

Source: Davis, K., Desrocher, M., & Moore, T. (2011). Fetal alcohol spectrum disorder: A review of neurodevelopmental findings and interventions. *Journal of Developmental and Physical Disabilities*, 23(2), 143–167; First Nations and Inuit Health Committee & Canadian Paediatric Society. (2012). *Position Statement: Fetal Alcohol Syndrome*. Retrieved May 26, 2012 from http://www.cps.ca/english/statements/II/ii02-01.htm; & Weiner, S. M., & Finnegan, L. P. (2011). Drug withdrawal in the neonate. In S. Gardner, B. Carter, M. Enzman-Hines, & J. Hernandez (Eds.), *Merenstein & Gardner's handbook of neonatal intensive care*. St. Louis, MO: Mosby Elsevier.

all newborns exposed to drugs, depending on the substance used (Weiner & Finnegan, 2011). Drug dependency acquired in utero is manifested by a constellation of neurologic and physical behaviours and is known as **neonatal abstinence syndrome**. Although often treated as a single entity, neonatal abstinence syndrome is not a single pathologic condition. The manifestations of withdrawal are a function of the drug's half-life, the specific drug or combination of drugs used, dosage, route of administration, timing of drug exposure, and length of drug exposure (Schechner, 2008). Typical newborn behaviours include CNS hypersensitivity, autonomic dysfunction, and GI disturbances (Marcellus, 2007). Neonatal absti-

nence syndrome has both medical and developmental consequences for the newborn.

Nursing Assessment

Several tools can be used to assess a drug-exposed newborn. Figure 24.5 shows an example. Regardless of the tool used for assessment, address these key areas:

- Maternal history to identify risk behaviours for substance abuse:
  - Previous unexplained fetal demise
  - Lack of prenatal care
  - History of missed prenatal appointments
  - Severe mood swings
  - Precipitous labour
  - Poor nutritional status
  - Abruptio placentae
  - Hypertensive episodes
  - History of drug abuse
- Laboratory test results (toxicology) to identify substances in mother and newborn
- Signs of neonatal abstinence syndrome
- Evidence of seizure activity and need for protective environment

The newborn's behaviour often prompts the health care provider or nurse to suspect intrauterine drug exposure (Box 24.4). The newborn physical examination may also reveal low birth weight for gestational age or drug- or alcohol-related birth defects and dysfunction.

▶ **Take** NOTE!

Cocaine-exposed newborns are typically fussy, irritable, and inconsolable at times. Cocaine-exposed infants demonstrate poor coordination of sucking and swallowing, making feeding time frustrating for the newborn and caregiver alike.

Assess the newborn for signs of neonatal abstinence syndrome, including CNS symptoms (high-pitched cry, poor sleep patterns, tremors, hypertonia, myoclonic jerks, excoriated skin, convulsions), metabolic symptoms (sweating, hyperthermia, nasal stuffiness, sneezing), GI symptoms (poor feeding, excessive sucking, regurgitation, projectile vomiting, loose and/or watery stools), and respiratory symptoms (tachypnea) (Weiner & Finnegan, 2011; Zimmermann-Baer, Nötzli, Rentsch, et al., 2010).

Assist with obtaining diagnostic studies to identify the severity of withdrawal. Toxicology screening of the newborn's blood, urine, and meconium identifies the substances to which the newborn has been exposed. A urine screen will only reveal recent newborn exposure to maternal use of drugs, while meconium testing provides evidence of longer-term patterns of drug misuse (Schechner, 2008).

CENTRAL NERVOUS SYSTEM DISTURBANCES													
SIGNS AND SYMPTOMS	SCORE	AM						PM				
Excessive high-pitched cry	2											
Continuous high-pitched cry	3											
Sleeps <1 hour after feeding	3											
Sleeps <2 hours after feeding	2											
Sleeps <3 hours after feeding	1											
Hyperactive Moro reflex	2											
Markedly hyperactive Moro refex	3											
Mild tremors disturbed	1											
Moderate–severe tremors disturbed	2											
Mild tremors undisturbed	1											
Moderate–severe tremors undisturbed	4											
Increased muscle tone	2											
Excoloration (specify area)	1											
Myoclonic jerks	3											
Generalized convulsions	5											
METABOLIC / VASOMOTOR/RESPIRATORY DISTURBANCES												
Sweating												
Fever <101 (99–100.8°F/37.2–38.2°C)	1											
Fever >101 (38.2°C and higher)	2											
Frequent yawning (>3– 4 times/interval)	1											
Mottling	1											
Nasal stuffiness	1											
Sneezing (>3–4 times/interval)	1											
Nasal flaring	2											
Respiratory rate >60 / min	1											
Respiratory rate >60 / min, with retractions	2											
GASTROINTESTINAL DISTURBANCES												
Excessive sucking	1											
Poor feeding	2											
Regurgitation	2											
Projectile vomiting	3											
Loose stools	2											
Watery stools	3											
TOTAL SCORE												

FIGURE 24.5 Neonatal abstinence scoring system (From: Cloherty, J. P., & Stark, A. P. [1998]. *Manual of neonatal care* [4th ed., pp. 26–27]. Boston: Little, Brown.)

BOX 24.4 Manifestations of Neonatal Abstinence Syndrome

CNS Dysfunction
- Tremors
- Generalized seizures
- Hyperactive reflexes
- Restlessness
- Hypertonic muscle tone, constant movement
- Shrill, high-pitched cry
- Disturbed sleep patterns

Metabolic, Vasomotor, and Respiratory Disturbances
- Fever
- Frequent yawning
- Mottling of the skin
- Sweating
- Frequent sneezing
- Nasal flaring
- Tachypnea (respiratory rate >60 beats/minute)
- Apnea

Gastrointestinal Dysfunction
- Poor feeding
- Frantic sucking or rooting
- Loose or watery stools
- Regurgitation or projectile vomiting (Marcellus, 2007)

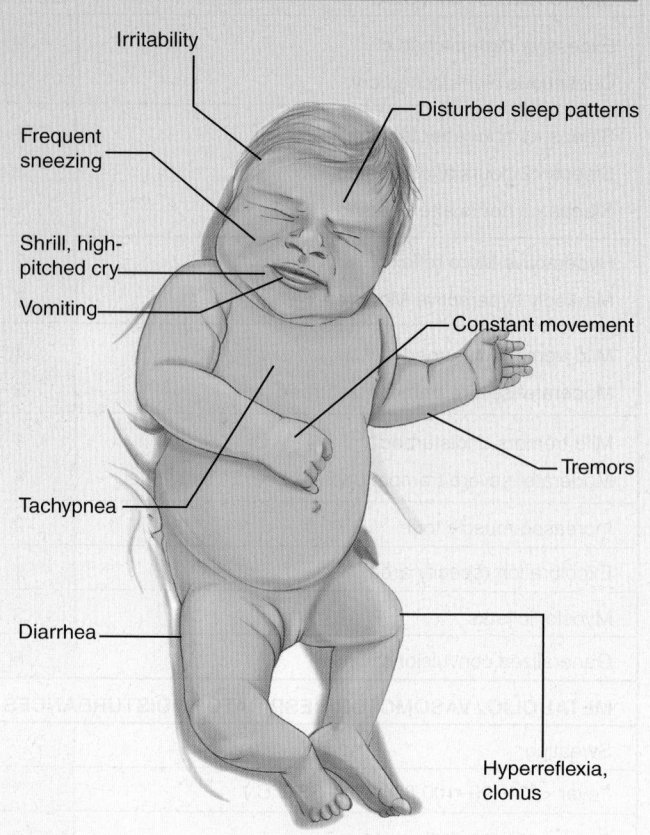

Nursing Management

The needs of the substance-exposed newborn are multiple, complex, and costly, both to the health care system and to society. Substance abuse takes place among people of all colours, sizes, shapes, incomes, cultures, and social living conditions. Many pregnant women are unaware of the adverse impact their substance use can have on the newborn.

Nurses are in a unique position to help because they interact with high-risk mothers and newborns in many settings, including the community, health care facilities, and family agencies. It is the responsibility of all nurses to identify, educate, counsel, and refer pregnant women with substance-abusing problems. For example, nurses can be instrumental in increasing the number of pregnant women who make a serious attempt to quit smoking by using the "5 A's" approach:

- Ask: ask all women if they smoke and would like to quit.
- Advise: encourage the use of clinically proven treatment plans.
- Assess: provide motivation by discussing the "5 R's":
  - Relevance of quitting to the woman
  - Risk of continued smoking to the fetus
  - Rewards of quitting for both

- Roadblocks to quitting
- Repeat at every visit
- Assist: help the woman to protect her fetus and newborn from the negative effects of smoking.
- Arrange: schedule follow-up visits to reinforce the woman's commitment to quit.

Although this approach is geared toward smoking cessation, nurses can adapt it to focus on cessation for any substance use. Early, supportive, ongoing nursing care is critical to the well-being of the mother and her newborn.

Caring for a substance-exposed newborn remains a major challenge to health care professionals. The major goals include providing comfort to the newborn by relieving symptoms, improving feeding and weight gain, preventing seizures, promoting mother–newborn interactions, and reducing the incidence of newborn mortality and abnormal development (Weiner and Finnegan, 2011).

Promoting Comfort

Keep environmental stimuli to a minimum. For example, decrease stimuli by dimming the lights in the nursery, and swaddle the newborn tightly to decrease irritability behaviours. Other techniques such as gentle rocking, using a flexed position, and offering a pacifier can help manage CNS irritability. A pacifier also helps satisfy the newborn's need for non-nutritive sucking. Use a calm, gentle approach when handling the newborn and plan activities to avoid overstimulating the newborn, allowing time for rest periods.

Meeting Nutritional Needs

When feeding the newborn, use small amounts and position the newborn upright to prevent aspiration and to facilitate rhythmic sucking and swallowing. Breastfeeding is encouraged unless the mother is still using drugs. Mothers who are on a well-monitored methadone maintenance program may also be encouraged to breastfeed (Jansson, Choo, Velez, et al., 2008). Monitor the newborn's weight daily to evaluate the success of food intake. Assess hydration; check skin turgor and fontanels. Assess the frequency and characteristics of bowel movements, and monitor the newborn's fluid and electrolyte levels and acid–base status.

Preventing Complications

Pharmacologic treatment is warranted if conservative measures, such as swaddling and decreased environmental stimulation, are not adequate. Newborns with confirmed drug exposure will require drug therapy if they have any combination of the following symptoms: seizures, diarrhea and vomiting resulting in excessive weight loss and dehydration, poor feeding, inability to sleep, and/or fever unrelated to infection. Common medications used in the management of newborn withdrawal include morphine, paregoric, phenobarbital, tincture of opium, methadone, clonidine, chlorpromazine, and diazepam (Marcellus, 2007); of these options, oral morphine is the withdrawal medication most commonly used in Canada. Administer the prescribed medication and document the newborn's behavioural responses.

The newborn is at risk for skin breakdown. Weight loss, diarrhea, dehydration, and irritability can contribute to this risk. Provide meticulous skin care and protect the newborn's elbows and knees against friction and abrasions.

Promoting Parent–Newborn Interaction

For a mother who abuses substances, the birth of a drug-exposed newborn is both a crisis and an opportunity. The mother may feel guilty about the newborn's condition. Many of these newborns are unresponsive and have disorganized sleeping and feeding patterns. When awake, they can be easily overstimulated and irritated. Such characteristics make parent–newborn interactions difficult and frustrating, leading to possible detachment and avoidance (Weiner & Finnegan, 2011). In addition, the mother may be single and a victim of physical or sexual abuse and may have a limited support system. Many of these mothers may have had poor parenting themselves, lack infor-

mation about characteristic infant behaviours, and have unrealistic expectations about the newborn's abilities (Weiner & Finnegan, 2011). Instruct the mother or caretaker in how to care for the newborn, including what to do after the newborn goes home (Teaching Guideline 24.1).

On the other hand, the newborn may be a powerful motivator for the mother to undergo treatment and seek recovery. The nurse can play a pivotal role in assisting her to abstain from drug use and to promote effective parenting skills. Infants with neonatal abstinence syndrome have significantly improved outcomes when their parents are able to provide a safe and supportive environment (Marcellus, 2007).

TEACHING GUIDELINE 24.1

Caring for Your Newborn at Home

- Hold your newborn with the head elevated to prevent choking.
- To aid your newborn's sucking and swallowing during feeding, position the chin downward and support it with your hand.
- Place your newborn flat on his or her back to sleep or nap, never on the stomach.
  - Provide "tummy time" during waking hours.
- If your newborn is fussy or crying, try these measures to help calm him or her:
  - Wrap your newborn snugly in a blanket and gently rock in rocking chair.
  - Take your baby for a ride in the car (secured in a newborn car seat).
  - Play soothing music and "dance" with the newborn.
  - Use a wind-up swing with music.
- To help your newborn get to sleep, try these measures:
  - Plan a bath with a gentle massage prior to bedtime.
  - Change diaper and clothes to make the baby comfortable.
  - Feed your baby just prior to bedtime.
  - If your newborn cries when put in the crib and all needs are met, it is OK to allow him or her to cry.
  - Use a rocking chair to feed and sing a soft lullaby.
- Call your primary care provider if you observe withdrawal behaviours such as:
  - Slight tremors (shaking) of hands and legs
  - Stiff posture when held in your arms
  - Irritability and frequent fussiness
  - High-pitched cry, excessive sucking motions
  - Erratic sleep pattern
  - Frequent yawning, nasal stuffiness, sweating
  - Prolonged time needed to feed
  - Frequent vomiting after feeding

Hyperbilirubinemia

Hyperbilirubinemia results when unconjugated bilirubin is deposited in the skin and mucous membranes. Hyperbilirubinemia is considered severe when the total serum bilirubin level exceeds 340 mmol/L in the first 28 days of life; the condition is considered critical when levels are above 425 mmol/L (Canadian Paediatric Society [CPS], 2007a).

Hyperbilirubinemia is exhibited as jaundice (yellowing of the body tissues and fluids). Newborn jaundice is one of the most common reasons for hospital readmission. It occurs in 60% to 80% of term newborns in the first week of life and in virtually all preterm newborns (Rodriguez, Fanaroff, & Lissauer, 2008).

Pathophysiology

Newborn jaundice results from an imbalance in the rate of bilirubin production and bilirubin elimination. This imbalance determines the pattern and degree of newborn hyperbilirubinemia.

During the newborn period, a rapid transition from the intrauterine to the extrauterine pattern of bilirubin physiology occurs. Fetal unconjugated bilirubin is normally cleared by the placenta and the mother's liver in utero, so total bilirubin at birth is low. After the umbilical cord is cut, the newborn must conjugate bilirubin (convert a lipid-soluble pigment into a water-soluble pigment) in the liver on his or her own. The rate and amount of bilirubin conjugation depend on the rate of red blood cell breakdown, the bilirubin load, the maturity of the liver, and the number of albumin-binding sites (Maisels, 2010). Bilirubin production increases after birth mainly because of a shortened red blood cell lifespan (70 days in the newborn versus 90 days in the adult) combined with an increased red blood cell mass. Therefore, the amount of bilirubin the newborn must deal with is large compared with that of an adult.

Bilirubin has two forms—unconjugated or indirect, which is fat-soluble and toxic to body tissues, and conjugated or direct, which is water-soluble and non-toxic. Elevated serum bilirubin levels are manifested as jaundice in the newborn.

Physiologic Jaundice

Physiologic jaundice is the manifestation of the normal hyperbilirubinemia seen in newborns, appearing during the third to fourth days of life as a result of the limitations and abnormalities of bilirubin metabolism. Most newborns have been discharged by the time this jaundice peaks (at about 72 hours).

Physiologic jaundice may result from an increased bilirubin load because of relative polycythemia, a shortened red blood cell lifespan, immature hepatic uptake and conjugation process, and increased enterohepatic circulation. Newborns with delayed passage of meconium are more likely to develop physiologic jaundice (Maisels, 2010).

Physiologic jaundice differs between breastfed and bottle-fed newborns with regard to the onset of symptoms. Breastfed newborns typically have peak bilirubin levels on the fourth day of life; levels for bottle-fed newborns usually peak on the third day of life. The rate of bilirubin decline is less rapid in breastfed newborns compared with bottle-fed newborns because bottle-fed newborns tend to have more frequent bowel movements. Jaundice associated with breastfeeding presents in two distinct patterns: early-onset breastfeeding jaundice and late-onset breastfeeding jaundice.

Early-Onset Breastfeeding Jaundice

Early-onset breastfeeding jaundice is probably associated with ineffective breastfeeding practices because of relative caloric deprivation in the first few days of life. Decreased volume and frequency of feedings may result in mild dehydration and the delayed passage of meconium. This delayed defecation allows reuptake of bilirubin into the enterohepatic circulation and an increase in the serum level of unconjugated bilirubin. To prevent this, strategies to promote early effective breastfeeding are important. Current guidelines recommend early and frequent breastfeeding without supplemental water unless medically indicated (CPS, 2007a). Early frequent feedings can provide the newborn with adequate calories and fluid volume (via colostrum) to stimulate peristalsis and passage of meconium to eliminate bilirubin.

Late-Onset Breastfeeding Jaundice

Late-onset breastfeeding jaundice occurs later in the newborn period, with the bilirubin level usually peaking in the 6th to 14th day of life, but the levels are not considered pathologic (De Luca, Carnielli, & Paolillo, 2009). The specific cause of late-onset breastfeeding jaundice is not entirely understood, but it may be related to a change in the milk composition resulting in enhanced enterohepatic circulation. Additional research is needed to determine the cause. Interrupting breastfeeding is not recommended unless bilirubin levels reach dangerous levels; rarely is this necessary.

Pathologic Jaundice

Pathologic jaundice is manifested within the first 24 hours of life when total bilirubin levels rise rapidly in full-term infants, reaching 340 to 425 mmol/L (CPS, 2007a). The CPS has outlined risk factors for the development of severe hyperbilirubinemia and created evidence-based treatment guidelines. Conditions that alter the production, transport, uptake, metabolism, excretion, or reabsorption of bilirubin can cause pathologic jaundice in the newborn. A few conditions that contribute to red blood cell breakdown and thus higher bilirubin levels include polycythemia, blood incompatibilities, and systemic acidosis. These altered conditions can lead to high levels of unconjugated bilirubin, possibly reaching toxic levels and resulting in a severe condition called kernicterus.

Kernicterus (yellow nucleus) or bilirubin encephalopathy is a preventable neurologic disorder characterized by encephalopathy, motor abnormalities, hearing and vision loss, and death (Maisels, 2010). Neurotoxicity develops because unconjugated bilirubin has a high affinity for brain tissue, and bilirubin not bound to albumin is free to cross the blood–brain barrier and damage cells of the CNS.

In the acute stage, the newborn becomes lethargic, irritable, and hypotonic and sucks poorly. If the hyperbilirubinemia is not treated, the newborn becomes hypertonic, with arching and seizures. A high-pitched cry may be noted. These changes can occur rapidly, so all newborns must be assessed for jaundice and tested if indicated so that treatment can be initiated.

The most common condition associated with pathologic jaundice is hemolytic disease of the newborn secondary to incompatibility of blood groups of the mother and the newborn. The most frequent conditions are Rh factor and ABO incompatibilities.

> ▶ **Take** NOTE!
>
> *Significant jaundice in the newborn less than 24 hours of age should be reported immediately to the physician, as it may indicate a pathologic process.*

Rh Isoimmunization

Rh incompatibility or isoimmunization develops when an Rh-negative woman who has experienced Rh isoimmunization subsequently becomes pregnant with an Rh-positive fetus. The maternal antibodies cross the placenta into the fetal circulation and begin to break down the red blood cells (Fig. 24.6). Destruction of the fetal red blood cells leads to fetal anemia and hemolytic disease of the new-

born. The severity of the fetal hemolytic process depends on the level and effectiveness of anti-D antibodies and the capacity of the fetal system to remove antibody-coated cells. Intrauterine transfusions with Rh-negative, type O blood may be life-saving if performed in time (March of Dimes, 2009).

Immune hydrops, also called hydrops fetalis, is a severe form of hemolytic disease of the newborn that occurs when pathologic changes develop in the organs of the fetus secondary to severe anemia. Hydrops fetalis results from fetal hypoxia, anemia, congestive heart failure, and hypoproteinemia secondary to hepatic dysfunction. ABO and Rh incompatibilities can both cause hydrops fetalis, but Rh disease is the more common cause. Fetuses with hydrops may die in utero from profound anemia and circulatory failure. The placenta is very enlarged and edematous.

ABO Incompatibility

ABO incompatibility is an immune reaction that occurs when the mother has type O blood and the fetus has type A, B, or AB blood. Although it occurs more frequently than Rh incompatibilities, it causes less severe problems and rarely results in hemolytic disease severe enough to be clinically diagnosed and treated. Enlargement of the spleen and liver may be found in newborns with ABO incompatibility, but hydrops fetalis is rare (Martin & Cloherty, 2008). Because the antibodies resulting in ABO incompatibility occur naturally, it is impossible to eliminate this type of incompatibility.

Women with type O blood develop anti-A or anti-B antibodies throughout their life through foods they eat and exposure to infections. Most species of anti-A and anti-B antibodies are immunoglobulin M (IgM), which cannot cross the placenta and thus cannot gain access to the fetal red blood cells. Some anti-A and anti-B antibodies from the mother may cross the placenta to the fetus during the first pregnancy and can cause hemolysis of fetal blood cells.

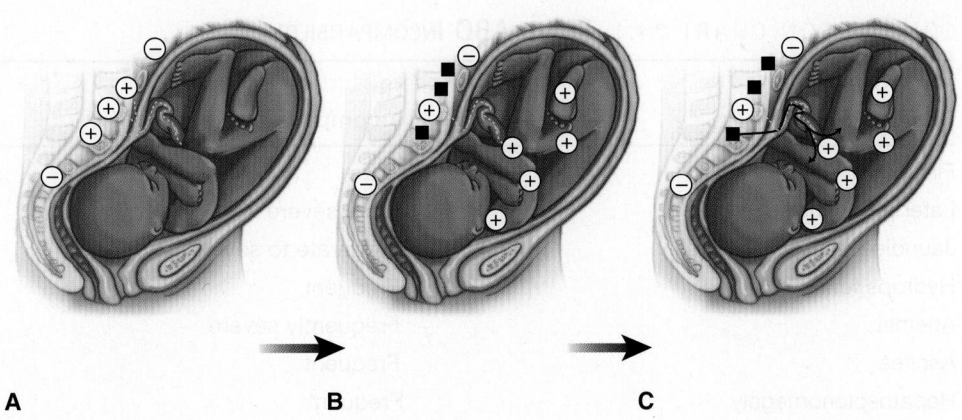

Subsequent Rh⊕fetus

FIGURE 24.6 Rh isoimmunization. (**A**) The Rh-negative mother is exposed to Rh-positive antigens. (**B**) Maternal antibodies form. (**C**) Rh antibodies are transferred to the fetus.

A   B   C

Nursing Assessment

Nurses play an important role in early detection and identification of jaundice in the newborn. Keen observation skills are essential.

Health History and Physical Examination

Review the medical record for factors that might predispose the newborn to hyperbilirubinemia, such as:

• Polycythemia
• Significant bruising or cephalhematoma, which increases bilirubin production
• Infections such as TORCH (toxoplasmosis, hepatitis B, rubella, cytomegalovirus, herpes simplex virus)
• Use of drugs during labour and birth such as diazepam (Valium) or oxytocin (Pitocin)
• Prematurity
• Gestational age of 34 to 36 weeks
• Hemolysis due to ABO incompatibility or Rh isoimmunization
• Macrosomic infant of a diabetic mother
• Delayed cord clamping, which increases the erythrocyte volume
• Decreased albumin binding sites to transport unconjugated bilirubin to the liver because of acidosis
• Delayed meconium passage, which increases the amount of bilirubin that returns to the unconjugated state and can be absorbed by the intestinal mucosa
• Siblings who had significant jaundice
• Inadequate breastfeeding leading to dehydration, decreased caloric intake, weight loss, and delayed passage of meconium
• Ethnicity, such as Asian, Mediterranean, or Aboriginal
• Male gender (Martin & Cloherty, 2008)

Perform a complete physical examination. Assess the skin, mucous membranes, sclerae, and bodily fluids (tears, urine) for a yellow colour. Detect jaundice by observing the infant in a well-lit room and blanching the skin with digital pressure over a bony prominence. Typically, jaundice begins on the head and gradually progresses to the abdomen and extremities. Also inspect for pallor (anemia), excessive bruising (bleeding), and dehydration (sluggish circulation), which may contribute to the development of jaundice and the risk for kernicterus.

Assess the newborn for Rh incompatibility. Be alert for clinical manifestations such as ascites, congestive heart failure, edema, pallor, jaundice, hepatosplenomegaly, hydramnios, thick placenta, and dilation of the umbilical vein (De Luca et al., 2009).

The hydropic newborn appears pale, edematous, and limp at birth and typically requires resuscitation. The newborn with immune hydrops exhibits severe generalized edema, organ hypertrophy and enlargement, and effusion of fluid into body cavities (Randenberg, 2010).

Laboratory and Diagnostic Testing

Determine maternal and fetal blood types, checking for incompatibilities (Comparison Chart 24.1). Assess laboratory values for bilirubin (both unconjugated and conjugated). Bilirubin levels establish the diagnosis of hyperbilirubinemia. The newborn with Rh incompatibility demonstrates a rapidly rising unconjugated bilirubin level at birth or in the first 24 hours. Also expect to obtain alkaline phosphatase, liver enzymes, and prothrombin time and partial thromboplastin time as well as:

• Direct Coombs test: to identify hemolytic disease of the newborn; positive results indicate that the newborn's red blood cells have been coated with antibodies and thus are sensitized
• Hemoglobin concentration: for evidence of anemia
• Blood type: to determine Rh status and any incompatibility of the newborn
• Total serum protein: to detect reduced binding capacity of albumin
• Reticulocyte count: to identify an elevated level indicating increased hemolysis

Assist with obtaining blood specimens. Use cord blood for hemoglobin concentration measurements; use a heel stick for direct Coombs testing and bilirubin levels. Prepare the parents and newborn for radiologic evaluation if necessary to determine abnormalities that may be causing the jaundice.

COMPARISON CHART 24.1   RH VS. ABO INCOMPATIBILITY

Clinical Picture	Rh Incompatibility	ABO Incompatibility
First-born	Rare	Common
Later pregnancies	More severe	No increase in severity
Jaundice	Moderate to severe	Mild
Hydrops fetalis	Frequent	Rare
Anemia	Frequently severe	Rare
Ascites	Frequent	Rare
Hepatosplenomegaly	Frequent	Common

Nursing Management

Nursing management of a newborn with hyperbilirubinemia requires a comprehensive approach. As members of the health care team, nurses share in the responsibility for early detection and identification, family education, management, and follow-up of the mother and the newborn. Documentation of the timing of onset of jaundice is essential to differentiate between physiologic (>24 hours) and pathologic (<24 hours) jaundice. Nurses can improve care by offering their presence and support.

Reducing Bilirubin Levels

Encourage early initiation of feedings to prevent hypoglycemia and provide protein to maintain the albumin levels to transport bilirubin to the liver. Ensure newborn feedings (breast milk or formula) every 2 to 3 hours to promote prompt emptying of bilirubin from the bowel. Encourage the mother to breastfeed (8 to 12 feedings per day) to prevent inadequate intake and thus dehydration. Supplement breast milk with formula only if bilirubin levels continue to increase with breastfeeding only. Monitor serum bilirubin levels frequently to reduce the risk for severe hyperbilirubinemia.

Phototherapy

For the newborn with jaundice, regardless of its etiology, phototherapy is used to convert unconjugated bilirubin to the less toxic water-soluble form that can be excreted. Phototherapy, via special lights placed above the newborn or a fibreoptic blanket placed under the newborn and wrapped around him or her, involves blue wavelengths of light to alter unconjugated bilirubin in the skin. For the newborn receiving phototherapy, place the infant under the lights or on the fibreoptic blanket, exposing as much skin as possible. Cover the newborn's genitals and shield the eyes to protect these areas from becoming irritated or burned when using direct lights. Assess the intensity of the light source to prevent burns and excoriation (Fig. 24.7). Turn the newborn every 2 hours to maximize the area of exposure, removing the newborn from the lights only for feedings. Maintain a neutral thermal environment to decrease energy expenditure, and assess the newborn's neurologic status frequently.

Assess the newborn's temperature every 3 to 4 hours as indicated. Monitor fluid intake and output closely and assess daily weights for gains or losses. Check skin turgor for dehydration.

With feedings, remove the newborn from the lights and remove the eye shields to allow interaction with the newborn. Encourage breast or bottle feedings every 2 to 3 hours. Follow agency policy about removing the eye shields periodically to assess the eyes for discharge or corneal irritation secondary to eye shield pressure.

Monitor stool for consistency and frequency. Unconjugated bilirubin excreted in the feces will produce a

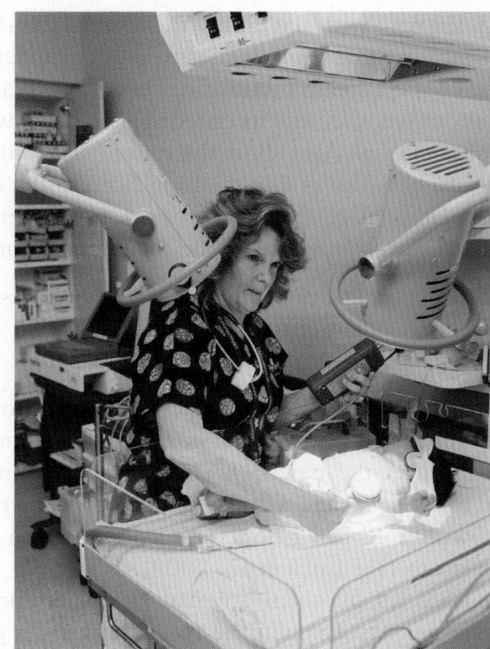

FIGURE 24.7 A newborn receiving phototherapy. Here the nurse is checking the intensity of the lights with a metre.

greenish appearance, and typically stools are loose. Lack of frequent green stools is a cause for concern.

Provide meticulous skin care. Assess skin surfaces frequently for dryness and irritation secondary to the dehydrating effects of phototherapy and irritation from highly acidic stool to prevent excoriation and skin breakdown (Martin & Cloherty, 2008). Monitor the newborn's skin turgor.

Exchange Transfusion

If the total serum bilirubin level remains elevated after intensive phototherapy, an exchange transfusion, the quickest method for lowering serum bilirubin levels, may be necessary (De Luca et al., 2009). In the presence of hemolytic disease, severe anemia, or a rapid rise in the total serum bilirubin level, an exchange transfusion is recommended. An exchange transfusion removes the newborn's blood and replaces it with nonhemolyzed red blood cells from a donor. During the transfusion, monitor the newborn's cardiovascular status continuously because serious complications can arise, such as acid–base imbalances, infection, hypovolemia, and fluid and electrolyte imbalances. Exchange transfusion is used only as a second-line therapy after phototherapy has failed to yield results. Intensive nursing care is needed.

Assist the physician with an exchange transfusion if necessary. Monitor the newborn's status closely for changes, especially in vital signs and heart rate and rhythm, before, during, and after the procedure.

Providing Parent Teaching and Support

Nurses can help the parents to understand the diagnostic tests and treatment modalities by offering individualized teaching. Explore with the family their understanding of jaundice and treatment modalities to reduce anxiety and gain their cooperation in monitoring the infant. Teach the parents about jaundice and its potential risk using written and verbal material. Also show the parents how to identify newborn behaviours that might indicate rising bilirubin levels. Emphasize the need to seek treatment from their pediatrician should any of the following occur:

- Lethargy, sleepiness, poor muscle tone, floppiness
- Poor sucking, lack of interest in feeding
- High-pitched cry

Teach the parents how to assess their newborn for signs of jaundice because physiologic jaundice may not occur until after the newborn is discharged. Reinforce the need for appropriate follow-up with the primary care provider within 48 to 72 hours after discharge to assess jaundice status (De Luca et al., 2009).

The need for phototherapy can be anxiety-producing for the parents. Explain the rationale for the procedure and demonstrate techniques that the parents can use to interact with their newborn. Additional education about phototherapy may be necessary when home phototherapy is used (Teaching Guideline 24.2).

Newborn Infections

Newborns are susceptible to infections because their immune system is immature and slow to react. The antibodies that newborns receive from their mother during pregnancy and from breast milk help protect them from invading organisms. However, these need time to reach optimal levels.

Bacterial infections of the newborn affect 1 to 4 of every 1,000 live births (Puopolo, 2008). Making the diagnosis of sepsis in newborns is difficult due to its nonspecific symptoms. The mortality rate from newborn sepsis may be as high as 50% if untreated. Infection is a major cause of death during the first month of life, contributing to 13% to 15% of all neonatal deaths (PHAC, 2008).

Pathophysiology

When a pathogenic organism overcomes the newborn's defenses, infection and sepsis result. **Neonatal sepsis** is the presence of bacterial, fungal, or viral microorganisms or their toxins in blood or other tissues. Infections that have an onset within the first month of life are termed newborn infections. Exposure to a pathogenic organism, whether a virus, fungus, or bacteria, occurs, and the organism enters the newborn's body and begins to multiply.

Newborn infections are usually grouped into three classes according to their time of onset: congenital infection, which is acquired in utero (intrauterine infections) by vertical transmission with onset before birth; early-onset infections, acquired by vertical transmission in the perinatal period, either shortly before or during birth; and late-onset infections, acquired by horizontal transmission in the nursery. As many as 80% to 90% of neonatal infections have their onset in the first 2 days of life (CPS, 2007b). Comparison Chart 24.2 compares the three classes of newborn infections.

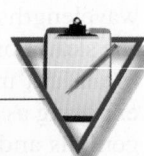

TEACHING GUIDELINE 24.2

Caring for Your Newborn Receiving Home Phototherapy

- Inspect your newborn's skin, eyes, and mucous membranes for a yellow colour.
- Remember that a public health nurse will come to visit and help you set up the light system.
- Keep the lights about 30.5 to 76 centimetres (12 to 30 inches) above your newborn.
- Cover your newborn's eyes with eye patches to protect them.
- Keep your newborn undressed except for the diaper area; fold the diaper down below your newborn's navel in the front and as far as possible in the back to expose as much skin area as possible.
- Turn your newborn every 2 hours so that all areas of the body are exposed.
- Remove your newborn from the lights only for feeding.
- Remove the eye patches during feedings so that you can interact with your newborn.

- Record your newborn's temperature, weight, and fluid intake daily.
- Document the frequency, colour, and consistency of all stools; the stools should be loose and green as the bilirubin is broken down.
- Keep the skin clean and dry to prevent irritation.
- Feed your newborn frequently, including supplemental glucose water if allowed, to provide added fluid, protein, and calories.
- Rock, cuddle, or hold your newborn to promote bonding when out of the lights.
- Contact your pediatrician or home health care agency with any questions or changes, including refusing feedings, fewer than five wet diapers in one day, vomiting of complete amounts of feeding, or elevated temperature.
- Keep appointments for follow-up laboratory testing to monitor bilirubin levels.

Nursing Assessment

Nursing assessment focuses on early identification of a newborn at risk for infection to allow for prompt treatment, thus reducing mortality and morbidity. Be aware of the myriad risk factors associated with newborn sepsis.

Among the factors that contribute to the newborn's overall vulnerability to infection are poor skin integrity, invasive procedures, exposure to numerous caregivers, and an environment conducive to bacterial colonization (Puopolo, 2008).

COMPARISON CHART 24.2   INTRAUTERINE VS. EARLY-ONSET VS. LATE-ONSET NEWBORN INFECTIONS

	Intrauterine (Congenital) Infections	Early-Onset Infections	Late-Onset Infections
Risk factors	• Immature immune system IgM, IgA, and T lymphocytes • Decreased gastric acid, which is needed to reduce organisms	• Prolonged rupture of membranes • Urinary tract infections • Preterm labour • Prolonged or difficult labour • Maternal fever • Colonization with group B streptococci • Maternal infections • Low birth weight • Prematurity • Meconium staining • Need for resuscitation • Birth asphyxia • Improper handwashing	
Common causative organisms	• Cytomegalovirus • Rubella • Toxoplasmosis • Syphilis	• *Escherichia coli* • Group B streptococci • *Klebsiella pneumoniae* • *Listeria monocytogenes* • Other enteric gram-negative bacilli	• *Candida albicans* • Coagulase-negative staphylococci • *Staphylococcus aureus* • *E. coli* • *Enterobacter* • *Klebsiella* • *Serratia* • *Pseudomonas* • Group B streptococci
Mechanism of infection	• Organism crossing placenta into fetal circulatory system; organism residing in amniotic fluid. • Ascent of organism via the vagina, ultimately infecting membranes and causing rupture and leading to respiratory and gastrointestinal tract infections.	Most occur during birthing process when newborn comes into contact with infected birth canal (newborn cannot defend against host organisms). • Newborn susceptibility to infection by exogenous organisms possibly due to inadequacy of physical barriers (thin, friable skin with little subcutaneous tissue). • Lack of gastric acidity, possibly resulting in easy colonization by environmental organisms • Aspiration of microorganisms during birth with development of pneumonia	More common in newborns undergoing invasive procedures such as endotracheal intubation or catheter insertion; break in skin or mucosal protection barrier.

Sources: Canadian Paediatric Society. (2007b). Position statement (FN2007–03): Management of the infant at increased risk for sepsis. *Pediatrics & Child Health*, *12*(10), 893–898. Retrieved March 14, 2012 from http://www.cps.ca/english/statements/FN/FN07–03.pdf; Kane, E., & Bretz, G. (2011). Reduction in coagulase-negative staphylococcus infection rates in the NICU using evidence-based research. *Neonatal Network*, *30*(3), 165–174; Puopolo, K. M. (2008). Bacterial and fungal infections. In J. Cloherty, E. C. Eichenwald, & A. R. Stark (Eds.), *Manual of neonatal care* (6th ed.). Philadelphia: Lippincott Williams & Wilkins; and Tappero, E., & Johnson, P. (2010). Laboratory evaluation of neonatal sepsis. *Newborn and Infant Nursing Reviews*, *10*(4), 209–217.

Few newborn infections are easy to recognize because manifestations usually are nonspecific. Early symptoms can be vague because of the newborn's inability to mount an inflammatory response. Often, the observation is that the newborn does not "look right." Assess the newborn for common nonspecific signs of infection, including:

- Hypothermia
- Pallor or duskiness
- Hypotonia
- Cyanosis
- Poor weight gain
- Irritability
- Seizures
- Jaundice
- Grunting
- Nasal flaring
- Apnea and bradycardia
- Lethargy
- Hypoglycemia
- Poor feeding (lack of interest in feeding)
- Abdominal distention (Tappero & Johnson, 2010)

Since infection can be confused with other newborn conditions, laboratory and radiographic tests are needed to confirm the presence of infection. Be prepared to coordinate the timing of the various tests and assist as necessary.

Evaluate the complete blood count with a differential to identify anemia, leukocytosis, or leukopenia. Elevated C-reactive protein levels may indicate inflammation. As ordered, obtain X-rays of the chest and abdomen, which may reveal infectious processes located there. Blood, cerebrospinal fluid, and urine cultures are indicated to identify the location and type of infection present. Positive cultures confirm that the newborn has an infection.

Nursing Management

To enhance the newborn's chance of survival, early recognition and diagnosis are the keys. Often the diagnosis of sepsis is based on a suspicious clinical picture. Antibiotic therapy is usually started before the laboratory results identify the infecting pathogen (see Evidence-based Practice 24.1). Along with antibiotic therapy, circulatory, respiratory, nutritional, and developmental support is important. Antibiotic therapy is continued for 7 to 21 days if cultures are positive and discontinued if cultures are negative after 48 hours (CPS, 2007b). The use of antibiotics, along with early recognition and supportive care, have greatly reduced mortality and morbidity related to sepsis (Tappero & Johnson, 2010).

Nurses possess the education and assessment tools to decrease the incidence and reduce the impact of infections on women (see Chapter 20 for additional information) and their newborns. Implement measures for prevention and early recognition, including:

- Formulating a sepsis prevention plan that includes education of all members of the health care team on identification and treatment of sepsis
- Screening all newborns daily for signs of sepsis
- Monitoring sepsis cases and outcomes to reinforce continued quality-improvement measures or to modify current practices
- Outlining and carrying out measures to prevent nosocomial infections, such as:
  - Thorough handwashing hygiene for all staff
  - Frequent oral care and inspections of mucous membranes
  - Proper positioning and turning to prevent skin breakdown
  - Use of strict aseptic technique for all wound care
  - Frequent monitoring of invasive catheter sites for signs of infection
- Identifying newborns at risk for sepsis by reviewing risk factors
- Monitoring vital sign changes and observing for subtle signs of infection
- Monitoring for signs of organ system dysfunction:
  - Cardiovascular compromise: tachycardia and hypotension
  - Respiratory compromise: respiratory distress and tachypnea
  - Renal compromise: oliguria or anuria
  - Systemic compromise: abnormal blood values
- Providing comprehensive sepsis treatment:
  - Circulatory support with fluids and vasopressors
  - Supplemental oxygen and mechanical ventilation
  - Obtaining culture samples as requested
  - Antibiotic administration as ordered, observing for side effects
  - Promoting newborn comfort
- Assessing the family's educational needs and providing instructions as necessary

Perinatal infections continue to be a public health problem, with severe consequences for those affected. By promoting a better understanding of newborn infections and appropriate use of therapies, nurses can lower the mortality rates associated with severe sepsis, especially with appropriate timing of interventions. The potential for nursing interventions to identify, prevent, and minimize the risk for sepsis is significant. Primary disease prevention must be a major focus for nurses. Family education plays a key role in the prevention of perinatal infections, in addition to following accepted practices in immunization.

Congenital Conditions

Congenital conditions can arise from many etiologies, including single-gene disorders, chromosome aberrations, exposure to teratogens, and many sporadic conditions of unknown cause. Congenital conditions may be inherited or sporadic, isolated or multiple, apparent or hidden,

EVIDENCE-BASED PRACTICE 24.1
Treating Neonatal Sepsis with Gentamicin Given as a Once-Daily Dose or as Multiple Doses per Day

● Study

Sepsis in a newborn can be fatal, and the signs and symptoms can be vague. Because of the high risk for morbidity when treatment is delayed, antibiotic therapy is usually initiated before the infection is confirmed by cultures. Gentamicin is a common antibiotic used to treat neonatal sepsis because of its effectiveness against gram-negative pathogens. However, gentamicin, like other aminoglycosides, can have adverse effects on hearing and kidney function, leading to questions about the most effective dosing regimen. Studies have shown that once-a-day dosing is most effective in older children and adults. In newborns, twice-daily dosing has been the common regimen for some time; however, recent studies have demonstrated effective treatment with reduced risk in longer-interval dosing, up to 48 hours in small premature infants.

A retrospective comparative study involving neonates with confirmed or suspected sepsis was completed to evaluate the effectiveness and safety of two types of dosing regimens: once-a-day dosing and multiple-doses-per-day dosing over a 28-month period. The population selected for the study included infants born at more than 28 weeks' gestation admitted to the NICU. Information about clinical effectiveness, pharmacokinetic effectiveness, ototoxicity, and nephrotoxicity was collected. The aim of the study was to contribute to building evidence of the effectiveness

of once-a-day dosing. Over the study period newborns were assigned to one of two groups, once-daily dosage of 4 mg/kg and twice-daily dosage of 2.5 mg/kg given via intravenous infusion.

▲ Findings

Regardless of the dosing regimen, gentamicin was shown to be effective in treating sepsis. The once-daily dosing regimen appeared to be more effective, with higher peak levels and lower trough levels of the drug in the single-dose group compared with the multiple-dose group. A high trough level in either group is related to higher incidence of ototoxicity and nephrotoxicity. However, the study suggests that daily dosing may be more therapeutic with less risk for ototoxicity or nephrotoxicity.

■ Nursing Implications

The study confirmed the effectiveness of gentamicin in the treatment of neonatal sepsis, but it did not determine whether a once-daily dose was more effective than multiple doses per day. Nurses can integrate the findings of this study into their practice when caring for newborns who are at risk for or have developed sepsis. Regardless of the regimen ordered, nurses can be diligent in ensuring that trough drug levels are monitored. Although the study showed no evidence of hearing and kidney adverse effects, nurses still need to monitor newborns for this possibility.

Source: Hagen, I., & Oymar, K. (2008). Pharmacologic differences between once daily and twice daily gentamicin dosage in newborns with suspected sepsis. *Pharmacy World and Science*, *31*, 18–23.

---

gross or microscopic. They cause nearly half of all deaths in term newborns and cause long-term sequelae for many. The incidence varies according to the type of defect. When a serious anomaly is identified prenatally, the parents can decide whether or not to continue the pregnancy. When an anomaly is identified at or after birth, parents need to be informed promptly and given a realistic appraisal of the severity of the condition, the prognosis, and treatment options so that they can participate in all decisions pertaining to their child.

Congenital conditions can affect virtually any body system. This chapter describes those congenital conditions that require immediate treatment or affect the newborn in the period immediately after birth. Other congenital conditions, such as congenital heart disease or CNS defects, are discussed in later chapters due to their long-term nature and ongoing effects.

Esophageal Atresia and Tracheoesophageal Fistula

Esophageal atresia and tracheoesophageal fistula are GI anomalies in which the esophagus and trachea do not sep-

arate normally during embryonic development. Esophageal atresia refers to a congenitally interrupted esophagus where the proximal and distal ends do not communicate; the upper esophageal segment ends in a blind pouch and the lower segment ends a variable distance above the diaphragm (Fig. 24.8).

Tracheoesophageal fistula is an abnormal communication between the trachea and esophagus. When associated with esophageal atresia, the fistula most commonly occurs between the distal esophageal segment and the trachea. The incidence of esophageal atresia is 1 per 3,000 to 4,500 live births (Lovvorn, Glenn, Pacceti, et al., 2011).

Pathophysiology

Several types of esophageal atresia exist, but the most common anomaly is a fistula between the distal esophagus and the trachea, which occurs in 86% of newborns with an esophageal defect. Esophageal atresia and tracheoesophageal fistula are thought to be the result of incomplete separation of the lung bed from the foregut during early fetal development (de Jong, Felix, de Klein, et al., 2010). A large percentage of these newborns have other congenital anomalies involving the vertebra,

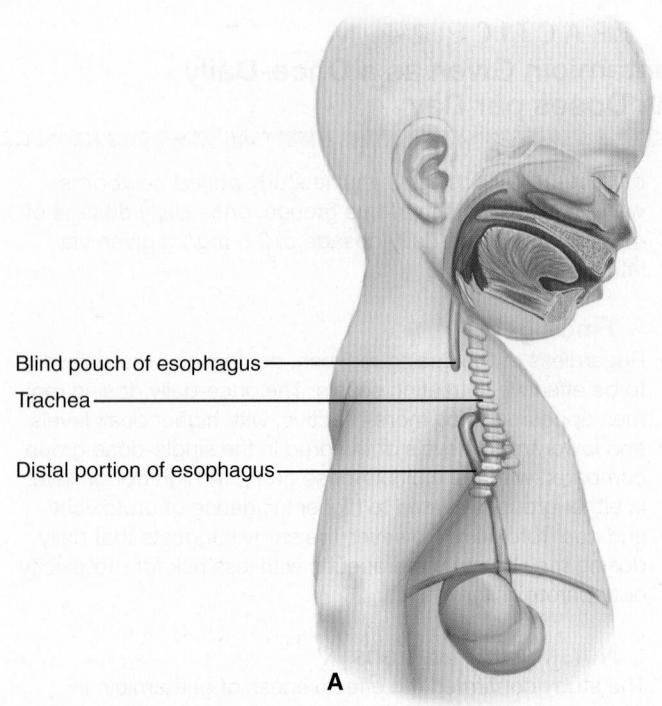

Blind pouch of esophagus

Trachea

Distal portion of esophagus

A

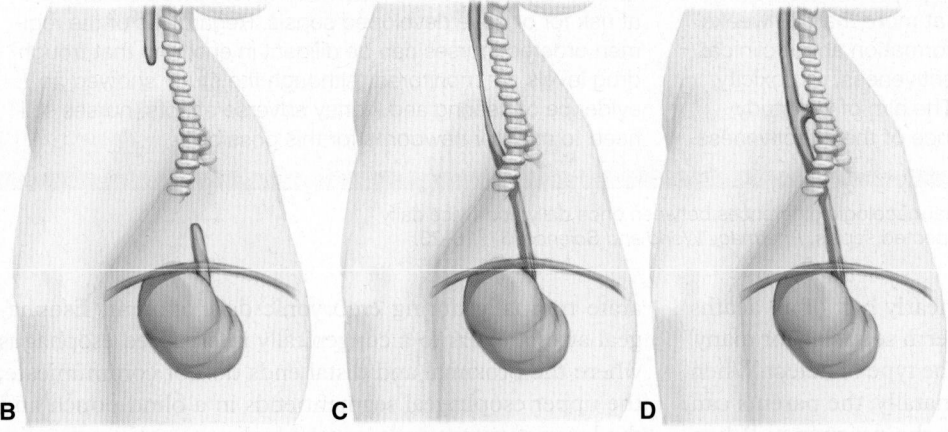

B   **C**   **D**

FIGURE 24.8 Esophageal atresia and tracheoesophageal fistula. (**A**) The most common type of esophageal atresia, in which the esophagus ends in a blind pouch and a fistula connects the trachea with the distal portion of the esophagus. (**B**) The upper and distal portions of the esophagus end in a blind pouch. (**C**) The esophagus is one segment, but a portion of it is narrowed. (**D**) The upper portion of the esophagus connects to the trachea via a fistula.

kidneys, heart, and musculoskeletal and GI systems (Lovvorn et al., 2011); most have several anomalies.

Nursing Assessment

Review the maternal history for polyhydramnios. Often this is the first sign of esophageal atresia because the fetus cannot swallow and absorb amniotic fluid in utero, leading to accumulation. Soon after birth, the newborn may exhibit copious, frothy bubbles of mucus in the mouth and nose, accompanied by drooling. Abdominal distention develops as air builds up in the stomach. In esophageal atresia, a gastric tube cannot be inserted beyond a certain point because the esophagus ends in a blind pouch. The newborn may have rattling respirations, excessive salivation and drooling, and "the three

C's" (coughing, choking, and cyanosis) if feeding is attempted. The presence of a fistula increases the risk for respiratory complications such as pneumonitis and atelectasis due to aspiration of food and secretions

▶ *Take* NOTE!

The "three C's" of choking, coughing, and cyanosis in conjunction with feeding are considered the classic signs of tracheoesophageal fistula and atresia.

Prepare the newborn and parents for radiographic evaluation. Diagnosis is made by X-ray: a gastric tube appears coiled in the upper esophageal pouch, and air in the GI tract indicates the presence of a fistula (Lovvorn et al., 2011). Once a diagnosis of esophageal atresia is established, begin preparations for surgery if the newborn is stable.

Nursing Management

Nursing management focuses on preparing the newborn and parents for surgery and providing meticulous postoperative care.

Providing Preoperative Care

Preoperative nursing interventions include the following measures:

- Initiate nothing by mouth (NPO) status.
- Elevate the head of the bed 30 to 45 degrees to prevent reflux and aspiration.
- Monitor hydration status and fluid and electrolyte balance; administer and monitor parenteral IV fluid infusions.
- Assess and maintain the patency of the orogastric tube; monitor the functioning of the tube, which is attached to low continuous suction; and avoid irrigation of the tube to prevent aspiration.
- Have oxygen and suctioning equipment readily available should the newborn experience respiratory distress.
- Assist with diagnostic studies to rule out other anomalies.
- Use comfort measures to minimize crying and prevent respiratory distress; provide non-nutritive sucking.
- Inform the parents about the rationales for the aspiration prevention measures.
- Document frequent observations of the newborn's condition.

Providing Postoperative Care

Surgery consists of closing the fistula and joining the two esophageal segments. Postoperative care involves closely observing all of the newborn's body systems to identify any complications. Expect to administer TPN and antibiotics until the esophageal anastomosis is proven intact and patent. Then begin oral feedings, usually within a week after surgery. Keep the parents informed of their newborn's condition and progress. Closely assess the newborn during feeding and report any difficulty with swallowing. Provide parent teaching. Demonstrate and reinforce all teaching prior to discharge.

Omphalocele and Gastroschisis

Omphalocele and gastroschisis are congenital anomalies of the anterior abdominal wall. An **omphalocele** is a defect of the umbilical ring that allows evisceration of the abdominal contents into an external peritoneal sac. Defects vary in size; they may be limited to bowel loops or may include the entire GI tract and liver (Fig. 24.9).

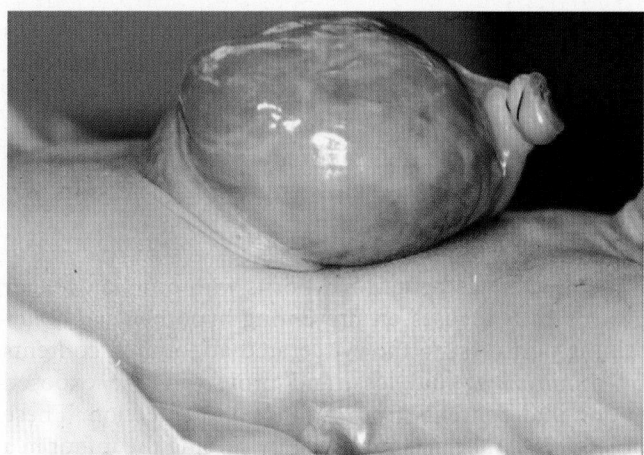

FIGURE 24.9 Omphalocele in a newborn. Note the large, protruding sac.

Bowel malrotation is common, but the displaced organs are usually normal. Omphaloceles are associated with other anomalies in more than 70% of cases. This anomaly is usually detected during routine prenatal ultrasound of the fetus or during investigation of an increased alpha-fetoprotein level (Lovvorn et al., 2011).

Gastroschisis is a herniation of the abdominal contents through an abdominal wall defect, usually to the left or right of the umbilicus (Lovvorn et al., 2011). Gastroschisis differs from omphalocele in that there is no peritoneal sac protecting the herniated organs, and thus exposure to amniotic fluid makes them thickened, edematous, and inflamed (Ringer & Hansen, 2008). Gastroschisis is associated with significant newborn morbidity and mortality rates. Despite surgical correction, feeding intolerance, failure to thrive, and prolonged hospital stays occur in nearly all newborns with this anomaly (Lovvorn et al., 2011).

Each of these diagnoses requires that a pediatric surgeon be available at delivery to determine the extent of the defect and complications.

Nursing Assessment

Review the maternal history for factors associated with high-risk pregnancies, such as maternal illness and infection, drug use, smoking, and genetic abnormalities. These factors are also associated with omphalocele and gastroschisis. They contribute to placental insufficiency and the birth of an SGA or preterm newborn, the populations in which both of these abdominal defects most commonly occur. The combined incidence of both congenital abdominal wall anomalies is 1 in 2,000 births (Lovvorn et al., 2011).

Omphalocele and gastroschisis are readily observed. Note the appearance of the protrusion on the abdomen and evidence of a sac. Inspect the sac closely for the presence of organs, most commonly the intestines but sometimes the liver. Also inspect the contents for any twisting of the intestines. Note the colour of the organs within the sac and measure the size of the omphalocele.

Also perform a complete physical examination of the newborn. Typically these congenital conditions are associated with other congenital anomalies, such as those involving the cardiovascular, genitourinary, and CNSs.

Nursing Management

Nursing management of newborns with omphalocele or gastroschisis focuses on preventing hypothermia, maintaining perfusion to the eviscerated abdominal contents by minimizing fluid loss, and protecting the exposed abdominal contents from trauma and infection. These objectives can be accomplished by placing the infant in a sterile drawstring bowel bag that maintains a sterile environment for the exposed contents, allows visualization, reduces heat and moisture loss, and allows heat from radiant warmers to reach the newborn. The newborn is placed feet-first into the bag and the drawstring is secured around the torso (Lovvorn et al., 2011). Strict sterile technique is necessary to prevent contamination of the exposed abdominal contents.

An orogastric tube attached to low suction is used to prevent intestinal distention. IV therapy is administered to maintain fluid and electrolyte balance and provide a route for antibiotic therapy. Monitor the newborn's fluid status frequently. Closely observe the exposed bowel for vascular compromise, such as changes in colour or a decrease in temperature, and report these immediately.

Providing Postoperative Care

Surgical repair of both defects occurs after initial stabilization and comprehensive evaluation for any other anomalies. It may have to occur in stages, depending on the defect (Box 24.5).

> **BOX 24.5   Surgery to Repair Omphalocele and Gastroschisis**
>
> Surgical repair of gastroschisis is an emergency due to the high risk for intestinal atresia, resulting in obstruction. Primary repair of gastroschisis is usually performed without incident, unless the contents are unable to fit into the abdominal cavity. This occurs more often with a large omphalocele, requiring the surgeon to do a staged closure. This involves covering the defect with a synthetic material that is sequentially squeezed like toothpaste to reduce the defect into the abdominal cavity. After enough of the defect is in the abdominal cavity, a surgical repair is then performed (Islam, 2008). If damage to the exposed organs occurs, such as necrosis, then the necrotic sections are removed during the repair. If a significant amount of small intestine is lost, then the complication of short bowel syndrome may occur.

Postoperative care involves providing pain management, monitoring respiratory and cardiac status, monitoring intake and output, assessing for vascular compromise, maintaining the orogastric tube to suction, documenting the amount and colour of drainage, and administering ordered medications and treatments (Lovvorn et al., 2011). Also be alert for complications, such as short bowel syndrome (see Chapter 41 for additional information).

Promoting Parent–Newborn Interaction

The parents need continued support and progress reports on their newborn. They may be distraught at the sight of the anomaly, and they may be frightened to touch their newborn. Encourage the parents to touch the newborn and participate in care as much as possible. Because of the nature of this defect, bonding opportunities will be limited initially. However, strongly encourage frequent visiting. In addition, provide information to the parents about the defect, treatment modalities, and prognosis. After surgery, instruct the parents in care measures and provide them with home care instructions. Anticipate the need for a referral to a home health care agency and community resources for support.

Imperforate Anus

An imperforate anus is a GI system malformation of the anorectal area that may occur in several forms. The rectum may end in a blind pouch that does not connect to the colon, or it may have fistulas (openings) between the rectum and the perineum, the vagina in girls or the urethra in boys (Fig. 24.10). The malformations occur during early fetal development and are associated with anomalies in other body systems.

Imperforate anus occurs in about 1 of every 5,000 live births (Lovvorn et al., 2011). The defect can be further classified as a high or low type, depending on its level. The level significantly influences the outcome in

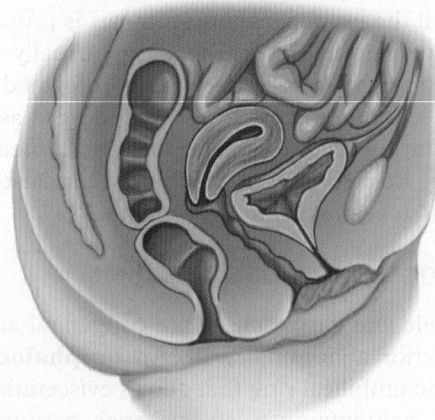

FIGURE 24.10 Imperforate anus, in which the rectum ends in a blind pouch.

terms of fecal continence as well as management (Lovvorn et al., 2011).

Surgical intervention is needed for both high and low types of imperforate anus. Surgery for a high type of defect involves a colostomy in the newborn period, with corrective surgery performed in stages to allow for growth. Surgery for the low type of anomaly, which frequently includes a fistula, involves closure of the fistula, creation of an anal opening, and repositioning of the rectal pouch into the anal opening. A major challenge for either type of surgical repair is finding, using, or creating adequate nerve and muscle structures around the rectum to provide for normal evacuation.

Nursing Assessment

In the newborn, observe for an appropriate anal opening. If the anal opening exists, observe for passage of meconium stool within the first 24 hours of life. Assess urine output to identify genitourinary problems. For the newborn with an imperforate anus, inspection of the perineal area would reveal absence of the usual opening. In addition, meconium generally is not passed or present within 24 hours of birth.

In the infant with suspected imperforate anus, assess for common signs of intestinal obstruction, which may occur as a result of the malformation. These include abdominal distention and bilious vomiting.

Prepare the newborn and family for radiographic studies that may be ordered to assess for complications associated with imperforate anus.

Nursing Management

Nursing management focuses on preparing the newborn and parent for surgery and providing postoperative care. Preoperatively, maintain the newborn's NPO status and provide gastric decompression. Administer IV therapy and antibiotic therapy as ordered and monitor the newborn's hydration status. Provide a full explanation of the defect, surgical options, potential complications, typical postoperative course, and long-term care needed to the parents. Make sure they are aware of the available treatment modalities. Prepare them for the possibility that the newborn may require an ostomy. Provide support to the parents and family.

Postoperative care includes ensuring adequate pain relief, maintaining NPO status and gastric decompression until normal bowel function is restored, and providing colostomy care if applicable.

Bladder Exstrophy

In bladder exstrophy, the bladder protrudes onto the abdominal wall because the abdominal wall failed to close during embryonic development. Wide separation of the rectus muscles and the symphysis pubis accompanies this defect. Virtually all affected male infants have associated epispadias. The upper urinary tract is usually normal. The incidence is approximately 1 in 10,000 to 50,000 live births (Tu, Chueh, & Kennedy, 2009). Initial bladder closure is completed within 48 hours after birth. Further surgical reconstruction is performed in several stages at about 2 to 3 years of age. (See Chapter 42 for more information.)

■■■ Key Concepts

- Asphyxia, the most common clinical insult in the perinatal period, results in brain injury and may lead to mental retardation, cerebral palsy, or seizures.
- TTN occurs when the liquid in the lung is removed slowly or incompletely.
- Common risk factors for RDS include young gestational age, perinatal asphyxia regardless of gestational age, cesarean birth in the absence of labour (related to the lack of thoracic squeeze), male gender, and maternal diabetes.
- Meconium aspiration has three major pulmonary effects: airway obstruction, surfactant dysfunction, and chemical pneumonitis.
- The management of persistent pulmonary hypertension of the newborn requires meticulous attention to detail, with continuous monitoring of oxygenation, blood pressure, and perfusion.
- Periventricular/intraventricular hemorrhage is bleeding that usually originates in the subependymal germinal matrix region of the brain with extension into the ventricular system.
- NEC is a serious GI disease of unknown etiology in newborns that can result in necrosis of a segment of the bowel.
- Infants of diabetic mothers are at risk for malformations most frequently involving the cardiovascular, skeletal, central nervous, GI, and genitourinary systems; cardiac anomalies are the most common.
- Factors that place the newborn at risk for birth trauma include cephalopelvic disproportion, maternal pelvic anomalies, oligohydramnios, prolonged or rapid labour, abnormal presentation, fetal prematurity, fetal macrosomia, and fetal abnormalities.
- Women who use drugs during their pregnancy expose their unborn child to the possibility of IUGR, prematurity, neurobehavioural and neurophysiologic dysfunction, birth defects, infections, and long-term developmental sequelae.
- Newborns of women who abuse tobacco, illicit substances, caffeine, and alcohol can exhibit withdrawal behaviour.
- Physiologic jaundice is a common, normal newborn phenomenon that appears during the second or third day of life and then declines over the first week after birth. Pathologic jaundice is manifested within the first 24 hours of life when total bilirubin levels increase

significantly and the total serum bilirubin level is higher than 350 mmol/L in a full-term infant.

■ Newborn infections are usually classified according to the time of onset and grouped into three categories: congenital infection, acquired in utero by vertical transmission with onset before birth; early-onset neonatal infections, acquired by vertical transmission in the perinatal period, either shortly before or during birth; and late-onset neonatal infections, acquired by horizontal transmission in the nursery.

■ Congenital conditions can arise from many etiologies, including single-gene disorders, chromosome aberrations, exposure to teratogens, and many sporadic conditions of unknown cause. Congenital structural anomalies may be inherited or sporadic, isolated or multiple, apparent or hidden, and gross or microscopic.

■ Esophageal atresia refers to a congenitally interrupted esophagus where the proximal and distal ends do not communicate; the upper esophageal segment ends in a blind pouch and the lower segment ends a variable distance above the diaphragm. Tracheoesophageal fistula is an abnormal communication between the trachea and esophagus.

■ Omphalocele and gastroschisis are congenital anomalies of the anterior abdominal wall. An omphalocele is a defect of the umbilical ring that allows evisceration of abdominal contents into an external peritoneal sac. Gastroschisis is a herniation of abdominal contents through an abdominal wall defect, usually to the left or right of the umbilicus.

REFERENCES

Acute Care of at-Risk Newborns (ACoRN) Neonatal Society. (2009). *ACoRN: Acute care of at-risk newborns.* ACoRN Neonatal Society. Vancouver, BC: Author.

Arenson, J., & Drake, P. (2007). *Maternal and newborn health.* Sudbury, MA: Jones and Bartlett Publishers.

Asenjo, M. (2011). *Imaging in transient tachypnea of the newborn.* Retrieved March 14, 2012 from http://www.emedicine.com/radio/topic710.htm

Askin, D. F. (2009). Fetal-to-neonatal transition—What is normal and what is not? Part 2: Red flags. *Neonatal Network, 28*(3), e37–e40.

Bhakti, K. Y. (2008). Respiratory distress syndrome. In J. Cloherty, E. C. Eichenwald, & A. R. Stark (Eds.), *Manual of neonatal care* (6th ed.). Philadelphia: Lippincott Williams & Wilkins.

Blackburn, S.T. (2007). *Maternal, fetal and neonatal physiology: A clinical perspective* (3rd ed.). St. Louis: Saunders Elsevier.

Bradshaw, W. T. (2009). Necrotizing enterocolitis: Etiology, presentation, management, and outcomes. *Journal of Perinatal and Neonatal Nursing, 23*(1), 87–94.

Canadian Paediatric Society. (2007a). Position statement (FN 2007–02): Guidelines for the detection, management and prevention of hyperbilirubinemia in term and late preterm newborn infants (35 or more weeks' gestation). *Pediatrics and Child Health, 12*(Suppl. B), 1B–12B. Retrieved March 14, 2012 from http://www.cps.ca/english/statements/fn/fn07–02.htm

Canadian Paediatric Society. (2007b). Position statement (FN2007–03): Management of the infant at increased risk for sepsis. *Pediatrics and Child Health, 12*(10), 893–898. Retrieved March 14, 2012 from http://www.cps.ca/english/statements/FN/FN07–03.pdf

Centers for Disease Control and Prevention. (2007). *Surgeon general's report: Women and smoking fact sheet: Tobacco use and reproduc-tive outcomes.* Retrieved March 14, 2012 from http://www.cdc.gov/tobacco/data_statistics/sgr/2001/highlights/outcomes/index.htm

Chertok, I. R., Raz, I., Shoham, I., Haddad, H., & Wiznitzer, A. (2009). Effects of early breastfeeding on neonatal glucose levels of term infants born to women with gestational diabetes. *Journal of Human Nutrition and Dietetics, 22,* 166–169.

Cleveland, L. M. (2009). Symbolic interactionism and nurse-mother communication in the neonatal intensive care. *Research and Theory for Nursing Practice, 23*(3), 216–229.

Consortium on Safe Labour. (2010). Respiratory morbidity in late preterm births. *Journal of the American Medical Association, 304*(4), 419–425.

Cooper, D. J. (2011). Induced hypothermia for neonatal hypoxic-ischemic encephalopathy: Pathophysiology, current treatment, and nursing considerations. *Neonatal Network, 30*(1), 30–35.

Davis, K., Desrocher, M., & Moore, T. (2011). Fetal alcohol spectrum disorder: A review of neurodevelopmental findings and interventions. *Journal of Developmental and Physical Disabilities, 23*(2), 143–167.

de Jong, E. M., Felix, J. F., de Klein, A., & Tibboel, D. (2010). Etiology of esophageal atresia and tracheoesophageal fistula: "mind the gap." *Current Gastroenterology Reports, 12*(3), 215–222.

De Luca, D., Carnielli, V. P., & Paolillo, P. (2009). Neonatal hyperbilirubinemia and early discharge from the maternity ward. *European Journal of Pediatrics, 168*(9), 1025–1030.

Finan, E., Aylward, D., Aziz, K., and Canadian Paediatric Society, Neonatal Resuscitation Program Executive Committee. (2011). Neonatal resuscitation guidelines update: A case-based review. *Paediatrics and Child Health, 16*(5), 289–291.

First Nations and Inuit Health Committee & Canadian Paediatric Society. (2012). *Position Statement: Fetal Alcohol Syndrome.* Retrieved May 26, 2012 from http://www.cps.ca/english/statements/II/ii02-01.htm

Gardner, S. L., Enzman-Hines, M., & Dickey, L. (2011). Respiratory diseases. In S. Gardner, B. Carter, M. Enzman-Hines, & J. Hernandez (Eds.), *Merenstein & Gardner's handbook of neonatal intensive care.* St. Louis, MO: Mosby Elsevier.

Gregory, K. E. (2008). Predictors of necrotizing enterocolitis in premature infants. *Nursing Research, 57*(4), 260–270.

Harris, L. L., & Stark, A. R. (2008). Meconium aspiration. In J. Cloherty, E. C. Eichenwald, & A. R. Stark (Eds.), *Manual of neonatal care* (6th ed.). Philadelphia: Lippincott Williams & Wilkins.

Hatfield, L., Shwoebel, A., & Lynyak, C. (2011). Caring for the infant of the diabetic mother. *Maternal/Child Nursing, 36*(1), 10–16.

Islam, S. (2008). Clinical care outcomes in abdominal wall defects. *Current Opinion in Pediatrics, 20*(3), 305–310.

Jansson, L. M., Choo, R., Velez, M. L., et al. (2008). Methadone maintenance and breastfeeding in the neonatal period. *Pediatrics, 121,* 106–114.

Kane, E., & Bretz, G. (2011). Reduction in coagulase-negative staphylococcus infection rates in the NICU using evidence-based research. *Neonatal Network, 30*(3), 165–174.

Kattwinkel, J., Perlman, J. M., Aziz, K., et al. (2010). Special report—Neonatal resuscitation: 2010 American Health Association guidelines for cardiopulmonary resuscitation and emergency cardiovascular care. *Pediatrics, 126*(5), e1400–e1411. Retrieved March 14, 2012 from http://pediatrics.aappublications.org/content/126/5/e1400.full.pdf

Laroia, N. (2010). *Birth trauma.* eMedicine. Retrieved March 16, 2012 at http://emedicine.medscape.com/article/980112-overview

Louis, N. A. (2008). Transient tachypnea of the newborn. In J. Cloherty, E. C. Eichenwald, & A. R. Stark (Eds.), *Manual of neonatal care* (6th ed.). Philadelphia: Lippincott Williams & Wilkins.

Lovvorn, H. N., Glenn, J. B., Pacceti, A. S., & Carter, B. S. (2011). Neonatal surgery. In S. Gardner, B. Carter, M. Enzman-Hines, & J. Hernandez (Eds.), *Merenstein & Gardner's handbook of neonatal intensive care.* St. Louis, MO: Mosby Elsevier.

Maisels, M. J. (2010). Screening and early postnatal management strategies to prevent hazardous hyperbilirubinemia in newborns of 35 or more weeks' gestation. *Seminars in Fetal Medicine, 15,* 129–135.

Marcellus, L. (2007). Neonatal abstinence syndrome: Reconstructing the evidence. *Neonatal Network, 26*(1), 33–40.

March of Dimes. (2007). *Illicit drug use during pregnancy.* MODQuick Reference: Fact Sheets. Retrieved March 15, 2012 from http://www.marchofdimes.com/pregnancy/alcohol_illicitdrug.html

March of Dimes. (2009). *Birth defects: Rh disease*. Retrieved March 14, 2012 from http://www.marchofdimes.com/baby/birthdefects_rh.html

Martin, J. B. (2011). Prevention of intraventricular hemorrhages and periventricular leukomalacia in the extremely low birth weight infant. *Newborn and Infant Nursing Reviews, 11*(3), 141. doi:10.1053/j.nainr.2011.07.006

Martin, C. R., & Cloherty, J. P. (2008). Neonatal hyperbilirubinemia. In J. Cloherty, E. Eichenwald, & A. Stark (Eds.), *Manual of neonatal care* (6th ed.). Philadelphia: Lippincott Williams & Wilkins.

National Center on Birth Defects and Developmental Disabilities, Centers for Disease Control and Prevention, & Department of Health and Human Services. (2004). *Fetal alcohol syndrome: Guidelines for referral and diagnosis*. Retrieved March 14, 2012 from http://www.cdc.gov/ncbddd/fasd/documents/fas_guidelines_accessible.pdf

Nicholson, L. (2007). Caput succedaneum and cephalohematoma: The Cs that leave bumps on the head. *Neonatal Network, 26*(5), 277–281.

Premji, S. S., & Semenic, S. (2009). Do Canadian prenatal record forms integrate evidence-based guidelines for diagnosis of a FASD? *Canadian Journal of Public Health, 100*(4), 274–280.

Public Health Agency of Canada. (2007). *Respiratory distress syndrome*. Retrieved March 14, 2012 from http://www.phac-aspc.gc.ca/publicat/2007/lbrdc-vsmrc/rds-sdr-eng.php

Public Health Agency of Canada. (2008). *Canadian perinatal health report, 2008 edition*. Retrieved March 14, 2012 from http://www.phac-aspc.gc.ca/publicat/2008/cphr-rspc/pdf/cphr-rspc08-eng.pdf

Puopolo, K. M. (2008). Bacterial and fungal infections. In J. Cloherty, E. C. Eichenwald, & A. R. Stark (Eds.), *Manual of neonatal care* (6th ed.). Philadelphia: Lippincott Williams & Wilkins.

Randenberg, A. L. (2010). Nonimmune hydrous fetalis. Part I: Etiology and pathophysiology. *Neonatal Network, 29*(5), 281–295.

Ringer, S. A., & Hansen, A. R. (2008). Surgical emergencies in the newborn. In J. Cloherty, E. C. Eichenwald, & A. R. Stark (Eds.), *Manual of neonatal care* (6th ed.). Philadelphia: Lippincott Williams & Wilkins.

Rodriguez, R., Fanaroff, A., & Lissauer, T. (2008). *Neonatology at a glance*. Malden, MA: John Wiley.

Rozance, P. J., & Hay, W. W. (2010). Describing hypoglycemia: Definition or operational threshold. *Early Human Development, 86*, 275–280.

Saugstad, O. D. (2010). Resuscitation of newborn infants: From oxygen to air. *Lancet, 276*(9757), 1970–1971.

Schechner, S. (2008). Drug abuse and withdrawal. In J. Cloherty, E. C. Eichenwald, & A. R. Stark (Eds.), *Manual of neonatal care* (6th ed.). Philadelphia: Lippincott Williams & Wilkins.

Siegel, R., Gardner, S. L., & Dickey, L. A. (2011). Families in crisis: Theoretical and practical considerations. In J. Cloherty, E. C. Eichenwald, & A. R. Stark (Eds.), *Manual of neonatal care* (7th ed.). Philadelphia: Lippincott Williams & Wilkins.

Soll, R., & Ozek, E. (2010). Prophylactic protein free synthetic surfactant for preventing morbidity and mortality in preterm infants. *Cochrane Database of Systemic Reviews, 1*, 1–13.

Spillers, J. (2010). PPHN: Is sildenafil the new nitric? A review of the literature. *Advances in Neonatal Care, 10*(2), 69–74.

Statistics Canada. (2011). *Births, estimates, by province and territory*. Retrieved March 14, 2012 from http://www40.statcan.ca/l01/cst01/demo04a-eng.htm

Steiker, L. K. H. (2009). A dialogue on fetal alcohol spectrum disorder (FASD) and the prenatal impact of substances on children: An interview with Elizabeth C. Pomeroy. *Journal of Social Work Practice in the Addictions, 9*(4), 417–422.

Tappero, E., & Johnson, P. (2010). Laboratory evaluation of neonatal sepsis. *Newborn and Infant Nursing Reviews, 10*(4), 209–217.

Thanh, N. X., & Jonsson, E. (2010). Drinking alcohol during pregnancy: Evidence from Canadian Community Health Survey 2007/2008. *Journal of Population Therapeutics and Clinical Pharmacology, 17*(2), e302–e307.

Tu, W., Chueh, J., & Kennedy, W. (2009). Dichorionic diamniotic twin pregnancy discordant for bladder exstrophy. *Advances in Urology, 2009*, Article ID 186483.

Vassilyadi, M., Tataryn, Z., Shamji, M. F., & Ventureyra, E. C. G. (2009). Functional outcomes among premature infants with intraventricular hemorrhage. *Pediatric Neurosurgery, 45*(4), 247.

Verklan, T. (2009). So, he's a little premature... What's the big deal? *Critical Care Clinics of North America, 21*, 149–161.

Verklan, T., & Lopez, S. M. (2011). Neurologic disorders. In S. Gardner, B. Carter, M. Enzman-Hines, & J. Hernandez (Eds.), *Merenstein & Gardner's handbook of neonatal intensive care*. St. Louis, MO: Mosby Elsevier.

Verklan, M. T., & Walden, M. (2004). *Core curriculum for neonatal intensive care nursing* (3rd ed.). St. Louis, MO: Elsevier Saunders.

Wiedemann, J. R., Saugstad, A. M., Barnes-Powell, L., & Duran, K. (2008). Meconium aspiration syndrome. *Neonatal Network, 27*(2), 81–87.

Weiner, S. M., & Finnegan, L. P. (2011). Drug withdrawal in the neonate. In S. Gardner, B. Carter, M. Enzman-Hines, & J. Hernandez (Eds.), *Merenstein & Gardner's handbook of neonatal intensive care*. St. Louis, MO: Mosby Elsevier.

Whyte, R. K., & Fetus & Newborn Committee. (2010). CPS position statement (FN 2010–01): Safe discharge of the late preterm infant. *Paediatrics and Child health, 15*(10), 655–660.

Wong, S., Ordean, A., & Kahan, M. (2011). SOGC clinical practice guideline: Substance use in pregnancy. *Journal of Obstetrics and Gynaecology Canada, 33*(4), 367–384. Retrieved March 14, 2012 from http://www.sogc.org/guidelines/documents/gui256CPG1104E.pdf

Zimmermann-Baer, U., Nötzli, U., Rentsch, K., & Bucher, H. U. (2010). Finnegan neonatal abstinence scoring system: Normal values for first 3 days and weeks 5–6 in non-addicted infants. *Addiction, 105*, 524–528.

RECOMMENDED READINGS

Acanthi, C. V., Li, S., Joseph, K. S., & Kramer, M. S., for the Fetal and Infant Health Study of the Canadian Perinatal Surveillance System. (2009). A comparison of foetal and infant mortality in the United States and Canada. *International Journal of Epidemiology, 38*, 480–489.

Cloherty, J. P., Eichenwald, E. C., Hansen, A. R., & Stark, A. R. (2011). *Manual of neonatal care* (7th ed.). Philadelphia: Lippincott Williams & Wilkins.

Elliott, E. J., Payne, J. (2008). Fetal alcohol syndrome: A prospective national surveillance study. *Archives of Disease in Childhood, 93*(9), 732–737.

Glasser, J. G. (2011). *Pediatric omphalocele and gastroschisis*. Retrieved March 14, 2012 from http://www.emedicine.com/ped/topic1642.htm

Hook, C. D., & Damos, J. R. (2008). Vacuum assisted vaginal delivery. *American Family Physician, 78*(8), 953–960.

Lao, O. B., Larison, C., Garrison, M., Waldhausen, J. H. T., & Goldin, A. B. (2009). Outcomes in neonates with gastroschisis in U.S. children's hospitals. *American Journal of Perinatology, 27*, 97–102.

March of Dimes. (2011). *Birth defects*. Retrieved March 14, 2012 http://www.marchofdimes.com/baby/birthdefects.html

Oberlander, T. F., & Jacobson, S. W. (2010). Prenatal alcohol exposure alters biobehavioral reactivity to pain in newborns. *Alcoholism: Clinical and Experimental Research, 34*(4), 681–692.

Selway, L. D. (2010). State of the science: Hypoxic ischemic encephalopathy and hypothermic intervention for neonates. *Advances in Neonatal Care, 10*(2), 60–66.

Ward, S. L., & Hisley, S. M. (2010). *Clinical pocket companion for maternal-child nursing care: Optimizing outcomes for mothers, children & families*. Philadelphia: F.A. Davis.

Wood, B. P. (2011). Necrotizing enterocolitis. *eMedicine*. Retrieved from http://www.emedicine.com/radio/topic469.htm

Yoo, H. J., Kim, W. S., Cheon, J., Yoo, S., Park, K., & Jung, S. (2010). Congenital esophageal stenosis associated with esophageal atresia/tracheoesophageal fistula: Clinical and radiologic features. *Pediatric Radiology, 40*(8), 1353–1359.

Zaichkin, J., & Weiner, G. M. (2011). Neonatal Resuscitation Program (NRP) 2011: New Science, New Strategies. *Neonatal Network, 30*(1), 5–13.

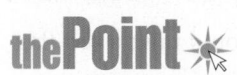

For additional learning materials, including Internet Resources, visit
http://thePoint.lww.com/Chow1e.

CHAPTER WORKSHEET

MULTIPLE CHOICE QUESTIONS

1. Which finding would lead the nurse to suspect that a newborn is experiencing respiratory distress syndrome?

    a. Abdominal distention

    b. Acrocyanosis

    c. Depressed fontanels

    d. Nasal flaring

2. When assessing the substance-exposed newborn, which finding would the nurse expect?

    a. Calm facial appearance

    b. Daily weight gain

    c. Increasing irritability

    d. Feeding and sleeping well

3. A newborn with tracheoesophageal fistula is likely to present with which assessment finding?

    a. Subnormal temperature

    b. Absent Moro reflex

    c. Inability to swallow

    d. Drooling from mouth

4. The nurse would be most alert for the development of transient tachypnea in a newborn who:

    a. Was born by cesarean birth

    b. Received no sedation

    c. Has a mother with heart disease

    d. Is small for gestational age

CRITICAL THINKING EXERCISES

1. As the nursery nurse, you receive a newborn from the labour and birth suite and place him under the radiant warmer. The nurse who gives you the report states that the mother couldn't remember when her membranes broke before labour and that she ran a fever during labour for the past few hours. The Apgar scores were good, but the newborn seemed lethargic. As you begin your assessment, you note that he is pale and floppy and has a subnormal temperature; heart rate is 180 beats/minute and respiratory rate is 70 breaths/minute.

    a. What in the mother's history should raise a red flag to the nurse?

    b. What condition is this newborn at high risk for?

    c. What interventions are appropriate for this condition?

2. Terry, a day-old baby girl, is very irritable and calming measures don't seem to work. As the nursery nurse you notice that she is losing weight and her formula intake is poor, even though she is manifesting hungry behaviour. The mother received no prenatal care and denied drug use, but her drug screen was positive for heroin.

    a. What additional information do you need to obtain from the mother?

    b. What additional laboratory work might be needed for Terry?

    c. What specific measures need to be made for her ongoing care?

3. Baby boy Sims, a term newborn, was brought to the nursery. His mother received no prenatal care, but the newborn's Apgar scores were fine. As the nurse carried out her newborn assessment, she noted an imperforate anus and palpated no testicles in the scrotal sac.

    a. What additional assessments should the nurse complete?

    b. Are anorectal agenesis and genitourinary tract anomalies common?

    c. What diagnostic tests might be ordered? What might be included in the treatment plan for this newborn?

STUDY ACTIVITIES

1. Arrange for a tour of a regional NICU to see the nurse's role in caring for sick neonates. Ask the nurse to give a quick history of each newborn's condition. Was the nurse's role like you imagined? What was your impression of the NICU, and how would you describe it to expectant parents?

2. Select a website from http://thePoint.lww.com/Chow1e. What kind of information is given? How helpful would it be for parents with an infant diagnosed with a specific condition?

3. A herniation of a newborn's abdominal contents present at birth describes _____.

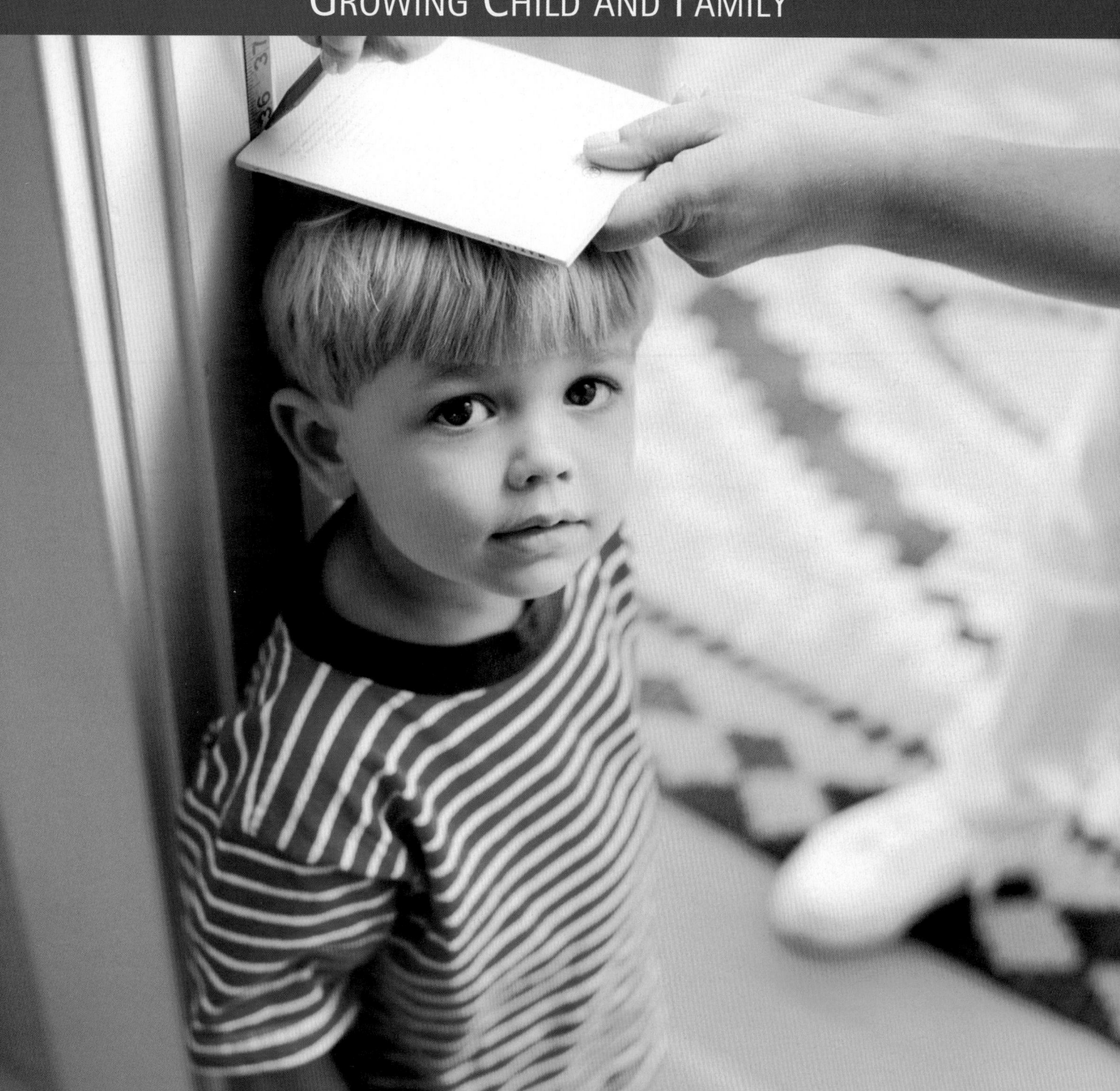

UNIT NINE

HEALTH PROMOTION FOR THE GROWING CHILD AND FAMILY

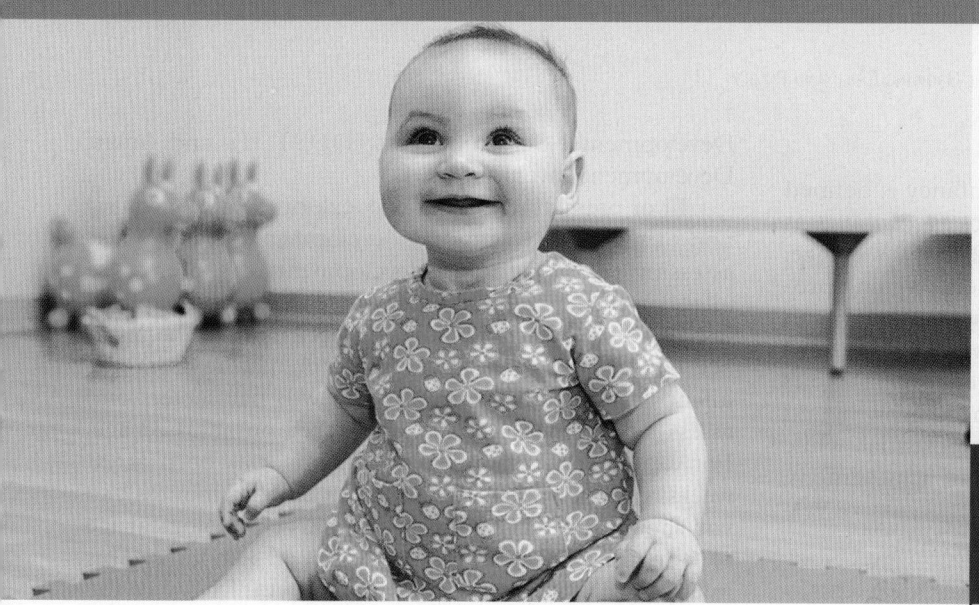

CHAPTER 25

Adapted by Christine A. Ateah

GROWTH AND DEVELOPMENT OF THE NEWBORN AND INFANT

KEY TERMS

anticipatory guidance
binocularity
cephalocaudal
colic
colostrum
development

discipline
foremilk
growth
hind milk
let-down reflex
maturation

object permanence
prolactin
proximodistal
shaken baby syndrome
stranger anxiety
temperament

LEARNING OBJECTIVES

Upon completion of the chapter, the learner will be able to:

1. Identify normal developmental changes occurring in the newborn and infant.
2. Identify the gross and fine motor milestones of the newborn and infant.
3. Express an understanding of language development in the first year of life.
4. Describe nutritional requirements of the newborn and infant.
5. Develop a nutritional plan for the first year of life.
6. Identify common issues related to growth and development in infancy.
7. Demonstrate knowledge of appropriate anticipatory guidance for common developmental issues.

Allison Johnson is a 6-month-old girl brought to the clinic by her mother and father for her 6-month check-up. As new parents, they have a list of questions and concerns. On assessment you find that Allison's weight is 7.3 kg, length 65 cm, and head circumference 42.5 cm. As the nurse caring for her, assess Allison's growth and development, and then teach the parents what changes to expect in Allison over the next few months.

Wow
Of all the joys that lighten our hearts, what joy is welcomed like a newborn child.

The newborn or neonatal period of infancy is defined as the period from birth until 28 days of age. Infancy is defined as the period from birth to 12 months of age. Growth and development are interrelated, ongoing processes in infancy and childhood. **Growth** refers to an increase in physical size. **Development** is the sequential process by which infants and children gain various skills and functions. Heredity influences growth and development by determining the child's potential, while environment contributes to the degree of achievement. **Maturation** refers to an increase in functionality of various body systems or developmental skills.

Growth and Development Overview

Growth and developmental changes in the first year of life are numerous and dramatic. Physical growth, maturation of body systems, and gross and fine motor skills progress in an orderly and sequential fashion. Though timing may vary from infant to infant, the order in which developmental skills are acquired is consistent. Infants also exhibit vast amount of learning in the psychosocial and cognitive, language and communication, and social/emotional domains. Adequate growth and development are indicative of health in the infant or young child. Nurses must be familiar with normal developmental milestones so that they can accurately assess the infant's development as well as provide age-appropriate anticipatory guidance to the parents.

Achievement of developmental milestones may be assessed in a variety of ways. While obtaining the health history, the nurse may ask the parent or caregiver if the skill is present and when it was attained. The infant may also demonstrate the skill during the interview or examination, or the nurse may elicit the skill from the infant. A number of screening tools are also used to assess development, such as the Ages & Stages Questionnaire (ASQ) (see Appendix G), Nipissing District Developmental Screen (NDDS), Prescreening Developmental Questionnaire (PDQ II), Infant–Toddler Checklist for Communication and Language Development (CCLD), Denver II Developmental Screening Test (DDST II), and Infant Development Inventory (IDI).

Ill or premature infants may exhibit delayed acquisition of physical growth and developmental skills. When assessing the growth and development of a premature infant, use the infant's adjusted age to determine expected outcomes. To determine adjusted age, subtract the number of weeks that the infant was premature from the infant's chronological age. Plot growth parameters and assess developmental milestones based on adjusted age. For example, a 6-month-old boy who was born at 28 weeks' gestation was born 12 weeks early (3 months), so you should subtract 3 months from his chronological age of 6 months to get an adjusted age of 3 months. This infant would demonstrate healthy growth if he were the size of a 3-month-old, and he should be expected to achieve the developmental milestones of a 3-month-old rather than a 6-month-old.

Physical Growth

Ongoing assessments of growth are important so that too-rapid or inadequate growth can be identified early. With early identification, the cause can be diagnosed and the potential for further appropriate growth maximized. Infants grow very rapidly over the first 12 months of life. Weight, length, and head and chest circumference are all indicators of physical growth in the newborn and infant (Table 25.1).

Weight

The average newborn weighs 3,400 g (7 pounds 5 ounces) at birth. Newborns lose up to 10% of their body weight over the first 5 days of life. The average newborn then gains about 20 to 30 g per day and regains his or her birth weight by 10 to 14 days of age. Most infants double their birth weight by 4 to 6 months of age and triple their birth weight by the time they are 1 year old (Hagan, Shaw, & Duncan, 2008).

Height

The average newborn is 48 to 53 cm (19 to 21 inches) long at birth. During the first 6 months, length increases

TABLE 25.1 AVERAGE MEASUREMENTS OF INFANTS AT BIRTH, 6, AND 12 MONTHS

Age	Weight (kg)	Length (cm)	Head Circumference (cm)
Birth	3.4	48–53	33–35
6 months	7.3	63.5–68.5	42–44.5
12 months	10.5	71–76	45–47.5

Source: Hagan, J. F., Shaw, J. S., & Duncan, P. (2008). *Bright futures guidelines for health supervision of infants, children, and adolescents* (3rd ed.). Elk Grove Village, IL: American Academy of Pediatrics.

by 2.5 cm (1 inch) per month, then by about 1.25 cm per month in the second 6 months (Hagan et al., 2008).

Head and Chest Circumference

Average head circumference of the full-term newborn is 33 to 35 cm (13 to 14 inches). The head circumference is about 2 to 3 cm greater than the chest circumference, which averages 30.5 to 33 cm (12 to 13 inches). The head circumference increases rapidly during the first 6 months: the average increase is about 1.5 cm per month. From 6 to 12 months of age, the head circumference increases an average of 0.5 cm monthly. The chest circumference is not routinely measured after the newborn period but does increase in size as the child grows (Hagan et al., 2008).

Organ System Maturation

The newborn and infant's organ systems undergo significant changes as the infant grows. Systems that undergo significant change include the neurologic system, the cardiovascular system, the respiratory system, the gastrointestinal (digestive) system, the renal system, the hematopoietic system, the immunologic system, and the integumentary system.

Neurologic System

The infant experiences tremendous changes in the neurologic system over the first year of life. Critical brain growth and continued myelination of the spinal cord are occurring. Involuntary movement progresses to voluntary control, and immature vocalizations and crying progress to the ability to speak as a result of maturational changes of the neurologic system.

States of Consciousness

The normal term newborn's ability to move sequentially through states of consciousness reassures parents and health care providers that the neurologic system, though immature, is intact. A normal newborn will ordinarily move through six states of consciousness (Brazelton & Nugent, 1995):

1. Deep sleep: the infant lies quietly without movement.
2. Light sleep: the infant may move a little while sleeping and may startle at noises.
3. Drowsiness: eyes may close; the infant may be dozing.
4. Quiet alert state: the infant's eyes are open wide, and the body is calm.
5. Active alert state: the infant's face and body move actively.
6. Crying: the infant cries or screams, and the body moves in a disorganized fashion.

Newborns usually progress through these states slowly, rather than going from deep sleep immediately into outright crying.

> ▶ **Take** NOTE!
>
> *The first period of reactivity (the first 15 minutes after birth) is a quiet alert state and is an opportune time to promote bonding and breastfeeding.*

Brain Growth

The nervous system continues to mature throughout infancy, and the increase in head circumference is indicative of brain growth. The brain undergoes tremendous growth during the first 2 years of life. By 6 months of age, the infant's brain weighs half that of the adult brain. At the age of 12 months, the brain has grown considerably, weighing 2½ times what it did at birth. Generally, the anterior fontanel remains open until 12 to 18 months of age to accommodate this rapid brain growth. However, the fontanel may close as early as 9 months of age, and this is not of concern in the infant with age-appropriate growth and development.

In general, the neurologic system matures a significant amount over the first year of life. Myelination of the spinal cord and nerves continues over the first 2 years. Maturation of the nervous system and continued myelination are necessary for the tremendous developmental skills that are achieved in the first 12 months. During the first few months of life, reflexive behaviour is replaced with purposeful action.

Reflexes

Primitive reflexes are subcortical and involve a whole-body response. Selected primitive reflexes present at birth include Moro, root, suck, asymmetric tonic neck, plantar and palmar grasp, step, and Babinski. Except for the Babinski, which disappears around 1 year of age, these primitive reflexes diminish over the first few months of life, giving way to protective reflexes. Protective reflexes (also termed postural responses or reflexes) are motor responses related to maintenance of equilibrium. These responses are prerequisites for appropriate motor development and remain throughout life once they are established. The protective reflexes include the righting and parachute reactions. Appropriate presence and disappearance of primitive reflexes, as well as development of protective reflexes, are indicative of a healthy neurologic system. Persistence of primitive reflexes beyond the usual age of disappearance may indicate an abnormality of the neurologic system and should be investigated.

Table 25.2 gives descriptions and illustrations of several primitive and protective reflexes as well as the timing of appearance and disappearance of these reflexes.

(text continues on page 807)

TABLE 25.2 SELECTED PRIMITIVE AND PROTECTIVE REFLEXES IN INFANCY

	Description	Age Reflex Appears	Age Reflex Disappears
Primitive Reflexes			
Root	When infant's cheek is stroked, the infant turns to that side, searching with mouth.	Birth	3 months
Suck	Reflexive sucking when nipple or finger is placed in infant's mouth.	Birth	2–5 months
Moro	With sudden extension of the head, the arms abduct and move upward and the hands form a "C."	Birth	4 months

	Description	Age Reflex Appears	Age Reflex Disappears
Asymmetric tonic neck	While lying supine, extremities are extended on the side of the body to which the head is turned and opposite extremities are flexed (also called the "fencing" position).	Birth	4 months
Palmar grasp	Infant reflexively grasps when palm is touched.	Birth	4–6 months
Plantar grasp	Infant reflexively grasps with bottom of foot when pressure is applied to the plantar surface.	Birth	9 months

(continued)

TABLE 25.2 SELECTED PRIMITIVE AND PROTECTIVE REFLEXES IN INFANCY (continued)

	Description	Age Reflex Appears	Age Reflex Disappears
Babinski	Stroking along the lateral aspect of the sole and across the plantar surface results in fanning and hyperextension of the toes.	Birth	12 months
Step	With one foot on a flat surface, the infant puts the other foot down as if to "step."	Birth	4–8 weeks

Protective Reflexes

	Description	Age Reflex Appears	Age Reflex Disappears
Neck righting	Neck keeps head in upright position when body is tilted.	4–6 months	Persists
Parachute (sideways)	Protective extension with the arms when tilted to the side in a supported sitting position.	6 months	Persists
Parachute (forward)	Protective extension with the arms when held up in the air and moved forward. The infant reflexively reaches forward to catch himself.	6–7 months	Persists
Parachute (backward)	Protective extension with the arms when tilted backward.	9–10 months	Persists

Source: Johns Hopkins Hospital, Custer, J. W., Rau, R. E., & Lee, C. K. (2008). *The Harriett Lane handbook* (18th ed.). St. Louis, MO: Mosby.

Respiratory System

The respiratory system continues to mature over the first year of life. The respiratory rate slows from an average of 30 to 60 breaths/minute in the newborn to about 20 to 30 breaths/minute in the 12-month-old. The newborn breathes irregularly, with periodic pauses. As the infant matures, the respiratory pattern becomes more regular and rhythmic.

In comparison with the adult, in the infant:

• The nasal passages are narrower.
• The trachea and chest wall are more compliant.
• The bronchi and bronchioles are shorter and narrower.
• The larynx is more funnel shaped.
• The tongue is larger.
• There are significantly fewer alveoli.

These anatomic differences place the infant at higher risk for respiratory compromise. The respiratory system does not reach adult levels of maturity until about 7 years of age. The lack of immunoglobulin A (IgA) in the mucosal lining of the upper respiratory tract also contributes to the frequent infections that occur in infancy.

Cardiovascular System

The heart doubles in size over the first year of life. As the cardiovascular system matures, the average pulse rate decreases from 120 to 140 beats/minute in the newborn to about 100 beats/minute in the 1-year-old. Blood pressure steadily increases over the first 12 months of life, from an average of 60/40 in the newborn to 100/50 in the 12-month-old. The peripheral capillaries are closer to the surface of the skin, thus making the newborn and young infant more susceptible to heat loss. Over the first year of life, thermoregulation (the body's ability to stabilize body temperature) becomes more effective: the peripheral capillaries constrict in response to a cold environment and dilate in response to heat.

Gastrointestinal System

Teeth

The vast majority of newborns do not have teeth at birth, nor do they develop them in the first month of life. Occasionally, an infant is born with one or more teeth (termed natal teeth) or develops teeth in the first 28 days of life (termed neonatal teeth). The presence of natal or neonatal teeth may be associated with other birth anomalies. On average, the first primary teeth begin to erupt between the ages of 6 and 8 months. The primary teeth (also termed deciduous teeth) are lost later in childhood and will be replaced by the permanent teeth. The gums around the emerging tooth often swell. The lower central incisors are usually the first to appear, followed by the upper central incisors (Fig. 25.1). An average 12-month-old has four to eight teeth.

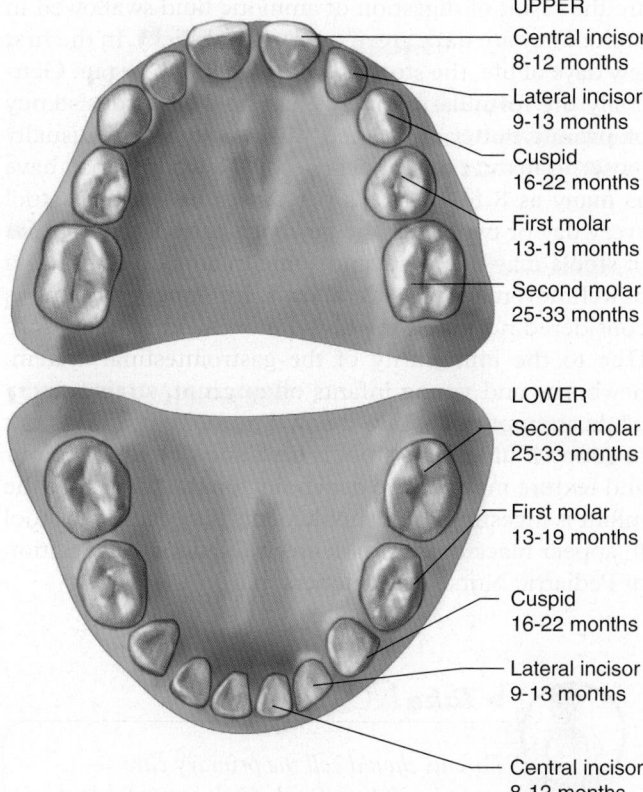

UPPER
Central incisor 8-12 months
Lateral incisor 9-13 months
Cuspid 16-22 months
First molar 13-19 months
Second molar 25-33 months

LOWER
Second molar 25-33 months
First molar 13-19 months
Cuspid 16-22 months
Lateral incisor 9-13 months
Central incisor 8-12 months

FIGURE 25.1 Sequence and average age of tooth eruption.

Digestion

The newborn's digestive system is not developed fully. Small amounts of saliva are present for the first 3 months of life, and ptyalin is present only in small amounts in the saliva. Gastric digestion occurs as a result of the presence of hydrochloric acid and rennin. The small intestine is about 270 cm long and grows to the adult length over the first few years of life (Wyllie, 2007). The stomach capacity is relatively small at birth, holding about 15 to 30 mL. However, by 1 year of age, the stomach can accommodate three full meals and several snacks per day. In the duodenum, three enzymes in particular are important for digestion. Trypsin is available in sufficient quantities for protein digestion after birth. Amylase (needed for complex carbohydrate digestion) and lipase (essential for appropriate fat digestion) are both deficient in the infant and do not reach adult levels until about 5 months of age.

The liver is also immature at birth. The ability to conjugate bilirubin and secrete bile is present after about 2 weeks of age. Conjugation of medications may remain immature over the first year of life. Other functions of the liver, including gluconeogenesis, vitamin storage, and protein metabolism, remain immature during the first year of life.

Stools

The consistency and frequency of stools change over the first year of life. The newborn's first stools (meconium) are the result of digestion of amniotic fluid swallowed in utero. They are dark green to black and sticky. In the first few days of life, the stools become yellowish or tan. Generally the formula-fed infant has stools the consistency of peanut butter. Breastfed infants' stools are usually looser in texture and appear seedy. Newborns may have as many as 8 to 10 stools per day or as few as 1 stool every day or two. After the newborn period, the number of stools may decrease, and some infants do not have a bowel movement for several days. Infrequent stooling is considered normal if the bowel movement remains soft. Due to the immaturity of the gastrointestinal system, newborns and young infants often grunt, strain, or cry while attempting to have a bowel movement. This is not of concern unless the stool is hard and dry. Stool colour and texture may change depending on the foods that the infant is ingesting. Iron supplements may cause the stool to appear black or very dark green (National Association of Pediatric Nurse Practitioners, n.d.).

> ▶ **Take** NOTE!
>
> *Parents should call the primary care provider if the infant's stools are red, white, or black; mucus-like; frequent and watery; frothy or foul-smelling; hard, dry, formed, or pellet-like; or if the baby is vomiting.*

Genitourinary System

In the infant, extracellular fluid (lymph, interstitial fluid, and blood plasma) accounts for about 35% of body weight and intracellular fluid accounts for 40%, compared with the adult quantities of 20% and 40%, respectively (Greenbaum, 2007). Thus, the infant is more susceptible to dehydration. Infants urinate frequently, and the urine has a relatively low specific gravity. The renal structures are immature, and the glomerular filtration rate, tubular secretion, and reabsorption as well as renal perfusion are all reduced compared with the adult. The glomeruli reach full maturity by 2 years of age.

Integumentary System

In utero, the fetus is covered with vernix caseosa, which protects the developing infant's skin. At birth, the infant may be covered with vernix (earlier gestational age) or vernix may be found in the folds of the skin, axilla, and groin areas (later gestational age). Production of vernix ceases at birth. Fine downy hair (lanugo) covers the body of many newborns. Often this hair is lost over time and is not replaced. Darker-skinned races tend to have more lanugo present at birth than those with light skin.

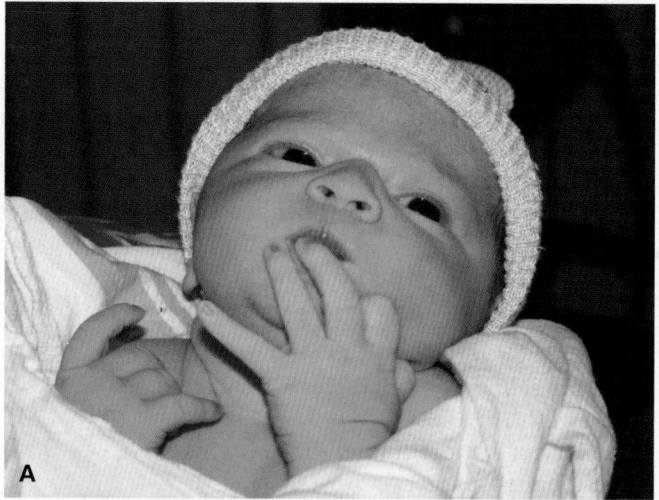

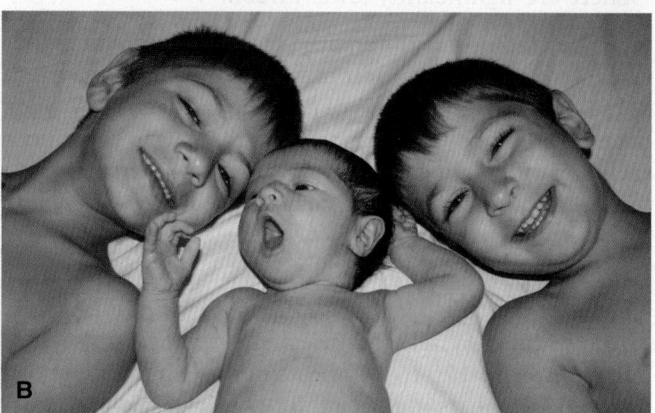

FIGURE 25.2 (**A**) Acrocyanosis. Note blueness of the hands. (**B**) Mottling of the skin in a young infant.

Acrocyanosis (blueness of the hands and feet) is normal in the newborn; it decreases over the first few days of life (Fig. 25.2). Newborns often experience mottling of the skin (a pink-and-white marbled appearance) because of their immature circulatory system (Fig. 25.2). Mottling decreases over the first few months of life.

The newborn and young infant's skin is relatively thinner than that of the adult, with the peripheral capillaries being closer to the surface. This may cause increased absorption of topical medications.

Hematopoietic System

Significant changes in the hematopoietic system occur over the first year of life. At birth, fetal hemoglobin (HbF) is present in large amounts. After birth, HbF production nearly ceases, and adult hemoglobin (HbA) is produced in steadily increasing amounts throughout the first 6 months. Since HbF has a shorter lifespan than HbA, infants may experience physiologic anemia at the age of 2 to 3 months (Glader, 2007). During the last 3 months of gestation, maternal iron stores are transferred to the fetus. The newborn typically has 0.3 to 0.5 g of iron stores available. As the high hemoglobin concentration of the newborn decreases over the first 2 to 3 months, iron is reclaimed and stored. These stores may be sufficient for the first 6 to 9 months of life but will become depleted if iron supplementation does not occur. Ongoing iron intake is required throughout the first 15 years of life in order to reach adult levels (American Academy of Pediatrics, 1999).

> ▶ *Take* NOTE!
>
> *Maternal iron stores are transferred to the fetus throughout the last trimester of pregnancy. Infants born prematurely miss all or at least a portion of this iron store transfer, placing them at increased risk for iron-deficiency anemia compared with term infants.*

Immunologic System

The fetus receives large amounts of immunoglobulin G (IgG) through the placenta from the mother. This confers immunity during the first 3 to 6 months of life for antigens to which the mother was previously exposed. Infants then synthesize their own IgG, reaching approximately 60% of adult levels at 12 months of age (Feigin, Cherry, Kaplan, & Demmler-Harrison, 2009). Immunoglobulin M (IgM) is produced in significant amounts after birth, reaching adult levels by 9 months of age. IgA, immunoglobulin D (IgD), and immunoglobulin E (IgE) production increases very gradually, maturing in early childhood (Feigin et al., 2009).

Psychosocial Development

Erikson (1963) identified the psychosocial crisis of infancy as Trust versus Mistrust. Development of a sense of trust is crucial in the first year, as it serves as the foundation for later psychosocial tasks. The parent or primary caregiver can have a significant impact on the infant's development of a sense of trust. When the infant's needs are consistently met, the infant develops this sense of trust. But if the parent or caregiver is inconsistent in meeting the infant's needs in a timely manner, then the infant develops a sense of mistrust. Table 25.3 lists activities that promote a sense of trust in infancy.

TABLE 25.3 **DEVELOPMENTAL THEORIES**

Theorist	Stage	Activities
Erikson	Trust vs. Mistrust (birth to 1 year)	Caregivers respond to the infant's basic needs by feeding, changing diapers, and cleaning, touching, holding, and talking to the infant. This creates a sense of trust in the infant. As the nervous system matures, infants realize they are separate beings from their caregivers. Over time, the infant learns to tolerate small amounts of frustration and trusts that although gratification may be delayed, it will eventually be provided.
Piaget	Sensorimotor (birth to 2 years) • Substage 1: use of reflexes (birth to 1 month) • Substage 2: primary circular reactions (1 to 4 months) • Substage 3: secondary circular reactions (4 to 8 months) • Substage 4: coordination of secondary schemes (8 to 12 months)	• Infant uses senses and motor skills to learn about the world. • Reflexive sucking brings the pleasure of ingesting nutrition. Infant begins to gain control over reflexes; recognizes familiar objects, odours, and sounds. • Thumb sucking may occur by chance; then the infant repeats it on purpose to bring pleasure. Imitation begins. Object permanence begins. Infant shows affect. • Infant repeats actions to achieve wanted results (e.g., shakes rattle to hear the noise it makes). The infant's actions are purposeful, but the infant does not always have an end goal in mind. • Infants coordinate previously learned schemes with previously learned behaviours. They may grasp and shake a rattle intentionally or crawl across the room to reach a desired toy. Infant can anticipate events. Object permanence is present at about 8 months of age. The infant begins to associate symbols with events (e.g., waving goodbye means someone is leaving).
Freud	Oral stage (birth to 1 year)	Pleasure is focused on oral activities: feeding and sucking.

Sources: Erikson, E. H. (1963). *Childhood and society* (2nd ed.). New York: W. W. Norton and Company; Goldson, E., & Reynolds, A. (2011). Child development and behavior. In W. W. Hay, M. J. Levin, J. M. Sondheimer, & R. R. Deterding (Eds.), *Current pediatric diagnosis and treatment* (20th ed.). New York: McGraw-Hill; and Piaget, J. (1969). *The theory of stages in cognitive development.* New York: McGraw-Hill.

Cognitive Development

The first stage of Jean Piaget's theory of cognitive development is referred to as the sensorimotor stage (birth to 2 years) (Piaget, 1969). Infants learn about themselves and the world through their developing sensory and motor capacities. Infants' development from birth to 1 year of age can be divided into four substages within the sensorimotor stage: reflexes, primary circular reaction, secondary circular reaction, and coordination of secondary schemes. Cause and effect guides most of the cognitive development seen in infancy (see Table 25.3).

The concept of **object permanence** begins to develop between 4 and 7 months of age and is solidified by about 8 months of age (Piaget, 1969). If an object is hidden from the infant's sight, he or she will search for it in the last place it was seen, knowing it still exists. This development of object permanence is essential for the development of self-image. By age 12 months, the infant knows he or she is separate from the parent or caregiver. Self-image is also promoted through the use of mirrors. By 12 months of age, infants can see themselves in the mirror. The 12-month-old will explore objects in different ways, such as throwing, banging, dropping, and shaking. He or she may imitate gestures and knows how to use certain objects correctly (e.g., puts phone to ear, turns up cup to drink, attempts to comb hair) (Piaget, 1969).

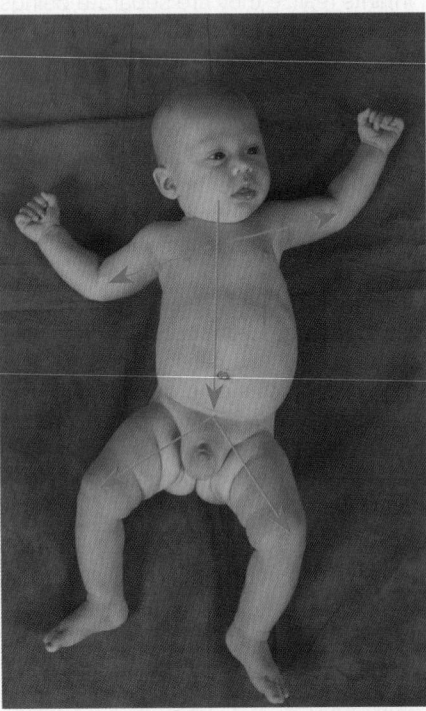

FIGURE 25.3 Gross motor skills develop in a cephalocaudal direction, fine motor skills in a proximodistal fashion.

Motor Skill Development

Infants exhibit phenomenal increases in their gross and fine motor skills over the first 12 months of life.

Gross Motor Skills

The term "gross motor skills" refers to those that use the large muscles (e.g., head control, rolling, sitting, and walking). Gross motor skills develop in a **cephalocaudal** fashion (from the head to the tail) (Fig. 25.3). In other words, the baby learns to lift the head before learning to roll over and sit (Goldson & Reynolds, 2011). At birth, babies have poor head control and need to have their necks supported when being held. They can lift their heads only slightly while in a prone position. Over the next several months, the infant's motor skills progress at a dramatic rate. First, the infant achieves head control, then the ability to roll over, sit,

TABLE 25.4 DEVELOPMENT OF GROSS MOTOR SKILLS IN INFANCY

Age	Gross Motor Skills
1 month	Lifts and turns head to side in prone position Head lag when pulled to sit Rounded back in sitting
2 months	Raises head and chest, holds position Improving head control
3 months	Raises head to 45 degrees in prone Slight head lag in pull to sit
4 months	Lifts head and looks around Rolls from prone to supine Head leads body when pulled to sit
5 months	Rolls from supine to prone and back again Sits with back upright when supported
6 months	Tripod sits
7 months	Sits alone with some use of hands for support
8 months	Sits unsupported
9 months	Crawls, abdomen off floor
10 months	Pulls to stand Cruises
12 months	Sits from standing position Walks independently

Sources: Feigelman, S. (2007). The first year. In R. M. Kliegman, R. E. Behrman, H. B. Jenson, & B. Stanton (Eds.). *Nelson textbook of pediatrics* (18th ed.). Philadelphia: Saunders; and Shelov, S. P., & Altmann, T. R. (Eds.). (2009). *Caring for your baby and young child: Birth to age 5* (5th ed.). New York: Bantam Books.

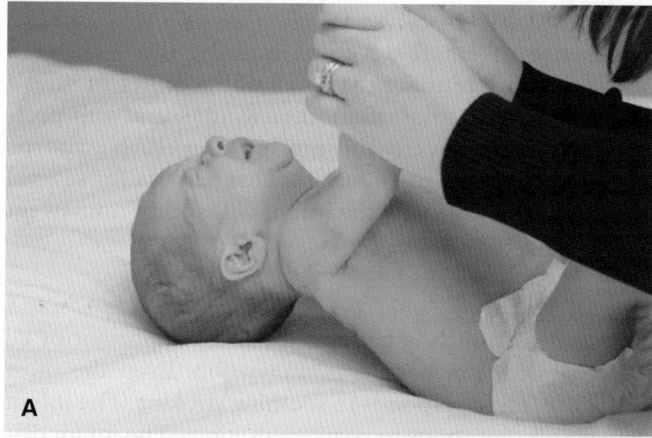

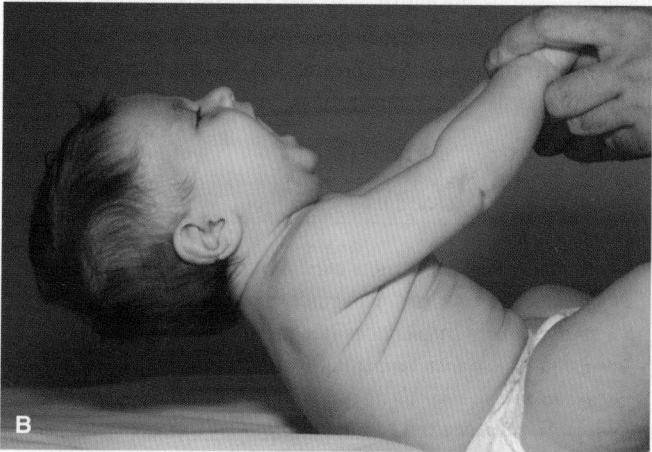

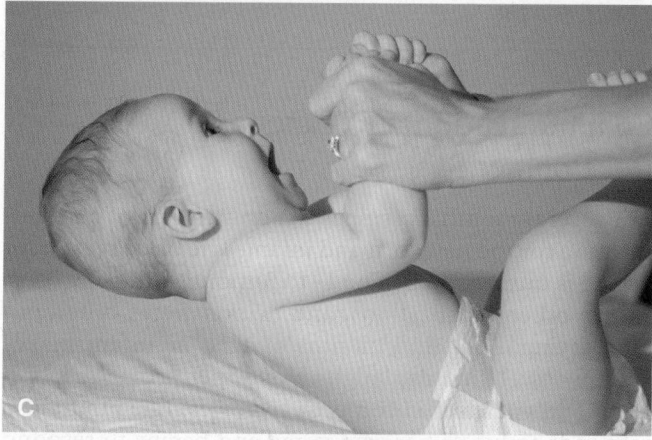

FIGURE 25.4 When pulled to sit, an infant shows (**A**) significant head lag (newborn; 2 or 3 weeks old), (**B**) improving head control (2 months old), and (**C**) no head lag (4 months old).

crawl, pull to stand, and, usually around 1 year of age, walk independently. Table 25.4 gives details on when the infant develops each specific gross motor skill. Progression of gross motor skills is illustrated in Figures 25.4 to 25.6.

▶ **Take** NOTE!

Warning signs that may indicate problems with motor development include the following: arms and legs are stiff or floppy; child cannot support head at 3 to 4 months of age; child reaches with one hand only; child cannot sit with assistance at 6 months of age; child does not crawl by 12 months of age; child cannot stand supported by 12 months of age.

Fine Motor Skills

Fine motor development includes the maturation of hand and finger use. Fine motor skills develop in a **proximodistal** fashion (from the centre to the periphery; see Fig. 25.3). In other words, the infant first bats with the whole hand, eventually progressing to gross grasping, before being capable of fine fingertip grasping (Fig. 25.7) (Goldson & Reynolds, 2011). The newborn's hand movements are involuntary in nature, whereas the 12-month-old is capable of feeding himself or herself with a cup and spoon. By 12 months of age, the infant should be able to eat with his or her fingers and assist with dressing (e.g., pushing an arm through the sleeve). Table 25.5 gives details on when the infant develops each specific fine motor skill.

Sensory Development

Though hearing should be fully developed at birth, the other senses continue to develop as the infant matures. Though they mature at different rates, sight, smell, taste, and touch all continue to develop after birth.

Sight

The newborn is nearsighted, able to view objects most clearly at a distance of 20 to 37.5 cm (8 to 15 inches). Newborns prefer the human face to other objects and may even imitate the facial expressions made by those caring for them. In addition to human faces, newborns show a preference for certain objects, particularly those with contrasts such as black-and-white stripes. The newborn's eyes wander and occasionally cross. At 1 month of age, the infant can recognize by sight the people he or she knows best. The infant will study objects within his or her visual range closely. The ability to fuse two ocular images into one cerebral picture (**binocularity**) begins to develop at 6 weeks of age and is well established by 4 months of age. Full colour vision develops by 7 months of age, as do distance vision and the ability to track objects.

Hearing

The newborn's hearing is intact at birth and as acute as that of an adult. Newborns prefer the sound of human voices to nonhuman sounds. By 1 month of age, the infant can recognize the sounds of those he or she knows best.

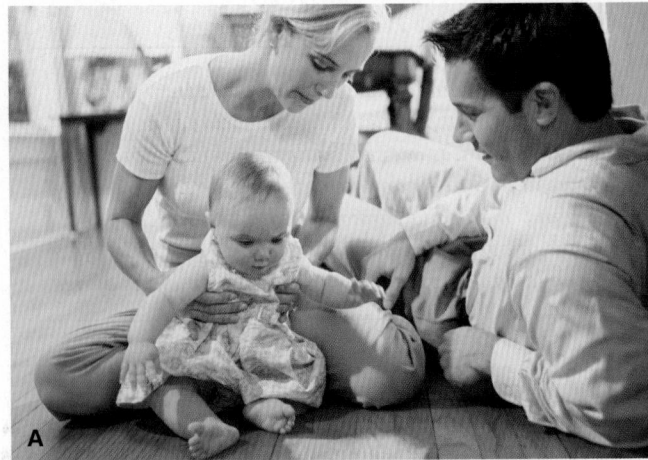

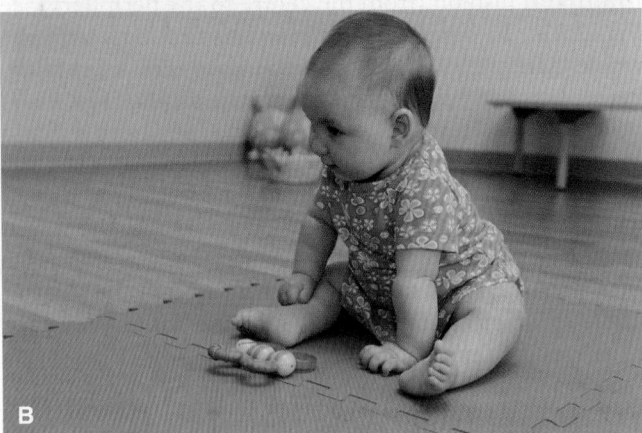

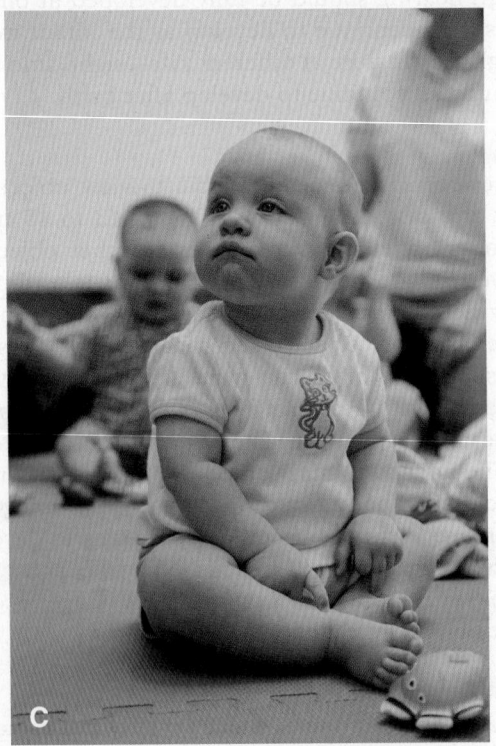

FIGURE 25.5 Development of sitting. (**A**) At 4 months, the infant requires significant support. (**B**) The 6-month-old infant sits in tripod fashion. (**C**) The 8-month-old sits alone.

Smell and Taste

The sense of smell develops rapidly: the 7-day-old infant can differentiate the smell of his or her mother's breast milk from that of another woman and will preferentially turn toward the mother's smell. Newborns prefer sweet tastes to all others. This persists for several months, and eventually the infant will accept non-sweet flavours.

Touch

The sense of touch is perhaps the most important of all the senses for newborn communication. Even the most immature infant responds to soothing stroking. The infant prefers soft sensations to coarse sensations. The infant dislikes rough handling and may cry. Holding, stroking, rocking, and cuddling calm infants when they are upset and make them more alert when they are drowsy. Infants learn to understand their caregiver's moods by the way they touch them.

> ▶ *Take* NOTE!
>
> *Warning signs that may indicate problems with sensory development include the following: young infant does not respond to loud noises; child does not focus on a near object; infant does not start to make sounds or babble by 4 months of age; infant does not turn to locate sound at the age of 4 months; infant crosses eyes most of the time at the age of 6 months.*

Communication and Language Development

For several months, crying is the only means of communication for the newborn and infant. The basic reason for crying is unmet needs. The 1- to 3-month-old baby coos, makes other vocalizations, and demonstrates differentiated crying. At 4 to 5 months of age, the infant makes simple vowel sounds, laughs aloud, performs "raspberries," and vocalizes in response to voices. The infant also responds to his or her own name and begins to respond to "no." Between 4 and 7 months, the infant begins to distinguish emotions based on tone of voice. Squealing and yelling begin around 6 months of age; these sounds may be used to express joy or displeasure. At the age of 7 to 10 months, babbling begins and progresses to strings (e.g., mamama, dadada) without meaning. The infant at this age is also able to respond to simple commands. At 9 to 12 months of age, the infant begins to attach meaning to "mama" and "dada" and starts to imitate other speech sounds. The average 12-month-old uses two or three recognizable words with meaning, recognizes objects by name, and starts to imitate animal sounds. At

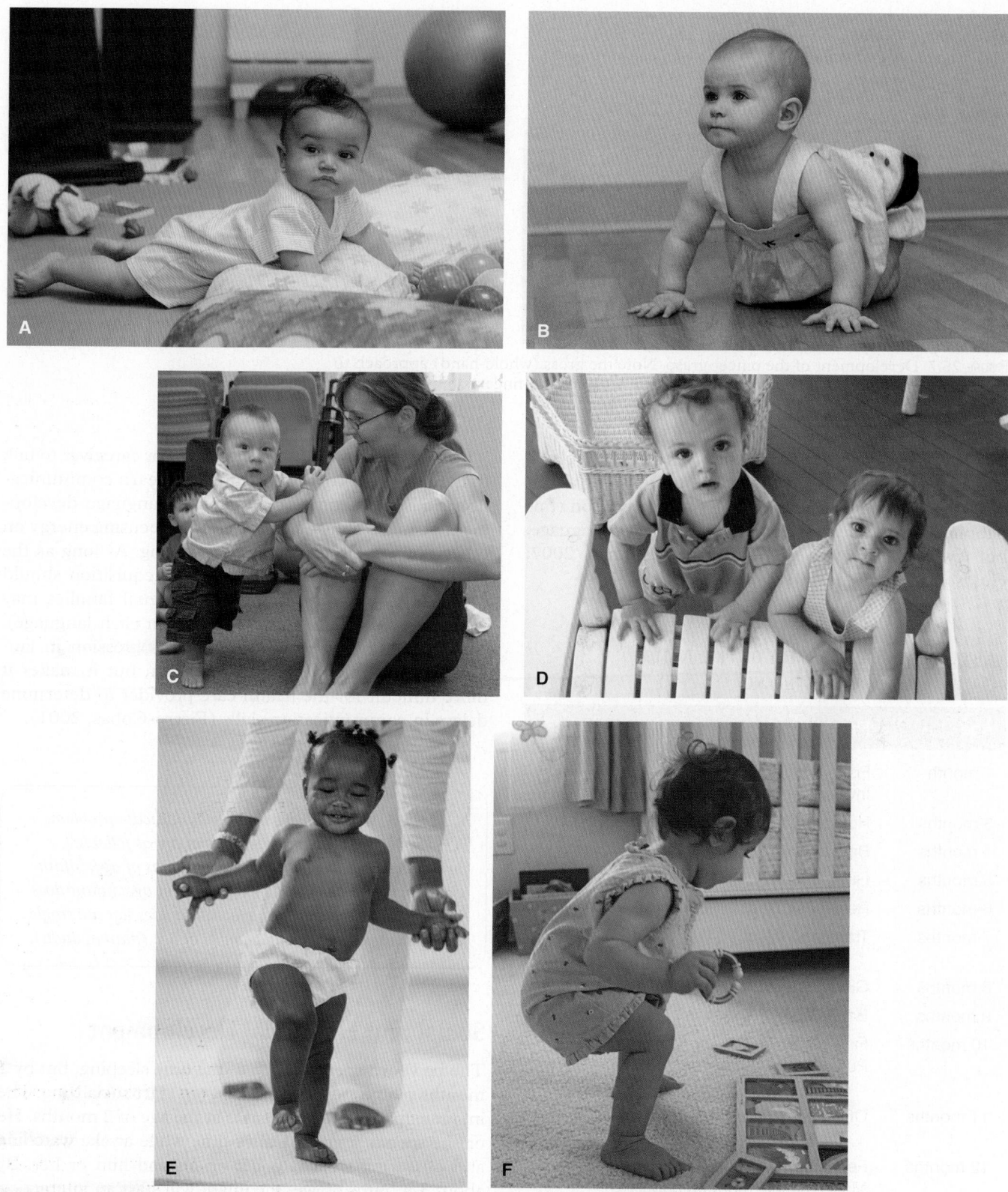

FIGURE 25.6 Development of locomotion. (**A**) At 4 months, the infant pushes up from a prone position. (**B**) At 8 months, the infant crawls with the abdomen off the floor. (**C**) The infant pulls to stand by 10 months of age. The infant (**D**) cruises along furniture or (**E**) takes steps with assistance at 10 to 11 months of age. (**F**) The infant independently stands from a crouched position and walks at around 12 months of age (plus or minus 3 months).

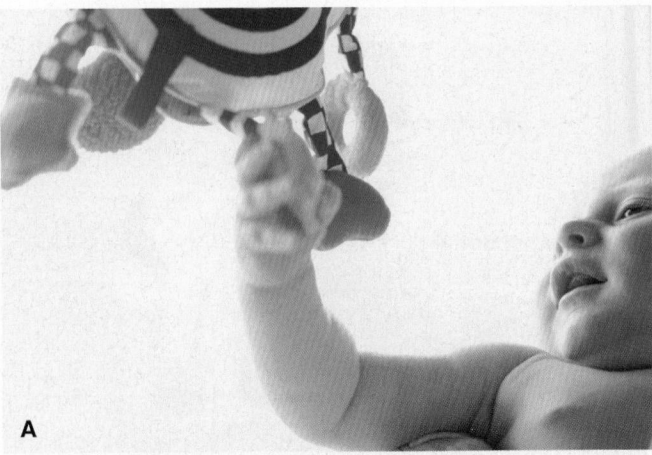
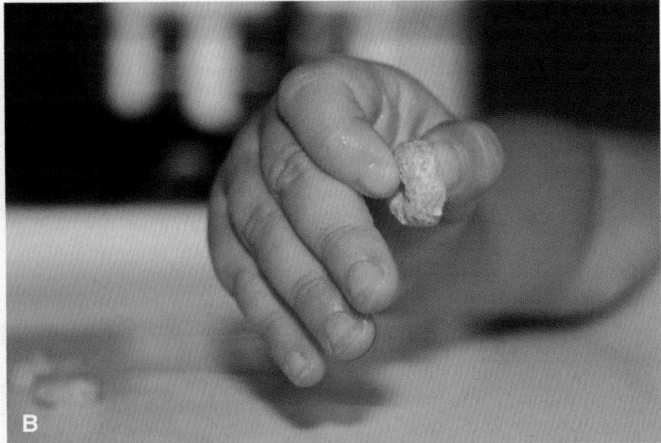

FIGURE 25.7 Development of the pincer grasp. Note the gross (whole-hand) approach to grasping a small object (**A**) compared with the fine (thumb-to-finger) ability (**B**).

this age, the infant pays increasing attention to speech and tries to imitate words; he or she may also say, "uh-oh." The 12-month-old also babbles with inflection (this babbling has the rhythm and timing of spoken language, but few of the "words" make sense) (Feigelman, 2007; Goldson & Reynolds, 2011).

TABLE 25.5 **DEVELOPMENT OF FINE MOTOR SKILLS IN INFANCY**

Age	Fine Motor Skills
1 month	Fists mostly clenched Involuntary hand movements
3 months	Holds hand in front of face, hands open
4 months	Bats at objects
5 months	Grasps rattle
6 months	Releases object in hand to take another
7 months	Transfers object from one hand to the other
8 months	Gross pincer grasp (rakes)
9 months	Bangs objects together
10 months	Fine pincer grasp Puts objects into container and takes them out
11 months	Offers objects to others and releases them
12 months	Feeds self with cup and spoon Makes simple mark on paper Pokes with index finger

Sources: Feigelman, S. (2007). The first year. In R. M. Kliegman, R. E. Behrman, H. B. Jenson, & Stanton, B. (Eds.). *Nelson textbook of pediatrics* (18th ed.). Philadelphia: Saunders; and Shelov, S. P., & Altmann, T. R. (Eds.). (2009). *Caring for your baby and young child: Birth to age 5* (5th ed.). New York: Bantam Books.

It is very important for the parent or caregiver to talk to the infant in order for the infant to learn communication skills. Sometimes regression in language development occurs briefly when the child is focusing energy on other skills, such as crawling or walking. As long as the infant's hearing is normal, language acquisition should continue to progress. Infants in bilingual families may "language mix" (use some words from each language). This is considered to be a normal progression in language development for these children, but it makes it more difficult for the health care provider to determine delays in communication skills (Fierro-Cobas, 2001).

▶ **Take** NOTE!

Warning signs that may indicate problems in language development are as follows: infant does not make sounds at 4 months of age; infant does not laugh or squeal by 6 months of age; infant does not babble by 8 months of age; infant does not use single words with meaning at 12 months of age (mama, dada).

Social and Emotional Development

The newborn spends much of the time sleeping, but by 2 months of age the infant is ready to start socializing. The infant exhibits a first real smile at the age of 2 months. He or she spends a great deal of time while awake watching and observing what is going on around him or her. By about 3 months of age, the infant will start an interaction with a caregiver by smiling widely and possibly gurgling. This prompts the caregiver to smile back and talk to the infant. The infant responds with more smiling, cooing, and gurgling as well as moving the arms and legs. The 3- to 4-month-old will also mimic the parent's facial movements, such as widening the eyes and sticking out the tongue. The baby may hesitate at first, but once the other person responds pleasantly to the infant, the infant engages and gets into the interaction. The infant may cry when the pleasant interaction stops. At 6 to 8 months of age, the infant may enjoy socially interactive games such as patty-cake and peek-a-boo (Feigelman, 2007; Goldson & Reynolds, 2011).

Stranger Anxiety

Around the age of 8 months, the infant may develop stranger anxiety. The previously happy and very friendly infant may become clingy and whiny when approached by strangers or people not well known. **Stranger anxiety** is an indicator that the infant is recognizing himself or herself as separate from others. As the infant becomes more aware of new people and new places, he or she may view an interaction with a stranger as threatening and may start crying, even if the parent is right there. Family members whom the child sees infrequently, as well as others the child does not spend a lot of time with, should approach the infant calmly and slowly, with the parent in sight. Sometimes this will prevent a sudden crying spell (Feigelman, 2007; Goldson & Reynolds, 2011).

Separation Anxiety

Separation anxiety may also start in the last few months of infancy. The infant becomes quite distressed when the parent leaves. The infant will eventually calm down and become engaged with the current caregiver. It is not until the infant is older that cognition and memory are sufficient for him or her to understand that the parent will come back (Feigelman, 2007; Goldson & Reynolds, 2011).

> ▶ **Take** NOTE!
>
> *Warning signs of possible problems with social/emotional development include the following: child does not smile at people at 3 months of age; child refuses to cuddle; child does not seem to enjoy people; child shows no interest in peek-a-boo at 8 months of age.*

Temperament

Temperament is an individual's nature; it is referred to as the "how" of behaviour (Child Development Institute, 2010). Temperament ranges from low or moderately active, regular, and predictable to highly active, more intense, and less adaptable. These are all considered normal along a continuum. An infant's innate temperament affects the way he or she responds to the environment. As parents take note of their infant's usual activity level, how intensely he or she reacts with others and the environment, and how stimulated the baby becomes with interactions, they start to learn about their infant's temperament.

The parent should note how adaptable and flexible the infant is as well as how predictable and persistent the baby is.

When parents are familiar with how the baby approaches life on a routine basis, they will be better able to recognize when the baby is not acting like himself or herself. Nurses can help parents interpret observations about their infant's temperament and recommend ways to support the infant's individual behaviour. Some infants are slower to warm up than others; those infants should be approached slowly and calmly. Some infants exhibit increased levels of activity compared with quieter, more passive babies; those infants generally require more direct play with the parent or caregiver and will be the type of older infant who is in constant motion. Some infants are loud and some are not. The quiet infant may become overwhelmed with excessive stimulation, whereas the very active baby may need additional stimulation to be satisfied (Child Development Institute, 2010). Becoming familiar with the infant's temperament also helps the parents describe the best approach to the infant by others (e.g., to child care workers or health care professionals).

Cultural Influences on Growth and Development

Many cultural differences have an impact on growth and development. For instance, certain ethnic groups tend to be shorter than others because of their genetic makeup (Ferry, 2010). These children will not grow to be as tall as those of another ethnic background. Cultural feeding practices in some cultures may lead to overweight in some children. Some cultures and certain religions advocate vegetarianism; those children need nutritional assessment to ensure they are getting enough protein intake for adequate growth.

Parenting styles and health promotion behaviours can also be significantly influenced by culture. Parents and extended family are the most significant influences in an infant's life in most cultures. Certain cultures place a high value upon independence and may encourage their infants to develop quickly, while other cultures "baby" their infants for longer periods. In most cultures, the mother takes primary responsibility for caring for the child, but in some cultures, major health-related decisions may be deferred to the father or grandparents.

Health beliefs are often strongly influenced by an individual's religious or spiritual background. Sometimes this creates conflict in the health care setting when the health care providers have a different value system than that of the infant's family.

The nurse should explore the family's cultural practices related to growth and development. Usually, these practices are not harmful and can be supported by the health care team, but safety must always be considered. The nurse should not make assumptions about a family's cultural practices based on their skin colour, accent, or name; rather, the nurse should perform an adequate assessment (Leininger & MacFarland, 2006).

> ▶ *Take* NOTE!
>
> *Many communities now include people from a variety of cultures, so it is important for nurses to practice transcultural nursing (nursing care that is directed by cultural aspects and that respects the individual's differences). Many nurse researchers are exploring the cultural aspects of health care and the impact that cultural diversity has upon health.*

Refer back to Allison Johnson, who was introduced at the beginning of the chapter. What developmental milestones would you expect Allison to have reached by this age? How would this be different if Allison had been born 6 weeks premature?

The Nurse's Role in Newborn and Infant Growth and Development

WATCH & LEARN

Growth and development affect every aspect of the infant's life. As infants progress through various stages of development, they do so in a predictable fashion. Growth and development are sequential and orderly, though some children develop at faster rates than others. It is important for the nurse to understand growth and development. Health care visits through infancy often focus primarily on **anticipatory guidance** (educating parents and caregivers about what to expect in the next phase of development). The purpose of anticipatory guidance is to give parents the tools they need to support their infant's development in a safe fashion.

Hospital nurses also need to use their knowledge of growth and development when caring for ill infants. Hospitalization often requires the infant to be confined to the crib or the hospital room. Nurses must support growth and development within the constraints imposed by the child's illness.

Nursing Process Overview

After the infant's current growth and development status has been assessed, problems related to growth and development may be identified. The nurse may then identify one or more nursing diagnoses, including:

- Ineffective breastfeeding
- Risk for disproportionate growth

- Imbalanced nutrition, less than body requirements
- Risk for impaired parent/infant attachment
- Delayed growth and development
- Risk for caregiver role strain

Nursing care planning for the infant with growth and development issues should be individualized based on the infant's and family's needs. Nursing Care Plan 25.1 can be used as a guide in planning nursing care for the infant with a growth and/or development problem. The nurse may choose the appropriate nursing diagnoses from the plan and individualize them as needed. The nursing care plan is intended to serve as a guide, not as an all-inclusive growth and development care plan.

Promoting Healthy Growth and Development

Adding a new person to the family produces both excitement and anxiety. Newborns are completely reliant upon their parents or caregivers to fill every need. It is quite a burden and precious responsibility that new parents are taking on. Many parents read the latest books about caring for newborns, while others rely on information received from family and friends. Newborns and their mothers spend only a short time in the hospital after delivery, so it is very important that parents can care for their newborn and know when to call the primary care provider with concerns.

Periodic screening for adequate growth and development is recommended for all infants and children. The prevention of devastating disease is another priority for infants and children. Immunizations are a very important part of the newborn's and infant's health care visits. Nurses caring for newborns and infants should be familiar with the recommended infant/child periodic screenings (checkups) as well as the current immunization schedule (see Chapter 30 for further information on immunizations).

Promoting Growth and Development Through Play

Experts in child development and behaviour have said repeatedly that play is the work of children. Infants practice their gross and fine motor skills and language through play (Goldson & Reynolds, 2011). Play is a natural way for infants and children to learn. Play is critical to infant development, as it gives infants the opportunity to explore their environment, practice new skills, and solve problems. The newborn prefers interacting with the parent to toys. Parents can talk to and sing to their newborns while participating in the daily activities that infants need, such as feeding, bathing, and changing diapers. Newborns and young infants love to watch people's faces and often appear to mimic the expressions they see.

As infants become older, toys may be geared toward the motor skills or language skills that the child is developing. Parents can promote fine motor development in

(text continues on page 819)

Nursing Care Plan 25.1

GROWTH AND DEVELOPMENT ISSUES IN THE NEWBORN AND INFANT

NURSING DIAGNOSIS: Breastfeeding, ineffective, related to lack of exposure, misconceptions, or knowledge deficit as evidenced by first baby, mother's verbalization, or nursing observations

Outcome Identification and Evaluation

Mother/infant dyad will experience successful breastfeeding: *Infant will latch on, suck and swallow at the breast; mother will not experience sore nipples.*

Interventions: Promoting Effective Breastfeeding

- Educate mother on recognition of and response to infant hunger cues *to promote on-cue breastfeeding, which will establish milk supply.*
- Educate mother on appropriate diet and fluid intake *to ensure ability to manufacture adequate supply of breast milk.*
- Demonstrate breastfeeding positions with infant at the breast *(appropriate positioning increases probability of successful latch).*
- Assess infant's latch technique, sucking motion, and audible swallowing *(an appropriately latched infant will take most of the areola in the mouth, suck in spurts, and demonstrate audible swallowing).*
- Assess infant voiding/stool patterns: *At least six voids per day and passage of stool ranging from one or more per day to one every several days is a normal pattern for breastfed infants.*
- Assess infant weight gain: *Gain of 15 to 30 g per day after the second week of life indicates infant is receiving appropriate nutrition.*
- Assess mother's nipples for redness or soreness; *if infant appropriately latches on nipples will not become sore.*

NURSING DIAGNOSIS: Risk for altered growth pattern (risk factors: Caregiver knowledge deficit, first infant, premature infant, or maladaptive feeding behaviours)

Outcome Identification and Evaluation

Infant will demonstrate adequate growth and appropriate feeding behaviours: *Steady increases in weight, length, and head circumference; infant feeds appropriately for age.*

Interventions: Promoting Adequate Growth

- Observe mother/infant dyad breastfeeding or bottle-feeding *to determine need for further education or identify infant difficulties with feeding.*
- Educate mother about appropriate breastfeeding or bottle-feeding *so that mother is aware of what to expect in normal feeding pattern.*
- When infant is old enough, provide education about addition of solid foods, spoon and cup feeding: *After 6 months of age, breast milk or formula needs to be supplemented with a variety of foods.*
- Determine need for additional caloric intake if necessary *(premature infants and infants with chronic illnesses or metabolic disorders often need adjustments in caloric intake to demonstrate adequate or catch-up growth).*
- Obtain daily weights (if hospitalized, weekly if outpatient) and weekly length and head circumference *to determine whether feeding pattern is sufficient to promote adequate growth.*

NURSING DIAGNOSIS: Nutrition, altered, less than body requirements, related to possible ineffective feeding pattern or inadequate caloric intake as evidenced by failure to gain weight or by inadequate increases in weight, length, and head circumference over time

Outcome Identification and Evaluation

Infant will take in adequate nutrients using effective feeding pattern: *Infant will demonstrate adequate weight gain (15 to 30 g per day) and steady increases in length and head circumference.*

Interventions: Promoting Adequate Nutritional Intake

- Assess current feeding pattern and daily intake *to determine areas of concern.*
- Increase frequency of breastfeeding or volume of bottle-feeding *if needed to meet caloric needs.*
- Introduce solid foods on age-appropriate schedule: *Introducing solids at the right time improves the chances that the child will learn to take solid foods.*

(continued)

Nursing Care Plan 25.1 (continued)

- Limit juice intake or discontinue altogether *(juice has little nutritive value and displaces nutrients from breast milk or formula).*
- Use human milk fortifier (if ordered) *to increase caloric density of breast milk.*
- Increase caloric density of formula (if ordered) by mixing to a more concentrated level or with additives (fats or carbohydrates) *to provide increased calories needed to support adequate growth.*
- If infant is taking solids already, choose higher calorie foods *to maximize nutrient intake.*

NURSING DIAGNOSIS: Parent/infant attachment, altered, risk for (risk factors: Premature infant, parental knowledge deficit about normal newborn activity and care, infant with difficult temperament or medical problems)

Outcome Identification and Evaluation

Parent and infant will demonstrate appropriate attachment via *eye contact, parental response to infant cues, parental verbalization of caring for infant, infant response to parent's caretaking behaviours.*

Interventions: Encouraging Appropriate Parent–Infant Attachment

- Assess parent's response to infant cues *to determine degree of attachment and level of parent's knowledge about infant care.*
- Assess infant's response to parent's caretaking behaviours *to determine degree of attachment.*
- Determine infant's temperament *to counsel parent effectively about responses appropriate for that type of temperament.*
- Encourage *en face* positioning for holding or feeding the young infant *to encourage give-and-take response between infant and parent.*
- Encourage parent to meet infant's needs promptly and with affection *to promote sense of trust in the infant.*
- Reinforce parent's attempts at improving attachment with infant *(positive reinforcement naturally encourages appropriate behaviours).*

NURSING DIAGNOSIS: Growth and development, altered, related to speech, motor, psychosocial, or cognitive concerns as evidenced by delay in meeting expected milestones

Outcome Identification and Evaluation

Development will be maximized: *Infant will make continued progress toward attainment of developmental milestones.*

Interventions: Maximizing Development

- Perform developmental evaluation of the infant *to determine infant's current level of functioning.*
- Offer age-appropriate play, activities, and toys *to encourage further development.*
- Carry out interventions as prescribed by developmental specialist, physical therapist, occupational therapist, or speech therapist *(repeated exposure to the activities or exercises is needed to make developmental progress).*
- Provide support to parents of infants with developmental concerns, *as developmental progress can be slow and it is difficult for families to stay motivated and maintain hope.*

NURSING DIAGNOSIS: Caregiver role strain, risk for (risk factors: First baby, knowledge deficit about newborn care, lack of prior exposure, fatigue if premature, ill, or developmentally delayed infant)

Outcome Identification and Evaluation

Parent will experience competence in role: *Will demonstrate appropriate caretaking behaviours and verbalize comfort in new role.*

Interventions: Preventing Caregiver Role Strain

- Assess parent's knowledge of newborn/infant care and the issues that arise as a part of normal development *to determine parent's needs.*
- Provide education on normal newborn/infant care *so that parents have the knowledge they need to appropriately care for their new baby.*
- Provide anticipatory guidance related to normal infant development *to prepare parents for what to expect next and how to intervene.*
- Encourage respite for parents *(even a few hours away from the demands of an infant's care can rejuvenate the parents).*

Nursing Care Plan 25.1 (continued)

NURSING DIAGNOSIS: Injury, risk for (risk factors: Developmental age, infant curiosity, rapidly progressing motor abilities)

Outcome Identification and Evaluation
Infant safety will be maintained: *Infant will remain free from injury.*

Interventions: Preventing Injury
* Encourage car seat safety *to decrease risk of injury related to motor vehicles.*
* Childproof home: *As infant becomes more mobile, he or she will want to explore everything, increasing risk of injury.*
* Parents should have the Poison Control Centre phone number available: *Should an accidental ingestion occur, Poison Control can give parents the best advice for appropriate intervention.*
* Never leave an infant unattended in the sink, bathtub, or swimming pool *to prevent drowning.*
* Teach parents first aid measures and infant CPR *to minimize consequences of injury should it occur.*
* Parents should watch the infant at all times *(no amount of childproofing can replace the watchful eye of a caring parent).*

infants by providing age-appropriate toys. For example, a rattle that a young infant can hold promotes reaching and attaining. The older infant builds fine motor skills by stacking cups or placing smaller toys inside of larger ones. Gross motor skills are reinforced and practiced over and over again when the infant wants to reach something he or she is interested in.

When playing with toys, the infant usually engages in solitary play; he or she does not share with other infants or directly play with other infants (Feigelman, 2007; Goldson & Reynolds, 2011). A wide variety of toys are available for infants, but infants often enjoy the most basic ones, such as plastic containers of various shapes and sizes, soft balls, and wooden or plastic spoons.

Books are also very important toys for infants. Reading to all ages of infants is appropriate, and the older infant develops fine motor skills by learning to turn book pages.

Table 25.6 lists age-appropriate toys.

Promoting Early Learning
Research has shown that reading aloud and sharing books during early infancy are critical to the development of neural networks that are important in the later tasks of reading and word recognition. Reading books increases listening comprehension. Infants demonstrate their excitement about picture books by kicking and waving their arms and babbling when looking at them. At 6 to 12 months, the infant reaches for books and brings them to the mouth. Over time, reading leads to acquisition of language skills. Reading picture books and simple stories to infants starts a good habit that should be continued throughout childhood (Zuckerman, 2009).

Promoting Safety
Although the leading causes of death for infants less than 1 year of age in Canada are immaturity and congenital anomalies, injury-related death is also a major concern

TABLE 25.6 APPROPRIATE TOYS FOR NEWBORNS AND INFANTS

Age	Appropriate Toys
Newborn to 1 month	• Mobile with contrasting colours or patterns • Unbreakable mirror • Soft music via tape or music box • Soft, brightly coloured toys
1–4 months	• Bright mobile • Unbreakable mirror • Rattles • Singing by parent or caregiver, varied music • High-contrast patterns in books or images
4–7 months	• Fabric or board books • Different types of music • Unbreakable mirror • Easy-to-hold toys that do things or make noise (fancy rattles) • Floating, squirting bath toys • Soft dolls or animals
8–12 months	• Plastic cups, bowls, buckets • Unbreakable mirror • Large building blocks • Stacking toys • Busy boxes (with buttons or knobs that make things happen) • Balls • Dolls • Board books with large pictures • Toy telephone • Push–pull toys (older infants)

Sources: Shelov, S. P., & Altmann, T. R. (Eds.). (2009). *Caring for your baby and young child: Birth to age 5* (5th ed.). New York: Bantam Books; and Schuman, A. T. (2007). The ABCs of toy safety: More than just child's play. *Contemporary Pediatrics, 24*(7), 49–57, 64.

(Public Health Agency of Canada, 2009). As infants become more mobile, they risk injury from falls down stairs and off chairs, tables, and other structures. Curiosity leads the infant to explore potentially dangerous items, such as electrical outlets, hot stove or furnace vents, mop buckets, and toilets. Since infants explore so much with their mouths, small objects or hard foods pose a choking hazard. The infant will invariably pick up any accessible object and bring it to the mouth. With increasing dexterity, poisoning from medications, household cleaning products, or other substances also becomes a problem.

Additional information about safety and injury prevention in childhood, including in the home and car, can be found on the Safe Kids Canada website (visit http://thePoint.lww.com/Chow1e for the direct link). Based at The Hospital for Sick Children in Toronto, Safe Kids Canada is a national program that promotes effective strategies to prevent unintentional injuries in childhood.

Safety in the Car

Motor vehicle accidents are one source of injury, particularly if the infant is improperly restrained. Infants should never be transported in a motor vehicle without proper restraint. Infant car seats should face the rear of the car until the infant is 12 months of age, weighs 10 kg (22 pounds), and is able to walk (Canadian Paediatric Society, 2008). The car seat should be secured tightly at the centre of the back seat. The infant should never be placed in a front seat that is equipped with an airbag.

Infants should never be left unattended in a motor vehicle. The temperature rises very quickly inside a closed vehicle, and an infant can suffocate from heat in a closed vehicle in the summer. Even during cooler weather, the heat generated within a closed vehicle can reach three to five times the exterior temperature. Kidnapping is also a concern if the baby is left unattended in a vehicle.

Safety in the Home

It is important that the baby's crib meets current government standards. The crib should have a firm mattress that is on a firm support and fits snugly on all four sides. The distance between crib bars should be 6 cm (2^3/$_8$ inches) or less to prevent injury (Government of Canada, 2010). All crib edges should be smooth. Only well-fitting crib sheets should be used, not sheets intended for large beds. Crib side rails should always be raised when the parent is not right next to the crib.

Even before the infant can roll over, he or she wiggles and pushes with the feet. The infant can easily fall from a changing table, sofa, or crib with the side rails down, so the infant should never be left unattended on any surface. If infant seats, bouncy seats, or swings are used, the infant should always be restrained in the seat with the appropriate straps.

Baby walkers have been prohibited in Canada since 2004 because of their great potential to cause serious injuries in children. The CPS does not recommend the use of infant walkers because the walker may tip over and the baby fall out of it or the infant may fall down the stairs while in it. Walkers allow infants access to things they may not otherwise be capable of reaching until they are able to walk alone, such as hot stoves and items on the edge of the countertop. Additional information about crib safety and baby walkers can be found at Health Canada's website; visit http://thePoint.lww.com/Chow1e for a direct link.

As the infant becomes more mobile, learning to crawl and walk, new safety issues arise. Safety gates should be used at the tops and bottoms of stairways. Gates may also be used to block curious infants from rooms that may pose physical danger to them because of sharp-edged furniture or decorative objects. Electrical outlets should be covered with approved safety covers. Cabinets and drawers should be secured with child safety latches. Medications, household cleaning supplies, and other potentially hazardous substances should be stored completely out of reach of infants (Safe Kids Canada, 2011).

Choking is a risk because infants immediately bring small items to the mouth for exploration. To avoid choking, recommend the following to parents:

- Use only toys recommended for children 0 to 12 months of age.
- Avoid stuffed animals with eyes or buttons that can be dislodged by the persistent infant.
- Keep the floor free of small items (accidentally dropped coins, paper clips, straight pins).
- Avoid feeding popcorn, nuts, carrot slices, grapes, and hot dog pieces to infants.

Suffocation is also a risk for infants. Cribs should not have pillows, comforters, stuffed animals, or other soft items in them. Keep plastic bags of any size away from infants. Avoid the risk of strangulation by keeping window blind and drapery cords out of the infant's reach (Safe Kids Canada, 2011).

Though no safety measure is as effective as close supervision by a watchful parent or caregiver, the above safety measures can be critical to the infant's well-being.

Safety in the Water

Infants can drown in a very small amount of water. Never leave an infant unattended in the sink, a baby bathtub or standard bathtub, a swimming or wading pool, or any other body of water, even if it is quite shallow. The bathroom door should be kept closed and the toilet lid down. Water should be emptied from tubs, pails, or buckets immediately after use. If the family has a swimming pool, a locked fence or locked screen enclosure should surround it. Exterior doors should be kept locked to prevent the older infant from wandering out to the pool (Safe Kids Canada, 2011).

TABLE 25.7   NUTRITIONAL REQUIREMENTS

Nutritional Requirements	Newborn	Infant
Fluid	140–160 mL/kg/day	100 mL/kg/day for first 10 kg, 50 mL/kg/day for next 10 kg
Calories	105–108 kcal/kg/day	1 to 6 months: 108 kcal/kg 6 to 12 months: 98 kcal/kg

Source: Johns Hopkins Hospital, Custer, J. W., Rau, R. E., & Lee, C. K. (2008). *The Harriett Lane handbook* (18th ed.). St. Louis, MO: Mosby.

Remember Allison Johnson, the infant described in the beginning of the chapter? What anticipatory guidance related to safety would you provide to Allison's parents?

Promoting Nutrition

Adequate nutrition is essential for growth and development. Breastfeeding and bottle-feeding of infant formula are both acceptable means of nutrition in the newborn and infant. Breast milk or formula supplies all of the infant's daily nutritional requirements until 4 to 6 months of age, at which time solid foods may be introduced (Shelov & Altmann, 2009).

Cultural Factors

Many dietary practices are affected by culture, both in the types of food eaten and in the approach to progression of infant feeding. Some ethnic groups tend to be lactose intolerant (particularly blacks, Aboriginal populations, and Asians); therefore, alternative sources of calcium must be offered. Explore the cultural practices of the family related to infant feeding so that you can support the family's cultural values.

Nutritional Needs

Newborns and infants are experiencing tremendous growth and need diets that support these rapid changes. Table 25.7 compares fluid and caloric needs in the newborn and infant.

Breastfeeding

Health Canada, CPS, and Dieticians of Canada all recommend breastfeeding as the natural and preferred method of newborn and infant feeding. In keeping with the World Health Organization (WHO) recommendation, Health Canada (2004) recommends breastfeeding exclusively for the first 6 months of life for healthy infants and encourages health care professionals to promote this recommendation. Health Canada (2004) advises that breastfeeding "....provides optimal nutritional, immunological and emotional benefits for the growth and development of infants."

Breast Milk Composition

Breast milk includes lactose, lipids, polyunsaturated fatty acids, and amino acids. The ratio of whey to casein protein in breast milk makes it readily digestible. The high concentration of fats and the balance of amino acids are believed to contribute to proper myelination of the nervous system. The concentration of iron in breast milk is less than that of formula, but the iron has increased bioavailability and is sufficient to meet the healthy infant's requirements for the first 6 months of life.

In addition to complete nutrition, immunologic protection is transferred from the mother to the infant via breast milk and maternal–infant bonding is promoted. The benefits of breastfeeding are listed in Box 25.1.

BOX 25.1   **Benefits of Breastfeeding**

Infant
- Increased bonding with mother
- Immunologic protection
- Breast milk has anti-infective properties
- Protection against gastrointestinal infections
- Decreased incidence of asthma, otitis media, bacterial meningitis, botulism, urinary tract infection
- Possible enhancement of cognitive development
- Decreased incidence of obesity in later childhood

Maternal
- Increased bonding with infant
- Lessens maternal blood loss in the postpartum period
- Decreased risk of ovarian and premenopausal breast cancer
- Reduced incidence of pregnancy-induced, long-term obesity
- Possible delay of return of ovulation in some women
- Always ready; no mixing!
- Economic advantage

Source: Heird, W. C. (2007). The feeding of infants and young children. In R. M. Kliegman, R. E. Behrman, H. B. Jenson, & B. Stanton (Eds.), *Nelson textbook of pediatrics* (18th ed.). Philadelphia: Saunders.

Breast Milk Supply and Demand

Frequent, on-demand breastfeeding of the newborn is necessary to establish an adequate milk supply. After delivery of the placenta, levels of progesterone drop dramatically, which stimulates the anterior pituitary to produce prolactin. **Prolactin** stimulates the production of milk in the acinar or alveolar cells of the breast. When the infant sucks at the breast, nervous impulses stimulate further production of breast milk.

The first "milk" to be produced by the breasts is termed **colostrum**. It is produced for the first 2 to 4 days after birth. Colostrum is a thin, watery, yellowish fluid that is easy to digest, as it is high in protein and low in sugar and fat. Colostrum provides complete nutrition, all that is needed by the newborn for the first 2 to 4 days of life (Shelov & Altmann, 2009). Transitional breast milk replaces colostrum on days 2 to 4 after birth. By day 10 after birth, mature breast milk is produced. Mature breast milk has a slightly bluish colour and appears thin.

The breastfeeding mother produces milk continually. **Foremilk** collects in the lactiferous sinuses, which are small tubules serving as reservoirs for milk located behind the nipples. The **let-down reflex** is responsible for the release of milk from these reservoirs. When the baby sucks at the breast, oxytocin is released from the posterior pituitary, causing the lactiferous sinuses to contract. This allows milk to "let down" into the nipples, and the infant then sucks the milk. The let-down reflex is triggered not only by suckling at the breast but also by thinking of the baby or by the sound of a baby crying. After the foremilk is let down, new, fattier milk is formed. This **hind milk** helps the breastfed infant to grow quickly (Shelov & Altmann, 2009). Mothers should be informed that the production of oxytocin during suckling may also cause uterine contractions and may cause afterpains during breastfeeding.

Breastfeeding Technique

Before each breastfeeding session, mothers should wash their hands. It is not necessary to wash the breast in most cases. The mother should be positioned comfortably. A number of positions are possible, and they should be varied throughout the day (Fig. 25.8). The mother may hold the breast in a "C" position if that is

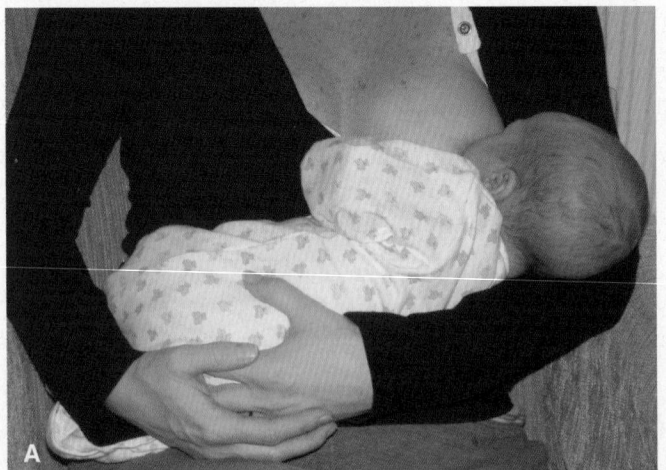
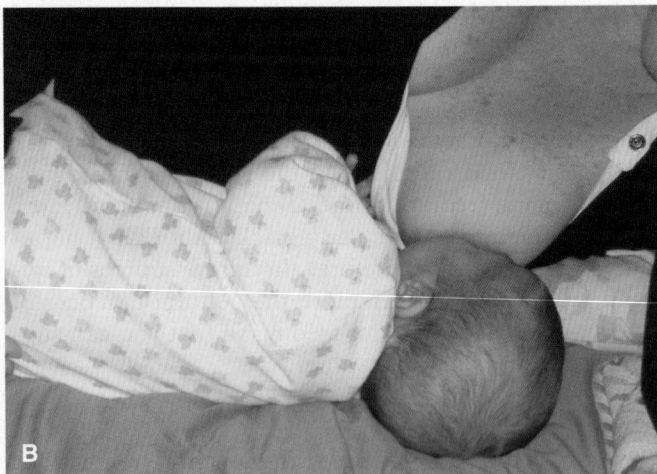
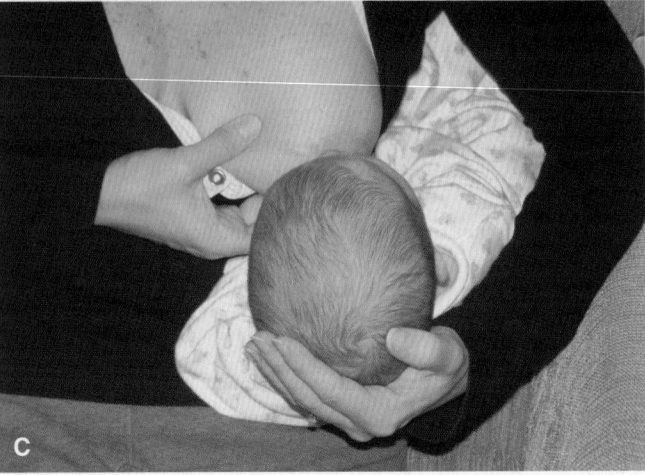

FIGURE 25.8 Various positions may be used during breastfeeding: (**A**) cradle hold, (**B**) side-lying, (**C**) football hold.

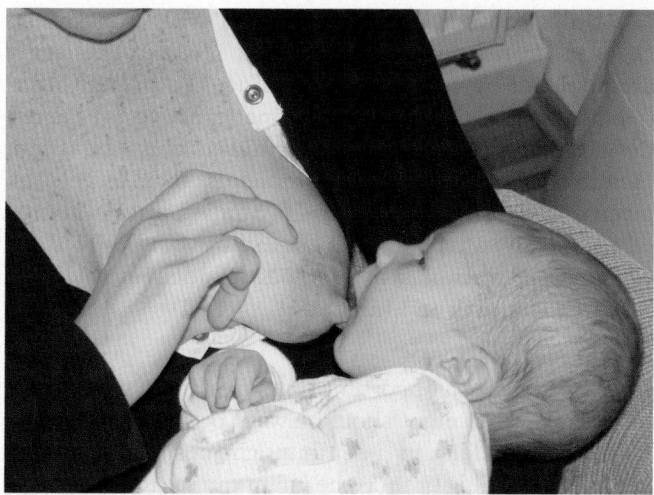

FIGURE 25.9 Stroking the infant's cheek with the nipple will elicit the rooting reflex.

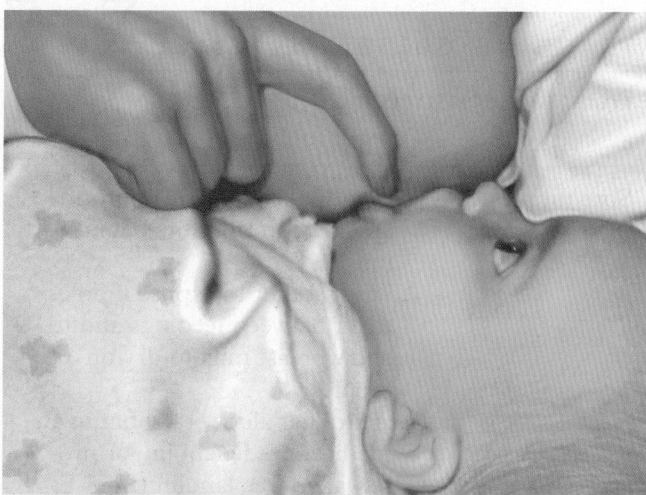

FIGURE 25.11 Inserting a finger between the areola and the infant's mouth helps to break the suction.

helpful to her. Stroke the nipple against the baby's cheek (Fig. 25.9). This should stimulate the infant to open the mouth widely. Bring the baby's wide-open mouth to the breast to form a seal around all of the nipple and areola (Fig. 25.10). When the infant has finished feeding, the mother can break the suction by inserting her finger into the baby's mouth, thus releasing the mouth from the nipple (Fig. 25.11). This technique may prevent the infant from pulling on the nipple, which can lead to soreness and cracking.

Watching and listening to the infant feed may help the nurse assess the adequacy of the baby's latch technique. The infant who is properly latched on to the

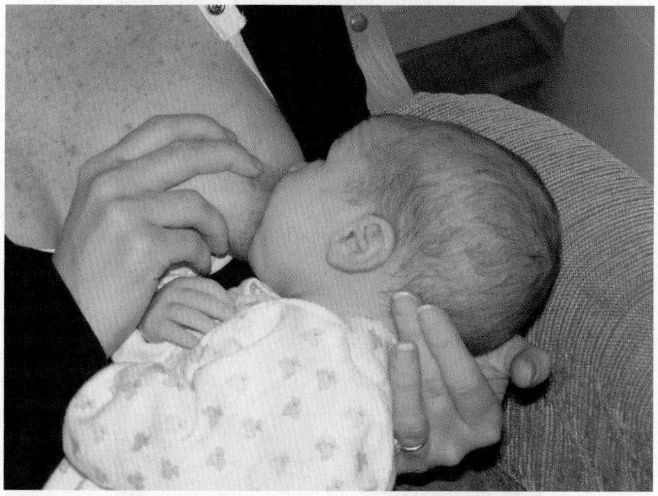

FIGURE 25.10 Bringing the infant's open mouth to the breast, rather than bringing the breast to the infant, helps the infant correctly latch on. The infant's mouth forms a seal around all of the nipple and areola. Note the "C" position for holding the breast during latching on.

breast will suck rhythmically, taking most or all of the areola into the mouth. Audible swallowing should be heard as milk is delivered into the infant's mouth. Assess the mother for pain related to breastfeeding. She should not be in pain if the baby is latched on properly.

Establishment of breastfeeding is best achieved if the infant is allowed to feed on demand, whenever he or she is hungry. This may be as often as every 1½ to 3 hours in the neonate. Infants may feed for 10 to 20 minutes on each breast at each feeding, or longer on just one breast, alternating the breast at each feeding. Both methods are acceptable.

The breastfeeding infant does not need supplementation with water or formula even in the first few days of life as long as he or she continues to wet six to eight diapers per day.

Teaching Guideline 25.1 offers solutions for breastfeeding problems. Additional information about breastfeeding support may be found on the La Leche League Canada website; visit http://thePoint.lww.com/Chow1e for a direct link.

Bottle-Feeding

For the mother who does not desire to, or cannot, breastfeed, commercially prepared formulas are available for bottle-feeding. These formulas are designed to imitate human milk. Standard infant formulas based on cow's milk provide 20 kcal/30 mL and use lactose as a source for carbohydrates (Shelov & Altmann, 2009). Vegetable oil is used as the source of fat; whey or casein provides protein. Newer cow's milk–based formulas contain long-chain polyunsaturated fatty acids that are thought to improve brain development. Ordinary cow's milk is not recommended for the first year of life.

TEACHING GUIDELINE 25.1

Promoting Breastfeeding

Problem	Solutions
Sore nipples	Prevention: encourage appropriate latch on from the beginning
	Advise mother to expose nipples to air between feedings and to allow breast milk to dry on nipples.
	Explain that aloe vera, vitamin E, medical-grade lanolin, or preservative-free lanolin (Lansinoh) may help to heal sore nipples.
Engorgement	Apply warm compresses or encourage the mother to take a warm shower prior to having the baby latch on. Warmth encourages some of the milk to be released, allowing the breast to soften and making it easier for the infant to latch on.
Poor sucking	Advise the mother to feed on cue, not on a schedule, and to encourage the sleepy infant by stroking the feet, undressing, and rubbing the head.
Inadequate milk supply	Decrease maternal stress.
	Encourage adequate maternal diet and fluid intake. Mothers who return to work must pump in order to keep up milk supply when away from infant.
Father feels left out	Encourage father to participate in other aspects of care.
Mother worries about adequacy of breast milk	Explain that if infant is voiding six times per day and gaining weight, then he or she is receiving enough milk and appropriate nutrition.

▶ *Take NOTE!*

Cow's milk does not provide an adequate balance of nutrients for the growing infant, especially iron. It may also overload the infant's renal system with inappropriate amounts of protein, sodium, and minerals.

Only formulas that are fortified with iron should be used. Iron stores that the infant received prenatally are depleted by 4 to 6 months of age. To prevent iron-deficiency anemia, poor growth patterns, and impaired development, iron-fortified formulas must be used. Health Canada (2005) recommends that infants be given iron-fortified commercial formulas until 12 months of age, ideally after 6 months of exclusive breastfeeding. Commercial formulas also provide an adequate blend of essential vitamins and minerals.

Feeding Patterns

Infant feeding is an opportune time to establish good eating behaviours. The infant should always be held while being bottle-fed. Cradling in a semi-upright position allows for additional bonding time, as the infant can see the caregiver's face while feeding (Fig. 25.12). Talking or singing during feeding time also increases bonding. As with breastfed infants, the bottle-fed infant should be fed on cue. Overfeeding with the bottle increases the incidence of gastroesophageal reflux, so families need to learn their baby's cues to hunger and satiety (Shelov & Altman, 2009).

It is important to feed the baby when he or she displays signs of hunger. Crying is a late sign of hunger; earlier signs include making sucking motions, sucking on hands, or putting the fist to the chin. The infant should be burped two or three times per feeding, when he or she slows feeding or stops sucking. Newborns may only take 15 to 30 mL (½ to 1 ounce) per feeding initially, working up to 60 to 90 mL (2 to 3 ounces) in the first few days. They need to feed about 6 to 10 times per day. The infant will gradually be able to ingest more milk per feeding. By 3 to 4 months of age, babies feed four or five times per

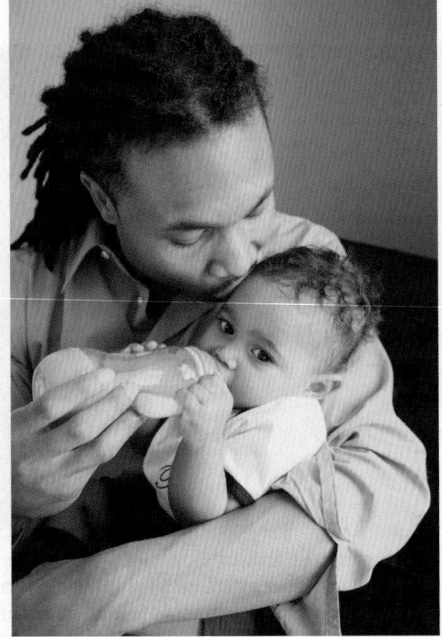

FIGURE 25.12 Technique for bottle-feeding the infant.

day and take 180 to 210 mL (6 to 7 ounces) per feeding. Most infants will not require specific amounts per feeding; the infant should be fed until full. To prevent overfeeding, healthy bottle-fed infants should be allowed to self-regulate the amount of formula ingested per feeding. When the baby is satiated, he or she might fall asleep, spit out the nipple or formula, play with the nipple, or lie quietly, only sucking once in a while (Shelov & Altmann, 2009).

Types of Formulas and Bottles

Parents may choose to use commercial formulas that are ready-to-feed or available as a concentrate or as a powder. Parents should follow the instructions for mixing the concentrate or powder to avoid dehydration or fluid and electrolyte imbalances. Ready-to-feed formula should be used as is and never diluted (Shelov & Altmann, 2009).

A wide variety of baby bottle and nipple types are available for formula feeding, and the choice is purely individual. Few infants require special nipples or bottles. Box 25.2 gives guidelines on preparation and storage of formula and care of bottles.

Special Formulas

Special formulas may be needed for an infant who is allergic to a particular component of standard formula or has a renal, hepatic, metabolic, or intestinal disorder. For example, lactose-free cow's milk formulas are available for the lactose-intolerant child. Formulas using soy as the base ingredient instead of whey or casein are also available. Soy formulas are necessary for infants with a milk allergy, and they may be appealing to the vegetarian family.

BOX 25.2 **Preparation and Storage of Bottles and Formula**

- Wash nipples and bottles in hot soapy water and rinse well OR
- Run nipples and bottles through the dishwasher.
- Store tightly covered ready-to-feed formula can after opening in refrigerator for up to 48 hours.
- After mixing concentrate or powdered formula, store tightly covered in refrigerator for up to 48 hours.
- Do not reheat and reuse partially used bottles. Throw away the unused portion after each feeding.
- Do not add cereal to the formula in the bottle.
- Do not sweeten formula with honey.
- Warm formula by placing bottle in a container of hot water.
- Do not microwave formula.

Source: Shelov, S. P., & Altmann, T. R. (Eds.) (2009). *Caring for your baby and young child: Birth to age 5* (5th ed.). New York: Bantam Books.

These special formulas are designed to meet the nutritional needs of infants, depending on the disorder. Infants who fail to gain weight may be placed on standard infant formula prepared to deliver a higher caloric density per ounce. Preterm infants (those born at less than 34 weeks' gestation) need adequate nutrition to exhibit catch-up growth. Good catch-up growth (quadrupling or even quintupling the birth weight) in the first year or so of life is critical for adequate head growth and avoidance of neurodevelopmental consequences. Premature infant follow-up formulas are designed to provide additional calories, protein, and a particular calcium-to-phosphorus ratio as well as the vitamins and minerals needed for adequate catch-up growth.

Progressing to Solid Foods

After 6 months of age, infants usually require the nutrients available in solid foods in addition to those in breast milk or formula. Progressing to feeding solid foods can be exciting and trying. Before solid foods are attempted, the infant should be assessed for readiness to progress. Parents need instruction in choosing appropriate solid foods and support in the progression process.

Assessing Infant Readiness

Several factors contribute to the appropriate timing of solid food introduction. The tongue extrusion reflex is necessary for sucking to be an automatic reaction—that is, when a nipple or other item is placed in the mouth, the tongue extrudes and sucking begins. This reflex disappears at about 4 to 6 months of age (Shelov & Altmann, 2009). Introducing solid food with a spoon prior to 4 to 6 months of age will result in extrusion of the tongue. The parent may think that the infant does not want the food and is spitting it out intentionally, but this is not the case; the infant simply must be mature enough to eat with a spoon (absence of extrusion reflex).

The ability to swallow solid food does not become completely functional until 4 to 6 months of age. Enzymes to appropriately digest food other than breast milk and formula are also not present in sufficient quantities until the age of 4 to 6 months.

Before the introduction of solid foods and the cup, the infant should be able to sit supported in a high chair. Solids should be fed with a spoon, with the infant in an upright position.

Choosing Appropriate Solid Foods

Iron-fortified rice cereal mixed with a small amount of breast milk or formula is a good choice for the first solid food. The cereal is easily digested, and its taste is generally well accepted. The cereal should be quite thin at first; it can be mixed to a thicker consistency as the infant gets older. Once the feeding of cereal with a spoon is successful, other single foods may be introduced. The

BOX 25.3 Foods to Avoid in Infancy

- Honey
- Egg yolks and meats (until 10 months of age)
- Excessive amounts of fruit juice
- Foods likely to cause choking
  - Peanuts
  - Popcorn
  - Other small, hard foods (e.g., raw carrot chunks)
  - Grapes and hot dog slices (must be cut into smaller pieces)
- Foods likely to result in allergic reaction
  - Citrus
  - Strawberries
  - Wheat
  - Cow's milk
  - Egg whites
  - Peanut butter

Source: Brown, J. (2011). *Nutrition now* (6th ed.). Florence, KY: Wadsworth Publishing.

foods should be puréed to a smooth consistency, whether prepackaged "baby food" or puréed at home.

The introduction of one new food every 4 to 7 days is recommended (Hagan et al., 2008; Shelov & Altmann, 2009). This allows for identification of food allergies (Box 25.3). No salt, sugar, or other seasoning should be added to these first foods.

Generally, by 8 months of age, the infant is ready for more texture in his or her foods. Soft, smashed table food without large chunks is appropriate. Finger foods such as Cheerios, soft green bean pieces, or soft peas may also be offered. Avoid hard foods that the infant may choke on. Strained, puréed, or mashed meats may be introduced at 10 to 12 months of age.

The cup should be introduced at 6 to 8 months of age. One ounce of breast milk or formula should be placed in the cup while the infant is learning. This will decrease the amount of mess should the cup be spilled. Old-fashioned sippy cups are generally acceptable for use, though older infants quickly learn to drink from an ordinary cup with assistance when they are thirsty. Newer "no-spill" sippy cups are not recommended for general home use. They require sucking, much like a bottle, and do not really encourage the child to learn cup drinking. They should be reserved for use on long trips in the car or other instances in which spills should be avoided (Rychnovsky, 2000).

Fruit juice is unnecessary and should not be introduced until 6 months of age. If juice is given, it should be limited to 120 to 180 mL (4 to 6 ounces) per day. Fruit itself is much more nutritious than fruit juice. If infants are allowed to consume larger quantities of juice, it can displace important nutrients from breast milk or formula (CPS, 2006).

Promoting Healthy Eating Habits

Infants and children learn about food within a social context, so the family plays an important role in creating healthy eating habits. Families "model" eating behaviours; infants and children learn about eating through watching others. Lifelong eating patterns are often established in childhood, so it is important to emphasize healthy eating practices beginning in infancy (Nicklaus & Fisher, 2003). Parents should not let infants eat whatever they want (permissive feeding style); this will lead to fights over eating in the future. Infants may require as many as 20 exposures to a new food before it is accepted. On the other hand, infants should not be coerced into eating all that is provided (authoritarian feeding style). Forcing an infant to eat when he or she is full sets the child up for overeating in the future and may lead to more power struggles (Shelov & Altmann, 2009). Parents need to find a balance between the permissive and authoritarian feeding styles to establish lifelong healthy eating patterns in their children. By providing education about appropriate diet and feeding behaviours, the nurse can help the family to accomplish this goal.

Think back to Allison Johnson. What questions should you ask Allison's parents related to her nutritional intake? What anticipatory guidance related to nutrition would be appropriate?

Teaching Newborn Care

Educate new parents (and re-educate parents with subsequent additions to the family) about the basics of newborn care. Refer to Teaching Guideline 25.2 for basic newborn care.

Promoting Healthy Sleep and Rest

Newborns sleep about 20 hours a day, waking frequently to feed and quickly returning to sleep. By 3 months of age, most infants sleep 7 to 8 hours per night without waking. They will continue to take about three naps a day. By 4 months of age, the infant is more active and alert and may have more trouble going to sleep in the evening. Night waking may occur, but the infant should be capable of sleeping through the night and does not require a night feeding. By 12 months of age, infants sleep 8 to 12 hours per night and take two naps per day (Feigelman, 2007).

Discuss safe sleeping practices with parents of newborns and infants; the baby should sleep on a firm mattress without pillows or comforters. The baby's bed should be placed away from air conditioner vents, open windows, and open heaters. Sudden infant death syndrome (SIDS) has been found to be more likely to occur if an infant is placed on his or her stomach (prone) than on his or her back (supine) to sleep (Shelov & Altmann, 2009). Therefore, parents and caregivers are advised to

TEACHING GUIDELINE 25.2

Routine Newborn Care

Primary care follow-up	• First visit within first week of life; also see provider if:
	  • Temperature below 36.0 °C or above 38.5 °C
	  • Poor feeding
	  • "Not acting right"
	  • Excessively sleepy
	  • Vomiting, diarrhea, or difficulty breathing

Weight gain/loss	• Weight loss first 5 to 10 days of life, then should gain weight routinely
Wet diapers	• Minimum of six per day if bottle-feeding or after milk comes in when breastfeeding
Bathing	• Sponge bathe until cord falls off. • Clean the soiled areas daily; full bath every few days. • Do not allow infant to become chilled with the bath.
Umbilical cord care	• Clean the base of cord with alcohol. • Dried cord falls off after 1 to 2 weeks. • Call provider if skin is red or cord has drainage, bleeding, or foul odour.
Illness prevention	• Practice good handwashing. • Limit exposure to individuals with contagious illness.
Dressing	• Newborns do not usually need additional bundling except in very cold weather. • Dress the infant in the amount of clothing that the parents are comfortable wearing (T-shirt is sufficient in summer, long pants and long-sleeved shirts in winter).
Sleep	• Put the infant to sleep on his or her back to decrease the risk for SIDS. The infant should sleep alone, in a crib that meets government standards, and in the same room as his or her parent(s) for the first 6 months.

place infants to sleep on their backs. This practice has been emphasized in Canada for over a decade as part of the "Back to Sleep" public health campaign. Due to the risks of suffocation or other injuries associated with infants sleeping with adults on adult beds or other areas such as couches (bed-sharing), Health Canada (2008) and CPS (2010) recommend that the safest place for an infant to sleep is alone in a crib that meets Health Canada's safety standards. It is recommended that the infant's crib be placed in the caregiver's room for the first 6 months (co-sleeping) to facilitate night-time breastfeeding. In addition, soft materials should be kept out of the baby's sleep environment, the baby should not be too warm, and the home environment should be a nonsmoking one (CPS, 2010).

In the newborn period, the primary caregiver should try to sleep when the baby is sleeping. Since newborns need to be fed every 1½ to 3 hours around the clock, parents may become exhausted quickly and are often eager for the infant to sleep through the night. Adding rice cereal to the evening bottle has not been proven to discourage night waking and is not recommended (Hagan et al., 2008). Provide support to parents of newborns and educate them on infant sleeping patterns.

It is important to establish a bedtime routine around 4 months of age due to the infant's increased alertness and activity level. The baby who is 4 months or older

needs time for calming and relaxation before going to sleep. A consistent bedtime routine should be established, perhaps a bath followed by rocking, singing, or reading. The infant should fall asleep in his or her own crib rather than being rocked to sleep or held until sleeping and then put in the crib. After 4 months of age, infants must learn to soothe themselves back to sleep following night waking. Older infants may exhibit head banging as a form of self-soothing and use it to fall asleep at night. Night feedings are unnecessary at this age and will create a routine of further night waking that will be difficult to break (Hagan et al., 2008). Parents should minimize attention and stimulation provided during a night waking. Briefly checking on the infant to ascertain his or her safety, followed by placing the infant back in a lying position and telling him or her good night, is all that is needed. This may have to be repeated several times before the infant falls back to sleep. It is important to keep interactions brief during the night waking so that the infant learns to fall back to sleep on his or her own. Continued issues with night waking should be discussed with the infant's primary care provider.

What anticipatory guidance should you provide to Allison's parents in relation to sleep?

Promoting Healthy Teeth and Gums

Healthy teeth and gums require proper oral hygiene and appropriate fluoride supplementation. Fluoride use is one of the most successful preventive dental health measures (Canadian Dental Association [CDA], 2008). The CDA supports fluoridation of drinking water at regulated standard levels. It is recommended that children younger than 3 years of age should have their teeth brushed by an adult with just a "smear" of fluoridated toothpaste. Excess fluoride ingestion can result in discolouration of the teeth (fluorosis).

Before tooth eruption, parents should clean the child's gums after feeding with a damp washcloth. After teeth have erupted, parents can continue to use a soft cloth for tooth cleaning and then eventually use a small soft-bristled toothbrush. Toothpaste is unnecessary in infancy. Infants should not be allowed to take milk or juice bottles to bed, as the high sugar content of the fluid in contact with the teeth all night leads to dental caries. Weaning from the bottle at 12 to 15 months of age may help prevent dental caries. No-spill sippy cups have also been implicated in the development of dental caries and should be avoided. The CDA recommends that infants receive their first dental visit within 6 months of the first tooth eruption or by the age of 1 year.

Guidance and Positive Discipline

Parenting requires ever-changing adaptations to the developing infant's needs. Unconditional love, patience, compassion, and awareness of expected infant behaviour are important. The infant's activities are based on the basic needs for food, security, warmth, love, and comfort (Ateah, Secco, & Woodgate, 2003).

As the infant is undergoing rapid changes in motor skills, safety needs increase. Nurses should encourage the parents to "childproof" their home so that the infant can develop physical skills without being at risk. In a childproof home, fewer restrictions need to be placed on the infant's behaviour, and he or she can explore.

Physical punishment such as spanking is associated with negative developmental outcomes and should never be used in infancy. Infants are at increased risk for injury from physical punishment and cannot make the connection between the punishment and the undesirable behaviour (Gottesman, 2000). Providing a safe environment, redirection away from undesirable behaviours, and expressing concern and explanations in appropriate instances are far more effective measures. Infants are not being "good" or "bad" on purpose. They do not understand danger. Therefore, until language and understanding develop, the onus is on the parent or other caregiver to ensure that the environment is safe for exploring and that the infant is closely supervised. This is particularly important once the infant becomes mobile.

Addressing Child Care Needs

Many mothers work outside the home, there are many single-parent families, and many families live a distance away from relatives. In all of these circumstances, infants may need to be cared for outside the home, often in professional child care settings or home day care centres.

Parents contemplating child care must consider a number of factors. Do they want a sitter to come to their home? Will they use a traditional day care centre or a home care situation with fewer children? How much can they afford? If families choose to use a freestanding day care centre or home-based day care centre, they should make sure that the provider is appropriately licensed. Parents should feel comfortable with the caregiver-to-child ratio. Are the caregivers trained in infant CPR and first aid? Families may need to visit or interview several facilities before finding one that meets their requirements.

When an older infant is attending a child care situation for the first time, it may be helpful to visit the centre once or twice beforehand so that the infant can get used to the caregivers from the comfort and security of the parent's lap. Warn parents that separation anxiety in late infancy can cause disturbing crying episodes when the parent leaves. Reassure parents that the crying will likely stop after the infant becomes used to the setting and caregivers and that the infant will not suffer harm due to the separation.

Addressing Common Developmental Concerns

Parents commonly have multiple concerns during normal infant growth and development. Although most of these issues are not actual disease states or behaviour problems, nurses must be aware of these issues to recognize them and to intervene appropriately.

Colic

Healthy 6-week-old infants cry for a total of about 3 hours every day. Crying and fussing is more prevalent in the evenings. By the age of 12 weeks, the total amount of crying is about 1 hour per day, and infants are better able to soothe themselves by this age. **Colic** is defined as inconsolable crying that lasts 3 hours or longer per day. It typically resolves by 3 months of age, coinciding with the age at which infants are better able to soothe themselves (e.g., by finger sucking). The cause of colic is unknown but is considered by some to be due to gastrointestinal or neurologic system immaturity or temperament. Some parents are overly anxious or overly attentive or, at the other extreme, may not give the infant the attention he or she needs. Any of these may contribute to a baby's fussing and crying.

Prolonged crying leads to increased stress among caregivers. Failure to stop the crying leads to frustration, and crying that prevents the parents from sleeping contributes to the exhaustion they are already experiencing. Unfortunately, in some cases, extreme frustration can lead to **shaken baby syndrome**, in which an infant is shaken hard enough to cause brain injury or death. This occurs most frequently in infants younger than 12 months of age and has been linked to a caregiver's exasperated response to an infant's crying. Infants are at risk for such injury due to the fact that their heads are disproportionately large relative to their bodies and their neck muscles are weak. Parents and caregivers are encouraged to seek respite when they are becoming frustrated with their infant and fear losing control. All caregivers of infants should be reminded to "Never shake a baby!" (CPS, 2001).

Educate parents that normal crying increases by the time the infant is 6 weeks old and diminishes by about 12 weeks. When faced with a colicky baby, parents should develop a stepwise approach to checking that all of the infant's basic needs are met. When these needs are met, attempts at soothing the infant may be used. Reducing stimulation may decrease the length of crying. Carrying the infant more may also be helpful. Some infants respond to the motion of an infant swing or a car ride. Vibration, white noise, or swaddling may also help to decrease fussing in some infants. Pacifiers can be soothing to babies who need additional non-nutritive sucking. Parents should try one intervention at a time, taking care not to stimulate the infant excessively in the process of searching for solutions. Nurses should provide ongoing support to the parents of a colicky infant and reassure them that this is a temporary condition that will resolve in time (Shelov & Altmann, 2009). More information on understanding crying and suggestions for soothing a crying infant can be found on the Prevent Shaken Baby Syndrome British Columbia website, sponsored by the BC Children's Hospital; visit http://thePoint.lww.com/Chow1e for a direct link.

Spitting Up

Spitting up (regurgitating small amounts of stomach contents) occurs in all infants. Approximately 50% of normal 2-month-olds spit up at least twice a day (Hobbie, Baker, & Bayerl, 2000). Although spitting up after feeding is normal, it can be a cause of great concern to parents. Overfed babies who feed based on a parent-designed schedule and those who burp poorly are more likely to spit up. For some infants, the amount and frequency of spitting up are significant, and it may indicate gastroesophageal reflux.

Teach parents that feeding smaller amounts on a more frequent basis may help to decrease spitting-up episodes. Always burp the baby at least two or three times per feeding. Keep the baby upright for 30 minutes after feeding and do not lay the infant prone after feeding. Avoid bouncing or excess activity immediately after feeding. Positioning in an infant seat compresses the stomach and is not recommended. When placing the baby in bed, position him or her on the side with the head of the bed slightly elevated (Shelov & Altmann, 2009).

Reassure parents that if the infant is wetting at least six diapers per 24 hours and gaining weight, then spitting up is normal. If the infant vomits one third or more of most feedings, chokes when vomiting, or experiences forceful emesis, the primary care provider should be notified.

Thumb Sucking, Pacifiers, and Security Items

Infants demonstrate a clear need for non-nutritive sucking: even fetuses can be observed sucking their thumbs or fingers in utero. Thumb sucking is a healthy self-comforting activity. Infants who suck their thumbs or pacifiers often are better able to soothe themselves than those who do not. Studies have not shown that sucking either thumbs or pacifiers leads to the need for orthodontic braces unless the sucking continues well beyond the early school-age period. However, pacifier use has been associated with the increased incidence of otitis media (Marter & Agruss, 2007), and hygiene is always a concern as pacifiers often fall on the floor. See Evidence-based Practice 25.1.

Infants may also become attached to a doll, stuffed animal, or blanket. Just like thumb sucking, the attachment item gives the infant the security to self-soothe when he or she is uncomfortable.

Families need to explore their feelings and cultural preferences about sucking habits and security items. Parents should not try to break the habit during a stressful time for the infant. When the infant is intensely trying to master a new skill such as sitting or walking, he or she may need the sucking or security item to self-soothe. Pacifiers and security items can be physically taken away at some point, but the thumb is attached. The infant who has become attached to thumb sucking should not have additional attention drawn to the issue, as that may prolong thumb sucking.

Families of infants who use pacifiers may want to wean the infant from the pacifier when the child approaches 1 year of age (Marter & Agruss, 2007). This is the time when the need for additional sucking naturally decreases. Attempts to wean the child from a security blanket or toy should probably be reserved for after infancy.

Teething

Discomfort is common as the tooth breaks through the periodontal membrane. Infants may drool, bite on hard objects, or increase finger sucking. Some infants may become very irritable, refuse to eat, and not sleep well. Fever, vomiting, and diarrhea are generally not considered a sign of teething but rather of illness.

Teething pain results from inflammation. Teach parents that application of cold may be soothing to the gums.

EVIDENCE-BASED PRACTICE 25.1
Benefits and Risks of Pacifier Use

● **Study**

The authors review the history of pacifier use and several recent research studies that attempted to determine the risks and benefits of pacifier use. The majority of the studies were performed within the early part of the 21st century.

▲ **Findings**

Upon analysis of the various research studies, the authors reached several conclusions. Pacifier use has been shown to lower the risk of SIDS when used at the time of sleep. Additional benefits include assistance in development of neurologic maturity in preterm infants and not shortening breastfeeding duration in preterm or term infants older than 1 month of age. Potential risks include shortening of breastfeeding duration if a pacifier is used before 1 month of age, increased incidence of otitis media when used after 1 year of age, and development of dental misalignment.

■ **Nursing Implications**

In light of the potential risks and benefits of pacifier use, nurses must be prepared to provide parents with accurate information related to the use of pacifiers. Educate parents to avoid introduction of the pacifier until breastfeeding is well established (4 weeks of age), to use pacifiers only during periods of sleep, and to never force a pacifier on an infant or replace a pacifier in a sleeping infant's mouth. Additionally, parents should begin to wean the infant from the pacifier in late infancy so that it is not used past 1 year of age.

Marter, A., & Agruss, J. C. (2007). Pacifiers: An update on use and misuse. *Journal for Specialists in Pediatric Nursing*, *12*(4), 278–285.

The infant may chew on a frozen teething ring, or parents can rub an ice cube wrapped in a washcloth on the gums. Over-the-counter topical anesthetics such as baby Orajel may also be helpful. Parents should apply the ointment correctly to the gums, avoiding the lips, as these ointments cause numbing. Occasionally, oral acetaminophen or ibuprofen may be given to relieve pain (Tinanoff, 2007).

*R*efer back to 6-month-old Allison Johnson. List some *common developmental concerns of 6-month-old infants. What anticipatory guidance related to these concerns would you provide to her parents?*

■■■ Key Concepts

■ Infancy encompasses the period from birth to the age of 12 months.

■ The infant exhibits tremendous growth, doubling the birth weight by 6 months of age and tripling it by 12 months of age.

■ Most organ systems are immature at birth and develop and mature over the first year of life.

■ Child development is orderly, sequential, and predictable, progressing in a cephalocaudal and proximodistal fashion.

■ The infant is mastering the psychosocial task of Trust versus Mistrust.

■ Cognitive development in infancy is sensorimotor; infants use their senses and progressing motor skills to master their environment.

■ The 12-month-old babbles expressively and uses two or three words with meaning.

■ Promotion of safety is of key importance throughout infancy.

■ Breastfeeding is the natural and preferred method for infant feeding.

■ Breastfed and bottle-fed infants should both be fed on cue rather than on a parent-designed schedule.

■ Solid foods should be introduced at the age of 4 to 6 months. A spoon should be used to feed the infant, and rice cereal should be the first food. New foods should be introduced no more frequently than every 4 to 7 days.

■ The cup may be introduced at 6 months of age. No-spill sippy cups are generally not recommended.

■ Spitting up is part of normal development in the otherwise thriving infant and does not require medical intervention.

■ The infant's activities are based on basic needs such as food, security, love, and comfort. Since the infant is not being "good" or "bad" on purpose, caregiver responses to infants should be based on meeting their needs and not as disciplinary responses.

REFERENCES

American Academy of Pediatrics, Committee on Nutrition. (1999). *Iron fortification of infant formulas.* Retrieved November 14, 2011 from http://aappolicy.aappublications.org/cgi/content/full/pediatrics;104/1/119

Ateah, C. A., Secco, L., & Woodgate, R. L. (2003). The risks and alternatives to physical punishment use with children. *Journal of Pediatric Health Care, 17*(3), 126–132.

Brazelton, T. B., & Nugent, J. K. (1995). *Neonatal behavioral assessment scale* (3rd ed.). London: MacKeith Press.

Brown, J. (2011). *Nutrition now* (6th ed.). Florence, KY: Wadsworth Publishing.

Canadian Dental Association. (2008). *CDA position on use of fluorides in caries prevention.* Retrieved August 14, 2011 from http://www.cda-adc.ca/_files/position_statements/fluorides.pdf

Canadian Paediatric Society. (2001). Joint statement on shaken baby syndrome. *Pediatrics & Child Health, 6,* 663–667.

Canadian Paediatric Society. (2006). Feeding your baby in the first year. Retrieved October 22, 2011 from http://www.caringforkids.cps.ca/pregnancybabies/Feeding.htm

Canadian Paediatric Society. (2008). *Transportation of infants and children in motor vehicles.* Retrieved October 22, 2011 from http://www.cps.ca/english/statements/ip/ip08-01.htm

Canadian Paediatric Society. (2010). *Safe sleep for babies.* Retrieved August 15, 2011 from http://www.caringforkids.cps.ca/pregnancybabies/safesleepforbaby.htm

Child Development Institute. (2010). *Temperament and your child's personality.* Retrieved August 15, 2011 from http://www.childdevelopmentinfo.com/development/temperament_and_your_child.htm

Erikson, E. H. (1963). *Childhood and society* (2nd ed.). New York: W. W. Norton and Company.

Feigelman, S. (2007). The first year. In R. M. Kliegman, R. E. Behrman, H. B. Jenson, & B. Stanton (Eds.), *Nelson textbook of pediatrics* (18th ed.). Philadelphia: Saunders.

Feigin, R. D., Cherry, J., Kaplan, S. L., & Demmler-Harrison, G. J. (2009). *Feigin and Cherry's textbook of pediatric infectious disease* (6th ed.). Philadelphia: Saunders.

Ferry, R. J. (2010). *Short stature.* Retrieved August 15, 2011 from http://emedicine.medscape.com/article/924411-overview

Fierro-Cobas, V. (2001). Language development in bilingual children: A primer for pediatricians. *Contemporary Pediatrics, 18*(7), 79–98.

Glader, B. E. (2007). Physiologic anemia of infancy. In R. M. Kliegman, R. E. Behrman, H. B. Jenson, & B. Stanton (Eds.), *Nelson textbook of pediatrics* (18th ed.). Philadelphia: Saunders.

Goldson, E., & Reynolds, A. (2011). Child development and behavior. In W. W. Hay, M. J. Levin, J. M. Sondheimer, & R. R. Deterding (Eds.), *Current pediatric diagnosis and treatment* (20th ed.). New York: McGraw-Hill.

Gottesman, M. M. (2000). Nurturing the social and emotional development of children, a.k.a. discipline. *Journal of Pediatric Health Care, 14*(2), 81–84.

Government of Canada. (2010). Cribs, cradles and bassinets. Retrieved October 22, 2011 from http://www.healthycanadians.gc.ca/init/kids-enfants/sleep-sommeil/cc-lb/index-eng.php

Greenbaum, L. A. (2007). Electrolyte and acid-base disorders. In R. M. Kliegman, R. E. Behrman, H. B. Jenson, & B. Stanton (Eds.), *Nelson textbook of pediatrics* (18th ed.). Philadelphia: Saunders.

Hagan, J. F., Shaw, J. S., & Duncan, P. (2008). *Bright futures guidelines for health supervision of infants, children, and adolescents* (3rd ed.). Elk Grove Village, IL: American Academy of Pediatrics.

Health Canada. (2004). *Exclusive breastfeeding duration.* Retrieved August 14, 2011 from http://www.hc-sc.gc.ca/fn-an/alt_formats/hpfb-dgpsa/pdf/nutrition/excl_bf_dur-dur_am_excl-eng.pdf

Health Canada. (2005). *Food and nutrition: Infant formulas.* Retrieved August 15, 2011 from http://www.hc-sc.gc.ca/fn-an/pubs/infant-nourrisson/nut_infant_nourrisson_term_4-eng.php#alt-inf

Health Canada. (2008). *Consumer product safety: Safe sleep practices for infants.* Retrieved August 15, 2011 from http://www.hc-sc.gc.ca/cps-spc/advisories-avis/aw-am/sleep-sommeil-eng.php

Heird, W. C. (2007). The feeding of infants and young children. In R. M. Kliegman, R. E. Behrman, H. B. Jenson, & B. Stanton (Eds.), *Nelson textbook of pediatrics* (18th ed.). Philadelphia: Saunders.

Hobbie, C., Baker, S., & Bayerl, C. (2000). Parental understanding of basic infant nutrition: misinformed feeding choices. *Journal of Pediatric Health Care, 14*(1), 26–31.

Johns Hopkins Hospital, Custer, J. W., Rau, R. E., & Lee, C. K. (2008). *The Harriett Lane handbook* (18th ed.). St. Louis, MO: Mosby.

Leininger, M. M., & MacFarland, M. R. (2006). *Culture, care, diversity and universality: A worldwide nursing theory* (2nd ed.). Sudbury, MA: Jones & Bartlett.

Marter, A., & Agruss, J. C. (2007). Pacifiers: An update on use and misuse. *Journal for Specialists in Pediatric Nursing, 12*(4), 278–285.

National Association of Pediatric Nurse Practitioners. (n.d.). *The scoop on babies' poop.* Retrieved August 15, 2011 from http://www.napnap.org/Files/poop_eng.pdf

Nicklaus, T. A., & Fisher, J. O. (2003). To each his own: Family influences on children's food preferences. *Pediatric Basics, 102,* 13–20.

Piaget, J. (1969). *The theory of stages in cognitive development.* New York: McGraw-Hill.

Public Health Agency of Canada. (2009). *Child and youth injury in review, 2009 Edition: Spotlight on consumer product safety.* Retrieved November 14, 2011 from http://www.phac-aspc.gc.ca/publicat/cyi-bej/2009/pdf/injrep-rapbles2009_eng.pdf

Rychnovsky, J. D. (2000). No-spill sippy cups. *Journal of Pediatric Health Care, 14*(5), 207–208.

Safe Kids Canada. (2011). *Home safety by the numbers.* Retrieved November 14, 2011 from http://www.safekidscanada.ca/Parents/Safety-Information/Home-Safety/Home-Safety.aspx

Schuman, A. T. (2007). The ABCs of toy safety: More than just child's play. *Contemporary Pediatrics, 24*(7), 49–57, 64.

Shelov, S. P., & Altmann, T. R. (Eds.). (2009). *Caring for your baby and young child: Birth to age 5* (5th ed.). New York: Bantam Books.

Tinanoff, N. (2007). Periodontal diseases. In R. M. Kliegman, R. E. Behrman, H. B. Jenson, & B. Stanton (Eds.), *Nelson textbook of pediatrics* (18th ed.). Philadelphia: Saunders.

Wyllie, R. (2007). Normal development, structure, and function. In R. M. Kliegman, R. E. Behrman, H. B. Jenson, & B. Stanton (Eds.). *Nelson textbook of pediatrics* (18th ed.). Philadelphia: Saunders.

Zuckerman, B. (2009). Promoting early literacy in pediatric practice: Twenty years of Reach Out and Read. *Pediatrics, 124,* 1660–1665.

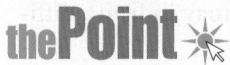

For additional learning materials, including Internet Resources, visit
http://thePoint.lww.com/Chow1e.

CHAPTER WORKSHEET

MULTIPLE CHOICE QUESTIONS

1. The mother of a 3-month-old boy asks the nurse about starting solid foods. What is the most appropriate response by the nurse?

   a. "It's okay to start puréed solids at this age if fed via the bottle."

   b. "Infants don't require solid food until 12 months of age."

   c. "Solid foods should be delayed until the age of 6 months, when the infant can handle a spoon on his own."

   d. "The tongue extrusion reflex disappears at the age of 4 to 6 months, making it a good time to start solid foods."

2. The father of a 2-month-old girl is expressing concern that his infant may be getting spoiled. The nurse's best response is:

   a. "She seems to be learning how to be the centre of attention."

   b. "Consistently meeting the infant's needs helps promote a sense of trust."

   c. "Infants need to be fed and kept clean; if you're sure those needs are met, just let her cry."

   d. "Consistency in meeting needs is important, but you're right, holding her too much will spoil her."

3. Parents of an 8-month-old girl express concern that she cries when left with the babysitter. How does the nurse best explain this behaviour?

   a. Crying when left with the sitter may indicate difficulty with building trust.

   b. Stranger anxiety should not occur until toddlerhood; this concern should be investigated.

   c. Separation anxiety is normal at this age; the infant recognizes parents as separate beings.

   d. Perhaps the sitter doesn't meet the infant's needs; choose a different sitter.

CRITICAL THINKING EXERCISES

1. The mother of an 11-month-old boy who was born at 24 weeks' gestation is concerned about his size and motor skills. What information should the nurse provide?

2. An infant's mother thinks there may be something wrong with him because "he spits up so much." What further information should the nurse obtain?

3. If you determine that the infant in the question above is experiencing normal spitting up associated with his developmental age, develop a brief teaching plan to review with the mother.

STUDY ACTIVITIES

1. A mother brings her 9-month-old boy to the clinic for a well-child check-up. She has questions about feeding, speech, and walking. Develop a teaching plan of anticipatory guidance for the 9-month-old infant.

2. Develop a safety plan for the 12-month-old infant.

3. In the clinical setting, observe two infants of the same age, one who is developing appropriately for his or her age and one who is delayed. Note the similarities and differences between the two infants.

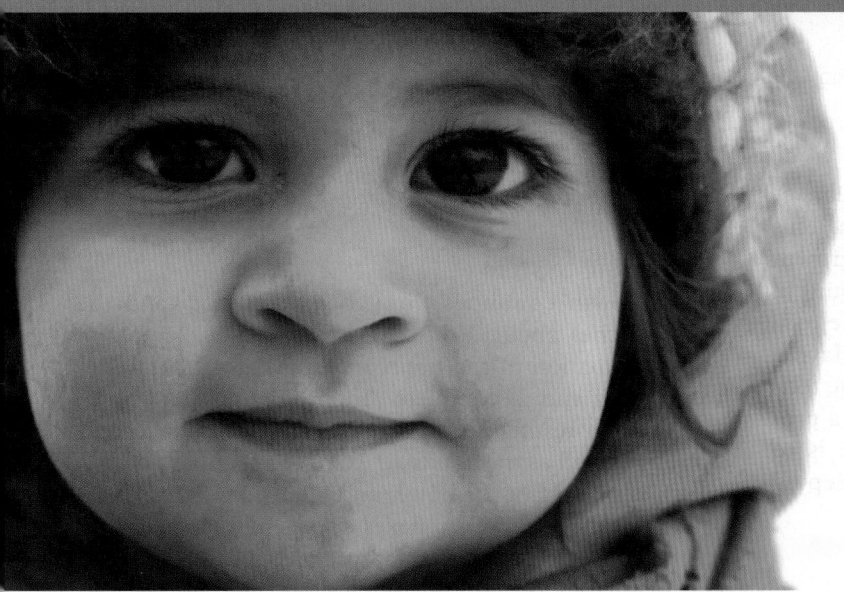

CHAPTER26

Adapted by Christine A. Ateah

GROWTH AND DEVELOPMENT OF THE TODDLER

KEY TERMS

animism
egocentrism
food jag
individuation

parallel play
physiologic anorexia
regression
separation

separation anxiety
sibling rivalry
telegraphic speech

LEARNING OBJECTIVES

Upon completion of the chapter, the learner will be able to:

1. Explain normal physiologic, psychosocial, and cognitive changes occurring in the toddler.
2. Identify the gross and fine motor milestones of the toddler.
3. Demonstrate an understanding of language development in the toddler years.
4. Discuss sensory development of the toddler.
5. Demonstrate an understanding of emotional/social development and moral development during toddlerhood.
6. Implement a nursing care plan to address common issues related to growth and development in toddlerhood.
7. Encourage growth and learning through play.
8. Develop a teaching plan for safety promotion in the toddler period.
9. Demonstrate an understanding of toddler needs related to sleep and rest, as well as dental health.
10. Develop a nutritional plan for the toddler based on average nutritional requirements.
11. Provide appropriate anticipatory guidance for common developmental issues that arise in the toddler period.
12. Demonstrate an understanding of appropriate methods of discipline for use during the toddler years.
13. Identify the role of the parent in the toddler's life and determine ways to support, encourage, and educate the parents about toddler growth, development, and concerns during this period.

Eugene Dupuis is a 2-year-old boy brought to the clinic by his mother and father for his 2-year-old check-up. During your assessment, you find that his weight is 13.6 kg, height 82.5 cm, and head circumference 48.5 cm. As the nurse caring for him, assess Eugene's growth and development, and then provide appropriate anticipatory guidance to the parents.

Wow

Toddlers will take risks and make many mistakes, but remember that both are an essential part of their growth.

The toddler period encompasses the second 2 years of life, from the age of 1 year to the age of 3 years. This period is a time of significant advancement in growth and development for the child. It can also be quite a challenging time for parents. The theme during the toddler years is one of holding on and letting go. Having learned that parents are predictable and reliable, the toddler is now learning that his or her behaviour has a predictable, reliable effect on others. The challenge is to encourage independence and autonomy while keeping the curious toddler safe.

▶ **Take** NOTE!

When grandparents assume the primary caregiver role for their grandchildren, nurses should be alert to the possibility of increased stress that is placed upon the older caregiver, particularly during the active and sometimes trying years of toddlerhood.

Growth and Development Overview

Infancy is a time of intense growth and development. Both physical growth and acquisition of new motor skills slow somewhat during the toddler years. Refinement of motor skills, continued cognitive growth, and acquisition of appropriate language skills are of prime importance during the toddler years. The nurse uses the knowledge of normal toddler development as a roadmap for behavioural assessment of the 1- to 3-year-old child.

Physical Growth

The toddler's height and weight continue to increase steadily, though the increase occurs at a slower velocity compared with infancy. Toddler gains in height and weight tend to occur in spurts rather than in a linear fashion. The average toddler weight gain is 1.4 to 2.3 kg per year. Length/height increases by an average of 7.5 cm per year. Toddlers generally reach about half of their adult height by 2 years of age. Head circumference increases about 2.5 cm between 1 and 2 years of age, then increases at an average of a 1.3 cm per year until the age of 5 years. The anterior fontanel should be closed by the time the child is 18 months old. Head size becomes more proportional to the rest of the body near the age of 3 years.

Organ System Maturation

Though not as pronounced as the changes occurring during infancy, the toddler's organ systems continue to grow and mature in their functioning. Significant functional changes occur within the neurologic, gastrointestinal, and genitourinary systems. The respiratory and cardiovascular systems undergo changes as well.

Neurologic System

Brain growth continues through toddlerhood, and the brain reaches about 90% of its adult size by 2 years of age. Myelination of the brain and spinal cord continues to progress and is complete around 24 months of age. Myelination results in improved coordination and equilibrium as well as the ability to exercise sphincter control, which is important for bowel and bladder training. Integration of the primitive reflexes occurs in infancy, allowing for the emergence of the protective reflexes near the end of infancy or early in toddlerhood. The forward or downward parachute reflex is particularly helpful when the child starts to toddle. Rapid increase in language skills is evidence of continued progression of cognitive development.

Respiratory System

The respiratory structures continue to grow and mature throughout toddlerhood. The alveoli continue to increase in number, not reaching the adult number until about 7 years of age. The trachea and lower airways continue to grow but remain small compared with the adult. The tongue is relatively large in comparison with the size of the mouth. Tonsils and adenoids are large and the Eustachian tubes are relatively short and straight.

Cardiovascular System

The heart rate decreases and blood pressure increases in toddlerhood. Blood vessels are close to the skin surface and so are compressed easily when palpated.

Gastrointestinal System

The stomach continues to increase in size, allowing the toddler to consume three regular meals per day. Pepsin production matures by 2 years of age. The small intestine continues to grow in length, though it does not reach the maximum length of 2 to 3 m until adulthood. Stool passage decreases in frequency to one or two per day, with as many as 25% of toddlers having a bowel movement every other day (Arias, Bennison, Justus, & Thurman, 2001). The colour of the stool may change (yellow, orange, brown, or green) depending upon the toddler's diet. Since the toddler's intestines remain somewhat immature, the toddler often passes whole pieces of difficult-to-digest food such as corn kernels. Bowel control is generally achieved by the end of the toddler period.

Genitourinary System

Bladder and kidney function reach adult levels by 16 to 24 months of age. The bladder capacity increases, allowing the toddler to retain urine for increased periods of time. Urine output should be about 1 mL/kg/hour. The

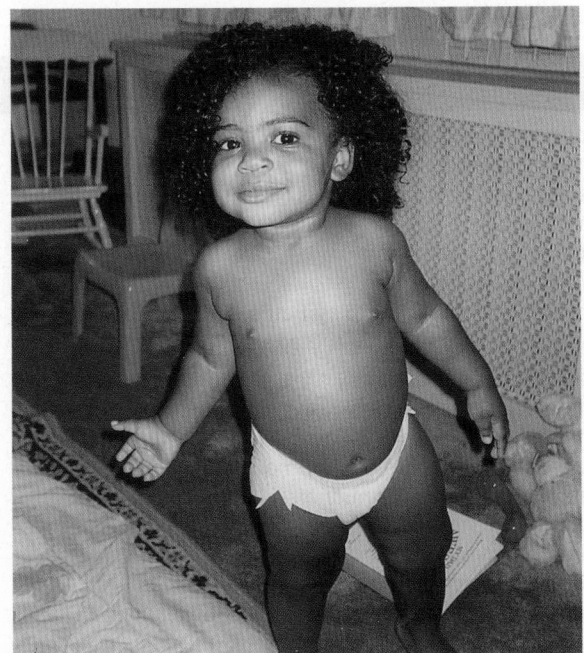

FIGURE 26.1 The typical toddler appearance is that of a rounded abdomen, a slight swayback, and a wide-based stance.

urethra remains short in both the male and female toddler, making them more susceptible to urinary tract infections compared with adults.

Musculoskeletal System

During toddlerhood, the bones increase in length and the muscles mature and become stronger. The abdominal musculature is weak in early toddlerhood, resulting in a pot-bellied appearance. The toddler appears to have a swayback along with the potbelly (Fig. 26.1). Around 3 years of age, the musculature strengthens and the abdomen is flatter in appearance.

Psychosocial Development

Erikson defines the toddler period as a time of autonomy versus shame and doubt. It is a time of exerting independence. Since the toddler developed a sense of trust in infancy, he or she is ready to give up dependence and to assert his or her sense of control and autonomy (Erikson, 1963). Toddlers struggle for self-mastery, to learn to do for themselves what others have been doing for them. Toddlers often experience ambivalence about the move from dependence to autonomy, and this results in emotional lability. The toddler may quickly change from happy and pleasant to crying and screaming. Exertion of independence also results in the toddler's favourite response, "no." The toddler will often answer "no" even when he or she really means "yes."

This negativism—always saying "no"—is a normal part of healthy development and is occurring as a result of the toddler's attempt to assert his or her indepen-

dence. Table 26.1 gives further information related to developing a sense of autonomy.

Cognitive Development

According to Jean Piaget (1969), toddlers move through the last two substages of the first stage of cognitive development, the sensorimotor stage, between 12 and 24 months of age (Table 26.1). Young toddlers engage in tertiary circular reactions and progress to mental combinations. Rather than just repeating a behaviour, the toddler is able to experiment with a behaviour to see what happens. By 2 years of age, toddlers are capable of using symbols to allow for imitation. With increasing cognitive abilities, toddlers may now engage in delayed imitation. For example, they may imitate a household task that they observed a parent doing several days ago.

Piaget identified the second stage of cognitive development as the preoperational stage. It occurs in children between ages 2 and 7 years. During this stage, toddlers begin to become more sophisticated with symbolic thought. The thinking of the older toddler is far more advanced than that of the infant or young toddler, who views the world as a series of objects. During the preoperational stage, objects begin to have characteristics that make them unique from one another. Objects are considered large or small, a particular colour or shape, or a unique texture. This moves beyond the connection of sensory information and physical action. Words and images allow the toddler to begin this process of developing symbolic thought by providing a label for the objects' characteristics. Toddlers also use symbols in dramatic play. First, they imitate life with appropriate toy objects, and then they are able to substitute objects in their play. A bowl may be used to pretend to eat from, but then later it can be used upside down on the head as a hat (Fig. 26.2). Human feelings and characteristics may also be attributed to objects (**animism**). See Table 26.1 for further explanation of cognitive development in toddlerhood.

▶Take NOTE!

Mothers who are depressed may not be as sensitive to their children as other mothers. For this reason, maternal depression is a risk factor in children's cognitive development. Be alert to the mental status of a toddler's mother so that appropriate referrals can be made if needed.

Motor Skill Development

Toddlers continue to gain new motor skills as well as refine others. Walking progresses to running, climbing, and jumping. Pushing or pulling a toy, throwing a ball,

TABLE 26.1 **DEVELOPMENTAL THEORIES**

Theorist	Stage	Activities
Erikson	Autonomy vs. Shame & Doubt Age: 1–3 years	Achieves autonomy and self-control Separates from parent/caregiver Withstands delayed gratification Negativism abounds Imitates adults and playmates Spontaneously shows affection Increasingly enthusiastic about playmates Cannot take turns in games until the age of 3 years

Piaget	Sensorimotor
	   Substage 5: Tertiary Circular
	      Reactions
	Age: 12–18 months
	Sensorimotor
	   Substage 6: Mental
	      Combinations
	Age: 18–24 months
	Preoperational
	Age: 2–7 years
		• Differentiating self from objects
		• Increased object permanence (knows that objects that are out of sight still exist [e.g., cookies in the cabinet])
		• Uses ALL senses to explore environment
		• Places items in and out of containers
		• Imitates domestic chores (domestic mimicry)
		• Imitation is more symbolic
		• Starting to think before acting
		• Understands requests and is capable of following simple directions
		• Has a sense of ownership (my, mine)
		• Time, space, and causality understanding is increasing
		• Uses mental trial and error rather than physical
		• Makes mechanical toys work
		• Plays make-believe with dolls, animals, and people
		• Increased use of language for mental representation
		• Understands the concept of "two"
		• Starting to make connections between an experience in the past and a new one that is currently occurring
		• Sorts objects by shape and colour
		• Completes puzzles with four pieces
		• Play becomes more complex

Adapted from: Erikson, E. H. (1963). *Childhood and society* (2nd ed.). New York: W.W. Norton and Company; Feigelman, S. (2007a). Preschool years. In R. M. Kliegman, R. E. Behrman, H. B. Jenson, & B. Stanton (Eds.), *Nelson textbook of pediatrics* (18th ed.). Philadelphia: Saunders; Feigelman, S. (2007b). The second year. In R. M. Kliegman, R. E. Behrman, H. B. Jenson, & B. Stanton (Eds.), *Nelson textbook of pediatrics* (18th ed.). Philadelphia: Saunders; and Piaget, J. (1969). *The theory of stages in cognitive development.* New York: McGraw-Hill.

and pedaling a tricycle are accomplished in toddlerhood. Fine motor skills progress from holding and pinching to managing utensils, holding a crayon, stringing a bead, and using a computer. Development of eyehand coordination is necessary for the refinement of fine motor skills. These increased abilities of mobility and manipulation help the curious toddler explore and learn more about his or her environment (Fig. 26.3). As the toddler masters a new task, he or she has confidence to conquer the next challenge. Thus, mastery in motor skill development contributes to the toddler's growing sense of self-esteem. The toddler who is eager to face challenges will likely develop more quickly than one who is reluctant. The senses of sight, hearing, and touch are useful in helping to coordinate gross and fine motor movement.

Gross Motor Skills

As gross motor skills are mastered and then used repeatedly, the large muscle groups in the toddler are strengthened. The "toddler gait" is characteristic of new walkers. The toddler does not walk smoothly and maturely. Instead, the legs are planted widely apart, toes are pointed forward, and the toddler seems to sway from side to side while moving forward (Fig. 26.4). Often the toddler seems to speed along, pitching forward, appearing ready to topple over at any moment. The toddler may fall often, but will use outstretched arms to catch himself or herself (parachute reflex). After about 6 months of practice walking, the toddler's gait is smoother and the feet are closer together. By 3 years of age, the toddler walks in a heel-to-toe fashion similar to that of adults. Toddlers often use physical actions such as running,

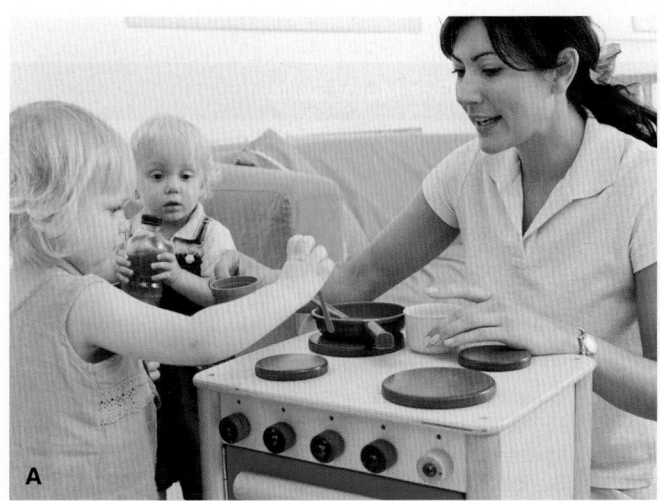

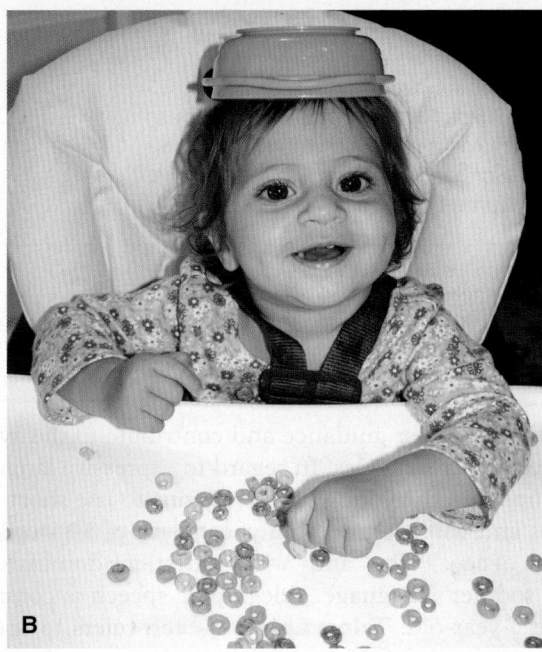

FIGURE 26.2 The toddler will (**A**) pretend with items in the way they are intended to be used as well as (**B**) find other creative uses for them.

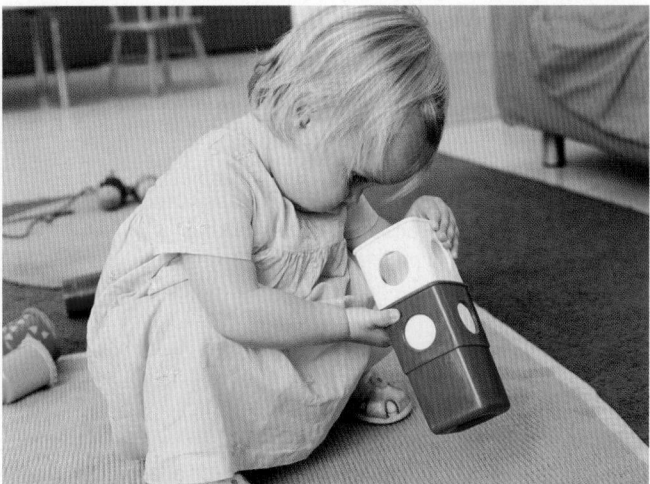

FIGURE 26.3 The toddler's curiosity about the world increases, as does his or her ability to explore it.

Sensory Development

Toddlers use all of their senses to explore the world around them. Toddlers examine new items by feeling them, looking at them, shaking them to hear what sound they make, smelling them, and placing them in their mouths. Toddler vision continues to progress and should be 20/50 to 20/40 in both eyes. Depth perception also continues to mature. Hearing should be at the adult

jumping, and hitting to express their emotions because they are only just learning to express their thoughts and feelings verbally. Table 26.2 lists motor skill expectations in relation to age.

Fine Motor Skills

Fine motor skills in the toddler period are improved and perfected. Holding utensils requires some control and agility, but even more is needed for buttoning and zipping. Adequate vision is necessary for the refinement of fine motor skills because eye–hand coordination is crucial for directing the fingers, hand, and wrist to accomplish small muscle tasks such as fitting a puzzle piece or stringing a bead. See Table 26.2 for age expectations for various motor skills.

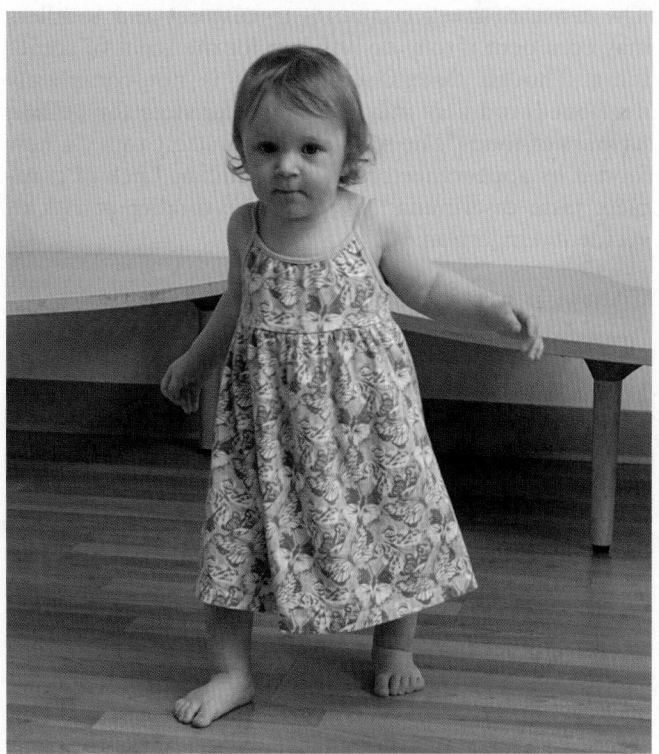

FIGURE 26.4 The young toddler (early walker) walks with a wide-based stance, feet pointing forward and arms out for support.

TABLE 26.2 MOTOR SKILL DEVELOPMENT

Age	Expected Gross Motor Skill	Expected Fine Motor Skills
12–15 months	Walks independently	Feeds self finger foods Uses index finger to point
18 months	Climbs stairs with assistance Pulls toys while walking	Masters reaching, grasping, and releasing: stacks blocks, puts things in slots Turns book pages (singly with board book, multiple if paper) Removes shoes and socks Stacks four cubes
24 months	Runs Kicks ball Can stand on tiptoe Carries several toys, or a large toy while walking Climbs onto and down from furniture without assistance	Builds tower of six or seven cubes Right- or left-handed Imitates circular and vertical strokes Scribbles and paints Starting to turn knobs Puts round pegs into holes
36 months	Climbs well Pedals tricycle Runs easily Walks up and down stairs with alternate feet Bends over easily without falling	Undresses self Copies circle Builds tower of nine or ten cubes Holds a pencil in writing position Screws/unscrews lids, nuts, bolts Turns book pages one at a time

Adapted from: Feigelman, S. (2007a). Preschool years. In R. M. Kliegman, R. E. Behrman, H. B. Jenson, & B. Stanton (Eds.), *Nelson textbook of pediatrics* (18th ed.). Philadelphia: Saunders; Feigelman, S. (2007b). The second year. In R. M. Kliegman, R. E. Behrman, H. B. Jenson, & B. Stanton (Eds.), *Nelson textbook of pediatrics* (18th ed.). Philadelphia: Saunders.

level, as infants are ordinarily born with hearing intact. The sense of smell continues to mature, and toddlers may comment if they do not care for the scent of something. Though taste discrimination is not completely developed, toddlers may exhibit preferences for certain flavours of foods. The toddler is more likely to try a new food if its appearance or smell is familiar. Lack of complete taste discrimination places the toddler at risk of accidental ingestion.

Communication and Language Development

Language development occurs rapidly during the toddler years. The acquisition of language is a dynamic and complex process. The child's age and social interactions and the types of language to which he or she has been exposed influence language development. Receptive language development (the ability to understand what is being said or asked) is typically far more advanced than expressive language development (the ability to communicate one's desires and feelings). In other words, the toddler understands language and is able to follow commands far sooner than he or she can actually use the words themselves. Language is a very important part of the toddler's ability to organize his or her world and actually make sense of it. Thoughtfully planned use of language can

provide behaviour guidance and contribute to the avoidance of power struggles. In regard to expressive language development, the young toddler begins to use short sentences and will progress to a vocabulary of 50 words by 2 years of age. "Why" and "what" questions dominate the older toddler's language. Telegraphic speech is common in the 3-year-old. **Telegraphic speech** refers to speech that contains only the essential words to get the point across, much like a telegram. Rather than "I want a cookie and milk," the toddler might say, "Want cookie milk." In telegraphic speech, the nouns and verbs are present and are verbalized in the appropriate order. Table 26.3 gives an overview of receptive and expressive language development in the toddler.

▶*Take* NOTE!

Stuttering usually has its onset at between 2 and 4 years of age. It occurs more often in boys than in girls. About 75% of all cases of stuttering resolve within 1 to 2 years after they start (Prasse & Kikano, 2008).

Early identification and referral of children with potential speech delays is critical. If a delay is identified, early intervention may increase the child's potential to

TABLE 26.3   LANGUAGE DEVELOPMENT IN TODDLERS

Age	Receptive Language	Expressive Language
12 months	Understands common words independent of context Follows a one-step command accompanied by gesture	Uses a finger to point to things Imitates or uses gestures such as waving goodbye Communicates desires with word and gesture combinations Vocal imitation First word
15 months	Looks at adult when communicating Follows a one-step command without gesture Understands 100–150 words	Repeats words that he or she hears Babbles in what sound like sentences
18 months	Understands the word "no" Comprehends 200 words Sometimes answers the question, "What's this?"	Uses at least 5–20 words Uses names of familiar objects
24 months	Points to named body parts Points to pictures in books Enjoys listening to simple stories Names a variety of objects in the environment Beginning to use "my" or "mine"	Vocabulary of 40–50 words Sentences of two or three words (me up, want cookie) Asks questions (what that?) Uses simple phrases Uses descriptive words (hungry, hot) Two thirds of what the child says should be understandable Repeats overheard words
30 months	Follows a series of two independent commands	Vocabulary of 150–300 words
36 months	Understands most sentences Understands physical relationships (on, in, under) Participates in short conversations May follow a three-part request	Speech usually understood by those who know the child, about half understood by those outside family Asks "why?" Three- to four-word sentences Talks about something that happened in the past Vocabulary of 1,000 words Can say name, age, and gender Uses pronouns and plurals

Adapted from: Feigelman, S. (2007a). Preschool years. In R. M. Kliegman, R. E. Behrman, H. B. Jenson, & B. Stanton (Eds.), *Nelson textbook of pediatrics* (18th ed.). Philadelphia: Saunders; Feigelman, S. (2007b). The second year. In R. M. Kliegman, R. E. Behrman, H. B. Jenson, & B. Stanton (Eds.), *Nelson textbook of pediatrics* (18th ed.). Philadelphia: Saunders; Goldson, E., & Reynolds. A. (2011). Child development and behavior. In W. W. Hay, M. J. Levin, J. M. Sondheimer, & R. R. Deterding (Eds.), *Current pediatric diagnosis and treatment* (20th ed.). New York: McGraw-Hill.

acquire age-appropriate receptive and expressive language skills.

Of special concern in the toddler years is the development of speech and language in potentially bilingual children. At the age of 1 to 2 years, the potentially bilingual child may blend two languages—that is, parts of the word in both languages are blended into one word. At the age of 2 to 3 years, the potentially bilingual toddler may mix languages within a sentence. Thus, the assessment of adequate language development is more complicated in bilingual children.

> ▶ *Take* NOTE!
>
> *Children with preexisting conditions such as genetic syndromes that are known to have an effect on language development should be referred to a speech–language pathologist as soon as the condition is recognized rather than waiting until the child exhibits a delay.*

> ▶ *Take* NOTE!
>
> *Bilingual children often mix languages, and thus speech delay may be more difficult to assess in this population. The bilingual child should have a command of 20 words (between both languages) by 20 months of age and should be making word combinations. If this is not the case, further investigation may be warranted (Abell & Ey, 2007).*

Emotional and Social Development

Emotional development in the toddler years is focused on **separation** and **individuation**. Seeing oneself as separate from the parent or primary caregiver is accompanied by forming a sense of self and learning to exert control over one's environment. As this need to feel in control of his or her world emerges, the toddler displays **egocentrism** (focus on self). This need for control results in emotional lability: very happy and pleasant at one moment, then overreacting to limit setting with a temper tantrum at the next moment. As toddlers identify the boundaries between themselves and the parent or primary caregiver, they learn to negotiate a balance between attachment and independence. Toddlers initially rely on the parents' communication and signals in order to initiate appropriate behaviour or inhibit undesirable behaviour. They have a difficult time choosing between sets of behaviours as they occur in different situations. Power struggles often occur in this age group, and it is important for parents and caregivers to thoughtfully and intentionally develop the rituals and routines that will provide stability and security for the toddler. Many toddlers rely upon a security item (blanket, doll, or bear) to comfort themselves in stressful situations (Fig. 26.5). This ability to self-soothe is a function of autonomy and is viewed as a sign of a nurturing environment, rather than, as one might suspect, one of neglect.

Children also begin to learn about gender differences in the toddler years. They observe the differences between male and female body parts if they are exposed to them.

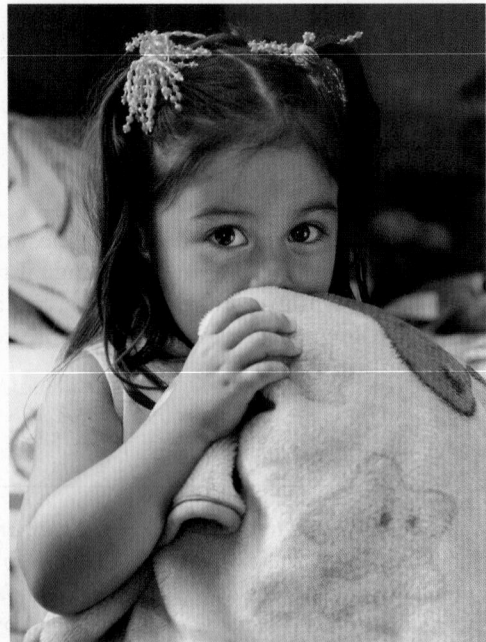

FIGURE 26.5 The toddler may be able to self-soothe and produce a sense of comfort during this stage of establishing autonomy by relying upon a security item such as a doll, toy bear, or blanket.

Toddlers may question parents about these differences and may begin to explore their own genitals. Toddlers also begin to understand and mimic social gender differences. They make observations about gender-specific behaviour dependent upon what they are exposed to.

Aggressive behaviours are typically displayed during the toddler years. Toddlers may hit, bite, or push other children and grab toys. Adults can assist the toddler in building empathy by pointing out when someone is hurt and explaining what happened. Toddlers should not be blamed for their impulsive behaviour; rather, they should be guided toward socially acceptable actions in order to foster the development of appropriate social judgment. It is particularly important for the parent or caregiver to serve as a role model for appropriate behaviour, rather than losing his or her own temper, in order for the toddler to be able to learn how to acceptably handle frustrations. Offering limited choices is one way of allowing toddlers some control over their environment and helping them to establish a sense of mastery. Since toddlers naturally have a short attention span, they will likely have a difficult time staying on task. As toddlers become more self-aware, they start to develop emotions of self-consciousness such as embarrassment and shame.

Though toddlers are becoming more self-aware, they still do not have clear body boundaries. They do not clearly understand the body's functions, though they are beginning to make appropriate connections. Bowel movements may be viewed as a part of the child, and the toddler may initially become upset at seeing it disappear in the toilet. The toddler will protect his or her body by resisting intrusive procedures such as temperature or blood pressure measurement.

Separation Anxiety

As toddlers become increasingly skilled at mobility, they realize that if they have the capability of leaving, then so does the parent. As self-awareness develops and conflicts over closeness versus exploration occur, **separation anxiety** may re-emerge in the 18- to 24-month period. Power struggles may escalate and distress at separating from the parent may increase. Again, a predictable routine with appropriate limit setting may help toddlers to feel safer and more secure during this period. From the age of 24 to 36 months, separation anxiety again eases. The older toddler begins to have a concept of object constancy: he or she has an internal representation of the parent or caregiver and is better able to tolerate separation, knowing that a reunion will occur.

Temperament

Temperament is the biological basis for personality. It is our emotional and motivational core, around which the personality develops over time. Temperament affects how the toddler interacts with the environment. The "easygoing" toddler may adapt more easily and not mind changes in routine as much as other toddlers. The easygoing toddler usually sleeps and eats well and has more predictable and regular behaviours. However, the toddler may still express frustration by having a temper tantrum. The "difficult" toddler is more likely to have intense reactions, negative or positive, with temper tantrums being more likely, more frequent, and more intense than in other toddlers. The structure and routine that toddlers need to feel secure are essential for the difficult toddler; otherwise, the child feels insecure and as a result is more likely to behave inappropriately. The difficult toddler is also the most active of the three temperament types. The "slow-to-warm-up" toddler may be very shy and not as likely to seek out other children. He or she may experience more difficulty with separation anxiety. The behaviour of the slow-to-warm-up toddler is more passive; the toddler may be very watchful and withdrawn and may take longer to mature. Changes in routine usually do not result in as much upset, since the toddler's natural reaction is one of passivity.

Based on the toddler's temperament, make suggestions to the parents for interacting with their child in various situations. For example, to avoid temper tantrums, suggest that the parent should be especially diligent about maintaining structure and routine as well as avoiding tantrum triggers such as fatigue and hunger. Explain to parents that they may need to exercise additional patience with new activities to which the slow-to-warm-up toddler may need extra time becoming accustomed.

Fears

Common fears of toddlers include loss of parents (which contributes to separation anxiety) and fear of strangers. Some toddlers may be very slow to warm up to people they do not know. The nurse caring for a toddler in the out-patient or hospital setting should take the time to establish a relationship with the toddler in order to allay the toddler's fears. Toddlers may be afraid of loud noises and large or unfamiliar animals. Going to sleep may be a scary time for toddlers as they may be afraid of the dark. A nightlight in the toddler's room may be very helpful.

Moral Development

Kohlberg's (1984) description of moral development places the older toddler in the preconventional level. The toddler is only just beginning to learn right from wrong and does not understand the larger concept of morality. Older toddlers begin to feel empathy for others, and acts of altruism may be seen in children as young as 18 months of age.

Environmental and Cultural Influences on Growth and Development

Poverty may directly influence the toddler's ability to grow adequately, as resources for the purchase and preparation of appropriate food may be lacking. Appropriate toys (safe ones) may also not be available in those situations. Food customs continue to have an impact on the child's diet and ability to ingest appropriate nutrients. Individual families' value systems have an impact on the toddler's development as well. Some parents desire to keep their child a "baby" for a longer period, thus delaying weaning or continuing to feed the child baby food or puréed food for a longer period. Other families may highly value independence and encourage the toddler to walk everywhere on his or her own rather than carrying the child.

Culture may also affect emotional development. Some families start at a very young age to discourage crying in boys, encouraging them to "act like a big boy" or "be a man." Ridicule for crying at this age may hurt the toddler's self-concept. Educating families about normal growth and development while continuing to value and support cultural practices is important.

Remember Eugene Dupuis, whom you met at the beginning of the chapter? What developmental milestones would you expect him to have reached at his age?

The Nurse's Role in Toddler Growth and Development

WATCH & LEARN

The toddler's growth and development affects his or her everyday life as well as the family's. Though some toddlers may grow more quickly or reach developmental milestones sooner than others, growth and development remains orderly and sequential. Health care visits throughout toddlerhood continue to focus on growth and development. The nurse must have a good understanding of the changes that occur during the toddler years in order to provide appropriate anticipatory guidance and support to the family.

When the toddler is hospitalized, growth and development may be altered. The toddler's primary task is establishing autonomy, and the toddler's focus is mobility and language development. Hospitalization removes most opportunities for the toddler to learn through exploration of the environment. Isolation for contagious illness further constrains the toddler's ability to find some control over the environment. The nurse caring for the hospitalized toddler must use knowledge of normal growth and development to be successful in interactions with the toddler, promote continued development, and recognize delays (see Chapter 32) (Fig. 26.6).

Nursing Process Overview

Upon completion of assessment of the toddler's current growth and development status, problems or issues related to growth and development may be identified.

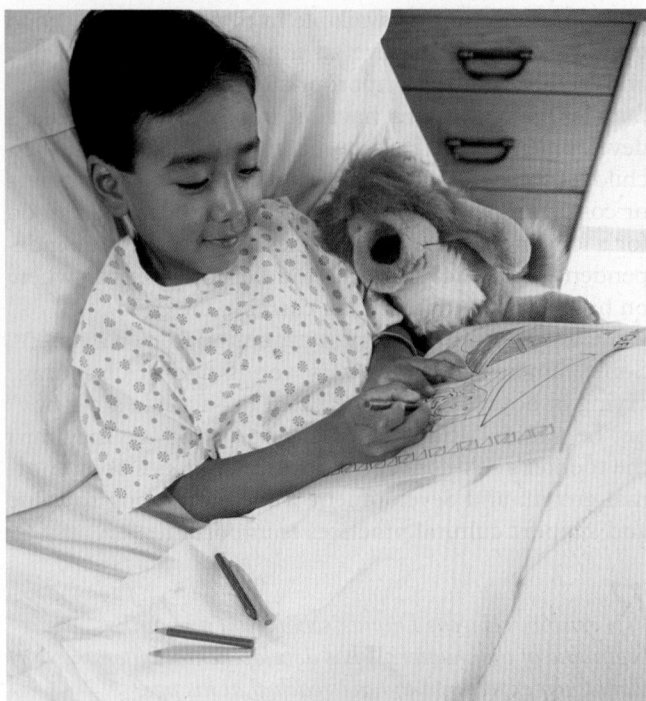

FIGURE 26.6 The hospitalized young child continues to enjoy developmental tasks appropriate for his or her age, such as colouring.

TABLE 26.4 SIGNS OF DEVELOPMENTAL DELAY

Age or Time Frame	Concern
After independent walking for several months	• Persistent tiptoe walking • Failure to develop a mature walking pattern
By 18 months	• Not walking • Not speaking 15 words • Does not understand the function of common household items
By 2 years	• Does not use two-word sentences • Does not imitate actions • Does not follow basic instructions • Cannot push a toy with wheels
By 3 years	• Difficulty with stairs • Frequent falling • Cannot build tower of more than four blocks • Difficulty manipulating small objects • Extreme difficulty in separation from parent or caregiver • Cannot copy a circle • Does not engage in make-believe play • Cannot communicate in short phrases • Does not understand simple instructions • Little interest in other children • Unclear speech, persistent drooling

The nurse may then identify one or more nursing diagnoses, including but not limited to:

• Delayed growth and development
• Imbalanced nutrition, less than body requirements
• Interrupted family processes
• Readiness for enhanced parenting
• Risk for caregiver role strain
• Risk for delayed development
• Risk for disproportionate growth
• Risk for injury

Nursing care planning for the toddler with growth and development issues should be individualized based on the toddler's and family's needs. The nursing care plan may be used as a guide in planning nursing care for the toddler with a growth or developmental concern. The nurse may choose the appropriate nursing diagnoses from Nursing Care Plan 26.1 and individualize them as needed. The nursing care plan is intended to serve as a guide only and is not intended to be an inclusive growth and development plan.

Promoting Healthy Growth and Development

Parents who give their toddler love, attention, and respect regardless of the child's gender, behaviour, or capabilities are helping to lay the foundation for self-esteem. Self-esteem is also built through familiarity with the daily rou-

tine. Routine and ritual help toddlers develop a conscience. Making expectations known through everyday routines helps to avoid confrontations. If the toddler knows the routine, he or she knows what to expect and how he or she is expected to act. When routine and limits are absent, the toddler develops feelings of uncertainty and anxiety. Limit setting (and remaining consistent with those limits) helps toddlers master their behaviour, develop self-esteem, and become successful participants in the family. Children then are able to learn about cooperation throughout the predictable flow of daily life. Nurses need to be aware of normal developmental expectations in order to determine whether the toddler is progressing appropriately. Table 26.4 lists potential signs of developmental delay. Any toddler with one or more of these concerns should be referred for further developmental evaluation.

Promoting Growth and Development Through Play

Play is the major socializing medium for toddlers. Parents should limit television viewing and encourage

(text continues on page 845)

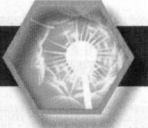

Nursing Care Plan 26.1

GROWTH AND DEVELOPMENT ISSUES IN THE TODDLER

NURSING DIAGNOSIS: Risk for injury related to curiosity, increased mobility, and developmental immaturity

Outcome Identification and Evaluation
Toddler safety will be maintained: *Toddler will remain free from injury.*

Interventions: Preventing Injury
- Teach and encourage appropriate use of forward facing car seat *to decrease risk of toddler injury related to motor vehicles.*
- Teach toddlers to stay away from the street and provide constant supervision *to prevent pedestrian injury.*
- Require bicycle helmet use while riding any wheeled toy *to prevent head injury and form habit of helmet use.*
- Childproof the home *to provide a developmentally safe environment for the curious and increasingly mobile toddler.*
- Post poison control centre phone number *in case of accidental ingestion.*
- Never leave a toddler unattended in a tub or pool or near any body of water *to prevent drowning.*
- Teach parents first-aid measures and child CPR *to minimize consequences of injury should it occur.*
- Provide close observation and keep side rails up on crib/bed in hospital *because toddlers are at particularly high risk for falling or becoming entangled in tubing as they attempt mobility.*

NURSING DIAGNOSIS: Imbalanced nutrition, less than body requirements, related to inappropriate nutritional intake to sustain growth needs (excess juice or milk intake, inadequate food variety intake) as evidenced by failure to attain adequate increases in height and weight over time

Outcome Identification and Evaluation
Toddler will consume adequate nutrients while using an appropriate feeding pattern: *Toddler will demonstrate weight gain and increases in height.*

Interventions: Promoting Appropriate Nutrition
- Assess current feeding schedule and usual intake, as well as methods used to feed, *to determine areas of adequacy versus inadequacy.*
- Determine toddler's ability to drink from cup, finger feed, swallow, and consume textures *to determine if additional exposure is needed or if further interventions such as speech or occupational therapy are required.*
- Weigh toddler daily on same scale if hospitalized, weekly on same scale if at home, and plot growth patterns weekly or monthly as appropriate on standardized growth charts *to determine if growth is improving.*
- Wean from bottle by 15 months of age *to discourage excess milk or juice intake in toddler who can carry bottle around.*
- Limit juice to 120 to 180 mL per day and milk to 500 to 750 mL per day *to discourage sense of fullness achieved with excess milk or juice intake, thereby increasing appetite for solid foods.*
- Provide three nutrient-dense meals and at least two healthy snacks per day *to encourage adequate nutrient consumption.*
- Feed toddler on a similar schedule daily, without distractions and with the family: *toddlers respond well to routine and structure and may eat better in the social context of meals, and they become distracted easily (TV should be off).*

NURSING DIAGNOSIS: Delayed growth and development related to motor, cognitive, language, or psychosocial concerns as evidenced by delay in meeting expected milestones

Outcome Identification and Evaluation
Development will be enhanced: *Toddler will make continued progress toward realization of expected developmental milestones.*

Interventions: Enhancing Growth and Development
- Screen for developmental capabilities *to determine toddler's current level of functioning.*
- Offer age-appropriate toys, play, and activities (including gross motor) *to encourage further development.*
- Perform interventions as prescribed by physical, occupational, or speech therapist: *participation in those activities helps to promote function and accomplish acquisition of developmental skills.*
- Provide support to families of toddlers with developmental delay *(progress in achieving developmental milestones can be slow and ongoing motivation is needed).*
- Reinforce positive attributes in the toddler *to maintain motivation.*
- Model age-appropriate communication skills *to illustrate suitable means for parenting the toddler.*

(continued)

Nursing Care Plan 26.1 (continued)

NURSING DIAGNOSIS: Risk for disproportionate growth related to excess milk or juice intake, late bottle weaning, and consumption of inappropriate foods or in excess amounts

Outcome Identification and Evaluation
Toddler will grow appropriately and not become overweight or obese: *Toddler will achieve weight and height within the 5th to 85th percentiles on standardized growth charts.*

Interventions: Promoting Proportionate Growth
- Wean from bottle and discourage use of no-spill sippy cups by 15 months of age *(will keep mobile toddler from carrying around and continually drinking from cup or bottle).*
- Provide juice (120–180 mL per day) and milk (500–750 mL per day) from a cup at meal and snack time *to encourage appropriate cup drinking and limit intake of nutrient-poor, high-calorie fluids.*
- Provide only nutrient-rich foods without high sugar content for meals and snacks; *even if the toddler won't eat, it is inappropriate to provide high-calorie junk food just so the toddler eats something.*
- Ensure adequate physical activity *to stimulate development of motor skills and provide appropriate caloric expenditure. This also sets the stage for forming life-long habit of appropriate physical activity.*

NURSING DIAGNOSIS: Interrupted family processes related to issues with toddler development, hospitalization, or situational crisis as evidenced by decreased parental visitation in hospital, parental verbalization of difficulty with current situation, possible crisis related to health of family member other than the toddler

Outcome Identification and Evaluation
Family will demonstrate adequate functioning: *Family will display coping and psychosocial adjustment.*

Interventions: Enhancing Family Functioning
- Assess the family's level of stress and ability to cope *to determine family's ability to cope with multiple stressors.*
- Engage in family-centred care *to provide a holistic approach to care of the toddler and family.*
- Encourage the family to verbalize feelings *(verbalization is one method of decreasing anxiety levels)* and acknowledge feelings and emotions.
- Encourage family visitation and provide for sleeping arrangements for a parent or caregiver to stay in the hospital with the toddler *(contributes to family's sense of control of situation).*
- Involve family members in toddler's care, *giving them a feeling of control and connectedness.*

NURSING DIAGNOSIS: Readiness for enhanced parenting related to parental desire for increased skills and success with toddler as evidenced by current healthy relationships and verbalization of desire for improved skills

Outcome Identification and Evaluation
Parent will provide safe and nurturing environment for the toddler.

Interventions: Increasing Parenting Skill Set
- Use family-centred care *to provide holistic approach.*
- Educate parent about normal toddler development *to provide basis for understanding the parenting skills needed in this time period.*
- Acknowledge and encourage parent's verbalization of feelings related to chronic illness of child or difficulty with normal toddler behaviour *to validate the normalcy of the parent's feelings.*
- Encourage positive parenting with respect to toddlers and their normal development *(helps parents develop approaches to toddlers that can be used in place of anger and frustration).*
- Acknowledge and provide positive feedback for positive parenting skills already present *to contribute to parents' confidence in their abilities to parent.*
- Role model appropriate parenting behaviours related to communicating and providing positive discipline with the toddler *(role modelling actually shows rather than just telling the parent what to do).*

Adapted from: Carpenito-Moyet, L. J. (2010). *Nursing diagnosis: Application to clinical practice* (13th ed.). Philadelphia: Lippincott Williams & Wilkins.

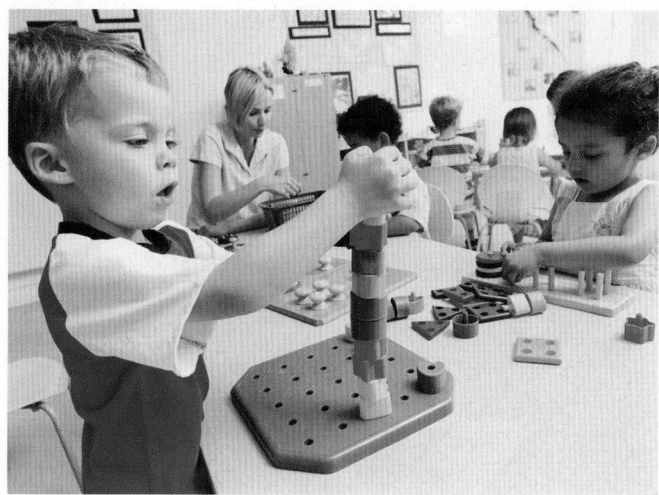

FIGURE 26.7 Parallel play. The toddler usually plays alongside another child rather than cooperatively.

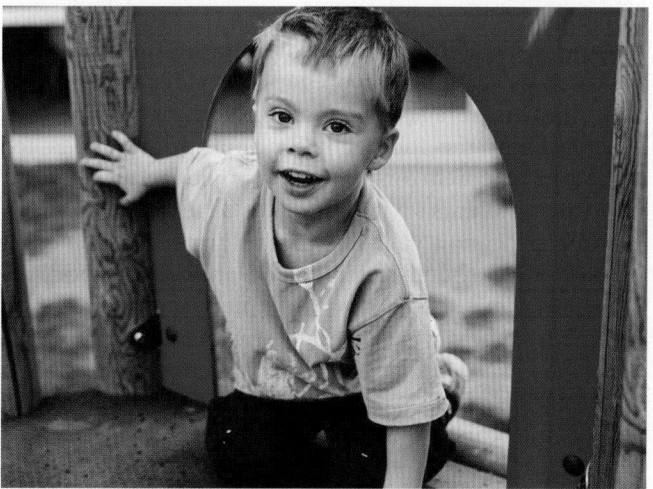

FIGURE 26.8 Toddlers love outdoor physical play, such as climbing on playground equipment. An adult should always supervise toddlers when they are playing outdoors.

creative and physical play instead. Toddlers typically play alongside another child (**parallel play**) rather than cooperatively (Fig. 26.7). The short attention span of the toddler will make him or her often change toys and types of play. It is important to provide a variety of safe toys to allow the toddler many different opportunities for exploring the environment. Toddlers do not need expensive toys; in fact, regular household items sometimes make the most enjoyable toys. Toddlers are egocentric, a normal part of their development. This makes it difficult for them to share. As they are developing a sense of self (who they are as a person), they may see their toys as an extension of themselves. Learning to share occurs in later toddlerhood. Toddlers also like dramatic play and play that recreates familiar activities in the home. Toddlers enjoy introduction to music and musical instruments. They like to listen to music of all kinds and will often dance to whatever they hear on the radio. Toddlers enjoy drums, xylophones, cymbals, and toy pianos. Musical instruments made at home are also enjoyed. A few pebbles or coins inside an empty water bottle with the top tightly secured is a great music maker; an empty butter tub with a lid and a pair of wooden spoons makes a nice drum.

Adequate physical activity is necessary for the development and refinement of movement skills. Toddlers need at least 30 minutes of structured physical activity and anywhere from 1 to several hours of unstructured physical activity per day. Indoor and outdoor play areas should encourage play activities that use the large muscle groups. The activity must occur within a safe environment. Outdoor play structures should be positioned over surfaces that are soft enough to absorb a fall, such as sand, wood chips, or sawdust (Fig. 26.8). Box 26.1 lists recommended age-appropriate toys.

Promoting Early Learning

The parent–child relationship and the interactions between parent and child form the context for the toddler's early learning.

BOX 26.1 Appropriate Toys for Toddlers

- Familiar household items such as plastic bowls and cups of various sizes, large plastic serving utensils, pots and pans, wooden spoons, cardboard boxes and tubes (from paper towel rolls), old magazines, baskets, purses, hats
- Child-size household item toys (kitchen, broom, vacuum cleaner, lawnmower, telephone, and so on)
- Blocks, cars and trucks, plastic animals, trains, plastic figures (family, community helpers), simple dolls, stuffed animals, balls, doll beds and carriages
- Manipulative toys with knobs, wind-ups and buttons that make things happen, putting large pegs or shapes into matching holes, stringing large beads on shoelaces, blocks and containers that stack, jigsaw puzzles with large pieces, toys that can be taken apart and put back together again
- Gross motor toys: play gym, push and pull toys, wagons, tricycle or other ride-on toys, tunnels
- CD players for music, various musical instruments
- Chalk, large crayons, finger paint, Play-Doh, washable markers
- Bucket, plastic shovel and other containers for sand and water play
- Squeaking, floating, squirting toys for the bath

Adapted from: Schuman, A. T. (2007). The ABCs of toy safety: More than just child's play. *Contemporary Pediatrics, 24*(7), 49–57, 64; Shelov, S. P., & Altmann, T. R. (Eds.) (2009). *Caring for your baby and young child: Birth to age 5* (5th ed.). New York: Bantam Books.

Promoting Language Development

Talking and singing to the toddler during routine activities such as feeding and dressing provides an environment that encourages conversation. Frequent, repetitive naming helps the toddler learn appropriate words for objects. The parent or caregiver should be attentive to what the toddler is saying as well as to his or her moods. Using clarification validates the toddler's emotions and ideas. Parents should listen to and answer the toddler's questions. They should sit down quietly with the toddler and gently repeat what the toddler is saying. Encouragement and elaboration convey confidence and interest to the toddler. The toddler needs time to complete his or her thoughts without being interrupted or rushed because he or she is just starting to be able to make the connections necessary to transfer thoughts and feelings into language.

Parents should not overreact to the child's use of the word "no." They can give the toddler opportunities to use the word "no" appropriately by asking silly questions such as, "Can a cat drive a car?" or "Is a banana purple?" When promoting language development, the parent or primary caregiver should teach the toddler appropriate words for body parts and objects and should help the toddler choose appropriate words to label feelings and emotions. Toddlers' receptive language and interpretation of body language and subtle signs far surpass their expressive language, especially at a younger age.

Parents should be careful when discussing very serious topics in the presence of the toddler, since the toddler is very adept at reading emotions.

If the parents speak a foreign language in addition to English, both languages should be used in the home.

Encouraging Reading

Reading to the toddler every day is one of the best ways to promote language and cognitive development (Fig. 26.9). Toddlers particularly enjoy homemade or purchased books about feelings, family, friends, everyday life, animals and nature, and fun and fantasy. Board books have thick pages that are easier for young toddlers to turn; older toddlers can turn paper pages one at a time. The toddler may also enjoy "reading" the story to the parent. The Canadian Paediatric Society (2008) offers tips for parents on how to nurture interest and skills in reading (see Teaching Guideline 26.1).

Choosing a Preschool

The older toddler may benefit from the structure and socialization provided by attending preschool. Attending preschool will help the toddler become more mature and independent and give the toddler a different source for a sense of accomplishment. At this age, toddlers need supervised play with some direction that fosters their cognitive development. A strict curriculum is not necessary in this age group. When choosing a preschool, the

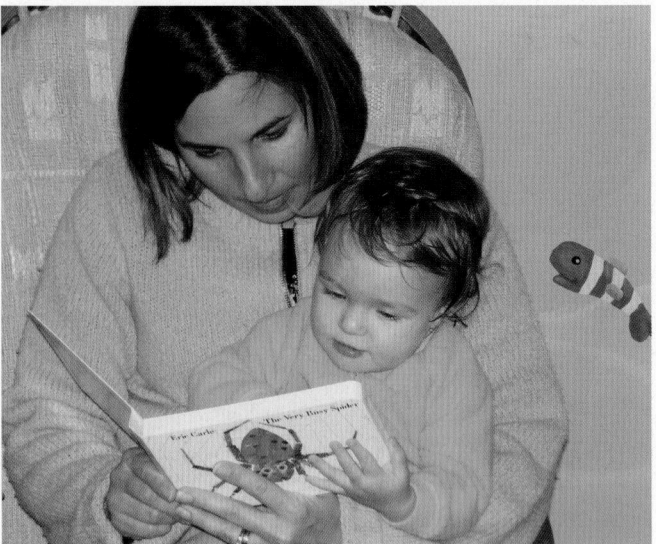

FIGURE 26.9 Reading to a toddler daily is one of the best ways to promote language development and school readiness.

parent or caregiver should look for an environment that has the following qualities:

- Goals and an overall philosophy with which the parents agree (promotion of independence and self-confidence through structured and free play)

TEACHING GUIDELINE 26.1

Tips to Nurture Reading Skills in Young Children

Make books, stories, and storytelling a part of your child's daily routine to help nurture a love of reading.

- **Use rhymes, games, and songs.**
- **Talk about what's going on.** You'll help your toddler develop vocabulary before he or she can even talk.
- **Once your toddler starts talking,** help him or her find the words for familiar things. By repeating words, you'll help your child remember them.
- **Ask questions.** When you say, "What's that?" and name the picture in a book, it teaches your toddler that things have names.
- **Sing songs.** Music makes the words easier to remember, and singing is a fun way to make language come alive.

Visit the public library. There are lots of free resources to encourage love of reading. Many libraries offer free programs for parents and babies and young children that use books, rhymes, and songs. Ask a librarian for more ideas.

Adapted from: Canadian Paediatric Society. (2008). *Read, speak, sing to your baby: How parents can promote literacy from birth.* Retrieved August 16, 2011 from http://www.caringforkids.cps.ca/growinglearning/Reading2Babies.htm.

- Teachers and assistants trained in early childhood development as well as child cardiopulmonary resuscitation (CPR)
- Small class sizes and an adult-to-child ratio with which the parent feels comfortable
- Disciplinary procedures consistent with the parents' values
- Parents can visit at any time
- School is childproofed inside and out
- Appropriate hygiene procedures, including prohibiting sick children from attending

Teach the parents how to ease the toddler's transition to attending preschool. Encourage parents to talk about going to preschool and visit the school a couple of times. On the first day, parents should calmly and in a matter-of-fact tone tell the toddler that they will return to pick him or her up. If the toddler expresses separation anxiety, the parent should remain calm and follow through with the plan for school attendance. After a few days of attendance, the toddler will be accustomed to the new routine and crying when parting from the parent should be minimal.

Promoting Safety

Safety is of prime concern throughout the toddler period. Curiosity, mobility, and lack of impulse control all contribute to the incidence of unintentional injury in toddlerhood. Even the most watchful and caring parents have toddlers who run into the street, otherwise disappear from parents, and fall down the stairs. Toddlers require direct observation and cannot be trusted to be left alone. A childproof environment provides a safe place for the toddler to explore and learn. Motor vehicle accidents, drowning, choking, burns, falls, and poisoning are the most common injuries suffered by toddlers. Safety and injury prevention focuses on these categories.

Safety in the Car

The safest place for the toddler to ride is in the middle of the back seat of the car. Parents should use the appropriate size and style of car seat for the child's weight and age as required by Transport Canada. At a minimum, all children who are 12 months of age and over weighing 10 to 18 kg should be in a forward-facing car seat with harness straps and a clip. Transport Canada (2005) stresses the importance of reading the manufacturer's instructions to help install a car seat correctly. The harness straps are installed using the slot positions at or slightly above the child's shoulders, and the straps must be fastened tightly (allowing only one finger between harness strap and child at the chest). The child seat is installed using either a tether strap and a seat belt or a tether strap and the Universal Anchorage System (UAS) (Fig. 26.10). Parents should be advised to check whether local fire, police, or public health departments have car seat clinics, information sessions, or other opportunities where car seats can be inspected for proper installation.

Drivers should not use their cell phone or attempt to intervene with children while they are driving. Excellent internet resources are available for both parents and professionals regarding car seat safety. Visit http://thePoint.lww.com/Chow1e for direct links to suggested Web resources.

Safety in the Home

Key areas of concern for keeping toddlers safe in the home include avoiding exposure to tobacco smoke, preventing injury, and preventing poisoning.

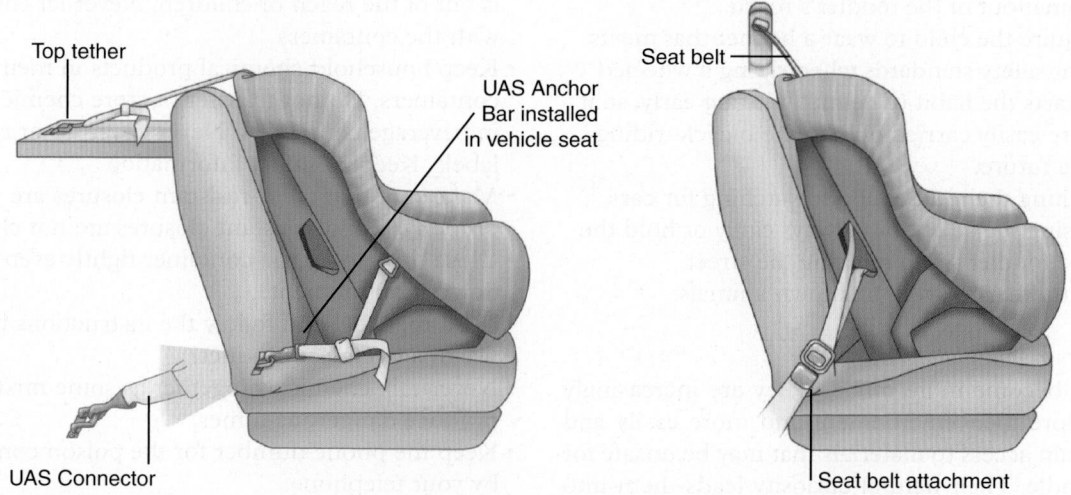

FIGURE 26.10 The top tether further secures the forward-facing car seat. Car seats manufactured after September 1, 2002 have two UAS connectors that attach to the UAS anchor bars in newer vehicles. (Transport Canada, 2005)

Avoiding Exposure to Tobacco Smoke

Environmental exposure to tobacco smoke has been associated with increased risk of respiratory disease and infection, decreased lung function, and increased incidence of middle ear effusion and recurrent otitis media. Parents should avoid cigarette smoking entirely to best protect their children. Even smoking outside the home is suboptimal because smoke lingers on parents' clothing and children who are often carried (such as younger toddlers) face more exposure. Counsel parents to stop smoking (optimal), but if they continue smoking never to smoke inside the home or car with children present.

Preventing Injury

The toddler is able to open drawers and doors, unlock deadbolts, and climb anywhere he or she wants to go. Toddlers have a limited concept of body boundaries and essentially no fear of danger. Toddlers may fall from any height to which they can climb (e.g., play structures, tables, counters). They may also fall from wheeled toys such as tricycles. As toddlers gain additional height and hand dexterity, they are able to reach potentially dangerous items on the counter or stove, leading to an accidental ingestion, burn, or cut.

To prevent injury in the home, stress the following to parents:

- Never leave a toddler unsupervised outdoors.
- Lock doors to dangerous rooms.
- Install safety gates at the top and bottom of staircases.
- Ensure that window locks are operable; if windows are left opened, then secure all window screens.
- Keep pot handles on the stove turned inward, out of an inquisitive toddler's reach.
- Teach the toddler to avoid the oven, stove, and iron.
- Keep electrical equipment, cords, and matches out of reach.
- Remove firearms from the home, or keep them in a locked cabinet out of the toddler's reach.
- Always require the child to wear a helmet that meets government safety standards when riding a wheeled toy. This starts the habit of helmet wearing early, so it can be more easily carried over to the bicycle-riding years of the future.
- Begin teaching the toddler about watching for cars when crossing the street, but always carry or hold the hand of the toddler when crossing the street.
- Teach the toddler to avoid unknown animals.

Preventing Poisoning

As toddlers become more mobile, they are increasingly able to explore their environment and more easily and efficiently gain access to materials that may be unsafe for them to handle. Their natural curiosity leads them into situations that may place them in danger. Poor taste discrimination in this age group allows for ingestion of chemicals or other materials that older children would

---

> ### BOX 26.2 **Potentially Dangerous Household Products**
>
> - Cleaning and bleaching agents (e.g., drain cleaners, ammonia)
> - Drugs and medicines (e.g., iron, narcotics)
> - Household chemicals (e.g., pesticides, antifreeze)
> - Polishers and waxes (e.g., furniture polish, car wax)
> - Cosmetic preparations (e.g., cologne, nail polish)
> - Solvents (e.g., turpentine, paint thinner)

Source: Children's Safety Association of Canada. (n.d.). *Potentially dangerous household products.* Retrieved August 16, 2011 from http://www.safekid.org/potent.htm.

find too unpleasant to swallow. Box 26.2 lists most potentially dangerous ingested poisons. Discuss poison prevention in the home at each well-child visit. Potentially poisonous substances (e.g., medications, cleaners, hair care products, car care products) should be stored out of the toddler's reach, out of the toddler's sight, and in a childproof, locked cabinet.

Health Canada (2009) reports that household chemical products, such as bleaches, paint thinners, ammonia, and abrasive cleaners, are among the top causes of injuries and deaths in children under the age of 5 years. Bad taste and odour do not keep children away from chemical products, and even a very small amount can be harmful. Chemical products can be poisonous, flammable, or corrosive, and the containers can be explosive. Health Canada (2009) advises families and caregivers to:

- Teach children that the hazard symbols on the containers mean DANGER! DO NOT TOUCH!
- Keep all chemical products in a locked cupboard that is out of the reach of children. Never let children play with the containers.
- Keep household chemical products in their original containers. Do not transfer or store chemical products in beverage containers. Never cover up or remove labels. Keep all safety information.
- Make sure that child-resistant closures are working properly. Child-resistant closures are not childproof.
- Close the cap on the container tightly even if you set it down for a moment.
- Read the label and follow the instructions before each use of a chemical product.
- Never mix chemicals together as some mixtures can produce dangerous fumes.
- Keep the phone number for the poison control centre by your telephone.
- Keep other harmful products, such as cosmetics, drugs, vitamins, and first-aid treatment products, out of the sight and reach of children.

BOX 26.3 Preventing Drowning

- Adult supervision is required in all bodies of water, including swimming pools, bathtubs, and open bodies of water. Children under the age of 5 years should be within arm's reach of an adult at all times.
- Adults supervising children near water should be trained in CPR, first aid, water rescue, and swimming.
- Backyard swimming pools should have four-sided fencing at least 1.2 m high and a self-closing, self-latching gate.
- Children under the age of 5 years should wear life jackets when they are in or near water. The life jacket label should indicate that it has been approved by at least one of the following: Transport Canada, Canadian Coast Guard, or Fisheries and Oceans Canada.
- Swimming lessons help give children confidence and comfort around water, but children under the age of 5 years do not have adequate physical skills to perform swimming strokes on their own.

Source: Safe Kids Canada. (2010). *Safety information: Drowning prevention.* Retrieved August 16, 2011 from http://www.safekidscanada. ca/Parents/Safety-Information/Drowning-Prevention/Index.aspx.

For more information, see "Stay Safe: An Education Program About Hazard Symbols!" on the Health Canada website. Visit http://thePoint.lww.com/Chow1e for the direct link.

Safety in the Water

Drowning is the second leading cause of injury-related death for Canadian children (Safe Kids Canada, 2010). Drowning may occur in very small volumes of water such as a toilet, bucket, or bathtub, as well as the obvious sites such as swimming pools and other bodies of water. Toddlers' large heads in relation to their body size place them at risk for toppling over into a body of water that they are inquisitive about. Toddlers should be supervised at all times when in or around the water. In general, most children do not have the physical and cognitive capabilities necessary to truly learn how to swim until 4 years of age. Parents who want to enrol a toddler in a swimming class should be aware that a water safety skills class would be most appropriate. However, even toddlers who have completed a swimming program still need *constant* supervision in the water. Box 26.3 gives recommendations for the prevention of drowning.

*R*emember Eugene Dupuis, the 2-year-old introduced at the beginning of the chapter? What anticipatory guidance related to safety should you provide to his parents?

Promoting Nutrition

The toddler's ability to chew and swallow is improving, and he or she learns to use utensils effectively to feed himself or herself. The early years lay a foundation for the future, and a great deal of parental and societal interest is focused upon nutrition and eating. Forming healthy eating habits has its foundation early in life, and diet has significant influence upon the child's future health status. By establishing healthier food choice patterns early in life, the child is better able to continue these healthy choices later in life. The child less than 2 years of age should not have his or her fat intake restricted, but this does not mean that unhealthy foods such as sweets should be eaten liberally. A diet high in nutrient-rich foods and low in nutrient-poor high-calorie foods such as sweets is appropriate for children of all ages.

Weaning

The timing of weaning from breastfeeding is influenced by a number of factors such as cultural beliefs, local and regional ethnic beliefs, the mother's work schedule, desired child spacing, or societal feelings about the nature of the mother–infant relationship. The extent and duration of breastfeeding are inversely related to the development of obesity later in life: children who breastfeed longer are less likely to become obese than those who breastfeed for shorter periods of time. The overall benefits of breastfeeding are well known. Thus, extending breastfeeding into toddlerhood is believed to be beneficial to the child. Extended breastfeeding provides nutritional, immunologic, and emotional benefits to the child. Contrary to popular belief, it is biologically possible to become pregnant while breastfeeding. Table 26.5 gives recommendations for breastfeeding duration.

Weaning is a highly individualized decision. Educate the mother about the benefits of extended breastfeeding and support her in her decision to wean at a given time.

Weaning from the bottle should occur by 12 to 15 months of age. Prolonged bottle-feeding is associated with the development of dental caries. No-spill "sippy cups" contain a valve that requires the toddler to suck in order to obtain fluid, thus functioning similar to a bottle. Hence, no-spill sippy cups can also be associated with dental caries and are not recommended. Cups with spouts that do not contain valves are acceptable. The

TABLE 26.5 RECOMMENDATIONS FOR BREASTFEEDING DURATION

Organization	Length of Time
World Health Organization	2 years
Health Canada	Up to 2 years and beyond
Canadian Paediatric Society	Up to 2 years and beyond

12- to 15-month-old is developmentally capable of consuming adequate fluid amounts using a cup.

Teaching About Nutritional Needs

Adequate calcium intake and appropriate exercise lay the foundation for proper bone mineralization. The toddler requires an average intake of 500 mg calcium per day. Dairy products are considered the primary sources of dietary calcium. One cup (250 mL) of milk or yogurt provides 300 mg of calcium. Broccoli, oranges, sweet potatoes, tofu, and dried beans or legumes are also good sources of calcium (35 to 120 mg calcium per serving).

▶ *Take* NOTE!

Though 125 g of cooked spinach contains 120 mg of calcium, it is essentially non-bioavailable, making spinach a poor source of calcium.

Iron-deficiency anemia in the first 2 years of life may be associated with developmental and psychomotor delays. Even after correction of the anemia, the effects can be long-lasting (Eden, 2002). Thus, although it is important for toddlers to consume adequate amounts of iron, they tend to have the lowest daily iron intake of any age group. When breastfeeding or formula feeding ends (most often at 1 year of age), it is often replaced with iron-poor cow's milk. Encourage the parents to provide iron-fortified cereals and other foods rich in iron and vitamin C.

▶ *Take* NOTE!

Toddlers who consume a strictly vegan diet (no food from animal sources) are at risk for deficiencies in vitamin D, vitamin B12, and iron. Supplementation with these nutrients should occur to promote adequate nutrition and growth.

The first 2 years of life require high energy intake because they are a time of very rapid growth and development. According to Canada's Food Guide, the percentage of total calories from fat should be 30% to 40% for young children between the ages of 1 and 3 years. Figure 26.11 gives guidance on serving sizes and daily nutritional needs for toddlers. Refer to the Nutrition Resource Centre website (visit http://thePoint.lww.com/Chow1e for the direct link) for more information and Appendix H for Canada's Food Guide. Box 26.4 lists common sources of several nutrients.

BOX 26.4 Key Nutrients Provided by Fruits and Vegetables

Dietary fibre: applesauce, carrots, corn, green beans, mangos, pears

Folate: avocados, broccoli, green peas, oranges, spinach and dark greens, strawberries

Vitamin A: apricots, cantaloupe, carrots, mangos, spinach and dark greens, sweet potatoes

Vitamin C: broccoli, cantaloupe, green peas, oranges, potatoes, strawberries, tomatoes

Adapted from: Brown, J. (2011). *Nutrition now* (6th ed.). Florence, KY: Wadsworth Publishing.

Parents should encourage toddlers to drink water. Juice intake should be limited to 180 mL per day.

Advancing Solid Foods

Parents should offer three full meals and two snacks daily. Portion sizes for toddlers are about one quarter the size of adult portions. Large portions of a new or different food on the toddler's plate may intimidate the toddler. Normal toddler behaviours of mouthing, handling, tasting, extruding the food from the mouth, and then resampling the food often occur. These behaviours are a normal part of toddler development. Parents need to understand and tolerate these behaviours rather than scolding the toddler for them. Toddlers are often afraid to try new things anyway, so the parent or caregiver should be flexible with the toddler's acceptance or rejection of new foods. If the toddler refuses healthy food choices at meal or snack time, parents should not substitute high-fat, high-sugar, processed food "just to make sure he's eating something." This sets the stage for future power struggles. The parent decides which foods will be served or offered. The toddler decides how much will be eaten. The toddler self-regulates the amount of food needed to sustain and allow further growth and development. The toddler may not eat well every day but generally, over the course of several days, will consume the foods he or she needs.

Foods should be served near room temperature. Some of the food on the plate should be soft and moist. Food should always be cut into bite-size pieces. Teaching Guideline 26.2 gives recommendations on ways to prevent choking.

Promoting Self-Feeding

Toddlers most often eat with their fingers, but they do need to learn to use utensils properly. The following are suggestions for parents:

- Use a child-sized spoon and fork with dull tines.
- Seat the toddler in a high chair or at a comfortable height in a secure chair. The toddler should have his or her feet supported rather than dangling (Fig. 26.12).

How much food does my toddler need?

Food guide for toddlers 12–24 months

Offer your toddler a variety of foods from each food group in Canada's Food Guide every day. For toddlers under 24 months old, there is no recommended number of servings for each food group. However, you can use the following chart as a guide on how much to offer. Let your toddler decide how much of it to eat.

Food group	Suggested serving sizes
Vegetables and Fruit	
Offer at least one dark green vegetable (such as bok choy, green beans, broccoli) and one orange vegetable (such as carrots, sweet potato, squash) or certain orange fruits (such as cantaloupe, apricots, peaches) each day.	¼–½ medium vegetable or fruit 15–60 mL (1–4 tbsp) cooked vegetables or fruit, or grated or chopped raw vegetables or fruit 30–60 mL (2 tbsp–¼ cup or 1–2 oz) 100% juice
Grain Products	
Offer whole grain products each day.	¼–½ slice bread ⅛–¼ bagel, pita, or tortilla 5–15 g cold cereal 30–100 mL (2 tbsp–½ cup) cooked cereal 15–60 mL (1–4 tbsp) cooked pasta, rice, bulgur or couscous
Milk and Alternatives	
Offer 500 mL (2 cups or 16 oz) of milk each day.	60–125 mL (¼–½ cup or 2–4 oz) homo (3.25% M.F.) milk 15–25 g (½–1 oz) cheese 30–100 g (2 tbsp–½ cup) yogurt
Meat and Alternatives	
Offer beans, lentils and tofu often. Offer fish at least two times a week.	10–35 g (1–4 tbsp or ¼–1¼ oz) cooked fish, poultry or lean meat 15–100 mL (1 tbsp–½ cup) tofu or cooked beans or lentils ¼–1 egg 5–15 mL (1 tsp–1 tbsp) peanut butter or other nut butters

Source: Feeding Your Toddler, Nutrition Services, York Region Community and Health Services Department, 2007.

GOOD TO KNOW:

Have a nutrition question?

For advice you can trust, speak to a registered dietitian about healthy eating. Call the EatRight Ontario toll-free information service at 1-877-510-510-2 or visit www.ontario.ca/eatright.

FIGURE 26.11 Food guide for toddlers 12 to 36 months. (From Nutrition Resource Centre. [2009]. *Eat right, be active: A guide for parents and caregivers of toddlers 12–36 months.* Retrieved August 16, 2011 from http://www.nutritionrc.ca/resources/pdfs/heal_erba-toddler-eng_09SE09.pdf.) *(continued)*

Food guide for toddlers 24–36 months

For children 24 months and older, Canada's Food Guide gives recommendations on the number of servings for each food group. Food Guide Servings can be divided into smaller amounts of food offered at different meal and snack times. You can get a copy of Canada's Food Guide from www.healthcanada.gc.ca/foodguide or by contacting your local public health unit.

Number of daily servings	How much is one Food Guide Serving?
Vegetables and Fruit	
4 Food Guide Servings	• 1 medium vegetable or fruit • 125 mL (½ cup) fresh, frozen, or canned vegetables or tomato sauce, fruit, or 100% juice • 250 mL (1 cup) leafy raw vegetables
Grain Products	
3 Food Guide Servings	• 1 slice of bread • ½ bagel • ½ pita or ½ large tortilla • 125 mL (½ cup) cooked rice, bulgur, quinoa, pasta, or couscous • 175 g (¾ cup) hot cereal • 30 g cold cereal
Milk and Alternatives	
2 Food Guide Servings	• Breastmilk • 250 mL (1 cup) milk or fortified soy beverage • 175 g (¾ cup) yogurt • 50 g (1½ oz) hard cheese
Meat and Alternatives	
1 Food Guide Serving	• 2 eggs • 30 mL (2 tbsp) peanut butter or other nut butters • 125 mL (½ cup) or 75 g (2½ oz) cooked fish, shellfish, poultry, or lean meat • 175 mL (¾ cup) cooked and canned beans, lentils, chickpeas, hummus, or tofu

Adapted from: Eating Well with Canada's Food Guide, Health Canada, 2007.

FIGURE 26.11 (continued)

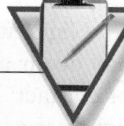

TEACHING GUIDELINE 26.2

Avoiding Choking

- Slowly add foods that are more difficult to chew as the toddler becomes more adept at chewing.
- Cut all foods into bite-sized pieces.
- Avoid foods that are hard to chew and may become lodged in the airway, such as:
  - Nuts
  - Gumdrops or other chewy candies
  - Raw carrots
  - Peanut butter (by itself)
  - Popcorn
- Cut hotdogs and grapes into quarters. Cook carrots until soft; if serving raw, then grate them.
- Always supervise the toddler while he or she is eating.

- Never leave the toddler unattended while eating.
- Minimize distractions during mealtime. Turn off the television and serve food to the toddler along with the other members of the family.

Promoting Healthy Eating Habits

Since the toddler's rate of growth has slowed somewhat compared with that in infancy, the toddler requires less caloric intake for his or her size compared with the infant. This tends to result in **physiologic anorexia**: toddlers simply do not require as much food intake for their size as they did in infancy. During a **food jag**, which is common for toddlers, the toddler may prefer only one

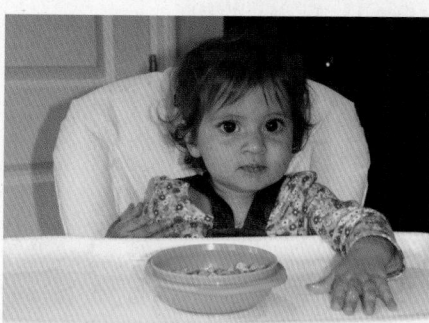

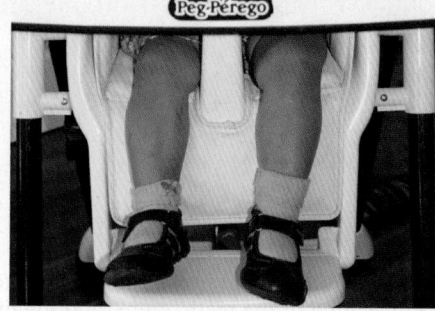

FIGURE 26.12 The toddler should be appropriately and safely seated in the high chair. The safety strap is secure, the toddler's feet are supported, and the tray table is locked in place.

particular food for several days, then not want it for weeks. Again, it is important for the parent to continue to offer healthy food choices during a food jag and not give in by allowing the toddler to eat foods that are preferred by the child but lacking in nutritional content.

The normal developmental issue of testing limits will also occur for the toddler at mealtime. Since toddlers still have limited ability to express their emotions with words, they use nonverbal behaviours to do so. While eating, the toddler may dislike the taste of a particular food or experience a feeling of fullness but will communicate that feeling by screaming or throwing food. When the child exhibits these behaviours, the parent must remain calm and remove the toddler from the situation. Meals should be eaten in a calm and pleasant environment. Parents should serve as role models for appropriate eating habits, but toddlers may also be willing to try more foods if they are exposed to other children who eat those foods. Praise the child for trying a new food, and never punish the toddler for refusing to try something new. A new food may need to be offered many times in a row before the toddler chooses to try it. Parents should be sure to include foods the child is familiar with and likes to eat at the same meal that the new food is being introduced. Teaching Guideline 26.3

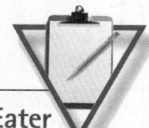

TEACHING GUIDELINE 26.3

Meeting Nutritional Needs of the Picky Eater

Alternative Food Choices for the Picky Eater

- Won't drink milk? Obtain calcium through yogurt (frozen or regular), cheese, pudding, and hot cocoa.
- Poor meat intake? Obtain iron through unsweetened iron-fortified cereals or breakfast bars, raisins; cook with an iron skillet.
- Loves processed white bread? Encourage fibre intake with fresh fruits and vegetables, bran muffins, beans or peas (can be in soup).
- Refuses vegetables? Encourage vitamin A intake with apricots, sweet potatoes, and vegetable juices.

Books for Parents of the Picky Eater

- *Coping with a Picky Eater: A Guide for the Perplexed Parent* by W. Wilkoff. New York: Simon & Schuster, 1998.
- *First Foods* by M. Stoddard. New York: Dorling-Kindersley Publishing, Inc., 1998.
- *How to Get Your Kid to Eat. But Not Too Much* by E. Satter. Boulder, CO: Bull Publishing Co., 1987.
- *The "Everything" Baby's First Food Book* by J. Tarlou. Holbrook, MA: Adams Media Corp., 2001.
- *The Family Nutrition Book* by W. Sears & M. Sears. Boston: Little Brown & Co., 1999.
- *The Healthy Baby Meal Planner* by A. Karmel. New York: Simon & Schuster, 2001.

lists alternative foods that meet nutritional needs and a list of books for parents of the picky eater.

Preventing Overweight and Obesity

In the child younger than 3 years of age, the greatest risk factor for the development of overweight or obesity is having an obese parent. The nurse can screen for overweight in the child over 2 years of age by calculating the body mass index (BMI) and plotting the BMI on the standardized age- and gender-appropriate growth charts (see Appendix F for growth charts and refer to Chapter 31 for BMI calculation instructions). Trends over time may be predictive of the development of overweight or obesity.

Another factor in the development of obesity in young children is juice intake. Since most young children like the sweet taste of juice, they may drink excessive amounts of it. Toddlers who drink excess fruit juice and eat well may develop overweight or obesity because of the high sugar content in the juice. On the other end of the spectrum, some children may actually feel full from juice consumption and decrease their intake of solid foods.

> ▶ **Take** NOTE!
>
> *Young children should consume only pasteurized juice, as unpasteurized juice consumption places the toddler at increased risk of Escherichia coli, Salmonella, and Cryptosporidium infection.*

Refer back to Eugene Dupuis. What questions should you ask his parents related to his nutritional intake? What anticipatory guidance related to nutrition would be appropriate?

Promoting Healthy Sleep and Rest

The 18-month-old requires 13.5 hours of sleep per day, the 24-month-old 13 hours, and the 3-year-old 12 hours. A typical toddler should sleep through the night and take one daytime nap. Most children discontinue daytime napping at around 3 years of age. Toddlers usually make the move from their crib to a youth or toddler bed or even a full-size bed. When the crib becomes unsafe (that is, when the toddler becomes physically capable of climbing over the rails), then he or she must make the transition to a bed.

Consistent bedtime rituals help the toddler prepare for sleep. Choose a bedtime and stick to it as much as possible. The nightly routine might include a bath followed by reading a story. The routine should be a calm period with minimal outside distractions. Toddlers often require a security item to help them get to sleep. Older toddlers may be afraid of the dark, so a nightlight is often helpful.

Night waking is a problem for some toddlers. This may occur as a result of change in routine or as a desire for contact. For some toddlers, night waking is caused by nightmares. As the imagination and capacity for make-believe grow, the toddler may not be able to distinguish between reality and pretend. The parent should hold and comfort the toddler after a nightmare. Limiting television viewing (especially shortly before bedtime) may be helpful in limiting nightmares.

Provide anticipatory guidance to Eugene Dupuis' parents in relation to his sleep.

Promoting Healthy Teeth and Gums

By 30 months of age, the toddler should have a full set of primary ("baby") teeth. Parents may not be aware of the importance of preventing cavities in primary teeth since they will eventually be replaced by the permanent teeth. Poor oral hygiene, prolonged use of a bottle or no-spill sippy cup, lack of fluoride intake, and delayed or absent professional dental care may all contribute to the development of dental caries. Cleaning of the toddler's teeth should progress from brushing with simply water to using a very small amount (pea-sized) of fluoridated toothpaste with brushing beginning at 2 years of age (Fig. 26.13). Weaning from the bottle no later than

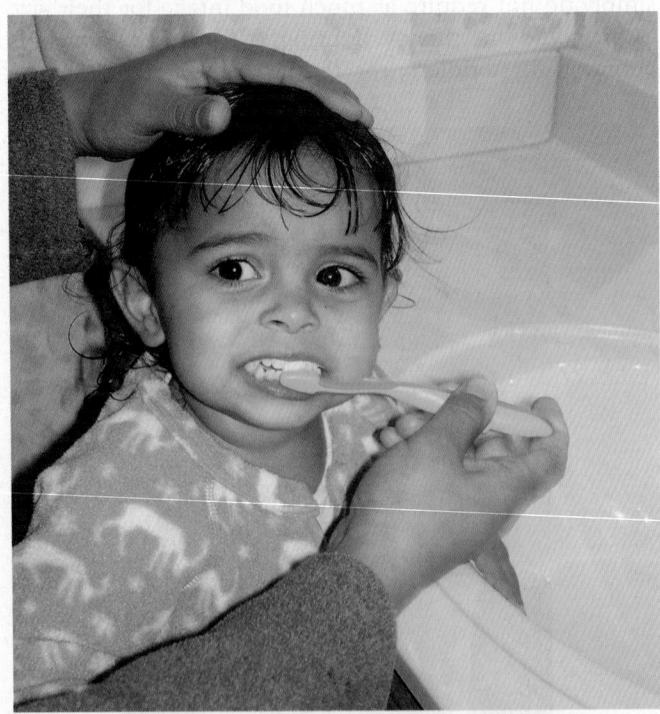

FIGURE 26.13 The parent should brush the toddler's teeth to ensure proper cleaning of the teeth, gums, and tongue. Use only water for brushing before 2 years of age and a pea-sized amount of fluoride-containing toothpaste after the age of 2 years.

15 months of age and severely restricting the use of a no-spill sippy cup (the kind that requires sucking for fluid delivery) are recommended.

At the age of 1 year, the toddler should have his or her first dentist visit to establish current health of the teeth and gums. Eating should be limited to meal and snack times, as "grazing" throughout the day exposes the teeth to food throughout the day. Carbohydrate-containing foods combined with oral bacteria create a decreased oral pH level that is optimal for the development of dental caries (cavities).

Public water fluoridation is a public health initiative that ensures that most children receive adequate fluoride intake to prevent dental caries. If the water supply contains adequate fluoride, no other supplementation is necessary other than brushing with a small amount of fluoride-containing toothpaste after the age of 2 years. Excess fluoride ingestion should be avoided, as it contributes to the development of fluorosis (mottling of the enamel). Fluorosis occurs most often in the toddler years. Risk factors for fluorosis development include:

- High fluoride levels in the local water supply
- Use of fluoride-containing toothpaste prior to the age of 2 years
- Excessive ingestion of fluoride either in toothpaste or in foods
  - Fluoride-containing foods: tea, ready-to-eat infant foods containing chicken, white or purple grape juice, and beverages, processed foods, and cereals that were manufactured with fluoride-containing water

Promoting Positive Discipline

Discipline is a common concern during toddlerhood. The toddler's intense emotional reactions can be difficult for parents to understand and cope with. The toddler needs firm, gentle guidance to learn what the expectations are and how to meet them. The parent's love and respect for the toddler teach the toddler to care about himself or herself and for others. Affection is as important as the guidance aspect of discipline. Having realistic expectations of what the toddler is capable of learning and understanding can help the parent with a positive discipline approach. The toddler's push for autonomy can often test a parent's limits. The easygoing infant may become more challenging in toddlerhood. The toddler's continual quest for new experiences often places the toddler at risk, and his or her negativism very often taxes the parent's patience.

In an effort to prevent the toddler from experiencing harm and in response to his or her continual testing of limits, some parents resort to the use of physical punishment such as spanking. The Canadian Paediatric Society (2004) recommends that all forms of physical punishment should be discouraged. Research points out the dangers and risks inherent in the use of physical or

---

BOX 26.5 Risks Associated with Physical Punishment

- **Child injury:** this may be due to caregiver anger or stress, which may result in the use of stronger force than intended and/or retaliation by the caregiver. Injury can also occur when the caregiver increases the intensity of the punishment if the child does not respond as expected. Young children in particular are no match for the strength of an adult.
- **Impaired parent–child relationship:** deliberately inflicted pain by a parent can lead to feelings in a child (e.g., fear and anxiety) that can negatively affect the parent–child relationship. Over time, parent–child communication may be impaired.
- **Poor child mental health outcome:** poorer outcomes in child mental health, including depression and anxiety, have been associated with physical punishment.
- **Negative child behaviour:** physical punishment has been associated with negative behaviours in childhood such as increased aggression, which may continue into adolescence.
- **Negative adult behaviour:** adults can continue to experience the negative effects of having received physical punishment as a child such as aggression, criminal and antisocial behaviour, tolerance of violence, and poorer mental health. The cycle of use of physical punishment may then continue with their own children.

Source: The complete listing of research studies and references on which these risks were based and determined can be found in Durrant, J. E., Ensom, R., and Coalition on Physical Punishment of Children and Youth. (2004). *Joint statement on physical punishment of children and youth.* Ottawa: Coalition on Physical Punishment of Children and Youth. Retrieved August 16, 2011 from http://www.cheo.on.ca/uploads/AboutUs/Files/joint_statement_e.pdf.

---

corporal punishment (Box 26.5). Of particular concern is the fact that physical punishment puts children, particularly very young children, at risk for injury and therefore physical child abuse. Young children are not capable of linking punishment with undesired behaviours and are often punished for doing what comes naturally. (See Evidence-based Practice 26.1.)

Normal toddler development includes natural curiosity, and this curiosity often results in dangerous or problematic activities for the toddler. Toddlers have a difficult time learning the rules and do not behave badly intentionally. Providing a childproof environment will allow the toddler to participate in safe exploration, which will meet his or her developmental needs and decrease the frequency of intervention needed on the part of the parents.

Discipline should be focused on limit setting, negotiation, and techniques to assist the toddler to learn problem solving. Effective and positive discipline focuses on

EVIDENCE-BASED PRACTICE 26.1
Corporal Punishment and Behaviour Problems in Early Childhood

● Study

A large volume of research indicates that there are few, if any, positive developmental outcomes associated with the use of corporal or physical punishment, such as spanking. In order to determine whether negative consequences resulted, the authors used data from the National Institute of Child Health and Human Development Study of Early Child Care and Youth Development, a large longitudinal ongoing multi-centre study. They reviewed the data from more than 100 children, performing analyses that specifically controlled for contextual and parenting variables as well as for partial child effects. The Home Observation for the Measurement of the Environment (HOME) was administered when the children were 15, 36, and 54 months of age. The HOME measurement determined the use of corporal punishment. To determine the presence of behaviour problems, the Child Behaviour Checklist was administered at 36 months of age and again when the child was in the first grade.

▲ Findings

Multiple regression analysis was performed on the data sets, controlling for variables such as the child's gender, ethnicity, and temperament as well as maternal sensitivity and depression. The results established a causal link between the use of corporal punishment and child adjustment, particularly an increase in behaviour problems during toddlerhood.

■ Nursing Implications

Targeted interventions may have a positive impact on decreasing the use of physical or corporal punishment in young children. Advise parents about the risks associated with physical punishment. Provide them with education about appropriate alternative methods of discipline, including limit setting with consistent follow-through, and extinction. Support parents' efforts to use alternative methods of discipline.

Mulvaney, M. K., & Mebert, C. J. (2007). Parental corporal punishment predicts behaviour problems in early childhood. *Journal of Family Psychology*, 21(3), 389–397.

teaching and guiding children and not forcing them to obey. Discipline should involve mutual respect, consistency, and fairness. The goal is to protect children from danger while helping them learn self-discipline, responsibility, and control. Offering realistic choices helps give the toddler a sense of mastery. Rules should be simple, limited in number, and provided with an age-appropriate explanation. Maintaining the toddler's schedule of meals and rest/sleep will help to prevent conflicts that occur as a result of hunger or fatigue. Toddlers should not be made to share, as this is a concept they do not understand. Parents should encourage simple activities enjoyed by the children involved and avoid confrontation over toys. Parents should offer toddlers appropriate choices to help them develop autonomy, but they should not offer a choice when none exists.

Positive reinforcement should be used as much as possible. "Catching" a child being good helps to reinforce appropriate or desirable behaviours (Gottesman, 2000). When the toddler is displaying appropriate behaviour, the parent should respond consistently with praise and encouragement.

Using "time-out" with younger toddlers is not recommended as they may fear abandonment from the parent. However, if the parent is very frustrated, a brief separation period may be needed for a cooling down period for the parent. "Extinction" may be a useful technique with 2- and 3-year-olds. Extinction involves systematic ignoring of the undesired behaviour. Par-

ents sometimes unknowingly contribute to the occurrence of an unwanted behaviour simply by their response to the toddler (even if it is negative in nature, it is still attention). Parents who want to extinguish a particular (non-dangerous) behaviour should resolve to ignore it every time it occurs. When the child withholds the behaviour or performs the opposite (appropriate) behaviour, the parents should respond in a positive manner. Teaching Guideline 26.4 provides tips on avoiding power struggles and offering appropriate guidance to toddlers.

Addressing Common Developmental Concerns

Common developmental concerns of the toddler period are toilet training, temper tantrums, thumb-sucking or pacifier use, sibling rivalry, and regression. An understanding of the normalcy of negativism, temper tantrums, and sibling rivalry will help the family cope with these issues. Prepare parents for these developmental events by giving appropriate anticipatory guidance.

Toilet Training

When myelination of the spinal cord is achieved around the age of 2 years, the toddler is capable of exercising voluntary control over the sphincters. Girls may be ready for toilet training earlier than boys. Toddlers are ready for toilet training when:

TEACHING GUIDELINE 26.4

Providing Toddlers with Guidance

- When giving the toddler instructions, tell the child what to do, NOT what not to do. This allows for a positive focus. If you must say "no," "don't," or "stop," then follow with a direction of what to do instead.
- Offer limited choices, when a choice is truly available. Say, "Do you want to wear your blue hat or your red hat?" NOT "Do you want to put on your hat?" This gives the toddler some, but not all, control.
- Role model appropriate communication and avoid yelling.
- Pay attention to the inflection in your voice. A statement or direction should not end in a questioning tone or with "Okay?" Be clear. Statements should sound like statements, and only questions should end in a questioning tone.
- When a toddler behaves aggressively, label the child's feelings calmly, but be firm and consistent with the expectation. For example, "I know you're mad at your friend, but it is not okay to hit. Hitting hurts, and that makes your friend sad."

Adapted from: American Academy of Pediatrics. (1998). *Guidance for effective discipline.* Retrieved August 16, 2011 from http://aappolicy. aappublications.org/cgi/content/full/pediatrics;101/4/723; Anderson, J. (2008). Discipline techniques: The 12-month-old. *Contemporary Pediatrics, 25*(9), 84–87.

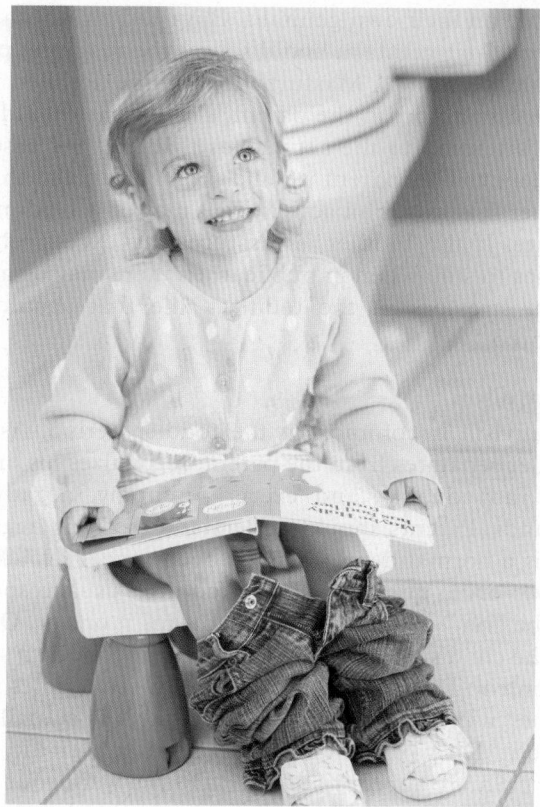

FIGURE 26.14 The toddler will feel most comfortable with a potty chair that sits on the floor.

- Bowel movements occur on a fairly regular schedule.
- The toddler expresses knowledge of the need to defecate or urinate. This may be through verbalization, change in activity, or gestures such as:
  - Looks into or grabs diaper
  - Squats
  - Crosses legs
  - Grimaces and/or grunts
  - Hides behind a door or the couch when defecating
- The diaper is not always wet (this indicates the ability to hold the urine for a period of time).
- The toddler is willing to follow instructions.
- The toddler walks well alone and is able to pull down his or her pants.
- The toddler follows caregivers to the bathroom.
- The toddler climbs onto the potty chair or toilet.

Parents should approach toilet training with a calm, positive, and nonthreatening manner. Start with the toddler fully clothed on the potty chair or toilet while the parent or caregiver talks about what the toilet is used for and when. The toddler will feel most comfortable with a toddler potty chair that sits on the floor (Fig. 26.14). If a potty chair is unavailable, facing toward the toilet tank may make the toddler feel more

secure, as the buttocks remain on the front of the seat rather than sinking through the toilet seat opening. After a week or longer, remove a dirty diaper and place the contents in the toilet. Next try having the toddler sit on the potty chair or toilet without pants or diaper on. The toddler may benefit from watching a same-sexed caregiver or friend use the toilet. Parents should always use gentle praise and no reproaches. Usually the best time to achieve success with defecation on the toilet is following a meal. When the toddler has achieved success with bowel control, bladder control will come next. It may be many months before nighttime bladder control is achieved, and the toddler may still require a diaper at night. Parents should use appropriate words for body parts, urination, and defecation, then use those words consistently so the toddler understands what to say and do.

After a couple of weeks of successful toileting, the toddler may start wearing training pants. When toddlers have an accident and don't make it to the toilet, gently remind them about toileting and let them help clean up. Toddlers should never be punished for bowel or bladder "accidents."

With so much attention focused on the genitalia during toilet training and the frequency of being without a diaper, it is natural for toddlers to become more focused on their own genitalia. Boys and girls both will explore their genitalia and discover the resulting pleasurable sensation. Masturbation in the toddler may cause discomfort in the parent. The parent should not draw attention to the activity, as that may increase its frequency. The parent should calmly explain to the toddler that this is an activity that may only be done in private. If the toddler is masturbating excessively or refuses to stop when in public, then there may be additional stressors in the toddler's life that should be explored.

Negativism

Negativism is common in the toddler period. As the toddler separates from the parent, recognizes his or her own individuality, and exerts autonomy, negativism abounds. Parents should understand that this negativism is a normal developmental occurrence. Avoid asking yes-or-no questions, as the toddler's usual response will be "no," whether he or she means it or not. Offering the child simple choices will give the toddler a sense of control. The parent should not ask the toddler if he or she "wants" to do something, if there is actually no choice. "Do you want to use the red cup or the blue cup?" is more appropriate than "Do you want your milk now?" When it is time to go outside, don't ask, "Do you want to put your shoes on?" Instead, state in a matter-of-fact tone that shoes must be worn outside and give the toddler a choice of the type of shoe or colour of socks. If the child continues with negative answers, then the parent should remain calm and make the decision for the child.

Temper Tantrums

Even children who displayed an easygoing personality as infants may lose their temper frequently during the toddler years (Fig. 26.15). A toddler who was more intense as an infant may have more temper tantrums. Temper tantrums are a natural result of the frustration that toddlers experience. Toddlers are eager to explore new things, but their efforts are often thwarted (usually for safety reasons). Toddlers do not behave badly on purpose. They need time and maturity to learn the rules and regulations. Some of their frustration may come from lack of language skills to express themselves. Toddlers are just starting to learn how to verbalize feelings and to use alternative actions rather than just "acting out." The temper tantrum may be manifested as a screaming and crying fit or a full-blown episode in which the toddler throws himself or herself on the floor kicking, screaming, and pounding, perhaps even holding the breath. Fatigue or hunger may limit the toddler's coping abilities and promote negative behaviour and temper tantrums.

Although tantrums are frustrating for parents and caregivers, they are a normal part of the toddler's quest

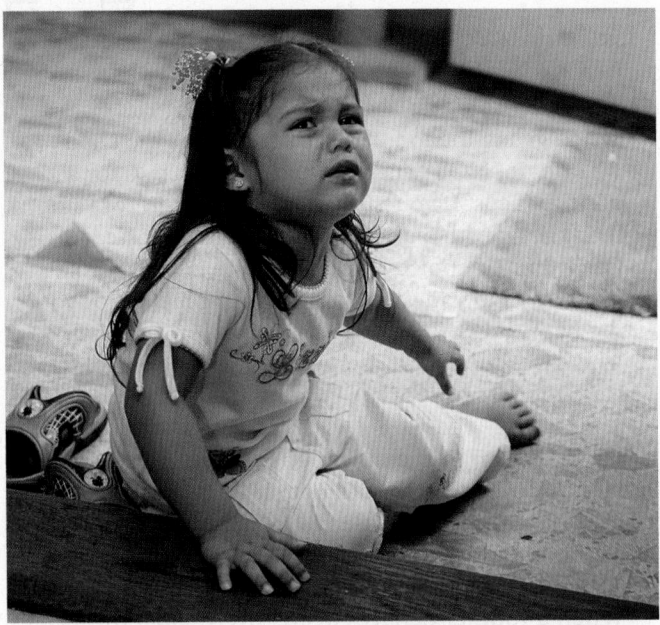

FIGURE 26.15 Tantrums are a normal component of toddler development.

for independence. As toddlers mature, they become better able to express themselves and to understand their environment.

Parents need to learn their toddler's behavioural cues in order to limit activity that is frustrating. When the parent notes the beginnings of frustration, a friendly warning might be given. Intervening early with an activity change might prevent a tantrum. Use distraction, refocusing, or removal from the situation.

When a temper tantrum does occur, the best course of action is to ignore the behaviour and ensure that the child is safe during the tantrum. Physical punishment is inappropriate and will probably just prolong the tantrum and produce more intense negative behaviour as well as put the child at risk for physical injury (Ateah, Secco, & Woodgate, 2003). It is very important for parents to model self-control. Since toddlers' tantrums most often result from frustration, the role-modelled behaviour of self-control helps to teach toddlers to control their temper when they can't get what they want.

Thumb-Sucking and Pacifiers

Infants bring their hands to their mouths and begin thumb-sucking as a form of self-soothing. This habit may continue into the toddler years and beyond. The pacifier is used for the same reason. Toddlers may calm themselves in a stressful situation by thumb-sucking or sucking on a pacifier. Opinions about thumb- and finger sucking and pacifier use are significantly affected by family history and culture. For most children, there is no need to worry about a sucking habit until it is time for the permanent teeth to erupt. It is recommended that if thumb-sucking or pacifier use continues beyond this point then the issue must be discussed with the child's dentist. Prolonged and frequent sucking in the withdrawn child is more likely to yield changes to the tooth and jaw structure than sucking that is primarily used for self-soothing. Parents must sort through their own feelings about thumb-sucking and pacifier use and then decide how they want to handle the habit.

To ensure safety with pacifier use:

• Use only one-piece pacifiers.
• Replace worn pacifiers with new ones.
• Never tie a pacifier around a toddler's neck.

Sibling Rivalry

Many families have subsequent children when their first child is a toddler. The toddler has been accustomed to being the baby and receiving a great deal of attention, both at home and with the extended family. Since toddlers are normally egocentric, bringing a new baby into the home may be quite disruptive. To minimize issues with **sibling rivalry**, parents should attempt to keep the toddler's routine as close to normal as possible. Spend individual time with the toddler on a daily basis. Involve the toddler in the care of the baby. The toddler is capable of fetching a diaper or T-shirt, entertaining the baby with a toy, or helping sing a song to calm the baby. "Helping" the parent care for the baby gives the toddler a sense of importance (Fig. 26.16). The toddler will need significant support while holding the baby.

Regression

Some toddlers experience **regression** during a stressful event (e.g., the birth of a sibling, hospitalization). Stress in a toddler's life affects his or her ability to master new developmental tasks. During regression, the toddler may want to go back to an earlier stage. He or she may desire a bottle or pacifier long ago forgotten. The toddler may stop displaying previously achieved language or motor skills. A significant stress in the toddler's life may also disrupt the toilet training process (e.g., toilet training may not be achieved near the time a sibling is born). When regression occurs, parents should ignore the regressive behaviour and offer praise for age-appropriate behaviour or attainment of skills.

Refer to Eugene Dupuis, the 2-year-old in the case study. List common developmental concerns of the toddler. What anticipatory guidance related to these concerns would the nurse provide to Eugene's parents?

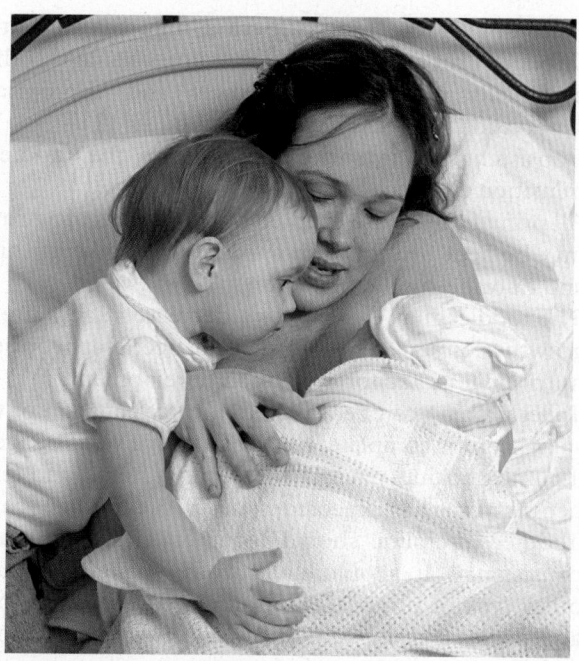

FIGURE 26.16 The toddler may be more likely to accept the new baby in a positive manner if he or she feels that this is "our baby," not just "mommy's baby." This toddler is meeting her new brother for the first time.

■ ■ ■ Key Concepts

■ The toddler's organ systems are continuing to mature, and growth slows during this period as compared with infancy.

■ The psychosocial task of the toddler years is to attain a sense of autonomy by experiencing separation and individuation.

■ Cognitive development in toddlerhood progresses from sensorimotor in nature to preoperational.

■ The toddler refines gross motor skills after learning to walk and builds fine motor skills through the use of utensils and various manipulative toys.

■ The toddler progresses from limited expressive language capabilities to a vocabulary of 1,000 words by the age of 3 years.

■ Toddlers use all of their senses to explore and learn about their environment.

■ Visual acuity progresses to at least 20/50 in the toddler period.

■ Negativism is likely in toddlers as they attempt to exert their independence.

■ Very ritualistic, toddlers feel safer and more secure when clear limits are enforced and a structured routine is followed.

■ Toddler development may be promoted through active gross motor play, books, music, and block building.

■ Safety is a primary concern in the toddler years as the child is more mobile, very curious, and experimenting with autonomy.

- Poisoning in the toddler period may be prevented through proper storage of medications and other potentially poisonous substances and appropriate supervision.
- Consistent bedtime rituals help ease the toddler's transition to sleep.
- All primary teeth are erupted by 30 months of age and may be kept healthy with appropriate tooth brushing and fluoride supplementation.
- The toddler may experience a decrease in appetite as growth slows, yet he or she still needs appropriate nutritional intake for continued development.
- Toilet training can be achieved after myelination of the spinal cord is complete, usually around 2 years of age.
- Thumb-sucking, pacifier use, security items, and temper tantrums are expected issues in the toddler years.
- Toddler discipline should focus on clear limits and consistency. It should not involve spanking or any other type of physical punishment. It should be balanced with a caring and nurturing environment along with frequent praise and encouragement for appropriate behaviour.
- Parental role modelling of appropriate behaviour, especially related to dealing with frustration, is beneficial to toddlers.
- Parents play an important role in toddler development, not only by providing a loving environment but also by role modelling appropriate behaviour in most areas of daily life.

REFERENCES

Abell, S., & Ey, J. L. (2007). Ask Dr. Sue. Bilingual child. *Clinical Pediatrics, 46*(7), 658–659.

Anderson, J. (2008). Discipline techniques: The 12-month-old. *Contemporary Pediatrics, 25*(9), 84–87.

Arias, A., Bennison, J., Justus, K., & Thurman, D. (2001). Educating parents about normal stool pattern changes in infants. *Journal of Pediatric Health Care, 15*(5), 269–274.

Ateah, C. A., Secco, L., & Woodgate, R. L. (2003). The risks and alternatives to physical punishment use with children. *Journal of Pediatric Health Care, 17*(3), 126–132.

Brown, J. (2011). *Nutrition now* (6th ed.). Florence, KY: Wadsworth Publishing.

Canadian Paediatric Society. (2004). Effective discipline for children. *Paediatric Child Health, 9*(1), 37–41.

Canadian Paediatric Society. (2008). *Read, speak, sing to your baby: How parents can promote literacy from birth.* Retrieved on August 16, 2011 from http://www.caringforkids.cps.ca/growinglearning/Reading2Babies.htm

Carpenito-Moyet, L. J. (2010). *Nursing diagnosis: Application to clinical practice* (13th ed.). Philadelphia: Lippincott Williams & Wilkins.

Children's Safety Association of Canada. (n.d.). *Potentially dangerous household products.* Retrieved August 16, 2011 from http://www.safekid.org/potent.htm

Durrant, J.E., Ensom, R., and the Coalition on Physical Punishment of Children and Youth. (2004). *Joint statement on physical punishment of children and youth.* Ottawa: Coalition on Physical Punishment of Children and Youth. Retrieved August 16, 2011 from http://www.cheo.on.ca/uploads/AboutUs/Files/joint_statement_e.pdf

Eden, A. (2002). The prevention of iron-deficiency anemia. *Archives of Pediatric and Adolescent Medicine, 156,* 519.

Erikson, E. H. (1963). *Childhood and society* (2nd ed.). New York: W.W. Norton and Company.

Feigelman, S. (2007a). Preschool years. In R. M. Kliegman, R. E. Behrman, H. B. Jenson, & B. Stanton (Eds.), *Nelson textbook of pediatrics* (18th ed.). Philadelphia: Saunders.

Feigelman, S. (2007b). The second year. In R. M. Kliegman, R. E. Behrman, H. B. Jenson & B. Stanton (Eds.), *Nelson textbook of pediatrics* (18th ed.). Philadelphia: Saunders.

Goldson, E., & Reynolds, A. (2011). Child development and behavior. In W. W. Hay, M. J. Levin, J. M. Sondheimer, & R. R. Deterding (Eds.), *Current pediatric diagnosis and treatment* (20th ed.). New York: McGraw-Hill.

Gottesman, M. M. (2000). Nurturing the social and emotional development of children, a.k.a. discipline. *Journal of Pediatric Health Care, 14*(2), 81–84.

Health Canada. (2009). *Is your child safe?* Retrieved August 16, 2001 from http://www.hc-sc.gc.ca/cps-spc/pubs/cons/child-enfant/index-eng.php

Kohlberg, L. (1984). *Moral development.* New York: Harper & Row.

Nutrition Resource Centre. (2009). *Eat right, be active: A guide for parents and caregivers of toddlers 12–36 months.* Retrieved August 16, 2011 from http://www.nutritionrc.ca/resources/pdfs/heal_erba-toddler-eng_09SE09.pdf

Piaget, J. (1969). *The theory of stages in cognitive development.* New York: McGraw-Hill.

Prasse, J. E., & Kikano, G. E. (2008). Stuttering: An overview. *American Family Physician, 77*(9), 1271–1276.

Safe Kids Canada. (2010). *Safety information: Drowning prevention.* Retrieved August 16, 2011 from http://www.safekidscanada.ca/Parents/Safety-Information/Drowning-Prevention/Index.aspx

Schuman, A. T. (2007). The ABCs of toy safety: More than just child's play. *Contemporary Pediatrics, 24*(7), 49–57, 64.

Shelov, S. P. & Altmann, T. R. (Eds.) (2009). *Caring for your baby and young child: Birth to age 5* (5th ed.). New York: Bantam Books.

Transport Canada. (2005). *Car Time – Stage 2: Safe travel in a forward-facing child seat.* Retrieved August 16, 2011 from http://www.tc.gc.ca/eng/roadsafety/safedrivers-childsafety-car-cartime-stage2-226.htm

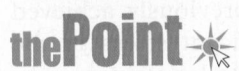

thePoint For additional learning materials, including Internet Resources, visit **http://thePoint.lww.com/Chow1e.**

CHAPTER WORKSHEET

MULTIPLE CHOICE QUESTIONS

1. The nurse is caring for a hospitalized 30-month-old who is resistant to care, angry, and yells "no" all the time. The nurse identifies this toddler's behaviour as

    a. problematic, as it interferes with needed nursing care.

    b. normal for this stage of growth and development.

    c. normal because the child is hospitalized and out of his routine.

    d. concerning, since toddlers should have more control of their emotions.

2. The mother of a 15-month-old is concerned about a speech delay. She describes her toddler as being able to understand what she says, sometimes following commands, but using only one or two words with any consistency. What is the nurse's best response to this information?

    a. The toddler should have a developmental evaluation as soon as possible.

    b. If the mother would read to the child, then speech would develop faster.

    c. Receptive language normally develops earlier than expressive language.

    d. The mother should ask her pediatrician for a speech therapy evaluation.

3. A 2-year-old is having a temper tantrum. What advice should the nurse give the mother?

    a. For safety reasons, the toddler should be restrained during the tantrum.

    b. Punishment should be initiated, as tantrums should be controlled.

    c. The mother should promise the toddler a reward if the tantrum stops.

    d. The tantrum should be ignored as long as the toddler is safe, and comfort should be provided afterward.

4. What is the best advice about nutrition for the toddler?

    a. Encourage cup drinking and give water between meals and snacks.

    b. Encourage unlimited milk intake, because toddlers need the protein for growth.

    c. Avoid sugar-sweetened fruit drinks and allow as much natural fruit juice as desired.

    d. Allow the toddler unlimited access to the sippy cup to ensure adequate hydration.

CRITICAL THINKING EXERCISES

1. Develop a teaching plan about safety to present to a toddler-age preschool class.

2. Construct a 3-day menu for a 2-year-old, one that is realistic and will provide the nutrients needed.

3. Develop a plan for educating the parent of a 34-month-old who has been resistant to toilet training. Include assessments the nurse will make as well as the plan for teaching.

STUDY ACTIVITIES

1. Visit a preschool that provides care for special-needs toddlers as well as typical toddlers. Perform a developmental assessment on a typical toddler and one with special needs (both the same age). Compare and contrast your findings.

2. Care for two average 2-year-olds in the clinical setting. Describe each toddler's behaviour, response to the parent, and response to the nurse and list strategies used to gain compliance and minimize stress to the toddler.

3. Observe in the toddler classroom of a typical preschool. Choose two toddlers of the same age with different temperaments. Record the toddlers' differences and similarities in response to structure and authority, interactions with classmates, attention levels, and language and activity levels.

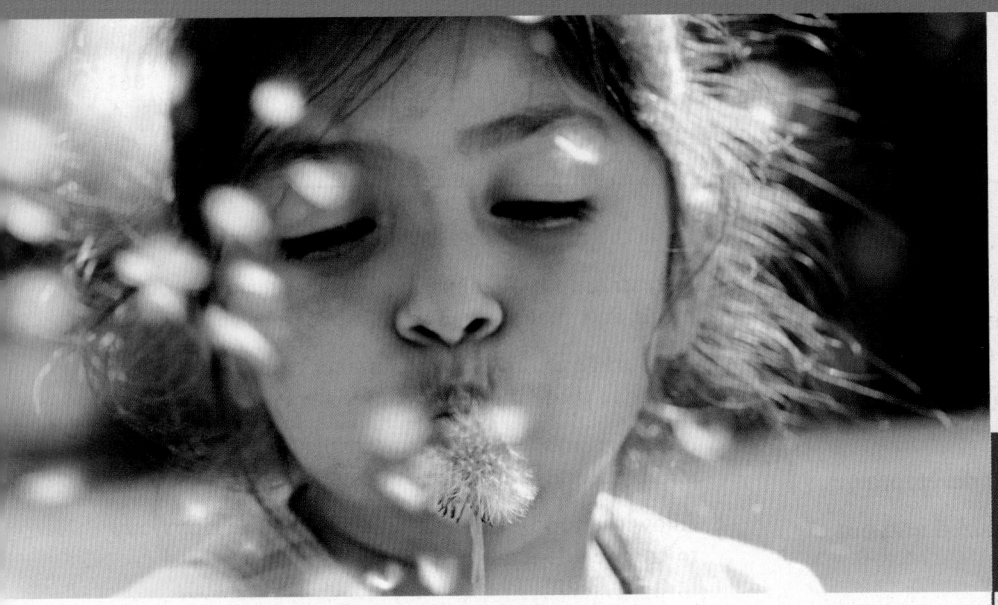

CHAPTER 27

Adapted by Christine A. Ateah

GROWTH AND DEVELOPMENT OF THE PRESCHOOLER

KEY TERMS

animism
empathy
imaginary friend

magical thinking
preoperational thought
school readiness

telegraphic speech
transduction

LEARNING OBJECTIVES

Upon completion of the chapter, the learner will be able to:

1. Identify normal physiologic, cognitive, and psychosocial changes occurring in the preschool-aged child.
2. Express an understanding of language development in the preschool years.
3. Implement a nursing care plan that addresses common concerns or delays in the preschooler's development.
4. Integrate knowledge of preschool growth and development with nursing care and health promotion of the preschool-age child.
5. Develop a nutritional plan for the preschool-age child.
6. Identify common issues related to growth and development during the preschool years.
7. Demonstrate knowledge of appropriate anticipatory guidance for common developmental issues that arise in the preschool period.

*N*ila Patel is a 4-year-old girl, brought to the clinic by her mother and father for her school check-up. During your assessment you measure her weight to be 20 kg and her height 100 cm. As the nurse caring for her, assess Nila's growth and development, and then provide appropriate anticipatory guidance to her parents.

WoW

Quality parenting is achieved only by example.

The preschool period is the period between 3 and 6 years of age. This is a time of continued growth and development. Physical growth continues much more slowly compared with earlier years. Gains in cognitive, language, and psychosocial development are substantial throughout the preschool period. Many tasks that began during the toddler years are mastered and perfected during the preschool years. The child has learned to tolerate separation from parents, has a longer attention span, and continues to learn skills that will lead to later success in the school-age period. Preparation for success in school occurs during the preschool period because most children enter elementary school by the end of the preschool period.

Growth and Development Overview

The healthy preschooler is slender and agile, with an upright posture. The formerly clumsy toddler becomes more graceful, demonstrating the ability to run more smoothly. Athletic abilities may begin to develop. Major development occurs in the area of fine motor coordination. Psychosocial development is focused on the accomplishment of initiative. Preconceptual thought and intuitiveness dominate cognitive development. The preschooler is an inquisitive learner and absorbs new concepts like a sponge absorbs water.

Physical Growth

The average preschool-age child will grow 6.5 to 7.8 cm per year. Average weight gain during this time period is about 2.3 kg per year (Feigelman, 2007). The average weight of a 3-year-old is 14.5 kg, increasing to an average weight of 18.6 kg by age 5. The loss of baby fat and the growth of muscle during the preschool years give the child a stronger and more mature appearance (Fig. 27.1). The length of the skull also increases slightly, with the lower jaw becoming more pronounced. The upper jaw widens through the preschool years in preparation for the emergence of permanent teeth, usually starting around age 6.

Organ System Maturation

Most of the body systems have matured by the preschool years. Myelination of the spinal cord allows for bowel and bladder control to be complete in most children by age 3 years. The respiratory structures are continuing to grow in size, and the number of alveoli continues to increase, reaching the adult number at about 7 years of age. The eustachian tubes remain relatively short and straight. Heart rate decreases and blood

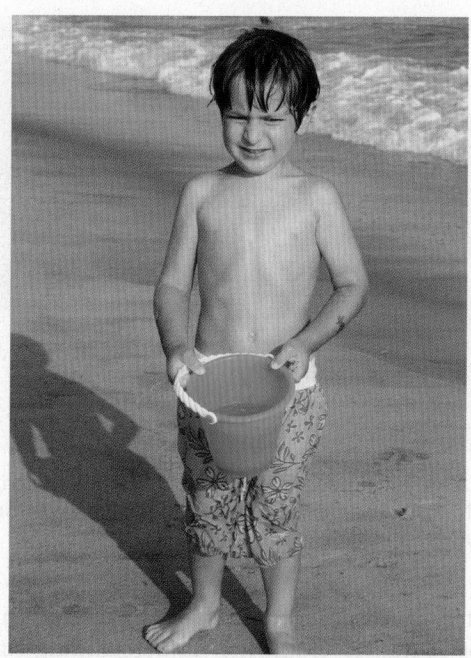

FIGURE 27.1 The preschool child has a more slender appearance and more erect posture than the toddler.

pressure increases slightly during the preschool years. An innocent heart murmur may be heard upon auscultation, and splitting of the second heart sound may become evident. The preschooler should have 20 deciduous teeth present.

The small intestine is continuing to grow in length. Stool passage usually occurs once or twice per day in the average preschooler. The 4-year-old generally has adequate bowel control. The urethra remains short in both boys and girls, making them more susceptible to urinary tract infections than adults. Bladder control is usually present in the 4- and 5-year-old child, but an occasional accident may occur, particularly in stressful situations or when the child is absorbed in an interesting activity.

The bones continue to increase in length and the muscles continue to strengthen and mature. However, the musculoskeletal system is still not fully mature, making the preschooler susceptible to injury, particularly with overexertion or excess activity.

Psychosocial Development

According to Erik Erikson, the psychosocial task of the preschool years is establishing a sense of initiative versus guilt (Erikson, 1963). The preschooler is an inquisitive learner, very enthusiastic about learning new things. Preschoolers feel a sense of accomplishment when succeeding in activities (Fig. 27.2), and feeling pride in one's accomplishment helps the child to use initiative. However, when the child extends him- or herself further than current capabilities allow, he or she may feel a sense of guilt. The superego or conscience development is

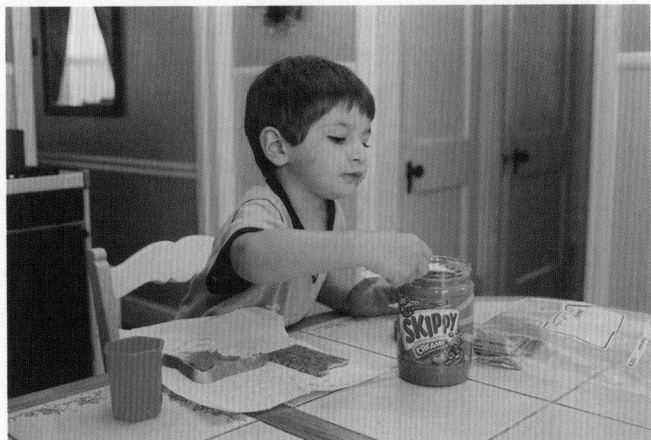

FIGURE **27.2** Allowing the preschooler to assist with simple household tasks such as preparing a sandwich encourages the development of initiative.

completed during the preschool period, and this is the basis for moral development (understanding right and wrong). Table 27.1 gives examples illustrating the stage of initiative versus guilt.

Cognitive Development

According to Jean Piaget's theory (1969), the preschool-age child continues in the preoperational stage. Preoperational thought dominates during this stage and is based on a self-centred understanding of the world. In the pre-conceptual phase of preoperational thought, the child remains egocentric and is able to approach a problem from a single point of view only. The young preschooler may understand the concept of counting and begins to engage in fantasy play (Papalia & Feldman, 2011).

Magical thinking is a normal part of preschool development. The preschooler believes that his or her thoughts are all-powerful. The fantasy experienced through magical thinking allows the preschooler to make room in his or her world for the actual or the real. Through make-believe and magical thinking, preschool children satisfy their curiosity about differences in the world around them (Papalia & Feldman, 2011).

The preschooler may have an **imaginary friend** as well. This friend serves as a creative way for the preschooler to sample different activities and behaviours and practice conversational skills (Brazelton & Sparrow, 2002). Despite this imagination, the preschooler is able to switch easily between fantasy and reality throughout the day.

The child in the intuitive phase can count 10 or more objects, correctly name at least four colours, and better understand the concept of time, and he or she knows about things that are used in everyday life, such as appliances, money, and food. The preschooler uses **transduction** when reasoning: he or she extrapolates from a particular situation to another, even though the

events may be unrelated. The preschooler also attributes life-like qualities to inanimate objects (**animism**) (Papalia & Feldman, 2011). Table 27.1 gives further examples illustrating this developmental stage.

The acquisition of language skills in the toddler period is enhanced in the preschool period. The expansion of vocabulary enables the preschooler to progress further with symbolic thought. At this age, children do not completely understand the concept of death or its permanence: they may ask when their grandparent or pet who died is returning.

Moral Development

The preschool child can understand the concepts of right and wrong and is developing a conscience. That inner voice that warns or threatens is developing in the preschool years. Kohlberg identified the stage between 4 and 10 years as the preconventional stage, which is characterized by a punishment-and-obedience orientation (Kohlberg, 1984). Preschool children see morality as external to themselves; they defer to authority (that of the adult). The child's moral standards are those of their parents or other adults who influence them, not necessarily their own. Preschoolers adhere to those standards to gain rewards or avoid negative consequences. Since the preschool child is facing the psychosocial task of initiative versus guilt, it is natural for the child to experience guilt when something goes wrong. The child may have a strong belief that if someone is ill or dying, then he or she may be at fault and the illness or death is punishment (Ford, 2007).

As the child's moral development progresses, he or she learns how to deal with angry feelings. Sometimes the way the child chooses to deal with those feelings may be inappropriate, such as fighting and biting. Preschoolers are so involved in imagination and fantasy that lying may begin to occur at this age (Brazelton & Sparrow, 2002). However, since young children are very imaginative, they may have difficulty telling the difference between reality and fantasy. Preschoolers also use their limited life experiences to make sense of and help them cope with crisis. They need to learn the socially acceptable limits of behaviour and are also learning the rewards of manners. The preschool child begins to help out in the family and begins to understand the concept of give-and-take in relationships.

Motor Skill Development

As the preschooler's musculoskeletal system continues to mature, existing motor skills become refined and new ones develop. The preschooler has more voluntary control over his or her movements and is less clumsy than the toddler. Significant refinement in fine motor skills occurs during the preschool period (Table 27.2).

TABLE 27.1 DEVELOPMENTAL THEORIES

Theorist	Stage	Activities
Erikson	Initiative vs. guilt Age 3–6 years	• Likes to please parents • Begins to plan activities, make up games • Initiates activities with others • Acts out the roles of other people (real and imaginary) • Develops sexual identity • Develops conscience • May take frustrations out on siblings • Likes exploring new things • Enjoys sports, shopping, cooking, working • Feels remorse when makes wrong choice or behaves badly • Cooperates with other children • Negotiates solutions to conflicts
Piaget	Preoperational substage: preconceptual phase Age: 2–4 years Preoperational substage: intuitive phase Age 4–7 years	• Exhibits egocentric thinking, which lessens as the child approaches age 4 • Short attention span • Learns through observing and imitating • Displays animism • Forms concepts that are not as complete or as logical as the adult's • Able to make simple classifications • By age 4 understands the concept of opposites (hot/cold, soft/hard) • Reasoning is that of specific to specific • Has an active imagination • Able to classify and relate objects • Has intuitive thought processes; knows if something is right or wrong, though cannot state why • Tolerates others' differences but doesn't understand them • Very curious about facts • Knows acceptable cultural rules • Uses words appropriately but often without true understanding of their meaning • Has a more realistic sense of causality • May begin to question parents' values
Kohlberg	Punishment–obedience orientation Age 2–4 years (preconventional morality)	• Determines good vs. bad depends on associated punishment • Children may learn inappropriate behaviour at this stage if parental intervention does not occur

Adapted from: Erikson, E. H. (1963). *Childhood and society* (2nd ed.). New York: W. W. Norton and Company; Feigelman, S. (2007). Preschool years. In R. M. Kliegman, R. E. Behrman, H. B. Jenson, & B. F. Stanton (Eds.). *Nelson textbook of pediatrics* (18th ed.). Philadelphia: Saunders; Kohlberg, L. (1984). *Moral development*. New York: Harper & Row; and Piaget, J. (1969). *The theory of stages in cognitive development*. New York: McGraw-Hill.

Gross Motor Skills

The preschooler is agile while standing, walking, running, and jumping (Fig. 27.3). He or she can go up and down stairs and walk forward and backward easily. Standing on tiptoes or on one foot still requires extra concentration. The preschooler seems to be in constant motion. He or she also uses the body to understand new concepts (such as using the arms in a "chug-chug" motion when describing how the train wheels work).

Fine Motor Skills

The 3-year-old can move each finger independently and is capable of grasping utensils and crayons in adult fashion, with the thumb on one side and the fingers on the other. He or she can also scribble freely, copy a circle, trace a square, and feed him- or herself without spilling much. These skills become refined over the next 2 years, and by 5 years of age the child can write letters, cut with scissors more accurately, and tie shoelaces (Fig. 27.4).

TABLE 27.2 MOTOR SKILL DEVELOPMENT

Age	Expected Gross Motor Skills	Expected Fine Motor Skills
4 years	• Throws ball overhand • Kicks ball forward • Catches bounced ball • Hops on one foot • Stands on one foot up to 5 s • Alternates feet going up and down steps • Moves backward and forward with agility	• Uses scissors successfully • Copies capital letters • Draws circles and squares • Traces a cross or diamond • Draws a person with two to four body parts
5 years	• Stands on one foot 10 s or longer • Swings and climbs well • May skip • Somersaults • May learn to skate and swim	• Prints some letters • Draws person with body and at least six parts • Dresses/undresses without assistance • Can learn to tie laces • Uses fork, spoon, and knife (supervised) well • Copies triangle and other geometric patterns • Mostly cares for own toileting needs

Adapted from: Feigelman, S. (2007). Preschool years. In R. M. Kliegman, R. E. Behrman, H. B. Jenson, & B. F. Stanton (Eds.). *Nelson textbook of pediatrics* (18th ed.). Philadelphia: Saunders; Goldson, E., & Reynolds. A. (2011). Child development and behavior. In W. W. Hay, M. J. Levin, J. M. Sondheimer, & R. R. Deterding (Eds.), *Current pediatric diagnosis and treatment* (20th ed.). New York: McGraw-Hill; and Papalia, D., & Feldman, R. (2011). *A child's world: Infancy through adolescence* (12th ed.). New York: McGraw Hill.

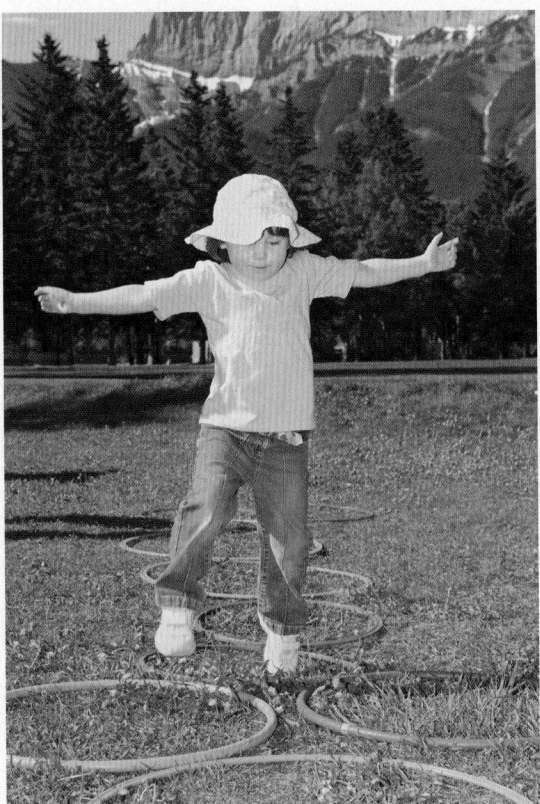

FIGURE 27.3 The preschool child is agile, capable of standing on one foot for several seconds and hopping on one foot.

Communication and Language Development

The acquisition of language allows the preschool child to express thoughts and creativity. The preschool years are a time of refinement of language skills. The 3-year-old exhibits **telegraphic speech**, using short sentences

Sensory Development

Hearing is intact at birth and should remain so throughout the preschool years. The senses of smell and touch continue to develop throughout the preschool years. The young preschooler may have a less discriminating sense of taste than the older child, putting him or her at increased risk for accidental ingestion. Visual acuity continues to progress and should be equal bilaterally. The typical 5-year-old has visual acuity of 20/40 or 20/30. Colour vision is intact at this age.

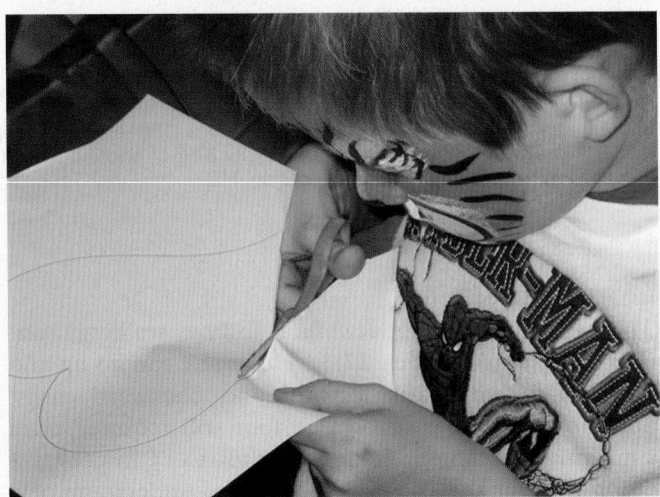

FIGURE 27.4 The 5-year-old has the fine motor dexterity to cut well with scissors.

TABLE 27.3 **COMMUNICATION SKILLS IN THE PRESCHOOL CHILD**

Age	Communication Abilities
4 years	• Speaks in complete sentences using adult-like grammar • Tells a story that is easy to follow • 75% of speech understood by others outside of family • Asks questions with "who," "how," "how many" • Stays on topic in a conversation • Understands the concepts of "same" and "different" • Asks many questions • Knows names of familiar animals • Names common objects in books and magazines • Knows at least one colour • Uses language to engage in make-believe • Follows a three-part command • Can count a few numbers • Vocabulary of 1,500 words
5 years	• Persons outside of the family can understand most of the child's speech • Explains how an item is used • Participates in long, detailed conversations • Talks about past, future, and imaginary events • Answers questions that use "why" and "when" • Can count to 10 • Recalls part of a story • Speech should be completely intelligible, even if the child has articulation difficulties • Speech is generally grammatically correct • Vocabulary of 2,100 words • Says name and address

Adapted from: Feigelman, S. (2007). Preschool years. In R. M. Kliegman, R. E. Behrman, H. B. Jenson, & B. F. Stanton (Eds.). *Nelson textbook of pediatrics* (18th ed.). Philadelphia: Saunders; Papalia, D., & Feldman, R. (2011). *A child's world: Infancy through adolescence* (12th ed.). New York: McGraw Hill; and Taylor, E. (2008). Providing developmentally based care for preschoolers. *AORN Journal, 88*(2), 267–273.

that contain only the essential information. Vocabulary at 3 years comprises about 900 words. The preschool child may acquire as many as 10 to 20 new words per day and at age 5 usually has a vocabulary of 2,100 words (Taylor, 2008). By the end of the preschool period, the child is using sentences that are adult-like in structure (Table 27.3).

The 3- to 6-year-old is starting to develop fluency (the ability to smoothly link sounds, syllables, and words when speaking). Initially, the child may exhibit dysfluency or stuttering. Speech may sound choppy, or the child may say repeated consonants or "um." Stuttering usually has its onset between 2 and 4 years of age, and most children will recover from it without therapy (Prasse & Kikano, 2008). Parents should slow down their speech and should give the child time to speak without rushing or interrupting. Some sounds remain difficult for the preschooler to enunciate properly: "f," "v," "s," and "z" sounds are usually mastered by age 5 years, but some children do not master the sounds of "sh," "l," "th," and "r" until age 6 or later.

Communication in preschool children is concrete in nature, as they are not yet capable of abstract thought. Despite its concrete nature, the preschooler's communication can be quite elaborate and involved; he or she may talk about dreams and fantasies. In addition to acquiring vocabulary and learning the correct use of grammar, the preschool child's receptive language skills are also becoming refined.

The preschooler is very much in tune with the parents' moods and easily picks up on negative emotions in conversations. If the preschooler hears parents discussing things that are frightening to the child, the preschooler's imagination may fuel the development of fears and lead to misinterpretation of what the child has heard.

In the potentially bilingual child, by 4 years of age the child will cease the language mixing exhibited during the toddler years and should be able to use each language as a separate system (Abell & Ey, 2007).

Emotional and Social Development

By the time a child enters kindergarten, he or she should have developed a useful set of social skills that will help him or her have successful experiences in the school setting as well as in life in general. These skills include cooperation, sharing (of things and feelings), kindness, generosity, affection display, conversation, expression of feelings, helping others, and making friends.

Preschoolers tend to have strong emotions. They can be very excited, happy, and giddy in one moment, then extremely disappointed in the next. The preschool child has a vivid imagination, and fears are very real to preschoolers. Most children of this age have learned to control their behaviours. They should be able to name the feelings they are having rather than acting on them. Strong feelings may be expressed through outlets such as clay or Play-Doh, water play, drawing or painting, or through dramatic play such as with puppets.

Preschoolers are developing a sense of identity. They recognize that they are boys or girls. They know that they belong to a particular family, community, or culture.

They take pride in using self-control rather than giving in to their impulses. The preschool child is capable of helping others and being involved in routines and transitions.

Parents can encourage and assist preschool children with developing the social and emotional skills that will be needed when the child enters school. Preschool children thrive on one-to-one communication with a parent. During interactive communication, children learn to express their feelings and ideas. Interactive communication fosters not only emotional and moral development but also self-esteem and cognitive development. Asking the preschool child questions requires the child to think out his or her own intention or motivation and encourages vocabulary development. Parents may use individual communication as a time to explore right and wrong, thus further contributing to moral development. Being listened to while answering parents' questions gives preschoolers a sense that they are valued, that what they think and have to say matters.

Establishing a few simple rules and enforcing them consistently gives preschoolers the structure and security they need while promoting moral development. Parents or caregivers can help the child give a name to the emotion that is being experienced. Fears are very real to preschoolers because of their active imaginations and may result in a variety of emotions. Parents should validate the feeling or emotion, then discuss with the child alternatives for dealing with the emotion.

Preschoolers are developing their sense of identity, and parents should encourage preschoolers to do simple things for themselves, like dressing and washing their hands and face (Fig. 27.5). Parents should give the child the time he or she needs to complete the task. This helps to establish a sense of accomplishment.

At this age, the child may begin to show an interest in basic sexuality (Papalia & Feldman, 2011). The preschooler may want to know why boys' and girls' bodies are different, how the reproductive organs function, and where babies come from. The parent should answer the child honestly and directly, using the correct anatomic terms. Long explanations are not necessary, just simple answers. This curiosity is a normal function of the preschool years, and the curiosity may also involve playing with the genitals (see the section on masturbation later in this chapter).

Friendships

Preschoolers need interactions with friends as well. Learning how to make and keep a friend is an important part of social development. Friends may be other children in the neighbourhood or those at preschool or day care. A special friend is someone the preschooler can care about, talk to, and play with (Fig. 27.6). The preschooler is more likely to agree to rules and wants to please friends and be like them. The preschooler loves to

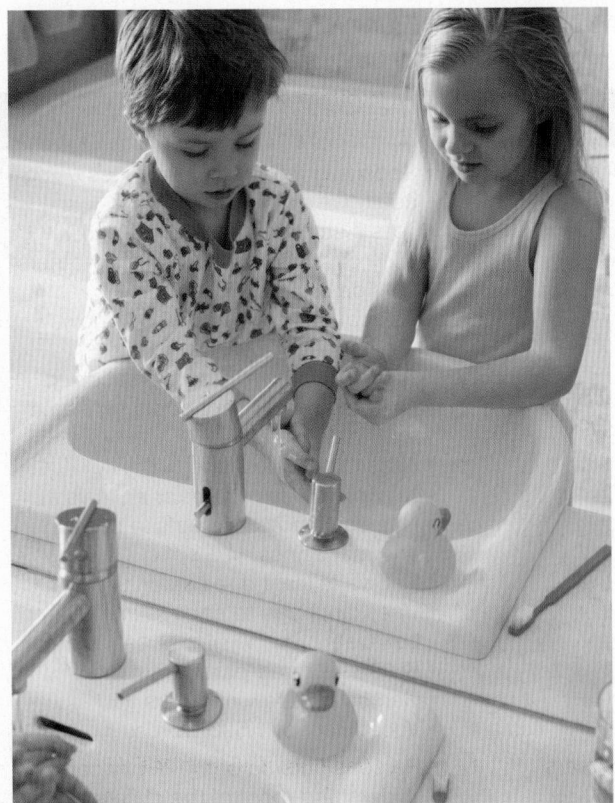

FIGURE 27.5 Encouraging the preschooler to complete simple tasks by himself or herself helps to build self-esteem.

sing, dance, and act and will enjoy these activities with friends. Disagreements may occur, but the parent can encourage the children to express their views, discuss and resolve conflicts, and continue being friends.

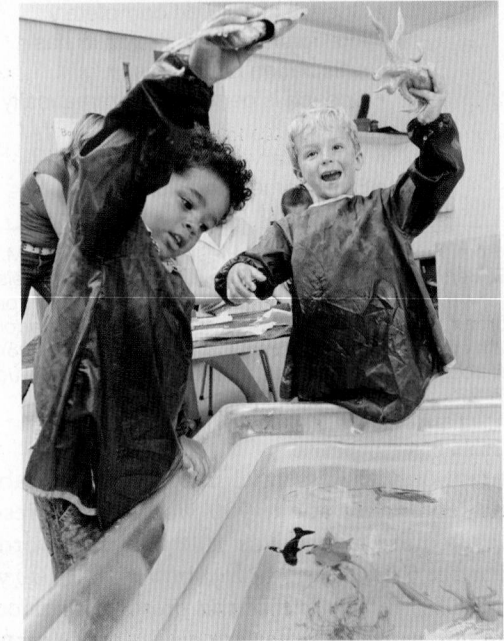

FIGURE 27.6 The preschool child begins to develop friendships.

Temperament

By the time children are 3 years old, they recognize that what they do actually matters. It is helpful for the parent to view the child as an active participant in the parent–child relationship. The child's temperament has become a reliable indicator of how a parent might expect the child to react in a certain situation. When the parent is in tune with the preschooler's temperament, it is easier to find ways to ease transitions and changes for that child. In the area of task orientation, temperament may range from the highly attentive and persistent to the more distractible and active (Child Development Institute, 2010).

A child's social flexibility is also evident by this age. A child who is quite adaptable will handle stimuli from the outside world in an approaching rather than a withdrawing manner. Temperament also determines the extent of reactivity (the child's sensory threshold of responsiveness, high versus low). This determines the quality of the child's mood and the intensity of reactions to stimuli, change, or situations. When the parents are familiar with the child's task orientation, social flexibility, and reactivity, they can better structure activities and situations for the child.

The 4-year-old is better at learning self-control and can use setbacks in appropriate behaviour as opportunities for growth. Temper tantrums should ease off by this age as the child's language skills are more capable of keeping up with complex ideas. The 4-year-old is able to see the rewards of growing up. This awareness of self-power may, however, lead to additional fears. The 5-year-old who has a more vulnerable type of temperament, as opposed to a confident temperament, may be more apt to experience fears.

Fears

With their vivid imaginations, preschoolers experience a variety of fears. Preschoolers may be scared of loud noises such as fire engine sirens or barking dogs. Imaginary monsters may scare the child. Preschoolers are often afraid of people they do not know as well as people who look or dress very differently from what they are accustomed to, such as on Halloween. Many preschoolers are afraid of the dark. Preschoolers may also fear insects as well as animals they are not familiar with. The preschooler's memory is long enough that he or she may fear returning to the doctor's office when a painful procedure occurred during the prior visit.

Parents should acknowledge fears rather than minimizing them. They can then collaborate with the child on strategies for dealing with the fear.

Cultural Influences on Growth and Development

As in the toddler period, the value that the family places on independence will affect the child's development of a healthy self-concept.

Some cultures value reading and education more than others. If reading is not valued in the home, the preschool child's first experience with books may not occur until he or she is in school.

Food served in the home is often very specific to the family's ethnic background. As the preschool child is exposed to persons of other cultures in school, he may or may not like the food that is served. Exploring customs or cultural practices that the family participates in is important so that these practices may be safely incorporated into the child's plan of care.

*R*efer back to Nila, who was introduced in the beginning of the chapter. What developmental milestones would you expect Nila to have reached at this age? Nila's mother expresses concerns about her child's imaginary friend, Sasha. How would you respond?

The Nurse's Role in Preschool Growth and Development
WATCH&LEARN

Growth and development in the preschool child remains orderly and sequential. Some preschoolers grow faster than others or reach various developmental milestones sooner than others. Nurses must be aware of the usual growth and development patterns for this age group so that they can assess preschool children appropriately and provide guidance to their families. The changes that the preschool child is experiencing affect not only the child but also the family. Health care visits throughout the preschool period continue to focus on expected growth and development and anticipatory guidance. An additional concern is the preparation for school entry (school readiness).

If the preschooler is hospitalized, growth and development may be altered. Hospitalization hinders the preschool child's ability to explore the environment and engage in make-believe play and thus presents a challenge for the curious and inquisitive child. If the child must be isolated for a contagious illness, the opportunities for exploration and experimentation are further restricted. In addition, a sick preschooler may feel a sense of guilt, worrying that maybe he or she caused the illness by negative thoughts or behaviours.

When caring for the hospitalized preschooler, the nurse must use knowledge of normal growth and development to recognize potential delays, promote continued appropriate growth and development, and interact successfully with the preschooler.

Nursing Process Overview

Upon completion of assessment of the preschool child's growth and development status, problems or issues related to growth and development may be identified.

The nurse may then identify one or more nursing diagnoses, including but not limited to:

- Delayed growth and development
- Imbalanced nutrition, less than body requirements
- Interrupted family processes
- Readiness for enhanced parenting
- Risk for caregiver role strain
- Risk for delayed development
- Risk for disproportionate growth
- Risk for injury

Planning nursing care for the preschool child with growth and development issues should take into account the preschooler's and family's individual needs. The nursing care plan may be used as a guide in planning nursing care for the preschooler with a growth or developmental concern. The nurse may choose the appropriate nursing diagnoses from Nursing Care Plan 27.1 and individualize them as needed. The nursing care plan is intended to serve as a guide only and is not intended to be an inclusive growth and development plan.

Promoting Healthy Growth and Development

The building of self-esteem continues throughout the preschool period. It is of particular importance during these years, as the preschooler's developmental task is focused on the development of initiative rather than guilt. A sense of guilt will contribute to low self-esteem, whereas a child who is rewarded for his or her initiative will have increased self-confidence. The parent who provides a loving and nurturing environment for the preschooler builds upon the earlier foundation.

Routine and ritual continue to be important throughout the preschool years, as they help the child to develop a sense of time as well as provide the structure for the child to feel safe and secure. Daily routine continues to assist with the development of conscience in the preschooler. As in toddlerhood, making expectations known through everyday routines helps to avoid confrontations. The preschooler is developing the maturity to know how to behave in various situations and is capable of learning manners.

Setting limits (and remaining consistent with those limits) continues to be important in the preschool period. Consistent limits provide the preschooler with expectation and guidance. As the preschooler increasingly participates in fantasy and imagination, the limits of routine and structure help guide his or her behaviour and ability to distinguish reality.

Nurses caring for preschoolers should have knowledge of normal developmental expectations so they can determine whether the preschool child is progressing appropriately. Table 27.4 lists potential signs of developmental delay. A preschool child with one or more of

TABLE 27.4 SIGNS OF DEVELOPMENTAL DELAY

Age	Concern
4 years	• Cannot jump in place or ride a tricycle • Cannot stack four blocks • Cannot throw ball overhand • Does not grasp crayon with thumb and fingers • Difficulty with scribbling • Cannot copy a circle • Does not use sentences with three or more words • Cannot use the words "me" and "you" appropriately • Ignores other children or does not show interest in interactive games • Will not respond to people outside the family; still clings or cries if parents leave • Resists using toilet, dressing, sleeping • Does not engage in fantasy play
By 5 years	• Unhappy or sad often • Little interest in playing with other children • Unable to separate from parent without major protest • Is extremely aggressive • Is extremely fearful or timid, or unusually passive • Cannot build tower of six to eight blocks • Easily distracted; cannot concentrate on single activity for 5 min • Rarely engages in fantasy play • Trouble with eating, sleeping, or using the toilet • Cannot use plurals or past tense • Cannot brush teeth, wash and dry hands, or undress efficiently

these concerns should be referred for further developmental evaluation.

Promoting Growth and Development Through Play

Providing sincere encouragement for the preschool child's efforts and accomplishments helps him or her develop a sense of initiative. Giving children opportunities to decide how and with whom they want to play also helps them develop initiative. Preschool children like to write, colour, draw, paint with a brush or their fingers, and trace or copy patterns (Fig. 27.7). They may start small collections that may be sorted. They like using toys for their intended purpose as well as for whatever invented purpose they can imagine.

(text continues on page 873)

Nursing Care Plan 27.1

GROWTH AND DEVELOPMENT ISSUES IN THE PRESCHOOL CHILD

NURSING DIAGNOSIS: Risk for injury related to developmental age, environment, and motor vehicle travel

Outcome Identification and Evaluation

Child's safety will be maintained: *Child will remain free from injury.*

Interventions: Preventing Injury

- Teach and encourage appropriate use of forward-facing car seat or booster seat if greater than 18 kg *to decrease risk of injury related to motor vehicles.*
- Teach preschoolers to stay away from street and to cross the street only when holding the hand of an adult *to prevent pedestrian injury.*
- Require bicycle helmet use while riding any wheeled toy *to prevent head injury and form habit of helmet use.*
- Teach the preschooler appropriate safety rules in the home (avoiding electric outlets, etc.): *the preschooler is able to follow simple directions and carry out directives. Limits help him or her to organize the environment.*
- Post poison control centre phone number *(in case of accidental ingestion; the preschool child is very curious).*
- Never leave a preschool child unattended in a tub or pool or near any body of water *to prevent drowning.*
- Provide swimming lessons for children age 4 or 5 *to encourage water safety, but not as a replacement for adult supervision.*
- Teach parents first-aid measures and child CPR *to minimize consequences of injury should it occur.*
- Provide close observation and keep side rails up on bed in hospital *because the preschool child continues to be at risk for falling or injuring self on equipment or tubing (because of curiosity).*

NURSING DIAGNOSIS: Imbalanced nutrition, less than body requirements, related to inappropriate nutritional intake to sustain growth needs (excess juice or milk intake, inadequate food variety intake) as evidenced by failure to attain adequate increases in height and weight over time

Outcome Identification and Evaluation

Child will consume adequate nutrients: *Child will demonstrate weight gain and increases in height.*

Interventions: Promoting Appropriate Nutrition

- Assess current feeding schedule and usual intake, as well as methods used to feed, *to determine areas of adequacy versus inadequacy.*
- Determine if the preschooler is unable to drink from a cup or does not finger feed or use utensils properly, or if the child has difficulty swallowing or tolerating certain textures of foods *to determine if further interventions such as speech or occupational therapy are required.*
- Weigh child daily on same scale if hospitalized, weekly on same scale if at home, and plot growth patterns weekly or monthly as appropriate on standardized growth charts *to determine if growth is improving.*
- Limit juice to 120 to 180 mL per day, milk to 500 to 750 mL per day, *to discourage sense of fullness achieved with excess milk or juice intake, thereby increasing appetite for appropriate solid foods.*
- Provide three nutrient-dense meals and at least two healthy snacks per day *to encourage adequate nutrient consumption.*
- Feed child on a similar schedule daily, without distractions and with the family: *preschool children continue to respond well to routine and structure. They are more interested in the social context of meals and are still apt to become distracted easily, so the TV should be off at mealtimes.*

NURSING DIAGNOSIS: Delayed growth and development related to motor, cognitive, language, or psychosocial concerns as evidenced by delay in meeting expected milestones

Outcome Identification and Evaluation

Development will be enhanced: *Child will make continued progress toward realization of expected developmental milestones.*

Interventions: Enhancing Growth and Development

- Screen for developmental capabilities *to determine child's current level of functioning.*
- Offer age-appropriate toys, play, and activities (including gross motor) *to encourage further development.*

(continued)

Nursing Care Plan 27.1 (continued)

- Perform interventions as prescribed by physical, occupational, or speech therapist: *participation in those activities helps to promote function and accomplish acquisition of developmental skills.*
- Provide support to families of preschoolers with developmental delay *(progress in achieving developmental milestones can be slow and ongoing motivation is needed).*
- Reinforce positive attributes in the child *to maintain motivation.*
- Model age-appropriate communication skills *to illustrate suitable means for parenting the preschooler.*

NURSING DIAGNOSIS: Risk for disproportionate growth related to excess milk or juice intake, consumption of inappropriate foods or in excess amounts

Outcome Identification and Evaluation
Child will grow appropriately and not become overweight or obese: *Child will achieve weight and height within the 5th to 85th percentiles on standardized growth charts.*

Interventions:
- Discourage use of no-spill sippy cups *(they contribute to dental caries and allow unlimited access to fluids, possibly decreasing appetite for appropriate solid foods).*
- Provide juice (120 to 180 mL per day) and milk (500 to 750 mL per day) from a cup at meal and snack time *to encourage appropriate cup drinking and limit intake of nutrient-poor, high-calorie fluids.*
- Provide only nutrient-rich foods without high sugar content for meals and snacks; *even if the preschooler is a picky eater, it is inappropriate to provide high-calorie junk food just so the child eats something.*
- Teach parents to role model appropriate eating (nutrient-rich, varied diet) *to encourage child to try/accept new foods, as well as become familiar with a variety of food.*
- Limit the intake of fast foods and foods with high sugar and fat content *to decrease intake of nutrient-poor, high-calorie foods.*
- Ensure adequate physical activity *to stimulate development of motor skills and provide appropriate caloric expenditure. This also sets the stage for forming life-long habit of appropriate physical activity.*
- Teach parents to limit television viewing to 1 to 2 hours per day *to encourage participation in physical activities.*

NURSING DIAGNOSIS: Interrupted family processes related to issues with preschool child's development, hospitalization, or situational crisis as evidenced by decreased parental visitation in hospital, parental verbalization of difficulty with current situation, possible crisis related to health of family member other than the preschool child

Outcome Identification and Evaluation
Family will demonstrate adequate functioning: *Family will display coping and psychosocial adjustment.*

Interventions: Enhancing Family Functioning
- Assess the family's level of stress and ability to cope *to determine family's ability to cope with multiple stressors.*
- Engage in family-centred care *to provide a holistic approach to care of the preschooler and family.*
- Encourage the family to verbalize feelings *(verbalization is one method of decreasing anxiety levels)* and acknowledge feelings and emotions.
- Use puppets or dramatic play with the child *to elicit the preschooler's feelings about the current situation.*
- Encourage family visitation and provide for sleeping arrangements for a parent or caregiver to stay in the hospital with the preschooler; *this contributes to family's sense of control in situation.*
- Involve family members in preschooler's care, *giving them a feeling of control and connectedness.*

NURSING DIAGNOSIS: Readiness for enhanced parenting related to parental desire for increased skill level and success with preschool child as evidenced by current healthy relationships and verbalization of desire for improved skills

Outcome Identification and Evaluation
Parent will provide safe and nurturing environment for the preschool child: *Parents will verbalize new skills they will employ in the family.*

Nursing Care Plan 27.1 (continued)

Interventions: Increasing Parenting Skill Set

- Use family-centred care *to provide holistic approach.*
- Educate parent about normal preschool development *to provide basis of understanding for parenting skills needed in this time period.*
- Acknowledge and encourage parent's verbalization of feelings related to chronic illness of child or difficulty with normal preschool behaviour; *this validates the normalcy of parents' feelings.*
- Encourage positive parenting and respect for preschooler and his/her normal development *(helps parents develop approaches to preschoolers that can be used in place of anger and frustration).*
- Acknowledge and admire positive parenting skills already present *to contribute to parents' confidence in their abilities to parent.*
- Role model appropriate parenting behaviours related to communicating with the child *(role modelling actually demonstrates rather than just verbalizes what the parent should strive for).*

Adapted from: Carpenito-Moyet, L. J. (2010). *Nursing diagnosis: Application to clinical practice* (13th ed.). Philadelphia: Lippincott Williams & Wilkins.

Preschoolers begin to play cooperatively with one another. Play may be focused around a distinct theme. They define roles, make up rules, and assign jobs. They are able to work together toward a common goal such as building a house or fort with discarded boxes. Cooperative play encourages the preschool child to learn to share, take turns and compromise, listen to others' opinions, consider the feelings of others, and use self-control and overcome fears.

Preschoolers have incredible imaginations and love to play "make-believe" (Fig. 27.8). Encouraging pretend play and providing props for dress-up stimulates curiosity and creativity. Fantasy play is usually cooperative in

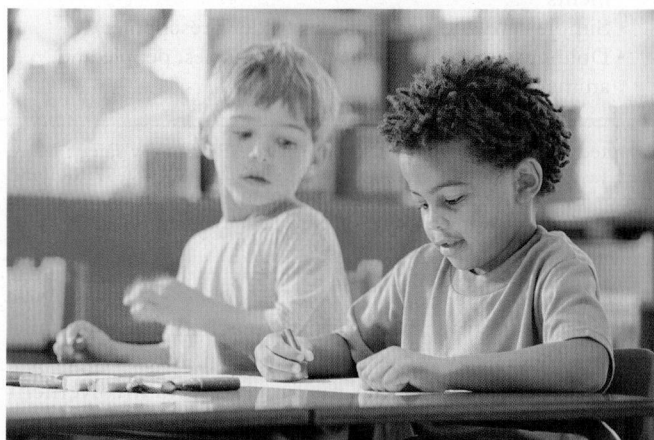

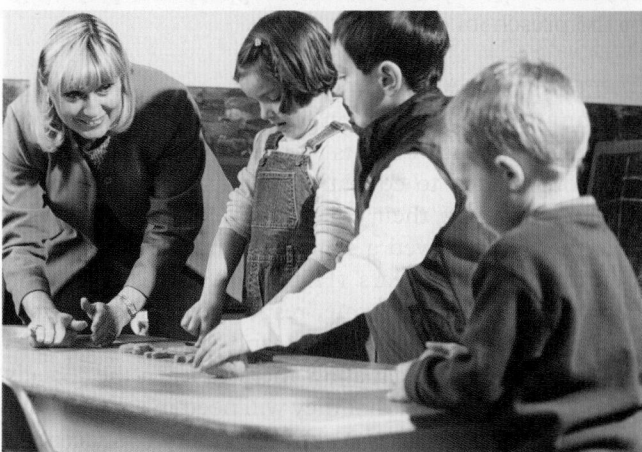

FIGURE 27.7 The preschool child loves to create things, so colouring and moulding clay are ideal activities for children this age.

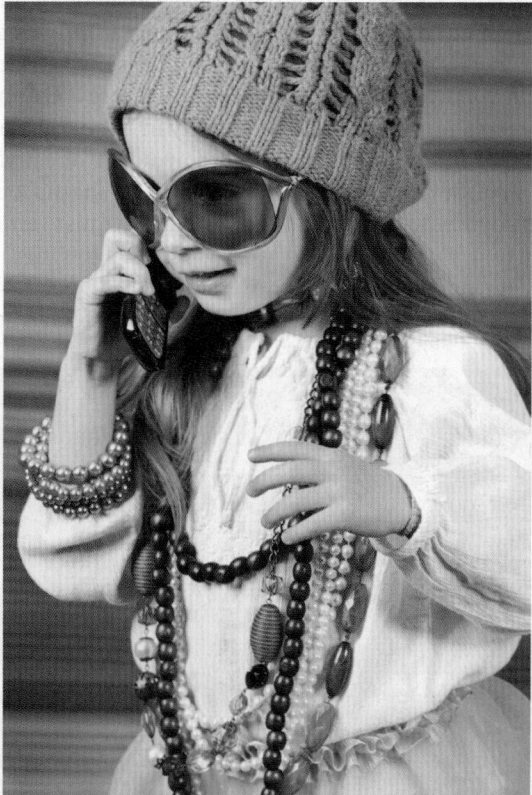

FIGURE 27.8 Preschool children enjoy imitative play.

nature. It encourages the preschooler to develop social skills such as taking turns, communication, paying attention, and responding to one another's words and actions. Fantasy play also allows preschoolers to explore complex social ideas such as power, compassion, and cruelty. Through role playing, children begin to develop their sexual identity as well.

Since preschool children have vivid imaginations, it is important to be careful about what television they watch. The preschooler should be limited to 1 to 2 hours per day of quality television (Christakis & Zimmerman, 2007). The violence in some television programs may scare the preschool child or inspire him or her to act out violent behaviour.

Most preschoolers also engage in dramatic play, fuelled by their innate curiosity and vivid imaginations. Three-year-olds may not realize that they are pretending. They run from scary creatures, make plans, and pack their backpacks (never intending to actually leave). Four-year-olds are more sophisticated with dramatic or pretend play: they know they are pretending, and they use dress-up clothes and props to act out more complex roles and scenarios (Fig. 27.9). Five-year-olds are capable of quite complex scenarios. They pretend they are real or fantasy characters. They often use dramatic play to express anxiety, try out negative feelings, or conquer their fears. For example, a child who is afraid of getting an injection at the doctor's office may work through that feeling with pretend play.

Parents should encourage physical activity in the preschool child. Regular physical activity improves gross motor skills, may enhance the child's self-confidence, and allows the child to expend excess energy. Establishing the habit of daily physical activity in the early years is important in the long-term goal of avoiding obesity. The main goal of organized sports at this age should be fun and enjoyment, although of course safety must remain a priority.

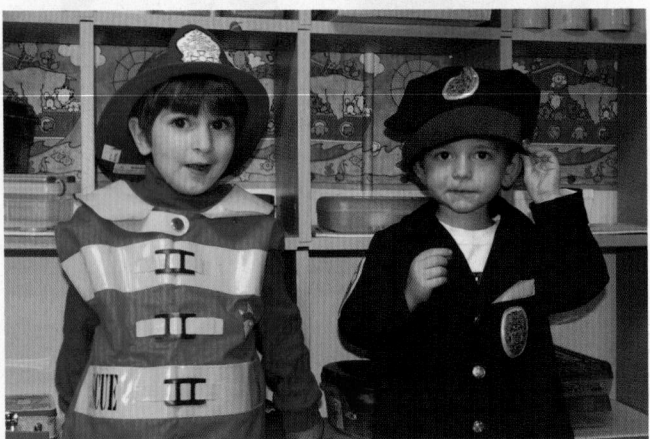

FIGURE 27.9 Preschool children love to dress up and pretend.

BOX 27.1   Appropriate Toys for Preschoolers

- Blocks, simple jigsaw puzzles (four to six large pieces), pegboards, wooden bead with string
- Supplies for creativity: chalk, large crayons, finger paint, Play-Doh or clay, washable markers, paper, paint and paintbrush, scissors, paste, or glue
- Puppets, dress-up clothes, and props for dramatic play
- Bucket, plastic shovel, and other containers for sand and water play
- Play kitchen with accessories and pretend food (empty food boxes can be recycled for kitchen play)
- Squeaking, floating, squirting toys for the bath
- Sandbox with shovel and various toys for building
- Dolls that can be dressed and undressed (large buttons, zippers, and snaps), doll care accessories (diapers, bottles, carriage, crib)
- Gross motor toys: tricycle or big wheel (with helmet), jungle gym or swing set (with supervision), hula hoop, tunnel, wagon
- Blocks, Legos, cars and trucks, plastic animals, trains, plastic figures (family, community helpers), stuffed animals, balls, sewing cards
- Tape or CD players for music, various musical instruments
- Simple card and board games (older preschooler)
- Dollhouse with furniture and accessories, people and animals

Adapted from: Schuman, A. T. (2007). The ABCs of toy safety: More than just child's play. *Contemporary Pediatrics*, *24*(7), 49–57, 64; and Shelov, S. P., & Altmann, T. R. (Eds.). (2009). *Caring for your baby and young child: Birth to age 5* (5th ed.). New York: Bantam Books.

Expensive toys that claim to teach the young child are not necessary. Toys that require interactive rather than passive play and that may include the involvement of the parent are recommended (Schuman, 2007; Shelov & Altmann, 2009). Box 27.1 lists appropriate playthings for the preschool child.

Promoting Early Learning

The family is the foundation for the child's early growth and development. Parents serve as role models for behaviour related to education and learning, as well as instilling values in their children. School readiness is a topic that has received a significant amount of national attention (High, 2008). To succeed in school, children need a safe, responsive home environment that allows them to learn and explore, as well as structure and limits that allow them to learn the socially acceptable behaviours that they will need in school. Language development is critical to the ability to succeed in school and can be encouraged through books and reading. Each of these components is important in readying the child for education in a more formal setting.

Promoting language development, choosing a preschool, and making the transition to kindergarten are discussed in more detail below.

Promoting Language Development

The parent serves as the child's first teacher. The interactions between parent and child in relation to books and other play activities model the types of interactions that the child will later have in school. Asking open-ended questions stimulates the development of thinking as well as language in the preschool child. The preschooler is a great imitator, so the parent should serve as a role model for appropriate language. Parents should avoid swearing, as the child is sure to repeat "bad words" likely in the same tone of voice as heard even if he or she does not understand what the words mean. Allowing children to pursue interests at their own pace will help them to develop the literacy and numeric skills that will enable them to later focus on academic skills.

Preschoolers enjoy books with pictures that tell stories (Fig. 27.10). Stories with repeated phrases help to keep the child's attention. Children like stories that describe experiences similar to their own. The preschool child demonstrates early literacy skills by reciting stories or portions of books. He or she also may retell the story from the book, pretend to read books, and ask questions about the story. The preschool child has enough focus and expanded attention to notice when a page is skipped during reading and will call it to the parent's attention.

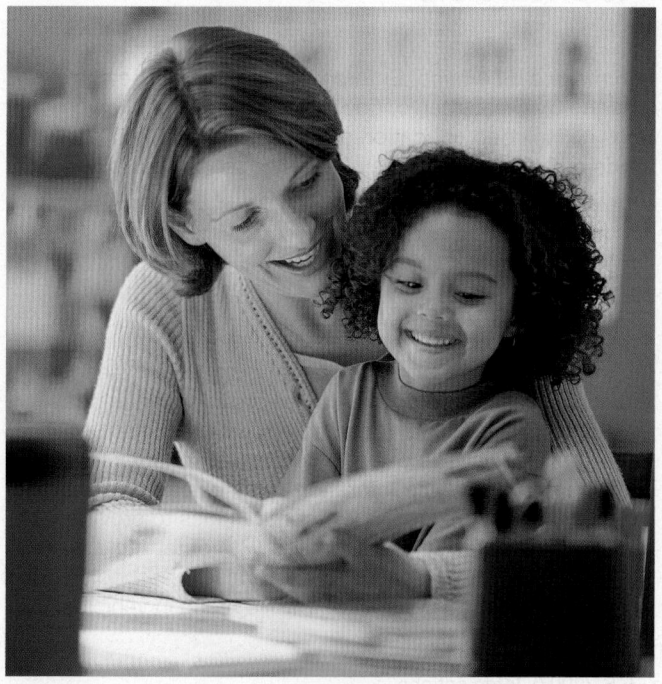

FIGURE 27.10 Preschool children enjoy being read to and looking at the pictures that go along with the story.

> ▶ *Take* NOTE!
>
> *Risk factors for lack of social and emotional readiness for school include insecure attachment in the early years, maternal depression, parental substance abuse, and low socioeconomic status. Nurses should screen for these factors and make referrals if appropriate.*

Choosing a Preschool/Starting Kindergarten

Many parents choose to enrol their child in preschool. Preschool should be used primarily as an opportunity to foster the child's social skills and accustom him or her to the group environment. When selecting a preschool, the parent may want to consider the accreditation of the school, the teachers' qualifications, and recommendations of other parents. The focus of the school environment is also important: What is the daily schedule of activities? Is the school very structured, or does it have a looser environment? The parents must decide how focused on curriculum they want the school to be. The parent should observe the classroom, evaluating the environment, noise level, and sanitary practices as well as how the children interact with each other and how the teachers interact with the children. As preschool is the foundation for later education, the child should have the opportunity to build self-esteem and the skills needed for the more formal setting of elementary school.

Whether or not the child attended preschool, kindergarten will be the next big step. Kindergarten hours may be longer than preschool hours, and kindergarten is usually held 5 days per week. This may be a significant change for some children. For most children, the setting and personnel in kindergarten will be new to the child. Rules and expectations are often very different as well. When discussing starting kindergarten with the preschool child, parents should do so in an enthusiastic fashion, keeping the conversation light and positive. Parents should meet with the child's teacher prior to the start of school, if possible, to discuss particular needs or concerns. Parents may want to schedule a tour of the school for the preschooler or attend the school's open house with the child to ease the transition. Practicing the new daily routine prior to the start of school will also be helpful.

Most provinces require up to date immunizations and a health screening of the child before he or she enters kindergarten, so advise parents to plan ahead and schedule these in a timely fashion so that school entrance is not delayed.

Promoting Safety

In Canada, accidental injury remains the leading cause of death for children between the ages of 1 and 14 years (Public Health Agency of Canada, 2009). Preschoolers

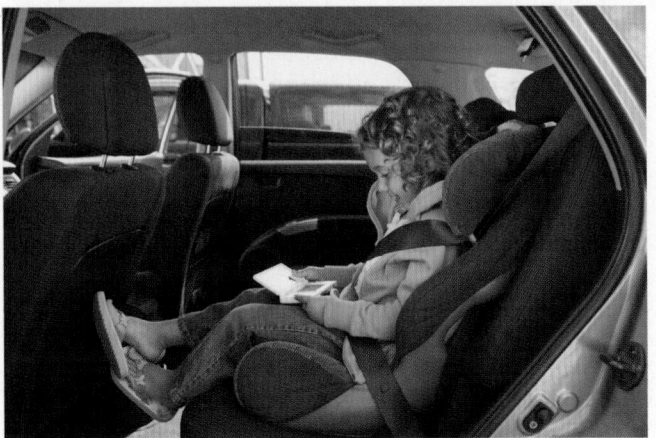

FIGURE 27.11 The preschool child who weighs less than 18 kg should use a forward-facing car seat that meets government regulations.

are at an ideal age to be taught about safety and safe behaviours. They are cognitively able to absorb concrete information and they desire to master the situations they are in, but they continue to display poor judgment related to safety issues. Their engagement in fantasy is so strong that it makes it difficult for them to master complicated cause-and-effect relationships. The preschool child is capable of learning safe behaviours but may not always be able to transfer those behaviours to a different situation.

Parents must continue to closely supervise preschool children to avoid accidental injury during this period.

Safety in the Car

The preschooler who weighs less than 18 kg should use a forward-facing car seat with harness and top tether. Although some province regulations allow children to move to a booster seat once they reach 18 kg, Transport Canada (2011) advises that use of a forward-facing car seat provides the best protection for young children and some are made to hold children up to 30 kg. Manufacturer's instructions and government regulations should be followed (Fig. 27.11, Evidence-based Practice 27.1).

▶ *Take* NOTE!

Although motor vehicle accidents remain a major cause of injury and death in the preschool-age group, many families do not use appropriate car seat/seat belt safety with their children. It is recommended that parents keep a copy of the manufacturer's instructions for the car/booster seat and that these instructions are followed carefully. Parents should be encouraged to check with their local fire, police, or other agency that may have a car seat clinic to determine proper installation and use.

EVIDENCE-BASED PRACTICE 27.1
Interventions Directed Toward Acquiring and Using Booster Seats for Children 4 to 8 Years Old

● **Study**

Children outgrow toddler car seats around the age of 4 years or when they weigh 18 kg. Regular seat belts do not fit children properly. The purpose of booster seats for the 4- to 8-year-old child is to raise him or her higher on the seat of the car in order for the adult seat belt to secure the child properly. Booster seats provide increased comfort and safety for this age group. Booster seat use in this age group has been shown to decrease injury and death via motor vehicle accident by nearly 60%. The authors reviewed five studies involving 3,070 subjects and performed a meta-analysis of the study results. Each of the randomized controlled trials reviewed assessed the efficacy of interventions directed toward increasing booster seat use.

▲ **Findings**

The author's meta-analysis of the studies revealed that interventions directed toward improving booster seat use

can make a difference. Enforcement of booster seat law was the weakest intervention. More successful interventions all included education of parents about the importance and appropriate use of booster seats. Providing a free booster seat upon completion of the training or an incentive coupon to receive a discount upon purchase were the most helpful interventions.

■ **Nursing Implications**

Parents want to protect their children from injury when riding in motor vehicles, but many may lack the knowledge or financial resources to do so. Nurses are in a unique position to provide ongoing, repeated education about the importance of booster seat use for the preschooler to families wherever they encounter them. Nurses can also seek out resources in their individual communities to provide financial incentives to assist families with obtaining a booster seat. Nurses should always praise preschoolers for complying with booster seat use while riding in vehicles.

Ehiri, J. E., Ejere, H. O. D., Magnussen, L., Emusu, D., King, W., & Osberg, J. S. (2007). Interventions for promoting booster seat use in four to eight year olds traveling in motor vehicles. *The Cochrane Library 2007, 4.*

Safety in the Home

Matches, bodies of water, bicycle riding, and poisons continue to be sources of potential injury during the preschool years. Motor vehicle accidents and drowning, especially for children under the age of 5 years, are the two leading causes of accidental death for Canadian children (Safe Kids Canada, 2010). There are a number of safeguards that parents of preschoolers can use to help prevent their children from becoming injured in and around the home.

Preventing Exposure to Tobacco Smoke

Parents should protect their preschoolers from second-hand tobacco smoke. Exposure to tobacco smoke is associated with an increased incidence of otitis media and respiratory infections, as well as increased symptoms and medication use in children with asthma. Other effects include decreased lung function and behavioural difficulties (World Health Organization, n.d.). The preschool child should never be in an enclosed space (such as a car) where tobacco smoke is present.

Preventing Injury

The preschool child who runs out into the street is at risk for being struck by a car. Teach preschoolers to stop at the curb and never go into the street without a grown-up. The preschooler may learn to ride a bicycle (with or without training wheels). The child must wear an approved bicycle helmet any time he or she rides the bicycle, even if it is just in the driveway. Requiring helmet use in the early years may lead to the habit of helmet use as the child gets older. Allowing the preschooler to choose his or her own helmet may encourage the child to use the helmet.

Bicycles should be safe for this age group. The size must be correct; the balls of the feet should reach both pedals while the child is sitting on the seat and has both hands on the handlebars. Children under 5 years of age have difficulty learning to use hand-operated brakes, so traditional pedal-back brakes are recommended in this age group. Preschoolers are not mature enough to ride a bicycle in the street even if they are riding with adults, so they should always ride on the sidewalk (Healthy Children, 2010b).

It is important to make the inside of the home safe for the preschool child. Parents should install and maintain smoke alarms in the home. Increased physical dexterity and refinement of motor skills enable the preschooler to strike matches or use a lighter and start a fire. The preschool child is capable of washing his or her hands independently, so the water heater should be set at a maximum of 49° C (120° F) to prevent scalding (Healthy Children, 2010a).

Preventing Poisoning

Though taste discrimination is continuing to develop, preschoolers still have unrefined taste discrimination, placing them at risk for accidental ingestion. Parents should never try to coax a child to take a vitamin supplement, tablet, or pill by calling it "candy." Dangerous fluids should be stored in their original containers and should be kept out of reach of preschoolers; they should not be poured into containers that look like ordinary drinking glasses or cups. Potentially dangerous cleaning or personal health and beauty products, gardening and pool chemicals, as well as automotive materials should be kept out of reach of preschoolers and in a locked cabinet if possible. Medications should have childproof caps and should be kept in a locked cabinet. The poison control telephone number should be posted on or near the home phone (Canadian Association of Poison Control Centres, 2011).

Safety in the Water

According to the Canadian Paediatric Society (2008), young children, particularly those who are preschool age and younger, cannot be considered "water safe" even if given basic water safety instruction and swimming lessons. Active adult supervision is required for young children because they do not have the developmental ability to learn the necessary skills to swim independently.

Starting at age 5, children are more likely to be physically capable of beginning to learn basic swim techniques and have the cognitive maturity to accomplish the task of swimming and basic water safety. Water activities and swimming programs should focus on building the child's confidence and teaching appropriate swim techniques as well as safety measures. Parents and caregivers should be trained in infant/child CPR. Homes with swimming pools should have lifesaving devices readily accessible. Preschoolers are still too young to be left unattended around any body of water, even if they know how to swim. Preschoolers should never be allowed to swim in any fast-moving water. Preschoolers who are riding in boats or fishing off riverbanks should wear a personal flotation device. Parents should also be cautioned about close supervision of young children walking, skating, or riding near thin or weak ice.

> ▶ **Take** NOTE!
>
> *Safe Kids Canada (2010) recommends that backyard swimming pools should have four-sided fencing at least 1.2 m high and a self-closing, self-latching gate.*

Recall Nila Patel, the 4-year-old presented at the beginning of the chapter. What anticipatory guidance related to safety should you provide to her parents?

Promoting Nutrition

The preschool child has a full set of primary teeth, is able to chew and swallow competently, and has learned to use utensils fairly effectively to feed himself or herself

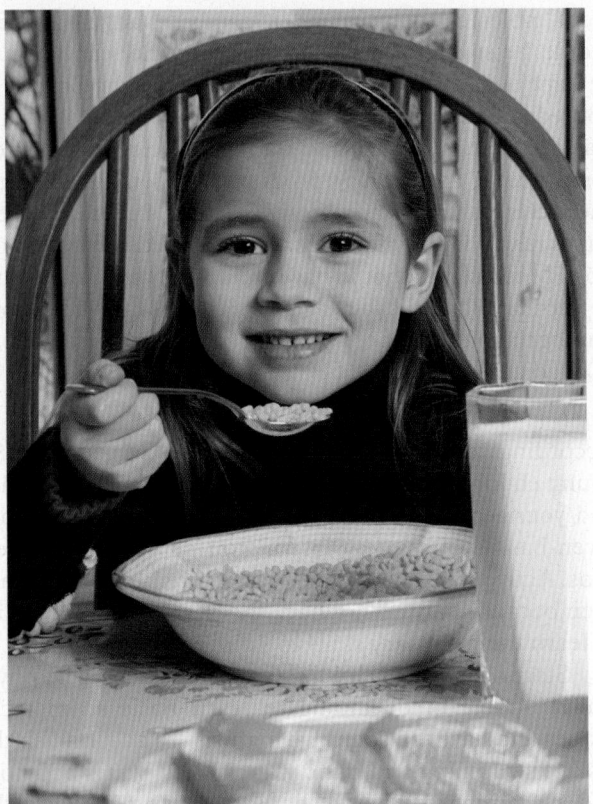

FIGURE **27.12** The preschool child has the manual dexterity to handle utensils appropriately and feed himself or herself independently.

(Fig. 27.12). As in the toddler years, it is important for the preschool child to continue to learn and build upon healthy eating habits. These habits will last throughout the child's life. A diet high in nutrient-rich foods such as whole grains, vegetables, fruits, appropriate dairy foods, and lean meats is appropriate for the preschooler. Nutrient-poor, high-calorie foods such as sweets and typical fast foods should be offered only in limited amounts.

Nutritional Needs

Preschool-aged children require 700 to 1000 mg calcium and 10 mg iron daily (Health Canada, 2010). Box 27.2 lists good calcium and iron sources. Canada's Food Guide recommends that 30% to 40% of the total caloric intake of young children up to the age of 3 years should come from fat, decreasing to 25% to 35% at 4 years of age and for the remainder of childhood (Health Canada, 2007).

> ▶ **Take** NOTE!
>
> *Drinking excess amounts of milk may lead to iron deficiency, as the calcium in milk blocks iron absorption.*

BOX 27.2 Daily Calcium and Iron Recommendations for Preschool Children

Calcium:
700 mg (3-year-old)
1000 mg (4- to 8-year-old)   Iron: 10 mg

Calcium in foods:
- 240 mL low-fat or whole milk: 300 mg
- 240 mL low-fat yogurt: 300 mg
- 47 g cheddar cheese: 300 mg
- 30 mL dried white beans (cooked): 160 mg
- 60 g tofu: 125 mg
- 1 medium orange: 50 mg
- 120 g mashed sweet potatoes: 44 mg
- 120 g cooked or 360 g raw broccoli: 35 mg

Iron in foods:
- 180 mL 100% fortified prepared cereal: 18 mg
- 180 mL 50% fortified prepared cereal: 9 mg
- 90 g beef: 3 mg
- 90 g chicken leg: 3 mg
- 120 g cooked lentils: 3 mg
- 90 g chicken breast: 2 mg
- 60 g fresh cooked spinach: 1.6 mg
- 60 g tofu: 0.9 mg
- 1 slice enriched bread: 0.8 to 0.9 mg
- 60 g frozen spinach, cooked: 0.7 mg

Adapted from: Health Canada. (2010). *Vitamin D and calcium: Updated dietary reference intakes.* Retrieved October 25, 2011 from http://www.hc-sc.gc.ca/fn-an/nutrition/vitamin/vita-d-eng.php; and United States Department of Agriculture. (2010). *USDA national nutrient database for standard reference, Release 23.* Retrieved August 18, 2011 from http://www.ars.usda.gov/research/publications/publications.htm?SEQ_NO_115=257886.

Promoting Healthy Eating Habits

Preschool children may be picky eaters. They may eat only a limited variety of foods or foods prepared in certain ways and may not be very willing to try new things. The 3- or 4-year-old may exhibit "food fads," eating only certain foods over a several-day period. As the child gets older, pickiness lessens. By 5 years of age the child is more focused on the social context of eating: table conversation and manners. The 5-year-old is generally more willing to at least try new foods and may like to help with meal preparation and clean-up as appropriate.

If the preschooler is growing well, then the pickiness is not a cause for concern. A larger concern may be the negative relationship that can develop between the parent and child relating to mealtime. The more the parent coaxes, cajoles, bribes, and threatens, the less likely the child is to try new foods or even eat the ones he or she likes that are served. The parent must maintain a positive and patient demeanour at mealtime. The child should be offered a healthy diet, with foods from all groups over the course of the day as recommended by

Canada's Food Guide (Health Canada, 2007) (See Appendix H). See Figure 26.11 in Chapter 26, and note the explanation of serving sizes. Refer also to the Nutrition Resource Centre website for more information (visit http://thePoint.lww.com/Chow1e for the direct link).

The parent should maintain a matter-of-fact approach, offer the meal or snack, and then allow the child to decide how much of the food, if any, he or she is going to eat. High-fat, nutrient-poor snacks should not be substituted for healthy foods just to coax the child to "eat something."

Preventing the Development of Overweight and Obesity

In Canada, the number of obese children at all ages is on the rise. Overweight and obese children are at risk for hypertension, hyperlipidemia, and the development of insulin resistance. Children whose weight is at or above the 95th percentile when 3 to 6 years old have a 50% chance of being obese as adults (Krebs, Collins, & Johnson, 2004). The risk is increased if one or both parents are overweight. Research has demonstrated that preschool children who are overweight or obese show a preference for higher-fat foods and tend to overeat (Neumark-Sztainer, 2003).

Parents are in an opportune position to exert a positive influence on their preschooler's nutritional intake and activity level. The habits learned in early childhood will likely carry over into the school-age, adolescent, and adult years. Children whose parents take an authoritarian approach to mealtime may learn to overeat, as they are encouraged to finish the entire meal ("Clean your plate!"). If they are offered appropriate, healthy food choices and access to high-calorie, nutrient-poor food is limited, preschoolers will learn to self-regulate (eat only until full). Food should not be used as either reward or punishment.

Parents should remain positive and patient at mealtime. Mealtimes should continue to be structured. Unstructured meals lead to an increase in fat and calorie consumption. To limit the chance that overeating will occur, preschoolers should be offered a variety of healthy foods at each meal. This may include one each of a protein source, grain, vegetable, and fruit. The preschool child's serving size is usually one third to one half of the recommended size of an adult serving. The preschool child may imitate the other eaters at the table. Parents have a prime chance to be good role models, setting an example of eating vegetables and fruits.

The Nutrition Resource Centre (2009) advises that 125 mL of unsweetened fruit juice a day is sufficient. Preschoolers should be encouraged to drink water.

Limiting television viewing and encouraging physical activity are also important strategies for the prevention of overweight and obesity.

Refer back to Nila Patel, the 4-year-old introduced at the beginning of the chapter. What questions should you ask Nila's parents related to nutritional intake? What anticipatory guidance related to nutrition would be appropriate? Nila's mother expresses concerns regarding obesity. How would you address these?

Promoting Healthy Sleep and Rest

The preschool child needs about 11 to 12 hours of sleep each day (Feigelman, 2007). Some preschool children continue to take a nap during the day. Unless very tired, many preschool children will resist going to bed from time to time. Bedtime rituals continue to be reassuring to children, and it is important to continue them in the preschool years. Having a time of relaxation with a decrease in stimulation will allow the child to fall asleep more easily. Some children continue to need a security item at bedtime or naptime. A nightlight in the bedroom may be necessary, as many children this age are afraid of the dark. Teaching Guideline 27.1 gives information about assisting parents to establish a bedtime routine.

Nightmares often occur in preschool children as a result of the child's struggle to distinguish what is real from what is not. When a child awakens from a nightmare, he or she is often crying and may be able to recount

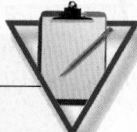

TEACHING GUIDELINE 27.1

Bedtime Routines

- Establish a bedtime as well as morning wake-up time, and enforce them consistently.
- Avoid sugar or caffeine consumption in the evening.
- Avoid stimulating activities such as roughhousing before bedtime.
- Do not allow television watching in bed.
- Make the child's bedroom an inviting and comfortable area of the home.
- Provide a nightlight in the child's bedroom if he or she is afraid of the dark.
- Conform to a nightly routine:
  - Television off at a certain time
  - Bath
  - Quiet game or story reading/telling
  - Bedtime prayer or song
- Maintain quiet in the bedroom and nearby to increase the child's ability to fall asleep.

Adaped from: Dowshen, S. (2008). *Sleep and your preschooler: Establishing a bedtime routine.* Retrieved August 18, 2011 from http://kidshealth.org/parent/general/sleep/sleep_preschool.html#; and Goldson, E., & Reynolds. A. (2011). Child development and behavior. In W. W. Hay, M. J. Levin, J. M. Sondheimer, & R. R. Deterding (Eds.), *Current pediatric diagnosis and treatment* (20th ed.). New York: McGraw-Hill.

what the dream was about. Parents should validate the child's fear rather than discounting it (Goldson & Reynolds, 2011). Saying, "Yes, I agree, monsters are scary; it's a good thing they aren't real" is more appropriate than, "Don't be silly: monsters aren't real." Sometimes children benefit from reading stories about dreams. Recommended books include:

• *Bedtime for Frances* by Russell Hoban
• *Ben's Dream* by Chris van Allsberg
• *In the Night Kitchen* by Maurice Sendak
• *There's a Nightmare in My Closet* by Mercer Mayer

Nightmares should not be confused with night terrors. After a nightmare, the child is aroused and interactive, but night terrors are different: a short time after falling asleep, the child seems to awaken and is screaming. The child usually does not respond much to the parent's soothing, but he or she eventually stops screaming and goes back to sleep. Night terrors are often frightening for parents because the child does not seem to be responding to them. One technique that may help to decrease the incidence of night terrors is to wake the child about 30 to 45 minutes into the sleep cycle. If continued nightly for about a week, the cycle of night terrors may be broken (Hopkins & Glaze, 2008). See Comparison Chart 27.1.

*T*hink back to Nila Patel. What anticipatory guidance would you provide to her parents in relation to sleep during the preschool years?

Promoting Healthy Teeth and Gums
Dental caries prevention continues to be important and can be achieved through daily brushing and flossing.

Parents should use only a pea-sized amount of toothpaste to prevent excess fluoride consumption, which can contribute to fluorosis (American Academy of Pediatrics, n.d.). The preschooler may brush his or her own teeth, but the parent must continue to supervise to ensure adequate brushing and help prevent overuse and possible ingestion of toothpaste. Parents must perform flossing because the preschool child cannot perform this task adequately.

Cariogenic foods should be avoided. If sugary foods are consumed, the mouth should be rinsed with water if it is not possible to brush the teeth immediately (Wagner & Oskouian, 2008). The preschool child should visit the dentist every 6 months.

▶ *Take* NOTE!

Dental caries prevention is important in the primary teeth, because loss of these teeth to caries may affect the proper formation of permanent teeth as well as the width of the dental arch.

Promoting Positive Discipline
Successful discipline results from a loving and nurturing environment in which the preschooler's self-esteem is fostered and where limits are well chosen and responded to in a consistent manner. The Canadian Paediatric Society (2004) recommends that all forms of physical punishment should be discouraged. The use of physical punishment has been associated with a number of risks in childhood, such as physical child abuse and aggression, as well as additional issues in adulthood, including

COMPARISON CHART 27.1 NIGHTMARES VERSUS NIGHT TERRORS

	Nightmare	Night Terror
Definition	Scary or bad dream followed by awakening	Partial arousal from deep sleep
When parents become aware	Child awakens parent after episode is over	Screaming and thrashing during the episode awakens the parent
Timing	Usually in the second half of the night	Usually about an hour after falling asleep
Behaviour	Crying, may be scared after awakening	Sits up, thrashes, cries, screams, talks, looks wild-eyed. Sweats may have racing heartbeat
Responsiveness	Responsive to parent's soothing and reassurances	Child unaware of parent's presence, may scream and thrash more if restrained
Return to sleep	Difficulty going back to sleep if afraid	Rapidly returns to sleep without full awakening
Memory of occurrence	May remember the dream and talk about it later	No memory of event

Information from: Hopkins, B., & Glaze, D. (2008). Disorders of arousal in children. *Pediatric Annals*, *37*(7), 481–487.

antisocial and criminal behaviours (Gershoff, 2002) (see Chapter 26).

If parents are consistent in their approach to discipline while encouraging the preschooler's normal growth and development of imagination and make-believe, the child will learn to understand the reasons certain things are not allowed. The sense of initiative can be preserved and guilt avoided if the rules are clear and enforced consistently (American Academy of Pediatrics, 1998).

Minimize the occurrence of undesired behaviours by anticipating conditions or situations likely to lead to them. For example, preschoolers still require close supervision while outside where there are many risks to their safety. When a situation becomes difficult, parents should use distraction to change the preschooler's focus when appropriate. To help preserve self-esteem, children should not be labelled in a negative way. When teaching preschoolers about undesired behaviour, parents should be sure they also understand the reason why the behaviour is wrong or unacceptable. This helps to encourage the child to use internal controls over behaviour. Parents should serve as role models for self-control, including their choice of words, the tone in which the words are delivered, and the actions that accompany them. Preschool children are becoming capable of understanding the concept of right and wrong. They start to understand each other's feelings (**empathy**) and are cognitively capable of remembering basic rules (American Academy of Pediatrics, 1998).

Although a short time away from the situation may be appropriate in an emotionally charged situation involving aggression, the experience of isolation and fear of abandonment can sometimes be emotionally difficult for children. The use of a calm explanation about why an action is wrong is the most useful response. For example, if a child draws on furniture or walls with markers, caregivers should explain that markers should be used only on paper because they damage furniture; and the child can assist in cleaning up the markings. If a situation is very emotionally charged, either for the child or the caregiver, and a period of quiet time is warranted, it is preferable that the caregiver stay with the young child during this time. It is very important to praise and encourage the child when he or she follows the rules and behaves appropriately.

Parents should talk about acceptable alternative strategies that the child can use in the future instead of the undesired behaviour. Preserving a child's self-esteem while helping him or her to fit into the real world and get along with others is of utmost importance. Effective and positive discipline is about teaching and guiding children, not forcing them to obey. Books and other media that are available to help educate parents about appropriate discipline and to help the child learn self-control are listed in Box 27.3.

BOX 27.3 **Selected Resources for Parents and Preschoolers**

Books for Parents (about discipline)
- *How to Talk so Kids Will Listen and Listen so Kids Will Talk* by A. Faber & E. Mazlish (Harper Resource)
- *Kids Are Worth It: Giving Your Children the Gift of Inner Discipline* by B. Colorosos (Harper Collins Publishers)
- *Positive Discipline A to Z: 1001 Solutions to Everyday Parenting Problems* by J. Nelson, L. Lott, & S. G. Glenn (Three Rivers Press)
- *Positive Discipline: What It Is and How to Do It* by Joan E. Durrant (Save the Children Sweden, Southeast Asia, and the Pacific; available in Canada through the Canadian Association of Family Resource Programs [visit http://thePoint.lww.com/Chow1e for a direct link])
- *The Case Against Spanking: How to Discipline Children without Hitting* by I. A. Hyman (Jossey-Bass)
- *The Nurturing Parent: How to Raise Creative, Loving, Responsible Children* by J. S. Dacey & A. J. Packer (Fireside)
- *Without Spanking or Spoiling: A Practical Approach to Toddler and Preschool Guidance* by E. Crary (Parenting Press)

Books for Preschoolers (About Dealing with Feelings and Learning how to Behave):
- *Hands Are Not for Hitting* by M. Agassi (Free Spirit Publishing)
- *I Can't Wait* by E. Crary (Parenting Press)
- *I Want It* by E. Crary (Parenting Press)
- *I Want to Play* by E. Crary (Parenting Press)
- *I Was so Mad* by M. Mayer (Golden Books)
- *I Was so Mad* by N. Simon & D. Leder (Albert Whitman & Company)
- *I'm Excited* by E. Crary (Parenting Press)
- *I'm Frustrated* by E. Crary (Parenting Press)
- *I'm Mad* by E. Crary (Parenting Press)
- *I'm Scared* by E. Crary (Parenting Press)
- *Feet Are Not for Kicking* by E. Verdick (Free Spirit Publishing)
- *Teeth Are Not for Biting* by E. Verdick (Free Spirit Publishing)
- *When Sophie Gets Angry . . . Really, Really Angry* by M. Bang (Blue Sky Press)
- *Words Are Not for Hurting* by E. Verdick (Free Spirit Publishing)

Addressing Common Developmental Concerns

Common developmental concerns of the preschool period include lying, sex education, and masturbation (Shelov & Altmann, 2009). Parents often express difficulty in dealing with these issues with their preschool children. Offering appropriate anticipatory guidance may give the parents the support and confidence they need to deal with these issues.

Lying

It is common for preschoolers to say things that are not truthful. It may occur because the child fears punishment, has gotten carried away with imagination, or is imitating what he or she sees the parent do. The parent should try to ascertain the reason for the lie before responding. The parent should remain calm and serve as a role model of an even temper.

The younger children are, the more likely it is that they may be unclear about what is truth and what is fantasy or imagination. If the child's lying is really just his or her imagination getting carried away, then the parent should guide the child in distinguishing between what is real and what is not real (Brazelton & Sparrow, 2002). The preschooler's imagination is very vivid, and the child needs direction in the use of that faculty. Parents should serve as role models of appropriate behaviour for their children to learn it.

Sex Education

Preschoolers are keen observers but are still not able to interpret all that they see correctly. The child may recognize, but not understand, sexual activity. Preschoolers are very inquisitive and want to learn about everything around them; therefore, they are very likely to ask questions about sex and where babies come from. Before attempting to answer questions, parents should try to find out first what the child is really asking and what the child already thinks about that subject. Then they should provide a simple, direct, and honest answer. The child needs only the information that he or she is requesting. Additional questions will occur in the future and should be addressed as they arise.

Masturbation

The normal curiosity of the preschool years often leads children to explore their own genitals (Shelov & Altmann, 2009). This behaviour may be upsetting to some parents, but masturbation is a healthy and natural part of normal preschool development if it occurs in moderation. If the parent overreacts to this behaviour, then it may occur more frequently. Masturbation should be treated in a matter-of-fact way by the parent. The child needs to learn certain rules about this activity: nudity and masturbation are not acceptable in public. Most importantly, the child should also be taught safety: no other person can touch the private parts unless it is the parent, doctor, or nurse checking to see when something is wrong.

*T*hink back to Nila Patel. What are some developmental concerns that are common during the preschool years? What anticipatory guidance related to these concerns would you provide to Nila's parents?

■■■ Key Concepts

- The preschool child grows at a slower rate and takes on a more slender and upright appearance than the toddler.
- The primary psychosocial task of the preschool period is developing a sense of initiative.
- Cognitive development moves from an egocentric approach to the world toward a more empathetic understanding of what happens outside of the self.
- The preschooler gains additional motor skills and displays significant refinement of fine motor abilities.
- Cognitive and language skills that develop in the preschool years help prepare the child for success in school.
- The vocabulary of a preschooler increases to about 2,100 words, and the child speaks in full sentences with appropriate use of tense and prepositions.
- Appropriate growth and development should be maintained in the ill or hospitalized child.
- Recognizing concerns or delays in growth and development is essential so that the appropriate referrals may be made and intervention can begin.
- The preschool child requires a well-balanced diet and not an overreliance on milk and/or fruit juice for calories. Food jags may occur.
- Adequate physical activity and provision of a nutrient-dense diet (rather than foods high in fat and sugar) are the foundation for obesity prevention in the preschool child.
- Adequate dental care is important for the health of the primary teeth.
- Preschoolers need about 12 hours of sleep per day and benefit from a structured bedtime routine.
- Due to the active imagination of the preschooler, nightmares and night terrors may begin during this period.
- Safety and injury prevention remain a focus in the preschool years.
- Structure, warmth, appropriate limit setting, and consistency are the keys for positive discipline in the preschool period.
- Effective and positive discipline is about teaching and guiding children while preserving their self-esteem and maintaining trust.
- Masturbation may occur as the preschooler discovers his or her body. If not excessive, it is considered as a normal part of growth and development.

REFERENCES

Abell, S., & Ey, J. L. (2007). Ask Dr. Sue. Bilingual child. *Clinical Pediatrics, 46*(7), 658–659.

American Academy of Pediatrics. (n.d.). *Protecting all children's teeth (PACT): A pediatric oral health training program.* Retrieved August 18, 2011 from http://www.aap.org/oralhealth/pact/pact-home.cfm

American Academy of Pediatrics. (1998). *Guidance for effective discipline.* Retrieved August 18, 2011 from http://aappolicy.aappublications.org/cgi/content/full/pediatrics;101/4/723

Brazelton, T. B., & Sparrow, J. (2002). *Touchpoints three to six: Your child's emotional and behavioral development.* New York: De Capo Publishing.

Canadian Association of Poison Control Centres. (2011). *National poison prevention week March 10-14, 2010.* Retrieved August 16, 2011 from http://www.capcc.ca/announcements/page36.html

Canadian Paediatric Society. (2004). Effective discipline for children. *Paediatrics & Child Health, 9*(1), 37–41.

Canadian Paediatric Society. (2008). Swimming lessons for infants and toddlers. *Paediatrics & Child Health, 8*(2), 113–114. Retrieved August 16, 2011 from http://www.cps.ca/english/statements/ip/ip03-01.htm

Carpenito-Moyet, L. J. (2010). *Nursing diagnosis: Application to clinical practice* (13th ed.). Philadelphia: Lippincott Williams & Wilkins.

Child Development Institute. (2010). *Is your child easy or difficult to raise?* Retrieved August 18, 2011 from http://www.childdevelopmentinfo.com/development/temp3.shtml

Christakis, D. A., & Zimmerman, F. J. (2007). Children & television: A primer for pediatricians. *Contemporary Pediatrics, 24*(3), 31–42.

Dowshen, S. (2008). *Sleep and your preschooler: Establishing a bedtime routine.* Retrieved August 18, 2011 from http://kidshealth.org/parent/general/sleep/sleep_preschool.html#

Erikson, E. H. (1963). *Childhood and society* (2nd ed.). New York: W. W. Norton and Company.

Feigelman, S. (2007). Preschool years. In R. M. Kliegman, R. E. Behrman, H. B. Jenson, & B. F. Stanton (Eds.), *Nelson textbook of pediatrics* (18th ed.). Philadelphia: Saunders.

Ford, G. S. (2007). Hospitalized kids: Spiritual care at their level. *Journal of Christian Nursing, 24*(3), 135–140.

Gershoff, E. T. (2002). Corporal punishment by parents and associated child behaviours and experiences: A meta-analytic and theoretical review. *Psychological Bulletin, 128*, 539–579.

Goldson, E., & Reynolds, A. (2011). Child development and behavior. In W. W. Hay, M. J. Levin, J. M. Sondheimer, & R. R. Deterding (Eds.), *Current pediatric diagnosis and treatment* (20th ed.). New York: McGraw-Hill.

Health Canada. (2007). *Eating well with Canada's Food Guide: A resource for educators and communicators.* Retrieved October 24, 2011 from http://www.peelregion.ca/health/eating/pdfs/canadafg-educators_e%5B1%5D-final.pdf

Health Canada. (2010). *Vitamin D and calcium: Updated dietary reference intakes.* Retrieved October 25, 2011 from http://www.hc-sc.gc.ca/fn-an/pubs/nutrition/guide-prenatal-eng.php

Healthy Children. (2010a). *Safety for your child: 2 to 4 years.* Retrieved August 18, 2011 from http://www.healthychildren.org/english/tips-tools/Pages/Safety-for-Your-Child-2-to-4-Years.aspx

Healthy Children. (2010b). *Safety for your child: 5 years.* Retrieved August 18, 2011 from http://www.healthychildren.org/english/tips-tools/Pages/Safety-for-Your-Child-5-Years.aspx

High, P. C. (2008). School readiness. *Pediatrics, 121*(4), e1008–e1015.

Hopkins, B., & Glaze, D. (2008). Disorders of arousal in children. *Pediatric Annals, 37*(7), 481–487.

Kohlberg, L. (1984). *Moral development.* New York: Harper & Row.

Krebs, N. F., Collins, J., & Johnson, S. L. (2004). Screen for and treat overweight in 2-to 5-year-olds? Yes! *Contemporary Pediatrics* [electronic version]. *Retrieved June 16, 2010 from* http://www.modernmedicine.com/modernmedicine/Cover+Article/Screen-for-and-treat-overweight-in-2--to-5-year-ol/ArticleStandard/Article/detail/128422

Neumark-Sztainer, D. (2003). Childhood and adolescent obesity. *Pediatric Basics: The Journal of Pediatric Nutrition and Development, 101*, 12–20.

Nutrition Resource Centre. (2009). *Eat right be active: A guide for parents and caregivers of preschoolers ages 3–5.* Retrieved November 14, 2011 from http://www.eatrightontario.ca/pdf/Eat%20Right%20Be%20Active%20Eng%203-5.pdf

Papalia, D., & Feldman, R. (2011). *A child's world: Infancy through adolescence* (12th ed.). New York: McGraw Hill.

Piaget, J. (1969). *The theory of stages in cognitive development.* New York: McGraw-Hill.

Prasse, J. E., & Kikano, G. E. (2008). Stuttering: An overview. *American Family Physician, 77*(9), 1271–1276.

Public Health Agency of Canada. (2009). *Child and youth injury in review, 2009 Edition: Spotlight on consumer product safety.* Retrieved October 22, 2011 from http://www.phac-aspc.gc.ca/publicat/cyi-bej/2009/pdf/injrep-rapbles2009_eng.pdf

Safe Kids Canada. (2010). *Safety information by topic.* Retrieved August 16, 2011 from http://www.safekidscanada.ca/Parents/Home/index.aspx

Schuman, A. J. (2007). The ABCs of toy safety: More than just child's play. *Contemporary Pediatrics, 24*(7), 49–57, 64.

Shelov, S. P., & Altmann, T. R. (Eds.). (2009). *Caring for your baby and young child: Birth to age 5* (5th ed.). New York: Bantam Books.

Taylor, E. (2008). Providing developmentally based care for preschoolers. *AORN Journal, 88*(2), 267–273.

Transport Canada. (2011). *Stage 2: Forward-facing seats.* Retrieved October 23, 2011 from http://www.tc.gc.ca/eng/roadsafety/safedrivers-childsafety-stage2-forward-facing-1085.htm

United States Department of Agriculture. (2010). *USDA national nutrient database for standard reference.* Retrieved August 18, 2011 from http://www.ars.usda.gov/Services/docs.htm?docid=8964

Wagner, R., & Oskouian, R. (2008). The ECC epidemic. *Contemporary Pediatrics, 25*(9), 60–80.

World Health Organization. (n.d.). *Passive smoking.* Retrieved August 18, 2011 from http://www.who.int/tobacco/en/atlas10.pdf

RECOMMENDED READINGS

American Academy of Pediatrics. (2007). *Policy statement: The use and misuse of fruit juice in pediatrics.* Retrieved August 18, 2011 from http://aappolicy.aappublications.org/cgi/content/full/pediatrics;107/5/1210

Centers for Disease Control and Prevention. (2010). *State vaccination requirements.* Retrieved August 18, 2011 from http://www.cdc.gov/vaccines/vac-gen/laws/state-reqs.htm

Ferber, R. (1985). *Solve your child's sleep problems.* New York: Simon & Schuster.

Healthy Children. (2011). *Car safety seats: Information for families 2011.* Retrieved August 18, 2011 from http://www.healthychildren.org/English/safety-prevention/on-the-go/Pages/Car-Safety-Seats-Information-for-Families.aspx

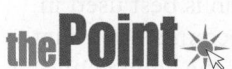

thePoint For additional learning materials, including Internet Resources, visit http://thePoint.lww.com/Chow1e.

CHAPTER WORKSHEET

MULTIPLE CHOICE QUESTIONS

1. The nurse is caring for a hospitalized 4-year-old who insists on having the nurse perform every assessment and intervention on her imaginary friend first. She then agrees to have the assessment or intervention done to her. The nurse identifies this preschooler's behaviour as:

   a. Problematic, because the child is old enough to begin to have a basis in reality

   b. Normal, because the child is hospitalized and out of her routine

   c. Normal for this stage of growth and development

   d. Problematic, as it interferes with needed nursing care

2. The mother of a 3-year-old is concerned about her child's speech. She describes her preschooler as hesitating at the beginning of sentences and repeating consonant sounds. What is the nurse's best response?

   a. Hesitancy and dysfluency are normal during this period of development.

   b. Reading to the child will help model appropriate speech.

   c. Expressive language concerns warrant a developmental evaluation.

   d. The mother should ask her pediatrician for a speech therapy evaluation.

3. The mother of a 4-year-old asks for advice on using time-out for discipline with her child. What advice should the nurse give the mother?

   a. The longer the time-out lasts, the more effective it is.

   b. Time-out away from the situation is best used in emotional situations, and it is recommended that the parent or caregiver stay with the young child

   c. Time-out is most effective without explanations.

   d. The child should stay in time-out until crying ceases.

4. A 5-year-old child is not gaining weight appropriately. Organic problems have been ruled out. What is the priority action by the nurse?

   a. Allow the child's unlimited access to the sippy cup to ensure adequate hydration.

   b. Encourage sweets for the extra caloric content.

   c. Teach the mother about nutritional needs of the preschooler.

   d. Assess the child's usual intake pattern at home.

CRITICAL THINKING EXERCISES

1. Teach a preschool class about bicycle and street safety. Be certain to design the content at an appropriate developmental level.

2. Construct a 3-day menu for a picky 4-year-old. Include three daily meals and two snacks. Follow the nutritional guidelines recommended in Canada's Food Guide.

3. Colour or draw with a preschool child. Analyze the drawings and interactions or discussions you have with the child, relating them to psychosocial and cognitive development expected at this age.

STUDY ACTIVITIES

1. Care for two average 3-, 4-, or 5-year-old children in the clinical setting (make sure both are the same age). Describe each child's development level, response to hospitalization, and family dynamics.

2. Visit a preschool that provides care for special needs children as well as typically developing children. Perform a development assessment on a typical child and one with special needs (both the same age). Compare and contrast your findings.

3. Observe in a 3-, 4- or 5-year-old classroom of a typical preschool. Choose two children who are the same age with different temperaments. Record the differences and similarities in their response to structure and authority, interactions with classmates, attention levels, and language and activity levels.

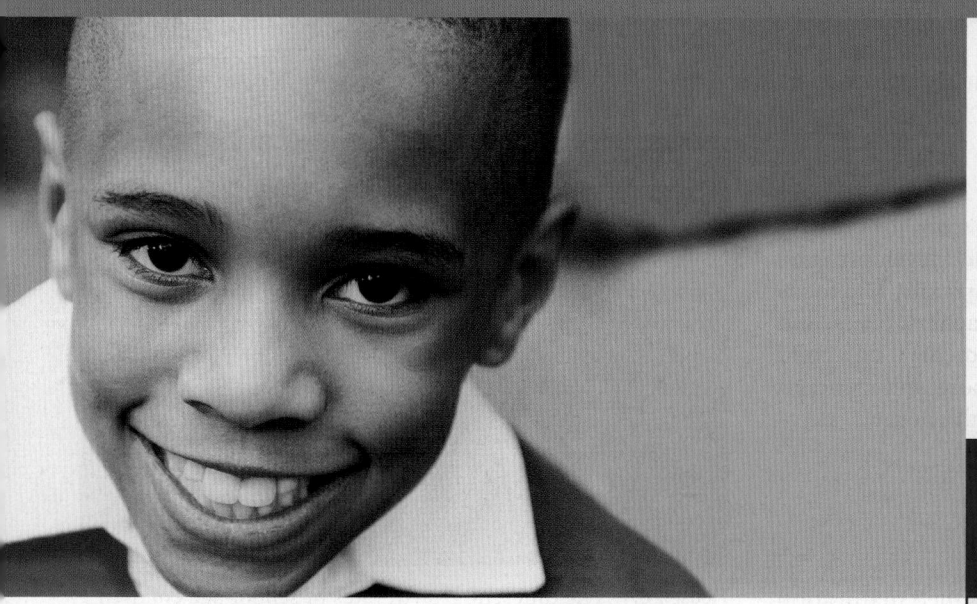

GROWTH AND DEVELOPMENT OF THE SCHOOL-AGE CHILD

KEY TERMS

bruxism
caries
industry
inferiority

malocclusion
prepubescence
principle of conservation
school-age child

school refusal
secondary sexual
characteristics
self-esteem

LEARNING OBJECTIVES

Upon completion of the chapter, the learner will be able to:

1. Identify normal physiologic, cognitive, and moral changes occurring in the school-age child.
2. Describe the role of peers and schools in the development and socialization of the school-age child.
3. Identify the developmental milestones of the school-age child.
4. Identify the role of the nurse in promoting safety for the school-age child.
5. Demonstrate knowledge of the nutritional requirements of the school-age child.
6. Identify common developmental problems in the school-age child.
7. Demonstrate knowledge of the appropriate nursing guidance for common developmental problems.

Lawrence Jones is a 10-year-old boy brought to the clinic by his mother for his annual school check-up. During your assessment you measure his weight at 28 kg and his height at 135 cm.

As the nurse caring for him, assess Lawrence's growth and development, and then provide appropriate anticipatory guidance to his mother.

Wow

Always give a hundred percent, and you will never doubt your ability to succeed.

School-age children, between the ages of 6 and 12 years, are experiencing a time of slow progressive physical growth, while their social and developmental growth accelerates and increases in complexity. The focus of their world expands from family to teachers, peers, and other outside influences (e.g., coaches, media). The child at this stage becomes increasingly more independent while participating in activities outside the home.

Growth and Development Overview

The school-age years are a time of continued maturation of the child's physical, social, and psychological characteristics. It is during this time that children begin abstract thinking and seek approval of peers, teachers, and parents. Their eye–hand–muscle coordination allows them to participate in organized sports in school or the community. The **school-age child** typically values school attendance and school activities. The nurse uses knowledge of normal growth and development of the school-age child to assist the child with coping with disruptions and changes during this time period.

Physical Growth

From 6 to 12 years of age, children grow an average of 5 cm per year, increasing their height by 30 to 60 cm. An increase of 3 to 3.5 kg per year in weight is expected (Feigelman, 2007a). In early school-age years, girls and boys are similar in height and weight and appear thinner and more graceful than in previous years. In later school-age years, most girls begin to surpass boys in both height and weight; during this time period there is an approximate 2-year difference between boys and girls. (See Appendix F for growth charts.)

Pre-adolescent boys and girls do not want to be different from peers of the same sex, although there are differences in physical and physiologic growth during the school-age years. These differences, especially **secondary sexual characteristics**, are concerning and often a source of embarrassment for both sexes. Girls' early development may be associated with concern about physical appearance and may lead to low **self-esteem**. Boys developing later may have a negative self-concept, which may be linked to future risk-taking behaviours such as early sexual activities, substance abuse, or reckless vehicle use.

The differences between girls and boys are more apparent at the end of the middle-school years and may become extreme and a source of emotional problems. These differences in height and weight relationships, and changes in growth patterns, should be explained to parents and children (Fig. 28.1). Physical maturity is not necessarily associated with emotional and social maturity. An

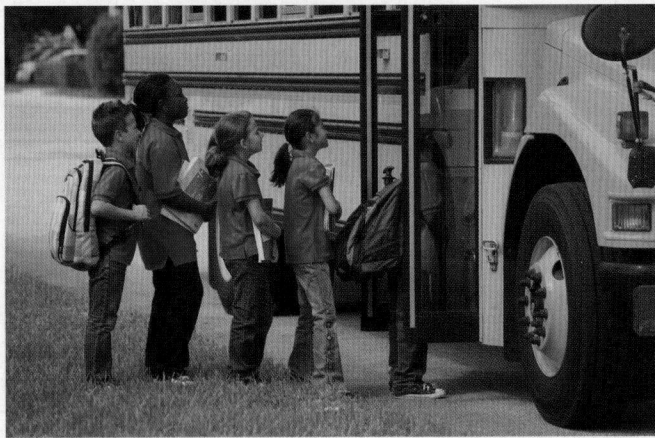

FIGURE 28.1 The different growth rates of school-age children are depicted by these same-age school-age children.

8-year-old who is the size of an 11-year-old will think and act like an 8-year-old. Many times, the expectations placed on these children are unrealistic and can impact the self-esteem and competence of the child. This can work in reverse, to similar effect, for an 11-year-old who is the size of an 8-year-old and is therefore treated as such.

Organ Systems Maturation

Maturation of organs may differ with age or gender. Maturation of organs remains fairly consistent until late school age. In late school-age years (10- to 12-year-olds), boys experience a slowed growth in height and increased weight gain, which may lead to obesity. During this time, girls may begin to have changes in the body that soften body lines. Preadolescence is a period of rapid growth, especially for girls.

Neurologic System

The brain and skull grow very slowly during the school-age years. Brain growth is complete by the time the child is 10 years of age. The shape of the head is longer and the growth of the facial bones changes facial proportions.

Respiratory System

The respiratory system continues to mature with the development of the lungs and alveoli, resulting in fewer respiratory infections. Respiratory rates decrease, abdominal breathing disappears, and respirations become diaphragmatic in nature. The frontal sinuses are developed by 7 years of age. Tonsils decrease in size from the preschool years, but they remain larger than in adolescents. The adenoids and tonsils may appear large normally, even in the absence of infection.

Cardiovascular System

The school-age child's blood pressure increases. Also, the pulse rate decreases. The heart grows more slowly during the middle years and is smaller in size in relation to the rest of the body than at any other development stage.

Gastrointestinal System

During the school-age years, all 20 primary deciduous teeth are lost, replaced by 28 of 32 permanent teeth, with the exception of the third molars. The school-age child experiences fewer gastrointestinal upsets compared with earlier years. Stomach capacity increases, which permits retention of food for longer periods of time. In addition, the caloric needs per kilogram of weight for the school-age child are lower than in the earlier years.

Genitourinary System

Bladder capacity increases but varies among individual children. Girls generally have a greater bladder capacity than boys. Urination patterns vary with the amount of fluids ingested, the time they were ingested, and the stress level of the child. The formula for bladder capacity is 30 mL times age in years plus 60 mL. Therefore, the bladder capacity of the 7-year-old would be 270 mL. The larger capacity of the bladder allows for the child to experience longer periods between voiding.

Prepubescence

The late school-age years are also referred to as *preadolescence* (the time between middle childhood and the 13th birthday). During preadolescence, **prepubescence** occurs. Prepubescence typically occurs in the 2 years before the beginning of puberty and is characterized by the development of secondary sexual characteristics, a period of rapid growth for girls, and a period of continued growth for boys. There is approximately 2 years' difference in the onset of prepubescence between boys and girls. Sexual development in both boys and girls can lead to a negative perception of physical appearance and lowered self-esteem. Early development in girls can lead to embarrassment, and delayed development in boys can lead to a negative self-concept. Early development may lead to risk-taking behaviours in both boys and girls. It is important for the nurse and parents to educate the late school-age child about body changes to decrease anxiety and promote comfort with these changes in the body.

Musculoskeletal System

Musculoskeletal growth leads to greater coordination and strength, yet the muscles are still immature and can be injured easily. Bones continue to ossify throughout childhood, but mineralization is not complete until maturity; children's bones resist pressure and muscle pull less than mature bones.

Immune System

Lymphatic tissues continue to grow until the child is 9 years old; immunoglobulins A and G (IgA and IgG) reach adult levels at around 10 years of age. Due to the lymphatic system becoming more competent in localizing infections and producing antibody–antigen responses, school-age children may have fewer infections. They may experience more infections during the first 1 to 2 years of school due to exposure to other children who may have infections.

Psychosocial Development

Erikson (1963) describes the task of the school-age years to be a sense of **industry** vs. **inferiority** (Feigelman, 2007a). During this time, the child is developing his or her sense of self-worth by becoming involved in multiple activities at home, at school, and in the community, which develops the child's cognitive and social skills. He or she is very interested in learning how things are made and work. The school-age child's satisfaction from achieving success in developing new skills leads him or her to an increased sense of self-worth and level of competence. It is the role of the parents, teachers, coaches, and nurses of the school-age child to identify areas of competency and to build on the child's successful experiences to promote mastery, success, and self-esteem. If the expectations of the parents, teachers, and nurses are set too high, the child will develop a sense of inferiority and incompetence that can affect all aspects of his or her life. See Table 28.1 for a further explanation of psychosocial development in school-age children.

Cognitive Development

Piaget's stage of cognitive development for the 7- to 11-year-old is the period of concrete operational thoughts (Feigelman, 2007a). In developing concrete operations, the child is able to assimilate and coordinate information about his or her world from different dimensions. She is able to see things from another person's point of view and think through an action, anticipating its consequences and the possibility of having to rethink the action. She is able to use stored memories of past experiences to evaluate and interpret present situations. The school-age child also develops the ability to classify or divide things into different sets and to identify their relationships to each other. The school-age child is able to classify members of four generations on a family tree vertically and horizontally, and at the same time see that one person can be a father, son, uncle, and grandson. It is at this time that the school-age child develops an interest in collecting objects. She starts out collecting multiple objects and becomes more selective as she gets older. Also, during concrete operational thoughts, the school-age child develops an understanding of the **principle of conservation**—that matter does not change when its form changes. For example, if the child pours a half-cup of water into a short, wide glass and into a tall, thin glass, she still only has a half-cup of water despite the fact that it looks like the tall, thin glass has more (Fig. 28.2). She

TABLE 28.1 DEVELOPMENTAL THEORIES

Theorist	Stage	Activities
Erikson	Industry vs. inferiority	Interested in how things are made and run Success in personal and social tasks Increased activities outside home—clubs, sports Increased interactions with peers Increased interest in knowledge Needs support and encouragement from important people in child's life Needs support when child is not successful Inferiority occurs with repeated failures with little support or trust from those who are important to the child
Piaget	Concrete operational	Learns by manipulating concrete objects Lacks ability to think abstractly Learns that certain characteristics of objects remain constant Understands concept of time Engages in serial ordering, addition, subtraction Classifies or groups objects by their common elements Understands relationships among objects Starts collections of items Can reverse thought process
Kohlberg	Conventional Stage 3: interpersonal conforming, "good child, bad child" Stage 4: "law and order"	An act is wrong because it brings punishment Behaviour is completely wrong or right Does not understand the reason behind rules If child and adult differ in opinions, the adult is right Can put self in another person's position Begins to exercise the "golden rule" Acts are judged in terms of intention, not just punishment

Adapted from: Erikson, E. (1963). *Childhood and society* (2nd ed.). New York: Norton; Kohlberg, L. (1984). *Moral development.* New York: Harper & Row; and Piaget, J. (1969). *The theory of stages in cognitive development.* New York: McGraw-Hill.

learns about conserving matter in a sequence ranging from the simplest to the more complex. See Table 28.1 for further information about cognitive development of school-age children.

Moral Development

During the school-age years, the child's sense of morality is constantly being developed. According to Kohlberg (1984), the school-age child is at the conventional stage

of moral development. The 7- to 10-year-old usually follows rules out of a sense of being a "good" person. At this age, children want to be good to their parents, friends, and teachers and to themselves. The adult is viewed as being right. This is stage 3: interpersonal conformity (good child, bad child), according to Kohlberg. Ten- to twelve-year-olds progress to stage 4: the "law and order" stage. At this stage, the child can determine if an action is good or bad based upon the reason for the action, not just on the possible consequences of the

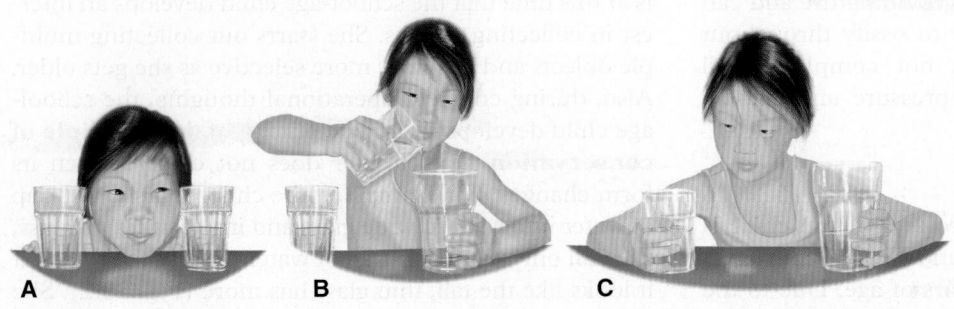

FIGURE 28.2 School-age children understand the theory of conservation (**A**). If you pour an equal amount of liquid into two glasses of unequal shape (**B**), the amount of water you have remains the same despite the unequal appearance in the two glasses (**C**).

A B C

action. The older school-age child's behaviour is guided by the child's desire to cooperate and by his or her respect for others. This leads to the child's ability to understand and incorporate into his or her behaviour the concept of the "golden rule" (Feigelman, 2007a). See Table 28.1 for additional information about the moral development of school-age children.

Motor Skill Development

Gross and fine motor skills continue to mature throughout the school-age years. Refinement of motor skills occurs, and speed and accuracy increase. To assess the motor skills of school-age children, ask questions about participation in sports and after-school activities, band membership, constructing models, and writing skills.

Gross Motor Skills

During the school-age years, coordination, balance, and rhythm improve, facilitating the opportunity to ride a two-wheel bike, jump rope, dance, and participate in a variety of other sports (Fig. 28.3). Older school-age children may become awkward due to their bodies growing faster than their ability to compensate.

School-age children between the ages of 6 and 8 enjoy gross motor activities such as bicycling, skating, and swimming. They are enthralled with the world and are in constant motion. Sometimes fear is limited due to the strong impulses of exploration. Children between 8

and 10 years of age are less restless, but their energy level continues to be high with activities more subdued and directed. These children exhibit greater rhythm and gracefulness of muscular movements, allowing them to participate in physical activities that require longer and more concentrated attention and effort, such as baseball or soccer.

Between the ages of 10 and 12 years (the pubescent years for girls), energy levels remain high but are more controlled and focused. Physical skills in this age group are similar to adults', with strength and endurance increasing during adolescence.

All school-age children should be encouraged to engage in physical activities and learn physical skills that contribute to their health for the rest of their lives. Cardiovascular fitness, weight control, emotional tension release, and development of leadership and following skills are enhanced through physical activity and team sports.

Fine Motor Skills

Myelination of the central nervous system is reflected by refinement of fine motor skills. Eye–hand coordination and balance improve with maturity and practice. Hand usage improves, becoming steadier and independent and granting an ease and precision that allows these children to write, print words, sew, or build models or other crafts. The child between 10 and 12 years of age begins to exhibit manipulative skills comparable to adults. School-age children take pride in activities that require dexterity and fine motor skills such as playing musical instruments (Fig. 28.4). Talent and practice become the keys to proficiency.

Sensory Development

All senses are mature early in the school-age years. The typical school-age child has 20/20 visual acuity (Jarvis, 2008). In addition, ocular muscular control, peripheral vision, and colour discrimination are fully developed by

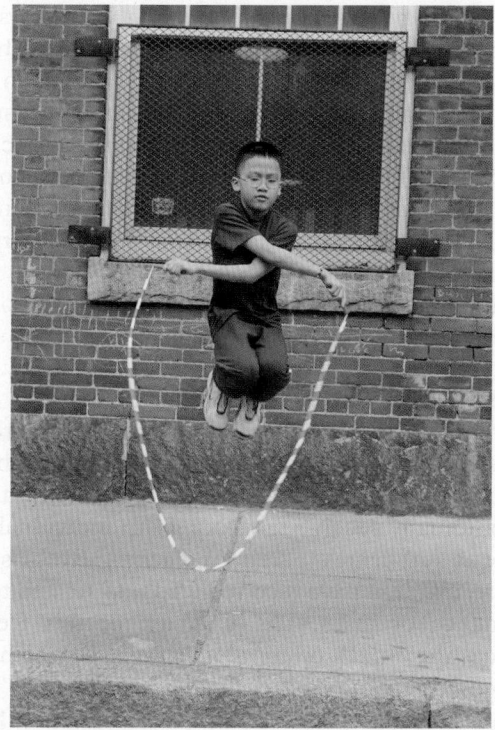

FIGURE 28.3 Jumping rope is an example of the increased development of gross motor skills of the school-age child.

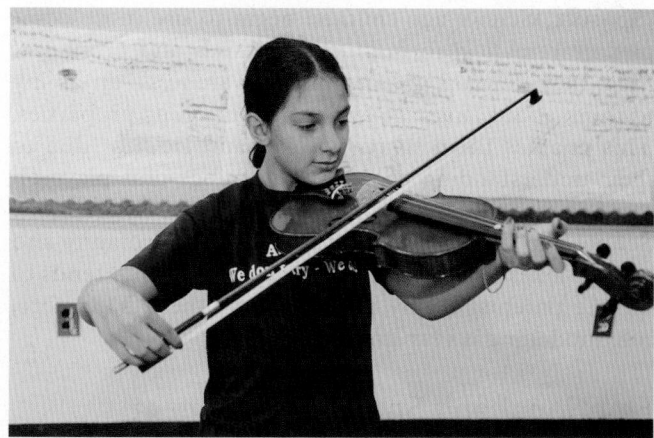

FIGURE 28.4 School-age children improve their fine motor skills so they can play musical instruments well.

the time the child is 7 years of age. Good vision is essential to the physical development and educational progression of school-age children. Vision screening identifies problems with vision and results in appropriate referrals when warranted. Some problems frequently identified include amblyopia, referred to in lay terms as "lazy eye," when the vision in one eye doesn't properly develop; uncorrected refractive errors or other eye defects; and malalignment of the eyes (called *strabismus*). Treatment for amblyopia is recommended by 6 years of age because by age 9, untreated amblyopia can cause irreversible vision loss. This condition is correctable prior to this time with glasses, patching, and/or exercises (Canadian Ophthalmological Society, 2007). Proper screening and referral, as well as notification to parents of the existing condition, are essential to the education and socialization of the school-age child.

Hearing deficits that are severe are usually diagnosed in infancy, but the less severe conditions may not be diagnosed until the child enters school and has difficulty learning or with speech. It is important to screen children for hearing deficits to ensure proper educational and social progression. With loud music heard over long periods of time each day, there are concerns about these environmental noises affecting hearing in the school-age and adolescent populations.

The sense of smell is mature and can be tested in the school-age child by using scents that children are familiar with, such as chocolate or other familiar odours. In addition, the school-age child may be tested for the sense of touch with objects to discriminate cold from hot, soft from hard, and blunt from sharp.

Communication and Language Development

Language skills continue to accelerate during the school-age years, and vocabulary expands. The school-age child learns to read and reading efficiency improves language skills. Reading skills are improved with increased reading exposure. School-age children begin to use more complex grammatical forms such as plurals and pronouns. Also, they develop metalinguistic awareness—an ability to think about language and comment on its properties. This enables them to enjoy jokes and riddles (due to their understanding of double meanings and plays on words and sounds) and begin to understand metaphors. School-age children may experiment with profanity and "dirty" jokes if exposed to them. This age group tends to imitate parents, family members, or others. Therefore, role modelling is very important.

Emotional and Social Development

Patterns of temperamental traits identified in infancy may continue to influence behaviour in the school-age child. Analyzing past situations may provide clues to the way a child may react to new or different situations. Children may react differently over time due to their experiences and abilities. Self-esteem is the child's view of his or her individual worth. This view is impacted by feedback from family, teachers, and other authority figures.

Temperament

Temperament has been described as the way individuals behave. Some descriptions of temperament are that the child is *easy, slow to warm,* or *difficult* (Feigelman, 2007b). These behaviours vary from the child who is easy (even-tempered and predictable) to the child labelled as difficult (due to high activity levels, irritability, and moodiness) (Alba-Fisch, n.d.). The child who is labelled as easy may adapt to school entry and other experiences smoothly and with little or no stress. The child labelled as slow-to-warm-up may be slow to adapt to changes. The slow-to-warm-up school-age child may exhibit discomfort when placed in different or new situations such as school. This child may need time to adjust to the new place or situation and may demonstrate frustration with tears or somatic complaints. The slow-to-warm-up child should be allowed time to adjust to new situations and people (such as teachers) within his or her own time frame. All of these factors may impact the younger school-age child upon entering the school environment, with changes in authority and the introduction of many peers. The difficult or easily distracted child may benefit from an introduction to the new experience and people by role-playing, by visiting the site and being introduced to the teachers, and by hearing stories or participating in conversations about the upcoming school experience. These children require patience, firmness, and understanding to make the transition into a new situation or experience such as school. The Behavioural Style Questionnaire (McDevitt & Carey, 1978) is a temperament questionnaire for children 3 to 7 years old; the Middle Childhood Temperament Questionnaire is another tool for children 8 to 12 years of age (Hegvik, McDevitt, & Carey, 1982). These tools may be useful for determining type of temperament and guiding interventions.

Self-Esteem Development

Self-esteem mirrors the child's individual self-worth and consists of both positive and negative qualities. Children strive to achieve internalized goals of attainment, although they continually receive feedback from individuals they perceive as authorities (parent or teacher). By the school-age years, children have received feedback related to their performance or tasks. The direction of this feedback influences the child's opinion of self-worth, which influences self-esteem and self-evaluation.

Children face the process of self-evaluation from a framework of either self-confidence or self-doubt. Children who have mastered the earlier developmental task of autonomy and initiative face the world with feelings of pride rather than shame (Erikson, 1963).

If school-age children regard themselves as worthwhile, they have a positive self-concept and high self-esteem. Significant adults in school-age children's lives can manipulate the environment to facilitate success. This success impacts the self-esteem of the child.

Body Image

Body image is how the school-ager perceives his or her body. School-age children are knowledgeable about the human body but may have different perceptions about body parts. School-age children are very interested in peers' views and acceptances of their body, body changes, and clothing. This age group may model themselves after parents, peers, and persons in movies or on television. It is important for late school-agers to feel accepted by peers. If they feel different and are teased, there may be lifelong effects.

School-Age Fears

School-age children are less fearful of harm to their body than in their preschool years, but can fear being kidnapped or undergoing surgery. They may continue to fear the dark and worry about their past behaviours. They may fear death and be fascinated by death and dying. They are less fearful of dogs and noises. The school-age child needs reassurance that his or her fears are normal for this developmental age. Parents, teachers, and other caretakers should discuss the fears and answer questions posed by the child (Hockenberry, Wilson, Winkelstein, & Kline, 2003).

Peer Relationships

The school-age child's concept of self is shaped not only by his or her parents but also by relationships with others. Peer relationships influence children's independence from parents. Peers play an important role in the approval and critiquing of skills of school-age children. Previously, only adults such as parents and teachers have been authorities; now, peers influence school-age children's perceptions of themselves. The support of peers helps to support the school-age child by providing enough security to risk the parental conflict brought about when establishing independence. School-age children associate with peers of the same sex most of the time. Although games and other activities are shared by both boys and girls, the child's concept of the appropriate sex role is influenced by his or her relationship with peers.

Continuous peer relationships provide the most important social interaction for school-age children. Valuable lessons are learned from interactions with children their own age. Children learn to respect differing points of view that are represented in their groups (Fig. 28.5). Peer groups establish norms and standards that signify acceptance or rejection. Children may modify behaviour to gain

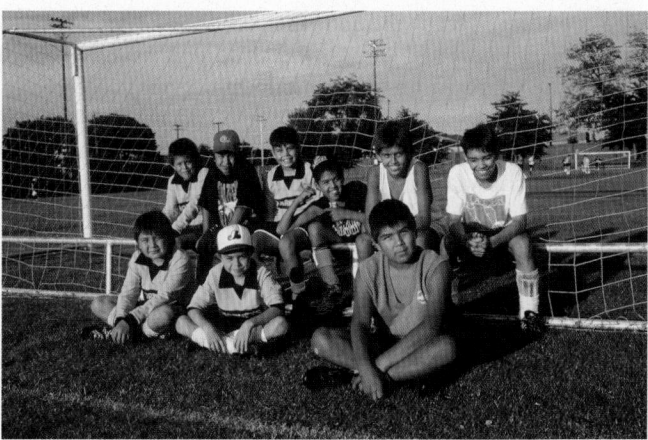

FIGURE 28.5 School-age children like to join teams, such as soccer teams (Chris Cheadle/ALL CANADA PHOTOS INC.).

acceptance. A characteristic of school-age children is their formation of groups with rules and values. Peer and peer-group identification are important to the socialization of the school-age child (Feigelman, 2007a).

Teacher and School Influences

School serves as a means to transmit values of society and to establish peer relationships. Secondary only to the family, school exerts a profound influence on the social development of the child. Often school requires changes for the child and parent. The child enters an environment that requires conforming to group activities that are structured and directed by an adult other than the parent. The parent's attitude and support influence the child's transition into the school setting. Parents who are positive and supportive promote a smooth entry into school. Parents who encourage clinging behaviours may delay a successful transition into school.

To facilitate the transition from home to school, the teacher must have the personality and knowledge of development that will allow him or her to meet the needs of young children. Even though the teacher's responsibilities are primarily to stimulate and guide intellectual development, teachers must share in shaping the child's attitudes and values. The system of awards and punishment or consequences administered by teachers affects the self-concept of children and influences their response to school. Teachers and school are important in shaping the socialization, self-concept, and intellectual development of children.

Family Influences

The school-age years are a time for peer relationships, questioning of parents, and the potential for parental conflict but continued respect for family values. School-age years are the beginning of the time of peer-group influence, with testing of parental and family values. Although the peer group is influential, the family's values usually predominate when parental and peer-group values come into conflict. Even though the school-age child may question the parents' values, the child will usually incorporate the values from parents into his or her values.

Many times in the late school-age and pre-adolescent period, the child may prefer to be in the company of peers and show a decreased interest in family functions. This may require an adjustment for parents. Parents' awareness of this developmental trend and their continuing support for the child are important while they continue to enforce restrictions and control of behaviours. The school-ager is beginning to strive for independence, but values and parental authority and controls continue to impact choices and values. School-age children continue to need parenting that provides structure and guidance and not parents as "pals."

Cultural Influences on Growth and Development

Culture influences habits, beliefs, language, and value. School-age children thrive on learning the music, language, traditions, holidays, games, values, gender roles, and other aspects of culture. Nurses must be aware of the effects on children of various groups' family structures and traditional values. The school-age child's cultural and ethnic backgrounds must be considered when assessing growth and development, including differences in growth in children of different racial and cultural backgrounds. Cultural implications must be considered for all children and families in order to provide appropriate care.

Refer back to Lawrence Jones, who was introduced at the beginning of this chapter. What developmental milestones would you expect him to have reached by this age?

The Nurse's Role in School-Age Growth and Development

WATCH & LEARN

The nurse's role in school-age growth and development includes assessing growth and development, promoting healthy growth and development, and addressing common developmental concerns. The nursing process overview would include an assessment of the individual child and identification of nursing diagnoses needing intervention or referral. The nurse promotes healthy growth and development through anticipatory guidance and goal attainment. Nursing care plans for individual children with common developmental concerns should be individualized considering the needs of the child and the family.

Nursing Process Overview

Upon completion of assessment of the school-age child's current growth and development status, problems or issues related to growth and development may be identified. The nurse may then identify one or more nursing diagnoses, including:

• Risk for disproportionate growth
• Imbalanced nutrition: more than body requirements
• Delayed growth and development
• Risk for caregiver role strain
• Risk for injury

Nursing care planning for the school-age child with growth and development issues should be individualized based on the school-age child's and family's needs. The nursing care plan can be used as a guide in planning nursing care for the school-age child with a growth and development concern. The nurse may choose the appropriate nursing diagnoses from Nursing Care Plan 28.1 and individualize them as needed. The nursing care plan is intended to serve as a guide, not to be an all-inclusive growth and development care plan.

Promoting Healthy Growth and Development

The family plays a critical role in promoting healthy growth and development of the school-age child. Respectful interchange of communication between the parent and child will foster self-esteem and self-confidence. This respect will give the child confidence in achieving personal, educational, and social goals appropriate for his or her age. The nurse should observe interactions between parents and school-age children to observe for this respect or lack of respect ("putting the child down"). The nurse can model appropriate behaviours by listening to the child and making appropriate responses. The nurse can be a resource for parents and an advocate for the child in promoting healthy growth and development.

Promoting Growth and Development Through Play

Cooperative play is exhibited by the school-age child. Play for the school-age child includes both organized cooperative activities (such as team sports) and solitary activities. School-age children have the coordination and intellect to participate with other children their age in sports such as soccer, baseball, football, and tennis. The school-age child comprehends that his or her cooperation with others will lead to a unified whole for the team. Additionally, the child learns rules and the value of playing by the rules.

School-age children also enjoy solitary activities including board, card, video, and computer games, and dollhouse and other small-figure play (Fig. 28.6). Many school-agers start collections of stamps, cars, or other valuable or not-so-valuable items. During the school-age years, children may also begin a scrapbook or keep a diary. They may participate in activities such as dance or

(text continues on page 894)

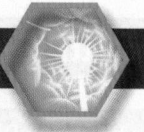

Nursing Care Plan 28.1

GROWTH AND DEVELOPMENT ISSUES OF THE SCHOOL-AGE CHILD

NURSING DIAGNOSIS: Risk for disproportionate growth (risk factors: caregiver knowledge deficit, frequent illnesses)

Outcome Identification and Evaluation
School-age child will demonstrate adequate growth: *appropriate weight gain for age and sex*

Interventions: Promoting Proportionate Growth
- Assess parent's knowledge of nutritional needs of school-age children *to determine need for further education.*
- Educate mother about appropriate serving sizes and foods *so that mother is aware of what to expect for school-age children.*
- Determine need for additional caloric intake if necessary *(if very active in sports, if have a chronic illness).*
- Plot out height, weight, and body mass index (BMI) *to detect possible pattern.*

NURSING DIAGNOSIS: Imbalanced nutrition, more than body requirements, related to lack of exercise, increased caloric intake, poor food choices

Outcome Identification and Evaluation
School-age child will lose weight at an appropriate rate: *increase amount of exercise, make appropriate eating choices, decrease caloric intake to appropriate amount for age and sex*

Interventions: Promoting Nutrition
- Assess knowledge of parents and child about nutritional needs of school-age children *to determine deficits in knowledge.*
- Have child keep food and exercise diary for 1 week *to determine current patterns of eating and exercise.*
- Interview parents in relationship to their eating habits and exercise habits *to determine where adjustments might need to be made.*
- Analyze preceding data, and base recommendations for changes on these data.
- Discuss ways to decrease temptation to overeat and to make good meal choices (see Teaching Guideline 28.2).
- Have child assist in meal planning and grocery shopping *to allow him some sense of control in process.*
- Incorporate increase in daily exercise, which will stress sense of self-improvement *to increase caloric expenditure and self-esteem.*
- Decrease TV/computer time *to increase caloric expenditure.*
- Develop reward system *to increase self-esteem.*
- Investigate joining healthy eating and activity programs for school-age children *to increase self-esteem and to increase awareness that other children have the same problem.*

NURSING DIAGNOSIS: Growth and development, delayed related to speech, motor, psychosocial, or cognitive concerns as evidenced by delay in meeting expected school performances

Outcome Identification and Evaluation
Development will be maximized: School-age child will make continued progress toward attainment of expected school performances.

Interventions: Promoting Growth and Development
- Perform scheduled evaluation of the school-age child by school and health care provider *to determine current functioning.*
- Develop realistic multidisciplinary plan *to ensure maximizing resources.*
- Carry out interventions as prescribed by developmental specialist, physical therapist, occupational therapist, or speech therapist at home and at school *to maximize benefit of interventions.*
- Have scheduled evaluation meetings *to be able to adapt interventions as soon as possible.*

(continued)

Nursing Care Plan 28.1 (continued)

NURSING DIAGNOSIS: Caregiver role strain, risk for (risk factors: new sibling in household, knowledge deficit about school-age issues, lack of prior exposure, fatigue, ill or developmentally delayed child)

Outcome Identification and Evaluation

Parent will experience competence in role: will demonstrate appropriate caretaking behaviours and verbalize comfort in caring for a school-age child

Interventions: Preventing Caregiver Role Strain

- Assess parent's knowledge of school-age children and the issues that arise as a part of normal development *to determine parent's needs.*
- Provide education on normal issues of school-age children *so that parents are armed with the knowledge they need to appropriately care for their school-age child.*
- Provide anticipatory guidance related to upcoming expected issues related to school-age development *to prepare parents for what to expect next and how to intervene.*

NURSING DIAGNOSIS: Injury, risk for (risk factors: curiosity, increasing cognitive skills and motor abilities)

Outcome Identification and Evaluation

School-age child's safety will be maintained: *will remain free from injury*

Interventions: Preventing Injury

- Discuss safety measures needed for the following: bikes, scooters, guns, skateboards, cars, water, and playground *to decrease risk of injury related to those areas.*
- Discuss and develop a fire safety plan *to decrease risk of injury related to fire.*
- Discuss appropriate safety equipment needed for each sport *to decrease risk of injury.*
- Discuss appropriate sports to participate in depending upon age, sex, and maturity of child *to prevent possible injury and to promote child's self-esteem.*
- Parents should have the poison control centre phone number available (*in the event of accidental ingestion, poison control can give parents the best advice for appropriate intervention*).
- Teach parents and child first-aid measures and child cardiopulmonary resuscitation (CPR) *to minimize consequences of injury should it occur.*
- Discuss influence of peers on actions of school-age children *to prevent possible injury due to mimicking behaviour.*

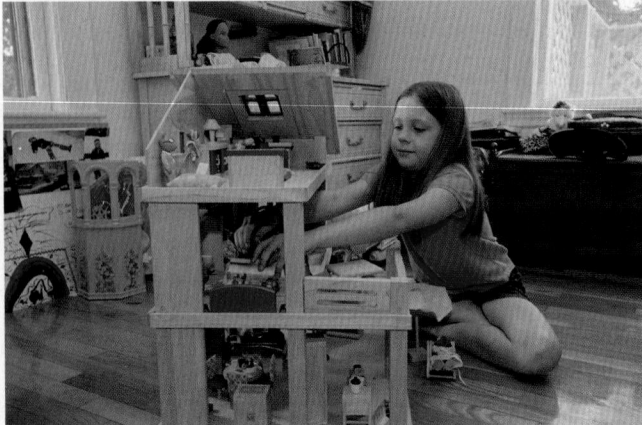

FIGURE 28.6 This school-age girl enjoys solitary play with her dollhouse and dolls.

karate. Girls and boys may join clubs, gangs, or special interest groups.

Active play has decreased in recent years as television viewing and computer game playing have increased. This trend has resulted in health risks such as obesity, type 2 diabetes, and cardiovascular problems.

Promoting Learning

School attendance and learning are very important to the school-age child. Parent–child, child–teacher, and child–peer relationships and activities influence the school-age child's learning.

Formal Education

Most children are excited about starting school and making new friends. They like the notion of getting books, having book bags, and having homework assignments. The reality of the work involved with school and homework may decrease the enthusiasm about school.

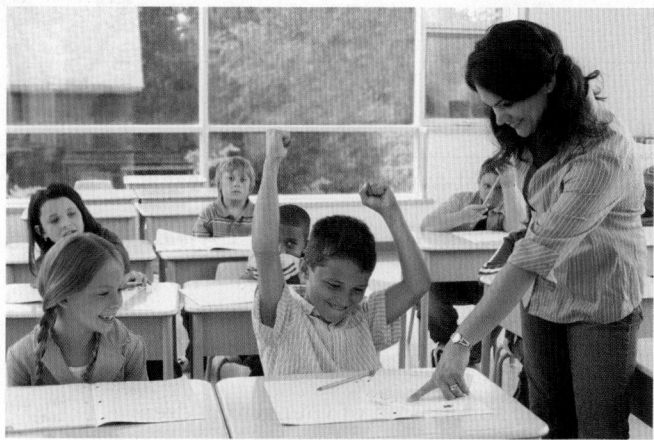

FIGURE 28.7 School is important to the school-age child.

Peers are very important within this age group. Both peers and teachers influence children. Attending school may be their first experience interacting with a large number of children their own age. Through this interaction, children learn cooperation, competition, and the importance of following the rules. Peer approval and influences grow as the child matures. Teachers have significant influences on children. They help to guide the child's intellectual development by rewarding successes and helping the child deal with failures. The student–teacher relationship is a key to success. Teachers play a role in fostering feelings of industry and preventing feelings of inferiority (Fig. 28.7). School-age children also learn skills, rules, values, and other ways to work with peers and other authority figures.

Parental support is important for school adjustment and achievement. Parents must collaborate with teachers and school personnel to ensure that the child is fulfilling the expectations and requirements for this age group in school. Parents must monitor the child's homework assignments and friends, and observe for any changes in behaviour that would indicate school or behavioural problems.

Reading

Encouraging reading is an excellent way to promote learning in the school-age child. Trips to the library and purchasing books help to promote a love of reading. School-age children enjoy being read to as well as reading on their own. Younger school-age children (6 to 8 years) enjoy books that are simple to read with few words on a page, such as the Dr. Seuss books. They enjoy books about animals and trains and simple mysteries. Children 8 to 10 years of age have more advanced reading skills and enjoy those books from early childhood, plus more classic novels and adventures such as the Harry Potter series. Older children enjoy horror stories, mysteries, romances, and adventure stories as well as classic novels. School-age children of all ages benefit from books on topics related to

things they may be experiencing, such as a visit to the hospital for a surgical procedure. See Box 28.1 for ideas for parents to promote reading in the school-age child.

Promoting Safety

School-age children become more independent with age. This independence leads to an increased self-confidence and decreased fears, which may contribute to accidents and injuries. School age is a time when the child may walk to school with peers who may influence his or her behaviour. Increased independence may also increase exposure to dangerous situations such as the approach of strangers or unsafe streets. Promotion of safe habits during the school-age years is important for parents and nurses. See Teaching Guideline 28.1 for additional information on safety education for nurses and parents.

Unintentional injuries are the leading cause of death in Canadian children between 1 and 19 years of age. In 2005, injuries caused 720 deaths and 29,000 hospitalizations among Canadians under the age of 20 (Public Health Agency of Canada, 2009). School-age children are very active at home, in the community, and at school. This increased mobility, activity, and time away from parents increase the risk for unintentional injuries. School-age children continue to need supervision and guidance. They need information and rules about car safety, pedestrian safety, bicycle and other sport safety, fire safety, and water safety.

Car Safety

Motor vehicle accidents are a common cause of injury in the school-age child. While travelling in the car, school-age children should always sit in the rear seat. The front seat is dangerous because of passenger-side airbags in most new-model cars. The school-age child should use a three-point

TEACHING GUIDELINE 28.1

Safety Issues and Interventions of the School-Age Child

Safety Issue	Interventions
Car safety	• Should wear seat belt or be in age- and weight-appropriate booster seat at all times. • Fasten seat belt before car is started. • Children under 13 years must sit in back seat. • Utilize childproof locks in back seat. • Establish rules of conduct in car.
Pedestrian safety	• Child should look right, left, then right again before crossing the street. • Cross only at safe crossings. • Older children and adults should provide supervision of younger children. • Should only walk on sidewalks. • Should not dart out between parked cars. • In parking lots, should watch for cars backing up. • If children are playing outside, drivers should be aware of their presence before backing up.
Bike safety: general	• Have a well-maintained and appropriate-size bike for child. • Parents should orient the child to the bike. • Child should demonstrate his or her ability to ride bike safely before being allowed to ride on street. • Safe areas for bike riding should be established as well as routes to and from area of activities. • Should not ride bike barefoot, with someone else on bike, or with clothing that might get entangled in the bike. • Should wear sturdy, well-fitting shoes. • Should wear CSA-approved helmets. • Bike should be inspected often to ensure it is in proper working order. • A basket should be used to carry heavy objects.
Bike safety in traffic	• All traffic signs and signals must be observed. • If riding at night, the bike should have lights and reflectors and the rider should wear light-colored clothes. • Should ride on the side of the road travelling with traffic. • Should keep close to the side of the road and in single file. • Should watch and listen for cars. • Should not wear headphones while riding a bike. • Never hitch a ride on any vehicles.
Sports safety	• Match sport to child's ability and desire. • Sports program should have warm-up procedure. • Coaches should be trained in CPR and first aid. • Child should wear appropriate protection devices for individual sport.
Skateboarding and inline skating safety	• Should wear helmet, and protective padding on knees, elbows, and wrists • Should not skate in traffic or on streets or highways. • Skating on homemade ramps could be dangerous—should assess ramps for any hazards before skating.
All-terrain vehicle safety	• Should not be operated by children less than 16 years of age. • Should wear helmet and protective coverings. • No nighttime riding. • Should not be used on public roads. • Should not stand up in the vehicle or ride in a person's lap.

TEACHING GUIDELINE 28.1 (continued)

Safety Issues and Interventions of the School-Age Child

Safety Issue	Interventions
Fire safety	• All homes should have working smoke detectors and fire extinguishers. Change the batteries at least twice a year. • Should have fire-escape plan. • Should practice fire-escape plan routinely. • Nobody should smoke in bed. • Should teach what to do in case of a fire: use fire extinguisher, call 911, and how to put out clothing fire. • Should wear flame-retardant clothing. • Should use stove and other cooking facilities under adult supervision. • All flammable materials and liquids should be stored safely. • Fireplaces should have protective gratings. • Teach children to avoid touching wires they might encounter while playing.
Water safety	• Teach children how to swim. • If swimming skill is limited, must wear life preserver at all times. • Never swim alone—should, if at all possible, swim only where there is a life guard. • Should be taught basic CPR. • Should not run or fool around at edge of pool. • Drains in pool should be covered with appropriate cover. • Should wear life jacket when on boat. • Make sure there is enough water to support diving.
Firearm safety	• Should teach never to touch gun—tell adult. • If have guns in household, need to secure them in safe place, use gun safety locks, store bullets in separate place. • Never point a gun at a person.
Toxin safety	• Teach child the hazards of accepting illegal drugs, alcohol, or dangerous drugs. • Store potential dangerous material in safe place.

Adapted from: Centers for Disease Control and Prevention. (2011). *Unintentional drowning: Fact sheet.* Retrieved August 19, 2011 from http://www.cdc.gov/HomeandRecreationalSafety/Water-Safety/waterinjuries-factsheet.html; Hagan, J. F., Shaw, J. S., & Duncan, P. (2008). *Bright futures guidelines for health supervision of infants, children, and adolescents* (3rd ed.). Elk Grove Village, IL: American Academy of Pediatrics; Healthy Children. (2010a). *Tips & tools: Safety for your child: 8 years.* Retrieved August 19, 2011 from http://www.healthychildren.org/english/tips-tools/Pages/Safety-for-Your-Child-8-Years.aspx; Healthy Children. (2010b). *Tips & tools: Safety for your child: 10 years.* Retrieved August 19, 2011 from http://www.healthychildren.org/english/tips-tools/Pages/Safety-for-Your-Child-10-Years.aspx; and Healthy Children. (2011c). *Tips & tools: Safety for your child: 6 years.* Retrieved August 19, 2011 from http://www.healthychildren.org/english/tips-tools/Pages/Safety-for-Your-Child-6-Years.aspx.

restraint system in the rear seat of the car with the shoulder strap and lap belt fitted snugly. Although some province regulations allow children to move to a booster seat once they reach 18 kg, Transport Canada (2011) advises that use of a forward-facing car seat provides the best protection for young children and some are made to hold children up to 30 kg. Manufacturer's instructions and government regulations should be followed. Regular seat belts should be used only when they fit the child correctly. This usually occurs when the child is approximately 36 kg and 145 cm tall. Children under 13 years of age should not ride in the front seat of a vehicle (Canadian Paediatric Society, 2011).

Pedestrian Safety

Due to the risk of pedestrian-related accidents, young school-age children should walk to school or the bus with an older friend, sibling, or parent. Darting out into the street without looking both ways or from between cars is a common occurrence in the school-age years. Children should be taught safe street and pedestrian practices.

Bicycle and Sport Safety

Bicycling, riding scooters, skateboarding, and inline skating or roller skating are common activities of school-age children. Laws in a number of provinces require helmets for riding bicycles. In addition, when skiing, skating,

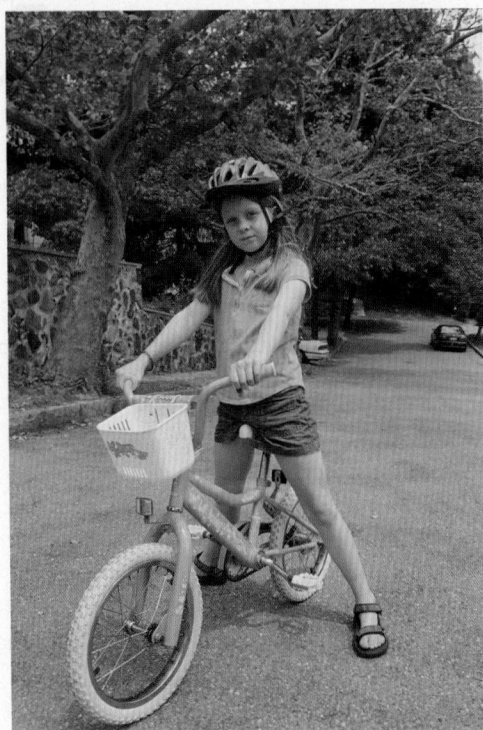

FIGURE 28.8 Wearing the appropriate safety equipment and having an appropriately sized bicycle are important to prevent injuries in school-age children.

or skateboarding, school-age children should wear a helmet, kneepads, and elbow pads.

Research has shown that head injuries due to bicycle accidents have been reduced by 85% when wearing a well-fitting helmet. It is important for children to wear helmets that fit and that do not obstruct their vision or hearing. Because school-age children have completed most of their skull growth, a helmet can be worn into adolescence. It is important for the child to have a bicycle that is appropriate for his or her size and age. The child should be able to plant both feet on the ground when sitting on the seat of the bike (Fig. 28.8). It is important to stress to parents the importance of appropriate size and not to get a bike for the child to "grow into." If older school-agers are using the bike for transportation on busy streets, they should be taught to use bike lanes and to give appropriate hand signals for turning.

Fire Safety

School-age children are eager to help parents with cooking and ironing. They are curious about fire and are drawn to play with fire, matches, and fireworks. Serious burns can occur from any exposure to fire. Educate children about the hazards of fire. In addition, teach children proper behaviour around fires at home and outdoors. Always supervise children in the use of matches. In the home setting, parents should develop a fire safety plan with their children, teach children what to do if their

clothes catch on fire, and practice evacuating the house in the event of a fire. In the school setting, children should be aware of the appropriate response to fire drills and fire drills should be conducted on a regular basis.

Water Safety

Teach school-age children swim and water safety. An adult should always supervise children when they are swimming to prevent water-related accidents.

Child Abuse

Child maltreatment or abuse, including physical abuse and sexual abuse, is a crime of violence against children. There were 114,607 cases of substantiated child abuse in Canada in 2003, including physical, emotional, and sexual abuse as well as exposure to domestic violence in the household (Trocmé et al., 2005). Physical abuse constituted 24% and sexual abuse 3% of substantiated abuse cases (Trocmé et al., 2005). The abusers of children can be family, friends, or strangers. It is important for parents to teach children the concept of "good touch" vs. "bad touch" prior to their school-age years. Whenever the school-age child's behaviour yields suspicion of physical or sexual abuse, the nurse is required to report to the appropriate provincial authorities.

*R*emember Lawrence Jones, the 10-year-old presented in the case study? What anticipatory guidance related to safety should you provide to his mother?

Promoting Nutrition

Growth, body composition, and body shape remain constant during late school-age years. Caloric needs decrease while the appetite increases. In preparation for adolescence, the body fat composition of school-age children increases. This tendency toward increased body fat occurs earlier in girls than in boys, with the amount of increase greater in girls. Boys have more lean body mass per inch of height than girls.

Diet preferences established in the preschool years continue during the school-age period. As the child grows older, influences of family, media, and peers can impact the eating habits of this age group. Some of these influences are parents' work schedule, outside activities, and exercise level of the child. Decreased exercise levels and poor nutritional choices lead to the mounting problem of obesity seen in this age group. See Box 28.2 for appropriate questions to ask the child and parent regarding nutritional status.

Nutritional Needs

School-age children should be directed and encouraged to follow Canada's Food Guide for the number of daily portions from all four food groups (see Appendix H). This is important so that the child ingests sufficient amounts of

BOX 28.2 Dietary Questions

Questions for the Child
- How often do you eat together with your family?
- What are the usual mealtimes?
- How often does the family eat out?
- Do you eat breakfast every morning?
- Where do you eat lunch?
- What do you drink/how much?
- What foods do you eat most often?
- What is your favourite food?
- How often do you eat fast foods?
- What type of exercise do you do?

Questions for the Parents
- How would you describe your child's usual appetite?
- Do you have any special cultural/religious practices regarding food?
- Has your child gained or lost weight recently?
- Do you have any concerns about his or her eating behaviours?
- How does your child exercise? Your family?
- Is there a family history of cancer, hypertension, diabetes, obesity, or heart disease?

essential nutrients such as protein and calcium for maintenance of growth and good nutrition. Calcium is needed for the development of strong bones and teeth. Milk, yogurt, and cheese provide protein, vitamins, and minerals and are an excellent source of calcium. Meat, poultry, fish, and eggs provide protein, vitamins, and minerals.

Nutritional Guidelines

School-age children should choose culturally appropriate foods and snacks from Canada's Food Guide. School-age children need to limit intake of fat and processed sugars (see Box 28.3). The Food Guide recommends choosing foods lower in fat (especially saturated and trans fats), sugar, and salt. However, a small amount of unsaturated fat should be included daily. Refer to the Nutrition Resource Centre website for more information (visit http://thePoint.lww.com/Chow1e for the direct link).

*R*egarding Lawrence Jones, what questions should you ask Lawrence's mother related to nutritional intake? What anticipatory guidance related to nutrition would be appropriate?

Promoting Healthy Sleep and Rest

The number of hours of sleep required for growth and development decreases with age. Children between the ages of 6 and 8 years require about 12 hours of sleep per night. Children between 8 and 10 years of age require 10

to 12 hours of sleep per night, and children between 10 and 12 years of age need 9 to 10 hours of sleep per night. Young school-age children may need an occasional brief nap for an energy boost after being in school for most of the day. Bedtime rituals and consistent schedules continue to be important throughout the school-age years. Parents must facilitate the bedtime schedule and quiet time before bed. Bedtime is a special time for parents and children to read together, listen to stories or soothing music, share events of the day, and exchange expressions of affection (Healthy Children, 2011b). Children should have bedtime expectations as well as wake-up times and methods for waking up (alarm, calling by parent, and so forth).

Night terrors or sleepwalking may occur in 6- to 8-year-olds but should be resolved between the ages of 8 and 10 years. In the older school-age child (11 to 12 years), encourage parents to allow a variation in the sleep schedule on the weekends and a regular schedule on weekdays.

*P*rovide anticipatory guidance to Lawrence Jones's mother in relation to proper sleep for her 10-year-old son.

Promoting Healthy Teeth and Gums

Dental care with emphasis on prevention of **caries** is important in this age group. Sometimes dental care is not considered to be important by parents of young children because the primary teeth will be replaced by permanent teeth. This misperception leads to complications of permanent teeth such as **malocclusion**.

Proper alignment of teeth is important to tooth formation, speech development, and physical appearance.

BOX 28.3 Canada's Food Guide Recommendations for School-Age Children

- Eat the recommended number of food group servings per day according to age. Eat at least one dark green and one orange vegetable each day.
- Have vegetables and fruit more often than juice.
- Make at least half of grain products whole grain each day.
- Drink skim, 1%, or 2% milk each day.
- Have meat alternatives such as beans, lentils, and tofu often.
- Eat at least two servings of fish each week.
- Include a small amount of unsaturated fat daily.
- Drink water when thirsty.
- Choose foods lower in fat, sugar, and salt.

Adapted from: Health Canada. (2011). *Canada's food guide: Children.* Retrieved November 16, 2011 from http://www.hc-sc.gc.ca/fn-an/food-guide-aliment/choose-choix/advice-conseil/child-enfant-eng.php.

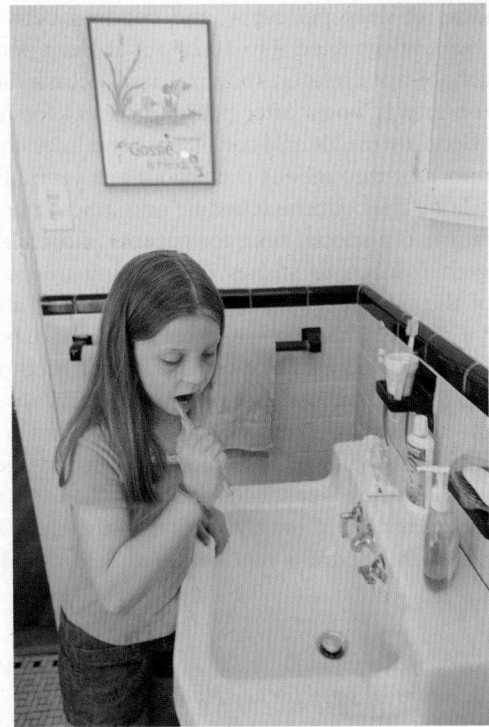

FIGURE 28.9 Using correct technique to brush the teeth is important for the prevention of cavities.

Many school-age children need braces or other orthodontic devices to correct malocclusion, a condition in which the teeth are crowded, crooked, or misaligned. **Bruxism** or teeth grinding while asleep may continue in the school-age years. Bruxism may result in grinding away of tooth enamel. Teeth grinding may be due to malalignment. A dental evaluation should be scheduled if persistent teeth grinding occurs.

School-age children need to brush their teeth with a soft toothbrush and fluoridated toothpaste two to three times per day for 2 minutes each time (Fig. 28.9) (Nield, Stenger, & Kamat, 2007). Parents should replace the toothbrush every few months (Peterson-Sweeney & Stevens, 2010). Flossing the teeth at least once daily is recommended by the Canadian Dental Association (2011). Parents must monitor teeth brushing, observe for abnormal alignment of their child's teeth, and schedule regular dental examinations every 6 months to ensure good dental health and prevent dental problems. Children may need help with brushing teeth until they are between 7 and 10 years of age. A general guideline is when children are able to write (not print) their name they should be able to manage brushing their teeth on their own.

Dental sealants may be recommended by dentists for school-age children. The sealant is a plastic coating applied to biting surfaces to seal out tooth decay on permanent back teeth. In addition, if fluoride is not in the community's water supply a dentist should be consulted

to determine if fluoride supplements should be given (Canadian Dental Association, 2011).

Children who wear braces are more prone to cavities; encourage them to brush their teeth after meals and snacks. In addition, the public health nurse should promote dental health through education on dental care and gum problems that result from lack of proper dental care. Diet can play a part in dental health. Limiting sticky, high-sugar, and high-carbohydrate foods will decrease the possibility of cavities.

Promoting Appropriate Discipline

Because of their increasing ability to view situations from different angles, school-age children should be able to see how their actions affect others. School-age children are aware of the cause and effect of their behaviours and realize that their behaviours have consequences. They should be able to express emotions without using physical force or violence.

In disciplining children, parents should teach them the rules established by the family, values, and social rules of conduct. Rules should provide the school-age child with guidelines about behaviour that is acceptable and unacceptable. School-age children look to their parents for guidance and as role models. Parents should role model appropriate expressions of feelings and emotions and allow the child to express emotions and feelings. Discuss the effects of the child's temperament on his or her behaviour, as well as what constitutes age-appropriate behaviour. Include how the parents' temperament can influence the child's temperament.

Effective guidance and discipline focus on the development of the child. They can preserve the child's self-esteem and dignity. Discuss with parents guidelines regarding discipline. Explain to parents that they should never belittle the child. Children may view parents and caretakers negatively if they are consistently belittled or insulted. These negative actions can inhibit learning and teach the child to react unkindly to others. Instead, parents should respond with praise as appropriate. Positive acknowledgments of progress are likely to encourage healthy development and appropriate behaviour (Barakat & Clark, 2007; Durrant, 2007). Discuss with parents how to be realistic when planning activities so as to not overwhelm the child, resulting in undesirable behaviour. Encourage parents to say "no" only when they mean it, to avoid a negative atmosphere in the home, and to avoid inconsistency.

When undesired behaviour occurs, the parent's response is based upon different factors:

- Developmental level of both the child and the parents
- Seriousness of the misbehaviour
- Established rules of the family
- Temperament of the child
- Response of the child to positive reinforcement

Addressing Common Developmental Concerns

The developmental task (according to Erikson) of the school-age child is industry (Erikson, 1963; Feigelman, 2007a). They are busy learning, achieving, and exploring. As the school-age child becomes more independent, forces other than the family such as television, video games, and peers influence them. Some of these influences are positive and others are negative. Some of the common developmental concerns for the school-age child are discussed in the following sections. Guidelines to assist the parents and nurses when encountering these concerns are included in Teaching Guideline 28.2.

Television and Video Games

The influence of television and video games upon the school-age child is a growing concern for parents and child specialists. The Canadian Paediatric Society (CPS, 2008) reports that although not all TV watching is harmful, the increasing amount of TV viewing and video game playing by children are cause for concern. There is evidence regarding the negative effects on children of exposure to violence, inappropriate sexuality, and offensive language. Although a school-age child can determine what is real from what is fantasy, research has shown that this amount of time in front of the TV—watching it or playing video games—can lead to aggressive behaviour, less physical activity, and altered body image (CPS, 2008).

Although some television shows and video games can have positive influences on children, teach parents guidelines on the use of TV and video games. Parents should set limits on how much TV watching the child can have. The CPS (2008) recommends a maximum of 2 hours of television viewing per day. The parent should establish guidelines on when the child can watch TV, for example, after homework or when chores are completed (KidsHealth, 2011). Television watching should not be used as a reward. The parents should be aware of what the child is watching. Watch the programs together and use that opportunity to discuss the subject matter with the child. There should be no TV during dinner and no TV in the child's room. The parents need to set an example for the child. Read instead of watching TV, or do a physical activity together as a family. It may be advisable for parents to obtain technology that allows filtering of TV programming.

Obesity

The CPS (2004) reports increasing numbers of overweight and obese children. Obesity occurs when the intake of calories and food exceeds the expenditures. Some factors linked to obesity include family role modelling, lack of exercise, and unstructured meals as well as cultural, genetic, environmental, and socioeconomic factors.

Children with low metabolic rates and increased numbers of fat cells tend to gain more weight. Obese children are at risk for cardiovascular conditions such as high cholesterol and hypertension; type 2 (non–insulin dependent) diabetes; respiratory complications such as obstructive sleep apnea; mental health issues such as depression, anxiety, and eating disorders; and orthopedic problems (Krebs, Primark, & Haemer, 2011; U.S. Department of Agriculture and U.S. Department of Health and Human Services, 2010). When parents lack knowledge about nutrition, do not monitor snacks or meals, and have unstructured meals, habits are established that lead to obesity.

Although obesity is increasing in all ethnic groups, some Aboriginal communities seem to be more at risk. Particular attention must be paid to this issue because there is a strong hereditary component to type 2 diabetes in addition to the social, behavioural, and environmental risk factors that increase the likelihood of its development (CPS, 2004).

Preventing obesity in childhood is important because the fat cells of childhood are carried into adulthood obesity and contribute to disease. Due to the risk of obesity, encourage parents to never use food as a reward. To prevent obesity, establish regular mealtimes and offer healthy foods and snacks. Encourage parents to praise their child's good food choices and to role model appropriate eating and exercise.

School Phobia

School refusal (also called *school phobia* or *school avoidance*) has been defined as frequent absences, dropping out of school, or academic disengagement or disruption (Ruggiero, 1999). School phobia needs to be defined both symptomatically and operationally as the cause for the anxiety. School avoidance occurs in approximately 5% of school-age children. These children may refuse to attend school or create reasons why they cannot go to school.

Some of the fears expressed by school-refusing children include tests, bullying, teacher reprimands, physical harm, or undressing in the locker room. Due to the emotional distress caused in these children when attending school, they are frequently classified as having school phobia. Young children may complain of stomachache or headache and older children may complain of palpitations or feeling faint.

It is important to investigate specific causes of school refusal/school phobia and take appropriate actions. The physician or nurse practitioner should conduct a physical examination of the child to rule out any physical illness. After these measures are taken, the parent, teacher, school counsellor, and school administrator may devise a plan to assist the student to overcome a specific fear. In uncomplicated cases, parents must return the child to school as soon as possible. There may be altered schedules (partial days or decreased hours) to help promote a successful transition back to school. Another idea to help

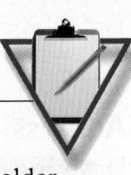

Addressing Common Developmental Concerns

Television and Video Games

- Limit television watching and video-game playing to less than 1 to 2 hours per day.
- Monitor television programs.
- Prohibit television or video games with violence.
- Do not put television or video games in children's bedrooms.
- Provide a schedule of accepted television programs for viewing each week.
- Co-view television and video games with the child.
- Encourage sports, interactive play, and reading.

Obesity

- Provide healthy meals and snacks.
- Schedule and encourage daily exercise.
- Encourage involvement in sports.
- Restrict TV and computer-game use.
- Limit the amount of fast-food intake.
- Provide education about healthy nutrition.
- Never use food as a reward.
- Be a good role model.

School Phobia

- Return child to school.
- Investigate cause of the fear.
- Support child.
- Collaborate with teachers.
- Praise success in school attendance.

Latchkey Kids

- Provide rules to follow and expectations, such as
  - Not answering the door or phone
  - No friends in the house when parents are not home
  - No playing with fire
- Teach child to call a trusted neighbour when help is needed and 911 in the event of emergency.
- Post all resource numbers, including after-school help lines if available, in a clearly viewable spot.
- Purchase caller ID for the phone system.
- Enroll the child in an after-school program if available.
- Discuss limitations of outside play.
- Discuss limitations of television viewing and video-game use.
- Make sure the child knows how to contact the parent.
- Set clear homework expectations.
- DO NOT keep guns in the home.

Lying

- Help parents in understanding why the child is lying.
- When the child lies, calmly confront the child and explain why the behaviour is not acceptable.
- Educate parents that their behaviour should reflect what they teach and expect from their child.
- Educate parents that punishments can decrease the child's sense of worth.
- Seek professional help if lying persists in the older school-age child, to rule out underlying problems.

Cheating

- Educate parents that the child must be mature enough to understand the concept of rules.
- Handle cheating situations openly.
- Help parents to understand why their child is cheating and to modify the trigger.
- Develop positive discipline techniques.
- Educate parents that their behaviour should reflect what they expect from their child.
- Seek professional help if cheating persists in the older school-age child, to rule out underlying problems.

Bullying

The Bullied Child

- Educate parents whose children are at risk for being bullied
  - Children who appear different from the majority
  - Children who act different from the majority
  - Children who have low self-esteem
  - Children with a mental or psychological problem
- Teach parents to role play different scenarios the child may face at school; show the child different ways to react to being bullied.
- Impress upon the child that he or she did not cause the bullying.
- Develop ways to increase the child's self-esteem at home.
- Discuss the situation with the teacher and develop a plan of care.

The Bullying Child

- Educate parents on reasons why it is important to correct the behaviour.
- Discuss ways the child can appropriately show his or her anger and feelings.
- Have parents help the child to feel empathy for those who are bullied.
- Do not allow fighting at home.
- Promote settling of conflicts without violence.

Tobacco and Alcohol Education

- Inquire about tobacco and alcohol use.
- Discuss the physical and social dangers of tobacco and alcohol use.
- Urge parents to be good role models.
- Discuss the influences of tobacco and alcohol use by peers.
- Educate the child on spit tobacco. Let them know it is just as dangerous as smoking tobacco.
- Advocate for a smoke-free environment in the home and other places frequented.
- Avoid having tobacco and alcohol products readily available in the home.

desensitize the child may be to have him or her spend part of the day in the counsellor's or school nurse's office.

Latchkey Children

With both parents in the work force, many children return home from school alone without adult supervision for a number of hours. There can be risks associated with children being on their own. Due to these risks, a number of provinces have a legal requirement that children younger than 12 years of age must be provided with supervision.

Most young children are not capable of handling stress or making decisions on their own before 11 or 12 years of age, although maturity levels vary. Despite the level of maturity, children who are unsupervised are more likely to participate in risky behaviors such as smoking, drinking, and drugs (Kroll & Nield, 2010). Children left alone have a higher incidence of injuries such as burns, falls, and poisoning than children who are supervised (Kroll & Nield, 2010). In addition, latchkey children may feel anxiety, fear, boredom, or loneliness (Kroll & Nield, 2010).

If children come home to no supervision, they should know the names, addresses, and phone numbers of parents and a neighbour, as well as emergency numbers. They should be given rules about answering the door and the phone. They should tell anyone who comes to the door or who calls that mom is home but busy at this time. Directions as to the handling of the house key and fire safety should be taught and demonstrated (see Teaching Guideline 28.2).

Stealing, Lying, and Cheating

It is during the school-age years that antisocial behaviours can emerge. Children who were previously well behaved may now exhibit behaviours such as stealing, lying, or cheating (Mannheim & Zieve, 2010). Parents are usually disturbed by this change in behaviour. In turn, they have difficulty in addressing these issues and need help in providing appropriate interventions.

Children between 6 and 8 years old do not fully understand the concepts of ownership and property rights. These children may steal things because they like the look of the item. By the age of 9, the child should respect others' possessions and property and understand that stealing is wrong (Children's Hospital Boston, n.d.). The school-age child may steal because he or she desires the item, feels peer pressure and is trying to impress peers, or has low self-esteem (Children's Hospital Boston, n.d.). Stealing becomes a concern if the child steals and does not have remorse, steals continually, or if stealing is accompanied by other behaviour problems (Children's Hospital Boston, n.d.).

The concept of cheating is not well understood until the child is 7 years old. Before this age, the desire to "win" is most important and rigid rules are hard to understand. Children between 8 and 12 years old fully understand the concept of cheating, and following of rules becomes more important (Children's Hospital Boston, n.d.). Cheating usually results from competition and strong pressure placed on the child to succeed (Healthy Children, 2011a). If cheating persists in older school-age children, parents should discuss the matter with a health care provider because the behaviour may indicate underlying problems.

In dealing with children who exhibit stealing, lying, or cheating behaviours, parents must first realize the importance of their own behaviours in those areas. Parents are role models to the school-age child. Therefore, when the child sees or hears that parents lie, steal, or cheat (e.g., parents bragging about cheating on their taxes), they think it is all right to mimic those behaviours. Secondly, parents must directly confront any stealing, lying, or cheating behaviours and discuss (and follow through consistently with) the consequences of such behaviours (see Teaching Guideline 28.2).

Bullying

Bullying, which is inflicting repeated verbal, emotional, or physical abuse upon others, is on the rise (Schoen & Schoen, 2010). Utilizing e-mail, text messages, social networking, and instant messaging—often referred to as cyber-bullying—is a growing concern. Bullies often look for victims who appear shy, weak, and defenseless. Children with disabilities are at an increased risk of being bullied (Schoen & Schoen, 2010).

Many children attending school are frightened and afraid most of the day. In Canada, 5% of boys and 7% of girls ages 4 to 11 have reported being bullied sometimes or very often (Peters, & Konarski, 1998, as cited in Public Safety Canada, 2011). Most bullying occurs at school (Augustyn & Zuckerman, 2007). Both boys and girls are bullied and can bully others; however, boys are twice as likely to be bullies and victims of bullying (Augustyn & Zuckerman, 2007). Boys usually bully other boys and use force more often, while girls can be bullied by both sexes using mainly verbal bullying, social alienation, and intimidation (Schoen & Schoen, 2010).

Being bullied as a child can have negative consequences throughout life. These children often have increased episodes of common childhood illnesses, such as headaches, stomachaches, and sleep problems, as well as anxiety, loneliness, depression, and suicidal tendencies (Schoen & Schoen, 2010). Parents and caregivers should be advised to listen and respond to all complaints from children about being bullied, even if they seem trivial in nature. After the problem of either being bullied or being the bully has been identified, parents must work with the child, the school, the teacher, and the health care provider to solve the problem (see Teaching Guideline 28.2 and Evidence-based Practice 28.1). Many helpful resources and programs address the issue of bullying, such as the Canadian Safe Schools Network. Visit http://thePoint.lww.com/Chow1e for a direct link.

EVIDENCE-BASED PRACTICE 28.1
Benefits of Bully-Prevention Education

● **Study**

Child conduct problems continue to pose a problem in elementary schools. In addition to the behavioural disruption that occurs as a result of bullying and victimization, research has demonstrated that child bullies and victims are at increased risk for mental health problems and antisocial behaviour. This study was performed over a 2-year period utilizing fourth-grade classrooms at 28 public elementary schools. The group-randomized trial assigned classrooms to receive either a program aimed at bullying and aggression prevention or no treatment at all. Self-reported bullying and victimization were then analyzed after the 2-year trial.

▲ **Findings**

Upon analysis of the findings, the researchers reported a mild decrease in bullying and a greater decrease in bullying victimization. It appears that bullying-prevention programs in elementary schools may be effective in decreasing aggression and violence in the school-age group.

■ **Nursing Implications**

Nurses should continue to educate parents and teachers about bullying. Encourage children to be involved in peer groups. Become actively involved in the local elementary school bullying-prevention program. When bullies are identified, refer them for education in alternative means of emotional expression such as social skills training.

Jensen, J. M., & Dieterich, W. A. (2007). Effects of a skills-based prevention program on bullying and bully victimization among elementary school children. *Prevention Science, 8,* 285–296.

Tobacco and Alcohol Education

School-age children are eager to grow up and be independent. Peers and acceptance are very important at this time. School-age children may be exposed to messages that are in conflict with their parents' values regarding smoking and alcohol. Peers often exert pressure for children to experiment with tobacco and alcohol.

School-age children are ready to absorb information that deals with drugs and alcohol. Information from parents or other adults who are major influences in the child's life is essential at this time to set clear rules and model behaviours for children to embrace. Discussions with children need to be based on facts and focused on the present. Some topics for discussion include:

• What alcohol and drugs are like and how they harm you
• Differences in medical use vs. illegal use of drugs
• How to think critically to interpret messages seen in advertising, media, sports, and entertainment personalities

See Teaching Guideline 28.2.

Recall Lawrence Jones, the 10-year-old presented at the beginning of the chapter. List potential developmental problems he may experience. What anticipatory guidance related to these concerns should you provide to his mother?

■■■ Key Concepts

■ Physical growth is slow and steady, with social and cognitive development progressing rapidly, during the school-age years of 6 to 12. Height increases approxi-

mately 5 cm per year, and weight gain is 3 to 3.5 kg per year.

■ With the entrance into the school system, school-age children have the influences of peers and teachers.

■ With the development of gross motor skills and involvement in sports at school and in the community, safety education and practices are required. Also, with the participation in cooperative sports, injuries occur.

■ Visual acuity is reaching maturation and 20/20 vision is expected by 7 years of age.

■ Increased independence leads to increased exposure to safety hazards.

■ The school-age child develops the cognitive ability to classify objects and to identify relationships among objects.

■ Dental care is very important to prevent dental caries, malocclusion, and other problems. In early school age, the first primary teeth will be lost.

■ The onset of puberty may occur by the later school-age years.

■ Erikson's developmental task for the age group is the development of a sense of industry.

■ Peers are very important, especially peers of the same sex. School-age children usually have a best friend and belong to clubs. They have collections of nonvaluable items such as rocks, clips, and so forth.

■ School-age children are capable of concrete operations, solving problems, and making decisions. They continue to need guidance, rules, and directions from parents.

■ The school-age child develops a conscience and knows cultural and social values. He can understand and obey rules.

- The nurse's role includes educating parents and school-age children in promoting health and safety.
- Nurses should inform the school-age child about expected developmental changes in the body to promote self-esteem and self-confidence.

REFERENCES

Alba-Fisch, M. (n.d). *Temperament: Miss or match.* Retrieved August 19, 2011 from http://www.taconicnet.com/articles/temperament.php

Augustyn, M., & Zuckerman, B. (2007). Impact of violence on children. In R. M. Kleigman, R. E. Behrman, H. B. Jenson, & B. F. Stanton (Eds.), *Nelson textbook of pediatrics* (18th ed.). Philadelphia: Saunders.

Barakat, I. S., & Clark, J. A. (2007). *Positive discipline and child guidance.* Retrieved August 18, 2011 from http://muextension.missouri.edu/xplor/hesguide/humanrel/gh6119.htm

Canadian Ophthalmological Society. (2007). *Amblyopia: Treat "lazy eye" in early childhood.* Retrieved August 19, 2011 from http://www.eyesite.ca/english/public-information/eye-conditions/pdfs/Amblyopia_e.pdf

Canadian Dental Association. (2011). *Dental care for children.* Retrieved October 30, 2011 from http://www.cda-adc.ca/en/oral_health/cfyt/dental_care_children/

Canadian Paediatric Society. (2004). Growth assessment in Aboriginal children: Is there need for change? *Paediatrics & Child Health, 9*(7), 477–479; Retrieved August 18, 2011 from http://www.ncbi.nlm.nih.gov/pmc/articles/PMC2720866/

Canadian Paediatric Society. (2008). *How to promote good television habits.* Retrieved November 14, 2011 from http://www.caringforkids.cps.ca/growinglearning/GoodTelevision.htm

Canadian Paediatric Society. (2011). *Car seat safety.* Retrieved February 18, 2012 from http://www.caringforkids.cps.ca/handouts/car_seat_safety

Centers for Disease Control and Prevention. (2011). *Unintentional drowning: Fact sheet.* Retrieved August 19, 2011 from http://www.cdc.gov/HomeandRecreationalSafety/Water-Safety/waterinjuries-factsheet.html

Children's Hospital Boston. (n.d.). *Lying and stealing.* Retrieved August 19, 2011 from http://www.childrenshospital.org/az/Site1254/mainpageS1254P0.html

Durrant, J. E. (2007). *Positive discipline: What it is and how to do it.* Retrieved August 18, 2011 from www.cheo.on.ca/uploads/AboutUs/Files/js_positive_discipline.pdf

Erikson, E. (1963). *Childhood and society* (2nd ed.). New York: Norton.

Feigelman, S. (2007a). Middle childhood. In R. M. Kleigman, R. E. Behrman, H. B. Jenson, & B. F. Stanton (Eds.), *Nelson Textbook of Pediatrics* (18th ed.). Philadelphia: Saunders.

Feigelman, S. (2007b). Overview and assessment variability. In R. M. Kleigman, R. E. Behrman, H. B. Jenson & B. F. Stanton (Eds.), *Nelson Textbook of Pediatrics* (18th ed.). Philadelphia: Saunders.

Hagan, J. F., Shaw, J. S., & Duncan, P. (2008). *Bright futures guidelines for health supervision of infants, children, and adolescents* (3rd ed.). Elk Grove Village, IL: American Academy of Pediatrics.

Health Canada. (2011). *Canada's food guide: Children.* Retrieved November 14, 2011 from http://www.hc-sc.gc.ca/fn-an/food-guide-aliment/choose-choix/advice-conseil/child-enfant-eng.php

Healthy Children. (2010a). *Tips & tools: Safety for your child: 8 years.* Retrieved August 19, 2011 from http://www.healthychildren.org/english/tips-tools/Pages/Safety-for-Your-Child-8-Years.aspx

Healthy Children. (2010b). *Tips & tools: Safety for your child: 10 years.* Retrieved August 19, 2011 from http://www.healthychildren.org/english/tips-tools/Pages/Safety-for-Your-Child-10-Years.aspx

Healthy Children. (2011a). *Family life: Competition and cheating.* Retrieved August 19, 2011 from http://www.healthychildren.org/English/family-life/family-dynamics/communication-discipline/pages/Competition-and-Cheating.aspx

Healthy Children. (2011b). *Family life: The importance of family routines.* Retrieved August 19, 2011 from http://www.healthychildren.org/English/family-life/family-dynamics/pages/The-Importance-of-Family-Routines.aspx

Healthy Children. (2011c). *Tips & tools: Safety for your child: 6 years.* Retrieved August 19, 2011 from http://www.healthychildren.org/english/tips-tools/Pages/Safety-for-Your-Child-6-Years.aspx

Hegvik, R., McDevitt, S., & Carey, W. (1982). The middle childhood temperament questionnaire/develop. *Journal of Developmental and Behavioral Pediatrics, 3*(4), 197–200.

Hockenberry, M., Wilson, D., Winkelstein, M. L., & Kline, N. (2003). *Wong's infant care of infants and children* (7th ed.). St. Louis, MO: Mosby.

Jarvis, C. (2008). *Physical examination and health assessment.* St. Louis, MO: Mosby.

KidsHealth. (2011). *How TV affects your child.* Retrieved November 14, 2011 from http://kidshealth.org/parent/positive/family/tv_affects_child.html#

Kohlberg, L. (1984). *Moral development.* New York: Harper & Row.

Krebs, N. R., Primark, L. E., & Haemer, M. (2011). Normal childhood nutrition & its disorders. In W. W. Hay, M. J. Levin, J. M. Sondheimer, & R. R. Deterding (Eds.), *Current pediatric diagnosis and treatment* (20th ed.). New York: McGraw-Hill.

Kroll, M. A., & Neild, L. S. (2010). *Home alone: At what age are children ready?* Retrieved August 19, 2011 from http://www.pediatricsconsultantlive.com/display/article/1803329/1562016

Mannheim, J. K., & Zieve, D. (2010). *School-age children development.* Retrieved November 15, 2011 from http://www.nlm.nih.gov/medlineplus/ency/article/002017.htm

McDevitt, S., & Carey, W. (1978). The measurement of temperament in 3–7 year old children. *Journal of Child Psychology and Psychiatry, 19*, 245–253.

Nield, L. S., Stenger, J. P., & Kamat, D. (2007). Dental disease: pearls about those pearly whites. *Consultant for Pediatricians, 6*(8), 449–454.

Peterson-Sweeney, K., & Stevens, J. (2010). Optimizing the health of infants and children: Their oral health counts! *Journal of Pediatric Nursing, 25*(4), 244–249.

Piaget, J. (1969). *The theory of stages in cognitive development.* New York: McGraw-Hill.

Public Health Agency of Canada. (2009). *Child and youth injury in review, 2009 edition—Spotlight on consumer product safety.* Retrieved August 18, 2011 from www.phac-aspc.gc.ca/publicat/cyi-bej/2009/index-eng.php

Public Safety Canada. (2011). *First steps to stop bullying: Adults helping children aged 4 to 11.* Retrieved August 18, 2011 from www.publicsafety.gc.ca/res/cp/bully_4211-eng.aspx

Ruggiero, M. (1999). Maladaptation to school. In M. Levine, W. Carey, & A. Croker (Eds.), *Developmental behavioral pediatrics.* Philadelphia: Saunders.

Schoen, S., & Schoen, A. (2010). Bullying and harassment in the United States. *The Clearing House, 83*(2), 68–73.

Transport Canada. (2011). *Keep kids safe—Stage 2: Forward-facing seats.* Retrieved October 23, 2011 from http://www.tc.gc.ca/eng/roadsafety/safedrivers-childsafety-stage2-forward-facing-1085.htm

Trocmé, N., Fallon, B. MacLaurin, B., Daciuk, J., Felstiner, C., et al. (2005). *Canadian incidencestudy of reported child abuse and neglect – 2003: Major findings.* Ottawa, ON: Minister of Public Works and Government Services Canada.

U.S. Department of Agriculture and U.S. Department of Health and Human Services. (2010). *Dietary guidelines for Americans, 2010* (7th ed.). Washington DC: U.S. Government Printing Office; retrieved August 19, 2011 from http://www.cnpp.usda.gov/DGAs2010-PolicyDocument.htm

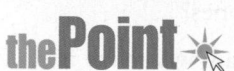

For additional learning materials, including Internet Resources, visit **http://thePoint.lww.com/Chow1e.**

CHAPTER WORKSHEET

MULTIPLE CHOICE QUESTIONS

1. The successful resolution of developmental tasks for the school-age child, according to Erikson, would be identified by:

   a. Learning from repeating tasks

   b. Developing a sense of worth and competence

   c. Using fantasy and magical thinking to cope with problems

   d. Developing a sense of trust

2. Which of the following are reasons that stealing occurs in school-age children? (Choose all that apply)

   a. To escape punishment

   b. High self-esteem

   c. Low expectations of family/peers

   d. Lack of sense of propriety

   e. Strong desire to own something

3. Which of the following will promote weight loss in an obese school-age child? (Choose all that apply)

   a. Unlimited computer and TV time

   b. Role modelling by family

   c. Becoming active in sports

   d. Eating unstructured meals

   e. Involving child in meal planning and grocery shopping

   f. Drinking three glasses of water per day

4. As the school nurse conducting screening for vision in a 6-year-old child, you would refer the child to a specialist if the visual acuity in both eyes is:

   a. 20/20

   b. 20/25

   c. 20/30

   d. 20/50

5. Ms. Jones has two sons, ages 6 and 9, who want to play on the same baseball team. As the school nurse, what advice would you give Ms. Jones?

   a. Having the boys on the same team will make it more convenient for the mother.

   b. Levels of coordination and concentration differ, so the boys need to be on different teams.

   c. Put the boys on the same team because they are both school-age children.

   d. It is best to avoid putting the boys on the same team to prevent sibling rivalry.

CRITICAL THINKING EXERCISES

1. Ms. Sams brings her 8-year-old son (Frank) to the pediatrician's office for his annual exam. She states that she is concerned about his recent behaviour. He went to the grocery store with his friend and his friend's mother and he came home with a Matchbox car. The friend's mother stated she had not purchased the car.

   a. What would be your response to Ms. Sams?

   b. Ms. Sams said she still has the car. What would you advise Ms. Sams to do to make Frank aware of consequences of his actions?

2. Sally's mother is asking the nurse advice about purchasing a two-wheeled bike for her 7-year-old. What guidance should the nurse offer this parent?

3. Ms. Shaw brings in her 12-year-old daughter for a well-child check. The school-ager says to the nurse, "I look different from my friends. I do not wear bras and my friends are already wearing bras." What would be an appropriate response to this school-ager?

4. Johnny is an 11-year-old whose mother and father both work during the day. He returns home alone after school. How should the parents prepare Johnny for this experience? What safety rules would be included in the education for Johnny?

STUDY ACTIVITIES

1. Attend a sporting event (such as soccer or baseball) with school-age teams. Describe the coordination and gross motor functioning of this group.

2. Attend a first-grade class. Observe the behaviours exhibited by the school-age children in this class. How do these behaviours compare with normal values for this age group?

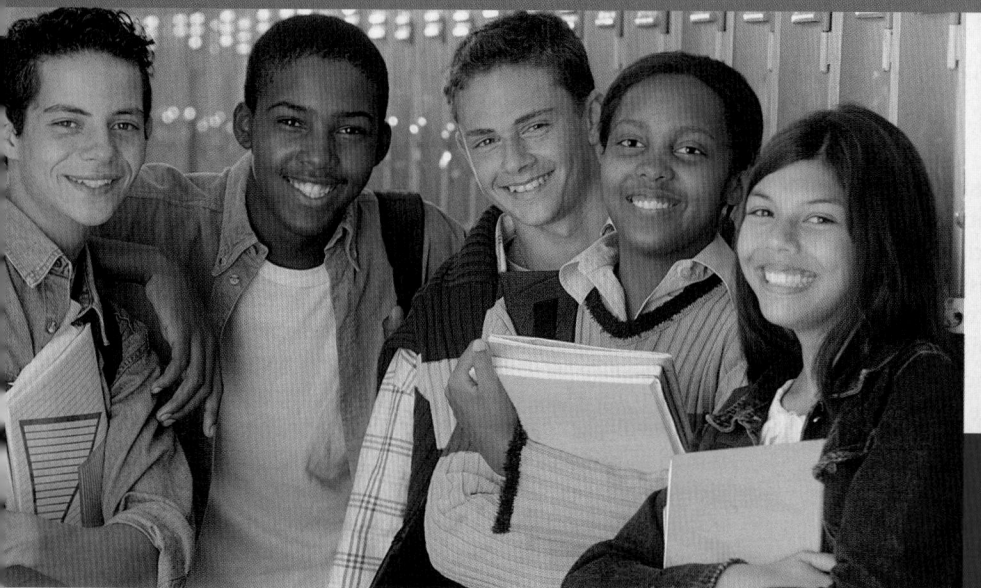

CHAPTER 29

Adapted by Christine A. Ateah

GROWTH AND DEVELOPMENT OF THE ADOLESCENT

KEY TERMS

adolescence
adolescent egocentrism
invincibility

menarche
peer groups
puberty

risk-taking behaviours
sexuality

LEARNING OBJECTIVES

Upon completion of the chapter, the learner will be able to:

1. Identify normal physiologic changes, including puberty, occurring in the adolescent.
2. Discuss psychosocial, cognitive, and moral changes occurring in the adolescent.
3. Identify changes in relationships with peers, family, teachers, and community during adolescence.
4. Describe interventions to promote safety during adolescence.
5. Demonstrate knowledge of the nutritional requirements of the adolescent.
6. Demonstrate knowledge of the development of sexuality and its influence on dating during adolescence.
7. Identify common developmental concerns of the adolescent.
8. Demonstrate knowledge of the appropriate nursing guidance for common developmental concerns.

Lisa Chung is a 15-year-old girl brought to the clinic by her mother for her annual school check-up. During your assessment, you measure Lisa's weight at 50 kg and her height at 150 cm. As the nurse caring for her, assess Lisa's growth and development, and then provide appropriate anticipatory guidance to her and her mother.

Wow

The only way to grow is to let go.

Adolescence spans the years of transition from childhood to adulthood, which is usually between the ages of 12 and 19 years. There is some overlap between late school age and adolescence. The adolescent experiences drastic changes in the physical, cognitive, psychosocial, and psychosexual areas. With this rapid growth during adolescence, the development of secondary sexual characteristics, and interest in the opposite sex, the adolescent needs the support and guidance of parents and nurses to facilitate healthy lifestyles and to reduce **risk-taking behaviours**.

Growth and Development Overview

Adolescence is a time of rapid growth with dramatic changes in body size and proportions. The magnitude of these changes is second only to the growth in infancy. During this time, sexual characteristics develop and reproductive maturity is achieved. The age of onset and the duration of the physiologic changes vary from individual to individual. Generally, girls enter **puberty** earlier (at 9 to 10 years of age) than boys (at 10 to 11 years). Adolescents will represent varying levels of identity formation and will offer unique challenges to the nurse (Table 29.1).

Physiologic Changes Associated with Puberty

The secretion of estrogen in girls and testosterone in boys stimulates the development of breast tissue in girls, pubic hair in both sexes, and changes in genitalia. These biological changes that occur during adolescence are known as *puberty*. Puberty is the result of triggers among the environment, the central nervous system, the hypothalamus, the pituitary gland, the gonads, and the adrenal glands. Gonadotropin-releasing hormone (GnRH), produced by the hypothalamus, travels through the capillaries to the anterior pituitary gland to stimulate the production and secretion of follicle-stimulating hormone (FSH) and luteinizing hormone (LH). The increased levels of FSH and LH stimulate the gonadal response. LH stimulates ovulation in girls and acts on testicular Leydig cells in boys, prompting maturation of the testicles and testosterone production. FSH with LH stimulates sperm production. Estrogen, progesterone, testosterone, and other androgens released from the gonads effect biological changes and changes in various organs, including alterations in muscles, bones, skin, and hair follicles. When serum sex hormones are decreased, the hypothalamus triggers the secretion of GnRH to initiate the proper gonadal responses.

Girls reach physical maturity before boys, and menstruation usually begins between the ages of 9 and 15 years

(most often between 12 and 13 years). Breast budding (thelarche) occurs at approximately age 9 to 11 years and is followed by the growth of pubic hair. The first sign of pubertal changes in boys is testicular enlargement in response to testosterone secretion, usually occurring in stage 2 of the Tanner scale of pubertal changes (Tanner, 1962) (see Chapter 31). As testosterone levels increase, the penis and scrotum enlarge, hair distribution increases, and scrotal skin texture changes. During late puberty, boys will typically experience their first ejaculation, which may occur while they are sleeping (nocturnal emissions). Nurses should provide anticipatory guidance to adolescent males regarding involuntary nocturnal emissions (wet dreams) to assure them that this is a normal occurrence.

Tanner stages 3 to 5—increased breast tissue and pubic hair distribution in girls, and scrotal and penile changes as well as hair distribution changes in boys—usually occur during adolescence (see Chapter 31). The nurse should provide guidance to adolescents about the normalcy of the sexual feelings and evolving body changes that occur during puberty.

Physical Growth

Diet, exercise, and hereditary factors influence the height, weight, and body build of the adolescent. Over the past three decades, adolescents have become taller and heavier than their ancestors and the beginning of puberty is earlier.

The rapid growth during adolescence is secondary only to that of the infant years and is a direct result of the hormonal changes of puberty. Both girls and boys experience changes in appearance and size. Height in girls increases rapidly after **menarche** and usually ceases 2 to 2½ years after menarche. Boys' growth spurt occurs later than girls' and usually begins between the ages of 10½ and 16 years and ends sometime between the ages of 13½ and 17½ years. Peak height velocity occurs at approximately 12 years of age in girls or at about 6 to 12 months after menarche. Boys reach peak height velocity at about 14 years of age. Peak weight velocity occurs about 6 months after menarche in girls and at about 14 years of age in boys. Muscle mass increases in boys and fat deposits increase in girls (Fig. 29.1).

Growth is rapid during early adolescence, but it decreases in middle and late adolescence. Height for adolescent boys who are between the 50th and 95th percentiles ranges from 132 to 176.8 cm. Weight of boys in these percentiles ranges from 35.3 to 95.8 kg. On average, boys will gain 10 to 30 cm in height and 7 to 30 kg in weight.

Height for girls who are between the 50th and 95th percentiles ranges from 144.8 to 173.6 cm, with weight ranging from 27.2 to 82.5 kg. On average, girls will grow 5 to 20 cm in height and gain 7 to 25 kg in weight during

TABLE 29.1 PHYSIOLOGIC CHANGES OF ADOLESCENCE

Stage of Adolescence	Puberty Changes in Females	Puberty Changes in Males	Physical Growth in Females	Physical Growth in Males
Early adolescence (10–13 years)	Pubic hair begins to curl and spread over mons pubis; pigmentation increases Breast bud and areola continue to enlarge; no separation of breast First menstrual period (average, 12 years; normal range, 9–16 years)	Pubic hair spreads laterally, begins to curl; pigmentation increases Growth and enlargement of testes in scrotum (scrotum reddish in colour) and continued lengthening of penis	Increase in percentage of body fat Head, neck, hands, and feet reach adult proportions Senses matured Respiratory rate decreases to 15–20 breaths/minute Heart grows in size and strength, heart rate decreases, blood pressure increases to adult level Full set of permanent teeth with exception of last four molars (wisdom teeth) Liver, kidneys, spleen, and digestive tract mature; enlarge during growth spurt Exocrine and apocrine sweat glands and sebaceous glands become fully functioning	Increase in percentage of body fat Head, neck, hands, and feet reach adult proportions Leggy look due to extremities growing faster than the trunk Senses matured Respiratory rate decreases to 15–20 breaths/minute Heart grows in size and strength, heart rate decreases, blood pressure increases Full set of permanent teeth with exception of last four molars (wisdom teeth) Liver, kidneys, spleen, and digestive tract mature; enlarge during growth spurt Exocrine and apocrine sweat glands and sebaceous glands become fully functioning
Middle adolescence (14–16 years)	Pubic hair becomes coarse in texture and continues to curl; amount of hair increases Areola and papilla separate from the contour of the breast to form a secondary mound	Pubic hair becomes coarser in texture and takes on adult distribution Testes and scrotum continue to grow; scrotal skin darkens; penis grows in width, and glans penis develops May experience breast enlargement	Reach peak height and weight velocity Muscle mass and strength increase Increase in shoulder, chest, and hip breadth	Voice changes; more masculine due to rapid enlargement of the larynx and pharynx as well as lung changes Growth spurt during this time Muscle mass and strength increase Increase in shoulder, chest, and hip breadth
Late adolescence (17–20 years)	Mature pubic hair distribution and coarseness	Mature pubic hair distribution and coarseness Breast enlargement disappears Adult size and shape of testes, scrotum, and penis; scrotal skin darkening Ejaculation occurs	Physically mature Ossification of skeletal system complete Eruption of last four molars BMR reaches adult levels	Physically mature Ossification of skeletal system complete Eruption of last four molars BMR reaches adult levels

BMR, basal metabolic rate.

Adapted from: Marcell, A. V. (2007). Adolescence. In R. M. Kleigman, R. E. Behrman, H. B. Jenson, & B. F. Stanton (Eds.), *Nelson Textbook of Pediatrics* (18th ed.). Philadelphia: Saunders.

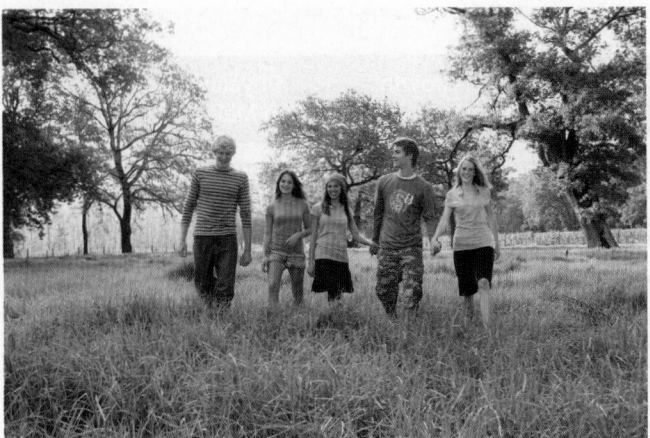

FIGURE 29.1 These adolescents reflect the differences in sizes and shapes seen in adolescents of the same age.

adolescence. See Appendix F for growth charts for this age group. Refer to Chapter 31 for instructions for calculating body mass index (BMI).

Organ System Maturation

Adolescence is a time of metabolic slowing and of increasing size of some organs.

Neurologic System

During adolescence, there is continued brain growth although the size of the brain does not increase significantly. Neurons do not increase in number, but growth of myelin sheath enables faster neural processing.

Respiratory System

The adolescent years see an increase in diameter and length of the lungs. Respiratory rate decreases and reaches the adult rate. Respiratory volume and vital capacity increase. Volume and capacity are greater in boys than girls, which may be associated with increased chest and shoulder size in boys. The growth of the laryngeal cartilage, larynx, and vocal cords produces the voice changes experienced in adolescence. Deepening of both male and female voices occurs but is more pronounced in boys (Edelman & Mandle, 2002).

Cardiovascular System

There is an increase in size and strength of the heart. Systolic blood pressure increases and heart rate decreases. Blood volume reaches higher levels in boys than girls, which may be due to boys' greater muscle mass.

Gastrointestinal System

The liver, spleen, kidneys, and digestive tract enlarge during the growth spurt in early adolescence, but do not change in function. These systems are functionally mature in early school age.

Musculoskeletal System

The ossification of the skeletal system is incomplete until late adolescence in boys. Ossification is more advanced in girls and occurs at an earlier age. During the growth spurt, muscle mass and strength increase. At similar stages of development, muscle development is generally greater in boys. Estrogen, progesterone, and testosterone (sex steroids) and other androgens are released from the gonads and effect changes in the muscles and bones. Low estrogen levels tend to stimulate skeletal growth, while higher levels inhibit growth.

Integumentary System

During adolescence the skin becomes thick and tough. Under the influence of androgens, the sebaceous glands become more active, particularly on the face, back, and genitals. Due to the increased levels of testosterone during Tanner stages 4 and 5 in both boys and girls, both sexes may have increased sebum production, which may lead to the development of acne and oily hair.

The exocrine and apocrine sweat glands function at adult levels during adolescence. The exocrine glands are all over the body and they produce sweat that helps to eliminate body heat through evaporation. The apocrine glands are found in the axillae, genital, and anal areas, and around the breasts. The apocrine sweat glands produce sweat in response to hair follicles. This sweat is produced continuously and is stored and released in response to emotional stimuli.

Psychosocial Development

According to Erikson (1963), it is during adolescence that teenagers achieve a sense of identity. As the adolescent is trying out many different roles in regard to his relationships with peers, family, community, and society, he is developing his own individual sense of self. If he is not successful in forming his own sense of self, he develops a sense of role confusion or diffusion. The adolescent culture becomes very important to the teenager. It is through his involvement with teenage groups that the adolescent finds support and help with developing his own identity.

Erikson (1963) believed that during the task of developing his own sense of identity, the adolescent revisits each of the previous stages of development. The sense of trust is encountered as the adolescent strives to find out whom and what ideals he can have faith in. In revisiting the stage of autonomy, the adolescent is seeking out ways to express his individuality in an effective manner. He would avoid behaviours that would "shame" or ridicule him in front of his peers. The sense of initiative is revisited as the adolescent develops his vision for what he might become. And the sense of industry is again encountered as the adolescent makes his choice to participate in different activities at school, in the community, and in the work force.

The ability of the adolescent to successfully form a sense of self is dependent upon how well the adolescent successfully completed the former stages of development. Erikson (1963) believed that if the adolescent has been successful, he could develop resources during adolescence to overcome any gaps in previous developmental stages. If the adolescent believes that he cannot express himself in any manner due to societal restrictions, he will develop role confusion. See Table 29.2 for additional information.

TABLE 29.2 DEVELOPMENTAL THEORIES

Theories	Stages	Activities
Erikson (psycho-social)	Identity vs. role confusion or diffusion	
	Early (11–14 years)	Focuses on bodily changes
		Experiences frequent mood changes
		Importance placed upon conformity to peer norms and peer acceptance
		Strives to master skills within peer groups
		Defining boundaries with parents and authority figures
		Early stage of emancipation—struggles to separate from parents while still desiring dependence upon them
		Identifies with same-sex peers
	Middle (14–16 years)	Takes more responsibility for own behaviours
		Continues to adjust to changed body image
		Tries out different roles within peer groups
		Need for acceptance by peer group; interested in attracting opposite gender
		Time of greatest conflict with parents/authority figures
	Late (17–20 years)	Able to understand implications of behaviour and decisions
		Roles within peer groups established
		Feels secure with body image
		Has matured sexual identity
		Has idealistic career goals
		Importance of individual friendships emerges
		Process of emancipation from family almost complete
Piaget (cognitive)	Formal operations	Limited abstract thought process
	Early (11–14 years)	Egocentric thinking
		Eager to apply limited abstract process to different situations and to peer groups
	Middle (14–17 years)	Increased ability to think abstractly or in more idealistic terms
		Able to solve verbal and mental problems using scientific methods
		Thinks he or she is invincible—risky behaviours increase
		Likes making independent decisions
		Becomes involved/concerned with society, politics
	Late (17–20 years)	Abstract thinking is established
		Developed critical thinking skills—tests different solutions to problems
		Less risky behaviours
		Develops realistic goals and career plans
Kohlberg	Postconventional level III	Morals based upon peer, family, religion-based, and societal morals
	Early (11–14 years)	Asks broad, usually unanswerable questions about life
		Developing own set of morals—evaluates individual morals in relation to peer, family, and societal morals
	Middle (14–17 years)	Internalizes own morals and values
		Continues to compare own morals and values with those of society
	Late (17–20 years)	Evaluates morals of others

Adapted from: Erikson, E. (1963). *Childhood and society* (2nd ed.). New York: Norton; Kohlberg, L. (1984). *Moral development.* New York: Harper & Row; and Piaget, J. (1969). *The theory of stages in cognitive development.* New York: McGraw-Hill.

Cognitive Development

According to Piaget (1969), the adolescent progresses from a concrete framework of thinking to an abstract one. It is the formal operational period. During this period, the adolescent develops the ability to think outside of the present; i.e., she can incorporate into her thinking concepts that do exist as well as concepts that might exist. Her thinking becomes logical, organized, and consistent. She is able to think about a problem from all points of view, ranking the possible solutions while solving the problem. Not all adolescents achieve formal operational reasoning at the same time.

In the early stages of formal operational reasoning, the adolescent's thinking is egocentric. She is very idealistic, constantly challenging the way things are and wondering why things cannot change. These activities lead to the adolescent's feeling of being omnipotent. The adolescent must undergo this way of thinking, even though it can frustrate adults, in her quest to reach formal operational reasoning. As the teenager progresses toward middle adolescence, her thinking becomes very introspective. She assumes others are just as interested in what interests her, which leads her to feel unique, special, and exceptional. That feeling of "being exceptional" leads to the risk-taking behaviours for which teenagers are well known. Also, the teenager feels very committed to her viewpoints. She tries very hard to convince others of her viewpoints and strongly embraces those causes that support her opinions. This idealism can cause the adolescent to reject her family, her culture, her church, and her community beliefs, which can cause conflict with her family, culture, church, and community. See Table 29.2 for additional information.

Moral Development

It is during the adolescent years that teenagers develop their own set of values and morals. According to Kohlberg (1984), adolescents are experiencing the postconventional stage of moral development. It is only because adolescents are developing their formal operational way of thinking that they can experience the postconventional stage of moral development. At the beginning of this stage, teenagers begin to question the status quo. The majority of their choices are based upon emotions while they are questioning societal standards. As they progress to developing their own set of morals, adolescents realize that moral decisions are based upon rights, values, and principles that are agreeable to a given society. They also realize that those rights, values, and principles can be in conflict with the laws of the given society, but they are able to reconcile the differences. Because adolescents undergo the process of developing their own set of morals at different rates, they might find that their friends view a situation differently. This difference can lead to conflicts and the forming of different friendships. See Table 29.2 for additional information.

Referring back to Lisa Chung, identify the stage of psychosocial development that she should be in according to Erikson. What approaches for assessment and teaching would be most effective based on the stage you identified?

Motor Skill Development

During adolescence, the teenager refines and continues to develop his or her gross and fine motor skills. Because of this period of rapid growth spurts, teenagers may experience times of decreased coordination and have a decreased ability to perform previously learned skills, which can be worrisome for the teenager.

Gross Motor Skills

It is usually during early adolescence that teenagers begin to develop endurance. Their concentration has increased so they can follow complicated instructions. Coordination can be a problem because of the uneven growth spurts. During middle adolescence, speed and accuracy increase while coordination also improves. Teenagers become more competitive with each other (Fig. 29.2). During late adolescence, the teenager usually narrows his or her areas of interest and concentrates on the needed relevant skills.

Fine Motor Skills

The use of computers has greatly increased the fine motor skills of teenagers (Fig. 29.3). In the early adolescent years, the teenager increases his ability to manipulate objects. His handwriting is neat and he increases his

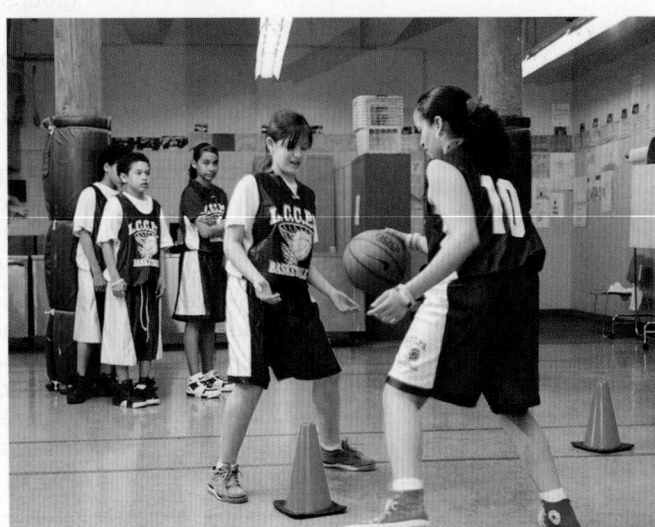

FIGURE 29.2 Adolescents become involved in competitive sports, which draw upon their gross motor skills.

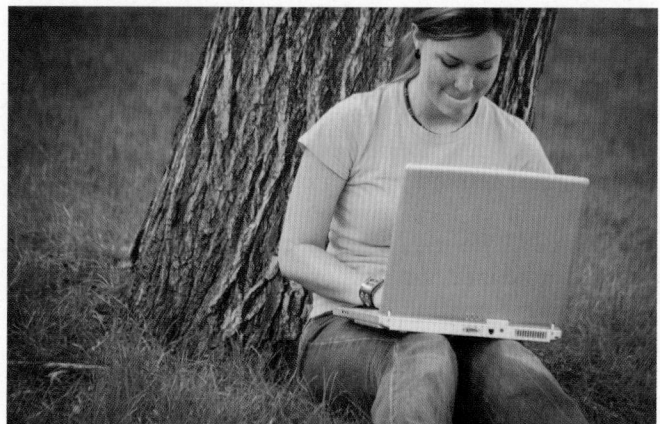

FIGURE 29.3 Using computers has increased the fine motor skills of adolescents.

finger dexterity. The middle adolescent years see the teenager refining his dexterity skills. By late adolescence, the teenager has developed precise eye–hand coordination and finger dexterity.

Communication and Language Development

Language skills continue to develop and be refined during adolescence. Adolescents have improved communication skills, using correct grammar and parts of speech. Vocabulary and communication skills continue to develop during middle adolescence. However, the usage of colloquial speech (slang) increases, causing communication with people other than peers to be difficult at times. By late adolescence, language skills are comparable to those of adults.

Emotional and Social Development

Adolescents undergo a great deal of change in the areas of emotional and social development as they grow and mature into adults. Areas that are affected include the adolescent's relationship with parents; self-concept and body image; importance of peers; and **sexuality** and dating.

Relationship with Parents

Families and parents of adolescents experience changes and conflict that require adjustments and the understanding of adolescent development. The adolescent is striving for self-identity and increased independence. She spends more time with peers and less time with family and attending family functions. Parents sense that they have less influence on the adolescent as she spends more time with peers, questions family values, and becomes more mobile. This may lead to family issues, and the parents may respond by setting stricter limits or asking questions about the teen's activities and friends.

BOX 29.1) Ways to Improve Communication with Teens

- Set aside appropriate amount of time to discuss subject matter without interruptions.
- Talk face to face. Be aware of body language.
- Ask questions to see why he feels that way.
- Ask her to be patient as you tell your thoughts.
- Choose words carefully so he understands you.
- Tell her exactly what you mean.
- Give praise and approval to your teenager often.
- Speak to him as an equal—don't talk down to him.
- Be aware of your tone of voice and body language.
- Don't pretend you know all the answers.
- Admit that you do make mistakes.
- Rules and limits should be set fairly.

Adapted from: Neinstein, L. S. (2011). *Interviewing and communicating with adolescents (A4)*. Available at http://www.usc.edu/student-affairs/Health_Center/adolhealth/content/a4.html.

Other parents may drop all rules and assume that the adolescent can manage herself. Both of these responses increase tension in the family. Box 29.1 offers tips nurses can provide to parents to improve communication with their teenager.

With the adolescent attempting to establish some level of independence—and the parents learning to let go while focusing on aging parents, their marriage, and other children—a state of disequilibrium occurs. The family may experience more stress than at any other time.

Some families have better outcomes with their adolescents than others. Families who listen to and continue to demonstrate affection for and acceptance of their adolescent have a more positive outcome. This does not mean that the family accepts all of the teen's ideas or actions, but they are willing to listen and attempt to negotiate some limits.

Siblings experience changes in the relationship with the adolescent brother or sister; the older sibling may attempt to parent and the younger sibling may regress in an attempt to avoid the family conflict. Understanding the status of the adolescent–family relationship is essential for the nurse.

Self-Concept and Body Image

Self-concept and self-esteem are tied to body image in many ways. Adolescents who perceive their body as being different than peers or as less than ideal may view themselves negatively. Adolescent girls often are influenced by peers and the media and want to weigh less and have smaller hips, waist, or thighs. Boys tend to view themselves as being too thin or not muscular enough.

Sexual characteristics are important to the adolescent's self-concept and body image. Boys are concerned about the size of their penis and whether they have facial hair while girls are concerned about breast size and the onset of menstruation. Larger breasts are considered more feminine and menstruation is considered the rite of passage into adulthood. All of these body changes are important to the adolescent's self-concept.

Importance of Peers

Peer groups play an essential role in the identity of the adolescent (Marcell, 2007). Adolescent peer relationships are very important in providing opportunities to learn about negotiating differences; for recreation, companionship, and someone to share problems with; for learning peer loyalty; and for creating stability during transitions or times of stress. Learning to work out differences with peers is a skill that is important throughout life. Peers serve as someone safe to discuss family issues with, as the teen emotionally moves away from the family while trying to find his or her identity. Due to changes that have taken place within family systems in society, peer groups play a significant role in the socialization of adolescents (Fig. 29.4).

Peers serve as credible sources of information, role model social behaviours, and act as sources of social reinforcement. Friends provide an opportunity for fun and excitement. Peers impact teens' appearance, dress, social behaviour, and language. Peers also can have positive influences on each other, such as promoting college attendance, or negative influences, such as involvement with alcohol, drugs, or gangs. Early and middle adolescence are periods when teens are prone to join gangs. Peer role modeling and peer acceptance may lead to the formation of a gang that provides a collective identity and gives a sense of belonging. Peer pressure, companionship, and protection are the most frequent reasons given for joining gangs, particularly those associated with criminal activity.

Parents must know their teen's friends and continue to be aware of potential problems while allowing the teen the independence to become his or her own person. Nurses must remind parents of the importance of peers and the impact they have on the teen's decisions and life choices. The transition to greater peer involvement requires guidance and support. Adolescents who do not have parental or adult supervision and opportunities for conversation with adults may be more susceptible to peer influences and at higher risk for poor peer selections.

Sexuality and Dating

Adolescence is a critical time in the development of sexuality. Sexuality includes the thoughts, feelings, and behaviours related to the adolescent's sexual identity. Adolescents usually begin experimentation with heterosexual and homosexual behaviours, although these behaviours may occur earlier in some cultures.

Most adolescents become interested in the opposite sex during this time period (Fig. 29.5). Some of the reasons cited for this developing interest are physical development and body changes, peer-group pressure, and curiosity. Teen dating can range from group dating to single dating to serious relationships. Most early adolescents spend more time in activities with mixed-sex groups, such as dances and parties, than they do dating as a couple. Popular dating activities today include going out to dinner or the movies, "hanging out" at the mall, or visiting each other's home. During this period of early adolescence, teens tend to date for fun and recreation. Also, they may

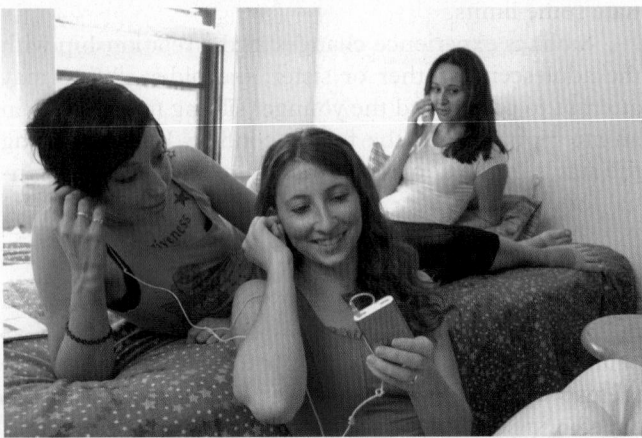

FIGURE 29.4 Peers play an important role in shaping the adolescent's identity.

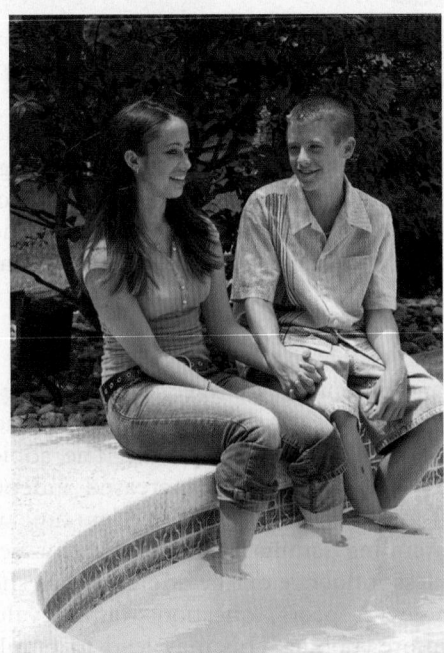

FIGURE 29.5 Dating becomes an important aspect of the teenager's life.

see dating as a way to upgrade social standing by being seen with a popular boy or an attractive girl.

Middle and late adolescents have group and single dates. Dating or spending time with a potential romantic partner is viewed as a major developmental marker for teens and is one of the most challenging adjustments. Lesbian, gay, or bisexual behaviour as a teen may or may not indicate that the adolescent will maintain that orientation into adulthood (Sass, 2011). Gay and lesbian adolescents face many challenges due to issues of nonacceptance and peer insensitivity. In Canada, public policies seek to identify and address the potential danger of psychological abuse directed at gay and lesbian youth (Saewyc, 2007). Nevertheless, these adolescents are at higher risk for mental health issues and suicide than heterosexual youth. It is vitally important that nurses be supportive, open, and accepting when working with all adolescents because nurses are frequently the "gatekeepers" of the clinical encounter and can be critical in determining the quality of their initial experience and satisfaction with their health care (Dysart-Gale, 2010).

Of frequent great concern to parents during the adolescent period of developing sexuality and dating are unwanted pregnancy, sexually transmitted infections (STIs), and teen feelings of despair over failed relationships. Adolescents may not worry about negative consequences of sexual activity, believing "it will not happen to me."

Lisa Chung's mother states that she is concerned about the changes that have occurred in her and Lisa's relationship over the past year. Lisa seems much more self-centred, always wants to be with her friends, is very critical of her mother and father, and seems to be constantly in conflict with them. Based on what you know about this stage of development, what guidance, including approaches and techniques, can you discuss with Mrs. Chung to address her concerns?

Cultural Influences on Growth and Development

Although the adolescent's culture continues to influence the teenager, the desire to be in harmony with peers becomes paramount. That desire can cause conflict with his family and culture. Today's adolescents live in a rapidly changing, increasingly culturally diverse world. They are exposed to many different cultures and ethnic groups.

Attitudes regarding adolescence vary among different cultures. Certain cultures may have more permissive attitudes toward issues facing adolescents, while others are more conservative, e.g., toward sexuality. Experiencing a rite of passage ceremony to signal the adolescent's movement to adult status varies among cultures. The North American culture does not universally have a rite of passage for teenagers. Some religious and social groups do have ceremonies that signal a movement toward the maturity of adulthood, e.g., the Jewish bar or bat mitzvah, the Catholic confirmation, and social debuts. In many parts of the world, separate "youth cultures" have developed in an attempt to blend traditional and modern worlds for the adolescent.

It is important for the nurse to recognize the ethnic background of each client. Research has shown that certain ethnic groups are at higher risk for certain diseases. For example, Aboriginal people are at higher risk for developing type 2 diabetes (Canadian Population Health Initiative, 2004). But the major barrier to the adolescent's health and successful achievement of the tasks of adolescence is socioeconomic status. Adolescents at a lower socioeconomic level are at higher risk for developing health care problems and risk-taking behaviours. In caring for adolescents, recognize the influence of their culture, ethnicity, and socioeconomic level upon them.

The Nurse's Role in Adolescent Growth and Development

During adolescence, the teenager faces many challenges. His or her fluctuating relationships with parents and other adult figures may limit him or her from seeking assistance in dealing with the common issues of adolescence. In dealing with adolescents, be aware that they have unpredictable behaviours, are inconsistent with their need for independence, have sensitive feelings, may interpret situations different from what they are, think friends are extremely important, and have a strong desire to belong. The following Nursing Process Overview will address promoting healthy growth and development and dealing with common developmental concerns.

Nursing Process Overview

Upon completion of assessment of the adolescent's current growth and development status, problems or issues related to growth and development may be identified. The nurse may then identify one or more nursing diagnoses, including:

- Risk for disproportionate growth
- Imbalanced nutrition: more than body requirements
- Delayed growth and development
- Risk for caregiver role strain
- Risk for injury
- Ineffective coping

Nursing care planning for the adolescent with growth and development issues should be individualized based on the adolescent's and family's needs. Nursing Care Plan 29.1 can be used as a guide in planning nursing care for the adolescent with a growth and

(text continues on page 918)

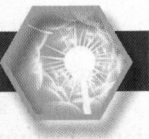

Nursing Care Plan 29.1

GROWTH AND DEVELOPMENT OF THE ADOLESCENT

NURSING DIAGNOSIS: Risk for disproportionate growth (risk factors: caregiver and adolescent knowledge deficit, low self-esteem, frequent illnesses)

Outcome Identification and Evaluation
Adolescent will demonstrate adequate growth: *appropriate weight gain for age and sex*

Interventions: Promoting Appropriate Physical Growth
- Assess parents' and adolescent's knowledge of nutritional needs of adolescents *to determine need for further education.*
- Educate parents and adolescent about appropriate serving sizes and foods *so that they are aware of what to expect for adolescents.*
- Determine need for additional caloric intake if necessary *(if very active in sports, if have a chronic illness).*
- Plot out height, weight, and body mass index (BMI) *to detect possible pattern.*
- Assess for risk factors for developing eating disorder *to refer to if needed and plan interventions.*

NURSING DIAGNOSIS: Nutrition, more than body requirements, imbalanced, related to lack of exercise, increased caloric intake, poor food choices, and stresses of adolescence

Outcome Identification and Evaluation
Adolescent will lose weight at an appropriate rate: *increase amount of exercise, make appropriate eating choices, decrease caloric intake to appropriate amount for age and sex*

Interventions: Promoting Appropriate Nutrition
- Assess knowledge of parents and adolescent about nutritional needs of teenagers *to determine deficits in knowledge.*
- Have adolescent keep a detailed food and exercise diary for 1 week *to determine current patterns of eating and exercise.*
- Interview family in relationship to their eating habits and exercise habits *to determine where adjustments might need to be made.*
- Discuss changes in a positive manner—talk about developing healthy eating habits instead of dieting *to promote compliance.*
- Analyse preceding data, and base recommendations for changes on these data *to promote compliance and to prioritize recommendations.*
- Discuss ways to decrease temptation to overeat, e.g., eat slowly, put down the fork between bites, serve food on smaller plates, and count mouthfuls *to allow time to realize that you are full.*
- Have adolescent create meal plans and grocery shop *to allow him or her some sense of control and decision-making.*
- Incorporate increase in daily exercise, which will stress sense of self-improvement *to increase caloric expenditure and self-esteem.*
- Decrease television/computer time *to increase caloric expenditure.*
- Encourage peer exercise activities *to increase peer interactions and to realize that others are like him or her.*
- Develop reward system *to increase self-esteem.*
- Investigate joining weight loss program for adolescents *to increase self-esteem and to increase awareness that other adolescents have the same problem.*

NURSING DIAGNOSIS: Growth and development, delayed, related to speech, motor, psychosocial, or cognitive concerns as evidenced by delay in meeting expected school performances

Outcome Identification and Evaluation
Development will be maximized: *Adolescent will make continued progress toward attainment of expected school performance.*

Interventions: Promoting Growth and Development
- Perform scheduled evaluation of the adolescent by school and health care provider *to determine current functioning.*
- Develop realistic multidisciplinary plan *to ensure maximizing resources.*
- Carry out interventions as prescribed by developmental specialist, physical therapist, occupational therapist, or speech therapist at home and at school *to maximize benefit of interventions.*
- Have scheduled evaluation meetings *to be able to adapt interventions as soon as possible.*

(continued)

Nursing Care Plan 29.1 (continued)

NURSING DIAGNOSIS: Caregiver role strain, risk for (risk factors: knowledge deficit about adolescent issues, lack of prior exposure, fatigue, ill or developmentally delayed child)

Outcome Identification and Evaluation

Parent will experience competence in role: *will demonstrate appropriate caretaking behaviours and verbalize comfort in caring for an adolescent*

Interventions: Preventing Caregiver Role Strain

- Assess parent's knowledge of adolescence and the issues that arise as a part of normal development *to determine parent's needs.*
- Provide education on normal issues of adolescence *so that parents are armed with the knowledge they need to appropriately care for their adolescents.*
- Provide anticipatory guidance related to upcoming expected issues related to adolescent development *to prepare parents for what to expect next and how to intervene in an appropriate manner.*

NURSING DIAGNOSIS: Injury, risk for (risk factors: increased motor and cognitive skills and feeling of invincibility)

Outcome Identification and Evaluation

Adolescent's safety will be maintained: *will remain free from injury*

Interventions: Preventing Injury

- Discuss safety measures needed for the following: bikes, scooters, guns, skateboards, cars, and water *to decrease risk of injury related to those areas.*
- Discuss and develop a fire safety plan *to decrease risk of injury related to fire.*
- Discuss appropriate safety equipment needed for each sport *to decrease risk of injury.*
- Discuss appropriate sports to participate in depending upon age, sex, and maturity of adolescent *to prevent possible injury.*
- Teach parents and adolescent first-aid measures and cardiopulmonary resuscitation (CPR) *to minimize consequences of injury should it occur.*
- Discuss influence of peers upon actions of adolescents *to prevent possible injury due to mimicking behaviour.*

NURSING DIAGNOSIS: Coping, ineffective, for coping with normal stress of adolescence (risk factors: low self-esteem, poor relationship with parents and peers, participating in risk-taking behaviours)

Outcome Identification and Evaluation

Adolescent will demonstrate adequate coping abilities *as evident by management of stress of adolescence and no evidence of participating in risk-taking behaviours.*

Interventions: Promoting Effective Coping

- Assess adolescent's knowledge of normal stress facing teenagers *to determine current knowledge.*
- Assess adolescent's present coping skills *to determine areas for improvement/support.*
- Encourage parents to accept teenager as a unique individual.
- Discuss with parents and adolescent normal developmental issues facing teens *to give them knowledge needed to cope.*
- Provide different situations the teen might be faced with and different solutions.
- Develop with adolescent different solutions to problems.
- Allow for increasing independence and opportunities to solve own problems.
- Encourage development of friends with same values.
- Parents provide unconditional love.
- Assess for any evidence of any risk-taking behaviours (drugs, smoking, suicide).

development concern. The nurse may choose the appropriate nursing diagnoses from this plan and individualize them as needed. The nursing care plan is intended to serve as a guide, not to be an all-inclusive growth and development care plan.

Promoting Healthy Growth and Development

WATCH & LEARN

It takes multiple groups who address multiple issues to promote healthy growth and development in the adolescent. Some of these groups include sports teams in the school or the community, peers, teachers, band and choir members, and so forth. Also, the family's support and love will influence growth and development.

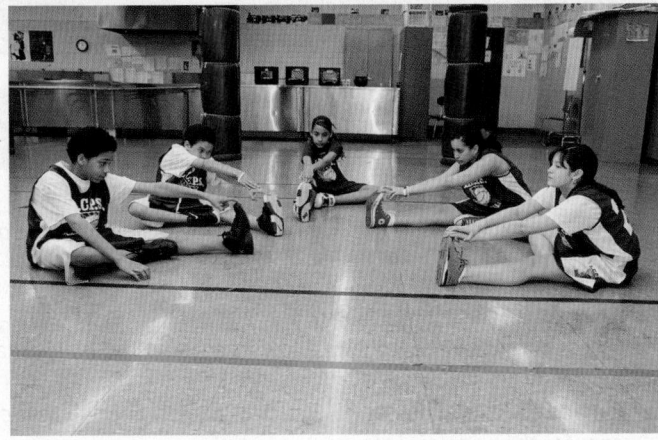

FIGURE 29.6 Stretching before exercise is an important part of exercise.

Promoting Growth and Development Through Sports and Physical Fitness

Many adolescents are involved in team sports that provide avenues for exercise. Adolescents probably spend more time and energy participating in sports than any other age group. Participation in sports contributes to the adolescent's development, educational process, and better health (Kelly, 2010; National Center for Chronic Disease Prevention and Health Promotion, 2010). Sports and games provide an opportunity to interact with peers while enjoying socially accepted stimulation and conflict.

Competition in sports activities helps the teenager in processing self-appraisal and in developing self-respect and concern for others. Every sport has some potential for injury. Rapidly growing bones, muscles, joints, and tendons are more vulnerable to unusual strains and fractures. Parents and coaches need to be aware of early warning signs of fatigue, dehydration, and injury. See Chapter 44 for a discussion of sports injuries. Also see Evidence-based Practice 29.1.

In relation to youth sports, the role of the nurse is to educate to prevent injuries (Fig. 29.6). This education

---

EVIDENCE-BASED PRACTICE 29.1
Interventions Directed Toward Prevention of Ankle Ligament Injury or Sprain

● **Study**

Adolescents are increasingly involved in organized sports that put them at risk for injury. Soccer and basketball, in particular, result in a very high incidence of ankle injuries, and ankle sprains are very commonly treated in the acute care setting. Inversion of the plantar-flexed foot is the most common mechanism of ankle injury resulting in damage to the lateral ligament complex. The authors analyzed 14 randomized or quasi-randomized trials that included data for a total of 8,279 participants. The interventions evaluated included use of modified footwear (high-top athletic shoes), external ankle supports, coordination training, and health education. The study evaluated the occurrence as well as the recurrence of ankle sprains.

▲ **Findings**

Ankle coordination and strength training may be beneficial in the prevention of ankle sprains, but the results from the

included studies were not powerful. However, the review provided sufficient evidence that the use of semi-rigid orthoses reduces the risk of ankle sprain in young and adult athletes. Use of these devices was shown to be particularly helpful in preventing reinjury of the ankle.

■ **Nursing Implications**

Nurses should recommend the use of semi-rigid ankle orthoses to adolescent athletes participating in sports such as soccer and basketball. Although physical conditioning of the ankle was not decisively proved to decrease the risk of ankle injury, it was not proved to be harmful so it should still be encouraged in student athletes. Exercises designed to improve coordination and proprioception should be included. At a minimum, adolescent athletes participating in high-risk sports should wear high-top athletic shoes in order to provide some protection against the occurrence of ankle injury.

Handoll, H. H. G., Rowe, B. H., Quinn, K. M., & de Bie, R. (2007). Interventions for preventing ankle ligament injuries. *The Cochrane Library 2007, 4.*

should include discouraging participation when the teen is tired or has an existing injury.

Adolescence is a good time to develop an exercise program. The Public Health Agency of Canada (PHAC, 2011) recommends that youth ages 12 to 17 years participate in at least 60 minutes of moderate- to vigorous-intensity physical activity per day, with vigorous exercise at least three times a week. High levels of physical activity may reduce cardiovascular disease risk factors during adolescence. Nurses should encourage all adolescents to be physically active on a daily basis.

Promoting Learning

School, teachers, family, and peers influence education and learning for the adolescent. Also, activities such as athletics and club membership enhance learning through interactions with peers, coaches, club leaders, and others.

School

School plays an essential part in preparing adolescents for the future. Completing school prepares the adolescent for college or employment to make an adequate income. It is important to realize that schools may not meet the developmental needs of all adolescents. School performance may also suffer due to lack of parental involvement. A number of factors, such as single parent families and both parents being in the work force, can mean that parents have less time to devote to involvement in their child's school activities.

There is evidence that the transition from elementary school to middle school at age 12 or 13, and then the transition to high school, both of which occur during times of physical changes, may have a negative effect on teens. It is important to observe for transition problems into middle or high school, which may be exhibited by failing grades or behaviour problems. Also, students who experience difficulties in school, resulting in negative evaluations and failing grades, may feel alienated from school. Students with failing grades and those repeating grades exhibit more emotional behaviour, such as violence, and are more likely to engage in risky behaviours, such as tobacco and alcohol use (National Center for Chronic Disease Prevention and Health Promotion, 2010). Schools that support peer-group relationships, promote health and fitness, encourage parental involvement, and strengthen community relationships have better student outcomes. Parents, teachers, and health care providers should provide guidance and support.

Promoting Safety

Unintentional and intentional injuries are the leading cause of death in Canadians under the age of 19. Motor vehicle accidents are the leading cause of death among Canadian adolescents, with suicide ranking second. Drowning also ranks as a major concern and cause of death in this age group (PHAC, 2009a).

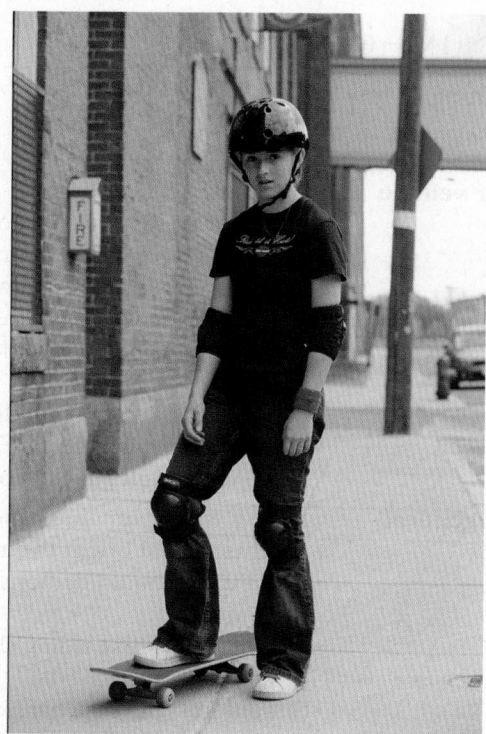

FIGURE 29.7 Wearing appropriate safety equipment can prevent injuries.

Influencing factors related to the prevalence of adolescent injuries include increased physical growth; insufficient psychomotor coordination for the task; abundance of energy; impulsivity; peer pressure; and inexperience. Impulsivity, inexperience, and peer pressure may place the teen in a vulnerable situation between knowing what is right and wanting to impress peers. On the other hand, teens have a feeling of invulnerability, which may contribute to negative outcomes. Alcohol and other drugs are contributing factors in accidents among adolescents. Most of the serious or fatal injuries in adolescents are preventable (Fig. 29.7). Nurses must educate parents and adolescents on car, gun, and water safety to prevent unintentional injuries. See Teaching Guideline 29.1 for information on promoting safety.

Motor Vehicle Safety

The largest numbers of adolescent injuries and deaths are due to motor vehicle accidents (PHAC, 2009a). When the adolescent passes his or her driving test, he or she is able to drive legally. However, driving is complex and requires judgments that the teen is often incapable of exhibiting. Also, the typical adolescent is opposed to authority and is interested in showing peers and others his or her independence.

It is essential to promote driver education, to teach about the importance of wearing seat belts, and to explain laws about teen driving and curfews (Fig. 29.8). See Teaching Guideline 29.1 for additional information.

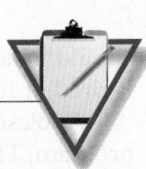

TEACHING GUIDELINE 29.1

Promoting Safety

Safety Issue	Activities
Motor vehicle	• Wear seat belt at all times. • Do not drive with someone who is impaired. • Take driver-education course. • Establish driving rules between parent and adolescent prior to getting license. • Have all passengers wear seat belts. • Do not use cell phone while driving. • Do not drink and drive. • Maintain car in good condition. • Do not drive when tired. • Drive with adult supervision for a certain period of time after receiving license.
Bike: general	• Have a well-maintained and appropriate-size bike for adolescent. • Parents should orient the adolescent to the bike. • Adolescent should demonstrate his or her ability to ride bike safely before being allowed to ride on street. • Safe areas for bike riding should be established as well as routes to and from area of activities. • Should not ride bike barefoot, with someone else on bike, or with clothing that might get entangled in the bike • Should wear sturdy, well-fitting shoes • Should wear Canadian Standards Association (CSA)–approved helmets • Bike should be inspected often to ensure it is in proper working order. • A basket should be used to carry heavy objects.
Bike: in traffic	• All traffic signs and signals must be observed. • If riding at night, the bike should have lights and reflectors and the rider should wear light-coloured clothes. • Should ride on the side of the road travelling with traffic • Should keep close to the side of the road and in single file • Should watch and listen for cars • Should not wear headphones while riding a bike • Never hitch a ride on any vehicles.
All-terrain vehicles	• Should not be operated by adolescent less than 16 years of age • Should wear helmet and protective coverings • No nighttime riding • Should not be used on public roads • Should not stand up in the vehicle or ride in a person's lap • Should not drive if drinking or using drugs
Skateboards/skates	• Should wear helmet, and protective padding on knees, elbows, and wrists • Should not skate in traffic or on streets or highways • Skating on homemade ramps could be dangerous—should assess ramps for any hazards before skating.
Water safety	• Learn how to swim. • If swimming skill is limited, must wear life preserver at all times • Never swim alone—should if at all possible, swim only where there is a life guard • Should be taught basic cardiopulmonary resuscitation (CPR) • Should not run or fool around at edge of pool • Drains in pool should be covered with appropriate cover. • Should wear life jacket when on boat • Make sure there is enough water to support diving. • Should not swim if drinking alcohol or using drugs

TEACHING GUIDELINE 29.1 (continued)

Promoting Safety

Safety Issue	Activities
Firearms	• Should never pick up a gun • If guns are in household, should take firearm safety class • If have guns in household, need to secure them in safe place, use gun safety locks, store bullets in separate place • Never point a gun at a person.
Fire safety	• All homes should have working smoke detectors and fire extinguishers. • Change the batteries at least twice a year. • Should have fire-escape plan • Should practice fire-escape plan routinely • Nobody should smoke in bed. • Should teach what to do in case of a fire: use fire extinguisher, call 911, and how to put out clothing fire • All flammable materials and liquids should be stored safely. • Fireplaces should have protective gratings. • Avoid touching any downed power lines.
Machinery	• Use safety devices. • Receive training on how to use equipment. • Do not use when alone.
Sports	• Match sport to adolescent's ability and desire. • Sports program should have warm-up procedure and hydration policy. • Should undergo sports physical before start of activity • Coaches should be trained in CPR and first aid. • Should wear appropriate protection devices for individual sport
Sun	• Use sunscreen with an SPF of 15 or higher. • Apply sunscreen prior to going out. • Reapply sunscreen often. • Limit sun exposure, especially between 10 AM and 4 PM. • Wear hat when working outside. • Wear sunglasses while outside.
Personal safety	• Never go with a stranger. • Do not enter a car when the driver has been drinking. • Notify adult where you are when out after dark. • Keep cell phone fully charged. • Never give out personal information over the Internet. • Say "no" to drugs, alcohol, smoking, or to being touched when you do not want to be touched.
Toxins	• Teach the hazards of accepting illegal drugs, alcohol, dangerous drugs. • Store potentially dangerous material in safe place.

Adapted from: American Academy of Pediatrics, Council on Environmental Health and Section on Dermatology (2011). *Policy statement—Ultraviolet radiation: A hazard to children and adolescents.* Retrieved February 22, 2012 from http://aappolicy.aappublications.org/cgi/reprint/pediatrics;127/3/588. pdf and Hagan, J. F., Shaw, J. S., & Duncan, P. (2008). *Bright futures guidelines for health supervision of infants, children, and adolescents* (3rd ed.). Elk Grove Village, IL: American Academy of Pediatrics.

Firearm Safety

In Canada, the rate of firearm-related offences among youth is increasing, with the highest rates of gun violence occurring in urban areas (Statistics Canada, 2008). Guns in the home must be kept locked in a safe location, with ammunition stored separately. The availability of guns to individuals who are at risk for suicide is a major issue. See Teaching Guideline 29.1 for additional information on gun safety.

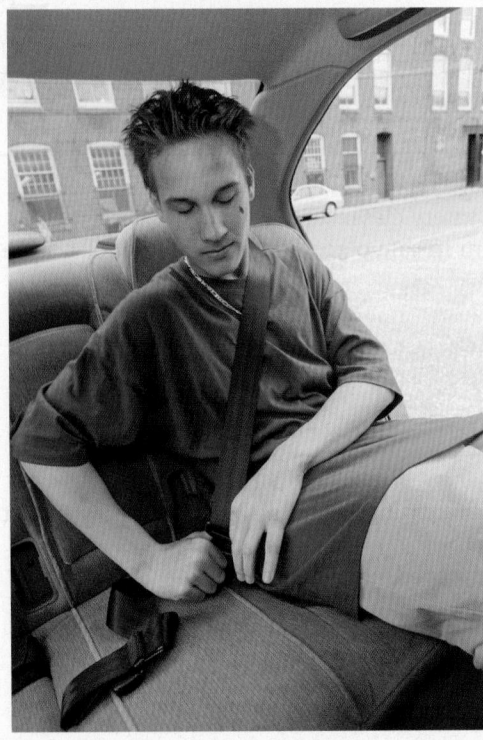

FIGURE 29.8 The use of seat belts has led to fewer fatal injuries in car accidents.

Water Safety

Drowning is a needless cause of death in adolescents. Many drownings are a result of risk-taking behaviours. With the growing independence of the adolescent, the lack of adult supervision could result in the teen taking a risk that results in drowning. Provide water safety education and proper supervision to decrease the incidence of risk taking. Teach about swimming lessons for nonswimmers. See Teaching Guideline 29.1 for additional information.

Remember Lisa Chung, the 15-year-old presented at the beginning of the chapter? What anticipatory guidance related to safety should you provide to Lisa and her mother?

Promoting Nutrition

Multiple factors influence the adolescent's diet and eating habits (Box 29.2). Dietary and lifestyle factors are two of the reasons cited for the increasing rates of overweight and obesity in Canadian adolescents. The overweight rate for

---

BOX 29.2 **Factors Influencing the Adolescent's Diet**

- Peer pressure
- Busy schedules
- Concern about weight control
- Convenience of fast food

Canadian adolescents is 26%, and the obesity rate is 9%. Over the past 25 years, the overweight rate has more than doubled and the obesity rate has tripled (Statistics Canada, 2005a).

Nutritional Needs

Nutritional needs are increased during adolescence due to accelerated growth and sexual maturation, with an increased need for zinc, calcium, and iron for growth. Adolescents may appear to be hungry constantly and need regular meals and snacks with adequate nutrients to meet the body's anaerobic requirements. However, the number of calories needed for adolescence depends on the teen's age and activity level as well as growth patterns. Teenage girls who are moderately active require about 2,000 calories per day, while moderately active teenage boys require between 2,400 and 2,800 calories per day (U.S. Department of Agriculture and U.S. Department of Health and Human Services, 2010). Canada's Food Guide emphasizes that calories are only one aspect of healthy eating and that a focus on calorie counting can result in making less healthy food choices. The amounts and types of food servings recommended for each age group were determined to meet all nutritional needs. According to Statistics Canada (2005a), almost 60% of children and adolescents reported consuming the five recommended daily servings of fruits and vegetables.

Nutritional Assessment

The nurse must understand normal growth and development of the adolescent in order to provide guidance that fits the quest for independence and the need for teens to make their own choices. Assess the eating habits and diet preferences of the adolescent. The assessment should include an evaluation of foods from the different food groups that the adolescent eats each day. Also, assess the number of times that fast foods, snacks, and other junk food are eaten per week. This assessment will help the nurse to guide the adolescent in making better food choices at home and in fast-food establishments. Many fast-food restaurants offer baked chicken sandwiches and salads with fewer calories and less fat. Adolescents may be guided in alternating hamburger and fries with more nutritious choices. Remember that planning should always include the adolescent.

Nutritional Guidelines

Canada's Food Guide was developed to meet the needs of people of all ages for vitamins, minerals, and other nutrients; to reduce the risk of obesity, type 2 diabetes, heart disease, certain types of cancer, and osteoporosis; and to contribute to overall health and vitality (see Appendix H). Table 29.3 outlines daily serving recommendations for children and adolescents between 9 and 18 years of age. Nurses may use the information in Table 29.3 and Box 29.3 to help teens plan a healthy diet for themselves.

TABLE 29.3 CANADA'S FOOD GUIDE: RECOMMENDED NUMBER OF SERVINGS FOR CHILDREN AND ADOLESCENTS (SEE APPENDIX H)

Food Group	Children Ages 9–13 Years	Teens Ages 14–18 Years	
		Females	Males
Vegetables and fruit	6	7	8
Grain products	6	6	7
Milk and alternatives	3–4	3–4	3–4
Meat and alternatives	1–2	2	3

Adapted from: Health Canada. (2007a). *Eating well with Canada's Food Guide*. Retrieved August 23, 2011 from http://www.hc-sc.gc.ca/fn-an/food-guide-aliment/order-commander/eating_well_bien_manger-eng.php.

What questions should you ask Lisa Chung and her mother related to nutritional intake? What anticipatory guidance related to nutrition would be appropriate?

Promoting Healthy Sleep and Rest

The average number of hours of sleep that teens require per night is 8.5 to 9.5 (KidsHealth, 2011). The adolescent often experiences a change in sleep patterns that leads to feeling more awake at night and the desire to sleep later in the morning (KidsHealth, 2011). Also, in this independence-seeking phase of adolescence, the teen may stay up later to do homework or to complete projects and may have difficulty awakening in the morning. Due to early school schedules and activities, the teen will often try to make up for needed sleep by sleeping longer hours on the weekend. Explain to parents the need to discourage late hours on school nights because it may affect school performance.

Rapid growth and increased activities may produce fatigue and the need for more rest. Parents may relate that the teen sleeps all the time and never has the time or energy to help with household chores. Provide advice to teens and parents about having realistic expectations; encourage them to agree on a level of normalcy and

adequate rest for the teen so that he or she can still fulfill responsibilities in the home.

Provide anticipatory guidance to Lisa Chung and her mother in relation to sleep during the adolescent years.

Promoting Healthy Teeth and Gums

Most permanent teeth have erupted with the possible exception of the third molars (wisdom teeth). These molars may become impacted and require surgical removal. The rate of cavities decreases but the need for routine dental visits every 6 months, daily flossing, and brushing two to three times per day is very important. Some of the conditions that occur during adolescence include malocclusion, gingivitis, and tooth evulsion (knocked-out teeth). Malocclusion occurs in approximately 50% of adolescents, resulting from facial and mandibular bone growth. The treatment includes braces and other dental devices. Teach the adolescent to brush the teeth more frequently if he or she has braces or other dental devices. Gingivitis is the inflammation of the gums and breakdown of gingival epithelium due to diet and hormonal changes. The use of dental devices/braces makes cleaning more difficult and contributes to gingivitis. Tooth evulsion may occur during sports activities and other incidents such as falls. The avulsed tooth should be reimplanted as soon as possible. The nurse may see the teen first so it is important that nurses know the proper procedure, which is to reinsert the tooth into its socket if possible or to store it in cool milk or normal saline for transport to the dentist.

Promoting Personal Care

Promotion of personal care during adolescence is an important topic to cover with the adolescent and his or her parents. Topics to discuss include general hygiene tips, caring for body piercings and tattoos, preventing suntanning, and promoting a healthy sexual identity.

General Hygiene Tips

Adolescents find that frequent baths and deodorant use are important due to apocrine sweat gland secretory activity. Also, to decrease oily skin due to sexual steroids

---

BOX 29.3 **Iron-Rich Foods**

- Liver, kidney, and other organ meats
- Mussels and clams
- Dried peas, beans, and lentils
- Wheat germ
- Sardines
- Blackstrap molasses
- Brown barley
- Currants, raisins, and other dried fruits
- Granola

Adapted from: Toronto Public Health. (2008). *Nutrition matters: Loading up with iron-rich foods*. Retrieved November 1, 2011 from http://www.toronto.ca/health/pdf/loadingup.pdf.

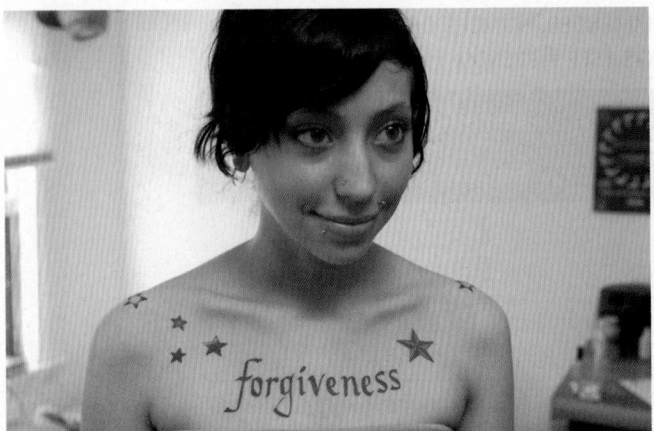

FIGURE 29.9 Having multiple piercings and tattoos can lead to certain health risks.

and hormones, the adolescent should be told to wash his or her face two to three times per day with plain unscented soap. Vigorous scrubbing should be discouraged because it could irritate the skin and lead to follicular rupture. The hair should be shampooed daily to remove excess oil from the hair and scalp. Many over-the-counter medications are available for beginning acne or acne with a few lesions. These preparations may cause drying or redness. Squeezing acne lesions should be discouraged to prevent further irritation and permanent scarring. If the adolescent has severe acne, encourage him or her to ask a parent to make an appointment with a dermatologist.

Caring for Body Piercings and Tattoos

It is not uncommon for a teen to experiment with body piercing on areas such as the tongue, lip, eyebrow, navel, and nipple (Fig. 29.9). Other sites, including the genitals, chin cleft, knuckles, and uvula, have also been used. Generally, body piercing is harmless, but nurses should caution teens about performing these procedures under nonsterile conditions and should educate them about complications. Qualified personnel using sterile needles should perform the procedure. Teach the adolescent to cleanse the pierced area twice a day and more often at some sites.

The complications of body piercing vary by site. Infections from body piercing usually result from unclean tools of the trade. Some of the infections that may occur as a result of unclean tools include hepatitis, tetanus, tuberculosis, and human immunodeficiency virus (HIV). Also, keloid formation and allergies to metal may occur. The navel is an area prone to infection because it is a moist area that endures friction from clothing. After a navel infection occurs, it may take up to a year to heal. Pierced ear cartilage also heals slowly and is prone to infection. Tongue piercings heal very quickly, usually within 4 weeks, probably due to the antiseptic effects of saliva. Other concerns with tongue piercing include tooth damage from biting on the jewelry or partial paralysis if the jewelry pierces a nerve.

Tattoos are continuing to grow in popularity among adolescents (U.S. Food and Drug Administration, 2009) and serve to define one's identity (see Fig. 29.9). Because of the invasiveness of the tattooing procedure, it should be considered a health-risk situation. Like piercings, tattoos are open wounds that are predisposed to infection (Centers for Disease Control and Prevention, 2006).

Nurses should educate adolescents about the risk of blood-borne infections, such as hepatitis B and C as well as HIV, skin infections, scarring, and allergic reactions to dyes used in the tattoo process (U.S. Food and Drug Administration, 2009). Teach teens to cleanse tattoos with an antibacterial soap and water several times a day and to keep the area moist with an ointment to prevent scab formation. Refer to Box 29.4 for additional information about tattoos.

Preventing Suntanning

Suntanning is popular among adolescents and is influenced by the media, which promotes a link between tan skin and beauty. However, tans and sunburns are both signs of ultraviolet (UV) radiation damage (Health Canada, 2011b). Most exposure to UV rays occurs during childhood and adolescence, thereby putting people at risk for the development of skin cancer. However, it is difficult to convince adolescents that tanning is harmful to their skin and puts them at risk for skin cancer later in life.

Educate teens about the benefits and effects of different sun protection products. Explain to them that sun damage and skin cancers can be prevented if sunscreens are used as directed on a regular basis. Encourage sunscreen or sunblock use for water sports, beach activities, and participation in outdoor sports. Also, make adolescents aware of allergies to some sunscreen products. See Teaching Guideline 29.1 for additional information.

Promoting a Healthy Sexual Identity

Encourage parents and teens to have discussions about sexuality. In addition, nurses should ensure that

---

BOX 29.4 **What Adolescents Need to Know About Tattooing**

- Infections occur as a result of nonsterile equipment used in the procedure.
- Tattoos are open wounds predisposing to infection; sites require proper care with antibacterial soap and water several times per day and application of ointment.
- For most people a tattoo is permanent; new procedures for removal are painful and expensive.

Adapted from: American Academy of Pediatrics. (2010). *Ages & stages: Tattoos.* Retrieved March 26, 2011, from http://www.healthy-children.org/English/ages-stages/teen/safety/pages/Tattoos.aspx

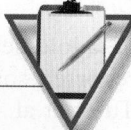

TEACHING GUIDELINE 29.2

Adolescent Sexuality

- It should be your choice to engage in sexual relations. Do not be influenced by peers. When you say "no," be firm and clear about your position.
- Pregnancy, sexually transmitted infections, and human immunodeficiency virus (HIV) infection can occur with any sexual encounter without the use of barrier methods of contraception. Use appropriate contraception if sexually active. Discuss abstinence as a contraceptive method.
- Sexual activity in a mature relationship should be pleasurable to both parties. If your sexual partner is not interested in your pleasure, you need to reconsider the relationship.
- "Sexting," or sending and receiving sexually explicit messages or pictures electronically, can result in this information being widely disseminated. Once such images exist in cyberspace, they may continue indefinitely and result in unintended social, psychological, and legal consequences (e.g., distribution of child pornography) (Katzman, 2010).

adolescents have the knowledge, skills, and opportunities that enable them to make responsible decisions regarding sexual behaviours. Education for the adolescent should include a discussion about media influences and the use of sexuality to promote products. This discussion should make the adolescent aware of the motives of the media and the need to be an individual and not be influenced by advertising. Encourage parents to be aware of who their adolescents are dating and where they go on their dates. Refer to Teaching Guideline 29.2 for information on counselling related to adolescent sexuality.

Promoting Positive Discipline

Adolescents may challenge or not follow the rules of the house possibly due to their egocentricity or feelings of invulnerability. Adolescents need to know the reasons for rules and expectations and should be part of the discussion of their development.

Offer guidance to parents related to positive discipline. Parents should acknowledge and offer reinforcement and support when the teen follows the rules and expectations. Consistency and predictability are important, and praise is a powerful reinforcer of learning.

Addressing Common Developmental Concerns

Adolescence is a time of rapid growth and development with maturation of sexuality. The adolescent period begins with a child and ends with the expectation of adulthood. There are many developmental concerns that present during this period, including obesity, violence, suicide, and homicide. The following is an overview of some of these concerns.

Obesity

From 1979 to 2004, the obesity rate for Canadian adolescents 12 to 17 years of age tripled from 3% to 9% (Statistics Canada, 2005a). Although obesity has increased in all segments of the Canadian population, there are differences specific to race, ethnicity, and other factors that contribute to obesity. The prevalence of obesity in Aboriginal adolescents is 20%, or more than 2½ times the national average (Statistics Canada, 2005a). Although lower socioeconomic status tends to be associated with obesity in adults, the same relationship is not as strong or as consistent in children (Statistics Canada, 2005a).

This increase in obesity in adolescents can lead to increases in hypertension, heart disease, and type 2 diabetes, although these related health problems are not usually evident until later in life. However, there is cause for concern because overweight and obesity are likely to persist into adulthood (Statistics Canada, 2005a). Influential factors causing obesity include poor food choices and eating practices in conjunction with lack of exercise. Adolescents are busy and eat on the run with many meals from fast-food facilities. A general decrease in physical activity has resulted in a more sedentary lifestyle leading to weight gain. Increased time spent playing computer games and watching television has decreased physical activity and exercise and further contributed to weight gain and obesity.

Nurses must make parents and adolescents aware of the factors leading to obesity. Nurses should recommend:

- Proper nutrition and healthy food choices according to Canada's Food Guide
- Good eating habits
- Decreased fast-food intake
- Exercising for 30 minutes on a daily basis
- Parents/adolescents exercising more at home
- Decreased computer use and television watching

Violence

PHAC (2009b) defines youth violence as any intentional assault on another person(s) by one or more individuals 12 to 19 years of age. Although a growing number of female youth are participating in violent acts, the perpetrators are most commonly young heterosexual males, who display more frequent and more severe types of violent behaviours. Most of the victims of youth violence are also youth, most commonly girlfriends of boyfriends, peers, family members, and members of ethnocultural groups or sexual minorities. Due to a lack of consensus on what constitutes youth violence and the fact that statistics do not give the whole picture of violence, the extent of the issue is difficult to determine (PHAC, 2009b). See Box 29.5 for factors contributing to adolescent violence.

BOX 29.5 Factors Contributing to Adolescent Violence

- Crowded conditions/housing
- Low socioeconomic status
- Limited parental supervision
- Single parent families/both parents in work force
- Access to guns or cars
- Drug or alcohol use
- Low self-esteem
- Racism
- Peer or gang pressure
- Aggression

Adapted from: Centers for Disease Control and Prevention. (2011). *Youth Violence: Risk and Protective Factors. Risk Factors for the Perpetration of Youth Violence.* Retrieved on December 13, 2011 at http://www.cdc.gov/ViolencePrevention/youthviolence/riskprotectivefactors.html

Homicide

Homicide is the fourth leading cause of death in Canada for youth and young adults between the ages of 15 and 24 years (Statistics Canada, 2009). Law enforcement data indicate that the use of guns in violent crimes among young people is increasing: between 2002 and 2006, fire-arm-related criminal offences rose 32% for youth 12 to 17 years of age (Statistics Canada, 2008). Refer to Box 29.5 for factors that contribute to violence among adolescents.

Suicide

After unintentional injuries (primarily motor vehicle accidents), suicide is the second leading cause of death among young Canadians between 15 and 24 years of age and the fourth leading cause of death in children up to 14 years of age (Statistics Canada, 2009). Of particular concern is the suicide rate among Aboriginal teens, which is five to six times higher than that of non-Aboriginal teens and among the highest in the world. The suicide rate among Inuit adolescents is 11 times higher than non-Aboriginal rates (Health Canada, 2006).

The causes of suicide are complex and may range from seemingly (to others) nonserious matters to overwhelming issues that overload a young person's coping mechanisms; suicide is ultimately about escape (Canadian Mental Health Association, 2011). Young people feel tremendous pressure from a number of sources, such as school, home, and social groups. Many more youth attempt suicide than die from it. Although suicidal youth are not likely to make a direct plea for help, and despite the fact that there is no comprehensive list of warning signs, the Canadian Mental Health Association (2011) provides some common warning signs as outlined in Box 29.6.

Dating Violence

Violent behaviour that takes place in a context of dating is not uncommon. Canadian research indicates that 29%

of adolescent females and 13% of adolescent males reported some incidence of abuse in their relationship. Tutty et al. (2005) reported that teen dating violence is similar to adult intimate partner violence, which exists on a continuum from verbal and emotional abuse to sexual assault and murder. Some of the reasons identified for dating violence include a way to show anger, self-defence, and control; the use of alcohol increases the likelihood of dating violence. Predictors of dating violence that have been identified for males include having witnessed violence within the family (O'Keefe, 1997; Tutty et al., 2005). There are a number of prevention programs in Canada that address youth dating violence. Information on such programs can be accessed through the School-Based Violence Prevention Programs website; the direct link can be accessed on http://thePoint. lww.com/Chow1e.

Gangs

According to the Canadian Research Institute for Law and the Family (2005), it appears that the number of gangs—and therefore gang-related activity such as homicides and drug incidents—is increasing. The formation and composition of youth gangs is influenced by factors such as age, ethnicity, and socioeconomic status. Generally, the degree of organization and the type of activities in which members engage tend to distinguish the different types of youth gangs. At-risk youth are frequently targeted for membership. There are both national and provincial programs and resources in place trying to address the numerous and complex issues associated with youth gangs.

BOX 29.6 Risk Factors for Suicide in Adolescents

- Sudden change in behaviour (for better or worse)
- Withdrawal from friends and activities
- Lack of interest
- Increased use of alcohol and other drugs
- Recent loss of a friend, family member, or parent, especially if from suicide
- Conflicting feelings or a sense of shame about being gay or straight
- Mood swings, emotional outbursts, high level of irritability or aggression
- Feelings of hopelessness
- Preoccupation with death, giving away valued possessions
- Talk of suicide (e.g., "No one cares if I live or die")
- Increased risk taking
- Writing or drawing about suicide (e.g., in a diary)
- "Hero worship" of people who have died by suicide

Adapted from: Canadian Mental Health Association. (2011). *Youth and suicide.* Retrieved February 22, 2012 from http://www.cmha.ca/bins/content_page.asp?cid=3-101-104.

Nursing Interventions to Decrease Youth Violence

Nurses working with adolescents should include violence prevention in anticipatory guidance. Violence is a learned behaviour that is often reinforced by the media, television, music, and personal example. Explain to parents, teachers, and peers the importance of being good role models. Parents should monitor video games, music, television, and other media to decrease their teen's exposure to violence. Parents need to know who their adolescent's friends are and monitor for negative behaviours and actions.

The identification of adolescents at risk for suicide is a very important task for nurses, parents, peers, and counsellors. See Box 29.6 for signs of risk factors.

Substance Use

Agents commonly abused by children and adolescents include alcohol, hallucinogens, sedatives, analgesics, anxiolytics, steroids, inhalants, and stimulants. The substance abused is related to its availability and cost. Two common substances that are more accessible and have the highest incidence of use are tobacco and alcohol. Research consistently supports the hypothesis that drug use progresses from beer or wine to cigarettes or hard liquor and then to marijuana, followed by illicit drugs.

Some of the long-term effects and consequences of drug and alcohol use include: possibility of overdose and death; unintentional injuries; irrational behaviours; inability to think clearly; unsafe driving and legal conse-quences; problems with relationships with family and friends; sexual activity and STIs; and health problems such as liver problems (hepatitis) and cardiac problems (sudden death with cocaine). Refer to Table 29.4 for commonly abused drugs and behaviours exhibited.

Tobacco

Tobacco is the primary risk factor for preventable death and disease in Canada, causing more than 45,000 deaths each year (Canadian Lung Association, 2011). The long-term consequences of youth smoking are reinforced by the fact that most young people who smoke regularly continue to do so throughout adulthood. Health Canada (2010) reports that the rate of smoking among adolescents 15 to 19 years of age is on the decline; it is currently 14%—the lowest rate recorded for youth in this age group. A higher percentage of male youth (16%) compared with female youth (12%) smoke. The Federal Tobacco Control Strategy aims to reduce the prevalence of smoking for this age group to 9% by 2011. Some reasons given by teens when asked why they started smoking are because their friends smoke, they just wanted to try it, they thought it was cool, or their parents smoke (Canadian Lung Association, 2011).

The short-term health effects of smoking include damage to the respiratory system, addiction to nicotine, and the associated risk of other drug use. In a study of Canadian young adults ages 15 to 24, rates of marijuana use were highest among current smokers and lowest

TABLE 29.4 DRUGS COMMONLY ABUSED

Drug	Manifestations	Considerations
Marijuana	Red eyes, dry mouth, euphoria, relaxation, decreased motivation, loss of inhibition, appetite stimulation	Considered a gateway drug
Cocaine	Weight loss, euphoria, elation, agitation, increased motor activity, pressured speech, tachycardia, hypertension, anorexia, insomnia	Psychotic behaviour with large doses; if combined with other drugs can be fatal
Opiates	Elation, euphoria, detachment, drowsiness, constricted pupils, slurred speech, impaired judgment	Self-neglect with malnutrition and dehydration; criminal behaviours to get drugs; infections at injection sites
Amphetamines	Euphoria, agitation, weight loss, insomnia, tachycardia, hypertension	Possible paradoxical effect of depression in children
Hallucinogens	Hallucinations, illusions, depersonalization, heightened awareness, dilated pupils, hypertension, increased salivation, distorted perceptions	Panic flashbacks long after use of drugs; psychotic behaviours
PCP	Euphoria, distorted perceptions, agitation, violence, antisocial behaviours, hypertension, increased salivation, increased pain response	Irrational behaviours, panic, psychosis
Barbiturates	Euphoria followed by depression or hostility; impaired judgment; decreased inhibitions; slurred speech; incoordination	Often used with stimulants; may have a paradoxical effect of hyperactivity in children

PCP, phencyclidine hydrochloride.

Adapted from: Jenkins, R. R., & Adger, A. (2007). Substance abuse. In R. M. Kleigman, R. E. Behrman, H. B. Jenson, & B. F. Stanton (Eds.), *Nelson Textbook of Pediatrics* (18th ed.). Philadelphia: Saunders.

among those who had never tried smoking (Leatherdale, Hammond, Kaiserman, et al., 2007). Smoking negatively impacts physical fitness and lung growth and increases the potential for addiction in adolescents. Smokeless tobacco may also cause many problems, including bleeding gums and mouth sores that never heal. Smokeless tobacco, although not as commonly used as cigarettes, also leads to discoloration of the teeth and eventually may lead to cancer.

Alcohol

Alcohol is the most commonly used substance among Canadian youth. In an expansive survey of substance use among youth, 91% of 15- to 24-year-olds reporting that they have consumed alcohol and 77% of 15- to 19-year-olds reporting drinking alcohol during the previous year (Health Canada, 2007b). For those young people who reported consuming alcohol during the previous year, more than one third reported doing so at least once a week and another third reported consuming five or more drinks in a typical drinking situation. The most common pattern of alcohol consumption among youth, reported by 40% of those surveyed, was light/infrequent drinking (Health Canada, 2007b).

Some of the problems associated with alcohol use in teens include impaired school or work performance; interpersonal problems with friends, family, teachers, and supervisors; physical and psychological impairment; unsafe sexual activity; and impaired driving. Alcohol use as an adolescent can lead to prevailing alcohol use as an adult and can contribute to physical health problems. Like tobacco, alcohol is considered a "gateway drug" that can lead to other types of substance use and abuse.

Illicit Drugs

Adolescents may also experiment with or abuse illicit drugs. Among Canadian teenagers, cannabis was the most frequently reported illicit drug used at 39.3%, followed by 5.2% reporting use of cocaine, speed, ecstasy, hallucinogens, and/or heroin (Health Canada, 2007b). The use of inhalants by young adolescents has been a more recent concern, particularly in northern Aboriginal communities as well as in urban areas, although; actual usage rates are unknown. Inhalants are often readily available and include model glue, contact cement, lacquers, and aerosols. In addition to the risks associated with other intoxicants, these substances can cause long-term neurological deficits (Health Canada, 2011a).

Data reveal that illicit use of individual drugs reflects rapidly changing determinants specific to that drug. Influencing factors include the psychoactive potential of the drug and the reported benefits, how risky the drug is to use, how acceptable it is to peer groups, and the accessibility of the drug (Johnston, O'Malley, & Bachman, 2002). Some teenagers are at greater risk for drug use than others, such as those who have mental health disor-

ders, those with a family member who has a drug or alcohol problem, and those who are involved in the legal system or are living on the street (Canadian Medical Association, 2008).

Nursing Interventions to Decrease Substance Use Among Teens

Nurses should educate the adolescent on the problems related to alcohol use and abuse. Topics that should be discussed include:

- Short- and long-term effects of alcohol, tobacco, and drugs on health
- Risk factors and implications for unintentional injuries and sexual activity
- Short- and long-term effects of alcohol, tobacco, and drugs on relationships and school performance and progression
- The how and why of chemical dependency
- Impact of substance abuse on society
- Importance of maintaining a healthy lifestyle
- Importance of resisting peer pressure to use drugs and alcohol
- Importance of having confidence in his or her own judgment
- Accurate and up to date drug information, such as that provided online by Health Canada's Not4Me program; visit http:thePoint.lww.com/Chow1e for the direct link to their website.

Sexually Transmitted Infections and Teen Pregnancy

The average age of first sexual intercourse in Canada is reported to be 16.5 years for both males and females. Oral sexual activity is reportedly about as common as sexual intercourse for sexually active teens. Oral sexual activity precedes the initiation of first sexual intercourse for up to 25% of adolescents (Maticka-Tyndale, 2008; Rottermann, 2008).

Although adolescence is known as a time of risk taking, with unprotected sex and multiple sex partners placing teens at risk for HIV infection, other STIs, and pregnancy, recent findings indicate that most Canadian adolescents are assuming responsibility for their sexual health by using condoms and other forms of contraception and seeking out abortion far more than any previous Canadian generation (Maticka-Tyndale, 2008). However, STIs and unwanted pregnancy continue to be issues for this age group.

Sexually Transmitted Infections

Some of the most prevalent STIs include chlamydia, gonorrhea, human papillomavirus (HPV), and herpes. In Canada, chlamydia is the most commonly reported STI, with rates increasing 73.6% from 1998 to 2007 and the female rate reportedly twice that of males (PHAC, 2007).

The highest chlamydia rates have been reported in Northern Canada, specifically Nunavut, the Northwest Territories, and Yukon (PHAC, 2007). Rates of gonorrhea have also been increasing overall over the past decade, particularly for females between the ages of 15 and 24 and males between the ages of 20 and 24. Like chlamydia, the distribution of gonorrhea cases varies across Canada, with the highest reported rates in the Northwest Territories and Nunavut, followed by Manitoba and Saskatchewan (PHAC, 2007). A number of geographical, social, and economic forces are responsible for the increased rates in these areas in comparison with other geographic areas of Canada.

Female adolescents are more susceptible to STIs due to their anatomy. During adolescence and young adulthood, women's columnar epithelial cells are especially sensitive to invasion by sexually transmitted organisms such as *Chlamydia* and *Gonococcus*. These cells extend out over the vaginal surface of the cervix during youth, where they are unprotected by cervical mucus, but recede to a more protected location as women age. STIs are covered in Chapter 36.

Exposure to the HIV virus most commonly occurs through unprotected vaginal, anal, or oral sex with someone who has the virus. Other methods of HIV exposure include sharing needles and syringes or using the same unsterilized tattoo or piercing needles that someone with the virus has used.

Certain groups of Canadian teens are at most risk for STIs. Geographical, social, and economic forces in rural and northern locations may create environments that increase the likelihood that youth will become sexually active early in their teens or become victims of sexual abuse, both of which make them more susceptible to STIs. In addition, they may not have the same kinds of social support and resources available to them as in urban areas. Other groups of adolescents at high risk are those who are gay, lesbian, bisexual, transgender, or questioning, as these teens may not feel comfortable seeking help as they struggle to make sense of their feelings and experiences, which may be at odds with those of their family and the prevailing culture (Maticka-Tyndale, 2008).

Health care providers may help these adolescents to understand their situation if:

• Confidentiality is ensured
• Information is explained clearly and at a level the adolescent understands
• Opportunities are provided for the adolescent to ask questions
• Success is emphasized with proper treatment and follow-up

Teen Pregnancy

In Canada, pregnancy rates among adolescents have been declining over the past few decades. The pregnancy rate is highest among 18- to 19-year-olds, many of whom have planned their pregnancies, whereas among 15- to 17-year-olds the rate is lower but includes a higher proportion of unplanned pregnancies (Canadian Paediatric Society, 2006; Statistics Canada, 2005b). Abortion rates are high, with just over 50% of adolescent pregnancies resulting in induced abortions performed in hospitals and clinics (Statistics Canada, 2005b).

Teen pregnancy rates are highest in the North and the prairie provinces, peaking among Aboriginal teenagers. Twenty-four percent of teenage mothers identified themselves as Aboriginal compared with 10% of other teenage mothers (Luong, 2008).

Adolescents are more likely to produce a low birth weight infant, which increases the incidence of infant mortality and childhood illness. Teen pregnancy can pose health risks for both mother and infant, particularly for younger adolescents. Pregnant teens are at risk for anemia, hypertension, renal disease, eclampsia, and depressive disorders (Combes-Orme, 1993; Turner, Grindstaff, & Phillips, 1990, as cited in Dryburgh, 2007). Infants born to teenage mothers are at risk for low birth weight and other issues that may result from lack of prenatal care, poor nutrition, smoking, use of illicit drugs, STIs, and inadequate parenting skills (Health Canada, 2011a).

Nursing Interventions to Prevent STIs and Teen Pregnancy

Talk to adolescents about sexuality and encourage discussions with parents. Nurses need to be open and respectful of the teen's decision about sexual activity. If adolescents are sexually active, they should be directed to teen clinics and contraceptive options should be explained. In areas where specialized teen clinics are not available, nurses should feel comfortable discussing sexuality, safety, and contraception with teenage patients. The adolescent's lack of abstract thinking may influence contraceptive practices, and feelings of invulnerability may lead to HIV, STIs, or unwanted pregnancies. Nurses in schools and community clinics are in a position to identify these at-risk teens and to provide guidance, suitable information, and appropriate referrals. Both males and females share the responsibility for birth control. If possible, it is best to meet with both partners when selecting a method of birth control. For information about adolescent contraceptive methods, visit the websites of the following organizations: Sexuality and U, Sexuality Education Resource Centre Manitoba, and Aboriginal Sexual Health (direct links available at http://thePoint.lww.com/Chow1e). All adolescents require frequent ongoing follow-up to maintain contraception behaviours.

If a teen pregnancy does occur, the Canadian Paediatric Society (2006) recommends that the following actions be taken by the primary care practitioner:

• Inquire about the physical and emotional effects of her pregnancy.

- Determine her knowledge of the options and her feelings about these options.
- Explore any family, cultural, or community issues that may play a role in her situation.
- When appropriate, explore her partner's opinion about the options and discuss his role in the young woman's decision-making process.
- Establish the extent of her support system. (Who has she told about the pregnancy? How have they reacted? Who may provide support during the decision-making process?)
- Assess for any underlying health issues and for any complications.
- Assess for current substance use and other high-risk health behaviours.
- Review housing and school status as well as the adolescent's personal and academic goals.

In cases in which the health care practitioner is unable to counsel and/or follow up with a pregnant teen about her options, she or he has a responsibility to refer the teen to appropriate professionals and resources.

Think back to Lisa, who was introduced at the beginning of the chapter. List common developmental concerns of the adolescent. What anticipatory guidance related to these concerns would you provide?

■■■ Key Concepts

- Adolescence is a period of rapid and variable growth in the areas of physical, psychosocial, cognitive, and moral development.
- The adolescent is developing his own identity, becoming an abstract thinker, and developing his own set of morals and values. Inability to successfully develop an individual identity leads to poor preparation for the challenges of adulthood.
- Relationships with parents fluctuate widely during adolescence. The teenager eventually becomes emancipated from her parents.
- Peers become important—guiding mainly the early and middle adolescent in his decisions, while the late adolescent can usually formulate his own decisions.
- Adolescence is a critical time in the development of sexuality. Sexuality includes the thoughts, feelings, and behaviours surrounding the adolescent's sexual identity.
- The egocentric and invincible thought processes of the adolescent can lead to injuries. Health care providers must emphasize safety regarding cars, bikes, water, firearms, and fire.
- Motor vehicle accidents are the number one cause of death in adolescents.

- The nutritional habits of the adolescent can lead to deficiency in the vitamins and minerals needed for rapid growth during this period.
- Obesity in adolescents is a growing health concern. Health care providers are facing increased numbers of adolescents with hypertension, type 2 diabetes, and hyperlipidemia.
- Substance abuse and experimentation are common during adolescence; it is associated with other risk-taking behaviours such as injuries and sexual activity.
- Health care providers must work collaboratively with the adolescent in the development of interventions to promote health.

REFERENCES

American Academy of Pediatrics, Council on Environmental Health and Section on Dermatology (2011). *Policy statement—Ultraviolet radiation: A hazard to children and adolescents.* Retrieved February 22, 2012 from http://aappolicy.aappublications.org/cgi/reprint/pediatrics;127/3/588.pdf

American Academy of Pediatrics. (2010). *Ages & stages: Tattoos.* Retrieved March 26, 2011, from http://www.healthychildren.org/English/ages-stages/teen/safety/pages/Tattoos.aspx

Canadian Lung Association. (2011). *Smoking & tobacco: Facts about smoking.* Retrieved November 1, 2011 from http://www.lung.ca/protect-protegez/tobacco-tabagisme/facts-faits/index_e.php

Canadian Medical Association. (2008). *CMAJ fact sheet: Alcohol and drug use among teenagers.* Retrieved August 23, 2011 from http://www.cmaj.ca/cgi/reprint/178/2/149

Canadian Mental Health Association. (2011). *Youth and suicide.* Retrieved February 22, 2012 from http://www.cmha.ca/bins/content_page.asp?cid=3-101-104

Canadian Paediatric Society. (2006, reaffirmed 2011). *Adolescent pregnancy.* Retrieved August 23, 2011 from http://www.cps.ca/english/statements/am/ah06-02.htm

Canadian Population Health Initiative. (2004). *Improving the health of Canadians.* Retrieved August 11, 2011 from http://secure.cihi.ca/cihiweb/products/IHC2004rev_e.pdf

Canadian Research Institute for Law and the Family. (2005). *Youth gangs in Canada: A preliminary review of programs and services.* Retrieved August 23, 2011 from http://people.ucalgary.ca/crilf/publications/Youth_Gang_Report.pdf

Centers for Disease Control and Prevention. (2006). *CDC's position on tattooing and HCV infection.* Retrieved November 14, 2011 from http://www.cdc.gov/ncidod/diseases/hepatitis/c/tattoo.htm

Centers for Disease Control and Prevention (2011). *Youth Violence: Risk and Protective Factors. Risk Factors for the Perpetration of Youth Violence.* Retrieved on December 13, 2011 at http://www.cdc.gov/ViolencePrevention/youthviolence/riskprotectivefactors.html

Combes-Orme, T. (1993). Health effects of adolescent pregnancy: Implications for social workers. *Families in Society: The Journal of Contemporary Human Services, 31*(1), 344–354.

Dryburgh, H. (2007). *Teenage pregnancy.* Retrieved August 23, 2011 from http://www.statcan.gc.ca/kits-trousses/preg-gross/preg-gross-eng.htm

Dysart-Gale, D. (2010). Social justice and social determinants of health: Lesbian, gay, bisexual, transgendered, intersexed and queer youth in Canada. *Journal of Child and Adolescent Psychiatric Nursing, 23*(1),23–28.

Edelman, C. L., & Mandle, C. L. (2002). *Health promotion throughout the lifespan* (5th ed.). St. Louis: Mosby.

Erikson, E. (1963). *Childhood and society* (2nd ed.). New York: Norton.

Health Canada. (2006). *First Nations, Inuit and Aboriginal health: Suicide prevention.* Retrieved November 15, 2011 from http://www.hc-sc.gc.ca/fniah-spnia/promotion/suicide/index-eng.php

Health Canada. (2007a). *Eating well with Canada's Food Guide.* Retrieved August 23, 2011 from http://www.hc-sc.gc.ca/fn-an/food-guide-aliment/order-commander/eating_well_bien_manger-eng.php

Health Canada. (2007b). *Substance use by Canadian youth – A national survey of Canadians' use of alcohol and other drugs: Canadian addiction survey.* Retrieved August 23, 2011 from http://www.hc-sc.gc.ca/hc-ps/pubs/adp-apd/cas_youth-etc_jeunes/index-eng.php

Health Canada. (2010). *Canadian Tobacco Use Monitoring Survey (CTUMS): CTUMS 2009 wave 1 survey results.* Retrieved August 23, 2011 from http://www.hc-sc.gc.ca/hc-ps/tobac-tabac/research-recherche/stat/_ctums-esutc_2009/w-p-1_sum-som-eng.php

Health Canada. (2011a). *First Nations, Inuit and Aboriginal health: Clinical Practice Guidelines for Nurses in Primary Care—Pediatric and Adolescent Care.* Retrieved November 14, 2011 from http://www.hc-sc.gc.ca/fniah-spnia/services/nurs-infirm/clini/pediat/index-eng.php

Health Canada. (2011b). *It's your health: Preventing skin cancer.* Retrieved November 16, 2011 from http://www.hc-sc.gc.ca/hl-vs/alt_formats/pdf/iyh-vsv/diseases-maladies/cancer-eng.pdf

Jenkins, R. R., & Adger, A. (2007). Substance abuse. In R. M. Kleigman, R. E. Behrman, H. B. Jenson, & B. F. Stanton (Eds.), *Nelson Textbook of Pediatrics* (18th ed.). Philadelphia: Saunders.

Johnston, L.D., O'Malley, P.M., & Bachman, J.G. (2002). *Monitoring the future: National results on adolescent drug use. National Institute on Drug Abuse.* Bethesda, MD: U.S. Department of Health and Human Servics.

Katzman, D.K. (2010). Sexting: Keeping teens safe and responsible in a technologically savvy world. *Paediatric and Child Health,* 15(1), 41–42.

Kelly, A. W. (2010). Non-contact sports: Running, swimming, and dance—Identifying common injuries. *Pediatric Annals,* 39(5), 279–284.

KidsHealth, M. L. (2011). *All about sleep.* Retrieved November 15, 2011 from http://kidshealth.org/parent/general/sleep/sleep.html#

Kohlberg, L. (1984). *Essays on moral development.* San Francisco: Harper & Row.

Leatherdale, S. T., Hammond, D. G., Kaiserman, M., & Ahmed, R. (2007). Marijuana and tobacco use among young adults in Canada: Are they smoking what we think they're smoking? *Cancer Causes & Control,* 18(4), 391–397.

Luong, M. (2008). *Life after teenage motherhood.* Retrieved August 23, 2011 from http://www.statcan.gc.ca/pub/75-001-x/2008105/pdf/10577-eng.pdf

Marcell, A. V. (2007). Adolescence. In R. M. Kleigman, R. E. Behrman, H. B. Jenson, & B. F. Stanton (Eds.), *Nelson Textbook of Pediatrics* (18th ed.). Philadelphia: Saunders.

Maticka-Tyndale, E. (2008). Sexuality and sexual health of Canadian adolescents: Yesterday, today and tomorrow. *The Canadian Journal of Human Sexuality,* 17 85–95.

National Center for Chronic Disease Prevention and Health Promotion. (2010). *Healthy youth! Student health and academic achievement.* Retrieved August 23, 2011 from http://www.cdc.gov/HealthyYouth/health_and_academics/#1

Neinstein, L. S. (2011). *Interviewing and communicating with adolescents (A4).* Available at http://www.usc.edu/student-affairs/Health_Center/adolhealth/content/a4.html

O'Keefe, M. (1997). Predictors of dating violence among high school students. *Journal of Interpersonal Violence,* 12(4), 546–568.

Piaget, J. (1969). *The theory of stages in cognitive development.* New York: McGraw-Hill.

Public Health Agency of Canada. (2007). *Brief report on sexually transmitted infections in Canada: 2007.* Retrieved August 23, 2011 from http://www.phac-aspc.gc.ca/publicat/2009/sti-its/index-eng.php

Public Health Agency of Canada. (2009a). *Leading causes of injury deaths in Canada, 2005.* Retrieved August 23, 2011 from http://dsol-smed.phac-aspc.gc.ca/dsol-smed/is-sb/leadcauses/leading_causes_inj_mort_2005-eng.pdf

Public Health Agency of Canada. (2009b). *Youth and violence.* Retrieved August 23, 2011 from http://www.phac-aspc.gc.ca/ncfv-cnivf/publications/nfntsyjviolence-eng.php?option=print

Public Health Agency of Canada. (2011). *Physical activity tips for youth (12–17 years).* Retrieved October 31, 2011 from http://www.phac-aspc.gc.ca/hp-ps/hl-mvs/pa-ap/06paap-eng.php

Rottermann, M. (2008). Trends in teen sexual behaviour and condom use. *Health Reports,* 19, 1–5.

Saewyc, E. (2007). Substance use among non-mainstream youth. In *Substance abuse in Canada: Youth in focus.* Ottawa, ON: Canadian Centre on Substance Abuse. Retrieved August 23, 2011 from http://www.ccsa.ca/Eng/KnowledgeCentre/OurPublications/Pages/SubstanceAbuseinCanada.aspx

Sass, A. E., & Kaplan, D. W. (2011). Adolescence. In W. W. Hay, M. J. Levin, J. M. Sondheimer, & R. R. Deterding (Eds.), *Current pediatric diagnosis and treatment* (20th ed.). New York: McGraw-Hill.

Statistics Canada. (2005a). *Nutrition: Findings from the Canadian Community Health Survey.* Issue no. 1. Ottawa, ON: Component of Statistics Canada Catalog no. 82–620-MWE2005001.

Statistics Canada. (2005b). *Pregnancy outcomes by age group.* Retrieved August 23, 2011 from http://www40.statcan.gc.ca/l01/cst01/hlth65a-eng.htm

Statistics Canada. (2008). *Study: Firearms and violent crime.* Retrieved August 23, 2011 from http://www.statcan.gc.ca/daily-quotidien/080220/dq080220b-eng.htm

Statistics Canada. (2009). *Ranking and number of deaths for the 10 leading causes by age group, Canada, 2005.* Retrieved August 23, 2011 from http://www.statcan.gc.ca/pub/84-215-x/2009000/tbl/tbl4-eng.htm

Tanner, J. (1962). *Growth at adolescence* (2nd ed.). Oxford, England: Blackwell Scientific Publications.

Toronto Public Health. (2008). *Nutrition matters: Loading up with iron-rich foods.* Retrieved November 1, 2011 from http://www.toronto.ca/health/pdf/loadingup.pdf

Turner, R. J., Grindstaff, C. F., Phillips, N. (1990). Social support and outcome in teenage pregnancy. *Journal of Health and Social Behavior,* 31(1), 43–57.

Tutty, L. M., Bradshaw, C., Thurston, W. E., et al. (2005). *School-based violence prevention programs: Preventing violence against girls and young women* (Revised Ed.). Calgary, AB: RESOLVE. Retrieved August 23, 2011 from www.ucalgary.ca/resolve/violenceprevention

U.S. Department of Agriculture and U.S. Department of Health and Human Services. (2010). *Dietary guidelines for Americans, 2010* (7th ed.). Retrieved August 23, 2011 from http://www.cnpp.usda.gov/DGAs2010-PolicyDocument.htm

U.S. Food and Drug Administration. (2009). *Think before you ink: Are tattoos safe?* Retrieved August 23, 2001 from http://www.fda.gov/downloads/ForConsumers/ConsumerUpdates/UCM143401.pdf.

RECOMMENDED READINGS

Advocates for Youth. (2010). *Gay, lesbian, bisexual transgender, and questioning (GLBTQ) youth.* Retrieved November 16, 2011 from http://www.advocatesforyouth.org/publications/424?task=view.

Alba-Fisch, M. (n.d.). *Temperament: miss or match.* Retrieved August 23, 2011 from http://www.taconicnet.com/articles/temperament.php.

Alford, S. (2003). *Adolescents: at risk for sexually transmitted infections.* Retrieved August 23, 2011 from http://www.advocatesforyouth.org/storage/advfy/documents/fssti.pdf.

Ball, J.W., & Bindler, R. C. (2006). *Child health nursing: Partnering with children and families.* Upper Saddle River, NJ: Prentice Hall.

Burstein, G. R., Lowry, R., Klein, J. D., & Santelli, J. S. (2003). Missed opportunities for sexually transmitted diseases, human immunodeficiency virus, and pregnancy prevention services during adolescent health supervision visits. *Pediatrics,* 111(Suppl. 1–1), 996–1001.

Children of Alcoholics Foundation. (n.d.). *How to help kids avoid alcohol and other drugs.* Retrieved August 23, 2011 from http://www.coaf.org/family/caregivers/avoid.htm.

Fox, J.A. (2002). *Primary health care of infants, children and adolescents* (2nd ed.). St. Louis: Mosby.

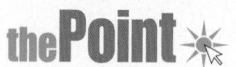

For additional learning materials, including Internet Resources, visit **http://thePoint.lww.com/Chow1e.**

CHAPTER WORKSHEET

MULTIPLE CHOICE QUESTIONS

1. When giving parents guidance for the adolescent years, the nurse would advise the parents to: (Choose all that apply)

   a. Accept the adolescent as a unique individual.

   b. Provide strict, inflexible rules.

   c. Listen and try to be open to the adolescent's views.

   d. Screen all of his or her friends.

   e. Respect the adolescent's privacy.

   f. Provide unconditional love.

2. In developing a weight-loss plan for an adolescent, which of the following would you include? (Choose all that apply)

   a. Have parents make all of the meal plans.

   b. Eat slowly and place the fork down between each bite.

   c. Have the family exercise together.

   d. Refer to an adolescent weight-loss program.

   e. Keep a food and exercise diary.

3. Which of the following is associated with early adolescence? (Choose all that apply)

   a. Uses scientific reasoning to solve problems

   b. Still at times wants to be dependent upon parents

   c. Incorporates own set of morals and values

   d. Is influenced by peers and values memberships in cliques

4. Which of the following has the most influence in deterring an adolescent from beginning to drink alcohol?

   a. Drinking habits of parents

   b. Drinking habits of peers

   c. Drinking philosophy of adolescent's culture

   d. Drinking philosophy of adolescent's religion

5. In developing a pregnancy prevention program at school for 15- to 17-year-olds, the school nurse must take into consideration that:

   a. Teenagers think that no harm will come to them.

   b. Teenagers will learn best from their parents.

   c. Teenagers can only think in the here and now.

   d. Teenagers will learn best from professionals.

CRITICAL THINKING EXERCISES

1. During a sports physical examination, Susan, a 16-year-old, tells her health care provider that she is overweight. What additional information would the health care provider obtain?

2. The parents of Joe, a 14-year-old, talk to the school nurse about Joe's behaviour at home. He is moody, fights with his younger siblings, only wants to be on his computer, and does not want to go on the family vacation. What advice would you give the parents?

3. Jane tells the school nurse that she might be homosexual. What additional information would you obtain?

4. Alicia's parents are worried because all of Alicia's friends wear heavy makeup and have multiple piercings and hair colours. What advice would you give Alicia's parents?

STUDY ACTIVITIES

1. Talk to an early, middle, and late adolescent. Compare and contrast their interactions with you. Identify what psychosocial, cognitive, and moral stage they are in, using examples from their conversations with you.

2. Have an adolescent keep a food and exercise diary for 1 week. Analyse the information. Develop with the adolescent any interventions needed to promote healthy eating and exercise habits.

3. Plan a class on the dangers of smoking for 15-year-olds.

4. Plan a class for parents on how to keep the lines of communication open for adolescents.

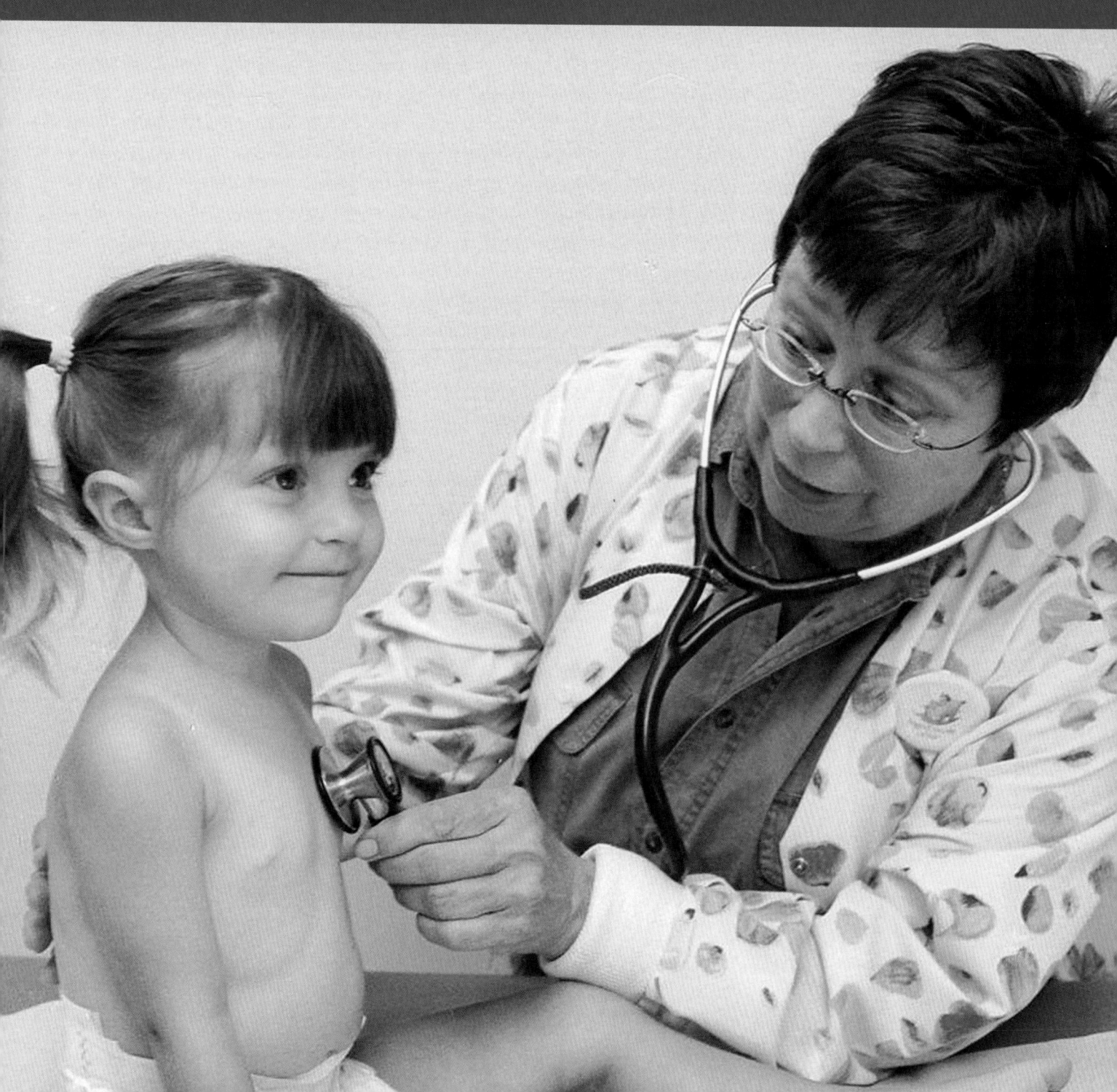

UNIT TEN

FOUNDATIONS OF PEDIATRIC NURSING

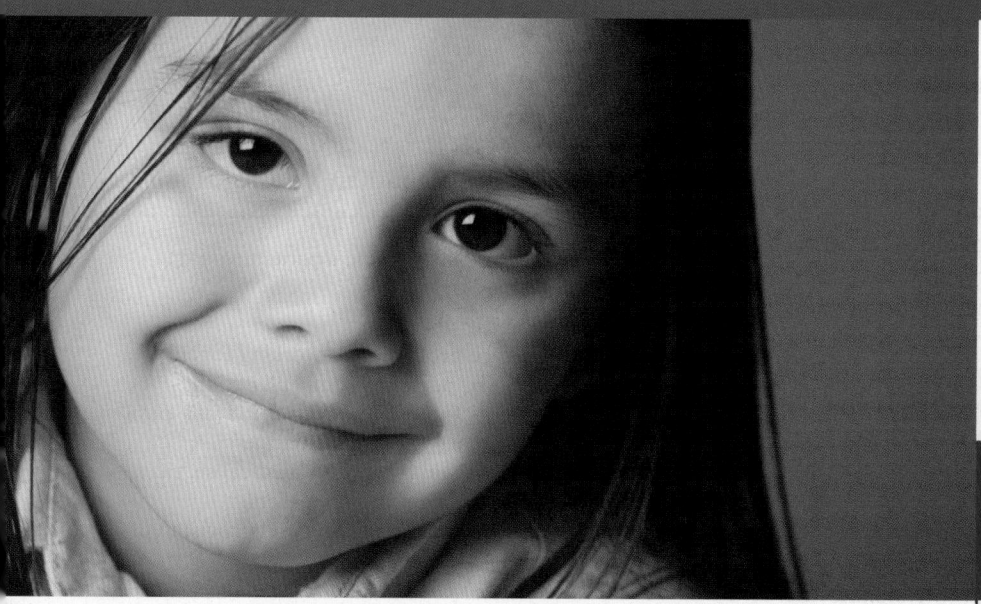

CHAPTER *30*

Adapted by Donna C. Meyer and
Deborah L. Olmstead

HEALTH SUPERVISION

KEY TERMS

active immunity
developmental screenings
developmental
   surveillance

immunity
medical home
pain management
passive immunity

risk assessment
screening tests
selective screening
universal screening

LEARNING OBJECTIVES

Upon completion of the chapter, the learner will be able to:

1. Describe the principles of health supervision.
2. List the three components of a health supervision visit.
3. Utilize instruments appropriately for developmental and functional testing of children.
4. Demonstrate knowledge of the principles of immunization.
5. Identify barriers to immunization.
6. Identify pain management strategies for immunizing infants and children.

The Robertson family is seen in the health clinic. Three-year-old Maya and 12-month-old Evan are brought in by their father. Maya was last seen in the clinic when she was 1 year old and Evan has never been seen. The father states that they have both been healthy so they did not need to come to the clinic before this. Currently, Maya is complaining of a sore throat, which is what prompted today's visit.

Wow

It is never too late to embrace prevention. It starts with a genuine desire for health improvement.

Principles of Health Supervision

Health supervision is the forward-looking provision of services with the goal of providing the child with an optimal level of functioning. Health supervision has three components around which this chapter is organized: developmental surveillance and screening, injury and disease prevention, and health promotion. Health supervision begins at birth and continues through the completion of adolescence. Health supervision is vital to every child and is most effective when the child has a centralized source of health care. Any place that provides access to children and families can be an appropriate setting for health supervision services. Some of the settings in which services can be provided include family physicians' or pediatricians' offices, community public health centres, homeless shelters, day care centres, and schools.

The framework for the health supervision visit is based on the Rourke Baby Record, which is an evidence-based health supervision guide for primary health care providers of children in the first 5 years of life (Canadian Paediatric Society [CPS], 2011), and the Greig Health Record, used by clinicians caring for children and adolescents 6 to 17 years of age (Greig, Constantin, Carsley, & Cummings, 2010). Both the Rourke Baby Record and the Greig Health Record are endorsed by the College of Family Physicians of Canada and the Canadian Paediatric Society (CPS).

Wellness

The focus of pediatric health supervision is wellness. The health supervision visit provides an opportunity to maximize health promotion for the child, family, and community. Nurses have the ability to guide clients to a state of optimal health during these encounters. Health supervision visits must be viewed as a continuum of care and not as isolated episodes of tasks to be accomplished.

Medical Home

A **medical home** is a team of professionals who provide continuous and comprehensive primary care and with whom the family has a strong therapeutic relationship (Cohen, Friedman, Nicholas, Adams, & Rosenbaum, 2008). Studies show that a medical home addresses population health, particularly the determinants of health (Canadian Institute for Health Information, 2009; College of Family Physicians of Canada, 2009). The medical home is the setting that allows the highest level of health supervision. To be effective, the medical home must be accessible, family centred, and community based. Features of a medical home are presented in Box 30.1.

Partnerships

The child is the focus of the health supervision visit. However, the child's health is linked to the needs and

---

BOX 30.1 **What is a Canadian Medical Home?**

A health care office or clinic where a patient would have:

- His or her own family physician
- A team of health care professionals working together with the patient's own personal family physician
- Timely appointments for all visits with the family physician and other primary care team members
- Arrangement and coordination of all medical services, including referrals to consulting specialists
- An active role in the decision making and provision of their ongoing care
- An electronic medical record

The medical home would include:

- Appropriate funding and resources
- Necessary funding supports for ongoing evaluation and quality management

Source: *College of Family Physicians of Canada.* (2011). *A vision for Canada: Family practice—The patient's medical home.* Retrieved November 22, 2011 from http://www.cfpc.ca/WorkArea/linkit.aspx?LinkIdentifier=id&ItemID=3753. Used with permission.

---

resources of the family and community of which the child is a member. If the family is in turmoil because of divorce, drug abuse, or parental health problems, the child may not receive the attention and energy needed to thrive. Likewise, a community with high levels of poverty, poor infrastructure, and lack of resources will not be able to provide the support services needed to allow children to blossom to their full potential. By recognizing the importance of these determinants of health, nurses can develop integrated approaches to address health concerns. Through interdisciplinary linkages, nurses can influence the impact of the determinants of health through the development of community-based programs that benefit the health of the entire community (Aston, Meagher-Stewart, Edwards, & Young, 2009).

The partnership between the child and the health supervision team is designed to allow the child to reach his or her optimal state of health. By its nature, this partnership develops over time. In infancy the family is the surrogate for the child in the partnership. The child's participation in the partnership increases at a rate that is developmentally appropriate. The partnership increases the child's sense of self-worth and competence. The child's increasing influence in the partnership allows the nurse to tailor health supervision to the child's needs. The partnership allows the child to take increasing responsibility for personal health and optimizes health promotion (Hagan, Shaw, & Duncan, 2008).

Nurses must validate and enhance the role of family members in the health supervision partnership. The family provides the framework that informs the child's concept of wellness. The health care community must involve the family to have a significant impact on a child's health. The family wants the best possible outcome for their child, and health care decisions are based on the knowledge they possess. When the nurse acknowledges that the family has unique insights to offer on their child's health, a trusting partnership can begin. Nurses can strengthen this partnership by recognizing the family's healthy practices, addressing their health issues, and strengthening their skills. The family's contributions to this partnership enhance the chance of success for health care plans. Families are the ones who must implement any health care strategy and know what expected outcomes are reasonable. They have intimate knowledge of the child's past responses to previous strategies. Their feedback is invaluable to formulating an effective long-term health supervision plan that optimizes their child's wellness.

▶ **Take** NOTE!

Observe the parent–child interaction during the health supervision visit. The nurse can learn much about the family dynamic by observing the family for behavioural clues:

- *Does the parent make eye contact with the infant?*
- *Does the parent anticipate and respond to the infant's needs?*
- *Are parents effective when dealing with a toddler's temper tantrum?*
- *Do the parents' comments increase the school-age child's sense of self-worth?*

Behavioural observations are crucial to a thorough assessment of the family's needs and issues.

Partnerships between the community and the health promotion team benefit individual clients and the community. When nurses develop partnerships with community agencies such as schools, churches, and ancillary health facilities, barriers to care can be eased. The nurse becomes aware of available resources in the community that will benefit an individual family. With input from community partners, the nurse can perform an assessment of the community's needs. The assessment then provides the foundation for the development of community-based health promotion programs. These programs expand the resources of the community, which in turn enhances the health of its members (Hagan et al., 2008).

Special Issues in Health Supervision

Special issues in health supervision include cultural influences, community influences, health supervision and the chronically ill child, and health supervision and the internationally adopted child.

Cultural Influences on Health Supervision

Canada is home to more than 200 different ethnic groups, including an estimated 5 million people, or 16.2% of the total population, who belong to visible minority groups (Statistics Canada, 2006). A family's understanding of health is informed by the culture they inhabit. Successful interactions result when the nurse is aware of the beliefs and interactive styles that are often present in members of a specific culture. If the goals of the health care plan are not consistent with the health belief system of the family, the plan has little chance for success. Optimal wellness for the child requires the nurse and the family to negotiate a mutually acceptable plan of care that balances the cultural beliefs and practices of the family with those of the health care establishment. The nurse must possess the attributes of cultural competence and sensitivity for the partnership to be successful. Culturally effective care is the result of a dynamic partnership between the nurse and the family.

Most health programs in Canada are designed in ways that are most accessible to the mainstream culture and generally ignore the beliefs and practices related to health and illness of diverse ethnic and cultural groups (Poureslami et al., 2007). Families who are visible minorities may have to deal with cultural as well as language barriers in accessing health care (Lyman, Loock, Scott, & Koushambi, 2008). The nurse must take the time to communicate openly with families about their beliefs, including how they view illness and treatment, and empower families to take charge of their health (Poureslami et al., 2007).

The decisions of particular population groups, such as Aboriginals, to access health care are influenced by factors such as how they have been treated in the health care system during previous encounters. Having a history of negative experiences influences when, where, and how people access health care (Lyman et al., 2008). Health care providers must reflect on their own assumptions about cultural and ethnic populations in order to be culturally competent.

Community Influences on Health Supervision

The child is a member of a community as well as a family and a culture. Each community is unique in its strengths, weaknesses, and values. A community can be a contributor to a child's health or be the cause of his or her illnesses. The child's health cannot be totally separated from the health of the surrounding community.

Ideally the child's medical home is within the family's community. Being within the family's community increases access to care. Barriers such as lack of transportation, expense of travel, and time away from the parents' work setting are reduced. The presence of the medical home within the community facilitates the bonds between the health team and schools, churches, and available support services and agencies. Community support and resources are necessary for children with significant problems. A close working relationship between the child's health care provider and community agencies is an enormous benefit to the child (see Partnerships section).

The community assessment may reveal problems that are causing or contributing to the child's health deficit. Deteriorating infrastructure can contribute to decreased access to care and increased risk of injury or illness. Poverty has been linked to low birth weight and premature birth, among other health problems (Shore & Shore, 2009). Substandard housing can be directly related to lead poisoning and asthma (Centers for Disease Control and Prevention [CDC], 2009). A thorough knowledge of the family's community is needed before a health surveillance program can be effective.

Health Supervision and the Child with Chronic Illness

Effective health supervision must be responsive to the individual child's situation. The child with a chronic illness needs to be assessed repeatedly to determine health maintenance needs. These assessments determine the frequency of visits and types of interventions needed. The illness' impact on the functional health patterns of the child determine whether standard health supervision visits need to be augmented.

An effective partnership among the child's medical home, family, and community is vital for a child with a chronic illness. Coordination of medical specialty care, community agencies, and family support networks enhances the quality of life and health of these children. Access to care and services minimizes the risk of injury from the illness. Support groups and community-based resources optimize the family's adaptation to the stressors of chronic illness.

Comprehensive health supervision includes frequent psychosocial assessments. Issues to be covered include:

- Transportation availability to health care facilities
- Financial stressors
- Family coping effectiveness
- School personnel response to the chronic illness

These are often stressful and emotionally charged issues. The nurse with a trusting and ongoing relationship with the child and family is in the best position to help with these issues. The nurse can assist the family to utilize community resources and participate in support groups. The nurse can also educate school personnel about the child's illnesses and assist them in maximizing the child's potential for academic success.

Health Supervision and the Child Adopted Internationally

About 2,000 foreign children are adopted by Canadian families every year, with the largest proportion of children being adopted from China, the United States, Ethiopia, and Haiti (Citizenship and Immigration Canada, 2008, as cited by the Adoption Council of Canada, 2009). Most internationally adopted children are younger than 5 years of age and frequently come from countries with poor health care infrastructure and few resources. Infectious diseases such as tuberculosis and intestinal parasitism are common. There is also little or no prenatal screening for syphilis, hepatitis B, or HIV infection. Many children have undergone prolonged deprivation or suffered through natural disasters. Medical records are often lacking or dubious, and immunization history may be unavailable or unreliable. Due to lack of resources in the home country, screening and treatment for these diseases are sporadic and ineffective. If testing is documented, it is likely to be unreliable (Shetty, 2010). Testing supplies may have been outdated or improperly stored. Also, the test may have been performed before the infection resulted in the child's development of antibodies in his or her blood (seroconversion).

For these reasons, health supervision of these children must include comprehensive infectious disease screening (Shetty, 2010). Proper screening is important not only for the child's health but also for the health of the adopting family and the larger community. Universal screening for tuberculosis upon arrival and a physical examination and medical history are recommended (Long & Boffa, 2007). Universal screening for hepatitis B, HIV, and syphilis infections are also recommended.

Components of Health Supervision

Developmental surveillance and screening, injury and disease prevention, and health promotion are the critical components of health supervision for children. Disease prevention and health promotion are concepts well established in adult health supervision. Injury prevention and developmental surveillance/screening are additional components of pediatric health supervision visits that help ensure every child achieves his or her optimum state of wellness.

Developmental Surveillance and Screening

Developmental surveillance is an ongoing collection of skilled observations made over time during health care visits. Components of this surveillance include:

- Noting and addressing parental concerns
- Obtaining a developmental history
- Making accurate observations
- Consulting with relevant professionals

Developmental screenings are brief assessment procedures that identify those children who warrant more intensive assessment and testing. Developmental screening assessments may be observational or by caregiver report (Fig. 30.1).

Development, the emergence of the child's abilities, is a longitudinal process. Within the trust and security of the medical home, family and health care providers can share observations and concerns. In collaboration, the family and the health care provider observe the child's accomplishments or milestones over time. Data collection for developmental surveillance of infants and young children is performed through developmental questionnaires, health care provider observations, and a thorough physical examination. Reviewing school records and testing can provide academic performance data for the older child. Input from teachers, coaches, and other adults involved with the child can give insight to the child's emotional and social development.

When developmental delay is suspected, frequent developmental surveillance is highly warranted. Reem-

phasizing parental roles and responsibilities fosters cooperation and compliance. It is therefore crucial that parents understand the need for frequent assessments. A pattern of developmental delays warrants a formal evaluation.

It is absolutely critical for the pediatric nurse to understand normal growth and development parametres and become proficient at screening for problems related to development. The historical information obtained from the parent or primary caregiver about developmental milestones may indicate warning signs or identify risk for developmental delay. Refer to Table 30.1 for developmental warning signs and possible deficiency areas.

One of the most important predictors of poor health in childhood is low birth weight (500 to 2,499 g) (Human Resources and Skills Development Canada, 2011). Low birth weight puts a child at risk for many chronic illnesses, such as childhood asthma and the development of type II diabetes as an adult (Johansson et al., 2008), as well as developmental delays resulting from learning difficulties and impaired hearing and vision. Low birth weight is an important population health indicator as it reflects determinants of health such as socioeconomic disadvantages, poor maternal health and nutrition, and tobacco use, substance abuse, and physical abuse during pregnancy (Canadian Institute for Health Information, 2007).

Depression in mothers is a significant risk factor for emotional and cognitive development problems in children (CPS, 2004). Women of child-bearing age who already suffer from depression (pre-pregnancy) are particularly at risk for postpartum mood disorders that range from postpartum blues (relatively common with few negative sequelae) to depression to psychosis (relatively rare with gross impairment functioning). The incidence of postpartum depression in Canada is 13%. The consequences of this condition are not limited to the infant but extend to development of the toddler, school-age child, and adolescent (CPS, 2004).

The Edinburgh Postnatal Depression Scale (EPDS) is a 10-item screening tool used to identify postpartum depression. The mother is asked to underline the response to each question that most describes how she has been feeling in the past 7 days. A score of 13 or more on the EPDS is considered an indicator of postpartum depression. A score of 10 to 12 indicates that the woman is at risk for postpartum depression. The EPDS may be administered at 6 to 8 weeks postpartum at a child health clinic, postnatal check-up, or home visit (Public Health Agency of Canada [PHAC], 2009b).

Risk factors for developmental delay can be organized in to four categories: child characteristics, parenting or interaction variables, parent characteristics, and sociodemographic factors (Box 30.2). Infants or children with any of these risk factors should be carefully screened for developmental delays. This screening should

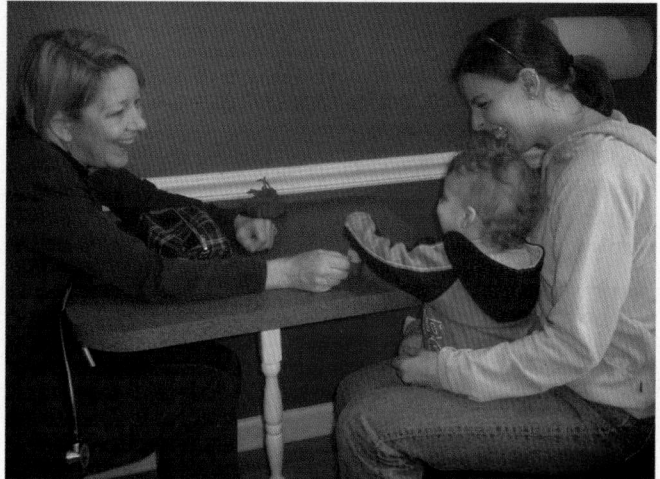

FIGURE 30.1 Developmental screening provides the opportunity for the nurse to identify problem areas in the child's development.

TABLE 30.1 Infant/Toddler Developmental Warning Signs

Age	Warning Sign	Possible Developmental Concern
Any age	No response to environmental stimulus	Sensory deficit
Any age	Persistently up on toes (longer than 30 s) in supported standing position	Cerebral palsy
Before 3 months	Rolls over	Hypertonia
After 2–3 months	Persistent fisting	Neurologic dysfunction
After 4 months	Persistent head lag	Hypotonia
5 months	Not reaching for toys	Motor, visual, or cognitive deficit
6 months	Lack of tripod sitting	Hypotonia
6 months	Not smiling	Visual deficit, attachment issue
6 months	Primitive reflex persistence	Neurologic dysfunction
6 months	Not babbling	Hearing deficit
9 months	No reciprocal vocalizations or facial expressions	Autism spectrum disorders
12 months	No spoon or crayon use	Fine motor delay
15–18 months	Not walking	Gross motor delay
18 months	No imitative play	Autism spectrum disorders
Prior to 18 months	Hand dominance present	Hemiplegia in opposite upper extremity
18 months	No first word	Hearing deficit, expressive language deficit
24 months	Echolalia (repetitive speech) or inability to follow simple commands	Social delay or autism spectrum disorders

---

BOX 30.2 Risk Factors for Developmental Delay

Child Characteristics
- Birth weight less than 2,499 g
- Gestational age less than 37 weeks
- Central nervous system abnormality
- Hypoxic–ischemic encephalopathy
- Hypertonia
- Hypotonia
- Hyperbilirubinemia requiring exchange transfusion
- Kernicterus
- Congenital malformations
- Symmetric intrauterine growth deficiency
- Perinatal or congenital infection
- Suspected sensory impairment
- Chronic (>3 months) otitis media with effusion
- Inborn error of metabolism
- HIV infection
- Exposure to lead

Parenting Variables
- Lack of sensitivity to infant's cues
- Lack of parental knowledge of expected milestones
- Sibling with developmental concerns

Parent Characteristics
- Parent with less than high school education
- Maternal prenatal alcohol or illicit drug abuse
- Lone parenting (this risk factor is associated with depression, poverty, and increased risk for low birth weight)
- Parent with developmental disability or mental illness (including depression)
- Criminality of parent(s)
- History of neglect or physical/sexual abuse in parent(s)

Sociodemographic Factors
- Adolescent parenting
- Poverty
- Severe family dysfunction
- Isolation and lack of social support

Sources: Canadian Institute for Health Information. (2007). *Number of low birth weight babies rising in Canada*. Retrieved November 18, 2011 from http://www.newswire.ca/en/story/36367/number-of-low-birth-weight-babies-rising-in-canada; Hwa-Froelich, D. A., Loveland Cook, C. A., & Flick, L. H. (2008). Maternal sensitivity and communication styles: Mothers with depression. *Journal of Early Intervention, 31,* 44–66; Ontario Association for Infant and Child Development. (2009). *Frequently asked questions. Retrieved November* 18, 2011 from http://www.oaicd.ca/faq; Ottawa Coalition for the Prevention of Low Birth Weight. (2007). *What is low birth weight?* Retrieved November 18, 2011 from http://www.successby6ottawa.ca/lbwfpn/english/; Tough, S., Siever, J. E., Leew, S., Johnston, D. W., Benzies, K., & Clark, D. (2008). Maternal mental health predicts risk of developmental problems at 3 years of age: Follow-up of a community-based trial. *BMC Pregnancy and Childbirth, 8,* 16; and Tough, S., Siever, J. E., Benzies, K., Leew, S., & Johnston, D. W. (2010). Maternal well-being and its association to risk of developmental problems in children at school entry. *BMC Pregnancy and Childbirth, 10,* 19.

occur in a prospective manner, with screenings occurring at frequent intervals to identify concerns early.

> ▶ **Take** NOTE!
>
> *Any child who loses a developmental milestone—for example, the child able to sit without support who now cannot—needs an immediate full evaluation. There is a high likelihood of a significant neurologic problem.*

A number of developmental screening tools are available to guide the nurse in assessing development. Refer to Table 30.2 for a summary of these assessment tools (Cairney, Clinton, & Dowling, 2011; Cappiello & Gahagan, 2009; Limbos & Joyce, 2011; Macy, 2011; University of British Columbia, 2009). Many screening methods assist the nurse to identify infants and children who may have developmental delays, thus allowing for prompt identification and referral for more definitive evaluation. The appropriateness of a school-age child's developmental level can be evaluated using additional information. This information can include handwriting samples, ability to draw, school performance, and social skills.

Injury and Disease Prevention

Disease prevention involves interventions performed to protect clients from a disease or identify it at an early stage and lessen its consequences. These interventions are determined by the results of the nurse's assessment, provincially and nationally accepted practice guidelines, and the family's goals. Components of disease prevention include screening tests and immunizations.

Unintentional injuries are the leading cause of mortality for Canadian children 1 to 19 years of age (PHAC, 2009a). Injury prevention is primarily accomplished through education, anticipatory guidance, and physical changes in the environment. Injuries can be unintentional (poisoning, falls, or drowning) or intentional (child abuse, homicide, or suicide). The types of injuries a child is most likely to encounter vary greatly among age groups.

The majority of childhood injuries are predictable and preventable (Safe Kids Canada, 2010). Safe Kids Canada, the national injury prevention body for the Hospital for Sick Children, partners with groups across the nation to conduct research, raise awareness, educate families, and advocate for safer environments to protect children from serious injury (PHAC, 2009a). Using these resources and in partnership with the family and community, the nurse can have an enormous impact on child safety. Specific interventions are discussed in Chapters 25 through 29.

Screening Tests

Screening tests are procedures or laboratory analyses designed to identify those who may have a treatable con-

dition. These tests are designed to assure that no person with the disorder is missed. They have a high sensitivity (a high false-positive rate) and a low specificity (a low false-negative rate). If a screening test result is positive, follow-up tests with higher specificity are performed. A **risk assessment** is performed by the health care professional in conjunction with the client and includes objective as well as subjective data to determine the likelihood of having a condition. **Universal screening** occurs when an entire population is screened regardless of the client's individual risk. This type of screening is performed when a reliable risk assessment procedure is not available. **Selective screening** is done when a risk assessment indicates the client has one or more risk factors for the disorder.

> ▶ **Take** NOTE!
>
> *To increase cooperation from young children during screenings, set up a reward system. Easy-to-do rewards include:*
>
> - *Stamping the back of the child's hand with a "smiley face" icon*
> - *Making an eye cover by placing two stickers back to back over a tongue blade and letting the child keep the cover after the screening*
> - *Copying a design onto a sheet of paper and letting the child take it home to colour*
> - *Letting the child play with a simple device such as a penlight or stethoscope*

Metabolic Screening

Universal newborn metabolic screening is under provincial jurisdiction, and the number of diseases screened for varies in each province. The types of diseases screened for include inherited metabolic diseases (phenylketonuria), endocrine diseases (congenital hypothyroidism), hematologic diseases (hemoglobinopathies), and organic and amino acid disorders (Hanley, 2005). Screening tests are performed by collecting drops of blood from the infant by a heel stick when the infant is between 24 hours and 5 days of age. Most provinces screen for the following diseases (Canadian Organization for Rare Disorders, 2010):

- Endocrine disorders (e.g., congenital hypothyroidism)
- Hemoglobinopathies (e.g., sickle cell)
- Fatty acid disorders (e.g., Carnitine–acylcarnitine translocase deficiency)
- Amino acid disorders (e.g., Benign hyperphenylalaninemia)
- Organic acid disorders (e.g., Isovaleric aciduria)
- Other metabolic disorders (e.g., Galactose epimerase deficiency)
- Other diseases (e.g., cystic fibrosis)

TABLE 30.2 **DEVELOPMENTAL SCREENING TOOLS**

Age	Screening Tool	Definition	Nursing Implications
Birth–6 years	Denver II	Assesses personal–social, fine motor–adaptive, language, and gross motor skills	Nurse administered. Requires props (such as ball, crayon, doll) available in the Denver II kit. Simple to learn to administer
Birth–6 years	Denver PRQ	Assesses personal–social, fine motor–adaptive, language, and gross motor skills	Parental report of all items on the Denver II
Birth–6 years	CDI	Simple questions about infant, toddler, or preschooler behaviours. Measures social, self-help, gross motor, fine motor, expressive language, language comprehension, letters, numbers, and general development as appropriate	A parental-report screening tool
Birth–6 years	ASQ	Assesses communication, gross motor, fine motor, personal–social, and problem-solving skills	A parental-report screening tool, scored by the nurse after completion to determine child's progress in each of the developmental areas
Birth–8 years	PEDS	Screens for a wide range of developmental, behavioural, and family issues	A parental-report screening tool that can also be used in nurse interview format. Also available in Spanish
12–96 months	Batelle Developmental Inventory Screening Test	Assesses fine and gross motor, adaptive, personal–social, receptive and expressive language, and cognitive skills	Direct elicitation, parental description, and examiner observation. Requires special training
1–42 months	Bayley Scales of Infant Development II	Provides a mental and motor scale for assessment of cognitive, language, personal–social, and fine and gross motor development. A behaviour rating scale is obtained during the testing.	Direct elicitation. Thorough. Requires special training
6–24 months	Infant/Toddler Checklist for Communication and Language Development	Screens for delays in language development as the first evidence that development is atypical	Parents complete multiple choice questions. Takes 5–10 min to complete
0–9 months	Brigance Screens	Tap speech-motor language readiness general knowledge and social–emotional skills	Takes 10 min to complete. Direct elicitation and observation.
1–72 months	Nipissing District Developmental Screen	Screens for vision, hearing, language, communication, gross and fine motor, self-help and cognitive, social and emotional function	Can be administered face-to-face with a parent at a physician's office or can be administered over the telephone
4–18 years	Pediatric Symptom Checklist	Includes 35 short statements about problem behaviours, including both externalizing (conduct, attention) and internalizing (depression, anxiety)	Two versions: parent-completed version and youth self-report. Requires a licensed practitioner to interpret

CDI, Child Development Inventory; ASQ, Ages and Stages Questionnaire; PEDS, Parents' Evaluation of Developmental Status.

The nurse needs to confirm that newborn metabolic screening was performed prior to discharge from the birthing unit during any initial health supervision visit. If a test was not performed or was performed when the infant was younger than 24 hours of age, the screening should be performed at that visit. Infants who have been in the neonatal intensive care unit for longer than 3 weeks must have the screen repeated in 3 to 6 weeks as some endocrine disorders may have been missed on the first screen in sick newborns.

Hearing Screening

Universal hearing screening of infants is inconsistent across Canada. Screening only those infants with risk factors for hearing loss limits the ability to identify hearing loss in the well-baby population (Canadian Association of Speech Language Pathologists and Audiologists [CASLPA], 2010).

Hearing loss in infants is fairly common, with an incidence ranging from 1 to 3 per 1,000 to 1,200 live births per year in Canada (CASLPA, 2010), and some congenital hearing loss may not be evident until the child is older. Hearing loss can be also acquired in later infancy or childhood due to meningitis, trauma to the nervous system, damaging noise levels, and ototoxic drugs (American Academy of Pediatrics [AAP], 2009).

Even mild hearing loss can cause serious delays in social and emotional development, language acquisition, and cognitive function. Identification of hearing loss by 3 months of age is crucial to prevent or reduce the impact on the child's development (Durieux-Smith, Fitzpatrick, & Whittingham, 2008). Accepted methodologies for screening newborn hearing are presented in Table 30.3.

Screening for hearing loss in older children begins with a history from the primary caregivers. If any concerns or problems are noted, objective audiometry should be performed. When the child is capable of following simple commands reliably, the nurse can perform some basic procedures to screen for hearing loss. The whisper test is easy to perform but does require a quiet room away from distractions in order to be valid. The Weber's and Rinne tests can be used to screen for sensorineural or conductive hearing loss. Refer to Table 30.3 for additional explanations of hearing screening tests. Screening for hearing loss is recommended if the parent or caregiver is concerned about a child's hearing, speech, or language; if a child has developmental delays; or if a child has risk factors for acquired hearing loss such as those listed in Box 30.3 (AAP, 2009).

Vision Screening

Newborns with ocular structural abnormalities are at high risk for vision impairment. Ongoing vision screening is performed at every scheduled health supervision visit. The screening procedures for children younger than 3 years of age or any nonverbal child involve evaluating the child's ability to fixate on and follow objects. The neonate should be able to fixate on an object 25 to 30 cm from the face. After fixation, the infant should be able to follow the object to the midline. By 2 months of age, the infant should be able to follow the object 180 degrees. The technique of photoscreening can help identify problems such as ocular malalignment, refractive error, and lens and retinal problems.

> ▶ *Take* NOTE!
>
> *Use objects with black and white patterns when performing vision screening on an infant less than 6 months of age. The infant's vision at this age is more attuned to high-contrast patterns than to colours. Try checkerboard patterns or concentric circles. Animal figures like pandas and Dalmatians also work well.*

After the age of 3 years, a variety of standardized age-appropriate vision screening charts are available. These charts include the "tumbling E" and Allen figures (Fig. 30.2A, B). These charts allow for a more precise vision assessment and aid the nurse in identifying preschool children with visual acuity problems (Dunfield & Keating, 2007). By age 5 or 6, most children know the alphabet well enough to use the traditional Snellen chart for vision screening (Fig. 30.2C). When using any vision-screening

---

BOX 30.3   Risk Factors for Hearing Impairment

- Family history of hearing loss
- Prenatal infection
- Anomalies of the head, face, or ears
- Low birth weight (less than 1,500 g)
- Hyperbilirubinemia requiring exchange transfusion
- Ototoxic medications
- Low Apgar scores: 4 or less at 1 min, or 6 or less at 5 min
- Mechanical ventilation lasting 5 days
- Syndrome associated with hearing loss
- Head trauma
- Bacterial meningitis
- Neurodegenerative disorders
- Persistent pulmonary hypertension
- Otitis media with effusion for 3 months

Adapted from: De Michele, A. M., & Ruth, R. A. (2010). *Newborn hearing screening*. Retrieved November 21, 2011 from http://emedicine.medscape.com/article/836646-overview.

TABLE 30.3 **HEARING SCREENING METHODS**

Test Name	Age Group	Characteristics	Nursing Implications
ABR	Newborn–6 months	Measures electroencephalo-graphic waves Test results may be affected by ear debris	Infant must be quiet (sedation may be needed)
EOAE	Newborn–6 months or developmentally delayed children at the infant's level of functioning	Machine produces clicks that stimulate cilia in the cochlea and measures the response.	Infant must be quiet. Test results may be inaccurate in first 24 h of life.
VRA	6 months–2 years	Visual reward linked to a tone signal Child looks to the visual reward in response to the tone Reward is activated, reinforcing the response	Child must be in an alert and happy state for best results. Schedule for after sleep/rest period. Allow child to sit in parent's lap.
Tympanometry	Over 7 months	Measures tympanic membrane mobility and determines middle ear pressure	The probe must form a seal with the canal. The child must remain still to obtain a valid result.
CPA	2–4 years	Similar to VRA except uses "listening games" Child does listening game at the tone. Receives social reward May be used when developmental age is 2 years	See Nursing Implications for VRA
Pure-tone (conventional) audiometry	4 years and older	Measures hearing acuity through a range of frequencies and intensities Child must wear earphones. Performed in a soundproof room if possible	Teach the child the desired motor response before screening. Administer conditioning trials. Offer two presentations of stimulus to ensure reliability. At a minimum, screen 1,000-, 2,000-, and 4,000-Hertz levels at 20 dB.
Whisper test	4 years and older	One ear is occluded. Examiner stands behind the child and whispers a word. The child must accurately repeat the whispered word.	The child must be in a quiet room and away from distractions. The child should be alert and well rested for accurate results. Consider a reward system to increase compliance.
Weber's test	6 years and older	Place a vibrating tuning fork in the middle of the top of the head. Ask if the sound is in one ear or both ears. The sound should be heard in both ears.	The child must understand the instructions and be able to cooperate.
Rinne test	6 years and older	Place a vibrating tuning fork on the mastoid process to assess bone conduction. The child signals when the sound is gone. Next place a vibrating tuning fork outside the ear to test air conduction. The child signals when the sound is gone. For a passing test, air conduction time should be twice as long as bone conduction time.	The child must understand the instructions and be able to cooperate.

ABR, auditory brain stem response; EOAE, evoked otoacoustic emissions; VRA, visual reinforcement audiometry; CPA, conditioned play audiometry.

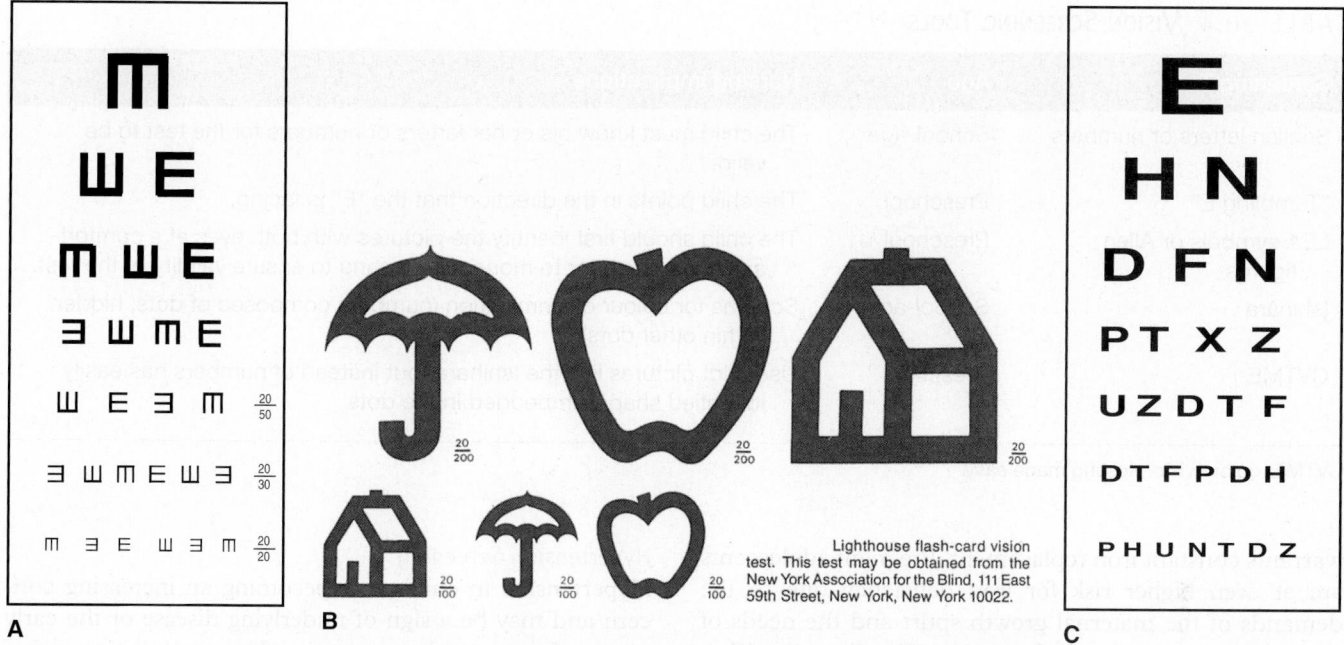

A   B   C

Lighthouse flash-card vision test. This test may be obtained from the New York Association for the Blind, 111 East 59th Street, New York, New York 10022.

FIGURE 30.2 (**A**) The "tumbling E" chart is appropriate for children who do not yet know the alphabet, but who can follow directions to indicate the direction that the arms of the "E" are pointing. (**B**) A picture chart similar to the Allen object recognition chart is appropriate for vision screening in the preschool-age child. (**C**) The Snellen eye chart may be used for children age 6 or older who know the alphabet.

chart, several simple steps need to be followed (Bowden & Greenberg, 2008).

1. Place the chart at the child's eye level.
2. Make sure there is sufficient lighting.
3. Place a mark on the floor about 6 m from the chart (distance depends on what the tool is calibrated for).
4. Align the child's heels on the mark.
5. The child reads each line with one eye covered and then with the other eye covered (Fig. 30.3). Explain

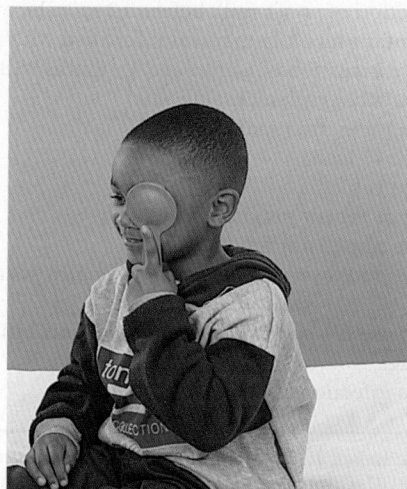

FIGURE 30.3 One eye must be covered while the other is tested in order to detect discrepancies in visual acuity between the two eyes and identify amblyopia early.

to the child that he or she should keep the eye covered but open.
6. The child reads each line with both eyes.

It is important that screenings are performed when children are alert and awake. Fatigue and disinterest can mimic poor vision. In addition to visual acuity screening, children should also be screened for colour discrimination. Any child with eye abnormalities or who has failed visual screening needs to be evaluated by a specialist appropriately trained to treat pediatric clients. Refer to Table 30.4 for further information about various vision screening tools (CPS, 2009b).

Iron–Deficiency Anemia Screening

Approximately 5% of Canadian children suffer from iron-deficiency anemia; among First Nations and Inuit children, this rate increases to 14% to 15% (Christofides, Schauer, & Zlotkin, 2005). The increased incidence of iron-deficiency anemia is directly associated with periods of diminished iron stores, rapid growth, and high metabolic demands. At 6 months of age, the in utero iron stores of a full-term infant are almost depleted, and the infant requires the introduction of complementary foods such as iron-fortified cereals and foods naturally rich in iron (AAP, 2010). Health Canada recommends breastfeeding infants exclusively up to 6 months of age followed by the addition of solid foods rich in iron with continued breastfeeding up to 2 years of age and beyond (Storr, Courant, & Friel, 2004). The adolescent growth spurt

TABLE 30.4 VISION SCREENING TOOLS

Screening Tool	Age	Nursing Implications
Snellen letters or numbers	School-age	The child must know his or her letters or numbers for the test to be valid.
"Tumbling E"	Preschool	The child points in the direction that the "E" is facing.
LEA symbols or Allen figures	Preschool	The child should first identify the pictures with both eyes at a comfortable distance prior to monocular testing to ensure validity of the test.
Ishihara	School-age	Screens for colour discrimination (numbers composed of dots, hidden within other dots)
CVTME	Preschool	Uses dot pictures like the Ishihara, but instead of numbers has easily identified shapes imbedded in the dots

CVTME, colour vision testing made easy.

warrants constant iron replacement. Pregnant adolescents are at even higher risk for iron deficiency due to the demands of the maternal growth spurt and the needs of the developing fetus (CDC, 2011a). The Canadian Task Force on the Periodic Examination recommends that all children at high risk for iron-deficiency anemia be screened at 9 months of age (Christofides et al., 2005). Risk factors for iron-deficiency anemia are presented in Box 30.4.

Lead Screening

Lead is a natural element that is found in many foods, in the air and soil, and in most homes (e.g., in paints or toys). Research suggests there is no safe blood level for lead, especially in children. Lead exposure in children is associated with intellectual, neurologic, and motor deficits such as deficiencies in reading and math skills, fine and gross motor skills, and distractibility and other characteristics of attention deficit hyperactivity disorder (ADHD) (Abelson & Sanborn, 2010; Payne, 2008). Lead screening is recommended for children who may have been exposed to lead in one of several ways:

1. In the past 6 months, lived in a house or apartment built before 1978
2. Live in a house with peeling or chipped paint
3. Have a sibling or playmate with a history of lead poisoning
4. Have been eating paint chips (Abelson & Sanborn, 2010)

Lead can also be found in the drinking water of homes, schools, or day care facilities built before 1960 (Abelson & Sanborn, 2010). Other sources of lead can include the soil around homes that have peeling outdoor paint, crayons, children's toys or jewelry, ethnic cosmetics (e.g., kohl, surma, ceruse), some imported spices, and the clothing of parents who work with lead (e.g., smelters or refineries) (Abelson & Sanborn, 2010; Health Canada, 2009). Box 30.5 presents a simple questionnaire the nurse can give to the parents of a child who may have been exposed to lead.

Hypertension Screening

Hypertension in children is becoming an increasing concern and may be a sign of underlying disease or the early onset of primary hypertension. Universal hypertension screening for children is recommended beginning at 3 years of age (Hagan et al., 2008). If the child has risk factors for

---

BOX 30.4 Risk Factors for Iron-Deficiency Anemia

Children at high risk for iron-deficiency anemia include those from low-income families, First Nations and Inuit children, and migrants or recently arrived refugees. Specific risk factors include:

- Periods of rapid growth
- Low birth weight or premature birth
- Low dietary intake of meat, fish, poultry, and ascorbic acid
- Macrobiotic diet
- Introduction of cow's milk before 12 months of age
- Use of infant formula that is not fortified with iron
- Exclusive breastfeeding after age 4 months without iron-fortified supplemental foods
- Meal skipping, frequent dieting
- Exposure to lead
- Feeding problems
- Current or recent pregnancy
- Intensive physical training
- Recent blood loss, including heavy/lengthy menstrual periods
- Chronic use of aspirin or nonsteroidal anti-inflammatory drugs
- Parasitic infections

Adapted from: Baker, R. D., Greer, F. R., & the Committee on Nutrition. (2010). Clinical report: Diagnosis and prevention of iron deficiency and iron-deficiency anemia in infants and young children (0–3 years of age). *Pediatrics, 126*(5), 1040–1050. Retrieved November 21, 2011 from http://aappolicy.aappublications.org/cgi/content/full/pediatrics;126/5/1040.

BOX 30.5 **A Basic Personal-Risk Questionnaire for Lead Exposure in Children**

1. Does your child live in or regularly visit a house or child care facility that was built before 1978?
2. Does your child live in or regularly visit a house or child care facility built before 1978 that is being or has recently been (within the past 6 months) renovated or remodelled?
3. Does your child have a sibling or playmate who has or had lead poisoning?

From: Centers for Disease Control and Prevention. (1997). *Screening young children for lead poisoning: Guidance for state and local health officials*. Atlanta, GA: US Department of Health and Human Services, National Center for Environmental Health.

---

systemic hypertension, such as preterm birth or congenital heart disease, then screening begins at the time the risk factor becomes apparent. Evaluation of hypertension in children should include a complete history, which may reveal symptoms such as headache, irritability, blurred vision, seizures, frequent epistaxis, and hematuria (Koshy, Grisaru, & Midgley, 2008). The increasing prevalence of childhood obesity has been associated with a greater incidence of prehypertension and hypertension (McCrindle, 2010).

The guidelines for determining hypertension in children and adolescents mirror the guidelines established for the adult population (Box 30.6). Pre-adolescent children whose blood pressure is in the 90th to 95th percentile are considered to have prehypertension. Adolescent children whose blood pressure is 120/80 mm Hg are categorized as being prehypertensive, even if their percentile ranking is below the 90th percentile. Anticipatory guidance on diet and lifestyle changes is appropriate for any child with prehypertension (National Heart, Lung, and Blood Institute, 2005).

Hyperlipidemia Screening

Hyperlipidemia screening of children can reduce the incidence of adult coronary disease. Atherosclerosis has been documented in children and a link exists between these lesions and high lipid levels. Selectively screening

---

BOX 30.6 **Pre-Adolescent Childhood Hypertension Guidelines**

Optimal	<90th percentile
Prehypertension	90th to 95th percentile
Stage I	>95th percentile up to 5 mm Hg above 99th percentile
Stage II	5 mm Hg above 99th percentile, or higher

BOX 30.7 **Hyperlipidemia Screening**

Screen if parents or grandparents, at <55 years of age, have/had documented:

- Coronary atherosclerosis
- Myocardial infarction
- Angina pectoris
- Peripheral vascular disease
- Cerebrovascular disease
- Sudden cardiac death

Screen if a parent's blood cholesterol level is 240 mg/dL or higher.

Screen at health care provider's discretion:

- Parental history is unobtainable.
- Child has diabetes or hypertension.
- Child has lifestyle risk factors:
  - Cigarette smoking
  - Obesity
  - Sedentary activity pattern
  - High-fat dietary intake

Adapted from: Hagan, J. F., Shaw, J. S., & Duncan, P. M. (Eds.). (2008). *Bright futures: Guidelines for health supervision of infants, children, and adolescents* (3rd ed.). Elk Grove Village, IL: American Academy of Pediatrics.

---

those children at high risk for hyperlipidemia can reduce their lifelong risk of coronary artery disease.

The risk assessment focuses on the child's family history. Children whose parents or grandparents had premature cardiovascular disease (before 55 years of age) or who have a parent with hypercholesterolemia are screened. If the child's family history is not available, screening is done at the discretion of the health care provider. The nurse also assesses for lifestyle factors that may contribute to hyperlipidemia such as sedentary lifestyle, cigarette smoking, obesity, and high-fat dietary intake. Children with diseases such as diabetes and hypertension are also candidates for hyperlipidemia screening. See Box 30.7 for details.

Remember Maya and Evan, the 3-year-old and 12-month-old from the beginning of the chapter? How would you assess Maya's and Evan's growth and development? Which screening tests are warranted for them and why? What further information would you need to determine which tests should be performed?

Immunizations

The development of effective vaccines, which began in the 1940s, revolutionized children's health care around the world. Immunization is the key component in disease prevention, saving more lives in the past century than any other health intervention. Despite World Health Organization (WHO) estimates that immunization programs prevent more than 2 million deaths worldwide each year, immunization is not currently mandatory in Canada.

Immunization has allowed the focus of disease to shift from treatment to prevention. It is important, therefore, for nurses to understand the principles of immunization, proper use of vaccines, appropriate management of children's distress and pain associated with immunizations, and potential barriers to immunization. Armed with this knowledge base, the nurse can partner with families to provide the highest level of disease protection for children.

Principles of Immunization

The immune system has the ability to recognize materials present in the body as "self" or "non-self." Foreign materials (non-self) are called *antigens*. When an antigen is recognized by the immune system, the immune system responds by producing antibodies (immunoglobulins) or directing special cells to destroy and remove the antigen.

Immunity is the ability to destroy and remove a specific antigen from the body. The acquisition of immunity can be active or passive. **Passive immunity** is produced when the immunoglobulins of one person are transferred to another. This immunity lasts only weeks or months and can be transferred from mothers to infants via the placenta or breast milk (colostrum). Passive immunity can also be achieved through the administration of preformed antibodies or immunoglobulins (e.g., hepatitis B immune globulin). **Active immunity** is acquired when a person's own immune system generates the immune response. Active immunity lasts for many years or for a lifetime. This long-term protection is the result of immunologic memory. After the initial immune response, specialized cells for that antigen continue to exist. When an antigen returns, these memory cells very rapidly produce a fresh supply of antibodies to re-establish protection. This immunity can occur after exposure to natural pathogens or after exposure to vaccines. Vaccines (biologicals) mimic the characteristics of the natural antigen and contain antigens designed to produce a protective immune response. They are used to induce an active, artificial immunity. The immune system mounts a response and establishes an immunologic memory as it would for an infection.

Vaccine classifications are based on the characteristics of the antigen(s) present in the biological. The antigen may be viral or bacterial. It may be live and attenuated (weakened) or it may be killed. The vaccine may contain a whole antigen or a portion of it (fractional/split cell). Several types of vaccines are currently available:

- Live attenuated vaccines contain whole, living viruses or bacteria that have been modified or weakened. These vaccines result in a prolonged, extensive immunity that most closely resembles natural immunity (even after one dose). The bacteria or viruses are attenuated, meaning they are weakened and produce an immune response without producing the complications of the illness itself.

- Killed or inactivated vaccines contain bacterial or viral organisms that have been killed by heat or chemical processes. Because the organisms in these vaccines are incapable of reproducing, a series of immunizations are needed to produce a lasting immune response.

- Toxoid vaccines contain bacterial toxins that have been weakened by heat or chemicals while retaining their ability to induce an immune response. These vaccines pose no risk for people who are immunocompromised and may provide broad immunity when the vaccine contains multiple antigens (e.g., tetanus diphtheria [Td]).

- Conjugate vaccines are created by attaching an antigen (bacteria) to a carrier protein. Linking bacterial polysaccharides with proteins dramatically increases the immune response. Conjugate vaccines are often used to prevent invasive bacterial disease (e.g., meningococcal conjugate vaccine). Polysaccharide vaccines cannot be used in children under the age of 18 months and generally tend to provide negligible and short-term protection in children and infants. Therefore, they are used mostly in adult populations.

- Recombinant vaccines make use of bacteria or yeast to produce large quantities of a bacterial or viral protein. A purified form of this protein is then created for use in a vaccine. Protection from the natural disease occurs when the child's immune system makes antibodies in response to the immunization. An example is the hepatitis B vaccine, which is produced by merging a gene portion of the virus with a gene of a yeast cell. This yeast cell subsequently produces hepatitis B surface antigen (HBsAg), which is used for the preparation of a vaccine.

Immunization Management

Numerous organizations participate in Canada's immunization programs (visit http://thePoint.lww.com/Chow1e for direct links to such organizations). The National Advisory Committee on Immunization (NACI) provides the PHAC with current scientific and medical advice with regard to immunization. NACI comprises experts from the fields of pediatrics, immunology, infectious disease, internal medicine, microbiology, and public health. Reporting to the chief public health officer of Canada, NACI works with the PHAC's Centre for Infectious Disease Prevention and Control to provide current and ongoing updates and public health advice. This committee provides recommendations related to vaccine-preventable disease and the use of both current and newly approved vaccines; it also identifies at-risk groups that immunization programs should target.

The *Canadian Immunization Guide* (CIG), produced by NACI every 4 years, is based on current scientific research and knowledge (NACI, 2008). It encompasses recommendations on vaccine use and immunization scheduling in Canada and addresses all components of immunization (Table 30.5). In addition to the recommended

TABLE 30.5 ROUTINE IMMUNIZATION SCHEDULES FOR CHILDREN FROM INFANCY THROUGH AGE 18

Infants and Children

Timing	DTaP-IPV	Hib	MMR	Var	HB	Pneu-C-7	Men-C	Tdap	Inf
Birth					Infancy 3 doses ★ or Pre-teen/teen 2–3 doses				
2 months	●	✦				■	◉		
4 months	●	✦				■	(◉)		
6 months	●	✦				■	◉ or		6–23 months ⊗ 1–2 doses
12 months			■	●		■ (12–15 months)	◉ if not yet given		
18 months	●	✦	■ or						
4–6 years	●		■						
14–16 years							◉ if not yet given	▲	

Children <7 Years of Age not Immunized in Early Infancy

Timing	DTaP-IPV	Hib	MMR	Var	HB	Pneu-C-7	Men-C	Tdap
First visit	●	✦	■	●	★	■	⊗	
2 months later	●	(✦)	■		★	(■)	(⊗)	
2 months later	●					(■)		
6–12 months later	●	(✦)			★			
4–6 years of age	(●)							
14–16 years of age								▲

Children ≥7 Years of Age up to 17 Years of Age not Immunized in Early Infancy

Timing	Tdap	IPV	MMR	Var	HB	Men-C
First visit	▲	⬟	■	●	★	◉
2 months later	▲	⬟	■	(●)	(★)	
6–12 months later	▲	⬟			★	
10 years later	▲					

( )   Symbols with brackets around them imply that these doses may not be required, depending on the age of the child or adult.

●   **Diphtheria, tetanus, acellular pertussis and inactivated polio virus vaccine (DTaP-IPV):** DTaP-IPV(± Hib) vaccine is the preferred vaccine for all doses in the vaccination series, including completion of the series in children who have received one or more doses of DPT (whole cell) vaccine (e.g., recent immigrants). The 4- to 6-year dose can be omitted if the fourth dose was given after the child's fourth birthday.

✦   ***Haemophilus influenzae* type b conjugate vaccine (Hib):** The Hib schedule shown is for the *Haemophilus* b capsular polysaccharide–polyribosylribitol phosphate (PRP) conjugated to tetanus toxoid (PRP-T). For catch-up, the number of doses depends on the age at which the schedule is begun. Not usually required past age 5 years.

(continued)

TABLE 30.5 ROUTINE IMMUNIZATION SCHEDULES FOR CHILDREN FROM INFANCY THROUGH AGE 18 (continued)

■	**Measles, mumps, and rubella vaccine (MMR):** A second dose of MMR is recommended for children at least 1 month after the first dose for the purpose of better measles protection. For convenience, options include giving it with the next scheduled vaccination at 18 months of age or at school entry (age 4–6 years) (depending on the provincial/territorial policy) or at any intervening age that is practical. In the catch-up schedule (i.e., children <7 years of age not immunized in early infancy), the first dose should not be given until the child is ≥12 months old. MMR should be given to all susceptible adolescents and adults.
●	**Varicella vaccine (Var):** Children aged 12 months to 12 years should receive one dose of varicella vaccine. Susceptible individuals ≥13 years of age should receive two doses at least 28 days apart.
★	**Hepatitis B vaccine (HB):** Hepatitis B vaccine can be routinely given to infants or pre-adolescents, depending on the provincial/territorial policy. For infants born to chronic carrier mothers, the first dose should be given at birth (with hepatitis B immunoglobulin); otherwise the first dose can be given at 2 months of age to fit more conveniently with other routine infant immunization visits. The second dose should be administered at least 1 month after the first dose, and the third at least 2 months after the second dose, but these may fit more conveniently into the 4- and 6-month immunization visits. A two-dose schedule for adolescents is an option.
■	**Pneumococcal conjugate vaccine-7-valent (Pneu-C-7):** Recommended for all children under 2 years of age. The recommended schedule depends on the age of the child when vaccination is begun.
◉	**Meningococcal C conjugate vaccine (Men-C):** Recommended for children <5 years of age, adolescents, and young adults. The recommended schedule depends on the age of the individual and the conjugate vaccine used. At least one dose in the primary infant series should be given after 5 months of age. If the provincial/territorial policy is to give Men-C to persons ≥12 months of age, one dose is sufficient.
▲	**Diphtheria, tetanus, acellular pertussis vaccine – adult/adolescent formulation (Tdap):** A combined adsorbed "adult type" preparation for use in people ≥7 years of age, contains less diphtheria toxoid and pertussis antigens than preparations given to younger children and is less likely to cause reactions in older people.
◒	**Influenza vaccine (Inf):** Recommended for all children 6–23 months of age and all persons ≥65 years of age. Previously unvaccinated children <9 years of age require two doses of the current season's vaccine with an interval of at least 4 weeks. The second dose within the same season is not required if the child received one or more doses of influenza vaccine during the previous influenza season.
⬢	**IPV Inactivated polio virus**

Source: *Canadian Immunization Guide* (7th ed.). Public Health Agency of Canada, 2006. Reproduced with the permission of the Minister of Health, 2011.

routine immunization schedules, NACI outlines "catch-up" schedules for children who have not been adequately immunized (see Table 30.5). Updates to the CIG are published yearly in the *Canada Communicable Disease Report*. Children's immunization records must be compared with the latest edition of the schedules in their area of residence when assessing the need for immunization. PHAC has an Immunization Schedule Tool for parents based on their province/territory of residence (PHAC, 2011b). This tool, based on the child's age, allows parents to check which immunizations their child is currently due to receive.

Seventeen guidelines define the "ideal" parametres for immunization practices, with the goal of maintaining the highest protection for Canadians against vaccine-preventable diseases. Canada's National Immunization Strategy, launched through the joint efforts of the federal, provincial, and territorial governments, addresses and responds to both current and future immunization needs of Canadians. Funded through the federal budget, its work addresses surveillance of vaccine-preventable diseases, vaccine safety, immunization coverage rates, research, and education.

▶ *Take* NOTE!

Vaccines are administered to Canadians at various ages, according to NACI recommendations and provincial/territorial immunization schedules.

Vaccine Administration

When preparing to immunize infants or children, obtaining a complete immunization history is essential in order to identify any contraindications to immunization and determine the appropriate vaccine to administer during the visit (Box 30.8).

▶ *Take* NOTE!

When obtaining an immunization history, ask the question, "When and where did your child receive his (or her) last immunization?" This question allows for more information gathering than the yes–no question, "Are your child's immunizations up to date?" The nurse can compare this information with that on the available immunization record; discover in what settings the child is getting health care; and use the information as a starting point in a discussion of any reactions to previous immunizations.

When present, contraindications—defined as conditions that "significantly increase the chance that a serious adverse event will occur if the vaccine is given"—require vaccines to be deferred (NACI, 2008, p. 73). In Canada, only three contraindications to vaccination exist: (1) anaphylaxis to some component of the biological (vaccine), (2) a state of significant immunocompromise (live vaccines), and (3) pregnancy (live vaccines) (Table 30.6). The CIG contains a comprehensive listing of the many conditions that are *not* contraindications to immunization for nurses to use as a resource. Temporarily postponing vaccinations is recommended when an infant or child has a severe illness with a high fever or has recently received blood products. Postponing vaccination is not required for a minor respiratory illness or

BOX 30.8 Obtaining an Immunization History: Questions for Parents

- How is your feeling child today? Does your child have a fever?
- Does your child have any allergies to food or medication?
- Has your child ever had any problems after his/her vaccines?
- Has your child ever had a seizure or convulsion related to a fever? (If yes, advise prophylactic acetaminophen for immunization.)

If the vaccine to be given is a live viral or live bacterial vaccine, add these questions:

- Does your child have any problems with his/her immune system?
- Has your child received any blood products or blood transfusions in the past year?

Source: *Canadian Immunization Guide* (7th ed.). Public Health Agency of Canada, 2006. Reproduced with the permission of the Minister of Health, 2011.

low-grade fever (Kroger, Sumaya, Pickering, & Atkinson, 2011).

Precautions are conditions that increase the risk of a child experiencing an adverse reaction following immunization or conditions that may impair the child's ability to acquire immunity from the vaccine. On an individual basis, nurses must weigh the benefits of immunization against the likelihood of an adverse event. A summary of precautions and contraindications for specific vaccines is presented in Table 30.7.

Storage and administration of vaccines are other key considerations in immunization and directly impact the efficacy of a vaccine given. Improperly stored or

TABLE 30.6 CONTRAINDICATIONS AND SELECTED PRECAUTIONS FOR VACCINE ADMINISTRATION

Issue of Concern	Type of Vaccine	
	Inactivated/Subunit	Live
Allergy to vaccine component	Contraindication if the specific vaccine contains that particular component	
Severely immunocompromised	Precaution	Contraindication
Pregnancy	None	Contraindication
Recent administration of blood product containing antibodies	None	Precaution
Recent administration of live virus vaccine	None	Precaution
Severe bleeding disorder	Precaution	Precaution

Source: *Canadian Immunization Guide* (7th ed.). Public Health Agency of Canada, 2006. Reproduced with the permission of the Minister of Health, 2011.

TABLE 30.7 Contraindications and Precautions for Commonly Used Vaccines

Vaccine	Contraindications	Precautions
Hepatitis B (HB)	Standard contraindications*	• Moderate or severe illness with or without acute fever • Infants <2,000 g if mother HBsAg negative
Diphtheria, Tetanus, acellular Pertussis (DTaP)	• Standard contraindications* • Previous encephalopathy within 7 days after Diphtheria, Tetanus, Pertussis (DTP) or DTaP vaccine	• Temperature 40.5° C within 48 h after previous dose • Continuous crying lasting 3 h within 48 h after previous dose • Convulsion within 3 days after previous immunization • Pale or limp episode or collapse within 48 h after previous dose • Unstable progressive neurologic problem • History of Guillain–Barré syndrome within 6 weeks
Measles, Mumps, Rubella (MMR)	• Standard contraindications*,† • Pregnancy or possibility of pregnancy within 4 weeks • Blood products within the past 5 months • Immunocompromised person • If not given same day as varicella and/or yellow fever, hold until spaced 28 days apart	• Thrombocytopenia or history of thrombocytopenic purpura
Varicella	• Standard contraindications*,† • Pregnancy or possibility of pregnancy within 4 weeks • Blood products received within the past 5 months • Immunocompromised person • If not given same day as MMR and/or yellow fever, hold until spaced 28 days apart	• Do not give within 24 h of antiviral medications. • Family history of congenital or hereditary immunodeficiency
Haemophilus influenzae type B (Hib)	Standard contraindications*	• Moderate or severe acute illness
Influenza	Standard contraindications*	• History of Guillain–Barré syndrome within 6 weeks
Pneumococcal conjugate vaccine (Pneu-C-7, Pneu-P-23)	Standard contraindications*	• Moderate or severe acute illness
Meningococcal conjugate (Men-C)	Standard contraindications*	• Moderate or severe acute illness
Human papillomavirus (HPV)	Standard contraindications*	• Moderate or severe acute illness

People with immune deficiencies and pregnant women should not receive live vaccines. (See CIG for guidelines.)

*(1) Do not administer if client has had an anaphylactic reaction to prior dose of vaccine or any of its components. (2) Do not administer if client has a moderate to severe acute illness. Minor illnesses are not a reason to postpone immunization.

†Inquire about neomycin or gelatin allergies.

Source: *Canadian Immunization Guide* (7th ed.). Public Health Agency of Canada, 2006. Reproduced with the permission of the Minister of Health, 2011.

TABLE 30.8   VACCINE ADMINISTRATION: NEEDLE AND SITE SELECTION

Client	Needle Size (gauge)	Needle Length (cm)	Site (Intramuscular)
Infants <1 year	25	2.2–2.5	Anterolateral thigh
Children ≥1 year	25	1.6	Deltoid*
Older children (larger muscle) and adolescents	22–25	2.5–3.8	Deltoid
All patients receiving subcutaneous injections	25	1.6	Upper arm

*Unless the muscle mass is not adequate, in which case the anterolateral thigh would be used with a 2.5 cm needle.

Source: *Canadian Immunization Guide* (7th ed.). Public Health Agency of Canada, 2006. Reproduced with the permission of the Minister of Health, 2011.

reconstituted vaccines can be rendered ineffective (CDC, 2011b), so proper vaccine storage is critical to efficacy. Administration of vaccines by the correct route and use of the correct needles are also imperative in providing safe and effective immunization (Table 30.8). The vaccine manufacturer's package insert is the best reference source for any vaccine.

Prior to administration of a vaccine(s), information sheets provided by each province or territory must be reviewed with parents/guardians. A discussion of any parental concerns about immunization, along with a review of the infant's or child's previous health and immunization history, are imperative. At this time the nurse also screens for precautions and contraindications for each vaccine to be administered. The parents must feel comfortable and acknowledge an understanding of the information presented. The use of a reliable translator to present immunization information in cases in which language barriers may exist is considered mandatory. Consent from parents/guardians to immunize must be accompanied by an understanding of the immunization information given and is a requirement of informed consent. Box 30.9 presents the requirements of immunization documentation.

Families should always be provided with a personal record of the child's immunizations. This record serves to reinforce the importance of the procedure and acts as a reminder for maintaining the currency of immunizations.

Vaccine Descriptions

This section reviews the vaccines most commonly being used in Canada for routine immunization of infants and children. These immunizations are recommended by NACI and are found in the CIG. Although immunization in Canada is currently not mandatory, each province or territory determines which immunizations are required for school admittance. This information can be found on the PHAC website, a direct link to which can be accessed by visiting http://thePoint.lww.com/Chow1e. Children who are not immunized are requested to remain out of school during any outbreaks of vaccine-preventable diseases.

Diphtheria, Pertussis, and Tetanus Vaccines

Immunizations against diphtheria, pertussis, and tetanus are given in a combination vaccine. The whole-cell pertussis vaccine was introduced in Canada in the 1940s. It was then replaced in the 1980s by the adsorbed

---

BOX 30.9   Requirements of Immunization Documentation

Vaccines administered to an individual should be recorded in three locations:

- The personal immunization record held by the client or his or her parent/guardian
- The record maintained by the health care provider who gave the immunization
- The local or provincial registry

Each method of recording should include the following:

- Documentation of informed consent
- Trade name of the product
- Disease(s) against which the vaccine protects
- Date given (day, month, and year)
- Dose
- Site and route of administration
- Manufacturer
- Lot number
- Name and title of person administering the vaccine

Source: *Canadian Immunization Guide* (7th ed.). Public Health Agency of Canada, 2006. Reproduced with the permission of the Minister of Health, 2011.

whole-cell vaccine and subsequently by an acellular vaccine in 1997 and1998. Only acellular vaccines are now available in Canada; whole-cell preparations are no longer in use. Acellular vaccines have decreased the frequency and severity of both local and systemic adverse reactions compared with whole-cell pertussis vaccines (NACI, 2008).

The vaccine currently used for children under age 7 is diphtheria, tetanus, acellular pertussis (DTaP). It contains diphtheria and tetanus toxoids and pertussis cell wall proteins. The older version of this vaccine—diphtheria, pertussis, tetanus (DPT)—contained killed whole cells of pertussis bacteria and caused more frequent and severe adverse reactions than DTaP. The diphtheria, tetanus (DT) vaccine is used for children under age 7 who have contraindications to pertussis immunization. In Canada, acellular pertussis vaccine is recommended for all children 2 months of age or older for whom there are no contraindications.

Full-strength diphtheria toxoid causes significant adverse reactions in people over the age of 7 years. For this group, the Tdap adolescent preparation vaccine is used. This vaccine contains tetanus toxoid, reduced diphtheria toxoid, and acellular pertussis vaccine. The lowercase "d" is used to designate the lower dose of diphtheria toxoid. NACI recommends that Tdap be used for all tetanus boosters in older children (11 to 12 years of age) and adolescents because it provides a boost to diphtheria and pertussis immunization. See Table 30.5 for routine schedules.

> ▶ *Take* NOTE!
>
> *Pertussis prevalence has risen steadily since the 1970s, with 31% of cases occurring in adolescents and adults (PHAC, 2011a). This increase prompted NACI's recommendation to change the tetanus booster for older children and adolescents from Td to Tdap beginning in 2006 in order to provide continuing protection against pertussis infection (NACI, 2008).*

Haemophilus influenzae Type B Vaccines

Haemophilus influenzae type B is a bacterium that causes several life-threatening illnesses in children under 5 years of age. These infections include meningitis, epiglottitis, and septic arthritis. *Haemophilus influenzae* type B conjugate vaccines (Hib) have been extremely effective in cutting the rates of these diseases in children. A total of three doses is necessary to complete the primary series in infants. The CIG recommends a booster dose at 15 to 18 months of age. Hib vaccine is not given to children 5 years of age or older.

Polio Vaccine

Inactivated polio vaccine (IPV) is the only polio vaccine currently recommended in Canada. It is a killed virus vaccine that poses no risk for vaccine-acquired disease. Oral polio vaccine (OPV), a live attenuated virus vaccine, was the preferred polio vaccine until 2000. At that time it became apparent that the only victims of poliomyelitis were people who had acquired it from OPV. NACI determined that in this country the risks associated with OPV outweighed the benefits and withdrew its recommendation for this vaccine.

Measles, Mumps, and Rubella Vaccines

Measles, mumps, and rubella (MMR) is a live attenuated virus combination vaccine. It is the one most commonly used in childhood immunizations. MMR can be given the same day as other live attenuated virus vaccines such as varicella vaccine (Var). However, if not given on the same day, the immunizations should be spaced at least 28 days apart (Kroger, Sumaya, Pickering, & Atkinson, 2011). Anaphylactic reactions are believed to be associated with the neomycin or gelatin components of the vaccine, rather than the egg component. The vaccine is not prepared from the allergenic albumen portion of the egg, so egg allergy is no longer a contraindication for measles vaccine (Kroger et al., 2011). Pregnancy in a child's mother is not a contraindication to the vaccination of the child (Kroger et al., 2011). Individual MMR vaccines are available if needed.

Hepatitis B Vaccine

Hepatitis B vaccine (HepB) is a recombinant vaccine. The vaccine is 80% to 90% effective in preventing hepatitis B infection. For infants, the mother's HBsAg status determines when immunization for hepatitis B begins. If the mother's status is positive or unknown, the neonate is immunized within the first 12 hours of life, at 1 to 2 months of age, and at 6 months of age. This is vital, because up to 90% of infected neonates develop chronic carrier status and will be predisposed to cirrhosis and hepatic cancer (CDC, 2010). If the mother's status is negative, immunizations are done routinely at 2, 4, and 6 months of age. Because hepatitis B is a sexually transmitted infection, it is important to verify the immunization status of all adolescents.

Varicella Vaccine

Var is a live attenuated virus vaccine. All children ages 12 months to 12 years who have not had varicella (chickenpox) should be immunized. Children 13 years of age or older who have not had varicella or the vaccine should receive two doses of the vaccine, at least 28 days apart (NACI, 2008). The vaccine is effective for varicella postexposure prophylaxis if administered within 3 to 5 days after exposure. Var may be given on the same day as other live attenuated virus vaccines. However, if not given on the same day, the immunizations should be spaced at least 28 days apart. Pregnancy in a child's mother is not a contraindication to the vaccination of the child.

Pneumococcal Vaccines

Streptococcus pneumoniae (pneumococcus) is the most common cause of pneumonia, sepsis, meningitis, and otitis media in young children (CDC, 2011c). The available pneumococcal vaccines are pneumococcal conjugate vaccine (PCV7) and pneumococcal polysaccharide vaccine (PPV). PCV7 contains seven strains of *S. pneumoniae*. It does stimulate an immune response in infants and is given at 2 months of age as part of the initial immunization series. Health Canada has recently approved Prevnar 13 (pneumococcal 13-valent conjugate vaccine) for use in children ages 6 weeks to 5 years for active immunization against invasive pneumococcal disease (*Health Canada approves...*, 2009).

PPV contains 23 strains of *S. pneumoniae*. It does not provoke an immune response in children less than 2 years of age. PPV is given to children over 2 years of age who are at high-risk for pneumococcal sepsis. This group includes children with anatomic/functional asplenia; sickle-cell disease; chronic cardiac, pulmonary, or renal disease; diabetes mellitus; HIV infection; immunosuppression; or children who have or are getting cochlear implants (CDC, 2011c).

Influenza Vaccines

Influenza immunization is recommended yearly for children between the ages of 6 and 59 months. Children 2 years old or older should be vaccinated if they have chronic health problems. It is also recommended that caregivers and household contacts of these children be immunized. Additionally, the vaccine can be given to anyone wishing to have immunity.

Human Papillomavirus Vaccine

Human papillomavirus (HPV) is a DNA tumour virus transmitted through direct skin-to-skin contact. HPV is contracted most often during vaginal or anal penetrative sexual acts. HPV infection is most common in adolescents and young adults ages 15 to 24 years who are sexually active (NACI, 2008). HPV causes genital warts and is responsible for the development of cervical cancer. In 2007, CPS recommended that the HPV vaccine be administered routinely to all girls between 9 and 13 years of age before the onset of sexual activity (thereby providing optimal protection against initial infection with the HPV). The vaccine is also recommended for all unimmunized females 13 years of age and older as a "catch-up program" within approved programs. The three-vaccine series should begin at age 9 to 13 years. The vaccine is anticipated to prevent most cases of genital warts and cervical cancer (CPS, 2007).

Meningococcal Vaccine

Meningococcal disease may manifest as meningitis or as a deadly blood infection (meningococcemia). It is caused by the bacterium *Neisseria meningitidis,* which is spread through direct contact or by air droplets. Invasive meningococcal disease is endemic in Canada and shows periods of increased activity approximately every 10 to 15 years. The incidence rates have been highest in children younger than 1 year of age, with a smaller peak in the 15- to 19-year age group. The meningococcal C conjugate vaccines have been approved for use in infants, children, and adults. They are recommended for the immunization of children 1 to 4 years of age and for adolescents and young adults to prevent the increased risk of serogroup C meningococcal disease. NACI recommends that these vaccines be used according to local routine immunization programs across the country. Polysaccharide vaccines are not recommended for routine use in childhood immunization.

Recall 3-year-old Maya and 12-month-old Evan, introduced at the beginning of the chapter. What immunizations would be appropriate for them to receive? Explain how you would administer the injections and discuss any contraindications or precautions that are necessary.

Vaccine Safety

While no vaccine can be 100% safe and effective, serious adverse events related to vaccines are rare. The safety and efficacy of existing vaccines nonetheless are under constant review. Research to improve vaccines is ongoing, with the goal of continuing to refine vaccines so that a maximum immune response is produced with the least amount of risk for the client. Because vaccines are being given to healthy infants and children, there is a low tolerance for any adverse events. Misconceptions around vaccine safety are a major barrier to optimizing immunization rates. Canada's vaccine safety surveillance system documents and closely monitors all reported adverse events as part of its mandate to keep immunizations as safe as possible.

If a clinically significant adverse event occurs following an immunization, it is reported to the infant's or child's provincial or territorial public health authorities as well as to the PHAC. A standard report form—available through public health units and the CPS—is used to report specific adverse events (e.g., anaphylaxis, injection-site reactions, neurologic events) as well as any severe, unusual, or unexpected adverse events that are of concern to the vaccine provider, health care provider, vaccine recipient, or parent(s)/guardian(s). Any severe adverse events following childhood immunizations are also monitored through the Immunization Monitoring Program ACTive (IMPACT). This pediatric, hospital-based network currently has 12 active sites across Canada. IMPACT has received more than 18,000 case reports to date and has concluded that these reports have been extremely beneficial in documenting "the rarity of harm from vaccinations" (CPS, 2009a).

Barriers to Immunization

A fully immunized child is protected from the discomforts and complications of many infectious diseases. Disease prevention spares the family the emotional and financial burdens that serious illnesses can cause. Effective immunization programs prevent devastating epidemics in a community. Health care dollars not spent treating preventable diseases can be used for other urgent issues. Despite the numerous advantages of an optimal immunization status, however, many children in Canada are not fully immunized, and many factors are related to this status.

Distress and Pain

Infants and children who are being immunized (as well as their parents) can experience significant anxiety and fear related to needle(s). Pain—be it the threat of pain or the pain itself—is always stressful for children and can be frightening. Pain associated with needles is described by children as being the most hurtful type of pain, and they report anticipatory stress and anxiety related to negative memories of previous painful events (Kortesluoma & Nikkonen, 2006; Stinson, Yamada, Dickson, Lamba, & Stevens, 2008; Taylor, Boyer, & Campbell, 2008; Uman, Chambers, McGrath, & Kisely, 2008; von Baeyer, Marche, Rocha, & Salmon, 2004; Walco, 2008). This leads to increased fear and noncompliance during future interventions, which is well documented throughout the pediatric literature (Kennedy, Luhmann, & Zempsky, 2008; Schechter et al., 2007). Avoidance of future medical care by children and families can be a consequence of these obstacles.

Safety Misconceptions

Parental and public concerns and controversies about vaccine safety are also a significant reason for inadequate immunization. Misconceptions about the safety of vaccines and about what constitutes a contraindication to vaccination are major contributors to inadequate immunization status, which in turn can lead to a resurgence of vaccine-preventable diseases and their negative sequelae (see Table 30.7). A telling example is the recent resolution to the long-term controversy regarding the unsubstantiated link between immunization and the development of autism in children. *The Lancet* recently retracted its 12-year-old publication of a "landmark study" that implied the existence of a link between MMR and autism by withdrawing the original research from within its archives (Eggertson, 2010). The consequence of this flawed research has been the reappearance of measles in unimmunized children, including outbreaks in the United Kingdom, United States, and

Canada. Concerns surrounding the use of a vaccine preservative thimerosal, which contains minute amounts of mercury, also generated public scrutiny and controversy. Thimerosal was subsequently removed from all vaccines used for children in Canada as of March 2001.

Other Factors

Other factors have been shown to impact immunization rates in Canada as well. For example, the number of children in a family can play a role. The more children in a family, the less likely they are to be fully vaccinated. This may be due to the family's hectic schedules, difficulty accessing public health units, and other related factors. The costs for vaccines can also deter families from obtaining immunizations. Although most provinces and territories have extensively funded immunization programs, there are exceptions. For example, if a young woman does not fit within the current schedule for receiving the HPV vaccine in the funded component of the program, the expense to receive the three doses (a complete series) would be substantial and unaffordable for many families. Finally, parents may want to postpone some of the scheduled immunizations due to concerns about the effects of multiple injections on their child. However, delaying a portion of the immunizations puts the child at risk for contracting disease. Disrupting the optimal spacing of the immunizations can also decrease the efficacy of vaccines, putting the child at further risk.

Easing Barriers to Immunization

According to the CIG, "providing vaccines in a climate of appropriate informed consent, including discussion of commonly held misconceptions etc. can help ensure that immunization will maintain its status as one of the most effective preventive measures in the history of medicine" (NACI, 2008, p. 30). In addition to the measures outlined below, NACI is an excellent resource for additional information on vaccination recommendations in Canada. Visit http://thePoint.lww.com/Chow1e for a direct link to NACI.

Fear of Needles

International organizations, including WHO, have declared unresolved pain in children to be *morally unjust*. The Canadian Nurses Association Code of Ethics for Registered Nurses (2008) mandates that nursing practices reflect "right behaviour and right knowledge." This makes it the responsibility of nurses to manage children's needle-related pain and anxiety based on current evidence-based practice. It is imperative, therefore, that these practices be incorporated into routine immunization care.

Empirical evidence shows that both pharmacologic and non-pharmacologic (non–drug related) methods currently exist to safely decrease needle-related pain and effectively manage infants' and children's distress and fear related to needles (Buscemi, Vandermeer, & Curtis, 2008; Stinson et al., 2008; Taddio et al., 2009a, Taddio, llersich, Ipp, Kikuta, & Shah, 2009b, Taddio et al., 2010; Uman et al., 2008; Walco, 2008). For example, pain experienced by infants receiving intramuscular or subcutaneous injections can be reduced by a variety of methods: (1) offering sweet-tasting suspensions such as oral sucrose during immunizations (Curtis, Jou, Ali, Vandermeer, & Klassen, 2007; Taddio et al., 2010), (2) breastfeeding or giving the infant a pacifier during immunizations (Taddio et al., 2010), (3) swaddling the upper body during immunizations, and (4) using topical anesthetics at immunization sites (this has been shown not to interfere with the immunologic response to vaccines; Halperin, Halperin, McGrath, Smith, & Houston, 2002). Distraction techniques such as books, bubbles (Fig. 30.4), and "blowing away the pain" have demonstrated the best outcomes for non-pharmacologic management of needle-related pain in children, and the positive effects of these techniques have been proven for anticipatory stages as well as during and following painful procedures in children (Buscemi et al., 2008; Uman et al., 2008). Distraction is an ideal tool for use by nurses managing immunization-related pain. The order in which vaccines

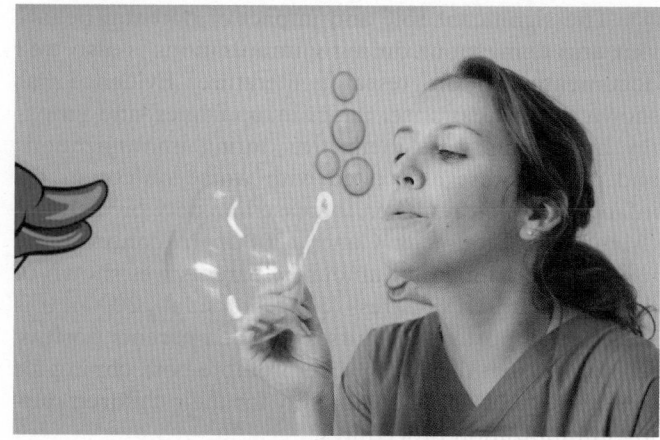

FIGURE 30.4 Blowing bubbles can be an effective distraction technique when immunizing children. Used with permission from the Children's Burns Trust, London.

are given can also impact the pain response, with recommendations that the most painful vaccine be administered last (Moshe, Parkin, Lear, Goldbach, & Taddio, 2009). See Evidence-based Practice 30.1.

EVIDENCE-BASED PRACTICE 30.1
Nursing Practice in Immunization Pain Management

● **Study**

Vaccine injections are the most common painful, iatrogenic procedures performed in childhood. Multiple injections routinely administered during a single immunization visit may affect the overall pain experience. Researchers wanted to determine whether acute pain response is affected by the order in which vaccines are given.

Study participants were healthy 2- to 6-month-old infants receiving routine immunizations. In this single-centre, double-blind, randomized clinical trial, infants received either DTap-Hib vaccine or pneumococcal vaccine (PCV) first, followed by the remaining vaccine. Infant pain during vaccine injection was assessed by the Modified Behavioural Pain Scale (MBPS) using a videotaped recording of the procedure. Parents also rated pain using a 10 cm visual analogue scale (VAS). Crying behaviour (yes/no) was also recorded. The study was conducted between 2006 and 2007 and enrolled a total of 120 infants. Sixty infants received the DTaP-Hib vaccine first, and the other 60 infants received the PCV vaccine first. Infant characteristics did not differ between groups.

▲ **Findings**

Overall mean pain scores per infant after receiving both vaccine injections were significantly lower when DTaP-Hib was administered first compared with when PCV was administered first. When given first, the DTaP-Hib vaccine

was also shown to cause significantly less pain ($P < 0.001$) than the PCV as assessed by the methods cited above. Because infants who received the less painful vaccine first (DTaP-Hib) experienced less pain overall, the researchers recommend that the order of vaccine injections administered should be the DTaP-Hib vaccine first followed by the PCV.

■ **Nursing Implications**

The importance of optimal management of pain and distress in infants, children, and their parents during the administration of vaccines is a key to addressing a significant barrier to the immunization. As discussed earlier in this chapter, vaccine injections are described in the research literature as being one of the most painful procedures infants and children experience. Because multiple injections are part of routine immunization schedules in Canada, the order of vaccine administration could potentially impact the overall pain experience.

As the findings from this Canadian study demonstrated, infants' pain responses during immunizations were affected by the order in which the vaccines were administered. These findings provide health care professionals with the unique opportunity to put evidence into practice simply by the order in which they administer vaccines, thus reducing the pain experienced by infants and children being immunized.

Moshe, I., Parkin, P. C., Lear, N., Goldbach, M., & Taddio, A. (2009). Order of vaccine injection and infant pain response. *Archives of Pediatric and Adolescent Medicine, 163*(5), 469–472.

The significant role and impact of parental behaviour and demeanour during immunizations is also well documented in the research literature. Evidence has shown that reassurance, criticism, apologies, and empathy by parents were ineffective during immunizations and in fact were associated with worse outcomes for infants and children (i.e., increased anxiety or distress) (Manimala, Blount, & Cohen, 2000). In contrast, the use of distraction and humour by parents was shown to decrease children's distress (Schechter et al., 2007). It is therefore important for nurses to teach parents positive techniques that they can use to promote both coping for themselves and coping and safety for their children during immunization procedures.

Vaccine Misconceptions

Addressing any myths or misconceptions that parents may hold about the risks versus benefits of immunizations requires that nurses' knowledge be current and based on available evidence. Taking time to discuss and provide reliable resources to parents about vaccine "truths" (pamphlets, websites) not only meets the knowledge needs of parents but also is a requirement in obtaining informed consent. Immunization information must be available in the language most understandable to the parents.

Establishing a medical home for every child can also be beneficial in ensuring optimal immunization status. Parents in a long-term, trust-based relationship with a health care provider are more likely to have their concerns about vaccine safety assuaged. Missed opportunities for immunizations can be reduced by:

• Maintaining a centralized immunization record
• Verifying immunization status at every visit, not just during health supervision visits
• Verifying the immunization status of siblings accompanying the child to the appointment
• Providing parents with up to date information on vaccines geared to their concerns and needs

*R*ecall Maya and Evan. Discuss potential barriers to Maya and Evan being fully immunized. As a nurse, how can you help ease these barriers?

Health Promotion

Health promotion is the process of enabling people to increase control over and improve their health (World Health Organization [WHO], 1986). It involves health education, nutrition, sanitation, immunization, and prevention and control of communicable diseases. The nurse implements health promotion through education and anticipatory guidance.

Partnership development is the key strategy for success when implementing a health promotion activity. Identifying key stakeholders from the community increases problem solving and provides additional venues for disseminating information. Nurses who work in community settings not only provide programs that focus on disease control and epidemiology, but they are in a unique position to provide client-centred care that considers health status and the determinants of health.

Providing Anticipatory Guidance

Anticipatory guidance is primary prevention. The nurse partners with the parents to build a roadmap to optimal health for the child. Although the challenges frequently encountered by most families form the skeleton of the guidance, the nurse fleshes out information provided to parents based on other factors such as results of risk assessments and screening tests, health concerns unique to the child, and the interests and concerns of the parents. Age-related anticipatory guidance information is provided in Chapters 25, 26, 27, 28, and 29 of this book.

*P*rovide appropriate anticipatory guidance for both 3-year-old Maya and 12-month-old Evan.

Promoting Oral Health Care

Effective oral health practices are essential to the overall health of children and adolescents. Poor oral health can have significant negative effects on systemic health. Children who suffer from untreated dental caries have an increased incidence of pain and infections and may have problems eating and playing, difficulty at school, and sleep pattern disturbances (CDC, 2011d). The Canadian Dental Association recommends that children have an assessment by a dentist within 6 months of the eruption of the first tooth or by 1 year of age (Dosani, Nguyen, & Farkouh, 2010).

Optimal oral health is not limited to prevention and treatment of dental caries. Oral health includes anticipatory guidance on the topics of non-nutritive sucking habits, injury prevention, oral cancer prevention, and intraoral/perioral piercing. Preventing and treating malocclusion can have a significant benefit for children. Comprehensive health care is not possible if oral health is not a priority in the health delivery system.

Optimizing oral health can benefit the community as well as the individual client. There has been a 60% reduction in early childhood caries over the past 50 years since community water supplies were fluoridated at optimal levels. The cost of pediatric oral health care could be reduced 50% with the proper use of fluoride treatments coupled with other preventive measures. These health care dollar savings will benefit community resources.

Launched on a test basis in 2004, the Children's Oral Health Initiative (COHI) was developed as a way to address the inequities between the oral health of First Nations and Inuit children and that of the general Canadian population. COHI focuses on the prevention of dental disease and promotion of good oral health practices. The goal of COHI is to shift the emphasis from a treatment-based approach to oral health to a balanced prevention and treatment focus. The initial focus for oral health promotion is directed at three target groups:

• Pregnant women and primary caregivers
• Preschool children, 0–4 years of age
• School-age children, 5–7 years of age

Expectations from Health Canada are that once COHI is fully implemented the result will be a significant improvement in the oral health of First Nation and Inuit children (Health Canada, 2011).

Promoting Healthy Weight

Childhood obesity is a growing problem. In 2004, one in four (26%) Canadian children and adolescents 2 to 17 years of age were overweight. In the past 15 years, the obesity rate in children has increased at an alarming rate—from 2% to 10% in boys and from 2% to 9% in girls. This increase is disturbing because obese children tend to become obese adults (Lau et al., 2007). The principal causes of this increase in obesity are unhealthy eating habits and decreased physical activity. Research has demonstrated that weight is best managed with a combination of diet and exercise (Healthy People, 2010). Nurses will have the maximum effect in promoting healthy weight in children by initiating activities that address both healthy eating patterns and physical fitness. Children, parents, and communities are all targets for healthy weight promotion by nurses.

The focus of healthy weight promotion should be health centred, not weight centred. Emphasizing the benefits of health through an active lifestyle and nutritious eating pattern creates a nurturing environment for the child. This allows the child to maintain self-esteem. Linking success to numbers on a scale increases the possibility of developing eating disorders, nutritional deficiencies, and body hatred. A health-centred orientation also allows the family to develop a lifestyle that respects cultural food patterns and traditions.

The nurse can stress the benefits of the mother's healthy nutritional habits to the fetus at prenatal visits. Parents who have a healthy eating pattern are likely to maintain and encourage those patterns in their children. The nurse provides parents with anticipatory guidance about age-related eating patterns during each health supervision visit. Parents with toddlers and preschoolers may need training in techniques that cope with the child's growing autonomy while providing a variety of nutritious options.

The nurse can begin directly advising young children on healthy foods. Information and teaching modalities need to be age appropriate. Using colourful posters and games, the preschool child can learn the difference between healthy and unhealthy food choices. As children enter school-age, group and peer-led activities can be very effective. The nurse must gear material toward the teen's growing autonomy in making self-care decisions. Before beginning education to school-age and teenage children, it is important to obtain nutritional histories directly from them. School-agers and teenagers are increasingly eating meals away from the family table. As they spend more time away from their parents, they need to develop the ability to make nutritious choices. The goal is to help older children develop strategies for implementing healthy choices within an increasingly independent lifestyle. Detailed anticipatory guidance is provided in Teaching Guideline 30.1 and in Chapters 25 to 29.

Healthy physical activity can take many forms. During the preschool years, nurses need to encourage parents to provide a wide variety of physical activities. This exposure to multiple exercise options allows the child to find the one that is most enjoyable and increases the chances of maintaining an active lifestyle. The focus should be on non-competitive, fun activities such as dance or gymnastics. When the child enters the school-age years, the lure of television and computers, collectively termed "screen time," can significantly diminish the amount of time spent in physical activity. Parents can influence their children to stay physically active in several ways. They can limit the amount of time spent in sedentary activities and actively encourage the child to pursue any exercise activity that he or she enjoys. In addition to verbal encouragement, parents can stimulate exercise activities by participating in exercise with the child. A simple family walk can increase physical fitness while providing time for increased interaction between parent and child. See Teaching Guideline 30.2 for additional suggestions for promoting physical activity.

Promoting Personal Hygiene

Handwashing is the first personal hygiene topic that needs to be introduced to children. Handwashing prevents disease by limiting a child's exposure to pathogens. The nurse can introduce the topic to preschool children with the use of cartoons and games. Have the child sing "Twinkle, Twinkle Little Star" while washing his or her hands; this encourages adequate cleansing time. Use soap containers and towels with colourful characters to make the experience more fun. The school-age child can understand the concepts of germs and disease. Slogans such as "Let's drown a germ" can serve as a reminder of the importance of handwashing. The Glo Germ tool is very effective in this age group. Placing Glo Germ, a non-toxic substance that shines under a black light, on the children's hands allows them to follow how germs travel from object to object. After washing their hands, the children can see if they did a good job (if the Glo Germ remains on the hands, the hands were not washed thoroughly enough). (Visit http://thePoint.lww.com/Chow1e for the direct link to the Glo Germ website.) In

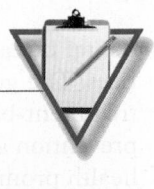

TEACHING GUIDELINE 30.1

Teaching Healthy Eating

Breakfast

1. Don't skip breakfast. You will not have enough energy to play well later in the day. Skipping breakfast can also lower your grades in school.
2. Avoid high-sugar foods at breakfast. They will make you sleepy during the day.
3. Start your breakfast with some fruit. Good choices include a small glass of juice, berries on your cereal, or a banana.
4. Protein is important at breakfast. Milk, either in a glass or on cereal, is a good source of protein. So is a serving of yogurt or some peanut butter.

Lunch

1. Prepare a healthy lunch to take to school each day.
2. Add a variety of healthy alternatives to your lunches.
   a. Try different types of breads. Pitas, wraps, bagels, and taco shells can be a good change of pace in the sandwich routine.
   b. Freeze fruits before putting them in the lunch box. This will keep the lunch items cool and the fruit fresh tasting. Canned pineapple and grapes freeze well. So do bananas.
   c. Try alternatives to high-fat chips. Dried fruits, baked pretzels, and animal crackers are just a few examples of tasty, healthy treats.
   d. Low-fat chocolate milk is more nutritious than prepackaged juice boxes, which have high sugar concentrations.

Snacks

1. Limit snacks to after school and bedtime. Light snacks such as yogurt or fruit provide good hunger management. A very hungry child will tend to overeat at meals.
2. Children need to learn to eat only when they are hungry. Children often eat out of boredom. Discourage nonstop grazing by planning activities to occupy the child.

Dinner

1. Plan your menu a week ahead. Planning ahead reduces the likelihood of eating out or getting "take-out." Restaurant foods are more likely to be high in fats and carbohydrates.
2. Prepare homemade healthy versions of take-out favourites. Top prepared pizza crust with cooked chicken, vegetables, mushrooms, and cheese. Serve the pizza with a salad for a complete and healthy meal. "Make your own tacos" nights, using lean hamburger and low-fat sour cream, can be a lot of fun for children.
3. Don't turn dinner into a battle zone. Forcing children to eat foods they do not like will only deepen their dislike of them. Give them the healthy foods they do enjoy and eventually they will explore more options.
4. Lead by example. Children eventually adopt the eating patterns of their parents. If they see their parents eat vegetables, they will eventually try them.

TEACHING GUIDELINE 30.2

Teaching Healthy Activity

1. Plan physical activities that your family can do as a group.
2. Write exercise activities on your family's daily schedule.
3. Look for activities that appeal to your child's interest such as dance, team sports, or swimming.
4. Place value on non-competitive as well as competitive activities.
5. Show your child you believe exercise is important. Exercise daily yourself.
6. Encourage the community to develop safe areas for spontaneous games and activities.

response to peer pressures, teenagers are usually stringent about personal hygiene. Young teens may need guidance in dealing with pubescent body changes such as adult-type body odour, susceptibility to fungal infections such as tinea pedis (athlete's foot), and acne.

Promoting Safe Sun Exposure

Skin cancers are a significant health problem in Canada. Blistering sunburns in children substantially increase the risk of melanoma and other skin cancers (National Cancer Institute, 2011). People with fair skin are at highest risk for skin cancers but anyone can become sunburned and develop skin cancer. When teaching clients about safe sun exposure it is very important to remind them that harmful ultraviolet (UV) rays can reflect off water, snow, sand, and concrete. Being under a shade awning does not guarantee protection. Adequate sun protection

TEACHING GUIDELINE 30.3

Teaching Safe Sun Exposure

Sunscreen

1. Use sunscreen lotions every day. Harmful UV rays penetrate clouds and cause damaging sunburns.
2. Use sunscreens with a sun protection factor (SPF) of 15 or higher. An adequate amount for an average-sized child is 15 mL
3. Apply sunscreens half an hour before sun exposure.
4. Reapply every hour if the child is perspiring heavily.
5. Reapply immediately after swimming.
6. Infants 6 months old or younger should not use sunscreens. Take steps to completely avoid sun exposure with this age group.

Clothing

1. Wear hats. The brim of the hat should be 10 cm greater and shade the ears. Straw hats need to have a sun proof liner to be effective. Children introduced to hats as young infants usually accept hats as part of the "outfit."
2. Wear UV-blocking sunglasses. The eye is the second most common site for melanoma.

3. Wear long, loose, and lightweight clothing for maximum sun protection.

Lifestyle

1. Avoid sun exposure between 10 AM and 4 PM. This is when UV rays are strongest.
2. Ask your health care provider if your medication will increase your sensitivity to UV rays. If the answer is yes, take extra precautions to reduce sun exposure.
3. Avoid tanning parlours. The devices emit UV rays just like the sun and can cause damage.
4. Check the UV index before going out. The higher the index, the more precautions you should take. UV index figures are available in newspaper, TV, and radio weather reports and on the Internet.
5. Advocate for safe-sun scheduling of recreational activities. Talk to others about scheduling outdoor activities before 10 AM, after 4 PM, or in the shade.
6. Consider UV-blocking plastic film for your house and car windows.

---

requires proper use of sunscreen lotions, avoiding peak sun hours, and wearing proper clothing. See Teaching Guideline 30.3 for more detailed instructions. With proper sun protection starting in infancy, 80% of skin cancers could be prevented.

▶ **Take** NOTE!

Give children the following physical reference when doing health promotion on safe sun exposure. Tell the child, "Only play outside when your shadow is taller than you are." The child's shadow will be "taller" before 10 AM and after 2 PM. The nurse can demonstrate this concept by placing a ruler on end and shining a bright light over it. As the nurse moves the light, the child will see the ruler's shadow lengthen.

■■■ Key Concepts

■ Health supervision for children is a dynamic process. Optimal wellness for the child can only occur if the nurse forms meaningful partnerships with the child, the family, and the community. These partnerships allow for free exchange of information and the estab-

lishment of mutually agreed upon goals. The medical home exists when there is a single primary care provider for the child. The medical home establishes a trusting long-term relationship with the child and family. This relationship leads to comprehensive, coordinated, and cost-effective care for the child.

■ Health supervision has three components: developmental surveillance and screening, injury and disease prevention, and health promotion.

■ Developmental surveillance is an ongoing process requiring a skilled observer and interviewer. To be effective, the nurse must understand normal growth and development expectations and be proficient at developmental screening procedures and techniques. Caregivers are most likely to reveal risk factors or warning signs for developmental delay when the nurse has a long-term and trusting relationship with the family.

■ Screening tests are part of injury and disease prevention. They are modalities that identify treatable disease in an early or asymptomatic state and allow for cure or lessening of the disease's injury.

■ Vision and hearing screening are functional testing modalities that the nurse must be proficient in administering in order for the child's results to be valid.

■ Immunizations are a cornerstone of pediatric disease prevention. The nurse increases the effectiveness of immunization by understanding the principles of immunization and applying them to the client's individual circumstances. Adhering to good immunization management practices, as outlined by the NACI and CIG, enhances the benefits and reduces the risks of immunization.

- Barriers to full immunization include fragmentation of health care, concerns about vaccine safety, pain and distress of immunizations for children and parents, and lack of knowledge. The nurse can be pivotal in ensuring that children and adolescents are fully immunized by serving as client educator and advocate.

- Children with chronic illnesses have a critical need for comprehensive and coordinated health supervision. Children with chronic illnesses require more frequent health supervision assessments. These children must have a medical home. The location of that medical home may be with a knowledgeable primary health care provider or at a multidisciplinary specialty facility. The location is determined by the child's needs and the family's preferences.

- The nurse incorporates frequent assessments of the many psychosocial stressors faced by families of children with chronic illnesses when establishing health care plans for them.

REFERENCES

Abelson, A., & Sanborn, M. (2010). Lead and children: Clinical management for family physicians [Clinical Review Environment and Health Series]. *Canadian Family Physician, 56,* 531–535.

Adoption Council of Canada (2009). *2008 International Adoption Statistics.* Retrieved April 19, 2012 from http://www.adoption.ca/2008%20International%20Adoption%20Stats.htm

American Academy of Pediatrics. (1998). Screening for elevated blood levels, *Pediatrics, 101,* 1072–1078.

American Academy of Pediatrics. (2009). Clinical report—Hearing assessment in infants and children: Recommendations beyond neonatal screening. *Pediatrics, 124,* 1252–1263. Retrieved November 18, 2011 from http://pediatrics.aappublications.org/content/124/4/1252.full.pdf

American Academy of Pediatrics. (2010). Clinical report—Diagnosis and prevention of iron-deficiency and iron deficiency anemia in infants and young children (0–3 years of age). *Pediatrics, 128,* 1040–1050. Retrieved November 18, 2011 from http://pediatrics.aappublications.org/content/124/4/1252.full.html

Aston, M., Meagher-Stewart, D., Edwards, N., & Young, L. (2009). Public health nurses primary care practice. Strategies for fostering citizen participation. *Journal of Community Health Nursing, 26,* 24–34.

Baker, R. D., Greer, F. R., & the Committee on Nutrition. (2010). Clinical report: Diagnosis and prevention of iron deficiency and iron-deficiency anemia in infants and young children (0–3 years of age). *Pediatrics, 126*(5), 1040–1050. Retrieved November 21, 2011 from http://aappolicy.aappublications.org/cgi/content/full/pediatrics;126/5/1040

Bowden, V. R., & Greenberg, C. S. (2008). *Pediatric nursing procedures.* Philadelphia: Lippincott Williams & Wilkins.

Buscemi, N., Vandermeer, B., Curtis, S. (2008). The Cochrane Library and procedural pain in children: An overview of reviews. *Evidence-Based Child Health: A Cochrane Review Journal, 3,* 260–279.

Cairney, J., Clinton, J., & Dowling, S-K. (2011). *International environmental scan of child development monitoring resources.* Retrieved February 22, 2012 from http://www.childdevelopmentmonitoring. net/files/download-files/International%20Environmental%20 Scan%20of%20Child%20Development%20Monitoring.pdf

Canadian Association of Speech Language Pathologists and Audiologists. (2010). *CASLPA position paper on universal newborn hearing screening.* Retrieved November 18, 2011 from http://www.caslpa.ca/english/resources/position.asp

Canadian Institute for Health Information. (2007). *Number of low birth weight babies rising in Canada.* Retrieved November 18, 2011 from http://www.newswire.ca/en/story/36367/number-of-low-birth-weight-babies-rising-in-canada

Canadian Institute for Health Information. (2009). *Analysis in brief. Experiences with primary health care in Canada.* Retrieved November 18, 2011 from http://secure.cihi.ca/cihiweb/products/cse_phc_aib_en.pdf

Canadian Nurses Association. (2008). *Code of ethics for registered nurses (2008 centennial edition).* Retrieved November 18, 2011 from http://www.cna-aiic.ca/CNA/practice/ethics/code/default_e.aspx

Canadian Organization for Rare Disorders. (2010). *Newborn screening in Canada status report.* Retrieved November 18, 2011 from http://www.raredisorders.ca/documents/CanadaNBSstatusupdated-Nov.112010.pdf

Canadian Paediatric Society. (2004). Position statement: Maternal depression and child development (revised). *Paediatrics & Child Health, 9,* 575–583. Retrieved November 18, 2011 from http://www.cps.ca/english/statements/pp/pp04–03.htm

Canadian Paediatric Society. (2007). Position statement: Human papillomavirus vaccine for children and adolescents. *Paediatrics & Child Health, 12*(7), 599–603. Retrieved November 18, 2011 from http://www.cps.ca/english/statements/ID/ID07–01.htm

Canadian Paediatric Society. (2009a). IMPACT after 17 years: Lessons learned about successful networking. *Paediatrics & Child Health, 14*(1), 33–35.

Canadian Paediatric Society (2009b). Position statement: Vision screening in infants, children and youth. *Paediatrics & Child Health, 14,* 246–248. Retrieved November 18, 2011 from http://www.cps.ca/english/statements/cp/cp09–02.htm

Canadian Paediatric Society. (2011). *Rourke Baby Record.* Retrieved November 18, 2011 from http://www.cps.ca/english/statements/CP/Rourke/Rourkebabyrecord.htm

Cappiello, M. M., & Gahagan, S. (2009). Early child development and developmental delay in indigenous communities. *Pediatric Clinics of North America, 56,* 1501–1517. doi:10.1016/j.pcl.2009.09.017

Centers for Disease Control and Prevention. (1997). *Screening young children for lead poisoning: Guidance for state and local health officials.* Atlanta, GA: US Department of Health and Human Services, National Center for Environmental Health.

Centers for Disease Control and Prevention (2009). *CDC's healthy homes initiative.* Retrieved November 21, 2011 from http://www.cdc.gov/nceh/lead/healthyhomes.htm

Centers for Disease Control and Prevention. (2010). *Hepatitis B information for health professionals.* Retrieved November 21, 2011 from http://www.cdc.gov/hepatitis/HBV/index.htm

Centers for Disease Control and Prevention. (2011a). *Nutrition for everyone: Iron and iron deficiency.* Retrieved November 21, 2011 from http://www.cdc.gov/nutrition/everyone/basics/vitamins/iron.html

Centers for Disease Control and Prevention. (2011b). *Recommendations and guidelines: Vaccine storage and handling.* Retrieved November 21, 2011 from http://www.cdc.gov/vaccines/recs/storage/default.htm

Centers for Disease Control and Prevention. (2011c). *Vaccines and preventable diseases: Pneumococcal disease – Q& A.* Retrieved November 21, 2011 from http://www.cdc.gov/vaccines/vpd-vac/pneumo/dis-faqs.htm

Centers for Disease Control and Prevention. (2011d). *Untreated dental caries (cavities) in children ages 2–19, United States.* Retrieved November 21, 2011 from http://www.cdc.gov/Features/dsUntreatedCavitiesKids/

Christofides, A., Schauer, C., & Zlotkin, S. H. (2005). Iron deficiency anemia among children: Addressing a global public health problem within a Canadian context. *Paediatrics & Child Health, 10,* 597–601.

Cohen, E., Friedman, J., Nicholas, D. B., Adams, S., & Rosenbaum, P. (2008). A home for medically complex children: The role of hospital programs. *Journal for Healthcare Quality, 30*(3), 7–15.

College of Family Physicians of Canada. (2009). *Patient-centered primary care in Canada: Bring it on home.* Retrieved November 18, 2011 from http://www.cfpc.ca/uploadedFiles/Resources/Resource_Items/Bring20it20on20Home20FINA L20ENGLISH.pdf

College of Family Physicians of Canada. (2011). *A vision for Canada: Family practice—The patient's medical home.* Retrieved November 22, 2011 from http://www.cfpc.ca/WorkArea/linkit.aspx?LinkIdentifier=id&ItemID=3753

Curtis, S. J., Jou, H., Ali, S., Vandermeer, B., & Klassen, T. (2007). A randomized controlled trial of sucrose and/or pacifier as analgesia for infants receiving venipuncture in a pediatric emergency department. *BMC Pediatrics, 7,* 27.

De Michele, A. M., & Ruth, R. A. (2010). *Newborn hearing screening.* Retrieved November 21, 2011 from http://emedicine.medscape.com/article/836646-overview

Dosani, F. Z., Nguyen, T. D., & Farkouh, D. R. (2010). *The infant oral exam.* Retrieved November 19, 2011 from http://www.oralhealthjournal.com/issues/story.aspx?aid=1000353810&type=Print%20Archive

Dunfield, L., & Keating, T. (2007). *Preschool vision screening* [Technology report number 73]. Ottawa, ON: Canadian Agency for Drugs and Technologies in Health.

Durieux-Smith, A., Fitzpatrick, E., & Whittingham, J. (2008). Universal newborn hearing screening: A question of evidence. *International Journal of Audiology, 47,* 1–10.

Eggertson, L. (2010). Lancet retracts 12-year-old article linking autism to MMR. *Canadian Medical Association Journal,182*(4), E199–E200.

Gold, R.M. (2006). *Your child's best shot: A parent's guide to vaccination* (3rd ed.). Ottawa, ON: Canadian Paediatric Society.

Greig, A., Constantin, E., Carsley, C., & Cummings, C. (2010). Preventative health care visits for children and adolescents aged six to 17 years: The Greig Health Record. [Executive Summary]. *Paediatrics & Child Health, 15*(3), 157–159.

Hagan, J. F., Shaw, J. S., & Duncan, P. (Eds.). (2008). *Bright futures: Guidelines for health supervision of infants, children and adolescents* (3rd ed.). Elk Grove Village, IL: American Academy of Pediatrics.

Halperin, B. A., Halperin, S. A., McGrath, P., Smith, B., & Houston, T. (2002). Use of lidocaine–prilocaine patch to decrease intramuscular injection pain does not adversely affect the antibody response to diphtheria-tetanus-acellular pertussis-inactivated poliovirus-Haemophilus influenzae type b conjugate and hepatitis B vaccines in infants from birth to six months of age. *The Pediatric Infectious Diseases Journal, 21*(5), 399–405.

Hanley, W. B. (2005). Newborn screening in Canada: Are we out of step? *Paediatrics & Child Health, 10,* 203–207.

Health Canada. (2009). *Lead information package: Some commonly asked questions about lead and human health.* Retrieved November 18, 2011 from http://www.hc-sc.gc.ca/ewh-semt/contaminants/lead-plomb/asked_questions-questions_posees-eng.php

Health Canada. (2011). *First Nations and Inuit health: Children's oral health initiative.* Retrieved November 18, 2011 from http://www.hc-sc.gc.ca/ahc-asc/activit/strateg/fnih-spni-eng.php#cohi-isbde

Health Canada approves Prevnar 13 vaccine for invasive pneumococcal disease. (December 22, 2009). Retrieved November 18, 2011 from http://www.news-medical.net/news/20091222/Health-Canada-approves-Prevnar-13-vaccine-for-invasive-pneumococcal-disease.aspx

Healthy People. (2010). *About healthy people.* Retrieved November 21, 2011 from http://www.healthypeople.gov/2020/about/default.aspx

Human Resources and Skills Development Canada. (2011). *Indicators of well-being in Canada. Low birth weight.* Retrieved November 18, 2011 from http://www4.hrsdc.gc.ca/.3ndic.1t.4r@-eng.jsp?iid=4

Hwa-Froelich, D. A., Loveland Cook, C. A., & Flick, L. H. (2008). Maternal sensitivity and communication styles: Mothers with depression. *Journal of Early Intervention, 31,* 44–66.

Johansson, S., Iliadou, A., Bergvall, N., et al. (2008). The association between low birth weight and type 2 diabetes: Contribution of genetic factors. *Epidemiology, 19,* 659–665.

Kennedy, R. M., Luhmann, J., & Zempsky, W. T. (2008). Clinical implications of unmanaged needle-insertion pain and distress in children. *Pediatrics, 122*(Suppl. 3), S130–S133.

Kortesluoma, R. L., & Nikkonen, M. (2006). "The most disgusting ever": Children's pain descriptions and views of the purpose of pain. *Journal of Child Health Care, 10*(3), 213–227.

Koshy, S., Grisaru, S., & Midgley, J. (2008). The diagnosis and management of hypertension in children. *Hypertension Canada,* Bulletin 95. Retrieved November 18, 2011 from http://www.stacommunications.com/customcomm/Back-issue_pages/Hyp_Can/hypcan-PDFs/eng/2008/June2008eng/01.pdf

Kroger, A. T., Sumaya, C. V., Pickering, L. K., & Atkinson, W. L. (2011). General recommendations on immunization: Recommendations of the Advisory Committee on Immunization Practices (ACIP). *Morbidity and Mortality Weekly Report, 60*(RR02), 1–60. Retrieved November 21, 2011 from http://www.cdc.gov/mmwr/preview/mmwrhtml/rr6002a1.htm?s_cid=rr6002a1_e

Lau, D. C. W., Douketis, J. D., Morrison, K. M., Hramiak, I. M., Sharma, A.M., & Ur, E. (2007). 2006 Canadian clinical practice guidelines on the management and prevention of obesity in adults and children [executive summary]. *Canadian Medical Association Journal, 176*(Suppl. 8). Retrieved November 18, 2011 from http://www.cmaj.ca/cgi/data/176/8/S1/DC1/1

Limbos, M. M., & Joyce, D. P. (2011). Comparison of the ASQ and PEDS in screening for developmental delay in children presenting for primary care. *Journal of Developmental & Behavioral Pediatrics, 32*(7), 499–511. doi:10.1097/DBP.0b013e31822552e9

Limbos, M. M., Joyce, D. P., & Roberts, G. J. (2010). Nipissing District Developmental Screen: Patterns of use by physicians in Ontario. *Canadian Family Physician, 56*(2), e66–e72.

Long, R., & Boffa, J. (2007). Why internationally adopted children should be screened for tuberculosis. *Canadian Medical Association Journal, 177,* 172–173.

Lyman, J. M., Loock, C. Scott, L., & Koushambi, B. K. (2008). Culture, health and inequalities: New paradigms, new practice imperatives. *Journal of Research in Nursing, 13,* 138–148.

Macy, M. (2011). The evidence behind developmental screening instruments. *Infants & Young Children, 25*(1), 19–61. doi: 10.1097/IYC.0b013e31823d37dd

Manimala, M. R., Blount, R. L., & Cohen, L. L. (2000). The effects of parental reassurance versus distraction on child distress and coping during immunizations. *Child Health Care, 29,* 161–177.

McCrindle, B.W. (2010). Assessment and management of hypertension in children and adolescents. *Nature Reviews Cardiology, 7,* 155–163.

Moshe, I., Parkin, P. C., Lear, N., Goldbach, M., & Taddio, A. (2009). Order of vaccine injection and infant pain response. *Archives of Pediatric and Adolescent Medicine, 163*(5), 469–472.

National Advisory Committee on Immunization. (2008). *Canadian immunization guide* (7th ed.). Retrieved April 2, 2011 from http://www.phac-aspc.gc.ca/publicat/cig-gci/index-eng.php

National Cancer Institute. (2011). *What you need to know about melanoma and other skin cancers.* Retrieved November 21, 2011 from http://www.cancer.gov/cancertopics/wyntk/skin

National Heart, Lung, and Blood Institute. (2005). *The fourth report on the diagnosis, evaluation and treatment of high blood pressure in children and adolescents* (NIH Publication No. 05–5267). Washington, DC: U.S. Department of Health and Human Services. Retrieved November 21, 2011 from http://www.nhlbi.nih.gov/health/prof/heart/hbp/hbp_ped.pdf

Ontario Association for Infant and Child Development. (2009). *Frequently asked questions.* Retrieved November 18, 2011 from http://www.oaicd.ca/faq

Ottawa Coalition for the Prevention of Low Birth Weight. (2007). *What is low birth weight?* Retrieved November 18, 2011 from http://www.successby6ottawa.ca/lbwfpn/english/

Payne, M. (2008). Lead in drinking water. *Canadian Medical Association Journal, 179,* 253–254.

Poureslami, I. M., Rootman, I., Balka, E., Devarakonda, R., Hatch, J., & FitzGerald, M. J. (2007). A systematic review of asthma and health literacy: A cultural-ethnic perspective in Canada. *MedScape General Medicine, 9*(3), 40. Retrieved November 18, 2011 from http://www.ncbi.nlm.nih.gov/pmc/articles/PMC2100106/

Public Health Agency of Canada. (2009a). *Child and youth injury review, 2009 edition – Spotlight on consumer product safety.* Retrieved November 18, 2011 from http://www.phac-aspc.gc.ca/publicat/cyi-bej/2009/pdf/injrep-rapbles2009_eng.pdf

Public Health Agency of Canada. (2009b). *What mothers say: The Canadian Maternity Experiences Survey.* Retrieved November 18, 2011 from http://www.phac-aspc.gc.ca/rhs-ssg/pdf/survey-eng.pdf.

Public Health Agency of Canada. (2011a). *Vaccine-preventable diseases: Pertussis.* Retrieved November 18, 2011 from http://www.phac-aspc.gc.ca/im/vpd-mev/pertussis-eng.php

Public Health Agency of Canada. (2011b). *Your immunization schedule.* Retrieved November 18, 2011 from http://www.phac-aspc.gc.ca/im/iyc-vve/is-cv-eng.php

Safe Kids Canada. (2010). *Annual review: Impact on injury 2009–2010.* Retrieved November 18, 2011 from http://www.safekidscanada.ca/Parents/About-Us/Annual-Review/Index.aspx

Schechter, N. L., Zempsky, W. T., Cohen, L. L., McGrath, P. J., McMurtry, C. M., & Bright, N.S. (2007). Pain reduction during pediatric immunizations: Evidence-based review and recommendations. *Pediatrics, 119*(5), e1184–e1198.

Shetty, S. (2010). *CDC commentary: Health of the internationally adopted child.* Retrieved April 11, 2011 from http://www.medscape.com/viewarticle/730225

Shore, R., & Shore, B. (2009). *KIDS COUNT indicator brief: Preventing low birthweight.* Retrieved November 21, 2011 from http://www.aecf.org/~/media/Pubs/Initiatives/KIDS%20COUNT/K/KID-SCOUNTIndicatorBriefPreventingLowBirthWeig/PreventingLowBirthweight.pdf

Statistics Canada. (2006). *Canada's ethnocultural mosaic, 2006 census: Findings.* Retrieved November 18, 2011 from http://www12.statcan.ca/census-recensement/2006/as-sa/97-562/index-eng.cfm

Stinson, J., Yamada, J., Dickson, A., Lamba, J., & Stevens, B. (2008). Review of systematic reviews on acute procedural pain in children in the hospital setting. *Pain Research & Management, 13*(1), 51–57.

Storr, G. B., Courant, G., Friel, J., & the Expert Advisory Panel on Exclusive Breastfeeding. (2004). *Exclusive breastfeeding duration – 2004 Health Canada recommendation.* Retrieved November 18, 2011 from http://www.hc-sc.gc.ca/fn-an/nutrition/infant-nourisson/excl_bf_dur-dur_am_excl-eng.php

Taddio, A., Chambers, C. T., Halperin, S. A., et al. (2009a). Inadequate pain management during routine childhood immunizations: The nerve of it. *Clinical Therapeutics, 31*(Suppl. B), S152–S167.

Taddio, A., Ilersich, A. L., Ipp, M., Kikuta, A., & Shah, V. (2009b). Physical interventions and injection techniques for reducing injection pain during routine childhood immunizations: Systematic review of randomized controlled trials and quasi-randomized controlled trials. *Clinical Therapeutics, 31*(Suppl. B), S48–S76.

Taddio, A., Appleton, M., Bortolussi, R., et al. (2010). Reducing the pain of childhood vaccination: An evidence-based clinical practice guideline. *Canadian Medical Association Journal, 182*(18), E843–E856.

Taylor, E. M., Boyer, K., & Campbell, F. A. (2008). Pain in hospitalized children: A prospective cross-sectional survey of pain prevalence, intensity, assessment and management in a Canadian pediatric teaching hospital. *Pain Research & Management, 13*(1), 25–32.

Tough, S., Siever, J. E., Leew, S., Johnston, D.W., Benzies, K., & Clark, D. (2008). Maternal mental health predicts risk of developmental problems at 3 years of age: Follow-up of a community-based trial. *BMC Pregnancy and Childbirth, 8*, 16.

Tough, S., Siever, J. E., Benzies, K., Leew, S., & Johnston, D.W. (2010). Maternal well-being and its association to risk of developmental problems in children at school entry. *BMC Pregnancy and Childbirth, 10*, 19.

University of British Columbia. (2009). Literature Review: Developmental Screening at Age 18 Months. Retrieved April 19, 2012 from http://www.childdevelopmentmonitoring.net/pan-canadian-18-months

Uman, L. S., Chambers, C. T., McGrath, P. J., & Kisely, S. (2008). A systematic review of randomized controlled trials examining psychological interventions for needle-related procedural pain and distress in children and adolescents: An abbreviated Cochrane review. *Journal of Pediatric Psychology, 33*(8):842–854.

von Baeyer, C. L., Marche, T. A., Rocha, E. M., & Salmon, K. (2004). Children's memory for pain: Overview and implications for practice. *Journal of Pain, 5*(5), 241–249.

Walco, G.A. (2008). Needle pain in children: Contextual factors. *Pediatrics, 122*(Suppl. 3), S125–S129.

World Health Organization. (1986). *The Ottawa charter for health promotion.* Retrieved November 18, 2011 from http://www.who.int/healthpromotion/conferences/previous/ottawa/en/

RECOMMENDED READINGS

Berberich, F. R., & Landman, Z. (2009). Reducing immunization discomfort in 4- to 6-year-old children: A randomized clinical trial. *Pediatrics, 124*, e203–e209.

Canadian Paediatric Society. (2008). *Immunization: Vaccine safety.* Retrieved November 18, 2011 from http://www.caringforkids.cps.ca/handouts/vaccine_safety

Chambers, C. T., Taddio, A., Uman, L. S., McMurtry, C. M., & HELPinKIDS Team. (2009). Psychological interventions for reducing pain and distress during routine childhood immunizations: A systematic review. *Clinical Therapeutics, 31*(Suppl. B), S77–S103.

National Network for Immunization Information. (2010). *Communicating with patients about immunization.* Retrieved November 18, 2011 from http://www.immunizationinfo.org/pressroom/nnii-factsheets/national-network-immunization-information-nnii-resource-kit

Public Health Agency of Canada. (2008). Healthy settings for young people in Canada. Retrieved November 18, 2011 from http://www.phac-aspc.gc.ca/hp-ps/dca-dea/publications/yjc/pdf/youth-jeunes-eng.pdf

Vibhuti Shah, V., Taddio, A., & Rieder, M. J. (2009). Effectiveness and tolerability of pharmacologic and combined interventions for reducing injection pain during routine childhood immunizations: Systematic review and meta-analyses. *Clinical Therapeutics, 31*(Suppl. B), S104–S151.

World Health Organization. (2010). *Vaccine safety net.* Retrieved August 9, 2010 from http://www.who.int/immunization_safety/safety_quality/vaccine_safety_websites/en/

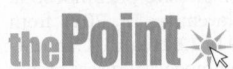

the Point For additional learning materials, including Internet Resources, visit **http://thePoint.lww.com/Chow1e.**

CHAPTER WORKSHEET

MULTIPLE CHOICE QUESTIONS

1. During the health interview, the mother of a 4-month-old client makes the statement, "I'm not sure my baby is doing what he should be." What is the nurse's best response?

   a. "I'll be able to tell you more after I do his physical."

   b. "Fill out this developmental screening questionnaire and then I can let you know."

   c. "Tell me more about your concerns."

   d. "All mothers worry about their babies. I'm sure he's doing well."

2. An infant male is at your facility for his initial health supervision visit. He is 2 months old and does not respond to a bell during his examination. What questions would you ask the mother?

   a. "Is there any family history of hearing problems in first-degree relatives?"

   b. "Is he vocalizing/making sounds at all?"

   c. "Have you noticed any abnormalities in his ear structure or notice any skin tags?"

   d. All of the above.

3. A 15-month-old girl is having her first health supervision visit at your facility. Her mother has not brought a copy of the toddler's immunization record but believes she is fully immunized. The mother states that her daughter "had immunizations 3 months ago at the local health unit." Which would be the best action by the nurse?

   a. Ask the mother to bring the records at the 18-month health supervision visit.

   b. Start the "catch-up" schedule because there are no immunization records.

   c. Keep the child at the facility while the mother returns home for the records.

   d. Contact the local public health unit where mom believes her daughter was last immunized and verify her immunization status.

4. A preschooler who has come to the clinic for his immunizations is yelling, "You're not giving me a needle today!" What strategies would you use to help manage this child's anxiety/distress around getting needles?

   a. Tell him everything will be fine and to not yell.

   b. Reassure him that the needles won't hurt.

   c. Address his feelings about getting immunized, and ask him what he would like to do to help feel better during his needles.

   d. Ignore his statement and begin talking with his mother about the immunizations.

   e. Acknowledge his fear about receiving a needle, and tell him the needle won't take long.

5. Which of the following facilities fulfils the characteristics of a medical home?

   a. An urgent care centre

   b. A primary care pediatric practice

   c. A mobile outreach immunization program

   d. A dermatology practice

6. The child's first examination by a dentist should occur by his or her:

   a. first birthday

   b. second birthday

   c. entry into kindergarten

   d. entry into first grade

CRITICAL THINKING EXERCISES

1. The client is a 5-year-old boy. During this health supervision visit, his mother states that she has concerns about his hearing. Your facility has been his medical home since birth. He was the product of a normal pregnancy and delivery. He has had frequent ear infections since the age of 8 months. Six months ago he had a ruptured appendix. He was treated with an aminoglycoside. He has been fully recovered for 4 months.

   a. During the health interview, what information does the nurse want to elicit from the mother?

   b. What information does the nurse want to verify from the permanent medical record?

   c. What risk factors for hearing loss does this child have?

   d. What is the best course of action at this time?

(question continues on page 966)

2. The nurse must examine a 4-year-old to determine his readiness for school. Describe the developmental, vision, and hearing screening tools that will assist the nurse to identify any problems.

STUDY ACTIVITIES

1. Develop an immunization plan for the following well children: a 2-month-old, an 18-month-old who has never been immunized, and a 5-year-old who was current with all immunizations at age 18 months.

2. This is the first health supervision visit, since arriving in this country 1 week ago, for a 3-year-old international adoptee from Haiti. Develop a health supervision plan for this visit.

3. Develop a healthy weight program for the following: a preschool class, a family in which the parents and the two school-age children are mildly overweight, and a teenage girl who is of normal weight but fears "becoming fat."

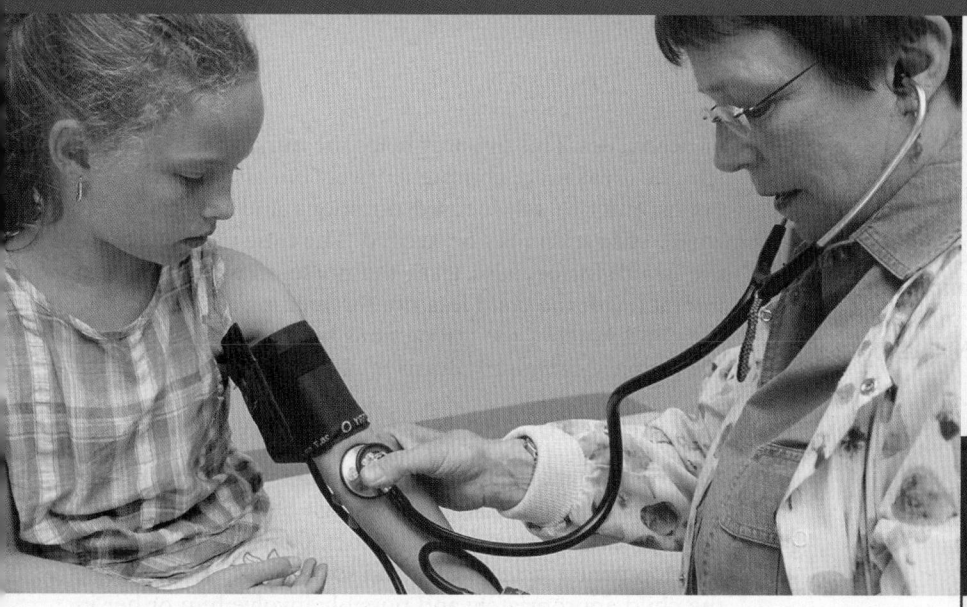

CHAPTER 31

Adapted by Debbie Fraser

Elliot Simmons, 3 years old, is brought to the clinic for his annual examination. His mother states that he is very fearful and anxious about this visit.

HEALTH ASSESSMENT OF CHILDREN

KEY TERMS

accommodation
acrocyanosis
auscultation
body mass index (BMI)
cerumen
chief concern

fontanel
inspection
lanugo
obligate nose breathing
palpation
PERRLA

point of maximal impulse (PMI)
stadiometer
Tanner stages
tympanometer

LEARNING OBJECTIVES

Upon completion of the chapter, the learner will be able to:

1. Demonstrate an understanding of the appropriate health history to obtain from the child and the parent or primary caregiver.
2. Individualize elements of the health history depending upon the age of the child.
3. Discuss important concepts related to health assessment in children.
4. Describe the appropriate sequence of the physical examination in the context of the child's developmental stage.
5. Perform a health assessment using approaches that relate to the age and developmental stage of the child.
6. Distinguish normal variations in the physical examination from differences that may indicate serious alterations in health status.
7. Determine the sexual maturity of females and males based upon evaluation of the secondary sex characteristics.

Wow

Growth and development is a journey, on which many children venture without a map.

Assessment of the child's health status involves many components: the health interview and history; observation of the parent–child interaction; physical examination; and the child's emotional, physiologic, cognitive, and social development. The nurse's skills are vital to the success of the assessment process. The nurse must (Mandleco, 2005):

• Establish rapport and trust
• Demonstrate respect for the child and the parent or caregiver
• Communicate effectively by actively listening, demonstrating empathy, and providing feedback
• Observe systematically
• Obtain accurate data
• Validate and interpret data accurately

The focus of the assessment process depends on the purpose of the visit and the needs of the patient. Assessment is an ongoing process and is repeated to varying degrees at every encounter. Expert nurses are constantly evaluating all of those in their care, whether directly or indirectly as part of conversation and play. Indeed, some of the subtlest developmental signs may express themselves only during relaxed and casual interaction with a child (Burns, Dunn, Brady, Starr, & Blosser, 2009). You can observe gait while watching a child run down the hall; assess fine motor skills and social adaptation while playing a board game; or observe balance and coordination when bouncing a ball. Playful activities such as tickling a child can give the nurse feedback related to upper body strength when the child attempts to push the nurse's arms away. Nurses must also learn to perform a comprehensive and thorough examination of a child in an efficient manner.

A thorough and thoughtful assessment of a child is the foundation upon which a nurse determines the needs of and plan of care for the patient. Nothing can replace it for giving the nurse a snapshot of the life and health of the child. A comprehensive history, a thorough examination, and developmental, functional, or cognitive testing as appropriate will provide practical information about the health of a child and guide the nurse's plan of care. The history and physical examination also provide a time for health education, teaching about expected growth and development, and discussing healthy lifestyle choices. The nurse uses critical thinking skills to analyze the data and establish priorities for nursing intervention or follow-up (Burns et al., 2009).

The health assessment may be documented using a number of formats. The information should be easily retrievable and available to all members of the child's health care team.

Health History

The health history provides the nurse with an overall picture of what the child has experienced, highlighting areas of concern such as recurrent upper respiratory infections or headaches. This not only helps the nurse to assess those specific areas more comprehensively but also provides the opportunity to ask focused questions and identify areas where education may be needed. The time used to obtain the health history also gives the nurse an opportunity to interact with the child in a nonthreatening manner, while the child watches the interactions between the nurse and the primary caregiver (Burns et al., 2009; Miller, 2011).

Preparing for the Health History

Appropriate materials and a suitable environment are needed when performing a thorough health history. Take into account family roles and values. Consider the age and developmental stage of the child so that you can approach the child appropriately and possibly involve him or her in the health history. Observe the child–parent interaction. Determine the extent of the health history that is needed in a given situation. Being well organized and staying flexible will help ensure success (Burns et al., 2009).

Gathering Materials and Preparing Yourself for the Health History

Before you begin, make sure you have materials to record your history data (either a computer or a chart paper and a pen), a private space with adequate lighting, chairs for adults and the nurse, and a bed or examination table for the child. The space should be safe for your patient's developmental stage and allow you uninterrupted time for your examination. Sit down for as much of the history taking as possible to demonstrate a relaxed and welcoming manner (Burns et al., 2009).

Approaching the Parent or Caregiver

Greet the parent or caregiver by name. While interviewing the parent, provide toys or books to occupy the child, allowing the parent to concentrate on your questions. Use open-ended questions and avoid making judgmental comments. Show respect by remaining approachable. Remember that the structure of the family and its roles and dynamics will affect how the family communicates and how they make decisions about health care. Demonstrate patience and help the parent stay on track when there are several children in the family. Throughout the interview, refer to the child by name and use the correct gender when referring to the child, demonstrating interest and competence.

▶ *Take* NOTE!

Illness can cause great stress in families and individuals, so nurses must remember to protect themselves from potentially threatening behaviour on the part of the family. Sit close to the door, and if you are uncomfortable with a family member, ask for assistance. You may need to keep the door open or have another nurse or security personnel present in certain cases (Griffin, 2003).

Approaching the Child

Show a professional demeanor while still being warm and friendly to the caregivers and child. A white examination coat or all-white uniform may be frightening to children, who may associate the uniform with painful experiences or find it too unfamiliar (Roohafza et al., 2009). The nurse can wear a variety of professional-looking outfits, whether colourful uniform tops or smocks worn over white uniforms, or everyday clothing, depending on the setting of the nurse's practice. Make eye contact if possible and address the child by name. Use slow deliberate gestures rather than very quick or grand ones, which may be frightening to shy children.

Some young children will warm up when given time to be invisible in the room, such as hiding behind a parent before they tentatively appear. Make physical contact with the child in a nonthreatening way at first. Briefly cuddling a newborn before returning him or her to the caregiver, warmly shaking the hand of older children and teens, and laying your hand on the head or arm of toddlers and preschoolers will convey a gentle demeanor. A joke, a puppet, a silly story, or even a simple magic trick may coax the child into warming up. Being at the same eye level as the child can also be more reassuring than standing over the child (Miller, 2011). This may require having extra seating for the nurse at the same level as the child and parent/caregiver. Aim to be seen as a trustworthy adult who is the child's partner in feeling better and staying healthy.

Elicit the child's cooperation by allowing him or her control over the pace, the order, or anything else that the child can control while still allowing you to obtain the information you need. All of this establishes a personal relationship with the child and helps gain his or her cooperation (Miller, 2011).

Communicating with the Child During the Health History

The child should be given opportunities to actively participate in the health history and assessment process. For young children, such as toddlers and preschoolers, ask them to point to where it hurts and allow them to answer questions. Validation of the information by the parent/caregiver is essential because of the limited comprehension and language use of children at these ages. The school-age child can be more accurate because of his or her increased language skills and maturity level.

Initially, address the child and obtain as much information from him or her as possible. School-age children should be able to answer questions about interactions with friends and siblings and school and activities they enjoy or are involved in. Ask the parent/caregiver if any additional information or observations should be included.

Adolescents may not feel comfortable addressing health issues, answering questions, or being examined in the presence of the parent/caregiver. The nurse must establish a trusting relationship with the adolescent to provide him or her with optimal health care. Ask adolescents whether they would be more comfortable answering questions alone in the examination area or whether they prefer for their parents to be present. Either way, the parent/caregiver will have an opportunity to talk with the nurse after the health history and assessment are completed (Burns et al., 2009).

Demonstrate an interest in the teen by asking questions about school, work, hobbies or activities, and friendships. Begin with these topics to make the teen feel comfortable in communicating with you. Communicate honestly with the adolescent and explain the rationale for various aspects of the health history. Teens are very sensitive to nonverbal communication, so be very aware of your gestures and expressions (Sass & Kaplan, 2011). Once a rapport has been established, move on to more emotionally charged questions that relate to sexuality, substance use, depression, and suicide.

Always assure the teen that complete confidentiality will be maintained to the extent possible. Current provincial law will determine the types of information that may be withheld from parents. If the information that the nurse receives indicates that the teen may be in danger, then the nurse must inform the teen that the information will be shared with other providers and/or the parents (Burns et al., 2009).

> ▶ **Take** NOTE!
>
> *Do not try to become the adolescent's peer. Remain in the role of the health care provider while demonstrating respect and acceptance toward the teen. Clarify the meaning of jargon or slang that the teen uses, but do not use these words yourself, as the teen will simply not accept you as a peer.*

Observing the Parent–Child Interaction

Observation of the parent–child interaction begins during the focused conversation of the health interview and continues throughout the physical examination. Explore the family dynamics, not only through questions but also by observing the family for behavioural clues. Does the parent make eye contact with the infant? Does the parent anticipate and respond to the infant's needs? Are the parents ineffective when dealing with a toddler's temper tantrum? The plan of care may need to be adjusted to teach appropriate responses to the infant's needs or toddler's behaviour. Do the parents' comments increase the school-age child's sense of self-worth? Behavioural observations are crucial to proper assessment of the family's needs (Burns et al., 2009; Columbia University College of Physicians and Surgeons, n.d.).

Does the parent seem to be coping with the health issue or does he or she appear overwhelmed? Is the parent's/caregiver's behaviour appropriate? Does the child look at the parent/caregiver before answering? Does the child seem relaxed and happy with the parent/caregiver, or is the child tense? The infant will appear calm and relaxed if his or her needs are generally met. Crying may occur when the baby is ill or frightened but may also indicate discomfort with the parent or caregiver. Use a calm and comforting voice with the infant. Infants respond well to higher-pitched and soothing voices.

When observing the relationship between the adolescent and the parent/caregiver, does the parent/caregiver allow the adolescent to speak, or does he or she frequently interrupt? Does the parent/caregiver contradict what is being said? Observe the body language of the adolescent. Does the adolescent seem relaxed or tense? Since adolescents are between childhood and adulthood, they have unique needs. They are in a time of multiple physical and emotional changes, many of which they cannot control. They need to know that the nurse is interested in what they have to say (Sass & Kaplan, 2011). The use of open-ended questions allows the adolescent to talk. "Tell me about your. . . ." or "What have you noticed about. . . ." are comfortable phrases to use to elicit the information needed.

Be aware of your reactions to the adolescent's questions or behaviours, such as your nonverbal and facial expressions. Talk with the adolescent using accurate language that is developmentally and age-appropriate.

Determining the Type of History Needed

The purpose of the examination will determine how comprehensive the history must be. If the health care provider rarely sees the child or if the child is critically ill, a complete and detailed history is in order, no matter what the setting. The child who has received routine health care and presents with a mild illness may need only a problem-focused history. In critical situations, some of the history taking must be delayed until after the child's condition is stabilized. Evaluate the situation to determine the best timing and the extent of the history (Burns et al., 2009). Also, be sensitive to repetitive interviews in hospital situations, and collaborate with physicians or other members of the health care team to ensure that a family already under stress does not need to undergo prolonged or repetitive questioning.

*R*emember Elliot, the 3-year-old being seen for his annual examination? When you enter the room, he is hiding behind his mother's legs. Considering his age and developmental level, how will you proceed with obtaining a health history?

Performing a Health History

The health interview is the foundation of an accurate health assessment. Information about the child's health will come not only from a physical examination, but also from a careful conversation or interview with the child and/or the caregiver (Burns et al., 2009). Depending on the intent of the health assessment, many of the questions will be direct, and many will require the caregiver or child to answer simply "yes" or "no." In other than emergency situations, though, asking open-ended questions offers an excellent opportunity to learn more about the patient's life. For example, "Are you happy at school?" may elicit a brief nod of the head, whereas "Tell me what it's like on your school playground" may result in a story about the child's friends, the kind of activities he or she enjoys, any bullying that goes on, and so forth. These stories will provide the nurse with clues to the child's stage of physical, emotional, and moral development as well as his or her functional status (Burns et al., 2009; Columbia University College of Physicians and Surgeons, n.d.).

Establish a therapeutic relationship with the child and family. Without the trust that comes from this therapeutic relationship, the family may not reveal vital information due to fear, embarrassment, or mistrust (Bunik, Brayden, & Fox, 2011). Use therapeutic communication techniques such as active listening, open-ended questions, and eliminating barriers to communication. Establishing a "medical home" where ongoing health supervision occurs encourages the formation of trust through continuity of care and the family's continuing relationships with health care providers (see Chapter 30).

Components of the Health Interview

The structure of the health interview is determined by the nature of the visit. At an initial visit, large amounts of historical data are collected. Having the family fill out a questionnaire can save time, but a questionnaire is not a substitute for the health interview. The questionnaire may serve as a springboard to begin structured conversations between the family and the nurse. At subsequent visits, the health interview can focus on the pertinent issues of that visit as well as any health issues that are being monitored.

The health history includes demographics, chief concern and history of present illness, past health history, review of systems, family health history, developmental history, functional history, and family composition, resources, and home environment.

▶ **Take** NOTE!

Any questionnaires used in the health care setting must be appropriate to the reading level and primary language of the person filling them out.

Demographics

Questions should start with simple and nonintrusive ones; once a rapport between the nurse and patient has started, sensitive questions can be asked. First obtain data such as the child's name, nickname, birth date, and gender. Determine the child's race or ethnicity, the language the child understands, and the language the child speaks. Record the child's address and home telephone number and the parent's or caregiver's work telephone number. Identify who the historian is (the child or the parent or caregiver), and note how reliable you consider this source of information to be. Do not assume that an adult with the child is the child's parent. Establish the relationship of the adult to the child, and ask who cares for the child if that person does not. Determine the composition of the household, including other children and other family members or other persons who live there.

Chief Concern and History of Present Illness

Next, ask about the **chief concern** (reason for the visit). The reason may not always be apparent to you. A question such as, "What can I help you with today?" or "What did you notice in your baby/child that you wanted to have checked today?" is very welcoming. The response from the child or parent may be a functional problem, a developmental concern, or a disease.

Record the chief concern in the child's or parent's own words.

Next, address the history related to the present illness. For each concern, determine its onset, duration, characteristics and course (location, signs, symptoms, exposures, and so on), previous episodes in patient or family, previous testing or therapies, what makes it better and what makes it worse, and what the concern means to the child and family. Inquire about any exposure to infectious agents.

Past Health History

Ask about the prenatal history (any problems with pregnancy), perinatal history (any problems with labour and delivery), past illnesses, or any other health or developmental problems. Document the child's prior history of illnesses (recurrent, chronic, or serious) and any accidents or injuries in the past. Inquire about any operations or hospitalizations the child has had. Document the child's diet. Note the child's allergies to foods, medications, animals, environmental or contact agents, or latex products. Determine the child's reaction to the allergen as well as its severity. Determine the child's immunization status (refer to Chapter 30 for further information on immunizations). Record any medications the child is taking, the dosage and schedule, as well as when the last dose was given. In pre-adolescent and adolescent females, determine menstrual history.

Family Health History

Obtaining information about the family's health is a key part of a health interview. Perform a three-generation family health history. This information may be documented in a genogram (Fig. 31.1). Asking about the age and health

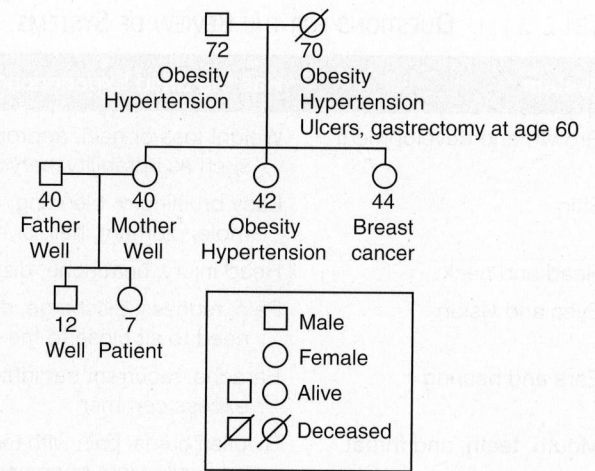

FIGURE 31.1 Genogram.

status of mother, father, siblings, and other family members helps to identify trends and specific health issues (Burns et al., 2009; Hagan, Shaw, & Duncan, 2008). For example, do the grandparents have early-onset coronary artery disease? If they do, the child may benefit from additional health screening. Siblings may exhibit a genetic disease or carry a trait for the disease. This family health information helps to guide future health planning.

Review of Systems

Inquire about current or past history of problems related to:

- Growth and development
- Skin
- Head and neck
- Eyes and vision
- Ears and hearing
- Mouth, teeth, and throat
- Respiratory system and breasts
- Cardiovascular system
- Gastrointestinal system
- Genitourinary system
- Musculoskeletal system
- Neurologic system
- Endocrine system
- Hematologic system

Table 31.1 gives specific questions related to each of these systems.

Developmental History

Determine the age when landmarks in gross motor control were achieved, such as sitting, standing, walking, pedalling, and so on. Ask whether the child has attained fine motor skills such as grasping, releasing, pincer grasp, crayon or utensil use, and handwriting skills. Note the child's age and extent of language acquisition. Document speech problems, such as a lisp or stuttering. The rate of

TABLE 31.1   QUESTIONS FOR THE REVIEW OF SYSTEMS

System	Has the Child Experienced:
Growth and development	Weight loss or gain, appropriate energy and activity levels, fatigue, behavioural changes such as irritability, nervousness, anger, or increased crying
Skin	Easy bruising or bleeding, rash, lesion, skin disease, pruritus, birthmarks, or change in mole, pigment, hair, or nails
Head and neck	Head injury, headache, dizziness, syncope
Eyes and vision	Pain, redness, discharge, diplopia, strabismus, cataracts, vision changes, reading difficulties, need to sit close to the board at school or close to the TV at home
Ears and hearing	Earache, recurrent ear infection, tubes in eardrums, discharge, difficulty hearing, ringing, excess cerumen
Mouth, teeth, and throat	Swollen gums, pain with teething, caries, tooth loss, toothache, sores, difficulty with chewing or swallowing, hoarseness, sore throat, mouth breathing, change in voice
Respiratory system and breasts	Nasal congestion or discharge, cough, wheeze, noisy breathing, snoring, shortness of breath or other difficulty breathing, problems with or changes in breasts
Cardiovascular system	Murmur, colour change (cyanosis), exertional dyspnea, activity intolerance, palpitations, extremity coldness, high blood pressure, high cholesterol
Gastrointestinal system	Nausea, vomiting, abdominal pain, cramping, diarrhea, constipation, stool-holding, anal pain or itching
Genitourinary system	Dysuria; polyuria; oliguria; narrow urine stream; dark, cloudy, or discoloured urine; difficulty with toilet training; bedwetting *Boys:* undescended testicles, pain in penis or scrotum, sores or lesions, discharge, scrotal swelling when crying, changes in scrotum or penis size, addition of pubic hair *Girls:* vaginal discharge, itching, rash, problems with menstruation or menstrual cycle
Musculoskeletal system	Joint or bone pain, stiffness, swelling, injury (e.g., broken bones or sprains), movement limitation, decreased strength, altered gait, changes in coordination, back pain, posture changes or spinal curvature
Neurologic system	Numbness, tingling, difficulty learning, altered mood or ability to stay alert, tremors, tics, seizures
Endocrine system	Increased thirst, excessive appetite, delayed or early pubertal changes, problems with growth
Hematologic system	Swelling of lymph nodes, pale colour, excessive bruising

Adapted from: Burns, C., Dunn, A., Brady, M., Starr, N., & Blosser, C. (2004). *Pediatric primary care: A handbook for nurse practitioners* (4th ed.). Philadelphia: WB Saunders; Jarvis, C. (2008). *Physical examination and health assessment* (5th ed.). St. Louis: Saunders; Weber, J., & Kelley, J. (2003). *Health assessment in nursing* (2nd ed.). Philadelphia: Lippincott Williams & Wilkins.

developmental skill acquisition may vary from child to child, but the sequence of skill attainment should remain the same. Inquire about self-care ability (e.g., tying shoes, dressing, brushing teeth) and, in the younger child, how toilet training is progressing. Assess feeding skills, including how well the child drinks from a cup and uses utensils or whether the child has any special requirements. Inquire about social skills and comfort articles (e.g., blankets, stuffed animals). Note whether the child has a habit of thumb or finger sucking or using a pacifier. Document day care attendance and preschool or school adjustment and achievements.

Functional History

The functional history should contain information about the child's daily routine. Inquire about:

- Safety measures (e.g., car seats and their placement, use of seat belts, smoke detectors, bike helmets)
- Routine health care and dental care (including dates of dental care and what was done)
- Nutrition, including a 24-hour dietary recall or week-long food diary, use of supplements and vitamins, feeding pattern and satisfaction with diet, amount of "junk food" consumed, food likes and dislikes, and the parent's perception of the child's nutrition (refer to Chapters 25 through 29 for nutritional needs at various ages)
- Physical activity and organized sports, play, and recreation
- Television and computer habits
- Sleep behaviour and bedtime
- Elimination patterns and any concerns

- Hearing or vision problems (dates of last screenings and results)
- Relationships with other family members and friends, coping and temperament, and attention or school behaviour problems
- Religious involvement and other spiritual practices
- Use of adaptive and assistive devices such as eyeglasses or contact lenses, hearing aids, walker, braces, or wheelchair
- Sexual practices (Burns et al., 2009; Hagan et al., 2008)

Family Composition, Resources, and Home Environment

Determine the marital status of the parents. Does the child live with the parents, a stepparent, or other family member? Is the child adopted or in foster care? Are the parents the primary caretakers for the child? If not, the primary caretaker should be included in the interview process if possible. Parents may not know some of the child's routines if the child spends much of the time being cared for by someone else. Working parents may learn about a health or behaviour issue only after being alerted by the child's day care centre or babysitter. It may be helpful to expand the family history to include the grandparents and their interaction with the child.

Determine the employment status of the parents and their occupations, as this could affect the child's overall well-being; for example, the parents' work schedule may not allow them to spend much time with the child. Assess family income and financial resources. Major family changes can also affect how the parents and child interact, so evaluate for relationship problems or changes.

Ask about the family's home and its age and the home environment. Is there a safe outdoor play area? If there is a pool, are safety features in place? Determine whether the home has electricity and an indoor water supply. Also determine whether the home has heating, air conditioning, and refrigeration. What pets does the family have? How are they housed? Are there infestations of insects or rodents in the home?

▶ **Take** NOTE!

Homes built before 1978 contain lead paint, which is of concern because paint is the cause of 70% of lead poisoning (Abelsohn & Sanborn, 2010). Since 1992, all interior and exterior house paints used in Canada have been lead free (Health Canada, 2011). Children who live in older homes are at increased risk for exposure to lead. For more information, visit Health Canada's website on this topic; visit http://thePoint.lww.com/Chow1e for the direct link.

The Physical Examination

After the history comes the physical examination. It should focus on the chief concern or any of the systems that engaged the nurse's critical thinking while taking the history. The examination will reflect the nurse's general practice style, the developmental stage and age of the child, the temperament of the child and caregiver, and the health status of the child. A very ill child will not waste energy protesting the examination, so the nurse can move quickly in that situation. A healthy child, however, will express his or her normal developmental stage and will show varying degrees of resistance to the examination (Columbia University College of Physicians and Surgeons, n.d.; Miller, 2011).

Preparing for the Physical Examination

When performing the physical examination, being prepared and organized ensures that you will obtain the needed information. The appropriate methods to use and ways to approach the child depend on the child's developmental stage.

Gathering Materials and Preparing for the Examination

The examination area should include an exam table or the child's hospital crib or bed. Appropriate lighting is necessary for adequate observation and inspection. Gather the equipment necessary for the examination such as clean gloves, stethoscope, thermometer, sphygmomanometer, tape measure, reflex hammer, penlight, otoscope/ophthalmoscope, tongue depressor, and cotton ball. An infant or adult scale is needed, as well as a **stadiometer** for children capable of standing independently. Young children may be frightened by seeing a large amount of equipment, so take out one piece of equipment at a time. Some children can be very resistant to what they see as a threat or an invasion of their privacy, so it may help to have washable toys in the examination area to use as distractions during the assessment (Burns et al., 2009; Hagan et al., 2008; Miller, 2011).

Children and their parents may be able to sense any frustration or anxiety on the part of the examiner, so display a confident and matter-of-fact approach. If the child is not cooperative, do not become discouraged; more time and explanation will usually do the trick.

Regardless of the child's age, if the examination room is cold, the child will be uncomfortable and possibly less cooperative. Provide appropriate covers to ensure the child's comfort, or have the child remain dressed until the time of the examination (Miller, 2011).

Approaching the Child

Approach the child according to his or her developmental age and stage. Table 31.2 outlines a general approach

TABLE 31.2 DEVELOPMENTAL CONSIDERATIONS FOR EXAMINATION

	Newborn	Infant	Toddler	Preschooler	School-ager	Early Teen	Late Teen
Place to perform examination	May lie on examination table or in caregiver's lap	In caregiver's lap or on exam table with caregiver right beside infant	Allow some freedom of movement where possible; child may stand between sitting caregiver's legs or sit on the lap.	Some may be willing to sit on exam table with caregiver standing close by with hand on the leg.	Sitting on examination table where they still have eye contact with caregiver	Some may be willing to have their caregiver wait outside the exam room.	Explain to the caregiver that the teen needs privacy and that he or she should wait outside the exam room.
Examination direction	Keep up a running dialogue with the caregiver, explaining each step as you do it.	Continue to explain each step to the caregiver; address child by name. Perform most invasive parts last.	Introduce yourself to caregiver and child; explain most steps to the child and all steps to caregiver; allow child to handle instruments. Perform most invasive parts last.	Allow child to decide the order of the examination; explain what the instruments do and let the child try them; speak to the caregiver before and after the examination.	Include the child in all parts of the examination; use head-to-toe approach with genital exam last. Speak to the caregiver before and after the examination.	Speak to the child using mature language; appeal to his or her desire for self-care. Use a head-to-toe approach, with genital exam last.	Explain confidentiality to caregiver and teen; allow time talking with them together and separately. Use a head-to-toe approach, with genital exam last.

Adapted from: Burns, C., Dunn, A., Brady, M., Starr, N. B., & Blosser, C. (2009). *Pediatric primary care* (4th ed.) Philadelphia: WB Saunders; Columbia University College of Physicians and Surgeons. (2011). *Points on the pediatric physical exam.* Retrieved March 24, 2011 from http://www.columbia.edu/itc/hs/medical/clerkships/peds/Student_Information/Reference_Materials/Pediatric_PE.html; and Miller, S. (2011). *Pediatric physical exam video.* Retrieved March 22, 2011 from http://www.columbia.edu/itc/hs/medical/clerkships/peds/Student_Information/Reference_Materials/PE_Video.html.

to the physical examination in each broad developmental category.

If several children are to be seen at the same time, begin with the child who will be most cooperative. If the other children do not see anything scary and realize that their sibling was examined without a problem, it sets the stage for better cooperation from the younger ones.

Newborns and Infants

If the infant is asleep, auscultate the heart, lungs, and abdomen first while the baby is quiet. Count the heart rate and respiratory rate before undressing the baby. Completely undress newborns and infants down to their diaper, removing it just at the end to examine the genitalia, anus, spine, and hips. It is best to examine the infant 1 to 2 hours before a feeding. Having the parent or caregiver hold the child during the examination can help to alleviate fears and anxieties (Fig. 31.2). Allow the parent or caregiver to be a nurturer rather than assisting with painful procedures, unless there are no other choices available (Miller, 2011).

Perform the assessment in a head-to-toe manner, leaving the most traumatic procedures, such as examination of the ears, nose, mouth, and throat, until last (Burns et al., 2009; Miller, 2011). Also delay eliciting the Moro reflex until the end of the examination, as the startling sensation may make the infant cry. Use firm, gentle handling while examining the infant. Make sure your hands and the stethoscope are warm. Perform the assessment as quickly and completely as possible. Use a soft and crooning voice, smile, and engage the infant in eye contact. If the baby is crying, a pacifier may be useful and brightly coloured objects may help distract him or her.

> ### ▶ Take NOTE!
>
> *Many older infants demonstrate stranger anxiety as a normal part of development. If the infant is not being held by the parent, make sure the parent is within the infant's view; this will increase the baby's comfort and cooperation (Bickley & Szilagyi, 2009; Burns et al., 2009; Miller, 2011).*

Toddlers and Preschoolers

Toddlers and preschoolers usually prefer to remove their clothing one item at a time as needed for the examination. After one area is examined, the child may feel more comfortable replacing that item of clothing before removing another one (Bunik et al., 2011). An examination gown is usually not necessary before school age. Again, make certain the room temperature is comfortable.

When the nurse enters the room, a child of this age is often sitting or standing by the parent. Incorporate play as appropriate during the health assessment. Remember your own facial expressions and tone. Use little touch at the beginning of the encounter with the child and the caregiver.

Introduce the equipment to be used slowly, explaining briefly what is going to happen. Let the child touch and hold the equipment whenever possible, even taking a parent's temperature or putting the blood pressure cuff on a teddy bear (Fig. 31.3). The toddler will prefer to sit on the caregiver's lap. When the toddler must be supine for the abdominal examination, sit in your chair knee-to-knee with the caregiver so the toddler may lie back on the caregiver's and your laps.

Praise the child for being cooperative during the examination. "You did such a good job holding still while I listened to your chest" and similar phrases give positive feedback to the child.

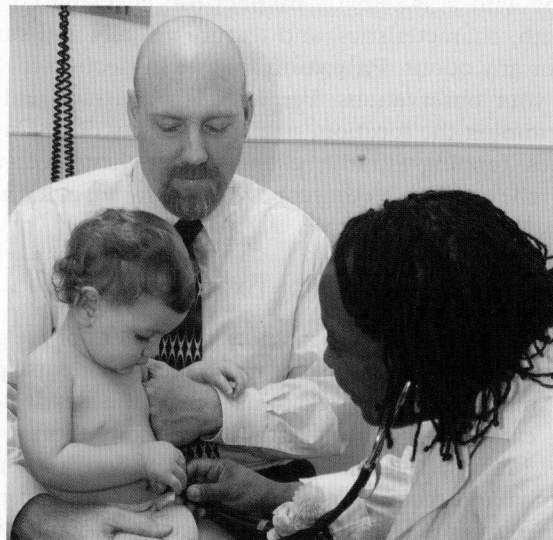

FIGURE 31.2 The infant or toddler may feel more comfortable and secure being examined while sitting in the parent's or caregiver's lap.

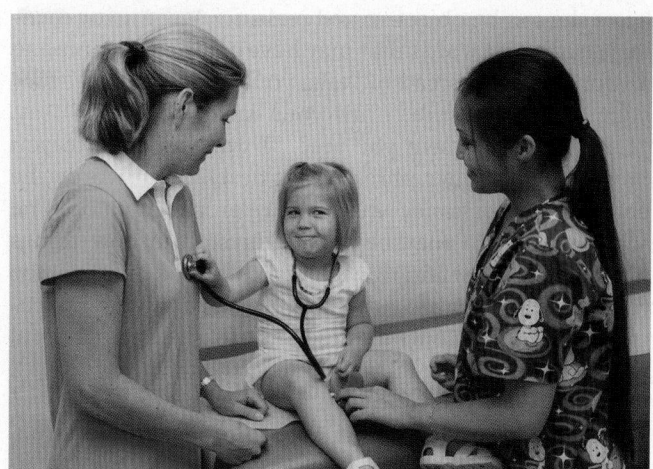

FIGURE 31.3 The preschooler enjoys listening to her mother's heart first.

If the child is uncooperative, assess as thoroughly as possible and move on to the next area to be assessed. The caregiver may need to place an arm around the toddler's body to provide restraint for invasive procedures. Use short phrases to tell the toddler what you are going to do, rather than asking if it is OK (Miller, 2011; Nettina, 2010).

> ▶ **Take** NOTE!
>
> *Toddlers are egocentric. Telling a toddler how well another child behaved probably will not be helpful in gaining the young child's cooperation.*

The preschooler may fear body invasion and mutilation and will withdraw from any procedure or assessment that is viewed as intrusive. Otherwise, the sense of initiative often leads the preschooler to be cooperative. The preschooler may be willing to undress completely, leaving just the underpants on. Use simple explanations to inform the child about each step of the examination, offering reassurance as appropriate. Allow him or her to "help" by holding the stethoscope or penlight. If choices are available, offer them to the child. Again, always compliment the child on his or her cooperation.

> ▶ **Take** NOTE!
>
> *Preschoolers like to play games. To encourage deep breathing during lung auscultation, hold up a finger or a lit penlight and instruct the child to "blow it out" (Miller, 2011).*

School-Age Children

The school-age child's thinking is still very concrete, but he or she can be objective and realistic. Avoid using medical jargon and words that may have a double meaning to a young child. Instead of "take your temperature," "take your blood pressure," "hit your knee," or "test," say, "Let's see how warm you are," "I want to listen to you breathe," and other phrases that describe, in words the child can understand, what you are preparing to do. The school-age child may be very interested in how things work and why certain things need to be done and will be responsive to truthful and simple explanations. Instruments that are colourful or look like toys are very helpful until adolescence (Burns et al., 2009; Miller, 2011), when teens are put off by childish things.

Always respect a child's desire to avoid pain and insult. Allow children to wear their underpants under the examination gown to provide a sense of security until the genitalia need to be examined. Allow the child to replace his or her clothing as soon as possible. Privacy and respect for the child's feelings are important to children of this age (Bunik et al., 2011).

> ▶ **Take** NOTE!
>
> *Describing and commenting on your findings during the physical examination is interesting to the school-age child, as children of this age like to learn about how the body works (Miller, 2011).*

Adolescents

Provide privacy while the adolescent is undressing and putting on a gown. Demonstrate an attitude of respect. Perform the assessment in a head-to-toe manner, exposing only the area to be examined. Provide information about physical changes in a matter-of-fact way, such as, "the hair on your legs is what is expected at this time." This provides information related to sensitive areas that the teen may be reluctant to ask about. It also provides the adolescent with information about the sexual development that is normal and expected. Allow opportunities for the teen to ask questions without the caregiver being present. Assure the adolescent that there are no "dumb questions" about the changes being experienced. Teenage girls should remove their bra so that you can do a breast examination, teach breast self-examination, and check for scoliosis. If the nurse is a male and the patient is an adolescent female, it is recommended that a female staff member be present during the breast and genital examination (Sass & Kaplan, 2011).

Steps of the Physical Examination

The physical examination of children, just as for adults, begins with a systematic **inspection**: checking colour, warmth, characteristics, and texture visually and smelling for any odour. **Palpation** follows inspection to validate your observations. Percussion is a useful tool for determining the location, size, and density of organs or masses. Tapping with the reflex hammer elicits deep tendon reflexes. The stethoscope is used to auscultate the heart, lungs, and abdomen.

Performing a Physical Examination

A complete examination includes assessment of the general appearance, vital signs, body measurements, pain assessment, as well as examination of the head, neck, eyes, ears, nose, mouth and throat, skin, thorax and lungs, breasts, heart and peripheral perfusion, abdomen, genitalia and rectum, musculoskeletal system, and neurologic system. The nurse in most settings will not be assessing the breasts, genitalia, or eyes or ears in detail. Be aware of the role of the nurse in different settings and how the nurse can facilitate the assessment process.

General Appearance

Never discount first impressions. As you become more comfortable performing physical examinations, you will develop an ability to describe what you see and hear. Does the child give an impression of being ill or well? What is the child's expression and energy level? Note lethargy, listlessness, excessive activity, or inappropriate attention span for the child's age. Observe the child's state of alertness and whether he or she is responding appropriately to the stress of the situation. Note the child's posture and positioning:

- The newborn's posture is flexed, with arms and legs tucked in.
- The older infant should have improving head and then trunk control.
- The toddler demonstrates lordosis (swayback) and bowlegs, with a relatively large head and protuberant belly.
- The preschooler is more slender and upright in appearance.
- The school-age child and adolescent should demonstrate an upright, straight, and well-balanced posture.

Note whether the child's development appears appropriate. Observing the child initially may yield a wealth of information about the child's development. Is the child active, moving about the room? Does the child's speech seem appropriate for his or her age? Notice whether the family interacts appropriately with one another and the child. Does the child appear clean and well cared for? Does the child appear well nourished or small for age or obese? Do you smell tobacco or alcohol on the family's clothing? Does the child have a toy or transitional object? Is there a baby bottle or pacifier nearby? Do the siblings appear equally well cared for? Is there tension in the room between adults or adolescents? This initial quick assessment of general appearance will serve the nurse well if it is objective; delay your interpretation of what you have assessed until you gather more data.

Measurement of Vital Signs

Measure, document, and interpret the vital signs of children using age-appropriate equipment and approaches. The child's age and size, as well as knowledge of underlying health conditions, will affect your analysis of the vital signs. Vital signs are the temperature, pulse rate, respiratory rate, and blood pressure. In terms of vital signs, there is greater fluctuation in what is considered normal in children compared to adults. Therefore, count the heart rate and respiratory rate for a full minute (this will require comforting an infant or distracting a young child). If possible, perform these measurements when the child is quiet; if the child is crying or otherwise active during the assessment, document this. Many acute care settings require continuous measurement of vital signs using specific monitoring equipment. Also assess the child's pain level when assessing the vital signs.

Temperature

Temperature is measured as it is in adults. Thermometers are available in glass, electronic, and digital types. Use the same type of equipment consistently to allow reliable comparisons to be made and to permit tracking of temperatures during the course of illness (Bowden & Greenberg, 2008). No matter which type of thermometer is used, ensure accuracy by carefully following the manufacturer's instructions.

The routes for taking the child's temperature are tympanic, temporal, oral, axillary, and rectal. Evidence is conflicting as to which method actually correlates best with the child's core, bladder, or arterial temperature, but recent studies support the use of a tympanic temperature as the most accurate, if it is appropriately obtained (El Radhi & Patel, 2006; Nimah, Bshesh, Callahan, & Jacobs, 2006). The Community Paediatrics Committee of the Canadian Paediatric Society (CPS) (2011) supports the use of tympanic thermometers for children over 2 years of age but suggests that rectal temperatures remain the gold standard when precise measurements are required.

> ▶ **Take** NOTE!
>
> *Because of the mercury in glass thermometers, the Canadian Paediatric Society does not recommend their use (Community Paediatrics Committee, CPS, 2011).*

Choosing a way of measuring temperature depends on what is available at the facility and the child's age and physical condition. Tympanic thermometers measure the temperature within seconds, so this route is ideal for most children. Tympanic temperature reflects the pulmonary artery temperature. Tympanic thermometers are now available with smaller speculums, more appropriate for the infant's or young child's ear canal. The accuracy of a tympanic temperature reading depends on the user's technique and on the fit of the probe in the ear canal (Nursing Procedure 31.1). The tympanic method may be affected by ear wax, otitis media, and crying (Community Paediatrics Committee, CPS, 2011).

Temporal scanning is a newer method of temperature measurement that uses infrared scanning on the skin over the temporal artery combined with a mathematical computation to determine the child's arterial temperature. Measure temperature on the exposed side of the head (not the side that has been lying on a pillow or covered by a hat). Slide the sensor tip externally in a horizontal line across the child's forehead, midway between the eyebrows and hairline and ending at the temporal artery. Hold it there until the device registers

Nursing Procedure 31.1

TYMPANIC TEMPERATURE

1. Note age of child. If younger than 3 years, pull the earlobe back and down.
2. Insert the tympanic thermometer gently into the ear canal with the infrared sensor beam directed toward the centre of the tympanic membrane rather than the sides of the ear canal.
3. Push the button to take the temperature and hold until a reading is obtained. The length of time required for the temperature to register varies per manufacturer but is only a few seconds at most.

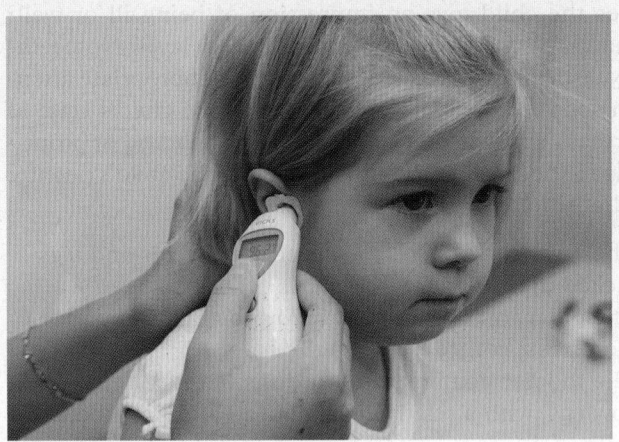

the temperature reading, which usually requires 1 second. Accuracy may be affected by excessive sweating (Exergen Corporation, 2007).

Oral temperature is highly reliable if the child can cooperate. By 4 years of age, the child can hold an electronic oral thermometer in the mouth well enough to obtain a reading. Place the probe under the tongue. The child's mouth remains closed until the device registers the temperature. Have the child sit or lie quietly while

the temperature is being taken. Electronic devices provide a temperature reading in as little as 4 seconds, but again the length of time varies with manufacturer. Oral intake, oxygen administration, and nebulized medications or treatments may affect oral temperature. (See Evidence-based Practice 31.1.)

The axillary method works well for children who are uncooperative, neurologically impaired, or immunosuppressed or have injuries or surgery to the oral cavity

EVIDENCE–BASED PRACTICE 31.1
Accuracy of Supralingual Temperature Measurement with Pacifier Thermometers

● **Study**

Nurses and parents are concerned with being able to measure temperature accurately with the least invasive method possible. Research trials on pacifier thermometry in the past have been limited. The purpose of this study was to determine the accuracy of measuring the supralingual temperature with a pacifier thermometer. The researchers conducted a prospective, cross-sectional study using a convenience sample of children ages 7 days to 24 months. Subjects were limited to those without gastrointestinal illness or contraindication to either the supralingual or rectal method of temperature measurement. Each child underwent pacifier temperature measurement with recordings at 3 and 6 minutes. The result was adjusted upward 0.5°F as recommended by the thermometer manufacturer. Rectal temperature was then taken.

▲ **Findings**

Analysis of the pairs of recorded temperatures for each subject revealed close agreement between the rectal

temperature and the adjusted 6-minute pacifier temperatures. Differences between the two were not statistically significant. Variations between measurements are certain to occur when temperature is measured at different sites, so the researcher does not recommend replacing rectal thermometers with pacifier thermometers when a rectal temperature is indicated. Rather, it is the researcher's recommendation to use the pacifier thermometer as a screening tool.

■ **Nursing Implications**

Pacifier thermometers are an acceptable tool for temperature screening in children 7 days to 24 months of age. Nurses must use the thermometer properly, as well as instruct parents in its appropriate use if it is to be used at home. Consistent use of one particular method is important for tracking trends in temperature management over time. The mathematical upward adjustment of 0.5°F must be included in the reporting of temperatures measured by pacifier thermometry. Note: This U.S. study reported Fahrenheit temperature only.

Braun, C. A. (2006). Accuracy of pacifier thermometers in young children. *Pediatric Nursing, 32*(5), 413–418.

(Bowden & Greenberg, 2008). However, this method provides an inaccurate estimate of core temperature because it is significantly influenced by environmental conditions. Place the tip of the electronic or digital thermometer in the axilla to obtain the reading. Make sure the tip is indeed in the axilla and not just between the arm and the child's side. Hold the thermometer parallel rather than perpendicular to the child's side to obtain the most accurate reading. Keep the child's arm pressed down to the side until the thermometer registers, which will be as little as 10 seconds with certain electronic models but 2 or 3 minutes with digital models commonly used at home.

Though long considered to reflect core temperature, the rectal route is invasive, not well accepted by children or parents, and probably unnecessary with the modern alternative methods now available. In addition to its intrusiveness, obtaining the rectal temperature runs the risks of damaging the rectal mucosa and inducing bradycardia in young infants. To take the rectal temperature, position the young infant supine with legs flexed. The older infant or child should be prone or side-lying. Small children may lie across the parent's lap for additional comfort. Apply a water-soluble jelly to the covered probe, insert the thermometer past the anal sphincter no more than 2.5 cm (1 inch), and hold it there until the temperature registers (as little as 15 seconds with certain electronic models but longer with digital models).

> ▶ **Take** NOTE!
>
> *Avoid the rectal route of temperature measurement in the immunosuppressed child, as well as the child who has diarrhea, a bleeding disorder, or a history of rectal surgery (Asher & Northington, 2008).*

Pulse

Assess the heart rate while the child is resting or sleeping. The heart rate in infants is much faster than in adults. It also varies in infants and children who are anxious, fearful, or crying. As the child grows, the heart rate slows and the range of normal values narrows. Table 31.3 lists normal heart rate ranges according to the child's age group. The radial pulse is difficult to palpate accurately in children less than 2 years of age because the blood vessels lie close to the skin surface and are easily obliter-

ated (Bickley & Szilagyi, 2009). For children younger than 10 years of age, auscultate the apical pulse with the stethoscope for a full minute (Jarvis, 2008). The **point of maximum intensity (PMI)**, the point on the chest wall where the heartbeat is heard most distinctly, is just above and outside the left nipple of the infant at the third or fourth intercostal space. The PMI moves to a more medial and slightly lower area until 7 years of age, when it is heard best at the fourth or fifth interspace at the midclavicular line (see the section below on chest examination for more information). Apical pulse rate should also be taken if the child has a cardiac problem such as an irregular heart rate or a congenital heart defect, as well as before administration of certain medications such as digoxin. During this procedure with children, allow the young child to examine or handle the stethoscope to become familiar with the equipment. In older children, palpate the radial pulse for a full minute. Note any irregularities in strength or rhythm.

Finally, document the method used to obtain pulse measurement as well as any activity of the child during the assessment and any action taken.

> ▶ **Take** NOTE!
>
> *In the infant and young child, the heart rate is often quite elevated due to fear or anxiety when the stethoscope is placed on the chest initially. For an accurate heart rate, wait several seconds until the rate slows, then count for 1 full minute.*

Respiratory Rate

Assess respirations when the child is resting or sitting quietly, since respiratory rate often changes when infants or young children cry, feed, or become more active. They also tend to breathe faster when they are anxious or scared. The most accurate respiratory rate is obtained before disturbing the infant or child (Bowden & Greenberg, 2008). This can often be done easily when the parent/caregiver is holding the child before any clothing is removed. Count the respiratory rate for a full minute to ensure accuracy. Infants' respirations are primarily diaphragmatic, so count the abdominal movements. After 1 year of age, count the thoracic movements. Table 31.3 gives ranges of respiratory rate according to the child's

TABLE 31.3 **HEART RATE AND RESPIRATORY RATE RANGES BY AGE GROUP**

	Newborn	Infant	Toddler	Preschooler	School-ager	Adolescent
Heart rate	80–160	80–150	80–140	80–130	75–120	70–100
Respiratory rate	30–70	20–40	20–40	20–30	16–22	15–20

Adapted from: Kliegman, R. M., Behrman, R. E., Jenson, H. B., & Stanton, B. F. (2007). *Nelson textbook of pediatrics* (18th ed.). Philadelphia: WB Saunders; and Schaider, J. (ed.). (2007). *Rosen & Barkin's 5-minute emergency medicine consult.* Philadelphia: Lippincott Williams & Wilkins.

Nursing Procedure 31.2

PULSE OXIMETRY MONITORING

1. Explain the procedure to the child and family (use a penlight to show how the sensor "looks through the skin").
2. Attach the probe to the child and connect to the monitor.
3. Set the parameters for the alarm if monitoring pulse oximetry continuously.
4. Observe and record pulse rate and oxygen saturation.
5. Record the activity level of the child and the percentage of oxygen in use.
6. Check skin condition and rotate sensor position every few hours.

Types of probes
a. infant continuous

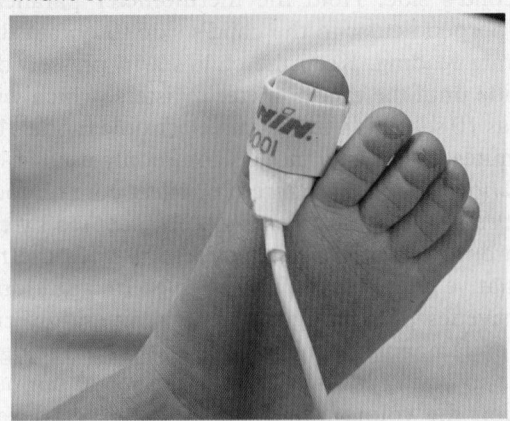

b. finger continuous

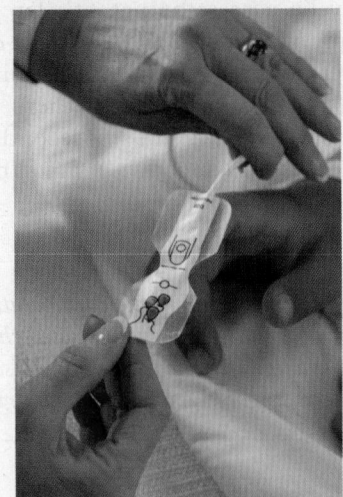

c. finger intermittent

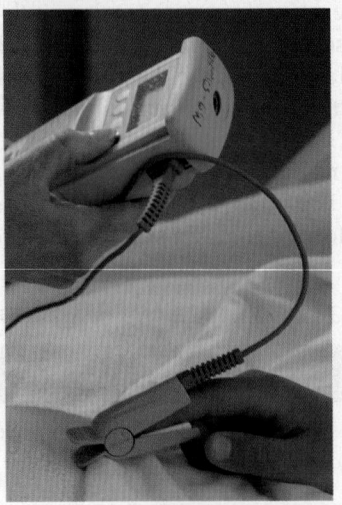

age group. Document the rate, activity of the child, any deviations from normal, and any action taken.

> ▶ *Take* NOTE!
>
> *Infants normally display an uneven or irregular breathing pattern, with short pauses between some breaths. This may be accentuated when they are ill (Bickley & Szilagyi, 2009).*

Measuring Oxygen Saturation

Since the incidence of respiratory dysfunction is high in children who are ill, pulse oximetry is often routinely included in the vital signs assessment. This method is reliable and noninvasive. Pulse oximetry determines the oxygen saturation (SaO_2) in blood by using a sensor that measures the absorption of light waves as they pass through highly perfused areas of the body. The pulse rate on the oximeter should coincide with the apical pulse rate to ensure that the oxygen saturation reading is accurate. Nursing Procedure 31.2 details how to use the pulse oximeter. Identify whether pulse oximetry monitoring will be continuous or intermittent (as with vital signs).

A few guidelines to follow when using pulse oximetry are as follows:

- The probe may be placed on the finger, toe, ear, or foot. Avoid placing the probe on the same extremity with a blood pressure cuff or an intravenous or other type of line.
- Use the physician's orders or health care agency guidelines to set parameters for high and low pulse rate as well as high and low oxygen saturation. Never turn off the alarm settings.
- Ensure that the probe is not applied too tightly, as this will prevent venous flow and cause inaccurate readings.

Potential sources of errors in pulse oximeter readings include abnormal hemoglobin value, hypotension, hypothermia, ambient light interference, motion artifact, and skin breakdown. Falsely low readings may be associated with a nonsecure connection (movement of child's foot or hand), cold extremities/hypothermia, and hypovolemia. Falsely high readings may be associated with carbon monoxide poisoning and anemia (DeMeulenaere, 2007).

Blood Pressure

Beginning at age 3, measure blood pressure yearly at well-child visits. In the hospital or outpatient setting when a child is ill or undergoing surgery or a procedure, the frequency of blood pressure measurement will depend on the child's physical status. Measurement of blood pressure can be frightening to a young child, so include an age-appropriate explanation and perform the procedure after obtaining the pulse rate and respirations. Accuracy of blood pressure measurement depends on the cuff size, as well as the operator's skill (if the heart sounds are auscultated) or accurate calibration of an electronic device. The Canadian Hypertension Education Program (2010) recommends that the cuff bladder width be at least 40% of the circumference of the upper arm at its midpoint. The cuff bladder length should cover 80% to 100% of the circumference of the upper arm. Various pediatric and infant cuffs are available, as well as larger thigh cuffs that may be used on an arm in an obese adolescent.

> ▶ *Take* NOTE!
>
> *Using an accurate cuff size is important: a wider cuff yields a lower reading and a narrower cuff yields a higher reading.*

Measure blood pressure in the upper arm, lower arm, thigh, or calf/ankle. The size of the cuff should match the extremity used. The measurement should be taken in the same limb, at the same place, and in the same position with each subsequent measurement to ensure consistency in tracking the blood pressure. To measure blood pressure using the upper arm, place the limb at the level of the heart, place the cuff around the upper arm, and auscultate at the brachial artery. When obtaining blood pressure in the lower arm, again, position the limb at the level of the heart, place the cuff above the wrist, and auscultate the radial artery. For measurement in the thigh, place the cuff above the knee and auscultate the popliteal artery. To obtain blood pressure on the calf or ankle, place the cuff above the malleoli or at the midcalf and auscultate the posterior tibial or dorsal pedal artery. Figure 31.4 shows appropriate cuff placement and auscultation points for the various sites.

The U.S. National Heart, Lung, and Blood Institute (NHLBI, 2005) recommends auscultation as the preferred method of obtaining blood pressure readings in children (Fig. 31.5). Systolic pressure in children is read at the moment you hear the first Korotkoff sound as you lower the manometer pressure (Kay et al., 2001). The point at which the sound disappears is the diastolic pressure. The systolic blood pressure sometimes can be heard to a measurement of zero, so document the reading as systolic pressure over "P" for pulse.

Due to the small arm vessels in infants and young children, it may be very difficult to hear the Korotkoff sounds by auscultation (Jarvis, 2008). Alternative methods for obtaining blood pressure measurements in children include the use of Doppler or oscillometric (Dinamap) devices. The Doppler ultrasound method uses high-frequency sound waves that bounce off body parts to obtain blood pressure. Apply the gel to the Doppler end and listen with the Doppler device where you would ordinarily auscultate.

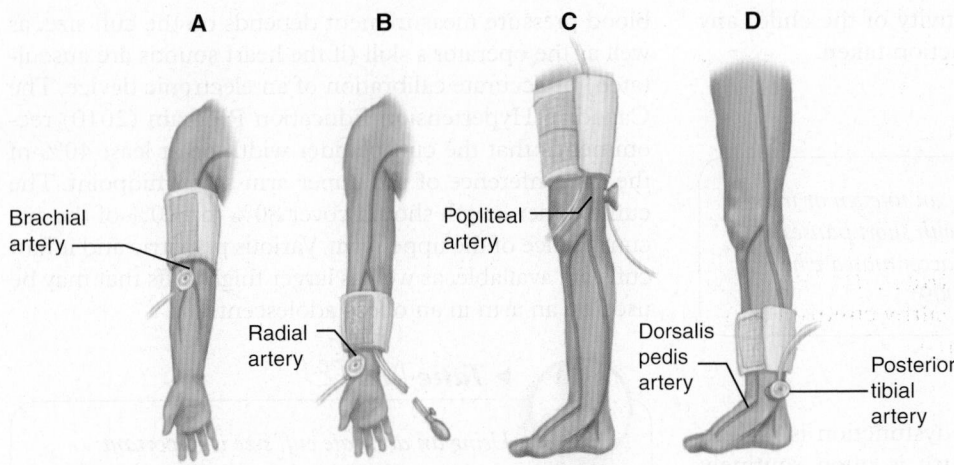

FIGURE 31.4 Various positions of cuff placement and auscultation area for obtaining blood pressure. (**A**) Upper arm. (**B**) Lower arm. (**C**) Thigh. (**D**) Calf/ankle.

With either the Doppler method or auscultation, inflate the cuff 20 mm Hg past the point where the distal pulse disappears. Oscillometric equipment measures the mean arterial pulse and then calculates the systolic and diastolic readings. The accuracy of this method depends heavily on ongoing validation and calibration. Also, the cuff inflates to a preset value often far higher than the infant or child's blood pressure, resulting in a tight, uncomfortable cuff being in place for a longer period of time.

▶ **Take NOTE!**

If the oscillometric device yields a blood pressure greater than the 90th percentile for gender and height, repeat the reading using auscultation.

In children older than 1 year, the systolic pressure in the thigh tends to be 10 to 40 mm Hg higher than in the arm; the diastolic pressure remains the same. Refer to Appendix I for the NHLBI blood pressure levels based on gender and height. Systolic blood pressure increases if the child is crying or anxious, so measure the blood pressure with the child quiet and relaxed. If the reading is lower in the leg than in the arm, always consider coarctation of the aorta or interference with circulation to the lower extremities. Also pay attention to the pulse pressure (the difference between the systolic and diastolic readings): unusually wide (more than 50 mm Hg) or narrow (less than 10 mm Hg) pulse pressure readings suggest a congenital heart defect (Burns et al., 2009).

Infants and children presenting with cardiac concerns should have blood pressures assessed in all four extremities and also in the sitting, lying, and standing positions. Document the method and site used, the activity of the child, any changes that may have occurred, and any actions or interventions performed.

Pain Assessment

Pain is considered to be the "fifth vital sign" (Jarvis, 2008). Use the FLACC (face, legs, activity, cry, and consolability) pain scale to measure pain in children who are too young to verbally or conceptually quantify their pain, or when there is a language barrier (Manworren & Hynan, 2003). The FLACC pain scale consists of a possible 10 points, with 0, 1, or 2 points given for each of five clinical signs (see Table 35.7 in Chapter 35).

Children who are older and can express that pain is worsening or improving should use the Pain Faces Scale (see Fig. 35.3 in Chapter 35). Explain that each face represents a person who is happy or sad, depending on how much or how little pain he has: 0 is for a person who is "very happy because he doesn't hurt at all"; 1 means "it hurts just a little bit"; 2, "it hurts a little more"; 3, "it hurts even more"; 4, "it hurts a whole lot"; and 5, "it hurts as much as you can imagine—but you don't have to be crying to feel this bad." Then ask the child to point to the face that best describes the amount of pain being felt (Wong & Baker, 1988).

For additional information related to pain assessment, refer to Chapter 35.

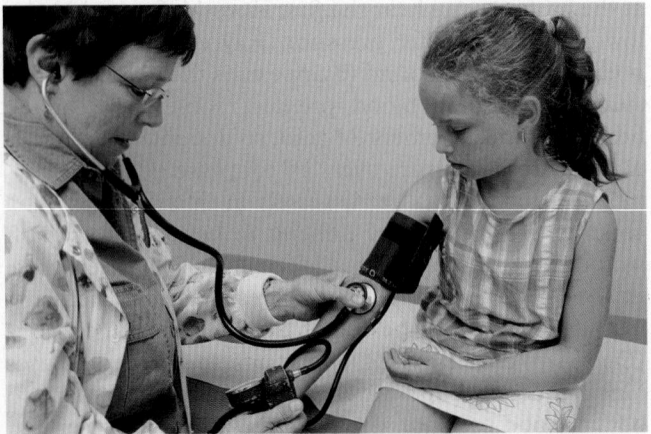

FIGURE 31.5 Auscultation is the preferred method for measuring blood pressure in children.

Body Measurements

Appropriate growth in children is usually an indicator of good health. A child who is not growing well may be in poor health, have inappropriate or inadequate dietary intake, or have a chronic disease (Bickley & Szilagyi, 2009). Accurate assessment of growth is a critical skill for the pediatric nurse.

Determine the child's height or length, weight, and weight for length or **body mass index (BMI)**. Measure the head circumference for healthy children under age 3. Plot these measurements on a graph so they can be compared with earlier measurements and those of the child's peers. Additional anthropometric measurements used in children may include the chest circumference, mid-upper arm circumference, and skinfold measurement at the triceps, abdomen, or subscapular regions, but these are not performed routinely and are usually used only when a nutritionist consultation is necessary.

The growth chart is a screening tool for nutritional problems as well as a useful screen for chronic illness. Record each measurement in ink with a small dot at the correct location for the child's age and the date of the measurement written above it. Then use a plastic straightedge to connect the previous measurement to the most current one. Children grow at variable rates; in infancy and pre-puberty, the growth velocity is normally more rapid. The growth chart allows the nurse to compare the patient with other children of the same age and gender while allowing for normal genetic variation. When measurements fall close to the same percentiles over time, growth is normal for that child. Children whose measurements fall within the 5th and 95th percentiles are generally considered within the normal growth range (Rebeshi & Brown, 2007).

Sudden or sustained changes in percentile may indicate a chronic disorder, emotional difficulty, or nutritional intake problem (Bickley & Szilagyi, 2009). These findings require further assessment of the physical status of the child as well as other types of evaluations such as dietary intake or serum laboratory measurements.

Appendix F gives growth charts for boys and girls, ages birth to 36 months and 2 to 20 years. Look for a trend over time of healthy growth that is neither too fast nor too slow.

▶ *Take* NOTE!

The Dieticians of Canada, CPS, College of Family Physicians of Canada, and Community Health Nurses of Canada (2010) recommend that pediatric body measurements be followed using the World Health Organization (2010) growth charts.

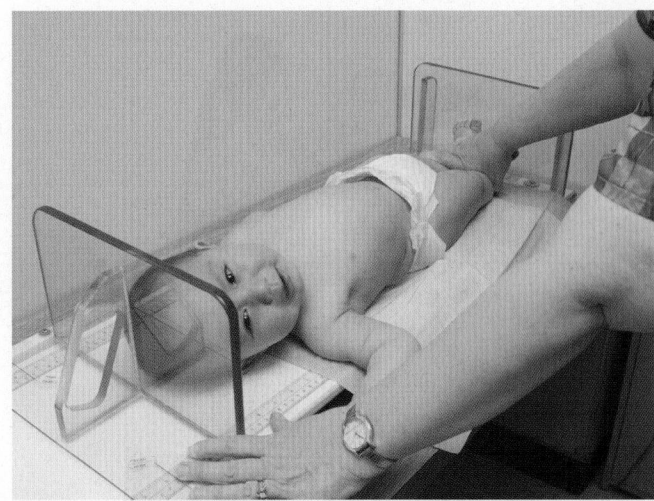

FIGURE 31.6 The recumbent measuring board is the most accurate method for obtaining a length measurement in infants and very young children.

Length or Height

Calculate the length of the infant and toddler in a lying position until the age of 24 months. Use a measuring board (Fig. 31.6) or a cloth or paper measuring tape. Stretch out the legs to get a full extension of the body. Marking the examination paper at the child's head and extended foot is an option. Make sure that the growth chart where the measurement is plotted is marked for length and not height, as the two measurements differ. Document the length in centimetres.

Once the child can cooperate and stand independently, begin measuring the standing height. Using a stadiometer (height bar) is best (Fig. 31.7), but a cloth or paper tape can be used. Ask the child to remove his or her shoes and check that the back, shoulders, buttocks, and heels are against the wall, with the pelvis tucked as much as possible to correct for lordosis. The chin should be parallel to the floor. Plot this measurement on a growth chart marked for height rather than length. Record the height in centimeters.

▶ *Take* NOTE!

Cloth and paper measuring tapes may stretch over time. Periodically replace or recalibrate all measuring tools.

Weight

Measure weight on a scale that is calibrated between every measurement. Just before placing the child on the electronic scale, press the "zero" or "tare" button and make sure the reading is 0. Calibrate the balance-type scale by setting the weight at zero, observing the beam balance, and making adjustments as necessary. Infants

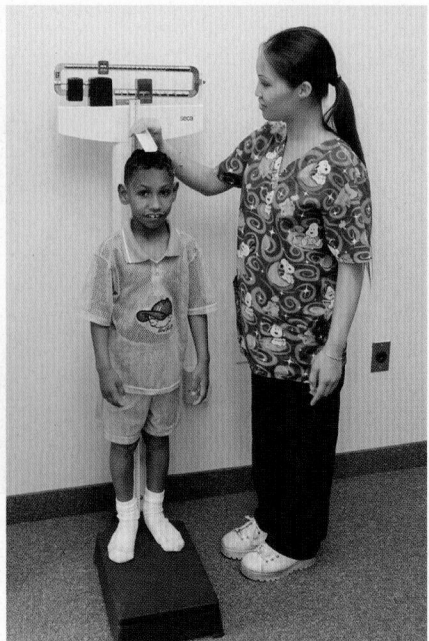

FIGURE 31.7 Standing height is most accurately measured with the stadiometer.

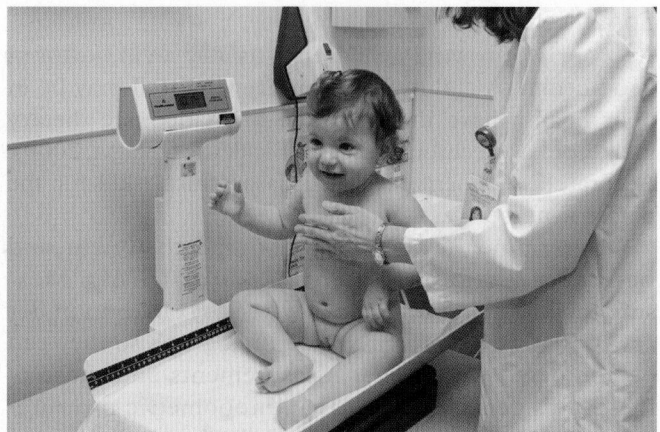

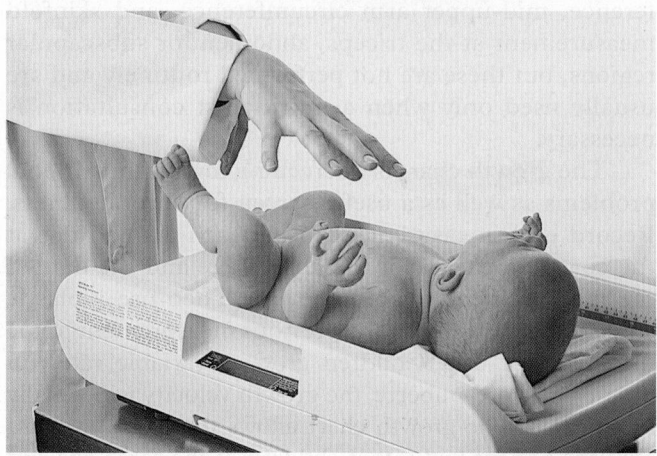

FIGURE 31.8 A nurse or caregiver should remain nearby while weighing the infant or toddler.

and toddlers should be weighed on a platform-type electronic or balance scale, with examination paper placed between the child and the scale surface. Calibrate the scale with the examination paper in place. Remove the infant's diaper immediately before placing him or her on the scale. Toddlers may sit on the scale with the nurse or caregiver nearby to avoid falls (Fig. 31.8). Weigh older children and adolescents on a standing scale (Fig. 31.9). They may keep their underpants on and wear a lightweight examination gown or lightweight clothing.

An alternate method for obtaining weight, though much less accurate, is to weigh the caregiver initially and then weigh the caregiver holding the child. The difference between the two weights is the child's weight.

Regardless of the method used, weigh the infant to the nearest 10 g and the toddler and older child to the nearest 100 g. Record the weight in kilograms.

Weight for Length

For children between the ages of newborn and 36 months, plot weight on the growth chart in comparison to the child's length. This allows the nurse to determine whether the child is a healthy weight for how long he or she is. Children placing in less than the 3rd percentile on the weight-for-length chart are considered underweight. Those placing greater than the 95th percentile are considered to be overweight.

Body Mass Index

With the recent increase in obesity in children, BMI is becoming an important measurement. BMI is a measure of body fat and is determined by comparing the child's

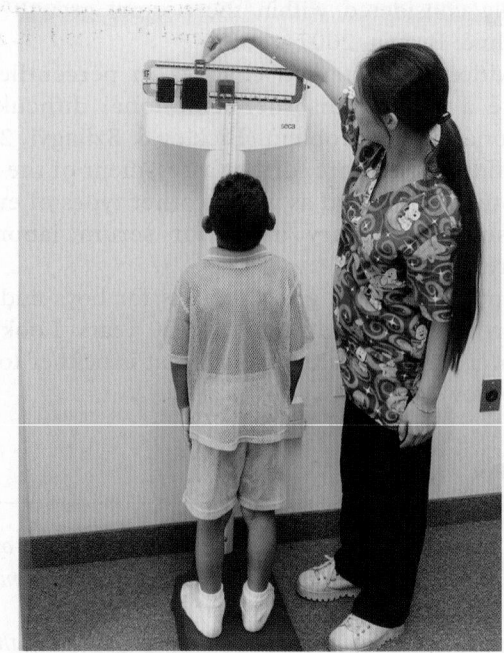

FIGURE 31.9 Children who can stand independently can be weighed on a regular standing balance scale.

BOX 31.1 Calculation of Body Mass Index (BMI)

$$\frac{\text{weight in kilograms}}{(\text{height in metres}) \times (\text{height in metres})} \times 10{,}000$$

height and weight (CDC, 2002). Calculate the BMI using the child's weight and height. Box 31.1 gives BMI calculation formulas. BMI is included on the charts for children ages 2 to 20 years. Plot the BMI on the growth chart according to the child's age. A child older than 5 years whose BMI for age plots at less than the 3rd percentile is considered to be underweight. BMI between the 85th and 97th percentiles indicates that the child is overweight, and BMI greater than the 97th percentile indicates that the child is obese. Children younger than 5 years of age are considered overweight if their BMI is greater than the 97th percentile and obese if it is greater than the 99.9th percentile.

The growth chart can indicate when a child is not growing adequately and can also be used to predict the development of overweight and obesity (CDC, 2002).

Head Circumference

Measure head circumference at well-child visits and upon hospital admission until the third birthday. Then measure it at the annual well-child visit until 6 years old if there are problems such as microcephaly or macrocephaly present at age 3. Measure the largest point across the skull, not including the ears, with a non-stretching cloth or paper tape. Begin at the forehead just above the eyebrows and bring the tape around the head in a taut circle just above the occipital prominence at the back of the head (Fig. 31.10). Plot this measurement in relation

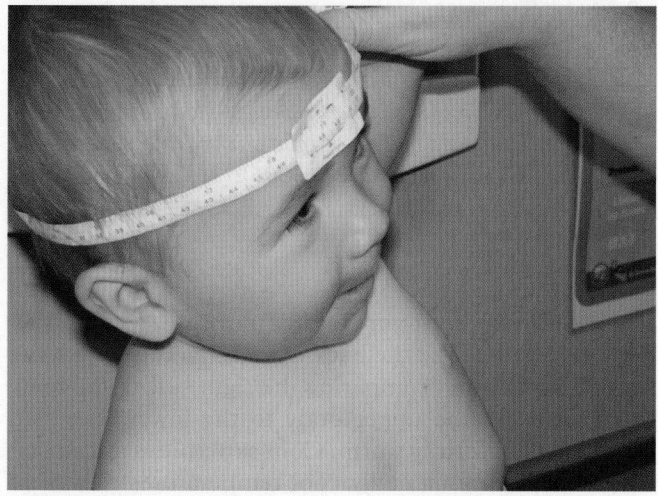

FIGURE 31.10 Measure occipito-frontal head circumference at the largest point.

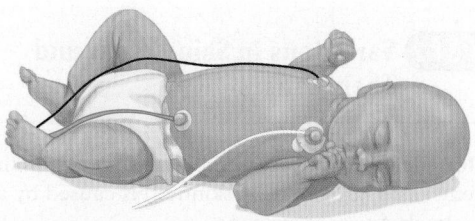

FIGURE 31.11 Placement of cardiac and apnea monitor leads: white on the right upper chest, black on the left upper chest, red on the abdomen (not over bone).

to the child's age on the appropriate standardized growth chart (usual growth charts include head circumference only up to age 3 years).

Monitoring Equipment

Sometimes children in acute care settings require continuous monitoring of vital signs. This monitoring could be via an apnea monitor or a cardiopulmonary monitor. The apnea monitor measures abnormal or irregular breathing in infants. The cardiopulmonary monitor generally measures heart rate and respiratory rate. Additional equipment on this monitor also allows for blood pressure and temperature monitoring. Set high and low alarm limits according to the health care facility's policies. Figure 31.11 indicates the placement of electrodes for the apnea and cardiopulmonary monitors. Assess the skin where the electrodes are placed to ensure there is no skin breakdown. If the alarm sounds, immediately check the child to ensure the leads are not disconnected or the child is not in distress.

Skin

The skin is the body's largest organ and reveals information about a child's nutrition, respiratory, cardiac, endocrine, and hydration status all at a glance. A careful skin examination provides an invaluable understanding of a child's health (Jarvis, 2008).

Inspection

Inspect the colour of the skin. The colour should be appropriate to the child's racial or ethnic background, with the nail beds, conjunctivae, soles of the feet, and palms of the hands appearing pink. Normal variations include the following:

- Blueness of the hands and feet, known as **acrocyanosis**, is normal in babies up to several days of age and results from an immature circulatory system completing the switch from fetal to extrauterine life (see Fig. 25.3 in Chapter 25).
- Cooling or warming the newborn and young infant may produce a vasomotor response that causes a mottling of the skin over the trunk and extremities (see Fig. 25.3 in Chapter 25).

BOX 31.2 Variations in Skin Colour and Their Causes

- **Pallor** (defined as decreased pinkness in light-skinned patients, ashy-grey in dark-skinned) is caused by anemia, shock, fever, or syncope.
- **Peripheral cyanosis** (blue discolouration) occurs in nails, soles, and palms and may be caused by anxiety or cold; also associated with central cyanosis.
- **Central cyanosis** (blueness of the lips, tongue, oral mucosa, and trunk) is caused by hypoxia or circulatory collapse.
- Overall yellow colour (**jaundice**) may be physiologic in the newborn or related to liver or hematopoietic disease in any age child.
- **Yellowing** of nose, palms, and soles may result from excess intake of yellow vegetables.
- **Redness** of the skin results from blushing, exposure to cold, hyperthermia, inflammation (localized), or alcohol ingestion.
- **Lack of colour** in skin, hair, and eyes is related to albinism.

Adapted from: Bickley, L., & Szilagyi, P. G. (2009). *Bates guide to physical examination and history taking* (10th ed.). Philadelphia: Lippincott Williams & Wilkins; and Jarvis, C. (2008). *Physical examination and health assessment* (5th ed.). St. Louis, MO: Saunders.

- Babies of darkly pigmented First Nations, African, and Asian parents will be paler than their parents for many months until the melanocytes in the epidermis begin production.
- Dark-skinned infants commonly have hyperpigmented areolas, genitals, and linea nigra.

Other variations related to skin colour are discussed in Box 31.2.

Inspect the skin for the presence of **lanugo**. All infants display some degree of lanugo (soft, downy hair on the body, particularly the face and back). Lanugo is more abundant in infants of First Nations descent and in premature infants and recedes over the first few weeks of life.

Inspect the entire body for nevi and vascular and other lesions. Note their location, size, distribution, characteristics, and colour. Pigmented nevi (also termed birthmarks) are indicated by a darker patch of skin and generally do not fade over time. Note the presence of hyperpigmented nevi (formerly called Mongolian spots), which appear as blue or grey, variably and irregularly shaped macules (Fig. 31.12). These are a common finding in dark-skinned infants. These nevi fade over months to years as the child's skin pigment darkens. Do not mistake hyperpigmented nevi for bruises. Inspect the skin for vascular lesions. Table 31.4 describes vascular lesions and their significance.

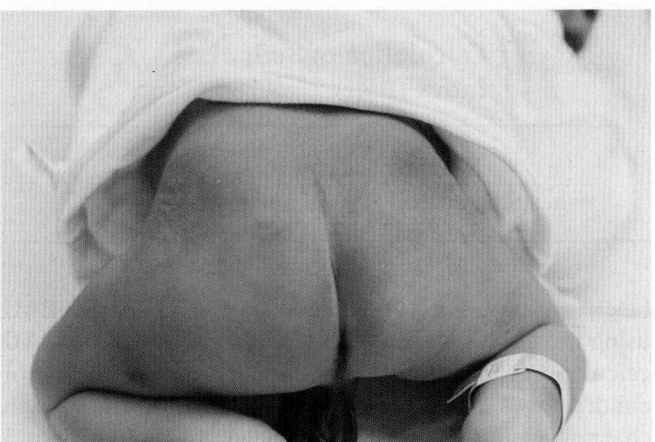

FIGURE 31.12 Transient hyperpigmentation most often occurs in darker-skinned infants.

Rashes are common in children and are often associated with communicable diseases. Describe the rash in detail, noting types of lesions, distribution, drying, scabbing, and any drainage. The newborn and young infant may display milia (small white papules) on the forehead, chin, nose, and cheeks. These recede spontaneously. In adolescents the skin examination may reveal open or closed comedones (pimples or blackheads) across the face, chest, and back. Teens may sport tattoos, brandings, or various body piercings; inspect these areas for signs of infection such as erythema or drainage.

Document the presence of any lacerations, abrasions, or burns. Note the distribution of the injury and whether it seems consistent with the mechanism described in the health history. Be alert to the possibility of child abuse if the type or number of burns, lacerations, or bruises seems unusual for the situation.

▶ *Take* NOTE!

Petechiae or ecchymoses may be found over areas traumatized by the birth process; these may take a few weeks to resolve. Certain cultures use "cupping" or "coining" when a child is ill, and these practices may yield bruises or mild burns (International Cupping Therapy Association, 2006).

Palpation

Palpate the skin for temperature, moisture, texture, turgor, and edema. Use the back of your hand to assess the skin's temperature, comparing the right side of the body to the left and the upper body to the lower. The skin should feel uniformly warm. Cool extremities are associated with environmentally cool temperatures as well as impending circulatory collapse and shock. Warm skin may be associated with fever or sunburn, or locally a

TABLE 31.4 VASCULAR LESIONS AND THEIR SIGNIFICANCE

Description	Significance
Salmon nevi: light pink macule usually on eyelids, nasal bridge, back of neck ("stork bite")	Usually fade over time, but may never go away completely. No complications.
Strawberry nevus: raised reddish papule made of blood vessels (hemangiomas)	Present at or develop after birth; recede over time, usually by age 9 years. Usually no complications.
Nevus flammeus: dark purple-red flat patch, grows with the child ("port-wine stain")	May be associated with Sturge-Weber syndrome. May be disfiguring; may be removed with laser therapy.
Ecchymosis: purplish discolouration, changing to blue, brown, black (bruise)	Common on lower extremities in young children. Should correlate with the injury.
Petechiae: pinpoint reddish purple macules that do not blanch when pressed	Broken tiny blood vessels; occur with coughing, bleeding disorders, meningococcemia
Purpura: larger purple macules	Bleeding under the skin; occur with bleeding disorders, meningococcemia

Adapted from: Bickley, L., & Szilagyi, P. G. (2009). *Bates guide to physical examination and history taking* (10th ed.). Philadelphia: Lippincott Williams & Wilkins; and Jarvis, C. (2008). *Physical examination and health assessment* (5th ed.). St. Louis, MO: Saunders.

burn or infectious process. The skin should feel fairly dry, occasionally moister in the creases. Dry, flaking skin may occur in the young infant, particularly if born postmaturely. Overall skin dryness in the well-hydrated child may occur with excess sun exposure, poor nutrition, or over-bathing. Moist skin occurs with perspiration, fever resolution, and shock. The infant's and young child's skin is very soft ordinarily. Older children should continue to have a smooth and even skin texture. The preadolescent and adolescent may have oily feeling skin on the face, shoulders, or back.

Assess skin turgor by elevating the skin on the abdomen in the infant or on the back of hand in the older child or teen. The "pinched-up" skin should quickly return to place. Skin that remains tented is strongly suggestive of moderate to severe dehydration. When edema is present, palpate the edematous area to determine its extent. Palpate any lumps or protrusions to determine firmness or tenderness. Palpate lesions or rashes with a gloved hand to document the size and extent of the lesions.

Hair and Nails

Inspect the hair and scalp, noting distribution of hair as well as colour, texture, amount, and quality. The young infant's hair may be absent entirely or quite thick; it will be replaced by hair that is of a texture and colour closer to what the child will have throughout childhood. Coarse, dry hair at any age may indicate a thyroid disorder or nutritional deficiency. Inspect the scalp thoroughly; it should be free from lesions and infestations. Note the presence of a greasy, scaly plaque on the scalp of infants; termed seborrheic dermatitis or cradle cap, it is benign and easily treated.

Inspect the nails for colour, shape, and condition. Full-term infants may have long, papery fingernails that can scratch their skin if not trimmed. Children should have healthy nails. Dry, brittle nails may indicate a nutritional deficiency. Inspect the skin around the nails to ensure that it is intact and without signs of infection. Many children (especially school-age children) have a nervous habit of nail biting or hangnail biting or pulling.

Inspect the school-age child's or adolescent's toenails to ensure they are trimmed in a horizontal fashion. Self-trimming of toenails either too low or in a curved fashion places the child at risk for the development of ingrown nails. Clubbing of the nails indicates chronic hypoxemia related to respiratory or cardiac disease. Nails that curve inward or outward may be hereditary or linked with injury, infection, or iron deficiency anemia.

Head

Examining the head is critical in the newborn and infant periods but should not be overlooked in older children as an opportunity to check for diseases of the scalp and functional and developmental problems that are reflected in poor hygiene of the head and scalp. Note hair distribution and any bald or thinning areas. Use of gloves may be indicated, depending on the overall scalp cleanliness and chance of infestation by head lice (seen as small greyish specks near the base of hair shafts).

Inspection

Examine the head and face for shape and symmetry. In newborns, the head may be temporarily misshapen from uterine positioning or a long vaginal delivery. Some infants have a slight flattening of the back of the head since the recommended sleeping position is supine. Note any irregularities or asymmetry. Observe the infant's head shape by looking down on it from above. Observe whether the head appears centred on the neck or tilts to one side. After 4 months of age, the infant should have achieved enough head control to hold the head erect and in midline when placed in a vertical position. Pull the infant from the supine position into sitting to determine the extent of head lag. To determine the extent of head control in older infants and children, ask the child to turn the head in different directions, either by simple commands or by following a colourful object.

Observe the infant's face when crying, smiling, or babbling for symmetry of muscle movement. In children who are old enough to follow directions, a game of "Simon Says" is a playful way to determine facial symmetry and strength; ask them to puff out their cheeks, make kisses, look surprised, stick out their tongue, and so on (effectively testing function of cranial nerve VII [facial]) (Bickley & Szilagyi, 2009).

> ▶ **Take** NOTE!
>
> *When you note a flattened occiput in an infant, encourage the parent or caregiver to allow the infant "tummy time" while awake and observed and to change the infant's head position frequently when upright in an infant seat (Dowshen, 2008).*

Palpation

Gently palpate the anterior and posterior **fontanels** (Fig. 31.13), which remain open in infancy to allow for rapid brain growth in the first months of life. Note the size of the fontanels. The anterior fontanel is about the size of a quarter at birth and slowly gets smaller until it

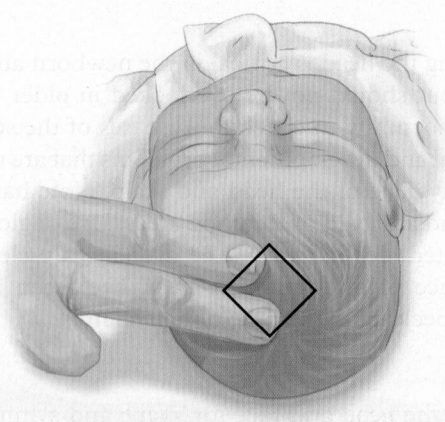

FIGURE 31.13 Note location and size of the anterior fontanel. The anterior fontanel usually closes between the ages of 9 and 18 months, while the posterior fontanel is usually closed by 2 months of age.

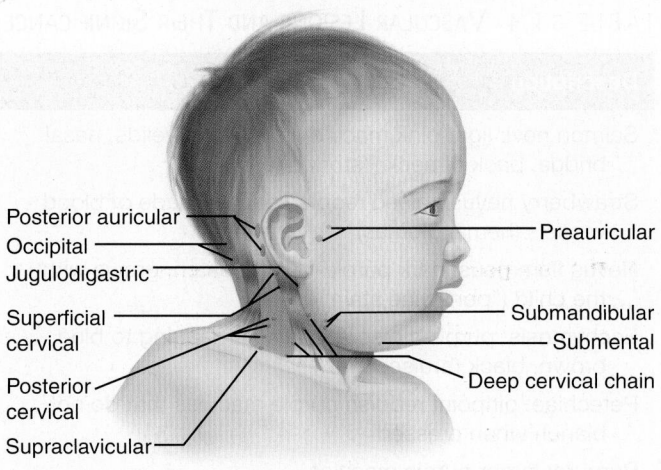

FIGURE 31.14 Location of lymph nodes.

can no longer be felt when it is closed by the age of 9 to 18 months. The posterior fontanel is much smaller and may close any time between shortly after birth and approximately 2 months of age. The fontanel should be neither depressed nor taut and bulging, though it is not uncommon to see it pulsate or briefly bulge if the baby cries. In an acutely ill infant, assess the fontanels while obtaining the vital signs. Dehydration can cause the fontanels to be sunken; increased intracranial pressure and overhydration can cause them to bulge. Palpate the skull for asymmetry, overriding or open sutures, and lumps or other deformities. Palpate the jaw joints as the child bites down to assess cranial nerve V (trigeminal). Use the fingertips to palpate for occipital, postauricular, preauricular, submental, and submandibular lymph nodes, noting their size, mobility, and consistency (Fig. 31.14).

> ▶ **Take** NOTE!
>
> *Large fontanels may be associated with Down syndrome or congenital hypothyroidism. A fontanel that becomes larger over time rather than smaller may indicate the development of hydrocephalus, especially if accompanied by an accelerated increase in head circumference (Bickley & Szilagyi, 2009).*

Neck

Inspect the neck for symmetry. The infant's neck is short, but by 4 years of age the child's neck should be similar in appearance to the adult's. Webbing or excessive neck skinfolds may be associated with Turner syndrome, and lax neck skin may occur with Down syndrome. Assess the flexibility of the neck through a full range of motion. Take younger children through a passive range of motion. Older children will be able to look in all directions on command and stretch their chins to the chests themselves. Test cranial nerve XI (accessory) in the older child by having the child attempt to turn the head against resistance. Assessment of neck mobility is particularly important when infections of the central nervous system are suspected. Pain or resistance to range of motion may indicate meningeal irritation. Do not assess neck mobility in the trauma victim.

Palpate the neck for masses and lymph nodes. Palpate the cervical and clavicular lymph nodes with the distal part of the fingers using gentle but firm pressure in a circular motion. Tilt the child's head upward slightly to allow better access. Assess the lymph nodes for swelling, mobility, temperature, and tenderness. In healthy infants and adolescents, the cervical lymph nodes are usually not palpable, whereas they are often found to be small, nontender, and mobile in healthy children from the ages of 1 to 11 years (see Fig. 31.14 for locations of lymph nodes). Enlarged cervical lymph nodes frequently occur in association with upper respiratory infections and otitis media. Significant enlargement should be reported to the physician or nurse practitioner. Palpate the trachea; the thyroid is usually palpable only in older children.

▶ **Take** NOTE!

The infant or child who has experienced trauma should have the cervical spine maintained completely immobile until a radiologist has determined that the spinal cord is not damaged.

Eyes

Assessment of the eyes includes evaluation of the external and internal structures as well as screening for visual acuity. Any nurse caring for a child should be adept at examining the external structures. Assessment of the internal structures will also be covered below but is usually performed only by the advanced practitioner. Refer to Chapter 30 for information on vision screening. Determination of visual acuity tests the function of cranial nerve II (optic).

External Structures

Observe the eyes for symmetry and spacing, even distribution of eyelashes and eyelids, and presence of epicanthal folds. Note the child's ability to blink, reporting inability to do so. The eyes should look symmetrical and both should be facing forward in the midline when the child is looking directly ahead. The iris should be perfectly round and the sclerae should be clear. The cornea should be uniformly transparent. Inspect the corners of the eye (medial and lateral canthus) and the conjunctiva (lining of the eyelids). They should be free of discharge, inflammation, or swelling. Epicanthal folds may be present

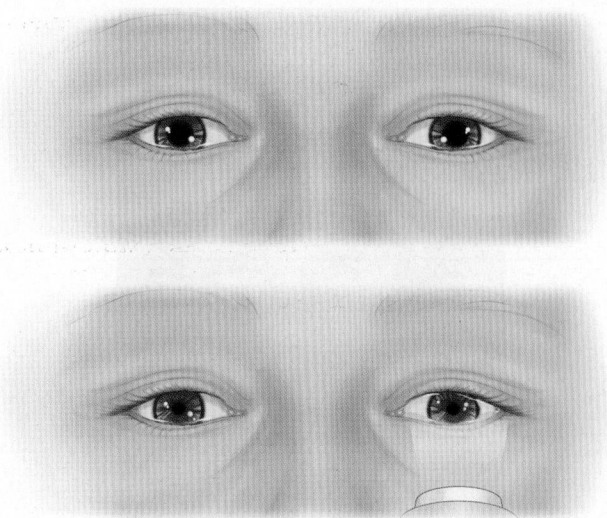

FIGURE 31.15 The pupils should be equal, round and reactive to light and accommodation (PERRLA).

in children of Asian descent, children with genetic abnormalities, or those with fetal alcohol spectrum disorder. Using a small penlight or ophthalmoscope, inspect the function and clarity of the pupil by putting your nondominant hand on the child's forehead and moving the light toward and away from each eye. This will elicit the blink reflex. Next observe whether the pupil contracts with the light and expands when the light is removed. Make the same motion with a small toy or object and direct the child to look at it. The eyes demonstrate **accommodation**, or focusing at different distances, if the pupil constricts as the object moves closer. If normal findings are present, report **PERRLA** (pupils are equal, round, reactive to light and accommodation) (Fig. 31.15). This is a particularly important assessment in head and eye injuries, as well as when other neurologic concerns are present. Absence of pupillary reflexive action after age 3 weeks may indicate blindness (Jarvis, 2008).

▶ **Take** NOTE!

The normal infant may exhibit intermittent strabismus (crossing of the eyes) until about 6 months of age. However, persistent strabismus at any age or intermittent strabismus after 6 months of age should be evaluated by a pediatric ophthalmologist (Burns et al., 2009).

Check extraocular muscle motility and function of cranial nerves III and VI (oculomotor and abducens) by instructing the child to follow the light through the six cardinal positions of gaze. Infants and very young children will follow an interesting object. This tests cranial nerve III (oculomotor). Instruct the older child to look downward and inward (testing cranial nerve IV [trochlear]). Assess

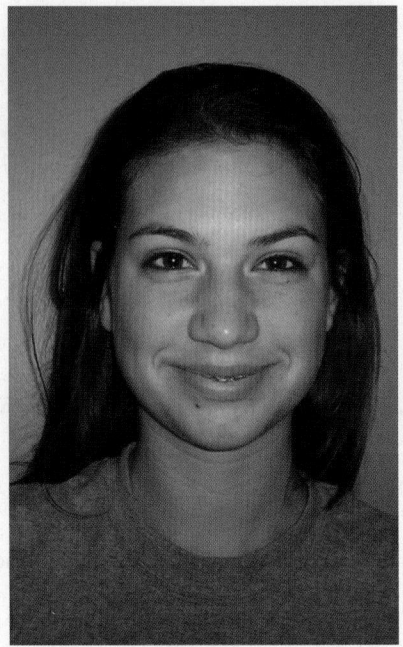

FIGURE 31.16 Note reflected light falling symmetrically on each pupil with the Hirschberg test.

eye muscle strength using two tests. Using the Hirschberg test, bring the penlight to the middle of your face and direct the child to look at it. The small dot of reflected light seen in the iris should be symmetrically placed in each eye (Fig. 31.16). The cover test also assesses eye muscle strength. Cover one of the child's eyes and instruct the child to focus on an interesting object. The eye should not waver. While the child is still focusing with the first eye, remove the cover from the second. Observe the uncovered eye for movement. Report any movement or drift.

To test peripheral vision, have the child focus on a specific point or object directly in front. Bring a finger or a small object from beyond the range of vision into the area of the peripheral vision. When the child sees the object from the side, while still focusing on the object or point in front, the child should say "stop." This also tests cranial nerve II (optic).

Internal Structures

Assessment of the internal structures of the eye is best accomplished by an advanced practitioner with experience in this type of assessment. An adequate assessment requires that the child cooperate. Restraint for eye examination does not usually prove fruitful, as movement and tearing of the eyes interfere with the accuracy of the examination. Use the ophthalmoscope to inspect the internal eye structures. Observe the glow of the pupil, which appears red (creamy-coloured in children with very dark eye colour). Inspect the optic disk, macula, fovea, and blood vessels. Refer any child with blurring or bulging of the optic disk or hemorrhage of vessels to a pediatric ophthalmologist for further evaluation.

▶ **Take** NOTE!

Immediately report absence of the red reflex in one or both eyes, as this may indicate the presence of cataracts (Bickley & Szilagyi, 2009).

Ears

Assessment of the ears includes evaluation of the external and internal structures as well as screening for hearing. Any nurse caring for a child should be adept at examining the external structures. Assessment of the internal structures will also be covered below but is usually performed only by the advanced practitioner. Refer to Chapter 30 for information on hearing screening. Testing of hearing also tests the function of cranial nerve VIII (acoustic).

External Structures

Assess the placement of the external ears on the head. They should be symmetrical and placed no lower than the eyes. The pinna should deviate no more than 10 degrees from an imaginary line that is perpendicular to a line drawn between the outer canthus of the eye and the top of the ear. Low-set ears may be associated with genetic abnormalities or syndromes (Fig. 31.17). Note

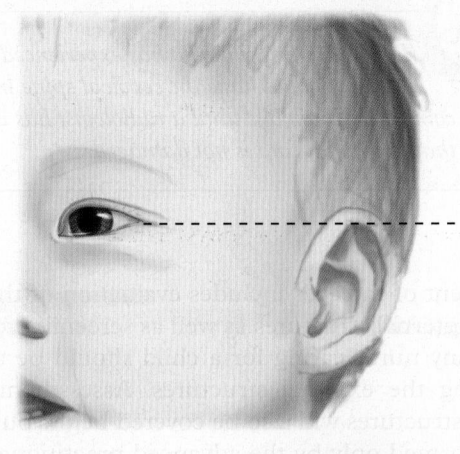

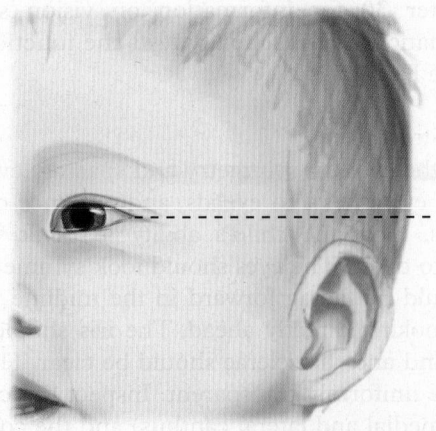

FIGURE 31.17 Low-set ears may be associated with chromosomal or other genetic anomalies.

protrusion or flattening of the ears, which may be normal for that child or may indicate inflammation (protrusion) or persistent side-lying (flattening). Note the presence of pits or skin tags in the preauricular area. Observe the exterior ear canal. A waxy **cerumen** that is soft and an orangish-brown colour is normally found lubricating and protecting the external ear canal and should be left in place or washed gently away when bathing. Note drainage from the ear canal, which is always considered abnormal. Pull on the auricle and palpate the mastoid process, neither of which should result in pain in the healthy child.

> ▶ *Take* NOTE!
>
> *Impacted and dry cerumen can be softened with a few drops of mineral or cooking oil and then gently irrigated from the canal with an ear syringe and warm water (Nettina, 2010).*

Internal Structures

Use a **tympanometer** to assess the mobility of the eardrum (tympanic membrane). Gently pull down on the earlobe of infants and toddlers and up on the outer edge of the pinna in older children to straighten the ear canal, and press the tip of the tympanometer over the external canal. A reading of air pressure is recorded by the instrument, and this is useful to assess middle ear disease. Many tympanometers record a wave pattern that may be printed to include in the child's chart.

A nurse practitioner or physician generally performs inspection of the ear canal and tympanic membrane with an otoscope (Fig. 31.18). The otoscopic examination is usually performed near the end of the physical assessment for infants and young children, as they are often quite resistant to this intrusive procedure. The

infant or toddler may require restraint in the parent's lap for the otoscopic evaluation. The preschooler may cooperate if the nurse uses a game such as looking for pretend puppies or potatoes in the child's ear. As with the tympanometer, gently pull down on the earlobe of the infant or toddler and up on the outer edge of the pinna in older children to straighten the ear canal. Use an otoscopic speculum appropriate to the size of the child's ear canal. Insert the speculum into the ear canal to visualize the canal and the tympanic membrane. The canal should be pink, should have tiny hairs, and should be free from scratches, drainage, foreign bodies, and edema. The tympanic membrane should appear pearly pink or grey and should be translucent, allowing visualization of the bony landmarks. It may be red if the child has been crying recently. Compress the pneumatic insufflator bulb to provide a puff of air; this causes motion of the tympanic membrane when the middle ear is healthy. Note abnormalities such as a fluid level, bubble or pus behind the tympanic membrane, tympanic membrane immobility, holes or perforations in the tympanic membrane, and the presence of tympanostomy tubes, scarring, or vesicles.

> ▶ *Take* NOTE!
>
> *Never attempt to flush a foreign object out with water until it has been identified, because small pieces of sponge, clay, or vegetative material like peas or beans swell with water, further obstructing the ear canal (Nettina, 2010).*

Nose and Sinuses

The nose, as with all facial features in a child, should be symmetrical, but it can be displaced temporarily by birth trauma in newborns. Children of Asian or African descent often display a flattened nasal bridge as a normal variation. Ensure that the nares provide unobstructed airflow by alternately occluding one nostril at a time and observing for air movement through the other nostril. If the child is breathing comfortably, there should be little nostril movement visible. Adolescents may have pierced their nose or nasal septum; ensure that the site is free from infection or loose jewelry that could migrate into the sinuses. Ideally the nose should not be draining, though clear mucus may be present if the child has been crying. Assess the amount, colour, thickness, and presence of any odour if drainage is present. Inspect the interior of the nose by tilting the child's head backward and pushing the tip of the nose upward. Direct the beam of a penlight in the nostril. The nasal mucosa should be uniformly firm, pink, and free from edema, excoriation, or masses. Test the older child's sense of smell by having the child close the eyes and identify a familiar scent such as

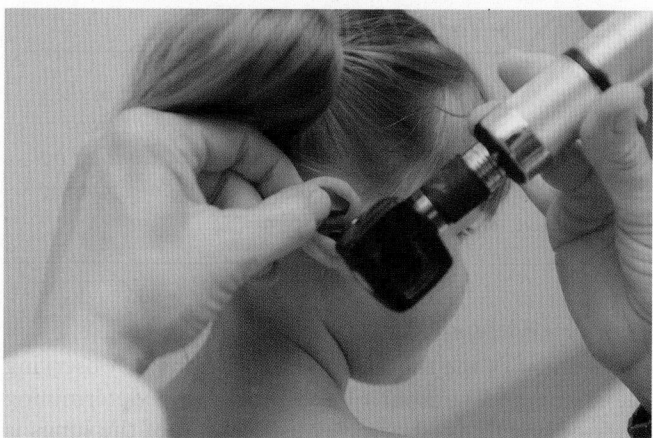

FIGURE 31.18 Otoscopic examination allows visualization of the internal structures of the ear.

peppermint or coffee (cranial nerve I [olfactory]). Palpate the sinuses for tenderness.

> ▶ *Take* NOTE!
>
> *Infants up to 3 to 6 months of age have traditionally been thought to be **obligate nose breathers** because of their long soft palate and relatively large tongue, which allows for swallowing without aspiration during breast or artificial nipple feeding. This lessens with age and as the infant becomes better able to breathe through the mouth when necessary (Bickley & Szilagyi, 2009).*

Mouth and Throat

Wear a powder-free glove to examine the mouth, teeth, and throat. Inspection of the exterior of the mouth may be done at any point in the examination. Infants and young children may find assessment of the mouth and particularly the pharynx and uvula to be quite intrusive, so delay that part of the assessment until the end of the examination, after otoscopic evaluation. Assess the character and quality of the child's voice and the infant's cry. It should be neither too hoarse nor too shrill.

Inspection of the Mouth

Observe the lips for colour, symmetry, and absence of inflammation or edema. Salivation in infants begins at about 3 months of age; drooling occurs because the infant does not learn to swallow saliva until several months later. Next, inspect the interior of the mouth. The mouth is the first part of the digestive system, and a pink, moist, healthy mucosal lining is indicative of a healthy gastrointestinal tract. In infants, the tongue should lie within the mouth at rest and should be capable of extending over the lower gum line to help the baby feed. The tongue extrusion reflex is normal in infants up until the age of 6 months and allows the infant to suckle easily from birth. Observe movement of the tongue when the infant or young child babbles or cries. Ask the older child to touch the tongue to the roof of the mouth and then stick out the tongue and move it from side to side (testing cranial nerve XII [hypoglossal]). Full movement should be present and the tongue should be free from lesions or exudate. Visualize the hard and soft palate (which should be intact) or palpate with the gloved finger.

Most infants have no teeth before the fifth to sixth month. When the teeth begin to erupt, they usually erupt symmetrically at the rate of about one a month, until toddlers have 20 teeth by 30 months of age. The infant may drool for several months before teething. During teething the gums will be swollen at the location of the impending tooth. In older children, the secondary teeth replace the primary teeth much more slowly and with little discomfort

from the 5th to the 20th year. Figure 31.19 shows the usual permanent tooth eruption pattern.

Look for dental caries or alignment problems and inspect the gums for signs of infection. Test cranial nerve IX (glossopharyngeal) by having the child identify taste with the posterior portion of the tongue.

> ▶ *Take* NOTE!
>
> *Natal (present at birth) or neonatal (erupting by 30 days of age) teeth should be evaluated by a pediatric dentist for potential extraction, as they may pose an aspiration risk (Bickley & Szilagyi, 2009).*

Inspection of the Throat

Inspect the tonsils, uvula, and oropharynx. Assess the infant's throat during a yawn or cry, as any forcible attempt to depress the tongue with a tongue depressor produces a strong reflex elevation of the base of the tongue that completely blocks the view of the pharynx. The young child will require restraint so that the nurse can depress the tongue and visualize the back of the mouth without injuring the child (Fig. 31.20). Asking the older child to open wide, stick out the tongue, and say "aaaah" simultaneously will allow for a quick look at the tonsils and pharynx without the need to use a tongue depressor, but the nurse must be very quick because the tongue rises rapidly after those manoeuvres are performed.

Tonsils usually cannot be seen in the infant. As the child becomes a toddler, the tonsils become dramatically larger and then begin to decrease in size again by the ninth year. The tonsils should be pink and often have crypts on their surfaces, which are sometimes filled with debris. Is the uvula at midline? Does it rise if the gag reflex is elicited (cranial nerve X [vagus])? Inspect the oropharynx, which should be pink and free from exudate.

> ▶ *Take* NOTE!
>
> *If a gag reflex is inadvertently elicited in the very ill child, the airway may become compromised. Therefore, the pharynx should be examined by asking the child to say "aaah" rather than by depressing the tongue with a tongue depressor.*

Thorax and Lungs

Assessment of the thorax and lungs begins by observing the shape and contour of the thorax and determining work of breathing. Accurate auscultation of the lungs is essential, since children often have respiratory infections and disorders and may exhibit alterations in respiratory

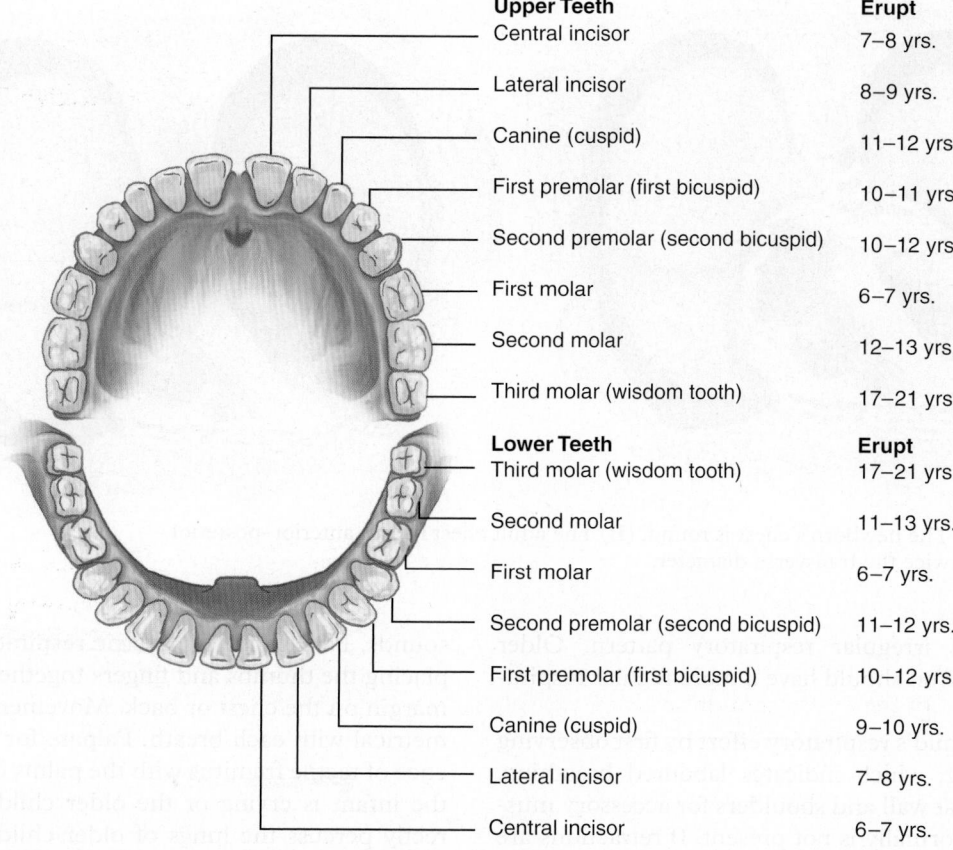

Upper Teeth	Erupt
Central incisor	7–8 yrs.
Lateral incisor	8–9 yrs.
Canine (cuspid)	11–12 yrs.
First premolar (first bicuspid)	10–11 yrs.
Second premolar (second bicuspid)	10–12 yrs.
First molar	6–7 yrs.
Second molar	12–13 yrs.
Third molar (wisdom tooth)	17–21 yrs.

Lower Teeth	Erupt
Third molar (wisdom tooth)	17–21 yrs.
Second molar	11–13 yrs.
First molar	6–7 yrs.
Second premolar (second bicuspid)	11–12 yrs.
First premolar (first bicuspid)	10–12 yrs.
Canine (cuspid)	9–10 yrs.
Lateral incisor	7–8 yrs.
Central incisor	6–7 yrs.

FIGURE 31.19 Sequence of permanent tooth eruption.

effort and breath sounds. Note the child's colour, which should be pink; cyanosis indicates hypoxia. Listen for audible stridor (inspiratory high-pitched sound), expiratory grunting or snoring, audible wheezing (heard with the naked ear), or cough. Document type and extent of cough. Observe the nail beds for clubbing, which occurs with diseases inducing chronic hypoxic states.

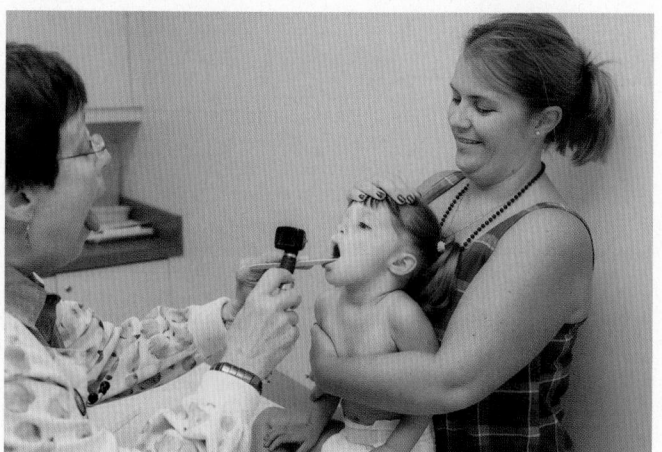

FIGURE 31.20 The young child may need to be restrained so that the throat examination can be done safely.

Thorax

Examine the chest with the head in a midline position to determine size and shape as well as symmetry, movement, and bony landmarks. The newborn's chest should be smooth and round, with the transverse diameter nearly equal to the anterior–posterior diameter. The shape of the chest progresses to that of the adult by age 5 to 6 years. At that time the anterior–posterior diameter is about half the transverse diameter (Fig. 31.21). At the point where the xiphoid process and the right and left costal margins meet, the costal angle should measure 90 degrees or less. Inspect for structural deformity such as pectus excavatum (depressed sternum) or pectus carinatum (protuberant sternum) (Fig. 31.22). Note symmetric movement of the chest wall with respiration. Infants and younger children are primarily diaphragmatic breathers, so the abdomen and chest will rise and fall together. Older children, particularly adolescent females, demonstrate thoracic breathing, yet the abdomen and chest should continue to rise and fall together. Asymmetry of chest wall movement is an abnormal finding.

Observe the depth and regularity of respirations, noting the length of the inspiratory and expiratory phases in relation to each other. The newborn and young infant

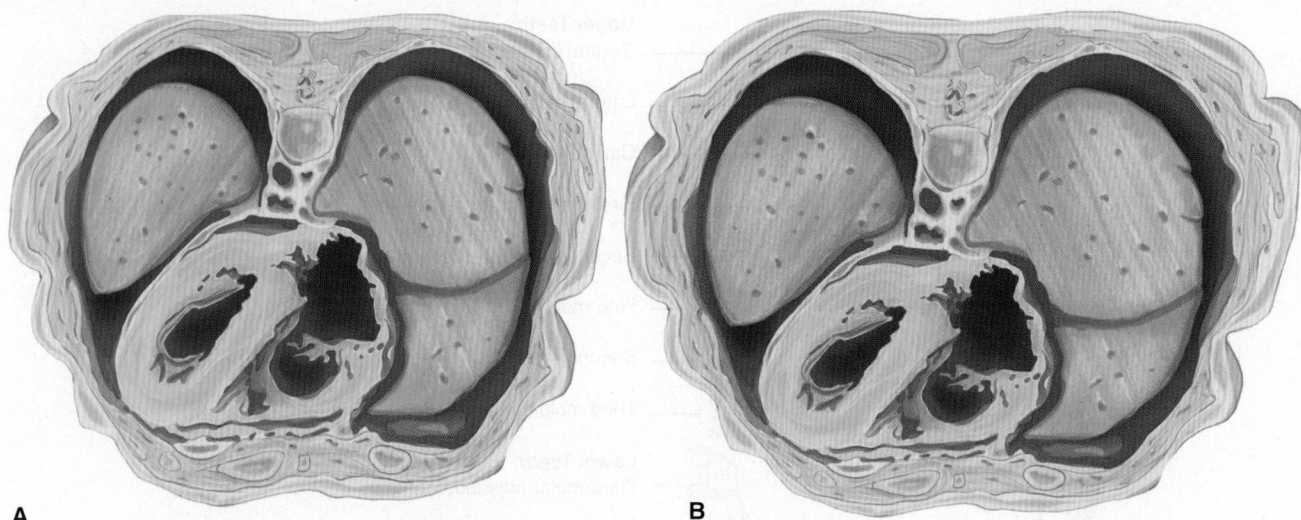

A   **B**

FIGURE 31.21 (**A**) The newborn's chest is round. (**B**) The adult chest has an anterior–posterior diameter about twice the transverse diameter.

demonstrate an irregular respiratory pattern. Older infants and children should have a more regular respiratory pattern.

Assess the child's respiratory effort by first observing for nasal flaring, which indicates laboured breathing. Observe the chest wall and shoulders for accessory muscle use, which normally is not present. If retractions are present, note their location and severity. Typical locations for retraction include the intercostal, subcostal, substernal, suprasternal, and clavicular regions (Fig. 31.23). Pay attention to the position the child naturally assumes to breathe comfortably: children in respiratory distress often sit forward and are uncomfortable lying down or talking (Jarvis, 2008).

Lungs

Experienced examiners may palpate and percuss the lungs before using **auscultation** to evaluate the breath sounds. Palpate for symmetric respiratory excursion by placing the thumbs and fingers together along the costal margin on the chest or back. Movement should be symmetrical with each breath. Palpate for the normal presence of tactile fremitus with the palms or fingertips while the infant is crying or the older child says "99." Indirectly percuss the lungs of older children, noting resonance over lung fields. Hyperresonance may be present in conditions resulting in hyperaeration of the lungs, such as asthma.

Auscultation

Use the bell of the stethoscope or switch to a small diaphragm to auscultate lung sounds in the infant or child. The adult-sized diaphragm may be used for the adolescent. Auscultate the lung fields with the infant or child in a sitting position, even if that requires propping the infant in a parent's lap. Infants and young children have

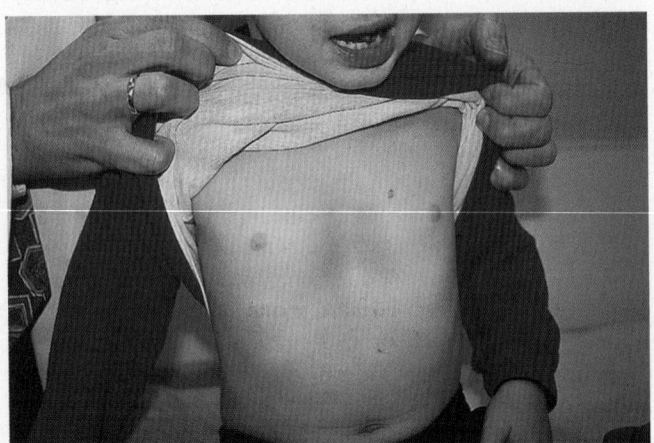

FIGURE 31.22 Pectus excavatum: note depression in xiphoid area.

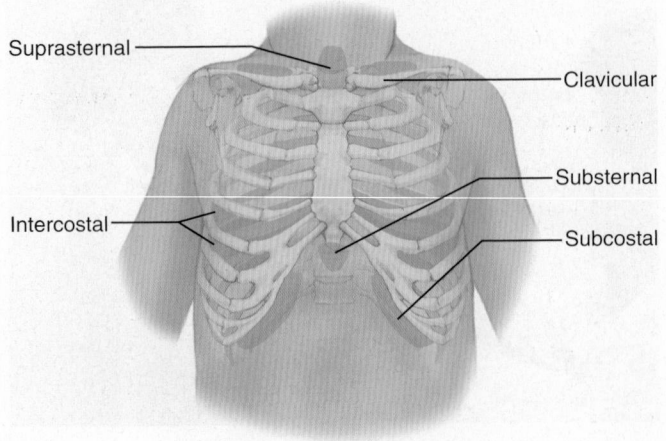

Suprasternal — — Clavicular

Substernal

Intercostal — — Subcostal

FIGURE 31.23 Location of retractions.

loud breath sounds because of their thin chest walls. Breath sounds should be clear with adequate aeration throughout all lung fields. Listen to a full inspiration and expiration at the apices of the lungs as well as symmetrically across the entire lung field, systematically comparing the right to the left side. Listen on the anterior chest and posterior chest and in the axillary regions.

Playing games may encourage younger children to cooperate with deep breathing during lung assessment. The child can blow a cotton ball up in the air, blow a pinwheel, or "blow out" the light of the penlight (Miller, 2011). Older children are capable of deep breathing when instructed to do so.

The child who has a respiratory disorder or who is experiencing respiratory distress may exhibit diminished breath sounds, most often in the lung bases. Diminished breath sounds are softer and quieter than lung sounds demonstrating adequate aeration. In the healthy infant or child, no adventitious sounds should be heard. If noisy breath sounds are heard in the infant or young child, particularly over all lung fields, compare the sound to the noises heard over the trachea or within the nose. Infants and young children with secretions in the nasopharyngeal area may have those sounds transmitted over the lung fields. These sounds usually clear with coughing or airway suctioning; they are not true adventitious sounds. Note adventitious breath sounds such as wheezes or crackles, documenting their location and whether they are present on inspiration, expiration, or both. It is most important to describe the abnormal breath sounds being heard rather than attempting to classify the sounds. Adventitious lung sounds are associated with a variety of disorders, and extensive experience is required to appropriately classify lung sounds. Adventitious breath sounds should be reported for further evaluation.

Breasts

Assess the breasts of children of all ages and both genders. Note the size of the breasts in relation to the age of the child. Palpate the axillary lymph nodes during the breast assessment.

Inspection

Observe the breasts for position, shape, size, symmetry, and colour. Newborns of both genders may have swollen nipples from the influence of maternal estrogen, but by several weeks of age the nipples should be flat and should continue to be so in all prepubertal children. In children the nipples are located lateral to the midclavicular line, usually between the fourth and fifth ribs. The areola becomes darker in colour as the child approaches puberty. Overweight children may appear to have enlarged breasts due to adipose tissue. Note the location of additional (supernumerary) nipples if present (usually located along the mammary ridge); they may appear as darkly pigmented elevated or nipple-like

spots. These are usually of no concern as they do not change over time, but they may be associated with renal disorders.

Inspect the breasts for the current stage of development: widening of the areola, elevation of the nipple, and increase in the breast size. Female breast development may begin as early as age 8 but starts by age 13 in most girls. Breast development then continues in a characteristic pattern but usually is asymmetric, with one breast larger than the other throughout the lifespan. The sexual maturity rating scale developed by Tanner in 1962 is used to describe breast development (**Tanner stages**; Fig. 31.24). Adolescent boys may develop gynecomastia (enlargement of the breast tissue) due to hormonal pubertal changes. When the hormone levels stabilize, male adolescents then have flat nipples. Occasionally gynecomastia is caused by marijuana use, anabolic steroids, or hormonal dysfunction (Jarvis, 2008).

Palpation

Palpate the breasts in a systematic fashion. A tender nodule palpated just under the nipple confirms pubertal changes. This change may be difficult to assess in girls with excessive adipose tissue. Normal breast tissue should feel smooth, firm, and elastic. Note masses or nodules if present. Palpate for axillary lymph nodes with the child's arms relaxed at the side but slightly abducted. Note size and texture of nodes if present.

Heart and Peripheral Perfusion

The examination of the heart in children is identical to that of adults except for the focus of the examiner's attention. Congenital heart defects are the most common cause of heart problems in children, and children with these defects present differently than adults with heart disease.

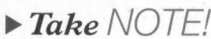

▶ *Take NOTE!*

The younger the child, the more responsive the heart rate is to activity changes. It increases with fever, fear, crying, or anxiety and decreases with sleep, sedation, or vagal stimulation (Jarvis, 2008).

Inspection

Observe the child's posture. Note the presence of pallor, cyanosis, mottling, or edema, which may indicate a cardiovascular problem. Inspect the anterior chest from the side or at an angle, noting symmetry in shape as well as movement. Observe for the apical impulse, which is visible in about half of children. It occurs at the PMI, which is located at the fourth intercostal space at the left midclavicular line in children less than 7 years of age and

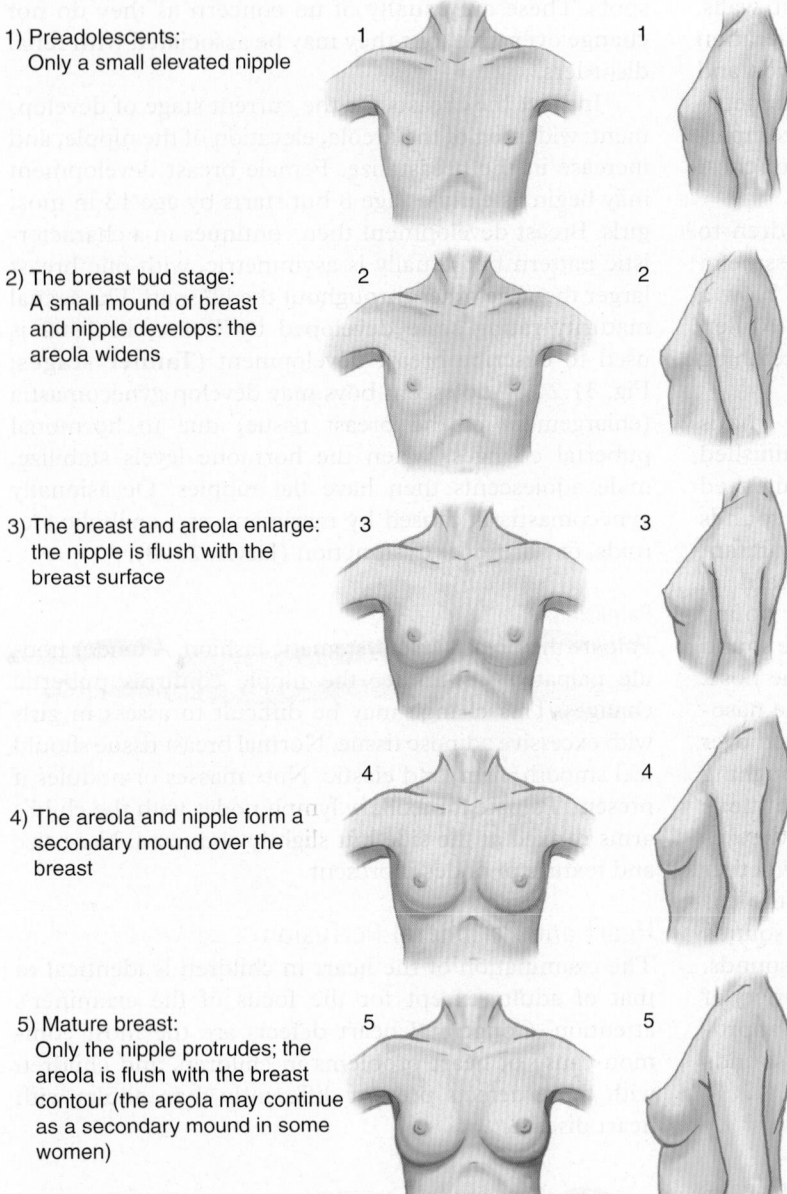

1) Preadolescents:
   Only a small elevated nipple

2) The breast bud stage:
   A small mound of breast
   and nipple develops: the
   areola widens

3) The breast and areola enlarge:
   the nipple is flush with the
   breast surface

4) The areola and nipple form a
   secondary mound over the
   breast

5) Mature breast:
   Only the nipple protrudes; the
   areola is flush with the breast
   contour (the areola may continue
   as a secondary mound in some
   women)

FIGURE 31.24 Tanner sexual maturity rating for breast development.

then lateral to the left midclavicular line at the fifth intercostal space in children ages 7 years and older (Fig. 31.25). Note clubbing of the fingertips or distention of neck veins, both of which may be associated with congenital heart disease.

Palpation

Using the fingertips, palpate the chest for lifts and heaves or thrills, which are not normal. Palpate the apical pulse in the area of the PMI (see Fig. 31.25). Check the pulses and compare the upper body to lower body pulses, as well as left versus right, noting strength and quality (Fig. 31.26). The pedal, brachial, and femoral pulses are usually easily palpated. The radial pulse is very difficult to

palpate in children less than 2 years of age. Note warmth of the distal extremities. To assess capillary refill time, place slight pressure on the nail beds and quickly release it. Observe the length of time required for refill and return to original colour. Compare capillary refill time of the fingers to the toes. A capillary refill time of less than 2 seconds indicates adequacy of perfusion.

Auscultation

Perform auscultation of the heart with the child in two different positions, upright and reclined (Fig. 31.27). Auscultate the heart rate in the area of the PMI (see Fig. 31.25). As you begin auscultation, listen first for respirations and note their timing so as not to confuse the heart

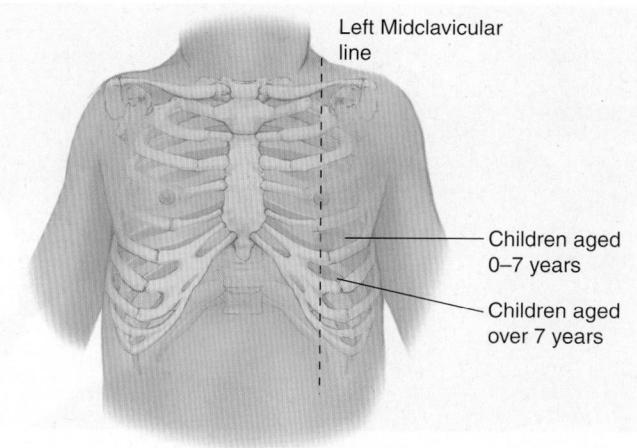

FIGURE 31.25 The point of maximal intensity (PMI) or apical impulse according to age.

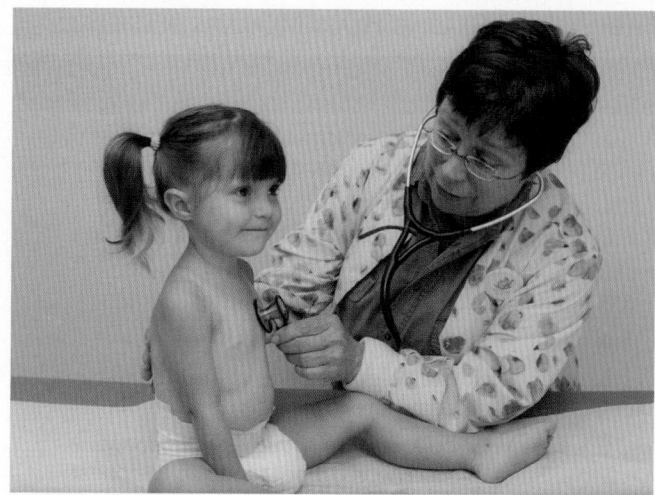

FIGURE 31.27 Auscultating the child's heart.

sounds with the lung sounds. A crying infant may help by briefly holding his or her breath between cries. Once you are confident that you are listening to the heart, be sure to listen for 1 to 3 minutes because of the irregularity of rhythms in some children. Count the heart rate, which should be consistent with the palpated pulse (either radial or brachial).

Develop a systematic approach to auscultation of the heart. Listen over all four valvular areas anteriorly (Fig. 31.28). In the infant or younger child, also auscultate the heart in the axillary region and posteriorly (certain murmurs radiate to these areas). Note S1, S2, extra heart sounds, or murmurs. S1 is usually loudest at the mitral and tricuspid areas and increases in intensity with fever, exercise, and anemia. S2 is usually most intense at the aortic and pulmonic areas. A split S2 heard at the apex occurs in many infants and young children. S3 may be heard in many healthy children and is considered normal, though the child with a chronic cardiac condition may develop an S3 when congestive heart failure is present. S4 is usually considered abnormal, most often occurring with cardiac disease.

Sinus arrhythmia is a common and normal finding in children and adolescents. It results in an irregular heart rhythm: the heart rate increases with inhalation and decreases with exhalation. If the child holds his or her breath, the rhythm becomes regular.

Auscultate for murmurs. Note the location (where it is heard best or loudest) and timing of the murmur. A systolic murmur occurs in association with S1 (closure of the atrioventricular valves), a diastolic murmur in association with S2 (closure of the semilunar valves). Also note the duration of murmur. Does it occur early or late in diastole or systole? Does it occur all the way across

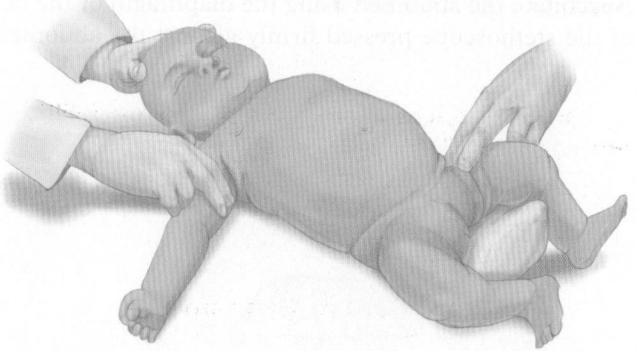

FIGURE 31.26 It is important to assess brachial and femoral pulses simultaneously to determine equality or differences in strength and intensity.

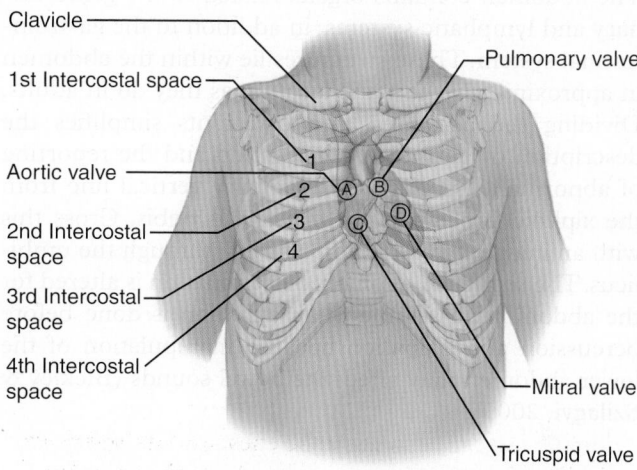

FIGURE 31.28 Areas where the sounds of heart valves radiate. A: Aortic valve—second intercostal space, just right of sternum. B: Pulmonary valve—second intercostal space, just left of sternum. C: Tricuspid valve—fourth intercostal space, just right of sternum. D: Mitral valve—fourth intercostal space at left midclavicular line.

TABLE 31.5 GRADING HEART MURMURS IN CHILDREN

Grade	Sound
1	Barely audible; sometimes heard, sometimes not. Usually heard only with intense concentration.
2	Quiet, soft; heard each time the chest is auscultated
3	Audible, intermediate intensity
4	Audible, with a palpable thrill
5	Loud, audible with edge of the stethoscope lifted off the chest
6	Very loud, audible with the stethoscope placed near but not touching the chest

Adapted from: Menashe, V. (2007). Heart murmurs. *Pediatrics in Review, 28*, e19–e22.

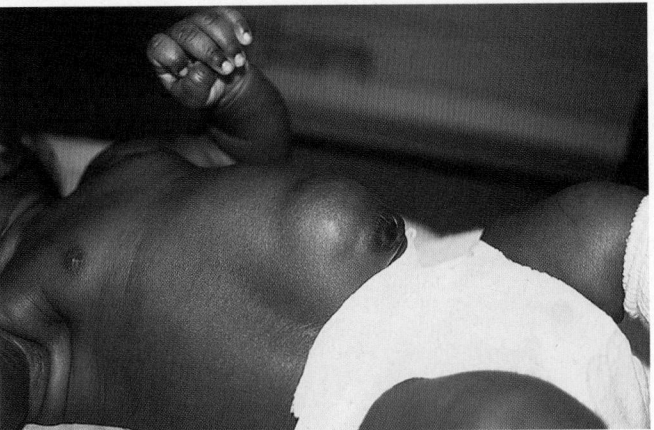

FIGURE 31.29 The umbilical hernia may increase in size when the infant cries.

systole (holosystolic)? Note the intensity of the murmur. Table 31.5 discusses grading of murmur intensity.

Innocent murmurs occur frequently in children because of the child's more dynamic circulation, thin chest wall, and angulated vessels (Menashe, 2007). An innocent murmur is most often heard at the second or fourth intercostal space, and its timing is systolic. The innocent murmur is usually medium-pitched and musical. Often an innocent murmur disappears when the child changes position. A venous hum that is heard in the supraclavicular area and possibly radiating down the chest is considered an innocent murmur. Refer any child with a murmur to an experienced practitioner for further evaluation.

Abdomen

The abdomen contains organs related to the genitourinary and lymphatic systems, in addition to the gastrointestinal system. These structures lie within the abdomen in approximately the same location as they do in adults. Dividing the abdomen into quadrants simplifies the description of normal organ location and the reporting of abnormalities. Draw an imaginary vertical line from the xiphoid process to the symphysis pubis. Cross this with an imaginary perpendicular line through the umbilicus. The sequence of physical examination is altered for the abdominal assessment: auscultation is done before percussion and palpation because manipulation of the lower abdomen may affect the bowel sounds (Bickley & Szilagyi, 2009).

Inspection

Inspect the abdomen for size, shape, and symmetry. The abdomen in the infant and toddler is rounded and protuberant until the abdominal musculature becomes well developed. Though rounded, the abdomen should not be distended (at any age). By adolescence, the stature is more erect and the abdomen begins to appear flat when standing and concave when supine. The thin skin of a young child may allow the visualization of superficial venous circulation across the abdomen. Inspect the abdomen for movement. At eye level with the abdomen, note abdomen and thorax movement occurring simultaneously. Visible peristaltic waves are abnormal and should be reported immediately.

Inspect the newborn's umbilicus for colour, bleeding, odour, and drainage. The umbilical stump should slowly dry, become black and hard, and fall away from the cutaneous navel by the end of the second week of life. Note drainage or granulation at the umbilical site indicating delayed drying of the umbilical stump. Inspect the umbilicus in older infants and young children for the presence of umbilical hernia. Because the umbilicus divides the rectus abdominis muscle, it is not uncommon to see an umbilical hernia protrude through and become larger when the infant or toddler strains or cries (Fig. 31.29). This is a benign finding and will usually disappear as the abdomen becomes stronger. Adolescents may have jewelry piercing the umbilicus (Fig. 31.30).

Auscultation

Auscultate the abdomen using the diaphragm or the bell of the stethoscope pressed firmly against the abdomen.

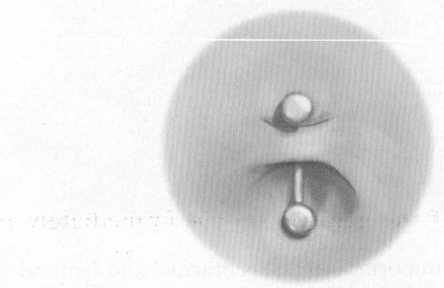

FIGURE 31.30 Navel piercing sites should be free from infection.

Count the bowel sounds in each of the four quadrants for a full minute. Bowel sounds should be present by a few hours after birth and should remain active throughout life. Note whether bowel sounds are normally active, hyperactive, hypoactive, or absent. Normal bowel sounds can be described as growls, gurgles, and clicking sounds. Hypoactive bowel sounds may occur postoperatively. Hyperactive bowels sounds are common with diarrhea. Classify bowel sounds as absent after listening for 5 full minutes in each area. Absent bowel sounds may indicate ileus or peritonitis.

Percussion

Indirectly percuss all areas of the abdomen. Normal findings include dullness along the costal margins and tympany over the remainder of the abdomen. A full bladder may yield dullness to percussion.

Palpation

Palpate the abdomen with the child in a supine position. If the child's legs are small enough, the knees may be brought up with the nondominant hand to flex the hips and relax the abdomen. Palpate all four quadrants of the abdomen in a systematic fashion, first lightly and then deeply. Apply light pressure with the fingertips to perform light palpation, assessing for tenderness and muscle tone (Fig. 31.31). Note skin turgor by gently elevating a piece of skin and allowing it to fall back into place. Perform deep palpation to assess the organs and any masses. Place one hand on top of the other and palpate from the lower quadrants to the upper (see Fig. 31.31). The edge of the liver may be felt at the right costal margin, and the tip of the spleen can be felt at the left costal margin. The descending colon may be felt in the left lower quadrant as a small column and the bladder as a soft balloon below the umbilicus. The kidneys are rarely palpable. The abdomen should be soft and nontender to palpation. Report firmness, tenderness, or masses. Palpate the inguinal area for the presence of hernia or enlarged lymph nodes.

> ▶ *Take* NOTE!
>
> *To decrease ticklishness with abdominal palpation, place a flat, warm, still hand on the abdomen while distracting the child before palpation begins. An alternate technique is to first palpate with the child's hand under the examiner's hand.*

Genitalia and Anus

Examination of the genitals should immediately follow the abdominal assessment in the younger child and should be reserved for the end of the assessment in the adolescent. Though the anus is part of the gas-

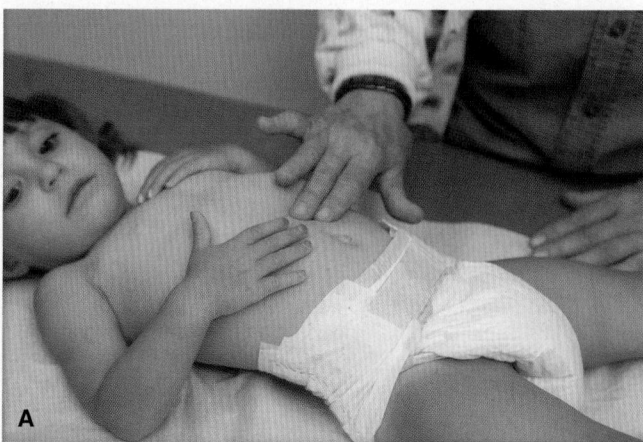

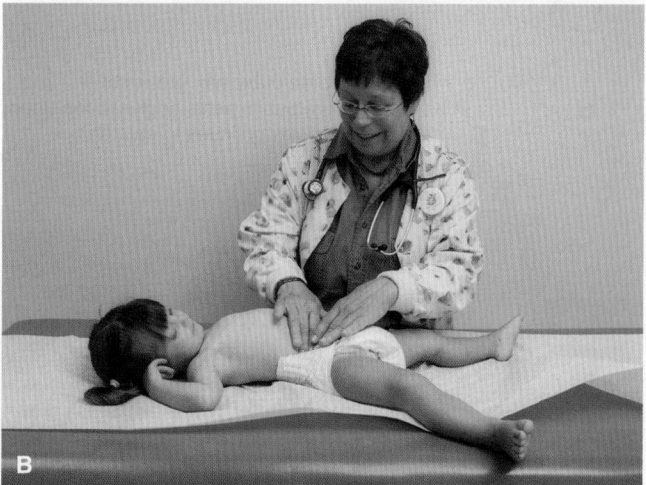

FIGURE 31.31 (**A**) Light and (**B**) deep palpation of the abdomen.

trointestinal tract, it is best assessed during the genital examination. Ensure privacy for the older child and adolescent. Keep the child covered as much as possible. Use a casual, matter-of-fact approach to place the child or teen at ease. During the genital examination, teach the child or adolescent about normal variations and changes with puberty, as well as issues related to health promotion.

Male

Inspect the penis and scrotum for size, colour, skin integrity, and obvious masses. The obese boy's penis may appear small because of additional skinfolds. Penis size should correlate with pubertal stage (Fig. 31.32). The penis may have a foreskin that covers the glans, protecting and lubricating it. If present, do not forcibly retract the foreskin. In circumcised males the urinary meatus is exposed and should be at the tip of the glans. Assess the meatus for absence of discharge. If possible, observe the stream of urine for strength of flow and patency of the urethral orifice. Skin lesions may indicate sexually

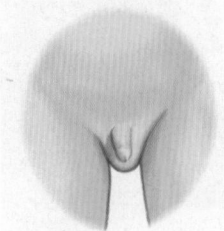

From top to bottom:

1) No pubic hair and scrotum size and proportion the same as during childhood

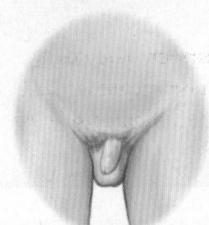

2) Few straight hairs at base of penis, little or no penis enlargement, testes/scrotum begin to enlarge

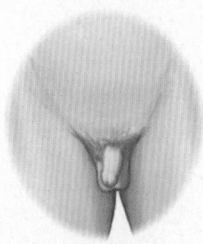

3) Sparse pubic hair growth over entire pubis, penis begins to lengthen, scrotum continues to enlarge

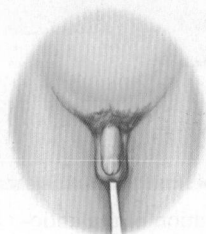

4) Thick pubic hair growth but not on thighs, penis grows in length and diameter, testes almost full grown

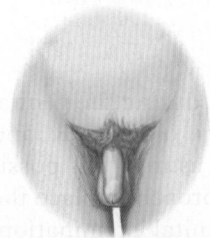

5) Pubic hair growth spread over medial thighs, penis and scrotum are adult size and shape

FIGURE 31.32 Tanner male sexual maturity rating for genitalia and pubic hair.

transmitted infection. A foreskin that cannot be retracted in a boy over 3 years of age may indicate phimosis. Report abnormal findings.

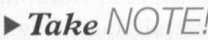

▶ *Take* NOTE!

When you first remove a male infant's diaper, this is the ideal time to assess the force of the urine stream and the erection reflex, as the cool air may make the infant void and briefly experience an erection.

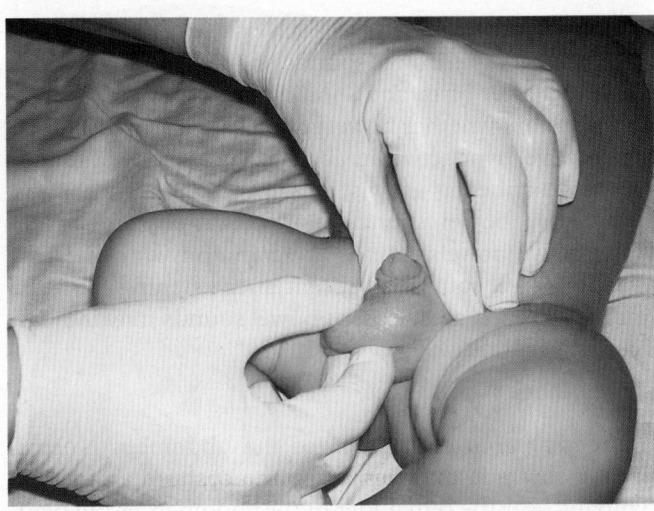

FIGURE 31.33 Placing a digit over the inguinal canal during testicular palpation prevents retraction of the testis into the canal.

Assess the presence and distribution of pubic hair. Inspect the scrotum for size, slight asymmetry, colour, and absence of edema. The scrotum may initially be swollen from birth trauma or maternal hormones, but this swelling should decrease in the first few days of life. The scrotum is ordinarily more deeply pigmented than the rest of the boy's skin. Figure 31.32 illustrates scrotal changes that occur with puberty. Assess the testicles by placing one finger over the inguinal canal and palpating the scrotum with the other. This prevents the retractile testes in a young child from slipping back up the inguinal canal. The testicles should be smooth, of similar size, and freely moveable. The infant's testicles may be palpated in the scrotum or in the inguinal canal, where they can be easily moved into the scrotum with gentle pressure from the examiner's nondominant hand (Fig. 31.33). Beyond infancy, allow the boy to sit cross-legged to reduce the cremasteric reflex that retracts the testicles during palpation. An adolescent boy may need to stand for the nurse to fully palpate the scrotum. Document the presence of both testicles in the scrotal sac, if they are retractile, or if they are absent. Report undescended testicle or other abnormal findings.

Female

In most cases, the female genitalia examination is limited to assessment of the external genitalia. Internal examination is not routinely performed before maturity unless the adolescent anticipates becoming or is sexually active or requests birth control or if pathology is suspected. If an internal examination is needed, refer the child or adolescent to the appropriate advanced practitioner or physician.

Position the infant in the parent's lap or on the examination table or crib. The toddler or preschooler should be examined in the parent's lap, in a frog-legged position. The school-age or adolescent girl should lie on the examination table or bed. Provide for privacy by keeping the genital area covered until it is time for the examination.

Perform the assessment of the external genitalia in a systematic fashion. First, determine the presence and distribution of pubic hair. Infants and young girls (particular those of dark-skinned races) may have a small amount of downy pubic hair. Otherwise, the appearance of pubic hair indicates the onset of pubertal changes, sometimes prior to breast changes. Pubic hair generally begins to appear by age 11 years, with age 13 being the latest. Figure 31.34 illustrates the development of pubic hair through puberty in girls.

Inspect the labia majora and minora for size, colour, and skin integrity. The newborn's labia minora are swollen from the effects of maternal estrogen but will decrease

in size and be hidden by the labia majora within the first weeks of life. Redness or swelling of the labia may occur with infection, sexual abuse, or masturbation. Lesions on the external genitalia may indicate sexually transmitted infection. Gently spread the labia to inspect the clitoris, urethral meatus, and vaginal opening. Some girls may prefer to spread the labia themselves. The urinary meatus and vaginal orifice should be visible and not occluded by the hymen. It is not uncommon to see a hymenal tag. Note clitoral size. Inspect the urinary meatus and vaginal opening for edema or redness, which should not be present. Observe for any vaginal discharge. A small amount of blood-tinged or mucoid discharge may be noted in the first few weeks of life as a result of maternal hormone exposure. A small amount of clear mucus-like discharge is normal in all females. If present, document labial adhesion or other abnormal findings.

Anus

Inspect the anal area for fissures, rash, hemorrhoids, prolapse, or skin tags. Examine the infant's anal area while examining the genitalia. The younger child may lie back in the parent's lap and flex the knees to the chest. The older child or adolescent may be prone or in a side-lying position. If the adolescent boy is already standing for the scrotal assessment, have him bend forward so that you can assess the anal area. The anus should appear moist and hairless. Gently stroke the anal area to elicit the anal reflex (quick contraction). If indicated, inspect anal sphincter tone by inserting a gloved finger lubricated with water-soluble jelly just inside the anal sphincter.

Musculoskeletal

Assessment of the musculoskeletal system includes examination of the clavicles and shoulders, spine, extremities, joints, and hips. Determining the child's ability to move all extremities through the full range of motion is also important.

Clavicles and Shoulders

Palpate the clavicles. In the newborn, tenderness or crepitus reveals a fracture sustained at birth. In the older infant or child, a bump indicates callus formation with clavicle fracture. Test shoulder strength and the function of cranial nerve XI (accessory) in the older child by requesting that the child shrug the shoulders while you apply downward pressure.

Spine

Observe the child's resting posture and alignment of the trunk. The newborn's position will look like the position the baby preferred in utero and is one of the general flexions. The older infant moves more and can sit unassisted in the second half of the first year. Toddlers stand with a wide-based gait, a slightly swayed back, and the abdomen slightly protruding. The posture straightens in the

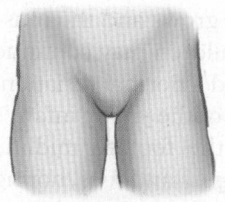
Stage 1 Preadolescents. No pubic hair. Mons and labia covered with fine vellus hair as on abdomen.

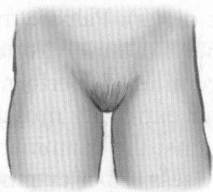
Stage 2 Growth sparse and mostly on labia. Long, downy hair, slightly pigmented, straight or only slightly curly.

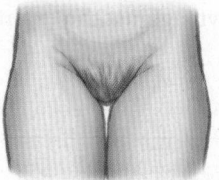
Stage 3 Growth sparse and spreading over mons pubis. Hair darker, coarser, curlier.

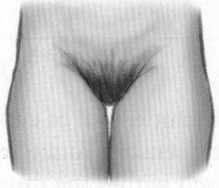
Stage 4 Hair is adult in type but over smaller area; none on medial thigh.

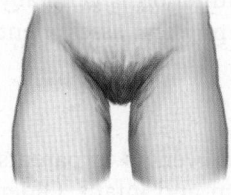
Stage 5 Adult in type and pattern; inverse triangle. Also on medial thigh surface.

FIGURE 31.34 Tanner female sexual maturity rating for pubic hair.

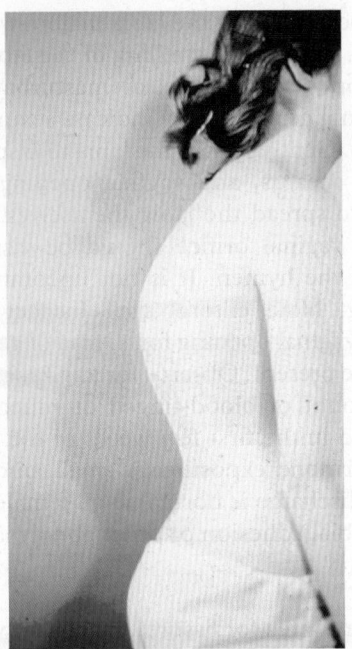

FIGURE 31.35 The teen's posture often demonstrates kyphosis.

preschool and school-age years. Adolescents often demonstrate kyphosis as the skeleton and muscles are both growing rapidly (Fig. 31.35).

Inspect the child's spine. The newborn's spine has a single C-shaped curve and remains rounded for the first 3 months of life. The cervical curve begins to develop around 3 to 4 months of age as the baby gains head control. By 12 to 18 months of age, the lumbar curve develops, which corresponds to the onset of walking. The S-shaped spine in older children and adolescents is similar to that of the adult's. The spine should be flexible, with good muscle tone and no rigidity. Assess the back, hips, and shoulders for symmetry.

Examine the pre-adolescent and adolescent for the development of scoliosis. Refer to Chapter 44 for information about scoliosis screening. Scoliosis screening is generally performed during well-child examinations by the physician or nurse practitioner or by the middle or high school nurse on a particular day of the school year.

Note mobility of the vertebral column by having the child bend forward and side to side. Flex the neck and move it from side to side. No resistance or pain should occur. Inspect the back for discolouration, tufts of hair, or dimples. A normal pilonidal dimple is sometimes seen at the base of the spine, but there should be no tuft of hair or nevi along the spine. Document and report abnormal findings.

Extremities

All children, even newborns, should be able to move all extremities spontaneously. Screen the infant younger than 6 months of age for developmental dysplasia of the hip by performing the Ortolani and Barlow manoeuvres

(refer to Chapter 44 for additional information). These manoeuvres are usually best performed by a proficient examiner. Inspect and palpate the child's upper and lower extremities. Assess for symmetry in size, contour, movement, warmth, and colour of the extremities. The infant's feet and legs appear bowed secondary to in utero positioning but can be straightened through passive range of motion. Observe the child in a standing position. Bowing of the lower legs (internal tibial torsion) lessens as the toddler begins to bear weight and usually resolves in the second or third year of life as the strength of the muscles and bones increases. When it persists past that time, it is termed genu varum (bow legs). Genu valgum (knock knee) is usually present until the child is 7 years old. Observe the child walking, noting any difficulty with leg position or balance. If the child is reluctant to walk, use play as a way to elicit the behaviour. The school-age child should have gait and leg appearance similar to that of the adult.

Note the normal flat foot in the toddler and young child. The arch develops as the child grows and the muscles become less lax, though some children may continue with flexible flat feet; this is considered a normal variation.

Perform passive range of motion of the young infant's extremities. Inability to straighten the foot to midline may indicate clubfoot. Count the fingers and toes, noting abnormalities such as polydactyly (increased number of digits) or syndactyly (webbing of the digits). Palpate the joints for warmth or tenderness. Check the mobility of the joints of the upper and lower extremities by performing range of motion. Determine lower extremity muscle strength by having the child push against the examiner's hands with the soles of the forefoot. Assess upper extremity strength by having the child squeeze the examiner's crossed fingers and/or push up or down against the examiner's outstretched hands.

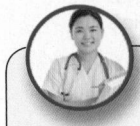

▶ *Take* NOTE!

Slight tremors may be noticed in the infant's extremities in the first month of life.

Neurologic

The neurologic examination should include level of consciousness, balance and coordination, sensory function, and reflexes. Motor function is assessed within the musculoskeletal section. Cranial nerve function is generally tested within other portions of the physical assessment as it applies to that section.

Level of Consciousness

Note the state of alertness and attentiveness to parents and the environment in the newborn and infant. Older infants become interactive with other people, as do toddlers and preschoolers. Younger children demonstrate orientation by positive interaction with family members and by crying or fussing when they feel threatened. By school age, the child should be oriented to name and place and a few years later should be able to state the date as well (even if only the day of the week).

Balance and Coordination

Balance and coordination are controlled by the cerebellum. Observe the child's gait to assess balance and coordination. Observe toddlers and older children rising and walking from a seated and supine position. They should be able to stand and balance without straining or holding on to objects. Continue to test cerebellar function by having the younger child skip or hop and requesting that the older child or adolescent walk heel to toe. Further tests of cerebellar function responsible for balance and coordination are discussed in Box 31.3. Demonstrate each test and make sure the child understands your instructions.

Sensory Testing

Portions of sensory testing related to most of the cranial nerves, vision, hearing, taste, and smell have already been incorporated into other sections as appropriate within the physical assessment. Test cranial nerve V (trigeminal) by lightly touching the child's cheek with a cotton ball. The young infant will root toward the side that is touched. With the child's eyes closed, ask the child to identify other locations where he or she is lightly touched (several different ones) to assess sensation. Ask the child to tell you when he or she is touched. Make a game of this activity to encourage cooperation in younger children. In the older child who knows the definitions of sharp and dull, test for these sensations with the child's eyes closed. Use the rounded end of a tongue blade for dull and the broken edge of a tongue blade for the sharp sensation. The child should be able to discriminate the sensations of sharp and dull.

Reflexes

Assess the infant's primitive and protective reflexes. The primitive reflexes involve a whole-body response and are subcortical in nature. Selected primitive reflexes present at birth include Moro, root, suck, asymmetric tonic neck, plantar and palmar grasp, step, and Babinski. Most of the primitive reflexes diminish over the first few months of life, giving way to protective or postural reflexes. Protective reflexes are motor responses related to maintenance of equilibrium. They are necessary for appropriate motor development and remain throughout life once they are established. The protective reflexes include the righting and parachute reactions.

Place one finger in each of the infant's hands to elicit the palmar grasp reflex (usually disappears by age 3 to 4 months). Touch the thumb to the ball of the infant's foot to elicit the plantar grasp reflex. The infant's toes will curl down (this reflex disappears by 8 to 10 months). Refer to Table 25.2 and Figures 25.1 through 25.6 in Chapter 25 for additional explanation of the other reflexes. Appropriate presence and disappearance of primitive reflexes, as well as development of protective reflexes, is indicative of a healthy neurologic system. Primitive reflexes that persist beyond the usual age of disappearance may indicate an abnormality of the neurologic system and should be further investigated (Bickley & Szilagyi, 2009).

Assess deep tendon reflexes in all infants and children. Appropriate responses indicate that the reflex arc is intact. Use the reflex hammer in all ages or the curved tips of the two first fingers to elicit the responses in infants. The limb must be relaxed and the muscle partly stretched. Use a snapping motion of the wrist to tap with the fingertips or the reflex hammer. Test the biceps, triceps, patellar, and Achilles reflexes as you would in the adult. It may help to place a finger under the infant's knee to encourage relaxation. Young children who tense up when their reflexes are being tested may relax the area if you have them focus on another area, so have the child clasp the hands while testing the Achilles and patellar

---

BOX 31.3 Cerebellar Function Testing

- **Romberg:** Ask the school-age or older child to stand still with eyes closed and arms down by the sides. Observe the child for leaning (stand close in case this does occur). This is considered a positive Romberg test, indicating cerebellar dysfunction.

For the following tests, the child should demonstrate accuracy and smoothness:

- **Heel-to-shin:** Have the child lie in a supine position, place one heel on the opposite knee, and run it down the shin.
- **Rapid alternating movements:** The child pats the thighs with the hands, lifts them, turns them over, pats the thighs with the back of the hands, and repeats the process multiple times. An alternate test is for the child to touch the thumb to each finger of the same hand starting at the index finger, then reverse the direction and repeat.
- **Finger-to-finger:** The child's eyes are open. The child touches the examiner's outstretched finger with the index finger, then touches his or her own nose. The examiner moves the finger to a different spot and the child repeats this process several times.
- **Finger-to-nose:** The child's eyes are closed. The child stretches the arm with the index finger extended, then touches his or her nose with that finger, keeping the eyes closed.

Adapted from: Bickley, L., & Szilagyi, P. G. (2009). *Bates guide to physical examination and history taking* (10th ed.). Philadelphia: Lippincott Williams & Wilkins; and Jarvis, C. (2008). *Physical examination and health assessment* (5th ed.). St. Louis, MO: Saunders.

reflexes. As the child focuses on the hands, the lower extremities relax (Jarvis, 2008). Distraction may also be helpful.

Grade the strength of the response using the standard scale from 0 to 4+:

• 0: no response
• 1+: diminished or sluggish
• 2+: average
• 3+: brisker than average
• 4+: very brisk, may involve clonus

The newborn's deep tendon reflexes are normally brisk (3+). They decrease to average (2+), usually by 4 months of age. Healthy children should have reflexes of 2+ if the reflex has been elicited properly. Absent, sluggish, or hyperreactive responses usually indicate disease (Bickley & Szilagyi, 2009).

Refer back to Elliot, the 3-year-old from the beginning of the chapter. What are some important considerations when performing his physical examination?

■■■ Key Concepts

■ The health history in children includes more than just the immediate concern, history of present illness, and past medical history; it is important to include the perinatal history and developmental milestones.

■ Allow the chief concern to determine which parts of the history require more in-depth investigation.

■ The developmental history will warrant more attention in the younger child, while school performance and adjustment will be more important in the school-age child and adolescent.

■ Though the parent will provide most of the health history for the infant and young child, allow the young verbal child to answer questions during the health history as appropriate.

■ Direct health history questions to the school-age child and adolescent, seeking clarification from the parents as needed.

■ Provide confidentiality and privacy for the adolescent during the health history.

■ Weight and length or height should be assessed at each well-child visit to determine adequacy of growth.

■ Measure head circumference until age 3 years to monitor brain growth.

■ Perform hearing and vision screenings for children of all ages.

■ BMI can be used to identify children who are overweight or at risk for being overweight.

■ The normal range of vital signs varies based on the child's age.

■ The sequence of the physical examination in children should be based on the child's developmental age, his

or her level of cooperation, and the severity of the illness.

■ Obtain heart rate and respiratory rate and auscultate the heart and lungs while the infant or young child is quiet.

■ Perform intrusive procedures such as examination of the ears, mouth, and throat last in the infant or young child.

■ Perform the health assessment in a head-to-toe fashion in the school-age child or adolescent, reserving the genitalia and anus examination for last.

■ Plan the health assessment in such a way as to minimize trauma to the child or adolescent.

■ Use age-appropriate measurement tools to assess pain in children.

■ Allow the infant or young child to remain in the parent's lap for as much of the assessment as possible so that the child feels secure.

■ Use age-appropriate games during the health assessment to gain cooperation in the younger child.

■ Having the young boy sit cross-legged for a testicular examination may reduce the cremasteric reflex.

■ The newborn may exhibit a wide variety of normal skin variations.

■ The infant's fontanels should be soft and flat; report a bulging fontanel immediately.

■ Jaundice (outside of the newborn period), pallor, cyanosis, and poor skin turgor indicate illness and may need immediate intervention.

■ Heart murmurs should be assessed for intensity, location, and duration. They may be innocent or may indicate a congenital heart defect.

■ The infant's chest wall is relatively thin, allowing upper airway sounds to be transmitted throughout the lung fields.

■ Substernal or xiphoid retractions indicate that the child is labouring to breathe, whereas a fixed, depressed sternum (pectus excavatum) is a structural abnormality.

■ The Tanner stages of sexual maturity provide a basis for assessing pubertal development in boys and girls. Use the breast and pubic hair charts for girls and the pubic hair and penis and scrotum size chart for boys.

REFERENCES

Abelsohn, A. R., & Sanborn, M. (2010). Lead and children: Clinical management for family physicians. *Canadian Family Physician, 56,* 531–535.

Asher, C., & Northington, L. K. (2008). Position statement for measurement of temperature/fever in children. *Journal of Pediatric Nursing, 23*(3), 234–236.

Bickley, L., & Szilagyi, P. G. (2009). *Bates guide to physical examination and history taking* (10th ed.). Philadelphia: Lippincott Williams & Wilkins.

Bowden, V. R., & Greenberg, C. S. (2008). *Pediatric nursing procedures* (2nd ed.). Philadelphia: Lippincott Williams & Wilkins.

Bunik, M., Brayden, R. M., & Fox, D. (2011). Ambulatory & office pediatrics. In W. W. Hay, M. J. Levin, J. M. Sondheimer & R. R. Deterding (Eds.), *Current pediatric diagnosis and treatment* (20th ed.). New York: McGraw-Hill.

Burns, C., Dunn, A., Brady, M., Starr, N., & Blosser, C. (2009). *Pediatric primary care: A handbook for nurse practitioners* (4th ed.). Philadelphia: WB Saunders.

Canadian Hypertension Education Program. (2010). *Canadian recommendations for the management of hypertension.* Retrieved August 18, 2011 from http://hypertension.ca/chep/wp-content/uploads/2010/03/CHEPbooklet_2010.pdf

Centers for Disease Control and Prevention. (2002). *2000 CDC growth charts for the United States: Methods and development.* Retrieved August 8, 2011 from http://www.cdc.gov/nchs/data/series/sr_11/sr11_246.pdf

Columbia University College of Physicians and Surgeons. (n.d.). *Points on the pediatric physical exam.* Retrieved November 14, 2011 from http://www.columbia.edu/itc/hs/medical/clerkships/peds/Student_Information/Reference_Materials/Pediatric_PE.html

Community Paediatrics Committee, Canadian Paediatric Society. (2011). *Temperature measurement in paediatrics.* Retrieved August 2, 2011 from http://www.cps.ca/english/statements/CP/cp00-01.htm

DeMeulenaere, S. (2007). Pulse oximetry: Uses and limitations. *The Journal for Nurse Practitioners, 3*(5), 312–317.

Dieticians of Canada, Canadian Paediatric Society, College of Family Physicians of Canada, Community Health Nurses of Canada. (2010). *Promoting optimal monitoring of child growth in Canada: Using the new WHO growth charts.* Retrieved August 8, 2011 from http://www.cps.ca/English/statements/N/growth-charts-statement-FULL.pdf

Dowshen, S. (2008). *Positional plagiocephaly (flattened head).* Retrieved August 8, 2011 from http://kidshealth.org/parent/growth/sleep/positional_plagiocephaly.html?tracking = P_RelatedArticle#[

El Radhi, A. S., & Patel, S. (2006). An evaluation of tympanic thermometry in a pediatric emergency department. *Emergency Medicine Journal, 23*(1), 40–41.

Exergen Corporation. (2007). *EXERGEN Temporal Scanner: Temporal artery thermometer consumer information center model TAT-2000C.* Retrieved August 8, 2011 from http://www.exergen.com/medical/TAT/tatconsumerpage.htm

Griffin, T. (2003). Facing challenges to family-centered care II: Anger in the clinical setting. *Pediatric Nursing, 29*(3), 212–215.

Hagan, J. F., Shaw, J. S., & Duncan, P. (2008). *Bright futures guidelines for health supervision of infants, children, and adolescents* (3rd ed.). Elk Grove Village, IL: American Academy of Pediatrics.

Health Canada. (2011). *Lead-based paint.* Retrieved November 2, 2011 from http://www.hc-sc.gc.ca/hl-vs/iyh-vsv/prod/paint-peinture-eng.php

International Cupping Therapy Association. (2006). *Cupping therapy.* Retrieved March 24, 2011 from http://www.cuppingtherapy.org/

Jarvis, C. (2008). *Physical examination and health assessment* (5th ed.). St. Louis, MO: Saunders.

Kay, J. D., Sinaiko, A. R., & Daniels, S. R. (2001). Pediatric hypertension. *American Heart Journal, 142*(3), 422–432.

Kliegman, R. M., Behrman, R. E., Jenson, H. B., & Stanton, B. F. (2007). *Nelson textbook of pediatrics* (18th ed.). Philadelphia: Saunders.

Mandleco, B. (2005). *Pediatric nursing skills and procedures.* Clifton Park, NY: Thomson Delmar.

Manworren, R., & Hynan, L. (2003). Clinical validation of FLACC: Preverbal patient pain scale. *Pediatric Nursing, 29*(2), 140–146.

Menashe, V. (2007). Heart murmurs. *Pediatrics in Review, 28,* e19–e22.

Miller, S. (2011). *Pediatric physical exam video.* Retrieved November 14, 2011. http://www.columbia.edu/itc/hs/medical/clerkships/peds/Student_Information/Reference_Materials/PE_Video.html

National Heart, Lung, and Blood Institute, National Institutes of Health, U.S. Department of Health and Human Services. (2005). *The fourth report on the diagnosis, evaluation, and treatment of high blood pressure in children and adolescents* (NIH Publication No. 05-5267). Washington, D.C.: U.S. Department of Health and Human Services.

Nettina, S. (2010). *Lippincott manual of nursing practice* (9th ed.). Philadelphia: Lippincott Williams & Wilkins.

Nimah, M. M., Bshesh, K., Callahan, J. D., & Jacobs, B. R. (2006). Infrared tympanic thermometry in comparison with other temperature measurement techniques in febrile children. *Pediatric Critical Care Medicine, 7*(1), 48–55.

Rebeshi, L. M., & Brown M. H. (2007). *The pediatric nurse's survival guide.* Clifton Park, NY: Thomson Delmar Learning.

Roohafza, H., Pirnia, A., Sadeghi, M., Toghianifar, Talaei, M., & Ashrafi, M. (2009). Impact of nurses clothing on anxiety of hospitalised children. *Journal of Clinical Nursing, 18,* 1953–1959.

Sass, A. E., & Kaplan, D. W. (2011). Adolescence. In W. W. Hay, M. J. Levin, J. M. Sondheimer & R. R. Deterding (Eds.), *Current pediatric diagnosis and treatment* (20th ed.). New York: McGraw-Hill.

Schaider, J. (ed.). (2007). *Rosen & Barkin's 5-minute emergency medicine consult.* Philadelphia: Lippincott Williams & Wilkins.

Weber, J., & Kelley, J. (2003). *Health assessment in nursing* (2nd ed.). Philadelphia: Lippincott Williams & Wilkins.

Wong, D., & Baker, C. (1988). Pain in children: Comparison of assessment scales. *Pediatric Nursing, 14,* 9–17.

World Health Organization. (2010). The WHO child growth standards. Retrieved August 2, 2011 from http://www.who.int/childgrowth/en/

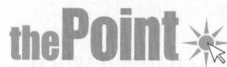

the Point For additional learning materials, including Internet Resources, visit **http://thePoint.lww.com/Chow1e.**

CHAPTER WORKSHEET

MULTIPLE CHOICE QUESTIONS

1. A 5-year-old boy visits the physician's office with an upper respiratory infection. Which approach would give the nurse the most information about the child's developmental level?

   a. Playing a game with the child

   b. Talking with the child about the teddy bear next to him

   c. Using a screening tool during a follow-up office visit

   d. Asking the 10-year-old sibling about the child

2. Which statement indicates the best sequence for the nurse to conduct an assessment in a non-emergency situation?

   a. Introduce yourself, ask about any problems, take a history, do the physical examination.

   b. Perform the physical examination and then ask the family if there are any problems in the child's life.

   c. Do the physical examination while at the same time asking about the child's previous illnesses; then talk about the family's concerns.

   d. Get a complete history of the family's health beliefs and practices, then assess the child.

3. What approach by the nurse would most likely encourage a child to cooperate with an assessment of physical and developmental health?

   a. Explain to the child what's going to happen when the child asks questions.

   b. Explain what is going to happen in words the child can understand.

   c. Force them to cooperate by having a parent hold them down.

   d. Give the child a sticker before beginning the examination.

4. A sleeping 5-month-old girl is being held by the mother when the nurse comes in to do a physical examination. What assessment should be done initially?

   a. Listening to the bowel sounds

   b. Counting the heart rate

   c. Checking the temperature

   d. Looking in the ears

5. Which assessment finding is considered normal in children?

   a. Irregular respiratory rate and rhythm

   b. Split S2 and sinus arrhythmia

   c. Decreased heart rate with crying

   d. Genu varum past the age of 5 years

CRITICAL THINKING EXERCISES

1. A soft and muffled heart murmur is heard in a 4-year-old patient. The mother states that she has never heard that the child has a murmur. What should the nurse do?

2. A nurse is helping a new mother breastfeed her 4-day-old baby. The mother notices that the baby has a bluish cast to the skin on his hands and that sometimes they have a tremor. She asks the nurse if the baby is cold, though the baby is swaddled and comfortably resting against the mother's skin. How might the nurse help teach this mother?

3. Devise a plan for encouraging cooperation of the toddler or preschooler during various parts of the physical examination.

STUDY ACTIVITIES

1. In the clinical setting, obtain a health history on an infant, child, or adolescent.

2. In the clinical setting, compare the approach you use for the physical examination of a toddler versus a school-age child or adolescent.

3. No matter how thoughtfully and appropriately you plan your assessment, odds are good that you will have difficulty assessing a 2-year-old. Discuss with your classmates the strategies that you have used for success and brainstorm with them about their ideas for assessing a crying or resistant young child.

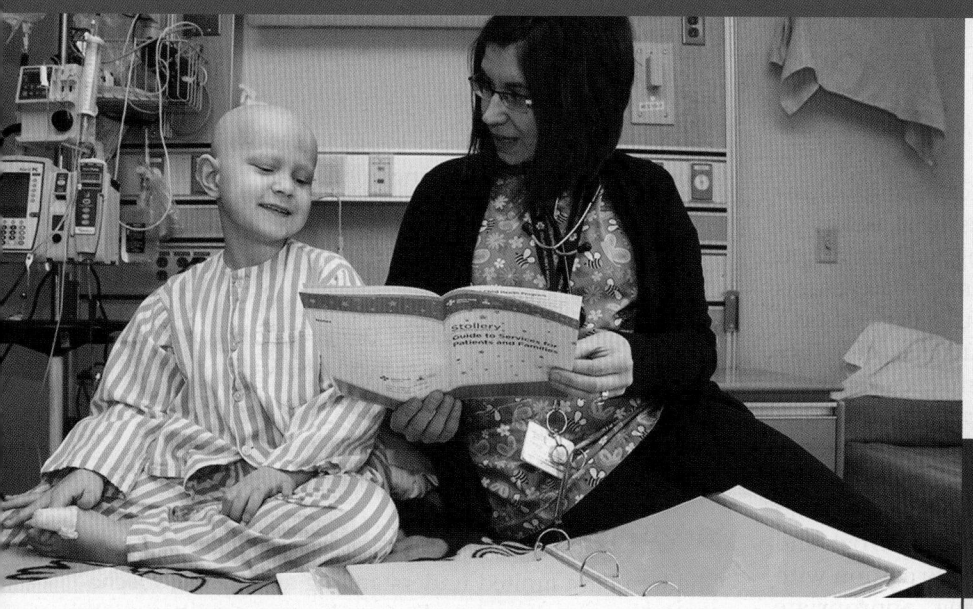

CHAPTER 32

Adapted by Jane Fryer and
Shirley Perry

NURSING CARE OF CHILDREN DURING ILLNESS AND HOSPITALIZATION

KEY TERMS

child life specialist
denial
magical thinking

regression
sensory deprivation
sensory overload

separation anxiety
therapeutic hugging
therapeutic play

LEARNING OBJECTIVES

Upon completion of the chapter, the learner will be able to:

1. Identify the major impact and stressors of illness and hospitalization for children in the various developmental stages.
2. Identify the reactions and responses of children and their families during illness and hospitalization.
3. Explain the factors that influence the reactions and responses of children and their families during illness and hospitalization.
4. Describe the nursing care that minimizes the stressors of children who are ill or hospitalized.
5. Examine the major components of admission for children to the hospital.
6. Outline the specific nursing interventions required for hospitalized children.
7. Use appropriate safety measures when caring for children of all ages.
8. Describe basic care procedures for children in various health care settings.
9. Review the major components and nursing responsibilities related to patient education and discharge from the hospital.

Jake Jorgenson, 8 years old, was brought to the clinic with a history of headaches, vomiting not related to feeding, and changes in his gait. Initial testing leads to a suspected brain tumour. Jake is to be admitted to the neurologic service at a pediatric hospital for further testing and treatment. Up until this point he has been a healthy child with no previous hospitalizations. He lives at home with his parents and two siblings, Jenny, age 11, and Joshua, age 5. As a nurse on this unit, think of ways you can help prepare Jake and his family for this hospitalization.

Wow

Sick children need love, hope, faith, and most of all a positive attitude from their nurse.

Illness, with the occasional consequence of hospitalization, affects children and their families in a variety of ways. Hospitalization is often confusing, complex, and overwhelming for children and their families. Reactions and responses to illness and hospitalization depend on a number of factors, including the unique characteristics and common situations associated with each developmental stage. The result requires nursing strategies that prepare children and their families for this experience while at the same time minimizing negative effects. These strategies include identifying the needs of children and families through astute assessment of nonverbal and verbal behaviours, then validating the information with accurate interpretation and providing appropriate responses and interventions.

Although the nurse implements these strategies throughout the interaction with the child and family, a critical time to ensure the best outcome for the child and family occurs during the admission process. A crucial aspect of these strategies and interventions involves assessing the learning needs and abilities of the child and family. For the interventions to be successful, the nurse must communicate and teach using the most effective method for the individual child and family. The nurse also evaluates the child's and family's competence in performing specific activities prior to discharge.

Hospitalization in Childhood

In today's health care environment, children receive much of their care for illnesses in community health settings such as physician's offices, walk-in clinics, or day surgery centres. As a result of this trend, fewer children may actually be admitted to a hospital unit. Children are hospitalized for acute or chronic illnesses, trauma, surgery, or palliation. Some children remain in the hospital while awaiting adequate services to be put in place to enable safe discharge.

According to the Public Health Agency of Canada, children comprise only 10.6% of all those who are hospitalized throughout the country. Birth-related problems and respiratory system disease account for 60% of all hospitalizations in children under 1 year of age. For children between 1 and 4 years of age, 40% of hospitalizations result from respiratory system diseases. Of children 5 to 9 years of age, 27% are hospitalized for respiratory system disease, 13% for unintentional injuries, and 12% for digestive system disease. Unintentional injuries and digestive and respiratory system disease are responsible for 45% of all hospitalizations in children between the ages of 10 and 14. In adolescents, mental disorders, unintentional injuries, and digestive system diseases account for 40% of all hospitalizations (Public Health Agency of Canada, 2008).

Other health problems begin before or immediately following birth, such as congenital heart disease or gastrointestinal atresia. Before getting used to the idea of having a new child, the family must now deal with illness and possible extended hospitalizations. Specific genetic or environmental factors also predispose some children to disease and injury, such as the genetic disorder cystic fibrosis or the environmental factors associated with poverty. Many of these factors or situations put the child and family at greater risk for chronic health conditions and long periods of illness, hospitalization, and even death.

Stressors of Hospitalization

Children have limited understanding and coping mechanisms to assist them in relieving the stressors that might occur during hospitalization. According to Bricher (2000), hospitalized children are vulnerable not only because of their illness but also because they have a limited understanding of their situation and very little control over what is happening to them. Hospitalization creates a series of traumatic and stressful events that produce uncertainty for all children and their families, whether the hospital stay involves an elective procedure or is an emergency situation. Specific factors will affect the overall hospital experience as well as the responses and reactions of children and their families.

Besides the physiologic effects of the health problem, the impact of illness and hospitalization on a child includes anxiety and fear related to the overall process and the potential for bodily injury and pain. In addition, children are separated from their homes, families, friends, and what is familiar to them, which may result in **separation anxiety** (distress related to removal from family and familiar surroundings). There is a general loss of control over their lives and sometimes their emotions and behaviours. The result may be anger, guilt, **regression** (return to a previous stage of development), acting out, and other types of defence mechanisms to cope with these effects. Children's typical coping strategies are tested during this experience.

Fear and Anxiety

For many children, hospitalization is like entering a foreign world, and the result is fear and anxiety. Often anxiety stems from the rapid onset of the illness or injury, particularly when the child has limited experiences with disease or injury. The child hears unfamiliar words and noises, smells unfamiliar odours and eats unfamiliar food, and sees ominous-looking equipment and strangers in unusual attire like surgical caps, masks, or gowns. He or she may hear other children crying. All of these things make hospitalization a difficult experience for children.

Normal fears of childhood include the fear of separation, loss of control, and bodily injury, mutilation, or harm, and all of these are particularly relevant during a

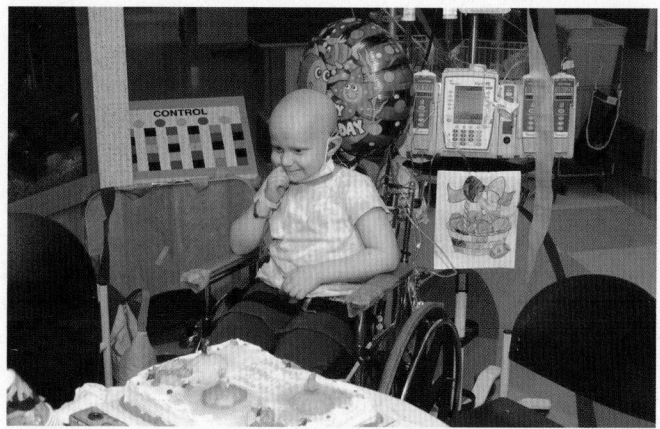

FIGURE 32.1 The presence of familiar objects and home routines normalizes the environment and helps the child cope with hospitalization. Celebrating a birthday in the hospital can be comforting. (Courtesy of Stephen Wreakes.)

hospital stay. Children's fears are similar to adult fears of the unknown, including fear of unfamiliar environments and losing control. Children may be exposed to equipment, people, situations, and procedures that may be new to them and cause them pain (Fig. 32.1). In addition, children of various developmental stages have specific reactions. For example, preschool children have an egocentric view of the environment and events that happen to them and participate in magical, fantasy-type thoughts, both of which may lead to additional fears. Although children are increasingly able to adapt as they grow older, lack of understanding about the need for hospitalization can make such adaptation difficult. Moreover, being hospitalized threatens the sense of control that children are striving for as they develop (Romino, Keatley, Secrest, & Good, 2005).

> ▶ *Take* NOTE!
>
> *Coyne (2006), in a grounded theory study, conducted in-depth interviews with 11 children, ages 7 to 14 years, to record the children's experiences of hospitalization in their own words. These children identified their concerns as "separation from family and friends; being in an unfamiliar environment; receiving investigations and treatments; and loss of self-determination" (p. 328). In one 9-year-old girl's words, "I don't like blood test things like that … I hate the needles and things 'cause … I was really good for one yesterday but they don't put the EMLA cream on" (p. 331).*

Separation Anxiety

Separation anxiety is a major stressor for children of certain ages. It usually begins around 8 months and ends as the child nears 3 years of age (Healthy Children, 2011).

Separation anxiety consists of three stages during which the child exhibits certain behavioural reactions to the stress of the separation. The first phase, protest, occurs when the child is separated from his or her parents or primary caretaker (Bowlby, 1960). This phase may last from a few hours to several days. The child reacts aggressively to this separation and exhibits great distress by crying, expressing agitation, and rejecting others who attempt to offer comfort. The child may also exhibit anger and inconsolable grief.

If the parents do not return within a short time, the child exhibits the second phase, despair (Bowlby, 1960). The child displays hopelessness by withdrawing from others, becoming quiet without crying, exhibiting apathy, depression, disinterest in play and food, and overall feelings of sadness. Today, health care providers primarily observe the first and second stages because of the shorter hospital stays and the more common use of a family-centred approach to care.

Detachment (also known as **denial**) is the third and final phase of separation anxiety (Bowlby, 1960). During this phase the child forms coping mechanisms to protect him- or herself from further emotional pain. This occurs more often during long-term separations. During this stage, the child shows interest in the environment, starts to play again, and forms temporary relationships with the nurses and other children. If the parents return, the child ignores them. A child in this phase of separation anxiety exhibits resignation, not contentment. It is more difficult to reverse this stage, and developmental delays may occur.

Loss of Control

When hospitalized, children experience a significant loss of control. This loss of control increases the perception of threat and affects their coping skills. They lose control over routine self-care, their usual tasks, and play as well as decisions related to the care of their own bodies. In the hospital, the child's usual routine is disrupted. He or she cannot choose what to do and at what time. The child can no longer accomplish simple tasks independently as he or she does at home or school. Confinement to the bed or crib worsens this loss of control. For example, if connected to tubes or intravenous lines, the child may not even be able to visit the bathroom alone.

Hospitalization also affects the child's control over decisions related to his or her own body. Many of the procedures and treatments that occur in the hospital are invasive or at least disturbing to children, and much of the time they do not have the option to refuse to undergo them. Adults are presumed to be competent to make health care decisions, but generally children are not (Bricher, 2000). Though parents and nurses of hospitalized children have the children's best interest in mind, children often feel powerless when in the hospital, not having their feelings and wishes respected and having minimal control over events.

▶ *Take* NOTE!

Always ask yourself, "Who speaks for the child?" If you do act as an advocate for a child, make sure you reflect the child's wishes, not what you think his or her wishes might or should be (Bricher, 2000).

Children's Responses to the Stressors of Hospitalization

The stressors that children experience during hospitalization may result in various reactions. Children react to the stresses of hospitalization before admission, during the hospital stay, and after discharge. Defence behaviours such as anger, guilt, regression, and acting out may occur. Many factors influence the amount and degree of reactions the child may experience, and these factors may increase or diminish the child's fears. Children with chronic illnesses who have experienced multiple hospitalizations may have different reactions. Chapter 35 gives additional information about the child with a chronic illness. Children's responses to the stressors of fear, separation anxiety, and loss of control will also vary depending on their age and developmental level.

▶ *Take* NOTE!

Quote from a child hospitalized for a short-term illness: "I was a little nervous because I believed they would cut around here (shows a quadrangle covering his stomach) . . . and then I thought they would take everything out and then they would sew all around with skin-thread . . . that's what I believed." (Forsner, Jansson, & Sorlie, 2005, p. 158)

Infants

Newborns and infants are adapting to life outside the womb with rapid growth and development and establishment of a healthy attachment to parents or primary caregivers. They are dependent on others for nurture and protection. They gain a sense of trust in the world through rhythmic and reciprocal patterns of contact and feeding, resulting in bonding to the primary caregiver. They need a secure pattern of restful sleep, satisfaction of oral and nutritional needs, relaxation of body systems, and spontaneous response to communication and gentle stimuli. The caregiver–infant attachment is critical for psychological health, especially during periods of illness and hospitalization.

Unfortunately, during illness and hospitalization, these critical patterns of feeding, contact, comfort, sleeping, elimination, and stimulation are disrupted, resulting

in fear and separation anxiety. By 5 to 6 months of age, infants have developed an awareness of self as separate from mother. As a result, infants of this age are acutely aware of the absence of their primary caregiver and become fearful of unfamiliar persons (Bowlby, 1988). Any situation that results in separation of an infant from the primary caregiver may result in separation anxiety. These situations could arise as a result of hospital policy regarding rooming-in, such as in the neonatal intensive care unit or pediatric intensive care unit (PICU). The infant's oral needs, the basic source of infant satisfaction, are often not met in the hospital due to the condition of the child or the procedures that must be performed. The infant is accustomed to having his or her basic needs met by the parent when the infant cries or gestures.

Toddlers

Toddlers are more aware of self and can communicate their desires. Because their autonomy is developing, toddlers need to master accomplishments to minimize the development of shame and doubt. Control becomes an issue for toddlers. Toddlers also need opportunities to explore, and they need consistent routines. In addition, toddlers are aware of the need for care and protection of others, so they need familiarity and closeness to the primary caregiver. When the toddler is hospitalized, disruption occurs in this development of autonomy.

Toddlers are often fearful of strangers and can recall traumatic events. Simply walking toward the treatment room where a traumatic procedure previously occurred may result in extreme upset in the toddler. A resurgence in separation anxiety often occurs during the toddler years. When the toddler is separated from his or her parents or caregivers in an unfamiliar environment, then separation anxiety is compounded. In response to this anxiety, toddlers may demonstrate behaviours such as pleading with the parents to stay, physically trying to go after the parents, throwing temper tantrums, and refusing to comply with usual routines. Any restrictions resulting in loss of mobility or interference with normal developmental progress can contribute to the loss of control experienced by toddlers. Disruption in usual routines also contributes to loss of control, and the toddler feels insecure. As a result, regression in toilet training and refusal to eat are common reactions in hospitalized toddlers.

Preschoolers

The preschooler has better verbal and developmental skills to adapt to various situations, but illness and hospitalization can still be stressful. Preschoolers may understand that they are in the hospital because they are sick, but they may not understand the cause of their illness. Preschoolers fear mutilation and are afraid of intrusive procedures since they do not understand the body's integrity. They interpret words literally and have an active imagination. Therefore, when the nurse says, "I need to take some blood," preschoolers' fantasies may run wild. They may not understand the concept of blood and may think everything will come out of their body. They may think that blood is "taken" the same way a child picks up a toy to take it out of the room. Preschoolers' thinking is egocentric; they believe that some personal deed or thought caused their illness, which can lead to guilt and shame. These feelings may be internalized. Overall, preschoolers' concrete, egocentric, and **magical thinking** (type of thinking that allows for fantasies and creativity) limits their ability to understand, so communication and interventions must be on their level.

Separation anxiety may not be as much of an issue as it is in toddlers, since preschoolers may already be spending time away from their parents in preschool. They are, however, still acutely aware of the comfort and security that their family provides for them, so disruptions in these relationships lead to challenges. The preschooler may constantly ask for his or her parents or ask to call the parents. He or she may quietly cry, refuse to eat or take medication, or generally be uncooperative.

In addition, the hospitalized preschooler loses control over the environment. The preschooler is naturally curious about his or her surroundings and learns best by observing and working with objects. This might be limited during hospitalization. Because the preschooler cannot participate in usual activities and explore the environment as usual, the child's normal creative, curious nature may give rise to a variety of fantasies that may present challenges.

School-Age Children

School-age children generally are hospitalized because of long-term illnesses or trauma. The general task of their developmental stage, to develop confidence through a sense of industry, can be disrupted during hospitalization. Even at this time, they generally want to continue to learn and maintain their skills and abilities. The stress of illness or anxiety related to diagnostic tests and therapeutic interventions may lead to inward or outward expressions of distress. If they have learned various coping skills, this distress may be minimized. After 11 years of age, there is an increased awareness of physiologic, psychological, and behavioural causes of illness and injury. Typically the school-age child has a more realistic understanding of the reasons for the illness and can better comprehend explanations. School-age children are concerned about disability and death and fear injury and pain. They want to know the reasons why procedures and tests are being performed. They can understand cause-and-effect and how it relates to their illness. They are often uncomfortable with any type of sexual examination.

Separation anxiety is not as much of an issue for school-age children. They are accustomed to periods of separation and may already be experiencing some separation anxiety related to being in school. At the same time,

they may be missing school and friends as they try to adjust to the unfamiliar environment. They may feel that friends will forget them if they remain in the hospital for a long time. Some school-age children may regress and become needy, demanding their parents' attention or playing with special "comfort toys" they used at a younger age.

Since school-age children are accustomed to controlling self-care and typically are highly social, they like being involved. They are accustomed to making choices about meals and activities and fill their days with activities. Hospitalization presents loss of control by limiting their activities, making them feel helpless and dependent. This may result in feelings of loneliness, boredom, isolation, and depression. The key is to give them opportunities to maintain independence, retain a sense of control, enhance self-esteem, and continue to work toward achieving a sense of industry.

Adolescents

Adolescents fear injury and pain. Since appearance is important to them, they are concerned with how the illness/injury will affect their body image. Anything that changes their perception of themselves has a major impact on their response. Typically, adolescents do not like to show fear or vulnerability because such expressions could cause them to "lose face" and therefore lose acceptance by their peers. They also may feel ambivalent about wanting their parents to be present. Adolescents typically do not experience separation anxiety related to being away from their parents; instead, their anxiety comes from being separated from friends.

Finally, loss of control is a key factor affecting the behaviour of adolescents who are hospitalized (Vessey, 2003). Anger, withdrawal, or general lack of cooperation may occur due to the feelings of loss of control. In addition, their desire to appear confident may lead them to question everything that is being done or that they are asked to do. Their feelings of invincibility may cause them to take risks and be noncompliant with treatment. Overall, adolescents strive for independence, self-assertion, and liberation while developing their identity. Nevertheless, for Aboriginal teens who live on reserves or in remote communities, being hospitalized in an urban centre far from their home and family may be particularly distressing (Blackstock, Bruyere, & Moreau, 2006).

*R*emember *Jake, the 8-year-old with a suspected brain tumour? What responses to hospitalization might you see in him and his family?*

Factors Affecting Children's Reaction to Hospitalization

Various factors have a great impact on the ability of children to handle illness and hospitalization. These factors

BOX 32.1 **Factors Affecting a Child's Response to Illness and Hospitalization**

- Developmental age
- Cognitive level
- Previous experience with illness, separation, and hospitalization
- Type and amount of preparation given
- Innate and acquired coping skills
- Seriousness of the diagnosis/onset of illness or injury (e.g., acute or chronic)
- Support systems available, including the family and health professionals
- Cultural background
- Parents' reaction to illness and hospitalization

include the amount of separation from the parents, the child's age, the cognitive or developmental level of the child, and any previous experience the child has had with illness and hospitalization (Box 32.1). Recent life stresses and changes may also reduce the child's coping abilities and increase his or her vulnerability to anxiety. The child's temperament and coping skills can contribute in a negative or positive way to his or her hospital experience. Finally, the parents' responses to the situation will shape the child's reactions. Because of all of these factors, each child will respond differently and will perceive the hospital experience differently.

Separation from Parents or Primary Caregivers

A widely researched factor associated with children's reactions to hospitalization is the effect of separation from parents. Over 50 years ago, researchers such as John Bowlby studied the impact that hospitalization has on immediate and long-term emotional distress for the child. Subsequent research led to today's liberal visitation and rooming-in policies of hospitals. These ideas continue to be important components in the care of the ill child and family (Bjork, Nordstrom, & Hallstrom, 2006; Dudley & Carr, 2004), but today's generally shorter stays in hospitals do not allow time for the various stages of separation anxiety.

Developmental Abilities and Perceptions

The age, cognitive level, and developmental level of children will affect their perceptions of events. This, in turn, will affect their reactions to illness and hospitalization. Younger children, with their limited life experience and immature intellectual capacities, have a more difficult time comprehending what is happening to them. This can be particularly true for toddlers and preschoolers, who perceive the intactness of their bodies to be violated

during invasive procedures. In addition, they frequently interpret illness as punishment for wrongdoing or hospital procedures as hostile, mutilating acts. Thus, children below the age of 5 are vulnerable to emotional distress from hospitalization.

Previous Experiences with Illness and Hospitalization

In general, children's lack of understanding and experience with illness, hospitalization, and hospital procedures increases their anxiety. However, previous experience with hospitalization and illness can make preparation either easier or more difficult (if the experiences were perceived as negative). For example, if the child associates going to the hospital with the birth of a sibling, he or she may view this experience as positive. On the other hand, if the child associates the hospital with the serious illness or death of a relative or close friend or with a previous personal hospitalization that was difficult, he or she will probably view the experience as negative.

Previous hospitalization experiences may influence the child's responses and reactions to his or her current hospitalization. For example, older children may cling to their parents, kick, or create a scene because of their previous experience. One research study compared the psychological responses of children hospitalized in a PICU with those hospitalized on a general unit. The children who were younger and more severely ill and who underwent more invasive procedures had significantly more medical fears, a lower sense of control over their health, and ongoing post-traumatic stress responses for 6 months after discharge (Rennick, Johnston, Dougerty, & Ritchie, 2002).

Present Experiences with Illness and Hospitalization

The effects of hospitalization on children are influenced by the nature and severity of the health problem, the condition of the child, and the degree to which activities and routines in the hospital differ from those of everyday life. Being in an unfamiliar environment elicits fear of the unknown, from the strange hospital environment to the large number of unfamiliar people (Coyne, 2006). Likewise, disruptions in the child's routine—including school attendance, peer relationships, and normal daily activities—that result when the child is separated from family and friends can be detrimental (Coyne, 2006). Losing the ability to take control over activities such as personal needs, sleeping and waking times, food choices, and mealtimes contributes to a loss of self-determination (Coyne, 2006). A lack of sensory stimulation in the hospital environment may produce listlessness, indifference, unhappiness, and even appetite changes. When the child's motor activity is restricted, anger and hyperactivity may result. Play, recreation, and educational opportunities

---

BOX 32.2 Children and Coping

Coping Behaviours/Methods
Ignore or negate the problem
Stoicism, passive acceptance
Acting out—yelling, kicking, screaming, crying
Anger, withdrawal, rejection
Intellectualizing

Suggestions for Promoting Coping
Breathing techniques, such as blowing bubbles,
  pinwheels, or party noise-makers
Distraction with books or games
Imagery
Music
Teaching, discussion, and encouragement that is age
  appropriate

---

provide an outlet to distract children from the illness, provide them with pleasant experiences, and help them understand their condition.

The ability to work through a situation for children and families will also affect their responses to illness and hospitalization. Of course, this ability depends on the age of child, perceptions of the event, previous situations, encounters with health care personnel, and support from significant others. Box 32.2 lists coping skills used by children and suggestions for promoting positive coping.

Parents' Response to Children's Hospitalization

Children sense their parents' anxiety and concern, and even hearing whispers can set off a child's imagination. For example, preschoolers may invent elaborate stories to explain what is happening to them. If parents do not tell the child the truth or do not answer his or her questions, the child will become confused and frightened and the child's trust in the parent may become weakened. It is important for children to believe that someone is in control and that the person can be trusted. Some parents, however, have their own fears and insecurities. Thus, how a child reacts often is shaped by the parents' response to the illness and hospitalization.

Parents show their commitment to caring for their ill child by their feelings of love, responsibility, involvement, and vigilant watching over them (Dudley & Carr, 2004). One child in a qualitative study illustrated this commitment to care: "I just couldn't picture anyone else staying. We had everyone here from Timbuktu and back say I'll come stay at the hospital and give you a break but no, it is just Dad and I" (Dudley & Carr, 2004, p. 271).

The relationship between the family and the hospital staff may also contribute to the stress of the child. These relationships contribute significantly to the quality of the environment. Hospital personnel must assume responsibility for the care of children who are hospitalized by maintaining good partnerships with families. Nurses can support parents by providing accurate, timely information and an explanation of treatment plans and by supporting the parents' ability to stay with their child at all times (Pagnamenta & Benger, 2008).

The Hospitalized Child's Family

Whether planned or unplanned, hospitalization increases the family's stress and anxiety level. The illness or serious injury of one family member affects all members of the family. The process disrupts the family's usual routines and may alter family roles. The disruption is typically more significant if specialized health care is needed far from home that requires the family members to be separated (Scott-Findlay & Chalmers, 2001). Parents and siblings have their own reactions to this experience.

Reactions of Parents

Watching a child in pain is difficult, especially when the parent is assisting with the procedure by holding the child. The parent may feel guilty for not seeking care sooner. Parents may also exhibit other feelings such as denial, anger, depression, and confusion. Parents may deny that the child is ill. They may express anger, especially directed at the nursing staff, another family member, or a higher power because of their loss of control in caring for the child. Depression may occur because of exhaustion and the psychological and physical requirements of spending long hours in a hospital caring for a child. Confusion may develop as a result of dealing with an unfamiliar environment or the loss of a parental role. Finally, the parents' marriage may be strained because of dual roles, long separation, and increased stress.

A qualitative study by Stratton (2004) indicates that parents have experiences in four categories: facing boundaries, attempting to understand, coping with uncertainty, and seeking reassurance from caregivers. First, parents feel helpless when they play a passive role in their child's care, such as when a medical procedure is required that hurts or traumatizes the child. Then parents attempt to understand by becoming informed and understanding the procedures. Next, they deal with the fear of uncertainty and attempt to promote a sense of comfort by interacting with the hospital staff. They seek reassurance from the caregivers.

Reactions of Siblings

Certain age groups, such as the preschooler, may feel they caused the illness. Their magical and egocentric thinking, combined with little information, contributes to their fears that they may have caused the illness or injury by their thoughts, wishes, or behaviours (Winch, 2001).

If the family roles or routines change significantly, the siblings may feel insecure or anxious. They may develop changes in behaviour or in school performance during this time.

The authors of a recent qualitative study reveal that children often feel uncertainty and difficulty expressing their own fears and needs when a sibling is ill or disabled: "Thinking about stuff, my sister, and thinking about her, you know, seizures and is that going to happen to me?" (Branstetter, Domian, Williams, Graff, & Piamjarijakul, 2008, p. 178). In this same study, sibling resentment was evident when parents placed greater expectations on the well child. Some siblings were more comfortable than others in taking on a caregiver role and participated in caregiving activities (Branstetter et al., 2008). For these children, anticipating their sibling's needs in a positive way validated their feelings and the realities of their experiences as the brother or sister of an ill child (Branstetter et al., 2008).

Factors Influencing Family Reactions

The parenting style and the family–child relationship can influence the hospital experience as well as the family members' coping skills. Cultural, ethnic, and religious variations, values and practices related to illness, general response to stress, and attitudes about the care of a sick child have a significant influence on the family's response and behaviours. For example, it is important to spend time with Aboriginal families as they have a rich storytelling tradition (Baltruschat, n.d.) through which their beliefs and concerns are often communicated. Patients and families from the far North and Native Reserves may find it difficult to adjust to the hospital culture given the differences in the traditional food they eat compared with the food offered in the hospital.

Jake's parents are very upset that he has to be hospitalized. His mother says to you, "I'm worried how Jake is going to react to all of this. What can we do to help him?" How would you address his mother's concerns?

The Nurse's Role in Caring for the Hospitalized Child

In most instances, the nurse is the primary person involved in the care of a hospitalized child. The nurse is probably the first one to see the child and family and will spend more time with them than other health care providers. Nurses are part of a medical community that makes decisions in the child's best interest, but the nurse needs to bear in mind the child's rights and must try to

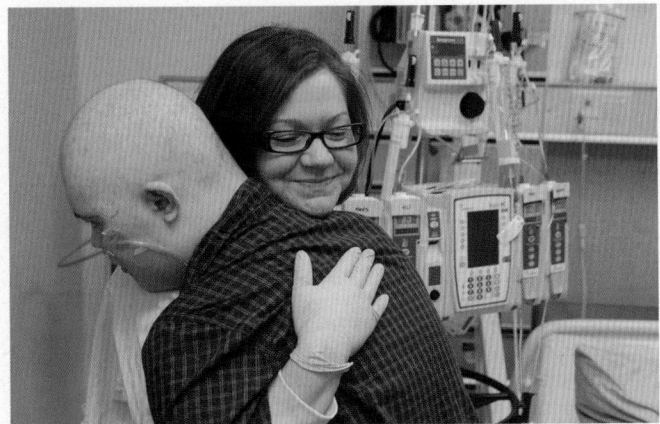

FIGURE 32.2 A teenager with Down syndrome receives a reassuring hug from his nurse. (Courtesy of Stephen Wreakes.)

minimize the distress of children so that the hospital stay may be as pleasant an experience as possible (Bricher, 2000). When establishing strategies to care for children in the hospital, nurses should examine the general effects of hospitalization on children in each developmental stage and should strive to understand the factors affecting hospitalization as well as the reactions of the child and family. Nursing Care Plan 32.1 summarizes the nursing care associated with a hospitalized child.

Bjork et al. (2006) have identified five themes to describe the needs of children in the hospital setting. They include (1) the need for physical and emotional closeness to parents; (2) the need to have fun, be happy, play, and have social interactions with other children and adults; (3) the need to be actively involved in making decisions about their care and participating in their own care when possible; (4) the need for positive relationships with health care staff (Fig. 32.2); and (5) to have their physical and emotional needs met. The initial contact with children and their families can serve as a foundation for a trusting relationship that helps to meet these needs. Each institution has its own criteria for admission and transfer of pediatric patients, formulated in light of its mission and abilities and limitations (Sigrest, Neff, Eichner, & Hardy, 2003).

The first encounter with a child should be unthreatening and friendly. Approach the child with open hands without any medical equipment. Allow the child to interact with you and get to know you before you begin any assessments, treatments, or procedures. Be genuine and listen to what the child has to say. Use favourite toys and common television shows to establish rapport. Allow the child to participate in the conversation without the pressure of having to comply with requests or undergo any procedures. A trusting relationship can be built by using appropriate language, games, and play such as singing a song during a procedure, preparing the child adequately

(text continues on page 1018)

Nursing Care Plan 32.1

OVERVIEW FOR THE HOSPITALIZED CHILD AND FAMILY

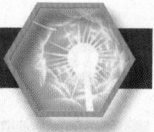

NURSING DIAGNOSIS: Anxiety related to hospital situation, fear of injury or bodily mutilation, separation from family or friends, changes in routine, painful procedures and treatments, and unfamiliar events and surroundings as evidenced by crying, fussing, withdrawal, or resistance

Outcome Identification and Evaluation
Child and family will exhibit a decrease in anxiety level as evidenced by positive coping strategies, verbalization or playing out of feelings, appropriate behaviours, positive interactions with staff, child and parent cooperation and participation, and absence of signs and symptoms of increasing anxiety and fear.

Interventions: Minimizing Anxiety
- Orient child and family to the unit and the child's room *to familiarize them with the facility.*
- Place the child in a room with another child of a similar age, developmental level, and condition severity *to promote sharing. Utilize the expertise of the CLS if available.*
- Explain all events, treatments, procedures, and activities to the parents and child (at level the child will understand) in a calm, relaxed manner *to help them prepare for what is to come and decrease fear of the unknown. A calm, relaxed manner helps to establish rapport and instill trust.*
- Encourage parents to room in if possible *to provide the child with support;* if parents cannot stay, encourage them to call *to reduce child's fear of being alone.*
- Urge parents to inform the child when they will be leaving and when they are expected to return *to help child cope with their absence and promote trust.*
- Assess child's usual routine at home and attempt to incorporate aspects of usual routine into hospital routine *to ease the transition to the hospital and promote child participation in routine.*
- Offer comfort measures such as holding, stroking, and rocking *to relieve distress.*
- Provide atraumatic care *to minimize exposure to distress, which would increase anxiety.*
- Encourage the child's participation in play (unstructured and therapeutic play as necessary) *to allow for expression of feelings and fears and promote energy expenditure.*
- Suggest that parents bring in a special toy or object from home *to promote feelings of security.*
- Provide positive reinforcement for participation in care activities *to foster self-esteem.*
- Assess for regression behaviours and inform parents that such behaviours are common *to help alleviate their concerns about this behaviour.*
- Provide consistency with care measures *to facilitate trust and acceptance.*

NURSING DIAGNOSIS: Risk for powerlessness related to lack of control over procedures, treatments, and care, and changes in usual routine

Outcome Identification and Evaluation
Child and family will demonstrate an increase in control over the situation as evidenced by participation in care activities, identification of needs and choices, and incorporation of appropriate aspects of child's usual routine with that of the hospital.

Interventions: Promoting Control
- Encourage child and parents to identify areas of concern *to help in determining priority needs.*
- Encourage parent and child to participate in care activities *to promote feelings of control.*
- Incorporate aspects of child's routine at home and use terms similar to those used at home *to foster a sense of normalcy.*
- Offer child choices as much as possible, such as options for foods, drinks, hygiene, activities, or clothing (if appropriate) *to promote feelings of individuality and control.*
- Allow child opportunities for being out of bed or room within limitations as appropriate *to foster independence.*
- Work with child, as age and development allow, and family to set up a schedule *to promote structure and routine.*

(continued)

Nursing Care Plan 32.1 (continued)

NURSING DIAGNOSIS: Deficient diversional activity related to confinement in bed or health care facility, limited mobility, activity restrictions, or equipment as evidenced by verbalization of boredom, lack of participation in play, reading, or schoolwork

Outcome Identification and Evaluation
Child will participate in diversional activities as evidenced by engagement in unstructured and therapeutic play that is developmentally appropriate and interaction with family, staff, and other children.

Interventions: Promoting Adequate Diversional Activities
- Question child and family about favourite types of activities *to establish a baseline for developing appropriate choices during hospitalization.*
- Assist with planning activities within the limits of the child's condition *to maintain muscle tone and strength without overexerting the child.*
- Spend time with the child *to provide stimulation and foster trust.*
- Enlist the aid of a CLS *to provide suggestions for appropriate activities.*
- Encourage interaction with other children *to promote sharing and avoid loneliness.*
- Provide developmentally appropriate opportunities for unstructured and therapeutic play *to facilitate expression of feelings.*
- Encourage short trips to the playroom or activity room *to provide a change of scenery and sensory stimulation.*
- Integrate play activities with nursing care *to achieve therapeutic effect.*

NURSING DIAGNOSIS: Interrupted family processes related to separation from child due to hospitalization, increased demands of caring for an ill child, changes in role function, and effect of hospitalization on other family members such as siblings as evidenced by parental verbalization of issues, parental presence in hospital, or child's hospitalization requiring parent to miss work

Outcome Identification and Evaluation
Family will demonstrate positive coping strategies as evidenced by visiting frequently and staying with the child as necessary, sharing of family responsibilities, obtaining assistance for relief or respite, and visiting by other members of the child's family and friends.

Interventions: Maximizing Family Functioning
- Encourage parents and family members to verbalize concerns related to child's illness, diagnosis, and prognosis *to promote family-centred care and identify areas where intervention may be needed.*
- Explain therapies, procedures, child's behaviours, and plan of care to parents *to promote understanding of the child's status and plan of care, which helps to decrease anxiety.*
- Encourage parental involvement in care *to promote feelings of the parents being needed and valued, providing them with a sense of control over their child's health.*
- Identify support system for family and child *to help identify resources available for coping.*
- Educate family and child on additional resources available *to promote a wider base of support to deal with the situation.*
- Suggest ways that parents can divide time between child and other siblings *to prevent feelings of guilt.*
- Provide support and positive reinforcement *to promote family coping and foster family strength.*
- Encourage frequent visits by family members, including siblings as appropriate, *to promote ongoing family functioning.*
- Stress the need for adequate rest, sleep, exercise, and nutrition for family members *to promote family health and minimize stress of hospitalization on family.*
- Assist with referrals for resources and help from additional family members and friends as necessary *to allow for respite or relief of care responsibilities.*
- Encourage family to maintain usual routine as much as possible *to minimize the effects of hospitalization on family functioning.*

Nursing Care Plan 32.1 (continued)

NURSING DIAGNOSIS: Self-care deficit related to immobility, activity restrictions, regression, or use of equipment, devices, or prescribed treatments as evidenced by inability to feed, bathe or dress self or accomplish other activities of daily living

Outcome Identification and Evaluation

Child will participate in self-care within limitations of condition as evidenced by assisting with bathing and hygiene, feeding, toileting, and dressing and grooming.

Interventions: Promoting Self-Care

- Assess child's usual routine for self-care and self-care abilities *to provide a baseline for individualizing interventions.*
- Provide child-sized equipment and devices *to promote child's ability to complete the self-care task.*
- Encourage parents and child to do as much self-care as possible, within limitations of the child's condition and developmental level, *to promote feelings of independence and foster growth and development.*
- Offer praise and encouragement for activities performed *to foster self-esteem, confidence, and competence.*
- Ensure adequate rest periods *to minimize energy expenditure associated with self-care activities.*

NURSING DIAGNOSIS: Risk for delayed growth and development related to stressors associated with hospitalization, current condition or illness, separation from family, and sensory overload or sensory deprivation

Outcome Identification and Evaluation

Child will demonstrate developmentally appropriate milestones as evidenced by age-appropriate behaviours and activities.

Interventions: Promoting Growth and Development

- Assess child's developmental stage *to establish a baseline and determine appropriate strategies.*
- Use unstructured and therapeutic play and adaptive toys *to promote developmental functioning.*
- Provide stimulating environment when possible *to maximize potential for growth and development.*
- Praise accomplishments and emphasize child's abilities *to foster self-esteem and encourage feelings of confidence and competence.*
- Include parents in techniques to foster growth and development *to promote feelings of control in their child's care.*

NURSING DIAGNOSIS: Deficient knowledge related to hospitalization, surgery, treatments, procedures, required care, and follow-up as evidenced by questioning and verbalization, lack of prior exposure

Outcome Identification and Evaluation

Child and family will demonstrate understanding of all aspects of child's current situation as evidenced by identification of child's and family's needs, verbal statements of understanding and/or need for additional information, return demonstration of procedures and treatments, and verbalization of instructions for follow-up and continued care.

Interventions: Providing Child and Family Teaching

- Assess child's and family's willingness to learn *to ensure effective teaching.*
- Provide family with time to adjust to diagnosis *to facilitate their ability to learn and participate in the child's care.*
- Repeat information *to promote multiple opportunities for child and family to learn.*
- Teach in short sessions *to prevent overloading the child and parents with information.*
- Gear teaching to a level of understanding for the child and the family (depends on age of child, physical condition, memory) *to promote learning.*
- Provide reinforcement and rewards *to help facilitate the teaching/learning process.*
- Use multiple modes of learning, such as written information, verbal instruction, demonstrations, and media, when possible *to facilitate learning and retention of information.*
- Provide the child and family with written step-by-step instructions for procedures or care *to allow for reference at a later date.*
- Have child and family provide return demonstrations of care procedures *to ensure effectiveness of teaching.*
- Arrange for trial home care during hospitalization and after discharge as appropriate *to ensure understanding and provide opportunities for additional teaching and learning.*

for procedures, and providing explanations and encouragement. Get down to the child's level and play on his or her terms.

Decisions must be made that will affect the trust the child has developed. For example, it is imperative to decide how much control the child will have during treatment, how much information to share with the child about upcoming events, and whether parents should participate. Reinforce the child's use of coping strategies that lead to healthy outcomes by providing options whenever it is safe to do so. Finally, provide comfort and reassurance through techniques such as praising the child and providing opportunities to cuddle with a favourite toy.

Preparing Children and Families for Hospitalization

When preparing children for hospitalization, be aware of the situations that may create distress in a child and try to minimize or eliminate them. Even the most minor situations may be frightening to young children. Fear of the unknown is often the most stressful factor associated with hospitalization. The American Academy of Pediatrics Child Life Council and Committee on Hospital Care policy statement (2006) on child life services proposes that "play and age-appropriate communication may be used to (1) promote optimal development, (2) present information, (3) plan and rehearse useful coping strategies for medical events or procedures, (4) work through feelings about past or impending experiences, and (5) establish therapeutic relationships with children and parents to support family involvement in each child's care" (p. 1757). Table 32.1 presents some hospital activities that may seem scary or stressful to a child and gives suggestions for preparing the child and family for these activities. Thoughtful preparation for these situations might relieve the associated stress. Educate children about what to expect so they can cope with their imagination and distinguish reality from fantasy. Describe the intervention and the sequence of steps that will occur, and include sensory information such as how the child will feel.

Good preparation can reduce the child's fears and increase his or her ability to cope with the hospital experience. Preparation should include exploring the child's perceptions, reviewing previous experiences, and identifying coping strategies. Useful techniques include:

- Practicing nursing care on stuffed animals or dolls and allowing the child to do the same
- Avoiding the use of medical terms
- Allowing the child to handle some equipment
- Teaching the child the steps of the procedure or informing him or her exactly what will happen during the hospital stay
- Showing the child the room where he or she will be staying
- Introducing the child to the health care personnel with whom he or she will come in contact
- Explaining the sounds the child may hear
- Letting the child sample the food that they will be served

TABLE 32.1 STRATEGIES TO REDUCE FEAR OF COMMON HOSPITALIZATION SITUATIONS

Situation	Strategies to Reduce Fear
Procedure involving intrusion into the body or use of equipment or technology	Describe the procedure and equipment in terms the child can understand. Review the steps of the procedure or steps involved with the use of the equipment. Explain what the child's role will be and what is or isn't allowed. If appropriate, have the child rehearse with the equipment or role play.
Darkness, such as with radiologic examinations or at night	Keep a light on in the examination area. Use a night light in the patient's room. If possible, allow the child to hold the caregiver's or nurse's hand or a favourite toy.
Transport to other areas of the hospital	Allow the caregiver to accompany the child if possible. Inform the child of where he or she is going, about how long he or she will be there and approximately when he or she will return. Introduce the child to the person who will be transporting the child.
Numerous personnel in and out of child's room	Identify all staff members working with the child (each shift and each day). Place a small board in the child's room with the name of the nurse caring for the child that shift or day. Inform the child how long the nurse will be caring for the child (adapt this information according to the child's cognitive level; for example, instead of saying that you'll be there for 8 hours, say, "I'll be your nurse until just before dinnertime" or "I'll be your nurse until you go for your test." Say good-bye to the child when leaving for the day; tell the child about his or her new nurse; inform the child of when you will return.

All hospital staff must share the responsibility of minimizing the stress and maximizing the coping abilities of the hospitalized child and his or her parents/ guardians (Sorensen, Card, Malley, & Strzelecki, 2009). All techniques used to prepare the child for hospitalization should emphasize the philosophy of atraumatic care. To help the child gain a better understanding of the coming procedure, provide a detailed explanation as well as a hands-on demonstration (Mansson & Dykes, 2004). Adapt all information to the cognitive and developmental level of the child. Identify what role the child will play in the situation; it is always helpful for children to have something to do, since it shows them that they are included. A rehearsal of what will occur in the hospital allows the child to become comfortable with the situation. If time permits, provide pamphlets that describe the procedure and suggest preparation activities for the child at home before admission.

The child and family may be able to take a tour of the hospital unit or the surgical facility. DVDs, photographs, and books on hospitalization and surgery can serve as resources for the family and child. Many institutions offer programs to familiarize children and families with the hospital experience (Fig. 32.3). Bloch and Toker (2008) conducted a study to examine the effects of the "teddy bear hospital" as a method to relieve the anxiety associated with hospitalization. Children attended a simulated hospital where they were given the opportunity to act as parents to their teddy bears, giving their bears a medical condition or illness of their own choosing. The results of this study showed significantly lower levels of anxiety in the group who participated in the "teddy bear hospital" experience (Bloch & Toker, 2008). Teddy bear hospitals have been utilized in several Canadian hospitals. As children "treat" and care for their teddy bears they internalize the feelings of love and care that nurses have for them when the nurses treat them.

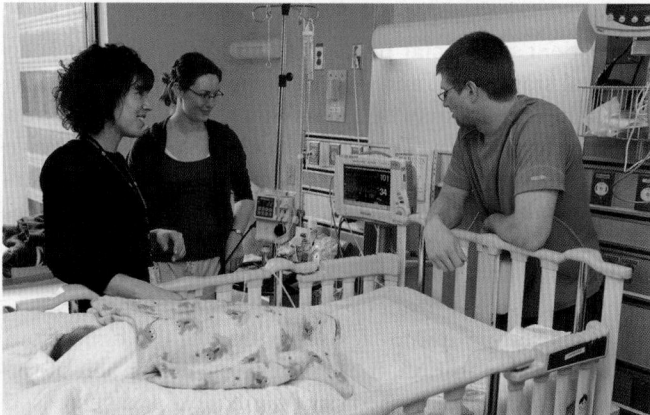

FIGURE 32.3 A nurse shows parents how the medical equipment works. It is important for children and parents to understand how medical equipment is used. (Courtesy of Stephen Wreakes.)

TEACHING GUIDELINE 32.1

Preparing Your Child for Hospitalization

- Read stories about experiences with hospital or surgery.
- Talk about going to the hospital and what it will be like coming home.
- Be honest and encourage your child to ask questions.
- Visit the hospital and go through the preadmission tour if time permits.
- Plan support to your child via your presence, telephone calls, and special items brought from home.
- Encourage your child to draw pictures to express how he or she is feeling.
- Include siblings in the preparation.

Parents are instrumental in preparing children by reviewing the materials that are given, answering questions, and being truthful and supportive. Teaching Guideline 32.1 provides suggestions for parents in preparing their child for hospitalization.

Admitting the Child to the Facility

Admitting the child to the facility involves preparing him or her for admission and introducing the child to the unit where he or she will be staying. Use the appropriate hospital forms. Chapter 2 gives general information about communicating with and teaching children and families.

In today's health care environment, the admission process occurs quickly, with little time for extensive preparation; this is why preparation before admission is so important. Of course, the urgency of the child's medical condition also may limit the amount of preparation that can be done in advance.

Types of Admissions and Nursing Care

The hospital units to which a child may be admitted include:

- General inpatient unit
- Emergency department
- PICU
- Outpatient or special procedures unit
- Rehabilitation unit or hospital

Regardless of the site of care, nursing care must begin by establishing a trusting, caring relationship with the child and family. Smile, introduce yourself, and give your title. Let the child and family know what will happen and what is expected of them. Ask the family and child what names they prefer to be called by. Maintain eye contact at the appropriate level. With a younger child, start with the family first so the child can see that the family trusts you. Communicate with children at age-appropriate levels.

The next step, as the child's medical condition allows, involves an orientation to the hospital unit. Briefly explain policies and routines and the personnel who will be involved in the care of the child.

During the nursing interview that follows, obtain information about the child's history, routines, and reason for admission. Obtain baseline vital signs, height and weight, and perform a physical assessment. Each health care setting has its own policies and procedures for this. Recognize the needs of the family and child during this process. If some of this information already exists, do not ask for it again, except to confirm vital information such as allergies, medications taken at home, and history of the illness. Typically, the information is collected immediately if the child's condition is urgent; otherwise, the information is collected within 8 hours, except for the information that is required for safe care.

General Inpatient Unit Stays

Today, general inpatient unit stays for children are shorter and involve more acute conditions, resulting in little time for admission preparation. Many times the admission procedure and treatment actually occur simultaneously. Sometimes the stay is in a special 23-hour observation unit so the child is in the setting for less than 24 hours. General hospital stays may be in a pediatric hospital, a pediatric unit in a general hospital, or a general unit that occasionally admits children. General units often lack child-oriented services, such as play areas, child-size equipment, and staff familiar with caring for children.

> ▶ *Take* NOTE!
>
> *When a child is admitted to a general unit, take extra time to orient and explain the routine and procedures to the child and family. Emphasize that the parents can stay with the child (if institutional policy permits). If possible, place the child in a room close to the nurses' station and order food appropriate for the child's age and developmental level.*

Emergency Departments

The number-one reason for illness and hospitalization in children is injuries from accidents. Many times a family's first experience with the acute care setting is the emergency department. Due to the situation, the child and family may experience increased anxiety, and it may become overwhelming as uncertainties develop and critical decisions must be made. The family may be frightened, insecure, and in a state of shock. Procedures and tests are performed quickly, with minimal time for preparation. The family is often ill prepared for the visit, having little money or clothing with them. Siblings may be present if the parents did not have time to get a sitter.

Due to the fast pace of the emergency department, the family may be hesitant to ask questions, so keep the family and child well informed. Allow the family to stay with the child, provide support, and allow the family, and when appropriate the child, to participate in decisions.

Families may have a strong fear of the unknown and may be terrified that the child will die or be permanently disabled. Help the family to identify their concerns and their support systems. Prepare them for what they will experience. Provide comfort such as holding, touching, talking softly, and other appropriate interventions according to age and developmental level.

Pediatric Intensive Care Units

The PICU specializes in caring for children in crisis. The same principles and concepts of general care of children apply to this setting, but everything is intensified. Families will be faced with an unfamiliar, high-tech environment and a large number of staff.

Families must deal with the critical situation that brought them to the PICU. The child will likely experience pain, unusual noises, and increased stimulation and will probably undergo uncomfortable procedures. Parents may face the possibility of losing their child. Sometimes the child cannot talk, eat, or display other appropriate developmental behaviours. **Sensory overload** (increased stimulation) or **sensory deprivation** (lack of stimulation) can affect both child and family.

Welcome families (if institutional policy permits) and encourage them to stay with the child and participate in care. Explain everything to the parents and, when appropriate, to the child. Frequently touch the child and encourage the parents to comfort him or her. Listen for clues about what the child and family need during the PICU stay.

Outpatient or Special Procedure Units

Outpatient or special procedure units are used to keep hospital stays short and decrease the cost of hospitalization. These units may be a part of a general hospital or a freestanding facility. Typically, the child and family arrive in the morning; the child has the procedure, test, or surgery and then goes home later that same day. Examples of surgeries performed in outpatient settings include tympanostomy tube placement, hernia repair, tonsillectomy, cystoscopy, bronchoscopy, and chemotherapy.

This setting minimizes separation of the child from the family. In addition, there is minimal disruption of the family pattern, a decreased risk of infection, and decreased cost. However, these units do not have the equipment for overnight stays, so if complications develop, the child will need to be transported to another facility or another area of the hospital.

Rehabilitation Units

The rehabilitation unit provides care for children beyond the initial period of illness or injury. The care involves an interdisciplinary approach that assists the child to reach his or her fullest potential and achieve developmental skills. For example, rehabilitation units help children regain abilities lost due to neurologic injuries or serious burns. The facilities often resemble a home environment, with special services to help children to relearn activities of daily living and to help them deal with the physical or mental challenges associated with the original illness or injury. Typically, families are encouraged to participate and are given support for their child's eventual return home. There is a balance of nurturing and firm discipline while the child reclaims independence.

Isolation Rooms

Isolation rooms are used for situations involving the risk for infection. When a child is admitted with an infectious disease, or to rule out an infectious disease, or if the child has impaired immune function, isolation will be instituted. Children in this setting may experience sensory deprivation due to the limited contact with others and the use of personal protective equipment such as gloves, masks, and gowns.

Encourage the family to visit often, and help them to understand the reason for the isolation and any special procedures that are required. Introduce yourself before entering the room and allow the child to view your face before applying a mask. Continue to have contact with the child and hold or touch the child often, especially if the parents are not present.

Preparing the Child and Family for Surgery

If the child is to undergo a surgical procedure, whether in the hospital or an outpatient setting, special interventions are necessary. The parents should be allowed to stay with the child until surgery begins. Parents should also be allowed to be with the child when he or she wakes up in the post-anaesthesia recovery area. A child life specialist (CLS) is invaluable in providing support to children and families as they prepare for surgery. (See Child Life Specialist section.) If available, the expert services of a CLS should be initiated as soon as possible, preferably before surgery. Collaboration between the nurse and the CLS is important in order to provide the CLS with accurate medical insight (Sorensen et al., 2009). If the assistance of a CLS is not available, the nurse can provide developmentally appropriate support, education, and resources based on the principles of family-centred care.

Preoperative Care

Preoperative care for the child who is to undergo surgery is similar to that for an adult. The major difference is that the

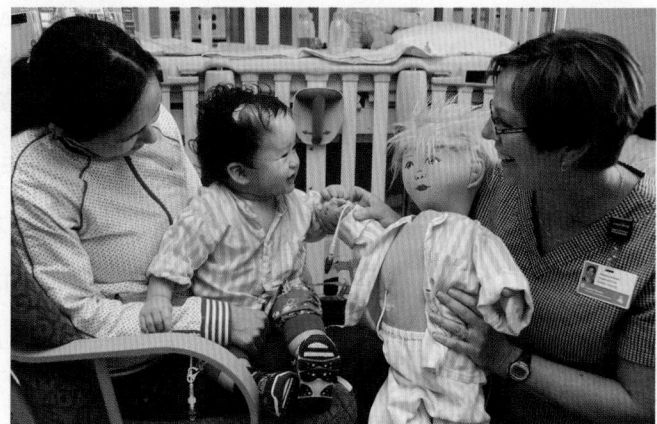

FIGURE 32.4 Dolls can be used to help children cope with the fear and anxiety of hospitalization. (Courtesy of Stephen Wreakes.)

preparation and teaching must be geared to the child's age and developmental level. Many facilities offer special programs to help prepare children and families for the surgical experience. Presurgical preparation programs allow children and their families to experience a "trial run" in a supportive environment to reduce anxiety, increase knowledge, and enhance coping skills (Justus et al., 2006).

Child and family teaching is essential. Like any intervention, adapt the teaching to the child's developmental level. Table 32.2 highlights key teaching strategies to reduce fear and anxiety in common hospitalization situations based on the child's developmental level. For example, when teaching a toddler or preschooler about breathing exercises, have the child blow a pinwheel or cotton balls across the table through a straw. The child can enjoy the activity while also reaping the respiratory benefits of the activity.

In preparation for surgery, use items such as stuffed animals or dolls to help children understand what is going to happen to them (Fig. 32.4). Allow the child to role-play various experiences with dolls. Dolls designed to simulate surgical experiences have been developed. For example, Shadow Buddies are custom-made dolls that have the same illness or surgery as the child; the doll may have an ostomy, scar, or catheter. The dolls were developed to help children cope with their illness or disease and send the message that it is okay to be different. These dolls also provide the child with a companion to talk to. Refer to http://thePoint.lww.com/Chow1e for a direct link to the Shadow Buddies' website.

Intraoperative Care

A major controversy is whether parents should be present during anaesthesia induction. Proponents argue that the presence of a parent during anaesthesia induction is comforting, so the child can remain calm and experience a decreased anxiety level, which in turn decreases

TABLE 32.2 COMMON HOSPITALIZATION-RELATED FEARS ACCORDING TO DEVELOPMENTAL LEVEL

Developmental Level	Common Fears/Anxieties	Implications for Teaching
Infants and toddlers	Separation	Remind parents to use positive facial expressions. Encourage the parent or caregiver to stay with the child as much as possible. Urge the parent or caregiver to use stroking or secure, comfortable holding positions to promote calm. Talk to the child and parents using a soft, comforting tone of voice with the parent or caregiver holding the child. Use terms that the child and parents can understand.
Preschoolers and school-age children	Pain Mutilation Separation Possible punishment for wrongdoings	Provide factual explanations using terms the child and parents can understand. Incorporate pictures and other visual aids in explanation. Allow time for children to play out their concerns and fears. Tailor the timing of education to meet the child's learning needs, allowing enough time for the child to ask questions. For toddlers, provide information as close to the day of surgery as possible to prevent undue anxiety. Some recommend that information be provided no more than 1 week beforehand (Justus et al., 2006).
Adolescents	Loss of independence Effects on body image	Acknowledge the adolescent's right to privacy. Allow as much independence as possible within the constraints of the diagnosis. Provide detailed explanations of the procedure at least 7 to 10 days beforehand. Answer questions honestly, ensuring privacy at all times. Remain available for questions or concerns arising before or after surgery.

catecholamine release and increases oxygenation. As a result, adverse effects such as breath-holding laryngospasm and long-term psychological effects are diminished (Romino et al., 2005). However, parents must receive thorough preparation; inadequate preparation increases the parents' anxiety, and children experience greater anxiety if accompanied by an anxious parent (Munro & D'Errico, 2000).

Studies have shown that being present at anaesthesia induction can also benefit parents. Parents experience high levels of stress when separated from their child during surgery, and allowing parents to be present for anaesthesia induction can decrease this stress (Romino et al., 2005).

Postoperative Care

Postoperative nursing care for a child is similar to that for an adult. However, due to anatomic differences, frequent, astute observation is a must. Assessment of the child's airway, breathing, and circulation is key. The surgical site is inspected and fluids and hydration are administered. If possible, allow parents to be present in the post-anaesthesia care unit as soon as possible to provide the child with support and a familiar face.

Pain management is crucial. Use an appropriate pain assessment tool to rate the child's pain. Frequently reassess the child's pain, and use atraumatic care. Expect to administer pharmacologic agents as ordered. Also encourage the use of non-pharmacologic methods. A research study (Huth, Broome, & Good, 2004) showed that distraction techniques such as guided imagery helped children cope with tonsillectomy and adenoidectomy pain. The children who received an educational program about imagery reported less sensory pain, distress, and anxiety while in the outpatient surgery unit, but no differences were found in the reports of pain at home or use of pain medications.

Maintaining Safety During Hospitalization

Safety is a critical aspect of care of the child in the hospital. Due to their age and developmental level, children are vulnerable to harm. Ensure the child has an identification band in place at all times. Sometimes in implementing interventions an armband is removed, so make sure it is attached to another extremity. Monitor children closely to avoid accidents such as a child pushing the wrong knob or picking up a piece of equipment or supplies left in the bed or room. Table 32.3 provides

TABLE 32.3 NURSING CONSIDERATIONS FOR PROVIDING SAFE, DEVELOPMENTALLY APPROPRIATE CARE

	Ensuring Safety	Promoting Healthy Growth and Development
Infants	• Maintain close supervision of the infant. • Keep one hand on the infant when crib sides are down. • Keep crib rails up all the way when the infant is in the crib. • Avoid leaving small objects that are harmful or that can be swallowed in the crib. • Avoid entanglement or strangulation by medical tubing. • Provide safe and appropriate toys for the infant. • Place infants in rooms close to the nurses' station. • Encourage a family member to stay with the infant at all times.	• Use the *en face* position when holding newborns. • Smile and talk to the infant during bathing, feeding, and other interactions. • Minimize the number of painful or uncomfortable procedures. • Provide comfort during and after procedures by holding or talking, using soothing tones and movements. • When handling the infant, use smooth, continuous movements. • Use gentle stroking and holding, which may reduce stress. • Use tube stabilizers on all medical tubing (e.g., intravenous lines, monitor lines, feeding tubes, oxygen tubing; Garros, King, Brady-Fryer, & Klassen, 2003). • Serve as a role model for first-time parents. • Encourage the family to maintain home routines while in hospital, planning nursing care around the usual feeding and sleep times. • Use the pacifier between feedings to satisfy non-nutritive sucking needs.
Toddlers	• Keep crib side rails up with overhead crib protection intact when the toddler is in the crib. • Never leave toddler alone in the room unless secured in the crib. • Use a bed only for the older toddler who has an adult present in the room at all times. • Avoid leaving small objects than can be swallowed or are harmful in the crib or bed. • Place crib out of reach of cords, equipment, and electrical outlets. • Provide safe and appropriate toys for the toddler. • Avoid entanglement or strangulation by medical tubing. • Always have someone with the toddler when ambulating.	• Encourage the parent to stay with the toddler to decrease separation anxiety. • To promote autonomy, allow the toddler to make appropriate choices, such as which juice to take the medicine with. • Written consent may be required when a toddler sleeps in a bed rather than a crib. Consent policies may vary according to hospital. • Encourage active play in the playroom or with push/pull toys in the hallway (accompanied by an adult). • Expect and plan for regression in areas of toilet training, eating, and other behaviours. • Expect increased temper tantrums in general and intense reactions to intrusive procedures. • Maintain home routine while in hospital, planning nursing care around the usual feeding and sleep times. • Give simple directions with choices appropriate to the hospital situation. • Place toddlers in rooms close to the nurses' station. • Use tube stabilizers on all medical tubing (e.g., intravenous lines, monitor lines, feeding tubes, oxygen tubing Garros et al., 2003). • Provide close supervision while encouraging independence.
Preschoolers	• Keep bed in low position with the side rails up when the preschooler is in the bed. • Instruct the child to call the nurse or caregiver for help getting out of bed. • Keep harmful objects out of reach of the child.	• Encourage parents to stay with the preschooler in the room as well as other areas of the hospital. • Encourage the preschooler to be involved in care by providing choices and opportunities for the child to help. • Use play as an opportunity to work through the preschooler's fears. • Explain activities in simple, concrete terms, being cautious with language you use because of the preschooler's fantasies and magical thinking. • Expect reactions to pain and bodily injury to be verbally aggressive and specific. • Try to maintain home routines while the child is in the hospital, working them into the plan of care when possible.

(continued)

TABLE 32.3 NURSING CONSIDERATIONS FOR PROVIDING SAFE, DEVELOPMENTALLY APPROPRIATE CARE (continued)

	Ensuring Safety	Promoting Healthy Growth and Development
School-agers	• Keep the bed in the low position with the side rails up while the child is in the bed, explaining that this is a hospital rule, not a punishment.	• Provide opportunities for the child to be involved in care. • Allow children to select their meals, assist with treatments, and keep their rooms neat. • Allow visits with other children if condition allows. • Encourage parents to tell the child when they will return. • Plan care around the child's usual home routines (meals, sleep). • Encourage the child to do schoolwork.
Adolescents	• Be aware of the adolescent's whereabouts. The teen may not wish to stay in the room but may become confused about where the room or unit is located in the hospital.	• Allow teens to interact with others. • Alter hospital routines as possible to allow the teen to sleep in or stay up later at night. • Provide others close to their age as roommates. • Encourage visits from friends. • Provide emotional support for feelings of being alone or away from friends; be alert for regression, which may result in the teen becoming emotional. • Answer questions honestly and with appropriate information. • Give the teen a sense of control by allowing choices. • Be sensitive to concerns about being "different."

nursing goals for ensuring safe, developmentally appropriate care for the hospitalized child. Make sure the crib is checked for loose items after a treatment or procedure, particularly sharp items such as needles or blades. Children can choke on small items such as small plastic caps that are inadvertently left in a crib or bed following a procedure.

Use of Restraints

When caring for children, some type of physical restriction may be necessary. The restriction, often referred to as a restraint, may be needed to ensure the child's safety, allow for a therapeutic or diagnostic procedure to be done, immobilize a body part or limit movement, or prevent disruption of prescribed therapy. However, restraints can be overused and can cause harm to the patient (Joint Commission Resources, 2008):

• Children can potentially be traumatized if they are restrained by adults in health care settings. Restrictive holds should be viewed as a last resort only when all other non-invasive approaches have been utilized. Comforting positions and holds can be taught to support children when a procedure must be done to further medical care (personal communication, Lois Wolgemuth, Certified Child Life Specialist, March 25, 2010).
• The best policy is one of "least restraint," in which a staff member utilizes all possible appropriate alternative interventions before deciding to use a restraint.

▶ **Take** NOTE!

Restraints can promote physical distress in a child. Children also may view restraints as punishment. When determining the need for restraining a child, the nurse needs to consider the child's age, developmental level, mental status, and threat to others and self. Applying the principles of atraumatic care, the nurse uses a restraint only when necessary and for the shortest time possible.

Before a restraint is used, other measures need to be tried. Explain why the child should not touch the intravenous site or should maintain a certain position so that the child has a basic understanding of what is necessary. This may be all that is necessary for an older child. See Figure 32.5 and Evidence-based Practice 32.1.

Therapeutic hugging (use of a holding position that promotes close physical contact between the child and a parent or caregiver) may be used for certain procedures or treatments where the child must remain still. For example, the parent can hold the child in his or her lap snugly to prevent the child from moving during an injection or venipuncture. This technique may be used to position a child for intravenous access, injections, an otoscopic examination, or a lumbar puncture. When using this technique, make sure the parent understands his or her role and knows which body parts to hold still in a safe manner.

EVIDENCE-BASED PRACTICE 32.1
Preventing Entanglement and Strangulation by Intravenous Tubing in the Hospitalized Child

Young children are at greater risk (than adults) for occlusion of their airways. Intravenous (IV) tubing presents a risk for entanglement and strangulation in children between the ages of 6 and 36 months. Interventions to prevent this risk include ongoing assessment of the need for continuous IV infusions, supervision based on the developmental requirements of the child, and modifications to the IV equipment itself.

● Case Reports
Pediatric specialists in one large Canadian children's hospital reported two cases of entanglement and strangulation with IV tubing, one of which resulted in a fatality.

Case One
An 11-month-old boy with a history of prematurity and mild respiratory distress syndrome was admitted to the hospital for pneumonia and dehydration requiring IV fluids and antibiotics. He was an active child who could roll, sit, and pull himself to a standing position in his crib. It was noted by his parents and the nursing staff that he became entangled in his IV lines on three or four occasions, with the lines usually encircling his abdomen or legs. Shortly before discharge and only 45 minutes after the most recent check by the nursing staff, he was found with the IV tubing wrapped around his neck three times; he was apnoeic and pulseless. Although the child was initially resuscitated, he was later removed from life support. Upon examination, erythematous marks consistent with strangulation were found around the child's neck.

Case Two
An 8.5-month-old boy was admitted to the hospital for a serious infection requiring percutaneous insertion of a central catheter line for the administration of antibiotics. Five minutes after being observed by the nursing staff, the child was found sitting in his crib, head forward, with his IV tubing wrapped tightly twice around his neck; he was pulseless and apnoeic. The child received full cardiopulmonary resuscitation with intubation, during which he experienced two generalized clonic seizures. He eventually made an uneventful recovery, but neuropsychological testing 2 weeks after the event revealed a mild cognitive and motor delay.

▲ Results
These two cases are the first to describe strangulation by IV tubing and require a proactive preventive response. A primary prevention strategy identified by the investigators in this report was the necessity to reduce the flexibility of the IV tubing. A Canadian entrepreneur developed a rigid, clear plastic sleeve that may be used to enclose the exposed portions of the IV tubing along with any other medical tubing or wires. The secondary prevention strategy identified in this report is the need for careful evaluation by the bedside nurse of the risk factors for entanglement. As a result of this report, changes were made to the policies at this Canadian hospital requiring tubing stabilizer devices to be used on all tubing or wiring for children between 6 and 36 months of age.

■ Nursing Implications
It is the responsibility of the bedside nurse to assess the risk of entanglement for each patient. Some children over the age of 36 months may also require tubing stabilizers to prevent injury, particularly if the older child does not have the cognitive ability to untangle him- or herself. The bedside nurse must also carefully document the use of tubing stabilizers as well as any adverse events involving entanglement of any kind.

The bedside nurse also needs to assess the need for continuous IV therapy. Is it possible to have intermittent IV access using a locking device when the IV is not infusing? Careful assessment and monitoring of any child with IV lines or other medical tubing is crucial to prevent entanglement and/or strangulation. Other sources of entanglement include oxygen tubing, monitoring wires, and feeding tubes.

Garros, D., King, J., Brady-Fryer, B., & Klassen, T. (2003). Strangulation with intravenous tubing: A previously undescribed adverse advent in children. *Pediatrics, 111*(6), 732–734.

Alternatively, distraction or stimulation (such as with a toy) can help to gain the child's cooperation. This is a good opportunity to collaborate with the CLS and utilize his or her expertise in this area. One-to-one supervision and behaviour modification techniques may be other alternatives to the use of restraints.

If it is determined that the child requires a restraint, select the most appropriate, least restrictive type of restraint (Disability Rights California, 2008). For example, if the child has an intravenous catheter in the antecubital space that stops flowing when the child bends the arm, an elbow restraint or arm board would be appropriate. With the elbow restraint or arm board, the child's arm flexion is restricted yet he or she can still move the shoulder and hands. Ensure that arm boards used to stabilize intravenous sites are secured with a minimal amount of tape; netting and gauze are better choices. Ask parents if the child has sensitivity to tape. Table 32.4 presents various types of restraints and the potential dangers associated with them. See also Figure 32.6.

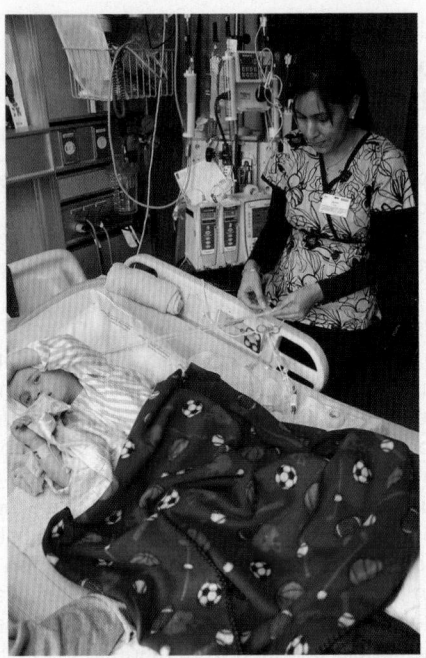

FIGURE 32.5 The use of rigid plastic sleeves on intravenous tubing reduces the risk of entanglement and strangulation. (Courtesy of Stephen Wreakes.)

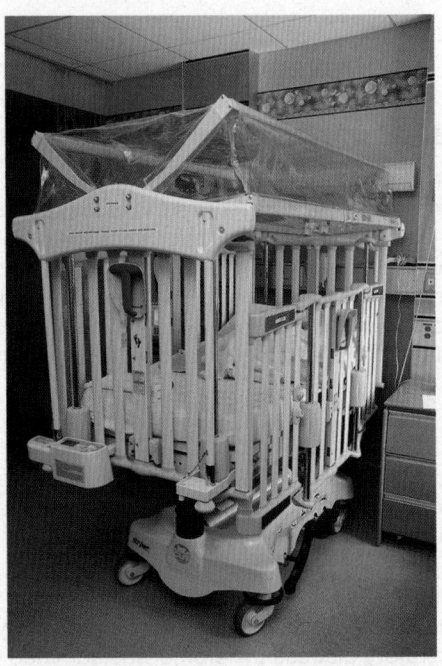

FIGURE 32.6 A bubble crib is used to keep a child from climbing out of the crib. (Courtesy of Stephen Wreakes.)

TABLE 32.4 TYPES OF RESTRAINTS AND ASSOCIATED SAFETY CONCERNS

Type of Restraint	Purpose	Safety Concerns
Clove hitch restraint	Wrist or ankle restraint to prevent range of motion of extremities	Check wrist or ankle for any sign of circulatory, integumentary, or neurologic compromise.
Elbow restraint	Prevents child from flexing and reaching face, head, IV and other tubes	Position the restraint so it does not rub against axilla. Check pulse, temperature, and capillary refill of the extremity.
Mummy restraint	Body restraint using a sheet folded in a square appropriate to size of infant or young child to secure the whole body of the child or every extremity except for one	Ensure that all extremities are secured within the sheet.
Jacket (vest) restraint	Jacket worn by child with ties attached to the child's back and to side of bed or chair. Used to keep children flat in bed, such as after surgery, or safe and comfortable in a chair.	Ensure the child can turn head to side and that the head of the bed is elevated. Place ties in back so child cannot manipulate them.
Crib top bubble restraint (Fig. 32.6)	Clear plastic cover over the bed to prevent older infant or young child from falling and climbing out of bed	Ensure that there are no tears or loose plastic.
Specially designed chairs/carts	Chairs/carts with tables or other devices to hold child in specific positions during transport or to prevent child from getting out of device	May need to use a vest or jacket restraints to help keep child in chair/cart. Never leave child unattended. Lock the wheels if the chair/cart is stationary.

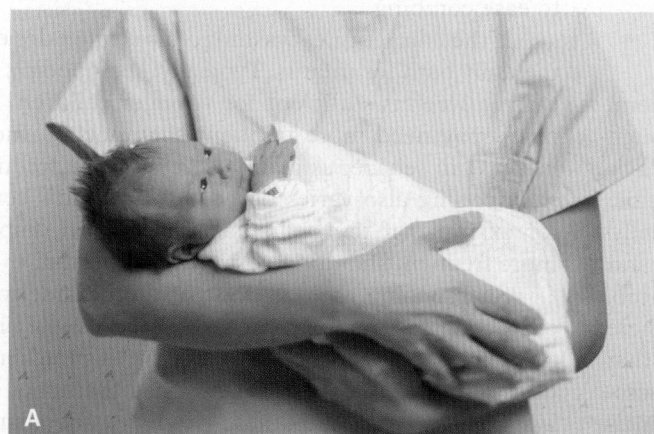
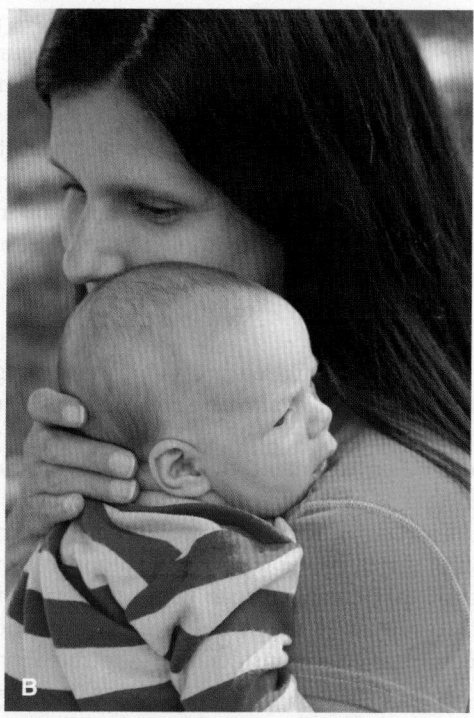

FIGURE 32.7 Methods for transporting the infant. (**A**) Cradle method for carrying infants up to 3 months of age. One hand grasps the infant's thighs; the other arm supports the infant's head and back. (**B**) The "over-the-shoulder method" for carrying infants up to 7 months of age. Support the head if the infant does not have head control.

▶ *Take* NOTE!

When selecting a restraint, the nurse must choose the least restrictive type of restraint and apply it for the shortest time necessary (Department of Health & Human Services, Centers for Medicare & Medicaid Services, 2006).

Before applying a restraint, explain the reason for the restraint to the child and the parents. Emphasize that the rationale is to maintain the child's safety; the restraint is not punishment. Having the child and parents state the reason for the restraint demonstrates their understanding.

Transport of the Child

Children may need to be transported to other units for diagnostic tests or surgery, to different areas in the same unit, such as the playroom or treatment room, or for discharge. When the child is transported to other areas, specific guidelines need to address safety issues, the age and developmental level of the child, the child's physical condition, and the destination. These factors need to be considered before transport so that the appropriate method can be used with the least amount of risk for the child. Various methods to transport children include carrying the infant and using strollers, wagons, or rolling beds

(Fig. 32.7). If possible, the parents should accompany the child to offer support and comfort.

When carrying an infant, good support of the back and head is vital. Rails should be up on all beds and wagons during transport. Use safety belts with strollers and wheelchairs.

▶ *Take* NOTE!

Never leave a child unattended during transport. Keep the child visible at all times during the transport.

Providing Basic Care for the Hospitalized Child

Basic care involves general hygiene measures, including bathing, hair care, oral care, and nutritional care. Young children are dependent on an adult for most, if not all, of their self-care needs. If parents are present, allow them to provide care for the child to decrease the child's stress. Older children may perform hygiene measures themselves but may need some assistance from the nurse.

General Hygiene Measures

General hygiene measures help to maintain healthy skin, hair, and teeth. Skin is a complex structure; its primary function is to protect the tissues that it encloses and to protect itself. Injury to the child's skin may occur when inserting and maintaining an intravenous line, removing a dressing, positioning a child in bed, changing a diaper, using and removing electrode patches, and maintaining restraints. Risk factors for potential problems include impaired mobility, protein malnutrition, edema, incontinence, sensory loss, anemia, and infection. A good time to assess the skin is during bath time.

Bathing

Bathing infants and children is a common daily general hygiene measure in the health care environment. Although a parent or primary caregiver often does this in today's family-centred environment, the nurse is still responsible for ensuring that bathing is done safely and hygienically. Adhere to safety principles to prevent falls, burns, and aspiration of water. Never leave a child alone in a bathtub. Use a gentle, pH-balanced soap with moisturizer if there is a need to rehydrate the skin. Note any condition that might require special considerations or further assessment, such as paralysis, loss of sensation, surgical incisions, skin traction/cast, external lines (intravenous lines, urinary catheters, or feeding tubes), or other alterations in skin integrity. Pay close attention to the ears, between skinfolds, the neck, the back, and the genital area for potential alterations in skin integrity. Table 32.5 highlights specific developmental considerations for bathing.

Before bathing and performing other hygiene measures, assess the family's preferences and home practices for the child, such as time of day, rituals, special equipment, and allergies to products. This is a good time to assess the amount of assistance that might be required by the parents and to address learning needs related to

TABLE 32.5 DEVELOPMENTAL CONSIDERATIONS FOR BATHING

Age of Child	Special Considerations
Infants	Use a sponge bath or tub bath to bathe young infants who cannot sit unaided. Support the infant's body at all times. Ensure appropriate water temperature. Avoid use of talcum powder.
Toddlers and preschoolers	Bathe older infants, toddlers and preschoolers at the bedside or in a regular bathtub, depending on their health condition.
School-age children and adolescents	Older children may prefer a shower if available and acceptable for their health condition. Assess whether a shower would be safe. Provide privacy.

hygiene. Follow general guidelines in bathing any patient with regard to equipment, room temperature, privacy, and use of products such as deodorant and lotion.

Hair Care

Lying in bed can make the hair matted and tangled. Avoid pulling on the child's hair when combing or brushing it. If necessary, use commercial detangling solutions to ease combing.

If the hair requires washing, this is often done during the daily bath for infants. Typically, shampooing once or twice a week is sufficient for younger children. Adolescents may need more frequent shampooing due to the increase in sebaceous gland secretion. The frequency of shampooing also varies based on the child's condition; for example, if the child has experienced diaphoresis, more frequent shampooing may be indicated.

Shampooing may be done at the bedside with specially adapted equipment, at a readily accessible sink while the child is sitting in a chair or lying on a stretcher, or in a tub or shower. Commercial no-rinse shampoos may be available for use. With these products, the shampoo is applied to the hair and then brushed or combed out.

If the child uses a tub or shower for hair care, monitor the child's safety throughout to ensure that the child does not slip and fall due to the slippery surface or is not burned due to improper water temperature.

Oral Hygiene

Oral hygiene is an important part of basic care. Wipe the infant's gums with a wet cloth after each feeding. Assist children in brushing and flossing their teeth after each feeding or meal and before bedtime. The child who is immunosuppressed needs special attention to oral hygiene, such as using soft toothbrushes and moistened gauze sponges to prevent bleeding and careful inspection of the oral cavity for areas of breakdown.

Nutritional Care

Adequate nutrition is necessary for growth and development and tissue repair, so it is an essential component of care for the ill or hospitalized child.

Frequently, the ill or hospitalized child experiences a loss of appetite, which can affect the child's nutritional status. This may be compounded by other problems such as nausea and vomiting and NPO restrictions for testing or surgery.

▶ *Take* NOTE!

Never attempt to force a child to eat. This can exacerbate nausea and vomiting and can lead to an aversion to food that extends past the hospital stay (Hockenberry, 2009).

TEACHING GUIDELINE 32.2

Promoting Nutrition for Your Hospitalized Child

- Check with the nurse about any restrictions related to your child's diet. Find out if intake and output are being monitored.
- Encourage your child to eat favourite foods.
- Assist your child with eating or drinking as necessary; be present at mealtimes to help promote socialization.
- Frequently offer small cups of fluid and finger foods; avoid giving large quantities at one time.
- Try offering fluids at different temperatures at different times to promote variety.
- Remember that children can ingest greater amounts of thin liquids (e.g., gelatine or carbonated drinks) than thicker liquids (e.g., cream soups or milkshakes).
- Include ice chips as fluid intake. Ice is approximately equivalent to half the same amount of water (e.g., 1 cup of ice [250 mL] equals a half-cup [125 mL] of water).
- Use straws (unless not allowed) and brightly coloured utensils, cups, or dishes to provide contrast and stimulation.
- Offer the child choices; when using a menu, allow the child to choose what he or she wants.
- Avoid spicy or highly seasoned foods.
- Talk with the dietician to see if any special preferences can be addressed.
- Offer praise to your child for what he or she eats or drinks.
- Never punish the child for not eating or drinking.
- Encourage the older child to help keep track of what he or she eats and drinks.

If possible, schedule procedures or treatments away from mealtimes. In younger children, refusing to eat may be related to the child's feeling of separation; in others, refusing to eat reflects the child's attempt to control the situation. Encourage parents to use gentle persuasion instead of force to assist with intake. They should give the child choices about what to eat; this reinforces the child's sense of control. Remind parents that the child's appetite will probably improve as his or her condition improves. Teaching Guideline 32.2 provides some tips for promoting nutrition in the hospitalized child. Although geared to parents, nurses also can incorporate these guidelines into the child's plan of care.

Developmentally Appropriate Approaches to Nursing Care

When addressing the fears, separation anxiety, and loss of control that occur in hospitalized children, the nurse should consider the child's age and cognitive or developmental level. Interventions are then based on how the child experiences these stressors at that age or developmental level. The content, timing, setting, and method of preparation are also based on the child's age and cognitive or developmental level. General guidelines for addressing fear and anxiety, separation anxiety, and loss of control are provided in Box 32.3.

Newborns and Infants

Assess the development or lack of development that is occurring in the infant, and assess the baby's attachment to the parents or primary caregivers. The infant's facial expression is the most consistent indicator of pain or bodily injury. To decrease fear and minimize separation anxiety, avoid separation from the primary caregiver if possible; this will also promote healthy attachment. If the parent or primary caregiver cannot stay with the infant,

---

BOX 32.3 **Guidelines to Address the General Effects of Hospitalization**

Minimizing Fear and Anxiety
- Know the developmental stages in which magical thinking occurs.
- Explain everything to children and their families before it occurs (see Chapter 34).
- Use age-appropriate communication techniques. Include the family in this process so they can help the child cope with these fears.

Addressing/Minimizing Separation Anxiety
- Know the stages of separation anxiety and be able to recognize them.
- Remember that behaviours demonstrated during the first stage do not indicate that the child is "bad."
- Encourage the family to stay with the child.
- Help the child cope, and intervene before the behaviours of detachment occur.
- Try guided imagery, using the child's imagination and enjoyment of play, to help the child relax (Bricher, 2000).

Addressing Loss of Control
- Minimize physical restrictions, altered routines and rituals, and dependency issues, because they produce loss of control.
- Recognize the child's inherent powerlessness in the hospital setting and explore strategies that give children an opportunity to participate in their own health care decisions (Bricher, 2000).

arrange for volunteers to provide consistent comfort to the baby.

Maintaining the infant's home routine related to sleep and feeding helps decrease feelings of loss of control. Weigh the infant daily, at the same time, on the same scale. Monitor intake and output closely. Be alert to signs of discomfort other than crying, such as a furrowed brow or tense body posture. Additional nursing goals related to promoting infant growth and development are presented in Table 32.3.

Toddlers

Key nursing concerns when caring for toddlers center on separation anxiety, adequate growth and development, and autonomy. Establishing a trusting relationship with the toddler through nonthreatening play may decrease the amount of fear the toddler feels. Be alert to subtle, nonverbal indicators of grief or discontent.

▶ **Take** NOTE!

Keep the bed or crib and playroom as "safe" places. Perform invasive procedures such as venipuncture in the treatment room if possible. Never perform any nursing interventions in the playroom, no matter how nonthreatening they may appear to the nurse (Leahy et al., 2008).

Encourage the parent or primary caregiver to stay with the toddler in the hospital to decrease separation anxiety. Maintaining the home routine related to meals and sleep or a nap provides similar structure and may help decrease the toddler's feelings of loss of control. If indicated, weigh the toddler daily. Closely monitor intake and output. Refer to Table 32.3 for additional nursing considerations related to promoting growth and development in the hospitalized toddler.

Preschoolers

Nursing care for the hospitalized preschooler focuses on their special needs, fears, and fantasies. When working with preschoolers, remember that they use magical thinking and fantasy. Be honest and specific, providing information just prior to the intervention to allay the child's fears. As with toddlers, encouraging parental involvement may decrease the amount of separation anxiety the preschooler experiences while in the hospital. Allowing the preschooler to make simple decisions such as which colour bandage to use or whether to take medicine from a cup or syringe helps the child to feel some sense of control. Table 32.3 gives specific nursing considerations related to promoting growth and development for the preschooler in the hospital.

School-Age Children

Provide honest information using concrete, meaningful words to the school-age child to minimize fear of the unknown. School-age children are still very attached to their parents, so encouraging parental involvement or rooming-in decreases separation anxiety. Involve the child in making simple decisions and planning the schedule as appropriate to give him or her a sense of control. Nursing considerations when caring for hospitalized school-age children include ensuring safety and promoting growth and development (see Table 32.3).

Adolescents

The adolescent may or may not express fears. Educate the teen honestly: younger teens require more concrete explanations, while older teens can process more abstract concepts. Respect the teen's need for privacy. Encourage visits from the adolescent's friends to minimize anxiety related to separation. Prepare a mutually agreeable schedule with the teen, as appropriate, that includes the teen's preferences while incorporating the required nursing care. Collaborating with the adolescent will provide the teen with increased control. Refer to Table 32.3 for additional nursing considerations related to care of the adolescent in the hospital.

Think back to Jake, the 8-year-old from the beginning of the chapter. Discuss nursing care you could provide that will help minimize stressors.

Providing Play, Activities, and Recreation for the Hospitalized Child

Play is an important component in the child's plan of care. Today many health care settings providing care for children have playrooms with age-appropriate toys, equipment, and other creative activities (Fig. 32.8). If the facility

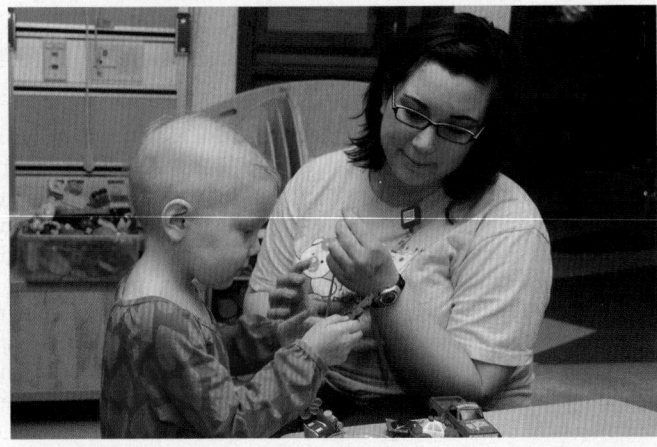

FIGURE 32.8 A child occupied in a hospital playroom. (Courtesy of Stephen Wreakes.)

is large enough, there may even be a separate area for teens where they can listen to music, play video games, and visit with peers. Obviously, some children will not be able to use these facilities if their activity level is restricted or if isolation is necessary. Children may also play in their rooms. Ensure that opportunities for unstructured play are provided to all children who can engage in play. Therapeutic play may be used to teach children about their health status or to allow them to work through issues in their lives.

> ▶ *Take* NOTE!
>
> *Avoid using the term "playroom" when caring for older school-age children and adolescents. Instead, call it the "activity room" or "social room." Doing so promotes a greater feeling of maturity and makes it more likely that they will use the area.*

Child Life Specialist

The **child life specialist** is a specially trained individual who provides programs that prepare children for hospitalization, surgery, and other procedures that could be painful (Child Life Council, 2010–2011). The CLS is a member of the multidisciplinary team and works in conjunction with the health care providers and parents to foster an atmosphere that promotes the child's well-being. Services provided by a CLS include:

- Nonmedical preparation for tests, surgeries, and other medical procedures
- Support during medical procedures
- Therapeutic play
- Activities to support normal growth and development
- Sibling support
- Grief and bereavement support
- Emergency room interventions for children and families
- Hospital preadmission tours and information programs
- Outpatient consultation with families (Child Life Council, 2010–2011)

When CLSs are part of the multidisciplinary team, they should be introduced to the child as early as possible. It is imperative that the CLS develops a trusting relationship with the child in order to provide the most effective care. Nurses need to be educated about the services and qualifications of the CLS and participate in collaboration.

Unstructured Play

Unstructured play allows children to control events, ideas, and relationships. Encourage parents to bring small toys and favourite stuffed animals from home to make the child feel more comfortable in the strange environment of the hospital. Children also enjoy receiving small new toys as surprises when they are hospitalized. Many children enjoy diversional activities such as playing board games or electronic games, reading books, and watching TV or DVDs. Quiet activities appropriate to the developmental level of the child provide the opportunity for play and encourage the use and development of fine motor skills even if the child is confined to bed. Infants and toddlers enjoy manipulating blocks and playing with stacking toys. The preschooler may enjoy colouring, dollhouses, or playing with plastic building blocks such as Legos. School-age children and adolescents may enjoy playing video games or building a model geared toward their developmental level.

Play as Part of Nursing Care

Play is also an important part of nursing care. Use play as appropriate while providing routine nursing care to the child (Fig. 32.9). An example of the use of play in nursing care involves the school-age child's love of competition and games. To increase range of motion in a school-age child who is hospitalized for traction due to a fracture, have the child throw a soft sponge ball or beanbag ball into hoops, and compete against the child. To increase deep breathing, encourage the child to blow bubbles or blow a whistle. To increase intake of fluids, help the child create a graph to chart the number of glasses of fluids he or she drinks over a period of time. Award the child a sticker, baseball card, special pencil, or other small item if he or she reaches a certain level.

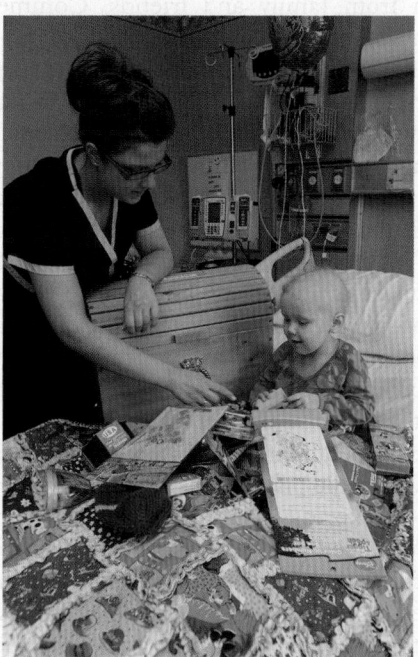

FIGURE 32.9 The nurse plays with the child and helps the child work through her feelings about being hospitalized. (Courtesy of Stephen Wreakes.)

When using play as part of nursing care, it is important to evaluate the outcome of play. Play used in the manner described above should enhance the child's outcome. For example, for the child blowing bubbles, determine whether this activity enhanced coughing and deep breathing.

Therapeutic Play

WATCH & LEARN

Another important aspect of play is **therapeutic play**. Health care professionals use therapeutic play to help the child deal with the physical and psychological challenges associated with illness and hospitalization. Therapeutic play is nondirected and focuses on helping the child cope with his or her feelings and fears. This type of play places greater emphasis on the developmental and psychosocial implications of illness and hospitalization and validation of the child's voice (Bricher, 2000). Supervised play with medical equipment in the hospital environment can help children work thorough their feelings about what has happened to them. In a hospital that is large enough or that is a children's hospital, the CLS typically coordinates these activities. Goals include maintaining normal living patterns, minimizing psychological trauma, and promoting optimal development of the child. If a CLS is not available at the facility, the nurse provides this type of activity.

In emotional outlet play or traumatic play, the child acts out or dramatizes real-life stressors. For example, using a wooden hammer and pegs, a soft sponge ball, or boxing gloves can allow the child to express anger over separation from family and friends. Commercial toys such as anatomically correct dolls and puppets have removable parts so children can see various organs of the body. Sometimes younger children "talk" to puppets and dolls, allowing them to express their feelings to a nonthreatening "person" about a specific situation or what they want from the health care provider. For example, the Shadow Buddies dolls mentioned earlier in the chapter provide a way of coping with a specific condition. For example, there is an ostomy buddy who has a stoma, a cancer buddy with thinning hair and a chest catheter for chemotherapy treatments, and a heart buddy who has a chest incision and a repaired heart. If the child has a dressing, the doll can also get one.

Other types of therapeutic play include drawing and supervised "needle play." Drawing is another method for the child to express his or her thoughts and feelings. Supervised "needle play" assists children who must undergo frequent bloodwork, injections, or intravenous procedures. A doll can receive an injection as the child works out his or her anger and anxiety. Keep in mind safety and the child's growth and development level before planning this type of directed play; an adult must always be present.

Promoting Schoolwork and Education During Hospitalization

Promote schoolwork and the child's typical activities while he or she is in the hospital. Determine the amount of this schoolwork by assessing the child's condition, the availability of teachers, and the family situation. Many children's hospitals have teachers at the hospitals; there may be classrooms too. These teachers work closely with the child's neighbourhood school to continue schoolwork as the child's condition permits. Hospitals without the educational staff will rely on parents to coordinate with the child's school. Parents may bring in schoolbooks and the child's routine work or homework for completion while in the hospital. This connection to the child's school as well as interactions with peers helps maintain normalcy for the child and minimizes the disruption of everyday life.

Addressing the Needs of Family Members

Assess the factors that may influence the family's reaction to their child's hospitalization and plan the care of the child to accommodate some of these issues. Encourage families to have support systems in place before, during, and after hospitalization. Basically, using good communication and tailoring your actions to the family's needs and preferences increase the parents' satisfaction with the health care setting (Marino, Marion, & Hayes, 2000).

Parents and Caregivers

As stated previously, the anxiety level of caregivers greatly affects the anxiety level of the child. Thus, it is important to help the family work through their feelings. Common sources of parental anger when a child is hospitalized include visiting restrictions, an unexpected change in the child's health status, confusion resulting from conflicting or insufficient information provided by the hospital staff, and feeling undervalued in the care of their child (Griffin, 2003).

The importance of family involvement to the well-being of the child is reflected in the philosophies, policies, procedures, and physical environments where care is delivered. The philosophy of family-centred care places the family at the core of care.

In a recent qualitative study exploring the support needs of parents during the hospitalization of a child, Sarajarvi, Haapamaki, and Paavilainen (2006) found the two main needs of parents to be emotional and informational support. A comment from one parent reveals the need for emotional support from nurses: "Although you can cope with the child's care alone, you hope that the nurse would be your companion, because you have a great need for support, like being listened to and talking" (Sarajarvi et al., 2006, p. 208). According to the parents in this study, support from nurses came in the form of discussion, listening, information, and time given to families (Sarajarvi et al., 2006).

Parents need to make sense of what's going on and need accurate, timely information about their child's condition and treatment (Sudbery & Blenkinship, 2005). They often feel vulnerable and experience opposing emotions where fear and despair contend with optimism and concern, and love for their child conflicts with the guilty feelings of self-regard (Sudbery & Blenkinship, 2005). One parent describes the experience of living in the hospital with a sick child in this way: "It's like living in a goldfish bowl, but where your every move is seen by other people..." (Sudbery & Blenkinship, 2005, p. 49).

The family is the primary and continuing provider of care for the child. Encourage parents to room in with the child throughout the hospital stay, if possible. Facilities can be designed to welcome family participation. For example, having electronic and Internet access and providing extra meals and sleeping arrangements for the parents can encourage parents to participate in care. View the parents as vital members of the health care team and partners in the care of the ill child.

Siblings

Family-centred care recognizes the need to treat the child in context of the family, including siblings. Important questions that will affect how siblings deal with the hospitalization of their brother or sister include:

- Was the admission an emergency?
- Were there previous admissions, and how did the siblings perceive those hospitalizations?
- How serious is the illness or trauma?
- Is the prognosis known?

Address the sibling's possible feelings of guilt. Use educational materials, allow time for visits, send photographs back and forth between siblings, and allow siblings to talk on the phone.

In a study by Hamama, Ronen, and Rahav (2008) that examined the emotional responses among siblings of a child with cancer, girls were found to report less anxiety than boys. This difference may be related to cultural expectations that allow girls to express emotions more readily than boys. This study also found that anxiety was greater in the siblings of large families.

Providing Patient and Family Teaching

Not all experiences with hospitalization are negative: in fact, the experience may enhance the child's and family's coping skills, bolster self-esteem, and provide new socialization experiences. It may allow the child to master self-care skills and provides an opportunity for the child and family to learn new information. Parents may learn more about their child's growth and development skills as well as additional parenting or caregiving skills, resulting in improvement in their parenting abilities.

The overall goals of patient and family teaching are to minimize the child's and family's stress, educate them about treatment and nursing care in the hospital, and ensure the family can provide appropriate care at home upon discharge. Providing support before, during, and after hospitalization may minimize stress. Preadmission programs can introduce the child and family to the setting. During the hospital stay, forming partnerships with the child and family, using strategies to promote coping, and providing appropriate preparation for procedures, tests, and surgery all serve to decrease stress.

Assess the child's and family's knowledge of the illness and hospital experience. This provides a baseline for teaching. Include hospital rules in child and family teaching. Behavioural changes in hospitalized children often disturb parents or caregivers. Determine the child's usual patterns of behaviour and explain to the parents about the child's reaction to hospitalization. Encourage the family to maintain consistent discipline even while in the hospital to provide structure for the child as well as prevent discipline issues after discharge. Also discuss how siblings may react to the hospitalization and provide appropriate teaching to the siblings. Every interaction the nurse has with the child or family provides an opportunity for teaching. Explain the purpose of even simple procedures such as vital signs assessment to the child and family. Provide ongoing information about the child's illness or trauma, treatment plan, and expected outcomes. Chapter 2 gives general principles related to teaching children and their families.

Preparing the Child and Family for Discharge

Discharge planning actually begins upon admission. The nurse assesses the family's resources and knowledge level to determine what education and referrals they may need. Upon discharge, children and their parents or caregivers receive written instructions about home care, and a copy is retained in the medical record. These instructions are individualized for the child. Generally, discharge instructions should include:

- Follow-up appointment information
- Guidelines about when to contact the physician or nurse practitioner (e.g., new or worsening symptoms or indications that the child is not improving)
- Diet
- Activity level allowed
- Medications, including dose, times to be given, route, adverse effects, and special instructions; any prescriptions should be included
- Information on additional treatments the child requires at home

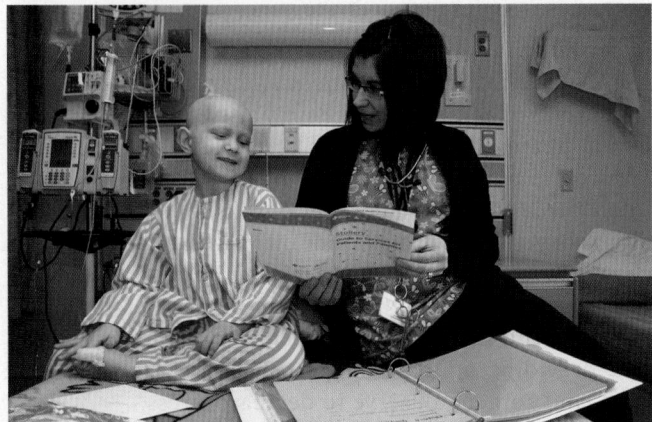

FIGURE 32.10 The nurse uses charts with pictures and books to perform patient teaching before the child goes home. (Courtesy of Stephen Wreakes.)

• Specific dates for when the child may return to school or day care
• Names and phone numbers of agencies the family has been referred to, such as medical equipment providers and home care nurse agencies

Provide and review educational booklets that give basic health information or general care for a child with a particular disease (Fig. 32.10). Electronic resources may also be used if available. The ability to watch a procedure over and over is helpful to some families. Explain, demonstrate, and request a return demonstration of any treatments or procedures to be done at home. Provide a written schedule if the child is to receive multiple medications, tube feedings, or other medical treatments. For complicated cases, a written teaching plan may be used to provide continuity of child/family education between various nurses. As the family attempts to perform each task, document whether the caregiver continues to require assistance or prompting with the task or whether he or she can perform the task independently.

Parents of children with multiple medical needs may benefit from a trial period of home care. This occurs while the child is still in the hospital, but the parents or caregivers provide all of the care that the child requires. Support the family and praise their accomplishments during this trial period.

■■■ Key Concepts

■ Stressors associated with hospitalization include separation from family and routines; fear of an unknown environment; potential for pain, bodily injury, or mutilation; and loss of control.
■ Responses of children to the general stressors of hospitalization include anxiety, fear, anger, guilt, and regression.
■ Parents may experience anger or guilt related to the hospitalization of their child.

■ The responses of children and families to hospitalization can be influenced by the age and developmental level of the child, their perceptions of the situation, previous experiences, separation from family and peers, coping skills, and the preparation and support provided by the family, facility, and health care providers.
■ Whatever the reason for admission, preparation is vital.
■ Upon admission to the hospital or outpatient unit, orient the child and family to the unit, discuss unit rules, and begin patient/family teaching.
■ Due to their age and developmental level, children may be vulnerable to harm, so nurses must use appropriate safety measures in caring for children (e.g., identification of children, use of restraints and transportation, basic hygiene measures).
■ Nursing care is directed toward meeting the child's needs related to self-care, separation anxiety, growth and development, diversion, family, control, teaching, pain relief, and coping.
■ Play, including therapeutic play, is an important strategy to prepare children for hospitalization and to help them adapt to the effects of illness and hospitalization. It provides an emotional outlet, opportunities for teaching and learning, and the ability to become familiar with a situation and improve physiologic abilities. A CLS is a specially trained individual who is a member of the child's multidisciplinary team. He or she works in conjunction with the child's health care providers and parents to foster an atmosphere that promotes the child's well-being.
■ Family-centred care and atraumatic care are philosophies that pay special attention to the concerns of the family and child during hospitalization.
■ Providing support to hospitalized children and their families is critical for minimizing stress.
■ Discharge planning begins upon admission. Each interaction with the family is an opportunity for patient teaching.

REFERENCES

American Academy of Pediatrics Child Life Council and Committee on Hospital Care. (2006). Policy statement: Child life services. *Pediatrics, 118*(4), 1757–1763. Retrieved September 19, 2011 from http://pediatrics.aappublications.org/content/118/4/1757.full.html

Baltruschat, D. (n.d.). Television and Canada's aboriginal communities – seeking opportunities through traditional storytelling and digital technologies. Available May 31, 2011 from http://web.mit.edu/cms/mit3/papers/baltruschat.pdf

Bjork, M., Nordstrom, B., & Hallstrom, I. (2006). Needs of young children with cancer during their initial hospitalization: An observational study. *Journal of Pediatric Oncology Nursing, 23*(4), 210–219.

Blackstock, C., Bruyere, D., & Moreau, E. (2006). *Many hands, one dream: Principles for a new perspective on the health of Frist Nations, Inuit and Metis children and youth.* Ottawa, ON: Canadian Pediatric Society.

Bloch, U., & Toker, A. (2008). Doctor, is my teddy bear okay? The "Teddy Bear Hospital" as a method to reduce children's fear of hospitalization. *Israel Medical Association Journal, 10*, 597–599.

Bowlby, J. (1960). Separation anxiety. *International Journal of Psychoanalysts, 41,* 89–113.

Bowlby, J. A. (1988). *A secure base: Parent-child attachment and healthy human development.* New York: Basic Books.

Branstetter, J., Domian, E., Williams, P., Graff, J., & Piamjarijakul, U. (2008). Communication themes in families of children with chronic conditions. *Issues in Comprehensive Pediatric Nursing, 31,* 171–184.

Bricher, G. (2000). Children in the hospital: Issues of power and vulnerability. *Pediatric Nursing, 26*(3), 277–282.

Child Life Council. (2010–2011). *CLC fact sheet.* Retrieved August 17, 2010 from http://www.childlife.org/files/CLCFactSheet2010-11.pdf

Coyne, I. (2006). Children's experiences of hospitalization. *Journal of Child Health Care, 10*(4), 326–336.

Department of Health & Human Services, Centers for Medicare & Medicaid Services. (2006). 42 CFR Part 482 Medicare & Medicaid Programs; hospital conditions of participation: Patients' rights: Final rule. *Federal Register, 71*(236). Retrieved September 19, 2011 from https://www.cms.gov/CFCsAndCoPs/downloads/finalpatientrightsrule.pdf

Disability Rights California. (2008). *Summary of select regulations regarding behavioral restraint and seclusion.* Retrieved September 19, 2011 from http://www.disabilityrightsca.org/pubs/545701.htm#_ftn5

Dudley, S., & Carr, J. (2004). Vigilance: The experience of parents staying at the bedside of hospitalized children. *Journal of Pediatric Nursing, 19*(4), 267–275.

Forsner, M., Jansson, L., & Sorlie, V. (2005). The experience of being ill as narrated by hospitalized children aged 7–10 years with short-term illness. *Journal of Child Health Care, 9*(2), 153–165.

Garros, D., King, J., Brady-Fryer, B., & Klassen, T. (2003). Strangulation with intravenous tubing: A previously undescribed adverse advent in children. *Pediatrics, 111*(6), 732–734.

Griffin, T. (2003). Facing challenges to family-centered care, II: Anger in the clinical setting. *Pediatric Nursing, 29*(3), 212–214.

Hamama, L., Ronen, T., & Rahav, G. (2008). "Self-control, self-efficacy, role overload, and stress responses among siblings of children with cancer." *Health and Social Work, 33,* 121–132.

Healthy Children. (2011). *Ages and stages: Soothing your child's separation anxiety.* Retrieved September 19, 2011 from http://www.healthychildren.org/English/ages-stages/toddler/pages/Soothing-Your-Childs-Separation-Anxiety.aspx

Hockenberry, M. (2009). *Wong's essentials of pediatric nursing* (8th ed.). St. Louis, MO: Mosby.

Huth, M. M., Broome, M. E., & Good, M. (2004). Imagery reduces children's post-operative pain. *Pain, 110*(1–2), 439–448.

Joint Commission Resources. (2008). Restraint reduction. In I. J. Chatman (Ed.), *Issues in provision of care, treatment, and services for hospitals* (2nd ed.). Oakbrook Terrace, IL: JCAHO.

Justus, R., Wyles, D., Wilson, J., Rode, D., Walther, V., & Lim-Sulit, N. (2006). Preparing children and families for surgery: Mount Sinai's multidisciplinary perspective. *Pediatric Nursing, 32*(1), 35–43.

Leahy, S., Kennedy, R. M., Hesselgrave, J., Gurwitch, K., Barkey, M., & Millar, T. F. (2008). On the front lines: Lessons learned in implementing multidisciplinary peripheral venous access pain-management programs in pediatric hospitals. *Pediatrics, 122,* S161–S170. Retrieved September 19, 2011 from http://pediatrics.aappublications.org/content/122/Supplement_3/S161.full.html

Mansson, M. E., & Dykes, A. (2004). Practices for preparing children for clinical examination and procedures in Swedish pediatric wards. *Pediatric Nursing, 30*(3), 182.

Marino, B. L., Marion, E. K., & Hayes, J. S. (2000). Parents' reports of children's hospital care: What it means for your practice. *Pediatric Nursing, 26*(2), 195–198.

Munro, H., & D'Errico, F. C. (2000). Parental involvement in perioperative anesthetic management. *Journal of PeriAnesthesia Nursing, 15,* 397–400.

Pagnamenta, R., & Benger, J. (2008). Factors influencing parent satisfaction in a children's emergency department: Prospective questionnaire-based study. *Emergency Medicine Journal, 25,* 417–419.

Public Health Agency of Canada. (2008). *Leading causes of death and hospitalization in Canada.* Retrieved August 11, 2011 from http://www.phac-aspc.gc.ca/publicat/lcd-pcd97/index-eng.php

Rennick, J. E., Johnston, C. C., Dougerty, G., & Ritchie, J. A. (2002). Children's psychological response after critical illness and exposure to invasive technology. *Journal of Developmental and Behavioral Pediatrics, 23*(3), 133–144.

Romino, S. L., Keatley, V. M., Secrest, J., & Good, K. (2005). Parental presence during anesthesia induction in children. *AORN Journal, 81*(4), 779–792.

Sarajarvi, A., Haapamaki, M., & Paavilainen, E. (2006). Emotional and informational support for families during their child's illness. *International Nursing Review, 53,* 205–210.

Scott-Findlay, S., & Chalmers, K. (2001). Exploring the experiences of rural families with a child with cancer. *Journal of Pediatric Oncology Nursing, 18*(5), 205–216.

Sigrest, T. D., Neff, J. M., Eichner, J. M., & Hardy, D. R. (2003). Facilities and equipment for the care of pediatric patients in a community hospital. *Pediatrics, 111*(5), 1120.

Sorensen, H. L., Card, C. A., Malley, M. T., & Strzelecki, J. M. (2009). Using a collaborative child life approach for continuous surgical preparation. *AORN: Association of Preoperative Registered Nurses Journal, 90*(4), 557–566.

Stratton, K. M. (2004). Parents' experiences of their child's care during hospitalization. *Journal of Cultural Diversity, 11*(1), 4.

Sudbery, J., & Blenkinship, A. (2005). 'Acting as a good parent would'? Psychosocial support for parents in a children's hospital. *Journal of Social Work Practice, 19*(1), 43–57.

Vessey, J. A. (2003). Children's psychological responses to hospitalization. *Annual Review of Nursing Research, 21,* 173–201.

Winch, A. (2001). Role play: A nurse's role in helping well children cope with a parent's serious illness and/or hospitalization. *Journal of the Society of Pediatric Nurses, 6*(1), 42–46.

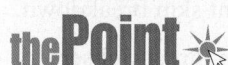

For additional learning materials, including Internet Resources, visit **http://thePoint.lww.com/Chow1e.**

Special thanks to Stephen Wreakes, Medical Photographer, University of Alberta Hospital, Alberta Health Services.

CHAPTER WORKSHEET

MULTIPLE CHOICE QUESTIONS

1. The nurse would most likely assess separation anxiety in which child?

   a. A 2-month-old infant

   b. A 15-month-old toddler

   c. A 4-year-old preschooler

   d. An 11-year-old child

2. When developing the preoperative plan of care for an adolescent, the nurse plans interventions to address the adolescent's anxieties and fears related to:

   a. Separation from parents

   b. Punishment for wrongdoings

   c. Changes in body image

   d. Magical thinking

3. The nurse is preparing a 5-year-old boy for surgery on his lower leg. His mother is helping him into the hospital gown and the boy fights removal of his underwear. What is the most appropriate nursing action?

   a. Allow the mother to remove the underwear.

   b. Tell the boy he is acting childishly.

   c. Notify the operating room that the underwear is on.

   d. Allow the boy to keep his underwear on.

4. A 6-month-old infant requires restraint to prevent removal of his nasogastric tube. What is the priority nursing intervention?

   a. Tie the restraint loosely to prevent skin breakdown.

   b. Leave the baby unrestrained when directly observed.

   c. Position the restrained infant prone to prevent aspiration.

   d. Place the infant in a room near the nurses' station.

5. A 10-year-old child on a regular diet refuses to eat the food on her meal tray. She requests chicken nuggets, French fries, and ice cream. What is the best nursing action?

   a. Ask that the child's desired foods be sent up from the kitchen.

   b. Negotiate with the child to eat at least part of the food on the tray.

   c. Remove a privilege.

   d. Offer the child cereal and milk from stock on the nursing unit.

CRITICAL THINKING EXERCISES

1. Becky, an 8-year-old, is admitted to the pediatric unit for an emergency surgery. She is in third grade and very active in after-school programs. Her mother is with her during the admission process but will have to return to work shortly after Becky returns from surgery to the pediatric unit. Would the nurse expect Becky to show separation anxiety? What are the three top nursing diagnoses for Becky?

2. A 6-year-old is admitted to the general pediatric unit after spending several hours in the emergency department with an acute asthma attack. Her mother and two younger siblings are present, but the mother plans to leave shortly to take the siblings home. The father will visit in about 2 hours, after work. What is the overall goal for this child's care? What could the nurse say to promote coping in this child? What would be the best answer if the mother asks if she should stay?

STUDY ACTIVITIES

1. Shadow a CLS in a hospital. Identify his or her role and how he or she works with the nursing staff.

2. Follow a child and family during the admission process, from preadmission to initial time on the unit, to identify the procedures and tasks involved. Examine the response of the child and family and how the nursing staff responds to their needs.

3. Spend a day in the radiology department or the emergency room to learn about the strategies used to prepare children for various procedures.

4. Develop a teaching plan to orient a toddler or preschooler and his or her family to a nursing unit. Include the resources, personnel, and techniques to include in the teaching plan.

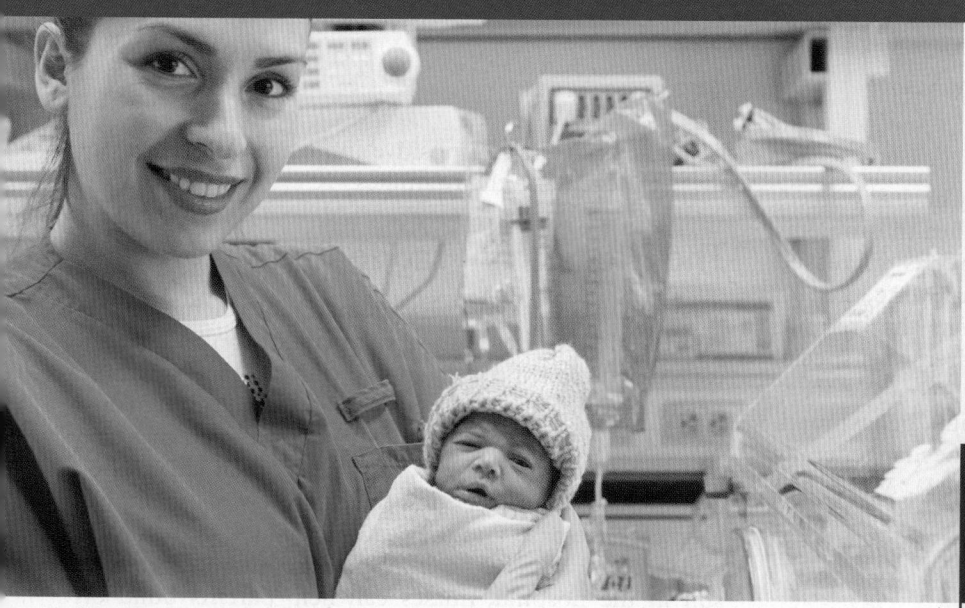

NURSING CARE OF THE CHILD WITH SPECIAL NEEDS

KEY TERMS

chronic illness
developmental delay

developmental disability
palliative care

respite care
terminal illness

LEARNING OBJECTIVES

Upon completion of the chapter, the learner will be able to:

1. Analyze the impact that being a child with special needs has on the child and family.
2. Describe ways that nurses assist children with special needs and their families to obtain optimal functioning.
3. Identify anticipated times when the child and family will require additional support.
4. Plan for transition of the special needs child from the inpatient facility to the home and from pediatric to adult medical care.
5. Discuss early intervention and public school education for the special needs child.
6. Differentiate developmental responses to death and appropriate interventions.
7. Discuss key elements related to pediatric end-of-life care.

*P*reet Singh, a 2-year-old boy, who was born at 27 weeks' gestation, is seen in your clinic for the first time. He has a history of hydrocephalus and developmental delay. During the examination, his mother states, "I'm concerned about finding a good, affordable preschool for Preet. His older brother attends public school, but I can't imagine Preet there." After further discussion with Preet's mother, you realize he has not been involved in an early intervention program.

Wow

The touch of a mother's hand and the sound of her voice bring comfort to her special child, and when you bring comfort, you strengthen both of them.

As medicine and scientific technology have advanced, the number of children surviving with health problems that require long-term interventions has increased significantly (Kepreotes, Keatinge, & Stone, 2010). Children are now living with conditions that require high-tech treatments for survival. Children with special health care needs are defined as those who have or are at risk for a chronic physical, developmental, behavioural, or emotional condition beyond the needs generally required by children (Jackson Allen, 2004). More than 200,000 children in Canada have special health care needs (Statistics Canada, 2006). Of those, about 75% have more than one disability and 40% are classified as living with severe to very severe disabilities (Statistics Canada, 2006).

In addition to the direct effects of their special needs, these children and their families often have inadequate insurance to cover medical expenses not covered through the Canadian health care system. Many of these families also have financial needs, unmet family support needs, or difficulty obtaining the specialty care their children require. Children with special health care needs generally require more intensive and diverse health services, as well as coordination of those services, than do their healthy peers (Srivastava, Stone, & Murphy, 2005). It can be challenging for the family of a child with special needs to navigate the system and obtain all of the services their child requires (Farmer, Marien, & Frasier, 2003).

Another difficult situation that families may encounter is losing a child to the disease process. A child's chronic illness may progress to the point of becoming terminal. Despite the increased survival rates for children with cancer as a result of improved treatment options and protocols, cancer remains the leading cause of death from disease in all children over the age of 1 year (Public Health Agency of Canada, 2011). Less frequently, other diseases and conditions also lead to **terminal illness** in children, with congenital defects and traumatic injuries being the more common causes. Caring for the dying child is a family-centred, multidisciplinary process. Nurses must respond to the child's and family's physiologic, emotional, and spiritual needs during this difficult time. Children display differing responses to the dying process and impending death depending on their developmental level. Children and their families need significant amounts of support throughout the process of dying.

For children with special needs, the pediatric nurse fills the critical role of child and family advocate and case manager. When a child is dying, nurses provide physical care for the child and also strive to meet the emotional needs of the child and family. Nurses are in a unique position, both in the inpatient and outpatient settings, to have a significant and positive influence on the lives of these children and their families.

The Medically Fragile Child

When an infant is born very prematurely, when a child is injured and requires long-term rehabilitation and special care, or when a child is diagnosed with a complex chronic health condition, the parents are often devastated initially. The parents of medically fragile children may feel they must adapt to the risk and protect their child. They are interested in preserving their family while compensating for the past, and they cautiously look to the future and become hopeful again. While the infant or child is still in the hospital, nurses can help parents build on their strengths, empowering them to care for their medically fragile infant or special needs child. Education is paramount and should begin as early in the hospitalization as possible. In many situations, particular discharge needs are known early in the course of the infant's or child's hospitalization. Nurses should provide anticipatory guidance about the course of treatment and the expected outcome (Lewis, 2007).

Most children with **chronic illness**, or those who are dependent on technology, progress through stages of growth and development just as typical children do, though possibly at a slower pace. The exception is the child with significant psychomotor delay, though some developmental progression may occur. Children with special health care needs have the same wants and needs as their peers, including the needs to communicate, play, enjoy leisure activities, develop friendships, and access education (Hewitt-Taylor, 2010).

Of particular concern is the growing subset of children who have emotional, behavioural, and developmental problems, either alone or in conjunction with other chronic illnesses (Hysing, Elgen, Gillberg, & Lundervold, 2009). Children with these needs have even greater difficulty receiving the care and services they require. Many children with emotional, behavioural, or developmental problems also have health problems. Often, these children's problems are not diagnosed early and treatment is difficult (Horowitz & Marchetti, 2010). Ongoing counselling and therapy can be difficult for some families to obtain. Ultimately, this has a negative impact on the child's physical and mental health and may result in decreased achievement and productivity as the child matures.

Effect of Special Needs on the Child and Family

The child with special needs and his or her family are both affected by the child's condition and way of living. Each member of the family experiences effects related to the child's special needs. Family members' experiences and their responses to the child's illness influence each other directly. They also affect the coping ability of the child with special needs. Children's ability to cope is significantly affected by the family's response to stressors.

Effects on the Child

Children with special health care needs experience differing effects of the chronic illness or disability based on their developmental level, which naturally changes over time for most children.

Infants may fail to develop a sense of trust or attach appropriately with the parents because of frequent hospitalizations, often with multiple caregivers involved, lack of consistency in nurturing, or parental detachment or grieving over the child's condition. The infant's ability to learn through sensorimotor exploration may be impaired due to lack of appropriate stimulation, confinement to a crib, or increased contact with painful experiences (Vessey & Sullivan, 2010).

The toddler may experience difficulty developing autonomy because of increased dependency on the parent or over-involvement by the parent. Motor and language skill development may be delayed if the toddler is not given adequate opportunities to test his or her limits and abilities (Vessey & Sullivan, 2010).

Limited opportunity also reduces the preschooler's development of a sense of initiative. The preschooler may experience limited opportunities for socialization, causing him or her to withdraw or to feel criticized. Body image development may be hindered due to painful exposures and anxiety. In preschoolers, magical thinking may lead to feelings of guilt for having caused their own disease or condition (Vessey & Sullivan, 2010).

The school-age child may have limited opportunities to achieve a sense of industry because of school absence and inability to participate in activities or competitive events. Lack of socialization limits the school-age child's ability to form peer relationships. The ability to learn via concrete operations is affected by the child's physical limitations or possibly the treatments required (Vessey & Sullivan, 2010).

Adolescents may feel as though they are different from their peers because of their lack of skills/abilities or their appearance. This may hinder the teen's ability to form a sense of personal identity. Since the teen with special health care needs often requires significant amounts of support from the parents, it may be difficult for the adolescent to achieve independence. If the earlier stages of cognitive development have been delayed, then reaching the level of abstract thinking may be blocked (Vessey & Sullivan, 2010).

The child with special health care needs may be able to focus on the positive experiences in his or her life as a method of coping, leading to as much independence as possible. Other children may always feel different from their peers (in a negative sense) and withdraw. Irritability and acting out may also occur. Some children may be compliant and/or seek support for themselves. The child's coping pattern may change over time or with certain situations, such as relapse or worsening of the condition. Children with overprotective parents may display marked dependence and may be very fearful. Children whose parents have been overly indulgent may be more independent and defiant. The nurse must assess the child's individual response to the current health care status and intervene as appropriate (Vessey & Sullivan, 2010). See Evidence-based Practice 33.1.

Effects on the Parents

Raising a child with special needs is generally not the life parents expected to have. Some parents may adapt over time and ultimately accept the child's illness or disability. Others may adapt but do not accept the child's condition and experience the continual fading and re-emergence of chronic sorrow. Denial of their child's problem may prevent parents from progressing through grief, but it also allows them to have hope (Knafl & Santacroce, 2010).

Caring for the special needs child at home (rather than having the child in a facility) may decrease the parents' feelings of anxiety and helplessness. As with typically developing children, parents enjoy witnessing the emotional and social growth of the child (Wang & Barnard, 2004). Parents of special needs children experience a multitude of emotions and changes in their lives; they report that they "live worried" (Coffey, 2006). They feel helpless and overwhelmed at discharge from the hospital. Though willing to carry the burden, they may experience fear, anger, sadness, guilt, frustration, or resentment. Many parents experience grief as a result of losing the "perfect child" they dreamed of (Knafl & Santacroce, 2010). See Evidence-based Practice 33.2.

Stressors of Daily Living

Families with a child who has special health care needs experience life differently than other families. They may have to change their housing situation to accommodate the child's needs (Moore, Anderson, Carter, & Coad, 2010). Their sleep is affected. Constant supervision of the technologically dependent child makes it difficult to carry out other basic household activities. In addition to basic child care and running of the household, medical and technical care must be incorporated into daily life (Fig. 33.1). The family's identity and the parents' employment may be altered radically. Holidays and vacations are affected, as it is difficult to plan activities. Visits from nurses and other health care professionals are disruptive to family life.

Mothers appear to carry the larger burden of care, though fathers are not unaffected. Somehow, parents eventually take charge, and though they fear failure, they

EVIDENCE-BASED PRACTICE 33.1
Life Skills Intervention for Children with Cystic Fibrosis and Effects of Intervention on Psychosocial Adjustment, Functional Health Status, and Physiological Status Over Time

● **Study**

Improved survival and an altered course for cystic fibrosis (CF) have led to a need to balance psychosocial and developmental needs in affected children. The authors performed a blinded, randomized controlled trial at four university CF centres. One hundred sixteen children participated in the study over a 9-month period. The intervention performed consisted of a home visit to assess each child's knowledge and management of CF. Information was provided using an educational problem-solving approach. Subsequent focus groups were held during which the children discussed how to deal with peer issues.

▲ **Findings**

Children who participated in the intervention group had greater improvements in loneliness, global self-worth, and

perceived illness experience than children who did not participate. The intervention did not demonstrate an impact upon physical or functional health status but did improve psychosocial status.

■ **Nursing Implications**

In addition to CF, many chronic and debilitating conditions affect children's quality of life. Any school-age or older child with a chronic condition that impairs physical functioning would benefit from interventions similar to those performed in this study. In particular, nurses who work in settings that allow them to have long-term relationships with these children have the potential to positively influence their lives. Nurses should help children learn communication and problem-solving skills that could lessen the impact of their chronic condition.

Christian, B. J., & D'Auria, J. P. (2006). Building life skills for children with cystic fibrosis: Effectiveness of an intervention. *Nursing Research, 55*, 300–307.

display vigilance, can negotiate and seek information, and become advocates for their child and experts on his or her care. Though parents may feel trapped, isolated, and experience a loss of freedom, their need to survive as a family continues to motivate them. Parents may feel a need to be with their child at all times and experience stress related to coping with the heavy load of caregiving (Kepreotes et al., 2010).

The extended burden of caregiving can also have adverse health effects on caregivers: only a small percentage of parents of children with special health care needs report that they routinely participate in health-promoting activities for themselves (Kuster, Badr, Chang, Wuerker, & Benjamin, 2004). Additionally, parents of children with special health care needs are at increased risk for the development of depression (Knafl & Santacroce, 2010).

EVIDENCE-BASED PRACTICE 33.2
The Health of Children with Cerebral Palsy and Stress in Their Parents

● **Study**

Children with CP tend to have more health issues than their able-bodied peers, and their parents are more likely to be stressed and have poorer health as well. A cross-sectional survey with home visits was completed. The children were compared with a normative sample.

▲ **Findings**

This study found that children with CP have significantly poorer physical health than non-CP children with respect to physical functioning, bodily pain, ability to participate in family activities, and general health. Psychological problems in children with CP were twice as common as in children without CP, with the most common problems being hyperactivity and emotional disorders. Psychological disorders are seen more frequently in children whose CP is

milder. These issues are a key predictor of high parenting stress and may be more important than the severity of the child's physical impairments.

■ **Nursing Implications**

Assessment of children with any complex health condition must include questions about physical pain and psychological problems. Both of these issues are treatable and have a large impact not only on the child's quality of life but on the emotional and physical health of their parents as well. Parents whose children have psychological issues in addition to physical impairments are more likely to experience high parental stress levels and require extra support. Using a family-centred approach to the care of children with special needs is essential in order to provide the optimal level of care to both the children and their parents.

Parkes, J., McCullough, N., Madden, A., & McCahey, E. (2009). The health of children with cerebral palsy and stress in their parents. *Journal of Advanced Nursing, 65*(11), 2311–2323.

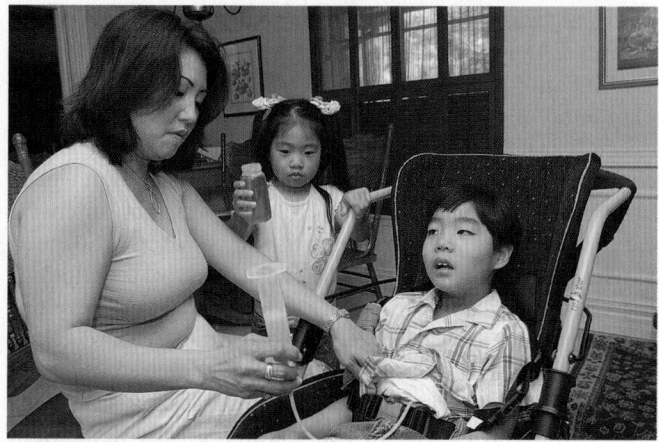

FIGURE 33.1 The special needs child often requires a significant amount of care at home.

In addition to the caregiving burden, parents experience role conflicts, financial burdens, and the struggle between independence in providing care and the isolation associated with it (Ratliffe, Harrigan, Haley, Tse, & Olson, 2002). It is very difficult to enjoy spontaneous events outside the home because so much planning is necessary (Case-Smith, 2004; Ratliffe et al., 2002).

The possibility of independence revolves around mobility issues, education, and assistive technology. Though education for all children is provincially and territorially mandated, parents have anxiety about educational decisions and also find it difficult to obtain the support and educational services the child needs.

Additional stress is associated with transition times in the care of a special needs child. These transition times include:

• Initial diagnosis or change in prognosis
• Increased symptoms
• When the child moves to a new setting (hospital, school)
• During a parent's absence
• During periods of developmental change (Knafl & Santacroce, 2010; Looman, O'Conner-Von, & Lindeke, 2008)

Vulnerable Child Syndrome

"Vulnerable child syndrome" is a clinical state in which the parents' reactions to a serious illness or event in the child's past continue to have long-term psychologically harmful effects on the child and parents for many years (Duncan & Caughy, 2009). The parents view the child as being at higher risk for medical, developmental, or behavioural problems (Kerruish, Settle, Campbell-Stokes, & Taylor, 2005). Parents exhibit excessive unwarranted concerns and seek health care for their child very frequently. Risk factors for the development of vulnerable

child syndrome include preterm birth, congenital anomaly, newborn jaundice, physical disability, an accident or illness from which the child was not expected to recover, or crying or feeding problems in the first 5 years of life (Pearson & Boyce, 2004). The parent has difficulty separating from the child, and the child senses that anxiety and then develops symptoms that reinforce the parent's fears. Alternatively (or additionally), the parents may to try to retain control, particularly at times of increasing independence, and fear disciplining the child as they do not want to "upset" the child (O'Connor & Szekely, 2001).

Effects on Siblings

The siblings of children with special health care needs are also affected dramatically. Their relationship with their parents is different than it would have been if they had a typical brother or sister. Parents often need to spend more time with the child with special needs and have less time with their healthy children. Children exhibit emotional and psychological responses to their sibling's long-term needs (Looman et al., 2008). Knowledge about the sibling's illness, attitude toward and adjustment to it, the sibling's own self-esteem, how socially supported the sibling is, and the parents' awareness of sibling's feelings are all related to how well the sibling adjusts (O'Brien, Duffy, & Nicholl, 2009).

Nursing Management of the Medically Fragile Child

Family-centred care provides the optimal framework for caring the medically fragile children and their families. Family-centred care minimizes the impact of chronic illness and maximizes the child's developmental potential. To provide the best nursing care for these children and their families, the nurse must first develop a trusting relationship with the family.

To ensure optimal functioning, children with special health care needs require comprehensive and coordinated services from multiple professionals. These professionals should work collaboratively to address the child's health, educational, psychological, and social service needs (Farmer et al., 2003). In addition to case management and advocacy, nursing management focuses on screening and ongoing assessment of the child, provision of home care, care of the technologically dependent child, education and support of the child and family, and referral for resources.

Developing a Therapeutic Relationship

Raising children is always challenging, but for the parent of a special needs child it is often overwhelming and exhausting. The parents' needs change continuously, so it is best if the family has a permanent relationship with a health care provider. This promotes trust and a more efficient two-way flow of information (Nuutila & Salanterä, 2006).

BOX 33.1 **Principles Related to Family Involvement**

Families

- Define who they are and their culture
- Need to have their basic needs met
- Need to have access to information and training
- Deserve to receive culturally competent care
- Can identify priorities and concerns that lead to policy change
- Know their strengths, limitations, and fears
- Share decision-making power and responsibility for outcomes

---

Adapted from: Federation of Families for Children's Mental Health. (n.d.). *FFCMH principles for family involvement*. Retrieved September 23, 2011 from http://ffcmh.org/wp-content/uploads/2010/06/FFCMH PrinciplesforFamilyInvolvement.pdf.

Respect the parents' range of emotions and work with them as a team to manage the child's care. Parents need to be recognized for complying with the treatment plan or for other small gains that are made (Jackson Allen, 2004). Empowering the family strengthens them and gives them self-confidence (Lindblad, Rasmussen, & Sandman, 2005). Feeling supported and invigorated gives parents strength, energy, and hope. Box 33.1 lists principles related to family involvement.

Screening and Ongoing Assessment

Nurses should perform routine health screening assessments as well as screening to identify children with unmet health care needs (Jackson Allen, 2004). It is important to remember that children with special health care needs may attain developmental milestones more slowly than typically developing children; therefore, development must be carefully monitored. If the Denver II is used for ongoing developmental surveillance of the young child, then the results should be compared from visit to visit to determine progress rather than using it as a screening tool (Ware, Sloss, Chugh, & Budd, 2002). Other developmental tools include the Ages and Stages Questionnaire (ASQ; see Appendix G) and the Nipissing District Developmental Screen (NDDS; Limbos, Joyce, & Roberts, 2010). Assess special needs children and their families for vulnerable child syndrome.

Promoting Home Care

Home is the most developmentally appropriate environment for all children, even those who are technologically dependent (Looman et al., 2008). The child's home provides an emotionally nurturing and socially stimulating environment. Children desire to be cared for at home, and those who are cared for at home display an improved physical, emotional, psychological, and social status (Wang & Barnard, 2004).

Technologically dependent children may require supplemental oxygen, assisted ventilation, tracheostomy care, assisted enteral or parenteral feeding, or parenteral medication administration. Traditionally, hospitalization would have been required for these children—in fact, intensive care would have been necessary for children who need assisted ventilation—but with advances in technology, today even children with extensive medical and developmental needs may be cared for at home (Moore et al., 2010; Spalding & Salib, 2008). Early discharge planning is important, and parents will need detailed instructions and support in caring for the technologically dependent child at home (Lewis, 2007).

Early Discharge Planning

Early discharge planning and ongoing inclusion and education of the family facilitates continuity of care (Lewis & Noyes, 2007). Box 33.2 provides information about preparing the medically fragile child for discharge.

BOX 33.2 **Preparing for Home Care Before Discharge**

- Promote liaison with community resources. Develop communication between various services. Plan appointments. Set up homecare support if applicable.
- Teach skills, encouraging active caregiving in the hospital setting to increase the parents' self-confidence.
- Discuss psychological and emotional issues with parents.
- Obtain/organize equipment and supplies (running out of supplies may cause significant stress on families).
- Refer the family for necessary financial resources.
- Ensure the family's home environment is adequate (enough room for equipment, electricity on, air conditioner for warm weather, heater for cold weather, and refrigeration for food).
- For the baby being discharged from the NICU:
  - Teach the parents about the infant's cues and behaviours and the preemie's different sleep–wake patterns.
  - Encourage kangaroo care and infant massage while in the NICU (as the infant's condition allows).
  - Educate the parents about possible effects on short- and long-term neurodevelopment.
  - Refer to local early intervention program.
  - Assist the family with finding a primary care provider who is experienced in the ongoing follow-up of high-risk infants.

Data from: American Academy of Pediatrics Committee on Fetus and Newborn (2008). Hospital discharge of the high-risk neonate. *Pediatrics*, 122(5), 1119–1126.

Caring for the Technologically Dependent Child at Home

Homecare nurses are often involved in the care of technologically dependent children. Caring for a technologically dependent child at home is a complex process, yet children thrive in the homecare setting with appropriate intervention and care. Many parents feel that rearing a technologically dependent child is different only because of the presence of the equipment. While nurses may tend to think that parents treat the technologically dependent child differently than the other children, generally speaking, parents value normalization and want to raise and provide discipline to all of their children in the same manner. To facilitate positive experiences, there needs to be clear communication between parents and nurses about parents' child-rearing expectations.

Improved collaboration between parents and homecare nurses may decrease the parents' stress and maximize opportunities for appropriate growth and development in the technologically dependent child (O'Brien & Wegner, 2002). Thus, a strong relationship and good communication and negotiation skills are assets to the family, child, and health care professionals involved.

To minimize the child's self-perception of being different, the nurse can help the family to incorporate the medical regimen into daily life (Green & Ray, 2006). Specific activities could include teaching families about technical issues, such as home and travel oxygen therapy, use of the ventilator, suctioning, chest percussion and postural drainage, tube feedings and care of the feeding tube, and medications. Nurses should also assist parents with the planning and management of routine care, respiratory treatments, nutritional support, and developmental interventions. As well, nurses have an important role in reinforcing exercises and techniques as prescribed by developmental therapists (Romanko, 2005). Refer to Chapter 2 for additional information about homecare nursing.

Providing Care Coordination

Once a child with special health care needs has been identified and has been discharged to the home setting, the nurse plays a vital role in care coordination. Any child with special health care needs benefits from having a "medical home," i.e., a team of professionals who provide continuous and comprehensive primary care and with whom the family has a strong therapeutic relationship (Cohen, Friedman, Nicholas, Adams, & Rosenbaum, 2008). The nurse in the medical home model is a critical team member, providing ongoing care coordination and follow-up. If such services are available in the local area, refer the child and family with special needs to an integrated health program that provides interdisciplinary, collaborative care for children who require complex, coordinated care. Box 33.3 lists nursing interventions for families of children with special health care needs.

> ### BOX 33.3 Nursing Interventions for Families of Children with Special Health Care Needs
>
> - Flag the special needs child's chart.
> - Develop written health plans.
> - Provide care coordination and collaboration with specialists in other disciplines, early intervention, schools, and public agencies.
> - Address needs for prior authorization for treatments, medication, or specialist referrals; retain copies in the child's chart of authorization forms and approvals.
> - Modify office routines to promote family and child comfort.
> - Assist parents with child care decisions. Help parents to understand the child's limits and abilities and the potential health issues (e.g., infections and injuries) associated with child care.
> - Know community resources available to children with special health care needs.
> - When the child is hospitalized, encourage high levels of parental participation (if desired by the parent).
> - Provide care coordination across multiple health settings.
> - Educate child care providers on child health needs.
> - Help parents get involved with parent support networks.

Data from: Looman, W. S., O'Conner-Von, S., & Lindeke, L. L. (2008). Caring for children with special health care needs and their families: What advanced practice nurses need to know. *Journal for Nurse Practitioners*, 4(7), 512–518, and McAllister, J. W., Presler, E., Turchi, R., & Antonelli, R. C. (2009). Achieving effective care coordination in the medical home. *Pediatric Annals*, 38(9), 491–497.

Providing Ongoing Follow-Up of the Former Premature Infant

Many former premature infants experience a myriad of medical and developmental problems throughout infancy, early childhood, and beyond. Upon or following discharge, many former premature infants display one or many of the following medical or developmental problems:

- Chronic lung disease (bronchopulmonary dysplasia)
- Cardiac changes such as right ventricular hypertrophy and pulmonary artery hypertension
- Growth retardation, poor feeding, anemia of prematurity, other nutrient deficiencies
- Apnea of prematurity, gastro-esophageal reflux disease, bradycardia
- Sudden infant death syndrome (SIDS)
- Rickets (osteopenia) of prematurity
- Hydrocephalus, ventriculomegaly, abnormal head MRI results, ventriculoperitoneal shunt
- Inguinal or umbilical hernias
- Retinopathy of prematurity, strabismus, decreased visual acuity

- Hearing deficits
- Delayed dentition
- Gross motor, fine motor, and language delay; sensory integration issues (Gargus et al., 2009)

Over the long term, former premature infants are at higher risk than typical infants for developing cognitive delay, cerebral palsy (CP), attention-deficit disorder, learning disabilities, difficulties with socialization, and vulnerable child syndrome (Duncan & Caughy, 2009; Gargus et al., 2009). Additionally, many former premature infants display alterations in muscle tone at or shortly after discharge from the neonatal intensive care unit (NICU) that require physical therapy intervention.

For these reasons, high-risk infants require special attention and thorough, appropriate assessment to discern subtle changes that may affect their long-term physical, cognitive, emotional, and social outcome. The pediatric nurse should have an understanding of the special concerns that former premature infants and children as well as their families may face.

From the beginning, encourage families to keep a binder that includes all of the infant's pertinent check-up, insurance, and medical and developmental information; this will serve as a resource for the parents, and they will be able to supply complete information when visiting various providers (Kelly, 2006c).

Providing Routine Well-Child Care of the Former Premature Infant

Former premature infants require similar well-child care as typical infants do, with additional visits for management of multiple complex medical issues and developmental screening/intervention. Teach families routine newborn care, including bathing, dressing, and avoidance of passive cigarette smoke. All visits for primary care follow-up will be scheduled based on the infant's chronological age.

Prior to discharge from the NICU, the infant will be tested for oxygen desaturation while seated in the car seat (Canadian Paediatric Society [CPS], 2000, reaffirmed in 2011). Clearance will be obtained prior to the infant's discharge. Former premature infants require car seat use just as other infants do, but their small size and potential for poor airway control place them at high risk for not being able to maintain an adequate airway while seated in the car seat. Help the parents to find methods of padding the car seat or placing an additional semi-firm cushion inside the seat for the infant to ride in the car safely. Some infants may need to continue cardiac/apnea monitoring while in the car seat.

Since the former premature infant is at increased risk for SIDS compared with the general population, it is critical to teach parents to put the infant on his or her back to sleep (although this is contraindicated with gastroesophageal disease) (Kelly, 2010).

Give immunizations according to the current recommended immunization schedule, based on the infant's chronological age (Public Health Agency of Canada, 2006; Woods & Riley, 2006). All former preemies should receive the flu vaccine as recommended after 6 months chronological age. Respiratory syncytial virus (RSV) prophylaxis is critical for certain groups of premature infants (Kelly, 2010). Administer palivizumab (Synagis) vaccine according to the recommended schedule (refer to Chapter 39 for additional information about RSV prophylaxis) (Kelly, 2006b; Romanko, 2005).

Assessing Growth and Development of the Former Premature Infant

When assessing growth and development of the infant or child who was born prematurely, determine the child's adjusted or corrected age so that you can perform an accurate assessment. The corrected or adjusted age should be used for evaluating progression in growth as well as development. For example, if a 6-month-old infant was born at 28 weeks' gestation (12 weeks or 3 months early), his growth and development expectations are those of a 3-month-old (corrected age). Continue to correct age for growth and development until the child is 3 years old.

Many former premature infants require special diets to foster catch-up growth (Kelly, 2010). Extra calories are needed for increased growth needs. Additional calcium and phosphorus are required for bone mineralization. For these reasons, former preemies should be fed breast milk fortified with additional nutrients or a commercially prepared formula specific for premature infants. When former preemies demonstrate consistent adequate growth (usually by 6 months corrected age), they may be switched to a "term infant formula" such as Similac or Enfamil, concentrated to higher caloric density if needed. Assess the infant's ability to suck efficiently and refer him or her to occupational or speech therapy if the infant is a slow feeder or has difficulty feeding.

All anticipatory guidance related to nutrition is based on the child's corrected age. In other words, begin solids at 6 months corrected age, not chronologic age, and delay the addition of whole milk until 12 months corrected age, rather than 1 year chronologic age (Kelly, 2010). Signs that the former premature infant may be ready to attempt spoon feeding include interest in feeding, decrease in tongue thrust, and adequate head control (Kelly, 2006a).

Early screening and intervention for issues related to development are critical to the attainment of optimal development in the former preemie. The co-morbidities that ex-preemies exhibit in the form of prior and current medical problems place these infants at high risk for **developmental delay** (Moddemann & Shea, 2006). Even mild developmental delays warrant evaluation and intervention. A number of screening tools are available for developmental assessment, although research has indicated that overall sensitivity to children born prematurely remains an issue (Rydz, Shevell, Majnemer, & Oskoui, 2005). Parent-report questionnaires can demonstrate fairly accurate estimations of developmental problems (American Academy of Pediatrics, 2001). Most importantly, assess the child's development based on corrected age until the child is 3 years old. Refer infants and children early if developmental concerns are suspected.

Identifying and Managing Failure to Thrive and Feeding Disorders in Children with Special Needs

Failure to thrive (FTT) is a term used to describe inadequate growth in infants and children. The child fails to demonstrate appropriate weight gain over a prolonged period of time. Length or height velocity and head circumference growth may also be affected. Typical children may experience FTT, but it is much more common in the child with special needs (CPS, 2009). Adequate nutrition is critical for appropriate brain growth in the first 2 years of life and obviously for growth in general throughout childhood and adolescence (Burns, Dunn, Brady, Starr, & Blosser, 2009). **Developmental disability** may contribute to FTT, as the child's ability to consume adequate nutrition is impaired because of sensory or motor delays, such as with CP. Other organic causes of FTT include inability to suck and/or swallow correctly, malabsorption, diarrhea, vomiting, or alterations in metabolism and caloric/nutrient needs associated with a variety of chronic illnesses. Infants and children with cardiac or metabolic disease, chronic lung disease (bronchopulmonary dysplasia), cleft palate, or gastro-esophageal reflux disease are at particular risk. Feeding disorders or food refusal may occur in infants or children who have required prolonged mechanical ventilation, long-term enteral tube feedings, or an unpleasant event such as a choking episode. Inorganic causes of FTT include neglect, abuse, behavioural problems, lack of appropriate maternal interaction, poor feeding techniques, lack of parental knowledge, or parental mental illness. Poverty is the single greatest contributing risk factor (Block, Krebs, the Committee on Child Abuse and Neglect, & the Committee on Nutrition, 2005).

The two categories of causes are not mutually exclusive. Organic causes of FTT may lead to behavioural problems that potentiate problems with adequate growth; hence FTT is thought of as a multifactorial problem (Locklin, 2005).

Screen all children for FTT to identify them early (CPS, 2009). In addition to poor growth, the infant or child with FTT may present with a history of developmental delay or loss of acquired milestones. Infants or children with feeding problems may display nipple, spoon, or food refusal; difficulty sucking; disinterest in feeding; or difficulty progressing from liquid to puréed to textured food. Perform a detailed dietary history and instruct the

---

> ### BOX 33.4 Nursing Interventions During Hospitalization for Failure to Thrive
>
> - Observe parent–child interactions, especially during feedings.
> - Develop an appropriate feeding schedule.
> - Provide feedings as prescribed (usually 120 kcal/kg/ day is needed to demonstrate proper weight gain).
> - Weigh the child daily and maintain strict records of intake and output.
> - Educate parents about proper feeding techniques and volumes.
> - Provide extensive support to alleviate parental anxiety related to the child's inability to gain weight.

Adapted from: Ayoob, K. T., & Barresi, I. (2007). Feeding disorders in children: Taking an interdisciplinary approach. *Pediatric Annals, 36*(8), 478–483 and Locklin, M. (2005). The redefinition of failure to thrive from a case study perspective. *Pediatric Nursing, 31*(6), 474–479.

parents to complete a 3-day food diary to identify what the child actually eats and drinks. Assess the parent–child interaction, with particular attention to the parent's ability to read and respond to the infant's or child's cues. Observe feeding, noting the child's oral interest or aversion, oral–motor coordination, and swallowing ability, as well as parent–child interactions before, during, and after the feeding (Block et al., 2005). Further aversion to eating may occur as the parent's anxiety over the thought of the child not eating or losing weight leads to attempts to force-feed the child (Ayoob & Barresi, 2007).

Significant FTT may require hospitalization for evaluation and management. Sometimes enteral tube feedings are necessary in order for children with FTT or feeding disorders to demonstrate adequate growth. Box 33.4 lists nursing interventions for the hospitalized child with FTT.

> ▶ *Take NOTE!*
>
> *Infants with FTT related to maternal neglect may be less interactive than other infants and avoid eye contact (Burns et al., 2009).*

Promoting Growth and Development

When caring for the infant with special health care needs in the hospital, provide consistent caregivers to encourage the infant to develop a sense of trust. Allow and encourage the parent to stay with the infant, providing a comfortable place for the parent to sleep. To promote attachment, emphasize the baby's positive qualities. Encourage developmentally appropriate skills and allow the infant to have pleasurable experiences through all of the senses (Vessey & Sullivan, 2010).

For the toddler, begin developmentally appropriate limit-setting and discipline. Encourage independence as the toddler is able. Modify gross motor and sensory activities to accommodate the toddler's limitations. To encourage a sense of control, offer the toddler simple choices. As the preschooler develops, encourage mastery of self-help skills as the child is able. Encourage socialization with same-age peers to develop a sense of friendship. Reinforce to the child that the illness or disability is not a punishment for wrongdoing or the child's fault in any way (Vessey & Sullivan, 2010).

Encourage the school-age child to attend school and make up work that must be missed for medical treatments or appointments. Provide education to the school staff and other students about the child's special needs. Promote involvement in appropriate sports activities; music, drama, or art activities; and clubs such as Boy Scouts or Girl Scouts. Educate the child about the illness or disability and the course of treatment (Vessey & Sullivan, 2010).

Inform parents of teens that those with chronic illness often demonstrate the same traits as typical teens, such as risk-taking, rebelling, and trying out different identities. Assist the teen with coping and interpersonal skills. Promote involvement in activities with other teens with special needs as well as typical adolescents. Ensure that the teen participates in rites of passage as able, such as attending the prom or obtaining a driver's license. Discuss future plans with the teen, such as college or vocation, as well as transition to an adult health care provider (Vessey & Sullivan, 2010).

Providing Resources to the Child and Family

Nurses should be familiar with the resources available to children with special health care needs in the community. Educational opportunities for children with special health care needs include early intervention programs and programs offered through the public school system. Financial resources, respite care, and complementary therapies are other areas the nurse should become familiar with.

Educational Opportunities for the Special Needs Child

The foundation for health and development in children is laid during the first years of life. Children with special health care needs often require multiple developmental interventions and special education in the early years in order to reach their developmental potential later in childhood. Children learn best when they are at the stage of maximal readiness, and the early years must not be missed as an opportunity for development.

Early intervention programs are intended to enhance the development of infants and toddlers who have, or are at risk for, disabilities, thereby minimizing educational costs and special education needs. Early intervention is also directed toward enhancing the capacity of families to meet their child's needs as well as to maximize the likelihood of independent living (Schulman, Meringolo,

& Scott, 2007). In Canada, early intervention programs fall under provincial and territorial jurisdiction. See your local ministry of health for resources.

Think back to Preet, the 2-year-old boy with a history of hydrocephalus and developmental delay, from the beginning of the chapter. Discuss with his mother the educational opportunities that are available for Preet. Explain what early intervention is and why it is important for Preet.

Schools may have a profound impact on the child's overall health and development. Some children with special needs do not require additional services to succeed in school. For these children, the nurse's role is to assess for school success or failure and determine the effect of the school environment on the child's health. Each province and territory has different programs in place, many provided within the public school system, to ensure that children with special needs receive appropriate education. There is a wide variety in funding options, however, and in many cases parents are required to pay for these services.

In some provinces, preschool special education is provided through the local public school system for children of ages 3 to 5 years. A child may be eligible for special needs preschool when a significant delay is present in the cognitive, language, adaptive, social-emotional, or motor development domains to the extent that it adversely affects the child's learning ability. The child receives (in the school setting) developmental therapy as needed to augment his or her ability to participate in the education process. The least restrictive environment is preferred, with special needs children participating in classes containing age-appropriate typical peers whenever possible. Special needs preschool services are often offered in the elementary school setting but may have additional fees associated with them. Check with your local board of education and ministries of education and health to find out more about available resources.

Financial and Insurance Resources

Canada has a predominantly publically funded and administered health care system. Comprises 13 interlocking provincial and territorial plans, the health insurance system is designed to ensure that all eligible Canadian residents have reasonable access to medically necessary hospital and physician services on a prepaid basis, without direct charges at the point of service (Health Canada, 2008). The Canada Health Act is the federal legislation for publically funded health insurance. It provides the provinces and territories with criteria and conditions that must be met to receive full federal cash contribution under the Canada Health Transfer. Additional services that are outside the scope of the Canada

Health Act are provided at provincial and territorial discretion and often vary from one province to another. These services are generally aimed toward specific populations, such as children.

With the provincial and territorial variations in funding for special programs, such as early intervention programs, families with children with special needs often are required to have private health insurance to cover additional costs. However, private health insurance plans often only cover medical expenses and not additional programming, such as educational assistance. Most provinces and territories have programs in place for low-income families who may not have private insurance or may not be able to afford other interventions their child may need.

Respite Care

Primary caregivers of children with special health care needs must be dedicated, skillful, vigilant, and knowledgeable. Constant care is a stress on the primary caregiver, who needs temporary relief from the daily caregiving demands. **Respite care** provides an opportunity for families to take a break from the daily intensive caregiving responsibilities. Respite care should meet the child's health care needs and offer the child developmental opportunities. Finding and using respite care that the family is comfortable with and trusts may decrease the family's stress and lead to an enhanced quality of life for special needs children and their families. Nurses can facilitate access to respite care, educate respite providers, and ensure quality respite care practices through involvement in community agencies.

Complementary Therapies

Adjuvant therapies are often used by families of children with special health care needs. These may include, among others, homeopathic and herbal medicine, pet therapy, hippotherapy, music, and massage. Many families desire to blend natural or Eastern medicine with traditional allopathic medicine for their special needs child in search of palliation or a cure. When obtaining the health history, ask specifically about homeopathy or herbal medications the child may be taking.

Pet therapy may be used to decrease stress or as a component of psychotherapy.

Hippotherapy is also referred to as horseback riding for the handicapped, therapeutic horseback riding, or equine-facilitated psychotherapy. Individuals with almost any cognitive, physical, or emotional disability may benefit from therapeutic riding or other supervised interaction with horses. The unique movement of the horse under the child helps the child with physical disabilities to achieve increased flexibility, balance, and muscle strength. Children with mental or emotional disabilities may experience increased self-esteem, confidence, and patience as a result of their unique relationship with the horse. A physical therapist or psychotherapist (depending on the situation)

BOX 33.5   Conditions Benefiting from Hippotherapy

- Muscular dystrophy
- CP
- Visual impairment
- Down syndrome
- Mental retardation
- Autism
- Multiple sclerosis
- Emotional disabilities
- Brain injury
- Myelomeningocele
- Spinal cord injury
- Amputation
- Attention-deficit disorder
- Learning disabilities
- Deafness
- Cerebrovascular accident (stroke)

Adapted from: American Hippotherapy Association. (2010). *Hippotherapy as a treatment strategy. Retrieved March* 27, 2011 from http://www.americanhippotherapyassociation.org/hippotherapy/hippotherapy-as-a-treatment-strategy/.

---

generally works very closely with specially trained equine staff (Gasalberti, 2006). Box 33.5 lists chronic medical conditions for which hippotherapy may be beneficial. Additional information may be obtained through the North American Riding for the Handicapped Association or the Canadian Therapeutic Riding Association. Visit http://thePoint.lww.com/Chow1e for the direct links to their websites.

Music may be used to induce positive behavioural changes or various other positive effects (Gasalberti, 2006).

Massage therapy may be beneficial to a wide variety of children. It may be used to reduce pain, promote relaxation, or demonstrate a specific positive effect related to the child's particular medical condition (Gasalberti, 2006).

▶ *Take* NOTE!

Become familiar with the risks and benefits of homeopathic and herbal medications, as many families use these treatments in an effort to improve their child's quality of life or outcome.

Providing Support and Education

At the time of initial diagnosis, allow and encourage the family to express their feelings. Parents of children with special health care needs require emotional, practical, economic, and social support. Encourage parents to obtain help with daily routines. Encourage stress reduction for the parents through exercise and allowing time for themselves. Be a supportive and encouraging listener, making sure to nurture the whole child, not just his or her special condition (Jackson Allen, 2004).

Parents value the peer support groups, sometimes feeling that only other parents of disabled or chronically ill children could understand the heartache, fear, and other emotions they often experience. Pediatric nurses should be proactive in helping families find support systems (Coffey, 2006).

Fathers may have the same concerns about their children as mothers do, but they may show this concern differently. It is important for nurses to involve them in the child's care. Teach skills to both parents, and actively involve fathers by asking about their observations and opinions (Ahmann, 2006).

Parents become the experts on their child's needs and care and they should be recognized as such. Parents want to be taken seriously and do not like being ignored (Lindblad et al., 2005). They should be viewed as having reliable and valuable information about their children. By being an active and reflective listener, the nurse can demonstrate to the parents that their opinion is valued, in addition to finding out what the child really needs. Some parents may hesitate to volunteer information, unsure about which information the nurse needs. Show respect for the parents' knowledge of their child's needs by seeking advice on the child's daily care, medical/physical needs, and current developmental level, no matter what the site of care is (Bowie, 2004).

Families may need additional support from the nurse at times of transition (discussed previously). As the child's health equipment or treatment needs change, adjust the teaching plan. Educate the child and family about the use of adaptive equipment. Ensure that families understand how specific activities must be modified to accommodate the child's needs. Provide anticipatory guidance related to expected developmental changes, including resources and laws related to education. Act as a liaison between the family and the day care centre or school. As the child grows and matures, encourage parents to relinquish caregiving tasks to the child as appropriate to encourage independence and promote self-esteem (Meleski, 2002).

Assisting the Adolescent with Special Health Needs Making the Transition to Adulthood

Adolescence is a time of physical changes, psychosocial challenges, and initiation of independence from parents. The adolescent with a chronic illness or one who is technologically dependent may experience this period differently than other teens. Puberty is often affected by chronic illness (either delayed or earlier). Chronic illness may lead to isolation from peers at a time when peer interaction is the core of psychosocial development. Teens

may struggle to fit in with their peers by hiding their illness or health care needs (ignoring them), complying poorly with treatment regimens, or engaging in risky behaviours. At a time when the child should be developing independence from the parents, he or she may be experiencing significant dependence related to the special health condition. Adolescents with chronic health disorders demonstrate mental illness at a rate three to four times higher than normally developing adolescents (Burns, Sadof, & Kamat, 2006). For these reasons, the adolescent with special health care needs may require increased amounts of support from the nurse.

With the tremendous advances in technology and health care, about 90% of all children with chronic illness or special health care needs live into adulthood (Lindeke, Krajicek, & Patterson, 2001). Making the transition to adult care for a child with special health care needs can be difficult. The initiation of the transition plan should be in early adolescence or at the start of puberty and is dependent on the severity and exacerbation of the condition, the physical and cognitive abilities of the adolescent, his or her psychological and emotional stability, and the family and social supports available (Paone, Wigle, & Saewyc, 2006). Advance planning leads to a smoother transition to adult care. Have ongoing conversations with the teen about this transition.

The CPS (2007) recommends the use of the ON TRAC model for transition (Paone et al., 2006). This model has three stages:

- Early transition (ages 10 to 12): the child and family are introduced to the transition process, and the child begins to participate in his or her own care.
- Middle transition (ages 13 to 15): the adolescent and family gain understanding of the transition process, and the adolescent practices skills, gathers information, and sets goals to participate in his or her own care.
- Late transition (ages 16 to 18): the adolescent and family prepare to leave the pediatric setting with confidence, and the adolescent uses independent health care behaviours and consumer skills into the adult system (Paone et al., 2006).

The ON TRAC model guides health care providers to address the following areas during the transition process:

- Evolving self-esteem and identity
- Fostering personal autonomy and independence
- Continued development in the sexual area
- Achieving psychosocial stability
- Continued educational, vocational, and financial planning
- Health and healthy lifestyle–promoting practices, including healthy active living (Paone et al., 2006)

Prior to moving to adult care (with an adult medical specialist), ensure that the adolescent understands the treatment rationale, symptoms of worsening condition, and in particular danger signs. Teach the adolescent about when to seek help from a health professional. Introduce the teen to the medical insurance process. At transition, coordinate a seamless transfer by providing a detailed written plan to the care coordinator or advanced practice nurse (after verbal collaboration).

After the transition, serve as a consultant to the adult office in relation to the teen's needs (Jalkut & Allen, 2009). Consult with a transition services coordinator or other service agency as available in the local community (Betz & Redcay, 2002).

The Dying Child

The idea that a child may die is simply unimaginable to most people, yet children die daily. In 2007, more than 3,600 children under the age of 19 died in Canada (Statistics Canada, 2010). More than half of these deaths were infants younger than 1 year of age. Pediatric nurses will inevitably encounter situations in which a child dies. These situations are extremely difficult for all persons involved, and the nurse plays a key role in caring for the dying child and his or her family.

Grieving

Anticipatory grief may be experienced by the family when the diagnosis of terminal illness is made. Families may deny the prognosis, become angry at the health care system or a higher power, or experience depression. Acute grief is an intense process that occurs around the time of the actual death. Family members may feel short of breath or as though the throat is tight. They may verbalize that the situation is unreal to them or search for reasons why the death was not prevented. Families may also display hostility or restlessness. Each individual will express grief in his or her own manner. Mourning the death of a loved one takes a long time, and families should be supported throughout the process.

Palliative Care of the Dying Child

Appropriate **palliative care** is essential for any child with a life-threatening or progressive incurable condition. The World Health Organization (2011) defines palliative care as "an approach that improves the quality of life of patients and their families facing problems associated with life-threatening illness, through the prevention and relief of suffering by means of early identification and impeccable assessment and treatment of pain and other problems, physical, psychosocial and spiritual." Whether palliative care is provided in the home, hospital, or hospice setting, the goal is to provide the best quality of life possible at the end of life while alleviating physical, psychological, emotional, and spiritual suffering. The Initiative for Pediatric Palliative Care from the Centre for Applied Ethics (2003)

has established principles on which palliative care of children should be based. These include:

- Maximizing family involvement in decision making and care planning in the ways and to the degree that each individual family finds comfortable
- Informing and involving children who have life-threatening illnesses in decisions regarding their care, and planning care as fully as possible given the child's developmental abilities and desires
- Reducing pain and distressful symptoms
- Providing emotional and spiritual support for children and their families as they cope with the multiple losses associated with life-threatening illnesses
- Facilitating resolution of the family's practical needs, such as the need for respite, through coordination in the community
- Facilitating continuity of care across care settings, both within and outside the hospital
- Offering bereavement support to the child and family before and after the child's death

Hospice Care

Hospice allows for family-centred care in either the child's home or a hospice facility. As with adult hospice care, the comfort of the entire family is important. Canada is home to the first free-standing pediatric hospice centre in North America, Canuck Place Children's Hospice in Vancouver, British Columbia (Straatman, Cadell, Davies, Siden, & Steele, 2008). The goal of pediatric hospice care is the enhancement of quality of life for the child and family through an individualized plan of care (Children's Hospice International, n.d.). The recommended standards for pediatric hospice care do not preclude involvement in ongoing treatment (this is in contrast to adult hospice), but certain eligibility criteria must be met (Children's Hospice International, n.d.). Parents are educated on ways to comfort and interact with their dying child, such as massage, movement, or singing. Spiritual support is available through a chaplain, social worker, or the family's minister. The nurse not only educates the family about the dying process but also assists them with providing basic care and pain management. The decision to withhold nutrition or hydration may be made in certain instances. Pain management is of utmost importance for the terminally ill child (Association of Pediatric Oncology Nurses, 2003). Ongoing bereavement care is also provided to the family by the hospice after the child's death (Ramer-Chrastek, Brunnquell, & Hasse, 2002).

Nursing Management of the Dying Child

Though interdisciplinary care is essential for quality care at the end of life, it is the nurse who plays the key role of child/family advocate and who is usually the constant presence throughout the dying process. Nursing management of the dying child focuses on end-of-life decision making, meeting the child's and family's needs, and assisting the family after the child's death. Throughout the process, focus on the family as the unit of care (Michelson & Steinhorn, 2007).

Assisting the Family with End-of-Life Decision Making

Parents are obligated not only to protect their children from harm but also to do as much good for them as possible, both from an ethical and legal standpoint (Rushton, 2004). When the time comes for end-of-life decision making, parents are often torn about the "right" course of action. Parents may be asked to make decisions about stopping treatment, withdrawing treatment, providing palliative care, or consenting to do not resuscitate (DNR) orders. Patients, parents, and health care providers are generally in agreement that continued suffering is not desired for any child with a terminal illness.

Nurses involved in this process must examine their own values related to dying and consider the Canadian Nurses Association's Code of Ethics (2008). The family's feelings must also be acknowledged. During the process of end-of-life decision making, health care providers must assure families that the focus of care is changing and that the child is not being abandoned (Michelson & Steinhorn, 2007). Emphasize to parents that no matter what their decision is, the health care team is dedicated to the comfort and expert care of their child (Rushton, 2004).

Ensure that communication is family-centred. Quality of life must be taken into consideration when making decisions to continue or withhold treatment (CPS, 2008). Provide parents facing end-of-life decisions with honest information and education from the time of the diagnosis/prognosis forward. Anticipate that parents may vacillate in the decision-making process. Clarify information for them and allow them private time to discuss the options. Do not make judgments about or question the parents' decision. Be sensitive to any ethnic, spiritual, or cultural preferences during the terminal stage of the illness. Encourage parents to interact with other parents who have a child with a terminal illness (Rushton, 2005).

Allowing Natural Death

The decision to institute a DNR order is one of the most difficult decisions a family may ever have to make. DNR refers to withholding cardiopulmonary resuscitation should the child's heart stop beating. Parents may initially feel like this means they are giving up on their child. Nurses must educate families that resuscitation may be inappropriate and lead to more suffering than if death were allowed to occur naturally. The parents need to understand that when a palliative care route is chosen, rather than continuing a curative or treatment route, the focus of the child's care is changing but that the child and family are not being abandoned. Families may wish to specify a certain extent of resuscitation that they feel more comfortable with (e.g., allowing supplemental oxygen but not providing chest compressions). Some institutions are now replacing the DNR terminology with "allow natural death" (AND), which may be more acceptable to families facing the decision to withhold resuscitation (CPS, 2008). Discussion of advanced care planning with the parents should be standard for all health care professionals caring for children with chronic life-threatening conditions.

Involving the Dying Child in the Decision-Making Process

End-of-life decision making often involves ethical dilemmas for the patient, family, and health care team. This is particularly true when the parents' wishes conflict with the child's or adolescent's desires. Children should be involved in decision making to the extent that they are able. Discuss intervention within the context of the child's condition and wishes. Children who are developmentally able (usually those over age 9) should be included in the discussion around the continuation or withdrawal of treatment (CPS, 2008). Be available to the older child or adolescent to provide support and information if he or she desires. Talk with the child or adolescent with the parents present, as well as in private. Maintain the child's comfort and dignity. Encourage the child to spend time with other children with a terminal illness. Assure the child that everything will be done to make him or her comfortable.

Consult parents about the timing and depth of end-of-life discussions. Just as parents do, the terminally ill child may vacillate in the decision-making process. Remain sensitive, and respect the child's decisions (Hinds et al., 2001).

Organ or Tissue Donation

With large numbers of organ transplant candidates on waiting lists and the shortage of viable organs, pediatric organ and tissue donation is a priority (Bratton et al., 2006). For many families, knowing that a child's organs or tissues may save another child's life provides a way to help others despite their own loss. A healthy child who dies unexpectedly is an excellent candidate for organ donation. Many chronic illnesses in children preclude the option of organ or tissue donation, though individual determinations of eligibility should be made.

The discussion of organ donation should be separated from the discussion of impending death or brain death notification. Written consent is necessary for organ donation, so the family must be appropriately informed and educated. Many families who never thought about it before may consider the option of donation if adequately educated about the process. Ask whether the dying child ever expressed a wish to donate organs and whether the parents have considered it.

Families need to know that procurement of the organs does not mar the child's appearance, so that an open casket at the child's funeral is still possible if the family desires. The donating child will not suffer further because of organ donation. The organs or tissues will be harvested in a timely fashion after the declaration of death, so the family need not worry about delay of the wake or funeral. The family's cultural and religious beliefs must be considered, and the team discussing organ donation with the family must do so in a sensitive and ethical manner (Bratton et al., 2006).

Managing Pain and Discomfort

Pain management is an essential component of care for the child with a terminal illness. Providing for comfort enhances the child's quality of life and minimizes suffering (Baker et al., 2008). Assess pain using a developmentally appropriate tool (see Chapter 35 for further information). Provide pain medication around the clock rather than on an "as needed" basis to prevent recurrence or escalation of pain. Determine the child's preferred comfort measures and use them to provide additional relief. Change the child's position frequently but gently to minimize discomfort. Limit nursing care to comfort measures that ease the child's discomfort. Maintain a calm environment, minimizing noise and light.

Easing Anxiety or Fears

Involve the parents and other family members in all phases of the child's care. Explain all aspects of care to the child to minimize anxiety related to nursing interventions. Answer the child's questions honestly. Involve the child in decision making whenever possible. Limit interventions to those related to palliation, rather than treatment, advocating for the child as needed. Remain with the child when a parent or family member is not in the room so the child will not fear dying alone.

Providing Nutrition

Since the body naturally requires less nutrition as the child is dying, do not excessively coax the child to eat or drink. Offer frequent small meals or snacks of the child's choosing. Soups and shakes require less energy to eat and so may be desirable. If the child desires a different food, provide that one. Keep strong odours away from the child to decrease nausea. Administer antiemetics as needed. Provide mouth care and keep the lips lubricated to keep the mouth feeling clean and prevent the discomfort associated with chapped lips. Make sure the environment is a pleasant one for eating.

Supporting the Dying Child and Family

To foster a holistic connection with the child and family, be attuned to the entire family's needs and emotions. Nurses provide physical care through specific tasks and interventions for the dying child, but they also need to be fully present with the child and family. In general, people are uncomfortable with the concept of a dying child. Nurses should work through their own feelings about the situation to be able to be "in the moment" with the child and family. Ask yourself: Can I be fully present with this family? If not, then what can I change to be so (Rushton, 2005)?

Families and dying children benefit from the presence of the nurse, not just the interventions he or she performs. Families report that the simple of act of being present with the family is very healing (Mellichamp, 2007). Listen to the child and family; be still and silent for a time to accomplish this. Foster respect for the whole child by attending to him or her as such.

Respect the parents of the dying child by helping them honour the commitments they have made to their child. Acknowledge that parents have diverse needs for information and participation in decision making. Allow and encourage family customs or rituals in relation to death and dying. Families may desire the pastor or priest to be present when the child's death is imminent. Certain rituals may be desired, depending on the family's religious or spiritual background. Ensure that these important events occur, and alter nursing care routines as needed to accommodate them. Respect the family's need to participate in these rituals and customs (Ethier, 2010).

Work collaboratively with the family and health care team to provide for the needs of the child and family (Michelson & Steinhorn, 2007). Resources for families of a dying child are listed in Box 33.6. The Make-a-Wish Foundation works to grant the wishes of terminally ill children, giving the child and family an experience of hope, strength, and love.

Meeting the Dying Child's Needs According to Developmental Stage

It is important to provide the type of support and education that the dying child needs according to his or her developmental stage. For the infant, unconditional love and trust are of utmost importance. Ensure that the infant's family is available to the child. The toddler, 1 to 3 years old, thrives on familiarity and routine. Maximize the toddler's time with parents, be consistent, provide favourite toys, and ensure physical comfort. Spirituality in the preschool years focuses on the concept of right versus wrong. The 3- to 5-year-old may see death as punishment for wrongdoing; correct this misunderstanding. Use honest and precise language. Help the parents to teach the child that though the family will miss the child, it will continue to function without him or her (Ethier, 2010).

The school-age child has a concrete understanding of death. Children who are 5 to 10 years old need specific, honest details (as desired). Encourage the child to help make decisions, and help the child to establish a sense of control (Ethier, 2010).

Resources for Families of a Dying Child

Organizations (Visit http://thePoint.lww.com/Chow1e for direct links to these organizations' websites.)

• Project Joy and Hope
• Canuck Place Children's Hospice
• Children's Hospice International
• Compassionate Friends

Books
• *Gentle Willow: A Story for Children about Dying* by Joyce Mills
• *35 Ways to Help a Grieving Child* by the Dougy Center for Grieving Children
• *Sad Isn't Bad* by Michaeline Mundy
• *A Child Asks. . . . What Does Dying Mean?* by Lake Pylant Monhollon
• *Choices—When Your Child Is Dying* by Shelia Lee
• *Lifetimes* by Bryan Mellonie and Robert Ingpen
• *The Fall of Freddie the Leaf: A Story of Life for All Ages* by Leo Buscaglia
• *The Worst Loss: How Families Heal from the Death of a Child* by Barbara Rosof
• *I Have No Intention of Saying Goodbye: Parents Share Their Stories of Hope and Healing After a Child's Death* by Sandy Fox
• *Stars in the Deepest Night: After the Death of a Child* by Genesse Gentry
• *The Bereaved Parent* by Harriet Schiff
• *You Are Special* by Max Lucado

The young adolescent (10 to 14 years old) will benefit from reinforcement of self-esteem, self-respect, and a sense of worth. Respect the child's need for privacy and time alone as well as time requested with peers. Support the need for independence and encourage the child to participate in decision making. The older teen (14 to 18 years of age) has a more adult-like understanding of death and will need further support through honest, detailed explanations and will want to feel truly involved and listened to (Ethier, 2010).

■■■ Key Concepts

■ Children with special health care needs are those who have, or are at risk for, a chronic physical, developmental, behavioural, or emotional condition that generally requires more intensive and diverse health services, as well as coordination of those services, than do typical children.

■ Most children with chronic illnesses or who are dependent on technology progress through stages of growth and development just as typical children do, though

possibly at a slower pace, and desire to be treated as normal children.

■ Parents of special needs children experience a multitude of emotions and changes in their lives, often carrying a heavy caregiving burden. They become the experts on their child's care and should be empowered and supported in their efforts.

■ Children with special health care needs are at increased risk for the development of vulnerable child syndrome, which may have psychologically harmful effects on the child and parents for many years.

■ Home is the most developmentally appropriate environment for children with special health care needs and those who are technologically dependent. Children display an improved physical, emotional, psychological, and social status when they are cared for at home.

■ Family-centred care provides the optimal framework for caring for children and families with special needs. Empowering the family strengthens it. A permanent relationship with the health care provider benefits the family, as care coordination and advocacy are provided.

■ Use adjusted (or corrected) age when assessing growth and development of the infant or child who was born prematurely. Provide early screening and intervention for issues related to development to maximize the former preemie's potential for growth and development.

■ Become familiar with the risks and benefits of adjuvant therapies used by some families of children with special health care needs.

■ Screen children with special health care needs for FTT or a feeding disorder.

■ Screening helps to identify children with unmet health needs early so that intervention may begin.

■ The child and family with special needs may require additional support during times of transition, such as at initial diagnosis or change in prognosis, when symptoms increase, when the child moves to new setting (hospital, school), during periods of developmental change, or during a parent's absence.

■ Early discharge planning and ongoing inclusion and education of the family facilitate continuity of care. During mid-adolescence, initiate a written plan to help the special needs child make the transition to adult care.

■ Early intervention provides care coordination (developmental services and special education), as well as an individualized family service plan for qualifying children and their families.

■ Younger children who are dying generally need for their families to be close and to trust their needs will be provided for. Older children require honest explanations given at a level appropriate for the child's age or developmental stage.

■ Support the dying child and the family throughout the end-of-life decision-making process, providing facts as desired about palliative care, hospice, and organ donation.

REFERENCES

Ahmann, E. (2006). Supporting fathers' involvement in children's health care. *Pediatric Nursing, 32*(1), 88–90.

American Academy of Pediatrics. (2001). Policy statement: Developmental surveillance and screening of infants and young children. *Pediatrics, 108,* 192–195.

American Academy of Pediatrics Committee on Fetus and Newborn. (2008). Hospital discharge of the high-risk neonate. *Pediatrics, 122*(5), 1119–1126.

American Hippotherapy Association. (2010). *Hippotherapy as a treatment strategy.* Retrieved September 23, 2011 from http://www.americanhippotherapyassociation.org/hippotherapy/hippotherapy-as-a-treatment-strategy/

Association of Pediatric Oncology Nurses. (2003). *Precepts of palliative care for children, adolescents and their families.* Retrieved September 23, 2011 from http://www.aphon.org/files/public/last_acts_precepts.pdf

Ayoob, K. T., & Barresi, I. (2007). Feeding disorders in children: Taking an interdisciplinary approach. *Pediatric Annals, 36*(8), 478–483.

Baker, J. N., Hinds, P. S., Spunt, S. L., et al. (2008). Integration of palliative care practices into the ongoing care of children with cancer: Individualized care planning and coordination. *Pediatric Clinics of North America, 55,* 223–250.

Betz, C. L., & Redcay, G. (2002). Lessons learned from providing transition services to adolescents with special health care needs. *Issues in Comprehensive Pediatric Nursing, 25,* 129–149.

Block, R. W., Krebs, N. F., the Committee on Child Abuse and Neglect, & the Committee on Nutrition. (2005). Failure to thrive as a manifestation of child neglect. *Pediatrics, 116*(5), 1234–1237.

Bowie, H. (2004). Mommy first. *Pediatric Nursing, 30*(3), 203–206.

Bratton, S. L., Kolovos, N. S., Roach, E. S., McBride, V., Geiger, J. L., & Meyers R. L. (2006). Pediatric organ transplantation needs: Organ donation best practices. *Archives of Pediatrics and Adolescent Medicine, 160*(5), 468–472.

Burns, C., Dunn, A., Brady, M., Starr, N. B., & Blosser, C. (2009). *Pediatric primary care* (4th ed.). Philadelphia: Saunders.

Burns, J. J., Sadof, M., & Kamat, D. (2006). The adolescent with a chronic illness. *Pediatric Annals, 35*(3), 207–216.

Canadian Nurses Association. (2008). *Code of Ethics for Registered Nurses.* Ottawa, ON: Author.

Canadian Paediatric Society. (2000, reaffirmed in 2011). Assessment of babies for car seat safety before hospital discharge. *Paediatrics & Child Health, 5*(1), 53–56.

Canadian Paediatric Society. (2007). Transition to adult care for youth with special needs. *Paediatrics & Child Health, 12*(9), 785–788.

Canadian Paediatric Society. (2008). Advanced care planning for paediatric patients. *Paediatrics & Child Health, 13*(9), 791–796.

Canadian Paediatric Society. (2009). Nutrition in neurologically impaired children. *Paediatrics & Child Health, 14*(6), 395–401.

Case-Smith, J. (2004). Parenting a child with a chronic medical condition. *American Journal of Occupational Therapy, 58,* 551–560.

Centre for Applied Ethics. (2003). *The initiative for pediatric palliative care.* Retrieved September 23, 2011 from http://www.ippcweb.org/module1.asp

Children's Hospice International. (n.d.). *About children's hospice, palliative and end-of-life care.* Retrieved September 23, 2011 from http://www.chionline.org/resources/about.php

Coffey, J. S. (2006). Parenting a child with chronic illness: A metasynthesis. *Pediatric Nursing, 32*(1), 51–59.

Cohen, E., Friedman, J., Nicholas, D. B., Adams, S., & Rosenbaum, P. (2008). A home for medically complex children: The role of hospital programs. *Journal for Healthcare Quality, 30*(3), 7–15.

Duncan, A. F., & Caughy, M. O. (2009). Parenting style and the vulnerable child syndrome. *Journal of Child and Adolescent Psychiatric Nursing, 22*(4), 228–234.

Ethier, A. M. (2010). Care of the dying child and the family. In D. Tomlinson & N. E. Kline (Eds.), *Pediatric oncology nursing.* New York: Springer.

Farmer, J. E., Marien, W. E., & Frasier, L. (2003). Quality improvements in primary care for children with special health care needs: Use of a brief screening measure. *Children's Health Care, 32*(4), 273–285.

Federation of Families for Children's Mental Health. (n.d.). *FFCMH principles for family involvement.* Retrieved September 23, 2011 from http://ffcmh.org/wp-content/uploads/2010/06/FFCMHPrinciples-forFamilyInvolvement.pdf

Gargus, R. A., Vohr, B. R., Tyson, J. E., et al. (2009). Unimpaired outcomes for extremely low birth weight infants at 18 to 22 months. *Pediatrics, 124*(1), 112–121.

Gasalberti, D. (2006). Alternative therapies for children and youth with special health care needs. *Journal of Pediatric Health Care, 20*(2), 133–136.

Green, A., & Ray, T. (2006). Attention to child development: A key piece of family-centered care for cardiac transplant recipients. *Journal for Specialists in Pediatric Nursing, 11*(2), 143–148.

Health Canada. (2008). *Canada Health Act Annual Report 2007–2008.* Retrieved September 23, 2011 from http://www.hc-sc.gc.ca/hcs-sss/pubs/cha-lcs/2008-cha-lcs-ar-ra/index-eng.php

Hewitt-Taylor, J. (2010). Supporting children with complex health needs. *Nursing Standard, 19*(24), 50–56.

Hinds, P. S., Oakes, L., Furman, W., et al. (2001). End-of-life decision making by adolescents, parents, and healthcare providers in pediatric oncology: Research to evidence-based practice guidelines. *Cancer Nursing, 24*(2), 122–136.

Horowitz, J. A., & Marchetti, C. M. (2010). Mood disorders. In P. J. Allen, J. A. Vessey, & N. A. Schapiro (Eds.), *Primary care of the child with a chronic condition* (5th ed.). St. Louis: Mosby.

Hysing, M., Elgen, I., Gillberg, C., & Lundervold, A. J. (2009). Emotional and behavioural problems in subgroups of children with chronic illness: Results from a large-scale population study. *Child: Care, Health and Development, 35*(4), 527–533.

Jackson Allen, P. L. (2004). Children with special health care needs: National survey of prevalence and health care needs. *Pediatric Nursing, 30*(4), 307–314.

Jalkut, M. K., & Allen, P. J. (2009). Transition from pediatric to adult health care for adolescents with congenital heart disease: A review of the literature and clinical implications. *Pediatric Nursing, 35*(6), 381–387.

Kelly, M. M. (2006a). Primary care issues for the healthy premature infant. *Journal of Pediatric Health Care, 20*(5), 293–299.

Kelly, M. M. (2006b). The basics of prematurity. *Journal of Pediatric Health Care, 20*(4), 238–244.

Kelly, M. M. (2006c). The medically complex premature infant in primary care. *Journal of Pediatric Health Care, 20*(6), 367–373.

Kelly, M. M. (2010). Prematurity. In P. J. Allen, J. A. Vessey, & N. A. Schapiro (Eds.), *Primary care of the child with a chronic condition* (5th ed.). St. Louis: Mosby.

Kepreotes, E., Keatinge, D., & Stone, T. (2010). The experience of parenting children with chronic health conditions: A new reality. *Journal of Nursing and Healthcare of Chronic Illness, 2*(1), 51–62.

Kerruish, N. J., Settle, K., Campbell-Stokes, P., & Taylor, B. J. (2005). Vulnerable Baby Scale: Development and piloting of a questionnaire to measure maternal perceptions of their baby's vulnerability. *Journal of Paediatrics and Child Health, 41*(8), 419–423.

Knafl, K. A., & Santacroce, S. J. (2010). Chronic conditions & the family. In P. J. Allen, J. A. Vessey, & N. A. Schapiro (Eds.), *Primary care of the child with a chronic condition* (5th ed.). St. Louis: Mosby.

Kuster, P. A., Badr, L. K., Chang, B. L., Wuerker, A. K., & Benjamin, A. E. (2004). Factors influencing health-promoting activities of mothers caring for ventilator-assisted children. *Journal of Pediatric Nursing, 19*(4), 276–287.

Lewis, M. (2007). Discharge management for children with complex needs. *Paediatric Nursing, 19*(4), 26–30.

Lewis, M., & Noyes, J. (2007). Discharge management for children with complex needs. *Paediatric Nursing, 19*(4), 26–30.

Limbos, M. M., Joyce, D. P., & Roberts, G. J. (2010). Nipissing district developmental screen. *Canadian Family Physician, 56,* 66–72.

Lindblad, B., Rasmussen, B. H., & Sandman, P. (2005). Being invigorated in parenthood: Parents' experiences of being supported by professionals when having a disabled child. *Journal of Pediatric Nursing, 20*(4), 288–297.

Lindeke, L. L., Krajicek, M., & Patterson, D. L. (2001). PNP roles and interventions with children with special needs and their families. *Journal of Pediatric Health Care, 15,* 138–143.

Locklin, M. (2005). The redefinition of failure to thrive from a case study perspective. *Pediatric Nursing, 31*(6), 474–479.

Looman, W. S., O'Conner-Von, S., & Lindeke, L. L. (2008). Caring for children with special health care needs and their families: What advanced practice nurses need to know. *Journal for Nurse Practitioners,* 4(7), 512–518.

McAllister, J. W., Presler, E., Turchi, R., & Antonelli, R. C. (2009). Achieving effective care coordination in the medical home. *Pediatric Annals, 38*(9), 491–497.

Meleski, D. D. (2002). Families with chronically ill children: A literature review examines approaches to helping them cope. *American Journal of Nursing, 102*(5), 47–54.

Mellichamp, P. (2007). End-of-life care for infants. *Home Healthcare Nurse, 25*(1), 41–44.

Michelson, K. N., & Steinhorn, D. M. (2007). Pediatric end-of-life issues and palliative care. *Clinical Pediatric Emergency Medicine, 8,* 212–219.

Moddemann, D., & Shea, S. (2006). The developmental pediatrician and neonatal follow-up. *Paediatrics & Child Health, 11*(5), 295–299.

Moore, A. J., Anderson, C., Carter, B., & Coad, J. (2010). Appropriated landscapes: The intrusion of technology and equipment into the homes and lives of families with a child with complex needs. *Journal of Child Health Care, 14*(1), 3–5.

Nuutila, L., & Salanterä, S. (2006). Children with a long-term illness: Parents' experiences of care. *Journal of Pediatric Nursing, 21*(2), 153–160.

O'Brien, I., Duffy, A., & Nicholl, H. (2009). Impact of childhood chronic illness on siblings: A literature review. *British Journal of Nursing, 18*(22), 1360–1365.

O'Brien, M. E., & Wegner, C. B. (2002). Rearing the child who is technology dependent: Perceptions of parents and home care nurses. *Journal for Specialists in Pediatric Nursing, 7*(1), 7–15.

O'Connor, M. E., & Szekely, L. J. (2001). Frequent breastfeeding and food refusal associated with failure to thrive: A manifestation of the vulnerable child syndrome. *Clinical Pediatrics, 40*(1), 27–33.

Paone, M. C., Wigle, M., & Saewyc, E. (2006). The ON TRAC model for transitional care of adolescents. *Progress in Transplantion, 16*(4), 291–302.

Pearson, S. R., & Boyce, W. T. (2004). The vulnerable child syndrome. *Pediatrics in Review, 25*(10), 345–349.

Public Health Agency of Canada. (2006). *Canadian Immunization Guide, Seventh edition – 2006.* Retrieved September 23, 2011 from http://www.phac-aspc.gc.ca/publicat/cig-gci/index-eng.php

Public Health Agency of Canada. (2011). Childhood cancers. Available November 7, 2011 at http://www.phac-aspc.gc.ca/cd-mc/cancer/childhood_cancer-cancer_enfants-eng.php

Ramer-Chrastek, J., Brunnquell, D., & Hasse, S. (2002). Letting nature take its course: One family's choice of hospice home care for their terminally ill infant. *American Journal of Nursing, 102*(10), 24CC-DD, FF, 24II-JJ.

Ratliffe, C. E., Harrigan, R. C., Haley, J., Tse, A., & Olson, T. (2002). Stress in families with medically fragile children. *Issues in Comprehensive Pediatric Nursing, 25,* 167–188.

Romanko, E. A. (2005). Caring for children with bronchopulmonary dysplasia in the home setting. *Home Healthcare Nurse, 23*(2), 95–102.

Rushton, C. H. (2004). Ethics and palliative care in pediatrics: When should parents agree to withdraw life-sustaining therapy for children? *American Journal of Nursing, 104*(4), 54–63.

Rushton, C. H. (2005). A framework for integrated pediatric palliative care: Being with dying. *Journal of Pediatric Nursing, 20*(5), 311–325.

Rydz, D., Shevell, M. I., Majnemer, A., & Oskoui, M. (2005). Topical review: Developmental screening. *Journal of Child Neurology, 20*(1), 4–21.

Schulman, L. H., Meringolo, D., & Scott, G. (2007). Early intervention: A crash course for pediatricians. *Pediatric Annals, 36*(8), 463–469.

Spalding, K., & Salib, D. (2008). *In focus fact sheet: Children and youth home care in Canada.* Retrieved September 23, 2011 from http://www.ryerson.ca/crncc/knowledge/factsheets/pdf/In_Focus_Children_and_Youth_Homecare_FINAL.pdf

Srivastava, R., Stone, B. L., & Murphy, N. A. (2005). Hospitalist care of the medically complex child. *Pediatric Clinics of North America, 52,* 1165–1187.

Statistics Canada. (2006). *Participation and activity limitation survey 2006: Analytical report.* Retrieved September 23, 2011 from http://www.statcan.gc.ca/pub/89-628-x/89-628-x2007002-eng.pdf

Statistics Canada. (2010). *Deaths 2007. Statistics Canada* [Catalogue no. 84F0211X]. Retrieved August 24, 2010 from http://dsp-psd.pwgsc.gc.ca/collection_2009/statcan/84F0211X/84f0211x2006000-eng.pdf

Straatman, L, Cadell, S., Davies, B., Siden, H., & Steele, R. (2008). Paediatric palliative care research in Canada: Development and progress of a new emerging team. *Paediatrics & Child Health, 13*(9), 591–594.

Vessey, J. A., & Sullivan, B. J. (2010). Chronic conditions and child development. In P. J. Allen, J. A. Vessey, & N. A. Schapiro (Eds.), *Primary care of the child with a chronic condition* (5th ed.). St. Louis: Mosby.

Wang, K. K., & Barnard, A. (2004). Technology-dependent children and their families: A review. *Journal of Advanced Nursing, 45*(1), 36–46.

Ware, C. J., Sloss, C. F., Chugh, C. S., & Budd, K. S. (2002). Adaptations of the Denver II scoring system to assess the developmental status of children with medically complex conditions. *Children's Health Care, 31*(4), 255–272.

Woods, S., & Riley, P. (2006). A role for community health care providers in neonatal follow-up. *Paediatrics & Child Health, 11*(5), 301–302.

World Health Organization. (2011). *WHO definition of palliative care.* Retrieved September 23, 2011 from http://www.who.int/cancer/palliative/definition/en

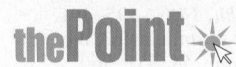

For additional learning materials, including Internet Resources, visit http://thePoint.lww.com/Chow1e.

CHAPTER WORKSHEET

MULTIPLE CHOICE QUESTIONS

1. The parents of a 5-year-old with special health care needs talk to the parents of a 10-year-old with a similar condition for quite a while each day. What is the nurse's interpretation of this behaviour?

   a. The nurse has not provided enough emotional support for the parents.

   b. This relationship between the children's parents is potentially unhealthy.

   c. Support between parents of special children is extremely valuable.

   d. Confidentiality is a pressing issue in this particular situation.

2. The nurse is caring for a child who has received all possible medical care for cancer yet continues to experience relapse and metastasis. It is time to make the transition from curative care attempts to palliative care. What is the most important nursing consideration at this time?

   a. The health care professionals should make the decision about the child's care.

   b. The family may lose a sense of hope, so cancer treatments should continue.

   c. Involve the family in the decision-making process regarding the shift to palliative care.

   d. Palliative care can take place only at home, so the child should be discharged.

3. The nurse is caring for a 3-year-old with a gastrostomy tube and tracheostomy who is on supplemental oxygen and multiple medications. The mother is rooming-in during this hospitalization. What is the priority nursing action?

   a. Incorporate the mother's assistance in care when convenient.

   b. Recognize the mother as the expert on her child's needs and care.

   c. Recommend that the mother go home to get some rest.

   d. Provide family-centred care since the mother is there.

4. The nurse is caring for a child with a developmental disability who is starting kindergarten this year. The mother is tearful and doesn't want the child to go to school. What is the best response by the nurse?

   a. "Do you need some time alone to collect yourself?"

   b. "You've known for a while this time would come."

   c. "Can I call your husband or a friend for you?"

   d. "It is normal to feel stressed or sad at this time."

5. The parents of a child with a developmental disability ask the nurse for advice about disciplining their child. What is the best response by the nurse?

   a. "You should choose methods that are most congruent with your values about discipline."

   b. "Children like this really can't follow directions, so they may be very hard to discipline."

   c. "Punish your child only for socially unacceptable or offending behaviours."

   d. "Spanking works well for this type of child, as they really don't like pain."

CRITICAL THINKING EXERCISES

1. A 15-year-old boy is dying of cancer after all medical care options have been exhausted. Describe the plan of care for this child and his family. What strategies should the nurse use to support the child and his family through this difficult process?

2. A 5-month-old infant who was born at 24 weeks' gestation is ready to be discharged from the NICU. She will be going home on oxygen, gastrostomy tube feedings, and eight medications. Develop a teaching plan for the family.

STUDY ACTIVITIES

1. In the clinical setting, care for a child with a terminal illness. Reflect in your clinical journal about the feelings you had during the care of the child, as well as the feelings and behaviours that you noticed in the child, siblings, parents, and nursing staff.

2. Visit a preschool that provides care for developmentally delayed and typical children. Choose two same-age children, one with a disability or impairment and the other a typical healthy child. Perform a developmental screening test (e.g., Denver II) on each of the two children. Compare and contrast your findings.

3. Spend the day with a homecare nurse providing care for a technologically dependent child. What obstacles has the family overcome to have this child at home? What adjustments does the nurse make to provide family-centred care in the home (as compared with the hospital setting)?

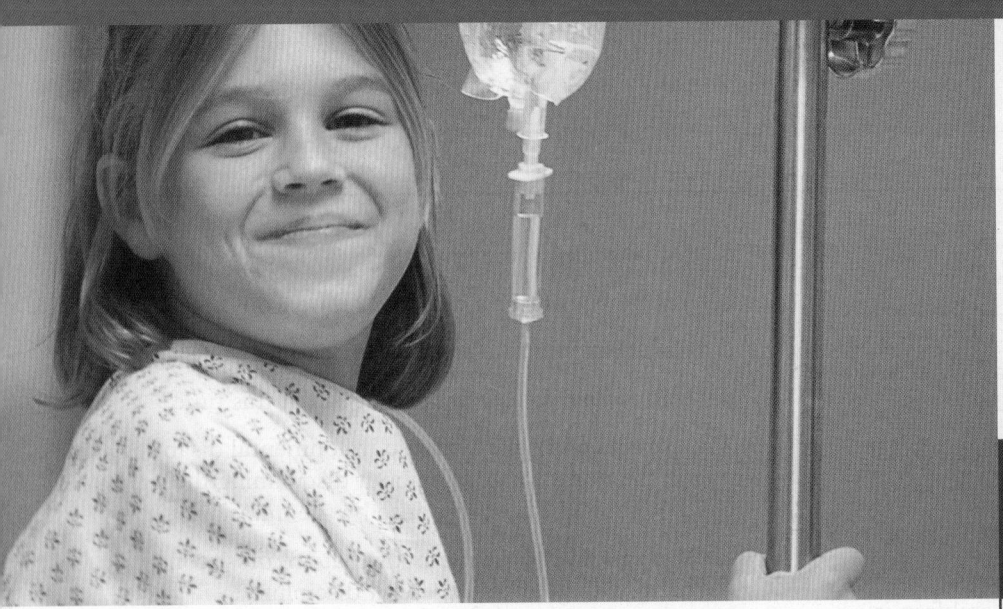

CHAPTER 34

Adapted by B. Nicole Harder

MEDICATION ADMINISTRATION, INTRAVENOUS THERAPY, AND NUTRITIONAL SUPPORT

KEY TERMS

biotransformation
bolus feeding
enteral nutrition
gastrostomy

gavage feedings
infiltration
parenteral nutrition
pharmacodynamics

pharmacokinetics
residual
total parenteral
nutrition

LEARNING OBJECTIVES

Upon completion of this chapter, the learner will be able to:

1. Describe atraumatic methods for preparing children for procedures.
2. Describe the eight "rights" of pediatric medication administration.
3. Explain the physiologic differences in children that affect a medication's pharmacodynamic and pharmacokinetic properties.
4. Accurately determine recommended pediatric medication doses.
5. Demonstrate the proper technique for administering medication to children via the oral, rectal, ophthalmic, otic, intravenous, intramuscular, and subcutaneous routes.
6. Integrate the concepts of atraumatic care in medication administration for children.
7. Identify the preferred sites for peripheral and central intravenous medication administration.
8. Describe nursing management related to maintenance of intravenous infusions in children, as well as prevention of complications.
9. Explain nursing care related to enteral tube feedings.
10. Describe nursing management of the child receiving total parenteral nutrition.

Lily Kline, a 9-month-old, is admitted to your unit for failure to thrive. The physician has ordered insertion of a nasogastric tube to begin gavage feedings. The parents are very nervous and upset about this. They ask, "What will this tube do for Lily? It sounds very uncomfortable. What do you have to do to insert it? Will it have to stay in all the time? Won't it move?" How would you address their concerns?

WOW

Parents judge us by our technical abilities and their child's outcome, not by what they believe nurses are capable of doing.

The ill child often requires medications, intravenous (IV) therapy, or enteral nutrition to restore health. These procedures occur most often in the inpatient setting, but with today's advanced technology many children may receive treatment in the home, day care centre, school, physician's office, or other community setting.

This chapter begins with an overview of the important aspects of caring for a child who is to undergo a procedure. The key elements of and guidelines for care related to medication administration, IV therapy, and nutritional support in children will be discussed. Child and parent education is emphasized. The chapter will focus on adapting and modifying nursing procedures based on the child's growth and development and providing these treatments using a family-centred, atraumatic approach.

Children and Procedures

Children undergo numerous diagnostic and therapeutic procedures in a wide range of settings during their development. Medication administration, IV therapy, and nutritional support are just three examples. These procedures may be performed in the community or out-patient setting or in a care facility (see Chapters 2 and 32 for additional information). Regardless of the procedure to be performed or the setting, children, like adults, need thorough preparation before the procedure and support during and after the procedure to promote the best outcome.

Before the Procedure

Appropriate preparation for procedures helps to decrease the child's and family's anxiety level, promote the child's cooperation, and support the child's and family's coping skills. Adequate preparation also helps to foster the child's feeling of mastery over a potentially stressful event, as undergoing invasive procedures in particular is extremely distressing for children.

Preparation may include psychological preparation (including explanation and education) as well as preparing the child physically. Employ the concept of atraumatic care when preparing children for a procedure. General guidelines for preparation include the following:

- Provide a description of and the reason for the procedure using age-appropriate language ("the doctor will look at your blood to see why you are sick").
- Describe where the procedure will occur ("the X-ray department has big machines that won't hurt you; it's a little cold there too").
- Introduce strange equipment the child may see ("you will lie on a special bed that moves in the big machine, but you can still see out").
- Describe how long the procedure will last ("you will be in the X-ray department until lunchtime").

- Identify unusual sensations that may occur during the procedure ("you may smell something different" [e.g., alcohol smell], "the MRI machine makes loud noises").
- Inform the child about any pain or other expected sensations that may be involved ("it might feel warm in your hand when the medicine goes in").
- Identify any special care required after the procedure ("you will need to lie quietly for 15 minutes afterward").

> ▶ **Take** NOTE!
>
> *In the hospital, perform all invasive procedures in the treatment room or a room other than the child's room. The child's room should remain a safe and secure area.*

A major aspect of preparation involves play. In general, young children respond better to play materials and older children benefit more from viewing peer modeling films. However, consider the child's temperament, coping strategies, and previous experiences as well as developmental needs and cognitive abilities. First, gain trust and provide support. Include the child's parents because parents are usually the greatest source of comfort for the child. Be brief, simple, and appropriate in explaining situations at the child's level of development. Explain what is to be done and what is expected of the child. Avoid terms that have double meanings or might be confusing. Table 34.1 lists alternative words or phrases to use for terms that may be confusing or misunderstood.

During the Procedure

Use a firm, positive, confident approach that provides the child with a sense of security. Encourage cooperation by involving the child in decision making and allowing the child to select from a list or group of appropriate choices. Allow the child to express feelings of anger, anxiety, fear, frustration, or any other emotions. Often this is how a child communicates and copes with the situation. Tell the child that it is okay to scream or cry, but that it is very important to hold still. Use distraction methods such as those listed in Box 34.1.

Toddlers and preschoolers often resist procedures despite preparation. Being held down or restrained is often more traumatizing to the young child than the procedure itself. Use alternative methods (positions that provide comfort for the child) to keep the child still during the procedure (Fig. 34.1).

After the Procedure

After the procedure, hold and comfort the child. Cuddle and soothe infants. Encourage children to express their

TABLE 34.1 ALTERNATIVES FOR CONFUSING OR MISUNDERSTOOD TERMS

Term to Avoid	How Children Might Interpret It	Use These Terms Instead
Catheter	Too technical	Tube
Deaden	Kill?	Make sleepy
Dye	"Die"	Special medicine to help the doctor see _____ (part of the body) better
Electrodes	Too technical	Stickers, ticklers, snaps
ICU	"I see you"	Special room with your own nurse
Incision, cut open, make a hole	Too explicit	Special or small opening
Monitor	Too technical	TV screen
Organ	Like a piano?	Special place in the body
Pain	May be too explicit	Child's word for hurt; "boo-boo"
Put to sleep, anesthesia	May confuse with putting a pet to sleep	Special kind of sleep
Shot	Children are scared of shots	Medication under the skin
Stool	Like you sit on?	"Poop" or child's word for it
Stretcher or gurney	"Stretch her"	Rolling bed or special bed on wheels
Take your temperature/blood pressure	Where are you going to "take" them?	See how warm you are/hug your arm
Test	Like at school? (the child will need to perform)	See how your heart is working
Tourniquet	Too technical	Special kind of rubber band
Urine	"You're in?"	"Pee" or child's word for it
X-ray	Don't understand	Picture or big camera to take pictures of the inside of your body

Partially adapted from Florida Children's Hospital, Child Life Department. (n.d.).

feelings through play, such as dramatic play or use of puppets. Gross motor activities such as pounding or throwing are also helpful for children to discharge pent-up feelings and energy. School-age children and adolescents may not outwardly demonstrate behaviour indicating the need for comforting; however, provide them with opportunities to express their feelings and be comforted. Remember to provide children with encouraging words

---

BOX 34.1 Distraction Methods During Procedures

- Have the child point toes inward and wiggle them.
- Ask the child to squeeze your hand.
- Encourage the child to count aloud.
- Sing a song and have the child sing along.
- Point out the pictures on the ceiling.
- Have the child blow bubbles.
- Play music that is appealing to the child.

---

during the procedure and after all interventions are completed.

Medication Administration

WATCH & LEARN

It is very likely that at one time or another, children will need to receive medication. As with adults, pediatric medication administration is a critical component of safe and effective nursing care. However, the need for safety takes on even greater importance due to the physiologic, psychological, and cognitive differences inherent in children. Therefore, the pediatric nurse must adapt administration principles and techniques to meet the child's needs. Medication administration, regardless of the route, requires a solid knowledge base about the drug and its action.

As with medication administration to any patient, the nurse must adhere to the "rights" of medication administration (Box 34.2). Confirming the child's identity and double-checking the dosage before administration of any medication are two critical safeguards that play a major role in preventing medication errors.

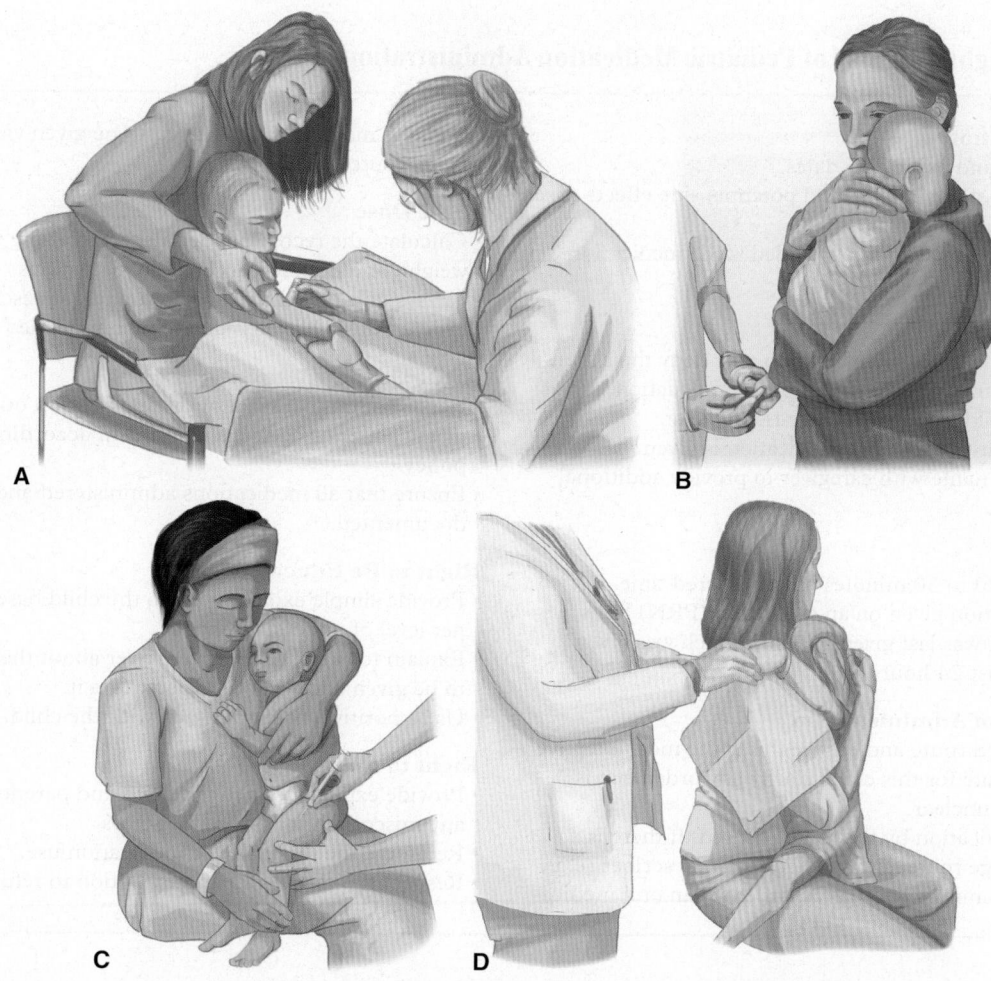

FIGURE 34.1 Positioning a child for comfort during a painful procedure. (**A**) Sitting on the parent's lap while undergoing allergy testing provides this toddler with a sense of comfort. (**B**) Position the infant cuddled over the parent's (preferable) or the nurse's shoulder when obtaining a heelstick. (**C**) Use "therapeutic hugging" to maintain a child's position while the child is having an IM medication administered. (**D**) Hold the older child while using a story or book for distraction.

Differences in Pharmacodynamics and Pharmacokinetics

Although a drug's mechanism of action is the same in any individual, the physiologic immaturity of some body systems in a child can affect a drug's **pharmacodynamics** (behaviour of the medication at the cellular level). As a result, the body may not respond to the drug as intended. The intended effect may be enhanced or diminished, necessitating a change in the dosage to ensure optimal effectiveness without increasing the child's risk for toxicity.

The child's age, weight, body surface area (BSA), and body composition also can affect the drug's **pharmacokinetics** (movement of drugs throughout the body via absorption, distribution, metabolism, and excretion). Drugs are administered to children via many of the same routes that are used for adults. However, this is the only similarity between the two.

During the absorption process, drugs move from the administration site into the bloodstream. In infants and young children, the absorption of orally administered medications is affected by slower gastric emptying, increased intestinal motility, a proportionately larger small intestine surface area, higher gastric pH, and decreased lipase and amylase secretion compared with adults. Intramuscular (IM) absorption in infants and young children is affected by amount of muscle mass, muscle tone and perfusion, as well as vasomotor instability. Similarly, decreased perfusion alters subcutaneous (SC) absorption. Absorption by these routes is erratic and may be decreased. In contrast, topical absorption of medications is increased in infants and young children because the stratum corneum is thinner and well hydrated (Lilley, Collins, Harrington, & Snyder, 2011; Woo, 2004).

The distribution of medications (movement of a drug from the blood to interstitial spaces and then into cells) is

---

BOX 34.2 Eight "Rights" of Pediatric Medication Administration

Right Medication
- Check order and expiration dates.
- Know action of medication and potential side effects (use pharmacy, drug formulary).
- Ensure that the medication provided is the medication that is ordered.

Right Patient
- Check identification, since children may deny their identity in an attempt to avoid an unpleasant situation, play in another child's bed, or remove ID bracelet.
- Confirm identity each time medication is given.
- Verify child's name with caregiver to provide additional confirmation.

Right Time
- Give within 20 to 30 minutes of the ordered time.
- For a medication given on an as-needed (PRN) basis, know when it was last given and how much was given during the past 24 hours.

Right Route of Administration
- Check ordered route and ensure this is the most effective and safest route for this child; clarify any order that is confusing or unclear.
- Give the medication by the route ordered. If there is a need to change route, always check with prescriber (e.g., if a child is vomiting and has an order for an oral medica-

tion, the medication may need to be given via the IV or rectal route).

Right Dose
- Calculate the recommended dose according to child's weight, and double-check your calculations.
- Always question the pharmacist and/or prescriber if the ordered dose falls outside the recommended dose range.

Right Documentation
- Record administration of the medication on the appropriate paper or computerized form according to agency policy.
- Ensure that all medications administered and refused are documented.

Right to Be Educated
- Provide simple explanations to the child based on his or her level of understanding.
- Explain to the parents or caregiver about the medication to be given and what to expect from it.
- Use a positive, firm approach with the child.

Right to Refuse
- Provide explanations to the child and parents to clarify any misconceptions or relieve fears.
- Reinforce the rationale for medication use.
- Respect the child's or parents' option to refuse.

---

also altered in infants and young children. Medication distribution in children is affected by the following:

- Higher percentage of body water than adults
- More rapid extracellular fluid exchange
- Decreased body fat
- Liver immaturity, altering first-pass elimination
- Decreased amounts of plasma proteins available for drug binding
- Immature blood–brain barrier, allowing permeation by certain medications (Lilley et al., 2011; Woo, 2004)

Metabolism of medications in children is altered because of differences in hepatic enzyme production and the child's increased metabolic rate. **Biotransformation** (the alteration of chemical structures from their original form, which allows for the eventual excretion of the substance) in children is affected by the same variations that affect distribution. In addition, the immaturity of the kidneys until the age of 1 to 2 years affects renal blood flow, glomerular filtration, and active tubular secretion. This results in a longer half-life and increases the potential for toxicity of drugs primarily excreted by the kidneys (Lilley et al., 2011; Woo, 2004).

Developmental Issues and Concerns

Children are constantly growing and developing. The specific psychosocial, cognitive, physical, and motor developmental levels of children are important. Nurses need a solid understanding of growth and development to ensure safe administration of medications to children. Table 34.2 details some key areas in administering medications to children. Always give developmentally appropriate, truthful explanations before administering medications to children. Explain why the drug is needed, what the child will experience, what is expected of the child, and how the parents can participate and support their child. Refer to Chapters 25 through 29 for further information about growth and developmental issues.

The child's past experiences with taking medications and the approaches that may have been used will often affect how the child reacts. Always approach children positively; let your manner convey the belief that they can accomplish the needed behaviour. Never label the child as "bad" if he or she does not fully cooperate in taking medication. When medications must be administered parenterally (e.g., IM or SC), assure the child that this method is not a consequence of the child's behaviour.

TABLE 34.2 GROWTH AND DEVELOPMENT ISSUES RELATED TO PEDIATRIC MEDICATION ADMINISTRATION

Stage of Development	Issue/Concern	Nursing Interventions
Infant	Development of trust, which is fostered by consistent care; development of stranger anxiety later in infancy	Involve parents in medication administration to reduce stress for infant Ensure that parents hold and comfort infant during intervention
Toddler	Development of autonomy with displays of negativism, rituals, routines, and choices necessary to maintain some sense of control	Follow routines and rituals from home in giving medications if these are safe and positive approaches Involve parents in medication administration Offer simple choices (e.g., "Do you want Mom or me to give you your medicine?") Allow child to touch or handle equipment as appropriate
Preschooler	Development of initiative, which is fostered when they sense they are helping	Provide an opportunity to play with the equipment and respond positively to explanations and comforting Provide choices that are possible and keep them simple (e.g., "Do you want juice or water with your medication?" or "Which medication do you want to take first?") Do not ask, "Will you take your medicine now?" Involve parents in medication administration Be aware that giving suppositories is particularly upsetting to this age group because of their fears of bodily intrusion and mutilation
School-age child	Development of industry, benefiting from being a part of their care; generally very cooperative	Explain to child in simple terms the purpose of the medication Seek their assistance, such as putting pills in cup or opening the packet, and allow a broader range of choices Establish a reward system to enhance their cooperation if necessary
Adolescent	Development of identity, benefiting from much more control over their care	Approach in same manner as adults, with respect and sensitivity to their needs Maintain the adolescent's privacy as much as possible

Help parents to work through the feelings of frustration that may result from the child's refusal to cooperate with medication administration. Provide parents with facts about growth and developmental issues and children's fears and anxiety related to medication administration. Model alternative ways for the parents to deal with undesirable behaviour.

▶ *Take* NOTE!

Always administer medications promptly, assist the child in holding still using a comforting position for the child, and reinforce positive behaviour.

Determination of Correct Dose

Administering the correct dose is a key component of medication administration. Many drug references list recommended pediatric dosages, and nurses are responsible for checking doses to ensure that they are appropriate for

the child. Two common methods for determining pediatric doses are based on the unit of drug per kilogram of body weight or BSA.

Dose Determination by Body Weight

The most common method for calculating pediatric medication doses is based on body weight. The recommended dosage is usually expressed as the amount of drug to be given over a 24-hour period (mg/kg/day) or as a single dose (mg/kg/dose). Differentiate between the 24-hour dosage and the single dose. Use these guidelines to determine the correct dose by body weight:

1. Weigh the child.
2. Check the drug reference for the safe dose range (e.g., 10 to 20 mg/kg of body weight).
3. Calculate the low safe dose (Box 34.3).
4. Calculate the high safe dose.
5. Determine if the dose ordered is within this range.

The pediatric dosage should not exceed the minimum recommended adult dosage. Generally, once a child or adolescent weighs 50 kg or greater, the adult dose is

BOX 34.3 **Dosage Calculation Using Body Weight-Proportion Method**

- Calculate the low safe dose range (e.g., 10 to 20 mg/kg and the child weighs 30 kg):
  - Set up a proportion using the low safe dose range
    10 mg/1 kg = x mg/30 kg
  - Solve for x by cross-multiplying:
    $1 \times x = 10 \times 30$
    $x = 300$ mg
- Calculate the high safe dose range:
  - Set up a proportion using the high safe dose range
    20 mg/1 kg = x mg/30 kg
  - Solve for x by cross-multiplying:
    $1 \times x = 20 \times 30$
    $x = 600$
- Compare the safe dose range (for this example, 300 to 600 mg) with the ordered dose. If the dose falls within the range, the dose is safe. If the dose falls outside the range, notify the prescriber.

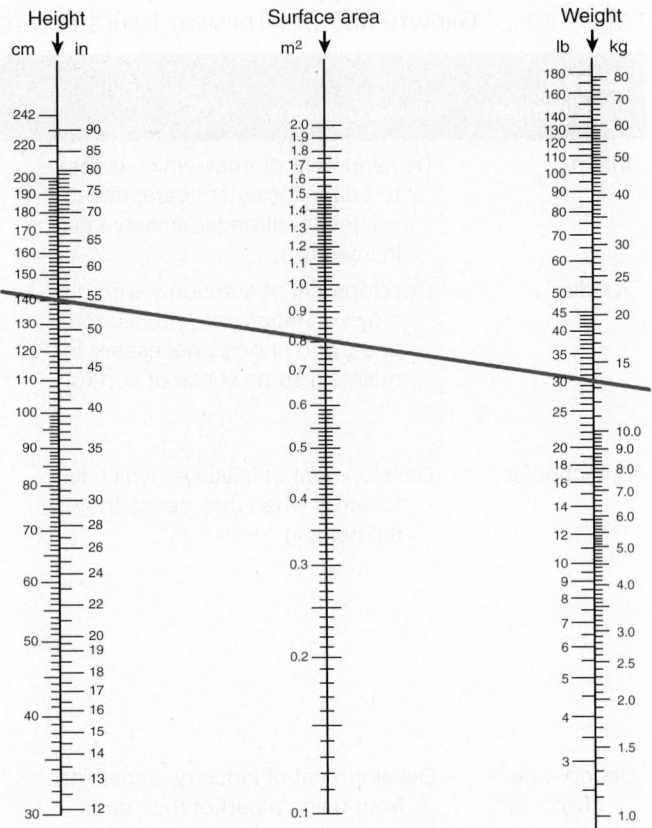

FIGURE 34.2 A nomogram to determine body surface area.

frequently prescribed (Bowden & Greenberg, 2008). However, always verify that the dose does not exceed the recommended adult dose.

Dose Determination by BSA

Calculating the dosage based on BSA takes into account the child's metabolic rate and growth. It is commonly used for chemotherapeutic agents. Some recommended medication doses may read "mg/BSA/dose." To determine the dose using BSA, you will need to know the child's height and weight, which will be plotted on a nomogram (Fig. 34.2). A nomogram is a graph divided into three columns: height (left column), surface area (middle column), and weight (right column). Use these guidelines to determine BSA:

1. Measure the child's height.
2. Determine the child's weight.
3. Using the nomogram, draw a line to connect the height measurement in the left column and the weight measurement in the right column.
4. Determine the point where this line intersects the line in the surface area column. This is the BSA, expressed in meters squared (m^2).

Once you have determined the BSA, use the recommended dosage range to calculate the safe dosage.

Oral Administration

Medications to be given via the oral route are supplied in many forms, such as liquids (elixirs, syrups, or suspensions), powders, tablets, and capsules. Generally, children under the age of 5 to 6 are at risk for aspiration because

they have difficulty swallowing tablets or capsules. Therefore, if a tablet or capsule is the only oral form available, it needs to be crushed or opened and mixed with a pleasant-tasting liquid or a small amount (generally no more than a tablespoon) of a nonessential food such as applesauce. However, never crush or open an enteric-coated or time-release tablet or capsule. The crushed tablet or inside of a capsule may taste bitter, so never mix it with formula or other essential foods. Otherwise, the child may associate the bitter taste with the food and later refuse to eat it.

Liquid medications, primarily suspensions, may be less concentrated at the top of the bottle than at the bottom of the bottle. Always shake the liquid to ensure even drug distribution. The key to administering liquid forms of oral medications is to use calibrated equipment such as a medicine cup, spoon, plastic oral syringe, or dropper (Fig. 34.3). If a dropper is packaged with a certain medication, never use it to administer another medication, since the drop size may vary from one dropper to another. If using a syringe for oral administration, only use the type intended for oral medications, not one designed for parenteral administration. When using a dropper or oral syringe (without a needle) for infants or young children, direct the liquid toward the posterior side of the mouth. Give the drug slowly in small amounts (0.2 to 0.5 mL) and allow the child to swallow before more medication is placed in the mouth. A nipple without the bottle attached

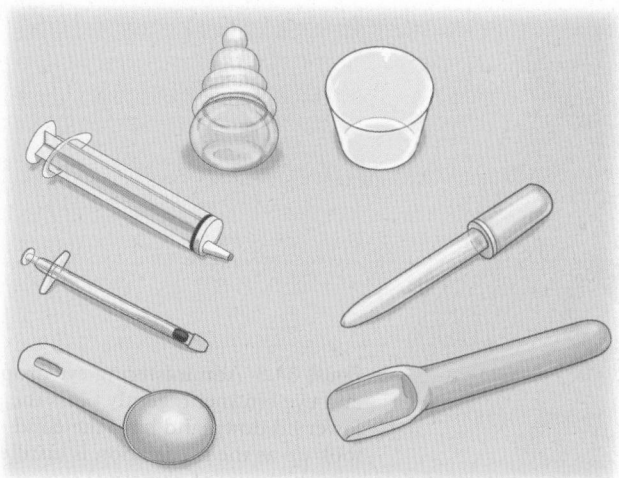

FIGURE 34.3 Devices used to administer oral medications to children.

is sometimes used to administer medication to infants. Place the medication directly in the nipple and keep the nipple filled with medication as the infant sucks so no air is taken in while the infant takes the medication. Always place the infant or young child upright (at least a 45-degree angle) to avoid aspiration (Fig. 34.4). The toddler or young preschooler may enjoy using the oral syringe to squirt the medicine into his or her mouth. Older children can take oral medication from a medicine cup or measured medicine spoon.

As children adapt to swallowing tablets or capsules, administration is similar to that of adults. When helping the younger child learn how to swallow medication, the tablet or capsule can be placed at the back of the tongue or in a small amount of food such as ice cream or applesauce. Always tell children if there is medicine in the food; otherwise they may not trust you.

▶ *Take* NOTE!

Use the medicine cup or syringe with proper calibration instead of household cups or measuring spoons, since they are not calibrated and may deliver an incorrect dose of medication.

When the child has a nasogastric, orogastric, **gastrostomy** (opening into the stomach) or nasojejunal tube, oral medications may be given via these devices. The tube allows for the medication to be placed directly into the stomach or jejunal area. Medication for administration via a tube must be supplied in a liquid form, or a crushed tablet or opened capsule can be mixed with a liquid (Box 34.4). Always check tube placement prior to administering the medication. After administration, flush the tube to maintain patency.

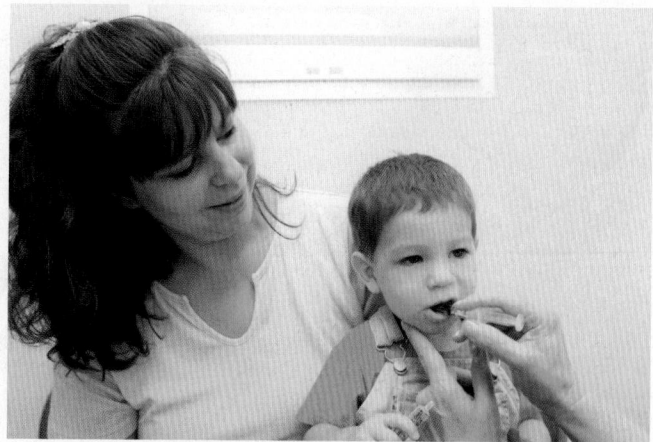

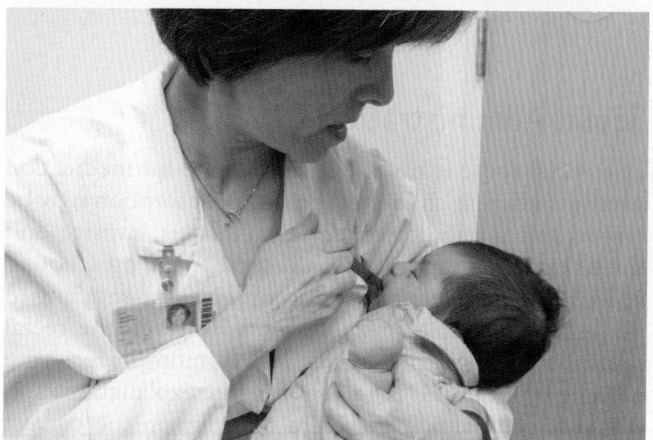

FIGURE 34.4 Position the infant or young child for safe medication administration.

▶ *Take* NOTE!

Never force an oral medication into a child's mouth or pinch the child's nose. Doing so increases the risk for aspiration and interferes with the development of a trusting relationship.

BOX 34.4 **Guidelines for Administering Medications Via Gastrostomy or Jejunostomy Tube**

- Give only liquid medications through the tube.
- Flush the tube before and after giving each medication.
- If the medication comes in a capsule, open the capsule and dissolve the contents in 10 to 20 mL of warm water to prevent tube occlusion.
- If the medication comes as a pill, ask the pharmacist if the medication can be crushed and mixed with water.
- Do not mix or crush medications together.

Adapted from McMaster Children's Hospital. (2006). *When your child has a gastrostomy tube: A guide for parents and families.* Hamilton, ON: Author.

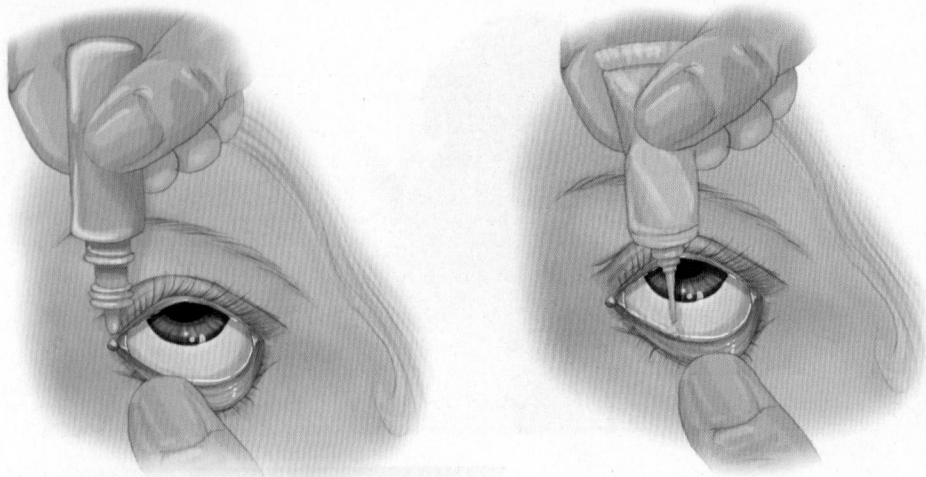

FIGURE 34.5 Administering eye drops and eye ointment: gently press the lower lid down and have the child look up as the medication is instilled into the lower conjunctival sac.

Rectal Administration

The rectal route is not a preferred route for medication administration in children. The drug's absorption may be erratic and unpredictable. The method is invasive and can be extremely upsetting to the toddler and preschooler because of age-related fears and may be embarrassing to the school-age child or adolescent. However, the rectal route may be used when the child is vomiting or receiving nothing by mouth. Use age-appropriate explanations and reassurance. Helping the child to maintain the correct position may be necessary to ensure proper insertion and safety.

Lubricate the suppository well with a water-soluble lubricant. With the child in the side-lying position, insert the suppository into the rectum quickly but gently. Wear gloves or use a finger cot to insert the suppository above the anal sphincter. For an infant or child under the age of 3, use the small finger for insertion. For an older child, use the index finger. To prevent expulsion of the suppository, hold the buttocks together for several minutes or until the child loses the urge to defecate. If the child has a bowel movement within 10 to 30 minutes after administration of the medication, examine the stool for the presence of the suppository. If it is observed, it will need to be determined whether the drug is to be administered again.

Ophthalmic Administration

Many children fear having anything placed in their eyes. Provide older children with an age-appropriate explanation to gain their cooperation. Ophthalmic medications are typically supplied in the form of drops or ointment. Ensure that the medication is at room temperature, as chilled medication may be uncomfortable to the child. Proper positioning of the child is necessary to control the child's head, keep the child's hands from interfering, and prevent injury to the eye. Attempt to administer the medication when the child is not crying to ensure that the medication reaches its intended target area.

Place the child in the supine position, slightly hyperextending the neck with the head lower than the body so the medication will be dispersed over the cornea. Rest the heel of your hand on the child's forehead to stabilize it. Retract the lower eyelid and place the medication in the conjunctival sac, being careful not to touch the tip of the tube or dropper to the sac. Wear gloves and maintain sterile technique. For eye drops, place the prescribed number of drops into the lower conjunctival sac (Fig. 34.5). For ointment, apply the medication in a thin ribbon from the inner canthus outward without touching the eye or eyelashes. If the child is old enough to cooperate, instruct the child to gently close the eyes to allow the medication to be dispersed.

Children often require ophthalmic medications at home. Parents or caregivers need instruction about how to administer this type of medication. Teaching Guideline 34.1 provides information on administering eye drops and eye ointments.

Otic Administration

Medications for otic administration are typically in the form of drops. This route of administration can be upsetting to the child because he or she cannot see what is happening. The child often receives otic drugs for an earache, and he or she may fear that the ear drops will increase the pain. Explain the procedure to the younger child in terms that he or she can understand to help allay these fears. Gain the older child's cooperation by explaining the purpose of the medication and the procedure for administration.

Reinforce the need for the child to keep the head still. Younger children may require assistance to do so. Be sure that the ear drops are at room temperature. If necessary, roll the container between the palms of your hands

TEACHING GUIDELINE 34.1

Applying Eye Medications

- Wash your hands with soap and water. Dry them thoroughly using paper towels or a clean cloth.
- Allow the eye drops or ointment to come to room temperature (if the medication was stored in the refrigerator). If necessary, warm the eye drop bottle or ointment tube in the palm of your hand. Keep the cap on to avoid any spillage.
- Remove the cap, placing it on a dry, clean surface.
- For young children (3 years or less), obtain assistance to keep their arms and fingers away during the procedure. If doing this procedure alone, wrap the child in a towel or blanket, keeping the arms inside.
- If you are applying eye drops, it may be easiest if you are standing or sitting behind the child, looking over the back of the child's head as he or she reclines. If you are applying an eye ointment, it may be easiest to face the child directly.
- Using one hand, hold the child's forehead in place while raising the eyelid with your thumb.
- With your other hand, hold the eye drop bottle or ointment tube above the eye, using an extended finger against the child's cheek, forehead, or nose to steady your hand.

- Gently squeeze the eye drop bottle, dispensing the proper number of drops, or gently squeeze the ointment tube, dispensing a small trail (about 2 cm) of ointment into the gap between the lower portion of the eye and bottom eyelid.
- Make sure the tip of the bottle or tube does not make contact with the eye or any other surface.
- For eye drops, gently press your finger against the inside corner where the eye meets the nose for about 1 minute, blocking the tears and medication from exiting through the tear duct. This will help the eye retain more of the medication. If your child is old enough, he or she may be able to do this unassisted.
- For ointment, have the child close his or her eye and not rub the area.
- Ask the child not to blink or squeeze the eye shut more than normal, as this may wash away the medication prematurely.
- Gently dab away any tears with a clean tissue.
- If necessary, clean the tip of the bottle or tube with a clean tissue and recap.
- Wash your hands again and dry them thoroughly.

Sources: Pediatric Glaucoma & Cataract Family Association. (2008a, 2008b).

---

to help warm the drops. Cold ear drops can cause pain and possibly vertigo when they reach the eardrum (Bowden & Greenberg, 2008).

Place the child in a supine or side-lying position with the affected ear exposed (Fig. 34.6). Pull the pinna downward and back in children under the age of 3 and

upward and back in older children. Instill the medication using a dropper. Then have the child remain in the same position for several minutes to ensure that the medication stays in the ear canal. Massage the area anterior to the affected ear to promote passage of the medication into the ear canal. If necessary, place a piece of cotton or

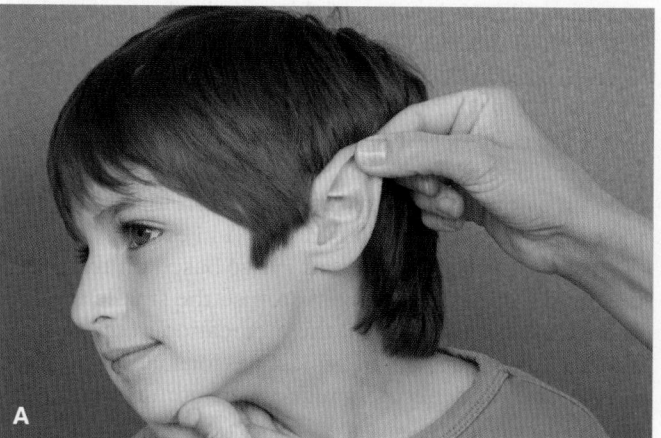
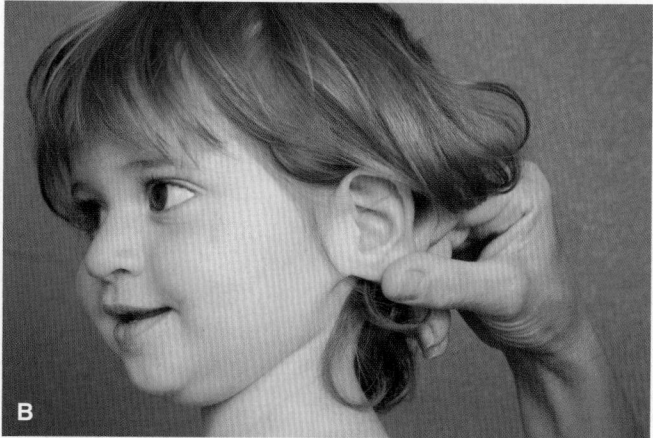

FIGURE 34.6 Administering ear drops. (**A**) For a child over 3 years of age, the nurse pulls the pinna of the affected ear up and back. (**B**) For a child less than 3 years of age, the nurse pulls the pinna of the ear down and back.

a cotton ball loosely in the ear canal to prevent the medication from leaking.

Nasal Administration

Nasally administered medications are typically drops and sprays. Administering nose drops to infants and young children may be difficult, and additional help may be needed to help maintain the child's position. For nose drops, position the child supine with the head hyperextended to ensure that the drops will flow back into the nares. A pillow or folded towel placed under the neck can be used to facilitate this hyperextension. Place the tip of the dropper just at or inside the nasal opening, taking care not to touch the nares with the dropper (Fig. 34.7). Doing so might stimulate the child to sneeze. Although the nasal membranes are not sterile, the drop solution is, and sneezing would contaminate the dropper, leading to contamination of the drop solution when the dropper is returned to the bottle. Once the drops are instilled, maintain the child's head in hyperextension for at least 1 minute to ensure that the drops have come in contact with the nasal membranes.

For nasal sprays, position the child upright and place the tip of the spray bottle just inside the nasal opening and tilted toward the back. Squeeze the container, providing just enough force for the spray to be expelled from the container. Using too great a force can push the spray solution and secretions into the sinuses or Eustachian tube.

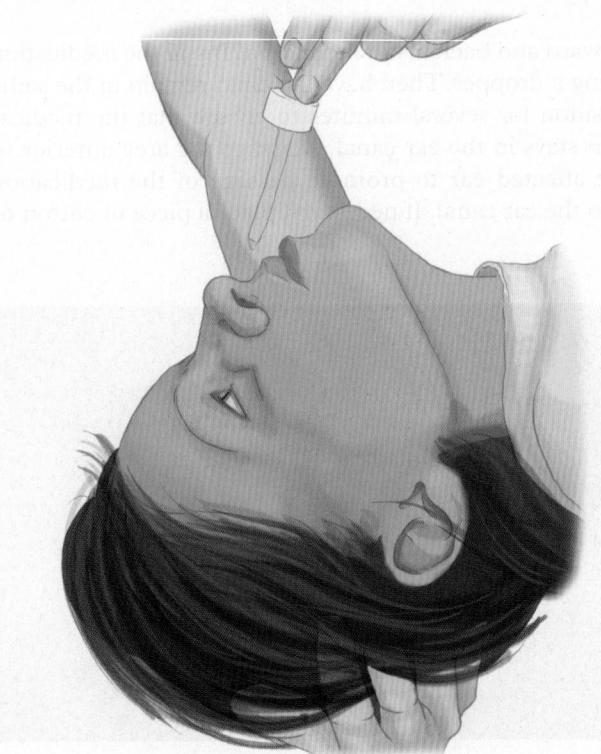

FIGURE 34.7 Administering nose drops. Tilt the head down and back.

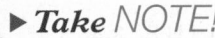

> ▶ *Take* NOTE!
>
> *In young infants, instill the medication in one naris at a time, since young infants are obligate nose breathers.*

IM Administration

IM administration delivers medication to the muscle. In children, this method of medication administration is used infrequently because it is painful and children often lack adequate muscle mass for medication absorption. However, IM administration is used to administer certain medications.

Muscle development and the amount of fluid to be injected determine IM injection sites in children. Needle size (gauge and length) is determined by the size of the muscle and the viscosity of the medication. For example, more viscous medications often require a larger-gauge needle. In addition, the needle must be long enough to ensure that the medication reaches the muscle.

The preferred injection site for infants is the vastus lateralis muscle (Immunization Action Coalition, 2010). To locate this muscle, first identify the greater trochanter and the lateral femoral condyle. The injection site is on the lateral aspect of the leg in the middle third of these two landmarks. An alternative site is the rectus femoris muscle, which is located in the same middle third as the vastus lateralis but on the anterior aspect of the leg. The ventrogluteal site, often used in adults, is not used in children until the child has been walking for at least a year as the muscle has not fully developed before this time. To find this site, first place the palm of the nondominant hand on the greater trochanter so the index finger points toward the anterosuperior iliac spine. Spread the middle finger to form a "V" and inject in the middle of the V. The dorsogluteal site is avoided in children younger than 5 years of age (Bowden & Greenberg, 2008) because the sciatic nerve occupies a larger portion of this area in the young child. The deltoid muscle, which is a small muscle mass, is used as an IM injection site in children only after the age of 4 to 5 years due to the small muscle mass before that age. To locate the deltoid, first find the lateral side of the humerus. Place the ring finger on the acromion process. One finger breadth below is the deltoid muscle. Inject in the middle in the muscle. Figure 34.8 illustrates IM injection sites.

Select the needle size and gauge based on the size of the child's muscle. The goal is to use the smallest length and gauge that will deposit the medication in the muscle. Table 34.3 provides general guidelines for solution amount, needle size, and needle gauge when administering IM medications.

Insert the needle into the skin at a 90-degree angle. If the child is a very small infant or has a small muscle mass, use a 45-degree angle.

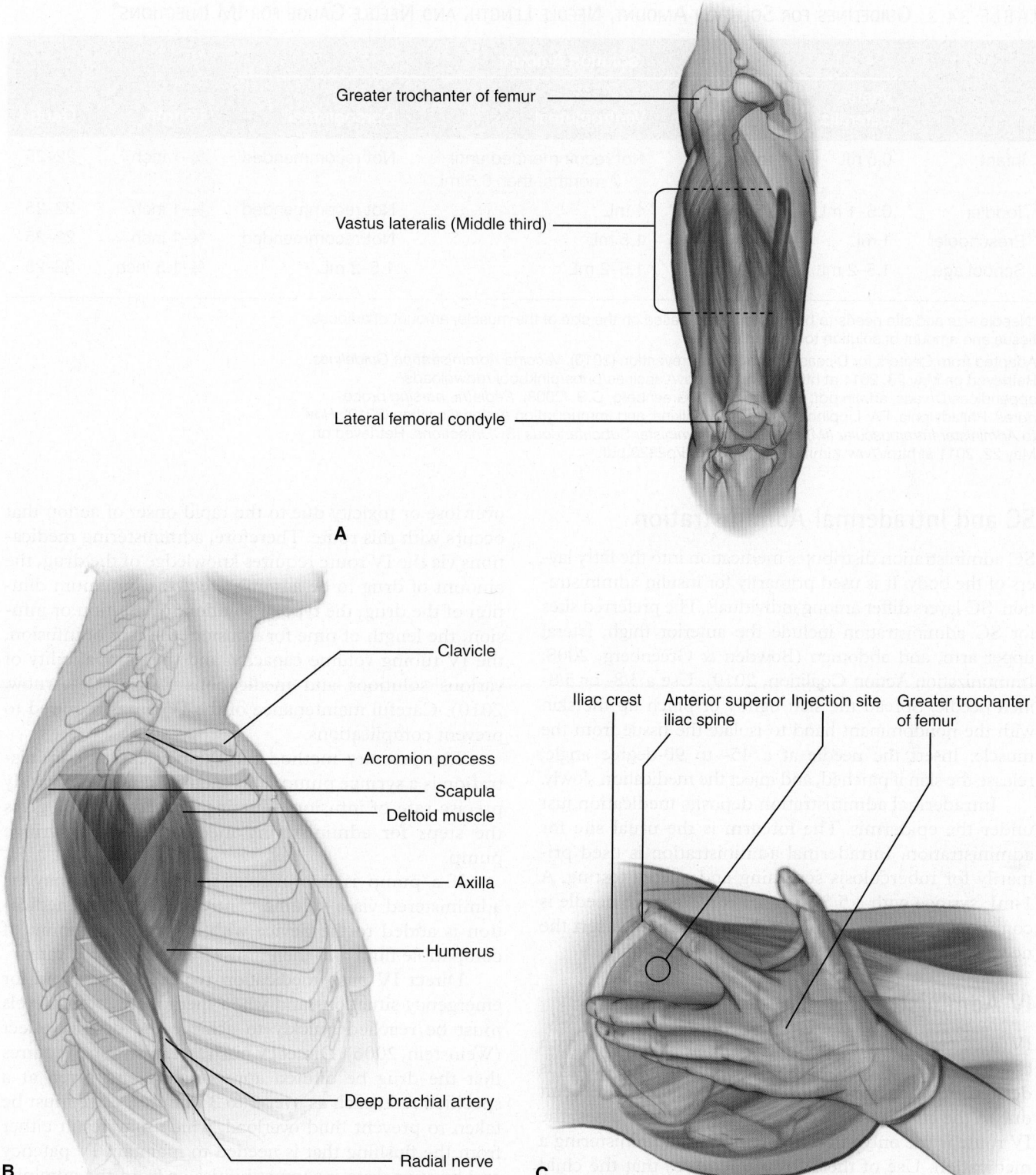

FIGURE 34.8 Locating IM injection sites. (**A**) Vastus lateralis: identify the greater trochanter and the lateral femoral condyle; inject in middle third and anterior lateral aspect. (**B**) Deltoid: locate the lateral side of the humerus, one fingerwidth below the acromion process. (**C**) Ventrogluteal: place the palm of the left hand on the right greater trochanter so the index finger points toward anterosuperior iliac spine; spread the middle finger to form a V and inject in the middle of the V.

TABLE 34.3 GUIDELINES FOR SOLUTION AMOUNT, NEEDLE LENGTH, AND NEEDLE GAUGE FOR IM INJECTIONS*

	Solution Amount					
	Vastus Lateralis	Deltoid	Ventrogluteal	Dorsogluteal	Length	Gauge
Infant	0.5 mL	Not recommended	Not recommended until 7 months; then 0.5 mL	Not recommended	⅝–1 inch	22–25
Toddler	0.5–1 mL	0.5 ml	1 mL	Not recommended	⅝–1 inch	22–25
Preschooler	1 mL	0.5 mL	1.5 mL	Not recommended	⅝–1 inch	22–25
School age	1.5–2 mL	0.5–1 mL	1.5–2 mL	1.5–2 mL	⅝–1.5 inch	22–25

*Needle size and site needs to be individualized based on the size of the muscle, amount of adipose tissue and amount of solution to be administered.

Adapted from Centers for Disease Control and Prevention (2010). *Vaccine Administration Guidelines.* Retrieved on May 23, 2011 at http://www.cdc.gov/vaccines/pubs/pinkbook/downloads/appendices/D/vacc_admin.pdf; Bowden, V.R. & Greenberg, C.S. (2008). *Pediatric nursing procedures.* Philadelphia, PA: Lippincott Williams & Wilkins; and Immunization Action Coalition (2010). *How to Administer Intramuscular (IM) and How To Administer Subcutaneous (SC) Injections.* Retrieved on May 22, 2011 at http://www.immunize.org/catg.d/p2020.pdf.

SC and Intradermal Administration

SC administration distributes medication into the fatty layers of the body. It is used primarily for insulin administration. SC layers differ among individuals. The preferred sites for SC administration include the anterior thigh, lateral upper arm, and abdomen (Bowden & Greenberg, 2008; Immunization Action Coalition, 2010). Use a 3/8- or 5/8-inch needle. Spread the skin tightly or pinch up the skin with the nondominant hand to isolate the tissue from the muscle. Insert the needle at a 45- to 90-degree angle, release the skin if pinched, and inject the medication slowly.

Intradermal administration deposits medication just under the epidermis. The forearm is the usual site for administration. Intradermal administration is used primarily for tuberculosis screening and allergy testing. A 1-mL syringe with a 5/8-inch, 25- or 27-gauge needle is commonly used to administer the medication. Insert the needle beneath the skin at a 5- to 15-degree angle.

IV Administration

IV medication administration is commonly used with children, especially when a rapid response to a drug is desired or when absorption via other routes is difficult due to the child's illness or condition. In some cases, the IV route is the only effective method for administering a medication. Use of the IV route requires that the child have an IV device inserted, peripherally or centrally. Although insertion of this device is invasive and traumatic for the child, IV medication administration is considered to be less traumatic when compared with the trauma associated with multiple injections. Unfortunately, the veins of a child are small and easily irritated.

Most medications given by the IV route must be given at a specified rate and diluted properly to prevent overdose or toxicity due to the rapid onset of action that occurs with this route. Therefore, administering medications via the IV route requires knowledge of the drug, the amount of drug to be administered, the minimum dilution of the drug, the type of solution for dilution or infusion, the length of time for infusion, the rate of infusion, the IV tubing volume capacity, and the compatibility of various solutions and medications (Algren & Arnow, 2010). Careful maintenance of the IV site is required to prevent complications.

The primary method for IV medication administration is a syringe pump. This method provides a highly precise rate of infusion. Nursing Procedure 34.1 gives the steps for administering medication via a syringe pump.

If a pump is unavailable, the medication may be administered via a volume control device. The medication is added to the device with a specified amount of compatible fluid and then infused at the ordered rate.

Direct IV push medication typically is reserved for emergency situations and when therapeutic blood levels must be reached quickly to achieve the desired effect (Weinstein, 2006). Direct IV push administration requires that the drug be diluted appropriately and given at a specified rate, such as over 2 to 3 minutes. Care must be taken to prevent fluid overload, which may result either from the flushing that is needed to maintain IV patency and prevent drug incompatibilities or from the administration of multiple drug therapies.

Providing Atraumatic Care

When administering any medication, including oral medications, use the principles of atraumatic care (see Chapters 1 and 35 for more information). Children can experience stress and fear or upset when they must take

Nursing Procedure 34.1

ADMINISTERING MEDICATION VIA A SYRINGE PUMP

Purpose: To provide accurate and safe administration of IV medication

1. Verify the medication order.
2. Gather the medication and necessary equipment and supplies.
3. Wash hands and put on gloves.
4. Attach the syringe pump tubing to the medication syringe and purge air from the tubing by gently filling the tubing with medication from the syringe.
5. Insert the syringe into the pump according to the manufacturer's directions.
6. Clean the appropriate port on the child's IV access device or tubing, flush the device or tubing if appropriate (e.g., an intermittent infusion device [saline lock]), and attach the syringe tubing to the IV tubing or device.

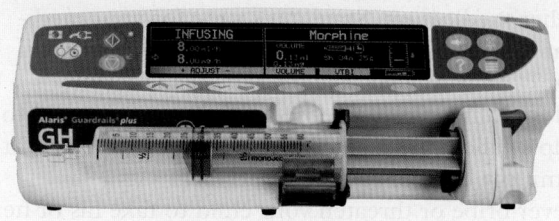

7. Set the infusion rate on the pump as ordered.
8. When the medication infusion is completed, flush the syringe pump tubing to deliver any medication remaining in the tubing, according to institution protocol.
9. Document the procedure and the child's response to it.

---

oral medications. The child may become upset or stressed when he or she must be secured snugly or positioned to minimize movement. The child may experience further discomfort if the medication has an unpleasant taste. Encourage the child to participate in care and provide developmentally appropriate options, such as which fluid to drink with the medication or which flavour of ice pop to suck on before or after the administration (Table 34.2).

To decrease discomfort and pain for the child who is to receive an injection, apply a topical anesthetic such as EMLA cream or vapocoolant spray to the site before injection (Kroger, Sumaya, Pickering, & Atkinson, 2011) (see Chapter 35 for additional information). When preparing the site for injection, clean it with alcohol or an antiseptic solution and allow this solution to dry.

Ensuring that the child doesn't move is essential to prevent injury. When administering an injection to a young child, at least two adults should hold him or her; this may also be necessary to help an older child to remain still. Use positions that are comforting to the child, such as those in Figure 34.1. After administration, encourage the parents or caregivers to hold and cuddle the child and offer praise.

Educating the Child and Parents

Teaching the child and parents or caregivers about medication administration is a key component of patient education. Many medications are given in home, making the parents or caregivers the persons responsible for administration. They need to know what medications they are giving and why, how to give them, and what to expect from the drug, including adverse effects. If the medication is to be given via injection, parents and caregivers need to learn how to administer the injection properly.

Parents and caregivers commonly need suggestions about the best ways to administer the medication to their child. Provide them with tips for administration, such as mixing unpleasant-tasting medications with applesauce or yogurt or offering a favourite liquid to drink afterward. Also teach the parents how to measure the amount of drug to be given. Encourage them to use a calibrated device and not a typical household spoon, which can vary in the amount that it holds. Teaching Guideline 34.2 gives pointers about oral medication administration.

IV Therapy

IV access provides a route for the administration of medications and fluids. It is commonly used for children because it is the quickest, and often the most effective, method of administration. As with adults, numerous sites and various devices and equipment may be used to provide IV therapy over a short or long period of time. When administering IV therapy, safety is crucial. The nurse must have a solid knowledge base about the fluids or medications to be given as well as a thorough understanding of the child's physical and emotional development. Venipuncture can be a terrifying and painful experience for children and their families. Nurses play a crucial role in providing support and education to the child and family before, during, and after the procedure (refer to p. 338 for additional information related to provision of atraumatic care with procedures).

Sites

IV therapy may be administered via a peripheral vein or a central vein. Peripheral IV therapy sites commonly include the hands, feet, and forearms (Fig. 34.9). In neonates and

TEACHING GUIDELINE 34.2

Administering Oral Medications

- Be firm when telling your child that it is time for his or her medication. State, "It's time for your medicine" instead of asking, "Will you take your medicine?" or "Can you take your medicine for me?"
- Allow your child to choose an appropriate liquid to help swallow the medication or drink after taking it. Limit the choices to two or three.
- Never bribe or threaten your child to take his or her medication.
- Never refer to the medication as "candy."
- Be honest about the taste of the medication. If necessary, mix it with another food such as applesauce, yogurt, or syrup to help mask the taste.
- If the medication's taste cannot be masked or disguised, have your child hold his or her nose while taking the medication (taste and smell are closely related).
- Do not mix the medication with formula or baby food.
- Always check with your health care provider and pharmacy about opening capsules or crushing tablets and mixing them with food. Some medications should not be opened or crushed.
- If you are giving a liquid using an oral syringe or dropper, place the medication slowly along the inside of the cheek. Never squirt the medication forcibly to the back of the child's throat. It may cause the child to gag and spit out the medication or aspirate it into his or her lungs.
- Always praise the child after taking the medication and provide comfort and cuddling.

young infants, the scalp veins may be used (O'Grady et al., 2011); these veins are covered only by a thin layer of SC tissue and so are easily visualized. The scalp veins do not have valves, so the device may be inserted in either direction, although the preference would be in the direction of blood flow. However, use of a scalp vein requires that that area of the infant's head be cleared of hair to enhance visualization. Thus, scalp veins are usually used only if attempts at other sites have been unsuccessful (Bergvall & Sawyer, 2009).

▶ **Take** NOTE!

When selecting an IV site in an extremity, always choose the most distal site. Doing so prevents injury to the veins superior to the site and allows additional access sites should complications develop in the most distal site.

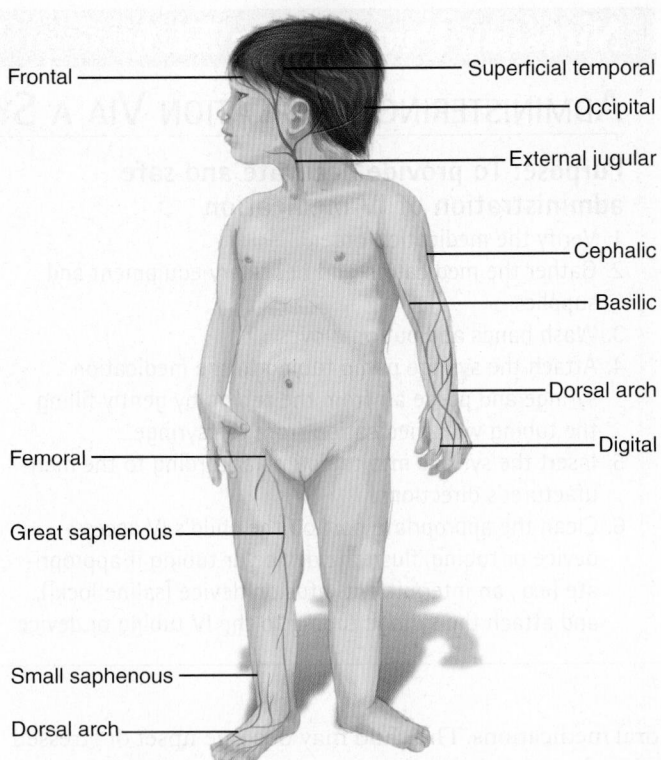

FIGURE 34.9 Preferred peripheral sites for IV insertion.

Central IV therapy usually is administered through a large vein, such as the subclavian, femoral, or jugular vein or the vena cava. The tip of the device lies in the superior vena cava just at the entrance to the right atrium. The device is inserted surgically or percutaneously and exits the body typically in the chest area, just below the clavicle. A device can be inserted via a peripheral vein, such as the median, cephalic, or basilic vein, and then be threaded into the superior vena cava.

In the neonate, the umbilical artery or vein may be used as the site for IV therapy. These sites are commonly used during the first few days after birth (Verheij, te Pas, Witlox, Smits-Wintjens, Walther, & Lopriore, 2010). The umbilical artery usually is used to administer IV fluids and to obtain arterial blood gases. The umbilical vein is commonly used to infuse IV fluids.

Equipment

The choice of equipment is determined by the solution or medication to be administered, the duration of the therapy, the age and developmental level of the child, the child's health status, and the condition of his or her veins. Various types of IV devices are commercially available. In addition, different types of tubing and infusion control devices may be necessary.

Peripheral Access Devices

Devices used for peripheral venous access in a child include over-the-needle catheters or winged-infusion sets, commonly referred to as "butterflies" or scalp vein needles. These devices are inserted into the vein and then connected to the IV solution via tubing to provide a continuous infusion of fluid. These devices can also be inserted for intermittent use if the child does not require a continuous fluid infusion. Typically, the hub of the device is capped or plugged to allow intermittent access, such as for administering medications or obtaining blood specimens. When used in this manner, these devices are termed peripheral intermittent infusion devices or saline or heparin locks.

Needle size on the device also varies. Typically, needle size ranges from 21 to 25 gauge, depending on the child's size. The rule of thumb is to use the smallest-gauge catheter with the shortest length possible to prevent traumatizing the child's fragile veins.

Central Access Devices

Numerous devices for central venous access are available. The type chosen depends on several factors, including the duration of the therapy, the child's diagnosis, the risks to the child from insertion, and the ability of the child and family to care for the device. The device may have one or multiple lumens. Although central venous access devices can be used short term, the majority are used for moderate- to long-term therapy.

Central venous access devices are indicated when the child lacks suitable peripheral access, requires IV fluid or medication for more than 3 to 5 days, or is to receive specific treatments, such as the administration of highly concentrated solutions or irritating drugs that require rapid dilution (Cook, 2007; Moureau, Bagnall-Trick, Nichols, & Moureau, 2007). Patient preference is also a consideration. Central venous access is advantageous because it provides vascular access without the need for multiple IV starts, thus decreasing discomfort and fear. However, central venous access devices are associated with complications such as thrombosis due to partial occlusion of the vessel and infection at the site as well as in the blood due to the direct access to the central circulation (de Jonge, Polderman, & Gemke, 2005). Typically, a chest X-ray is performed after a central venous access device is inserted to verify proper placement. No fluids are administered until correct placement is confirmed. Table 34.4 describes the major types of central venous access devices.

TABLE 34.4 TYPES OF CENTRAL VENOUS ACCESS DEVICES

Device	Description
Nontunnelled central venous catheter	Usually used short term One or more lumens Surgical or percutaneous insertion most commonly via the subclavian, internal jugular, or femoral vein with the tip of the catheter at the top of the superior vena cava just above the right atrium Useful for emergency situations Catheter sutured in place at the exit site
Peripherally inserted central catheters (PICC)	Short- to moderate-term therapy Insertion via a peripheral vein such as antecubital, basilic, cephalic, or medial antecubital vein Catheter typically threaded into superior vena cava; distal tip terminates in the superior vena cava, inferior vena cava, or proximal right atrium Insertion via saphenous vein with tip terminating in inferior vena cava above the diaphragm for infants Single or multiple lumens PICC insertion requires additional training and advanced skill
Tunnelled central venous catheter (e.g., Groshong, Hickman/Broviac)	Usually for long-term use Catheter inserted by a physician via small incision in jugular or subclavian vein and tunnelled in the subcutaneous tissue under the skin Initially sutured in place to stabilize position; sutures removed after approximately 1 to 2 weeks when cuff on catheter attaches to subcutaneous tissue Single or multiple lumens Some have valves that prevent backflow of blood and air entrance
Implanted ports (e.g., Port-a-Cath)	Surgically inserted by a physician Stainless-steel port with a polyurethane or silicone catheter attached Catheter tip lying in subclavian or jugular vein; port implanted under skin in a subcutaneous pocket, usually on the upper chest wall Port covered completely by skin and visible only as a slight bulging on the chest; possibly more appealing to the older child and adolescent because there are no visible parts or dressings Access to port via a specially angled, non-coring needle (Huber needle) Site preparation and pain relief measures necessary before accessing the port

Adapted from Cook, L. S. (2007). Choosing the right intravascular catheter. *Home Healthcare Nurse, 25*(8), 523–531; and Bowden, V. R., & Greenberg, C. S. (2008). *Pediatric nursing procedures.* Philadelphia, PA: Lippincott Williams & Wilkins.

Infusion Control Devices

Infants and young children are at increased risk for fluid volume overload compared with adults. Also, malfunction at the IV insertion site, such as infiltration, may result in much greater injury than a similar incident would cause in an adult. Therefore, IV fluids must be carefully administered and monitored. To ensure accurate fluid administration, infusion control devices such as infusion pumps, syringe pumps, and volume control sets may be used.

Infusion pumps used for children are similar to those used for adults. Typically, the IV solution bag is attached to a calibrated volume control set that has been filled with a specified amount of IV solution (Fig. 34.10). The fluid chamber holds a maximum of 100 to 150 mL of fluid that can be infused over a specified period of time as ordered. Usually, a maximum of a 2-hour infusion amount in the chamber avoids accidental fluid overload in the pediatric population. This chamber can be filled every 1 to 2 hours so that only small amounts of ordered quantities of fluid can infuse and the child is protected from receiving too much fluid volume.

In addition, syringe pumps may be used to deliver fluid and medications to children. These pumps can be programmed to deliver minute amounts of fluid over controlled periods of time (see discussion on p. 350 for additional information about syringe pumps).

Fluid Administration

Administering IV fluids to an infant or child requires close attention to the child's fluid status. Typically, the amount of fluid to be administered in a day (24 hours) is determined by the child's weight (in kilograms) using the following formula:

- 100 mL/kg of body weight for the first 10 kg
- 50 mL/kg of body weight for the next 10 kg
- 20 mL/kg of body weight for the remainder of body weight in kg

Table 34.5 gives examples of calculating a child's fluid requirements using body weight. Once the 24-hour total fluid requirement is determined, this amount is divided by 24 hours to arrive at the correct hourly rate of infusion.

Inserting Peripheral IV Access Devices

Typically, peripheral IV devices are used for short-term therapy, usually averaging 3 to 5 days. Review the child's diagnosis and medical history for information that may affect therapy, such as site selection or insertion. For example, a child who has a history of chronic illness may have heightened fears and anxieties related to insertion due to his or her previous experiences or difficulty in accessing IV sites. Typically, the nondominant extremity should be used for insertion, but this may not be

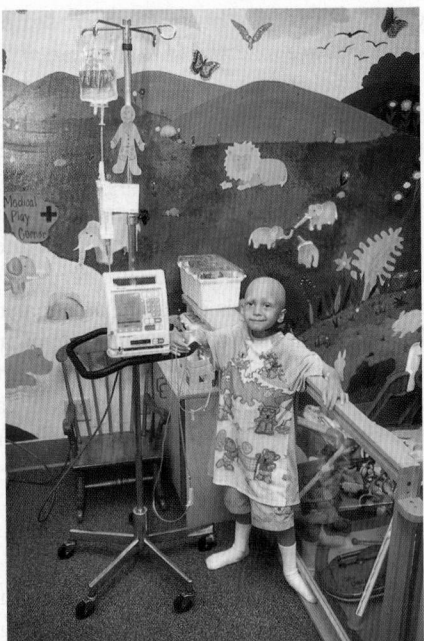

FIGURE 34.10 Volume control infusion device.

possible if a right-handed child has a cast on the left arm.

Check the orders for the prescribed therapy. Determine the purpose and length of the IV therapy and the type of fluid or medication that is to be administered. This information aids in selecting the best device and insertion site. For example, the device needs to be of an adequate

TABLE 34.5 INTRAVENOUS MAINTENANCE FLUID CALCULATIONS BY BODY WEIGHT

<10 kg in weight	100 mL per kg of weight = # mL for 24 hours Example: A child weighs 7.4 kg 7.4 × 100 = 740 mL (daily requirement) 740/24 = 30.8 or 31 mL/hour
11–20 kg in weight	100 mL per kg of weight for the first 10 kg + 50 mL/kg for the next 10 kg = # mL for 24 hours Example: A child weighs 16 kg (10 × 100 = 1,000) plus (6 × 50 = 300) Total = 1,300 mL (daily requirement) 1,300/24 = 54 mL/hour
>20 kg in weight	100 mL/kg for the first 10 kg + 50 mL/kg for the next 10 kg + 20 mL/kg for each kg >20 kg = # mL for 24 hours Example: A child weighs 30 kg (10 × 100 = 1,000) plus (10 × 50 = 500) plus (10 × 20 = 200) Total = 1,700 mL (daily requirement) 1,700/24 = 70.8 or 71 mL/hr

gauge to allow the solution or medication to infuse into the vein while at the same time allowing enough blood flow around the device to promote dilution of the infusion.

Establish rapport with the child and parents. Inform them about IV therapy and what to expect. Be honest with the child. Explain that the venipuncture will hurt but only for a short time. Provide the child with a time frame that he or she can understand, such as the time it takes to brush the teeth or eat a snack. If possible, use therapeutic play to assist the child in coping (see Chapter 32 for more information).

Insertion of an IV therapy device is traumatic. Follow the principles of atraumatic care, including the following:

• Gather all equipment needed before approaching the child.
• If possible, select a site using hand veins rather than wrist or upper arm veins to reduce the risk of phlebitis. Avoid using lower extremity veins if possible because these are associated with an increased risk of infection (Public Health Agency of Canada, 2002).
• Ensure adequate pain relief using pharmacologic and nonpharmacologic methods prior to insertion of the device (see Chapter 35 for more information about management of pain related to procedures).
• Allow the antiseptic used to prepare the site to dry completely before attempting insertion.
• Use a barrier such as gauze or a washcloth or the sleeve of the child's gown under the tourniquet to avoid pinching or damaging the skin.
• If the child's veins are difficult to locate, use a device to transilluminate the vein (shows the vein's size and direction of travel).
• Make only two attempts to gain access; if you are unsuccessful after two attempts, allow another individual two attempts to access a site. If still unsuccessful, evaluate the need for insertion of another device.
• Encourage parental participation as appropriate in helping to position the child or to provide comfort positioning, such as therapeutic hugging.
• Coordinate care with other departments such as the laboratory for blood specimen collection to minimize the number of venipunctures for the child.
• Secure the IV line using a minimal amount of tape or transparent dressing.
• Protect the site from bumping by using a security device such as an IV dressing (Fig. 34.11).

Maintaining IV Fluid Therapy

Throughout the course of therapy, monitor the fluid infusion rate and volume closely, as often as every hour. If a volume control set is used to administer the IV infusion, fill the device with the allotted amount of fluid that the child is to receive in 1 hour. Doing so prevents inadvertent administration of too much fluid. Never assume that just because an infusion pump is in use, the infusion is being

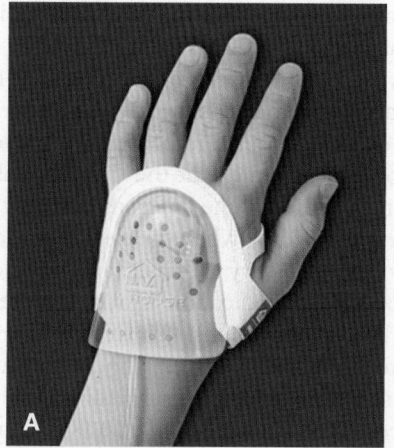

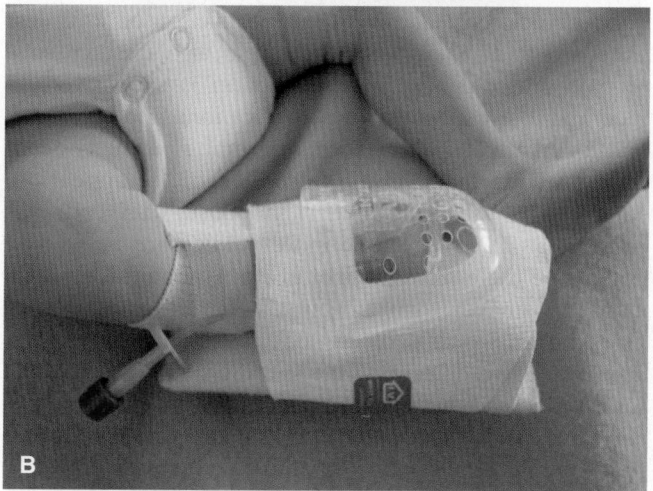

FIGURE 34.11 (**A**) IV dressing over the IV site on a child's hand. (**B**) IV dressing over the site on an infant's foot.

administered without problems. Pumps can malfunction. The tubing can become blocked or the IV device can move out of the vein lumen. Not enough fluid, fluid overload, or infiltration of the solution into the tissues can occur.

In addition to monitoring the fluid infusion, closely monitor the child's output. Expected urine output for children and adolescents is 1 to 2 mL/kg/hour (Weinstein, 2006).

▶ *Take* NOTE!

When measuring the output of an infant or child who is not toilet-trained or who is incontinent, weigh the diaper to determine the output. Remember that 1 g of weight is equal to 1 mL of fluid.

Historically, padded armboards and footboards were used to prevent movement of the IV device, but today these are considered mechanical restraints and as such should be used only as a last resort when no less restrictive method is available or effective. Padded boards can interfere with inspection of the insertion site. They also restrict movement, increasing the risk of contractures; they may be uncomfortable; and they can irritate the underlying tissue, leading to excoriation and infection. Moreover, research has failed to demonstrate that the use of armboards promotes patency of the IV line (Algren & Arnow, 2010).

Flushing the IV line when the device is used intermittently may be necessary to maintain patency, such as before and/or after medication is administered and after obtaining blood specimens. However, there is much debate as to how often flushing should be done and the best flush solution to use, heparin or saline (Hepzibha, 2010; Pryce, 2009; Tripathi et al., 2008). Saline has been found to be more compatible with numerous solutions and medications administered intravenously and less expensive and less irritating to the vein; also, the incidence of pain and phlebitis is less. Heparin is expensive and incompatible with numerous medications and solutions, and it can affect clotting time, depending on the concentration of the flush solution used. Evidence appears to support the use of normal saline flush with catheters larger than 22 gauge, but more studies are needed to determine the effectiveness of normal saline flushes with catheters smaller than 22 gauge (Alexander, Corrigan, Gorski, Hankins, & Perucca, 2010). Additional research is also needed to determine the specific frequency interval for flushing and the volume and concentration of the flush solution to use (Knue, Doellman, & Jacobs, 2006). Always follow your agency's policy for flushing IV lines.

If the child is receiving IV therapy via a central venous access device, provide site care using sterile technique and flush the device according to agency policy. Note the exit site for the device and inspect it frequently for signs of infection. If the device has multiple lumens, label each lumen with its use (i.e., blood specimen, medication, or fluid). Always check the compatibilities of solutions and medications being given simultaneously.

▶ *Take* NOTE!

When flushing or administering medications through a peripherally inserted central catheter (PICC) line, use a 5-mL syringe or larger because PICC lines are fragile. Using a larger-volume syringe exerts less pressure on the PICC, thereby reducing the risk of complications (Bowden & Greenberg, 2008).

Preventing Complications

IV therapy is invasive and associated with numerous complications. Strict aseptic technique is necessary when inserting the device and caring for the site. Adherence to standard precautions is key. Inspect the insertion site every 1 to 2 hours for inflammation or **infiltration** (inad-

vertent infusion of a nonirritant solution or medication into the surrounding tissue) (Weinstein, 2006). Note signs of inflammation such as warmth, redness, induration, or tender skin. Check closely for signs of infiltration such as cool, blanched, or puffy skin. Use of a transparent dressing or IV dressing provides easy access for assessing the IV insertion site. These types of dressings also help to prevent movement of the catheter hub, thus minimizing the risk of mechanical irritation and complications such as phlebitis or infection.

In adults, an IV site is typically changed every 72 to 96 hours and at any time when the integrity of the system has been compromised or contamination is suspected (O'Grady et al., 2011; Weinstein, 2006). However, with children, the 72- to 96-hour time frame may need to be adjusted to minimize the child's exposure to the repeated trauma of insertion. Follow the agency's policies and procedures related to site changes. Consider an alternative route for fluid and medication administration or the insertion of an alternative IV device, such as a PICC line.

Discontinuing IV Therapy

Prepare the child for removal of the IV device in much the same manner as for insertion. Many children may fear the removal of the device to the same extent that they feared its insertion. Explain what is to occur and enlist the child's help in the removal. If appropriate, allow the child to assist in removing the tape or dressing. This gives the child a sense of control over the situation and also encourages his or her cooperation. In addition, practice atraumatic care by doing the following:

- Use water or adhesive remover to help loosen the tape.
- If a transparent dressing is in place, gently lift off the dressing by pulling up opposite corners using a motion parallel to the skin surface.
- Avoid using scissors to cut the tape, but if cutting the tape is necessary, be sure that the child's fingers are clear of the tape and scissors.
- Turn off the infusion solution and pump.
- Once all tape and dressings are removed, gently slide the IV device out using a motion opposite to that used for the insertion.
- Apply pressure to the site with a dry gauze dressing and then cover with a small adhesive bandage. If possible, allow the child to choose the bandage.

▶ *Take* NOTE!

If the IV site was in the arm at or near the antecubital space, do not have the child bend his or her arm after removal of the device. Doing so increases the risk for hematoma formation (Johnson, 2007).

Nutritional Support

Adequate nutrition is important for all individuals but especially for children. The quality of a child's nutrition during the growing years has a major effect on his or her overall health and development (Klossner & Hatfield, 2009). The presence of a chronic illness, disease, or trauma can increase the child's nutritional demands; if the child cannot meet these even with oral supplementation, other measures may be necessary to provide nutritional support. Such measures may include **enteral nutrition** (delivery of nutrition into the gastrointestinal [GI] tract via a tube) and **parenteral nutrition** (IV delivery of nutritional substances). The nutritional plan is determined by the child's age, developmental level, and health status.

Enteral Nutrition

Enteral nutrition, commonly called tube feedings, involves the insertion of a tube so that feedings can be delivered directly into the child's GI tract. The tube may be inserted via the nose or mouth or through an opening in the abdominal area, with the tube ending in the stomach or jejunum. Nasogastric or orogastric tube feedings are commonly referred to as **gavage feedings**. Gastrostomy feedings involve the insertion of a gastrostomy tube through an opening in the abdominal wall and into the stomach. Jejunostomy feedings are similar to gastrostomy feedings except that the tube lies in the jejunum.

Enteral nutrition is indicated for children who have a functioning GI tract but cannot ingest enough nutrients orally. The child may be unconscious or have a severely debilitating condition that interferes with his or her ability to consume adequate food and fluids. Other conditions that may warrant the use of enteral nutrition include the following:

• Failure to thrive
• Inability to suck or tiring easily during sucking
• Abnormalities of the throat or esophagus
• Swallowing difficulties or risk for aspiration
• Respiratory distress
• Metabolic conditions
• Severe gastroesophageal reflux disease
• Surgery
• Severe trauma

Enteral feedings may be given via nasogastric, orogastric, gastrostomy, or jejunostomy tubes (Fig. 34.12). Table 34.6 provides additional information about these types of feeding tubes. Enteral feedings are less costly than parenteral feedings; they are considered a safer alternative for nutritional support and are associated with improved outcomes (Westhus, 2004). Tube misplacement is a serious

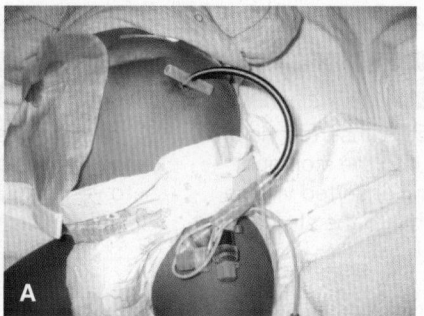

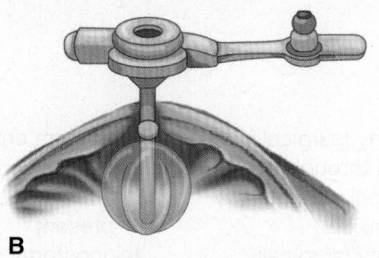

FIGURE 34.12 (**A**) Gastrostomy tube. (**B**) Low-profile (button) gastrostomy tube. The filled balloon keeps the tube in place inside the stomach.

complication of enteral feeding. See Evidence-Based Practice 34.1.

> ▶ *Take* NOTE!
>
> *Small-diameter feeding tubes, though more comfortable, may easily become dislodged if the child coughs vigourously or vomits (Bowden & Greenberg, 2008; Florida State Hospital, 2009).*

Inserting a Nasogastric or Orogastric Feeding Tube

Tubes for gavage feeding can be inserted via the nose or mouth. For infants, who are obligate nose breathers, insertion via the mouth may be appropriate. Oral insertion also promotes sucking in the infant. For the older child, nasal insertion is usually the preferred method. If the tube is to remain in place, the nose also is considered to be more comfortable. Nursing Procedure 34.2 gives the steps for inserting a gavage feeding tube.

Once the gavage feeding tube is inserted, checking for placement is essential. Tube placement must be confirmed each time the tube is inserted and prior to each use. Radiologic confirmation of tube placement is considered the most accurate method, but the risks associated with repeated radiation exposure to verify tube placement prohibit its use (Westhus, 2004). Several methods have been proposed as reliable for checking

TABLE 34.6 TYPES OF ENTERAL FEEDING TUBES

Type of Tube	Indication	Nursing Implications
Nasogastric (inserted via the nose into the stomach) Orogastric (inserted via the mouth into the stomach)	Short-term enteral feeding Orogastric usually limited to young infants only	• Long-term use or repeated insertion causes irritation and discomfort • Silicone and polyurethane tubes are very flexible and more comfortable; they require a stylet or guidewire for insertion • Length of long-term use varies according to the type of tube used and the institution protocol. Periodically a nasogastric tube is removed and reinserted via the opposite nostril to prevent pressure on the nasal mucosa • Maintaining orogastric placement between feedings can be difficult due to oral secretions
Gastrostomy (surgically inserted through the abdominal wall into the stomach) Jejunostomy (surgically inserted through the abdominal wall into the jejunum)	Long-term enteral feeding or when esophageal atresia or stricture is present Jejunostomy tubes are indicated when gastric feeding is not tolerated	• The inner section of the tube is below the skin surface with the tip located in the stomach or jejunum (may be balloon, winged or mushroom-shaped). The outer section appears above the skin surface at the insertion site and has an opening or feeding port to which the feeding solution is attached • Low-profile gastrostomy device (gastrostomy button) is flush with the abdominal surface. The flip-top opening is anchored by a dome that fits against the stomach wall. Less conspicuous, it allows the child to be more active and mobile • After initial insertion, the tube length is measured from the insertion site to the far end of the tube and recorded. This measurement is checked at least daily to ensure that the tube has not moved • For any gastrostomy or jejunostomy tube, the type and size of tube inserted as well as the amount required to fill the balloon, if present, should be known

tube placement. Research has shown the following methods to be acceptable:

• Testing the pH of the feeding tube aspirate (pH less than 6 indicates gastric placement; pH over 6 indicates intestinal placement)
• Inspecting the colour of the aspirate (clear, tan, or green indicates gastric placement; yellow or bile-stained indicates intestinal placement [Westhus, 2004])

Even with these methods, tube malpositioning can occur. Research also has suggested using measurements of bilirubin, trypsin, and pepsin levels to enhance assessment of tube placement, but no methods are available for bedside testing of these levels (Huffman et al., 2004). Therefore, nurses need to be vigilant in checking for tube placement using the recommended methods and be cautious and proactive if there is any suspicion that the tube may be misplaced.

If the gavage feeding tube is to remain in place, secure it to the child's cheek. Do not tape the tube to the child's forehead because this could lead to irritation and pressure on and possible breakdown of the nasal mucosa. Also measure the length of the tube extending from the

nose or mouth to the end and record this information. Double-check this measurement before administering each intermittent tube feeding to verify that the feeding tube is in the proper position. Once the position of the gavage feeding tube is confirmed, the feeding solution or medication can be administered.

▶ *Take* NOTE!

Instilling air into the tube and then auscultating for the sound is no longer considered a viable method for checking tube placement. Air instilled into a tube that is positioned above the gastroesophageal sphincter can still be auscultated as air in the stomach, thereby giving a false-positive result.

Remember Lily, the 9-month-old infant diagnosed with failure to thrive who is to receive gavage feedings with a nasogastric tube? What equipment will be needed, and what steps will you take to complete the procedure?

EVIDENCE-BASED PRACTICE 34.1
Feeding Tube Aspirates, pH, and Enzyme Content as Accurate Predictors of Proper Feeding Tube Placement in Children

Nutritional support is essential in the care of ill children. Many patients require enteral feedings to obtain proper nutrition during illness. Feeding tube placement errors can have a negative impact. Tubes inadvertently placed in the esophagus or in the stomach when they should have been in the intestines increase the risk for aspiration. Tubes placed in the intestines that were intended to be in the stomach can lead to malabsorption and diarrhea. Tubes placed in the lungs can have catastrophic, even fatal results. Extreme care needs to be taken to ensure correct positioning of a feeding tube prior to use. Radiography is the most accurate way to determine that a feeding tube is in the desired location and not inadvertently in the lung. The risk of repeated exposure to radiation makes it unrealistic to use radiography every time feeding tube placement needs to be confirmed.

● Study

A prospective descriptive clinical study was performed at a university-based children's hospital. A convenience sample of 56 children, from birth to 14 years, who required feeding tubes—nasogastric, orogastric, or nasointestinal—was used. Placement of the feeding tube was checked 30 minutes after radiologic confirmation by aspirating 2.5 mL of fluid. The appearance of the fluid was described, pH was determined by two methods, and the aspirate was assayed for pepsin and trypsin content.

▲ Findings

Mean gastric pH was significantly lower than mean intestinal pH. Colour of the gastric aspirate (clear and colourless, green, off-white, or brown) was significantly different than the intestinal aspirate (yellow or bile-stained). Both enzymes, pepsin and trypsin, were statistically significant discriminators between gastric and intestinal tube placement. Aspirating fluids from feeding tubes, visually examining the fluid, and assaying the fluid for aspirate characteristics were found to be adaptable from adults to children.

■ Nursing Implications

Nurses need to utilize accurate assessment skills when verifying feeding tube placement. Nurses can feel more confidence that simple bedside tests, such as pH and visual appearance of aspirate, can provide evidence that a feeding tube is placed properly in the stomach. When pH is >6 and the aspirate's visual appearance is yellow or bile-coloured, this may indicate intestinal placement, but further assessment and verification is still warranted. Refer to p. 359 for further explanation.

Westhus, N. (2004). Methods to test feeding tube placement in children. *American Journal of Maternal Child Nursing, 29*(5), 290–291.

Administering Enteral Feedings

Enteral feedings can be given continuously or intermittently, regardless of the type of tube used. Intermittent feedings are commonly called **bolus feedings**. With a bolus feeding, a specified amount of feeding solution is given at specific intervals, usually over a short period of time such as 15 to 30 minutes. Given via a syringe, feeding bag, or infusion pump, bolus feedings most closely resemble regular meals. Continuous feedings are given at a slower rate over a longer period of time. In some cases, the feeding may be given during the night so that the child can be free to move about and participate in activities during the day. For continuous feedings, an enteral feeding pump is used to administer the solution at a prescribed rate.

Checking for tube placement is a priority before administering any intermittent tube feeding and periodically during continuous tube feedings, regardless of the type of tube being used. Once placement is confirmed, the feeding can be given. Also, measure the gastric **residual** (the amount remaining in the stomach; indicates gastric emptying time) by aspirating the gastric contents with a syringe, measuring it, and then replacing the contents. Check the residuals periodically,

according to the facility's policy, such as every 4 to 6 hours, and before each intermittent feeding. If the residual volume exceeds the amount specified by the physician's order, hold the feeding and notify the physician.

Begin the feeding by placing the child in a supine position with the head and shoulders elevated approximately 30 degrees so that the feeding will remain in the stomach area (Springhouse, 2007). Flush the tube with a small amount of water to clear it and prevent occlusion. This is not necessary for a gavage feeding if the tube is being inserted each time a feeding is given. Ensure that the feeding solution is at room temperature. Administer the feeding as per the facility's policy.

Feeding solutions may be placed into the barrel of a syringe or into a feeding bag attached to the feeding tube and allowed to flow by gravity. The rate of flow for gravity-assisted feedings can be increased or decreased by raising or lowering the feeding solution container, respectively. Typically, intermittent feedings last from 15 to 30 minutes. A feeding bag also may be attached to a pump to control the rate of flow. Monitor the child's tolerance to the feeding.

Once the feeding is complete but before the formula completely empties from the container, flush the tube

Nursing Procedure 34.2

INSERTING A GAVAGE FEEDING TUBE

Purpose: To provide a means for delivering nutrition to the child's functioning GI tract

1. Verify the order for gavage feeding.
2. Explain the procedure to the child and parents using appropriate language geared to the child's development level.
3. Gather the necessary equipment; remove formula for feeding from refrigerator if appropriate and allow it to come to room temperature.
4. Wash hands and put on gloves.
5. Inspect the child's nose and mouth for deformities that may interfere with passage of the tube.
6. Position the infant supine with the head slightly elevated and with the neck slightly hyperextended so that the nose is pointed upward. If necessary, place a rolled towel or blanket under the neck to help in maintaining this position. Assist the older child to a sitting position if appropriate. Alternatively, have the parent or another person hold the child to promote comfort and reassurance. Enlist the aid of additional persons, such as a parent or other health care team member, to assist in maintaining the child's position.
7. Determine the tubing length for insertion: measure from the tip of the nose to the earlobe to the middle of the area between the xiphoid process and umbilicus. Mark this measurement on the tube with an indelible pen or with a piece of tape.

8. Lubricate the tube with a generous amount of sterile water or water-soluble lubricant to promote passage of the tube and minimize trauma to the child's mucosa.
9. Insert the tube into one of the nares or the mouth. Direct a nasally inserted tube straight back toward the occiput; direct an orally inserted tube toward the back of the throat.
10. Advance the tube slowly to the designated length; encourage the child (if capable) to swallow frequently to assist with advancing the tube.
11. Watch for signs of distress, such as gasping, coughing, or cyanosis, indicating that the tube is in the airway. If these signs develop, withdraw the tube and allow the child to rest before attempting reinsertion.
12. Check for proper placement of the tube by attaching a bulb syringe to the end of the tube and aspirating stomach contents; the pH of the aspirate should be less than 6 (indicating gastric acid) and the colour of the aspirate should be clear, tan, or green (indicating gastric secretions); return any aspirated contents to the stomach.
13. Document the type of tube inserted, length of tubing inserted, measurement of external tubing length after insertion, and confirmation of placement.

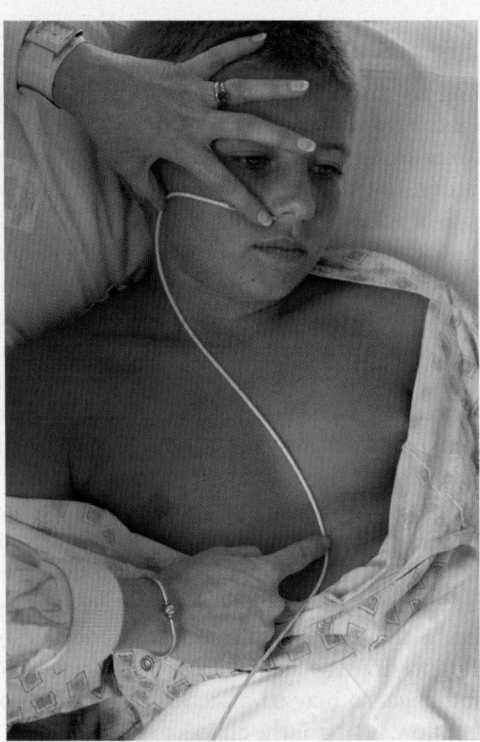

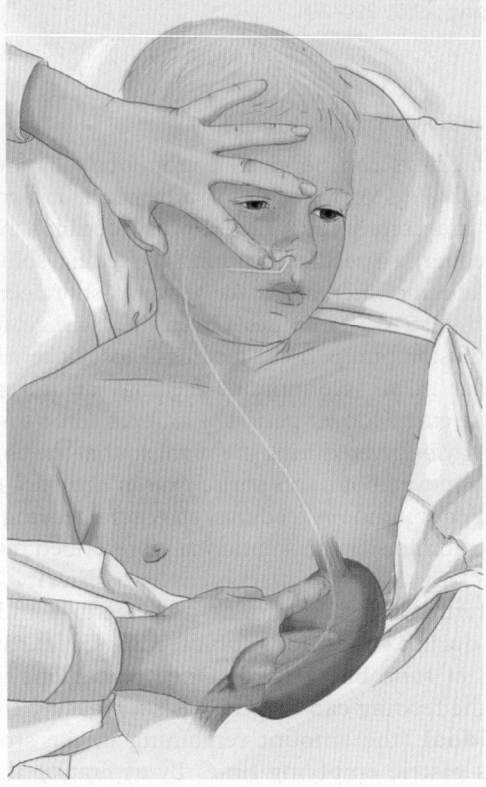

with water. As the water leaves the syringe or tubing, clamp the tube to prevent air from entering the stomach. Then disconnect the syringe or tube-feeding bag from the tube (McMaster Children's Hospital, 2006).

> ▶ **Take** NOTE!
>
> *If the child vomits during the feeding, stop the feeding immediately and turn the child onto his or her side or sit the child up.*

If the child has a gastrostomy button, open the cap and connect an adaptor or insert extension tubing through the one-way valve. This allows access to the gastric conduit. The feeding solution container is connected to the extension tubing or adaptor and the feeding is given as described previously. After the feeding is completed, the extension tubing or adaptor is flushed with water and the flip-top opening is closed.

Burp the infant during and after any type of tube feeding in the same manner as for an infant who is bottle- or breast-fed. Also, position the child on his or her right side with the head slightly elevated, approximately 30 degrees, for about 1 hour after the feeding to facilitate gastric emptying and reduce the risk of aspiration and regurgitation. Weigh the child daily throughout enteral nutrition therapy to determine the effectiveness of the therapy.

Providing Skin and Insertion Site Care

Skin around the insertion gastrostomy or jejunostomy site may become irritated from movement of the tube, moisture, or leakage of stomach or intestinal contents; it may also be irritated by the adhesive device holding the tube in place. Keeping the skin clean and dry will help prevent most of these problems (McMaster Children's Hospital, 2006). Routine site care includes gentle cleansing with soap and water followed by rinsing or cleaning with water alone.

The skin around a gastrostomy or jejunostomy tube requires cleaning at least once a day. Ordinary soap and water are sufficient to clean about the tube site to prevent build-up. To clean under an external disc or bumper, a cotton-tipped applicator may be used. Diluted hydrogen peroxide is not recommended for cleaning the site because it is irritating and cytotoxic (Burd & Burd, 2003). During insertion site care, rotate the gastrostomy tube or button a quarter-turn to prevent skin adherence and irritation (McMaster Children's Hospital, 2006). Assess the insertion site and condition of the surrounding skin for signs and symptoms of infection, such as erythema, induration, foul drainage, or pain.

Preventing movement of the tube also helps reduce skin irritation. Check the volume of the balloon with a balloon-tipped device about once or twice a week and reinflate the balloon to the initial volume if needed. Measure the external length of the mushroom-tipped device daily and ensure that the tube is stabilized (Burd & Burd, 2003). Tube stabilization methods help prevent the tube from moving around and sliding farther into the stomach or jejunum. Stabilize the tube by pulling gently on the tubing and sliding the stabilizer bar or disc snugly against the abdomen. Then, measure and record the length of the tube from the exit site of the abdominal wall to the end of the tube. All future measurements should be the same unless the tube length is changed. For tubes without a stabilizer bar or disc or for additional stabilization needs, several other methods may be used, including nipples, tape, tension loops, and hydroactive dressings.

Promoting Growth and Development

Some children receive all of their nutritional needs through tube feedings, whereas other children use tube feedings as a supplement to eating by mouth. Feeding time is a special time for infants and children. Occasionally, babies who are fed solely through an enteral feeding tube may forget or lose the desire to eat by mouth. Use a pacifier to help avoid this, allowing the infant to associate the nipple in his or her mouth with a feeding (Sexton & Natale, 2009). The sucking motion will also exercise the jaw and promote the flow of the feedings. The saliva produced during sucking aids in digestion. Combined with holding the infant and cuddling, rocking, and talking to him or her, this promotes a more normal feeding time.

Talking with children, playing music, or reading a story promotes an active feeding time. At home, encourage parents to include the feeding as a part of regular family mealtime together to provide socialization for the child. Allow the child to participate in the feedings by gathering supplies and administering the actual feeding so that the child may experience independence and adaptation. If the child also eats food by mouth, feed him or her by mouth first and then administer the tube feeding. During tube feedings in bed, make sure the head of the bed is elevated at least 30 degrees to help prevent vomiting and aspiration (Springhouse, 2007).

Children with feeding tubes should be allowed as normal a routine as possible. For example, they can crawl, walk, and jump just like children of the same age and developmental level. However, in some cases, contact sports such as football, hockey, and wrestling should be avoided because of the higher risk of injury. Securing the tubing under the child's clothing will prevent it from becoming accidentally dislodged. Dressing younger children in one-piece outfits helps to prevent them from playing with the gastrostomy or jejunostomy tube and helps to protect the insertion site (Fidanza, 2003).

Educating the Child and Family

Educate children receiving enteral feedings and their parents thoroughly about this method of nutritional support.

Reinforce the reason for the therapy and provide the child and parents with opportunities to verbalize their concerns and ask questions. Ensure that the parents understand the risks and benefits of the therapy and the expected duration.

Provide the child, if developmentally appropriate, and parents with opportunities to participate in the feeding sessions. This helps allay some of their fears and anxieties and promotes a sense of control over the situation. They will also gain valuable practice in learning the skill should the feedings be required at home. Teaching Guideline 34.3 identifies important topics to include in the teaching plan for a child receiving enteral nutrition at home. Education also involves helping the family develop appropriate coping strategies to adapt, solve problems, and negotiate for the support and services they will need after discharge (Burd & Burd, 2003).

Remember Lily from the beginning of the chapter? She is to be discharged home after having a gastrostomy tube inserted to continue feedings at home.

What teaching is needed for her family prior to discharge?

Parenteral Nutrition

Nutritional support can be administered intravenously through a peripheral or central venous catheter. The concentration and components of the solution determine the type of parenteral nutrition. Parenteral nutrition given via a central venous access is termed **total parenteral nutrition (TPN)**. Comparison Chart 34.1 gives information about peripheral and central parenteral nutrition.

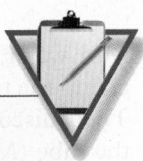

TEACHING GUIDELINE 34.3

Topics to be Covered for Home Enteral Nutrition

- Type of nutritional support
- Rationale for therapy
- Expected results from therapy
- Duration of therapy
- Frequency of feedings
- Feeding solution and equipment
- Tube insertion technique (if appropriate)
- Methods to check for correct placement
- Steps for administering the feeding (and medication if ordered)
- Procedure for flushing tube
- Frequency of weighing the child
- Signs and symptoms of complications and when to notify the health care provider
- Troubleshooting problems, such as clogging of the tube
- Daily tube care (e.g., cleaning the site, rotating tube)
- Site assessment
- Technique for reinsertion/replacement of tube as appropriate
- Equipment suppliers
- Resources for support
- Follow-up visits and referrals

Administering TPN

Typically, the health care provider determines the concentration and components of the TPN solution based on a thorough assessment of the child's status, including

COMPARISON CHART 34.1 PERIPHERAL PARENTERAL NUTRITION VERSUS TOTAL PARENTERAL NUTRITION

	Peripheral Parenteral Nutrition	Total Parenteral Nutrition
Indications/use	Primarily supplemental Short-term use to supply additional calories and nutrients	Provides all nutrients to meet child's needs Enough calories supplied to maintain a positive nitrogen balance
Route	Peripheral vein	Central venous access to allow rapid dilution of hypertonic solution
Child's status	Nutritional status usually within acceptable parameters Oral intake decreased or absent	Child with a nonfunctioning GI tract, such as a congenital or acquired GI disorder Severe failure to thrive Multisystem trauma or organ involvement Preterm newborns
Components	Fluid, electrolytes, and carbohydrates (dextrose); usually no protein or fats Carbohydrate concentration usually limited to 10% (Weinstein, 2006)	Highly concentrated solution of carbohydrates, electrolytes, vitamins, and minerals Lipid emulsion to supply need for essential fatty acids Total nutrient admixture with components of TPN plus lipids and other additives in one container

Weinstein, S. M. (2006). *Plumer's principles and practice of intravenous therapy* (8th ed.). Philadelphia, PA: Lippincott Williams & Wilkins.

the results of laboratory testing. This information is used as a baseline for evaluating the effectiveness of therapy.

The solution is prepared under sterile conditions in the pharmacy. For TPN, a central venous access device is inserted and secured, if one is not already in place. Use specialized tubing with an in-line filter (0.22 μm) to prevent small microparticles from entering the circulation. If total nutrient admixture is being administered, the use of a 1.2-μg filter is recommended.

The infusion of the solution is initiated at a slow rate that is gradually increased as ordered based on how the child tolerates the therapy. TPN solutions are highly concentrated glucose solutions that can cause hyperglycemia if given too rapidly. Use of an infusion pump is essential to control the rate of infusion. TPN solutions may be refrigerated until they are to be used. Once started, a single solution of TPN should hang for no longer than 24 hours (Springhouse, 2007). Fat emulsions are administered periodically to meet the child's need for essential fatty acids. These solutions are given as a piggyback solution into the TPN line, but below the in-line filter.

Throughout TPN therapy, be vigilant in monitoring the infusion rate and report any changes in the infusion rate to the health care provider immediately. Adjustments may be made to the rate, but only as ordered by the provider. The infusion rate should never be adjusted more than 10% higher or lower than the current rate (Weinstein, 2006).

Check blood glucose levels frequently, such as every 4 to 6 hours, initially to evaluate for hyperglycemia. These levels can be obtained with a bedside glucose meter. Minimize the trauma and discomfort associated with frequent invasive procedures by using the principles of atraumatic care. If blood glucose levels are elevated, SC administration of insulin may be needed. Once the child's glucose level stabilizes, the frequency of blood glucose level determinations decreases, such as every 8 to 12 hours, based on the facility's policy.

> ▶ **Take** NOTE!
>
> If for any reason the TPN infusion is interrupted or stops, be prepared to begin an infusion of a 5% to 10% dextrose solution at the same infusion rate as the TPN (Bowden & Greenberg, 2008). This helps to prevent rebound hypoglycemia that may occur due to the increased insulin secretion by the child's body in response to the use of the highly concentrated TPN solution.

Perform catheter site care, tubing and filter changes, and dressing changes according to the facility's policy. Inspect the insertion site closely for signs of infection. Also monitor the child's vital signs, daily weights, and intake and output closely for changes. In addition, review laboratory test results, which can aid in early detection of problems, such as infection or electrolyte excesses or deficits.

TPN can be administered continuously over a 24-hour period, or after initiation it may be given on a cyclic basis, such as over a 12-hour period during the night. When administering cycled TPN, the solution is infused at half the prescribed rate for the first and last hour to prevent hyper- and hypoglycemia.

Preventing Complications

Nurses play a key role in minimizing the risk for complications related to use of central venous access devices and TPN. Box 34.5 describes these complications. Key measures to reduce the risk of complications include the following:

- Monitor the child's vital signs closely for changes.
- Adhere to strict aseptic technique when caring for the catheter and administering TPN.
- Ensure that the system remains a closed system at all times. Secure all connections, use occlusive dressings, and clamp the catheter or have the child perform the Valsalva manoeuver during tubing and cap changes.
- Adhere to agency policy for flushing of the catheter and maintaining catheter patency.
- Assess intake and output frequently.
- Monitor blood glucose levels and obtain laboratory tests as ordered to evaluate for changes in fluid and electrolytes.

> ▶ **Take** NOTE!
>
> Never administer any medication, blood, or other solution through the TPN lumen. Doing so increases the risk for contamination of the system and subsequent infection (Springhouse, 2007).

Promoting Growth and Development

Meals are a time for meeting nutritional needs as well as a time for love, comfort, support, and socialization. TPN meets the child's nutritional needs, but the child's need for love and support also must be met. Implement measures similar to those for children receiving enteral nutrition (see discussion earlier in this chapter). Also provide opportunities for holding and cuddling the child. Allow the older child to participate in activities that can help to occupy the time associated with meals. Encourage the child and parents to participate in the care to promote a sense of independence as well as a sense of control over the situation.

Educating the Child and Family

Children who require long-term TPN therapy may receive TPN in the home. Administering TPN at home

---

BOX 34.5 Complications That Can Occur with Central Venous Access Devices and TPN

- Air embolism from inadvertent entry of air into the system during tubing or cap changes or accidental disconnection
- Cardiac tamponade due to catheter advancement with movement of the arm, neck, or shoulder
- Catheter occlusion from the development of a fibrin sheath or thrombus at the catheter tip, malpositioning or kinking, or the deposition of precipitates or a blood clot
- Venous thrombosis from injury to the vessel wall during insertion or movement of the catheter after insertion or from chemical irritation due to administration of concentrated solutions, vesicants, and other medications through the catheter
- Hyperglycemia, typically with too rapid an infusion of TPN
- Hypoglycemia, which may occur with rapid cessation
- Dehydration as the child's body attempts to rid itself of excess glucose through renal excretion
- Electrolyte imbalance (particularly potassium, sodium, calcium, magnesium, and phosphorus)
- Infection at the skin insertion site, along the catheter pathway, or in the bloodstream. Organisms can arise from the skin, hands of caregivers, or other areas such as wound drainage, droplets from the lungs, or urine. For example, connection sites can be contaminated during tubing or dressing changes.

---

requires thorough education of the child and parents. This teaching can occur in the health care agency or in the child's home. The amount of information to be taught can be overwhelming, so ensure that ample time is available. Allow time for questions and concerns. Offer emotional support and guidance whenever necessary.

Provide written and verbal instructions about the care involved. Have the child (if appropriate) and parents demonstrate the care needed, including care of the central venous access device. Review with them the measures for obtaining, storing, and handling the solutions and supplies. Develop plans for troubleshooting problems with devices and equipment and give instructions on how to recognize and treat complications. Also teach them about danger signs and symptoms that require immediate notification. Be sure they have the name and number of a contact person in case of emergency situations.

Initiate the appropriate referrals for support. Specialized home care infusion services are available for follow-up in the home. In addition, social services can be helpful in providing assistance with finances, health insurance reimbursement, scheduling, transportation, emotional support, and community resources.

■■■ Key Concepts

- Children and families need appropriate explanation and education before a procedure is performed. Preparation may include explaining the procedure as well as physically preparing the child. Appropriate preparation helps to decrease the child's and family's anxiety, promote the child's cooperation, and support the child's and family's coping skills.
- The "eight rights" of pediatric medication administration are the right drug, right dose, right route, right time, right patient, right documentation, right to be educated, and right to refuse.
- The physiologic immaturity of some body systems in children can affect a drug's pharmacodynamics, leading to differences in the body's response to the drug and thus enhancing or diminishing the drug's effects. The child's age, weight, BSA, and body composition can affect the drug's pharmacokinetics.
- The two most common methods for determining pediatric drug doses involve the use of the child's body weight and BSA.
- Children under the age of 5 to 6 years are at risk for aspiration when receiving tablets or capsules because they have difficulty swallowing them; liquids may be more appropriate. When administering oral medications to children, always tell them whether a medication is being mixed with food.
- Medication administration via the rectal route is not preferred because the drug's absorption may be erratic and unpredictable and children find this route extremely upsetting or embarrassing.
- When administering otic medications, pull the pinna downward and back if the child is under age 3 years, up and back for older children.
- IM administration is used infrequently in children because it is painful and children often lack the adequate muscle mass. When used with infants, the preferred site is the vastus lateralis muscle.
- Administration of medication via the IV route is common with children, especially when a rapid response to the drug is desired or when absorption via other routes is difficult or impossible. The primary method for IV medication administration is via an infusion pump.
- Preferred sites for peripheral IV therapy include the veins of the hands, feet, and forearms. The scalp vein may be used in infants but only if attempts at other sites have been unsuccessful. The general rule for insertion of any peripheral devices is to use the smallest-gauge catheter for the shortest length of time possible to prevent trauma to the child's fragile veins.
- Central venous therapy usually is administered through a large vein, such as the subclavian, femoral, or jugular vein or vena cava. The tip of the device lies in the superior vena cava just at the entrance to the right atrium. Devices include single- or multiple-lumen short- and

long-term catheters, PICCs, tunnelled catheters, and vascular access ports.

- Monitoring intake and output is important when a child is receiving IV therapy. Site inspection, proper care of the site, and proper dressing changes are key to preventing complications.

- Nutritional support can be administered enterally via a nasogastric or orogastric tube (gavage feeding) or via a gastrostomy or jejunostomy device or administered parenterally through a peripheral or central venous access device.

- Enteral nutrition is indicated for children who have a functioning GI tract but cannot consume adequate amounts of nutrients orally.

- Prior to any enteral feeding, placement of the feeding tube must be confirmed. The gold standard for confirming placement is with an X-ray. At the bedside, checking the colour and pH of the aspirate is used to confirm placement.

- Children receiving TPN require close monitoring of the infusion rate and volume, intake and output, vital signs, and blood glucose levels. Strict aseptic technique is necessary when caring for the central venous access site and TPN infusion.

REFERENCES

Alexander, M., Corrigan, A., Gorski, L., Hankins J., & Perucca, R. (Eds.). (2010). *Infusion Nurses Society. Infusion nursing: An evidenced-based approach* (3rd ed.). St. Louis, MO: Saunders Elsevier.

Algren, C., & Arnow, D. (2010). Pediatric variations of nursing interventions. In M. J. Hockenberry (Ed.), *Wong's essentials of pediatric nursing* (8th ed.). St. Louis, MO: Mosby.

Bergvall, E., & Sawyer, T. L. (2009). *Catheterization, scalp vein.* Retrieved November 27, 2011 from http://emedicine.medscape.com/article/1348863-overview#a16

Bowden, V. R., & Greenberg, C. S. (2008). *Pediatric nursing procedures.* Philadelphia, PA: Lippincott Williams & Wilkins.

Burd, A., & Burd, R. S. (2003). The who, what, why, and how-to guide for gastrostomy tube placement in infants. *Advances in Neonatal Care, 3*(4), 197–205.

Cook, L. S. (2007). Choosing the right intravascular catheter. *Home Healthcare Nurse, 25*(8), 523–531.

de Jonge, R. C., Polderman, K. H., & Gemke, R. J. (2005). Central venous catheter use in the pediatric patient: Mechanical and infectious complications. *Pediatric Critical Care Medicine, 6*(3), 329–339.

Fidanza, S. (2003). *Gastrostomy care.* Broomfield, CO: McKesson Health Solutions LLC.

Florida State Hospital. (2009). *Operating procedure 150–15: Health: Tube feeding.* Retrieved November 27, 2011 from http://www.dcf.state.fl.us/facilities/fsh/FSHOPS/150–15.pdf

Florida Children's Hospital, Child Life Department. (n.d.). *Suggested vocabulary to use with children.* Orlando, FL: Author.

Hepzibha, A. (2010). Heparin versus normal saline as a flush solution. *International Source for the Advancement of Science & Arts, 1*(1), 63–75.

Huffman, S., Jarczyk, K. S., O'Brien, E., et al. (2004). Methods to confirm feeding tube placement: Application of research in practice. *Pediatric Nursing, 30*(1), 10–13.

Immunization Action Coalition. (2010). *How to administer intramuscular (IM) vaccine injections; how to administer subcutaneous (SC) injections.*
Retrieved November 27, 2011 from http://www.immunize.org/catg.d/p2020.pdf

Johnson, L. (2007). *Phlebotomy & age related competencies.* Retrieved November 27, 2011 from http://www.aspnedu.org/classwork/homework_assignments/PhlebotomyandAgeRelated_Competencies.pdf

Klossner, N. J., & Hatfield, N. (2009). *Introductory maternity and pediatric nursing* (2nd ed.). Philadelphia, PA: Lippincott Williams & Wilkins.

Knue, M., Doellman, D., & Jacobs, B. R. (2006). Peripherally inserted central catheters in children: A survey of practice patterns. *Journal of Infusion Nursing, 29*(1), 28–33.

Kroger, A. T., Sumaya, C. V., Pickering, L. K., & Atkinson, W. L. (2011). General recommendations on immunization: Recommendations of the Advisory Committee on Immunization Practices (ACIP). *Morbidity and Mortality Weekly Report (MMWR), 60*(RR02), 1–60. Retrieved November 27, 2011 from http://www.cdc.gov/mmwr/preview/mmwrhtml/rr6002a1.htm?s_cid=rr6002a1_e

Lilley, L. L., Collins, S. C., Harrington, S., & Snyder, J. S. (2011). *Pharmacology and the nursing process* (6th ed.). St. Louis, MO: Mosby, Inc.

McMaster Children's Hospital. (2006). *When your child has a gastrostomy tube: A guide for parents and families.* Hamilton, ON: Author.

Moureau, N. L., Bagnall-Trick, N., Nichols, H., & Moureau, G. (2007). Follow an intentional process for early assessment of vascular access selection for patients requiring intravenous therapy. *Nursing Critical Care, 2*(6), 28–36.

O'Grady, N. P., Alexander, M., Burns, L. A., et al. (2011). Guidelines for the prevention of intravascular catheter-related infections. *Clinical Infectious Diseases, 52*(May 1), e1–e32.

Pediatric Glaucoma & Cataract Family Association. (2008a). *How to apply eye drops.* Retrieved November 27, 2011 from http://www.pgcfa.org/drops.htm

Pediatric Glaucoma & Cataract Family Association. (2008b). *How to apply eye ointment.* Retrieved November 27, 2011 from http://www.pgcfa.org/ointment.htm

Pryce, R. (2009). Question 3. Cannula patency: should we use flushes or continuous fluids, or heparin? *Archives of Diseases in Childhood, 94*(12), 992–994.

Public Health Agency of Canada. (2002). *Infection control guidelines: Preventing infections associated with indwelling intravenous access devices.* Retrieved October 16, 2010 from http://www.phac-aspc.gc.ca/publicat/ccdr-rmtc/97vol23/23s8/iiadp_e.html

Sexton, S., & Natale, R. (2009). Risks and benefits of pacifiers. *American Family Physician, 15*(79), 681–685. Retrieved November 27, 2011 from http://www.aafp.org/afp/2009/0415/p681.html

Springhouse. (2007). *Best practices: Evidence-based nursing procedures* (2nd ed.). Ambler, PA: Lippincott Williams & Wilkins.

Tripathi, S., Kaushik, V., & Singh, V. (2008). Peripheral IVs: Factors affecting complications and patency—A randomized controlled trial. *Journal of Infusion Nursing, 31*(3), 182–188.

Verheij, G. H., te Pas, A. B., Witlox, R. S. G. M., Smits-Wintjens, V. E. J. H., Walther, F. J., & Lopriore, E. (2010). Poor accuracy of methods currently used to determine umbilical catheter insertion length. *International Journal of Pediatrics.* Retrieved October 15, 2010 from http://www.hindawi.com/journals/ijped/2010/873167.html

Weinstein, S. M. (2006). *Plumer's principles and practice of intravenous therapy* (8th ed.). Philadelphia, PA: Lippincott Williams & Wilkins.

Westhus, N. (2004). Methods to test feeding tube placement in children. *MCN: The American Journal of Maternal Child Nursing, 29*(5), 282–291.

Woo, T. M. (2004). Pediatric pharmacology update, essentials for prescribing. *Advance for Nurse Practitioners, 12*(6), 22–28.

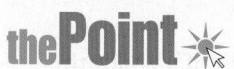

the Point For additional learning materials, including Internet Resources, visit **http://thePoint.lww.com/Chow1e.**

CHAPTER WORKSHEET

MULTIPLE CHOICE QUESTIONS

1. A nurse is preparing to administer an IM injection to an infant. What is the most appropriate site for this injection?

   a. Deltoid muscle

   b. Vastus lateralis

   c. Dorsogluteal

   d. Rectus femoris

2. A 3-year-old child is to receive a medication that is supplied as an enteric-coated tablet. What is the best nursing action?

   a. Crush the tablet and mix it with applesauce.

   b. Dissolve the medication in the child's milk.

   c. Place a pill in the posterior part of the pharynx and tell the child to swallow.

   d. Check with the prescriber to see if an alternative form can be used.

3. The nurse is caring for an infant who weighs 9.2 kg and is nothing by mouth and receiving IV fluid therapy. What rate does the nurse calculate as meeting the child's daily fluid requirements?

   a. 82 mL/hour

   b. 41 mL/hour

   c. 38 mL/hour

   d. 22 mL/hour

4. When administering ear drops to a 2-year-old, which action would be most appropriate?

   a. Tell the child that the drops are to treat his infection.

   b. Pull the pinna of the child's ear down and back.

   c. Have the child turn his head to the opposite side after giving the drops.

   d. Massage the child's forehead to facilitate absorption of the medication.

CRITICAL THINKING EXERCISES

1. When reviewing the medical record of a child, the nurse notes that the ordered dose of medication is different from the recommended dose. How should the nurse proceed?

2. While caring for a 5-year-old child who is receiving IV fluid therapy at a rate of 50 mL/hour, the nurse notes that the infusion is running slowly. The insertion site appears slightly reddened and swollen. What should the nurse do next?

3. A school-age child is to be discharged, continuing TPN therapy at home. The child lives with his parents and two younger siblings. How would the nurse prepare this child and family for discharge? How could the nurse promote growth and development for this child during TPN therapy?

STUDY ACTIVITIES

1. Review the medical records of several children who are on a pediatric unit in your agency. Note the type of medication, route ordered, and what specific interventions are needed for each child related to the medication administration and developmental age of the child. Compile a list of the most commonly used routes.

2. Interview several parents about their experiences in giving medications to their children. From these interviews, develop a teaching sheet that provides tips to facilitate oral medication administration to children.

3. Create a chart that compares and contrasts the SC, IM, and IV methods of medication administration. Include examples of medications given via these routes, onset of action, appropriate sites, and necessary safety measures for each.

4. An infant is to receive intermittent gavage feedings via a nasogastric tube every 6 hours. The feeding tube was inserted with a previous feeding and remains in place. The nurse is preparing to administer the next scheduled feeding. Place the events in the proper sequence.

   _____ a. Check the placement of the feeding tube.

   _____ b. Position the infant on his right side with the head of the bed slightly elevated.

   _____ c. Allow the feeding to come to room temperature.

   _____ d. Flush the tube with water.

   _____ e. Clamp the tube to prevent air from entering the stomach.

   _____ f. Pour the solution into the barrel of the syringe.

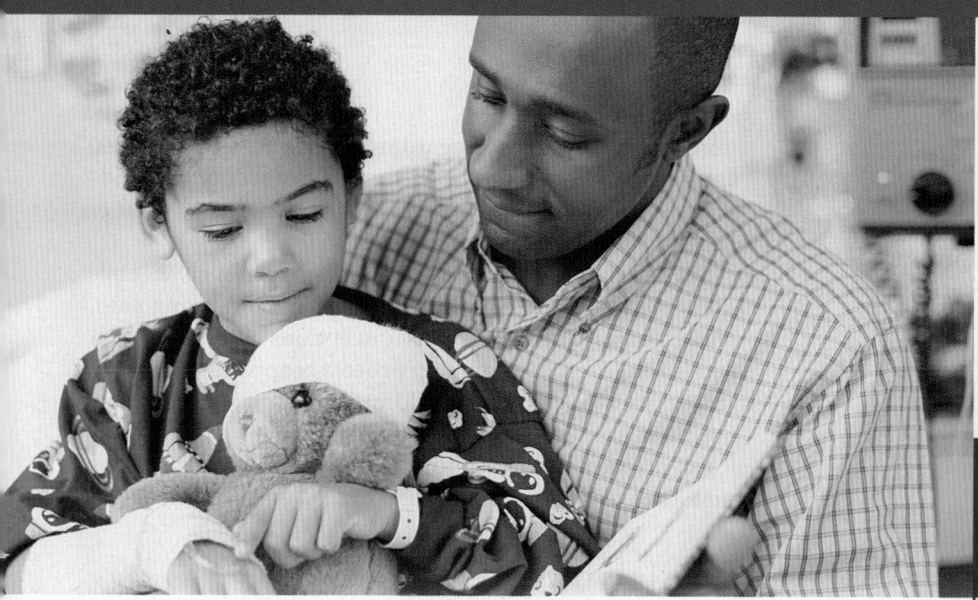

PAIN MANAGEMENT IN CHILDREN

KEY TERMS

acute pain
chronic pain
conscious sedation
drug tolerance
epidural
neuromodulators

neuropathic
   pain
nociceptive pain
nociceptors
pain
pain threshold

patient-controlled
   analgesia
physical dependence
somatic pain
transduction
visceral pain

LEARNING OBJECTIVES

Upon completion of the chapter, the student will be able to:

1. Identify the major physiologic events associated with the perception of pain.
2. Discuss the factors that influence the pain response.
3. Identify the developmental considerations of the effects and management of pain in the infant, toddler, preschooler, school-age child, and adolescent.
4. Explain the principles of pain assessment as they relate to children.
5. Understand the use of the various pain rating scales and physiologic monitoring for children.
6. Establish a nursing care plan for children related to management of pain, including pharmacologic, physical, and psychological techniques and strategies.

Aiden Russell is a 6-year-old on the pediatric unit admitted for a wound infection. He requires BID dressing changes. In report you are told that Aiden cries and fights during the dressing change but otherwise seems to be playing and not experiencing much pain. The reporting nurse states, "Aiden's mother keeps requesting pain medication for Aiden. She states he's complaining of pain most of the time. I'm not sure if I believe her: When I see Aiden, he's playing Nintendo games or watching television and seems to be fine. I've tried to hold off on his pain medication as long as I can."

Wow

All of our patients in pain deserve as much comfort as we can give.

Pain is a highly individualized experience that can affect any person of any age. It is a complex phenomenon that involves multiple components and is influenced by a myriad of factors. Pain often has been described as a subjective experience that involves both sensory and emotional factors. The International Association for the Study of Pain (2011) defines **pain** as "an unpleasant sensory and emotional experience that is associated with actual or potential tissue damage." Pain in children occurs across a spectrum of conditions, including everyday pains (bumps and bruises), acute injuries and medical events, recurrent or chronic pain, and pain related to disease processes. One commonly used definition is that pain is whatever the person says it is, existing whenever the person says it does (Frampton & Hughes-Webb, 2011; McCaffery & Pasero, 2011)—that is, pain is present when the person says that it is. The person experiencing the pain is the only one who can identify his or her pain and know what the pain is like.

Pain is a universal experience. The assessment and management of pain are an individual's right and an important part of basic clinical care for all patients. This is supported by the Canadian Pain Coalition in its charter outlining the rights and responsibilities of pain patients. To view this website, visit http://thePoint.lww.com/Chow1e for a direct link.

Pain affects adults and children alike, but children may lack the verbal capacity to describe their pain accurately. In addition, many caregivers and health care providers have misconceptions about pain in children; it is difficult to assess the complex nature of the pain experience; and limited resources and research are available related to pain relief strategies for children compared with adults. All this makes pain management a critical element in the plan of care for children.

Pain is a major source of distress for children and their families as well as for health care providers. Pain affects children of all ages, even preterm infants. Various provincial health associations have issued position papers and guidelines related to the need to treat pain and suffering in children (Registered Nurses' Association of Ontario, 2007). Effective pain management involves initial pain assessment, therapeutic interventions, and reassessment for all children in any health care setting.

Despite increased evidence of effective ways to assess and manage pain in children, it remains undertreated. Untreated pain in children can lead to serious physical and emotional consequences, such as increased oxygen consumption and alterations in blood glucose metabolism as well as increased anxiety (e.g., needle phobias). In addition, the experience of pain early in life may lead to long-term consequences for the child (Kennedy, Luhmann, & Zempsky, 2008). Treating pain reduces anxiety and decreases the need for physical restraints during procedures, reduces anxiety regarding subsequent procedures, and prevents short- and long-term consequences of inadequately treated pain, particularly in newborns (Cohen & Baxter, 2008; Kennedy et al., 2008).

This chapter describes the pain experience in children, including the types of pain, factors influencing pain, and common myths and misconceptions associated with pain in children. The nursing process is applied to provide an overview of care for a child in pain. Various pain management strategies are described, including pharmacologic, physical, and psychological interventions as well as measures to address procedure-related and chronic pain.

Physiology of Pain

The sensation of pain is a complex phenomenon that involves a sequence of physiologic events in the nervous system. These events are transduction, transmission, perception, and modulation.

Transduction

Peripheral nerve fibres extend from the spinal cord to various locations in and throughout the body's tissues, such as skin, joints, bones, and membranes covering the internal organs. At the end of these fibres are specialized receptors, called **nociceptors**, which become activated when they are exposed to noxious stimuli. The noxious stimuli can be mechanical, chemical, or thermal. Mechanical stimuli may include intense pressure to an area, a strong muscular contraction, or extensive pressure due to muscular overstretching. Chemical stimulation may involve the release of mediators, such as histamine, prostaglandins, leukotrienes, or bradykinin, as a response to tissue trauma, ischemia, or inflammation. Thermal stimuli typically involve extremes of heat and cold. This process of nociceptor activation is called **transduction**.

Transmission

When nociceptors are activated by noxious stimuli, the stimuli are converted to electrical impulses that are relayed along the peripheral nerves to the spinal cord and brain. Specialized afferent nerve fibres are responsible for moving the electrical impulse along. Myelinated A-delta fibres are large fibres that conduct the impulse at very rapid rates. The pain transmitted by these fibres is often referred to as fast pain, most commonly associated with mechanical or thermal stimuli (Cavanaugh & Basbaum, 2011). Pain also is transmitted by unmyelinated small C fibres. These fibres transmit the impulse slowly and are often activated by chemical stimuli or continued mechanical or thermal stimuli (Cavanaugh & Basbaum, 2011). These fibres carry the impulse to the spinal cord via the dorsal horn. Neurotransmitters are released to facilitate the transmission process to the brain.

Several theories have been proposed in an attempt to explain the process of pain transmission. The best known of these is the gate-control theory. According to this theory, the dorsal horn of the spinal cord contains interneuronal or interconnecting fibres. These fibres, when stimulated, close the gate or pathway to the brain, thereby inhibiting or blocking the transmission of the pain impulse. Subsequently, the impulse does not reach the brain where it would be interpreted as pain.

Perception

Once in the dorsal horn of the spinal cord, the nerve fibres divide and then cross to the opposite side and rise upward to the thalamus. The thalamus responds quickly and sends a message to the somatosensory cortex of the brain, where the impulse is interpreted as the physical sensation of pain. The impulses carried by the fast pain A-delta fibres lead to the perception of sharp, stabbing, localized pain that also commonly involves a reflex response to withdraw from the stimulus. The impulses carried by the slow C fibres lead to the perception of diffuse, dull, burning, or aching pain. The point at which the person first feels the lowest intensity of the painful stimulus is termed the **pain threshold** (Fig. 35.1). In addition to sending a message to the cerebral cortex, the thalamus also sends a message to the limbic system, where the sensation is interpreted emotionally, and to the brain stem centres, where autonomic nervous system responses begin.

Modulation

Research has identified substances called **neuromodulators** that appear to modify the pain sensation. These substances have been found to change a person's perception of pain. Examples of these neuromodulators include serotonin, endorphins, enkephalins, and dynorphins.

Pain perception can be modified peripherally or centrally. In the peripheral nerve fibres, chemical substances are released that either stimulate the nerve fibres or sensitize them. Peripheral sensitization allows the nerve fibres to react to a stimulus that is of lower intensity than would be needed to cause pain. As a result, the person perceives more pain. Actions that block or inhibit the release of these substances can lead to a decrease in pain perception.

Modification of pain perception can occur centrally in the spinal cord at the dorsal horn. Substances released by the excited interneurons can potentiate the pain sensation. Other neurochemicals, through their binding to specific receptors, can inhibit the perception of pain.

Types of Pain

Many different systems can be used to classify pain. Most commonly, pain is classified based on its duration, etiology, or source or location.

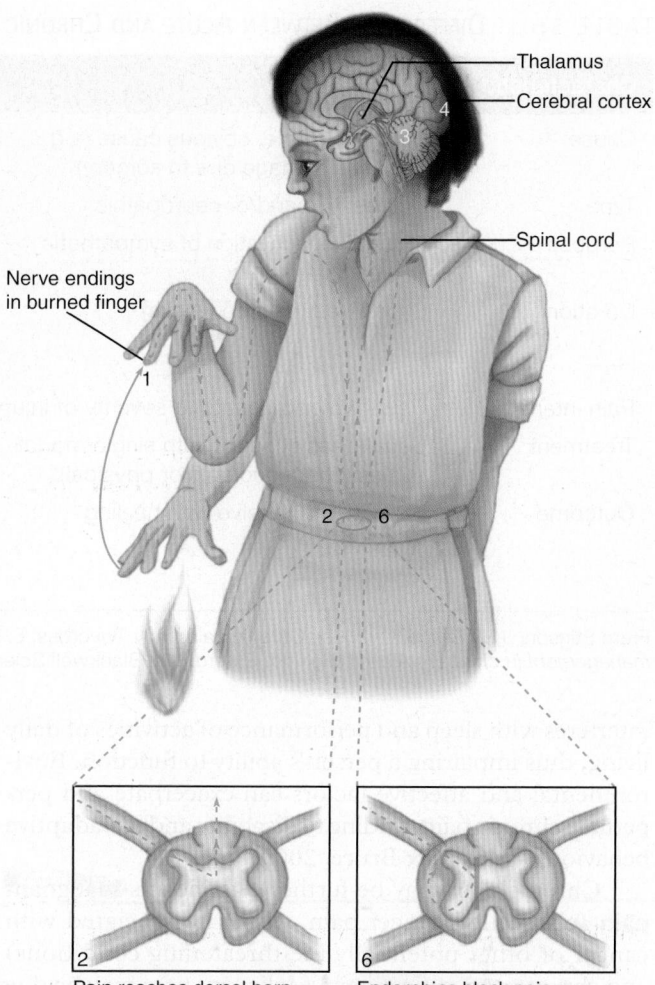

FIGURE 35.1 The transmission of pain stimulus.

Classification by Duration

Pain is classified by duration as acute or chronic (Table 35.1). **Acute pain** is defined as pain that is associated with a rapid onset of varying intensity. It usually indicates tissue damage and resolves with healing of the injury. Acute pain reflects stimulation of nociceptors and serves a protective function (i.e., alerting the person to a problem). Examples of causes of acute pain include trauma, invasive procedures, acute illnesses such as sore throat or appendicitis, and surgery. This type of pain is usually short in duration, generally lasting a few days. Children also experience acute pain associated with various procedures performed in health care settings.

Chronic pain is defined as pain that continues beyond the normal time expected for resolution of the problem or persists or recurs for other reasons. Chronic pain provides no protective function and may be part of a medical condition (arthritis); develop following surgery, illness, or injury (phantom limb pain); or have no obvious cause. It may be continuous or intermittent, with and without periods of exacerbation or remission. It often

TABLE 35.1 DIFFERENCES BETWEEN ACUTE AND CHRONIC PAIN

Characteristic	Acute Pain	Chronic Pain
Cause	Usually a single, obvious cause (e.g., tissue damage due to surgery)	Usually multiple causative or triggering factors Neuronal or CNS abnormality (plasticity, sensitization)
Type	Nociceptive and/or neuropathic	Nociceptive, neuropathic, or mixed; psychosocial factors
Purpose	Protective; activation of sympathetic nervous system	No protective function; rarely accompanied by signs of activation of sympathetic nervous system
Duration	Short-lived (days to weeks)	Long lasting (>6 weeks to 3 months) or recurring beyond time of normal healing; may be associated with chronic disease
Pain intensity	Usually proportionate to severity of injury	Often out of proportion to objective physical findings
Treatment	Usually easy to treat with single modalities (pharmacologic or physical)	More difficult to treat, requiring multidisciplinary, multimodal treatment approach
Outcome	Expected to resolve with healing	Pain persists in significant proportion of patients (30%–62%), with smaller proportion developing pain-associated disability syndrome (5%–8%)

From Stinson, J., & Bruce, L. (2009). Chronic pain. In A. Twycross, L. Bruce, & S. Dowden (Eds.). *Pain management in children: A clinical guide*. Oxford, UK: Blackwell Science.

interferes with sleep and performance of activities of daily living, thus impairing a person's ability to function. Environmental and affective factors can exacerbate and perpetuate chronic pain, leading to disability and maladaptive behaviour (Stinson & Bruce, 2009).

Chronic pain may be further classified as malignant pain (also called cancer pain, which is associated with cancer or other potentially life-threatening conditions) and chronic non-cancer pain. Malignant pain may be due to the disease itself or due to its effects on the body or the procedures and treatments used. Chronic non-cancer pain may be the result of numerous conditions, such as juvenile idiopathic arthritis, sickle cell disease, or inflammatory bowel disease.

In children, recurrent pain is most commonly associated with headache and abdominal, limb, or chest pain, with only a small percentage of this pain found to have an organic etiology (Stanford, Chambers, Biesanz, & Chen, 2008). The signs and symptoms that indicate a possible organic etiology include constant pain, pain that wakes the child from sleep, well-localized pain, and other physical findings such as fever, weight loss, changes in colour, consistency, or frequency of stools, and urinary tract symptoms (Hershey, Powers, Winner, & Kabbouche, 2009). This type of pain lasts for longer periods of time or comes and goes over time.

▶ *Take* NOTE!

Acute and chronic pain may occur concurrently. Acute pain that is not properly treated may become chronic.

Classification by Etiology

Pain can be classified by etiology as nociceptive or neuropathic. **Nociceptive pain** reflects pain due to activation of the A-delta fibres and C fibres by noxious stimuli. The pain perceived often correlates closely with the degree or intensity of the stimulus and the extent of real or possible tissue damage (Bingham, Ajit, Blake, & Samad, 2009). With nociceptive pain, nervous system functioning is intact. Reports of nociceptive pain vary depending on the location of the nociceptors being stimulated, ranging from sharp or burning to dull, aching, or cramping to deep aching or sharp stabbing. Examples of conditions that result in nociceptive pain include chemical burns, sunburn, cuts, appendicitis, and bladder distention.

Neuropathic (or nerve) **pain** is pain due to malfunctioning of the peripheral or central nervous system. It may be continuous or intermittent and is commonly described as burning, tingling, shooting, or stabbing. It may be spontaneous or evoked (i.e., having a trigger factor such as touch or change in temperature). There may also be motor abnormalities, such as tremor, spasms, atrophy, dystonia, and weakness, and autonomic disturbances such as cyanosis, erythema, mottling, increased sweating, swelling, and poor capillary refill. Examples of neuropathic pain in children include complex regional pain syndrome and phantom limb pain, which is pain that is felt in the area of a limb that has been amputated. Children with cancer also experience neuropathic pain, which may be due to either the cancer treatment (chemotherapy or radiotherapy) or the underlying cancer itself (e.g., due to the tumour impinging on a spinal nerve root). Children can also experience a combination of nociceptive and neuropathic pain (called mixed pain).

Classification by Source or Location

Pain also may be classified by the source or location of the area involved as somatic pain (superficial and deep) or visceral pain. These classifications typically indicate nociceptive pain. **Somatic pain** refers to pain that develops in the tissues. It can be further divided into two groups: superficial and deep. Superficial somatic pain, often called cutaneous pain, involves stimulation of nociceptors in the skin, subcutaneous tissue, or mucous membranes. Typically the pain is well localized and described as a sharp, pricking, or burning sensation. Superficial somatic pain may be due to external mechanical, chemical, or thermal injury or skin disorders. Tenderness commonly is present. The individual also experiences hyperalgesia (an increased response to noxious stimulus) and allodynia (a painful response to a normally nonpainful or non-noxious stimulus (Stinson & Bruce, 2009).

Deep somatic pain typically involves the muscles, tendons, joints, fasciae, and bones. It can be localized or diffuse and is usually described as dull, aching, or cramping. Deep somatic pain may be due to strain from overuse or direct injury, ischemia, and inflammation. Tenderness and reflex spasm may be present. Additionally, the person may exhibit sympathetic nervous system activation such as tachycardia, hypertension, tachypnea, diaphoresis, pallor, and pupillary dilation.

Visceral pain is pain that develops within organs such as the heart, lungs, gastrointestinal tract, pancreas, liver, gallbladder, kidneys, or bladder. It can be well or poorly localized and is described as a deep ache or a sharp stabbing sensation that may be referred to other areas. Visceral pain may be due to distention of the organ, organ muscular spasm or pulling, ischemia, or inflammation. Tenderness, nausea, vomiting, and diaphoresis may be present.

Factors Influencing Pain

Many factors influence a child's perception of pain and the ways children behave when in pain. Research has found that environmental and psychological factors may exert a greater influence on the child's perception of pain compared with adults (McGrath & Hillier, 2003). Certain factors such as age, gender, cognitive level, temperament, previous pain experiences, and family and cultural background cannot be changed. However, situational factors involving behavioural, cognitive, and emotional aspects can be modified. Certain situational factors can intensify pain and distress, while others can eventually trigger pain episodes and prolong pain-related disability or maintain the cycle of repeated pain episodes in recurrent pain syndromes (Auvray, Mylin, & Spence, 2010; Ruskin, Amaria, Warnock, & McGrath, 2011).

Age and Gender

Research has demonstrated that the nervous system structures needed for pain impulse transmission and perception are present by the 24th week of gestation. Therefore, children of any age, including preterm newborns, are capable of experiencing pain (Finley, Franck, Grunau, & von Baeyer, 2005). Early on, children can interpret pain as an unpleasant sensation, but this interpretation is based on their comparison with other sensations. As they get older, they learn to use words to describe their pain more fully.

Gender also may play a role in a child's perception of pain (Hurley & Adams, 2008). For example, gender differences are beginning to emerge in relation to chronic pain in older school-age children and adolescents. Researchers have found that chronic pain is more common in girls, who also report more intense, more frequent, and more prolonged pain than boys (Stinson & Bruce, 2009). Differences in coping styles also exist, with girls using more emotional coping styles such as catastrophizing (Stinson & Bruce, 2009).

Cognitive Level

Cognitive level is a key factor affecting a child's pain perception and response and usually goes hand in hand with the child's age. Cognitive level typically increases with age, thereby influencing the child's understanding of the pain and its impact and his or her choices for coping strategies. In addition, as the child's cognitive level increases, his or her ability to communicate information about pain increases. However, this increased understanding and ability to communicate with advancing age may not apply to the child experiencing developmental delays. For example, a developmentally delayed school-age child or adolescent may have the cognitive level of a toddler or preschooler. Health care providers need to be cognizant of this difference when caring for the child in pain. Numerous research studies have revealed that young children often describe pain in concrete terms, whereas older children use more abstract terms that involve both physical and psychological components (Auvray et al., 2010).

Temperament

Temperament affects how a child will respond to a situation. Previous experience with a situation or the method used to cope with a new or a threatening or harmful situation along with the child's coping style will affect the child's pain experience. Even mild symptoms of negative mood may affect the perceptions and persistence of pain (Valrie, Gill, Redding-Lallinger, & Daeschner, 2008). A child with a "difficult temperament" is more likely to have an increased response to pain.

Previous Pain Experiences

A child identifies pain based on his or her experiences with pain in the past. The number of episodes of pain, the type of pain, the severity or intensity of the previous pain experience, and how the child responded all affect how the child will perceive and respond to the current experience. For example, research studies have demonstrated that neonates who had undergone painful procedures such as circumcision and heel lancing showed a stronger negative response to routine immunizations and venipuncture weeks to months later (Kennedy et al., 2008).

Family and Culture

The child's cultural and family background will influence how he or she expresses and manages pain. Some cultures transmit the standard of accepting pain stoically; others allow outward expression. The parents have a strong influence on the child's ability to cope. For example, if a parent reacts to the child's pain in a positive manner and offers comfort measures, the child may have an easier time coping. If the parent shows anger or disapproval, the pain experience may be intensified for the child.

Situational Factors

Situational factors involve factors or elements that interact with the child and his or her current situation involving the experience of pain. These factors are highly variable and dependent on the specific situation. Examples of situational factors are highlighted in Table 35.2.

Developmental Considerations

Since children of various developmental ages respond differently to pain and perceive pain in different ways, it is important to review developmental considerations. Refer to Chapters 25 through 29 for a more complete understanding of childhood development. Nurses must understand how children of various ages respond to painful stimuli and what behaviours may be expected based on their developmental level. By understanding these developmental considerations, the nurse can appropriately assess the child's pain and provide effective interventions.

Infants

Research has demonstrated that infants, including preterm infants, experience pain and can distinguish pain from other tactile experiences (Weissman, Aranovitch, Blazer, & Zimmer, 2009). Much of this research focuses on pain related to invasive procedures, such as heelsticks and intravenous catheter insertion. However, there is new evidence that pain in infants exists beyond acute procedural and postoperative pain and includes pain that may be due to inflammatory, visceral, and central sources. Research suggests that neonates, especially preterm infants, actually experience pain at a greater intensity (due to greater sensitivity and lower behavioural thresholds to acute pain) than their older counterparts and adults (American Medical Association [AMA], 2010; Codipietro, Ceccarelli, & Ponzone, 2008). This greater intensity is due to the immaturity in preterm infants of the inhibitory and facilitatory mechanisms in the central nervous system, which develop at a later time during fetal development. The most important caveat with premature and older infants is that noxious information is processed in a pain-processing system that is in constant change (plasticity) during development (Johnston, Fernandes, & Campbell-Yeo, 2011).

In preterm and term newborns, behavioural and physiologic indicators are used for determining pain. Behavioural indicators include facial expression, body

TABLE 35.2 SITUATIONAL FACTORS AFFECTING A CHILD'S PAIN EXPERIENCE

Cognitive	Behavioural	Emotional
Information about condition and pain problem, including cause and prognosis	Distress responses; specific behaviours and actions	Anticipatory anxiety
Knowledge about available therapy	Use of therapies	Heightened distress; feelings about scheduled possibly painful treatments
Expectations about the effectiveness of therapy and about the future	Child's or family's response to pain condition	Fear about undiagnosed condition and continuing pain; impact of pain and illness on family
Ability to identify pain triggers	Resolution of stressful situation	Situation-specific stress such as school, sports
Knowledge about stress reduction	Participation in routine activities	Frustration related to interruption in activities Underlying anxiety and depression

Adapted from McGrath, P. A., & Hillier, L. M. (2003). Modifying the psychologic factors that intensify children's pain and prolong disability. In N. L. Schecter, C. B. Berde, & M. Yaster (Eds.), *Pain in infants, children, and adolescents* (2nd ed., Fig. 6.1, p. 87). Philadelphia, PA: Lippincott Williams & Wilkins.

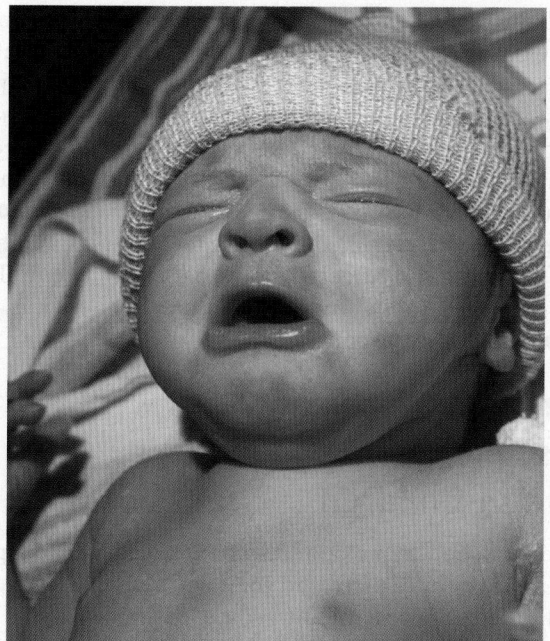

FIGURE 35.2 In the younger infant, facial expression is the most common response to pain.

movements, and crying (American Academy of Pediatrics [AAP] et al., 2010; Henry, Haubold, & Dobrzykowski, 2004). Physiologic indicators include changes in heart rate, respiratory rate, blood pressure, oxygen saturation levels, vagal tone, palmar sweating, and plasma cortisol or catecholamine levels (AAP et al., 2010; Stevens, Pillai Riddel, Oberlander, & Gibbins, 2007).

In the younger infant, facial expression is the most common response to pain (Fig. 35.2). The brows may be lowered and drawn together, with the eyes tightly closed. The mouth is open, often forming a square. The body may be stiff, and thrashing may be seen. When the area is stimulated, the infant may demonstrate a generalized reflex withdrawal. The infant may exhibit a high-pitched, shrill cry.

The older infant often displays similar behavioural manifestations of pain. The older infant may display an angry facial expression, but the eyes are open. He or she often demonstrates a definite withdrawal response when the area is stimulated. The older infant cries loudly and tries to push away the stimulus that is causing the pain. Other manifestations include irritability, restless sleeping, and poor feeding.

▶ *Take* NOTE!

Although an infant usually exhibits typical behaviours indicating pain, absence of these manifestations does not indicate a lack of a pain; the response to pain is highly variable (Ranger, Johnston, & Anand, 2007; Weissman et al., 2009).

Infants are preverbal, so facial expression, diffuse body movements, and other signs, as indicated above, provide helpful feedback that the infant is in pain.

Infants also demonstrate physiologic responses to pain. These may include the following:

Increased heart rate, usually averaging approximately 10 beats/min; possibly bradycardia in preterm newborns
Decreased vagal tone
Decreased oxygen saturation
Palmar or plantar sweating (as measured by skin conductivity testing); not reliable in infants born at less than 37 weeks' gestation

Research has identified short- and long-term consequences of inadequately treated pain in newborns (Spence et al., 2010). These include hyperalgesia around a wound from such situations as repeated heelsticks; an increased risk of developing intraventricular hemorrhage with repeated painful stressors; and a change in the pattern of response to subsequent pain. Children's memories of painful experiences can have long-term consequences for their reaction to later painful events and their acceptance of later health care interventions. Moreover, preterm infants may be at greater risk for experiencing memories of pain due to the often long hospitalizations involving numerous invasive and painful procedures (AAP et al., 2010).

Toddlers

Toddlers can react to painless procedures as intensely as painful ones, with intense emotional upset and physical resistance or aggression (Hockenberry et al., 2011). They may bite, hit, scream, or kick. Other behaviours may include being very quiet, pointing to where it hurts, or saying such words as "owww." Facial grimacing and teeth clenching may be noted. Toddlers may also react with fear and try to hide or leave the room. They often have limited vocabularies, so it may be difficult for them to express pain. Toddlers may also demonstrate regressive behaviours, such as clinging to the parent or crying loudly.

Preschoolers

Since preschoolers may differentiate poorly between themselves and the external world, the physical and verbal aggression is more goal-directed. They also may become quiet or try to withdraw and hide: the child may say he or she needs to go to the bathroom or needs to get something from another room. Because of their magical type of thinking, preschoolers may believe pain is a punishment for misbehaving or having bad thoughts. Preschoolers may not verbally report their pain, thinking that pain is something to be expected or that the adults are aware of their pain. They can tell someone where it hurts and can use various tools to describe the severity of pain; however, because they may have limited experience with pain, they may have difficulty distinguishing between types of pain (sharp or dull), describing the intensity of the pain, and determining whether the pain is worse or better.

School-Age Children

School-age children can communicate the type, location, and severity of pain. Children over the age of 8 years can use specific words, such as "sharp as a knife," burning, or pulling, to describe their pain. However, they may deny pain in an attempt to appear brave or to avoid further pain related to a procedure or intervention. They may be more concerned with their fear about the illness and its effects rather than the pain. They also may fear being embarrassed by acting-out behaviours. Thus, a typical response might be to withdraw by staring at the television. Other behaviours may include muscular rigidity, such as clenching the fists, stiffening the body, closing the eyes, wrinkling the forehead, or gritting the teeth.

Adolescents

Adolescents are concerned primarily about body image and fear losing control over their behaviour. This may result in denial or refusal of medications. Their mood and what they think is expected of them will also affect their response. Adolescents often ask numerous questions and pay close attention to how others respond to them. Fearing that their behaviour may be viewed as juvenile, they may attempt to remain stoic, not exhibiting any emotion. Subtle changes such as increased muscle tension with clenched fists and teeth, rapid breathing, and guarding the affected body part may occur. They may also show lack of interest in everyday activities or a decreased ability to concentrate.

Common Myths and Misconceptions about Pain in Children

In general, children respond to pain based on the type of pain, the extent of pain, and their age and developmental level. Table 35.3 highlights some common myths and misconceptions related to pain in children. Because of these myths, children continue to be medicated less than

TABLE 35.3 MYTHS AND MISCONCEPTIONS ABOUT CHILDREN AND PAIN

Myth or Misconception	Fact
Newborns do not feel pain	Newborns, including preterm newborns, do feel pain The neurologic and hormonal systems needed for the transmission of painful stimuli are sufficiently developed
Exposure to pain at an early age has little to no effect on the child	Prolonged or severe pain can lead to increased newborn morbidity. Infants who have experienced pain during the neonatal period respond differently to subsequent painful events (American Academy of Pediatrics and Canadian Paediatric Society, 2000)
Infants and small children have little memory of pain	Repeated exposure to painful procedures and events can have long-term consequences Memories of pain may be stored in the child's nervous system, influencing later reactions to painful stimuli (Johnston et al., 2011)
The intensity of a child's behavioural reaction indicates the intensity of the child's pain	Numerous factors affect a child's response to pain. Each child is an individual, with his or her own set of responses
A child who is sleeping is not in pain	Sleep may be a coping strategy for the child in pain, or it may reflect exhaustion of the child who is coping with pain
Children are truthful when they are asked if they are experiencing pain	Often children deny pain to avoid a painful situation or procedure, embarrassment, or loss of control Children may assume that others know how they are feeling and thus will not verbalize their complaints
Children learn to adapt to pain and painful procedures	Repeated exposure to pain or painful procedures can result in an increase in behavioural manifestations
Children experience more adverse effects of narcotic analgesics than adults do	The risk of adverse effects of narcotic analgesics is the same for children as for adults
Children are more prone to addiction to narcotic analgesics	Addiction to narcotics when used in children is very rare

Adapted from The Hospital for Sick Children (2005). *Myths vs facts of children's pain*. Retrieved June 4, 2011 from http://www.iasp-pain.org/AM/Template.cfm?Section=Home&Template=/CM/Content-Display.cfm&ContentID=2998.

adults with a similar diagnosis, leading to inadequate pain management (Dowden, McCarthy, & Chalkiadis, 2008; Taylor, Boyer, & Campbell, 2008).

NURSING PROCESS OVERVIEW FOR THE CHILD IN PAIN

WATCH & LEARN

Nursing care of the child with pain includes nursing assessment, nursing diagnosis, planning, interventions, and evaluation. Each step of this process must be individualized for each patient. A general understanding of the physiology of pain, factors that influence pain, comprehensive pain assessment, and effective pain management techniques can help to individualize the child's plan of care.

Assessment

A thorough assessment is fundamental to understand the pain experience and to assess and monitor treatment responses. Assessment of pain in children consists of both subjective and objective data collection. The acronym **QUESTT** is an excellent way to remember the key principles of pain assessment (Stinson, 2009):

Question the child.
Use a reliable and valid pain scale.
Evaluate the child's behaviour and physiologic changes to establish a baseline and determine the effectiveness of the intervention. The child's behaviour and motor activity may include irritability and protection as well as withdrawal of the affected painful area.
Secure the parent's involvement.
Take the cause of pain into account when intervening.
Take action.

Health History

Conducting a thorough history of the child's prior pain experiences and current pain complaints is the first step in pain assessment. When assessing pain in children, tailor the assessment to the child's developmental level and ask questions geared to the child's cognitive ability. During the health history, determine the child's previous exposure to pain, if any, and how the child responded. This information will provide clues about how the child copes and his or her current response. Attempt to determine what word the child uses to denote pain. Some children may not understand the term "pain" but do understand terms such as "ouchie" or "boo-boo."

The health history also includes questioning the parents about their cultural beliefs related to pain and their child's usual responses. This information aids in planning developmentally and culturally appropriate family-centred care.

Questioning the Child

When questioning the child, phrase the questions in a manner that the child will be able to understand based on his or her developmental level. Some input from the child's family may be helpful in determining where best to focus the questions.

Ask the child what pain means to him or her. Use words that the child may comprehend more easily, such as "hurt," "boo-boo," or "ouch," as appropriate. Inquire about similar experiences in the past and how he or she responded. Determine whether the child let others know that he or she was hurting and how this message was conveyed (e.g., crying, acting out, or pointing to the hurting area).

To assess pain of relatively brief duration, the focus is on determining the 1) severity, location, and quality of the pain; 2) associated symptoms; 3) alleviating and aggravating factors; and 4) treatments tried and their effectiveness. Continue the health history by inquiring about what the child wants others, including the nurse, to do when the child hurts. Conversely, ask the child what he or she doesn't want others to do. Ask if there is anything special the child wants to tell the nurse, such as a special pain-relief technique or a specific comfort object.

For a child with chronic pain, a more detailed pain history needs to be taken (Table 35.4). If the child is experiencing chronic or recurrent pain, suggest the child and family record information in a symptom diary. Explain that this will be helpful in identifying potential triggers (e.g., stressors, change in weather) and the best ways to manage the pain.

Questioning the Parents

Parents play a key role in assessing pain in children. Often it is the parents who provide information about the child's current and past experiences with pain. In addition, parents can provide information about how the child exhibits and responds to pain. Parents may be aware of subtle changes in the child's behaviour that may precede the pain, occur with the pain, or indicate relief of pain. Including the parents in this process helps create a positive experience for all involved and promotes feelings of control over the situation.

The questions posed to the parents are similar in focus to those posed to the child. However, more detailed information may be obtained from the parents because they are usually able to describe events more fully or in greater detail due to their higher cognitive level. Parents typically know their child best.

TABLE 35.4 PAIN HISTORY QUESTIONS FOR CHILDREN WITH CHRONIC PAIN AND THEIR PARENTS/CAREGIVERS

Description of pain	**Type of pain**—*Is the pain acute (e.g., medical procedures, postoperative pain, accidental injury), recurrent (e.g., headaches), or chronic (e.g., juvenile idiopathic arthritis)?* **Onset of Pain**—*When did the pain begin? What were you doing before the pain began? Was there any initiating injury, trauma, or stressor?* **Duration**—*How long has the pain been present?* (e.g., hours, days, weeks, months) **Frequency**—*How often is pain present? Is the pain always there or is it intermittent? Does it come and go?* **Location** *Where is the pain located? Can you point to the part of the body that hurts?* (Body outlines can be used to help children indicate where they hurt.) Children older than 3 to 4 years of age can mark an "X" to indicate painful areas, shade in with crayons areas of pain, or choose different colours to represent varying degrees of pain intensity *Does the pain go anywhere else?* (e.g., radiates up or down from the site that hurts). Pain radiation can also be indicated on body diagrams **Intensity** *What is your pain intensity at rest? What is your pain intensity with activity?* (Use an appropriate pain assessment tool.) *Over the past week, what is the least pain you have had? What is the worst pain you have had? What is your usual level of pain?* **Quality of Pain** School-age children can communicate about pain in more abstract terms *Describe the quality of your pain?* (e.g., word descriptors such as sharp, dull, achy, stabbing, burning, shooting, or throbbing) Word descriptors can provide information on whether the pain is nociceptive or neuropathic in nature or a combination of both
Associated symptoms	*Are there any other symptoms that go along with or occur just before or immediately after the pain?* (e.g., nausea, vomiting, light-headedness, tiredness, diarrhea, or difficulty ambulating) *Are there any changes in the colour or temperature of the affected extremity or painful area?* (These changes most often occur in children with conditions such as complex regional pain syndromes)
Temporal or seasonal variations	*Is the pain affected by changes in seasons or weather?* *Does the pain occur at certain times of the day?* (e.g., after eating or going to the toilet)
Impact on daily living	*Has the pain led to changes in daily activities and/or behaviours?* (e.g., sleep disturbances, change in appetite, decreased physical activity, change in mood, or a decrease in social interactions or school attendance) *What level would the pain need to be so that you could do all your normal activities?* (e.g., tolerability) *What level would the pain need to be so that you won't be bothered by it?* (Rated on similar scale as pain intensity) *What brings on the pain or makes the pain worse?* (e.g., movement, deep breathing and coughing, stress, etc.)?
Pain relief measures	*What has helped to make the pain better?* *Have you taken medication to relieve your pain? If so, what was the medication and did it help? Were there any side effects?* It is important to also ask about the use of physical, psychological, and complementary and alternative treatments tried and how effective these methods were in relieving pain. The degree of pain relief or intensity of pain after a pain-relieving treatment/intervention should be determined

From Stinson J. (2009). Pain assessment. In A. Twycross, L. Bruce, & S. Dowden (Eds.), *Pain management in children: A clinical guide.* Oxford, UK: Blackwell Science.

When questioning the parents, use the following examples as a guide for assessing the child's pain:

Has your child ever been in pain before? If so, what was the cause of the pain? How long did he or she have the pain? Where was the pain located?

How did your child react to the pain? What did you do to lessen the pain?

Did your child let you know that he or she was in pain? Did he or she tell you or did you notice something?

Are there any special signs that let you know that your child is hurting? If so, what are they?

Is there anything that your child does or that you do when he or she is hurting that helps relieve the pain?

Does one thing work better than another when your child is hurting?

Is there any special information that you want to tell me about your child?

Approaches to Measuring Pain in Children

The three approaches to measuring pain are self-report (what the child says), behavioural indicators (how the child behaves), and physiologic indicators (how the child's body reacts). These measures are used separately (unidimensional) or in combination (multidimensional or composite) in a range of pain assessment tools that are available for use in practice. The ideal would be a multidimensional measure that includes self-report and one or more of these other approaches. However, this approach would not be applicable for preverbal, non-verbal, or cognitively impaired children for whom behavioural observation must be the source for pain measurement (Stinson, 2009).

Children's self-report of their pain is the preferred approach and should be used with children who are old enough to understand and use a self-report scale (usually 3 years of age and older) and are not overtly distressed. With infants, toddlers, preverbal, cognitively impaired, and sedated children who are unable to self-report, an appropriate behavioural or composite pain assessment tool should be used. No meaningful self-report can be obtained if the child is overtly distressed (e.g., due to pain, anxiety, or some other stressor). The child's pain can be estimated using a behavioural pain assessment tool until the child is less distressed.

Tools for Assessing Pain in Children

In adults, pain intensity is most often assessed by asking patients to rate their pain on a numeric rating scale, with 0 indicating no pain and 10 indicating the worst pain possible. Because of children's more limited understanding of number concepts, a variety of other pain rating scales have been developed.

Self-report Tools

The types of self-report tools that have been designed for use with school-age children and adolescents are outlined below.

Faces Pain Scales. Faces pain scales present the child with drawings or photographs of facial expressions representing increasing levels of pain intensity. The child is asked to select which face best represents his or her pain intensity. The nurse then documents the number (rank order) corresponding to the written description and expression chosen. Faces scales have been well validated for use in children 5 to 12 years of age. There are two types of faces scales: line drawings (e.g., the Faces Pain Scale–Revised [FPS–R], which is available in more than 30 languages; Fig. 35.3) and photographs (e.g., Oucher; Fig. 35.4). Three different Oucher scales have been

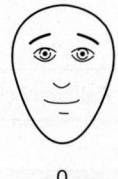 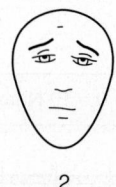 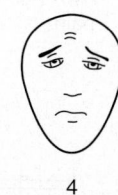 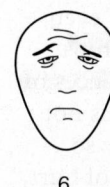 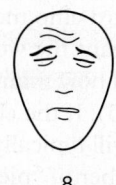 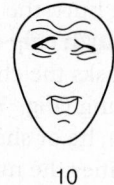

0   2   4   6   8   10

FIGURE 35.3 Faces Pain Scale–Revised (FPS–R). Numbers are for reference and are not shown to children. This scale and instructions in many languages are available online for clinical and research use (visit http://thePoint.lww.com/Chow1e for a direct link). (Reprinted from Hicks, C. L., von Baeyer, P. A. Spafford, I. van Korlaar, B. Goodenough, The FPS–R: Toward a common metric in pediatric pain measurement. *Pain*, *93*, 173–183, Copyright (2001) with permission from Elsevier and the International Association for the Study of Pain.)

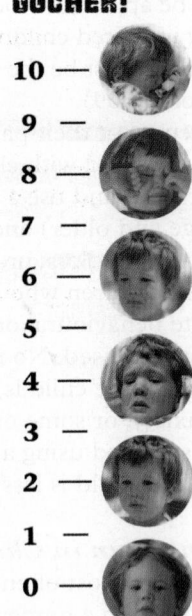

FIGURE 35.4 Oucher Pain Rating Scale. (Used with permission from Beyer, J. E., Denyes, M. J., & Villarruel, A. M. (1992). The creation, validation, and continuing development of the Oucher: A measure of pain intensity in children. *Journal of Pediatric Nursing, 7*(5), 335–346.)

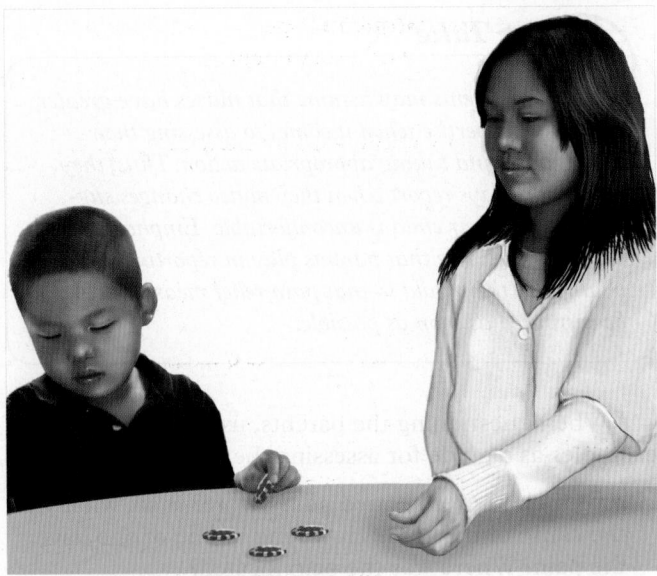

FIGURE 35.5 The Pieces of Hurt Tool. Here the nurse asks the child to identify the pieces of hurt (number of chips) that indicate his degree of pain.

developed for use with white, Hispanic, and black children (Cohen et al., 2008). Faces pain scales that show a happy and smiling no pain face or faces with tears for most pain possible have been found to affect the pain scores recorded (e.g., Wong–Baker FACES Pain Rating Scale). Therefore, faces pain scales with neutral expressions for no pain are generally recommended (Stinson, Yamada, Kavanagh, Gill, & Stevens, 2006).

Graphic Rating Scales. The most commonly used graphic rating scale is the Pieces of Hurt Tool, which is used in preschool children (4 years of age or older). This tool uses four red poker chips to quantify the child's level of pain. The chips are arranged in a horizontal line on a surface in front of the child. The nurse starts by pointing to the chip closest to the child's left side and explains that this first chip means a little hurt, the second chip means more hurt, the third chip means even more hurt, and the fourth chip means the worst hurt ever. Then the nurse asks the child how many "pieces of hurt" he or she is having (Fig. 35.5). If the child is not experiencing any pain, he or she will typically say so. When the child identifies the number of "pieces of hurt," the nurse follows up by asking the child to tell the nurse more about his or her hurt.

Verbal Rating Scales. Verbal rating scales consist of a list of simple word descriptors or phases to denote varying degrees or intensities of pain. Each word or phrase has an associated number. Children are asked to select a

single word or phrase that best represents their level of pain intensity, and the score is the number associated with the chosen word. One example of a verbal rating scale is using word descriptors of not at all = 0, a little bit = 1, quite a lot = 2, and most hurt possible = 3.

Numeric Rating Scale. A numeric rating scale consists of a range of numbers (e.g., 0 to 10 or 0 to 100) that can be represented in verbal or graphic format. Children are told that the lowest number represents no pain and the highest number represents the worse pain (Fig. 35.6). The child is instructed to circle, record, or state the number that best represents his or her level of pain intensity. In clinical practice, verbal numeric rating

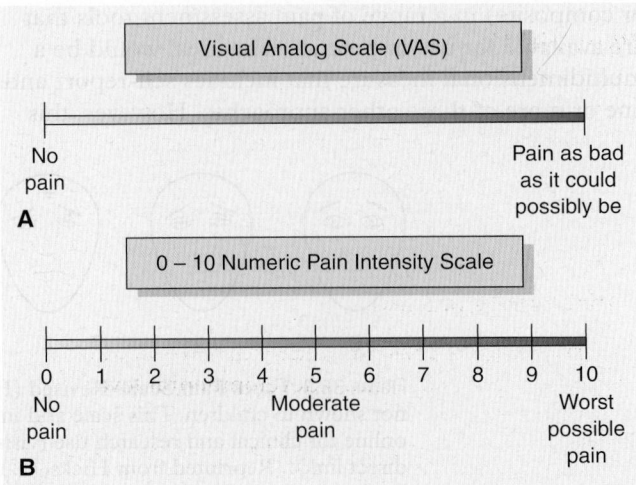

FIGURE 35.6 (**A**) Visual analog scale. (**B**) Numeric pain intensity scale.

scales are the most frequently used pain intensity measure with children over 8 years of age.

Visual Analog Scales.   Visual analog scales involve a horizontal or vertical line with marked endpoints. The endpoints are identified as no pain and worst pain (Fig. 35.6). The nurse explains the scale to the child, and the child makes a line that best describes the level of pain. The nurse then measures the distance from the "no pain" endpoint to the child's mark and records this as the pain score. The visual analog scale is most often used in research with children over 8 years.

Adolescent Pediatric Pain Tool.   The Adolescent Pediatric Pain Tool is a useful self-report tool for older children, usually from ages 8 to 17 years (Bowden & Greenberg, 2008). The tool involves three aspects of assessment. In the first assessment the child identifies the location of the pain on two illustrations of the body, front and back views (Fig. 35.7). The child is instructed to colour the areas where he or she is hurting. The child is also instructed to colour the area as big or as small as how much he or she is hurting. For example, if the hurt is mild or moderate, the child would colour a moderate area of the location; if the pain was severe, he or she would colour a much larger area. The second portion of the tool involves a scale that ranges from "no pain" to "worst possible pain"; the child is instructed to identify the severity of his or her pain. The third assessment is a list of words that may be used to describe pain, such as throbbing, pounding, stabbing, or sharp. The child is asked to point to or circle the words that describe the current pain. Children with limited reading skills or vocabulary may have difficulty with some of the words listed to describe pain. Work with the child and encourage the parents to help the child understand the various descriptive words. Parental participation fosters control over the situation and gives the parents some insight into what their child is experiencing.

Physical Examination

Physical examination of the child for pain primarily involves the skills of observation and inspection. These skills are used to assess for physiologic and behavioural changes that indicate pain. Auscultation also may be used to assess for changes in vital signs, specifically heart rate and blood pressure.

Manifestations of Pain

Observe for physical signs and symptoms of pain, keeping in mind the child's developmental level. Look for facial expressions of discomfort, grimacing, or crying. Be alert for movements that may suggest pain. For example, an infant or toddler may pull on the ear when experiencing ear pain. The child may move the head from side to side, suggesting head pain. Typically, children with abdominal pain will lie on one side and draw their knees up to the abdomen. Inspect the child's gait: a limp or avoidance of weight bearing may suggest leg pain. Immobility, guarding of a particular body area, or refusal to move an area may be observed. Inspect the skin for flushing or diaphoresis, possible indicators of pain. Also monitor vital signs for changes. Pulse or heart rate, respiratory rate, and blood pressure may increase. Other physiologic parameters suggesting pain may include elevated intracranial pressure and pulmonary vascular resistance and decreased oxygen saturation levels.

> ▶ **Take** NOTE!
>
> *The body responds to acute pain via the sympathetic nervous system, leading to stimulation and subsequently the increase in vital signs. However, if the child has persistent or chronic pain, the body adapts and these changes may be less noticeable (Bowden & Greenberg, 2008; Oakes, 2011).*

The child also may exhibit behavioural changes indicating pain. Be alert for irritability and restlessness. Watch for clenching of teeth or fists, body stiffening, or increased muscle tension. Note any changes in the child's behaviour—for example, a child who previously was talkative and playful who becomes quiet and almost withdrawn. In addition, pay close attention to the child's cultural background and how these beliefs may be affecting the behavioural response to pain.

Each child is an individual with unique responses to pain, so the nurse must ensure that observations of behaviour do indeed reflect the child's pain level. Several physiologic and behavioural assessment tools have been developed to help quantify and ensure the accuracy of the observations.

Behavioural Tools

The tools developed to assess pain in infants and young children generally use behavioural indicators of pain. A wide range of specific, expressive behaviours have been identified in infants and young children that are indicative of pain. These include individual behaviours (e.g., crying and facial expression), large movements (e.g., withdrawal of the affected limb, touching the affected area, and moving or tensing the limbs and torso), changes in social behaviour or appetite, and changes in sleep–wake state or cognitive functions.

Observational tools are used for children who are too young to understand and use self-report scales (younger than 4 years of age), too distressed to

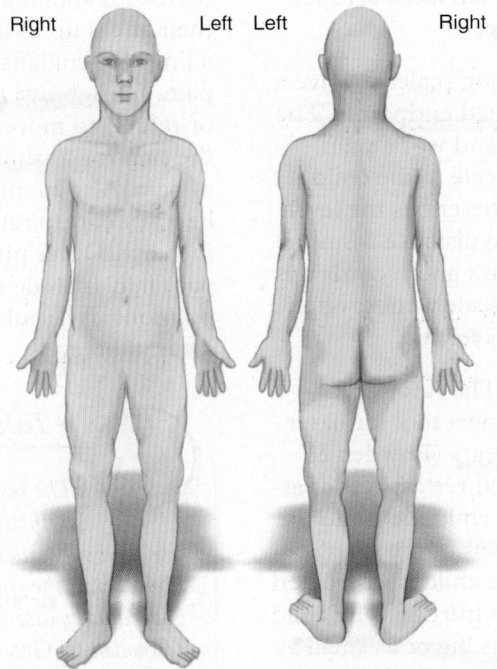

Right   Left   Left   Right

Sensory

Aching ("pain all over")

Hurting ("pain all over")

Sore ("like a cut")

Beating (procedural pain "spots")

Pounding ("gets on your nerves")

Cutting ("hurts more than a cut")

Like a sharp knife ("stabbing and sharp")

Sharp (no meaning)

Stabbing (no meaning)

Cramping ("everywhere like a plane crash")
Crushing (no meaning)
Pressure ("pushing all over")
Itching ("all over")
Scratching ("helps sometimes")
Shocking (pain "surprises" her)
Splitting ("splitting in half" her body)
Numb ("knows pain is there"/ procedural pain)
Stiff ("cannot move")
Swollen ("meds do not help")
Tight ("cannot move")

Affective

Awful ("cannot do anything")

Crying ("hurts so bad")

Frightening ("scared it won't stop")

Screaming (afraid of "going to the hospital")

Terrifying ("cannot sleep," "really tired," "not going to live")

Dizzy ("don't know where I am")

Evaluative

Annoying ("cannot sleep")

Bad ("cannot stop the hurting")

Miserable ("cannot sleep or do stuff")

Terrible ("don't like it")

Uncomfortable ("can't stay in one spot")

Uncontrollable ("cannot stop it")

Temporal

Always ("pain always there")

Comes and goes ("always pain")

Comes on all of a sudden ("no warning")

Constant ("never goes away")

Continuous ("pain not going away")

Forever ("never will go away")

Once in a while ("in a month sometimes pain; sometimes not")

Sneaks up ("don't know when the pain will happen")

Sometimes ("goes away sometimes; sometimes not")

FIGURE 35.7 Adolescent Pediatric Assessment Tool. (*Top*) Adolescent Pediatric Pain Tool (APPT): body outline. (*Bottom*) Pain quality: words chosen and meaning of words. (Used with permission from Crandall, M., & Savedra, M. (2005). Multidimensional assessment using the adolescent pediatric pain tool: A case report. *Journal for Specialists in Pediatric Nursing, 10*(3), 115–123.)

use self-report scales, impaired in their cognitive or communicative abilities, or very restricted by bandages, surgical tape, mechanical ventilation, or paralyzing drugs. They are also used for children whose self-report ratings are considered to be exaggerated, minimized, or unrealistic due to cognitive, emotional, or situational factors.

Physiologic Indicators

Neonates and children clearly display metabolic, hormonal, and physiologic responses to pain. These physiologic reactions all indicate the activation of the sympathetic nervous system, which is part of the autonomic nervous system and is responsible for the fight or flight response associated with stress. Physiologic changes can include changes in heart rate, respiratory rate, blood pressure, and oxygen saturation as well as sweating and dilated pupils. These indicators usually reflect stress reactions and are only loosely correlated with self-report of pain. They can occur in response to other states, such as exertion, fever, and anxiety, or in response to medications. On their own, physiologic indicators do not constitute a valid clinical pain measure for children. Therefore, a multidimensional measure that incorporates physiologic and behavioural indicators in addition to self-report is preferred whenever possible.

Multidimensional Pain Tools for Infants and Young Children

Premature Infant Pain Profile. The Premature Infant Pain Profile (PIPP) is a composite tool that is useful for measuring pain in preterm and term neonates (28 to 40 weeks' gestation). The PIPP consists of three behavioural (facial actions: brow bulge, eye squeeze, and nasolabial furrow), two physiologic (heart rate and oxygen saturation), and two contextual (gestational age and behavioural state) indicators of infant pain (Table 35.5). Each indicator is evaluated on a four-point scale (0, 1, 2, 3) for a possible total score of 18 to 21 based on the gestational age of the infant. A total score of 6 or less generally indicates minimal or no pain, while scores higher than 12 indicate moderate to severe pain.

CRIES Scale for Neonatal Postoperative Pain Assessment. The CRIES scale is another composite tool that was developed to quantify postoperative pain in full-term infants. The tool also may be used to monitor the infant's progress over time during recovery or after interventions. The tool assesses five parameters: *c*ry, *r*equires increased oxygen, *i*ncreased vital signs, *e*xpression, and *s*leeplessness (Table 35.6). Each parameter is scored as 0, 1, or 2 and then totalled. As with other assessment tools, the higher the score, the greater the infant's pain.

FLACC Behavioural Scale for Postoperative Pain in Young Children. The FLACC behavioural scale is useful in assessing a child's pain when the child cannot report his or her level of pain accurately. It has been demonstrated to be a reliable tool for children aged 2 months to 7 years (Oakes, 2011). This tool measures five parameters: *f*acial expression, *l*egs, *a*ctivity, *c*ry, and *c*onsolability (Table 35.7). Observe the child with the legs and body uncovered. If the child is awake, observe him or her for 2 to 5 minutes; if sleeping, observe the child for 5 minutes or longer. Each parameter is scored as 0, 1, or 2; the scores are totalled, with a maximum achievable score of 10 (indicating greater pain).

Non-Communicating Children's Pain Checklist–Revised. The most well-validated measure is the Non-Communicating Children's Pain Checklist–Revised (Box 35.1).

Choosing the Right Pain Assessment Measure

Many reliable, valid, and clinically useful tools are available for assessing pain in neonates, infants, children, and adolescents. However, no single, easily administered, widely accepted technique exists for assessing pain in all children. Typically, different pain rating scales are appropriate for children of different developmental levels. Because a child may regress when in pain, a simpler tool may be needed to ensure that he or she understands what is being asked. Regardless of the tool selected, nurses need to be consistent in using the tool so that appropriate comparisons can be made and effective interventions can be planned and implemented. Perhaps the most important consideration is to choose a single set of tools for a given institution and then to use those tools consistently.

Frequency of Pain Assessment and Documentation

Effective pain management depends on regular assessment of the presence and severity of pain and the child's response to pain management interventions. Many health care facilities have specific policies and procedures in place related to pain assessment, including the frequency of assessment, the rating tool to use for each age group, and nursing interventions to be instituted based on the rating. For example, many facilities require assessment of the child using a specific tool with documentation at least once a shift and 30 minutes to 1 hour after a nonpharmacologic or pharmacologic pain-relief intervention. This process provides a more objective method to determine whether the pain is increasing or decreasing and whether pain-relief methods are effective.

Regular assessment and documentation facilitate effective treatment and communication among members of the health care team, patient, and family. Pain is

TABLE 35.5   PREMATURE INFANT PAIN PROFILE

Infant ID Number:_____

Date:/Time:_____

Event:_____

Process	Indicator	0	1	2	3	Score
Chart	Gestational age (at time of observation)	36 weeks and more	32 weeks to 35 weeks, 6 days	28 weeks to 35 weeks, 6 days	Less than 28 weeks	
Observe infant 15 seconds before procedure Heart rate____ Oxygen saturation____	Behavioural state	Active/awake Eyes open Facial movements Crying (with eyes open or closed)	Quiet/awake Eyes open No facial movements	Active/sleep Eyes closed Facial movements	Quiet/sleep Eyes closed No facial movements	
Observe infant 30 seconds after procedure	Heart rate max.____	0 to 4 beats/min increase	5 to 14 beats/min increase	15 to 24 beats/min increase	25 beats/min or more increase	
	Oxygen saturation Min.____	<2% decrease	2% to 4% decrease	5% to 7% decrease	≥7% decrease	
	Brow bulge	None	Minimum	Moderate	Maximum	
	Eye squeeze	None	Minimum	Moderate	Maximum	
	Nasolabial furrow	None	Minimum	Moderate	Maximum	

Total Score

Scoring method for PIPP

1. Familiarize yourself with each indicator and how it is scored.
2. Score gestational age (from medical record) before you begin.
3. Score behavioural state by observing the infant for 15 seconds immediately before the event.
4. Record baseline heart rate and oxygen saturation.
5. Observe the infant for 15 seconds immediately following the event, looking between the monitor and the infant. Score each indicator for the 30-second period of time, noting changes from baseline.
6. Add all indicators to calculate the final score.

From Stevens, B. J., Hohnson, C., Petryshen, P, & Taddio, A. (1996). Premature infant pain profile: Initial development and validation. *Clinical Journal of Pain, 12,* 13–22.

considered the fifth vital sign and, therefore, should be assessed and documented along with the other vital signs (American Pain Society, 1995). Putting mechanisms in place that make documentation of pain easy for nurses helps ensure consistent documentation. Standardized forms and tools for documenting pain (e.g., admission assessment forms, vital signs chart) allow for the initial assessment and ongoing re-assessment and can also be used to document the efficacy of pain-relieving interventions. Including pain intensity as part of the vital signs record allows for pain to be assessed, documented, and taken as seriously as other vital signs.

Nursing Diagnoses, Goals, Interventions, and Evaluation

After the assessment is completed, the nurse identifies appropriate nursing diagnoses. The most commonly identified nursing diagnosis would be acute or chronic pain. However, the related factors and defining characteristics can vary widely. Nursing diagnoses will focus on the effects of pain on the child—for example, the stress incurred as a result of the pain or the fear or anxiety associated with the pain or events causing the pain. Moreover, pain can affect physiologic functions, such as sleep, nutrition, mobility, and elimination. Examples of common nursing diagnoses may include the following:

TABLE 35.6 THE CRIES SCALE FOR NEONATAL POSTOPERATIVE PAIN ASSESSMENT

Assessment	0	1	2
Crying	No	High-pitched, but consolable	High-pitched, inconsolable
Oxygen required for saturation above 95%	No	<30%	>30%
Increased vital signs	Heart rate and blood pressure within 10% of preoperative values	Heart rate or blood pressure 11% to 20% higher than preoperative values	Heart rate or blood pressure 21% or more above preoperative values
Expression	No grimace	Grimace	Grimace with grunt
Sleeplessness	No	Waking at frequent intervals	Constantly awake
Total infant score			

Used with permission from Krechel, S. W., & Bildner, J. (1995). CRIES: A new neonatal postoperative pain measurement score. Initial testing of validity and reliability. *Paediatric Anaesthesia, 5*, 53–61.

Acute pain related to repeated need for invasive procedures, surgical experience, recent trauma, or infection

Chronic pain related to prolonged illness or injury, effects of cancer on surrounding tissues, or treatment-related effects

Fear related to the unknown, separation from family, anticipation of invasive procedures, or effects of treatment

Anxiety related to the stress and uncertainty of the situation

Deficient knowledge related to current condition and appropriate methods for managing pain

Disturbed sleep pattern related to inability to manage pain effectively

Impaired mobility related to increased episodes of pain

Risk for constipation related to potential adverse effects of narcotic analgesic agents

When caring for a child experiencing pain, the ultimate goal is that the child will be free of pain as evidenced by participation in age-appropriate activities of daily living and that vital signs will be within age-appropriate parameters. However, this may be unrealistic at times, especially if the child is experiencing chronic pain. Therefore, a more appropriate goal would be that the child reports that his or her pain has decreased to a tolerable level or, in the case of chronic pain, that the child's functioning has improved (e.g., attending school, increased physical, and social activity). Pain assessment tools can be used to quantify the amount by which the child's pain has decreased. For example, if the child has rated the pain as 7 out of 10, a realistic goal might be that the child reports a pain rating of no more than 4 out of 10. Additional goals would reflect improvement or resolution of the identified problem. For example, a short-term goal for a child experiencing disturbed sleep due to the pain might be that the child sleeps for a minimum of 4 consecutive hours through the night. A long-term goal might be that the child sleeps for 7 to 8 hours undisturbed through the night.

TABLE 35.7 FLACC BEHAVIOURAL SCALE

Category	Scoring		
	0	1	2
Face	No particular expression or smile	Occasional grimace or frown, withdrawn, disinterested	Frequent to constant frown, clenched jaw, quivering chin
Legs	Normal position or relaxed	Uneasy, restless, tense	Kicking or legs drawn up
Activity	Lying quietly, normal position, moves easily	Squirming, shifting back and forth, tense	Arched, rigid, or jerking
Cry	No cry (awake or asleep)	Moans or whimpers, occasional complaint	Crying steadily, screams or sobs, frequent complaints
Consolability	Content, relaxed	Reassured by occasional touching, hugging, or being talked to, distractable	Difficult to console or comfort

Each of the five categories is scored from 0 to 2, which results in a total score between 0 and 10.

BOX 35.1 **Non-Communicating Children's Pain Checklist—Revised**

How often has this child shown these behaviours in the last 2 hours? Please circle a number for each item. If an item does not apply to this child (e.g., this child does not eat solid food or cannot reach with his/her hands), then indicate "not applicable" for that item.

0 = Not at All   1 = Just a Little   2 = Fairly Often   3 = Very Often   NA = Not Applicable

I. Vocal

1.	Moaning, whining, whimpering (fairly soft)	0	1	2	3	NA
2.	Crying (moderately loud)	0	1	2	3	NA
3.	Screaming/yelling (very loud)	0	1	2	3	NA
4.	A specific sound or word for pain (e.g., a word, cry, or type of laugh)	0	1	2	3	NA

II. Social

5.	Not cooperating, cranky, irritable, unhappy	0	1	2	3	NA
6.	Less interaction with others, withdrawn	0	1	2	3	NA
7.	Seeking comfort or physical closeness	0	1	2	3	NA
8.	Being difficult to distract, not able to satisfy or pacify	0	1	2	3	NA

III. Facial

9.	A furrowed brow	0	1	2	3	NA
10.	A change in eyes, including: squinching of eyes, eyes opened wide, eyes frowning	0	1	2	3	NA
11.	Turning down of mouth, not smiling	0	1	2	3	NA
12.	Lips puckering up, tight, pouting, or quivering	0	1	2	3	NA
13.	Clenching or grinding teeth, chewing or thrusting tongue out	0	1	2	3	NA

IV. Activity

14.	Not moving, less active, quiet	0	1	2	3	NA
15.	Jumping around, agitated, fidgety	0	1	2	3	NA

V. Body and Limbs

16.	Floppy	0	1	2	3	NA
17.	Stiff, spastic, tense, rigid	0	1	2	3	NA
18.	Gesturing to or touching part of the body that hurts	0	1	2	3	NA
19.	Protecting, favouring, or guarding part of the body that hurts	0	1	2	3	NA
20.	Flinching or moving the body part away, being sensitive to touch	0	1	2	3	NA
21.	Moving the body in a specific way to show pain (e.g., head back, arms down, curls up, etc.)	0	1	2	3	NA

VI. Physiological

22.	Shivering	0	1	2	3	NA
23.	Change in colour, pallor	0	1	2	3	NA
24.	Sweating, perspiring	0	1	2	3	NA
25.	Tears	0	1	2	3	NA
26.	Sharp intake of breath, gasping	0	1	2	3	NA
27.	Breath holding	0	1	2	3	NA

VII. Eating/Sleeping

28.	Eating less, not interested in food	0	1	2	3	NA
29.	Increase in sleep	0	1	2	3	NA
30.	Decrease in sleep	0	1	2	3	NA

Score Summary:

Category: I   II   III   IV   V   VI   VII   TOTAL

Score:

From Dr. Lynn Breau. Version 01.2009 © 2009 Lynn Breau, Patrick McGrath, Allen Finley, Carol Camfield.

Various interventions can be used for pain management. These interventions include pharmacologic, physical, and psychological (cognitive and behavioural) measures (the 3 P's). A guiding principle when caring for the child experiencing pain is the provision of atraumatic care (see Chapter 32 for more information). For example, apply a topical anesthetic cream to a site early enough before a venipuncture that it becomes effective. Use an intermittent infusion device to obtain multiple blood specimen samples rather than performing repeated venipunctures. Consider the use of sedation with analgesics for more painful procedures. In addition to pharmacologic measures, physical (e.g., heat and cold, massage) and cognitive and behavioural approaches are appropriate for pain management, including pain management related to procedures.

Throughout the child's care, be sure to discuss specific goals and interventions with the child and family as appropriate. Include the family in developing appropriate interventions so that they can continue to support the child. Education of the child and family about interventions, including various therapies, is key. Play therapy may be helpful in allowing the child to express his or her feelings and adapt to the stressors of the current situation. Ongoing assessment is needed to determine the effectiveness of the pain relief measures in achieving the desired goals.

Nursing Care Plan 35.1 can be used as a guide in planning nursing care for the child experiencing pain. The nursing care plan should be individualized based on the child's symptoms and needs. Specific information related to pain management and the nurse's role will be discussed later in the chapter.

When you enter Aiden's room, he is crying and says his leg hurts. What will be your initial action? What will be your plan of care to manage Aiden's pain (refer to QUESTT assessment)? How would you address the statements made by the nurse in report? What approaches can you use to change staff behaviour about pain management?

Management of Pain

Three general principles guide pain management in children:

1. Individualize interventions based on the type of pain (acute or chronic), the amount of pain experienced, and the child's personality.
2. Use pharmacologic, physical, and psychological approaches to ease or eliminate the pain.
3. Use aggressive pharmacologic treatment with the first procedure.

Strategies for pain management include psychological interventions such as distraction, relaxation, and guided imagery, physical therapies (heat and cold, massage, exercise), and pharmacologic interventions such as analgesics, patient-controlled analgesia (PCA), local analgesia, epidural analgesia, and conscious sedation.

Nonpharmacologic Management

Various physical and psychological techniques may be available to assist in managing mild pain in children or augment the effectiveness of medications for moderate or severe pain. Many of these nonpharmacologic techniques assist children in coping with pain and give them an opportunity to feel a sense of mastery or control over the situation. Two types of techniques are cognitive-behavioural strategies and physical strategies. With these techniques as well as administration of medications, parents need to be involved in this process. See Evidence-Based Practice 35.1.

Cognitive-Behavioural Strategies
Cognitive-behavioural strategies are used to improve the way the child copes and manages his or her pain. These strategies help to change the interpretation of the painful stimuli, reducing pain perception or making pain more tolerable. In addition, these strategies help to decrease negative attitudes, thoughts (catastrophizing), and anxieties, thereby improving the child's coping mechanisms. Typically, these interventions work well with older children, but some younger children also benefit from these techniques if they are adapted to the child's age and developmental level. Common cognitive-behavioural strategies include relaxation, distraction, imagery, biofeedback, thought stopping, and positive self-talk.

Relaxation
Relaxation aids in reducing muscle tension and anxiety. A wide variety of techniques can be used. Relaxation can be as simple as holding an infant or young child closely while stroking the child or speaking in a soft soothing manner or having the child inhale and exhale slowly using rhythmically controlled deep breathing. It also can involve more sophisticated techniques such as progressive muscle relaxation. With this technique the child is asked to focus on one area of the body, tense the muscles in that area, and then let that body part go limp. In an organized fashion, usually working from the toes to the head or vice versa, the child is then asked to focus on another body part, alternately tensing and relaxing the muscles. Eventually the exercises work through all body areas, leading to relaxation of the entire body.

Distraction
Distraction involves having the child focus on another stimulus, thereby attempting to shift his or her attention

(text continues on page 1106)

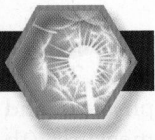

Nursing Care Plan 35.1

OVERVIEW FOR THE CHILD IN PAIN

NURSING DIAGNOSIS: Acute pain related to need for invasive procedures, surgery, recent trauma, or infection as evidenced by pain rating scale, facial grimacing, crying, irritability, withdrawal activity, or changes in vital signs

Outcome Identification and Evaluation
Child will achieve adequate comfort level as evidenced by a decrease in rating number (3 or less) on a pain rating scale, quietness, calm resting behaviours, decrease in crying and irritability, and vital signs within acceptable parameters.

Intervention: Promoting Pain Relief
- Assess pain level using a developmentally appropriate pain rating tool *to establish a baseline.*
- Assess for verbal and nonverbal indicators of pain; question parents about child's typical behaviours and previous experiences with pain *to determine factors that may be influencing child's response to pain.*
- Institute nonpharmacologic methods for pain control based on the child's age and cognitive level; encourage parental participation in use of methods *to provide additional support for the child.*
- Administer pharmacologic agents as ordered using the least traumatic route possible *to alter pain impulse transmission and minimize distress while promoting effective pain relief.*
- Explain the action of the drug and what the child should expect from the medication at a level that the child can understand *to promote trust and reduce fear.*
- Give analgesics around the clock if pain is continuous and can be predicted *to maintain steady blood levels of the drug, thereby maximizing the drug's effect.*
- Perform atraumatic care at all times *to minimize the child's exposure to physical and psychological distress.*
- If a procedure is to be done, explain the purpose of the medication before the procedure and what to expect *to help minimize fear of the unknown.*
- Anticipate timing of procedures or situations that may lead to pain and provide appropriate analgesic therapy as ordered *to ensure that therapy is most effective at the time of the procedure.*
- Ensure that the child's environment is quiet and conducive to rest, dim the lights, close the door or curtain *to reduce sensory overload that would increase the child's pain sensation.*
- Encourage the parents to stroke, touch, caress, and hold the child *to promote feelings of security.*
- Reassess child's pain level after use of nonpharmacologic and pharmacologic methods *to determine effectiveness;* anticipate the need to modify or adapt nonpharmacologic methods or adjust analgesic dosage, route, or frequency *to promote maximum pain relief.*
- Perform nursing care activities after administering analgesic *to prevent exacerbating the child's pain.*
- Use diversional activities, distraction, and play appropriate to the child's age and cognitive level *to promote additional pain relief.*

NURSING DIAGNOSIS: Anxiety related to stress and uncertainty of the situation, unknown cause of pain, lack of familiarity with procedures, testing, and health care facility, and painful procedures, as evidenced by crying, irritability, withdrawal, stoic, or aggressive behaviours

Outcome Identification and Evaluation
Child and family will demonstrate a decrease in anxiety level as evidenced by age-appropriate positive coping behaviours, verbalization of feelings, playing out of feelings, child and family cooperation with plan of care, and absence of signs and symptoms associated with escalating anxiety.

Intervention: Minimizing Anxiety
- Assess child's and parents' understanding of the situation, including their understanding of what may be causing the pain and the reasons for the procedures and testing, *to provide baseline information about the child's and parents' knowledge and possible clues to anxiety.*
- Spend time with the child and parents discussing what they think might be happening, encouraging child and parents to talk openly about their feelings, *to facilitate continued expressions and communication.* Allow time for questions and answer questions honestly *to establish rapport and build trust.*

Nursing Care Plan 35.1 (continued)

- Approach the child and family in a calm, relaxed manner *to foster trust and communication.*
- Allow the child options related to pharmacologic agent administration as much as possible, such as fluid to drink or snack to eat, extremity to use for venipuncture (right or left), colour of bandage, or holding tape or dressing, *to foster feelings of control.*
- Provide atraumatic care *to reduce exposure to distress, which would exacerbate the child's anxiety level.*
- Explain any procedures, tests, and activities at a level the child can understand *to reduce fear of the unknown.*
- Incorporate aspects of the child's routine at home as much as possible *to reduce feelings of separation and promote feelings of normalcy.*
- Ensure consistency in care *to facilitate trust and acceptance.*
- Encourage parents in the use of comfort measures such as stroking, cuddling, holding, and rocking *to promote feelings of security and minimize stress.*
- Provide positive reinforcement for choices, participation in activities, and use of appropriate coping methods *to foster self-esteem.*
- Encourage the child's participation in play (unstructured and therapeutic play as needed) *to promote expression of feelings and fears.*

NURSING DIAGNOSIS: Deficient knowledge related to current condition and appropriate methods for managing pain as evidenced by crying, irritability, pushing away, questions, and verbalizations about pain and relief methods

Outcome Identification and Evaluation
Child and parents will demonstrate adequate knowledge about the child's current condition and use of pain relief methods as evidenced by statements about the cause of the child's pain, demonstration of chosen nonpharmacologic relief methods, use of pharmacologic agents, and statements related to signs and symptoms of increased and decreased pain.

Intervention: Providing Child and Family Teaching
- Assess child's and parents' knowledge and understanding of child's current condition and current pain level *to establish a baseline for teaching.*
- Provide time for child and parents to ask questions; answer questions honestly and in terms they can understand *to promote learning.*
- Explain in simplified terms how the child's condition is associated with pain or the rationale for procedures needed that may contribute to pain *to promote understanding and foster trust.*
- Teach in short sessions *to prevent overloading the child and parents with information.*
- Provide reinforcement and rewards *to help facilitate the teaching/learning process.*
- Use multiple modes of learning, such as written information, verbal instruction, demonstrations, and media when possible, *to facilitate learning and retention of information.*
- Instruct parents and child as appropriate in nonpharmacologic methods for pain relief; encourage practice and participation by parents in methods chosen *to foster independence and use of method when necessary.*
- Teach child as appropriate and parents about pharmacologic methods for pain relief; review specific information about drug to be used, including action, duration, administration, possible adverse effects, and care necessary when drug is used, *to promote learning;* have child and parents report back information or demonstrate administration *to evaluate effectiveness of teaching.*
- Provide parents with written information about pain relief methods for use at home if indicated *to allow for reference at a later date.*

NURSING DIAGNOSIS: Disturbed sleep patterns related to inability to manage pain effectively as evidenced by frequent waking by child during night, signs and symptoms of pain including irritability and restlessness, statements about being tired, pain rating scale.

Outcome Identification and Evaluation
Child will exhibit increased ability to sleep during night as evidenced by increasing periods of calm and restfulness (initially starting at 2 hours and gradually increasing to 7 to 8 hours), decreased pain level on pain rating scale, and statements of decreased fatigue.

(continued)

Nursing Care Plan 35.1 (continued)

Intervention: Promoting Sleep and Rest

- Assist child in using nonpharmacologic methods of pain relief, such as imagery, distraction, and muscle relaxation, *to promote relaxation.*
- Administer pharmacologic pain relief as ordered *to minimize pain interfering with sleep;* anticipate a change in drug therapy if pain relief is inadequate.
- Cluster nursing care activities *to minimize energy expenditure and disruptions in child's ability to rest.*
- Help child with a nighttime routine similar to the one he or she uses at home *to promote feelings of security.*
- Offer child back rub, warm bath, or warm liquids, reading a story, or listening to music *to facilitate relaxation;* provide stroking, hugging, cuddling, rocking, and light touch *to promote a sense of security and calm.*
- Dim the lights and close the curtain or door to the room *to provide a quiet, restful environment.*
- Ensure round-the-clock pain relief for the child through the night *to minimize the risk of pain.*

NURSING DIAGNOSIS: Risk for injury related to possible adverse effects of analgesics.

Outcome Identification and Evaluation

Child will remain free of any injury related to signs and symptoms of adverse effects of analgesic therapy as evidenced by respiratory rate appropriate for age, no complaints of GI upset, dizziness, or sedation or episodes of constipation, nausea, vomiting, or pruritus.

Intervention: Promoting Safety

- Ensure that the child's call light is within reach to allow for notification of health care personnel should problems arise.
- Administer analgesic exactly as prescribed to reduce the risk of error and development of adverse effects.
- Assess child's respiratory status closely for changes to allow for early detection of respiratory depression.
- If an opioid analgesic is being given, have naloxone readily available to reverse the action of the narcotic if respiratory depression occurs.
- Monitor appetite and assess bowel sounds for changes; note any abdominal distention or decreased bowel sounds, which would suggest decreased peristalsis.
- Ensure adequate fluid and fibre intake to reduce risk of constipation.
- Offer small frequent meals and give medication with food to minimize risk of GI upset.
- Assess for nausea and vomiting; if necessary withhold food and fluids to rest the GI tract and administer antiemetics until nausea and vomiting resolve.
- Instruct the child to remain in bed after receiving analgesic, raise crib or side rails as appropriate, and instruct the child and parents to have someone accompany the child to the bathroom if allowed to reduce the risk of falls from sedation.
- Assess for complaints of itching and observe for rash or reddened areas; if pruritus occurs, urge the child not to scratch and expect to administer antihistamine as ordered to reduce pruritus.
- Provide the child with distraction to assist in helping to reduce effects of pruritus.

---

away from pain. This technique does not eliminate the pain but does help to make it more tolerable. Various methods can be used for distraction, including

- counting
- repetition of specific phrases or words, such as "ouch"
- listening to music or singing
- playing games, including computer games
- blowing bubbles or blowing pinwheels or party favours
- listening to favourite stories (Fig. 35.8)
- watching cartoons, television shows, or movies
- visiting with friends
- humour

Humour has been demonstrated to be an effective distraction technique for pain management. However,

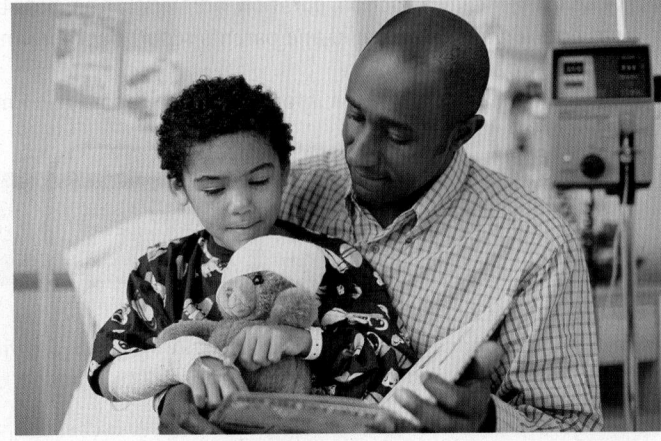

FIGURE 35.8 A child using distraction for pain management.

EVIDENCE-BASED PRACTICE 35.1
What Are the Effects of a Combination of Hypnosis and EMLA for Venipuncture in Children with Cancer?

Children with cancer undergo multiple procedures, and many describe these procedures as the most distressing part of their disease. A variety of psychological and pharmacologic interventions can help decrease procedural pain, behavioural distress, and anxiety (before and during the procedure) by redirecting the child from threatening to nonthreatening stimuli, resulting in a therapeutic benefit.

● Study
This study, from a large university-affiliated pediatric medical centre, used a randomized controlled trial design to determine whether the addition of self-hypnosis as a distraction technique would alleviate venipuncture pain more than the use of EMLA cream alone. A convenience sample of 45 children with cancer, ranging from 7 to 16 years of age, was randomly assigned to one of the following groups: 1) EMLA alone, 2) EMLA plus self-hypnosis (taught by a therapist prior to venipuncture), or 3) EMLA plus attention (time with therapist discussing nonmedical issues to control for therapist time); groups 2 and 3 served as controls.

Two oncology nurses performed all port access or venipunctures per institutional guidelines. All three groups received standard care, with the intervention (self-hypnosis) group receiving a brief (15-minute) training session on self-hypnosis (1 to 3 minutes of hypnotic involvement, followed by analgesic suggestions [magic glove] and then post-hypnotic suggestion [hypnotic experience would be repeated and provide comfort during actual procedure]) prior to the procedure. Children's pain, anxiety (before

and during the procedure), and behavioural distress as well as the parents' anxiety during the procedure were measured during the first venipuncture and then again during follow-up venipunctures approximately 3 and 6 months later.

▲ Findings
Scores for pain, anticipatory and procedure-related anxiety, and behavioural distress were lower in the intervention group compared with the control groups. Parents whose children were randomized to the EMLA plus self-hypnosis group experienced less anxiety during their child's procedure than did parents whose children were in the control groups. The benefits experienced by the EMLA plus self-hypnosis group were maintained over time (up to 6 months following the first procedure).

■ Nursing Implications
This study demonstrated that the use of local anesthetic plus self-hypnosis is effective in reducing pain, anxiety, and behavioural distress in children undergoing venipuncture. It also supports the notion that children can be easily taught to use self-hypnosis in a short period of time before painful medical procedures. Nurses need to encourage the use of self-hypnosis and other distraction strategies because they have been shown to positively enhance procedure outcomes. The nurse needs to facilitate and encourage parent participation in the use of distraction strategies such as supporting their child using self-hypnosis.

Liossi, C., White, P., & Hatira, P. (2009). A randomized clinical trial of a brief hyponosis intervention to control venipuncture-related pain of pediatric cancer patients. *Pain, 142,* 255–263.

make sure that the technique is age-appropriate and be sure to determine what or who will make the child laugh. If possible, allow the child and family to choose the materials that they consider humourous.

The type of distraction used depends on the age of the child. For example, a younger child may enjoy blowing pinwheels and blowing bubbles. He or she also will enjoy listening to favourite stories or books. Older children may enjoy computer games, listening to favourite music, or visiting with friends.

Imagery
Imagery involves helping children to focus their attention away from their pain or the feared components of a procedure and focus instead on an imaginative experience that is viewed as comforting, safe, fun, or intriguing. This mental image usually is a positive, pleasurable image, but it need not be real. The child is encouraged to include details and sensations that are associated with the image, such as

specific descriptions of the image, colours, sounds, feelings, and smells. In some instances, the child may write down or record the image on a tape or compact disc. When pain occurs, the child is encouraged to create the mental image or read or listen to the description.

Biofeedback
Biofeedback involves having the child gain an awareness of his or her body functions (e.g., muscle tension) and learning ways to modify them voluntarily (e.g., using relaxation). The child usually is taught specific skills about how to modify body functions using an apparatus that measures pain-related changes in muscle tone or physiologic data, such as blood pressure or pulse rate. This teaching usually occurs over several sessions, in advance of the pain experience. With practice, the child learns to control the changes without the apparatus. This technique can be used by older children, such as adolescents, who can concentrate for longer periods of time.

Thought Stopping

Thought stopping involves substituting a pleasurable or positive thought for the negative thoughts and feelings associated with a painful experience. Examples of positive thoughts might be, "It's only for a short time" or "It's important so I get better." The negative component of the pain is not ignored or suppressed; rather, it is transformed into something positive. Thought stopping also can involve the use of short, positive phrases. For example, the child may repeat "quick stick, feel better, go home soon" when he or she anticipates pain or experiences pain.

Thought stopping is a useful method for reducing anxiety before and during events associated with pain. Children can be taught to use this technique any time they experience anxiety related to a painful experience. Doing so helps to promote the child's sense of control over the situation.

Positive Self-Talk

Positive self-talk is similar to thought stopping in that it involves the use of positive statements. With positive self-talk the child is taught to say positive statements when he or she is experiencing pain. For example, the child may be taught to say, "I will feel better and be able to go home and play with my friends."

Physical Interventions

Physical interventions focus on interfering with the transmission of pain impulses reaching the brain. The interventions involve some type of cutaneous stimulation near the site of the pain. This stimulation decreases the ability of the A-delta and C fibres to transmit pain impulses. Examples of physical interventions include application of heat and cold, massage and pressure, and transcutaneous electrical nerve stimulation.

A particular intervention for infants is non-nutritive sucking, which reduces pain behaviours in neonates undergoing painful procedures (Weissman et al., 2009). Infants derive satisfaction from sucking. In addition, they show reduced pain behaviours after ingestion of sucrose or other sweet-tasting solutions such as glucose, since these substances are mediated through the opioid pathways (Cohen, 2008; Harrison, Louhgnan, Maniasm Gordon, & Johnston, 2009; Shah, Taddio, Reider, & HELPinKIDS Team, 2009; Stevens, Yamada, & Ohlsson, 2010; Taddio, Yiu, Smith, Katz, McNair, & Shah, 2009). Nonnutritive sucking is recommended as a technique for providing atraumatic care, but this method must be used with caution in infants with unstable blood glucose levels.

Heat and Cold (Thermal Stimulation) Applications

Heat and cold applications alter physiologic mechanisms associated with pain. Cold results in vasoconstriction and alters capillary permeability, leading to a decrease in edema at the site of the injury. Due to vasoconstriction, blood flow is reduced and the release of pain-producing substances such as histamine and serotonin also is decreased. Moreover, transmission of painful stimuli via peripheral nerve fibres is decreased.

> ▶ **Take** NOTE!
>
> Ice should never be applied directly to the skin, nor should the weight of a limb rest on an ice pack. Both of these actions may burn the skin. The ice pack should be applied for up to 10 minutes at a time and then removed. Wait 1 hour, and then reapply if necessary.

Heat results in vasodilation and increases blood flow to the area. It also leads to a decrease in nociceptive stimulation and removal of chemical substances that can stimulate nociceptive fibres. The increase in blood flow alters capillary permeability, leading to a reduction in swelling and pressure on nociceptive nerve fibres. Heat may also trigger the release of endogenous opioids, which mediate the pain response.

> ▶ **Take** NOTE!
>
> Heat should not be used on soft-tissue injuries that are still acutely painful, on open wounds, on areas of the body with reduced sensation or feeling, or on areas of bleeding or swelling. Care should always be taken when using heat treatments to make sure the child remains safe from further injury. Children should not be left alone with a hot pack. The hot pack should feel warm, not hot. Check the child's skin after 5 minutes for any sign of redness, blisters, or burning. Remove the hot pack after 20 minutes, wait for an hour, and then reapply if helpful.

Massage and Pressure

Massage and pressure, like other physical interventions, are believed to inhibit stimulation of the A-delta and C fibres. These methods are helpful in relaxing muscles and reducing tension. In addition, these techniques can aid in distracting the child. Massage can be as simple as rubbing a body part or pressing on an area such as an injection site for about 10 seconds, or it can be more involved, requiring the use of another person to perform the massage. Lotion or ointment can be used during the massage and may provide a comforting effect. Contralateral pressure or massage (i.e., of the opposite area) may be used, especially if the area of pain cannot be accessed or if the affected area is too painful to touch.

A more formal method of pressure application is acupressure. In acupressure the fingertip, thumb, or a blunt instrument is used to apply gentle, firm pressure to specifically designated sites to control pain. The pressure

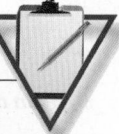

may be applied in one circular motion for several minutes and then released, or a vibrating motion can be created using the fingertips. The motion of applying and then releasing pressure is thought to facilitate the release of endogenous endorphins and enkephalins. The techniques of pressure and massage can be taught to children and parents. The techniques are easy to learn and use.

The Nurse's Role in Nonpharmacologic Pain Intervention

The nurse plays a major role in teaching the child and family about nonpharmacologic pain interventions, helping them choose the most appropriate and most effective methods, and ensuring that the child and parents use the method before pain occurs as well as before the pain increases. Teaching Guideline 35.1 lists some helpful instructions for the parents and child about nonpharmacologic pain management.

The nurse also assists the child and parents when using the technique, ensuring that they are using the technique correctly and offering suggestions for modifications or adaptations as necessary.

Parents are important components of the pain management program. Give them the option to stay with the child or let them know that someone else will support the child if they opt not to stay. Offer simple, concrete ways to assist and help the child to manage pain. Many of the nonpharmacologic techniques can be done by parents, and children may respond better if their parents demonstrate the technique and encourage them to use it. Invite parents to participate in decisions as well as act as a coach to their child during procedures. Prepare the parents and explain the most appropriate pain management approaches and strategies. Discuss the type and amount of pain expected as well as the potential complications associated with pain management approaches. Ask how the parent predicts the child will react to a painful situation. Finally, offer techniques and strategies to the parents as they act as the coach during these situations.

▶ *Take* NOTE!

Although parents want to help their children and some are able to act as coaches, the response of the child to pain and stress and to their parents' distraction interventions is highly variable. Some children appear to be soothed by their parents' distraction actions; others appear to become distressed. Be alert to factors that may influence the child's response, including age, sex, diagnosis, ethnicity, previous experience, temperament, anxiety, and coping style. Also be aware of parental factors, including ethnicity, gender, previous experience, belief in the helpfulness of the intervention, parenting style, and parental anxiety (Rony, Fortier, Chorney, Perret, & Kain, 2010).

TEACHING GUIDELINE 35.1

Teaching to Manage Pain without Drugs

- Review the methods available and choose the method(s) that your child and you find best for your situation.
- Learn to identify the ways in which your child shows pain or demonstrates that he or she is anxious about the possibility of pain—for example, does he or she get restless, make a face, or get flushed in the face?
- Begin using the chosen technique before your child experiences pain or when your child first indicates he or she is anxious about or beginning to experience pain.
- Practice the technique with your child and encourage the child to use the technique when he or she feels anxious about pain or anticipates that a procedure or experience will be painful.
- Perform the technique with your child; for example, take a deep breath in and out or blow bubbles with him or her; listen to the music or play the computer game with your child.
- Avoid using terms such as "hurt" or "pain" that suggest or cause your child to expect pain.
- Use descriptive terms such as "pushing," "pulling," "pinching," or "heat."
- Avoid overly descriptive or judgmental statements, such as "this will really hurt a lot" or "this will be terrible."
- Stay with your child as much as possible; speak softly and gently stroke or cuddle your child.
- Offer praise, positive reinforcement, hugs, and support for using the technique even when it was not effective.

Pharmacologic Management

Research overwhelmingly supports the appropriate use of analgesics to reduce the perception of pain in children (Mancuso & Burns, 2009). Analgesics may be administered using a wide variety of methods, the choice of which is determined by the drug being administered; the child's age and developmental status; the type, intensity, and location of the pain; and any factors that may be influencing the child's pain, such as past pain experiences and the meaning of pain for the child and family. Analgesic dosing should be calculated based on the child's weight. Neonates and some infants who were born preterm are more sensitive to opioids, and dosing should be adjusted appropriately.

Medications Used for Pain Management

Analgesics (medications for pain relief) typically fall into one of two categories: nonopioid analgesics and opioid analgesics. Drugs such as anesthetics, sedatives, and

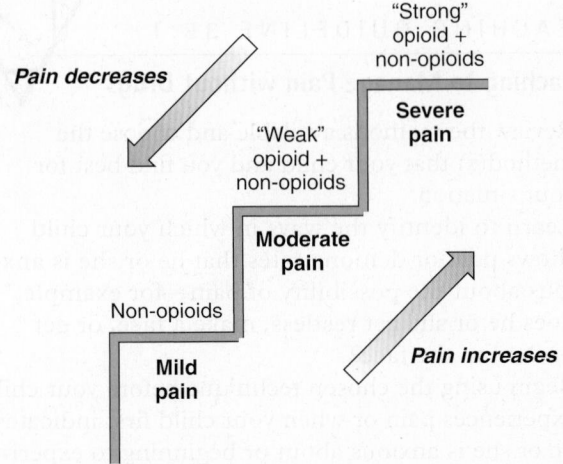

FIGURE 35.9 Stepped approach to pharmacologic pain management. (Used with permission from the World Health Organization.)

hypnotics also may be used as adjuvant medications to help minimize anxiety and assist with pain relief. However, sedatives should not be used on their own for painful procedures.

The World Health Organization (2011) recommends the use of more than one class of analgesic to promote better pain relief, reduce the amount of opioid required, and minimize side effects. It is important to match the analgesia to the severity of pain as outlined in Figure 35.9.

Nonopioid Analgesics

Nonopioid analgesics include acetaminophen and nonsteroidal anti-inflammatory drugs (NSAIDs) such as ibuprofen, ketorolac, naproxen, indomethacin, diclofenac, and celecoxib (Drug Guide 35.1). These agents may be used to treat mild to moderate pain, often for conditions such as arthritis; joint, bone, and muscle pain; headache; dental pain; and menstrual pain. Nonopioid analgesics are also used in combination with opioids for relief of moderate to severe pain, as recommended for balanced analgesia. Acetaminophen, probably the most widely known nonopioid analgesic, also is commonly used to treat fever in children, as is ibuprofen.

> ▶ **Take** NOTE!
>
> *Aspirin should not be used in children for analgesic and antipyretic purposes because of the high risk of Reye's syndrome.*

Nonopioid agents are typically administered orally or rectally. In some cases, such as with postoperative pain, they may be administered intravenously as a continuous infusion or as bolus doses (Durrmeyer, Vutskits, Anand, & Rimensberger, 2010). Administration via intramuscular injection is not recommended because the injection can cause significant pain and the onset of pain relief is more rapid.

Adverse effects associated with these agents include gastrointestinal irritation, blood clotting problems, and renal dysfunction. However, research has demonstrated that children experience only mild gastrointestinal upset and negligible effects on a healthy, well-functioning renal system. Blood clotting problems arise primarily when these agents are given perioperatively before primary hemostasis has occurred (Durrmeyer et al., 2010). Nonopioids are relatively safe, have few incompatibilities with other medications, and do not depress the central nervous system. Unfortunately, they exhibit a ceiling effect for analgesia: after a certain level, they do not provide increasing pain relief even when administered at increased doses. As a result, they may be combined with opioids for more effective pain relief.

Opioid Analgesics

Opioid analgesics are the medications of choice for moderate to severe pain. They are classified as either agonists (when they act as the neurotransmitter at the receptor site) or antagonists (when they block the action at the receptor site). Opioid agents that act as agonists include morphine, codeine, fentanyl, meperidine, hydromorphone, and oxycodone (see Drug Guide 35.1). Opioids can be administered orally, rectally, intramuscularly, or intravenously. In addition, some agents such as fentanyl can be administered transdermally or transmucosally. Morphine is considered the "gold standard" for all opioid agonists; it is the drug to which all other opioids are compared and is usually the drug of choice for severe pain (Oakes, 2011).

Opioid agonists, such as morphine, are associated with numerous adverse effects, resulting primarily from their depressant action on the central nervous system. Because opioids also stimulate the chemoreceptor trigger zone, leading to nausea and vomiting, prevention and management of side effects should always be considered.

Mixed agonist–antagonists (such as nalbuphine) are associated with less respiratory depression than agonists. Unfortunately, unlike agonists, this group has a ceiling effect, leading to inadequate effectiveness even with increased dosages. When this occurs, increasing the dosage of the mixed agonist–antagonist or combining it with an agonist provides no additional pain relief.

> ▶ **Take** NOTE!
>
> *Meperidine, an opioid agonist, is not recommended as a first-choice agent for pain relief in children. Meperidine's metabolite, normeperidine, is associated with the development of restlessness, irritability, twitching, agitation, tremors, and most importantly, seizures (AMA, 2010). Normeperidine is a central nervous system stimulant whose effects cannot be reversed by an opioid antagonist such as naloxone (AMA, 2010).*

DRUG GUIDE 35.1   COMMON DRUGS FOR PAIN MANAGEMENT IN CHILDREN

Drug	Action	Indication	Nursing Implications
Acetaminophen (Tylenol)	Possible inhibition of cyclooxygenase in the central nervous system Direct action on hypothalamic heat-regulating centre	Mild to moderate pain: arthritis, musculoskeletal pain, headache	• Administer orally or rectally. Do not exceed recommended dosing per weight—may cause liver toxicity • Caution parents to read labels of other over-the-counter (OTC) drugs carefully; some may contain acetaminophen and if given in conjunction may lead to overdose.
Ibuprofen (Motrin, Advil)	Inhibition of prostaglandin synthesis	Mild to moderate pain, fever	• Administer orally. • Give with food or after meals if GI upset occurs. • Assess for easy bruising, bleeding gums, or frank or occult blood in urine or stool. • Monitor for nausea, vomiting, GI upset, diarrhea or constipation, dizziness or drowsiness. • Caution parents to read labels of OTC medications closely; some may contain ibuprofen or other NSAIDs and if given in conjunction may lead to overdose
Other NSAIDs: ketorolac (Toradol), diclofenac (Voltaren), indomethacin (Indocin), naproxen (Naprosyn)	Inhibition of prostaglandin synthesis	Mild to moderate pain	• Administer oral form with food or after meals if GI upset occurs • Monitor for headache, dizziness, nausea, vomiting, constipation, or diarrhea • Assess for signs and symptoms of bleeding, such as bruising, epistaxis, gingival bleeding, or frank or occult blood in urine or stool • Ketorolac: May also be given IV or IM. In children 2–16 years, recommended as single dose only • Naproxen: Also available in combination products (caution parents to read OTC labels carefully) • Indomethacin: When administering IV, report oliguria or anuria • Diclofenac: May also be given rectally
Opioid agents: morphine, codeine, fentanyl (Sublimaze, Duragesic), hydromorphone (Dilaudid), oxycodone (Oxycontin)	Opioid agonist acting primarily at mu-receptor sites (morphine, codeine, fentanyl, hydromorphone, oxycodone)	Moderate to severe acute and chronic pain Morphine: intractable pain, preoperative sedation Codeine: also suppresses cough reflex Fentanyl: pain associated with short procedures such as bone marrow aspiration, fracture reductions, suturing	• Assess respiratory status frequently, noting any decrease in ventilatory rate or changes in breathing patterns; have naloxone readily available in case of respiratory depression (particularly morphine, fentanyl, hydromorphone) • Monitor for sedation dizziness, lethargy, confusion • Educate parents and child that the drug may make the child sleepy, drowsy, or lightheaded • Institute safety measures to prevent injury to the child • Assess bowel sounds for decreased peristalsis; observe for abdominal distention • Ensure adequate fiber intake and administer stool softeners as prescribed to minimize risk for constipation • Monitor urine output for changes and report • Morphine: May cause itching, particularly facial • Codeine: May cause nausea, vomiting, and abdominal pain. IV administration results in apnea and severe hypotension. Most commonly administered orally in combination with acetaminophen • Fentanyl: Observe for chest wall rigidity, which can occur with rapid IV infusion • Oxycodone is the opioid component of Percocet

(continued)

DRUG GUIDE 35.1   COMMON DRUGS FOR PAIN MANAGEMENT IN CHILDREN (continued)

Drug	Action	Indication	Nursing Implications
Mixed opioid agonist–antagonist: pentazocine (Talwin), butorphanol (Stadol), nalbuphine (Nubain)	Pentazocine: antagonist at mu-receptor sites, agonist at kappa-receptor sites Butorphanol: high affinity for kappa-receptor sites, minimal affinity for sigma-receptor sites Nalbuphine: partial agonist at kappa-receptor sites, antagonist at mu-receptor sites	Moderate to severe pain Relief of migraine headache (butorphanol) Preoperative analgesia (nalbuphine)	• Monitor the child for sedation. Educate child and parents that the drug may make the child sleepy, drowsy, or lightheaded • Institute safety measures to prevent injury to the child • Pentazocine, butorphanol: Monitor for diaphoresis, dizziness. Assess for tachycardia and hypertension • Butorphanol is given intranasally for migraine headaches

Adapted from Karch, A. (2010). *2010 Lippincott's nursing drug guide*. Philadelphia, PA: Wolters Kluwer Health/Lippincott Williams & Wilkins; and Taketomo, C. K., Hodding, J. H., & Kraus, D. M. (2010). *Lexi-comp's drug reference handbook: Pediatric & neonatal dosage handbook* (18th ed.). Hudson, OH: Lexi-comp, Inc.

▶ **Take** NOTE!

Codeine is no longer recommended for the treatment of pain in children. Because codeine has a very low affinity for opioid receptors, its analgesic effect is dependent on its conversion to morphine, which occurs through the cytochrome P-450 enzyme (CYP2D6). About 10% of the population has poor CYP2D6 drug metabolism, thereby making codeine an ineffective analgesic agent. Ultra-rapid CYP2D6 metabolism has been reported recently in certain individuals, causing growing concern over the safety of codeine.

▶ **Take** NOTE!

When administering parenteral or epidural opioids, always have naloxone (Narcan) readily available to reverse the opioid's effects should respiratory depression occur.

Tolerance, Dependence, and Addiction

Drug tolerance (increased dosage required for the same pain relief previously achieved with a lower dose) and **physical dependence** (the need for continued administration of the drug to prevent withdrawal symptoms) can occur when opioids are given over a prolonged period of time. Several factors, including the duration of therapy, type of drug, age of the child, and gender differences, have been shown to affect the development of these phenomena (Anand et al., 2010).

▶ **Take** NOTE!

Physical dependence can occur after as few as 5 days of continuous use of an opioid drug; symptoms of withdrawal begin if the drug is stopped suddenly (Oakes, 2011).

Addiction (psychological dependence) is a primary, chronic, neurobiologic disease with genetic, psychosocial, and environmental factors that influence its development and manifestations. Addiction is characterized by behaviours that include one or more of the following: loss of control over drug use, continued use despite knowledge of harm, and compulsive use and craving. Drug Guide 35.1 gives additional information related to the use of opioid analgesics.

Adjuvant Drugs

Adjuvant drugs are drugs that are used to promote more effective pain relief, either alone or in combination with opioids. These agents are not classified as analgesics. Benzodiazepines, such as diazepam and midazolam, help to relieve anxiety as well as muscle spasms. Midazolam also produces amnesia. Anticonvulsants, such as gabapentin and pregabalin, and tricyclic antidepressants, such as amitriptyline and nortriptyline, are used to treat neuropathic pain.

Local Anesthetics

Local anesthetics are commonly used to provide analgesia for procedures. They are effective in providing successful pain relief with only minimal risk of systemic adverse effects. However, local anesthetics such as lidocaine historically were not used in children because they need to be injected; the belief was that children feared needles and use of a local anesthetic subjected the child to two needle-sticks instead of one. Advances in technology have led to the development of improved methods of delivery such as topical ointments and iontophoresis for administration of local anesthetics, thereby promoting atraumatic care. (For more detailed discussion, see the next section on drug administration methods and later in the chapter on the nurse's role in managing procedure-related pain).

Drug Administration Methods

With any medication administered for pain management, the timing of administration is vital. Timing depends on the type of pain. For continuous pain, the current recommendation is to administer analgesia around the clock at scheduled intervals to achieve the necessary effect (Oakes, 2011). Scheduled dosing has been associated with decreased pain intensity ratings for children (Sutters et al., 2010). As-needed or PRN dosing is not recommended. This method can lead to inadequate pain relief because of the delay before the drug reaches its peak effectiveness, and as a result the child continues to experience pain, possibly necessitating a higher dose of analgesic to achieve relief; this then places the child at risk for overmedication and toxic effects.

For pain that can be predicted or considered temporary, such as with a procedure, analgesia is administered so that the peak action of the drug matches the time of the painful event.

Opioid dose should be titrated to pain intensity. A maximum or "ceiling" dose does not exist for opioids. They can be titrated safely for increased analgesic effect; however, side effects may be a limiting factor.

There are various methods for administering pain medications to children. The preferred methods are the oral, rectal, intravenous, topical, or local nerve block routes. Epidural administration and conscious sedation also can be used.

Oral Method

The oral method is often preferred because it is simple, easy, and convenient. The medication may be in the form of a pill, capsule, tablet, syrup, or elixir. Oral administration provides relatively steady blood levels of the drug when administered as a scheduled dose. Peak effectiveness typically occurs 1 to 2 hours after administration.

Rectal Method

The rectal method may be used when the child cannot take the medication orally, such as when he or she has difficulty swallowing or is experiencing nausea and vomiting. It is a viable alternative for drug administration. Some analgesics are available in suppository form; for others that are not, the drug can be compounded into a suppository form. The absorption rate varies with rectal administration, and children may find insertion of a suppository uncomfortable and embarrassing (Bowden & Greenberg, 2008).

Intravenous Method

Intravenous analgesia administration is the method of choice in emergency situations and when pain is severe and quick relief is needed. With intravenous administration, the drug usually takes effect within 5 minutes. Intravenous administration can be accomplished with bolus injections or continuous infusions. Continuous infusions may be preferred over bolus doses because steady blood levels are more easily maintained, thereby enhancing the drug's effect in relieving pain. Typically, opioids such as morphine, hydromorphone, and fentanyl are used due to their short half-life and decreased risk for toxicity.

Transdermal Method

Certain pain medications, such as fentanyl, can be administered transdermally using a patch. Special attention needs to be taken to monitor patch integrity (e.g., the edges of patch are not lifting, thereby affecting delivery or absorption of the drug). The skin should also be monitored for breakdown and the patch discontinued should this occur. Follow manufacturers' recommendations for application, with patch changes recommended every 72 hours.

Patient-Controlled Analgesia

In **patient-controlled analgesia**, a computerized pump is programmed to deliver an infusion of analgesics via a catheter inserted intravenously or subcutaneously. PCA enables children to administer analgesic doses according to their pain level. The analgesic may be given as a continuous infusion, as a continuous infusion supplemented by patient-delivered bolus doses, or as patient-delivered bolus doses only. Typically the child presses a button to administer a bolus dose. The pump has a lockout function that is preset with the dose and time interval: if the child presses the button before the preset time, he or she will not receive an overdose of medication. By delivering small, frequent doses of opioids, the child can experience pain relief without the effects of oversedation. The child also experiences a sense of control over the pain experience.

The child must have the necessary intellect, manual dexterity, and strength to operate the device. PCA has a high degree of safety, results in less overall opioid use, and is considered a standard for the delivery of analgesia in children over the age of 5 years (Franson, 2010).

PCA has been used to control postoperative pain and the pain associated with trauma, cancer, and sickle cell crisis. It can be used in acute care settings or in the home. Most commonly, morphine, hydromorphone, and fentanyl are the drugs used with PCA. The dosage is based on the child's response. Initial bolus doses of morphine commonly range from 0.01 to 0.03 mg/kg. Dosages for infusions depend on the child's age, the opioid used, and the type of pain. A commonly used range for morphine infusion to treat postoperative pain ranges from 0.01 to 0.04 mg/kg/hour. Higher dosage ranges have been used to treat the pain associated with sickle cell crisis and cancer (Field, Knight-Perry, & Debaun, 2009).

Nurse-Controlled Analgesia

Nurse-controlled analgesia allows the nurse to press the button only after a thorough pain assessment has been made. The main advantage of this method is the timeliness of dose administration. For sudden, intermittent pain in a child who is too young to press the button or is cognitively or physically unable to control the device, the nurse may do so without the delay associated with dose preparation. Reduced pain scores, increased pain management satisfaction, and decreased opioid utilization have been reported with nurse-controlled analgesia (Howard et al., 2010).

Local Anesthetic Application

A local anesthetic may sometimes be used to alleviate the pain associated with procedures such as venipuncture, injections, wound repair, lumbar puncture, or accessing implanted ports. Local anesthesia is a type of regional analgesia that blocks or numbs specific nerves in a region of the body. Medications called local anesthetics include topical forms, such as creams, agents delivered by iontophoresis, vapocoolants and skin refrigerants, and injectable forms.

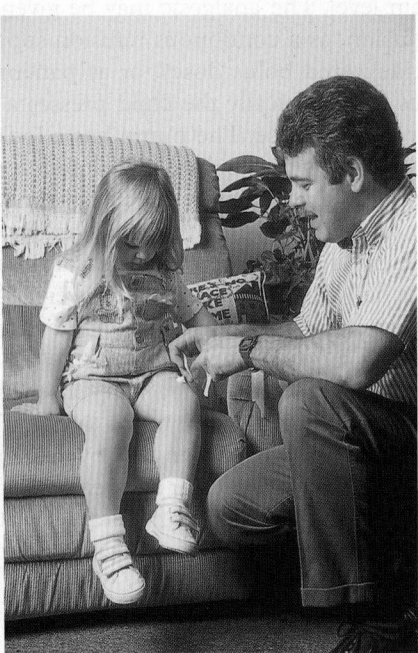

FIGURE 35.10 A parent applies Maxilene cream to the child at home in preparation for a procedure.

Topical Forms

Topical anesthetics should be used to reduce pain and distress for immunizations, intravenous cannulation, or venipuncture whenever possible. In a comparison of EMLA cream (eutectic mixture of local anesthetics [lidocaine and prilocaine]) and Ametop (amethocaine 4% gel) for intravenous cannulation or venipuncture in children aged 3 months to 15 years, amethocaine provided greater reduction in self- and observer-reported pain scores for needle pain (Lander, Weltman, & So, 2010). Maxilene (liposomal lidocaine 4% cream) has also been found to be highly effective in reducing the pain associated with intravenous cannulation in children (Shah et al., 2009) (Fig. 35.10, Box 35.2) due to its quick onset of action (30 minutes) and minimal vascular effects. Liposomal encapsulation prevents the anesthetic from being metabolized too quickly (Shah et al., 2009).

BOX 35.2 Applying Maxilene

Follow these guidelines when applying Maxilene:

- Explain the purpose of the medication to the child and parents, reinforcing that it will help the pain hurt less.
- Check the scheduled time for the procedure; plan to apply the cream at least 30 minutes before procedures such as a heelstick, venipuncture, lumbar puncture, or bone marrow aspiration.
- Place a thick layer of the cream on the skin at the intended site of the procedure, making sure that the area where the cream is being applied is free of any breaks. Do not rub the cream in once it is applied to the skin.
- Use approximately one-third to one half of a 5-g tube per application.
- Cover the site with a transparent dressing such as Tegaderm or OpSite, and secure it so that the dressing is occlusive. Alternatively, use plastic film wrap and tape the edges to secure the dressing.
- Instruct the child not to touch the dressing once it is secured. If necessary, cover the occlusive dressing with a protection device or a loosely applied gauze or elastic bandage.
- After the allotted time, remove the occlusive dressing and wipe the cream from the skin. Inspect the skin for a change in colour (blanching or redness), which indicates that the medication has penetrated the skin adequately.
- Verify that sensation is absent by lightly tapping or scratching the area. Use this technique also to demonstrate to the child that the anesthetic is effective. If sensation is present, reapply the cream.
- Prepare the child for the procedure. Assess the child's pain after the procedure to evaluate for pain and to differentiate pain from fear and anxiety.

> **Take** NOTE!

EMLA is used with caution in children younger than 3 months of age and in other susceptible persons because it may be associated with methemoglobinemia (Oakes, 2011; Zempsky, 2008). It is contraindicated in children who have congenital or idiopathic methemoglobinemia (OpenAnesthesia. org, 2011). It must be used cautiously in those under age 12 months who are receiving methemoglobin-inducing agents, such as sulfonamides, phenytoin, phenobarbital, and acetaminophen. Use of these agents in combination with EMLA increases the child's risk for methemoglobinemia, a condition that could lead to cyanosis and hypoxemia (OpenAnesthesia.org, 2011).

TAC (tetracaine, epinephrine, cocaine) and LET (lidocaine, epinephrine, tetracaine) are other examples of topical anesthetics. These are commonly used for lacerations that require suturing. The agent is applied directly to the wound with a cotton ball or swab for 20 to 30 minutes until the area is numb. These methods are not used in patients with known sensitivity to any of these medications.

Vapocoolant spray, another type of local analgesia, can be sprayed onto the skin or administered using a cotton ball soaked in liquid. The depth of anesthesia is not known, but it appears to provide immediate pain control. It is inexpensive and requires no waiting time. The effect lasts for approximately 1 to 2 minutes.

Injectable Forms

Injectable forms of lidocaine or procaine can be administered subcutaneously or intradermally around the procedural area approximately 5 to 10 minutes before the procedure. Common problems with injectable anesthesia include the pain associated with subcutaneous injection, some burning associated with lidocaine administration, as well as blanching of the skin.

> **Take** NOTE!

The burning that lidocaine causes on injection may be diminished by buffering lidocaine with sodium bicarbonate, using 10 parts lidocaine and 1 part sodium bicarbonate (1 mL of 1% to 2% lidocaine and 0.1 mL of 8.4% sodium bicarbonate). Then inject 0.1 mL or less of the solution intradermally at the site of venipuncture. Anesthetic action is almost immediate. The solution is stable only for approximately 1 week if not refrigerated.

Epidural Analgesia

Epidural anesthesia is commonly used for intraoperative and postoperative pain management in patients undergoing urologic, orthopedic, and general surgical procedures below the T-4 dermatome level (nipple line). The goal of epidural analgesia is regional pain relief in the form of segmental analgesia, which is achieved by intermittent or continuous injection of drugs into the epidural space to selectively block transmission of pain signals at the level of the spinal cord while leaving motor and sensory function intact.

For epidural analgesia, a catheter is inserted into the epidural space. The site of surgery will determine the dermatome level and thus the level of catheter placement. The three most common approaches to the epidural space in children are thoracic, lumbar, and caudal. The approach selected is based not only on the site of surgery but also on the age and anatomic considerations of the patient. For example, the spinal cord in infants ends at L-3 rather than L-1; therefore, care must be taken to avoid injury to the spinal cord in this region when lumbar punctures are performed.

Drug choice and dosing are based on long duration of action and spread through the epidural space to optimize the analgesic effect. Longer-acting anesthetic agents such as bupivacaine can be combined with analgesics such as fentanyl or morphine. These drugs diffuse into the cerebrospinal fluid, cross the dura mater to the spinal cord, and bind with the opioid receptors located at the dorsal horn. The drugs can be administered as bolus injections or as a continuous infusion.

Epidural analgesia is typically used postoperatively, providing analgesia to the lower body for up to 72 hours. The small amount of medication used with this type of analgesia causes less sedation, thereby allowing the child to participate more actively in postoperative care activities. This type of analgesia also is effective for children undergoing upper or lower abdominal surgeries because it controls localized intense pain, somatic pain, and visceral pain.

When epidural analgesia is being administered, additional narcotic analgesics are not given in order to prevent complications such as respiratory depression, pruritus, nausea, vomiting, and urinary retention.

> **Take** NOTE!

Respiratory depression, although rare when epidural analgesia is used, is always a possibility. When it does occur, it usually occurs gradually over a period of several hours after the medication is initiated. This allows adequate time for early detection and prompt intervention.

Constant assessment is essential because insertion of an epidural catheter and epidural analgesia can lead to infection at the site of the insertion, epidural hematoma, arachnoiditis, neuritis, or spinal headache (rare) due to a cerebrospinal fluid leak. An occlusive dressing is required over the insertion site.

Conscious Sedation

Conscious sedation is a medically controlled state of depressed consciousness that allows protective reflexes to be maintained so the child has the ability to maintain a patent airway and respond to physical or verbal stimulation. This procedure requires adherence to specific protocols as outlined by Accreditation Canada and Health Canada. The depressed state is obtained by using various agents such as morphine, fentanyl, midazolam, or diazepam and other adjuvants such as pentobarbital and ketamine. Administration of conscious sedation should be atraumatic—that is, by using the oral, topical, or existing intravenous routes. Midazolam and fentanyl often are the drugs of choice for conscious sedation because they act quickly, last only a short time, and are available in oral and intravenous formulations (Box 35.3).

Conscious sedation is used for procedures that are painful and stressful. For example, conscious sedation is suggested, especially for toddlers and preschool children who are undergoing frightening or invasive procedures and who are manifesting extreme anxiety and behavioural upset (AAP et al., 2008). Other indications include situations involving the following:

Evidence that the child is experiencing a heightened stress reaction—attempting to flee, crying inconsolably, or flailing

Verbalization by the child that he or she is frightened and does not want to be touched

Inability to remain immobilized, such as during laceration repair or computed tomography

Any procedure that is painful and fear-provoking

Personnel administering conscious sedation must be specially trained, and emergency equipment and medications must be readily available.

The Nurse's Role in Pharmacologic Pain Intervention

The nurse plays a major role in providing pharmacologic pain relief. As with any medication, the nurse is responsible for adhering to the five rights of medication administration: right drug, right dose, right route, right time, and right patient. The nurse also must have a solid knowledge base about the medications used for pain relief. This knowledge includes information about the drug's pharmacokinetics (absorption, distribution, metabolism, and excretion) and pharmacodynamics (mechanism of action, including adverse effects).

Assessment is crucial when pharmacologic pain interventions are used. An initial assessment of pain provides a baseline from which options for relief can be chosen. Factors that can affect the choice of analgesic, such as the child's age, pain intensity, physiologic status, or previous experiences with pain, also need to be considered. The nurse acts as an advocate for the child and the family to ensure that the most appropriate pharmacologic agent is chosen for the situation.

Assessment is ongoing once the agent is administered. The nurse must monitor physiologic parameters such as level of consciousness, vital signs, oxygen saturation levels, and urinary output for changes that might indicate an adverse reaction to the agent. More intensive monitoring is needed when agents are administered intravenously or epidurally or by conscious sedation. For example, if the child is receiving conscious sedation, interventions include the following:

Ensuring that emergency equipment is readily available

Maintaining a patent airway

Monitoring the child's level of consciousness and responsiveness

Assessing the child's vital signs (especially pulse rate, heart rate, blood pressure, and respiratory rate)

Monitoring oxygen saturation levels

Typically, a specially trained health care provider is specifically designated to perform these activities during

---

BOX 35.3 Oral Forms of Midazolam and Fentanyl

Two of the most commonly used agents for conscious sedation are midazolam and fentanyl. Each of these is available in oral form, which promotes atraumatic care.

Oral Midazolam Syrup
- Clear, purplish-red, cherry-flavoured syrup
- Syrup containing 2 mg/mL
- Recommended dosage: 0.25 to 0.5 mg/kg to a maximum dose of 20 mg
- Action usually within 10 to 20 minutes
- Major adverse effects: respiratory depression and arrest

Fentanyl Oralet
- Oral transmucosal formulation
- Candy-type lozenge on a plastic holder
- Available in 200, 300, and 400 mg
- Recommended dose: 5 to 15 µg/kg
- Not recommended for use in children weighing less than 15 kg
- Onset of action within about 15 minutes of sucking lozenge; duration of action approximately 1 hour

TABLE 35.8 INTERVENTIONS FOR COMMON OPIOID-INDUCED ADVERSE EFFECTS

Adverse Effect	Nursing Interventions
Constipation	Encourage fluid intake unless contra-indicated Ensure intake of high-fibre foods, including fruits, if allowed Encourage activity, including ambulation if possible Obtain order for stool softener Administer laxative as ordered
Pruritus	Apply cool compresses and lotions Administer antihistamine as ordered
Nausea and vomiting	Inform child and parents that these symptoms usually subside in 1 to 2 days Encourage small frequent meals with bland foods Administer antiemetic if ordered Note: If side effects persist, child may require opioid rotation and/or consideration of low-dose naloxone infusion

the administration of the sedation. Afterward, the nurse is responsible for ongoing monitoring of the child's status.

Monitor the child closely for evidence of adverse effects. Table 35.8 describes the interventions useful for responding to potential adverse effects. Be alert for signs and symptoms of respiratory depression secondary to opioid administration. Have an opioid antagonist such as naloxone (Narcan) and the benzodiazepine antagonist flumazenil (Romazicon) readily available should the child experience respiratory depression.

In addition to assessing physiologic parameters, the nurse must assess the child's and parents' emotional status before and after the agent is administered. For example, increased anxiety and fear may necessitate a change in method of administration, such as topical application instead of an intradermal injection of a local anesthetic. Nonpharmacologic methods may be employed to help lessen anxiety, thereby promoting more effective relief from the drug.

Nurses also are responsible for ensuring that the child and parents are adequately prepared for the use of the pharmacologic agent. The nurse educates the child and parents about the drug, why it is being used, its intended effects, and possible adverse effects, tailoring the teaching to the child's cognitive level. Provide opportunities for the child and parents to ask questions, offering support and guidance throughout the experience. Provide a demon-

stration or use visual aids so that the child and parents know exactly what to expect. Encourage the use of play to help the child express fears and anxieties related to the administration.

Management of Procedure-Related Pain

One of the most common causes of pain in children is procedure-related pain. The procedure may be minor, such as an intramuscular injection, heelstick, or venipuncture, or it may be more involved, such as lumbar puncture, bone marrow aspiration, or wound care. Regardless, pain is real for children and painful procedures are often extremely distressing to them. Variables that affect the pain experience include the type of procedure, the skill of the health care provider performing the procedure, and previous experiences with pain.

The Nurse's Role in Managing Procedure-Related Pain

Through the use of cognitive-behavioural and pharmacologic approaches, nurses can significantly reduce the pain and distress of procedures. The guiding principle is the provision of atraumatic care to the child, which includes the following:

- Using topical Maxilene, iontophoretic lidocaine, vapo-coolant spray, or buffered lidocaine at the intended site of a skin or vessel puncture
- Incorporating the use of nonpharmacologic strategies for pain relief in conjunction with pharmacologic methods
- Preparing the child and parents ahead of time about the procedure
- Using therapeutic hugging (see Chapter 32) to secure the child
- Using the smallest-gauge needle possible or an automated lancet device to puncture the skin
- Using an intermittent infusion device or peripherally inserted central catheter if multiple or repeated blood samples are necessary; coordinating care so that several tests can be performed from one sample if possible
- Opting for venipuncture in newborns instead of heelsticks if the amount of blood needed would require much squeezing
- Using kangaroo care (skin-to-skin contact) for newborns before and after heelstick
- Provide 24% oral sucrose to reduce procedural pain in neonates and young infants. Sucrose is a sugar commonly found in food. It is most effective in newborn and young infants but may help reduce pain in infants up to 12 months of age. It is administered as an oral solution (dissolved in water) either via a syringe or on a pacifier. The addition of a pacifier enhances the analgesic effect, which lasts for about 5 to 8 minutes. See Table 35.9 for oral sucrose dosing in infants.

TABLE 35.9 **DOSING OF 24% ORAL SUCROSE IN INFANTS**

Age	Maximum Oral Dose	Contraindications
23–32 weeks' gestational age	Up to 0.5 mL	Necrotizing enterocolitis
33–37 weeks' gestational age	Up to 1.0 mL	Short bowel syndrome with carbohydrate intolerance
>37 weeks' gestational age up to 18 months	Up to 2.0 mL	Unconsciousness or heavily sedated with absent gag reflex, unable
All infants who are NPO	Up to 0.5 mL	

Other dosing instructions include the following (Harrison, 2008; Taddio et al., 2008):

- The dose can be given in aliquots throughout the procedure, or the total amount can be given before the procedure.
- Place the dose on the infant's tongue 2 minutes prior to the painful procedure. Offer a pacifier if it is part of the infant's care routine.
- The dose may be administered in 2-minute intervals for prolonged procedures to the maximum daily dose.
- The maximum daily dose is four in 24 hours.

▶ **Take** NOTE!

Individualize interventions based on the painfulness of the procedure and the child's developmental age and personality. Use cognitive-behavioural approaches and pharmacologic interventions. For example, encouraging the school-age child to assist during painful procedures in age-appropriate ways may actually help ease some of the pain related to a heightened state of anxiety or at least assist the child in coping with the situation. Always use appropriate pharmacologic treatment for the first procedure to provide a painless experience for the child.

Nursing care for the child with procedure-related pain includes the child as well as the parents. Be sure to prepare them for the procedure using an appropriate developmental approach. Provide support and information to the parents on their role before, during, and after the procedure, including how to position the child for comfort and how to use simple distraction techniques and positive coping statements (Cohen, 2008).

Some controversy exists as to whether all procedures should be performed in a treatment room. Research findings suggest that taking a child to a treatment room may be neither feasible nor desirable in all situations and for all procedures. Attention needs to be directed toward the individual needs of the child, the demands of the procedure, and the situational conditions to facilitate the best outcome. The ultimate goal is to do whatever is best for the child.

Unless contraindicated, encourage the parents to be present before, during, and after the procedure to provide comforting support to the child. Also encourage the child and parents to use nonpharmacologic methods to help maximize pain relief and reduce anxiety. For example, nonpharmacologic methods that are helpful for the toddler and preschooler may include positioning the child on the lap and hugging the child, distracting the child with toys or interactive books, and blowing bubbles.

Play therapy can be useful when preparing children for painful procedures. Encourage children to make decisions about their care related to pain management if their condition or procedure allows. It is also helpful to anticipate and recognize painful situations and provide pain medication before the actual procedure to ensure comfort. Many nonpharmacologic strategies can be enhanced and better implemented with the help of the child life specialist or play therapist, both of whom have specialized training in these techniques.

Recall Aiden from the beginning of the chapter. What are some interventions that may be helpful prior to, during, and after his dressing change?

Management of Chronic Pain

Pain in children is typically acute, but chronic pain is also a significant problem in the pediatric population, affecting approximately 15% to 20% of children (Kozlowska, Rose, Khan, Kram, Lane, & Collins, 2008). Historically, chronic pain was defined by the duration of the pain, such as longer than 3 to 6 months. However, research has identified elements associated with chronic pain as occurring much earlier in time. Currently, chronic pain is identified as the interplay of biological, psychological, social, and cultural factors addressed within a developmental framework (Kozlowska et al., 2008). Chronic pain has been reported in children as young as 3 years of age but is most prevalent in young teenagers and is more commonly reported by girls. While many children and adolescents experience persistent or recurrent pain, only a small proportion becomes disabled by it. Chronic pain negatively impacts all aspects of the child's life and results in frequent use of health care services. It is associated with significant levels of functional impairment in areas such as academic performance and school attendance, emotional functioning, sleep disturbance, peer and social functioning, and parental burden (parenting stress and dysfunctional family roles).

Unlike acute pain, which usually has an identifiable cause, most chronic pain conditions in children are idiopathic in nature. This often results in patients and families continuing their search for an underlying cause for the pain, which leads to prolonged and involved multiple medical investigations (vicious cycle of doctor shopping to find a diagnosis and cure). During this process the child often receives little, if any, appropriate pain management. This process elevates the child's fear and the parent's stress and anxiety, which may further contribute to pain symptoms and disability.

> ▶ *Take* NOTE!
>
> *Once serious or treatable physical causes are ruled out, most children and parents need and are willing to accept an explanation based on both physical (sensitization of pain receptors) and psychological (stress or worry) factors. This helps prevent or reduce the continued search for the cause of the pain.*

The Nurse's Role in Managing Chronic Pain

The nurse's role in managing chronic pain in children is similar to that for the child experiencing acute pain or procedure-related pain. Assessment of the child's pain is key and requires a more comprehensive assessment than that required for acute pain. Review past physical examination findings for clues to the underlying problem. Observe the child's overall appearance, gait, and posture. Assess the child's cognitive level and emotional response, especially related to the experience of pain. Expect to complete a neurologic examination and observe for muscle spasms, trigger points, and increased sensitivity to light touch. Abnormal body postures assumed by the child resulting from chronic pain may lead to the development of secondary pain in the muscles and fascia. When children tense their muscles due to fear of examination, somatic pain may occur.

Various strategies are used to manage chronic pain (Table 35.10). A multidisciplinary, multimodal approach that incorporates the three P's (physical, psychological, and pharmacologic interventions) is likely to be most effective in addressing pain relief as well as the pain's impact on other areas of life, such as sleep or school functioning. In children, physical and psychological interventions are the mainstay of treatment for many types of chronic pain, with drug treatments often being used only when physical and psychological interventions alone are insufficient. When pharmacologic agents are used, the oral form is the dosing method of choice. As with any pain management strategy, education of the child and family is paramount.

The main goal of treatment is to return the child to a functional state that will enable him or her to participate in daily activities and return to school, rather than focusing solely on reducing or controlling the pain. Decisions regarding the most appropriate treatments should be individualized based on the assessment of the child. Wherever possible, interventions should be aimed at treating any trigger factors as well as the underlying cause(s) of the pain. Many children and adolescents with chronic pain can be managed effectively by their family doctor. Referral to a multidisciplinary pediatric pain program should be considered for children with complex

TABLE 35.10   AN OVERVIEW OF INTERVENTIONS FOR CHRONIC PAIN MANAGEMENT IN CHILDREN

Pharmacologic Interventions	Physical Interventions	Psychological Interventions
Simple analgesics	Exercise	Education (about pain experience and pain problem)
Opioids	Thermal stimulation (heat, cold, desensitization)	Sleep hygiene
Anticonvulsants	Physiotherapy	Relaxation
Antidepressants	Occupational therapy	Biofeedback
Anti-arrhythmics (alpha-adrenergic blockers)	Massage	Behavioural therapies
Anxiolytics	Transcutaneous electrical nerve stimulation	Cognitive therapies
Hypnotics	Acupuncture	Cognitive-behavioural therapy
Anaesthetics	Nerve blocks	Acceptance and commitment therapy
Cannabinoids		Family therapies
		Psychotherapy

Used with permission from Twycross, Downden, & Bruce (Eds.) (2009). Managing Pain in Children: A Clinical Guide. Wiley-Blackwell.

or ongoing chronic pain. Treatment should also address pain-related disability, with the goal of maximizing functioning and improving quality of life. This approach includes specific treatment that targets possible underlying pain mechanisms as well as symptom-focused management that addresses pain, sleep disturbance, anxiety, or depressive feelings.

■■■ Key Concepts

■ Pain is a highly individualized, subjective experience affecting persons of any age. It is a universal experience and is considered the fifth vital sign.

■ Pain management is a critical element in a child's plan of care for several reasons: children may lack the verbal capacity to describe their pain experience; caregivers and health care providers often have misconceptions about pain in children; assessment of the complex nature of the pain experience is difficult; and, despite effective ways to treat it, pain in children remains undertreated.

■ The sensation of pain involves a sequence of physiologic events: transduction, transmission, perception, and modulation.

■ Pain can be classified by duration as acute or chronic, by etiology as nociceptive or neuropathic, or by source or location as somatic or visceral.

■ Factors influencing a child's perception of pain include age and gender, cognitive level, temperament, previous pain experiences, and family and cultural background, none of which can be changed. Situational factors involve behavioural, cognitive, and emotional aspects and can be changed.

■ Infants, including preterm infants, experience pain. Behavioural and physiologic indicators are used to assess pain. Toddlers commonly react with intense emotional upset and physical resistance or aggression. Preschoolers may feel that pain is a punishment for misbehaving or having bad thoughts. School-age children can communicate the type, location, and severity of pain but may deny having pain to appear brave or avoid further pain. Adolescents, with their focus on body image and fear of loss of control, often ask numerous questions and may attempt to remain stoic to avoid being viewed as childish.

■ Assessment of pain in children includes both subjective and objective data. Nurses need to tailor the assessment to the child's developmental level and ask appropriate questions geared to the child's cognitive level. Parental questioning during the health history also is important.

■ Self-report pain rating scales are valuable assessment tools that allow the child's level of pain to be quantified. Examples include the Face Pain Scale–Revised, the Oucher pain rating scale, the Pieces of Hurt Tool, the word-graphic rating scale, visual analog and numeric scales, and the Adolescent Pediatric Pain Tool.

■ Different pain rating scales are appropriate for different developmental levels. However, children may regress when in pain, so a simpler tool may be needed to make sure that the child understands what is being asked. Consistency in using the same tool is essential so that appropriate comparisons can be made and effective interventions can be planned and implemented.

■ Physical examination of the child for pain primarily involves the skills of observation and inspection. These skills are used to assess for physiologic and behavioural changes that indicate pain. Auscultation also may be used to assess for changes in vital signs, specifically heart rate and blood pressure. Physiologic and behavioural pain assessment tools, such as the PIPP for preterm and term neonates, the CRIES Scale for Neonatal Postoperative Pain Assessment, the FLACC Behavioural Scale for Postoperative Pain in Young Children, and the Non-Communicating Children's Pain Checklist–Revised, measure specific parameters and changes that would indicate that the child is in pain.

■ Nonpharmacologic pain management strategies aim to assist children in coping with pain and to give them a sense of mastery or control over the situation. These strategies may be categorized as cognitive-behavioural, in which the child focuses on a specific area or aspect rather than the pain (e.g., relaxation, distraction, imagery, biofeedback, thought stopping, and positive self-talk), or physical, in which the focus is on interfering with the transmission of pain impulses reaching the brain (e.g., heat and cold applications, massage and pressure).

■ The nurse plays a major role in teaching the child and family about available nonpharmacologic pain interventions, helping them choose the most appropriate and most effective methods, and ensuring that the child and parents use the method before the pain occurs as well as before it increases.

■ Pharmacologic interventions involve the administration of drugs for pain relief, most commonly nonopioids and opioid analgesics. The selection of administration method is determined by the drug being administered; the child's status; the type, intensity, and location of the pain; and any factors that may be influencing the child's pain. The preferred methods for administering analgesics include the oral, rectal, intravenous, or local nerve block routes; epidural administration; and conscious sedation.

■ Nonopioid analgesics used to treat mild to moderate pain include acetaminophen and NSAIDs such as ibuprofen, ketorolac, naproxen, and less commonly, indomethacin, diclofenac, and piroxicam.

■ Morphine is considered the "gold standard" for all opioid agonists; it is the drug with which all other opioids are compared and is usually the drug of choice for severe pain.

■ Local anesthetics are commonly used to provide analgesia for procedures. They are effective in providing successful pain relief with only minimal risk of systemic adverse effects. The first choice for the most effective, painless local anesthesia is Maxilene. It achieves anesthesia to a depth of 2 to 4 mm, so it reduces the pain of phlebotomy, venous cannulation, and intramuscular injections up to 24 hours after injection.

■ Epidural analgesia involves the insertion of a catheter into the epidural space through which drugs can be administered as bolus injections (a one-time bolus or on an intermittent schedule), as a continuous infusion, or as PCA. Usually an opioid, such as morphine, fentanyl, or hydromorphone, is given in conjunction with a long-acting local anesthetic, such as bupivacaine.

■ Conscious sedation is a medically controlled state of depressed consciousness that allows protective reflexes to be maintained so that the child has the ability to maintain a patent airway and respond to physical or verbal stimulation.

■ When providing pharmacologic pain relief, the nurse must adhere to the five rights of medication administration and have a solid knowledge base about the medications used for pain relief and the drug's pharmacokinetics (absorption, distribution, metabolism, and excretion) and pharmacodynamics (mechanism of action, including adverse effects). Initial and ongoing assessment is crucial.

■ The principles of atraumatic care guide nursing interventions for providing pain relief, especially for procedure-related pain.

■ Chronic pain in children can significantly affect the child's daily life and activities as well as the family's life.

REFERENCES

American Academy of Pediatrics and Canadian Paediatric Society. (2000). Prevention and management of pain and stress in the neonate. *Pediatrics, 105*(2), 454–461.

American Academy of Pediatrics, Committee on Fetus and Newborn and Section on Surgery, Section on Anesthesiology and Pain Medicine, Canadian Paediatric Society, Fetus and Newborn Committee. (2010). Policy Statement. Prevention and management of pain in the Neonate: An update. *Pediatrics, 118*(5), 2231–2240. Retrieved June 4, 2011 from http://aappolicy.aappublications.org/cgi/content/full/pediatrics;118/5/2231

American Academy of Pediatrics, American Academy of Pediatric Dentistry, Cote, C. J., Wilson, S., & Work Group on Sedation. (2008). Guidelines for monitoring and management of pediatric patients during and after sedation for diagnostic and therapeutic procedures: An update. *Paediatric Anaesthesia, 18*(1), 9–10. doi: 10.1111/j.1460-9592.2007.02404.x

American Medical Association. (2010). *Pain management series: Module 6: Pediatric pain management (continuing medical education)*. Retrieved December 3, 2011 from http://www.ama-cmeonline.com/pain_mgmt/module06/index.htm

American Pain Society. (1995). *Pain: The fifth vital sign*. Los Angeles, CA: American Pain Society.

Anand, K., Willson, D., Berger, J., Harrison, R., Meert, K., Zimmerman, J., et al. (2010). Tolerance and withdrawal from prolonged opioid use in critically ill children. *Pediatrics, 125*, e1208–e1225.

Auvray, M. A., Mylin, E. B., & Spence, C. A. (2010). The sensory-discriminative and affective-motivational aspects of pain. *Neuroscience and Biobehavioral Reviews, 34*, 214–223.

Bingham, B., Ajit, S. K., Blake, D. R., & Samad, T. A. (2009). The molecular basis of pain and its clinical implications in rheumatology. *Nature Clinical Practice Rheumatology, 5*(1), 28–37.

Bowden, V. R., & Greenberg, C. S. (2008). *Pediatric nursing procedures*. Philadelphia, PA: Lippincott Williams & Wilkins.

Cavanaugh, D.J., & Basbaum, A.I. (2011). Basic mechanisms and pathophysiology. In M. E. Lynch, K. D. Graig, & P. W. H. Peng (Eds.), *Clinical pain management: A practical guide*. Hoboken, NJ: Wiley-Blackwell.

Codipietro, L., Ceccarelli, M. & Ponzone, A. (2008). Breastfeeding or oral sucrose solution in term neonates receiving heel lance: A randomized, controlled trial. *Pediatrics, 122*(3), e716–e721. Retrieved December 4, 2011 from http://pediatrics.aappublications.org/cgi/content/full/122/3/e716

Cohen, L. L. (2008). Behavioral approaches to anxiety and pain in venous access. *Pediatrics, 122*(Suppl 3), S134–S139.

Cohen, L.L., & Baxter, A. L. (2008). Distraction techniques for procedural pain in children. Retrieved June 3, 2011 from http://www.medscape.org/viewarticle/583976

Cohen, L. L., Lemanek, K., Blount, R. L., Dahlquist, L.M., et al. (2008). Pediatric pain assessment: Review of measure. *Journal of Pediatric Psychology, 33*(9), 939–955.

Dowden, S., McCarthy, M., & Chalkiadis, G. (2008). Achieving organizational change in pediatric pain management. *Pain Research & Management, 13*(4), 321–326.

Durrmeyer, X., Vutskits, L., Anand, K. J., & Rimensberger, P. C. (2010). Use of analgesic and sedative drugs in the NICU: Integrating clinical trials and laboratory data. *Pediatric Research, 67*(2), 117–127.

Field, J. J., Knight-Perry, J. E., & Debaun, M. R. (2009). Acute pain in children and adults with sickle cell disease: Management in the absence of evidences-based guidelines. *Current Opinion in Hematology, 16*(3), 173–178.

Finley, G. A., Franck, L. S., Grunau, R. E., & von Baeyer, C. L. (2005). Why children's pain matters. *International Association for the Study of Pain. Pain: Clinical Updates, XIII*(4), 1–6. Retrieved December 3, 2011 from http://www.iasp-pain.org/AM/AMTemplate.cfm?Section=Home&CONTENTID=2265&TEMPLATE=/CM/ContentDisplay.cfm&SECTION=Home

Frampton, C. L., & Hughes-Webb, P. (2011). The measurement of pain. *Clinical Oncology, 23*(6), 381–386. doi:10.1016/j.clon.2011.04.008

Franson, H. E. (2010). Postoperative patient-controlled analgesia: A literature review. *American Association of Nurse Anesthetists Journal, 78*(5), 374–378.

Harrison, D. (2008). Oral sucrose for pain management in infants: myths and misconceptions. *Journal of Neonatal Nursing, 14*, 39–46.

Harrison, D., Louhgnan, P., Maniasm, E., Gordon, I., & Johnston, L. (2009). Repeated doses of sucrose in infants continue to reduce procedural pain during prolonged hospitalizations. *Nursing Research, 58*(6), 427–434.

Henry, P. R., Haubold, K., & Dobrzykowski, T. M. (2004). *Pain in the healthy full-term neonate: Efficacy and safety of interventions*. Retrieved June 4, 2011 from http://www.medscape.com/viewarticle/481612

Hershey, A. D., Powers, S. W., Winner, P., & Kabbouche, M. A. (2009). *Pediatric headaches in clinical practice*. Oxford, UK: Wiley.

Hockenberry, M. J., McCarthy, K., Taylor, O., Scarberry, M., Franklin, Q., Louis, C. U., et al. (2011). Managing painful procedures in children with cancer. *Journal of Pediatric Hematology Oncology, 33*(2), 119–127.

Hockenberry, M. J., & Wilson, D. (2009). *Wong's essentials of pediatric nursing* (8th ed.). St. Louis, MO: Elsevier Mosby.

Howard, R. F., Lloyd-Thomas, A., Thomas, M., Williams, D.G., Saul, R., Bruce, E., et al. (2010). Nurse-controlled analgesia (NCA) following major surgery in 10,000 patients in a children's hospital. *Paediatric Anaesthesia, 20*(2), 126–134.

Hurley, R. W., & Adams, M. C. B. (2008). Sex, gender, and pain: An overview of a complex field. *International Anesthesia Research Society, 107*(1), 309–317.

International Association for the Study of Pain. (2011). *IASP pain terminology*. Retrieved December 3, 2011 from http://www.iasp-pain.org/AM/Template.cfm?Section=General_Resource_Links&Template=/CM/HTMLDisplay.cfm&ContentID=3058#Pain

Johnston, C. C., Fernandes, A. M., & Campbell-Yeo, M. (2011). Pain in neonates is different. *Pain, 152*(3 Suppl), S65–S73. doi:10.1016/j.pain.2010.10.008

Johnston, C. C., Stevens, B., Boyer, K & Porter, F. (2002). Development of psychologic responses of pain and assessment of pain in infants and toddlers. In N. Schecter, C. Berde, M. Yaster (Eds). *Pain in infants, children and adolescents* (pp. 105–127). New York: Lippincott, Williams & Wilkins.

Kennedy, R. M., Luhmann, J., & Zempsky, W. T. (2008). Clinical implications of unmanaged needle-insertion pain and distress in children. *Pediatrics, 122*(Suppl 3), S130–S133. doi:10.1542/peds.2008-1055e

Kozlowska, K., Rose, D., Khan, R., Kram, S., Lane, L., & Collins, J. (2008). A conceptual model and practice framework for managing chronic pain in children and adolescents. *Harvard Review of Psychiatry, 16*(2), 136–150.

Lander, J. A., Weltman, B. J., & So, S.S. (2010). EMLA and Amethocaine for reduction of children's pain associated with needle insertion: Update. *Cochrane Database of Systematic Reviews, 11*, CD004236. DOI: 10.1002/14651858.CD004236.pub2.

Liossi, C., White, P., & Hatira, P. (2009). A randomized clinical trial of a brief hyponosis intervention to control venipuncture-related pain of paediatric cancer patients. *Pain, 142*, 255–263.

Mancuso, T., & Burns, J. (2009). Ethical concerns in the management of pain in the neonate. *Paediatric Anaesthesia, 19*(10), 953–957.

McCaffery, M., & Pasero, C. (2011). *Pain assessment and pharmacologic management.* St. Louis, MO: Mosby.

McGrath, P. A., & Hillier, L. M. (2003). Modifying the psychologic factors that intensify children's pain and prolong disability. In N. L. Schecter, C. B. Berde, & M. Yaster, *Pain in infants, children, and adolescents* (2nd ed.). Philadelphia, PA: Lippincott Williams & Wilkins.

Oakes, L. (2011). *Compact clinical guide to infant and child pain management. An evidence-based approach for nurses.* Y. D'Arcy (Series Ed.). New York: Springer.

OpenAnesthesia.org. (2011). *EMLA contraindications.* Retrieved June 5, 2011 from http://openanesthesia.org/index.php?title=EMLA_contraindications

Ranger, M., Johnston, C. C., & Anand, K. J. S. (2007). Current controversies regarding pain assessment in neonates. *Seminars in Perinatology, 31*(5), 283–88. doi:10.1053/j.semperi.2007.07.003

Registered Nurses' Association of Ontario. (2007, Revised). *Nursing best practice guideline: Assessment and management of pain.* Retrieved December 3, 2011 from http://www.rnao.org/Page.asp?PageID=924&ContentID=720

Rony, R. Y., Fortier, M. A., Chorney, J. M., Perret, D., & Kain, Z. N. (2010). Parental postoperative pain management: Attitudes, assessment, and management. *Pediatrics, 125*(6), e1372–e1378. doi:10.1542/peds.2009-2632.

Ruskin, D. A., Amaria, K. A., Warnock, F. F., & McGrath, P. A. (2011). Assessment of pain in infants, children and adolescents. In D.C. Turk & R. Melzack (Eds.), *Handbook of pain assessment* (3rd ed.). New York: The Guilford Press.

Shah, V., Taddio, A., Reider, M. J., & HELPinKIDS Team. (2009). Effectiveness and tolerability of pharmacologic and combined interventions for reducing injection pain during routine childhood immunizations: systematic review and meta-analysis. *Clinical Therapeutics, 31*(Suppl 2), S104–S1051.

Spence, K., Henderson-Smart, D., New, K., Evans, C., Whitelaw, J., Woolnough, R., et al. (2010). Evidenced-based clinical practice guideline for management of newborn pain. *Journal of Paediatrics and ChildHealth, 46*(4),184–192.doi:10.1111/j.1440-1754.2009.01659.x

Stanford, E. A., Chambers, C. T., Biesanz, J. C., & Chen, E. (2008). The frequency, trajectories and predictors of adolescent recurrent pain: A population-based approach. *Pain, 138*(1), 11–21.

Stevens, B. J., Pillai Riddel, R. R., Oberlander, T. E., & Gibbins, S. (2007). Assessment of pain in neonates and infants. In K. J. S. Anand, B. J. Stevens, & P. J. McGrath (Eds.), *Pain in neonates and infants* (3rd ed.). Philadelphia, PA: Elsevier.

Stevens, B., Yamada, J., & Ohlsson A. (2010). Sucrose for analgesia in newborn infants undergoing painful procedures. *Cochrane Database of Systematic Reviews, 20*(1), CD001069.

Stinson, J. (2009). Pain Assessment. In A. Twycross, L. Bruce, & S. Dowden (Eds.), *Pain in children: A clinical guide.* London: Blackwell Science.

Stinson, J., & Bruce, L. (2009). Chronic pain. In A. Twycross, L. Bruce, & S. Dowden (Eds.), *Pain management in children: A clinical guide.* Oxford, UK: Blackwell Science.

Stinson, J., Yamada, J., Kavanagh, T., Gill, N., & Stevens, B. (2006). Systematic review of the psychometric properties and feasibility of self-report pain measures for use in clinical trials in children and adolescents. *Pain, 125*(1–2), 143–157.

Sutters, K. A., Miaskowski, C., Holdridge-Zeuner, D., Waite, S., Paul, S. M., et al. (2010). A randomized clinical trial of the efficacy of scheduled dosing of acetaminophen and hydrocodone for the management of postoperative pain in children after tonsillectomy. *Clinical Journal of Pain, 26*(2), 95–103.

Taddio, A., Chah, V., Hancosk, R., et al. (2008). Effectiveness of sucrose analgesia in newborns undergoing painful medical procedures. *Canadian Medical Association Journal, 179*(1), 37–43.

Taddio, A., Yiu, A., Smith, R. W., Katz, J., McNair, C., & Shah, V. (2009). Variability in clinical practice guidelines for sweetening agents in newborn infants undergoing painful procedures. *Clinical Journal of Pain, 25*(2), 153–155.

Taylor, E. M., Boyer, C., & Campbell, F. (2008). Pain in hospitalized children: A prospective cross-sectional survey of pain prevalence, intensity, assessment and management in a Canadian pediatric teaching hospital. *Pain Research & Management, 13*(1), 25–32.

Valrie, C. R., Gill, K. M., Redding-Lallinger, R., & Daeschner, C. (2008). Daily mood as a mediator of the pain-sleep relationship in children with sickle-cell disease. *Journal of Pediatric Psychology, 33*(3), 317–322.

Weissman, A., Aranovitch, M., Blazer, S., & Zimmer, E. Z. (2009). Heel-lancing in newborns: behavioral and spectral analysis assessment of pain control methods. *Pediatrics, 124*(5), e921–e926.

World Health Organization. (2011). *WHO's pain ladder.* Retrieved December 3, 2011 from http://www.who.int/cancer/palliative/painladder/en/

Zempsky, W.T. (2008). Pharmacologic Approaches for Reducing Venous Access Pain in Children. *Pediatrics, 122*, S140–S153. Retrieved December 4, 2011 from http://pediatrics.aappublications.org/cgi/content/full/122/Supplement_3/S140

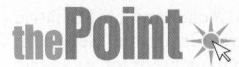

For additional learning materials, including Internet Resources, visit http://thePoint.lww.com/Chow1e.

CHAPTER WORKSHEET

MULTIPLE CHOICE QUESTIONS

1. The nurse is preparing to assess the pain of a 3-year-old child who had surgery the day before. Which pain rating scale would be most appropriate for the nurse to use?

   a. FPS–R

   b. Pieces of Hurt Tool

   c. Word-graphic rating scale

   d. Visual analog scale

2. When developing the plan of care for a child in pain, the nurse identifies appropriate strategies aimed at modifying which factors influencing pain?

   a. Gender

   b. Cognitive level

   c. Previous pain experiences

   d. Anticipatory anxiety

3. An adolescent who is a competitive swimmer comes to the emergency department complaining of localized aching pain in his shoulder. He states, "I've been practicing really hard and long to get myself ready for my meet this weekend." The area is tender to the touch. The nurse determines that the adolescent is most likely experiencing which type of pain?

   a. Cutaneous pain

   b. Deep somatic pain

   c. Visceral pain

   d. Neuropathic pain

4. After teaching a child's parents about the different methods of distraction that can be used for pain management, which statement by the parents indicates a need for additional teaching?

   a. "We'll have her focus on her hand and count each finger slowly."

   b. "We'll read some of her favourite stories to her."

   c. "We'll have her imagine that she's at the beach this summer."

   d. "She likes to play video games, so we'll bring in some from home."

5. A child is scheduled for a bone marrow aspiration at 4 p.m. The nurse would plan to apply Maxilene cream to the intended site at which time?

   a. 1:30 p.m.

   b. 3:00 p.m.

   c. 3:30 p.m.

   d. 4:00 p.m.

CRITICAL THINKING EXERCISES

1. The nurse asks a 12-year-old girl if she is having pain. She denies pain, even though she is lying on her left side holding her abdomen with her knees flexed up to it. What might be some underlying factors leading the adolescents to deny her pain? How would the nurse go about assessing this adolescent's pain?

2. The nurse comes into the room of a 6-year-old who is sleeping. His mother states, "He's asleep, so he's not in pain." How should the nurse respond?

3. A child who is receiving ibuprofen is experiencing increased pain. The dosage of ibuprofen is increased but is no longer effective in providing adequate pain relief. What is occurring? What would be most likely happen next?

STUDY ACTIVITIES

1. Interview nurses who work on a pediatric unit about their experiences with managing pain in children. Ask them how they assess pain in children and the major methods they use to assist the children in managing their pain.

2. Interview families of children with chronic illnesses who deal with pain. Ask the parents how they assess their children's pain level and what methods they have used in assisting their children in managing pain.

3. Compare and contrast the drugs fentanyl and midazolam when used for conscious sedation in terms of onset of action, duration, primary effects, and antidotes.

4. A child is receiving epidural analgesia with morphine. The nurse would be alert for which of the following adverse effects? Select all that apply.

   _____ a. Respiratory depression

   _____ b. Pruritus

   _____ c. Constipation

   _____ d. Vomiting

   _____ e. Amnesia

   _____ f. Hematoma

UNIT ELEVEN

NURSING CARE OF THE CHILD WITH A HEALTH DISORDER

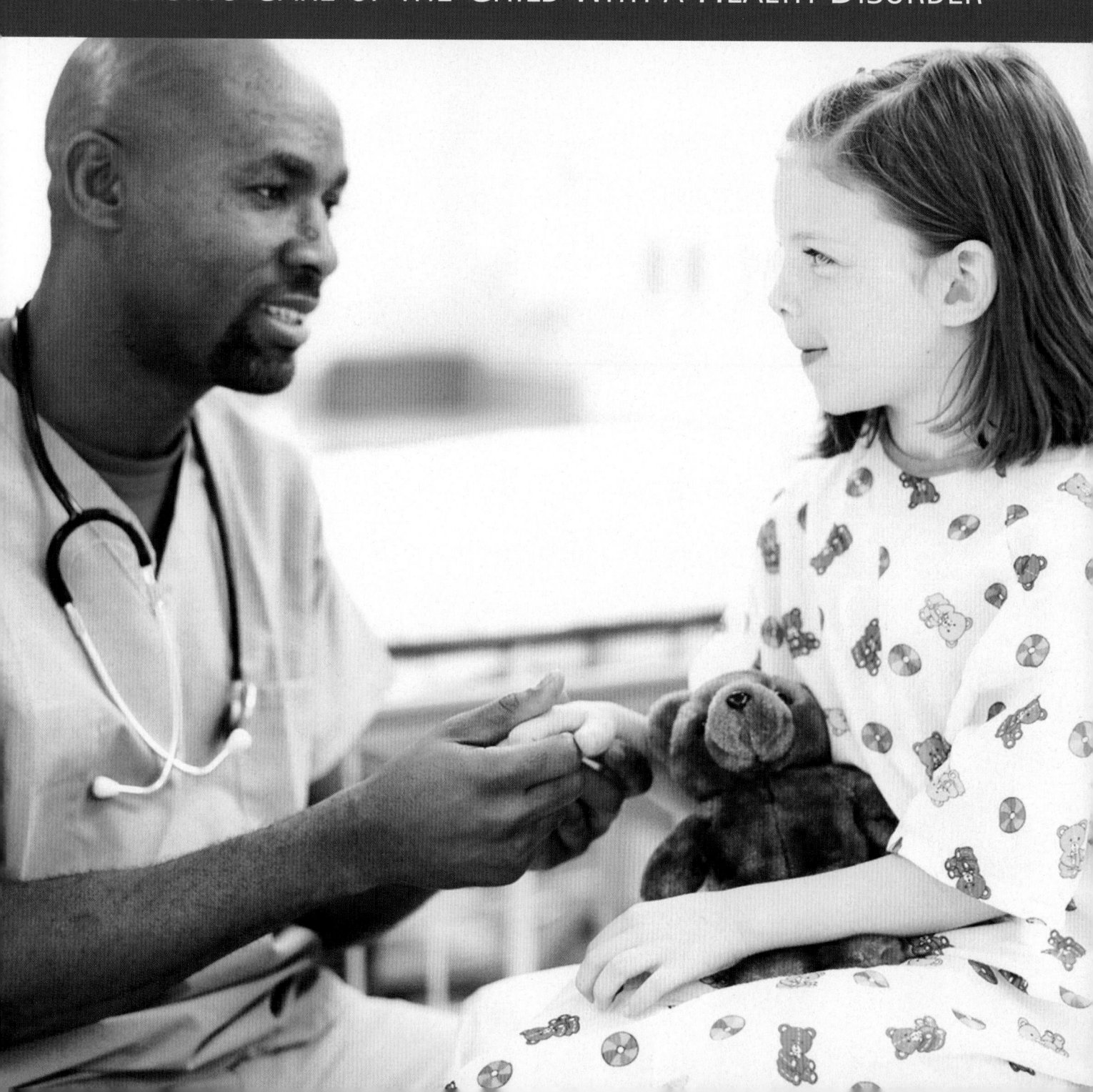

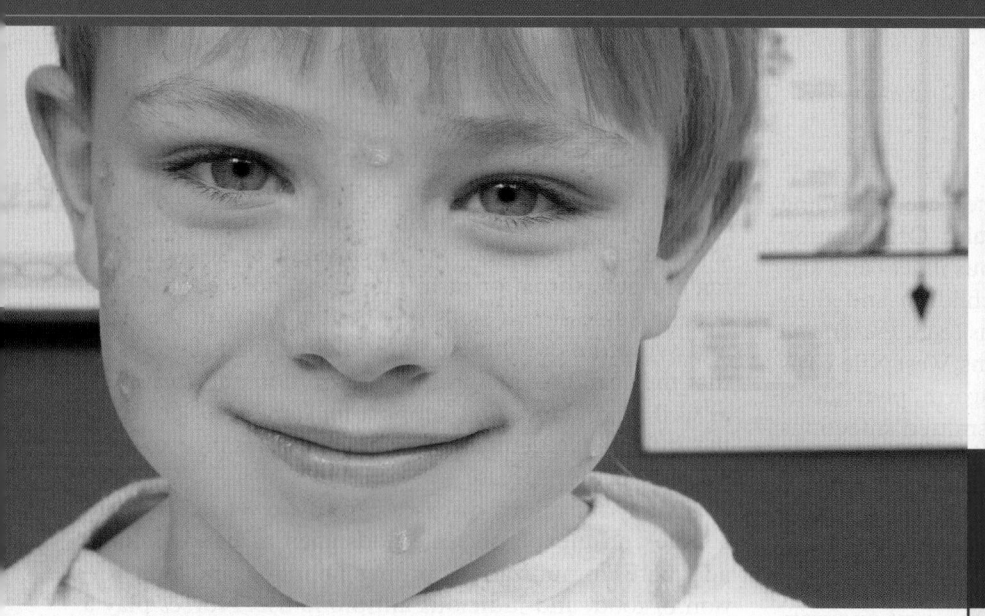

CHAPTER 36

Adapted by Debbie Fraser

NURSING CARE OF THE CHILD WITH AN INFECTIOUS OR COMMUNICABLE DISORDER

KEY TERMS

antigen
antibody
chain of infection
communicability

endogenous pyrogens
exanthem
fomite
pathogen

phagocytosis
SIRS

LEARNING OBJECTIVES

Upon completion of the chapter, the learner will be able to:

1. Discuss anatomic and physiologic differences in children versus adults in relation to the infectious process.
2. Identify nursing interventions related to common laboratory and diagnostic tests used in the diagnosis and management of infectious conditions.
3. Identify appropriate nursing assessments and interventions related to medications and treatments for childhood infectious and communicable disorders.
4. Distinguish various infectious illnesses occurring in childhood.
5. Devise an individualized nursing care plan for the child with an infectious or communicable disorder.
6. Develop patient/family teaching plans for the child with an infectious or communicable disorder.

Samuel Goldberg, 3 months old, is brought to the clinic by his mother. He presents with a history of fever and nasal congestion. His mother states, "He's been very irritable and crying more than usual."

WOW

Complete and lasting freedom from infectious disease remains a dream, but one worth fighting a hard battle for.

Infectious and communicable diseases are a leading cause of death worldwide (World Health Organization [WHO], 2011b). They can lead to serious illness and significantly affect the lives of affected children and their families. They include bacterial infections (e.g., *Escherichia coli*), viral infections (e.g., viral exanthems, West Nile virus [WNV]), parasitic infections (e.g., pinworm, pediculosis capitis [head lice]), and sexually transmitted infections (STIs) (e.g., chlamydia, gonorrhea).

There has been a dramatic decrease in the incidence and severity of infections and communicable diseases since the advent of vaccines, antibiotics, antiviral drugs, and antitoxins (Global Health Council, 2011). Some diseases have been effectively controlled, but the vast majority could not be eliminated. New diseases emerge and old diseases are reappearing, sometimes in a drug-resistant form. The Public Health Agency of Canada (PHAC) tracks a number of infectious diseases. This list of nationally reportable diseases is revised periodically to add new pathogens or remove diseases as their incidence declines (Box 36.1). Individual provinces may also mandate reporting of additional diseases. Weekly communicable disease reports are provided by PHAC and can be found online; visit http://thePoint.lww.com/Chow1e for a direct link.

Nurses, particularly those working in schools, child care centres, and out-patient settings, are often the first to see the signs of infectious or communicable diseases in children. These signs are often vague at first, consisting of a sore throat or rash. Therefore, nurses must have accurate assessment skills and be familiar with the signs and symptoms of these common childhood diseases so that they can provide prompt recognition and treatment as well as guidance and support for families. Identifying the infectious agent is of primary importance to help prevent further spread.

Many infectious diseases can be prevented through simple and inexpensive methods such as handwashing, adequate immunization, proper handling and preparation of food, and judicious antibiotic use. Nurses play a key role in educating parents and the community on ways to prevent infectious and communicable diseases.

Infectious Process

Infection occurs when an organism enters the body and multiplies, causing damage to the tissues and cells. The body's response to this damage due to infection or injury is inflammation. The body delivers fluid, blood, and nutrients to the area of infection or injury and attempts to

---

BOX 36.1 **Current List of Nationally Notifiable Diseases**

Acquired immunodeficiency syndrome (AIDS)	Invasive meningococcal disease
Acute flaccid paralysis	Invasive pneumococcal disease
Amoebiasis	Legionellosis
Anthrax	Leprosy
Botulism	Malaria
Brucellosis	Measles
Campylobacteriosis	Mumps
Chickenpox	Pertussis
Chlamydia, genital	Plague
Cholera	Poliomyelitis
Creutzfeldt-Jakob disease	Rabies
Cryptosporidiosis	Rubella
Cyclosporiasis	Salmonellosis
Diphtheria	Shigellosis
Giardiasis	Smallpox
Gonorrhea	Syphilis
Group B streptococcal disease of the newborn	Tetanus
Hantavirus pulmonary syndrome	Tuberculosis
Hepatitis A	Tularemia
Hepatitis B	Typhoid
Hepatitis C	Verotoxigenic *E. coli*
HIV	Viral hemorrhagic fevers (Crimean Congo, Ebola, Lassa, Marburg)
Influenza, laboratory-confirmed	West Nile virus, asymptomatic infection
Invasive *Haemophilus influenzae* type b disease	West Nile virus
Invasive group A streptococcal disease	

For the direct link to this list of nationally notifiable diseases in Canada, visit http://thePoint.lww.com/Chow1e.

TABLE 36.1 FUNCTION OF WHITE BLOOD CELLS BY LEUKOCYTE TYPE

Cell	Cell's Function Is to Combat
Neutrophils (bands and segs)	Pyogenic infection (bacterial)
Eosinophils	Allergic disorders and parasitic infections
Basophils	Parasitic infections, some allergic disorders
Lymphocytes	Viral infections (measles, rubella, chickenpox, infectious mononucleosis)
Monocytes	Severe infections, by phagocytosis

Adapted from Fischbach, F. T., & Dunning III, M. B. (2009). *A manual of laboratory and diagnostic tests* (8th ed.). Philadelphia, PA: Lippincott Williams & Wilkins.

eliminate the pathogens and help repair the tissues. The body does this through vascular and cellular reactions. The vascular response is an initial period of vasoconstriction followed by vasodilation. This vasodilation allows for the increase of fluids, blood, and nutrients to the area.

The cellular response involves the arrival of white blood cells to the area. White blood cells are the body's defense against infection or injury. The types of white blood cells are neutrophils, lymphocytes, basophils, eosinophils, and monocytes. Elevations in certain portions of the white blood cell count reflect different processes occurring in the body, such as infection, allergic reaction, or leukemia. Table 36.1 gives further explanation of the function of each type of white blood cell. Each type is generally present in a balanced state; the types are reported as a percentage of the total white blood cell count or as the number per certain volume of blood.

The white blood cells use **phagocytosis** to ingest and destroy the **pathogen**. If bacteria escape the action of phagocytosis, they enter the bloodstream and lymph system and the immune system is activated. With activation of the immune system, B lymphocytes (humoral immunity) and T lymphocytes (cell-mediated immunity) are matured and activated. B and T cells recognize and attack infectious pathogens. B cells, which mature in the bone marrow, produce specific antibodies to a specific offending **antigen** (a substance that the body recognizes as foreign). T cells, which mature in the thymus, attack the antigen directly. Once B and T cells have been exposed to an antigen, some cells will remember the antigen: thus, if the particular antigen invades again, the body will act faster.

Infection or inflammation caused by bacteria, viruses, or other pathogens stimulates the release of **endogenous pyrogens** (interleukins, tumour necrosis factor, and interferon) and results in fever. The pyrogens act on the hypothalamus, where they trigger prostaglandin produc-

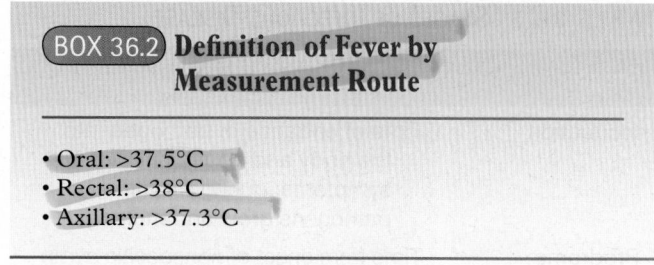

BOX 36.2 Definition of Fever by Measurement Route

- Oral: >37.5°C
- Rectal: >38°C
- Axillary: >37.3°C

Source: Canadian Paediatric Society. (2009b, reaffirmed 2011). *Temperature measurement in pediatrics.* Retrieved September 26, 2011 from http://www.cps.ca/english/statements/CP/cp00-01.htm.

tion and increase the body's temperature set point. This triggers the cold response, resulting in shivering, vasoconstriction, and a decrease in peripheral perfusion to help decrease heat loss and allow the body's temperature to rise to the new set point. Fever, defined as a temperature greater than 38°C, then occurs. Box 36.2 gives specific parameters for fever based on the measurement route.

Antipyretics are often used to lower fever and increase the comfort of the patient. They decrease the temperature set point by inhibiting the production of prostaglandins, leading to sweating and vasodilation and therefore heat loss and a drop in temperature.

It is important to distinguish between fever and hyperthermia. Hyperthermia occurs when normal thermoregulation fails, resulting in an unregulated rise in core temperature. Hyperthermia may occur if the central nervous system of the child becomes impaired by disease, drugs, or abnormalities of heat production or thermal stressors, such as being left in a hot automobile or exertional heat stroke. In the absence of hyperthermia and in the normally neurologic child, the body does not allow fever to rise to lethal levels. The body actually produces a natural antipyretic, called cryogen. If there is no hyperthermic insult, it is rare to see a child's temperature rise to greater than 41.4°C (Crocetti & Serwint, 2005).

Stages of Infectious Disease

Infectious diseases follow a similar pattern. They progress through certain stages (Table 36.2) in which **communicability** (ability to spread to others) can be predicted. It is important for nurses to understand these stages to help control and manage infectious diseases.

Chain of Infection

The **chain of infection** is the process by which an organism is spread. Behaviour of infants and young children, mainly pertaining to hygiene, increases their risk of infection by promoting the chain of infection. Poor hygiene habits, including lack of handwashing, placing toys and hands in the mouth, drooling, and leaking diapers, all can contribute to the spread of infection and communicable diseases. Table 36.3 reviews the chain of infection and nursing implications related to it.

TABLE 36.2 STAGES OF INFECTIOUS DISEASE

Stage	Explanation
Incubation	Time of entrance of pathogen into the body and appearance of first symptoms; during this time, pathogens grow and multiply.
Prodrome	Time from onset of nonspecific symptoms, such as fever, malaise, and fatigue, to more specific symptoms
Illness	Time during which patient demonstrates signs and symptoms specific to an infection type
Convalescence	Time when acute symptoms of illness disappear

Preventing the Spread of Infection

Nurses play a key role in breaking the chain of infection and preventing the spread of diseases. It is very important that nurses not only follow infection control and prevention practices but also educate parents and children on the measures they can take to prevent the spread of infection.

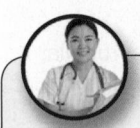 ▶ *Take* NOTE!

Frequent handwashing is the single most important way to prevent the spread of infection.

TABLE 36.3 CHAIN OF INFECTION

Chain Link	Explanation	Nursing Implications

Infectious agent	Any agent capable of causing infection: bacteria, viruses, rickettsiae, protozoa, and fungus	• Control or eliminate infectious agents through
		  • Handwashing
		  • Wearing gloves
		  • Cleaning, disinfection, or sterilization of equipment

Reservoir	A place where the pathogen can thrive and reproduce: human body, animals, insects, food, water, inanimate objects (e.g., stethoscopes)	• Control or eliminate reservoirs • Control sources of body fluids, drainage, or solutions that may harbour pathogens • Follow institution guidelines for disposing of infectious wastes • Provide proper wound care; change dressings or bandages when soiled • Assist clients to carry out appropriate skin and oral care • Keep linens clean and dry
Portal of exit	A way for the pathogen to exit the reservoir: skin and mucous membranes, respiratory tract, urinary tract, gastrointestinal tract, reproductive tract	• Control portals of exit and educate patients and families • Cover mouth and nose when sneezing or coughing • Avoid talking, coughing, or sneezing over open wounds or sterile fields • Use personal protective equipment
Modes of transmission	Direct transmission: body-to-body contact Indirect transmission: transferred by **fomite** or vector; spread by droplet or airborne transmission	• Wash hands before and after patient contact, invasive procedures, or touching open wounds • Use personal protective equipment when necessary • Urge patients and family to wash hands frequently, especially before eating or handling food, after eliminating, and after touching infectious material.
Portal of entry	A way for the pathogen to enter the host: skin and mucous membranes, respiratory tract, urinary tract, gastrointestinal tract, reproductive tract	• Use proper sterile technique during invasive procedures • Provide appropriate wound care • Dispose needles and sharps in puncture-resistant containers • Provide all patients with their own personal care items
Susceptible host	Any person who cannot resist the pathogen	• Protect susceptible host by promoting normal body defenses against infection • Maintain integrity of the patient's skin and mucous membranes • Protect normal defenses by regular bathing and oral care, adequate fluid intake and nutrition, proper immunization

Isolation precautions help nurses break the chain of infection and provide strategies to prevent the spread of pathogens among hospitalized patients. Guidelines for preventing nosocomial and occupational infections can be found on the PHAC website; visit http://thePoint. lww.com/Chow1e for a direct link. Additional guidelines are available from various provincial health departments and organizations such as colleges of registered nurses.

In 2008, the Canadian Pediatric Society (CPS, 2008a) updated its practice guideline for infection control in the pediatric office setting. These guidelines can be found online; visit http://thePoint.lww.com/Chow1e for a direct link. Additionally, the PHAC (1999) produced guidelines for infection control for hospitalized children. These guidelines include both routine practices, which are designed for care of all patients in the hospital regardless of their diagnosis, and additional precautions that address the care of patients who are known or suspected to be infected by epidemiologically important pathogens. Transmission of pathogens can occur through the air, by droplets, or by contact. Box 36.3 gives an overview of standard and transmission-based precautions for hospitalized patients.

When caring for children, modifications of these guidelines may be appropriate. For instance, diaper changing is routine in the pediatric setting. Since it does not usually soil hands, it is not mandatory to wear gloves (except if gloves are required due to transmission-based precautions). According to the standard precaution guidelines, single rooms are required for those who are incontinent and cannot control bodily excretions. Since the majority of young children are incontinent, obviously this guideline is inappropriate in the pediatric setting. Pediatric units often have common rooms, such as playrooms and schoolrooms. Children placed on transmission-based isolation are not allowed to leave their rooms and therefore are not allowed to use these common rooms.

Variations in Pediatric Anatomy and Physiology

Normal immune function is an amazing protective response by the body. It involves complex responses including phagocytosis, humoral immunity, cellular immunity, and activation of the complement system. Blood and lymph are responsible for transporting the agents of the immune system. Due to the immature responses of the immune system, infants and young children are more susceptible to infection. The newborn displays a decreased inflammatory response to invading organisms, contributing to an increased risk of infection. Cellular immunity is generally functional at birth, and humoral immunity occurs when the body encounters and then develops immunity to new diseases. Since the young infant has had limited exposure to disease and is

losing the passive immunity acquired from maternal antibodies, the risk of infection is higher. Young children continue to have an increased risk of infection and communicable disorders because disease protection from immunizations is not complete. (Refer to Chapter 47 for further details.)

Common Medical Treatments

Various medications as well as other medical treatments are used to treat infectious disorders in children. Most of these treatments will require a physician's order when the child is in the hospital. The most common treatments and medications are listed in Common Medical Treatments 36.1 and Drug Guide 36.1. The nurse caring for the child with an infectious disorder should be familiar with what the procedures are, how they work, and common nursing implications related to use of these modalities.

NURSING PROCESS OVERVIEW FOR THE CHILD WITH A COMMUNICABLE DISORDER

Care of the child with an infectious disorder includes assessment, nursing diagnosis, planning, interventions, and evaluation. There are a number of general concepts related to the nursing process that may be applied to the care of children with infectious disorders. From a general understanding of the care involved for a child with an infectious disorder, the nurse can then individualize the care based on the patient's specifics.

*R*emember Samuel, the 3-month-old with fever, congestion, and irritability? What additional health history and physical examination assessment information should you obtain?

Assessment

Assessment of the child with a communicable or infectious disorder includes health history, physical examination, and laboratory and diagnostic testing.

Health History

The health history comprises past medical history, including the mother's pregnancy history, family history, and history of present illness (when the symptoms started and how they have progressed), as well as treatments used at home. The past medical history might be significant for lack of recommended immunizations, prematurity, maternal infection during pregnancy or labour, prolonged difficult delivery, or immunocompromise. Family history might be significant for lack of

BOX 36.3 Standard Precautions and Isolation Precautions

Standard Precautions
- Apply to all patients
- Apply to all body fluid secretions and excretions except sweat, non-intact skin, and mucous membranes
- Designed to reduce the risk of transmission of microorganisms from recognized and unrecognized sources
- Techniques and equipment include:
  - Handwashing before and after direct contact with a patient
  - Clean, non-sterile gloves when touching blood, body fluid secretions or excretions, non-intact skin, and contaminated items
  - Masks, eye protection, and face shields when patient care may include splashing or sprays of blood or body fluid secretions or excretions
  - Fluid-resistant nonsterile gowns to protect skin and clothing when patient care may include splashing or sprays of blood or body fluid secretions or excretions
  - Single rooms not necessary in routine care
  - Patient care equipment handled in a manner that prevents skin or mucous membrane exposure and contamination of clothing
  - Reusable equipment cleaned and reprocessed after direct patient contact
  - Precautions taken to prevent injury when using, cleaning, or disposing of needles and sharps
  - Mouthpieces, resuscitation bags, and other ventilation devices readily available

Additional Precautions
- Designed for patients with known or suspected infection with pathogens for which additional precautions are warranted to interrupt transmission

Airborne
- Designed to reduce the risk of infectious agents transmitted by airborne droplet nuclei or dust particles that may contain the infectious agent
- Examples of such illnesses include measles, varicella, tuberculosis
- Techniques and equipment include standard precautions as well as
  - Single room (If unavailable, consider cohorting patients with the same disease and consult with an infection control professional.)
  - Room with negative air pressure ventilation, with air externally exhausted or high-efficiency particulate air filtered if recirculated
  - If infectious pulmonary tuberculosis is suspected or proven, wear a respiratory protective device, such as an N95 respirator, while in the patient's room
  - Susceptible health care personnel should not enter the room of patients with measles or varicella zoster infections. Those with proven immunity to these viruses need not wear a mask

Droplet
- Designed to reduce the risk of transmission of infectious agents by contact of the conjunctivae or the mucous membranes of the nose or mouth of a susceptible person with large-particle droplets containing pathogens generated from a person (generally through coughing, sneezing, talking, or procedures such as suctioning) who has a clinical disease or who is a carrier of the disease
- Examples of such illnesses include viral respiratory infections, pertussis, streptococcal group A, influenza, meningitis, rubella, and scarlet fever
- Techniques and equipment include standard precautions as well as
  - Single room (If unavailable, consider cohorting patients with the same disease. If this is not possible, separation of at least 1 m between patient and other patients and visitors should be maintained.)
  - Wear a mask if within 1 m of the patient.
  - Eye protection may be indicated if within 1 m of a coughing child or for procedures that may result in coughing

Contact
- Most important and most common route of transmission of health care-associated infections
- Designed to reduce the risk of infectious agents transmitted by direct or indirect contact. Direct-contact transmission involves skin-to-skin contact and physical transfer of pathogens between a susceptible host and an infected or colonized person. Examples include patient care activities that involve physical contact such as turning and bathing. Direct-contact transmission also can occur between two patients, where one serves as the source of infectious pathogen and the other as a susceptible host. Indirect-contact transmission involves contact of a susceptible host with a contaminated intermediate object, usually inanimate, in the patient's environment
- Examples of such illnesses include infectious diarrhea, pediculosis, scabies, viral respiratory infections,* and multidrug-resistant bacteria.
- Techniques and equipment include standard precautions as well as
  - Single room (If unavailable, consider cohorting patients with the same disease.)
  - Gloves (clean or sterile) should be used at all times
  - Proper hand hygiene after glove removal
  - Use gowns, unless the patient is continent and contact of clothing with patient and patient environmental surfaces is not anticipated. Remove gowns before leaving the patient's room.
  - Patient care equipment should be cleaned and disinfected before use with another patient
  - Toys should not be shared with other patients

Prevention standards are applied in all health care settings and are modified to meet each setting's unique needs. Health care workers must practice within the specific institution's guidelines.

---

*Certain infections require more than one precaution.

Source: Siegel, J. D., Rhinehart, E., Jackson M., Chiarello, L., & the Healthcare Infection Control Practices Advisory Committee. (2007). *Guideline for isolation precautions: Preventing transmission of infectious agents in healthcare settings.* Retrieved September 25, 2011 from http://www.cdc.gov/hicpac/pdf/isolation/Isolation2007.pdf.

COMMON MEDICAL TREATMENTS 36.1

Treatment	Explanation	Indication	Nursing Implications
Hydration	Promoting proper fluid balance either orally or intravenously	Child who can't replace insensible loss due to fever, child who is vomiting or has diarrhea	• Encourage oral fluids, if possible • Offer child fluid he or she prefers; try ice pops or games to promote fluid intake • If administering IV fluids, ensure proper fluid and rate per order and assess IV site and fluid intake every hour • Maintain strict record of intake and output
Fever reduction	Reducing temperature by use of antipyretics or nonpharmacologic interventions	Febrile child who is uncomfortable or who can't keep up with the increased metabolic demands associated with fever	• Administer antipyretics, such as ibuprofen and acetaminophen • Avoid aspirin use in children and adolescents • Use nonpharmacologic interventions such as dressing lightly, removing blankets, use of a fan, tepid bath, and cooling blanket • Some nonpharmacologic interventions remain controversial • Make sure that nonpharmacologic measures do not induce shivering or discomfort. If they do, they should be stopped immediately

DRUG GUIDE 36.1   COMMON DRUGS FOR COMMUNICABLE DISORDERS

Medication	Action	Indication	Nursing Implications
Antibiotics	Kill and prevent the growth of bacteria	Treatment of bacterial infections such as sepsis	• Check for antibiotic allergies • Give as prescribed for the length of time prescribed
Antivirals (e.g., acyclovir)	Kill and prevent the growth of viruses	Treatment of viral infections such as herpes simplex II	• Observe infusion site for signs of tissue damage • If administering topically, clean and dry area before application and wear gloves • Give as prescribed for the length of time prescribed
Antipyretics (acetaminophen, ibuprofen)	Decrease the temperature set point (only in a child with a raised temperature) by inhibiting the production of prostaglandins, leading to heat loss (through vasodilation and sweating) and resulting in a reduction in fever	Febrile child who is uncomfortable or who can't keep up with the increased metabolic demands associated with fever	• Ensure proper dosing, concentration, and dosing interval • Avoid aspirin use in children and adolescents • Avoid ibuprofen use in children with a bleeding disorder • Assess fever and any related symptoms such as tachycardia, shivering, diaphoresis • Proper education to caregivers on appropriate dosing, concentration, dosing interval, and use of proper measuring device is essential
Antipruritics (usually antihistamines)	Agents that relieve itching may be given topically or orally	Relief of discomfort secondary to itching	• When applying topically, wear gloves • Do not apply to open wounds • Oral antihistamines may cause drowsiness

Adapted from Karch, A. (2010). *2010 Lippincott's nursing drug guide.* Philadelphia, PA: Wolters Kluwer Health/ Lippincott Williams & Wilkins; and Taketokmo, C. K., Hodding, J. H., & Kraus, D. M. (2010). *Lexi-comp's Drug Reference Handbook: Pediatric & Neonatal Dosage Handbook* (18th ed.). Hudson, OH: Lexi-comp, Inc.

immunization or recent infectious or communicable disease. When eliciting the history of the present illness, inquire about the following:

- Any known exposure to infectious or communicable disease
- Immunization history
- History of having any common childhood communicable diseases
- Fever
- Sore throat
- Lethargy
- Malaise
- Poor feeding or appetite
- Vomiting
- Diarrhea
- Cough
- Rash (in the older child ask for a description of how it feels; is it painful, does it itch?)

▶ **Take** NOTE!

Many childhood infectious and communicable diseases involve a rash. Rashes can be difficult to identify; therefore, a thorough description and history from the caregiver are extremely important.

Physical Examination

Physical examination of the child with an infectious disorder includes inspection, observation, and palpation.

Inspection and Observation

The physical examination should begin with inspection and observation. Assess the child's skin, mouth, throat, and hair for lesions or wounds. Note the colour, shape, and distribution of any lesions or wounds. Assess whether there is any exudate from the lesions or wounds. Observe for scratching, restlessness, and avoidance of the use of a body part or guarding of a body part. A thorough and accurate description is important to assist in identifying the rash and causative organism. Observe the child's affect, energy level, and interaction with caregiver. Lethargy can indicate serious infection or sepsis. Observe for discharge from the nose, cough, or respiratory difficulty.

Assess hydration status. Inspect oral mucosa; dry and pale mucous membranes can indicate dehydration. Observe for other signs of dehydration, such as sunken eyes and no tears with crying.

Assessment of vital signs can provide more information about the child's condition. Elevated temperature can indicate infection. Often tachypnea and tachycardia accompany fever. Hypotension may also occur, but it is usually a late sign with sepsis.

▶ **Take** NOTE!

Neonates may not present with fever; some may be hypothermic (Anderson-Berry, Bellig, & Ohning, 2011).

Palpation

Palpate the skin to assess temperature, moisture, texture, and turgor. In a child with an infectious or communicable disease the skin may be warm and moist due to fever. Turgor may be decreased secondary to dehydration. In infants, palpate the fontanels; if sunken, the infant may be dehydrated. Palpate the rash to determine if it is raised or flat. A thorough picture of the presenting rash can help identify the child's illness. Palpate the lymph nodes and note any that are swollen and tender.

Laboratory and Diagnostic Testing

Common Laboratory and Diagnostics Tests 36.1 offers an explanation of the laboratory and diagnostic tests used most commonly when considering communicable disorders. The tests can assist the physician in diagnosing the disorder and/or be used as guidelines in determining ongoing treatment. Laboratory or non-nursing personnel obtain some of the tests, while the nurse might obtain others. In either instance the nurse should be familiar with how the tests are obtained, what they are used for, and normal versus abnormal results. This knowledge will also be necessary when providing patient and family education related to the testing.

Performing Venipuncture

Obtaining a blood specimen may be very frightening to children because of the fear of needles, pain, and blood loss. Incorporate the concept of atraumatic care in the performance of all venipunctures or other needlesticks for children. Whether the laboratory technician or the nurse is drawing the blood, the procedure should be performed in an area other than the child's bed, such as the treatment room; the child's bed should be kept as a "safe" area. Provide teaching about the procedure based upon the child's developmental level and readiness to learn. In infants and younger children, additional assistance with positioning and restraint will be needed to perform the procedure safely and to ensure proper collection. Use a topical anesthetic cream or gel, refrigerant spray, or iontophoresis prior to venipuncture. In young infants, administer oral sucrose beginning 1 to 2 minutes prior to the procedure and throughout the course of the venipuncture (Hatfield, Chang, Bittle, Deluca, & Polomano, 2011). Refer to Chapter 34 for additional information related to decreasing the incidence of pain related to venipuncture in infants and children.

COMMON LABORATORY AND DIAGNOSTIC TESTS 36.1

Test	Explanation	Indication	Nursing Implications
Complete blood count (CBC)	Evaluate white blood cell count (particularly the percentage of individual white cells)	Detect the presence of inflammation, infection	• Normal values vary according to age and gender • White blood cell count differential is helpful in evaluating source of infection • May be affected by myelosuppressive drugs
Erythrocyte sedimentation rate (ESR)	Nonspecific test used in conjunction with other tests to determine the presence of infection or inflammation	Detect the presence of inflammation, infection	• Send to laboratory immediately; specimens allowed to stand for longer than 3 hours may produce a falsely low result
C-reactive protein (CRP)	Nonspecific test that measures a type of protein produced in the liver that is present during episodes of acute inflammation or infection Usually used to diagnose bacterial infections; does not consistently rise with viral infections	Detect the presence of infection	• Presence of an intrauterine device may cause positive test results because of tissue inflammation • Exogenous hormones, such as oral contraceptives, may cause increased levels • Nonsteroidal anti-inflammatories, salicylates, and steroids may cause decreased levels • CRP is a more sensitive and rapidly responding indicator than ESR
Blood culture and sensitivity	Deliberate growing of microorganism in a solid or liquid medium. Once it has grown, it is tested against various antibiotics to determine which antibiotics will kill it	Detect the presence of bacteria or yeast, which may have spread from a certain site in the body into the bloodstream. Determine which antibiotics the bacteria or yeast is sensitive to	• Follow aseptic technique and hospital protocol to prevent contamination • Two cultures obtained from two different sites are preferred • Ideally obtain before administering antibiotics; if patient is taking antibiotics, notify laboratory and draw specimen shortly before next dose • Smaller volumes are available for pediatric use • Deliver to laboratory immediately (within 30 minutes)
Stool culture (including stool for ova and parasites [O&P])	To determine if a bacteria or parasite has infected the intestines	Detect pathogens, including parasites or overgrowth of normal flora in the bowel. Indicated for patients with diarrhea, fever, or abdominal pain	• Stool must be free of urine, water, and toilet paper • Do not retrieve out of toilet water • Deliver to laboratory immediately • Mineral oil, barium, and bismuth interfere with the detection of parasites; specimen collection should be delayed for 7 to 10 days • Often a minimum of three specimens on three separate days are required for adequate examination, since many parasites and worm eggs are shed intermittently

(continued)

COMMON LABORATORY AND DIAGNOSTIC TESTS 36.1 (continued)

Test	Explanation	Indication	Nursing Implications
Urine culture	Collection of urine to detect the presence of bacteria in the urine	Detect the presence of bacteria in the urine. Indicated for patients with fever of unknown origin, dysuria, frequency or urgency, or if urinalysis suggests infection	• Should be obtained by midstream clean-catch, catheterization, or suprapubic aspiration. Avoid contamination with stool, vaginal secretions, hands, or clothing • Placing bags on the perineum is not acceptable due to high chance of contamination (CPS, 2004) • Obtain before antibiotics are administered • Deliver to laboratory immediately or refrigerate
Genital tract culture	Specimens from the genital tract include urethral, cervical, and anorectal swabs to detect the presence of invasive organisms	Detect the presence of sexually transmitted infections. Indicated in patients with vaginal discharge, pelvic pain, urethritis, or penile discharge and those at high risk of sexually transmitted infections	• Menses may alter test • Female patients should avoid douching or tub bathing 24 hours before a cervical culture (may make fewer organisms available) • Obtain urethral cultures from male patients before voiding, preferably before the first morning void (voiding 1 hour before urethral culture washes secretions out of the urethra) • Fecal material may contaminate a rectal culture • Transport specimens to laboratory as soon as possible • Advise patients to avoid intercourse and all other sexual contact until test results are available
Throat culture	Vigorous swabbing of the tonsillar area and posterior pharynx to detect the presence of invasive organisms	Most reliable method of detecting group A streptococcal pharyngitis Will also detect *Bordetella pertussis, Corynebacterium diphtheriae* Also may be used to detect sexually transmitted infections in those who have engaged in oral intercourse May be performed in those with fever of unknown origin	• Ensure specimen is of secretions in the pharyngeal or tonsillar area • When performing on young children, have adult hold child in lap • Health care worker needs to stabilize head by placing hand on the child's forehead

Adapted from Fischbach, F. T., & Dunning III, M. B. (2009). *A manual of laboratory and diagnostic tests* (8th ed.). Philadelphia, PA: Lippincott Williams & Wilkins.

The usual sites for obtaining blood specimens via venipuncture are the superficial veins of the dorsal surface of the hand or the antecubital fossa, although other locations may also be used. In specific situations, the jugular or femoral vein may be used and either the physician or advanced practice nurse will perform the venipuncture. Capillary puncture of the child's fingertip, the great toe, or the infant's heel may also be used to obtain blood specimens. Fingertip puncture is similar to that in the adult, directed to the sides of the fingertip. Great toe puncture is performed in the same way. Capillary heel puncture must be performed in the proper location to avoid striking the medial plantar artery or periosteum. Nursing Procedure 36.1 gives instructions related to capillary heel puncture. Automatic lancet devices are used to deliver a more precise puncture

Nursing Procedure 36.1

CAPILLARY HEEL PUNCTURE

1. Choose the collection site and apply a commercial heel warmer or warm pack for several minutes prior to specimen collection.
2. Assemble equipment:
   - Gloves
   - Automatic lancet
   - Antiseptic wipe
   - Cotton ball or dry gauze
   - Capillary blood collection tube
   - Band-aid
3. Don gloves. Remove the warm pack.
4. Cleanse the site with antiseptic prep pad and allow to dry.
5. Hold the dorsum of the foot with the nondominant hand; with the dominant hand, pierce the heel with the lancet.
6. Wipe away the first drop of blood with the cotton ball or dry gauze.
7. Collect the blood specimen with a capillary specimen collection tube. Avoid squeezing the foot during specimen collection if possible, as it may contribute to hemolysis of the specimen.
8. Hold dry gauze over the site until bleeding stops, then apply a Band-aid.

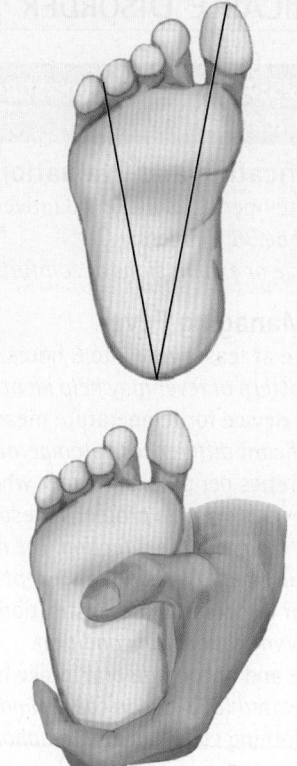

For additional information and guidelines, refer to the *WHO Guidelines on Drawing Blood: Best Practices in Phlebotomy*, available online at http://whqlibdoc.who.int/publications/2010/9789241599221_eng.pdf.

---

depth. The young infant may benefit from the use of oral sucrose via pacifier before and during the capillary puncture (Hatfield et al., 2011) (see Chapter 35).

Children with indwelling venous access devices may be spared the trauma of puncture for blood specimens. Follow your institution's guidelines for withdrawing blood from peripherally inserted venous catheters or central venous catheters. The initial blood will be discarded to prevent contamination with intravenous fluids or medications such as heparin. The discard amount depends on the size of the catheter, the weight of the child, and the institution's guidelines. After aspiration of the specimen, flush the venous access device with normal saline to prevent clogging. The device may then be reconnected to the intravenous fluid or flushed according to the institution's protocol.

Performing Arterial Puncture

Occasionally, blood samples may be obtained from an artery rather than a vein or capillary. Blood gases in particular are usually obtained by arterial puncture. Arterial puncture requires additional training and in many institutions is performed only by the respiratory therapist, physician, or nurse practitioner.

Nursing Diagnoses, Goals, Interventions, and Evaluations

Upon completion of a thorough assessment, the nurse might identify several nursing diagnoses, including the following:

- Altered body temperature: fever
- Impaired comfort
- Impaired skin integrity
- Risk of infection
- Fluid volume deficit
- Social isolation
- Knowledge deficit

After completing an assessment of Samuel, you note the following: rectal temperature of 39°C, poor sucking, and lethargy. Based on these assessment findings, what would your top three nursing diagnoses be for Samuel?

Nursing goals, interventions, and evaluation for the child with a communicable or infectious disorder are based on the nursing diagnoses. Nursing Care Plan 36.1

(text continues on page 1140)

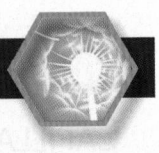

Nursing Care Plan 36.1

OVERVIEW FOR THE CHILD WITH AN INFECTIOUS OR COMMUNICABLE DISORDER

NURSING DIAGNOSIS: Altered body temperature: fever related to infectious disease process as evidenced by rectal temperature greater than 38°C

Outcome Identification and Evaluation
Child will maintain temperature within adaptive levels and be comfortable and remain hydrated.
Temperature will be 38°C or less.
Child will verbalize or exhibit signs of comfort during febrile episode; child will demonstrate adequate signs of hydration.

Interventions: Managing Fever
- Assess temperature at least every 4 to 6 hours, 30 to 60 minutes after antipyretic is given and with any change in condition; *recognizing the pattern of fever may help identify source.*
- Use same site and device for temperature measurement *to reflect a more accurate trend in temperature, since different sites can result in significant differences in temperature reading.*
- Administer antipyretics per physician order when the child is experiencing discomfort or cannot keep up with the metabolic demands of the fever. *Fever is a protective response of the body to fight infection. Antipyretics provide symptomatic relief but do not change the course of the infection. The major benefits to decreasing fever are increasing comfort in the child and decreasing fluid requirements, helping to prevent dehydration.*
- Notify physician of temperature per institution or specific order guidelines; *increases in temperature may indicate worsening infection and relevant changes in condition.*
- Assess fluid intake and encourage oral intake or administer intravenous fluids per physician order; *increased metabolic rate and diaphoresis related to fever can cause fluid loss and lead to fluid volume deficit.*
- Keep linens and clothing clean and dry; *diaphoresis can leave clothing and linen soaked and increases discomfort for the child.*
- Use of nonpharmacologic measures such as tepid bath and removal of clothing and blankets is controversial. If used, discontinue if shivering begins.

NURSING DIAGNOSIS: Impaired comfort related to infectious and/or inflammatory process as evidenced by hyperthermia, pruritus, rash or skin lesions, sore throat, or joint pain

Outcome Identification and Evaluation
Pain or discomfort will be reduced to level acceptable to child.
Child will verbalize absence or decrease of pain using a pain scale (FLACC, faces, or linear pain scale), will verbalize decrease in uncomfortable sensations such as itching and aches; infants will exhibit decreased crying and ability to rest quietly.

Interventions: Improving Comfort
- Assess pain and response to interventions frequently with use of pain scales or other pain measurement tools; *provides baseline of pain and allows for evaluation of effectiveness of interventions.*
- Administer analgesics and antipruritics as ordered *to relieve pain via interruption of CNS pathways and to decrease discomfort related to itching.*
- Apply cool compresses to areas of pruritus or provide a cool bath *to decrease inflammation and soothe pruritus.*
- Keep child's fingernails short (use mitts, gloves, or socks over hands if necessary); *short fingernails can help prevent injury to the skin, which leads to increased pain.*
- Encourage child to press on rather than scratch the area of pruritus; *pressing on the area that itches can help soothe the itching and prevent scratching, which can lead to injury to the skin.*
- Provide frequent fluids and offer warm fluids such as soup or cold foods such as ice pops *to help ease the discomfort of a sore throat.*
- Provide cool mist humidification *to help ease the discomfort of a sore throat.*
- Dress the child in light clothing; *restrictive clothing and diaphoresis can lead to increased pruritus.*
- Use diversional activities and distraction appropriate to developmental level: *distraction from pain can reduce the need for pharmacologic agents, and distraction from pruritus can minimize scratching.*

Nursing Care Plan 36.1 (continued)

NURSING DIAGNOSIS: Impaired skin integrity related to mechanical trauma secondary to infectious disease process as evidenced by rash, pruritus, and scratching

Outcome Identification and Evaluation
Child will maintain or regain skin integrity.
   Child will not demonstrate increased skin breakdown. Child or parent will be able to describe or demonstrate measures to protect and heal skin and proper care for any lesions.

Interventions: Promoting Skin Integrity
- Monitor skin for colour changes, temperature, redness, swelling, warmth, pain or signs of infection, changes in rash lesions, distribution, or size *to help identify problems early and allow for prevention of infection; can also provide information regarding the course of the illness.*
- Encourage fluid intake and proper nutrition *to promote wound healing.*
- Keep child's fingernails short (use mitts, gloves, or socks over hands if necessary); *short fingernails can help prevent injury to the skin, which leads to increased pain.*
- Encourage child to press on rather than scratch the area of pruritus; *pressing on the area that itches can help soothe the itching and prevent scratching, which can lead to injury to the skin.*
- Use antipruritics and topical ointments or creams as ordered *to minimize scratching to prevent injury to skin; can aid in healing.*

NURSING DIAGNOSIS: Risk of infection related to insufficient knowledge regarding measures to avoid exposure to pathogens, increased environmental exposure to pathogens, transmission to others secondary to contagious organism or presence of infectious organisms

Outcome Identification and Evaluation
Child will exhibit no signs or symptoms of local or systemic infection. Child will not spread infection to others. *Symptoms of infection will decrease over time; others will remain free of infection. Child and family will demonstrate appropriate hygiene measures using proper technique, such as handwashing to prevent the spread of infection.*

Interventions: Preventing and Controlling Infection
- Monitor vital signs; *elevation in temperature may indicate infection.*
- Monitor skin lesions for signs of local infection: *redness, warmth, drainage, swelling, and pain at lesions can indicate infection.*
- Maintain aseptic technique and practice good handwashing *to prevent introduction of further infectious agents and prevent transmission to others.*
- Administer antibiotics as prescribed *to prevent or treat bacterial infection.*
- Encourage nutritious diet and proper hydration according to child's preferences and ability to feed orally *to assist body's natural defenses against infection.*
- Isolate child as required based on transmission-based precautions *to prevent nosocomial spread of infection.*
- Teach child and family preventive measures such as good handwashing, covering mouth and nose with cough or sneeze, and adequate disposal of used tissues *to prevent nosocomial or community spread of infection.*

NURSING DIAGNOSIS: Fluid volume deficit, risk of, related to increased metabolic demands and insensible loss due to fever, vomiting, poor feeding or intake

Outcome Identification and Evaluation
Fluid volume will be maintained and balanced. *Oral mucosa will remain moist and pink, skin turgor is elastic, urine output is at least 1 to 2 mL/kg/hr.*

Interventions: Promoting Adequate Fluid Balance
- Administer IV fluids if ordered *to maintain adequate hydration in children who are NPO, unable to tolerate oral intake, or unable to keep up with fluid losses.*
- When oral intake is allowed and tolerated, encourage oral fluids *to promote intake and maintain hydration.*
- Assess for signs of adequate hydration such as pink and moist oral mucosa, elastic skin turgor, adequate urine output; *discrepancies may identify fluid imbalance.*

(continued)

Nursing Care Plan 36.1 (continued)

- Monitor intake and output *to identify fluid imbalance.*
- Assess urine specific gravity, urine and serum electrolytes, blood urea nitrogen, creatinine, and osmolality and daily weights; *these are reliable indicators of fluid status.*

NURSING DIAGNOSIS: Social isolation related to required isolation from peers secondary to transmission-based precautions, as evidenced by disruption in usual play secondary to inability to leave hospital room, activity intolerance, and fatigue

Outcome Identification and Evaluation
Child will participate in stimulating activities. *Child is able to verbalize reason for isolation and length of isolation (if developmentally appropriate); child verbalizes interest in activities.*

Interventions: Preventing Social Isolation
- Explain reasons for transmission-based precautions and length of time; *this helps increase understanding and decrease anxiety about isolation. Children sometimes mistake isolation as punishment. Explaining length of time gives child an end point he or she can work toward.*
- Visit child frequently, at least every hour, and try to spend some uninterrupted time to play and allow child time to verbalize feelings about separation from others; *helps establish a therapeutic relationship and demonstrates caring.*
- Let child see caregiver's face before applying mask if appropriate *to help child identify and relate to those caring for him or her and minimize anxiety about strangers and the unknown.*
- Consult child life specialist *to arrange for stimulating activities child enjoys; can help child to better understand reasons for isolation.*
- Contact volunteers to spend time with child, if appropriate: *gives child attention and support, which will assist child with coping and decrease stress.*

NURSING DIAGNOSIS: Knowledge deficit related to lack of information regarding medical condition, prognosis, and medical needs as evidenced by verbalization, questions, or actions demonstrating lack of understanding regarding child's condition or care.

Outcome Identification and Evaluation
Child and family will verbalize accurate information and understanding about condition, prognosis, and medical needs. *Child and family demonstrate knowledge of condition and prognosis and medical needs, including possible causes, contributing factors, and treatment measures.*

Interventions: Providing Patient and Family Teaching
- Assess child's and family's willingness to learn: *child and family must be willing to learn in order for teaching to be effective.*
- Provide family with time to adjust to diagnosis *to help facilitate adjustment and ability to learn and participate in child's care.*
- Repeat information: *allows family and child time to learn and understand.*
- Teach in short sessions; *many short sessions are found to be more helpful than one long session.*
- Gear teaching to level of understanding of the child and family (depends on age of child, physical condition, memory) *to ensure understanding.*
- Provide reinforcement and rewards *to facilitate the teaching/learning process.*
- Use multiple modes of learning involving many senses (provide written, verbal demonstration, and videos) when possible; *the child and family are more likely to retain information when it is presented in different ways using many senses.*

---

provides a general guide for planning care for a child with an infectious or communicable disorder. Additional information about nursing management will be included later in the chapter as it relates to specific disorders.

Managing Fever
Fever is one of the most common reasons parents seek medical attention for their children (Sullivan, Farrar, &

the AAP's Section on Clinical Pharmacology and Therapeutics, and Committee on Drugs, 2011). Most infections or communicable diseases are accompanied by fever. Many parents have great concerns about fever: they fear febrile seizures, neurologic complications, and a potential serious underlying disease. Many health care providers may share these fears. This leads to the common recommendation to intervene and reduce fever.

EVIDENCE-BASED PRACTICE 36.1
The Effect of Physical Methods Such as Sponging on Decreasing Body Temperature in Children

Health care providers commonly recommend physical methods such as sponging to decrease elevated temperature in children.

● Study
The authors reviewed seven randomized and quasi-randomized studies that evaluated the effects of sponging alone or in combination with antipyretic drugs. Study participants included children between the ages of 1 month and 15 years.

▲ Findings
Tepid water sponging alone was found to have limited usefulness but may decrease fever in some children if used along with antipyretic drugs. Adverse effects, including excess shivering, goose pimples, increased irritability, and febrile seizures, occurred more frequently when ice water or alcohol was used for sponge bathing.

■ Nursing Implications
To alleviate parental concerns about fever, nurses should educate parents about why fever occurs. Discourage parents from using alcohol baths or ice water to decrease body temperature in children. Counsel parents to administer appropriate doses of antipyretics when fever causes discomfort in the child or if the child is at risk of febrile seizures. Advise parents that tepid bathing in a warm room may be used safely in conjunction with antipyretics to decrease fever in children.

Meremikwu, M.M., Oyo-Ita A. (2003). Physical methods versus drug placebo or no treatment for managing fever in children. *Cochrane Database of Systematic Reviews* 2003, Issue 2. Art. No.: CD004264. DOI: 10.1002/14651858.CD004264. [Edited (no change to conclusions), published in Issue 2, 2009.]

These fears and misconceptions about fever can lead to mismanagement of fever, such as inappropriate dosing of antipyretics, awakening the child during sleep to give antipyretics, or inappropriate use of nonpharmacologic treatments such as sponging the child with alcohol or cold water (Crocetti & Serwint, 2005; Sullivan et al., 2011). See Evidence-based Practice 36.1.

Health care providers need to educate parents that fever is a protective mechanism the body uses to fight infection. Evidence exists that an elevated body temperature actually enhances various components of the immune response (Crocetti & Serwint, 2005; Sullivan et al., 2011). Fever can slow the growth of bacteria and viruses and increase neutrophil production and T-cell proliferation (Crocetti & Serwint, 2005). Studies have shown that the use of antipyretics may prolong illness (Crocetti & Serwint, 2005; Sullivan et al., 2011). Concern also exists that reducing fever may hide signs of serious bacterial illness (Crocetti & Serwint, 2005; Sullivan et al., 2011).

▶ *Take* NOTE!

Parents should be made aware that infants less than 6 months of age with a temperature higher than 38°C should be seen by a physician or nurse practitioner. These infants are considered at risk of sepsis until proven otherwise due to their immature immune system and inability to localize or handle infection very well (Powell, 2007a).

In infants over 3 months of age, fever less than 39°C usually does not require treatment (Powell, 2007b). Antipyretics provide symptomatic relief but do not change the course of the infection. The major benefits to decreasing fever are increasing comfort in the child and decreasing fluid requirements, which helps to prevent dehydration. Children with certain underlying conditions, such as cardiovascular disease or pulmonary disease, also benefit from treating fever because such treatment decreases demands on the body.

Home Management of Fever

Management of fever typically occurs at home. Therefore, it is important that guidance and instruction are given at child visits and reviewed at subsequent visits. Written and video materials related to fever management have been effective in increasing caregivers' knowledge (Broome, Dokken, Broome, Woodring, & Stegelman, 2003). The CPS consumer website (visit http://thePoint.lww.com/Chow1e for a direct link) provides a number of fact sheets relating to infections, including specific guidelines for parents for temperature taking and home fever management (Caring for Kids, 2008). Parents can refer to the written instructions when needed (see Teaching Guideline 36.1). The use of acetaminophen and ibuprofen to reduce fever in children has been shown to be safe and effective when the appropriate dose is administered at the appropriate interval (Crocetti & Serwint, 2005). Box 36.4 gives dosing recommendations.

TEACHING GUIDELINE 36.1

Fever Management

- Fever is a sign of illness, not a disease; it is the body's weapon to fight infection.
- Diurnal variation may allow temperature changes as much as 1°C over a 24-hour period, peaking in the evening.
- In some children fever can be associated with a seizure or dehydration, but this will not lead to brain damage or death. Discuss the facts about febrile seizures (see Chapter 37 for further information on febrile seizures).
- Watch for the signs and symptoms of dehydration; it is important to provide oral rehydration by increasing fluid intake.
- Dress the child lightly and avoid warm, binding clothing or blankets.
- The use of sponging with tepid water is controversial; if used, encourage the parent to give an antipyretic prior to sponging. Ensure the sponging does not produce shivering (which causes the body to produce heat and maintain the elevated set point), and reinforce the importance of using tepid water, not cold water or alcohol. Instruct the parent to stop if the child experiences discomfort.
- Seek medical assistance or guidance for any child
  - Younger than 6 months who has a fever
  - Who is lethargic or listless or is excessively irritable or cranky, regardless of temperature
  - With wheezing or persistent coughing
  - With a fever lasting more than 3 days
  - With a fever greater than 40.6°C
  - Who is immunocompromised by illness, such as cancer or HIV

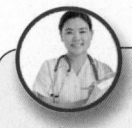

▶ *Take* NOTE!

Never give aspirin to children to reduce fever due to the risk of Reye's syndrome.

Acetaminophen Use

Acetaminophen is widely used and accepted, but toxic reactions can be seen in children (American Academy of Pediatrics [AAP] Committee on Drugs, 2009). Unintentional causes of acetaminophen toxicity include overdosing or incorrect dosing due to failure to read and understand the label instructions, use of an incorrect measuring device or concentration, and co-administration with an over-the-counter fixed-dose combination medication (the parent may not recognize that it has acetaminophen in it).

▶ *Take* NOTE!

The CPS (1998) has stated that both acetaminophen and ibuprofen have been shown to be effective in treating fever provided that appropriate dosing schedules are followed, although this guideline is currently under review. The American Academy of Pediatrics (2001) recommends against the practice of alternating doses of acetaminophen and ibuprofen.

BOX 36.4 Dose Recommendations for Acetaminophen and Ibuprofen

Acetaminophen, 10 to 15 mg/kg/dose
- No more than every 4 hours
- No more than five doses in a 24-hour period

Ibuprofen, 5 to 10 mg/kg/dose
- Only children older than 6 months of age
- Daily dose should not exceed 40 mg/kg
- No more than four doses in a 24-hour period

Adapted from Gal, P., & Reed, M. D. (2007). Medications. In R. M. Kliegman, R. E. Behrman, H. B. Jenson, & B. F. Stanton (Eds.), *Nelson's textbook of pediatrics* (18th ed.). Philadelphia: Saunders.

Managing Skin Rashes

Many infectious or communicable diseases are accompanied by skin rashes. These rashes can be very uncomfortable and irritating for the child. Management often occurs at home, so parents need to be educated on ways to relieve the discomfort and protect and maintain skin integrity. Antipruritics, including oral medications or topical creams or ointments, may be prescribed by the physician (see Drug Guide 36.1). Parents need to be instructed on the importance of maintaining skin integrity to prevent infection or scarring. Teach parents to keep their child's fingernails short and hands clean. Explain the importance of discouraging scratching, and discuss distraction techniques they can use with the child. Cool compresses or cool baths can help relieve itching. Encouraging the child to press rather than scratch the itchy area can help relieve discomfort while maintaining skin integrity. Refer to Chapter 45 for more information on managing skin rashes.

Based on your top three nursing diagnoses for Samuel, describe appropriate nursing interventions.

Sepsis

Sepsis is a systemic overresponse to infection resulting from bacteria (most common), fungi, viruses, or parasites. It can lead to septic shock, which results in hypotension, low blood flow, and multisystem organ failure. Septic shock is a medical emergency, and patients are usually admitted to an intensive care unit (see Chapter 52). The cause of sepsis may not be known, but common causative organisms include *Escherichia coli, Listeria monocytogenes,* group B streptococcus, enteroviruses, and herpes simplex virus in neonates and *Neisseria meningitidis, Streptococcus pneumoniae,* and *Staphylococcus aureus* in older children (Enrione & Powell, 2007). Sepsis can affect any age group but is more common in neonates and young infants (Santhanam & Tolan, 2011). Neonates and young infants have a higher susceptibility due to their immature immune system, inability to localize infections, and lack of immunoglobulin M (IgM), which is necessary to protect against bacterial infections.

The prognosis for sepsis is variable and depends on the child's age and the cause of the sepsis. Mortality rate may be as high as 40% to 60% for certain types of infections (Behrman, Kliegman, Jenson, & Stanton, 2007). Neonates are at the highest risk, and 50% of neonatal deaths result from serious bacterial infections in the first month of life (Crawford, 2006). Due to this high mortality rate, when a febrile neonate presents, a full workup is indicated (Powell, 2007b) and admission to the hospital to rule out sepsis is usually the standard of practice.

Pathophysiology

Sepsis results in **systemic inflammatory response syndrome (SIRS)** due to infection. The pathophysiology of sepsis is complex. It results from the effects of circulating bacterial products or toxins, mediated by cytokine release, occurring as a result of sustained bacteremia. The pathogens cause an overproduction of proinflammatory cytokines, previously termed endotoxins, which are responsible for the clinically observable effects of the sepsis. Impaired pulmonary, hepatic, or renal function may result from excessive cytokine release during the septic process.

Therapeutic Management

Therapeutic management of sepsis in infants, especially neonates, is more aggressive than for older children. Neonates and infants with sepsis or even suspected sepsis are treated in the hospital. The infant is admitted for close monitoring along with antibiotic therapy. Intravenous antibiotics are started immediately after the blood, urine, and cerebrospinal fluid cultures have been obtained. The length of therapy and the specific antibiotic used will be determined based on the source of the positive culture and the results of the culture and sensitivity. Common treatment length for positive cultures is 7 to 14 days. If final culture reports are negative and symptoms have subsided, antibiotics may be discontinued (usually after 72 hours of treatment). If the child is not responding to therapy and symptoms worsen, sepsis may be progressing to shock. Management of the child with septic shock is usually done in the intensive care unit.

Nursing Assessment

For a full description of the assessment phase of the nursing process, refer to page 1131. Assessment findings pertinent to sepsis are discussed below.

Health History

Elicit a description of the present illness and chief complaint. Signs of sepsis can vary with each child. Some common signs and symptoms reported during the health history might include the following:

- Child just does not look or act "right"
- Crying more than usual, inconsolable
- Fever
- Hypothermia (in the neonate and those with severe disease)
- Lethargic and less interactive or playful
- Increased irritability
- Poor feeding or poor suck
- Rash (e.g., petechiae, ecchymosis, diffuse erythema)
- Difficulty breathing
- Nasal congestion
- Diarrhea
- Vomiting
- Decreased urine output
- Hypotonia
- Changes in mental status (confused, anxious, excited)
- Seizures
- Older child may complain of heart racing

Explore the patient's current and past medical history for risk factors such as

- Prematurity
- Lack of immunizations
- Immunocompromise
- Exposure to communicable pathogens

In neonates and young infants, discuss pregnancy and labour risk factors such as

• Premature rupture of membranes or prolonged rupture
• Difficult delivery
• Maternal infection or fever, including STIs
• Resuscitation and other invasive procedures
• Positive maternal group beta streptococcal vaginosis

Sepsis may occur in the hospitalized child. Assess for risk factors such as

• Intensive care unit stay
• Presence of central line or other invasive lines or tubes
• Immunosuppression

Physical Examination

Perform a thorough physical examination of the infant or child with proven or suspected sepsis. Specific findings related to inspection and observation are noted below.

Inspection and Observation

Observe the child's general appearance, colour, level of arousal, and hydration status. The child with sepsis may appear lethargic and pale and show signs of dehydration. In neonates and infants, observe the quality of their cry and reaction to parental stimulation, noting weak cry, lack of smile or facial expression, or lack of responsiveness. Inspect the skin for petechiae or other skin lesions. Petechiae may indicate a serious bacterial infection (often *N. meningitidis*), and other skin lesion patterns may help identify the cause of the fever. Observe respiratory effort and rate. The infant or child with sepsis may demonstrate tachypnea and increased work of breathing, such as nasal flaring, grunting, and retractions.

Assess vital signs, noting abnormalities. Note elevation in temperature or hypothermia in the young infant. Note tachypnea or tachycardia in the child or apnea or bradycardia in the infant. Document blood pressure. Hypotension, especially when accompanied by signs of poor perfusion, can be a sign of worsening sepsis with progression to shock (refer to Chapter 52).

▶ **Take** NOTE!

Listen to the parents' descriptions of the neonate's or infant's behaviour and appearance, as well as changes they have observed. Many times they are the first to notice when their child is not acting right, even before clinical signs of infection are seen.

Laboratory and Diagnostic Tests

Symptoms of sepsis can be vague in infants. Therefore, laboratory tests play a crucial role in confirming or ruling out sepsis. Common laboratory and diagnostic studies ordered for the assessment of sepsis include the following:

• Complete blood count (CBC): white blood cells will be elevated; in severe cases they may be decreased (this is an ominous sign)
• C-reactive protein (CRP): elevated
• Blood culture: positive in septicemia, indicating bacteria is present in the blood
• Urine culture: may be positive, indicating presence of bacteria in the urine
• Cerebrospinal fluid analysis: may reveal increased white blood cells and protein and low glucose
• Stool culture: may be positive for bacteria or other infectious organisms
• Culture of tubes, catheters, or shunts suspected to be infected: the fluid inside those tubes may be tested to detect the presence of bacteria
• Chest X-ray: may reveal signs of pneumonia such as hyperinflation and patchy areas of atelectasis or infiltration

Nursing Management

Monitor the infant or child closely for changes in condition, especially the development of shock. Administer antibiotics as ordered. Refer to Nursing Care Plan 36.1 for nursing diagnoses and related interventions. In addition to these interventions, reducing risk of infection and providing education to the child and family should be noted.

Preventing Infection

Sepsis is a potentially life-threatening illness, and prevention is important. Handwashing is the most effective intervention against nosocomial infection. Nurses play a key role in minimizing environmental sources through proper cleaning of equipment and disposal of soiled linens and dressings as well as adhering to proper aseptic technique with all invasive procedures. Following your institution's policies and using evidence-based practice guidelines for interventions such as invasive line dressing changes and intravenous tubing changes can help reduce the risk of infection. Encourage immunization as recommended. To reduce group B streptococcal infection in neonates, screen pregnant woman; if the results are positive, administer intrapartum antibiotics.

▶ **Take** NOTE!

There has been a dramatic reduction in invasive Haemophilus influenzae *type b (Hib) infections since the widespread use of the Hib vaccine (Centers for Disease Control and Prevention [CDC], 2008).*

Educating the Child and Family

Early recognition of the signs of sepsis is essential in preventing morbidity and mortality. Educate parents about the importance of fever, especially in neonates and infants less than 3 months old. Instruct parents to contact their health care provider if their infant or neonate has a fever. A health care provider should see any child with a fever accompanied by lethargy, poor responsiveness, or lack of facial expressions. Signs and symptoms of sepsis can be vague and vary from child to child. Parents need to be encouraged to contact their health care provider if they feel their febrile child is "just not acting right."

Bacterial Infections

Bacteria are one-celled organisms that can live, grow, and reproduce. They exist everywhere. Most are completely harmless, and some are very useful. Others can lead to disease either because they are in the wrong place in the body or they are designed to invade and cause disease in humans and animals. Children are at a high risk of developing bacterial infections, which can result in life-threatening illness. Fortunately, many bacterial diseases, such as diphtheria, pertussis, and tetanus, can be prevented by immunization (see Chapter 30 for more information related to immunizations).

Scarlet Fever

Scarlet fever is an infection resulting from a group A *Streptococcus*. The bacteria produce a toxin that causes a rash. Not all children with a group A streptococcal infection will develop the rash of scarlet fever. Only those who are infected with streptococci that produce pyrogenic exotoxins but who lack antitoxin antibodies, making them sensitive to the bacterial toxin, will develop scarlet fever (Gerber, 2007). It is usually seen in children less than 18 years of age, with the peak incidence between the ages of 4 and 8 years; it is rare in children less than 2 years (Balentine & Lombardi, 2010). Transmission is airborne and follows contact with respiratory tract secretions. Close contact that occurs in schools and child care centres facilitates transmission. Foodborne outbreaks have occurred due to human contamination of food. After exposure, the incubation period is 2 to 5 days (Gerber, 2007). Communicability is highest during acute infection, and the child is no longer contagious 24 hours after the initiation of appropriate antimicrobial therapy (Gerber, 2007). There has been a dramatic decrease in the mortality from scarlet fever due to antibiotic use, but complications such as rheumatic fever and glomerulonephritis still exist (Balentine & Lombardi, 2010; Gerber, 2007).

Nursing Assessment

Symptoms of scarlet fever begin abruptly. The history may reveal a fever greater than 38.5°C, chills, body aches, loss of appetite, nausea, and vomiting. Inspect the pharynx, which is usually very red and swollen. The tonsils may have yellow or white specks of pus, and cervical lymph nodes may be swollen. Inspect the skin for the most striking symptom of scarlet fever, which is an erythematous rash appearing on the face, trunk, and extremities. The rash is typically absent from the palms of the hands and soles of the feet. It looks like a sunburn but feels like sandpaper (Fig. 36.1). The rash lasts

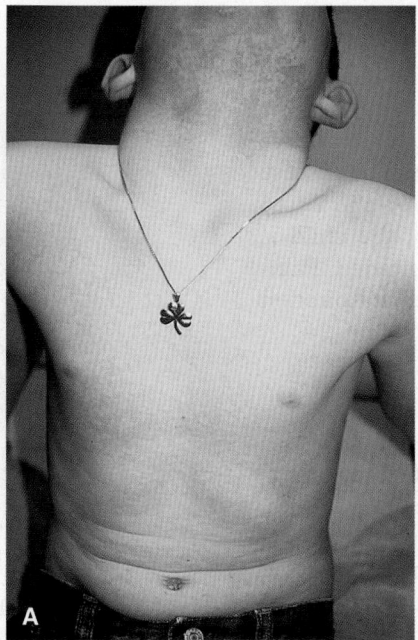
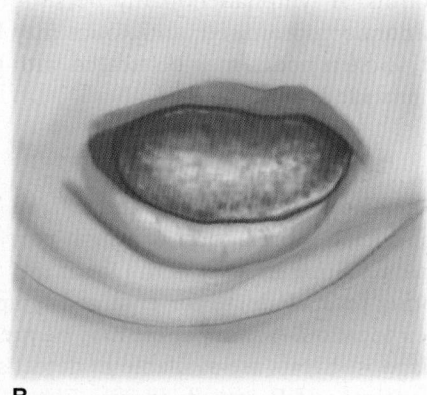

FIGURE 36.1 (**A**) Rash of scarlet fever. (**B**) Strawberry tongue.

approximately 5 days and is followed by desquamation, typically on the fingers and toes. Early in the illness the tongue develops a thick coat with a strawberry appearance. The tongue will later lose the coating and become bright red (see Fig. 36.1).

Diagnosis is made by identification of group A *Streptococcus* on throat culture. Several rapid tests for group A streptococcal pharyngitis are available. The accuracy of these tests depends on the quality of the specimen. It is important that the secretions obtained are pharyngeal or tonsillar (refer to Common Medical Treatments 36.1 for more information on throat cultures).

Nursing Management

Care of the child with scarlet fever will usually occur at home. Penicillin V is the antibiotic of choice. In those sensitive to penicillin, erythromycin may be used. Educate the family on the importance of taking the antibiotic as directed and finishing all the medicine.

Encourage fluid intake to maintain adequate hydration due to fever. Teach parents ways to provide comfort for the child. A cool mist humidifier can help soothe the child's sore throat. Soft foods, warm liquids like soup, or cold foods such as ice pops may also be helpful. If the child is hospitalized, droplet precautions, along with standard precautions, are necessary.

Cat Scratch Disease

Cat scratch disease is a relatively common and occasionally serious disease caused by the bacteria *Bartonella henselae*. It occurs in both children and adults but is more frequent in children (KidsHealth, 2009). Cats can carry the bacteria in their saliva, and in 90% of cases the child has had a recent interaction with cats and often kittens (AAP, 2006). No evidence exists to support person-to-person transmission (KidsHealth, 2009). *B. henselae* is transmitted between cats via the cat flea. The incubation period is 7 to 12 days, with lymphadenopathy appearing in 5 to 50 days. Therapeutic management is supportive and is aimed at management of symptoms. The disease itself is usually self-limiting resolving on its own in 2 to 4 months. If lymphadenopathy persists or if the child is immunocompromised, antibiotics may be needed. Painful, swollen nodes may be treated with needle aspiration to provide symptom relief.

Nursing Assessment

Note history of headaches and fatigue. The history may also include interaction or rough play with cats or kittens, resulting in a scratch. Document the temperature, noting fever. Palpate for enlarged lymph nodes, noting their location. A skin papule may be present or reported. Diagnostic tests are available to detect serum antibodies to antigens of *Bartonella* species.

Nursing Management

Administer antibiotics if ordered. No transmission-based isolation is required; standard precautions are sufficient. Educate the child and family about prevention and control measures. Teach children to avoid rough play with cats and kittens. Teach parents and children to immediately wash any bites or scratches with soap and running water. Explain that cats should never lick open wounds on the child. Control of fleas in cats is important to prevent the spread of *B. henselae*.

Diphtheria

Diphtheria is caused by infection with *Corynebacterium diphtheriae* and may affect the nose, larynx, tonsils, or pharynx. Tonsillar and pharyngeal infections are the most common and will be the focus of this discussion. A pseudomembrane forms over the pharynx, uvula, tonsils, and soft palate (Fig. 36.2). The neck becomes edematous and lymphadenopathy develops. The pseudomembrane causes airway obstruction and suffocation. Diphtheria generally occurs in children less than 15 years old who are unimmunized. Routine infant immunization can prevent the disease from occurring. Therapeutic management involves administration of antibiotics and antitoxin, as well as airway management.

Nursing Assessment

Children at risk of diphtheria are those who are unimmunized. Note history of sore throat and fever, usually less than 38.9°C. As the pseudomembrane forms, swallowing becomes difficult and signs of airway obstruction

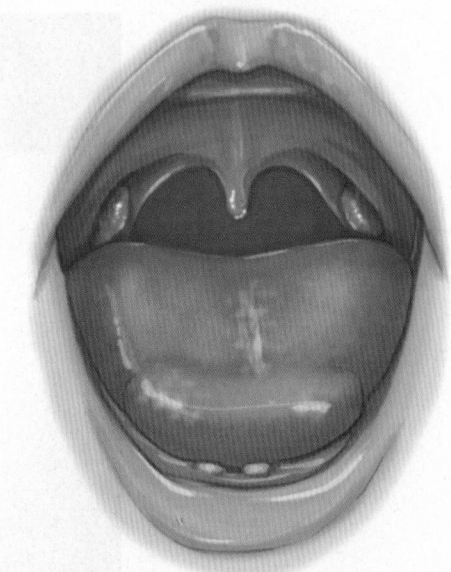

FIGURE 36.2 In diphtheria a pseudomembrane forms over the pharynx, uvula, tonsils, and soft palate.

become apparent. A specimen of the membrane may be cultured for *C. diphtheriae*.

Nursing Management

Close observation of respiratory status is of utmost importance. Administration of antibiotics and the antitoxin is critical to encourage sloughing of the membrane. The child should remain on strict droplet precautions in addition to standard precautions and should maintain bed rest.

Pertussis

Pertussis is an acute respiratory disorder characterized by paroxysmal cough (whooping cough) and copious secretions. The highest incidence is seen in children less than 1 year of age, with children less than 6 months of age at greatest risk of severe disease and death (CDC, 2010b). The disease is caused by *Bordetella pertussis*. The incubation period is 6 to 21 days, usually 7 to 10 days. Pertussis usually starts with 7 to 10 days of cold symptoms. The paroxysmal coughing spells then begin and can last 1 to 4 weeks. Convalescence occurs over the course of several weeks to months. Immunization has decreased the incidence of pertussis, but the increasing numbers of unimmunized children, particularly immigrants, contribute to the incidence of the disease. Additionally, the efficacy of the pertussis vaccine is reported to be about 85%; therefore, some individuals who have been vaccinated will still contract the disease (PHAC, 2006). Complications include seizures, pneumonia, encephalopathy, and death.

Therapeutic Management

Therapeutic management of pertussis focuses on eradication of the bacterial infection and respiratory support. Guidelines developed by the National Consensus Conference on Pertussis (PHAC, 2003) include antimicrobial treatment. Recommended drugs include erythromycin, clarithromycin, or azithromycin.

Nursing Assessment

The most important risk factor for the development of pertussis is the lack of immunization against it. The history may reveal cold and cough symptoms, progressing to paroxysmal coughing spells. During the paroxysms, the child might cough 10 to 30 times in a row, followed by a whooping sound. This might be accompanied by redness in the face, progressive cyanosis, and protrusion of the tongue. Saliva, mucus, and tears flow from the mouth, nose, and eyes. Between the paroxysmal episodes, the child might rest well and appear relatively unaffected. Auscultate the lungs to assess air exchange. The diagnosis may be confirmed by a variety of laboratory tests accompanied by clinical history. Culture is considered the gold standard, but polymerase chain reaction is used by some laboratories due to its increased sensitivity and faster results (CDC, 2011a).

Nursing Management

Nursing care will focus on providing a high-humidity environment and suctioning frequently to mobilize secretions. Observe for signs of airway obstruction. Encourage fluids to keep secretions thin and maintain adequate hydration. Offer reassurance to the child and family; the coughing episodes can be very frightening. Droplet precautions along with standard precautions are necessary for the hospitalized child.

Tetanus

Tetanus is an acute, often fatal neurologic disease caused by the toxins produced by *Clostridium tetani*. Tetanus is rare in Canada but continues to be significant worldwide due to lack of routine immunization. It is characterized by increased muscle tone and spasm. *C. tetani* spores can live anywhere but are found most commonly in soil, dust, and feces from humans or animals, such as sheep, cattle, chickens, dogs, cats, and rats. The spores can enter the body through a wound that is contaminated, through a burn or by injecting contaminated street drugs. Once it enters the body, an anaerobic environment allows it to multiply and a poisonous toxin is released.

There are four forms of tetanus. Neonatal tetanus is the most common worldwide, affecting newborns in the first week of life secondary to an infected umbilical stump or unsterile surgical technique during circumcision (Arnon, 2007). Most women in Canada have been immunized and will pass the immunity to their fetus. Maternal immunization along with proper hygiene during delivery and adequate cord care make this type of tetanus rare in Canada, but in underdeveloped countries it remains a significant problem. The second form is local tetanus. This rare form is characterized by local muscle spasms within the area of a wound. The third type is cephalic tetanus, which is associated with recurrent otitis media or head trauma. It is also rare and affects the cranial nerves, especially facial nerves. Generalized tetanus is the most common form and results in spasms that progress in a descending fashion beginning at the jaw. The most profoundly affected muscles are those of the neck and back. In Canada, the fatality rate associated with tetanus has declined and cases are rare; the last tetanus-related death in Canada was reported in 1997 (PHAC, 2006). The general incubation period is 3 to 21 days; it averages 8 days. Recovery can be long and difficult, and children with tetanus may have to spend several weeks in the hospital in an intensive care setting. It has been suggested that the shorter the incubation period, the higher the risk of more severe illness and the poorer the prognosis will be. Complications associated with tetanus include breathing problems, fractures, elevated blood pressure, dysrhythmias, clotting in the blood vessels of the lung, pneumonia, and coma.

Therapeutic management is directed toward supporting respiratory and cardiovascular function. Tetanus immunoglobulin may be given as well as the tetanus vaccine. Removal of the offending organism, by debridement of the wound, may occur, and intravenous antibiotics such as metronidazole may be initiated. In severe cases, the child may require intensive nursing care with mechanical ventilation.

Nursing Assessment

Note history of initial signs such as headache, spasms, crankiness, and cramping of the jaw (lockjaw), which are followed by difficulty swallowing and a stiff neck. Tetanus progresses in a descending fashion to other muscle groups, causing spasms of the neck, arms, legs, and stomach; seizures may result. Document the presence of fever along with an elevated blood pressure and tachycardia. Opisthotonos may be noted due to severe spasms of the neck and back. The spasms or muscle contractions in children may be strong enough to result in fractures. The diagnosis of tetanus is based on the clinical findings of the history and physical examination.

Nursing Management

Nursing management focuses on observing for signs of respiratory distress. Provide a quiet environment with reduced external stimuli to decrease the incidence of spasms. Appropriately manage pain. Encourage adequate nutrition and hydration. Administer sedatives and muscle relaxants as ordered to reduce the pain associated with the muscle spasms and to prevent seizures. Encourage the parents to stay with their child. The child's mental status is unaffected by the disease, and therefore he or she is aware of what is happening. Efforts need to be made to reduce the child's anxiety and to provide reassuring, sympathetic care to the child and family.

Tetanus is a preventable but potentially fatal disease. Education is essential regarding the importance of receiving this routine immunization (refer to Chapter 30 for immunization schedule) as well as a booster every 10 years. Instructing parents on proper wound care can also help prevent tetanus. All wounds should be cleaned thoroughly and a proper antiseptic used. If a wound is deep and contamination is suspected, the child should be seen by a health care professional. If it has been more than 5 years since the last tetanus dose, a booster may be needed. This can help to neutralize the poison and prevent it from entering the nervous system.

Viral Infections

Viruses are very small particles that infect cells. They cannot multiply on their own and require a living host, such as humans, animals, or plants. They can reproduce only by invading and taking over the host cells. Young children are highly sensitive to viruses. Their resistance is low and

exposure is high. Viruses are hard to destroy without damaging or killing the living cells they infect. This is why drugs are not used to control them. Many viral diseases, including measles, rubella, varicella, mumps, and poliomyelitis, can be prevented by immunization (see Chapter 30 for more information on immunizations).

Viral Exanthems

Many viral infections of the skin in childhood are called viral exanthems. **Exanthem** means rash or skin eruption. Viral exanthems of childhood often present with a distinct rash pattern that assists in the diagnosis of the virus. Table 36.4 discusses common childhood exanthems.

Typically, children with viral exanthems are cared for at home, but there are times when a child may be hospitalized or may develop the disease while being hospitalized. Appropriate transmission-based precautions must be taken.

Immunizations have led to a decrease in the incidence of certain viral exanthems, such as measles, rubella, and varicella (refer to Chapter 30 for immunization information).

Therapeutic management of the viral exanthems focuses on fever management and relief of discomfort.

Nursing Assessment

Obtain the history of the present illness, noting the onset of rash in relation to the onset of fever. Note accompanying symptoms such as respiratory complaints. Document known exposure to childhood diseases. Note immunization status. Inspect the skin for rash, noting the distribution, type, and extent of lesions. Table 36.4 describes the rash as well as accompanying symptoms for each of the viral exanthems.

Nursing Management

Nursing management of viral exanthems focuses on fever reduction, relief of discomfort, and protection of skin integrity. Encourage hydration. Administer antipyretics and antipruritics as needed (refer to Drug Guide 36.1). Nonpharmacologic interventions to reduce fever, such as tepid sponging and cool compresses, may be used. Refer to Nursing Care Plan 36.1 for additional information; care should be individualized based on the child's and family's response to the illness.

> ▶ *Take NOTE!*
>
> *Trim the child's fingernails or cover hands with mitts, gloves, or socks (which work well with younger infants and children) if the rash itches to help prevent breaks in the skin, which can lead to discomfort and infection.*

(text continues on page 1154)

TABLE 36.4 COMMON VIRAL EXANTHEMS OF CHILDHOOD

Disease	Causative Organism	Source	Transmission	Incubation Period	Period of Communicability
Rubella (German measles)	Rubella virus	Primarily nasopharyngeal secretions; also present in blood, stool, and urine of infected persons Peak incidence during late winter and early spring	Usually direct or indirect contact with droplets Mother to fetus	14 to 23 days, usually 16 to 18	7 days before to 7 days after onset of rash
Rubeola (measles)	Measles virus	Nasopharyngeal secretions, blood, and urine of infected persons	Highly contagious Usually direct or indirect contact with droplets	10 to 12 days	1 to 2 days before the onset of symptoms (3 to 5 days before onset of rash) to 5 days after rash has appeared
Varicella zoster virus (chickenpox)	Varicella zoster, human herpes virus (HHV) 3	Nasopharyngeal secretions Peak occurrence late fall, winter, and spring	Highly contagious Direct contact with infected persons or airborne spread, to a lesser degree contact with lesions (scabbed lesions are not infectious) Can be transmitted transplacentally from mother to fetus	14 to 21 days, usually 14 to 16	1 to 2 days before onset of rash until all vesicles have crusted over (about 3 to 7 days after onset of rash)
Exanthem subitum (roseola infantum or sixth disease)	HHV-6; less frequently HHV-7	Unknown, but most adults secrete HHV-6 and HHV-7 in saliva, so may serve as primary source Usually limited to children <3 years old; peak incidence 6 to 15 months of age	Little is known; suspected to be from saliva of infected person and enters the host through the oral, nasal, or conjunctival mucosa	5 to 15 days, average of 10 days	Unknown, but most likely contagious during fever stage

(continued)

TABLE 36.4 COMMON VIRAL EXANTHEMS OF CHILDHOOD (continued)

Disease	Causative Organism	Source	Transmission	Incubation Period	Period of Communicability
Erythema infectiosum (fifth disease)	Human parvovirus B19	Infected person Seasonal peaks are in late winter and early spring.	Respiratory route Large droplet spread from nasopharyngeal viral shedding Percutaneous exposure to blood and blood products Mother to fetus	4 to 21 days, average 16 to 17 days	Uncertain, but most children are no longer infectious by the time the rash appears and diagnosis is made Isolation or exclusion from school, once child is diagnosed, is unnecessary Those with aplastic crisis may be communicable up to 1 week after onset of symptoms Those who are immuno-suppressed with chronic infection and severe anemia may be communicable for months to years
Hand, foot and mouth disease, or herpan-gina (if only mouth) involvement	Coxsackie A viruses (espe-cially A16)	Spread via fecal–oral route, particularly in children who wear diapers (1- to 4-year-olds) Most common during spring and summer	Direct contact with infected fecal, oral secretions; spread mostly through saliva	3 to 6 days	From time of infection until fever resolves; virus is shed for several weeks after the infection begins

Disease		Clinical Manifestations	Management/Complications	Nursing Implications
Rubella (German measles)	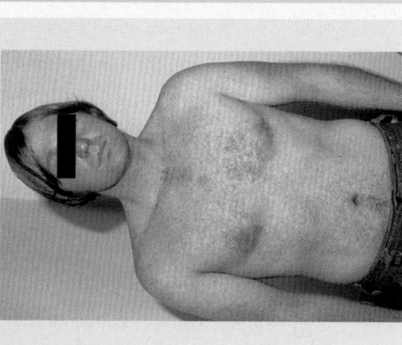	• Characteristic sign is lymphadenopathy (retroauricular, posterior cervical, postoccipital) 24 hours before the onset of the rash; may last up to 1 week • Rash begins on face and spreads quickly down the neck, trunk, and extremities; on the second day the rash may appear pinpoint and resemble the rash of scarlet fever • Mild pruritus may occur • The rash disappears in the same order it spread and is usually cleared by the third day. Desquamation is minimal • Rubella without a rash has been noted • Polyarthralgia and polyarthritis are rare in children but common in adolescents	• Disease is usually mild and self-limiting • Treatment is mainly supportive • Complications: encephalitis and thrombocytopenia are rare • Maternal rubella during pregnancy can result in miscarriage, fetal death, or congenital malformations	• Institute comfort measures, such as antipyretics, antipruritics, and analgesics for joint pain • Contact precautions in addition to standard precautions for the duration of the illness in the hospitalized child • Avoid exposure to pregnant women
Rubeola (measles)	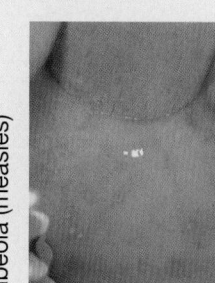 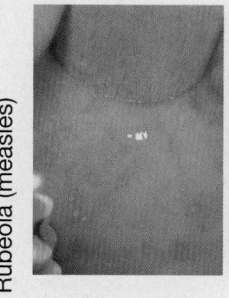	• Prodromal phase: 3 to 5 days, consisting of fever, cough, coryza (inflammation of the mucous membranes lining the nose), conjunctivitis • Followed by Koplik spots • Erythematous maculopapular rash appears 3 to 4 days after the onset of the prodromal phase	• AAP recommends consideration of vitamin A supplementation in children 6 months to 2 years hospitalized for measles or its complications or those with measles and immunodeficiency (Behrman et al., 2007) • In developing countries, treatment with vitamin A can reduce morbidity and mortality • Treatment is mainly supportive; may include antipyretics, bed rest, maintenance of adequate fluid intake • Complications: otitis media bronchopneumonia, laryngotracheobronchitis (croup), and diarrhea common in young children; acute encephalitis	• Institute comfort measures, such as antipyretics and antipruritics • Provide eye care: clean eyes with warm, moist cloth to remove secretions • Soothe coryza and cough using cool mist humidification to alleviate symptoms • Droplet precautions until fifth day of rash in addition to standard precautions

(continued)

TABLE 36.4 **COMMON VIRAL EXANTHEMS OF CHILDHOOD** (continued)

Disease	Clinical Manifestations	Management/Complications	Nursing Implications
Varicella zoster virus (chickenpox) 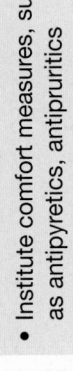	• Prodromal symptoms may be present 24 to 48 hours before the onset of the rash, such as fever, malaise, anorexia, headache, and mild abdominal pain • Lesions often appear first on scalp, face, and trunk; initially intensely pruritic erythematous macules that evolve to papules and then form clear, fluid-filled vesicles • Vesicles eventually erupt, and then lesions scab and crust • More severe in adolescents and adults than in young children	• Treatment: antiviral therapy and varicella zoster immune globulin may be used in those considered to be at high risk, such as the immunocompromised, pregnant women, and newborns exposed to maternal varicella • PHAC does not recommend routine antiviral therapy for treatment of uncomplicated varicella infection in otherwise healthy children • In most cases, varicella infection is self-limiting • Treatment is mainly supportive: fever reduction, antipruritics to relieve itching, and skin care to prevent infection of lesions • Complications: bacterial superinfection of skin lesions, thrombocytopenia, arthritis, hepatitis, cerebellar ataxia, encephalitis, meningitis, pneumonia, and glomerulonephritis • Congenital infection and life-threatening perinatal infection • Varicella zoster results in a lifelong latent infection. Reactivation results in herpes zoster (shingles), uncommon in childhood	• Institute comfort measures, such as antipyretics and antipruritics • Airborne and contact precautions, in addition to standard precautions in the hospitalized child for a minimum of 5 days after onset of rash and as long as vesicular lesions are present • For those with exposure to susceptible persons, airborne and contact precautions, in addition to standard precautions from 8 to 21 days after exposure • Children may return to school or child care once lesions have crusted
Exanthem subitum (roseola infantum)	• Prodromal phase: usually asymptomatic but may include upper respiratory signs • Clinical illness: high fever ranging from 37.9° to 40°C for 3 to 5 days; resolves abruptly; rash appears 12 to 24 hours later; rash usually lasts 1 to 3 days	• Generally benign; children generally are quite comfortable • In children who are uncomfortable or irritable or have a history of febrile seizures, antipyretics may be warranted • Complications: may be responsible for some febrile seizures • Can progress to central nervous system involvement, encephalitis, and meningoencephalitis (rare)	• Institute comfort measures, such as antipyretics, antipruritics • Standard precautions are sufficient in the hospitalized child

| Erythema infectiosum (fifth disease) | 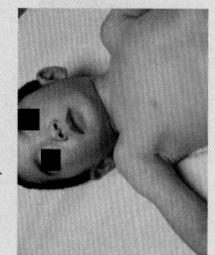 | • Prodromal phase: mild symptoms, low-grade fever, headache, mild upper respiratory infection
• Characteristic rash presents in three stages:
• Begins with erythematous flushing and often described as "slapped-cheek" appearance, often with circumoral pallor
• Spreads to trunk
• Moves peripherally, presenting as a maculopapular, lace-like appearance
• Palms and soles are usually spared; rash often is pruritic.
• Rash fluctuates in intensity and will disappear and reappear with environmental changes such as exposure to sunlight
• Rash resolves spontaneously over 1 to 3 weeks
• Children with preexisting anemias may develop aplastic crisis
• In children with aplastic crisis rash is usually absent, but may present with prodromal symptoms of fever, malaise, and myalgia | • Disease in usually benign and self-limiting
• Supportive treatment: antipyretics and antipruritics to improve comfort
• Children with hemolytic disease, such as sickle cell, or immunodeficiency are at risk of aplastic crisis
• Blood transfusion may be necessary in children with aplastic crisis
• Complications: arthritis and arthralgia
• May result in fetal loss if mother is infected during pregnancy (greatest risk seems to be in second trimester). Can also result in congestive heart failure (hydrops fetalis). The risk of transplacental infection is 30% if the woman is infected during pregnancy (Weir, 2005) | • Institute comfort measures, such as antipyretics, antipruritics
• Droplet precautions in addition to standard precautions are required in the hospitalized child
• Pregnant women (including health care workers) need to be informed of the potential risks to the fetus and preventive measures to decrease these risks (strict infection control practices, not caring for those likely to be contagious, such as immunocompromised patients with chronic parvovirus infection or patients with parvovirus-associated aplastic crisis)
• Routine exclusion from a workplace where an outbreak is occurring is not recommended |
| Hand, foot, and mouth disease | | • Vesicles on tongue and oral mucosa erode to shallow ulcers; vesicles on hands and feet are football-shaped with erythematous rims. Fever usually occurs first. Extensive mouth lesions may lead to anorexia, dehydration, and drooling | • Disease is usually mild and self-limiting, resolving within 1 week
• Treatment is mainly supportive
• Dehydration may occur if mouth lesions are significant. Meningitis, encephalitis, and pulmonary edema are rare complications | • Contact precautions and good hand hygiene are necessary.
Encourage oral fluids of preference, ice pops. Provide analgesics such as acetaminophen as needed |

Adapted from Siegel, J. D., Rhinehart, E., Jackson, M., Chiarello, L., & the Healthcare Infection Control Practices Advisory Committee. (2007). *Guideline for isolation precautions: Preventing transmission of infectious agents in healthcare settings*. Retrieved June 8, 2011, from http://www.cdc.gov/hicpac/pdf/isolation/Isolation2007.pdf; Mason, W. H. (2007). Rubella. In R. M. Kliegman, R. E. Behrman, H. B. Jenson, & B. F. Stanton (Eds.), *Nelson's textbook of pediatrics* (18th ed., pp. 1337–1341). Philadelphia, PA: Saunders; Mason, W. H. (2007). Measles. In R. M. Kliegman, R. E. Behrman, H. B. Jenson, & B. F. Stanton (Eds.), *Nelson's textbook of pediatrics* (18th ed., pp. 1331–1336). Philadelphia, PA: Saunders; Myers, M. G., Seward, J. F., & LaRussa, P. S. (2007). Varicella-zoster virus. In R. M. Kliegman, R. E. Behrman, H. B. Jenson, & B. F. Stanton (Eds.), *Nelson's textbook of pediatrics* (18th ed., pp. 1366–1372). Philadelphia, PA: Saunders; Leach, C. T. (2007). Roseola (human herpes viruses 6 and 7). In R. M. Kliegman, R. E. Behrman, H. B. Jenson, & B. F. Stanton (Eds.), *Nelson's textbook of pediatrics* (18th ed., pp. 1380–1383). Philadelphia, PA: Saunders; Koch, W. C. (2007). Parvovirus B19. In R. M. Kliegman, R. E. Behrman, H. B. Jenson, & B. F. Stanton (Eds.), *Nelson's textbook of pediatrics* (18th ed., pp. 1357–1360). Philadelphia, PA: Saunders; Abzug, M. J. (2007). Nonpolio enteroviruses. In R. M. Kliegman, R. E. Behrman, H. B. Jenson, & B. F. Stanton (Eds.), *Nelson's textbook of pediatrics* (18th ed., pp. 1350–1356). Philadelphia, PA: Saunders; and Centers for Disease Control and Prevention. (2010). *Hand, foot and mouth disease (HFMD)*. Retrieved June 20, 2011 from http://www.cdc.gov/ncidod/dvrd/revb/enterovirus/hfht.htm

Varicella

Varicella or chickenpox is caused by the herpes virus varicella zoster. Varicella is spread both by airborne droplets and through contact with skin lesions. Following a primary infection (chickenpox), the virus becomes dormant in the sensory nerve ganglia and can become reactivated in the form of herpes zoster or shingles. The incubation period for varicella is 10 days to 3 weeks; individuals are contagious for 1 to 2 days before the outbreak of the vesicular rash and remain infectious until all lesions have crusted. The incidence of chickenpox has decreased dramatically since the introduction of universal vaccinations. Today, chickenpox occurs primarily in unvaccinated children, with 90% of all susceptible children having the disease by age 12 (PHAC, 2006). Complications of chickenpox include scarring, secondary bacterial infections, otitis media, pneumonia, endocarditis, osteomyelitis, and septic arthritis. Complications are more common in adolescents and pregnant women. Congenital varicella, while rare, can cause scarring, limb atrophy, cerebellar atrophy, and eye abnormalities.

Nursing Assessment

Inquire about exposure to infected individuals and immunization status. Note history of fever, malaise, anorexia, headache, cough, and coryza. Examine the skin for the characteristic rash: whose lesions appear first on the trunk or face and then spread to the limbs. Lesions begin as red macules; they then progress to form vesicles and pustules and then finally crust over. Lesions in various stages are usually seen at the same time; this is a classic finding in chickenpox.

Nursing Management

Nursing management is primarily supportive and directed at reducing the intense pruritus that accompanies varicella lesions. Acetaminophen is used to manage fever, and oral fluids should be encouraged to prevent dehydration. The child's fingernails should be kept short to discourage scratching. Cool compresses or frequent baths can be used to relieve itching. Baking soda may be added to the bath water for additional relief. Hospitalized patients should be placed in respiratory isolation. Immunocompromised children exposed to chickenpox should be treated prophylactically with varicella zoster immunoglobulin. The CPS (2008c) recommends that children with mild cases of chickenpox be allowed to return to school or day care when they are well enough to participate in normal activities. In Canada, the varicella vaccine is currently recommended for children between 12 and 18 months of age (see Chapter 30 for information related to varicella vaccination).

Mumps

Mumps, a contagious disease caused by *Paramyxovirus,* is characterized by fever and parotitis (inflammation and swelling of the parotid gland). Mumps is spread via contact with infected droplets. Infected individuals are contagious for 1 to 7 days prior to onset of symptoms and for 7 to 9 days after parotid swelling begins. The PHAC (2006) recommends immunization against mumps for all children. Mumps occurs most frequently in unimmunized children between 5 and 19 years of age. About one third of all infected prepubertal boys also develop orchitis (inflammation of the testicle). Complications of mumps include meningoencephalitis with seizures and auditory neuritis, which can result in deafness. Therapeutic management is supportive.

Nursing Assessment

Note history of exposure to infected individuals as well as immunization status. Determine history of low-grade fever and onset and progression of parotid swelling. History may also include malaise, anorexia, headache, and abdominal pain. The parotid swelling is easily observed as swelling of the neck either bilaterally or unilaterally (Fig. 36.3). In boys, note orchitis. The diagnosis is usually based on the history and clinical presentation, but serum may be tested for the presence of mumps immunoglobulin G (IgG) or IgM **antibody**.

Nursing Management

Nursing management of mumps is primarily supportive. Acetaminophen is used for fever management, and occasionally narcotic analgesics may be required for pain management. Oral fluids are encouraged to prevent dehydration. If orchitis is present, ice packs to the testicles and gentle testicular support may be helpful. Hospitalized patients

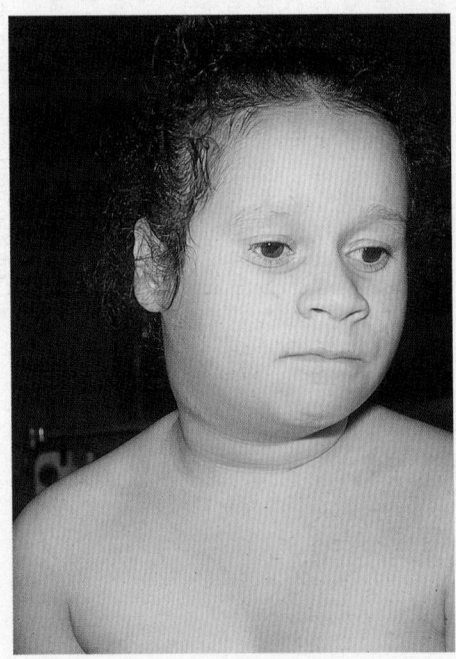

FIGURE 36.3 Parotitis associated with mumps.

should be confined to respiratory isolation to prevent spread of the disease. Infected children are considered no longer contagious 9 days following onset of parotid swelling. Current recommendations include first mumps immunization on or after the child's first birthday followed by a second vaccine between 4 and 6 years of age (see Chapter 30 for information related to mumps vaccination).

> ▶ *Take* NOTE!
>
> *Mumps outbreaks have occurred in recent years, mainly in under-immunized communities or on university campuses. The mumps vaccine is not 100% effective, and mumps infection can be seen in vaccinated individuals. According to the CDC (2011b), one dose of the measles mumps rubella vaccine is estimated to prevent 62% to 91% of cases and two doses prevent 76% to 95% of cases. By 1995, high numbers of two-dose childhood vaccinations reduced the rate of mumps in the United States by 99%. During an outbreak it is essential to define the population at risk and the transmission setting, identify and isolate suspected cases, and identify and vaccinate susceptible individuals.*

Poliomyelitis

Poliomyelitis is an infection caused by the highly infectious poliovirus, which is an enterovirus. The virus invades the central nervous system and can progress to total paralysis. Transmission occurs through direct or indirect contact. The poliovirus is spread most commonly via the fecal–oral route or by the oral–oral route. Polio most commonly occurs in young children and is also referred to as infantile paralysis. This disease is rare due to effective immunization programs but is still seen in developing countries in the eastern Mediterranean region, India, and Africa.

Nursing Assessment

Initial signs and symptoms include fever, fatigue, headache, vomiting, neck stiffness, and limb pain. Symptoms then progress to tremors of the extremities and possible paralysis. Kernig's sign will be positive and deep tendon reflexes will be hyperactive initially and then diminished. Paralysis is asymmetric and generally affects the legs more than the arms. Respiratory problems can occur if the respiratory centre of the brain is involved. The poliovirus can be isolated in feces or the pharynx of infected individuals, and cerebrospinal fluid evaluation will generally show elevated leukocytes and protein.

Nursing Management

Nursing management is aimed at providing supportive care, focusing on maintaining respiratory status and nutritional status until the illness has run its course. Bed rest will usually be ordered, so skin care is a priority. Encouragement to maintain self-care (as appropriate) and mobility are also important nursing functions. Long-term care, including physical therapy and bracing to help strengthen muscles, may be needed during and after hospitalization.

No cure for polio exists, but it can be prevented by the polio vaccine, which is routinely administered in developed countries (refer to the immunization schedule in Chapter 30). Oral polio vaccine (OPV) is a live strain, and thus the virus is shed in the stool for up to 6 weeks after immunization, leading to the risk of vaccine-acquired polio in caregivers. For this reason, OPV has been replaced in Canada by inactivated polio vaccine, an injectable form. However, OPV is still used in developing countries, so immigrants or travelers whose children were recently immunized in their home country should take precautions if they are immunocompromised or unvaccinated. Areas where polio is endemic, including Afghanistan, Egypt, India, Niger, Nigeria, and Pakistan, agreed to a massive immunization campaign in 2004 and hope to make polio the first eradicated disease of the 21st century (Stephenson, 2004).

Rabies

Rabies is a preventable viral infection of the central nervous system. It is transmitted to other animals and humans through close contact with the saliva of a rabid animal, usually by a bite. The number of human cases of rabies has steadily declined in Canada (Grill, 2009). It is rare in North America and Western Europe due to routine vaccination of domestic animals, such as dogs, and the availability of effective postexposure prophylaxis. Today, most cases of rabies in these areas are due to wild animals such as raccoons, skunks, foxes, and increasingly, bats (Immunization Action Coalition, 2010). Rabies continues to be a major health problem in other parts of the world, especially in areas where dogs are not controlled.

Most cases of rabies occur in children younger than 15 years of age, and most human deaths occur in Asia and Africa (WHO, 2011a). Children have an increased susceptibility to rabies due to their fearlessness around animals, eagerness to play with animals, shorter stature, and inability to protect themselves. The incubation period for rabies is extremely variable. Typically it is several weeks to months but can range from days to years (Immunization Action Coalition, 2010). The incubation period tends to be shorter in children. Once symptoms of rabies have developed the prognosis is poor: death usually occurs within days of the onset of symptoms. Prevention is paramount, and eliminating infection in animal vectors is essential. Successful animal vaccination and animal control campaigns in Canada have led to a very low rate of human rabies cases (Grill, 2009). Rabies among cats and dogs in Canada has been virtually eliminated. Recently, rabies transmitted from other animals, especially through bat bites, has become a cause for concern (Immunization Action Coalition, 2010).

The decision to provide postexposure prophylaxis can be complex. The local medical officer of health should be notified and the suspected case referred to the nearest Canadian Food Inspection Agency veterinarian. Several factors need to be considered, such as local epidemiology, the type of animal involved, the availability of the responsible animal for testing or quarantine, and the circumstances around the exposure, such as a provoked versus unprovoked attack. In Canada, concurrent use of passive and active immunoprophylaxis is recommended (Grill, 2009). This consists of a regimen of one dose of immune globulin and five doses of human rabies vaccine over a 28-day period. Rabies immune globulin and the first dose of rabies vaccine should be given as soon as possible after exposure, ideally within 24 hours. Additional doses of rabies vaccine should be given on days 3, 7, 14, and 28 after the first vaccination. Rabies immune globulin is infiltrated into and around the wound, with any remaining volume administered intramuscularly at a site distant from the vaccine inoculation. Human rabies vaccine is administered intramuscularly into the anterolateral thigh or deltoid, depending on the age and size of the child. Administration into the gluteus muscle should be avoided, since this site has been associated with vaccine failure (Rupprecht et al., 2010; Toltzis, 2007).

Nursing Assessment

Note history of an animal bite, especially if it was unprovoked, and exposure to bats. Document history of early symptoms of rabies infection, which are nonspecific and flu-like, such as fever, headache, and general malaise. The child may complain of pain, pruritus, and paresthesia at the bite site. As the virus spreads to the central nervous system, encephalitis develops. The disease will have progressive neurologic manifestations, which may include insomnia, confusion, anxiety, changes in behaviour, agitation or excitation, hallucinations, hypersalivation, dysphagia, and hydrophobia, which results from aspiration when swallowing liquid or saliva. In some cases progressive paralysis may be present. The patient may have periods of lucidity alternating with these neurologic changes.

Laboratory testing may include hair and saliva specimens from which the virus may be isolated. Serum and cerebrospinal fluid can be tested for antibodies to the rabies virus. Direct fluorescent antibody testing can be done to diagnose rabies in a suspected animal. The test can only be done postmortem and requires brain tissue from the potentially rabid animal.

Nursing Management

Few patients survive once symptomatic rabies infection develops. Intensive supportive care is required, but recov-

ery is extremely rare. Therefore, it is vital to educate children and families about the importance of seeking medical care after any animal bite to prevent death from rabies infection. Also, teach children to avoid wild animals, stray animals, and any animal with unusual behaviour. Teach children not to provoke or attempt to capture wild or stray animals.

Regardless of whether immunoprophylaxis is initiated, appropriate wound management is necessary in all victims of a bite from a potentially rabid animal. This includes a thorough cleansing of all wounds with soap and water. Irrigation of wounds for at least 10 minutes with a virucidal agent, such as povidone–iodine solution, is recommended (Toltzis, 2007).

When caring for a child requiring postexposure prophylaxis, provide support and education to the child and family. Due to the seriousness and urgency surrounding this disease and treatment, the child and family are often very frightened. Consider comfort measures, such as EMLA cream and positioning, when giving immunization.

Vector–Borne Infections

Children are at particular risk of contracting vector-borne diseases, which are diseases transmitted by ticks, mosquitoes, or other insect vectors (Table 36.5). Young children are unaware of the health risks around them and cannot take protective measures. Their immature immune system leads to a decreased capacity to resist vector-borne diseases. These diseases can be severe and even fatal, though most are treatable if identified early. Many times the child presents initially with nonspecific symptoms. Coupled with the fact that there are few definitive diagnostic tests available, this can lead to difficulty in promptly recognizing and treating these diseases.

Tick-borne diseases are becoming more prevalent in Canada. Lyme disease in particular has been reported in a number of provinces.

Lyme Disease

Lyme disease is caused by the spirochete *Borrelia burgdorferi*. It is transmitted to humans via the bite of an infected black-legged tick. Lyme disease has been reported in more than 50 countries, including Canada, and is now seen in parts of southern and southeastern Quebec, southern and eastern Ontario, southern Manitoba, New Brunswick, and Nova Scotia as well as much of southern British Columbia (PHAC, 2010). Most cases are seen between April and October. Lyme disease can affect any age group, but the reported incidence is highest among children 5 to 10 years of age (Behrman et al., 2007). The prognosis for recovery in children who are treated is excellent.

TABLE 36.5 OTHER VECTOR-BORNE ILLNESSES

Disease	Causative Organism	Geographic Distribution	Vector of Transmission	Manifestations
Mediterranean spotted fever (boutonneuse fever)	Rickettsia conorii	Africa, Mediterranean region, India, Middle East	Tick bite	• Fever, headache, maculopapular rash • Eschar may be present at tick bite
Rickettsial pox	Rickettsia akari	Northeastern cities in United States, Europe, and Asia, mainly urban settings	Mouse mite bite	• Bite becomes a papule, then pustule, then ulcerates and forms eschar at site. Fever, local adenopathy, headache, myalgia, maculopapular rash that may become vesicular
Epidemic typhus	Rickettsia prowazekii	Africa, South America, Central America, Mexico, Asia; occasional cases seen in United States Cases in United States associated with louse or flea of flying squirrel	Louse feces (typically from the body louse) that are rubbed into broken skin or mucous membranes	• Abrupt onset of high fever, chills, and myalgia with severe headache and malaise • Rash appears 4 to 7 days after onset of symptoms, beginning on the trunk and spreading to the extremities • Maculopapular rash becomes petechial or hemorrhagic, then develops brown pigmented areas • Changes in mental status may occur • Flying squirrel–related disease typically presents as a milder illness
Endemic typhus (murine typhus)	Rickettsia typhi and Rickettsia felis	Worldwide, especially warm coastal ports. In United States, most prevalent in southern Texas and southern California	Rat flea or cat flea feces	• Headache, myalgia, and chills that slowly worsen • Fever for 10 to 14 days • Rash appears after 3 to 8 days; it is macular or maculopapular with sparse lesions and no hemorrhage
Scrub typhus	Orientia tsutsugamushi	Southern Asia, Japan, Indonesia, Australia, Korea, Asiatic Russia, India, China	Chigger bite	• Possible necrotic eschar at site of bite, fever, headache, myalgia, cough, and gastrointestinal symptoms • Lymphadenopathy, maculopapular rash on trunk and extremities
Ehrlichiosis	3 pathogens: Ehrlichia chaffeensis, Anaplasma phagocytophilum, Ehrlichia ewingii	Mostly in southeastern and south-central United States	Tick	• Fever with clinical signs similar to Rocky Mountain spotted fever. Rash is less commonly associated • May also present with leukopenia, anemia, and hepatitis
Q fever	Coxiella burnetii	Worldwide	Inhalation of infected aerosols, ingestion of contaminated dairy products	• Most cases are initially asymptomatic. Occurs in two forms: • Acute: follows initial exposure and presents with abrupt onset of fever, chills, weakness, headache, and loss of appetite • Chronic: occurs years after initial exposure and may present with endocarditis (in patients with underlying heart disease), hepatitis, or fever of unknown origin
Malaria	Plasmodium (four species exist that infect humans: P. falciparum, P. vivax, P. ovale, P. malariae)	Endemic in tropical areas of the world Highest risk in sub-Saharan Africa, Papua New Guinea, the Solomon Islands, and Vanuatu Other areas of risk: Haiti and Indian subcontinent	Bite of Anopheles species of mosquito	• High fever with chills, rigours, sweats, and headache, which may be paroxysmal • Nausea, vomiting, diarrhea, cough, arthralgia; abdominal and back pain may also occur • Anemia and thrombocytopenia with pallor and jaundice may be seen • May occur in a cyclic pattern, and depending on the species fever may occur every other day or every third day

Therapeutic Management

In most cases Lyme disease can be cured by antibiotics, especially if they are started early in the illness. Doxycycline is the drug of choice for children older than 8 years (Shapiro, 2007). Because doxycycline can cause permanent discolouration of the teeth, children younger than 8 should be treated with amoxicillin (Shapiro, 2007). For patients allergic to penicillin, ceftriaxone or erythromycin can be used. Duration of treatment is usually 2 to 4 weeks.

Nursing Assessment

The clinical signs of Lyme disease are divided into three stages: early localized disease, early disseminated disease, and late disease. Untreated patients may progress through the three stages or may present with early disseminated or late disease without having any symptoms of the other stages. If children are treated in the early stage, it is uncommon to see them with late disease. Nursing assessment for Lyme disease includes an accurate health history as well as physical examination.

Health History

Explore the health history for a tick bite. Document onset of rash. In early localized disease, the rash usually occurs 7 to 14 days after the tick bite (though it can appear between 3 and 32 days after the bite). In early disseminated disease, the rash usually begins 3 to 5 weeks after the tick bite. Note complaints of fever, malaise, mild neck stiffness, headache, fatigue, myalgia, and arthralgia or pain in the joints. In late disease, note recurrent arthritis of the large joints, such as the knees, beginning weeks to months after the tick bite. The child with late disease may or may not have a history of earlier stages of the disease, including erythema migrans.

Physical Examination

Observe for a rash. Early local disease is characterized by a ring-like rash at the site of the tick bite (erythema migrans) (Fig. 36.4). If untreated, the rash gradually expands and will remain for 1 to 2 weeks. Early disseminated disease should be suspected if multiple areas of erythema migrans are found. The multiple lesions are usually smaller than the primary lesions. Note cranial nerve palsies (especially cranial nerve VII), conjunctivitis, or signs of meningeal irritation, which occur in early disseminated disease.

Laboratory and Diagnostic Testing

Immunoglobulin-specific antibody tests may not be positive in the early stage of Lyme disease but may be useful in the later stages. PHAC (2010) recommends a two-step approach to blood testing that includes an initial screening test followed by more blood testing on those samples that initially tested positive.

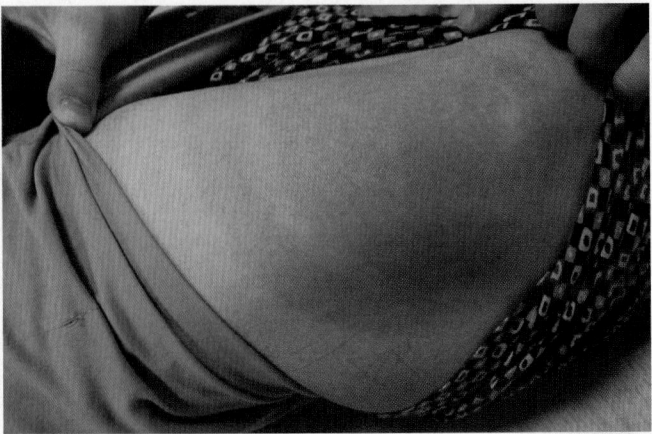

FIGURE 36.4 Erythema migrans, a ring-like rash at the site of the tick bite, occurs in Lyme disease.

Nursing Management

Administer antibiotics as ordered. In the hospitalized patient, no transmission-based precautions are necessary. Educate the patient and family on the importance of taking the antibiotic as directed and finishing all the medicine. Another important nursing function is educating the patient, family, and community on prevention measures (Box 36.5). For infection to occur, the tick must be attached for 36 to 48 hours (CDC, 2011c), so prompt removal of ticks is essential to the prevention of Lyme disease. Teaching Guideline 36.2 gives information on removal of ticks.

West Nile Virus

WNV is a potentially severe illness that in North America presents as a seasonal epidemic, flaring up in the summer and continuing into the fall. It is termed an "arbovirus" in that it is usually transmitted through the bite of mosquitoes, which have in turn acquired the virus via blood meal from infected birds. There is some suggestion that WNV can also be transmitted in utero, via blood transfusions, and during organ transplantation (Hayes & O'Leary, 2004). A single-stranded RNA virus,

---

BOX 36.5 ▶ Prevention of Tick-Borne Illnesses

- Wear appropriate protective clothing when entering possible tick-infested areas. Clothing should fit tightly around wrists, waist, and ankles. Tuck pants into socks if possible.
- After leaving the area, check for ticks and remove them promptly.
- Insect repellent may provide temporary relief but may produce toxicity, especially in children, if used frequently or in large doses.

TEACHING GUIDELINE 36.2

Tick Removal

- Use fine-tipped tweezers.
- Protect fingers with a tissue, paper towel, or latex gloves.
- Grasp tick as close to the skin as possible and pull upward with steady, even pressure.
- Do not twist or jerk the tick.
- Once the tick is removed, clean site with soap and water and wash your hands.
- Save the tick for identification in case the child becomes sick. Place in a sealable plastic bag and put it in the freezer. Write date of bite on the bag.

WNV is thought to replicate in dendritic cells at the portal of entry, from which it travels to lymph nodes and other organs. The incubation period can range from 2 to 14 days, and approximately 20% of children who become infected develop an illness attributable to the infection. The first confirmed case of WNV in Canada occurred in Ontario in 1999. Since then, there has been an increase in symptomatic cases, from 414 in 2002 (Quebec and Ontario) to 2,361 across Quebec, Ontario, Manitoba, Saskatchewan, and Alberta in 2007 (Artsob et al., 2009).

In cases in which illness does develop, symptoms typically include abrupt-onset fever (38° to 40°C), headache, myalgia, and anorexia. Abdominal pain, nausea, vomiting, and diarrhea are also frequently associated with WNV, whereas maculopapular rash, lymphadenopathy, sore throat, and cough are more variable symptoms (Petersen, Marfin, & Gubler, 2003). In uncomplicated cases, WNV infection typically resolves in less than 1 week; however, severe illness may result in myocarditis, pancreatitis, and fulminant hepatitis. In less than 1% of cases, patients may develop severe neurologic complications, including encephalitis and meningitis, although this is more common in adults than children. Encephalitis accounts for approximately 60% of neurologic cases, with severe muscle weakness and paresis commonly seen; flaccid paralysis and axonal neuropathy are noted in approximately 10% of such cases (CPS Infectious Diseases and Immunization Committee, 2003).

Therapeutic Management

Treatment is supportive. There are no effective antiviral agents for WNV, although several are being investigated. Killed viral vaccines are also being tested.

Nursing Assessment

WNV should be considered in any child who presents with a sudden-onset febrile episode or acute neurologic illness and who has had exposure to mosquitoes, blood transfusion, or organ transplantation. Definitive diagno-

sis of WNV can only be made via serum and/or cerebrospinal fluid laboratory testing, in which an enzyme-linked immunosorbent assay is used to detect IgM antibodies to the virus.

Nursing Management

Supportive nursing care for children with WNV is based on the severity and type of symptoms. Prevention is the best course, and nurses should educate families about possible strategies for avoiding infection. The first principle is avoidance, especially in areas where WNV-infected mosquitoes have been detected. Wearing clothing to cover exposed skin is a generally accepted preventive measure, as is judicious application of mosquito repellant. However, CPS advises the use of repellant formulations that contain no more than 10% *N,N*-diethyl-m-toluamide in children younger than 12 years of age and recommends against using *N,N*-diethyl-m-toluamide in infants younger than 6 months. Care should be taken to avoid the mouth and eyes when applying repellant. Mosquito bites may also be reduced by having children avoid outside play during times of peak mosquito activity (generally, dawn and dusk).

Parasitic and Helminthic Infections

Parasites are organisms larger than yeast or bacteria that can cause infection. They live in or on a host. Parasites receive nourishment from the host without benefiting or killing the host. Parasites frequently seen in children are scabies and head lice. A helminth is a parasitic intestinal worm. Helminthic infections seen in children include pinworms, roundworms, and hookworms. Children are at increased risk of parasitic or helminthic infections due to poor hygiene practices: they are typically more careless about handwashing, and they tend to put things in their mouths and share toys and objects with other children.

Nursing Assessment and Management

Parents are often embarrassed when they find out that their child has a parasitic or helminthic infection. Reassure them that these infections can occur in any child. Tables 36.6 and 36.7 give nursing assessment and management information related to specific common parasitic and helminthic infections in children.

▶ *Take* NOTE!

The head louse is becoming increasingly resistant to pediculicides (Diamantis, Morrell, & Burkhart, 2009). This may lead parents to resort to home remedies. Parents need to be informed that these remedies are unproven and can be toxic.

(text continues on page 1164)

TABLE 36.6 COMMON PARASITIC INFECTIONS SEEN IN CHILDREN

Infection	Causative Organism	Transmission	Clinical Manifestations	Diagnosis/Treatment	Isolation/Control Measures
Pediculosis capitis (head lice)	*Pediculus humanus capitis* (head louse)	Direct contact with hair of infested people, less commonly with personal belongings such as combs and hats of those infested Incubation period from laying of eggs to hatching of nymph is 6 to 10 days; adult lice will appear 2 to 3 weeks later	Extreme pruritus is the most common symptom Adult eggs (nits) or lice may be seen, especially behind the ears and at the nape of the neck	Diagnosis by identification of eggs, nymph, and lice with the naked eye is possible; adult lice are rarely seen Treatment: Washing hair with a pediculicide such as permethrin, pyrethrin, or lindane Careful instructions on proper use of any product should be given and strict adherence to application instructions encouraged Detection of living lice 24 hours after treatment suggests incorrect use, a very heavy infestation, reinfestation, or resistance to treatment Removal of nits after treatment is not necessary to prevent spread but may be done for aesthetic reasons (AAP, 2006)	Contact precautions in addition to standard precautions Control measures: Household and other close contacts should be examined and if infested treated. Bedmates should be treated prophylactically Children should not be excluded or sent home from school Importance of environmental measures is controversial Most children can be treated effectively without treating their clothing and bedding If needed, dry-cleaning clothing or simply sealing it in a plastic bag for 10 days is effective Disinfection of headgear, pillowcases, and towels by washing in hot water and drying on the hot cycle may be helpful, even though fomites do not play a role in transmission Soaking combs and hairbrushes in pediculicide shampoo or hot water can also be done Temperatures above 66°C are lethal to lice (CPS, 2008b) Lice is not a sign of poor hygiene; all socioeconomic groups are affected
Pediculosis pubis (pubic lice)	*Phthirus pubis*	Transmission usually occurs through sexual contact; also can be through contaminated items such as towels	Pruritus of anogenital area; other hairy areas of the body, including eyelashes, eyebrows, axilla, beard, can be affected	Diagnosis by identification of eggs, nymph, and lice with the naked eye is possible; adult lice are rarely seen Same as treatment with pediculicides to treat head lice Retreatment is recommended 7 to 10 days later Petroleum oil is used to treat eyelashes and eyebrows	Contact precautions in addition to standard precautions All sexual contacts should be treated

| Scabies | *Sarcoptes scabiei* | Transmission usually occurs through prolonged, close personal contact

Incubation period in those without previous exposure is 4 to 6 weeks

People who were previously infested can develop symptoms in 1 to 4 days | Intense pruritus (especially at night) with presence of erythematous, papular rash with excoriations. The lesions are generally distributed but often are concentrated on the hands and feet and in body folds. May be found on head and neck, which is usually spared in adults

In infants and young children and those who are immunocompromised, the rash may include vesicles, pustules, or nodules | Diagnosis can be made by a history of itching (especially at night), classic rash, and reports of itching in household or sexual contacts

Mites can be seen on microscopic examination of skin scrapings to confirm diagnosis

Treatment: A scabicide, such as 5% permethrin, should be applied to the entire body below the head. Treatment of infants and young children should include the head, neck, and body. The cream is left on for a specified time (usually 8 to 14 hours) depending on the type of scabicide (CPS, 2009a, reaffirmed 2010)

Careful instructions on proper use of any product should be given and strict adherence to application instructions should be urged

Itching may not subside for several weeks, even after successful treatment | Contact precautions in addition to standard precautions

Prophylactic therapy for household members and health care workers in close contact with the patient

Bedding and clothing worn the 4 days prior to treatment should be laundered in hot water and dried on the hot cycle (mites do not survive more than 3 to 4 days without skin contact) |

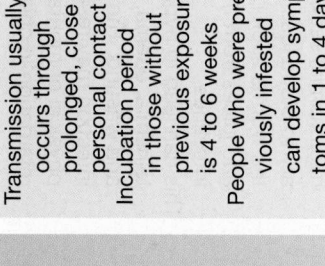

Adapted from Centers for Disease Control and Prevention. (2010a). *Parasites: Lice: Head lice.* Retrieved September 25, 2011 from http://www. cdc.gov/parasites/lice/head/index.html; Centers for Disease Control and Prevention. (2010c). *Scabies.* Retrieved September 25, 2011 from http:// www.cdc.gov/scabies/index.html; Diamantis, S. A., Morrell, D. S., & Burkhart, C. N. (2009). Pediatric infestations. *Pediatric Annals, 38*(6), 326–331; and Siegel, J. D., Rhinehart, E., Jackson M., Chiarello, L., & the Healthcare Infection Control Practices Advisory Committee. (2007). *2007 Guideline for isolation precautions: Preventing transmission of infectious agents in healthcare settings.* Retrieved September 25, 2011 from http://www.cdc.gov/hicpac/pdf/isolation/Isolation2007.pdf.

TABLE 36.7 COMMON HELMINTHIC INFECTIONS IN CHILDREN

Infection	Causative Organism	Clinical Manifestations	Transmission	Diagnosis/Treatment	Isolation/Control Measures
Roundworm (ascariasis)	*Ascaris lumbricoides*, common in temperate and tropical areas	Loss of appetite, nausea, vomiting, and abdominal pain may be seen In significant infestation, partial or complete intestinal obstruction may occur. The more worms, the worse the symptoms	Human feces are the major source of infected eggs Hand to mouth is the usual route of transmission. The eggs are swallowed due to unclean hands or contaminated food. They pass into the intestine; larvae then hatch, penetrate the intestinal wall, enter the circulatory system, and migrate to any body tissue	Diagnosis: once female worms are in the intestine, eggs can be visualized by microscopic evaluation of the stool Occasionally a worm may be visualized in vomit or stool Treatment is with mebendazole, albendazole, or pyrantel pamoate	• Standard precautions are sufficient • Sanitary disposal of feces • Proper hand hygiene
Hookworm	*Ancylostoma duodenale* (Old World hookworm) (found mainly in Europe, Africa, China, Japan, India, and the Pacific Islands) and *Necator americanus* (New World hookworm) (found mainly in the Americas, Caribbean, Africa, Asia, and the Pacific)	Most often people are asymptomatic until significant worms are established May see pruritic, erythematous, papular rash at entry site (referred to as ground itch) or pulmonary symptoms as the larvae migrate One of the greatest concerns in chronic infection is anemia (microcytic hypochromic anemia) secondary to blood loss as the worms suck blood and juices from the intestines This can lead to hypoproteinemia, edema, pica, and wasting. The infection may result in physical or mental retardation in children	Hookworms are found in soil and enter the host through pores, hair follicles, and even intact skin (hands and feet are major sites of entry) The maturing larvae travel through the circulatory system into the lungs and then up the bronchial tree and are swallowed with secretions. They then migrate into the intestinal tract and attach to the wall of the small intestines, where they feed and reproduce Transmission via ingested soil has been seen with *A. duodenale* only	Diagnosis is made through microscopic examination of feces that reveals hookworm eggs Treatment: Albendazole, mebendazole, and pyrantel pamoate. Iron supplementation and possible blood transfusion in severe cases	• Standard precautions are sufficient • Proper sanitation and disposal of feces • Treatment of all known infested people • Screening of high-risk individuals • Encourage the wearing of shoes and avoiding being barefoot

Pinworm				
Enterobius vermicularis	Some people are asymptomatic May cause anal itching (pruritus ani), especially at night Other clinical findings may include teeth grinding at night, weight loss, and enuresis	Fecal–oral route directly, indirectly, or inadvertently by contaminated hands or shared toys, bedding, clothing, toilet seats Incubation period is 1 to 2 months or longer	Diagnosis is made when adult worms are visualized in the perianal region; they are best viewed when the child is sleeping. Very few ova are present in stool, so examination of stool is not recommended Transparent tape pressed to perianal area and then viewed under a microscope may reveal eggs. Three consecutive specimens should be obtained when the child first awakens in the morning Treatment: Drug of choice is mebendazole, usually given as a single dose and repeated in 2 weeks. Pyrantel pamoate and albendazole may also be used In children less than 2, experience with these drugs is limited; therefore, risks and benefits need to be weighed before administration All family members should be treated since transmission from person to person is very easy	Standard precautions are sufficient Reinfection occurs easily Infected people should bathe in the morning, which will remove a large portion of the eggs. Frequent changing of underclothes and bedding. Personal hygiene measures such as keeping fingernails short, avoiding scratching of perianal area and nail biting Good hand hygiene is the most effective preventive measure, especially after using the bathroom and before eating

TABLE 36.8 EFFECTS OF SEXUALLY TRANSMITTED INFECTIONS ON THE FETUS OR NEWBORN

STI	Effects on Fetus or Newborn
Chlamydia	Newborn can be infected during delivery Eye infections (neonatal conjunctivitis), pneumonia, low birth weight, preterm birth, stillbirth
Gonorrhea	Newborn can be infected during delivery Rhinitis, vaginitis, urethritis, inflammation of sites of fetal monitoring Ophthalmia neonatorum can lead to blindness and sepsis (including arthritis and meningitis)
Herpes type II (genital herpes)	Contamination can occur during birth Neurodevelopmental delay, premature birth, low birth weight, death
Syphilis	Can be passed in utero Can result in fetal or infant death Congenital syphilis symptoms include skin ulcers, rashes, fever, weakened or hoarse cry, swollen liver and spleen, jaundice and anemia, various deformities
Trichomoniasis	Fever, irritability, preterm birth, low birth weight
Venereal warts	May develop warts in throat (laryngeal papillomatosis); uncommon but life-threatening

Adapted from March of Dimes. (2008). *Sexually transmitted infections.* Retrieved June 21, 2011 from http://www.marchofdimes.com/complications_stis.html.

▶ *Consider* THIS!

As the nurse at a pediatric clinic, you receive a call from a frantic mother. She tells you, "The school sent my daughter home and told me she has lice! We are clean people! I don't understand how this could happen!" How would you address her concerns? Discuss the plan of care for this child. What education and interventions will be necessary to prevent the spread of pediculosis capitis?

Sexually Transmitted Infections

STIs, commonly called sexually transmitted diseases, are infectious diseases transmitted through sexual contact, including oral, vaginal, or anal intercourse. Certain infections can be transmitted in utero to the fetus or during childbirth to the newborn. Table 36.8 gives information on specific STIs and their effects on the fetus or newborn.

STIs are a major health concern for adolescents. The rates of many STIs are highest in adolescents (CDC, 2010d). The incidence of STIs in adolescents may be significantly underestimated because only those adolescents who have had sexual intercourse are included in the calculation of cases (AAP Committee on Infectious

Diseases, 2006). Adolescents are at greater risk of developing STIs for a variety of reasons: they frequently have unprotected intercourse, they are biologically more susceptible to infection, and they engage in partnerships of limited duration (CDC, 2010d).

Detection of STIs also serves as an important warning sign of potential sexual abuse in infants and children. Due to the serious implications that a diagnosis of an STI can have in children, only tests that have high specificities and that can isolate an organism should be used. Also, treatment for the child with a suspected STI may be held until a definitive diagnosis can be made. Chapter 47 provides information related to the human immunodeficiency virus.

Nursing Assessment

Many health care providers fail to assess sexual behaviour and STI risks, to screen for asymptomatic infection during clinic visits, or to counsel patients on STI risk reduction. Nurses need to remember that they play a key role in the detection, prevention, and treatment of STIs in adolescents and children. All states allow adolescents to give consent to confidential STI testing and treatment. Table 36.9 discusses common clinical manifestations of the specific STIs in adolescents.

(text continues on page 1168)

TABLE 36.9 SEXUALLY TRANSMITTED INFECTIONS COMMON IN ADOLESCENTS

Disease	Causative Organism	Transmission Mode	Diagnostic Testing	Female Symptoms	Male Symptoms	Treatment
Chlamydia Curable STI Seen frequently among sexually active adolescents and young adults Sexually active adolescents should be screened at least annually	*Chlamydia trachomatis* (bacteria)	Vaginal, anal, oral sex, and by childbirth	Culture fluid from urethral swabs in males or endocervical swabs for females and conjunctival secretions in neonates	May be asymptomatic Dysuria Vaginal discharge (mucus or pus) Endocervicitis May lead to pelvic inflammatory disease, ectopic pregnancy, infertility Can cause inflammation of the rectum and conjunctiva Can infect the throat from oral sexual contact with an infected partner	May be asymptomatic Dysuria Penile discharge (mucus or pus) Urethral tingling May lead to epididymitis and sterility Can cause inflammation of the rectum and conjunctiva Can infect the throat from oral sexual contact with an infected partner	Preferred treatment: Azithromycin (Zithromax) Doxycycline (Vibramycin) Second-line treatment: Erythromycin (EES) Ofloxacin (Floxin) Sexual partners also need evaluation, testing, and treatment
Gonorrhea Curable STI Patient often co-infected with *Chlamydia trachomatis*	*Neisseria gonorrhoeae* (bacteria)	Vaginal, anal, oral sex, and by childbirth	Staining samples directly for the bacterium, detection of bacterial genes or DNA in urine and growing the bacteria in laboratory cultures; more than one test may be used	May be asymptomatic or no recognizable symptoms until serious complications such as pelvic inflammatory disease Dysuria Urinary frequency Vaginal discharge (yellow and foul) Dyspareunia Endocervicitis Arthritis May lead to pelvic inflammatory disease, ectopic pregnancy, infertility Symptoms of rectal infection include discharge, anal itching, and occasional painful bowel movements with fresh blood	Most produce symptoms but can be asymptomatic Dysuria Penile discharge (pus) Arthritis May lead to epididymitis and sterility Symptoms of rectal infection include discharge, anal itching, and occasional painful bowel movements with fresh blood	Usually a single dose of one of the following: Preferred treatment: Cefixime (Suprax) as a single dose Second-line treatment: Ceftriaxone (Rocephin) Azithromycin (Zithromax) Usually will be treated for co-infection with *Chlamydia*, so a combination is given (such as ceftriaxone and doxycycline) Sexual partners also need evaluation, testing, and treatment Note: many cases of gonorrhea in Canada are resistant to quinolones (ciprofloxacin and ofloxacin); therefore, these drugs are only used if susceptibility testing has been done

(continued)

TABLE 36.9 SEXUALLY TRANSMITTED INFECTIONS COMMON IN ADOLESCENTS (continued)

Disease	Causative Organism	Transmission Mode	Diagnostic Testing	Female Symptoms	Male Symptoms	Treatment
Herpes type II (genital herpes) Lifelong recurrent viral disease Most people have not been diagnosed There is no cure	Herpes simplex virus II (HSV II)	Having sexual contact (vaginal, oral, or anal) with someone who is shedding the herpes virus either during an outbreak or during a period with no symptoms Can be transmitted through close contact such as close skin-to-skin contact	Visual inspection and symptoms or culture Virologic and type-specific serologic tests can tell if HSV II is present; does not confirm genital herpes, though most providers will assume a positive HSV II means genital herpes	Blister-like genital lesions Dysuria Fever, headache, muscle aches	Blister-like genital lesions Dysuria Fever, headache, muscle aches	Acyclovir (Zovirax) Famciclovir or valacyclovir Does not cure; just controls symptoms Sexual partners benefit from evaluation and counseling. If symptomatic, need treatment If asymptomatic, offer testing and education
Syphilis	*Treponema pallidum* (spirochete bacteria)	Sexual contact with an infected person	Blood tests Venereal Disease Research Laboratory, rapid plasma reagin, and treponemal tests (e.g., fluorescent treponemal antibody absorbed) can lead to a presumptive diagnosis Darkfield examination and direct fluorescent antibody tests of lesion exudate or tissue provide definitive diagnosis of early syphilis	Course of disease divided into four stages **Primary infection:** • Chancre on place of entrance of bacteria (usually vulva or vagina but can develop in other parts of the body) **Secondary infection:** • Maculopapular rash (hands and feet) • Sore throat • Lymphadenopathy • Flu-like symptoms **Latent infection:** • No symptoms • No longer contagious • Many people if not treated will suffer no further signs or symptoms Some people will go on to develop tertiary or late syphilis	Course of disease divided into four stages **Primary infection:** • Chancre on place of entrance of bacteria (usually on penis but can develop in other parts of the body) **Secondary, latent, and tertiary infections:** All similar to female symptoms	Penicillin G injection (if penicillin allergy, doxycycline or ceftriaxone) Sexual partners need evaluation and testing

Infection	Transmission	Diagnosis	Signs and Symptoms	Treatment
Trichomoniasis *Trichomonas vaginalis* (protozoa)	Vaginal intercourse with an infected partner. May be picked up from direct genital contact with damp or moist objects, such as towels, wet clothing, or a toilet seat	Microscopic evaluation of vaginal secretions or culture	Many women have symptoms but some may be asymptomatic Dysuria Urinary frequency Vaginal discharge (yellow, green, or grey and foul odour) Dyspareunia Irritation or itching of genital area	Metronidazole (Flagyl) Sexual partners need evaluation, testing, and treatment also. Note: patients taking metronidazole should be counselled to avoid alcohol for 24 hours after therapy.
			Tertiary infections: • Tumours of skin, bones, and liver • Central nervous system symptoms • Cardiovascular symptoms • Usually not reversible at this stage	
			Most infected men are asymptomatic. Dysuria Penile discharge (watery white)	
Venereal warts (condylomata acuminata) One of the most common STIs in Canada Could lead to cancers of the cervix, vulva, vagina, anus, or penis No cure; warts can be removed but virus remains	Vaginal, anal, oral sex with an infected partner	Visual inspection Abnormal Pap smear may indicate cervical infection of HPV	Wart-like lesions that are soft, moist, or flesh coloured and appear on the vulva and cervix, and inside and surrounding the vagina and anus. Sometimes appear in clusters that resemble cauliflower-like bumps and are either raised or flat, small or large	Preventative vaccine May disappear without treatment Treatment is aimed at removing the lesions rather than HPV itself No optimal treatment has been identified, but several ways to treat depending on size and location Most methods rely on chemical or physical destruction of the lesion: Imiquimod cream 20% Podophyllin antimitotic solution 0.5% Podofilox solution 5% 5-fluorouracil cream trichloroacetic acid Small warts can be removed by • Freezing (cryosurgery) • Burning (electrocautery) • Laser treatment Large warts that have not responded to treatment may be removed surgically
			Wart-like lesions that are soft, moist, or flesh-coloured and appear on the scrotum or penis. They sometimes appear in clusters that resemble cauliflower-like bumps and are either raised or flat, small or large	

Adapted from Centers for Disease Control and Prevention. (2010). *Sexually transmitted diseases treatment guidelines, 2010. Morbidity and Mortality Weekly Report (MMWR)*, 59(RR-12), 1–116. Retrieved June 19, 2011 from http://www.cdc.gov/std/treatment/2010/STDtreatment-2010-RR5912.pdf; and Mehring, P. M. (2009). Sexually transmitted infections. In C. M. Porth & G. Matfin (Eds.), *Pathophysiology: Concepts of altered health states* (8th ed.., pp. 1167–1180). Philadelphia, PA: Wolters Kluwer Health/Lippincott Williams & Wilkins.

TEACHING GUIDELINE 36.3

Proper Condom Use

- Use latex or polyurethane condoms.
- Use a new condom with each act of sexual intercourse. Never reuse a condom.
- Handle condoms carefully to avoid damaging the condom.
- Ensure condom has been stored in a cool, dry place away from direct sunlight. Do not store condoms in wallet or automobile or anywhere they would be exposed to extreme temperatures.
- Check the expiration date and discard if expired. Do not use a condom if it appears brittle, sticky, or discoloured. These are signs of aging.
- Put condom on before any genital contact.

- Expel the air from the tip of the condom. Leaving enough space for the semen, pinch the condom tip and unroll over the erect penis. Cover as much of the penis as possible.
- Ensure adequate lubrication during intercourse. Use only water-based lubricants such as K-Y Jelly with latex condoms. Oil-based or petroleum-based lubricants, such as body lotion, massage oil, or cooking oil, can weaken latex condoms.
- Withdraw while penis is still erect, and hold condom firmly against base of penis.
- After use tie the open end of the condom and discard in the garbage. Do not place in the toilet.

Adapted from American Academy of Pediatrics Committee on Infectious Diseases [2006] and Public Health Agency of Canada. (2008). *Canadian guidelines on sexually transmitted infections,* Appendix B. Retrieved September 24, 2011 from http://www.phac-aspc.gc.ca/std-mts/sti-its/guide-lignesdir-eng.php.

Nursing Management

Encourage the patient to complete the antibiotic prescription. Prevention of STIs among children and adolescents is critical, and health care providers have a unique opportunity to provide counselling and education. Adapt the style, content, and message to the patient's developmental level. Identify risk factors and risk behaviours and help the patient develop specific individualized actions for prevention. This conversation needs to be direct and nonjudgmental.

If adolescents choose to have sexual intercourse explain the need to use barrier methods, such as male and female condoms. For teens who have already had

TABLE 36.10 BARRIERS TO CONDOM USE AND MEANS TO OVERCOME THEM

Perceived Barrier	Intervention Strategy
Decreases sexual pleasure (sensation) Note: Often perceived by those who have never used a condom	• Encourage the patient to try • Put a drop of water-based lubricant or saliva inside the tip of the condom or on the glans of the penis before putting on the condom • Try a thinner latex condom or a different brand or more lubrication
Decreases spontaneity of sexual activity	• Incorporate condom use into foreplay • Remind patient that peace of mind may enhance pleasure for self and partner
Embarrassing, juvenile, "unmanly"	• Remind patient that it is "manly" to protect himself and others
Poor fit (too small or too big, slips off, uncomfortable)	• Smaller and larger condoms are available
Requires prompt withdrawal after ejaculation	• Reinforce the protective nature of prompt withdrawal and suggest substituting other postcoital sexual activities
Fear of breakage may lead to less vigorous sexual activity	• With prolonged intercourse, lubricant wears off and the condom begins to rub. Have a water-soluble lubricant available to reapply.
Non-penetrative sexual activity	• Condoms have been advocated for use during fellatio; unlubricated condoms may prove best for this purpose due to the taste of the lubricant • Other barriers, such as dental dams or an unlubricated condom, can be cut down the middle to form a barrier; these have been advocated for use during certain forms of non-penetrative sexual activity (e.g., cunnilingus and anilingus)

Source: *Canadian Guidelines on Sexually Transmitted Infections.* Public Health Agency of Canada, 2008. Minister of Public Works and Government Services Canada, 2011.

sexual intercourse explain the benefits of minimizing their lifetime number of sexual partners, how to use barrier methods consistently and correctly, and the need to be aware of the connection between drug and alcohol use and STIs (see Teaching Guideline 36.3 and Table 36.10).

■■■ Key Concepts

■ Infants and young children are more susceptible to infection due to their immature immune system. Young children continue to have an increased risk of infections and communicable disorders because disease protection from immunizations is not complete.

■ When obtaining blood cultures, follow aseptic technique and hospital protocol to prevent contamination. Obtain the specimen before administering antibiotics.

■ When administering antipyretics, proper education must be given to caregivers on appropriate dosing, concentration, dosing interval, and use of proper measuring device.

■ Promoting proper fluid balance and reducing temperature in a febrile child are important nursing interventions when caring for a child with an infection or communicable illness.

■ Many childhood infectious and communicable diseases involve a rash. Rashes can be difficult to identify, so a thorough description and history from the caregiver are important.

■ Sepsis, a systemic overresponse to infection resulting from bacteria, fungi, viruses, or parasites, can lead to septic shock. Any infant less than 3 months old with a fever or any child with a fever accompanied by extreme lethargy, unresponsiveness, or lack of facial expressions should be seen by a health care provider.

■ Many bacterial and viral infections, such as diphtheria, tetanus, pertussis, mumps, measles, rubella, varicella, and poliomyelitis, can be prevented by vaccination.

■ Children are at a particular risk of contracting vector-borne diseases, which are diseases transmitted by ticks, mosquitoes, or other insect vectors. Two of the most commonly seen are Lyme disease and WNV.

■ Viral exanthems of childhood often present with a distinct rash pattern that assists in the diagnosis of the virus. Common childhood exanthems include exanthem subitum (roseola infantum), rubella (German measles), rubeola (measles), varicella (chickenpox), and erythema infectiosum (fifth disease).

■ Nurses play a key role in educating the public on the importance of immunizations.

■ Health care providers need to remember and educate parents that fever is a protective mechanism the body uses to fight infection.

REFERENCES

American Academy of Pediatrics. (2001). Policy statement: Acetaminophen toxicity in children. *Pediatrics, 108*, 1020–1024.

American Academy of Pediatrics Committee on Drugs. (2009). Acetaminophen toxicity in children. *Pediatrics, 108*(4), 1020–1024. Retrieved September 26, 2011 from http://aappolicy.aappublications.org/cgi/reprint/pediatrics;108/4/1020.pdf

American Academy of Pediatrics Committee on Infectious Diseases. (2006). *Red book: 2006 report of the committee on infectious diseases* (27th ed.). Elk Grove Village, IL: American Academy of Pediatrics.

Anderson-Berry, A. L., Bellig, L. L., & Ohning, B. L. (2011). *Neonatal sepsis.* Retrieved on September 26, 2011 from http://emedicine.medscape.com/article/978352-overview

Arnon, S. S. (2007). Tetanus (Clostridium tetani). In R. M. Kliegman, R. E. Behrman, H. B. Jenson, & B. F. Stanton (Eds.), *Nelson's textbook of pediatrics* (18th ed.). Philadelphia, PA: Saunders.

Artsob, H., Gubler, D. J., Enria, D. A., et al. (2009). West Nile virus in the New World: Trends in the spread and proliferation of West Nile Virus in the Western hemisphere. *Zoonoses Public Health, 56*, 357–369.

Balentine, J., & Lombardi, D. P. (2010). *Scarlet fever in emergency medicine.* Retrieved September 26, 2011 from http://emedicine.medscape.com/article/785981-overview#a0199

Behrman, R. E., Kliegman, R. M., Jenson, H. B., & Stanton, B. F. (Eds.). (2007). *Nelson's textbook of pediatrics* (18th ed.). Philadelphia, PA: Saunders.

Broome, M. E., Dokken, D. L., Broome, C. D., Woodring, B., & Stegelman, M. F. (2003). A study of parent/grandparent education for managing a febrile illness using the CALM approach. *Journal of Pediatric Health Care, 17*, 176–183.

Canadian Paediatric Society. (1998). Acetaminophen and ibuprofen in the management of fever and mild to moderate pain in children. *Paediatrics and Child Health, 3*(4), 273–274.

Canadian Pediatric Society. (2004). PID Note: Bag urine specimens still not appropriate in diagnosis urinary tract infections in infants. *Paediatrics and Child Health, 9*(6), 377–378.

Canadian Paediatric Society. (2008a). Infection control in paediatric office settings. *Paediatrics and Child Health, 13*(5), 408–419.

Canadian Paediatric Society. (2008b). Head lice infestations: A clinical update. *Paediatrics and Child Health, 13*(8), 692–696.

Canadian Paediatric Society. (2008c). *School and daycare exclusion policies for chickenpox: A rational approach.* Retrieved September 26, 2011 from http://www.cps.ca/english/statements/id/id99-01.htm

Canadian Paediatric Society. (2009a, reaffirmed 2010). *Scabies management.* Retrieved September 26, 2011 from http://www.cps.ca/english/statements/II/ii01-01.htm#Control%20measures

Canadian Paediatric Society. (2009b, reaffirmed 2001). *Temperature measurement in pediatrics.* Retrieved September 26, 2011 from http://www.cps.ca/english/statements/CP/cp00-01.htm

Canadian Paediatric Society Infectious Diseases and Immunization Committee. (2003). West Nile virus – Mosquitoes no longer just an annoyance! *Canadian Journal of Infectious Diseases, 14*(3), 150–153.

Caring for Kids. (2008). *When your child is sick: Fever and temperature taking.* Retrieved September 25, 2011 from http://www.caringforkids.cps.ca/whensick/Fever.htm

Centers for Disease Control and Prevention. (2008). Haemophilus influenzae *Serotype b (Hib) Disease.* Retrieved September 26, 2011 from http://www.cdc.gov/ncidod/dbmd/diseaseinfo/haeminfluserob_t.htm

Centers for Disease Control and Prevention. (2010a). *Parasites: Lice: Head lice.* Retrieved September 26, 2011 from http://www.cdc.gov/parasites/lice/head/index.html

Centers for Disease Control and Prevention. (2010b). *Pertussis (whooping cough): Surveillance & reporting.* Retrieved September 26, 2011 from http://www.cdc.gov/pertussis/surv-reporting.html

Centers for Disease Control and Prevention. (2010c). Scabies. Retrieved September 26, 2011 from http://www.cdc.gov/scabies/index.html

Centers for Disease Control and Prevention. (2010d). Sexually transmitted diseases treatment guidelines, 2010. *Morbidity and Mortality Weekly Report, 59*(RR-12), 1–116. Retrieved September 26, 2011 from http://www.cdc.gov/std/treatment/2010/STD-Treatment-2010-RR5912.pdf

Centers for Disease Control and Prevention. (2011a). Epidemiology and prevention of vaccine-preventable diseases. In W. Atkinson, S. Wolfe, & J. Hamborsky (Eds.). (12th ed.). Washington, DC: Public Health Foundation.

Centers for Disease Control and Prevention. (2011b). *Mumps vaccination*. Retrieved September 25, 2011 from http://www.cdc.gov/mumps/vaccination.html

Centers for Disease Control and Prevention. (2011c). *NIOSH workplace safety and health topics: Tick-borne diseases*. Retrieved September 26, 2011 from http://www.cdc.gov/niosh/topics/tick-borne/

Crawford, M. B. (2006). Pediatrics, bacteremia and sepsis. *eMedicine*. Retrieved July 22, 2006 from http://www.emedicine.com/EMERG/topic364.htm#section~author_information

Crocetti, M. T., & Serwint, J. R. (2005). Fever: Separating fact from fiction. *Contemporary Pediatrics*. Retrieved September 26, 2011 from http://contemporarypediatrics.modernmedicine.com/contpeds/content/printContentPopup.jsp?id = 143315

Diamantis, S. A., Morrell, D. S., & Burkhart, C. N. (2009). Pediatric infestations. *Pediatric Annals, 38*(6), 326–331.

Enrione, M. A., & Powell, K. R. (2007). Sepsis, septic shock, and systemic inflammatory response syndrome. In R. M. Kliegman, R. E. Behrman, H. B. Jenson, & B. F. Stanton (Eds.), *Nelson's textbook of pediatrics* (18th ed.). Philadelphia, PA: Saunders.

Fischbach, F. T., & Dunning, M. B. III. (2009). *A manual of laboratory and diagnostic tests* (8th ed.). Philadelphia, PA: Lippincott Williams & Wilkins.

Gal, P., & Reed, M. D. (2007). Medications. In R. M. Kliegman, R. E. Behrman, H. B. Jenson, & B. F. Stanton (Eds.), *Nelson's textbook of pediatrics* (18th ed.). Philadelphia, PA: Saunders.

Gerber, M. A. (2007). Group A streptococcus. In R. M. Kliegman, R. E. Behrman, H. B. Jenson, & B. F. Stanton (Eds.), *Nelson's textbook of pediatrics* (18th ed.). Philadelphia, PA: Saunders.

Global Health Council. (2011). *The impact of infectious diseases*. Retrieved September 26, 2011 from http://www.globalhealth.org/infectious_diseases/

Grill, A. K. (2009). Approach to management of suspected rabies exposures: What primary care physicians need to know. *Canadian Family Physician, 55*, 247–251.

Hatfield, L. A., Chang, K., Bittle, M., Deluca, J., & Polomano, R. C. (2011). The analgesic properties of intraoral sucrose: An integrative review. *Advances in Neonatal Care, 11*(2), 83–92. doi: 10.1097/ANC.0b013e318210d043.

Hayes, E. B., & O'Leary, D. R. (2004). West Nile virus infection: A pediatric perspective. *Pediatrics, 113*, 1375–1381.

Immunization Action Coalition. (2010). *Rabies questions and answers. Information about the disease and vaccines*. Retrieved September 26, 2011 from http://www.immunize.org/catg.d/p4216.pdf

KidsHealth. (2009). *Infections: Cat scratch disease*. Retrieved September 26, 2011 from http://kidshealth.org/parent/infections/bacterial_viral/cat_scratch.html#

Petersen, L. R., Marfin, A. A., & Gubler, D. J. (2003). West Nile virus. *Journal of the American Medical Association, 290*, 524–528.

Powell, K. R. (2007a). Fever. In R. M. Kliegman, R. E. Behrman, H. B. Jenson, & B. F. Stanton (Eds.), *Nelson's textbook of pediatrics* (18th ed.). Philadelphia, PA: Saunders.

Powell, K. R. (2007b). Fever without a focus. In R. M. Kliegman, R. E. Behrman, H. B. Jenson, & B. F. Stanton (Eds.), *Nelson's textbook of pediatrics* (18th ed.). Philadelphia, PA: Saunders.

Public Health Agency of Canada. (1999). *Canada Communicable Disease Report: Infection Control Guidelines [supplement]*. Retrieved November 24, 2010 from http://www.phac-aspc.gc.ca/publicat/ccdr-rmtc/99pdf/cdr25s4e.pdf

Public Health Agency of Canada. (2003). *National Consensus Conference on Pertussis*. Ottawa, ON: Author. Retrieved November 24, 2010 from http://www.phac-aspc.gc.ca/publicat/ccdr-rmtc/03vol29/29s3/index.html

Public Health Agency of Canada. (2006). *Canadian immunization guide* (7th ed.). Ottawa, ON: Author. Retrieved November 24, 2010 from http://www.phac-aspc.gc.ca/publicat/cig-gci/index-eng.php

Public Health Agency of Canada. (2008). *Canadian guidelines on sexually transmitted infections*. Retrieved September 24, 2011 from http://www.phac-aspc.gc.ca/std-mts/sti-its/guide-lignesdir-eng.php

Public Health Agency of Canada. (2010). *Lyme disease fact sheet*. Retrieved September 24, 2011 from http://www.phac-aspc.gc.ca/id-mi/lyme-fs-eng.php#s8

Rupprecht, C. E., Briggs, D., Brown, C. M., et al. (2010). Use of a reduced (4-dose) vaccine schedule for postexposure prophylaxis to prevent human rabies. *Morbidity and Mortality Weekly Report, 59*(2), 1–9. Retrieved September 26, 2011 from http://www.cdc.gov/mmwr/preview/mmwrhtml/rr5902a1.htm#tab3

Santhanam, S., & Tolan, R. W. Jr. (2011). *Pediatric sepsis*. Retrieved September 26, 2011 from http://emedicine.medscape.com/article/972559-overview#a1

Shapiro, E. D. (2007). Lyme disease (*Borrelia burgdorferi*). In R. M. Kliegman, R. E. Behrman, H. B. Jenson, & B. F. Stanton (Eds.), *Nelson's textbook of pediatrics* (18th ed.). Philadelphia, PA: Saunders.

Siegel, J. D., Rhinehart, E., Jackson M., Chiarello, L., & the Healthcare Infection Control Practices Advisory Committee. (2007). *2007 Guideline for isolation precautions: Preventing transmission of infectious agents in healthcare settings*. Retrieved September 26, 2011 from http://www.cdc.gov/hicpac/pdf/isolation/Isolation2007.pdf

Stephenson, J. (2004). Polio eradication plan. *Journal of the American Medical Association, 291*(7), 813.

Sullivan, J. E., Farrar, H. C., & the AAP's Section on Clinical Pharmacology and Therapeutics, and Committee on Drugs. (2011). Clinical report: Fever and antipyretic use in children. *Pediatrics, 127*(3), 580–587. doi: 10.1542/peds.2010-3852.

Toltzis, P. (2007). Rabies. In R. M. Kliegman, R. E. Behrman, H. B. Jenson, & B. F. Stanton (Eds.), *Nelson's textbook of pediatrics* (18th ed.). Philadelphia, PA: Saunders.

Weir, E. (2005). Parvovirus B19 infection: Fifth disease and more. *Canadian Medical Association Journal, 172*(6), 743.

World Health Organization. (2011a). Rabies fact sheet. Retrieved September 26, 2011 from http://www.who.int/mediacentre/factsheets/fs099/en/

World Health Organization. (2011b). *World health statistics 2011*. Retrieved September 26, 2011 from http://www.who.int/whosis/whostat/2011/en/index.html

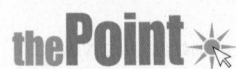

thePoint

For additional learning materials, including Internet Resources, visit
http://thePoint.lww.com/Chow1e.

CHAPTER WORKSHEET

MULTIPLE CHOICE QUESTIONS

1. Compared with adults, why are infants and children at increased risk of infection and communicable diseases?

   a. The infant has had limited exposure to disease and is losing the passive immunity acquired from maternal antibodies.

   b. The infant demonstrates an increased inflammatory response.

   c. Cellular immunity is not functional at birth.

   d. Infants are at an increased risk of infection until they receive their first set of immunizations.

2. A mother calls the clinic because her 2-year-old daughter has a rectal temperature of 37.8°C. She wonders how high a fever should be before she should give medications to reduce it. What is the best response by the nurse?

   a. "All fevers should be treated to prevent seizures."

   b. "Antipyretics should be used with any rise in temperature. They can help change the course of the infection."

   c. "Give your child aspirin when her fever is above 38°C."

   d. "In a normal healthy child, if your child is not uncomfortable, fevers less than 39°C do not require medication."

3. A neonate should be evaluated by a physician if which signs and symptoms are present?

   a. Acting fussier than normal

   b. Refusing the pacifier

   c. Rectal temperature above 38°C

   d. Mottling is present during bathing

4. As the nurse in a public health department, you have been asked to provide information to local child care centres on controlling the spread of infectious diseases. What is the best information you can provide?

   a. The etiology of common infectious diseases

   b. Proper handwashing techniques

   c. The physiology of the immune system

   d. Why children are at a higher risk of infection than adults

CRITICAL THINKING EXERCISES

1. A 12-year-old child presents with complaints of a very sore throat and fever. On assessment you find an erythematous rash on his face that feels like sandpaper. You obtain a throat culture that is positive for group A *Streptococcus*. What instructions would you give the parents regarding his care at home?

2. A 1-month-old infant is admitted to the hospital to rule out sepsis. What would be your priority nursing interventions?

3. A 4-year-old child presents with a fever and rash. What three items should the nurse obtain during the health history?

   a. Immunization history

   b. Any exposure to communicable or infectious diseases

   c. Whether the child takes a daily vitamin

   d. Thorough description and history of the rash

   e. Mother's immunization history

STUDY ACTIVITIES

1. The 4-year-old presented in question number 3 above was diagnosed with varicella zoster virus. Write a nursing care plan for a child with varicella.

2. You are asked to give a presentation to a group of adolescents on STIs, including transmission, symptoms, treatment, and prevention. What information would you include?

3. A child is brought to the office of the school nurse with intense itching. Upon assessment the nurse finds an erythematous, papular rash with excoriations on the child's hands and feet. As suspected, the diagnosis of scabies is confirmed. What teaching is necessary for the parents, family, and classmates of the child?

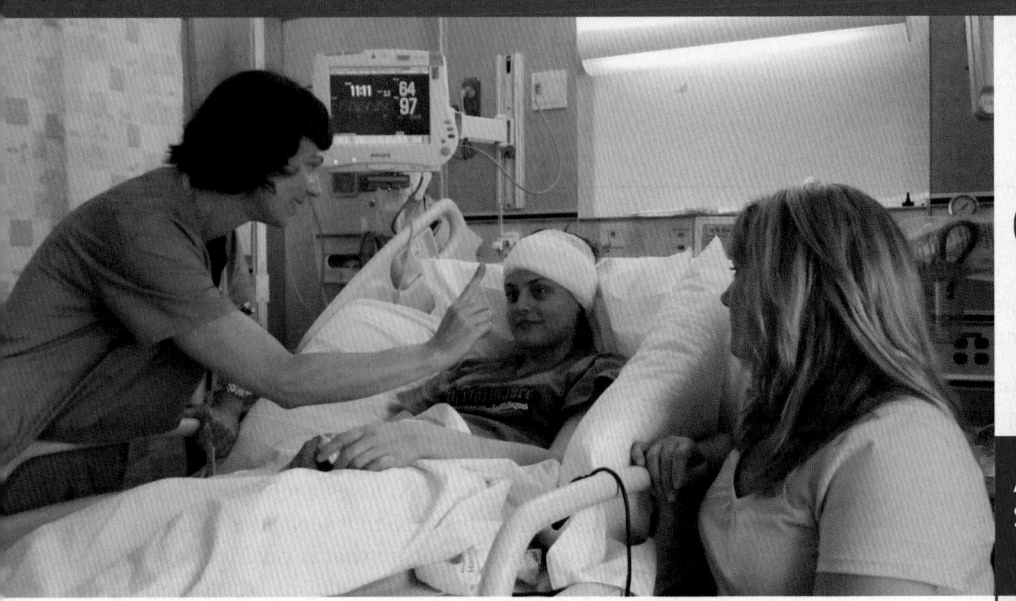

CHAPTER 37

Adapted by Keith E. Aronyk and Susan Neufeld

NURSING CARE OF THE CHILD WITH A NEUROLOGIC DISORDER

KEY TERMS

central nervous system (CNS)
cerebrospinal fluid (CSF)
decorticate posturing
decerebrate posturing

head circumference
intracranial pressure (ICP)
lumbar puncture (LP)
myelination
myoclonic

neural tube
postictal
syringomyelia
status epilepticus
teratogen
tonic–clonic

LEARNING OBJECTIVES

Upon completion of the chapter, the learner will be able to:

1. Compare how the anatomy and physiology of the neurologic system in children differ from those in adults.
2. Identify various factors associated with neurologic disease in infants and children.
3. Discuss common laboratory and other diagnostic tests useful in the diagnosis of neurologic conditions.
4. Discuss common medications and other treatments used for treatment and palliation of neurologic conditions.
5. Recognize risk factors associated with various neurologic disorders.
6. Distinguish among different neurologic illnesses based on the signs and symptoms associated with them.
7. Discuss nursing interventions commonly used for neurologic illnesses.
8. Devise an individualized nursing care plan for the child with a neurologic disorder.
9. Develop client and family teaching plans for the child with a neurologic disorder.
10. Describe the psychosocial impact of chronic neurologic disorders on children.

Antonio Chapman, 3 months old, has had increased irritability, poor sucking and feeding, and a fever for the past 24 hours. Today he is lethargic with a weak high-pitched cry and is vomiting his feeds.

Wow

We worry about what a child will become tomorrow, yet we forget that he is someone today.   —Stacia Tauscher

Neurologic disorders in children can be divided into several categories, including structural disorders, seizure disorders, infectious disorders, trauma to the neurologic system, blood flow disruption disorders, and chronic headaches.

Nurses must be familiar with neurologic conditions affecting children in order to provide prevention, prompt treatment, guidance, and support to families. Due to the potentially devastating effects that neurologic disorders can have on children and their families, nurses need to be skilled in assessment and interventions in this area and must be able to provide support throughout the course of the illness and beyond.

Variations in Pediatric Anatomy and Physiology

Neurologic disorders can result from congenital problems as well as from infection or trauma. Certain neurologic conditions occur in children more often than adults. In addition, the location and type of brain tumours that occur in children are different than those in adults. Growth and development of a child with a neurologic deficit must be taken into consideration and future problems anticipated. Additionally, transition to adult care, a system that is not well suited to neurologic disorders traditionally seen in childhood, must be considered as more children with neurologic disorders survive and thrive with advances in research and clinical care.

Brain and Spinal Cord Development

Development of the brain and spinal cord occurs early in gestation, in the first 3 to 4 weeks, beginning with **neural tube closure**. During early fetal development, genetic disorders, infection, **teratogens**, and malnutrition can result in malformations in the developing brain and spinal cord and impair **central nervous system (CNS)** development.

At birth, most of the cranial bones are not yet fused to form a solid skull structure. These bones are also soft and pliable, enabling the cranium to pass through the birth canal. "Ping-pong" fractures (an indentation of a cranial bone) are sometimes seen in infants due to the pliability of these bones.

Premature infants have more capillaries in the periventricular area, which is the brain tissue that lines the outside of the lateral ventricles. These fragile capillaries are at greater risk for rupture, leading to intraventricular hemorrhage. The cranial bones are so soft in premature infants that external pressure from positioning can change the shape of the skull. For example, a premature infant who is turned only side to side may develop a long narrow (scaphocephalic) skull shape.

Nervous System

Development of the nervous system is complete but immature at birth. The neurons in the brain are not fully myelinated. The speed and accuracy of nerve impulses increase as **myelination** increases. This process accounts for the acquisition of fine and gross motor movements and coordination in early childhood. Myelination proceeds in a cephalocaudal direction. For example, infants are able to control the head and neck before the trunk and extremities. More than myelination, synaptic connections among neurons hold the key to learning and the development of higher cognitive functions.

The immaturity of the CNS in preterm infants can result in delayed development of motor skills. Premature newborns may have difficulty coordinating sucking and swallowing, leading to feeding and growth issues. Also, episodes of apnea and bradycardia can be problematic in the preterm newborn due to the underdevelopment of the nervous system.

Head Size

The head of the infant and young child is large in proportion to the body. The head of an infant accounts for a quarter of the body height while in adults it accounts for one eighth of the body height (Fig. 37.1). The head is the fastest growing body part during infancy, with the growth rate levelling off around 5 years of age. Generally, a healthy child's head circumference continues along the same percentile on the standardized growth chart. Overall head size and shape are much more important to assess than the size and shape of specific structures. For example, prominent cranial sutures or a barely palpable anterior fontanel mean very little in the context of a healthy baby who is meeting developmental milestones and has a normal skull size and shape.

The neck muscles in infants and toddlers are not well developed. The combination of a large head in proportion to body and weaker neck muscles puts infants and toddlers at greater risk for head injury from falls. Additionally, infants are at particular risk for severe acquired brain injury from violent shaking, impact, or both.

Common Medical Treatments

A variety of interventions, including medical treatments and medications, are used to treat neurologic illness in children. The most common medical treatments and medications used for neurologic disorders are listed in Common Medical and Surgical Treatments 37.1 and Drug Guide 37.1.

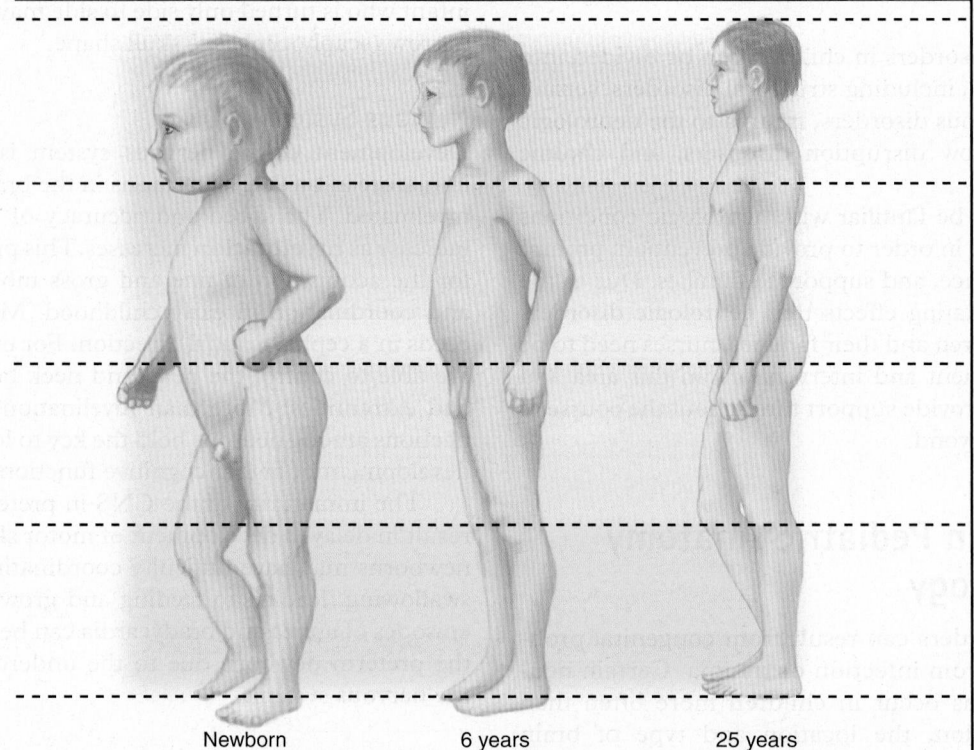

Newborn   6 years   25 years

FIGURE 37.1 Proportion of head to body height in the newborn, child, and adult.

COMMON MEDICAL AND SURGICAL TREATMENTS 37.1

Treatment	Explanation	Indications	Nursing Implications
NPO	Withholding oral food and fluids	Child presenting with a neurologic problem that might require surgery	Put a sign on the door and remove all fluids and food from the room.
Craniotomy	Opening of the skull either above or below the tentorium	Decompress or repair brain structures	Educate caregivers. Maintain fluid balance with IV balanced salt solution. Monitor for signs and symptoms of: • Intracranial hemorrhage (rapid decrease in LOC, hemiplegia, third nerve palsy, apnea) • Incisional hemorrhage (bulging incisions, bleeding through incision onto head dressing, tachycardia, hypotension, decreased urine output) CSF leak (boggy swelling under the scalp near the incision; for posterior fossa craniotomy this is called a "pseudomeningocele")

Treatment	Explanation	Indications	Nursing Implications

Shunt placement or ventriculoscopic third ventriculostomy	For shunt placement, a catheter is placed in a cerebral ventricle or spinal subarachnoid space to pass the CSF to the peritoneal cavity, atrium of the heart, or pleural spaces. (Ventriculoperitoneal shunts are commonly used.)
	For ventriculoscopic third ventriculostomy, under endoscopic guidance, the floor of the third ventricle is fenestrated to allow CSF to circulate in the subarachnoid space. This is for obstructions that occur below the third ventricle.
		Hydrocephalus, increased ICP	Monitor:
			• For signs and symptoms of increased ICP
			• Neurologic status closely
			• LOC and vital signs
			  • For signs and symptoms of infection
			  • Signs of CSF leak: bulging along shunt tract (closed leak) or fluid leaking through incisions (i.e., child waking up with wet hair or fluid stain on pillow case)

Intubation and ventilation	Adequate oxygenation to prevent hypoxia and further damage to the brain	Increased ICP	Monitor: • Arterial blood gases • For signs and symptoms of increased ICP • Pulse oximetry
Balance fluid and electrolytes	Intravenous access with a balanced salt solution to ensure normovolemia and normal serum electrolytes	Increased ICP	Monitor: • Blood work for glucose, sodium, potassium, chloride Meticulous monitoring
External ventricular drainage (EVD) or spinal drainage	A catheter is temporarily placed in the ventricle or spinal subarachnoid space and CSF is drained in a closed system to an external reservoir	Most commonly used with shunt infections until CSF is sterile and shunt can be replaced; treats acute-onset hydrocephalus, meningitis, encephalitis, tumours that cause blockage of CSF, closed head injury, subarachnoid hemorrhage, increased ICP; also can be used to monitor ICP. Spinal drainage is used to temporarily decrease CSF pressure to protect tenuous dural closure in children at high risk for CSF leak	Monitor: • For signs and symptoms of increased ICP • Neurologic status closely • LOC and vital signs • For signs and symptoms of infection • For signs of CSF leak at catheter insertion site. • Level of collection container when drain is unclamped. Double secure collecting system to avoid unexpected changes in position. • Colour of CSF (should progress pink to yellow–xanthochromic) • CSF volume drained hourly and daily; include in output. Maintain an intact closed, sterile system.
PT/OT/ST	Used to improve motor function and ability of clients with neurologic disorders	Traumatic brain injury/spinal cord injury	Ensure adequate communication exists within the interdisciplinary team. Recognize the need for a swallowing assessment.

DRUG GUIDE 37.1

Medication	Action/Indication	Nursing Implications
Antibiotics (oral, parenteral, intrathecal)	Treatment of bacterial meningitis and shunt infections/kill and prevent the growth of bacteria	Check for antibiotic allergies. Monitor serum levels to ensure therapeutic dosing if indicated. Give as prescribed for the length of time prescribed.
Anticonvulsants (oral, parenteral)	Used with epilepsy, head trauma, neurosurgical procedures Treatment and prevention of seizures	Maintain seizure precautions. Monitor for drug interactions and long-term adverse effects. Monitor and document all seizure activity. Many are used in combination, but need to be aware of interactions and long-term adverse effects. Stopping drug abruptly may precipitate seizures or even status epilepticus.
Benzodiazepines Diazepam (oral, rectal, or parenteral) Lorazepam (parenteral or oral)	Anticonvulsants; enhance the inhibition of γ-aminobutyric acid (GABA) Treatment for status epilepticus	Diazepam is available in rectal form to stop prolonged seizures in children. Useful for home management; nurses must educate family members on administration and when to call MD. Monitor sedation level and for cessation of seizure activity.
Analgesics (acetaminophen, ibuprofen, ketorolac, opioids)	Diminish pain and provide sedation effect. Used to treat pain. Used to help avoid increase in ICP	Monitor for improvements in pain. Monitor sedation and respiratory status with narcotics. Monitor neurologic status closely. Used cautiously because loss of accurate neurologic evaluation can occur
Osmotic diuretics (i.e., mannitol)	Increases plasma osmolality, therefore inducing diffusion back into plasma and extravascular space/ reduces ICP	Monitor electrolytes. Monitor I/O closely. Monitor vital signs. Monitor for signs and symptoms of increased ICP.
Corticosteroids (i.e., dexamethasone)	Suppresses inflammation and normal immune response/reduces cerebral edema. In conjunction with a $5HT_3$ antagonist, may decrease postoperative vomiting	Give oral doses with food. Dosage must be tapered before discontinuing.
Antiemetics ($5HT_3$ receptor antagonists, dimenhydrinate)	Used to prevent and treat vomiting. May not be as efficacious for nausea/vomiting. Can result in ICP spikes in the setting of neurologic disorders, puts pressure on surgical incisions and increases the child's discomfort	Observe for signs and symptoms of nausea and vomiting. Monitor effectiveness of medication, and in the postoperative setting, consider using a preventive approach with intermittent administration of an antiemetic.

Adapted from: Karch, A. (2010). *2010 Lippincott's nursing drug guide*. Philadelphia: Wolters Kluwer Health/Lippincott Williams & Wilkins; and Taketokmo, C. K., Hodding, J. H., & Kraus, D. M. (2010). *Lexi-comp's drug reference handbook: Pediatric & neonatal dosage handbook* (18th ed.). Hudson, OH: Lexi-comp, Inc.

NURSING PROCESS OVERVIEW FOR THE CHILD WITH A NEUROLOGIC DISORDER

Care of the child with a neurologic disorder includes assessment, nursing diagnosis, planning, interventions, and evaluation. A number of general concepts related to the nursing process can be applied to the management of neurologic disorders. From a general understanding of the care involved for a child with neurologic dysfunction, nurses can then individualize the care based on the child's needs.

*R*emember Antonio, the 3-month-old with lethargy, a weak, high-pitched cry, and vomiting? What additional health history and physical examination assessment information should the nurse obtain?

Assessment

Neurologic assessment in children includes health history, physical examination, and laboratory and diagnostic testing.

> ▶ *Take* NOTE!
>
> *Neurologic assessment should proceed from least invasive to most invasive. A period of distant observation of the child can provide invaluable information. The use of toys and familiar objects, as well as incorporating play, will help promote cooperation from the child. Whenever possible, keep the child with his or her parents or primary caregiver.*

Health History

The health history consists of the past medical history (including the mother's pregnancy history), family history, and history of present illness (when the symptoms started and how they have progressed) as well as allergies, medications, and treatments used at home. The past medical history might be significant for prematurity, difficult birth, infection during pregnancy, failure to meet developmental milestones, nausea, vomiting, headaches, irritability, gait changes, falls, visual disturbances, or trauma. Family history might be significant for genetic disorders with neurologic manifestations, seizure disorders, or headaches. When eliciting the history of the present illness, inquire about the following:

- Nausea
- Vomiting
- Changes in gait
- Visual disturbances
- Complaints of headaches: headache behaviour in young children may include general irritability or more specific behaviours such as head banging or pressing the forehead to the floor or cold surface. The timing of headaches is also important (e.g., a child with hydrocephalus may wake up in the morning with a severe headache and nausea, followed by some relief after vomiting).
- Recent trauma
- Changes in school performance
- Change in consciousness, including any loss of consciousness
- Poor feeding
- Lethargy
- Increased irritability
- Fever
- Neck pain
- Altered muscle tonicity
- Delays in growth and development
- Ingestion or inhalation of neurotoxic substances or chemicals

Physical Examination

Physical examination of the nervous system consists of inspection and observation, palpation, and auscultation.

Inspection and Observation

Specific areas to inspect and observe include level of consciousness (LOC); vital signs; head, face, and neck; cranial nerve function; motor function; reflexes; sensory function; and **intracranial pressure (ICP)**.

Level of Consciousness. Begin the physical examination with inspection and observation. Observe the child's LOC, noting a decrease or significant changes. LOC is the earliest indicator of improvement or deterioration of neurologic status. Extreme irritability or lethargy is considered an abnormal finding. Consciousness consists of alertness and cognition. Alertness is a wakeful state and includes the ability to respond to stimuli. Cognition includes the ability to process stimuli and demonstrate a verbal or motor response. Five different states constitute the levels of consciousness:

1. *Full consciousness* is defined as a state in which the child is awake and alert. The child is oriented to time, place, and person as developmentally appropriate and exhibits age-appropriate behaviours.
2. *Confusion* is defined as a state in which disorientation exists. The child may be alert but responds inappropriately to questions.
3. *Obtunded* is defined as a state in which the child has limited responses to the environment and falls asleep unless stimulation is provided.
4. *Stupor* exists when the child only responds to vigorous stimulation.
5. *Coma* defines a state in which the child cannot be aroused, even with painful stimuli.

The Glasgow Coma Scale (Teasdale & Jennett, 1974) is commonly used to standardize LOC. It consists of three parts: eye opening, verbal response, and motor response. An example of an adaptation of the Glasgow Coma Scale for children into a neurologic assessment tool is shown in Figure 37.2. When assessing LOC in children, consider that the infant or child may not respond to unfamiliar voices in an unfamiliar environment. Therefore, it may be helpful to observe the parents interacting with the child. It is also important to record the infant or child's best response and note any use of sedation that may affect the child's response.

> ▶ *Take* NOTE!
>
> *Many times parents will be the first to notice changes in their child's LOC. Listen to parents and respond to their concerns.*

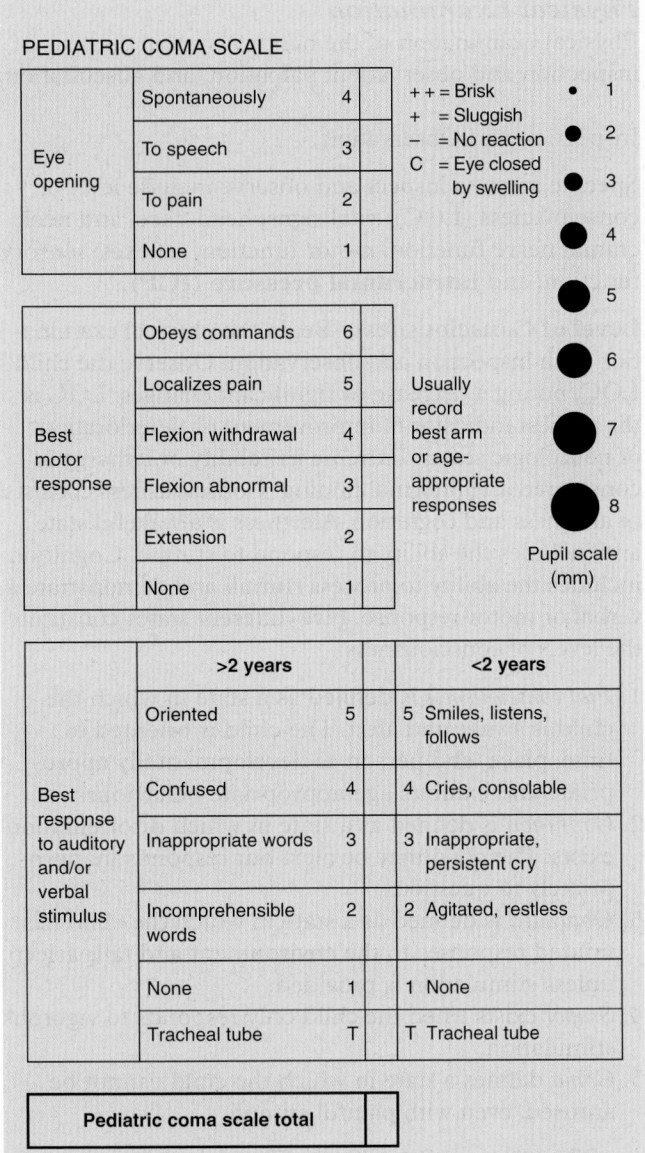

PEDIATRIC COMA SCALE

Eye opening	Spontaneously	4
	To speech	3
	To pain	2
	None	1

+ + = Brisk
+ = Sluggish
− = No reaction
C = Eye closed by swelling

Best motor response	Obeys commands	6
	Localizes pain	5
	Flexion withdrawal	4
	Flexion abnormal	3
	Extension	2
	None	1

Usually record best arm or age-appropriate responses

Pupil scale (mm)

Best response to auditory and/or verbal stimulus	>2 years		<2 years
	Oriented	5	5 Smiles, listens, follows
	Confused	4	4 Cries, consolable
	Inappropriate words	3	3 Inappropriate, persistent cry
	Incomprehensible words	2	2 Agitated, restless
	None	1	1 None
	Tracheal tube	T	T Tracheal tube

| Pediatric coma scale total | |

FIGURE 37.2 Example of a pediatric neurologic assessment tool. The adapted pediatric Glasgow Coma Scale in this tool provides for developmentally appropriate cues to assess level of consciousness (LOC) in infants and children. Numeric values are assigned to the levels of response and the sum provides an overall picture, as well as an objective measure, of the child's LOC.

▶ *Take* NOTE!

Lack of response to painful stimuli is abnormal and can indicate a life-threatening condition. Report this finding immediately.

Vital Signs. Certain neurologic conditions such as cerebral infections, increased ICP, coma, brain stem injury, or head injuries can cause alterations in the pediatric client's vital signs. The classic Cushing's triad (bradycardia, hypertension, and bradypnea) that indicates

pending demise in adults is not often seen in children. Any bradycardia, even sustained mild bradycardia, is an ominous sign in children after neurosurgery or with a neurologic deficit and should be investigated immediately.

Head, Face, and Neck. Inspect and observe the head for size and shape. Abnormal skull shape can result from head positioning or, rarely, premature closure of cranial sutures. Inspect and observe the face for symmetry. Asymmetry may occur due to paralysis of certain cranial nerves, position in utero, or swelling caused by trauma. Observe the child's neck movements and preferred position at rest (i.e., does the child have a head tilt). If CNS infection such as meningitis is suspected, neck stiffness will be observed.

All children younger than 3 years of age and any child whose head size is questionable should have their head circumference measured and plotted on a growth chart (see Appendix F for growth charts). Assessment of the growth trend of the head is important in detecting potential neurologic conditions. Report and investigate any variation in head circumference percentiles over time. A rapid increase in head size could indicate hydrocephalus, mass lesion, or a genetic megalencephaly syndrome, while a rapid decrease may indicate a congenital or perinatal brain insult or a genetic microencephaly syndrome. It is the pattern of growth over time that is important as most children with large or small heads that follow a normal growth curve do not have an underlying problem. Indeed, one parent may also have a large or small head just like their child does.

▶ *Take* NOTE!

Any assessment that involves movement of the head and neck should not be attempted in cases of trauma or suspected trauma until cervical injury is ruled out. Maintain complete immobilization of the cervical spine until that time.

Cranial Nerve Function. Techniques for assessing cranial nerve function in children are similar to adult assessment techniques. The method of obtaining responses may vary based on the age and developmental level of the child. Certain elements of the adult assessment may be omitted. Alterations in cranial nerve function can be the result of compression of a specific nerve, infection, or trauma leading to brain injury. Refer to Table 37.1 for an explanation of cranial nerve assessment in children. Watching the child play, laugh, and interact with his or her parents and listening to the child talk before any examination provides valuable information.

Use the doll's eyes manoeuvre to evaluate cranial nerves III, IV, and VI. This manoeuvre can be helpful when assessing an infant, uncooperative child, or comatose client. It examines horizontal and vertical eye movements by turning the head in one direction and assessing

TABLE 37.1 ASSESSMENT OF CRANIAL NERVES IN INFANTS AND CHILDREN

Cranial Nerve	Function	Assessment Procedure
I (olfactory) II (optic)	Sense of smell Vision	Not evaluated in infants and young children. In children, assess child's ability to recognize common smells (e.g., an orange) while eyes are closed. Do not use strong alcohol-based scents as they can be a sensory stimulant instead of an olfactory stimulant. It is important to assess these nerves after a frontal head or facial injury as they can be severed. Ophthalmoscopic exam is important in assessing damage to retina and retinal vessels (retinal hemorrhage often seen in shaken baby syndrome). Papilledema is especially important in children at risk for increased ICP such as children with hydrocephalus, shunt malfunction, brain tumours, or trauma. The normally sharp optic disk margins become blurred. A skilled clinician can quickly assess for papilledema in an active infant or child by darkening the room and coming in from side of child before he or she can blink. Assess vision fields and visual acuity in the older child. Talk to the child or have the parent in the visual field while applying stimulus.
III (oculomotor), IV (Trochlear), VI (Abducens)	Motor control and sensation of eye muscles, movement of major eye muscles	Assess extraocular eye movement by having child follow object (toy or brightly coloured object) in the shape of an H to cover the six cardinal directions. The abducens nerve has a long subarachnoid course and is the most sensitive indicator of intracranial hypertension. Assess pupil reaction (oculomotor) the same as in an adult.
V (trigeminal)	Mastication muscles and facial sensation	Note strength of infant's suck on pacifier, examiner's thumb, or bottle. In children, assess strength of bite and ability to discern light touch on face.
VII (facial)	Facial muscles, salivation, and taste	Note symmetry of facial expressions; in infant, monitor during spontaneous cries or smiles. Ask child to show you his or her teeth, close eyes tight, and whistle. In older child, test as in adults. Assess taste by asking to discern certain common tastes (salt, sugar).
VIII (acoustic)	Hearing	In infant, note response to voice. In children, use whisper test or a Weber's or Rinne test. Ask child to talk to parents using a cell phone, alternating ears. Consult audiologist if further assessment is required.
IX (glossopharyngeal), X (vagus)	Motor impulses to heart and other organs, swallowing, and gag reflex	Watch for soft palate and uvula movement when a child says "ah." Note voice quality such as hoarseness or whispering and problems with articulation. Ask parents if they have noticed any changes in child's speech sounds. Gag reflex and swallowing are tested as in adults. Check time of last feeding, especially in the infant, to avoid vomiting when gag reflex is tested (do not test gag reflex if not necessary). Consult a speech language therapist if further assessment is required.
XI (accessory)	Impulses to muscles of shoulders and pharynx	In infants, note symmetry of head position when placed in the sitting position. In children, same as adults: have them turn their head in both directions and shrug their shoulders against resistance. This can be made into a game of strength!
XII (hypoglossal)	Motor impulses to tongue and skeletal muscles	In infants, note spontaneous tongue movements. Have child stick out the tongue after testing (i.e., show me your teeth, close your eyes tight, stick out your tongue) and observe for symmetry.

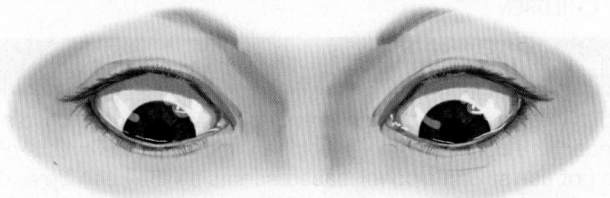

FIGURE 37.3 Sunsetting of the eyes is a sign of dilation of the third ventricle as seen in chronic untreated hydrocephalus.

whether the eyes move symmetrically in the other direction. For example, if you suddenly turn the child's head to the right, the child's eyes should look to the left symmetrically. Assess vertical eye movements in a similar manner by flexing or extending the neck (do not perform this manoeuvre if there is any worry about the cervical spine). Absence of expected eye movements may indicate increased ICP. When assessing oculomotor function, be sure to note nystagmus or sunset appearance of the eyes. Observe for nystagmus by looking for involuntary, rapid, rhythmic eye movements that may be present at rest or with eye movement. Horizontal nystagmus may occur with lesions in the brain stem and can be the result of certain medications (phenytoin in particular). Vertical nystagmus indicates brain stem dysfunction. *Sunsetting* is when the sclera of the eyes is showing over the top of the iris (Fig. 37.3). With sunsetting, the infant or child is unable to look up when the head is held still and an interesting object is moved above the child's gaze; they will lift their eyebrows and eyelids in an attempt to follow the object but will be unable to lift their eyes. Sunset eyes may indicate hydrocephalus with third ventricle dilation as vertical eye movements are coordinated near the back of the third ventricle. Finally, pupillary response may be abnormal when a neurologic disorder is present. Figure 37.4 demonstrates varied pupillary responses.

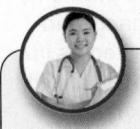

▶ *Take* NOTE!

Report immediately the sudden presence of one or both fixed and dilated pupils.

Motor Function. Alterations in motor function, such as changes in gait, muscle tone, or strength, may result from increased ICP, head injury, and cerebral infections. Observe muscle strength, bulk, and tone in the infant or child. Assess bilaterally and compare. Observe spontaneous activity, posture, and balance and assess for asymmetrical movements. In the infant, observe resting posture, which will normally be a slightly flexed posture. The infant should be able to extend extremities to a normal stretch. Because cortical control of motor function is lost in certain neurologic disorders, postural reflexes reemerge and are directly related to the area of the brain that is damaged. Therefore, it is important to assess for two distinct types of posturing that may

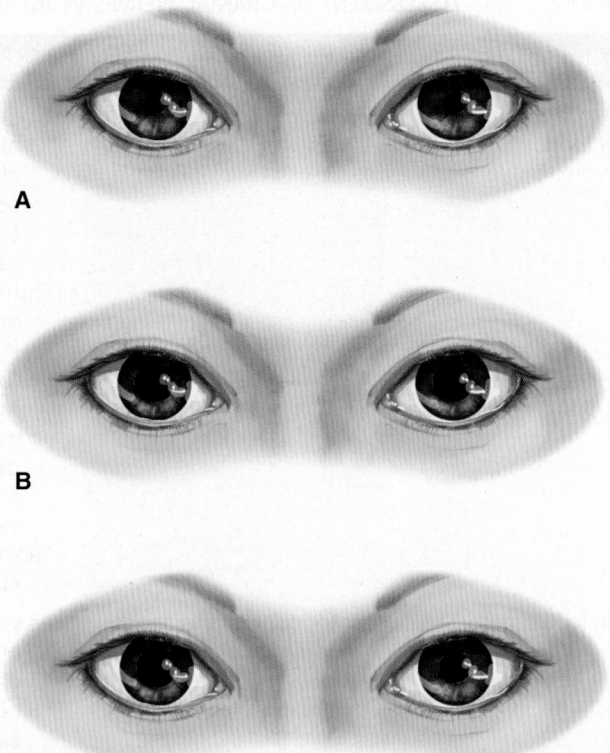

A

B

C

FIGURE 37.4 Assessing pupil size and reaction: (**A**) *Pinpoint* is commonly observed in poisonings, brain stem dysfunction, and opiate use. (**B**) *Dilated but reactive* is seen in the dark or occasionally after seizures. *Fixed and dilated* is associated with brain stem herniation secondary to increased ICP. (**C**) *One dilated and fixed* may indicate ipsilateral uncal herniation with third nerve compression. Note that anisocoria (unequal pupil size) is a normal variant.

occur. **Decorticate posturing** occurs with damage of the cerebral cortex (Fig. 37.5A).

Decerebrate posturing occurs with damage at the level of the brain stem (Fig. 37.5B). Both types of posturing are characterized by extremely rigid muscle tone and lower limb extension.

Reflexes. Testing of deep-tendon reflexes is part of the neurologic assessment, just as it is in adults. Testing of primitive and protective reflexes in the infant is important because infants cannot perform tasks on command. The Moro, tonic neck, and withdrawal reflexes are important in assessing neurologic health in infants. Refer to Chapter 25 (Table 25.2) for a further explanation of primitive and protective reflexes in infants. Absence of certain reflexes, asymmetry of reflexes, persistence of primitive reflexes after the age of normal disappearance, or increases in reflexes may be present in specific neurologic conditions.

Sensory Function. Alterations in sensory function can result from brain or spinal cord lesions. Assessment of sensory function is often difficult in children under the age of 12. When assessing sensory function, the child should be able to distinguish between light touch, pain, vibration, heat, and cold. When assessing

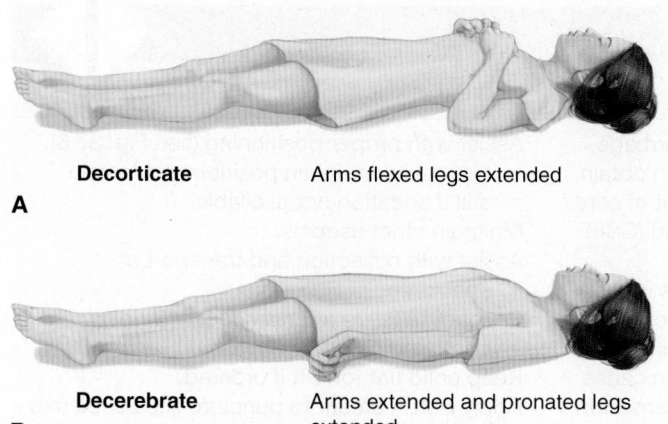

Decorticate Arms flexed legs extended

A

Decerebrate Arms extended and pronated legs extended

B

FIGURE 37.5 (**A**) Decorticate posturing occurs with damage of the cerebral cortex and includes adduction of the arms, flexion at the elbows with arms held over chest, and flexion of the wrists with hands fisted. Lower extremities are adducted and extended. (**B**) Decerebrate posturing occurs with damage that includes the midbrain and includes extension and pronation of the arms with legs extended.

an infant, limit the examination to responses to touch or pain. The normal response in a 4-month-old infant will be movement away from the stimulus. In the child, techniques similar to those used in the adult assessment are followed. Make sure to explain what you are doing to the child, especially before the pin-prick test, to gain continued cooperation.

Increased Intracranial Pressure. Increased ICP may occur with many neurologic disorders. It may result from head trauma, hydrocephalus, infection, brain tumours, and intracranial hemorrhage. Observe for signs and symptoms associated with increased ICP while caring for a child with a potential or suspected neurologic disorder. Refer to Comparison Chart 37.1 for early versus late signs and symptoms of increased ICP. As ICP increases, LOC decreases and the signs and symptoms will become more pronounced. It is

essential to recognize early signs and symptoms of increased ICP and intervene immediately to prevent long-term damage and possible death.

Palpation

Palpation of the newborn and infant skull and fontanels is an important function of the neurologic examination. Changes in size or fullness of the fontanels may exist in certain neurologic conditions and must be noted. A bulging fontanel can be a sign of increased ICP and is seen in such neurologic disorders as hydrocephalus and head trauma. It is normal for the fontanels to be full or bulging during crying; take this into consideration during assessment.

The posterior fontanel normally closes by 2 months of age, and the anterior fontanel normally closes by 12 to 18 months of age. In children with hydrocephalus, widening of the fontanels may be noted, along with palpable tension and a resulting increase in **head circumference**. Non-palpable fontanels in the presence of a skull that is otherwise normal in size and shape is not a cause for concern. In craniosynostosis (premature fusion of skull bones), skull growth continues parallel to the fused suture and is restricted perpendicular to the fused sutures resulting in an abnormal skull shape (Virchow, 1851).

Auscultation

If the clinician suspects an intracranial vascular disorder, the skull may be auscultated in the temporal regions. The finding of a loud or localized bruit is usually significant and requires immediate further investigation (i.e., angiogram). Benign symmetric bruits may be auscultated in children less than 4 years of age or in children with acute febrile illness.

Laboratory and Diagnostic Testing

Common Laboratory and Diagnostic Tests 37.1 offers explanations of the most commonly used laboratory

COMPARISON CHART 37.1 EARLY VS. LATE SIGNS OF INCREASED INTRACRANIAL PRESSURE

Early Signs	Late Signs

• Headache
• Vomiting, possibly projectile
• Blurred vision, double vision (diplopia)
• Dizziness
• Decreased pulse and respirations
• Increased blood pressure or pulse pressure
• Pupil reaction time decreased, unequal, or both
• Changes in LOC, irritability
• In infant, will also see:
  • Bulging, tense fontanel
  • Wide sutures and increased head circumference
  • Dilated scalp veins
  • High-pitched cry
	• Decreased LOC
	• Bradycardia
	• Irregular respirations
	• Cheyne–Stokes respirations
	• Decerebrate or decorticate posturing
	• Fixed and dilated pupils

(text continues on page 464)

COMMON LABORATORY AND DIAGNOSTIC TESTS 37.1

Test	Explanation	Indications	Nursing Implications
Lumbar puncture (LP)	Withdraw CSF from the subarachnoid space for analysis	Diagnose hemorrhage, infection. Can obtain measurement of cerebrospinal fluid (CSF) pressure LP is dangerous in the context of increased intracranial pressure (ICP) as it can cause downward herniation of the brain.	Assist with proper positioning (see Fig. 37.6). Help child maintain position and remain still if sedation not available. Maintain strict asepsis. Assist with collection and transport of specimen. Encourage fluids after procedure if not contraindicated. Keep child flat for 1 h if ordered. Apply EMLA cream to puncture site 30–60 min before procedure to reduce pain, if ordered.
Head and neck X-ray	Radiographic image of the head and neck	Detect skull and spinal fractures Show location and course of ventricular catheters reveal information about increased ICP and skull defects. In tertiary care hospitals, plain films are largely replaced by computed tomography (CT) or magnetic resonance imaging (MRI)	Children may be afraid. Allow a parent or family member to accompany the child. If the child is unable or unwilling to stay still for the X-ray, restraint may be necessary. The time of restraint should be limited to the amount of time needed for the X-ray.
Cerebral angiography	X-ray study of cerebral blood vessels. Involves injection of a contrast medium and use of fluoroscopy (continuous biplanar X-ray to show live images)	Show vessel abnormalities or space-occupying lesions	Same as head and neck X-rays. Assess for allergy to contrast medium. Push fluids following procedure, if not contraindicated, to help flush out contrast medium. Assess arterial puncture site for hematoma. Assess circulation of the limb distal to the puncture.
Ultrasound	Use of sound waves to locate the depth and structure within soft tissues and fluid	Assess intracranial hemorrhage in newborns and determine ventricular size	Better tolerated by nonsedated children than CT or MRI Can be performed at bedside
Computed tomography (CT)	X-ray study that looks at tissue density and structures. Images only a "slice" of tissue at a time.	Used when emergency scans are needed in the absence of an available MRI unit.	Machine is large and can be frightening to children. Sedation may be necessary. Can be performed with or without the use of contrast medium; if contrast used, assess for allergy and encourage fluids postprocedure if not contraindicated.
Electroencephalogram (EEG)	Measures electrical activity of the brain. Can be measured over the course of days using a cap-like electrode array	Diagnose seizures Can be used to investigate coma or brain death	Inform technician of what anticonvulsants the client is taking. Morning anticonvulsants may need to be withheld.

Test	Explanation	Indications	Nursing Implications
Magnetic resonance imaging (MRI)	Use of a high-intensity magnetic field and radio-frequency energy to show different tissue characteristics	Assess tumours and inflammation Diagnose congenital abnormalities, such as neural tube defects Shows normal versus abnormal brain tissue	Client may not have any metal devices, internal or external, while undergoing MRI (ensure hospital gown does not have metal snaps). Procedure can be lengthy and child must remain still. Child is placed in long narrow tube and the machine makes a banging noise when it is turned on and off during the procedure; therefore, can be difficult to gain cooperation. If the child is unable to remain still, sedation may be necessary. Can be performed with or without contrast medium. If contrast medium is used, assess for allergy and renal problems and encourage fluids postprocedure if not contraindicated.
Positron emission tomography (PET)	Similar to CT or MRI but radioisotope is added. Measures physiologic function	Provides information on brain functional development Assist in identifying seizure foci Assess tumours and brain metabolism	Procedure can be lengthy and child must remain still. If unable to do so, sedation may be necessary. IV access will be needed for the procedure. Encourage fluids postprocedure if not contraindicated, to help body eliminate radioisotopes.
Intracranial pressure (ICP) monitoring (intraventricular catheter, subarachnoid screw or bolt, epidural sensor, anterior fontanel pressure monitor)	A sensing device is placed in the head to monitor ICP.	Monitor ICP resulting from hydrocephalus, acute head trauma, and brain tumours. Ventricular catheter also allows for draining of CSF to help reduce ICP.	Usually monitored in critical care setting. Monitor for signs and symptoms of increased ICP. Monitor for infection. Keep head of bed elevated 15°–30° Alarms for monitoring device should remain on at all times. Reduce stimulation and avoid interventions that may cause pain or stress and result in an increased ICP.
Video electroencephalogram (EEG)	Measure electrical activity of the brain continuously along with recorded video of actions and behaviours	Help determine precise localization of seizure area before surgery. Assist in diagnosis and management of seizures by correlating behaviours with abnormal EEG activity	Ensure that seizure precautions are in place. Parent or caregiver must be with client at all times. Client movements are limited and usually confined to the room. When client changes position, ensure that he or she is still seen by video camera. Boredom can be a problem. Must notify nurse if seizure activity occurs; push the alert button to highlight attack on EEG recoding. Nurse must immediately go to the room, expose as much of the client as possible (remove covers; if at night, turn on light), and avoid blocking the camera. Ask questions (e.g., what is your name, can you raise your left arm, remember the word banana) to help assess responsiveness more accurately. Stay with the client until full recovery has occurred. Ask the client what word you asked him or her to remember, and document all findings and time of the event.

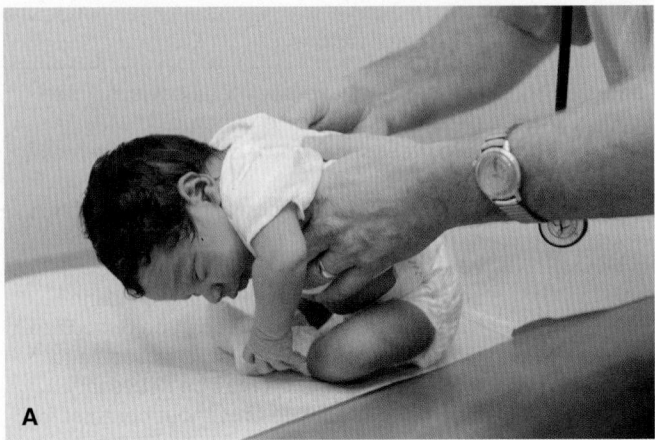
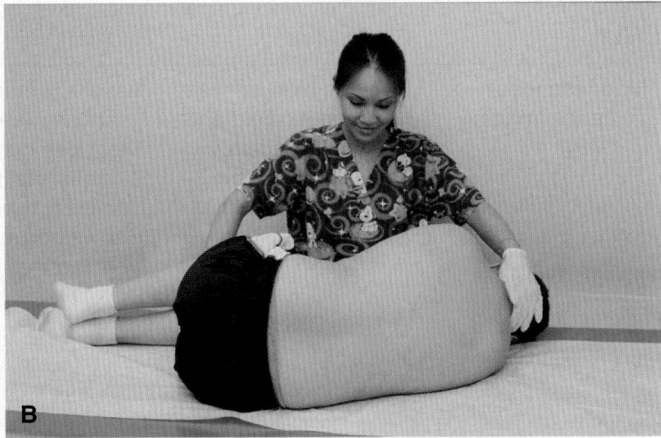

FIGURE 37.6 Proper positioning for a LP. (**A**) The newborn is positioned upright with head flexed forward. (**B**) The child or older infant is positioned on the side with head flexed forward and knees flexed to abdomen.

and diagnostic tests when considering neurologic disorders. The tests can assist the physician in diagnosing the disorder and/or serve as guidelines in determining ongoing treatment. Laboratory or non-nursing personnel obtain some of the tests, while a nurse might obtain others. In either instance, nurses should be familiar with how the tests are obtained, what they are used for, and normal versus abnormal results. This knowledge will also be necessary when providing child and family education related to the testing. Many of these tests, such as **lumbar puncture** (LP; Fig. 37.6), can be frightening to parents and the child. Prepare the family and the child and provide support and reassurance during and after the test or procedure.

After completing an assessment of Antonio, the nurse noted the following: a full, taut anterior fontanel; when being held, Antonio was inconsolable; when lying still, he was calmer.

Nursing Diagnoses and Related Interventions

Upon completion of a thorough assessment, the nurse might identify several nursing diagnoses, including:

- Risk for increased ICP
- Pain
- Impaired physical mobility
- Imbalanced nutrition: less than body requirements
- Risk for deficient fluid volume
- Interrupted family processes

Nursing goals, interventions, and evaluation for the child with a neurologic disorder are based on the nursing diagnoses.

Based on the assessment findings, what would be your top three prioritized nursing diagnoses for Antonio?

Nursing Care Plan 37.1 may be used as a guide in planning nursing care for the child with a neurologic disorder. It should be individualized based on the client's symptoms and needs. Additional information will be included later in this chapter related to specific disorders.

Based on your top three nursing diagnoses for Antonio, describe appropriate nursing interventions.

Seizure Disorders

Mikati (2011) identifies that only 30% of people who have a first afebrile seizure are later diagnosed with epilepsy. Underlying causes of seizures include electrolyte imbalance, meningitis, metabolic disorders, head trauma, brain lesions, and cardiorespiratory problems. Seizure disorders discussed below include epilepsy, febrile seizures, and neonatal seizures.

Epilepsy

Epilepsy is a condition in which seizures are triggered recurrently from within the brain. Epilepsy is a common neurologic disorder discovered in childhood, although brain injury or infection can cause epilepsy at any age. Epilepsy Canada (visit http://thePoint.lww.com/Chow1e for a direct link) indicates that "when repeated seizures continue to occur for unknown reasons (idiopathic) or because of an underlying problem that cannot be corrected (symptomatic), the condition is known as epilepsy." The prognosis for most children with seizures associated with epilepsy is good. Many children will outgrow epilepsy, but some children will have persistent seizures that are difficult to manage and may be unresponsive to pharmacologic interventions. Living with a seizure disorder may impact on the quality of life of the child and family.

(text continues on page 1189)

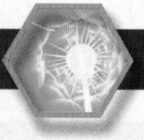

Nursing Care Plan 37.1

OVERVIEW FOR THE CHILD WITH A NEUROLOGIC DISORDER

NURSING DIAGNOSIS^a: At risk for increased ICP, which could result in downward herniation of brain structures due to accumulation of CSF in the ventricles, cerebral edema secondary to brain injury or infection, space-occupying lesions, as evidenced by vomiting, headache, complaints of visual disturbances, decreased pulse and respirations, elevated blood pressure or widening pulse pressure, changes in level of consciousness, decreased pupillary response, increased head circumference, or bulging fontanel in an infant.

Outcome Identification and Evaluation

Child will remain free of signs and symptoms of increased ICP as evidenced by remaining free of headache, vomiting, vision disturbances, vital signs within parameters for age, no signs of altered LOC, free of excessive irritability or lethargy, head circumference and anterior fontanels are within parameters for age, and pupils equal and responsive to light.

Interventions: Monitoring and Maintaining Normal Intracranial Pressure

- Assess neurologic status closely, monitor for signs and symptoms of increased ICP: *Changes in LOC, signs of irritability or lethargy, and changes in pupillary reaction can indicate changes in ICP.*
- Monitor vital signs: *Decreased pulse and respiratory rate and increased blood pressure or pulse pressure can indicate increased ICP.*
- Measure head circumference in children <3 years of age: *Increases in head circumference outside parameters for age can indicate increased ICP.*
- Elevate head of bed 15 to 30 degrees *to facilitate venous return and can help to reduce ICP.*
- Minimize environmental stimuli and noise, and avoid pain-producing procedures if possible: *All can increase ICP.*
- Have emergency equipment ready and available: *Increased ICP can result in respiratory or cardiac arrest.*
- Notify physician immediately if changes in assessment are noted: *Early intervention is critical to prevent neurologic damage and death.*
- Follow ordered parameters for EVD, including the height of the reservoir that is open to drainage, and monitor for normal ICP (0–15 mm Hg) *to ensure that actions can be taken for increased ICP.*

NURSING DIAGNOSIS: Risk for ineffective (cerebral) tissue perfusion related to increased ICP, alteration in blood flow secondary to hemorrhage, vessel malformation, cerebral edema

Outcome Identification and Evaluation

Child will exhibit adequate cerebral tissue perfusion through course of illness and childhood: Child will remain alert and oriented with no signs of altered LOC; vital signs will be within parameters for age; motor, sensory, and cognitive function will be within parameters for age; head circumference remains within parameters for age.

Interventions: Promoting Adequate Tissue Perfusion

- Assess neurologic status closely, monitor for signs and symptoms of increased ICP: *Changes in LOC, signs of irritability or lethargy, changes in pupillary reaction can indicate decreased cerebral tissue perfusion.*
- Monitor vital signs: *Decreased pulse and respiratory rate and increased blood pressure or pulse pressure can indicate increased ICP, which can lead to decreased cerebral perfusion.*
- Monitor serum NaCl *to detect over-secretion or under-secretion of antidiuretic hormone.* (See Chapter 48 for information on syndrome of inappropriate antidiuretic hormone [SIADH] and diabetes insipidus [DI].)
- Avoid hypovolemia, maintain adequate blood pressure, control ICP with CSF drainage if the child has an EVD system, and use osmotic diuretics (i.e., mannitol) appropriately *to maintain cerebral perfusion pressure as ordered.*
- Have emergency equipment ready and available: *Decreased cerebral perfusion can result in respiratory or cardiac failure.*
- Notify physician immediately if changes in assessment are noted: *Early intervention with appropriate brain imaging is critical to prevent neurologic damage and death.*

(continued)

Nursing Care Plan 37.1 (continued)

NURSING DIAGNOSIS: Risk for injury related to altered level of consciousness, weakness, dizziness, ataxia, loss of muscle coordination secondary to seizure activity

Outcome Identification and Evaluation
Child will remain free of injury as evidenced by no signs of aspiration or traumatic injury.

Interventions: Preventing Injury
- Ensure child has patent airway and adequate oxygenation (have suction, oxygen available at bedside) and place child in side-lying position if possible: *A child with altered LOC may not be able to manage secretions and is at risk for aspiration and ineffective airway clearance; providing suction and oxygenation can help ensure an open airway and the side-lying position can help secretions drain and prevent obstruction of airway or aspiration.*
- Protect child from hurting self during seizures or changes in LOC by removing environmental obstacles, easing child to lying position, and padding side rails *to help keep the environment safe.*
- Institute seizure precautions for any child at risk for seizure activity (see Box 37.2) *to help prevent injury that can result from acute seizure activity.*
- Do not insert a tongue blade or restrain child during a seizure *to avoid injury to caregiver and child.*
- Administer anticonvulsant medications as ordered *to help promote cessation and prevention of seizure activity.*
- Assist child with ambulation *to help prevent injury in child with weakness, dizziness, or ataxia.*
- Allow for periods of rest *to prevent fatigue and decrease risk of injury.*

NURSING DIAGNOSIS: Disturbed sensory perception related to presence of neurologic lesion or pressure on sensory or motor nerves secondary to increased ICP, presence of tumour, swelling postoperatively as evidenced by visual disturbances (i.e., reports of double vision), pupillary changes, nystagmus, ataxia, balance disturbances, or loss of response to stimuli

Outcome Identification and Evaluation
Child will be free of changes in sensory perception or will remain at baseline as evidenced by no complaints of double vision, PERRLA, no disturbances of gait or balance noted, and no increased in loss of responses to stimuli. Observe for changes if these are present and communicate the child's baseline sensory disturbances to the health care team.

Interventions: Managing Disturbed Sensory Perception
- Assess for changes in sensory perception *to provide baseline data and allow nurse to recognize change in sensory perception early.*
- Monitor child for risk of injury secondary to changes in sensory perception: *Visual changes and disturbances of gait or balance increase child's risk for injury.*
- Notify physician of changes in sensory perception: *Can indicate increased ICP and medical emergency.*
- Assist child to learn to use adaptive methods to live with permanent changes in sensory perception (i.e., use of prism eyeglasses or eye patches for diplopia) and maximize the use of intact senses: *Adaptive devices can enhance sensory input and intact senses can often compensate for impaired senses.*
- Provide familiar sounds (voices, music) *to help relieve anxiety related to changes in sensory perception, especially visual changes.*
- Work with OT/PT/SLP to establish a rehabilitation program *to promote optimal fine motor, gross motor, and speech-language rehabilitation outcomes.*

NURSING DIAGNOSIS: Risk for infection related to surgical interventions, presence of foreign body (i.e., shunt), trauma to skull, nutritional deficiencies, stasis of pulmonary secretions and urine, presence of infectious organisms as evidenced by fever, poor feeding, decreased responsiveness, and presence of virus or bacteria on laboratory screening

Outcome Identification and Evaluation
Child will exhibit no signs or symptoms of local or systemic infection and will not spread infection to others: Symptoms of infection will decrease over time; others will remain free of infection.

Nursing Care Plan 37.1 (continued)

Interventions: Preventing Infection
- Monitor vital signs: *Elevation in temperature can indicate presence of infection.*
- Monitor incision sites for signs of local infection: *Redness, warmth, drainage, swelling, pain at incision site can indicate presence of infection.*
- Maintain aseptic technique—practice good handwashing and use proper technique when managing postoperative incisions and external shunts *to prevent introduction of further infectious agents.*
- Administer antibiotics as prescribed *to prevent or treat bacterial infection.*
- Encourage nutritious diet and proper hydration according to child's preferences and ability to feed orally *to assist body's natural defenses against infection.*
- Isolate child as required *to prevent nosocomial spread of infection.*
- Often a shunt infection will require removal of the entire shunt and extraventricular drainage until infection clears *to preventing recurring infection as the microorganisms may not be completely eliminated from colonized shunt hardware.*
- Teach child and family preventive measures such as good handwashing, covering mouth and nose upon cough or sneeze, and adequate disposal of used tissues *to prevent nosocomial or community spread of infection.*

NURSING DIAGNOSIS: Self-care deficit related to neuromuscular or cognitive impairments; as evidenced by an inability to perform hygiene care and transfer self independently

Outcome Identification and Evaluation
Child will demonstrate ability to care for self within age parameters and limits of disease: Child is able to feed, dress, manage elimination within limits of disease and age.

Interventions: Maximizing Self–Care
- Introduce child and family to self-help methods as soon as possible *to promote independence from the beginning.*
- Encourage family and staff to allow child to do as much as possible *to allow child to gain confidence and independence.*
- Teach specific measures for bowel and urinary elimination as needed (e.g., self-catheterization for spina bifida or spinal cord injuries) *to promote independence and increase self-care abilities and self-esteem.*
- Collaborate with physical therapy, occupational therapy, and speech therapy departments to provide child and family with appropriate tools to modify environment and methods to promote transferring and self-care *to allow for maximum functioning.*
- Praise accomplishments and emphasize child's abilities *to help improve self-esteem and encourage feelings of confidence and competence.*
- Balance activity with periods to rest *to reduce fatigue and increase energy for self-care.*

NURSING DIAGNOSIS: Impaired physical mobility related to muscle weakness, hypertonicity, impaired coordination, loss of muscle function or control as evidenced by an inability to move extremities, to ambulate without assistance, to move without limitations

Outcome Identification and Evaluation
Child will be able to engage in activities within age parameters and limits of disease: Child is able to move extremities, move about environment, and participate in exercise programs within limits of age and disease.

Interventions: Maximizing Physical Mobility
- Encourage gross and fine motor activities *to facilitate motor development.*
- Collaborate with physical therapy, occupational therapy, and speech therapy departments to strengthen muscles and promote optimal mobility *to facilitate motor development.*
- Use passive and active ROM and teach child and family how to perform these exercises *to help increase mobility by preventing contractures and facilitating joint mobility and muscle development (active ROM).*
- Praise accomplishments and emphasize child's abilities *to help improve self-esteem and encourage feelings of confidence and competence.*

(continued)

NURSING DIAGNOSIS: Risk for delayed development related to physical disability, cognitive deficits, activity restrictions

Outcome Identification and Evaluation

Child will demonstrate developmental milestones within age parameters and limits of disease: Child expresses interest in the environment and people around him or her and interacts with environment age appropriately.

Interventions: Maximizing Development

- Use therapeutic play and adaptive toys *to help facilitate developmental functioning.*
- Provide stimulating environment when possible *to maximize potential for growth and development.*
- Praise accomplishments and emphasize child's abilities *to help improve self-esteem and encourage feelings of confidence and competence.*
- Establish a relationship with the child's school for discharge planning in individual program planning *to promote optimal reintegration into the school system, including advocacy for adequate support for disabilities.*

NURSING DIAGNOSIS: Nutrition, imbalanced: Less than body requirements related to vomiting and difficulty feeding secondary to increased ICP; difficulty sucking, swallowing, or chewing; surgical incision pain or difficulty assuming normal feeding position; inability to feed self as evidenced by decreased oral intake, impaired swallowing, weight loss

Outcome Identification and Evaluation

Child will exhibit signs of adequate nutrition: Weight will remain within parameters for age, skin turgor will be good, intake and output will be within normal limits, adequate calories will be ingested, vomiting will cease or decrease.

Interventions: Promoting Adequate Nutrition

- Monitor height and weight: *Insufficient intake will lead to impaired growth and weight loss.*
- Monitor hydration status (moist mucous membranes, elastic skin turgor, adequate urine output): *Insufficient intake can lead to dehydration.*
- Use and teach the family techniques to promote caloric and nutritional intake (i.e., positioning, modified utensils, soft or blended foods, allow extra time) *to facilitate intake.*
- Assess respiratory system frequently *to assess for aspiration.*
- Monitor for nausea and vomiting and medicate if ordered *to help reduce vomiting and increase intake.*
- Monitor for pain and medicate if ordered *to help reduce pain related to surgical incisions and trauma, and increase intake.*
- Assist family to assume as normal a feeding position as possible *to help increase oral intake.*
- Monitor child's ability to manage secretions, keep oral suction available at bedside and teach child and/or family how to use it. Children at risk for impaired swallowing also require a swallowing assessment by an OT or SLP *to identify risk for aspiration and allow for secretion management by the child and family.*
- Provide short-term or long-term enteral feeding as required and implement appropriate family teaching *to ensure adequate nutrition that the family can maintain at home.*

NURSING DIAGNOSIS: Fluid volume deficit, risk for, related to vomiting, altered level of consciousness, poor feeding or intake, insensible loss due to fever, failure of regulatory mechanisms (as in diabetes insipidus) as evidenced by dry oral mucosa, decreased skin turgor, sudden weight loss, hypotension, and tachycardia

Outcome Identification and Evaluation

Fluid volume will be maintained and balanced: Oral mucosa moist and pink, skin turgor elastic, urine output at least 1 to 2 mL/kg/hour

Interventions: Promoting Adequate Fluid Balance

- Administer IV fluids if ordered *to maintain adequate hydration in children who are NPO or unable to tolerate oral intake.*
- When oral intake is allowed and tolerated, encourage oral fluids *to promote intake and maintain hydration.*
- Strictly monitor intake and output *to help identify fluid imbalance and detect signs of abnormal pituitary secretions resulting in conditions such as SIADH and DI (see Chapter 48 for further information).*
- Maintain normal hydration and avoid over-hydration in children in whom cerebral edema is a concern: *Fluid overload can contribute to cerebral edema.*
- Monitor serum electrolytes (especially serum sodium), urea nitrogen, creatinine, and osmolality; measure urine specific gravity and take daily weights: *These are reliable indicators of fluid status and can also detect signs of abnormal pituitary secretions resulting in conditions such as SIADH and DI.*

Nursing Care Plan 37.1 (continued)

NURSING DIAGNOSIS: Knowledge deficit related to lack of information regarding complex medical condition, prognosis, and medical needs as evidenced by verbalization, questions, or actions demonstrating lack of understanding regarding child's condition or care

Outcome Identification and Evaluation

Child and family will verbalize accurate information and understanding about condition, prognosis, and medical needs: Child and family demonstrate knowledge of condition and prognosis and medical needs, including possible causes, contributing factors, and treatment measures.

Interventions: Providing Client and Family Teaching

• Assess child's and family's willingness to learn: *Child and family must be willing to learn for teaching to be effective.*
• Provide family with time to adjust to diagnosis *to help facilitate adjustment and ability to learn and participate in child's care.*
• Repeat information *to allow family and child time to learn and understand.*
• Teach in short sessions: *Many short sessions are found to be more helpful than one long session.*
• Gear teaching to a level of understanding of the child and also the family (depends on age of child, physical condition, memory) *to ensure understanding.*
• Provide reinforcement and rewards *to help facilitate the teaching–learning process.*
• Use multiple modes of learning involving many senses (provide written, verbal, demonstration, and videos) when possible: *Child and family more likely to retain information when presented in different ways using many senses.*

NURSING DIAGNOSIS: Family processes, interrupted related to child's illness, hospitalization, diagnosis of chronic illness in child and potential long-term effects of illness as evidenced by family's presence in hospital, missed work, demonstration of inadequate coping

Outcome Identification and Evaluation

Family will maintain functional system of support and demonstrate adequate coping, adaptation of roles and functions, and decreased anxiety: Parents are involved in child's care, ask appropriate questions, express fears and concerns, and are able to discuss child's care and condition calmly.

Interventions: Promoting Adequate Family Processes

• Encourage parents and family members to verbalize concerns related to child's illness, diagnosis, and prognosis *to allow the nurse to identify concerns and areas where further education may be needed and to demonstrate family-centred care.*
• Explain therapies, procedures, child's behaviours, and plan of care to parents: *Understanding the child's current status and plan of care helps decrease anxiety.*
• Encourage parental involvement in care: *Allows parents to feel needed and valued with a sense of control over their child's health.*
• Identify family and child support systems *to identify needs and resources available for coping.*
• Educate family and child on additional resources available, such as community resources, support groups, and funding agencies, *to help them develop a wide base of support.*

ᵃNote that this is not approved NANDA terminology. All other Nursing Diagnoses included in the Nursing Care Plans are from Nursing Diagnoses: Definitions and Classification 2009–2011.

Pathophysiology

Epilepsy is a complex disorder of the CNS in which brain function is affected. Recurrent or unprovoked seizures are the clinical manifestation of epilepsy and result from a disruption of electrical communication among the neurons of the brain. This disruption results from an imbalance between the excitatory and inhibitory mechanisms in the brain, causing the neurons to either fire when they are not supposed to or not fire when they should. Epilepsy may be acquired and related to brain injury or it may be a familial tendency, but in many cases the cause is unknown (Centers for Disease Control and Prevention [CDC], 2010c).

There are two major categories of seizures: partial and generalized. In partial seizures only one area of the brain is involved, while general seizures involve the entire brain. Partial seizures account for a large portion of childhood seizures and are classified as *simple* or *complex*. Generalized seizures include infantile spasms, absence seizures, **tonic–clonic** seizures, myoclonic seizures, and

TABLE 37.2 COMMON TYPES OF SEIZURES

Type	Description	Characteristics
Infantile spasms	Uncommon type of generalized seizure seen in an epilepsy syndrome of infancy and childhood Usually seen at 3–12 months of age and usually stop by 2–4 years of age	Presents as a sudden jerk followed by stiffening May see: • Head flexed, arms extended, and legs drawn up • Arms fling out, knees are pulled up, and the body bends forward (referred to as "jackknife seizures") • Cry may precede or follow Majority of infants have some brain disorder before seizures begin. The infant seems to stop developing and may lose skills that he or she has already attained after the onset of infantile spasms. Steroid therapy and anticonvulsants are common forms of treatment.
Absence (formerly *petit mal*)	Type of generalized seizure Occurs more frequently in girls than boys Uncommon before age 5	Sudden cessation of motor activity or speech with a blank facial expression or rhythmic twitching of the mouth or blinking of the eyelids Complex absence seizure consists of **myoclonic** movements of the face, fingers, or extremities and possible loss of body tone. Lasts less than 30 s Child may experience countless seizures in a day. Not associated with a postictal state May go unrecognized or mistaken for inattentiveness because of subtle change in child's behaviour
Tonic–clonic (formerly *grand mal*)	Common generalized seizures Most dramatic seizure type	Associated with an aura Loss of consciousness occurs and may be preceded by a piercing cry. Presents with entire body experiencing tonic contractions followed by rhythmic clonic contractions alternating with relaxation of all muscle groups. Cyanosis may be noted due to apnea. Saliva may collect in the mouth due to inability to swallow. Child may bite tongue. Loss of sphincter control, especially the bladder, is common. Postictal phase: child will be semicomatose or in a deep sleep for approximately 30 min to 2 h; usually responds only to painful stimuli. Child will have no memory of the seizure; may complain of headache and fatigue. Safety of the child is a primary concern. See Teaching Guideline 37.1.
Myoclonic	Type of generalized seizure that involves the motor cortex of the brain May occur along with other seizure forms	Sudden, brief, massive muscle jerks that may involve the whole body or one body part. Child may or may not lose consciousness.
Atonic	Type of generalized seizure often referred to as "drop attacks" Seen in children with Lennox–Gastaut syndrome	Sudden loss of muscle tone. In children, may only be a sudden drop of the head. Child will regain consciousness within a few seconds to a minute. Can result in injury related to violent fall

Type	Description	Characteristics
Simple partial	Type of partial seizure that occurs in part of the brain The symptoms seen will depend on which area of the brain is affected.	Motor activity characterized by clonic or tonic movements involving the face, neck, and extremities. Can include sensory signs such as numbness, tingling, paresthesia, or pain Usually persists for 10–20 s Child remains conscious and may verbalize during the seizure. No postictal state
Complex partial	Common type of partial seizure May begin with a simple partial seizure then progress	May or may not have a preceding aura. Consciousness will be impaired. Automatisms and complex purposeful movements are common features in infants and children. Infants will present with behaviours such as lip smacking, chewing, swallowing, and excessive salivation; can be difficult to distinguish from normal infant behaviour. In older children, will see picking or pulling at bed sheets or clothing, rubbing objects, or running or walking in a nondirective and repetitive fashion. These seizures can be difficult to control.
Status epilepticus	Common neurologic emergency in children Can occur with any seizure activity In children with epilepsy, it commonly occurs early in the course of epilepsy. Can be life threatening	Prolonged or clustered seizures in which consciousness does not return between seizures. The age of the child, cause of the seizures, and duration of **status epilepticus** influence prognosis. Prompt medical intervention is essential to reduce morbidity and mortality. Treatment includes: • Basic life support—ABCs (airway, breathing, circulation) • Administration of anticonvulsants to cease seizures is crucial. Common medications include benzodiazepines such as lorazepam and diazepam, and phenytoin (see Drug Guide 37.1 and Table 37.3). • Blood glucose levels and electrolytes along with evaluation of the underlying cause should be initiated.

Adapted from: Cavazos, J. E., & Spitz, M. (2011). *Seizures and epilepsy: Overview and classification.* Retrieved December 3, 2011 from http://emedicine.medscape.com/article/1184846-overview; Johnston, M. V. (2007). Seizures in children. In R. M. Kliegman, R. E. Behrman, H. B. Jenson, & B. F. Stanton (Eds.), *Nelson's textbook of pediatrics* (18th ed.). Philadelphia: Saunders; and Zak, M., & Chan, V. W. (2010). Pediatric neurologic disorders. In S. M. Nettina (Ed.), *Lippincott manual of nursing practice* (9th ed.). Philadelphia: Lippincott Williams & Wilkins.

atonic seizures. There are many different types of seizures, and the classification of the type of seizure is crucial in assisting with the management and control of seizures. Not all cases are easily classified. The most common seizure types are discussed in Table 37.2.

Therapeutic Management

Management of epilepsy focuses on controlling seizures or reducing their frequency and helping the child with recurrent seizures and his or her family to cope with and adapt to the seizure disorder. The primary mode of treatment is the use of anticonvulsants. There have been significant advances in the treatment of epilepsy due to the many new anticonvulsant medications that have become available in recent years (Table 37.3). Most anticonvul-

sants are taken orally and are often used in combination. Different medications control different types of seizures, which may be due to individual variation. It can take time to find the right combination to best control an individual's seizures, and modifications in medications across the lifespan are often required.

If seizures remain uncontrolled, another option for managing them is surgery. Depending on the area of the brain that is affected, it may be possible to remove the area that is responsible for the seizure activity or to interrupt the impulses from spreading and therefore stop or reduce the seizures. The adverse effects range from mild to severe, depending on the area of the brain that is affected. Other non-pharmacologic treatments that may be considered in children with intractable seizures

TABLE 37.3 COMMON ANTICONVULSANT MEDICATIONS

Medication	Nursing Implications
Phenytoin (IV and PO; IM administration is contraindicated)	Monitor serum levels to ensure therapeutic dosing. Be aware that gingival hyperplasia appears most commonly in children and adolescents. If on prolonged therapy, ensure adequate intake of vitamin D–containing foods. Monitor serum calcium and magnesium levels.
Phenobarbital	Assess for excessive sedation. Monitor serum levels to ensure therapeutic dosing. Monitor for drug interactions. Increase vitamin D–fortified foods or administer supplement if prescribed. Withdrawal symptoms will occur if drug is stopped abruptly. Valproic acid interferes with this drug, causing increased phenobarbital levels.
Carbamazepine	Monitor serum levels to ensure therapeutic dosing; toxicity can occur even with levels slightly above therapeutic range. Plasma concentration decreased by phenytoin, phenobarbital, and valproic acid.
Valproic acid (divalproex sodium, sodium valproate)	Monitor serum levels to ensure therapeutic dosing. Depakote sprinkles are available and useful for children who are unable to tolerate valproate suspension, tablets, or capsules. The contents can be sprinkled on food that does not require chewing.
Gabapentin	Do not administer within 2 h of antacids. Rapidly absorbed in the gastrointestinal tract
Topiramate	Dilantin, Tegretol, and valproic acid decrease concentration of topiramate.
Lamotrigine	Valproate inhibits metabolism; therefore, monitor serum blood values and decrease the dose if necessary.
Clobazam	A benzodiazepine; monitor for sedation.
Levetiracetam	Generally well tolerated, occasionally decreased red and white blood cell counts may be seen.
Vigabatrin	Observe for sedation or blurred vision.

Adapted from: Johnston, M. V. (2007). Seizures in children. In R. M. Kliegman, R. E. Behrman, H. B. Jenson, & B. F. Stanton (Eds.), *Nelson's textbook of pediatrics* (18th ed.). Philadelphia: Saunders; and Karch, A. (2010). *2010 Lippincott's nursing drug guide.* Philadelphia: Wolters Kluwer/Lippincott Williams & Wilkins.

include placing a vagal nerve stimulator and avoiding environmental trigger factors such as sleep deprivation, photic stimulation, and febrile illness. Refer to Common Medical and Surgical Treatments 37.1.

Nursing Assessment

For a full description of the assessment phase of the nursing process, refer to page 456. Assessment findings pertinent to epilepsy are discussed below.

Health History

Elicit a description of the present illness and chief complaint, which will usually involve a seizure episode. Gain information to help characterize the episode as a seizure or as a nonepileptic event (see Box 37.1 for a list of nonepileptic events). It is rare to actually observe the child having a seizure; therefore, a complete, accurate, and detailed history from a reliable source is essential. *Questions should include:*

- Where did the event occur—while sleeping, eating, playing, or just after waking?
- Description of child's behaviour during the event— what types of movements, progression, length, respiratory status, apnea?
- How did the child act after the event?

BOX 37.1 **Nonepileptic Events**

- Syncope
- Breath holding
- Pseudoseizures
- Apnea
- Gastro-esophageal reflux
- Cardiac conduction abnormalities
- Migraines
- Tics

- Have the episodes been recurrent? If so, how frequent?
- Any precipitating factors such as a fever, head trauma, infection, sleep deprivation, or exposure to strong stimuli such as flashing lights or loud noises?

Explore the child's current and past medical history for risk factors such as:

- Family history of seizures or epilepsy
- Any complications during the prenatal, perinatal, or postnatal periods
- Changes in developmental status or delays in developmental milestones
- Any recent illness, fever, trauma, or toxin exposure

Children known to have epilepsy are often admitted to the hospital for other health-related issues or complications and treatment of their seizure disorder. The health history should include questions related to:

- Age at onset of seizures
- Seizure control—what medications is the child taking and has he or she been able to take them; when was his or her last seizure?
- Description and classification of seizures—does the child lose consciousness; does the child become apneic?
- Precipitating factors that may contribute to onset of seizures
- Adverse effects related to anticonvulsant medications
- Compliance with medication regimen

Physical Examination

Perform a complete neurologic examination. Careful assessment of the child's mental status, language, learning, behaviour, and motor abilities can help provide information about any neurologic deficits. If you directly observe seizure activity, provide a thorough and accurate description of the event. This description needs to include:

- Time of onset and length of seizure activity
- Alterations in behaviour such as a cry or changes in facial expression, motor abilities, or sensory alterations prior to the seizure that may indicate an aura
- Precipitating factors such as fever, anxiety, just waking, or eating
- Description of movements and any progression
- Description of respiratory effort and any apnea noted
- Changes in colour (pallor or cyanosis) noted
- Position of mouth, any injury to mouth or tongue, inability to swallow, or excessive salivation
- Loss of bladder or bowel control
- State of consciousness during seizure and **postictal** (after seizure) state—during the seizure, the nurse may ask the child to remember a word; after the seizure, assess whether child is able to recall it, to help accurately establish current mental state

- Assessment of orientation to person, place, and time; motor abilities; speech; behaviour; alterations in sensation postictally
- Duration of postictal state

Laboratory and Diagnostic Tests

Laboratory and diagnostic tests are used to evaluate the cause of, and also aid in identifying the type of, seizure activity (refer to Common Laboratory and Diagnostic Tests 37.1). Common laboratory and diagnostic studies ordered for the diagnosis and assessment of epilepsy include:

- Serum glucose, electrolytes, and calcium—to rule out metabolic causes such as hypoglycemia and hypocalcemia
- LP—to analyze **cerebrospinal fluid (CSF)** to rule out meningitis or encephalitis
- Skull X-ray examinations—to evaluate for the presence of fracture or trauma
- Computed tomography (CT) and magnetic resonance imaging (MRI) studies—to identify abnormalities and intracranial bleeds and rule out tumours
- Electroencephalograms (EEGs)—EEG findings may be noted with certain seizure types, but a normal EEG does not rule out epilepsy because seizure activity rarely occurs during the actual testing time. EEGs are useful in evaluating seizure type and assisting in medication selection. They can be useful in differentiating seizures from nonepileptic activity
- Video EEGs—provide the opportunity to see the child's actual behaviour on video, accompanied with EEG changes; can improve the chance of catching a seizure because the monitoring is done over a period of time

Nursing Management

Nursing management focuses on preventing injury during seizures; administering appropriate medication and treatments to prevent or reduce seizures; and providing education and support to the child and family to help them cope with the challenges of living with a chronic seizure disorder. See Box 37.2 for a list of basic seizure

---

BOX 37.2 Seizure Precautions

- Padding of side rails and other hard objects
- Side rails raised on bed at all times when child is in bed
- Oxygen and suction at bedside
- Supervision, especially during bathing, ambulation, or other potentially hazardous activities
- Use of a protective helmet during activity may be appropriate.
- Child should wear a medical alert bracelet.

precautions. In addition to the nursing diagnoses and related interventions discussed in Nursing Care Plan 37.1, interventions common to epilepsy follow.

Relieving Anxiety

Seizures produce fear and anxiety due to their unpredictable nature along with the uncontrolled, forceful, and sometimes violent appearance. Instruct parents and family members, along with those in the community who may care for the child, on how to respond in case of a seizure (see Teaching Guideline 37.1). This will help to empower the parents, family, and other caregivers, and in turn alleviate some of the anxiety they may feel.

Managing Treatment

Provide child and family teaching and instruction regarding the administration of anticonvulsant therapy and its importance. Included in this discussion should be common adverse effects, the need to continue the medication unless instructed otherwise by the physician, and the need to call the physician if the child is ill and vomiting and unable to take his or her medication. Encourage

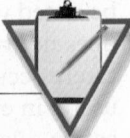

TEACHING GUIDELINE 37.1

How to Respond When Your Child has a Seizure

Instruct parents and caregivers:

- Remain calm.
- Time the seizure episode.
- If the child is standing or sitting, ease him or her to the ground if possible.
- Loosen tight clothing and jewelry around the neck if possible.
- Place the child on one side and open the airway if possible.
- Do not restrain the child.
- Remove hazards in the area.
- Do not forcibly open the jaw with a tongue blade or fingers.
- Document the length of seizure and movements noted, as well as cyanosis or loss of bladder or bowel control and any other characteristics.
- Remain with the child until he or she is fully conscious.
- Call EMS if:
  - The child stops breathing
  - Any injury has occurred
  - Seizure lasts for more than 5 minutes
  - This is the child's first seizure
  - Child is unresponsive to painful stimuli after seizure

parents to discuss unwanted adverse effects with the physician so that they can be addressed and noncompliance with the medication regimen can be reduced. The most common cause of breakthrough seizures is noncompliance.

Providing Family Support and Education

Having a child with a chronic seizure disorder can place stress and anxiety on the family that is often due to fears and misconceptions they may have. An important nursing function is to educate not only the child and family but also the community, including the child's teachers and caregivers, on the reality and facts about the disorder. Encourage parents to be involved in the management of their child's seizures but to allow the child to learn about the disorder and its management as soon as he or she is old enough. Encourage parents to treat the child with epilepsy just as they would a child without this disorder. Children who are brought up no differently than children without epilepsy will be more likely to develop a positive self-image and have increased self-esteem. Any activity restrictions, such as limiting swimming or participation in sports, will be based on the type, frequency, and severity of seizures the child has. Educate parents and children on any restrictions and encourage parents to place only the necessary restrictions on the child.

The needs of the child and family will change as the child grows and develops. The nurse needs to recognize these changes and provide appropriate education and support. Referral to support groups such as Epilepsy Canada is appropriate (visit http://thePoint.lww.com/Chow1e for a direct link).

Febrile Seizures

Febrile seizures are the most common type of seizure seen during childhood (American Academy of Pediatrics, 2008; Johnston, 2007). They usually affect children who are less than 5 years of age, with the peak incidence occurring in children between 18 and 24 months old. It is rare to see febrile seizures in children younger than 6 months and older than 7 years of age. This type of seizure is more commonly seen in boys and there is an increased risk for children who have a family history of febrile seizures. Febrile seizures are associated with a fever, usually related to a viral illness. These seizures are usually benign but can be very frightening for both the child and family. The prognosis is generally excellent for febrile seizures. However, febrile seizures may indicate a serious underlying infectious disease, such as meningitis or sepsis. Other than a recurrence rate of 30% to 50%, depending on the age of the child, there do not appear to be any long-term adverse effects associated with simple febrile seizures (Duffner, Baumann, Berman, Green, & Schneider, 2008).

Therapeutic Management

Treatment includes determination of the cause of the fever and interventions to control the fever. It is important to note that the use of antipyretics does not prevent febrile seizures. Anticonvulsant prophylaxis is no longer recommended (Duffner et al., 2008). Intermittent use of anticonvulsants at the time of a fever may be used in exceptional circumstances.

Nursing Assessment

A febrile seizure is usually associated with rapid rise in core temperature to 39°C or higher. The seizure usually presents as a generalized tonic–clonic seizure that lasts a few seconds to 10 minutes and is followed by a brief postictal period of drowsiness. A simple febrile seizure is defined as a generalized seizure lasting less than 15 minutes (usually a few seconds to 10 minutes) that occurs once in a 24-hour period and is accompanied by a fever without any CNS infection present (American Academy of Pediatrics, 2008; Johnston, 2007). It is likely to have stopped by the time a child receives medical attention. Diagnosis is made based on a thorough history and physical examination, accompanied by a determination of the source of the fever. In some cases an LP may be performed to rule out meningitis or encephalitis. This will be based on the age and the clinical presentation of the child.

Risk factors for recurrence of a febrile seizure include young age at first febrile seizure and family history of febrile seizures and high fever. Children who experience one or more febrile seizures are at no greater risk for developing epilepsy than the general population. No evidence exists that febrile seizures cause structural damage or cognitive declines (Duffner et al., 2008).

Nursing Management

Observing a febrile seizure can be very upsetting for the family. A primary goal of nursing management is to provide parental support and education regarding febrile seizures. Reassure parents of the benign nature of febrile seizures. Counsel parents on controlling fever and discuss how to keep a child safe during a seizure. Instruct parents when to call their physician and when to take their child to the emergency room. Reinforce that any recurrent seizure activity will require prompt medical attention.

Neonatal Seizures

There is a high incidence of seizures in the neonatal period. The immature brain is more prone to seizure activity, and metabolic, infectious, structural, and toxic diseases are more likely to be seen in this age group (Johnston, 2007). Excluding premature infants, neonatal seizures are seizures that occur within the first 4 weeks of life and are most commonly seen within the first 10 days. They are different from those in the child or adult because generalized tonic–clonic seizures tend not to occur during the first month of life (Johnston, 2007). Seizures in newborns are associated with underlying conditions such as hypoxic-ischemic encephalopathy, metabolic disorders (hypoglycemia and hypocalcemia), neonatal infection (meningitis and encephalitis), and intracranial hemorrhage. The prognosis depends mainly on the underlying cause of the seizures and the severity of the insult. There is increasing evidence that neonatal seizures have an adverse effect on neurodevelopment and may predispose the infant to cognitive, behavioural, or epileptic complications later in life.

Therapeutic Management

Acute neonatal seizures should be treated aggressively because repeated seizure activity may result in injury to the brain. Treatment focuses on ensuring adequate ventilation; correcting any underlying metabolic disturbance that may exist, such as hypoglycemia; and possibly administering anticonvulsant therapy. Phenobarbital is often used in the initial management of neonatal seizures. The dosage of anticonvulsants may be higher in the neonate because neonates metabolize drugs more rapidly than older infants.

Nursing Assessment

The characteristics of seizures seen in the neonatal period differ from those seen in older children. Neonatal seizures may be difficult to recognize clinically. Several clinical features may help distinguish seizures from nonepileptic activity, such as tremors or jitteriness in neonates. Autonomic changes such as tachycardia and elevated blood pressure are common with seizures in neonates, and these changes do not occur with nonepileptic events. Also, nonepileptic movements can be suppressed by gently restraining the limb; in true seizures this is not the case. Ocular deviation may be seen with seizure activity but will not be present with nonepileptic activity. Recent advances in EEG and video monitoring guide the diagnosis, characterization, and management of neonatal seizures (Johnston, 2007). Five major seizure types have been recognized in the neonatal period. See Table 37.4 for information on types of seizures seen in newborn infants.

Laboratory and diagnostic tests including serum testing (e.g., serum glucose, electrolytes, calcium), LP (to analyze CSF), cranial ultrasound, CT, and MRI may be performed to help determine the cause of the seizures. EEGs and video EEGs may assist in the characterization of neonatal seizures and their medical management.

Nursing Management

Nursing management will focus on carrying out interventions to cease seizure activity; monitoring neurologic status closely; recognizing the seizures; preventing injury during seizure activity; and providing support and education to the parents and family.

TABLE 37.4 Types of Seizures Seen in Newborn Infants

Type	Age Affected	Characteristics
Subtle	Preterm and full term	Chewing motions, excessive salivation, alterations in respiratory rate, apnea, blinking, pedalling movements
Tonic	Preterm	Rigid posturing of the extremities and trunk May be associated with fixed deviation of the eyes
Focal clonic	Full term	Rhythmic twitching of local muscle groups such as the extremities or face.
Multifocal clonic	Full term	Similar to focal clonic, except many muscle groups are involved, frequently simultaneously
Myoclonic	Preterm and full term	Brief focal jerks, involving one extremity; or multifocal jerks, involving several body parts

Source: Johnston, M. V. (2007). Seizures in childhood. In R. M. Kliegman, R. E. Berman, H. B. Jenson, & B. F. Stanton (Eds.), *Nelson's textbook of pediatrics* (18th ed., pp. 2457–2475). Philadelphia: Saunders.

Structural Defects

Due to the sensitivity of the development of the neurologic system in the first weeks of embryonic life, there exists a potential for defects to occur. These structural defects include neural tube defects, Chiari malformation, hydrocephalus, microcephaly, craniosynostosis, and intracranial vascular malformations.

Neural Tube Defects

Neural tube defects account for the majority of congenital anomalies of the CNS (Kinsman & Johnston, 2007). They are serious congenital malformations of the spine and the brain and include disorders such as spina bifida, anencephaly, and encephalocele. Because the neural tube closes between the third and fourth weeks in utero, a mother may not even know she is pregnant before the defect occurs (thus the importance of prenatal folic acid). The cause of neural tube defects is not known but many factors such as drugs, malnutrition, chemicals, and genetics can adversely affect normal CNS development.

A number of population research studies indicate that prenatal supplementation of folic acid decreases the risk of neural tube defects by 60% to 70% (Canadian Paediatric Society [CPS], 1997). CPS (1997) recommends that all women of childbearing age who are capable of becoming pregnant take 0.4 mg (400 μg) of folic acid daily. Prenatal screening of maternal serum for alpha-fetoprotein and ultrasound examination at 16 to 18 weeks' gestation can help identify fetuses at risk. Anencephaly and encephalocele are discussed below. Refer to Chapter 43 for information on spina bifida.

Anencephaly

Anencephaly is a defect in brain development resulting in small or missing brain hemispheres, skull, and scalp. It occurs when the cephalic or upper end of the neural tube fails to close during the third to fourth week of gestation. These infants are born without both a forebrain and a cerebrum, and the condition is incompatible with life. The remaining brain tissue may be exposed. The incidence of anencephaly reported in Canada for 1999 was 0.9 in 10,000 live births (Health Canada, 2002).

Nursing Assessment

Anencephalic infants have a distinctive appearance, with a large defect noted in the vault of the skull. The mother may have had a difficult labour due to the malformation of the head not allowing it to engage in the cervix. The majority of anencephalic infants will be stillborn. Most others die within hours to several days of birth (Kinsman & Johnston, 2007). There have been a few cases in which the infant has lived for several months. The infant is usually blind, deaf, unconscious, and unable to feel pain. Some infants born with anencephaly may be born with a brain stem, but the lack of cerebrum rules out the possibility of gaining consciousness. Reflex actions such as respirations, reactions to sound and touch, and ability to suck may be present.

Nursing Management

The prognosis is extremely poor. Nursing management is supportive in nature and focuses on comfort measures for the dying infant. Some parents may have been aware of the diagnosis prenatally due to screening tests such as alpha-fetoprotein and ultrasonography. Termination of pregnancy with early diagnosis is something parents may choose when they learn of their infant's prognosis. Parents and family will need support and understanding from all health care professionals during this difficult time. Fear of what the child will look like may be overwhelming. Use of an infant cap can be helpful and allow parents to feel more comfortable holding and comforting their infant. Assisting with anticipatory grieving and decision making related to end-of-life care will also be key nursing interventions.

Encephalocele

Encephalocele is a protrusion of the brain and meninges through a skull defect. It results from failure of the anterior portion of the neural tube to close. The prognosis, including the extent of complications and cognitive deficits, will depend on the size and location of the encephalocele and involvement of other brain structures. Encephaloceles are often accompanied by craniofacial and other abnormalities such as hydrocephalus, microcephaly, spastic quadriplegia, ataxia, visual problems, developmental delay, and seizures; however, the child may also display normal development. Treatment consists of surgical repair, including removal of the herniated contents of the encephalocele and closure of the dura mater and skin. Many infants require shunt placement to correct associated hydrocephalus and corrective repair of any of the craniofacial abnormalities that are related to nasofrontal encephaloceles.

Somewhat related to encephalocele, cranial dermal sinus tracts present as a small dimple in the midline of the cranium on the bridge of the nose or the base of the occiput. Often these small defects go undiagnosed until the child presents with complications such as recurrent meningitis.

Nursing Assessment

Initial assessment post-delivery will reveal a visible external sac protruding from the skull area. It occurs most commonly in the occipital region but can occur elsewhere, such as frontally or nasofrontally. Generally the lesion is covered by skin, but it may also be open. Therefore, assessment to ensure that the sac covering is intact remains important. Assess neurologic status carefully. Before surgical correction, the infant will be examined thoroughly to determine brain tissue involvement or associated anomalies. Diagnostic procedures such as CT, MRI, and ultrasound may be performed.

Nursing Management

Nursing management will consist of preoperative and postoperative care, along with symptomatic and supportive care. Preoperative and postoperative care will be similar to that for the child with myelomeningocele, with a focus on preventing rupture of the sac, preventing infection, and providing adequate nutrition and hydration. Infants with an encephalocele are at an increased risk for developing hydrocephalus. Therefore, monitor for signs and symptoms of increased ICP and head circumference. More importantly, ensure the infant's parents watch for signs of increased ICP at home, including changes in behaviour, irritability, and vomiting (i.e., not tolerating feeds).

Microcephaly

Microcephaly is defined as a head circumference that is more than three standard deviations below the mean for the age and sex of the infant (Kinsman & Johnston, 2007). It may be congenital, in which case the infant will have a small head at birth, or it may be acquired, with the child's head size failing to follow a normal growth curve the first few years of life. There are many causes of microcephaly. In utero, microcephaly can be caused by abnormal development of the brain during gestation or be acquired through maternal infections such as rubella, toxoplasmosis, and cytomegalovirus. Congenital microcephaly can also be related to chromosomal abnormalities and other syndromes. Postnatal acquired microcephaly may occur due to severe malnutrition, infection, or anoxia in early infancy.

Nursing Assessment

Microcephalic infants will present at birth with a normal or reduced head size. As the child ages, head growth will fail while the face may continue to grow at a normal rate. As the child grows older, this smallness of the skull becomes more pronounced. Development of motor functions and speech may be delayed. The degree of mental retardation varies, but it is a common occurrence. Depending on the cause of the microcephaly, convulsions may be present, and motor deficit ranges from clumsiness to spastic quadriplegia.

Nursing Management

There is no medical treatment required for microcephaly. Nursing care will be supportive and focus on determining the extent of neurologic and cognitive deficits, as well as teaching parents the care of a child with such impairments. Engagement in multidisciplinary early intervention programs for the child is the key to optimizing child development and providing family support.

Chiari Malformation

The term *Chiari malformation* encompasses a number of cerebellar and brain stem anomalies (Table 37.5). The two most common types are Chiari I and Chiari II. In Chiari I malformation, symptoms differ depending on the age at presentation. In infants and young children, Chiari I symptoms are often more severe and include swallowing difficulties, gastro-esophageal reflux, and respiratory problems (Albert, Menezes, Hansen, Greenlee, & Weinstein, 2010). In older children and adolescents, symptoms may include occipital cervical headache, **syringomyelia** (excessive CSF present in the central canal of the spinal cord), hand weakness, and scoliosis. Chiari I malformations are usually not associated with hydrocephalus. Although the brain and cerebellum are normally developed in Chiari I malformations, the cerebellar tonsils herniate through the foramen magnum and

TABLE 37.5 CHIARI MALFORMATIONS

Type	Characteristics	Possible Symptoms
Chiari 0	Abnormal CSF flow at the level of the foramen magnum without significant cerebellar tonsillar herniation. Syringomyelia and scoliosis usually present	Hand weakness, gait disorder (cervical myelopathy)
Chiari I	Cerebellar tonsillar herniation >5 mm below the foramen magnum Often associated with syringomyelia and scoliosis Not associated with brain stem herniation or hydrocephalus	Occipital cervical headaches (often associated with coughing or straining), breathing difficulties, feeding and swallowing problems, hand weakness, and gait disorder (cervical myelopathy)
Chiari II	Major cerebellar and medullary anomaly associated with spina bifida Cerebral anomalies include medullary kinking, breaking of the tectum, abnormal tentorium, interdigitation of the parietal lobes, and hydrocephalus.	Asymptomatic Chiari II is not uncommon, but when symptoms are manifest they are severe and include apnea, bradycardia, and total bulbar palsy (paralysis of pharyngeal and laryngeal musculature resulting in the inability to swallow and absence of voice).
Chiari III	Rare congenital cerebellar and brain stem anomaly associated with occipital encephalocele Hydrocephalus, syringomyelia, and tethered spinal cord may also be present.	Symptoms vary from mild to severe, depending on how much of the brain stem and cerebellum are in the occipital encephalocele. May include bulbar symptoms (not usually a full palsy but the child has difficulties with feeding and swallowing), bradycardia, and apnea.
Chiari IV	Rare, hypoplasia or aplasia of the cerebellum.	Symptoms are highly variable but usually associated with significant developmental and cognitive disabilities.

disturb the normal flow of CSF around the spinal cord. Chiari II malformations are associated with hydrocephalus and myelomeningocele. The deformity results from a small posterior fossa forcing the cerebellum, the medulla oblongata, and the fourth ventricle to herniate through the foramen magnum into the cervical canal. This herniation results in an obstruction of CSF flow and causes hydrocephalus. Many children with Chiari II malformations have no symptoms. Symptomatic type II Chiari malformations, although rare, are the leading cause of death in infants and young children with myelomeningocele (Stevenson, 2004). Treatment of symptomatic Chiari I and Chiari II malformations include surgical decompression and restoration of normal CSF flow patterns.

Nursing Assessment

Preoperative nursing assessment for Chiari I and II malformations includes taking a history of headache, breathing difficulties (snoring and sleep apnea), and feeding and swallowing problems. Assessment of cranial nerve function and motor sensory function in the extremities is essential to establish a baseline. Postoperative nursing assessment includes cardiorespiratory monitoring, pupillary reaction, LOC, and motor sensory assessment of the extremities. The incision should be assessed regularly for evidence of a CSF leak (bulging, leaking, or both). Urgent

neurosurgical assessment and intervention are required for bradycardia, apnea, and decreased LOC.

Nursing Management

Nursing management will focus on preoperative and postoperative care. Often, early nursing management of any posterior fossa surgery, including Chiari I and Chiari II decompressions, is carried out in an intensive care environment. Early recognition of signs and symptoms of brain stem compression and increased ICP is critical. Additionally, preventing infection, watching for CSF leak, and observing for improvement of preoperative symptoms are important in the postoperative period. Parent and family teaching includes care of the incision at home, signs of infection and CSF leak, and the importance of long-term follow-up as neurologic improvement may be slow.

Hydrocephalus

Hydrocephalus is not a specific illness but rather is due to an underlying brain disorder. It is a frequently seen disorder of the nervous system, occurring in 0.5 to 4 per 1,000 live births (Zak & Chan, 2010). It results from an abnormality in the circulation of CSF or an imbalance in the production and absorption of CSF. In hydrocephalus, CSF usually accumulates within the ventricular system and causes the ventricles to enlarge. Common disorders or illnesses associated with hydrocephalus include myelo-meningocele; intraventricular hemorrhage in premature infants; meningitis; intrauterine viral infections; lesions the brain such as posterior fossa brain tumours; malformations of the brain such as aqueductal stenosis; and brain injury. Hydrocephalus may be congenital or acquired. Causes of congenital hydrocephalus include myelomeningocele, aqueductal stenosis, and intrauterine infections. Acquired hydrocephalus can result from trauma, hemorrhage, neoplasms, or infections.

Hydrocephalus is also classified as obstructive or non-communicating versus non-obstructive or communicating. Obstructive or non-communicating hydrocephalus occurs when CSF is unable to pass between the ventricles and the subarachnoid space. Neural tube defects, neonatal meningitis, trauma, tumours, or Chiari malformations usually result in this type of hydrocephalus. One of the most common causes of obstructive or non-communicating hydrocephalus in children is aqueductal stenosis, which results from the narrowing of the aqueduct of Sylvius (a passageway between the third and fourth ventricles in the midbrain) (Kinsman & Johnston, 2007). Non-obstructive or communicating hydrocephalus occurs when passage of CSF between the ventricles and the subarachnoid space does occur but CSF reabsorption is impaired. Examples include hydrocephalus that results from subarachnoid hemorrhage and meningeal infections.

Prognosis for the child with hydrocephalus depends mainly on the underlying cause. Advances in the monitoring, diagnosis, care, and treatment of children with hydrocephalus have decreased the number of children with brain damage sustained prior to recognition of their hydrocephalus. Children with hydrocephalus require monitoring for developmental disabilities, visual problems, and cognitive impairment. Long-term follow-up and multidisciplinary care are necessary, often in specialized clinics.

Anatomy and Pathophysiology

CSF is formed primarily in the ventricular system by the choroid plexus, although there is a smaller contribution from the brain parenchyma itself. CSF flows from the two lateral ventricles through each foramen of Monro into the third ventricle, then through the aqueduct of Sylvius to the fourth ventricle, then through the lateral foramina of Luschka or the midline foramen of Magendie into the subarachnoid space. It then flows down, dorsal to the spinal cord and backup toward the brain, ventral to the cord, and into the basal cisterns of the brain. From there CSF flows up over the cerebral convexities to the arachnoid granulations in the cranial venous sinuses where it is absorbed into the bloodstream. Overall, this flow of CSF is a result of slow bulk flow combined with a more rapid "to and fro" pulsatile flow. Any disturbance in the orderly flow pattern of CSF may result in increases in

CSF pressure leading to compression or distortion of the brain. Most commonly, this disturbance leads to enlarged ventricles (hydrocephalus) requiring diversion or shunting of CSF.

Therapeutic Management

Hydrocephalus must be identified early. Early therapeutic intervention is necessary to prevent macrocephaly or brain injury. Specific treatment will depend on the cause of the hydrocephalus. The goals of treatment include relieving hydrocephalus and managing complications associated with the underlying disorder. With few exceptions, most cases of hydrocephalus are treated with surgical placement of an extracranial shunt, most often a ventriculoperitoneal shunt (Fig. 37.7). In many cases, however, a ventriculoscopic third ventriculostomy, in which an opening is made in the third ventricle so that CSF can bypass the aqueduct of Sylvius, will obviate the need for an extracranial shunt. Often, the child will undergo shunt revision surgery at various times during

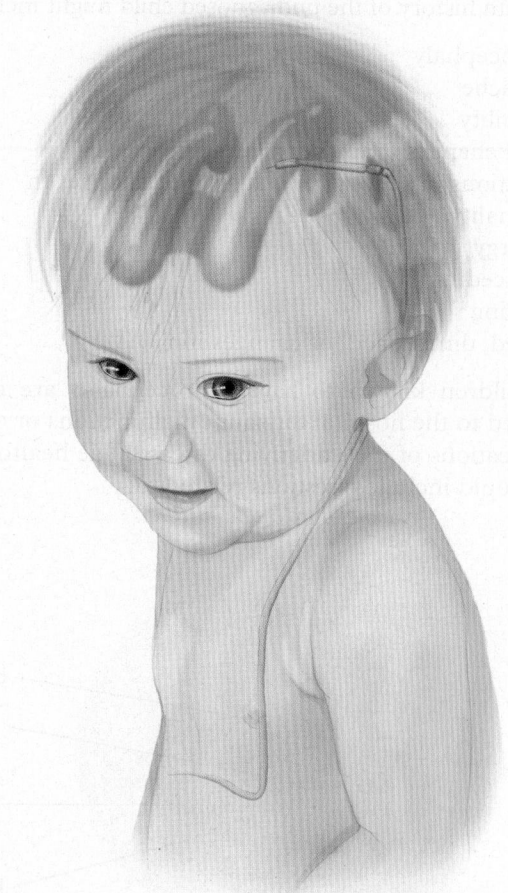

FIGURE 37.7 To treat hydrocephalus, a ventriculoperitoneal shunt catheter is placed in an enlarged ventricle. The shunt diverts the flow of CSF within the ventricular system to the peritoneum, where CSF is now absorbed across the peritoneal membrane into the body's circulation.

his or her life. It is important for health care professionals and parents to be able to recognize signs and symptoms of shunt malfunction.

Nursing Assessment

For a full description of the assessment phase of the nursing process, refer to page 456. Assessment findings pertinent to hydrocephalus are discussed below.

Health History

Explore the maternal pregnancy history for:

• Intrauterine infections
• Premature labour and delivery

Explore the child's medical history for:

• Prematurity with intracranial hemorrhage
• Meningitis
• Trauma
• Congenital syndromes

Elicit a description of the present illness and chief complaint. Common signs and symptoms reported during the health history of the undiagnosed child might include:

• Macrocephaly
• Headache
• Irritability
• Visual changes (papilledema or diplopia)
• Alterations in school performance or changes in personality
• Lethargy
• Poor feeding
• Vomiting
• Altered, diminished, or changes in LOC

Children known to have hydrocephalus are often admitted to the hospital for shunt malfunctions or other complications of the underlying disease. The health history should include questions related to:

• Neurologic status—have there been changes or decreases in LOC; changes in personality; deterioration in school performance?
• Complaints of headache, often with a typical pattern of morning headache followed by vomiting and improvement over the day.
• Vomiting
• Visual disturbances
• Any other changes in physical or cognitive state

Physical Examination

Physical examination of the infant or child with hydrocephalus will include inspection, observation, and palpation.

Inspection and Observation

Observe the infant's or child's general appearance and affect. Pay particular attention to the size of the skull, the prominence of the forehead, and the presence of dilated scalp veins. Nurses who work in pediatric neurosciences need to acquire funduscopy skills and be able to recognize papilledema in infants and children. Signs and symptoms associated with increased ICP may be seen (see Comparison Chart 37.1). Note LOC and motor function. Changes or decreases in LOC may be noted along with brisk reflexes and spasticity of the lower extremities. Symptoms seen vary by age, primarily due to the fact that the infant's skull is able to accommodate the build-up of CSF with expansion of the cranial sutures. In the infant, the most obvious indication of hydrocephalus is a rapid increase in head circumference (Fig. 37.8). In the older child, headache, developmental decline, and changes in personality may be seen.

Palpation

In the infant with hydrocephalus, palpation of the skull may reveal spilt cranial sutures and wide-open, bulging fontanels. The fontanels will be nonpulsatile and feel tense and very full.

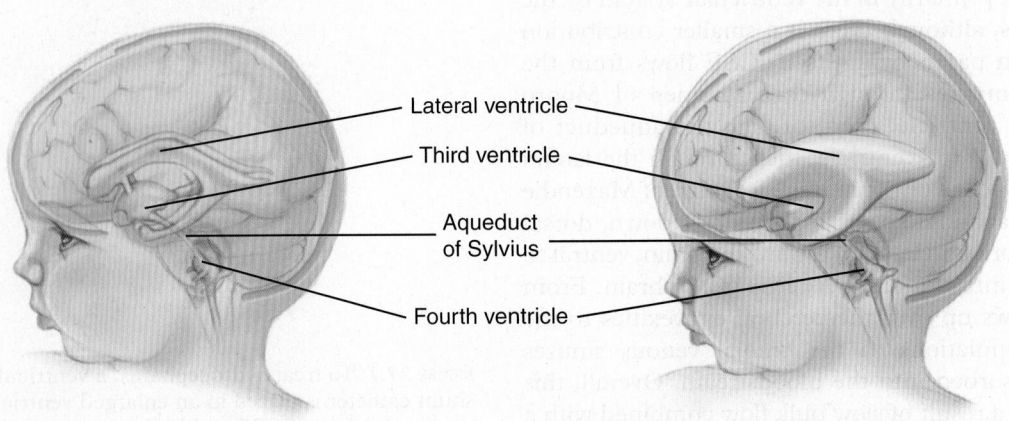

FIGURE 37.8 Infant with hydrocephalus. Note broadening of the forehead and large head size.

Labels: Lateral ventricle, Third ventricle, Aqueduct of Sylvius, Fourth ventricle

Laboratory and Diagnostic Tests

Common laboratory and diagnostic tests ordered for the diagnosis and assessment of hydrocephalus include:

• Skull X-ray studies (may reveal separation of sutures). Also, children with shunts may require plain X-rays of the shunt hardware in the skull, chest, and abdomen ("shunt series").
• CT
• MRI

CT and MRI are used to evaluate the presence of hydrocephalus and can also aid in identifying the cause of hydrocephalus. Refer to Common Laboratory and Diagnostic Tests 37.1.

▶ *Consider THIS!*

Sandra and Michael Graham have brought their 6-month-old son, Thomas, to the pediatric unit for observation. Thomas's head circumference has increased from the 50th percentile at the 4-month check-up to the 95th percentile at the 6-month check-up. Upon assessment, the nurse notes a bulging anterior fontanel, sunsetting eyes, and persistent primitive reflexes.

What do you think is going on?
Identify early signs.
Identify late signs.
Describe nursing care for Thomas.
What teaching will the nurse do with Sandra and Michael?

Nursing Management

Nursing management of the child with hydrocephalus will focus on maintaining cerebral perfusion, minimizing neurologic complications, maintaining adequate nutrition, promoting growth and development, and supporting and educating the child and family. In addition to the nursing diagnoses and related interventions discussed in Nursing Care Plan 37.1, interventions common to hydrocephalus are discussed below.

Preventing and Recognizing Shunt Infection and Malfunction

The major complications associated with shunts are infection and malfunction. Due to the serious nature and potentially devastating effects of shunt infection or malfunction, parents and health professionals need to be aware of the signs and symptoms to provide early recognition and prompt treatment. Signs and symptoms of a shunt infection include fever, abdominal pain (infected CSF irritating the peritoneum), meningeal signs (infected CSF circulating around the meninges), poor feeding, vomiting, decreased responsiveness, and signs of local inflammation anywhere along the shunt tract. Even minor evidence of infection (e.g., a small pustule) or failure at the surgical sites

BOX 37.3 Nursing Management of External Ventricular Drainage (EVD) Device

• Maintain sterile technique and follow the manufacturer's instructions when setting up the system.
• Ensure that all connections are secure and label the line as an EVD.
• Regularly check that the drip chamber of the manometer is set at the height prescribed in relation to the child (i.e., zero at mid head with laser levels).
• Clamp the drain in the event of movement or anticipated movement with care. Re-zero and open the clamps when done.
• Accurately document the volume and colour of CSF every hour (CSF is normally clear and colourless; cloudiness indicates infection). Notify the physician or charge nurse of any significant increase in amount of drainage (if exceeds 10 mL more than previous volumes).
• If minimal or no drainage, check tubing for kinks, blockage, or closed clamps. Check to see whether CSF is pulsating in the tubing. If blockage is suspected, notify the neurosurgery department immediately.
• Dress the entry site into skull using a sterile dressing, and change the dressing using sterile technique if it becomes soiled. Notify neurosurgery of any CSF leak, swelling, or purulent drainage from the site.
• Routine CSF samples may be sent for culture and analysis as ordered by the physician. Never open the line; if a sample needs to be taken, use appropriate access ports and maintain sterile technique.
• A small amount of blood in the CSF drainage is not uncommon, especially with repositioning. Frank bleeding that does not clear rapidly should be reported.

can indicate a shunt infection. Shunt infection can occur at any time but is most common from 1 to 2 months after placement or revision of a shunt. Usually the shunt will be removed and an external ventricular drainage (EVD) system placed until the CSF is sterile and there are no longer signs of peritoneal or meningeal irritation (Box 37.3; also see Common Medical and Surgical Treatments 37.1). Intravenous antibiotics will be used based on the type of organism present in the CSF. It is important that the CSF be sampled prior to initiation of antibiotics to ensure that the correct pathogens are targeted. The process of treating a shunt infection can take up to 2 weeks.

▶ *Take NOTE!*

Rapid drainage of CSF, which may occur if the child sits up without the EVD system being clamped, will decrease ICP and might lead to extreme headache. In rare cases, persistent over-drainage can lead to collapse of the ventricles, possible formation of subdural hematomas, and resultant neurologic deterioration.

A new shunt will be placed after the infection has cleared. Keeping the peritoneal surgical incision free of feces and urine can help prevent infection. Additionally, inspect surgical incisions after shunt placement for signs and symptoms of infection and any signs of leaking CSF (if the CSF can get out, pathogens can get in).

Signs and symptoms of shunt malfunction include headache, vomiting, and drowsiness. More subtle signs such as deterioration in school performance or changes in personality may also occur. Signs and symptoms of increased ICP, as listed in Comparison Chart 37.1, can also be indicative of shunt problems. Malfunction of the shunt occurs primarily due to obstruction but may result from separation of the tubing, suboptimal valve function (i.e., too fast or too slow for the child's CSF drainage needs), or poor placement of the ventricular or distal catheters. A shunt that has been placed within the past year is at higher risk for malfunction. Early recognition and operative intervention are essential. It is a skilled clinician, in collaboration with knowledgeable parents and timely imaging, who can differentiate a shunt malfunction from common childhood illnesses such as gastroenteritis and seasonal influenza.

Supporting and Educating the Child and Family

Hydrocephalus will require lifelong follow-up and regular evaluations. It requires early recognition of shunt malfunction and infection to prevent neurologic damage. Children will require future surgeries and hospitalizations, which can place a strain on the family. Potential developmental disabilities are an additional strain. The support of the family in establishing realistic goals and helping the child to achieve his or her developmental and educational potential is important.

The family should be involved in the child's care from the time of diagnosis. Initially, parents may be frightened because shunt placement involves entering the brain. Provide parents with accurate information regarding the procedure, and be available to listen to parents' concerns and answer their questions. Ongoing education about hydrocephalus and its treatment are important, including signs and symptoms of shunt problems. As the family becomes more comfortable with the diagnosis and treatment, they will become experts in the child's care and will often recognize subtle changes in the child that may indicate shunt problems. Referral to support groups such as Spina Bifida & Hydrocephalus Canada and the Hydrocephalus Association can be helpful for both the family and the child. (Visit http://thePoint.lww.com/Chow1e for direct links to these organizations' websites.)

Intracranial Arteriovenous Malformation

Intracranial arteriovenous malformation (AVM) is a rare congenital disorder. It is caused by abnormal development of blood vessels and can occur in the cerebral hemispheres, cerebellum, or brain stem. Very rarely, an AVM may occur in the spinal cord. AVMs that hemorrhage can lead to serious neurologic deficits and even death. However, some AVMs never cause problems. AVMs account for 30% to 50% of hemorrhagic strokes in children (Ogilvy et al., 2001).

Therapeutic Management

More aggressive treatment strategies are used for intracranial AVMs in children than adults because of higher lifetime risk of complications. Treatment is often multistage using multiple treatment modalities, including surgical decompression or occlusion, endovascular embolization, and radiosurgery. The treatment approach will be based on the age of the child and the size and location of the AVM. The child will usually require intensive care monitoring following treatment to observe for re-bleeding, cerebral swelling, or ischemic stroke.

Nursing Assessment

Presentation of an intracranial AVM may involve seizures, headaches, decreased LOC, or progressive neurologic deficits. In children less than 2 years of age, presentation may also include high output cardiac failure due to arteriovenous shunting, macrocephaly from hydrocephalus, or intractable seizure activity. Diagnosis is made using imaging procedures such as MRI, CT, and/or cerebral or spinal angiography. Due to advances in neuroimaging techniques, an increasing number of AVMs are detected before they rupture.

Nursing Management

Nursing management for these children is aimed at supportive care. Monitor for changes in neurologic status, noting any seizure activity, signs or symptoms of increased ICP, or signs and symptoms of intracranial hemorrhage. Hydrocephalus may occur as a result of intracranial hemorrhage secondary to the AVM. An EVD and eventual shunt placement may be necessary (refer to the Hydrocephalus section).

Craniosynostosis

Craniosynostosis is the premature closure of one or more cranial sutures (Fig. 37.9). Complete closure of all sutures does not normally occur until late in childhood. Premature closure of the various sutures either alone or in combination results in a characteristic craniofacial appearance (Table 37.6). In cases in which only one suture is fused, neurologic impairments are rarely seen. The incidence of craniosynostosis is approximately 1 in 2,000 births (Kinsman & Johnston, 2007). The cause is unknown, but in 10% to 20% of cases a genetic disorder such as Saethre-Chotzen, Crouzon, Apert, Pfeiffer, or Carpenter syndrome is present (Kinsman & Johnston,

TABLE 37.6   TYPES OF CRANIOSYNOSTOSIS

Types	Description	
Sagittal synostosis (scaphocephaly)	Sagittal suture is closed. Head grows long and narrow in anteroposterior direction. Broad forehead and a prominent occiput are present. Most common form	
Metopic synostosis (trigonocephaly)	Metopic suture is closed. Usually a ridge down the forehead can be seen or felt. Triangular-shaped forehead Eyebrows may appear "pinched" on either side. Eyes may also appear close together.	
Unilateral coronal synostosis (anterior plagiocephaly)	Early closure of one side of the coronal suture Forehead and orbital rim (eyebrow) have a flattened appearance on that side.	

(continued)

TABLE 37.6 TYPES OF CRANIOSYNOSTOSIS (continued)

Types	Description	
Bicoronal synostosis (brachycephaly)	Very flat, recessed forehead Skull is shortened in the anteroposterior direction. Commonly seen in Apert and Crouzon syndromes	
Lambdoid (posterior plagiocephaly)	Early closure of one lambdoid suture Trapezoid-shaped head in craniosynostosis. Similar to shape found in positional moulding or positional plagiocephaly	

Photos courtesy of Stephen Wreakes, Medical Photographer, Alberta Health Services (University of Alberta Hospital).
Skull models courtesy of Medical Modelling, Inc. http://www.medicalmodeling.com/craniofacialmodels

2007). The prognosis is good for the majority of infants presenting with craniosynostosis, and normal brain development will occur. Exceptions to this are the infant or child who has associated genetic disorders that involve brain function and development.

Surgical correction of craniosynostosis allows for normal skull growth and acceptable appearance of the head and face. Surgical intervention is currently evolving toward earlier and more minimally invasive procedures.

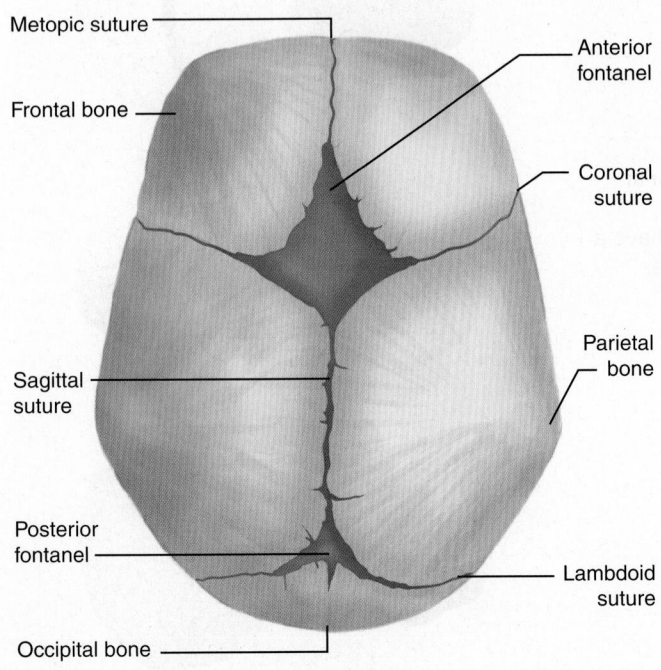

FIGURE 37.9 Skull sutures in the infant.

Metopic suture
Frontal bone
Anterior fontanel
Coronal suture
Parietal bone
Sagittal suture
Posterior fontanel
Lambdoid suture
Occipital bone

Nursing Assessment

Most cases of craniosynostosis are evident at birth. As the brain continues to grow despite a fused suture, skull growth is inhibited perpendicular to the suture and the skull is elongated parallel to the fused suture. There may also be a palpable bony ridge along the suture. If the sagittal or metopic suture is fused there is usually a prominent, palpable bony ridge. Diagnostic imaging studies will confirm fusion of the sutures. Note that true lambdoidal craniosynostosis is very rare and that any posterior skull flattening is most likely due to positioning.

Nursing Management

Following cranial remodelling surgery for craniosynostosis, nursing management includes observing hemoglobin and hematocrit levels due to large volumes of blood loss that can occur and managing pain. Significant facial swelling may be present. This can result in an inability of the child to open his or her eyes for a few days postoperatively. Parents need to know about facial swelling before they see their child after surgery; pictures of other infants as they recover often help. Encourage the parents to talk to, hold, and comfort their child during this time as he or she is often very irritable not only from pain but also from not being able to see. Provide support and education to the parents before, during, and after the procedure.

Positional Plagiocephaly

The CPS (2004) currently recommends that infants sleep on their backs to decrease the risk of sudden infant death syndrome. With more infants sleeping on their backs, there has been a dramatic increase in the incidence of positional plagiocephaly (KidsHealth, 2011). Positional plagiocephaly refers to asymmetry in head shape without fused sutures. It results from gravitational force exertion on the developing cranium. Positional plagiocephaly in the infant is often associated with either torticollis or tightness of the neck muscles on one side.

Intervention for positional plagiocephaly is generally conservative, such as changing the infant's position, encouraging "tummy time," and avoiding excessive use of the car seat for infant seating outside the automobile. Switching the direction the infant lies in the crib and on the changing table can help him or her to turn the head in the other direction. Exercises for tight neck muscles are also essential, and referral to a pediatric physiotherapist may also be appropriate. Because positional plagiocephaly is becoming so common, these interventions can be taught to parents soon after delivery or even in prenatal classes for healthy infant development. Finally, if the infant's skull shape continues to be malformed despite conservative intervention, a skull moulding helmet that holds skull growth in the prominent areas and encourages skull growth in flat areas may be appropriate (Fig. 37.10). Because moulding helmets capitalize on normal skull growth, they are most effective in the first year of life when skull growth is most rapid.

Nursing Assessment

The infant will have a history of a preferred head position when supine, favouring the flat side of the skull. View the infant's head from the top, noting asymmetry ranging from flattening on one side posteriorly to posterior flattening associated with ipsilateral anterior bulging (Fig. 37.11). Another telltale sign of positional plagiocephaly is a forward shift of the ear on the flat side. Assess neck range of motion to determine whether torticollis is also present. Palpate the cranial sutures, which will not

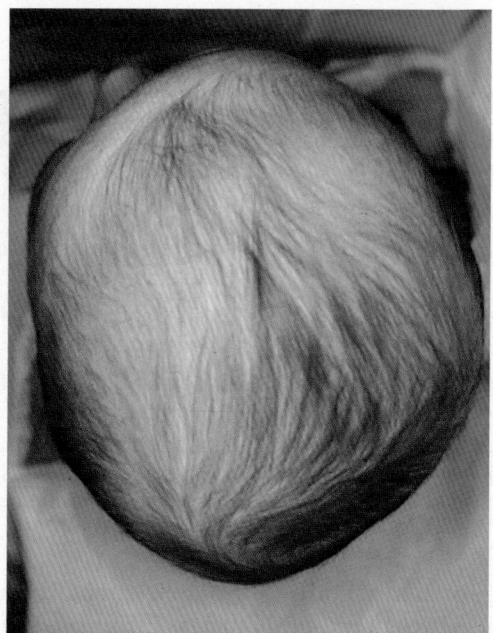

FIGURE 37.11 Note flattening of the right posterior parietal and occipital regions of the skull as well as contralateral flattening (or same-sided prominence) of the left frontal region in this infant with positional plagiocephaly.

feel as prominent as they do when they are fused. If the diagnosis is uncertain, skull X-ray examination or three-dimensional cranial CT scans determine whether craniosynostosis is present.

Nursing Management

Nursing management is directed toward repositioning the infant to decrease time spent with the flattened area in the dependent position. Position the infant so that turning away from the affected side is necessary for him or her to view objects of interest. Place the infant on the abdomen when awake and supervised. Discourage use of the car seat outside the automobile. Place a rolled washcloth along the affected side of the head to discourage turning the head in that direction. Following these recommendations will prevent the development or progression of positional plagiocephaly.

Infectious Disorders

The most common infectious disorders of the neurologic system include bacterial meningitis, aseptic meningitis, and encephalitis.

Bacterial Meningitis

Bacterial meningitis is an infection of the meninges, the lining that surrounds the brain and spinal cord. It is a serious illness in children and can lead to brain damage, nerve damage, deafness, stroke, and even death. It requires rapid assessment and treatment. The leading cause of bacterial

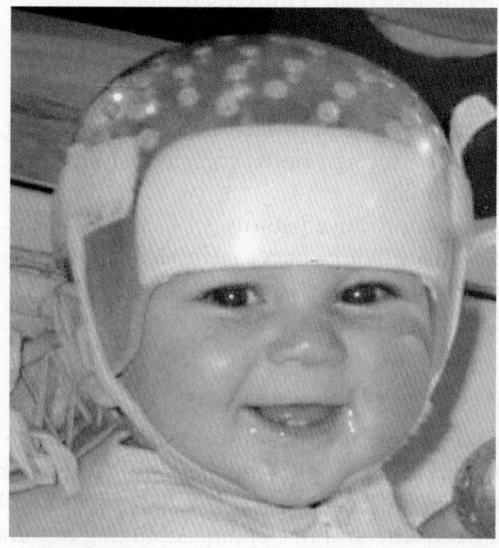

FIGURE 37.10 Moulding helmet for positional plagiocephaly.

TABLE 37.7   COMMON CAUSES OF MENINGITIS IN DIFFERENT AGE GROUPS

Causative Organism	Age Affected
E. coli	Newborns and infants
Streptococcus group B	Infants <1 month
H. influenzae type B	1 month–6 years, typically 6–9 months old
S. pneumoniae	Children >3 months of age and adults
N. meningitidis	Children >3 months of age and adults

Adapted from: Zak, M., & Chan, V. W. (2010). Pediatric neurologic disorders. In S. M. Nettina (Ed.), *Lippincott manual of nursing practice* (9th ed.). Philadelphia: Lippincott Williams & Wilkins.

meningitis in newborns is group B streptococcus and gram-negative enteric bacilli such as *Escherichia coli* (Spiro & Spiro, 2004). The leading causative agents of bacterial meningitis in Canada for infants and children (six weeks of age and older) are *Neisseria meningitidis* and *Streptococcus pneumoniae* (CPS, 2008). See Table 37.7 for the common causes of meningitis seen in different age groups. The incidence of *Haemophilus influenzae* type B (Hib), once a common cause of bacterial meningitis in children, has dramatically decreased with the introduction of the Hib vaccine (CPS, 2008).

Pathophysiology

Bacterial meningitis causes inflammation, swelling, purulent exudates, and tissue damage to the brain. It can occur secondary to upper respiratory tract infections, sinus infections, or ear infections. Basal skull fracture, neurosurgical intervention, or congenital structural abnormalities may also cause meningitis. When an infant or child presents with repeated episodes of meningitis, look for a deep dimple anywhere along the midline from the bridge of the nose to the lumbosacral area.

Therapeutic Management

Bacterial meningitis is a medical emergency and requires prompt hospitalization and treatment. Deterioration may be rapid and can occur in less than 24 hours, leading to long-term neurologic damage and even death. If bacterial meningitis is suspected, intravenous antibiotics will be started immediately after LP has been performed and blood cultures have been obtained. Ideally, a CT scan to rule out an intracranial mass lesion should be obtained prior to the LP. The length of therapy and specific antibiotic will be determined based on the analysis and the culture and sensitivity of the CSF. Corticosteroids may be ordered to help reduce the inflammatory process. Specific medical treatment varies based on the suspected causative organism.

Nursing Assessment

For a full description of the assessment phase of the nursing process, refer to page 456. Assessment findings pertinent to bacterial meningitis are discussed below.

Health History

Elicit a description of the present illness and chief complaint. Common signs and symptoms reported during the health history might include:

- Sudden onset of symptoms
- Preceding respiratory illness or sore throat
- Presence of fever and chills
- Headache
- Vomiting
- Photophobia
- Stiff neck
- Rash
- Irritability
- Drowsiness
- Lethargy
- Muscle rigidity
- Seizures

Symptoms in infants can be more subtle and atypical, but the history may reveal:

- Poor sucking and feeding
- Weak cry
- Lethargy
- Vomiting
- Seizures

Explore the child's current and past medical history for risk factors such as:

- Young age: 1 month to 5 years, with most cases in children less than 1 year of age and young adults 15 to 24 years of age
- Any fever or illness during pregnancy or around delivery (for infants less than 3 months of age)
- Exposure to ill persons
- Exposure to tuberculosis
- Travel history
- Recent neurosurgical procedure or head trauma
- Presence of a foreign body, such as a shunt or a cochlear implant
- Immunocompromised status
- Close-contact living spaces such as dormitories or military bases
- Day care attendance

Physical Examination

Observe the general appearance of the child. The infant with bacterial meningitis appears ill (fever, irritable, inconsolable, stiff neck), and the older child will complain of headache and neck pain. A bulging fontanel may be present in the infant. Presence of positive Kernig's

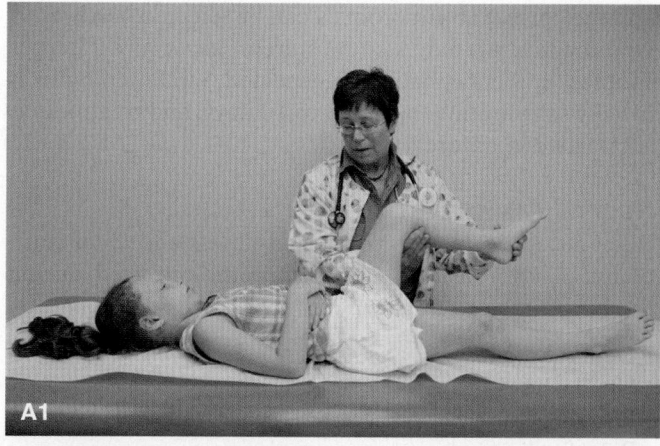
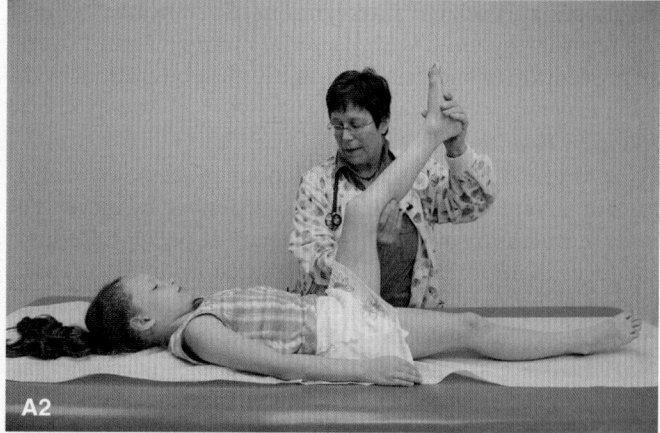
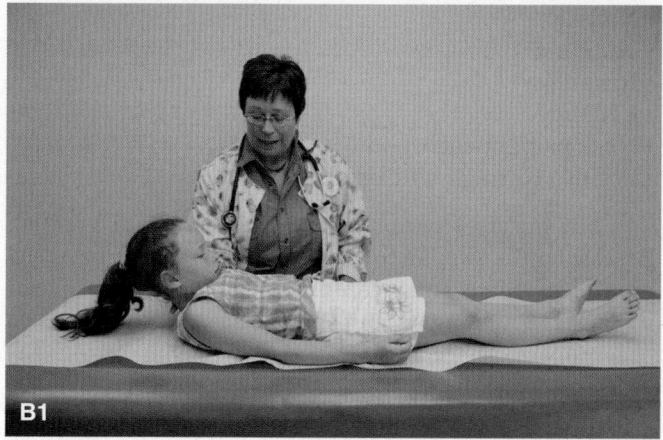
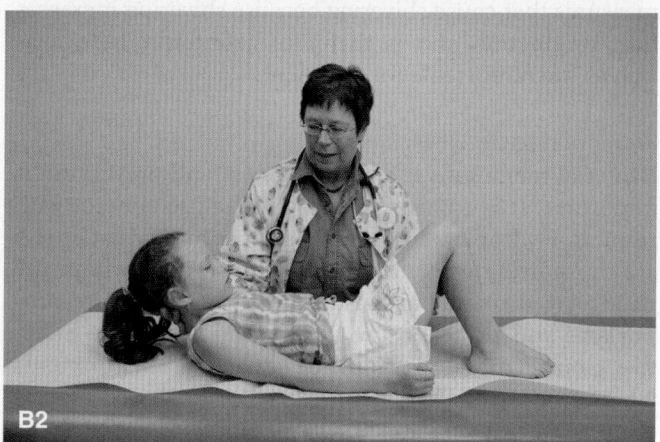

FIGURE 37.12 (**A**) Kernig's sign is tested by flexing each leg at the hip and knee (**A1**), then extending the leg (**A2**). A positive report of pain along the vertebral column is a positive sign that indicates irritation of meninges. (**B**) Brudzinski's sign is tested with the child lying supine with the neck flexed (**B1**). A positive sign occurs if resistance or pain is met. The child may also passively flex the hip and knees in reaction, indicating meningeal irritation (**B2**). Note that false-negatives results are common for these signs.

and Brudzinski's signs can also indicate irritation of the meninges (Fig. 37.12). Inspect the child for the presence of a petechial, vesicular, or macular rash.

▶ *Take* NOTE!

Abrupt eruption of a petechial or purplish rash can be indicative of meningococcemia (infection with N. meningitidis*). Immediate medical attention is warranted.*

Laboratory and Diagnostic Tests

Common laboratory and diagnostic studies ordered for the assessment of bacterial meningitis include:

- LP—fluid pressure will be measured and a sample is obtained for analysis and culture. CSF will reveal increased white blood cells, increased protein, and low glucose (the bacteria present feed on the glucose).

Polymerase chain reaction analysis will reveal the DNA in the causative organism (bacterial or viral).
- Complete blood count—white blood cell count will be elevated.
- Blood culture—performed to rule out sepsis. Blood culture will be positive in cases of septicemia.

Nursing Management

Quickly initiate supportive measures to ensure proper ventilation, reduce the inflammatory response, and help prevent injury to the brain. Interventions are aimed at reducing ICP and maintaining cerebral perfusion along with treating fluid volume deficit, controlling seizures, and preventing injury that may result from altered LOC or seizure activity. Initiate appropriate isolation precautions. In addition to standard precautions, infants and children diagnosed with bacterial meningitis will be placed on droplet isolation until 24 hours of antibiotics have been received in order to help prevent transmission to others. Refer to Nursing Care Plan 37.1 for nursing diagnoses and related interventions. Specifically, reducing fever in the child with bacterial meningitis and overall prevention of bacterial meningitis must be emphasized.

Reducing Fever

Hyperthermia related to the infectious process, increased metabolic rate, and dehydration as evidenced by increased body temperature and tachycardia may be present. Reducing fever is important to help maintain optimal cerebral perfusion by reducing the metabolic needs of the brain. Administer antipyretics such as acetaminophen and NSAIDs such as ibuprofen. Reduction of environmental temperature and the use of cooling blankets, fans, and cold compresses may be helpful in reducing fever. Avoid measures that cause shivering because shivering increases heat production and is therefore counterproductive as well as uncomfortable for the client.

Preventing Bacterial Meningitis

Bacterial meningitis is a serious illness and prevention is important. It is transmitted by direct close contact with respiratory droplets from the nose or throat. Most at risk are those living with the child or anyone with whom the child played or was in close contact. Postexposure prophylaxis and postexposure immunization may be effective. Control measures should be initiated in environments where risk exists. Disinfect toys and other shared objects to decrease transmission of the microorganisms to others.

To reduce group B streptococcus infection in neonates, screen pregnant women; if the screening results are positive, administer intrapartal antibiotics. Vaccines are available for some specific causative organisms, but complete vaccination prevention is not possible at this time. The Hib vaccine is routine starting at 2 months of age and all children should be immunized to continue the reduction of bacterial meningitis caused by *H. influenzae* type B. The pneumococcal and meningococcal conjugate vaccines are also routine for all children starting at 2 months of age in Canada.

Aseptic Meningitis

Aseptic meningitis is the most common type of meningitis, and the majority of children affected are younger than 5 years of age (CDC, 2010a). If the causative organism can be identified, it is usually a virus. Enteroviruses, such as echovirus and coxsackievirus, account for many cases of aseptic meningitis. Less common causes include mumps, herpes virus, HIV, measles, varicella, and polio.

Therapeutic Management

Prompt diagnosis and treatment are essential to improve outcomes. Even if viral meningitis is suspected, the child is also treated aggressively for bacterial meningitis until the diagnosis is confirmed. Antibiotics are administered and continued until the causative organism is recognized and the correct antimicrobials can be selected. Early antiviral medication may also be started, especially if herpes simplex viral encephalitis is suspected. Viral meningitis is usually self-limiting, lasting 3 to 10 days, and treatment is supportive in nature.

Nursing Assessment

Elicit a description of the present illness and chief complaint. Common signs and symptoms reported during the health history might include:

- General malaise
- Headache
- Photophobia
- Poor feeding
- Nausea
- Vomiting
- Irritability
- Lethargy
- Neck pain, nuchal rigidity
- Positive Kernig's and Brudzinski's signs

The onset of symptoms may be abrupt or gradual. Assessment is similar to that of the child with bacterial meningitis. Signs and symptoms are similar to those seen in bacterial meningitis, but the child is usually less ill.

Nursing Management

Nursing management is similar to the nursing care of the child with bacterial meningitis and will focus on comfort measures to reduce pain and fever. Aseptic meningitis can be managed successfully at home if the child's neurologic status is stable and he or she is tolerating oral intake.

Encephalitis

Encephalitis is an inflammation of the brain that may also include an inflammation of the meninges (meningoencephalitis). It can be caused by protozoan, bacterial, fungal, or viral invasion of the nervous system. In children it is most often associated with a viral illness. In Canada, most confirmed cases of encephalitis are associated with enterovirus, herpes simplex virus, human herpes virus 6, Epstein-Barr virus, or arbovirus (Ford-Jones et al., 1998). Other notable causes include *Mycoplasma pneumoniae* and *Bartonella henselae*. Arthropod-borne viruses (e.g., West Nile virus, St. Louis encephalitis) are spread by the bites of insects, especially mosquitoes and ticks. Recovery from encephalitis can occur in a few days or may be complicated and involve severe neurologic damage with residual effects. Prognosis depends on the age of the child and the causative organism. Prompt diagnosis and treatment are essential. The child suspected of having encephalitis should be hospitalized. Treatment is mainly supportive in nature and focuses on maintaining optimal cerebral perfusion; hydration and nutrition; and injury prevention.

Nursing Assessment

For a full description of the assessment phase of the nursing process, refer to page 456. Assessment findings pertinent to encephalitis are discussed below.

Health History

Elicit a description of the present illness and chief complaint. Common signs and symptoms reported during the health history might include:

• Fever
• Flu-like symptoms
• Altered LOC
• Headache
• Lethargy
• Drowsiness
• Generalized weakness
• Seizure activity

Explore the client's current history for risk factors such as:

• Recent travel
• Recreational activities, such as hiking and camping
• Contact with animals

Physical Examination

Perform a neurologic examination to distinguish between encephalitis and viral meningitis. In encephalitis, a neurologic examination will reveal changes in LOC such as lethargy, behaviour and speech disturbances, and memory loss (CPS, 1998). Neurologic findings vary and reflect the areas of the brain that are involved.

Laboratory and Diagnostic Tests

LP may be performed, and the CSF may show elevated leukocyte, elevated protein, and normal glucose levels. In some cases, levels may be normal. MRI, CT, and EEG may be performed to help identify early changes and provide useful clues in developing a diagnosis.

Nursing Management

Nursing management is similar to nursing care for the child with meningitis. Importantly, the child's LOC, fever, orientation, seizures, increased ICP, speech changes, and motor disturbances should be monitored closely. Deterioration in the child's neurologic status may lead to full supportive care in an intensive care setting.

Nurses play an important role in prevention of some forms of encephalitis. Encephalitis can result from complications of childhood illnesses such as measles, mumps, or chickenpox. Explaining the importance of keeping children up to date in their immunizations is the key to preventing related viral encephalitis. Vector control and avoiding mosquito and tick bites are the best ways to reduce the risk of infection with arthropod-borne viruses. This can be accomplished by using insect repellent (repellents containing *N,N*-diethyl-*meta*-toluamide [DEET] should be used cautiously in children less than 12 years of age and not at all in children less than 1 year of age), wearing clothing that covers the arms and legs, controlling mosquito populations by eliminating areas of standing water where mosquitoes can breed, and using insect traps. Public measures such as sprayed insecticides to reduce the mosquito population can also be effective.

Reye Syndrome

Reye syndrome is a disease that primarily affects children less than 15 years of age who are recovering from a viral illness. The exact cause of Reye syndrome is unknown. It has been found that Reye syndrome is a reaction that is triggered by the use of salicylates or salicylate-containing products to treat a viral infection. This reaction causes brain swelling, liver failure, and death in hours if treatment in not initiated. In the 1980s, the adverse effects of salicylates used to treat viral illnesses began to be publicized and parents were warned not to give these products to children and teenagers. Since then there has been a dramatic decrease in the occurrence of Reye's syndrome. Health Canada, under the Food and Drug Act, has collaborated with manufacturers to label all over-the-counter acetylsalicylate-containing products with warnings that they should not be given to children and teenagers for fever (Health Canada, 2006).

Trauma

In Canadian children over 1 year of age, unintentional injury (trauma) is the leading cause of mortality and one of the leading causes of hospitalization (Public Health Agency of Canada, 2008). Children face significant risk of trauma to their developing neurologic system, often leading to neurologic disorders with life-threatening and lasting effects. Neurologic trauma may include head trauma, abusive head trauma, birth trauma, and near drowning.

Head Trauma

In Canada, injury causes more death in children than disease (Statistics Canada, 2007). Of these injuries, head injury is the most common cause of death and disability in childhood. Common causes of head trauma in children include falls, motor vehicle collisions, pedestrian and bicycle injuries, and child abuse. Many factors make children more susceptible to head trauma than adults. Larger head size in relation to the body, coupled with a higher centre of gravity, causes the child to hit his or her head more readily when involved in motor vehicle collisions, bicycle injuries, and falls. Children are also at risk for injury related to psychosocial factors such as their high activity level, curiosity, incomplete motor development, and lack of knowledge and judgment. Also, their dependence on others to care for them places them at risk for injuries caused by child abuse.

TABLE 37.8 COMMON HEAD INJURIES SEEN IN CHILDREN

Injury	Description	Characteristics
Skull fractures	A break in one or more bones encasing the brain	In infants and children less than 2 years old, a great deal of force is needed to produce a skull fracture. Due to the flexibility of the immature skull, it is able to withstand a great degree of deformation before a fracture will occur. Skull fractures can result in little or no brain damage but may have serious consequences if the underlying blood vessels, dura mater, or brain tissue is injured.
Linear skull fracture	A simple break in the skull that follows a relatively straight line	Most common skull fracture. Can result from a direct blow or fall. Not usually serious unless there is additional injury to the dura mater or brain.
Depressed skull fracture	The bone is locally broken and pushed inward, causing pressure on the brain.	Can result from forceful impact from a blunt object, such as a hammer or another heavy but fairly small object. Rarely, a dural tear from a depressed skull fracture will result in a post-traumatic, pulsatile, accumulation of CSF, which results in a growing skull fracture. Surgery is often required to elevate the bony pieces and inspect the dura mater for evidence of injury.
Diastatic skull fracture	A fracture through the skull sutures	Usually associated with a blow to the top of the head causing coronal/sagittal suture separation or a blow to the back of the head causing lambdoidal suture separation (refer to Fig. 37.9 for location of sutures) Usually treatment is not required but observation will be necessary.
Compound skull fracture	A laceration of the skin and splintering of the bone	The fracture can be linear or depressed. Generally is the result of blunt force Requires skin closure and antibiotics. Surgery may be necessary if associated with depressed skull fracture or dural laceration.
Basal skull fracture	A fracture of the bones that form the base of the skull	Usually results from blunt head trauma such as falls. Findings include CSF rhinorrhea and otorrhea, bleeding from the ear, and orbital or postauricular ecchymosis (bruising behind ear is referred to as Battle's sign). Most of these are minor head injuries, not requiring admission to hospital. Only with CSF leak or cranial nerve injury (CN VI, VII, VIII) will hospitalization be required.
Concussion	A mild brain injury that is caused by rotational forces involving the brain and brain stem structures.	Most common head injury. Results from a blow or jolt to the head caused by sports injuries, motor vehicle collisions, and falls. Confusion and amnesia after the head injury are seen. Loss of consciousness may or may not occur. Noted symptoms may include headache, vomiting, memory loss, and poor concentration. Treatment includes rest and monitoring for neurologic changes that could indicate a more severe injury, such as increased sleepiness, worsening headache, increased vomiting, worsening confusion, difficulty walking or talking, changes in LOC, and seizures.

Injury	Description	Characteristics
Contusion	Bruising of cerebral tissue	Results from a blow to the head from incidents such as a motor vehicle collisions, falls, or abuse. There are some typical patterns of contusions in the brain. A direct blow results in a contusion at the site of impact (coup injury). A moving skull striking a stationary object results in a coup-contrecoup contusion (two or more contusions at opposite ends of the brain). Coup-contrecoup injuries occur most commonly with impact to the back of the head. May cause focal disturbances in vision, strength, and sensation. The signs and symptoms will vary based on the location of the injury and extent of vascular injury and can range from mild weakness to prolonged unconsciousness and paralysis. Treatment includes close monitoring for neurologic changes. Surgery is usually not necessary, although anticonvulsants may be required.
Acute subdural hematoma	Collection of blood between the dura and cerebrum	Not usually associated with skull fractures. Subdural hematomas arise from injuries to the bridging veins that pass from the brain surface to the superior sagittal sinus in the dura mater. Associated with a more severe brain injury, brain swelling, and increased ICP. Treatment depends on clinical symptoms, size of clot, and area of the brain involved. In some cases, the bleed may be closely monitored for resolution. In other cases, treatment may include burr hole drainage or surgical evacuation by craniotomy. Close monitoring of neurologic status and for signs of increased ICP is indicated.
Epidural hematoma	Collection of blood between the skull and outside surface of the dura mater.	Often results from skull fracture with an injury to the middle meningeal artery in the fronto-temporal region. Most epidural hematomas are neurosurgical emergencies. Arterial bleeding is usually present; therefore, brain compression occurs rapidly and can result in impairment of the brain stem and respiratory or cardiovascular function. Characteristic of an epidural hematoma is a temporary lucid interval, with the child beginning to recover from the traumatic incident, followed by rapid deterioration. Symptoms include vomiting, headache, and lethargy. Treatment depends on clinical symptoms, the size of the clot, and the area of the brain involved. Prompt surgical evacuation and control of the bleeding are usually necessary. The earlier the bleed is recognized and treated, the more favourable the outcome. Close monitoring of neurologic status is indicated.

Children younger than 3 years of age have a very mobile spine, especially in the cervical region, along with weak neck muscles. This places them at risk for acceleration/deceleration injuries, which result in excessive forces passing back and forth through the brain and skull, causing cerebral contusions and deep white matter micro-hemorrhages (diffuse axonal injuries). These brain injuries can occur at the point of impact and at distant points opposite the point of impact (i.e., coup-contrecoup phenomenon).

Head trauma is a broad term that can include specific patterns of injury. See Table 37.8 for descriptions of common head injuries seen in children. Head trauma in children is serious because it can cause an immediate threat to the child's life as well as a number of complications that can lead to lifelong impairment of physical, cognitive, and psychosocial functioning. Prognosis for the child who has suffered a head injury depends on the extent and severity of the injury.

Nursing Assessment

For a full description of the assessment phase of the nursing process, refer to page 456. Assessment findings pertinent to head trauma are discussed below.

Health History

Take a detailed history, including past medical history along with details of the events surrounding the injury, such as mental status at the time of the injury, any loss of consciousness, irritability, lethargy, abnormal behaviour, vomiting, any seizure activity, and any complaints of headache, vision changes, or neck pain.

Physical Examination

Perform a thorough physical examination. Initial physical assessment will focus on the ABCs (airway, breathing, and circulation) (refer to Chapter 52 for further information on emergency management). All children who experience head trauma need an assessment of their neurologic function as soon as they are seen (see Fig. 37.2). This includes the pediatric Glasgow Coma Scale, vital signs, pupillary response, outward evidence of trauma to the face and head such as lacerations, bleeding, CSF leak, bruising, and seizure activity. Fixed and dilated pupils, fixed and constricted pupils, or sluggish pupillary reaction to light warrant prompt intervention.

> ▶ **Take** NOTE!
>
> *A child's spine must remain stabilized after a head injury until spinal cord injury is ruled out.*

Laboratory and Diagnostic Tests

Diagnostic tests that may be used include X-ray examinations of the head and neck as well as CT and MRI scans. These procedures can assist in providing a more definitive diagnosis of the severity and type of trauma. Laboratory tests are essential to determine the extent of blood loss and prepare for possible blood transfusion (complete blood count, electrolytes, cross-match).

> ▶ **Take** NOTE!
>
> *If clear liquid fluid is noted draining from the ears or nose, notify the physician or advanced practitioner. If the fluid tests positive for glucose, this is indicative, but not definitive, of leaking CSF.*

Osmond et al. (2010) have developed a clinical decision rule for the use of CT scans in the examination of minor head injury in children presenting to the emergency department. While further research is required before using the decision rule in clinical practice, the authors have identified key factors that help identify whether or not the seemingly minor head injury is potentially more serious. Having any one of four high-risk factors was related to the need for neurosurgical intervention: (1) failure to reach a score of 15 on the Glasgow Coma Scale within 2 hours, (2) suspicion of an open skull fracture, (3) worsening headache, and (4) irritability, and having any one of three additional medium-risk factors was related to having a brain injury that could be seen on CT: (1) large, boggy hematoma of the scalp; (2) signs of basal skull fracture (hemotympanum, "raccoon eyes," otorrhea or rhinorrhea of CSF, and/or battle sign); and (3) dangerous mechanism of injury (e.g., motor vehicle crash, fall from a minimum of 91 cm or five stairs, or fall from bicycle with no helmet).

Nursing Management

Nursing management of the child with head trauma depends on the seriousness of the injury. Until the extent of the injury has been determined, the child should be NPO (nil per os, Latin for "nothing by mouth"). Nurses play a critical role in identifying neurologic deterioration to ensure timely medical or surgical intervention.

Caring for the Child with Mild to Moderate Head Injury

Most children with mild to moderate head injury with no loss of consciousness and normal behavioural patterns can be cared for and observed at home. Provide parents and caregivers with clear instructions regarding the care of their child at home. Explain that they must seek medical attention if the child's condition worsens at any time during the first several days after the injury. See Teaching Guideline 37.2.

Children with mild head injury may exhibit some cognitive and behavioural symptoms, such as difficulty paying attention, problems making sense of what has been seen or heard, and forgetting things, in the early days after the injury. The majority make a full recovery. However, some may experience ongoing cognitive and behavioural difficulties, including slow information processing and attention difficulties. Children must be symptom free, which usually takes 2 to 3 weeks, before returning to sports after even a mild head injury due to the potential for second impact syndrome.

Caring for the Child with Severe Head Injury

Children with more severe head injuries may require intensive care initially until stabilized. The focus will be on maintaining the child's airway; monitoring breathing, circulation, and neurologic status closely; preventing and controlling seizure activity; and treating any other injuries that may have occurred as a result of the trauma. Nursing management will continue to focus on ongoing evaluation of neurologic status.

Monitoring the Child with Head Injury at Home

Instruct parents and caregivers:

- Stay with the child for the first 24 hours and be ready to take the child to the hospital if necessary.
- Closely observe the child for a few days.
- Wake the child every 2 hours to ensure that he or she moves normally, wakes enough to recognize the caregiver, and responds to the caregiver appropriately.
- Call the medical provider or bring child to the emergency room if the child exhibits any of the following:
  - Headache that gets worse
  - Slurred speech
  - Dizziness that does not go away or happens repeatedly
  - Extreme irritability or other abnormal behaviour
  - Vomiting more than two times
  - Clumsiness or difficulty walking
  - Oozing blood or watery fluid from ears or nose
  - Difficulty waking up
  - Unequal-sized pupils
  - Seizures
- Review signs and symptoms of increased ICP and provide parents with a number they can call if they have questions or concerns.

Individualize care to the specific needs of the child (see Common Medical and Surgical Treatments 37.1). Maintain a quiet environment to help reduce restlessness and irritability. Manage pain and administer sedation as ordered. Observe the level of sedation closely to ensure that any sedation does not hinder the ability to assess adequately for neurologic changes. Monitor for the development of hemorrhage, infection, cerebral edema, and transtentorial herniation.

▶ **Take** NOTE!

Parents are extremely helpful resources in evaluating a child's behaviour for changes or abnormalities. They can provide insight into whether a behaviour seen is normal or abnormal for this child. Examples include the ease with which a child is normally aroused, how much the child normally sleeps during the day, and what is the child's normal visual and hearing acuity.

Head injuries can range from a temporary unconsciousness that resolves quickly to a prolonged coma. Nursing management of the comatose child encompasses total supportive care and monitoring of the child.

Providing Support and Education

Provide support and education for the family of a child who has suffered head trauma. Encourage involvement in the child's care. The extent of residual neurologic damage and recovery may be unclear for the child with a head injury. This can be frustrating and stressful for parents and family. Encourage verbalization of their feelings and concerns. Rehabilitation of the child with permanent brain damage is an essential component of his or her care. It should begin as soon as possible in the hospital setting and may continue for months to years. This can place a strain on the family and its finances. Families need to be involved in the rehabilitation process. The nurse will be a key member in ensuring the parents and family are involved with the interdisciplinary team.

Preventing Head Injuries

Prevention of head injuries provides the greatest benefit to children and the community. Nurses play a key role in educating the public on topics such as helmet use with certain sports, bicycle and motorcycle safety, seat belt use, and providing adequate supervision of children to help prevent injuries and accidents.

Abusive Head Trauma

Abusive head trauma, also referred to as shaken baby syndrome. The infant's large head and weak neck muscles place him or her at increased risk for brain injury due to violent shaking or cranial impact. This form of head injury is most often seen in children less than 9 months of age. There are many precipitating factors to abusive head trauma, but frustration with infant crying is likely the most significant.

The full impact of neurologic deficits resulting from abusive head trauma may take several years to be identified, and recovery can be very slow. Long-term outcomes are often poor. The majority of infants and children with abusive head trauma have some impairment of motor and cognitive abilities, language, vision, and behaviour. However, many exhibit severe neurologic problems such as profound mental retardation, spastic quadriparesis, and cortical blindness.

Nursing Assessment

The infant who has been a victim of abusive head trauma can present in many ways. Symptoms and physical findings may be similar to those seen in children with accidental head trauma, epilepsy, or increased ICP related to infection. A high degree of suspicion is warranted for infants presenting with decreased LOC. Nurses are mandatory reporters of abuse (for further information on this, see Chapter 52), and early recognition of suspected child abuse is essential to prevent death and disability from repetitive abusive head trauma.

Health History

It is important that nurses and other health care providers review the infant's history closely and pay particular attention to the caregiver's explanation of the injury. As soon as abusive head trauma is suspected, enlist the help of a team of child abuse experts. Carefully document any discrepancies between the physical injuries and the history of injury given by the parent, if the stories among those involved in the infant's care are conflicting, or if the caregivers are unable to give an explanation for the injury. Also, any previous intracranial or skeletal injuries that cannot be explained should be noted.

In less severe cases, common signs and symptoms may include:

• Poor feeding or sucking
• Vomiting
• Lethargy or irritability
• Failure to thrive
• Increased sleeping
• Difficulty arousing

In more severe cases, the symptoms will be more acute and may consist of:

• Seizure activity
• Apnea
• Bradycardia
• Decreased LOC
• Bulging fontanel

Physical Examination

In many cases of abusive head trauma, there will be no external evidence of trauma. The classic presentation includes retinal hemorrhages, acute subdural hematoma, and multiple fractures of ribs and long bones.

Laboratory and Diagnostic Tests

Diagnostic tests including CT, MRI, ophthalmologic examination to confirm retinal hemorrhages, and skeletal survey X-rays to determine other injuries may be performed to help determine the extent and type of injury. Laboratory work is required to ensure coagulation studies are normal and to rule out congenital metabolic disorders.

Nursing Management

Treatment and nursing management will be similar to that for the child with accidental head trauma (see section on Head Trauma). Prevention of abusive head trauma is a major concern for all health care professionals. Be aware of risk factors related to the potential for abusive head trauma to occur. Recognizing these risk

---

> **BOX 37.4** **Risk Factors Associated with Abusive Head Trauma**
>
> • Single parent
> • Young parent
> • Substance abuse by a parent
> • Any external factors present such as financial, social, or physical burdens that place stress on the parent
> • Premature or sick infant
> • Infant crying

factors will allow appropriate intervention and protection of the child to take place. See Box 37.4 for risk factors related to abusive head trauma.

Educating parents and caregivers on appropriate ways to handle stress and ways to cope with a crying infant can help to prevent non-accidental head trauma (Teaching Guideline 37.3). Many parents and caregivers

---

> **TEACHING GUIDELINE 37.3**
>
> **Tips to Calm a Crying Baby**
>
> Instruct parents and caregivers:
>
> • Try to figure out what is upsetting the baby.
>   • Is the baby hungry?
>   • Is the baby's diaper dry?
>   • Is the baby cold or hot?
>   • Is the baby overtired or overstimulated?
>   • Is the baby in pain?
>   • Is the baby sick or running a fever?
> • Try to help the baby relax.
>   • Turn down the lights.
>   • Swaddle the baby.
>   • Walk the baby.
>   • Rock the baby.
>   • Give the baby a breast, bottle, or pacifier.
>   • Shhh, talk to, or sing to the baby.
>   • Take the baby for a stroller or car ride.
> • Sometimes the baby may continue to cry after all your efforts. If you feel overwhelmed, frustrated, or angry, focus on keeping the baby safe.
>   • Stop what you are doing, take a deep breath, and count to 10.
>   • Place the baby in a safe place, such as the crib or playpen.
>   • Leave the room and shut the door, and find a quiet place for yourself.
>   • Check on the baby every 5 to 15 minutes.
>   • Do not be afraid to call for help; call a friend, relative, or neighbour.

may perceive shaking a child as a less violent way to react than other means of enforcing discipline. They need to be aware that shaking a baby, even for only a few seconds, can cause serious brain damage and death. Decreasing mortality and morbidity associated with abusive head trauma and non-accidental injury through early preventive education is an essential nursing concern. Information about the dangers of shaking a baby should be a part of prenatal care and standard discharge teaching on postpartum units. In addition, this information should be provided to the community and in health education classes to reach young potential child care providers.

Perinatal Head Injuries

Perinatal head trauma may result from excessive forces before or during the birth process, especially from a prolonged labour, an abnormal or difficult presentation, cephalopelvic disproportion, or the use of mechanical forces such as forceps or vacuum during delivery. Risk factors include multiple-gestation pregnancies, large-for-date infants, extreme prematurity, macrocephaly, or congenital anomalies. Most perinatal head injuries are minor and resolve without treatment.

Nursing Assessment

Inspect the head for lumps, bumps, or bruises. Note if swelling or bruising crosses suture lines. See Comparison Chart 37.2 and Figure 37.13 for a comparison of caput succedaneum and cephalohematoma, common types of head trauma resulting from the birth process.

Nursing Management

Nursing management will be mainly supportive and will focus on assessing for resolution of the trauma or any associated complications, along with providing support and education to the parents. Provide parents with explanation and reassurance that these injuries are harmless. It can be very alarming and concerning to parents to see swelling or bruising on their child's head. Provide parents with education regarding the length of time until resolution and when and if they need to seek further medical attention for the condition.

Near Drowning

Worldwide, drowning remains a significant cause of death for children. However, in Canada adult males have higher rates of death from drowning than children (World Health Organization, 2010).

Near drowning is described as an incident in which a child has suffered a submersion injury and has survived for at least 24 hours. Near-drowning events result in a significant number of injured children and can result in long-term neurologic deficits. In children between the ages of 1 and 4 years, most drowning and near-drowning incidents occur in residential swimming pools (CDC, 2010b). Most incidents are accidental and result from inadequate supervision or lack of use of personal flotation devices.

Nursing Assessment

Hypoxia is the primary problem resulting from near drowning. The child requires rapid assessment of airway, breathing, and circulation followed by appropriate resuscitative measures. The child may be comatose,

COMPARISON CHART 37.2 CAPUT SUCCEDANEUM VS. CEPHALOHEMATOMA

	Caput Succedaneum (see Fig. 37.13A)	Cephalohematoma (see Fig. 37.13B)
Description	An edematous area of the scalp of the newborn	Collection of blood between the skull bone and periosteum
Cause	Pressure from the uterus or vaginal wall during a head-first delivery or as a result of vacuum extraction	Pressure against the mother's pelvis results in bleeding. Common with forceps births
Characteristics	The swelling may be on any portion of the scalp and may cross the midline and suture lines. Mild discolouration may be present.	Does not cross the midline or suture lines
Treatment	None necessary (only observation)	In most cases only observation is necessary and resolution occurs within 2–9 weeks.
Complications	Usually heals spontaneously within a few days and without complication, but if extensive bruising is present hyperbilirubinemia may occur.	Anemia, hypotension, underlying skull fracture, rarely leads to an infection such as meningitis. Due to the resolving hematoma, hemolysis of red blood cells occurs and the infant may develop hyperbilirubinemia.

Adapted from: Adams-Chapman, I., & Stoll, B. J. (2007). Nervous system disorders. In R. M. Kliegman, R. E. Behrman, H. B. Jenson, & B. F. Stanton (Eds.), *Nelson's textbook of pediatrics* (18th ed.). Philadelphia: Saunders.

Caput succedaneum

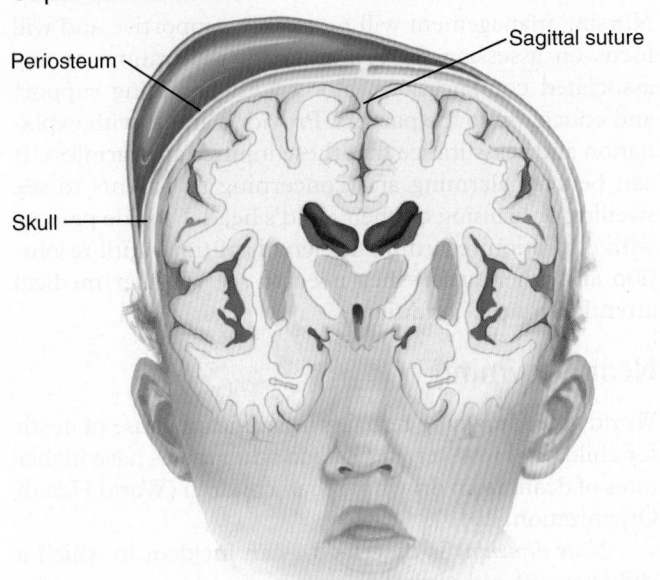

Cephalohematoma

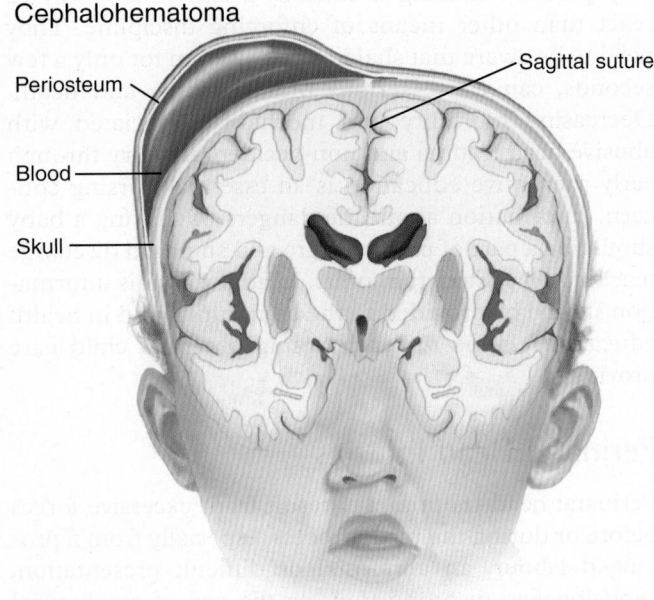

A

B

FIGURE 37.13 (**A**) Infant with caput succedaneum. Edema is noted at birth and crosses the suture line. (**B**) Infant with cephalohematoma. Bleeding appears within the first 2 to 3 days of birth and does not cross the suture line. It can become calcified into a hardened area over time.

hypothermic, lack spontaneous respirations, and present with hypoxia and acidosis. Gain information about the site and time of submersion, the water temperature, and how long before the child received interventions such as cardiopulmonary resuscitation (CPR) and emergency medical services (EMS).

Nursing Management

Resuscitative measures should be started as soon as the child is pulled from the water, and the child should be transported to a hospital immediately. If a diving injury is suspected, c-spine precautions should be initiated. Management will be based on the degree of cerebral insult that has occurred. The child who has been successfully resuscitated will usually require intensive nursing care and monitoring. Promotion of oxygenation and monitoring for infection related to aspiration of water are primary nursing concerns. Chronic neurologic damage occurs in many near drownings secondary to hypoxia. As with all severe brain injuries, the child may need rehabilitation and long-term follow-up. Provide parents with support and education relating to their child's condition. Educating children, families, and the community is an important nursing intervention to help prevent drowning (see Teaching Guideline 37.4).

Blood Flow Disruption

Cerebrovascular disorders are among the top 10 causes of death in children and occur most frequently in the first year of life (Lynch, Hirtz, DeVeber, & Nelson, 2002). Although they occur less often than in adults, they are still an important cause of mortality and chronic morbidity in children. Many children will develop lifelong cognitive and motor impairments. Improvements in imaging techniques have led to an increase in the reported incidence and prevalence of cerebrovascular disorders in children in recent years (Roach, deVeber, Riela, & Wiznitzer, 2008). Childhood cerebrovascular disorders (stroke) are usually seen after the first month of life. Periventricular/intraventricular

---

TEACHING GUIDELINE 37.4

Teaching to Prevent Drowning

Instruct parents and caregivers:

- Install proper pool fencing.
- Start water safety training at a young age.
- Never leave an infant or young child without adult supervision in or near water (this includes bathtubs).
- Empty water from all containers, such as 5-gallon buckets, immediately after use.
- Ensure that the child wears personal flotation devices at all times when near water.
- Learn CPR and keep emergency numbers handy (make sure babysitters are CPR qualified).
- Know the depth of water before permitting a child to jump or dive.

COMPARISON CHART 37.3   RISK FACTORS AND CAUSES OF STROKE IN THE PEDIATRIC CLIENT VS. THE ADULT CLIENT

Type of Stroke	Risk Factors and Causes in Children	Risk Factors and Causes in Adults
Ischemic stroke	Cardiac disorders and intracardiac defects (congenital, such as ventricular septal defect, atrial septal defect, aortic stenosis, or acquired, such as rheumatic heart disease) Coagulation abnormalities that lead to thrombosis Sickle-cell disease Infection, such as meningitis Arterial dissection Genetic disorders	Cardiac disease, including atherosclerosis Diabetes mellitus Hyperlipidemia Hypercoagulability states Polycythemia Sickle-cell disease Smoking Increased age Male gender Obesity Excessive alcohol consumption
Hemorrhagic stroke	Vascular malformations such as intracranial arteriovenous malformation (AVM) Aneurysms Warfarin therapy Cavernous malformations Malignancy Trauma Coagulation disorders such as hemophilia Thrombocytopenia Liver failure Leukemia Intracranial tumours such as medulloblastoma	Hypertension Aneurysms Use of anticoagulant medications Smoking Increased age Male gender Obesity Excessive alcohol consumption

hemorrhage is seen in preterm infants and in infants up to 1 month of age.

Cerebrovascular Disorders (Stroke)

A cerebrovascular disorder is a sudden disruption of the blood supply to the brain. It affects neurologic functioning, such as movement and speech. Two major types of cerebrovascular disorders are seen in children just as in adults: ischemic stroke and hemorrhagic stroke. In children, ischemic stroke is more common than hemorrhagic stroke. There is a wide array of risk factors and causes of stroke in children as compared with adults (Comparison Chart 37.3), but in many cases the cause remains unidentified. The outcomes reported for cerebrovascular disorders in children vary, but many children will develop some neurologic or cognitive deficit.

Nursing Assessment

The clinical presentation will vary according to age, the underlying cause, and the location of the stroke. Signs and symptoms of acute stroke are similar to those seen in the adult and depend on the area of the brain that has been affected. Common signs of ischemic stroke include:

• Weakness on one side or hemiplegia
• Facial droop
• Slurred speech
• Speech dysphagias

In hemorrhagic stroke, the child develops a severe headache that is associated with vomiting, focal neurologic deficits, and rapid deterioration in LOC.

Strokes in children are diagnosed in the same manner as strokes in adults using clinical examination, CT (which may be normal in early stroke), and MRI. However, the child may need further tests, such as metabolic studies, coagulation tests, echocardiography, and LP to help identify the cause of the stroke.

Nursing Management

Historically, children have been excluded from adult stroke studies. Therefore, many treatments used in children have had to be adapted from adult studies. Acute treatment depends on the results of diagnostic imaging with interventions provided by the neurovascular team. The child often requires intensive care with management of increased ICP. The exact treatment will depend on the underlying cause. Nursing management will be similar to that for the adult client who has suffered a stroke. Following the acute phase, care will focus on assessing neurologic status, increasing mobility, providing adequate nutrition and hydration, and encouraging self-care. Rehabilitative care may be initiated, depending on the long-term deficits, to help the child attain optimal function. Parental support and education will be essential in helping them care for a child who has new disabilities.

Periventricular/Intraventricular Hemorrhage (PVH/IVH)

Intraventricular hemorrhage (IVH), which is bleeding into the ventricles, is most commonly seen in preterm infants, especially very low birth weight infants (less than 1500 g) (Adams-Chapman & Stoll, 2007). Due to the preterm infant's fragile capillaries in the periventricular area (germinal matrix), immature cerebrovascular development, and poorly supported vascular bed, these infants are at an increased risk for intracranial bleeds. Causes of rupture of the capillaries leading to IVH vary and include fluctuations in systemic and cerebral blood flow, increases in cerebral blood flow from hypertension, seizure activity, hypoxia, sepsis, and respiratory distress. The smaller the neonate is, and the more premature, the higher the risk of developing IVH.

Complications of IVH include development of hydrocephalus, periventricular leukomalacia (an ischemic injury resulting from inadequate perfusion of the white matter adjacent to the ventricles), cerebral palsy, and severe neurodevelopmental delay. The size and severity of the IVH is measured using a grading system that was developed by Burstein, Papile, and Burstein (1979):

- Grade 1: small hemorrhage that is confined to the periventricular germinal matrix
- Grade 2: hemorrhage extends into the lateral ventricles without hydrocephalus
- Grade 3: hemorrhage extends into the lateral ventricles always with hydrocephalus
- Grade 4: major parenchymal (in the brain) periventricular hemorrhage usually with hydrocephalus

Infants who experience mild IVH may have negligible neurologic deficits. Those with higher grades of IVH are more likely to demonstrate neurologic and cognitive deficits.

Therapeutic Management

Infants with a documented IVH will receive follow-up with scans to monitor the lesion for evidence of progression or resolution. Supportive care includes the correction of underlying medical disturbances that might be related to the development of IVH as well as cardiovascular, respiratory, and neurologic support. Correction of anemia, hypotension, and acidosis along with ventilatory support may be necessary in some cases. A temporary ventricular catheter system, which may be connected to a reservoir placed under the scalp, may be used to manage early hydrocephalus. If hydrocephalus persists, placement of a ventricular shunt may be necessary (see Hydrocephalus section).

Nursing Assessment

The signs and symptoms seen with IVH vary significantly, and there may be no clinical signs evident. Closely monitor newborns who are at an increased risk, such as premature and low birth weight infants. Daily occipital frontal head circumference measures are critical and should be documented in chart form for all neonates with suspected IVH. Some signs that may be seen include:

- Apnea
- Bradycardia
- Respiratory distress
- Weak suck
- Seizure activity
- High-pitched cry
- Bulging fontanel, split sutures
- Anemia

Premature and low birth weight neonates may have head ultrasonography in the first 10 days of life to assess the presence of an IVH. Diagnostic tests such as CT and MRI also may be performed to document the presence of an IVH and provide more accurate assessment of the severity and size of the bleed.

Nursing Management

Nursing management will include monitoring for signs and symptoms of increased ICP, rapid increases in head circumference, neurologic changes, and delays in attainment of developmental milestones. In addition, provide education and support to the parents.

Chronic Headaches

Headaches, including migraines, are common reasons why children miss school, visit their primary care physician, and receive subsequent referrals to neurologists. Children with reports or symptoms of headaches need to be examined thoroughly. Headaches may result from sinusitis or eyestrain or can be indicative of more serious conditions such as brain tumours, acute meningitis, or increased ICP. Migraines are a specific type of headache. They are benign, recurrent, throbbing headaches often accompanied by nausea, vomiting, visual auras, and photophobia. Acute migraines can occur in children as young as 3 to 4 years old (Rosenblum & Fisher, 2001). The cause of migraine headaches is not well understood.

Therapeutic Management

After other acute or chronic conditions are ruled out, management of chronic headaches will focus on treating the child's pain. Pharmacologic measures may be used in the treatment of chronic headaches and migraines (Rosenblum & Fisher, 2001). Medications used in children to treat and prevent headaches are similar to the medications used to treat adults. Headaches may also be caused by medication overuse (Reimschisel, 2003). The child may have a primary headache disorder that is exacerbated by the frequent use of medications. Although medication overuse headaches are common in children, they are frequently under-recognized and under-diagnosed.

Nursing Assessment

Elicit a description of the present illness and chief complaint. Important health history information to obtain is onset of the pain, aggravating and alleviating factors, frequency and duration of the pain, time of day the pain usually occurs, location of the pain, and quality and intensity of the pain.

In young children, symptoms of headache may be hard to recognize. However, common signs and symptoms may include:

- Irritability
- Lethargy
- Head holding
- Head banging or other repetitive self stimulating behaviours
- Sensitivity to sound or light

Assessment also includes a thorough physical examination to rule out any life-threatening illness, such as a brain tumour or increased ICP. A detailed neurologic exam is warranted. Neuroimaging may be performed based on the child's history and physical exam, if needed, to rule out a brain tumour or mass lesion as the cause of the headaches (Rosenblum & Fisher, 2001).

Nursing Management

Nursing measures will focus on support and education. Reassure the child and family that no serious medical or neurologic disease is present. Because headaches are recurring and the cause may be unknown, pain management can be difficult. Provide education to help the child and parents gain control over the headaches. Teach the child and family to keep a very accurate record of headaches and activities surrounding the headaches to help

---

BOX 37.5 Potential Headache Triggers

- Foods, such as chocolate, caffeine, or monosodium glutamate (MSG)–containing foods
- Changes in hormone levels, around menses and ovulation
- Changes in:
  - Weather
  - Season
  - Sleep patterns
  - Meal schedule
- Stress
- Intense activity
- Bright or flickering lights
- Odours, such as strong perfumes

---

establish a pattern of occurrence and identify triggering factors. Encourage parents and the child to recognize the triggering factors and to avoid them (Box 37.5). Teach the child and family about pain medications and how to use them. Teach other management techniques, which may include exercise, regular attendance at school, use of biofeedback, stress reduction techniques, and possible psychiatric assessment (Rosenblum & Fisher, 2001).

▪▪▪ Key Concepts

- Development of the brain and spinal cord occurs in the first 3 to 4 weeks of gestation. Infection, trauma, teratogens, and malnutrition during this period can result in malformations and may affect normal CNS development.
- The brain of the newborn is highly vascular, leading to an increased risk for hemorrhage.
- The head of the infant and young child is large in proportion to the body and the neck muscles are not well developed, which places the infant at an increased risk for head injury from falls and accidents.
- Neurologic disorders in children can result from congenital problems as well as infections or trauma.
- LP and CSF analysis can be useful in the diagnosis of hemorrhage or infection.
- CT and MRI studies can be useful in diagnosing congenital abnormalities such as neural tube defects, hemorrhage, tumours, fractures, demyelinating diseases, or inflammation.
- EEGs measure the electrical activity of the brain and can be used in diagnosing seizures or brain death.
- Antibiotics are used in the treatment of bacterial meningitis and shunt infections.
- Anticonvulsants are used in the treatment and prevention of seizures and are often used in combination.
- Corticosteroids are used to reduce cerebral edema and must be tapered before discontinuing.
- Risk factors associated with neurologic disorders include prematurity, perinatal insult, infection during pregnancy, family history of genetic disorders with a neurologic manifestation, seizure disorders, and headaches.
- Alterations in motor function, such as changes in gait or muscle tone or strength, may indicate certain neurologic problems such as increased ICP, head injury, and cerebral infections.
- Increased ICP is a sign that may occur with many neurologic disorders. It may result from head trauma, perinatal insult, hydrocephalus, infection, and brain tumours. It is essential that the nurse observes for signs and symptoms associated with increased ICP while caring for a child with a potential or suspected neurologic disorder. Recording changes from baseline is essential.

- A bulging fontanel in an infant can be a sign of increased ICP and is seen in such neurologic disorders as hydrocephalus and head traumas.
- Increased ICP can result in downward herniation of brain structures, leading to cranial nerve compression (fixed dilated pupil) or medullary compression (cardiorespiratory depression and death).
- Cortical control of motor function is lost in certain neurologic disorders; postural reflexes reemerge and are directly related to the area of the brain that is damaged. Decorticate posturing occurs with damage of the cerebral cortex. Decerebrate posturing includes damage to the brain stem.
- Hydrocephalus results from a disturbance in the flow pattern of CSF but may result from an imbalance in the production and absorption of CSF. Key assessment findings include a rapid increase in head circumference seen in the infant, or headache and vomiting in the older child. Signs and symptoms associated with increased ICP may be seen.
- Bacterial meningitis requires rapid assessment and treatment. On assessment, the nurse may find the infant with bacterial meningitis irritable, lethargic, or febrile with nuchal rigidity. The older child may complain of severe headache and neck pain.
- Nursing management of seizures focuses on preventing injury during seizures, instituting seizure precautions, maintaining a patent airway, administering appropriate medication and treatments to prevent or reduce seizures, and providing education and support to the child and family to help them cope with the challenges of living with a chronic seizure disorder.
- Nursing management of the child with hydrocephalus will focus on maintaining cerebral perfusion, minimizing neurologic complications, recognizing and preventing shunt infection and malfunction, maintaining adequate nutrition, promoting growth and development, and supporting and educating the child and family.
- Nursing management of the child with bacterial meningitis will include administering intravenous antibiotics, reducing ICP, and maintaining cerebral perfusion along with treating fluid volume deficit, controlling seizures, and preventing injury that may result from altered LOC or seizure activity.
- Nurses play a key role in educating the public on topics such as helmet use with certain sports, bicycle and motorcycle safety, seat belt use, and providing adequate supervision of children to help prevent injuries and accidents and resultant head trauma from occurring.
- Many neurologic disorders affect multiple body systems with lifelong deficits that require long-term rehabilitation. Adjusting to the demands this condition places on the child and family is difficult. Parents may need time to accept their child's condition but as soon as possible they should be involved in the child's care.
- Children with neurologic disorders and their families need education and support throughout the child's lifetime. As the child grows, the needs of the family and child will change. Nurses need to provide ongoing education and support.
- Some neurologic disorders require complete intensive daily care. Adjusting to these demands can be difficult for the family. Encourage respite care and provide meaningful education programs that emphasize independence for the child in the least restrictive educational environment possible. Refer caregivers to local resources, including education services and support groups.

REFERENCES

Adams-Chapman, I., & Stoll, B. J. (2007). Nervous system disorders. In R. M. Kliegman, R. E. Behrman, H. B. Jenson, & B. F. Stanton (Eds.), *Nelson's textbook of pediatrics* (18th ed.). Philadelphia: Saunders.

Albert, G. W., Menezes, A. H., Hansen, D. R., Greenlee, J. D., & Weinstein, S. L. (2010). Chiari malformation type I in children younger than age 6 years: Presentation and surgical outcome. *Journal of Neurosurgery: Pediatrics, 5,* 554–561.

American Academy of Pediatrics. (2008). Febrile seizures: Clinical practice guideline for the long-term management of the child with simple febrile seizures. *Pediatrics, 121*(6), 1281–1286; retrieved December 5, 12011 from http://pediatrics.aappublications.org/cgi/reprint/121/6/1281

Burstein, J., Papile, L. A., & Burstein, R. (1979). Intraventricular hemorrhage and hydrocephalus in premature newborns: A prospective study with CT. *American Journal of Roentgenology, 132*(4), 631–635.

Canadian Paediatric Society. (1997). Periconceptional use of folic acid for reduction of the risk of neural tube defects. *Paediatrics & Child Health, 2*(2), 114–119.

Canadian Paediatric Society. (1998). Acute childhood encephalitis and meningoencephalitis. *Paediatrics & Child Health, 3*(1), 45–46.

Canadian Paediatric Society. (2004). Recommendations for safe sleeping environments for infants and children. *Paediatrics & Child Health, 9*(9), 659–663.

Canadian Paediatric Society. (2008). Therapy of suspected bacterial meningitis in Canadian children six weeks of age and older. *Paediatrics & Child Health, 13*(4), 309.

Cavazos, J. E., & Spitz, M. (2011). *Seizures and epilepsy: Overview and classification.* Retrieved December 3, 2011 from http://emedicine.medscape.com/article/1184846-overview

Centers for Disease Control and Prevention. (2010a). *Meningitis questions and answers.* Retrieved December 3, 2011 from http://www.cdc.gov/meningitis/about/faq.html

Centers for Disease Control and Prevention. (2010b). *Unintentional drowning: Fact sheet.* Retrieved December 3, 2011 from http://www.cdc.gov/HomeandRecreationalSafety/Water-Safety/waterinjuries-factsheet.html

Centers for Disease Control and Prevention. (2010c). *Frequently asked questions: Epilepsy.* Retrieved December 3, 2011 from http://www.cdc.gov/epilepsy/basics/faqs.htm#5

Duffner, P. K., Baumann, R. J., Berman, P., Green, J. L., & Schneider, S. (2008). Febrile seizures: Clinical practice guidelines for the long-term management of the child with simple febrile seizures. *Pediatrics, 212*(6), 1281–1286.

Fischbach, F. T., & Dunning, M. B., III. (2009). *A manual of laboratory and diagnostic tests* (8th ed.). Philadelphia: Lippincott Williams & Wilkins.

Ford-Jones, E. L., MacGregor, D., Richardson, S., Jamieson, F., Blaser, S., & Artsob, H. (1998). Acute childhood encephalitis and meningoencephalitis: Diagnosis and management. *Paediatrics & Child Health, 3*(1), 33–41.

Health Canada. (2002). *Congenital anomalies in Canada: A perinatal health report.* Ottawa, ON: Minister of Public Works and Government Services Canada.

Health Canada. (2006). *Reye's syndrome.* Retrieved December 4, 2011 from http://www.hc-sc.gc.ca/hl-vs/iyh-vsv/diseases-maladies/reye-eng.php

Johnston, M. V. (2007). Seizures in childhood. In R. M. Kliegman, R. E. Berman, H. B. Jenson, & B. F. Stanton (Eds.), *Nelson's textbook of pediatrics* (18th ed.). Philadelphia: Saunders.

Karch, A. (2010). *2010 Lippincott's nursing drug guide.* Philadelphia: Wolters Kluwer/Lippincott Williams & Wilkins.

KidsHealth. (2011). *Positional plagiocephaly (flattened head).* Retrieved December 5, 2011 from http://kidshealth.org/parent/general/sleep/positional_plagiocephaly.html#

Kinsman, S. L., & Johnston, M. V. (2007). Congenital anomalies of the central nervous system. In R. M. Kliegman, R. E. Behrman, H. B. Jenson, & B. F. Stanton (Eds.), *Nelson's textbook of pediatrics* (18th ed.). Philadelphia: Saunders.

Lynch, J. K., Hirtz, D. G., DeVeber, G., & Nelson, K. B. (2002). Report of the National Institute of Neurologic Disorders and Stroke workshop on perinatal and childhood stroke. *Pediatrics, 109*(1), 116–123.

Mikati, M. A. (2011). Seizures in childhood. In R. M. Kliegman, B. F. Stanton, J. W. St. Geme III, N. F. Schor, & R. E. Behrman (Eds.), *Nelson's textbook of pediatrics* (19th ed.). Philadelphia: Elsevier Saunders.

Ogilvy, C. S., Stieg, P. E., Awad, I., et al. (2001). Recommendations for the management of intracranial arteriovenous malformations: A statement for healthcare professionals from a special writing group of the Stroke Council, American Stroke Association. *Stroke, 32*(6), 1458–1472.

Osmond, M. H., Klassen, T. P., Wells, G. A., et al. (2010). CATCH: A decision rule for the use of computed tomography in children with minor head injury. *Canadian Medical Association Journal, 182*(4), 341–348.

Public Health Agency of Canada. (2008). Leading causes of death and hospitalization in Canada. Retrieved December 4, 2011 from http://www.phac-aspc.gc.ca/publicat/lcd-pcd97/index-eng.php

Reimschisel, T. (2003). Breaking the cycle of medication overuse headache. *Contemporary Pediatrics, 20*(101), 101–102.

Roach, E. S., deVeber, G., Riela, A. R., & Wiznitzer, M. (2008). Recognition and treatment of stroke in children. Retrieved December 5, 2011 from http://www.ninds.nih.gov/news_and_events/proceedings/stroke_proceedings/childneurology.htm

Rosenblum, R., & Fisher, P. (2001). A guide to children with acute and chronic headaches. *Journal of Pediatric Health Care, 15*(5), 229–235.

Spiro, C. S., & Spiro, D. M. (2004). Acute meningitis. *Clinician Reviews, 14*(3), 54–58.

Statistics Canada. (2007). *Ten leading causes of death by selected age groups, by sex, Canada, 2003 to 2007.* Retrieved December 4, 2011 from http://www.statcan.gc.ca/pub/84-215-x/2010001/tbls-eng.htm

Stevenson, K. L. (2004). Chiari type II malformation: Past, present, and future. *Neurosurgery Focus, 16*(2), 1–7.

Teasdale, G., & Jennett, B. (1974). Assessment of coma and impaired consciousness. *Lancet, 2*(7872), 81–84.

Virchow, R. (1851). Uber den Cretinismus, namentlich in Franken, und uber pathologische Schadelformen. *Verh Phys Med Gesell Wurzburg, 2*, 230.

World Health Organization. (2010). Drowning fact sheet number 347. Retrieved December 4, 2011 from www.who.int/mediacentre/factsheets/fs347/en/index.html

Zak, M., & Chan, V. W. (2010). Pediatric neurologic disorders. In S. M. Nettina (Ed.), *Lippincott manual of nursing practice* (9th ed.). Philadelphia: Lippincott Williams & Wilkins.

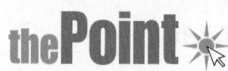

For additional learning materials, including Internet Resources, visit http://thePoint.lww.com/Chow1e.

CHAPTER WORKSHEET

MULTIPLE CHOICE QUESTIONS

1. When compared with adults, why are infants and children at an increased risk for head trauma?

   a. The head of the infant and young child is large in proportion to the body, and the neck muscles are not well developed.

   b. The development of the nervous system is complete at birth but remains immature.

   c. The spine is very immobile in infants and young children.

   d. The skull is more flexible due to the presence of sutures and fontanels.

2. At a well-child visit, hydrocephalus may be suspected in an infant if upon assessment the nurse finds:

   a. Narrow sutures

   b. Sunken fontanels

   c. A rapid increase in head circumference

   d. An increase in weight since the last visit

3. A 10-year-old child is admitted to the hospital due to a history of seizure activity. As his nurse, you are called into the room by his mother who states that he is having a seizure. What would be the priority nursing intervention?

   a. Prevention of injury by removing the child from his bed

   b. Prevention of injury by placing a tongue blade in the child's mouth

   c. Prevention of injury by restraining the child

   d. Prevention of injury by placing the child on his side and opening his airway

CRITICAL THINKING EXERCISES

1. A child is seen in the doctor's office after hitting his head while skateboarding. The child suffered no loss of consciousness and has no external injuries or significant past medical history. He is acting appropri-ately at this time. His only complaint is a dull headache. What instructions would you give the parents regarding his care at home? Include when they should seek further medical care.

2. A 10-year-old child is admitted to the pediatric unit after experiencing a seizure. A complete, accurate, and detailed history from a reliable source is essen-tial. What information would you ask for while obtaining the history?

3. A 6-year-old child is admitted to the hospital because of a possible seizure. The child's mother calls the nurse to the room because the child is "jerking all over" and won't respond when she calls the child's name. List appropriate nursing interventions for this child. Prioritize the list of interventions.

4. Describe the impact of cerebrovascular accident in the child as compared with the adult. How does it affect the child's future? How will the nurse provide care differently for the child stroke victim as com-pared with the adult?

STUDY ACTIVITIES

1. A 4-month-old child with a history of hydrocephalus has undergone surgery for placement of a ventriculo-peritoneal shunt. What information would you include in the teaching plan?

2. Develop an example of a "headache log" that could be used by the family for chronicling the child's headaches, including triggers, relieving factors, and precipitating events. Ensure that the log is developed at a 6th-grade reading level to make it practical for low literacy parents.

3. In the clinical setting, interview the parent of a child who has suffered significant brain trauma or injury (such as head trauma, IVH, or stroke). Talk with the family about the types of care the child requires. Reflect upon this interview in your clinical journal, and compare how the ongoing care for this child compares with that for a typical child.

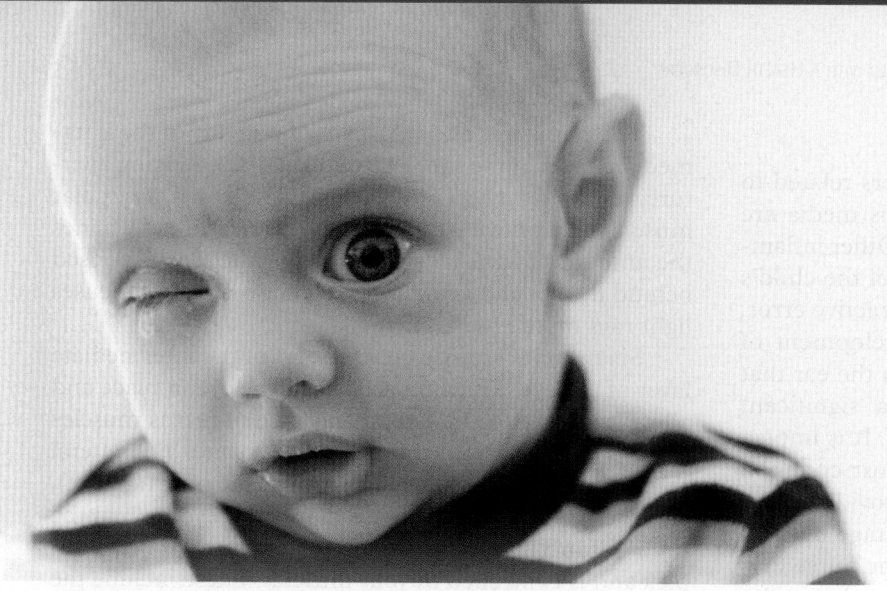

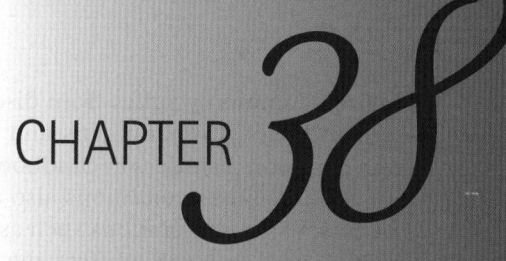

NURSING CARE OF THE CHILD WITH A DISORDER OF THE EYES OR EARS

KEY TERMS

acuity
amblyopia
blindness
conductive hearing loss
deaf
decibel

hearing impairment
nystagmus
pressure-equalizing tubes
   (PE tubes)
ptosis
sensorineural hearing loss

strabismus
tympanometry
tympanostomy
vision impairment

LEARNING OBJECTIVES

Upon completion of the chapter, the learner will be able to:

1. Differentiate between the anatomic and physiologic differences of the eyes and ears in children as compared with adults.
2. Identify various factors associated with disorders of the eyes and ears in infants and children.
3. Discuss common laboratory and other diagnostic tests useful in the diagnosis of disorders of the eyes and ears.
4. Discuss common medications and other treatments used for treatment and palliation of conditions affecting the eyes and ears.
5. Recognize risk factors associated with various disorders of the eyes and ears.
6. Distinguish between different disorders of the eyes and ears based on the signs and symptoms associated with them.
7. Discuss nursing interventions commonly used in regard to disorders of the eyes and ears.
8. Devise an individualized nursing care plan for the child with a sensory impairment or other disorder of the eyes or ears.
9. Develop patient/family teaching plans for the child with a disorder of the eyes or ears.
10. Describe the psychosocial impact of sensory impairments on children.

Matthew Baxter, a 9-month-old, is brought to the clinic by his mother. His mother tells you, "Matthew has been fussy and not eating or sleeping well for the past 2 days."

Wow

With the help of a nurse's knowledge and teaching, the child's senses provide him or her with an antenna to the universe.

Children commonly suffer from disorders related to the eyes and ears. Conjunctivitis and otitis media are two very common disorders in childhood. Other inflammatory and infectious conditions also affect the child's eyes or ears. Various alterations such as refractive error, strabismus, and amblyopia affect the development of visual **acuity** in children. Any alteration in the ear that contributes to hearing loss may have a significant impact on the child's language acquisition. It is important for nurses to be familiar with the most common disorders of the eyes and ears in order to provide appropriate care to these children and to encourage optimal development in all children. In addition, the nurse may be caring for a child with another problem who is also either visually or hearing impaired. The nurse must take these developmental differences into account when planning care for these children.

It is important for the nurse to understand the impact of eye and ear disorders on the child's development. Some children may be born with anomalies of the eyes or ears that will have a significant impact on vision and hearing as well as on psychomotor development. On the other hand, disorders affecting the eyes or ears, particularly if chronic or recurrent, can have a significant impact on the development of visual acuity or may cause **hearing impairment**. Nurses should be familiar with the most common disorders of the eyes and ears in order to provide appropriate care to these children and to encourage optimal development in all children. A basic understanding of normal anatomy and physiology of the eye and ear will enhance the nurse's ability to care for these children.

Anatomy and Physiology of the Eye

The eyebrow, eyelid, and eyelash serve to protect the eye by keeping particles out of the eye. Tears lubricate the eyes and protect them from dirt and infection. The lacrimal gland produces the watery part of tears, while the tarsal gland produces the oily part of tears. Tears exit the eye through the puncta in the upper and lower lids. The nasolacrimal duct carries tears from the lacrimal sac into the nasal cavity.

The cornea, sclera, and conjunctiva are important features of the external layer of the eye. The cornea, the first and most powerful lens of the eye, is a transparent sphere-shaped dome that covers both the pupil and the iris. Its dual purpose is to protect the eye and refract light as it enters the eye. The spherical shape of the cornea allows it to refract light. The sclera or "white of the eye" forms the supporting wall of the eyeball. The conjunctiva is a thin, transparent tissue on the inside of the eyelids, the surface of the eyeball, and the sclera. The conjunctiva secretes oils and mucus, which moisten and lubricate the eye.

The pupil, iris, and lens are components of the intermediate layer of the eye. The pupil, a black-looking aperture, allows light to enter the eye. The iris is a circular muscle that controls the size of the pupil and determines the amount of light entering the eye. The lens is housed behind the iris and is the second component that focuses light rays on the retina.

Six muscles are also components of the intermediate layer of the eye. These muscles hold the eye in place and allow it to rotate. The lateral and medial rectus muscles move the eye only in the horizontal plane. The lateral rectus muscle moves the eye away from the nose (abduct), and the medial rectus muscle moves the eye toward the nose (adduct). Vertical eye motion is a little more complex and is controlled by four muscles. These include the superior rectus, inferior rectus, superior oblique, and inferior oblique muscles. When the eye is fully abducted, only the superior and inferior rectus muscles can elevate and depress the eye. When the eye is fully adducted, only the inferior and superior oblique muscles can elevate and depress the eye. When the eye is neither fully abducted nor adducted, all of the four muscles contribute a percentage of the vertical motion.

The retina, optic nerve, macula, and fovea are responsible for producing sharp, detail vision and colour vision (van de Pol, 2009).

Age-Appropriate Visual Milestones

Most white newborns have blue eyes because of the lack of pigmentation in the iris at birth. The iris becomes pigmented over time, and the eye colour is usually determined by 6 to 12 months of age but may continue to change for several years as a normal phenomenon. The newborn's sclera may be slightly bluish-tinged but becomes white within weeks. The eyeball of the infant and the young child occupies a relatively larger space within the orbit than the adult's does, making the infant's and child's eyeball more susceptible to injury (Fig. 38.1).

The spherical shape of the newborn's lens does not allow for distance accommodation, so the newborn sees best at a distance of about 8 to 10 inches (Graven & Browne, 2008). The optic nerve is not completely myelinated, so colour discrimination is incomplete. Visual acuity develops over the first several years of the child's life. At birth, acuity ranges from 20/100 to 20/400, with 20/20 achieved by age 6 to 7 years (Weber & Kelley, 2010). The rectus muscles are uncoordinated at birth and mature over time so that binocular vision (the ability to focus with both eyes simultaneously) may be achieved by 4 months of age (Weber & Kelley, 2010). In the very preterm infant, retinal vascularization is incomplete, so visual acuity may be affected (American Academy of Pediatrics, 2006). Box 38.1 provides visual milestones from birth to about 1 year of age.

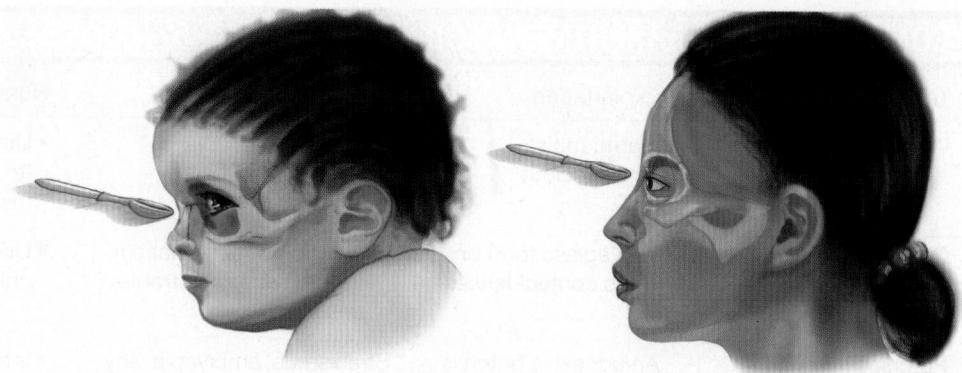

FIGURE 38.1 The relatively larger space that the infant's and young child's eyeball occupies within the orbit makes it more susceptible to injury as compared with the adult's eye.

Common Medical Treatments

A variety of interventions are used to treat disorders of the eyes and ears in children. The treatments listed in Common Medical Treatments 38.1 and Drug Guide 38.1 usually require a physician's order when a child is hospitalized.

NURSING PROCESS OVERVIEW FOR THE CHILD WITH A DISORDER OF THE EYES OR EARS

Care of the child with a disorder of the eyes and ears includes assessment, nursing diagnosis, planning, interventions, and evaluation. A number of general concepts related to the nursing process can be applied to disor-

ders of the eyes and ears. From a general understanding of the care involved for a child with alterations in the eyes and ears, the nurse can then individualize the care based on client specifics.

Assessment

Assessment of disorders of the eyes and ears in children includes health history, physical assessment, and laboratory or diagnostic testing.

Remember Matthew, the 9-month-old, with fussiness and poor feeding who was not sleeping well? What additional health history and physical examination assessment information should you obtain?

BOX 38.1 Eye Development Milestones

Birth
• Poor eyesight, blinks in response to bright light or touching of the eye
• Eyes are sometimes uncoordinated, may look crossed-eyed
• Able to stare at object if held 8 to 10 inches away
• Initially fixes eyes on a face or light, then begins to follow a moving object

1 Month
• Looks at faces and pictures with contrasting black and white images
• Can follow an object up to 90 degrees
• Watches parent closely
• Tears begin to work

2 to 3 Months
• Begins to be able to see an object as one image
• Looks at hands
• Follows light, faces, object

4 to 5 Months
• Beginning to reach hands to objects
• Can stare at block

• Recognizes bottles
• Will look at self in mirror
• Will look at own hand

5 to 7 Months
• Has full colour vision, able to see at longer distances
• Can pick up a toy that is dropped
• Will turn head to see an object
• Will touch image of self in mirror

7 to 11 Months
• Can stare at small objects
• Begins to have depth perception
• Plays peek-a-boo

11 to 12 Months
• Can watch objects that are moving fast

12 to 14 Months
• Able to place shapes in proper holes
• Becomes interested in pictures
• Recognizes familiar objects and pictures in books
• Points and gestures for objects and actions, recognizes own face in mirror

COMMON MEDICAL TREATMENTS 38.1

Treatment	Explanation	Indication	Nursing Implications
Warm compress	Warm, moist washcloth	Conjunctivitis	• Use very warm water from the tap (to avoid risk of burning, do not microwave).
Corrective lenses	In eyeglass form or as contact lenses	Correction of astigmatism, refractive error, strabismus	• Use a safety strap to help young children wear their eyeglasses.
Patching	An adhesive patch is applied to the healthier eye for several hours each day.	Strabismus, amblyopia, any other eye condition that results in one eye being weaker than the other	• Inform parents that though difficult to obtain, compliance with patching is critical. • A "pirate patch" may coax preschoolers into compliance.
Eye muscle surgery	Surgical alignment of the eyes	Strabismus	• Protect the operative site with patching. • Use elbow restraints if necessary.
Pressure-equalizing (PE) tubes (tympanostomy tubes)	Tiny plastic tubes inserted in the tympanic membrane	Chronic otitis media with effusion	• Teach parents "dry ears" precautions if prescribed or preferred by the surgeon.
Hearing aids	Amplification device worn in the ear	Hearing impairment	• Ensure appropriate fit and adequate amplification. • Direct families to outfitters that provide loaner aids of various brands and styles to determine best fit and amplification for the child.
Cochlear implants	Surgically inserted electronic prosthetic device	Sensorineural hearing loss	• Inform families that the usual minimum age for this procedure is 12 months.

Adapted from: Goller, Y. (2006). Cochlear implantation in children: Implications for the primary care provider. *Journal of the American Academy of Nurse Practitioners*, *18*(9), 397–408; and Yoon, P. J., Kelley, P. E., & Friedman, N. R. (2011). Ear, nose, & throat. In W. W. Hay, M. J. Levin, J. M. Sondheimer, & R. R. Deterding (Eds.), *Current pediatric diagnosis and treatment* (20th ed.). New York: McGraw-Hill.

DRUG GUIDE 38.1   COMMON DRUGS FOR EAR AND EYE DISORDERS

Medication	Action	Indication	Nursing Implications
Antibiotics (oral, otic, ophthalmic)	Treatment of bacterial infections of the eyes and ears	Acute otitis media, otitis externa, conjunctivitis	Teach families to complete the entire course as prescribed. Check for drug allergies prior to administration.
Antihistamines	Block histamine reaction	Allergic conjunctivitis	Topical drops used. Oral agents usually prescribed if allergic rhinitis accompanies the conjunctivitis.
Analgesics	Pain relief	Otitis media, otitis externa, after eye or ear surgery	Narcotic analgesics may be necessary in some instances.

Adapted from: Taketokmo, C. K., Hodding, J. H., & Kraus, D. M. (2010). *Lexi-comp's pediatric dosage handbook* (17th ed.). Hudson, Ohio: Lexi-comp.

Health History

The health history comprises past medical history, family history, history of present illness (when the symptoms started and how they have progressed), as well as treatments used at home. The past medical history may be significant for prematurity, genetic defects, eye or ear deformities, visual acuity deficit or **blindness**, hearing impairment or deafness, recurrent ear infections, or ear surgeries. Family history might be significant for eye or ear deformities or vision or hearing impairment or may reveal contacts for infectious exposure.

When eliciting the history of the present illness, inquire about its onset and progression and the presence of fever, nasal congestion, eye or ear pain, eye rubbing, ear pulling, headache, lethargy, or behavioural changes. Document if the child has corrective lenses or hearing aids prescribed and to what extent these devices are actually used.

Physical Examination

When assessing the eyes and ears, begin with inspection and observation. Palpation is also used when assessing for ear disorders. Testing of visual acuity and hearing is also performed.

Inspection and Observation

The physical examination should begin with inspection or observation. Note whether the child uses eyeglasses, corrective lenses, or a hearing aid. Observe the eyes: note their positioning and symmetry, presence of strabismus, nystagmus, and squinting. The eyelids should open equally (failure to open fully is termed **ptosis**). Note variations in eye slant and the presence of epicanthal folds. Assess the eyes for presence of eyelid edema, sclera colour, discharge, tearing, and pupillary equality, as well as size and shape of the pupils. Evert the eyelid to inspect the palpebral conjunctivae for redness. Test for extraocular movements and pupillary light response and accommodation. Note symmetry of corneal light reflex. Note presence of red reflex with an ophthalmoscope. Perform an age-appropriate visual acuity test. Refer to Chapter 30 for more detailed information related to visual acuity testing.

▶ **Take** NOTE!

Attempts to inspect the palpebral conjunctivae may be frightening to children. Ask the older, cooperative child to evert the eyelid himself or herself while the nurse inspects the conjunctivae.

▶ **Take** NOTE!

Though the sclerae are bluish in newborns, they become white in the first few weeks of life. Blue sclerae that persist beyond a few weeks of life may be an indicator of osteogenesis imperfecta type I, an inherited connective tissue disorder (Weber & Kelley, 2010).

Inspect the Ears. Note their size and shape, position, and the presence of skin tags, dimples, or other anomalies. Upon otoscopic examination, note presence of cerumen, discharge, inflammation, or a foreign body in the ear canal. Visualize the tympanic membrane and observe its colour, landmarks, and light reflex, as well as presence of perforation, scars, bulging, or retraction. Tympanic membrane mobility may be tested with pneumatic otoscopy. Auditory acuity is tested via the whisper test, audiometry, or other age-appropriate test (refer to Chapter 30 for a more detailed explanation of hearing testing).

Palpation

Usually, the eyes are not palpated. In the case of injury, the upper eyelid may be everted for examination purposes. Palpate the ear for tenderness over the tragus or pinna. Note the presence of tenderness over the mastoid area (tenderness may be present when otitis media progresses to mastoiditis). Palpate for enlarged cervical lymph nodes (this occurs when the eyes or ears are infected).

Laboratory and Diagnostic Testing

Common Laboratory and Diagnostic Tests 38.1 offers an explanation of the laboratory and diagnostic tests most commonly used for disorders of the eyes and ears. These tests can assist the physician in diagnosing the disorder and/or can be used as guidelines in determining ongoing treatment. Laboratory or non-nursing personnel obtain some of the tests, while the nurse may obtain others. In either instance, the nurse should be familiar with how the tests are obtained, what they are used for, and normal versus abnormal results. This knowledge will also be necessary when providing patient and family education related to the testing.

Nursing Diagnoses and Related Interventions

Upon completion of a thorough assessment, the nurse might identify several nursing diagnoses, including:

- Disturbed sensory perception
- Risk for infection
- Pain
- Delayed growth and development

COMMON LABORATORY AND DIAGNOSTIC TESTS 38.1

Test	Explanation	Indication	Nursing Implications
Culture of eye or ear discharge	Fluid draining from the eye or ear is cultured.	To find appropriate antibiotic coverage for a particular infection	Easy to collect, relatively pain free. If drainage must be removed from within the ear canal, more likely to be painful.
Tympanic fluid culture	Culture of fluid aspirated from the middle ear	To find appropriate antibiotic coverage for a particular infection	Painful; usually performed only by specially trained physicians
Tympanometry	Probe in ear canal measures movement of the eardrum	Determines extent of effusion of the middle ear	Quick and easy to perform (seconds) Requires accurate-sized probe for adequate seal of the ear canal

Adapted from: Yoon, P. J., Kelley, P. E., & Friedman, N. R. (2011). Ear, nose, & throat. In W. W. Hay, M. J. Levin, J. M. Sondheimer, & R. R. Deterding (Eds.), *Current pediatric diagnosis and treatment* (20th ed.). New York: McGraw-Hill.

- Impaired verbal communication
- Deficient knowledge
- Interrupted family processes
- Risk for injury

After completing an assessment of Matthew, the nurse noted the following: fever, tugging at his ears, and increased crying when lying down. Based on the assessment findings, what would your top three nursing diagnoses be for Matthew?

Nursing goals, interventions, and evaluation for the child with an eye or ear disorder are based on the nursing diagnoses. Nursing Care Plan 38.1 may be used as a guide in planning nursing care for the child with an eye or ear disorder, but it should be individualized based on the patient's symptoms and needs. Refer to Chapter 35 for the nursing care plan for pain management. Additional information will be included later in the chapter as it relates to specific disorders.

Based on your top three nursing diagnoses for Matthew, describe appropriate nursing interventions.

Childhood Visual Disorders

Refractive Errors

The most common cause of visual difficulties in children is refractive errors. Refractive errors (disorders) are noted in 5% to 7% of preschoolers (Tingley, 2007). Refractive errors occur when the light that enters the lens does not bend appropriately to allow it to fall directly on the retina. Refractive disorders include myopia (nearsightedness), hyperopia (farsightedness), and astigmatism (both nearsightedness and farsightedness).

Myopia results when the cornea is too steep or is more rounded than normal, causing the light to bend unusually. Light enters the cornea and stops short of focusing directing on the retina, causing blurry vision at a distance. Children who are nearsighted may see well at close range but have difficulty focusing on the blackboard or other objects at a distance. Prescription glasses with concave lens will re-focus the light and correct this refractive disorder. Young children naturally have hyperopia because the depth of the eye globe is not fully developed until about age 5 years (Braverman, 2011). These children may have blurriness at close range, but by school age this blurriness usually resolves. True hyperopia occurs when the developed cornea is too flat. Light enters the cornea and extends beyond the retina for focusing, causing up-close vision to be blurry. Treatment of hyperopia includes prescription glasses with a convex lens to re-focus the light.

Generally, a child 12 years of age can demonstrate the responsibility necessary to wear and care for contact lenses. Contact lenses may be used in younger children but are lost or damaged more readily. Because of the continuing refractive development in the child's vision through adolescence, laser surgery for vision correction is not recommended by the Canadian Ophthalmological Society until 18 years of age, although it may be performed experimentally in some children (Canadian Ophthalmological Society, 2007).

Nursing Assessment

Elicit the health history, noting blurred vision, complaints of eye fatigue with reading, or complaints of eye strain (headache, pulling sensation, or eye burning). Note

(text continues on page 1231)

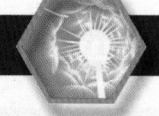

Nursing Care Plan 38.1

OVERVIEW FOR THE CHILD WITH A DISORDER OF EYES OR EARS

NURSING DIAGNOSIS: Sensory perception, disturbed (visual) related to visual impairment or blindness as evidenced by lack of reaction to visual stimuli, squinting, holding items close

Outcome Identification and Evaluation
Child will reach maximal vision potential: *Child uses corrective lenses appropriately and is able to participate in play and schoolwork.*

Intervention: Improving Vision
• Encourage corrective lens use *for enhancement of vision.*
• For the severely impaired or blind child, identify yourself via voice and name items in environment for the child *so that the child is aware of his or her surroundings.*
• Support the family's efforts at vision therapy and other habilitation programs *to promote vision enhancement.*
• Engage the parents in bedside caregiving *because the parents' voice and presence are reassuring to the child.*

NURSING DIAGNOSIS: Sensory perception, disturbed (auditory) related to hearing loss as evidenced by lack of reaction to verbal stimuli, delayed attainment of language milestones

Outcome Identification and Evaluation
Child will reach maximal hearing and speech potential: *Child uses aids appropriately and communicates effectively.*

Intervention: Improving Hearing
• Assess hearing ability frequently *because early detection of hearing loss allows for earlier intervention and correction.*
• Assess language development at each visit *to allow for early detection of hearing loss (earlier intervention and correction).*
• Encourage hearing aid use *for amplification of sound.*
• Teach about hearing aid battery safety *to avoid aspiration of battery.*
• Assist child with focusing on sounds in the environment *to encourage listening skills.*
• Refer for and encourage attendance at communication habilitation program *to maximize communication potential.*

NURSING DIAGNOSIS: Risk for infection related to presence of infectious organisms as evidenced by fever, presence of virus or bacteria on laboratory screening

Outcome Identification and Evaluation
Child will exhibit no signs of secondary infection and will not spread infection to others: *Symptoms of infection decrease over time, and others remain free from infection.*

Intervention: Reducing Infection Risk
• Maintain aseptic technique and practice good handwashing *to prevent introduction of further infectious agents.*
• Limit number of visitors, screening for recent illness, *to prevent further infection.*
• Administer antibiotics if prescribed *to prevent or treat bacterial infection.*
• Encourage nutritious diet according to child's preferences *to assist body's natural infection-fighting mechanisms.*
• Isolate the child as required *to prevent nosocomial spread of infection.*
• Teach child and family preventive measures such as good handwashing, covering mouth and nose when coughing or sneezing, adequate disposal of used tissues, *to prevent nosocomial or community spread of infection.*

(continued)

Nursing Care Plan 38.1 (continued)

NURSING DIAGNOSIS: Growth and development delay, related to sensory impairment as evidenced by delay in attainment of developmental milestones

Outcome Identification and Evaluation

Child will achieve optimum independence for age: *Child participates in age-appropriate developmental activities.*

Intervention: Encouraging Growth and Development

- Encourage attainment of developmental milestones with use of assistive devices as needed *for timely developmental achievements.*
- Foster independence in ADLs *to promote sense of accomplishment.*
- Encourage participation in play with another child or within a group *to promote socialization.*
- Assist family to set limits and apply discipline *because structure and routine provide a secure environment in which the developing child can grow.*
- Encourage friendships with other children with a sensory impairment *to promote socialization and let the child know that he or she is not the only one with these challenges.*

NURSING DIAGNOSIS: Impaired verbal communication related to hearing loss as evidenced by lack of or inarticulate speech, lack of alternate communication channel

Outcome Identification and Evaluation

The child will communicate effectively with the method chosen by the family (this may be sign language, oral/deaf speech, cued speech, or augmentative alternative communication device).

Intervention: Improving Communication

- Encourage choice of and attendance at communication habilitation program *to promote continued learning.*
- Provide consistency between home and hospital with regard to communication style/devices *to promote continued learning.*
- Support the child's efforts at correct speech *to promote speech development through reinforcement and praise.*
- Encourage family to use spoken language and read books at home *to continue to promote appropriate language development.*

NURSING DIAGNOSIS: Deficient knowledge related to sensory impairment (vision or hearing) as evidenced by new diagnosis and parents' questions

Outcome Identification and Evaluation

Parents express understanding of diagnosis and care of child: *Parents verbalize understanding, demonstrate use of assistive devices, or independently perform medical treatments.*

Intervention: Educating the Family

- Review diagnosis and plan of care with the parents *to promote understanding of the disease process.*
- Refer family to resources available for sensory-impaired children *to provide further education and support to the parents.*
- Demonstrate medical treatments prescribed or use of assistive devices, requiring a return demonstration, *which shows the parents' ability to provide the prescribed care for the child.*
- Encourage exploration of different communication and learning modes available for the sensory-impaired child *to allow the child and family to find the right educational and communication style fit.*

Nursing Care Plan 38.1 (continued)

NURSING DIAGNOSIS: Family processes, interrupted, related to child's sensory impairment as evidenced by parent verbalization, nonverbal language, altered coping

Outcome Identification and Evaluation

Parents demonstrate adequate coping and decreased anxiety: *Parents are involved in child's care, ask appropriate questions, and are able to discuss child's care and condition calmly.*

Intervention: Encouraging Appropriate Family Interactions

- Encourage parents' verbalization of grief if child is hearing or vision impaired. *Parents must deal with their own feelings of loss to successfully care for the child with an impairment.*
- Encourage parents' verbalization of concerns related to child's illness. *This allows for identification of concerns and demonstrates to the family that the nurse also cares about them, not just the child.*
- Explain therapy, procedures, and child's behaviour to parents; *developing an understanding of the child's current status helps decrease anxiety.*
- Encourage parental involvement in care *so that parents may continue to feel needed and valued.*

NURSING DIAGNOSIS: Risk for injury related to vision loss as evidenced by difficulty navigating surroundings

Outcome Identification and Evaluation

The infant or child will remain free from injury.

Intervention: Preventing Injury

- Orient the child to hospital surroundings *because awareness is the first step to preventing injury.*
- Encourage parent to be at bedside *so that the child feels more comfortable.*
- Encourage use of assistive devise *to promote safety.*

---

complaints of difficulty concentrating on or maintaining a clear focus on objects up close, avoidance of up-close work, or poor work performance (hyperopia). Note the risk factor of family history of myopia. Observe for squinting when the child looks at objects at a distance. Observe the hyperopic child for the presence of esotropia. Readily observable physical findings are not noted in the myopic child. Test visual acuity using an age-appropriate screening tool (for more information related to visual acuity screening, refer to Chapter 30). Hyperopia is usually not identified with visual acuity screening alone; it usually requires a retinal examination by an ophthalmologist.

Nursing Management

Nursing management of the child with a refractive error focuses on providing education about corrective lens use and monitoring for the need for new eyeglasses or contact lenses.

Educating About Eyeglass Use

Children may or may not be compliant with wearing eyeglasses. Glasses still carry a stigma, and the child may be teased or bullied. However, many children enjoy the improved vision they achieve when wearing their eyeglasses, and this can help them overcome the teasing they might suffer. Encourage the child with newly prescribed

eyeglasses to wear them by having the parent spend "special time" with the child doing an activity that requires the glasses (such as reading or drawing). Teach the parent and child to remove eyeglasses with both hands and to lay them on their side (not directly on the lens on any surface). Instruct the child and family about cleaning the glasses daily with mild soap and water or a commercial cleansing agent provided by the optometrist. Use a soft cloth to clean the glasses, not paper towels, tissues, or toilet paper.

Educating About Contact Lens Use

Teach the older child or adolescent how to care for the contact lenses properly, including lens hygiene and lens insertion and removal. Inform the child and parents that protective eyewear should be worn when the child is participating in contact sports. If the eye becomes inflamed, remove the contact lens and wear eyeglasses until the eye is improved. Consult with the child's eye care provider to determine whether medications prescribed for an eye problem can be used while the contact lens is in.

Monitoring for Fit and Visual Correction

Encourage the family to complete visual assessments as scheduled. Since the child's vision is continuing to develop and refraction is not stable, the corrective lens prescription may change more frequently than it does in an adult

(American Academy of Ophthalmology, 2008). As the young child in particular is continuing to grow at a rapid rate, the head size is also changing. Eyeglass frames may hurt or pinch the child as the child's head becomes larger. Teach families to check the fit of the glasses monthly. Monitor for signs of ill fit, such as constant removal of the glasses in an older child or rubbing at the glasses or eyes in the very young child. Monitor for squinting, eye fatigue or strain, and complaints of headache or dizziness, which may indicate the need for a change in the lens prescription.

Astigmatism

Astigmatism develops when the cornea is shaped more like a football. The oblong or oval shape causes light rays to focus on two points in the back of the eye rather than just one due to the astigmatic cornea having a steeper curve and a flatter one. Prescription glasses will also correct this refractive defect.

Nursing Assessment

Explore the health history for symptoms of astigmatism. Children with astigmatism often have blurry vision and difficulty seeing letters as a whole, so their ability to read is affected. They may have headaches or dizziness. Older children may complain of eye fatigue or strain. Children with astigmatism often learn to tilt their heads slightly so that they can focus more effectively. This may lead to "normal" vision screenings, but the headache and dizziness still warrant further examination by an eye specialist (Braverman, 2011). The diagnosis of astigmatism requires not only a visual acuity test but also a refractive error evaluation by an optometrist or ophthalmologist.

Nursing Management

Corrective lenses can help to, in effect, smooth out the curvature of the cornea, making the light ray refraction occur smoothly. As with refractive errors, encourage the child who requires corrective lenses for astigmatism to wear the eyeglasses or contact lenses regularly.

Strabismus

Strabismus is a condition in which one eye cannot focus with the other eye on an object because of the imbalance of the eye muscles. It is common and occurs in about 4% of children (Optometrists Network, 2010). The most common types of strabismus are exotropia and esotropia. In exotropia, the eyes turn outward; in esotropia they turn inward. Because of this unequal alignment, visual development may proceed at a different rate in each eye. Diplopia (double vision) may result, so vision in one eye may be "turned off" by the brain to avoid diplopia. Many infants have strabismus intermittently, but this usually resolves by 3 months of age. Intermittent strabismus that persists past 6 months of age or constant strabismus at any age warrants referral to an ophthalmologist for further evaluation (Burns, Dunn, Brady, Starr, & Blosser, 2009).

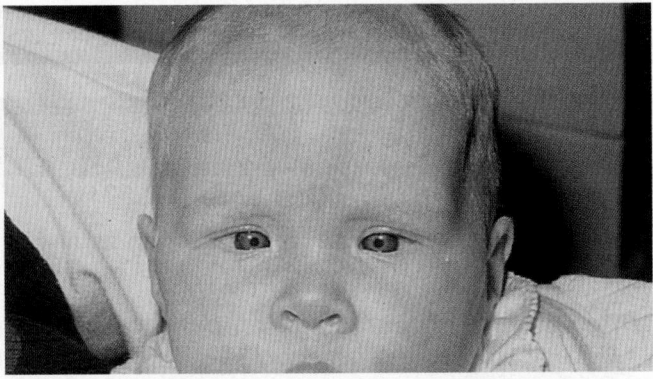

FIGURE 38.2 Esotropia. Test for strabismus by observing symmetry of the corneal light reflex. The reflex falls in the centre of one pupil and to the left or right of the pupil of the other eye.

If the strabismus is mild or asymptomatic, no treatment may be necessary. Patching can be helpful, however, particularly if one eye sees more poorly than the other. As well, glasses to improve vision or correct refractive error may straighten the eyes. Eye muscle exercises are rarely helpful. Therapeutic management of strabismus may include patching of the stronger eye or eye muscle surgery. Complications of strabismus include amblyopia and visual deficits.

Nursing Assessment

Parents may be the first persons to notice that the child's eyes do not face in the same direction. Question parents about the onset of the problem and whether it is continuous or intermittent. If intermittent, does it occur more often when the child is tired? Elicit the health history, noting complaints of blurred vision, tired eyes, squinting or closing one eye in bright sunlight, tilting the head to focus on an object, or a history of bumping into objects (depth perception may be limited).

Observe the child's eyes for obvious exotropia or esotropia. In the absence of an obvious finding, assessment of the symmetry of the corneal light reflex is extremely helpful (Fig. 38.2). The "cover test" is also a useful tool for the identification of strabismus.

True strabismus should not be confused with pseudostrabismus. In pseudostrabismus, the eyes may appear slightly crossed (as in the child with wide nasal bridge and epicanthal folds), but the corneal light reflex remains symmetric (Weber & Kelley, 2010).

Nursing Management

It is extremely important to treat strabismus appropriately in the developing years so that equal visual acuity may be achieved in both eyes. When patching is prescribed, encourage the family to comply with this modality. Encourage eyeglass wearing if prescribed. Provide appropriate postoperative care by protecting the operative site with eye patching.

Amblyopia

Amblyopia is an ocular condition in an otherwise healthy eye in which there is an abnormal cortical response in the occipital lobe of the brain due to insufficient or inadequate stimulation of the fovea, neural pathway, and cortex. If untreated, amblyopia may result in unilateral vision loss. It is caused by anything that prevents a clear image from being focused inside the eye. Amblyopia develops within the first decade of life and is more severe the earlier it develops (Bacal & Wilson, 2000). If left untreated, it is the most common cause of vision loss in children and young adults (Doshi & Rodriguez, 2007). It occurs in about 5% of children (Ruben, 2003). The vision in one eye is reduced because the eye and the brain are not working together properly. While the eyes are fighting to focus differently because of their differences in visual acuity, one eye becomes stronger than the other. This is why amblyopia is often referred to as "lazy eye."

Amblyopia may be caused by any disorder that affects normal visual development, including strabismus and differences in visual acuity or astigmatism between the two eyes. It may also result from eye trauma, ptosis, or cataract. Children with amblyopia, if untreated, will have worsening of the poorer eye and strain in the better eye, which may also lead to worsening of acuity in that eye. Eventually, blindness will result in one or both eyes.

Therapeutic management of amblyopia focuses on strengthening the weaker eye. This may be achieved through patching for several hours per day for a few weeks to as long as a year, atropine drops in the better eye (once daily), vision therapy, or eye muscle surgery if the cause is strabismus or cataracts.

Nursing Assessment

One of the most important functions of the nurse is to identify on screening the preschool child with amblyopia. Begin visual acuity testing using an age-appropriate tool by 3 years of age. Observe for asymmetry of the corneal light reflex in the child of any age. This may be the only sign in the preverbal child.

Nursing Management

It is very important for children with amblyopia to receive appropriate treatment during the early years of visual development. Patching the better eye for several hours each day encourages the eye with poorer vision to be used appropriately and promotes visual development in that eye. The once-daily use of atropine drops in the better eye results in blurring in that eye, similarly encouraging use and development of the weaker eye (Doshi & Rodriguez, 2007). Support and encourage children and parents to comply with the patching protocol or atropine drop use. Promoting eye safety is extremely important for the child with amblyopia; if the better eye suffers a serious injury, both eyes may become blind.

Vision Screening

Adequate visual development requires appropriate sensory stimulation to both eyes over the first few years of life (Graven & Browne, 2008). When one or both eyes are deprived of this stimulation, visual development does not progress appropriately, and visual impairment or blindness may result. This may occur when the eyes are not aligned properly, when visual acuity between the eyes is disparate, or when other problems with the eyes exist (Graven & Browne, 2008). If vision disorders are diagnosed at an early age and treatment is initiated, then vision may progress normally. However, when these disorders go untreated, the young child's developing vision may be significantly reduced. Children must be appropriately screened for these disorders.

> ▶ **Take** NOTE!
>
> *Impoverished children often do not have access to appropriate vision care. The range of services for vision care coverage varies throughout the provinces.*

Based on recommendations from the American Academy of Ophthalmology, the Canadian Paediatric Society (CPS) (CPS, 2009) recommends several stages for pediatric visual screening (Table 38.1). A variety of vision screening practices are used throughout Canada.

All eye examinations should incorporate a detailed history that includes the following:

- Chief complaint and/or reason for the eye evaluation
- Systematic history, including birth weight and pertinent prenatal, perinatal, and postnatal medical factors
- Past hospitalizations and operations
- General health and development
- Review of systems
- Family and social history
- Existing eye conditions and relevant systemic diseases
- Current medications and allergies
- Risk factors, such as family history of congenital cataract, glaucoma, retinoblastoma, metabolic disease, or genetic disease

Eye Conditions of the Newborn

Nasolacrimal Duct Obstruction

Stenosis or simple obstruction of the nasolacrimal duct (dacryostenosis) is a common disorder of infancy, occurring in about 5% to 20% of the general infant population (Gross, 2002). It is unilateral in about 65% of cases (Gross, 2002). Dacryostenosis symptoms include pooling or draining tears, mucous or yellowish discharge, and reddening that results from rubbing. Over 90% of cases usually resolve by 1 year of age (American Association for

TABLE 38.1 RECOMMENDED SCREENING STAGES

Newborn to 3 Months	6 to 12 Months	3 to 5 Years	6 to 18 Years
Conduct a complete examination of the skin and external eye structures	Conduct a complete examination of the external eye structures. Assess for fix and follow abilities of each eye.	Conduct a complete examination of the external eye structures. Perform visual acuity testing with age-appropriate tool. • HOTV chart from 36 months and • LogMAR LH chart from 42 months	Conduct a complete examination of the external eye structures. Screen whenever routine health examinations are conducted. Perform visual acuity testing.
Check for eye infections	Check ocular alignment to detect strabismus	Check corneal light reflex	Check corneal light reflex
Inspect the red reflex	Check corneal light reflex	Cover/uncover	Cover/uncover
High-risk newborns (e.g., children with retinopathy of prematurity) should be examined by an ophthalmologist.	Check the red reflex Check how the eyes work together	Check the red reflex Check how the eyes work together	Check the red reflex Check how the eyes work together

Adapted from: Canadian Paediatric Society. (2009). Vision screening in infants, children and youth. *Paediatrics & Child Health, 14*(4), 246–248.

Pediatric Ophthalmology and Strabismus [AAPOS], 2011) but will require the parents to milk or massage the nasolacrimal duct two to three times per day. If secondary bacterial infection is suspected or confirmed, antibiotic ointment or drops may be ordered. If the obstruction does not resolve by 12 months of age, then the pediatric ophthalmologist may probe the duct with the infant under general anesthesia to relieve the obstruction (a brief outpatient procedure) (Casady, Meyer, Simon, Stasior, & Zobal-Ratner, 2006).

Nursing Assessment

Tearing or discharge from one or both eyes is often first noted at the 2-week check-up. Obtain a thorough history about the eye drainage to distinguish it from neonatal conjunctivitis. Determine the onset and progression of symptoms, as well as the newborn's response to any interventions attempted so far. Upon physical examination, note redness of the lower lid of the affected eye. If drainage is present, note its consistency, colour, and quantity. Nasolacrimal duct obstruction is usually a medical diagnosis based upon clinical presentation (Fig. 38.3), but culture of the eye drainage (ordered by a physician or advanced practice nurse) may be used to rule out conjunctivitis or secondary bacterial infection.

Nursing Management

As previously stated, the majority of cases of nasolacrimal duct stenosis resolve spontaneously by 12 months of age (AAPOS, 2011). Nevertheless, the continual

tearing and discharge are quite upsetting to the parents. Teach parents to clean the eye area frequently with a moist cloth. In addition, teach parents to massage the nasolacrimal duct, which may change the pressure and cause it to open, allowing drainage to occur. Refer to Teaching Guideline 38.1 for appropriate nasolacrimal

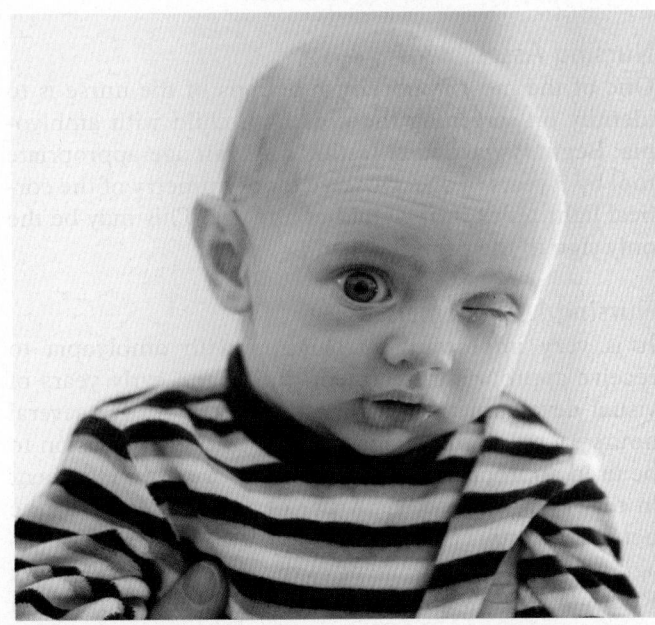

FIGURE 38.3 Mild eyelid redness and tearing are present in the infant with nasolacrimal duct stenosis. Note the presence of obstruction.

Nasolacrimal Duct Massage

- Using the forefinger or little finger, push on top of the bone (the puncta must be blocked).

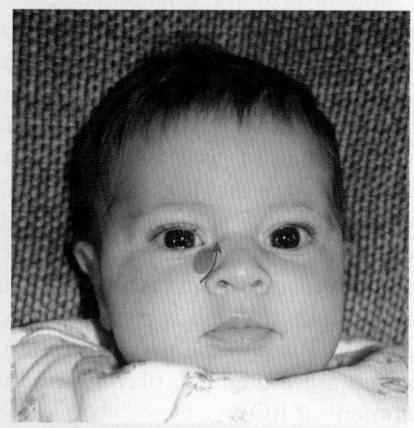

A

- Gently push in and up.

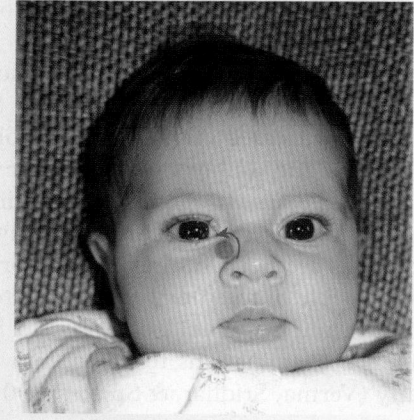

B

- Then gently push downward along the side of the nose.

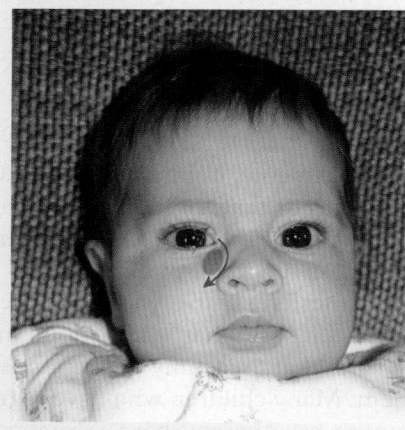

C

Adapted from: American Association for Pediatric Ophthalmology and Strabismus. (2011). Nasolacrimal duct obstruction. Retrieved October 20, 2011 from http://www.aapos.org/terms/conditions/72.

duct massage technique. Ensure that parents are educated about when and how to administer antibiotic eye drops if ordered.

Congenital Cataract

Congenital cataract occurs infrequently, but early diagnosis and treatment are essential in order to prevent permanent visual loss. The condition presents as a black spot or opacity of the lens of the eye that is present at birth. The cause can be heredity dominant, recessive, or X-linked. The condition can also result from intrauterine rubella, cytomegalovirus (CMV), or a metabolic disorder such as diabetes or galactosemia. Sensory amblyopia will result if the condition goes untreated. Complications include visual developmental delay related to amblyopia. Worldwide, congenital cataract causes 16% of the cases of legal blindness in children younger than 5 years of age (Lighthouse International, 2011). Surgery to remove the opaque lens can be performed on infants as early as 2 weeks of age. The infant is then fitted with a contact lens. Intraocular lens implants are also being used (Watkinson & Graham, 2005). The best visual outcomes occur when cataracts are removed prior to 3 months of age. Glaucoma may occur as a complication after cataract surgery.

Nursing Assessment

Note history of lack of visual awareness. Observe the eyes for apparent cloudiness of the cornea (not always visible). Upon ophthalmoscopic examination, the red reflex will not be observed in the affected eye.

Nursing Management

Postoperative care focuses on protecting the operative site and providing developmentally appropriate activities. Ensure that the protective eye patch is secure. Elbow restraints may be necessary in the older infant to prevent accidental injury to the operative site. Teach families how to administer antibiotic or corticosteroid ophthalmic drops if prescribed for postoperative use. Once the surgical site is healed, the "good" eye may be patched for several hours a day to promote visual development in the eye with the contact or intraocular lens. Regular visual assessments are critical for determining the adequacy of visual development after cataract removal. Instruct parents about the importance of using sunglasses that block ultraviolet rays in the child who has had a lens removed.

Infantile Glaucoma

Infantile glaucoma is an autosomal recessive disorder that is more common in children born to interrelated couples. It occurs in about 1 of 10,000 live births (Lighthouse International, 2011) and is often associated with other genetic disorders. Infantile glaucoma is characterized by obstruction of aqueous humour flow and increased intraocular pressure that results in large, prominent eyes.

Vision loss may occur as a result of corneal scarring, optic nerve damage, or, most commonly, amblyopia.

Unlike adult glaucoma, in which medical management is the first step, treatment of infantile glaucoma is focused on surgical intervention. Infantile glaucoma is treated surgically via goniotomy (removal of obstruction of the aqueous humour). Laser surgery is being used as well. Sometimes several surgeries may be necessary to correct the problem. Ongoing medical therapy may also be required.

Nursing Assessment

Note any family history of infantile glaucoma or other genetic disorders. Elicit the health history, noting a history of the infant keeping the eyes closed most of the time or rubbing the eyes. Observe the eye for corneal enlargement and clouding; the eye may appear enlarged. Photophobia may occur, so bright light may bother the infant. Tearing or conjunctivitis and eyelid squeezing or spasm may also occur. The pediatric ophthalmologist may use a tonometer to measure the intraocular pressure during the diagnostic phase.

Nursing Management

The main goal of nursing care for the infant with glaucoma is postoperative care. Family education will also be important.

Providing Postoperative Care

The eye will be patched postoperatively, and the child should be maintained on bed rest. Nursing care focuses on protection of the surgical site. Infants and toddlers may require elbow restraints to prevent them from rubbing the affected eye. These children may be quite anxious with one or both eyes patched, since their ability to see will be affected. Use a calm and soothing approach with these children as well as distraction and developmentally appropriate play activities.

Educating the Family

Instruct parents and children to make sure that the child avoids roughhousing and contact sports for at least 2 weeks after surgery (Ho & Walton, 2004). Before the first surgery occurs, prepare parents for the possibility that three or four operations may be necessary. Teach families how to administer postoperative medications. Encourage parents to comply with ongoing recommended visual assessments.

Nystagmus

Nystagmus refers to a very rapid, irregular eye movement. It is described by some as "bouncing" of the eyes. It may occur in children with congenital cataracts, but the most common cause is a neurologic problem. It is difficult for the brain and eyes to communicate when the eyes are in continuous motion; thus, visual development

may be affected. Children with nystagmus must receive further evaluation by an ophthalmologist and possibly a neurologist.

Retinopathy of Prematurity

Retinopathy of prematurity (ROP) is a disorder characterized by rapid growth of retinal blood vessels in the premature infant. In the fetus, retinal vascularization begins at 4 months' gestation and progresses until completion at 9 months' gestation or shortly after birth. The premature infant is born with incomplete retinal vascularization, yet new vessels continue to grow between the vascularized and nonvascularized retina. Risk factors include low birth weight, early gestational age, sepsis, high light intensity, and hypothermia. Changes in oxygen tension resulting from hypoxia, oxyhemoglobin dissociation curve changes that occur when adult blood is transfused to the premature infant, and the duration/concentration of supplemental oxygen are thought to play an important role in the development of ROP.

Premature infants should have serial examinations by an ophthalmologist until the ROP has regressed and normal vascularization is seen. If ROP continues to progress, laser surgery may be necessary to prevent blindness (Hack & Klein, 2006). Complications of ROP include myopia, glaucoma, and blindness. Strabismus may occur even in cases of regressed (resolved) ROP. Refractive errors and amblyopia may occur as early as 3 months corrected age. In the first year of life, ophthalmologic examinations may occur frequently so that if corrective lenses are needed, they may be prescribed at the earliest possible time. After 1 year corrected age, former premature infants should continue to have yearly ophthalmologic examinations to detect and treat visual deficits early (Verma, Sridhar, & Spitzer, 2003).

Nursing Assessment

Ensure that all former premature infants are routinely screened for visual deficits. Discuss developmental progress with the parents. Observe for the development of strabismus, manifested by an asymmetric corneal light reflex.

Nursing Management

Nursing management of infants with ROP mainly focuses on ensuring that the family is compliant with the ophthalmologist's follow-up recommendations. Recurrent illness or rehospitalization of premature infants may interfere with scheduled eye follow-up appointments. Ensure that these appointments are rescheduled and that the family understands the importance of them. Many children who have regressed ROP or who require cryotherapy have refractive errors, so even when the ROP is considered resolved, these children should still maintain appropriate ophthalmology follow-up.

Infectious and Inflammatory Disorders of the Eyes

Infectious and inflammatory disorders of the eyes include conjunctivitis, nasolacrimal duct obstruction, eyelid lesions, and periorbital cellulitis.

Conjunctivitis

Inflammation of the bulbar or palpebral conjunctiva is referred to as conjunctivitis. It can be infectious, allergic, or chemical in nature. Viruses or bacteria may cause infectious conjunctivitis. Adenoviruses and influenza account for the bulk of cases of viral conjunctivitis. The most common bacterial cause is *Staphylococcus aureus*, but many cases are also caused by *Streptococcus pneumoniae, Haemophilus influenzae,* and other bacteria (Yoon, Kelley, & Friedman, 2011). In the newborn, *Chlamydia trachomatis* and *Neisseria gonorrhoeae* are more common causes. Infectious conjunctivitis is very contagious, so epidemics are common, particularly in young children. Risk factors for acute infectious conjunctivitis include age less than 2 weeks; day care, preschool, or school attendance; concomitant viral upper respiratory infection; pharyngitis; and otitis media. Concurrent acute otitis media may occur depending upon the bacterial cause (Natal & Chao, 2011). Complications from simple infectious conjunctivitis are uncommon. Neonates with chlamydial conjunctivitis may be at risk for the development of chlamydial pneumonia.

Allergic conjunctivitis results from exposure to particular allergens. Allergic conjunctivitis may be a seasonal or year-round complaint. A genetic predisposition to allergic conjunctivitis exists, just as it does for asthma, allergic rhinitis, and atopic dermatitis. Allergic conjunctivitis occurs more frequently in school-age children and adolescents than it does in infants and young children because of repeat exposure to allergens over time. In the case of seasonal allergic conjunctivitis, the severity of symptoms and the number of children affected are directly related to the pollen count in the area.

Therapeutic Management

Therapeutic management of conjunctivitis is prescribed depending upon the cause. Bacterial conjunctivitis is generally treated with an ophthalmic antibiotic preparation (drops or ointment). Viral conjunctivitis is a self-limiting disease and does not require topical medication. Eye drops with an antihistamine or mast cell stabilization effect may be helpful in alleviating symptoms of allergic conjunctivitis. If other allergy signs and symptoms are also present, an oral antihistamine may also be prescribed. Table 38.2 compares bacterial, viral, and allergic conjunctivitis.

Pathophysiology

When bacteria or viruses come in contact with the bulbar or palpebral conjunctiva, they are recognized as foreign antigens and an antigen–antibody immune reaction occurs, resulting in inflammation. Allergic conjunctivitis occurs through a different mechanism. Contact with the allergen results in an allergic response (overreaction of the immune response). The mast cell and histamine mediators are then activated, resulting in inflammation.

Nursing Assessment

Nursing assessment of the child with conjunctivitis, regardless of the cause, is similar. It includes health history, physical examination, and, in rare instances, laboratory testing.

Health History

Elicit a description of the present illness and chief complaint. Common signs and symptoms reported during the health history might include:

- Redness
- Edema
- Tearing
- Discharge
- Eye pain
- Itching of the eyes (usually with allergic conjunctivitis)

TABLE 38.2 TYPES OF CONJUNCTIVITIS

Type of Conjunctivitis	Conjunctivae	Discharge	Additional Findings	Eyelid Edema	Treatment
Bacterial	Inflamed	Purulent, mucoid	Mild pain	Occasional	Antibiotic drops or ointment
Viral	Inflamed	Watery, mucoid	Lymphadenopathy, photophobia, tearing	Usually present	Symptom relief; antiherpetic agent if cause is herpes virus
Allergic	Inflamed	Watery or stringy	Itching	Usually present	Antihistamine and/or mast cell stabilizer drops

Adapted from: Braverman, R. S. (2011). Eye. In W. W. Hay, M. J. Levin, J. M. Sondheimer, & R. R. Deterding (Eds.), *Current pediatric diagnosis and treatment* (20th ed.). New York: McGraw-Hill.

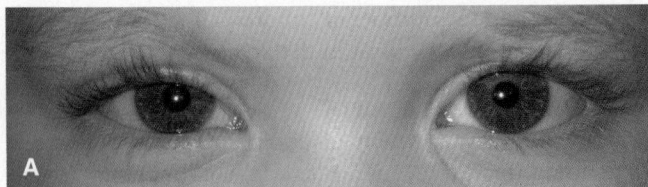

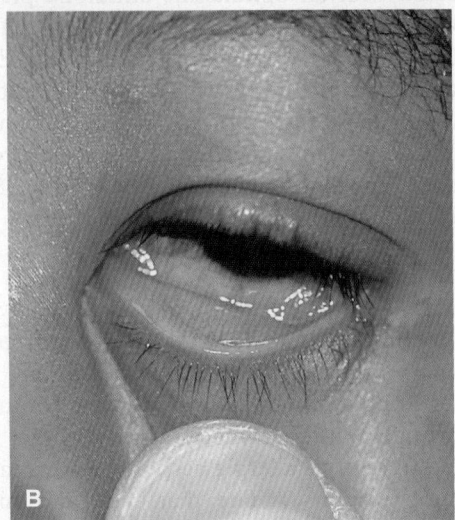

FIGURE 38.4 (**A**) Bacterial conjunctivitis: note redness of conjunctiva, copious discoloured drainage with matting, and eyelid swelling. (**B**) Allergic conjunctivitis: note redness of conjunctiva, clear watery discharge, rubbing of the eyes.

Determine the onset of symptoms and their progression as well as response to treatments used at home. Assess for risk factors for infectious conjunctivitis, such as day care or school attendance. Note any history of an upper respiratory infection, sore throat, or earache. Question parents about possible infectious exposures. Review the health history for risk factors for allergic conjunctivitis such as a family history and a history of asthma, allergic rhinitis, or atopic dermatitis. Determine seasonality related to the symptoms and whether the symptoms occur after exposure to particular allergens, such as pollen, hay, or animals.

Physical Examination

Observe for eyelid swelling or redness. Inspect the conjunctivae for redness (Fig. 38.4). Note quantity, colour, and consistency of discharge. Bacterial infections generally result in a thick, coloured discharge, whereas a clear or white discharge is generally seen with viral conjunctivitis. Allergic conjunctivitis often results in a watery discharge, sometimes profuse, which is usually present bilaterally. Contact with an allergen rubbed into one of the eyes may result in unilateral symptoms. Observe the child for other signs of allergic or atopic disease and document the presence of a runny nose or cough as well.

Laboratory and Diagnostic Tests

Cases of bacterial, viral, and allergic conjunctivitis are generally diagnosed based on history and clinical pre-

sentation. Cases of viral and allergic conjunctivitis do not warrant laboratory testing. If bacterial conjunctivitis is suspected, then a bacterial culture of the eye drainage may be performed to determine the exact causative organism, thus allowing the most appropriate antibiotic to be prescribed.

Nursing Management

Nursing management of the various types of conjunctivitis focuses on alleviating symptoms and, for infectious causes, preventing spread.

Alleviating Symptoms

Teach parents how to apply eye drops or ointment (antibiotic for bacterial causes and antihistamine or mast cell stabilizer for allergic). Warm compresses may be used to help loosen the crust that accumulates on the eyelids overnight when drainage is copious, particularly with bacterial conjunctivitis.

The child with allergic conjunctivitis may experience perennial or seasonal allergies (or both). Encourage the child to avoid perennial allergens once the offending allergen is determined (refer to Chapter 39 for additional information related to education about perennial allergen avoidance). Seasonal allergies may include tree pollen in the winter or spring, grass pollen in the summer, and ragweed or flower pollen in the fall.

It is impossible to completely eliminate seasonal allergic responses, partly because it is important for children to participate in physical activity outdoors. Teach families to minimize seasonal allergens on the child's skin and hair. Educate families to:

• Encourage the child not to rub or touch the eyes.
• Rinse the child's eyelids periodically with a clean washcloth and cool water.
• When the child comes in from outdoors, wash the child's face and hands.
• Ensure that the child showers and shampoos before bedtime.

▶ **Take** NOTE!

The itching of allergic conjunctivitis may be relieved with cool compresses. An easy way to accomplish this is to have the child hold a tube of yogurt over the affected eye.

Preventing Infectious Spread

Since infectious conjunctivitis is extremely contagious, the parent must wash hands diligently after caring for the child. Teach parents and children about appropriate handwashing and discourage them from sharing towels and washcloths. Children with viral conjunctivitis may return to school or day care when symptoms lessen.

When mucopurulent drainage is no longer present (usually after 24 to 48 hours of treatment with a topical antibiotic), the child with bacterial conjunctivitis may safely return to day care or school (Ohnsman, 2007).

> ▶ *Take* NOTE!
>
> *Avoid the use of vasoconstricting eye drops such as Visine to rid the eyes of redness. Rebound vasodilation may occur, and with it the redness returns. This leads to repeated frequent use of the drops to keep the eyes from being red but does not treat the actual cause of the redness (Taketokmo, Hodding, & Kraus, 2010).*

Eyelid Disorders

Disorders of the eyelid include hordeolum (stye), chalazion, and blepharitis. Hordeolum is a localized infection of the sebaceous gland of the eyelid follicle, usually caused by bacterial invasion. Chalazion is a chronic painless infection of the meibomian gland. Blepharitis refers to chronic scaling and discharge along the eyelid margin. Chalazion may resolve spontaneously. Therapeutic management of hordeolum and blepharitis usually involves the use of antibiotic ointment.

Nursing Assessment

Determine the child's health history, noting onset of symptoms, extent and character of eye discharge, and presence of pain (hordeolum is usually painful). Inspect the eyelids, noting redness along the eyelid margin and the presence of eyelid edema (hordeolum, blepharitis). Hordeolum may also be quite visible as an enlarged lesion along the lid margin, with purulent drainage present

(Fig. 38.5). Chalazion may be visible as a small nodule on the lid margin. The conjunctivae remain clear with all three of these disorders.

Nursing Management

For hordeolum and blepharitis, instruct parents in the administration of antibiotic ointment. Encourage the use of hot, moist compresses. Inform parents that the stye may require several weeks to resolve completely. Also inform parents that chalazion will usually resolve spontaneously; if it does not, minor surgical drainage may be required.

Periorbital Cellulitis

Periorbital cellulitis is a bacterial infection of the eyelids and tissue surrounding the eye. The bacteria may gain entry to the skin via an abrasion, laceration, insect bite, foreign body, or impetiginous lesion. Periorbital cellulitis may also result from a nearby bacterial infection, such as sinusitis. *S. aureus, Streptococcus pyogenes,* and *S. pneumoniae* are the most commonly implicated bacteria. The bacteria produce either an enzyme or endotoxins that initiate the inflammatory response. Redness, swelling, and infiltration of the skin by the inflammatory mediators occur.

Therapeutic management of periorbital cellulitis focuses on intravenous antibiotic administration during the acute phase followed by completion of the course with oral antibiotics. Complications of periorbital cellulitis include bacteremia and progression to orbital cellulitis, which is a more extensive infection involving the orbit of the eye.

Nursing Assessment

Note the onset and duration of symptoms, as well as any treatment used so far. Document any history of fever. The child may complain of pain around the eye as well as restricted movement of the eye area. Inspect the eye, noting marked eyelid edema as well as a purplish or red colour of the eyelid (Fig. 38.6). Usually, the conjunctivae

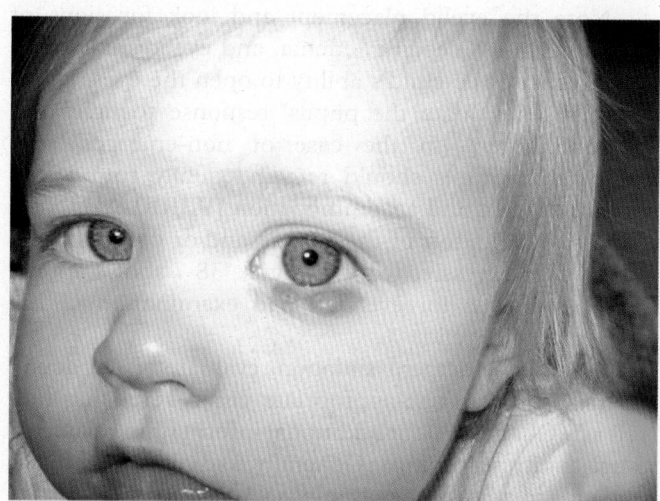

FIGURE 38.5 Hordeolum.

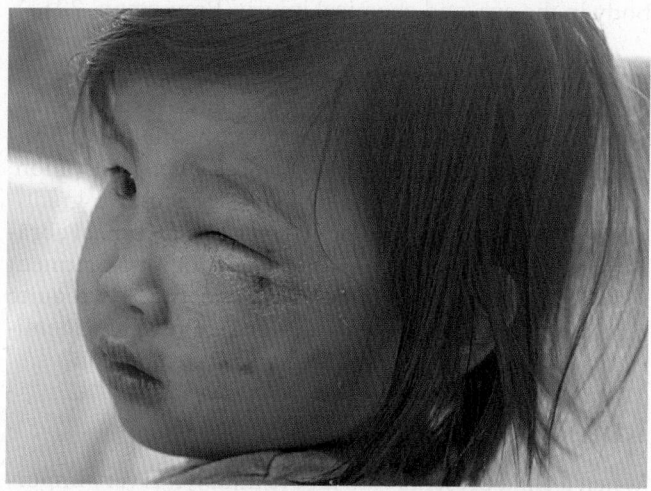

FIGURE 38.6 Periorbital cellulitis.

are clear and no discharge is present. If the extent of the edema allows the child to open the eye, assess visual acuity, which should be normal.

> ▶ *Take* NOTE!
>
> *Notify the physician immediately if any of these signs of progression to orbital cellulitis occur: conjunctival redness, change in vision, pain with eye movement, eye muscle weakness or paralysis, or proptosis.*

Nursing Management

Apply warm soaks to the eye area for 20 minutes every 2 to 4 hours. Administer intravenous antibiotics as prescribed. Teach families the importance of completing the entire course of oral antibiotic treatment at home. Instruct parents to call the physician or have the child evaluated again if:

• The child is not improving.
• The child reports inability to move the eye.
• Visual acuity changes.
• Ptosis occurs.

Eye Injuries

As mentioned earlier, infants and young children are more susceptible to eye injuries than adults since the eyeball is relatively larger in relation to the space within the orbit. Developmental maturity may also play a part in eye injuries. For example, as infants and toddlers learn to walk and run, they do not have the awareness and maturity to avert potential hazards, mishaps, or accidents. Older children involved in sports and school science experiments are also at risk for eye injuries. A few of the more common eye injuries are eyelid injuries, contusion, scleral hemorrhage, corneal abrasion, a foreign body in the eye, and chemical injury (Braverman, 2011).

Therapeutic management depends on the type of injury. Eyelid lacerations may require suturing. Deep lacerations may result in ptosis at a later date, so these patients should be referred to an ophthalmologist. Simple contusions (black eye) usually need only observation, ice, and analgesics. Scleral hemorrhages resolve gradually without intervention over a few weeks. Corneal abrasions may be allowed to self-heal, or antibiotic ointment may be prescribed. Foreign bodies in the eye require removal to prevent further irritation or abrasion. Chemical injuries require irrigation and vision evaluation.

Nursing Assessment

When a child presents with an eye injury, it is very important to obtain an accurate history related to the injury, followed by a focused physical examination, which consists mostly of inspection and observation. The nurse must determine whether an eye injury is non-emergent or emergent in order to provide rapid and appropriate treatment in the case of an emergency so that vision may be preserved.

Health History

Obtain an accurate history. Determine the mechanism of injury and obtain as much detail about the injury as possible. Questions that should be asked during the health history include:

• When did the injury occur?
• What exactly happened?
• Was an object involved? If so, what type of object, and how fast was it going?
• Was it a splash injury?
• Was the child wearing eye protective gear or eyeglasses when the injury occurred?

Determine the extent of pain if present. Document photosensitivity, sensation of a foreign body in the eye, and blurry or lost vision. Inquire about past medical history, including previous eye injury or surgery or vision problems. Determine the child's immunization status.

Physical Examination

Regardless of the type of eye injury, examination of the child's eye can be quite difficult. The nurse plays an important role in assisting the child and family to cope with the examination. Children with an eye injury often are in acute pain. The area surrounding the eye swells quickly after blunt trauma. The edema and tearing make the eye examination more difficult. Children are very frightened because of the pain and difficulty seeing. Approach the child in a calm and gentle manner. Soothe and coax the child as the eye is examined. Younger children may need to be restrained briefly in order for the examination to proceed safely.

Note the eyelid placement and look for signs of trauma such as bleeding, edema, and eyelid malformation. Evaluate the child's ability to open the eyes. Use a penlight to evaluate the pupils' response to light and accommodation (in the case of non-emergent eye trauma, the pupils should remain equally round and reactive to light and accommodation [PERRLA]). Note redness or irritation of the sclerae and/or conjunctivae. Observe for excessive tearing. Figure 38.7 shows appropriate technique for eversion and examination of the interior of the eyelid.

In a non-emergent situation, evaluate visual acuity via the use of an age-appropriate vision screening tool (refer to Chapter 30 for additional information related to visual acuity screening). Generally, radiologic testing is used only in emergency situations (Augsburger & Asbury, 2008). Table 38.3 gives assessment information specific

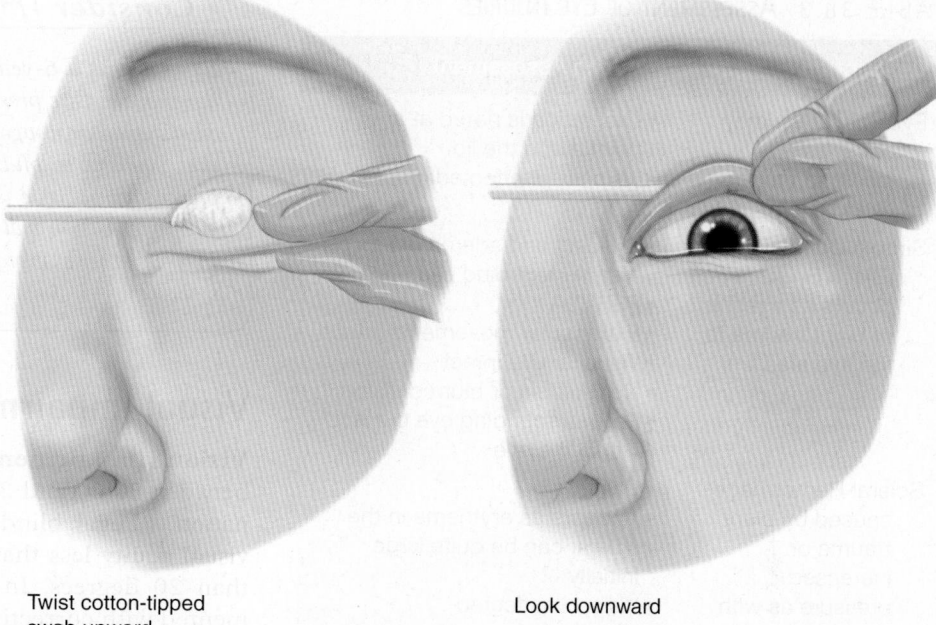

FIGURE 38.7 Eversion of the eyelid for examination. Place a cotton-tipped applicator over the eyelid. Pull the eyelid outward and up over the applicator.

Twist cotton-tipped swab upward

Look downward

> ▶ *Take* NOTE!
>
> *If pupillary reaction is abnormal, vision is affected (decreased acuity from the child's norm, diplopia, or blurriness), or extraocular movements are affected, the child should be immediately referred to an ophthalmologist for further evaluation (Braverman, 2011).*

to eyelid laceration, simple contusion, scleral hemorrhage, corneal abrasion, and foreign body in the eye.

Nursing Management

Children with urgent or emergent conditions must be referred to an ophthalmologist immediately to preserve vision. Urgent and emergent conditions include:

- Traumatic hyphema
- Blowout fracture
- Ruptured globe
- Thermal/chemical injury
- Extensive animal bite
- Lid laceration with underlying structural involvement
- Corneal abrasion in which corneal penetration is suspected
- Foreign body imbedded in the globe (Augsburger & Asbury, 2008; Braverman, 2011)

Managing Non-Emergent Eye Injuries

Non-emergent eye injuries usually need only simple management. Assist the physician with positioning and distraction of the child for eyelid laceration suturing. The child may require sedation or pain medication for this procedure.

To decrease edema in the child with a black eye (simple contusion), instruct the parent to apply an ice pack to the area for 20 minutes, then remove it for 20 minutes, and continue to repeat the cycle. Tell the parents and child that bruising of the surrounding eye area may take up to 3 weeks to resolve.

The appearance of a scleral hemorrhage may be frightening. Instruct the parents and child about the benign nature of the hemorrhage and its natural history of resolution without intervention over a period of a few weeks.

If the child with a corneal abrasion has pain, analgesics may be helpful. Tell parents that most corneal abrasions heal on their own. If an antibiotic ointment is prescribed, instruct the parents in appropriate administration of the ointment.

Foreign bodies may be removed from the eye by gently everting the eyelid and wiping the foreign body away with a sterile cotton-tipped applicator. Irrigation with normal saline may also wash the foreign body away.

For chemical injury, irrigate the eye with copious amounts of water. Consult an ophthalmologist for further evaluation and management.

> ▶ *Take* NOTE!
>
> *Refer the child with a large foreign body in the eye or one that is imbedded in the globe of the eye to the ophthalmologist for appropriate, safe removal.*

TABLE 38.3 ASSESSMENT OF EYE INJURIES

Description of Injury	Nursing Assessment
Eyelid Injuries: may occur as laceration to the eyelid	• Laceration is noted at any point along the lid. • Vision is unaffected.
Simple Contusion (Black Eye): occurs as a result of blunt trauma to the eye area	• Bruising and edema of lids or area surrounding eye • PERRLA • Extraocular movements intact • Visual acuity intact • No diplopia or blurred vision • Pain surrounding eye but not within the eye
Scleral Hemorrhage: caused by blunt trauma or increased pressure as with coughing	• Painless • Appears as erythema in the sclera; can be quite large initially • Vision unaffected
Corneal Abrasion: results from foreign body such as sand, grit, or other small object scratching the cornea	• May have tearing • Eye pain • PERRLA • Vision may be blurry. • Photophobia may be present.
Foreign Body: may be dirt, glass, or other small particle	• Tearing • Complaint of "something in the eye" • PERRLA • Vision may be blurry.

Adapted from: Augsburger, J., & Asbury, T. (2008). Ocular and orbital trauma. In P. Riordan-Eva, & J. P. Whitcher (Eds.), *Vaughan & Asbury's general ophthalmology* (17th ed.). New York: McGraw-Hill; and Braverman, R. S. (2011). Eye. In W. W. Hay, M. J. Levin, J. M. Sondheimer, & R. R. Deterding (Eds.), *Current pediatric diagnosis and treatment* (20th ed.). New York: McGraw-Hill.

Eye injuries can be prevented, and nurses play a vital role in educating the public about prevention of eye injuries and use of appropriate safety equipment. See Evidence-Based Practice 38.1 at the end of the chapter.

▶ **Take** *NOTE!*

Patching of the eye with a corneal abrasion is no longer recommended, as children are often able to open the eye under the patch, which causes drying of the eye and further irritation, possibly contributing to prolonged recovery from the abrasion (Turner & Rabiu, 2006).

▶ **Consider** *THIS!*

Bryn Carle, a 6-year-old, is brought to the clinic by her mother. She presents with redness of the left eye, edema, and drainage. What other assessment information would be helpful? Based on the history and clinical presentation, Bryn is diagnosed with conjunctivitis. What education will be necessary for the family to assist in alleviating symptoms and preventing infectious spread?

Visual Impairment

Vision impairment in children refers to acuity between 20/60 and 20/200 in the better eye on examination. "Legal blindness" is a term used to refer to visual acuity less than 20/200 or peripheral vision less than 20 degrees. In most cases, vision may be augmented with corrective lenses. Some blind children can differentiate light versus dark, while others live in total darkness.

Visual impairment in children may result from a number of different causes. In the United States, visual impairment and blindness are most often caused by refractive error, astigmatism, strabismus, amblyopia, nystagmus, infantile glaucoma, congenital cataract, ROP, and retinoblastoma (Lighthouse International, 2011). Factors that increase the risk for developing visual impairment include prematurity, developmental delay, genetic syndrome, family history of eye disease, African-American heritage, previous serious eye injury, diabetes, HIV, and chronic corticosteroid use. Trauma is also an important cause of blindness in children.

Children with visual impairments often exhibit motor and cognitive delays as well (Carter, 2011). With one less sense with which to experience their environment, these children may lag behind in developmental milestones. Visual impairments are associated with many other syndromes. For example, many children with genetic syndromes have visual impairments, and albinism is associated with blindness (Lighthouse International, 2011).

▶ **Take** *NOTE!*

Worldwide, 500,000 children become blind each year. Seventy percent of these cases result from the preventable condition xerophthalmia, caused by vitamin A deficiency. Ten to fifteen percent of cases are caused by trachoma, a treatable infection caused by C. trachomatis.

▶ *Take* NOTE!

Laser pointers pose a risk for retinal damage in infants and young children. Damage occurs if the child stares at the red light for longer than 10 seconds. Laser pointers should not be used as toys (U.S. Food and Drug Administration, 2010).

Nursing Assessment

Nursing assessment for infant and child visual impairment includes a careful health history, physical examination, and visual acuity testing.

Health History

Parents and nurses alike should be alert to signs of potential visual impairment. One of the most important functions of the nurse is to recognize signs of visual impairment as early as possible. These signs may include:

At any Age:
• Dull, vacant stare

Infants:
• Does not "fix and follow"
• Does not make eye contact
• Unaffected by bright light
• Does not imitate facial expression

Toddlers and Older Children:
• Rubs, shuts, covers eyes
• Squints
• Blinks frequently
• Holds objects close or sits close to television
• Bumps into objects
• Head tilt or forward thrust

Physical Examination

Assess for symmetry or asymmetry of corneal light reflex. Perform the "cover test." Use an age-appropriate visual acuity screening tool (refer to Chapter 30 for additional information on visual acuity screening).

Nursing Management

Important nursing functions in relation to visual impairment and blindness are supporting the child and family and promoting socialization, development, and education. In addition, when the child with a visual impairment is hospitalized for any reason, the nurse must plan appropriate care for that child, taking into consideration his or her level of disability. Box 38.2 gives tips on working with the visually impaired child, and these tips should also be taught to families.

BOX 38.2 Tips for Interacting with the Visually Impaired Child

• Use the child's name to gain attention.
• Identify yourself and let the child know you are there before you touch the child.
• Encourage the child to be independent while maintaining safety.
• Name and describe people/objects to make the child more aware of what is happening.
• Discuss upcoming activities with the child.
• Explain what other children or individuals are doing.
• Make directions simple and specific.
• Allow the child additional time to think about the response to a question or statement.
• Use touch and tone of voice appropriate to the situation.
• Use parts of the child's body as reference points for the location of items.
• Encourage exploration of objects through touch.
• Describe unfamiliar environments and provide reference points.
• Use the sighted-guide technique when walking with a visually impaired child.

Adapted from: Delta Gamma Center for Children with Visual Impairments. (2011). *Interacting with visually impaired.* Retrieved October 17, 2011 from http://dgckids.org/resources/interacting-with-visually-impaired/.

Supporting the Child and Family

Provide emotional support to the family with a visually impaired child. Ensure that the child's environment provides familiarity and security. Encourage activities that stimulate development; these activities will vary from child to child depending upon whether the child also demonstrates impairment in other areas, such as hearing or motor skills. The blind infant will not provide the eye contact that parents are looking for, so educate the parents about other indicators that the infant is acknowledging the parents' presence, such as:

• Increased motor activity
• Eyelid movement
• Changes in breathing pattern
• Making sounds

Encourage the family of a visually impaired child to display affection through touch and tone of voice. Refer families to support networks and other resources for the blind and visually impaired. Box 38.3 lists some online resources for families of children who are visually impaired or blind.

Promoting Socialization, Development, and Education

Blind children, since they lack the visual stimulation that children usually receive, may develop self-stimulatory

---

BOX 38.3 **Resources for Families of Children with Visual Impairments**

- American Association of Pediatric Ophthalmology and Strabismus—Mainly for health care providers, some information and resources for laypersons
- American Council of the Blind—The nation's leading membership organization of blind and visually impaired people
- American Foundation for the Blind—Product resource for people with visual deficits
- American Optometric Association—Education and resources for parents
- Canadian National Institute for the Blind—Resources within Canada
- Helen Keller Services for the Blind—Serves blind, deaf–blind, and visually impaired persons in the New York metropolitan area
- International Council for Education of People with Visual Impairment—Promotes equal access to appropriate education for all visually impaired children and youths
- Lighthouse International—Information on visual disorders, statistics, resources available for families; resource for products for people with visual deficits
- National Association for Parents of Children with Visual Impairments—Information, referrals, financial resources; also in Spanish
- National Eye Institute, a division of the National Institutes of Health—Conducts and supports vision research; information for the lay person or health care provider for eye examinations and financial resources
- National Federation of the Blind—Information, education, and support for the blind
- National Dissemination Center for Children with Disabilities—Provides information, education, and resources for families and educators; also in Spanish
- Prevent Blindness America—Resources for lay persons
- Recording for the Blind and Dyslexic—Texts and tapes of books
- Association for Retinopathy of Prematurity and Related Diseases—Resources for families and health care providers
- Sight for Students—Provides vision examinations and glasses to uninsured children across the country
- Vision 2020: the Right to Sight—Information, education, goals for prevention and treatment of blindness worldwide

---

For direct links to these resources, visit http://thePoint.lww.com/Chow1e.

actions in compensation ("blindisms"). Examples of blindisms are eye pressing, rocking, spinning, bouncing, and head banging. These repetitive behaviours may indicate an effort to communicate or, alternatively, they may interfere with the child's ability to socialize (Hammer, 1998). Work

with the parents to plan a strategy for the development of alternative behaviours specific to the individual child.

Refer the blind or visually impaired child who is younger than 3 years of age to the local early intervention program to establish case management services for the child's developmental needs. In some provinces (e.g., Alberta), parents can self-refer their child for early intervention if he or she has two or more disabilities. An individualized education plan (IEP) should be developed to maximize the child's learning ability. Nurses may be one of the professionals involved in the development of the IEP.

The severely visually impaired or blind child will need to learn to read Braille and will also need to learn to navigate the environment with the use of a cane or via another method.

Basic Anatomy of the Ear

The external ear, the auricle or pinna, is composed of elastic cartilage and is covered with closely adherent skin. The auricle collects and amplifies sound waves and directs them toward the tympanic membrane, which is 1 cm in diameter and 1 mm thick. The tympanic membrane protects the middle ear space from the external environment and conducts and amplifies sound through the middle ear by way of the ossicles (malleus, incus, and stapes), which are the three tiniest bones in the body. The stapes footplate fills the oval window, which allows sound vibration to enter the inner ear. These sound vibrations cause the fluid in the cochlea to move, which in turn causes the hair cells of the cochlea to bend. The hair cells create neural signals that are picked up by the auditory nerve, sent to the brain, and there interpreted as sound (Irwin, 2006).

Congenital deformities of the ear are often associated with other body system anomalies and genetic syndromes. The presence of ear anomalies may lead to the search for and subsequent diagnosis of the other anomalies or syndromes. The infant's relatively short, wide, and horizontally placed eustachian tubes allow bacteria and viruses to gain access to the middle ear easily, resulting in increased numbers of ear infections as compared with the adult (Yoon et al., 2011). As the child matures, the tubes assume a more slanted position, so older children and adults generally have fewer cases of middle ear effusion and infection (Fig. 38.8). Sometimes enlargement of the adenoids contributes to obstruction of the eustachian tubes, leading to infection.

Otitis Media

Otitis media is defined as inflammation of the middle ear with the presence of fluid. It can be subdivided into two categories. Acute otitis media (AOM) refers to an acute infectious process of the middle ear that may produce a rapid onset of ear pain and possibly fever. Otitis media with effusion (OME) refers to a collection of fluid in the

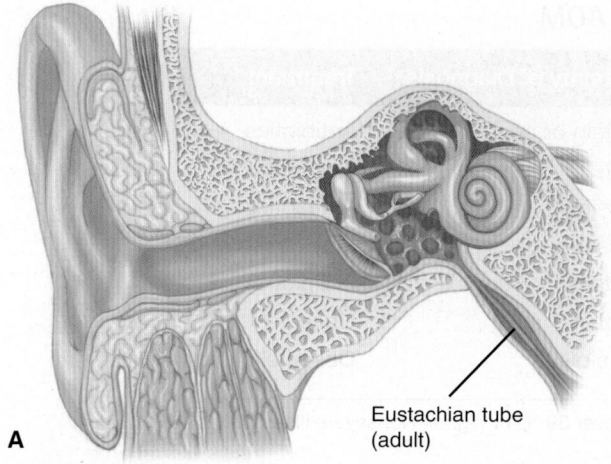

A Eustachian tube (adult)

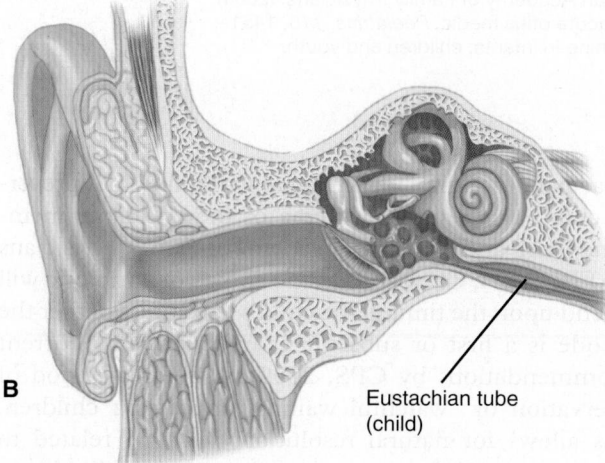

B Eustachian tube (child)

FIGURE 38.8 Note the child's relatively shorter, wider eustachian tubes and their horizontal positioning (**B**) as compared with the adult's (**A**).

middle ear space without signs and symptoms of infection. Chronic otitis media with effusion (chronic OME) is defined as OME lasting longer than 3 months.

Acute Otitis Media

AOM is a common illness in children, resulting from infection (bacterial or viral) of fluid in the middle ear. AOM has a peak incidence in the first 2 years of life, especially between 6 and 12 months of age, although its incidence is increasing in all age groups (Carlson, 2007). Increased susceptibility in infants may be partly explained by the short length and horizontal positioning of the eustachian tube, limited response to antigens, and lack of previous exposure to common pathogens (Yoon et al., 2011). AOM occurs mostly in the fall through spring, with the highest incidence in the winter. AOM often recurs in infants and young children when the fluid in the middle ear becomes reinfected. The most significant risk factors for AOM are

| BOX 38.4 | Risk Factors for Acute Otitis Media |

- Eustachian tube dysfunction
- Recurrent upper respiratory infection
- First episode of AOM before 3 months of age
- Day care attendance (increases exposure to viruses causing upper respiratory infections)
- Previous episodes of AOM
- Family history
- Passive smoking
- Crowding in the home or large family size
- Native American, Inuit, or Australian Aborigine ethnicity
- Absence of infant breastfeeding
- Immunocompromise
- Poor nutrition
- Craniofacial anomalies
- Presence of allergies (possibly)

Adapted from: American Academy of Pediatrics and American Academy of Family Physicians. (2004). Clinical practice guidelines: Diagnosis and management of acute otitis media. *Pediatrics, 113*, 1451–1465; Carlson, L. (2007). Inside and out: A review of otitis in children. *Advance for Nurse Practitioners, 15*(5), 51–58; and Yoon, P. J., Kelley, P. E., & Friedman, N. R. (2011). Ear, nose, & throat. In W. W. Hay, M. J. Levin, J. M. Sondheimer, & R. R. Deterding (Eds.), *Current pediatric diagnosis and treatment* (20th ed.). New York: McGraw-Hill.

eustachian tube dysfunction and susceptibility to recurrent upper respiratory infections (Box 38.4).

Pathophysiology

An upper respiratory infection frequently precedes AOM. Fluid and pathogens travel upward from the nasopharyngeal area, invading the middle ear space. Fluid behind the eardrum has difficulty draining back out toward the nasopharyngeal area because of the horizontal positioning of the eustachian tube. A viral upper respiratory infection may cause AOM or may place the child at risk for bacterial invasion. Pathogens gain access to the eustachian tube, where they proliferate and invade the mucosa. Fever and pain occur acutely. Increased pressure behind the tympanic membrane may result in perforation, which could lead to decreased pain and yield drainage in the ear canal. Most perforations heal spontaneously and are completely benign.

AOM is most commonly caused by viral pathogens and resolve spontaneously. However, bacterial AOM is usually caused by one of the following organisms: *S. pneumoniae, H. influenzae,* and *Moraxella catarrhalis.* Bacterial AOM symptoms are often more severe and frequently require antibiotics to resolve.

After clearance of the infection, fluid remains in the middle ear space behind the tympanic membrane, sometimes for several months (OME). This may occur because of the positioning of the eustachian tubes, which results

TABLE 38.4 TREATMENT RECOMMENDATIONS FOR AOM

Age and Severity of Illness[a]	Certainty of Diagnosis	Treatment
Less than 6 months old	Certain or possible	Antibiotics
6 months to 2 years	Certain	Antibiotics
6 months to 2 years with severe illness	Possible	Antibiotics
6 months to 2 years with nonsevere illness	Possible	May observe[b]
Greater than 2 years with severe illness	Certain	Antibiotics
Greater than 2 years with nonsevere illness	Certain	Observe[b]
Greater than 2 years	Possible	Observe[b]

[a]Severe illness is defined as moderate to severe otalgia or fever 39 °C or higher. Nonsevere illness is defined as mild otalgia and fever less than 39 °C.

[b]Observation is appropriate only when follow-up can be ensured. If symptoms are persistent or become worse, antibiotics may then be started.

Adapted from: American Academy of Pediatrics and American Academy of Family Physicians. (2004). Clinical practice guidelines: Diagnosis and management of acute otitis media. *Pediatrics*, *113*, 1451–1465; and Canadian Paediatric Society. (2009). Vision screening in infants, children and youth. *Paediatrics & Child Health*, *14*(4), 246–248.

in difficulty in draining fluid back to the nasopharyngeal area, and/or the high frequency of upper respiratory infections in infants and young children, which again results in backup of fluid from the nasopharyngeal area.

The most common complications of AOM include:

- Reversible hearing loss
- Expressive speech delay
- Tympanosclerosis (scarring of the tympanic membrane; usually has no effect on hearing)
- Tympanic membrane perforation (acute with resolution or chronic)
- Chronic suppurative otitis media (chronic drainage via perforation or **tympanostomy** tubes)
- Acute mastoiditis (infection of the mastoid process)
- Intracranial infections, including bacterial meningitis and abscesses

Therapeutic Management

It is unreasonable to obtain a culture of middle ear fluid with every episode of AOM to determine the specific cause. Scientific studies of fluid obtained via tympanostomy in children with AOM have been performed, and clinical decision making is based upon this research. There is great concern in the health care community about the development of antibiotic resistance due to the overuse of antibiotics (Sheppard, 2008). For this reason, clinical practice guidelines have been developed for a number of disorders based upon large quantities of research.

Certain diagnosis of AOM is based upon rapid onset of symptoms, signs of fluid in the middle ear, and signs or symptoms of inflammation in the middle ear, including a bulging tympanic membrane with marked discolouration (hemorrhagic, red, grey, or yellow), rapid onset

of ear pain (otalgia), unexplained irritability in a preverbal child, and visible erythema of the tympanic membrane (AAP and American Academy of Family Physicians [AAFP], 2004; CPS, 2009). The choice of antibiotic will depend upon the timing, the child's age, and whether the episode is a first or subsequent infection. The current recommendations by CPS, 2009 allow for a period of observation or "watchful waiting" in certain children. This allows for natural resolution of AOM related to viral causes and decreases the overuse of antibiotics in the pediatric population (AAP and AAFP, 2004). Table 38.4 provides treatment recommendations for AOM.

Recommendations for AOM treatment in previously healthy children include watchful waiting and observation for 48 to 72 hours without antimicrobial agents in the following instances:

- The child is older than 6 months of age.
- The child does not have immunodeficiency, chronic cardiac or pulmonary disease, anatomic abnormalities of the head or neck, a history of complicated otitis media (otitis media accompanied by suppurative complications or chronic perforation), or Down syndrome.
- The illness is not severe—otalgia appears to be mild and fever is lower than 39°C in the absence of antipyretics.
- Parents are capable of recognizing signs of worsening illness and can readily access medical care if the child does not improve.

If the child's status worsens or does not improve during the observation period, antimicrobial therapy must be started. Pain management is also an important component of AOM treatment, as is appropriate follow-up to ensure disease resolution (CPS, 2009).

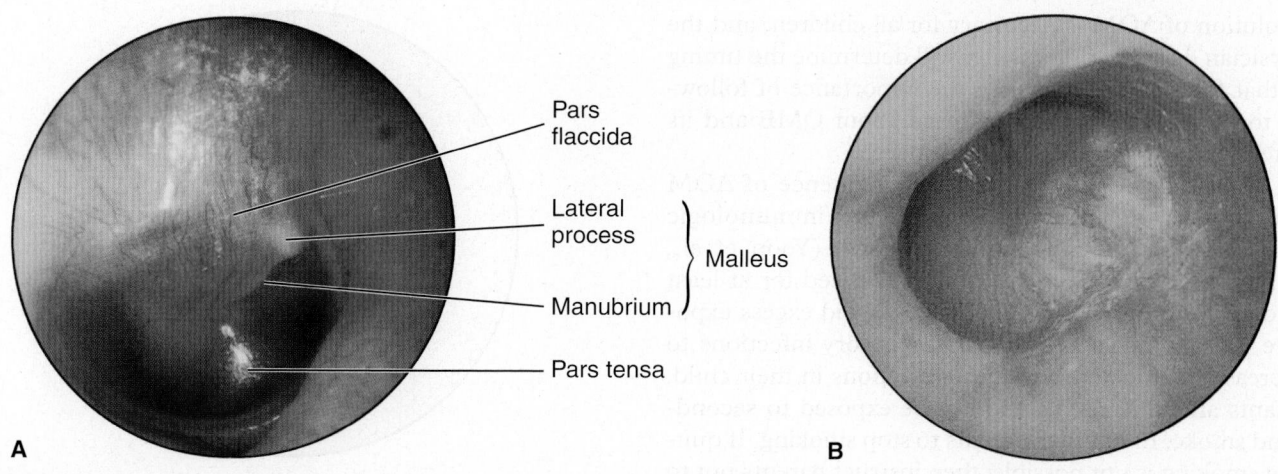

FIGURE 38.9 (**A**) Normal tympanic membrane. (**B**) Acute otitis media: note erythema and opacity of the tympanic membrane.

Nursing Assessment

Nursing assessment of the child with AOM consists of health history and physical examination.

Health History

Elicit a description of the present illness and chief complaint. Note acute, abrupt onset of signs and symptoms. Common signs and symptoms reported during the health history might include:

- Fever (may be low grade or higher)
- Complaints of otalgia (ear pain)
- Fussiness or irritability
- Crying inconsolably, particularly when lying down
- Batting or tugging at the ears (may also occur with teething or OME, or may be a habit)
- Rolling the head from side to side
- Poor feeding or loss of appetite
- Lethargy
- Difficulty sleeping or awakening crying in the night
- Fluid draining from the ear

Determine the child's response to any treatments used thus far. Explore the child's current and past medical history for risk factors such as:

- Young age
- Day care attendance
- Previous history of AOM or OME
- Bottle feeding
- Bottle propping
- Pacifier use
- Passive smoke exposure
- Antecedent or concurrent upper respiratory infection

Physical Examination and Diagnostic Testing

The child may complain of pain when the ear is examined. On otoscopic examination, the tympanic membrane will have a dull or opaque appearance and is bulging and/or red (Fig. 38.9). Sometimes pus (greenish or yellowish) may be visible behind the eardrum. Upon pneumatic otoscopy, the eardrum will be immobile. (A physician or nurse practitioner usually performs otoscopic examination.) If the tympanic membrane has become perforated, drainage may be present in the ear canal, but the canal will otherwise appear normal. Palpate for possible cervical lymphadenopathy. **Tympanometry** is not as useful in the diagnosis of AOM as it is with OME.

Nursing Management

Nursing management of the child with AOM is mainly supportive in nature. It focuses on pain management, family education, and prevention of AOM.

Managing Pain Associated with AOM

Analgesics such as acetaminophen and ibuprofen have been shown to be effective at managing mild to moderate pain associated with AOM. They have the added benefit of reducing fever. Narcotic analgesics such as codeine may be prescribed for severe pain. Application of heat or a cool compress may also be helpful. Instruct the family to have the child lie on the affected side with the heating pad or covered ice pack placed on that ear (AAP and AAFP, 2004).

Educating the Family

If the treatment selected for AOM is observation or watchful waiting, explain the rationale for this to the family. Ensure that the family understands the importance of returning for re-evaluation if the child is not improving or if the AOM progresses to severe illness. When antibiotics are prescribed, the family must understand the importance of completing the entire course of antibiotics. Families are tempted to stop giving the antibiotic because the child is usually vastly improved after taking the medication for 24 to 48 hours. Follow-up for resolution of AOM is necessary for all children, and the physician or nurse practitioner will determine the timing of that follow-up. Emphasize the importance of follow-up to the parents, educating them about OME and its potential impact on hearing and speech.

Breastfed infants have a lower incidence of AOM than do formula-fed infants, and the immunologic benefits of breast milk are well known (Yoon et al., 2011), so encourage mothers to breastfeed for at least 6 to 12 months. Instruct families to avoid excess exposure to individuals with upper respiratory infections to decrease the incidence of these infections in their child. Infants and children should not be exposed to second-hand smoke. Encourage parents to stop smoking. If quitting smoking is not possible, then instruct parents not to smoke inside the house or automobile. Encourage the parents to have the child immunized with Prevnar and, when appropriate, influenza vaccine.

Otitis Media with Effusion

OME refers to the presence of fluid within the middle ear space, without signs or symptoms of infection. It may occur independent of AOM or may persist after the infectious process of AOM has resolved. Risk factors for OME include passive smoking, bottle feeding, frequent viral upper respiratory infections, allergy, young age, male gender, adenoid hypertrophy, eustachian tube dysfunction, and certain congenital disorders (Yoon et al., 2011). Severe complications of OME include AOM, hearing loss, and deafness. However, the hearing loss associated with these conditions is usually reversible.

Nursing Assessment

Nursing assessment of the child with OME includes health history, physical examination, and diagnostic testing.

Health History

Determine the extent of symptoms. Children may be asymptomatic or may experience a popping sensation or fullness behind the eardrum. Explore the health history for risk factors such as passive smoking, absence of breastfeeding, frequent viral upper respiratory infections, allergy, or recent history of AOM.

Physical Examination

Otoscopic examination may reveal a dull, opaque tympanic membrane that may be white, grey, or bluish (Fig. 38.10). If the tympanic membrane is not opaque, a fluid level or air bubble may be visualized. Mobility may be absent or diminished upon pneumatic otoscopy. Tympanometry may be used to confirm the diagnosis of OME.

Nursing Management

OME may take several months to resolve. Nursing management during the resolution phase focuses on education and monitoring for hearing loss.

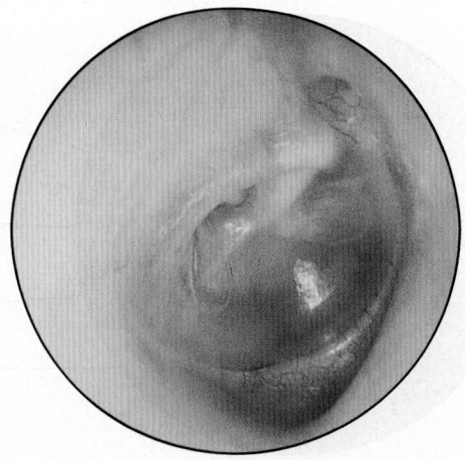

FIGURE 38.10 Otitis media with effusion; note the dull white tympanic membrane.

Educating the Family

Educate the family about the natural history of OME and the anatomic differences in young children that contribute to OME. Inform parents that antihistamines, decongestants, antibiotics, and corticosteroids have not been proven to hasten the resolution of OME and thus are not recommended. OME usually resolves spontaneously, but children should be rechecked every 4 weeks while this resolution is occurring. Teach parents not to feed infants in a supine position and to avoid bottle propping.

Monitoring for Hearing Loss

When OME persists, the primary concern is its effect on hearing. In the infant or toddler who should be experiencing rapid language development, impaired hearing can depress language acquisition significantly (AAP, 2004). Children with OME who are at risk for speech, language, or learning problems may be referred for evaluation of hearing earlier than a child with OME who isn't at risk. Risk factors for speech, language, or learning disabilities are presented in Box 38.5. Children with chronic OME (persistent OME of 3 months' duration or longer) should

---

BOX 38.5 **Risk Factors for Speech, Language, or Learning Difficulties in Children**

- Permanent hearing loss (without OME)
- Speech/language delay (suspected or diagnosed)
- Craniofacial disorder that may interfere with speech
- Any pervasive developmental disorder
- Genetic disorders or syndromes associated with speech or learning problems
- Cleft palate
- Blindness or significant visual impairment

Adapted from: American Academy of Pediatrics. (2004). Clinical practice guideline: Otitis media with effusion. *Pediatrics, 113*, 1412–1429.

be referred to a specialist for hearing evaluation (AAP, 2004). Children who are not already at risk for speech concerns and are not experiencing difficulty with language acquisition may be reassessed every 3 to 6 months as long as hearing loss is not identified. At-risk children may require treatment earlier.

To communicate more effectively with children with OME who have hearing loss:

- Turn off music or television.
- Position yourself within 3 feet of the child before speaking.
- Face the child while speaking.
- Use visual cues.
- Increase the volume of your speech only slightly.
- Speak clearly.
- Request preferential classroom seating.
- Use an FM (frequency-modulated) system in the classroom.

> ▶ **Take** NOTE!
>
> *Evaluation of hearing is recommended when OME lasts 3 months or longer in children in whom language delay, hearing loss, or a learning problem is suspected (AAP, 2004).*

Providing Postoperative Care for the Child With Pressure-Equalizing Tubes

The standard treatment for persistent or problematic OME is surgical insertion of **pressure-equalizing (PE) tubes** into the tympanic membrane (via myringotomy). The tubes usually stay in place for at least several months and generally fall out on their own (Fig. 38.11). The procedure is usually done on an outpatient basis, and the child returns home in the evening. Teach

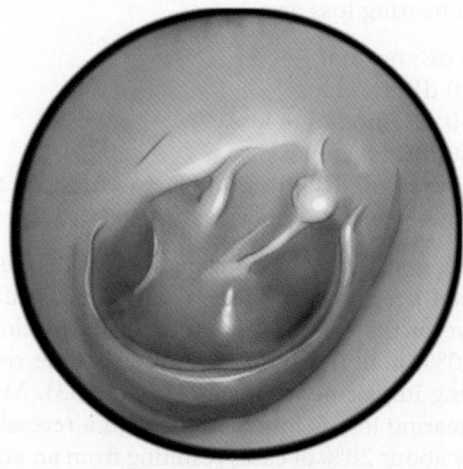

FIGURE 38.11 Pressure-equalizing tubes in place in the tympanic membrane.

the parents to administer ear drops postoperatively if prescribed. After PE tube placement, the surgeon may recommend avoiding water entry into the ears. If recommended, advise parents to have the child wear earplugs in the bathtub or while swimming.

Placement of the PE tubes allows for adequate hearing, which in turn encourages appropriate speech development. Placement of PE tubes does not prevent middle ear infection. If the middle ear becomes infected with PE tubes in place, the tubes allow infected fluid to drain from the ear. Tell parents to contact their pediatrician if drainage from the ear is noted. After PE tubes are placed, young children often have rapid increases in language acquisition, and parents should observe for this (KidsHealth, 2009a).

> ▶ **Take** NOTE!
>
> *Children with PE tubes who swim in a lake must wear earplugs, as lake water is contaminated with bacteria and entry of that water into the middle ear should be avoided (Cincinnati Children's, 2009).*

Otitis Externa

Otitis externa is defined as infection and inflammation of the skin of the external ear canal. *Pseudomonas aeruginosa* and *S. aureus* are typical causative agents, although fungi such as *Aspergillus* and other bacteria also may be implicated. Moisture in the canal contributes to pathogen growth (Yoon et al., 2011). Otitis externa is commonly known as "swimmer's ear" since it occurs more frequently in those who swim often (and thus have wet ear canals). Changing the pH in the ear canal contributes to the inflammatory process (Zoltan, Taylor, & Achar, 2005).

Nursing Assessment

Nursing assessment of the child with otitis externa focuses on the health history and physical examination.

Health History

Elicit a description of the present illness and chief complaint. Note history of ear itching or pain, ear drainage, or a feeling of fullness in the ear canal, with possible difficulty hearing. Note onset and progression of symptoms as well as the child's response to treatments. Explore the child's current and past medical history for risk factors such as previous episodes of otitis externa or history of recent swimming in a pool, lake, or ocean.

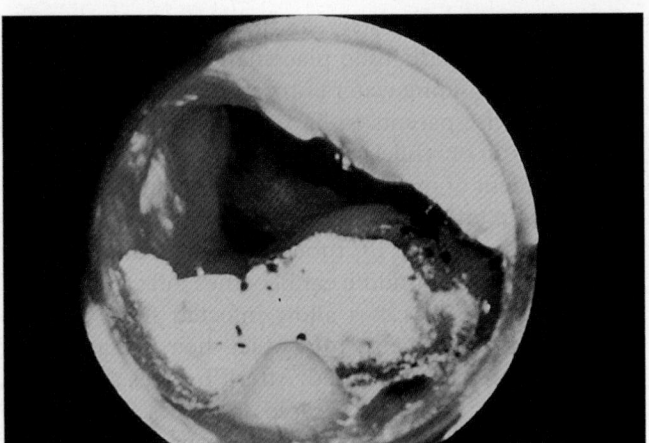

FIGURE **38.12** Note edema and erythema of the ear canal as well as purulent discharge in the child with otitis externa.

▶ *Take* NOTE!

The child with otitis externa usually has significant ear pain. Pressure on the tragus should be avoided, as it can worsen the pain.

Physical Examination

Typically a white or coloured discharge can be seen in the ear canal or running from the ear. On otoscopy, the canal is red and edematous, often too swollen for insertion of the speculum and viewing of the tympanic membrane (Fig. 38.12). Diagnosis is based on clinical findings. Occasionally, the ear drainage is cultured for bacteria or fungus, particularly if otitis externa is not improving with treatment.

Nursing Management

The primary goals of nursing management are pain relief, treatment of the infection, and prevention of recurrence.

Managing Pain

Analgesics (often narcotics) may be administered to manage the pain. A warm compress or heating pad to the affected ear is helpful in some children.

Treating the Infection

Antibiotic or antifungal ear drops should be administered as prescribed. In some cases, a wick is placed in the ear canal. The wick keeps the antibiotic drops in contact with the skin of the ear canal and promotes healing. Wick insertion can be extremely painful, and younger children will need to be restrained during insertion for their safety.

Preventing Reinfection

Once the infection has resolved, children and their parents should be educated about prevention of further episodes. Since moisture contributes to otitis externa, the ear canals should be kept dry. Encourage the child and parents to use one of the methods described in Teaching Guideline 38.2 after swimming or showering.

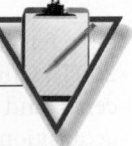

TEACHING GUIDELINE 38.2

Preventing Otitis Externa

1. Avoid the use of cotton swabs, headphones, and earphones.
2. Wear earplugs when swimming.
3. Promote ear canal dryness and alternate pH. Use one or more of the following methods:
   • Dry the ear canals using a hair dryer set on a lower setting.
   • Administer solutions that have a drying effect on the auditory canal skin and change the pH of the canal to discourage organism growth in susceptible children. The following solutions can be used:
   • A few drops of Domeboro solution can be placed in the canal and then allowed to run out.
   • A mixture of half rubbing alcohol and half vinegar (squirted into the canal and then allowed to run out). The alcohol solution should be used only when the ear canals are healthy. Using it while the canals are inflamed will cause stinging and increased pain.

Adapted from: Kids Health (2009b). Swimmer's ear. Retrieved October 17, 2011 from http://kidshealth.org/parent/infections/ear/swimmer_ear.html#.

Hearing Loss and Deafness

Infants are ordinarily born with the sense of hearing fully developed. Language development in infancy and early childhood is dependent upon adequate hearing, and even the fluctuating hearing loss associated with intermittent bouts of AOM can hinder language development (AAP, 2004). Hearing loss may be unilateral (involving one ear) or bilateral (involving both ears). The extent of hearing loss is defined based on the softest intensity of sound that is perceived, described in **decibels** (dB). Levels of hearing loss are:

• 0 to 20 dB: normal
• 20 to 40 dB: mild loss
• 40 to 60 dB: moderate loss
• 60 to 80 dB: severe loss
• Greater than 80 dB: profound loss (American Speech-Language-Hearing Association, 2011)

Hearing loss may be congenital or of delayed onset. Congenital hearing loss affects about 1 to 6 infants per 1,000 live births (Gifford, Holmes, & Bernstein, 2009). About 10% of all newborns have at least one risk factor for hearing impairment (Verma et al., 2003). Most congenital hearing loss is inherited through a recessive gene, with only about 20% of cases resulting from an autosomal dominant trait (Kaye and The Committee on Genetics, 2006). Congenital hearing loss accounts for about one half of all cases of hearing impairment; the remainder are acquired. Premature infants and those with persistent pulmonary hypertension of the newborn are at increased risk for hearing loss compared with other infants (Verma et al., 2003). Hearing loss commonly occurs with a large number of congenital or genetic syndromes, as well as in association with anomalies of the head and face. Most Canadian provinces (except Manitoba and Alberta) have passed a variety of newborn universal hearing screening laws, thus allowing for earlier identification of infants with congenital hearing loss (Personal communication, McNiven, M., May 26, 2010).

Delayed-onset hearing loss may be conductive, sensorineural, or mixed. **Conductive hearing loss** results when transmission of sound through the middle ear is disrupted, as in the case of OME. When fluid fills the middle ear, the tympanic membrane is unable to move properly, and partial or complete hearing loss occurs. **Sensorineural hearing loss** is caused by damage to the hair cells in the cochlea or along the auditory pathway. This may result from kernicterus, use of ototoxic medication, intrauterine infection with CMV or rubella, neonatal or postnatal infection such as meningitis, severe neonatal respiratory depression, or exposure to excess noise. Mixed hearing loss occurs when the cause may be attributed to both conductive and sensorineural problems.

Regardless of the cause of hearing loss, early intervention can make a difference in the child's ability to communicate. Once the hearing loss has been determined, intervention can begin. Hearing aids, cochlear implants, communication devices, and speech education may enable these children to communicate verbally. Improved communication beginning in infancy and early childhood may also improve the child's school achievement.

> ▶ *Take NOTE!*
>
> *The earplugs or covers used to block ambient noise in premature infants in the NICU may decrease the preemie's risk for hearing loss and improve developmental outcomes (Turk, Williams, & Lasky, 2009).*

Nursing Assessment

Nursing assessment of the child with hearing loss or impairment focuses on the health history, physical examination, and hearing testing.

Health History

Common signs and symptoms reported during the health history might include:

Infant:
- Wakes only to touch, not environmental noises
- Does not startle to loud noises
- Does not turn to sound by 4 months of age
- Does not babble at 6 months of age
- Does not progress with speech development

Young Child:
- Does not speak by 2 years of age
- Communicates through gestures
- Does not speak distinctly, as appropriate for age
- Displays developmental (cognitive) delays
- Prefers solitary play
- Displays immature emotional behaviour
- Does not respond to ringing of the telephone or doorbell
- Focuses on facial expressions when communicating

Older Child:
- Often asks for statements to be repeated
- Is inattentive or daydreams
- Performs poorly at school
- Displays monotone or other abnormal speech
- Gives inappropriate answers to questions except when able to view the face of the speaker

At any Age:
- Speaks loudly
- Sits very close to TV or radio, or adjusts volume too loud
- Responds only to moderate or loud voices

Signs of hearing loss should be investigated as early as possible in order for appropriate communication intervention to begin.

Explore the child's current and past medical history for risk factors such as congenital anomalies, genetic syndrome, infection, family history, kernicterus, neonatal ventilator use, ototoxic medication, or exposure to excess noise. Note whether newborn hearing screening was done, along with the results.

Physical Examination and Laboratory and Diagnostic Tests

Determine the child's level of interaction with the environment. For preschoolers and older children, administer the whisper test, keeping in mind that this is a gross screening test only. Conduct the Weber and Rinne tests (see Chapter 31 for further explanation). If further evaluation is needed, the nurse may be responsible for administering an otoacoustic emission test or auditory brain stem evoked response test, either in the hospital or in the outpatient office.

Nursing Management

The primary goal of nursing care for the child with a hearing impairment is to provide education and support to the family and child. Individualize care for the child with a hearing impairment and the family based on their specific responses to the hearing impairment.

TABLE 38.5 COMPARING COMMUNICATION OPTIONS FOR THE HEARING IMPAIRED

Spoken Language	
Oral deaf education (auditory–verbal therapy)	Uses technology to boost auditory potential; teaches children to notice sound and give it meaning. Develops oral speech
Cued speech	A system using hand signs to clarify lip-reading; gives the person clues about the sounds the speaker is making
Signed Language	
American Sign Language (ASL)	Entirely communicated through hand signs, gestures, and facial expressions. Has its own grammar and syntax
Combination: Total communication	Combines auditory training and teaching of spoken language with SEE ("signing exact English"; corresponds to the words and syntax of English)
Augmentative and Alternative Communication (AAC)	
May use gestural communication	Can also include physical devices such as notebooks, communication boards, charts, or computers. Ranges from very low-tech to technologically complex

Adapted from: American Speech-Language-Hearing Association. (20011). *Augmentative and alternative communication (AAC)*. Retrieved October 17, 2011 from http://www.asha.org/public/speech/disorders/AAC.htm.

Augmenting Hearing

Compliance with hearing aids and communication curricula is critical so that the child can develop hearing and speech. Hearing aids should be cleaned daily with a damp cloth. Batteries are usually changed weekly. Ensure that parents are aware of the dangers of accidental ingestion of hearing aid batteries, which include severe chemical burn and damage to the child's mucosa if the battery becomes lodged. Ingestion and damage are not uncommon due to the small size of these batteries, which makes them interesting objects to a small child, as well as their caustic nature. When inserting a hearing aid, the volume should be turned down and then adjusted to the appropriate level after insertion. As the infant or child grows, the hearing aid will need to be reassessed for proper fit. Many schools for the **deaf** and other organizations provide loaner hearing aids so that the best fit and amplification may be determined prior to purchase. Assist the family in exploring this type of option in the local community. Also, help the family access government and/or local agencies that can help them defray the cost of the child's hearing aids.

When cochlear implants are used, the nurse focuses on postoperative care of the incision site and pain management.

Promoting Communication and Education

Families and children need to learn how to communicate effectively with one another. If the child learns American Sign Language (ASL), for instance, the parents and siblings should as well. Table 38.5 gives information on communication options for hearing-impaired children and their families. Communication may also be enhanced by the use of text telephone service and closed-caption television in the home. Bells and alarms in the home may use lights rather than sound to alert the child. Provide a sign language interpreter for the child at health care visits if the parent is not present for interpretation.

Encouraging Education

Refer the child less than 3 years of age to the local early intervention program for case management of

---

BOX 38.6 Resources for Families of Children with Hearing Impairments

- Alexander Graham Bell Association for the Deaf and Hard of Hearing—Wide range of programs and services, advocating independence through listening and talking
- American Speech–Language–Hearing Association (ASHA)—Information, education, referrals, and resources for the hearing impaired
- American Academy of Audiology (AAA)—Education, referrals for audiologists, resources
- Auditory–Verbal International (AVI)—Advocates for listening, amplification of hearing, and learned speech
- Canadian Hearing Society—Resources within Canada
- Cochlear Implant Association—Support, information, advocacy for rights and services
- National Cued Speech Association—Promotes and supports the effective use of cued speech
- American Academy of Otolaryngology—Head and Neck Surgery—Education and resources
- International Hearing Society—Education, referrals, information on hearing aids
- John Tracy Clinic—Worldwide free service for families of preschool children with hearing loss
- League for the Hard of Hearing—Hearing rehabilitation and human services agency
- Oral Deaf Education—Promotes spoken language use in the hearing impaired for effective communication

For direct links to these resources, visit http://thePoint.lww.com/Chow1e.

EVIDENCE-BASED PRACTICE 38.1
The Effect of Patching for Corneal Abrasion on Healing and Decreased Pain

● Study

Simple corneal abrasions are a common eye complaint. Eye patching with or without antibiotic ointment has often been used despite a lack of evidence for its use. Additionally, patches are difficult to keep on young children and may be associated with corneal erosion. The authors included quasi-randomized and randomized studies evaluating patching versus no patching for treatment of simple corneal abrasion. Eleven trials with a total of 1,014 participants were included in the review.

▲ Findings

The authors found that patching for simple corneal abrasions did not improve healing on day 1, nor did it decrease the amount of pain experienced. Additionally, binocular vision is lost when one eye is patched. Based on these results, it is not recommended that patching be used for treatment of simple corneal abrasions.

■ Nursing Implications

Parents worry significantly when their child experiences even a very mild eye injury. Teach parents about the ability of the cornea to heal quickly from a minor abrasion. Emphasize that nonpatched corneal abrasions have been shown to heal more rapidly than those that are patched.

Turner, A., & Rabiu, M. (2006). Patching for corneal abrasion. *Cochrane Database of Systematic Reviews,* Issue 2, Article No: CD004764.

developmental needs. At 3 years of age and beyond, provincial laws provide for public education and related services for children with disabilities. An IEP should be developed to maximize the child's learning ability. Nurses may be involved in the development of the IEP.

Some children attend schools specifically geared toward deaf students. The choice of school will depend upon the family's preferences and resources.

Providing Support

The diagnosis of a significant disability can be extremely stressful for the family. Encourage families to express their feelings and provide emotional support. Ensure that the needs of any siblings are also attended to. When the family is ready, encourage them to network with other families who have children with similar needs. Educate the family about the child's prescribed plan of care. Refer families to resources and support groups (Box 38.6).

■■■ Key Concepts

- Although hearing is fully developed at birth, visual development continues to progress until about age 7 years.
- The relatively short and horizontally positioned eustachian tubes of infants and young children make them more susceptible than adults to otitis media.
- Binocular vision develops by age 4 months; visual acuity progresses to 20/50 by age 3 years and usually reaches 20/20 by age 7 years.
- To maximize speech and language development, hearing loss should be identified early and intervention begun immediately.
- The corneal light reflex test and cover test are useful tools for identifying strabismus and amblyopia.
- Tympanometry is used to determine the presence of fluid behind the eardrum (such as with OME).

- Topical ophthalmic medications are used to treat certain infectious eye disorders.
- Systemic antibiotics are used for the treatment of periorbital cellulitis and AOM.
- Very premature infants are at high risk for developing visual deficits related to ROP and are also at increased risk for hearing impairment compared with other infants.
- Children with genetic syndromes or family history are at increased risk for visual and hearing impairments.
- Strabismus, glaucoma, and cataracts may all lead to visual impairment if left untreated.
- Recurrent or constant nasal congestion contributes to OME.
- Asymmetry of the corneal light reflex occurs with true strabismus.
- A cloudy cornea indicates the presence of cataract.
- Eye strain, eye rubbing, and headaches may indicate a visual deficit.
- Delay in language acquisition may occur when hearing loss is present.
- Appropriate handwashing is the single most important factor in reducing the spread of acute viral or bacterial conjunctivitis.
- Otitis externa can be prevented by keeping the ear canal dry and altering canal pH.
- Children with visual disorders should be encouraged to use prescribed corrective lenses.
- The child with hearing loss should receive early intervention with hearing aids or other augmentative devices.
- Hearing and/or vision impairment can significantly hinder developmental progress.
- The fluctuating hearing loss associated with recurrent AOM and the hearing loss associated with chronic OME can both significantly hinder language development in the infant and toddler.

■ Amblyopia must be identified early and treated with patching, corrective lenses, or surgery to prevent visual deterioration and promote appropriate vision development.

REFERENCES

American Academy of Ophthalmology. (2008). *Is LASIK for me? A patient's guide to refractive surgery.* Retrieved October 17, 2011 from http://www.geteyesmart.org/eyesmart/glasses-contacts-lasik/upload/LASIK-patient-guide.pdf

American Academy of Pediatrics. (2004). Clinical practice guideline: Otitis media with effusion. *Pediatrics, 113,* 1412–1429.

American Academy of Pediatrics. (2006). Screening examination of premature infants for retinopathy of prematurity. *Pediatrics, 117,* 572–576.

American Academy of Pediatrics and American Academy of Family Physicians. (2004). Clinical practice guidelines: Diagnosis and management of acute otitis media. *Pediatrics, 113,* 1451–1465.

American Association for Pediatric Ophthalmology and Strabismus. (2011). *Nasolacrimal duct obstruction.* Retrieved October 20, 2011 from http://www.aapos.org/terms/conditions/72

American Speech-Language-Hearing Association. (2011). *Types of hearing loss.* Retrieved October 17, 2011 from http://www.asha.org/public/hearing/disorders/types.htm

Augsburger, J., & Asbury, T. (2008). Ocular and orbital trauma. In P. Riordan-Eva & J. P. Whitcher (Eds.), *Vaughan & Asbury's general ophthalmology* (17th ed.). New York: McGraw-Hill.

Bacal, D. A., & Wilson, M. C. (2000). Strabismus: Getting it straight. *Contemporary Pediatrics, 17*(2), 49–60.

Braverman, R. S. (2011). Eye. In W. W. Hay, M. J. Levin, J. M. Sondheimer, & R. R. Deterding (Eds.), *Current pediatric diagnosis and treatment* (20th ed.). New York: McGraw-Hill.

Burns, C., Dunn, A., Brady, M., Starr, N. B., & Blosser, C. (2009). *Pediatric primary care* (4th ed.). Philadelphia: Saunders.

Canadian Ophthalmological Society. (2007). *Laser surgery of the eye. A safe, precise technique.* Retrieved October 17, 2011 from www.eyesite.ca/english/public-information/eye-conditions/pdfs/LaserSurgery_e.pdf

Canadian Paediatric Society. (2009). Vision screening in infants, children and youth. *Paediatrics & Child Health, 14*(4), 246–248.

Carlson, L. (2007). Inside and out: A review of otitis in children. *Advance for Nurse Practitioners, 15*(5), 51–58.

Carter, S. L. (2011). *Sensory impairment.* Retrieved October 17, 2011 from http://www.pediatrics.emory.edu/divisions/neonatology/dpc/sensory.html

Casady, D. R., Meyer, D. R., Simon, J. W., Stasior, G. O., & Zobal-Ratner, J. L. (2006). Stepwise treatment paradigm for congenital nasolacrimal duct obstruction. *Ophthalmic Plastic and Reconstructive Surgery, 22*(4), 243–247.

Cincinnati Children's. (2009). *Pressure equalizer (PE) tube insertion.* Retrieved October 17, 2011 from http://www.cincinnatichildrens.org/health/info/ent/procedure/pe-tube.htm

Delta Gamma Center for Children with Visual Impairments. (2011). *Interacting with visually impaired.* Retrieved October 17, 2011 from http://dgckids.org/resources/interacting-with-visually-impaired/

Doshi, N. R., & Rodriguez, M. L. (2007). Amblyopia. *American Family Physician, 75*(3), 361–367.

Gifford, K. A., Holmes, M. G., & Bernstein, H. H. (2009). Hearing loss in children. *Pediatrics in Review, 30,* 207–216.

Goller, Y. (2006). Cochlear implantation in children: Implications for the primary care provider. *Journal of the American Academy of Nurse Practitioners, 18*(9), 397–408.

Graven, S. N., & Browne, J. V. (2008). Visual development in the human fetus, infant, and young child. *Newborn and Infant Nursing Reviews, 8*(4), 194–201.

Gross, R. D. (2002). Case study: Nasolacrimal-duct obstruction. *Infectious Diseases in Children* (Suppl.), 18–19.

Hack, M., & Klein, N. (2006). Young adult attainments of premature infants. *Journal of the American Medical Association, 295*(6), 695–696.

Hammer, E. (1998). Self-stimulation: Dr. Hammer responds. *News from Advocates for Deaf-Blind, 2*(1); retrieved October 17, 2011 from http://www.nfb.org/images/nfb/Publications/fr/fr17/Issue3/F170308.htm

Ho, C. L., & Walton, D. S. (2004). Primary congenital glaucoma: 2004 update. *Journal of Pediatric Ophthalmology and Strabismus, 41,* 271–288.

Irwin, J. (2006). Basic anatomy and physiology of the ear. In V. E. Newton & P. J. Vallely (Eds.), *Infection and Hearing Impairment.* Hoboken, NJ: John Wiley & Sons Ltd.

Kaye, C. I., & The Committee on Genetics. (2006). Newborn screening fact sheets. *Pediatrics, 118,* 934–963.

KidsHealth. (2009a). *Middle ear infections and ear tube surgery.* Retrieved October 17, 2011 from http://kidshealth.org/parent/medical/ears/ear_infections.html?tracking=P_RelatedArticle#

KidsHealth. (2009b). *Swimmer's ear.* Retrieved October 17, 2011 from http://kidshealth.org/parent/infections/ear/swimmer_ear.html#

Lighthouse International. (2011). *Childhood causes of blindness, worldwide.* Retrieved October 17, 2011 from http://www.lighthouse.org/about-low-vision-blindness/causes-of-blindness/

Natal, B. L., & Chao, J. H. (2011). Emergent management of acute otitis media. Retrieved October 17, 2011 from http://www.emedicine.com/emerg/topic351.htm

Ohnsman, C. M. (2007). Exclusion of students with conjunctivitis from school: Policies of state departments of health. *Journal of Pediatric Ophthalmology and Strabismus, 44*(2), 101–105.

Optometrists Network. (2010). *Strabismus.* Retrieved October 17, 2011 from http://www.strabismus.org/

Ruben, J. R. (2003). *Vision testing in children: An interactive primer.* Retrieved June 7, 2010 from http://www.aapos.org

Sheppard, J. (2008). Keeping an eye on topical ocular antibiotics in the age of bacterial resistance. *Contemporary Pediatrics, 25*(Suppl. 7), 2–5.

Taketokmo, C. K., Hodding, J. H., & Kraus, D. M. (2010). *Lexi-comp's pediatric dosage handbook* (17th ed.). Hudson, OH: Lexi-comp.

Tingley, D. H. (2007). Vision screening essentials: Screening today for eye disorders in the pediatric patient. *Pediatrics in Review, 28*(2), 54–61; retrieved May 24, 2010 from http://pedsinreview.aappublications.org/content/28/2/54.extract

Turk, C., Williams, A. L., & Lasky, R. E. (2009). A randomized clinical trial evaluating silicone earplugs for very low birth weight newborns in intensive care. *Journal of Perinatology, 29*(5), 358–363.

Turner, A., & Rabiu, M. (2006). Patching for corneal abrasion. *Cochrane Database of Systematic Reviews,* Issue 2, article No: CD004764.

U.S. Food and Drug Administration. (2010). *FDA safety notification: Risk of eye and skin injuries from high-powered, hand-held lasers used for pointing or entertainment.* Retrieved October 17, 2011 from http://www.fda.gov/MedicalDevices/Safety/AlertsandNotices/ucm237129.htm

van de Pol, C. (2009). *Basic anatomy and physiology of the human visual system.* Retrieved October 17, 2011 from http://www.usaarl.army.mil/publications/HMD_Book09/files/Section%2013%20%20Chapter%206%20Anatomy%20and%20Structure%20of%20the%20Eye.pdf

Verma, R. P., Sridhar, S., & Spitzer, A. R. (2003). Continuing care of NICU graduates. *Clinical Pediatrics, 42*(4), 299–315.

Watkinson, S., & Graham, S. (2005). Visual impairment in children. *Nursing Standard, 19*(51), 58–65.

Weber, J., & Kelley, J. H. (2010). *Health assessment in nursing* (4th ed.). Philadelphia: Lippincott Williams & Wilkins.

Yoon, P. J., Kelley, P. E., & Friedman, N. R. (2011). Ear, nose, & throat. In W. W. Hay, M. J. Levin, J. M. Sondheimer, & R. R. Deterding (Eds.), *Current pediatric diagnosis and treatment* (20th ed.). New York: McGraw-Hill.

Zoltan, T. B., Taylor, K. S., & Achar, S. A. (2005). Health issues for surfers. *American Family Physician, 71*(12), 2313–2317.

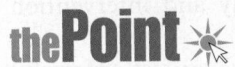

thePoint For additional learning materials, including Internet Resources, visit **http://thePoint.lww.com/Chow1e.**

CHAPTER WORKSHEET

MULTIPLE CHOICE QUESTIONS

1. Which situation would cause the nurse to become concerned about possible hearing loss?

   a. A 12-month-old who babbles incessantly, making no sense

   b. An 8-month-old who says only "da"

   c. A 3-month-old who startles easily to sound

   d. A 3-year-old who drops the letter "s"

2. A 4-year-old complains of extreme pain when the tragus is touched. Though not diagnostic, this sign is most indicative of which disorder?

   a. Acute otitis media

   b. Acute tympanic effusion

   c. Otitis interna

   d. Otitis externa

3. The nurse is caring for an infant who has undergone surgery for infantile glaucoma. What is the priority nursing intervention?

   a. Place the child prone postoperatively for comfort.

   b. Teach the family about use of the contact lens.

   c. Place elbow restraints on the infant.

   d. Provide a mobile for optical stimulation.

4. A 2-year-old with strabismus has been prescribed eye patching for 6 hours per day. What teaching does the nurse provide for the mother?

   a. Try to patch 6 hours per day, but if you miss some it is OK.

   b. Patching is necessary to strengthen vision in the weaker eye.

   c. Patching will keep the eye from turning in.

   d. Since the child is so young, patching can be delayed until school age.

CRITICAL THINKING EXERCISES

1. A 16-month-old toddler is being seen for his sixth ear infection. What particular information about his growth and development must the nurse ask about? Be specific about the questions you would ask.

2. How would you distinguish allergic conjunctivitis from acute bacterial conjunctivitis?

3. A 13-month-old has been diagnosed with severe visual impairment. Develop a list of sample nursing diagnoses for this situation.

STUDY ACTIVITIES

1. Develop a sample plan for teaching a low-literacy parent about the etiology, treatment, and complications of recurrent acute otitis media.

2. While in the pediatric clinical setting, compare the play styles of a sighted child with those of a visually impaired child.

3. Research hearing and vision resources in your local community.

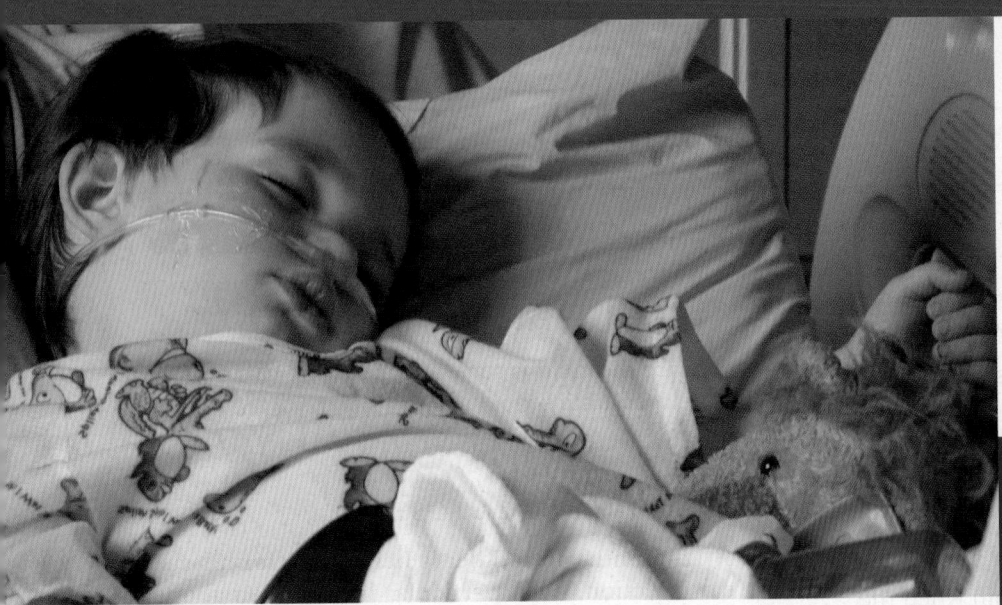

CHAPTER 39

Adapted by Jannell A. Plouffe

NURSING CARE OF THE CHILD WITH A RESPIRATORY DISORDER

KEY TERMS

atelectasis	inspiration	rhinorrhea
atopy	laryngitis	stridor
clubbing	oxygenation	subglottic stenosis
coryza	pharyngitis	suctioning
cyanosis	pulmonary	tachypnea
expiration	pulse oximetry	tracheostomy
hypoxemia	rales	ventilation
hypoxia	retractions	wheezing
infiltrate	rhinitis	work of breathing

LEARNING OBJECTIVES

Upon completion of the chapter, the learner will be able to:

1. Compare how the anatomy and physiology of the respiratory system in children differs from that of adults.
2. Identify various factors associated with respiratory illness in infants and children.
3. Discuss common laboratory and other diagnostic tests useful in the diagnosis of respiratory conditions.
4. Discuss common medications and other treatments used for treatment and palliation of respiratory conditions.
5. Recognize risk factors associated with various respiratory disorders.
6. Distinguish different respiratory illnesses based on the signs and symptoms associated with them.
7. Discuss nursing interventions commonly used for respiratory illnesses.
8. Devise an individualized nursing care plan for the child with a respiratory disorder.
9. Develop patient/family teaching plans for the child with a respiratory disorder.
10. Describe the psychosocial impact of chronic respiratory disorders on children.

Alexander Roberts, 4 months old, is brought to the clinic by his mother. He presents with a cold and has been coughing a great deal for 2 days. Today he has had difficulty taking the bottle and is breathing very quickly. Mrs. Roberts says he seems tired.

Wow

Restoring a full breath allows a child to participate fully in life's adventures.

Respiratory disorders are the most common causes of illness and hospitalization in children. These illnesses range from mild, non-acute disorders (such as the common cold or sore throat), to acute disorders (such as bronchiolitis), to chronic conditions (such as asthma), to serious life-threatening conditions (such as epiglottitis). Chronic disorders, such as allergic rhinitis, can affect quality of life, but frequent acute or recurrent infections also can interfere significantly with quality of life for some children.

Respiratory infections account for the majority of acute illness in children (Brady, 2009). The child's age, pre-existing health status, living conditions, and the season of the year can influence the etiology of respiratory disorders as well as the course of illness. For example, infants are more likely to deteriorate quickly than older children. Lower socioeconomic status dictates the conditions of the home environment and nutritional status and places children at higher risk for increased severity or frequency of disease (Quinn, Kaufman, Siddiqi, & Yeats, 2010). Certain viruses have increased prevalence in the winter, whereas allergen-related respiratory diseases are more prevalent in the spring and fall. Children with chronic illness such as diabetes, congenital heart disease, neuromuscular disorders, and cystic fibrosis tend to be more severely affected with respiratory disorders. Parents might have difficulty in determining the severity of their child's condition and may seek care in the very early or mild phase of the illness or they may wait, presenting to the health care setting at a late stage when the child is very ill.

Nurses must be familiar with respiratory conditions affecting children in order to provide guidance and support to families. When children become ill, families often encounter nurses in out-patient settings first. Nurses must be able to ask questions to determine the severity of the child's illness and whether they must seek care at a health facility. Since respiratory illness accounts for the majority of pediatric hospital admissions, nurses caring for children require expert assessment and intervention skills in this area. Early detection of worsening respiratory status allows for timely treatment and the possibility of preventing a minor problem from becoming a critical illness. Difficulty with breathing can be very frightening for both the child and parents. The child and the family need the nurse's support throughout the course of a respiratory illness.

Nurses are also in the unique position of being able to have a significant impact upon the burden of respiratory illness in children by the appropriate identification of, education about, and encouragement of prevention of respiratory illnesses.

Variations in Pediatric Anatomy and Physiology

Respiratory conditions often affect both the upper and lower respiratory tract, though some affect primarily one or the other. Respiratory dysfunction in children tends to be more severe than in adults. Several differences in the infant's or child's respiratory system account for the increased severity of these diseases in children compared with adults. See Figure 39.1.

Nose

Newborns are obligatory nose breathers until at least 4 weeks of age. The young infant cannot automatically open his or her mouth to breathe if the nose is obstructed, which can lead to apnea or cessation of respiration. The nares must be patent for breathing to allow the infant to be successful while feeding. Newborns breathe through their mouths only while crying.

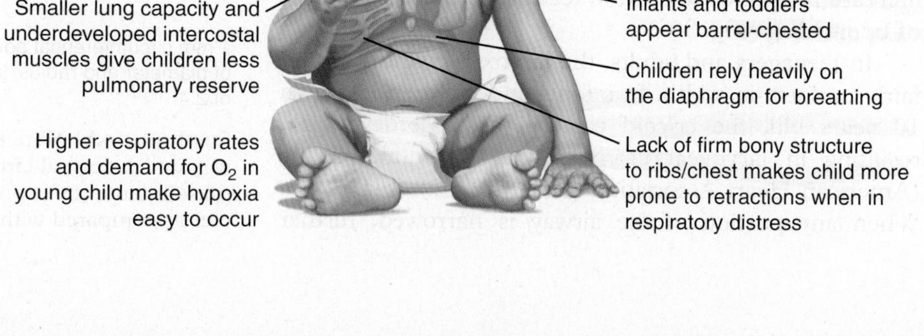

Infants up to 4-6 weeks are obligate nose breathers

The tongue is larger in proportion to the mouth, making airway obstruction more likely in unconscious child

Smaller lung capacity and underdeveloped intercostal muscles give children less pulmonary reserve

Higher respiratory rates and demand for O_2 in young child make hypoxia easy to occur

Airway is smallest at the cricoid in children younger than 8 years

Smaller, narrower airway; make children more susceptible to airway obstruction and respiratory distress

Infants and toddlers appear barrel-chested

Children rely heavily on the diaphragm for breathing

Lack of firm bony structure to ribs/chest makes child more prone to retractions when in respiratory distress

FIGURE 39.1 Developmental and biological variances in the respiratory system.

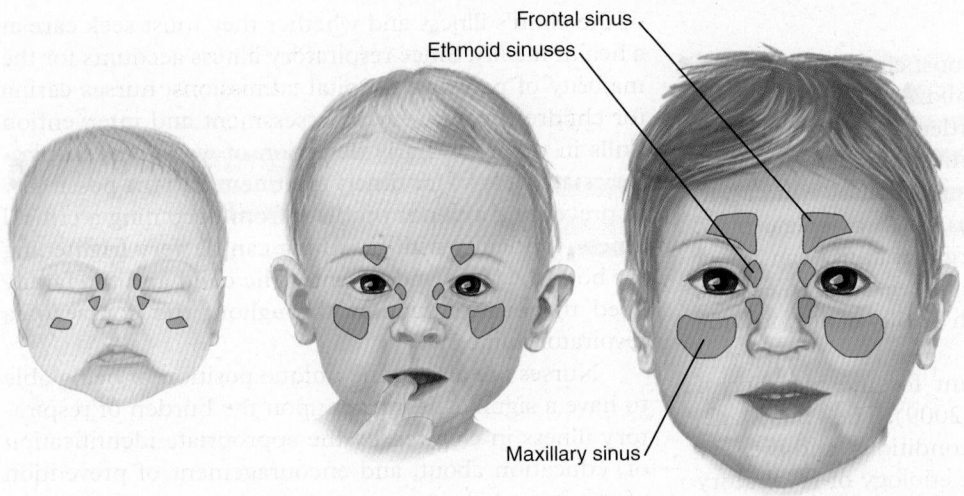

Frontal sinus
Ethmoid sinuses
Maxillary sinus

FIGURE 39.2 Development of the frontal, ethmoid, and maxilliary sinuses.

The upper respiratory mucus serves as a cleansing agent, yet newborns produce very little mucus, making them more susceptible to infection. However, the newborn and young infant may have very small nasal passages, so excess mucus can cause partial or complete airway obstruction.

Infants are born with maxillary and ethmoid sinuses present. The frontal sinuses (most often associated with sinus infection) and the sphenoid sinuses develop by age 6 to 8 years, so younger children are less apt to acquire sinus infections than adults. See Figure 39.2.

Throat

The tongue of the infant relative to the oropharynx is larger than in adults. Posterior displacement of the tongue can quickly lead to severe airway obstruction; this can be accentuated by the infant lying supine. Through early school age, children tend to have enlarged tonsillar and adenoidal tissue even in the absence of illness. This can contribute to an increased likelihood of airway obstruction when the tonsils become enlarged.

Trachea

The airway lumen is smaller in infants and children than in adults. The infant's trachea is approximately 4 mm wide compared with the adult width of 20 mm. When edema, mucus, or bronchospasm is present, the capacity for air passage is greatly diminished. A small reduction in the diameter of the pediatric airway can significantly increase resistance to airflow, leading to increased **work of breathing** (Fig. 39.3).

In teenagers and adults, the larynx is cylindrical and fairly uniform in width. In infants and children less than 10 years old, the cricoid cartilage is underdeveloped, resulting in laryngeal narrowing and a funnel shape (American Heart Association [AHA], 2007) (Fig. 39.4). When any portion of the airway is narrowed, further

narrowing from mucus or edema will result in an exponential increase in resistance to airflow and work of breathing. In infants and children, the larynx and glottis are placed higher in the neck, increasing the chance of aspiration of foreign material into the lower airways. Congenital laryngomalacia occurs in some infants and results in the laryngeal structure having increased pliability due to structural weakness, yielding greater collapse on **inspiration**. Box 39.1 gives details related to congenital laryngomalacia.

The child's airway is highly compliant, making it quite susceptible to dynamic collapse in the presence of airway obstruction (AHA, 2007). The muscles supporting the airway are less functional than those in the adult. Children

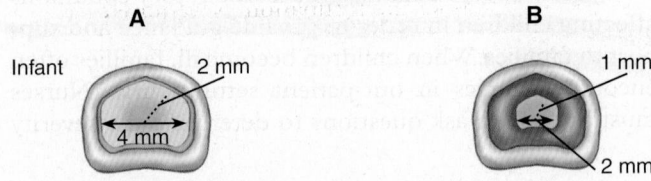

A Infant — 2 mm — 4 mm

B 1 mm — 2 mm

1 mm circumferential edema causes 50% reduction of diameter and radius, increasing pulmonary resistance by a factor of 16.

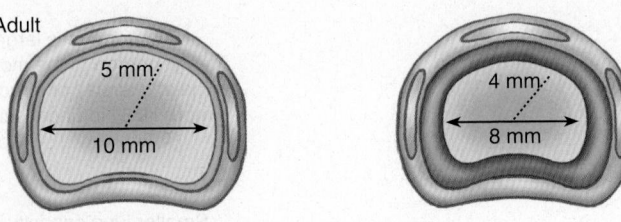

Adult — 5 mm — 10 mm — 4 mm — 8 mm

1 mm circumferential edema causes 20% reduction of diameter and radius, increasing pulmonary resistance by a factor of 2.4.

FIGURE 39.3 (**A**) Note the smaller diameter of the child's airway under normal circumstances. (**B**) With 1 cm of edema present, note the exponential decrease in airway lumen diameter as compared with the adult.

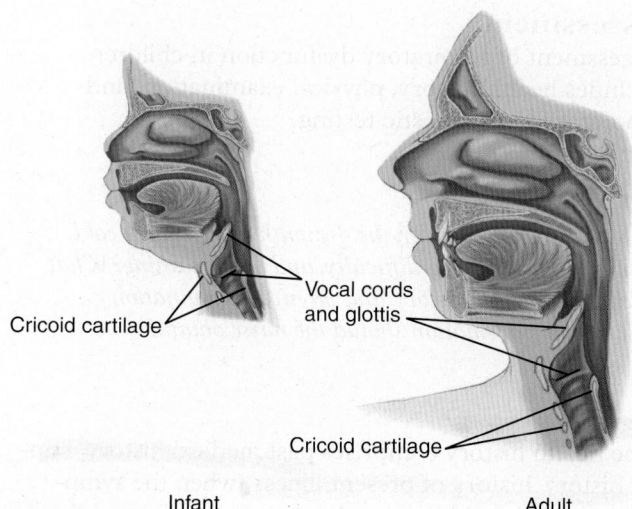

Cricoid cartilage

Vocal cords
and glottis

Cricoid cartilage

Infant   Adult

FIGURE 39.4 Differences in the upper airway between a child and an adult.

have a large amount of soft tissue surrounding the trachea, and the mucous membranes lining the airway are less securely attached compared with adults. This increases the risk for airway edema and obstruction. Upper airway obstruction resulting from a foreign body, croup, or epiglottitis can result in tracheal collapse during inspiration.

Lower Respiratory Structures

The bifurcation of the trachea occurs at the level of the third thoracic vertebra (T3) in children, compared with the level of the sixth thoracic vertebra in adults. This anatomic difference is important when suctioning children and when endotracheal intubation is required (AHA,

---

BOX 39.1 Congenital Laryngomalacia

- Inspiratory stridor is present and is intensified with certain positions.
- Suprasternal retractions may be present, but the infant exhibits no other signs of respiratory distress.
- Congenital laryngomalacia is generally a benign condition that improves as the cartilage in the larynx matures. It usually disappears by age 1 year.
- The crowing noise heard with breathing can make parents very anxious. Reassure parents that the condition will improve with time.
- Parents become very familiar with the "normal" sound their infant makes and are often able to identify intensification or change in the stridor. Airway obstruction may occur earlier in infants with this condition, so intensification of stridor or symptoms of respiratory illness should be evaluated early by the primary care provider.

2007) (see Chapter 52 for further discussion). This difference also contributes to risk for aspiration of foreign bodies or gastric contents. The bronchi and bronchioles of infants and children are also narrower in diameter than the adult's, placing them at increased risk for lower airway obstruction (see Fig. 39.3). Lower airway obstruction during exhalation often results from bronchiolitis or asthma or foreign body aspiration into the lower airway.

Alveoli develop by approximately 24 weeks' gestation, to a level that sustains extrauterine life, but with not without ventilator support. Term infants are born with about 50 million alveoli. After birth, alveolar growth slows until 3 months of age and then progresses until the child reaches 7 or 8 years of age, at which time the alveoli reach the adult number of around 300 million. Alveoli make up most of the lung tissue and are the major sites for gas exchange. Oxygen moves from the alveolar air to the blood, while carbon dioxide moves from the blood into the alveolar air. Smaller numbers of alveoli, particularly in the premature and/or young infant, place the child at a higher risk for **hypoxemia** and carbon dioxide retention as there are fewer overall gas exchange units.

Chest Wall

In older children and adults the ribs and sternum support the lungs and help keep them well expanded. The movement of the diaphragm and intercostal muscles alters volume and pressure within the chest cavity, resulting in air movement into the lungs. Infants' chest walls are highly compliant (pliable); in diseased states, when respiratory effort is increased to meet metabolic needs, retractions are visible. Functional residual capacity can be greatly reduced if either respiratory effort is diminished or work of breathing increases, since retractions decrease the aspiratory volume as the chest wall collapses decreasing the lung volume. This lack of lung support also makes the tidal volume of infants and toddlers almost completely dependent upon movement of the diaphragm. If diaphragm movement is impaired (as in states of hyperinflation such as asthma), the intercostal muscles cannot lift the chest wall and respiration is further compromised.

Metabolic Rate and Oxygen Need

Children have a significantly higher metabolic rate than adults. Their resting respiratory rates are faster and their demand for oxygen is higher. Adult oxygen consumption is 3 to 4 L/min, while infants consume 6 to 8 L/min. In any situation of respiratory distress, infants and children will develop hypoxemia more rapidly than adults (AHA, 2007). This may be attributed not only to the child's increased oxygen requirement but also to the effect that certain conditions have on the oxyhemoglobin dissociation curve.

Normal oxygen transport relies upon binding of oxygen to hemoglobin in areas of high pO_2 (pulmonary arterial beds) and release of oxygen from hemoglobin

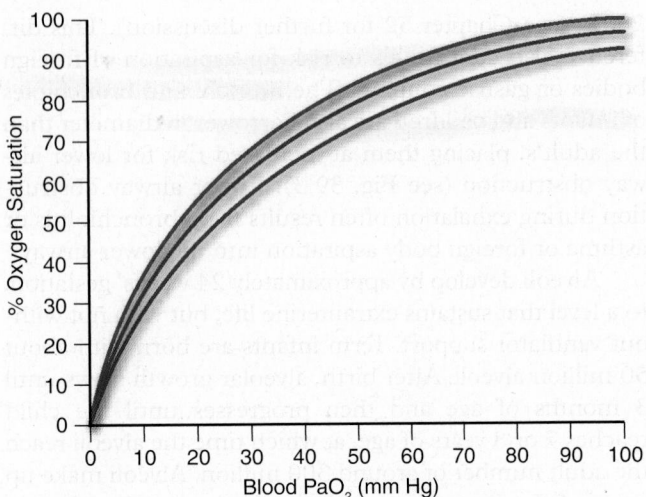

FIGURE 39.5 Normal hemoglobin dissociation curve (*green*), shift to the right (*red*), and shift to the left (*black*).

when the pO_2 is low (peripheral tissues). Normally, a pO_2 of 95 mm Hg results in an oxygen saturation of 97%. A decrease in oxygen saturation results in a disproportionate (much larger) decrease in pO_2 (Fig. 39.5). Thus, a small decrease in oxygen saturation is reflective of a larger decrease in pO_2. Conditions such as alkalosis, hypothermia, hypocarbia, anemia, and fetal hemoglobin cause oxygen to become more tightly bound to hemoglobin, resulting in the curve shifting to the left. Conditions common to pediatric respiratory disorders such as acidosis, hyperthermia, and hypercarbia cause hemoglobin to decrease its affinity for oxygen, further shifting the curve to the right, meaning that oxygen is more readily released to the tissues for cellular functions.

Common Medical Treatments

A variety of interventions are used to treat respiratory illness in children. The treatments listed in Common Medical Treatments 39.1 and Drug Guide 39.1 usually require a physician's order when a child is hospitalized.

NURSING PROCESS OVERVIEW FOR THE CHILD WITH A RESPIRATORY DISORDER

Care of the child with a respiratory disorder includes assessment, nursing diagnosis, planning, interventions, and evaluation. There are a number of general concepts related to the nursing process that can be applied to respiratory disorders. From a general understanding of the care involved for a child with respiratory dysfunction, the nurse can then individualize the care based on client specifics.

Assessment

Assessment of respiratory dysfunction in children includes health history, physical examination, and laboratory or diagnostic testing.

Remember Alexander, the 4-month-old with the cold, cough, fatigue, feeding difficulty, and fast breathing? What additional health history and physical examination assessment information should the nurse obtain?

Health History

The health history comprises past medical history, family history, history of present illness (when the symptoms started and how they have progressed) as well as medications and treatments used at home. The past medical history might be significant for recurrent colds or sore throats, allergies, **atopy** (such as asthma or atopic dermatitis), prematurity, respiratory dysfunction at birth, poor weight gain, or history of recurrent respiratory illnesses, or chronic lung disease. Family history might be significant for chronic respiratory disorders such as asthma or might reveal contacts for infectious exposure. When eliciting the history of the present illness, inquire about onset and progression, fever, nasal congestion, noisy breathing, presence and description of cough, rapid respirations, increased work of breathing, ear, nose, sinus, or throat pain, ear pulling, headache, vomiting with coughing, poor feeding, and lethargy. Also inquire about exposure to secondhand smoke. Children exposed to environmental smoke have an increased incidence of respiratory illnesses such as asthma, bronchitis, and pneumonia (Wipfli et al., 2008).

Physical Examination

Physical examination of the respiratory system includes inspection and observation, auscultation, percussion, and palpation.

Inspection and Observation

Colour. Observe the child's colour, noting pallor or cyanosis (circumoral or central). Pallor (pale appearance) occurs as a result of peripheral vasoconstriction in an effort to conserve oxygen for vital functions. **Cyanosis** (a bluish tinge to the skin) occurs as a result of **hypoxia**. It might first present circumorally (just around the mouth) and progress to central cyanosis. Newborns might have blue hands and feet (acrocyanosis), a normal finding. The infant might have pale hands and feet when cold or when ill, as peripheral circulation is not well developed in early infancy. It is important, then, to note if the cyanosis is central (involving the midline), as this is a true sign of hypoxia. Children with low red blood cell counts might not demonstrate cyanosis as early in the

COMMON MEDICAL TREATMENTS 39.1   RESPIRATORY DISORDERS

Treatment	Explanation	Indication	Nursing Implications
Oxygen	Supplemented via mask, nasal cannula, hood, or tent or via endotracheal or nasotracheal tube	Hypoxemia, respiratory distress	Monitor response via work of breathing and pulse oximetry.
High humidity	Addition of moisture to inspired air	Common cold, croup, tonsillectomy	Infant may require extra blankets with cool mist, and frequent changes of bedclothes under oxygen hood or tent as they become damp.
Suctioning	Removal of secretions via bulb syringe or suction catheter	Excessive airway secretions (common cold, flu, bronchiolitis, pertussis)	Should be done carefully and only as far as recommended for age or tracheostomy tube size, or until cough or gag occurs
Chest physiotherapy (CPT) and postural drainage	Promotes mucus clearance by mobilizing secretions with the assistance of percussion or vibration accompanied by postural drainage (see Chapter 34 for more information about CPT and postural drainage)	Bronchiolitis, pneumonia, cystic fibrosis, or other conditions resulting in increased mucus production. Not effective in inflammatory conditions without increased mucus.	May be performed by respiratory therapist in some institutions, by nurses in others. In either case, nurses must be familiar with the technique and able to educate families on its use.
Saline gargles	Relieves throat pain via salt water gargle	Pharyngitis, tonsillitis	Recommended for children old enough to understand the concept of gargling (to avoid choking)
Saline lavage	Normal saline introduced into the airway, followed by suctioning	Common cold, flu, bronchiolitis, any condition resulting in increased mucus production in the upper airway	Very helpful for loosening thick mucus; child may need to be in semi-upright position to avoid aspiration
Chest tube	Insertion of a drainage tube into the pleural cavity to facilitate removal of air or fluid and allow full lung expansion	Pneumothorax, empyema	Should tube become dislodged from container, the chest tube must be clamped immediately to avoid further air entry in to the chest cavity.
Bronchoscopy	Introduction of a bronchoscope into the bronchial tree for diagnostic purposes. Also allows for bronchiolar lavage.	Removal of foreign body, cleansing of bronchial tree	Watch for postprocedure airway swelling, complaints of sore throat.

course of hypoxemia as children with normal hemoglobin levels. Therefore, absence of cyanosis or the degree of cyanosis present is not always an accurate indication of the severity of respiratory involvement.

▶ *Take NOTE!*

Note the rate and depth of respiration as well as work of breathing. Often the first sign of respiratory illness in infants and children is **tachypnea.**

▶ *Take NOTE!*

A slow or irregular respiratory rate in an acutely ill infant or child is an ominous sign (AHA, 2007). See Chapter 52.

Nose and Oral Cavity. Inspect the nose and oral cavity. Note nasal drainage and redness or swelling in the nose. Note the colour of the pharynx, presence of exudates, tonsil size and status, and presence of lesions anywhere within the oral cavity.

(text continues on page 1264)

DRUG GUIDE 39.1   COMMON DRUGS FOR RESPIRATORY DISORDERS

Medication	Action	Indication	Nursing Implications
Expectorant (guaifenesin)	Reduces viscosity of thickened secretions by increasing respiratory tract fluid	Common cold, pneumonia, other conditions requiring mobilization and subsequent expectoration of mucus	Encourage deep breathing before coughing in order to mobilize secretions. Maintain adequate fluid intake. Assess breath sounds frequently. Only suitable in older children.
Cough suppressants (dextromethorphan, codeine, hydrocodone)	Relieves irritating, nonproductive cough by direct effect on the cough centre in the medulla, which suppresses the cough reflex	Common cold, sinusitis, pneumonia, bronchitis	Should be used only with non-productive coughs in the absence of wheezing. Not recommended in children less than 2 years and caution in all pediatrics.
Antihistamines	Treatment of allergic conditions	Allergic rhinitis, asthma	May cause drowsiness or dry mouth
Antibiotics (oral, parenteral)	Treatment of bacterial infections of the respiratory tract	Pharyngitis, tonsillitis, sinusitis, bacterial pneumonia, cystic fibrosis, empyema, abscess, tuberculosis	Check for antibiotic allergies. Should be given as prescribed for the length of time prescribed.
Antibiotics (inhaled)	Treatment of bacterial infections of the respiratory tract	Used in cystic fibrosis	Can be given via nebulizer
Beta$_2$ adrenergic agonists (short-acting) (i.e., albuterol, levalbuterol)	May be administered orally or via inhalation. Relax airway smooth muscle, resulting in bronchodilation. Inhaled agents result in fewer systemic side effects.	Acute and chronic treatment of wheezing and bronchospasm in asthma, bronchiolitis, cystic fibrosis, chronic lung disease. Prevention of wheezing in exercise-induced asthma.	Can be used for acute relief of bronchospasm. May cause nervousness, tachycardia and jitteriness
Beta$_2$ adrenergic agonists (long-acting) (i.e., salmeterol)	Administered via inhalation. Long-acting bronchodilator does not produce an acute effect so should not be used for an asthma attack.	Long-term control in chronic asthma. Prevention of exercise-induced asthma.	Used only for long-term control or for exercise-induced asthma. Not for relief of bronchospasm in an acute wheezing episode.
Racemic epinephrine	Produces bronchodilation	Croup, bronchiolitis	Assess lung sounds and work of breathing. Observe for rebound bronchospasm. Score pre- and post-mask to determine effectiveness.
Anticholinergic (ipratropium)	Administered via inhalation to produce bronchodilation without systemic effects	Chronic or acute treatment of wheezing in asthma and chronic lung disease	In children, generally used as an adjunct to beta$_2$ adrenergic agonists for treatment of bronchospasm
Antiviral agents (amantadine, rimantadine, zanamivir, oseltamivir)	Treatment and prevention of influenza A	Influenza A, H1N1 influenza	Amantadine, rimantadine: monitor for confusion, nervousness, and jitteriness. Zanamivir, oseltamivir: well tolerated but expensive

Medication	Action	Indication	Nursing Implications
Corticosteroids (inhaled)	Exert a potent, locally acting anti-inflammatory effect to decrease the frequency and severity of asthma attacks. May also delay pulmonary damage that occurs with chronic asthma.	Maintenance program for asthma, chronic lung disease. Acute treatment of croup syndromes.	Not for treatment of acute wheezing. Rinse mouth after inhalation to decrease incidence of fungal infections, dry mouth, and hoarseness. Minimal systemic absorption makes inhaled steroids the treatment of choice for asthma maintenance program.
Corticosteroids (oral, parenteral)	Suppress inflammation and normal immune response. Very effective, but long-term or chronic use can result in peptic ulceration, altered growth, and numerous other side effects.	Treatment of acute exacerbations of asthma or wheezing with chronic lung disease. Acute treatment of severe croup.	May cause hyperglycemia. May suppress reaction to allergy tests. Consult physician if vaccinations are ordered during course of systemic corticosteroid therapy. Short courses of therapy are generally safe. Children on long-term dosing should have growth assessed. If child suffers an acute illness after steroid therapy attention must be taken to assure adequate stress response and may necessitate a serum cortisol serum level be obtained
Decongestants (e.g., pseudoephedrine)	Treatment of runny or stuffy nose	Common cold, limited but possible usefulness in sinusitis and allergic rhinitis	Assess child periodically for nasal congestion. Some children react to decongestants with excessive sleepiness or increased activity. Caution should be utilized as decongestants have been shown to pose risk in pediatric populations.
Leukotriene receptor antagonists (montelukast, zafirlukast, zileuton)	Decrease inflammatory response by antagonizing the effects of leukotrienes (which mediate the effects of airway edema, smooth muscle constriction, altered cellular activity)	Long-term control of asthma in children age 1 year and older. Montelukast: for allergic rhinitis in children 6 months and older. Decreases the duration of cough post bronchiolitis infection and emergency room or seeking help from health care providers.	Given once daily, in the evening. Not for relief of bronchospasm during an acute wheezing episode, but may be continued during the episode.
Mast-cell stabilizers (cromolyn, nedocromil)	Administered via inhalation. Prevent release of histamine from sensitized mast cells, resulting in decreased frequency and intensity of allergic reactions.	Maintenance program for asthma and chronic lung disease, pre-exposure treatment for allergens	For prophylactic use, not to relieve bronchospasm during an acute wheezing episode. Can be used 10–15 min prior to exposure to allergen, to decrease reaction to allergen.

(continued)

DRUG GUIDE 39.1 COMMON DRUGS FOR RESPIRATORY DISORDERS (continued)

Medication	Action	Indication	Nursing Implications
Methylxanthines (theophylline, aminophylline)	Administered orally or intravenously. To provide for continuous airway relaxation. Sustained-release oral preparation can be used to prevent nocturnal symptoms. Requires serum level monitoring.	Used rarely in current-day practice. Used late in the course of treatment for moderate or severe asthma in order to achieve long-term control. Also indicated for apnea of prematurity (see "Caffeine").	Monitor drug levels routinely. Report signs of toxicity immediately: tachycardia, nausea, vomiting, diarrhea, stomach cramps, anorexia, confusion, headache, restlessness, flushing, increased urination, seizures, arrhythmias, insomnia.
Caffeine	Stimulates the respiratory centre	Apnea of prematurity	See "Methylxanthines."
Pulmozyme (dornase alfa)	Enzyme that hydrolyzes the DNA in sputum, reducing sputum viscosity.	Cystic fibrosis	Monitor for dysphonia and pharyngitis.
Synagis (palivizumab)	Monoclonal antibody used to prevent serious lower respiratory RSV disease	For certain high-risk groups of children	Should be administered monthly during the RSV season. Given intramuscularly only.

Adapted from: Taketokmo, C. K., Hodding, J. H., & Kraus, D. M. (2010). *Lexi-comp's pediatric dosage handbook* (17th ed.). Hudson, OH: Lexi-comp.

Cough and Other Airway Noises. Note the sound of the cough (is it wet, productive, dry and hacking, tight?). If noises associated with breathing are present (grunting, stridor, or audible wheeze) these should also be noted. Grunting occurs on **expiration** and is produced by premature glottic closure. It is an attempt to preserve or increase functional residual capacity and an ominous sign of pending respiratory failure. Grunting might occur with alveolar collapse or loss of lung volume, such as in atelectasis, pneumonia, and pulmonary edema. **Stridor**, a high-pitched, readily audible inspiratory noise, is a sign of upper airway obstruction as the air flowing through the narrowed portion of the airway generates turbulent flow or stridor. Sometimes wheezes can be heard with the naked ear; these are referred to as audible wheezes.

Respiratory Effort. Assess respiratory effort for depth and quality. Is breathing laboured? Does the chest rise and fall equally on both sides? Infants and children with significant nasal congestion may have tachypnea, which usually resolves when the nose is cleared of mucus. Mouth breathing also may occur when a large amount of nasal congestion is present. Increased work of breathing, particularly if associated with restlessness and anxiety, usually indicates lower respiratory involvement. Assess for the presence of nasal flaring, retractions, or head bobbing. Nasal flaring can occur early in the course of respiratory illness and is an effort to inhale greater amounts of oxygen.

Retractions (the inward pulling of soft tissues with respiration) can occur in the intercostal, subcostal, substernal, supraclavicular, or suprasternal regions (Fig. 39.6). Document the severity of the retractions: mild, moderate, or severe. Also note the use of accessory neck muscles. Note the presence of paradoxical breathing (lack of simultaneous chest and abdominal rise with the inspiratory phase; Fig. 39.7). Bobbing of the head with each breath is also a sign of increased respiratory effort.

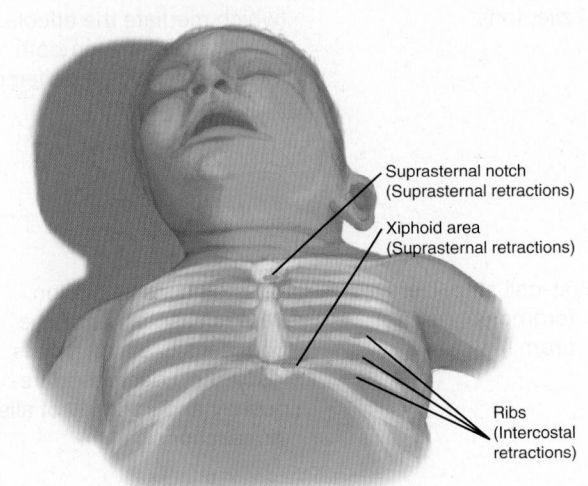

Suprasternal notch (Suprasternal retractions)

Xiphoid area (Suprasternal retractions)

Ribs (Intercostal retractions)

FIGURE 39.6 Location of retractions.

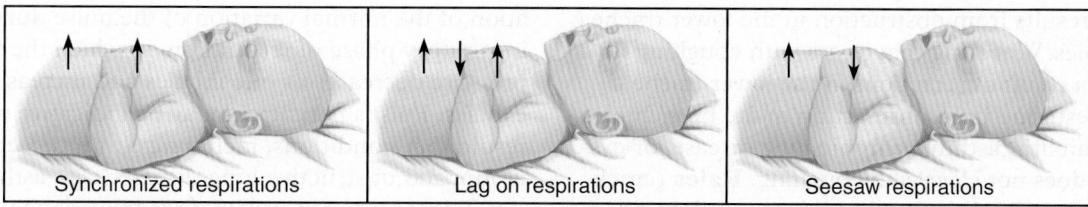

Synchronized respirations | Lag on respirations | Seesaw respirations

FIGURE 39.7 Seesaw respirations.

> ▶ *Take* NOTE!
>
> *Seesaw (or paradoxical) respirations are very ineffective for ventilation and oxygenation. The chest falls on inspiration and rises on expiration. Seesaw respiratory pattern and head bobbing are warning signs of severe respiratory distress and pending respiratory failure.*

Anxiety and Restlessness. Is the child anxious or restless? Restlessness, irritability, and anxiety result from difficulty in securing adequate oxygen. These might be very early signs of respiratory distress, especially if accompanied by tachypnea. Restlessness might progress to listlessness and lethargy if the respiratory dysfunction is not corrected. The change in level of consciousness (obtundation), where the listless infant or child may appear to the unknowing parent as sleeping or just tired is due to an alteration in gas exchange. This alteration is due to carbon dioxide accumulating and or hypoxia occurring to the degree that the brain is not receiving significant oxygen for vital cellular metabolism.

Clubbing. Inspect the fingertips for the presence of **clubbing**, an enlargement of the terminal phalanx of the finger, resulting in a change in the angle of the nail to the fingertip (Fig. 39.8). Clubbing might occur in children with a chronic respiratory illness. It is the result of increased capillary growth as the body attempts to supply more oxygen to distal body cells.

Hydration Status. Note the child's hydration status. The child with a respiratory illness is at risk for dehydration due to increased insensible fluid loss associated with tachypnea and decreased fluid intake. Pain related to sore throat or mouth lesions may prevent the child from drinking properly. Nasal congestion interferes with the infant's ability to suck effectively at the breast or bottle. Tachypnea and increased work of breathing

interfere with the ability to safely ingest fluids, as the tachypnea may pose some degree of an aspiration risk.

Assess the oral mucosa for colour and moisture. Note skin turgor, presence of tears, and adequacy of urine output.

Auscultation

Assess lung sounds via auscultation. Evaluate breath sounds over the anterior and posterior chest, as well as in the axillary areas. Note the adequacy of aeration. Breath sounds should be equal bilaterally. The intensity and pitch should be equal throughout the lungs; document diminished breath sounds. In the absence of concurrent lower respiratory illness, the breath sounds should be clear throughout all lung fields. During normal respiration, the inspiratory phase is usually softer and longer than the expiratory phase.

Prolonged expiration is a sign of bronchial or bronchiolar obstruction. Bronchiolitis, asthma, pulmonary edema, and an intrathoracic foreign body can cause prolonged expiratory phases.

Infants and young children have thin chest walls. When the upper airway is congested (as in a severe cold), the noise produced in the upper airway might be transmitted throughout the lung fields. When upper airway congestion is transmitted to the lung fields, the congested-sounding noise heard over the trachea is the same type of noise heard over the lungs but is much louder and more intense. To ascertain if these sounds are truly adventitious lung sounds or if they are transmitted from the upper airway, auscultate again after the child coughs or his or her nose has been suctioned. Another way to discern the difference is to compare auscultatory findings over the trachea to the lung fields to determine if the abnormal sound is truly from within the lung or is actually a sound transmitted from the upper airway.

Note adventitious sounds heard on auscultation. **Wheezing**, a high-pitched sound that usually occurs on

FIGURE 39.8 **(A)** Normal fingertip. **(B)** Early clubbing. **(C)** Advanced clubbing.

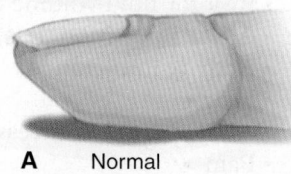 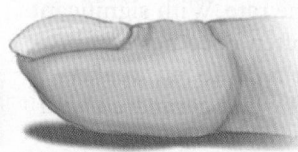 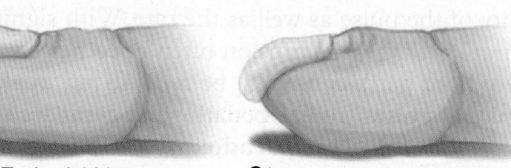

A Normal | **B** Early clubbing | **C** Advanced clubbing

expiration, results from obstruction in the lower trachea or bronchioles. Wheezing that clears with coughing is most likely a result of secretions in the lower trachea. Wheezing resulting from obstruction of the bronchioles, as in bronchiolitis, asthma, chronic lung disease, or cystic fibrosis, does not clear with coughing. **Rales** (crackling sounds) result when the alveoli become fluid-filled, such as in pneumonia or pulmonary edema. Note the location of the adventitious sounds as well as the timing (on inspiration, expiration, or both). Tachycardia might also be present. An increase in heart rate often initially accompanies hypoxemia.

Percussion

When percussing, note sounds that are not resonant in nature. Flat or dull sounds might be percussed over partially consolidated lung tissue, as in pneumonia. Tympany might be percussed with a pneumothorax. Note the presence of hyperresonance (as might be apparent with asthma). Percussion is challenging to perform in children since all the structures are in such close proximity. It is even more challenging in a moving, uncooperative child, and a great deal of skill and practice are required to become proficient.

Palpation

Palpate the sinuses for tenderness in the older child. Assess for enlargement or tenderness of the lymph nodes of the head and neck. Document alterations in tactile fremitus detected on palpation. Increased tactile fremitus might occur in a case of pneumonia or pleural effusion. Fremitus might be decreased in the case of barrel chest, as with cystic fibrosis. Absent fremitus might be noted with pneumothorax or atelectasis. Pneumothorax can lead to **subcutaneous emphysema**, sometimes abbreviated **SCE** or **SE** and also called **tissue emphysema**, which is caused when gas or air is present in the subcutaneous layer of the skin. Subcutaneous refers to the tissue beneath the cutis of the skin, and emphysema refers to trapped air. Since the air generally comes from the chest cavity, subcutaneous emphysema usually occurs on the chest, neck, and face, where it is able to travel from the chest cavity along the fascia. Subcutaneous emphysema has a characteristic crackling feel to the touch, a sensation that has been described as similar to touching crispy rice-type cereal. This sensation of air under the skin is known as subcutaneous crepitation.

Compare central and peripheral pulses. Note the quality of the pulse as well as the rate. With significant respiratory distress, perfusion often becomes compromised. Poor perfusion might be reflected in weaker peripheral pulses (radial, pedal) when compared with central pulses. **Pulsus paradoxus**, also known as **paradoxic pulse** or **paradoxical pulse**, is an exagger-

ation of the normal variation of the pulse during the inspiratory phase of respiration, in which the blood pressure decreases as one inhales and increases as one exhales. Pulsus paradoxus may be indicative of several respiratory conditions, including chronic sleep apnea, croup, and obstructive lung disease (e.g., asthma).

The paradox in pulsus paradoxus is that beats may be detected on cardiac auscultation during inspiration that cannot be palpated at the radial pulse. It results from an accentuated decrease in the blood pressure, which causes the (radial) pulse to not be palpable. As it usually occurs with inspiration, the heart rate may be slightly increased due to decreased cardiac output.

Laboratory and Diagnostic Testing

Common Laboratory and Diagnostic Tests 39.1 explains the laboratory and diagnostic tests most commonly used for a child with a respiratory disorder. The tests can assist the physician or nurse practitioner in diagnosing the disorder and/or be used as guidelines in determining ongoing treatment. Laboratory or non-nursing personnel obtain some of the tests, while the nurse might obtain others. In either instance the nurse should be familiar with how the tests are obtained, what they are used for, and normal versus abnormal results. This knowledge will also be necessary when providing patient and family education related to the testing.

> ▶ *Take NOTE!*
>
> *Ambient light may interfere with pulse oximetry readings. When the pulse oximeter probe is placed on the infant's foot or young child's toe, covering the probe and foot with a sock may help to ensure an accurate measurement (DeMeulenaere, 2007).*

Nursing Diagnoses, Goals, Interventions, and Evaluation

Upon completion of a thorough assessment, the nurse might identify several nursing diagnoses, including:

- Ineffective airway clearance
- Ineffective breathing pattern
- Impaired gas exchange
- Risk for infection
- Pain
- Risk for fluid volume deficit
- Altered nutrition, less than body requirements
- Activity intolerance
- Fear
- Altered family processes
- Pain

COMMON LABORATORY AND DIAGNOSTIC TESTS 39.1   RESPIRATORY DISORDERS

Test	Explanation	Indication	Nursing Implications
Allergy skin testing	Suggested allergen is applied to skin via scratch, pin or prick. A wheal response indicates allergy to the substance. Carries risk of anaphylaxis. (Nursing note: antihistamines must be discontinued before testing, as they inhibit the test.)	Allergic rhinitis, asthma	Close observation for anaphylaxis is necessary. Epinephrine and emergency equipment should be readily available. Some children react to the skin test almost immediately; others take several minutes.
Arterial blood gases	Invasive method (requires blood sampling) of measuring arterial pH, partial pressure of oxygen and carbon dioxide, and base excess in blood	Usually reserved for severe illness, the intubated child, or suspected carbon dioxide retention	Hold pressure for several minutes after a peripheral arterial stick to avoid bleeding. Radial arterial sticks are common and can be very painful. Note if the child is crying excessively during the blood draw, as this affects the carbon dioxide level.
Chest X-ray	Radiographic image of the expanded lungs: can show hyperinflation, atelectasis, pneumonia, foreign body, pleural effusion, abnormal heart or lung size	Bronchiolitis, pneumonia, tuberculosis, asthma, cystic fibrosis, bronchopulmonary dysplasia	Children may be afraid of the X-ray equipment. If a parent or familiar adult can accompany the child, often the child is less afraid. If the child is unable or unwilling to hold still for the X-ray, restraint may be necessary. Restraint should be limited to the amount of time needed for the X-ray.
Fluorescent antibody testing	Determines presence of respiratory syncytial virus (RSV), adenovirus, influenza, parainfluenza or Chlamydia in nasopharyngeal secretions	Bronchiolitis, pneumonia	To obtain a nasopharyngeal specimen instill 1–3 mL of sterile normal saline into one nostril, aspirate the contents using a small sterile bulb syringe, place the contents in sterile container, and immediately send them to the lab.
Fluoroscopy	Radiographic examination that uses a fluorescent screen—"real-time" imaging	Identification of masses, abscesses	Requires the child to lay still. Equipment can be frightening. Children may respond to presence of parent or familiar adult.
Gastric washings for AFB	Determines presence of AFB (acid-fast bacilli) in stomach (children often swallow sputum)	Tuberculosis	Nasogastric tube is inserted and saline is instilled and suctioned out of the stomach for the specimen.
Peak expiratory flow	Measures the maximum flow of air that can be forcefully exhaled in 1 s. Measured in litres per second.	Daily use can indicate adequacy of asthma control.	It is important to establish the child's "personal best" by taking twice-daily readings over a 2-week period while well. The average of these is termed "personal best." Charts based on height and age are also available to determine expected peak expiratory flow.

(continued)

COMMON LABORATORY AND DIAGNOSTIC TESTS 39.1 RESPIRATORY DISORDERS (continued)

Test	Explanation	Indication	Nursing Implications
Pulmonary function tests (PFTs)	Measures respiratory flow and lung volumes	Asthma, cystic fibrosis, chronic lung disease	Usually performed by a respiratory therapist trained to do the full spectrum of tests. Spirometry can be obtained by the trained nurse in the out-patient setting.
Pulse oximetry	Non-invasive method of continuously (or intermittently) measuring oxygen saturation	Can be useful in any situation in which a child is experiencing respiratory distress	Probe must be applied correctly to finger, toe, foot, hand, or ear in order for the machine to appropriately pick up the pulse and oxygen saturation.
Rapid flu test	Rapid test for detection of influenza A or B	Influenza	Should be done in first 24 h of illness so that medication administration can begin. Have the child gargle with sterile normal saline and then spit into a sterile container. Send immediately to the lab.
Rapid strep test	Instant test for presence of strep A antibody in pharyngeal secretions	Pharyngitis, tonsillitis	Results in 5–10 min. Negative tests should be backed up with throat culture.
RAST (radioallergosorbent test)	Measures minute quantities of immunoglobulin E in the blood. Carries no risk of anaphylaxis but is not as sensitive as skin testing.	Asthma (food allergies)	Blood test that is usually sent out to a reference laboratory
Sinus X-rays, computed tomography (CT), or magnetic resonance imaging (MRI)	Radiologic tests that may show sinus involvement	Sinusitis, recurrent colds	X-ray results are usually received more quickly than CT or MRI results.
Sputum culture	Bacterial culture of invasive organisms in the sputum	Pneumonia, cystic fibrosis, tuberculosis	Must be true sputum, not mucus from the mouth or nose. Child can deep breathe, cough, and spit, or specimen may be obtained via suctioning of the artificial airway.
Sweat chloride test	Collection of sweat on filter paper after stimulation of skin with pilocarpine. Measures concentration of chloride in the sweat.	Cystic fibrosis	May be difficult to obtain sweat in a young infant
Throat culture	Bacterial culture (minimum of 24–48 h required) to determine presence of streptococcus A or other bacteria	Pharyngitis, tonsillitis	Can be obtained on separate swab at same time as rapid strep test to decrease trauma to the child (swab both applicators at once). Do not perform immediately after the child has had medication or something to eat or drink.
Tuberculin skin test	Mantoux test (intradermal injection of purified protein derivative)	Tuberculosis, chronic cough	Must be given intradermally; not a valid test if injected incorrectly

Adapted from: Pagana, K. D., & Pagana, T. J. (2010). *Mosby's manual of diagnostic and laboratory tests* (4th ed.). St. Louis, MO: Mosby.

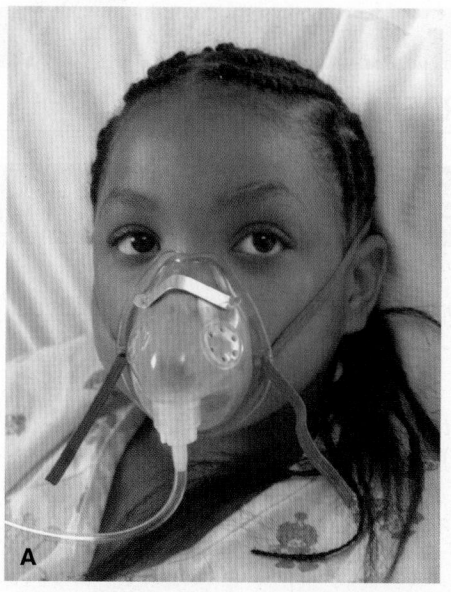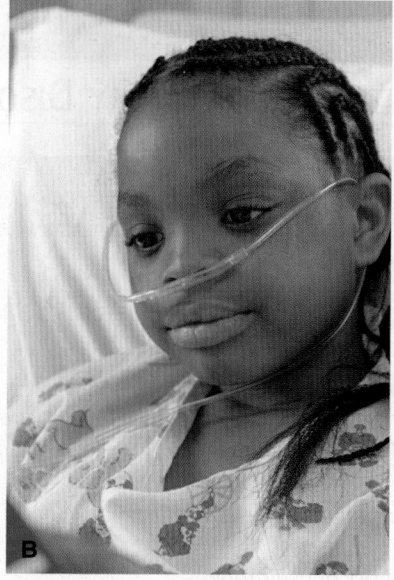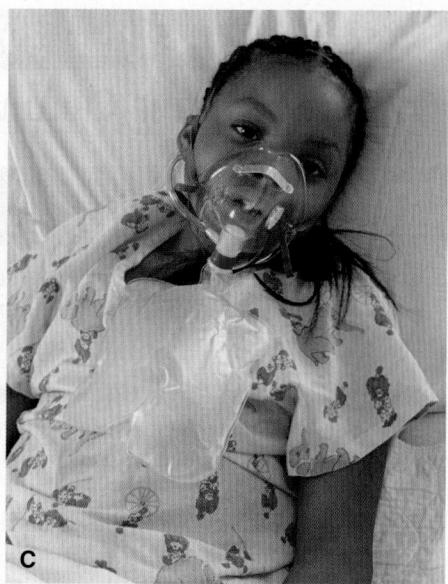

FIGURE 39.9 (**A**) Simple oxygen mask provides about 40% oxygen. (**B**) The nasal cannula provides an additional 4% oxygen per 1 L of oxygen flow (i.e., 1 L will deliver 25% oxygen). (**C**) The nonrebreather mask provides 80% to 100% oxygen.

After completing an assessment of Alexander, the nurse notes the following: lots of clear secretions in the airway, child appears pale, respiratory rate 68, retractions, nasal flaring, wheezing, and diminished breath sounds. Based on these assessment findings, what would your top three nursing diagnoses be for Alexander?

Nursing goals, interventions, and evaluation for the child with a respiratory disorder are based on the nursing diagnoses. Nursing Care Plan 39.1 can be used as a guide in planning nursing care for the child with a respiratory disorder. The nursing care plan should be individualized based on the patient's symptoms and needs; refer to Chapter 35 for detailed information on pain management. Additional information will be included later in the chapter as it relates to specific disorders.

Based on your top three nursing diagnoses for Alexander, describe appropriate nursing interventions.

Oxygen Supplementation

Oxygen may be delivered to the child by a variety of methods (Fig. 39.9). Since oxygen administration is considered a drug, it requires a physician's order, except when following emergency protocols outlined in a health care facility's policies and procedures. Many health care settings develop specific guidelines for oxygen administration that are often coordinated by respiratory therapists, yet the nurse still remains responsible for ensuring that oxygen is administered properly and

assessments are performed to determine the effect of oxygen delivery on the patient.

Oxygen sources include wall-mounted systems as well as cylinders. The supply of oxygen available from a wall-mounted source is limitless, but use of a wall-mounted source restricts the child to the hospital room. Cylinders are portable oxygen tanks; the D-cylinder holds a little less than 400 L of oxygen, and the E-cylinder holds about 650 L of oxygen. Cylinders turn on with a metal key that is kept with the tank. The tank empties relatively quickly if the child requires a high flow of oxygen, so this is not the best oxygen source in an emergency. The cylinder is useful for the child on low-flow oxygen because it allows mobility.

Respiratory therapists usually maintain the respiratory equipment that is found in the emergency room or hospital. However, in an out-patient setting the nurse may be responsible for maintaining respiratory equipment and checking the level of oxygen in the office's oxygen tanks each day.

▶ *Take* NOTE!

Oxygen itself is not a fuel; thus it does not burn on its own. However, oxygen can be extremely dangerous as the application of oxygen to a fire will cause the fire to burn hotter and more vigorously. Post signs ("Oxygen in Use"), and inform the family to avoid matches, lighters, and other flammable or volatile materials and to use only facility-approved equipment during respiratory therapy sessions.

(text continues on page 1272)

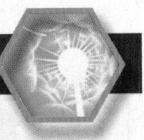

Nursing Care Plan 39.1

OVERVIEW FOR THE CHILD WITH A RESPIRATORY DISORDER

NURSING DIAGNOSIS: Ineffective airway clearance related to inflammation, increased secretions, mechanical obstruction, or pain as evidenced by presence of secretions, productive cough, tachypnea, and increased work of breathing

Outcome Identification and Evaluation

Child will maintain patent airway, *free from secretions or obstruction, easy work of breathing, respiratory rate within parameters for age.*

Interventions: Maintaining a Patent Airway

- Position with airway open (sniffing position if supine): *Open airway allows adequate ventilation.*
- Humidify oxygen or room air and ensure adequate fluid intake (intravenous or oral) *to help liquefy secretions for ease in clearance.*
- Suction with bulb syringe or via nasopharyngeal catheter as needed, particularly prior to bottle-feeding *to promote clearance of secretions.*
- If tachypneic, maintain NPO status *to avoid risk of aspiration.*
- In older child, encourage expectoration of sputum with coughing *to promote airway clearance.*
- Perform chest physiotherapy if ordered *to mobilize secretions.*
- Ensure emergency equipment is readily available *to avoid delay should airway become unmaintainable.*

NURSING DIAGNOSIS: Ineffective breathing pattern related to inflammatory or infectious process as evidenced by tachypnea, increased work of breathing, nasal flaring, retractions, diminished breath sounds

Outcome Identification and Evaluation

Child will exhibit adequate ventilation: *Respiratory rate within parameters for age, easy work of breathing (absence of retractions, accessory muscle use, grunting), clear breath sounds with adequate aeration, oxygen saturation >94% or within prescribed parameters.*

Interventions: Promoting Effective Breathing Patterns

- Assess respiratory rate, breath sounds, and work of breathing frequently *to ensure progress with treatment and so that deterioration can be noted early.*
- Use pulse oximetry to monitor oxygen saturation in the least invasive manner *to note adequacy of oxygenation and ensure early detection of hypoxemia.*
- Position for comfort with open airway and room for lung expansion and use pillows or padding if necessary to maintain position *to ensure optimal ventilation via maximum lung expansion.*
- Administer supplemental oxygen and/or humidity as ordered to *improve oxygenation.*
- Allow for adequate sleep and rest periods *to conserve energy.*
- Administer antibiotics as ordered: *May be indicated in the case of bacterial respiratory infection.*
- Encourage incentive spirometry and coughing with deep breathing (can be accomplished through play) *to maximize ventilation (play enhances the child's participation).*

NURSING DIAGNOSIS: Gas exchange, impaired, related to airway plugging, hyperinflation, atelectasis as evidenced by cyanosis, decreased oxygen saturation, and alterations in arterial blood gases

Outcome Identification and Evaluation

Gas exchange will be adequate: *Pulse oximetry reading on room air is within normal parameters for age, blood gases within normal limits, absence of cyanosis.*

Interventions: Promoting Adequate Gas Exchange

- Administer oxygen as ordered *to improve oxygenation.*
- Monitor oxygen saturation via pulse oximetry *to detect alterations in oxygenation.*
- Encourage clearance of secretions via coughing, expectoration, chest physiotherapy, and suctioning: *Mobilization of secretions may improve gas exchange.*

Nursing Care Plan 39.1 (continued)

- Administer bronchodilators if ordered (albuterol, levalbuterol, and racemic epinephrine) *to treat bronchospasm and improve gas exchange.*
- Provide frequent contact and support to the child and family *to decrease anxiety, which increases the child's oxygen demands.*
- Assess and monitor mental status (confusion, lethargy, restlessness, combativeness): *Hypoxemia can lead to changes in mental status.*

NURSING DIAGNOSIS: Risk for infection related to presence of infectious organisms as evidenced by fever or presence of virus or bacteria on laboratory screening

Outcome Identification and Evaluation
Child will exhibit no signs of secondary infection and will not spread infection to others: *Symptoms of infection decrease over time; others remain free from infection.*

Interventions: Preventing Infection
- Maintain aseptic technique, practice good handwashing, and use disposable suction catheters *to prevent introduction of further infectious agents.*
- Limit number of visitors and screen them for recent illness *to prevent further infection.*
- Administer antibiotics if prescribed *to prevent or treat bacterial infection.*
- Encourage nutritious diet according to child's preferences and ability to feed orally *to assist body's natural infection-fighting mechanisms.*
- Isolate the child as required *to prevent nosocomial spread of infection*
- Teach child and family preventive measures such as good handwashing, covering mouth and nose when coughing or sneezing, adequate disposal of used tissues *to prevent nosocomial or community spread of infection.*

NURSING DIAGNOSIS: Fluid volume deficit, risk for, related to decreased oral intake, insensible losses via fever, tachypnea, or diaphoresis

Outcome Identification and Evaluation
Fluid volume will be maintained: *Oral mucosa moist and pink, skin turgor elastic, urine output at least 1 to 2 mL/kg/hour.*

Interventions: Maintaining Adequate Fluid Volume
- Administer intravenous fluids if ordered to maintain adequate hydration in NPO state.
- When allowed oral intake, encourage oral fluids. Popsicles, favourite fluids, and games can be used *to promote intake.*
- Assess for signs of adequate hydration (elastic skin turgor, moist mucosa, adequate urine output).
- Strict intake and output monitoring *can help identify fluid imbalance.*
- Urine specific gravity, urine and serum electrolytes, blood urea nitrogen, creatinine, and osmolality *are reliable indicators of fluid status.*

NURSING DIAGNOSIS: Nutrition, altered: Less than body requirements related to difficulty feeding as evidenced by poor oral intake, tiring with feeding

Outcome Identification and Evaluation
Child will maintain adequate nutritional intake: *Weight gain or maintenance occurs. Child consumes adequate diet for age.*

Interventions: Promoting Adequate Nutritional Intake
- Weigh on same scale at same time daily: *Weight gain or maintenance can indicate adequate nutritional intake.*
- Calorie counts over a 3-day period *are helpful in determining if caloric intake is sufficient.*
- Assist family and child to choose higher-calorie, protein-rich foods *to optimize growth potential.*
- Coax young children to eat better by playing games and offering favourite foods *resulting in improved intake.*

(continued)

Nursing Care Plan 39.1 (continued)

NURSING DIAGNOSIS: Activity intolerance related to high respiratory demand as evidenced by increased work of breathing and requirement for frequent rest when playing

Outcome Identification and Evaluation
Child will resume normal activity level: *Activity is tolerated without difficulty breathing. Pulse oximetry readings and vital signs within parameters for age and activity level.*

Interventions: Increasing Activity Tolerance
- Provide rest periods balanced with periods of activity. Group nursing activities and visits to allow for sufficient rest. *Activity increases myocardial oxygen demand so must be balanced with rest.*
- Provide small, frequent meals to prevent overtiring (*energy is expended while eating*).
- Encourage quiet activities that do not require exertion *to prevent boredom.*
- Allow gradual increase in activity as tolerated, keeping pulse oximetry reading within normal parameters, *to minimize risk for further respiratory compromise.*

NURSING DIAGNOSIS: Fear related to difficulty breathing, unfamiliar personnel, procedures, and environment (hospital) as evidenced by clinging, crying, fussing, verbalization, or lack of cooperation

Outcome Identification and Evaluation
Fear/anxiety will be reduced: *Decreased episodes of crying or fussing, happy and playful at times.*

Interventions: Relieving Fear
- Establish trusting relationship with child and family *to decrease anxiety and fear.*
- Explain procedures to child at developmentally appropriate level *to decrease fear of unknown.*
- Provide favourite blanket or soft toy to patient, as well as comfort measures preferred by client such as rocking or music *for added security.*
- Involve parents in care *to give child reassurance and decrease fear.*

NURSING DIAGNOSIS: Family processes, altered, related to child's illness or hospitalization as evidenced by family's presence in hospital, missed work, demonstration of inadequate coping

Outcome Identification and Evaluation
Parents demonstrate adequate coping and decreased anxiety: *Parents are involved in child's care, ask appropriate questions and are able to discuss child's care and condition calmly.*

Interventions: Promoting Adequate Family Processes
- Encourage parents' verbalization of concerns related to child's illness: *Allows for identification of concerns and demonstrates to the family that the nurse also cares about them, not just the child.*
- Explain therapy, procedures, and child's behaviour to parents; *developing an understanding of the child's current status helps decrease anxiety.*
- Encourage parental involvement in care *so that parents may continue to feel needed and valued.*

The efficiency of oxygen delivery systems is affected by several variables, including the child's respiratory effort, the litre flow of oxygen delivered, and whether the equipment is being used appropriately. In general, oxygen facemasks come in infant, child, and adult sizes. Select the mask that best fits the child. In addition, ensure that the mask is sealed properly to decrease the amount of oxygen that escapes from the mask. Ensure that the litre flow is set according to the manufacturer's recommendations for use with that particular delivery method. The oxygen flow rate or concentration is usually determined by the physician's order. Whichever method of delivery is used, provide humidification during oxygen delivery to prevent drying of nasal passages and to assist with liquefying secretions. Table 39.1 gives details on oxygen delivery methods.

▶ *Take* NOTE!

Monitor vital signs, colour, respiratory effort, pulse oximetry, and level of consciousness before, during, and after oxygen therapy to evaluate its effectiveness.

TABLE 39.1 OXYGEN DELIVERY METHODS

Delivery Method	Description	Nursing Implications
Simple mask	Provides 35%–60% oxygen with a flow rate of 6–10 L/min. Oxygen delivery percentage affected by respiratory rate, inspiratory flow, and adequacy of mask fit.	• Must maintain oxygen flow rate of at least 6 L/min to maintain inspired oxygen concentration and prevent rebreathing of carbon dioxide • Mask must fit snugly to be effective but should not be so tight as to irritate the face. • Running at a flow rate of less than 5 L may risk rebreathing exhaled air and lead to hypercarbia and respiratory failure.
Venturi mask	Provides 24%–50% oxygen by using a special gauge at the base of the mask that allows mixing of room air with oxygen flow	• Set oxygen flow rate according to percentage of oxygen desired as indicated on the gauge/dial. • As with simple mask, must fit snugly
Nasal cannula	Provides low oxygen concentration (22%–44%) but needs patent nasal passages	• Must be used with humidification to prevent drying and irritation of airways • Can provide very small amounts of oxygen (as low as 25 mL/min) • Maximum recommended litre flow in children is 3 L/min. • Children can eat or talk while on oxygen. • Inspired oxygen concentration affected by mouth breathing • Requires patent nasal passages • Can deliver a high concentration of oxygen in an infant who is an obligatory nose breather due to the small amount of air inspired with each breath. This must be taken into consideration. For example, nasal prongs set at a flow of 2 L of oxygen, is 2,000 mL of oxygen per minute. An infant's volume of ventilation is around 5 mL/kg; thus a 5 kg infant would inspire 25 mL of air per breath. Therefore, with a tight fit of nasal prongs the infant could receive 100% oxygen.
Oxygen tent	Provides high-humidity environment with up to 50% oxygen concentration	• Oxygen level drops when tent is opened. • Must change linen frequently as it becomes damp from the humidity • Secure edges of tent with blankets or by tucking edges under mattress. • Young children may be fearful and resistant. • Mist may interfere with visualization of child inside the tent. • Careful cleaning required to prevent hospital-acquired bacterial infections such as *Pseudomonas*.
Oxygen hood	Provides high concentration (up to 80%–90%) for infants only. Allows easy access to chest and lower body.	• Litre flow must be set at 10–15 L/min. • Good method for infant but need to remove for feeding • Can and should be humidified
Partial rebreathing mask	Simple facemask with an oxygen reservoir bag. Provides 50%–60% oxygen concentration.	• Must set litre flow rate at 10–12 L/min to prevent rebreathing of carbon dioxide • The reservoir bag does not completely empty when child inspires if flow rate is set properly.
Nonrebreathing mask	Simple facemask with valves at the exhalation ports and an oxygen reservoir bag with a valve to prevent exhaled air from entering the reservoir. Provides 95% oxygen concentration.	• Must set litre flow rate at 10–12 L/min to prevent rebreathing of carbon dioxide • The reservoir bag does not completely empty when child inspires if flow rate is set properly.

Adapted from: American Heart Association. (2007). *Pediatric advanced life support provider manual*. Dallas, TX: American Heart Association; and Bowden, V. R., & Greenberg, C. S. (2008). *Pediatric nursing procedures* (2nd ed.). Philadelphia: Lippincott Williams & Wilkins.

Acute Infectious Disorders

Acute infectious disorders include the common cold, sinusitis, influenza, pharyngitis, tonsillitis, laryngitis, pertussis, croup syndromes, respiratory syncytial virus (RSV), pneumonia, and bronchitis.

Common Cold

The common cold is also referred to as a viral upper respiratory infection (URI) or nasopharyngitis. Colds can be caused by a number of different viruses, including rhinoviruses, parainfluenza virus, RSV, enteroviruses, and adenoviruses. Viral particles spread through the air or from person-to-person contact. Colds occur more frequently in winter. The Respiratory Virus Detection Surveillance System reports on respiratory viruses in Canada. Each week, selected laboratories report numbers of tests performed and numbers positive for influenza, RSV, parainfluenza, and adenovirus to the Public Health Agency of Canada (PHAC), Centre for Immunization and Respiratory Infectious Diseases (CIRID). Colds affect children of all ages and have a higher incidence among day care attendees and school-age children (Yoon, Kelley, & Friedman, 2011). It is not unusual for a child to have six to nine colds per year. Spontaneous resolution occurs after about 7 to 10 days. Potential complications include secondary bacterial infections of the ears, throat, sinuses, or lungs.

Therapeutic management of the common cold is directed toward symptom relief. Nasal congestion may be relieved via humidity and use of normal saline nasal wash or spray followed by suctioning. Antihistamines are not indicated, as they dry secretions further. Over-the-counter cold preparations are no longer recommended for use in children (Lokker et al., 2009; Vassilev, Chu, Ruck, Adams, & Marcus, 2009).

Nursing Assessment

The child may have either a stuffy or runny nose. Nasal discharge is usually thin and watery at first but may become thicker and discoloured. The colour of nasal discharge is not an accurate indicator of viral versus bacterial infection. The child may be hoarse and complain of a sore throat. Cough usually produces very little sputum. Fever, fatigue, watery eyes, and appetite loss may also occur. Symptoms are generally at their worst over the first few days and then decrease over the course of the illness.

Assess for risk factors such as day care or school attendance. Inspect for edema and vasodilation of the mucosa. Diagnosis is based on clinical presentation rather than lab or X-ray studies. Comparison Chart 39.1 differentiates causes of nasal congestion.

Nursing Management

Nursing management of the child with a common cold consists of promoting comfort, providing family education, and preventing spread of the cold.

Promoting Comfort

Nursing care of the common cold is aimed at supportive measures. Nasal congestion may be relieved with the use of normal saline nose drops, followed by bulb syringe suctioning in infants and toddlers. Older children may use a normal saline nose spray to mobilize secretions. A cool mist humidifier also helps with nasal congestion. Generally, other over-the-counter nose sprays are not recommended for use in children and should be used with caution in consultation with physician or nurse practitioner. Promotion of adequate oral fluid intake is important to liquefy secretions.

Educate parents about the use of cold and cough medications. Cough and cold medications are used with caution in select populations as emerging evidence

COMPARISON CHART 39.1 **CAUSES OF NASAL CONGESTION**

Sign or Symptom	Allergic Rhinitis	Common Cold	Sinusitis
Length of illness	Varies, may have year-round symptoms	10 days or less	Longer than 10–14 days
Nasal discharge	Thin, watery, clear	Thick, white, yellow, or green; can be thin	Thick, yellow or green
Nasal congestion	Varies	Present	Present
Sneezing	Varies	Present	Absent
Cough	Varies	Present	Varies
Headache	Varies	Varies	Varies
Fever	Absent	Varies	Varies
Bad breath	Absent	Absent	Varies

demonstrates potential harm. Although these medications are available over the counter, they should be used in consultation with a physician or nurse practitioner. Although they may offer some symptomatic relief, these medications have not been proven to shorten the length of cold symptoms. Products containing acetaminophen combined with other "cold symptom" medications may mask a fever in the child who is developing a secondary bacterial infection. As with all viral infections in children, teach parents that aspirin use should be avoided because of its association with Reye syndrome (KidsHealth, 2011).

Providing Family Education

Currently there are no medications available to treat the viruses that cause the common cold, so symptomatic treatment is all that is necessary. Antibiotics are not indicated unless the child also has a bacterial infection. Explain to parents the importance of reserving antibiotic use for appropriate illnesses. Provide education about the use of normal saline nose drops and bulb suctioning to clear the infant's nose of secretions. Normal saline nasal wash using a bulb syringe to instill the solution is also helpful for children of all ages with nasal congestion. Though normal saline for nasal administration is available commercially, parents can also make it at home (Box 39.2). Teaching Guideline 39.1 gives instructions on use of the bulb syringe.

Counsel parents about symptoms of complications of the common cold. These include:

- Prolonged fever
- Increased throat pain or enlarged, painful lymph nodes
- Increased or worsening cough, cough lasting longer than 10 days, chest pain, difficulty breathing
- Earache, headache, tooth or sinus pain
- Unusual irritability or lethargy
- Skin rash

If complications do occur, tell parents to notify the health care provider for further instruction or reassessment. Most infants and children do not develop complications and can be managed safely in the home without a visit to a health care provider or emergency room.

BOX 39.2 Homemade Salt Water Nose Drops

Mix 240 mL distilled water, 2.5 mL sea salt, and 1.25 mL baking soda. Keeps for 24 hours in the refrigerator, but should be allowed to come to room temperature prior to use.

Preventing the Common Cold

Teaching about ways to prevent the common cold is a vital nursing intervention. Explain that frequent handwashing helps to decrease the spread of viruses that cause the common cold. Teach parents and family to avoid secondhand smoke as well as crowded places, especially during the winter. Avoid close contact with individuals known to have a cold. Encourage parents and families to consume a healthy diet and get enough rest.

▶ *Consider THIS!*

Corey Davis, a 3-year-old, is brought to the clinic by her mother. She presents with a runny nose, congestion, and a nonproductive cough. Her mother says, "She is miserable."

What other assessment information would be helpful? Based on the history and clinical presentation, Corey is diagnosed with a common cold. What education would be helpful for this family? Include ways to improve Corey's comfort and ways to prevent the common cold.

Sinusitis

Sinusitis (also called rhinosinusitis) generally refers to a bacterial infection of the paranasal sinuses. The disease may be either acute or chronic in nature, with the treatment approach varying with chronicity. Approximately 5% of URIs are complicated with acute sinusitis (DeMuri & Wald, 2010). In young children the maxillary and ethmoid sinuses are the main sites of infection. After age 10 years, the frontal sinuses may be more commonly involved (Yoon et al., 2011). Mucosal swelling, decreased ciliary movement, and thickened nasal discharge all contribute to bacterial invasion of the nose. Nasal polyps also place the child at risk for bacterial sinusitis. Complications include orbital cellulitis and intracranial infections such as subdural empyemas.

Symptoms lasting less than 30 days generally indicate acute sinusitis, whereas symptoms persisting longer than 4 to 6 weeks usually indicate chronic sinusitis. Sinusitis is managed with antibiotic treatment. The course of treatment is a minimum of 10 days but often extends for 2 to 3 weeks. To eradicate the infection, it is recommended that antibiotics should be continued for 7 days after the child is symptom-free (Taylor & Adam, 2006). Naturally, chronic sinusitis requires a longer course of treatment than acute sinusitis. Surgical therapy may be indicated for children with chronic sinusitis, particularly if it is recurrent or if nasal polyps are present.

Nursing Assessment

The most common presentation of sinusitis is persistent signs and symptoms of a cold. Rather than improving

TEACHING GUIDELINE 39.1

Using the Bulb Syringe to Suction Nasal Secretions

- Hold the infant on your lap or on the bed with head tilted slightly back.

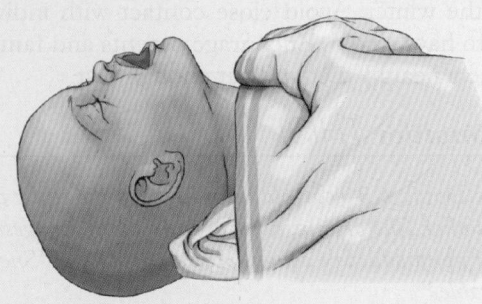

- (If using saline) Instill several drops of saline solution in one of infant's nostrils.

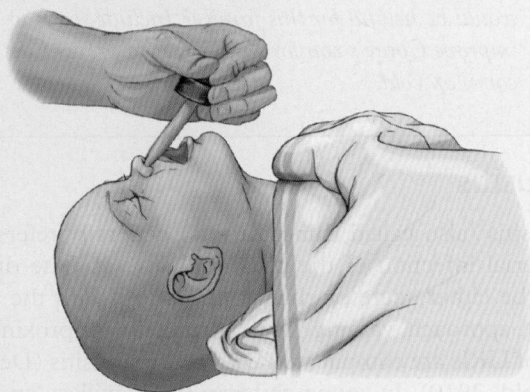

- Compress the sides of the bulb syringe completely. Use only a rubber-tipped bulb syringe.

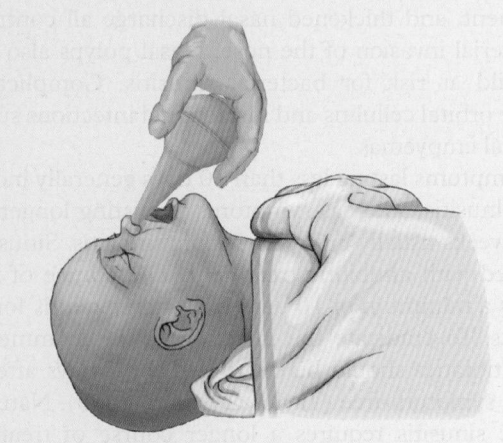

- Place rubber tip in infant's nose and release pressure on the bulb as you compress the opposite nare to create a seal.

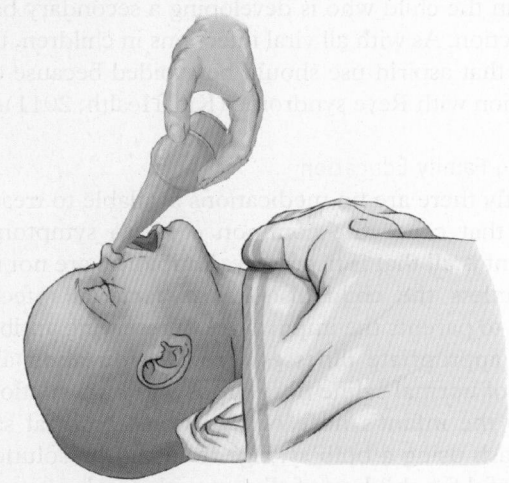

- Remove the syringe and squeeze bulb over tissue or the sink to empty it of secretions.

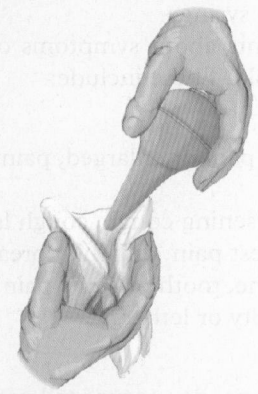

- Repeat on alternate nostril if necessary. Using a bulb syringe prior to bottle-feeding or breastfeeding may relieve congestion enough to allow the infant to suck more efficiently.
- Clean the bulb syringe thoroughly with warm water after each use and allow to air dry.

after 7 to 10 days, nasal discharge persists. Explore the history for:

• Cough
• Fever
• In preschoolers or older children, halitosis (bad breath)
• Facial pain may or may not be present, so is not a reliable indicator of disease.
• Eyelid edema (in the case of ethmoid sinus involvement)
• Irritability
• Poor appetite

Cold symptoms that are severe and not improving over time may also indicate sinusitis (Taylor & Adam, 2006). Assess for risk factors such as a history of recurrent cold symptoms or a history of nasal polyps.

On physical examination, note eyelid swelling, extent of nasal drainage, and halitosis. Inspect the throat for evidence of postnasal drainage. Inspect the nasal mucosa for erythema. Palpate the sinuses, noting pain with mild pressure. The diagnosis may be made based on the history and clinical presentation, augmented by X-ray, computed tomography scan, or magnetic resonance imaging findings in some cases. (Refer to Comparison Chart 39.1, which differentiates the causes of nasal congestion.)

Nursing Management

Normal saline nose drops or spray, cool mist humidifiers, and adequate oral fluid intake are recommended for children with sinusitis. Teach families the importance of continuing the full course of antibiotics to eradicate the cause of infection. Also educate the family that using decongestants, antihistamines, and intranasal steroids as adjuncts in the treatment of sinusitis has not been shown to be beneficial (DeMuri & Wald, 2010). Normal saline nose spray or nasal washes may promote drainage.

Influenza

Influenza viral infection occurs primarily during the winter. "The flu" is spread through inhalation of droplets or contact with fine-particle aerosols. Infected children shed the virus for 1 to 2 days before symptoms begin. Average annual infection rates in children range from 35% to 50% (Public Health Agency of Canada [PHAC], 2010a). Influenza viruses primarily affect the upper respiratory epithelium but can cause systemic effects as well. Children with chronic heart or lung conditions, diabetes, chronic renal disease, or immune deficiency are at higher risk than other children for more severe influenza infection.

Bacterial infections of the respiratory system commonly occur as complications of influenza infection, severe secondary bacterial pneumonia in particular (American Academy of Pediatrics [AAP], 2009). Otitis media occurs in 30% to 50% of all influenza cases (AAP, 2009). Less common complications include Reye syndrome and acute myositis. Reye syndrome is an acute

encephalopathy that has been associated with aspirin use in the influenza-infected child (KidsHealth, 2011). Acute myositis is particular to children. A sudden onset of severe pain and tenderness in both calves causes the child to refuse to walk. Due to the potential for complications, a prolonged fever or a fever that returns during convalescence should be investigated.

Nursing Assessment

Children who attend day care or school are at higher risk for influenza infection than those who are routinely at home. Note the presence of risk factors for severe disease, such as chronic heart or lung disease (such as asthma), diabetes, chronic renal disease, or immune deficiency or children with cancer receiving chemotherapy. School-age children and adolescents experience the illness similarly to adults. Abrupt onset of fever, facial flushing, chills, headache, myalgia, and malaise are accompanied by cough and **coryza**. About half of infected individuals have a dry or sore throat. Ocular symptoms such as photophobia, tearing, burning, and eye pain are common.

Infants and young children exhibit symptoms similar to other respiratory illnesses. Fever greater than 39.5°C is common. Infants may be mildly toxic in appearance and irritable and have a cough, coryza, and pharyngitis. Wheezing may occur, as influenza also can cause bronchiolitis. An erythematous rash may be present, and diarrhea may also occur. Diagnosis may be confirmed by a rapid assay test.

Nursing Management

Nursing management of influenza is mainly supportive. Symptomatic treatment of cough and fever and maintenance of hydration are the focus of care. Oseltamivir (Tamiflu), amantadine hydrochloride (Symmetrel), and other newer antiviral drugs can be effective in reducing symptoms associated with influenza if started within the first 24 to 48 hours of the illness (Canadian Paediatric Society [CPS], 2010).

Preventing Influenza Infection

Yearly vaccination against influenza is recommended for high-risk groups. Vaccine recommendations are proposed annually after extensive review of the literature and prediction based on worldwide prevalence. These recommendations are first presented as a national immunization plan. Each provincial jurisdiction then determines the specific strategy and coverage for the region. Children who are 6 months or older and considered high risk are those who:

• Have chronic heart or lung conditions
• Have sickle-cell anemia or other hemoglobinopathy
• Are under medical care for diabetes, chronic renal disease, or immune deficiency
• Are on long-term aspirin therapy (risk of developing Reye syndrome after the flu)

Among otherwise healthy children, infants and toddlers are at highest risk for developing severe disease. Refer to the annual provincial guidelines for influenza vaccine that are released late in the fall of each year. Refer to Chapter 30 for more information on immunizations.

Pharyngitis

Inflammation of the throat mucosa (pharynx) is referred to as **pharyngitis**. A sore throat may accompany nasal congestion and is often viral in nature. A bacterial sore throat most often occurs without nasal symptoms. Group A streptococci account for 15% to 30% of cases, with the remainder being caused by other viruses or bacteria (Jaggi & Shulman, 2006).

Complications of group A streptococcal infection include acute rheumatic fever (see Chapter 40) and acute glomerulonephritis (see Chapter 42). An additional complication of streptococcal pharyngitis is peritonsillar abscess; this may be noted by asymmetric swelling of the tonsils, shift of the uvula to one side, and palatal edema. Retropharyngeal abscess may also follow pharyngitis and is most common in young children (Lander, Lu, & Shah, 2008). It can progress to the point of airway obstruction and requires careful evaluation and appropriate treatment.

Viral pharyngitis is usually self-limited and does not require therapy beyond symptomatic relief. Group A streptococcal pharyngitis requires antibiotic therapy. If either the rapid diagnostic test or throat culture (described below) is positive for group A streptococci, penicillin is generally prescribed. Appropriate alternative antibiotics include amoxicillin and, for those allergic to penicillin, macrolides and cephalosporins (Allen & Moore, 2010).

> ▶ **Take** NOTE!
>
> A "strep carrier" is a child who has a positive throat culture for streptococci when asymptomatic. Strep carriers are not at risk for complications from streptococci as are those who are acutely infected with streptococci and are symptomatic (Martin, 2010).

Nursing Assessment

Onset of the illness is often quite abrupt. The history may include a fever, sore throat and difficulty swallowing, headache, and abdominal pain, which are quite common. Inquire about recent incidence of viral or strep throat in the family, day care, or school setting.

Inspect the pharynx and tonsils, which may demonstrate varying degrees of inflammation (Figs. 39.10, 39.11, and 39.12). Exudate may be present but is not diagnostic of bacterial infection. Note the presence of petechiae on the palate. Inspect the tongue for a strawberry appearance. Palpate for enlargement and tenderness of the

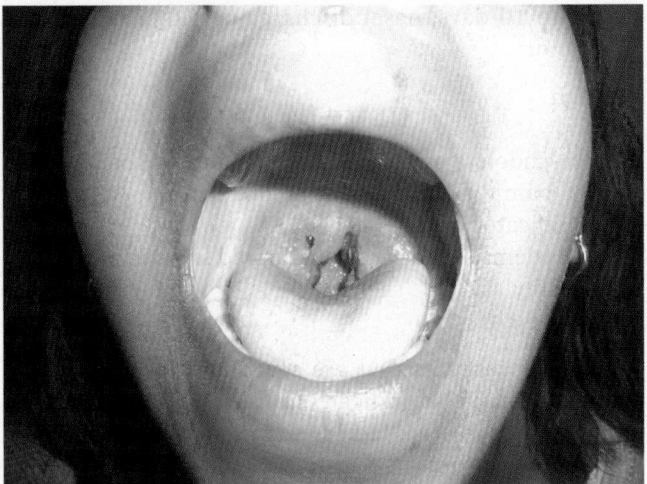

FIGURE 39.10 Note the red colour of the pharynx, as well as redness and significant enlargement of the tonsils.

anterior cervical nodes. Inspect the skin for the presence of a fine, red, sandpaper-like rash (called scarlatiniform), particularly on the trunk or abdomen, a common finding with streptococcus A infection.

The nurse may obtain a throat swab for rapid diagnostic testing and throat culture. (The only contraindication for taking a throat swab is the suspicion of epiglottitis, as any instrumentation of the airway in this condition could precipitate complete airway obstruction.) If both tests are being obtained, the applicators may be swabbed simultaneously to decrease perceived trauma to the child. The rapid strep test is a sensitive and reliable measure that rarely results in false-positive readings (Blosser, Brady, & Mueller, 2009). If the rapid strep test is negative, the second swab may be sent for a throat culture.

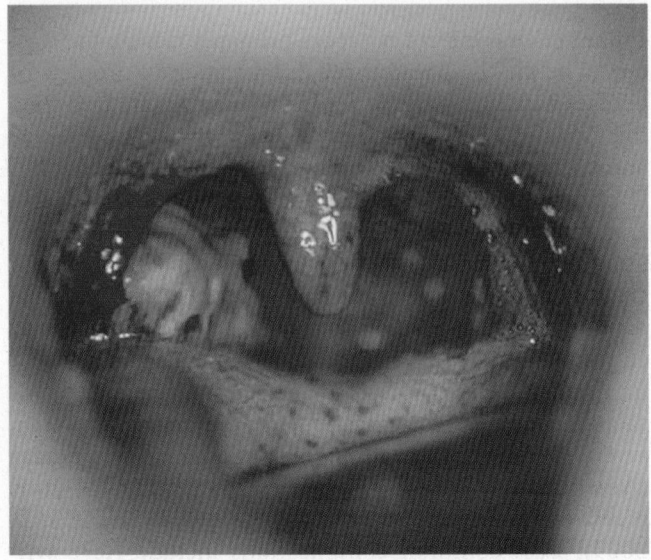

FIGURE 39.11 Pharyngitis.

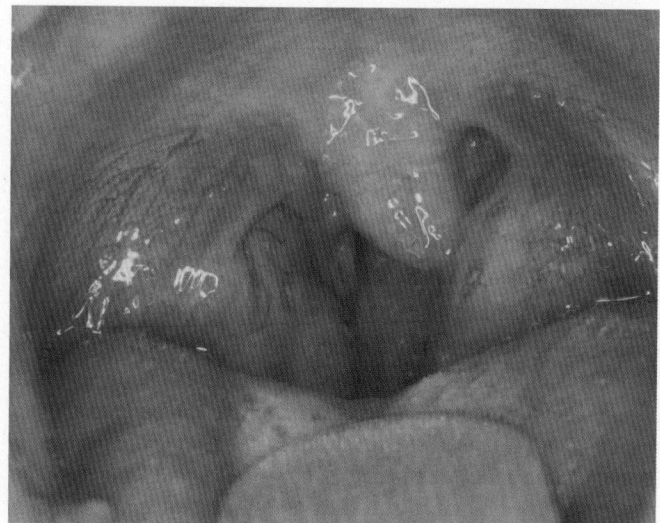

FIGURE 39.12 "Kissing tonsils" occur when the tonsils are so enlarged that they touch the uvula and/or each other, greatly narrowing the airway.

Nursing Management

Nursing management of the child with pharyngitis focuses on promoting comfort and providing family education.

Promoting Comfort

Saline gargles (made with 8 oz of warm water and a half-teaspoon of table salt) are soothing for children who are old enough to cooperate. Analgesics such as acetaminophen and ibuprofen may ease fever and pain. Sucking on throat lozenges or hard candy may also ease pain. The risk for aspiration of a foreign body must be considered, however, and use of hard lozenges should be restricted to the older school-age child. Cool mist humidity helps to keep the mucosa moist in the event of mouth breathing. Encourage the child to ingest ice pops, cool liquids, and ice chips to maintain hydration.

Providing Family Education

Parents may be accustomed to "sore throats" being treated with antibiotics, but in the case of a viral cause antibiotics will not be necessary and the pharyngitis will resolve in a few days. For the child with streptococcal pharyngitis, urge parents to have the child complete the entire prescribed course of antibiotics. After 24 hours of antibiotic therapy, instruct the parents to discard the child's toothbrush to avoid reinfection. Children may return to day care or school after they have been receiving antibiotics for 24 hours, as they are considered noncontagious at that point.

Tonsillitis

Inflammation of the tonsils often occurs with pharyngitis and thus may also be viral or bacterial in nature. Viral infections require only symptomatic treatment. Treatment for bacterial tonsillitis is the same as for bacterial pharyngitis. Peritonsillar abscess may follow a bout of tonsillitis and requires incision and drainage of the pus-containing mass followed by a course of intravenous antibiotics (Galioto, 2008). Occasionally, surgical intervention is warranted. Tonsillectomy (surgical removal of the palatine tonsils) may be indicated for the child with recurrent streptococcal tonsillitis, massive tonsillar hypertrophy, or other reasons. When hypertrophied adenoids obstruct breathing, then adenoidectomy (surgical removal of the adenoids) may be indicated.

Nursing Assessment

Note whether fever is present currently or by history. Inquire about the history of recurrent pharyngitis or tonsillitis. Note if the child's voice sounds muffled or hoarse. Inspect the pharynx for redness and enlargement of the tonsils. As the tonsils enlarge, the child may experience difficulty breathing and swallowing. When tonsils touch at the midline ("kissing tonsils" or 4+ in size), the airway may become obstructed (see Fig. 39.12). Also, if the adenoids are enlarged, the posterior nares become obstructed. The child may breathe through the mouth and may snore. Palpate the anterior cervical nodes for enlargement and tenderness. Rapid test or culture may be positive for streptococcus A.

Nursing Management

Tonsillitis that is medically treated requires the same nursing management as pharyngitis. Nursing care for the child after tonsillectomy is described below.

Promoting Airway Clearance

Until fully awake, place the child in a side-lying or prone position to facilitate safe drainage of secretions. Once alert, he or she may prefer to sit up or have the head of the bed elevated. Suctioning, if necessary, should be done carefully to avoid trauma to the surgical site. Dried blood may be present on the teeth and the nares, with old blood present in emesis. Since the presence of blood can be very frightening to parents, alert them to this possibility.

Maintaining Fluid Volume

Hemorrhage is unusual postoperatively but may occur any time from the immediate postoperative period to as late as 10 days after surgery. Inspect the throat for bleeding. Mucus tinged with blood may be expected, but fresh blood in the secretions indicates bleeding. Early bleeding may be identified by continuous swallowing of small amounts of blood while awake or sleeping. Other signs of hemorrhage include tachycardia, pallor, restlessness, frequent throat clearing, and emesis of bright red blood.

To avoid trauma to the surgical site, discourage the child from coughing, clearing the throat, blowing the nose, and using straws. Upon discharge, instruct the parents to immediately report any sign of bleeding to the physician. To maintain fluid volume postoperatively, encourage children to take any fluids they desire; ice pops and ice chips are particularly soothing. Citrus juice and brown or red fluids should be avoided: the acid in citrus juice may irritate the throat, and red or brown fluids may be confused with blood if vomiting occurs.

Relieving Pain

For the first 24 hours after surgery, the throat is very sore. Adequate pain relief is essential to establish adequate oral fluid intake. An ice collar may be prescribed, as well as analgesics with or without narcotics. Counsel parents to maintain pain control for their child upon discharge from the facility, not only to ensure his or her comfort but also to enable the child to continue to drink fluids. Most centres performing tonsillectomies offer this procedure as a day surgery, restricting an overnight admission postoperatively to only those children with other co-morbid conditions or obstructive sleep apnea.

Infectious Mononucleosis

Infectious mononucleosis is a self-limited illness caused by the Epstein-Barr virus. It is characterized by fever, malaise, sore throat, and lymphadenopathy. Mononucleosis is commonly called the "kissing disease" since it is transmitted by oropharyngeal secretions. It can occur at any age but is most often diagnosed in adolescents and young adults (Blosser et al., 2009). Some infected individuals may have concomitant streptococcal pharyngitis. Complications include splenic rupture, Guillain–Barré syndrome, and aseptic meningitis (Stephenson & DuBois, 2007).

Nursing Assessment

Note any history of exposure to infected individuals. Determine history of fever and onset and progression of sore throat, malaise, and other complaints. Observe for periorbital edema. Inspect the pharynx and tonsils for inflammation and the presence of patches of grey exudate. Petechiae may be present on the palate. Palpate for bilateral nontender enlargement of the posterior cervical lymph nodes. After 3 to 5 days of illness, the pharynx may become edematous and the tonsillar exudate more extensive. Lymphadenopathy may progress to include the anterior cervical nodes, which may become tender. Palpate the abdomen for the presence of splenomegaly or hepatomegaly. Splenic enlargement indicates potentially more severe illness; to avoid splenic injury, patients are generally restricted from playing contact sports. An erythematous maculopapular rash may appear as the illness progresses. Definitive diagnosis may be made by Monospot or Epstein-Barr virus titers.

> ▶ **Take** NOTE!
>
> The Monospot test is usually negative if obtained within the first 7 to 10 days of illness with infectious mononucleosis. Epstein-Barr virus titer is reliable at any point in the illness (Blosser et al., 2009).

Nursing Management

Nursing management of mononucleosis is primarily symptomatic. The throat may be very sore, so analgesics and salt-water gargles are recommended. Bed rest should be encouraged while the child is febrile. Frequent rest periods may be necessary for several weeks after the onset of illness, as fatigue may persist as long as 6 weeks. During the acute phase, if tonsillar or pharyngeal edema threatens to obstruct the airway, then corticosteroids may be given to decrease the inflammation. In the presence of splenomegaly or hepatomegaly, strenuous activity and contact sports should be avoided (CPS, 2007). Appearance of rash or jaundice should be reported to the physician.

> ▶ **Take** NOTE!
>
> Concomitant strep throat in the presence of infectious mononucleosis should be treated with an antibiotic other than ampicillin, as it may cause an allergic-type rash if used in the presence of mononucleosis.

Laryngitis

Inflammation of the larynx is termed **laryngitis**. It may occur alone or in conjunction with other respiratory symptoms. It is characterized by a hoarse voice or loss of the voice (so soft as to make it difficult to hear). Oral fluids might offer relief, but resting the voice for 24 hours will allow the inflammation to subside. Laryngitis alone requires no further intervention.

Croup

Children between 3 months and 3 years of age are the most likely to be affected with croup, though croup may affect any child (KidsHealth, 2009). Croup is also referred to as laryngotracheobronchitis because inflammation and edema of the larynx, trachea, and bronchi occur as a result of viral infection. Parainfluenza is responsible for the majority of cases of croup (Wald, 2010). Other causes include adenovirus, influenza virus A and B, RSV, and rarely, measles virus or *Mycoplasma pneumoniae* (Bjornson et al., 2004). The inflammation and edema obstruct the airway, resulting in symptoms.

COMPARISON CHART 39.2 CROUP VS. EPIGLOTTITIS

	Spasmodic Croup	Epiglottitis
Preceding illness	None or minimal coryza	None or mild upper respiratory infection
Usually affects age:	3 months to 3 years	1–8 years
Onset	Usually sudden, often at night	Rapid (within hours)
Fever	Variable	High
Barking cough, hoarseness	Yes	No
Dysphagia	No	Yes
Toxic appearance	No	Yes
Cause	Viral	*Haemophilus influenzae* type B

Mucus production also occurs, further contributing to obstruction of the airway. Narrowing of the subglottic area of the trachea results in audible inspiratory stridor. Edema of the larynx causes hoarseness. Inflammation in the larynx and trachea causes the characteristic barking cough of croup. Symptoms occur most often at night, and croup is usually self-limited, lasting only about 3 to 5 days (CPS, 2010).

Croup often presents suddenly at night, with resolution of symptoms in the morning. Complications of croup are rare but may include worsening respiratory distress, hypoxia, or bacterial superinfection (as in the case of bacterial tracheitis). Croup is usually managed on an out-patient basis, with only 1% to 2% of cases requiring hospitalization (Alberta Medical Association, 2005).

Corticosteroids (usually a single dose) are used to decrease inflammation and racemic epinephrine aerosols demonstrate the alpha-adrenergic effect of mucosal vasoconstriction, helping to decrease edema (Johnson, 2009). Children with croup may be hospitalized if they have significant stridor at rest or severe retractions after a several-hour period of observation. Comparison Chart 39.2 gives information comparing croup to epiglottitis.

Nursing Assessment

Note the age of the child; children between 3 months and 3 years of age are most likely to present with viral croup (laryngotracheobronchitis). History may reveal a cough that developed during the night (most common presentation) and that sounds like barking (or a seal). Inspect for presence of mild URI symptoms. Temperature may be normal or elevated mildly. Listen for inspiratory stridor and observe for suprasternal retractions. Auscultate the lungs for adequacy of breath sounds. Various scales are available for scoring croup severity, though these are of limited value in the clinical assessment and treatment of croup (Alberta Medical Association, 2005). Croup is usually diagnosed based on history and clinical presentation, but a lateral neck X-ray may be obtained to rule out epiglottitis.

> ▶ *Take* NOTE!
>
> *The child with fever, a toxic appearance, and increasing respiratory distress despite appropriate croup treatment may have bacterial tracheitis (Huang et al., 2009). Notify the physician of these findings in a child with croup.*

Nursing Management

If the child's care is being managed at home, advise parents about the symptoms of respiratory distress and instruct them to seek treatment if the child's respiratory condition worsens. Teach parents to expose their child to humidified air (via a cool mist humidifier or steamy bathroom). Though never clinically proven, the use of humidified air has long been recommended for alleviating coughing jags and anecdotally reported as helpful. If ordered, administer dexamethasone or teach parents about home administration. Explain to parents that the effects of racemic epinephrine last about 2 hours and the child must be observed closely as occasionally a child will worsen again, requiring another aerosol. Teaching Guideline 39.2 gives information about home care of croup.

Epiglottitis

Epiglottitis (inflammation and swelling of the epiglottis) is most often caused by *Haemophilus influenzae* type B. Extensive use of the Hib vaccine since the 1980s has resulted in a significant decrease in the incidence of epiglottitis (Brady, 2009). Epiglottitis usually occurs in children between the ages of 2 and 7 years and can be life threatening (Brady, 2009). Respiratory arrest and death may occur if the airway becomes completely occluded. Additional complications include pneumothorax and pulmonary edema. Therapeutic management focuses on airway maintenance and support. Intravenous antibiotic therapy is necessary (Guldfred, Lyhne, & Becker, 2008). Affected children will most likely be managed in the

TEACHING GUIDELINE 39.2

Home Care of Croup

- Keep the child quiet and discourage crying.
- Allow the child to sit up (in your arms).
- Encourage rest and fluid intake.
- If stridor occurs, take the child into a steamy bathroom for 10 minutes.
- Administer medication (corticosteroid) as directed.
- Watch the child closely. Call the physician if:
  - The child breathes faster, has retractions, or has any other difficulty breathing
  - The nostrils flare or the lips or nails have a bluish tint
  - The cough or stridor does not improve with exposure to moist air
  - Restlessness increases or the child is confused
  - The child begins to drool or cannot swallow
- If there is any colour change such as cyanosis to the face or lips, contact emergency services as the child may be in imminent respiratory failure.

Adapted from: KidsHealth. (2009). *About croup.* Retrieved December 5, 2011 from http://kidshealth.org/parent/infections/lung/croup.html.

pediatric intensive care unit. Comparison Chart 39.2 gives information comparing croup with epiglottitis.

Nursing Assessment

Carefully assess the child with suspected epiglottitis. Note sudden onset of symptoms and high fever. The child has an overall toxic appearance. He or she may refuse to speak or may speak only with a very soft voice. The child may refuse to lie down and may assume the characteristic position, sitting forward with the neck extended. Drooling may be present. Note anxiety or a frightened appearance. Note the child's colour. Cough is usually absent. A lateral neck X-ray may be performed to determine the presence of epiglottitis. This is done cautiously, so as not to induce airway obstruction with changes in position of the child's neck (Guldfred et al., 2008).

Nursing Management

Do not leave the child unattended. Keep the child and parents as calm as possible. Allow the child to assume a position of comfort. *Do not* place the child in a supine position, as airway occlusion may occur. Provide 100% oxygen in the least invasive manner that is most acceptable to the child. Do not under any circumstance attempt to visualize the throat: reflex laryngospasm may occur, precipitating immediate airway occlusion. If the child with epiglottitis experiences complete airway occlusion, an emergency tracheostomy may be necessary. Ensure that emergency equipment is available and that personnel specifically trained in intubation of the pediatric occluded airway and percutaneous tracheostomy are notified of the child's presence in the facility.

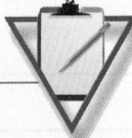

▶ *Take* NOTE!

Epiglottitis is characterized by dysphagia, drooling, anxiety, irritability, and significant respiratory distress. Prepare for the event of sudden airway occlusion.

Bronchiolitis (RSV)

Bronchiolitis is an acute inflammatory process of the bronchioles and small bronchi. Nearly always caused by a viral pathogen, RSV accounts for the majority of cases of bronchiolitis, with adenovirus, parainfluenza, and human meta-pneumovirus also being important causative agents. This discussion will focus on RSV bronchiolitis.

The peak incidence of bronchiolitis is in the winter and spring, coinciding with RSV season. RSV season in the United States and Canada generally begins in September or October and continues through April or May. Virtually all children will contract RSV infection within the first few years of life. RSV bronchiolitis occurs most often in infants and toddlers, with a peak incidence around 6 months of age (Goodman, 2011). The severity of disease is related inversely to the age of the child, with the most severe cases occurring between 1 and 3 months of age. Repeated RSV infections occur throughout life but are usually localized to the upper respiratory tract after toddlerhood.

Therapeutic Management

Management of RSV focuses on supportive treatment. Supplemental oxygen, nasal and/or nasopharyngeal suctioning, oral or intravenous hydration, and inhaled bronchodilator therapy are used. Many infants are managed at home with close observation and adequate hydration. Hospitalization is required for children with more severe disease. The infant with tachypnea, significant retractions, poor oral intake, or lethargy can deteriorate quickly, to the point of requiring ventilatory support, and thus warrants hospital admission.

Pathophysiology

RSV is a highly contagious virus and may be contracted through direct contact with respiratory secretions or from particles on objects contaminated with the virus (CPS, 2010; PHAC, 2010b). RSV invades the nasopharynx, where it replicates and then spreads down to the lower airway via aspiration of upper airway secretions. RSV infection causes necrosis of the respiratory epithelium of small airways, peribronchiolar mononuclear infiltration, and plugging of the lumens with mucus and exudate. The small

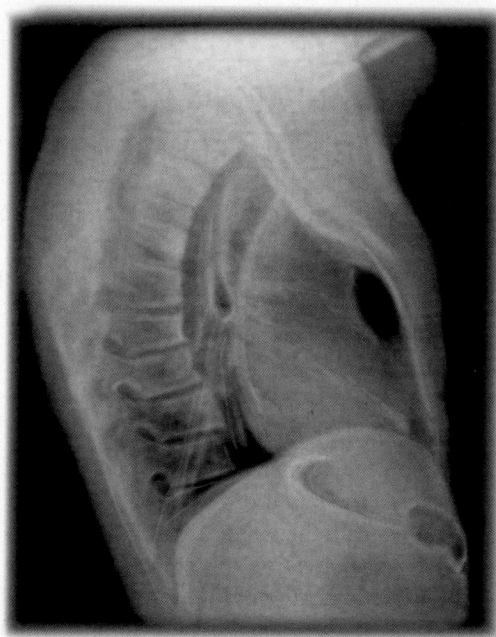

FIGURE 39.13 Hyperinflation with atelectasis is noted upon chest X-ray.

airways become variably obstructed; this allows adequate inspiratory volume but prevents full expiration. This leads to hyperinflation and atelectasis (Morrow & Argent, 2008) (Fig. 39.13). Serious alterations in gas exchange occur, with arterial hypoxemia and carbon dioxide retention resulting from mismatching of pulmonary ventilation and perfusion. Hypoventilation occurs secondary to markedly increased work of breathing.

Nursing Assessment

For a full description of the assessment phase of the nursing process, refer to page 1260. Assessment findings pertinent to bronchiolitis are discussed below.

Health History

Elicit a description of the present illness and chief complaint. Common signs and symptoms reported during the health history might include:

- Onset of illness with a clear runny nose (sometimes profuse)
- Pharyngitis
- Low-grade fever
- Development of cough 1 to 3 days into the illness, followed by a wheeze shortly thereafter
- Poor feeding

Explore the child's current and past medical history for risk factors such as:

- Young age (less than 2 years old), more severe disease in a child less than 6 months old
- Prematurity

- Multiple births
- Birth during April to September
- History of chronic lung disease (bronchopulmonary disease)
- Cyanotic or complicated congenital heart disease
- Immunocompromise
- Male gender
- Exposure to passive tobacco smoke
- Crowded living conditions
- Day care attendance
- School-age siblings
- Low socioeconomic status
- Lack of breastfeeding

Physical Examination

Examination of the child with RSV involves inspection, observation, and auscultation.

Inspection and Observation

Observe the child's general appearance and colour (centrally and peripherally). The infant with RSV bronchiolitis might appear air-hungry, exhibiting various degrees of cyanosis and respiratory distress, including tachypnea, retractions, accessory muscle use, grunting, and periods of apnea. Cough and audible wheeze might be heard. The infant might appear listless and disinterested in feeding, surroundings, or parents.

Auscultation

Auscultate the lungs, noting adventitious sounds and determining the quality of aeration of the lung fields. Earlier in the illness, wheezes might be heard scattered throughout the lung fields. In more serious cases, the chest might sound quiet and without wheeze. This is attributed to significant hyperexpansion with very poor air exchange.

Laboratory and Diagnostic Tests

Common laboratory and diagnostic studies ordered for the assessment of RSV bronchiolitis include:

- Pulse oximetry: oxygen saturation might be significantly decreased.
- Chest X-ray: although not recommended in most situations, chest X-ray might reveal hyperinflation and patchy areas of atelectasis or infiltration.
- Blood gases: might show carbon dioxide retention and hypoxemia.
- Nasal-pharyngeal washings: positive identification of RSV can be made via enzyme-linked immunosorbent assay (ELISA) or immunofluorescent antibody (IFA) testing.

Nursing Management

RSV infection is usually self-limited, and nursing diagnoses, goals, and interventions for the child with bronchiolitis are aimed at supportive care. Children with less severe disease might require only antipyretics, adequate hydration, and close observation. They can often be successfully managed at home, provided the primary caregiver is reliable and comfortable with close observation. Parents or caregivers should be educated to watch for signs of worsening and must understand the importance of seeking care quickly should the child's condition deteriorate.

Hospitalization is required for children with more severe disease, and children admitted with RSV bronchiolitis warrant close observation. In addition to the nursing diagnoses and related interventions discussed in Nursing Care Plan 39.1 for respiratory disorders, interventions common to bronchiolitis follow.

▶ *Take* NOTE!

Currently no safe and effective antiviral drug is available for definitive treatment of RSV. Routine antibiotic use is discouraged in RSV bronchiolitis treatment because the secondary bacterial infection rate of the lower airway is very low (Checchia, 2011).

Maintaining Patent Airway

Infants and young children with RSV tend to have copious secretions. Position the child with the head of the bed elevated to facilitate an open airway. These children often require frequent assessment and suctioning to maintain a patent airway (Nettina, 2010). Use a Yankauer or tonsil-tip suction catheter to suction the mouth or pharynx of older infants or children, rinsing the catheter after each suctioning. Nasal bulb suctioning may be sufficient to clear the airway in some infants, while others will require nasopharyngeal suctioning with a suction catheter. Nursing Procedure 39.1 gives further information. The routine use of sterile normal saline is not indicated in all children, as its use has been demonstrated to result in decreased oxygen saturations for up to 2 minutes after suctioning is complete (Morrow & Argent, 2008). Adjust the pressure ranges for suctioning infants and children between 60 and 100 mm Hg, 40 and 60 mm Hg for premature infants.

Promoting Adequate Gas Exchange

Infants and children with bronchiolitis might deteriorate quickly as the disease progresses. In the child ill enough to require oxygen, the risk is even greater. Assessment should include work of breathing, respiratory rate, and oxygen saturation. The percentage of inspired oxygen (FiO_2) should be adjusted as needed to maintain oxygen saturation within the desired range. There is evolving literature warning of the potentially toxic effects of oxygen delivered in concentrations of 50% or greater, especially in the young infant. Positioning the infant with the head of the bed elevated may also improve gas exchange. Frequent assessment is necessary for the hospitalized child with bronchiolitis (Nettina, 2010).

Nursing Procedure 39.1

NASOPHARYNGEAL OR ARTIFICIAL AIRWAY SUCTION TECHNIQUE

1. Check to ensure the suction equipment works properly before starting.
2. After washing your hands, assemble the equipment needed:
   - Appropriate-size sterile suction catheter
   - Clean gloves
   - Supplemental oxygen
   - Sterile saline as a lubricant
3. Don gloves, keeping dominant hand clean.
4. Preoxygenate the infant or child.
5. Apply lubricant to the end of the suction catheter if using the nasopharyngeal route.
6. Insert the suction catheter into the child's nostril or airway. Use the no-touch sterile technique for an artificial airway, and the clean technique for the nose or mouth.
   - Insert only to the posterior portion of the oral pharynx if inserting via the nostril to avoid eliciting gagging which may increase the risk for vomiting and reflux.
   - Insert only 0.5 cm farther than the length of the artificial airway.
7. Intermittently apply suction for no longer than 10 seconds, while twisting and removing the catheter.
8. Supplement with oxygen after suctioning.

▶ *Take* NOTE!

In the tachypneic infant, slowing of the respiratory rate does not necessarily indicate improvement: often, a slower respiratory rate is an indication of tiring, and carbon dioxide retention may soon be followed by apnea (AHA, 2007).

Reducing Risk for Infection

Since RSV is easily spread through contact with droplets, in-patients should be isolated according to hospital policy to decrease the risk of nosocomial spread to other patients. Patients with RSV can safely room share. Attention to handwashing is necessary, as droplets might enter the eyes, nose, or mouth via the hands.

Providing Family Education

Educate parents to recognize signs of worsening distress. Tell parents to call their physician or nurse practitioner if the breathing is rapid or becomes more difficult or if the child cannot eat secondary to tachypnea. Children who are less than 1 year of age or who are at higher risk (those who were born prematurely or who have chronic heart or lung conditions) might have a longer course of illness. Instruct parents that cough can persist for several days to weeks after resolution of the disease, but infants usually act well otherwise.

Preventing RSV Disease

Strict adherence to handwashing policies in day care centres and when exposed to individuals with cold symptoms are important for all groups. Though generally benign in healthy older children, RSV can be devastating in young infants or children with pre-existing risk factors. Palivizumab (Synagis) is a monoclonal antibody effective in the prevention of severe RSV disease in those who are most susceptible (Checchia, 2011). It is given as an intramuscular injection once a month throughout the RSV season. The use of palivizumab in Canada is based on provincial criteria and usually focused on select high-risk population groups. Qualifying factors may include:

- Prematurity
- Chronic lung disease (bronchopulmonary dysplasia) requiring medication or oxygen
- Certain congenital heart diseases
- Immunocompromise
- Residing in a remote geographic community (Samson, 2009)

Pneumonia

Pneumonia is an inflammation of the lung parenchyma. It can be caused by a virus, bacteria, *Mycoplasma,* or fungus. It may also result from aspiration of foreign material into the lower respiratory tract (aspiration pneumonia). Pneumonia occurs more often in winter and early spring. It is common in children but is seen most frequently in infants and young toddlers. Viruses are the most common cause of pneumonia in younger children and the least common cause in older children (Table 39.2). Viral pneumonia is usually better tolerated in children but can be severe in infants less than 1 year of age due to many of the anatomic and physiologic differences. Children with bacterial pneumonia are more apt to present with a toxic appearance, but rapid recovery generally occurs if appropriate antibiotic treatment is instituted early.

> ▶ **Take** NOTE!
>
> *Community-acquired pneumonia (CAP) refers to pneumonia in a previously healthy person that is contracted outside of the hospital setting.*

Pneumonia is usually a self-limited disease. A child who presents with recurrent pneumonia should be evaluated for chronic lung disease such as asthma or cystic

TABLE 39.2 COMMON CAUSES OF PNEUMONIA ACCORDING TO AGE

Age Group	Most Common Causative Agents
1–3 months	RSV, other respiratory viruses (parainfluenza, influenza, adenovirus); *Streptococcus pneumoniae, Chlamydia trachomatis*
4 months to 5 years	Respiratory viruses, *Streptococcus pneumoniae, Chlamydia pneumoniae, Mycoplasma pneumoniae*
5–18 years	*Mycoplasma pneumoniae, Chlamydia pneumoniae, Streptococcus pneumoniae*

Adapted from: Nield, L. S., Mahajan, P., & Kamat, D. M. (2005). Pneumonia: Update on causes and treatment options. *Consultant for Pediatricians, 4*(8), 365–370.

fibrosis. Potential complications of pneumonia include bacteremia, pleural effusion, empyema, lung abscess, and pneumothorax (Sectish & Prober, 2007). Excluding bacteremia, these may require treatment with thoracentesis and/or chest tubes as well as antibiotics. Pneumatoceles (thin-walled cavities developing in the lung) might occur with certain bacterial pneumonias and usually resolve spontaneously over time.

Therapeutic management of children with less severe disease includes antipyretics, adequate hydration, and close observation. Even bacterial pneumonia can be successfully managed at home if the work of breathing is not severe and oxygen saturation is within normal limits. However, hospitalization is required for children with more severe disease. The child with tachypnea, significant retractions, poor oral intake, or lethargy might require hospital admission for the administration of supplemental oxygen, intravenous hydration, and antibiotics.

> ▶ **Take** NOTE!
>
> *Haemophilus influenzae type B has been nearly eliminated as a cause of pneumonia in North America and other developed countries as a result of universal immunization with Hib vaccine.*

Pathophysiology

Pneumonia occurs as a result of the spread of infectious organisms to the lower respiratory tract from either the upper respiratory tract or the bloodstream. In bacterial pneumonia, mucus stasis occurs as a result of vascular engorgement. Cellular debris (erythrocytes, neutrophils, and fibrin) accumulates in the alveolar space. Relative hyperexpansion with air trapping follows. Inflammation of the alveoli results in atelectasis. **Atelectasis** is defined as a collapsed or airless portion of the lung, so gas exchange becomes impaired. The inflammatory response further impairs gas exchange (Sectish & Prober, 2007).

Viral pneumonia usually results in an inflammatory reaction limited to the alveolar wall. Aspiration of food, fluids, or other substances into the bronchial tree can result in aspiration pneumonia. Aspiration is the most common cause of recurrent pneumonia in children and often occurs as a result of gastro-esophageal reflux disease. Secondary bacterial infection often occurs following viral or aspiration pneumonia and requires antibiotic treatment.

Nursing Assessment

For a full description of the assessment phase of the nursing process, refer to page 1260. Assessment findings pertinent to pneumonia are discussed below.

Health History

Elicit a description of the present illness and chief complaint. Note onset and progression of symptoms. Common signs and symptoms reported during the health history include:

- Antecedent viral URI
- Fever
- Cough (note type and whether productive or not)
- Increased respiratory rate
- History of lethargy, poor feeding, vomiting, or diarrhea in infants
- Chills, headache, dyspnea, chest pain, abdominal pain, and nausea or vomiting in older children

Explore the child's past and current medical history for risk factors known to be associated with an increase in the severity of pneumonia, such as:

- Prematurity
- Malnutrition
- Passive smoke exposure
- Low socioeconomic status
- Day care attendance
- Underlying cardiopulmonary, immune, or nervous system disease (Brady, 2009)

Physical Examination

Physical examination consists of inspection, auscultation, percussion, and palpation.

Inspection

Observe the child's general appearance and colour (centrally and peripherally). Cyanosis might accompany coughing spells. The child with bacterial pneumonia may appear ill. Assess work of breathing. Children with pneumonia might exhibit substernal, subcostal, or intercostal retractions. Tachypnea and nasal flaring may be present. Describe cough and quality of sputum if produced.

Auscultation

Auscultation of the lungs might reveal wheezes or rales in the younger child. Local or diffuse rales may be present in the older child. Document diminished breath sounds.

Percussion and Palpation

In the older child, percussion might yield local dullness over a consolidated area. Percussion is much less valuable in the infant or younger child. Tactile fremitus felt upon palpation may be increased with pneumonia.

Laboratory and Diagnostic Tests

Common laboratory and diagnostic studies ordered for the assessment of pneumonia include:

- Pulse oximetry: oxygen saturation might be significantly decreased or within normal range
- Chest X-ray: varies according to patient age and causative agent. In infants and young children, bilateral air trapping and perihilar **infiltrates** are the most common findings. Patchy areas of consolidation might also be present. In older children, lobar consolidation is seen more frequently.
- Sputum culture: limited usefulness in determining causative bacteria in older children and adolescents due to contamination by oral bacterial flora
- White blood cell count: might be elevated in bacterial pneumonia or decreased in viral pneumonia

Nursing Management

Nursing diagnoses, goals, and interventions for the child with pneumonia are primarily aimed at providing supportive care and education about the illness and its treatment. Prevention of pneumococcal infection is also important. Children with more severe disease will require hospitalization. Refer to the Nursing Care Plan 39.1 for nursing diagnoses and related interventions. In addition, the following should be noted.

Providing Supportive Care

Ensure adequate hydration and assist in thinning of secretions by encouraging oral fluid intake in the child whose respiratory status is stable. In children with increased work of breathing, intravenous fluids may be necessary to maintain hydration. Allow and encourage the child to assume a position of comfort, usually with the head of the bed elevated to promote aeration of the lungs. If pain due to coughing or pneumonia itself is severe, administer analgesics as prescribed. Provide supplemental oxygen to the child with respiratory distress or hypoxia as needed. Oxygen saturation goals will need to be determined and the concentration of oxygen adjusted accordingly.

Providing Family Education

Educate the family about the importance of adherence to the prescribed antibiotic regimen. Antibiotics may be given intravenously if the child is hospitalized, but upon discharge or if the child is managed on an out-patient basis, oral antibiotics will be used.

Teach the parents of a child with bacterial pneumonia to expect that following resolution of the acute illness, for 1 to 2 weeks, the child might continue to tire easily and the infant might continue to need small, frequent feedings. Cough may also persist after the acute recovery period but should lessen over time.

If the child is diagnosed with viral pneumonia, parents might not understand that their child does not require an antibiotic. Pneumonia is often perceived by the public as a bacterial infection, so most parents will need an explanation related to treatment of viral infections. As with bacterial pneumonia, the child may experience a week or two of weakness or fatigue following resolution of the acute illness.

The young child is at risk for the development of aspiration pneumonia. Parents need to understand that the child might be at risk for injury related to his or her age and developmental stage. To prevent recurrent or further aspiration, teach the parents the safety measures in Teaching Guideline 39.3.

Preventing Pneumococcal Infection

Children at high risk for severe pneumococcal infection should be immunized against it. Although provincial guidelines for immunizations may vary with regard to

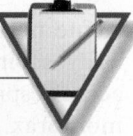

TEACHING GUIDELINE 39.3

Preventing Aspiration

• Keep toxic substances such as lighter fluid, solvents, and hydrocarbons out of reach of young children. Toddlers and preschoolers cannot distinguish safe from unsafe fluids due to their developmental stage.
• Avoid oily nose drops and oil-based vitamins or home remedies to avoid lipid aspiration into the lungs.
• Avoid oral feedings if the infant's respiratory rate is 60 breaths/minute or faster to minimize the risk of aspiration of the feeding.
• Do not "force-feed" in the event of poor oral intake or severe illness to minimize the risk of aspiration of the feeding.
• Do not prop bottles for infants while they are alone in the crib.
• Certain car seats may promote reflux in premature infants. If possible, have a hospital staff member assess the premature infant's car seat prior to discharge from hospital.
• Position infants and ill children on their right side after feeding to minimize the possibility of aspirating emesis or regurgitated feeding.

timing, cost, and eligibility, the high-risk category includes all children between 0 and 23 months of age as well as children between 24 and 59 months of age with certain conditions such as immune deficiency, sickle-cell disease, asplenia, chronic cardiac conditions, chronic lung problems, cerebrospinal fluid leaks, chronic renal insufficiency, diabetes mellitus, and organ transplants. For additional information refer to Chapter 30.

Bronchitis

Bronchitis is an inflammation of the trachea and major bronchi. It is often associated with a URI. Bronchitis is usually viral in nature, though *Mycoplasma pneumoniae* and other bacterial organisms are causative in about 10% of cases (Carolan, 2011). Recovery usually occurs within 5 to 10 days. Therapeutic management involves mainly supportive care. Expectorants may be administered with caution, and adequate hydration is important. If bacterial infection is the cause, antibiotics are indicated.

Nursing Assessment

The illness might begin with a mild URI. Fever develops, followed by a dry, hacking cough that might become productive in older children. The cough might wake the child at night. Auscultation of the lungs might reveal coarse rales. Respirations remain unlaboured. The chest X-ray might show diffuse alveolar hyperinflation and perihilar markings.

Nursing Management

Nursing management is aimed at providing supportive care. Teach parents that expectorants will help loosen secretions and antipyretics will help reduce the fever, making the child more comfortable. Encourage adequate hydration. Antibiotics are prescribed only in cases believed to be bacterial in nature. Discourage the use of cough suppressants: it is important for accumulated sputum to be raised.

Tuberculosis

Tuberculosis is a highly contagious disease caused by inhalation of droplets of *Mycobacterium tuberculosis* or *Mycobacterium bovis*. Children usually contract the disease from an immediate household member. Prevalence in Canada varies, with tuberculosis occurring most frequently in First Nations communities and among certain immigrant populations (Health Canada, 2010; PHAC, 2010a). In addition, children with chronic illness or malnutrition are more susceptible to infection. After exposure to an infected individual, the incubation period is 2 to 10 weeks. The inhaled tubercle bacilli multiply in the alveoli and alveolar ducts, forming an inflammatory exudate. The bacilli are spread by the bloodstream and lymphatic system to various parts of the body. Though pulmonary tuberculosis is the most common, children may also have infection in other parts of the body, such as the gastrointestinal tract or central nervous system.

In the case of drug-sensitive tuberculosis, the PHAC (2011a) recommends a 6-month course of oral therapy. The first 2 months consist of isoniazid, rifampin, and pyrazinamide given daily. This is followed by twice-weekly isoniazid and rifampin; administration must be observed directly (usually by a public health nurse). In the case of multidrug-resistant tuberculosis, ethambutol or streptomycin is given via intramuscular injection (PHAC, 2011a).

Nursing Assessment

Routine screening for tuberculosis infection is not recommended for low-risk individuals, but children considered to be at high risk for contracting tuberculosis should be screened using the Mantoux test. Children considered to be at high risk are those who:

- Are infected with HIV
- Are incarcerated or institutionalized
- Have a positive recent history of latent tuberculosis infection
- Are immigrants from or have a history of travel to endemic countries
- Are exposed at home to HIV-infected or homeless persons, illicit drug users, migrant farm workers, or nursing home residents (Federico, 2011)

Children with chronic illnesses (except HIV infection) are not more likely to become infected with tuberculosis but should receive special consideration and be screened prior to initiation of immunosuppressant therapies (Reznik & Ozuah, 2005).

The presentation of tuberculosis in children is quite varied. Children can be asymptomatic or exhibit a broad range of symptoms. Symptoms may include fever, malaise, weight loss, anorexia, pain and tightness in the chest, and rarely hemoptysis. Cough might or might not be present and usually progresses slowly over several weeks to months. As tuberculosis progresses, the respiratory rate increases and the lung on the affected side is poorly expanded. Dullness to percussion might be present, as well as diminished breath sounds and crackles. Fever persists and pallor, anemia, weakness, and weight loss are present. Diagnosis is confirmed with a positive Mantoux test, positive gastric washings for acid-fast bacillus, and/or a chest X-ray consistent with tuberculosis (Reznik & Ozuah, 2005).

Nursing Management

Hospitalization of children with tuberculosis is necessary only for the most serious cases. Nursing management is aimed at providing supportive care and encouraging adherence to the treatment regimen. Most nursing care for childhood tuberculosis is provided in out-patient clinics, schools, or a public health setting. Supportive care includes ensuring adequate nutrition and adequate rest, providing comfort measures such as fever reduc-

tion, preventing exposure to other infectious diseases, and preventing reinfection.

Providing Care for the Child with Latent Tuberculosis Infection

Children who test positive for tuberculosis but who do not have symptoms or radiographic/laboratory evidence of disease are considered to have latent infection. These children should be treated with isoniazid for 9 months to prevent progression to active disease. Follow-up and appropriate monitoring can be achieved via the child's primary care provider or local health department.

Preventing Infection

Tuberculosis infection is prevented by avoiding contact with the tubercle bacillus. Thus, hospitalized children with tuberculosis must be isolated according to hospital policy to prevent nosocomial spread of tuberculosis infection. Promotion of natural resistance through nutrition, rest, and avoidance of serious infections does not prevent infection. Pasteurization of milk has helped to decrease the transmission of *Mycobacterium bovis*. Administration of bacille Calmette–Guérin (BCG) vaccine can provide some protection against tuberculosis and is recommended for administration to First Nations newborns prior to discharge from the hospital.

Acute Noninfectious Disorders

Acute noninfectious disorders include epistaxis, foreign body aspiration, respiratory distress syndrome (RDS), acute respiratory distress syndrome (ARDS), and pneumothorax.

Epistaxis

Epistaxis (a nosebleed) occurs most frequently in children younger than adolescent age. Bleeding of the nasal mucosa occurs most often from the anterior portion of the septum. Epistaxis may be recurrent and idiopathic (meaning there is no cause). The majority of cases are benign, but in children with bleeding disorders or other hematologic concerns, epistaxis should be further investigated and treated.

▶ **Take** NOTE!

The child with recurrent epistaxis or epistaxis that is difficult to control should be further evaluated for underlying bleeding or platelet concerns.

Nursing Assessment

Explore the child's history for initiating factors such as local inflammation, mucosal drying, or local trauma (usually nose picking). Inspect the nasal cavity for blood.

Nursing Management

The presence of blood often frightens children and their parents. The nurse and parents should remain calm. The child should sit up and lean forward (lying down may allow aspiration of the blood). Apply continuous pressure to the anterior portion of the nose by pinching it closed. Encourage the child to breathe through the mouth during this portion of the treatment. Ice or a cold cloth applied to the bridge of the nose may also be helpful. The bleeding usually stops within 10 to 15 minutes. Apply petroleum jelly or water-soluble gel to the nasal mucosa with a cotton-tipped applicator to moisten the mucosa and prevent recurrence.

Foreign Body Aspiration

Foreign body aspiration occurs when any solid or liquid substance is inhaled into the respiratory tract. It is common in infants and young children and can present in a life-threatening manner. The object may lodge in the upper or lower airway, causing varying degrees of respiratory difficulty. Small, smooth objects such as peanuts are the most frequently aspirated, but any small toy, article, or piece of food smaller than the diameter of the young child's airway can potentially be aspirated: popcorn, vegetables, hot dogs, fruit snacks, coins, latex balloon pieces, pins, and pen caps are commonly seen (Gregori et al., 2008).

Foreign body aspiration occurs most frequently in children ages 6 months to 4 years (Federico, 2011). Children this age are growing and developing rapidly. They tend to explore things with their mouths and can easily aspirate small items.

The child often coughs out foreign bodies from the upper airway. If the foreign body reaches the bronchus, then it may need to be surgically removed via bronchoscopy. Postoperative antibiotics are used if an infection is also present. Complications of foreign body aspiration include pneumonia or abscess formation, hypoxia, respiratory failure, and death (Gregori et al., 2008).

Nursing Assessment

The infant or young child might present with a history of sudden onset of cough, wheeze, or stridor. Stridor suggests that the foreign body is lodged in the upper airway. Sometimes the onset of respiratory symptoms is much more gradual. When the item has travelled down one of the bronchi, then wheezing, rhonchi, and decreased aeration can be heard on the affected side. A chest X-ray will demonstrate the foreign body only if it is radiopaque (Fig. 39.14).

Nursing Management

The most important nursing intervention related to foreign body aspiration is prevention. Anticipatory guidance for families with 6-month-olds should include a discus-

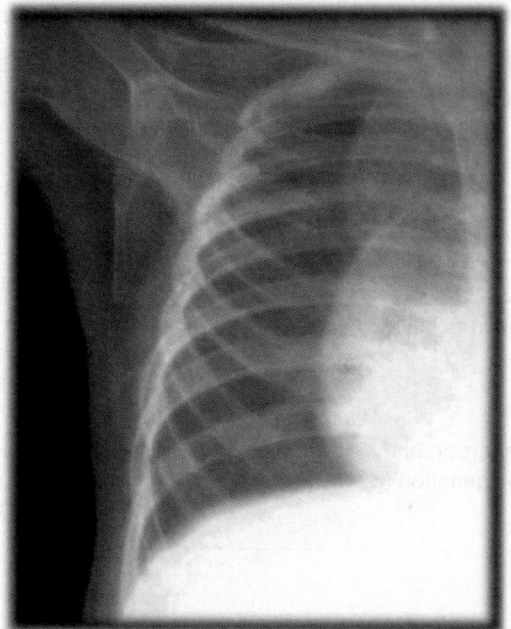

FIGURE 39.14 Foreign body is noted in the bronchus upon chest X-ray.

sion of aspiration avoidance. This information should be reiterated at each subsequent well-child visit through age 5 years. Tell parents to avoid letting their child play with toys with small parts and to keep coins and other small objects out of the reach of children. Teach parents not to feed peanuts and popcorn to their child until he or she is at least 3 years old (Federico, 2011). When children progress to table food, teach parents to chop all foods so that they are small enough to pass down the trachea should the child neglect to chew them up thoroughly. Carrots, grapes, and hot dogs should be cut into small pieces. Harmful liquids should be kept out of the reach of children (AAP, 2010).

> ▶ **Take** NOTE!
>
> *Items smaller than 3.2 cm (1.25 inches) can be aspirated easily. A simple way for parents to estimate the safe size of a small item or toy piece is to gauge its size against a standard toilet paper roll, which is generally about 3.8 cm (1.5 inches) in diameter (Safe Kids USA, 2009).*

Respiratory Distress Syndrome

RDS is a respiratory disorder that is specific to neonates. It results from lung immaturity and a deficiency in surfactant, so it is seen most often in premature infants. Other infants who might experience RDS include infants of diabetic mothers, those delivered via cesarean section

TABLE 39.3 ALTERNATIVES TO TRADITIONAL MECHANICAL VENTILATION

Mode	Description	Additional Information
High-frequency ventilators (high frequency, oscillating, or jet)	Provide very high respiratory rates (up to 1,200 breaths/minute) and very low tidal volumes	May decrease risk of barotraumas and volutrauma associated with ventilator pressures
Nitric oxide	Causes pulmonary vasodilation if pulmonary hypertension is an issue, helping to increase blood flow to alveoli	Safe; no long-term developmental risks
Liquid ventilation	Perfluorocarbon liquid acts as a surfactant. Provides an effective medium for gas exchange and increases pulmonary function.	Virtually no reported physiologic sequelae
Extracorporeal membrane oxygenation (ECMO)	Blood is removed from body via catheter, warmed and oxygenated in the ECMO machine, and then returned to infant.	Labour-intensive. Risk of bleeding is great. Not available at all centres in Canada.

without preceding labour, and those experiencing perinatal asphyxia (Thilo & Rosenberg, 2011). It is believed that each of these conditions has an impact on surfactant production, thus resulting in RDS in the term infant.

The administration of surfactant via endotracheal tube shortly after delivery helps to decrease the incidence and severity of RDS (Stevens, 2007). Management of RDS focuses on intensive respiratory care, usually with mechanical ventilation. Newer techniques for ventilatory support are also available (Engle, 2008; Seger & Soll, 2009) (Table 39.3).

Pathophysiology

The lack of surfactant in the affected newborn's lungs results in stiff, poorly compliant lungs with poor gas exchange. Right-to-left shunting and hypoxemia result. As the disease progresses, fluid and fibrin leak from the pulmonary capillaries cause hyaline membrane to form in the bronchioles, alveolar ducts, and alveoli. Presence of the membrane further decreases gas exchange. Complications of RDS include air leak syndrome, bronchopulmonary dysplasia, patent ductus arteriosus and congestive heart failure, intraventricular hemorrhage, retinopathy of prematurity, necrotizing enterocolitis, complications resulting from intravenous catheter use (infection, thrombus formation), and developmental delay or disability (Sweet et al., 2007).

Nursing Assessment

The onset of RDS is usually within several hours of birth. The newborn exhibits signs of respiratory distress, including tachypnea, retractions, nasal flaring, grunting, and varying degrees of cyanosis. Auscultation reveals fine rales and diminished breath sounds. If untreated, RDS progresses to seesaw respirations, respiratory failure, and shock.

Nursing Management

Rarely, mucus plugging can occur in the neonate placed on a ventilator after surfactant administration. Therefore, close observation and assessment for adequate lung expansion are critical. In addition to expert respiratory intervention, other crucial nursing goals include maintenance of normothermia, prevention of infection, maintenance of fluid and electrolyte balance, and promotion of adequate nutrition (parenterally or via gavage feeding). Nursing care of the infant with RDS generally occurs in the intensive care unit.

Acute Respiratory Distress Syndrome

ARDS occurs following a primary insult such as sepsis, viral pneumonia, smoke inhalation, or near-drowning. Acute onset of respiratory distress and hypoxemia occur within 72 hours of the insult in infants and children with previously healthy lungs (Thilo & Rosenberg, 2011). The alveolar–capillary membrane becomes more permeable and pulmonary edema develops. Hyaline membrane formation over the alveolar surfaces and decreased surfactant production cause lung stiffness. Mucosal swelling and cellular debris lead to atelectasis. Gas diffusion is impaired significantly. ARDS can progress to respiratory failure and death, though some individuals recover completely or have residual lung disease.

Medical treatment is aimed at improving **oxygenation** and **ventilation**. Mechanical ventilation is used with special attention to lung volumes and positive end-expiratory pressure (PEEP). Newer treatment modalities show promise for improving outcomes of ARDS.

Nursing Assessment

Tachycardia and tachypnea occur over the first few hours of the illness. Significantly increased work of breathing with nasal flaring and retractions develops. Auscultate

EVIDENCE-BASED PRACTICE 39.1
Various Body Positions and their Effects on Hospitalized Infants and Young Children with Acute Respiratory Distress

● Study

Prone positioning has been found to improve ventilation in some adults with acute respiratory distress and in premature infants with RDS, but due to the risk of SIDS, infants are generally positioned supine. The authors reviewed 21 studies that evaluated the effect of positioning (supine, prone, lateral, elevated, and flat positions) on respiratory function (oxygen saturation, partial pressure of arterial oxygen, oxygenation index, thoraco-abdominal synchrony, and episodes of oxygen desaturation) in infants and young children with acute respiratory distress.

▲ Findings

The only position found to produce a statistically significant improvement in respiratory function was the prone position. The prone position was better in terms of improving ventilation and oxygenation. The other positions did not demonstrate statistically significant differences.

■ Nursing Implications

Nurses should critically consider the result of this review. Certainly, if an alternate position is used, the infant must be closely monitored and the position changed should any level of deterioration occur. If hospitalized infants with acute respiratory distress are placed in the prone position, continuous cardiopulmonary and oxygenation saturation monitoring must be provided because of the risk of SIDS in this age group. Do not encourage families to use the prone position at home when an infant is ill with a respiratory condition.

Wells, D. A., Gillies, D., & Fitzgerald, D. A. (2010). Positioning for acute respiratory distress in hospitalised infants and children. *Cochrane Database of Systematic Reviews, 18*, CD003645.

for breath sounds, which might range from normal to high-pitched crackles throughout the lung fields. Hypoxemia develops. Bilateral infiltrates can be seen on a chest X-ray.

Nursing Management

Nursing care of the child with ARDS is mainly supportive and occurs in the intensive care unit. Closely monitor respiratory and cardiovascular status. Comfort measures such as hygiene and positioning as well as pain and anxiety management, maintenance of nutrition, and prevention of infection are also key nursing interventions. The acute phase of worsening respiratory distress can be frightening for a child of any age, and the nurse can be instrumental in soothing the child's fears. As the disease worsens and progresses, especially when ventilatory support is required, psychological support of the family as well as education about the intensive care unit procedures will be especially important. See Evidence-based Practice 39.1 for information about positioning of infants and children with acute respiratory distress.

Pneumothorax

A collection of air in the pleural space is called a pneumothorax. It can occur spontaneously in an otherwise healthy child, or as a result of chronic lung disease, cardiopulmonary resuscitation, surgery, or trauma. Trapped air consumes space within the pleural cavity, and the affected lung suffers at least partial collapse. Needle aspiration and/or placement of a chest tube is used to evacuate the air from the chest. Some small pneumothoraces resolve independently, without intervention.

Nursing Assessment

Primary pneumothorax (spontaneous) occurs most often in adolescence (Gluckman & Forti, 2011) (Fig. 39.15). The infant or child with a pneumothorax might have a sudden or gradual onset of symptoms. Chest pain might be present as well as signs of respiratory distress such as tachypnea, retractions, nasal flaring, or grunting. Assess potential risk factors for acquiring a pneumothorax, including chest trauma or surgery, intubation and mechanical ventilation, or a history of chronic lung disease such as cystic fibrosis. Inspect the child for a pale or cyanotic appearance. Auscultate for increased heart rate (tachycardia) and absent or diminished breath sounds on the affected side. The X-ray reveals air within the thoracic cavity.

Nursing Management

The child with a pneumothorax requires frequent respiratory assessments. Pulse oximetry might be used as an adjunct, but clinical evaluation of respiratory status is most useful. In some cases, administration of 100% oxygen hastens the reabsorption of air, but it is generally used only for a few hours (Gluckman & Forti, 2011). If a chest tube connected to a water seal or suction is present, provide care of the drainage apparatus as appropriate (Fig. 39.16). A pair of hemostats should be kept at the bedside to clamp the tube should it become dislodged from the drainage container. The dressing around the chest tube is occlusive and is not routinely changed. If the tube becomes dislodged from the child's chest, apply Vaseline gauze and an occlusive dressing, immediately perform appropriate respiratory assessment, and notify the physician.

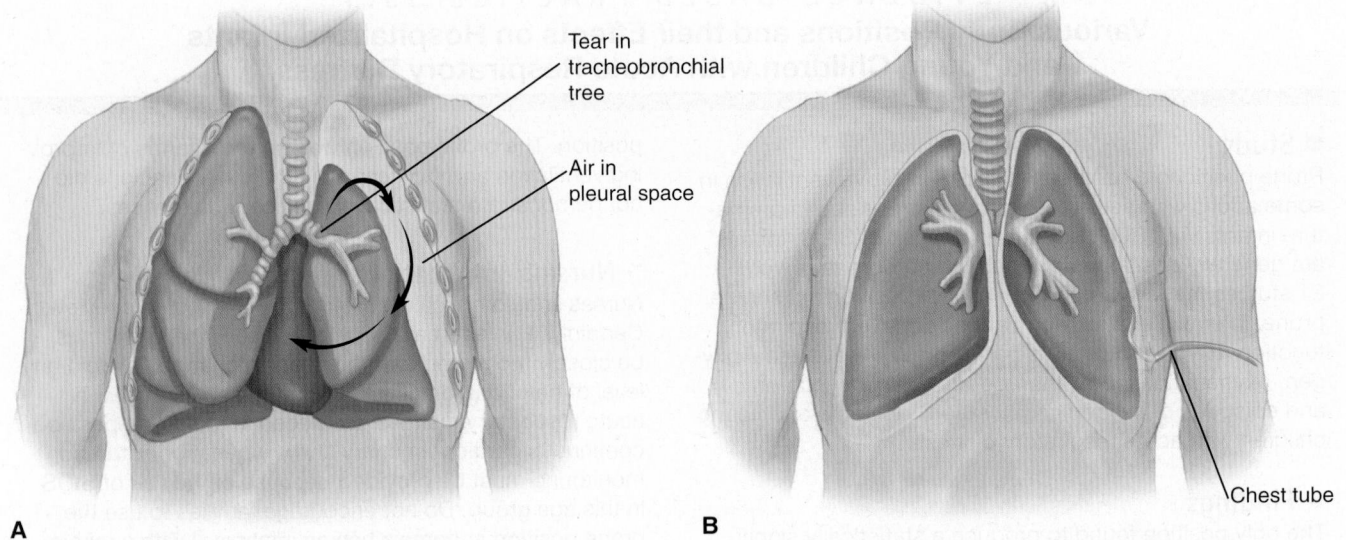

A

B

Chest tube

FIGURE 39.15 Pneumothorax.

Chronic Diseases

Chronic respiratory disorders include allergic rhinitis, asthma, chronic lung disease (bronchopulmonary dysplasia), cystic fibrosis, and apnea.

Allergic Rhinitis

Allergic **rhinitis** is a common chronic condition in childhood, affecting up to 40% of children (Hagemann, 2005).

Allergic rhinitis is associated with atopic dermatitis and asthma, with as many as 80% of asthmatic children also suffering from allergic rhinitis (Thomas, Kocevar, Zhang, Yin, & Price, 2005). Perennial allergic rhinitis occurs year-round and is associated with indoor environments. Allergens commonly implicated in perennial allergic rhinitis include dust mites, pet dander, cockroach antigens, and molds. Seasonal allergic rhinitis is caused by elevations in outdoor levels of allergens. It is typically caused by certain pollens, trees, weeds, fungi, and molds.

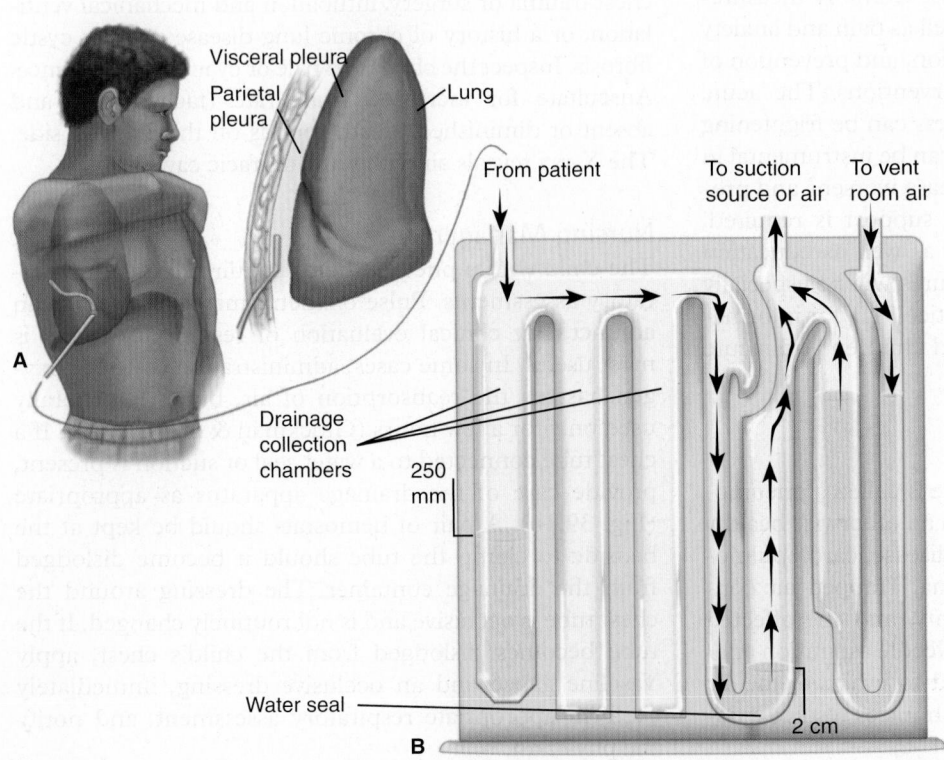

Visceral pleura

Parietal pleura

Lung

A

From patient

To suction source or air

To vent room air

Drainage collection chambers

250 mm

Water seal

2 cm

B

FIGURE 39.16 The chest tube is connected to suction or water seal via a drainage container.

Complications from allergic rhinitis include exacerbation of asthma symptoms, recurrent sinusitis and otitis media, and dental malocclusion.

Pathophysiology

Allergic rhinitis is an intermittent or persistent inflammatory state that is mediated by immunoglobulin E (IgE). In response to contact with an airborne allergen protein, the nasal mucosa mounts an immune response. The antigen (from the allergen) binds to a specific IgE on the surface of mast cells, releasing the chemical mediators of histamine and leukotrienes. The release of mediators results in acute tissue edema and mucous production (Banasiak & Meadows-Oliver, 2005). Late-phase mediators are released and more inflammation results. IgE binds to receptors on the surfaces of mast cells and basophils, creating the sensitization memory that causes the reaction with subsequent allergen exposures. Allergen exposure then results in mast cell degranulation and release of histamine and other chemotactic factors. Histamine and other factors cause nasal vasodilation, watery mucous called **rhinorrhea**, and nasal congestion. Irritation of local nerve endings by histamine produces pruritus and sneezing (Hagemann, 2005). Treatment of allergic rhinitis is aimed at decreasing response to these allergic mediators as well as treating inflammation.

Nursing Assessment

For a full description of the assessment phase of the nursing process, refer to page 1260. Assessment findings pertinent to allergic rhinitis are discussed below.

Health History

Elicit a description of the present illness and chief complaint. Common signs and symptoms reported during the health history might include:

- Mild, intermittent to chronic nasal stuffiness
- Thin, runny nasal discharge
- Sneezing
- Itching of nose, eyes, palate
- Mouth breathing and snoring

Determine the seasonality of symptoms. Are they perennial (year-round) or do they occur during certain seasons? What types of medications or other treatments have been used, and what was the child's response?

Explore the history for the presence of risk factors such as:

- Family history of atopic disease (asthma, allergic rhinitis, or atopic dermatitis)
- Known allergy to dust mites, pet dander, cockroach antigens, pollens, or molds
- Early childhood exposure to indoor allergens
- Early introduction to foods or formula in infancy
- Exposure to tobacco smoke
- Environmental air pollution
- Recurrent viral infections (Sheikh & Najib, 2011)

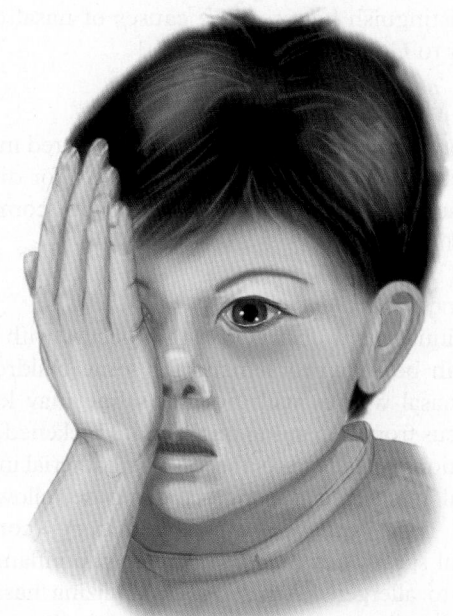

FIGURE 39.17 Allergic shiners beneath the eyes and allergic salute across the nose.

Nonwhite race and higher socioeconomic status have also been noted as risk factors (Hagemann, 2005).

Physical Examination

Physical examination of the child with allergic rhinitis includes inspection, observation, and auscultation.

Inspection and Observation

Observe the child's facies for red-rimmed eyes or tearing, mild eyelid edema, "allergic shiners" (bluish or greyish cast beneath the eyes; Fig. 39.17), and "allergic salute" (a transverse nasal crease between the lower and middle thirds of the nose that results from repeated nose rubbing). Inspect the nasal cavity. The turbinates may be swollen and grey/blue in colour. Clear mucoid nasal drainage may be observed. Inspect the skin for rash. Listen for nasal phonation with speech.

Auscultation

Auscultate the lungs for adequate aeration and clarity of breath sounds. In the child who also has asthma, exacerbation with wheezing often occurs with allergic rhinitis.

Laboratory and Diagnostic Tests

The initial diagnosis is often made based on the history and clinical findings. Common laboratory and diagnostic studies ordered for the assessment of allergic rhinitis may include:

- Nasal smear (positive for eosinophilia)
- Positive allergy skin test
- Positive radioallergosorbent test (RAST)

To distinguish between the causes of nasal congestion, refer to Comparison Chart 39.1.

Nursing Management

In addition to the nursing diagnoses and related interventions discussed in Nursing Care Plan 39.1 for disorders of the nose, mouth, and throat, interventions common to allergic rhinitis follow.

Maintaining Patent Airway

The continual nasal obstruction that occurs with allergic rhinitis can be very problematic for some children. Performing nasal washes with normal saline may keep the nasal mucus from becoming thickened. Thickened, immobile secretions often lead to a secondary bacterial infection. The nasal wash also decongests the nose, allowing for improved nasal airflow. Anti-inflammatory (corticosteroid) nasal sprays can help to decrease the inflammatory response to allergens. A mast cell stabilizing nasal spray such as cromolyn sodium may decrease the intensity and frequency of allergic responses. Oral antihistamines are now available in once-daily dosing, providing convenience for the family. Some children may benefit from a combined antihistamine/nasal decongestant if nasal congestion is significant. Leukotriene modifiers such as montelukast may also be beneficial for some children (Banasiak & Meadows-Oliver, 2005).

Providing Family Education

One of the most important tools in the treatment of allergic rhinitis is learning to avoid known allergens. Teaching Guideline 39.4 gives information on educating families about avoidance of allergens. Children may be referred to a specialist for allergen desensitization (allergy shots). Products helpful with control of allergies are available from a number of vendors (visit http://thePoint.lww.com/Chow1e for a direct link to one such site).

Asthma

Asthma is a chronic inflammatory airway disorder characterized by airway hyperresponsiveness, airway edema, and mucus production. Airway obstruction resulting from asthma might be partially or completely reversed. Severity ranges from long periods of control with infrequent acute exacerbations in some children to the presence of persistent daily symptoms in others (Subbarao, Mandhane, & Sears, 2009). It is the most common chronic illness of childhood. A small percentage of children with asthma account for a large percentage of health

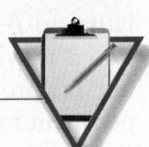

TEACHING GUIDELINE 39.4

Controlling Exposure to Allergens

Tobacco

- Avoid all exposure to tobacco smoke (this includes self-smoking).
- If parents cannot quit, they must not smoke inside the home or car.

Dust Mites

- Use pillow and mattress covers.
- Wash sheets, pillowcases, and comforters once a week in 54°C water.
- Use blinds rather than curtains in bedroom.
- Remove stuffed animals from bedroom.
- Reduce indoor humidity to <50%.
- Remove carpet from bedroom.
- Clean solid surface floors with wet mop each week.

Pet Dander

- Remove pets from home permanently.
- If unable to remove them, keep them out of bedroom and off carpet and upholstered furniture.

Cockroaches

- Keep kitchen very clean.
- Avoid leaving out food or drinks.
- Use pesticides if necessary, but ensure that the asthmatic child is not inside the home when it is sprayed.

Indoor Molds

- Repair water leaks.
- Use dehumidifier to keep basement dry.
- Reduce indoor humidity to <50%.

Outdoor Molds, Pollen, and Air Pollution

- Avoid going outdoors when mold and pollen counts are high.
- Avoid outdoor activity when pollution levels are high.

Adapted from: National Asthma Education and Prevention Program. (2007). *Expert panel report 3: Guidelines for the diagnosis and management of asthma* (NIH Publication No. 07-4051). Bethesda, MD: National Institutes of Health, National Heart, Lung and Blood Institute; and Ratcliffe, M. M. & Kieckhefer, G. M. (2010). Asthma. In P. J. Allen, J. A. Vessey, & N. A. Schapiro (Eds.), *Primary care of the child with a chronic condition* (5th ed.). St. Louis, MO: Mosby.

care use and expense. Asthma accounts for about 12 million lost school days per year and a significant number of lost workdays on the part of parents (Kovesi et al., 2010). The incidence and severity of asthma are increasing; this may be attributed to increased urbanization, increased air pollution, and more accurate diagnostics.

Severity ranges from symptoms associated only with vigorous activity (exercise-induced bronchospasm) to daily symptoms that interfere with quality of life. Though uncommon, childhood death related to asthma is also on the rise worldwide. Air pollution, allergens, family history, and viral infections might all play a role in asthma (Ratcliffe & Kieckhefer, 2010). Many children with asthma also have gastro-esophageal disease, though the relationship between the two diseases is not clearly understood.

Complications of asthma include chronic airway remodelling, status asthmaticus (where progressively worsening reactive airways are unresponsive to usual therapy), and respiratory failure. Children with asthma are also more susceptible to serious bacterial and viral respiratory infections (Ratcliffe & Kieckhefer, 2010).

Current goals of medical therapy are avoidance of asthma triggers and reduction or control of inflammatory episodes. An asthma management continuum of recommended pharmacotherapy has been developed by the Canadian Thoracic Society for children ages 6 years and older (Fig. 39.18) (Lougheed et al., 2010). This continuum is used to guide management of diagnosed asthma. For example, fast-acting bronchodilators are used to treat acute symptoms, inhaled corticosteroids are used for initial maintenance therapy, and leukotriene receptor antagonists are used as second-line monotherapy for mild asthma. Additional agents such as long-acting beta$_2$ agonists may be added if adequate control is not obtained (Lougheed et al., 2010). Although children under the age of 6 years may be prescribed similar medications as older children, there are important differences in the types of asthma and the symptom patterns for younger children that must be considered in treatment strategies (Kovesi

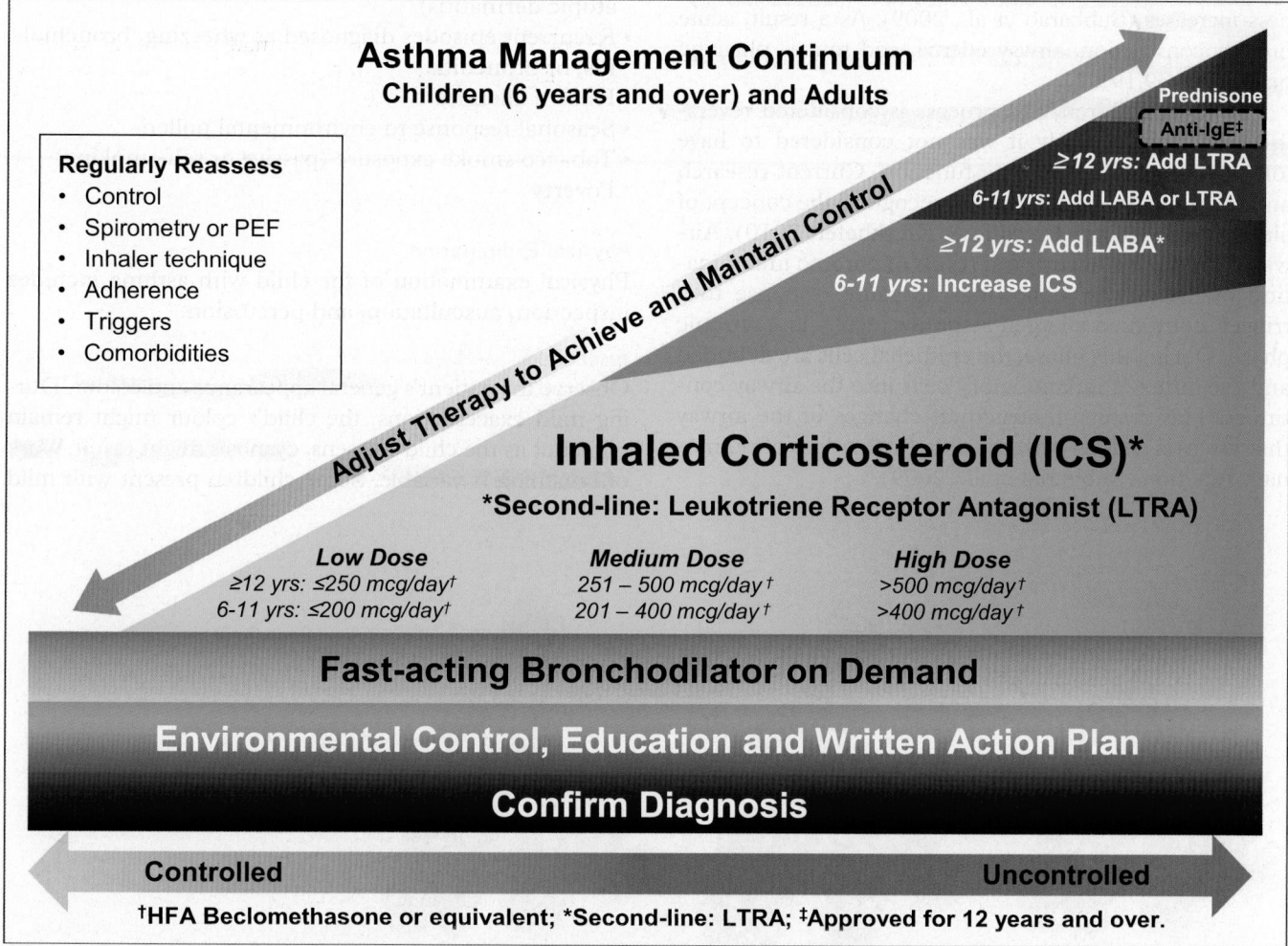

FIGURE 39.18 Asthma management continuum. HFA, hydrofluoroalkane; ICS, inhaled corticosteroids; IgE, immunoglobulin E; LABA, long-acting beta$_2$ agonists; LTRA, leukotriene receptor antagonists; PEF, peak expiratory flow.

et al., 2010). For example, it is difficult in young children to differentiate between wheezing and noisy breathing due to retained upper airway secretions, and it is not feasible to conduct conventional pulmonary lung function tests (Kovesi et al., 2010).

Pathophysiology

In asthma, the inflammatory process contributes to increased airway activity. Thus, control or prevention of inflammation is the core of asthma management. Asthma results from a complex variety of responses in relation to a trigger. When the process begins, mast cells, T lymphocytes, macrophages, and epithelial cells are involved in the release of inflammatory mediators. Eosinophils and neutrophils migrate to the airway, causing injury. Chemical mediators such as leukotrienes, bradykinin, histamine, and platelet-activating factor also contribute to the inflammatory response. The presence of leukotrienes contributes to prolonged airway constriction (Banasiak & Meadows-Oliver, 2005). Autonomic neural control of airway tone is affected, airway mucus secretion is increased, mucociliary function changes, and airway smooth muscle responsiveness increases (Subbarao et al., 2009). As a result, acute bronchoconstriction, airway edema, and mucus plugging occur (Fig. 39.19).

In most children, this process is considered reversible and until recently it was not considered to have longstanding effects on lung function. Current research and scientific thought, however, recognize the concept of airway remodelling (Ratcliffe & Kieckhefer, 2010). Airway remodelling occurs as a result of chronic inflammation of the airway. Following the acute response to a trigger, continued allergen response results in a chronic phase. During this phase, the epithelial cells are denuded and the influx of inflammatory cells into the airway continues. This results in structural changes of the airway that are irreversible, with possible further loss of pulmonary function (Subbarao et al., 2009).

Nursing Assessment

For a full description of the assessment phase of the nursing process, refer to page 1260. Assessment findings pertinent to asthma are discussed below (Registered Nurses' Association of Ontario, 2008).

Health History

Elicit a description of the present illness and chief complaint. Common signs and symptoms reported during the health history might include:

- Cough, particularly at night: hacking type of cough that is initially nonproductive, becoming productive of frothy sputum
- Difficulty breathing: shortness of breath, chest tightness or pain, dyspnea with exercise
- Wheezing

Explore the child's current and past medical history for risk factors such as:

- History of allergic rhinitis or atopic dermatitis
- Family history of atopy (asthma, allergic rhinitis, atopic dermatitis)
- Recurrent episodes diagnosed as wheezing, bronchiolitis, or bronchitis
- Known allergies
- Seasonal response to environmental pollen
- Tobacco smoke exposure (passive or self-smoking)
- Poverty

Physical Examination

Physical examination of the child with asthma includes inspection, auscultation, and percussion.

Inspection

Observe the patient's general appearance and colour. During mild exacerbations, the child's colour might remain pink, but as the child worsens, cyanosis might result. Work of breathing is variable. Some children present with mild

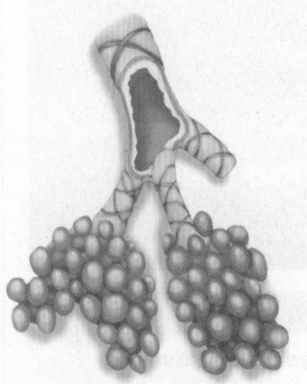
Normal airway

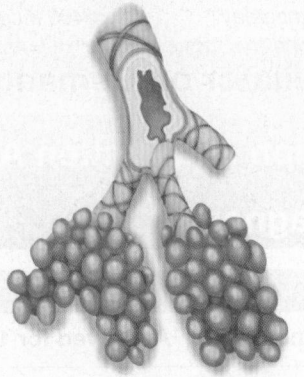
Airway with inflammation

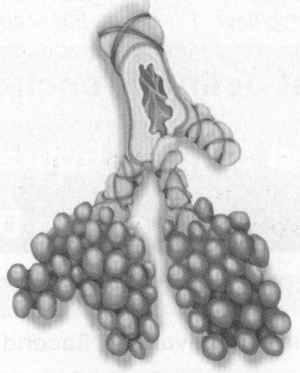
Airway with inflammation, bronchospasm, and mucus production

FIGURE 39.19 Note airway edema, mucus production, and bronchospasm occurring with asthma.

retractions, while others demonstrate significant accessory muscle use and eventually head-bobbing if not effectively treated. The child may appear anxious and fearful or be lethargic and irritable. An audible wheeze might be present. Children with persistent severe asthma may have a barrel chest and routinely demonstrate mildly increased work of breathing.

Auscultation and Percussion

A thorough assessment of lung fields is necessary. Wheezing is the hallmark of airway obstruction and might vary throughout the lung fields. Coarseness might also be present. Assess the adequacy of aeration. Breath sounds might be diminished in the bases or throughout. A quiet chest in an asthmatic child can be an ominous sign. With severe airway obstruction, air movement can be so poor that wheezes might not be heard upon auscultation. Percussion may yield hyperresonance.

Laboratory and Diagnostic Tests

Laboratory and diagnostic studies commonly ordered for the assessment of asthma include:

- Pulse oximetry: oxygen saturation may be significantly decreased or normal during a mild exacerbation
- Chest X-ray: usually reveals hyperinflation
- Blood gases: might show carbon dioxide retention and hypoxemia
- Pulmonary function tests (PFTs): can be very useful in determining the degree of disease but are not useful during an acute attack. Children as young as 5 or 6 years might be able to comply with spirometry.
- Peak expiratory flow rate (PEFR): is decreased during an exacerbation
- Allergy testing: skin test or RAST can determine allergic triggers for the asthmatic child

Nursing Management

Initial nursing management of the child with an acute exacerbation of asthma is aimed at restoring a clear airway and effective breathing pattern as well as promoting adequate oxygenation and ventilation (gas exchange). Refer to Nursing Care Plan 39.1. Additional considerations are reviewed below.

Educating the Child and Family

Asthma is a chronic illness and needs to be understood as such. Teach families of children with asthma, and the children themselves, how to care for the disease. Symptom-free periods (often very long) are interspersed with episodes of exacerbation. Parents and children often do not understand the importance of maintenance medications for long-term control. They may view the episodes of exacerbation (sometimes requiring hospitalization or emergency room visits) as an acute illness and are simply relieved when they are over. Frequently during the periods between acute episodes, children are viewed as disease-free and

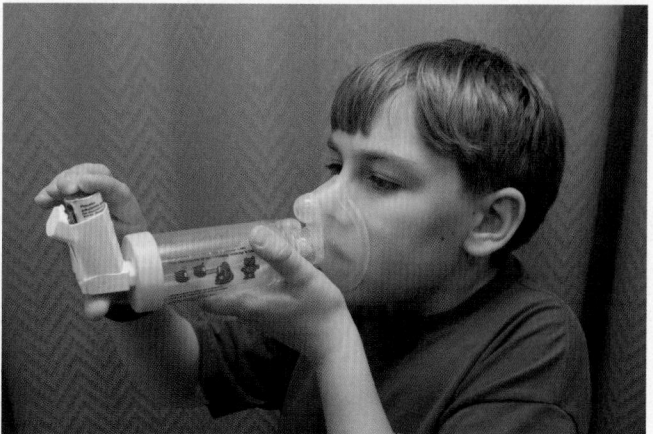

FIGURE 39.20 Commercial spacer device.

long-term maintenance schedules are abandoned. The prolonged inflammatory process occurring in the absence of symptoms, primarily in children with moderate to severe asthma, can lead to airway remodelling and eventual irreversible disease.

To provide appropriate education to the child and family, determine the severity of the asthma as outlined by the National Asthma Education and Prevention Program (NAEPP, 2007). Stress the concept of maintenance medications for the prevention of future serious disease in addition to controlling or preventing current symptoms.

Educate families and children on the appropriate use of nebulizers, metered-dose inhalers, spacers, dry-powder inhalers, and Diskus, as well as the purposes, functions, and side effects of the medications they deliver. Require return demonstration of equipment use to ensure that children and families can use the equipment properly (Teaching Guideline 39.5).

> ▶ *Take* NOTE!
>
> *The NAEPP (2007) recommends use of a spacer or holding chamber with metered-dose inhalers to increase the bioavailability of medication in the lungs. See Figure 39.20.*

Each child should have a management plan in place to determine when to step up or step down treatment. Figure 39.21 provides an example by the Asthma Society of Canada of a written format that may be helpful to families in the management of asthma. This written action plan should also be kept on file at the child's school, and relief medication should be available to the child at all times. Children who experience exercise-induced bronchospasm may still participate in physical education or athletics but may need to be allowed to use their medicine before the activity.

(text continues on page 1301)

TEACHING GUIDELINE 39.5

Using Asthma Medication Delivery Devices

Nebulizer

• Plug in the nebulizer and connect the air compressor tubing.

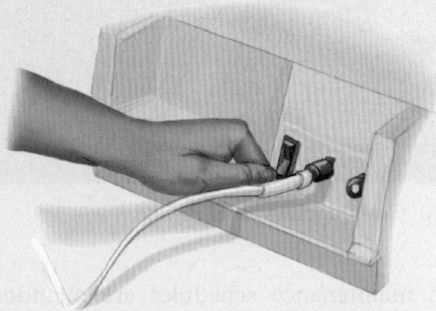

• Add the medication to the medicine cup.

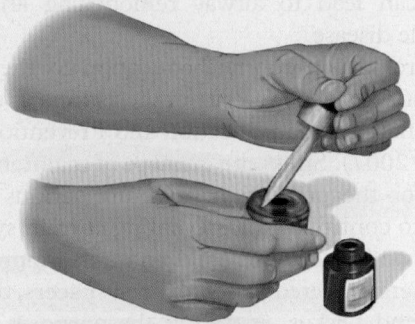

• Attach the mask or the mouthpiece and hose to the medicine cup.

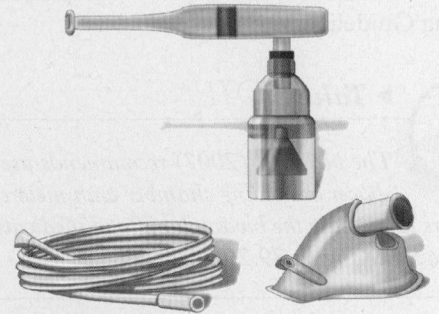

• Place the mask on the child OR

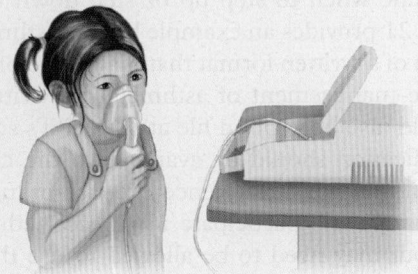

• Instruct the child to close the lips around the mouthpiece and breathe through the mouth.

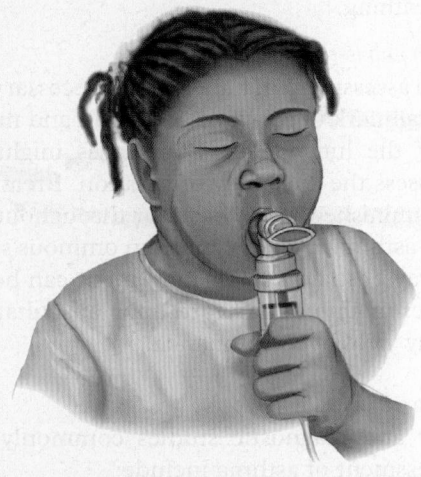

• After use, wash the mouthpiece and medicine cup with water and allow to air dry.

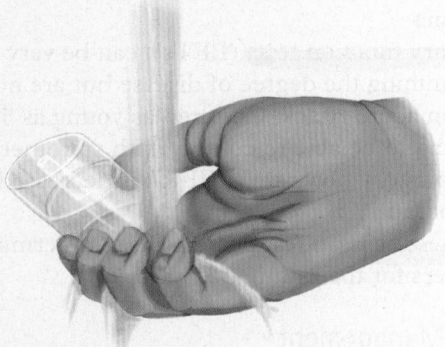

Metered–Dose Inhaler

• Shake the inhaler and take off the cap.

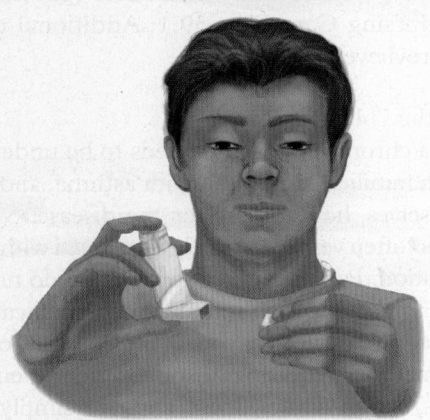

TEACHING GUIDELINE 39.5 (continued)

• Attach the inhaler to the spacer or holding chamber.
• Breathe out completely.

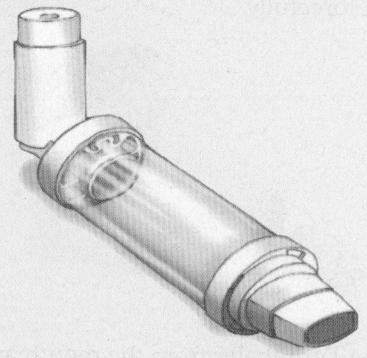

• Put the spacer mouthpiece in the mouth (or place the mask over the child's nose and mouth, ensuring a good seal).

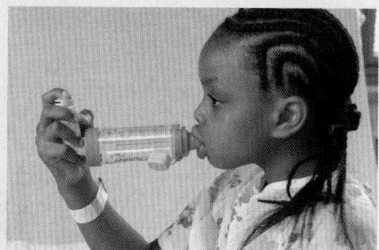

• Compress the inhaler and inhale slowly and deeply. Hold the breath for a count of 10.

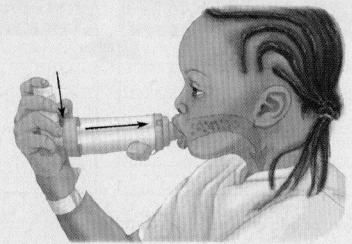

Diskus

• Hold the Diskus in a horizontal position in one hand and push the thumbgrip with the thumb of your other hand away from you until mouthpiece is exposed.

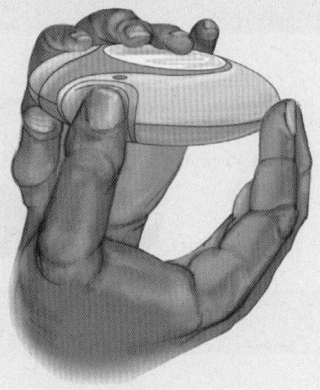

• Push the lever until it clicks (the dose is now loaded).

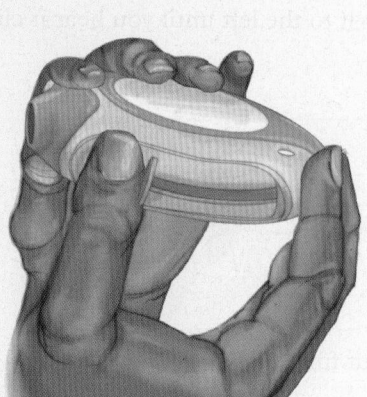

• Breathe out fully.
• Place your mouth securely around the mouthpiece and breathe in fully and quickly through your mouth.

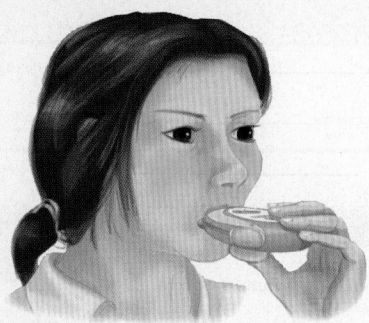

• Remove the Diskus, hold the breath for 10 seconds, and then breathe out.

Turbuhaler

• Hold the Turbuhaler upright. Load the dose by twisting the brown grip fully to the right.

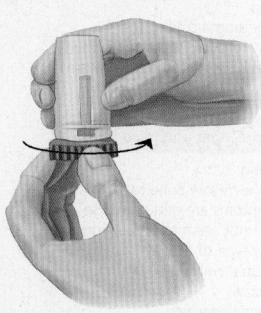

(continued)

TEACHING GUIDELINE 39.5 (continued)

Turbuhaler (*Continued*)

• Then twist it to the left until you hear it click.

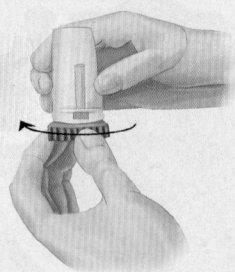

• Breathe out fully.

• Holding the Turbuhaler horizontally, place the mouth firmly around the mouthpiece and inhale deeply and forcefully.

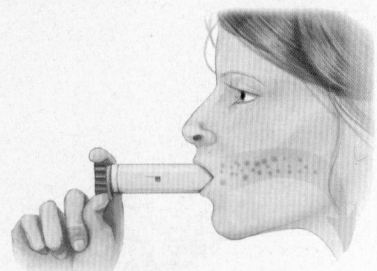

• Remove the Turbuhaler from the mouth and then breathe out.

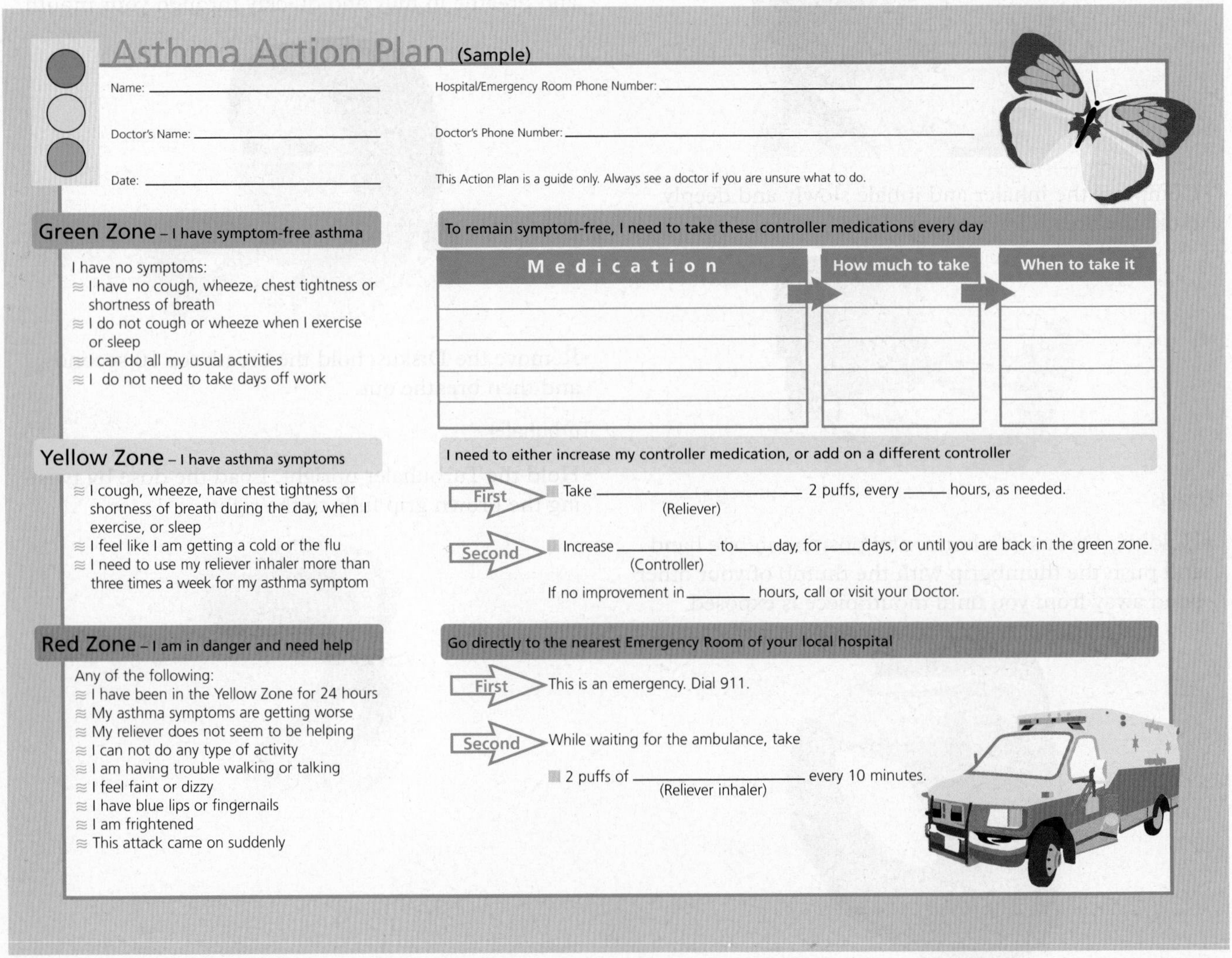

Asthma Action Plan (Sample)

Name: _____

Doctor's Name: _____

Date: _____

Hospital/Emergency Room Phone Number: _____

Doctor's Phone Number: _____

This Action Plan is a guide only. Always see a doctor if you are unsure what to do.

Green Zone – I have symptom-free asthma

I have no symptoms:
≋ I have no cough, wheeze, chest tightness or shortness of breath
≋ I do not cough or wheeze when I exercise or sleep
≋ I can do all my usual activities
≋ I do not need to take days off work

To remain symptom-free, I need to take these controller medications every day

Medication	How much to take	When to take it

Yellow Zone – I have asthma symptoms

≋ I cough, wheeze, have chest tightness or shortness of breath during the day, when I exercise, or sleep
≋ I feel like I am getting a cold or the flu
≋ I need to use my reliever inhaler more than three times a week for my asthma symptom

I need to either increase my controller medication, or add on a different controller

First ▸ ▪ Take _____ 2 puffs, every _____ hours, as needed.
(Reliever)

Second ▸ ▪ Increase _____ to ____ day, for ____ days, or until you are back in the green zone.
(Controller)

If no improvement in _____ hours, call or visit your Doctor.

Red Zone – I am in danger and need help

Any of the following:
≋ I have been in the Yellow Zone for 24 hours
≋ My asthma symptoms are getting worse
≋ My reliever does not seem to be helping
≋ I can not do any type of activity
≋ I am having trouble walking or talking
≋ I feel faint or dizzy
≋ I have blue lips or fingernails
≋ I am frightened
≋ This attack came on suddenly

Go directly to the nearest Emergency Room of your local hospital

First ▸ This is an emergency. Dial 911.

Second ▸ While waiting for the ambulance, take

▪ 2 puffs of _____ every 10 minutes.
(Reliever inhaler)

FIGURE 39.21 Sample Asthma Action Plan.

▶ *Consider* THIS!

Young children with asthma receiving inhaled medications via a nebulizer should use a snugly fitting mask to ensure accurate deposition of medication to the lungs. "Blow-by" via nebulizer should be discouraged, as medication delivery is variable and unreliable (NAEPP, 2007).

In addition to the presence or absence of symptoms, the Canadian consensus guidelines suggest that a written action plan is superior to use of peak flow meter for asthma control. (Teaching Guideline 39.6 gives instructions on peak flow meter use).

Avoidance of allergens is another key component of asthma management. Avoiding known triggers helps to prevent exacerbations as well as long-term inflammatory changes. This can be a difficult task for most families, particularly if the affected child suffers from several allergies. Teaching Guideline 39.4 outlines strategies for allergen avoidance.

Research has found a lag in parent/child education in relation to asthma management (Horner, 2004). Asthma education is not limited to the hospital or clinic setting. Nurses can become involved in community asthma education: community-centred education in schools, churches, and day care centres or through peer educators has been shown to be effective. Education should include pathophysiology, asthma triggers, and prevention and treatment strategies. With such a large number of children affected by this chronic disease, community education has the potential to make a broad impact. Many excellent websites are available for educational guidance in the home and in the community; visit http://thePoint.lww.com/Chow1e for direct links.

TEACHING GUIDELINE 39.6

Using a Peak Flow Meter

- Slide the arrow down to "zero."
- Stand up straight.
- Take a deep breath and close the lips tightly around the mouthpiece.
- Blow out hard and fast.
- Note the number the arrow moves to.
- Repeat three times and record the highest reading.
- Keep a record of daily readings, being sure to measure peak flow at the same time each day.

Adapted from: Ratcliffe, M. M., & Kieckhefer, G. M. (2010). Asthma. In P. J. Allen, J. A. Vessey, & N. A. Schapiro (Eds.), *Primary care of the child with a chronic condition* (5th ed.). St. Louis, MO: Mosby.

Promoting the Child's Self-Esteem

Fear of an exacerbation and feeling "different" from other children can harm a child's self-esteem. In qualitative research studies, children have made such statements as "my body shuts down" and "I feel like I'm going to die" (Yoos, Kitzman, McMullen, Sidora-Arcelo, & Anson, 2005). The fatigue and fear associated with chronic asthma may reduce the child's confidence and sense of control over his or her body and life. In addition to coping with a chronic illness, the asthmatic child often also has to cope with school-related issues. Moodiness, acting out, and withdrawal correlate with increases in school absence, which can contribute to poor school performance. To live in fear of an exacerbation or to be unable to participate in activities affects the child's self-esteem (Yoos et al., 2005).

Through education and support, the child can gain a sense of control. Children need to learn to master their disease. Accurate evaluation of asthma symptoms and improvement of self-esteem may help the child to experience less panic with an acute episode. Improved self-esteem might also help the child cope with the disease in general and with being different from his or her peers. The school-age child has the cognitive ability to begin taking responsibility for asthma management, with continued involvement on the part of the parents. Transferring control of asthma care to the child is an important developmental process that will contribute to the child's feeling of control over the illness (Buford, 2004).

Promoting Family Coping

Parent denial is an issue in many families. The family, through education and encouragement, can become the experts on the child's illness as well as advocates for the child's well-being. The resilient child is better able to cope with difficulties presented to him or her, including asthma. Cohesiveness and warmth in the family environment can improve a child's resiliency as well as contribute to family hardiness. Parents need to be allowed to ask questions and voice their concerns. A nurse who understands the family's issues and concerns is better able to plan for support and education. Provide culturally sensitive education and interventions that focus on increasing the family's commitment to and control of asthma management. As the child and parents become confident in their ability to recognize asthma symptoms and cope with asthma and its periodic episodes, the family's ability to cope will improve (Svavarsdottir & Rayens, 2005).

Chronic Lung Disease

Chronic lung disease (formerly termed bronchopulmonary dysplasia [BPD]) is often diagnosed in infants who have experienced RDS and continue to require oxygen at 28 days of age. Although it is a chronic respiratory condition seen most commonly in premature infants, the incidence of chronic lung disease has decreased in the past decade with advances in care of premature infants. Chronic lung disease results from a variety of factors, including pulmonary immaturity, acute lung injury, barotrauma, inflammatory mediators, and volutrauma. Epithelial stretching, macrophage and polymorphonuclear cell invasion, and airway edema affect the growth and development of lung structures. Cilia loss and airway lining denudation reduce the normal cleansing abilities of the lung. The number of normal alveoli is reduced by one third to one half. Lower birth weights, white race, and male gender pose increased risk for development of chronic lung disease. Complications include pulmonary artery hypertension, cor pulmonale, congestive heart failure, and severe bacterial or viral pneumonia (Harvey, 2004; Stoll & Kliegman, 2004).

Anti-inflammatory inhaled medications are used for maintenance, and short-acting bronchodilators are used as needed for wheezing episodes. Supplemental long-term oxygen therapy may be required in some infants.

Nursing Assessment

Tachypnea and increased work of breathing are characteristic of chronic lung disease. After discharge from the NICU, these symptoms can continue. Exertion such as activity or oral feeding can cause dyspnea to worsen. Failure to thrive might also be evident. Auscultation might reveal breath sounds that are diminished in the bases. These infants have reactive airway episodes, so wheezing might be present during times of exacerbation. If fluid overload develops, rales may be heard.

Nursing Management

If the infant is oxygen dependent, provide education to the parents about oxygen tanks, nasal cannula use, pulse oximetry use, and nebulizer treatments. Often these children require increased-calorie formulas to grow adequately. Fluid restrictions and/or diuretics are necessary in some infants. Follow-up echocardiograms might be used to determine resolution of pulmonary artery hypertension prior to weaning from oxygen. Encourage developmentally appropriate activities. It might be difficult for the oxygen-dependent infant or toddler to reach gross motor milestones or explore the environment because the length of his oxygen tubing limits him or her.

Parental support is also a key nursing intervention. After a long and trying period of ups and downs with their newborn in the intensive care unit, parents find themselves exhausted caring for their medically fragile infant at home.

Cystic Fibrosis

Cystic fibrosis is an autosomal recessive disorder that occurs in Canada at a rate of 2.8 per 10,000 births (Dupuis, Hamilton, Cole, & Corey, 2005). A deletion occurring on the long arm of chromosome 7 at the cystic fibrosis transmembrane regulator (CFTR) is the responsible gene mutation. DNA testing can be used prenatally and in newborns to identify the presence of the mutation. Currently there are no Canadian recommendations for prenatal screening for cystic fibrosis in the general population. Newborn screening is completed in those with a related family history.

Cystic fibrosis is the most common debilitating disease of childhood among those of European descent. Medical advances in recent years have greatly increased the length and quality of life for affected children. Whereas many children previously died before the age of 20 years, the median age of survival in Canada today is 37 years (PHAC, 2007). Complications include hemoptysis, pneumothorax, bacterial colonization, cor pulmonale, volvulus, intussusception, intestinal obstruction, rectal prolapse, gastro-esophageal reflux disease, diabetes, portal hypertension, liver failure, gallstones, and decreased fertility.

Therapeutic Management

Therapeutic management of cystic fibrosis is aimed toward minimizing pulmonary complications, maximizing lung function, preventing infection, and facilitating growth. All children with cystic fibrosis who have pulmonary involvement require chest physiotherapy with postural drainage several times daily to mobilize secretions from the lungs. Physical exercise is encouraged. Recombinant human DNase (Pulmozyme) is given daily using a nebulizer to decrease sputum viscosity and help clear secretions. Inhaled bronchodilators and anti-inflammatory agents are prescribed for some children. Aerosolized antibiotics are often prescribed and may be given at home as well as in the hospital. Choice of antibiotic is determined by sputum culture and sensitivity results. Pancreatic enzymes and supplemental fat-soluble vitamins are prescribed to promote adequate digestion and absorption of nutrients and optimize nutritional status. Increased-calorie, high-protein diets are recommended, and sometimes supplemental high-calorie formula, either orally or via feeding tube, is needed. Some children require total parenteral nutrition to maintain or gain weight (McMullen, 2004). Lung transplantation has been successful in some children with cystic fibrosis, but the availability of lungs suitable for transplantation in children is a limiting factor, and most lung transplants occur in early adulthood.

Pathophysiology

In cystic fibrosis, the CFTR mutation causes alterations in epithelial ion transport on mucosal surfaces, resulting in generalized dysfunction of the exocrine glands. The epithelial cells fail to conduct chloride, and water transport abnormalities occur. This results in thickened, tenacious secretions in the sweat glands, gastrointestinal tract, pancreas, respiratory tract, and other exocrine tissues. The increased viscosity of these secretions makes them difficult to clear. The sweat glands produce a larger amount of chloride, leading to a salty taste of the skin and alterations

TABLE 39.4 PATHOPHYSIOLOGY OF CYSTIC FIBROSIS AND RESULTANT RESPIRATORY AND GASTROINTESTINAL CLINICAL MANIFESTATIONS

Defect in the CFTR Gene Affects	Pathophysiology	Clinical Manifestations
Respiratory tract	• Infection leads to neutrophilic inflammation. • Cleavage of complement receptors and immunoglobulin G leads to opsonophagocytosis failure. • Chemoattractant interleukin-8 and elastin degradase contribute to inflammatory response. • Thick, tenacious sputum that is chronically colonized with bacteria results. • Air trapping related to airway obstruction • Pulmonary parenchyma is eventually destroyed.	• Airway obstruction • Difficulty clearing secretions • Respiratory distress and impaired gas exchange • Chronic cough • Barrel-shaped chest • Decreased pulmonary function • Clubbing • Recurrent pneumonia • Hemoptysis • Pneumothorax • Chronic sinusitis • Nasal polyps • Cor pulmonale (right-sided heart failure)
Gastrointestinal tract	• Decreased chloride and water secretion into the intestine (causing dehydration of the intestinal material) and into the bile ducts (causing increased bile viscosity) • Reduced pancreatic bicarbonate secretion • Hypersecretion of gastric acid • Insufficiency of pancreatic enzymes necessary for digestion and absorption • Pancreas secretes thick mucus.	• Meconium ileus • Retention of fecal matter in distal intestine, resulting in vomiting, abdominal distention and cramping, anorexia, right lower quadrant pain • Sludging of intestinal contents may lead to fecal impaction, rectal prolapse, bowel obstruction, intussusception. • Obstructive cirrhosis with esophageal varices, and splenomegaly • Gallstones • Gastro-esophageal reflux disease (compounded by postural drainage with chest physiotherapy) • Inadequate protein absorption • Altered absorption of iron and vitamins A, D, E, and K • Failure to thrive • Hyperglycemia and development of diabetes later in life

Adapted from: Federico, M. J. (2011). Respiratory tract & mediastinum. In W. W. Hay, M. J. Levin, J. M. Sondheimer, & R. R. Deterding (Eds.), *Current pediatric diagnosis and treatment* (20th ed.). New York: McGraw-Hill; and Hazle, L. A. (2010). *Cystic fibrosis*. In P. J. Allen, J. A. Vessey, & N. A. Schapiro (Eds.) *Primary care of the child with a chronic condition* (5th ed.). St. Louis, MO: Mosby.

in electrolyte balance and dehydration. The pancreas, intrahepatic bile ducts, intestinal glands, gallbladder, and submaxillary glands become obstructed by viscous mucus and eosinophilic material. Pancreatic enzyme activity is lost and malabsorption of fats, proteins, and carbohydrates occurs, resulting in poor growth and large, malodorous stools. Excess mucus is produced by the tracheobronchial glands. Abnormally thick mucus plugs the small airways, and then bronchiolitis and further plugging of the airways occur. Secondary bacterial infection with *Staphylococcus aureus*, *Pseudomonas aeruginosa*, and *Burkholderia cepacia* often occurs. This contributes to obstruction and inflammation, leading to chronic infection, tissue damage, and respiratory failure. Nasal polyps and recurrent sinusitis are common. Boys have tenacious seminal fluid and experi-

ence blocking of the vas deferens, often making them infertile (Hazle, 2010). In girls, thick cervical secretions might limit penetration of sperm (Boat & Acton, 2007). Table 39.4 gives further details of the pathophysiology and resulting respiratory and gastrointestinal clinical manifestations of cystic fibrosis.

Nursing Assessment

For a full description of the assessment phase of the nursing process, refer to page 1260. Assessment findings pertinent to cystic fibrosis are discussed below.

Health History

Elicit a description of the present illness and chief complaint. Common signs and symptoms reported during the health history in the undiagnosed child might include:

- A salty taste to the child's skin (resulting from excess chloride loss via perspiration)
- Meconium ileus or late, difficult passage of meconium stool in the newborn period
- Abdominal pain or difficulty passing stool (infants or toddlers might present with intestinal obstruction or intussusception at the time of diagnosis)
- Bulky, greasy stools
- Poor weight gain and growth despite good appetite
- Chronic or recurrent cough and/or upper or lower respiratory infections

Children known to have cystic fibrosis are often admitted to the hospital for pulmonary exacerbations or other complications of the disease. The health history should include questions related to:

- Respiratory status: has cough, sputum production, or work of breathing increased?
- Appetite and weight gain
- Activity tolerance
- Increased need for pulmonary or pancreatic medications
- Presence of fever
- Presence of bone pain
- Any other changes in physical state or medication regimen

Physical Examination

The physical examination includes inspection, auscultation, percussion, and palpation.

Inspection

Observe the child's general appearance and colour. Check the nasal passages for polyps. Note respiratory rate, work of breathing, use of accessory muscles, position of comfort, frequency and severity of cough, and quality and quantity of sputum produced. The child with cystic fibrosis often has a barrel chest (anterior–posterior diameter approximates transverse diameter) (Fig. 39.22). Clubbing of the nail beds might also be present. Note whether rectal prolapse is present. Does the child appear small or thin for his or her age? The child might have a protuberant abdomen and thin extremities, with decreased amounts of subcutaneous fat present. Observe for the presence of edema (sign of cardiac or liver failure). Note distended neck veins or the presence of a heave (signs of cor pulmonale).

Auscultation

Auscultation may reveal a variety of adventitious breath sounds. Fine or coarse crackles and scattered or localized wheezing might be present. With progressive obstructive pulmonary involvement, breath sounds might be diminished. Tachycardia might be present. Note the presence of a gallop (might occur with cor pulmonale). Note the adequacy of bowel sounds.

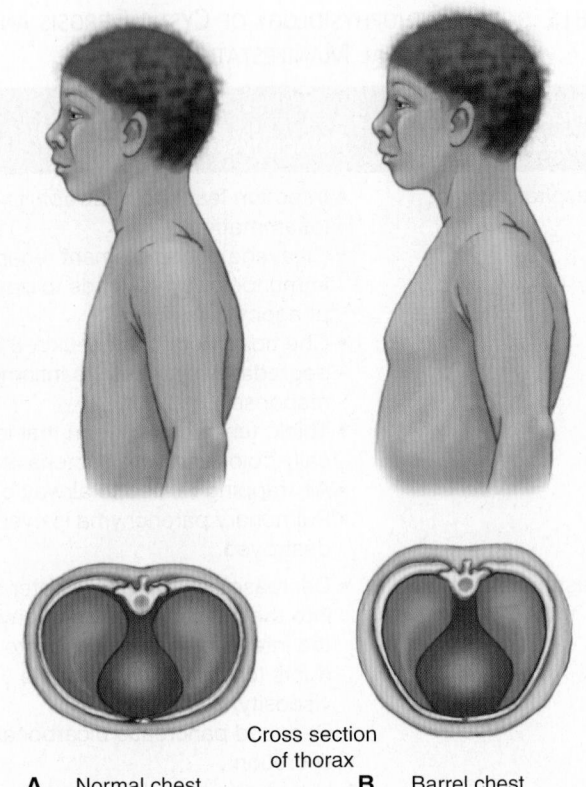

Cross section of thorax

A Normal chest   **B** Barrel chest

FIGURE 39.22 (**A**) Normal chest shape—transverse diameter > anterior–posterior diameter. (**B**) Barrel chest—transverse diameter = anterior–posterior diameter.

Percussion

Percussion over the lung fields usually yields hyperresonance due to air trapping. Diaphragmatic excursion might be decreased. Percussion of the abdomen might reveal dullness over an enlarged liver or mass related to intestinal obstruction.

Palpation

Palpation might yield a finding of asymmetric chest excursion if atelectasis is present. Tactile fremitus may be decreased over areas of atelectasis. Note if tenderness is present over the liver (might be an early sign of cor pulmonale).

Laboratory and Diagnostic Tests

Common laboratory and diagnostic studies ordered for the diagnosis and assessment of cystic fibrosis include:

- Sweat chloride test: considered suspicious if the level of chloride in collected sweat is above 50 mEq/L and diagnostic if the level is above 60 mEq/L
- Pulse oximetry: oxygen saturation might be decreased, particularly during a pulmonary exacerbation
- Chest X-ray: may reveal hyperinflation, bronchial wall thickening, atelectasis, or infiltration
- PFTs: might reveal a decrease in forced vital capacity and forced expiratory volume, with increases in residual volume (Boat & Acton, 2007; McMullen, 2004)

Nursing Management

Management of cystic fibrosis focuses on minimizing pulmonary complications, promoting growth and development, and facilitating coping and adjustment of the child and family. In addition to the nursing diagnoses and related interventions discussed in Nursing Care Plan 39.1 for respiratory disorders, interventions common to cystic fibrosis follow.

Maintaining Patent Airway

Chest physiotherapy is often used as an adjunct therapy in respiratory illnesses, but for children with cystic fibrosis it is a critical intervention. Chest physiotherapy involves percussion, vibration, and postural drainage, and either it or another bronchial hygiene therapy must be performed several times a day to assist with mobilization of secretions. Nursing Procedure 39.2 gives instructions on the chest physiotherapy technique.

For older children and adolescents, the flutter-valve device, positive expiratory pressure therapy, or a high-frequency chest compression vest may also be used. The flutter valve device provides high-frequency oscillation to the airway as the child exhales into a mouthpiece that contains a steel ball. Positive expiratory pressure therapy involves exhaling through a flow resistor, which creates positive expiratory pressure. The cycles of exhalation are repeated until coughing yields expectoration of secretions. The vest airway clearance system provides high-frequency chest wall oscillation to increase airflow velocity to create repetitive cough-like shear forces and to decrease the viscosity of secretions. Breathing exercises are also helpful in promoting mucus clearance. Encourage physical exercise, as it helps to promote mucus secretion as well as providing cardiopulmonary conditioning. Ensure that Pulmozyme is administered, as well as inhaled bronchodilators and anti-inflammatory agents if prescribed.

Preventing Infection

Vigorous pulmonary hygiene for mobilization of secretions is critical to prevent infection. Aerosolized antibiotics can be given at home as well as in the hospital. Children with frequent or severe respiratory exacerbations might require lengthy courses of intravenous antibiotics.

Maintaining Growth

Pancreatic enzymes must be administered with all meals and snacks to promote adequate digestion and absorption of nutrients. The number of capsules required depends on the extent of pancreatic insufficiency and the amount of food being ingested. The dosage can be adjusted until an adequate growth pattern is established and the number of stools is consistent at one or two per day. Children will need additional enzyme capsules when high-fat foods are being eaten. In the infant or young child, the enzyme capsule can be opened and sprinkled on cereal or applesauce. A well-balanced, high-calorie, high-protein diet is necessary to ensure adequate growth. Some children require up to 1.5 times the recommended daily allowance of calories for children their age. A number of commercially available nutritional formulas and shakes are available for diet supplementation.

In infants, breastfeeding should be continued with enzyme administration. Some infants will require fortification of breast milk or supplementation with high-calorie

---

Nursing Procedure 39.2

PERFORMING CHEST PHYSIOTHERAPY

1. Provide percussion via a cupped hand or an infant percussion device. Appropriate percussion yields a hollow sound (not a slapping sound).
2. Percuss each segment of the lung for 1 to 2 minutes.

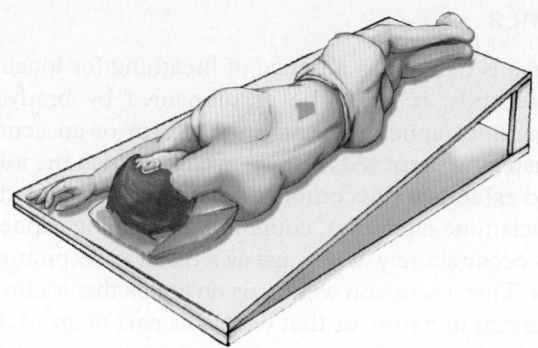

3. Place the ball of the hand on the lung segment, keeping the arm and shoulder straight. Vibrate by tensing and relaxing your arms during the child's exhalation. Vibrate each lung segment for at least five exhalations.

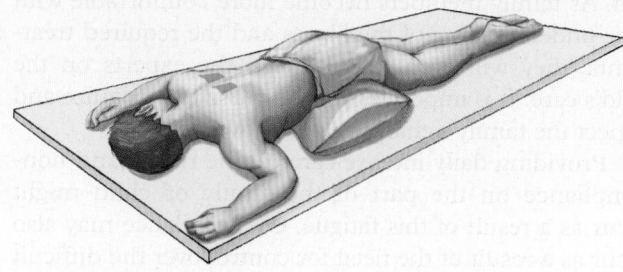

4. Encourage the child to deep breathe and cough.
5. Change drainage positions and repeat percussion and vibration.

formulas. Commercially available infant formulas can continue to be used for the formula-fed infant and can be mixed to provide a larger amount of calories if necessary. Supplementation with vitamins A, D, E, and K is necessary. Administer gavage feedings or total parenteral nutrition as prescribed to provide for adequate growth.

Promoting Family Coping

Cystic fibrosis is a serious chronic illness that requires intervention on a daily basis. It can be hard to maintain a schedule that requires pulmonary hygiene several times daily as well as close attention to appropriate diet and enzyme supplementation. Adjusting to the demands that the illness places on the child and family is difficult. Continual ongoing adjustments within the family must occur. Children are frequently hospitalized, and this may place an additional strain on the family and its finances. Children with cystic fibrosis may express fear or feelings of isolation, and siblings may be worried or jealous (Carpenter & Narsavage, 2004). The family should be encouraged to lead a normal life through involvement in activities and school attendance during periods of wellness.

> ▶ *Take* NOTE!
>
> *Massage therapy performed by the parent, nurse, or licensed massage therapist may help to decrease anxiety or relieve pain in the child with cystic fibrosis. It may have the added benefit of improving respiratory status, but it does not replace chest physiotherapy (Lee, Holdsworth, Holland, & Button, 2009).*

Starting at the time of diagnosis, families often demonstrate significant stress as the severity of the diagnosis and the significance of disease chronicity become real for them. The family should be involved in the child's care from the time of diagnosis, whether in the out-patient setting or in the hospital. Ongoing education about the illness and its treatments is necessary. Once the initial shock of diagnosis has passed and the family has adjusted to initial care, the family usually learns how to manage the requirements of care. Powerlessness gives way to adaptation. As family members become more comfortable with their understanding of the illness and the required treatments, they will eventually become the experts on the child's care. It is important for the nurse to recognize and respect the family's changing needs over time.

Providing daily intense care can be tiring, and noncompliance on the part of the family or child might occur as a result of this fatigue. Over-vigilance may also occur as a result of the need for control over the difficult situation as well as a desire to protect the child. Families welcome support and encouragement. Most families will eventually progress past the stages of fear, guilt, and powerlessness. They move beyond those feelings to a way

of living that is different than what they anticipated but is something that they can manage.

Refer parents to a local support group for families of children with cystic fibrosis. The Cystic Fibrosis Foundation and the Canadian Lung Association have chapters throughout Canada.

Parents of children with a terminal illness might face the death of their child at an earlier age than expected. Assisting with anticipatory grieving and making decisions related to end-of-life care are other important nursing interventions.

Preparing the Child and Family for Adulthood with Cystic Fibrosis

With current technological and medication advances, many more children with cystic fibrosis are surviving to adulthood and into their 30s and 40s (Cystic Fibrosis Foundation, 2011). Lung transplantation is now being used in some patients with success, thus prolonging life expectancy (barring transplant complications) (Hazle, 2010). Children should have the goal of independent living as an adult, as other children do. Making the transition from a pediatric medical home to an adult medical home should be viewed as a rite of passage (Tuchman, Schwartz, Sawicki, & Britto, 2010). Pediatric clinics are focused on family-centred care that heavily involves the child's parents, but adults with cystic fibrosis need a different focus, one that views them as independent adults.

Adults with cystic fibrosis can make the transition from pediatric to adult care with thoughtful preparation and coordination. They desire and deserve a smooth transition in care that will result in appropriate ongoing medical management of cystic fibrosis provided in an environment that is geared toward adults rather than children.

Adults with cystic fibrosis are able to find rewarding work and pursue relationships. Most men with cystic fibrosis are capable of sexual intercourse, though unable to reproduce. Females might have difficulty conceiving, and when they do they should be cautioned about the additional respiratory strain that pregnancy causes. All children of parents with cystic fibrosis will be carriers of the gene.

Apnea

Apnea is defined as absence of breathing for longer than 20 seconds; it might be accompanied by bradycardia. Sometimes apnea presents in the form of an acute life-threatening event (ALTE), an event in which the infant or child exhibits some combination of apnea, colour change, muscle tone alteration, coughing, or gagging. Apnea may also occur acutely at any age as a result of respiratory distress. This discussion will focus on apnea that is chronic or recurrent in nature or that occurs as part of an ALTE.

Apnea in infants may be central (unrelated to any other cause) or occur with other illnesses such as sepsis

Sudden Infant Death Syndrome (SIDS)

Definition

Sudden death of an infant <1 year of age that remains unexplained after investigation (PHAC, 2011b).

Modifiable Risk Factors

- Place infants in the supine position to sleep.
- Place infants to sleep in a crib, cradle, or bassinet that meets current Canadian regulations. Infants should not share a sleep surface with an adult or another child.
- Infants should share a room, **but not a sleep surface**, with a parent or caregiver for the first 6 months.
- Avoid overbundling or overdressing the infant.
- Breastfeeding for any duration has a protective effect for SIDS.
- Pacifiers have demonstrated a protective effect against SIDS.
- Avoid maternal prenatal smoking and exposure of the infant to secondhand smoke.

Visit http://thePoint.lww.com/Chow1e for Internet resources for more information on safe sleep for infants.

and respiratory infection. Apnea in newborns might be associated with hypothermia, hypoglycemia, infection, or hyperbilirubinemia. Apnea of prematurity occurs secondary to an immature respiratory system. Apnea should not be considered as a predecessor to sudden infant death syndrome (SIDS). Current research has not proven this theory, and SIDS generally occurs in otherwise healthy young infants (AAP, 2005). Box 39.3 gives more information about SIDS and its prevention (CPS, 2004).

Therapeutic management of apnea varies depending upon the cause. When apnea occurs as a result of another disorder or infection, treatment is directed toward that cause. In the event of apnea, stimulation may trigger the infant to take a breath. If breathing does not resume, rescue breathing or bag-valve-mask ventilation is necessary. Infants and children who have experienced an ALTE or who have chronic apnea may require ongoing cardiac/apnea monitoring. Caffeine or theophylline is sometimes administered, primarily in premature infants, to stimulate respirations (Kelly, 2010).

Nursing Assessment

Question the parents about the infant's position and activities preceding the apneic episode. Did the infant experience a colour change? Did the infant self-stimulate (breathe again on his or her own), or did he or she require stimulation from the caretaker? Assess risk factors for apnea, which may include prematurity, anemia, and history of metabolic disorders. Apnea may occur in association with cardiac or neurologic disturbances,

respiratory infection, seizures, sepsis, child abuse, or poisoning.

In the hospitalized infant, note absence of respiration, position, colour, and other associated findings, such as emesis on the bedclothes. If an infant who is apneic fails to be stimulated and does not breathe again, pulselessness will result.

Nursing Management

When an infant is noted to be apneic, gently stimulate him or her to take a breath again. If gentle stimulation is unsuccessful, then rescue breathing or bag-valve-mask ventilation must be started.

To avoid apnea in the newborn, maintain a neutral thermal environment. Avoid excessive vagal stimulation and taking rectal temperatures (the vagal response can cause bradycardia, resulting in apnea) (Jarvis, 2008). Administer caffeine or theophylline if prescribed and teach families about the use of these medications. Use of these medications requires careful monitoring, as the risk for apnea may return as the drug levels decrease.

Infants with recurrent apnea or ALTE may be discharged on a home apnea monitor (Fig. 39.23). Provide education on use of the monitor, guidance for when to notify the physician or monitor service about alarms, and training in infant CPR. The monitor is usually discontinued after 3 months without a significant event of apnea or bradycardia. In some ways the monitor gives parents peace of mind, but in others it can make them more nervous about the well-being of their child. Parents often experience disrupted sleep and some may display negative coping patterns as a result of the alarm (Scollan-Koliopoulos & Koliopoulos, 2010). Providing appropriate education to the parents about the nature of the child's disorder as well as action to take in the event of apnea may give the family a sense of mastery over the situation, thus decreasing their level of anxiety. Refer families to local area support groups such as those offered by Parent to Parent and Parents Helping Parents.

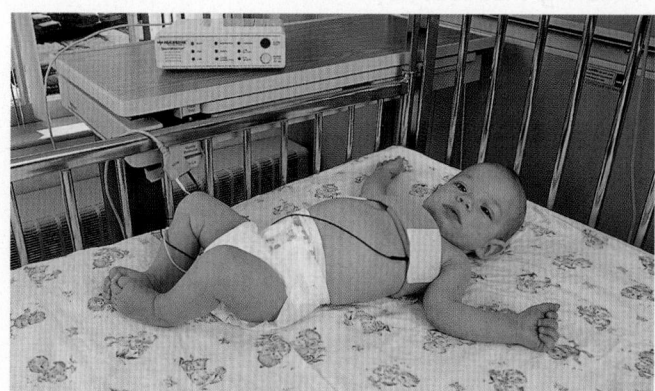

FIGURE 39.23 The home apnea monitor uses a soft belt with Velcro attachment to hold two leads in the appropriate position on the chest.

Tracheostomy

A **tracheostomy** is an artificial opening in the airway; usually a plastic tracheostomy tube is in place to form a patent airway. Tracheostomies are performed to relieve airway obstruction, such as with **subglottic stenosis** (narrowing of the airway sometimes resulting from long-term intubation). They are also used for pulmonary hygiene and in the child who requires chronic mechanical ventilation. The tracheostomy facilitates secretion removal, reduces work of breathing, and increases patient comfort. In some cases the tracheostomy facilitates mechanical ventilation weaning. It may be permanent or temporary depending on the condition that leads to the tracheostomy. The tracheostomy tube varies in size and type depending on the child's airway size and health and the length of time the child will require the tracheostomy. Silastic tracheostomy tubes are soft and flexible; they are available with a single lumen or may have an outer and inner lumen. Both types have an obturator (the guide used during tube changes). Typically, the tubes with inner cannulas are used with older children and in children with increased mucus production. Cuffed tracheostomy tubes are generally used in older children also. The cuff is used to prevent air from leaking around the tube. The funnel-shaped airway in younger children acts a physiological cuff and prevents air leak. Figure 39.24 shows various types of tracheostomy tubes.

Complications immediately postoperatively include hemorrhage, air entry, pulmonary edema, anatomic damage, and respiratory arrest. At any point in time the tracheostomy tube may become occluded and ventilation compromised. Complications of chronic tracheostomy include infection, cellulitis, and formation of granulation tissue around the insertion site (Russell, 2005). Placement of a tracheostomy tube, with or without ventilator support, may require families to temporarily or permanently relocate to the vicinity where the expertise for care and management of an infant or child with a tracheostomy can be found.

Nursing Assessment

When obtaining the history for a child with a tracheostomy, note the reason for the tracheostomy, as well as the

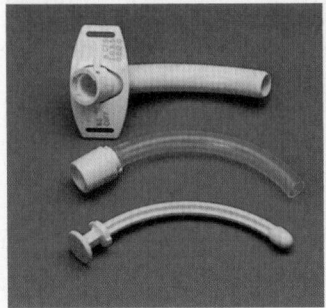
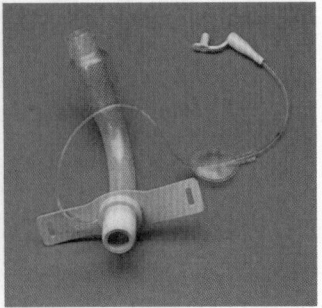

FIGURE 39.24 Note smaller size and absence of inner cannula on particular brands of pediatric tracheostomy tubes.

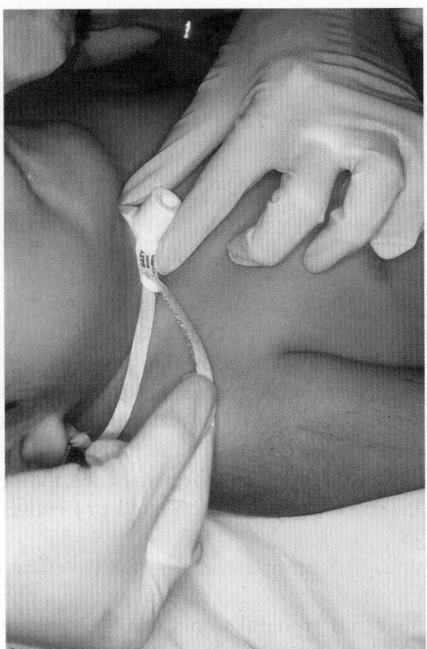

FIGURE 39.25 Properly fitting tracheostomy ties. One finger width fits between the ties and the child's neck.

size and type of tracheostomy tube. Inspect the site. The stoma should appear pink and without bleeding or drainage. The tube itself should be clean and free from secretions. The tracheostomy ties should fit securely, allowing one finger to slide beneath the ties (Fig. 39.25). Inspect the skin under the ties for rash or redness. Observe work of breathing.

When caring for the infant or child with a tracheostomy, whether in the intensive care unit, the patient floor, or the home, a thorough respiratory assessment is necessary. Note presence of secretions and their colour, thickness, and amount. Auscultate for breath sounds, which should be clear and equal throughout all lung fields. Pulse oximetry may also be measured. When infection is suspected or secretions are discoloured or have a foul odour, a sputum culture may be obtained.

▶ **Take** *NOTE!*

Keep small toys (risk of aspiration), plastic bibs or bedding (risk of airway occlusion), and talcum powder (risk of inhalation injury) out of reach of the child with a tracheostomy.

Nursing Management

In the immediate postoperative period the infant or child may require restraints to avoid accidental dislodgment of the tracheostomy tube. Infants and children who have had a tracheostomy for a period of time become accustomed to it and usually do not attempt to remove the

BOX 39.4 **Emergency Equipment (Available at Bedside)**

- Two spare tracheostomy tubes (one the same size and one a size smaller)
- Suction equipment
- Stitch cutter (new tracheostomy)
- Spare tracheostomy ties
- Saline as a lubricant
- Bag-valve-mask device
- Call bell within child's/parent's reach

tube. Since air inspired via the tracheostomy tube bypasses the upper airway, it lacks humidification, and this lack of humidity can lead to a mucus plug in the tracheostomy and hypoxia. Provide humidity to either room air or oxygen via a tracheostomy collar or ventilator, depending upon the child's need. Box 39.4 lists the equipment that should be available at the bedside of any child who has a tracheostomy.

Tracheostomies require frequent suctioning to maintain patency (Fig. 39.26). The appropriate length for insertion of the suction catheter depends on the size of the tracheostomy and the child's needs. Place a sign at the head of the child's bed indicating the suction catheter size and length (in centimetres) that it should be inserted for suctioning. Keep an extra tracheostomy tube of the same size and one size smaller at the bedside in the event of an emergency.

Most pediatric tracheostomy tubes do not have an inner cannula due to the small internal lumen, so the tracheostomy tube must be changed and cleaned to prevent secretion build-up and potential airway obstruction. If present, an inner cannula requires periodic removal and cleaning. Clean the removed tracheostomy tube with half-strength hydrogen peroxide and pipe cleaners or according to institutional policy. Rinse with distilled

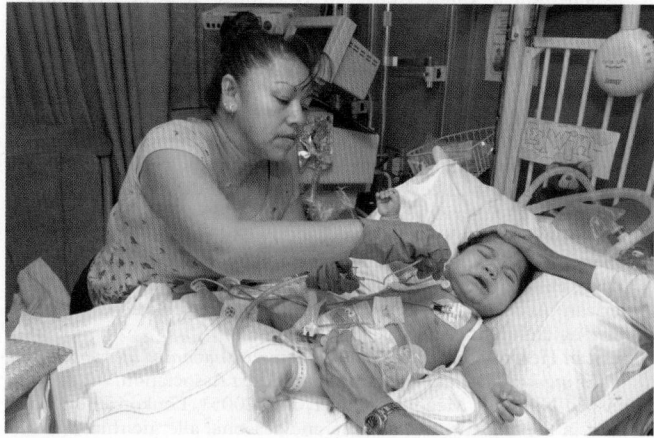

FIGURE 39.26 Suctioning is required to remove secretions.

Nursing Procedure 39.3

TRACHEOSTOMY CARE

1. Gather the necessary equipment:
   - Cleaning solution
   - Gloves
   - Precut gauze pad only necessary if fresh tracheostomy and for the first week thereafter.
   - Cotton-tipped applicators
   - Clean tracheostomy ties
   - Scissors
   - Extra tracheostomy tube in case of accidental dislodgement
2. Position the infant/child supine with a blanket or towel roll to extend the neck. The infant may need bundling to prevent him or her from interfering.
3. Open all packaging and cut tracheostomy ties to appropriate length if necessary.
4. Cleanse around the tracheostomy site with prescribed solution (half-strength hydrogen peroxide or acetic acid, normal saline or soap and water if at home) and cotton-tipped applicators working from just around the tracheostomy tube outward.
5. Rinse with sterile water and cotton-tipped applicator in similar fashion.
6. Place the precut sterile gauze under the tracheostomy tube.
7. With the assistant holding the tube in place, cut the ties and remove from the tube.
8. Attach the clean ties to the tube and tie or secure in place with Velcro.

water and allow it to dry. The tracheostomy tube can be reused many times if adequately cleaned between uses.

Perform tracheostomy care every 8 hours or per institution protocol. Change the tracheostomy tube only as needed or per institution protocol. Nursing Procedure 39.3 gives information about tracheostomy care.

If the older child or teen has a tracheostomy tube with an inner cannula, provide care of the inner cannula similar to that of an adult. Involve parents in care of the tracheostomy and begin education about caring for the tracheostomy tube at home as soon as the child is stable. Refer the family to local support groups or other resources for families with a child who has a tracheostomy (visit http://thePoint.lww.com/Chow1e for direct links to Internet Resources). The child with a tracheostomy may require home care by a nursing aide or registered nurse.

Assessment of the tracheostomy for impact on speech and communication is essential. It is suggested these infants learn sign language, as most small tracheostomy tubes do not allow for air to flow by the vocal cords. In older children, depending on the overall stability, a speech valve is sometimes used to divert airflow up through the vocal cords. The ability to use a speech valve safely must be determined by those with expertise in tracheostomies.

> ▶ *Take* NOTE!
>
> *Always change tracheostomy ties with an assistant to avoid the tube becoming accidentally dislodged.*

■■■ Key Concepts

■ Respiratory infections account for the majority of acute illnesses in children.

■ The upper and lower airways are smaller in children than adults, making them more susceptible to obstruction in the presence of mucus, debris, or edema.

■ Newborns are obligatory nose breathers.

■ The child's highly compliant airway is quite susceptible to dynamic collapse in the presence of airway obstruction.

■ Because they have fewer alveoli, children have a higher risk for hypoxemia than adults.

■ Generally, disorders of the nose and throat do not result in increased work of breathing or affect the lungs. Thus, if the lungs are involved, lower respiratory disease must be considered.

■ Wheezing may be associated with a variety of lower respiratory disorders, such as asthma, bronchiolitis, and cystic fibrosis.

■ Pulse oximetry is a useful tool for determining the extent of hypoxia. Findings should be correlated with the child's clinical presentation.

■ Rapid streptococcus and rapid flu tests are very useful for the quick diagnosis of strep throat or influenza so that appropriate treatment may be instituted early in the illness.

■ Supplemental oxygen is often necessary in the child who is hospitalized (particularly with lower respiratory disease). Oxygen should be humidified to prevent drying of secretions.

■ Suctioning, whether with a bulb syringe or suction catheter, is very effective at maintaining airway patency, especially in the younger child or infant.

■ Normal saline nasal wash is an inexpensive, simple, and safe method for decongesting the nose in the case of the common cold, allergic rhinitis, and sinusitis.

■ Infants who were born prematurely, children with a chronic illness such as diabetes, congenital heart disease, sickle cell anemia, or cystic fibrosis, and children with developmental disorders such as cerebral palsy tend to be more severely affected with respiratory disorders.

■ Passive cigarette smoke exposure increases the infant's and child's risk for respiratory disease.

■ Continual swallowing while awake or asleep is an indication of bleeding in the postoperative tonsillectomy patient.

■ Positioning to ease work of breathing and maintaining a patent airway are priorities for the child with a respiratory disorder.

■ To avoid Reye syndrome, aspirin should not be given to treat fever or pain in the infant or child with a viral infection.

■ Infants and children at high risk for serious RSV disease should be immunized with Synagis each RSV season. Children 6 to 23 months of age should be immunized against influenza yearly.

■ Children at high risk for exposure to tuberculosis should be screened for infection.

■ Promoting airway clearance and maintenance, effective breathing patterns, and adequate gas exchange is the priority focus of nursing intervention in pediatric respiratory disease.

■ Children with any degree of respiratory distress require frequent assessment and early intervention to prevent progression to respiratory failure.

■ Avoidance of allergens is critical in the treatment plan for the child with allergic rhinitis.

■ Avoidance of allergic triggers, control of the inflammatory process, and education of the child and family are the focus of asthma management.

■ Chest physiotherapy is extremely useful for mobilizing secretions in any condition resulting in an increase in mucus production and is required in children with cystic fibrosis.

■ Children with chronic respiratory disorders and their families often need large amounts of education and psychosocial support: children often experience fear and isolation, while families must learn to balance care of the chronically ill child with other family life.

REFERENCES

Alberta Medical Association. (2005). *Guideline for the diagnosis and management of croup.* Retrieved December 5, 2011 from http://www.albertadoctors.org/bcm/ama/ama-website.nsf/AllDoc/87256DB000705C3F87256E05005534E2/$File/CROUP.PDF

Allen, U., & Moore, D. (2010). Invasive group A streptococcal disease: Management and chemoprophylaxis. *Canadian Journal of Infectious Diseases and Medical Microbiology, 21*(3), 115–118.

American Academy of Pediatrics. (2005). The changing concept of sudden infant death syndrome: Diagnostic coding shifts, controversies regarding the sleeping environment, and new variables to consider in reducing risk. *Pediatrics, 116*(5), 1245–1255.

American Academy of Pediatrics. (2009). Policy statement: Recommendations for the prevention and treatment of influenza in children. *Pediatrics, 124*(4), 1–11.

American Academy of Pediatrics. (2010). Prevention of choking among children. *Pediatrics, 125*, 601–607.

American Heart Association. (2007). *Pediatric advanced life support provider manual.* Dallas, TX: American Heart Association.

Banasiak, N. C., & Meadows-Oliver, M. (2005). Leukotrienes: Their role in the treatment of asthma and seasonal allergic rhinitis. *Pediatric Nursing, 31*(1), 35–38.

Bjornson, C. L., Klassen, T. P., Williamson, J., et al. (2004). A randomized trial of a single dose of oral dexamethasone for mild croup. *New England Journal of Medicine, 351,* 1306–1313.

Blosser, C. G., Brady, M. A., & Mueller, W. J. (2009). Infectious diseases and immunizations. In C. A. Burns, A. M. Dunn, M. A. Brady, N. B. Starr, & C. G. Blosser (Eds.), *Pediatric primary care* (4th ed.). St. Louis, MO: Saunders.

Boat, T. F., & Acton, J. D. (2007). Cystic fibrosis. In R. M. Kliegman, R. E. Behrman, H. B. Jenson, & J. E. Stanton (Eds.), *Nelson textbook of pediatrics* (18th ed.). Philadelphia: WB Saunders.

Bowden, V. R., & Greenberg, C. S. (2008). *Pediatric nursing procedures* (2nd ed.). Philadelphia: Lippincott Williams & Wilkins.

Brady, M. A. (2009). Respiratory disorders. In C. A. Burns, A. M. Dunn, M. A. Brady, N. B. Starr, & C. G. Blosser (Eds.), *Pediatric primary care* (4th ed.). St. Louis, MO: Saunders.

Buford, T. A. (2004). Transfer of asthma management responsibility from parents to their school-age children. *Journal of Pediatric Nursing, 19*(1), 3–12.

Canadian Paediatric Society. (2004). Recommendations for safe sleeping environments for infants and children. *Paediatrics & Child Health, 9*(9), 659–663.

Canadian Paediatric Society. (2007). Exercise and febrile illnesses. *Paediatrics & Child Health, 12*(10):885–887.

Canadian Paediatric Society. (2010). *Information on influenza for health professionals.* Retrieved December 5, 2011 from http://www.cps.ca/english/Influenza_IllnessAntiviral.htm

Carolan, P. L. (2011). *Pediatric bronchitis.* Retrieved December 5, 2011 from http://emedicine.medscape.com/article/1001332-overview#aw2aab6b2b3aa

Carpenter, D. R., & Narsavage, G. L. (2004). One breath at a time: Living with cystic fibrosis. *Journal of Pediatric Nursing, 19*(1), 25–32.

Checchia, P. A. (2011). Current and emerging therapeutics and immunoprophylaxis for RSV. *Infectious Diseases in Children,* March, 7–9.

Cystic Fibrosis Foundation. (2011). *About cystic fibrosis.* Retrieved December 5, 2011 from http://www.cff.org/AboutCF/

DeMeulenaere, S. (2007). Pulse oximetry: Uses and limitations. *Journal for Nurse Practitioners, 3*(5), 312–318.

DeMuri, G. P., & Wald, E. R. (2010). Acute sinusitis: Clinical manifestations and treatment approaches. *Pediatric Annals, 39*(1), 34–40.

Dupuis, A., Hamilton, D., Cole, D. E. C., & Corey, C. (2005). Cystic fibrosis rates in Canada: A decreasing trend since the onset of genetic testing. *Journal of Pediatrics, 147,* 312–315.

Engle, W. A. (2008). Surfactant-replacement therapy for respiratory distress in the preterm and term neonate. *Pediatrics, 121,* 419.

Federico, M. J. (2011). Respiratory tract & mediastinum. In W. W. Hay, M. J. Levin, J. M. Sondheimer, & R. R. Deterding (Eds.), *Current pediatric diagnosis and treatment* (20th ed.). New York: McGraw-Hill.

Galioto, N. J. (2008). Peritonsillar abscess. *American Family Physician, 77*(2), 199–202.

Gluckman, W., & Forti, R. J. (2011). *Pediatric pneumothorax.* Retrieved December 5, 2011 from http://emedicine.medscape.com/article/1003552-overview#a0156

Goodman, F. (2011). RSV: The burden of disease and seasonal variability. *Infectious Diseases in Children,* March, 3–6.

Gregori, D., Salerni, L., Scarinzi, C., et al. (2008). Foreign bodies in the upper airways causing complications and requiring hospitalization in children aged 0–14 years: Results from the ESFBI study. *European Archives of Otorhinolaryngology, 265*(8), 971–978.

Guldfred, L. A., Lyhne, D., & Becker, B. C. (2008). Acute epiglottitis: Epidemiology, clinical presentation, management and outcome. *Journal of Laryngology Otology, 122*(8), 818–823.

Hagemann, T. M. (2005). Pediatric allergic rhinitis drug therapy. *Journal of Pediatric Health Care, 19,* 238–244.

Harvey, K. (2004). Bronchopulmonary dysplasia. In P. L. Jackson & J. A. Vessey (Eds.), *Primary care of the child with a chronic condition.* St. Louis, MO: Mosby.

Hazle, L. A. (2010). Cystic fibrosis. In P. J. Allen, J. A. Vessey, & N. A. Schapiro (Eds.), *Primary care of the child with a chronic condition* (5th ed.). St. Louis, MO: Mosby.

Health Canada. (2010). *First Nations, Inuit and Aboriginal Health: Tuberculosis (TB).* Retrieved on December 15, 2011 from http://www.hc-sc.gc.ca/fniah-spnia/diseases-maladies/tuberculos/index-eng.php

Horner, S. D. (2004). Effect of education on school-age children's and parents' asthma management. *Journal for Specialists in Pediatric Nursing, 9*(3), 95–102.

Huang, Y. L., Peng, C. C., Chiu, N. C., et al. (2009). Bacterial tracheitis in pediatrics: 12 year experience at a medical center in Taiwan. *Pediatric Intensive, 51*(1), 110–113.

Jaggi, P., & Shulman, S. T. (2006). Group A streptococcal infections. *Pediatrics in Review, 27,* 99–105.

Jarvis, C. (2008). *Physical examination and health assessment* (5th ed.). St. Louis, MO: Saunders.

Johnson, D. W. (March, 2009). Croup. *Clinical Evidence (Online).* Retrieved December 5, 2011 from http://www.ncbi.nlm.nih.gov/pmc/articles/PMC2907784/

Kelly, M. M. (2010). Prematurity. In P. J. Allen, J. A. Vessey, & N. A. Schapiro (Eds.), *Primary care of the child with a chronic condition* (5th ed.). St. Louis, MO: Mosby.

KidsHealth. (2009). *About croup.* Retrieved December 5, 2011 from http://kidshealth.org/parent/infections/lung/croup.html

KidsHealth. (2011). *Reye syndrome.* Retrieved December 5, 2011 from http://kidshealth.org/parent/infections/bacterial_viral/reye.html#

Kovesi, T., Schuh, S., Spier, S., et al. (2010). Achieving asthma control in preschoolers. *Canadian Medical Association Journal, 182*(4), 172–183.

Lander, L., Lu, S., & Shah, R. K. (2008). Pediatric retropharyngeal abscesses: A national perspective. *International Journal of Pediatric Otorhinolaryngology, 72*(12), 1837–1843.

Lee, A., Holdsworth, M., Holland, A., & Button, B. (2009). The immediate effect of musculoskeletal physiotherapy techniques and massage on pain and ease of breathing in adults with cystic fibrosis. *Journal of Cystic Fibrosis, 8*(1), 79–81.

Lokker, N., Sanders, L., Perrin, E. M., et al. (2009). Parental misinterpretations of over-the-counter pediatric cough and cold medication labels. *Pediatrics, 123*(6), 1464–1471.

Lougheed, M. D., Lemeire, C., Dell, S., et al. (2010). Canadian Thoracic Society Asthma Management Continuum – 2010 consensus summary for children 6 years and over and adults. *Canadian Respiratory Journal, 17*(1), 15–24.

Martin, J. M. (2010). Pharyngitis and streptococcal throat infections. *Pediatric Annals, 39*(1), 22–27.

McMullen, A. H. (2004). Cystic fibrosis. In P. L. Jackson & J. A. Vessey (Eds.), *Primary care of the child with a chronic condition* (4th ed.). St. Louis, MO: Mosby.

Morrow, B., & Argent, A. (2008). A comprehensive review of pediatric endotracheal suctioning: Effects, indications, and clinical practice. *Pediatric Critical Care Medicine, 9*(5), 465–477.

National Asthma Education and Prevention Program. (2007). *Expert panel report 3: Guidelines for the diagnosis and management of asthma* (NIH Publication No. 07-4051). Bethesda, MD: National Institutes of Health, National Heart, Lung and Blood Institute.

Nield, L. S., Mahajan, P., & Kamat, D. M. (2005). Pneumonia: Update on causes and treatment options. *Consultant for Pediatricians, 4*(8), 365–370.

Nettina, S. M. (2010). Pediatric respiratory disorders. In *Lippincott manual of nursing practice* (9th ed.). Philadelphia: Lippincott Williams & Wilkins.

Public Health Agency of Canada. (2007). *Cystic fibrosis.* Retrieved December 5, 2011 from http://www.phac-aspc.gc.ca/publicat/2007/lbrdc-vsmrc/fibrosis-fibrose-eng.php

Public Health Agency of Canada. (2010a). *Guidance: Infection prevention and control measures for healthcare workers in acute care and long-term care settings.* Retrieved December 12, 2011 from http://www.phac-aspc.gc.ca/nois-sinp/guide/ac-sa-eng.php

Public Health Agency of Canada. (2010b). *Respiratory syncytial virus.* Retrieved December 12, 2011 from http://www.phac-aspc.gc.ca/lab-bio/res/psds-ftss/pneumovirus-eng.php

Public Health Agency of Canada. (2011a). *Tuberculosis: Drug resistance in Canada – 2010.* Ottawa: Minister of Public Works and Government Services Canada.

Public Health Agency of Canada. (2011b). *Joint statement on safe sleep: Preventing sudden infant deaths in Canada.* Retrieved December 5, 2011 from http://www.phac-aspc.gc.ca/hp-ps/dca-dea/stages-etapes/childhood-enfance_0-2/sids/pdf/jsss-ecss2011-eng.pdf

Quinn, K., Kaufman, J. S., Siddiqi, A., & Yeats, K. B. (2010). Stress and the city: Housing stressors are associated with respiratory health among low socioeconomic status Chicago children. *Journal of Urban Health, 87*(4), 699–702.

Ratcliffe, M. M., & Kieckhefer, G. M. (2010). Asthma. In P. J. Allen, J. A. Vessey, & N. A. Schapiro (Eds.), *Primary care of the child with a chronic condition* (5th ed.). St. Louis, MO: Mosby.

Registered Nurses' Association of Ontario. (2008). *Promoting asthma control in children: Nursing best practice guideline* [supplement]. Retrieved December 5, 2011 from http://www.rnao.org/Storage/39/3376_Asthma-child_Supplement_-_2008_FINAL.pdf

Reznik, M., & Ozuah, P. O. (2005). A prudent approach to screening for and treating tuberculosis. *Contemporary Pediatrics, 22*(11), 73–88.

Russell, C. (2005). Providing the nurse with a guide to tracheostomy care and management. *British Journal of Nursing, 14*(8), 428–433.

Safe Kids USA. (2009). *Choking, suffocation and strangulation prevention.* Retrieved December 5, 2011 from http://www.safekids.org/safety-basics/safety-resources-by-risk-area/choking-suffocation-and-strangulation/

Samson, L. (2009). Prevention of respiratory syncytial virus infection. *Paediatrics & Child Health, 14*(8), 521–526.

Scollan-Koliopoulos, M., & Koliopoulos, J. S. (2010). Evaluation and management of apparent life-threatening events in infants. *Pediatric Nursing, 36*(2), 77–83.

Sectish, T. C., & Prober, C. G. (2007). Pneumonia. In R. M. Kliegman, R. E. Behrman, H. B. Jenson, & J. E. Stanton (Eds.), *Nelson textbook of pediatrics* (18th ed.). Philadelphia: WB Saunders.

Seger, N., & Soll, R. (2009). Animal derived surfactant extract for treatment of respiratory distress syndrome. *Cochrane Database of Systematic Reviews, 15*, CD007836.

Sheikh, J., & Najib, U. (2011). *Allergic rhinitis.* Retrieved December 5, 2011 from http://emedicine.medscape.com/article/134825-overview

Stephenson, J. T., & DuBois, J. J. (2007). Nonoperative management of spontaneous splenic rupture in infectious mononucleosis: A case report and review of the literature. *Pediatrics, 120*(2), e432–e435. doi:10.1542/peds.2006-3071

Stevens, T. P. (2007). Surfactant replacement therapy. *Chest, 131*(5), 1577–1582.

Stoll, B. J., & Kliegman, R. M. (2004). Hyaline membrane disease (respiratory distress syndrome). In R. E. Behrman, R. M. Kliegman, & H. B. Jenson (Eds.), *Nelson textbook of pediatrics* (17th ed.). Philadelphia: WB Saunders.

Subbarao, P., Mandhane, P. J., & Sears, M. R. (2009). Asthma: Epidemiology, etiology and risk factors. *Canadian Medical Association Journal, 181*(9), 181–190.

Svavarsdottir, E. K., & Rayens, M. K. (2005). Hardiness in families of young children with asthma. *Journal of Advanced Nursing, 50*(4), 381–390.

Sweet, D., Bevilacqua, G., Carnielli, V., et al. (2007). European consensus guidelines on the management of neonatal respiratory distress syndrome. *Journal of Perinatal Medicine, 35*, 175.

Taketokmo, C. K., Hodding, J. H., & Kraus, D. M. (2010). *Lexi-comp's pediatric dosage handbook* (17th ed.). Hudson, OH: Lexi-comp.

Taylor, A., & Adam, H. M. (2006). Sinusitis. *Pediatrics in Review, 27*, 395–397.

Thilo, E. H., & Rosenberg, A. A. (2011). The newborn infant. In W. W. Hay, M. J. Levin, J. M. Sondheimer, & R. R. Deterding (Eds.), *Current pediatric diagnosis and treatment* (20th ed.). New York: McGraw-Hill.

Thomas, M., Kocevar, V. S., Zhang, Q., Yin, D. D., & Price, D. (2005). Asthma-related health care resource use among asthmatic children with and without concomitant allergic rhinitis. *Pediatrics, 115*(1), 129–134.

Tuchman, L. T., Schwartz, L. A., Sawicki, G. S., & Britto, M. T. (2010). Cystic fibrosis and transition to adult medical care. *Pediatrics, 125*, 566–573.

Vassilev, Z. P., Chu, A. F., Ruck, B., Adams, E. H., & Marcus, S. M. (2009). Adverse reactions to over-the-counter cough and cold products among children: The cases managed out of hospitals. *Journal of Clinical Pharmacy Therapy, 34*(3), 313–318.

Wald, E. L. (2010). Croup: Common syndromes and therapy. *Pediatric Annals, 39*(1), 15–21.

Wells, D. A., Gillies, D., & Fitzgerald, D. A. (2010). Positioning for acute respiratory distress in hospitalised infants and children. *Cochrane Database of Systematic Reviews, 18*, CD003645.

Wipfli, H., Avila-Tang, E., Navas-Acien, A., et al. (2008). Secondhand smoke exposure among women and children: Evidence from 31 countries. *American Journal of Public Health, 98*(4), 672–679.

Yoon, P. J., Kelley, P. E., & Friedman, N. R. (2011). Ear, nose, & throat. In W. W. Hay, M. J. Levin, J. M. Sondheimer, & R. R. Deterding (Eds.), *Current pediatric diagnosis and treatment* (20th ed.). New York: McGraw-Hill.

Yoos, H. L., Kitzman, H., McMullen, A., Sidora-Arcelo, K., & Anson, E. (2005). The language of breathlessness: Do families and health care providers speak the same language when describing asthma symptoms? *Journal of Pediatric Health Care, 19*(4), 197–205.

RECOMMENDED READINGS

Bhogal, S. K., Zemek, R. L., & Ducharme, F. (2009). Written actions plans for asthma in children [review]. *Cochrane Collaboration, 1.* Indianapolis, IN: John Wiley & Sons.

Bourgeois, F. T., Valim, C., McAdam, A. J., & Mandl, K. D. (2009). Relative impact of influenza and respiratory syncytial virus in young children. *Pediatrics, 124*(6), e1072–e1080.

Carpenito-Moyet, L. J. (2009). *Nursing care plans and documentation: Nursing diagnosis and collaborative problems.* Philadelphia: Lippincott Williams & Wilkins.

Custer, R. W., & Row, J. E. (2009). *The Harriet Lane handbook: A manual for pediatric house officers* (18th ed.). Philadelphia: Mosby.

Harper, S. A., Bradley, J. S., Englund, J. A., et al. (2009). Seasonal influenza in adults and children: Diagnosis, treatment, chemoprophylaxis, and institutional outbreak management: Clinical practice guidelines of the Infectious Diseases Society of America. *Clinical Infectious Diseases, 48*(8), 1003–1032.

Long, S. S. (2008). *Principles and practice of pediatric infectious diseases* (3rd ed.). Philadelphia: Churchill Livingston.

MacDonald, N., Onyett, H., Bortolussi, R., & the Canadian Paediatric Society, Infectious Diseases and Immunization Committee. (2010). *Managing seasonal and pandemic influenza in infants, children and youth.* Retrieved December 5, 2011 from http://www.cps.ca/english/publications/SeasonalPandemicFlu.pdf

Mannino, D. M., Homa, D. M., & Redd, S. C. (2002). Involuntary smoking and asthma severity in children. *Chest, 122*, 409–415.

National Safety Council. (2008). *Injury facts: 2008 Edition.* Retrieved December 5, 2011 from https://www.usw12775.org/uploads/InjuryFacts08Ed.pdf

Tipping, C. J., Scholes, R. L., & Cox, N. S. (2010). A qualitative study of physiotherapy education for parents of toddlers with cystic fibrosis. *Journal of Cystic Fibrosis, 3*, 10–16.

Watson, T. A., Gillespie, C., Thomas, N., et al. (2009). Small group, interactive education and the effect on asthma control by children and their families. *Canadian Medical Association Journal, 18*(5), 257–263.

Zemek, R. L., Bhogal, S. K., & Ducharme, F. (2008). Systematic review of randomized controlled trials examining written action plans in children: What is the plan? *Archives of Pediatric and Adolescent Medicine, 162*(2), 157–163.

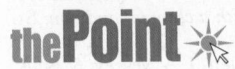

CHAPTER WORKSHEET

MULTIPLE CHOICE QUESTIONS

1. A 5-month-old infant with RSV bronchiolitis is in respiratory distress. The baby has copious secretions, increased work of breathing, cyanosis, and a respiratory rate of 78. What is the most appropriate *initial* nursing intervention?

   a. Attempt to calm the infant by placing him in his mother's lap and offering him a bottle.

   b. Alert the physician to the situation and ask for an order for a stat chest X-ray.

   c. Suction secretions, provide 100% oxygen via mask, and anticipate respiratory failure.

   d. Bring the emergency equipment to the room and begin bag-valve-mask ventilation.

2. A toddler has moderate respiratory distress, is mildly cyanotic, and has increased work of breathing, with a respiratory rate of 40. What is the priority nursing intervention?

   a. Airway maintenance and 100% oxygen by mask

   b. 100% oxygen and pulse oximetry monitoring

   c. Airway maintenance and continued reassessment

   d. 100% oxygen and provision of comfort

3. The nurse is caring for a child with cystic fibrosis who receives pancreatic enzymes. The nurse realizes that the child's mother understands the instructions related to giving the enzymes when the mother makes which of the following statements?

   a. "I will stop the enzymes if my child is receiving antibiotics."

   b. "I will decrease the dose by half if my child is having frequent, bulky stools."

   c. "Between meals is the best time for me to give the enzymes."

   d. "The enzymes should be given at the beginning of each meal and snack."

4. Which of these factors contributes to infants' and children's increased risk for upper airway obstruction as compared with adults?

   a. Underdeveloped cricoid cartilage and narrow nasal passages

   b. Small tonsils and narrow nasal passages

   c. Cylinder-shaped larynx and underdeveloped sinuses

   d. Underdeveloped cricoid cartilage and smaller tongue

5. Which is the most appropriate treatment for epistaxis?

   a. With the child lying down and breathing through the mouth, apply pressure to the bridge of the nose.

   b. With the child lying down and breathing through the mouth, pinch the lower third of the nose closed.

   c. With the child sitting up and leaning forward, apply pressure to the bridge of the nose.

   d. With the child sitting up and leaning forward, pinch the lower third of the nose closed.

CRITICAL THINKING EXERCISES

1. A 10-month-old girl is admitted to the pediatric unit with a history of recurrent pneumonia and failure to thrive. Her sweat chloride test confirms the diagnosis of cystic fibrosis. She is a frail-appearing infant with thin extremities and a slightly protuberant abdomen. She is tachypneic, has retractions, and coughs frequently. Based on the limited information given here and your knowledge of cystic fibrosis, choose three of the categories below as priorities to focus on when planning her care:

   a. Prevention of bronchospasm

   b. Promotion of adequate nutrition

   c. Education of the child and family

   d. Prevention of pulmonary infection

   e. Balancing fluid and electrolytes

   f. Management of excess weight gain

   g. Prevention of spread of infection

   h. Promoting adequate sleep and rest

2. A child with asthma is admitted to the pediatric unit for the fourth time this year. The mother expresses frustration that the child is getting sick so often. Besides information about onset of symptoms and events leading up to this present episode, what other types of information would you ask for while obtaining the history?

(question continued on page 1314)

3. The mother of the child in the previous question tells you that she smokes (but never around the child), the family has a cat that comes inside sometimes, and she always gives her child the medication prescribed. She gives salmeterol and budesonide as soon as the child starts to cough. When he is not having an episode, she gives him albuterol before his baseball games. Diphenhydramine helps his runny nose in the springtime. Based on this new information, what advice/instructions would you give the mother?

4. A 7-year-old presents with a history of recurrent nasal discharge. He sneezes every time he visits his cousins, who have pets. He lives in an older home that is carpeted. Tobacco smokers live in the home. His mother reports that he snores and is a mouth breather. She says he has symptoms nearly year-round, but they are worse in the fall and the spring. She reports that diphenhydramine is somewhat helpful with his symptoms, but she doesn't like to give it to him on school days because it makes him drowsy. Based on the history above, develop a teaching plan for this child.

5. The nurse is caring for a 4-year-old girl who returned from the recovery room after a tonsillectomy 3 hours ago. She has cried off and on in the past 2 hours and is now sleeping. What areas in particular should the nurse assess and focus on for this patient?

STUDY ACTIVITIES

1. While caring for children in the pediatric setting, compare the signs and symptoms of a child with asthma to those of an infant with bronchiolitis. What are the most notable differences? How does the history of the two children differ?

2. The nurse is caring for a child with asthma. The child has been prescribed Advair (fluticasone and salmeterol), albuterol, and prednisone. Develop a sample teaching plan for the child and family. Include appropriate use of the devices used to deliver the medications, as well as important information about the medications (uses and side effects).

3. While caring for children in the pediatric setting, compare the signs and symptoms and presentation of a child with the common cold to those of a child with either sinusitis or allergic rhinitis.

4. While caring for children in the pediatric setting, review the census of clients and identify those at risk for severe influenza and thus those who would benefit from annual influenza vaccination.

5. Compare the differences in oxygen administration between a young infant and an older child.

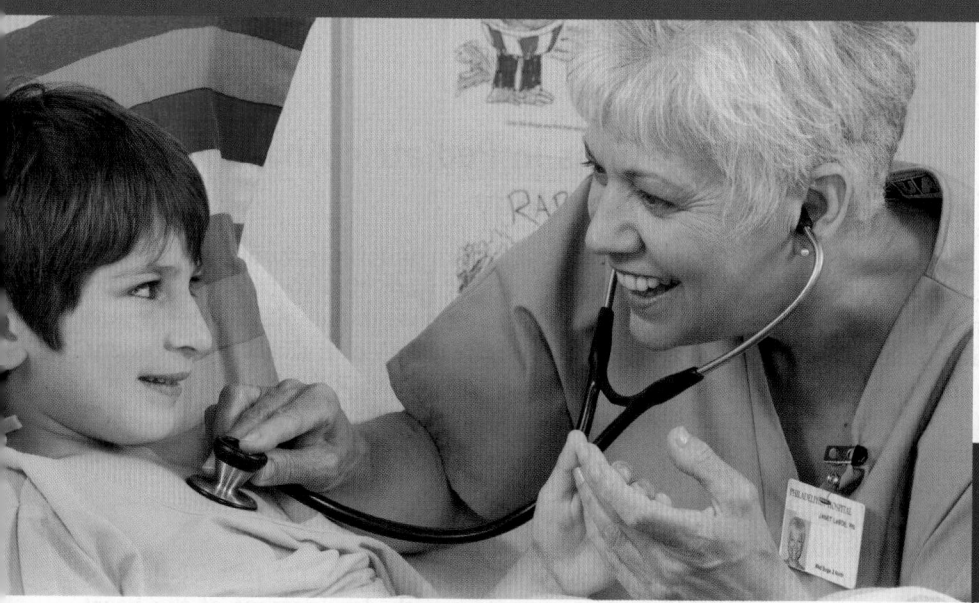

CHAPTER 40

Adapted by Lois E. Hawkins and
Gwen R. Rempel

NURSING CARE OF THE CHILD WITH A CARDIOVASCULAR DISORDER

KEY TERMS

arrhythmia
bradycardia
cardiac output
cardiomegaly
clubbing
congenital heart defect

congestive heart failure
cyanosis
echocardiography
electrocardiogram (ECG,
    EKG)
orthotopic

polycythemia
tachycardia
tetralogy of Fallot

LEARNING OBJECTIVES

Upon completion of the chapter, the learner will be able to:

1. Compare anatomic and physiologic differences of the cardiovascular system in infants and children versus adults.
2. Describe nursing care related to common laboratory and diagnostic tests used in the medical diagnosis of pediatric cardiovascular conditions.
3. Distinguish cardiovascular disorders common in infants, children, and adolescents.
4. Identify appropriate nursing assessments and interventions related to medications and treatments for pediatric cardiovascular disorders.
5. Develop an individualized nursing care plan for the child with a cardiovascular disorder.
6. Describe the psychosocial effects of chronic cardiovascular disorders on children.
7. Devise a nutrition plan for the child with a cardiovascular disorder.
8. Develop patient/family teaching plans for the child with a cardiovascular disorder.

*L*ogan Bernstein, 6 weeks old, is brought to the clinic by his mother. He presents with poor feeding. His mother states, "Logan falls asleep while breastfeeding, and he sweats so much."

Wow

The heart of the matter is healing the child's heart so he or she can embrace life to its fullest.

Cardiovascular disease is a significant cause of chronic illness and death in children. Typically, cardiovascular disorders in children are divided into two major categories: congenital heart disease (CHD) and acquired heart disease. CHD is defined as structural anomalies that are present at birth; however, some **congenital heart defects** may not be diagnosed until later in life. In Canada, congenital heart defects are present in about 1% of live births and are the most frequent congenital malformation in newborns (Heart and Stroke Foundation of Alberta, NWT & Nunavut, 2010; Marelli, Ionescu-Ittu, Rahme, & Pilote, 2007). In most cases, there is no known cause. In other cases, causes may include viral infections such as rubella (measles), certain genetic conditions such as Down syndrome, and drug or alcohol use during pregnancy (Heart and Stroke Foundation, 2010; Marelli et al., 2007).

Acquired heart disease includes disorders that occur after birth. These disorders develop from a wide range of causes, or they can occur as a complication or long-term effect of CHD. More than 100 genes have been identified that may be involved in the development of CHD (Cunningham, Leveno, & Bloom, 2010). Additional noncardiac anomalies, including chromosomal abnormalities such as Down syndrome, occur in about 28% of children with CHD (Park, 2008). Globally, CHD occurs at a rate of about 3% in children with first-degree relatives who have CHD (Oyen, Poulsen, Boyd, Wohlfahrt, Jensen, & Melbye, 2009).

The diagnosis of a cardiovascular disorder in any person can be extremely frightening and overwhelming. This is even truer for the child and his or her parents. Early on, children learn that the heart is necessary for life; so knowing that there is a heart problem can promote feelings of dread. These feelings are compounded by the child's age, the view of the child as being vulnerable and defenseless, and the stressors associated with the disorder itself. The child and parents need much support and reassurance (Cook & Higgins, 2010).

Nurses need to have a sound knowledge base about cardiovascular conditions affecting children so that they can provide appropriate assessment, intervention, guidance, and support to the child and family. Cardiovascular disorders require acute interventions that often have long-term implications for the child's health and growth and development (Snookes, Gunn, & Eldridge, 2010). Due to the potentially overwhelming and devastating effects that cardiovascular disorders can have on children and their families, nurses need to be skilled in assessment and interventions in this area and able to provide support throughout the course of the illness and beyond (Moons, Sluysmans, & De Wolf, 2009). This chapter describes the nursing management of children with congenital and acquired cardiovascular disorders, highlighting the common procedures used for treatment.

Variations in Pediatric Anatomy and Physiology

The cardiovascular system undergoes numerous changes at birth. Structures that were vital to the fetus are no longer needed. Circulation via the umbilical arteries and vein is replaced with the child's own closed independent circulation. Changes in the size of the heart, pulse rate, and blood pressure (BP) also occur.

Circulatory Changes from Gestation to Birth

The fetal heart is developed within the first 21 days of gestation in conjunction with development of the heart rate and fetal blood circulation. The four chambers of the heart and arteries are formed during gestational months 2 through 8. During fetal development, oxygenation of the fetus occurs via the placenta; the lungs, though perfused, do not perform oxygenation and ventilation. The foramen ovale, an opening between the atria, allows blood flow from the right to the left atrium. The ductus arteriosus allows blood flow between the pulmonary artery and the aorta, shunting blood away from the pulmonary circulation (Cunningham et al., 2010). Figure 40.1 illustrates fetal and newborn circulation.

With the first breath, several changes in the cardiopulmonary system enable the newborn to make the transition from fetal circulation to normal circulation. As the newborn breathes for the first time, the lungs inflate, reducing pulmonary vascular resistance to blood flow. As a result, pulmonary artery pressure drops. Subsequently, pressure in the right atrium decreases. Blood flow to the left side of the heart increases the pressure in the left atrium. This change in pressure leads to closure of the foramen ovale. The change in circulating oxygen levels promotes closure of the ductus arteriosus, which is located between the aorta and pulmonary artery. The ductus venosus, located between the left umbilical vein and the inferior vena cava, closes because of a lack of blood flow and vasoconstriction. The closed ductus arteriosus and ductus venosus eventually become ligaments. With the lack of blood flow through the umbilical arteries and vein, these structures atrophy (Cunningham et al., 2010; Martchenke & Blosser, 2009).

Structural and Functional Differences from Infancy to Adolescence

The structure and function of the infant's and child's cardiovascular system differ from those of adults, depending on age. Before the age of 7, the heart lies more horizontally. As a result, the apex is higher, below the fourth intercostal space. In the infant, the heart lies higher in the chest and occupies over half of the chest width. As the lungs

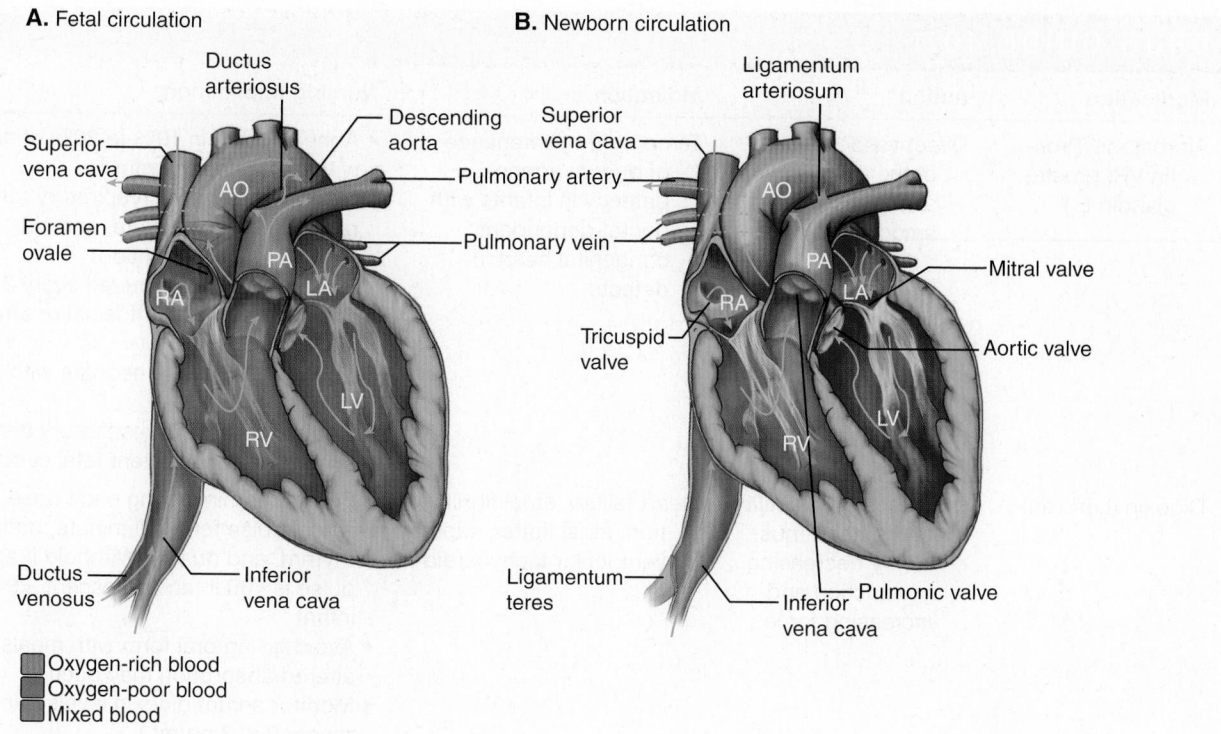

A. Fetal circulation

Ductus arteriosus

Descending aorta

Superior vena cava

Foramen ovale

AO

PA

RA

LA

LV

RV

Ductus venosus

Inferior vena cava

B. Newborn circulation

Ligamentum arteriosum

Superior vena cava

Pulmonary artery

Pulmonary vein

AO

PA

RA

LA

Mitral valve

Tricuspid valve

Aortic valve

LV

RV

Ligamentum teres

Pulmonic valve

Inferior vena cava

Oxygen-rich blood
Oxygen-poor blood
Mixed blood

FIGURE 40.1 Fetal (**A**) and newborn (**B**) circulation.

grow, the heart is displaced downward. The toddler/preschooler (between 1 and 5 years) has a heart four times the birth size. By school age (between 6 and 12 years) the child's heart is 10 times the size it was at birth. However, the heart is smaller proportionally at this time than at any other stage in life. During the school-age years, the heart grows more vertically within the thoracic cavity. During adolescence, the heart continues to grow in relation to the teen's rapid growth.

At birth, the ventricle walls are similar in thickness, but with time the left ventricular wall thickens. The immature myocytes of the infant's heart are thinner and less compliant than those of the adult. Right ventricular function dominates at birth, but over the first few months of life left ventricular function becomes dominant. The infant's heart at rest exhibits a greater resting tension than the adult's, so volume loading or increased stretch may actually lead to decreased **cardiac output**. The infant's sarcoplasmic reticulum is less well organized than the adult's, making the infant dependent on serum calcium for cardiac contraction. Inotropic response to calcium in the actin and myosin (contractile proteins) increases with age (Craig, Fineman, Moynihan, & Baker, 2001).

In addition to the small chamber size, the normal heart rate is higher in infancy than in adulthood, limiting the infant's ability to increase cardiac output by increasing the heart rate. The heart's efficiency increases as the child ages and the heart rate drops over time. The normal infant heart rate averages 120 to 130 beats/minute,

decreasing to 80 to 105 beats/minute in the toddler and preschooler, 70 to 80 beats/minute in the school-age child, and 60 to 68 beats/minute in the adolescent. Innocent murmurs and physiologic splitting of heart sounds may be noted in infancy or childhood (Park, 2008). These findings are related to the change in the size of the heart in relation to the thoracic cavity. The infant's and child's blood vessels widen and increase in length over time. The normal infant's BP is about 80/40 mm Hg. The BP increases over time to the adult level. The toddler's or preschooler's BP averages 80 to 100/64 mm Hg, the school-age child's 94 to 112/56 to 60 mm Hg, and the adolescent's 100 to 120/50 to 70 mm Hg (Martchenke & Blosser, 2009).

Common Medical Treatments

A variety of medications as well as other medical treatments, most commonly oxygenation and surgical procedures, are used to treat cardiovascular problems in children. Most of these treatments will require a physician's order when the child is in the hospital. The most common treatments and medications are listed in Common Medical Treatments 40.1 and Drug Guide 40.1. The nurse caring for the child with a cardiovascular disorder should be familiar with what the procedures and medications are and how they work as well as common nursing implications related to use of these modalities.

DRUG GUIDE 40.1

Medication	Action	Indication	Nursing Implications
Alprostadil (Prostin VR: prostaglandin E₁)	Direct vasodilation of the ductus arteriosus smooth muscle	Temporary maintenance of ductus arteriosus patency in infants with ductal-dependent congenital heart defects	• Apnea occurs in 10% to 20% of neonates within first hour of infusion • Monitor arterial BP, respiratory rate, heart rate, EKG, temperature, and pO₂; watch for abdominal distention • Fresh IV solution required every 24 hours • Reposition catheter if facial or arm flushing occurs • Use with caution in neonate with bleeding tendency • Contraindicated in respiratory distress syndrome or persistent fetal circulation
Digoxin (Lanoxin)	Increases contractility of the heart muscle by decreasing conduction and increasing force	Heart failure, atrial fibrillation, atrial flutter, supraventricular tachycardia	• Prior to administering each dose, count apical pulse for 1 full minute, noting rate, rhythm, and quality. Withhold if apical pulse is <60 in an adolescent, <90 in an infant • Avoid giving oral form with meals, as altered absorption may occur • Monitor serum digoxin levels (therapeutic range: 0.8–2 ng/mL) • Notes signs of toxicity: nausea, vomiting, diarrhea, lethargy, bradycardia • Ginseng, hawthorn, and licorice intake increases risk of drug toxicity • Note contraindications (ventricular fibrillation and hypersensitivity to digitalis) • Avoid rapid IV administration, as this may lead to systemic and coronary artery vasoconstriction
Furosemide (Lasix)	Inhibits resorption of sodium and chloride in ascending loop of Henle	Management of edema associated with heart failure or management of hypertension in combination with antihypertensives	• Administer with food or milk to decrease GI upset • Monitor BP, renal function, electrolytes (particularly potassium), and hearing • May cause photosensitivity
Heparin	Interferes with conversion of prothrombin to thrombin, preventing clot formation	Prophylaxis and treatment of thromboembolic disorders, especially after cardiac surgery	• Administer SQ, not IM • Dose is adjusted according to coagulation test results • Monitor for signs of bleeding, platelet counts • Ensure that the antidote, protamine sulfate, is available • Do not administer with uncontrolled bleeding or if subacute bacterial endocarditis is suspected
Indomethacin (Indocin)	Inhibits prostaglandin synthesis	To close patent ductus arteriosus	• Monitor heart rate, BP, EKG, urine output; monitor for murmur • Monitor serum sodium, glucose, platelet count, BUN, creatinine, potassium, and liver enzymes • May mask signs of infection • Note development of edema

Medication	Action	Indication	Nursing Implications
Spironolactone (Aldactone)	Competes with aldosterone to result in increased water and sodium excretion (spares potassium)	Management of edema due to heart failure, treatment of hypertension	• Administer with food • Monitor serum potassium, sodium, and renal function • May cause drowsiness, headache, arrhythmia • May cause false elevations in digitalis level • Teach patients to avoid high-potassium diets, salt substitutes, and natural licorice • Contraindicated in hyperkalemia, renal failure, and anuria
Antibiotics Penicillin G benzathine (PCN-G) Penicillin V potassium (Pen-VK)	Inhibits bacterial wall synthesis in susceptible gram-positive organisms, such as streptococci, pneumococci, and staphylococci	Mild to moderate infections, prophylaxis of endocarditis and rheumatic fever	• Contraindications include hypersensitivity to penicillins • Report hypersensitivity reactions (chills, fever, wheezing, pruritus, anaphylaxis) immediately • PCN-G: administer IM • Pen-VK: administer orally on empty stomach 1 hour prior to or 2 hours after a meal
Erythromycin	Inhibits RNA transcription in susceptible organisms, such as streptococci, pneumococci, and staphylococci	Children with penicillin allergy, mild to moderate infections, endocarditis, and rheumatic fever prophylaxis	• Contraindicated in pre-existing liver disease • IV administration may result in cardiovascular abnormalities • Abdominal distress common with oral use • Fever, dizziness, rash may occur.
Antihypertensive Drugs Angiotensin-converting enzyme (ACE) inhibitors (captopril [Capoten], enalapril [Vasotec])	Competitive inhibition of ACE	Management of hypertension; heart failure management in conjunction with digitalis and diuretics	• Monitor BP, renal function, WBC count, serum potassium • Discontinue if angioedema occurs • Captopril: administer orally on empty stomach 1 hour before or 2 hours after meals • Enalapril: may administer orally without regard to food
Beta-adrenergic blockers (propranolol [Inderal], atenolol [Tenormin], sotalol [Betaspace])	Competitively blocks response to beta₁- and beta₂-adrenergic stimulation (propranolol, sotalol), beta₁ only (atenolol), decreasing heart rate and force of contraction	Management of hypertension, arrhythmias; prevention of myocardial infarction (propranolol, atenolol); arrhythmia management (sotalol)	• Monitor EKG and BP • Propranolol: administer with food • Atenolol, sotalol: administer without regard to food. Do not stop drug abruptly • May result in bradycardia, dizziness, nausea and vomiting, dyspnea, hypoglycemia (propranolol) • Contraindications: heart block, uncompensated heart failure, cardiogenic shock, asthma, or hypersensitivity
Hydralazine (Apresoline)	Directs vasodilation of arterioles	Management of moderate to severe hypertension, heart failure	• Monitor heart rate, BP • Closely monitor BP with IV use • Administer oral dose with food • May cause palpitations, flushing, tachycardia, dizziness, nausea, and vomiting • Notify physician if flu-like symptoms occur • Contraindicated in rheumatic valvular disease

Taketokmo, C. K., Hodding, J. H., & Kraus, D. M. (2010). *Lexi-comp's pediatric dosage handbook* (17th ed.). Hudson, OH: Lexi-comp.

COMMON MEDICAL TREATMENTS 40.1

Treatment	Explanation	Indication	Nursing Implications
Oxygen	Supplemented via mask, nasal cannula, hood, tent, or endotracheal/nasotracheal tube	Hypoxemia, respiratory distress, heart failure	Monitor response via work of breathing and pulse oximetry
Chest physiotherapy (CPT) and postural drainage	Promotes mucus clearance by mobilizing secretions with the assistance of percussion or vibration accompanied by postural drainage (refer to Chapter 34 for additional information related to CPT and postural drainage)	Mobilization of secretions, particularly in postoperative period or with heart failure	May be performed by respiratory therapist in some institutions, by nurses in others. In either case, nurses must be familiar with the technique and able to educate families on its use
Chest tube	Drainage tube is inserted into the pleural cavity to facilitate removal of air or fluid and allow full lung expansion	After open heart surgery, pneumothorax	If tube becomes dislodged from container, the chest tube must be clamped immediately to avoid further air entry into the chest cavity
Pacing	External wiring connected to a small generator used to electrophysiologically correct cardiac arrhythmias or heart block (temporary). Permanent pacing is achieved with an implantable internal pacemaker	Bradyarrhythmias, heart block, cardiomyopathy, sinoatrial or atrioventricular node malfunction	Provide close observation of the child, pacing unit, and EKG Maintain asepsis at pacing lead insertion site Explain to child and family that the permanent pacemaker may be felt under the skin Advise against participation in contact sports. (Skippen, Sanatina, Froese, & Gow, 2010)

▶ *Take* NOTE!

*Give digoxin at regular intervals, every 12 hours, such as at 8 AM and 8 PM, 1 hour before or 2 hours after a feeding. If a digoxin dose is missed and more than 4 hours have elapsed, withhold the dose and give the dose at the next regular time; if less than 4 hours have elapsed, give the missed dose. If the child vomits digoxin, **do not** give a second dose. Monitor potassium levels, as a decrease enhances the effects of digitalis, causing toxicity (Taketokmo et al., 2010).*

NURSING PROCESS OVERVIEW FOR THE CHILD WITH A CARDIOVASCULAR DISORDER

Care of the child with a cardiovascular disorder includes all of the typical steps of the nursing process: assessment, nursing diagnosis, planning, interventions, and evaluation. There are a number of general concepts related to the nursing process that may be applied to any child with a cardiovascular disorder. The nurse should be knowl-

edgeable about the procedures, treatments, and medication as well as familiar with the nursing implications related to these interventions. With an understanding of these concepts, the nurse can individualize the care based on the patient's and family's needs.

*R*emember Logan, the 6-week-old with poor feeding? *What additional health history and physical examination assessment information should the nurse obtain?*

Assessment

When assessing a child with a cardiovascular disorder, expect to obtain a health history, perform a physical examination, and prepare the child for laboratory and diagnostic testing.

Health History

The health history comprises a history of the present illness, past medical history, and family history. Depending on his or her age, the child should be included in the health history interview; the child's age will determine the degree of involvement and the terminology used. Table 40.1 gives examples of typical questions that can be used when obtaining the child's health history.

TABLE 40.1 EXAMPLES OF QUESTIONS FOR OBTAINING A CHILD'S HEALTH HISTORY

Questions	Provides Information About
• What types and amounts (dosages) of medications has the child received? What were they used for? • Who prescribed them? • Were they effective? Did the child experience any adverse effects? • To whom does the child go for medical evaluation? How often? Were the visits for regular health check-ups or for situational problems? Were there previous hospitalizations? What for? • Has the child experienced any growth delay? Does the child have any problems with activity and coordination? • Does the child's skin colour change when crying? If so, what colour do you see? • Does the child stop frequently during play to sit or squat? • Does the child have feeding difficulty? Does the child sweat when feeding or sleeping? Does the child tire easily or sleep excessively? • Does the child frequently develop strep throat?	• Possible underlying conditions that may be related to the child's current status • Other health care personnel involved in the child's care as well as the parents' health care beliefs and patterns • How the medications may be affecting the child's health • The child's health status and the parents' health care knowledge, practices, and beliefs • Problems that may result from impaired cardiac output, adequacy of tissue oxygenation, and concomitant disorders associated with heart disease • Effectiveness of tissue oxygenation. A blue or grey skin colour may be due to cyanosis. • The child's exercise tolerance and tissue oxygenation • The child's energy expenditure, ability to tolerate activity, and tissue oxygenation • Child's risk of developing rheumatic fever and heart disease

Source: Park, M. K. (2008). *Pediatric cardiology for practitioners* (5th ed.). St. Louis, MO: Mosby.

History of Present Illness

Elicit the history of the present illness, which addresses when the symptoms started and how they have progressed. Inquire about any treatments and medications used at home. Ask parents about history of orthopnea, dyspnea, activity intolerance, growth delays, **cyanosis**, edema, dizziness, syncope, and/or frequent occurrences of pneumonia, which can be significant signs of pediatric heart disease. The history of present illness may reveal poor feeding, including fatigue, lethargy, and/or vomiting, or failure to thrive, even with adequate caloric intake. The parents may report diaphoresis, which is often seen in early heart failure. Delays in gross motor development, cyanosis (possibly reported by the parents as more of a grey colour than blue), and tachypnea (indicative of heart failure) may also be reported by the parent or caregiver.

Past Medical History

The past medical history includes information about the child as well as the mother's pregnancy history.

Assess the child's medical history for

- Problems occurring after birth (history of the child's condition after birth may reveal evidence of an associated congenital malformation or other disorder)
- Frequent infections
- Chromosomal abnormalities
- Prematurity
- Autoimmune disorders
- Use of medications, such as corticosteroids

Assess the mother's pregnancy, labour, and delivery history. Be sure to include information about the status of the neonate at birth. Also inquire about maternal use of medications, including illicit or over-the-counter drugs and alcohol, exposure to radiation; presence of hypertension, and maternal viral illnesses such as coxsackievirus, cytomegalovirus, influenza, mumps, or rubella. A history of significant problems related to labour and delivery is also important: stress or asphyxia at birth may be related to cardiac dysfunction and pulmonary hypertension in the newborn (Archer & Manning, 2009).

Assess for additional family risk factors such as

- History of heart disease or CHD (investigate the history further if heart disease occurred in a first-degree relative)
- Diabetes mellitus
- Sudden death or premature myocardial infarction (before age 50)
- Obesity, inactivity
- Stress
- Hypercholesterolemia (Martchenke & Blosser, 2009)

▶ **Take** NOTE!

Medications, such as isotretinoin (Accutane) for acne, lithium, and some antiseizure medications, taken by pregnant women may be linked to the development of congenital heart defects. In addition, smoking during pregnancy, febrile illness in the first trimester, rubella infection during pregnancy, exposure of the pregnant woman to strong cleaning products, repeated X-rays, and any harmful or poisonous material can increase the risk of CHD (Archer & Manning, 2009).

Physical Examination

Physical examination of the child with a cardiovascular condition consists of inspection, palpation, and auscultation. In addition, obtain the child's vital signs and measure the child's height and weight. Plot this information on a standard growth chart to evaluate nutritional status and growth. If the child is less than 3 years of age, measure and plot the head circumference also.

Inspection

Assess the child's overall appearance. Inspect the colour of the skin, noting mottling or cyanosis. Inspect the skin for edema. In infants, peripheral edema occurs first in the face, then the presacral region, and then the extremities. Edema of the lower extremities is characteristic of right ventricular heart failure in older children.

▶ **Take** NOTE!

CHD should be suspected in the cyanotic newborn whose colour does not improve with oxygen administration (Martchenke & Blosser, 2009).

Inspect the fingers and toes for **clubbing**. Clubbing (which usually does not appear until after 1 year of age) implies severe CHD due to chronic hypoxia. The first sign of clubbing is softening of the nail beds, followed by rounding of the fingernails, followed by shininess and thickening of the nail ends (see Fig. 39.6 in Chapter 39) and loss of the angle on the nail bed

Obtain the child's temperature; fever would suggest infection. Assess respirations, including rate, rhythm, and effort. Note location and severity of retractions if present. Inspect the chest configuration, noting any prominence of the precordial chest wall, which is often seen in infants and children with **cardiomegaly**. Note visible pulsations, which may indicate increased heart activity. Also inspect the neck veins for engorgement or abnormal pulsations. Note abdominal distention (Martchenke & Blosser, 2009; Park, 2008).

▶ **Take** NOTE!

Children with cardiac conditions resulting in cyanosis will often have baseline oxygen saturations that are relatively low because of the mixing of oxygenated with deoxygenated blood.

Palpation

Palpate the right and left radial or brachial pulse to assess cardiac rate and rhythm. Throughout infancy and childhood, the rate may vary. Palpate the femoral pulse; it should be readily palpable and equal in amplitude and strength to the brachial or radial pulse. A femoral pulse that is weak or absent in comparison with the brachial pulse is associated with coarctation of the aorta. Palpate apical pulses for rate, rhythm, and quality. Significant variations in pulse occur with activity, so the most accurate heart rate may be determined during sleep. In older children, exercise and emotional factors may influence the heart rate. A bounding pulse is characteristic of patent ductus arteriosus or aortic regurgitation. Narrow or thready pulses may occur in children with heart failure or severe aortic stenosis (Menashe, 2007). Note **tachycardia**, **bradycardia**, irregularities in rhythm, diminished peripheral pulses, or thready pulse. Palpate the child's abdomen for hepatomegaly, a sign of right-sided heart failure in the infant and child.

Auscultation

Auscultate the apical pulse for a full minute to determine heart rate and rhythm. Note irregularities in rhythm, tachycardia, or bradycardia. Auscultate the heart for murmurs. Many children have functional or innocent murmurs, but all murmurs must be evaluated on the basis of the following characteristics:

- Location
- Relation to the heart cycle and duration
- Intensity: grade I, soft and hard to hear; grade II, soft and easily heard; grade III, loud without thrill; grade IV, loud with a precordial thrill; grade V, loud, audible with a stethoscope barely touching the chest; grade VI, very loud, audible with a stethoscope held off the chest or with the naked ear
- Quality: harsh, musical, or rough; high, medium, or low pitch
- Variation with position (sitting, lying, standing) (Martchenke & Blosser, 2009; Park, 2008)

Auscultate for the character of heart sounds. Note distinct, muffled, or distant heart sounds. Abnormal splitting or intensifying of S2 sounds occurs in children with major heart problems. Ejection clicks, which are high-pitched, are related to problems with dilated vessels and/or valve abnormalities. Heard throughout systole, they can be early, moderate, or late. Clicks on the upper left sternal border are related to the pulmonary area. Aortic clicks are best heard at the apex and can be mitral or aortic in origin. A mild to late ejection click at the apex is typical of a mitral valve prolapse. The S3 heart sound may be heard in children and is associated with cardiac abnormalities. The S4 heart sound is not normally heard and is always associated with cardiac abnormalities (Martchenke & Blosser, 2009; Park, 2008).

Auscultate the BP in the upper and lower extremities and compare the findings; there should be no major differences between the upper and lower extremities. Determine the pulse pressure by subtracting the diastolic pressure from the systolic pressure. A pulse pressure of 20 to 50 mm Hg is normal in childhood (Martchenke & Blosser, 2009). A widened pulse pressure, which usually is accompanied by a bounding pulse, is associated with patent ductus arteriosus, aortic insufficiency, fever, anemia, or complete heart block. A narrowed pulse pressure is associated with aortic stenosis. Note hypotension or hypertension.

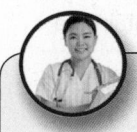

▶ *Take* NOTE!

Children and parents must be alerted if a heart murmur is detected, even if it is benign.

Laboratory and Diagnostic Testing

Common Laboratory and Diagnostic Tests 40.1 explains the laboratory and diagnostic tests most commonly used when considering cardiovascular disorders in children. The tests can assist the physician in diagnosing the disorder or can be used as guidelines in determining ongoing treatment. Laboratory or non-nursing personnel obtain some of the tests, while the nurse might obtain others. In either instance the nurse should be familiar with how the tests are obtained, what they are used for, and normal versus abnormal results. This knowledge will also be necessary when providing patient and family education related to the testing.

Cardiac Catheterization

Cardiac catheterization is a definitive study for infants and children with cardiac disease. However, it is highly invasive and not without risks, especially in sick infants and children. Indications for cardiac catheterization include the following:

• Questionable anatomic, physiologic, or electrophysiologic abnormalities
• Progressive monitoring related to pulmonary hypertension
• Periodic assessment both preoperatively and postoperatively
• Therapeutic interventions such as septostomy, valvuloplasty, stents, and transcutaneous valve replacement

Cardiac catheterization may be categorized as diagnostic, interventional, or electrophysiologic. Diagnostic cardiac catheterization typically is used to identify structural defects. Interventional cardiac catheterization is used as a treatment measure to dilate occluded or stenotic structures or vessels or close some defects. Electrophysiologic cardiac catheterization involves the use of electrodes to identify abnormal rhythms and destroy sites of abnormal electrical conduction. The

procedure lasts from 1 to 3 hours (Mullins, 2006; Park, 2008). Improvements in magnetic resonance imaging (MRI) have enabled access to necessary information without need for the child to undergo an invasive procedure such as a cardiac catheterization.

Performing Cardiac Catheterization

In cardiac catheterization, a radiopaque catheter is insertezd into a blood vessel and is then guided through the vessel to the heart with the aid of fluoroscopy. For a right-sided catheterization, the catheter is threaded to the right atrium via a major vein such as the femoral vein. With a left-sided catheterization, the catheter is threaded to the aorta and heart via an artery. Once the tip of the catheter is in the heart, contrast material is injected via the catheter and radiographic images are taken.

While the catheter is in the heart, several procedures can be performed. Measurements of BP and oxygen saturation are taken in each heart chamber and major blood vessels. Changes in cardiac output or stroke volume are also recorded. With the injection of contrast material, information is revealed about the heart anatomy, ventricular wall motion and ejection fraction, cardiac valve function, and structural abnormalities. The movement of the contrast material is filmed so that the details of the cardiac procedure are recorded. Endomyocardial biopsy samples of heart tissue to evaluate for infection, muscular dysfunction, or rejection after a transplant may also be obtained (Driscoll, 2006).

Nursing Management

Although cardiac catheterization may be considered nearly routine, for the child and parents or guardians, the procedure can be a source of much anxiety. Therefore, the nurse needs to educate the parents and, if appropriate for age, the child about all aspects of the procedure. Timing and type of catheterization will determine whether the child requires a hospital stay. Nursing management of the child undergoing cardiac catheterization includes preprocedural nursing assessment and preparation of the child and family, postprocedural nursing care, and discharge teaching.

Before the Procedure

A thorough history and physical examination are necessary to establish a baseline. Obtain vital signs. Note fever or other signs and symptoms of infection, which may necessitate rescheduling the procedure. Obtain the child's height and weight to aid in determining medication dosages. Assess the child for any allergies, especially to iodine and shellfish, because some contrast materials contain iodine as a base. Review the child's medications: medications such as anticoagulants are

COMMON LABORATORY AND DIAGNOSTIC TESTS 40.1

Test	Explanation	Indication	Nursing Implications
Angiography (visualization of arteries or veins)	Radiopaque contrast solution is injected through a catheter and into the circulation. X-rays are then taken to visualize the structure of the heart and blood vessels	To observe blood flow to parts of body and detect lesions; to confirm a diagnosis. Catheters can be used to remove plaques	• Make sure the parent signs a consent form • Administer premedication as ordered • Obtain child's weight to determine amount of dye needed • Keep the child NPO before the procedure according to institutional protocol • After the procedure, maintain the child on bed rest • Observe the puncture site for bleeding • Monitor vital signs frequently and check the pulse distal to the site
Ambulatory EKG monitoring (Holter)	Monitoring of the heart's electrical patterns for 24 hours using a portable compact unit	To identify and quantify arrhythmias in a 24-hour period during normal daily activities	• Instruct the child and parent to push the "event button" whenever chest pain, syncope, or palpitations occur. • Normal daily activities should be carried out during the testing period. • Having the child wear a snug undershirt over the leads helps to keep them in place.
Chest X-ray	A radiographic film of the chest area; will determine size of the heart and its chambers and pulmonary blood flow	Serves as a baseline for comparison with films taken after surgery; used to identify abnormalities of the lungs, heart, and other structures in the chest	• Instruct patient not to wear jewelry or any metal around neck or on the hospital gown • Explain to the child and family that no pain or discomfort should result • If a portable X-ray at bedside is done, remove electrodes temporarily
Echocardiogram	Non-invasive ultrasound procedure used to assess heart wall thickness, size of heart chambers, motion of valves and septa, and relationship of great vessels to other cardiac structures	Specific diagnosis of structural defects; determines hemodynamics and detects valvular defects	• Assure the child that the echo does not hurt • Instruct the child about EKG lead placement and use of gel on the scope's wand during the procedure • Encourage the child to lie still throughout the test
Electrocardiogram (EKG)	A graphic record produced by an electrocardiograph (device used to record the electrical activity of the myocardium to detect transmission of the cardiac impulse through the conductive tissues of the muscle). Facilitates evaluation of the heart rate, rhythm, conduction, and musculature	To detect heart rhythm and chamber overload; also serves as a baseline for measuring postoperative complications	• Assure the child that monitoring is a painless procedure • Place electrodes in the appropriate location • The child must lie still during the EKG recording period (usually about 5 minutes) • Wipe electrode paste or jelly off after procedure
Exercise stress test	Monitoring of heart rate, blood pressure, EKG, and oxygen consumption at rest and during exercise	Quantifies exercise tolerance; can be used to provoke symptoms or arrhythmias	• Child should be NPO for 4 hours prior to test • Obtain baseline EKG and vital signs • Instruct child to verbalize symptoms during testing • Usually takes about an hour

Test	Explanation	Indication	Nursing Implications
Hemoglobin (Hgb) and hematocrit (Hct)	Measures the total amount of hemoglobin in the blood (HgB) and indirectly measures the red blood cell number and volume (Hct)	To detect anemia or polycythemia (may occur with CHD resulting in cyanosis)	• False elevations occur with dehydration • May be obtained quickly via capillary puncture • Normal values vary with age
Magnetic resonance imaging (MRI)	Non-invasive imaging technique to detail internal structure and function	Specific diagnosis of structural defects: determines hemodynamics and detects vascular defects	Make sure the parent signs a consent form Screen patient for implanted devices that may contain metal (e.g., pacemakers) Younger children may require general anesthesia Monitor for allergic reaction to contrast material
Partial pressure of oxygen (pO₂)	Measures the amount of oxygen in the blood	To determine the presence and degree of hypoxia	• Most accurate result is with arterial specimen (venous and capillary specimens demonstrate lower levels) • Observe child for cyanosis • Supplement with oxygen per protocol

Abdallah, H. (2011). *Pediatric cardiac testing.* Retrieved October 18, 2011 from http://www.children-heartinstitute.org/testing/testhome.htm; and Pagana, K. D., & Pagana, T. J. (2010). *Mosby's manual of diagnostic and laboratory tests* (4th ed.). St. Louis, MO: Mosby.

typically withheld for several days prior to the procedure to reduce the child's risk of bleeding. Check the results of any laboratory tests, such as hemoglobin and hematocrit levels.

Perform a complete physical examination. Pay particular attention to assessing the child's peripheral pulses, including pedal pulses. Use an indelible pen to mark the location of the child's pedal pulses so they can be easily assessed after the procedure. Document the location and quality in the child's medical record.

Teach the parents and child, if appropriate, about the procedure, including what the procedure involves, how long it will take, and any special instructions from the health care provider. Use a variety of teaching methods as appropriate, such as online resources, DVDs, books, and pamphlets. Adapt these teaching methods to the child's developmental stage. For example, introduce the younger child to equipment through play therapy. For school-age and older children and their parents, offer a tour of the cardiac catheterization laboratory. Mention sounds and sights they may experience during the procedure. Explain the use of intravenous fluid therapy, sedation, and, if ordered, anesthesia to the child and parents. Tell the child that he or she may feel a sensation of the heart racing when the catheter is inserted. Also warn the older child that he or she may experience a feeling of warmth or stinging when the contrast material is injected. Encourage the child to

use familiar ways to relax. If necessary, teach the child simple relaxation measures.

Typically, food and fluid are withheld for 4 to 6 hours before the procedure. Prescribed medications may be taken with a sip of water. On the day of the procedure, check to ensure that a signed informed consent form is in the child's medical record and that all necessary assessment data have been included. Just before the procedure, ask the child to void and administer a sedative, as ordered. Whenever possible, have the parents accompany the child to the catheterization area.

Teach the child and family what to expect after the procedure is completed. Inform the parents of the possible complications, such as bleeding, low-grade fever, loss of pulse in the extremity used for the catheterization, and arrhythmias. Tell the child about the catheter site dressing and the need to keep that leg straight for several hours after the procedure. Teach the child and parent that frequent monitoring will be required after the procedure (Axton & Fugate, 2009).

After the Procedure

Throughout the postprocedural period, closely monitor the child for complications of bleeding, **arrhythmia**, infection, hematoma, and thrombus formation. After the procedure, evaluate the child's vital signs, the neurovascular status of the lower extremities, and the pressure dressing over the catheterization site every 15 minutes for the first hour and then every 30 minutes for the next hour. Vital signs should remain within acceptable parameters. Hypotension may signify hemorrhage due to perforation of the heart muscle or bleeding from the insertion site. Expect to monitor cardiac rhythm and oxygen saturation levels via pulse oximetry for the first few hours after the procedure to help identify possible complications.

Assess the child's distal pulses bilaterally for presence and quality. The pulse of the affected extremity may be slightly less than that of the other extremity in the initial postprocedure period, but it should gradually return to baseline. Also assess the colour and temperature of the extremity; pallor or blanching would indicate an obstruction in blood flow. Check capillary refill and sensation to evaluate blood flow to the area.

Maintain bed rest in the immediate post procedure period. Ensure that the child maintains the extremity in a straight position for approximately 4 to 8 hours, depending on the approach used and the facility's policy. Some facilities require straight positioning for 4 to 6 hours after a right-sided catheterization and for 6 to 8 hours after a left-sided catheterization to ensure healing of the vessel. Inspect the pressure dressing frequently. Check to make sure that it is dry and intact, without evidence of bleeding. Reinforce the dressing as necessary and report any evidence of drainage on the dressing. If there is a risk of the dressing becoming soiled or wet, cover it with a waterproof dressing.

▶ *Take* NOTE!

If arterial bleeding occurs after a cardiac catheterization, apply pressure 1 inch above the site to create pressure over the vessel, thereby reducing the blood flow to the area.

Monitor the child's intake and output closely to ensure adequate hydration. The contrast material has a diuretic effect, so assess the child for signs and symptoms of dehydration and hypovolemia. Typically, children resume oral intake as tolerated, beginning with sips of clear liquids and progressing to the preprocedure diet. Continue intravenous fluids as ordered and encourage oral fluid intake as tolerated to promote elimination of the contrast material.

Allow the child to talk about the experience and how and what he or she felt. Provide positive reinforcement for the child's actions.

Provide patient and family education before the child is discharged home (Teaching Guideline 40.1). Areas to address include site care and signs and symptoms of early complications such as fever, bleeding or bruising at the catheterization site, or changes in colour, temperature, or sensation in the extremity used. Also discuss diet and activity level (Axton & Fugate, 2009).

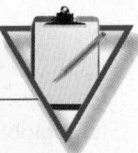

TEACHING GUIDELINE 40.1

Providing Care After a Cardiac Catheterization

- Change the pressure dressing as ordered. When doing so, inspect the insertion site for redness, irritation, swelling, drainage, and bleeding. Report any of these to the health care provider.
- Check the temperature, colour, sensation, and pulses on the child's extremities and compare. Report any changes to the health care provider.
- Resume the child's usual diet after the procedure; report any nausea or vomiting.
- Check the child's temperature at least once a day for approximately 3 days after the procedure. Report any temperature of 38°C or greater.
- Avoid giving the child a tub bath for approximately 3 days; use sponge baths or showers instead.
- Discourage strenuous exercise or activity for approximately 3 days.
- Watch for changes in the child's appearance, such as changes in skin colour, reports of the heart "fluttering" or "skipping a beat," fever, or difficulty breathing.
- Give acetaminophen (Tylenol) or ibuprofen (Motrin) for complaints of pain.
- Schedule a follow-up appointment with the health care provider in the time specified.

From Axton, S. E., & Fugate, T. (2009). *Pediatric nursing care plans for the hospitalized child* (3rd ed.). Upper Saddle River, NJ: Pearson; and Children's Mercy Hospitals & Clinics. (2011). *Cardiac catheterization.* Retrieved October 20, 2011 from http://www.childrens-mercy.org/Content/view.aspx?id=4890.

Nursing Diagnoses and Related Interventions

Upon completion of a thorough assessment, the nurse might identify several nursing diagnoses. These may include but are not limited to

- Decreased cardiac output related to structural defect, congenital anomaly, or ineffective heart pumping
- Ineffective tissue perfusion related to inadequate cardiac function or cardiac surgery
- Imbalanced nutrition, less than body requirements, related to increased energy expenditure and fatigue
- Risk of delayed growth and development related to effects of cardiac disease and treatments, inadequate nutrition, or frequent separation from caregivers secondary to illness
- Risk of infection related to need for multiple invasive procedures or cardiac surgery
- Excess fluid volume related to ineffective cardiac muscle function

EVIDENCE-BASED PRACTICE 40.1
Effects of Chronic or Intermittent Hypoxia on Cognition in Children

● Study

It is well known that significant hypoxia has an adverse effect on cognition, yet little is known about the effects of chronic or intermittent hypoxia on cognition in children. Many children with CHD suffer either chronic or intermittent hypoxia. The authors performed a systematic literature review to study this question. Fifty-five studies were included, a significant proportion of which addressed hypoxia associated with CHD.

▲ Findings

About 80% of the studies reported adverse effects on cognition in children who suffered chronic or intermittent hypoxia, including developmental and academic achieve-

ment. Adverse effects were noted at all childhood age levels except premature infants. The effects were noted even with mild oxygen desaturation.

■ Nursing Implications

It is critical that the developing child be afforded the opportunity to develop optimal cognition. Know the child's normal oxygen saturation so that decreases may be quickly acted upon. Use supplemental oxygen judiciously and within the physician order parameters. Since many children experience improved oxygenation after CHD repair, encourage adequate nutrition so that, in turn, the infant or child will demonstrate growth adequate for safe surgical intervention.

Bass, J. L., Corwin, M., Gozal, D., Moore, C., et al. (2004). The effect of chronic or intermittent hypoxia on cognition in childhood: A review of the evidence. *Pediatrics, 114*(3), 805–816.

• Interrupted family process related to crisis associated with heart disease, frequent need for testing and hospitalizations, or stresses associated with care demands
• Activity intolerance related to ineffective cardiac muscle function, increased energy expenditure, or inability to meet increased oxygen or metabolic demands
• Pain

fter completing Logan's assessment, the nurse noted the following: poor weight gain, tachypnea with occasional nasal flaring, crackles heard on auscultation, and edema noted in the face, presacral area, and extremities. Based on these assessment findings, what would your top three nursing diagnoses be for Logan?

Nursing goals, interventions, and evaluation for the child with a cardiovascular disorder are based on the nursing diagnoses. Nursing Care Plan 40.1 can be used as a guide in planning nursing care for the child with a cardiovascular disorder. The nursing care plan should be individualized based on the patient's symptoms and needs. Refer to Chapter 35 for detailed information about pain assessment and management. Additional information will be included later in the chapter as it relates to specific disorders.

ased on your top three nursing diagnoses for Logan, describe appropriate nursing interventions.

Congenital Heart Disease

In North America, more than 1% of newborn infants have CHD resulting from numerous causes (Hoffman &

Kaplan, 2002). The prevalence of CHD varies from study to study (Hoffman & Kaplan, 2002) yet is about 8 per 1,000 live births, with premature infants more commonly affected than term infants (Fixler, 2006). Many chromosomal disorders are associated with CHD, including Down syndrome, deletion 22q11, Turner syndrome, trisomy 13, trisomy 18, Williams syndrome, Prader–Willi syndrome, and cri-du-chat (Martchenke & Blosser, 2009). About one third of infants with CHD will have disease serious enough to result in death or will require cardiac catheterization or cardiac surgery within the first year of life. Complications of CHD include heart failure, hypoxemia, growth retardation, developmental delay, and pulmonary vascular disease. As many as 13% of children with CHD experience severe failure to thrive (Chen, Li, & Wang, 2004).

With advances in palliative and corrective surgery in the past 20 years, many more children with CHD are now able to survive into adulthood. In fact, a recent study in Quebec found that as of the year 2000 there was an equal number of children and adults with CHD (Marelli et al., 2007). As many as 85% of children with CHD grow to be adults, yet many have problems related to education, health insurance, and employment (Hetherington, 2009). Hypothermia and cardiopulmonary bypass required during cardiac surgery for CHD may have a long-term impact on the child's cognitive ability and academic function (Griffin, Elkin, & Smith, 2003; Mahle, Clancy, & Moss, 2000; Mahle, Visconti, & Freier, 2006). Due to the potential long-term effects that CHD may have on these children, nurses must be expertly equipped to care for them. See Evidence-based Practice 40.1.

(text continues on page 1331)

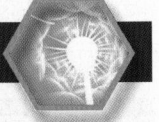

Nursing Care Plan 40.1

OVERVIEW FOR THE CHILD WITH A CARDIOVASCULAR DISORDER

NURSING DIAGNOSIS: Decreased cardiac output related to structural defect, congenital anomaly, or ineffective heart pumping as evidenced by arrhythmias, edema, murmur, abnormal heart rate, or abnormal heart sounds

Outcome Identification and Evaluation

Child or infant will demonstrate adequate cardiac output; *will have elastic skin turgor, brisk capillary refill, demonstrate pink colour, pulse and blood pressure within normal limits for age, regular heart rhythm, adequate urinary output.*

Interventions: Increasing Cardiac Output

- Monitor vital signs closely, especially BP and heart rate, *to detect increases or decreases.*
- Monitor cardiac rhythm via cardiac monitor *to detect arrhythmias quickly.*
- Observe for signs of hypoxia such as tachypnea, cyanosis, tachycardia, bradycardia, dizziness, and/or restlessness *to identify this change early.*
- Administer oxygen as needed *to correct hypoxia.*
- Place child in knee-to-chest or squatting position as needed *to increase systemic vascular resistance.*
- Administer antiarrhythmics, vasopressors, ACE inhibitors, beta blockers, corticosteroids, or diuretics as prescribed *to improve cardiac output.*
- Monitor for signs of thrombosis such as restlessness, seizure, coma, oliguria, anuria, edema, hematuria, or paralysis *to identify this condition early.*
- Administer adequate hydration *to decrease possibility of thrombosis formation.*
- Cluster nursing care and other activities *to allow adequate periods of rest.*
- Anticipate child's needs *to decrease the child's stress, thereby decreasing oxygen consumption requirement.*

NURSING DIAGNOSIS: Excess fluid volume related to ineffective cardiac muscle function as evidenced by weight gain, edema, jugular vein distention, dyspnea, shortness of breath, abnormal breath sounds, or pulmonary congestion

Outcome Identification and Evaluation

Child will attain appropriate fluid balance, *will lose weight (fluid), edema or bloating will decrease, lung sounds will be clear and heart sounds normal.*

Interventions: Encouraging Fluid Loss

- Weigh daily on same scale in similar amount of clothing; *in children weight is the best indicator of changes in fluid status.*
- Monitor location and extent of edema (measure abdominal girth daily if ascites is present); *decrease in edema indicates positive increase in oncotic pressure.*
- Protect edematous areas from skin breakdown: *edema leads to increased risk of alterations in skin integrity.*
- Auscultate lungs carefully to identify crackles *(indicating pulmonary edema).*
- Assess work of breathing and respiratory rate *(increased work of breathing is associated with pulmonary edema).*
- Assess heart sounds for gallop *(presence of S3 may indicate fluid overload).*
- Maintain fluid restriction as ordered *to decrease intravascular volume and workload on the heart.*
- Strictly monitor intake and output *to quickly note discrepancies and provide intervention.*
- Provide sodium-restricted diet as ordered *(restricting sodium intake allows better renal excretion of extra fluid).*
- Administer diuretics as ordered and monitor for adverse effects. *Diuretics encourage excretion of fluid and elimination of edema, reduce cardiac filling pressures, and increase renal blood flow. Adverse effects include electrolyte imbalance as well as orthostatic hypotension.*

NURSING DIAGNOSIS: Imbalanced nutrition, less than body requirements, related to increased energy expenditure and fatigue as evidenced by weight loss or height and weight below accepted standards

Outcome Identification and Evaluation

Child will improve nutritional intake resulting in *steady increase in weight and length/height, will feed without tiring easily.*

Interventions: Promoting Adequate Nutrition

- Determine body weight and length/height norm for age *to determine goal to work toward.*
- Assess child for food preferences that fall within dietary restrictions: *child will be more likely to consume adequate amounts of foods that he or she likes.*
- Weigh child daily or weekly (according to physician order or institutional standard) and measure length/height weekly *to monitor for increased growth.*
- Offer highest-calorie meals at the time of day when the child's appetite is the greatest *(to increase likelihood of increased caloric intake).*
- Provide increased-calorie shakes or puddings within diet restriction *(high-calorie foods increase weight gain).*
- Consult with the pediatric dietician *to provide optimal caloric intake within dietary restrictions.*
- Provide small, frequent feedings *to discourage tiring with feeding.*
- Feed infants with special nipple as needed *to decrease amount of energy expended for sucking.*
- Administer vitamin and mineral supplements as prescribed *to attain/maintain vitamin and mineral balance in the body.*

NURSING DIAGNOSIS: Ineffective tissue perfusion related to inadequate cardiac function or cardiac surgery as evidenced by pallor, cyanosis, edema, changes in mental status, prolonged capillary refill, clubbing, or diminished pulses

Outcome Identification and Evaluation

Child will demonstrate adequate tissue perfusion: *Child will be alert, not restless or lethargic, will have pink colour, decrease in edema, normal perfusion, and strong pulses.*

Interventions: Promoting Tissue Perfusion

- Assess level of consciousness, pulse, BP, peripheral perfusion, and skin colour frequently *to determine baseline and ongoing improvement.*
- Administer cardiac glycosides or vasodilators as ordered *to promote cardiac output necessary for proper perfusion.*
- Monitor pulse oximetry and arterial blood gas results *to assess ability to appropriately oxygenate.*
- Supplement oxygen as needed *to provide oxygen to organs for proper functioning.*
- Monitor hemoglobin and hematocrit *to identify blood loss.*
- Strictly assess intake and output *to determine adequacy of renal perfusion.*
- Position with head of bed elevated *to decrease blood volume returning to heart.*
- Change position every 2 to 4 hours *to promote circulation and avoid skin breakdown in areas of poor perfusion.*

NURSING DIAGNOSIS: Risk of delayed growth and development related to effects of cardiac disease and necessary treatments, inadequate nutrition, or frequent separation from caregivers secondary to illness

Outcome Identification and Evaluation

Child will display development appropriate for age, *will display evidence of cognitive and motor function within normal limits (individualized for each child).*

Interventions: Promoting Appropriate Development

- Promote adequate caloric intake *to stimulate growth and provide adequate energy.*
- Provide age-appropriate developmental activities *to stimulate development.*
- Consult with the physical or occupational therapist or child life specialist *to determine activities most appropriate for the child within the constraints of the child's illness.*
- Schedule daily activities to allow for essential rest periods *for energy conservation.*
- Encourage parents, teachers, and playmates to be sensitive to child's self-image, using positive comments, *to improve the child's self-concept.*
- As energy allows, encourage participation in all activities as feasible *to allow the child to feel normal.*

NURSING DIAGNOSIS: Risk of infection related to need for multiple invasive procedures or cardiac surgery as evidenced by break in skin integrity, decreased hemoglobin, or inadequate nutritional intake

Outcome Identification and Evaluation

Child will remain free from infection: *vital signs will be within normal limits, white blood cell count normal, cultures negative. Child will exhibit no signs or symptoms of infection.*

(continued)

Nursing Care Plan 40.1 (continued)

Interventions: Preventing Infection

- Maintain strict hand hygiene *to prevent spread of infectious organisms to the child.*
- Assess temperature *to detect elevation early in the course of infection.*
- Avoid contact with persons with known infections *to prevent risk of becoming ill.*
- Ensure appropriate immunization, including pneumococcal and influenza vaccinations, *to prevent development of common childhood illness.*
- Administer prophylactic antibiotics prior to all dental procedures, surgery, and many invasive procedures *to prevent subacute bacterial (infective) endocarditis.*
- Encourage good dental hygiene *to reduce the risk of endocarditis.*

NURSING DIAGNOSIS: Interrupted family processes related to crisis associated with heart disease, frequent need for testing and hospitalizations, or stresses associated with care demands, as evidenced by inadequate parental coping, frequent separations of parent and child, or inadequate support

Outcome Identification and Evaluation

Family will maintain functional system of support and will demonstrate adequate coping, adaptation of roles and functions, and decreased anxiety: *Parents are involved in child's care, ask appropriate questions, express fears and concerns, and can discuss child's care and condition calmly.*

Interventions: Promoting Family Processes

- Provide ongoing support to the child and family *to help them cope.*
- Encourage parents and family members to verbalize concerns related to child's illness, diagnosis, and prognosis: *allows the nurse to identify concerns and areas where further education may be needed. Demonstrates family-centred care.*
- Allow families to grieve over the loss of a "perfect" child: *parents must work through those grief feelings so they can be fully "present" for this chronically ill child.*
- Explain therapies, procedures, child's behaviours, and plan of care to parents: *understanding the child's current status and plan of care helps decrease anxiety.*
- Encourage parents to be involved in care: *allows parents to feel needed and valued and gives them a sense of control over their child's health.*
- Identify support system for family and child: *helps nurse identify needs and resources available for coping.*
- Educate family and child on additional resources available *to help them develop a wide base of support.*
- Encourage parents to seek genetic counselling *to provide them with the information required to make an informed decision about having another child.*

NURSING DIAGNOSIS: Activity intolerance related to ineffective cardiac muscle function, increased energy expenditure, or inability to meet increased oxygen or metabolic demands as evidenced by squatting positions, shortness of breath, cyanosis, or fatigue

Outcome Identification and Evaluation

Child will increase activity level as tolerated: *child participates in play and activities (specify particular activities and level as individualized for each child).*

Interventions: Promoting Activity

- Assess level of fatigue and activity tolerance *to determine baseline for comparison.*
- Note extent of dyspnea, oxygen requirement, or colour change with exertion *to provide baseline for comparison.*
- Cluster care activities, allowing rest periods in between, *to conserve child's energy.*
- Work with the parent and child to determine a mutually satisfactory daily schedule *to allow adequate rest and energy conservation.*
- Instruct family and child in prescribed activity restrictions *to prevent fatigue while allowing some activity.*
- In the infant, avoid long periods of crying or prolonged nipple feeding *(expends excessive calories).*
- Provide neutral thermal environment *to avoid increased oxygen and energy needs associated with excessive heat or cold.*

Axton, S. E., & Fugate, T. (2009). *Pediatric nursing care plans for the hospitalized child* (3rd ed.). Upper Saddle River, NJ: Pearson; and Carpenito-Moyet, L. J. (2010). *Nursing diagnosis: Application to clinical practice* (13th ed.). Philadelphia, PA: Lippincott Williams & Wilkins.

Pathophysiology

The exact cause of CHD is unknown. However, the belief is that it results from an interplay of several factors, including genetics (e.g., chromosomal alterations) and maternal exposure to environmental factors (e.g., toxins, infections, chronic illnesses, and alcohol).

Congenital heart defects result from some interference in the development of the heart structure during fetal life. Subsequently, the septal walls or valves may fail to develop completely or vessels or valves may be stenotic, narrowed, or transposed. Structures that formed to allow fetal circulation may fail to close after birth, altering the pressures necessary to maintain adequate blood flow.

After birth, with the change from fetal to newborn circulation, pressures within the chambers of the right side of the heart are less than those of the left side and pulmonary vascular resistance is less than that for the systemic circulation. These normal pressure gradients are necessary for adequate circulation to the lungs and the body. However, these pressure gradients become disrupted if a structure has failed to develop, a fetal structure has failed to close, or a narrowing stenosis, or transposition of a vessel has occurred. For example, blood typically flows from an area of higher pressure to lower pressure. If the ductus arteriosus fails to close, blood will move from the aorta to the pulmonary artery, ultimately increasing pulmonary artery pressure. With this shunting of blood, highly oxygenated blood can mix with less oxygenated blood, interfering with the amount available to the tissues via the systemic circulation. Some of the defects may result in significant hypoxemia, the sequelae of which include clubbing, polycythemia, exercise intolerance, hypercyanotic spells, brain abscess, and cerebrovascular accident (CVA) (Park, 2008).

The traditional approach to categorizing CHD has been in terms of whether the child exhibits cyanosis as a clinical manifestation—cyanotic versus acyanotic defects. However, children with acyanotic defects may exhibit cyanosis, and children with cyanotic defects may not demonstrate cyanosis unless they are seriously ill. Many children with congenital heart defects shift between cyanotic and acyanotic states depending on their hemodynamic status (Suddaby, 2001). Therefore, this chapter categorizes the disorders based on hemodynamic characteristics (blood flow patterns in the heart):

- Disorders with decreased pulmonary blood flow: tetralogy of Fallot, tricuspid atresia
- Disorders with increased pulmonary blood flow: patent ductus arteriosus (PDA), atrial septal defect (ASD), ventricular septal defect (VSD)
- Obstructive disorders: coarctation of the aorta, aortic stenosis, pulmonary stenosis
- Mixed disorders: transposition of the great arteries (vessels) (TGA), total anomalous pulmonary venous return (TAPVR), truncus arteriosus, and hypoplastic left heart syndrome (HLHS) (Suddaby, 2001)

Therapeutic Management

Prenatal education about avoiding certain substances or infection is essential to promote optimal outcomes for the fetus. Parents of children with CHD are encouraged to receive genetic counselling because of the increased risk of having subsequent children with a congenital heart defect. Children with small septal defects are urged to lead a normal life and often require no medical intervention. Therapeutic management of other forms of CHD focuses on palliative or corrective surgery. In newborns and very young infants with severe cyanosis (tricuspid atresia, TGA), a prostaglandin infusion will maintain patency of the ductus arteriosus, improving effective pulmonary blood flow. Definitive correction of structural disorders requires surgical intervention. Table 40.2 describes the surgical procedures used for the various congenital heart defects and the relevant nursing measures. Nursing management for the child with CHD will be provided following the disorders section.

Disorders with Decreased Pulmonary Blood Flow

Defects involving decreased pulmonary blood flow occur when there is some obstruction of blood flow to the lungs. As a result of the obstruction, pressure in the right side of the heart increases and becomes greater than that in the left side of the heart. Blood from the higher-pressure right side then shunts to the lower-pressure left side through a structural defect. Subsequently, deoxygenated blood mixes with oxygenated blood on the left side of the heart. This mixed blood, which is low in oxygen, is pumped via the systemic circulation to the body tissues.

Defects with decreased pulmonary blood flow are characterized by mild to severe oxygen desaturation. Typically, the child exhibits oxygen saturation levels ranging from 50% to 90%, producing mild to severe cyanosis. To compensate for low blood oxygen levels, the kidneys produce the hormone erythropoietin to stimulate the bone marrow to produce more red blood cells (RBCs). This increase in RBCs is called **polycythemia**. Polycythemia can lead to an increase in blood volume and blood viscosity, further taxing the workload of the heart. Although the number of RBCs increases, there is no change in the amount of blood that reaches the lungs for oxygenation (Chamberlain, 2008; Park, 2008; Suddaby, 2001). Disorders within this classification include tetralogy of Fallot and tricuspid atresia.

Tetralogy of Fallot

Tetralogy of Fallot is a congenital heart defect that actually comprises four heart defects: pulmonary stenosis (a narrowing of the pulmonary valve and outflow tract, creating an obstruction of blood flow from the right ventricle to the pulmonary artery), VSD, overriding aorta (enlargement of the aortic valve to the extent that it

TABLE 40.2 COMMON SURGICAL PROCEDURES AND NURSING MEASURES FOR CONGENITAL HEART DEFECTS

Disorder	Surgical Procedure	Nursing Measures
Tetralogy of Fallot	Palliation with systemic-to-pulmonary anastomoses: • Blalock-Taussig shunt: an end-to-side anastomosis (or connection with a small Gore-tex tube) of the subclavian artery and the pulmonary artery • Waterston shunt: anastomosis of the ascending aorta and the pulmonary artery • Definitive correction involves patch closure of the ventricular septal defect and repair of the pulmonary valve and right ventricular outflow tract	• Avoid BP measurements and venipunctures in the affected arm after a Blalock-Taussig shunt. Pulse will not be palpable in that arm because of use of the subclavian artery for the shunt. • Monitor for ventricular arrhythmias after corrective repair
Tricuspid atresia	• Palliation with Blalock-Taussig shunt or pulmonary artery banding may be performed • At 3 to 6 months of age, the superior vena cava is detached from the heart and connected to the pulmonary artery (Glenn procedure) • By age 2 to 5 years, a modified Fontan procedure may be performed. Systemic venous return is redirected to the pulmonary artery directly	• Monitor for atrial arrhythmias, left ventricular dysfunction, and protein-losing enteropathy • Some children may eventually require a pacemaker
Atrial septal defect	• If small, the defect may be sutured closed. Larger defects may require a patch of pericardium or synthetic material. • Ostium secundum ASD may be repaired percutaneously via cardiac catheterization with an Amplatzer septal occluder (other brands are also available)	• Monitor for atrial arrhythmias (lifelong) after surgical closure • With the Amplatzer device, strenuous activity should be avoided for 1 month after the procedure (AGA Medical Corporation, 2011)
Ventricular septal defect	• If surgical closure is required, it should be performed before permanent pulmonary vascular changes develop • Surgical closure may be in the form of suture closure of the VSD, transcatheter placement of a device in the defect, or Dacron patch closure	• Monitor for ventricular dysrhythmias or AV block • With the clamshell occluding or Amplatzer device, strenuous activity should be avoided for 1 month after the procedure (AGA Medical Corporation, 2011)
Atrioventricular canal defect	• Pulmonary artery banding as palliation in very young infants • Surgical correction by 3 to 18 months of age • Patch closure of the septal defects and suturing of the valve leaflets or valve reconstruction are performed	• Monitor for complete heart block postoperatively • Teach parents that mitral regurgitation is a long-term complication and may require valve replacement
Patent ductus arteriosus	• PDA is closed by coil embolization or device via cardiac catheterization • May also be surgically ligated	• Monitor for bleeding and laryngeal nerve damage
Coarctation of the aorta	• Balloon angioplasty via cardiac catheterization is possible in some children • Most common surgical repair is resection of the narrowed portion of the aorta, followed by end-to-end reanastomosis	• Preoperatively, administer prostaglandin medications as ordered to relax the ductal tissue • Postoperatively, measure and compare BP in all four extremities and quality of upper vs. lower pulses
Aortic stenosis	• Balloon dilation is accomplished via the umbilical artery in the newborn or the femoral artery via cardiac catheterization in the older child	• Provide routine post-catheterization care • Teach parents that long-term aortic regurgitation requiring valve replacement may occur
Pulmonary stenosis	• Balloon dilation valvuloplasty is performed via cardiac catheterization to dilate the valve. This is effective in all but the most severe cases, which will require surgical valvotomy	• Provide routine post-catheterization care for balloon dilation • Explain to parents that prognosis is excellent

Disorder	Surgical Procedure	Nursing Measures
Transposition of the great vessels (arteries)	• Balloon atrial septotomy is usually done as soon as the diagnosis is made. A balloon-tipped catheter is passed through the atrial septum to enlarge the atrial septum • Surgical correction involves switching the arteries into their normal anatomic positions	• Administer prostaglandin to maintain the open state of the ductus arteriosus, which will allow the mixing of poorly oxygenated blood with well-oxygenated blood • Monitor for rapid respirations and cyanosis • Administer oxygen as needed preoperatively
Total anomalous pulmonary venous return	The pulmonary vein is repositioned to the back of the left atrium and the ASD is closed	Monitor for dysrhythmias, heart block, and persistent heart failure
Truncus arteriosus	VSD repair, separation of the pulmonary arteries from the aorta, with subsequent connection to the right ventricle with a valve conduit	Preoperatively, administer prostaglandin infusion to prevent closing of the ductus arteriosus
Hypoplastic left heart syndrome	• Heart transplantation is the treatment of choice • Palliative staged treatment. First, Norwood procedure, reconstruction of the aorta and pulmonary arteries includes a cardiac transplant. Second, bidirectional Glenn procedure, connection of the superior vena cava to the right pulmonary artery to increase the blood flow to the lungs. Third, modified Fontan procedure.	• Preoperatively, administer prostaglandin infusion to prevent closing of the ductus arteriosus • After palliative repairs, monitor for dysrhythmias or worsening ventricular function
Valve disorders	• The incompetent valve is replaced with a valve prosthesis	• Lifelong anticoagulation therapy is necessary with prosthetic valves • Monitor prothrombin times • Monitor heart sounds for alterations

Sources: Fulton, D. R. (2008). Congenital heart disease in children and adolescents. In V. Fuster, R. A. O'Rourke, R. A. Walsh, & P. Poole-Wilson (Eds.), *Hurst's the heart* (12th ed). New York: McGraw-Hill Companies; and Miyamoto, S. D. Sondheimer, H. M., Fagan, T. E., & Collins, K. K. (2011). Cardiovascular diseases. In W. W. Hay, M. J. Levin, J. M. Sondheimer, & R. R. Deterding (Eds.), *Current pediatric diagnosis and treatment* (20th ed.) New York: McGraw-Hill.

appears to arise from the right and left ventricles rather than the anatomically correct left ventricle), and right ventricular hypertrophy (the muscle walls of the right ventricle increase in size due to continued overuse as the right ventricle attempts to overcome a high-pressure gradient). Surgical intervention is usually required during the first year of life (Fulton, 2008; Miyamoto, Sondheimer, Fagan, & Collins, 2011). The survival rate for adults who were treated surgically for tetralogy of Fallot 30 years ago is higher than 85% (Balliard & Anderson, 2009).

Pathophysiology

With pulmonary stenosis, the blood flow from the right ventricle is obstructed and slowed, resulting in a decrease in blood flow to the lungs for oxygenation and a decrease in the amount of oxygenated blood returning to the left atrium from the lungs. The obstructed flow also increases the pressure in the right ventricle. This blood, which is poorly oxygenated, is then shunted across the VSD into the left atrium. Poorly oxygenated blood also travels through the overriding aorta (if it extends to both ventricles). When

the VSD is large, the pressure in the right ventricle may be equal to that in the left ventricle. In this case, the path of blood shunting depends on which circulation is exerting the higher pressure, pulmonary or systemic.

Regardless of which way shunting occurs, a mixing of oxygenated and poorly oxygenated blood occurs, with this blood ultimately being pumped into the systemic circulation. The oxygen saturation of the blood in the systemic circulation is reduced, leading to cyanosis. The degree of cyanosis depends on the extent of the pulmonary stenosis, the size of the VSD, and the vascular resistance of the pulmonary and systemic circulations. In some children, cyanosis is so severe that it leads to severe hypoxia, dysrhythmias, and sudden death (Betz & Sowden, 2008).

Tetralogy of Fallot is usually diagnosed during the first weeks of life due to the presence of a murmur and/or cyanosis. Some newborns may be acutely cyanotic while others may exhibit only mild cyanosis that gradually becomes more severe, particularly during times of stress. Most often, infants with tetralogy of Fallot have PDA at

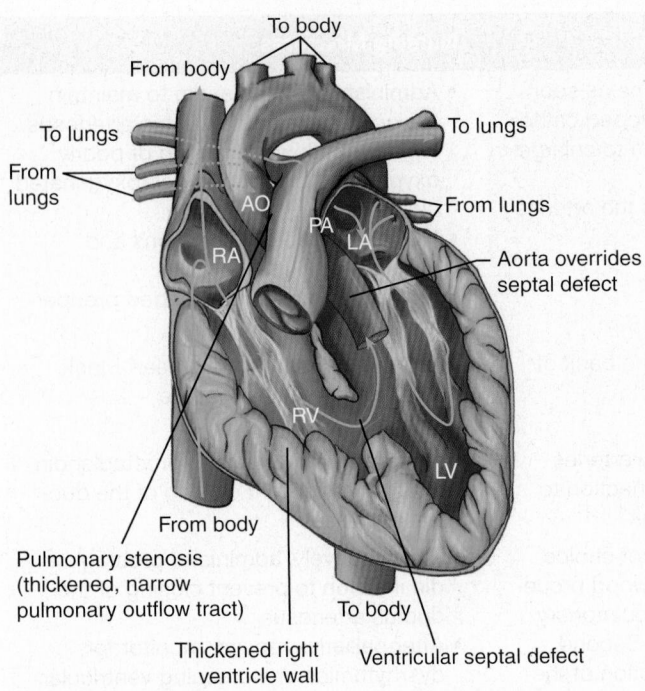

To body
From body
To body
To lungs
From lungs
To lungs
From lungs
AO
PA
RA
LA
Aorta overrides
septal defect
RV
LV
From body
Pulmonary stenosis
(thickened, narrow
pulmonary outflow tract)
To body
Thickened right
ventricle wall
Ventricular septal defect

■Oxygen-rich blood
■Oxygen-poor blood
☐Mixed blood

FIGURE 40.2 Tetralogy of Fallot.

birth, providing additional pulmonary blood flow and thereby decreasing the severity of the initial cyanosis. Later, as the ductus arteriosus closes, more severe cyanosis can occur (Fig. 40.2) (Fulton, 2008; Miyamoto et al., 2011).

Nursing Assessment

Nursing assessment consists of health history, physical examination, and laboratory and diagnostic tests.

Health History and Physical Examination

Obtain the health history, noting a history of colour changes associated with feeding, activity, or crying. Determine whether the infant or child is demonstrating hypercyanotic spells. Hypercyanosis develops suddenly and is manifested as increased cyanosis, hypoxemia, dyspnea, and agitation. If the infant's oxygen demand is greater than the supply, such as with crying or during feeding, then the spell progresses to severe hypoxia. When the degree of cyanosis is severe and persistent, the infant may become unresponsive. As the infant gets older, he or she may use specific postures, such as bending at the knees or assuming the fetal position to relieve a hypercyanotic spell. The walking infant or toddler may squat periodically. These positions improve pulmonary blood flow by increasing systemic vascular resistance. Ask the parents if they have noticed any of these unusual positions (Balliard & Anderson, 2009). Note history of irritability, sleepiness, or difficulty breathing.

During the physical examination, observe the skin colour and note any evidence of cyanosis. Also observe for changes in skin colour with positional changes and inspect the fingers for clubbing. Note whether the child has a hypercyanotic spell during the assessment. Count the child's respiratory rate and observe work of breathing, noting retractions, shortness of breath, or noisy breathing. Document oxygen saturation via pulse oximetry; it will likely be decreased. Auscultate the chest for adventitious breath sounds, which may suggest the development of heart failure. Auscultate the heart, noting a loud, harsh murmur characteristic of this disorder.

Laboratory and Diagnostic Tests

Note increased hematocrit, hemoglobin, and RBC count associated with polycythemia. Additional testing may include the following:

• Echocardiography, possibly revealing right ventricular hypertrophy, decreased pulmonary blood flow, and reduced size of the pulmonary artery
• **Electrocardiogram** (EKG), indicating right ventricular hypertrophy
• Cardiac catheterization and angiography, which reveal the extent of the structural defects

▶ Consider THIS!

Ava Gardener, 2 weeks old, is brought to the clinic by her mother. She presents with trouble feeding. Her mother states, "When Ava eats, she seems to have trouble breathing, and recently I've noticed a bluish colour around her lips." What other assessment information would you obtain?

Ava is to be admitted to the hospital secondary to suspected tetralogy of Fallot. What education and interventions may be necessary for this child and family? How can you assist the family to cope?

Tricuspid Atresia

Tricuspid atresia is a congenital heart defect in which the valve between the right atrium and right ventricle fails to develop. As a result, there is no opening to allow blood to flow from the right atrium to the right ventricle and subsequently through the pulmonary artery into the lungs (Fulton, 2008; Miyamoto et al., 2011).

Pathophysiology

In tricuspid atresia, blood returning from the systemic circulation to the right atrium cannot directly enter the right ventricle due to agenesis of the tricuspid valve. Subsequently, deoxygenated blood passes through an opening in the atrial septum (either an ASD or through a patent foramen ovale) into the left atrium, never entering the pulmonary vasculature. Thus, deoxygenated blood mixes

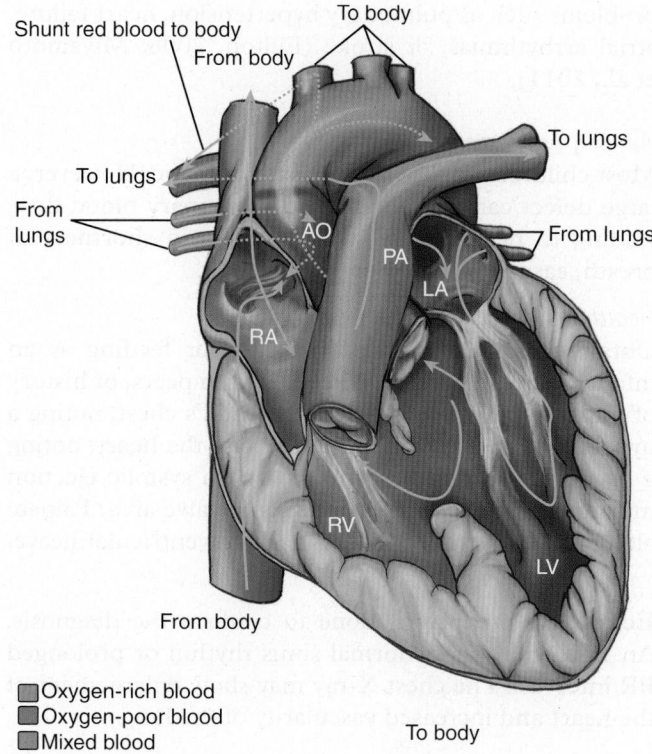

Shunt red blood to body
To body
From body
To lungs
To lungs
From lungs
From lungs
AO
PA
LA
RA
RV
LV
From body

■ Oxygen-rich blood
■ Oxygen-poor blood
■ Mixed blood
To body

FIGURE 40.3 Tricuspid atresia (with no PDA).

with oxygenated blood in the left atrium. Upon entering the left ventricle, the blood may cross a VSD or travel to the lungs through PDA. The foramen ovale, ductus arteriosus, and/or VSD must remain open for the newborn to maintain minimally adequate oxygenation (Fig. 40.3) (Fulton, 2008; Miyamoto et al., 2011).

Nursing Assessment

Nursing assessment consists of health history, physical examination, and laboratory and diagnostic tests.

Health History and Physical Examination

Note the infant's history since birth. Document history of cyanosis either at birth or a few days later when the ductus arteriosus closed. Note history of rapid respirations and difficulty with feeding. Inspect the skin for cyanosis or a pale grey colour. Observe the apical impulse, noting overactivity. Evaluate the baby's sucking strength (will usually have a weak or poor suck). Count the respiratory rate, noting tachypnea. Note increased work of breathing. Auscultate the lungs, noting crackles or wheezes if heart failure is beginning to develop. Auscultate the heart, noting a murmur. Palpate the skin, noting coolness and clamminess of the extremities. Document the presence of clubbing in the older infant or child.

Laboratory and Diagnostic Testing

Laboratory and diagnostic testing is similar to that for tetralogy of Fallot. A complete blood count (CBC) is needed to assess compensatory increases in hematocrit,

hemoglobin, and erythrocyte (RBC) count indicating the development of polycythemia. Oxygen saturation levels (typically reduced) may be determined by pulse oximetry or arterial blood gases. Additional testing may include the following:

- Echocardiography, revealing absence of tricuspid valve, underdeveloped right ventricle
- EKG
- Cardiac catheterization and angiography, which reveal the extent of the structural defects

Disorders with Increased Pulmonary Flow

Most congenital heart defects involve increased pulmonary blood flow. Normally, the left side of the heart has a higher pressure than the right side. Defects with connections involving the left and right sides will shunt blood from the higher-pressure left side to the lower-pressure right side. Even a small pressure gradient difference (e.g., 1 to 3 mm Hg) between the left and right sides will produce a movement of blood from the left to the right. In turn, the increase of blood on the right side of the heart will cause a greater amount of blood to move through the heart. If the amount of blood flowing to the lungs is large, the child may develop heart failure early in life. In addition, right ventricular hypertrophy may result. Sometimes with ventricular hypertrophy the right side of the heart pumps so forcefully that left-to-right shunting is reversed to right-to-left shunting. If this occurs, deoxygenated blood mixes with oxygenated blood, thereby lowering the overall blood oxygen saturation level.

Excessive blood flow to the lungs can produce compensatory responses such as tachypnea and tachycardia. Tachypnea increases caloric expenditure; poor cellular nutrition from decreased peripheral blood flow leads to feeding problems. Subsequently, the infant experiences poor weight gain, which retards overall growth and development. Increased pulmonary blood flow results in decreased systemic blood flow, so sodium and fluid retention may occur. Increased pulmonary blood flow also places the child at higher risk of pulmonary infections. As the child grows, the continuous increased pulmonary blood flow will cause vasoconstriction of the pulmonary vessels, actually decreasing the pulmonary blood flow. Over time, the pulmonary vasoconstriction causes pulmonary hypertension and may lead to pulmonary vascular disease. Surgical correction is essential before pulmonary disease develops (Park, 2008).

For children with congenital defects with increased pulmonary blood flow, oxygen supplementation may not be helpful. Oxygen acts as a pulmonary vasodilator. If pulmonary dilation occurs, pulmonary blood flow is even greater, causing tachypnea, increasing lung fluid retention, and eventually causing a greater problem with

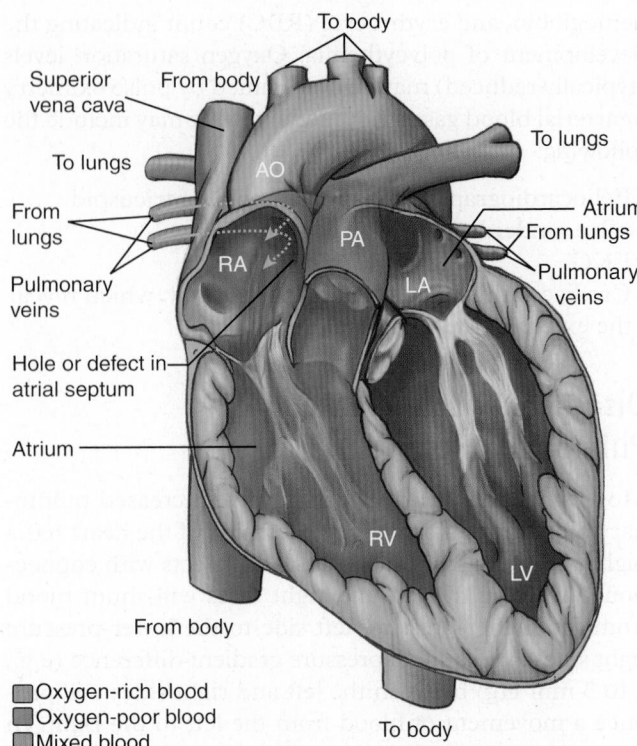

FIGURE 40.4 Atrial septal defect; note the opening between the two atria.

oxygenation. Examples of defects with increased pulmonary blood flow are ASD, VSD, atrioventricular septal defect (AVSD), and PDA.

Atrial Septal Defect

An ASD is a passageway or hole in the wall (septum) that divides the right atrium from the left atrium (Fig. 40.4). Three types of ASDs are identified based on the location of the opening:

- Ostium primum (ASD1): the opening is at the lower portion of the septum
- Ostium secundum (ASD2): the opening is near the centre of the septum
- Sinus venosus defect: the opening is near the junction of the superior vena cava and the right atrium

In as many as 80% of infants who have a small ASD, spontaneous closure of the defect occurs within the first 18 months of life. If not spontaneously closed by age 3, the child will most likely need an intervention or corrective surgery to close the defect (Fulton, 2008; Miyamoto et al., 2011).

Pathophysiology

With ASD, blood flows between the opening from the left atrium to the right atrium due to pressure differences. The shunting increases the blood volume entering the right atrium. This, in turn, leads to increased blood flow into the lungs. If untreated, the defect can cause

problems such as pulmonary hypertension, heart failure, atrial arrhythmias, or stroke (Fulton, 2008; Miyamoto et al., 2011).

Nursing Assessment

Most children with ASDs are asymptomatic. However, a large defect can cause increased pulmonary blood flow, leading to heart failure, which results in shortness of breath, easy fatigability, or poor growth.

Health History and Physical Examination

Obtain the health history, noting poor feeding as an infant, decreased ability to keep up with peers, or history of difficulty growing. Observe the child's chest, noting a hyperdynamic precordium. Auscultate the heart, noting a fixed split second heart sound and a systolic ejection murmur, best heard in the pulmonic valve area. Palpate along the left sternal border for a right ventricular heave.

Laboratory and Diagnostic Tests

Echocardiography is done to confirm the diagnosis. An EKG may show normal sinus rhythm or prolonged PR intervals. The chest X-ray may show enlargement of the heart and increased vascularity of the lungs.

Ventricular Septal Defect

VSD is an opening between the right and left ventricular chambers of the heart (Fig. 40.5). It is one of the most common congenital heart defects, with a prevalence of

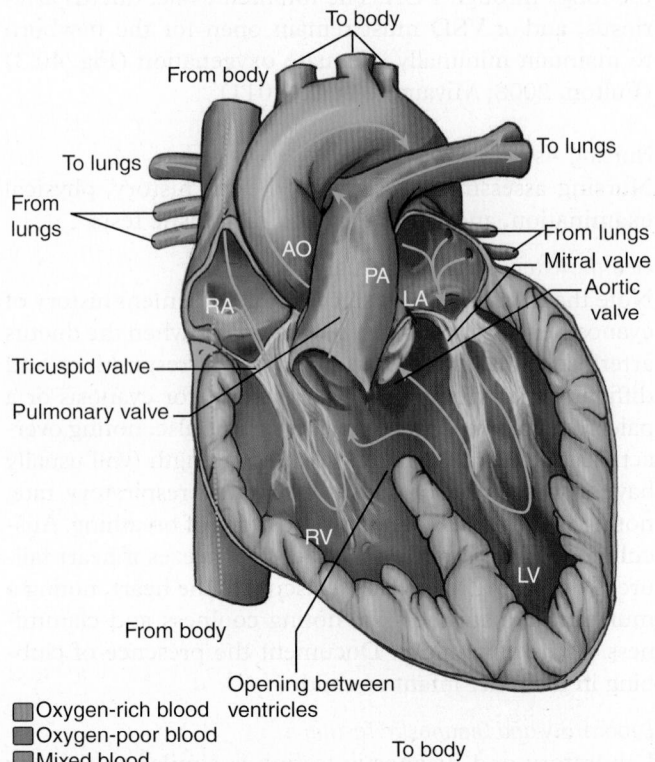

FIGURE 40.5 Ventricular septal defect; note the opening between the ventricles.

1.5 to 2.5 per 1,000 live births. VSD accounts for nearly one third of all congenital heart defects (Park, 2008). Spontaneous closure of the VSD occurs in 30% to 40% of children by 6 months of age (Park, 2008). Long-term outcomes for surgically repaired VSD are good, though the risk of sudden death is increased in those who develop pulmonary hypertension (Roos-Hesselink, Meijboom, & Spitaels, 2004).

Pathophysiology

In VSD, there is an abnormal opening between the right and left ventricles. The opening varies in size, from as small as a pinhole to a complete opening between the ventricles so that the right and left sides are as one. VSD size, pulmonary vascular resistance, and systemic vascular resistance determine the degree and direction of blood flow. A left-to-right shunt results when pulmonary vascular resistance is low. Increased amounts of blood flowing into the right ventricle are then pumped to the pulmonary circulation, causing heart failure and eventually an increase in pulmonary vascular resistance. Increased pulmonary vascular resistance leads to increased pulmonary artery pressure (pulmonary hypertension) and right ventricular hypertrophy. When the pulmonary vascular resistance exceeds the systemic vascular resistance, right-to-left shunting of blood across the VSD occurs, resulting in Eisenmenger syndrome (irreversible pulmonary hypertension and cyanosis). Children with small VSDs may remain asymptomatic. Heart failure commonly occurs in children with moderate to severe VSD. Children with VSD are also at risk of the development of aortic valve regurgitation as well as infective (bacterial) endocarditis (Miyamoto et al., 2011; Park, 2008).

Nursing Assessment

The newborn may not exhibit any signs and symptoms because left-to-right shunting through the VSD is minimal until the neonate's high pulmonary resistance drops.

Health History and Physical Examination

Determine the health history, which commonly reveals signs of heart failure around 4 to 8 weeks of age. Note history of tiring easily, particularly with exertion or feeding. Document the child's growth history, noting difficulty thriving. Ask the parent about colour change or diaphoresis with nipple feeding in the infant. Note history of frequent pulmonary infections, shortness of breath, and possibly periorbital edema. Note degree of tachypnea.

Auscultate the heart, noting a characteristic holosystolic harsh murmur along the left sternal border. Adventitious lung sounds may be auscultated if the child is experiencing heart failure. Palpate the chest for a thrill.

Laboratory and Diagnostic Tests

MRI or echocardiography with colour flow Doppler may reveal the opening as well as the extent of left-to-right shunting. These studies also may identify right ventricular

hypertrophy and dilation of the pulmonary artery resulting from the increased blood flow. Cardiac catheterization may be used to evaluate the extent of blood flow being pumped to the pulmonary circulation and to evaluate hemodynamic pressures.

Atrioventricular Septal Defect

AVSD (also known as AV canal or endocardial cushion defect) accounts for 4% to 5% of CHD and occurs in 2 of every 10,000 live births. Forty percent of children with Down syndrome and CHD have this defect (Miyamoto et al., 2011; Park, 2008).

Pathophysiology

AVSD occurs as a result of failure of the endocardial cushions to fuse (Fig. 40.6). These cushions are needed to separate the central parts of the heart near the tricuspid and mitral (AV) valves. The complete AVSD involves atrial and VSDs as well as a common AV orifice and a common AV valve. Partial and transitional forms of AVSD may also occur.

The complete AVSD permits oxygenated blood from the lungs to enter the left atrium and left ventricle, crossing over the atrial or ventricular septum and returning to the lungs via the pulmonary artery. This recirculation problem, which typically involves a left-to-right shunt, is inefficient because the left ventricle must pump blood back to the lungs and also meet the body's peripheral demand for oxygenated blood. Subsequently, the left

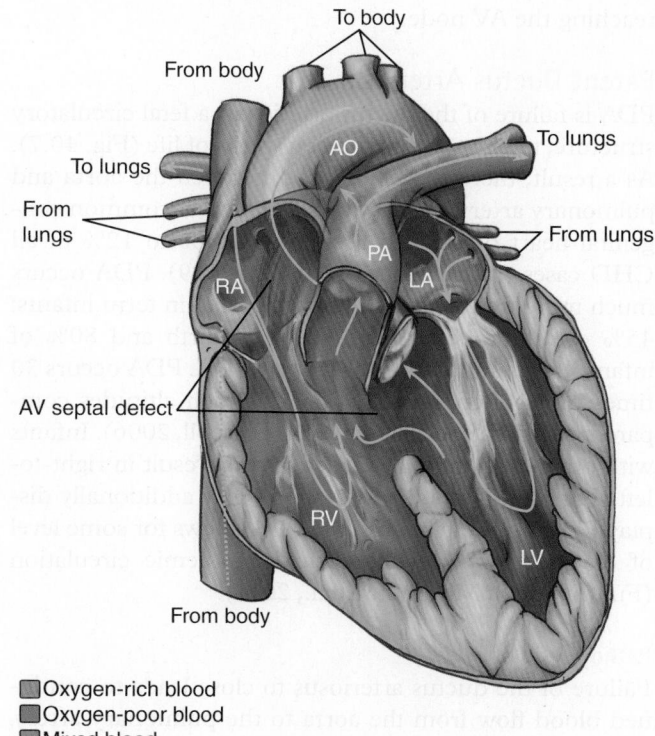

Oxygen-rich blood
Oxygen-poor blood
Mixed blood

FIGURE 40.6 Atrioventricular septal defect.

ventricle must pump two to three times more blood than in a normal heart. Therefore, this specific type of cardiac defect causes a large left-to-right shunt, an increased workload of the left ventricle, and high pulmonary arterial pressure, resulting in an increased amount of blood in the lungs, **congestive heart failure**, and pulmonary edema (Miyamoto et al., 2011; Park, 2008). There is the potential for bidirectional shunting.

Nursing Assessment

The infant with an AVSD commonly exhibits moderate to severe signs and symptoms of heart failure. However, for infants with partial or transitional AVSD, the signs and symptoms will be more subtle.

Health History and Physical Examination

Obtain the health history, noting frequent respiratory infections and difficulty gaining weight. Ask the parent if the infant has been experiencing difficulty feeding or increased work of breathing.

Inspect the skin, fingernails, and lips for cyanosis. Observe for retractions, tachypnea, and nasal flaring. Auscultate the lungs and heart, noting rales and a loud murmur. The murmur is commonly noted within the first 2 weeks of life. Infants with partial or transitional AVSD may display more subtle signs.

Laboratory and Diagnostic Tests

Echocardiography will reveal the extent of the defect and shunting as well as right ventricular hypertrophy. EKG may indicate right ventricular hypertrophy and possible first-degree heart block due to impulse blocking before reaching the AV node.

Patent Ductus Arteriosus

PDA is failure of the ductus arteriosus, a fetal circulatory structure, to close within the first weeks of life (Fig. 40.7). As a result, there is a connection between the aorta and pulmonary artery. PDA is the second most common congenital heart defect and accounts for 9% to 12% of all CHD cases (Martchenke & Blosser, 2009). PDA occurs much more frequently in premature than in term infants: 45% of infants less than 1,750 g at birth and 80% of infants less than 1,200 g will display PDA. PDA occurs 30 times more often in infants born at high altitudes compared with those born at sea level (Driscoll, 2006). Infants with other congenital heart defects that result in right-to-left shunting of blood and cyanosis may additionally display PDA. In these infants, the PDA allows for some level of oxygenated blood to reach the systemic circulation (Fulton, 2008; Miyamoto et al., 2011).

Pathophysiology

Failure of the ductus arteriosus to close leads to continued blood flow from the aorta to the pulmonary artery. Blood returning to the left atrium passes to the left ventricle, enters the aorta, and then travels to the pulmonary

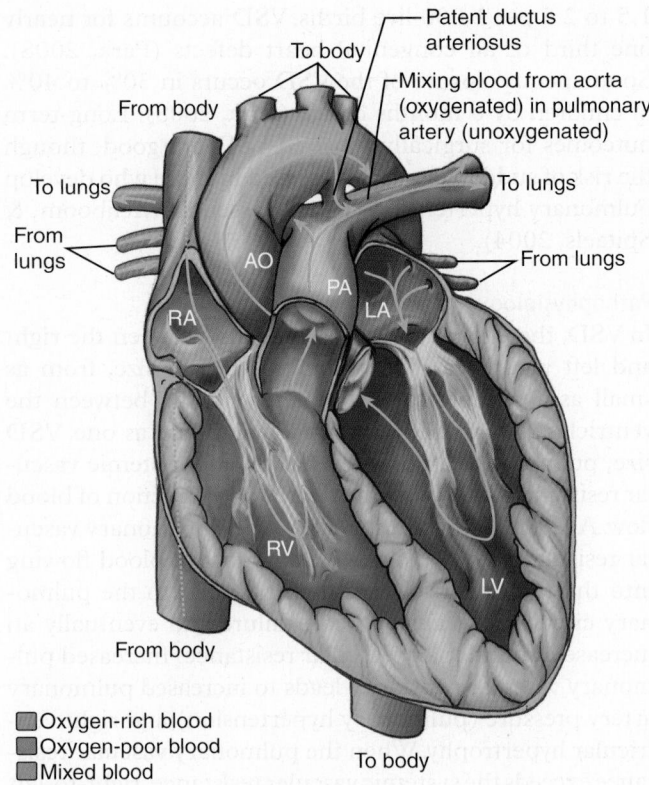

FIGURE 40.7 Patent ductus arteriosus.

artery via the PDA instead of entering the systemic circulation. This altered blood flow pattern increases the workload of the left side of heart. Pulmonary vascular congestion occurs, causing an increase in pressure. Right ventricular pressure increases in an attempt to overcome this increase in pulmonary pressure. Eventually, right ventricular hypertrophy occurs (Fulton, 2008; Miyamoto et al., 2011).

Nursing Assessment

The symptoms of PDA depend on the size of the ductus arteriosus and the amount of blood flow it carries. If it is small, the infant may be asymptomatic. Some infants demonstrate signs and symptoms of heart failure.

Health History and Physical Examination

Determine the health history, which may reveal frequent respiratory infections, fatigue, and poor growth and development. On physical examination, note tachycardia, tachypnea, bounding peripheral pulses, and a widened pulse pressure. The diastolic BP typically is low due to the shunting. Auscultate the lungs and heart, noting wheezes or crackles if heart failure is present. Note a harsh, continuous, machine-like murmur, usually loudest under the left clavicle at the first and second intercostal spaces.

Laboratory and Diagnostic Tests

Echocardiography reveals the size of the defect and confirms the diagnosis. An EKG may be normal or it may indicate ventricular hypertrophy, especially if the PDA is large. Chest X-ray demonstrates cardiomegaly.

Obstructive Disorders

Another group of congenital heart defects is classified as obstructive disorders. These disorders involve some type of narrowing of a major vessel (systemic or pulmonary), interfering with the ability of the blood to flow freely through the vessel. As a result, peripheral circulation or blood flow to the lungs is affected. Increased pressure backing up toward the heart causes an increased workload on the heart. Examples of defects in this group include coarctation of the aorta, aortic stenosis, and pulmonary stenosis.

Coarctation of the Aorta

Coarctation involves narrowing of the aorta, the major blood vessel carrying highly oxygenated blood from the left ventricle of the heart to the rest of the body (Fig. 40.8). It is the third most common congenital heart defect. Coarctation is more common in males than in females and is associated with Turner syndrome (Martchenke & Blosser, 2009).

Pathophysiology

Coarctation of the aorta occurs most often in the area near the ductus arteriosus. The narrowing can be preductal (between the subclavian artery and ductus arteriosus) or postductal (after the ductus arteriosus). As a result of the narrowing, blood flow is impeded, causing pressure

to increase proximal to the defect and to decrease distal to it. Thus, BP is increased in the heart and upper portions of the body and decreased in the lower portions of the body. Left ventricular afterload is increased, and in some children this may lead to heart failure. Collateral circulation also may develop as the body attempts to ensure adequate blood flow to the descending aorta. Due to the elevation in BP, the child is also at risk of aortic rupture, aortic aneurysm, and CVA (Fulton, 2008; Miyamoto et al., 2011).

Nursing Assessment

The extent of the symptoms depends on the severity of the coarctation. Young infants may present with severe cardiorespiratory distress. Some children with coarctation of the aorta grow well into the school-age years before the defect is discovered.

Health History and Physical Examination

Determine the health history, noting problems with irritability and frequent epistaxis. In older children, there also may be reports of leg pain with activity, dizziness, fainting, and headaches. Assess pulses throughout, noting full, bounding pulses in the upper extremities with weak or absent pulses in the lower extremities. Determine BP in all four extremities. BP in the upper extremities may be higher than that in the lower extremities. Auscultate the heart for a soft or moderately loud systolic murmur, most often heard at the base of the heart.

Laboratory and Diagnostic Tests

Diagnosis of coarctation of the aorta is based primarily on the history and physical examination. In addition, an echocardiogram may disclose the extent of narrowing and evidence of collateral circulation. Chest X-ray may reveal left-sided cardiac enlargement and rib notching indicative of collateral arterial enlargement. Other tests, such as EKG, computed tomography, or MRI, may be done to provide additional evidence about the extent of the coarctation and subsequent effects.

Aortic Stenosis

Aortic stenosis is a condition causing obstruction of the blood flow between the left ventricle and the aorta. Aortic stenosis accounts for 5% of all congenital heart defects, occurring four times more commonly in males. Twenty percent of patients with aortic stenosis have associated cardiac defects (Martchenke & Blosser, 2009).

Pathophysiology

Aortic stenosis can be caused by a muscle obstruction below the aortic valve, an obstruction at the valve itself, or an aortic narrowing just above the valve (Fig. 40.9). Supravalvar aortic stenosis is associated with Williams syndrome (Park, 2008). The most common type is an obstruction of the valve itself, called aortic valve stenosis. The aortic valve consists of three pliable leaflets. Normally the leaflets of

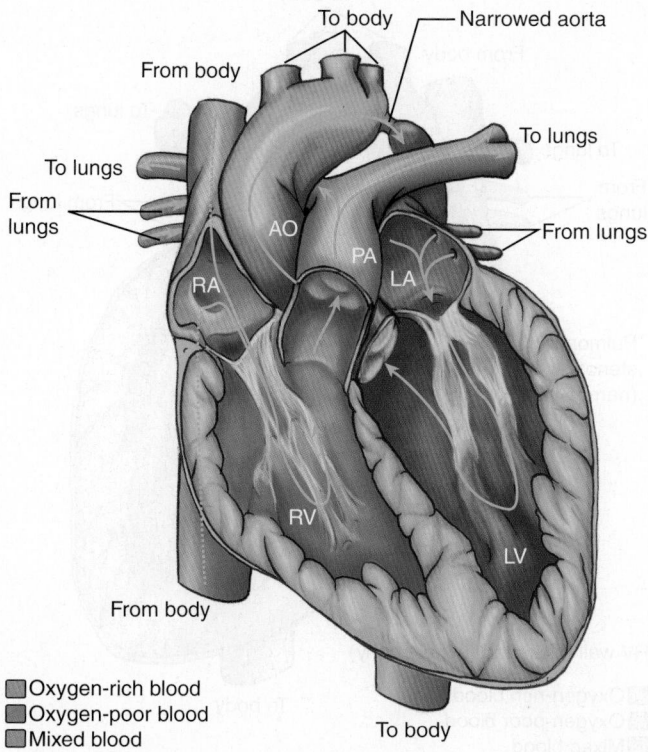

Oxygen-rich blood
Oxygen-poor blood
Mixed blood

FIGURE 40.8 Coarctation of the aorta.

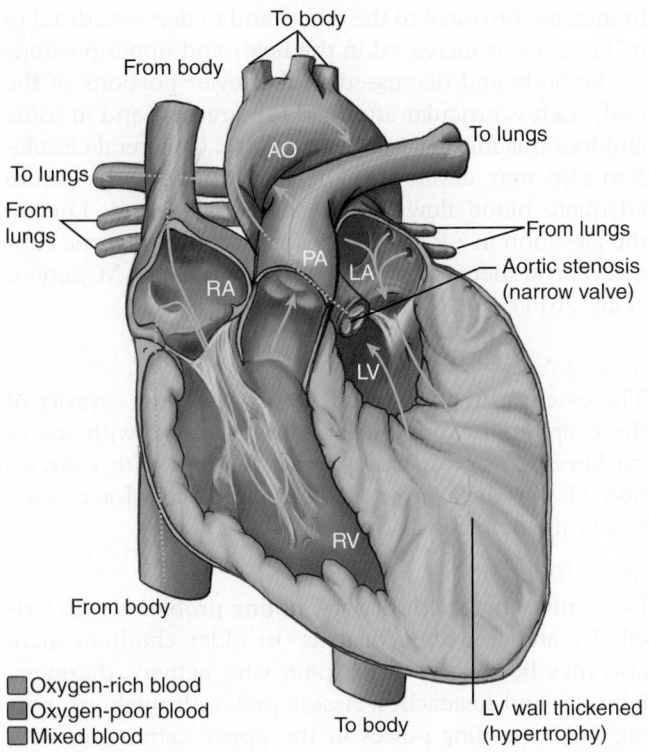

FIGURE 40.9 Aortic stenosis.

the aortic valve spread open easily when the left ventricle ejects blood into the aorta. When the aortic valve does not function properly, the left ventricle must work harder to pump blood into the aorta. Because of the increased workload, the left ventricular muscle hypertrophies and cardiac output may be compromised. Left ventricular failure can occur, leading to a backup of pressure in the pulmonary circulation and pulmonary edema. Heart failure is most commonly seen in the infant (Park, 2008; Ren, Aggarwal, & Balentine, 2011).

Nursing Assessment

Typically, the child with aortic stenosis is asymptomatic. However, it is important to obtain an accurate health history and perform a physical examination. Young infants may present in severe cardiorespiratory distress.

Health History and Physical Examination

Obtain the child's health history, noting easy fatigability or complaints of chest pain similar to anginal pain when active. Dizziness with prolonged standing may also be reported. In the infant, note difficulty with feeding. Palpate the child's pulse; if aortic stenosis is severe, the pulses may be faint. Palpate the child's chest, noting a thrill at the base of the heart. Auscultate the heart, noting a systolic murmur best heard along the left sternal border with radiation to the right upper sternal border.

Laboratory and Diagnostic Tests

The echocardiogram is the most important non-invasive test to identify aortic stenosis. An EKG may be normal

in children with mild to moderate forms of aortic stenosis. For children with severe aortic stenosis, left ventricular hypertrophy may be determined from the EKG. For children experiencing easy fatigability and chest pain, an exercise stress test may be done to evaluate the degree of cardiac compromise.

Pulmonary Stenosis

Pulmonary stenosis is a condition that causes an obstruction in blood flow between the right ventricle and the pulmonary arteries. Pulmonary stenosis accounts for 6% to 8% of all cases of CHD, and 1% to 2% of affected patients may have other cardiac malformations as well (Martchenke & Blosser, 2009). It can be associated with syndromes such as Noonan syndrome (Park, 2008). Children may be asymptomatic, although some children with severe stenosis may exhibit dyspnea and fatigue with exertion (Rao & Pflieger, 2010).

Pathophysiology

Pulmonary stenosis may occur as a muscular obstruction below the pulmonary valve, an obstruction at the valve, or a narrowing of the pulmonary artery above the valve (Fig. 40.10). Valve obstruction is the most common form of pulmonary stenosis. Normally the pulmonary valve is constructed with three thin and pliable valve leaflets; they spread apart easily, allowing the right ventricle to eject blood freely into the pulmonary artery. The most

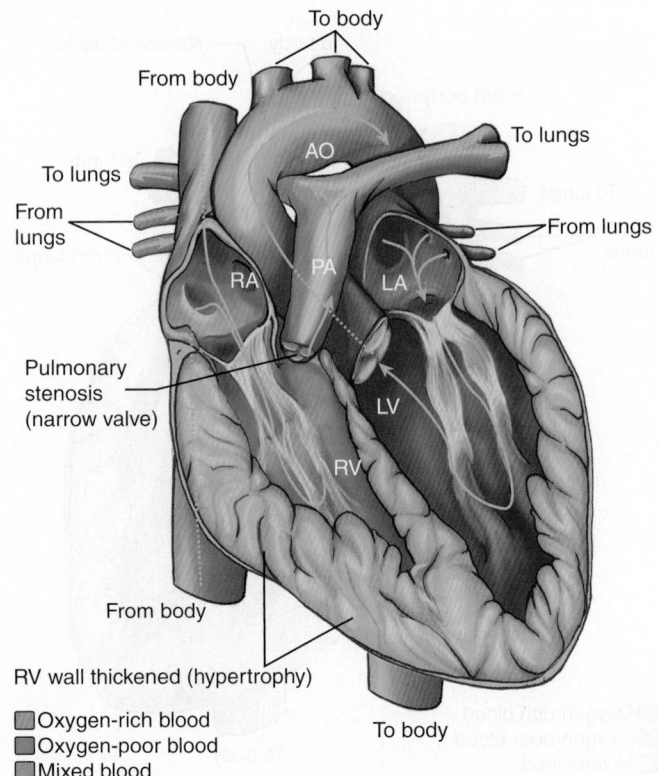

FIGURE 40.10 Pulmonary stenosis.

common problem causing pulmonary stenosis is that the pulmonary valve leaflets are thickened and fused together along their separation lines, causing obstruction to blood flow. The right ventricle has an additional workload, causing the muscle to thicken, resulting in right ventricular hypertrophy and decreased pulmonary blood flow. When the pulmonary valve is severely obstructed, the right ventricle cannot eject sufficient blood into the pulmonary artery. As a result, pressure in the right atrium increases, which can lead to a reopening of the foramen ovale. If this occurs, deoxygenated blood passes through the foramen ovale into the left side of the heart and is pumped to the systemic circulation. In some cases, PDA may be present, thus allowing for some compensation by shunting blood from the aorta to the pulmonary circulation for oxygenation (Fulton, 2008; Rao & Pflieger, 2010).

Nursing Assessment

The child with pulmonary stenosis may be asymptomatic or may exhibit signs and symptoms of mild heart failure. If the stenosis is severe, the child may demonstrate cyanosis. Therefore, it is important for the nurse to obtain an accurate health history and physical examination.

Health History and Physical Examination

Elicit the health history, noting mild dyspnea or cyanosis with exertion. Document the child's growth history, which is typically normal. Carefully palpate the sternal border for a thrill (not always present). Auscultate the heart, noting a high-pitched click following the second heart sound and a systolic ejection murmur loudest at the upper left sternal border.

Laboratory and Diagnostic Tests

An echocardiogram reveals the extent of obstruction present at the valve, as well as right ventricular hypertrophy. An EKG also helps to detect right ventricular hypertrophy.

Mixed Defects

Mixed defects are congenital heart defects that involve a mixing of well-oxygenated blood with poorly oxygenated blood. As a result, systemic blood flow contains lower oxygen content. Cardiac output is decreased, and heart failure occurs. Examples of mixed defects include TGA, TAPVR, truncus arteriosus, and HLHS.

Transposition of the Great Arteries (Vessels)

TGA is a congenital heart defect in which the pulmonary artery and the aorta arise from the opposite ventricle. Thus, the vessels are transposed from their normal positions. The aorta arises from the right ventricle instead of the left ventricle and the pulmonary artery arises from the left ventricle instead of the right ventricle. TGA accounts for approximately 5% to 7% of all CHD cases and is more common in boys (Park, 2008). It is

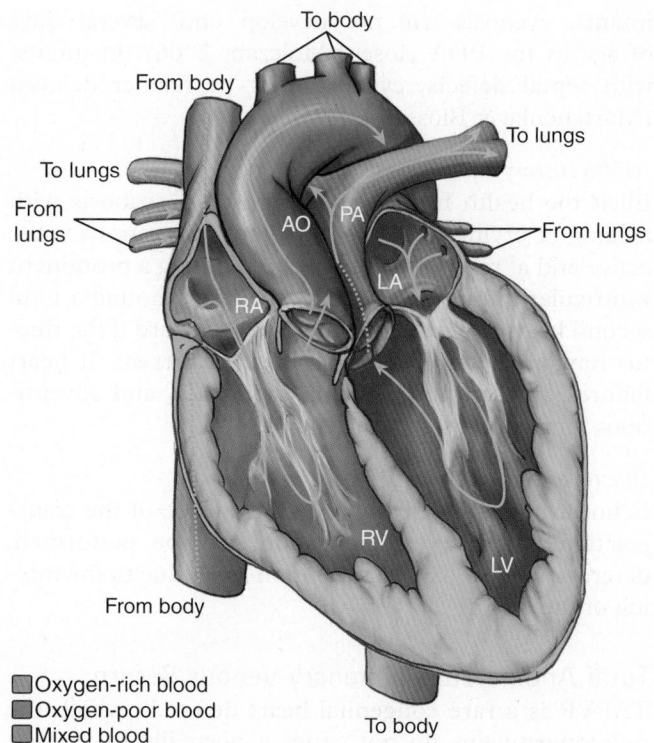

FIGURE 40.11 Transposition of the great arteries.

most often diagnosed in the first few days of life when the child manifests cyanosis, which indicates decreased oxygenation. As the ductus arteriosus closes, the symptoms will worsen. Heart failure may also be present in the first weeks to months of life. If untreated, 50% of affected infants will die in the first month of life and 90% in the first year (Martchenke & Blosser, 2009).

Pathophysiology

TGA creates a situation in which poorly oxygenated blood returning to the right atrium and ventricle is then pumped out to the aorta and back to the body. Oxygenated blood returning from the lungs to the left atrium and ventricle is then sent back to the lungs through the pulmonary artery (Fig. 40.11). Unless there is a connection somewhere in the circulation where the oxygen-rich and oxygen-poor blood can mix, all the organs of the body will be poorly oxygenated. Often the ductus arteriosus remains patent, allowing for some mixing of blood. Similarly, if a VSD is also present, mixing of blood may occur and cyanosis will be delayed. However, these associated defects can lead to increased pulmonary blood flow that increases pressure in the pulmonary circulation. This predisposes the child to heart failure (Fulton, 2008; Miyamoto et al., 2011).

Nursing Assessment

Significant cyanosis without a murmur in the newborn period is highly indicative of TGA. In about 10% of infants, cyanosis will not develop until several days of age as the PDA closes (Molczan, 2006). In infants with septal defects, cyanosis may be further delayed (Martchenke & Blosser, 2009).

Health History and Physical Examination

Elicit the health history, noting onset of cyanosis with feeding or crying. Observe the infant for cyanosis while active and at rest. Observe the chest, noting a prominent ventricular impulse. Auscultate the heart, noting a loud second heart sound. A murmur may be heard if the ductus remains open or a septal defect is present. If heart failure is present, note edema, tachypnea, and adventitious lung sounds.

Laboratory and Diagnostic Tests

Echocardiography clearly reveals evidence of the transposition. Cardiac catheterization may be performed, determining low oxygen saturation levels due to the mixing of the blood.

Total Anomalous Pulmonary Venous Return

TAPVR is a rare congenital heart defect in which the pulmonary veins do not connect normally to the left atrium; instead, they connect to the right atrium, often by way of the superior vena cava. TAPVR accounts for 1% of all congenital heart defects, and males exhibit this disorder three times more often than females (Park, 2008).

Pathophysiology

Oxygenated blood that would normally enter the left atrium now enters the right atrium and passes to the right ventricle. As a result, the pressure on the right side of the heart increases, leading to hypertrophy. TAPVR is incompatible with life unless there is an associated defect present that allows for shunting of blood from the highly pressured right side of the heart. A patent foramen ovale or an ASD is usually present. Since none of the pulmonary veins connect normally to the left atrium, the only source of blood to the left atrium is blood that is shunted from the right atrium across the defect to the left side of the heart (Fig. 40.12). The highly oxygenated blood from the lungs completely mixes with the poorly oxygenated blood returning from the systemic circulation. This causes an overload of the right atrium and right ventricle. The increased blood volume going into the lungs can lead to pulmonary hypertension and pulmonary edema (Fulton, 2008; Miyamoto et al., 2011).

Nursing Assessment

The degree of cyanosis present with TAPVR depends on the extent of the associated defects. For example, if the foramen ovale closes or the ASD is small, significant cyanosis will be present. The physical examination findings will vary depending on the type of TAPVR the infant

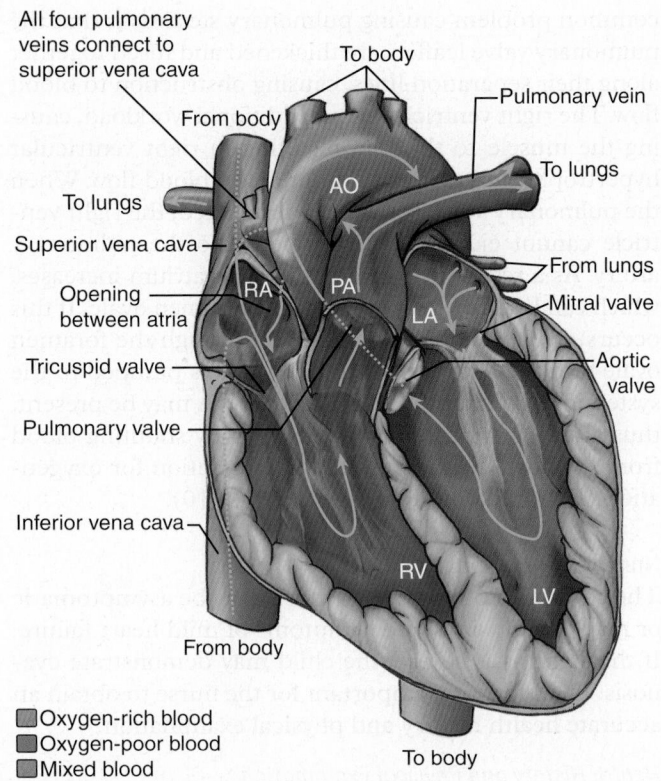

Oxygen-rich blood
Oxygen-poor blood
Mixed blood

FIGURE 40.12 Total anomalous pulmonary venous return.

has, whether obstruction is present and which other associated cardiac anomalies are present.

Health History and Physical Examination

Note history of cyanosis, tiring easily and difficulty feeding. Observe the chest for prominence of the right ventricular impulse and retractions with tachypnea. Auscultate the heart, noting fixed splitting of the second heart sound and a murmur. Palpate the abdomen for hepatomegaly.

Laboratory and Diagnostic Tests

An echocardiogram will reveal the abnormal connection of the pulmonary veins, enlargement of the right atrium and right ventricle, and an ASD if present. The chest X-ray will demonstrate an enlarged heart and pulmonary edema. Cardiac catheterization and MRI can also be useful to visualize the abnormal connection of the pulmonary veins, particularly if an obstruction is present.

Truncus Arteriosus

Truncus arteriosus is a congenital heart defect in which only one major artery leaves the heart and supplies blood to the pulmonary and systemic circulations. It affects males and females equally and accounts for 1% to 2% of all CHD cases (Hoffman, 2009; Miyamoto et al., 2011). About 10% to 20% of babies born with truncus arteriosus have other associated congenital heart malformations, and there is a strong association with DiGeorge syndrome and 22q11 deletion (Hoffman, 2009).

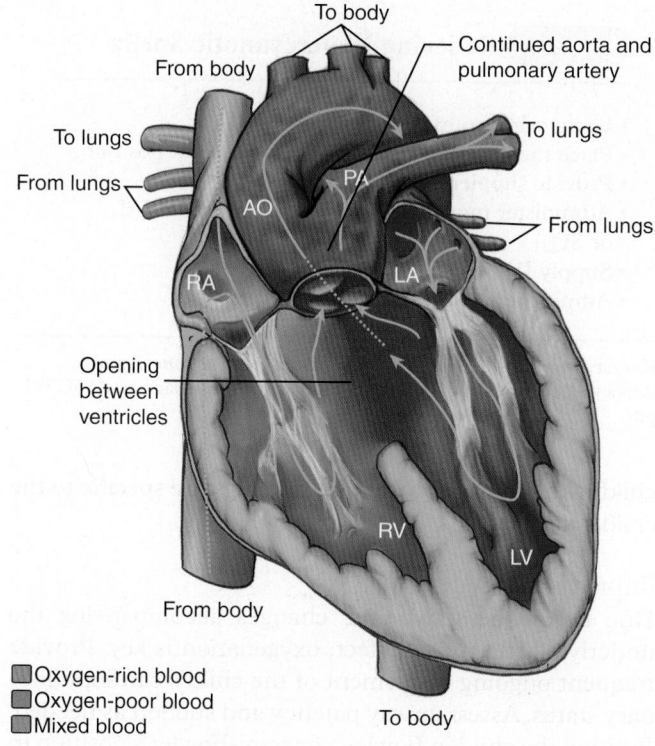

FIGURE 40.13 Truncus arteriosus.

Oxygen-rich blood
Oxygen-poor blood
Mixed blood

Pathophysiology

The one great vessel contains a single valve that comprises two to five leaflets and is positioned over both the left and right ventricles above a large VSD (Fig. 40.13). The common trunk gives rise to both the aorta and the pulmonary artery. There is complete mixing of pulmonary and systemic blood. Pressure in the pulmonary circulation typically is less than that in the systemic circulation, leading to increased blood flow to the lungs. As a result, systemic blood flow is decreased. Over time, the increased pulmonary blood flow can lead to pulmonary vascular disease (Fulton, 2008; Miyamoto et al., 2011).

Nursing Assessment

Typically, the infant demonstrates cyanosis in varying degrees depending on the extent of pulmonary over-circulation and the degree of compromise in the systemic circulation. Obtain an accurate health history and perform a physical examination.

Health History and Physical Examination

Elicit the health history, noting history of cyanosis that increases with periods of activity such as feeding. Also note history of tiring easily, difficulty in feeding, and poor growth. Count the respiratory rate, which may be elevated. Observe for nasal flaring, grunting or noisy breathing, retractions, and restlessness. Auscultate the lungs, noting adventitious breath sounds, and the heart, noting a murmur associated with a VSD.

Laboratory and Diagnostic Tests

An echocardiogram will confirm the presence of truncus arteriosus as the anatomy of the great arteries, the single truncal valve, and the VSD will be seen. On rare occasions a cardiac catheterization may be done to determine pressures in the pulmonary arteries.

Hypoplastic Left Heart Syndrome

HLHS is a congenital heart defect in which all of the structures on the left side of the heart are severely underdeveloped (Fig. 40.14). The mitral and aortic valves are small or atretic. The left ventricle is non-functional. Thus, the left side of the heart is completely unable to supply blood to the systemic circulation. HLHS is the fourth most common congenital heart defect, accounting for 1% of all CHD cases and 9% of critically ill newborns (Park, 2008). It appears to have a multifactorial and autosomal recessive inheritance pattern. Almost 30% of infants with HLHS also have a definable genetic or other congenital anomaly in addition to the heart defect (Hoffman, 2009). The options for treatment include reconstructive surgery, which consists of three stages beginning within days to weeks of birth, compassionate care, and cardiac transplantation (Hoffman, 2009). Some argue that compassionate care should no longer be offered for infants born with HLHS, whereas others advocate for continuing to offer this option to parents of infants diagnosed with HLHS (Friedman Ross & Frader, 2009).

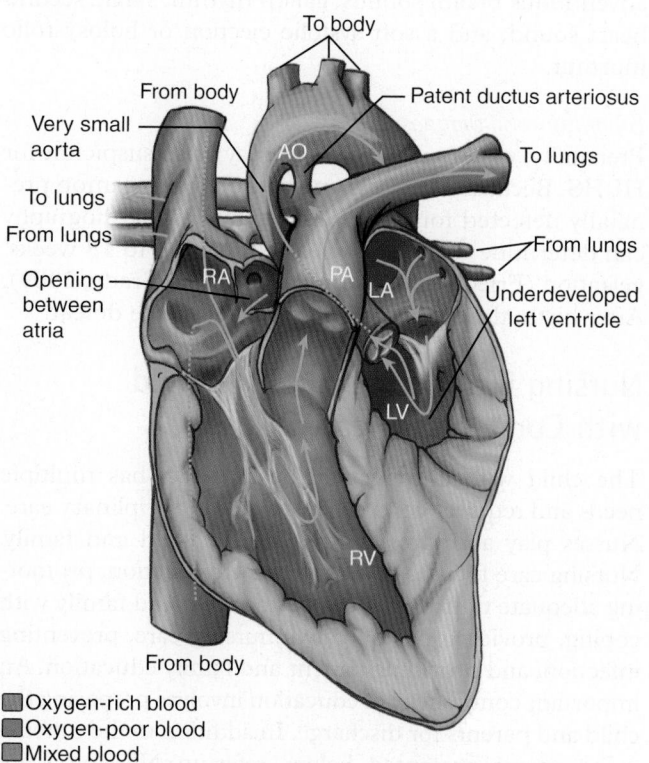

Oxygen-rich blood
Oxygen-poor blood
Mixed blood

FIGURE 40.14 Hypoplastic left heart syndrome.

Pathophysiology

With HLHS, the right side of the heart is the main working part of the heart. Blood returning from the lungs into the left atrium must pass through an ASD to the right side of the heart. The right ventricle must then pump blood to the lungs and also to the systemic circulation through the PDA. When the ductus arteriosus closes, the heart cannot pump blood into the systemic circulation, causing poor perfusion of the vital organs and shock. Death will occur rapidly without intervention (Fulton, 2008; Miyamoto et al., 2011).

Nursing Assessment

Those neonates who do not get diagnosed prenatally will usually present in the first days to weeks of life. Initially after birth, the newborn may be asymptomatic because the ductus arteriosus is still patent. However, as the ductus begins to close at a few days of age, the newborn will begin to exhibit cyanosis. Some infants may present with circulatory collapse (shock) and must be resuscitated emergently (Cantor & Sadowitz, 2010).

Health History and Physical Examination

Obtain the health history, noting onset of cyanosis. Note poor feeding and history of tiring easily. Evaluate the vital signs, noting tachycardia, tachypnea, and hypothermia. Observe for increased work of breathing and gradually increasing cyanosis. Note pallor of the extremities and decreased oxygen saturation via pulse oximetry and poor peripheral pulses. Auscultate the heart and lungs. Note adventitious breath sounds, gallop rhythm, single second heart sound, and a soft systolic ejection or holosystolic murmur.

Laboratory and Diagnostic Tests

Prenatally, maternal ultrasound may raise suspicion for HLHS. Because HLHS is one of the most common prenatally detected forms of CHD, fetal echocardiography can determine this diagnosis as early as 16 to 18 weeks' gestation (Friedberg, Silverman, & Moon-Grady, 2009). After birth, the echocardiogram confirms the defect.

Nursing Management of the Child with Congenital Heart Disease

The child with a congenital heart defect has multiple needs and requires comprehensive, multidisciplinary care. Nurses play a key role in helping the child and family. Nursing care focuses on improving oxygenation, promoting adequate nutrition, assisting the child and family with coping, providing postoperative nursing care, preventing infection, and providing patient and family education. An important component of education involves preparing the child and parents for discharge. In addition to the nursing management presented below, refer to Nursing Care Plan 40.1 for additional interventions appropriate for the

---

> **BOX 40.1 Relieving Hypercyanotic Spells**
>
> - Use a calm, comforting approach.
> - Place the infant or child in a knee-to-chest position.
> - Provide supplemental oxygen.
> - Administer morphine sulfate (0.1 mg/kg IV, IM, or SQ).
> - Supply IV fluids.
> - Administer propranolol (0.1 mg/kg IV).

Kargar, M. (2009). *Hypercyanotic spells tet spells and nursing care.* Retrieved October 20, 2011 from http://www.icrj.ir/iacc/arts%5C391.pdf.

child with CHD. Individualize nursing care specific to the child's needs.

Improving Oxygenation

Due to the hemodynamic changes accompanying the underlying structural defect, oxygenation is key. Provide frequent ongoing assessment of the child's cardiopulmonary status. Assess airway patency and suction as needed. Position the child in Fowler's or semi-Fowler's position to facilitate lung expansion. Monitor vital signs, including heart rate and respiratory rate and effort. Monitor the child's colour and oxygen saturation levels closely, using these to guide oxygen administration. Observe for tachypnea and other signs of respiratory distress, such as nasal flaring, grunting, and retractions. Auscultate the lungs for adventitious sounds. Provide humidified supplemental oxygen as ordered. Anticipate the need for assisted ventilation if the child has difficulty maintaining the airway or experiences deterioration in oxygenation capacity. Box 40.1 lists interventions related to relief of hypercyanotic spells.

Promoting Adequate Nutrition

Adequate nutrition is critical to foster growth and development as well as to reduce the risk of infection. Children with congenital heart defects typically have increased nutritional needs due to the increased energy expenditure associated with increased cardiac and respiratory workloads. In addition, many of the defects lead to heart failure, which may affect the child's fluid balance status.

Infants with cardiac disease have higher energy or calorie requirements related to their high metabolic rates (Meeks, Hallsworth, & Yeo, 2010). Nutrition may be provided orally, enterally, or parenterally. For example, for the newborn or infant, nutrition via breast milk or formula may be provided orally or by gavage feedings. Breastfeeding is usually associated with decreased energy expenditure during the act of feeding, yet some infants in intensive care are not stable enough to breastfeed. Gavage with breast milk is possible, and the use of human milk fortifier (either with breastfeeding or added to the gavage feed) adds additional calories that the infant requires. Formula-fed infants may also require increased-calorie formula, which may be achieved by more concentrated mixing of the formula or through the use of additives such as Polycose or vegetable oil. Consult the nutritionist to determine the individual infant's caloric needs and prescription of appropriate feeding.

Cutting a large hole in the nipple or "cross-cutting" the nipple decreases the work of feeding for some infants. Generally, nipple feedings should be limited to 20 minutes, as feeding for longer periods results in excess caloric expenditure. Many infants may feed orally for 20 minutes, receiving the remainder of that feeding via orogastric or nasogastric tube. Offer older children small, frequent feedings to reduce the amount of energy required to feed or eat and to prevent overtiring the child. When needed, administer and monitor total parenteral nutrition as prescribed.

> ▶ *Take* NOTE!

Breastfeeding a child before and after cardiac surgery may boost the infant's immune system, which can help fight postoperative infection. If breastfeeding is not possible, mothers can pump milk and the breast milk may be given via bottle, dropper, or gavage feeding.

Assisting the Child and Family to Cope

The diagnosis of CHD is especially overwhelming for the child and the parents. The numerous examinations, diagnostic tests, and procedures are sources of stress for the infant or child regardless of age and for the parents. Studies of children with chronic illness have shown that high levels of stress increase the risk of developing adjustment problems such as anxiety and depression (Brown, Daly, & Rickel, 2007). Parents may fear long-term disability or death or may worry that allowing the child to engage in any activity will worsen his or her status. Thus, the parents may tend to overprotect the child. It is important for the parents to continue parenting the child, even when the child requires extended hospitalizations or intensive care (Fernandes, 2005). Additionally, lower levels of parental stress have been correlated with lower levels of anxiety in children with CHD (Roberts & MacMath, 2006). Explain all that is happening with the child, using language the parents and child can understand. Allow the parents and child to voice their feelings, concerns, or questions. Provide ample time to address these questions and concerns. Encourage the parents and child, as developmentally appropriate, to participate in the child's care.

If the child is a newborn or infant, encourage attachment and bonding. Emphasize the child's positive attributes, including the normal aspects of the infant. Increased parental focus on the child's CHD can increase anxiety and maladjustment in the child (Roberts & MacMath, 2006). Assist the family in becoming more child-focused than illness-focused by encouraging discussion about the child's interests, activities, and friendships rather than the illness and its treatment. Help the parents to experience the joy of a new infant, seeing the beauty of the child, no matter how ill the infant is (Fernandes, 2005). Urge the parents to touch, stroke, pat, and talk to the infant. Encourage them to hold the infant close, using kangaroo care as appropriate. Evidence suggests that early physical contact can aid in promoting maternal attachment, reducing abandonment, and increasing breastfeeding success (Meeks et al., 2010). Benefits of early physical contact have also been related to fathers (Meeks et al., 2010). If the child is older, offer suggestions as to how the parents can meet the child's emotional needs. For example, encourage parents to bring a favourite toy or object from home while hospitalized.

Provide developmentally appropriate explanations to the child. Encourage play therapy to help the child understand what is happening.

Preventing Infection

Teach parents proper hand hygiene. Provide appropriate dental care. Make sure the child receives prophylaxis for bacterial endocarditis as needed (American Heart Association [AHA], 2008). Ensure that children 24 months or younger who have hemodynamically significant heart defects receive respiratory syncytial virus prophylaxis as recommended during respiratory syncytial virus season (Sorce, 2009).

Providing Care for the Child Undergoing Cardiac Surgery

Cardiac surgery may be necessary to correct a congenital defect or to provide symptomatic relief. The surgery may be planned as an elective procedure or done as an emergency. Open-heart surgery involves an incision of the heart muscle to repair the internal structures. This may require cardiopulmonary bypass. Closed-heart surgery involves structures related to the heart but not the heart muscle itself and may be performed with or without cardiopulmonary bypass (Gazit, Huddleston, Checchia, Fehr, & Pezzella, 2010a,b).

Providing Preoperative Care

The preoperative nursing assessment complements the history and physical examination and provides important baseline information for comparison during the postoperative period. Establish a relationship with the child and parents. Identify problems that may require particular nursing interventions during the postoperative period. Before cardiac surgery, interview the parents and, if age-appropriate, the child. Focus the interview on the history of the present illness; cardiac risk factors; the child's present physical, functional, and developmental status; additional medical problems; current medications and drug allergies; the child's and family's understanding of the illness and planned procedure; and the family support system.

The preoperative physical assessment includes the following:

- Temperature and weight measurements
- Examination of extremities for peripheral edema, clubbing, and evaluation of peripheral pulses
- Auscultation of the heart (rate, rhythm, heart sounds, murmurs, clicks, and rubs)
- Respiratory assessment, including respiratory rate, work of breathing, and auscultation of the lungs for breath sounds

Obtain necessary laboratory and diagnostic tests to establish a baseline. In addition, review the results of any tests done previously. Testing may include CBC, electrolyte levels, clotting studies, urinalysis, cultures of blood and other body secretions, renal and hepatic function tests, chest X-ray, EKG, echocardiogram, and diagnostic imaging. In most non-emergent cases, preoperative assessment is performed in an out-patient setting and the patient is admitted to the hospital on the day of surgery. Nursing care during this phase focuses on thorough patient and parent education. If the surgery is an emergency, patient teaching must be done quickly, emphasizing the most important elements of the child's care (Beke, Braudis, & Lincoln, 2005).

Child and parent education typically includes the following topics:

- Heart anatomy and its function, including what area is involved with the defect that is to be corrected
- Events before surgery, including any testing or preparation such as a skin scrub
- Day of surgery events, including accompanying the child to the operating room, planning for waiting during the operation, setting up an online care page for communication with family and friends
- Location of the child after surgery, such as a pediatric intensive care unit, which may include a visit to the unit if appropriate and explanation of the sights and sounds that may be present
- Appearance of the child after surgery (equipment or devices used for monitoring, such as oxygen administration, EKG leads, pulse oximeter, chest tubes, pacer wires, mechanical ventilation, or intravenous lines)
- Approximate location of the incision and coverage with dressings
- Postoperative activity level, including measures to reduce the risk of complications, such as coughing and deep-breathing exercises, incentive spirometry, early ambulation, and leg exercises

- Nutritional restrictions, such as nothing by mouth for a specified time before surgery and use of intravenous fluids
- Medications such as anesthesia, sedation, and analgesics as well as medications the child is taking now that need to be continued or withheld (Beke et al., 2005)

Prepare and educate the child at an age- and developmentally appropriate level. Advise parents to read books with their child about CHD and hospitalization such as

- *Clifford Visits the Hospital,* by N. Bridwell, 2000 (Scholastic Inc.)
- *Franklin Goes to the Hospital,* by P. Bourgeois, 2000 (Scholastic Paperbacks)
- *Pump the Bear,* by G. O. Whittingon, 2000 (Brown Books)
- *Blue Lewis and Sasha the Great,* by C. D. Newell, 2005 (Cally Press)
- *Cardiac Kids: A Book for Families Who Have a Child with Heart Disease,* by V. Elder, 1994 (Dayton Area Heart and Cancer Association)
- *When Molly Was in the Hospital: A Book for Brothers and Sisters of Hospitalized Children,* by D. Duncan, 1994 (Rayve Productions) (siblings)
- *A Night Without Stars,* by J. Howe, 1993 (Camelot) (older children)

Additionally, parents may download *Heart and Soul, Your Guide to Living with Congenital Heart Disease,* a parent resource book, free of charge from the Heart and Stroke Foundation of Canada. (Visit http://thePoint.lww.com/Chow1e for a direct link to their website.)

Parents may also help their child by buying a small thrift-store suitcase, spray-painting it, and allowing the child to decorate it with his or her name, pictures of family, stickers, or favourite story characters. This will be the child's "hospital suitcase" that the child may pack with toys and handheld video devices to bring to the hospital. Hospital tours are appropriate for school-age children, and older children and teens may benefit from an intensive care unit tour before surgery.

Instruct parents to stop food and liquids at the designated time, depending on the child's age, and to give all medications as directed. Some medications may be withheld before surgery. If the child's nutritional status is poor or questionable, nutritional supplementation may be ordered for a period of time preoperatively to ensure that the child has the best possible nutritional status before surgery. When it is time for the child to be transported to the surgical area, ensure that the parents accompany the child as far as possible, depending on the institution's policy. Also reinforce with the child that the parents will be present at the bedside when he or she awakens from surgery (Beke et al., 2005).

Providing Postoperative Care

The child will usually be transported from the operating room to the intensive care unit. Depending on the age, postoperative stability, and type of surgery, the child may stay in the intensive care unit for several hours up to several days. Vigilant nursing care is the key to the child's recovery after surgery and reduces the risk of complications. Nurses also play a vital role in supporting the parents.

Postoperative nursing interventions include the following:

- Assess vital signs frequently, as often as every 1 hour, until stable.
- Assess the colour of the skin and mucous membranes, check capillary refill, and palpate peripheral pulses.
- Observe cardiac rate and rhythm via electronic monitoring and auscultate heart rate, rhythm, and sounds frequently.
- Monitor hemodynamic status via arterial and/or central venous lines (left and right atrial, and pulmonary artery pressures, pulmonary artery oxygen saturation).
- Provide site care and tubing changes according to the institution's policy.
- Auscultate lungs for adventitious, diminished, or absent breath sounds.
- Assess oxygen saturation levels via pulse oximetry and arterial blood gases as well as work of breathing and level of consciousness frequently.
- Administer supplemental oxygen as needed.
- Monitor mechanical ventilation and suction as ordered.
- Inspect chest tube functioning, noting amount, colour, and character of drainage.
- Inspect the dressing (incision and chest tube) for drainage and intactness. Reinforce or change the dressing as ordered.
- Assess the incision for redness, irritation, drainage, or separation.
- Monitor intake and output hourly.
- Maintain an accurate intravenous infusion rate; restrict fluids as ordered to prevent hypervolemia.
- Assess for changes in level of consciousness. Report restlessness, irritability, or seizures.
- Obtain ordered laboratory tests, such as CBC, coagulation studies, cardiac enzyme levels, and electrolyte levels. Report abnormal results.
- Administer medications, such as digoxin or inotropic or vasopressor agents, as ordered, watching the child closely for possible adverse effects.
- Encourage the child to turn, cough, deep breathe, use the incentive spirometer, and splint the incisional area with pillows.
- Assess the child's pain level and administer analgesics as ordered. Allow time for the child to rest and sleep.

BOX 40.2   Possible Complications After Cardiac Surgery

- Atelectasis
- Bacterial (infective) endocarditis
- Cardiac arrhythmias
- Cardiac tamponade
- CVA
- Heart failure
- Hemorrhage
- Pleural effusion
- Pneumonia
- Pneumothorax
- Postperfusion syndrome
- Postcardiac surgery syndrome
- Pulmonary edema
- Seizures
- Wound infection

Bronicki, R. A., & Chang, A. C. (2011). Management of the postoperative pediatric cardiac surgical patient. In Sevransky, J. E. (Ed.), *MHS Critical Care Medicine, 39*(8), 1974–1984.

- Assist the child to get out of bed as soon as possible and as ordered.
- Assess daily weights.
- Administer small, frequent feedings or meals when oral intake is allowed.
- Position the child in a comfortable position, one that maximizes chest expansion. Change position frequently.
- Assess the child for complications (Box 40.2).
- Provide emotional and physical support to the child and family, making appropriate referrals such as to social services for assistance.
- Prepare the patient and family for discharge (Cook & Langton, 2009; Meeks et al., 2010).

▶ *Take NOTE!*

Abrupt cessation of chest tube output accompanied by an increase in heart rate and increased filling pressure (right atrial) may indicate cardiac tamponade (Ascenzi & Kane, 2007).

Providing Patient and Family Education

Provide patient and family education throughout the child's stay. Initially, teaching focuses on the underlying defect and measures to treat or control the problem. If the child requires surgery, teaching shifts to preoperative and postoperative events. Emphasize discharge teaching for each admission. Teaching Guideline 40.2 highlights

TEACHING GUIDELINE 40.2

Caring for the Child with a Congenital Heart Disease

- Give medications, if ordered, exactly as prescribed.
- Weigh the child at least once a week or as ordered, at approximately the same time of the day with the same scale and with the child wearing the same amount of clothing.
- Allow the child to engage in activity as directed. Provide time for the child to rest frequently throughout the day to prevent overexertion.
- Provide a nutritious diet, taking into account any restrictions for fluids or foods.
- Use measures to prevent infection, such as frequent handwashing, prophylactic antibiotics, and skin care.
- Adhere to schedule for follow-up diagnostic tests and procedures.
- Support the child's growth and development needs.
- Use available community support services.
- Notify the primary care provider if the child has increasing episodes of respiratory distress, cyanosis, or difficulty breathing; fever; increased edema of the hands, feet, or face; decreased urinary output; weight loss or difficulty eating or drinking; increased fatigue or irritability; decreased level of alertness; or vomiting or diarrhea.

Axton, S. E., & Fugate, T. (2009). *Pediatric nursing care plans for the hospitalized child* (3rd ed.). Upper Saddle River, NJ: Pearson; and Cook, E. H., & Higgins, S. S. (2010). Congenital heart disease. In P. J. Allen, J. A. Vessey, & N. A. Schapiro (Eds.), *Primary care of the child with a chronic condition* (5th ed.). St. Louis, MO: Mosby.

the major areas to be addressed in patient and family education.

Acquired Cardiovascular Disorders

Acquired cardiovascular disorders occur in children as a result of an underlying cardiovascular problem or may refer to other cardiac disorders that are not congenital. The most common type of acquired cardiovascular disorder in children is heart failure. Other acquired disorders include rheumatic fever, cardiomyopathy, bacterial endocarditis, hyperlipidemia, hypertension, and Kawasaki disease.

Heart Failure

Heart failure occurs most often in children with CHD and is the most common reason for admission to the hospital for children with CHD. Eighty percent of all cases of heart failure in children with CHD occur by the age of 1 year (Martchenke & Blosser, 2009). Heart failure also occurs secondary to other conditions such as myocardial dysfunction following surgical intervention for CHD, cardiomyopathy, myocarditis, fluid volume overload, hypertension, anemia, or sepsis or as a toxic effect of certain chemotherapeutic agents used in the treatment of cancer. Heart failure refers to a set of clinical signs and symptoms that reflect the heart's inability to pump effectively to provide adequate blood, oxygen, and nutrients to the body organs and tissues (Barker, Williams, & Tulloh, 2009; Miyamoto et al., 2011).

The child experiencing heart failure requires a multidisciplinary approach to care. Collaboration is necessary to achieve improved cardiac function, restored fluid balance, decreased cardiac workload, and improved oxygen delivery to the tissues.

Pathophysiology

Cardiac output is controlled by preload (diastolic volume), afterload (ventricular wall tension), myocardial contractility (inotropic state), and heart rate. Protracted alterations in any of these factors may lead to heart failure. In the event of reduced cardiac output, multiple compensatory mechanisms are activated. When the ventricular contraction is impaired (systolic dysfunction), reduced ejection of blood occurs, and therefore cardiac output is reduced. Diminished ability to receive venous return (diastolic dysfunction) occurs when high venous pressures are required to support ventricular function. As a result of decreased cardiac output, the renin-angiotensin-aldosterone system is activated as a compensatory mechanism. Fluid and sodium retention as well as increased contractility and vasoconstriction then occur. Initially BP is supported and organ perfusion is maintained, but increased afterload worsens systolic dysfunction. As the heart chambers dilate, myocardial oxygen consumption increases and cardiac output is limited by excessive wall stretch. Over time, the capacity of the heart to respond to these compensatory mechanisms fails, and cardiac output is further decreased (Barker et al., 2009; Miyamoto et al., 2011). Figure 40.15 shows the clinical manifestations that occur related to the mechanisms of heart failure.

Therapeutic Management

Management of heart failure is supportive. While augmenting nutrition and ensuring adequate rest are key, promotion of oxygenation and ventilation is of utmost importance. Many children with heart failure require intensive care until they are stabilized. Digitalis, diuretics, inotropic agents, vasodilators, antiarrhythmics, and antithrombotics have been widely used in children for symptom management (Barker et al., 2009; Martchenke & Blosser, 2009; Park, 2008). Recent technological advancements in ventricular assist devices allow their use in children, either in the short term as a bridge to

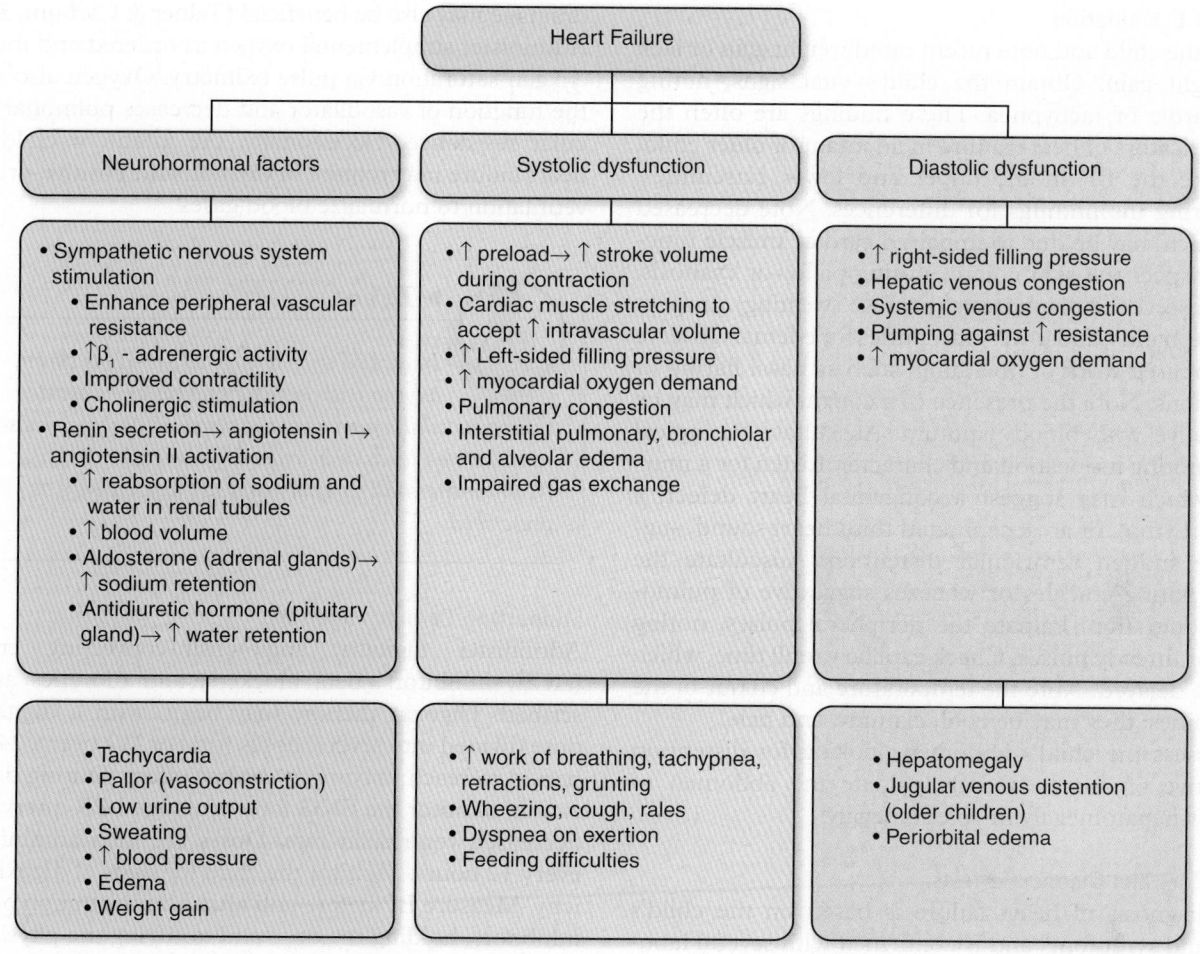

FIGURE 40.15 Pathophysiology of heart failure. (Adapted from Francis, G. S., Sonnenblick, E. H., Wilson Tang, W. H., & Poole-Wilson, P. (2008). Pathophysiology of heart failure. In Fuster, V., O'Rourke, R. A., Walsh, R., et al. (Eds.), *Hurst's the heart* (12th ed.). New York: McGraw-Hill.)

recovery to heart transplant or as palliative therapy (Pauliks & Ündar, 2008).

Nursing Assessment

For a full description of the assessment phase of the nursing process, refer to page 1320. Specific assessment findings related to heart failure are discussed below.

Health History

When obtaining the health history, elicit a description of the present illness and chief complaint. Common complaints reported during the health history might include

- Failure to gain weight or rapid weight gain
- Failure to thrive
- Difficulty feeding
- Fatigue
- Dizziness, irritability
- Exercise intolerance
- Shortness of breath
- Sucking and then tiring quickly

- Syncope
- Decreased number of wet diapers

Infants with heart failure often display subtle signs such as difficulty feeding and tiring easily. Pay close attention for reports of these problems from the parents. Also be alert for statements such as "the baby drinks a small amount of breast milk (or formula) and stops, but then wants to eat again very soon afterwards"; "the baby seems to perspire a lot during feedings"; or "the baby seems to be more comfortable when he's sitting up or on my shoulder than when he's lying flat." In addition, the parents may report episodes of rapid breathing and grunting.

The child's current and past medical history also provides additional clues. Question the parents about any history of congenital heart defects and treatments such as surgery to repair the defect. Determine the current medication regimen. Also ask about any recent or past infections, such as streptococcal infections or fever.

Physical Examination

Weigh the child and note recent rapid weight gain or lack of weight gain. Obtain the child's vital signs, noting tachycardia or tachypnea. These findings are often the first indicators of heart failure in an infant or older child. Measure the BP in the upper and lower extremities, comparing the findings for differences. Note decreased BP, which may be due to impaired cardiac muscle function. Inspect the skin colour, noting pallor or cyanosis. Also observe for diaphoresis (profuse sweating). Inspect the face, hands, and lower extremities for edema. Observe for increased work of breathing, such as nasal flaring or retractions. Note the presence of a cough, which may be productive with bloody sputum. Auscultate the apical pulse, noting its location and character. Listen for a murmur, which may suggest a congenital heart defect, a gallop rhythm, or an accentuated third heart sound, suggesting sudden ventricular distention. Auscultate the lungs, noting crackles or wheezes suggestive of pulmonary congestion. Palpate the peripheral pulses, noting weak or thready pulses. Check capillary refill time, which may be delayed. Note the temperature and colour of the extremities; they may be cool, clammy, and pale.

Assess the child's abdomen, looking for distention indicative of ascites. Gently palpate the abdomen to identify hepatomegaly or splenomegaly.

Laboratory and Diagnostic Tests

The diagnosis of heart failure is based on the child's signs and symptoms and is confirmed with several laboratory and diagnostic tests. These include

- Chest X-ray, revealing an enlarged heart and/or pulmonary edema
- EKG, indicating ventricular hypertrophy
- Echocardiogram, revealing the underlying cause of heart failure, such as a congenital heart defect

Other tests may be done to support the diagnosis. For example, the CBC may show evidence of anemia or infection. Electrolyte levels may reveal hyponatremia secondary to fluid retention and hyperkalemia secondary to tissue destruction or impaired renal function. Arterial blood gas results may demonstrate respiratory alkalosis in mild heart failure or metabolic acidosis. Tissue hypoxia may be evidenced by increased lactic acid and decreased bicarbonate levels.

Nursing Management

Nursing management of the child with heart failure focuses on promoting oxygenation, supporting cardiac function, providing adequate nutrition, and promoting rest.

Promoting Oxygenation

Position the infant or child in a semi-upright position to decrease work of breathing and lessen pulmonary congestion. Suction as needed. Chest physiotherapy and postural drainage may also be beneficial (Talner & Carboni, 2003). Administer supplemental oxygen as ordered and monitor oxygen saturation via pulse oximetry. Oxygen also serves the function of vasodilator and decreases pulmonary vascular resistance. Occasionally, the infant or child with heart failure may require intubation and positive-pressure ventilation to normalize blood gases.

> ▶ **Take** NOTE!
>
> *In a child with a large left-to-right shunt, oxygen will decrease pulmonary vascular resistance while increasing the systemic vascular resistance, which leads to increased left-to-right shunting. Monitor the child carefully and use oxygen only as prescribed.*

Supporting Cardiac Function

Administer digitalis, angiotensin-converting enzyme (ACE) inhibitors, beta blockers, and diuretics as prescribed. Digoxin therapy may begin with a digitalizing dose divided into several doses (oral or IV) over a 24-hour period to reach maximum cardiac effect. During digitalization, monitor the EKG for a prolonged PR interval and decreased ventricular rate. Doses are then administered every 12 hours. Monitor the child for signs of digoxin toxicity. Measure BP before and after administration of ACE inhibitors, holding the dose and notifying the physician if the BP falls more than 15 mm Hg. Observe for signs of hypotension such as lightheadedness, dizziness, or fainting. Weigh the child daily to determine fluid loss. Maintain accurate records of intake and output, restricting fluid intake if ordered. Carefully monitor potassium levels, administering potassium supplements if prescribed. Sodium intake is not usually restricted in the child with heart failure (Barker et al., 2009).

Providing Adequate Nutrition

Due to the increased metabolic rate associated with heart failure, the infant may require as much as 150 calories/kg/day. Older children will also require higher caloric intake than typical children. Offer small, frequent feedings if the child can tolerate them. During the acute phase of heart failure, many infants in particular will require continuous or intermittent gavage feeding to maintain or gain weight. Concentrate infant formula to 24 to 30 kcal/30 mL as instructed by the nutritionist (Medoff-Cooper & Irving, 2009; Talner & Carboni, 2003).

Promoting Rest

Minimize metabolic needs to decrease cardiac demand. The infant or older child with heart failure will usually limit activities based upon energy level. Ensure adequate time for sleep and attempt to limit disturbing interventions. Provide age-appropriate activities that can be performed quietly, such as books, drawing, and electronic or board games. The older child or adolescent with significant heart failure may require home schooling. As the child improves, a rehabilitation program may be helpful for maximizing activity within the child's cardiovascular status limits (Cook & Langton, 2009; Talner & Carboni, 2003).

Bacterial (Infective) Endocarditis

Bacterial (infective) endocarditis is a microbial infection of the endothelial surfaces of the heart's chambers, septum, or valves (most common). Children with congenital heart defects (septum or valve defects) or prosthetic valves are at increased risk of acquiring bacterial endocarditis, which is potentially fatal in these children. Other risk factors for endocarditis include central venous catheters and intravenous drug use. Endocarditis occurs when bacteria or fungi gain access to a damaged epithelium. Turbulence in blood flow associated with narrowed or incompetent valves or with a communication between the systemic and pulmonary circulation leads to damage of the endothelium. Thrombi and platelets then adhere to the endothelium, forming vegetations. When a microbe gains access to the bloodstream, it colonizes the vegetation, using the thrombi as a breeding ground. Clumps may separate from the vegetative patch and travel to other organs of the body, causing significant damage (septic emboli). Fungi or, more commonly, bacteria (particularly alpha-hemolytic streptococcus or *Staphylococcus aureus*) are frequently implicated in bacterial endocarditis (Brusch, Conrad, & Marill, 2011; Miyamoto et al., 2011).

Complete antibiotic or antifungal treatment of the causative organism is necessary, and treatment may last for 4 to 7 weeks. Prevention of bacterial endocarditis in the susceptible child with CHD or a valvular disorder is of utmost importance (Baltimore, 2008; Brusch et al., 2011; Miyamoto et al., 2011).

Nursing Assessment

For a full description of the assessment phase of the nursing process, refer to page 1320. Assessment findings related to endocarditis are discussed below.

Health History

Obtain the health history, noting intermittent, unexplained low-grade fever. Document history of fatigue, anorexia, weight loss, or flu-like symptoms (arthralgia, myalgia, chills, night sweats). Note history of CHD, valve disorder, or heart failure.

Physical Examination

Measure the child's temperature, noting low-grade fever. Observe for edema if heart failure is also present. Note petechiae on the palpebral conjunctiva, the oral mucosa, or the extremities. Inspect for signs of extracardiac emboli:

- Roth's spots: splinter hemorrhages with pale centres on sclerae, palate, buccal mucosa, chest, fingers, or toes
- Janeway lesions: painless flat red or blue hemorrhagic lesions on the palms or the soles
- Osler's nodes: small, tender nodules on the pads of the toes or fingers
- Black lines (splinter hemorrhages) under the nails (Brusch et al., 2011; Miyamoto et al., 2011)

Evaluate the EKG for a prolonged PR interval or dysrhythmias. Auscultate the heart for a new or changing murmur. Auscultate the lungs for adventitious breath sounds. Palpate the abdomen for splenomegaly (Martchenke & Blosser, 2009; Park, 2008).

Laboratory and Diagnostic Tests

Diagnosis is usually based on the clinical presentation. Laboratory tests and potential findings are as follows:

- Blood culture: positive for bacteria or fungus
- CBC: anemia, leukocytosis
- Urinalysis: microscopic hematuria
- Echocardiogram: cardiomegaly, abnormal valve function, area of vegetation

Nursing Management

Nursing management focuses on maintaining IV access for at least 4 weeks to appropriately administer the antibiotic or antifungal course of therapy. Monitor the child's temperature and subsequent blood culture results.

Ideally, endocarditis in children should be prevented. Children at increased risk of the development of bacterial endocarditis include those with

- Valvular dysfunction or prosthetic valves
- Mitral valve prolapse with regurgitation
- Most congenital heart defects (certain simple septal defects are excluded)
- Surgically constructed systemic-to-pulmonary shunts
- Hypertrophic cardiomyopathy

Children at high risk should practice good oral hygiene, including regular tooth brushing and flossing. Instruct parents or the older child to carry emergency medical identification at all times. A wallet card is available from the AHA (2008). The card may be presented to any health care provider and includes the recommended antibiotic prophylactic regimen. Instruct the parents to notify the primary care provider or cardiologist if the child develops flu-like symptoms or a fever.

High-risk children (as noted above) who are undergoing procedures that increase the risk of the introduction of the types of bacteria responsible for endocarditis

Procedures for Which Bacterial (Infective) Endocarditis Prophylaxis is Recommended

Dental Procedures
- Tooth extractions
- Periodontal procedures
- Dental implant placement
- Replacement of avulsed tooth
- Root canal or surgery
- Intraligamentary local anesthetic injections
- Any prophylactic dental procedure during which bleeding is anticipated

Respiratory Tract Procedures
- Tonsillectomy, adenoidectomy
- Rigid bronchoscopy
- Surgery involving the respiratory mucosa

Gastrointestinal Tract Procedures
- Esophageal varices sclerotherapy
- Dilation of esophageal stricture
- Endoscopic retrograde cholangiography for biliary obstruction
- Other biliary tract surgery
- Surgery involving the gastrointestinal mucosa

Genitourinary Tract Procedures
- Cystoscopy
- Urethral dilation
- Surgery involving the prostate

Data from American Heart Association. (2010). *Infective endocarditis (previously referred to as bacterial endocarditis)*. Retrieved June 13, 2011 from http://www.americanheart.org/presenter.jhtml?identifier=4436; American Heart Association. (2008). *Infective (bacterial) endocarditis wallet card*. Retrieved June 13, 2011 from http://www.heart.org/HEARTORG/General/Infective-Bacterial-Endocarditis-Wallet-Card_UCM_311659_Article.jsp; Greenberg, J. D., Bonwit, A. M., & Roddy, M. G. (2005). Subacute bacterial endocarditis prophylaxis: A succinct review for pediatric emergency physicians and nurses. *Clinical Pediatric Emergency Medicine, 6*(4), 266–272; and Yee, C. A. (2005). Endocarditis: The infected heart. *Nursing Management, 36*(2), 25–30.

should receive prophylaxis as recommended by the AHA. Usual antibiotics for prophylaxis may include ampicillin, amoxicillin, gentamicin, or vancomycin. Box 40.3 lists procedures for which antibiotic prophylaxis in high-risk children is recommended.

Acute Rheumatic Fever

Acute rheumatic fever (ARF) is a delayed sequela of group A streptococcal pharyngeal infection. In a developed country such as Canada, this disease occurs more often in school-age children between 5 and 15 years of age in areas where streptococcal pharyngitis is more prevalent, especially during the colder months (Simmons, 2010). It usually develops 2 to 3 weeks after the initial streptococcal infection. ARF has also been observed more commonly in Aboriginal communities (Steer & Carapetis, 2009). Current understanding of the disease process of ARF is that the child develops an antibody response to surface proteins of the bacteria. The antibodies then cross-react with antigens in cardiac muscle and neuronal and synovial tissues, causing carditis, arthritis, and chorea (involuntary random, jerking movements). ARF affects the joints, central nervous system, skin, and subcutaneous tissue and causes chronic, progressive damage to the heart and valves. Most attacks of ARF last 6 to 12 weeks and then are resolved, but rheumatic fever may recur with subsequent streptococcal infections (Parillo & Parillo, 2010).

Diagnosis of ARF is based on the modified Jones criteria (Box 40.4). Therapeutic management is directed toward managing inflammation and fever, eradicating the bacteria, preventing permanent heart damage, and preventing recurrences. Treatment includes a full 10-day course of penicillin (or equivalent) therapy as well as corticosteroids and nonsteroidal anti-inflammatory drugs. Long-term prophylaxis to prevent a new streptococcal infection and recurrent ARF involves monthly intramuscular injections of penicillin G benzathine. The most recent guidelines recommend prophylaxis for patients with a history of ARF, but without carditis, for a minimum of 10 years or until age 21, whichever is longer, with even longer duration for those with valvular disease (Steer & Carapetis, 2009).

Modified Jones Criteria (American Heart Association)

Diagnosis of acute rheumatic fever requires the presence of either two major criteria or one major plus two minor criteria.

Major Criteria
- Carditis
- Migratory polyarthritis
- Subcutaneous nodules
- Erythema marginatum
- Sydenham chorea

Minor Criteria
- Arthralgia
- Fever
- Elevated erythrocyte sedimentation rate or C-reactive protein
- Prolonged PR interval

Data from Miyamoto, S. D. Sondheimer, H. M., Fagan, T. E., & Collins, K. K. (2011). Cardiovascular diseases. In W. W. Hay, M. J. Levin, J. M. Sondheimer, & R. R. Deterding (Eds.), *Current pediatric diagnosis and treatment* (20th ed.). New York: McGraw-Hill; and Parrillo, S. J., & Parrillo, C. V. (2010). *Rheumatic fever in emergency medicine*. Retrieved October 20, 2011 from http://www.emedicine.com/emerg/topic509.htm.

Nursing Assessment

Elicit a description of the present illness and chief complaint, noting fever and joint pain. Explore the patient's recent medical history for risk factors such as documented streptococcal infection or sore throat within the past 2 to 3 weeks, or for past history of ARF. Observe the child for Sydenham chorea, a movement disorder of the face and upper extremities. Inspect the skin for evidence of the classic rash, erythema marginatum, which is a maculopapular red rash with central clearing and elevated edges. Auscultate the heart, noting a murmur. Palpate the surfaces of the wrists, elbows, and knees for firm, painless, subcutaneous nodules. Note prolonged PR interval on the EKG. Throat culture will provide definitive diagnosis of current streptococcal infection, while streptococcal antibody tests may yield evidence of recent infection. Echocardiogram is required to determine whether carditis is present.

Nursing Management

Nursing management of the child with ARF focuses on promoting adherence with both the acute course of antibiotics and ongoing prophylaxis following initial recovery. Invite the child to verbalize the frustration he or she may be feeling in relation to chorea symptoms. Offer support for dealing with the abnormal movements. Educate the child and others that the sudden jerky movements of chorea will eventually disappear, though they may last for several months. Some children may require a neuroleptic agent such as haloperidol (Haldol) for management of chorea. Administer corticosteroids or nonsteroidal anti-inflammatory agents for control of joint pain and swelling.

Cardiomyopathy

Cardiomyopathy is a condition in which the myocardium cannot contract properly (Batcheler & Dixon, 2009; Park, 2008). The incidence of cardiomyopathy among children is increasing; it occurs at a rate of 1 per 100,000 (AHA, 2011b). While idiopathic cardiomyopathy is the most common form, cardiomyopathy may occur in children with genetic or metabolic disorders, congenital heart defects, as a result of an inflammatory or infectious process or hypertension, or after cardiac transplantation or surgery. Cardiomyopathy clusters in infancy and adolescence. Three types of cardiomyopathy exist (Park, 2008). Restrictive cardiomyopathy is rare in children and results in atrial relaxation (Batcheler & Dixon, 2009; Park, 2008). Dilated cardiomyopathy is the most common type in childhood and may result in heart failure because of ventricular dilation with decreased contractility (Kantor, Abraham, Dipchand, Benson, & Redington, 2010). There is some familial tendency toward dilated cardiomyopathy, and it is also associated with Duchenne and Becker muscular dystrophy (Kaspar,

Allen, & Montanaro, 2009). Children with dilated cardiomyopathy may present with heart failure (Kantor et al., 2010). Hypertrophic cardiomyopathy, which is more common in adolescence and young adulthood, results in hypertrophy of the heart muscle, particularly the left ventricle, affecting the heart's ability to fill (Batcheler & Dixon, 2009; Park, 2008). It is the most common heart-related cause of sudden death in those under 35 years of age (Batcheler & Dixon, 2009). About two thirds of all cases of hypertrophic cardiomyopathy are familial, with some inherited in an autosomal dominant fashion (Batcheler & Dixon, 2009; Park, 2008).

There is no cure for cardiomyopathy, meaning that heart muscle function cannot be restored. Therapeutic management is directed toward improving heart function and BP. Mechanical ventilation and vasoactive medications are needed in many children, but these medications must be used judiciously; otherwise, they are ineffective and can worsen symptoms (Park, 2008). ACE inhibitors, beta blockers, antiarrhythmics, digoxin, or calcium-channel blockers may be used (Simmons, 2010). While combination therapy with ACE inhibitors and beta blockers is gaining more popularity than digoxin-based medical treatment, there is little evidence of obvious or sustained improvement in transplantation-free survival using combination therapy (Kantor et al., 2010). Pacemakers or surgery is helpful in some children (Park, 2008). In the presence of irreversible damage and persistent poor function, heart transplantation may be required (Kantor et al., 2010; Wilkinson, Sleepner, Alvarez, Bublik, & Lipshultz, 2008). Depending on the cause and degree of damage to the myocardium, one third of patients will have persistent poor function, one third will improve, and one third will recover completely (Simmons, 2010).

Nursing Assessment

Explore the health history for risk factors such as

- Congenital heart defect, cardiac transplantation or surgery
- Duchenne or Becker muscular dystrophy
- History of myocarditis, HIV infection, or Kawasaki disease (Park, 2008)
- Hypertension
- Drug, alcohol, or radiation exposure
- Connective tissue, autoimmune, or endocrine disease
- Maternal diabetes
- Familial history of sudden death (Park, 2008)

Inquire about a history of respiratory distress, fatigue, poor growth, chest pain, dizziness, or syncope (hypertrophic and dilated) (Batcheler & Dixon, 2009; Park, 2008). Observe the child for peripheral edema and abdominal distention (dilated and restrictive) (Batcheler & Dixon, 2009). Note increased work of breathing. Auscultate the heart, noting tachycardia, irregular rhythm, and murmurs

(Batcheler & Dixon, 2009; Simmons, 2010). Evaluate heart rhythm via EKG, noting dysrhythmias or indications of left ventricular hypertrophy (Batcheler & Dixon, 2009; Park, 2008).

Chest X-ray may reveal cardiomegaly or congested lungs. Echocardiogram demonstrates increased heart size, poor contractility, decreased ejection fraction, or asymmetric septal hypertrophy (Batcheler & Dixon, 2009; Park, 2008). Cardiac catheterization and/or MRI aids the diagnosis.

Nursing Management

Many children with cardiomyopathy require intensive care initially. Monitor for complications such as blood clots or arrhythmias, which could lead to cardiac arrest (Batcheler & Dixon, 2009). Refer to the prior section on heart failure for nursing interventions related to heart failure, which may be present with dilated cardiomyopathy. Administer vasoactive and other medications as prescribed, monitoring the child closely for response to these therapies as well as for complications (Park, 2008). Support the child in choosing activities that fit within the prescribed restrictions (Park, 2008). Provide extensive emotional support to the child and family, who may experience significant stress as they realize the severity of this illness (Simmons, 2010).

Hypertension

Hypertension affects only 1% to 3% of children and adolescents but often leads to long-term health consequences such as cardiovascular disease and left ventricular hypertrophy (Falkner, 2010). In children, acceptable BP values are based on gender, age, and height (AHA, 2011a). Hypertension is defined as BP persistently higher than the 95th percentile for gender, age, and height (National High Blood Pressure Education Program Working Group on High Blood Pressure in Children and Adolescents [NHBPEP], 2004). Prehypertension refers to BP that is persistently between the 90th and 95th percentiles (NHBPEP, 2004). BP is considered normal when the systolic and diastolic values are less than the 90th percentile for gender, age, and height (NHBPEP, 2004). However, some researchers claim that the recommendation of BP values according to age and height may be statistically and logically unsound and impractical (Falkner, 2010; Park, 2008).

Childhood hypertension may be further defined as primary or secondary (Anglum, 2009; Park, 2008). Primary hypertension in children is rare, but its incidence increases with age, so it is more common in adolescence than in early childhood. Hypertension in children most frequently occurs secondary to an underlying medical problem (most often renal disease) (Martchenke & Blosser, 2009; Park, 2008). Mild to moderate hypertension in childhood is usually asymptomatic and usually is determined only upon BP screening during a well-child visit or during follow-up for known risk factors (Casteel, 2010; Park, 2008).

Therapeutic management depends on the extent of the hypertension and the length of time it has existed. Weight reduction, appropriate diet, and increased physical activity are important components of management of prehypertensive and asymptomatic hypertensive children (Anglum, 2009; Casteel, 2010). Some children are candidates for and require antihypertensive medications or diuretics (Casteel, 2010).

Pathophysiology

The balance between cardiac output and vascular resistance determines the BP. An increase in either of these variables, in the absence of a compensatory decrease in the other, increases the mean BP (Casteel, 2010). Factors regulating cardiac output and vascular resistance include changes in electrolyte balance, particularly sodium, calcium, and potassium (Brady, Siberry, & Solomon, 2008; Hollis, 2009).

Nursing Assessment

Elicit the health history, determining the presence of risk factors for hypertension, such as

- Family history (Park, 2008)
- Obesity (Park, 2008)
- Hyperlipidemia (Park, 2008)
- Renal disease (including frequent urinary tract infections) (Park, 2008)
- Systemic lupus erythematosus
- CHD
- Neurofibromatosis, Turner syndrome, and other genetic disorders
- Prematurity
- Prolonged neonatal ventilation (Martchenke & Blosser, 2009)
- Umbilical artery catheterization (Martchenke & Blosser, 2009)
- Diabetes mellitus (Martchenke & Blosser, 2009; Park, 2008)
- Increased intracranial pressure
- Malignancy
- Solid organ transplant
- Medications known to raise BP (e.g., corticosteroids, amphetamines, antiasthmatics) (Martchenke & Blosser, 2009; Park, 2008)

Signs and symptoms reported during the health history might include growth retardation (with certain chronic medical conditions), obesity, and, particularly in older children, headache, subtle behavioural or school performance changes, fatigue, blurred vision, nosebleed, or Bell's palsy.

Determine the child's weight and height/length. Plot these growth parameters on the gender-appropriate chart for the child's age. Note the percentile for height/length, as it will be used to determine the BP percentile (see Appendix F). Measure the BP in all four extremities (to rule out coarctation of the aorta). Ensure that the child is relaxed and sitting or reclined. Refer to Chapter 31 for specific information related to accurate BP measurement in children.

Physical Examination

Inspect the skin for

- Acne, hirsutism, or striae (associated with anabolic steroid use)
- Café-au-lait spots (associated with neurofibromatosis)
- Malar rash (associated with lupus) (Martchenke & Blosser, 2009)
- Pallor, diaphoresis, or flushing (associated with pheochromocytoma)

Observe the extremities for edema (renal disease) or joint swelling (lupus). Inspect the chest for apical heave (ventricular hypertrophy) or wide-spaced nipples (Turner syndrome). Auscultate heart sounds, noting tachycardia (associated with primary hypertension) or murmur (associated with coarctation of the aorta). Palpate the abdomen for a mass or enlarged kidney (Flynn, 2001).

Laboratory and Diagnostic Testing

Though diagnosis of hypertension is based upon BP measurements, additional laboratory or diagnostic tests may be used to evaluate the underlying cause of secondary hypertension, including the following:

- Urinalysis, blood urea nitrogen, and serum creatinine: may determine presence of renal disease
- Renal ultrasound or angiography: may reveal kidney or genitourinary tract abnormalities
- Echocardiogram: may show left ventricular hypertrophy
- Lipid profile: determines the presence of hyperlipidemia (USDHHS, NHLBI, 2005)

Nursing Management

Salt restriction and potassium or calcium supplements have not been scientifically shown to decrease BP in children (Kay, Sinaiko, & Daniels, 2001). However, certain children may benefit from salt restriction, as some children seem to be sensitive to salt intake (Flynn, 2001). Assist the child and family to develop a plan for weight reduction if the child is overweight or obese (Martchenke & Blosser, 2009). Encourage the child and family to control portion sizes, decrease the intake of sugary beverages (juices and soft drinks) and snacks, eat more fresh fruits and vegetables, and eat a healthy breakfast (Martchenke & Blosser, 2009; NHBPEP, 2004). Consult the nutritionist for additional assistance with meal planning. To increase physical activity, the child should find a sport or type of exercise in which he or she is interested. Aerobic activities involving running, walking, or cycling are particularly helpful. When a child requires antihypertensive therapy, teach the child and family how to administer the medication (Casteel, 2010). Caution the parents about side effects related to antihypertensives (Casteel, 2010). Teach the parent to measure the child's BP as determined by the primary care physician or specialist as well as to keep appointments for BP follow-up (Casteel, 2010).

Kawasaki Disease

Kawasaki disease is an acute systemic vasculitis occurring mostly in infants and young children. It is one of the leading causes of acquired heart disease among children and occurs more frequently in the winter and spring (Simmons, 2010). Kawasaki disease affects all ethnic groups, yet it occurs more frequently in those of Asian or Pacific descent (Han, Sinclair, & Newman, 2000; Martchenke & Blosser, 2009; Newburger, Takahashi, & Gerber, 2004). Recent evidence suggests that Ontario has one of the highest incidences of Kawasaki disease outside of Asia (Lin, Manlhiot, & Ching, 2010). It is a self-limited syndrome but causes serious cardiovascular sequelae in up to 25% of affected children (Newburger et al., 2004; Park, 2008; Simmons, 2010). Coronary artery aneurysm results in myocardial infarction and death in some children (Simmons, 2010). Therapeutic management of acute Kawasaki disease focuses on reducing inflammation in the walls of the coronary arteries and preventing coronary thrombosis. Long-term management of children developing aneurysms during the initial phase is directed toward preventing myocardial ischemia (Martchenke & Blosser, 2009; Newburger et al., 2004; Park, 2008; Simmons, 2010). In the acute phase, high dose aspirin divided into four doses daily and a single infusion of intravenous immunoglobulin (IVIG) are used. Children whose fever persists longer than 48 hours after initiation of aspirin therapy may receive a second dose of IVIG. Pulsed-dose corticosteroid therapy may also be used to prevent or halt coronary dilation and inhibit progression to aneurysm (Rowley & Shulman, 2010).

Pathophysiology

Though the etiology is still unknown, Kawasaki disease may result from an infectious cause (Martchenke & Blosser, 2009; Park, 2008; Simmons, 2010). Current thought is that some infectious organism (as yet unidentified) causes disease in genetically susceptible people. Kawasaki disease appears to be an autoimmune response mediated by cytokine-induced endothelial cell surface antigens that leads to vasculitis. Neutrophils, followed by mononuclear cells, T lymphocytes, and immunoglobulin A–producing plasma cells, infiltrate the vessels. Inflammation then occurs in all three layers of the small and medium-sized blood vessels. Edema and smooth muscle necrosis occur within the vessel wall in severe cases. Generalized systemic vasculitis occurs in the blood vessels throughout the body due to the inflammation and edema. As elastin and collagen fibres fragment, the structural integrity of the vessel wall is impaired. This mechanism leads to coronary dilation (ectasia) or aneurysm. Some children never develop coronary artery changes, while others develop aneurysm in either the acute phase or as a long-term sequela. Infants are at the highest risk of coronary aneurysm (Rowley & Shulman, 2010).

Nursing Assessment

Nursing assessment consists of determining the health history, physical examination, and laboratory and diagnostic testing.

Health History

Elicit the health history, noting any of the following:

- Fever
- Chills
- Headache
- Malaise
- Extreme irritability
- Vomiting
- Diarrhea
- Abdominal pain
- Joint pain

Of particular note is a history of high fever (39.9°C) lasting at least 5 days that is unresponsive to antibiotics.

Physical Examination

Observe for significant bilateral conjunctivitis without exudate. Inspect the mouth and throat for dry, fissured lips, strawberry (cracked and reddened) tongue, and pharyngeal and oral mucosa erythema. Note hyperdynamic precordium. Evaluate the skin for

- Diffuse, erythematous, polymorphous rash
- Edema of the hands and feet
- Erythema and painful induration of the palms and soles
- Desquamation (peeling) of the perineal region, fingers, and toes, extending to the palms and soles
- Possible jaundice

Palpate the neck for cervical lymphadenopathy (usually unilateral) and the joints for tenderness. Palpate the abdomen for liver enlargement. Auscultate the heart, noting tachycardia, gallop, or murmur (Newburger et al., 2004; Rowley, 2004).

Laboratory and Diagnostic Testing

The CBC may reveal mild to moderate anemia, elevated white blood cell count during the acute phase, and significant thrombocytosis (elevated platelet count [500,000 to 1 million]) in the later phase. The erythrocyte sedimentation rate and the C-reactive protein level are elevated. Echocardiogram is performed as soon as possible after the diagnosis is confirmed to provide a baseline of a healthy heart or to evaluate for coronary artery involvement (Martchenke & Blosser, 2009). Echocardiograms may be repeated during the illness and as part of long-term follow-up. Occasionally cardiac involvement warrants cardiac catheterization.

Nursing Management

In addition to the administration of aspirin and immunoglobulin, nursing management of the child with Kawasaki disease focuses on monitoring cardiac status, promoting comfort, and providing family education.

Monitoring Cardiac Status

Administer intravenous and oral fluids as ordered, evaluating intake and output carefully. Prepare the child for the echocardiogram (Martchenke & Blosser, 2009). Assess frequently for signs of developing heart failure such as tachycardia, gallop, decreased urine output, or respiratory distress. Evaluate quality and strength of pulses. Provide cardiac monitoring as ordered, reporting arrhythmias.

Promoting Comfort

Provide acetaminophen for fever management and apply cool cloths as tolerated. Keep the environment quiet and cluster nursing care activities to decrease stimulation and hence irritability. Teach parents that irritability is a prominent feature of Kawasaki disease, and support their efforts to console the child. Apply petroleum jelly or another lubricating ointment to the lips. Encourage the older child to suck on ice chips; the younger child may suck on a cool, moist washcloth. Popsicles are also soothing. Provide comfortable positioning, particularly if the child has joint pain or arthritis.

Providing Patient and Family Education

Teach parents to continue to monitor the child's temperature after discharge until the child has been afebrile for several days. Children with prolonged or recurrent fever may require a second dose of IVIG. Inform parents that irritability may last for up to 2 months after initial diagnosis of Kawasaki disease. Toxic effects of aspirin therapy such as headache, confusion, dizziness, or tinnitus should be reported to the primary care provider. Nonsteroidal anti-inflammatory agents should be avoided while aspirin therapy is ongoing. For children with continued arthritis (which resolves in several weeks), range-of-motion exercises with a morning bath may help to decrease stiffness. Instruct parents to avoid measles and varicella vaccination for 11 months after high-dose IVIG administration (Martchenke & Blosser, 2009; Newburger et al., 2004). It is critical that the family comply with regularly scheduled cardiology follow-up appointments to determine development or progression of coronary artery ectasia or aneurysm. If the child has severe cardiac involvement, teach the parents about infant and/or child cardiopulmonary resuscitation before discharge from the hospital.

Hyperlipidemia

Hyperlipidemia refers to high levels of lipids (fats/cholesterol) in the blood (Burchett, Hanna, & Steiner, 2009; Manlhiot, Larsson, & Gurofsky, 2009). High lipid levels are a risk factor for the development of atherosclerosis, which can result in coronary artery disease, a serious cardiovascular disorder occurring in adults (Burchett et al., 2009). Children with high lipid levels, though remaining asymptomatic, are likely to have high levels as adults, which increases their risk of coronary artery disease. Therefore, detection, screening, and early intervention are important, especially if there is a family tendency toward heart disease (Burchett et al., 2009).

Pathophysiology

Cholesterol is a building block for hormones and cell membranes. It occurs naturally in foods derived from animals such as eggs, dairy products, meat, poultry, and seafood. Cholesterol is also manufactured in the body. Together, cholesterol and triglycerides are known as lipids. Very-low-density lipoprotein (VLDL) is a lipoprotein composed mainly of triglycerides with only small amounts of cholesterol, phospholipid, and protein. VLDLs are easily converted to low-density lipoproteins (LDLs). Cholesterol is expressed in terms of LDL cholesterol or high-density lipoprotein (HDL) cholesterol. LDLs contain relatively more cholesterol and triglycerides than protein. HDLs contain about 50% protein, with the rest being cholesterol, triglyceride, and phospholipid. High levels of cholesterol and triglycerides place a person at risk of atherosclerosis. Elevated VLDL and LDL levels and decreased HDL levels produce a particular increase in the risk of atherosclerosis (Daniels, Greer, & the Committee on Nutrition, 2008).

Therapeutic Management

Screening children for hyperlipidemia is of prime importance for early detection, intervention, and subsequent prevention of adult atherosclerosis. The U.S. National Cholesterol Education Program recommends screening for hyperlipidemia in children over 2 years of age if

• The parent has a total cholesterol level above 240 mg/dL

• There is a family history of cardiovascular disease in a parent or grandparent before age 55 years
• The family history is unavailable (Burchett et al., 2009)

All children should eat a diet with the appropriate amount of fats (see the section on nursing management below) and should participate in physical activity (Burchett et al., 2009; Manlhiot et al., 2009). When diet and exercise are not enough to lower cholesterol to appropriate levels, medications such as resins, fibric acid derivatives, statins, or niacin may be used (Manlhiot et al., 2009).

Nursing Assessment

Elicit the health history, noting risk factors such as family history of hyperlipidemia, early heart disease, hypertension, diabetes or other endocrine abnormality, CVA, or sudden death. Note prior lipid levels if available. Measure the child's height and weight, plotting them on standardized growth charts. Note overweight or obesity, as these are risk factors associated with hyperlipidemia. Typically, there are no other particular physical findings associated with hyperlipidemia. Table 40.3 gives details about the interpretation of cholesterol levels.

Nursing Management

Instruct families that the child must fast for 12 hours before lipid screening (initially and on follow-up samples). Dietary management is the first step in the prevention and management of hyperlipidemia in children over 2 years of age (Burchett et al., 2009; Manlhiot et al., 2009). The diet should consist primarily of fruits, vegetables, low-fat dairy products, whole grains, beans, lean meat and poultry, and fish. As in adults, fat should account for no more than 30% of daily caloric intake. Fat intake may vary over a period of days, as many young children are picky eaters. Limit saturated fats by choosing lean meats, removing skin from poultry before cooking, and avoiding palm, palm kernel, and coconut oils as well as hydrogenated fats. Teach families to read nutrition labels to determine the content of the food. Limit

TABLE 40.3   INTERPRETATION OF CHOLESTEROL LEVELS FOR CHILDREN AGE 2 TO 19 YEARS

Total Cholesterol (mg/dL)	LDL Cholesterol (mg/dL)	Interpretation
<170	<100	Normal
170–200	100–130	Borderline
>200	>130	High

Daniels, S. R., Greer, F. R., & the Committee on Nutrition. (2008). Lipid screening and cardiovascular health in childhood. *Pediatrics*, 122(91), 198–208.

intake of processed or refined foods as well as high-sugar drinks; these products provide minimal nutrition and significant calories. Children over 2 years of age should have 60 minutes per day of vigourous play or physical activity. Refer parents to *Healthy Habits for Healthy Kids—A Nutrition and Activity Guide for Parents* published by the American Dietetic Association (visit http://thePoint.lww.com/Chow1e for a direct link).

If medications are required, teach the child and family about the dose, administration, and possible adverse effects (Burchett et al., 2009). Assist the family to develop a medication dosing plan that is compatible with school and work schedules to increase compliance.

Heart Transplantation

Heart transplantation is indicated in children with end-stage heart disease related to cardiomyopathy or inoperable CHD (Park, 2008; Simmons, 2010). Candidates for heart transplantation are infants and children whose medical and surgical options have been exhausted and who have a 12- to 24-month life expectancy (Gabrys, 2005). Worldwide, between 350 and 390 children have received a heart transplant each year since 1991 (Boucek, Waltz, & Edwards, 2006). The overall 20-year survival rate for all pediatric heart transplant recipients is 40%, with 1-, 5- and 10-year survival reported as 80%, 68%, and 58%, respectively (Kirk et al., 2009). Humpl, Furness, Gruenwald, Hyslop, & van Arsdell's (2010) retrospective case series study suggests that the use of a ventricular assist device is effective in bridging children with advanced dilated cardiomyopathy or heart failure to transplantation.

A comprehensive evaluation is performed to determine whether the child is a candidate for heart transplantation and is the most important determinant of a favourable outcome (Park, 2008; Simmons, 2010). The evaluation includes

- Chest X-ray, EKG, echocardiogram, exercise stress test, cardiac catheterization, pulmonary function tests (Park, 2008);
- CBC with differential, prothrombin and partial thromboplastin times, serum chemistries and electrolytes, blood urea nitrogen, and creatinine (Simmons, 2010)
- Urinalysis and urine creatinine clearance
- Blood, throat, urine, stool, and sputum cultures for bacteria, viruses, fungi, and parasites
- Epstein-Barr virus, cytomegalovirus, varicella, herpes, hepatitis, and HIV titers
- HLA typing and panel reactive antibody typing and titer
- Computed tomography or MRI, electroencephalogram
- Consults with neurology, psychology, genetics, social work, nutritionist, physical and occupational therapy,

and financial coordinator or case manager (Conway & Dipchand, 2010)

Children with irreversible lung, liver, kidney, or central nervous system disease, recent malignancy (past 5 years), or chronic viral infection may be excluded as candidates.

Once candidacy is determined, the transplant centre registers the child as a potential recipient with the United Network for Organ Sharing (Gabrys, 2005). Blood type, body size, length of time on the waiting list, and medical urgency are used to evaluate compatibility (Berg, 2002). Children awaiting transplantation may need continuous or intermittent hospitalization. Coordination of organ procurement and the transplantation procedure is essential (Gabrys, 2005).

Surgical Procedure and Postoperative Therapeutic Management

Most transplantation procedures are **orthotopic**, which means that the recipient's heart is removed and the donor heart is implanted in its place in the normal anatomic position (del Rio, 2000). Cardiopulmonary bypass and hypothermia are used to maintain circulation, protect the brain, and oxygenate the recipient during the procedure. Postoperatively, the child may have near-normal heart function and capacity for exercise and may be able to return to school.

Immunosuppressive therapy is necessary for the rest of the child's life to avoid rejection of the transplanted heart. Usually a three-drug regimen is used that includes calcineurin inhibitors (cyclosporine, tacrolimus), cell toxins (mycophenolate mofetil, azathioprine), and corticosteroids. Ongoing follow-up is provided by the cardiologist and transplant surgeon. Complications of heart transplantation include bacterial, fungal, and viral infection and heart rejection. Neoplasm may occur as a result of chronic immunosuppression.

Nursing Management

Preoperative nursing care for the child undergoing heart transplantation is similar to that for children undergoing other types of heart surgery. In addition, the nurse should assist with the comprehensive pre-transplant evaluation (Humpl et al., 2010). Care for the child in the post-transplant period is intense and complex. Evaluate the family's ability to perform the tasks that will be necessary. Teach families about the evaluation and transplantation process as well as the waiting period (Gabrys, 2005). In the immediate preoperative period, perform a thorough history and physical examination and obtain last-minute bloodwork. Provide preoperative teaching similar to other cardiac surgeries. Older children, adolescents, and parents may enjoy the book *Future Conditional* by J. Hatton (1996, Yorkshire Art Circus), which was written by one of the first heart transplant survivors.

Postoperatively, provide frequent assessments and routine care for cardiac surgery patients. In addition, monitor the child closely for infection or signs of rejection (Gabrys, 2005). Acute rejection may be indicated by low-grade fever, fatigue, tachycardia, nausea, vomiting, abdominal pain, and decreased activity tolerance, though some children will be asymptomatic. Maintain strict handwashing techniques and isolate the child from other children with infections. Though live vaccines are contraindicated in immunosuppressed children, inactivated vaccines should be given as recommended (Centers for Disease Control and Prevention, 2011). Teach children and families that the child may return to school and usual activities about 3 months after the transplant. Provide emotional support to the child related to body image changes such as hair growth, gum hyperplasia, weight gain, moon facies, acne, and rashes that occur due to long-term immunosuppressive therapy.

■■■ Key Concepts

- At birth, when the umbilical cord is cut and the neonate's first breath occurs, the ductus venosus closes with the foramen ovale and the ductus arteriosus closes shortly thereafter. Pulmonary vascular resistance decreases and systemic vascular resistance increases.
- The infant's heart rate averages 120 to 130 beats/min and decreases throughout childhood, reaching the adult rate in adolescence. Conversely, the infant and child's BP is significantly lower than the adult's, increasing as the child ages.
- Check the infant's apical pulse prior to digoxin administration and hold the dose if the heart rate is less than 90.
- Poor weight gain, failure to thrive, and increased fatigability commonly occur with congestive heart failure.
- Clubbing of the fingernails occurs as a result of chronic hypoxia in the child with severe CHD.
- Children with cardiac conditions resulting in cyanosis often have baseline oxygen saturations that are relatively low due to the mixing of oxygenated blood with deoxygenated blood.
- Document the presence of a murmur by grading its intensity (I–IV), describing where it occurs within the cardiac cycle, and noting the location where the murmur is best heard.
- CHD should be suspected in the cyanotic newborn who does not improve with oxygen administration.
- Cardiac catheterization post-procedure care focuses on evaluation of the child's vital signs and condition of the pressure dressing, as well as assessment of the distal pulses bilaterally for presence and quality.
- Congenital heart disorders resulting in decreased pulmonary blood flow (tetralogy of Fallot, tricuspid atresia) lead to cyanosis.

- Disorders with increased pulmonary blood flow (patent ductus arteriosus, ASD, and VSD) may result in pulmonary edema if the defect is severe.
- A decrease in the lower extremity pulses or BP as compared with the upper extremities may be indicative of coarctation of the aorta.
- It is important to remain calm when an infant or child demonstrates a hypercyanotic spell. Place the child in a knee-chest position, administer oxygen and/or morphine or propranolol, and supply intravenous fluids.
- Children with certain congenital heart defects and/or heart failure require additional calories in order to display adequate growth.
- Children with hypertrophic cardiomyopathy, certain congenital heart defects, valve dysfunction, or prosthetic valves require prophylaxis for bacterial (infective) endocarditis when undergoing procedures or invasive dental work.
- Hypertension in the child or adolescent often leads to long-term health consequences such as cardiovascular disease and left ventricular hypertrophy.
- Kawasaki disease may result in severe cardiac sequelae, so these children need ongoing cardiac follow-up to screen for development of problems.
- It is important to screen for hyperlipidemia in high-risk children.
- Abrupt cessation of chest tube output, accompanied by an increase in the heart rate and increased filling pressure, may indicate cardiac tamponade.

REFERENCES

Abdallah, H. (2011). *Pediatric cardiac testing.* Retrieved October 18, 2011 from http://www.childrenheartinstitute.org/testing/testhome.htm

American Heart Association. (2008). *Prevention of infective (bacterial) endocarditis wallet card.* Retrieved October 23, 2011 from http://www.heart.org/idc/groups/heart-public/@wcm/@private/@hcm/documents/downloadable/ucm_311661.pdf

American Heart Association. (2010). *Infective endocarditis (previously referred to as bacterial endocarditis).* Retrieved June 13, 2011 from http://www.americanheart.org/presenter.jhtml?identifier=4436

American Heart Association. (2011a). *High blood pressure in children.* Retrieved October 23, 2011 from http://www.heart.org/HEARTORG/Conditions/HighBloodPressure/UnderstandYourRiskforHighBloodPressure/High-Blood-Pressure-in-Children_UCM_301868_Article.jsp

American Heart Association. (2011b). *Youth and cardiovascular diseases—statistics.* Retrieved October 23, 2011 from http://www.amhrt.org/idc/groups/heart-public/@wcm/@sop/@smd/documents/downloadable/ucm_319577.pdf

Anglum, A. (2009). Primary care management of childhood and adolescent hypertension. *Journal of the American Academy of Nurse Practitioners, 21*(10), 529–534.

Archer, N., & Manning, N. (2009). *Fetal cardiology.* Oxford, UK: Oxford University Press.

Ascenzi, J. A., & Kane, P. L. (2007). Update on complications of pediatric cardiac surgery. *Critical Care Nursing Clinics of North America, 19*(4), 361–369.

Axton, S. E., & Fugate, T. (2009). *Pediatric nursing care plans for the hospitalized child* (3rd ed.). Upper Saddle River, NJ: Pearson.

Bacha, E. A., Cooper, D., Thiagarajan, R., et al. (2008). Cardiac complications associated with the treatment of patients with congenital cardiac disease: consensus definitions from the Multi-Societal Database Committee for Pediatric and Congenital Heart Disease. *Cardiology in the Young, 18*(supplement 2), 196–201.

Bailliard, F., & Anderson, R. H. (2009). Tetralogy of Fallot. *Orphanet Journal of Rare Diseases, 4*(2). doi:10.1186/1750-1172-4-2.

Baltimore, R. (2008). New recommendations for the prevention of infective endocarditis. *Current Opinion in Pediatrics, 20*(1), 85–89.

Barker, J., Williams, C., & Tulloh, R. (2009). Understanding and treatment of heart failure. *Paediatrics and Child Health, 19*(1), 1–8.

Batcheler, S., & Dixon, M. (2009). Cardiac. In M. Dixon, D. Crawford, D. Teasdale, & J. Murphy (Eds.), *Nursing the highly dependent child or infant: A manual of care.* Des Moines, IA: Wiley-Blackwell.

Beke, D. M., Braudis, N. J., & Lincoln, P. (2005). Management of the pediatric postoperative cardiac surgery patient. *Critical Care Nursing Clinics of North America, 17*(4), 405–416.

Berg, A. B. (2002). Pediatric heart transplantation: A clinical overview. *Critical Care Nursing Quarterly, 25*, 79–87.

Betz, C. L., & Sowden, L. A. (2008). *Mosby pediatric nursing reference* (6th ed.). St. Louis, MO: Mosby.

Boucek, M. M., Waltz, D. A., Edwards, L. B., et al. (2006). Registry of the International Society for Heart and Lung Transplantation: Ninth official pediatric heart transplantation report, 2006. *Journal of Heart and Lung Transplantation, 25*, 893–903.

Brady, T., Siberry, G. K., & Solomon, B. (2008). Pediatric hypertension: A review of proper screening, diagnosis, evaluation, and treatment. *Contemporary Pediatrics, 25*(11), 46–56.

Brown, R. T., Daly, B. P., & Rickel, A. U. (2007). *Chronic illness in children and adolescents.* Cambridge, MA: Hogrefe.

Brusch, J. L., Conrad, S., & Marill, K. A. (2011). *Infective endocarditis.* Retrieved October 24, 2011 from http://emedicine.medscape.com/article/216650-overview

Burchett, M. L. R., Hanna, C. E., & Steiner, R. D. (2009). Endocrine and metabolic diseases. In C. E. Burns, A. M. Dunn, M. A. Brady, N. B. Starr, & C. G. Blosser (Eds.), *Pediatric primary care* (4th ed.). Philadelphia, PA: WB Saunders.

Cantor, R. M., & Sadowitz, P. D. (2010). *Neonatal emergencies.* New York: McGraw-Hill Medical.

Carpenito-Moyet, L. J. (2010). *Nursing diagnosis: Application to clinical practice* (13th ed.). Philadelphia, PA: Lippincott Williams & Wilkins.

Casteel, C. (2010). Care of the child with altered renal function. In W. Votroubek & A. Tabacco (Eds.), *Pediatric home care for nurses: A family-centered approach* (3rd ed.). Toronto, ON: Jones and Bartlett Publishers.

Centers for Disease Control and Prevention. (2011). *The pink book: Epidemiology and prevention of vaccine-preventable diseases* (12th ed.). Retrieved October 21, 2011 from http://www.cdc.gov/vaccines/pubs/pinkbook/pink-chapters.htm

Chamberlain, R. S. (2008). Pediatric cardiovascular disorders. In S. M. Nettina (Ed.), *Lippincott manual of nursing practice.* Philadelphia, PA: Lippincott Williams & Wilkins.

Chen, C.-W., Li, C.-Y., & Wang, J.-K. (2004). Growth and development of children with congenital heart disease. *Journal of Advanced Nursing, 47*(3), 260–269.

Children's Mercy Hospitals & Clinics. (2011). *Cardiac catheterization.* Retrieved October 20, 2011 from http://www.childrensmercy.org/content/uploadedFiles/Care_Cards/CMH-99-181p.pdf

Conway, J., & Dipchand, A. I. (2010). Heart transplantation in children. *Pediatric Clinics of North America, 57*(2), 353–373.

Cook, E. H., & Higgins, S. S. (2010). Congenital heart disease. In P. J. Allen, J. A. Vessey, & N. A. Schapiro (Eds.), *Primary care of the child with a chronic condition* (5th ed.). St. Louis, MO: Mosby.

Cook, K., & Langton, H. (2009). *Cardiothoracic care for children and young people. A multidisciplinary approach.* West Sussex, UK: Wiley-Blackwell.

Craig, J., Fineman, L. D., Moynihan, P., & Baker, A. L. (2001). Cardiovascular critical care problems. In M. A. Q. Curley & P. A. Moloney-Harmon (Eds.), *Critical care nursing of infants and children* (2nd ed.). Philadelphia, PA: WB Saunders.

Cunningham, F. G., Leveno, K. L., Bloom, S. L., et al. (2010). *Williams obstetrics* (23rd ed.). New York: McGraw-Hill.

Daniels, S. R., Greer, F. R., & the Committee on Nutrition. (2008). Lipid screening and cardiovascular health in childhood. *Pediatrics, 122*(91), 198–208.

del Rio, M. J. (2000). Transplantation in complex congenital heart disease. *Progress in Pediatric Cardiology, 11*(2), 107–113.

Driscoll, D. J. (2006). *Fundamentals of pediatric cardiology.* Philadelphia, PA: Lippincott Williams & Wilkins.

Falkner, B. (2010). Hypertension in children and adolescents: Epidemiology and natural history. *Pediatric Nephrology, 25*(7), 1219–1224.

Fernandes, J. R. H. (2005). The experience of a broken heart. *Critical Care Nursing Clinics of North America, 17*(4), 319–327.

Fixler, D. E. (2006). Epidemiology of congenital heart disease. In J. A. McMillan (Ed.), *Oski's pediatrics: Principles and practice.* Philadelphia, PA: Lippincott Williams & Wilkins.

Flynn, J. T. (2001). Evaluation and management of hypertension in childhood. *Progress in Pediatric Cardiology, 12*(2), 177–188.

Friedberg, M. K., Silverman, N. H., Moon-Grady, A. J., et al. (2009). Prenatal detection of congenital heart disease. *Journal of Pediatrics, 155*(1), 26–31.e1.

Friedman Ross, L. F., & Frader, J. (2009). Hypoplastic left heart syndrome: a paradigm case for examining conscientious objection in pediatric practice. *Journal of Pediatrics, 155*(1), 12–15.

Fulton, D. R. (2008). Congenital heart disease in children and adolescents. In V. Fuster, R. A. O'Rourke, R. A. Walsh, & P. Poole-Wilson (Eds.), *Hurst's the heart* (12th ed). New York: McGraw-Hill Companies.

Gabrys, C. A. (2005). Pediatric cardiac transplants: A clinical update. *Journal of Pediatric Nursing, 20*(2), 139–143

Gazit, A. Z., Huddleston, C. B., Checchia, P. A., Fehr, J., & Pezzella, A. T. (2010a). Care of the pediatric cardiac surgery patient—Part 1. *Current Problems in Surgery, 47*(3), 185–250.

Gazit, A. Z., Huddleston, C. B., Checchia, P. A., Fehr, J., & Pezzella, A. T. (2010b). Care of the pediatric cardiac surgery patient—Part 2. *Current Problems in Surgery, 47*(4), 261–376.

Greenberg, J. D., Bonwit, A. M., & Roddy, M. G. (2005). Subacute bacterial endocarditis prophylaxis: A succinct review for pediatric emergency physicians and nurses. *Clinical Pediatric Emergency Medicine, 6*(4), 266–272.

Griffin, K. J., Elkin, T. D., & Smith, C. J. (2003). Academic outcomes in children with congenital heart disease. *Clinical Pediatrics, 42*(5), 401–409.

Han, R. K., Sinclair, B., Newman, A., et al. (2000) Recognition and management of Kawasaki disease. *Canadian Medical Association Journal, 162*(6), 807–812.

Heart and Stroke Foundation of Alberta, NWT & Nunavut. (2010). *Congenital heart disease.* Retrieved October 24, 2011 from http://www.heartandstroke.ab.ca/site/c.lqIRL1PJJtH/b.3650945/k.E8F4/Heart_Disease_Congenital_Heart_Disease.htm

Hetherington, R. (2009). *The adult with congenital heart disease: Education and employment.* Retrieved October 24, 2011 from Available August 31, 2011 from http://www.aboutkidshealth.ca/en/resource-centres/congenitalheartconditions/lookingahead/the adultwithcongenitalheartdisease/pages/education-employment.aspx

Hoffman, J. I. E. (2009). *The natural and unnatural history of congenital heart disease.* Chichester, UK; Hoboken, NJ: Wiley-Blackwell.

Hoffman, J., & Kaplan, S. (2002). The incidence of congenital heart disease. *Journal of American College of Cardiology, 39*(12), 1890–1900.

Hollis, K. (2009). Hypertension in children and adolescents. *ADVANCE for Nurse Practitioners, 17*(6), 52–54.

Humpl, T., Furness, S., Gruenwald, C., Hyslop, C., & van Arsdell, G. (2010). The Berlin Heart EXCOR Pediatrics—The Sick Kids Experience 2004–2008. *Artificial Organs, 34*(12), 1082–1086.

Kantor, P. F., Abraham, J. R., Dipchand, A. I., Benson, L. N., & Redington, A. N. (2010). The impact of changing medical therapy on transplantation-free survival in pediatric dilated cardiomyopathy. *Journal of the American College of Cardiology, 55*(13), 1377–1384.

Kargar, M. (2009). *Hypercyanotic spells tet spells and nursing care.* Retrieved October 20, 2011 from http://www.icrj.ir/iacc/arts%5C391.pdf

Kaspar, R. W., Allen, H. D., & Montanaro, F. (2009). Current understanding and management of dilated cardiomyopathy in Duchenne and Becker muscular dystrophy. *Journal of the American Academy of Nurse Practitioners, 21*(5), 241–249.

Kay, J. D., Sinaiko, A. R., & Daniels, S. R. (2001). Pediatric hypertension. *American Heart Journal, 142*(3), 422–432.

Kirk, R., Edwards, L.B., Aurora, P., et al. (2009). Registry of the International Society for Heart and Lung Transplantation: Twelfth Official Pediatric Heart Transplantation report—2009. *The Journal of Heart and Lung Transplantation, 28*(10), 993–1006.

Lin, Y. T., Manlhiot, C., Ching, J. C., et al. (2010). Repeated systematic surveillances of Kawasaki disease in Ontario from 1995 to 2006. *Pediatrics International, 114*(2), e160–e165.

Mahle, W. T., Clancy, R. R., Moss, E. M., et al. (2000). Neurodevelopmental outcome and lifestyle assessment in school-aged and adolescent children with hypoplastic left heart syndrome. *Pediatrics, 100*(5), 1082–1089.

Mahle, W. T., Visconti, K. J., Freier, M. C., et al. (2006). Relationship of surgical approach to neurodevelopmental outcomes in hypoplastic left heart syndrome. *Pediatrics, 117*(1), e90–e97.

Manlhiot, C., Larsson, P., Gurofsky, R. C., et al. (2009). Spectrum and management of hypertriglyceridemia among children in clinical practice. *Pediatrics, 123*(2), 458–465.

Marelli, A., Mackie, A., Ionescu-Ittu, R., Rahme, E., & Pilote, L. (2007). Congenital heart disease in the general population. *Circulation, 115*, 163–172.

Martchenke, J., & Blosser, C. G. (2009) Cardiovascular disorders. In C. E. Burns, A. M. Dunn, M. A. Brady, M. B. Starr, C. G. Blosser (Eds.), *Pediatric primary care* (4th ed.). St. Louis, MO: Saunders Elsevier.

Medoff-Cooper, B., & Irving, S. Y. (2009). Innovative strategies for feeding and nutrition in infants with congenitally malformed hearts. *Cardiology in the Young, 19*(Suppl 2), 90–95.

Meeks, M., Hallsworth, M., & Yeo, H. (2010). *Nursing the neonate* (2nd ed.). West Sussex, UK: Wiley-Blackwell.

Menashe, V. (2007). Heart murmurs. *Pediatrics in Review, 28*, e19–e22.

Miyamoto, S. D., Sondheimer, H. M., Fagan, T. E., & Collins, K. K. (2011). Cardiovascular diseases. In W. W. Hay, M. J. Levin, J. M. Sondheimer, & R. R. Deterding (Eds.), *Current pediatric diagnosis and treatment* (20th ed.). New York: McGraw-Hill.

Molczan, K. (2006). Cardiac anomalies in the neonate: High index of suspicion important. *Journal of Emergency Nursing, 32*, 94–97.

Moons, P., Sluysmans, T., De Wolf, D., et al. (2009). Congenital heart disease in 111,225 births in Belgium: birth prevalence, treatment and survival in the 21st century. *Acta Paediatrica, 98*, 472–477.

Mullins, C. E. (2006). Therapeutic cardiac catheterization. In J. A. McMillan (Ed.), *Oski's pediatrics: Principles and practice.* Philadelphia, PA: Lippincott Williams & Wilkins.

National High Blood Pressure Education Program Working Group on High Blood Pressure in Children and Adolescents. (2004). The fourth report on the diagnosis, evaluation, and treatment of high blood pressure in children and adolescents. *Pediatrics, 114*(Suppl 2 of 3), 555–576.

Newburger, J. W., Takahashi, M., Gerber, M. A., et al. (2004). Diagnosis, treatment and long-term management of Kawasaki disease: A statement for health professionals from the Committee on Rheumatic Fever, Endocarditis, and Kawasaki Disease, Council on Cardiovascular Disease in the Young, American Heart Association. *Pediatrics, 114*(6), 1708–1733.

Oyen, N., Poulsen, G., Boyd, H. A., Wohlfahrt, J., Jensen, P. K., & Melbye, M. (2009). Recurrence of congenital heart defects in families. *Circulation, 120*(4), 295–301. doi: CIRCULATIONAHA. 109.857987 [pii]

Pagana, K. D., & Pagana, T. J. (2010). *Mosby's manual of diagnostic and laboratory tests* (4th ed.). St. Louis, MO: Mosby.

Park, M. K. (2008). *Pediatric cardiology* (5th ed.). Philadelphia, PA: Mosby Elsevier.

Parrillo, S. J., & Parrillo, C. V. (2010). *Rheumatic fever in emergency medicine.* Retrieved October 20, 2011 from http://www.emedicine.com/emerg/topic509.htm

Pauliks, L. B., & Ündar, A. (2008). New devices for pediatric mechanical circulatory support. *Current Opinion in Cardiology, 23*(2), 91–96.

Rao, P. S., & Pflieger, K. (2010). *Pulmonary stenosis, valvar.* Retrieved October 24, 2011 from http://emedicine.medscape.com/article/891729-overview

Ren, X. (M.), Aggarwal, K., Balentine, J., et al. (2011). *Aortic stenosis.* Retrieved October 24, 2011 from http://www.emedicine.com/emerg/topic40.htm

Roberts, J., & MacMath, S. (2006). *Starting a conversation. School children with congenital heart disease.* Calgary, AB: Detselig Enterprises Ltd.

Roos-Hesselink, J. W., Meijboom, F. J., Spitaels, S. E. C., et al. (2004). Outcome of patients after surgical closure of ventricular septal defect at young age: Longitudinal follow-up of 22–34 years. *European Heart Journal, 25*, 1057–1062.

Rowley, A. H. (2004). The etiology of Kawasaki disease: A conventional infectious agent. *Progress in Pediatric Cardiology, 19*(2), 109–113.

Rowley, A. H., & Shulman, S. T. (2010). Pathogenesis and management of Kawasaki disease. *Expert Review of Anti-infective Therapy, 8*(2), 197–203.

Simmons, F. J. (2010). Care of the child with altered cardiac function. In W. Votroubek & A. Tabacco (Eds.), *Pediatric home care for nurses: A family-centered approach.* (3rd ed.). Toronto, ON: Jones and Bartlett Publishers.

Skippen, P., Sanatina, S., Froese, N, & Gow, R. M. (2010). Pacemaker therapy of postoperative arrhythmias after pediatric cardiac surgery. *Pediatric Critical Care Medicine, 11*, 113–138.

Snookes, S., Gunn, J., Eldridge, B., et al. (2010). A systematic review of motor and cognitive outcomes after early surgery for congenital heart disease. *Pediatrics, 125*, e818–e827.

Sorce, L. R. (2009). Respiratory syncytial virus: From primary care to critical care. *Journal of Pediatric Healthcare, 23*(2), 101–108.

Steer, A. C., & Carapetis, J. R. (2009). Acute rheumatic fever and rheumatic heart disease in indigenous populations. *Pediatric Clinics of North America, 56*(6), 1401–1419.

Suddaby, E. C. (2001). Contemporary thinking for congenital heart disease. *Pediatric Nursing, 27*(3), 233–238, 270.

Taketokmo, C. K., Hodding, J. H., & Kraus, D. M. (2010). *Lexi-comp's pediatric dosage handbook* (17th ed.). Hudson, OH: Lexi-comp.

Talner, N. S., & Carboni, M. P. (2003). Congestive heart failure. In C. D. Rudolph, A. M. Rudolph, M. K. Hostetter, et al., *Rudolph's pediatrics* (21st ed.). New York: McGraw-Hill.

U. S. Department of Health and Human Services (USDHHS), National Institute of Health & National Heart Lung and Blood Institute (NHLBI) (2005). *The fourth report on the Diagnosis, Evaluation, and Treatment of High Blood Pressure in Children and Adolescents.* Retrieved March 14, 2012 from http://www.nhlbi.nih.gov/health/prof/heart/hbp/hbp_ped.pdf

Wilkinson, J. D., Sleepner, L. A., Alvarez, J. A., Bublik, N., & Lipshultz, S. E. (2008). The Pediatric Cardiomyopathy Registry: 1995–2007. *Progress in Pediatric Cardiology, 25*, 31–36.

Yee, C. A. (2005). Endocarditis: The infected heart. *Nursing Management, 36*(2), 25–30.

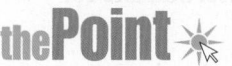

For additional learning materials, including Internet Resources, visit http://thePoint.lww.com/Chow1e.

CHAPTER WORKSHEET

MULTIPLE CHOICE QUESTIONS

1. The nurse is caring for a 5-year-old child with a congenital heart anomaly causing chronic cyanosis. When performing the history and physical examination, what is the nurse least likely to assess?

    a. Obesity from overeating

    b. Clubbing of the nail beds

    c. Squatting during play activities

    d. Exercise intolerance

2. A 2-day-old infant was just diagnosed with aortic stenosis. What is the most likely nursing assessment finding?

    a. Gallop and rales

    b. Blood pressure discrepancies in the extremities

    c. Right ventricular hypertrophy on EKG

    d. Heart murmur

3. Sam, age 11, has a diagnosis of rheumatic fever and has missed school for a week. What is the most likely cause of this problem?

    a. Previous streptococcal throat infection

    b. History of open heart surgery at 5 years of age

    c. Playing too much soccer and not getting enough rest

    d. Exposure to a sibling with pneumonia

4. The nurse is caring for a child after a cardiac catheterization. What is the nursing priority?

    a. Allow early ambulation to encourage activity participation.

    b. Check pulses above the catheter insertion site for strength and quality.

    c. Assess extremity distal to the insertion site for temperature and colour.

    d. Change the dressing to evaluate the site for infection.

5. While assessing a 4-month-old infant, the nurse notes that the baby experiences a hypercyanotic spell. What is the priority nursing action?

    a. Provide supplemental oxygen by face mask.

    b. Administer a dose of IV morphine sulfate.

    c. Begin cardiopulmonary resuscitation.

    d. Place the infant in a knee-to-chest position.

CRITICAL THINKING EXERCISES

1. A baby boy was born at 26 weeks' gestation to 15-year-old unmarried parents who abuse drugs. The infant weighed 1.5 kg at birth and was diagnosed with AVSD and Down syndrome. Discuss some of the major issues in planning for care. Include a care plan and a list of teaching needs for the family.

2. A 4-year-old boy has parents with little education, and the child has Medicaid coverage. Another child is 7 years old and has well-educated parents with private insurance coverage. Both of these children need a heart transplant, and a heart is available that is a very good match for both children. Discuss some of the issues involved in deciding which child should receive the heart.

3. A 13-year-old boy was diagnosed with hypertension over 2 years ago. He is noncompliant with his anti-hypertensive medication regimen. He is 5 feet tall and weighs 170 pounds. His favourite activity is video games. Develop a teaching plan for this teen, providing creative approaches at the appropriate developmental level.

STUDY ACTIVITIES

1. Teach a class of sixth graders about healthy activities to prevent high cholesterol levels, hypertension, and heart disease. Use visual materials.

2. Spend the day with a nurse practitioner in the pediatric cardiology clinic. Report to the clinical group your observations about the children's quality of life, growth, and development.

3. Observe in the pediatric cardiothoracic intensive care unit or telemetry unit. Note the different cardiac rhythms displayed by children with a variety of cardiovascular disorders.

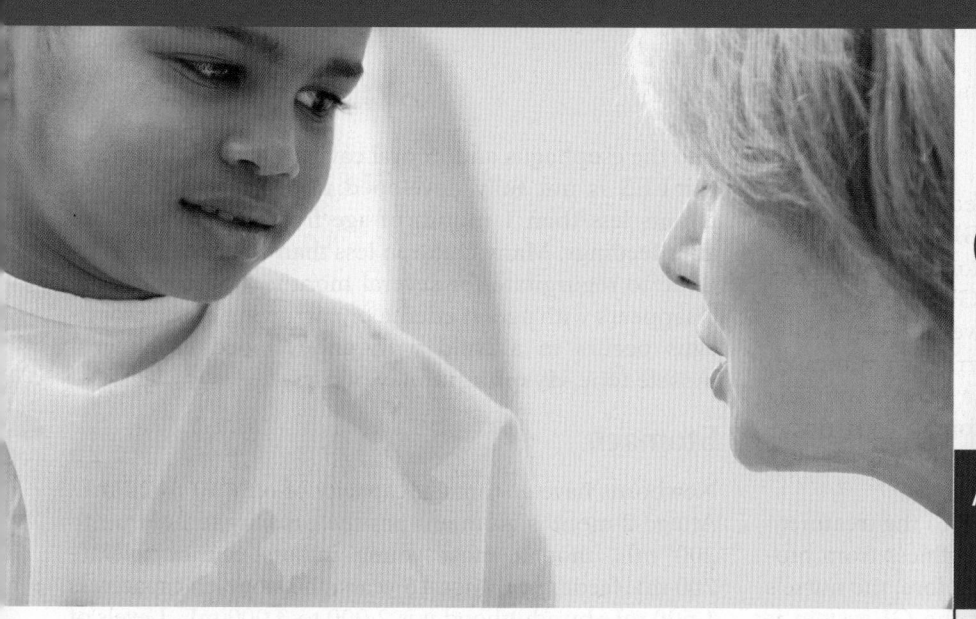

CHAPTER 41

Adapted by Cindy Holland

NURSING CARE OF THE CHILD WITH A GASTROINTESTINAL DISORDER

KEY TERMS

ALTE	dysphagia	lethargy
anal fissure	encopresis	protuberant
anastomosis	enteral	pylorus
atresia	fecal impaction	rebound tenderness
cholestasis	fibrosis	regurgitation
cirrhosis	guarding	steatorrhea
cleft	icteric	

LEARNING OBJECTIVES

Upon completion of the chapter, the learner will be able to:

1. Compare the differences in the anatomy and physiology of the gastrointestinal system between children and adults.
2. Discuss common medical treatments for infants and children with gastrointestinal disorders.
3. Discuss common laboratory and diagnostic tests used to identify disorders of the gastrointestinal tract.
4. Discuss medication therapy used in infants and children with gastrointestinal disorders.
5. Recognize risk factors associated with various gastrointestinal illnesses.
6. Differentiate between acute and chronic gastrointestinal disorders.
7. Distinguish common gastrointestinal illnesses of childhood.
8. Discuss nursing interventions commonly used for gastrointestinal illnesses.
9. Devise an individualized nursing care plan for infants/children with a gastrointestinal disorder.
10. Develop teaching plans for family/patient education for children with gastrointestinal illnesses.
11. Describe the psychosocial impact that chronic gastrointestinal illnesses have on children.

Ethan Richardson, 2 months old, is brought to the clinic by his mother. He has been vomiting for the past 3 days. His mother states she switched formula to see if that would help, but the vomiting worsened. Since last night she has attempted to feed him only Pedialyte. Mrs. Roberts says, "He can't keep anything down and he's very irritable." His weight at birth was 3.9 kg, length 52.5 cm, and head circumference 37 cm. At his 2-month check-up last week he weighed 5.9 kg.

WoW

Children instinctively eat to live, and the nurse can help them devour the joys that life brings.

Gastrointestinal (GI) disorders affect children of all ages. The most common result of a GI illness is dehydration, requiring fluid therapy at home or, in more extreme cases, in a hospital setting. GI illnesses range from acute to chronic problems. However, even acute, non–life-threatening illnesses (e.g., diarrhea or vomiting) can become life-threatening without proper nursing assessment and interventions. Therefore, all GI disorders should be taken seriously until symptoms are well controlled.

Patient and family education related to the treatment of GI disorders is key to preventing the illness from progressing to an emergency situation. Therefore, the nurse's knowledge of the disorders that affect the GI system is crucial. Most often, the parents or patient will contact the primary care provider in an out-patient setting to seek help. The nurse is usually the person to triage the phone call to determine the next step in the situation, which may be determining whether the patient should be managed at home, brought to the office for assessment, or sent directly to an emergency room for evaluation. The majority of GI disorders can be handled in an out-patient setting to avoid unnecessary hospitalizations, but some life-threatening problems (e.g., bowel obstruction) require emergency care in the hospital. Again, the knowledge base of the nurse is instrumental in obtaining the proper information by taking a thorough and accurate health history from the caregiver or patient.

Variations in Pediatric Anatomy and Physiology

The GI tract includes all of the structures from the mouth to the anus. The primary functions of the GI system are the digestion and absorption of nutrients and water, elimination of waste products, and secretion of various substances required for digestion. Babies are born with a GI tract that is not fully mature until age 2. Due to this immaturity, there are many differences between the digestive tract of the young child and that of the older child or adult.

Mouth

The mouth is highly vascular, making it a common entry point for infectious invaders. In addition, infants and young child repeatedly bring objects to their mouths and explore them in that fashion. This behaviour increases the infant's and young child's risk for contracting infectious agents via the mouth.

Esophagus

The esophagus provides a passageway from the mouth to the stomach for food. The lower esophageal sphincter (LES) prevents **regurgitation** of stomach contents up into the esophagus and/or oral cavity. The muscle tone of the LES is not fully developed until age 1 month, so infants less than 1 month of age frequently regurgitate after feedings. Many children less than 1 year of age continue to regurgitate for several months, but this usually disappears with age. If edema or narrowing of the esophagus occurs in a child with undeveloped esophageal muscle tone, **dysphagia** may occur.

Stomach

Newborns have a stomach capacity of only 10 to 20 mL. At age 2 months an infant has the capacity to hold up to 200 mL, though most young infants cannot tolerate 200 mL feedings. By age 16 years, the stomach capacity is 1,500 mL; by adulthood it is 2,000 to 3,000 mL. Levels of hydrochloric acid, which is found in gastric contents to aid in digestion, reach adult levels by age 6 months.

Intestines

A full-term infant has approximately 250 cm of small intestine; an adult has up to 600 cm. The function of the small intestine is not fully developed at birth. Fat losses may be up to 20% of intake for a newborn, as opposed to 7% for an adult. Intestinal growth occurs in rapid spurts, usually between the ages of 1 and 3 years and again between 15 and 16 years. Infants who have small bowel loss during early infancy have more problems with absorption and diarrhea than adults who have the same amount of small bowel loss.

Biliary System

The liver is relatively large at birth, accounting for 5% of the infant's body weight, compared with 2% in an adult. This allows the smooth edge of the liver to be easily palpated in infancy, as much as 2 cm below the costal margin. The pancreatic enzymes all develop at certain postnatal times, not reaching adult levels until 2 years of age (Hamilton, 2000).

Fluid Balance and Losses

Children exhibit differences compared with adults that affect the ways that fluid volume is maintained. These differences are evident in body fluid balance and insensible fluid losses.

Body Fluid Balance
Infants and children have a proportionately greater amount of body water than do adults. Infants and young children require a relatively greater fluid intake and excrete a relatively greater amount of fluid than adults. This places them at higher risk for fluid loss with illness compared with adults. Until age 2 years, the extracellular fluid makes up about half of the child's total body water. Since extracellular fluid has a larger proportion of sodium and chloride,

when potential fluid-loss states occur, water loss occurs more rapidly and in larger amounts than in adults.

Insensible Fluid Losses

Fever increases fluid loss at a rate of about 7 mL/kg/day for every sustained 1°C rise in temperature. Since children become febrile with illness more readily and their fevers are higher than those of adults, infants and young children are more apt than adults to experience insensible fluid loss with fever when ill.

Fluid loss via the skin accounts for about two thirds of insensible fluid loss. Infants have a relatively larger body surface area (BSA) than older children and adults. The newborn's BSA is about two or three times greater than the adult's, and the preterm infant's BSA is about five times greater than the adult's. This places infants, especially young infants, at increased risk for insensible fluid loss as compared with older children and adults.

The basal metabolic rate in infants and children is higher than that in adults in order to support growth. This higher metabolic rate, even in states of wellness, accounts for increased insensible fluid losses and an increased need for water for excretory functions. The young infant's renal immaturity does not allow the kidneys to concentrate urine as well as in older children and adults. This puts infants at particular risk for dehydration or overhydration, depending upon the circumstances.

Common Medical Treatments

There are many different forms of medical treatment for GI disorders. In the hospital setting, most medical treatments will require a physician's order. The most common treatments and medications used for GI disorders are listed in Common Medical Treatments 41.1 and Drug Guide 41.1. Both tables provide essential information about medical treatments and medications used in pediatric GI disorders. These tables should be referred to as needed while completing the remainder of the chapter.

NURSING PROCESS OVERVIEW FOR THE CHILD WITH A GI DISORDER

Nursing care of the child with a GI disorder includes nursing assessment, nursing diagnosis, planning, interventions, and evaluation. Each step of this process must be individualized for each patient. A general understanding of the GI tract and the most common disorders can help to individualize these nursing care plans.

Remember Ethan, the 2-month-old with vomiting and irritability? What additional health history and physical examination assessment information should you obtain?

Assessment

The assessment of the child with a GI disorder includes a health history, physical examination, and laboratory and diagnostic testing.

Health History

A thorough health history is very important in the assessment of a child with a GI disorder. The health history includes past history (previous illnesses/surgeries), past family history, present illness (when the symptoms began and how this differs from the patient's normal status), and how the patient's symptoms have been managed up to this point (relevant medical records/home treatments). Detailed knowledge of the past medical and surgical history of the patient may reveal bowel resection, previous intestinal infections, and dietary issues and problems. The patient's growth patterns can also be an instrumental part of the health history and may help to generate a timeline for when the current problems appeared. The family history is also extremely important in identifying common genetic/familial GI symptoms or disorders such as irritable bowel syndrome, inflammatory bowel disease, or food allergies. The history of the present illness and symptoms can often distinguish chronic problems from acute disorders. All of these pieces of the health history require descriptive questions and answers from both nurses and patients. The person providing the history must be able to provide accurate details of the health history.

Physical Examination

The physical examination of the child should be done from the least invasive part of the examination to the most invasive. It is important for the child to remain as relaxed as possible during this part of the assessment.

Inspection and Observation

Inspect and observe the child's colour, hydration status, abdominal size and shape, and mental status.

Colour. First observe the patient's skin, eye, and lip colour. Pale skin or lips in a patient with a GI disorder may be a sign of anemia or dehydration. During liver dysfunction, the bilirubin levels can rise, causing the skin to look jaundiced (yellow). The eyes can also become **icteric**, further indicating that the liver is not functioning correctly. Inspect the abdomen for signs of distended veins, which can indicate abdominal or vascular obstruction or distention. As in any part of a physical assessment, watch for areas of ecchymosis, which may be a sign of abuse.

Hydration Status. The child's hydration status often indicates how severe the current GI illness is. Dehydration can occur rapidly in children, especially in infants

(text continues on page 1368)

COMMON MEDICAL TREATMENTS 41.1   Gastrointestinal Disorders

Treatment	Explanation	Indications	Nursing Implications
Cleansing enema	Insertion of fluid into the rectum to soften the stool and stimulate bowel activity	Fecal impaction, severe constipation	Explain procedure to child prior to enema With multiple enemas, observe for electrolyte imbalances
Bowel preparation	Use of highly osmotic fluids to induce severe diarrhea to cleanse the entire bowel	Preparation for colonoscopy or bowel surgery	Some children may need to have a nasogastric tube placed so they can consume the needed amounts of fluids. Observe for signs and symptoms of dehydration/electrolyte imbalances
Feeding tubes	Flexible tubes used for enteral feeding when the infant or child is incapable of swallowing safely or for augmenting nutrition. May be orogastric, nasogastric, gastrostomy, or jejunostomy	Feeding difficulties, failure to thrive, gastroesophageal reflux disease, chronic illness	Orogastric and nasogastric tubes must be checked for placement prior to each use. If required long term, use a softer, flexible tube intended for long-term use. A barrier applied to the cheek may decrease risk of skin breakdown from tape Gastrostomy tubes vary in type Keep insertion site clean and dry
Intravenous therapy	Administration of fluids via a catheter that delivers electrolytes and fluids into the venous system	Dehydration, bowel rest, NPO status	Monitor intravenous site for redness, swelling, and pain Assess urine output to evaluate hydration status
Ostomy	A portion of the intestine is brought to the level of the skin to allow passage of stool	Imperforate anus, gastroschisis, omphalocele, Hirschsprung's disease, necrotizing enterocolitis, Crohn's disease, ulcerative colitis, trauma	Ostomy contents may be acidic and irritate the skin. Use a barrier paste or strip under the pouch to protect the peristomal skin Pouch should fit the stoma correctly Assess stoma for pinkness and moist appearance
Oral rehydration therapy	Administration by mouth of fluids that contain certain amounts of electrolytes and glucose to prevent dehydration and/or promote rehydration	Diarrhea, acute gastroenteritis, vomiting	Fluid administration should begin prior to the onset of dehydration Urine output should be monitored to evaluate hydration status
Probiotics (*Lactobacillus acidophilus*)	Food supplement containing dormant bacteria that when activated may alter the intestinal microflora	Treatment/prevention of diarrhea	Particularly helpful in preventing or decreasing the incidence of antibiotic-induced diarrhea
Total parenteral nutrition (TPN)	Intravenous complete nutrition that provides glucose, protein, lipids, vitamins, and minerals	Long-term NPO status, swallowing difficulties, difficulties tolerating enteral feeding (short bowel syndrome, necrotizing enterocolitis)	Higher glucose and protein concentrations and solutions containing calcium require central venous access Monitor blood glucose levels with initiation, rate changes, and discontinuation Blood chemistries should be monitored on a regular basis

DRUG GUIDE 41.1   COMMON DRUGS FOR GI DISORDERS

Classification	Action	Indications	Nursing Implications
Histamine-2 (H₂) blockers (ranitidine, famotidine, cimetidine, nizatidine)	Decrease histamine production, thereby reducing gastric acid secretion	Heartburn, esophagitis, GERD, benign duodenal or gastric ulcers	May cause drowsiness or dizziness
Proton pump inhibitors (omeprazole, lansoprazole, esomeprazole, pantoprazole, rabeprazole)	Block the pump that produces gastric acids	Erosive esophagitis, symptomatic GERD, *H. pylori* eradication	Adverse effects include headache, nausea, abdominal pain, or diarrhea
Prokinetics (metoclopramide, cisapride)	Stimulate GI motility to help empty the stomach faster and promote intestinal motility	Delayed gastric emptying, intestinal dysmotility	Metoclopramide may have adverse CNS effects. Cisapride is available only in limited-access protocol studies
Antibacterials/antibiotics (metronidazole, vancomycin)	Treat bacterial infections of the GI tract	Suspected or proven bacterial infections of the GI tract, such as *C. difficile* or parasitic infections	May cause GI upset, diarrhea. Very important to finish entire course of treatment
Immunosuppressants (6-mercaptopurine, azathioprine)	Suppress the immune system to keep autoimmune disorders in remission	Crohn's disease, ulcerative colitis, autoimmune hepatitis	Drug levels should be checked to determine drug metabolite levels and potential for hepatotoxicity or bone marrow suppression
Stimulants (senna, docusate sodium)	Stimulate peristalsis in the large intestine to produce a bowel movement	Constipation associated with slow transit through the colon	May cause cramping or diarrhea. Stool patterns should be assessed continually
Laxatives (polyethylene glycol, milk of magnesia, lactulose)	Softens the stool to allow for easier passage through the colon	Constipation	Stool patterns should be monitored. Dose may need to be readjusted frequently to find the correct dose for the patient
Antidiarrheals (loperamide, diphenoxylate/atropine)	Decrease peristalsis, thus prolonging transit time of stool through the intestines	Diarrhea related to short bowel syndrome, chronic nonspecific diarrhea, irritable bowel syndrome	May cause drowsiness or constipation
Corticosteroids (prednisone)	Act systemically to reduce inflammation and suppress the normal immune response	Inflammatory bowel disease, autoimmune disorders	Systemic adverse effects include hirsutism, osteoporosis, GI upset, cushingoid appearance, increased intraocular pressure, irritability, and personality changes. Should be taken as directed. Stopping the medication suddenly may cause adrenal insufficiency
Antiemetics (metoclopramide, dimenhydrinate, ondansetron)	Act on the central nervous system transmitters to prevent vomiting	Severe nausea and/or vomiting	May have adverse CNS effects, such as drowsiness or irritability

(continued)

DRUG GUIDE 41.1 COMMON DRUGS FOR GI DISORDERS (continued)

Classification	Action	Indications	Nursing Implications
Anticholinergics/antispasmodics (hyoscyamine, dicyclomine, glycopyrrolate)	Used to control abdominal spasms and cramping	Irritable bowel syndrome, functional bowel disorders	May cause excessive thirst or dizziness Encourage plenty of fluids while taking these medications
Anti-inflammatories (mesalamine, balsalazide, hydrocortisone enemas/suppositories, olsalazine, sulfasalazine)	Reduce inflammation in the colon	Ulcerative colitis, proctitis	Stool output should be monitored to assess for presence of oral medications (indicating poor absorption)

Adapted from: Taketokmo, C. K., Hodding, J. H., & Kraus, D. M. (2010). *Lexi-comp's pediatric dosage handbook* (17th ed.). Hudson, OH: Lexi-comp.

and young children. The oral mucosa should be pink and moist. Skin turgor should be elastic. Decreased turgor and tenting indicate dehydration. During crying, especially in infants, the absence of tears may indicate dehydration. Assess the amount of urine output the patient has had in the past 24 hours.

Abdominal Size and Shape. Inspect the size and shape of the abdomen while the child is standing and while lying supine. The abdomen should be flat when the child is supine. An especially **protuberant** abdomen suggests the presence of ascites, fluid retention, gaseous distention, or even a tumour, but many children (toddlers in particular) have a prominent "potbellied" abdomen as a normal variation of their anatomy (Weber & Kelley, 2010). A depressed or concave abdomen could indicate a high abdominal obstruction or dehydration. Inspect the umbilicus for colour, odour, discharge, inflammation, and herniation.

Mental Status. Perform a brief mental status examination of all GI patients. Mental status changes can occur in many instances, such as when ammonia levels are elevated with severe liver disease, severe dehydration, anaphylactic reactions to foods/medicines, tumours, and other metabolic disorders. Irritability and restlessness are usually the early signs of mental status changes. **Lethargy** and listlessness can occur much more rapidly in children than in adults and should be identified promptly and treated emergently.

Auscultation

As with all patients, both pediatric and adult, auscultate bowel sounds in all four quadrants. Hyperactive bowel sounds may be noted in children with diarrhea or gastroenteritis. Hypoactive or absent bowel sounds may signify an obstructive process and should be reported to the physician immediately. Absence of bowel sounds

can be determined after a 5-minute period of auscultation. This can be extremely difficult to perform with children and infants, who may be uncooperative during the examination.

Percussion

Dullness or flatness is normally found along the right costal margin and 1 to 3 cm below the costal margin of the liver. The area above the symphysis pubis may be dull in young children with full bladders, which is a normal finding. Percussion of the remainder of the abdomen should reveal tympany. Note abnormal findings.

Palpation

Palpation should be reserved for last in the sequence of abdominal examination. First, lightly palpate the abdomen to assess for areas of tenderness, lesions, muscle tone, turgor, and cutaneous hyperesthesia (a finding in acute peritonitis). Then perform deep palpation from the lower quadrants upward to best feel the liver edge, which should be firm and smooth. In infants and children, palpate the liver during inspiration below the right costal margin. The tip of the spleen may also be palpated during inspiration; it should be 1 to 2 cm below the left costal margin. Palpable kidneys, except in neonates, may indicate tumour or hydronephrosis. The sigmoid colon can be palpated in the left lower quadrant. The cecum may be felt in the right lower quadrant as a soft mass. Areas of firmness or masses in the abdomen may indicate tumour or stool.

Tenderness in the abdomen is not a normal physical finding. Right upper quadrant tenderness could indicate liver enlargement or cholecystitis (Browne, Flanigan, McComiskey, & Pieper, 2007). Right lower quadrant pain, including **rebound tenderness**, can be a warning sign of appendicitis and should be reported to a physician immediately. Palpate the external inguinal canals

TEACHING GUIDELINE 41.1

Stool Specimen Collection Variations

- If the child is in diapers, use a tongue blade to scrape a specimen into the collection container.
- If the child has runny stool, a piece of plastic wrap in the diaper may catch the stool specimen. Very liquid stool may require application of a urine bag to the anal area to collect the stool.
- The older ambulatory child may first urinate in the toilet, and then the stool specimen may be retrieved from a new or clean collection container that fits under the seat at the back of the toilet.
- For the bedridden child, collect the stool specimen from a clean bedpan (do not allow urine to contaminate the stool specimen).
- Send the specimen to the laboratory immediately for accuracy of results.

Adapted from: Berman, J. (2003). Heading off the dangers of acute gastroenteritis. *Contemporary Pediatrics, 20*(7), 57–74.

for the presence of inguinal hernias, often elicited by having the child either turn the head and cough or blow up a balloon (Katz, 2001).

Laboratory and Diagnostic Testing

Common Laboratory and Diagnostic Tests 41.1 gives information about the tests most often ordered by physicians for children with GI illnesses. Some of these tests are ordered in the hospital setting; others are done on an out-patient basis. Typically, the nurse is involved directly in the laboratory tests while a specifically trained person performs the diagnostic tests. Regardless of who performs the test, nurses must be familiar with preparation guidelines for the patient, how each test is performed, and normal and abnormal findings and their significance so that they can provide patient and family education. Teaching Guideline 41.1 gives tips on collecting stool specimens.

Nursing Diagnoses, Goals, Interventions, and Evaluation

Upon completion of a thorough assessment, the nurse might identify several nursing diagnoses, including:

- Risk for deficient fluid volume
- Diarrhea
- Constipation
- Risk for impaired skin integrity
- Imbalanced nutrition: less than body requirements
- Pain
- Ineffective breathing pattern
- Risk for caregiver role strain
- Disturbed body image

After completing an assessment on Ethan, you note the following: weight 4.5 kg, length 59.5 cm, and head circumference 40.8 cm. The head is round with a sunken anterior fontanel, the eyes appear sunken, mucous membranes are dry, heart rate is 158, breath sounds are clear with a respiratory rate of 42, there are positive bowel sounds in all four quadrants, and it is difficult to palpate the abdomen due to the infant's crying. Based on these assessment findings, what would your top three nursing diagnoses be for Ethan?

Nursing goals, interventions, and evaluation for the child with a GI disorder are based on the nursing diagnoses. Nursing Care Plan 41.1 can be used as a guide in planning nursing care for the child with a GI disorder. The nursing care plan should be individualized based on the patient's symptoms and needs. Refer to Chapter 35 for detailed information about pain management. Additional information will be included later in the chapter as it relates to specific disorders.

Based on your top three nursing diagnoses for Ethan, describe appropriate nursing interventions.

Stool Diversions

Children may undergo stool diversions for a variety of GI disorders. Surgical procedures include the creation of an ostomy, which involves bringing a portion of the small intestine (ileostomy) or large intestine (colostomy) to the surface of the abdomen (Fig. 41.1).

Ostomy pouches are worn over the ostomy site to collect stool. The pouch must be of an appropriate size and placed at the mucocutaneous junction (where the stoma connects to the skin). Proper fit helps prevent the skin around the stoma from breaking down (Registered Nurses' Association of Ontario [RNAO], 2009) (Fig. 41.2). The pouch may be tucked inside the diaper or underwear or angled to fit outside the diaper or underwear. Pouches cannot be seen under most clothing because they are designed to lie flat against the body. Avoid tight or constricting clothing around the stoma site. Teach families to store ostomy supplies in a dry place. Educate parents to inform school staff that the child should be allowed to use the water fountain and the bathroom without restriction, and the school nurse should have extra ostomy supplies available.

Ostomy care for a child can be challenging due to the child's normal growth and development as well as activity. Empty the ostomy pouch when it is one third full. In the hospital the stool output is measured several times per day. The stool may be semisolid (colostomy) to very liquid

(text continues on page 1372)

COMMON LABORATORY AND DIAGNOSTIC TESTS 41.1

Test	Explanation	Indications	Nursing Implications
Abdominal ultrasonography	Visualizes abdominal organs and related vessels, fluid collections	Abdominal pain, vomiting, pregnancy, abnormal liver tests, abdominal mass, enlarged organs on palpation	Barium decreases visualization of organs on ultrasound
Abdominal X-ray (KUB)	Plain X-ray of the abdomen without contrast media	Constipation, abdominal pain, abdominal distention, ascites, foreign body, palpable mass, trauma	Usually ordered as flat and upright to allow for free air and fluid levels in the bowel to be detected
Amylase (serum)	An enzyme that changes starch to sugar, which enters the blood with inflammation of the pancreas	Acute pancreatitis, pancreatic trauma, acute cholecystitis	Increased levels are seen after 3–6 h of the onset of abdominal pain
Barium enema	After instillation of barium, fluoroscopically allows visualization of the colon	Constipation, bleeding, suspected lower bowel obstruction or stricture	Bowel preparation prior to examination may be ordered Stool will be light-coloured due to barium for a few days
Electrolytes (serum)	Sodium, potassium, CO_2, chloride, blood urea nitrogen (BUN), creatinine	To determine extent of dehydration	BUN and creatinine may be elevated with dehydration Sodium, potassium, chloride, and CO_2 levels can be greatly affected with dehydration
Barium swallow/ upper GI series	Visualizes the form, position, mucosal folds, peristaltic activity, and motility of the esophagus, stomach, and upper GI tract	Foreign body ingestion, abdominal pain, vomiting, dysphagia, malrotation	Females of reproductive age must be screened for pregnancy. Infants may need to be given barium via bulb syringe or NG tube
Small bowel series	Done in conjunction with upper GI series to visualize the small intestine contour, position, and motility	Suspected inflammatory bowel disease (bowel wall thickening), intussusception, feeding intolerance related to strictures	It is very important to encourage large amounts of water/fluids after test to avoid barium-induced constipation
Endoscopic retrograde cholangio-pancreatography (ERCP)	A fibreoptic endoscope is used to view the hepatobiliary system by instilling contrast to outline the pancreatic and common bile ducts	Pancreatitis, jaundice, pancreatic tumours, common duct stones, biliary tract disease	Monitor for infection, urinary retention, cholangitis, or pancreatitis after the procedure Performed only occasionally in children
Esophageal manometry	Tests the esophagus for normal contractile activity and effectiveness of swallowing by measurement of intraluminal pressures and acid sensors	Abnormal esophageal muscle function, dysphagia, chest pain of unknown cause, esophagitis, vomiting	Often done in conjunction with pH probe The manometric catheter is placed through the nose into the esophagus, which may cause nasal irritation/sore throat
Esophageal pH probe	A single- or double-channeled probe placed into the esophagus to monitor the pH of the contents that are regurgitated into the esophagus from the stomach	Vomiting, gastro-esophageal reflux, correlation of symptoms to gastro-esophageal reflux events, and high risk for problems, as in asthma, apparent life-threatening event, sinusitis, or choking/gagging episodes	A 24-hour study is most accurate A special diet during study is often used. Keeping an accurate diary of symptoms and feedings during the study is essential May cause nasal irritation/sore throat

Test	Explanation	Indications	Nursing Implications
Gastric emptying scan	Assesses the rate at which the stomach empties food into the small intestine by adding isotopes to food and visualizing with scans	Unexplained nausea, vomiting, diarrhea, abdominal cramping	Medications may alter gastric emptying times. Crying or stress during the examination may cause delay in emptying and should be documented
Hemoccult	Checks for occult blood in the stool	Crohn's disease, ulcerative colitis, malabsorption syndromes, diarrhea, abdominal pain	
Hepatobiliary iminodiacetic acid scan	Visualizes the gallbladder and determines patency of the biliary system by use of a radionuclide. The amount of radionuclide ejected from the gallbladder (ejection fraction) is calculated	Differentiate between biliary atresia and neonatal hepatitis; assess liver trauma, right upper quadrant pain, and congenital malformations	Intravenous line will be established to give radionuclide Pain during injection should be assessed and documented
Lactose tolerance test	After ingesting lactose, this tests the hydrogen levels in the breath, which will increase with lactose build-up in the intestines	Postprandial diarrhea, gassiness, bloating, abdominal pain	May produce similar symptoms during the test itself A positive test will require diet modification and education regarding lactose intolerance
Lipase (serum)	An enzyme that changes fat to fatty acids and glycerol appearing in the blood with pancreatic change	Pancreatitis, pancreatic carcinoma, cholecystitis, peritonitis	Lipase levels stay elevated longer with acute pancreatitis
Liver biopsy	A test done to evaluate the microscopic hepatic structures	Hyperbilirubinemia, jaundice, chronic liver disease, hepatitis	Monitor after procedure for bleeding complications Must maintain strict bed rest for up to 8 h
Liver function tests (LFTs) (AST/ALT/GGT)	Enzymes that have high concentrations in the liver	Elevations may indicate the severity of liver disease	May be affected by drugs or viral illnesses
Lower endoscopy (colonoscopy)	Allows visualization and biopsies of the lower GI tract from the anus to the terminal ileum with a fibreoptic instrument	Rectal bleeding, lower abdominal pain, suspected tumours or strictures, foreign body removal	The child must undergo a bowel cleansing prior to the examination Encourage fluids to prevent dehydration. Provide monitoring related to conscious sedation or anesthesia Monitor for possible complications of perforation, bleeding, increased abdominal pain
Meckel's scan	A gamma camera is used to identify gastric mucosa seen in the distal portion of the ileum after injection of radiopharmaceuticals	Rectal bleeding, anemia, used only to identify a Meckel's diverticulum	Gloves are worn by nurse during and after scan when radiopharmaceuticals are given
Oropharyngeal motility study (OPMS)	A study done with different textures to evaluate the dynamics of swallowing and reveal transient abnormalities	Dysphagia, recurrent aspiration	Usually done in combination with therapists and nutritionist

(continued)

COMMON LABORATORY AND DIAGNOSTIC TESTS 41.1 (continued)

Test	Explanation	Indications	Nursing Implications
Rectal biopsy	Biopsy taken of the rectum at different levels to assess for the presence of ganglion cells	Absence of ganglion cells indicates Hirschsprung's disease	Infants/children should be assessed for rectal bleeding after examination. A small amount of bloody streaks is normal the first 24 h
Stool culture	Stool is smeared on culture medium and assessed for growth of bacteria over a period of days	To determine bacterial cause of diarrhea	Requires minimum of 48 h for growth, several days to weeks in some cases Can be done with a small amount of stool
Stool for ova and parasites (O&P)	Checks for the presence of parasites or their eggs in the stool	To determine cause of diarrhea or abdominal pain	Requires about 2 tablespoons of stool
Upper endoscopy	Allows visualization and biopsies of the upper GI tract (mouth to upper jejunum) with a fibreoptic instrument	Dysphagia, foreign body removal, epigastric/abdominal pain, suspected celiac disease, hematemesis	Provide monitoring related to conscious sedation or anesthesia Monitor for complications of perforation/bleeding
Urea breath test	Used to detect the presence of *H. pylori* in the exhaled breath	*H. pylori* infection	Patient must not take proton pump inhibitors for 5 days, all antibiotic therapy and Pepto-Bismol for 14 days

From: Fischbach, F. (2003). *A manual of laboratory & diagnostic tests* (7th ed.). Philadelphia: Lippincott Williams & Wilkins.

(ileostomy) in consistency depending on the location of the stoma. Liquid stool output can be acidic, causing irritation and breakdown of the surrounding skin if the skin is not properly protected by the barrier of the pouch. Special attention to skin care around the ostomy site is essential. Products such as barriers and pastes or strips are available to help protect the skin (RNAO, 2009).

The stoma should be moist and pink or red, demonstrating proper circulation to the intestine (RNAO, 2009) (Fig. 41.3). Immediately notify the physician if

the stoma is not moist and pink/red or if it has separated from the skin or is prolapsed or retracted. Also notify the physician if the volume of stool output is greatly increased.

Perform ostomy care as needed; pouches usually need to be changed every 1 to 4 days or when leakage occurs. The word "stoma" can be used as a mnemonic for the steps for changing an ostomy pouch as outlined in Nursing Procedure 41.1.

(text continues on page 1376)

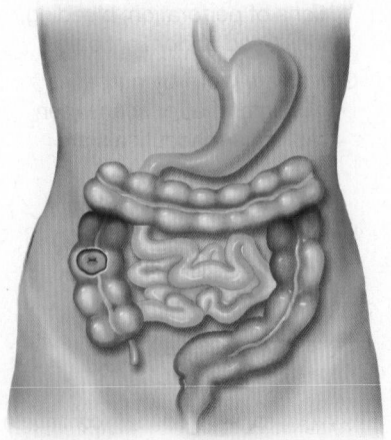
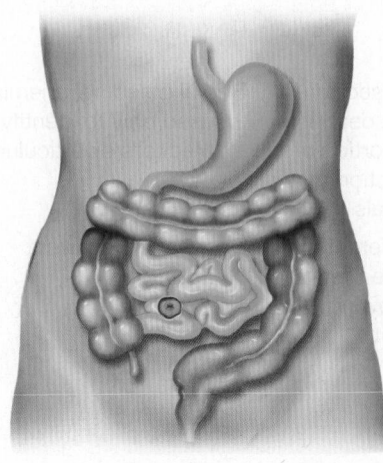

Figure 41.1 A colostomy is a stoma from the colon; an ileostomy is a stoma from the ileum.

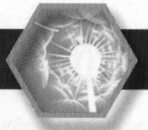

Nursing Care Plan 41.1

OVERVIEW FOR THE CHILD WITH A GI DISORDER

NURSING DIAGNOSIS: Fluid volume, risk for deficit: Risk factors may include excessive losses through vomiting or diarrhea, inadequate oral intake, possible NPO status (particularly in the surgical patient)

Outcome Identification and Evaluation
Child will maintain adequate fluid volume as evidenced by *elastic skin turgor; moist, pink oral mucosa; presence of tears; urine output 1 mL/kg/hour or more.*

Intervention: Maintaining Fluid Balance
- Maintain IV line and administer IV fluid as ordered *to maintain fluid volume.*
- Offer small amounts of oral rehydration solution frequently *to maintain fluid volume. Small amounts are usually well tolerated by children with diarrhea and vomiting.*
- When symptoms have lessened or resolved, reintroduce regular diet *to reduce number of stools, provide adequate nutrition, and shorten duration of effects of illness.*
- Avoid high-carbohydrate fluids such as Kool-aid and fruit juice, *as they are low in electrolytes, and increased simple carbohydrate consumption can decrease stool transit time.*
- Assess hydration status (skin turgor, oral mucosa, presence of tears) every 4 to 8 hours *to evaluate maintenance of adequate fluid volume.*
- Assess adequacy of urine output *to assess end-organ perfusion.*
- Maintain strict intake and output record and weigh child daily *to evaluate effectiveness of rehydration.*
- Weigh child daily: *Accurate weight is one of the best indicators of fluid volume status in children.*
- Discourage fluids and milk products that contain high levels of sugar during the acute phase of illness, *as these products may worsen diarrhea.*

NURSING DIAGNOSIS: Diarrhea: May be related to inflammation of small intestines, presence of infectious agents or toxins, possibly evidenced by loose liquid stools, hyperactive bowel sounds, or abdominal cramping

Outcome Identification and Evaluation
Child will experience decrease in diarrhea: *Will have bulkier stool as per normal routine.*

Intervention: Relieving Diarrhea
- Maintain clear liquid diet no longer than 24 hours, *as prolonged clear liquids will result in continued liquid ("starvation") stools.*
- Avoid milk products until diarrhea improves: *Temporary poor absorption from villus injury follows viral diarrhea.*
- Encourage complex carbohydrate foods *to bulk up the stools.*
- Add fat to carbohydrates *to increase intestinal transit time to encourage water absorption (bulks up stool).*

NURSING DIAGNOSIS: Constipation, related to GI obstructive lesions, pain on defecation, diagnostic procedures, inadequate toileting, or behavioural stool holding, possibly evidenced by change in character or frequency of stools, feeling of abdominal or rectal fullness or pressure, changes in bowel sounds, abdominal distention, and pain

Outcome Identification and Evaluation
Child will experience improvement in constipation *by passing daily soft bowel movement without pain or straining.*

Intervention: Relieving Constipation
- Palpate for abdominal distention, pain, and masses; percuss for dullness; and auscultate for bowel sounds *to assess for signs of constipation.*
- Encourage adequate fluid intake *to soften the stool.*
- Administer medications as ordered *to keep stool soft and moving on daily basis.*
- Encourage activity as tolerated: *Immobility contributes to constipation.*
- The child with stool withholding should sit on the toilet twice daily, preferably after breakfast and dinner, *to maximize chances for successful stool passage by taking advantage of the gastrocolic reflex.*
- For behavioural stool holding, demonstrate a positive and supportive approach with age-appropriate explanations *to encourage appropriate toileting.*

(continued)

Nursing Care Plan 41.1 (continued)

NURSING DIAGNOSIS: Skin integrity, risk for impaired: Risk factors include frequent loose stools, poor nutritional status, presence of stoma, acidic gastric contents contact with skin if gastrostomy present

Outcome Identification and Evaluation
Infant's skin will remain intact: *Buttocks skin will be free from rash, excoriation.*
In the child with an ostomy, skin surrounding stoma will remain intact: *Free from redness, rash, excoriation.*

Intervention: Maintaining Skin Integrity
- Change diapers frequently *to limit acidic stool content contact with skin.*
- Use barrier diaper cream *to protect skin.*
- Assess skin integrity at every diaper change *to recognize skin changes early so that corrective measures can begin.*
- Leave diaper area open to air several times a day if redness is present *so that air can circulate and skin healing can be facilitated.*
- Use plain water or only mild soap to cleanse the skin with diaper changes *to avoid pH changes that contribute to diaper area skin breakdown.*
- Avoid diaper wipes that contain fragrance or alcohol if the skin is red or has a rash, *as both alcohol and perfume cause stinging if used on non-intact skin and can worsen skin breakdown.*

For the child with an ostomy:
- Ensure proper fit of the ostomy appliance/pouch *to avoid acidic stool contact with skin.*
- Use a barrier (e.g., paste or strip) to attach appliance *to avoid repeated pulling of adhesive tape from skin.*
- If redness occurs, use stomadhesive powder on skin around stoma *to promote healing and prevent further skin breakdown.*
- Consult enterostomal therapy nurse as needed *to provide additional support.*

NURSING DIAGNOSIS: Nutrition: Imbalanced, less than body requirements; may be related to inability to ingest, digest, or absorb nutrients; intestinal pain after eating; decreased transit time through bowel; or psychosocial factors, possibly evidenced by lack of appropriate weight gain or growth, weight loss, aversion to eating, poor muscle tone, NPO status, or observed lack of intake

Outcome Identification and Evaluation
Nutritional status will be maximized: *Child will maintain or gain weight appropriately.*

Intervention: Maintaining Appropriate Nutrition
- Encourage favourite foods (within prescribed diet restrictions if present) *to maximize oral intake.*
- Administer enteral tube feedings as ordered *to maximize caloric intake.*
- Add butter, gravy, cheese as appropriate to foods (if allowed within diet restrictions) *to increase caloric intake.*
- Encourage high-quality, high-calorie snacks between meals, *so as not to interfere with meal intake.*
- Document response to feeding *to determine feeding tolerance.*
- Limit intake of calorie-free beverages: *Beverages should contain nutrients and calories.*
- Consult nutritionist *for appropriate diet supplementation recommendations.*
- Maintain calorie counts *to determine adequacy of intake.*

NURSING DIAGNOSIS: Breathing pattern, ineffective, risk for: Risk factors include postoperative immobility, abdominal distention or pain interfering with breathing, use of narcotic analgesics

Outcome Identification and Evaluation
Child will demonstrate effective breathing pattern: *Respiratory rate normal for age, absence of accessory muscle use, adequate aeration with clear breath sounds throughout all lung fields.*

Intervention: Promoting Effective Breathing Patterns
- Turn, cough, deep breathe every 2 hours *to encourage adequate aeration and discourage fluid pooling in lungs.* In the infant or toddler, turn every 2 hours and use percussor or chest physiotherapy *to prevent pooling of secretions.*
- Play games to encourage deep breathing (blow out penlight, blow cotton ball across bedside table with straw, etc.): *Children are more likely to cooperate with interventions if play is involved.*
- In the developmentally able child, encourage incentive spirometer use every 2 hours *to improve lung aeration.*
- Demonstrate/encourage use of pillow splinting with coughing *to decrease abdominal pain and stress on incision.*
- Administer analgesics as required *to relieve pain.*

Nursing Care Plan 41.1 (continued)

NURSING DIAGNOSIS: Caregiver role strain, risk for: Risk factors may include infant with congenital defect, child with chronic illness, problematic caregiver coping patterns, long-term stress, complexity and quantity of care child requires

Outcome Identification and Evaluation
Caregiver will exhibit emotional health: *Verbalizes concerns calmly, participates in child's care, and demonstrates knowledge of resources.*

Intervention: Easing Caregiver Role Strain
- Assess parental behaviour *to identify role strain.*
- Interview caregiver *to identify stressors and coping strategies.*
- Provide emotional support and encourage talking about feelings, fears, and concerns *to promote trust in nurse as a source of emotional support.*
- Arrange for and/or encourage respite care for child to *provide parent with time away from continual care.*
- Consult social services *to identify community resources available for caregiver support (home health, support group, etc.).*
- Encourage parent to meet own needs and find personal time *to increase energy level and self-esteem, ultimately enhancing the quality of care given.*
- Educate caregivers regarding child's pathology and medical management plan *to increase their understanding of the disease process and treatment, ultimately helping to address their fear of the unknown, encouraging their active and knowledgeable role in caregiving and promoting family-centred care.*

NURSING DIAGNOSIS: Body image disturbance; may be related to presence of stoma, loss of control of bowel elimination, scars from multiple surgical procedures, or effects of treatment regimen, possibly evidenced by verbalization of negative feelings about body, refusal to look at stoma, or participate in care.

Outcome Identification and Evaluation
Child or teen will demonstrate acceptance of change in body image *by verbalization of adjustment; looking at, touching, caring for body; returning to previous social involvement.*

Intervention: Promoting Proper Body Image
- Observe child's coping mechanisms *to reinforce their use in times of stress.*
- Acknowledge denial, anger, and other feelings as normal *to support child/teen through difficult transition.*
- Allow child gradual introduction to stoma *to ease transition.*
- Encourage child/teen to participate in care, *as this sense of control will contribute to positive self-esteem.*
- Allow adolescent or child decision-making opportunities *to increase a sense of control.*

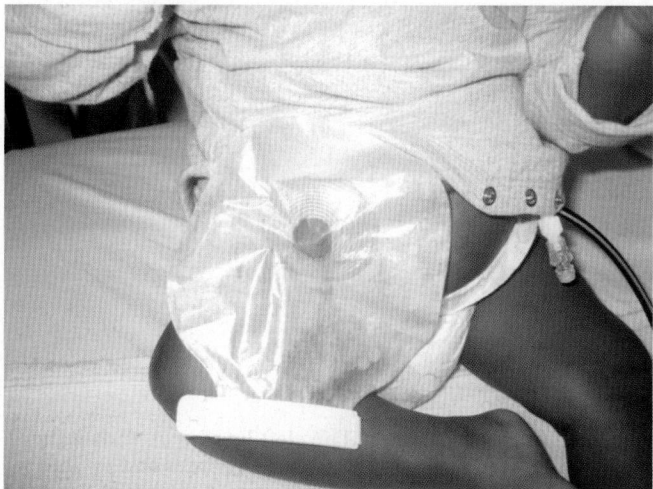

FIGURE 41.2 Ensure that the ostomy pouch fits closely around the stoma to prevent irritation of the surrounding skin.

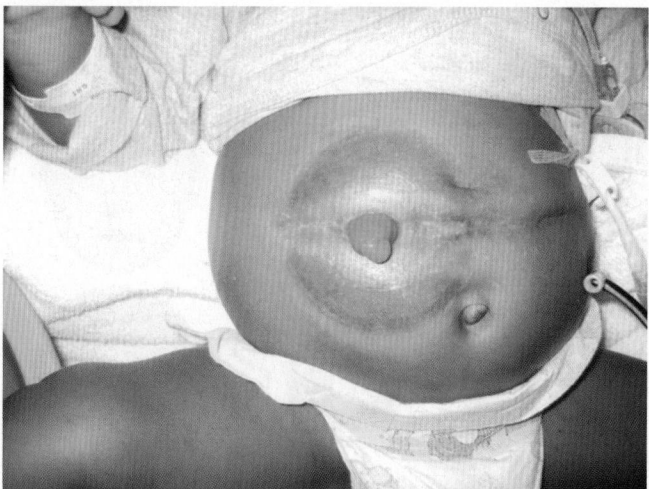

FIGURE 41.3 The healthy stoma is pink and moist.

Nursing Procedure 41.1

PERFORMING OSTOMY CARE

1. Set up the equipment:
   - Warm, wet washcloths or paper towels
   - Clean pouch and clamp
   - Skin barrier powder, paste, and/or sealant
   - Pencil or pen
   - Scissors
   - Pattern to measure stoma size
2. Take off the pouch (may need to use adhesive remover or wet washcloth to ease pouch removal).
3. Observe the stoma and surrounding skin. Clean the stoma and skin as needed, allowing it to dry thoroughly.
4. Measure the stoma, mark the new pouch backing, and cut the new backing to size.
5. Apply the new pouch.

Adapted from: Children's Hospital Boston. (2011). *Home care instructions for changing an ostomy pouch (bag or appliance)*. Boston: Author.

Ostomy surgery in the pediatric population brings challenges to both caregiver and child. There may be altered body image and other psychological issues. Depression and anxiety should be assessed when caring for a child with ostomy. Data suggest that assistance with coping strategies to manage these challenges is important in the postoperative period (RNAO, 2009).

Structural Anomalies of the GI Tract

Structural anomalies of the GI tract include cleft lip and palate, omphalocele and gastroschisis, hernias (inguinal and umbilical), and anorectal malformations.

Cleft Lip and Palate

Cleft lip and palate (Fig. 41.4) is the most common congenital craniofacial anomaly, occurring once in every 700 births (Mitchell & Wood, 2000). It occurs frequently in association with other anomalies and has been identified in more than 300 syndromes (Curtin & Boekelheide, 2010). The most common anomalies associated with cleft lip and palate include heart defects, ear malformations, skeletal deformities, and genitourinary abnormalities.

Complications of cleft lip and palate include feeding difficulties, altered dentition, delayed or altered speech development, and otitis media. The infant with cleft lip may have difficulty forming an adequate seal around a nipple in order to create the necessary suction for feeding and may also experience excessive air intake. Gagging, choking, and nasal regurgitation of milk may occur in babies with cleft palate. Excessive feeding time, inadequate intake, and fatigue contribute to insufficient growth (Cahill & Wagner, 2002). Primary or permanent teeth may be missing, malformed, or unusually positioned. Children with cleft palate may have slight delays in speech development, a nasal quality to the speech, and difficulty saying certain consonants correctly (Sharp, Dailey, & Moon, 2003). The opening in the cleft palate contributes to build-up of fluid in the middle ear (otitis media with effusion), which can lead to an acute infection (acute otitis media). Long-lasting otitis media with effusion leads to temporary and sometimes permanent hearing loss (Curtin & Boekelheide, 2010).

Pathophysiology

Development of the **cleft** occurs during the embryonic state of prenatal development. The tissue that forms the lip ordinarily fuses by 5 to 6 weeks of gestation, and the palate closes between 7 and 9 weeks of gestation. If either the lip or palate does not fuse, then the infant is born with a cleft. Cleft lip and cleft palate may occur in isolation

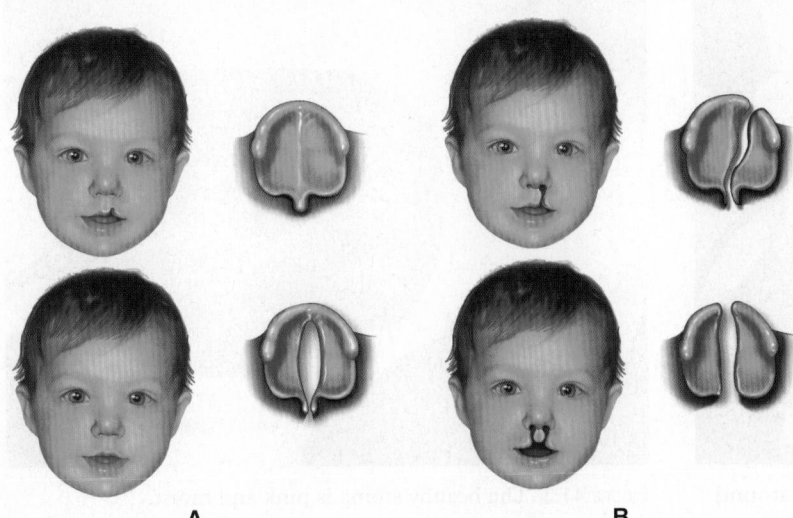

A   B

FIGURE 41.4 (**A**) The cleft lip may extend all the way through the vermilion border and up into the nostril, or it may be significantly smaller. (**B**) The cleft palate may be a small opening or may involve the entire palate.

from one another, but 50% of infants born with cleft lip also have cleft palate (Curtin & Boekelheide, 2010). The cleft may be unilateral (the left side is affected more often) or bilateral, complete or incomplete.

Therapeutic Management

Babies with cleft lip and palate are usually managed by a specialized team that may include a plastic surgeon or craniofacial specialist, oral surgeon, dentist or orthodontist, prosthodontist, psychologist, otolaryngologist, nurse, social worker, audiologist, and speech–language pathologist. Many children's hospitals offer these services in one location, such as a craniofacial specialty centre. Historically, cleft lip has been repaired surgically around the age of 2 to 3 months and cleft palate at 9 to 18 months, but institutions with an experienced craniofacial team have successfully repaired clefts in the neonatal period (Sandberg, Magee, & Denk, 2002). Early repair of the cleft lip restores a normal appearance to the child's face and may improve parent–infant bonding. Regardless of the timing of the surgical repair, however, surgical revision of the palate may be required as the child grows.

Nursing Assessment

For a full description of the assessment phase of the nursing process, refer to page 1365. Assessment findings pertinent to cleft lip and palate are discussed below.

Health History

For the newborn, explore pregnancy history for risk factors for development of cleft lip and palate, which include:

- Maternal smoking
- Diabetes
- Prenatal infection
- Poor prenatal nutrition
- Advanced maternal age
- Use of anticonvulsants, steroids, and other medications during early pregnancy

When an infant or child with cleft lip or palate returns for a clinic visit or hospitalization, inquire about feeding difficulties, weight gain and growth, respiratory difficulties, speech development, and otitis media.

Physical Examination

Observe the infant for the presence of the characteristic physical appearance of cleft lip. The cleft may involve the lip only or extend up into the nostril (Fig. 41.5). Cleft palate may be visualized on examination of the mouth. Palpate with a gloved finger to discover mild clefts.

Laboratory and Diagnostic Tests

Cleft lip may be diagnosed by prenatal ultrasound, but it is diagnosed most commonly at birth by the classic physical appearance.

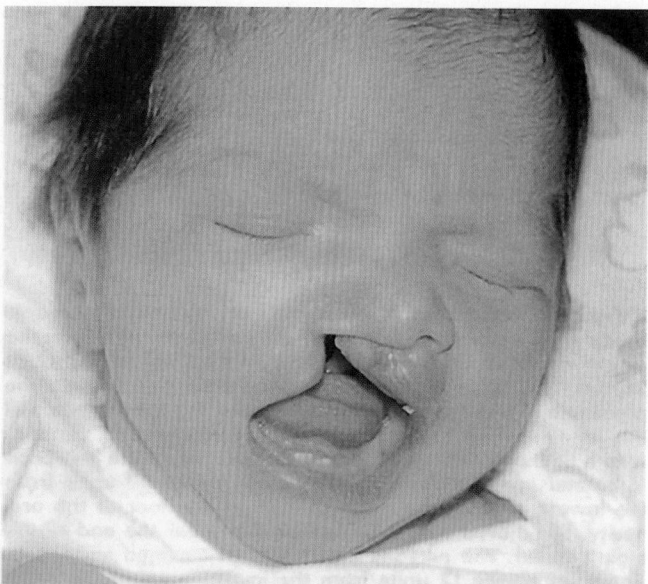

FIGURE 41.5 Cleft lip.

Nursing Management

Refer to the Nursing Care Plan 41.1 for nursing diagnoses and interventions related to airway maintenance, pain alleviation, fluid balance promotion, and restoration of family processes. These should be individualized for the particular situation. In addition to the nursing diagnoses and related interventions discussed in Nursing Care Plan 41.1, interventions common to cleft lip and palate follow.

Preventing Injury to the Suture Line

It is critical to prevent injury to the facial suture line or to the palatal operative sites. Do not allow the infant to rub the facial suture line. To prevent this, position the infant in a supine or side-lying position. It may be necessary to use arm restraints to stop the hands from touching the face or entering the mouth. Care for and protect the palate operative site by avoiding placing items in the mouth that might disrupt the sutures (e.g., suction catheter, spoon, straw, pacifier, or plastic syringe).

Prevent vigourous or sustained crying in the infant, because this may cause tension on either suture line. Ways to prevent crying include administering prescribed analgesics as needed for pain and providing other comfort or distraction measures, such as cuddling, rocking, and anticipation of needs.

Promoting Adequate Nutrition

Preoperatively, growth of the baby with a cleft lip may be optimized by breastfeeding. The contour of the breast against the lip may allow for a better seal to be maintained for adequate sucking (Reilly, Reid, Skeat, & the Academy of Breastfeeding Medicine Clinical Protocol Committee, 2007). A lactation consultant may be contacted to assist with breastfeeding techniques. Postoperatively, many

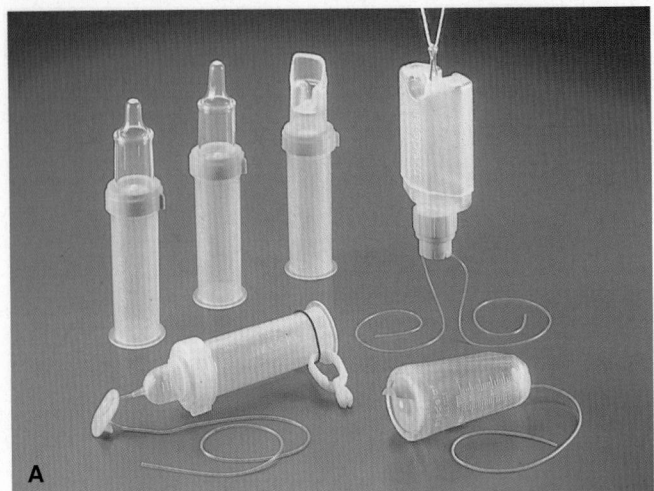

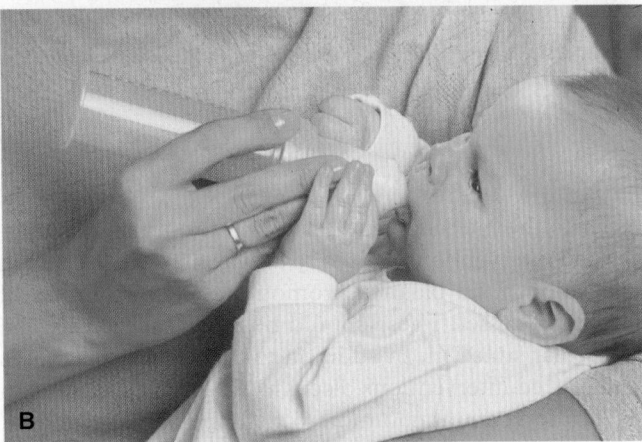

FIGURE 41.6 (**A**) Specialty feeding devices used for infants with cleft lip and cleft palate. (**B**) An infant uses a Haberman Feeder.

surgeons will allow breastfeeding almost immediately. Some infants will be fed with a special cleft lip nipple (Fig. 41.6). Parent and surgeon preference will determine the method of feeding. Burp the infant well to expel excess air taken in during difficulty with sucking.

The infant with cleft palate is at risk for aspiration with oral feeding and may have difficulty breastfeeding. In some instances a prosthodontic device may be created to form a false palate covering. This device may prevent breast milk or formula from being aspirated. In the bottle-fed infant, special nipples or feeders may have to be used. When the suture line is healed, ordinary feeding may resume.

Encouraging Infant–Parent Bonding

For some parents, the appearance of a cleft lip is shocking (Curtin & Boekelheide, 2010). Encourage parents to hold the medically stable infant immediately after delivery to encourage bonding. Acknowledge normal feelings of guilt, anger, and sadness. Support the parents in providing care for the infant, particularly feeding, which is a

viewed as a significant nurturing function. Provide education about the anticipated surgical procedure and eventual normal appearance of the child's lip.

Providing Emotional Support

Many families will benefit from support in addition to that received from the craniofacial team. Visit http://thePoint.lww.com/Chow1e for a list of websites that offer professional and parent-to-parent support for families of children with cleft lip or palate.

Meckel's Diverticulum

Meckel's diverticulum results from the persistence of the yolk sac or omphalomesenteric duct. The residual protuberant sac is usually located 100 cm from the ileocecal valve. Although usually asymptomatic, this sac may be present in 2% of the population (Browne et al., 2007) (Fig. 41.7). Meckel's diverticulum is the most common congenital anomaly of the GI tract (Rabinowitz & Hongye, 2010). The risk of associated complications decreases with advancing age; thus infants under the age of 1 year are at the greatest risk for complications (21%). The rule of twos is often applied to Meckel's diverticulum: it occurs in 2% of the population, it is located 2 feet (60 cm) from the ileocecal valve, it is usually 2 cm in both length and diameter, it involves two different types of tissue (gastric and pancreatic), males are twice as likely to have it, and it is usually symptomatic before 2 years of age (Browne et al., 2007).

The diverticulum contains all the layers of the intestinal wall, and peptic ulceration of the ileal mucosa adjacent to the ectopic gastric tissue of the diverticulum causes bleeding. Presentation is usually painless rectal bleeding (up to 60% of cases), anemia, intestinal obstruction (25%) (most commonly seen as volvulus and intussusception in

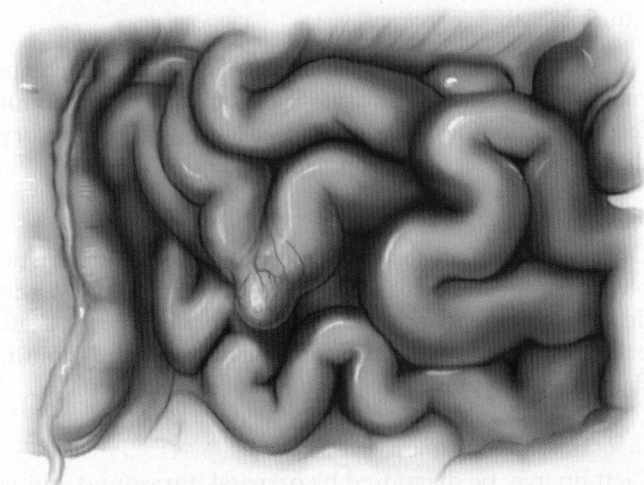

FIGURE 41.7 A Meckel's diverticulum is usually found within 100 cm of the ileocecal valve.

children) (Rabinowitz & Hongye, 2010), and diverticulitis (25%) (Browne et al., 2007).

Surgical correction of Meckel's diverticulum is necessary in patients who have complications. The surgery is usually done to remove the diverticulum itself. At times, ileal resection is necessary.

Nursing Assessment

For a full description of the assessment phase of the nursing process, refer to page 1365. Assessment findings pertinent to Meckel's diverticulum are discussed below.

Health History

Elicit a description of the present illness and chief complaint. Common signs and symptoms reported during the health history might include:

- Bleeding
- Anemia
- Severe colicky abdominal pain (in children with associated intestinal obstruction)

Physical Examination

Assess the child for an acute abdomen. Observe for abdominal distention, palpate for an abdominal mass, assess for abdominal **guarding** and rebound tenderness, and auscultate for hypoactive bowel sounds. Infants with painless rectal bleeding without obstruction will most likely present with a benign abdomen.

Laboratory and Diagnostic Tests

Common laboratory and diagnostic tests ordered for assessment of Meckel's diverticulum include the following:

- Abdominal X-rays to rule out an acute obstructive process
- Meckel's scan (conclusive)
- Stool tests for colour, consistency, and occult blood (usually positive in Meckel's diverticulum)
- Complete blood count (CBC) to assess for anemia
- Colonoscopy

Nursing Management

If anemia is significant, administer ordered blood products (packed red blood cells) to stabilize the patient before surgery. Administer intravenous fluids and maintain NPO status for symptomatic patients while further evaluation is being performed. Immediately report an acute abdomen to a physician. Postoperative care will vary depending on the surgery that was performed. Provide patient and family education as necessary to relieve anxiety related to the diagnosis and surgical intervention. Refer to the Nursing Care Plan 41.1 for additional information.

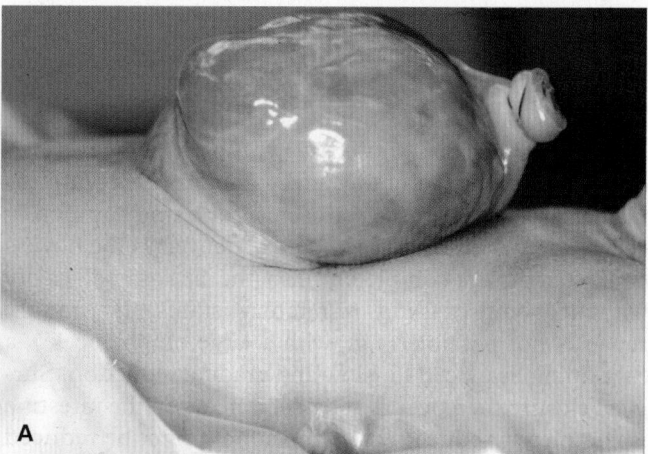

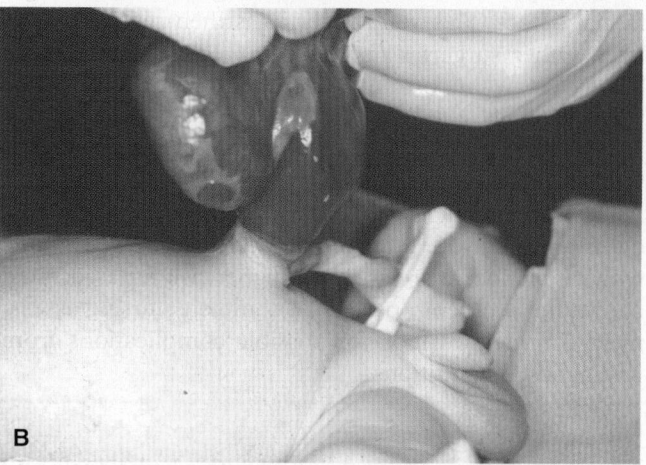

FIGURE 41.8 (**A**) Omphalocele: a membranous sac covers the exposed organs. (**B**) In gastroschisis, the organs are not covered by a membrane.

Omphalocele and Gastroschisis

Anterior abdominal wall defects, such as omphalocele and gastroschisis, occur in some infants (Fig. 41.8). The diagnosis of omphalocele and gastroschisis is usually made during a prenatal ultrasound examination. Omphaloceles are associated with an abnormal karyotype or genetic syndrome in more than 50% of the cases (Thilo & Rosenberg, 2011).

Gastroschisis tends to be associated with other anomalies less frequently. Omphalocele results from failure of the intestines to return to the abdominal cavity during 8th to 10th week of gestation. The intestine and other viscera, covered by a sac, herniate into the umbilical cord. This amnion covering protects the intestine. The defect may be large (>10 cm). In gastroschisis, the intestine and other abdominal contents herniate through the abdominal wall laterally and to the right of the normal umbilical cord (Lockridge, Caldwell, & Jason, 2002). The defect is usually small, less than 4 cm, and its cause is unknown. Unlike the omphalocele, the lack of a protective covering in gastroschisis results in inflammation and thickening of the bowel. This may lead to motility issues or intestinal strictures (Browne et al., 2007).

Therapeutic Management

A pediatric surgeon should see the baby at delivery to determine the extent of the defect and possible complications. Surgical repair of gastroschisis or a small omphalocele is completed within 24 hours of delivery if the bowels can be reduced completely into the abdominal cavity without compromising respiratory status. If primary repair is not possible (e.g., with a large omphalocele), a Silastic silo is placed for slow and gradual reduction. Surgical closure then occurs at a later date when the intestine is completely reduced. If the intestine cannot be reduced completely, the wound is allowed to granulate, leaving a fascial defect. This ventral hernia is then repaired years later. Other surgeries may be required to resect atretic bowel, create an ostomy, or place a gastrostomy tube (Browne et al., 2007).

Nursing Assessment

Assess infants born with either omphalocele or gastroschisis repeatedly for proper hydration status. Since infants with omphalocele are at much higher risk for associated congenital problems, perform a complete nursing assessment routinely to look for possible complications from undiagnosed conditions.

Nursing Management

Nursing management of the child with omphalocele and gastroschisis consists primarily of providing preoperative and postoperative care and family education.

Providing Preoperative Care

Nursing management in the postnatal/preoperative period should be focused on preventing infection and hypothermia, protecting the bowel, and providing fluid therapy and respiratory support (Browne et al., 2007). The infant is placed NPO and intravenous fluids, including total parenteral nutrition (TPN), are started. Before surgery, or if a staged reduction occurs, nursing care is aimed at keeping the infant sufficiently warmed, usually under a radiant warmer. Cover the abdominal wall defect with a plastic film and wrap it with a sterile dressing. A nasogastric tube will be inserted to decompress the stomach before repair. If ordered, administer intravenous antibiotics to prevent infection. Assess respiratory status as reduction of the defect and increased abdominal pressure may compromise respiratory efforts.

Providing Postoperative Care

Postoperatively, nursing care focuses on fluid and electrolyte maintenance. Administer TPN through a central venous catheter to provide nutrition while the bowel rests and the surgical site heals. The amount of time that the infant receives TPN will depend on progress to oral feedings once bowel motility occurs. Infants may require mechanical ventilation during this time. Administer antibiotics to prevent or treat infection (Lockridge et al., 2002). Dressing changes will be ordered based on the surgeon's preference.

Providing Family Education

Most cases of omphalocele or gastroschisis are diagnosed prenatally, so the parents have usually been educated on the diagnosis and what to expect during the pre- and postoperative courses. However, these infants usually have prolonged hospital stays due to the nature of these disorders. Mechanical ventilation and prolonged NPO status may lead to oral feeding issues, which may further complicate the infant's postoperative recovery. Bowel irritation from gastroschisis may result in dysmotility and a very slow titration of feeds. Teach the family about all aspects of care to help decrease their anxiety. Refer families to a support network; online resources can be found at http://thePoint.lww.com/Chow1e.

Small Bowel Atresia and Stenosis

Small bowel **atresia** (congenital) is a complete obstruction of the bowel lumen, while stenosis is a narrowing of the lumen. Atresias account for 20% of all neonatal small bowel obstructions. Forty percent are duodenal, 35% are ileal, and 20% are jejunal in location. Atresia occurs equally in males and females. Duodenal atresias are most often associated with other anomalies. Once the infant is stable, surgical repair is done to return bowel continuity. The atretic segment is resected and an anastomosis is done to connect the bowel ends.

Nursing Assessment

Assess the neonate for signs of intestinal obstruction (distention, bilious emesis, abdominal pain, and failure to pass gas or stool).

Nursing Management

Nursing management of the child with intestinal atresia consists primarily of providing preoperative and postoperative care, family education, and support.

Providing Preoperative Care

After the diagnosis has been made by radiologic imaging, the infant with an intestinal atresia requires gastric decompression with a nasogastric tube and suction. The infant is NPO, intravenous fluids are started, and bloodwork is monitored. The family requires education on the defect and management plan as well as support during this stressful period.

Providing Postoperative Care

Postoperative management includes gastric decompression with a nasogastric tube, TPN, intravenous fluids, monitoring of daily bloodwork, analgesia, antibiotics, and assessment of return of bowel function. Once bowel function returns, oral feeding may begin. Infants with less than 20 cm of small bowel remaining are classified as having a "short gut," which is associated with a poor prognosis (Browne et al., 2007).

Inguinal and Umbilical Hernias

Inguinal and umbilical hernias are defects that occur during fetal development. Either may be visible at birth, and inguinal hernias may be noted later in life (Sundaram, Hoffenberg, Kramer, Sondheimer, & Furuta, 2011).

Inguinal Hernia

In most cases of inguinal hernia, the processus vaginalis fails to close completely, which then allows the abdominal or pelvic viscera to enter the patent processus and travel through the internal inguinal ring into the inguinal canal. The hernia sacs that develop most often contain bowel in males and fallopian tubes or ovaries in females. Boys are more likely than girls to develop inguinal hernia and premature infants are particularly susceptible, with an incidence of up to 30% (Sundaram et al., 2011). Surgical correction of the inguinal hernia is performed soon after presentation of the defect to avoid incarceration and organ compromise.

Nursing Assessment

Assess infants and children with an inguinal hernia for the presence of a bulging mass in the lower abdomen or groin area (Fig. 41.9). It may be possible to visualize the mass, but often the mass is seen only during crying or straining, making it difficult to identify in the clinic setting. Groin thickening can be palpated, indicating that the inguinal canal is patent. The sac sliding over the cord is known as the silk glove sign (Browne et al., 2007). With a hernia, the testicle is palpable low in the scrotum below the defect; with a hydrocele, by contrast, the testicle is within the defect.

Nursing Management

A hernia that does not cause the infant or child pain does not require reduction. However, if the infant or child displays signs of severe pain and the large mass is palpable and not reducible, it may be incarcerated (Sundaram et al., 2011). A segment of bowel or gonad may be stuck in the canal, compromising blood supply to the organ. This requires immediate reduction or surgery if reduction is not possible. If reduced, surgical repair will occur usually within 48 hours to prevent repeated incarceration (Browne et al., 2007).

Contact the surgeon immediately if the hernia becomes irreducible. Routine pre- and postoperative care is expected during inguinal hernia surgical repair. Provide patient and family education to relieve anxiety.

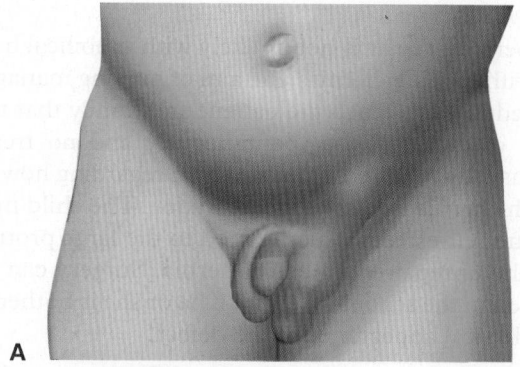

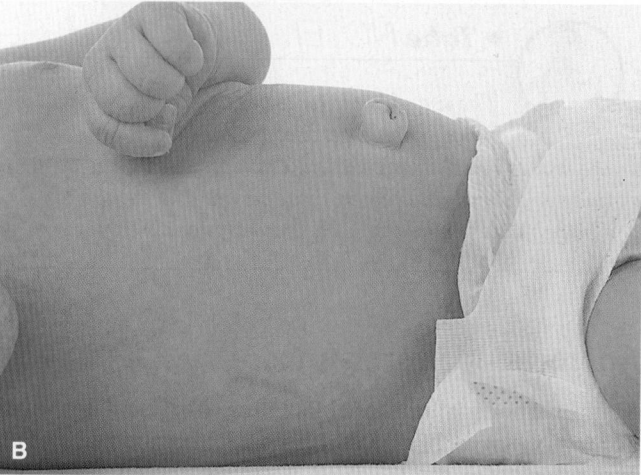

FIGURE 41.9 (**A**) Inguinal hernia: note the bulge in the inguinal (groin) area. (**B**) Umbilical hernia: note the protrusion in the umbilical area.

Umbilical Hernia

Umbilical hernia occurs in 10% to 30% of term infants but in up to 75% of preterm infants (Katz, 2001). Umbilical hernia is caused by incomplete closure of the umbilical ring, allowing the intestine to herniate through the opening. Unlike inguinal hernias, most umbilical hernias are not corrected surgically. Instead, most children will have spontaneous closure of the umbilical hernia by age 5 years (Sundaram et al., 2011). Surgical correction is necessary only for the largest umbilical hernias that have failed to close by age 5 years.

Nursing Assessment

The umbilical skin will bulge, which increases with crying. The defect can be measured by placing a finger into the umbilicus and palpating the ring defect in the fascia. Hernias may vary in size from 1 mm to 3 cm (Browne et al., 2007). Assess whether the hernia can be reduced. Notify the surgeon if the hernia will not reduce and the child appears to be in pain. Incarceration is extremely rare, but when it does occur the child will display signs of abdominal pain, tenderness, or redness at the umbilicus (see Fig. 41.9).

Nursing Management

Since operative repair is not as likely with umbilical hernias as with inguinal hernias, the aim of nursing management is education. Teach the patient and family that the majority of defects close spontaneously and no treatment is usually required. Educate them regarding how to reduce the hernia in case of incarceration. The child may have some self-esteem issues related to the large protrusion of the unrepaired umbilical hernia. Surgery can be performed in the school-age child if he or she is bothered by the physical appearance of the defect.

> ▶ *Take* NOTE!
>
> *The use of home remedies to reduce umbilical hernia should be discouraged because of the risk of bowel strangulation. This includes taping a quarter over a reduced umbilical hernia and the use of "belly bands" (Children's Hospital Boston, 2010).*

Anorectal Malformations

Malformations of the anal opening (imperforate anus) occur as often as 1 in 5,000 births. The obvious lack of an anal opening in the newborn is simple to recognize, but imperforate anus also occurs as a blind rectal opening. Frequently, a fistula accompanies the malformation from the distal part of the rectum into the perineum or genitourinary system. Numerous other congenital anomalies may be associated with imperforate anus (Sundaram et al., 2011).

Imperforate anus can be characterized as either high or low, depending on where the lesion ends relative to the levator ani muscle complex (Fig. 41.10). High lesions may end with a fistula from the bowel to the bladder, urethra, or vagina. Imperforate anus without a fistula has the rectum ending blindly about 2 cm from the skin. No stool will be passed. This type of imperforate anus neces-

---

BOX 41.1 **Anomalies Associated with Anorectal Malformations**

- VACTERL syndrome: **v**ertebral, **a**norectal, **c**ardiovascular, **t**racheo**e**sophageal, **r**enal, and **l**imb
- Esophageal atresia
- Intestinal atresia
- Malrotation
- Renal agenesis
- Hypospadias
- Vesicoureteral reflux
- Bladder exstrophy
- Cardiac anomalies
- Skeletal anomalies

---

sitates a colostomy to divert the colon to a stoma for a period of time after anorectoplasty is performed in order to allow healing to occur. This defect is frequently associated with Down syndrome (Browne et al., 2007). Low lesions have a perineal fistula, and dilation of the fistula can be performed to correct the lesion. Some infants require a staged repair in which the bowel is connected to the anal opening or an anal opening is created. Often several corrective surgeries must be performed to correct the genitourinary problems associated with imperforate anus (Peña, 2004; Wesson & Haddock, 2000).

Nursing Assessment

In the infant suspected of having an imperforate anus, assess for the common signs and symptoms of intestinal obstruction that occur when a fistula is not present. These include abdominal distention and bilious vomiting. In the newborn, observe for an appropriate anal opening. If the anal opening exists there is a fistula present. Observe for a meconium stool to be passed within the first 24 hours of life. Assess urine output to identify genitourinary problems. Radiographic studies are needed to further assess for complications associated with imperforate anus.

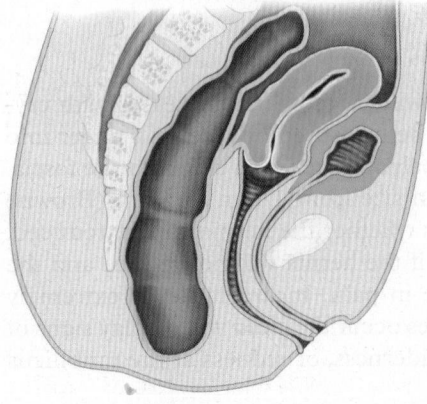 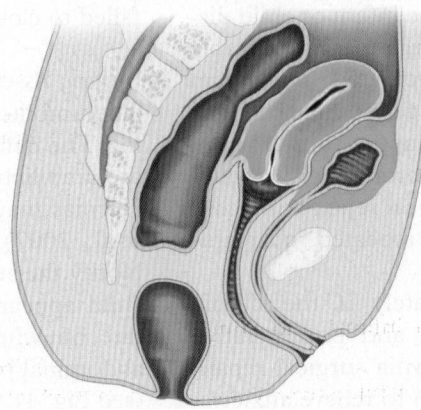

FIGURE 41.10 In imperforate anus, there is not an obvious anal opening from the rectum.

Nursing Management

When a fistula is not present, intravenous fluids are provided and the infant is NPO. Educate the family on the defect and the management plan. Postoperatively, teach colostomy care to the family whose child requires a permanent or temporary colostomy for passage of stool. Assess for and teach the parents about postoperative complications, including strictures, prolapse, constipation, or incontinence. Review long-term care regarding bowel continence with the family; the child with a high lesion may have problems with fecal incontinence up to school age.

For infants with low defects or fistulas, an anoplasty is performed. The anal opening is moved to the correct position and a larger opening is created. Nothing should be inserted rectally for two weeks to allow healing. Anal dilations are then initiated on a daily basis to prevent anal stricturing. Educate the caregivers on how and how often to use the dilators.

For the infant with a colostomy, anoplasty is done at a later date. Some surgeons may choose to do a pull-through procedure when the infant is several months old. Others prefer to leave the colostomy in place to allow healing and surgically close the colostomy at a later date. Still others will close the colostomy at the same time as the pull-through procedure. Regardless, it will be the first time that stool has passed through the anal sphincter. The stool may be quite loose depending on the severity of the imperforate anus. The perianal skin is at significant risk for breakdown, so a barrier cream should be used on that area and it should be cleaned once daily with soap and water. Otherwise, wipe liquid stool off the barrier cream with mineral oil and cotton balls. Most of the barrier cream will remain intact, protecting the infant's perianal area.

▶ **Take** NOTE!

To decrease the drying associated with frequent cleaning, avoid baby wipes and frequent use of soap and water.

Acute GI Disorders

Acute GI disorders include dehydration, vomiting, diarrhea, oral candidiasis, oral lesions, hypertrophic pyloric stenosis, necrotizing enterocolitis (NEC), intussusception, malrotation and volvulus, appendicitis, and Meckel's diverticulum.

Dehydration

Dehydration occurs more readily in infants and young children than it does in adults. The risk is increased in infants and young children because they have an increased extracellular fluid percentage and a relative increase in body water compared with adults. Increased basal metabolic rate, increased BSA, immature renal function, and increased insensible fluid loss through temperature elevation also contribute to the increased risk for dehydration in infants and young children as compared with adults. Dehydration left unchecked leads to shock, so early recognition and treatment of dehydration is critical to prevent progression to hypovolemic shock. The goals of therapeutic management of dehydration are to restore appropriate fluid balance and to prevent complications.

Nursing Assessment

For a full description of the assessment phase of the nursing process, refer to page 1365. Assessment findings pertinent to dehydration are discussed below.

Health History

Elicit a description of the present illness and chief complaint. Common signs and symptoms reported during the health history are included in Comparison Chart 41.1, which compares the clinical manifestations of mild, moderate, and severe dehydration.

Explore the patient's current and past medical history for risk factors for dehydration, such as:

- Diarrhea
- Vomiting
- Decreased oral intake
- Sustained high fever
- Diabetic ketoacidosis
- Extensive burns

▶ **Take** NOTE!

Nurses must be able to assess a child's hydration status accurately and intervene quickly. Children are at higher risk than adults for hypovolemic shock. Dehydrated children may deteriorate very quickly and experience shock.

Physical Examination and Laboratory and Diagnostic Tests

Assess the child's hydration status: heart rate, blood pressure, skin turgor, fontanels, oral mucosa, eyes, temperature and colour of extremities, mental status, and urine output. Children usually compensate well initially; their heart rate increases in moderate dehydration, but blood pressure remains normal until it decreases in severe dehydration.

Nursing Management

Nursing goals for the infant or child with dehydration are aimed at restoring fluid volume and preventing progression to hypovolemia. Provide oral rehydration to children

COMPARISON CHART 41.1 DEHYDRATION

	Mild	Moderate	Severe
Mental status	Alert	Alert to listless	Alert to comatose
Fontanels	Soft and flat	Sunken	Sunken
Eyes	Normal	Mildly sunken orbits	Deeply sunken orbits
Oral mucosa	Pink and moist	Pale and slightly dry	Dry
Skin turgor	Elastic	Decreased	Tenting
Heart rate	Normal	May be increased	Increased, progressing to bradycardia
Blood pressure	Normal	Normal	Normal, progressing to hypotension
Extremities	Warm, pink, brisk capillary refill	Delayed capillary refill	Cool, mottled or dusky, significantly delayed capillary refill
Urine output	May be slightly decreased	<1 mL/kg/h	Significantly <1 mL/kg/h

Adapted from: Johns Hopkins Hospital, Custer, J. W., Rau, R. E., & Lee, C. K. (2008). *The Harriett Lane handbook* (18th ed.). St. Louis, MO: Mosby; and Takayesu, J. K., & Lozner, A. W. (2010). *Pediatrics, dehydration*. Retrieved April 20, 2011 from http://emedicine.medscape.com/article/801012-overview.

for mild to moderate states of dehydration (Centers for Disease Control and Prevention [CDC], 2003; Dale, 2004) (Teaching Guideline 41.2). Continue breastfeeding, avoid sugary drinks, and offer oral rehydration solutions frequently. Children with severe dehydration should receive intravenous fluids (Khanna, Lakhanpaul, Burman-Roy, & Murphy, 2009). Initially, administer 20 mL/kg of normal saline or lactated Ringer's solution, and then reassess the hydration status (refer to Chapter 52 for further specifics regarding hypovolemic shock).

Once initial fluid balance is restored, the physician may order intravenous fluids at the maintenance rate or as much as 1.5 times maintenance. Maintenance fluid requirements refer to the amount needed under conditions of normal hydration. Maintenance fluid requirements may be determined with the use of the formula found in Box 41.2. In the example provided in Box 41.2, a 23 kg child will need maintenance fluid equivalent to 65 mL/hour.

The same anatomic and physiologic differences that make infants and young children susceptible to dehydration also make them susceptible to overhydration. Thus, continuously evaluate hydration status and be aware of the appropriateness of intravenous fluid orders.

Vomiting

Vomiting is the forceful expulsion of gastric contents through the mouth (Ulshen, 2004). It occurs as a reflex with three different phases:

TEACHING GUIDELINE 41.2

Oral Rehydration Therapy

- Oral rehydration solution (ORS) should contain 50 mmol/L sodium and 20 g/L glucose (standard ORSs include Pedialyte, Infalyte, and Ricelyte).
- Tap water, milk, undiluted fruit juice, soup, and broth are NOT appropriate for oral rehydration.
- Children with mild to moderate dehydration require 50 to 100 mL/kg of ORS over 4 hours.
- After re-evaluation, oral rehydration may need to be continued if the child is still dehydrated.
- When rehydrated, the child can resume a regular diet.

Adapted from: Stanton, B., Evans, J. B., & Batra, B. (2011). *Oral rehydration therapy*. Retrieved March 18, 2012 from http://www.uptodate.com/contents/oral-rehydration-therapy

BOX 41.2 Formula for Fluid Maintenance

- 100 mL/kg for first 10 kg
- 50 mL/kg for next 10 kg
- 20 mL/kg for remaining kg
- Add together for total mL needed per 24-hour period
- Divide by 24 for mL/hour fluid requirement

Thus, for a 23 kg child:
- $100 \times 10 = 1000$
- $50 \times 10 = 500$
- $20 \times 3 = 60$
- $1000 + 500 + 60 = 1560$
  $1560/24 = 65$ mL/hour

Adapted from: Johns Hopkins Hospital, Custer, J. W., Rau, R. E., & Lee, C. K. (2008). *The Harriett Lane handbook* (18th ed.). St. Louis, MO: Mosby.

TABLE 41.1 CAUSES OF VOMITING BY TEMPORAL PATTERN

Category	Acute	Chronic	Cyclic
Infectious	Gastroenteritis, otitis media, pharyngitis, sinusitis (acute), hepatitis, pyelonephritis, meningitis	*H. pylori, Giardia,* sinusitis (chronic)	Chronic sinusitis
GI	Intussusception, malrotation with volvulus, appendicitis, cholecystitis, pancreatitis	GERD, gastritis, peptic ulcer disease	GERD, malrotation with volvulus
Genitourinary	Ureteropelvic junction obstruction, pyelonephritis	Pregnancy, pyelonephritis	Hydronephrosis
Endocrine/metabolic	Diabetic ketoacidosis	Adrenal hyperplasia	Diabetic ketoacidosis, Addison's disease, acute intermittent porphyria
Neurologic	Concussion, subdural hematoma, brain tumour	Brain tumour, Arnold–Chiari malformation	Migraine, Arnold–Chiari malformation, brain tumour
Other	Food poisoning, toxic ingestion	Bulimia, rumination	Cyclic vomiting syndrome

- Prodromal period: nausea and signs of autonomic nervous system stimulation
- Retching
- Vomiting

Vomiting in infants and children has many different causes and is considered to be a symptom of some other condition. Table 41.1 lists common causes of vomiting.

Therapeutic management of vomiting most often involves slow oral rehydration and at times may require administration of antiemetics.

Nursing Assessment

For a full description of the assessment phase of the nursing process, refer to page 1365. Assessment findings pertinent to vomiting are discussed below.

Health History

Elicit a description of the present illness and chief complaint. Note onset and progression of symptoms. The assessment of an infant or child with vomiting should include a history of the vomiting events, including:

- Contents/character of the emesis
- Effort and force of vomiting episodes
- Timing

Contents and character of the vomitus may give clues to the cause of vomiting. Bilious vomiting is never considered normal and suggests an obstruction, whereas bloody emesis can signify esophageal or GI bleeding (Sundaram et al., 2011). Assess the effort and force of vomiting to identify whether the episodes are effortful and projectile, as with pyloric stenosis, or effortless, as is often seen in gastro-esophageal reflux (GER). The timing of the vomiting also is helpful in determining the cause.

Vomiting that occurs several hours past meals could signify delayed gastric emptying. When vomiting occurs upon waking or in the middle of the night, particularly if it is associated with headaches, an intracranial lesion or tumour may be suspected. Note any associated events, such as diarrhea or pain.

Diarrhea may occur with viral gastroenteritis or food poisoning. Pain in the epigastric area could signify peptic ulcer disease (PUD), pancreatitis, or cholecystitis. Assess the patient's past medical history to identify preexisting illnesses, drug abuse, trauma, prescribed medications, and previous abdominal surgery (Ulshen, 2004). Risk factors for vomiting include exposure to viruses, certain medication use, and overfeeding in an infant.

Physical Examination

Perform a physical examination, noting the child's general appearance. Note hydration status as well as mental status changes. Assess the abdomen for signs of trauma or distention. Note the quality of bowel sounds upon auscultation. Palpate the abdomen for the presence of abdominal masses, firmness, or tenderness.

Laboratory and Diagnostic Tests

Laboratory studies may be ordered to assess the child's hydration status or to rule out certain causes of vomiting, such as urinary tract infection, pancreatitis, or an acute infectious process. Common laboratory and diagnostic tests ordered for assessment of the cause of vomiting include:

- Abdominal ultrasound
- Upper GI series
- Plain abdominal radiographs

Nursing Management

Nursing management focuses on promoting fluid and electrolyte balance. Oral rehydration is accomplished successfully in most out-patient cases of simple vomiting. Teach the primary caregiver about oral rehydration (refer to Teaching Guideline 41.2). In the child with mild to moderate dehydration resulting from vomiting, oral feeding should be withheld for 1 to 2 hours after emesis, after which time oral rehydration can begin. Give the infant or child 15 to 60 mL of oral rehydration solution every 15 minutes, depending on the child's age and size. Most infants and children can retain this small amount of fluid if fed the restricted amount every 15 minutes. As the child improves, larger amounts will be tolerated (CDC, 2003; Dale, 2004).

> ▶ **Take** NOTE!
>
> *Homemade oral rehydration solution can be made by combining 1 L of water (can be water poured from cooking rice if desired), 8 teaspoons sugar, and 1 teaspoon salt.*

If oral rehydration is not possible due to continued nausea and vomiting, intravenous fluids will likely be ordered. In some cases, antiemetics may be used to help control the vomiting. Some antiemetics can cause drowsiness or other side effects and should not be used until a definitive diagnosis is made or severe pathologic processes can be excluded (Sundaram et al., 2011). Educate the family regarding the prevention of vomiting and use of antiemetic therapy.

> ▶ **Take** NOTE!
>
> *Ginger capsules, ginger tea, and candied ginger are generally useful in reducing nausea, are safe for use in children, and usually produce no side effects (White, 2007). Most commercially produced "ginger ale" no longer contains real ginger and so is of limited usefulness (Gardiner & Kemper, 2005).*

Diarrhea

Diarrhea is either an increase in the frequency or a decrease in the consistency of stool (Ulshen, 2004). Diarrhea in children can be either acute or chronic. Acute infectious diarrhea (gastroenteritis) remains the leading cause of death for children worldwide. In the United States, the incidence of diarrhea varies between 1 and 2.5 episodes per child per year, leading to 220,000 hospitalizations annually (Berman, 2003). The incidence rates are comparable in Canada; additionally, diarrhea and malnutrition are primary causes of morbidity and mortality in Aboriginal populations (Canadian Paediatric Society, 2006).

Pathophysiology

Acute diarrhea in children is most commonly caused by viruses, but it may also be related to bacterial or parasitic enteropathogens. Viruses injure the absorptive surface of mature villous cells, resulting in decreased fluid absorption and disaccharidase deficiency. Bacteria produce intestinal injury by directly invading the mucosa, damaging the villous surface, or releasing toxins (Berman, 2003). Acute diarrhea may be bloody or nonbloody. The viral, bacterial, and parasitic causes of acute infectious diarrhea are discussed in Box 41.3. Diarrhea may also occur in relation to antibiotic use. Risk factors for acute diarrhea include recent ingestion of undercooked meats, foreign travel, day care attendance, and well water use (Tablang, Grupka, & Wu, 2009).

Though most cases of diarrhea in children are of acute origin, it may also occur chronically. Chronic diarrhea is diarrhea that lasts for more than 2 weeks. This type of diarrhea is not usually caused by serious illnesses. Acute diarrhea usually resolves in 5 to 7 days, with most cases resolving in 2 weeks (Khanna et al., 2009). The causes of chronic diarrhea are listed in Box 41.4 according to age group.

Since most cases of diarrhea are acute and viral in nature, therapeutic management of diarrhea is usually supportive (maintaining fluid balance and nutrition). Probiotic supplementation may decrease the length and extent of diarrhea (Iannitti & Palmieri, 2010) (see Evidence-based Practice 41.1). Bacterial and parasitic causes of diarrhea may be treated with antibiotics or antiparasitic medications, respectively.

Nursing Assessment

For a full description of the assessment phase of the nursing process, refer to page 1365. Assessment findings pertinent to diarrhea are discussed below.

Health History

Elicit a description of the present illness and chief complaint. Important information related to the course of the diarrhea includes:

- Number and frequency of stools
- Duration of symptoms
- Stool volume
- Associated symptoms (abdominal pain, cramping, nausea, vomiting, fever)
- Presence of blood or mucus in the stool

Explore the patient's current and past medical history for risk factors such as:

- Likelihood of exposure to infectious agents (well water, farm animals, day care attendance)
- Dietary history

BOX 41.3 Causes of Acute Infectious Diarrhea

Viral	Bacterial	Parasitic
Rotavirus: characterized by acute onset of fever and vomiting, followed by loose, watery stools; most common cause of viral diarrhea	*Salmonella:* usually from ingestion of poultry, meats, or dairy products. Infants are at highest risk. Bacteria are excreted for up to 1 year. Severe cases are treated with antibiotics	*Giardia lamblia:* oral–fecal transmission; sudden onset of watery, foul-smelling stool; often causes gassiness and belching; treated with antiparasitic medications
Adenoviruses 40 and 41: second most common cause of viral diarrhea illnesses; similar characteristics to rotavirus	*Escherichia coli* 0157:H7: most often associated with gross bloody stools and abdominal cramping; may lead to hemolytic–uremic syndrome	*Entamoeba histolytica:* oral–fecal transmission; colitis symptoms common
Norwalk virus: more common in older children and adults; characterized by vomiting, nausea, and cramping abdominal pain	*Campylobacter:* symptoms vary from mild diarrhea to dysentery; severe cases may be treated with antibiotics	*Cryptosporidium:* spread via farm animals and people; fecal–oral transmission; watery diarrhea, nausea, vomiting, and flu-like symptoms. No definitive treatment
Caliciviruses: affected age is usually 3 months to 6 years; seen in day care settings	*Shigella:* high fevers and bloody stools are common; may cause seizures with fever. Treatment with antibiotics is recommended	
Astrovirus: affected age is usually 1–3 years; causes vomiting, diarrhea, fever, and abdominal pain	*Clostridium difficile:* usually related to antibiotic use; may cause pseudomembranous colitis in severe cases. Infants may be carriers of the bacteria and asymptomatic. Treatment with anti-infective medications may be helpful. Probiotic therapy is usually recommended	
Cytomegalovirus (CMV): causes other medical problems but may cause diarrhea with colitis	*Yersinia enterocolitica:* usually affects children less than 5 years of age; watery or mucoid diarrhea is common, occasionally with gross blood	

Adapted from: Sundaram, S., Hoffenberg, E., Kramer, R., Sondheimer, J. M., & Furuta, G. T. (2011). Gastrointestinal tract. In W. W. Hay, M. J. Levin, J. M. Sondheimer, & R. R. Deterding (Eds.), *Current pediatric diagnosis and treatment* (20th ed.). New York: McGraw-Hill; and Tablang, M. V., Grupka, M. J., & Wu, G. (2009). *Gastroenteritis, viral.* Retrieved April 20, 2011 from http://www.emedicine.com/med/topic856.htm.

- Family history of similar symptoms
- Recent travel
- Patient age (to identify common etiology for that age group)
- Use of antibiotics

Physical Examination

Inspection

Assess the child with diarrhea for dehydration. Observe the child's general appearance and colour. In mild dehydration, the child may appear normal. In moderate

BOX 41.4 Causes of Chronic Diarrhea by Age

Infants	Toddlers	School-Age Children
Intractable diarrhea of infancy	Chronic nonspecific diarrhea	Inflammatory bowel disease
Milk and soy protein intolerance	Viral enteritis	Appendiceal abscess
Infectious enteritis	*Giardia*	Lactase deficiency
Hirschsprung's disease	Tumours (secretory diarrhea)	Constipation with encopresis
Nutrient malabsorption	Ulcerative colitis	
	Celiac disease	

EVIDENCE-BASED PRACTICE 41.1
Effects of Probiotic Use on the Course of Diarrhea

● **Study**

Diarrhea (more than three loose, watery stools in a 24-hour period) occurs frequently in children. Most cases of diarrhea are caused by viruses, and symptomatic treatment is the only available therapy. The authors reviewed 23 randomized controlled studies that included a total of more than 1,900 participants. The studies evaluated the use of probiotics as compared with placebo or no treatment in relation to the severity and length of diarrhea.

▲ **Findings**

A variety of probiotics were noted to reduce diarrhea in infants and children as well as adults. Several of the studies demonstrated a shortened course of diarrhea when probiotics were used. The results were statistically significant, leading the authors to determine that probiotic therapy during acute diarrhea may be beneficial.

■ **Nursing Implications**

Probiotics are available as supplements: Capsules or powder that may be sprinkled on food. Additionally, live culture yogurt contains probiotics. Recommend these additions to the diet of older infants or children with acute diarrhea.

Allen, S. J., Okoko, B., Martinez, E., Gregorio, G., & Dans, L. F. (2007). Probiotics for treating infectious diarrhoea. *The Cochrane Library 2007, 4*. Indianapolis, IN: John Wiley & Sons.

dehydration, the eyes may have decreased tear production or sunken orbits. Mucous membranes may also be dry. Children with dehydration appear unwell overall. Mental status may be compromised with moderate to severe dehydration, as evidenced by listlessness or lethargy. Skin may be non-elastic or exhibit tenting, signifying lack of proper hydration. Abdominal distention or concavity may be present. Urine output is decreased if the child is dehydrated. Stool may be very loose or watery, resulting in anal redness or excoriation. Children with severe dehydration will also have pale or mottled skin, weak peripheral pulses, and delayed capillary refill time and will be tachycardic and hypotensive (Khanna et al., 2009).

Auscultation

Auscultate bowel sounds to assess for presence of hypoactive or hyperactive bowel sounds. Hypoactive bowel sounds may indicate obstruction or peritonitis. Hyperactive bowel sounds may indicate diarrhea/gastroenteritis.

Percussion

Percuss the abdomen. Note any abnormalities; the presence of abnormalities on examination for a diagnosis of acute or chronic diarrhea would indicate a pathologic process.

Palpation

Tenderness in the lower quadrants may be related to gastroenteritis. Tenderness with a mass in the left lower quadrant could be constipation. Rebound tenderness or pain should not be found on palpation; if found, it could indicate appendicitis or peritonitis.

Laboratory and Diagnostic Tests

Common laboratory and diagnostic studies ordered for the assessment of diarrhea include the following:

- **Stool culture:** may indicate presence of bacteria
- **Stool for ova and parasites (O& P):** may indicate presence of parasites
- **Stool viral panel or culture:** to determine presence of rotavirus or other viruses
- **Stool for occult blood:** may be positive if inflammation or ulceration is present in the GI tract
- **Stool for leukocytes:** may be positive in cases of inflammation or infection
- **Stool pH/reducing substances:** to see if the diarrhea is caused by carbohydrate intolerance
- **Electrolyte panel:** may indicate dehydration
- **Abdominal X-rays (KUB):** presence of stool in colon may indicate constipation or **fecal impaction**; air–fluid levels with dilated bowel loops may indicate intestinal obstruction

Nursing Management

Nursing management of the child with diarrhea focuses on restoring fluid and electrolyte balance and providing family education.

Restoring Fluid and Electrolyte Balance

Continue the child's regular diet if the child is not dehydrated. Initial nursing management of the dehydrated child with diarrhea is focused on fluid and electrolyte balance restoration. Refer to Nursing Care Plan 41.1. Probiotic supplementation while a child is taking antibiotics for other disorders may reduce the incidence of antibiotic-related diarrhea (Iannitti & Palmieri, 2010). After rehydration is achieved, it is important to encourage the child to consume a regular diet to maintain energy and growth (Diggins, 2008) (see Common Medical Treatments 41.1). The recommended algorithm for fluid management of children with gastroenteritis is outlined in Figure 41.11 (Khanna et al., 2009).

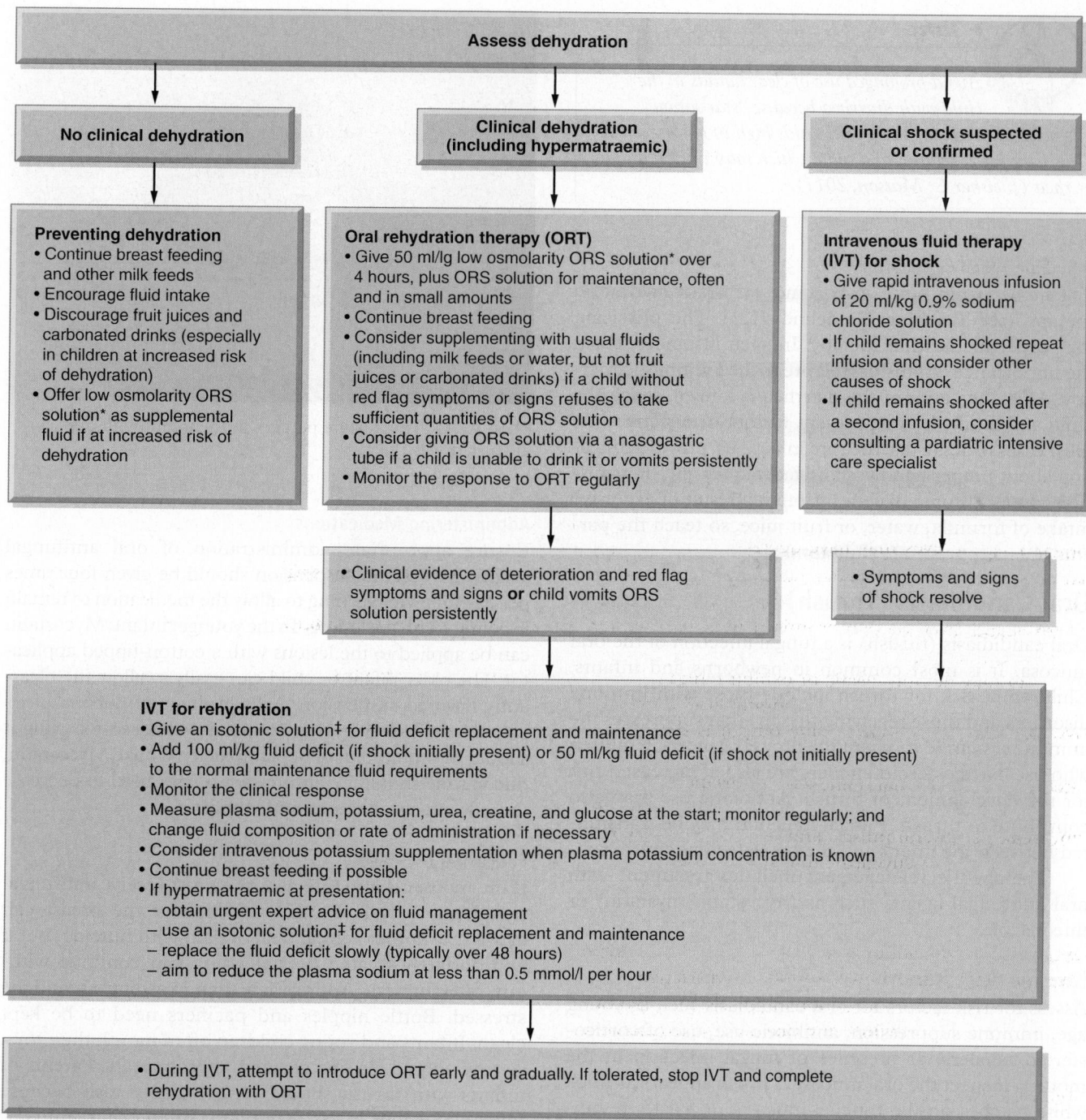

Assess dehydration

No clinical dehydration

Clinical dehydration (including hypermatraemic)

Clinical shock suspected or confirmed

Preventing dehydration
- Continue breast feeding and other milk feeds
- Encourage fluid intake
- Discourage fruit juices and carbonated drinks (especially in children at increased risk of dehydration)
- Offer low osmolarity ORS solution* as supplemental fluid if at increased risk of dehydration

Oral rehydration therapy (ORT)
- Give 50 ml/lg low osmolarity ORS solution* over 4 hours, plus ORS solution for maintenance, often and in small amounts
- Continue breast feeding
- Consider supplementing with usual fluids (including milk feeds or water, but not fruit juices or carbonated drinks) if a child without red flag symptoms or signs refuses to take sufficient quantities of ORS solution
- Consider giving ORS solution via a nasogastric tube if a child is unable to drink it or vomits persistently
- Monitor the response to ORT regularly

Intravenous fluid therapy (IVT) for shock
- Give rapid intravenous infusion of 20 ml/kg 0.9% sodium chloride solution
- If child remains shocked repeat infusion and consider other causes of shock
- If child remains shocked after a second infusion, consider consulting a pardiatric intensive care specialist

- Clinical evidence of deterioration and red flag symptoms and signs **or** child vomits ORS solution persistently

- Symptoms and signs of shock resolve

IVT for rehydration
- Give an isotonic solution‡ for fluid deficit replacement and maintenance
- Add 100 ml/kg fluid deficit (if shock initially present) or 50 ml/kg fluid deficit (if shock not initially present) to the normal maintenance fluid requirements
- Monitor the clinical response
- Measure plasma sodium, potassium, urea, creatine, and glucose at the start; monitor regularly; and change fluid composition or rate of administration if necessary
- Consider intravenous potassium supplementation when plasma potassium concentration is known
- Continue breast feeding if possible
- If hypermatraemic at presentation:
  – obtain urgent expert advice on fluid management
  – use an isotonic solution‡ for fluid deficit replacement and maintenance
  – replace the fluid deficit slowly (typically over 48 hours)
  – aim to reduce the plasma sodium at less than 0.5 mmol/l per hour

- During IVT, attempt to introduce ORT early and gradually. If tolerated, stop IVT and complete rehydration with ORT

*240-250 mOsm/l. The BNFC 2008 edition lists the following products with this composition: Dioralyte, Dioralyte Relief, Electrolade, and Rapolyte
‡Such as 0.9% sodium chloride, or 0.9% sodium chloride with 5% glucose

FIGURE 41.11 Algorithm to treat dehydration. (Reproduced from: Khana et al. Diarrhoea and vomiting caused by gastroenteritis in children under 5 years: Summary of NICE guidance. *British Medical Journal,* 338(7701), Figure 2, © 2009) with permission from BMJ Publishing Group Ltd.

> ▶ **Take** *NOTE!*

Avoid prolonged use of clear liquids in the child with diarrhea because "starvation stools" may result. Also avoid fluids high in glucose, such as fruit juice, gelatin, and soda, which may worsen diarrhea (Fleisher & Matson, 2011).

Providing Family Education

Teach the parents the importance of oral rehydration therapy (see Teaching Guideline 41.2). The physician may order medication therapy. In such instances, teach the importance of finishing all prescribed antibiotic therapy. After the cause of the diarrhea is known, teach the child and family how to prevent further occurrences. As most cases of acute diarrhea are infectious, provide education about proper handwashing techniques and transmission route. Chronic diarrhea is often a result of excessive intake of formula, water, or fruit juice, so teach the parents about appropriate fluid intake.

Oral Candidiasis (Thrush)

Oral candidiasis (thrush) is a fungal infection of the oral mucosa. It is most common in newborns and infants. Children at risk for thrush include those with immune disorders and those receiving therapy that suppresses the immune system (e.g., chemotherapy for cancer). Children who use corticosteroid inhalers are also at increased risk for the development of thrush. Antibiotic use may also contribute to thrush. Fungal infection may be transmitted between the infant and the breastfeeding mother.

Therapeutic management includes treatment with oral antifungal agents such as Mycostatin (nystatin) or fluconazole.

Nursing Assessment

Assess for risk factors for oral candidiasis such as young age, immune suppression, antibiotic use, use of corticosteroid inhalers, or presence of fungal infection in the mother. Inspect the oral mucosa. Thrush appears as thick white patches on the tongue, mucosa, or palate, resembling curdled milk (Fig. 41.12). Unlike milk retained in the mouth, the patches are not easily wiped off with a swab or washcloth. Also assess for presence of candidal diaper rash (beefy-red rash with satellite lesions). Determine the extent to which the presence of the lesions is interfering with the infant's ability to feed. The lesions may cause significant discomfort.

Diagnosis is usually based on clinical presentation, though a careful scraping of the lesions can be sent out for fungal culture.

Nursing Management

Nursing management of the patient with thrush includes administering medications and providing family education.

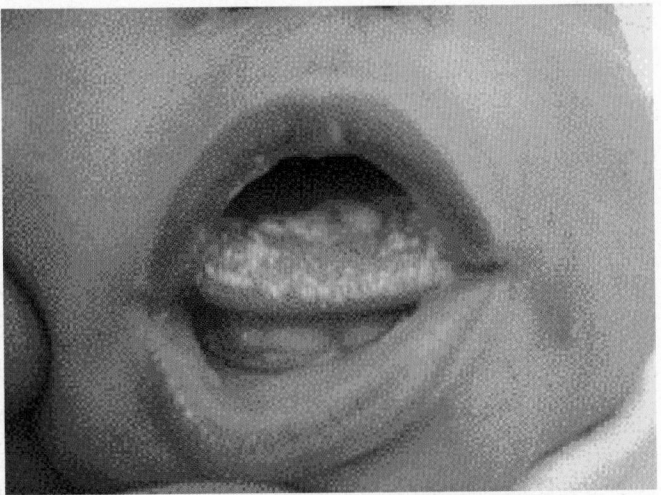

FIGURE 41.12 Thick white patches in the infant with oral candidiasis (thrush).

Administering Medications

Ensure appropriate administration of oral antifungal agents. Mycostatin suspension should be given four times per day following feeding to allow the medication to remain in contact with the lesions. In the younger infant, Mycostatin can be applied to the lesions with a cotton-tipped applicator. The older infant or child can easily swallow the pleasantly flavored suspension. An advantage of fluconazole is its once-daily dosing, but infants and children receiving it should be monitored for hepatotoxicity. Unlike Mycostatin, fluconazole should be administered with food to decrease the side effects of nausea and vomiting.

Educating the Family

If the mother is also infected, she must receive antifungal treatment as well. Fungal infection of the breast can cause the mother a great deal of pain with nursing, but if appropriately treated breastfeeding can continue without interruption. Appropriate handwashing should be stressed. Bottle nipples and pacifiers need to be kept clean. Infants and young children often mouth their toys, so toys should also be cleaned appropriately. Parents of infants with thrush should report diaper rash because fungal infections in the diaper area often occur concomitantly with thrush and also need to be treated.

> ▶ **Take** *NOTE!*

Geographic tongue is a benign, noncontagious condition. A reduction in the filiform papillae (bumps on the tongue) occurs in patches that migrate periodically, thus giving a map-like appearance to the tongue, with darker and lighter, higher and lower patches. Do not confuse the lighter patches of geographic tongue with the thick white plaques that form on the tongue with thrush.

TABLE 41.2 **ORAL LESIONS**

	Aphthous Ulcers	Gingivostomatitis	Herpangina
Cause	Trauma, vitamin deficiency, celiac disease, Crohn's disease	Herpes simplex virus	Enterovirus (coxsackie)
Appearance	Erythematous border, often yellow appearance to the ulcer, anywhere on oral mucosa or lips	Vesicular lesions on erythematous base, anywhere in oral cavity, including lips	Bright-red ulcers, generally in posterior oral cavity
Fever	Generally absent	May have high fever with initial outbreak	Abrupt onset of high fever (up to 39.4°–40.6°C), lasting 1–4 days
Length of illness	Generally heals within 7–14 days; may recur	10–12 days initially; may recur with stress, febrile illness, or intense sunlight exposure (as virus lies dormant in system)	Generally resolves within 5–7 days
Therapeutic management	Topical corticosteroid in dental paste may help	Acyclovir	Supportive treatment only

Adapted from: Gompf, S. G., Casanas, B. C., Carrington, M., & Cunha, B. A. (2010). *Herpangina.* Retrieved April 20, 2011 from http://emedicine.medscape.com/article/218502-overview and Plewa, M. C. (2010). *Pediatric aphthous ulcers.* Retrieved April 20, 2011 from http://emedicine.medscape.com/article/909213-overview.

Oral Lesions

A number of oral lesions may affect infants and children. A few of the most common are aphthous ulcers, gingivostomatitis (from herpes simplex virus [HSV]), and herpangina (Blevins, 2003; Leung & Kao, 2003). Table 41.2 lists the causes of common oral lesions. Regardless of type, oral lesions are often painful and can interfere with the child's ability to eat. Therapeutic management of oral lesions varies depending on the cause.

Nursing Assessment

Explore the health history for the presence of risk factors such as immune deficiency, cancer chemotherapy treatment, exposure to infectious agents, trauma, stress, or celiac or Crohn's disease. Note the onset of the lesion(s) and progression over time. Question the parent or child about the presence of sore throat or dysphagia (occurs with herpangina). Inspect the oral cavity, including the tongue, buccal mucosa, palate, and hypoglossal area. Note presence of lesions and their distribution. Refer to Table 41.2 for descriptions and illustrations of various oral lesions. Inspect the pharynx, which may be red with herpangina. Generally the diagnosis is based on the history and clinical presentation, but occasionally oral lesions are cultured for HSV.

Nursing Management

The primary concerns with oral lesions are pain management and maintenance of hydration. A corticosteroid-containing dental paste used for aphthous ulcers is formulated to "stick" to mucous membranes, so the lesion area should be as dry as possible prior to application of the paste. Children do not care for having the paste applied and will often resist. Older children with herpangina or stomatitis can "swish and spit" various formulations of "magic mouthwash" (typically a combination of liquid diphenhydramine, liquid acetaminophen, and milk of magnesia); these products may offer some pain relief. Common over-the-counter medications may be helpful for topical pain relief, though oral analgesics are often necessary.

The child with herpangina is typically a toddler or preschooler (Gompf, Casanas, Carrington, & Cunha, 2010).

It may be very difficult to coach a young child to drink fluids when his or her mouth is hurting. Playing games and offering favourite fluids and ice pops may encourage adequate oral intake. Carbonated beverages and citrus juices should be avoided when oral lesions are present as they can cause further stinging and burning.

> ▶ *Take* NOTE!
>
> *Viscous lidocaine should be used with caution as a topical treatment for numbing the lesions or as a swish-and-spit treatment, as younger children may swallow the lidocaine (Taketokmo, Hodding, & Kraus, 2010).*

Hypertrophic Pyloric Stenosis

Hypertrophic pyloric stenosis is one of the most common conditions requiring surgery in the first 2 months of life (Singh & Kass, 2010). Signs and symptoms typically present in the first 3 weeks of life but may present as late as 3 months after birth. In pyloric stenosis, the circular muscle of the **pylorus** becomes hypertrophied and elongated, obliterating the pyloric channel. A high-grade gastric obstruction results, and hyperperistalsis of the stomach causes projectile emesis (Browne et al., 2007) (Fig. 41.13). Many theories exist regarding the etiology of this condition, including trait transmission from the mother. The incidence is higher in males than females (4:1), and it occurs in whites more commonly than in children of any other race (Browne et al., 2007; Letton, 2001).

Pyloric stenosis requires surgical intervention once the infant's electrolyte imbalance has been managed. A pyloromyotomy is performed either through a small incision in the mid upper abdomen or laparoscopically. The pylorus muscle is cut, leaving the mucosa intact. This opens the pyloric channel and relieves the gastric outlet obstruction (see Fig. 41.13). Postoperative complications are rare.

Nursing Assessment

For a full description of the assessment phase of the nursing process, refer to page 1365. Assessment findings pertinent to hypertrophic pyloric stenosis are discussed below.

Health History

Elicit a description of the present illness and chief complaint. Common signs and symptoms reported during the health history might include the following:

- Forceful, nonbilious vomiting, unrelated to feeding position
- Hunger soon after vomiting episode
- Weight loss due to vomiting
- Progressive dehydration with subsequent lethargy

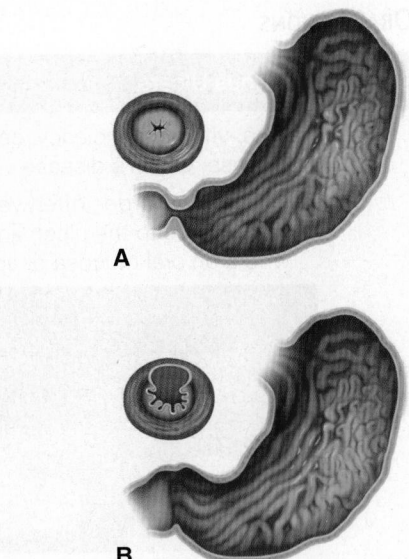

FIGURE 41.13 (**A**) Hypertrophied pylorus muscle and narrowed stomach outlet. (**B**) In pyloromyotomy, the pylorus is incised, thus increasing the diameter of the pyloric outlet.

Risk factors include a positive family history. The disorder occurs most frequently in first-born males.

Physical Examination and Laboratory and Diagnostic Tests

Palpate for a hard, moveable "olive" in the right upper quadrant (hypertrophied pylorus). If an easily palpable mass is felt, no further testing is necessary and a surgical consult is called. If no mass is identified, a pyloric ultrasound may be ordered to identify a thickened and elongated pylorus measuring greater than 3 by 15 mm. An upper GI series may identify pyloric stenosis as well, but an ultrasound is less invasive and is considered more diagnostic of pyloric stenosis. A peristaltic wave may be seen moving across the abdomen. Bloodwork may demonstrate hypochloremia, hypocalcemia, hypoglycemia, and unconjugated hyperbilirubinemia. The loss of fluids and gastric acids causes metabolic alkalosis (Browne et al., 2007). Assess laboratory values to determine if the infant has metabolic alkalosis resulting from dehydration.

> ▶ *Take* NOTE!
>
> *It may be difficult to examine the infant's abdomen when pyloric stenosis is suspected because of the infant's extreme irritability. A pacifier or nipple dipped in glucose water may soothe the infant long enough to obtain the abdominal examination.*

Nursing Management

Preoperative management of infants with pyloric stenosis is aimed at fluid management and correcting abnormal electrolyte values. Family anxiety is high during this time because of the impending surgery and the inability to feed an otherwise healthy infant. Provide emotional support to the family. Teach them about the surgical procedure and what to expect postoperatively. Ad lib feeding is recommended soon after surgery, with most infants going home within 24 hours (Adibe, Nichol, Lim, & Mattei, 2007).

Necrotizing Enterocolitis

NEC is characterized by ulcerations and necrosis of the distal ileum and proximal colon. It is the most common and most serious acquired GI disorder among hospitalized preterm neonates and is associated with significant acute and chronic morbidity and mortality (Stoll & Kliegman, 2004). The incidence of NEC is 1 to 3 per 1,000 live births; it affects 1% to 5% of all infants in intensive care units (Stoll & Kliegman, 2004).

The pathophysiology of NEC is unknown, but it involves inflammation and intestinal ischemia (Christensen, Gordon, & Besner, 2010). Immaturity of GI function is thought to be a predisposing factor. The lower the birth weight of the neonate, the more likely it is that he or she will develop NEC (it affects 11% of infants weighing 501 to 750 g compared to 3% of infants weighing 1,251 to 1,500 g) (Christensen et al., 2010). Three factors that play a role in the development of NEC are intestinal ischemia, **enteral** feedings, and bacterial infections. Christensen et al. (2010) report that a drastic reduction in NEC can be achieved through the implementation of feeding guidelines that promote initiating feeds earlier, avoidance of too rapid acceleration of feeds, and consistent care. The majority of infants with NEC may be managed non-operatively. Therapeutic goals include managing infection, supporting ventilation, managing fluid, and decreasing the workload of the bowel (Browne et al., 2007). Serial KUB X-rays determine resolution or progression of NEC. If medical treatment fails to stabilize the patient or if free air is present on a left lateral decubitus film, surgical intervention will be necessary to insert an abdominal drain or resect the portion of necrotic bowel. There may be a proximal enterostomy until the **anastomosis** site is ready for reconnection. Multiple surgeries may be required to remove stenotic bowel segments.

Nursing Assessment

For a full description of the assessment phase of the nursing process, refer to page 1365. Assessment findings pertinent to NEC are discussed below.

Health History

Elicit a description of the present illness and chief complaint. Common signs and symptoms reported during the health history might include the following:

• Abdominal distention, tenderness, and discolouration of the abdominal wall

• Bloody stools
• Feeding intolerance characterized by bilious vomiting
• Signs of sepsis
• Lethargy
• Apnea
• Shock

Risk factors include prematurity, advancing enteral feedings too quickly, and a history of anoxia/hypoxia or shock.

Physical Examination

Always keep in mind the possibility of NEC when dealing with premature infants, especially when enteral feedings are being administered. Perform a GI assessment on the infant. Consider infants with noticeable abdominal distention and/or high residual gastric volumes to be suspicious for NEC. Assess perfusion to all vital organs and monitor closely for circulatory collapse.

Laboratory and Diagnostic Tests

Common laboratory and diagnostic tests ordered for assessment of NEC include the following:

• KUB X-rays of the abdomen to confirm the presence of pneumatosis intestinalis (air in the bowel wall) or free air indicating perforation of the bowel
• Blood laboratory values to assess for increases in the white blood cell count, thrombocytopenia, or neutropenia

Nursing Management

Nursing management of the child with NEC focuses on maintaining fluid and nutritional status, caring for the patient having surgery, and teaching the family about the prognosis.

Maintaining Fluid and Nutritional Status

If NEC is suspected, immediately stop enteral feedings until a diagnosis is made. Administer intravenous fluids initially to restore proper fluid status and TPN to keep the infant supported nutritionally. Administer prescribed intravenous antibiotics to prevent sepsis from the necrotic bowel. If surgery is required, antibiotics may be needed for an extended time. Restart enteral feedings once the disease has resolved (normal abdominal examination and KUB negative for pneumatosis), bowel function has resumed, or as determined postoperatively by the surgeon.

Teaching the Family About the Prognosis

The diagnosis of NEC may cause significant family anxiety. If an extensive amount of bowel has necrosed, the infant is more likely to have long-term medical problems. Short bowel syndrome may result from a large resection (short bowel syndrome is discussed later in this chapter). Provide education about ostomy care if surgery

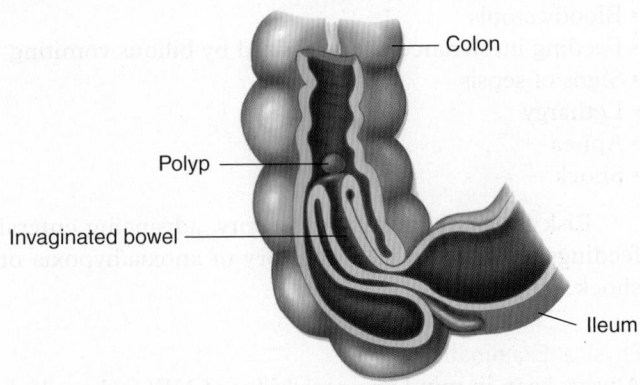

FIGURE 41.14 In intussusception, the intestine telescopes upon itself.

is required (refer to page 1369 for a discussion of ostomy care).

Intussusception

Intussusception is a process that occurs when a proximal segment of bowel "telescopes" into a more distal segment, causing edema, vascular compromise, and ultimately partial or total bowel obstruction (Fig. 41.14). This most commonly occurs in the ileocecal region with the ileum intussuscepting into the cecum (Browne et al., 2007).

Intussusception usually occurs in otherwise healthy infants under age 2. It is three times more likely in males than females. Seventy-five percent to ninety percent of cases of intussusception occur with no specified "lead point" (i.e., pathologic point) that causes the telescoping. When a lead point is identified, it is usually in a child over age 5. The most common type of lead point is Meckel's diverticulum, but other lead points may include duplication cysts, polyps, hemangiomas, tumours, the appendix, or even lymphomas (Wyllie, 2004b).

A barium or air enema is often successful at reducing intussusception in a large percentage of cases. If unsuccessful, reduction is attempted manually by the surgeon following a laparotomy. If the segment cannot be reduced or appears compromised, the segment is resected.

Nursing Assessment

For a full description of the assessment phase of the nursing process, refer to page 1365. Assessment findings pertinent to intussusception are discussed below.

Health History

Elicit a description of the present illness and chief complaint. Common signs and symptoms reported during the health history might include the following:

- Sudden onset of intermittent, cramping abdominal pain
- Severe pain (children usually draw up their knees and scream)
- Vomiting
- Diarrhea
- Currant-jelly stools, gross blood, or Hemoccult-positive stools
- Lethargy

Typically, symptoms exacerbate and then resolve. Between episodes, children may have no symptoms of intussusception. This return to a normal state is due to the intussusception reducing on its own. Assess the severity of pain, length of time the symptoms have been present, presence of vomiting, and stool patterns and colour. Immediately report the presence of bilious vomiting, which occurs only in an obstructive situation. Also assess for signs and symptoms of acute peritonitis. Explore the patient's current and past medical history for risk factors, such as cystic fibrosis or celiac disease.

Physical Examination

Palpate the abdomen for the presence of a sausage-shaped mass in the upper midabdomen; this is a hallmark sign of intussusception and will be accompanied by significant abdominal pain. Note any mental status changes.

Laboratory and Diagnostic Tests

Ultrasound is commonly used to diagnose intussusception (Browne et al., 2007). A barium or air enema is often successful at identifying and reducing a large percentage of intussusception cases. A pediatric surgeon should be available at the time of the enema in case the enema is unsuccessful or perforation (rare) occurs. If the segment cannot be reduced or appears compromised, it is resected. White blood cell elevation may occur, and electrolytes may show signs of dehydration.

Nursing Management

Administer intravenous fluids and antibiotics before the diagnostic laboratory and radiographic studies are performed. A nasogastric tube is placed for gastric decompression. An appropriate pain assessment tool should be utilized. Close attention to fluid balance and vital signs is imperative (Browne et al., 2007). Refer to the Nursing Care Plan 41.1 for nursing management of the postoperative child.

The parents may be very fatigued after dealing with a crying infant. They are often quite anxious about surgery in an otherwise healthy child. Offer emotional support and provide appropriate preoperative and postoperative education to the family.

Malrotation and Volvulus

Intestinal malrotation, a failure of the bowel to normally rotate and attach itself, occurs during the 10th week of embryonic development. At week 10, the intestine is anchored to the abdominal wall by the base of the mesentery in a specific pattern to avoid kinking or twisting

(Wyllie, 2004c). It can be asymptomatic unless the bowel twists or kinks resulting in a volvulus, which is a surgical emergency (Browne et al., 2007). If the volvulus involves the entire small bowel, it is termed a midgut volvulus.

The main symptom of malrotation with midgut volvulus is bilious vomiting. Many children also have abdominal pain, shock symptoms, abdominal distention, tachycardia, and grunting respirations. Bloody stools are a late sign, indicating a critical situation (Browne et al., 2007). Most cases of malrotation with volvulus will present in the first few weeks of life, but symptoms may not occur until the patient is well into adulthood.

Therapeutic management of malrotation and volvulus is accomplished surgically. A Ladd procedure is performed, during which the intestine is straightened out and bands contributing to the misalignment are divided. If the twisted segment (volvulus) is compromised and necrotic, it is resected and an ostomy may be necessary.

Nursing Assessment

For a full description of the assessment phase of the nursing process, refer to page 1365. Assessment findings pertinent to malrotation and volvulus are discussed below.

Health History

Elicit a description of the present illness and chief complaint. Common signs and symptoms reported with malrotation include intermittent vomiting and abdominal pain, failure to thrive, constipation, bloody diarrhea, and hematemesis. Infants with a midgut volvulus will present more emergently and show signs of shock. Since obstruction can occur with resulting necrosis of the bowel, inform the physician immediately if obstruction is suspected.

Physical Examination and Diagnostic and Laboratory Tests

Observe for severity of pain, palpate for abdominal guarding and rebound tenderness, and auscultate for hypoactive bowel sounds. Common laboratory and diagnostic studies ordered for the assessment of malrotation and volvulus include the following:

- KUB X-rays to reveal obstruction or double bubble, dilated loops
- Upper GI series to identify the location of the duodenojejunal junction and corkscrew appearance of the twisted bowel; the cecum will be on the left side (if compromised bowel is not suspected)
- Ultrasound
- Abdominal computed tomography (CT)

Nursing Management

When diagnostic testing reveals malrotation/volvulus, administer ordered intravenous fluids and intravenous antibiotics. A nasogastric tube is placed to decompress the stomach. Surgery is performed as soon as possible.

After surgery, provide postoperative care for the child (see Nursing Care Plan 41.1). Provide continuous emotional support and family education.

Appendicitis

Appendicitis, an acute inflammation of the appendix, is the most common cause of emergent abdominal surgery in children (Sundaram et al., 2011). It occurs in all age groups; the age range for occurrence in the pediatric population is 4 to 15 years (Albanese & Sylvester, 2010).

Pathophysiology

Appendicitis is due to a closed-loop obstruction of the appendix (Fig. 41.15). It is thought that the obstruction is due to fecal material impacted into the relatively narrow appendix, though other causes such as ingested foreign bodies may exist. This obstruction causes a subsequent increase in the intraluminal pressure of the appendix, resulting in mucosal edema, bacterial overgrowth, and eventual perforation. Due to the fecal material in the appendix, perforation causes inflammatory fluid and bacterial contents to leak into the abdominal cavity, resulting in peritonitis. Diffuse peritonitis is more likely in younger children. Older children and adolescents have a more developed omentum, which walls off the inflamed or perforated appendix, often causing a focal abscess.

Therapeutic Management

Appendicitis is considered a surgical emergency because if left uncorrected, the appendix may perforate, causing serious medical issues. Surgical removal of the appendix is necessary and is accomplished via open procedure or minimally invasive laparoscopic technique. In the case of perforation, lavage of the abdominal cavity is performed to cleanse it of the infected fluid released from the appendix. Antibiotics are administered postoperatively to prevent abscess formation.

Nursing Assessment

Early diagnosis and intervention are the key elements to avoid perforation. For a full description of the assessment phase of the nursing process, refer to page 1365. Assessment findings pertinent to appendicitis are discussed below.

Health History

Elicit a description of the present illness and chief complaint. Symptoms of appendicitis may begin as a vague abdominal complaint that persists and always becomes worse. It does not come and go. Common signs and symptoms reported during the health history might include the following:

- Vague midabdominal pain in the initial stages, localizing to the right lower quadrant over a few hours
- Anorexia

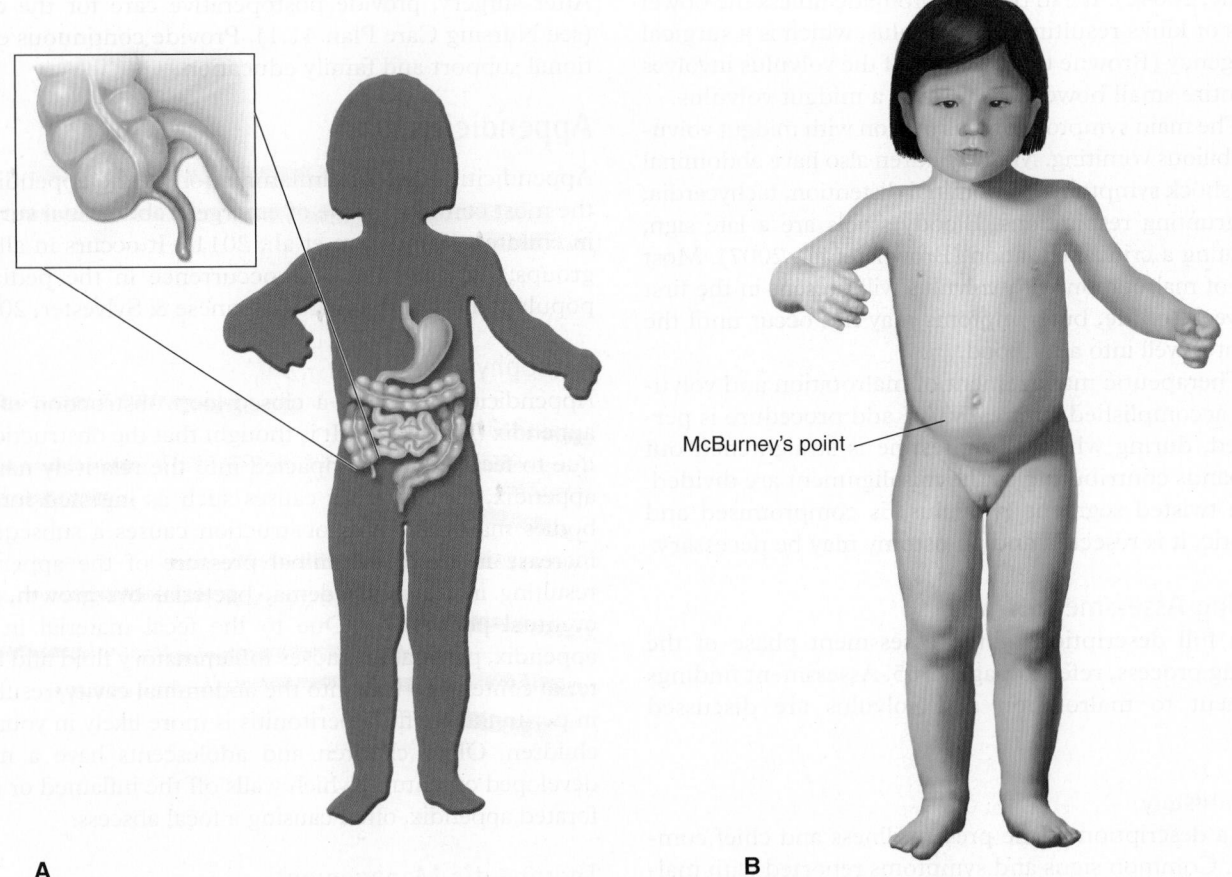

A

B

McBurney's point

FIGURE 41.15 (**A**) In appendicitis, the lumen of the appendix is obstructed, resulting in edema and compressed blood vessels. (**B**) As appendicitis progresses, pain may become localized at McBurney's point (a point midway between the anterosuperior iliac crest and the umbilicus).

- Nausea and vomiting (which usually develop after the onset of pain)
- Small-volume, frequent, soft stools, often confused with diarrhea
- Fever/chills (usually low-grade fever unless perforation occurs, which results in high fever)

Physical Examination

Children with early appendicitis may appear only mildly unwell. As the condition progresses, they often appear quite ill. They prefer side lying with their knees drawn up and often cannot walk or climb up onto the examination table without assistance. Any movement intensifies the pain. Upon palpation, maximal tenderness occurs over McBurney's point in the right lower quadrant (Minkes et al., 2011) (see Fig. 41.15). Assess the abdomen for acute peritonitis, as indicated by diffuse abdominal tenderness, rebound tenderness, distention, and guarding. Immediately report positive findings to a physician.

Laboratory and Diagnostic Tests

Common laboratory and diagnostic studies ordered for the assessment of appendicitis include the following:

- Abdominal ultrasound to identify an enlarged appendix with fluid around it
- Abdominal CT scan to visualize the appendix for further evaluation if it cannot be seen on ultrasound
- Laboratory testing: may reveal an elevated white blood cell count

Nursing Management

Provide pre- and postoperative care and patient and family education (see Nursing Care Plan 41.1). Preoperative antibiotics will be administered, and the child is made NPO (Browne et al., 2007). Care depends on what was found during surgical exploration. If the appendix is non-ruptured and nongangrenous, removal is considered a simple procedure with a length of hospital stay of 1 to 2 days. Routine postsurgical care should be provided. For a gangrenous or perforated appendix, intravenous antibiotics are usually given for a number of days followed by oral antibiotics (Browne et al., 2007) to decrease the risk of postoperative infection. Provide family teaching as it is important that the child complete the entire prescription of oral antibiotics.

Chronic GI Disorders

Chronic GI disorders include GER, PUD, constipation/encopresis, Hirschsprung's disease, short bowel syndrome, inflammatory bowel disease, celiac disease, recurrent abdominal pain, failure to thrive, and chronic feeding problems.

Gastro-esophageal Reflux

GER is passage of gastric contents into the esophagus. It is considered a normal physiologic process that occurs in healthy infants and children. However, when complications develop from the reflux of gastric contents back into the esophagus or oropharynx, it becomes more of a pathologic process known as gastro-esophageal reflux disease (GERD). GER occurs frequently during the first year of life; 85% of infants outgrow reflux by age 12 months (Sundaram et al., 2011). GER is particularly common in premature infants. Other possible diagnoses that can be mistaken for GER include food allergies, formula enteropathies, gastric outlet obstruction, malrotation, cyclic vomiting, or central nervous system lesions.

Pathophysiology

The process of GER occurs during episodes of transient relaxation of the LES, which can occur during swallowing, crying, or other Valsalva manoeuvres that increase intra-abdominal pressure. Delayed esophageal clearance and gastric emptying, highly acidic gastric contents, hiatal hernia (protrusion of the stomach upward into the mediastinal cavity through the esophageal hiatus of the diaphragm), or neurologic disease may also be contributing factors associated with reflux.

Symptoms of GERD in infants and children are listed below in the health history section. The signs and symptoms of GERD are often seen as a result of the damaging components of the refluxate (the pH of the gastric contents, bile acids, and pepsin). The longer the pH of the refluxate is below 4, the higher the risk for development of severe GERD (Weill, 2008).

As a result of GERD, other systems may be at risk for damage. These complications include esophagitis, esophageal stricture, Barrett's esophagus (a precancerous condition), laryngitis, recurrent pneumonia, asthma, or anemia from chronic esophageal erosion.

Therapeutic Management

Conservative medical management begins with appropriate positioning, such as elevating the head of the bed and keeping the infant or child upright for 30 minutes after feeding. Smaller, more frequent feedings may be helpful. If reflux does not improve with these measures, medications are prescribed to decrease acid production and stabilize the pH of the gastric contents. Also, prokinetic

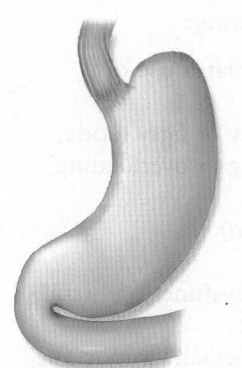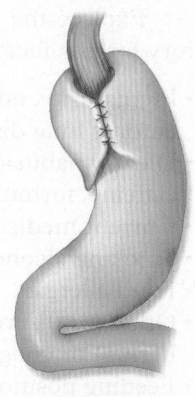

FIGURE 41.16 In the Nissen fundoplication, the fundus (upper portion of the stomach) is wrapped around the lower segment of the esophagus.

agents may be used to help empty the stomach more quickly, minimizing the amount of gastric contents in the stomach that the child can reflux.

If the GERD cannot be medically managed effectively or requires long-term medication therapy, surgical intervention may be necessary. A Nissen fundoplication is the most common surgical procedure performed for antireflux therapy. The gastric fundus is wrapped around the lower 2 to 3 cm of the esophagus (Fig. 41.16). This tightens the gastro-esophageal junction, reducing or eliminating the reflux of gastric contents. Laparoscopic fundoplications are being performed as a way to minimize the recovery period and reduce potential complications.

Nursing Assessment

For a full description of the assessment phase of the nursing process, refer to page 1365. Assessment findings pertinent to GER are discussed below.

Health History

Elicit a description of the present illness and chief complaint. Note onset and progression of symptoms. Common signs and symptoms reported during the health history include the following:

• Recurrent vomiting or regurgitation
• Weight loss or poor weight gain
• Irritability in infants
• Respiratory symptoms (chronic cough, wheezing, stridor, asthma, apnea)
• Hoarseness/sore throat
• Halitosis (mostly in older children)
• Heartburn or chest pains
• Abdominal pain
• Abnormal neck posturing (Sandifer syndrome)
• Hematemesis
• Dysphagia or feeding refusal
• Chronic sinusitis, otitis media
• Poor dentition (caused by acid erosion)

Explore the patient's current and past medical history for risk factors such as the following:

- Prematurity, noting prolonged ventilator use or chronic lung disease
- Dietary habits (e.g., chocolate, spicy or fatty foods, caffeine, formula feeding, overeating or overfeeding)
- Current medications
- Smoking/alcohol use (older children)
- Food allergies
- Other GI disorders (gastric outlet dysfunction/hiatal hernia) or congenital abnormalities
- Feeding positions and patterns (especially important in infants)
- Sleeping positions and patterns
- Other medical history, such as asthma, recurrent infections/pneumonia

Physical Examination

The physical examination consists of inspection, auscultation, percussion, and palpation.

Inspection

Observe the child's general appearance and colour. Infants and children with uncontrolled GER for a period of time may appear underweight or malnourished. Infants may be irritable due to painful regurgitation/reflux events. Note breathing patterns, because reflux-induced asthma may have developed. **Acute life-threatening events (ALTE)** and apnea have been associated with severe GERD (Sundaram et al., 2011). Observe the child for cyanosis, altered mental status, and alterations in tone. Inspect emesis for blood or bile.

Auscultation

Evaluate the lung fields for the presence of complications related to GERD, such as wheezing or pneumonia. No further pathologic findings related to GERD should be auscultated on examination.

Percussion

Perform routine abdominal percussion, noting any abnormalities. No specific findings should be noted.

Palpation

Use caution when palpating the abdomen, especially with infants with GER, because it may induce vomiting. No abnormalities should be palpated.

▶ **Take** NOTE!

Not all infants with GERD actually vomit. Those with "silent" GERD may only demonstrate irritability associated with feeding or posturing (arching back during or after feeding) and grimacing. Episodes of GERD often cause bradycardia, so if the above signs occur, they should be reported to the physician, even if the baby is not vomiting (Weill, 2008).

Laboratory and Diagnostic Tests

Common laboratory and diagnostic studies ordered for the assessment of GER include the following:

- Upper GI series: though not sensitive or specific to GER, it may show some reflux; used to narrow down the differential diagnosis
- Esophageal pH probe study: quantifies GER episodes as they correlate to symptoms
- Esophagogastroduodenoscopy: shows esophageal and gastric tissue damage from GERD
- CBC: may demonstrate anemia if chronic esophagitis or hematemesis is present
- Hemoccult: may be positive if chronic esophagitis is present

Nursing Management

As with most GI disorders, initial nursing management is aimed at restoring proper fluid balance and nutrition. Refer to Nursing Care Plan 41.1. Additional considerations are reviewed below.

Promoting Safe Feeding Techniques and Positioning

Feeding adjustments are an essential part of reflux management. Give infants smaller, more frequent feedings using a nipple that controls flow well. Frequently burp the infant during feeds to control reflux. Thickening of the formula with products such as rice or oatmeal cereal can significantly help keep the formula and gastric contents down. Positioning after feedings is important. Keep infants upright for 30 to 45 minutes after feeding. For infants, elevate the head of the crib 30 degrees. Placing in infant seats or swings is not recommended as this increases intra-abdominal pressure (Weill, 2008). For older children, elevate the head of the bed as much as possible and restrict meals for several hours before bedtime. However, individual physicians may have specific preferences about sleeping positions for infants with GERD.

Maintaining a Patent Airway

GERD symptoms often involve the airway. Maximize reflux precautions to keep the risk of airway involvement to a minimum. In rare instances, GERD causes apnea or an ALTE (Sundaram et al., 2011). In these cases, use an apnea or bradycardia monitor to monitor for such episodes. The monitor requires a physician's order and can be ordered through a home health company. Teach parents how to deal with these episodes, as their anxiety is very high. Provide CPR instruction to all parents whose children have had an ALTE previously.

Educating the Family and Child

The goals for the infant and child with GER are a decrease in symptoms, a decrease in the frequency and duration of reflux episodes, healing of the injured mucosa, and prevention of further complications of GERD. Teach the parents the signs and symptoms of complications. Explain that reflux is usually limited to the first year of life, though in some cases it persists. If medications are prescribed, thoroughly explain their use and their side effects (see Drug Guide 41.1).

Providing Postoperative Care

Following fundoplication, the child will usually not be fed for a number of days to reduce retching and decrease the possibility of tearing the wrap. Feeds are introduced very slowly and limited to pureed food for several weeks. Occasionally, a gastrostomy tube is placed simultaneously as required for feeding. In the immediate postoperative period, assess for pain, abdominal distention, retching, and return of bowel sounds. If a gastrostomy tube is placed, it is open to straight drain for a period of time postoperatively to keep the stomach empty and allow for the internal incision to heal. When bowel sounds have returned and the infant or child is stable, introduce feedings slowly either orally or via the gastrostomy tube if present. Assess for tolerance of feedings (absence of abdominal distention or pain, minimal residual, and passage of stool). If the abdomen does become distended or the child has discomfort, open the gastrostomy tube to air to decompress the stomach. Assess the insertion site of the gastrostomy tube for redness, edema, or drainage. Keep the site clean and dry per surgeon or hospital protocol. Teach the parents how to care for the gastrostomy tube and insertion site and how to use the tube for feeding.

Promoting Family and Patient Coping

Parents can feel a great deal of anxiety. Teach the family about all aspects of GERD to help promote coping. School-age children often have reflux episodes exhibited by postprandial vomiting, which can be very embarrassing for the children. Notify the school about the medical issues related to GER to minimize the situations for the child.

Peptic Ulcer Disease

PUD is a term used to describe a variety of disorders of the upper GI tract that result from the action of gastric secretions (Fig. 41.17). Mucosal inflammation and subsequent ulceration occur as a result of either a primary or a secondary factor. In children, duodenal ulcers are more common than gastric ulcers (Sundaram et al., 2011). Primary peptic ulcers are usually associated with *Helicobacter pylori,* a gram-negative organism that causes mucosal inflammation and in some cases more severe disease (Sundaram et al., 2011). *H. pylori* is found mostly in the duodenum.

Secondary peptic ulcers may occur as a result of an identifiable factor, such as excess acid production, stress, medications, or the presence of other underlying condi-

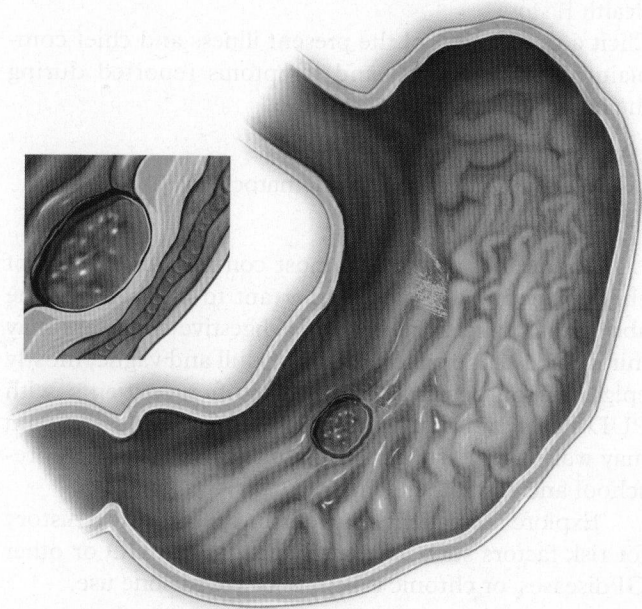

FIGURE 41.17 Peptic ulcer disease.

tions. Secondary ulcers tend to be gastric as opposed to duodenal in location.

Primary PUD is more common in children over age 10. There is a higher incidence of secondary PUD in patients under age 6, though it can be found in children of all ages (Herbst, 2004).

> ▶ *Take NOTE!*
>
> *Severe stress, such as burns or another illness necessitating critical care, can contribute to the development of a peptic ulcer in children (Sundaram et al., 2011).*

Therapeutic Management

PUD may be treated with antibiotics (if *H. pylori* is verified), histamine agonists, and/or proton pump inhibitors. If the child presents with a severe esophageal or gastric hemorrhage, a nasogastric tube may be placed to decompress the stomach. Gastroscopy allows for visualization of tissue changes and ulceration. The patient may require intravenous infusion of a histamine-2 (H_2) receptor antagonist or a proton pump inhibitor initially until the bleeding has stopped and the disease is stabilized.

Nursing Assessment

For a full description of the assessment phase of the nursing process, refer to page 1365. Assessment findings pertinent to PUD are discussed in following page.

Health History

Elicit a description of the present illness and chief complaint. Common signs and symptoms reported during the health history might include:

- Abdominal pain
- GI bleeding/hematemesis, hematochezia
- Nausea and vomiting

Abdominal pain is the most common complaint of children with PUD. It is important to characterize the abdominal pain, as many other digestive disorders may mimic PUD. The pain tends to be dull and vague, mostly epigastric or periumbilical. Most often, patients with PUD have pain that worsens after meals, and the pain may wake them at night. Vomiting may be noted in preschool and school-age children.

Explore the patient's current and past medical history for risk factors such as a family history of PUD or other GI diseases, or chronic salicylate or prednisone use.

> ▶ **Take** NOTE!
>
> *Adolescents at increased risk for the development of PUD include those who use tobacco, alcohol, and caffeine (Sundaram et al., 2011).*

Physical Examination and Laboratory and Diagnostic Tests

Palpate the abdomen for the location of the pain, which is usually epigastric or periumbilical. Note the presence of blood in emesis or stools (melena), as GI bleeding may occur (Anand et al., 2011). Common laboratory and diagnostic studies ordered for the assessment of PUD include the following:

- Laboratory studies: to identify anemia or *H. pylori* antibodies
- Urea breath test: to identify *H. pylori* gastritis
- Upper GI series: to detect presence of ulcerations
- Upper endoscopy: the definitive diagnostic test to look for ulceration and nodularity in the upper GI tract
- Biopsies: to assess for *H. pylori*, granulomas, eosinophils, or corrosive agents to identify the primary cause of the PUD

Nursing Management

Hemodynamic stabilization should be the focus of nursing management if significant GI bleeding occurs. Once patients are stabilized and tolerating oral feeds, they may be discharged to home. Provide discharge instructions on the following topics:

- Medications
- Dietary management (especially when allergic gastroenteropathy is found)
- Safety precautions (in cases of ingested substances)

- Stressors
- Prevention of disease recurrence

Constipation and Encopresis

Constipation is a very common problem seen in pediatric practice, reportedly representing 3% to 10% of all pediatric out-patient visits (Montgomery & Navarro, 2008). It accounts for 25% of the referrals made to a pediatric gastroenterologist for further management of the condition (Castiglia, 2001).

Constipation is usually defined as failure to achieve complete evacuation of the lower colon. It is usually associated with difficulty in passing hard, dry stools but can sometimes be seen as small stools, the size of marbles. Term newborns should pass a meconium stool within the first 24 hours of life. If this does not occur, the newborn is at risk for developing an underlying GI disorder. The bowel habits of both infants and children vary widely, so assess and treat each child on an individual basis. Breastfed infants may produce a stool with each feeding, though some will skip a few days between stools. Most bottle-fed babies will produce a stool one or two times per day, but they may go 2 to 3 days without producing a stool.

Encopresis is a term used to describe soiling of fecal matter beyond the age range of expected toilet training (4 to 5 years of age). Encopresis is often seen as a result of chronic constipation and withholding of stool. As stool is withheld in the rectum, the rectal muscle can stretch over time, and this stretching of the rectum causes fecal impactions. Patients who have a stretched rectal vault may experience diarrhea, where leakage occurs around a fecal mass. This is often an embarrassing issue that occurs with school-age children, and the child may hide his or her underwear due to *feeling shame or fearing punishment*. Many psychological issues can arise from chronic constipation and encopresis as the child may experience ridicule and shame (Burns, Dunn, Brady, Starr, & Blosser, 2009).

Pathophysiology

As stool passes through the colon, water is reabsorbed into the colon, resulting in a formed stool by the time it reaches the rectum. At this point, the anal sphincter relaxes to allow the passage of stool from the anus. In constipation, however, this relaxation does not occur.

Most causes of constipation are functional in nature (inorganic) (Montgomery & Navarro, 2008). Children with functional constipation usually present with this problem during the toilet-training years. Children have a painful experience during defecation, which in turn creates a fear of defecation, resulting in further withholding of stool. Organic causes of constipation rarely occur in children; however, this may be a sign of a disease such as spina bifida or sacral agenesis. The causes of pediatric constipation are discussed in Box 41.5.

BOX 41.5 Causes of Pediatric Constipation by Age

Newborn/Infant	Toddler and Preschool (Ages 2–4 Years)	School Age	Adolescent	Any Age
• Meconium plug • Hirschsprung's disease • Cystic fibrosis • Congenital anorectal malformations • Pseudo-obstruction • Endocrine: hypothyroidism • Metabolic: diabetes insipidus, renal tubular acidosis • Withholding • Dietary changes	• Anal fissures • Withholding • Toilet refusal • Short-segment Hirschsprung's disease • Neurologic disorders • Spinal cord: meningomyelocele, tumours, tethered cord	• Toilet or bathroom access limited or unavailable • Limited ability to recognize physiologic cues, preoccupation with other activities • Spinal cord tethering • Withholding	• Spinal cord injury (accidents, trauma) • Dieting • Anorexia • Pregnancy • Idiopathic slow transit constipation, particularly in females • Laxative abuse • Irritable bowel syndrome, constipation variant	• Medication side effect, dietary, postoperative state • Previous anorectal surgery • Withholding and overflow from chronic rectal distention • Relatively rapid change to sedentary state, dehydration • Hypothyroidism

Therapeutic Management

Once any organic process is ruled out as a cause for constipation, the condition may be managed initially with dietary manipulation such as increasing fibre and fluids. Behaviour modification is necessary for most children. Children need to relearn to allow bowel evacuation when stool is present. Children with severe constipation and withholding behaviours may not benefit from dietary management and may require laxative therapy. Bowel cleansing (e.g., pediatric dose enema) or, in severe cases, mechanical disimpaction may be required.

Nursing Assessment

For a full description of the assessment phase of the nursing process, refer to page 1365. Assessment findings pertinent to constipation/encopresis are discussed below.

Health History

Elicit a description of the present illness and chief complaint. Note the onset of symptoms as described by the parent/child. Common signs and symptoms reported during the health history may include the following:

• Altered stooling patterns (size, frequency, amount, colour)
• Pain and straining with defecation
• Withholding behaviours (postures to try to withhold the stool, such as crossing the legs, squatting or hiding in a corner, or "dancing")
• Complaints of abdominal pain and cramping and poor appetite
• Diarrhea leakage
• Soiling of undergarments

It is important to note the duration of the symptoms to determine an acute onset versus a chronic disorder.

Explore the patient's past and current medical history for risk factors such as

• Family history of GI disorders
• History of rectal bleeding or **anal fissures**
• Report of first meconium stool after 24 hours of age
• History of sexual abuse
• Poor diet (processed foods)

An accurate dietary history as well as a history of fluid intake should be taken. Current medication or laxative use should also be explored.

Physical Examination

Physical examination of the child with constipation consists of inspection, auscultation, percussion, and palpation.

Inspection

Observe the child's general appearance and signs of failure to thrive. Note whether the abdomen appears distended or rounded. Observe the lower back for a deep pilonidal dimple with hair tuft, which is suggestive of spina bifida occulta. Flat buttocks may be suggestive of sacral agenesis. Inspect the anus for signs of fissures or soiling. Inspect the child's underwear for stains or smears, which are indicative of soiling (Ulshen, 2004).

Auscultation

Auscultate bowel sounds to determine the possibility of an obstruction (hypoactive or absent bowel sounds) in the child with an acute case of constipation.

Percussion

Percuss the abdomen to reveal dullness, which would indicate a fecal mass.

Palpation

Palpate the abdomen for any tenderness or masses. A hard mass in the left lower quadrant may indicate hard stool in the descending colon. The nurse may assist the physician or practitioner with the performance of a rectal examination to assess for rectal tone, hard stool, and rectal vault size.

Laboratory and Diagnostic Tests

Laboratory and diagnostic tests are not routine with the diagnosis of functional constipation, but if an organic cause is suspected, the following laboratory and diagnostic tests would be ordered:

- Stool for occult blood: the presence of blood could indicate some other disease process
- Abdominal X-ray: large quantities of stool may be seen in the colon
- Sitz marker study: to detect colonic dysmotility
- Barium enema: to rule out a stricture or Hirschsprung's disease
- Rectal manometry: to evaluate rectal musculature dysfunction
- Rectal biopsy: to rule out Hirschsprung's disease

Nursing Management

Nursing management for the infant or child with constipation is aimed at educating the patient and family and promoting patient and family coping. Refer to Nursing Care Plan 41.1. Additional considerations are reviewed below.

Educating the Family and Patient

Teach parents how to assess for signs of constipation and withholding behaviours. Also provide guidelines on scheduling and supervising bowel habits in reconditioning the child to use the toilet regularly. Teach parents to use positive reinforcement techniques: for example, when the child produces an adequate-volume bowel movement, reward him or her with stickers, extra play time or television time, and so on (Schmitt, 2004).

Dietary changes may help some children. High-fibre diets help to regulate bowel activity, and reducing the consumption of processed foods may also help. Increasing fluid intake may also aid in bringing extra water into the bowel, thereby softening the stool. Infants and toddlers with constipation may experience constipation from formula or milk changes. Manipulating the formula or milk may result in better bowel habits.

Educate families about the importance of compliance with medication use, if medication is ordered. Parents often are very anxious about the use of these medications, but stress to them that compliance is essential. Assess for improper laxative use based on the history of stool patterns.

Many children present to their doctor with fecal impaction or partial impaction. Teach parents how to

---

Nursing Procedure 41.2

ADMINISTERING AN ENEMA

1. Gather supplies (enema bag, lubricant, enema solution).
2. Wash hands and apply gloves.
3. Position the child:
   - Infant or toddler on abdomen with knees bent
   - Child or adolescent on left side with right leg flexed toward chest
4. Clamp the enema tubing, remove the cap, and apply lubricant to the tip.
5. Insert the tube into the rectum:
   - 2.5 to 4 cm (1 to 1.5 inches) in the infant
   - 5 to 7.5 cm (2 to 3 inches) in the child
6. Unclamp the tubing and administer the prescribed volume of enema solution at a rate of about 100 mL per minute. Recommended volumes:
   - 250 mL or less for the infant
   - 250 to 500 mL for the toddler or preschooler
   - 500 to 1000 mL for the school-age child
7. Hold the child's buttocks together if needed to encourage retention of the enema solution for 5 to 10 minutes.

---

disimpact their children at home; this often requires an enema or stimulation therapy. Nursing Procedure 41.2 gives instructions on enema administration in children. Explain the procedure to the child in developmentally appropriate terms. Enema administration can be uncomfortable, but calming measures, such as distraction and praise, provide a comforting environment. After the impaction is removed, promote regular bowel habits to keep the impaction from recurring.

Promoting Patient and Family Coping

Childhood constipation can be a very stressful process for both the child and family. To facilitate daily bowel evacuation, the child should be encouraged to sit on the toilet twice a day (after breakfast and dinner) for 5 to 10 minutes. Instruct the family to gently encourage and provide support to the child by explaining why sitting on the toilet at regular intervals can encourage bowel movement regularity. Weeks to months may be required to change the stooling pattern (Burns et al., 2009).

Many parents seek counsellors to help the entire family deal with the issues. Counselling is geared toward allaying the fears of a child who is afraid to defecate due to pain. Also, children who are older may have other behavioural issues that need to be addressed. Psychological evaluation and possible behavioural therapy may need to be implemented if constipation becomes a power struggle.

▶ *Consider* THIS!

Jung Kim, 3 years old, is brought to the clinic by his parents with abdominal pain and a poor appetite. His mother states, "He cries when I put him on the toilet." What other assessment information would you obtain? What education and interventions may be necessary for this child and family?

Hirschsprung's Disease (Congenital Aganglionic Megacolon)

Hirschsprung's disease is the most common cause of neonatal intestinal obstruction (Lee, Shekherdimian, & Dubois, 2009) (Fig. 41.18). The disease is most commonly characterized by constipation in newborns; however, in milder cases, constipation may not present until early childhood. This is due to a lack of ganglion cells in the bowel, which causes inadequate motility in part of the intestine. The severity of the disease depends on the extent of the aganglionic segment. These ganglion cells can be absent from the rectosigmoid colon all the way into the small intestine. Approximately 75% of cases affect only the rectosigmoid colon (short-segment Hirschsprung's), but in 8% of cases, total colonic involvement is seen (long-segment Hirschsprung's). Hirschsprung's disease occurs in 1 in 5,400 to 7,200 newborns (Lee et al., 2009). Hirschsprung's disease usually occurs in the absence of other associated anomalies, but there is an association with Down syndrome (Wyllie, 2004a).

Therapeutic Management

Surgical resection of the aganglionic bowel and reanastomosis of the remaining intestine are necessary to promote proper bowel function. Rectal irrigation and dilators for anal stimulation may be used prior to surgical repair to allow for growth of the infant. There are several types of surgical procedures to correct this condition. A pull-through procedure may be done as a single-stage primary repair, or a temporary ostomy may be required to divert stool. The ostomy is closed at a later date when the colon is resected and the final repair done.

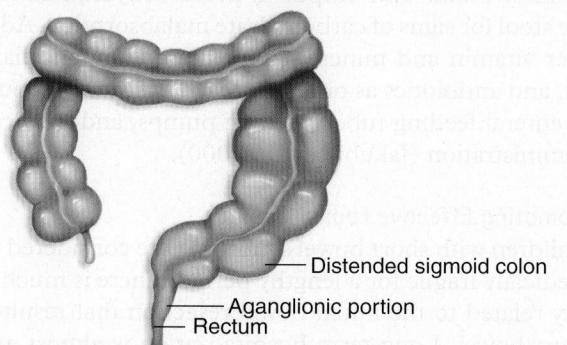

FIGURE 41.18 Enlarged megacolon of Hirschsprung's disease.

Distended sigmoid colon
Aganglionic portion
Rectum

Nursing Assessment

For a full description of the assessment phase of the nursing process, refer to page 1365. Assessment findings pertinent to Hirschsprung's disease are discussed below.

Health History

Elicit a description of the present illness and chief complaint. Newborn stool patterns are a key element in recognizing this diagnosis. Assess whether the newborn passed a meconium stool: most children with Hirschsprung's disease do not pass a meconium stool within the first 24 to 48 hours of life. Also, newborns who required rectal stimulation to pass their first meconium stool or who passed a meconium plug should be evaluated for Hirschsprung's.

Explore the child's current and past medical history for risk factors such as a family history of Hirschsprung's disease, Down syndrome, or intestinal atresia (lack of a normal opening) (Lee et al., 2009).

Physical Examination

Inspect and palpate the abdomen. The abdomen is typically distended, and often stool masses can be palpated in the abdomen. Perform a rectal examination to assess for rectal tone and the presence of stool in the rectum. Often with Hirschsprung's, although no stool may be present in the rectum, at the end of the rectal examination, when the finger is being withdrawn, the child may have a forceful expulsion of fecal material.

Laboratory and Diagnostic Tests

Common laboratory and diagnostic studies ordered for the assessment of Hirschsprung's disease include the following:

• Barium enema: to look for a narrowing of the intestine
• Rectal biopsy: to demonstrate an absence of ganglion cells (definitive diagnosis)

Nursing Management

Nursing management includes providing postoperative care, performing ostomy care, and providing patient and family education.

Providing Postoperative and Ostomy Care

Provide routine postoperative care and observe for the complication of enterocolitis (see Nursing Care Plan 41.1). Observe for the following signs and symptoms of enterocolitis:

• Fever
• Abdominal distention
• Chronic diarrhea
• Explosive stools
• Rectal bleeding
• Straining
• Bowel dilation on abdominal X-ray

If any of the above signs or symptoms are noted, immediately notify the physician, maintain bowel rest, and administer intravenous fluids and antibiotics to prevent the development of shock and possibly death.

The patient with Hirschsprung's may have either a colostomy or ileostomy, depending on the extent of disease in the intestine. In either case, perform proper ostomy care to avoid skin breakdown. Accurately measure stool output to assess the child's fluid volume status.

Providing Patient and Family Education

The family may be anxious and fearful about upcoming surgeries and possible complications. Help to relieve their anxiety by providing information about the diagnosis and the stages of surgical procedures the patient will undergo. If rectal irrigations or anal dilations are required, educate caregivers on appropriate techniques. Provide postoperative teaching to educate parents on proper stoma care as well as medication management (to avoid dehydration, most Hirschsprung's patients will be prescribed medications to slow stool output). Arrange for the family to consult with a wound care nurse to help them deal with the anxieties and care of newly placed stomas. Provide education about possible postsurgical problems, emphasizing the importance of prompt medical treatment for signs of enterocolitis.

Short Bowel Syndrome

Short bowel syndrome is a clinical syndrome of nutrient malabsorption and excessive intestinal fluid and electrolyte losses that occurs following massive small intestinal loss or surgical resection. The degree of malabsorption is usually related to the extent of resection of small bowel (Cuffari, 2009). The most common causes of short bowel syndrome are NEC, small intestinal atresia, gastroschisis, malrotation with volvulus, and trauma to the small intestine. A child can lose as much as 75% of the small intestine without serious long-term problems, as long as the duodenum, terminal ileum, and ileocecal valve are still functioning. However, even a 25% intestinal loss can result in significant problems if the terminal ileum and ileocecal valve are not spared (Jakubik, Colfer, & Grossman, 2000). If the terminal ileum is lost, vitamin B12 deficiency and bile salt malabsorption may occur. If the ileocecal valve is lost, small bowel bacterial overgrowth is likely to occur, as well as poor intestinal motility.

Therapeutic Management

The child with short bowel syndrome is at risk for chronic complications. The goals of therapeutic management are to minimize bacterial overgrowth and maximize the child's nutritional status. Antibiotics may be used to control bacterial overgrowth. Vitamin and mineral supplementation is necessary because the small intestine is usually where fat-soluble vitamins, calcium,

magnesium, and zinc are absorbed. Many children with short bowel syndrome require TPN for extended periods to achieve adequate growth. Progression to enteral feeding may occur extremely slowly, depending upon the intestine's response. Despite a markedly improved prognosis for these patients, some will not do as well and may ultimately require intestinal and liver transplantation due to irreversible liver damage from long-term use of TPN (Jakubik et al., 2000).

Nursing Assessment

Elicit the health history, noting diarrhea, which is the primary symptom of short bowel syndrome. Note past history of bowel loss or resection as noted above. Assess the child's hydration state and overall growth. Inspect the stool for consistency, colour, odour, and volume. Review laboratory results, particularly chemistries, to evaluate hydration status, and liver function tests, which may reveal evolving **cholestasis** secondary to long-term TPN use.

Nursing Management

Nursing management focuses on encouraging adequate nutrition and promoting effective family coping.

Encouraging Adequate Nutrition

Treatment for short bowel syndrome can be a slow and tedious process. Most patients will require TPN until they can tolerate enteral feeds without significant malabsorption. TPN is usually required for a lengthy time, so most children will require long-term intravenous access. Long-term intravenous access places the child at high risk for infection and resulting sepsis, so utilize sterile technique and closely monitor for signs and symptoms of infection. Immediately report to the physician any fevers or redness or drainage at the intravenous access site.

When started, enteral feeding must be administered very slowly to avoid further malabsorption. Usually the feeding is started continuously, 24 hours per day, via a feeding pump. Most patients have long-term feeding tubes, usually gastrostomy tubes, and will require special formulas to promote absorption. Assess for feeding tube residuals and abdominal distention or discomfort. Strictly monitor intake and output to avoid dehydration. Assess the stool for signs of carbohydrate malabsorption. Administer vitamin and mineral supplementation, antidiarrheals, and antibiotics as ordered. Teach the family about use of enteral feeding tubes, feeding pumps, and medication administration (Jakubik et al., 2000).

Promoting Effective Family Coping

Children with short bowel syndrome are considered to be medically fragile for a lengthy period. There is much anxiety related to the initial bowel resection that resulted in short bowel. Long-term hospitalization is almost always required, causing parents to miss work and cutting down on the time they have to spend with other children. This can lead to even more anxiety about finances and relationships. Encourage families to become the experts on their child's needs and condition via education and participation in care. Provide teaching so that the family is better able to care for the child in an out-patient setting. Education focuses on information about TPN and central line care, enteral feedings, assessing for hydration status, and managing medications.

> ▶ **Take** NOTE!

Maintaining long-term central venous access for TPN in infants can present a challenge. One-piece clothing with the central venous line tubing exiting and secured on the back of the outfit can help discourage the infant from pulling on (and subsequently dislodging) the line.

Inflammatory Bowel Disease

Crohn's disease and ulcerative colitis are the two major idiopathic inflammatory bowel diseases of children. The causes are unknown, but they may be due to an abnormal or uncontrolled genetically determined immunologic or inflammatory response to an environmental antigenic trigger, possibly a virus or bacterium (Haas-Beckert & Heyman, 2010). The features of Crohn's disease and ulcerative colitis are listed in Comparison Chart 41.2.

Therapeutic Management

Medication is used to control inflammation and symptoms. Medications commonly used include 5-aminosalicylates, antibiotics, immunomodulators, immunosuppressives, and anti-tumour necrosis antibody therapy. Dietary manipulation is also very important.

Failure to respond to medical therapy may result in surgical intervention. Many patients with ulcerative colitis eventually undergo a total proctocolectomy, with resulting ostomy, as a curative measure. Approximately 70% of Crohn's disease patients will require surgery to relieve obstruction, drain an abscess, or relieve intractable symptoms (Sundaram et al., 2011).

Nursing Assessment

For a full description of the assessment phase of the nursing process, refer to page 1365. Assessment findings pertinent to Crohn's disease and ulcerative colitis are discussed below.

Health History

Elicit a description of the present illness and chief complaint. Common signs and symptoms reported during the health history include:

- Abdominal cramping
- Nighttime symptoms, including waking due to abdominal pain or urge to defecate
- Fever
- Weight loss
- Poor growth
- Delayed sexual development

Children may be reluctant or unwilling to talk about their bowel movements, so explain the importance of doing so. Assess stool pattern history, including frequency, presence of blood or mucus, and duration of symptoms.

Explore the patient's current and past medical history for risk factors, such as:

- Family history of inflammatory bowel disease
- Family history of colon cancer
- Family history of immunologic disorders

Physical Examination

Assess the child's growth using growth charts to identify any poor growth patterns. Perform a full abdominal examination, noting tenderness, masses, or fullness. Inspect the perianal area to look for skin tags or fissures, which would be highly suspicious for Crohn's disease. Assist the physician in performing a rectal examination to further assess the rectal area for blood or other lesions.

Laboratory and Diagnostic Tests

Laboratory test results may be normal. Results for children with Crohn's disease and ulcerative colitis are found in Comparison Chart 41.2. Common laboratory and diagnostic studies ordered for the assessment of inflammatory bowel disease include the following:

- Radiologic studies such as upper GI series with small bowel series: may identify evidence of intestinal inflammation, estimate distribution and extent of disease, and help distinguish between Crohn's disease and ulcerative colitis
- CT scan: to rule out suspected abscess
- Colonoscopy and biopsy: to diagnose inflammatory bowel disease
- Upper endoscopy: to rule out affected mucosal tissue between the mouth and anus in children with upper abdominal complaints

Nursing Management

Nursing management focuses on teaching about disease management, teaching about nutritional management, teaching about medication therapy, and promoting family and child coping.

Teaching About Disease Management

The diagnosis of Crohn's disease or ulcerative colitis can be very difficult for the patient and family to comprehend.

COMPARISON CHART 41.2 FEATURES OF CROHN'S DISEASE AND ULCERATIVE COLITIS

Feature	Crohn's Disease	Ulcerative Colitis
Age at onset	10–20 years	10–20 years
Incidence	4 to 6 per 100,000	3 to 15 per 100,000
Area of bowel affected	Oropharynx, esophagus, and stomach, rare: small bowel only, 25% to 30%; colon and anus only, 25%; ileocolitis, 40%; diffuse disease, 5%	Total colon, 90%; proctitis, 10%
Distribution	Segmental; disease-free skip areas common	Continuous; distal to proximal
Pathology	Full-thickness, acute, and chronic inflammation; noncaseating granulomas (50%), extraintestinal fistulas, abscesses, stricture, and fibrosis may be present	Superficial, acute inflammation of mucosa with microscopic crypt abscess
X-ray findings	Segmental lesions; thickened, circular folds, cobblestone appearance of bowel wall secondary to longitudinal ulcers and transverse fissures; fixation and separation of loops; narrowed lumen; "sting sign"; fistulas	Superficial colitis; loss of haustra; shortened colon and pseudopolyps (islands of normal tissue surrounded by denuded mucosa) are late findings
Intestinal symptoms	Abdominal pain, diarrhea (usually loose with blood if colon involved), perianal disease, enteroenteric or enterocutaneous fistula, abscess, anorexia	Abdominal pain, bloody diarrhea, urgency, tenesmus
Extraintestinal symptoms:		
Arthritis/arthralgia	15%	9%
Fever	40% to 50%	40% to 50%
Stomatitis	9%	2%
Weight loss	90% (mean 5.7 kg)	68% (mean 4.1 kg)
Delayed growth and sexual development	30%	5% to 10%
Uveitis, conjunctivitis	15% (in Crohn's colitis)	4%
Sclerosing cholangitis	—	4%
Renal stones	6% (oxalate)	6% (urate)
Pyoderma gangrenosum	1% to 3%	5%
Erythema nodosum	8% to 15%	4%
Laboratory findings	High erythrocyte sedimentation rate; microcytic anemia; low serum iron and total iron-binding capacity; increased fecal protein loss; low serum albumin; antineutrophil cytoplasmic antibodies present in 10% to 20%; *Saccharomyces cerevisiae* antibodies positive in 60%	High erythrocyte sedimentation rate; microcytic anemia; high white blood cell count with left shift; antineutrophil cytoplasmic antibodies present in 80%

Adapted from: Haas-Beckert, B., & Heyman, M. B. (2010). Inflammatory bowel disease. In P. J. Allen, J. A. Vessey, & N. A. Schapiro (Eds.), *Primary care of the child with a chronic condition* (5th ed.). St. Louis, MO: Mosby; and Sundaram, S., Hoffenberg, E., Kramer, R., Sondheimer, J. M., & Furuta, G. T. (2011). Gastrointestinal tract. In W. W. Hay, M. J. Levin, J. M. Sondheimer, & R. R. Deterding (Eds.), *Current pediatric diagnosis and treatment* (20th ed.). New York: McGraw-Hill.

Provide teaching about the disease process and medication therapy to help the child and family understand the seriousness of the disease. The physician may discuss surgical options during uncontrolled flare-ups, but the nurse may be the person to whom the family members or patient address their questions regarding surgery. Provide the family with information to help answer some of their questions and allay fears.

Teaching About Nutritional Management

Teach the child and family about nutritional management of the disease. For example, adequate nutrition with a high-protein and high-carbohydrate diet may be recommended; when the disease is active, lactose may be tolerated poorly; and vitamin and iron supplements will most likely be recommended. Explain that in severe cases enteral feeding tubes or TPN may be needed; this is rare but often induces remission.

Teaching About Medication Therapy

Medications are extremely important in controlling inflammatory bowel disease. Provide information about the following common medications used to control the disease:

• 5-aminosalicylates: used to prevent relapse (usually used in ulcerative colitis)
• Antibiotics (usually metronidazole and ciprofloxacin): typically used in patients who have perianal Crohn's disease
• Immunomodulators (usually 6-mercaptopurine [6-MP] or azathioprine): used to help maintain remission. Monitor patients for neutropenia and hepatotoxicity.
• Cyclosporine or tacrolimus: used occasionally in conjunction with 6-MP or azathioprine to maintain remission in fulminant ulcerative colitis
• Methotrexate: sometimes used to manage severe Crohn's disease
• Anti-tumour necrosis antibody therapy: widely used for children with Crohn's disease; occasionally used for children with ulcerative colitis

Promoting Family and Child Coping

Inflammatory bowel disease is a chronic and often debilitating illness. Many children with this diagnosis can lead normal lives, but frequent illnesses can cause school absences, which in turn add stress to the situation. Because schools have become much less tolerant of absences and tardiness, it may be necessary to write letters to the school explaining the frequent absences or in-school needs. Bathroom privileges should be very flexible for children during flare-ups. Children with inflammatory bowel disease tend to be of small stature due to the illness itself and steroid use, which stunts growth; this may cause psychological issues, especially for older boys (Haas-Beckert & Heyman, 2010). Children with ostomies as a result of

surgical resection may have self-esteem issues related to the presence and care of the ostomy. Arrange for counselling for both the child and family to discuss fears and anxiety related to a chronic disease.

Celiac Disease

Celiac disease, also known as celiac sprue, is an immunologic disorder in which gluten, a product most commonly found in grains, causes damage to the small intestine. The villi of the small intestine are damaged due to the body's immunologic response to the digestion of gluten. The function of the villi is to absorb nutrients into the bloodstream. When the villi are blunted or damaged, malnutrition occurs.

Celiac disease is one of the most common chronic disorders in Europe and the United States, affecting about 1% of the population (Runge & Nguyen, 2010). In Canada, the estimated incidence of celiac disease is 1 in 133 persons (Canadian Celiac Association, 2011). The incidence is higher in those with a family history of celiac disease and in persons with autoimmune or genetic disorders (Runge & Nguyen, 2010). Relatives of those diagnosed with celiac disease are often screened for the disorder, especially in the presence of GI symptoms.

The only current treatment for celiac disease is a strict gluten-free diet. Eliminating gluten will cause the villi of the intestines to heal and function normally, with subsequent improvement of symptoms. Even very small amounts of gluten introduced back into the diet can cause damage to the villi, so the patient must adhere to the diet throughout life (Runge & Nguyen, 2010).

Nursing Assessment

For a full description of the assessment phase of the nursing process, refer to page 1365. Assessment findings pertinent to celiac disease are discussed below. The child with symptoms of celiac disease often presents for evaluation by age 2.

Health History

Elicit a description of the present illness and chief complaint. The symptoms of celiac disease are very broad and are easily confused with other GI disorders. The classic symptoms of children with celiac disease are as follows:

• Diarrhea
• **Steatorrhea**
• Constipation
• Failure to thrive or weight loss/anorexia
• Abdominal distention or bloating
• Abdominal pain
• Vomiting
• Poor muscle tone
• Irritability and listlessness
• Dental disorders

- Anemia (unresponsive to therapy)
- Delayed onset of puberty or amenorrhea
- Nutritional deficiencies

Explore the child's current and past medical history for risk factors such as being white and having a family history of celiac disease (Allen, 2004). Down syndrome, Turner syndrome, Williams syndrome, and selective IgA deficiencies are also linked genetically to celiac disease (Buzby, 2010).

Physical Examination

Assess for the typical appearance of children with celiac disease: distended abdomen, wasted buttocks, and very thin extremities (Allen, 2004) (Fig. 41.19).

Laboratory and Diagnostic Tests

Common laboratory and diagnostic studies ordered for the assessment of celiac disease include IgA serological antibody screening and intestinal biopsy for confirmation

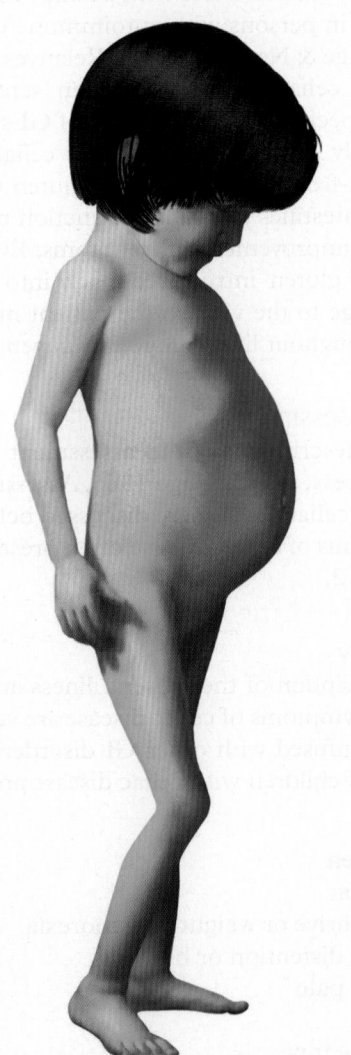

FIGURE 41.19 The child with celiac disease typically displays a distended abdomen and wasted extremities.

and genetic testing. The serum antibody markers look for antibodies in the bloodstream that are specific to a patient's response to gluten. The intestinal biopsy is the gold standard for confirming the diagnosis. (Buzby, 2010). It is taken from the duodenum during an upper endoscopic procedure performed by a gastroenterologist. Pathology from the biopsy reveals partial or subtotal villous atrophy or blunting of the villi of the small intestine. Genetic testing is also available for celiac disease, looking for certain human leukocyte antigen types (Runge & Nguyen, 2010). This may rule out celiac disease with 99% accuracy in people who are genetically predisposed to celiac disease, obviating the need for an intestinal biopsy (Allen, 2004).

Nursing Management

Providing patient and family education is the key nursing role in managing children with celiac disease. The patient must adhere to a strict gluten-free diet for his or her entire life. This is often very challenging because gluten is found in most wheat products, rye, barley, and possibly oats. Encourage the parents and child to maintain this gluten-free diet. Often, families consult a dietitian to learn about the gluten-free diet (Teaching Guideline 41.3). Symptoms usually resolve within days to weeks of eliminating gluten from the diet (Buzby, 2010).

Provide educational materials and resources to the parents. Many resources are available today about celiac disease because it is becoming more commonly diagnosed (Box 41.6).

Recurrent Abdominal Pain

Recurrent abdominal pain is a common GI complaint of children and adolescents. It affects children of all ages. The etiology remains unclear. A community-based study of middle- and high-school students showed that 13% to 17% have weekly abdominal pain (Jarrett, Heitkemper, Czyzewski, & Shulman, 2003). The Rome Committee is a group of specialists who are focusing on the identification, management, and treatment of both adults and children with these functional GI disorders. The three categories of recurrent abdominal pain in children are functional abdominal pain, nonulcer dyspepsia, and irritable bowel syndrome. Box 41.7 outlines the Rome Committee's criteria for distinguishing different features of irritable bowel syndrome (Longstreth, 2009).

Pathophysiology

The etiology of recurrent abdominal pain is controversial but most likely multifactorial. The two primary mechanisms are thought to be the autonomic nervous system, which controls the body's response to emotions and stress, and intestinal motility. Symptoms may result from an alteration in the transmission of messages between the enteric nervous system and the central nervous system, leading to visceral hypersensitivity. Information from the

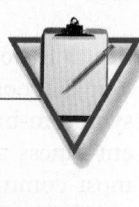

TEACHING GUIDELINE 41.3

Dietary Considerations in a Gluten-Free Diet

Foods Allowed	Foods to Avoid
Potato, soy, rice, or bean flour; rice bran; cornmeal; arrowroot; corn or potato starch; sago; tapioca; buckwheat; millet; flax; teff; sorghum; amaranth; quinoa	Wheat flour; rye; triticale; barley; oats; wheat germ or bran; graham, gluten, or durum flour; wheat starch; oat bran; bulgur; farina; spelt; kamut; malt extract; hydrolyzed vegetable protein
Plain, fresh, frozen, or canned vegetables made with allowed ingredients	Any creamed or breaded vegetables, canned baked beans, some French fries
All fruits and fruit juices	Some commercial fruit pie fillings and dried fruit
All milk and milk products except those made with gluten additives, aged cheese	Malted milk, flavored or frozen yogurt
All meat, poultry, fish, and shellfish; dried peas and beans; nuts; peanut butter; soybean; cold cuts; frankfurters or sausage without fillers	Any meats or poultry prepared with wheat, rye, oats, barley, gluten stabilizers, or fillers for meats; canned meats; self-basting turkey; some egg substitutes
Butter, margarine, salad dressings, sauces, soups, and desserts with allowable ingredients; sugar; honey; jelly; jam; hard candy; plain chocolate; coconut; molasses; marshmallows; meringues; pure instant or ground coffee; tea; carbonated drinks; wine	Commercial salad dressings; prepared soups, condiments, sauces, and seasonings made with avoided products; nondairy cream substitutes; flavored instant coffee; alcohol distilled from cereals; licorice

From: National Digestive Diseases Information Clearinghouse (NDDIC) (2008). *Celiac disease.* http://www.digestive.niddk.nih.gov/ddiseases/pubs/celiac/index.htm.

GI tract is transmitted through bidirectional nerve pathways to the brain. Most neurotransmitters are found in both the brain and the gut, suggesting the potential for integrated effects of pain modulation (Jarrett et al., 2003). As different possibilities exist for the pathophysiology of recurrent abdominal pain, it is clear that there are no structural or biochemical abnormalities that are identifiable.

Therapeutic management most often focuses on increasing the child's coping skills. Some children may need dietary manipulation or medications to control diarrhea (irritable bowel syndrome).

Nursing Assessment

For a full description of the assessment phase of the nursing process, refer to page 1365. Assessment findings pertinent to recurrent abdominal pain are discussed in following page.

BOX 41.6 Resources for Parents of Children with Celiac Disease

Visit http://thePoint.lww.com/Chow1e *for the direct links to the websites and phone numbers for these organizations.*

- American Celiac Society
- Canadian Celiac Association
- Celiac Disease Foundation
- Celiac Sprue Association
- Gluten Intolerance Group (GIG)
- R.O.C.K. (Raising Our Celiac Kids) support group

These resources can offer information on all aspects of celiac disease, including dietary guidelines and resources for food shopping and eating in restaurants.

From: Korn, D. (2002). *Wheat-free, worry-free: The art of happy, healthy gluten-free living.* Carlsbad, CA: Hay House, Inc.

BOX 41.7 Rome Committee Criteria for Irritable Bowel Syndrome

12 weeks or more of the following symptoms:

- Abdominal pain relieved by defecation
- Onset of pain or discomfort associated with a change in frequency of stool
- Onset of pain or discomfort associated with a change in form of the stool
- No structural or metabolic explanation for this abdominal pain

From: Longstreth, G. F. [updated by Drossman, D. A.] (2009). *Current approach to the diagnosis of irritable bowel syndrome* [electronic version]. Milwaukee, WI: International Foundation for Functional Gastrointestinal Disorders. Retrieved December 6, 2011 from http://www.aboutgimotility.org/store/viewproduct/163.

Health History

The diagnosis of recurrent abdominal pain is made on a symptom-based approach. Elicit a description of the present illness and chief complaint. The symptom reported most commonly during the health history is abdominal pain. The child may have difficulty providing a good description of the pain. It is usually periumbilical and commonly described as attacks of pain. It is uncommon for the child to wake up in the middle of the night with this type of pain. In cases of irritable bowel syndrome, the pain may be relieved by defecation. Because diet may play a large role in the symptoms, obtain a dietary history. Take a detailed medication history, because abdominal pain may be an adverse effect of some medications. Identifying social and school stressors is essential (Jarrett et al., 2003).

Physical Examination

Note the child's body positioning and facial expressions. Interactions with family members during the interview may provide more details regarding social stressors. Palpate the abdomen for tenderness.

Laboratory and Diagnostic Tests

Common laboratory and diagnostic studies ordered for the assessment of recurrent abdominal pain include the following:

- CBD: to rule out organic causes of abdominal pain
- Erythrocyte sedimentation rate: to rule out organic causes of abdominal pain
- Urinalysis: to rule out organic causes of abdominal pain
- Complete metabolic panel: to rule out organic causes of abdominal pain
- Stool studies: to assess for routine pathogens
- Gastro-duodenoscopy or colonoscopy: to identify a source
- Small bowel follow-through contrast study
- Abdominal CT scan
- Diagnostic laparoscopy

Nursing Management

Once the diagnosis of recurrent abdominal pain with no organic cause is made, the majority of the nursing management is focused on promoting coping skills. Often the physician performs a battery of tests to rule out organic causes, especially when patient and family anxiety is high. After these tests are complete, teach the family about the factors that exacerbate the pain and how to deal with these factors.

Diet changes may need to be implemented. High-fibre diets help with bowel regulation by keeping motility regular.

Often medications are used to relieve abdominal cramps. Antidiarrheals may be used for patients with irritable bowel syndrome that is manifested by diarrhea.

Acid-reducing medications may be tried for epigastric complaints. Occasionally pain modulators and antidepressants are used to help block the neurotransmitters in the brain–gut connection that cause pain. Encourage compliance with the medication regimen: compliance is needed to achieve beneficial results with many of these medications.

Arrange for counselling, if necessary, for children with social stressors. Children with recurrent abdominal pain may become so debilitated that they cannot function in school, possibly requiring homebound instruction. Provide education to the school, with parental permission, regarding the child's illness and how to best deal with it. Explain that this recurrent abdominal pain is a true pain that children feel and is not "in their minds" (Jarrett et al., 2003).

Hepatobiliary Disorders

Hepatobiliary disorders include pancreatitis, gallbladder disease, jaundice, biliary atresia, hepatitis, cirrhosis and portal hypertension, and liver transplantation.

Pancreatitis

Pancreatitis is increasingly being recognized as a childhood problem (Sokol & Narkewicz, 2011). It is classified into two categories: acute and chronic. Acute pancreatitis is an acute inflammatory process that occurs within the pancreas, with variable involvement of localized tissues and remote organ systems. Most common causes of acute pancreatitis include abdominal trauma, drugs and alcohol (though probably rare in children), multisystem disease (such as inflammatory bowel disease or systemic lupus erythematosus), infections (usually viruses such as cytomegalovirus [CMV] or hepatitis), congenital anomalies (ductal or pancreatic malformations), obstruction (most likely gallstones or tumours in children), or metabolic disorders. Chronic pancreatitis is defined based on the structural and/or functional permanent changes that occur in the pancreas (Werlin, 2004).

When pancreatitis is suspected, the child is placed on immediate bowel rest (NPO). Often, a nasogastric tube placed for suction will be needed to keep the stomach decompressed (Werlin, 2004). Normally, an oral diet may be resumed once the clinical signs and symptoms have resolved, usually within 3 to 7 days in mild pancreatitis. There is some research to support the early introduction of enteral feeds. TPN may supplement enteral feeds until the ileus has resolved (Al Samaraee, McCallum, Coyne, & Seymour, 2009).

Nursing Assessment

For a full description of the assessment phase of the nursing process, refer to page 1365. Assessment findings pertinent to pancreatitis are discussed in following page.

Health History

Elicit a description of the present illness and chief complaint. Common signs and symptoms reported during the health history include the following:

- Acute onset of persistent midepigastric and periumbilical abdominal pain, often with radiation to the back or chest
- Vomiting, especially after meals
- Fever

Explore the child's current and past medical history for risk factors such as:

- Cystic fibrosis
- History of gallstones
- Traumatic injury
- Family history of hereditary pancreatitis
- Alcohol ingestion (adolescents)

Physical Examination

On abdominal assessment, the bowel sounds may be diminished, suggesting peritonitis. The abdomen is very tender, and distention may occur in younger children and infants. In severe cases, jaundice, ascites, or pleural effusions may occur. Bluish discolouration around the umbilicus or flanks is seen in the most severe cases of pancreatitis when hemorrhage is present.

Laboratory and Diagnostic Tests

Common laboratory and diagnostic studies ordered for the assessment and monitoring of pancreatitis include the following:

- Serum amylase and/or lipase: levels three times the normal values are extremely indicative of pancreatitis (Werlin, 2004)
- Liver profile: often done to check for increased liver functions and/or bilirubin levels
- Bloodwork: leukocytosis is common with acute pancreatitis. Hyperglycemia and hypocalcemia may also be noted
- C-reactive protein: levels may be elevated

Diagnostic imaging studies performed to identify malformations or cysts on the pancreas include the following:

- Plain abdominal X-ray: may show a localized ileus
- Ultrasound or CT scan: allows direct visualization of the pancreas and surrounding structures and identification of cholelithiasis. Ultrasound is used most frequently with children as it is less invasive than a CT scan. A CT scan is usually reserved for use when there is difficulty in determining the cause of the pancreatitis during ultrasonography.
- Endoscopic retrograde cholangiopancreatography (ERCP): used in some children who may have ductal anomalies, usually with chronic pancreatitis or gallstones stuck in the biliary ducts, though complications from this procedure may occur.

Nursing Management

Maintain NPO status and nasogastric tube suction and patency. Administer intravenous fluids to keep the patient hydrated and correct any alterations in fluid and electrolyte balance. Pain management is crucial in children with pancreatitis. If hemorrhagic pancreatitis has occurred, blood products and/or intravenous antibiotics may be needed.

Surgery is rarely needed in patients with pancreatitis, except in those with severe abdominal trauma or major ductal abnormalities.

Though chronic pancreatitis is rare in children, provide patient and family education regarding the signs and symptoms of recurrence and complications.

Gallbladder Disease

Cholelithiasis is the presence of stones in the gallbladder. Cholesterol stones are usually associated with hyperlipidemia, obesity, pregnancy, birth control pill use, or cystic fibrosis (Schwarz, Hebra, & Miller, 2011). They are seen more often in females than males, and risk increases with age and onset of puberty (Schwarz et al., 2011). These stones occur in the gallbladder and may be found in the common bile duct. Pigment stones are found in prepubertal children and occur about equally in males and females. They are usually found in the common bile duct (associated with bacterial or parasitic infections) or the gallbladder itself (associated with hemolytic anemia or liver cirrhosis). Cholecystitis is an inflammation of the gallbladder that is caused by the chemical irritation due to the obstruction of bile flow from the gallbladder into the cystic ducts (Fig. 41.20). This inflammation is typically associated

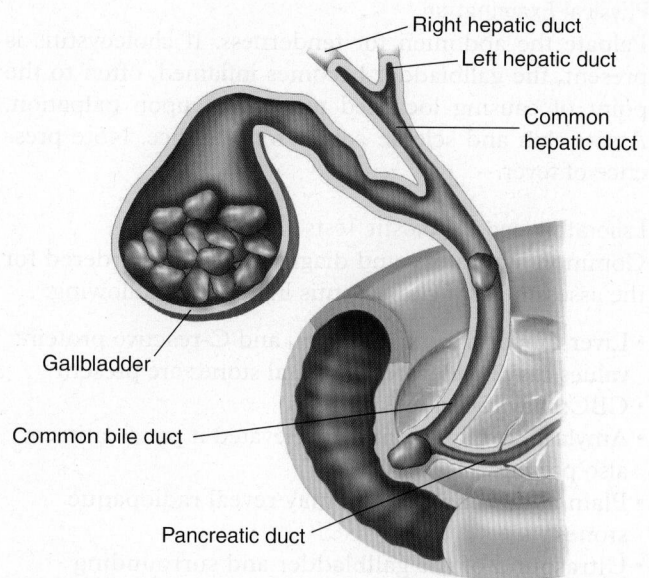

FIGURE 41.20 When gallstones block the flow of bile through the ducts, cholecystitis results.

with gallstones in children. The most common complication in children with gallstone disease is pancreatitis (Suchy, 2004).

If cholelithiasis results in symptomatic cholecystitis, then surgical removal of the gallbladder (cholecystectomy) will be necessary. Surgeons may also choose to remove the gallbladder with coincidental findings of cholelithiasis to prevent pancreatitis. This is often accomplished laparoscopically.

Nursing Assessment

For a full description of the assessment phase of the nursing process, refer to page 1365. Assessment findings pertinent to gallbladder disease are discussed below.

Health History

Elicit a description of the present illness and chief complaint. Common signs and symptoms reported during the health history include the following:

- Right upper quadrant pain, often radiating substernally or to the right shoulder, usually following the ingestion of fatty foods
- Nausea and vomiting
- Jaundice and fever (with cholecystitis)

Document a detailed diet history as it relates to the presenting symptoms. Pain episodes usually occur after meals (postprandially), especially after the ingestion of fatty or greasy foods. Younger children may present with more nonspecific symptoms, most often due to their lack of ability to communicate their symptoms to others. Explore the patient's current and past medical history for risk factors such as chronic TPN use or sickle-cell disease.

Physical Examination

Palpate the abdomen for tenderness. If cholecystitis is present, the gallbladder becomes inflamed, often to the point of causing localized tenderness upon palpation. Assess skin and sclerae colour for jaundice. Note presence of fever.

Laboratory and Diagnostic Tests

Common laboratory and diagnostic studies ordered for the assessment of cholecystitis include the following:

- Liver function tests, bilirubin, and C-reactive protein: values may be elevated if ductal stones are present
- CBC: may reveal leukocytosis
- Amylase and lipase: may be elevated if pancreatitis is also present
- Plain abdominal X-rays: may reveal radiopaque stones
- Ultrasound of the gallbladder and surrounding structures: to assess the intraluminal contents of the gallbladder as well as any anatomic alterations
- ERCP: to manage ductal stones

- Hepatibiliary iminodiacetic acid scan: to evaluate the function of the gallbladder (rare)

Nursing Management

The child with symptomatic cholecystitis will usually be hospitalized. Administer intravenous fluids, maintain NPO status and gastric decompression if vomiting, and administer pain medications. If ordered, administer intravenous antibiotics to treat clinically worsening symptoms of cholangitis, such as persistent fever and an elevated white cell count. Provide routine postoperative care after cholecystectomy is performed. Provide pre- and postoperative teaching for families of children undergoing gallbladder removal.

Jaundice

Jaundice is the most common clinical problem in newborns and is the most common reason for infant readmission to the hospital in the first week of life (American Academy of Pediatrics, 2004; Maisels, 2005a, 2005b, 2005c, 2005d). It may also occur in older infants and children as a symptom of another disease process. Jaundice is a condition in which the skin, sclerae, body fluids, and other tissues have a yellow discolouration caused by the deposition of bile pigment resulting from excess bilirubin in the blood. It may be caused by obstruction of bile passageways, excess destruction of red blood cells (hemolysis), or disturbances in functioning of liver cells (Maisels, 2005a, 2005b, 2005c, 2005d).

Newborn jaundice can be divided into two categories: physiologic and pathologic. Physiologic jaundice is the more common type, occurring usually after the first 24 hours of life. It usually lasts no longer than 1 week, and the infant shows no signs of illness. Physiologic jaundice occurs because the newborn cannot excrete bilirubin due to immaturity. Normally, the level of indirect or unconjugated bilirubin peaks at 85 to 102 µmol/L on day 3 or 4 of life. These levels may be higher in breast-fed infants.

Pathologic jaundice may appear at less than 24 hours of age and lasts for longer than 1 week. In some cases, the jaundice may disappear and reappear after a period of time, as in biliary atresia. In pathologic jaundice, the conjugated or direct bilirubin value is greater than 20% of the total bilirubin value (Maisels, 2005a, 2005b, 2005c, 2005d). There may be several causes for pathologic jaundice (Table 41.3).

► **Take** NOTE!

Significant jaundice in a newborn less than 24 hours of age should be immediately reported to the physician, as it may indicate a pathologic process.

TABLE 41.3 CAUSES OF PATHOLOGIC JAUNDICE

Cause	Laboratory Values	Possible Explanations	Notable Facts
Hemolysis	Indirect bilirubin levels are elevated in the first 24 h of life	Rh incompatibility, sickle-cell anemia, drug-induced, hemolytic–uremic syndrome, Wilson's disease, deficiencies of red blood cell enzymes (G6PD deficiency), hereditary spherocytosis	Unconjugated hyperbilirubinemia
Obstructive disorders	Direct hyperbilirubinemia, usually elevations in alkaline phosphatase, serum GGT, liver enzymes, occasionally pancreatic enzymes	Biliary atresia, cholelithiasis, choledochal cysts, tumours, bile duct stenosis	Surgical correction is necessary in all obstructive disorders to avoid long-term damage to vital organs
Infectious causes	Specific to different causes of infection	Hepatitis A, B, C, D, E, and G, cytomegalovirus, herpes simplex virus 1, 2, and 6, Epstein-Barr virus, measles, varicella, human parvovirus, toxoplasmosis, syphilis, bacterial sepsis/urinary tract infection, cholecystitis	Treatment options differ with causes; bacterial causes should be identified and treated immediately
Metabolic disorders	Specific to different disorders; elevations in conjugated bilirubin seen	Wilson's disease, alpha-1 antitrypsin deficiency, tyrosinemia, galactosemia, fructosemia, Zellweger syndrome, neonatal iron storage disease, cystic fibrosis, bile acid synthesis defects	Considered rare but should not be excluded from differential diagnosis of infant with hyperbilirubinemia
Toxic disorders	Elevations in conjugated bilirubin as well as drug levels and liver enzymes	TPN, drug overdose (such as acetaminophen and ethanol), toxic drug levels (phenytoin, valproic acid)	Patients receiving hepatotoxic drugs should be monitored for toxic blood levels periodically and with dosage changes
Idiopathic	Elevations in serum conjugated bilirubin levels	Idiopathic neonatal hepatitis, Alagille syndrome, familial intrahepatic cholestasis, cholestasis with lymphedema (Aagenaes syndrome), cholestasis with hypopituitarism	Can be infectious or hereditary

Therapeutic Management

Physiologic jaundice is initially managed by increasing oral feedings to enhance bilirubin excretion. Phototherapy is indicated when jaundice fails to resolve within an acceptable time frame. In babies with hemolytic disorders, exchange therapy may be necessary to remove the sensitized red blood cells and bilirubin and exchange them with bilirubin-free blood. This is usually accomplished in the intensive care unit. Pathologic jaundice requires further investigation to determine the cause; treatment is based on the cause.

Nursing Assessment

For a full description of the assessment phase of the nursing process, refer to page 1365. Assessment findings pertinent to jaundice are discussed below.

Health History

Elicit a description of the present illness and chief complaint. Typically, the parents report that the infant is sleepier than usual or feeding poorly. Explore the patient's current and past medical history for risk factors such as family history of metabolic or hepatic disease; exposure to drugs, toxins, or infectious agents; Rh or ABO incompatibility; presence of large cephalhematoma or significant bruising; and polycythemia. Assess the infant's feeding history.

Physical Examination

Assess the skin, mucous membranes, sclerae, and bodily fluids (tears, urine) for a yellow colour. Observe stool colour; stools may appear acholic (white and chalky). Use digital skin blanching to determine the presence of jaundice. Infants with jaundice will appear icteric initially in the face, and then the yellowish discolouration will spread caudally to the trunk and then the extremities. Inspect the abdomen for distention (liver enlargement or ascites).

Laboratory and Diagnostic Studies

Assess laboratory values for bilirubin (both unconjugated and conjugated), alkaline phosphatase, liver enzymes, gamma-glutamyl transpeptidase (GGT), and prothrombin time (PT) and partial thromboplastin time (PTT). Many infants and children will need radiologic evaluation to determine abnormalities that may be causing the jaundice.

Nursing Management

Nursing management of the infant or child with jaundice is specific to the underlying cause. However, in all cases, proper nutrition is essential to increase bilirubin clearance. For newborns with physiologic jaundice, encourage mothers of breastfeeding infants to nurse up to 12 times in a 24-hour period (Maisels, 2005a, 2005b, 2005c, 2005d). If this does not reduce jaundice, the infant's diet may need to be supplemented with formula for a specific period of time. Administer phototherapy as ordered, ensuring that appropriate precautions are taken to shield the eyes from the ultraviolet light (Fig. 41.21). Explain to parents that this therapy is used to expose the infants to light (sun or artificial) to help alter the bilirubin to a readily excreted form. Reassess the stools and feeding history of infants receiving phototherapy to ensure proper hydration. Help to relieve family anxiety regarding jaundice in the newborn or child by explaining when to notify the physician (increasing jaundice, lethargy, poor feeding, vomiting, or acute changes in the child's condition).

▶ *Take* NOTE!

The American Academy of Pediatrics does not recommend the use of sunlight as a treatment for physiologic jaundice because of the risk for sunburn and the difficulty with regulating light exposure.

Biliary Atresia

Biliary atresia is an absence of some or all of the major biliary ducts, resulting in obstruction of bile flow. It is one of the leading causes of end-stage liver disease in the pediatric population (Schreiber, Barker, Roberts, Martin, & the Canadian Pediatric Hepatology Research Group, 2010). The resultant obstruction to bile flow causes cholestasis and progressive fibrosis with end-stage cirrhosis of the liver (Balistreri, 2004). In approximately 80% of the cases, biliary atresia presents around 4 weeks of age in term, healthy infants who have resolved physiologic jaundice. In approximately 20% of cases, biliary atresia presents with persistent jaundice that never disappeared from the physiologic period. This second type of biliary atresia often is associated with other congenital anomalies, such as situs inversus, malrotation, polysplenia, and cardiovascular defects (Balistreri, 2004). The etiology of biliary atresia is unknown, but there are several theories, including infectious, autoimmune, or ischemic causes.

Therapeutic Management

If there is a high suspicion of biliary atresia, the infant will undergo exploratory laparotomy. If biliary atresia is found, a Kasai procedure (hepatoportoenterostomy) is performed to connect the bowel lumen to the bile duct remnants found at the porta hepatis. In Canada, the chance of survival is 50% if the surgery is performed within the first month of life, dropping to 20% when surgery is performed as late as 90 days after birth (Schreiber et al., 2010). Infants who are not identified early enough or those who have failed to respond to the Kasai procedure will need to undergo liver transplantation, usually by age 2 (Schwarz, 2009).

Nursing Assessment

For a full description of the assessment phase of the nursing process, refer to page 1365. Assessment findings pertinent to biliary atresia are discussed below.

Health History

Elicit a description of the present illness and chief complaint. Persistent or recurring jaundice is the most common symptom reported during the health history.

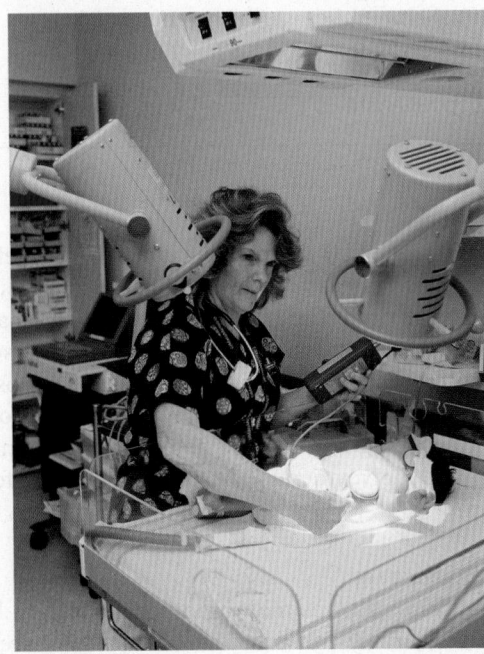

FIGURE 41.21 When receiving phototherapy, the infant's eyes must be covered to protect them from the ultraviolet light.

Physical Examination

In the initial assessment of an infant with cholestasis of unknown origin, assess the stool character. In biliary atresia, stools will be acholic (chalky and white due to the lack of bile pigment). During the physical assessment, the liver will feel enlarged and hardened. Splenomegaly may occur. In the absence of other congenital malformations, the infant will otherwise appear healthy.

Laboratory and Diagnostic Studies

Common laboratory and diagnostic studies ordered for the assessment of biliary atresia include the following:

- Serum bilirubin, alkaline phosphatase, liver enzymes, GGT: elevated
- Ultrasound: to identify anomalies
- Biliary scan: to distinguish whether the cholestasis is intrahepatic or extrahepatic
- Liver biopsy: to confirm the diagnosis (Balistreri, 2004)

Nursing Management

Nursing management of infants who have biliary atresia will focus on vitamin and caloric support. Administer fat-soluble vitamins A, D, E, and K. Special formulas containing medium-chain triglycerides are used because significant fat malabsorption occurs when cholestasis is present. Administer feedings via nasogastric tube as needed to ensure increased caloric intake. Identify infections as quickly as possible and administer intravenous antibiotics as ordered. Manage ascites with diuretics and dietary restrictions. Preoperative management before a Kasai procedure is focused on preparation for surgery; infants who have suspected biliary atresia require immediate surgery to optimize outcomes. Postoperative management involves controlling pain, administering fluids, maximizing nutrition, and monitoring bloodwork.

Parents and family members of these infants will have extreme anxiety due to the implications of the diagnosis and outcomes. Focus education on the diagnosis and postoperative care. Nursing Care Plan 41.1 gives information about routine postoperative care.

Hepatitis

Hepatitis is an inflammation of the liver that is caused by a variety of agents, including viral infections, bacterial invasion, metabolic disorders, chemical toxicity, and trauma. The most common viral causes of hepatitis are listed in Table 41.4. Other viruses that may cause hepatitis

TABLE 41.4 HEPATITIS VIRUSES A–E

	Hepatitis A Virus (HAV)	Hepatitis B Virus (HBV)	Hepatitis C Virus (HCV)	Hepatitis D Virus (HDV)	Hepatitis E Virus (HEV)
Transmission route	Oral–fecal route, poor sanitation, waterborne	Sexual, intravenous drug use, blood transfusion, perinatally transmitted from mother to infant	Blood product transfusion, intravenous drug use	Same as HBV; HBV markers in serum must be present	Oral–fecal, possible contact
Incubation period	15–30 days	50–150 days	30–160 days	50–150 days	15–65 days
Signs and symptoms	Flu-like symptoms Preicteric phase: headache, fatigue, fever, anorexia Icteric phase: jaundice, dark urine, tender liver (right upper quadrant pain)	Some cases are asymptomatic; others present with anorexia, abdominal pain, fatigue, rash, slight fever, visible jaundice, enlarged liver	Chronic cases usually present asymptomatically; others with flu-like symptoms, jaundice, hepatosplenomegaly	Same as HBV	Same as HAV; more severe in pregnant women
Prognosis	Rarely develops into fulminant liver failure; 95% of children recover without sequelae	Chronic disease state likely; increased risk of hepatic cancer	Many will develop chronic hepatitis and cirrhosis	Same as HBV, but increased likelihood of chronic active hepatitis and cirrhosis	Same as HAV; high mortality in pregnant women

Adapted from: Sokol, R., & Narkewicz, M. (2011). Liver & pancreas. In W. W. Hay, M. J. Levin, J. M. Sondheimer, & R. R. Deterding (Eds.), *Current pediatric diagnosis and treatment* (20th ed.). New York: McGraw-Hill.

are CMV, Epstein-Barr virus, and adenovirus. Fulminant hepatitis is thought to be caused by a non-A, non-B, non-C virus. Children who present with fulminant hepatitis have acute massive hepatic necrosis, resulting in death without liver transplantation. The disease progresses rapidly to severe jaundice, coagulopathy, elevated ammonia levels, significantly elevated liver enzyme levels (AST and ALT), and progressive coma. Autoimmune hepatitis is a chronic disorder, affecting mostly adolescent females. The clinical presentation of a child with autoimmune hepatitis includes hepatosplenomegaly, jaundice, fever, fatigue, and right upper quadrant pain.

Therapeutic Management

Acute hepatitis is treated with rest, hydration, and nutrition. Control of bleeding may also be necessary. Chronic hepatitis often eventually requires liver transplantation. Corticosteroids and immunosuppressants may be used for autoimmune hepatitis. The child with fulminant hepatitis usually requires intensive care with cardiorespiratory support.

Nursing Assessment

For a full description of the assessment phase of the nursing process, refer to page 1365. Assessment findings pertinent to hepatitis are discussed below. The nursing assessment for any child who presents with suspected hepatitis should be the same.

Health History

Elicit a description of the present illness and the chief complaint. Common signs and symptoms reported during the health history include the following:

- Jaundice
- Fever
- Fatigue
- Abdominal pain

Explore the patient's current and past medical history for risk factors such as:

- Recent foreign travel
- Sick contacts
- Medication use
- Abdominal trauma
- Sexual activity
- Intravenous drug use
- Blood product transfusion

Document onset of symptoms as well as all signs and symptoms the patient has been experiencing.

Physical Examination

Observe the skin for jaundice and the sclerae for icterus. Palpate the abdomen to reveal abnormal liver and spleen size or tenderness.

Laboratory and Diagnostic Studies

Common laboratory and diagnostic studies ordered for the assessment of hepatitis include the following:

- Liver enzymes, GGT: elevated
- PT/PTT: prolonged
- Ammonia: elevated in the presence of encephalopathy
- Autoimmune studies, such as antinuclear antibodies, anti-smooth muscle antibodies, and liver–kidney microsomal antibodies: may be used to diagnose autoimmune hepatitis
- Viral studies: to identify viral causes of hepatitis, such as hepatitis A–E antigens and antibodies, CMV, and Epstein-Barr virus
- Ultrasound: to assess liver or spleen abnormalities
- Liver biopsy: to determine the type of hepatitis and to assess for damage that has already been done to the liver

Nursing Management

Acute hepatitis requires rest, hydration, and nutrition. If the child develops vomiting, dehydration, elevated bleeding times (PT/PTT), or mental status changes (encephalopathy), hospitalization may be required. When caring for patients with infectious hepatitis, provide education about transmission and prevention, including proper hygiene, safe sexual activity, careful handwashing techniques, and blood/bodily fluid precautions.

Fulminant hepatitis treatment is aggressive and will require NPO status, nasogastric tube administration of lactulose to decrease ammonia levels that lead to encephalopathic conditions, TPN administration, vitamin K injections to help with coagulopathies, and, ultimately, liver transplantation. Fear and anxiety of the patient and parents will likely be very high. Teach the child and family about the diagnosis and what to expect during treatment. Provide immunoglobulin therapy and vaccinations to close contacts of infectious hepatitis patients.

Cirrhosis and Portal Hypertension

Cirrhosis of the liver occurs as a result of the destructive processes that occur during liver damage, leading to the formation of nodules. These nodules can be small (micronodular [<3 mm]) or large (macronodular [>3 mm]) and distort the vasculature of the liver, leading to further complications. Causes of cirrhosis in children include biliary malformations, alpha-1 antitrypsin deficiency, Wilson's disease, galactosemia, tyrosinemia, chronic active hepatitis, and prolonged TPN use (Sokol & Narkewicz, 2011). Major complications may exist due to cirrhosis of the liver, including portal hypertension. In portal hypertension, the blood flow to, through, or from the liver meets resistance, causing portal blood flow pressures to rise. As these pressures rise, collateral veins form between the portal and systemic venous circulations. The most significant complication of portal hypertension is

GI bleeding, from shunting to submucosal veins (varices) in the stomach and esophagus. Esophageal varices may be treated with sclerotherapy during endoscopy to stop acute bleeding. Often blood product administration and vasopressive drugs are needed. In the long term, the only cure for cirrhosis is liver transplantation.

Nursing Assessment

For a full description of the assessment phase of the nursing process, refer to page 1365. Assessment findings pertinent to cirrhosis and portal hypertension are discussed below.

Health History

Elicit a description of the present illness and chief complaint. Common signs and symptoms reported during the health history include the following:

- Nausea and vomiting
- Jaundice
- Weakness
- Swelling
- Weight loss

Explore the patient's current and past medical history for risk factors such as hepatitis, cystic fibrosis, Wilson's disease, hemochromatosis, and biliary atresia. Assess the past medical history to identify possible causes for liver disease.

Physical Examination

Inspect for jaundice, ascites, spider angiomas, and palmar erythema. Gynecomastia is often seen in males. Palpate the liver; typically it is enlarged and hard, but occasionally it is small and shrunken. Evaluate mental status to determine the presence of hepatic encephalopathy.

Laboratory and Diagnostic Studies

Laboratory and diagnostic testing will be similar to that of a child with hepatitis. Common laboratory and diagnostic studies ordered for the assessment of cirrhosis or portal hypertension include the following:

- Liver biopsy: reveals regenerating nodules and surrounding **fibrosis**
- Upper endoscopy: reveals varices and bleeding (Fig. 41.22)

Nursing Management

Nursing management is very similar to the care of the patient with hepatitis. In cases of cirrhosis causing portal hypertension and bleeding varices, GI bleeding must be controlled. This is usually done by replacing blood loss and providing vasopressive therapy to constrict the shunted blood flow. As with all liver disorders and GI bleeding, address and manage family and patient anxiety. Be honest about the child's treatment plan and

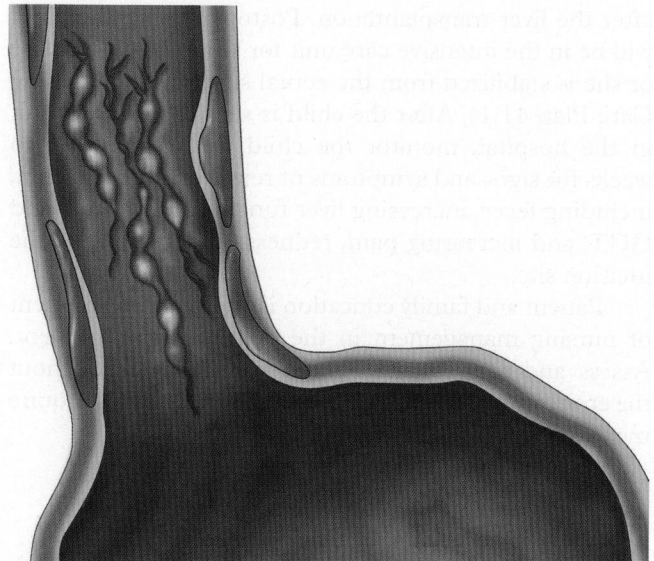

FIGURE 41.22 Esophageal varices.

prognosis. Involve the family in the care of the child and educate them as needed.

Liver Transplantation

Hepatobiliary disorders that result in failure of the liver to function result in the need for liver transplantation. Liver transplantation in children has become increasingly successful in the past several years due to advances in immunosuppression, better selection of transplant candidates, and improvements in surgical techniques and postoperative care (Boudi, 2011). Transplant centres now offer both cadaveric and living-related liver transplants for children. Rejection of the transplanted liver is the most significant complication. Most children will require immunosuppressive therapy for a lifetime, putting them at risk for infections.

Nursing Assessment

Many children will be admitted to a transplant centre for a preoperative workup to determine the best possible tissue and blood match for the patient. There is much anxiety among family members when a cadaveric transplant is the only possibility for survival. This puts a child on a waiting list that is prioritized based on several criteria. Because there are a limited number of pediatric liver transplant centres throughout the country, there may be many issues regarding transportation, finances, job loss, and lodging. Assess the need for social work intervention; a social worker is almost always involved with these patients. A liver transplant coordinator will assist with coordinating the care for pre- and post-transplant patients.

Nursing Management

Preoperatively, assist with the transplant workup and teach the child and family what to expect during and after the liver transplantation. Postoperatively, the child will be in the intensive care unit for several days until he or she is stabilized from the actual surgery (see Nursing Care Plan 41.1). After the child is sent to a regular unit in the hospital, monitor the child for several days to weeks for signs and symptoms of rejection and infection, including fever, increasing liver function test results and GGT, and increasing pain, redness, and swelling at the incision site.

Patient and family education is an important element of nursing management in the post-transplant patient. Assess and reassess medication knowledge throughout the entire hospitalization, as these children usually require medications for a lifetime.

▪▪▪ Key Concepts

- The esophagus of the young child exhibits underdeveloped muscle tone compared with the adult.
- A major difference between children and adults is the reduced stomach capacity in the child and the significantly shorter length of the small intestine (250 cm in the child versus 600 cm in the adult).
- Infants and children have a proportionately greater amount of body water than adults, resulting in a relatively greater fluid intake requirement than adults and placing infants and children at higher risk for fluid loss as compared with adults.
- The most common result of GI illnesses in infants and children is dehydration.
- The mildly or moderately dehydrated child must be identified and receive rehydration therapy to prevent progression to hypovolemic shock.
- Rehydration is a key medical treatment for dehydration as a result of many different GI disorders. Oral rehydration is most common, but in cases requiring hospitalization intravenous fluid therapy is key.
- Promotion of adequate nutrition is another significant treatment component. The child with a chronic GI disorder may require intravenous TPN or enteral tube feedings to exhibit appropriate growth.
- Surgical intervention is necessary for many acute or congenital GI disorders, such as pyloric stenosis, omphalocele, gastroschisis, cleft lip and palate, appendicitis, Hirschsprung's disease, and intestinal malrotation with midgut volvulus.
- Abdominal ultrasound is the diagnostic test of choice when evaluating for pyloric stenosis.
- Monitoring the blood count, electrolyte levels, and liver function tests is necessary in many pediatric GI disorders.
- H_2 blockers, proton pump inhibitors, and prokinetic agents are used to treat disorders in which gastric acid is a problem, such as esophagitis, GERD, and ulcers.
- Close monitoring for infection is important in children with inflammatory bowel disease, autoimmune hepatitis, or liver transplant who are being treated with immunosuppressants and/or corticosteroids.
- GI stimulants and laxatives may be necessary for treating constipation and encopresis.
- Diarrhea, vomiting, decreased oral intake, sustained high fever, diabetic ketoacidosis, and extensive burns place the infant or child at risk for the development of dehydration.
- Risk factors for vomiting include exposure to viruses, use of certain medications, and overfeeding in the infant.
- Risk factors for acute diarrhea include recent ingestion of undercooked meats, foreign travel, day care attendance, and well water ingestion.
- Vomiting is a symptom and should be characterized in terms of volume, colour, relation to meals, duration, and associated symptoms.
- Bleeding may occur as a result of a GI disorder, particularly from the intestine with Meckel's diverticulum and from esophageal varices with portal hypertension.
- Acute GI disorders are those that usually have a rapid onset and a short course, which at times may be severe. Examples include dehydration, vomiting, diarrhea, hypertrophic pyloric stenosis, and appendicitis.
- Chronic GI disorders are those that are long lasting or recur over time. Examples include constipation, GER, inflammatory bowel disease, recurrent abdominal pain, and failure to thrive.
- Right lower quadrant pain and rebound tenderness of the abdomen found on physical examination are telltale signs of appendicitis, which is considered a surgical emergency.
- Bilious vomiting is the main symptom of conditions resulting in bowel obstruction, such as malrotation with volvulus.
- The focus of nursing management of the child with diarrhea or vomiting is restoring proper fluid and electrolyte balance through oral rehydration therapy or intravenous fluids if necessary.
- Reduction of inguinal and umbilical hernias should be attempted; if reduction of the hernia is impossible, immediately notify the physician.
- Small, frequent, and thickened feedings and proper positioning after feedings are key elements in the treatment of GER.
- A crucial nursing intervention related to cleft lip and palate repair is protection of the surgical site while it is healing.
- Palpation of the abdomen should be the last part of the physical examination of an infant or child.
- A key element of nursing care for the child with a GI disorder is promotion of appropriate bowel elimination.
- Maximizing nutritional status is a critical nursing function for the child with a GI disorder.
- For the child who has undergone surgical repair or correction of a GI disorder, promoting effective

breathing patterns and managing pain are important nursing goals.

■ Counselling families about how to manage the child with vomiting or diarrhea at home, including oral rehydration therapy, is a key component of patient/family education.

■ Education of the child and family regarding the importance of medication compliance for management of inflammatory bowel disease is critical.

■ Behavioural therapy and counselling may be necessary for children who have functional constipation and stool withholding.

■ The child or adolescent with ineffective bowel control, poor growth, or an ostomy may have poor self-esteem and body image.

REFERENCES

Adibe, O., Nichol, P., Lim, F., & Mattei, P. (2007). Ad libitum feeds after laparoscopic pyloromyotomy: A retrospective comparison with a standardized feeding regimen in 227 infants. *Journal of Laparoendoscopic & Advanced Surgical Techniques. Part A, 17*(2), 235–237.

Albanese, C. T., & Sylvester, K. G. (2010). Pediatric surgery. In G. M. Doherty & L. W. Way (Eds.), *Current surgical diagnosis and treatment* (13th ed.). New York: McGraw-Hill.

Allen, P. L. J. (2004). Guidelines for the diagnosis and treatment of celiac disease in children. *Pediatric Nursing, 30*(6), 473–476.

Al Samaraee, A., McCallum, I., Coyne, P., & Seymour, K. (2009). Nutritional strategies in severe acute pancreatitis: A systematic review of the evidence. *The Surgeon, 8*(2010), 105–110.

American Academy of Pediatrics. (2004). Clinical practice guideline: Management of hyperbilirubinemia in the newborn infant 35 or more weeks of gestation. *Pediatrics, 114*(1), 297–316.

Anand, B. S., Bank, S., Qureshi, W. A., et al. (2011). Peptic ulcer disease. Retrieved December 8, 2011 from www.emedicine.com/ped/topic2341.htm

Balistreri, W. F. (2004). Cholestasis. In R. E. Behrman, R. M. Kliegman, & H. B. Jenson (Eds.), *Nelson textbook of pediatrics* (17th ed.). Philadelphia: WB Saunders.

Berman, J. (2003). Heading off the dangers of acute gastroenteritis. *Contemporary Pediatrics, 20*(7), 57–74.

Blevins, J. Y. (2003). Primary herpetic gingivostomatitis in young children. *Pediatric Nursing, 29*(3), 199–201.

Boudi, F. B. (2011). *Pediatric liver transplantation.* Retrieved April, 20, 2011 from http://emedicine.medscape.com/article/1012910-overview

Browne, N., Flanigan, L., McComiskey, C., & Pieper, P. (2007). *Nursing Care of the Pediatric Surgical Patient* (2nd ed.). Boston, MA: Jones and Bartlett Publishers Inc.

Burns, C., Dunn, A., Brady, M., Starr, N. B., & Blosser, C. (2009). *Pediatric primary care* (4th ed.). Philadelphia: Saunders.

Buzby, M. (2010). Celiac disease: The endocrine connection. *Journal of Pediatric Nursing, 25*(4), 311–313.

Cahill, J., & Wagner, C. (2002). Challenges in breastfeeding: Neonatal concerns. *Contemporary Pediatrics, 5*, 113.

Canadian Celiac Association. (2011). About Celiac Disease. Retrieved on December 17, 2011 from http://www.celiac.ca/index.php/about-celiac-disease-2/symptoms-treatment-cd/

Canadian Paediatric Society. (2006). Oral rehydration therapy and early refeeding in the management of childhood gastroenteritis. *Paediatrics & Child Health, 11*(8), 527–531.

Castiglia, P. (2001). Constipation in children. *Journal of Pediatric Health Care, 15*, 200–202.

Centers for Disease Control and Prevention. (2003). Managing acute gastroenteritis among children: Oral rehydration, maintenance, and nutritional therapy. *MMWR. Morbidity and Mortality Weekly Report, 52*(No. RR-16), 1–16.

Children's Hospital Boston. (2010). *Hernia (umbilical or inguinal).* Retrieved April 18, 2011 from http://www.childrenshospital.org/az/Site1018/mainpageS1018P0.html

Children's Hospital Boston. (2011). *Home care instructions for changing an ostomy pouch (bag or appliance).* Boston, MA: Author.

Christensen, R., Gordon, P., & Besner, G. (2010). Can we cut the incidence of necrotizing enterocolitis in half—today? *Fetal and Pediatric Pathology, 29*, 185–198.

Cuffari, C. (2009). *Short bowel syndrome.* Retrieved April 20, 2011 from http://emedicine.medscape.com/article/931855-overview

Curtin, G., & Boekelheide, A. (2010). Cleft lip and cleft palate. In P. J. Allen, J. A. Vessey, & N. A. Schapiro (Eds.), *Primary care of the child with a chronic condition* (5th ed.). St. Louis, MO: Mosby.

Dale, J. (2004). Oral rehydration solutions in the management of acute gastroenteritis among children. *Journal of Pediatric Health Care, 18*, 211–212.

Diggins, K. (2008). Treatment of mild to moderate dehydration in children with oral rehydration therapy. *Journal of the Academy of Nurse Practitioners, 20*, 402–406.

Fischbach, F. (2003). *A manual of laboratory & diagnostic tests* (7th ed.). Philadelphia: Lippincott Williams & Wilkins.

Fleisher, G. R., & Matson, D. O. (2011). *Patient information: Acute diarrhea in children.* Retrieved April 20, 2011 from http://www.uptodate.com/contents/patient-information-acute-diarrhea-in-children

Gardiner, P., & Kemper, K. J. (2005). For GI complaints, which herbs and supplements spell relief? *Contemporary Pediatrics, 22*(8), 51–55.

Gompf, S. G., Casanas, B. C., Carrington, M., & Cunha, B. A. (2010). *Herpangina.* Retrieved April 20, 2011 from http://emedicine.medscape.com/article/218502-overview

Hamilton, J. (2000). The pediatric patient: Early development and the digestive system. In W. Walker, P. Durie, J. Hamilton, J. Walker-Smith, & J. Watkins (Eds.), *Pediatric GI disease.* Hamilton, ON: BC Decker, Inc.

Haas-Beckert, B., & Heyman, M. B. (2010). Inflammatory bowel disease. In P. J. Allen, J. A. Vessey, & N. A. Schapiro (Eds.), *Primary care of the child with a chronic condition* (5th ed.). St. Louis, MO: Mosby.

Herbst, J. J. (2004). Primary (peptic) ulcers. In R. E. Behrman, R. M. Kliegman, & H. B. Jenson (Eds.), *Nelson textbook of pediatrics* (17th ed.). Philadelphia: WB Saunders.

Iannitti, T., & Palmieri, B. (2010). Therapeutical use of probiotic formulations in clinical practice. *Clinical Nutrition, 29*(6), 701–725.

Jakubik, L. D., Colfer, A., & Grossman, M. B. (2000). Pediatric short bowel syndrome: Pathophysiology, nursing care, and management issues. *Journal of the Society of Pediatric Nurses, 5*(3), 111–121.

Jarrett, M., Heitkemper, M., Czyzewski, D. I., & Shulman, R. (2003). Recurrent abdominal pain in children: Forerunner to adult irritable bowel syndrome? *Journal for Specialists in Pediatric Nursing, 8*(3), 81–89.

Johns Hopkins Hospital, Custer, J. W., Rau, R. E., & Lee, C. K. (2008). *The Harriett Lane handbook* (18th ed.). St. Louis, MO: Mosby.

Katz, D. A. (2001). Evaluation and management of inguinal and umbilical hernias. *Pediatric Annals, 30*(12), 729–735.

Khanna, R., Lakhanpaul, M., Burman-Roy, S., & Murphy, S. (2009). Diarrhoea and vomiting caused by gastroenteritis in children under 5 years: summary of NICE guidelines. *British Medical Journal, 338*(7701), 1009–1012.

Lee, S. L., Shekherdimian, S., & Dubois, J. J. (2009). *Hirschsprung disease.* Retrieved April 20, 2011 from http://emedicine.medscape.com/article/178493-overview

Letton, R. (2001). Pyloric stenosis. *Pediatric Annals, 30*(12), 745–749.

Leung, A. K., & Kao, C. P. (2003). Oral lesions in children. *Consultant for Pediatricians, 2*(2), 81–84.

Lockridge, T., Caldwell, A. D., & Jason, P. (2002). Congenital neonatal surgical emergencies: Stabilization and management. *Journal of Obstetric, Gynecologic, and Neonatal Nursing, 31*, 328–339.

Longstreth, G. F. [updated by Drossman, D. A.] (2009). *Current approach to the diagnosis of irritable bowel syndrome* [electronic version]. Milwaukee, WI: International Foundation for Functional Gastrointestinal Disorders. Retrieved December 6, 2011 from http://www.aboutgimotility.org/store/viewproduct/163

Maisels, J. (2005a). A primer on phototherapy for the jaundiced newborn. *Contemporary Pediatrics, 22*(6), 38–57.

Maisels, J. (2005b). Jaundice. In M. G. MacDonald, M. M. K. Seshia, & M. D. Mullett (Eds.), *Avery's neonatology: Pathophysiology and management of the newborn.* Philadelphia: Lippincott Williams & Wilkins.

Maisels, J. (2005c). Jaundice in a newborn: Answers to questions about a common clinical problem. *Contemporary Pediatrics, 22*(5), 34–40.

Maisels, J. (2005d). Jaundice in a newborn: How to head off an urgent situation. *Contemporary Pediatrics, 22*(5), 41–54.

Minkes, R., Bechtel, K. A., Billmire, D., et al. (2011). *Pediatric appendicitis.* Retrieved December 8, 2011 from www.emedicine.com/ped/topic127.htm

Mitchell, J., & Wood, R. (2000). Management of cleft lip and palate in primary care. *Journal of Pediatric Health Care, 14*(1), 13–19.

Montgomery, D. F., & Navarro, F. (2008). Management of constipation and encopresis in children. *Journal of Pediatric Health Care, 22*, 199–204.

Peña, A. (2004). Anorectal malformations. In R. E. Behrman, R. M. Kliegman, & H. B. Jenson (Eds.), *Nelson textbook of pediatrics* (17th ed.). Philadelphia: WB Saunders.

Plewa, M. C. (2010). *Pediatric aphthous ulcers.* Retrieved April 20, 2011 from http://emedicine.medscape.com/article/909213-overview

Rabinowitz, S. S., & Hongye, L. (2010). *Pediatric Meckel diverticulum.* Retrieved April 7, 2011 from http://www.emedicine.com/ped/topic1389.htm

Registered Nurses' Association of Ontario. (2009). *Nursing best practice guidelines: Ostomy care and management.* Retrieved December 6, 2011 from http://www.rnao.org/Page.asp?PageID=122& ContentID=3012

Reilly, S., Reid, J., Skeat, J., & the Academy of Breastfeeding Medicine Clinical Protocol Committee. (2007). ABM clinical protocol #17: Guidelines for breastfeeding infants with cleft lip, cleft palate, or cleft lip and palate. *Breastfeeding Medicine, 2*(4), 243–250.

Runge, K., & Nguyen, K. K. (2010). Celiac disease. In P. J. Allen, J. A. Vessey, & N. A. Schapiro (Eds.), *Primary care of the child with a chronic condition* (5th ed.). St. Louis, MO: Mosby.

Sandberg, D., Magee, W., & Denk, M. (2002). Neonatal cleft lip and cleft palate repair. *AORN Journal, 72*(3), 490–508.

Schmitt, B. D. (2004). Toilet training problems: Underachievers, refusers, and stool holders. *Contemporary Pediatrics, 21*(4), 71–80.

Schreiber, R., Barker, C., Roberts, E., Martin, S., & the Canadian Pediatric Hepatology Research Group. (2010). Biliary atresia in Canada: The effect of centre caseload experience on outcome. *Journal of Pediatric Gastroenterology and Nutrition, 51*(1), 61–65.

Schwarz, S. M. (2009). *Biliary atresia.* Retrieved April 20, 2011 from http://emedicine.medscape.com/article/927029-overview

Schwarz, S. M., Hebra, A., & Miller, M. (2011). *Pediatric cholecystitis.* Retrieved April 20, 2011 from http://emedicine.medscape.com/article/927340-overview

Sharp, H. M., Dailey, S., & Moon, J. B. (2003). Speech and language development disorders in infants and children with cleft lip and palate. *Pediatric Annals, 32*(7), 476–480.

Singh, J., & Kass, D. A. (2010). *Pediatrics, pyloric stenosis.* Retrieved April 20, 2011 from http://emedicine.medscape.com/article/803489-overview

Sokol, R., & Narkewicz, M. (2011). Liver & pancreas. In W. W. Hay, M. J. Levin, J. M. Sondheimer, & R. R. Deterding (Eds.), *Current pediatric diagnosis and treatment* (20th ed.). New York: McGraw-Hill.

Stanton, B., Evans, J. B., & Batra, B. (2011). *Oral rehydration therapy.* Retrieved March 18, 2012 from http://www.uptodate.com/contents/oral-rehydration-therapy

Stoll, B. J., & Kliegman, P. M. (2004). Neonatal necrotizing enterocolitis (NEC). In R. E. Behrman, R. M. Kliegman, & H. B. Jenson (Eds.), *Nelson textbook of pediatrics* (17th ed.). Philadelphia: WB Saunders.

Suchy, F. J. (2004). Diseases of the gallbladder. In R. E. Behrman, R. M. Kliegman, & H. B. Jenson (Eds.), *Nelson textbook of pediatrics* (17th ed.). Philadelphia: WB Saunders.

Sundaram, S., Hoffenberg, E., Kramer, R., Sondheimer, J. M., & Furuta, G. T. (2011). Gastrointestinal tract. In W. W. Hay, M. J. Levin, J. M. Sondheimer, & R. R. Deterding (Eds.), *Current pediatric diagnosis and treatment* (20th ed.). New York: McGraw-Hill.

Tablang, M. V., Grupka, M. J., & Wu, G. (2009). *Gastroenteritis, viral.* Retrieved April 20, 2011 from http://www.emedicine.com/med/topic856.htm

Takayesu, J. K. & Lozner, A. W. (2010). *Pediatrics, dehydration.* Retrieved April 20, 2011 from http://emedicine.medscape.com/article/801012-overview

Taketomko, C. K., Hodding, J. H., & Kraus, D. M. (2010). *Lexi-comp's pediatric dosage handbook* (17th ed.). Hudson, OH: Lexi-comp.

Thilo, E. H., & Rosenberg, A. A. (2011). The newborn infant. In W. W. Hay, M. J. Levin, J. M. Sondheimer, & R. R. Deterding (Eds.), *Current pediatric diagnosis and treatment* (20th ed.). New York: McGraw-Hill.

Ulshen, M. (2004). Major symptoms and signs of digestive tract disorders. In R. E. Behrman, R. M. Kliegman, & H. B. Jenson (Eds.), *Nelson textbook of pediatrics* (17th ed.). Philadelphia: WB Saunders.

Weber, J., & Kelley, J. H. (2010). *Health assessment in nursing* (4th ed.). Philadelphia: Lippincott Williams & Wilkins.

Weill, V. (2008). Gastroesophageal reflux in infancy. *Advance for Nurse Practitioners, 16*(1), 47–50.

Werlin, S. L. (2004). Pancreatitis. In R. E. Behrman, R. M. Kliegman, & H. B. Jenson (Eds.), *Nelson textbook of pediatrics* (17th ed.). Philadelphia: WB Saunders.

Wesson, D., & Haddock, G. (2000). Congenital anomalies. In W. Walker, P. Durie, J. Hamilton, J. Walker-Smith, & J. Watkins (Eds.), *Pediatric GI disease.* Hamilton, ON: BC Decker, Inc.

White, B. (2007). Ginger: An overview. *American Family Physician, 75*(11), 1689–1691.

Wyllie, R. (2004a). Congenital aganglionic megacolon (Hirschsprung disease). In R. E. Behrman, R. M. Kliegman, & H. B. Jenson (Eds.), *Nelson textbook of pediatrics* (17th ed.). Philadelphia: WB Saunders.

Wyllie, R. (2004b). Intussusception. In R. E. Behrman, R. M. Kliegman, & H. B. Jenson (Eds.), *Nelson textbook of pediatrics* (17th ed.). Philadelphia: WB Saunders.

Wyllie, R. (2004c). Malrotation. In R. E. Behrman, R. M. Kliegman, & H. B. Jenson (Eds.), *Nelson textbook of pediatrics* (17th ed.). Philadelphia: WB Saunders.

RECOMMENDED READING

March of Dimes. (2011). *Cleft lip and cleft palate.* Accessed December 6, 2011 from http://www.marchofdimes.com/baby/birthdefects_cleftpalate.html

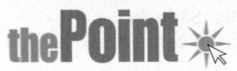

the Point For additional learning materials, including Internet Resources, visit **http://thePoint.lww.com/Chow1e.**

CHAPTER WORKSHEET

MULTIPLE CHOICE QUESTIONS

1. A mother brings her 6-month-old infant to the clinic. The child has been vomiting since early morning and has had diarrhea since the day before. His temperature is 38°C, pulse 140, and respiratory rate 38. He has lost 180 g since his well-child visit 4 days ago. He cries before passing a bowel movement. He will not breast-feed today. What is the priority nursing diagnosis?

   a. Thermoregulation alteration

   b. Pain (abdominal) related to diarrhea

   c. Fluid volume deficit related to excessive losses and inadequate intake

   d. Alteration in nutrition, less than body requirements, related to decreased oral intake

2. A child presents with a 2-day history of fever, abdominal pain, occasional vomiting, and decreased oral intake. Which finding would the nurse prioritize for immediate reporting to the physician?

   a. Temperature 38.8°C

   b. Rebound tenderness and abdominal guarding

   c. Parents will be leaving the child alone in the hospital

   d. Child can tolerate only sips of fluid without nausea

3. A 3-day-old infant presenting with physiologic jaundice is hospitalized and placed under phototherapy. Which response indicates to the nurse that the parent needs more teaching?

   a. "My infant is at risk for dehydration."

   b. "My infant needs to stay under the lights, except during feeding time."

   c. "My infant can continue to breastfeed during this time."

   d. "My infant has a serious liver disease."

4. A 3-month-old infant presents with a history of vomiting after feeding. The plan for the infant is to rule out GERD. What information from the history would lead the nurse to believe that this infant may need further intervention?

   a. Poor weight gain

   b. Has small "spits" after feeding

   c. Sleeps through the night

   d. Is difficult to burp

5. The nurse is caring for a child who has had diarrhea and vomiting for the past several days. What is the priority nursing assessment?

   a. Determine the child's weight.

   b. Ask if the family has traveled outside of the country.

   c. Assess circulation and perfusion.

   d. Send a stool specimen to the lab.

CRITICAL THINKING EXERCISES

1. A 6-month-old baby is brought to the pediatrician's office with a history of diarrhea. She has had six watery stools in the past 18 hours. She is vomiting her formula. Her mother states that she has had no fever.

   a. Upon completion of the history and physical examination, what signs and symptoms would you expect to find that would indicate that the baby is experiencing mild dehydration?

   b. What is the priority nursing diagnosis for this infant?

   c. Identify a plan for this nursing diagnosis; include a teaching plan for the mother.

2. A 14 kg child with moderate dehydration has received two boluses of normal saline in the emergency room prior to being admitted to the pediatric nursing unit. The physician orders D5 ½ NS @ 1½ maintenance.

   a. What would the intravenous fluid rate be?

   b. What will the nurse assess for to determine whether the child is becoming overhydrated?

3. An infant requires a temporary colostomy. What discharge instructions would you provide the parents about how to take care of the colostomy and when to call their health care provider?

STUDY ACTIVITIES

1. In the clinical setting, compare the growth records of a child with celiac disease with those of a similar-age child without disease.

2. While caring for children in the clinical setting, compare and contrast the medical history, signs and symptoms of illness, and prescribed treatment for a child with Crohn's disease and one with ulcerative colitis.

3. In the clinical setting, observe the behavioural responses of an infant or young child with inorganic failure to thrive.

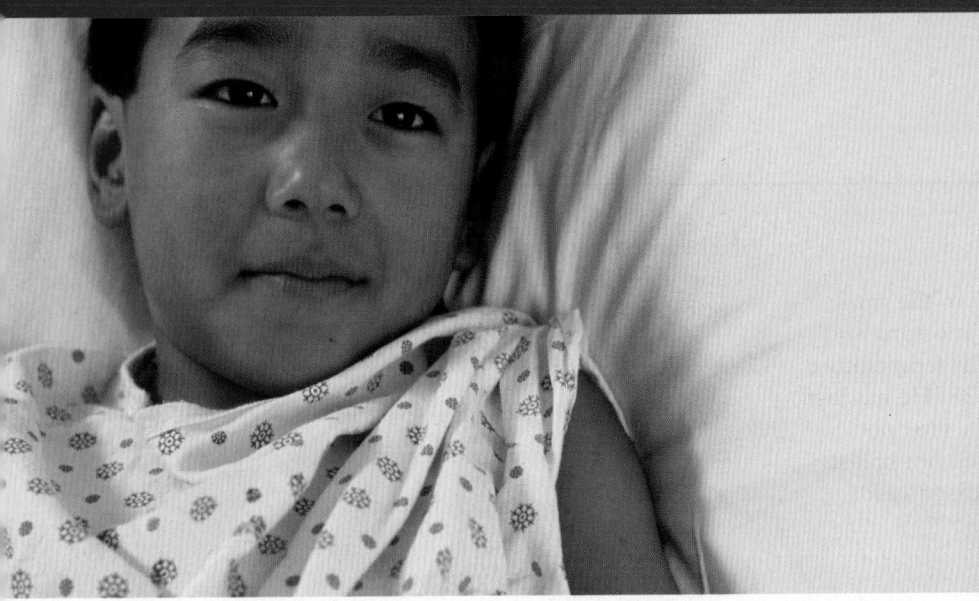

CHAPTER 42

Adapted by Julie Strong

NURSING CARE OF THE CHILD WITH A GENITOURINARY DISORDER

KEY TERMS

amenorrhea	dysmenorrhea	oliguria
anasarca	enuresis	proteinuria
anuria	hematuria	sepsis
azotemia	hyperlipidemia	urgency
bacteriuria	menorrhagia	urinary frequency

LEARNING OBJECTIVES

Upon completion of the chapter, the learner will be able to:

1. Compare anatomic and physiologic differences of the genitourinary system in infants and children versus adults.
2. Describe nursing care related to common laboratory and diagnostic testing used in the medical diagnosis of pediatric genitourinary conditions.
3. Distinguish genitourinary disorders common in infants, children, and adolescents.
4. Identify appropriate nursing assessments and interventions related to medications and treatments for pediatric genitourinary disorders.
5. Develop an individualized nursing care plan for the child with a genitourinary disorder.
6. Describe the psychosocial impact of chronic genitourinary disorders on children.
7. Devise a nutrition plan for the child with chronic kidney disease.
8. Develop patient/family teaching plans for the child with a genitourinary disorder.

Corey Bond, 5 years old, is brought to the clinic by her mother. She presents with fever and lethargy for the past 24 hours. Her mother states, "Corey has had a few accidents in her pants over the past few days, which is unusual for her. She also has been getting up at night more often to use the bathroom."

Wow *A child's essential bodily processes of elimination can be a major event of wonder and creative accomplishment.*

Genitourinary (GU) disorders in children and adolescents may occur as a result of abnormalities in fetal development, infectious processes, trauma, neurologic deficit, genetic influences, or other causes. Congenital disorders account for a large proportion of GU disorders in infants, while enuresis and urinary tract infection (UTI) also occur in a significant number of children. Some of the disorders directly involve the kidney from the outset, while others involve other parts of the urinary tract and may have a long-term effect on the kidneys and renal function, particularly if left untreated or treated inadequately. Disorders affecting the reproductive organs often require early diagnosis and management to preserve future reproductive capabilities.

Nurses must be knowledgeable about pediatric GU conditions to provide prompt recognition, nursing care, education, and support to children and their families. Though some disorders are acute and resolve quickly, many have a long-term effect on quality of life and will require more intense, extended support.

Management of acute or common pediatric GU disorders may be provided in the pediatric or family practice out-patient setting, while specialists such as pediatric nephrologists or urologists usually manage chronic involved GU disorders.

Variations in Pediatric Anatomy and Physiology

Though all of the urinary tract and reproductive organs are present at birth, their functioning is immature initially. Many pediatric GU disorders are congenital (present at birth). External GU malformations are easily identified at birth, but internal structural defects may not be identified until later in infancy or childhood when symptoms or complications arise. In children, chronic kidney disease (CKD) is most often the result of congenital structural defects or infectious, inflammatory, or immune processes that damage the kidney, whereas in adults it usually results from hypertension or diabetes. The infant or child is at increased risk for the development of certain GU disorders because of the anatomic and physiologic differences between children and adults.

Urinary Concentration

Blood flow through the kidneys (glomerular filtration rate [GFR]) is slower in the infant and young toddler compared with the adult (Lum, 2011). The kidney is less able to concentrate urine and reabsorb amino acids, placing the infant and young toddler at increased risk for dehydration during times when fluid loss or decreased fluid intake occurs. The normal range for serum blood urea nitrogen (BUN) and creatinine of the healthy infant or young toddler is usually less than that of the older child or adult. The renal system usually reaches functional maturity between 1 and 2 years of age.

Structural Differences

The kidney is large in relation to the size of the abdomen until the child reaches adolescence. Due to this increased size, the kidneys of the child are less well protected from injury by the ribs and fat padding than are those of the adult. The urethra is naturally shorter in females of all ages than in males, placing females at increased risk for the entrance of bacteria into the bladder via the urethra. In the female infant or young child, this risk is compounded by the physical proximity of the urethral opening to the rectum. The young male's urethra is much shorter than the adult male's, placing the male infant or young child at increased risk of UTI compared with the adult male.

Urine Output

Bladder capacity is about 30 mL in the newborn; it increases to the usual adult capacity of about 270 mL by 1 year of age. The expected urine output in the infant and child is 0.5 to 2 mL/kg/hour, with the average 1-year-old voiding about 400 to 500 mL per day. The average urine output for a teenager is about 800 to 1,400 mL per day. The infant and toddler may void as often as 9 or 10 times per day. By age 3, the average number of voids per day is the same as the adult's (three to eight).

Reproductive Organ Maturity

The reproductive organs are also immature at birth. The gonads are not mature until adolescence in most children. The hormonal changes that occur with puberty account for some of the reproductive concerns, particularly for female adolescents.

Common Medical and Surgical Treatments

A variety of medications as well as other medical treatments and surgical procedures are used to treat GU problems in children. Most of these treatments will require a physician's order when the child is in the hospital. The most common treatments and medications are listed in Common Medical Treatments 42.1 and Drug Guide 42.1. The nurse caring for the child with a GU disorder should be familiar with what the procedures are, how the treatments and medications work, and common nursing implications related to use of these modalities.

(text continues on page 1427)

COMMON MEDICAL TREATMENTS 42.1 GENITOURINARY DISORDERS

Treatment	Explanation	Indication	Nursing Implications
Urinary diversion	Surgical diversion of ureters to the abdominal wall. Continent diversion uses a piece of intestine to create a bladder that can be catheterized. Non-continent diversion involves a stoma on the abdominal wall that requires use of an ostomy pouch.	Any situation in which the bladder needs to be removed or does not function correctly (bladder exstrophy or prune belly)	Meticulous skin care is necessary to prevent breakdown around stoma. Teach families how to care for ostomy pouch or how to catheterize continent stoma. Expect mucus in urine if intestine is used for urinary reservoir. Monitor for signs of UTI.
Foley catheter	An indwelling urinary catheter stays in place by means of an inflated balloon.	Usually used only during the postoperative period	Monitor for urethral drainage or irritation. Keep area clean and dry. Monitor colour, consistency, clarity, and amount of urine in drainage bag. Monitor for infection, checking results of urinalysis and urine cultures.
Ureteral stent	A thin catheter temporarily placed in the ureter to drain urine. Removed via cystoscopy when it is time for discontinuation.	Urinary tract anomalies, post kidney transplant	Monitor urine output carefully. Check for bleeding postoperatively.
Nephrostomy tube	Tube placed directly into the kidney to drain urine externally to a bag	Urinary tract anomalies	Monitor urine output carefully.
Suprapubic tube	Catheter placed in the bladder via the abdominal wall above the symphysis pubis	Postoperative urine drainage with reconstructive surgeries	Monitor for blood in urine, adequate urine output. Minimize manipulation of suprapubic tube to avoid triggering bladder spasms.
Vesicostomy	Stoma in the abdominal wall to the bladder	Urinary tract anomalies, neurogenic bladder	Constant urine drainage requires diaper use. Monitor urine output. Assess skin around stoma for breakdown.
Appendicovesicostomy (Mitrofanoff procedure)	Uses appendix to create a stoma on the abdominal wall that allows for catheterization of the bladder	Urinary tract anomalies, neurogenic bladder	Allows for urinary continence, which improves the child's self-esteem. Teach family and child how to catheterize stoma.
Bladder augmentation	Uses a piece of stomach or intestine to enlarge bladder capacity	Decreased bladder capacity	Since a portion of the GI tract is used, urine is often mucus-like.

DRUG GUIDE 42.1 COMMON DRUGS FOR GU DISORDERS

Medication	Action	Indication	Nursing Implications
Anticholinergic agents (oxybutynin, propantheline bromide, belladonna & opium suppository)	Cause smooth muscle relaxation of the bladder	Urinary tract spasms or contractions related to surgical procedure or use of catheters. Control of nocturnal enuresis.	Increase fluid intake (limit to daytime use in the child with nocturnal enuresis). Avoid use in febrile patients.
Antibiotics (oral, parenteral)	Kill bacteria or arrest their growth	UTI, pelvic inflammatory disease, toxic shock syndrome	Check for antibiotic allergies. Should be given as prescribed for the length of time indicated.
Desmopressin (DDAVP)	Antidiuretic hormone effects by causing renal tubule to absorb more water, decreasing volume of urine	Nocturnal enuresis	Available as oral tablets and rapid-acting disintegrating wafers. Nasal DDAVP is no longer recommended in Canada.
Human chorionic gonadotropin (hCG)	Stimulates production of gonadal steroids	To precipitate testicular descent	Monitor for signs of precocious puberty if used long term.
Corticosteroids	Anti-inflammatory and immunosuppressive action	Induce remission and promote diuresis in nephrotic syndrome. High-dose intravenous therapy used when nephrotic syndrome is resistant to conventional doses. Prevent organ rejection following kidney transplantation.	Administer with food to decrease GI upset. May mask signs of infection. Do not stop treatment abruptly, or acute adrenal insufficiency may occur. Monitor for Cushing syndrome. Doses may be tapered over time. Monitor for hypertension during infusion.
Cytotoxic drugs (cyclophosphamide [Cytoxan] and chlorambucil [Leukeran])	Interfere with normal function of DNA by alkylation	Induction of prolonged remission in nephrotic syndrome	Causes bone marrow suppression. Monitor for signs of infection. Cyclophosphamide: administer in the morning; provide adequate hydration; have child void frequently during and after infusion to decrease risk of hemorrhagic cystitis. Chlorambucil: administer with nonspicy, non-acidic foods; rarely seizures occur.
Immunosuppressant drugs (cyclosporin A [CyA], azathioprine, tacrolimus, mycophenolate, sirolimus)	Inhibit production and release of interleukin-2. Inhibit T-cell activation by inhibiting calcineurin phosphatase activity. Inhibit T- and B-cell proliferation (mycophenolate). Inhibit response to interleukin-2, thus blocking T and B cells.	Prevention of rejection of kidney transplants. CyA and tacrolimus may be used for steroid-dependent nephrotic syndrome.	Monitor complete blood count, serum creatinine, potassium, and magnesium. Monitor blood pressure and observe for signs of infection. Give at regular intervals to maintain consistent drug levels. Blood levels should be drawn prior to morning dose. CyA: do not give with grapefruit juice as this inhibits the metabolism of drug. Azathioprine and mycophenolate: give on empty stomach; do not open capsule or crush tablet. Tacrolimus: give on empty stomach; assess for development of hyperglycemia. Sirolimus: do not take with grapefruit juice. Relapse of nephrotic syndrome may occur after withdrawal of CyA or tacrolimus therapy.

(continued)

DRUG GUIDE 42.1 COMMON DRUGS FOR GU DISORDERS (continued)

Medication	Action	Indication	Nursing Implications
Anti-thymocyte globulin (ATG, Thymo-globulin)	Suppress T-cell activity	Treatment of acute kidney transplant rejection	Monitor for signs and symptoms of anaphylaxis: fever, chills, chest tightness, wheezing, hypotension, nausea, and vomiting.
Angiotensin-converting enzyme (ACE) inhibitors (captopril, enalapril)	Potent vasoconstrictors, prevent conversion of angiotensin I to angiotensin II	Renal causes of hypertension Prevention of progression of CKD	Monitor blood pressure frequently. May cause cough, hyperkalemia. Captopril: administer on empty stomach. Enalapril: administer without regard to food.
Angiotensin receptor blockers (ARBs) (losartan, valsartan)	Block the angiotensin receptor causing vasodilation	Prevention of progression of CKD Hypertension	Monitor for elevated serum potassium. Monitor for hypotension, worsening or new cough, signs and symptoms of allergic reaction, and signs of hyperkalemia. Provide instruction to avoid high-potassium foods.
Diuretics: furosemide (Lasix), hydrochlorothiazide (HCTZ)	Inhibit resorption of sodium and chloride in ascending loop of Henle (furosemide) or inhibit reabsorption of sodium in distal tubules (HCTZ), leading to increased excretion of water and electrolytes	Nephrotic syndrome, acute glomerulonephritis, hemolytic-uremic syndrome or other instances of fluid overload with renal sufficiency	Administer with food or milk to decrease GI upset. Monitor blood pressure, kidney function, and electrolytes (particularly potassium). May cause photosensitivity.
Vasodilators: hydralazine (Apresoline), minoxidil	Direct vasodilation of arterioles, resulting in decreased systemic resistance	Renal causes of hypertension	May cause fluid retention. Hydralazine: administer with food. Monitor heart rate and blood pressure (closely with intravenous use). Minoxidil: may be administered without regard to food. May cause dizziness.
Calcium-channel blocker: nifedipine (Procardia)	Prevents calcium from entering voltage-sensitive channels, resulting in coronary vasodilation	Renal causes of hypertension	Administer with food; avoid grapefruit juice. Insoluble shell of extended-release tablet may pass in stool. Use caution and monitor blood pressure when administering liquid-filled capsule sublingually or by bite and swallow method, as significant hypotension may occur.
Albumin (intravenous)	Increases intravascular oncotic pressure, resulting in movement of fluid from interstitial to intravascular space	Nephrotic syndrome in the case of severe fluid overload	May require a filter depending upon brand used. Rapid infusion can result in vascular overload. Monitor vital signs; observe for pulmonary edema and cardiac failure.

Adapted from: Taketokmo, C. K., Hodding, J. H., & Kraus, D. M. (2010). *Lexi-comp's pediatric dosage handbook* (17th ed.). Hudson, OH: Lexi-comp.

NURSING PROCESS OVERVIEW FOR THE CHILD WITH A GU DISORDER

Care of the child with a GU disorder includes assessment, nursing diagnosis, planning, interventions, and evaluation. There are a number of general concepts related to the nursing process that may be applied to GU disorders. From a general understanding of the care involved for a child with urinary, renal, or reproductive dysfunction, the nurse can then individualize the care based on patient specifics.

Assessment

Assessment of urinary tract, kidney, or reproductive dysfunction includes health history, physical examination, and laboratory and diagnostic testing.

*R*emember Corey, the 5-year-old, with fever and *lethargy? What additional health history and physical examination assessment information should you obtain?*

Health History

The health history comprises past medical history, including the mother's pregnancy history, family history, and history of present illness (when the symptoms started and how they have progressed), as well as medications and treatments used at home. The past medical history may be significant for maternal polyhydramnios, oligohydramnios, diabetes, hypertension, or alcohol or cocaine ingestion. Neonatal history may include the presence of a single umbilical artery or an abdominal mass, chromosome abnormality, or congenital malformation. Document past medical history of UTI or other problems with the GU tract. Family history may be significant for kidney disease or uropathology, chronic UTIs, renal calculi, or a history of parental enuresis. Determine age of successful toilet training, pattern of incontinent episodes (having "accidents"), and toileting hygiene self-care routines. Note myelomeningocele or other spinal disturbance that may affect the child's ability to urinate. Note previous urologic surgeries or ongoing renal supportive therapy (e.g., dialysis). For the adolescent girl, obtain a thorough menstrual history, including sexual behaviour and pregnancy history.

When determining the history of the present illness, inquire about the following:

- Burning on urination
- Changes in voiding patterns
- Foul-smelling urine
- Vaginal or urethral discharge
- Genital pain, irritation, or discomfort
- Blood in the urine
- Edema
- Masses in the groin, scrotum, or abdomen

- Flank or abdominal pain
- Cramps
- Nausea and/or vomiting
- Poor growth
- Weight gain
- Fever
- Infectious exposure (particularly streptococcus A or *Escherichia coli*)
- Trauma

Record medications used for acute or chronic conditions or for contraception.

Physical Examination

Physical examination of the GU system includes inspection and observation, auscultation, percussion, and palpation.

Inspection and Observation

Observe the child's general appearance, noting growth delay or unusual weight gain. Inspect the skin for presence of pruritus, edema (generalized or periorbital), or bruising. Note pallor of the skin or dysmorphic features (associated with genetic conditions). Document presence of lethargy, fatigue, rapid respirations, confusion, or developmental delay. Observe the external genitalia area for infant diaper rash, constant urine dribble, displaced urethral opening, reddened urethral opening, or discharge. In females note vaginal irritation or labial fusion. In males observe the scrotal sac for enlargement or discolouration. Note the condition of a urinary stoma or diversion if present. With the child lying flat, observe the abdomen for distention, ascites, or slack abdominal musculature. In a child who receives peritoneal dialysis check the exit site for redness, swelling, or discharge.

Auscultation

Listen carefully to heart sounds, as a flow murmur may be present in the anemic child with a renal disorder (Klein, 2010). Note elevated heart rate. Auscultate blood pressure with the appropriate-size cuff, noting elevation or depression (use of the incorrect cuff size can falsely elevate or reduce the true blood pressure). In the edematous child, carefully auscultate the lungs, noting presence of adventitious sounds. Note absence of bowel sounds, as this may indicate peritonitis. In the child who receives chronic hemodialysis, auscultate the fistula for presence of a bruit (desired normal finding).

▶ *Take* NOTE!

Use the bell of the stethoscope when auscultating the infant's or child's blood pressure so that you can hear the softer Korotkoff sounds more accurately.

Percussion

Percuss the abdomen. Note unusual dullness or flatness (dullness is usually heard over the spleen at the right costal margin, over the kidneys, and 1 to 3 cm below the left costal margin). A full bladder may yield dullness above the symphysis pubis.

Palpation

Palpate the abdomen. Note presence of palpable kidneys (indicating enlargement or mass, as they are usually difficult to palpate in the older infant or child). Note presence of abdominal masses or a distended bladder. Document tenderness to palpation or along the costovertebral angle. Palpate the scrotum for the presence of descended testicles, masses, or other abnormalities. Note whether the foreskin, if present, can be retracted. In the child who receives chronic hemodialysis, palpate the fistula or graft for the presence of a thrill (desired normal finding).

Laboratory and Diagnostic Testing

Common Laboratory and Diagnostic Tests 42.1 offers an explanation of the laboratory and diagnostic tests most commonly used for a child suspected of having a GU disorder. The test results can help the physician to diagnose the disorder or to determine treatment. Laboratory or non-nursing personnel obtain some of the tests, while the nurse might obtain others. In either instance the nurse should be familiar with how the tests are obtained, what they are used for, and normal versus abnormal results. This knowledge will also be necessary when providing patient and family education related to the tests and results.

Urine specimens may be collected using a variety of different methods in infants and children. Suprapubic aspiration is a useful method for obtaining a sterile urine specimen from the neonate or young infant. A sterile needle is inserted into the bladder through the anterior wall of the abdomen and the urine is then aspirated. This method is generally performed by the physician or advanced practitioner. Infants and toddlers who are not toilet trained may require a urine bag for urine collection. A sterile urine bag is required for a urine culture, a clean bag for routine urinalysis. A 24-hour urine-collection bag is also available. The diagnosis of a UTI from a bag specimen in young infants should be confirmed with either suprapubic aspiration or urethral catheterization prior to treatment and radiologic investigation (Etoubleau et al., 2009). Refer to the Canadian Pediatric Society (CPS, 2004) for current recommendations. Nursing Procedure 42.1 gives details on the use of the urine bag.

Sterile urinary catheterization is performed like that in adults. The size of the catheter varies depending on the size of the child. If a small urinary catheter is not available, a sterile 5- or 8-French feeding tube is sometimes used.

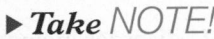

> **▶ Take NOTE!**
>
> *Use familiar terms such as "pee-pee," "tinkle," or "potty" to explain to the child what is needed and to gain his or her cooperation.*

Nursing Diagnoses and Related Interventions

Upon completion of a thorough assessment, the nurse might identify several nursing diagnoses, such as:

- Impaired urinary elimination
- Fluid volume excess/deficit
- Imbalanced nutrition, less (or more) than body requirements
- Risk for infection
- Deficient knowledge of the child or family
- Urinary retention
- Activity intolerance
- Interrupted family process
- Disturbed body image

After completing an assessment of Corey, you note the following: foul-smelling urine, abdominal tenderness, redness in her perineal area, and slightly blood-tinged, cloudy urine. Based on these assessment findings, what would your top three nursing diagnoses be for Corey?

Nursing goals, interventions, and evaluation for the child with a GU disorder are based on the nursing diagnoses. Nursing Care Plan 42.1 can be used as a guide in planning nursing care for the child with a GU disorder. The care plan overview includes nursing diagnoses and interventions for urinary tract disorders as well as genital (or reproductive system) disorders. The care plan should be individualized based on the patient's symptoms and needs. Refer to Chapter 35 for detailed information about pain management. Additional information will be included later in the chapter as it relates to specific disorders.

Based on your top three nursing diagnoses for Corey, describe appropriate nursing interventions.

Urinary Tract and Renal Disorders

The urinary tract and renal disorders discussed below include structural disorders, UTI, enuresis, and acquired disorders that result in altered renal function.

COMMON LABORATORY AND DIAGNOSTIC TESTS 42.1   GENITOURINARY DISORDERS

Test	Explanation	Indication	Nursing Implications
Complete blood count	Evaluates hemoglobin and hematocrit, white blood cell count, and platelet count	Any condition in which anemia, infection, or thrombocytopenia is suspected	Normal values vary according to age and gender. White blood cell count differential is helpful in evaluating source of infection.
Blood urea nitrogen (BUN) (serum)	Indirect measurement of kidney function and glomerular filtration in the presence of adequate liver function	Nephrotic syndrome, hemolytic-uremic syndrome, AKI, CKD, ESRD, acute glomerulonephritis, or other kidney diseases	BUN may be elevated with high-protein diet or dehydration, may be decreased with overhydration or malnutrition.
Creatinine (serum)	A more direct measurement of kidney function, only minimally affected by liver function. Generally, doubling of the creatinine level is suggestive of a 50% reduction in glomerular filtration rate.	Used to screen for impaired kidney function	A diet high in meat may cause a transient though not pronounced increase in creatinine. There are also slight diurnal variations in levels. Draw at same time each day if serial evaluations are ordered.
Creatinine clearance (urine and serum)	A 24-hour urine collection is evaluated for the presence of creatinine and compared with the serum creatinine level to determine creatinine clearance.	Used to diagnose impaired kidney function	Discard the first void and then begin the 24-hour urine collection. Keep the specimen on ice during the collection period. Collect all urine passed in the 24-hour period. Ensure that a venous blood sample is drawn during the 24-hour period. The urine specimen should be sent promptly to the laboratory at the end of the 24-hour period.
Potassium (serum)	Measures the concentration of potassium in the blood	Any suspected kidney disease; followed routinely in CKD and ESRD	Avoid hemolysis and allowing child to open and close the hand with a tourniquet in place, as these can cause an elevation in potassium levels. Evaluate the child with increased or decreased potassium levels for cardiac arrhythmias. Immediately notify physician of critically high potassium levels.
Total protein, globulin, albumin (serum)	Protein electrophoresis separates the various components into zones according to their electrical charge.	Used to diagnose, evaluate, and monitor CKD	Significantly low levels of albumin contribute to extent of edema, as albumin is necessary in the blood to maintain colloidal osmotic pressure.
Calcium (serum)	Measurement of calcium level in the blood; half of all calcium is protein-bound, so the level will decrease with hypoalbuminemia.	Kidney diseases associated with hypoalbuminemia and edema	Avoid prolonged tourniquet use during blood draw, as this may falsely increase the calcium level.

(continued)

COMMON LABORATORY AND DIAGNOSTIC TESTS 42.1 GENITOURINARY DISORDERS (continued)

Test	Explanation	Indication	Nursing Implications
Phosphorus (serum)	Measurement of phosphate level in the blood. Phosphorus levels are inversely related to calcium levels (they increase when calcium levels decrease).	Kidney disease, ongoing monitoring, particularly in the patient with hypocalcemia	Avoid hemolysis, as it can falsely elevate the phosphate level.
Urinalysis (urine)	Evaluates colour, pH, specific gravity, and odour of urine. Also assesses for presence of protein, glucose, ketones, blood, leukocyte esterase, red and white blood cells, bacteria, crystals, and casts.	Reveals preliminary information about the urinary tract. Useful in children with fever, dysuria, flank pain, urgency, or hematuria. Proteinuria may be noted in kidney disorders.	Be aware of the many drugs affecting urine colour and notify laboratory if child is taking one. Notify laboratory if female is menstruating. Refrigerate specimen if not processed promptly. While proteinuria may occur with various kidney disorders, it may also occur as either transient or orthostatic proteinuria, both of which are benign events.
Cystoscopy	Endoscopic visualization of the urethra and bladder	Evaluate hematuria, recurrent UTI; determine ureteral reflux; measure bladder capacity	Encourage fluids. Monitor vital signs. Child may feel burning with voiding after procedure. Pink tinge to urine is common after procedure.
Urine culture and sensitivity	Urine is plated in the laboratory and evaluated every day for the presence of bacteria. A final report is usually issued after 48–72 h. Sensitivity testing is performed to determine the best choice of antibiotic.	Used to diagnose UTI	Obtain culture specimen prior to starting antibiotics if at all possible. Avoid contamination of the specimen with stool. May be obtained by catheterization, clean-catch specimen, or sterile U-bag. In some institutions, suprapubic tap is performed in neonates and young infants by the physician or nurse practitioner.
Urodynamic studies	Measure the urine flow during micturition via a urine flow meter	Dysfunctional voiding	The child must have a full bladder. The child then urinates into the urine flow meter. There is no discomfort associated with the test.
Voiding cystourethrogram (VCUG)	The bladder is filled with contrast material via catheterization. Fluoroscopy is performed to demonstrate filling of the bladder and collapsing after emptying.	Hematuria, UTIs, vesicoureteral reflux, suspected structural anomalies	Just prior to the test, insert the Foley catheter. Ensure that the adolescent female patient is not pregnant. After the test, encourage the child to drink fluids to prevent bacterial accumulation and aid in dye elimination.

Test	Explanation	Indication	Nursing Implications
Intravenous pyelogram (IVP)	Radiopaque contrast material is injected intravenously and filtered by the kidneys. X-ray films are obtained at set intervals to show passage of the dye through the kidneys, ureters, and bladder.	Urinary outlet obstruction, hematuria, trauma to the renal system, suspected kidney tumour	Contraindicated in children allergic to shellfish or iodine. If the dye infiltrates at the intravenous site, hyaluronidase (Wydase) may be used to speed absorption of the iodine. Ensure adequate hydration before and after the test. Some institutions require enema or laxative evacuation of the bowel prior to the study to ensure adequate visualization of the urinary tract.
Glomerular filtration rate (GFR) Kidney biopsy	Radioactive material or Iohexol is injected intravenously. Blood sampling is done at timed intervals to measure clearance of substance from blood by kidney. Usually a percutaneous specimen is obtained by inserting a needle through the skin and into the kidney. The sample of kidney tissue obtained is then microscopically examined.	Determine stage of kidney function Diagnosis of kidney disease or assessment of kidney transplant rejection	Monitor urine output after procedure. Ensure that child returns to nuclear medicine department to complete all blood samples. After the biopsy, carefully assess for signs or symptoms of bleeding: increased heart rate, pale colour, flank pain or backache, shoulder pain, lightheadedness. Inspect urine for gross hematuria. Follow institutional policy regarding the length of bed rest. Contact sports should be avoided for several weeks.
Renal ultrasound	Reflected sound waves allow visualization of the kidneys, ureters, and bladder.	Useful in determining kidney size (as with hydronephrosis and polycystic kidney), presence of cysts or tumours, or rejection of kidney transplant	No fasting is required prior to the procedure. Does not require contrast material. The child should feel no discomfort during the ultrasound.

Adapted from: Pagana, K. D., & Pagana, T. J. (2010). *Mosby's manual of diagnostic and laboratory tests* (4th ed.). St. Louis, MO: Mosby.

Structural Disorders

Numerous urologic conditions occur as a result of altered fetal development. Many of these defects are apparent at birth, while others are not recognized until later in infancy or childhood.

Bladder Exstrophy

In classic bladder exstrophy, a midline closure defect occurs during the embryonic period of gestation, leaving the bladder open and exposed outside of the abdomen. The bony pelvis may also be malformed, resulting in an opening in the pelvic arch. Bladder exstrophy may be diagnosed by prenatal ultrasound. Complications include UTI from ascending organisms. Treatment of bladder exstrophy involves surgical repair.

Nursing Assessment

On physical examination of the infant or child, note the red appearance to the bladder seen on the abdominal

Nursing Procedure 42.1

APPLYING THE URINE BAG

1. Cleanse the perineal area well and pat dry (Fig. A). If a culture is to be obtained, cleanse the genital area with povidone–iodine (Betadine) or per institutional protocol.
2. Apply benzoin (or per institutional protocol) around the scrotum or the vulvar area to aid with urine bag adhesion.
3. Allow the benzoin to dry.
4. Apply the urine bag.
   - For boys: Ensure that the penis is fully inside the bag; a portion of the scrotum may or may not be inside the bag, depending upon scrotal size.
   - For girls: Apply the narrow portion of the bag on the perineal space between the anal and vulvar areas first for best adhesion, then spread the remaining adhesive section (Fig. B).

5. Tuck the bag downward inside the diaper to discourage leaking.
6. Check the bag frequently for urine (Fig. C).

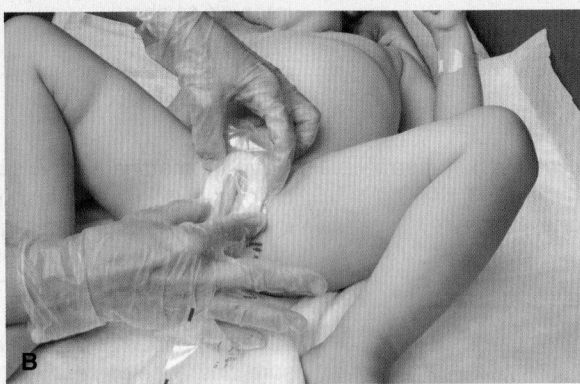

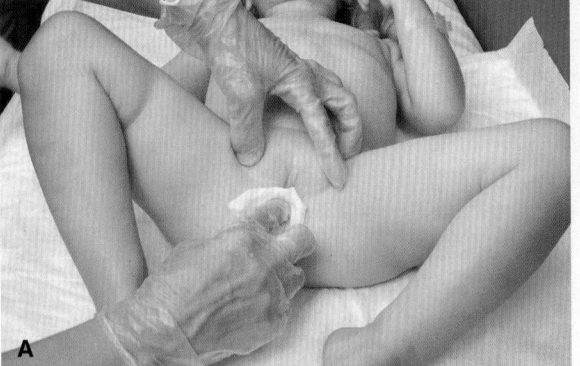

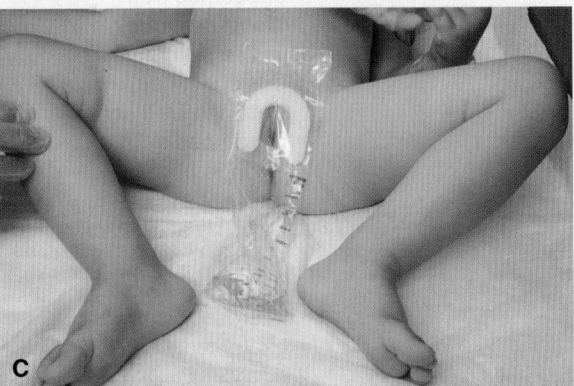

wall (Fig. 42.1). Draining urine will be visible. Note excoriation of abdominal skin around the bladder resulting from contact with urine. A malformed urethra may be present in females, while males may have an unformed or malformed penis or a normal penis with an epispadias.

Nursing Management

Nursing management consists of preventing infection and skin breakdown, providing postoperative care, and catheterizing the stoma.

Preventing Infection and Skin Breakdown

Bladder exstrophy requires surgical repair. In the preoperative period, care is focused on protecting the exstrophied bladder and preventing infection. Keep the infant in a supine position; keep the bladder moist and cover it with a sterile plastic bag. Change soiled diapers immediately to prevent contamination of the bladder with feces. Sponge-bathe the infant rather than immersing him or her in water to prevent pathogens in the bath

water from entering the bladder. Prevent breakdown of the surrounding abdominal skin by applying protective barrier creams. In some instances it may be necessary to

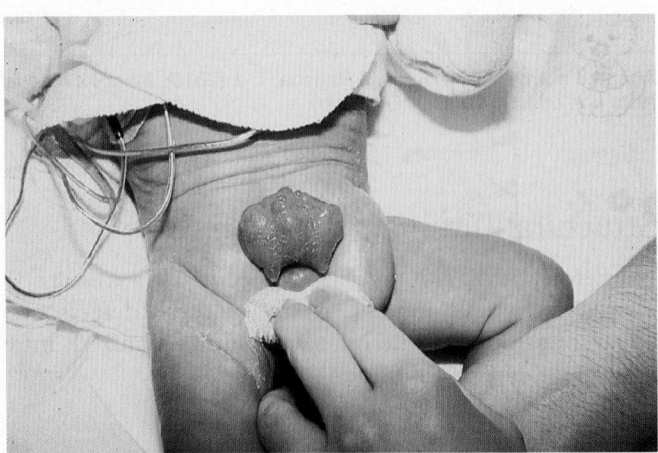

FIGURE 42.1 Note the bright-red colour of the bladder exstrophy.

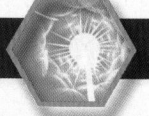

Nursing Care Plan 42.1

OVERVIEW FOR THE CHILD WITH A GENITOURINARY DISORDER

NURSING DIAGNOSIS: Activity intolerance related to generalized edema, anemia, or generalized weakness as evidenced by verbalization of weakness or fatigue, elevated heart rate, respiratory rate, or blood pressure with activity, complaint of shortness of breath with play or activity

Outcome Identification and Evaluation

Child will display increased activity tolerance, *desire to play without developing symptoms of exertion.*

Intervention: Promoting Activity

- Encourage activity or ambulation per physician's orders: *Early mobilization results in better outcomes.*
- Observe child for symptoms of activity intolerance such as pallor, nausea, lightheadedness, or dizziness or changes in vital signs *to determine level of tolerance.*
- If child is on bed rest, perform range-of-motion exercises and frequent position changes, as *negative changes to the musculoskeletal system occur quickly with inactivity and immobility.*
- Cluster nursing care activities and plan for periods of rest before and after exertional activities *to decrease oxygen need and consumption.*
- Refer the child to physical therapy *for exercise prescription to increase skeletal muscle strength.*

NURSING DIAGNOSIS: Excess fluid volume related to decreased protein in the bloodstream, decreased urine output, sodium retention, possible inappropriate fluid intake, or altered hormone levels inducing fluid retention as evidenced by edema, bloating, weight gain, oliguria, azotemia, or changes in heart and lung sounds

Outcome Identification and Evaluation

Child will attain appropriate fluid balance, *will lose weight (fluid), edema or bloating will decrease, lung sounds will be clear and heart sounds normal.*

Intervention: Encouraging Fluid Loss

- Weigh child daily on same scale in similar amount of clothing; *in children, weight is the best indicator of changes in fluid status.*
- Monitor location and extent of edema (measure abdominal girth daily if ascites present): *Decrease in edema indicates positive increase in oncotic pressure.*
- Auscultate lungs carefully to determine presence of crackles *(indicating pulmonary edema).*
- Assess work of breathing and respiratory rate *(increased work of breathing is associated with pulmonary edema).*
- Assess heart sounds for presence or absence of gallop *(presence of S3 may indicate fluid overload).*
- Maintain fluid restriction as ordered *to decrease intravascular volume and workload on the heart.*
- Strictly monitor intake and output *to quickly note discrepancies and provide intervention.*
- Provide sodium-restricted diet as ordered *(restricting sodium in the diet allows for better kidney excretion of extra fluid).*
- Administer diuretics as ordered and monitor for side effects of those medications. *Diuretics encourage excretion of fluid and elimination of edema, reduce cardiac filling pressures, and increase kidney blood flow. Side effects include electrolyte imbalance as well as orthostatic hypotension.*

NURSING DIAGNOSIS: Imbalanced nutrition: Less than body requirements related to anorexia and protein loss as evidenced by weight, length/height, and/or BMI below average for age

Outcome Identification and Evaluation

Child will improve nutritional intake, resulting in *steady increase in weight and length/height.*

Intervention: Promoting Adequate Nutrition

- Determine body weight and length/height norm for age, *to determine goal to work toward.*
- Assess child for food preferences that fall within dietary restrictions, *as the child will be more likely to consume adequate amounts of foods that he or she likes.*
- Weigh daily or weekly (according to physician order or institutional standard) and measure length/height weekly, *to monitor for increased growth.*

(continued)

Nursing Care Plan 42.1 (continued)

- Offer highest-calorie meals at the time of day when the child's appetite is the greatest (*to increase likelihood of increased caloric intake*).
- Provide increased calorie shakes or puddings within diet restriction (*high-calorie foods increase weight gain*).
- Administer vitamin and mineral supplements as prescribed *to attain/maintain vitamin and mineral balance in the body*.
- Consult dietitian *to assist in nutritional assessment and make recommendations based on KDOQI guidelines*.

NURSING DIAGNOSIS: Imbalanced nutrition: More than body requirements related to increased appetite secondary to steroid therapy as evidenced by weight greater than 95th percentile for age or recent increase in weight

Outcome Identification and Evaluation
Child will demonstrate balanced nutritional intake, *will maintain current weight or steadily lose excess weight*.

Intervention: Encouraging Appropriate Nutritional Intake
- Determine ideal body weight and body mass index for age *to determine goal to work toward*.
- Consult dietitian *for guidance in planning nutrient-rich diet in context of restrictions*.
- Evaluate for emotional/psychological reasons for overeating *to address these concerns*.
- Formulate a contract with the child *to involve him/her in the planning process and encourage adherence to the plan*.
- With the child, plan for daily exercise/activity *to expend excess calories*.
- Instruct the child/parent about appropriate nutrient-rich foods to choose within the constraints of diet and fluid restrictions *to provide basis for ongoing diet management at home*.
- Weigh child twice weekly on same scale *to determine progress toward goal*.

NURSING DIAGNOSIS: Impaired urinary elimination related to UTI or other urologic condition, or other factors such as ignoring urge to void at appropriate time as evidenced by urinary retention or incontinence, dribbling, urgency, or dysuria

Outcome Identification and Evaluation
Child will maintain continence; *will void in the toilet*.

Intervention: Promoting Adequate Urinary Elimination
- Assess the child's usual voiding pattern and success within that pattern *to determine baseline*.
- Develop a schedule for bladder emptying *to encourage voiding in the toilet*.
- Maintain adequate hydration, *as dehydration irritates the bladder*.
- Avoid constipation, *as constipation is associated with inability to adequately empty bladder*.
- Teach parents to restrict child's fluid intake after dinner *to avoid bedwetting*.
- Ensure child voids prior to going to bed *to avoid bedwetting*.
- Teach bladder-stretching exercises as prescribed per physician *to increase bladder capacity*.

NURSING DIAGNOSIS: Urinary retention related to anatomic obstruction, sensory motor impairment or dysfunctional voiding as evidenced by dribbling, inadequate bladder emptying

Outcome Identification and Evaluation
Child's bladder will empty adequately; *according to pre-established quantities and frequencies individualized for the child (usual urine output is 0.5 to 2 mL/kg/hour)*.

Intervention: Promoting Successful Bladder Emptying
- Assess child's ability to adequately empty bladder via history focused on character and duration of lower urinary symptoms *to establish baseline*.
- Assess for history of fecal impaction or encopresis, *as alterations in bowel elimination may have a negative impact on urinary elimination*.
- Assess for bladder distention by palpation or urinary retention by post-void residual obtained via catheterization or bladder ultrasound *to determine extent of retention*.
- Maintain adequate hydration *to avoid irritating effects of dehydration on the bladder*.
- Schedule voiding *to decrease bladder overdistention*.
- In the child with significant urinary retention, teach parents/child the technique of clean intermittent catheterization, *which allows for regular complete bladder emptying*.

Nursing Care Plan 42.1 (continued)

NURSING DIAGNOSIS: Disturbed body image related to anatomic differences, short stature, or effects of long-term corticosteroid use as evidenced by verbalization of dissatisfaction with the child's or adolescent's looks

Outcome Identification and Evaluation
Child or adolescent will display appropriate body image, *will look at self in mirror and participate in social activities.*

Intervention: Promoting Body Image
* Acknowledge feelings of anger over body changes and illness: *Venting feelings is associated with less body image disturbance.*
* Support the child's or teen's choices of comfortable, fashionable clothing *that may disguise anatomic abnormalities and dialysis tubing.*
* Involve the child and especially the teen in the decision-making process, *as a sense of control of their own body will improve body image.*
* Encourage children or teens to spend time with others their own age who have short stature or other effects of kidney disorders: *A peer's opinions are often better accepted than those of persons in authority, such as parents or health care professionals.*

NURSING DIAGNOSIS: Knowledge deficit related to lack of information regarding complex medical condition, prognosis, and medical needs as evidenced by verbalization, questions, or actions demonstrating lack of understanding regarding child's condition or care

Outcome Identification and Evaluation
Child and parents will verbalize accurate information and understanding about condition, prognosis, and medical needs: *Child and parents demonstrate knowledge of condition and medications and will demonstrate therapeutic procedures the child requires.*

Intervention: Educating the Child and Parents
* Assess child's and parents' willingness to learn: *Child and parents must be open to learning for teaching to be effective.*
* Provide parents with time to adjust to diagnosis: *Will facilitate adjustment and ability to learn and participate in child's care.*
* Teach in short sessions: *Many short sessions are found to be more helpful than one long session.*
* Repeat information: *Allows parents and child time to learn and understand.*
* Individualize teaching to the parents' and child's level of understanding (depends on age of child, physical condition, memory) *to ensure understanding.*
* Provide reinforcement and rewards *to facilitate the teaching/learning process.*
* Use multiple modes of learning involving many senses (written, verbal, demonstration, and videos) when possible: *Child and parents are more likely to retain information when presented in different ways using many senses.*

---

consult the ostomy nurse for advice on dealing with the abdominal skin excoriation. If an orthopedic surgeon is involved due to the malformed pubic arch, follow through with recommended positioning or bracing to prevent further separation of the pubic arch (Phillips & Gearhart, 2009).

Providing Postoperative Care

Nursing management in the postoperative period again focuses on preventing infection. Keep the infant supine and quickly change soiled diapers to prevent contamination of the incision with stool. Surgical reconstruction of the bladder within the pelvic cavity and reconstruction of a urethra are done if enough bladder tissue is present. An indwelling urethral catheter or suprapubic tube will allow urinary drainage, allowing the bladder to rest in the initial postoperative period. Ensure that catheters are well secured, drain freely, and do not become kinked. Sometimes tubes or catheters used in the postoperative period require irrigation. Refer to the institution's policy and the surgeon's orders for specifics related to urinary catheter irrigation.

Manage bladder spasms with oxybutynin (Ditropan) or belladonna and opioid (B & O) suppositories as ordered. Note blood-tinged urine upon return from surgery, with clearing of urine within hours to days.

Catheterizing the Stoma

If bladder tissue is insufficient for repair, then the bladder is removed and a continent urinary reservoir created.

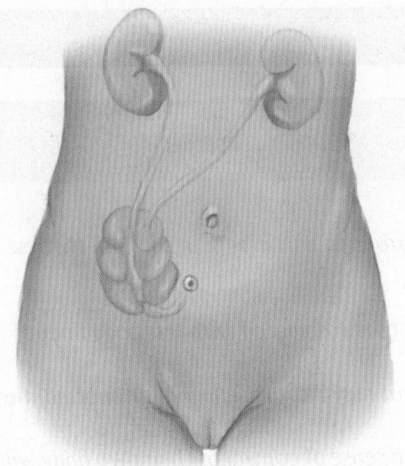

FIGURE 42.2 The abdominal stoma allows for urinary continence and requires catheterization.

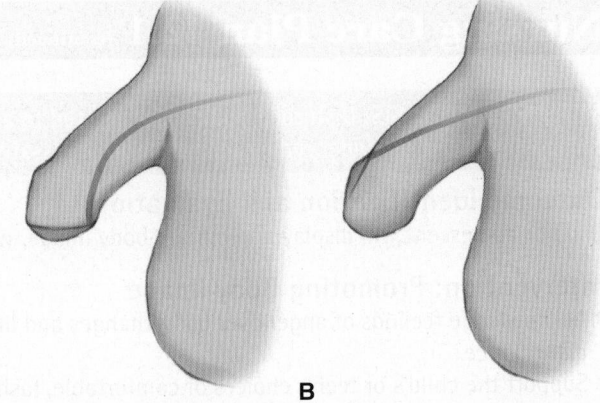

A   **B**

FIGURE 42.3 (**A**) Hypospadias: the urethral opening is located on the ventral side of the penis. (**B**) Epispadias: the urethral opening is located on the dorsal side of the penis.

The ureters are connected to a portion of the small intestine that is separated from the gastrointestinal (GI) tract, thus creating a urinary reservoir. The intestines are reanastomosed to leave the GI tract intact and separate from the GU tract. A stoma is created on the abdominal wall; it provides access to the urinary reservoir (Fig. 42.2). The stoma is catheterized about four to six times per day to empty the reservoir of urine. Urine from an intestine-based urinary reservoir tends to be mucus-like and is often cloudier than urine from a urinary bladder. Teach parents the procedure for catheterizing the urinary reservoir and instruct them to call the child's urologist or pediatrician if signs or symptoms of UTI occur.

> ▶ *Take* NOTE!
>
> *Children with congenital urologic malformations are at high risk for the development of latex allergy (Behrman & Howarth, 2011). Latex allergy can result in anaphylaxis. Primary prevention of latex allergy is warranted in all children with urologic malformations, so use latex-free gloves, tubes, and catheters in these children.*

Hypospadias/Epispadias

Hypospadias is a urethral defect in which the opening is on the ventral surface of the penis rather than at the end of the penis (Fig. 42.3). Epispadias is a urethral defect in which the opening is on the dorsal surface of the penis. In either case, the opening may be near the glans of the penis, midway along the penis, or near the base. If left uncorrected, the boy may not be capable of appropriately aiming a urinary stream from a standing position. The abnormal placement of the urethral opening may interfere with the deposition of sperm during inter-

course, leaving the man infertile. Also, if left uncorrected, the boy's self-esteem and body image may be damaged by the abnormal appearance of his genitalia (Schast & Reiner, 2010). For these reasons, the defect is usually repaired sometime during the child's first year of life. The goal of surgical correction for either condition is to provide for an appropriately placed meatus that allows for normal voiding and ejaculation (Kraft, Shulka, & Canning, 2010). The meatus is moved to the glans penis and the urethra is reconstructed as needed. Most repairs are accomplished in one surgery. More extensive reconstructions may require two stages.

Nursing Assessment

Note history of an unusual urine stream. Inspect the penis for placement of the urethral meatus: it may be slightly off centre of the glans or may be present somewhere along the shaft of the penis. Inspect for chordee, a fibrous band causing the penis to curve downward. Palpate for presence or absence of testicles in the scrotal sac because cryptorchidism (undescended testicles) often occurs with hypospadias, as do hydrocele and inguinal hernia.

Nursing Management

The newborn with hypospadias or epispadias should not undergo circumcision until after surgical repair of the urethral meatus. In more extreme cases, the surgeon may need to use some of the excess foreskin while reconstructing the meatus. Nursing management of the infant who has undergone a hypospadias or epispadias repair focuses on providing routine postoperative care and parent education.

Providing Postoperative Care

Postoperatively, assess urinary drainage from the urethral stent or drainage tube, which allows for discharge of urine without stress along the surgical site. Ensure that the urinary drainage tube remains carefully taped with the penis in an upright position to prevent stress on the urethral incision. The penile dressing is usually a compression type, used to decrease edema and bruising. Administer antibiotics if prescribed. Assess for pain, which is usually not extensive, and administer analgesics or antispasmodics (oral oxybutynin or B & O suppository) as needed for bladder spasms.

> ▶ **Take** NOTE!
>
> *Bladder spasms may also be managed effectively through the use of epidural analgesia, which is being used more frequently in the postoperative period in the pediatric population (Ellis, Martelli, LaMontagne, & Splinter, 2007).*

Double diapering is a method used to protect the urethra and stent or catheter after surgery; it also helps keep the area clean and free from infection. The inner diaper contains stool and the outer diaper contains urine, allowing separation between the bowel and bladder output. Nursing Procedure 42.2 details the double-diapering technique. Change the outside (larger) diaper when the child is wet; change both diapers when the child has a bowel movement.

Educating the Family

If the child is to be discharged with the urinary catheter in place, teach the parents how to care for the catheter and drainage system. Have parents demonstrate their ability to irrigate the catheter should a mucus plug occur.

Tub baths are generally prohibited until it is time to remove the penile dressing. Roughhousing, ride-on toys, or any activity involving straddling is not allowed for 2 to 3 weeks.

Obstructive Uropathy

Obstructive uropathy is an obstruction at any level along the upper or lower urinary tract. This discussion will focus on congenital structural defects, though obstruction can also occur as a result of other disease processes (acquired obstructive uropathy). The most common sites of obstruction are listed in Table 42.1. The defect may be unilateral or bilateral and can cause partial or complete obstruction of urine flow, resulting in dilation of the affected kidney (hydronephrosis). Complications include recurrent UTI, acute kidney injury (AKI), and progressive damage to the kidney resulting in CKD and end-stage kidney failure.

Nursing Assessment

For a full description of the assessment phase of the nursing process, refer to page 1427. Assessment findings pertinent to obstructive uropathy are discussed below.

Health History

Elicit a description of the present illness and chief complaint. Common signs and symptoms reported during the health history might include:

• Recurrent UTI
• Incontinence
• Fever
• Foul-smelling urine
• Flank pain

Nursing Procedure 42.2

DOUBLE DIAPERING

1. Cut a hole or a cross-shaped slit in the front of the smaller diaper. Ensure hole is large enough to prevent trauma to penis and traction to any tubing.
2. Unfold both diapers and place the smaller diaper (with the hole) inside the larger one.
3. Place both diapers under the child.
4. Carefully bring the penis (if applicable) and catheter/stent through the hole in the smaller diaper and close the diaper.
5. Close the larger diaper, making sure the tip of the catheter/stent is inside the larger diaper.

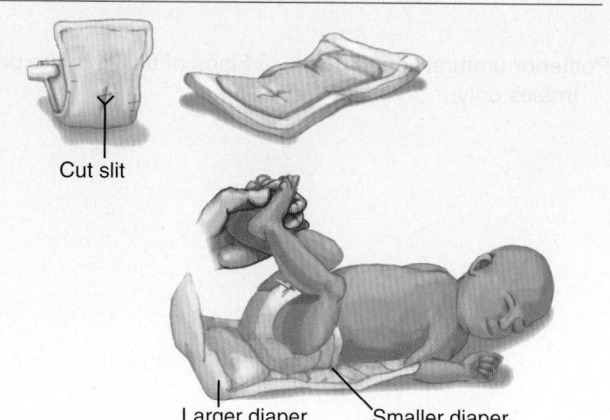

Cut slit

Larger diaper   Smaller diaper

Pictures and text adapted from: Children's Healthcare of Atlanta. (2004). *Double diapering.* Atlanta, GA: Author.

TABLE 42.1 COMMON SITES OF OBSTRUCTIVE UROPATHY

Disorder	Site	Illustration
Ureteropelvic junction (UPJ) obstruction	Junction of the upper ureter with the pelvis of the kidney	Urinary tract with unilateral hydronephrosis and narrowing of the UPJ on that side
Ureterovesical junction (UVJ) obstruction	Junction of the lower ureter and the bladder	Urinary tract with unilateral hydronephrosis and dilated tortuous ureters with narrowing of the UVJ on that side
Ureterocele	Ureter swells into the bladder	Bladder with cystic pouch where ureters insert (unilateral)
Posterior urethral valves (males only)	Flaps of tissue in the proximal urethra	Distended proximal urethra, bladder, ureters, and hydronephrosis

- Abdominal pain
- **Urinary frequency**
- Urinary **urgency**
- Dysuria
- **Hematuria**

Explore the child's current and past medical history for risk factors such as:

- "Prune belly" syndrome
- Chromosome abnormalities
- Anorectal malformations
- Ear defects

Physical Examination and Laboratory and Diagnostic Tests

Palpate the abdomen for the presence of an abdominal mass (hydronephrotic kidney). Assess the blood pressure; elevation may occur if kidney insufficiency is present. Many cases of obstructive uropathy may be diagnosed with prenatal ultrasound if the obstruction has been significant enough to cause hydronephrosis or dilation elsewhere along the urinary tract.

Nursing Management

Surgical correction is specific to the type of obstruction and generally consists of removal of the obstruction, reimplantation of the ureters as necessary, and occasionally creation of a urinary diversion. Postoperatively, assess urine output via vesicostomy, nephrostomy, suprapubic tube, or urethral catheter for colour, clots, clarity, and amount. Encourage fluids once the child can tolerate them orally. Administer analgesics and/or antispasmodics as needed for bladder spasms. Teach parents care of vesicostomy or drainage tubes, with which the child may be discharged.

> ▶ **Take** NOTE!
>
> Upon return from surgery, most children have intravenous fluids without added potassium infusion. Potassium is withheld from the intravenous fluid until adequate urine output is established postoperatively to avoid the development of hyperkalemia should the kidneys fail to function properly (Browne, Flanigan, McComiskey, & Pieper, 2007).

Hydronephrosis

Hydronephrosis is a condition in which the pelvis and calyces of the kidney are dilated (Fig. 42.4). Hydronephrosis may occur as a congenital defect, as a result of obstructive uropathy, or secondary to vesicoureteral reflux (VUR). Congenital hydronephrosis may be revealed on prenatal ultrasound and is the most common fetal GU anomaly (Carr & Kim, 2010). Children

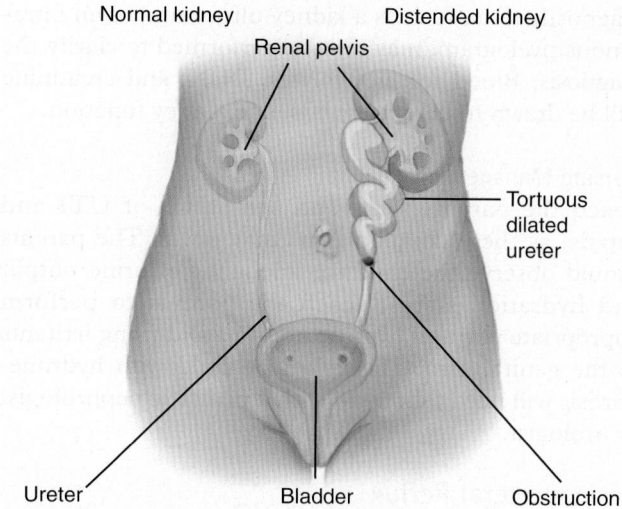

FIGURE **42.4** Hydronephrosis.

diagnosed antenatally with hydronephrosis should have a postnatal kidney ultrasound to confirm the cause of the hydronephrosis (Psooy & Pike, 2008). Complications of hydronephrosis include CKD, hypertension and, eventually, end-stage kidney failure.

Nursing Assessment

For a full description of the assessment phase of the nursing process, refer to page 1427. Assessment findings pertinent to hydronephrosis are discussed below.

Health History

Elicit a description of the present illness and chief complaint. The infant may be asymptomatic, but signs and symptoms reported during the health history might include:

- Failure to thrive
- Intermittent hematuria
- Presence of an abdominal mass
- Signs and symptoms associated with a UTI such as fever, vomiting, poor feeding, and irritability

Explore the child's current and past medical history for risk factors such as:

- Maternal oligohydramnios or polyhydramnios (congenital hydronephrosis)
- Elevated levels of serum alpha-fetoprotein (congenital hydronephrosis)

Physical Examination and Diagnostic and Laboratory Tests

Monitor the blood pressure of infants and children suspected of having hydronephrosis. Palpation of the abdomen may reveal enlarged kidney(s) or a distended bladder. A voiding cystourethrogram (VCUG) will be performed to determine the presence of a structural defect that may be causing the hydronephrosis. Other diagnostic tests, such as a kidney ultrasound or an intravenous pyelogram, may also be performed to clarify the diagnosis. Blood for electrolytes, BUN, and creatinine will be drawn to determine baseline kidney function.

Nursing Management

Teach the parents signs and symptoms of UTI and **sepsis**, as these complications may occur. The parents should observe the child for adequacy of urine output and hydration status. Teach the parents to perform appropriate perineal hygiene and to avoid using irritants in the genital area. The infant or child with hydronephrosis will need follow-up with a pediatric nephrologist or urologist.

Vesicoureteral Reflux

VUR is a condition in which urine from the bladder flows backup the ureters. This reflux of urine occurs during bladder contraction with voiding (Fig. 42.5). Reflux may occur in one or both ureters. If reflux occurs when the urine is infected, the kidney is exposed to bacteria and pyelonephritis may result. The increased pressure placed upon the kidney with reflux can cause kidney scarring and lead to hypertension later in life and, if severe, CKD and end-stage kidney failure.

Primary VUR results from a congenital abnormality at the vesicoureteral junction that results in incompetence of the valve (Ellsworth, Cendron, & McCullough, 2000). Secondary VUR is related to other structural or functional problems such as neurogenic bladder, bladder dysfunction, or bladder outlet obstruction (Roth, Koo, Spottswood, & Chan, 2002). As many as 30% to 40% of all children diagnosed with UTI have primary VUR (Thompson, Simon, Sharma, & Alon, 2005).

VUR is graded according to its severity: grade I results in minor dilation of the proximal ureter, and grade V is reflux into the kidney collecting system with severe calyceal blunting and severe dilation and tortuosity of the ureter (Wald, 2006). Grade I and II VUR cases

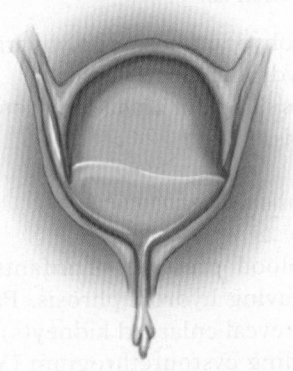

FIGURE 42.5 Note retrograde flow of urine up the ureter upon bladder contraction.

usually resolve spontaneously, but without intervention grade III to V cases are generally associated with recurrent UTIs, hydronephrosis, and progressive kidney damage (Nelson & Koo, 2011).

The goal of therapeutic management of VUR is prevention of pyelonephritis and subsequent kidney scarring, which may contribute to the development of hypertension later in life (Nelson & Koo, 2011). Management includes antibiotic prophylaxis and hygiene/voiding practices to prevent UTI. Serial urine cultures are used to determine recurrence of UTI. Biannual, annual, or biennial radionuclide VCUGs are performed to determine the status of VUR.

Grade III, IV, and V cases warrant surgical intervention. The ureters are resected from the bladder and reimplanted elsewhere in the bladder wall to regain functionality. Endoscopic injection of a biomaterial called dextranomer/hyaluronic acid (Deflux) via the urethra is becoming a common procedure to treat VUR in select patients (Routh, Inman, & Reinberg, 2010), including post kidney transplant (Williams, Giel, & Hasting, 2008). Deflux is associated with fewer postoperative side effects and is more effective in lower grades of VUR (Austin & Cooper, 2010).

▶ **Take** NOTE!

The keys to prevention of long-term sequelae such as hypertension in children with urologic conditions are early diagnosis and intervention, prevention of infection, and close clinical follow-up. Nurses play a key role in monitoring and education.

Nursing Assessment

For a full description of the assessment phase of the nursing process, refer to page 1427. Assessment findings pertinent to VUR are discussed below.

Health History

Elicit a description of the present illness and chief complaint. Common signs and symptoms reported during the health history might include:

• Fever
• Dysuria
• Frequency or urgency
• Nocturia
• Hematuria
• Pain in the back, abdomen, or flank

Explore the child's current and past medical history for risk factors such as:

• Recurrent UTI in the female
• Single episode of UTI in the male

• Congenital defect
• Family history of VUR

For the child who is receiving ongoing follow-up for VUR, determine whether UTIs have occurred since the last visit, as well as the name and dose of prophylactic antibiotic.

Physical Examination

Monitor the blood pressure for elevation. Palpate the abdomen for presence of a mass (if hydronephrosis is present). Renal ultrasound and VCUG are used to diagnose VUR.

Nursing Management

Nursing management for the child with VUR includes preventing infection and providing postoperative care.

Preventing Infection

When VUR is present, the goal is to avoid urine infection so that infected urine cannot gain access to the kidneys. Initially, most cases of VUR are managed medically. Teach the child to empty the bladder completely. Teach the child and parents appropriate perineal hygiene as well as toileting hygiene to prevent recurrence of UTI. Teach parents about the antibiotic therapy prescribed: the child will be maintained on a low daily dose to prevent UTI. The drug is most effective when given at bedtime because of urinary stasis overnight. Inform parents of the schedule for serial urine cultures and follow-up VCUG.

Providing Postoperative Care

If VUR is severe or if UTI is recurrent, surgical correction will be necessary. In the first 24 to 48 hours after surgery, maintain the intravenous fluid rate at 1.5 times maintenance to encourage a high urinary output. Monitor urine output via the Foley catheter; urine should be bloody initially, clearing within 2 to 3 days. If ureteral stents are present, monitor urine output from those as well. Administer analgesics for incisional pain relief and antispasmodics or B & O suppositories as needed for bladder spasms. Encourage ambulation and advancement of diet as ordered to promote return of appropriate bowel function. Teach parents that prophylactic antibiotics will be given until 1 to 2 months after surgery, when the VCUG demonstrates absence of reflux (Ellsworth et al., 2000).

▶ *Take* NOTE!

When caring for the child who has undergone urologic surgery, avoid manipulating the Foley or suprapubic catheter: catheter manipulation contributes to bladder spasms.

Urinary Tract Infection

UTI occurs most often as a result of bacteria ascending to the bladder via the urethra. UTI is the most common serious bacterial infection in children (Bauer & Kogan, 2008), with lower tract infection (cystitis) being less serious than upper tract infection (pyelonephritis). As many as 7% of females and 2% of males will experience a UTI by age 6 years (Alper & Curry, 2005). UTI is most common in infants and young children. It occurs more frequently in uncircumcised males younger than 3 months of age and in females less than 12 months of age (Shaikh, Morone, Bost, & Farrell, 2008), but after 1 year of age it is more common in females. One explanation for the more common occurrence in females is that the female's shorter urethra allows bacteria to have easier access to the bladder. The urethra is also located quite close to the vagina and anus in females, allowing spread of bacteria from those areas. The sexually active female adolescent is at risk for the development of cystitis, as bacteria may be forced into the urethra by pressure from intercourse. The male may be somewhat protected from UTI by the antibacterial properties of prostate secretions.

UTI presents differently in infants than it does in children. Infants may exhibit fever, irritability, vomiting, failure to thrive, or jaundice. Children may also experience fever and vomiting and may have dysuria, frequency, hesitancy, urgency, or pain (Alper & Curry, 2005).

Pathophysiology

E. coli accounts for approximately 70% to 90% of all UTIs in young children and is the source of most primary and recurrent UTIs due to colonization of the perineal area with this intestinal flora (Shah & Upadhyay, 2005). The bacteria colonizing this area then ascend into the sterile bladder causing UTI. In contrast, in infants less than 12 weeks of age, UTIs are thought to be secondary to a hematogenous source (Schlager, 2001). Other organisms include *Klebsiella, Staphylococcus aureus, Proteus, Pseudomonas,* and *Haemophilus.* Group B streptococcal infection is more common in neonates (Clark, Kennedy, & Shortliffe, 2010). Numerous factors may contribute to bacterial proliferation. Urinary stasis contributes to the development of a UTI once the bacteria have gained entry. Urine that remains in the bladder after voiding allows bacteria to grow rapidly. Decreased fluid intake also contributes to bacterial growth, as the bacteria become more concentrated. If the urine is alkaline, bacteria are better able to flourish. Untreated bladder infection may allow reflux of infected urine up the ureters to the kidneys and result in pyelonephritis, a more serious infection.

Therapeutic Management

UTIs are treated with either oral or intravenous antibiotics, depending on the severity of the infection. Urine

EVIDENCE-BASED PRACTICE 42.1
Antibiotics and Urinary Tract Infections in Children

● **Study**

UTIs commonly occur in children, causing frequent and painful urination. Traditionally, 7- to 10-day courses of antibiotics have been recommended for treating UTI in children. In the search for options to decrease side effects and improve costs, short courses of antibiotics may provide the solution. The authors included 10 randomized and quasi-randomized trials with a total of 652 participants. Participants included were low-risk, between the ages of 3 months and 18 years with culture-proven UTI. The studies assessed the benefits and harms of short-course (2 to 4 days) antibiotic treatment compared with that of standard duration (7 to 14 days).

▲ **Findings**

The authors found that a 2- to 4-day course of oral antibiotics appears to be as effective as the traditional long course (7 to 14 days) in eradicating UTI in children. Additionally, there was no statistical significance demonstrated in terms of repeat UTI within 1 to 15 months after the original infection.

■ **Nursing Implications**

Shorter courses of antibiotic treatment are much easier for families to comply with and complete, yet families may be accustomed to longer courses of antibiotic treatment and need further education. Educate families that the shorter course is indeed effective in treating UTI. Nurses should advocate for short-course antibiotic treatment in low-risk children with UTI.

Michael, M., Hodson, E. M., Craig, J. C., Martin, S., & Voyer, V. A. (2007). Short versus standard duration oral antibiotic therapy for acute urinary tract infection in children. *The Cochrane Library 2007, 4.* Indianapolis: John Wiley & Sons.

culture and sensitivity testing determines the appropriate antibiotic. Current treatment recommendations call for a 7- to 14-day course of antibiotics; this is in contrast to adult treatment, which may involve only 1 to 3 days of antibiotics in certain cases (Daniels & DiCenso, 2003). See Evidence-based Practice 42.1. Adequate fluid intake is necessary to flush the bacteria from the bladder. Fever management may also be needed.

Nursing Assessment

For a full description of the assessment phase of the nursing process, refer to page 1427. Assessment findings pertinent to UTI are discussed below.

Health History

Elicit a description of the present illness and chief complaint. Common signs and symptoms reported during the health history might include:

• Fever
• Nausea or vomiting
• Chills
• Abdomen, back, or flank pain
• Lethargy
• Jaundice (in the neonate)
• Poor feeding or "just not acting right" (in the infant)
• Urinary urgency or frequency
• Burning or stinging with urination (the infant may cry with urination, the toddler may grab the diaper)
• Foul-smelling urine

• Poor appetite (child)
• Enuresis or incontinence in a previously toilet-trained child
• Blood in the urine

Explore the child's current and past medical history for risk factors such as:

• Previous UTI
• Obstructive uropathy
• Inadequate toileting hygiene (often occurs with preschool girls)
• VUR
• Constipation
• Urine holding or dysfunctional voiding
• Neurogenic bladder
• Uncircumcised male
• Sexual intercourse
• Pregnancy
• Chronic illness

Physical Examination

In the neonate or young infant, observe for jaundice or increased respiratory rate. In infants and children, inspect the perineal area for redness or irritation. Observe the urine for visible blood, cloudiness, dark colour, sediment, mucus, or foul odour. Note pallor, edema, or elevated blood pressure. Palpate the abdomen. Note distended bladder, abdominal mass, or tenderness, particularly in the flank area.

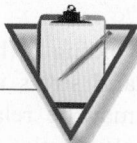

Laboratory and Diagnostic Tests

Common laboratory and diagnostic studies ordered for the assessment of UTI include:

- Urinalysis (clean-catch, suprapubic, or catheterized): may be positive for blood, nitrites, leukocyte esterase, white blood cells, or bacteria (**bacteriuria**)
- Urine culture: will be positive for infecting organism
- Renal ultrasound: may show hydronephrosis if child also has a structural defect
- VCUG: not usually performed until the child has been treated with antibiotics for at least 48 hours, as infected urine tends to reflux up the ureters anyway. VCUG performed once the urine has regained sterility may be positive for VUR.

Renal ultrasound, VCUG, and other nuclear medicine scans such as the DMSA renal scan may be indicated in certain populations. The physician or nurse practitioner will determine the need for radiologic testing.

Nursing Management

Goals for nursing management include eradicating infection, promoting comfort, preventing complications, and preventing recurrence of infection.

Eradicating Infection

The child who can tolerate oral intake will be prescribed an oral antibiotic. The child who has protracted vomiting related to the UTI or who has suspected pyelonephritis will require hospitalization and intravenous antibiotics. Any infant less than 3 months of age with fever and suspected UTI should also be hospitalized for administration of intravenous antibiotics, although ambulatory treatment has been successful (Doré-Bergeron et al., 2009). Administer oral or intravenous antibiotics as prescribed. Urge the parent to complete the entire course of oral antibiotic at home, even though the child is feeling better. Administer intravenous fluids as ordered or encourage generous oral fluid intake to help flush the bacteria from the bladder.

Promoting Comfort

Administer antipyretics such as acetaminophen or ibuprofen to reduce fever. A heating pad or warm compress may help relieve abdomen or flank pain. If the child is afraid to urinate due to burning or stinging, encourage voiding in a warm sitz or tub bath.

Preventing Recurrence of Infection

Encourage the parents to return as ordered for a repeat urine culture after completion of the antibiotic course to ensure eradication of bacteria. Teaching Guideline 42.1 gives further information on preventing UTIs in girls.

TEACHING GUIDELINE 42.1

Preventing Urinary Tract Infection in Females

- Drink enough fluid (to keep urine flushed through bladder).
- Drink cranberry juice to acidify the urine. Avoid colas and caffeine, which irritate the bladder.
- Urinate frequently and do not "hold" urine (to discourage urinary stasis).
- Avoid bubble baths (they contribute to vulvar and perineal irritation).
- Wipe from front to back after voiding (to avoid contaminating the urethra with rectal material).
- Wear cotton underwear (to decrease the incidence of perineal irritation).
- Avoid wearing tight jeans or pants.
- Wash the perineal area daily with soap and water.
- While menstruating, change sanitary pads frequently to discourage bacterial growth.
- Void immediately after sexual intercourse.

Enuresis

Enuresis is continued incontinence of urine past the age of toilet training. Box 42.1 gives further definitions related to enuresis. Nocturnal enuresis generally subsides by 6 years of age; if it does not, further investigation and treatment may be warranted. Occasional daytime wetting or dribbling of urine is usually not a cause for concern, but frequent daytime wetting concerns both the child and the parents. Nocturnal enuresis may persist in some children into late childhood and adolescence, causing significant distress for the affected child and family (Cox, 2009).

In some children, enuresis may occur secondary to a physical disorder such as diabetes mellitus or insipidus, sickle-cell anemia, ectopic ureter, or urethral obstruction. Other causes common to both diurnal and nocturnal enuresis include a urine-concentrating defect, UTI, constipation, and emotional distress (sometimes serious). The most frequent cause of daytime enuresis is dysfunctional

---

BOX 42.1 Definitions Related to Enuresis

- **Primary enuresis:** enuresis in the child who has never achieved voluntary bladder control
- **Secondary enuresis:** urinary incontinence in the child who previously demonstrated bladder control over a period of at least 3 to 6 consecutive months
- **Diurnal enuresis:** daytime loss of urinary control
- **Nocturnal enuresis:** nighttime bedwetting

voiding or holding of urine, though giggle incontinence and stress incontinence also occur. Nocturnal enuresis may be related to a high fluid intake in the evening, obstructive sleep apnea, sexual abuse, a family history of enuresis, or inappropriate family expectations. Physical causes of enuresis must be treated; further management of the disorder focuses on behavioural training, which may be augmented with the use of enuresis alarms or medications (Ellsworth & Caldamone, 2008).

Nursing Assessment

Elicit a description of the present illness and chief complaint. Determine the age of toilet training and when or if the child achieved successful daytime and nighttime dryness. Inquire about urine-holding behaviours such as squatting, dancing, or staring as well as rushing to the bathroom (diurnal enuresis). Inquire about the amount and types of fluid the child typically consumes before bedtime (nocturnal enuresis). Assess for risk factors such as:

• Family disruption or other stressors
• Chronic constipation (carefully assess bowel movement patterns)
• Excessive family demands related to toileting patterns
• History of being difficult to arouse from sleep
• Family history of enuresis

Assess the child's cognitive status: developmentally delayed children may take significantly longer to achieve urine continence than their typical same-age peers. Assess for short stature or elevated blood pressure, as these may occur when renal abnormalities are present.

Nursing Management

For the child with diurnal enuresis, encourage him or her to increase the amount of fluid consumed during the day in order to increase the frequency of the urge to void. Set a fixed schedule for the child to attempt to void throughout the day. These practices will usually be sufficient to retrain the child's voiding patterns. The child with nocturnal enuresis without a physiologic cause for bedwetting may require a varied approach (Cox, 2009).

Educating the Child and Family About Nocturnal Enuresis

Teach the family that the child is not lazy, nor does he or she wet the bed intentionally. Encourage the child and family to read books such as *Dry All Night: The Picture Book Technique That Stops Bedwetting* by Alison Mack or *Waking Up Dry: A Guide to Help Children Overcome Bedwetting* by Dr. Howard Bennett. Encourage the parents to limit intake of bladder irritants such as chocolate and caffeine. Teach parents to limit fluid intake after dinner and ensure that the child voids just before going to bed. Waking the child to void at 11 PM. may also be helpful. Teach the parents to use bed pads and to make the bed with two sets of sheets and pads to decrease the work-

load in the middle of the night. When sleeping at home, the child should wear his or her usual underwear or pajamas. If away on a family vacation, pull-ups may decrease the stress on both the child and the parents. The CPS (2005) offers a position statement on enuresis (reaffirmed in 2011).

Providing Support and Encouragement

It is important for the child to understand that he or she is not alone. According to the CPS (2005), 10% to 15% of 5-year-old children and 6% to 8% of 8-year-old children have enuresis. It is not only "little kids" who wet the bed, and all kids who wet the bed need help overcoming this problem. Parents should include the child in plans for nighttime urinary control; this helps to increase the child's motivation to become dry. Parents should include the child in bed linen changes, if age-appropriate, when he or she does wet the bed but should do so in a matter-of-fact manner rather than in a punitive way; in fact, punishment for bedwetting should *always be avoided*.

With patience, consistency, and time, dryness will be achieved. Provide ongoing emotional support and positive reinforcement to the child and family.

Decreasing Nighttime Voiding

Teach the family using an enuresis alarm system how to use the alarm as well as the previously mentioned techniques (Fig. 42.6). Visit http://thePoint.lww.com/Chow1e for a list of related websites. Most of these devices work by sounding an alarm when the first few drops of urine appear; the child then awakens and stops the urine flow. Over time the child becomes conditioned to either awaken when the bladder is full or stop the urine flow when sleeping.

When behavioural and motivational therapies are unsuccessful, particularly in the older child, medications

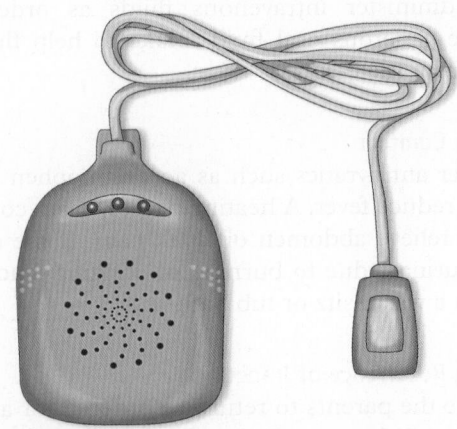

FIGURE 42.6 Some children and families find success with the use of an enuresis alarm. The alarm wakes the child at the first sign of wetness. Over time, the child learns to awaken at night in response to the sensation of a full bladder.

may be prescribed (Wolfish & Phan, 2009). Teach the child and parents about the use of desmopressin (DDAVP) if prescribed (refer to Drug Guide 42.1).

> ▶ **Take** NOTE!
>
> *Enuresis is a source of shame and embarrassment for children and adolescents. It affects the child's life emotionally, behaviourally, and socially. The family's life is also significantly affected. Treatment failures for enuresis have been correlated with adolescent low self-esteem (Martin & Volkmar, 2007).*

> ▶ **Consider** THIS!
>
> *Antonio Cruise, a 7-year-old boy, is brought to the clinic by his mother for his annual examination. During your assessment the mother brings up concerns that Antonio continues to wet the bed at night. She states, "I was hoping this would end on its own, but now I'm concerned that there is a problem."*
>
> *What further assessment information would you obtain?*
>
> *What education and interventions may be necessary for this child and family?*
>
> *What can you do to provide support and encouragement for Antonio and his family?*

Acquired Disorders Resulting in Altered Kidney Function

A number of acquired disorders are responsible for alterations in kidney function. They may occur as an autoimmune response or in relation to a bacterial infection. Kidney dysfunction may also occur as a result of obstructive disorders or repeated VUR, as discussed earlier. Left untreated, these disorders may lead to AKI. Even when treated appropriately, the desired response is sometimes not achieved and CKD and end-stage kidney disease develop. Kidney disorders are the most frequent cause of hypertension in children.

> ▶ **Take** NOTE!
>
> *Severe hypertension (blood pressure higher than the 99th percentile for age and sex) may lead to damage of the eye or vital organs (kidney, brain, or heart), or even death (Flynn & Tullus, 2009). Pediatric nurses must be adept at accurately measuring blood pressure in children.*

Nephrotic Syndrome

Nephrotic syndrome occurs as a result of increased glomerular basement membrane permeability, which allows abnormal loss of protein in the urine. Nephrotic syndrome generally occurs in three forms: congenital, idiopathic, and secondary. Congenital nephrotic syndrome is an inherited disorder; it is rare and occurs primarily in families of Finnish descent. The prognosis is poor, though some success has occurred with early, aggressive treatment and with the advances in kidney transplantation in infants (Jalanko, 2009). Nephrotic syndrome may occur secondary to another condition such as systemic lupus erythematosus, Henoch–Schonlein purpura, or diabetes. Idiopathic nephrotic syndrome is the most commonly occurring type in children and is often termed minimal change nephrotic syndrome (MCNS) (Lane, 2011). MCNS occurs more frequently in males than females, with 70% of cases occurring by age 5 years (Lane, 2011). This discussion will focus primarily on MCNS. Complications of nephrotic syndrome include anemia, infection, poor growth, peritonitis, thrombosis, and kidney failure.

Pathophysiology

Increased glomerular permeability results in the passage of larger plasma proteins through the glomerular basement membrane. This results in excess loss of protein (albumin) in the urine (**proteinuria**) and decreased protein and albumin (hypoalbuminemia) in the bloodstream. Protein loss in nephrotic syndrome tends to be almost exclusively albumin. Hypoalbuminemia results in a change in osmotic pressure, and fluid shifts from the bloodstream into the interstitial tissue (causing edema). This decrease in blood volume triggers the kidneys to respond by conserving sodium and water, leading to further edema. The liver senses the protein loss and increases production of lipoproteins. **Hyperlipidemia** then develops as the excess lipids cannot be excreted in the urine. Hyperlipidemia associated with nephrotic syndrome may be quite severe, yet cholesterol levels may decrease when the nephrotic syndrome is in remission, only to rise significantly again with a relapse.

Children with nephrotic syndrome are at increased risk for clotting (thromboembolism) because of the decreased intravascular volume. They are also at increased risk for the development of serious infection, most commonly pneumococcal pneumonia, sepsis, or spontaneous peritonitis. Steroid-resistant nephrotic syndrome may result in acute kidney failure.

Therapeutic Management

Medical management of MCNS usually involves the use of corticosteroids. Intravenous albumin may be used in the severely edematous child. Diuretics are also required in the edematous phase. Long-term therapy is usually required to induce remission. The nephrologist will determine the length of therapy based on the child's response. Children who have steroid-responsive MCNS generally have a favourable prognosis. Some children with MCNS exhibit a minimal response to steroid therapy or experience remissions and the MCNS is steroid-resistant (Lane, 2011). Immunosuppressive therapy such as cyclophosphamide, cyclosporin A, or mycophenolate mofetil may be necessary.

Nursing Assessment

For a full description of the assessment phase of the nursing process, refer to page 1427. Assessment findings pertinent to MCNS are discussed below.

Health History

Elicit a description of the present illness and chief complaint. Common signs and symptoms reported during the health history might include:

- Nausea or vomiting (may be related to ascites)
- Recent weight gain
- History of periorbital edema upon waking, progressing to generalized edema throughout the day (labial edema in girls and scrotal edema in boys)
- Weakness or fatigue
- Irritability or fussiness

Explore the child's current and past medical history for risk factors such as:

- Intrauterine growth retardation
- Young age (less than 3 years)
- Male sex

Physical Examination

The physical assessment of the child with nephrotic syndrome includes inspection and observation, auscultation, and palpation.

Observe the child for edema (periorbital, generalized [**anasarca**], or abdominal ascites). As the disease progresses, the edema also progresses to become more generalized, eventually becoming severe. Inspect the skin for a stretched, tight appearance, pallor, or skin breakdown related to significant edema (Fig. 42.7). Document height (or length) and weight. Note increased respiratory rate or increased work of breathing related to ascites and edema.

Note the blood pressure; it may be elevated in the child with nephrotic syndrome, though it is most often either normal or decreased unless the child is progressing to kidney failure. Auscultate heart and lung sounds, noting abnormalities related to fluid overload. Palpate the skin, noting tautness. Palpate the abdomen and document the presence of ascites.

Laboratory and Diagnostic Tests

Urine dipstick will reveal marked proteinuria. Infrequently, mild hematuria is also present. Serum protein

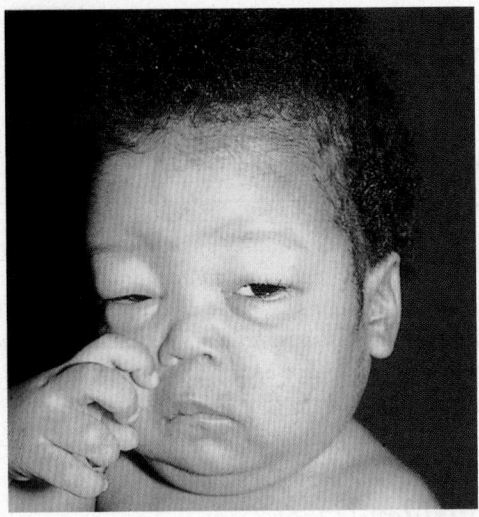

FIGURE 42.7 Note marked edema associated with nephrotic syndrome.

and albumin levels will be low (often markedly so). Serum cholesterol and triglyceride levels are elevated. With continued nephrotic syndrome, creatinine and BUN may become elevated.

Nursing Management

Goals for nursing management include promoting diuresis, preventing infection, promoting adequate nutrition, and educating the parents about ongoing care at home. As with other chronic disorders, provide ongoing emotional support to the child and family.

Promoting Diuresis

Administer corticosteroids as ordered. Tapering or weaning doses are required when the time comes to stop corticosteroid therapy. Administer diuretics if ordered, usually furosemide (Lasix). Children may develop hypokalemia because of potassium loss as an adverse effect of furosemide. Those children may require potassium supplementation or a diet higher in potassium-containing foods. Monitor urine output and the amount of protein in the urine (by dipstick). Weigh the child daily on the same scale either naked or wearing the same amount of clothing. Assess for resolution of edema. Measure pulse rate and blood pressure every 4 hours to detect hypovolemia resulting from excessive fluid shifts. Enforce oral fluid restrictions if ordered.

In cases of severe edema due to marked hypoalbuminemia, intravenous albumin may be administered. Increases in the serum albumin level cause fluid to shift from the subcutaneous spaces back into the bloodstream. A diuretic such as furosemide administered midway through or immediately after the albumin infusion allows for optimal diuresis and prevents fluid overload. Refer to Drug Guide 42.1 for the nursing implications related to use of these medications.

Preventing Infection

Monitor the child's temperature. Administer pneumococcal vaccine as prescribed (see Chapter 30 for information on immunizations). Administer prophylactic antibiotics, if prescribed. Live vaccines should be delayed until at least 2 weeks after corticosteroid or other immunosuppressive medication therapy ceases. Teach parents that if the child is unimmunized and is exposed to chickenpox, the pediatrician or nephrologist should be notified immediately so that the child may receive varicella zoster immunoglobulin.

Encouraging Adequate Nutrition and Growth

Encourage a nutrient-rich diet within prescribed restrictions. Fluid restriction is reserved for children with massive edema. Sodium intake may be restricted in the edematous child in an effort to prevent further fluid retention. Consultation with the dietitian is often helpful in meal planning because many of the foods that children like are high in sodium and because children who are taking steroids have an increased appetite, putting them at risk for rapid weight gain. Encourage protein-rich snacks. Consult with the child and family in planning meals and snacks that the child likes and will be likely to consume. Use of nutritional supplement shakes may be helpful in some children.

Educating the Family

Teach parents how to give medications and monitor for adverse effects. Demonstrate the urine dipstick technique for detecting protein, and encourage the family to keep a chart of dipstick results. The child may return to school but should avoid contact with sick playmates. If the child is exposed to another child with an infectious illness, the parents should monitor temperature and urine dipstick results more frequently to identify a relapse in nephrotic syndrome early so that treatment can begin.

Providing Emotional Support

Nephrotic syndrome is often a chronic condition, and children who are responsive to steroid treatment may enter remission only to experience relapse. This cycle of relapse and remission takes an emotional toll on the child and family. Frequent hospitalizations require the child to miss school and the parents to miss work; this creates further stress for the family. The child may experience social isolation because he or she must avoid exposure to infections or because of self-esteem problems. The child may be dissatisfied with his or her appearance because of edema and weight gain, short stature, and the classic "moon face" associated with chronic steroid use.

Provide emotional support to the child and family. Encourage them in their efforts to maintain the treatment plan. Introduce the child to other youngsters with chronic kidney conditions. Refer families to the Kidney Foundation of Canada for information about local support groups and resources.

Acute Glomerulonephritis

Acute glomerulonephritis is a condition in which immune processes injure the glomeruli. Immune mechanisms cause inflammation, which results in altered glomerular structure and function in both kidneys. It often occurs following an infection, usually an upper respiratory or skin infection. The most common form is acute post-streptococcal glomerulonephritis (APSGN), and the following discussion will focus on this type. APSGN is caused by an antibody–antigen reaction secondary to an infection with a nephritogenic strain of group A beta-hemolytic streptococcus. APSGN occurs more frequently in males than females, with a peak prevalence around 5 to 6 years of age (Bhimma, 2011). The most serious complication is progression to uremia and kidney failure (either acute or chronic).

There is no specific medical treatment for APSGN. Treatment is aimed at maintaining fluid volume and managing hypertension. If there is evidence of a current streptococcal infection, antibiotic therapy will be necessary.

Nursing Assessment

For a full description of the assessment phase of the nursing process, refer to page 1427. Assessment findings pertinent to acute glomerulonephritis are discussed below.

Health History

Elicit a description of the present illness and chief complaint. Common signs and symptoms reported during the health history might include:

- Fever
- Lethargy
- Headache
- Decreased urine output
- Abdominal pain
- Vomiting
- Anorexia
- Tea-coloured urine

Assess the child's current and past medical history for risk factors such as a recent episode of pharyngitis or other streptococcal infection, age over 2 years, or male sex.

Physical Examination and Laboratory and Diagnostic Tests

Assess the child's blood pressure for elevation, which is common. Note the presence of mild edema. Observe for signs of cardiopulmonary congestion such as increased work of breathing or cough. Auscultate the lungs for crackles and the heart for gallop. The urine dipstick test will reveal proteinuria as well as hematuria. Inspect the urine for gross hematuria, which will cause the urine to appear tea-coloured, cola-coloured, or even a dirty green colour. Serum creatinine and BUN may be normal or elevated, the serum complement level is depressed, and the erythrocyte sedimentation rate is elevated. Laboratory findings specific to streptococcus include an elevated anti-streptolysin (ASO) titer and an elevated DNAase B antigen titer.

Nursing Management

Administer antihypertensives such as labetalol or nifedipine and diuretics as ordered. Monitor blood pressure frequently. Maintain sodium and fluid restrictions as prescribed during the initial edematous phase. Weigh the child daily on the same scale, at the same time of day, and wearing the same amount of clothing each time. Monitor increasing urine output and note improvement in the urine colour. Document resolution of edema. Provide careful neurologic evaluation, as hypertension may cause encephalopathy and seizures. Children with APSGN generally are fatigued and choose bed rest during the acute phase. Provide the child with age-appropriate activities and cluster care to allow rest periods.

Some children may be managed at home if edema is mild and they are not hypertensive. Teach the family to monitor urine output and colour, take blood measurements, and restrict the diet as prescribed. The child cared for at home should not participate in strenuous activity until proteinuria and hematuria are resolved.

If kidney involvement progresses, dialysis may become necessary.

▶ *Take NOTE!*

Avoid use of nonsteroidal anti-inflammatory drugs (NSAIDs) in children with questionable renal function, as the antiprostaglandin action of NSAIDs may cause a further decrease in the GFR (Solomon, 2011).

Hemolytic–Uremic Syndrome

Hemolytic–uremic syndrome (HUS) is defined by three features: hemolytic anemia, thrombocytopenia, and acute kidney failure. In 90% of cases of HUS, an illness featuring diarrhea precedes the onset of the syndrome. Other causes include idiopathic, inherited, drug-related, association with malignancies, transplantation, and malignant hypertension. This discussion will focus on typical HUS, the type preceded by a diarrheal illness. Watery diarrhea progresses to hemorrhagic colitis, then to the triad of HUS. The features of HUS, as well as effects on other organs, are caused primarily by microthrombi and ischemic changes within the organs. The thrombotic events in the small blood vessels of the glomerulus lead to occlusion of the glomerular capillary loops and glomerulosclerosis, resulting in kidney failure.

A verotoxin-producing strain of *E. coli* 0157:H7, causes the majority of cases, though *Streptococcus pneu-moniae, Shigella dysenteriae,* and other bacteria may also be the cause (Tan & Silverberg, 2011). It is thought that antibiotic treatment for the aforementioned bacteria may contribute to release of the verotoxin. Undercooked ground beef accounts for most cases of *E. coli* 0157:H7 infection, but it is also transmitted via the feces of numerous animals as well as unpasteurized dairy and fruit products (McLaine, Rowe, & Orrbine, 2009). Transmission also occurs via human feces, and cases have been linked to public swimming pools. HUS occurs most often in children ages 6 months to 4 years (Tan & Silverberg, 2011). Complications include chronic kidney failure, seizures and coma, pancreatitis, intussusception, rectal prolapse, cardiomyopathy, congestive heart failure, and acute respiratory distress syndrome (Varade, 2000).

Therapeutic management of HUS is directed toward maintaining fluid balance; correcting hypertension, acidosis, and electrolyte abnormalities; replenishing the circulation of red blood cells; and providing dialysis if needed.

Nursing Assessment

For a full description of the assessment phase of the nursing process, refer to page 1427. Assessment findings pertinent to HUS are discussed below.

Health History

Elicit a description of the present illness and chief complaint. Common signs and symptoms reported during the health history might include watery diarrhea accompanied by cramping and sometimes vomiting. After several days, the diarrhea becomes bloody and eventually improves.

Explore the child's current and past medical history for risk factors such as ingestion of ground beef, visits to a water park or to a petting zoo before the onset of the diarrheal illness, or use of antidiarrheal medications or antibiotics.

Physical Examination

Observe the child for pallor, toxic appearance, edema, **oliguria**, or **anuria**. Assess for elevated blood pressure and tenderness in the abdomen. Assess the child for neurologic involvement, which may include irritability, altered level of consciousness, seizures, posturing, or coma.

Laboratory and Diagnostic Tests

Urinalysis may reveal the presence of blood, protein, pus, and/or casts. Serum laboratory abnormalities are numerous and may include:

- Elevated BUN and creatinine
- Moderate to severe anemia (with the presence of Burr cells, schistocytes, spherocytes, or helmet cells), mild to severe thrombocytopenia
- Increased reticulocyte count
- Increased bilirubin and lactic dehydrogenase (LDH) levels

- Negative Coombs' test (except in cases of *S. pneumoniae* infection)
- Leukocytosis with left shift
- Hyponatremia
- Hyperkalemia
- Hyperphosphatemia
- Metabolic acidosis

Nursing Management

Nursing management of the child with HUS focuses on supportive therapy and close observation and monitoring of the child's status. Institute and maintain contact precautions to prevent spread of *E. coli* 0157:H7 to other children (bacteria are shed for up to 17 days after resolution of the diarrhea). Close attention must be paid to fluid volume status. Prevention of HUS is also an important nursing function.

Maintaining Appropriate Fluid Volume Balance

Maintain strict intake and output monitoring and recording to evaluate the progression toward kidney failure. Carefully monitor intravenous infusions and blood chemistries. Administer diuretics as ordered. Assess blood pressure frequently and report elevations to the physician. Administer antihypertensives as ordered and monitor their effectiveness. Encourage adequate nutritional intake within the constraints of prescribed dietary restrictions. Monitor for bleeding as well as for fatigue and pallor. Follow the institutional protocol for transfusion of packed red blood cells and/or platelets (platelets are usually transfused only if active bleeding or severe thrombocytopenia occurs). Report progressive deterioration in laboratory findings to the physician. About 50% of children with HUS will require dialysis for at least several days.

Preventing HUS

Proper handwashing is necessary. Teach children to wash their hands after using the bathroom, before eating, and after petting farm animals. Encourage the use of "swim diapers," which contain feces, for children who are not toilet trained. Teach parents to thoroughly cook all meats to a core temperature of 68.3°C, or until the meat is grey or brown throughout and the juices from the meat are clear rather than pink. Wash all fruits and vegetables thoroughly. Ensure that drinking water and water used for recreation is appropriately treated. Avoid unpasteurized dairy products and fruit juices (including cider).

Kidney Failure

Kidney failure is a condition in which the kidneys cannot concentrate urine, conserve electrolytes, or excrete waste products. As in adults, kidney failure in children may occur as an acute injury or chronic condition. Some cases of AKI resolve without further complications, while dialysis is necessary in other children. When AKI continues to progress, it becomes CKD and finally end-stage renal disease (ESRD) (Auron & Brophy, 2010). GFR is a marker for kidney function; a decline in GFR represents worsening kidney function (Staples & Wong, 2010). For further information on the classification of CKD, see the National Kidney Foundation Kidney Dialysis Outcome Quality Initiative (KDOQI). (Visit http://thePoint.lww.com/Chow1e for a direct link to the website.) Dialysis and kidney transplantation are treatment modalities used for CKD and ESRD.

Acute Kidney Injury

AKI is defined as a sudden, often reversible decline in kidney function that results in the accumulation of metabolic toxins (particularly nitrogenous wastes) as well as fluid and electrolyte imbalance. Fluid overload may lead to hypertension, pulmonary edema, and congestive heart failure. Additional complications include hyperkalemia, metabolic acidosis, hyperphosphatemia, and uremia. In children, AKI most commonly occurs as a result of decreased kidney perfusion, as occurs in hypovolemic or septic shock. It may also occur in children with hemolytic anemia or as a result of nephrotoxicity from medications. Complications include anemia, hyperkalemia, hypertension, pulmonary edema, cardiac failure, and altered level of consciousness or seizures, and AKI may also progress to a chronic state.

Therapeutic management is aimed at treating the underlying cause and managing the fluid and electrolyte disturbances, as well as decreasing blood pressure.

> ▶ *Take* NOTE!
>
> *Medications commonly used in children can reduce renal function. Cephalosporins may cause a transient increase in BUN and creatinine. Truly nephrotoxic drugs often used in children include aminoglycosides, sulfonamides, vancomycin, and NSAIDs. Make sure that potentially nephrotoxic drugs are administered according to published safe guidelines (dosage, frequency, rate of administration) (Taketokmo, Hodding, & Kraus, 2010).*

Nursing Assessment

For a full description of the assessment phase of the nursing process, refer to page 1427. Assessment finding pertinent to AKI are discussed below.

Health History

Elicit a description of the present illness and chief complaint. Common signs and symptoms reported during the health history might include:

- Nausea
- Vomiting
- Diarrhea

• Lethargy
• Fever
• Decreased urine output

Assess the child's current and past medical history for risk factors such as history of shock, trauma, burns, urologic abnormalities, kidney disease, use of nephrotoxic medications, or severe blood transfusion reaction.

Physical Examination and Laboratory and Diagnostic Tests

Note decreased skin elasticity, dry mucous membranes, or edema. Auscultate the lungs for crackles, which may occur with pulmonary edema. Document tachypnea. Note cardiac rhythm disturbances. Evaluate the child's level of consciousness. Laboratory tests will reveal increased serum creatinine levels and possible electrolyte disturbances, such as hyperkalemia or hypocalcemia. Urinalysis may reveal proteinuria or hematuria.

> ▶ **Take** NOTE!
>
> *Monitor the infant or child with kidney failure carefully for signs of congestive heart failure, such as edema accompanied by bounding pulse, presence of an S3 heart sound, adventitious lung sounds, and shortness of breath.*

Nursing Management

Nursing care focuses on managing hypertension, restoring fluid and electrolyte balance, and educating the family.

Managing Hypertension

Carefully monitor the child's blood pressure. Administer antihypertensives as prescribed. When a fast-acting drug such as nifedipine (Procardia) sublingually or labetalol intravenously is used, stay with the child and monitor blood pressure frequently. Immediately notify the physician if high blood pressure is resistant to medication and the blood pressure remains elevated.

Restoring Fluid and Electrolyte Balance

Monitor vital signs frequently and assess urine specific gravity. Maintain strict records of intake and output. Weigh the child daily on the same scale either naked or wearing the same amount of clothing each time. Administer diuretics as ordered. When urine output is restored, diuresis may be significant. Monitor for signs of hyperkalemia (weak, irregular pulse; muscle weakness; abdominal cramping) and hypocalcemia (muscle twitching or tetany). Administer polystyrene sulphonate (Kayexalate) as ordered orally, rectally, or through a nasogastric tube to decrease potassium levels. Kayexalate removes potassium primarily by exchanging sodium for it, which is then eliminated in the feces. Administer packed red blood cell transfusions as ordered (may need to be followed by a dose of diuretic). Dialysis may become necessary if oliguria is sustained and leads to significant fluid overload, the electrolyte imbalance reaches dangerous levels, or uremia results in depression of the central nervous system.

Providing Family Education

Educate the family about the plan of care and the need for fluid restriction if ordered. Instruct the family to save all voids for observation and measurement by the nurse. Provide education about the use of dialysis if relevant.

End-Stage Renal Disease

ESRD is CKD that requires long-term renal supportive therapy (Auron & Brophy, 2010), such dialysis or renal transplantation. CKD in children most often results from congenital structural defects such as obstructive uropathy (Klein, 2010). It may also be caused by an inherited condition such as familial nephritis or may result from an acquired problem such as glomerulonephritis; it may also follow an infectious process such as pyelonephritis or HUS (Klein, 2010). This is in contrast to CKD in adults, which primarily results from diabetes or hypertension. Uremia, hypocalcemia, hyperkalemia, and metabolic acidosis occur. Complications of CKD and ESRD are many. Uremic toxins deplete erythrocytes and the failing kidneys cannot produce erythropoietin, so severe anemia results. Hypertension is common and may lead to left ventricular hypertrophy; ultimately, heart failure may occur. Hypocalcemia results in renal rickets (brittle bones). Growth is delayed, and sexual maturation may be delayed or absent. Many children with CKD and ESRD experience depression, anxiety, impaired social interaction, and poor self-esteem (Klein, 2010).

Nursing Assessment

For a full description of the assessment phase of the nursing process, refer to page 1427. Assessment findings pertinent to CKD and ESRD are discussed below.

Health History

Explore the health history for low birth weight (associated with kidney dysfunction and anatomic alterations), poor growth (weight, length/height, and head circumference), and regimen of dialysis. Note decreased appetite or energy level, dry or itchy skin, or bone or joint pain.

Physical Examination and Laboratory and Diagnostic Tests

Perform a thorough physical assessment, noting any abnormalities (may vary from child to child). If present, assess the peritoneal catheter site for absence of drainage, bleeding, or redness (desired findings). If the child undergoes hemodialysis, assess the fistula or graft site for the presence of a bruit and a thrill. Laboratory tests may reveal low hemoglobin and hematocrit levels, increased serum phosphorus and potassium levels, and decreased sodium, calcium, and bicarbonate levels. BUN, uric acid, and creatinine levels will be elevated. A 24-hour urine creatinine clearance test will show increased amounts of creatinine in the urine and reflects decreasing kidney function.

▶ **Take** NOTE!

Carefully assess children with CKD or ESRD for worsening uremia or metabolic acidosis. Uremia may result in central nervous system symptoms such as headache or coma, or GI or neuromuscular disturbances. Metabolic acidosis causes lethargy, dull headache, and confusion.

Nursing Management

Nursing goals for the child with CKD and ESRD include promoting growth and development, removing waste products and maintaining fluid balance via dialysis, encouraging psychosocial well-being, and supporting and educating the family. The National Kidney Foundation guidelines for care of children with CKD is an excellent resource for nurses caring for children with CKD and those on dialysis. See the section for professionals on its website; the direct link is available at http://thePoint. lww.com/Chow1e.

Promoting Growth and Development

Encourage the child to choose foods he or she likes that are within the imposed dietary restrictions. Daily protein requirements for adequate growth range from 0.85 to 2.1 g/kg/day and are dependent on the child's stage of CKD or whether the child is on hemodialysis or peritoneal dialysis. Sodium and/or potassium restrictions may also be necessary. Enforce fluid restrictions if prescribed. Administer medications such as erythropoietin, growth hormone, and vitamin and mineral supplements to augment nutritional status and promote growth. Table 42.2 lists medications and supplements used to support growth in children with CKD and ESRD.

Encouraging Psychosocial Well-Being

Children with CKD and particularly ESRD often suffer from depression and anxiety. Refer children and their families to the hospital social worker or counsellor as needed for depression or anxiety issues. The chronic need for dialysis (daily with peritoneal dialysis or three or four times per week with hemodialysis) confers long-term stress on the child and family. The child usually demonstrates poor growth and often suffers from body image disturbance. Frequent medical appointments and hospitalizations interfere with the child's scholastic achievements. Introduce the child to other children with CKD or ESRD (this often happens anyway at the hemodialysis centre).

TABLE 42.2 MEDICATIONS AND SUPPLEMENTS COMMONLY USED TO TREAT CKD AND ESRD COMPLICATIONS

Medication or Supplement	Purpose
Vitamin D and calcium	Correct hypocalcemia and hyperphosphatemia
Ferrous sulphate	Treat anemia
Bicitra or sodium bicarbonate tablets	Correct acidosis
Multivitamin	Augment nutritional status
Erythropoietin injections	Stimulate red blood cell growth
Growth hormone injections	Stimulate growth in stature
Antihypertensive	Treat high blood pressure; prevent CKD progression

Adapted from: Klein, M. S. (2010). Kidney disease, chronic. In P. J. Allen, J. A. Vessey, & N. A. Schapiro (Eds.), *Primary care of the child with a chronic condition* (5th ed.). St. Louis, MO: Mosby.

Refer the family to a renal social worker to ensure that they are aware of financial and support resources available within the community. Branches of the Kidney Foundation of Canada provide financial aid for kidney patients. Many hospitals across Canada partner with their local Kidney Foundation branch in providing summer camps for children with kidney problems. Camp is an excellent way for children to demonstrate that they have mastered some of the loss-of-control issues related to their disease.

Several websites provide forums for children and teens with kidney failure or transplantation so they can learn about their disease, access resources, and/or communicate with other children. Visit http://thePoint.lww.com/Chow1e for direct links to the websites.

Dialysis and Transplantation

Peritoneal dialysis or hemodialysis is considered a bridge to transplantation for children with ESRD. Kidney transplantation is needed for the child to progress with growth and development.

Peritoneal Dialysis

Peritoneal dialysis uses the child's abdominal cavity as a semipermeable membrane to help remove excess fluid and waste products (Figs. 42.8 and 42.9). The parent or caregiver performs peritoneal dialysis at home after completing a training course. The process is completed either overnight with the use of a machine (automated continuous cyclic peritoneal dialysis) (Fig. 42.10) or in increments throughout the day for a total of 4 to 8 hours (continuous ambulatory peritoneal dialysis). Most Canadian children

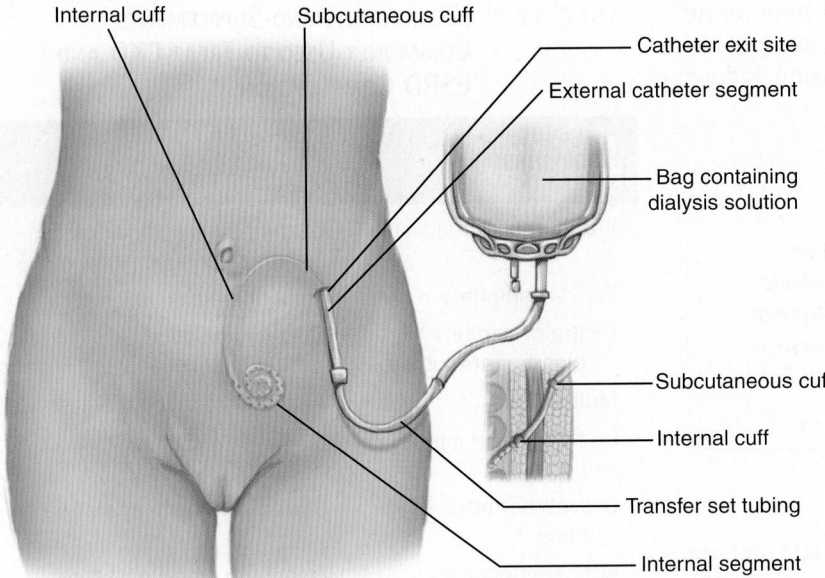

FIGURE 42.8 The peritoneal dialysis catheter is tunnelled under the skin into the peritoneal cavity.

who require peritoneal dialysis use automated peritoneal dialysis. Comparison Chart 42.1 compares these two methods of peritoneal dialysis.

The advantages of peritoneal dialysis over hemodialysis include improved growth as a result of more dietary freedom, increased independence in daily activities, and a steadier state of electrolyte balance. However, the risk for infection (peritonitis and sepsis) is a continual concern with peritoneal dialysis (Klein, 2010). Dialysate exchange protocols, care of the catheter in the abdomen, and dressing changes must all be performed using sterile technique to avoid introducing microorganisms into the peritoneal

Manual Ambulatory Peritoneal Dialysis

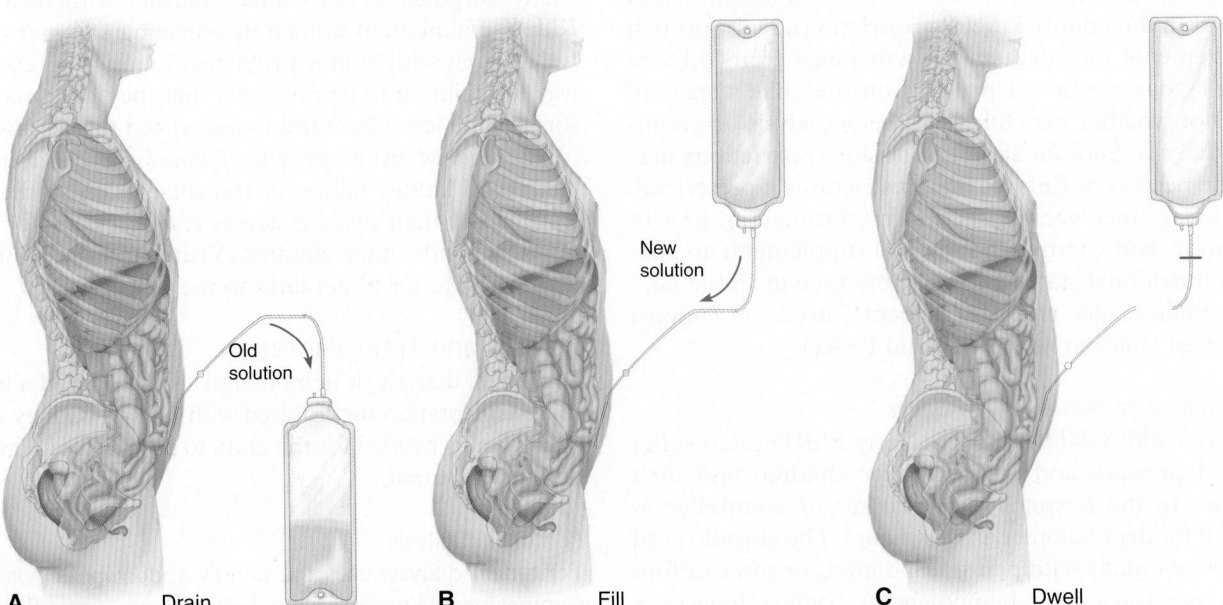

FIGURE 42.9 A cycle of manual ambulatory peritoneal dialysis includes drain, fill, and dwell phases. (**A**) During the "drain" phase, dialysis effluent is drained from the peritoneal cavity by gravity. Effluent contains the waste products and excess fluid (called ultrafiltration). After draining, the dialysis bag is weighed or the effluent volume is measured to determine the amount of ultrafiltration. (**B**) During the "fill" phase, dialysate fluid is instilled into the peritoneal cavity. (**C**) During the "dwell" phase, the child is disconnected from the bag and a sterile cap is placed on the catheter, freeing the child to pursue normal activities until the next cycle is initiated.

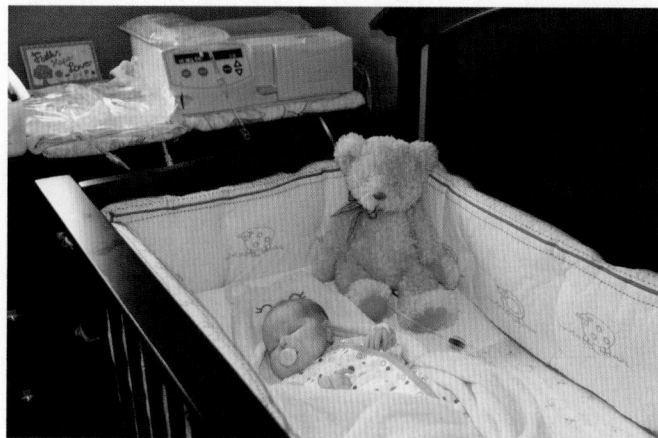

FIGURE 42.10 Automated continuous cyclic peritoneal dialysis.

BOX 42.2 **Risks Associated with Peritoneal Dialysis**

• Hypertension and other cardiac complications
• Seizures
• Obstructed or malpositioned catheter
• Dialysate leakage
• Hyperglycemia
• Increased triglyceride levels
• Increased protein loss
• Parental stress and burnout related to repetitive nature of daily intervention
• Constipation
• Infection (exit site, tunnel, or peritonitis)

cavity. Box 42.2 lists additional risks associated with peritoneal dialysis.

Hemodialysis

Hemodialysis removes toxins and excess fluid from the blood by pumping the child's blood through a hemodialysis machine and then reinfusing the blood into the arteriovenous fistula or graft. Children whose vessels are too small for the creation of a fistula or graft will be dialyzed via a central venous catheter. Needles to remove and reinfuse the blood are inserted into an arteriovenous fistula or graft, usually located in the child's arm (Fig. 42.11).

Hemodialysis frees the parent from the need to perform daily dialysis, but the procedure, which takes 3 to 6 hours, must be done two to four times per week (usually three) at a pediatric hemodialysis centre (Fig. 42.12). This requires time away from school and other activities for the child and from work and other family responsibilities for the parent. Since hemodialysis is usually performed only every other day, larger amounts of waste products build up in the child's blood (uremia), placing the child at higher risk for seizures. The access site may become infected, and occlusion is also possible. The child must follow a stricter diet between hemodialysis treatments, though dietary restrictions are usually lifted while the child is actually undergoing the treatment.

Nursing Assessment

Refer to the section on nursing assessment of the child with CKD/ESRD, as it is similar to assessment of the child undergoing dialysis. Assess for alterations in blood

COMPARISON CHART 42.1 METHODS OF PERITONEAL DIALYSIS

	Continuous Ambulatory Peritoneal Dialysis (CAPD)	Automated Continuous Cyclic Peritoneal Dialysis (CCPD)
When performed	Throughout the day, with exchanges every 3–6 h. Fluid is usually allowed to dwell overnight to allow child to sleep.	Usually overnight while child is sleeping
Method	Manual instillation and draining and changing of dialysate bags with each exchange	Automated via CCPD machine; bags and tubing are attached when started, then disconnected in the morning
Dwell time (based on child's peritoneal membrane characteristics; i.e., how quickly waste and water are removed)	3–6 h	Usually 30 min to 1 h
Mobility	Allows for mobility and permits child to participate in activities between exchanges	Child is confined to bed during the night while CCPD is ongoing but completely mobile while off CCPD during the day.

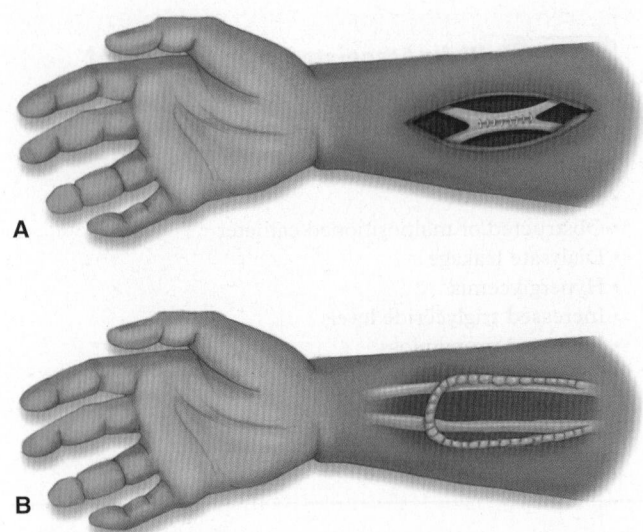

FIGURE 42.11 (**A**) Arteriovenous fistula. (**B**) Arteriovenous graft.

pressure and laboratory values following dialysis. Monitor for signs and symptoms of infection.

Assess the child receiving peritoneal dialysis for toleration of the fluid volume instilled within the peritoneum. The abdomen will remain distended while the fluid is indwelling and will be significantly flatter when the fluid is drained. Assess the Tenckhoff catheter exit and tunnel site for signs of infection. Monitor the child's temperature. Inspect the dialysate effluent for fibrin or cloudiness, which may indicate infection. Weigh the child daily (in the drain phase if on peritoneal dialysis).

For the child who receives hemodialysis, assess the arteriovenous fistula or graft site with each set of vital signs. Auscultate the site for the presence of a bruit and palpate for the presence of a thrill. Notify the physician immediately if either is absent.

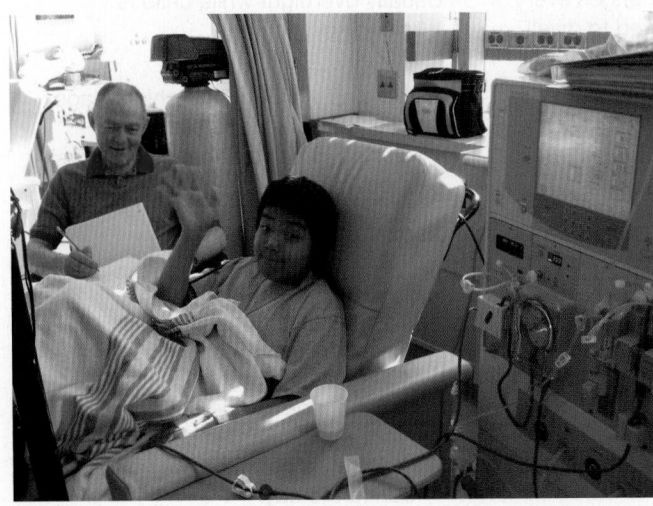

FIGURE 42.12 Pediatric hemodialysis.

▶ *Take* NOTE!

Avoid taking blood pressure, performing venipuncture, or using a tourniquet in the extremity with the arteriovenous fistula or graft: these procedures may cause occlusion and subsequent malfunction of the fistula or graft. Teach parents and children to inform all health care providers they come in contact with about the presence of the fistula or graft.

Nursing Management

Both peritoneal dialysis and hemodialysis are performed by specially trained and certified nurses. The general pediatric nurse's role is related to the ongoing care of the child. The child undergoing peritoneal dialysis usually is allowed a more liberal diet and intake of fluid than the child undergoing hemodialysis. Peritoneal dialysis removes waste and excess fluids on a daily basis, whereas hemodialysis occurs about every other day. Most routine medications are withheld on the morning that hemodialysis is scheduled, since they would be filtered out through the dialysis process anyway. Administer these medications as soon as the child returns from the dialysis unit.

Kidney Transplantation

Kidney transplantation is the optimal treatment for CKD/ESRD and offers the best opportunity for the child to live a normal life. Where possible, transplantation prior to the initiation of renal supportive therapy is the goal for children. Vigilant medication administration is necessary after the transplant to prevent organ rejection. The child may achieve 40% to 80% kidney function with the transplant and demonstrate improved growth, enhanced cognitive development, and improved psychosocial development and quality of life (Milliner, 2004).

Kidneys are obtained from a deceased donor (DD; a patient declared brain-dead who had previously given consent to organ donation) or from a live donor (LD) who may or may not be a relative. The transplanted kidney must match the child's blood type and the child's human leukocyte antigens (HLAs). The DD or LD kidney is implanted surgically in the abdomen and the blood vessels are anastomosed to the aorta and superior vena cava.

Generally, LD transplants have a lower rejection rate compared with DD transplants (Klein & Martin, 2010). LD kidney donation and subsequent transplantation can be planned ahead and scheduled in advance. In contrast, DD kidneys become available suddenly, leaving less time for preoperative preparation. For either type, last-minute blood tissue typing (HLA matching) is required before the final decision is made to move forward with transplantation.

Nursing Assessment

A thorough physical assessment is warranted for any kidney transplant patient, whether in the initial postoperative period, at a clinic visit, or when admitted to the hospital to rule out transplant rejection. Note recent health history, medications and their doses, and any symptoms the child has been having. In the initial postoperative period, assess the incision for redness, edema, or drainage; if any of these signs of infection or rejection occur, notify the transplant surgeon and nephrologist immediately. Monitor blood pressure and other vital signs closely. Document resolution of edema. Record intake and output accurately. Assess for signs and symptoms of transplant rejection such as malaise, fever, unexplained weight gain, or pain over the transplant area.

Nursing Management

Postoperative care focuses on preventing rejection, monitoring kidney function, maintaining fluid and electrolyte balance, and educating the child and family.

Preventing Rejection and Promoting Kidney Function

Administer immunosuppressants accurately and in a timely fashion. Obtain and monitor serum levels of these medications per protocol. Immediately report significant alterations in vital signs or edema at the surgical site, as they may indicate transplant rejection. Maintain strict documentation of intake and output. Once adequate urine output is established, intake is usually liberalized.

Educating the Child and Family

Develop a schedule to cluster care so that the child may receive the rest needed for recovery despite the many and frequent assessments and interventions. With the family, develop a medication schedule that will be compatible with the family's life at home as well as the restrictions related to some medications. Begin teaching with the family as soon as the child's condition is stable. Accurate medication administration and home monitoring are

necessary to prevent rejection. Immunosuppressants are taken on a regular schedule (every 8 to 12 hours) in order to maintain consistent blood levels. The child may return to school usually within 6 to 8 weeks after discharge from the hospital, but the family will need to communicate closely with the school nurse about the child's immunosuppressed status.

Reproductive Organ Disorders

A number of disorders may occur within the female or male genitalia and internal reproductive organs in children. These problems may be structural, infectious, or related to menstruation (in females).

Female Disorders

Disorders of the female reproductive organs that occur in children and adolescents include structural disorders, infectious disorders, and menstrual disorders.

Labial Adhesions

Labial adhesion or labial fusion is partial or complete adherence of the labia minora (Fig. 42.13). UTI may result from urinary stasis behind the labia; if the adhesions are left untreated, the vaginal orifice may become inaccessible, presenting difficulty with sexual intercourse in the future.

Nursing Assessment

Younger girls (3 months to 4 years of age) are at higher risk for adhesions (Nepple, Cooper, & Alagiri, 2011). Assess the history for dysuria or urinary frequency. Inspect the genitalia for fusion or adherence of the labia minora.

Nursing Management

Administer topical estrogen cream as prescribed, usually once or twice daily. Teach the parents to continue cream application until the labia separate. Encourage use of

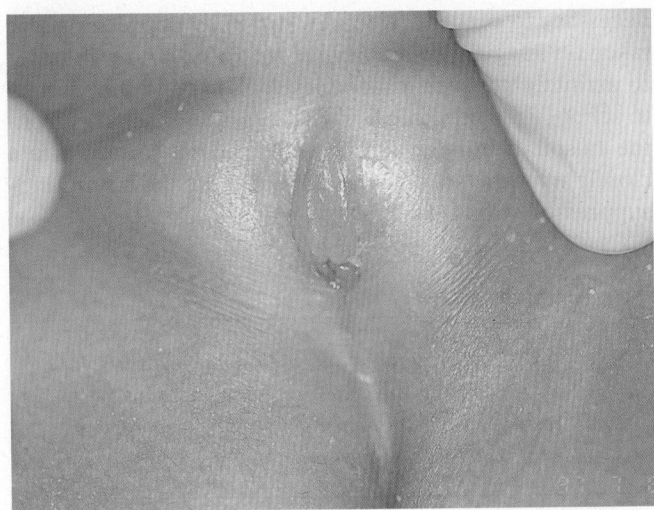

FIGURE 42.13 Labial adhesions. Note fusion of the upper portion of the labia minora. Copyrighted 2011. UBM Medica LLC. 82486:1111JM

petroleum jelly daily for 1 month following labial separation to prevent recurrence of adhesion.

Vulvovaginitis

Vulvovaginitis is inflammation of the vulva and vagina. Inflammation may occur as a result of bacterial or yeast overgrowth or from chemical factors such as bubble bath, soaps, or perfumes found in personal care products. Poor hygiene may also cause vulvovaginitis. Tight clothing may cause a heat rash in the perineal area. Persistent scratching of the irritated area may result in the complication of superficial skin infection.

Nursing Assessment

Elicit a description of the present illness and chief complaint. Common signs and symptoms reported during the health history may include itching or burning in the perineal area. Explore the patient's current and past medical history for risk factors, which may include:

- Young age (toilet-trained preschooler)
- Poor hygiene
- Sexual activity
- Immune disorders
- Diabetes mellitus

Inspect the perineum for redness, edema, irritation, rash, or vaginal discharge (note colour, consistency, and odour).

Nursing Management

Teach appropriate hygiene (daily and toileting). Girls (or their parents) should wash the genital area thoroughly on a daily basis with mild soap and water. Rinse the area well. Encourage girls to wipe after urinating and to wipe in a front-to-back motion after bowel movements. The girl should wear cotton underwear and should change it at least once a day. Administer topical or oral medications as ordered. Table 42.3 lists treatments related to specific types of vulvovaginitis.

Pelvic Inflammatory Disease

Pelvic inflammatory disease (PID) is an inflammation of the upper female genital tract and nearby structures. The fallopian tubes, ovaries, or peritoneum may be involved, and endometriosis may also be present. PID results from bacterial invasion through the cervix and vagina, ascending into the uterus and fallopian tubes. The most common causes of PID are *Chlamydia trachomatis* and *Neisseria gonorrhoeae*, although other bacteria and normal vaginal flora may be implicated. PID may result in fever, abdominal pain, dyspareunia (pain with intercourse), **dysmenorrhea**, and abnormal uterine bleeding. Long-term

TABLE 42.3 VULVOVAGINITIS: TYPES AND TREATMENTS

Cause	Assessment Findings	Treatment
Unhygienic practices	Irritation of labia and vaginal opening May have foul brownish-green discharge if infected with bacteria from rectum	Good hygiene Sometimes a mild anti-inflammatory cream is prescribed. Assess for signs and symptoms of UTI, which may occur as a complication.
Candida albicans	Red bumpy perineal rash in infants White cottage-cheese–like discharge Intense itching	Antifungal cream or vaginal suppository Prevent by ingesting probiotics (found in yogurt and kefir) daily and supplementing with a probiotic such as Lactinex when taking antibiotics.
Bordetella, Gardnerella	Thin grey vaginal discharge with fishy odour	Flagyl (metronidazole) orally
Trichomonas vaginalis	Foul yellow-grey or green vaginal discharge	Flagyl (metronidazole) orally. Sexually transmitted, so can be prevented with the use of condoms.

Adapted from: Neinstein, L. S., Gordon, C. M., Katzman, D. K., Rosen, D. S., & Woods, E. R. (2009). *Handbook of adolescent health care.* Philadelphia: Lippincott Williams & Wilkins.

complications include chronic pelvic pain, ectopic pregnancy, and infertility related to scarring.

Nursing Assessment

For a full description of the assessment phase of the nursing process, refer to page 1427.

When discussing any problem related to the reproductive organs or menstruation with the pre-teen or teen, it is necessary to discuss sexuality. The girl may be reluctant to share this information with the nurse. Approaches to discussing sexuality with the adolescent that may increase the likelihood of obtaining a truthful history include the following:

- Discuss the girl's general health, menarche, and menstrual cycle first, and then work toward discussing sexual behaviour.
- Start with questions about the girl's friends and social life, moving the conversation toward sexual behaviour.
- Always discuss sexual behaviour one-on-one with the adolescent (without the parent present), and then ask the adolescent's permission to discuss concerns with the parent. If the adolescent does not consent to parental involvement, then confidentiality must be maintained.

Assessment findings pertinent to PID are discussed below.

Health History

Elicit a description of the present illness and chief complaint. Common signs and symptoms reported during the health history might include:

- Abdominal pain (ranging from mild to severe)
- Prolonged or increased menstrual bleeding
- Dysmenorrhea
- Dysuria
- Painful sexual intercourse (dyspareunia)
- Nausea
- Vomiting

Explore the girl's current and past medical health history for risk factors such as:

- Multiple sexual partners
- Lack of consistent condom use
- Lack of contraceptive use
- History of prior sexually transmitted infection
- Douching
- Prostitution
- Alcohol or drug use (particularly if associated with sexual activity)

Physical Examination

Inspect for fever (usually over 38.3°C) or vaginal discharge. Palpate the abdomen, noting tenderness over the uterus or ovaries. An elevated C-reactive protein level and an elevated erythrocyte sedimentation rate indicate

---

TEACHING GUIDELINE 42.2

Preventing Pelvic Inflammatory Disease

- Insist that sexual partners use condoms.
- Do not use a vaginal douche routinely as this may lead to bacterial overgrowth.
- Get screened regularly for sexually transmitted infections.
- Make sure that each sexual partner also receives antibiotic treatment.

---

an inflammatory process. Cervical culture reveals the causative bacterial organism.

Nursing Management

PID is often treated in the out-patient setting with intramuscular or oral antibiotic regimens. If the adolescent is severely ill or has a very high fever or protracted vomiting, then she may be hospitalized. Antibiotics are needed to eradicate the infection. Maintain hydration via intravenous fluids if necessary and administer analgesics as needed for pain. Semi-Fowler's positioning promotes pelvic drainage. A key element to treatment of PID is education to prevent recurrence (Teaching Guideline 42.2).

Menstrual Disorders

Menstruation begins in most girls about 2 years after breast development starts, around the time of Tanner stage 4, breast and pubic hair development and on average at around 12 to 13 years of age. Menstruation has many effects on girls and women, including emotional and self-image issues. Adolescents may suffer from a variety of menstrual disorders, including premenstrual syndrome and several different disorders related to menstrual bleeding and cramping (Table 42.4).

In healthy girls, the heaviness of menstrual flow varies. Periods may occur irregularly for up to 2 years after menarche (the onset of menstruation), but after that the regular menstrual cycle should be established. The normal cycle can vary from 21 to 45 days in length, with the period usually lasting 2 to 7 days. Girls who take oral contraceptives usually have very regular 28-day cycles, with lighter bleeding than those who do not take contraceptives.

Pathophysiology

Premenstrual syndrome is a collection of physical and/or affective symptoms that occur predictably during the luteal phase of the menstrual cycle. Symptoms begin 5 to 10 days before each period and usually resolve by the time the period begins or shortly thereafter (the timing may vary by adolescent but is consistent with each cycle). Disorders of bleeding and cramping are summarized in Table 42.4.

TABLE 42.4 COMMON MENSTRUAL DISORDERS

Disorder	Definition	Cause
Primary amenorrhea	Lack of menarche within 2 years of reaching Tanner stage 4 breast development, or by 16 years of age	• Imperforate hymen • Agenesis of vulva or vagina • Turner syndrome • Chronic illness associated with delayed pubertal development (e.g., cystic fibrosis, Crohn's disease, sickle-cell disease, CKD) • Suppressed levels of follicle-stimulating hormone (FSH) or luteinizing hormone (LH), as occurs with eating disorders, intense athletics, severe psychological stress, or extreme weight loss
Secondary amenorrhea	Absence of menses for 6 months in the girl who has been menstruating regularly	• Pregnancy (most common cause) • Anovulation (resulting from lack of hypothalamic–pituitary axis maturity) • Polycystic ovary syndrome (PCOS) • Suppressed levels of FSH or LH, as occurs with eating disorders, intense athletics, severe psychological stress, or extreme weight loss
Mittelschmerz	Abdominal pain, usually unilateral, that varies from a few sharp cramps to several hours of crampy pain	Usually occurs midway through the menstrual cycle, around the time of ovulation; is thought to be a result of egg release from the ovary
Dysmenorrhea	Pain associated with menstruation, usually abdominal cramps ranging from mild to severe	• Prostaglandin release is responsible for the smooth muscle contraction of the uterus during menstruation (primary) • Fibroids, adenomyosis, endometriosis, scar tissue (secondary)
Menorrhagia	Excessive menstrual bleeding	• Anovulatory cycles • Endometriosis • Blood dyscrasias, bleeding disorders, or use of anticoagulants • Reproductive system neoplasms
Metrorrhagia	Bleeding between menstrual periods	• Improper use of oral contraceptives • Intrauterine device • Endometriosis • Reproductive system neoplasms • Miscarriage or ectopic pregnancy

Adapted from: Sass, A. E., & Kaplan, D. W. (2011). Adolescence. In W. W. Hay, M. J. Levin, J. M. Sondheimer, & R. R. Deterding (Eds.), *Current pediatric diagnosis and treatment* (20th ed.). New York: McGraw-Hill.

Nursing Assessment

For a full description of the assessment phase of the nursing process, refer to page 1427. When girls present for evaluation of menstrual concerns, a focused yet thorough nursing assessment is necessary.

Health History

Obtain a thorough and accurate menstrual history; determine age at menarche, usual length of menstrual period, usual menstrual flow, number of pads or tampons used per day, date of last normal menstrual period, premenstrual symptoms, and any pain related to the menstrual cycle. Obtain a description of the pain, what relief mea-

sures have been tried, and what the success of those measures has been. If pain occurs with menstrual periods, assess for associated symptoms such as nausea, vomiting, dizziness, or loose stools. Explore the history for symptoms of bloating, water retention, weight gain, headache, muscle aches, abdominal pain, food cravings, or breast tenderness. Determine the extent of emotional symptoms related to the menstrual cycle, such as anxiety, insomnia, mood swings, tension, crying spells, or irritability. Note the timing of these symptoms within the menstrual cycle.

Note past medical history, including any chronic illnesses and family history of gynecologic concerns. Elicit a sexual behaviour history, including the type of sexual activity (oral, anal, or vaginal), number and gender of sexual partners, frequency and most recent sexual contact, history of molestation or sexual abuse, and use of contraceptives (noting type) and/or condoms.

Take a medication history, including prescription medications and contraceptives, and determine whether the girl uses anabolic steroids, tobacco, or marijuana, cocaine, or other illegal drugs.

Physical Examination

The physical assessment related to menstrual disorders includes inspection and observation, auscultation, and palpation. The bimanual pelvic examination and Pap smear are usually indicated only for more severe menstrual disorders and are usually performed by the physician or advanced practice nurse.

Inspect the breasts and pubic hair distribution to determine Tanner stage. Observe the external genitalia for vaginal discharge, redness, or irritation. Note pallor or weight gain. Document presence and extent of clots in menstrual flow. Measure orthostatic blood pressure and orthostatic pulse; decreases with position change may occur in girls with anemia. Palpate the abdomen, noting distention or tenderness.

Laboratory and Diagnostic Tests

Common laboratory and diagnostic studies ordered for the assessment of menstrual disorders include:

- Complete blood count: to determine presence of anemia with **menorrhagia** or metrorrhagia
- Human chorionic gonadotropin: to assess for pregnancy with **amenorrhea**

Nursing Management

Nursing goals for the girl with a menstrual disorder focus on normalizing menstrual flow and restoring blood volume, providing comfort, and encouraging independence in self-care.

Normalizing Menstrual Flow and Restoring Blood Volume

For the girl with mild anemia related to menorrhagia, administer iron supplements as ordered. For moderate menorrhagia, oral contraceptives may also be prescribed, since altering hormone levels decreases menstrual flow. If the contraceptive contains a high dose of estrogen, the girl may experience nausea. Administer antiemetics as ordered and encourage the girl to eat small, frequent meals to alleviate nausea. Adolescents with severe anemia may require hospitalization and blood transfusion.

Providing Comfort

Provide a heating pad or warm compress to help alleviate menstrual cramps. Administer NSAIDs such as ibuprofen or naproxen to inhibit prostaglandin synthesis, which contributes to menstrual cramps. Advise girls that beginning NSAID therapy at the first sign of menstrual discomfort is the best way to minimize discomfort. If NSAIDs

are unsuccessful, oral contraceptives may be ordered; teach the girl appropriate use of oral contraceptives.

The adolescent experiencing premenstrual syndrome should keep a diary of her symptoms, their severity, and when they occur in the menstrual cycle. Like all adolescents, girls with premenstrual syndrome should eat a balanced diet that includes nutrient-rich foods so they can avoid hypoglycemia and associated mood swings. Encourage adolescent girls to participate in aerobic exercise three times a week to promote a sense of well-being, decrease fatigue, and reduce stress. Administer calcium (1,200 to 1,600 mg/day), magnesium (400 to 800 mg/day), and vitamin B6 (50 to 100 mg/day) as prescribed. In some studies, these nutrients have been shown to decrease the intensity of premenstrual symptoms (Moreno & Giesel, 2009). NSAIDs may be useful for painful physical symptoms, and spironolactone (Aldactone) may help reduce bloating and water retention. Herbs such as chasteberry or ginkgo may be recommended; though not found to be harmful, studies are inconclusive about their effectiveness (Dell, 2004). A recent research review proposes calcium (1,600 mg/day) and vitamin D (400 IU/day) supplementation in adolescents and women in an effort to prevent the development of premenstrual syndrome (Bertone-Johnson et al., 2005).

> ▶ *Take* NOTE!
>
> *Adolescents who experience more extensive emotional symptoms with premenstrual syndrome should be evaluated for premenstrual dysphoric disorder, as they may require anti-depressant therapy (Htay, Aung, Carrick, Papica, 2011).*

Encouraging Independence in Self-Care

Establishing a trusting relationship with the adolescent may make education about self-care more successful. Some girls have open relationships with their mothers and can discuss issues related to menses and sexuality with them, but many others cannot discuss such "embarrassing" issues with their mothers, and the nurse or other health care provider may be the only source of reliable information. Provide the adolescent with accurate information about menstruation and sexuality. Educate her about normal menstruation, the menstrual cycle, and the risk for pregnancy if sexual intercourse occurs (refer to Chapter 29 for information related to contraception). Refer girls to reliable websites if they are not comfortable with receiving information from the nurse; for a list of websites visit http://thePoint.lww.com/Chow1e. Encourage the girl to call or visit the office if she has additional questions.

Male Disorders

Male reproductive disorders include structural disorders and disorders caused by infection or inflammation. Circumcision will also be discussed in following page.

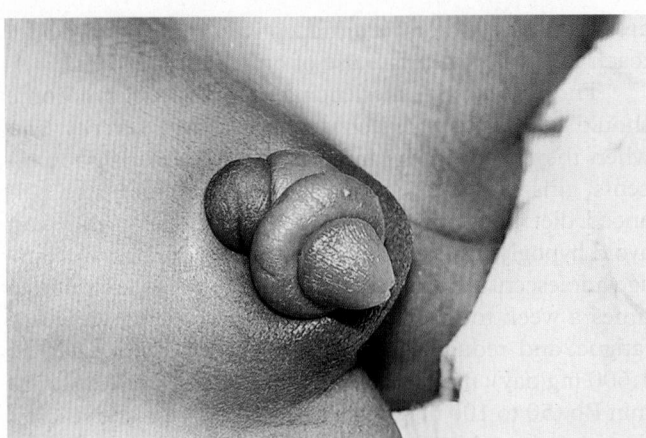

FIGURE 42.14 Paraphimosis: note the swollen prepuce. Copyrighted 2011. UBM Medica LLC. 82486:1111JM

Phimosis and Paraphimosis

In phimosis, the foreskin of the penis cannot be retracted. Although this is normal in the newborn, it can be pathologic later. Over time, the prepuce (foreskin) naturally becomes retractable. Local irritation, balanitis, or UTI may occur if urine is retained within the foreskin after voiding. Paraphimosis (Fig. 42.14) is a more serious disorder characterized by retraction of the phimotic prepuce, which causes a constricting band behind the glans of the penis and results in incarceration if left untreated.

Topical steroid cream applied twice a day for 1 month may be prescribed for phimosis. Paraphimosis requires reduction of the prepuce or a small dorsal incision to release the foreskin. Circumcision may be used to treat either condition.

Nursing Assessment

Elicit a description of the present illness and chief complaint. Common signs and symptoms reported during the health history might include:

- Irritation or bleeding from the opening of the prepuce (phimosis)
- Dysuria (phimosis)
- Pain (paraphimosis)
- Swollen penis (paraphimosis)

Determine the onset of symptoms and inspect the penis for irritation, erythema, edema, or discharge.

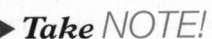

▶ *Take* NOTE!

A swollen, reddened penis (paraphimosis) is a medical emergency and can quickly result in necrosis of the tip of the penis if left untreated.

Nursing Management

Apply topical steroid medication as prescribed for phimosis, following gentle retraction to stretch the foreskin

back. Topical vitamin E cream may also help to soften the phimotic ring. When surgical intervention is necessary, provide routine postprocedural care and pain management (refer to the section on circumcision below). Teach the parents and uncircumcised boy proper hygiene, which will help to prevent phimosis and paraphimosis (Teaching Guideline 42.3).

Circumcision

Circumcision is the removal of the excess foreskin of the penis. Some newborn boys are circumcised shortly after birth before going home from the hospital. Some parents elect not to have their newborn boy circumcised at that time but may desire it later. Neonatal circumcision may be performed in the newborn nursery, hospital unit treatment room, or out-patient office. Circumcision is indicated later for the conditions of phimosis and paraphimosis. Circumcision done after the newborn period usually requires general anesthesia.

The benefits of circumcision include a decreased incidence of UTI, sexually transmitted diseases, acquired immune deficiency syndrome, and penile cancer, and in female partners a decreased occurrence of cervical cancer. Complications of circumcision include alterations in the urinary meatus, unintentional removal of excessive amounts of foreskin, or damage to the glans penis (American Academy of Pediatrics [AAP], 2005).

Whether to circumcise or not is a personal decision and often based on religious beliefs or social or cultural customs. The CPS (1996) does not recommend routine neonatal circumcision. Nurses should support and educate the parents in either case. Visit http://thePoint.lww.com/Chow1e for links to online information for families on circumcision.

Nursing Assessment

Prior to the procedure, assess for normal placement of the urinary meatus on the glans penis (in boys with hypospadias, circumcision should be delayed until evaluation by the pediatric urologist). After the circumcision, assess for redness, edema, or active bleeding. Note signs of infection, such as purulent drainage. Assess pain level.

Nursing Management

Nursing care of the boy undergoing circumcision focuses on managing pain, providing postprocedural care, and educating the parents.

Managing Pain

Whether circumcision is performed in the obstetric area of the hospital before newborn discharge or in the outpatient setting at a few days of age, pain management during the procedure must not be neglected. Advocate for appropriate pain management for the infant undergoing circumcision. The CPS follows the AAP recommendations for the use of a subcutaneous ring block with lidocaine or a dorsal nerve block to the penis. The AAP (2005) also recommends the use of EMLA (eutectic mixture of local anesthetic) cream topically to decrease pain during the circumcision. Playing calming music during the procedure may also help to soothe the infant, providing distraction. A sucrose-dipped pacifier may also be used as adjuvant therapy for pain management. To increase a sense of comfort during the procedure, restrain the infant in a padded circumcision chair with blankets covering the legs and upper body (Kraft, 2003). This allows the infant to be in a semi-upright position during the procedure while still allowing for a sterile procedural field. If a padded restraint chair is not available, provide atraumatic care by padding the circumcision board and covering the infant as previously described.

Providing Postprocedural Care

Usual care after circumcision depends on the type of appliance used (Gomco or Mogen clamp or Plastibell apparatus). Cleanse the penis with clear water for the first few days and avoid using alcohol-containing wipes. To avoid irritation to the penis, fasten diapers loosely. Notify the physician if excessive redness, active bleeding, or purulent discharge occurs. Assess for the first void following the procedure or, if performed in the out-patient setting, instruct parents to call the physician if the infant has not voided by 6 to 8 hours after the circumcision. Apply antibiotic ointment or petroleum jelly to the penile head with each diaper change as prescribed, based on the circumcision method used and the preference of the health care provider.

▶ **Take** NOTE!

If excess bleeding occurs after the circumcision, apply direct pressure and notify the health care provider immediately.

Educating the Parents

Instruct parents to give sponge baths until the circumcision is healed. Describe the normal granulation tissue that will be present during the healing process. Teach parents to apply ointment or petroleum jelly if indicated. Instruct the parents to call the health care provider if any of the following occur:

- The infant does not urinate within 6 to 8 hours after the procedure.
- Heavy bleeding occurs (more than small spots on the diaper or bleeding that requires direct pressure to stop it).
- There is purulent or serous drainage from the circumcised area.
- There is redness or swelling of the penile shaft.

▶ **Take** NOTE!

If the Plastibell is used, teach parents NOT to use petroleum jelly, as it may cause the ring to be dislodged. A yellowish crust may form that should be allowed to fall off on its own after several days.

Cryptorchidism

Cryptorchidism (also known as undescended testicles) occurs when one or both testicles do not descend into the scrotal sac. Ordinarily the testes, which in the fetus develop in the abdomen, make their descent into the scrotal sac during the seventh month of gestation. The cause for this failure to descend may be mechanical, hormonal, chromosomal, or enzymatic. The disorder may occur unilaterally or bilaterally. Up to 1% to 4% of term male infants and as many as 45% of all preterm male infants exhibit cryptorchidism (Ashley, Barthold, & Kolon, 2010).

Complications associated with cryptorchidism that is allowed to progress into the school-age years include sterility and an increased risk for testicular cancer in adolescence or the young adult years. Therapeutic management is surgical. An orchiopexy is performed to release the spermatic cord, and the testes are then pulled into the scrotum and tacked into place.

Nursing Assessment

Explore the health history for risk factors such as:

- Prematurity
- First-born child
- Cesarean birth
- Low birth weight
- Hypospadias

Palpate for the presence (or absence) of both testes in the scrotal sac.

▶ **Take** NOTE!

A retractile testis is one that may be brought into the scrotum, remains for a time, and then retracts backup the inguinal canal. This should not be confused with true cryptorchidism.

Nursing Management

If the testes are not descended by 6 months of age, the infant should be referred for surgical repair (Ashley et al., 2010). Postoperatively, observe the incision for signs of bleeding or infection.

Hydrocele and Varicocele

Hydrocele (fluid in the scrotal sac) is usually a benign and self-limiting disorder. It is usually noted early in infancy and often resolves spontaneously by 1 year of age. Varicocele (a venous varicosity along the spermatic cord) is often noted as a swelling of the scrotal sac. Varicocele is rare in boys before the onset of puberty (Robinson, Hampton, & Koo, 2010). Complications of varicocele include low sperm count or reduced sperm motility, which can result in infertility.

Nursing Assessment

Elicit a description of the present illness and chief complaint. The boy with hydrocele will have an enlarged scrotum that may decrease in size when he is lying down. Inspect the scrotum for a fluid-filled appearance.

The boy with varicocele will have a mass on one or both sides of the scrotum, bluish discolouration and may experience pain. Inspect the scrotum for masses; the spermatic vein feels worm-like on palpation.

Nursing Management

Both hydrocele and painless varicocele require watchful waiting, as these conditions will usually resolve spontaneously. If they do not resolve, or if the difference in testicular volume is marked in the boy with varicocele, refer the child to a urologist, as surgery may be indicated. Reassure parents that hydrocele is not associated with the development of infertility. Varicocele may lead to infertility if left untreated, so instruct parents to seek care if pain occurs or if there is a large difference in testicular size. Either condition may be surgically corrected on an outpatient basis. Provide routine postoperative care following either surgery.

Testicular Torsion

In testicular torsion, a testicle is abnormally attached to the scrotum and twisted. It requires immediate attention because ischemia can result if the torsion is left untreated, leading to infertility. Testicular torsion may occur at any age but most commonly occurs in boys of ages 12 to 18 years (Burns, Dunn, Brady, Starr, & Blosser, 2004).

Nursing Assessment

Elicit a description of the present illness and chief complaint. Signs and symptoms of testicular torsion include sudden, severe scrotal pain. Inspect the affected side for significant swelling, which may appear hemorrhagic or blue-black.

Nursing Management

Surgical correction is necessary immediately. Administer pain medication prior to surgery. Reassure the child and family that surgery will alleviate the problem and is performed to restore adequate blood flow to the testicle. After surgical repair, provide routine postoperative care.

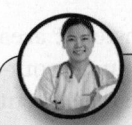

▶ *Take* NOTE!

Testicular torsion is considered a surgical emergency, as necrosis of the testis may occur and gangrene may set in.

Epididymitis

Epididymitis (inflammation of the epididymis) is caused by infection with bacteria. It is the most common cause of pain in the scrotum. It rarely occurs before puberty, but if it does it may occur as a result of a urethral or bladder infection related to a urogenital anomaly (Burns et al., 2004). Therapeutic management is directed toward eradicating the bacteria. If left untreated, a scrotal abscess, testicular infarction, or infertility may occur.

Nursing Assessment

Note history of painful swelling of the scrotum, which may be gradual or acute. If the boy is sexually active, explore history of sexual encounters prior to the onset of symptoms. Document history of dysuria or urethral discharge. Note fever, which may last from days to weeks. On inspection, note edema and erythema of the scrotum. Gently palpate the scrotum for a hardened and tender epididymis. Note urethral discharge if present. Palpate the inguinal lymph nodes for enlargement. Urinalysis may be positive for bacteria and white blood cells. The culture of urethral discharge may be positive for a sexually transmitted infection such as gonorrhea or chlamydia. The complete blood count may reveal an elevated white blood cell count.

Nursing Management

Encourage the boy to rest in bed with the scrotum elevated. Ice packs to the scrotum may help with pain relief. Administer pain medications such as NSAIDs or other analgesics as needed.

Administer antibiotics as prescribed. Educate the boy and his family to complete the entire course of antibiotics as prescribed to eradicate the infection. Advise the child and family to notify the physician if the condition is not improving or if the pain and swelling worsen.

Visit http://thePoint.lww.com/Chow1e for a direct link to printable pamphlets on pediatric urological issues from the Canadian Urological Association.

■■■ Key Concepts

- The urinary tract is immature in infants and young children, with a slower GFR and a decreased ability to concentrate urine and reabsorb amino acids compared with the adult.

- In children, CKD is most often the result of congenital structural defects or infectious, inflammatory, or immune processes that damage the kidney, whereas in adults it usually results from hypertension or diabetes.

- The short length of the urethra in girls and its proximity to the vagina and anus place the young girl at higher risk for the development of UTIs compared with the adult.

- The expected urine output in the infant and child is 0.5 to 2 mL/kg/hour.

- Though present at birth, the reproductive organs do not reach functional maturity until puberty.

- Obtaining a sterile urine specimen is necessary for accurate urine culture results.

- A urinary catheter must be inserted just prior to the VCUG.

- Close monitoring of serum blood counts and electrolytes is a critical component of nursing care related to kidney disorders.

- Certain congenital urologic anomalies may require multiple surgeries as well as urinary diversion; urine drains through a stoma on the abdominal wall that is either pouched or catheterized.

- The treatment for nocturnal enuresis may include the use of DDAVP nasal spray and/or an enuresis alarm to train the child to awaken to the sensation of a filling bladder.

- Nephrotic syndrome results in significant proteinuria and edema.

- Acute glomerulonephritis most often follows a group A streptococcal infection and commonly results in hematuria, proteinuria, and hypertension.

- The most common cause of HUS is infection with *E. coli* 0157:H7. It can be prevented by adequately cooking ground meat, washing hands and produce well, and making sure that an appropriate chemical balance is maintained in public recreational water sources such as swimming pools and water parks.

- Corticosteroids can cause GI upset. If used on a long-term basis, they should be tapered rather than discontinued abruptly to avoid adrenal crisis.

- Children taking immunosuppressants for nephrotic syndrome or for kidney transplantation are at increased risk for the development of overwhelming infection.

- Peritoneal dialysis may be accomplished at home by the parent. Close attention to sterile technique is needed.

- Hemodialysis requires central venous access or an arteriovenous fistula or graft that is accessed with needles three or four times per week at a hemodialysis centre. This is disruptive to the academic, social, and personal lives of the patient and family.

- Kidney transplantation is the best option for the treatment of end-stage kidney disease in children, but vigilant medication administration is needed to prevent organ rejection.

- Children with CKD experience anemia, poor growth, depression, anxiety, and low self-esteem.

- The diet for a child with a renal disorder must be individualized according to prescribed sodium, fluid, and/or protein restrictions.

- Postoperative care for the child undergoing urologic surgery includes pain management, avoidance or treatment of bladder spasms, and monitoring of urine output.

REFERENCES

Alper, B. S., & Curry, S. H. (2005). Urinary tract infection in children. *American Family Physician, 72*(12), 2483–2488.

American Academy of Pediatrics. (2005). *Circumcision policy statement.* Retrieved May 29, 2011 from http://aappolicy.aappublications.org/cgi/content/full/pediatrics%3b103/3/686

Ashley, R. A., Barthold, J. S., & Kolon, T. F. (2010). Cryptorchidism: Pathogenesis, diagnosis, treatment and prognosis. *Urological Clinics of North America, 37*, 183–193.

Auron, A., & Brophy, P. D. (2010). Pediatric renal supportive therapies: The changing face of pediatric renal replacement approaches. *Current Opinion in Pediatrics, 22*, 183–188.

Austin, J. C., & Cooper, C. S. (2010). Vesicoureteral reflux: Who benefits from correction. *Urological Clinics of North America, 37*, 243–252.

Bauer, R., & Kogan, B. A. (2008). New developments in the diagnosis and management of pediatric UTIs. *Urology Clinics of North America, 35*(1), 47–58.

Behrman, A. J., & Howarth, M. (2011). *Latex allergy.* Retrieved December 10, 2011 from http://emedicine.medscape.com/article/756632-overview#a0101

Bertone-Johnson, E. R., Hankinson, S. E., Bendich, A., Johnson, S. R., Willett, W. C., & Manson, J. E. (2005). Calcium and vitamin D intake and risk of incident premenstrual syndrome. *Archives of Internal Medicine, 165*, 1246–1252.

Bhimma, R. (2011). *Acute poststreptococcal glomerulonephritis.* Retrieved December 10, 2011 from http://emedicine.medscape.com/article/980685-overview

Browne, N. T., Flanigan, L. M., McComiskey, C. A., & Pieper, P. (2007). *Nursing care of the pediatric surgical patient.* Sudbury, MA: Jones Bartlett Publishers.

Burns, C. E., Dunn, A. M., Brady, M. A., Starr, N. B., & Blosser, C. (2004). *Pediatric primary care: A handbook for nurse practitioners* (3rd ed.). Philadelphia: Saunders.

Canadian Pediatric Society. (1996, review in progress 2009). Neonatal circumcision revisited. *Paediatrics & Child Health, 154*(6), 769–780. Retrieved December 10, 2011 from http://www.cps.ca/english/statements/fn/fn96-01.htm

Canadian Pediatric Society. (2004). PID note: Bag urine specimens still not appropriate in diagnosing urinary tract infections in infants. *Paediatrics & Child Health, 9*(6), 377–378. Retrieved December 10, 2011 from http://www.cps.ca/english/statements/ID/PIDNoteUTI.htm

Canadian Pediatric Society. (2005, reaffirmed February 2011). Management of primary nocturnal enuresis. *Paediatrics & Child Health, 10* (10), 611–614. Retrieved December 10, 2011 from http://www.cps.ca/english/statements/cp/cp05-02.htm

Carr, M. C., & Kim, S. S. (2010). Prenatal management of urogenital disorders. *Urological Clinics of North America, 37*, 149–158.

Children's Healthcare of Atlanta. (2004). *Double diapering.* Atlanta, GA: Author.

Clark, C. J., Kennedy, W. A., & Shortliffe, L. D. (2010). Urinary tract infection in children: When to worry. *Urological Clinics of North America, 37*, 229–241.

Cox, E. (2009). Managing childhood enuresis: An overview. *British Journal of School Nursing, 4*(9), 434–438.

Daniels, J., & DiCenso, A. (2003). Review: Antibiotic treatment for 2–14 days reduces treatment failure in children with urinary tract infection. *Evidence-Based Nursing, 6*, 15. Retrieved April 20, 2011 from http://ebn.bmjjournals.com/cgi/reprint/6/1/15

Dell, D. (2004). Premenstrual syndrome, premenstrual dysphoric disorder, and premenstrual exacerbation of another disorder. *Clinical Obstetrics and Gynecology, 47*(3), 568–575.

Doré-Bergeron, M.-J., Gauthier, M., Chevalier, I., McManus, B., Tapiero, B., & Lebrun, S. (2009). Urinary tract infections in 1- to 3-month-old infants: Ambulatory treatment with intravenous antibiotics. *Pediatrics, 124*(1), 16–24.

Ellis, J. A., Martelli, B., LaMontagne, C., & Splinter, W. (2007). Evaluation of a continuous epidural analgesia program for postoperative pain in children. *Pain Management Nursing, 8*(4), 146–155.

Ellsworth, P., & Caldamone, A. (2008). Pediatric voiding dysfunction: Current evaluation and management. *Urologic Nursing, 28*(4), 249.

Ellsworth, P., Cendron, M., & McCullough, M. (2000). Surgical management of vesicoureteral reflux. *AORN Journal, 71*(3), 498–513.

Etoubleau, C., Reveret, M., Brouet, D., et al. (2009). Moving from bag to catheter for urine collection in non-toilet-trained children suspected of having urinary tract infection: A paired comparison of urine cultures. *Journal of Pediatrics, 154*(6), 803–806.

Flynn, J. T., & Tullus, K. (2009). Severe hypertension in children and adolescents: Pathophysiology and treatment. *Pediatric Nephrology, 24*(6), 1101–1112.

Htay, T. T., Aung, K., Carrick, J., Papica, R., II (2011). *Premenstrual dysphoric disorder.* Retrieved December 10, 2011 from http://www.emedicine.com/med/topic3357.htm

Jalanko, H. (2009). Congenital nephrotic syndrome. *Pediatric nephrology, 24*(11), 2121–2128.

Klein, M. S. (2010). Kidney disease, chronic. In P. J. Allen, J. A. Vessey, & N. A. Schapiro (Eds.), *Primary care of the child with a chronic condition* (5th ed.). St. Louis, MO: Mosby.

Klein, M. S., & Martin, K. (2010). Organ transplantation. In P. J. Allen, J. A. Vessey, & N. A. Schapiro (Eds.), *Primary care of the child with a chronic condition* (5th ed.). St. Louis, MO: Mosby.

Kraft, N. L. (2003). A pictorial and video guide to circumcision without pain. *Advances in Neonatal Care, 3*(2), 50–64.

Kraft, K. H., Shulka, A. R., & Canning, K. A. (2010). Hypospadias. *Urological Clinics of North America, 37*, 167–181.

Lane, J. C. (2011). *Pediatric nephrotic syndrome.* Retrieved December 10, 2011 from http://emedicine.medscape.com/article/982920-overview

Lum, G. M. (2011). Kidney & urinary tract. In W. W. Hay, M. J. Levin, J. M. Sondheimer, & R. R. Deterding (Eds.), *Current pediatric diagnosis and treatment* (20th ed.). New York: McGraw-Hill.

Martin, A., & Volkmar, F. R. (2007). *Lewis's child and adolescent psychiatry* (4th ed.). Philadelphia: Lippincott Williams & Wilkins.

McLaine, P. N., Rowe, P. C., & Orrbine, E. (2009) Experiences with HUS in Canada: What have we learned about childhood HUS in Canada? *Kidney International, 75*, S25–S28.

Milliner, D. S. (2004). Pediatric renal-replacement therapy: Coming of age. *New England Journal of Medicine, 350*(26), 2637.

Moreno, M. A., & Giesel, A. E. (2009). *Premenstrual syndrome.* Retrieved May 29, 2011 from http://emedicine.medscape.com/article/953696-overview

Neinstein, L. S., Gordon, C. M., Katzman, D. K., Rosen, D. S., & Woods, E. R. (2009). *Handbook of adolescent health care.* Philadelphia: Lippincott Williams & Wilkins.

Nelson, C. P., & Koo, H. P. (2011). *Pediatric vesicoureteral reflux.* Retrieved October 9, 2011, from http://emedicine.medscape.com/article/1016439-overview

Nepple, K. G., Cooper, C. S., & Alagiri, M. (2011). *Labial adhesions.* Retrieved May 29, 2011 from http://emedicine.medscape.com/article/953412-overview

Pagana, K. D., & Pagana, T. J. (2010). *Mosby's manual of diagnostic and laboratory tests* (4th ed.). St. Louis, MO: Mosby.

Phillips, T. M., & Gearhart, J. P. (2009). Surgery illustrated – Surgical atlas primary closure of bladder exstrophy. *BJU International, 104*(9), 1308–1322.

Psooy, K., & Pike, J. (2008). Investigation and management of antenatally detected hydronephrosis. Retrieved June 14, 2010 from http://www.ncbi.nlm.nih.gov/pmc/articles/PMC2645869/

Robinson, S. P., Hampton, L. J., & Koo, H. P. (2010). Treatment strategy for the adolescent varicocele. *Urological Clinics of North America, 37*, 269–278.

Roth, K. S., Koo, H. P., Spottswood, S. E., & Chan, J. C. M. (2002). Obstructive uropathy: An important cause of chronic renal failure in children. *Clinical Pediatrics, 41*, 309–314.

Routh, J. C., Inman, B. A., & Reinberg, Y. (2010). Dextranomer/hyaluronic acid for pediatric vesicoureteral reflux: Systematic review. *Pediatrics, 125*(5), 1010–1019.

Sass, A. E., & Kaplan, D. W. (2011). Adolescence. In W. W. Hay, M. J. Levin, J. M. Sondheimer, & R. R. Deterding (Eds.), *Current pediatric diagnosis and treatment* (20th ed.). New York: McGraw-Hill.

Schast, A. P., & Reiner, W. G. (2010). Pediatric psychology in genitourinary anomalies. *Urological Clinics of North America, 37*, 299–305.

Schlager, T. A. (2001). Urinary tract infections in children younger than 5 years of age: Epidemiology, diagnosis, treatment, outcomes and prevention. *Paediatric Drugs, 3*(3), 219–227.

Shah, G., & Upadhyay, J. (2005). Controversies in the diagnosis and management of urinary tract infections in children. *Paediatric Drugs, 7* (6), 339–346.

Staples, A., & Wong, C. (2010). Risk factors for progression of chronic kidney disease. *Current Opinion in Pediatrics, 22*, 161–169.

Shaikh, N., Morone, N. E., Bost, J. E., & Farrell, M. H. (2008). Prevalence of urinary tract infection in childhood: A meta-analysis. *Pediatric Infectious Disease Journal, 4*, 302–308.

Solomon, D. H. (2011). *Patient information: Nonsteroidal anti-inflammatory drugs (NSAIDs).* Retrieved December 10, 2011 from http://www.uptodate.com/contents/patient-information-nonsteroidal-antiinflammatory-drugs-nsaids

Taketokmo, C. K., Hodding, J. H., & Kraus, D. M. (2010). *Lexi-comp's pediatric dosage handbook* (17th ed.). Hudson, OH: Lexi-comp.

Tan, A. J., & Silverberg, M. A. (2011). *Hemolytic uremic syndrome in emergency medicine.* Retrieved May 29, 2011 from http://emedicine.medscape.com/article/779218-overview

Thompson, M., Simon, S. D., Sharma, V., & Alon, U. S. (2005). Timing of follow-up voiding cystourethrogram in children with primary vesicoureteral reflux: Development and application of a clinical algorithm. *Pediatrics, 115*(2), 426–434.

Varade, W. (2000). Hemolytic uremic syndrome: Reducing the risks. *Contemporary Pediatrics, 9*, 54.

Wald, E. R. (2006). Vesicoureteral reflux: The role of antibiotic prophylaxis. *Pediatrics, 117*(3), 919–922.

Williams, M. A., Giel, D. W., & Hasting, M. C. (2008). Endoscopic Deflux® injection for pediatric transplant reflux: A feasible alternative to open ureteral reimplant. *Journal of Pediatric Urology, 4*, 341–344.

Wolfish, N. M., & Phan, C. (2009) Management of nocturnal enuresis in children. *Canadian Pharmacists Journal, 142*(2), 76–80. Retrieved June 22, 2010 from http://www.cpjournal.ca/doi/pdf/10.3821/1913-701X-142.2.76

RECOMMENDED READINGS

Canadian Institute for Health. (2010). *Treatment of end-stage organ failure in Canada 1999–2008 - Canadian Organ Replacement Register 2010 Annual Report.* Retrieved December 10, 2011 from http://secure.cihi.ca/cihiweb/products/corr_annual_report_2010_e.pdf

National Kidney Foundation. (2009). KDOQI clinical practice guideline for nutrition for children with CKD: 2008 Update. *American Journal of Kidney Diseases, 53*(3 Suppl. 2), S1–S124. Retrieved December 10, 2011 from http://www.kidney.org/professionals/KDOQI/guidelines_updates/pdf/CPGPedNutr2008.pdf

Wühl, E., & Schaefer, F. (2010). Can we slow the progression of chronic kidney disease? *Current Opinion in Pediatrics, 22*, 170–175.

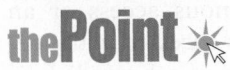

For additional learning materials, including Internet Resources, visit **http://thePoint.lww.com/Chow1e.**

CHAPTER WORKSHEET

MULTIPLE CHOICE QUESTIONS

1. The nurse is performing patient education for the parents of an infant with bladder exstrophy. Which statement by the parents would indicate an understanding of the child's future care?

   a. "Care will be no different than that of any other infant."

   b. "My infant will only need this one surgery."

   c. "My child will wear diapers all his life."

   d. "We will need to care for the urinary diversion."

2. A 4-year-old girl presents with recurrent UTI. A prior workup did not reveal any urinary tract abnormalities. What is the priority nursing action?

   a. Obtain a sterile urine sample after completion of antibiotics.

   b. Teach appropriate toileting hygiene.

   c. Prepare the child for surgery to reimplant the ureters.

   d. Administer antibiotics intramuscularly.

3. A 5-year-old who had a kidney transplant 9 months ago and has no history of chickenpox presents to the pediatric clinic for his vaccinations. Which is the most appropriate set to give?

   a. DTaP, IPV

   b. DTaP, IPV, MMR, varicella

   c. DTaP, IPV, varicella

   d. IPV only

4. When the nurse is caring for a child with HUS or acute glomerulonephritis and the child is not yet toilet trained, which action by the nurse would best determine fluid retention?

   a. Test urine for specific gravity.

   b. Weigh child daily.

   c. Weigh the wet diapers.

   d. Measure abdominal girth daily.

CRITICAL THINKING EXERCISES

1. Develop a teaching plan for an adolescent with premenstrual syndrome and dysmenorrhea.

2. Devise a meal plan for a 5-year-old child with a renal disorder that requires a 2 to 3 g sodium restriction per day. Keep in mind the child's developmental level and feeding idiosyncrasies at this age.

3. Develop a discharge teaching plan for a 3-year-old with nephrotic syndrome who will be taking corticosteroids long term.

4. Devise a developmental stimulation plan for an 11-month-old who has had significant urinary tract reconstructive surgery and is facing a prolonged period of confinement to the crib.

STUDY ACTIVITIES

1. In the clinical setting, compare the growth and development of two children the same age, one with CKD and one who has been healthy.

2. While caring for children in the clinical setting, compare and contrast the medical history, signs and symptoms of illness, and prescribed treatments for a child with nephrotic syndrome and one with acute glomerulonephritis.

3. Observe peritoneal dialysis or hemodialysis in a hospital or out-patient setting. Record observations about the children's psychosocial and developmental status.

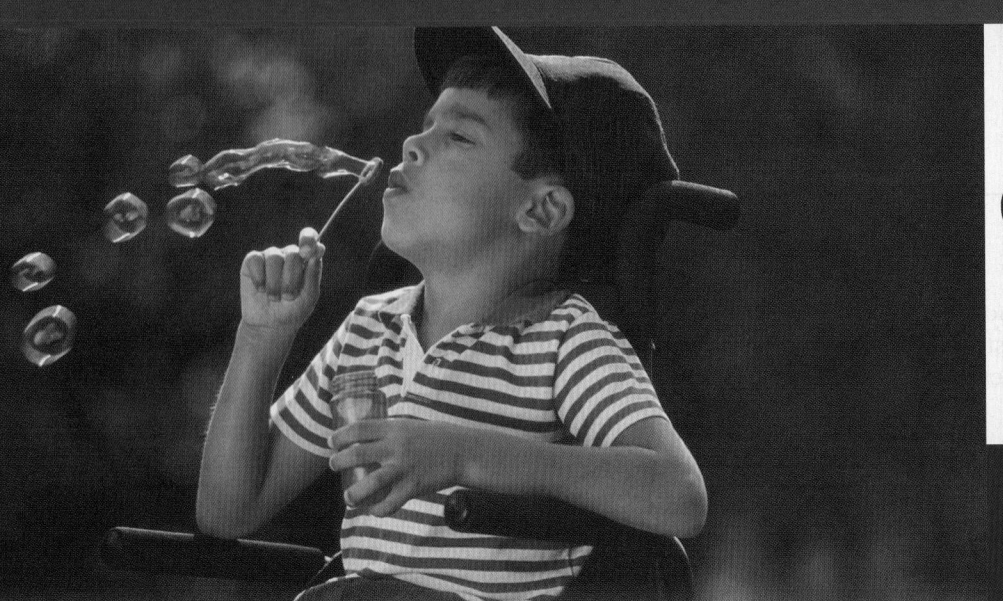

CHAPTER 43

Adapted by Donna Martin and
Doris Sawatzky-Dickson

NURSING CARE OF THE CHILD WITH A NEUROMUSCULAR DISORDER

KEY TERMS

atrophy
clonus
contracture
dystrophy

hypertonicity
hypotonia
neurogenic
neurotoxic

peripheral neuropathy
spasticity
teratogen

LEARNING OBJECTIVES

Upon completion of the chapter, the learner will be able to:

1. Compare differences between the anatomy and physiology of the neuromuscular system in children versus adults.
2. Identify nursing interventions related to common laboratory and diagnostic tests used in the diagnosis and management of neuromuscular disorders.
3. Identify appropriate nursing assessments and interventions related to medications and treatments used for childhood neuromuscular disorders.
4. Distinguish various neuromuscular illnesses occurring in childhood.
5. Devise an individualized nursing care plan for the child with a neuromuscular disorder.
6. Develop patient/family teaching plans for the child with a neuromuscular disorder.
7. Describe the psychosocial impact of chronic neuromuscular disorders on the growth and development of children.

*F*redrick Stevens, 4 years old, seems to be falling often and has started to have difficulty climbing the stairs on his own. His mother states, "Recently he hasn't been able to keep up with his 6-year-old sister when we're playing at the park. He usually ends up sitting on the bench with me." She is concerned about the changes she has seen in her son.

*W*ow

Enhancing a child's abilities may enhance his or her strength to overcome anything.

According to Muscular Dystrophy Canada (2009), "neuromuscular disorders" is a general term that refers to diseases that affect any part of the nerve or muscle. A variety of neuromuscular disorders may affect children, but the result of each disorder is muscular dysfunction. Neuromuscular disorders can result from congenital or **inherited** causes, including the muscular dystrophies and spinal muscle atrophies, or **acquired** causes, including dermatomyositis, infant botulism, Guillain–Barré syndrome, and **neurotoxicity** from lead or mercury exposures (Yang & Finkel, 2010). Some disorders such as cerebral palsy (CP) result from an insult to the central nervous system (CNS) such as birth trauma or hypoxia to the brain or spinal cord. **Spinal cord disorders** include neural tube defects such as spina bifida occulta, meningocele, and myelomeningocele. Neuromuscular disorders may also originate at the neuraxis at the muscle, neuromuscular junction, peripheral nerve, or motor neuron. Many of the neurologic motor disorders are chronic in nature, lasting the child's entire life and resulting in special needs for the child and family.

The nurse caring for a child with a neuromuscular dysfunction or disorder plays an important role in managing a variety of special needs. Not only must the nurse provide direct intervention in response to health alterations, but the nurse is often part of the larger multidisciplinary team and may serve as the coordinator of many specialists or interventions. Understanding the most common responses to these disorders gives the nurse the foundation required to plan care for any child with any neuromuscular disorder.

Variations in Pediatric Anatomy and Physiology

Neuromuscular disorders in children may occur as a congenital malformation or a genetic disorder that is present from birth but may not be identified until later in childhood or adolescence. They may also result from trauma or hypoxia or develop following a viral illness or exposure to a heavy metal such as lead or mercury. The neurologic and musculoskeletal systems in infants and children are immature compared with those in adults, placing children at increased risk for the development of a neuromuscular disorder.

Brain and Spinal Cord Development

Early in gestation, around 3 to 4 weeks, the neural tube of the embryo begins to differentiate into the brain and spinal cord. If the fetus suffers infection, trauma, malnutrition, or **teratogen** exposure during this critical period of growth and differentiation, brain or spinal cord development may be altered. During the early phases of life, dis-

ruption in the nervous system could cause irreversible damage to the circuits, preventing signals from occurring normally between brain regions and resulting in cognitive, behavioural, or motor dysfunctions (Fraser, Muckle, & Després, 2006). Compared with the adult, the child's spine is very mobile, especially the cervical spine region, resulting in a higher risk for cervical spine injury. The premature infant's CNS is less mature than the term newborn's. Such immaturity in the preterm infant places him or her at a higher risk for CNS insult during the neonatal period, which may result in delayed motor skill attainment or CP.

> ▶ *Take NOTE!*
>
> *Neurotransmitters appear early on in brain development and serve a crucial function in the development of synapses and dendrites, which in turn create cortical circuits for the transmission of signals from one area of the brain to another. Synaptogenesis is a process that initiates in the first weeks of life, proliferates in the first 3 years, and continues until late adolescence (Fraser et al., 2006).*

Myelination

Though development of the structures of the nervous system is complete at birth, myelination is incomplete. Myelination continues to progress and is complete by about 2 years of age. Myelination proceeds in a cephalocaudal and proximodistal fashion, allowing the infant to gain head and neck control before becoming able to control the trunk and the extremities. As myelination proceeds, the speed and accuracy of nerve impulses increase.

Muscular Development

The muscular system, including tendons, ligaments, and cartilage, arises from the mesoderm in early embryonic development. At birth (term or preterm), the muscles, tendons, ligaments, and cartilage are all present and functional. The newborn infant is capable of spontaneous movement but lacks purposeful control. Full range of motion is present at birth. Healthy infants and children demonstrate normal muscle tone; **hypertonia** or **hypotonia** is an abnormal finding. Deep tendon reflexes are present at birth and are initially brisk in the newborn and progress to average over the first few months. Sluggish deep tendon reflexes indicate an abnormality. As the infant matures and becomes mobile, the muscles develop further and become stronger. The adolescent boy, in response to testosterone release, experiences a growth spurt, particularly in the trunk and legs, and develops bulkier muscles at that time.

COMMON MEDICAL TREATMENTS 43.1

Treatment	Explanation	Indication	Nursing Implications
Skeletal or cervical traction	Traction is used to immobilize the cervical spine. Halo traction will be applied in stable injuries and allows the patient greater mobility. Cervical traction is applied by a jacket-like apparatus, and the patient can get out of bed, use a wheelchair, and even ambulate	To minimize or prevent trauma to the spinal cord	Monitor neurologic status closely Assess for signs and symptoms of infection or impaired skin integrity Provide appropriate pin site care
Physical therapy, occupational therapy, or speech therapy	Physical therapy focuses on attainment or improvement of gross motor skills. Occupational therapy focuses on refinement of fine motor skills, feeding, and activities of daily living. Speech therapy is warranted for the child with a speech impairment or feeding difficulty related to oral muscular issues	Cerebral palsy, spina bifida, spinal cord injury, muscular dystrophy, spinal muscular atrophy	Provide follow-through with prescribed exercises or supportive equipment Success of therapy is dependent upon continued compliance with the prescribed regimen Ensure that adequate communication exists within the interdisciplinary team
Orthotics, braces	Adaptive positioning devices specially fitted for each child by the physical or occupational therapist or orthotist. Used to maintain proper body or extremity alignment, improve mobility, and prevent contractures	Cerebral palsy, spinal cord injury, spina bifida, muscular dystrophy, spinal muscular atrophy	Provide frequent assessments of skin covered by the device to avoid skin breakdown Follow the therapist's schedule of recommended "on" and "off" times. Encourage families to comply with use

Common Medical Treatments

A variety of pharmaceuticals as well as other medical treatments are used to treat neuromuscular disorders in children. Most of these treatments will require a physician's order when the child is in the hospital. The most common treatments and medications are listed in Common Medical Treatments 43.1 and Drug Guide 43.1. The nurse caring for the child with a neuromuscular disorder should become familiar with what these procedures are and how they work as well as common nursing implications related to use of these modalities.

NURSING PROCESS OVERVIEW FOR THE CHILD WITH A NEUROMUSCULAR DISORDER

Care of the child with a neuromuscular disorder includes assessment, nursing diagnosis, planning, interventions, and evaluation. A number of general concepts related to the nursing process may be applied to neuromuscular dysfunction in children. From a general understanding of the care involved for a child with a neuromuscular disorder, the nurse can then individualize the care based on patient specifics.

Assessment

Assessment of neuromuscular dysfunction in children includes a detailed health history, physical examination, and laboratory and diagnostic testing.

*R*emember Fredrick, the 4-year-old who has been falling, having difficulty climbing stairs, and seems to tire easily when playing with his sister? What additional health history and physical examination assessment information should the nurse obtain?

Health History

The health history comprises past medical history, including the mother's pregnancy history, family history, and history of present illness (when the symptoms started and how they have progressed) as well as treatments used at home. The past medical history might be significant for prematurity, difficult birth, infection during pregnancy, changes in gait, falls, delayed development, or poor growth. Family history might be significant for neuromuscular disorders that are genetic. When eliciting the history of the present illness, inquire about the following:

• Changes in gait
• Recent trauma

DRUG GUIDE 43.1 COMMON DRUGS FOR NEUROMUSCULAR DISORDERS

Medication	Action	Indication	Nursing Implications
Benzodiazepines (diazepam, lorazepam)	Anticonvulsants; enhance the inhibition of GABA	Used adjunctively for relief of skeletal muscle spasm associated with cerebral palsy and paralysis resulting from spinal cord injury	Monitor sedation level Assess for improvements in spasticity
Baclofen (oral or intrathecal)	Central-acting skeletal muscle relaxant; precise mechanism unknown	Used to treat painful spasms and decrease spasticity in children with motor neuron lesions, such as cerebral palsy and spinal cord injury	Assess motor function Monitor for a decrease in spasticity Observe for mental confusion, depression, or hallucinations Dosage must be tapered before discontinuing because withdrawal symptoms may occur
Corticosteroids	Anti-inflammatory and immunosuppressive action	Duchenne muscular dystrophy, myasthenia gravis, dermatomyositis	Administer with food to decrease GI upset. May mask signs of infection Do not stop treatment abruptly or acute adrenal insufficiency may occur Monitor for Cushing syndrome Dosage may be tapered over time
Botulin toxin	Neurotoxin produced by *Clostridium botulinum* that blocks neuromuscular conduction	Relief of spasticity in cerebral palsy, occasionally for torticollis	Injected into the muscle by an advanced provider. May cause dry mouth

Adapted from: Karch, A. (2010). *2010 Lippincott's nursing drug guide.* Philadelphia: Wolters Kluwer Health/Lippincott Williams & Wilkins; and Taketokmo, C. K., Hodding, J. H., & Kraus, D. M. (2010). *Lexi-comp's Drug Reference Handbook: Pediatric & Neonatal Dosage Handbook* (18th ed.). Hudson, OH: Lexi-comp, Inc.

- Poor feeding
- Lethargy
- Fever
- Weakness
- Alteration in muscle tone

Determine the child's history of attainment of developmental milestones. Note the age that milestones such as sitting, crawling, and walking were attained, and determine whether the pace of attainment of milestones has decreased. Some children may progress normally at first and then demonstrate decreased velocity of development of achievements or even loss of abilities. Obtain a clear description of weakness; is it fatigue or is the child truly not as strong as he or she was in the past?

Physical Examination

Physical examination of the nervous and musculoskeletal systems consists of inspection, observation, and palpation and should also include auscultation of the heart and lungs, as the function of these organs may be affected by certain neuromuscular conditions. The most common classes of neuromuscular disorders with cardiac manifestations are the muscular dystrophies (Hsu, 2010).

Inspection and Observation

Observe the infant or child playing with toys, crawling, or walking to obtain significant information about cranial nerve, cerebellar, and motor function. Observe the child's general appearance, noting any asymmetry in muscle development. Lack of use of extremities leads to muscular **atrophy**, so a shortened limb may indicate chronic hemiparesis. Monitor weight, linear height in ambulatory patients (sometimes measured every 6 months), and arm span/segmental length in non-ambulatory patients. Note symmetry of spontaneous movement of extremities as well as facial muscles. Determine cranial nerve function. Inspect the spine for cutaneous abnormalities such as dimples or hair tufts, which may be associated with spinal cord abnormalities. Observe the child's level of consciousness, noting decreases or significant changes. Note presence of lethargy. Refer to Chapter 37 for a complete description of evaluation of level of consciousness.

Motor Function. Observe spontaneous activity, posture, and balance, and assess for asymmetric movements. In the infant, observe resting posture, which will normally be slightly flexed. The infant should be able to extend extremities to a normal stretch. Note position of comfort of the infant's or child's neck.

Reflexes. Note sluggish or brisk deep tendon reflexes. Note persistence of primitive reflexes in the older infant or child, such as Moro or tonic neck. Assess for development of protective reflexes, which is often delayed in infants with motor disorders.

Sensory Function. Alterations in sensory function accompany many neuromuscular disorders. Assess sensory function in a similar fashion to that used in the adult. The sensory functions of light touch, pain, vibration, heat, and cold are distinguishable by a child. Gentle tickling may be a useful strategy to determine sensory function. In the infant, assess for response to light touch or pain. The usual response to pain will be withdrawal from the stimulus. Always prepare the child for the sensory examination in order to gain cooperation. The pinprick test may be particularly frightening, but most children will cooperate if educated appropriately.

Palpation

Assess muscle strength and tone in the infant or child. Compare strength and tone bilaterally. Evaluate neck tone by pulling the infant from a supine position to a sitting position (Fig. 43.1). By 4 to 5 months of age, the infant should be able to maintain the head in a neutral position. Perform passive range of motion of the neck. Alterations in range of motion may indicate a neuromuscular disorder or torticollis. Note trunk tone in the infant by holding the infant under the axillae and palpating for trunk tone. The hypotonic infant will feel as though he or she is slipping through the examiner's hands. The hypertonic infant will feel rigid, extending the trunk and legs. Assess leg tone in the infant by placing the infant in the vertical position with the feet on a flat surface; the 4-month-old infant should be able to momentarily support his or her weight (Fig. 43.2).

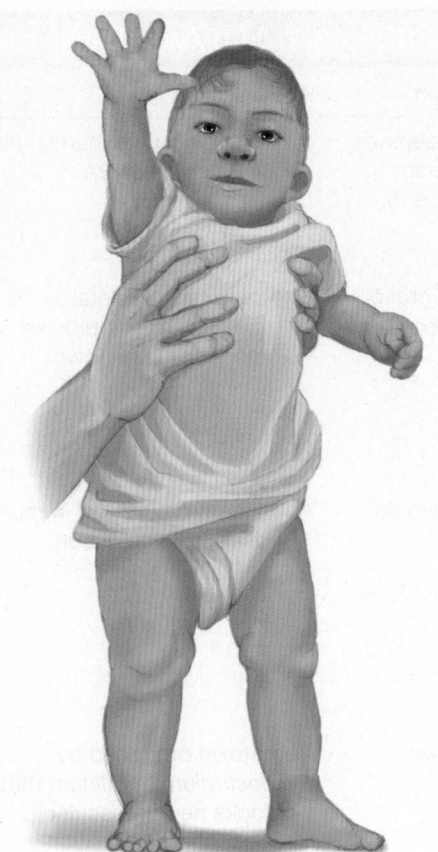

FIGURE 43.2 Assessing leg tone in an infant.

Assess the strength of the infant or child by noting ability to move the muscles against gravity. Note any **hypertonicity** or **spasticity**, which may be an early indication of CP or other neuromuscular disorder.

> ▶ **Take** NOTE!
>
> *In cases of trauma or suspected trauma, do not perform any assessment that involves movement of the head and neck until cervical injury is ruled out. Maintain complete immobilization of the cervical spine until that time.*

Auscultation

Auscultate the child's lung and heart sounds; adventitious lung sounds are often present when respiratory muscle function is impaired.

Laboratory and Diagnostic Testing

Common Laboratory and Diagnostic Tests 43.1 offers an explanation of the laboratory and diagnostic tests most commonly used in the assessment of neuromuscular disorders. The tests can assist the physician in diagnosing the disorder and/or be used as guidelines in determining

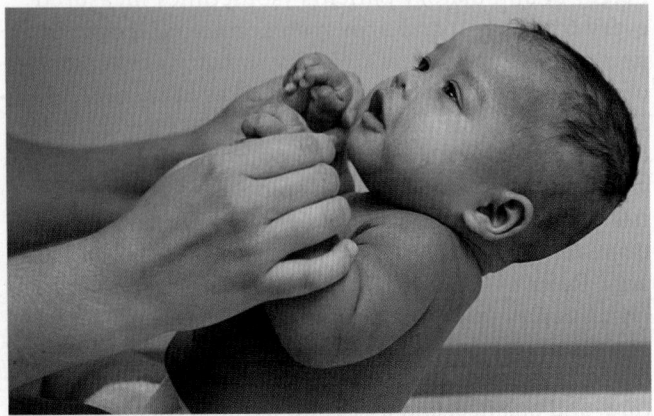

FIGURE 43.1 Assessing neck tone in an infant.

COMMON LABORATORY AND DIAGNOSTIC TESTS 43.1

Test	Explanation	Indication	Nursing Implications
Cervical spine X-rays	Radiographic image of the cervical spine	Detection of spinal fractures	In the trauma victim, the cervical spine should remain immobilized until cleared after cervical spine X-rays
Ultrasound	Use of sound waves to locate the depth and structure within soft tissues and fluid	Assessment of spinal abnormalities	Better tolerated by nonsedated children than CT or MRI Can be performed with a portable unit at bedside
Computed tomography (CT)	Non-invasive X-ray study that looks at tissue density and structures. Images a "slice" of tissue	Evaluation of congenital abnormalities such as neural tube defects, fractures, demyelination, or inflammation	Machine is large and can be frightening to children Procedure can be lengthy and child must remain still. If unable to do so, sedation may be necessary If performed with contrast medium, assess for allergy Encourage fluids after procedure if not contraindicated
Magnetic resonance imaging (MRI)	Based on how hydrogen atoms behave in a magnetic field when disturbed by radio-frequency signals. Does not require ionizing radiation. Provides a 3D view of the body part being scanned	Assessment of inflammation, congenital abnormalities such as neural tube defects	Remove all metal objects from the child Child must remain motionless for entire scan; parent can stay in room with child. Younger children will require sedation in order to be still A loud thumping sound occurs inside the machine during the procedure, which can be frightening to children
Creatine kinase	Reflects muscle damage: it leaks from muscle into plasma as muscles deteriorate	Diagnosis of muscular dystrophy, spinal muscular atrophy	Draw sample before electromyogram or muscle biopsy, as those tests may lead to release of creatine kinase
Electromyography	A recording electrode is placed in the skeletal muscle and electrical activity is recorded	Differentiates muscular disorders from those that are neurologic in origin	Requires insertion of short needles into the muscles
Nerve conduction velocity	Measures the speed of nerve conduction	Differentiation of muscular disorders	Feels like mild electric shocks
Muscle biopsy	Removal of a piece of muscular tissue either by needle or by open biopsy	Determination of type of muscular dystrophy or spinal muscular atrophy	Post-biopsy care is similar to that for other types of biopsy Involves a small incision with one or two sutures
Dystrophin	A normal intracellular plasma membrane protein in the muscle	Determination of specific type of muscular dystrophy	Absent in Duchenne muscular dystrophy, decreased in Becker muscular dystrophy
Genetic testing	Tests for presence of the gene for the disease or for carrier status	Determination of disease or carrier status of inherited muscular disorder	Entire family should be tested, even those unaffected, because carrier status should be determined and genetic counselling related to reproduction provided

Adapted from: Fischbach, F. T., & Dunning, M. B., III (2009). A manual of laboratory and diagnostic tests (8th ed.). Philadelphia: Lippincott Williams & Wilkins.

ongoing treatment. Laboratory or non-nursing personnel perform some of the tests, while the nurse might perform others. In either instance the nurse should be familiar with how the tests are performed, what they are used for, and normal versus abnormal results. This knowledge will also be necessary when providing patient and family education related to the testing.

It can be expected that children and adolescents with muscular dystrophies will undergo a cardiac workup because the "most common cardiac findings include dilated or hypertrophic cardiomyopathy, atrioventricular conduction defects, atrial fibrillation and ventricular arrhythmias" (Hsu, 2010, p. 35) that may result in an abnormal heart rate and diminished cardiac output.

Nursing Diagnoses, Goals, Interventions, and Evaluations

Upon completion of a thorough assessment, the nurse may identify several nursing diagnoses, including the following:

- Impaired physical mobility related to spasticity, neuromuscular impairment, or weakness
- Ineffective airway clearance related to respiratory muscle weakness
- Acute pain related to fracture or other injury
- Chronic pain related to muscle weakness, limited range of motion, or vertebral fracture
- Imbalanced nutrition, less than body requirements, related to spasticity, feeding, or swallowing difficulties
- Imbalanced nutrition, more than body requirements, related to immobility
- Urinary retention related to anatomic obstruction, sensory motor impairment, or dysfunctional voiding as evidenced by dribbling, inadequate bladder emptying
- Constipation related to immobility, loss of sensation
- Self-care deficit related to neuromuscular impairment, sensory deficits
- Risk for impaired skin integrity related to immobility, braces, or adaptive devices
- Chronic sorrow related to presence of chronic disability
- Risk for injury related to muscle weakness, **peripheral neuropathy**, osteoporosis
- Deficient knowledge related to lack of information regarding complex medical condition, prognosis, and medical needs
- Family processes, interrupted, related to child's illness, hospitalization, diagnosis of chronic illness in child, and potential long-term effects of illness

After completing an assessment of Fredrick, the nurse noted the following: he started walking at 2 years of age, he has difficulty jumping, his gait has a waddling appearance, and he does not rise from the floor in the usual fashion. Based on these assessment findings, what would your top three nursing diagnoses be for Fredrick?

Nursing goals, interventions, and evaluation for the child with neuromuscular dysfunction are based on the nursing diagnoses presented in Nursing Care Plan 43.1, which may be used as a guide in planning nursing care for the child with a neuromuscular disorder. The care plan includes many nursing diagnoses that are applicable to an infant, child, or adolescent. Children's responses to neuromuscular dysfunction and its treatment will vary, and nursing care should be individualized based on the child's and family's responses to illness as well as their culture. Additional information about nursing management will be included later in the chapter as it relates to specific disorders. Visit http://thePoint.lww.com/Chow1e for a list of Internet resources for families of children with neuromuscular disorders.

Based on your top three nursing diagnoses for Fredrick, describe appropriate nursing interventions.

Congenital Neuromuscular Disorders

Several disorders with neuromuscular effects are congenital in nature. These include the neural tube defects and genetic neuromuscular disorders. The structural disorders are spina bifida occulta, meningocele, and myelomeningocele (neural tube defects). The genetic neuromuscular disorders include the various types of muscular dystrophy (MD) and spinal muscular atrophy (SMA). These disorders are not always recognized at birth, as signs and symptoms are not evident until months or even years after birth, but they are still considered to be congenital as they have a genetic basis.

Neural Tube Defects

Neural tube defects account for the majority of congenital anomalies of the CNS. The neural tube closes between the third and fourth weeks of gestation. The cause of neural tube defects is not known, but many factors, such as drugs, malnutrition, chemicals, and genetics, can hinder normal CNS development. Strong evidence exists that folate deficiency is the main cause of neural tube defects (Oakley, 2009). In addition to increasing dietary folate intake (sources include cereals, baked goods, salad greens, some fruits, and legumes), Health Canada (2009) recommends that women who could become pregnant take a daily vitamin supplement containing 0.4 mg of folic acid. Despite progress toward increasing folic acid additives in common foods and encouraging women to take vitamin supplements, it is estimated that only about 10% of these types of birth defects have been prevented (Oakley, 2009). Prenatal screening of maternal serum for alpha-fetoprotein (AFP) and ultrasound at 16 to 18 weeks of gestation can

(text continues on page 1476)

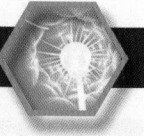

Nursing Care Plan 43.1

OVERVIEW FOR THE CHILD WITH A NEUROMUSCULAR DISORDER

NURSING DIAGNOSIS: Impaired physical mobility related to muscle weakness, hypertonicity, impaired coordination, loss of muscle function or control as evidenced by an inability to move extremities, to ambulate without assistance, to move without limitations

Outcome Identification and Evaluation

Child will be able to engage in activities within age parameters and limits of disease: *Child is able to move extremities, move about environment, and participate in exercise programs within limits of age and disease.*

Intervention: Maximizing Physical Mobility

- Encourage gross and fine motor activities *to facilitate motor development.*
- Collaborate with physical therapy, occupational therapy, and speech therapy to strengthen muscles and promote optimal mobility *to facilitate motor development.*
- Use passive and active range-of-motion exercises and teach child and family how to perform them *to prevent contractures, facilitate joint mobility and muscle development (active ROM), and help increase mobility.*
- Praise accomplishments and emphasize child's abilities *to improve self-esteem and encourage feeling of confidence and competence.*

NURSING DIAGNOSIS: Nutrition, imbalanced, less than body requirements, related to difficulty feeding secondary to deficient sucking, swallowing, or chewing; difficulty assuming normal feeding position; inability to feed self as evidenced by decreased oral intake, impaired swallowing, weight loss or plateau.

Outcome Identification and Evaluation

Child will exhibit signs of adequate nutrition *as evidenced by appropriate weight gain, intake and output within normal limits, and adequate ingestion of calories.*

Intervention: Promoting Adequate Nutrition

- Monitor height and weight: *Insufficient intake will lead to impaired growth and weight gain.*
- Monitor hydration status (moist mucous membranes, elastic skin turgor, and adequate urine output): *Insufficient intake can lead to dehydration.*
- Use techniques to promote caloric and nutritional intake and teach family about these techniques (e.g., positioning, modified utensils, soft or blended foods, allowing extra time) *to facilitate intake.*
- Assess respiratory system frequently *to assess for aspiration.*
- Assist family to help child assume as normal a feeding position as possible *to help increase oral intake.*

NURSING DIAGNOSIS: Urinary retention related to sensory motor impairment as evidenced by dribbling, inadequate bladder emptying

Outcome Identification and Evaluation

Child's bladder will empty adequately, *according to pre-established quantities and frequencies individualized for the child (usual urine output is 0.5 to 2 mL/kg/hour).*

Intervention: Promoting Successful Bladder Emptying

- Assess child's ability to empty bladder via history focused on character and duration of lower urinary symptoms *to establish baseline.*
- Assess for history of fecal impaction or constipation, *as alterations in bowel elimination may hinder urinary elimination.*
- Assess for bladder distention by palpation or urinary retention by post-void residual obtained via catheterization or bladder ultrasound *to determine extent of retention.*
- Maintain adequate hydration *to avoid irritating effects that dehydration has on the bladder.*
- Schedule voiding *to decrease bladder overdistention.*
- Teach the family of the child with significant urinary retention (and the child if old enough) the technique of clean intermittent catheterization *to allow regular, complete bladder emptying.*

(continued)

Nursing Care Plan 43.1 (continued)

NURSING DIAGNOSIS: Risk for constipation related to immobility, loss of sensation

Outcome Identification and Evaluation
Child will demonstrate adequate stool passage, *will pass soft, formed stool every 1 to 3 days without straining or other adverse effects.*

Intervention: Promoting Appropriate Bowel Elimination
- Assess usual pattern of stooling *to determine baseline and identify potential problems with elimination.*
- Palpate for abdominal fullness and auscultate for bowel sounds *to assess for bowel function and presence of constipation.*
- Encourage fibre intake *to increase frequency of stools.*
- Ensure adequate fluid intake *to prevent formation of hard, dry stools.*
- Encourage activity within child's limits or restrictions: *Even minimal activity increases peristalsis.*
- Administer medications or enemas as ordered *to promote bowel training/evacuation (especially in child with myelomeningocele or spinal cord injury).*

NURSING DIAGNOSIS: Self-care deficit related to neuromuscular impairments, cognitive deficits as evidenced by an inability to perform hygiene care and transfer self independently

Outcome Identification and Evaluation
Child will demonstrate ability to care for self within age parameters and limits of disease: *Child is able to feed, dress, and manage elimination within limits of disease and age.*

Intervention: Maximizing Self-Care
- Introduce child and family to self-help methods as soon as possible *to promote independence from the beginning.*
- Encourage family and staff to allow child to do as much as possible *to allow child to gain confidence and independence.*
- Teach specific measures for bowel and urinary elimination as needed *to promote independence and increase self-care abilities and self-esteem.*
- Collaborate with physical therapy, occupational therapy, and speech therapy to provide child and family with appropriate tools to modify environment and methods to promote transferring and self-care *to allow for maximum functioning.*
- Praise accomplishments and emphasize child's abilities *to improve self-esteem and encourage feelings of confidence and competence.*
- Balance activity with periods to rest *to reduce fatigue and increase energy for self-care.*

NURSING DIAGNOSIS: Risk for impaired skin integrity related to immobility, use of braces or adaptive devices

Outcome Identification and Evaluation
Child's skin will remain intact, *without evidence of redness or breakdown.*

Intervention: Promoting Skin Integrity
- Monitor condition of entire skin surface at least daily *to provide baseline and allow for early identification of areas at risk.*
- Avoid excessive friction or harsh cleaning products *that may increase risk of breakdown in child with susceptible skin.*
- Keep child's skin free from stool and urine *to decrease risk of breakdown.*
- Change child's position frequently *to decrease pressure to susceptible areas.*
- Monitor skin condition affected by braces or adaptive equipment frequently *to prevent skin breakdown related to poor fit.*

NURSING DIAGNOSIS: Chronic sorrow related to presence of chronic disability as evidenced by child's or family's expression of sadness, anger, disappointment, or feeling overwhelmed

Outcome Identification and Evaluation
Child and/or family will accept situation; *child/family will appropriately identify feelings, function at a normal developmental level, and plan for the future.*

Intervention: Easing Sorrow
- Assess degree of sorrow *to provide baseline for intervention.*
- Identify problems with eating or sleeping, *often affected when grief or sorrow is present.*
- Spend time with the child and family; *an empathetic presence is valued by suffering families.*

Nursing Care Plan 43.1 (continued)

- Encourage the use of positive coping techniques; *taking action, expressing feelings, intentional attempts at coping are help-ful techniques.*
- Refer for spiritual counselling as desired; *many families experience grief resolution in a more timely fashion if spiritual needs are addressed.*

NURSING DIAGNOSIS: Risk for injury related to muscle weakness

Outcome Identification and Evaluation
Child will remain free from injury; *child will not fall or experience other injury.*

Intervention: Preventing Injury
- Ensure that side rails of bed are elevated when caregiver is not directly at bedside *to prevent fall from bed.*
- Use appropriate safety restraints with adaptive equipment and wheelchairs *to prevent fall or slipping from equipment.*
- Do not leave child unattended in tub *as weakness may cause the child to slip under the water.*
- Avoid restraint use if at all possible; *close observation is more appropriate.*

NURSING DIAGNOSIS: Deficient knowledge related to lack of information regarding complex medical condition, prognosis, and medical needs as evidenced by verbalization, questions, or actions demonstrating lack of understanding regarding child's condition or care

Outcome Identification and Evaluation
Child and family will verbalize accurate information and understanding about condition, prognosis, and medical needs: *Child and family demonstrate knowledge of condition and prognosis and medical needs, including possible causes, contributing factors, and treatment measures.*

Intervention: Providing Patient and Family Teaching
- Assess child's and family's willingness to learn: *Child and family must be willing to learn for teaching to be effective.*
- Provide family with time to adjust to diagnosis *to facilitate adjustment and ability to learn and participate in child's care.*
- Repeat information *to allow family and child time to learn and understand.*
- Teach in short sessions: *Many short sessions are more helpful than one long session.*
- Gear teaching to the level of understanding of the child and family (depends on age of child, physical condition, memory) *to ensure understanding.*
- Provide reinforcement and rewards *to facilitate the teaching/learning process.*
- Use multiple modes of learning involving many senses (provide written, verbal demonstration and videos) when possible: *Child and family are more likely to retain information when it is presented in different ways using many senses.*

NURSING DIAGNOSIS: Family processes, interrupted, related to child's illness, hospitalization, diagnosis of chronic illness in child, and potential long-term effects of illness as evidenced by family's presence in hospital, missed work, demonstration of inadequate coping

Outcome Identification and Evaluation
Family will maintain functional system of support, demonstrate adequate coping, adaptation of roles: *Parents are involved in child's care, ask appropriate questions, express fears and concerns, and are able to discuss child's care and condition calmly.*

Intervention: Promoting Appropriate Family Functioning
- Encourage parents and family to verbalize concerns related to child's illness, diagnosis, and prognosis: *Allows the nurse to identify concerns and areas where further education may be needed; demonstrates family-centred care.*
- Explain therapies, procedures, child's behaviours, and plan of care to parents: *Understanding of the child's current status and plan of care helps decrease anxiety.*
- Encourage parental involvement in care *to allow parents to feel needed and valued and to have a sense of control over their child's health.*
- Identify support system for family and child: *Support system is often needed by stressed families to assist with coping.*
- Educate family and child on additional resources available *to help them develop a wide base of support.*

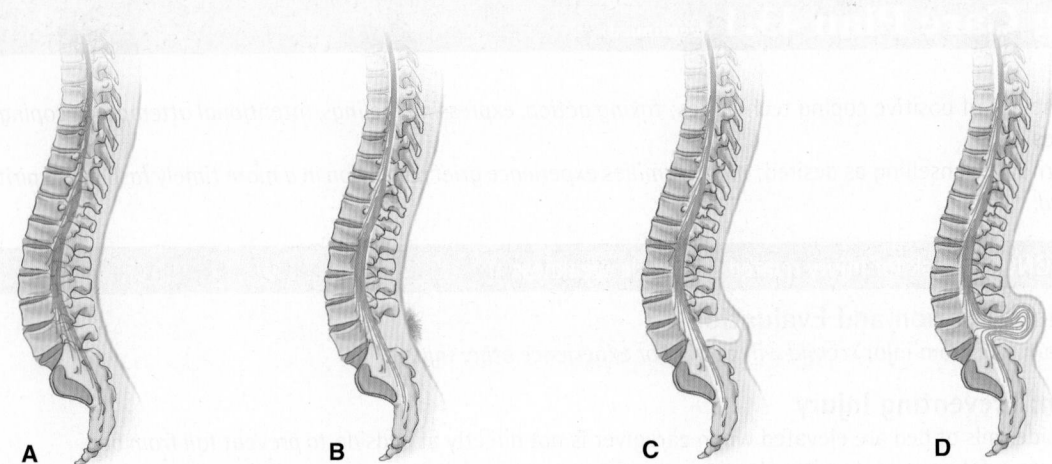

FIGURE 43.3 (**A**) Normal spine. (**B**) Spina bifida occulta. (**C**) Meningocele. (**D**) Myelomeningocele.

help identify fetuses at risk. Neural tube defects primarily affecting spinal cord development are also referred to as "spinal dysraphism" and are categorized as closed (spina bifida occulta) and open (meningocele and myelomeningocele) defects (Fig. 43.3). Neural tube defects primarily affecting brain development are discussed in Chapter 37.

Spina Bifida Occulta

Spina bifida is a term that is often used to refer to all neural tube disorders that affect the spinal cord. This can be confusing and a cause of concern for parents. There are well-defined degrees of spinal cord involvement in neural tube disorders; therefore, the use of the correct terminology is important for health care professionals.

Spina bifida occulta is a defect of the vertebral bodies without protrusion of the spinal cord or meninges. This defect is not visible externally and in most cases has no adverse affects (see Fig. 43.3). Spina bifida occulta is a common anomaly: it is estimated to affect one fifth of the population (Oakley, 2009). Children with spina bifida occulta need no immediate medical intervention.

Nursing Assessment

In most cases, spina bifida occulta is benign and asymptomatic and produces no neurologic signs; it may be considered a normal variant (Spina Bifida Association, 2011). The defect, which is usually present in the lumbosacral area, often goes undetected. However, there may be noticeable dimpling, abnormal patches of hair, or discolouration of skin at the defect site. As part of a newborn assessment, the spinal column should be checked for these signs. If present, further investigation, including magnetic resonance imaging (MRI), may be warranted.

Nursing Management

Nursing care will focus on educating the family. Inform parents of its presence and what the diagnosis means.

Many times parents will confuse this diagnosis with spina bifida cystica, a much more serious defect. Occasionally, children with spina bifida occulta eventually need surgical intervention due to degenerative changes or involvement of the spine and nerve roots resulting in complications such as tethered cord, syringomyelia, or diastematomyelia. When these associated problems occur, the condition is often termed "occult spinal dysraphism" to avoid confusion.

Meningocele

Meningocele, the less serious form of spina bifida cystica, occurs when the meninges herniate through a defect in the vertebrae. The spinal cord is usually normal and there are typically no associated neurologic deficits. Treatment for meningocele involves surgical correction of the lesion (see Fig. 43.3).

Nursing Assessment

Initial assessment after delivery will reveal a visible external sac protruding from the spinal area. It is most often seen in the lumbar region but can be anywhere along the spinal canal. Most are covered with skin and pose no threat to the patient. However, assessment to ensure that the sac covering is intact remains important. Assess neurologic status carefully: most children will be asymptomatic, with no neurologic deficits (Kinsman & Johnson, 2007; Liptak, 2008). Before surgical correction the infant will be thoroughly examined to determine whether there is any neural involvement or associated anomalies. Diagnostic procedures such as computed tomography (CT), MRI, and ultrasound may be performed.

Nursing Management

If the skin covering the sac is intact and the child has normal neurologic functioning, surgical correction may be delayed (Kinsman & Johnson, 2007). However, as in a child with myelomeningocele, immediately report any evidence of leaking cerebrospinal fluid (CSF) to ensure prompt intervention to prevent infection. Nursing management will be supportive. Provide preoperative and postoperative care similar to the child with myelomeningocele to prevent rupture of the sac and to prevent infection, and provide adequate nutrition and hydration. Monitor for symptoms of constipation or bladder dysfunction that may result due to increasing size of the lesion. Resulting hydrocephalus has been associated with some cases of meningocele (Kinsman & Johnson, 2007); therefore, monitor head circumference and watch for signs and symptoms of increased intracranial pressure (ICP).

Myelomeningocele

Myelomeningocele is the most severe form of neural tube defect. The prevalence rate in Canada is 2.6 per 10,000 total births, with varying rates between provinces and territories possibly reflecting the availability of screening and diagnostics (Public Health Agency of Canada, 2008). Myelomeningocele is a type of spina bifida cystica, and clinically the term "spina bifida" is often used to refer to myelomeningocele. It may be diagnosed in utero via ultrasound; otherwise it is visually obvious at birth. The newborn with myelomeningocele is at increased risk for meningitis, hypoxia, and hemorrhage.

In myelomeningocele, the spinal cord often ends at the point of the defect, resulting in absent motor and sensory function beyond that point (see Fig. 43.3). Therefore, the long-term complications of paralysis, orthopedic deformities, and bladder and bowel incontinence are often seen in children with myelomeningocele. The presence of **neurogenic** bladder and frequent catheterization puts the child at an increased risk for urinary tract infections, pyelonephritis, and hydronephrosis, which may result in long-term renal damage if managed inappropriately. Accompanying hydrocephalus associated with type II Chiari defect is seen in 80% of patients with myelomeningocele (Behrman, Kliegman, & Jenson, 2004). Due to the improper development and the downward displacement of the brain into the cervical spine, CSF flow is blocked, resulting in hydrocephalus. The lower the deformity is on the spine, the lower the risk of developing hydrocephalus (Kinsman & Johnson, 2007).

These children usually require multiple surgical procedures and, due to frequent catheterizations, are at increased risk for developing latex allergy (Kinsman & Johnson, 2007; Zak & Chan, 2010). Learning problems and seizures are more common in these children than in the general population, but 70% of those with myelomeningocele have normal intelligence (Behrman et al., 2004). Ambulation is possible for some children, depending on the level of the lesion. Due to advances in medical treatment, the life expectancy of children with this disorder has increased. For children born with myelomeningocele who receive aggressive treatment, the mortality rate is 10% to 15%; most deaths occur before the age of 4 years (Behrman et al., 2004).

Pathophysiology

The cause of myelomeningocele is unknown, but risk factors are consistent with other neural tube defects, such as maternal drug use, malnutrition, and a genetic predisposition (Kinsman & Johnson, 2007). In myelomeningocele, the neural tube fails to close at the end of the fourth week of gestation. As a result, an external sac-like protrusion that encases the meninges, spinal fluid, and in some cases nerves is present on the spine (see Fig. 43.3). A myelomeningocele can be located anywhere along the spinal cord, but 75% are located in the lumbosacral region (Behrman et al., 2004). The degree of neurologic deficit will depend on the location (Kinsman & Johnson, 2007). An increase in neurologic deficit is seen as the myelomeningocele extends into the thoracic region.

Therapeutic Management

Surgical closure will be performed as soon as possible after birth, especially if a CSF leak is present or if there is a danger of the sac rupturing. The goal of early surgical intervention is to prevent infection and to minimize further loss of function, which can result from the stretching of nerve roots as the meningeal sac expands after birth. A new option is becoming available but remains experimental. In utero fetal surgery to repair the myelomeningocele has been performed in the United States (Adzick, 2010), with the first randomized trial showing improved outcomes for the fetuses compared with postnatal surgery (Robinson, 2011). Ongoing management of this disorder remains complex; a multidisciplinary approach involving specialists in neurology, neurosurgery, urology, orthopedics, therapy, and rehabilitation is needed, along with intense nursing care. The chronic nature of this disorder necessitates lifelong follow-up.

Nursing Assessment

For a full description of the assessment phase of the nursing process, refer to page 1468. Assessment findings pertinent to myelomeningocele are discussed below.

Health History

High-risk deliveries should be identified. Explore the pregnancy history and past medical history for risk factors such as:

- Lack of prenatal care
- Lack of preconception and/or prenatal folic acid supplementation
- Previous child born with neural tube defect or family history of neural tube defects
- Maternal consumption of certain drugs that antagonize folic acid, such as anticonvulsants (carbamazepine and phenobarbital)

The older infant or child with a history of myelomeningocele requires numerous surgical procedures and lifelong follow-up. In an infant or child returning for a clinic visit or hospitalization, the health history should include questions related to:

• Current mobility status and any changes in motor abilities
• Genitourinary function and regimen
• Bowel function and regimen
• Signs or symptoms of urinary tract infections
• History of hydrocephalus with presence of shunt
• Signs or symptoms of shunt infection or malfunction (refer to section on hydrocephalus)
• Latex sensitivity
• Nutritional status, including changes in weight
• Any other changes in physical or cognitive state
• Resources available and used by the family

Physical Examination

Initial assessment after delivery will reveal a visible external sac protruding from the spinal area (Fig. 43.4). Observe the baby's general appearance and assess whether the sac covering is intact. Assess neurologic status and look for associated anomalies. Assess for movement of extremities and anal reflex, which will help determine the level of neurologic involvement. Flaccid paralysis, absence of deep tendon reflexes, lack of response to touch and pain stimuli, skeletal abnormalities such as club feet, constant dribbling of urine, and a relaxed anal sphincter may be found.

In the older infant or child, perform a thorough physical examination and focus on the functional assessment. Note level of paralysis or paresthesia. Inspect skin for breakdown. Determine the child's motor capabilities.

Laboratory and Diagnostic Tests

A myelomeningocele may be detected prenatally at around 16 to 18 weeks' gestation by ultrasound, by a blood test that detects AFP increases, or by analysis of amniotic fluid for AFP increases. Common laboratory and diagnostic studies ordered for the assessment of myelomeningocele include:

• MRI
• CT
• Ultrasound

These diagnostic tests are used to evaluate brain and spinal cord involvement (refer to Common Laboratory and Diagnostic Tests 43.1).

Nursing Management

Initial nursing management of the child with myelomeningocele involves preventing trauma to the meningeal sac and preventing infection before surgical repair of the defect. Refer to Nursing Care Plan 43.1. Additional considerations are reviewed below.

Preventing Infection

Risk for infection related to the presence of the meningeal sac and potential for rupture is a central nursing concern in the newborn with myelomeningocele. Until surgical intervention occurs, the goal is to prevent rupture or leakage of CSF from the sac. Keeping the sac from drying out is important, as is preventing trauma or pressure on the sac. Use sterile saline-soaked non-adhesive gauze or antibiotic-soaked gauze to keep the sac moist. Immediately report any seepage of clear fluid from the lesion, as this could indicate an opening in the sac and provide a portal of entry for microorganisms. Position the infant in the prone position or supported on the side to avoid pressure on the sac. To maintain warmth, place the infant in an appropriate infant incubator or warmer; avoid the use of blankets, which could exert too much pressure on the sac. Pay special attention while the infant is in a warmer because the radiant heat can cause drying and cracking of the sac.

Keep the lesion free of feces and urine to help avoid infection. Position the infant so that urine and feces flow away from the sac (e.g., prone position or place a folded towel under the abdomen) to help prevent infection. Placing a piece of plastic wrap below the meningocele is another way of preventing feces from coming into contact with the lesion. After surgery, position the infant in the prone or side-lying position to allow the incision to heal. Continue with precautions to prevent urine or feces from coming into contact with the incision.

Promoting Urinary Elimination

Children with myelomeningocele often have bladder incontinence, though some children may achieve normal urinary continence. The level of the lesion will influence the amount of dysfunction. Myelomeningocele remains one of the most common causes of neurogenic bladder in children. Therefore, evaluation of renal function by a pediatric urologist should be performed in each child with myelomeningocele.

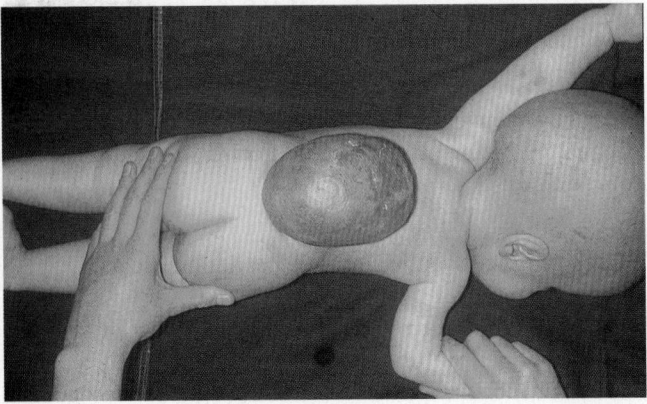

FIGURE 43.4 Usually a sac covers the deformity of myelomeningocele and is visible at birth.

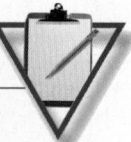

Neurogenic bladder refers to the failure of the bladder to either store urine or empty itself of urine. Children with neurogenic bladder have loss of control over voiding. The spastic type of neurogenic bladder is hyperreflexive and yields frequent release of urine but with incomplete emptying. The hypotonic neurogenic bladder is flaccid and weak and becomes stretched out; it can hold very large amounts of urine, resulting in continuous dribbling of urine from the urethra. Urinary stasis and retention occur in both types, placing the child at risk for urinary tract infection as well as reflux of bladder contents backup into the ureters and kidneys, resulting in renal scarring and insufficiency.

The goals of neurogenic bladder management are to promote optimal urinary continence and maintain low bladder pressure to prevent renal complications. Interventions for neurogenic bladder include clean intermittent catheterization (CIC) to promote bladder emptying, administration of medications such as oxybutynin chloride to improve bladder capacity, prompt recognition and treatment of infections and the use of prophylactic antibiotics such as trimethoprim, and in some children, surgical interventions such as bladder neck suspension, creation of a catheterization stoma, or detrusorectomy of the bladder to facilitate urinary elimination (de Jong, Chrzan, Klijn, & Dik, 2008). CIC is addressed below. In the child with a spastic or rigid bladder, teach parents how to administer antispasmodic medications such as oxybutynin. Teach the parents that the medications are used to increase bladder capacity and reduce the potential for reflux and infection. Refer to Chapter 42 for additional information on nursing care related to the surgical procedures.

Assessing Urinary Function

Determine the child's pattern and success of toilet training, both for bladder and bowel. Assess the child's cognitive/developmental level. Observe the genital area for dribbling of urine from the urethra, noting odour of urine if present. Note redness of the urethra or excoriation in the diaper area. Inspect the abdomen for scars from prior surgeries and the presence of urinary diversion or continent stoma. Palpate the abdomen for presence of distended bladder, fecal mass, or enlarged kidneys. Determine the child's level of paralysis or paresthesia.

Clean Intermittent Catheterization

Depending on the level of paralysis at birth in the child with myelomeningocele, CIC may be started at that time. In other children with spina bifida and in children who suffer spinal cord injury, catheterization may be started at a later age. Teach parents the technique of CIC via the urethra, unless a urinary diversion or continent stoma has been created (Teaching Guideline 43.1).

Teaching the parents the techniques of CIC is an important step in preserving renal function and preventing infection and helping the family gain some control

---

TEACHING GUIDELINE 43.1

Clean Intermittent Catheterization

- Wash hands with soap and water.
- Apply water-based lubricant to catheter.
- Perform catheterization. Insert catheter only as far as needed to obtain urine flow.
- Wash reusable catheter after use with soapy water; rinse and allow drying.
- When dry, store in zip-top plastic bag or other clean storage container.
- Weekly, soak the catheter in a 1:1 vinegar and water solution, rinsing well before next use.
- When developmentally ready, teach the child to self-catheterize.

---

over the child's physical condition. Until the child is able to self-catheterize, the parents will be responsible for this procedure. Children with normal intelligence and upper extremity motor skills usually learn to self-catheterize at the age of 6 or 7 years (Zak & Chan, 2010). Urinary incontinence is associated with poor self-esteem, particularly as the child gets older (Moore, Kogan, & Parekh, 2004). Educating the child to self-catheterize the urethra or stoma as appropriate empowers the child, gives him or her a sense of control, and allows for appropriate urinary elimination when the child is away from the parents (e.g., at school). See Evidence-based Practice 43.1.

Offer support and appropriate referrals to the child and family. Refer families to vendors in the local area for catheterization supplies.

▶ **Take** NOTE!

Over time, bacterial colonization of the bladder may occur; however, antibiotic prophylaxis is not recommended for these children because of the increased risk for development of antibiotic resistance.

▶ **Take** NOTE!

Use only latex-free catheters and gloves for catheterization of children with myelomeningocele and/or neurogenic bladder, as these children exhibit a high incidence of latex allergy (Zak & Chan, 2010).

Promoting Bowel Elimination

Children with myelomeningocele often have bowel incontinence as well; the level of the lesion affects the amount of dysfunction. Many children with myelomeningocele can achieve some degree of bowel continence.

EVIDENCE-BASED PRACTICE 43.1
Self-Intermittent Catheterization Among Female Children with Myelomeningocele and the Potential for Increased Complications

● Study
The authors reviewed the medical records of 31 females with myelomeningocele followed from the start of clean intermittent catheterization (CIC). Between all subjects, CIC was used for 459 patient-years. In all cases, the girls used noncoated polyvinyl chloride catheters.

▲ Findings
Over the total 459 patient-years, 13 patients experienced a total of 20 episodes of complications among them. These included hematuria, urethral polyps, and difficulties in catheterization. Complications were increased if assisted CIC was used or if a smaller-bore catheter was utilized.

■ Nursing Implications
There are few complications occurring in females with myelomeningocele who self-catheterize using clean technique. Encourage the use of large-size noncoated polyvinyl catheters. Teach females when developmentally capable to perform self-CIC. This function is safe and yields greater independence in this special population.

Source: Lindehall, B., Abrahamsson, K., Jodal, U., Olsson, I., & Sillen, U. (2007). Complications of clean intermittent catheterization in young females with myelomeningocele: 10 to 19 years of followup. *Journal of Urology, 178*(3), 1053–1055.

Bowel training with the use of timed enemas or suppositories along with diet modifications can allow for defecation at predetermined times once or twice a day. Although bowel incontinence can be difficult for children as they grow older due to social concerns and self-esteem and body image disturbances, it does not pose the same health risks as urinary incontinence.

Promoting Adequate Nutrition
The risk for altered nutrition, less than body requirements, related to the restrictions on positioning of the infant before and after surgery is another nursing concern. Assist the family in assuming as normal a feeding position as possible. Preoperatively, the risk of rupture may be too high to warrant holding. Therefore, the infant's head can be turned to the side or the infant can be placed in the side-lying position to facilitate feeding. If the infant is held, special care needs to be taken to avoid pressure on the sac or postoperative incision. Encourage the parents to interact as much as possible with the infant by talking and touching the infant during feeding to help promote intake. If the mother was planning on breastfeeding the infant, assist her in meeting this goal, if possible. If the infant can be held, encourage her to do this, or assist her in pumping and saving breast milk to be given to the infant via bottle until the infant is able to be held. Feeding an infant in an unusual position can be difficult, and it is the nurse's role to provide support, education, and modeling for the parents and family when needed.

Preventing Latex Allergic Reaction
Sensitivity to latex or natural rubber is very common among children with myelomeningocele due to the multiple exposures to latex products during surgical procedures and bladder catheterizations. Research has shown that up to 70% of children who require repeat surgeries due to spina bifida or bladder exstrophy are sensitive to latex (Kaplan, 2003). A latex-free environment should be created for all procedures performed on children with myelomeningocele to prevent latex allergy. Be familiar with those products and equipment at your facility that contain latex and those that are latex-free. The Food and Drug Administration now requires that all medical supplies be labelled if they contain latex, but this is not the case for consumer products. Many resources provide lists of latex-free products, and each hospital should have such a list readily available to health care professionals. Spina Bifida & Hydrocephalus Canada offers an updated list of latex-containing products and other helpful information for parents regarding consumer products; for a direct link, visit http://thePoint.lww.com/Chow1e.

Children who are at a high risk for latex sensitivity should wear medical alert identification. Education programs regarding latex sensitivity and ways to prevent it need to be directed at those who care for high-risk children, including teachers, relatives, babysitters, and all health care professionals.

Maintaining Skin Integrity
Address the risk for altered skin integrity related to the infant's prone position and impaired mobility. The prone position puts constant pressure on the knees and elbows, and it may be difficult to keep the infant clean of urine and feces. Diapering may be contraindicated preoperatively to avoid pressure on the sac. Therefore, ensure that the infant is kept as clean and dry as possible. This is made more difficult by the constant dribbling of stool and urine that may be present. Placing a pad beneath the diaper area and changing it frequently is important. Perform meticulous skin care. Place the infant on a special care mattress and place synthetic sheepskin under the infant to help reduce friction. Special attention to the

infant's legs is needed when positioning them, since paralysis may be present. Placing a folded diaper between the legs can help reduce pressure and friction from the legs rubbing together.

Educating and Supporting the Child and Family

Myelomeningocele is a serious disorder that affects multiple body systems and produces varying degrees of deficits. It is a disorder that has lifelong effects. Thanks to medical advances and technology, most children born with myelomeningocele can expect a normal life expectancy, but challenges remain for the family and child as they learn to cope and live with this physical condition. Adjusting to the demands this condition places on the child and family is difficult. Parents may need time to accept their infant's condition, but as soon as possible they should be involved in the infant's care.

Teaching should begin immediately in the hospital. Teaching should include positioning, preventing infection, feeding, promoting urinary elimination through CIC, preventing latex allergy, and understanding the signs and symptoms of complications such as increased ICP. Due to the chronic nature of this condition, long-term planning needs to begin in the hospital. These children usually require multiple surgical procedures and hospitalizations, which can place stress on the family and their finances. The nurse has an important role in providing ongoing education about the illness and its treatments and the plan of care. As the family becomes more comfortable with the condition, they will become the experts in the child's care. Respect and recognize the family's changing needs. Providing intense daily care can take its toll on a family, and continual support and encouragement are needed. Referral to Spina Bifida & Hydrocephalus Canada for families of children with myelomeningocele to locate contact information for provincial associations and a local support group is appropriate; visit http://thePoint.lww.com/Chow1e for a direct link to this organization.

▶ *Consider* THIS!

> *A newborn has an obvious defect on his spine. Upon assessment, the nurse notes flaccid extremities and a distended bladder. The parents are devastated.*
> *Identify additional assessments the nurse should make.*
> *Describe nursing care for this neonate.*
> *What teaching will the nurse do with this infant's family?*

Muscular Dystrophies

Muscular **dystrophy** refers to a group of more than 30 rare genetic diseases characterized by progressive muscle weakness and wasting. Some forms of MD present in infancy or childhood, while others may not appear until middle age or later. These disorders also differ in terms of distribution and extent of muscle weakness, rate of progression, and pattern of inheritance. All include muscle weakness over the lifetime; MD is progressive in all cases but more severe in some. The inheritance pattern for MD differs for each type but may be X-linked, autosomal dominant, or recessive. The genetic mutation in MD results in defects in muscle proteins that prevent normal function of the muscle. The skeletal muscle fibres are affected, yet there are no structural abnormalities in the spinal cord or the peripheral nerves.

Although a number of types of MD have been identified, Duchenne muscular dystrophy (DMD) is the most common childhood form of MD. DMD is an X-linked recessive disease (see Chapter 50) that is universally fatal, with an incidence of about 1 in 3,600 to 6,000 live male births (Bushby et al., 2009). Therefore, this discussion is focused on DMD.

Pathophysiology

In the 1860s, descriptions of boys who grew progressively weaker, lost the ability to ambulate, and died at an early age became prominent in the medical literature. A neurologist named Guillaume Duchenne studied 13 boys with this presentation, and the disease now carries his name. The molecular basis of DMD has been known for over two decades (Bushby et al., 2009). The gene mutation results in the absence of or defect in dystrophin, a protein that is critical for maintenance of muscle cells. Dystrophin is part of a complex structure involving several other protein components. The "dystrophin–glycoprotein complex" helps anchor the structural skeleton within the muscle cells. Due to defects in this assembly, contraction of the muscle leads to disruption of the outer membrane of the muscle cells and eventual weakening and wasting of the muscle. The gene is X-linked recessive, meaning that mainly boys are affected and they receive the gene from their mothers (women are carriers but have no symptoms). Girls in these families have a 50% chance of inheriting and passing the defective gene to their children.

Typically, the first signs and symptoms of DMD develop between the ages of 2 and 5 years, and most patients are diagnosed by 5 years of age when their physical abilities differ significantly from those of their peers (Bushby et al., 2009). The hips, thighs, pelvis, and shoulders are affected initially; as the disease progresses, all voluntary muscles as well as cardiac and respiratory muscles are affected with increasing weakness and wasting.

Boys with DMD are often late in learning to walk (older than 18 months). As toddlers, they may display pseudohypertrophy (enlarged appearance) of the calves. During the preschool years, they fall often and appear to be quite clumsy. The affected child has difficulty climbing stairs and running and cannot get up from the floor in the usual fashion. Boys with DMD display Gowers' sign,

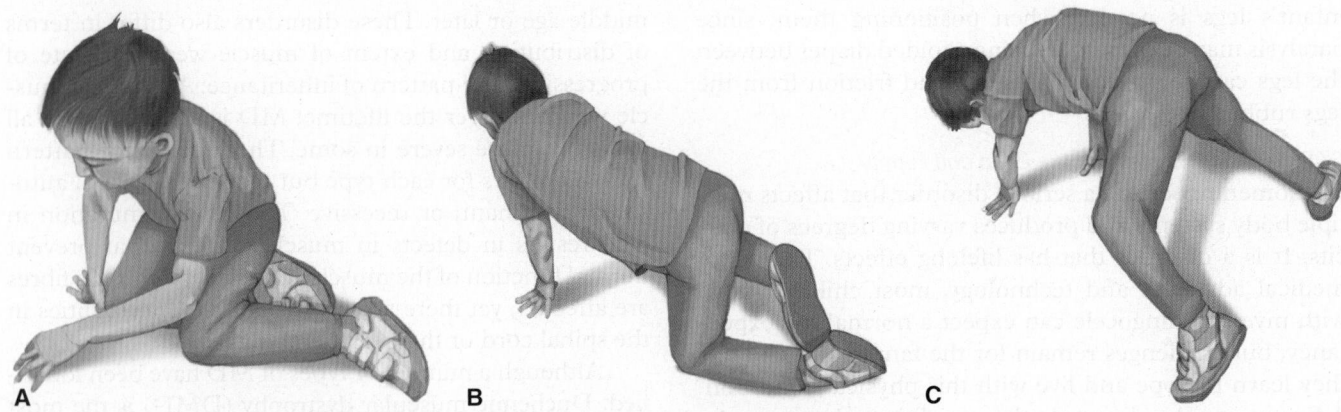

FIGURE 43.5 Gowers' sign: (**A**) First the child must roll onto his hands and knees. (**B**) Then he must bear weight by using his hands to support some of his weight, while raising his posterior. (**C**) The boy then uses his hands to "walk" up his legs to assume an upright position.

which is a medical sign indicating weakness of the leg muscles. Demonstration of Gowers' manoeuvre occurs when a patient uses the hands and arms to move from a squatting to standing position due to weakness in the hip and thigh muscles (Fig. 43.5). The school-age child walks on the toes or balls of the feet with a rolling or waddling gait. Balance is disturbed significantly, and the child's belly may stick out when the shoulders are pulled back in order to stay upright and keep from falling over. During the school-age years it also becomes difficult for the child to raise his arms. Sometime between the ages of 7 and 13 years, nearly all boys with DMD lose the ability to ambulate independently, and by the teen years any activity of the arms, legs, or trunk requires assistance or support (Muscular Dystrophy Association [MDA], 2009a). The most predictive factor for losing the ability to ambulate is loss of strength in hip extension and ankle dorsiflexion (Bakker, de Groot, Beelen, & Lankhorst, 2002). Most boys with DMD have normal intelligence, but many may exhibit a specific learning disability (Cotton, Voudouris, & Greenwood, 2005).

Acute respiratory illness leading to respiratory insufficiency was the most common cause of an unplanned admission to a pediatric intensive care unit among children with neuromuscular disorders (Panitch, 2006). With DMD, secretions in the lung are normal in quality and quantity (Kravitz, 2009). Several factors contribute to ineffective airway clearance, including inspiratory and expiratory muscle weakness, any type of dysfunction in the glottis, and the presence of scoliosis.

Therapeutic Management

Many promising therapeutic strategies for DMD have been developed in animal models over the past two decades (Bushby et al., 2009). Human trials using these strategies have begun, preserving the hope of future successful treatments for this currently incurable disease (Bushby et al., 2009). Though there is no cure for DMD, the use of glucocorticoids as well as respiratory, cardiac,

orthopedic, and rehabilitative interventions has led to improvements in function, quality of life, health, and longevity (MDA, 2009a; Sarant, 2007; Zak & Chan, 2010). Children who are diagnosed with DMD today have the possibility of life expectancy into their 40s (Bushby et al., 2009). Glucocorticoids are thought to help by protecting muscle fibres from damage to the sarcolemma (defective in the absence of dystrophin). Numerous studies have shown that boys treated with glucocorticoids demonstrate slowed decline in the progression of muscle weakness, which in turn reduces the risk of scoliosis and stabilizes cardiac and pulmonary function (Bushby et al., 2009). Families should be provided with a card or medical alert bracelet indicating that their child is on steroids, listing emergency-care considerations in the event of an acute illness or injury (Bushby et al., 2009). The side effects of glucocorticoids are many, including weight gain, osteoporosis, glucose intolerance, delayed puberty, and mood changes (Carter & McDonald, 2000; Davidson & Truby, 2009). Possible strategies to enhance bone health may include administration of vitamin D (for proven deficiencies) and increased calcium intake with possible supplementation in consultation with a dietician. "Nutritional issues have taken a back seat in the past; however, as the life expectancy slowly inches forward with improvements in medical management, such concerns warrant immediate attention" (Davidson & Truby, 2009, p. 384).

Braces or orthoses and mobility and positioning aids are necessary. As the muscles deteriorate, joints may become more fixated, resulting in **contractures**. Contractures restrict flexibility and mobility and cause discomfort. Sometimes contractures require surgical tendon release; however, muscle strength and range of motion around individual joints should be considered before health care teams and families consider the use of surgery (Bushby et al., 2010). Spinal curvatures result over time. Individuals with DMD who can still walk may develop lordosis. More frequently, scoliosis or kyphosis develops with this disorder. Monitoring for scoliosis should be conducted by clinical observation through the ambulatory phase, with spinal radiography warranted only if spinal curvature is observed. Spinal radiography is indicated as a baseline assessment when children come to rely upon wheelchairs for ambulation. Spinal fusion may be performed to straighten the spine, prevent further worsening of the deformity, eliminate pain (due to vertebral fractures), and slow the rate of respiratory decline (Bushby et al., 2010). Further complications include alterations in nutrition; pulmonary (aspiration pneumonias), urinary, or systemic infections; depression; learning or behavioural disorders; cardiac dysrhythmias; and eventually respiratory insufficiency and failure (as weakness of the chest muscles and diaphragm progresses).

Nursing Assessment

For a full description of the assessment phase of the nursing process, refer to page 1468. Assessment findings pertinent to DMD are discussed below.

Health History

Perform a standard family and child health history, being mindful of a family history of neurologic motor disorders. Note pregnancy and delivery history, as this information may be useful in ruling out a pregnancy problem or birth trauma as a cause for the motor dysfunction. Determine status of developmental milestone achievement. Children with DMD learn to walk but over time become unable to do so. If the child was previously diagnosed with MD, determine progression of disease. Inquire about functional status and the need for assistive or adaptive equipment such as braces or wheelchairs. Determine skills related to activities of daily living. Note history of cough or frequent respiratory infections, which occur as the respiratory muscles weaken. Consult respiratory therapy to conduct pulmonary function studies.

While talking with the child and family, determine whether psychosocial issues such as decreased self-esteem, depression, alterations in socialization, or altered family processes might be present.

Chronic pain was found to be a significant problem in youths with a neurologic motor disorder (Engel, Kartin, Carter, Jensen, & Jaffe, 2009). In this study, more than 70% of parents reported chronic pain in their children and more than half of the youths self-reported chronic pain. Therefore, it is prudent for the nurse to conduct a pain assessment. The best pain management strategies entail an individualized, multimodal approach (Engel et al., 2009).

Physical Examination

Perform a thorough physical examination of the child with suspected DMD or a known history of the disorder.

Particular findings related to inspection, observation, auscultation, and palpation are presented below.

Inspection and Observation

Observe the child's ability to rise from the floor. A hallmark finding of DMD is the presence of Gowers' sign: the child cannot rise from the floor in standard fashion because of increasing weakness (see Fig. 43.5). Observe the child's gait. Monitor for scoliosis. Determine effectiveness of cough and obtain results of cough peak flow and the maximal expiratory pressure (Kravitz, 2009). Monitor the trend in the child's weight and height.

Auscultation and Palpation

Auscultate the heart and lungs. Note tachycardia, which develops as the heart muscle weakens. Note adequacy of breath sounds, which may diminish with decreasing respiratory function. Note muscle strength with resistance testing and range of motion. Palpate muscle tone.

Laboratory and Diagnostic Tests

Serum creatine kinase levels are elevated early in the disorder, when significant muscle wasting is actively occurring. Muscle biopsy and genetic testing provides definitive diagnosis, demonstrating the absence of or defect in dystrophin. Following a positive muscle biopsy, genetic testing is mandatory (Bushby et al., 2009).

Pulmonary function studies will be performed on a child with DMD to determine the effectiveness of the cough. A maximal expiratory pressure of less than 45 cm H_2O is associated with ineffective cough and warrants use of cough-assistance techniques (Kravitz, 2009).

Nursing Management

Optimum management of DMD requires a multidisciplinary approach (Bushby et al., 2010). Nursing management is aimed at promoting mobility, maintaining cardiopulmonary function, preventing complications, and maximizing quality of life. Interventions directed at maintaining mobility and cardiopulmonary function also help to prevent complications. Refer to Nursing Care Plan 43.1 and individualize nursing care based upon the child's and family's response to the illness. Additional specifics related to care of the child with DMD are discussed below.

Promoting Mobility

Administer glucocorticoids as ordered. Daily use of a glucocorticoid is preferred to alternative regimens (Bushby et al., 2009). Patients not treated with glucocorticoids have a 90% chance of developing significant scoliosis (Bushby et al., 2010). Boys treated with glucocorticoids also have improved functional capacity and better pulmonary function than boys who are not treated with these medications (Davidson & Truby, 2009).

Encourage at least minimal weight-bearing in a standing position to promote improved circulation, healthier bones, and a straight spine. Individuals with DMD may use a standing walker or standing frame to maintain an upright position. Use orthotic supports such as hand braces or ankle–foot orthoses (AFOs) to prevent joint contractures. AFOs are contraindicated during ambulation because they typically limit compensatory movements needed for efficient ambulation, add weight that can compromise ambulation, and make it difficult to rise from the floor. Resting AFOs used at night can help to prevent or minimize progressive equinus contractures and are appropriate throughout life (Bushby et al., 2010). AFOs should be custom moulded and constructed for comfort and optimum foot and ankle alignment. Use of AFOs during the daytime may be appropriate for patients requiring full-time wheelchair use.

Schedule activities during the part of the day when the child has the most energy. Teach parents the use of positioning, exercises, orthoses, and adaptive equipment.

Decreased muscle extensibility and joint contractures occur as a result of various factors, including loss of the ability to actively move a joint through its range of motion, static flexed positioning, muscle imbalance surrounding a joint, and fibrotic changes in muscle tissue (Bushby et al., 2009). The maintenance of optimal ranges of motion and the management of joint contractures requires input from physical therapists. Active, active-assisted, or passive stretching should be performed 4 to 6 days per week (Bushby et al., 2010).

Maintaining Cardiopulmonary Function

The aim of cardiorespiratory care in DMD is to facilitate prevention or quick management of complications (Bushby et al., 2010). A well-planned, structured, proactive approach using assisted cough and nocturnal ventilation has prolonged survival (Bushby et al., 2010). Assess respiratory rate, depth of respirations, and work of breathing. Auscultate the lungs to determine whether aeration is sufficient and to assess clarity of breath sounds. Position the child for maximum chest expansion, usually in the upright position. Respiratory muscle weakness alters lung function and efficiency of breathing and leads to an inability to protect the lungs from recurrent pneumonia because of ineffective cough (Panitch, 2010).

Cough is the chief mechanism responsible for clearing the airways of secretions when the mucociliary escalator is ineffective, overwhelmed by infection and increased mucus production. Cough in patients with DMD may be compromised by respiratory muscle weakness. Assistance with airway clearance is a critical component of the care of children with DMD (Panitch, 2006). Alteration in breathing during sleep occurs well before sudden respiratory failure in these children (Panitch, 2010). Teach the child and family deep-breathing exercises to strengthen or maintain respiratory muscles and encourage coughing to clear the airways. In the ambulatory stage, minimum assessment of pulmonary function (forced vital capacity)

annually facilitates the child's and family's familiarity with the equipment.

The time when pulmonary care is truly needed is in the period following loss of independent ambulation. Monitor the results and trends of pulmonary function testing and pulse oximetry. When forced vital capacity is less than 40% predicted, volume recruitment or deep lung inflation is indicated by self-inflating manual ventilation bag or mechanical insufflation–exsufflation (Bushby et al., 2010). Manual or mechanically assisted cough techniques may be indicated during a respiratory infection or when baseline maximal expiratory pressure diminishes. There are a variety of ways to maximally insufflate the lungs to an adequate precough volume (Kravitz, 2009). Glossopharyngeal breathing (air-stacking or "frog breathing") is an effective technique for inflating the lungs one gulp at a time. Another way to achieve sufficient lung volumes is with the use of a self-inflating ambu bag (Kravitz, 2009). Acquire direct feedback from the patient to ensure that lungs are inflated to a sufficient yet comfortable volume (Kravitz, 2009).

Nocturnal ventilation is indicated in patients with signs and symptoms of hypoventilation. Optimally, use of lung volume recruitment and assisted cough techniques should always precede initiation of non-invasive ventilation (Bushby et al., 2010).

Use of intermittent positive-pressure ventilation and mechanically assisted coughing will become necessary in the teen years for some boys, possibly later for others (Gomez-Merino & Bach, 2002). The CoughAssist (a mechanical insufflator–exsufflator) is an effective means to clear airways in patients with neurologic motor disorders. This device is well tolerated with no increased risk for complications such as pneumothorax, gastro-esophageal reflux, or pulmonary hemorrhage (Kravitz, 2009). Teach parents monitoring and use of these modalities in conjunction with the respiratory therapist. Once assisted coughing is recommended, it should be used as a twice-daily preventive therapy.

The use of chest physiotherapy in patients with DMD is controversial and not fully established, although it may prove useful in DMD patients who have focal atelectasis from mucus plugging (Kravitz, 2009). There are not enough adequate studies to recommend the daily use of chest physiotherapy in patients with DMD (Kravitz, 2009).

Monitor cardiac status closely to identify heart failure early. Baseline assessment of cardiac function (including EKG and echocardiographic screening) should be performed at diagnosis or by the age of 6 years. Annual complete cardiac assessments should begin at 10 years or at the onset of cardiac signs and symptoms such as edema, weight gain, or crackles.

Maintaining good nutritional status, defined as weight or body mass index for age from the 10th to 85th percentiles, is essential (Bushby et al., 2010). Poor nutrition can potentially have a negative effect on every organ system. Anticipatory guidance and prevention of underweight or overweight status should be goals from the time of diagnosis and before commencing glucocorticoid treatments and then throughout life (Davidson & Truby, 2009). Referral to a dietician/nutritionist is recommended.

Maximizing Quality of Life

The best place to care for a child with a disability is in the child's home and community. Nurses must attend to sibling experiences and well-being with an awareness of siblings' increased risk for negative behaviours (Dauz Williams et al., 2010).

Long periods of bed rest may contribute to further weakness in the patient with DMD. Work with the family and child and occupational therapist to develop a schedule for diversional activities that provide appropriate developmental stimulation but avoid overexertion or frustration (related to inability to perform the activity). Periods of adequate rest must be balanced with activities. In Engel et al.'s study (2009), 80% of children with a neuromuscular disorder reported a sleep disorder. Walking or riding a stationary bike is appropriate for the child who has upper-extremity involvement. For the child with lower-extremity involvement, a wheelchair may become necessary for mobility, and the child may participate in crafts, drawing, and computer activities. Wheelchair sports can provide opportunities for physical activity as well as social interaction (Fig. 43.6). Participating in the Special Olympics or other such events may be appropriate for some children.

Provide emotional support to the child and family and referrals for parent education (e.g., positive discipline), group therapy, or family therapy as needed. Long-term direct care is stressful for families and becomes more complex as the child gets older (Chen, Chen, Jong, Yang, & Chang, 2002). In one study, one troubling aspect of caring for ventilator-dependent children at home was the mental health of mothers who are caring for these children (Sarvey, 2008). Families often need respite from continual caregiving duties. When a child is hospitalized, the family caregiver may or may not feel comfortable allowing nurses and other health care professionals to assume more of the child's daily care; this can be promoted as an opportunity for the caregiver to obtain respite from daily care. Respite care may also be offered in the home by various community services, so explore these resources with families. Families caring for children with chronic conditions face many challenges, including financial and time pressures, concerns over the well-being of the child, anxieties about lifelong care, social reaction and stigma, and aspects of future prognosis (Yantzi, Rosenberg, Burke, & Harrison, 2001). "Coping with the added challenge of traveling a far distance for health care may be the 'tipping' factor that topples the family over the threshold that they can manage" (Yantzi et al., 2001, p. 1789).

Assess the child's educational status. Some children attend school; others may opt for home-schooling. Administer antidepressants as ordered. Managing depression may increase the child's desire to participate in activities and self-care. Refer the child and family to Muscular Dystrophy Canada, which provides information and local support to families across Canada; visit http://thePoint. lww.com/Chow1e for a direct link to this organization. Ensure that families receive genetic counselling for family planning purposes as well as determining which family members may be carriers.

Spinal Muscular Atrophy

SMA is a genetic motor neuron disease that affects the spinal nerves' ability to communicate with the muscles. It is inherited via an autosomal recessive mechanism. The motor neuron protein SMN (survival of motor neurons) is deficient as a result of a faulty gene on chromosome 5. The motor neurons are located mostly in the spinal cord. Without adequate SMN, the signals from the neurons to the muscles instructing them to contract are ineffective, so the muscles lose function and over time atrophy. The proximal muscles, those closer to the body's centre, are usually more affected than the distal muscles. Emotional and mental development as well as sensation are unaffected by the disease (MDA, 2009c).

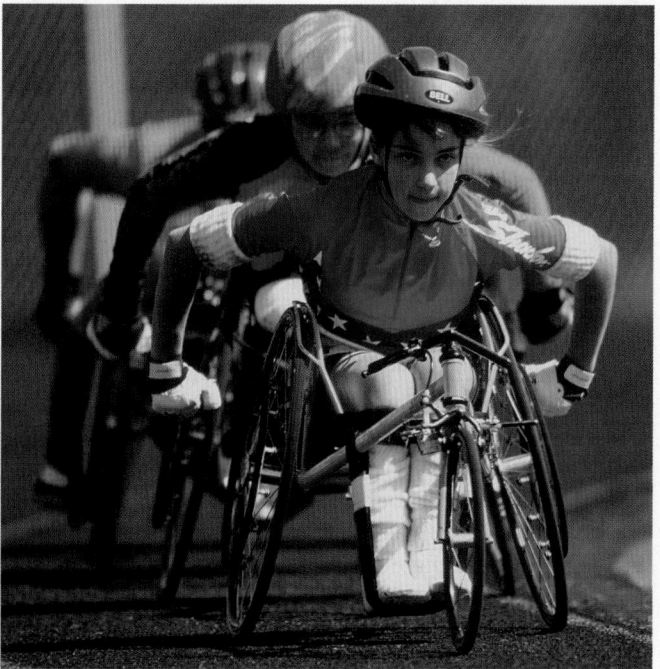

FIGURE 43.6 Wheelchair sports allow children with muscular dystrophy to experience physical activity and social interaction. (From: Bowden, V. R., & Greenberg, C. S. (2010). *Children and their families: A continuum of care* (4th ed.). Lippincott Williams & Wilkins.)

TABLE 43.1 **FEATURES OF SPINAL MUSCULAR ATROPHY**

Features	Type 1 SMA (Werdnig–Hoffman Disease, Infantile SMA)	Type 2 SMA (Intermediate SMA)	Type 3 SMA (Kugelberg–Welander Disease, Juvenile SMA)
Onset	Before birth to 6 months of age	6 to 18 months of age	After 18 months of age; child has started walking or has taken at least five independent steps
Symptoms	• Generalized weakness; cannot sit without support • Weak cry • Difficulty sucking, swallowing, and breathing	• Weakness that is most severe in the shoulders, hips, thighs, and upper back • Respiratory muscles may be involved • Scoliosis may occur	• Weakness that is most severe in the shoulders, hips, thighs, and upper back • Respiratory muscles may be involved • Scoliosis may occur
Progression	Rapidly progresses to early childhood death. Use of ventilators and gastrostomy feeding tubes may prolong life expectancy	Slower progression. Survival into adulthood common if respiratory status maintained appropriately	Slow progression. Lifespan usually unaffected. Walking ability maintained until at least adolescence; may need wheelchair later in life

Adapted from: Muscular Dystrophy Association. (2009c). *Facts about spinal muscular atrophy (SMA)*. Retrieved December 16, 2011 from http://www.mda.org/publications/PDFs/FA-SMA.pdf.

There are several types of SMA: type 1 (Werdnig–Hoffmann disease, infantile SMA), type 2 (intermediate), and type 3 (Kugelberg–Welander disease or juvenile SMA). Table 43.1 compares these three types, their usual progression, and their prognosis.

Respiratory muscle weakness may occur with all types of SMA and is usually the cause of death in type 1 and type 2 SMA (MDA, 2009c). Upper respiratory tract infections and aspiration related to dysphagia or gastro-esophageal reflux often develop into pneumonia and eventual respiratory failure, as the affected child cannot effectively cough independently in order to clear the airway. Many children with severe type 1 SMA are ventilator-dependent. The chest wall appears collapsed in children with type 1 and type 2 SMA because the ineffective intercostal muscles do not provide opposition against the diaphragm. The chest becomes bell-shaped and the xiphoid process is retracted (pectus excavatum), further restricting respiratory development. This respiratory compromise leads to poor clearance of airway secretions, sleep hypoventilation, underdevelopment of lungs and chest wall, and recurrent respiratory infections that exacerbate muscle weakness and lung integrity (Schroth, 2009). Inability to appropriately suck and swallow leads to difficulty in feeding the child with type 1 SMA. Weak back muscles affect the developing spine, resulting in the complications of scoliosis, kyphosis, or both.

Therapeutic management of SMA is supportive, aimed at promoting mobility, maintaining adequate nutrition and pulmonary function, and preventing complications. Spinal fusion may be performed in older children with significant scoliosis. Drugs that have been studied for use in type 2 and type 3 SMA include creatine, phenylbu-tyrate, gabapentin, and thyrotropin-releasing hormone, none of which has been proven beneficial (Bosboom, Vrancken, van den Berg, Wokke, & Iannaccone, 2009b). Pharmaceuticals have also not been proven to benefit patients with type 1 SMA (Bosboom, Vrancken, van den Berg, Wokke, & Iannaccone, 2009a).

Nursing Assessment

Note history of attainment of developmental milestones, as well as loss of milestones. SMA should be suspected in a child showing symmetrical weakness that is more proximal than distal and greater in the legs than arms, diminished or absent tendon reflexes, and preserved sensation (Wang et al., 2007). In the infant or child with known SMA, assess for recent hospitalizations or respiratory illness. Determine the respiratory support regimen used at home (if any). Note level of motor ability and identify the orthoses or adaptive equipment used. Elicit history related to feeding patterns at home. Assess for floppy appearance in the infant with SMA. Note decreased ability to initiate spontaneous muscle movement. In the infant or young child with SMA, note narrow chest with decreased excursion, relatively protuberant abdomen, and paradoxical breathing pattern. Observe chest for formation of pectus excavatum. Auscultate lungs for diminished or adventitious breath sounds. Monitor laboratory testing, which may include the following:

• Creatine kinase: elevated when muscular damage is occurring
• Genetic testing: identifies presence of gene for SMA
• Muscle biopsy: shows the muscle abnormality

- Nerve conduction velocity test and electromyelogram: to determine extent of involvement
- Polysomnography: overnight studies to determine respiratory insufficiency during sleep

Nursing Management

Nursing management of type 2 and type 3 SMA focuses on promoting mobility, maintaining pulmonary function, and preventing complications. Children with type 1 SMA need additional interventions related to prevention of complications from immobility and assistance with nutrition. Refer to Nursing Care Plan 43.1 for interventions related to these areas. Individualize the nursing plan of care based on the individual child's responses to the disorder.

Promote mobility through the use of range-of-motion exercises, lightweight orthotics, standing frames, and wheelchair use as appropriate. Support parents in their efforts to comply with physical and occupational therapy regimens. Older children may exercise with assistance in a warm pool. Position the child in a fashion that maintains appropriate body alignment.

Provide chest physiotherapy to assist with coughing and clearance of secretions. Use of a mechanical insufflator–exsufflator may provide better airway clearance (Chatwin & Simonds, 2009). In collaboration with respiratory therapy, teach families the use of non-invasive ventilation support, in which positive pressure is delivered to the lungs through a nasal or oronasal mask (Boitano, 2009). Provide routine tracheostomy care if the child has a tracheostomy (refer to tracheostomy sections of Chapter 34 and Chapter 39).

Administer gastrostomy tube feedings if ordered, and teach families gastrostomy tube care. Use bracing as prescribed to prevent spinal curvature. Inspect the skin frequently for breakdown in areas affected by bracing.

Cerebral Palsy

CP includes a number of disorders related to the development of movement and posture. Activity limitations are attributed to disturbances that occurred in the developing fetal or infant brain that affect sensation, cognition, communication, and behaviour (Rosenbaum et al., 2005). In the majority of cases, CP occurs before delivery but can also occur in the natal and postnatal periods (Johnston, 2007; Jones, Morgan, & Shelton, , 2007; Zak & Chan, 2010) (Box 43.1). Often no specific cause can be identified (Jones et al., 2007). CP is the most common movement disorder of childhood; it is a lifelong condition and one of the most frequent causes of physical disability in children (Johnston, 2007; Jones et al., 2007). In developed countries, the incidence is 1 to 2 in every 1,000 live births (O'Shea, 2008). The incidence is higher in premature and low birth weight infants (Hirtz et al., 2007; Jones et al., 2007).

BOX 43.1 Causes of Cerebral Palsy

Prenatal
- Congenital malformation
- Maternal seizures
- Maternal bleeding
- Exposure to radiation
- Environmental toxins
- Genetic abnormalities
- Intrauterine growth restriction
- Intrauterine infection, such as cytomegalovirus or toxoplasmosis
- Nutritional deficits
- Pre-eclampsia
- Multiple births
- Prematurity
- Low birth weight
- Malformation of brain structure
- Abnormalities of blood flow to the brain

Perinatal
- Prematurity (<32 weeks)
- Asphyxia
- Hypoxia
- Breech position
- Sepsis or central nervous system infection
- Placental complications
- Electrolyte disturbance
- Cerebral hemorrhage
- Kernicterus (a type of brain damage that may result from neonatal hyperbilirubinemia)
- Chorioamnionitis (infection of the placental tissues and amniotic fluid)

Postnatal
- Head trauma (e.g., motor vehicle accidents, abuse)
- Seizures
- Toxins
- Viral or bacterial infection of the central nervous system (e.g., meningitis)

Most affected children will develop symptoms in infancy or early childhood. There is a large variation in symptoms and disability. For some children it may be as mild as a slight limp; for others it may result in severe motor and neurologic impairments (National Institute of Neurologic Disorders and Stroke [NINDS], 2011a). Its primary signs include motor impairments such as spasticity, muscle weakness, and ataxia. Complications include epilepsy, visual and hearing abnormalities, sleep abnormalities, pain, gastric motility issues, esophageal dysmotility, gastro-esophageal reflux, delayed gastric emptying, sialorrhea (drooling), dental enamel erosion, respiratory disorders, and urodynamic abnormalities (Pruitt, 2009). Most children can survive into adulthood, but function and quality of life can vary from near normal to substantial impairments (NINDS, 2011a).

Pathophysiology

CP is a disorder caused by abnormal development of, or damage to, the motor areas of the brain. It results in a disruption in the brain's ability to control movement and posture. It is difficult to establish an exact location of the neurologic lesion, and the lesion itself does not change; thus, the disorder is considered nonprogressive since the brain injury does not progress. However, the clinical manifestations of the lesion change as the child grows. Some children may improve, but many either plateau in their attainment of motor skills or demonstrate worsening of motor abilities, as it is difficult to maintain the ability to move over time.

CP is classified in several ways, such as by the type of movement disturbance. Components of CP classification and a standardized classification system for CP are described in Box 43.2 and Table 43.2.

Therapeutic Management

Management involves multiple disciplines, including a primary physician, specialty physicians such as a neurologist and orthopedic surgeon, nurses, physical therapists, occupational therapists, speech therapists, dietitian, psychologist, counsellors, teachers, and parents. Spasticity management will be a primary concern and will be determined by clinical findings. There is no standard treatment for all children. The overall focus of therapeutic management will be to assist the child to gain optimal development and function within the limits of the disease. Treatment is mainly symptomatic, preventive, and supportive.

Medical management is focused on promoting mobility through the use of therapeutic modalities and medications. Many children will require surgical procedures to correct deformities related to spasticity. Multiple corrective surgeries may be required; they usually are orthopedic or neurosurgical. Surgery may be used to correct contractures that are severe enough to cause movement limitations. Common orthopedic procedures include tendon lengthening procedures, correction of hip and adductor muscle spasticity, and fusion of unstable joints to help improve locomotion, correct bony deformities, decrease painful spasticity, and maintain, restore, or stabilize a spinal deformity. Neurosurgical interventions may include placement of a shunt in children who have developed hydrocephalus. Another type of surgery, selective dorsal root rhizotomy, is used to decrease spasticity in the lower extremities by reducing the amount of stimulation that reaches the muscles via nerves.

Physical, Occupational, and Speech Therapy

The use of therapies such as physical therapy, occupational therapy, and speech therapy will be essential in promoting mobility and development in the child with CP. The earlier the treatment begins, the better chance the child has of overcoming developmental disabilities (NINDS, 2011a).

Physical therapists work with children to assist in the development of gross motor movements such as walking and positioning, and they help the child develop independent movement. They also assist in preventing contractures, and they instruct children and caregivers in the use of assistive devices such as walkers and wheelchairs. Occupational therapists may be responsible for fashioning orthotics and splints. AFOs are the most common orthotic used by children with CP (Cervasio, 2011) (Fig. 43.7). AFOs help prevent deformity from conditions such as contractures and help reduce the effects of existing deformities. They can help improve a child's mobility by assisting in control of alignment and helping to increase the

---

BOX 43.2 Components of Cerebral Palsy Classification

Motor Abnormalities
- *Nature and typology of the motor disorder:* the observed tonal abnormalities assessed on examination (e.g., hypertonia or hypotonia) as well as the diagnosed movement disorders present, such as spasticity, ataxia, dystonia, or athetosis
- *Functional motor abilities:* the extent to which the individual is limited in his or her motor function in all body areas, including oromotor and speech function

Associated Impairments
- The presence or absence of associated non-motor neurodevelopmental or sensory problems, such as seizures, hearing or vision impairments, or attentional, behavioural communicative, and/or cognitive deficits, and the extent to which impairments interact in individuals with CP

Anatomic and Radiologic Findings
- *Anatomic distribution:* the parts of the body (such as limbs, truck, or bulbar region) affected by motor impairments or limitations
- *Radiologic findings:* the neuroanatomic findings on computed tomography or magnetic resonance imaging, such as ventricular enlargement, white matter loss, or brain anomaly

Causation and Timing
- Whether there is a clearly identified cause (e.g., meningitis or head injury), as is usually the case with postnatal CP or when brain malformations are present, and the presumed time frame during which the injury occurred, if known

From: Paneth, N., Damiano, D., Rosenbaum, P., Leviton, A., Goldstein, M., & Bax, M. (2005). The classification of cerebral palsy. *Developmental Medicine and Child Neurology, 47*, 574–576.

TABLE 43.2   **CLASSIFICATION OF CEREBRAL PALSY**

Type	Description	Characteristics
Spastic	Hypertonicity and permanent contractures; different types based on which limbs are affected: • Hemiplegia: both extremities on one side • Quadriplegia: all four extremities • Diplegia or paraplegia: lower extremities	• Most common form • Poor control of posture, balance, and movement • Exaggeration of deep tendon reflexes • Hypertonicity of affected extremities • Continuation of primitive reflexes • In some children, failure to progress to protective reflexes
Athetoid or dyskinetic	Abnormal involuntary movements	• Infant is limp and flaccid • Uncontrolled, slow, worm-like, writhing, or twisting movements • Affects all four extremities and possible involvement of face, neck, and tongue • Movements increase during periods of stress • Dysarthria and drooling may be present
Ataxic	Affects balance and depth perception	• Rare form • Poor coordination • Unsteady gait • Wide-based gait
Mixed	Combination of the above (most commonly spastic and athetoid)	

efficiency of the child's gait. Spinal orthotics such as braces are used in young children with CP to combat scoliosis that develops due to spasticity. These braces are used to delay surgical management of the scoliosis until the child reaches skeletal maturity. Splinting is used to main-tain muscle length. Serial casting may also be used to increase muscle and tendon length.

Occupational therapy also assists in the development of fine motor skills and will help the child to perform optimal self-care by working on skills such as activities of daily living. Speech therapy assists in the development of receptive and expressive language and addresses the use of appropriate feeding techniques in the child who has swallowing problems. Speech therapists may teach aug-mented communication strategies to children who are nonverbal or who have articulation problems. Many chil-dren may not communicate verbally but can use alterna-tive means such as communication books or boards and computers with voice synthesizers to make their desires known or to participate in conversation.

Pharmacologic Management

Various pharmacologic options are available to manage spasticity. Medications are also used to treat seizure dis-orders in children with CP (refer to Chapter 37 for infor-mation related to seizure management). Oral medications used to treat spasticity include baclofen and diazepam (see Drug Guide 43.1). Anticholinergics may be pre-scribed to help decrease abnormal movements.

Parenterally administered medications such as botu-lin toxins and baclofen are also used to manage spastic-ity. Botulinum toxin is injected into the spastic muscle to balance the muscle forces across joints and decrease spasticity. It is useful in managing focal spasticity that is interfering with function, producing pain, or contributing

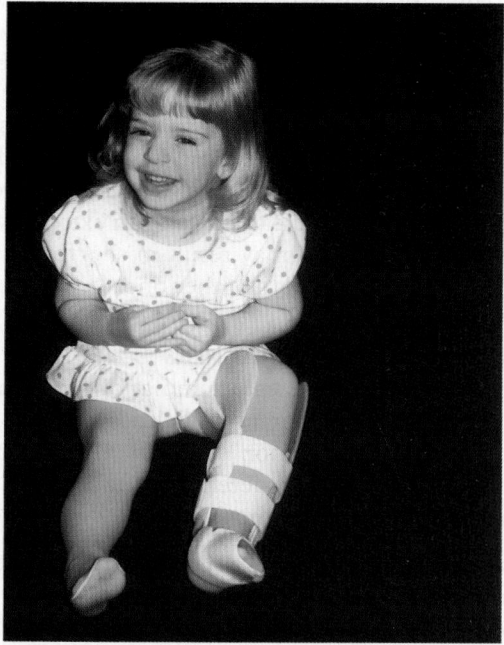

FIGURE 43.7 The child with cerebral palsy may benefit from wearing ankle–foot orthotics to provide the support needed for independent or assisted walking.

to a progressive deformity. Botulin toxin injection is performed by the physician or advanced practitioner and can be done in the clinic or out-patient setting.

Intrathecal administration of baclofen has been shown to decrease muscle tone, but it must be infused continuously due to its short half-life. Surgical placement of a baclofen pump will be considered in children with general spasticity that is limiting function, comfort, activities of daily living, and endurance. To test whether it is a suitable option, an intrathecal test dose of baclofen will be administered. If the trial is successful, a baclofen pump will be implanted. Once inserted, delivery of the drug can be individualized to meet the patient's unique needs. The pump needs to be replaced every 5 to 7 years and must be refilled with medication approximately every 3 months, depending on the type of pump. Complications with baclofen pump placement include infection, rupture, dislodgement, or blockage of the catheter.

Nursing Assessment

For a full description of the assessment phase of the nursing process, refer to page 1468. Assessment findings pertinent to CP are discussed below.

Health History

Elicit a description of the present illness and chief complaint. Obtain a detailed account of gestation and perinatal events (refer to Box 43.1). Common signs and symptoms reported during the health history of the undiagnosed child might include:

- Intrauterine infections
- Prematurity with intracranial hemorrhage
- Difficult, complicated, or prolonged labour and delivery
- Multiple births
- History of possible anoxia during prenatal life or birth
- History of head trauma
- Delayed attainment of developmental milestones
- Muscle weakness or rigidity
- Poor feeding
- Hips and knees feel rigid and unbending when child is pulled to a sitting position
- Seizure activity
- Subnormal learning
- Abnormal motor performance, scoots on back instead of crawling on abdomen, walks or stands on toes

Children known to have CP are often admitted to the hospital for corrective surgeries or other complications of the disease, such as aspiration pneumonia and urinary tract infections. The health history should include questions related to the following:

- Respiratory status: has a cough, sputum production, or increased work of breathing developed?
- Motor function: has there been a change in muscle tone, increase in spasticity?
- Presence of fever
- Feeding and weight loss
- Any other changes in physical state or medication regimen

Physical Examination

Observe general appearance. Pay close attention to the neurologic assessment and motor assessment. Assess for delayed development, size for age, and sensory alterations such as strabismus, vision problems, and speech disorders. Abnormal postures may be present. While lying supine, the infant may demonstrate scissor crossing of the legs with plantar flexion. In the prone position the infant may raise his or her head higher than normal due to arching of the back, or the opisthotonic position may be noted. The infant may also abnormally flex the arms and legs under the trunk. Primitive reflexes may persist beyond the point at which they disappear in a healthy infant. Evolution of protective reflexes may be delayed. Watch the infant or child play, crawl, walk, or climb to determine motor function and capability. Note any movement disorder. Infants with CP may demonstrate abnormal use of muscle groups such as scooting on their back instead of crawling or walking.

Assess active and passive range of motion. Pay particular attention to muscle tone. Though an increased or decreased resistance may be noted with passive movements, **hypertonicity** is most often seen. Increased resistance to dorsiflexion and passive hip abduction are the most common early signs. Sustained **clonus** may be present after forced dorsiflexion. Lift the child by placing your hands in the infant's or child's axillary area to assess shoulder girdle function and tone. Infants with CP often demonstrate prolonged standing on their toes when supported in an upright standing position in this fashion. Lift the young child off the ground while the child holds your thumbs to test hand strength. Observe for presence of limb deformity, as decreased use of an extremity (as in the case of hemiparesis) may result in shortening of the extremity compared with the other one.

Laboratory and Diagnostic Tests

A complete history, physical examination, and ancillary investigations are the primary modalities for establishing a diagnosis of CP. Common supplementary laboratory and diagnostic studies ordered for the diagnosis and assessment of CP include the following:

- Electroencephalogram: usually abnormal but the pattern is highly variable
- Cranial X-rays or ultrasound: may show cerebral asymmetry
- MRI or CT: may show area of damage or abnormal development but may be normal

• Screening for metabolic defects and genetic testing may be performed to help determine the cause of CP.

These tests will help determine whether CP is the likely cause of the child's symptoms or whether another condition is involved. These tests also will be important in evaluating the severity of the child's physical disabilities.

Nursing Management

Nursing management focuses on promoting growth and development by promoting mobility and maintaining optimal nutritional intake. Providing support and education to the child and family is also an important nursing function. In addition to the nursing diagnoses and related interventions discussed in Nursing Care Plan 43.1, interventions common to caring for a child with CP follow.

Promoting Mobility

Mobility is critical to childhood development. Treatment modalities to promote mobility include physiotherapy, pharmacologic management, and surgery. Surgical procedures are discussed above. Physical or occupational therapy as well as medications may be used to address musculoskeletal abnormalities, to facilitate range of motion, to delay or prevent deformities such as contractures, to provide joint stability, to maximize activity, and to encourage the use of adaptive devices. The nurse's role in relation to the various therapies is to provide ongoing follow-through with prescribed exercises, positioning, or bracing.

> ▶ **Take** NOTE!
>
> *Therapeutic horseback riding has been demonstrated to improve gross motor function in children with CP. If available in the local area, refer the child and family to the North American Riding for the Handicapped Association (Sterba, 2004; Sterba, Rogers, France, & Vokes, 2002).*

When casting, splinting, or orthotics are used, assess skin integrity frequently. Pain management may also be necessary. Nursing management of children receiving botulin toxin focuses on assisting with the procedure and providing education and support to the child and family. Nursing interventions related to baclofen include assisting with the test dose, providing preoperative and postoperative care if a pump is placed, and providing support and education to the child and family. Teaching Guideline 43.2 gives information related to baclofen pump insertion.

Promoting Nutrition

Children with CP may have difficulty eating and swallowing due to poor motor control of the throat, mouth, and

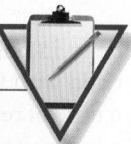

TEACHING GUIDELINE 43.2

Baclofen Pump: Patient/Family Education

• Check the incisions daily for redness, drainage, or swelling.
• Notify the physician if the child has a temperature greater than 38.5°C or if the child has persistent incision pain.
• Avoid tub baths for 2 weeks.
• Do not allow the child to sleep on the stomach for 4 weeks after pump insertion.
• Discourage twisting at the waist, reaching high overhead, stretching, or bending forward or backward for 4 weeks.
• When the incisions have healed, normal activity may be resumed.
• Wear loose clothing to prevent irritation at the incision site.
• Carry implanted device identification and emergency information cards at all times.

tongue. This may lead to poor nutrition and problems with growth. The child may require a longer time to eat because of poor motor control. Special diets, such as soft or puréed, may make swallowing easier. Proper positioning during feeding is essential to facilitate swallowing and reduce the risk of aspiration. Speech or occupational therapists can assist in working on strengthening swallowing muscles as well as assisting in developing accommodations to facilitate nutritional intake. Consult a dietitian to ensure adequate nutrition for children with CP. In children with severe swallowing problems or malnutrition, a feeding tube such as a gastrostomy tube may be placed.

Providing Support and Education

CP is a lifelong disorder that can result in severe physical and cognitive disability. In some cases disability may require complete intensive daily care of the child. Adjusting to the demands of this multifaceted illness is difficult. Children are frequently hospitalized and need numerous corrective surgeries, which places strain on the family and its finances. From the time of diagnosis, the family should be involved in the child's care. It is important to include parents in the planning of interventions and care of this child. In most cases they are the primary caregivers and will assist the child in development of functioning and skills as well as providing daily care. They will provide essential information to the health care team and will be advocates for their child throughout his or her life. It is important that nurses provide ongoing education for the child and family.

As the child grows, the needs of the family and child will change. Recognize and respect these needs. Providing daily intense care can be demanding and tiring. When a child with CP is admitted to the hospital, this may serve as a time of respite for family and primary caregivers. Encourage respite care and provide support and encouragement. Because CP is a lifelong condition, children will need meaningful education programs that emphasize independence in the least restrictive educational environment. Refer caregivers to the Cerebral Palsy Support Foundation of Canada, which provides information about local resources such as education services and support groups; visit http://thePoint.lww.com/Chow1e for a direct link to this organization. Refer children under age 3 years to the local early intervention program and services. Early intervention provides case management of developmental services for children with special needs.

Acquired Neuromuscular Disorders

A number of neuromuscular disorders may be acquired during childhood or adolescence. These include disorders resulting from trauma as well as those that are autoimmune, infectious, or toxic in nature. Unintentional injury continues to be the leading cause of childhood morbidity and mortality in Canada, with Aboriginal children experiencing a disproportionately higher rate of mortality and morbidity due to unintentional injury (Canadian Population Health Initiative, 2004). Children are at increased risk for trauma based on the developmental factors of physical and emotional immaturity. Adolescents are at increased risk due to the normal adolescent belief of invincibility. The developing neuromuscular system, if injured, may be irreparable, so the injury may have life-threatening or lifelong effects.

Neurologic trauma includes spinal cord injury and birth trauma or perinatal asphyxia. Autoimmune neuromuscular disorders include Guillain–Barré syndrome, congenital myasthenic syndromes, and dermatomyositis. Botulism, though uncommon in developed countries, is an important neuromuscular disorder resulting from food-borne infection. Environmental exposure to neurotoxins such as lead and mercury is associated with many cognitive and motor deficits in children (Abelsohn & Sanborn, 2010).

Spinal Cord Injury

Spinal cord injury is damage to the spinal cord that results in loss of function. Frequent causes are trauma (such as motor vehicle accidents), falls, diving into shallow water, gunshot or stab wounds, sports injuries, child abuse, or birth injuries. Spinal cord injuries are relatively uncommon in children, but when they do occur they have a devastating impact on the child's physical and functional status, social and emotional development, and family functioning. More spinal cord injuries are seen in adolescents due to their increased incidence of accidents, particularly motor vehicle accidents and diving into shallow water.

Spinal cord injury is an emergency that requires immediate medical attention. Cervical traction is often used initially, and surgical intervention is sometimes necessary. Ongoing medical treatment will be based on the child's age and overall health as well as the extent and location of the injury. Therapeutic management focuses on rehabilitation and prevention of complications. Spinal cord injury in children is managed similarly to that in adults.

Nursing Assessment

Symptoms vary based on the location and severity of the injury. Common signs and symptoms associated with spinal cord injury include:

- Inability to move or feel extremities
- Numbness
- Tingling
- Weakness

The higher the injury location in the spinal cord, the more extensive the damage and the greater the loss of function will be. High cervical injury will result in damage to the phrenic nerve, which innervates the diaphragm. Damage to this nerve will leave the child unable to breathe without assistance. Paralysis depends on the location of the injury in the spinal cord.

The diagnosis of spinal cord injury is made by clinical signs and diagnostic tests, which may include X-rays, CT, and MRI.

Nursing Management

Any child who requires hospitalization due to trauma should be considered at risk for a spinal cord injury, and immobilization of the spine is essential until full evaluation of the injury is complete and spinal cord damage is ruled out. Nursing management will be similar to management of the adult with a spinal cord injury and will focus on optimizing mobility, promoting bladder and bowel management, promoting adequate nutritional status, preventing complications associated with extreme immobility such as contractures and muscle atrophy, managing pain, and providing support and education to the child and family. Refer to the myelomeningocele section of this chapter for information related to urinary and bowel elimination.

The nurse plays an important role not only in the acute care of children with spinal cord injury but also during rehabilitation. Recovery from a spinal cord injury requires long-term hospitalization and rehabilitation. An interdisciplinary team of physicians, nurses, therapists, social workers, and case managers will work to manage the child's complex and long-term needs. Promoting communication among the interdisciplinary team is

TABLE 43.3 **COMMON TYPES OF INJURIES FROM NEUROMUSCULAR BIRTH TRAUMA**

Types	Description
Brachial plexus injury	• Occurs primarily in large babies, babies with shoulder dystocia or breech delivery • Results from stretching, hemorrhage within a nerve, or tearing of the nerve or the roots associated with cervical cord injury • Associated traumatic injuries include fracture of the clavicle or humerus or subluxations of the shoulder or cervical spine • Erb's palsy is an upper brachial plexus injury, and the involved extremity usually presents adducted, prone, and internally rotated. • Moro, bicep, and radial reflexes are absent, but the grasp reflex is usually present • Treatment consists of prevention of contractures, which involves immobilization of the limb gently across the abdomen for the first week and then the use of passive range-of-motion exercises • There is usually no associated sensory loss, and this condition usually improves rapidly • In some cases deficits persist, so observation is warranted
Cranial nerve injury	• Most common is facial nerve palsy • Frequently attributed to pressure resulting from forceps • May also result from pressure on the nerve in utero, related to fetal positioning such as the head lying against the shoulder • Physical findings include asymmetry of the face when crying; mouth may be drawn toward the normal side • The paralyzed side may be smooth, with a swollen appearance • Most infants begin to recover in the first week, but full resolution may take up to several months • In most cases, treatment is not necessary, only observation • In cases in which the eye is affected and unable to close, protection with the use of patches and synthetic tears may be necessary

essential and will be a key nursing function. Rehabilitation will need to focus on the ever-changing developmental needs of the child as he or she grows.

Prevention of spinal cord injuries is an important nursing consideration. Educate the public on vehicular safety, including seat belt use and the proper use of age-appropriate safety seats. Additional education topics include bicycle, sports, and recreation safety; prevention of falls; violence prevention, including gun safety; and water safety, including the risks associated with diving. This education can help decrease the incidence of spinal cord injury in children. Because socioeconomic differences in Canada parallel mortality and morbidity gradients in childhood injury, there is a strong need for targeted injury prevention efforts among children from economically disadvantaged populations (Faelker, Pickett, & Brison, 2000).

Birth Trauma

Birth traumas are injuries sustained by the newborn during the birthing process. They may result from the pressure of birth, especially in a prolonged or abrupt labour, abnormal or difficult presentation, cephalopelvic disproportion, or mechanical forces, such as forceps or vacuum used during delivery. Newborns at risk include multiple deliveries, large-for-dates infants, extreme prematurity, large fetal head, or newborns with congenital anomalies.

Most injuries are minor and resolve without treatment (Table 43.3).

Nursing Assessment

Assess the eyes and face for facial paralysis, observing for asymmetry of the face with crying or appearance of the mouth being drawn to the unaffected side. Ensure that the infant spontaneously moves all extremities. Note any absence of or decrease in deep tendon reflexes or abnormal positioning of extremities.

Nursing Management

Nursing management will be mainly supportive and will focus on assessing for resolution of the trauma or any associated complications, along with providing support and education to the parents. Provide parents with explanation and reassurance that these injuries are harmless. Parents are alarmed when their newborn cannot move an extremity or demonstrates asymmetric facial movement. Reassure parents and offer support. Provide parents with education regarding the length of time until resolution and when and if they need to seek further medical attention for the condition.

Guillain–Barré Syndrome

Guillain–Barré syndrome is a rare disorder in which the body's immune system attacks the peripheral nervous system. While Guillain–Barré syndrome occurs only in 0.6 to 4 per 100,000 people annually throughout the world, it is the most common form of acute neuromuscular paralysis in developed countries (Hughes & Cornblath, 2005; Pountney, 2009). There are at least four subtypes of Guillain–Barré syndrome (Hughes & Cornblath, 2005), and the incidence is lower in children than in adults (Alshekhlee, Hussain, Sultan, & Katirji, 2008). Although the reason for this is not fully understood, Guillain–Barré syndrome is believed to be an autoimmune condition triggered by a previous viral or bacterial infection, usually described as an influenza-like upper respiratory tract infection or an acute gastroenteritis with fever (NINDS, 2011b; Sivadon-Tardy et al., 2009). In rare cases, it has occurred after the patient has received an immunization or had surgery (NINDS, 2011b). Box 43.3 lists antecedent infections and events. In many cases the causative agent remains unidentified (Sivadon-Tardy et al., 2009).

Therapeutic Management

Treatment of Guillain–Barré syndrome is symptomatic and focuses on lessening the severity and speeding recovery. CSF filtration, plasma exchange, and administration of intravenous immunoglobulins may occur, especially in severe cases (Lugg, 2010). The goal of treatment is to keep the body functioning until the nervous system recovers. Guillain–Barré syndrome is a life-threatening condition, and some children will die during the acute phase as a result of respiratory failure. Up to 30% of patients have respiratory insufficiency, requiring mechanical ventilation (Lugg, 2010). The possibility of gastrointestinal pseudo-obstruction and urinary retention should be considered. Eighty percent of patients with Guillain–

Barré syndrome will make a full recovery, but a few may have a lengthy rehabilitation period.

Nursing Assessment

Early diagnosis and prompt treatment are essential since the disorder can quickly lead to respiratory failure and death from muscle paralysis. For a full description of the assessment phase of the nursing process, refer to page 1468. Assessment findings pertinent to Guillain–Barré syndrome are discussed below.

Health History

Elicit a description of the present illness and chief complaint. The clinical presentation is fairly similar in children and adults. It can occur a few days or weeks after the causative infection or event. Guillain–Barré syndrome has a quick onset and begins with muscle weakness and paresthesias such as numbness and tingling. In children, pain, especially of the lower extremities, has been reported as the initial presentation preceding motor involvement. Children with Guillain–Barré syndrome present with motor weakness and sensory loss beginning in the lower extremities. Typically, muscle weakness and sensory loss ascend in a symmetric fashion to the upper extremities over a period of several hours or days (Lee, Sung, & Rew, 2008; Pountney, 2009). This may be accompanied by discomfort or pain. Loss of reflex, such as the knee-jerk, is also commonly observed, and deep tendon reflexes disappear within the first few days of symptom onset. The onset phase has been arbitrarily defined as lasting up to 1 month (Hughes & Cornblath, 2005).

Other symptoms seen during the course of the illness include:

- Fairly symmetric flaccid weakness or paralysis
- Ataxia

Physical Examination and Laboratory and Diagnostic Tests

Physical examination findings may include decreased or absent tendon reflexes. Facial weakness or difficulty swallowing may also be present. Diagnosis is usually based on clinical findings of paralysis. In 80% of patients, CSF analysis reveals an increased level of protein, but this may not be evident until after the first few days of the illness. CSF should be analyzed before treatment with intravenous immunoglobulin. Neurophysiologic studies are important for diagnosis and subtype classification (Hughes & Cornblath, 2005).

BOX 43.3 **Antecedent Infections and Events Related to Guillain–Barré Syndrome**

Viral Infections
- Cytomegalovirus
- Epstein-Barr virus
- Herpes virus
- Human immunodeficiency virus

Bacterial Infections
- *Mycoplasma pneumoniae*
- Typhoid
- Paratyphoid
- Tuberculosis

Events
- Post-rabies vaccine and swine influenza vaccine
- Post-combined diphtheria, pertussis, and tetanus (DPT) vaccine
- Post-rubella, tetanus, cholera, and typhoid vaccines

Source: Joseph, S. A., & Tsao, C. (2002). Guillain–Barré syndrome. *Adolescent Medicine, 13*(3), 487.

▶ *Take NOTE!*

Tickling may be a successful technique for assessing the level of paralysis in the child with Guillain–Barré syndrome, either initially or in the recovery phase.

Nursing Management

Nursing management is supportive. In severe cases, the child may require intensive nursing care along with mechanical ventilation. Observe the child closely for the extent of paralysis and monitor for respiratory involvement. Nursing care focuses on the same concerns as in any patient with extreme immobility or paralysis.

Prevention of complications associated with immobility is a central concern and involves maintaining skin integrity, preventing respiratory complications and contractures, maintaining adequate nutrition, and managing pain. Interventions include turning and repositioning every 2 hours, assessing the skin for redness or breakdown, performing range-of-motion exercises, keeping the skin clean and dry, encouraging intake of fluids to maintain hydration status, and encouraging coughing and deep breathing every 2 hours and as needed. Enteral feeding or parenteral nutrition may be indicated if swallowing becomes impaired. Physical therapy may be helpful in preventing complications and promoting motor skill recovery. Provide support and education to the parents and child. The rapid onset and long recovery can be difficult and can cause strain on the family. If residual disability occurs or the recovery phase is longer than usual, the family will need help adjusting and caring for their child.

▶ **Take** NOTE!

Serial measurement of tidal volumes may reveal respiratory deterioration in the child with Guillain–Barré syndrome.

Myasthenia Gravis

In myasthenia gravis (MG) the immune system makes antibodies that inhibit the acetylcholine receptor (AChR) sites at the neuromuscular junction, thereby inhibiting normal neuromuscular transmission. The result is progressive weakness and fatigue of the skeletal muscles. Three types of myasthenic symptoms have been identified in children: neonatal, congenital, and juvenile.

- **Neonatal:** in 12% of pregnancies in which the mother has MG, she passes the antibodies to her infant through the placenta, causing neonatal MG. The symptoms will start in the first 2 days of life and disappear within a few weeks after birth. It is common for the mother's symptoms to improve during pregnancy, but they might worsen after labour.
- **Congenital:** children of a healthy mother can, very rarely, develop myasthenic symptoms beginning at birth. This is called congenital myasthenic syndrome (CMS). CMS is not caused by an autoimmune process but is due to synaptic malformation, which in turn is caused by genetic mutations. Thus, CMS is a hereditary disease. More than 11 different mutations have been identified, and the inheritance pattern is typically autosomal recessive.
- **Juvenile:** juvenile MG occurs in childhood but after the peripartum period.

A diagnosis of CMS is based on the following:

- Weakness that progresses as muscles tire
- A decremental electromyographic response, on low frequency, of the compound muscle action potential
- No anti-AChR or anti-muscle-specific kinase antibodies
- No response to immunosuppressant therapy
- Family history of symptoms that resemble CMS

Symptoms of CMS usually begin within the first 2 years of life, although in a few forms patients can develop their first symptoms as late as the seventh decade of life. The symptoms can vary from mild to severe. It is common for patients with the same form, even members of the same family, to be affected to differing degrees. In most forms of CMS weakness does not progress, and in some forms the symptoms may diminish as the patient gets older. Only rarely do symptoms of CMS become worse with time.

Therapeutic Management

Therapeutic management generally involves the use of anticholinesterase medications such as pyridostigmine, which blocks the breakdown of acetylcholine at the neuromuscular junction. Additional medications and treatments may include corticosteroids and other immunosuppressants, plasmapheresis, intravenous immunoglobulin, and in children who have reached puberty, thymectomy (Armstrong & Schumann, 2003). MG usually reaches maximum severity within 1 to 3 years of onset, and with proper treatment children can remain physically active. The condition may be aggravated by stress, exposure to extreme temperatures, and infections, resulting in a myasthenic crisis. Early diagnosis is a strong predictor of remission.

Nursing Assessment

Note history of fatigue and weakness; difficulty chewing, swallowing, or holding up the head; or pain with muscle fatigue. In the verbal child, note complaints of double vision. Observe the child for ptosis (droopy eyelids) or altered eye movements from partial paralysis. The neonate may display inadequate suck, weak cry, floppy extremities, and possibly, respiratory insufficiency. Note increased work of breathing. Laboratory testing may involve the edrophonium (Tensilon) test, in which a short-acting cholinesterase inhibitor is used. AChR antibodies may be present in elevated quantities in the serum.

Nursing Management

Administer anticholinergic or other medications as ordered, teaching children and families about the use of these drugs. Anticholinergic drugs should be given 30 to 45 minutes before meals, on time, and exactly as ordered. Encourage families to seek prompt medical treatment for suspected infections. Encourage appropriate stress management and avoidance of extreme temperatures. Teach families that physical activities should be performed during times of peak energy; rest periods are needed for energy conservation. Teach families to call their neurologist immediately if signs and symptoms of myasthenic crisis or cholinergic crisis appear. Encourage children to wear a medical alert bracelet.

> ▶ *Take* NOTE!
>
> *Signs and symptoms of myasthenic crisis include severe muscle weakness, respiratory difficulty, tachycardia, and dysphagia. Signs and symptoms of cholinergic crisis include severe muscle weakness, sweating, increased salivation, bradycardia, and hypotension.*

Dermatomyositis

Juvenile dermatomyositis is an autoimmune disease that results in inflammation of the muscles or associated tissues. It occurs more often in girls and is generally diagnosed between the ages of 5 and 14 years (MDA, 2009b). The autoimmune response may be triggered by exposure to a virus or to certain medications (MDA, 2009b). As with other autoimmune diseases, a genetic predisposition is present. The inflammatory cells of the immune system cause vasculitis that affects the skin, muscles, kidneys, retinas, and gastrointestinal tract.

First-line therapy includes high-dose daily corticosteroids, with emerging options in methylpredisolone and methotrexate. Second-line therapies are used for refractory patients, those considered to have severe features, or those with unacceptable medication toxicities. Options include intravenous gammaglobulin, cyclosporine, azathioprine, cyclophosphamide, mycophenolate mofetil, tacrolimus, rituximab, and anti-tumour necrosis factor–alpha agents (Wedderburn & Rider, 2009).

Nursing Assessment

Elicit a health history, which commonly involves history of fever, fatigue, and rash, usually followed by muscle pain and weakness. Determine onset and progression of muscle weakness. Inspect the skin for presence of rash involving the upper eyelids and extensor surfaces of the knuckles, elbows, and knees. The rash is initially a reddish-purplish colour, and then progresses to scaling with resulting rough-

ness of the skin. Test muscle strength, noting particularly weakness in the pelvic and shoulder girdles. Laboratory and diagnostic testing may include muscle enzyme levels, a positive antinuclear antibody test, and an electromyelogram to distinguish muscular weakness from other causes.

Nursing Management

Administer medications as ordered and teach families about their use; instruct them to monitor for side effects. Educate the family about the importance of maintaining the medication regimen in order to prevent calcinosis (calcium deposits) and joint deformity in the future. Encourage compliance with physical therapy regimens. Ensure that children are excused from physical education classes while the disease is active.

Infant Botulism

Botulism is a disease that is caused by a toxin produced in the immature intestines of young children following infection with the bacterium *Clostridium botulinum*. It is rare but can cause serious paralytic illness. According to Weir (2001), there are three main clinical forms of botulism: food-borne, intestinal, and wound related.

C. botulinum is an anaerobic, gram-positive, spore-forming bacillus common in the soil. The most frequent source in Canada is home-prepared products such as canned foods, fermented Inuit food, and improperly stored marine meat (Weir, 2001). Intestinal botulism occurs when spores are ingested and germinate in the gastrointestinal system. The gastrointestinal tract in the infant lacks the protective normal flora and *Clostridium*-inhibiting bile acids found in the normal adult gut. Botulism generally occurs in infants younger than 6 months of age (Arnon, 2007) and may be associated with feeding untreated honey to infants. Thus, honey should be avoided in children younger than 1 year of age (Vorvick, Vyas, & Zieve, 2011). Honey should never be added to baby food or used on a soother to quiet a fussy or "colicky" infant.

The disease is not infectious; to become infected, the child must ingest the bacterial spores. These spores then multiply in the intestinal tract and produce the toxin, which is absorbed in the immature intestines of the infant. It is generally not a problem for older children because the bacteria do not grow well in mature intestines due to the presence of the normal intestinal flora. Prognosis is good, but if treatment is not initiated, paralysis of the arms, legs, trunk, and respiratory system can develop. Therapeutic management is usually supportive but may involve administration of botulinum toxin in older children and teens.

Nursing Assessment

For a full description of the assessment phase of the nursing process, refer to page 1468. Assessment findings pertinent to botulism are discussed on following page.

Health History

Elicit a description of the present illness and chief complaint. Signs and symptoms usually occur soon after ingestion of the bacteria. Common signs and symptoms in infants reported during the health history might include:

• Constipation
• Poor feeding (due to poor swallowing)
• Poor sucking reflex
• Listlessness or irritability
• Generalized weakness
• Weak cry
• Loss of head control

Common signs and symptoms in older children reported during the health history might include:

• Double vision
• Blurred vision
• Drooping eyelids
• Difficulty swallowing
• Slurred speech
• Muscle weakness

Physical Examination and Laboratory and Diagnostic Tests

Assess for a diminished gag reflex, which is indicative of botulism. Diagnostic tests include cultures of stool and serum. Botulism is a rare disease and is difficult to diagnose since its symptoms are similar to those of other neuromuscular diseases. Therefore, assessment may include diagnostic tests to help rule out other diseases, such as Guillain–Barré syndrome, stroke, and MG. Laboratory proof of botulism is established with detection of the toxin or through culture of *C. botulinum* from gastric aspirate or stool (Weir, 2001).

Nursing Management

The local public health unit or a member of Health Canada's Botulism Reference Service should be contacted immediately when a case of botulism is suspected (Weir, 2001). One case of food-borne botulism represents a public health emergency.

Treatment is mainly supportive and focuses on maintaining respiratory and nutritional status. Antitoxin is not indicated in cases of infant intestinal botulism but may be indicated in older children (Weir, 2001).

Neurotoxins: Lead and Mercury Exposure

Lead and mercury exposures have been a major public health issue in Canada in recent decades (Fraser et al., 2006). Lead and mercury occur naturally in the earth's crust. Environmental sources include mining, smelting, fossil fuel burning, and waste incineration (Dewailly et al., 2001). These heavy metals can be transported from distant sources by water or air. Public health initiatives to remove environmental sources of lead and mercury have lessened childhood exposure to these toxic metals. For example, removal of lead from gasoline and paint and control of emissions from industrial sources have been successful in reducing the effects of lead in Canadian children (Tsekrekos & Buka, 2005). In the United States, lead-based paint in the home accounts for 70% of childhood cases of lead exposure. The remaining 30% of childhood lead exposures are from non-paint sources such as crayons, raisins, blinds, children's jewellery, and toys (Abelsohn & Sanborn, 2010; Tsekrekos & Buka, 2005). Lead was eliminated from all paint in 1991, but half of Canadian dwellings pre-date 1970 and still contain lead paint (Health Canada, 2011).

Exposure to mercury vapour is most commonly from dental amalgam, and exposure to organic mercury results from fish consumption (Brodkin et al., 2007). Occupational exposure to mercury is generally to mercury vapour and can occur in dentistry, mining, or manufacturing of electrical or medical equipment (Brodkin et al., 2007). Of special note is that many of Canada's indigenous peoples rely on seafood and waterfowl for subsistence and, therefore, may be exposed to unusually high doses of heavy metals (Dewailly et al., 2001; Harada et al., 2005). One study identified that a significant proportion of Inuit women in their reproductive years had lead and mercury blood concentrations that exceeded those levels associated with future mild neuro-developmental deficits in their infants and children (Dewailly et al., 2001). Lead and mercury negatively impact cognitive, behavioural, sensory, and motor capabilities. Recent studies suggest that prenatal and early postnatal exposure to very low levels of lead and mercury can adversely affect the child's development, including motor function, memory, learning, and behaviour (Fraser et al., 2006).

Children are more vulnerable to the effects of these heavy metal neurotoxins because children

• Are exposed more often by hand–mouth behaviours
• Spend more time on dusty floors
• Absorb neurotoxins more efficiently through their gastrointestinal tract
• May have a concurrent iron or calcium deficiency that increases absorption of neurotoxins
• Have biologically immature blood–brain barriers and liver detoxification systems (Abelsohn & Sanborn, 2010)

Currently, there is little evidence to support active treatment for mildly elevated blood lead levels (Tsekrekos & Buka, 2005). In 1994, the Canadian Task Force on the Periodic Health Examination concluded that there was limited evidence to recommend or not recommend chelation therapy in children aged 33 months to 12 years with blood levels between 1 and 2 μmol/L.

Nursing Assessment

For a full description of the assessment phase of the nursing process, refer to page 1468. Assessment findings pertinent to lead and mercury exposure are discussed below.

Health History

Signs and symptoms of lead toxicity include:

- Developmental disabilities, including speech deficits, learning disabilities (deficiencies in reading and math skills), attention-deficit/hyperactivity disorder, and aggressive behaviour
- Deficiencies in fine and gross motor skills
- Failure to grow
- Hearing loss
- Sleep disturbances
- Ataxia

Signs and symptoms of mercury toxicity include:

- Gingivitis
- Stomatitis and excessive salivation
- Metallic taste
- Sensory peripheral neuropathy
- Irritability
- Fatigue
- Ataxia
- Difficulties with memory and concentration

The American Academy of Pediatrics developed screening questions for parents to identify children who may be at risk for lead exposure, and these questions have been recommended for use in Canada. Ask parents these questions:

- Do you and your child live in or regularly visit a house/facility built before 1950?
- Do you and your child live in or regularly visit a house/facility built before 1978 that has been renovated within the past 6 months?
- Does your child have a sibling or playmate with a history of lead poisoning?
- Have you seen your child play with or eat paint chips?
- Do you live near lead smelting or processing plants or battery recycling facilities?
- Do you have a lead-related occupation or hobby (pottery, furniture refinishing)?

All refugee children aged 6 months to 6 years must be screened for lead poisoning within 3 months of arrival in Canada and again 3 to 6 months later (Abelsohn & Sanborn, 2010).

Physical Examination and Laboratory and Diagnostic Tests

Take a careful exposure history. When exposure to lead or mercury has been determined or suspected, appropriate blood tests should be completed. In the event that the serum lead or mercury level exceeds the recommended level, retest the blood immediately. Elevated blood lead levels (higher than 0.48 µmol/L) must be reported to the local public health department. Abelsohn and Sanborn (2010) propose that health care teams act upon levels higher than 0.24 µmol/L. A thorough neuropsychological evaluation and follow-ups are suggested for children with lead levels exceeding 0.20 µmol/L.

Nursing Management

Separate or remove the lead source from the child. If the child is iron deficient, iron supplementation can be neuroprotective by reducing gastrointestinal absorption of lead. Calcium and zinc supplements might also be indicated.

Chelation therapy is indicated when blood lead levels exceed 2.16 µmol/L and should be done by a health care team experienced in such treatment (Brodkin et al., 2007). Blood levels decline over time, but the half-life of lead is long and variable.

■■■ Key Concepts

- ■ Muscles, tendons, ligaments, and cartilage are all present and functional at birth, though intentional, purposeful movement develops only as the infant matures.
- ■ The spine is very mobile in the newborn and infant, especially the cervical spine region, resulting in a high risk for cervical spine injury.
- ■ The nurse's role in laboratory and diagnostic testing for neuromuscular disorders is mainly that of educating the child and family about and preparing the child for the test or procedure.
- ■ Assessment of range of motion and muscle tone is critical in the child with a neuromuscular disorder. Hypertonia or hypotonia is an abnormal finding in the infant or child.
- ■ Determining attainment of developmental milestones and subsequent progression or loss of those milestones is useful in distinguishing various neuromuscular disorders.
- ■ The nurse reinforces and carries out the exercise plans and adaptive equipment use as prescribed by the physical or occupational therapist in order to maintain muscle and joint function and to prevent complications.
- ■ Nursing management of a child with myelomeningocele focuses on preventing infection, promoting bowel and urinary elimination, promoting adequate nutrition, preventing latex allergy reaction, maintaining skin integrity, providing education and support to the family, and recognizing complications, such as hydrocephalus or increased ICP, associated with the disorder.
- ■ CP may result in significant motor impairment. Children with CP require ongoing physical therapy as well as nutritional intervention.

- Boys with DMD initially learn to walk at 18 months of age or older but later lose this ability.
- Respiratory compromise occurs in MD and SMA and eventually leads to death.
- Children with spinal cord injury require intense nursing management and lengthy rehabilitation to maintain or regain function.
- Children with neuromuscular disorders often experience pain, sleep disorders, and depression related to the chronic nature of the disorder.
- School attendance and participation in activities such as the Special Olympics are important for children with neuromuscular disorders.
- Because of biological and developmental factors, children are more prone to the neurotoxic effects of lead and mercury exposure, resulting in cognitive, behavioural, and motor disorders.

REFERENCES

Abelsohn, A., & Sanborn, M. (2010). Lead and children: Clinical management for family physicians. *Canadian Family Physician, 56,* 531–535.

Adzick, N. S. (2010). Fetal myelomeningocele: Natural history, pathophysiology, and in-utero intervention. *Seminars in Fetal & Neonatal Medicine, 15,* 9–14.

Alshekhlee, A., Hussain, Z., Sultan, B., & Katirji, B. (2008). Guillain-Barré syndrome: Incidence and mortality rates in US hospitals. *Neurology, 70,* 1608–1613.

Armstrong, S. M., & Schumann, L. (2003). Myasthenia gravis: Diagnosis and treatment. *Journal of the American Academy of Nurse Practitioners, 15*(2), 72–78.

Arnon, S. S. (2007). Botulism (*Clostridium botulinum*). In R. M. Kliegman, R. E. Behrman, H. B. Jenson, & B. F. Stanton (Eds.), *Nelson's textbook of pediatrics* (18th ed.). Philadelphia: Saunders.

Bakker, J. P. J., de Groot, I. J. M., Beelen, A., & Lankhorst, G. J. (2002). Predictive factors of cessation of ambulation in patients with Duchenne muscular dystrophy. *American Journal of Physical Medicine & Rehabilitation, 81*(12), 906–912.

Behrman, R. E., Kliegman, R. M., & Jenson, H. B. (2004). *Nelson's textbook of pediatrics* (17th ed.). Philadelphia: Saunders.

Boitano, L. J. (2009). Equipment options for cough augmentation, ventilation, and noninvasive interfaces in neuromuscular respiratory management. *Pediatrics, 123*(Suppl. 4), S226–S230.

Bosboom, W. M. J., Vrancken, A. F. J. E., van den Berg, L. H., Wokke, J. H. J., & Iannaccone, S. T. (2009a). Drug treatment for spinal muscular atrophy type 1. *Cochrane Database of Systematic Reviews,* Issue 1, Article No. CD006281.

Bosboom, W. M. J., Vrancken, A. F. J. E., van den Berg, L. H., Wokke, J. H. J., & Iannaccone, S. T. (2009b). Drug treatment for spinal muscular atrophy types II and III. *The Cochrane Database of Systematic Reviews [Computer File],* Issue 1, Article No. CD006282.

Brodkin, E., Copes, R., Mattman, A., Kennedy, J., Kling, R., & Yassi, A. (2007). Lead and mercury exposures: Interpretation and action. *Canadian Medical Association Journal, 176*(1), 59–63.

Bushby, K., Finkel, R., Birnkrant, D., et al. (2009). Diagnosis and management of Duchenne muscular dystrophy, part 1: Diagnosis, and pharmacological and psychosocial management. *The Lancet, 9,* 1–17.

Bushby, K., Finkel, R., Birnkrant, D., et al. (2010). Diagnosis and management of Duchenne muscular dystrophy, part 2: Implementation of multidisciplinary care. *The Lancet, 9,* 177–189.

Canadian Population Health Initiative. (2004). Improving the health of Canadians. Retrieved on December 23, 2011 from http://secure.cihi.ca/cihiweb/products/IHC2004_ch4_e.pdf

Carter, G. T., & McDonald, C. M. (2000). Preserving function in Duchenne dystrophy with long-term pulse prednisone therapy. *American Journal of Physical Medicine & Rehabilitation, 79*(5), 455–458.

Cervasio, K. (2011). Lower extremity orthoses in children with spastic quadriplegic cerebral palsy: Implications for nurses, parents, and caregivers. *Orthopedic Nursing, 30*(3), 155–159. doi 10.1097/NOR0b013e31821b6c18

Chatwin, M., & Simonds, A. K. (2009). The addition of mechanical insufflation/exsufflation shortens airway-clearance sessions in neuromuscular patients with chest infection. *Respiratory Care, 54*(11), 1473–1479.

Chen, J., Chen, S., Jong, Y., Yang, Y., & Chang, Y. (2002). A comparison of the stress and coping strategies between the parents of children with Duchenne muscular dystrophy and children with fever. *Journal of Pediatric Nursing, 17*(5), 369–379.

Cotton, S. M., Voudouris, N. J., & Greenwood, K. M. (2005). Association between intellectual functioning and age in children and young adults with Duchenne muscular dystrophy: Further results from a meta-analysis. *Developmental Medicine & Child Neurology, 47*(4), 257–265.

Dauz Williams, P., Piamjariyakul, U., Graff, J. C., et al. (2010). Developmental disabilities: Effects on well siblings. *Issues in Comprehensive Pediatric Nursing, 33,* 39–55.

Davidson, Z., & Truby, H. (2009). A review of nutrition in Duchenne muscular dystrophy. *Journal of Human Nutrition and Dietetics, 22,* 383–393.

deJong, T. P. V. M., Chrzan, R., Klijn, A., & Dik, P. (2008). Treatment of the neurogenic bladder in spina bifida. *Pediatric Nephrology, 23,* 889–896.

Dewailly, E., Ayotte, P., Bruneau, S., Lebel, G., Levallois, P., & Weber, J. P. (2001). Exposure of the Inuit population of Nunivak (Arctic Quebec) to lead and mercury. *Archives of Environmental Health, 56*(4), 350–357.

Engel, J., Kartin, D., Carter, G., Jensen, J., & Jaffe, K. (2009). Pain in youths with neuromuscular disease. *American Journal of Hospice and Palliative Medicine, 26*(5), 405–412.

Faelker, T., Pickett, W., & Brison, R. (2000). Socioeconomic differences in childhood injury: A population based epidemiologic study in Ontario, Canada. *Injury Prevention, 6,* 203–208.

Fischbach, F. T., & Dunning, M. B., III (2009). *A manual of laboratory and diagnostic tests* (8th ed.). Philadelphia: Lippincott Williams & Wilkins.

Fraser, S., Muckle, G., & Després, C. (2006). The relationship between lead exposure, motor function and behavior in Inuit preschool children. *Neurotoxicity and Teratology, 28,* 18–27.

Gomez-Merino, E., & Bach, J. R. (2002). Duchenne muscular dystrophy: Prolongation of life by noninvasive ventilation and mechanically assisted coughing. *American Journal of Physical Medicine & Rehabilitation, 81*(6), 411–415.

Harada, M., Fujino, T., Oorui, T., et al. (2005). Followup study of mercury pollution in Indigenous tribe reservations in the province of Ontario, Canada, 1975–2002. *Bulletins in Environmental Contamination and Toxicology, 74,* 689–697.

Health Canada. (2009). *Prenatal nutrition guidelines for health professionals: Folate contributes to a healthy pregnancy.* Retrieved December 16, 2011 from www.hc-sc.gc.ca/fn-an/pubs/nutrition/folate-eng.php

Health Canada. (2011). *Lead based paint.* Retrieved December 16, 2011 from http://www.hc-sc.gc.ca/hl-vs/iyh-vsv/prod/paint-peinture-eng.php

Hirtz, D., Thurman, D. J., Gwinn-Hardy, K., Mohamed, M., Chaudhuri, A. R., & Zalutsky, R. (2007). How common are the "common" neurologic disorders? *Neurology, 68*(5), 326–337.

Hsu, D. (2010). Cardiac manifestations of neuromuscular disorders in children. *Paediatric Respiratory Reviews, 11,* 35–38.

Hughes, R., & Cornblath, D. (2005). Guillain–Barré syndrome. *The Lancet, 366,* 1653–1666.

Johnston, M. V. (2007). Encephalopathies. In R. M. Kliegman, R. E. Behrman, H. B. Jenson, & B. F. Stanton (Eds.), *Nelson's textbook of pediatrics* (18th ed.). Philadelphia: Saunders.

Jones, M. W., Morgan, E., & Shelton, J. E. (2007). Cerebral palsy: Introduction and diagnosis: Part I. *Journal of Pediatric Healthcare, 21*(3), 146–152.

Joseph, S. A., & Tsao, C. (2002). Guillain–Barré syndrome. *Adolescent Medicine, 13*(3), 487.

Kaplan, M. S. (2003). Impact of repeated surgical procedures on the incidence and prevalence of latex allergy: A prospective study of 1263 children. *Pediatrics, 112*(2), 463.

Kinsman, S. L., & Johnston, M. V. (2007). Congenital anomalies of the central nervous system. In R. M. Kliegman, R. E. Behrman, H. B. Jenson, & B. F. Stanton (Eds.), *Nelson's textbook of pediatrics* (18th ed.). Philadelphia: Saunders.

Kravitz, R. (2009). Airway clearance in Duchenne muscular dystrophy. *Pediatrics, 123*(4), S231–S235.

Lee, J. H., Sung, I. Y., & Rew, I. S. (2008). Clinical presentation and prognosis in childhood Guillain–Barré syndrome. *Journal of Paediatrics and Child Health, 44,* 449–454.

Liptak, G. S. (2008). *Spotlight on spina bifida.* Retrieved December 16, 2011 from http://www.spinabifidaassociation.org/site/c.liKWL7PLLrF/b.2642343/k.8D2D/Fact_Sheets.htm

Lugg, J. (2010). Recognising and managing Guillain–Barré syndrome. *Emergency Nurse, 18*(3), 27–30.

Moore, C., Kogan, B. A., & Parekh, A. (2004). Impact of urinary incontinence on self-concept in children with spina bifida [abstract]. *Journal of Urology, 171*(4), 1659–1662. Retrieved December 16, 2011 from http://www.jurology.com/article/S0022-5347%2805%2962384-1/abstract

Muscular Dystrophy Association. (2009a). Facts about Duchenne and Becker muscular dystrophies. Retrieved December 16, 2011 from http://www.mda.org/publications/PDFs/FA-DMD.pdf

Muscular Dystrophy Association. (2009b). *Facts about inflammatory myopathies (myositis).* Retrieved December 16, 2011 from http://www.mda.org/publications/PDFs/FA-IM.pdf

Muscular Dystrophy Association. (2009c). *Facts about spinal muscular atrophy (SMA).* Retrieved December 16, 2011from http://www.mda.org/publications/PDFs/FA-SMA.pdf

Muscular Dystrophy Canada. (2009). *Comprehensive list of neuromuscular disorders covered by Muscular Dystrophy Canada.* Retrieved December 16, 2011 from http://www.muscle.ca/fileadmin/National/Muscular_Dystrophy/Disorders/Disorder_List_0903E.pdf

National Institute of Neurological Disorders and Stroke. (2011a). *NINDS cerebral palsy information page.* Retrieved December 16, 2011 from http://www.ninds.nih.gov/disorders/cerebral_palsy/cerebral_palsy.htm#What_research_is_being_done

National Institute of Neurological Disorders and Stroke. (2011b). *Guillain–Barré syndrome fact sheet.* Retrieved December 16, 2011 from http://www.ninds.nih.gov/disorders/gbs/detail_gbs.htm

Oakley, G. P. (2009). The scientific basis for eliminating folic acid-preventable spina bifida: A modern miracle from epidemiology. *Annals of Epidemiology, 19,* 226–230.

O'Shea, T. M. (2008). Diagnosis, treatment and prevention of cerebral palsy. *Clinical Obstetrics and Gynecology, 51*(4), 816–827.

Paneth, N., Damiano, D., Rosenbaum, P., et al. (2005). The classification of cerebral palsy. *Developmental Medicine & Child Neurology, 47,* 574–576.

Panitch, H. (2006). Respiratory issues in the management of children with neuromuscular disease. *Respiratory Care, 51*(8), 885–895.

Panitch, H. (2010). Paediatric neuromuscular diseases: The future is now. *Paediatric Respiratory Reviews, 11,* 1–2.

Pountney, D. (2009). Identifying and managing Guillain–Barré syndrome. *British Journal of Neuroscience Nursing, 5*(8), 381–383.

Pruitt, D. (2009). Common medical comorbidities association with cerebral palsy. *Physical Medicine and Rehabilitation Clinics of North America, 20,* 453–467.

Public Health Agency of Canada. (2008). *Canadian perinatal health report, 2008 edition.* Ottawa, ON: Author.

Robinson, R. (2011). Prenatal surgery to correct spina bifida found to improve fetal outcomes. *Neurology Today, 11*(6), 1, 6, 7. doi: 10.1097/01.NT.0000396251.38853.8d

Rosenbaum, P., Dan, B., Leviton, A., et al. (2005). The definition of cerebral palsy. *Developmental Medicine & Child Neurology, 47,* 571–573.

Sarant, H. B. (2007). Part XXVII: Neuromuscular disorders. In R. M. Kliegman, R. E. Behrman, H. B. Jenson, & B. F. Stanton (Eds.), *Nelson's textbook of pediatrics* (18th ed.). Philadelphia: Saunders.

Sarvey, S. (2008). Living with a machine: The experience of the child who is ventilator dependent. *Issues in Mental Health Nursing, 29,* 179–196.

Schroth, M. K. (2009). Special considerations in the respiratory management of spinal muscular atrophy. *Pediatrics, 123*(Suppl. 4), S245–S249.

Sivadon-Tardy, V., Orlikowski, D., Porcher, R., et al. (2009). Guillain–Barré syndrome and influenza virus infection. *Clinical Infectious Diseases, 48*(1), 48–56. doi: 10.1086/594124

Spina Bifida Association. (2011). *Spina bifida occulta.* Retrieved December 16, 2011 from http://www.spinabifidaassociation.org/site/c.liKWL7PLLrF/b.2700275/k.5F64/Spina_Bifida_Occulta.htm

Sterba, J. A. (2004). Effect of horseback riding therapy on gross motor function measure for each level of disability for children with cerebral palsy. *Developmental Medicine & Child Neurology, 46,* 47.

Sterba, J. A., Rogers, B. T., France, A. P., & Vokes, D. A. (2002). Horseback riding in children with cerebral palsy: Effect on gross motor function. *Developmental Medicine & Child Neurology, 44*(5), 301–308.

Tsekrekos, S., & Buka, I. (2005). Lead levels in Canadian children: Do we have to review the standard? *Paediatrics & Child Health, 10*(4), 215–220.

Vorvick, L., Vyas, J. M., & Zieve, D. (2011). *Botulism.* Retrieved December 16, 2011 from http://www.ncbi.nlm.nih.gov/pubmedhealth/PMH0001624/

Wang, C. H., Finkel, R. S., Bertini, E. S., et al. (2007). Consensus statement for standard of care in spinal muscular atrophy. *Journal of Child Neurology, 22*(8), 1027–1049. doi: 10.1177/0883073807305788

Wedderburn, L. R., & Rider, L. G. (2009). Juvenile dermatomyositis: New developments in pathogenesis, assessment and treatment. *Best Practice & Research Clinical Rheumatology, 23,* 665–678.

Weir, E. (2001). Botulism in Canada. *Canadian Medical Association Journal, 164*(4), 538.

Yang, M. L., & Finkel, R. S. (2010). Overview of paediatric neuromuscular disorders and related pulmonary issues: Diagnostic and therapeutic considerations. *Paediatric Respiratory Reviews, 11*(1), 9–17.

Yantzi, N., Rosenberg, M., Burke, S., & Harrison, M. (2001). The impacts of distance to hospital on families with a child with a chronic condition. *Social Science & Medicine, 52,* 1777–1791.

Zak, M., & Chan, V. W. (2010). Pediatric neurologic disorders. In S. M. Nettina (Ed.), *Lippincott Manual of Nursing Practice* (9th ed.). Philadelphia: Lippincott Williams & Wilkins.

RECOMMENDED READING

Arens, R., & Muzumdar, H. (2009). Sleep, sleep disordered breathing, and nocturnal hypoventilation in children with neuromuscular diseases. *Paediatric Respiratory Reviews, 11,* 24–30.

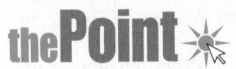

thePoint ✳ For additional learning materials, including Internet Resources, visit http://thePoint.lww.com/Chow1e.

CHAPTER WORKSHEET

MULTIPLE CHOICE QUESTIONS

1. A boy with DMD is admitted to the pediatric unit. He has an ineffective cough. Lung auscultation reveals diminished breath sounds. What is the priority nursing intervention?

   a. Apply supplemental oxygen.

   b. Notify the respiratory therapist.

   c. Monitor pulse oximetry.

   d. Position for adequate airway clearance.

2. A 7-year-old child with CP has been admitted to the hospital. Which information is most important for the nurse to obtain in the history?

   a. Age that the child learned to walk

   b. Parents' expectations of the child's development

   c. Functional status related to eating and mobility

   d. Birth history to identify cause of CP

3. The nurse is caring for a 2-year-old with myelomeningocele. When teaching about care related to neurogenic bladder, what response by the parent would indicate that additional teaching is required?

   a. "Routine catheterization will decrease the risk of infection from urine staying in the bladder."

   b. "I know it will be important for me to catheterize my child for the rest of her life."

   c. "I will make sure that I always use latex-free catheters."

   d. "I will wash the catheter with warm soapy water after each use."

4. The nurse is caring for a child with CP who requires a wheelchair to attain mobility. Which intervention would help the child achieve a sense of normality?

   a. Encourage follow-through with physical therapy exercises.

   b. Restrict the child to a special needs classroom.

   c. Encourage after-school activities within the limits of the child's abilities.

   d. Ensure the school is aware of the child's capabilities.

5. What is the priority nursing intervention for the child recently admitted with Guillain–Barré syndrome?

   a. Perform range-of-motion exercises.

   b. Take temperature every 4 hours.

   c. Monitor respiratory status closely.

   d. Assess skin frequently.

6. An 18-month-old lives in an old house with peeling paint on the porch. Renovations are in progress. The boy was walking at 13 months of age, but now he is experiencing difficulty with his balance and falls frequently. You are discussing the course of action with the parents and physician. What blood test is indicated?

   a. Iron

   b. Lead

   c. Calcium

   d. Mercury

CRITICAL THINKING EXERCISES

1. A 5-year-old girl, diagnosed with myelomeningocele, is admitted to the hospital for a corrective surgical procedure. Choose four questions from below that the nurse should ask when obtaining the health history that would assist in planning the child's care.

   a. What is the child's current mobility status?

   b. Is there a family history of myelomeningocele?

   c. What is the child's genitourinary and bowel function and regimen?

   d. Does this child have a history of hydrocephalus with presence of shunt?

   e. Does she have known latex sensitivity?

   f. Were there any complications during the pregnancy or birth of this child?

   g. Did the mother take prenatal folic acid supplementation?

(question continued on page 1502)

2. Based on the case in the above question, develop a nursing care plan for the child with myelomeningocele.

3. A 5-year-old child is admitted to the pediatric unit with a history of CP sustained at birth. The child is admitted for a scheduled tendon lengthening procedure. Based on your knowledge about the effects of CP, list three priorities to focus on when planning her care. Compare the care of this child with that of a child admitted for surgical correction of a broken femur with no significant past medical history.

4. A 3-year-old Inuit child is admitted with a history of gingivitis, ataxia, and peripheral neuropathy. The child's mother is present while the father stayed with the other 2 children in the home community. Based upon your knowledge of the negative effects of neurotoxins on motor, sensory, and cognitive function, list three priorities when planning care for this child and his family.

STUDY ACTIVITIES

1. In the clinical setting, compare the growth of a child with muscular dystrophy, spinal muscular atrophy, or CP with the growth of a similar-age child who has been healthy. What differences or similarities do you find? What are the explanations for your findings?

2. Identify the role of the registered nurse in the multidisciplinary care of the child with a debilitating neuromuscular disorder.

3. In the clinical setting, interview the parent of a child with DMD, myelomeningocele, spinal muscular atrophy, or severe CP. Determine the parent's feelings about the ongoing care for which he or she is responsible. Reflect upon this interview in your clinical journal.

4. In the clinical setting, compare the cognitive abilities of two children with a severe neurologic disorder. What are the reasons for the similarities or differences that you find?

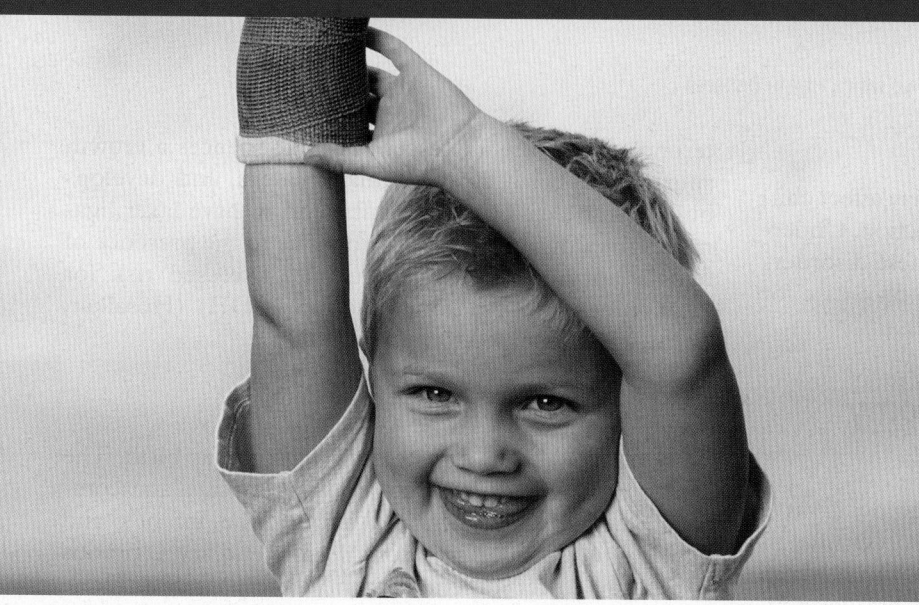

CHAPTER 44

Adapted by Sarah Southon and Kathleen Firth

NURSING CARE OF THE CHILD WITH A MUSCULOSKELETAL DISORDER

KEY TERMS

compartment syndrome
distraction
epiphysis
external fixation

immobilize
kyphosis
lordosis
ossification

splinting
traction
Trendelenburg gait

LEARNING OBJECTIVES

Upon completion of the chapter, the learner will be able to:

1. Compare the anatomy and physiology of the musculoskeletal system in children versus adults.
2. Identify nursing interventions related to common laboratory and diagnostic tests used in the diagnosis and management of musculoskeletal disorders.
3. Identify appropriate nursing assessments and interventions related to medications and treatments for common childhood musculoskeletal disorders.
4. Distinguish various musculoskeletal disorders occurring in childhood.
5. Devise an individualized nursing care plan for the child with a musculoskeletal disorder.
6. Develop patient/family teaching plans for the child with a musculoskeletal disorder.
7. Describe the psychosocial impact of chronic musculoskeletal disorders on the growth and development of children.

Dakota Dawes, 2 years old, is brought to the clinic by his mother. She states, "Last night Dakota said his arm hurt, but he didn't have any complaints during the day. Today when he was playing I noticed he wasn't using his right arm."

Wow

Nursing care that heals children to take wobbly steps, run, jump, fall, and get up again provides life itself in a child's world.

A variety of musculoskeletal disorders may affect children, but the result of each is motor dysfunction. Understanding the most common responses to these disorders gives the nurse the foundation required to plan care for any child with any musculoskeletal disorder.

Variations in Pediatric Anatomy and Physiology

Musculoskeletal disorders in children may occur as a congenital malformation or a genetic disorder that is present from birth but may not be identified until later in childhood or adolescence. Some disorders are developmental; others result from trauma. The infant and young child have resilient soft tissue, so sprains and strains are less common in this age group. Older school-age children and adolescents often participate in sports, resulting in an increased risk of injuries such as sprains, fractures, and torn ligaments. The musculoskeletal system in infants and children is immature compared with that in adults; thus, when a musculoskeletal problem occurs in childhood, the child's growth may be hindered. The immobility associated with most musculoskeletal disorders may affect the child's development and acquisition of motor skills.

Myelination

Myelination of the central nervous system continues to progress after birth and is complete by about 2 years of age. Myelination proceeds in a cephalocaudal and proximal–distal fashion, allowing voluntary muscle control to progress as myelination occurs. As myelination proceeds, the speed and accuracy of nerve impulses increase. Primitive reflexes are replaced with voluntary movement.

Muscle Development

The muscular system, including tendons, ligaments, and cartilage, arises from the mesoderm in early embryonic development. At birth (term or preterm), the muscles, tendons, ligaments, and cartilage are all present and functional. The newborn infant is capable of spontaneous movement but lacks purposeful control. Full range of motion is present at birth. Healthy infants and children demonstrate normal muscle tone. As the infant matures and becomes mobile, the muscles develop further and become stronger and their mass increases. The infant's muscles account for approximately 25% of total body weight, as compared with the adult's muscle mass, which accounts for about 40% of total body weight (Bechard, Wroe, & Ellis, 2008). Muscles grow rapidly in adolescence; this contributes to clumsiness, which places the teen at increased risk for injury. In response to testos-

terone release, the adolescent boy experiences a growth spurt, particularly in the trunk and legs, and develops bulkier muscles. Female infants tend to have laxer ligaments than male infants, possibly due to the presence of female hormones, placing them at increased risk for developmental dysplasia of the hip (DDH) (Hosalkar, Horn, Friedman, & Dormans, 2007b).

Skeletal Development

The infant's skeleton is not fully ossified at birth. The skeleton contains increased amounts of cartilage compared with adolescents and adults. The infant's and young child's bones are more flexible and more porous and have a lower mineral content than the adult's. These structural differences of a young child's bones allow for greater shock absorption, so the bones will often bend rather than break when an injury occurs. The thick, strong periosteum of the child's bones allows for a greater absorption of force than is seen in adults. As a result, the cortex of the bone does not always break, sometimes buckling or bending only. **Ossification** and conversion of cartilage to bone continue throughout childhood and are complete at adolescence.

During fetal development the spine displays **kyphosis**. Cervical **lordosis** develops as the infant starts to hold the head up. When the infant or toddler assumes an upright position, the primary and secondary curves of the spine begin to develop. The balance of the curves allows the head to be centred over the pelvis. During the toddler years, the period of early walking, lumbar lordosis may be significant (also termed toddler lordosis), and the toddler appears quite swaybacked and potbellied. As the child develops, the spine takes on more adult-like curves. During adolescence thoracic kyphosis may become evident. This is most often a postural effect, and as the teen matures, the posture appears similar to that of an adult.

Growth Plate

The ends of the bones in young children are composed of the **epiphysis** and the physis, in combination termed the growth plate. In infants, the epiphyses are cartilaginous and ossify over time. In children, the epiphysis is the secondary ossification centre at the end of the bone. The physis is a cartilaginous area between the epiphysis and the metaphysis. Growth of the bones occurs primarily in the epiphyseal region. This area is vulnerable and structurally weak. Traumatic force applied to the epiphysis during injury may result in fracture in that area of the bone. Epiphyseal injury may result in early, incomplete, or partial closure of the growth plate, leading to deformity or shortening of the bone. Epiphyseal growth continues until skeletal maturity is reached during adolescence. Production of androgens in adolescence gradually causes the growth plates to fuse, and thus long bone growth is complete (Fig. 44.1).

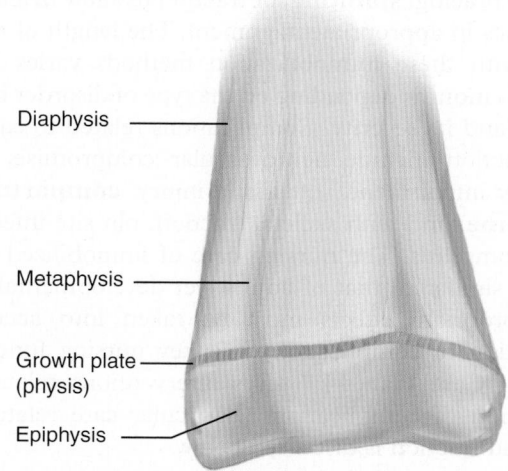

FIGURE 44.1 Anatomic areas of growing bone.

Diaphysis

Metaphysis

Growth plate
(physis)

Epiphysis

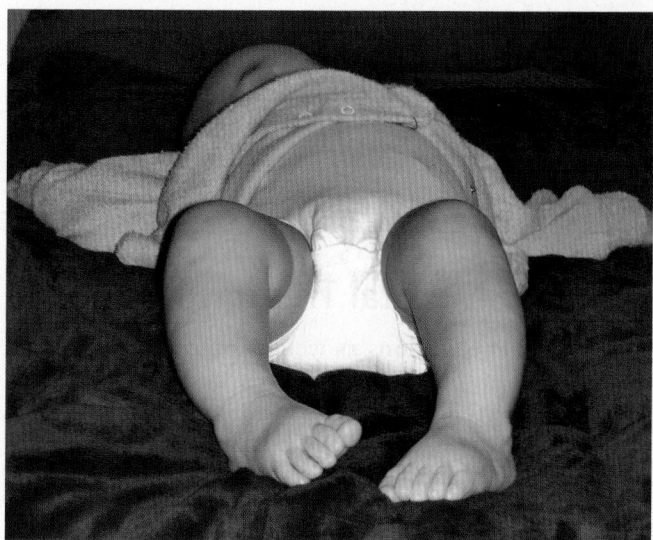

FIGURE 44.2 Internal tibial torsion with metatarsus adductus—normal findings in the infant.

Bone Healing

The child's bones have a thick, strong periosteum with an abundant blood supply. Bone healing occurs in the same fashion as in the adult, but because of the rich nutrient supply to the periosteum, it occurs more quickly in children. Children's bones produce callus more rapidly and in larger quantities than do adults'. As new bone cells quickly form, a bulge of new bone growth occurs at the site of the fracture. The younger the child, the more quickly the bone heals. Also, the closer the fracture is to the growth plate (epiphysis), the more quickly the fracture heals. The capacity for remodeling (the process of breaking down and forming new bone) is increased in children as compared with adults. This means that straightening of the bone over time occurs more easily in children who have not achieved skeletal maturity.

Positional Alterations

The lower extremities of the infant tend to have a bowed appearance, attributed to in utero positioning. In utero, the fetus' hips are usually flexed, abducted, and externally rotated, with the knees also flexed and the lower limbs inwardly rotated (Fig. 44.2). This normal developmental variation is termed internal tibial torsion. The legs straighten with passive motion, and internal tibial torsion should not be confused with "bowlegs." Internal tibial torsion usually resolves independently sometime in the second or third year of life as the toddler bears weight and the lower extremity muscles and bones mature. The bowlegged appearance is sometimes also referred to as genu varum. As internal tibial torsion or genu varum resolves, physiologic genu valgum occurs. Children usually demonstrate symmetric genu valgum (knock-knees) by the age of 2 to 3 years. In genu valgum, when the knees are touching the ankles are significantly separated, with the lower portion of the legs

angled outward (Fig. 44.3). By age 7 or 8 years, genu valgum gradually resolves in most children.

The newborn's feet also display in-toeing (metatarsus adductus) as a result of in utero positioning (see Fig. 44.2). The feet remain flexible and may be passively moved to midline and in a straight position. This also resolves as the infant's musculoskeletal system matures. Pes planus (flat feet) is noted in infants when they begin to walk. The long arch of the foot is not yet developed and makes contact with the floor, resulting in a medial bulge. As the child grows and the muscles become less lax, the arch generally develops. Some children may continue with flexible flat feet, and this is considered a normal variation.

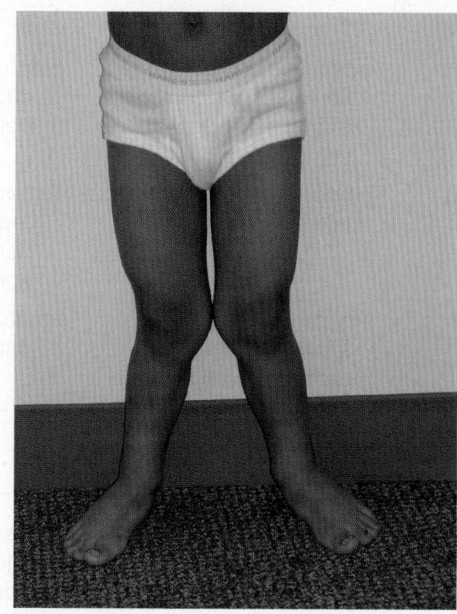

FIGURE 44.3 Genu valgum (knock-knees): note knees touching at midline and outward angle of the lower half of the legs.

▶ *Take* NOTE!

Fractures are rare in children less than 1 year of age. The infant who presents with a fracture should be carefully evaluated for child abuse or an underlying musculoskeletal disorder (Grewal & Ahier, 2010).

Common Medical Treatments

A variety of medications as well as other medical treatments are used to treat musculoskeletal disorders in children. Most of these treatments will require a physician's order when the child is in the hospital. The most common treatments and medications are listed in Common Medical Treatments 44.1 and Drug Guide 44.1. The nurse caring for the child with a musculoskeletal disorder should become familiar with what the procedures are, how they work, as well as common nursing implications related to use of these modalities. The treatment of musculoskeletal disorders often involves immobilization via casting, bracing, **splinting**, or traction to allow healing in the bones in appropriate alignment. The length of treatment with these immobilization methods varies from weeks to months depending on the type of disorder being treated and its severity. Complications related to casting and traction include neurovascular compromise, skin integrity impairment, soft tissue injury, **compartment syndrome**, and with skeletal traction, pin site infection or osteomyelitis. The nursing care of immobilized children is similar to that of adults, yet developmental and age-appropriate effects must be taken into account. Prevention of complications is a key nursing function. Nursing Care Plan 44.1 gives interventions related to prevention of complications. Particular care related to casts and traction is discussed below.

Casts

Casts are used to **immobilize** a bone that has been injured or a diseased joint. When a fracture has occurred, a cast

(text continues on page 1509)

COMMON MEDICAL TREATMENTS 44.1

Treatment	Explanation	Indication	Nursing Implications
Traction	Application of a pulling force on an extremity or body part	Fracture reduction, dislocations, correction of deformities	To maintain even, constant traction: • Ensure weights hang free at all times and ropes remain in the pulley grooves • Keep weights out of child's reach • Maintain prescribed weight • Elevate head or foot of bed only with physician's order Monitor for complications: • Perform neurovascular checks at least every 4 h • Assess for skin impairment
Casting	Application of plaster or fibreglass material to form a rigid apparatus to immobilize a body part	Fracture reduction, dislocations, correction of deformities	Assess frequently for neurovascular compromise, skin impairment at cast edges Protect cast from moisture Teach family how to care for cast at home
Splinting	Temporary stiff support of injured area	Temporary fracture reduction, immobilization and support of sprains	Similar to cast care. Some splints are removable and are replaced when the child is out of bed Teach family appropriate use of splints
Fixation	Surgical reduction of a fracture or skeletal deformity with an internal or external pin or fixation device	Fractures, skeletal deformities	No additional care for internal fixation External fixation: perform pin care as prescribed by the surgeon Assess for excess drainage or pin slippage, notifying physician if this occurs Velcro or snaps on sleeves and pant legs help with dressing
Cold therapy	Application of ice bags, commercial cold packs, or cold compresses	Most often used in acute injuries to cause vasoconstriction, thereby decreasing pain and swelling	Apply for 20–30 min, then remove for 1 h, then reapply for 20–30 min Discontinue when numbness occurs Place a towel between the cold pack and the skin to prevent thermal injury

Treatment	Explanation	Indication	Nursing Implications
Crutches	Ambulatory devices that transfer body weight from lower to upper extremities	Used whenever weight-bearing is contraindicated	Top of crutch should reach two to three finger-breadths below the axillae to prevent nerve palsy Teach child appropriate ambulation with crutches or reinforce teaching if performed by physical therapist
Physical therapy, occupational therapy	Physical therapy focuses on attainment or improvement of gross motor skills. Occupational therapy focuses on refinement of fine motor skills, feeding, and activities of daily living	Restore function after injury or surgery; promote developmental activities when limb use is compromised, as in limb deficiency	Provide follow-through with prescribed exercises or supportive equipment. Success of therapy is dependent upon continued compliance with the prescribed regimen Ensure adequate communication exists within the interdisciplinary team
Orthotics, braces	Adaptive positioning devices specially fitted for each child by the physical or occupational therapist or orthotist. Used to maintain proper body or extremity alignment, improve mobility, and prevent contractures	Used to immobilize a body part or prevent deformity through positioning. Used to treat developmental dysplasia of the hip and scoliosis; also may be used for a period of time after cast removal	Provide frequent assessments of skin covered by the device to avoid skin breakdown Cotton undergarment worn under the brace helps to maintain skin integrity Follow the therapist's schedule of recommended "on" and "off" times Encourage families to comply with use

DRUG GUIDE 44.1   COMMON DRUGS FOR MUSCULOSKELETAL DISORDERS

Medication	Action	Indication	Nursing Implications
Benzodiazepines (diazepam, lorazepam)	Antianxiety drugs that also have the effect of skeletal muscle relaxation	Treatment of muscle spasms associated with traction or casting	Monitor sedation level May cause dizziness Paradoxical excitement may occur Assess for improvements in spasms
Acetaminophen	Blocks pain impulses in response to inhibition of prostaglandin synthesis	Relief of mild pain if used alone, moderate or severe pain if used with a narcotic analgesic	Often combined with a narcotic such as codeine or oxycodone for increased analgesic effect Monitor pain levels and response to medication
Narcotic analgesics	Act on receptors in the brain to alter perception of pain	Relief of moderate to severe pain associated with injuries, orthopedic procedures	Assess pain location, quality, intensity, and duration Assess respiratory rate prior to and periodically after administration Monitor sedation level May cause nausea, vomiting, constipation, pupil constriction
Nonsteroidal anti-inflammatory drugs (NSAIDs: ibuprofen, ketorolac)	Inhibit prostaglandin synthesis, having a direct inhibitory effect on pain perception	Relief of mild to moderate pain. Treatment of Legg–Calvé–Perthes disease	Monitor for nausea, vomiting, diarrhea, constipation Administer with water or food to decrease GI upset
Bisphosphonate: IV—pamidronate, zoledronic acid; oral—alendronate, risedronate	Increase bone mineral density	Decrease incidence of fractures in moderate to severe osteogenesis imperfecta	IV: given at 4-month intervals, causes a decrease in serum calcium level, influenza-like reaction with first IV dose Oral: side effects include heartburn, regurgitation, upper abdominal discomfort

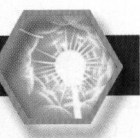

Nursing Care Plan 44.1

OVERVIEW FOR THE CHILD WITH A MUSCULOSKELETAL DISORDER

NURSING DIAGNOSIS: Impaired physical mobility related to injury, pain, or weakness as evidenced by inability to move an extremity, to ambulate, or to move without limitations

Outcome Identification and Evaluation

Child will engage in physical activities within limits of injury or disease: *Child will assist with transfers and positioning in bed and/or participate in prescribed bed exercises.*

Intervention: Maximizing Physical Mobility

- Assess child's ability to move based upon injury or disease and within limits of prescribed treatment *to determine baseline.*
- Prior to prescribed exercise or major position changes, ensure that pain medication is given: *Relief of pain increases child's ability to tolerate and participate in activity.*
- Use passive and active range-of-motion exercises and teach child and family how to perform them *to facilitate joint mobility and muscle development (active ROM) and to help increase mobility (within limits of restrictions related to injury or prescribed treatment).*
- Praise accomplishments and emphasize child's abilities *to improve self-esteem and encourage feelings of confidence and competence.*
- Teach child and family necessary care related to mobility issues *so the family can continue with these measures at home.*

NURSING DIAGNOSIS: Risk for constipation related to immobility and/or use of narcotic analgesics

Outcome Identification and Evaluation

Child will demonstrate adequate stool passage, *will pass soft, formed stool every 1 to 3 days without straining or other adverse effects.*

Intervention: Promoting Appropriate Bowel Elimination

- Assess usual pattern of stooling *to determine baseline and identify potential problems with elimination.*
- Palpate for abdominal fullness and auscultate for bowel sounds *to assess for bowel function and presence of constipation.*
- Encourage fibre intake *to increase frequency of stools.*
- Ensure adequate fluid intake *to prevent formation of hard, dry stools.*
- Encourage activity within child's limits or restrictions *as even minimal activity increases peristalsis.*

NURSING DIAGNOSIS: Self-care deficit related to immobility as evidenced by inability to perform hygiene care and transfer self independently

Outcome Identification and Evaluation

Child will demonstrate ability to care for self within age parameters and limits of disease: *Child is able to feed, dress, and manage elimination within limits of injury or disease and age.*

Intervention: Maximizing Self-care

- Introduce child and family to self-help methods as soon as possible *to promote independence from the beginning.*
- Encourage family and staff to allow child to do as much as possible *to allow child to gain confidence and independence.*
- Collaborate with physical therapy and occupational therapy as needed to provide child and family with appropriate tools to modify environment and methods to promote transferring and self-care *to allow for maximum functioning.*
- Praise accomplishments and emphasize child's abilities *to improve self-esteem and encourage feelings of confidence and competence.*
- Balance activity with periods to rest *to reduce fatigue and increase energy available for self-care.*

NURSING DIAGNOSIS: Risk for impaired skin integrity related to immobility, casting, traction, use of braces or adaptive devices

Outcome Identification and Evaluation

Child's skin will remain intact, *without evidence of redness or breakdown.*

Intervention: Promoting Skin Integrity

- Monitor condition of entire skin surface at least daily *to provide baseline and allow for early identification of areas at risk.*

Nursing Care Plan 44.1 (continued)

- Avoid excessive friction or harsh cleaning products *that may increase risk of breakdown in child with susceptible skin.*
- Keep child's skin free from stool and urine *to decrease risk of breakdown.*
- Keep linen free from food crumbs and wrinkles *to prevent pressure areas from forming.*
- Change child's position frequently *to decrease pressure on susceptible areas.*
- Monitor condition of skin affected by braces or adaptive equipment frequently *to prevent skin breakdown related to poor fit.*

For the child in traction:
- Pad bony prominences with cotton padding before applying traction *to protect skin from injury.*
- Gently massage child's back and sacrum with lotion *to stimulate circulation.*

For the child in a spica cast:
- Apply plastic wrap to the perineal edges of the cast *to prevent soiling of cast edges, which can contribute to cast breakdown.*
- Use a fracture bedpan *to facilitate toileting without soiling cast.*
- For the child still in diapers, tuck a smaller diaper under the perineal edges of cast and cover with a larger diaper *to prevent cast soiling.*

NURSING DIAGNOSIS: Deficient knowledge related to cast care, activity restrictions, or other prescribed treatment as evidenced by verbalization, questions, or actions demonstrating lack of understanding regarding child's condition or care

Outcome Identification and Evaluation

Child and family will demonstrate accurate understanding about condition and course of treatment *through verbalization and return demonstration.*

Intervention: Providing Patient and Family Teaching

- Assess child's and family's willingness to learn: *Child and family must be willing to learn for teaching to be effective.*
- Provide teaching at an appropriate level for the child and family (depends on age of child, physical condition, memory) *to ensure understanding.*
- Teach in short sessions: *Many short sessions are more helpful than one long session.*
- Repeat information *to give family and child time to learn and understand.*
- Provide reinforcement and rewards *to facilitate the teaching/learning process.*
- Use multiple modes of learning involving many senses (provide written, verbal, demonstration, and videos) when possible: *Child and family are more likely to retain information when presented in different ways using many senses.*

NURSING DIAGNOSIS: Risk for delayed development related to immobility, alterations in extremities

Outcome Identification and Evaluation

Development will be enhanced; *child will make continued progress toward developmental milestones and will not show regression in abilities.*

Intervention: Promoting Development

- Screen for developmental capabilities *to determine child's current level of functioning.*
- Offer age-appropriate toys, play, and activities (including gross motor) *to encourage further development.*
- Perform exercises or interventions as prescribed by physical or occupational therapist: *Repeat participation in those activities helps to promote function and acquisition of developmental skills.*
- Provide support to families: *Immobility and extremity deficits may lead to slow progress in achieving developmental milestones, so ongoing motivation is needed.*

---

serves to hold the bone in reduction, thus preventing deformity as the fracture heals. Casts are constructed of a hard material, traditionally plaster but now more commonly fibreglass. The hard nature of the cast keeps the bone aligned so that healing may occur more quickly. In a fracture that would heal on its own without specific immobilization, a cast may be used to reduce pain and to allow the child increased mobility. The choice of cast material and type of cast will be determined by the pediatrician or orthopedic surgeon. Table 44.1 shows selected casts used in children.

Cast Application

Before cast or splint application, perform baseline neurovascular assessment for comparison after immobilization. Include:

TABLE 44.1 SELECTED CASTS USED IN CHILDREN

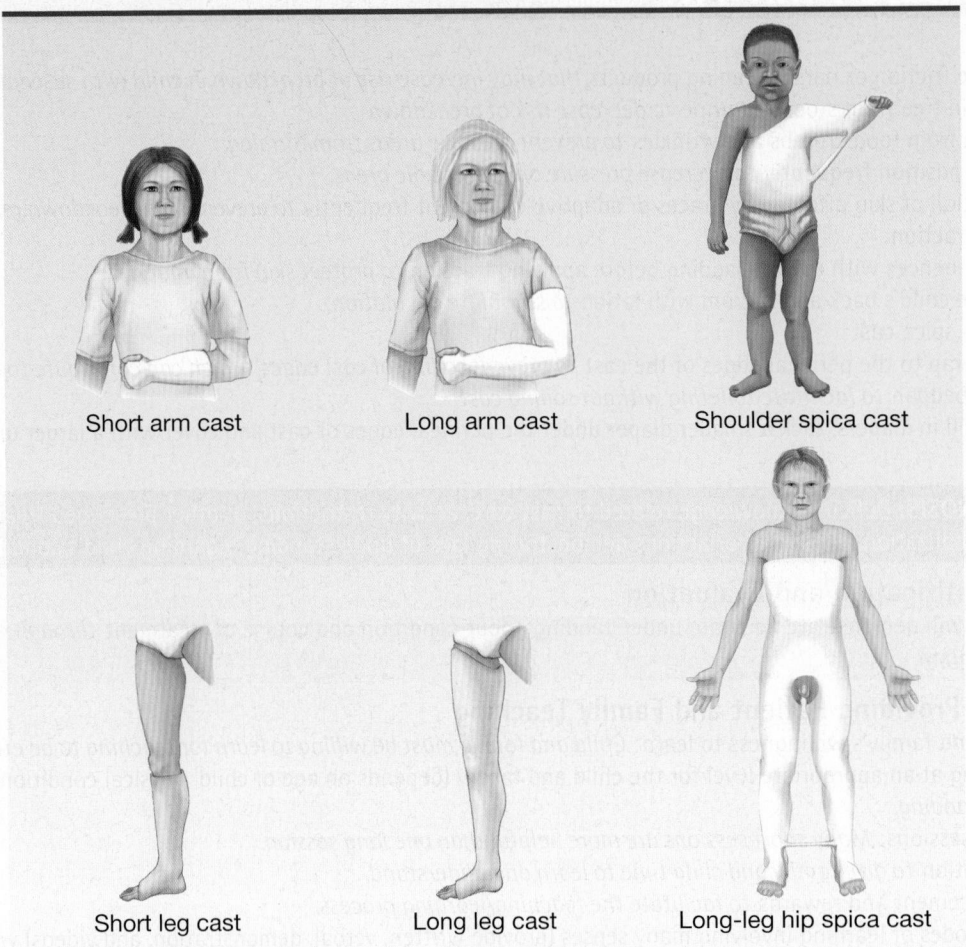

Short arm cast   Long arm cast   Shoulder spica cast

Short leg cast   Long leg cast   Long-leg hip spica cast

- Colour (note cyanosis or other discolouration)
- Movement (note inability to move fingers or toes, including each joint in the fingers and the ability to move the thumb in a "hitchhiking" position, to assess whether the nerves are functioning)
- Sensation (note whether loss of sensation is present)
- Edema
- Quality of pulses

Enlist the cooperation of the child and reduce his or her fear by showing the child the cast materials and using an age-appropriate approach to describe cast application. Premedicate as ordered to reduce pain when manual traction is applied to align the bone. Use **distraction** throughout cast application and assist with application of the cast or splint (Fig. 44.4).

▶ *Take* NOTE!

Modern fibreglass cast materials are available in a variety of colours, as well as a few patterns. Allowing the child to choose the colour will increase the child's cooperation with the procedure.

After the cast or splint is applied, drying time will vary based on the type of material used. Splints and fibreglass casts usually take only a few minutes to dry and will cause a very warm feeling inside the cast, so warn the child that it will begin to feel very warm. Plaster requires 24 to 48 hours to dry. Take care not to

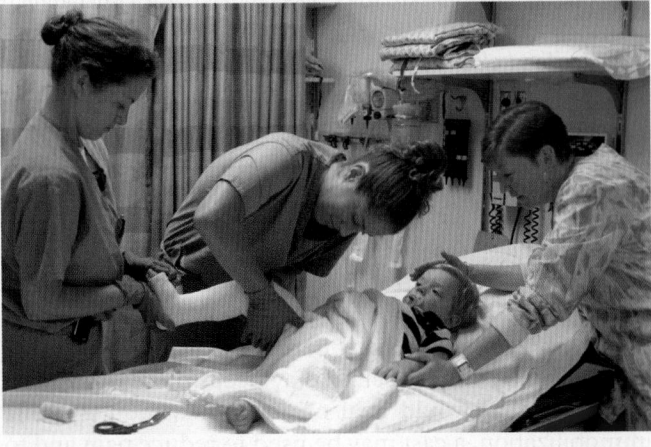

FIGURE 44.4 Assist with cast application by distracting or comforting the child.

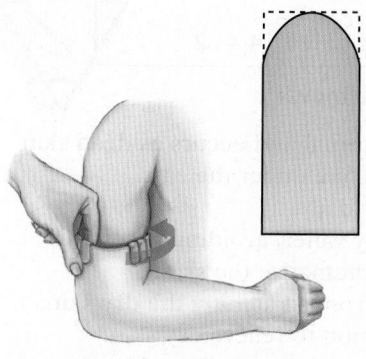

To petal a cast:

1. Cut several strips of adhesive tape or moleskin 3 to 4 inches in length. Use 1 inch tape for smaller areas (e.g., infant's foot) and 2 inch tape for larger areas (e.g., adolescent's waist).

2. Round one end of each strip to keep the corners from rolling.

3. Apply the first strip by tucking the straight end inside the cast and by bringing the rounded end over the cast edge to the outside.

4. Repeat the procedure, overlapping each additional strip, until all rough edges are completely covered.

FIGURE 44.5 Petaling the cast.

cause depressions in the plaster cast while drying, as those may cause skin pressure and breakdown. Instruct the child and family to keep the cast still, positioning it with pillows as needed. Fibreglass casts usually have a soft fabric edge, so they usually do not cause skin rubbing at the edges of the cast. On the other hand, plaster casts require special treatment of the cast edge to prevent skin rubbing. This may be accomplished through a technique called petaling: cut rounded-edge strips of moleskin or another soft material with an adhesive backing and apply them to the edge of cast, as shown in Figure 44.5.

Caring for the Child with a Cast

Perform frequent neurovascular checks of the casted extremity to identify signs of compromise early. These signs include:

• Increased pain
• Increased edema
• Pale or blue colour
• Skin coolness
• Numbness or tingling
• Prolonged capillary refill
• Decreased pulse strength (or absence of pulse)

Notify the physician of changes in neurovascular status or odour or drainage from the cast.

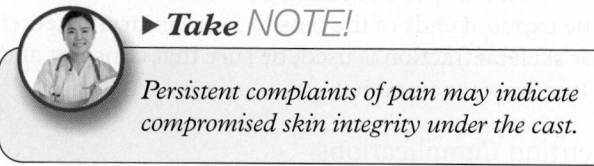

▶ **Take** NOTE!

Persistent complaints of pain may indicate compromised skin integrity under the cast.

Position the child with the casted extremity elevated on pillows. Ice may be applied during the first 24 to 48 hours after casting if needed. Teaching the child to use crutches is an important nursing intervention for any child with lower extremity immobilization so that the child can maintain mobility (Fig. 44.6). Provide homec-

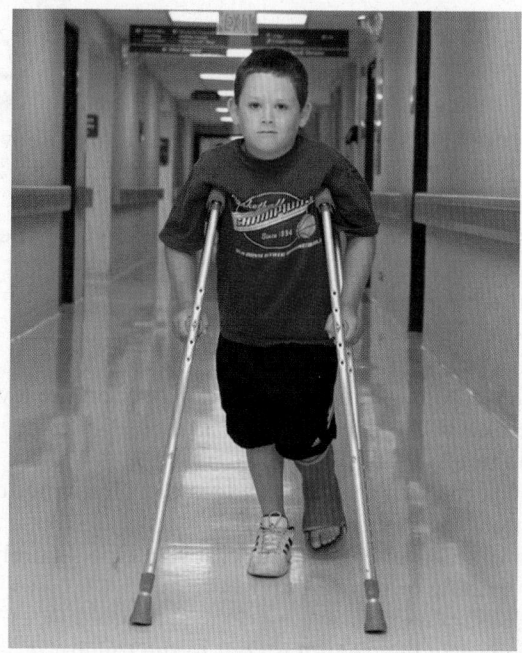

FIGURE 44.6 Reinforce appropriate crutch walking for children with lower extremity immobilization.

are instructions to the family about cast care (Teaching Guideline 44.1).

Assisting with Cast Removal

Children may be frightened by cast removal. Prepare the child using age-appropriate terminology:

• The cast cutter will make a loud noise (Fig. 44.7).

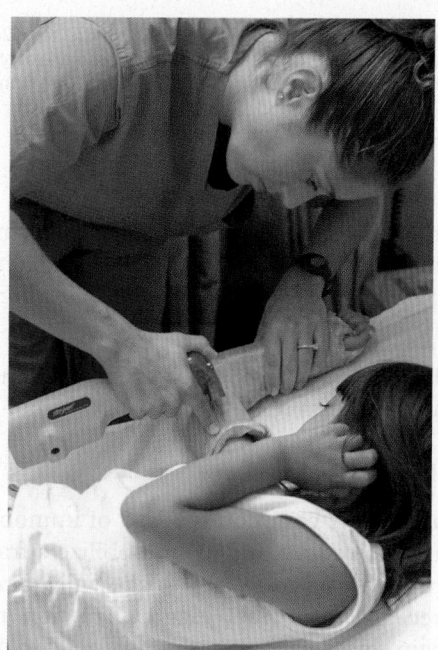

FIGURE 44.7 The loud noise of the cast saw may frighten the child.

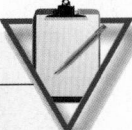

TEACHING GUIDELINE 44.1

Home Cast Care

• For the first 48 hours, elevate the extremity above the level of the heart and apply cold therapy for 20 to 30 minutes, then off 1 hour, and repeat.
• Assess for swelling, and have the child wiggle the fingers or toes hourly.
• For itching inside the cast:
  • Never insert anything into the cast for the purposes of scratching.
  • Blow cool air in from a hair dryer set on the lowest setting or tap lightly on the cast.
  • Do not use lotions or powders.
• Check the skin at the cast edges daily for irritation.
• Protect the cast from wetness.
• Apply a plastic bag around cast and tape securely for bathing or showering.
• Call the physician if:
  • The casted extremity is cool to the touch.
  • The child cannot move the fingers or toes.
  • Severe pain occurs when the child attempts to move the fingers or toes.
  • Persistent numbness or tingling occurs.
  • Drainage or a foul smell comes from under the cast.
  • Severe itching occurs inside the cast.
  • The child runs a fever greater than 38.6°C for longer than 24 hours.
  • Skin edges are red and swollen or exhibit breakdown.
  • The cast gets wet or is cracked, split, or softened.

Adapted from: American Academy of Family Physicians. (2010). *Cast care.* Retrieved September 22, 2011 from http://familydoctor.org/online/famdocen/home/healthy/firstaid/after-injury/094.html; and Bowden, V. R., & Greenberg, C. S. (2008). *Pediatric nursing procedures.* Philadelphia: Lippincott Williams & Wilkins.

• The skin or extremity will not be injured (demonstrate by touching the cast cutter lightly to your palm).
• The child will feel warmth or vibration during cast removal.

Teaching Guideline 44.2 gives instructions related to skin care after cast removal.

Traction

Traction, another common method of immobilization, may be used to reduce and/or immobilize a fracture, to align an injured extremity, and to allow the extremity to be restored to its normal length. Traction may also reduce pain by decreasing the incidence of muscle spasm. In running traction, the weight pulls directly on the extremity in only one plane. This may be achieved

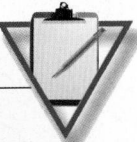

TEACHING GUIDELINE 44.2

Skin Care After Cast Removal

• Brown, flaky skin is normal and occurs as dead skin and secretions accumulate under the cast.
• Soak with warm water daily.
• Wash with warm soapy water, avoiding excessive rubbing, which may traumatize the skin.
• Discourage the child from scratching the dry skin.
• Apply moisturizing lotion to relieve dry skin.
• Encourage activity to regain strength and motion of extremity.

with either skin or skeletal traction. In balanced suspension traction, additional weights are used to provide a counterbalance to the force of traction. This allows for constant pull on the extremity even if the child changes position somewhat. Table 44.2 describes the various types of traction and nursing implications specific to each type. Comparison Chart 44.1 discusses skin versus skeletal traction.

Caring for the Child in Traction

Nursing care of the child in any type of traction focuses not only on appropriate application and maintenance of traction but also on promoting normal growth and development and preventing complications. Apply skin traction over intact skin only so that the pull of the traction is effective. Prepare the skin with an appropriate adhesive before applying the traction tapes to ensure that the tapes adhere well, preventing skin friction. After application of the traction tapes, apply the elastic bandage or use the foam boot. Attach the traction spreader block and then apply the prescribed amount of weight via a rope attached to the spreader block. Ensure that the rope moves without obstruction and that the weights hang freely without touching the floor.

In skeletal traction, apply weight via ropes attached to the skeletal pins. The pin sites should be treated as surgical wounds (see Providing Pin Care section). Protect the exposed ends of the pins to avoid injury. Whether skin or skeletal traction is used, be sure that constant and even traction is maintained.

Preventing Complications

Refer to Nursing Care Plan 44.1 for interventions related to pain management and prevention of complications of immobility such as skin integrity impairment. To prevent contractures and atrophy that may result from disuse of muscles, ensure that unaffected extremities are exercised. Assist the child to exercise the unaffected joints and to use the unaffected extremity if this does not

TABLE 44.2 TYPES OF TRACTION AND NURSING IMPLICATIONS

Type of Traction	Description	Nursing Implications
Bryant's traction Knees slightly flexed Buttocks slightly elevated and clear of bed	Both legs are extended vertically, with child's weight serving as countertraction. Skin traction is applied to both legs. Used for infants with femur fracture or developmental dysplasia of the hip	Maintain appropriate position. Ensure heels and ankles are free from pressure. Rewrap elastic bandages as ordered
Russell's traction 	Skin traction for femur fracture, hip and knee contractures. Uses a knee sling. In split Russell's traction, a portion of the traction weight may be redistributed via a pulley from the sling to the head of the bed (used for femur fracture, Legg–Calvé–Perthes disease, slipped capital femoral epiphysis)	Wrap bandages from ankle to thigh on children less than age 2 years, from ankle to knee on children older than 2 years. Use a foot support to prevent foot drop. Ensure heel is free from bed. Assess popliteal region for skin breakdown from the sling. Mark leg to ensure proper replacement of sling
Buck's traction 	Skin traction for hip and knee contractures, Legg–Calvé–Perthes disease, slipped capital femoral epiphysis Traction force delivered in straight line	Remove traction boot every 8 h to assess skin. Leg may be slightly abducted
Cervical skin traction 	Skin traction applied with a skin strap (head halter). Used for neck sprains/strains, torticollis, or nerve trauma	Ensure that head halter or skin strap does not place pressure on ears or throat. Limit of 2.3 Kg to 3.2 Kg weight
Side-arm 90–90 	Skin traction for humerus fractures and injuries to the shoulder girdle. Used to treat fractures of the humerus and injuries in or around the shoulder girdle	Maintain elbow flexed at 90°. Fingers and hand may feel cool because of elevation. Child may turn to affected side only

(continued)

TABLE 44.2   Types of Traction and Nursing Implications (continued)

Type of Traction	Description	Nursing Implications
Dunlop side-arm 00–90	Skeletal traction through an olecranon screw or pin in distal humerus. Lower arm is held in balanced suspension	See side-arm 90–90. In addition, provide appropriate pin site care
90–90 traction	For femur fracture reduction when skin traction is inadequate. Skeletal traction with force applied through pin in distal femur	A foam boot may be used for suspension of the lower leg. Force of traction applied to femur via the pin. The amount of weight used is just enough to hold lower limb suspended
Cervical skeletal tongs	Tongs attached to skull via pins. Used with fractures or dislocations of the cervical or high thoracic vertebrae	Assess frequently for increased pain, respiratory distress, and cranial nerve or brachial plexus injury. Place on Stryker frame or specially equipped bed to ease positioning without disruption of alignment
Halo traction	Metal halo attached to skull via pins. Used for cervical or high thoracic vertebrae fracture or dislocation and for postoperative immobilization following cervical fusion	Refer to nursing implications for cervical tongs Tape small wrench to front of brace so that front panel can be quickly removed in an emergency. May become ambulatory in this type of traction; will be top-heavy so may need assistance with balance
Balanced suspension traction	Used for femur, hip, or tibial fracture. Thomas splint suspends the thigh while the Pearson attachment allows knee flexion and supports the leg below the knee	Avoid pressure to popliteal area

COMPARISON CHART 44.1 SKIN VERSUS SKELETAL TRACTION

	Skin Traction	Skeletal Traction
Application of force	To the skin via strips or tapes secured with Ace bandages or traction boots	To the body part directly by fixation into or through the bone
Length of treatment	Usually limited	Allows for longer periods of traction
Amount of force	Less	More

disrupt traction alignment. Promote use of a trapeze if not contraindicated to involve the child in repositioning and assist with movement. Encourage deep-breathing exercises to prevent the pulmonary complications of long-term immobilization.

Promote normal growth and development by:

• Placing age-appropriate toys within the child's reach
• Encouraging visits from friends
• Providing diversional activities such as drawing, colouring, or video games (Fig. 44.8)

> ▶ **Take** *NOTE!*
>
> *Avoid sudden bumping or movement of the bed: this can disturb traction alignment and cause additional pain to the child as the weights are jostled.*

> ▶ **Take** *NOTE!*
>
> *Ongoing, careful neurovascular assessments are critical in the child with a cast or in skeletal traction. Notify the physician immediately if these signs of compartment syndrome occur: extreme pain (out of proportion to the situation), pain with passive range of motion of digits, distal extremity pallor, inability to move digits, loss of pulses.*

External Fixation

External fixation may be used for complicated fractures, especially open fractures with soft tissue damage. If the fracture is difficult to stabilize with the other methods of fixation, external fixation is chosen. A series of pins or wires are inserted into bone and then attached to an external frame. The fixator apparatus may be adjusted as needed by the health care provider. Once the desired level of correction is achieved, no further adjustment occurs and the bone is allowed to heal. Advantages of external fixation include increased patient comfort and improved function of muscles and joints when complicated fracture occurs. The externally fixated limb often takes longer to heal.

Caring for the Child with an External Fixator

In addition to routine neurovascular assessment, elevate the extremity to prevent swelling. The fixator may be moved by grasping the frame, as the fixator can tolerate ordinary movement. Encourage weight-bearing as prescribed. Provide appropriate education to the child and family. Encourage the child to look at the apparatus.

Providing Pin Care

Whether pins are inserted for skeletal traction or as part of an external fixator (see Fracture section), keeping the pin sites clean is important to prevent infection. Perform pin site care according to institutional policy or the physician's orders. Cleaning of the pin sites prevents infection by promoting comfort and preventing healing skin from adhering to the metal pin. Notify the orthopedic surgeon if signs of pin site infection are present, if pins are loose, or if pin slippage occurs.

Thus far, attempts to obtain evidence supporting the various types of pin site care have been unsuccessful. Certain physicians prefer the site to be cleaned with normal saline; others choose a solution with antibacterial properties. Some institutions recommend removal of all

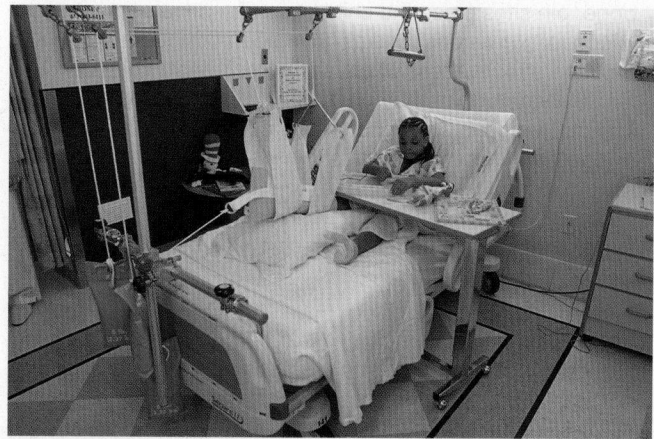

FIGURE 44.8 Provide age-appropriate diversional activities and schoolwork for children confined to bed in traction.

crusts formed on the skin around the pin; others do not. The rationale for crust removal is to promote free drainage and prevent the surrounding skin from adhering to the pin. A keyhole dressing may be necessary around the pin if drainage is present. No matter which procedure is ordered or preferred, perform pin care as necessary to prevent infection at the pin site. The Ilizarov fixator uses wires that are thinner than ordinary pins, so simply cleansing by showering is usually sufficient to keep the pin site clean. If drainage is present, the skin around the wires can be cleansed with a dry gauze pad. See Evidence-based Practice 44.1.

NURSING PROCESS OVERVIEW FOR THE CHILD WITH A MUSCULOSKELETAL DISORDER

Care of the child with a musculoskeletal disorder includes assessment, nursing diagnosis, planning, interventions, and evaluation. There are a number of general concepts related to the nursing process that may be applied to musculoskeletal dysfunction in children. From a general understanding of the care involved for a child with a musculoskeletal disorder, the nurse can then individualize the care based on patient specifics.

Assessment

Assessment of musculoskeletal dysfunction in children includes health history, physical examination, and laboratory and diagnostic testing.

*R*emember Dakota, the 2-year-old with right arm pain and refusal to use his arm? What additional health history and physical examination assessment information should the nurse obtain?

Health History

The health history comprises past medical history, family history, and history of present illness (when the symptoms started and how they have progressed) as well as treatments used at home. The past medical history might be significant for musculoskeletal congenital anomaly or orthopedic injury during the birthing process. Breech delivery may be associated with DDH. Determine history related to attainment of developmental milestones, such as walking and whether or not the child participates in sports. Inquire about the child's usual level of physical activity, participation in sports, and use of protective equipment. Family history may be positive for orthopedic problems. When eliciting the history of the present illness, inquire about the following:

• Limp or other changes in gait
• Recent trauma (determine the mechanism of injury)
• Recent strenuous exercise
• Fever
• Weakness
• Alteration in muscle tone
• Areas of redness or swelling

EVIDENCE-BASED PRACTICE 44.1
Pin Site Cleaning Methods and Infection Prevention

● Study

External fixation (metal pins) is used to immobilize bones while fractures heal. By the nature of pin insertion into the bone, pin sites place the child at risk for development of an infection. Numerous studies have been conducted to evaluate the effectiveness of pin site care. To date, pin site care is usually determined by physician or institution preference. The authors reviewed randomized controlled studies that evaluated the management of pin sites. The interventions reviewed included any type of cleaning method versus no cleaning, sterile versus non-sterile technique, use of massage, and whether or not a dressing was used.

▲ Findings

The results were inconclusive. No particular method of pin site care was determined to be statistically significant in reducing infection from orthopedic pins.

■ Nursing Implications

Despite the lack of clear insight from this study, it remains important for nurses to continue vigilance regarding pin site care. Ongoing assessment of pin sites for signs of infection and monitoring of the child's temperature are particularly important. Provide pin site care according to the physician's preference or institution's protocol. With the lack of conclusive evidence related to pin site care, nurses caring for pediatric orthopedic patients are in a prime position to develop and execute a well-designed research study related to pin site care.

Temple, J., & Santy, J. (2007). Pin site care for preventing infections associated with external bone fixators and pins. *The Cochrane Library 2007, 4.* Indianapolis: John Wiley & Sons.

Physical Examination

Physical examination of the musculoskeletal system consists of inspection, observation, and palpation.

Inspection and Observation

Observe the child's posture and alignment of the trunk. Inspect extremities for symmetry and positioning and for absence, duplication, or webbing of any digits. Note any obvious extremity deformity or limb-length discrepancy. Inspect skin for redness, warmth, bruises, and puncture sites. Observe gait in the child who has achieved the developmental skill of walking. Note refusal to walk, limp, in-toeing, out-toeing, or foot slap. Inspect injured joints for ecchymosis or swelling. In the injured extremity, note colour of fingertips or toes. Observe spontaneous range of motion. Perform scoliosis screening to determine spinal alignment. Note symmetry of thigh folds.

Palpation

Palpate the clavicles in the newborn or young infant for tenderness or a bump that indicates callus formation with clavicle fracture. Perform active range of motion to determine if a joint position is fixed (e.g., clubfoot). Palpate the affected joint or extremity to detect warmth or tenderness. In the injured child or the child with a cast or splint, thoroughly assess the neurovascular status of the affected extremities. Palpate the fingers or toes for warmth. Determine the capillary refill time. Note presence of sensation or motion. Evaluate muscle strength. Palpate pulses distal to the injury, noting their strength and quality. Perform the Ortolani and Barlow manoeuvres to assess for DDH.

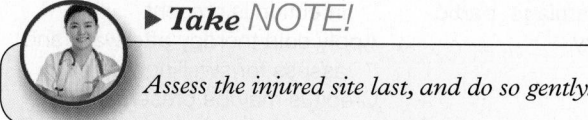

▶ *Take* NOTE!

Assess the injured site last, and do so gently.

Laboratory and Diagnostic Testing

Common Laboratory and Diagnostic Tests 44.1 explains the laboratory and diagnostic tests most commonly used when considering musculoskeletal disorders. The tests can assist the physician in diagnosing a disorder and/or be used as guidelines in determining ongoing treatment. Some of the tests are obtained by laboratory or non-nursing personnel while others might be obtained by the nurse. In either instance the nurse should be familiar with how the tests are obtained, what they are used for, and normal versus abnormal results. This knowledge will also be necessary when providing patient and family education related to the tests.

Nursing Diagnoses, Goals, Interventions, and Evaluation

Upon completion of a thorough assessment, the nurse might identify several nursing diagnoses, including:

- Pain related to trauma, edema, or muscle spasm (see Chapter 35)
- Impaired physical mobility related to injury, pain, or weakness
- Risk for constipation related to immobility
- Self-care deficit related to immobility
- Risk for impaired skin integrity related to immobility, braces, or adaptive devices
- Deficient knowledge related to cast care, activity restrictions, or other prescribed treatment
- Risk for developmental delay related to immobility, alterations in extremities

After completing an assessment of Dakota, the nurse noted the following: the history revealed he had been sledding with his older brother the day before. Upon examination, bruising and swelling of the right arm are noted, with point tenderness at the wrist. Based on the assessment findings, what would your top three nursing diagnoses be for Dakota?

Nursing goals, interventions, and evaluation for the child with musculoskeletal dysfunction are based on the nursing diagnoses (see Nursing Care Plan 44.1). The nursing care plan may be used as a guide in planning nursing care for the child with a musculoskeletal disorder. The care plan includes many nursing diagnoses that are applicable to the child or adolescent. Children's responses to musculoskeletal dysfunction and its treatment will vary, and nursing care should be individualized based on the child's and family's responses to illness.

The nursing care of immobilized children is similar to that of adults, but developmental and age-appropriate effects must be taken into account. Prevention of complications is a key nursing function. Refer to Nursing Care Plan 44.1 for interventions related to prevention of complications. Additional information about nursing care related to certain disorders will be included later in the chapter as it relates to specific disorders. Refer to Chapter 35 for nursing interventions related to pain management. Particular care related to casts, traction, and external fixation is discussed below.

Based on your top three nursing diagnoses for Dakota, describe appropriate nursing interventions.

COMMON LABORATORY AND DIAGNOSTIC TESTS 44.1

Test	Explanation	Indication	Nursing Implications
X-rays	Radiographic image; usually two views are obtained of the affected extremity (lateral and anteroposterior)	To detect fractures and other anomalies	Child must cooperate and hold still. Enlist the family's help in calming the child.
Ultrasound	Use of sound waves to locate the depth and structure within soft tissues and fluid	To diagnose toxic synovitis, Legg–Calvé–Perthes disease, slipped capital femoral epiphysis, osteomyelitis, fractures, ligament or soft tissue injuries. Monitoring and follow-up of fractures and remodeling	Better tolerated by nonsedated children than CT or MRI. Can be performed with a portable unit at bedside
Computed tomography (CT)	Non-invasive X-ray study that looks at tissue density and structures. Images a "slice" of tissue	To evaluate the extent of osteomyelitis, Legg–Calvé–Perthes disease, or slipped capital femoral epiphysis or to rule out other problems	Machine is large and can be frightening to children. Procedure can be lengthy and child must remain still. If unable to do so, sedation may be necessary. If performed with contrast medium, assess for allergy. Encourage fluids after the procedure if not contraindicated
Magnetic resonance imaging (MRI)	Based on how hydrogen atoms behave in a magnetic field when disturbed by radio-frequency signals. Does not require ionizing radiation. Provides a 3D view of the body part being scanned	To assess hard and soft tissue, as well as bone marrow, to evaluate extent of osteomyelitis, Legg–Calvé–Perthes disease, or slipped capital femoral epiphysis, or to rule out other problems	Remove all metal objects from the child. Child must remain motionless for entire scan; parent can stay in room with child. Younger children will require sedation in order to be still. A loud thumping sound occurs inside the machine during the scan procedure, and this can be frightening to children
Arthrography	X-ray of a joint after direct injection with a radiopaque substance	To assess ligaments, muscles, tendons, and cartilage, particularly after injury	Should not be performed if joint infection is present. Apply cold therapy afterward and assess for swelling and pain. Crepitus may be present in the joint for 1 to 2 days after procedure
Complete blood count	Evaluates hemoglobin and hematocrit, white blood cell count, platelet count	To evaluate hemoglobin and hematocrit with fracture with potential bleeding. To determine infection in osteomyelitis, septic arthritis, and toxic synovitis	Normal values vary according to age and gender. White blood cell count differential is helpful in evaluating source of infection. May be affected by myelosuppressive drugs
Erythrocyte sedimentation rate	Nonspecific test used to determine presence of infection or inflammation	To evaluate for osteomyelitis or septic arthritis	Send sample to laboratory immediately; if allowed to stand for longer than 3 h, may produce falsely low result

Test	Explanation	Indication	Nursing Implications
C-reactive protein	Measures acute-phase reactant protein indicative of inflammatory process	To evaluate for osteomyelitis or septic arthritis	Anti-inflammatory drugs may cause decreased levels More sensitive and rapidly responsive than erythrocyte sedimentation rate
Blood culture	To determine presence of bacteria in blood	May be positive with septic arthritis or osteomyelitis	Transport specimen to laboratory within 30 min Avoid skin contamination of specimen while obtaining it Cultures should usually be drawn before starting antibiotics, as partial antibiotic treatment may result in negative culture
Joint fluid aspiration	Aspirated joint fluid is examined for presence of pus and white blood cells; culture is performed	To evaluate for septic arthritis	Use cold therapy to decrease swelling after aspiration Apply pressure dressing to prevent hematoma formation or fluid re-collection Assess for fever and joint pain or edema, which may indicate infection Positive fluid culture indicates a bacterial infection in the joint. May also be used to relieve pressure in the joint space

Adapted from: Fischbach, F. T., & Dunning, M. B., III (2009). *A manual of laboratory and diagnostic tests* (8th ed.). Philadelphia: Lippincott Williams & Wilkins.

Congenital and Developmental Disorders

Congenital anomalies of the musculoskeletal system are usually readily identified at birth. Congenital structural anomalies involving the skeleton include pectus excavatum, pectus carinatum, limb deficiencies, polydactyly or syndactyly, metatarsus adductus, congenital clubfoot, and osteogenesis imperfecta. A developmental anomaly that may be diagnosed at birth or later in life is DDH. A muscular condition, torticollis, most often presents as a congenital condition but may also develop after birth. Tibia vara is a developmental disorder affecting young children. Rarely, a developmental positional alteration such as genu varum, genu valgum, or pes planus will persist past the usual age of resolution or cause the child pain. If those situations occur, bracing, orthotics, or surgical correction may become necessary.

Pectus Excavatum

Pectus excavatum and pectus carinatum are anterior chest wall deformities. Pectus excavatum, a funnel-shaped chest, accounts for 87% of anterior chest wall deformities (Goretsky, Kelly, Croitoru, & Nuss, 2004). A depression that sinks inward is apparent at the xiphoid process (Fig. 44.9). Pectus carinatum, a protuberance of the chest wall, accounts for only 5% of anterior chest wall deformities. The remainder are mixed deformities.

Pectus excavatum does not resolve as the child grows; rather, it progresses with growth. The chest depression may be minimal or marked. When the pectus is more pronounced, cardiac and pulmonary compression occurs. Symptoms of this compression most often present during puberty, when the pectus quickly worsens. Children may complain of shortness of breath, withdraw from physical activities, and have a poor body image.

Therapeutic Management

Therapeutic management of pectus excavatum involves surgical correction, preferably before puberty, when the skeleton is more pliable. Various surgical techniques may be used and generally involve either the placement of a surgical steel bar or use of a piece of bone in the rib cage to lift the depression. This discussion will focus on care of the child who undergoes surgical steel bar placement for pectus correction.

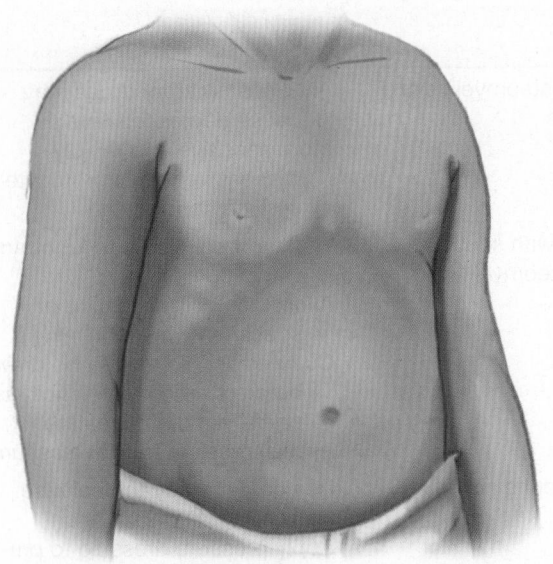

FIGURE 44.9 Pectus excavatum: note the depression in the chest wall at the xiphoid process.

Nursing Assessment

Elicit the health history, noting progression of the defect and effects on the child's cardiopulmonary function. Note shortness of breath, exercise intolerance, or chest pain. Observe the child's chest for anterior wall deformity, noting depth and severity. Auscultate the lungs to determine the adequacy of aeration. X-rays, computed tomography (CT), or magnetic resonance imaging (MRI) may be used to determine the extent of the anomaly and compression of inner structures.

Nursing Management

Prepare the child preoperatively by allowing a tour of the surgical area and the pediatric intensive care unit. Introduce the child to the pain scale that will be used in the postoperative period.

Postoperatively, nursing management focuses on assessment, protection of the surgical site, and pain management. Auscultate lung sounds frequently to determine the adequacy of aeration and to monitor for development of the complication of pneumothorax. Assess for signs of wound infection that would necessitate removal of the curved bar. Do not allow the child to lie on either side and do not log-roll the child (these positions may disrupt the bar's position). Administer analgesics as needed either intravenously or via the epidural catheter. Teach families that the child should not be allowed to lie on his or her side at home for 4 weeks after the surgery to ensure that the band does not shift. Encourage aerobic activity at home after clearance by the surgeon (this will increase the child's vital capacity, previously hindered by the pectus). The bar will be removed 2 to 4 years after the initial placement.

Limb Deficiencies

Limb deficiencies, either complete absence of a limb or a portion of it or deformity, occur as the fetus is developing. These defects are attributed to an amniotic band constricting the limb, resulting in either incomplete development or amputation of the limb. Many children born with limb deformities also have congenital deformities, such as craniofacial abnormalities and cardiac and genitourinary defects (Morrissy, Giavedoni, & Coulter-O'Berry, 2006; Polousky & Eilert, 2009).

Therapeutic management is aimed at improving the child's functional ability. Physical therapy and occupational therapy may be helpful. Adaptive equipment such as a prosthesis may also be prescribed.

Nursing Assessment

Note the extent of limb deformity, providing an accurate description of the presence or absence of a portion of the arm or leg, or missing fingers or toes. Assess the child's ability to use the extremity as a helper (arms) or in ambulation (legs). Determine status of acquisition of developmental skills.

Nursing Management

Reinforce prescribed activities that are meant to improve the child's function. Provide activities in which the child is capable of participating. If the limb deficiency is significant, refer the infant to the local early intervention office as soon as possible after birth. Early intervention is designed to promote development from birth to age 3 years. Absence of a limb or a significant portion of a limb will have a considerable impact on the child's ability to meet developmental milestones as expected.

Polydactyly/Syndactyly

Polydactyly is the presence of extra digits on the hand or foot (Fig. 44.10). It affects blacks more frequently than other ethnic groups (Kaneshiro, 2009). In one third of cases, polydactyly occurs in both the hand and foot (Gore & Spencer, 2004). It usually involves digits at the border of the hand or foot but can also affect a central digit (Hosalker et al., 2007a). Syndactyly is webbing of the fingers and toes. Both polydactyly and syndactyly can be

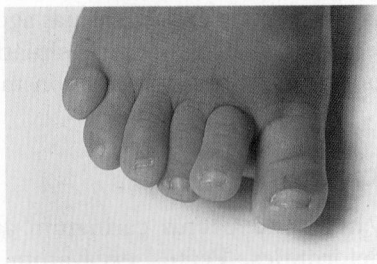

FIGURE 44.10 Note additional digits (toes) of polydactyly.

inherited and associated with other genetic syndromes (Cornwall, 2007; Hosalkar, Spiegel, & Davidson, 2007c; Kaneshiro, 2009).

Treatment includes tying off the additional digit until it falls off or surgical removal of the digit. No treatment is usually required for syndactyly, though surgical repair is sometimes performed for cosmetic reasons.

Nursing Assessment

Inspect the hands and feet for the presence of extra digits. Note whether the additional digits are soft (without bone) or are full or partial digits with bone present. Note location of webbing.

Nursing Management

If the digit is tied off, observe for expected necrosis of tissue and eventually loss of the extra digit. When surgical removal is necessary, provide routine preoperative and postoperative care as appropriate.

Metatarsus Adductus

Metatarsus adductus, a medial deviation of the forefoot, is one of the most common foot deformities of childhood (Fig. 44.11). It occurs as a result of in utero positioning (Hosalkar et al., 2007c). It occurs in one in 1,000 live births, affects boys and girls equally, and is bilateral in half of all cases and unilateral in the remainder (Gilmore & Thompson, 2003). Type I and type II are usually benign deformities, resolving spontaneously by the age of 3 years. Children with type III deformity usually require manipulation and serial casting, preferably before the age of 8 months. Surgical intervention is rarely needed.

Nursing Assessment

The deformity is usually noted at birth. Note inward deviation of the forefoot. The great and second toes might be separated. Determine forefoot flexibility. Range of

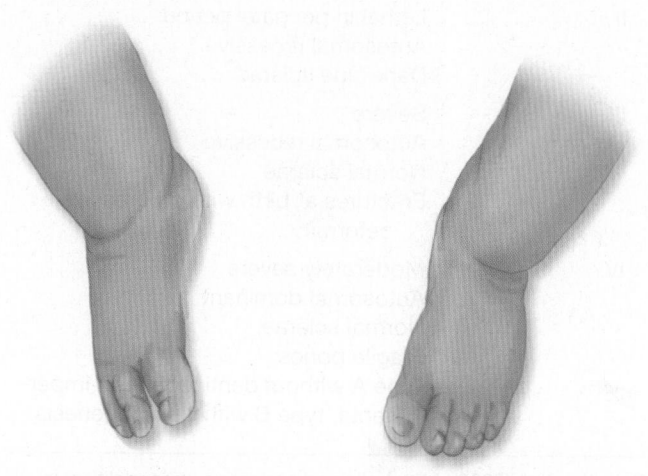

FIGURE 44.11 Metatarsus adductus: note medial deviation of the forefoot.

> **BOX 44.1** **Types of Metatarsus Adductus**
>
> • Type I: forefoot is flexible past neutral actively and passively.
> • Type II: forefoot is flexible passively past neutral, but only to midline actively.
> • Type III: forefoot is rigid and does not correct to midline even with passive stretching.

motion of the ankle, hindfoot, and midfoot is normal in all three types. Accompanying hip dysplasia may be seen; therefore, careful examination of the hips is warranted (Hosalkar, Gholve, & Wells, 2007a). Box 44.1 describes the three types based on flexibility of the forefoot.

Nursing Management

Nursing care for children with type I and type II metatarsus adductus is aimed at education and reassurance of the parents. The nursing care for the child with type III is similar to that of the child with clubfoot (see below).

Congenital Clubfoot

Congenital clubfoot (also termed congenital talipes equinovarus) is a congenital anomaly that occurs in one in 1,000 live births (Gilmore & Thompson, 2003). Clubfoot consists of:

• Talipes varus (inversion of the heel)
• Talipes equinus (plantarflexion of the foot; the heel is raised and would not strike the ground in a standing position)
• Cavus (plantarflexion of the forefoot on the hindfoot)
• Forefoot adduction with supination (the forefoot is inverted and turned slightly upward) (Mosca, 2006)

The foot resembles the head of a golf club (Fig. 44.12). Half of all cases occur bilaterally (Hosalkar et al., 2007c). Males are affected more frequently than females (Gunta, 2009; Hosalkar et al., 2007c). The exact etiology of clubfoot is unknown.

Clubfoot may be classified into four categories: postural, neurogenic, syndromic, and idiopathic. Postural clubfoot often resolves with a short series of manipulative casting. Neurogenic clubfoot occurs in infants with myelomeningocele. Clubfoot in association with other syndromes (syndromic) is often resistant to treatment. Idiopathic clubfoot occurs in otherwise normal healthy infants. The approach to treatment is similar regardless of the classification.

Therapeutic Management

The goal of therapeutic management of clubfoot is achievement of a functional foot; treatment starts as soon after

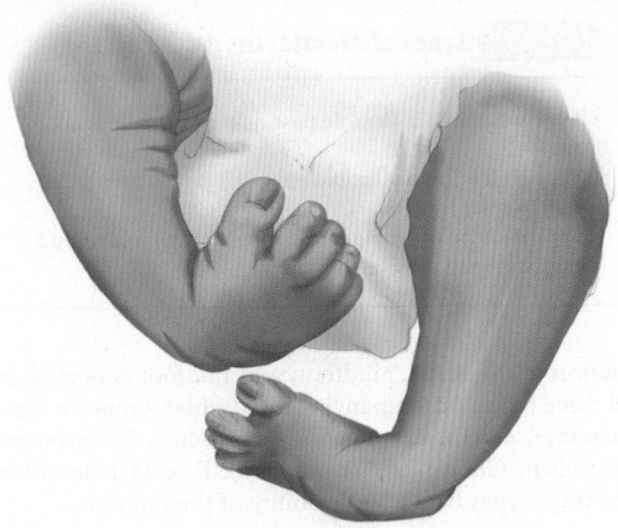

FIGURE 44.12 Note inverted heel, ankle equinus, and forefoot adduction in this infant with bilateral clubfoot.

birth as possible. Weekly manipulation with serial cast changes is performed; later, cast changes occur every 2 weeks. This approach is successful in about half of all cases. The other infants require corrective shoes or bracing; in some infants, surgical release of soft tissue may be necessary. Following surgery, the foot is immobilized with a cast for up to 12 weeks, and then ankle–foot orthoses or corrective shoes are used for several years.

Complications of clubfoot and its treatment include residual deformity, rocker-bottom foot, awkward gait, weight-bearing on the lateral portion of the foot if uncorrected, and disturbance to the epiphysis.

Nursing Assessment

Note family history of foot deformities and obstetric history of breech position. Inspect the foot for position at rest. Perform active range of motion, noting inability to move the foot into normal positioning at midline. X-rays are obtained to determine bony abnormality and note progress during treatment.

Nursing Management

Perform neurovascular assessment and cast care as for any disorder requiring casting. Provide emotional support, as treatment often begins in the newborn period and families may have a difficult time adjusting to the diagnosis and treatment required for their new baby. Teach families cast care and later the use of orthotics or braces as prescribed.

Osteogenesis Imperfecta

Osteogenesis imperfecta is a genetic bone disorder that results in low bone mass, increased fragility of the bones, and other connective tissue problems such as joint hyper-

mobility, resulting in instability of the joints that may further contribute to fracture occurrence. Dentinogenesis imperfecta may also occur: the tooth enamel wears easily and the teeth become discoloured.

The disorder usually occurs as a result of a defect in the collagen type 1 gene, usually through an autosomal recessive or dominant inheritance pattern. The types of osteogenesis imperfecta range from mild to severe connective tissue and bone involvement (Table 44.3). In children with moderate to severe disease, fractures are more likely to occur, and short stature is common. In addition to multiple fractures, additional complications include early hearing loss, acute and chronic pain, scoliosis, and respiratory problems.

▶ **Take** NOTE!

Blue sclerae are not diagnostic of osteogenesis imperfecta, but it is a common finding (Gunta, 2009). The sclerae of newborns tend to be bluish, progressing to white over the first few weeks of life. There are some individuals with blue sclerae who do not have osteogenesis imperfecta.

TABLE 44.3 **CLASSIFICATION OF OSTEOGENESIS IMPERFECTA**

Classification	Characteristics
I	Common and mild Autosomal dominant Blue sclerae Fragile bones, early fractures (by preschool age) Type A without dentinogenesis imperfecta, type B with dentinogenesis
II	Lethal in perinatal period Autosomal recessive Dark-blue sclerae
III	Severe Autosomal recessive Normal sclerae Fractures at birth with progressive deformity
IV	Moderately severe Autosomal dominant Normal sclerae Fragile bones Type A without dentinogenesis imperfecta, type B with dentinogenesis

Zaleske, D. J. (2006). Metabolic and endocrine abnormalities. In R. T. Morrissy & S. L. Weinstein (Eds.), *Lovell & Winter's pediatric orthopaedics* (6th ed.). Philadelphia: Lippincott Williams & Wilkins.

Therapeutic Management

The goal of medical and surgical management is to decrease the incidence of fractures and maintain mobility. Bisphosphonate administration is used for moderate to severe disease. Fracture care is often required. Physical therapy and occupational therapy prevent contractures and maximize mobility. Standing with bracing is encouraged. Lightweight splints or braces may allow the child to bear weight earlier. Severe cases may require surgical insertion of rods into the long bones.

Nursing Assessment

Elicit a health history, which may reveal a family history of osteogenesis imperfecta, a pattern of frequent fractures, or screaming associated with routine care and handling of the newborn. Inspect the eyes for sclerae that have a blue, purple, or grey tint. Note abnormalities of the primary teeth. Inspect skin for bruising and note joint hypermobility with active range of motion. Laboratory tests may include a skin biopsy (which reveals abnormalities in type 1 collagen) or DNA testing (locating the genetic mutation).

Nursing Management

Handle the child carefully and teach the family to avoid trauma (Teaching Guideline 44.3). Refer families to the Osteogenesis Imperfecta Foundation (visit http://thePoint. lww.com/Chow1e for a direct link), which provides access to multiple resources as well as clinical trials. An excellent book for families of children with osteogenesis imperfecta is *Children with Osteogenesis Imperfecta: Strategies to Enhance Performance* by H. L. Cintas and L. H. Gerber.

Encourage safe mobility. Reinforce physical and occupational therapists' recommendations for promotion of fine motor skills and independence in activities of daily living, as well as use of adaptive equipment and appropriate promotion of mobility. Adapted physical education is important to promote mobility and maintain bone and muscle mass. If the child is ambulatory, even with adaptive equipment use, walking is a good form of exercise. Swimming and water therapy are appropriate, allowing independent movement with little fracture risk.

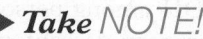 ▶ *Take* NOTE!

Use caution when inserting an intravenous line or taking a blood pressure measurement, as pressure on the arm or leg can lead to bruising and fractures.

Developmental Dysplasia of the Hip

DDH refers to abnormalities of the developing hip that include dislocation, subluxation, and dysplasia of the hip joint. In DDH, the femoral head has an abnormal relationship to the acetabulum. Frank dislocation of the hip may occur, in which there is no contact between the femoral head and acetabulum. Subluxation is a partial dislocation, meaning that the acetabulum is not fully seated within the hip joint. Dysplasia refers to an acetabulum that is shallow or sloping instead of cup-shaped. DDH may affect just one or both hips. The dysplastic hip may be provoked to subluxation or dislocated and then reduced again. DDH affects females eight times more often than males (Fig. 44.13).

Pathophysiology

While dislocation may occur during a growth period in utero, the laxity of the newborn's hip allows dislocation and relocation of the hip to occur. The hip can develop normally only if the femoral head is appropriately and deeply seated within the acetabulum. If subluxation and periodic or continued dislocation occur, then structural changes in the hip's anatomy occur. Continued dysplasia

---

TEACHING GUIDELINE 44.3

Preventing Injury in Children with Osteogenesis Imperfecta

- Never push or pull on an arm or leg.
- Do not bend an arm or leg into an awkward position.
- Lift a baby by placing one hand under the legs and buttocks and one hand under the shoulders, head, and neck.
- Do not lift a baby's legs by the ankles to change the diaper.
- Do not lift a baby or small child from under the armpits.
- Provide supported positioning.
- If fracture is suspected, handle the limb minimally.

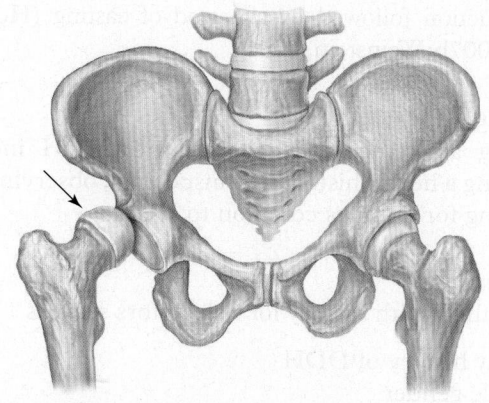

FIGURE 44.13 Developmental dysplasia of the hip.

of the hip leads to limited abduction of the hip and contracture of muscles. DDH is more common in females, probably due to the greater susceptibility of the female newborn to maternal hormones that contribute to laxity of the ligaments (Hosalkar et al., 2007b). Mechanical factors such as breech positioning or the presence of oligohydramnios also contribute to the development of DDH. Genetic factors also play a role: there is an increased incidence of DDH among persons of Native American and Eastern European descent, with very low rates among people of African or southern Chinese heritage (Hosalker et al., 2007b). Complications of DDH include avascular necrosis of the femoral head, loss of range of motion, recurrently unstable hip, femoral nerve palsy, leg-length discrepancy, and early osteoarthritis.

Therapeutic Management

The goal of therapeutic management is to maintain the hip joint in reduction so that the femoral head and acetabulum can develop properly.

Treatment varies based upon the child's age and the severity of DDH. Infants younger than 4 to 6 months of age may be treated with a Pavlik harness, which reduces and stabilizes the hip by preventing hip extension and adduction and maintaining the hip in flexion and abduction (Hosalkar et al., 2007b; Polousky & Eilert, 2009). The Pavlik harness is successful in the treatment of DDH in the majority of infants less than 6 months of age if it is used on a full-time basis and applied properly (Weinstein, 2006). Children from 4 months to 2 years of age often require closed reduction (Hosalkar et al., 2007b; Polousky & Eilert, 2009). Skin or skeletal traction may be used first to gradually stretch the associated soft tissue structures. Closed reduction occurs under general anesthesia, with the hip being gently manoeuvred back into the acetabulum. A spica cast worn for 12 weeks maintains reduction of the hip. After the cast is removed, the child must wear an abduction brace full-time (except for baths) for 2 months (Hosalkar et al., 2007b). Then the brace is worn at night and during naps until development of the acetabulum is normal. Children over 2 years of age or those who have failed to respond to prior treatment require an open surgical reduction followed by a period of casting (Hosalkar et al., 2007b; Weinstein, 2006).

Nursing Assessment

Nursing assessment of children with DDH includes obtaining a health history and inspecting, observing, and palpating for findings common to DDH.

Health History

Assess the health history for risk factors such as

- Family history of DDH
- Female gender
- Oligohydramnios or breech birth

- Native American or Eastern European descent
- Associated lower limb deformity or other congenital musculoskeletal deformity

Previously undiagnosed older children may complain of hip pain.

Physical Assessment

The physical examination for DDH includes inspection, observation, and palpation. Since DDH is a developmental process, ongoing screening assessments are required throughout at least for the first several months of the infant's life.

Inspection and Observation

Ensure that the infant is on a flat surface and is relaxed. Note asymmetry of thigh or gluteal folds with the infant in a prone position. Document shortening of affected femur observed as limb-length discrepancy. Older children may exhibit **Trendelenburg gait**. Figure 44.14 illustrates these assessments.

Palpation

Note limited hip abduction when passive range of motion is performed. Abduction should ordinarily occur to 75 degrees and adduction to within 30 degrees with the infant's pelvis stabilized. Perform Barlow and Ortolani tests, noting a "clunk" as the femoral head dislocates or reduces back into the acetabulum. Force is not necessary when performing the Barlow and Ortolani manoeuvres (American Academy of Pediatrics, 2000) (see Fig. 44.14).

> ▶ **Take** NOTE!
>
> *A higher-pitched "click" may occur with flexion or extension of the hip. When assessing for DDH, do not confuse this benign, adventitial sound with a true "clunk."*

Diagnostic Testing

Ultrasound of the hip allows for visualization of the femoral head and the outer edge of the acetabulum. Plain hip X-rays may be used in the infant or child over 6 months of age.

Nursing Management

Earlier recognition of hip dysplasia with earlier harness use results in better correction of the anomaly (Hosalkar et al., 2007b). Excellent assessment skills and reporting of any abnormal findings are critical. Initially, the infant will need to wear the Pavlik harness continuously (Fig. 44.15). The physician makes all appropriate adjustments to the harness when applied so that the hips are held in the optimal position for appropriate development. Teach parents use of the harness and assessment of the baby's skin. If started early, harness use usually continues for about

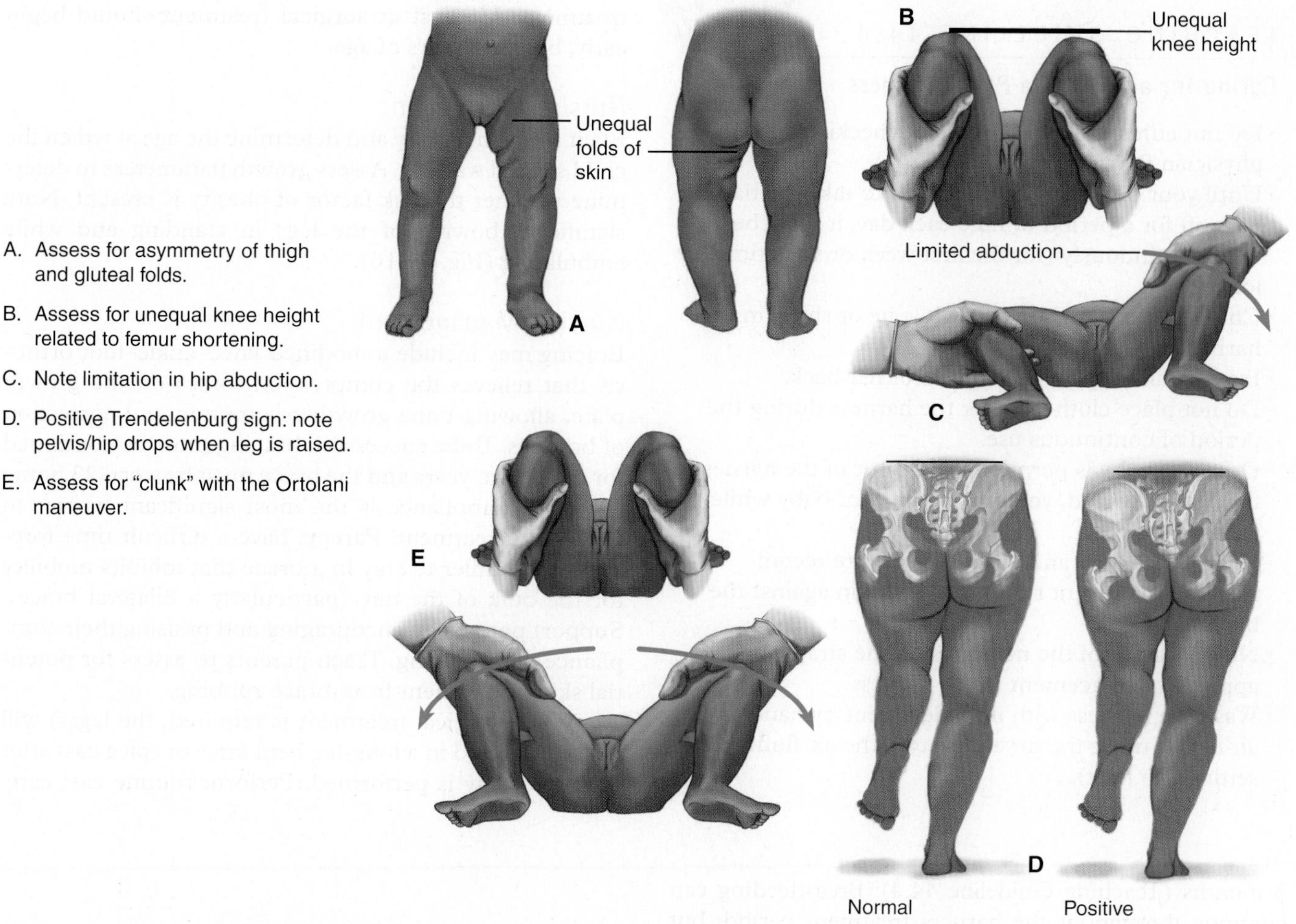

A. Assess for asymmetry of thigh and gluteal folds.

B. Assess for unequal knee height related to femur shortening.

C. Note limitation in hip abduction.

D. Positive Trendelenburg sign: note pelvis/hip drops when leg is raised.

E. Assess for "clunk" with the Ortolani maneuver.

Unequal folds of skin

Unequal knee height

Limited abduction

Normal   Positive

FIGURE 44.14 Assessment techniques for developmental dysplasia of the hip.

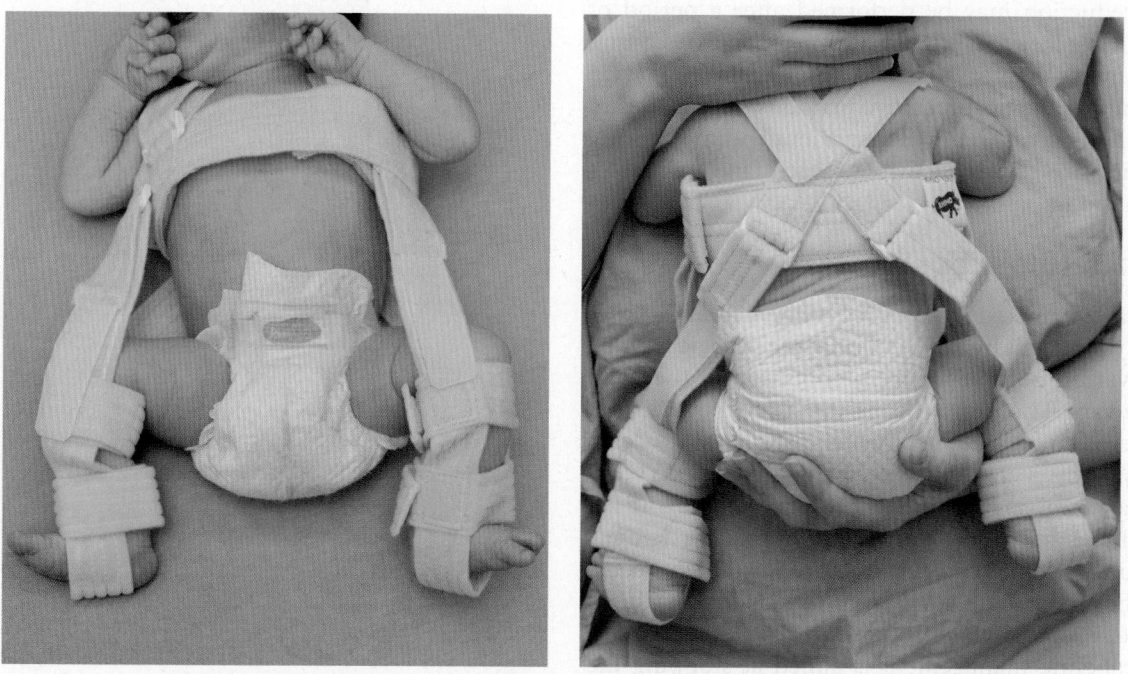

FIGURE 44.15 Pavlik harness for treatment of developmental dysplasia of the hip.

TEACHING GUIDELINE 44.4

Caring for a Child in a Pavlik Harness

- Do not adjust the straps without checking with the physician first.
- Until your physician instructs you to take the harness off for a period of time each day, it must be used continuously (for the first week or sometimes longer).
- Change your baby's diaper while he or she is in the harness.
- Place your baby to sleep on his or her back.
- Do not place clothes under the harness during the period of continuous use.
- Once the baby is permitted to be out of the harness for a short period, you may bathe your baby while the harness is off.
- Long knee socks and an undershirt are recommended to prevent rubbing of the skin against the brace.
- Note location of the markings on the straps for appropriate placement of the harness.
- Wash the harness with mild detergent by hand and air dry. If using the dryer, use *only* the air fluffing setting (no heat).

3 months (Teaching Guideline 44.4). Breastfeeding can continue throughout the harness treatment period, but creative positioning of the infant may be needed.

For infants or children diagnosed later than 6 months of age or those who do not improve with harness use, surgical reduction may be performed after a period of traction (Hosalker et al., 2007b). Postoperative casting followed by bracing or orthotic use is common. Caring for the child in the postoperative period is similar to care of any child in a cast. Pain management and monitoring for bleeding are priority activities. Teach families care of the cast at home.

Tibia Vara (Blount's Disease)

Tibia vara (Blount's disease) is a developmental disorder affecting young children. The normal physiologic bowing or genu varum becomes more pronounced in the child with tibia vara. The cause of tibia vara is unknown, but it is considered to be a developmental disorder as it occurs most frequently in children who are early walkers. In addition to early walking, obesity is also a risk factor. If left untreated, the growth plate of the upper tibia ceases bone production. Asymmetric growth at the knee then occurs and the bowing progresses. Severe degenerative arthritis of the knee is an additional long-term complication.

Therapeutic management is aimed at stopping the progression of the disease through bracing or surgical

treatment. Medical or surgical treatment should begin early, before 4 years of age.

Nursing Assessment

Elicit a health history and determine the age at which the child started walking. Assess growth parameters to determine whether the risk factor of obesity is present. Note significant bowing of the legs in standing and while ambulating (Fig. 44.16).

Nursing Management

Bracing may include a modified knee–ankle–foot orthosis that relieves the compression forces on the growth plate, allowing bone growth resumption and correction of bowlegs. To be successful, bracing must be continued for months to years and the brace must be worn 23 hours per day. Compliance is the most significant barrier to successful treatment. Parents have a difficult time forcing their toddler to stay in a brace that inhibits mobility for the bulk of the day (particularly a bilateral brace). Support parents by encouraging and praising their compliance with bracing. Teach parents to assess for potential skin impairment from brace rubbing.

When surgical treatment is required, the leg(s) will be immobilized in a long-leg bent knee or spica cast after the osteotomy is performed. Perform routine cast care.

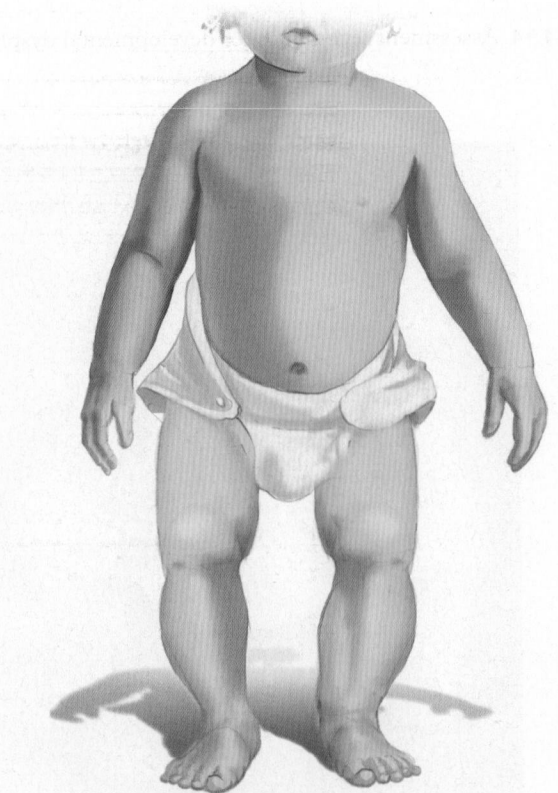

FIGURE 44.16 Note extreme bowing of the legs in tibia vara.

Refer to Nursing Care Plan 44.1 for additional interventions related to care of the immobilized child.

Torticollis

Torticollis is a painless muscular condition presenting in infants or in children with certain syndromes. Congenital muscular torticollis may result from in utero positioning or difficult birth. Preferential turning of the head to one side while in the supine position after birth may also lead to torticollis. Torticollis results from tightness of the sternocleidomastoid muscle, resulting in the infant's head being tilted to one side.

Medical treatment involves passive stretching exercises, which are effective in 90% of affected infants (Luther, 2002). Botulinum toxin injection has been used recently with success in cases of torticollis that have not improved with stretching exercises. Plagiocephaly may result from the continued pressure on the side of the skull to which the neck is turned.

Nursing Assessment

Note history of head tilt and infant's lack of desire to turn the head in the opposite direction. Observe the infant for wry-neck (tilting of the head to one side; Fig. 44.17). Note limited movement of the neck when passive range of motion is performed. Palpate the neck, noting a mass in the sternocleidomastoid muscle on the affected side.

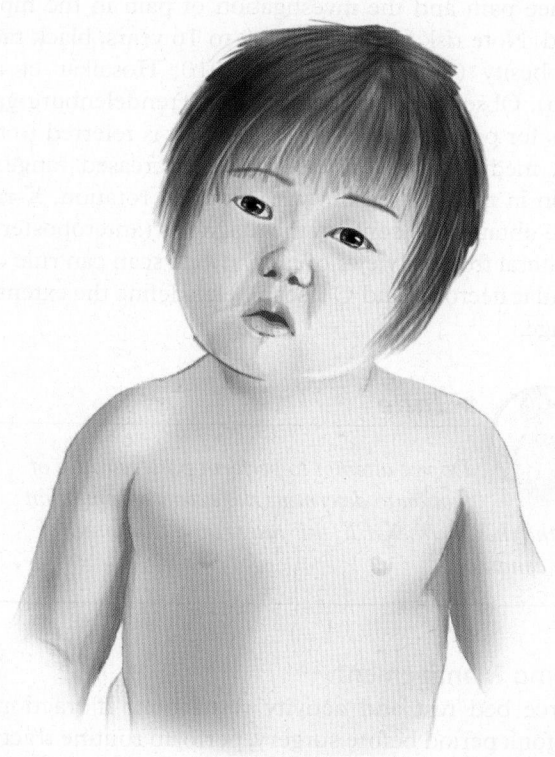

FIGURE 44.17 Note wry-neck or head tilt in the infant with torticollis.

Examine the head for evidence of plagiocephaly. In 20% of cases, accompanying hip dysplasia is seen; therefore, careful examination of the hips is warranted (Polousky & Eilert, 2009).

Nursing Management

Teach parents gentle neck-stretching exercises to be performed several times a day. While immobilizing the shoulder on the affected side, gently sustain a side-to-side stretch toward the unaffected side, holding the stretch for 10 to 30 seconds. Repeat 10 to 15 times per session. Perform an ear-to-shoulder stretch in a similar fashion. To prevent the development of torticollis in the unaffected infant, positional plagiocephaly must be prevented. Prevent flatness of one side of the head by varying the baby's head position, and do not always turn the head to one side while in the infant seat or swing or lying supine. Refer families to the National Infant Torticollis Foundation, a parent support network (visit http://thePoint.lww.com/Chow1e for a direct link).

Acquired Disorders

Several acquired musculoskeletal disorders may affect children. Nutritional deficits or malabsorption of fats may lead to rickets. Slipped capital femoral epiphysis (SCFE) and Legg–Calvé–Perthes disease affect mainly school-age and adolescent boys. Osteomyelitis, septic arthritis, and toxic synovitis are common infectious musculoskeletal disorders. Spinal curvature may occur as a result of a neuromuscular disorder or idiopathically.

Rickets

Rickets is a condition in which there is softening or weakening of the bones. Childhood rickets may occur as a result of nutritional deficiencies such as inadequate consumption of calcium or limited exposure to sunlight (required for adequate production of vitamin D). Rickets may also occur if the body cannot regulate calcium and phosphorus in the appropriate balance, such as in chronic renal disease. Gastrointestinal disorders in which fat absorption is altered (e.g., Crohn's disease and cystic fibrosis) may lead to rickets, as vitamin D is a fat-soluble vitamin. Vitamin D regulates calcium absorption from the small intestine and levels of calcium and phosphate in the bones. Calcium is primarily laid down in the bones of the fetus during the third trimester. Premature infants miss this period of calcium accumulation and also suffer from inadequate calcium intake in the neonatal period and often demonstrate rickets of prematurity. When calcium and phosphate levels in the blood are imbalanced, then calcium is released from the bones into the blood, resulting in loss of the supportive bony matrix. Rickets is most likely to occur during periods of rapid growth.

Therapeutic Management

Treatment of rickets is aimed at correcting the calcium imbalance so that the skeleton may develop properly and without deformity. Calcium and phosphorus supplements are given, and some children also require vitamin D supplements. If rickets is not corrected while the child is still growing, permanent skeletal deformities and short stature may result.

> ▶ **Take** NOTE!
>
> *Children who do not receive adequate daily exposure to sunlight require supplementation with 5 µg of vitamin D per day.*

Nursing Assessment

Obtain a health history, determining risk factors such as:

- Limited exposure to sunlight
- Strict vegetarian diet or lactose intolerance (either one without milk product ingestion)
- Exclusive breastfeeding by a mother who has a vitamin D deficiency
- Dark-pigmented skin
- Prematurity
- Malabsorptive gastrointestinal disorder
- Chronic renal disease

Note history of fractures or bone pain. Observe for dental deformities and bowlegs. Decreased muscle tone may also be present. Note low serum calcium and phosphate levels and high alkaline phosphatase levels. X-rays may show changes in the shape and structure of the bone.

Nursing Management

Administer calcium and phosphorus supplements at alternate times to promote proper absorption of both of these supplements. Encourage exposure to moderate amounts of sunlight and administer vitamin D supplements as prescribed. Teach families that good dietary sources of vitamin D are fish, liver, and processed milk.

Slipped Capital Femoral Epiphysis

SCFE is a condition in which the femoral head dislocates from the neck and shaft of the femur at the level of the epiphyseal plate. The epiphysis slips downward and backward. SCFE occurs most frequently in obese boys 9 to 16 years of age; it is more common in black boys than in white boys (Hosalkar et al., 2007b; Leung & Lemay, 2004). The exact cause is unknown, but it is thought that during the teenage growth spurt the femoral growth plate weakens and becomes less resistant to stressors. Hormonal alterations during this period may also play a role (Hosalkar et al., 2007b).

SCFE is classified based upon its severity and whether the slip is acute or chronic. Chronic SCFE may lead to shortening of the affected leg and thigh atrophy.

Therapeutic Management

Promptly refer the child with SCFE to an orthopedic surgeon, as early surgical intervention will decrease the risk of long-term deformity. The goals of therapeutic management are to prevent further slippage, minimize deformity, and avoid the complications of cartilage necrosis (chondrolysis) and avascular necrosis of the femoral head. Surgical intervention may include in situ pinning, in which a pin or screw is inserted percutaneously into the femoral head to hold it in place. Osteotomy may be used for more severe cases. Osteoarthritis may be a long-term complication of SCFE. If the child has one SCFE, he is at risk for the other hip to slip. The child should appear in the emergency department if the other hip develops acute pain. In a very young child (less than 9 years of age), the orthopedic surgeon may decide to pin the unaffected hip prophylactically. Children younger than 9 years of age are usually sent for an endocrine workup.

Nursing Assessment

Elicit a health history, determining the onset and extent of pain. In acute SCFE, the pain is usually sudden in onset and results in the inability to bear weight. Chronic SCFE may present with an insidious onset of pain and limp. Sometimes the pain in the child with SCFE is mistaken for knee pain and the investigation of pain in the hip is missed. Note risk factors of age 9 to 16 years, black race, and obesity (Grewal & Ahier, 2010; Hosalkar et al., 2007b). Observe ambulation, noting Trendelenburg gait. Assess for pain that is in the hip or that is referred to the groin, medial thigh, or knee. Note decreased range of motion in the affected hip with external rotation. X-rays will be obtained to confirm the diagnosis (anteroposterior and lateral frog-leg views of hips). Bone scan can rule out avascular necrosis, and CT scan helps define the extent of slippage.

> ▶ **Take** NOTE!
>
> *Do not attempt to perform passive range of motion to determine the extent of limitation in the child with SCFE; this may cause worsening of the condition.*

Nursing Management

Enforce bed rest and activity restriction. If traction is used for a period before surgery, perform routine traction care and neurovascular assessments. Assess pain and administer analgesics as needed. After in situ pinning, assist the child with crutch walking. Teach the family that weight-bearing is usually resumed about a week after the surgery and that the pin will be removed later. Prolonged immobility may isolate the adolescent from usual peer interactions, so encourage phone calls and visits with friends. Provide books, games, electronic devices, and magazines for distraction during the period of immobility. Provide family support.

Legg–Calvé–Perthes Disease

Legg–Calvé–Perthes disease is a self-limiting condition that involves avascular necrosis of the femoral head. It occurs most often in small, active white boys or those of Asian descent, usually between the ages of 4 and 10 years, with peak incidence between 6 and 9 years of age (Gunner & Scott, 2001). The disease affects girls much less frequently (Grewal & Ahier, 2010). The etiology is unknown, but the interruption of the blood supply to the femoral head results in bone death, and the spherical shape of the femoral head may be lost. Swelling of the soft tissues around the hip may occur. As new blood vessels develop, the area is supplied with circulation, allowing bone resorption and deposition to take place. During this period of revascularization, which takes 18 to 24 months, the bone is soft and more likely to fracture. Over time, the femoral head re-forms.

Therapeutic Management

The goal of therapeutic management is to maintain normal femoral head shape and to restore appropriate motion. Treatment of Legg–Calvé–Perthes disease includes anti-inflammatory medication to decrease muscle spasms around the hip joint and to relieve pain. Activity limitation may be prescribed, and sometimes traction followed by bracing is recommended to contain the femoral head. Serial X-ray follow-up determines progress of the disease. If surgery becomes warranted, then osteotomy may be performed. Complications include joint deformity, early degenerative joint disease, persistent pain, loss of hip motion or function, and gait disturbance.

Nursing Assessment

Explore the health history for short stature, delayed bone maturation, or a family history of Legg–Calvé–Perthes disease. Note painless limp, which may be intermittent over a period of months. Mild hip pain may result and may be referred to the knee or the thigh. Pain may be aggravated by exercise. Observe the child walking and note Trendelenburg gait. Perform range of motion, noting internal rotation of the hip and limited abduction. Muscle spasm may result with hip extension and rotation. Hip X-rays are obtained to evaluate the extent of epiphyseal involvement. MRI or bone scan may also be used to differentiate Legg–Calvé–Perthes disease from other disorders.

Nursing Management

Nursing care of Legg–Calvé–Perthes disease is highly variable and depends on the stage of the disease and its severity. Administer anti-inflammatory medications, noting their effect on pain. If activities are restricted, exercise the unaffected body parts. Assist families with use of the brace if prescribed. The brace may be wiped with a damp cloth if it becomes dirty. Some children will be prescribed no treatment other than avoidance of contact or high-impact sports. Swimming and bicycle riding help to maintain range of motion with little risk. If mobility equipment is needed, educate the child and family on its use. If osteotomy is performed, provide routine postoperative care, with education and support of the child and family.

Osteomyelitis

Osteomyelitis is a bacterial infection of the bone and soft tissue surrounding the bone. The long bone metaphysis is the most common location (Grewal & Ahier, 2010). Children usually present for evaluation within a few days to a week of onset of symptoms, though some may present later. Osteomyelitis is most often diagnosed in children between the ages of 3 and 12 years. Infection with *Staphylococcus aureus* accounts for 90% of cases in infants and children who are otherwise healthy (Carek, Dickerson, & Sack, 2001). Additional causes in infants include group B streptococcus and *Escherichia coli;* in children, *Streptococcus pyogenes* and *Haemophilus influenzae* are also implicated (although infection with *H. influenzae* is now rare due to improvements in immunizations).

Osteomyelitis is acquired hematogenously. Bacteria from the bloodstream mainly invade the most rapidly growing portion of the bone. The invading bacteria trigger an inflammatory response, formation of pus and edema, and vascular congestion. Small blood vessels thrombose and the infection extends into the metaphyseal marrow cavity. As the infection progresses, the inflammation extends throughout the bone and blood supply is disrupted, resulting in death of the bone tissues (Fig. 44.18).

Therapeutic Management

Treatment includes a 4- to 6-week course of antibiotics. Some children may receive 1 to 2 weeks of intravenous antibiotics and then be switched to oral antibiotics for the remainder of the course. Surgical debridement is rarely necessary. Early treatment may prevent the complications of bone destruction, fracture, and growth arrest. Additional complications include recurrent infection, septic arthritis, and systemic infection.

Nursing Assessment

For a full description of the assessment phase of the nursing process, refer to page 1516. Assessment findings pertinent to osteomyelitis are discussed here. Explore the health history for risk factors and symptoms. Risk factors

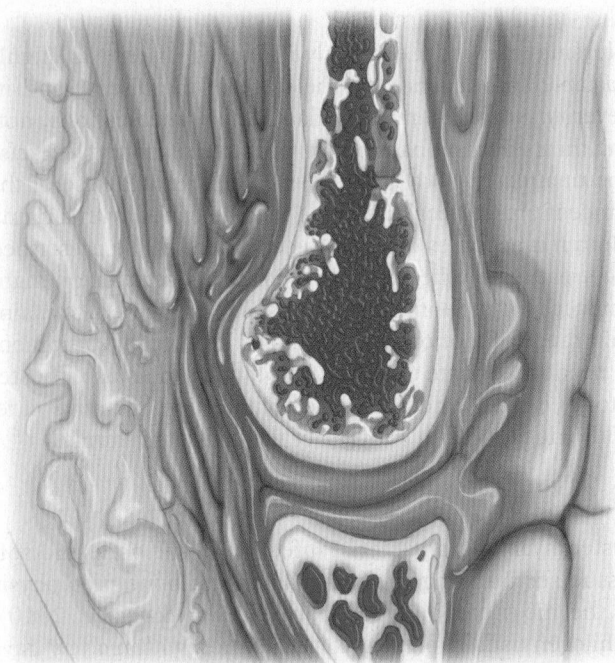

FIGURE 44.18 In osteomyelitis, bacterial invasion leads to infection within the bone.

include impetigo, infected varicella lesions, furunculosis, infected burns, and prolonged intravenous line use. Note history of irritability, lethargy, possible fever, and onset of pain or change in activity level. The child usually refuses to walk and demonstrates decreased range of motion in the affected extremity. Inspect the affected extremity for swelling. Palpate for local warmth and tenderness. Note point tenderness over affected bone.

Laboratory and diagnostic testing may reveal:

- Elevated white blood cell count, erythrocyte sedimentation rate, and C-reactive protein level
- Positive blood cultures (present in 50% of children; Carek et al., 2001)
- Deep soft tissue swelling on X-ray
- Changes on ultrasound or CT scan

Nursing Management

Nursing management of osteomyelitis focuses on assessment, pain management, and maintenance of intravenous access for administration of antibiotics. Individualize care based on the child's and family's response to the illness; see Nursing Care Plan 44.1. Maintain bed rest initially to prevent injury and promote comfort. Administer antipyretics as ordered if the child is febrile in the initial stage of the illness. Encourage use of unaffected extremities by providing developmentally appropriate toys and games. Instruct child and family on safe and proper use of crutches or walker if prescribed. Some children will be discharged home on intravenous antibiotics, while others will finish an

oral antibiotic course. Teach parents proper administration of medications and maintenance of a peripherally inserted central catheter or central line at home if the child is finishing the antibiotic course intravenously.

Septic Arthritis

Acute septic arthritis is a condition in which bacteria invade the joint space, most often the hip. It can occur at any age but usually occurs in children younger than 3 years of age (Dugdale, Vyas, & Zieve, 2011). Bacteria gain access to the joint in one of three ways:

- Directly from a puncture of the joint or via venipuncture or wound infection
- Seeding from a distal infection site (e.g., otitis media or respiratory infection)
- Compression of the joint capsule from adjacent osteomyelitis

S. aureus and various streptococci are the most common responsible organisms (Schwentker, 2009). *H. influenzae* used to be a common cause but is now rare due to improvements in immunizations (Schwentker, 2009). Sepsis of the hip joint may cause avascular necrosis of the femoral head due to pressure on blood vessels and cartilage within the joint space. Septic arthritis is considered a medical emergency, as this destruction may occur within just a few days. Additional complications of septic arthritis include permanent deformity, leg-length discrepancy, and long-term decreased range of motion and disability.

The goals of treatment of septic arthritis are to prevent destruction of the joint cartilage and maintain function, motion, and strength. Septic arthritis is treated rapidly with joint aspiration or arthrotomy, followed by intravenous antibiotic therapy while in the hospital and oral antibiotics at home.

Nursing Assessment

Note history of predisposing factors such as respiratory infection or otitis media, skin or soft tissue infections, or, in the neonate, traumatic puncture wounds and femoral venipunctures. The history is usually significant for sudden onset of fever and moderate to severe pain.

Upon physical examination, the infant or child appears ill. Note extent of fever, refusal to bear weight or straighten the hip, and limited range of motion (the child usually maintains the joint in flexion and will not allow the leg to be straightened). Palpate the affected joint for warmth and swelling.

Laboratory findings may include the following:

- White blood cell count normal or elevated with elevated neutrophil counts
- Elevated erythrocyte sedimentation rate and C-reactive protein levels

- Fluid from joint aspiration demonstrates elevated white blood cell count; culture determines responsible organism.
- Joint X-ray may show subtle soft tissue changes or increase in the joint space.
- Positive blood culture for the causative organism (15% of cases)

Nursing Management

Refer to Nursing Care Plan 44.1 for interventions related to musculoskeletal disorders. Assess aspiration wound for signs of infection. Monitor vital signs for resolution of fever. Pain management with ibuprofen or acetaminophen will be sufficient for some children; others may initially require morphine. The use of codeine has started to be discouraged in pediatrics as it is metabolized ultra-rapidly in some children. Assess the affected joint for a decrease in swelling, increasing range of motion, and decreasing or absent pain. The child may be discharged after 72 hours of intravenous antibiotics following joint aspiration if he or she is improving and can tolerate oral antibiotics. At discharge, if the child cannot ambulate, physical therapy may be consulted for short-term use of crutches or a wheelchair. Teach families how to assess for signs and symptoms of wound infection, how to administer oral antibiotics and pain medication, and how to assist their child with crutch walking.

Transient Synovitis of the Hip

Transient synovitis of the hip (also termed toxic synovitis) is the most common cause of hip pain in children (Kehl, 2006). It occurs in children as young as 9 months of age through adolescence, most commonly affecting children 3 to 8 years old (Hosalker et al., 2007b). Boys are affected twice as often as girls (Polousky & Eilert, 2009), and blacks exhibit the lowest incidence. The exact cause is unclear, but it is thought to be associated with recent or active infection, trauma, or allergic hypersensitivity (Hosalker et al., 2007b). A self-limiting disease, most cases resolve within a week, but it may last as long as 4 weeks. Therapeutic management involves nonsteroidal anti-inflammatory medications and bed rest to relieve weight-bearing on the affected hip joint.

Nursing Assessment

Explore the health history for risk factors such as antecedent trauma, concurrent or recent upper respiratory tract infection, pharyngitis, or otitis media. Note sudden acute onset of moderate to severe pain of one hip. Sometimes pain is referred to the anterior thigh or knee. Pain is usually the worst upon arising in the morning, and the child refuses to walk, with pain decreasing throughout the day. Temperature will be normal or low-grade (<38°C). Observe for a limp or for refusal to bear weight. Observe position of the affected hip: it will be held in a flexed and externally rotated position. Note restricted range of motion for abduction and internal rotation.

Nursing Management

Nursing care focuses on educating the family. Parents are very concerned when their child refuses to walk, and they will need significant support and reassurance.

Scoliosis

Scoliosis is a lateral curvature of the spine that exceeds 10 degrees. It may be congenital, associated with other disorders, or idiopathic. Table 44.4 explains the types of scoliosis. Idiopathic scoliosis accounts for more than 80% of all cases, with the majority of those occurring during adolescence (Scoliosis Research Society, 2011). Hence, this discussion focuses on adolescent idiopathic scoliosis. The etiology of idiopathic scoliosis is not known, but genetic factors, growth abnormalities, and bone, muscle, disc, or central nervous system disorders may contribute to its development. Adolescent idiopathic scoliosis affects 1% to 3% of children between the ages of 10 and 16 years (Weinstein, Dolan, Cheng, Danielsson, & Morcuende, 2008).

Pathophysiology

In the rapidly growing adolescent, the involved vertebrae rotate around a vertical axis, resulting in lateral curvature. The vertebrae rotate to the convex side of curve, with the spinous processes rotating toward the concave side. The spinal deformity begins with wedging of the intervertebral discs leading to asymmetrical forces on the growing vertebrae, decreasing growth of the vertebrae on the concave side (Will, Stokes, Qiu, Walker, & Sanders, 2009).

TABLE 44.4 **TYPES OF SCOLIOSIS**

Type	Associated Factors
Idiopathic	Unknown cause Infantile: occurs in the first 3 years of life Juvenile: diagnosed between ages 4 and 10 years, or prior to adolescence Adolescent: age 11 to 17 years
Neuromuscular	Associated with neurologic or muscular disease such as cerebral palsy, myelomeningocele, spinal cord tumours, spinal muscular atrophy
Myopathic	Associated with certain types of muscular dystrophy
Congenital	Results from anomalous vertebral development

| BOX 44.2 | **Types of Braces Used to Treat Scoliosis** |

- Underarm (Boston, Wilmington): less conspicuous, no visible neckpiece
- Milwaukee: traditional standard, has a visible neckpiece
- Nighttime bending (Charleston): creates a curve so severe that walking is not possible, so can be worn only at night

As the curve progresses, the shape of the thoracic cage changes, leading to visible signs of scoliosis that include waist and shoulder asymmetry, rib hump, and uneven scapulae. If scoliosis progresses to a severe degree (>100 degrees), cardiovascular and respiratory compromise may occur.

Therapeutic Management

Treatment of scoliosis is aimed at preventing progression of the curve and decreasing the impact on pulmonary and cardiac function. Treatment is based on the age of the child, expected future growth, and severity of the curve. Observation with serial examinations and spine X-rays is used to monitor curve progression. Bracing may be sufficient to decrease progression in curves of 20 to 45 degrees. Some curves will progress despite appropriate bracing and compliance. Box 44.2 describes types of scoliosis braces and Figure 44.19 shows examples. The choice of brace will depend on the location and severity of the curve.

Surgical correction is often required for curves greater than 45 degrees; it is achieved with rod placement and bone grafting (Grewal & Ahier, 2010; Spiegel, Hosalkar, Dormans, & Drommond, 2007). Partial spinal fusion accompanies many of the corrective surgeries. Multiple surgical approaches and techniques exist for fusion and rod placement. The surgical approach may be anterior, posterior, or both. Traditional rod placement (Harrington rod) involved a single rod fused to the vertebrae, resulting in curve correction but also a flat-backed appearance. Newer rod instrumentation allows for scoliosis curve correction with maintenance of normal back curvature. The rods are shorter, and several are wired or grafted to the appropriate vertebrae to achieve correction. Figure 44.20 shows one example of surgical rod instrumentation.

Nursing Assessment

For a full description of the assessment phase of the nursing process, refer to page 1516. Assessment findings pertinent to scoliosis are discussed below.

Health History

Determine why the child is presenting for evaluation of scoliosis. Often the family or primary care physician observes asymmetry in the hips or shoulders. The child may or may not have a history of back pain. It is important to determine whether there are any "red flags" in the history such as loss of bowel or bladder control, arm or leg numbness or tingling, weight loss, night sweats, or night pain. Explore the patient's current and past medical history for risk factors such as

- Family history of scoliosis
- Recent growth spurt
- Physical changes related to puberty

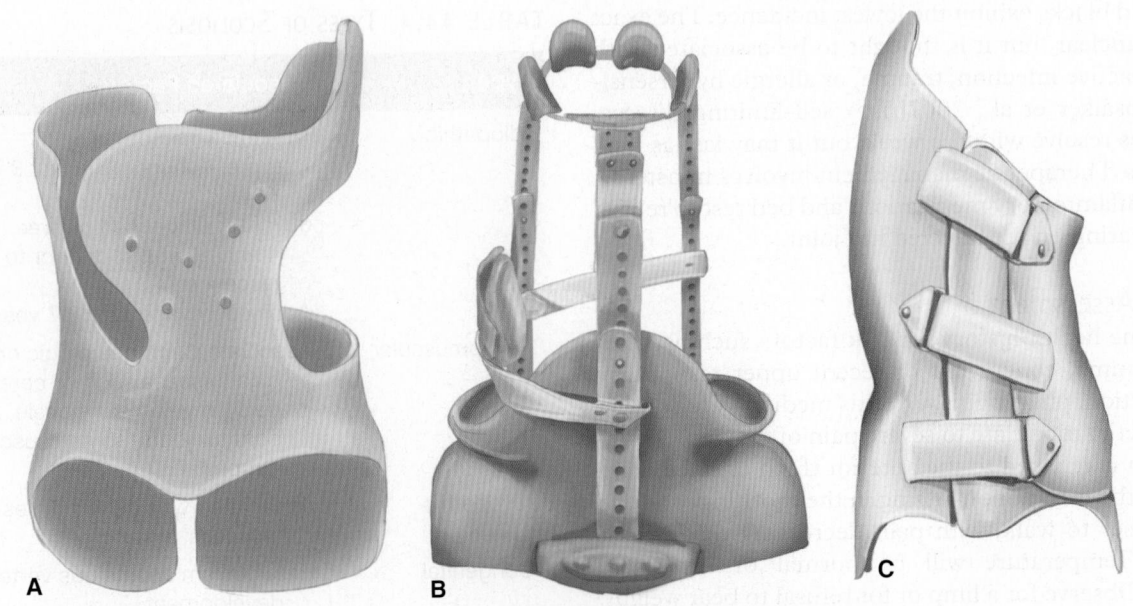

FIGURE 44.19 (**A**) Boston brace. (**B**) Milwaukee brace. (**C**) Nighttime bending brace.

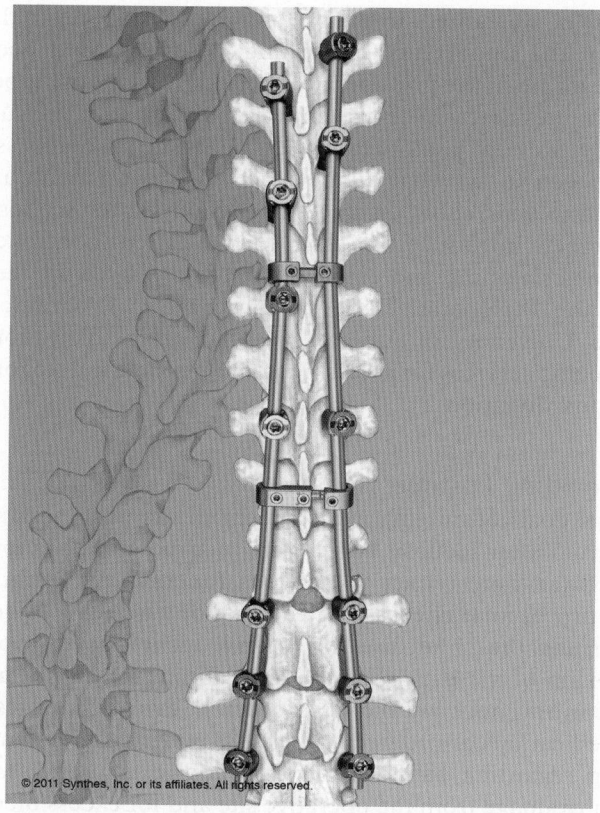

FIGURE 44.20 Spinal instrumentation involving a series of titanium screws connected to rods that are fused to the spine. ©Synthes, Inc. or its affiliates. All rights reserved.

Determine the age of development of secondary sex characteristics and the age of menarche, as these signs of pubertal development indicate the expected velocity and length of remaining growth.

Physical Examination

The physical assessment of a child with possible or actual scoliosis involves observing physical characteristics and identifying potentially serious neurologic abnormalities that may be causing the scoliosis.

Observe the child sitting, standing, and walking for evidence of asymmetry and gait abnormalities. Inspect and palpate the child's back in a standing position. Note asymmetries such as shoulder elevation, prominence of one scapula, uneven curve at the waistline, or a rib hump on one side. Measure shoulder levels from the floor to the acromioclavicular joints. Note the difference between the height of the high and low shoulder in centimetres. Measure the heights of the anterior and posterior iliac spines and note the difference in centimetres. View the patient from the side, noting abnormalities in the spinal curve. Perform the Adam's forward bend test: with the child bending forward, arms hanging freely, note asymmetry of the back (pronounced hump on one side). Figure 44.21 shows scoliosis noted upon visual inspection. Assess for leg-length discrepancy and measure if present. During the neurologic examination, balance, motor strength, sensation, and reflexes should all be normal.

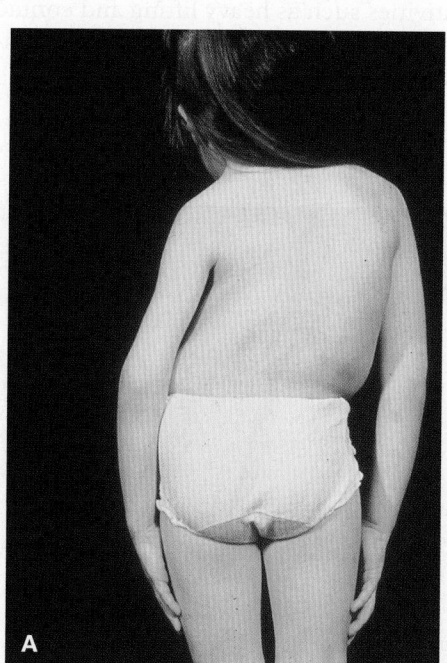

A

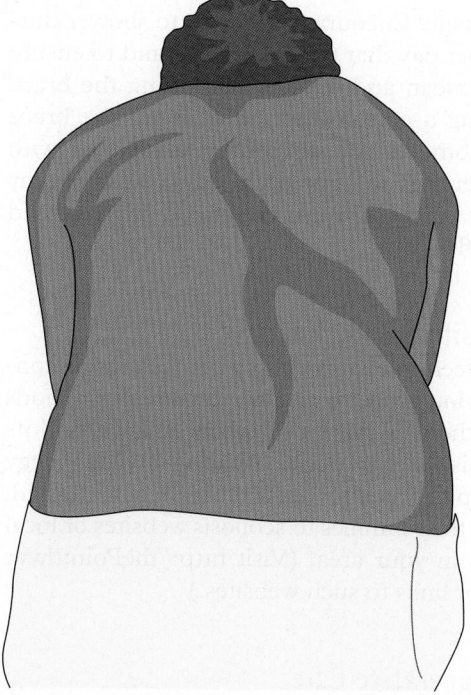

B

FIGURE 44.21 (**A**) Note right shoulder, scapula, and hip elevation as well as discrepancy in waist curvature. (**B**) Note right upper back hump.

Laboratory and Diagnostic Tests

Full-spine X-rays are necessary to determine the degree of curvature. The radiologist will determine the extent of the curve based on specific formulas and techniques of measurement. Abnormal neurologic signs or symptoms should be further investigated with MRI.

Nursing Management

Nursing Care Plan 44.1 lists general interventions; nursing care should be tailored based on the adolescent's response to the disease and its treatment. Additional nursing interventions specific to scoliosis are discussed here.

Encouraging Compliance with Bracing

Bracing is intended to prevent progression of the curve but does not correct the current curve. Although modern braces display an improved appearance, with no visible neckpiece, and can be worn under clothes, many adolescents are not compliant with brace wear. Many factors may contribute to noncompliance, including the discomforts associated with brace wear such as pain, heat, and poor fit. The family environment may not be conducive to compliance with brace wear, and teenagers are very concerned about body image. There are various types of braces for scoliosis; some need to be worn full-time (23 hours/day), while others are designed for nighttime wear only.

Inspect the skin for evidence of rubbing by the brace that may impair skin integrity. Teach families appropriate skin care and recommend they check the brace daily for fit and breakage. Encourage the teen to shower during the 1 hour per day that the brace is off and to ensure that the skin is clean and dry before putting the brace back on. Wearing a cotton undershirt under the brace may decrease some of the discomfort associated with brace wear. Exercises to strengthen back muscles may prevent muscle atrophy from prolonged bracing and maintain spine flexibility.

Promoting Positive Body Image

Encourage the teen to express his or her feelings or concerns about having scoliosis and the treatment methods involved. Give the teen ways to explain scoliosis and its treatment to his or her peers. Wearing stylish baggy clothes may help the teen to conceal the brace if desired. Refer teens and their families to scoliosis websites or local support groups in your area. (Visit http://thePoint.lww.com/Chow1e for links to such websites.)

Providing Preoperative Care

If the curve progresses despite bracing or causes pulmonary or cardiac compromise, surgical intervention may be warranted. In the preoperative period, teach the teen the importance of turning, coughing, and deep breathing in the postoperative period. Explain the tubes and lines that will be present immediately after the surgery. Review postoperative mobilization protocols, so the teen knows what will be expected. Most patients are able to walk short distances 2 or 3 days after scoliosis surgery. Introduce the child to the patient-controlled analgesia pump and explain pain scales. Refer the teen to the Perioperative Blood Conservation Program at the University of Alberta Hospital or to institution-specific services for assessment and possible autologous blood donation.

Providing Postoperative Care

The goals of nursing management in the postoperative period after scoliosis surgery are to avoid complications and facilitate return to previous functioning. Perform neurovascular checks with each set of vital signs. When turning the child, use the log-roll technique to avoid flexion of the back (Fig. 44.22). Administer prophylactic intravenous antibiotics if ordered. Provide analgesic medications as ordered and ensure patient understanding regarding patient-controlled analgesia use. Assess for drainage from the operative site and for excess blood loss via the Hemovac or other drainage tube. Maintain Foley patency and strict recording of fluid intake and output. Administer IV fluids and transfusions of packed red blood cells if ordered. Ambulation, once ordered, should be done slowly with the assistance of at least two people. The hospitalization period is typically less than 1 week, with another 3 to 6 weeks at home for recovery. Activities such as heavy lifting and contact sports will be restricted for 6 to 12 months according to the surgeon's recommendations.

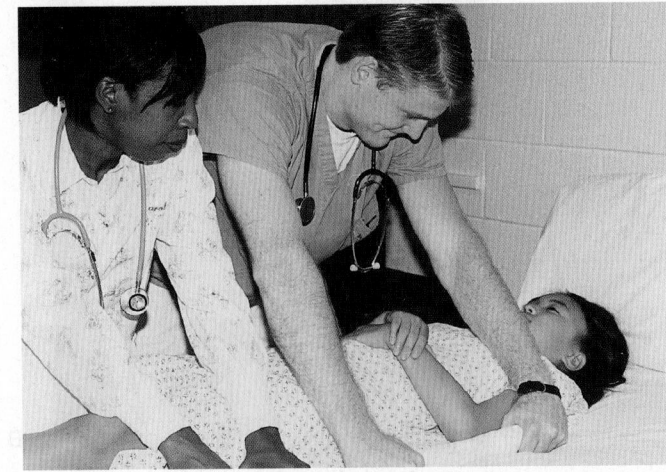

FIGURE 44.22 Log-roll the postoperative spinal fusion patient to prevent pain and spine flexion.

▶ *Consider* THIS!

Angela Hernandez, a 15-year-old girl, is being seen in the clinic after her dance teacher noticed unevenness in her posture. Upon assessment the nurse notes asymmetry of the hips, with shoulder elevation and prominence of one scapula. She is visibly upset and wants to know what caused this and what can be done. How would you address her concerns?

Angela's plan of care will include wearing of a brace. What education will be necessary and how can you promote compliance?

Describe nursing care for Angela if surgical correction is necessary.

Injuries

Injuries throughout childhood are inevitable. Trauma often occurs as a result of motor vehicle injury. The bulk of trauma resulting from physical activity or sports in children is due to running, skateboarding, and climbing trees. Only about one third of sports injuries in children occur during organized sports; the rest occur in physical education class or non-organized sports (Busch, 2006). Younger children tend to suffer contusions, sprains, and simple upper extremity fractures; adolescents more frequently experience lower-extremity trauma. As the number of children participating in youth sports increases and the intensity of training and level of competition also increase, the incidence of injury is also likely to rise.

Many types of musculoskeletal injuries exist. This discussion focuses on fractures, sprains, overuse syndromes, and dislocated radial head.

▶ *Take* NOTE!

Fracture in the newborn or infant should raise a high index of suspicion for abuse, as fractures are very unusual in children who cannot yet walk.

Fracture

Fractures occur frequently in children and adolescents; 40% of boys and 25% of girls will suffer a fracture by age 16 years. Most common fractures in children occur in the forearm and wrist (Grewal & Ahier, 2010). Greenstick and buckle fractures account for about half of pediatric fractures, and only about 20% of childhood fractures require reduction (Price, Phillips, & Devito, 2006).

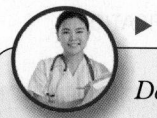

▶ *Take* NOTE!

Do not attempt to straighten or manipulate an injured limb.

Pathophysiology

Fractures result most frequently from accidental trauma (Grewal & Ahier, 2010). Nonaccidental trauma (child abuse) and other disease processes are the other causes of fractures. The growth plate is the most vulnerable portion of the child's bone and is frequently the site of injury. The Salter–Harris classification system is used to describe fractures involving the growth plate (Table 44.5). The thicker, more elastic periosteum in children yields to the force encountered with trauma, resulting more frequently in nondisplaced fractures in children. The increased vascularity and decreased mineral content make the child's bones more flexible. Plastic or bowing deformities and buckle and greenstick fractures are the result. Complete fractures do occur in children, but they tend to be more stable than in the adult, resulting in improved healing and function. Spiral, pelvic, and hip fractures are rare in children. Table 44.6 explains common types of fractures in children.

Plastic deformity and Salter–Harris type IV fractures may result in an angular deformity. Though healing of fractures is usually quick and without incident in children, delayed union, nonunion, or malunion can occur. Additional complications include infection, avascular necrosis, bone shortening from epiphyseal arrest, vascular or nerve injuries, fat embolism, reflex sympathetic dystrophy, and compartment syndrome, which is an orthopedic emergency. Later in life, osteoarthritis may occur as a long-term complication of childhood fracture (Dugdale, 2010).

▶ *Take* NOTE!

Any type of fracture can be the result of child abuse, but spiral femur fractures, rib fractures, and humerus fractures, particularly in the child younger than 2 years of age, should always be thoroughly investigated to rule out the possibility of abuse (Gholve, Hosalkar, & Wells, 2007).

Therapeutic Management

The vast majority of childhood fractures would heal well with splinting only, but casting of these fractures is performed to provide further comfort to the child and to allow for increased activity while the fracture is healing. Displaced fractures require manual traction to align the bones, followed by casting. More severe fractures may require traction for a period of time, usually followed by casting. Severe or complicated fractures may alternatively require open reduction and internal fixation for

TABLE 44.5 THE SALTER–HARRIS CLASSIFICATION SYSTEM

Type	Description	Illustration
I	Fracture is through the physis, widening it	
II	Fracture is partially through the physis, extending into the metaphysis	
III	Fracture is partially through the epiphysis, extending into the epiphysis	
IV	Fracture is through the metaphysis, physis, and epiphysis	
V	Crushing injury to the physis	

healing to occur. Complex fractures are often treated with external fixation (Fig. 44.23).

▶ **Take** NOTE!

Significant swelling may occur initially after immobilization with a splint. Splinting and then delaying casting for a few days provides time for some of the swelling to subside, allowing for successful casting a few days after the injury.

Nursing Assessment

For a full description of the assessment phase of the nursing process, refer to page 1516. Assessment findings pertinent to fractures are discussed below.

Health History

Elicit a description of the present illness and chief complaint. Common signs and symptoms reported during the health history might include recent trauma or fall, complaint of pain, difficulty bearing weight, limp, or refusal to use an extremity. Young children often demonstrate sudden onset of irritability and refusal to bear weight. Ask about the mechanism of injury and obtain a description of the traumatic event. Be alert to inconsistencies between the history and the clinical picture or mechanism of injury, as such inconsistency may be an indicator of child abuse. Explore the patient's current and past medical history for risk factors such as:

- Rickets
- Renal osteodystrophy
- Osteogenesis imperfecta
- Participation in sports, particularly contact sports
- Failure to use protective equipment as recommended for various physical activities and sports (e.g., wrist guards while rollerblading)

Physical Examination

Perform the physical examination of the child with a potential fracture carefully, so as not to cause further pain or trauma. The physical examination particular to fractures includes inspection, observation, and palpation.

Inspection and Observation

Inspect the skin for bruising, erythema, or swelling. Observe the extremities for deformity. Note neglect of an extremity or inability to bear weight. If ambulating, note any limp.

Palpation

Carefully palpate the joint or injured part. Distract the young child with a toy or activity while palpating. Note point tenderness, which is a reliable indicator of fracture in children. Assess neurovascular status, noting distal extremity temperature, spontaneous movement, sensation, numbness, capillary refill time, and quality of

TABLE 44.6 TYPES OF FRACTURES IN CHILDREN

Fracture Type	Description	Illustration
Plastic or bowing deformity	Significant bending without breaking of the bone	A
Buckle fracture	Compression injury; the bone buckles rather than breaks	B
Greenstick fracture	Incomplete fracture of the bone	C
Complete fracture	Bone breaks into two pieces	D

pulses. The neurovascular assessment is critical to providing a baseline so that any changes associated with compartment syndrome can be quickly identified.

Laboratory and Diagnostic Tests
Usually plain X-ray films are all that is required to identify a simple fracture. Complicated fractures that require

surgical intervention may require further evaluation with CT or MRI.

Nursing Management
Immediately after the injury, immobilize the limb above and below the site of injury in the most comfortable position with a splint. Use cold therapy to reduce swelling in the first 48 hours after injury. Elevate the injured extremity above the level of the heart. Perform frequent neurovascular checks. Assess pain level and administer pain medications as needed. Administer tetanus vaccine in the child with an open fracture if he or she has not received a tetanus booster within the past 5 years.

> ▶ **Take** NOTE!
>
> *Assess the injured, splinted, or casted extremity frequently for the "5 P's," which may indicate compartment syndrome: pain (increased out of proportion), pulselessness, pallor, paresthesia, and paralysis. Report these findings immediately.*

Providing Family Education
Unless bed rest is prescribed, children with upper extremity casts and "walking" leg casts can resume increased levels of activity as the pain subsides. Children who require crutches while in a cast may return to school, but those in spica casts will be at home for several weeks. Providing distraction and finding ways to keep up with school work are important. Families must also learn to care for the cast (see Teaching Guideline 44.1).

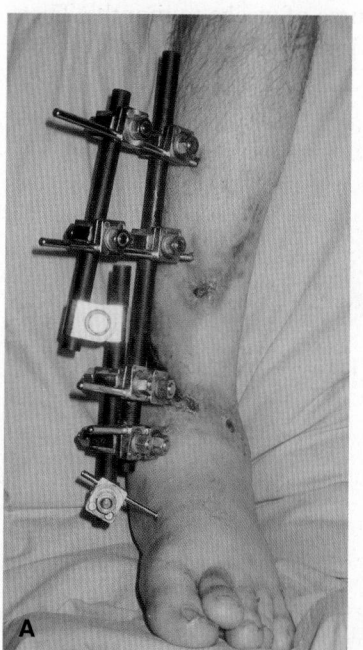
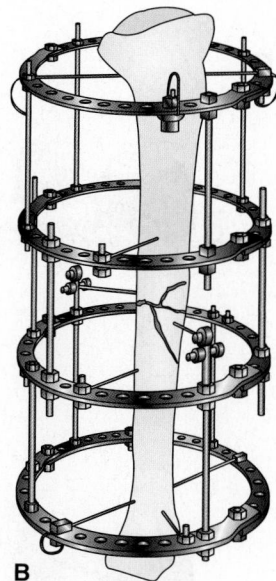

FIGURE 44.23 (**A**) External fixation is required for complicated fractures. (**B**) The Ilizarov fixator is a circular apparatus usually used for complicated lower extremity fractures. The pins are smaller in diameter, more like wires, than those used in other fixators.

Preventing Fractures

Discourage risky behaviour such as climbing trees and performing tricks on bicycles. Provide appropriate supervision, particularly with outdoor activity. Encourage appropriate use of protective equipment, such as wrist guards with rollerblading and shin guards with soccer. Ensure that playground equipment is in good working order and intact; there should not be protruding screws or unbalanced portions of equipment, which may increase the risk for falling.

Sprains

Sprains result from a twisting or turning motion of the affected body part. The tendons and ligaments stretch excessively and may tear slightly. They may occur at any joint, but the most common are ankle and knee sprains. Therapeutic management of sprains includes rest, ice, compression, and elevation (RICE). On initial evaluation, sprains need to be differentiated from torn ligaments and meniscal tears, as those conditions are more serious and may require surgical intervention.

Nursing Assessment

Elicit a health history, determining the mechanism of injury (whether it occurred during sports or simply a misstep or fall). Determine what treatment the family has used so far. Inspect the affected body part for edema, which is frequently present, and bruising, which sometimes occurs. Note limp or inability to bear weight. Do not attempt to perform passive range of motion on the affected body part. Assess neurovascular status distal to the injury (usually normal).

Nursing Management

Instruct the child and family in appropriate treatment of sprains, which includes:

- Rest: limit activity.
- Ice: apply cold packs for 20 to 30 minutes, remove for 1 hour, and repeat (for the first 24 to 48 hours).
- Compression: apply an Ace wrap or other elastic bandage or brace; check skin for alterations when rewrapping.
- Elevation: elevate the injured extremity above the level of the heart to decrease swelling (Fig. 44.24).

The child may require instruction in crutch walking as well. Teach families that to prevent sprains during sports, it is important for the child to perform appropriate stretching and warm-up activities.

▶ **Take** NOTE!

If the child's fingers or toes become increasingly swollen or discoloured, remove the Ace wrap immediately.

Overuse Syndromes

The term "overuse syndrome" refers to a group of disorders that result from repeated force applied to normal tissue. The connective tissues fail in response to repetitive stress, leading to a small amount of tissue breakdown. They develop over the course of weeks to months. There is usually no identifiable injury associated with overuse

RICE

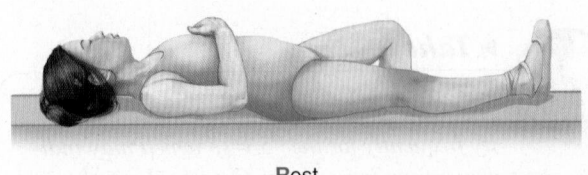

Rest

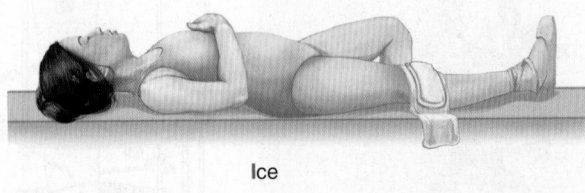

Ice

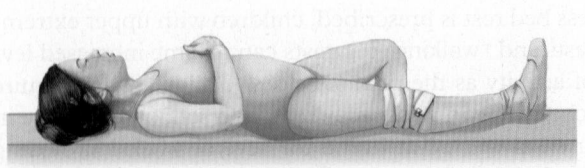

Compression

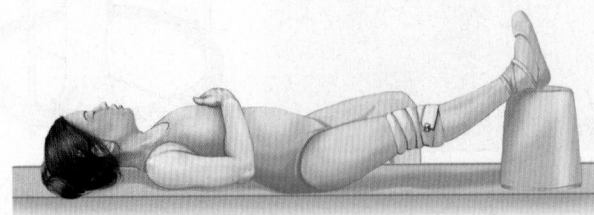

Elevation

FIGURE **44.24** RICE (rest, ice, compression, elevation) is the appropriate treatment for sprains.

TABLE 44.7 OVERUSE DISORDERS

Disorder	Anatomic Area Affected	Most Commonly Affected Activities and Age Groups	Symptoms
Osgood–Schlatter disease	Partial avulsion of the ossification centre of the tibial tubercle	Usually occurs in active adolescents, most often boys, and most frequently during periods of rapid growth	• Mild to moderate pain, activity-related • Tibial tubercle is tender when palpated • Painful swelling or prominence of the anterior portion of the tibial tubercle
Epiphysiolysis of proximal humerus	Proximal humerus (widening of growth plate)	Occurs with rigourous upper extremity activity, such as baseball pitching	• Tenderness in the shoulder or proximal humerus • Pain with active internal rotation • Full shoulder range of motion continues
Epiphysiolysis of distal radius	Distal radius (widening of growth plate)	Occurs with overuse of the distal radius, such as in gymnasts	• Wrist pain that worsens with activity
Sever's disease (calcaneal apophysitis)	Calcaneus (heel)	Usually occurs in 9- to 14-year-olds	• Pain over the posterior aspect of the calcaneus • Limited active and passive dorsiflexion of foot
Shin splints	Refers to a variety of overuse syndromes associated with the shin (stress fracture, tibial stress, muscular issues)	Occurs with activities that place repeated exertion on the lower leg, as in runners, ballerinas, elite soccer players	• Exercise-induced pain of the anterior aspect of the middle part of the lower leg • May be sharp pain • Worsens with exercise • With stress fracture, may have a limp that worsens with activity

syndromes, although they can occur in children who are in competitive activities such as ballet or gymnastics. Pain is usually associated with the activity and worsens with continued participation in the activity. Table 44.7 gives details on several common overuse syndromes. Therapeutic management is aimed at reassurance, pain management, and limiting rather than eliminating activity.

Nursing Assessment

Elicit a health history to determine the extent of involvement in sports. Note onset of pain, duration, intensity, aggravating factors, and treatments used at home. Examine the painful part, noting findings similar to those noted for each syndrome in Table 44.7.

Nursing Management

Initially, apply ice when pain is severe. Anti-inflammatory medications such as ibuprofen may be helpful. The child should limit exercise and participate in a different activity. After a few weeks, most overuse syndromes resolve; at that point, the athlete may resume the prior activity.

Osgood–Schlatter disease is the exception and may require 12 to 24 months to resolve (Gunta, 2009). Using pads or braces that are appropriate to the painful body part is also helpful. Supporting the arm with a sling may relieve stress on the proximal humerus when epiphysiolysis occurs. Heel cups used in athletic shoes help relieve stress on the heels associated with Sever's disease. To prevent overuse syndromes, encourage athletes to perform appropriate stretching exercises during a 20- to 30-minute warm-up period before each practice or game. Also encourage several weeks of conditioning training before the season begins.

▶ *Take* NOTE!

"Energy healing" such as therapeutic touch and Reiki may provide a non-pharmacologic adjunct to pain management for musculoskeletal injuries.

Dislocated Radial Head

Dislocation of the radial head ("nursemaid's elbow") occurs when a pulling motion on the arm causes the ligament surrounding the radial head to become entrapped within the joint. It usually occurs in children younger than 7 years of age and is a common injury in children of ages 2 to 5 (Rodts, 2009). To reduce the injury, the elbow is flexed to 90 degrees and then the forearm is fully and firmly supinated, causing the ligament to snap back into place. With appropriate reduction of the radial head, no complications result.

Nursing Assessment

The child will hold the arm slightly flexed at the side and refuse to move it. When the arm is still, the child apparently has no discomfort. Assess neurovascular status (intact).

Nursing Management

After treatment, usually hyperpronation to reduce the dislocation, assess the child's ability to use the arm without pain. Teach parents to avoid pulling up on the child's arm, particularly in an abrupt jerking fashion, to prevent recurrence.

■■■ Key Concepts

- The bones of the infant and young child are more flexible and have a thicker periosteum and more abundant blood supply than the adult's; as a result, bending occurs more frequently than breaking of the bone, and the fractured bone heals more quickly.
- The epiphysis of long bones is the growth centre of the bones in children. Injury to this area may result in long-term extremity deformity.
- Rapid muscle growth in the adolescent years places the teenager at increased risk for injury compared with other age groups.
- Plain radiographs are usually sufficient for diagnosing injuries in children. If CT or MRI is required, the nurse may need to help the child stay calm and still during the procedure.
- Apply a pressure dressing following joint aspiration to prevent hematoma formation or fluid recollection.
- Perform frequent assessments of pain status and the effect of pain medication in the child with a musculoskeletal disorder.
- Diazepam (Valium) may be helpful in relieving muscle spasm associated with traction.
- Fractures may occur as a result of unintentional or intentional injury, or because the bones are fragile, as in rickets or osteogenesis imperfecta.
- Congenital or developmental disorders such as DDH or clubfoot require bracing or casting for correction and to prevent deformity later in life.

- Sprains, fractures, and overuse syndromes occur frequently in young athletes. Appropriate warm-up and stretching may help prevent some of these injuries.
- Assessment of neurovascular status is an essential component of care for a child with a neuromuscular disorder.
- To prevent complications after a spinal fusion for scoliosis correction, use the log-roll method for turning the child so that back flexion is avoided.
- RICE is the appropriate treatment for sprains.
- Maintain traction and the appropriate amount of weight as ordered.
- The bulk of cast care occurs in the home. Teach the family of a child with a cast to perform neurovascular assessments, prevent the cast from getting wet, and care for the skin appropriately.
- Torticollis may be treated by teaching the family to perform daily neck muscle stretching exercises.
- Children with chronic disorders such as osteogenesis imperfecta may demonstrate slower or lesser growth than other children and may also be unable to participate in certain activities because of bone fragility.

REFERENCES

American Academy of Family Physicians. (2010). *Cast care.* Retrieved September 22, 2011 from http://familydoctor.org/online/famdocen/home/healthy/firstaid/after-injury/094.html

American Academy of Pediatrics. (2000). Clinical practice guideline: Early detection of developmental dysplasia of the hip. *Pediatrics, 105*(4), 896–905.

Bechard, L. W., Wroe, E., & Ellis, K. (2008). Body composition & growth. In C. Duggan, J. B. Watkins, & W. A. Walker (Eds.), *Nutrition in pediatrics. Basic science clinical application* (4th ed.). Hamilton, ON: BC Decker Inc.

Bowden, V. R., & Greenberg, C. S. (2008). *Pediatric nursing procedures.* Philadelphia: Lippincott Williams & Wilkins.

Busch, M. T. (2006). Sports medicine in children and adolescents. In R. T. Morrissy & S. L. Weinstein (Eds.), *Lovell & Winter's pediatric orthopaedics* (6th ed.). Philadelphia: Lippincott Williams & Wilkins.

Carek, P. J., Dickerson, L. M., & Sack, J. I. (2001). Diagnosis and management of osteomyelitis. *American Family Physician, 63*(12), 2413–2420.

Cornwall, R. (2007). Upper limb. In R. M. Kliegman, R. E. Behrman, H. B. Jenson, & B. F. Stanton (Eds.), *Nelson's textbook of pediatrics* (18th ed.). Philadelphia: Saunders.

Dugdale, D. C., III (2010). *Osteoarthritis.* Retrieved September 22, 2011 from http://www.nlm.nih.gov/medlineplus/ency/article/000423.htm

Dugdale, D. C., III, Vyas, J. M., & Zieve, D. (2011). *Septic arthritis.* Retrieved September 22, 2011 from http://www.nlm.nih.gov/medlineplus/ency/article/000430.htm

Fischbach, F. T., & Dunning, M. B., III (2009). *A manual of laboratory and diagnostic tests* (8th ed.). Philadelphia: Lippincott Williams & Wilkins.

Gholve, P. A., Hosalkar, H. S., & Wells, L. (2007). Common fractures. In R. M. Kliegman, R. E. Behrman, H. B. Jenson, & B. F. Stanton (Eds.), *Nelson's textbook of pediatrics* (18th ed.). Philadelphia: Saunders.

Gilmore, A., & Thompson, G. H. (2003). Common childhood foot deformities. *Consultant for Pediatricians, 2*(2), 63–71.

Gore, A. I., & Spencer, J. P. (2004). The newborn foot. *American Family Physician, 69*(4), 865–872.

Goretsky, M. J., Kelly, R. E., Croitoru, D., & Nuss, D. (2004). Chest wall anomalies: Pectus excavatum and pectus carinatum. *Adolescent Medicine Clinics, 15*(3), 455–471.

Grewal, P., & Ahier, J. (2010). Pediatric orthopedic problems. In S. M. Nettina (Ed.), *Lippincott manual of nursing practice* (9th ed.). Philadelphia: Lippincott Williams & Wilkins.

Gunner, K. B., & Scott, A. C. (2001). Evaluation of the child with a limp. *Journal of Pediatric Health Care, 15,* 38–40.

Gunta, K. E. (2009). Disorders of musculoskeletal function: Developmental and metabolic disorders. In C. M. Porth & G. Matfin (Eds.), *Pathophysiology concepts of altered health states* (8th ed.). Philadelphia: Wolters Kluwer/Lippincott Williams & Wilkins.

Hosalkar, H. S., Gholve, P. A., & Wells, L. (2007a). Torsional and angular deformities. In R. M. Kliegman, R. E. Behrman, H. B. Jenson, & B. F. Stanton (Eds.), *Nelson's textbook of pediatrics* (18th ed.). Philadelphia: Saunders.

Hosalkar, H. S., Horn, D., Friedman, J. E., & Dormans, J. P. (2007b). The hip. In R. M. Kliegman, R. E. Behrman, H. B. Jenson, & B. F. Stanton (Eds.), *Nelson's textbook of pediatrics* (18th ed.). Philadelphia: Saunders.

Hosalkar, H. S., Spiegel, D. A., & Davidson, R. S. (2007c). The foot and toes. In R. M. Kliegman, R. E. Behrman, H. B. Jenson, & B. F. Stanton (Eds.), *Nelson's textbook of pediatrics* (18th ed.). Philadelphia: Saunders.

Kaneshiro, N. K. (2009). *Polydactyly.* Retrieved July 7, 2011 from http://www.nlm.nih.gov/medlineplus/ency/article/003176.htm

Kehl, D. K. (2006). Developmental coax vara, transient synovitis and idiopathic chondrolysis of the hip. In R. T. Morrissy & S. L. Weinstein (Eds.), *Lovell & Winter's pediatric orthopaedics* (6th ed.). Philadelphia: Lippincott Williams & Wilkins.

Leung, A. K. C., & Lemay, J. F. (2004). The limping child. *Journal of Pediatric Health Care, 18,* 219–223.

Luther, B. L. (2002). Congenital muscular torticollis. *Orthopedic Nursing, 21*(3), 21–28.

Morrissy, R. T., Giavedoni, B. J., & Coulter-O'Berry, C. (2006). The limb-deficient child. In R. T. Morrissy & S. L. Weinstein (Eds.), *Lovell & Winter's pediatric orthopaedics* (6th ed.). Philadelphia: Lippincott Williams & Wilkins.

Mosca, V. S. (2006). The foot. In R. T. Morrissy & S. L. Weinstein (Eds.), *Lovell & Winter's pediatric orthopaedics* (6th ed.). Philadelphia: Lippincott Williams & Wilkins.

Polousky, J. D., & Eilert, R. E. (2009). Orthopedics. In W. W. Hay, M. J. Levin, J. M. Sondheimer, & R. R. Deterding (Eds.), *Current pediatric diagnosis and treatment* (19th ed.). New York: McGraw-Hill.

Price, C. T., Phillips, J. H., & Devito, D. P. (2006). Management of fractures. In R. T. Morrissy & S. L. Weinstein (Eds.), *Lovell & Winter's pediatric orthopaedics* (6th ed.). Philadelphia: Lippincott Williams & Wilkins.

Rodts, M. F. (2009). Nursemaid's elbow: A preventable pediatric injury. *Orthopaedic Nursing, 28*(4), 163–66.

Schwentker, E. P. (2009). *Pediatric septic arthritis surgery.* Retrieved September 22, 2011 from http://emedicine.medscape.com/article/1259337-overview

Scoliosis Research Society. (2011). *Common scoliosis questions: What is scoliosis?* Retrieved November 16, 2011 from http://www.srs.org/patient_and_family/scoliosis/

Spiegel, D. A., Hosalkar, H. S., Dormans, J. P., & Drommond, D. S. (2007). The neck. In R. M. Kliegman, R. E. Behrman, H. B. Jenson, & B. F. Stanton (Eds.), *Nelson's textbook of pediatrics* (18th ed.). Philadelphia: Saunders

Weinstein, S. L. (2006). Developmental hip dysplasia and dislocation. In R. T. Morrissy & S. L. Weinstein (Eds.), *Lovell & Winter's pediatric orthopaedics* (6th ed.). Philadelphia: Lippincott Williams & Wilkins.

Weinstein, S. L., Dolan, L. A., Cheng, J. C., Danielsson, A., & Morcuende, J. A. (2008). Adolescent idiopathic scoliosis. *Lancet, 371,* 1527–1537.

Will, R. E., Stokes, I. A., Qiu, X., Walker, M. R., & Sanders, J. O. (2009). Cobb angle progression in adolescent scoliosis begins at the intervertebral disc. *Spine, 34*(25), 2782–2786.

Zaleske, D. J. (2006). Metabolic and endocrine abnormalities. In R. T. Morrissy & S. L. Weinstein (Eds.), *Lovell & Winter's pediatric orthopaedics* (6th ed.). Philadelphia: Lippincott Williams & Wilkins.

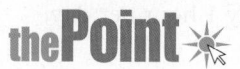

the Point For additional learning materials, including Internet Resources, visit **http://thePoint.lww.com/Chow1e.**

Chapter Worksheet

Multiple Choice Questions

1. The nurse is evaluating a parent's understanding of treatment for torticollis. Which response best indicates that the parent understands the appropriate treatment?

   a. Encourages the infant to turn the head to the unaffected side

   b. States that prone positioning for sleep will be needed

   c. Places the infant on the affected side

   d. Stretches the infant's neck to the opposite side and holds it for 5 seconds

2. The nurse is providing patient education related to use of a full-time brace that the orthopedic surgeon has ordered as treatment for idiopathic scoliosis in an adolescent girl. Which statement by the teen best indicates an understanding of appropriate use of the brace?

   a. "I can take my brace off only for special occasions."

   b. "I will take my brace off for only 1 hour per day, for showering."

   c. "I do not need to wear my brace at night while I am sleeping."

   d. "It is most important for me to wear my brace during the day, while I am upright."

3. The nurse is caring for a child with a fractured left femur who has been in skeletal traction for several days. Upon assessment, she notes that the left foot is pale, with a non-palpable pedal pulse. What is the priority nursing intervention?

   a. Release the traction, as there may be too much weight on it.

   b. Nothing; alterations in circulation are expected with skeletal traction.

   c. Immediately notify the physician of this abnormal finding.

   d. Massage the foot immediately to increase circulation.

Critical Thinking Exercises

1. Develop a teaching plan for the family of an infant with DDH or clubfoot.

2. Develop a discharge teaching plan for a 2-year-old who will be in a hip spica cast for 10 more weeks at home.

3. Devise a developmental/education plan for a child who will be confined to traction for 6 weeks. Choose a child in the clinical area whom you have cared for or choose a particular age group and develop the plan.

Study Activities

1. In the clinical setting, compare the growth and development of a child with osteogenesis imperfecta or rickets with that of typical healthy child. What differences or similarities do you find? What are the explanations for your findings?

2. Attend a pediatric orthopedic clinic and identify the role of the registered nurse in this setting.

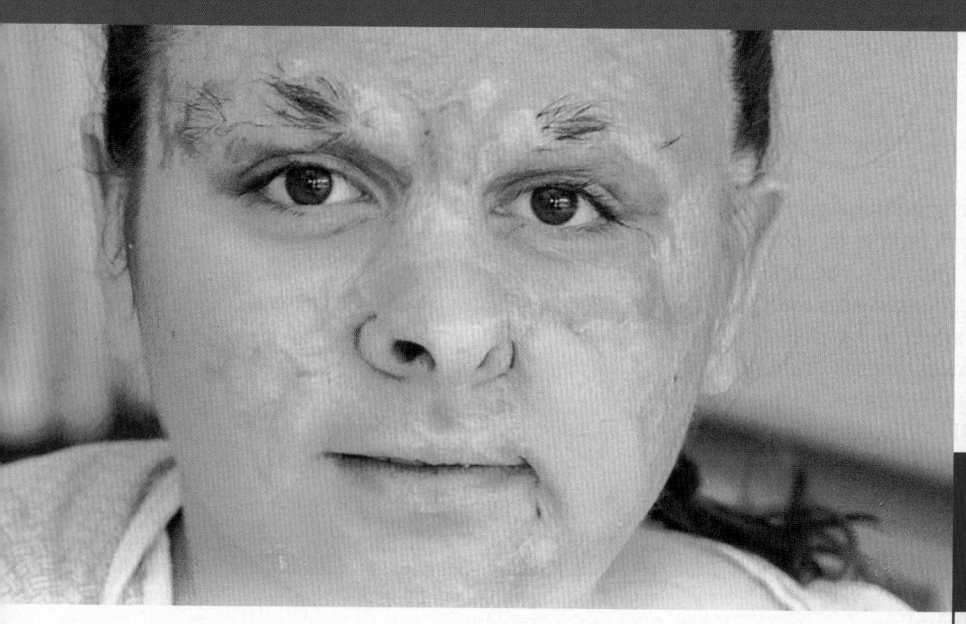

CHAPTER 45

Adapted by Tracy Lynne Mackie

NURSING CARE OF THE CHILD WITH AN INTEGUMENTARY DISORDER

KEY TERMS

annular
dermatitis
erythema
macule
papule
pruritus
scaling
vesicle

LEARNING OBJECTIVES

Upon completion of the chapter, the learner will be able to:

1. Compare anatomic and physiologic differences of the integumentary system in infants and children versus adults.
2. Describe nursing care related to common laboratory and diagnostic tests used in the medical diagnosis of integumentary disorders in infants, children, and adolescents.
3. Distinguish integumentary disorders common in infants, children, and adolescents.
4. Identify appropriate nursing assessments and interventions related to pediatric integumentary disorders.
5. Develop an individualized nursing care plan for the child with an integumentary disorder.
6. Describe the psychosocial impact of a chronic integumentary disorder on children or adolescents.
7. Develop patient/family teaching plans for the child with an integumentary disorder.

Eva Long, 1-year-old, is brought to the clinic by her mother, who states, "Eva has dry patches of skin, her wrists bleed from her scratching, and she's having trouble sleeping at night."

Wow

To a nurse the child's skin is life's gift wrapping, but to the child the skin is the space suit for life.

Integumentary disorders occur often in children. If they are severe or chronic, these disorders can have a significant impact on the child. Infants and children are exposed to a multitude of infectious microorganisms and allergens, and their skin is sometimes affected by these exposures. Some integumentary disorders are as mild and self-limited as a minor abrasion, while others, such as atopic dermatitis, are chronic. Any skin disorder that is severe or could become so can have a major impact on the child's physiologic or psychological status (Magin, Adams, Heading, et al., 2008). Nurses who care for children need to be familiar with common skin disorders of infancy, childhood, and adolescence so they can effectively intervene with children and their families.

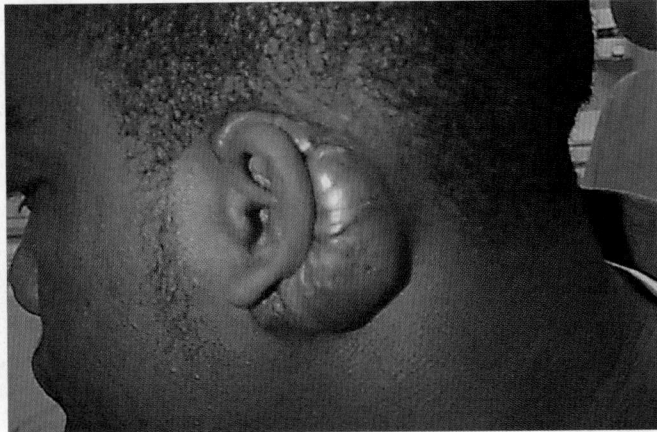

FIGURE 45.1 Keloid formation is more common in dark-skinned than light-skinned children.

Variations in Pediatric Anatomy and Physiology

The skin is the largest organ of the body, accounts for approximately one fifth of the body's total weight, and serves many functions. Skin is designed to protect the underlying tissues from trauma and invasion by microorganisms, to prevent the loss of body fluids, to synthesize vitamin D, and to function as an excretory organ. The skin is also important for the perception of pain, heat, and cold and for the regulation of body temperature.

Differences in the Skin Between Children and Adults

Throughout life, many skin changes occur: from embryonic development and fetal differentiation into different layers and features (e.g., hair, nails, glands), to thin and fragile neonatal skin, to skin thickening from childhood into adolescence (Vernon, Brady, & Starr, 2009). The infant's epidermis is thinner than the adult's, and the blood vessels lie closer to the surface because there is a decreased amount of subcutaneous fat. Thus, the infant loses heat more readily through the skin's surface than the older child or adult does. The thinness of the infant's skin also allows substances to be absorbed through the skin more readily than they would be in an adult. Bacteria can gain access via the infant's and younger child's skin more readily than they can through the adult's skin. The infant's skin contains more water compared with the adult's, and the epidermis is loosely bound to the dermis. The infant's skin is also less pigmented than that of the adult (in all races), placing the infant at increased risk for skin damage from ultraviolet radiation. Over time, the infant's skin toughens and becomes less hydrated and thus is less susceptible to microorganism invasion. By adolescence, many of the skin's changes are complete, resulting in thick skin with the epidermis and dermis bound and firm, fully functional sweat and apocrine

glands, and colour darkening to that of the adult ethnicity (Anonymous, 2009).

Differences in Dark-Skinned Children

Children with dark skin tend to have more obvious and pronounced cutaneous reactions compared with children with lighter skin (Vernon et al., 2009). Hypopigmentation or hyperpigmentation in the affected area following healing of a dermatologic condition is common in dark-skinned children. This change in pigmentation may be temporary (a few months following a superficial skin disorder) or permanent (following a more involved skin condition). Dark-skinned children tend to have more prominent papules, follicular responses, lichenification, and vesicular or bullous reactions than lighter-skinned children with the same disorders. Hypertrophic scarring and keloid formation (Fig. 45.1) occur more often in dark-skinned children (Burns, Dunn, Brady, et al., 2009).

Sebaceous and Sweat Glands

Sebaceous glands function immaturely at birth and they can be sensitive to the effects of hormones acquired from the mother during pregnancy. Milia, white bumps on the face under the surface of the skin, are quite common in infants. They are caused by retention of old skin cells and oily material within hair follicles. They occur in up to half of all infants and typically resolve spontaneously within the first month of life. The sebum secreted serves to lubricate the skin and hair. Sebum production increases in the preadolescent and adolescent years, which is why acne develops during this time. The infant's eccrine sweat glands are somewhat functional and will produce sweat as a response to emotional stimuli and heat. They become fully functional in the middle childhood years. Until that time, temperature regulation is less effective compared with that in older children and adults. The apocrine sweat glands are small and non-functional in the infant. They

COMMON MEDICAL TREATMENTS 45.1

Treatment	Explanation	Indication	Nursing Implications
Wet dressing	Dressing moistened with lukewarm water (sterile water may be required in certain cases)	In the presence of itching, crusting, or oozing—helps to remove crusts	Some people may prepare wet dressings with Burow's solution (pharmacologic preparation made of aluminium acetate dissolved in water) or Domeboro powder, but tap water dressings (and normal saline) have proven just as effective (Morelli, 2007b). Provide atraumatic care by giving pre-medication before dressing changes.
Bathing	Use of lukewarm water (with or without soap) to bathe	Itchy and irritating skin conditions	Recommend fragrance-free, dye-free soaps such as Dove, Aveeno, Basis, Lubriderm. Colloids (oatmeal baths) are especially helpful. Pat the child dry; do not rub the skin. Leave the child moist before applying medication, dressing, or moisturizer. Be sure to monitor safety in the bath if using lubricating substances as risk of serious injury increases.

mature during puberty, at which time body odour develops in response to the fluid secreted by these glands.

Common Medical Treatments

A variety of medications as well as other medical treatments are used to treat integumentary disorders in children. Most of these treatments will require a physician's order when the child is in the hospital. The most common treatments and medications are listed in Common Medical Treatments 45.1 and Drug Guide 45.1. The nurse caring for the child with an integumentary disorder should be familiar with the procedures and medications, how they work, as well as common nursing implications related to their use.

NURSING PROCESS OVERVIEW FOR THE CHILD WITH AN INTEGUMENTARY DISORDER

Nursing management of the child with an integumentary disorder requires astute assessment skills, development of accurate nursing diagnoses and expected outcomes, implementation of appropriate interventions, and evaluation of the entire process. Many skin rashes may be associated with other, often serious, illnesses, so the nurse must use comprehensive and excellent assessment skills when evaluating rashes in children. Certain integumentary conditions are chronic and require ongoing care related to health maintenance, education, and psychosocial needs.

Assessment

Nursing assessment of the child with an integumentary disorder includes obtaining the health history and performing a physical examination. Assisting with or obtaining laboratory tests may also be necessary. The College of Registered Nurses of British Columbia (2010) has published *Pediatric Decision Support Tools: Integumentary Assessment* to guide nurses through the process of assessing skin disorders.

*R*emember Eva, the 1-year-old with the dry patches, itching, and trouble sleeping? What additional health history and physical examination assessment information should the nurse obtain?

Health History

Determine the child's or parent's chief complaint, which is most often related to **pruritus**, **scaling**, or a cosmetic disruption. Document the history of the present illness, noting onset, location, duration, characteristics, other symptoms, and relieving factors, particularly as related to a rash or lesion. Ask about changes in skin texture, colour, or pigmentation as well as dryness/oiliness, bruises, petechiae, or changes in birthmarks or moles (Health Canada, 2001). Also ask about the quantity and quality of any discharge from the rash or lesions, and document any accompanying symptoms. Note the child's general state of health, history of chronic medical conditions, recent surgeries, hospitalizations, current medications, and immunization status. Is there a family history of chronic or acute skin conditions? Has there been a recent change in the child's

DRUG GUIDE 45.1 COMMON DRUGS FOR INTEGUMENTARY DISORDERS

Medication	Action	Indication	Nursing Implications
Antibiotics (topical)	Decrease skin colonization with bacteria	Mild acne vulgaris, impetigo, folliculitis	Apply as prescribed to clean skin or a cleansed wound. Be alert for neomycin allergy. Ointment is preferred over cream or lotion.
Antibiotics (systemic)	Bactericidal and bacteriostatic against a variety of organisms, depending on the preparation	Moderate to severe acne vulgaris, extensive impetigo, cellulitis, scalded skin syndrome	Check for medication allergies prior to administration. Teach families to finish entire course of antibiotics.
Corticosteroids (topical)	Anti-inflammatory and antipruritic effects	Atopic dermatitis, certain kinds of contact dermatitis	Grouped into four basic categories (based upon potency): low, moderate, high, and highest. Do not use moderate- or high-potency corticosteroid preparations on the face or genitals. Do not cover with an occlusive dressing. Absorption is increased in the young infant.
Antifungals (topical)	Fungicidals	Tinea, candidal diaper rash	Available as powders, lotions, creams, and ointments. Apply a thin layer as prescribed. Comply with length of treatment as prescribed to prevent re-emergence of the rash.
Antifungals (systemic): itraconazole, fluconazole, ketoconazole, terbinafine	Kill fungus; binds to human keratin, making it resistant to fungus	Tinea capitis, tinea versicolor, *Candida* infection, severe or widespread fungal skin infections	Some regimens require up to a 4-week course (e.g., for treatment of tinea capitis). Monitor liver function tests, potassium, and complete blood count (CBC). May cause photosensitivity.
Benzoyl peroxide	Antimicrobial; decreases colonization of *P. acnes*	Comedonal to mild acne vulgaris	A topical retinoid in combination with topical antibiotics works well. All topical applications must be used for 6 to 8 weeks before effectiveness is seen. Avoid contact with eyes and mucous membranes.
Retinoids (topical): tretinoin, adapalene, tazarotene	Anticomedogenic activity	Moderate to severe acne vulgaris	Adverse effects: dryness, burning, photosensitivity. Instruct child to use SPF 15 or higher sunscreen.
Topical immune modulators (tacrolimus, pimecrolimus)	Inhibit T-lymphocyte action at the skin level	Moderate to severe atopic dermatitis, or in conditions resistant to topical steroids	Use only in children over 2 years of age. Avoid sunlight exposure. May cause burning, pruritus, flu-like symptoms, or headache.
Antihistamines (diphenhydramine, chlorpheniramine, hydroxyzine)	Antihistaminic effect, result in sedation	Hypersensitivity reactions, atopic dermatitis, or contact dermatitis that is severely pruritic	May give three or four times a day unless sedation effect interferes with activities of daily living or school

Medication	Action	Indication	Nursing Implications
Systemic corticosteroids (prednisone, dexamethasone, methylprednisolone)	Anti-inflammatory and immunosuppressive action	Severe contact dermatitis	Administer with food to decrease GI upset. May mask signs of infection. Monitor blood pressure, urine for glucose. Monitor for Cushing syndrome. Doses may be tapered over time. Do not stop treatment abruptly or acute adrenal insufficiency may occur.
Isotretinoin (Accutane)	Reduces sebaceous gland size, decreases sebum production, and regulates cell proliferation and differentiation	Cystic acne or severe acne that is resistant to 3 months of treatment with oral antibiotics	Ensure that the adolescent girl is not pregnant and does not become pregnant. Monitor CBC, lipid profiles, liver function tests, and beta-human chorionic gonadotropin monthly. Monitor for suicide risk.
Coal tar preparations	Antipruritic and anti-inflammatory effect	Psoriasis, atopic dermatitis	May stain fabrics; strong and unpleasant odour Apply at bedtime and rinse off in the morning to improve compliance.
Silver sulfadiazine 1% (Flamazine)	Bactericidal against gram-positive and gram-negative bacteria and yeasts	Burns	Cover with occlusive dressing. Apply BID (twice a day). Do not use in patients with sulfa or peanut allergy. Forms a gel on the burn that is painful to remove. May cause transient neutropenia. Do not use on the child's face or on an infant less than 2 months of age.

Adapted from: Taketokmo, C. K., Hodding, J. H., & Kraus, D. M. (2010). *Lexi-comp's pediatric dosage handbook* (17th ed.). Hudson, OH: Lexi-comp.

food intake or environment? Does anyone in the home have a similar concern at this time? Does the child share a bed with anyone? Where is the child's home (i.e., urban, rural, reserve, isolated community, single-family dwelling, high-density housing)? Does the family have pets that go outdoors? Does the child play in the woods or garden? Note usual skin care routines, including the types of soaps, cosmetics, or other skin care products used, as well as recent changes in products. Determine the amount of daily sun exposure and whether the child consistently uses sunscreen.

Physical Examination

Perform a complete physical examination, noting any abnormalities. Perform a focused and thorough examination of the skin. The best lighting for examination of the skin is natural daylight. Look at the skin in general, noting distribution of any obvious lesions. Inspect the mucous membranes, noting and describing lesions if present. Examine all surfaces of the skin and scalp

carefully. Note temperature, moisture, texture, and fragility of the skin. If a rash or lesions are present, note their location and provide a detailed description of them. Describe whether a rash is macular, papular, pustular, or vesicular. Provide a description of vascular lesions if present (refer to Chapter 31 for additional information on vascular lesions). Describe lesions according to the following criteria:

- Linear: are the lesions in a line?
- Shape: are the lesions round, oval, or **annular** (ring around central clearing)?
- Morbilliform: are the lesions a rosy colour or in the form of a maculopapular rash?
- Target lesions: do the lesions resemble a bull's-eye?

If lesions are present on the scalp, has hair loss in that region occurred? If drainage is present, describe it as clear, purulent, honey-coloured, or otherwise. Note scaling or lichenification of the skin. Palpate for regional lymphadenopathy.

COMMON LABORATORY AND DIAGNOSTIC TESTS 45.1

Test	Explanation	Indication	Nursing Implications
Complete blood count (CBC) with differential	Evaluates hemoglobin and hematocrit, WBC count (particularly the percentage of individual WBCs), and platelet count	Infection or inflammatory process	Normal values vary according to age and gender. WBC differential is helpful in evaluating source of infection. May be affected by myelosuppressive drugs. Eosinophils may be elevated in the child with atopic dermatitis.
Erythrocyte sedimentation rate (ESR)	Nonspecific test used to detect presence of infection or inflammation	Infection or inflammatory process	Send sample to laboratory immediately; if allowed to stand for longer than 3 h, may result in falsely low result.
Potassium hydroxide (KOH) prep	Reveals branching hyphae (fungus) when viewed under microscope	To identify fungal infection	Place skin scrapings on a microscope slide and add a drop of 20% KOH solution.
Culture of wound or skin drainage	Allows for microbial growth and organism identification	Identification of specific organism	Note sensitivities.
Immunoglobulin E (IgE)	Measurement of serum IgE	Atopic dermatitis	Often elevated in allergic or atopic disease, though this is a nonspecific finding. May be increased if the child takes systemic corticosteroids.
Patch or skin testing	Needle prick testing with allergens	Atopic or contact dermatitis	Have emergency equipment available in the event of anaphylaxis (rare).

Adapted from: Pagana, K. D., & Pagana, T. J. (2010). *Mosby's manual of diagnostic and laboratory tests* (4th ed.). St. Louis, MO: Mosby.

Laboratory and Diagnostic Testing

Common Laboratory and Diagnostic Tests 45.1 details the laboratory and diagnostic tests most commonly used when considering integumentary disorders. The tests can assist the health care provider in diagnosing the disorder or can be used as guidelines in determining ongoing treatment. Some of the tests are obtained by laboratory or non-nursing personnel, while others might be obtained by the nurse. In either instance the nurse should be familiar with how the tests are obtained, what they are used for, and normal versus abnormal results. This knowledge will also be necessary when providing patient and family education related to the testing.

Nursing Diagnoses and Related Interventions

Upon completion of a thorough assessment, the nurse might identify several nursing diagnoses, such as:

- Impaired skin integrity
- Pain
- Risk for infection
- Disturbed body image
- Risk for fluid volume deficit
- Altered nutrition

fter completing an assessment of Eva, the nurse noted the following: hypopigmentation of the skin behind her knees, dry patches on her wrists and face, and slight wheezing heard bilaterally on auscultation. Based on these assessment findings, what would your top three nursing diagnoses be for Eva?

Desired outcomes and interventions are based on the nursing diagnoses. Nursing Care Plan 45.1 can be used as a guide in planning nursing care for the child with an integumentary disorder. Individualize the plan of care based on the child's and family's responses to the health alteration; see Chapter 35 for information about pain management. Additional information will be included later in the chapter as it relates to specific disorders.

ased on your top three nursing diagnoses for Eva, describe appropriate nursing interventions.

Infectious Disorders

Infectious disorders of the skin include those caused by viral, bacterial, or fungal infection. The viral exanthems

Nursing Care Plan 45.1

OVERVIEW FOR THE CHILD WITH AN INTEGUMENTARY DISORDER

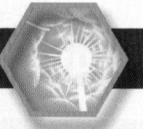

NURSING DIAGNOSIS: Impaired skin integrity related to infectious process, hypersensitivity reaction, injury, or mechanical factors as evidenced by rash, inflammation, abrasion, laceration, or disrupted epidermis

Outcome Identification and Evaluation

Integrity of skin surface will be restored; *rash, abrasion, laceration, or other skin disruption will heal.*

Interventions: Restoring Skin Integrity

- Assess site of skin impairment *to determine extent of involvement and plan care.*
- Monitor skin impairment every shift for changes in colour, warmth, edema, drainage, or other signs of infection *to identify problems early.*
- Determine the child's and family's skin care practices *to determine need for education related to skin care.*
- Individualize the child's skin care regimen depending on the child's particular skin condition *to most appropriately care for skin in light of the child's disorder.*
- In the immobile child, use a risk assessment tool (such as a modified Norton or Braden scale) *to identify risk for skin breakdown.*
- Position the child on the opposite side of the skin impairment *to avoid further skin breakdown.*
- Encourage appropriate nutritional intake *as adequate nutrients are necessary for appropriate immune function and skin healing.*
- Consult the wound and ostomy care nurse specialist *to determine best approach for individualized wound care.*
- Provide dressing change and wound care as prescribed *to promote wound or burn healing.*

NURSING DIAGNOSIS: Risk for infection related to disruption in protective skin barrier

Outcome Identification and Evaluation

Child will remain free of local or systemic infection, *will remain afebrile, without additional redness or warmth at skin disruption site.*

Interventions: Preventing Infection

- Use appropriate hand hygiene *to decrease transmission of infectious organisms.*
- Assess the skin impairment site for increased warmth, redness, edema, discharge, or new purulence *to identify infection early.*
- Assess temperature every 4 hours or more frequently if needed, *as infants may become hypothermic and children develop fever quickly in response to infection.*
- Note WBC and culture results, *reporting unexpected values to the primary care provider so that appropriate treatment may be started.*
- Follow prescribed therapies for skin alteration *to maintain skin moisture and prevent further breakdown, which may lead to infection.*
- Encourage appropriate nutritional intake *as adequate nutrients are necessary for appropriate immune function and skin healing.*

NURSING DIAGNOSIS: Disturbed body image related to chronic skin changes caused by disease process, burns, or other skin alteration as evidenced by child's verbalization, reluctance to participate in activities, or social withdrawal

Outcome Identification and Evaluation

Child will verbalize or demonstrate acceptance of alteration in body, *will return to previous level of social involvement.*

Interventions: Promoting Appropriate Body Image

- Assess child or teen for feelings about alteration in skin *to determine baseline.*
- Acknowledge feelings of anger or depression related to skin changes *to provide an outlet for feelings, and normalize the condition within the context of child health.*
- Encourage the child or teen to participate in skin care *to give some sense of control over what is occurring.*
- Help the child or teen to accept self *as the perception of self is tied to knowing oneself and identifying what the self values.*

(continued)

Nursing Care Plan 45.1 (continued)

NURSING DIAGNOSIS: Risk for deficient fluid volume related to burns

Outcome Identification and Evaluation
Fluid volume status will be balanced, *child will maintain a minimum urine output of 1 to 2 mL/kg/hour (minimum of 0.5 mL/kg/hour in late adolescent/adult) oral mucosa will be moist and pink, heart rate will remain within age- and situation-specific parameters.*

Interventions: Promoting Fluid Balance
• Assess fluid volume status at least every shift, more frequently if disrupted, *to obtain baseline for comparison.*
• Strictly monitor intake and output *to detect imbalance or need for additional fluid intake.*
• Weigh the child daily on the same scale, at the same time, in the same amount of clothing *as changes in weight are an accurate indicator of fluid volume status in children.*
• Provide intravenous fluid resuscitation in initial period, followed by encouragement of oral fluid intake in the burned patient, *to compensate for fluid loss through burned areas.*

NURSING DIAGNOSIS: Imbalanced nutrition, less than body requirements, related to increased metabolic state (burns) as evidenced by poor wound healing, difficulty gaining or maintaining body weight

Outcome Identification and Evaluation
Child will demonstrate balanced nutritional state, *will maintain or gain weight as appropriate for situation, and will demonstrate improvement in wound healing.*

Interventions: Promoting Nutrition
• Assess the child's food preferences and ability to eat *to provide a baseline for planning nursing care.*
• Consult the nutritionist *because nutritional needs are increased related to altered metabolic state as a result of burns.*
• Collaborate with the nutritionist, child, and parents to plan meals that appeal to the child *to increase variety of foods offered and increase the child's intake.*
• Administer vitamin and mineral preparations as prescribed *to supplement nutrients.*
• Provide smaller, more frequent meals and snacks *to promote increased intake.*
• Weigh the child daily *to determine progress.*

---

are discussed in Chapter 36. Bacterial and fungal infections of the skin are discussed below.

Bacterial Infections

Bacterial infections of the skin include bullous and non-bullous impetigo, folliculitis, cellulitis, and staphylococcal scalded skin syndrome. These bacterial skin infections are often caused by *Staphylococcus aureus* and group A beta-hemolytic *Streptococcus*, which are ordinarily normal flora on the skin. Impetigo, folliculitis, and cellulitis are usually self-limited disorders that rarely become severe.

Impetigo is a readily recognizable skin rash (Fig. 45.2). Nonbullous impetigo generally follows some type of skin trauma or may arise as a secondary bacterial infection of another skin disorder, such as atopic **dermatitis**. Bullous impetigo demonstrates a sporadic occurrence pattern and develops on intact skin, resulting from toxin production by *S. aureus*.

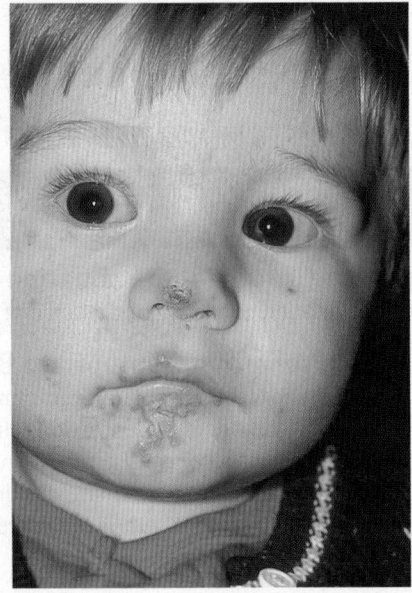

FIGURE 45.2 Note honey-coloured crusting with impetigo.

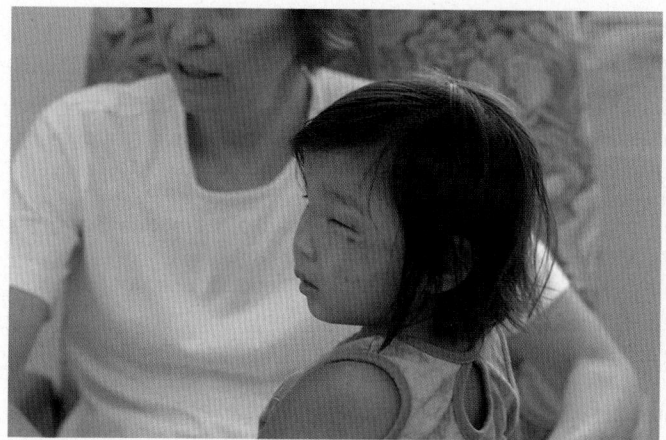

FIGURE 45.3 Note erythema and edema associated with cellulitis.

Folliculitis, infection of the hair follicle, most often results from occlusion of the hair follicle. It may occur as a result of poor hygiene, prolonged contact with contaminated water, maceration, or a moist environment or from use of occlusive emollient products.

Cellulitis is a localized infection and inflammation of the skin and subcutaneous tissues and is usually preceded by skin trauma of some sort (Fig. 45.3).

Staphylococcal scalded skin syndrome results from infection with *S. aureus* that produces a toxin, which then causes exfoliation. It has an abrupt onset and results in diffuse erythema and skin tenderness. Scalded skin syndrome is most common in infants and children before 5 years of age and can present as a localized infection or systemic illness (Morelli, 2007b).

Of particular concern are bacterial skin infections caused by methicillin-resistant *S. aureus* (MRSA) (So & Farrington, 2008). Rates of MRSA in Canada increased 10-fold between 1995 and 2006 (Canadian Paediatric Society [CPS], 2006). In children, MRSA can be acquired following a skin disruption such as cellulitis, an insect or spider bite, or chicken pox as well as in conjunction with turf burns, towel-sharing, shaving, improper disinfection of sports protective equipment and locker rooms, and poor hand hygiene (Barton, Hawkes, Moore, et al., 2006). Therefore, families, teachers, day care centre attendants, and coaches are the most important people to aid in the prevention of MRSA. Community outbreaks of MRSA were first reported between 1986 and 1989 in an Aboriginal community in Alberta and have since been noted across the country (Barton et al., 2006). Those from Aboriginal backgrounds are at higher risk for contracting MRSA due to crowding, lack of good quality water, and heavy antibiotic use (CPS, 2005). CPS guidelines (2005) state that awareness is the most important first-line management of MRSA in First Nations communities, followed by prevention, control, and treatment. If a child presents with a moderate to severe skin infection, new Canadian guidelines suggest culturing the wound for MRSA, especially if the child is from a community or area with known MRSA (Barton et al., 2006; CPS, 2006, 2007b).

Therapeutic management of bacterial skin infections includes topical or systemic antibiotics and appropriate hygiene (Table 45.1).

Nursing Assessment

Obtain the history as noted in the nursing process overview section. Note history of skin disruption such as a cut, scrape, or insect or spider bite (nonbullous impetigo and cellulitis). Note body piercing in the adolescent, which can lead to impetigo or cellulitis. Measure the child's temperature: fever may occur with bullous impetigo or cellulitis and is common with scalded skin syndrome. Inspect the skin, noting abnormalities, documenting their location and distribution, and describing drainage if present. Table 45.1 gives specific clinical manifestations of the various bacterial skin infections. Palpate for regional lymphadenopathy, which may be present with impetigo or cellulitis. Blood cultures are indicated in the child with cellulitis with lymphangitic streaking and in all cases of periorbital or orbital cellulitis.

Nursing Management

Administer antibiotics topically or systemically as prescribed. Teach the family about antibiotic administration and care of the lesions or rash. Soak impetiginous lesions with cool wet compresses to remove crusts before applying topical antibiotics. Children with mild infections should not attend school or day care until they have been treated for 24 hours, while children with more severe infections should stay home from school until the systemic symptoms (e.g., weakness, fever, diarrhea) have resolved (Vernon et al., 2009). Prevent transmission of nosocomial MRSA by appropriately isolating children according to the institution's policy when the child is hospitalized.

Educate the family about prevention of bacterial skin infections. Stress the importance of cleanliness and hygiene. Teach the family to keep the child's fingernails cut short and to clean the nails with a nail brush at bath time. When a skin disruption such as a cut, scrape, or insect bite occurs, teach the family to clean the area well to prevent the development of cellulitis. Folliculitis may be prevented with diligent hygiene and avoidance of occlusive emollients. Table 45.1 gives additional information about specific treatments for bacterial skin infections.

Fungal Infections

Fungi also cause infections on children's skin. Tinea is a fungal disease of the skin occurring on any part of the body. The part of the body affected determines the second word in the name; for instance, tinea pedis refers to

TABLE 45.1 MANIFESTATIONS AND MANAGEMENT OF BACTERIAL SKIN INFECTIONS

Disorder	Skin Findings	Usual Treatment
Nonbullous impetigo	• **Papules** progressing to **vesicles**, then painless pustules with a narrow erythematous border • Honey-coloured exudate when the vesicles or pustules rupture, forming a crust on the ulcer-like base (see Fig. 45.2)	• Limited amount: treat topically with mupirocin ointment three times daily for 7 to 10 days. • If lesions are numerous, oral first-line therapy is cloxacillin or cephalexin. • Vancomycin may be needed for a noscomial MRSA infection. • Remove honey-coloured crust twice daily with cool compresses.
Bullous impetigo	• Red **macules** and bullous eruptions on an erythematous base • Lesions may range in size from a few millimetres to several centimetres.	• Oral first-line therapy is cloxacillin • Maintain good hygiene.
Folliculitis	• Red, raised hair follicles	• Treat with aggressive hygiene: warm compresses after washing with soap and water several times a day. • Topical mupirocin is indicated; occasionally oral antibiotics are required.
Cellulitis	• Localized reaction: **erythema**, pain, edema, warmth at site of skin disruption (see Fig. 45.3)	• Mild cases are usually treated with cephalexin. • More severe cases and periorbital or orbital cellulitis require IV cephalosporins.
Staphylococcal scalded skin syndrome	• Flattish bullae that rupture within hours • Red, weeping surface is left, most commonly on face, groin, neck, and axillary region.	• Mild to moderate cases are treated with cloxacillin or cephalexin. • Severe cases are managed similar to burns with aggressive fluid management and IV cefazolin and gentamicin.

Adapted from: Burch, J. M., & Morelli, J. G. (2011). Skin. In W. W. Hay, M. J. Levin, J. M. Sondheimer, & R. R. Deterding (Eds.), *Current pediatric diagnosis and treatment* (20th ed.) New York: McGraw-Hill; and Lewis, L., & Friefman, A. D. (2011). *Impetigo*. Retrieved December 17, 2011 from http://emedicine.medscape.com/article/783562-overview.

a fungal infection on the feet. The three organisms most often responsible for tinea are *Epidermophyton*, *Microsporum*, and *Trichophyton*, although *Malassezia furfur* causes tinea versicolor. *Candida albicans* may cause an infection of the skin and should be suspected in a diaper rash that lasts longer than 4 days. All fungal skin infections may occur year-round, but tinea versicolor is more common in warm weather.

Therapeutic management of fungal infections involves appropriate hygiene and administration of an antifungal agent. Table 45.2 gives further information about treatment. Also see Evidence-based Practice 45.1.

Nursing Assessment

Elicit the health history, noting exposure to another person with a fungal infection or exposure to a pet (fungi are often carried by pets). Note onset of the rash and whether it is itchy. Determine whether the child has recently had a

haircut (tinea capitis). Note contact with damp areas such as locker rooms and swimming pools, use of nylon socks or non-breathable shoes, or minor trauma to the feet (tinea pedis). Document a history of wearing tight clothing or participating in a contact sport such as wrestling (tinea cruris). Inspect the skin and scalp, noting the location, description, and distribution of the rash or lesions (Figs. 45.4, 45.5, and 45.6). Table 45.2 describes the clinical findings associated with various types of tinea.

Scraping and potassium hydroxide (KOH) preparation show branching hyphae. For tinea capitis, Wood's lamp will fluoresce yellow-green if it is caused by *Microsporum* but not with *Trichophyton*. A fungal culture of a plucked hair is more reliable for diagnosis of tinea capitis.

Nursing Management

Maintain appropriate hygiene and administer antifungal agents as prescribed (see Table 45.2). Additional

TABLE 45.2 MANIFESTATIONS AND MANAGEMENT OF FUNGAL INFECTIONS

Disorder	Skin Findings	Usual Treatment
Tinea corporis (ringworm)	• Annular lesion with raised peripheral scaling and central clearing (looks like a ring) (see Fig. 45.4)	• Topical antifungal cream is required for at least 4 weeks. Avoid use of corticosteroids.
Tinea capitis	• Patches of scaling in the scalp with central hair loss • Risk of kerion development (inflamed, boggy mass that is filled with pustules) (see Fig. 45.5)	• Oral ketoconazole, fluconazole, terbinafine, or itraconazole • Selenium sulphide shampoo may be used to decrease contagiousness (adjunct only). • No school or day care for 1 week after treatment initiated
Tinea versicolor	• Superficial tan or hypopigmented oval scaly lesions, especially on upper back and chest and proximal arms • More noticeable in the summer with tanning of unaffected areas	• Topical antifungals (clotrimazole or ketoconazole) may be used, or selenium sulphide shampoo may be applied daily for 15 min for 7 to 14 days then once per month for 3 months.
Tinea pedis (athlete's foot)	• Red, scaling rash on soles and between the toes	• Topical antifungal cream, powder, or spray • Appropriate foot hygiene
Tinea cruris	• Erythema, scaling, maceration in the inguinal creases and inner thighs (penis/scrotum spared)	• Topical antifungal preparation for 4 to 6 weeks
Diaper candidiasis (also called monilial diaper rash)	• Fiery red lesions, scaling in the skin folds, and satellite lesions (located further out from the main rash) (see Fig. 45.6)	• Frequent diaper changes to keep skin clean and dry • Topical nystatin with diaper changes for several days • See section on diaper dermatitis for additional information.

Adapted from: Burch, J. M., & Morelli, J. G. (2011). Skin. In W. W. Hay, M. J. Levin, J. M. Sondheimer, & R. R. Deterding (Eds.), *Current pediatric diagnosis and treatment* (20th ed.). New York: McGraw-Hill.

EVIDENCE-BASED PRACTICE 45.1
Effectiveness of Various Systemic Antifungal Drugs in Treating Tinea Capitis in Children

● **Study**

Tinea capitis (fungal infection of the scalp) affects a large number of children. Until recently, conventional treatment involved a 6- to 8-week course of oral griseofulvin to eradicate the infection. However, griseofulvin was recently made unavailable in Canada and several other countries around the world. The authors evaluated data from 21 randomized controlled studies that included a total of 1,812 participants to determine the effectiveness of alternative treatments, such as terbinafine, itraconazole, and fluconazole, in eradicating dermatophytes in tinea capitis.

▲ **Findings**

The authors found that shorter courses (2 to 4 weeks) with terbinafine, itraconazole, or fluconazole were as effective at treating tinea capitis as the traditional longer course with griseofulvin.

■ **Nursing Implications**

Shorter courses of treatment will improve compliance, although the drugs may be more expensive. Educate families that the shorter course will be simpler to complete and result in fewer side effects and decreased need for laboratory evaluation of their child. Assist families with any paperwork needed to encourage insurance coverage for these drugs if needed.

González, U., Seaton, T., Bergus, G., Jacobson, J., & Martínez-Monzón, C. (2007). Systemic antifungal therapy for tinea capitis in children. *The Cochrane Library 2007*, 4. Indianapolis: John Wiley & Sons.

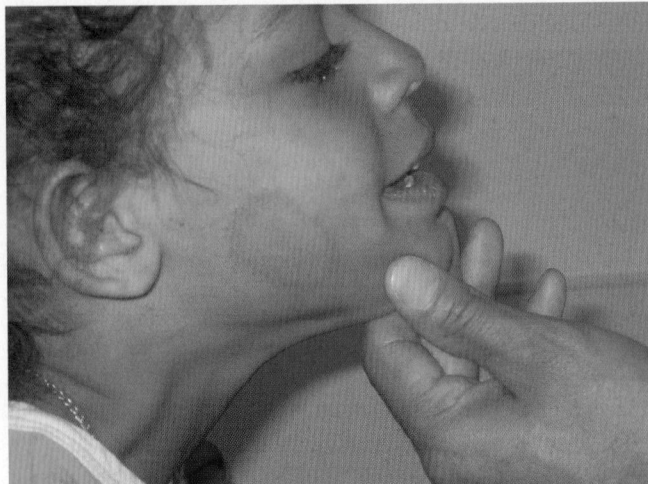

FIGURE 45.4 Tinea corporis: note raised scaly border with clearing in centre.

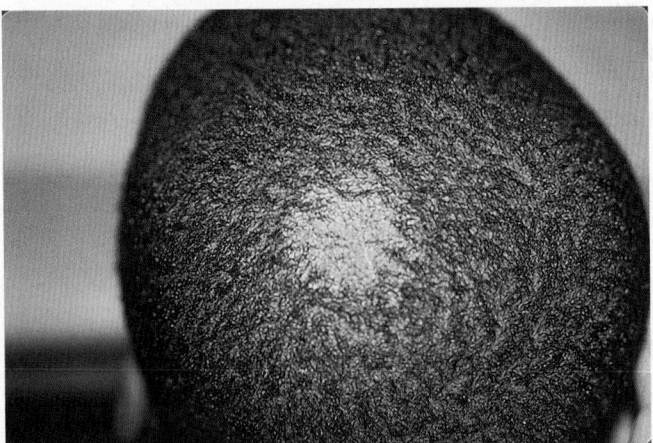

FIGURE 45.5 Note hair breakage and loss with tinea capitis.

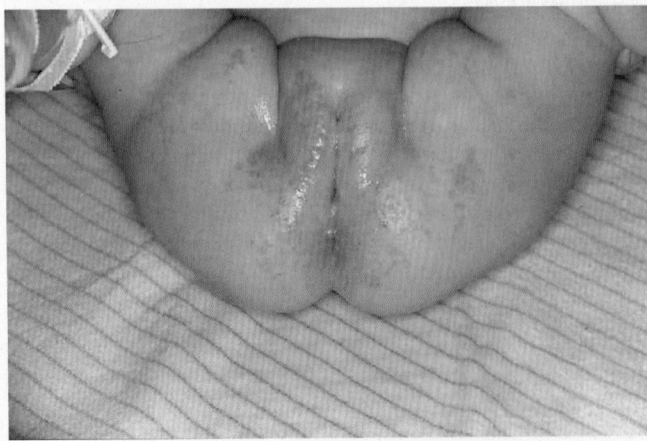

FIGURE 45.6 A bright red rash with satellite lesions occurs with diaper candidiasis.

specifics related to the individual fungal disorders are as follows:

- Tinea corporis is contagious, but the child may return to day care or school once treatment has begun. Identify and treat family members or other contacts.
- Counsel the child with tinea capitis and parents that hair will usually regrow in 3 to 12 months. Wash sheets and clothes in hot water to decrease the risk of the infection spreading to other family members.
- Instruct the child with tinea pedis to keep the feet clean and dry. Feet should be rinsed with water or a water/vinegar mixture and dried well, especially between the toes. The child should wear cotton socks and shoes that allow the feet to breathe. Going barefoot at home is allowed, but flip-flops should be worn around swimming pools and in locker rooms.
- Inform the child with tinea versicolor that return to normal skin pigmentation may take several months.
- Counsel the boy with tinea cruris to wear cotton underwear and loose clothing. It is important to maintain good hygiene, particularly after sports practice or a sporting event.
- For management of diaper candidiasis, follow the suggestions listed below in the section on diaper dermatitis.

Hypersensitivity Reactions

Skin disorders caused by hypersensitivity reactions include diaper dermatitis, atopic dermatitis, contact dermatitis, erythema multiforme, and urticaria. Drug reactions may result in skin rashes, erythema multiforme, or urticaria.

Diaper Dermatitis

Diaper dermatitis is an inflammatory reaction of the skin in the area covered by a diaper and is common in 2- to 4-month-olds (CPS, 2007a). Prolonged exposure to urine and feces may lead to skin breakdown (Fig. 45.7) as *C. albicans* is present in the feces of 90% of healthy newborns (CPS, 2007a) (see Fig. 45.6 and the section

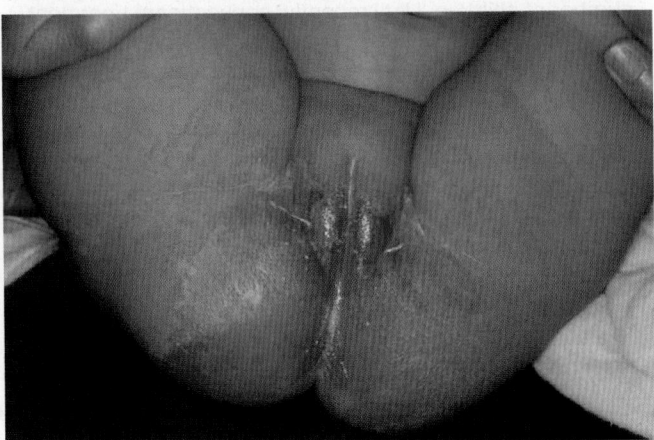

FIGURE 45.7 Diaper dermatitis.

TEACHING GUIDELINE 45.1

Diaper Dermatitis

- Change diapers frequently. Stool-soiled diapers should be changed as soon as possible.
- Gently wash the diaper area with a soft cloth, avoiding harsh soap.
- Baby wipes may be used in most children, but avoid wipes that contain fragrance or preservatives.
- Once the rash has occurred, allow the infant or child to play in the home without a diaper for a period of time each day to allow the rash to air dry and heal.
- Avoid rubber pants.

on fungal infections). Diaper wearing increases the skin's pH, activating fecal enzymes that further contribute to skin maceration.

Nursing Assessment

Determine from the history whether the infant or child wears diapers. Ask about the onset and progression of the rash, as well as any treatments and response. Inspect the skin in the diaper area for erythema and maceration (see Fig. 45.7). Ordinary diaper dermatitis does not usually result in a bumpy rash but starts as a flat red rash in the convex skin creases. It may appear red and shiny and may or may not also have papules. Untreated, it may become more widespread or severe.

Nursing Management

Prevention is the best management. Topical products such as ointments or creams containing vitamins A, D, and E, zinc oxide, or petrolatum are helpful to provide a barrier to the skin. Teaching Guideline 45.1 gives further information on diaper dermatitis. See above for treatment of diaper rash caused by *C. albicans* infection.

▶ **Take** NOTE!

Discourage parents from using any type of baby powder because aspiration; inhalation of talcum-containing powders may result in pneumonitis (Garlich & Nelson, 2011).

Atopic Dermatitis

Atopic dermatitis (eczema) usually presents in early childhood; half of the children who present with atopic dermatitis will do so in their first year of life, and a third of children will present between 1 and 5 years of age (Anonymous, 2009). Worldwide, approximately 5% to 20% of children are affected, with prevalence being notably higher in developed countries. Prevalence rates in Canada are 8.5% in children between 6 and 7 years of age and 9.4% in children of ages 13 and 14 (Barbeau & Lalonde, 2006). Atopic dermatitis is one of the disorders in the atopy family (along with asthma and allergic rhinitis). It is important to elicit patient and family history of asthma and asthma-like symptoms and to investigate allergies and other triggers for sickness.

The chronic itching associated with atopic dermatitis causes a great deal of psychological distress. The child's self-image may be affected, particularly if the rash is extensive. Difficulty sleeping may occur because of the itching, leading to irritability, decreased concentration, compromised immune status, and possible secondary infections. Parents' stress related to the child's condition may increase the child's anxiety and lead to an increase in itching and scratching. The child may outgrow atopic dermatitis or its severity may decrease as the child approaches adulthood, but many adults continue to toil with worries of dry skin as they age.

Therapeutic management includes good skin hydration, application of topical corticosteroids or immune modulators, oral antihistamines for sedative effects, and antibiotics if secondary infection occurs.

Pathophysiology

Atopic dermatitis is a chronic disorder characterized by acute and chronic periods of itching, inflamed, reddened, and swollen skin (Goodhue & Brady, 2009). The skin reaction occurs in response to specific allergens, usually food (especially eggs, wheat, milk, and peanuts) or environmental triggers (e.g., moulds, dust mites, cat dander). Other factors, such as high or low ambient temperatures, perspiring, scratching, skin irritants, or stress, may contribute to flare-ups. When the child encounters a triggering antigen, antigen-presenting cells stimulate interleukins to begin the inflammatory process. The skin begins to feel pruritic and the child starts to scratch. The sensation of itchiness comes first, and then the rash becomes apparent. The itching causes the rash to appear. Sweating causes atopic dermatitis to worsen, as do excessively humid or dry environments.

Nursing Assessment

For a full description of the assessment phase of the nursing process, refer to page 1545. Assessment findings pertinent to atopic dermatitis are discussed below.

Health History

Elicit a description of the present illness and chief complaint. Common signs and symptoms reported during the health history might include:

- Wiggling or scratching
- Dry skin
- Scratch marks noticed by the parents
- Disrupted sleep
- Irritability

Explore the child's current and past medical history for risk factors such as:

• Family history of atopic dermatitis, allergic rhinitis, or asthma
• Child's history of asthma or allergic rhinitis
• Food or environmental allergies

Determine the onset of the rash, its location, progression, severity, and response to treatments used so far. Note medications used to treat the rash, as well as other medications the child may be taking.

Physical Examination

Physical examination consists of inspection and observation and auscultation.

Inspection and Observation

Observe whether the infant is wiggling or the child is actively scratching. Carefully inspect the skin. Document dry, scaly, or flaky skin as well as hypertrophy and lichenification (Fig. 45.8). If lesions are present they may be dry lesions or weepy papules or vesicles. In children under 2 years old, the rash is most likely to occur on the face, scalp, wrists, and extensor surfaces of the arms or legs. In older children it may occur anywhere on the skin but is found more commonly on the flexor areas. Note erythema or warmth, which may indicate associated secondary bacterial infection. Document areas of hyperpigmentation or hypopigmentation, which may have resulted from a prior exacerbation of atopic dermatitis or its treatment. Inspect the eyes, nose, and throat for symptoms of allergic rhinitis.

Auscultation

Auscultate the lungs for wheezing (commonly found in the associated condition of asthma).

Laboratory and Diagnostic Tests

Serum IgE levels may be elevated in the child with atopic dermatitis. Skin prick allergy testing may determine the

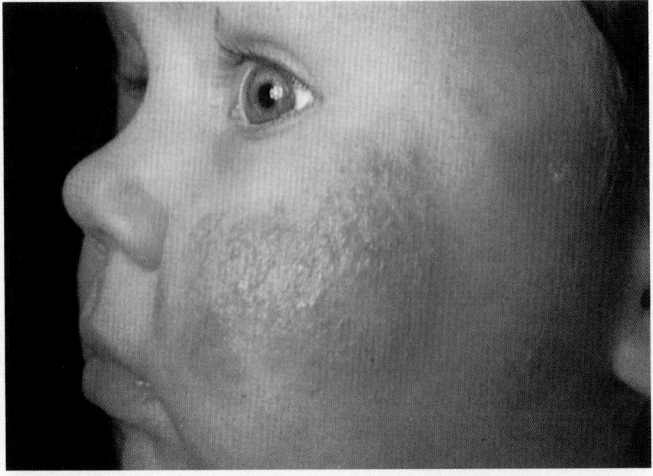

FIGURE 45.8 Atopic dermatitis rash is red, dry, and scaly.

food or environmental allergen to which the child is sensitive.

Nursing Management

Nursing management of the child with atopic dermatitis focuses on promoting skin hydration, maintaining skin integrity, and preventing infection.

Promoting Skin Hydration

First and foremost, avoid hot water and any skin or hair product containing perfumes, dyes, or fragrance. Bathe the child twice daily in warm (not hot) water. Use a mild soap to clean only the dirty areas. Recommended mild soaps or cleansing agents include:

• Unscented Dove or Dove for Sensitive Skin
• Tone
• Caress
• Oil of Olay
• Cetaphil

Lightly pat the child dry after the bath, but do not rub with the towel. Leave the child moist. Apply topical ointments or creams as prescribed to the affected area. Apply fragrance-free moisturizer over the prescribed topical medication and all over the child's body. Recommended moisturizers include:

• Eucerin, Moisturel, Curel (cream or lotion)
• Aquaphor
• Vaseline

Apply moisture multiple times throughout the day. Avoid clothing made of synthetic fabrics or wool. Avoid triggers known to exacerbate atopic dermatitis.

Following consultation with a pharmacist, evening primrose oil and other essential fatty acid supplements applied over a period of at least 6 weeks may produce an improvement in the atopic dermatitis (Senapati, Banerjee, & Gangopadhyay, 2008). Chamomile preparations for topical use may also be effective and are generally considered safe.

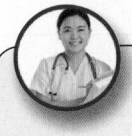

▶ *Take* NOTE!

Vaseline or generic petrolatum is an inexpensive, readily available moisturizer.

Maintaining Skin Integrity and Preventing Infection

Cut the child's fingernails short and keep them clean. Avoid tight clothing and heat. Use 100% cotton bed sheets and pajamas. In addition to keeping the child's skin well moisturized, it is extremely important to prevent the child from scratching. Scratching causes the rash to appear, and further scratching may lead to secondary infection. Antihistamines given at bedtime may sedate the child enough to allow him or her to sleep without awakening because of itching.

During the waking hours, behaviour modification may help to keep the child from scratching. Have the parent keep a diary for 1 week to determine the pattern of scratching. Help the parent to determine specific strategies that may raise the child's awareness of scratching. A hand-held clicker or counter may help to identify the scratching episode for the child, thus raising awareness. The use of diversion, imagination, and play may help to distract the child from scratching. The parent and child may create a game together in which the child participates in a behaviour other than scratching, such as pressing the skin or clenching the fist. It is important for the child to stay active to distract his or her mind from the itching.

Contact Dermatitis

Contact dermatitis is a cell-mediated response to an antigenic substance exposure. The first exposure is the sensitization phase. The antigen attaches to cells that migrate to regional lymph nodes and have contact with T lymphocytes, where recognition of antigen is developed. During the second phase, elicitation, contact with the antigen results in T-lymphocyte proliferation and release of inflammatory mediators. The rash will occur as a result of this cascade, usually within 1 to 2 days of contact, and its severity will depend on the length of exposure to and the concentration of the substance (Vernon et al., 2009).

One of the more common causes of contact dermatitis in children results from exposure to highly allergenic plants and thus will be the focus of this discussion. *Toxicodendron radican* (poison ivy), *Toxicodendron quercifolium* (Eastern poison oak), *Toxicodendron diversilobum* (Western poison oak), and *Toxicodendron vernix* (poison sumac) are the typical offenders. Contact with the plant's oil (urushiol), which is found in the leaves, stems, and roots, results in an allergic reaction in most people. Even contact with dormant plants or plants perceived to be dead may cause an allergic response. The rash is extremely pruritic and may last for 2 to 4 weeks, and lesions continue to appear during the illness.

Contact dermatitis is not contagious and does not spread either to other parts of the affected child's skin or to other people. Scratching does not spread the rash, but it may cause skin damage or secondary infection. Complications of contact dermatitis include secondary bacterial skin infections and lichenification or hyperpigmentation, particularly in dark-skinned people.

Therapeutic management is directed toward management of itching and the use of topical corticosteroids. Moderate-potency topical glucocorticoid cream or ointment is used for mild to moderate contact dermatitis, and high-potency preparations are used for more severe cases. Some severe cases of contact dermatitis may require the use of systemic steroids.

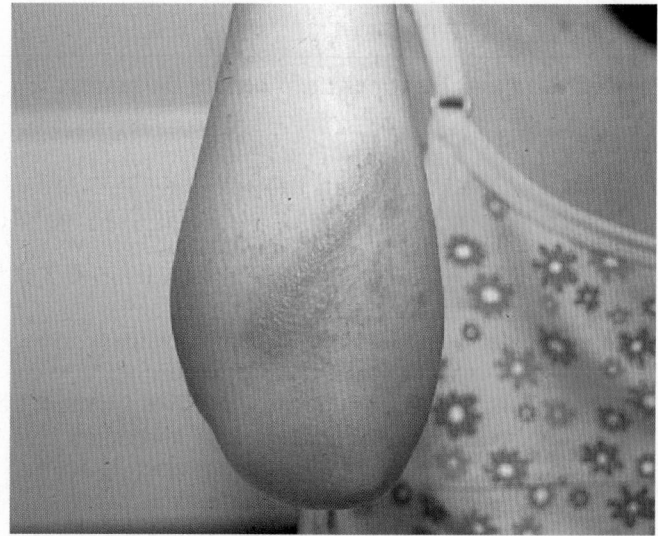

FIGURE 45.9 Note vesicular rash in linear formation characteristic of poison ivy.

Nursing Assessment

Elicit the health history, noting time spent in the woods or non-cultivated areas within 1 to 2 days before the onset of the rash. Note contact with a family pet that spends time outdoors. Note onset, description, location, and progression of the rash, which will be intensely pruritic in most children (Fig. 45.9). Document any treatment that has been used thus far, and the child's response. Examine the skin, noting an erythematous papulovesicular rash at the site of contact. Some lesions may be weeping; others erupt and form a crust. The lesions are often distributed in an asymmetric linear pattern on exposed body parts. If the child's shirt came in contact with the plant and then the shirt was removed by pulling it over the head, there may be widespread lesions over both sides of the face. Lesions near the eyes often cause significant eyelid edema.

▶ **Take** NOTE!

Nickel dermatitis may occur from contact with jewelry, eyeglasses, belts, or clothing snaps. Infants may display a small red circle with scaling at the site of contact with sleeper snaps.

Nursing Management

Contact dermatitis may be prevented by avoiding contact with the allergen. When the condition does occur, nursing management focuses on relieving the discomfort associated with the rash. Administer topical or systemic corticosteroids as prescribed and teach the family about use of the medications. Teaching Guideline 45.2 gives more information about the treatment and prevention of contact dermatitis.

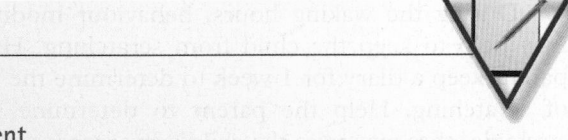

TEACHING GUIDELINE 45.2

Prevention and Treatment of Contact Dermatitis

Prevention

- Wear long sleeves and long pants on outings in the woods.
- Identify offending plants in the yard, and remove them by using a commercial weed or underbrush killer.
- Wear vinyl gloves (not rubber or latex) when working in the yard as vinyl is an effective barrier.
- Wash clothes, pets, garden items, sports equipment, and toys well using soap and water as natural oil residue from plants may be on these items.
- If contact occurs with skin, wash vigorously with soap and water as soon as possible.
- Ivy Block (an organoclay) is the only FDA-approved preventive treatment for contact dermatitis related to poison ivy, oak, or sumac. It is applied to the skin before possible exposure.

Treatment

- Wash lesions daily with mild soap and water.
- Mildly debride crusted lesions. Wet compresses twice daily will help soften and moisturize skin.
- Tepid baths (colloidal oatmeal such as Aveeno) are helpful to decrease itching. Avoid hot baths or showers, as they dry skin and will increase itching.
- Apply corticosteroid preparations topically as directed (if using high-potency preparations, do not cover with an occlusive dressing).
- Weeping lesions may be wrapped lightly; avoid occlusion. Burow's or Domeboro solutions with a dressing applied twice daily for 20 minutes may help to dry weepy lesions. Over-the-counter preparations such as calamine lotion or Ivy Rest may reduce itching and help the lesions to dry.
- Do not use topical antihistamines, benzocaine, or neomycin because of the potential for sensitization.

Data from: Allen, P. L. J. (2004). Leaves of three, let them be: If it were only that easy! *Pediatric Nursing*, *30*(2), 129–135; and Guin, J. D., & Bruckner, A. L. (2005). Compendium on poison ivy dermatitis: The insidious plants, the resulting lesions, the treatment options. *Contemporary Pediatrics*, *22*(Suppl. 1), 4–15.

Erythema Multiforme

Erythema multiforme, though uncommon in children, is an acute, self-limiting hypersensitivity reaction. It may occur in response to viral infections, such as adenovirus or Epstein-Barr virus, *Mycoplasma pneumoniae* infection, or a drug (especially sulfa drugs, penicillin, or immunizations) or food reaction. Stevens–Johnson syndrome is the most severe form of erythema multiforme and most often occurs in response to certain medications or to *Mycoplasma* infection (Box 45.1). Therapeutic management of erythema multiforme is generally supportive, as it resolves on its own.

Nursing Assessment

Note history of fever, malaise, and aches (myalgia). Determine onset and progression of rash, and presence of **pruritus** and burning. Document the child's temperature upon assessment. Inspect the skin for lesions, which most commonly occur over the hands and feet and extensor surfaces of the extremities, with spread to the trunk. Lesions progress from erythematous macules to papules, plaques, vesicles, and target lesions over a period of days (hence the name *multiforme*) (Fig. 45.10).

Nursing Management

Discontinue the medication or food if it is identified as the cause. Ensure that treatment for *Mycoplasma* is instituted if present. Encourage oral hydration. Administer analgesics and antihistamines as needed to promote comfort. If oral lesions are present, encourage soothing mouthwashes or use of topic oral anesthetics in the older child or teen. Oral lesions may be debrided with hydrogen peroxide.

Urticaria

Urticaria, commonly called hives, is a type I hypersensitivity reaction caused by an immunologically mediated

---

BOX 45.1 Stevens–Johnson Syndrome

- 1- to 14-day history of fever, malaise, headache, generalized aching, emesis, and diarrhea
- Sudden onset of high fever with rash appearing
- Rash is characteristic of erythema multiforme with the addition of inflammatory bullae on at least two types of mucosa (lips, oral mucosa, bulbar conjunctivae, or anogenital region).
- Mortality is determined by the extent of skin sloughing; less than 10% of body surface area affected gives an estimated mortality rate of 1% to 5%, greater than 30% of body surface area affected results in 25% to 35% mortality (Foster, Fola, & Letko, 2011).
- Treatment: hospitalization, isolation, fluid and electrolyte support, treatment of secondary infection of the lesions
- Ophthalmologic consult to determine if corneal ulceration, keratitis, uveitis, or panophthalmitis is present

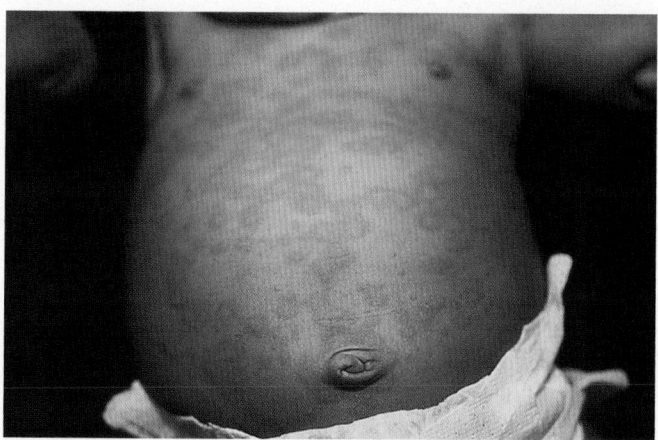

FIGURE 45.10 Erythema multiforme.

antigen–antibody response of histamine release from mast cells. Vasodilation and increased vascular permeability result, and erythema and wheals then occur. Urticaria usually begins rapidly and may disappear in a few days or may take up to 6 or 8 weeks to resolve. The most common causes of this reaction are foods, drugs, animal stings, infections, environmental stimuli (e.g., heat, cold, sun, tight clothes), and stress. Therapeutic management focuses on identifying and removing the cause as well as providing antihistamines or steroids.

Nursing Assessment

Obtain a detailed history of new foods, medications, symptoms of a recent infection, changes in environment, or unusual stress. Inspect the skin, noting raised, edematous hives anywhere on the body or mucous membranes. The hives are pruritic, blanch when pressed, and may migrate. Angioedema may also be present and is identifiable as subcutaneous edema and warmth, occurring most frequently on the extremities, face, or genitalia. Carefully assess airway and breathing, as hypersensitivity reactions may affect respiratory status.

Nursing Management

Identify and remove the offending trigger. Discontinue antibiotics. Administer antihistamines, corticosteroids, and topical antipruritics as prescribed. Inform the child and family that the episode should resolve within a few days. If it lasts up to 6 weeks, the child should be re-evaluated (Burns et al., 2009). Advise the family to obtain a medical alert bracelet for the child if the reaction is severe.

> ▶ *Take NOTE!*
>
> *In an emergency situation when airway and breathing are compromised, subcutaneous epinephrine followed by IV diphenhydramine and steroids is necessary.*

Seborrhea

Seborrhea is a chronic inflammatory dermatitis that may occur on the skin or scalp. In infants, it occurs most often on the scalp and is commonly referred to as cradle cap, usually resolving by 1 year of age. Infants may also manifest seborrhea on the nose or eyebrows, behind the ears, or in the diaper area. Adolescents manifest seborrhea on the scalp (dandruff) and on the eyebrows and eyelashes, behind the ears, and between the shoulder blades. Skin lesions are treated with corticosteroid creams or lotions. Anti-dandruff shampoos containing selenium sulphide, ketoconazole, or tar are used to treat the scalp. It is thought that seborrhea is related to an overproduction of sebum (from maternal or teenage hormones) and may be an inflammatory reaction to the fungus *Pityrosporum ovale* (Vernon et al., 2009).

Nursing Assessment

Elicit the health history, determining onset and progression of skin and scalp changes. Note response to treatment used so far. In the infant, inspect the scalp and forehead, behind the ears, and the neck, trunk, and diaper area for thick or flaky greasy yellow scales (Fig. 45.11). In the adolescent, note mild flakes in the hair with yellow greasy scales on the scalp, forehead, and eyebrows, behind the ears, or between the scapulae.

Nursing Management

Wash or shampoo the affected areas with a mild soap. Apply anti-inflammatory cream to skin lesions if prescribed. In the infant, apply mineral oil to the scalp, massage it in well with a washcloth, and then shampoo 10 to 15 minutes later, using a brush to gently lift the crusts;

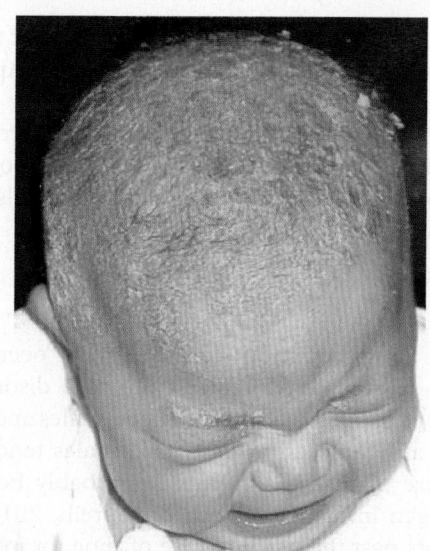

FIGURE 45.11 Severe cradle cap (yellow, greasy-appearing plaques).

do not forcibly remove the crusts. If needed, selenium sulphide shampoo may safely be used on the infant, following the aforementioned procedure. The adolescent may require daily shampooing with an anti-dandruff shampoo.

Psoriasis

Psoriasis is a chronic skin disease manifested by thick silvery scales that have spontaneous exacerbations and remissions. Psoriasis is immune-mediated and, although related to environmental factors, is genetically passed from parent to child. Psoriasis does occur in children, but the peak onset is between 15 and 25 years of age (Wong & Rogers, 2006).

Hyperproliferation of the epidermis occurs, with a rash developing at sites of mechanical, thermal, or physical trauma. Therapeutic management includes skin hydration, use of tar preparations, ultraviolet light, or tazarotene (a topical retinoid).

Nursing Assessment

Note family history of psoriasis. Determine onset and progression of rash, as well as treatments used and the response to treatment. Question the child about pruritus, which is usually absent with psoriasis. Inspect the skin for erythematous papules that coalesce to form plaques, most frequently found on the face, scalp, elbows, genital area, and knees. The plaques have a silvery or yellow-white scale and sharply demarcated borders. Layers of scale may be present, which, when removed, result in pinpoint bleeding (referred to as the Auspitz sign). Plaques on the scalp may result in alopecia. Examine the palms and soles, noting fissures and scaling.

Nursing Management

Exposure to sunlight may promote healing, but take care not to allow the child to become sunburned. Apply skin moisturizers or emollients daily to prevent dry skin and flare-ups. Apply topical anti-inflammatory creams as prescribed during flare-ups. Apply tar shampoos or skin preparations. Use mineral oil and warm towels to soak and remove thick plaques.

Acne

Acne, the most common skin condition occurring in childhood (Burch & Morelli, 2011), is a disorder that affects the pilosebaceous unit. It affects males and females as well as all ethnic groups. Overall, males tend to have more severe disease than females, probably because of the androgen influence (Burch & Morelli, 2011). Acne that persists past the usual course of time for infantile or adolescent acne may be caused by endocrine abnormalities. It may also occur in response to the use of certain types of drugs such as corticosteroids, androgens, phenytoin, and others. The usual presentation and nursing management of acne neonatorum and acne vulgaris are presented below.

Acne Neonatorum

Acne neonatorum is described as inflammatory erythematous papules and pustules distributed mostly on the infant's head (face, cheeks, scalp) with no comedones (Lucky, 2008). There has been recent discussion about the etiology of neonatal acne, including a proposed name change to "neonatal cephalic pustulosis" (Lucky, 2008). The cause of acne in the first month of life is hypothesized to be likely due to an inflammatory reaction to *Pityrosporum* species. Acne in the second or third month of life is usually termed infantile acne and often does have comedones (Lucky, 2008). It is believed that acne neonatorum occurs as a response to the presence of maternal androgens and affects about 20% of newborns (Holmes & Krusinski, 2006); it resolves spontaneously by 6 to 12 months of age (Lucky, 2008).

Nursing Assessment

Note oily face or scalp. Examine the face (especially the cheeks), upper chest, and back for inflammatory papules and pustules. Document absence of fever.

Nursing Management

Instruct parents to avoid picking or squeezing the pimples as that can place the infant at risk for secondary bacterial infection and cellulitis. Teach parents to wash the affected areas daily with clear water. Avoid using fragranced soaps or lotions on the area with acne. Inform the parents that as the newborn's hormones stabilize over time, the acne usually resolves without additional intervention.

Acne Vulgaris

Acne vulgaris occurs in up to 80% of adolescents at the onset of puberty, often between the ages of 12 and 16 years. Because it is caused by endogenous androgens, it often affects males more than females (Morelli, 2007a). Acne vulgaris may also continue into the 20s and 30s. It occurs most frequently on the face, chest, and back. There is little evidence to prove that diet affects acne outbreaks, but outbreaks have been shown to occur more frequently in winter than in summer, likely linked to stress levels and relaxation cycles.

Pathophysiology

The sebaceous gland produces sebum and is connected by a duct to the follicular canal that opens on the skin's surface. Androgynous hormones stimulate sebaceous gland proliferation and production of sebum. These hormones exhibit increased activity during the pubertal years. Abnormal shedding of the outermost layer of the skin (the stratum corneum) occurs at the level of the follicular opening, resulting in a keratin plug that fills the follicle. The sebaceous glands increase sebum production. Bacterial overgrowth of *Propionibacterium acnes* occurs because the presence of sebum and keratin in the follicular canal creates an excellent environment for growth. Inflammation occurs when the comedone ruptures and the contents sit in the dermis, initiating a neutrophilic inflammatory response. If the inflammation is close to the surface, a papule or pustule develops; if the inflammation is deeper, a nodule forms (Morelli, 2007a).

Therapeutic Management

Therapeutic management focuses on reducing *P. acnes*, decreasing sebum production, normalizing skin shedding, and eliminating inflammation (Morelli, 2007a). The skin should be cleansed gently twice a day. Medication therapy may include a combination of benzoyl peroxide, salicylic acid, retinoids, and topical or oral antibiotics. Isotretinoin (Accutane) may be used in severe cases. Drug Guide 45.1 gives further information on these medications. In girls, specific types of oral contraceptives may help lessen acne by decreasing the effects of androgens on the sebaceous glands.

Nursing Assessment

Note history of onset of acne lesions, as well as family history of acne. Determine medication use; certain medications may hasten the onset of acne or worsen it when already present. In particular, note use of corticosteroids, androgens, lithium, phenytoin, and isoniazid. Document history of an endocrine disorder, particularly one that results in hyperandrogenism. In girls, note worsening of acne 2 to 7 days before the start of the menstrual period. Inspect the skin for lesions (particularly on the face and upper chest and back, which are the areas of highest sebaceous activity). Note presence, distribution, and extent of noninflammatory lesions, such as open and closed comedones, as well as inflammatory lesions such as papules, pustules, nodules, or cysts (open comedones are commonly referred to as blackheads and closed comedones as whiteheads; Fig. 45.12). Examine the skin for hypertrophic scarring resulting from inflammatory lesions. Table 45.3 explains the acne classification. Note oily skin and oily hair, which result from increased sebum production. Determine remedies that have been used and the extent of success of those treatments. Assess the child's or teen's feelings about the disorder.

Nursing Management

Avoid oil-based cosmetics and hair products, as their use may block pores, contributing to noninflammatory lesions. Look for cosmetic products labelled as non-comedogenic. Headbands, helmets, and hats may exacerbate the lesions by causing friction. Dryness and peeling may occur with

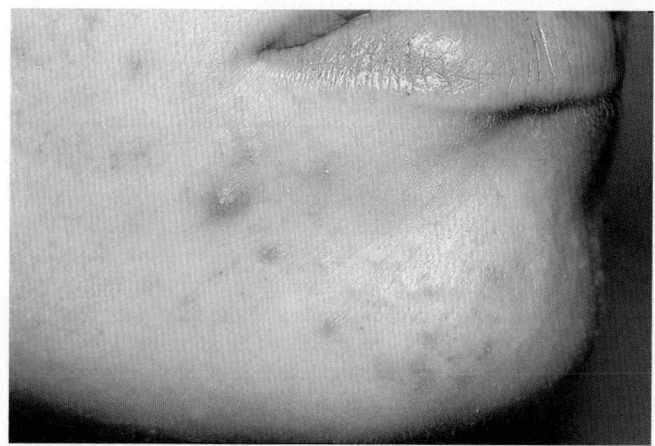

FIGURE 45.12 Acne vulgaris.

acne treatment, so encourage the child to use a moisturizer. Avoid picking or squeezing the lesions as this can result in secondary infections. Mild cleansing with soap and water twice daily is appropriate; excessive scrubbing and harsh chemical or alcohol-based cleansers should be avoided. Teach adolescents that the prescribed topical medications must be used daily and that it may take 4 to 6 weeks to see results. Boys should shave gently and avoid using dull razors so as not to further irritate the condition. Adolescent girls taking isotretinoin (Accutane) who are sexually active must be on a pregnancy prevention program because the drug causes defects in fetal development (Fulton, 2011) (Box 45.2).

Patients interested in complementary medicine approaches may try topical use of a tea tree oil preparation as there may be fewer adverse effects than with benzoyl peroxide preparations, but local reactions may still occur (Griffin, 2011).

If the acne is severe, depression may occur as a result of body image disturbances. Provide emotional support to adolescents undergoing acne therapy. Refer teens for counselling if necessary.

TABLE 45.3 CLASSIFICATION OF ACNE

Classification	Manifestations
Mild acne	Primarily noninflammatory lesions (comedones)
Moderate acne	Comedones plus inflammatory lesions such as papules or pustules (localized to face or back)
Severe acne	Lesions similar to moderate acne, but more widespread, and/or presence of cysts or nodules. Associated more frequently with scarring.

BOX 45.2 **Decreasing Risk of Fetal Exposure to Isotretinoin (ACCUTANE)**

- In Canada, there is no compulsory Accutane registry for prescribers or patients. Health Canada requires women to give informed written consent, receive education about drug effects to a fetus, and use two forms of contraception. Health Canada monitors the numbers of Accutane prescriptions and the resulting "fetal disorders" that are likely related. The Toronto Hospital for Sick Children reports an average of 10 to 20 pregnancy exposures per year and has developed Motherisk, a program that suggests mandatory Web-based education and certifies physicians to be allowed to prescribe isotretinoin.

Adapted from: Anderson, M. (2006). Accutane registry compulsory in US, but not Canada. *Canadian Medical Association Journal, 174* (12), 1701–1702; Cuzzell, J. Z. (2005). FDA approves mandatory risk management program for isotretinoin. *Dermatology Nursing, 17*(5), 383; U.S. Food and Drug Administration (2010b). *Isotretinoin (marketed as Accutane) capsule information.* Retrieved December 17, 2011 from http://www.fda.gov/Drugs/DrugSafety/PostmarketDrugSafety InformationforPatientsandProviders/ucm094305.htm.

▶ *Consider THIS!*

Paxton Herman, age 16, comes to the clinic with complaints of acne on his face and back. What assessment information should the nurse obtain? What education will be important for Paxton?

Injuries

With their inquisitive natures, developmental immaturity, and delicate skin properties, children are prone to experience a variety of skin injuries. Pressure ulcers are most likely to occur in hospitalized or otherwise immobile children. Typical healthy, active children are likely to suffer cuts, abrasions, foreign body penetration, burns and other thermal injuries, bites, and stings. Health Canada notes (2007) that the drowning rate in the Aboriginal population is six times higher than the Canadian average due to the proximity of Northern reserves (especially in Manitoba) to bodies of water. Other specific increased risks for injury among Aboriginal people include:

- Being involved in motor vehicle accidents as a result of the large distances travelled for regular activities
- Inability to receive necessary treatment following an injury due to distance from emergency facilities
- Vehicular injury resulting from use of all-terrain vehicles and snowmobiles (especially in the North)
- Hypothermia, especially in Northern climates where the water temperature is low

- Drowning due to the infrequent use of flotation devices and increased use of alcohol.
- Burns as a result of wood frame house construction, lack of smoke detectors in many homes, and smoking habits

Pressure Ulcers

Pressure ulcers result from prolonged pressure on an area of skin, leading to damage to the skin, subcutaneous layers, and deeper tissues. Injuries from unrelieved pressure may range from blanchable erythema to deep sores or ulcers (Colwell, 2009). Pressure ulcers can develop from a combination of factors, including immobility or decreased activity, decreased sensory perception, increased moisture, impaired nutritional status, inadequate tissue perfusion, and the forces of friction and shear. Common sites of pressure ulcers in hospitalized children include the occiput and toes, while children who require wheelchairs for mobility more often have pressure ulcers in the sacral or hip areas.

Nursing Assessment

Note history of immobility (chronic, related to a condition such as paralysis) or lengthy hospitalization, particularly in intensive care. Inspect the skin for areas of erythema or warmth. Note ulceration of the skin. Use the facility's wound assessment scale to document the extent of the ulcer. Many hospitals have a medical photographer and consent can be obtained from the parents to take a photo of the ulcer for reference as healing progresses. Many wound classification systems are available for pressure ulcer assessment, but they are out of scope for this textbook.

Nursing Management

Position the child to alleviate pressure on the area of the ulcer. Use specialized beds or mattresses to prevent further pressure areas from developing. Perform prescribed wound care meticulously, noting the formation of granulation tissue as the ulcer begins to heal. Prevent pressure ulcers in the child who is hospitalized for long periods of time by turning the child frequently, assessing the entire surface of the child's skin at least every shift, using pressure-alleviating beds and mattresses, and maintaining the child's nutritional status.

Minor Injuries

Children suffer minor injuries very frequently. These include minor cuts and abrasions as well as skin penetration of foreign bodies such as splinters or glass fragments. Due to developmental immaturity and inquisitive nature, children often attempt tasks they are not yet capable of or take risks that an adult would not, often resulting in a fall or other accident. The break in the skin allows an entry point for bacteria, and the complication of cellulitis may occur. Treatment is directed at cleaning the wound and preventing infection.

Nursing Assessment

Obtain the history from the child or caregiver to determine whether dirt, a foreign object, or other substance may be present in the wound. Inspect the wound, noting depth of injury, characteristics of the wound edges, a foreign body, and bleeding or swelling.

Nursing Management

Cleanse the wound with mild soap and water or with an antibacterial cleanser. Wet gauze helps to scrub away fine and large sand particles. Remove pieces of loose skin with sterile scissors, foreign particles with sterile forceps, and road tar with petrolatum. Small abrasions and minor, well-approximated cuts may be left open to the air. Apply a small amount of antibacterial ointment and cover large abrasions with a loose dressing. Change the dressing 12 hours later, and redress after cleaning the wound. Leave it open to air after 24 hours have passed from the time of injury. Assess the wound daily for signs of infection, which include purulence, warmth, edema, increasing pain, and erythema that extends past the margin of the cut or abrasion.

Calendula preparations are presumed to be safe for topical use and may speed wound healing. Chamomile may help to dry a weeping wound, and allergic reactions to the herb are rare (Ehrlich, 2010). Topical tea tree oil has natural antiseptic, antibacterial, antifungal, and antiviral properties and can help keep wounds clean and aid in the healing process.

Burns

Burns are one of the main causes of accidental death in children in Canada (Safe Kids Canada, 2010). A 10-year study of fatal and nonfatal burn injuries in Canadian children showed that more than 10,000 children were admitted to Canadian hospitals for burn injuries during the study period and almost 500 of those children died from their injuries (Spinks, Wasiak, Cleland, et al., 2008). The age group with the highest incidence of hospitalization and fatalities was children of ages 1 to 4, but children over 5 years of age suffered from more severe full-thickness burns (mostly in the 10- to 14-year-old age group) (Spinks et al., 2008).

Most pediatric burn-related injuries do not result in death, but injuries from burns often cause extreme pain and extensive burns can result in serious disfigurement. While most pediatric burns are tragic unintentional injuries, more than half are scald injuries (Spinks et al., 2008). Health Canada reported 212,437 emergency room visits due to scald burn injuries over a 4-year period, with 84% of the injuries occurring in the child's own home and more than 70% of these injuries occurring the bathroom or kitchen (Children's Safety Association of Canada, n.d.).

Great advances have been made in the care of children with serious burns. As a result, children who in the past would have died as a result of burns over large body surface areas have a much greater chance of survival (Quilty, 2010). These improved outcomes for seriously burned children are thought to be the result of refinements in:

- Resuscitation
- Operative techniques
- Critical care (mechanical ventilation, monitoring, and vascular access)
- Pain control
- Nutritional support
- Skin and blood banking
- Antibiotic therapy

Burns are classified according to the extent of injury. Superficial burns involve only epidermal injury and usually heal over the period of a week, without scarring or other sequelae. In partial-thickness burns, injury occurs not only to the epidermis but also to portions of the dermis. These burns usually heal within about 2 weeks and carry a minimal risk of scar formation. Deep partial-thickness burns take longer to heal, may scar, and result in changes in nail and hair appearance as well as sebaceous gland function in the affected area. They may require surgical intervention. Full-thickness burns result in significant tissue damage as they extend through the epidermis, dermis, and hypodermis, leading to extensive scarring. Hair follicles and sweat glands are destroyed as well. Full-thickness burns require a significant time to heal. If underlying tendons and/or bone are involved, the burn may be termed fourth degree. Contractures and limited function may occur as a complication of full-thickness burns. Skin grafting is usually necessary. Full or partially circumferential burns may result in ischemia from loss of blood flow related to progressive swelling of the area.

Pathophysiology

Burned tissue begins to coagulate after the injury, and direct coagulation and microvascular reactions in the adjacent dermis may extend the burn. The blood vessels demonstrate increased capillary permeability, resulting in vasodilation. This leads to increased hydrostatic pressure in the capillaries, causing water, electrolytes, and protein to leak out of the vasculature and result in significant edema. Edema forms very rapidly in the first 18 hours after the burn, peaking at around 48 hours. Capillary permeability then returns to normal between 48 and 72 hours after the burn and the lymphatic system can reabsorb the edema. Diuresis then occurs, as there is 5 to 10 times more fluid loss from burned areas than in normal tissues. This puts patients (especially children) at higher risks for dehydration and electrolyte imbalances as their bodies react to the burns and then slowly heal.

Initially, the severely burned child experiences a decrease in cardiac output, with a subsequent hypermetabolic response during which cardiac output increases dramatically. During this heightened metabolic state, the child is at risk for insulin resistance and increased protein catabolism. Children who are burned during an indoor or chemical fire are at increased risk for respiratory injury. Carbon monoxide poisoning often occurs in conjunction with burns as a result of smoke inhalation, and infants and children are at greater risk for carbon monoxide poisoning than adults. Children who have aspirated hot liquids are particularly at risk for airway-altering edema due to trauma to their esophagus and/or trachea.

Therapeutic Management

Health Canada (2001) states the goals of burn treatment as:

• Promoting healing and restoration of the tissues
• Preventing complications
• Preventing recurrences

Therapeutic management of burns focuses on fluid resuscitation, wound care, prevention of infection, and restoration of function. Burn infections are treated with antibiotics specific to the causative organism. If invasive burn damage occurs, surgery may be necessary. Children with partial-thickness burns over more than 10% of their total body surface area; burns that involve the face, hands, feet, genitalia, perineum, or major joints; electrical burns (including lightning injury); chemical burns; inhalation injury; pre-existing conditions that might affect recovery; or children who require special social, emotional, or long-term rehabilitative care should be hospitalized on a specific burn unit to receive specialized burn care.

Nursing Assessment

For a full description of the assessment phase of the nursing process, refer to page 1545. Upon arrival, the pediatric burn client should be evaluated to determine whether he or she will require intensive management. Assess airway, breathing, and circulation while someone else removes any smouldering clothing. Obtain a brief history of the burn circumstances while you are assessing the child and providing care.

Health History

If the burn is severe or there is a potential for respiratory compromise, ensure that airway, breathing, and circulation are adequate to stabilize the patient. Obtain a brief history while simultaneously evaluating the child and providing further emergency care. Elicit a description of how the burn occurred (exact mechanism of injury and surrounding circumstances), noting date and time. Determine whether smoke inhalation or an associated fall may have occurred. Document treatment that the

---

BOX 45.3 **Signs of Child Abuse–Induced Burns**

• Inconsistent history given when caregivers are interviewed separately
• Delay in seeking treatment by caregiver
• Uniform appearance of the burn, with clear delineation of burned and non-burned area (as with a hot object applied to the skin), or old burn scars in similar distribution as new burns
• In the case of a scald-induced burn, lack of spattering of liquid but evidence of so-called "porcelain-contact sparing," where the portion of the child's skin that was in contact with the tub or sink is not burned (commonly seen when forced immersion in extremely hot water is used as punishment).
• Flexor-sparing burns or burns that involve the dorsum of the hand
• A stocking/glove pattern on the hands or feet (circumferential ring appearing around the extremity, resulting from a caregiver forcefully holding the child under extremely hot water)

Adapted from: Jenkins, J. A., & Schraga, E. D. (2011). *Thermal burns in emergency medicine*. Retrieved December 17, 2011 from http://emedicine.medscape.com/article/769193-overview.

---

parent or caregiver has provided to the child's burn so far. Note the child's recent health status, medical history, current medications, allergies, recent illness, and immunization status, in particular noting the date of the most recent tetanus vaccination. Determine whether the history being given sounds consistent with the type of burn injury that has occurred. Inquire about what caused the burn and if the event was witnessed by anyone. Spatter-type burns resulting from the child pulling a source of hot fluid onto him- or herself usually yield a non-uniform, asymmetric distribution of injury. In contrast, intentional scald injuries usually yield a uniform "stocking" or "glove" distribution when the child's extremity is held under very hot water as punishment (Jenkins & Schraga, 2011). It is important for the nurse to pick up on clues in the health history that may indicate that the burn is a result of child abuse rather than an accident (Box 45.3). Children are also burned by curling irons, gasoline, fireworks, room heaters, ovens, and ranges. Obtain a detailed history about the circumstances surrounding these types of burns. Ask the parent what temperature the hot water heater is set for at home.

Physical Examination

Emergency examination of the burned child consists of a primary survey followed by a secondary survey. The primary survey includes evaluation of the child's airway, breathing, and circulation; the secondary survey focuses

BOX 45.4 **Emergency Assessment of the Burned Child**

Primary Survey
- Assess the child's airway, noting whether it is patent, maintainable, or un-maintainable.
- Suspect airway injury from burn or smoke inhalation if any of the following are present: burns around the mouth, nose, or eyes; carbonaceous (black-coloured) sputum; hoarseness; or stridor.
- Evaluate the child's skin colour, respiratory effort, symmetry of breathing, and breath sounds.
- Determine the pulse strength, perfusion status, and heart rate.
- Note extent and location of edema.

Secondary Survey
- Determine burn depth.
- Estimate burn extent by determining the percentage of body surface area affected. Use a chart for estimation (see Fig. 45.16) or rapidly estimate by using the child's palm size, which is equivalent to about 1% of the child's body surface area.
- Inspect the child for other traumatic injuries (children who have jumped or fallen from a house fire may suffer cervical spine or internal injuries).

Adapted from: Jenkins, J. A., & Schraga, E. D. (2011). *Thermal burns in emergency medicine.* Retrieved December 17, 2011 from http://emedicine.medscape.com/article/769193-overview.

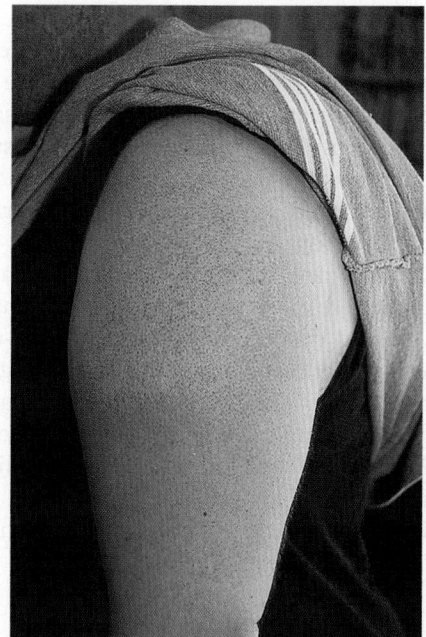

FIGURE 45.13 Superficial burn—painful but without blisters.

on evaluation of the burns and other injuries. Box 45.4 gives information about emergency assessment of the burned child. Inspect the child's skin, noting erythema, blistering, weeping, or eschar (charred skin).

The old terms used to describe the depth of burns as first, second, and third degree have been replaced by the contemporary terminology. Classify the burn according to its severity. Superficial burns are painful, red, dry, and possibly edematous (Fig. 45.13). Partial-thickness and deep partial-thickness burns are very painful and edematous and have a wet appearance or blisters (Fig. 45.14). Full-thickness burns may be very painful or numb or pain-free in some areas. They appear red, edematous, leathery, dry, or waxy and may display peeling or charred skin (Fig. 45.15). Note whether the burn is circumferential (encircling a body part) or partially circumferential.

> ▶ *Take NOTE!*
>
> *Due to overlying blistering, it is difficult to accurately distinguish between partial- and full-thickness burns. In addition, in the case of third-degree (full-thickness) burns, it is difficult to estimate burn depth during the initial evaluation.*

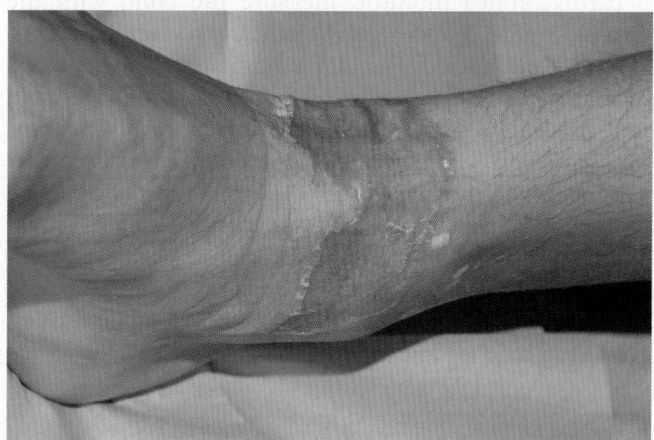

FIGURE 45.14 Partial-thickness burn—very painful, with blistering.

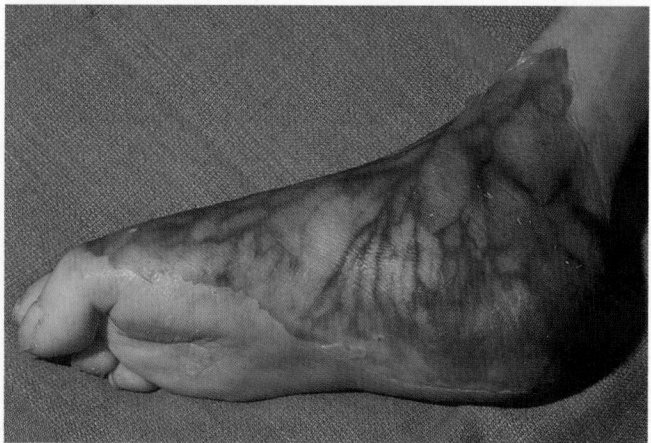

FIGURE 45.15 Full-thickness burn—colour ranges from red to charred, or white, minimal pain, marked edema.

Laboratory and Diagnostic Tests

In the child with more extensive burns, electrolyte level and complete blood count are used to measure fluid and electrolyte balance and to determine the possibility of infection, respectively. If wound infection is suspected, culture of the drainage will determine the particular bacteria. Nutritional indices such as albumin, transferrin, carotene, retinol, copper, cholesterol, calcium, thiamine, riboflavin, pyridoxine, and iron may be evaluated when the child has severe or extensive burns. Pulmonary status may be evaluated via pulse oximetry and end-tidal CO_2 monitoring, arterial blood gases, carboxyhemoglobin levels, and chest X-ray. Fibreoptic bronchoscopy and xenon ventilation–perfusion scanning may be used to evaluate inhalation injury. Electrocardiographic monitoring is important for the child who has suffered an electrical burn to identify cardiac arrhythmias, which can be noted for up to 72 hours after injury.

Nursing Management

Nursing management of the child who has been burned focuses first on stabilizing the child. Place the child on a cardiac/apnea monitor, measure the child with the Broselow tape, monitor pulse oximetry, and apply an end-tidal CO_2 monitor if the child is ventilated. Further management focuses on cleansing the burn, pain management, and prevention and treatment of infection. Fluid status and nutrition are important components of burn care, particularly in the early stages. Rehabilitation of the child with severe burns is also an important nursing function. Providing patient and family education about the prevention of burns as well as care of burns at home is critical. Nursing Care Plan 45.1 gives additional interventions related to fluid and nutritional management.

Promoting Oxygenation and Ventilation

Institute emergency airway management as needed. If the child requires intubation, make sure that the tracheal tube is taped in a very secure manner, as re-intubations in these patients will become increasingly difficult as the edema spreads over the first 48 hours. The burned child's respiratory status warrants vigilant evaluation and re-evaluation, as airway edema that is secondary to a burn may not become evident until 2 days after the injury. All children with severe burns should receive 100% oxygen via non-rebreather mask or bag-valve-mask ventilation. Continue to reassess the child's pulmonary status, adjusting the interventions as necessary (refer to Chapter 52 for further information about respiratory emergency care).

▶ *Take* NOTE!

High levels of carboxyhemoglobin as a result of smoke inhalation may contribute to falsely high pulse oximetry readings (Jenkins & Schraga, 2011).

Restoring and Maintaining Fluid Volume

Several formulas are available for the calculation of resuscitative fluids in children. Most experts recommend that pediatric burn therapy include:

- Fluid calculation based on the body surface area burned (Fig. 45.16)
- Use of a crystalloid (normal saline or lactated Ringer's solution) during the first 24 hours; in smaller children, a small amount of dextrose may be added

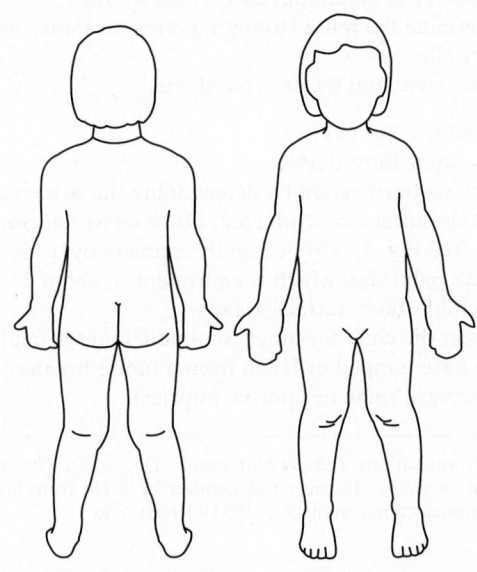

Area	Birth 1 yr (%)	1-4 yrs (%)	5-9 yrs (%)	10-14 yrs (%)	15 yrs (%)
Head	19	17	13	11	9
Neck	2	2	2	2	2
Ant. Trunk	13	13	13	13	13
Post. Trunk	13	13	13	13	13
R. Buttock	2 1/2	2 1/2	2 1/2	2 1/2	2 1/2
L. Buttock	2 1/2	2 1/2	2 1/2	2 1/2	2 1/2
Genitalia	1	1	1	1	1
R.U. Arm	4	4	4	4	4
L.U. Arm	4	4	4	4	4
R.L. Arm	3	3	3	3	3
L.L. Arm	3	3	3	3	3
R. Hand	2 1/2	2 1/2	2 1/2	2 1/2	2 1/2
L. Hand	2 1/2	2 1/2	2 1/2	2 1/2	2 1/2
R. Thigh	5 1/2	6 1/2	8	8 1/2	9
L. Thigh	5 1/2	6 1/2	8	8 1/2	9
R. Leg	5	5	5 1/2	6	6 1/2
L. Leg	5	5	5 1/2	6	6 1/2
R. Foot	3 1/2	3 1/2	3 1/2	3 1/2	3 1/2
L. Foot	3 1/2	3 1/2	3 1/2	3 1/2	3 1/2

FIGURE **45.16** Calculate total body surface area (TBSA) affected by using the child's age and the area affected. (McCance, K., & Huether, S. (2002). *Pathophysiology: Biologic basis for disease in adults and children* (4th ed.). St. Louis, MO: Mosby.)

- Administration of at least half of the volume deficit during the first 8 hours (amounts and timing of fluid volume resuscitation will vary from child to child) with close electrolyte monitoring
- Reassessment of the child and adjustment of the fluid rate accordingly; fluid requirements greatly decrease after 24 hours and should be adjusted
- Administration of a colloid fluid later in therapy once capillary permeability is less of a concern
- Monitoring of the child's urine output as part of ongoing assessment of response to therapy, expecting at least 1 mL/kg/hour
- Daily weights obtained at the same time each day (the best indicator of fluid volume status)
- Monitoring of electrolyte levels (particularly sodium and potassium) for their return to normal levels

Preventing Hypothermia

Due to loss of the protective dermis, children who are burned are at high risk for hypothermia and secondary infection. Therefore, care should be taken to keep the child warm. Warm intravenous fluids prior to administering them. Maintain a neutral thermal environment, and monitor the child's temperature frequently.

Cleansing the Burn

Initially, burning must be stopped, so remove charred clothing. Wash and rinse the burn thoroughly with mild soap and tap water. Cool water may be used, but ice should never be applied. Children who are burned with tar require special care. Tar can be removed with cool water and mineral oil. Blisters that are intact should not routinely be removed as they provide a protective barrier; however, debridement is recommended in certain cases where large blisters impede wound care. Wounds that are open require debridement. Debridement involves the removal of loose skin and eschar (dead, charred skin). This procedure is usually performed with sterile scissors and a pair of forceps or with a gauze sponge. The burned area should be gently cleansed; there is no advantage to aggressive scrubbing, and this technique only makes the pain more intense for the child. The nurse should wear a gown, mask, head covering, and gloves during dressing changes. Debridement is a necessary but often excruciatingly painful procedure, so the pain management needs of the child are of utmost importance (refer to the pain management section below).

When children return for evaluation of a wound that was previously seen in your facility, the dressing must be removed. Soak the dressing in lukewarm tap water to ease the removal of gauze, which may be stuck to the wound. The nurse plays an important role in ensuring that the dressing change goes smoothly. Be sure to:

- Have all dressing supplies ready.
- Provide pain medication as ordered.
- Promote good infection control technique among your colleagues.
- Assist with restraining young children, using the positions of comfort previously discussed in relation to atraumatic care.
- Encourage participation by the child's parents.
- Talk soothingly to the child, explain what you are going to do, and provide distraction during the procedure.

Preventing Infection

Prevention of infection is critical to successful outcomes for burned children. If the child's immunization status is unknown or if it has been 5 years or longer since the child's last tetanus vaccine, administer the tetanus vaccine (Jenkins & Schraga, 2011). Children who have never received tetanus vaccination should receive one as soon as they are stabilized. Apply antibiotic ointment in conjunction with burn dressing changes. Refer to Drug Guide 45.1 for information about topical antibiotics. Membrane dressings such as porcine xenograft and hydrocolloid dressings are alternatives to topical antibiotics and sterile dressings. Evaluate the child's wound during dressing changes, looking for wound redness, swelling, odour, or drainage. Strictly adhere to infection control procedures and hand hygiene to decrease the risk for burn infection. Maximize the child's nutritional status to decrease his or her susceptibility to a burn infection. Monitor the child's temperature for the development of fever. Upon discharge, instruct the parents about the signs of a wound infection.

Managing Pain

Pain management is of the utmost importance, and several options are available for the treatment of burn-related pain. Local anesthesia, sedatives, and systemic analgesics are commonly used. Children who have less severe burns that are managed at home can be given oral medications such as acetaminophen with codeine 30 to 45 minutes before dressing changes. In burns that result in more severe pain, the child should be hospitalized and given intravenous pain control with medications such as morphine sulphate. Depending on the child's age and situation and the type of health care facility, there are many effective medications that can be used in conjunction with narcotics for pain control and relief (e.g., benzodiazepines [intranasal midazolam], nonsteroidal anti-inflammatory drugs [NSAIDs: ibuprofen or ketorolac], antibiotics [topical flamazine]).

Pain may also occur at any time of the day or night, not just in relation to dressing changes. Assess the child's pain status frequently using an age-appropriate pain assessment scale. Administer pain medications as prescribed, and use non-pharmacologic techniques to alleviate or decrease the child's perception of pain. Age-appropriate non-pharmacologic interventions such as deep breathing, imagination, play, distraction, or virtual-reality therapy have been shown to alleviate pain during painful procedures such as dressing changes (Stinson, Yamada, Dickson, et al., 2008).

Treating Infected Burns

The potential for burn infection increases if the child has a large, open burn wound and if there are other potential sources of infection. In addition, children who are immunocompromised are at increased risk for burn infection. *S. aureus* is the usual bacterium implicated in burn cellulitis and burn impetigo (Quilty, 2010). In burn wound cellulitis, the area around the burn becomes increasingly red, swollen, and painful early in the course of burn management. With invasive burn cellulitis, the burn develops a dark brown, black, or purplish colour, with a discharge and foul odour. Burn impetigo is characterized by multifocal small superficial abscesses. Burn impetigo causes marked destruction of skin-grafted areas.

When an infection is suspected, antibiotics are usually started, pending wound culture results. Administer antibiotics as prescribed (or antifungals if an extensive burn injury becomes infected with a fungus).

Providing Burn Rehabilitation

Children who have suffered a significant burn injury face a myriad of physical and psychological challenges that extend well beyond the acute injury phase. Burned children most often exhibit anxiety and attention or behavioural problems (Pardo, Garcia, & Gomez-Cia, 2010). Skin grafting or special burn dressings are required for some children (Box 45.5). Children who have suffered extensive burns often require multiple skin-grafting surgeries. Figures 45.17 and 45.18 show healed skin grafts. Extensive burns may also result in the need for pressure garments to decrease the risk of extensive scarring. Pressure garments are not comfortable and they must be

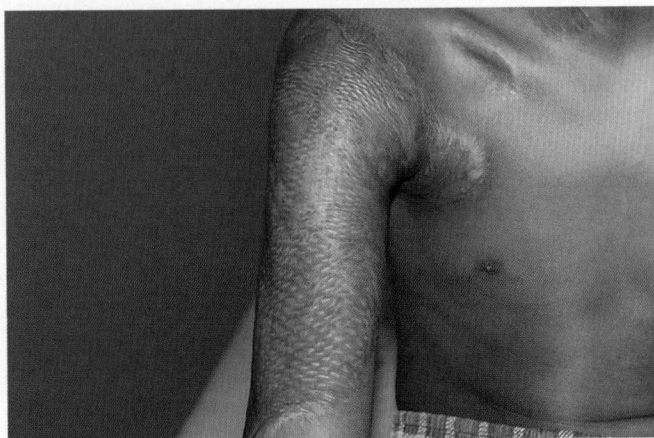

FIGURE 45.17 Healed mesh graft.

worn continuously for at least 1 year, but they have been shown to be very effective in reducing hypertrophic scarring resulting from significant burn injury.

Physical therapy will usually be initiated in the critical care setting and will continue long after hospital discharge, sometimes throughout life. Limb positioning, exercise, and range of motion are necessary to regain and maintain joint flexibility; splints and other supports provided by physiotherapists aid comfort and support during healing.

Nurses play a key role in smoothing the transition from the acute care phase of life-saving interventions and frequent dressing changes to normal activities such as school and play. Body image considerations may have a significant impact on the child when he or she returns to school and should be addressed. Children with altered

---

BOX 45.5 Skin Grafting and Special Burn Care

- Biologic skin coverings are used for extensive burns or in cases of no donor.
- Auto-graft allows for permanent coverage of a deep partial-thickness or full-thickness burn.
  - Consists of patient's own skin
- Split-thickness consists of epidermis and superficial layers of dermis. The donor site heals completely.
- Full-thickness consists of full dermal thickness. Cover the donor site with fine-mesh gauze or synthetic wound coverings to allow the site to heal.
- Kaltostat (calcium alginate dressing) is a brown seaweed extract that is spun into a fibre that is highly absorbent. It reacts with exudate on the wound to form a protective gel.

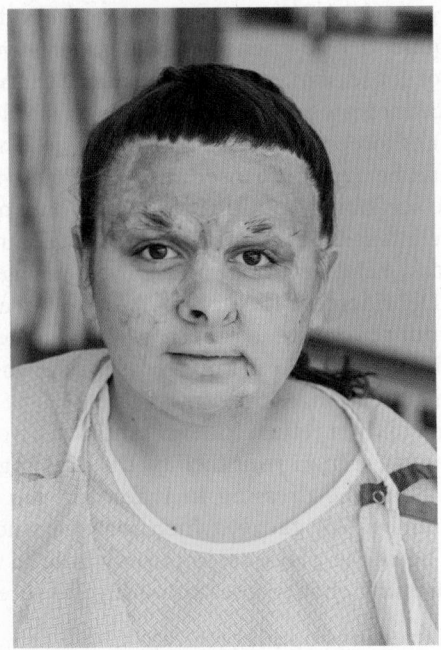

FIGURE 45.18 Extensive grafting to the face.

body image as a result of a burn might benefit from regular counselling and group therapy. Parents often need assistance with the behavioural challenges of caring for a child who is recovering from a burn injury. Visit http://thePoint. lww.com/Chow1e for direct links to websites that are available for support of persons who are burned.

Navigating through life after suffering a serious burn injury can be difficult for the child and family, and a skilled nurse can provide valuable assistance to families during the equally important but less acute phase of the journey.

Preventing Burns and Carbon Monoxide Poisoning

Instruct parents about prevention of burns. All homes should have working smoke detectors, and batteries should be changed twice a year. All homes should be equipped with fire extinguishers, and adults and older teenagers should be taught how to operate them. Children should sleep in fire-retardant sleepwear. Parents should not smoke in the house or the car, and they should keep lighters and matches out of children's reach. Young children are particularly susceptible to burns that occur in the kitchen, such as scalds from hot liquids and foods and burns from contact with hot burners or oven doors. Although fireworks are not legal in most parts of Canada, they are available. Caution parents about the extreme danger that fireworks present to children. Teaching Guideline 45.3 gives additional information for parents related to burn prevention. The booklet "Burn Prevention Tips," which includes a colouring book, is available from the Shriners Hospitals for Children.

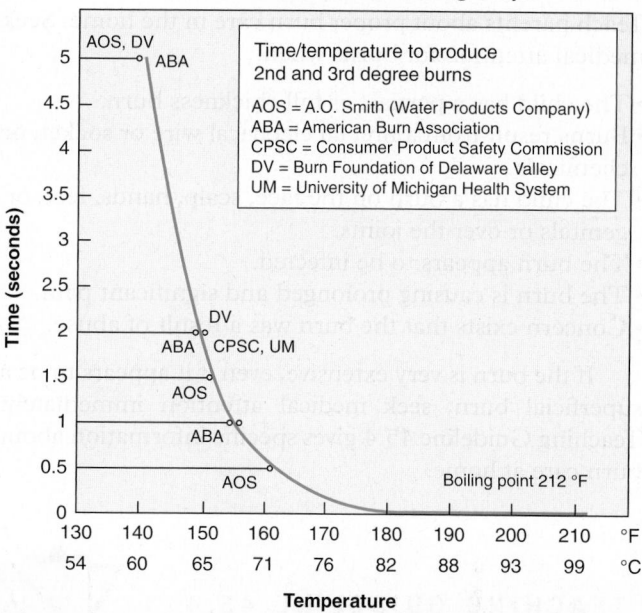

Hot Water Burn and Scalding Graph

FIGURE 45.19 Length of hot water exposure that results in significant burns based on water temperature. Used with permission of Accurate Building Inspectors. (2011). *Water temperature thermometry.* Retrieved December 17, 2011 from http://www.accuratebuilding.com/services/legal/charts/hot_water_burn_scalding_graph.html.

Children are at significant risk for burns related to hot water. Scald burns can occur when hot water comes into contact with the child's skin, even for a relatively short time. Since hot water presents such a serious risk to children, the temperature on all hot water heaters should be 48°C (120°F) or lower. Figure 45.19 shows how long a child can be exposed to water of various temperatures before a burn occurs. For example:

- If the water is 65°C (150°F), a child can receive a third-degree (full-thickness) burn within 2 seconds.
- If the water is 60°C (140°F), it takes 6 seconds of exposure to cause a significant burn.
- If the water is 54°C (130°F), a child can be burned significantly in only 30 seconds.
- At 48°C (120°F), the recommended maximum home hot water heater temperature, it takes as long as 5 minutes of exposure to burn a person (plenty of time to get out of the tub!) (Accurate Building Inspectors, 2011).

Instruct parents about prevention of carbon monoxide poisoning. All homes should have working carbon monoxide detectors, and batteries should be changed twice a year. Teach parents the signs of carbon monoxide poisoning: headaches, dizziness, disorientation, and nausea. If the carbon monoxide detector sounds, turn off any potential sources of combustion, if possible, and evacuate all occupants immediately. Do not attempt to re-enter the home until a qualified professional repairs the source of the carbon monoxide leak.

TEACHING GUIDELINE 45.3

Burn Prevention

- Keep hot water heater temperature lower than 48°C (120°F).
- Test bath water temperature with wrist or elbow before bathing children.
- Keep children away from open flames, stoves, and candles.
- Cook with pots on the inside of the stove with the handles turned in.
- Keep children away from the stove while cooking.
- Place hot liquids out of reach of children.
- Avoid drinking hot beverages while holding a child.
- Keep curling irons out of reach of children.
- Teach older children how to safely get out of the house in case of fire.
- Practice fire drills.
- Teach children to "stop, drop, and roll" if their clothes catch on fire.

Providing Burn Care at Home

Teach parents about proper burn care in the home. Seek medical attention for burns when:

- The child has a partial- or full-thickness burn.
- Burns result from a fire, an electrical wire or socket, or chemicals.
- The child has a burn on the face, scalp, hands, feet, or genitals or over the joints.
- The burn appears to be infected.
- The burn is causing prolonged and significant pain.
- Concern exists that the burn was a result of abuse.

If the burn is very extensive, even if it appears to be a superficial burn, seek medical attention immediately. Teaching Guideline 45.4 gives specific information about burn care at home.

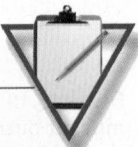

TEACHING GUIDELINE 45.4

Providing Immediate Burn Care

For First-Degree (Superficial) Burns

- Run cool water over the burned area until the pain lessens.
- Do not apply ice to the skin.
- Do not apply butter, ointment, or cream.
- Cover the burn lightly with a clean, non-adhesive bandage.
- Administer acetaminophen or ibuprofen for pain.
- Have the child seen by the primary care provider within 24 hours.
- Ongoing care: clean in tub or shower with fragrance-free mild soap; pat or air dry.
  - Apply a thin layer of antibiotic ointment.
  - Cover with a non-adherent dressing, then cover with dry gauze.

For More Extensive Burns

- Check the child's airway, breathing and compressions (ABCs) and perform cardiopulmonary resuscitation (CPR) if necessary. Please check the Heart and Stroke Foundation of Canada for recent changes to pediatric resuscitation guidelines.
- Remove clothing only if it comes off easily or if it is still smouldering.
- Do not apply butter, ointment, or any other type of cream.
- Cover the burn with a clean, lint-free bandage or sheet.
- Avoid applying large, wet sheets, as this can cause the child to become too cold.
- Do not attempt to break any blisters.
- If the child appears to be in shock, elevate the legs while protecting the burn and call 911.

Sunburn

Although tanning bed use has been much discussed in Canadian news in recent years, there is not much published literature to guide health care workers when educating parents, teens, and children about the effects of UV exposure. There is also much debate about the effects of natural sunlight versus ultraviolet (UV)B-induced erythema (Land & Small, 2009). Sunburn occurs as a result of overexposure to the UV rays of the sun. Depending on the child's age and type of skin, as well as the amount and intensity of the exposure, burns and blisters can occur within hours. It has been established and widely accepted that excessive sun exposure (with resultant skin damage) has been linked to the development of skin cancer later in life (Burns et al., 2009).

Nursing Assessment

Obtain the health history, noting recent sun exposure. Determine length of exposure and whether any type of sunscreen or sun block product was used. Note redness of the skin on the exposed areas. More severe areas will have a darker red, slightly purple hue. Blisters may be noted with more severe sunburn.

Nursing Management

Sunburn is usually treated with cool water, cool compresses, cooling lotions, oral NSAIDs, increased fluid intake, and (if prescribed) local anesthetic sprays. Administration of anesthetic sprays for sunburn should be dictated by the patient's symptoms, not by protocols (Land & Small, 2009). Cool compresses with aloe vera gel applied topically may provide significant soothing with very few adverse effects. NSAIDs (such as ibuprofen) can be very helpful with pain management in the early stages. Discourage hot showers or baths. Instruct the child to wear loose clothing and to ensure that burned areas are covered when going outside (until they are healed). If skin flaking occurs, discourage the child from "peeling" the flaked skin in order to prevent further injury. Refer to Chapter 30 for further information about safe sun exposure.

All children over the age of 6 months should use a sunscreen with a minimum SPF 15 whenever they are outdoors. Sun avoidance is advised between late morning and early afternoon if possible as the sun's rays are hottest at that time and risk of burning increases. The use of tanning beds should be limited or avoided, and parents should engage in ongoing discussion with the child's health care provider about the literature emerging on this topic.

Cold Injury

The term "frostbite" implies freezing of the tissues. It is described on a continuum from first to fourth degree. When a child is exposed to an extremely cold environment, changes in cutaneous circulation help to maintain the core body temperature. As circulation is shunted to the core, the most peripheral body parts are those at highest risk for frostbite. Local damage occurs when the tissue temperature drops to 0°C (32°F). Initially skin sensation is lost, the vasculature constricts, and plasma leakage occurs. Ice crystals develop in the extracellular fluid, and eventually vascular stasis leads to endothelial cell damage, necrosis, and sloughing of dead tissue. In Canada, cold injury can result from prolonged water exposure, especially in First Nations communities in Northern Canada.

Nursing Assessment

Note history of cold exposure. Inquire about pain or numbness. Examine the skin for indications of frostbite. First-degree frostbite results in superficial white plaques with surrounding erythema. Second-degree frostbite demonstrates blistering with erythema and edema. In third-degree frostbite, hemorrhagic blisters occur, progressing to tissue necrosis and sloughing in fourth-degree frostbite.

Nursing Management

Remove wet or tight clothing. Avoid vigorous massage to decrease the chance of damaging the skin further. When the child is in the hospital, with supports in place, immerse the affected part in warm water (not to exceed 40°C [104°F]) for 15 to 30 minutes. Thawing may cause significant pain, so administer analgesics. Keep the thawed part loosely covered, warm, and dry. Splinting may be used to help decrease associated edema. Consult the wound care specialist or plastic surgeon for further management.

Preventing frostbite may be achieved by:

- Dressing warmly in layers, and keeping warm and dry
- Avoiding exertion
- Remaining inside when cold weather or wind chill advisories are in effect
- Locking doors with high locks to prevent toddlers from going outside, and providing adequate supervision to children both indoors and outdoors.

Human and Animal Bites

Roughly 1% of emergency department visits in Canada are due to bite injuries. Dog bites are the most common, followed by cat bites and human bites. In 2005, the Public Health Agency of Canada reported that 43% of bite injuries occur to the face, 34% to the upper extremities, 18% to the lower extremities, and 4% to the trunk. The average age of Canadian children presenting to an emergency department with a dog bite is 7 years (Lang & Klassen, 2005), and the injury typically occurs when the child hits, kicks, threatens, plays with, hugs, grabs, or chases the dog (Lang & Klassen, 2005).

Therapeutic management involves cleansing and irrigating the wound, wound suturing or stapling if necessary, and topical and/or systemic antibiotic therapy. Rabies prophylaxis is indicated in animal bite injuries if the rabies status of the animal is unknown. Secondary bacterial infection of the bite wound with streptococci, staphylococci, or *Pasteurella multocida* may occur. Cat and human bites are the most likely to become infected with various bacteria or viruses (Hansen & Ahmed, 2010).

Nursing Assessment

Determine the history of the attack and whether it was provoked. Determine the child's tetanus vaccination status. Inspect the bite to determine the extent of laceration, avulsion, or crushing injury. Be sure to examine the child fully in case there are secondary injuries (e.g., from a fall while running).

Nursing Management

With dog bites, provide rabies immunoprophylaxis and a tetanus booster vaccination if indicated. Thoroughly cleanse the wound with soap and water or a povidone–iodine solution, then irrigate the wound well with normal saline. If the animal may be rabid, cleanse the wound for at least 10 minutes with a virucidal agent such as povidone–iodine solution. Administer antibiotics as prescribed.

Prevention of animal bites is important. Teach children the following:

- Never provoke a dog with teasing or roughhousing.
- Get adult permission before interacting with a dog, cat, or other animal that is not your pet.
- Do not bother an animal (especially a dog) that is eating or sleeping.
- Avoid high-pitched talking or screaming around dogs.
- Display a closed fist first for a dog to sniff.
- If a cat hisses or lashes out with a paw, leave it alone.

Never leave a child under 5 years of age alone with a dog (Centers for Disease Control and Prevention, 2009). Contact the local humane society for a dog bite prevention program that is appropriate for school-age children.

While very few human bites break skin, CPS (2008) published a position statement on managing human bites that discusses the risks of possible transmission of infections such as viral hepatitis and HIV from human bites.

Children may suffer significant emotional distress after being bitten. Nightmares and increased anxiety are common (National Health Service, 2010), and children will need much help working through the trauma by talking about the incident or reading books about this type of event.

Insect Stings and Spider Bites

Members of the Hymenoptera class of insects sting. This class includes bees, wasps, ants, yellow jackets, and hornets.

Spiders inject their venom when they bite. Stings and bites usually result in a local reaction. A systemic or anaphylactic reaction to a Hymenoptera sting may also occur, possibly resulting in airway compromise (refer to Chapter 47 for additional information on anaphylaxis). In North America, serious reactions may occur with three types of spiders: brown recluse (Southern and Midwestern United States), hobo (Western United States and Western Canada), or black widow (throughout the United States and in Southern Ontario) (Brehm, 2009).

Local reactions to insect stings and spider bites include pruritus, pain, and edema. A hypersensitivity reaction thought to be mediated by immunoglobulin E occurs in response to the venom. This may be a physiologic response to the antigens present in the insect's or spider's saliva and other fluids that are transmitted during stinging or biting. Bacterial superinfection may occur as a complication of the bite or sting or as a result of scratching.

Therapeutic management includes antihistamines to decrease itching and in some cases corticosteroids to decrease inflammation and swelling.

Nursing Assessment

Obtain the history of the bite or sting. Children are usually acutely aware when they have been stung by an insect, but spiders are generally not observed when the bite occurs. Inspect the bite or sting, noting an urticarial wheal or papular reaction. A large local reaction may be mistaken for cellulitis. Note whether a stinger remains present. Assess the child's work of breathing to determine if a systemic reaction or anaphylaxis is occurring (refer to Chapter 47).

Nursing Management

Remove jewelry or constrictive clothing if the sting or bite is on an extremity. Wounds that are not severe can be cleansed with mild soap and water. If the stinger is present, scrape it away with your fingernail or a credit card. Apply ice to decrease pain and edema and to localize the venom. Administer diphenhydramine as soon as possible after the sting in an attempt to minimize the reaction. Severe bites need to be assessed by qualified medical personnel.

Black widow spider bites often need to be treated with a specific antivenin, muscle relaxants, pain medications, tetanus prophylaxis, and sometimes antibiotics (Brehm, 2009). Venom from the brown recluse spider can be hemolytic and necrotizing if the bite is severe and not treated (Brehm, 2009).

Prevent insect stings and spider bites by wearing protective clothing and shoes when outdoors. Use insect repellents (with a maximum concentration of 30% *N,N*-Diethyl-*meta*-toluamide [DEET] in infants and children older than 2 months) (U.S. Food and Drug Administration, 2010a). Teach children never to disturb a bee or wasp nest or an ant hill. Careful attention must be paid around spiders as many spiders bite in self-defense.

Scabies

Scabies is caused by the mite *Sarcoptes scabiei* and is passed from person to person (direct contact) via contaminated articles for up to 48 hours. Scabies infection rates are high on many reserves in Canada due to overcrowding, sharing bed linens and clothing, a large pediatric population, failure to recognize infestation, reduced access to medical care, and improper treatment and follow-up. On some reserves, decreased access to running water increases the risk of secondary skin infections. Skin eruptions associated with scabies consists variably of wheals, papules, vesicles, burrows, and superimposed eczematous dermatitis. The lesions are intensely pruritic, especially at night or after a warm bath, which leads to marked excoriation. In infants, the face, scalp, palms, and soles are most commonly involved. In adolescents, the lesions often appear as thread-like burrows between the fingers, groin and genitalia, umbilicus, axillae, wrists, elbows, ankles, and buttocks. The symptoms may take 3 to 6 weeks to develop after initial contact with mite (the incubation period is 3 to 6 weeks). Complications of scabies include possible cellulitis and impetigo (CPS, 2001).

Nursing management consists of educating the family on the treatment of scabies to eradicate the mites, control for secondary infection, and relieve symptoms (Health Canada, 2001). Scabicide cream or lotion (typically Nix) will need to be applied to the entire body (chin to toes). The scabicide must be applied in skin creases, between fingers and toes, between buttocks, under breasts, and on external genitalia (Health Canada, 2001) and must be left on the skin for 8 to 14 hours. Typically, a single application is usually curative, but it may be re-applied after 1 week if symptoms persist. The safety of scabicide cream has not been established for infants less than 3 months of age; therefore, other treatments may be administered in these situations. As scabies may not appear for 1 to 2 months after the infection is acquired, prophylactic therapy is essential for all household members. All bed linen and clothing worn should be laundered in a hot, soapy wash and dried with a hot drying cycle. If hot water is not available, all bed linen and clothing should be placed into plastic bags and stored away from the family for 5 to 7 days, as the parasite cannot survive beyond 4 days without skin contact. Children may return to day care or school the day after treatment is completed.

■■■ Key Concepts

■ The infant's epidermis is thinner, loses heat more readily, absorbs substances more easily, and is more accessible to bacterial invasion than the skin of the adult. The increased water content of the infant's skin compared with that of the adult places the infant at increased risk of blister development and other skin alterations.

■ The child's skin thickness and characteristics reach adult levels in the late teenage years.

■ Children with dark skin tend to have more pronounced cutaneous reactions than children with lighter skin.

■ Sebum production increases in the preadolescent and adolescent years, contributing to the development of acne at that time.

■ Skin scrapings placed on a slide and prepared with potassium chloride may be evaluated microscopically to determine the presence of fungus.

■ Most bacterial skin infections are caused by *Staphylococcus aureus* and group A beta-hemolytic streptococcus.

■ Fungal skin infections, referred to collectively as tinea, may require up to several weeks of treatment.

■ Contact dermatitis and atopic dermatitis both present as pruritic rashes, whereas psoriasis is generally nonpruritic.

■ Hypersensitivity responses may result in erythema multiforme or urticaria.

■ Scaling may occur with atopic dermatitis and psoriasis, whereas honey-coloured crusting is common with impetigo. Erythema is a common finding with many skin disorders in children.

■ Burns may result in significant weeping and fluid loss.

■ Keeping the skin well moisturized is a key intervention in the management of atopic dermatitis and psoriasis.

■ Appropriate hygiene is of particular importance in integumentary disorders.

■ Pain management, prevention of infection, and rehabilitation are the focus of nursing management for the burned child.

■ The constant itch–rash–itch cycle of atopic dermatitis may have a considerable impact on the child's sleep, school functioning, and self-esteem.

■ Acne vulgaris, particularly if moderate or severe, may have a significant negative effect on the teen's self-esteem.

■ Teach children with chronic disorders such as atopic dermatitis, psoriasis, and acne (and their parents) to cleanse and moisturize the skin properly, avoid particular skin irritants, and use medications appropriately.

■ Many skin disorders are preventable. Teach families how to prevent contact dermatitis, burns, sunburn, frostbite, and bites and stings.

■ Educate children and families about the importance of good soap-and-water cleansing of all minor skin injuries.

■ Scabies rates are high on many reserves in Canada due to many factors including overcrowding and a high incidence of children.

REFERENCES

Accurate Building Inspectors. (2011). *Water temperature thermometry.* Retrieved December 17, 2011 from http://www.accuratebuilding.com/services/legal/charts/hot_water_burn_scalding_graph.html

Allen, P. L. J. (2004). Leaves of three, let them be: If it were only that easy! *Pediatric Nursing, 30*(2), 129–135.

Anderson, M. (2006). Accutane registry compulsory in US, but not Canada. *Canadian Medical Association Journal, 174*(12), 1701–1702.

Anonymous. (2009). Caring for the child with an integumentary condition. In S. L. Ward & S. M. Hisley (Eds.), *Maternal-child nursing care: Optimizing outcomes for mothers, children & families.* Philadelphia: FA Davis.

Barbeau, M., & Lalonde, H.,(2006). Burden of atopic dermatitis in Canada. *International Journal of Dermatology, 45,* 31–36.

Barton, M., Hawkes, M., Moore, D., et al. (2006). Guidelines for the prevention and management of community-associated methicillin-resistant *Staphylococcus aureus:* A perspective for Canadian health care practitioners. *Canadian Journal of Infectious Diseases & Medical Microbiology, 17*(Suppl. C), 4c–24c.

Brehm, C. B. (2009). Common injuries. In C. E. Burns, A. M. Dunn, M. A. Brady, N. B. Starr, & C. G. Blosser (Eds.), *Pediatric primary care* (4th ed.). St. Louis, MO: Saunders Elsevier.

Burch, J. M., & Morelli, J. G. (2011). Skin. In W. W. Hay, M. J. Levin, J. M. Sondheimer, & R. R. Deterding (Eds.), *Current pediatric diagnosis and treatment* (20th ed.). New York: McGraw-Hill.

Burns, C. E., Dunn, A. M., Brady, M. A., Starr, N. B., & Blosser, C. (2009). *Pediatric primary care* (4th ed.). Philadelphia: Saunders.

Canadian Paediatric Society. (2001). Scabies management. *Pediatric Child Health Journal, 6*(10), 775–757.

Canadian Paediatric Society. (2005). Methicillin-resistant *Staphylococcus aureus* in First Nations communities in Canada. *Paediatrics & Child Health, 10*(9), 557–560.

Canadian Paediatric Society. (2006). Control and treatment of methicillin-resistant *Staphylococcus aureus* in Canadian pediatric health care institutions. *Paediatrics & Child Health, 11*(3), 163–165.

Canadian Paediatric Society. (2007a). Antifungal agents for common pediatric infections. *Paediatrics & Child Health, 12*(10), 875–878.

Canadian Paediatric Society. (2007b). Community-associated methicillin-resistant *Staphylococcus aureus:* Implications for the care of children. *Paediatrics & Child Health, 12*(4), 323–324.

Canadian Paediatric Society. (2008). A bite in the playroom: Managing human bites in child care settings. *Paediatrics & Child Health, 13*(6), 515–521.

Centers for Disease Control and Prevention. (2009). *Dog bite prevention.* Retrieved October 11, 2011, from http://www.cdc.gov/homeandrecreationalsafety/dog-bites/biteprevention.html

Children's Safety Association of Canada. (n.d.). *Health Canada scald burn injuries: Statistics children, ages 0–6 years.* Retrieved December 17, 2011 from http://www.safekid.org/scaldstat.htm

College of Registered Nurses of British Columbia. (2010). *Pediatric decision support tools: Integumentary assessment.* Retrieved December 17, 2011 from https://www.crnbc.ca/Standards/CertifiedPractice/Documents/RemotePractice/765IntegumentaryAssessmentPediatricDST.pdf

Colwell, J. C. (2009). Skin integrity and wound care. In P. A. Potter & A. G. Perry (Eds.), *Fundamentals of nursing* (7th ed., pp. 1278–1341). St. Louis, MO: Mosby Elsevier.

Cuzzell, J. Z. (2005). FDA approves mandatory risk management program for isotretinoin. *Dermatology Nursing, 17*(5), 383.

Ehrlich, S. D. (2010). *Calendula.* Retrieved December 17, 2011 from http://www.umm.edu/altmed/articles/calendula–000228.htm

Foster, C. S., Fola, B., & Letko, E. (2011). *Stevens–Johnson syndrome.* Retrieved December 17, 2011 from http://emedicine.medscape.com/article/756523-overview

Fulton, J. (2011). *Acne vulgaris.* Retrieved December 17, 2011 from http://emedicine.medscape.com/article/1069804-overview

Garlich, F. M., & Nelson, L. S. (2011). Inhalation of baby powder. *Emergency Medicine, 43*(1), 17–20.

González, U., Seaton, T., Bergus, G., Jacobson, J., & Martínez-Monzón, C. (2007). Systemic antifungal therapy for tinea capitis in children. *The Cochrane Library, 4.* Indianapolis, IN: John Wiley & Sons.

Goodhue, C. J., & Brady, M. A. (2009). Atopic and rheumatic disorders. In C. E. Burns, A. M. Dunn, M. A. Brady, N. B. Starr, & C. G. Blosser (Eds.), *Pediatric Primary Care* (4th ed.). St. Louis, MO: Saunders Elsevier.

Griffin, R. M. (2011). *Vitamin supplements and lifestyle guide: Tea tree oil.* Retrieved December 17, 2011 from http://www.webmd.com/vitamins-and-supplements/lifestyle-guide-11/supplement-guide-tea-tree-oil

Guin, J. D., & Bruckner, A. L. (2005). Compendium on poison ivy dermatitis: The insidious plants, the resulting lesions, the treatment options. *Contemporary Pediatrics, 22*(Suppl. 1), 4–15.

Hansen, J. J., & Ahmed, A. (2010). Emergent management of bite wounds. *Emergency Medicine, 42*(6), 6–11.

Health Canada. (2001). *First Nations, Inuit and Aboriginal health: Pediatric clinical practice guidelines for nurses in primary care—Skin.* Retrieved December 17, 2011 from http://www.hc-sc.gc.ca/fniah-spnia/pubs/services/_nursing-infirm/2001_ped_guide/chap_16a-eng.php#_16–1

Health Canada. (2007). *First Nations, Inuit and Aboriginal Health: Water safety and drowning prevention.* Retrieved December 17, 2011 from http://www.hc-sc.gc.ca/fniah-spnia/promotion/injury-bless/surround-environ/drown-noyades-eng.php

Holmes, T. E., & Krusinski, P. A. (2006). Dermatologic diseases. In J. A. McMillan (Ed.), *Oski's pediatrics: Principles and practice.* Philadelphia: Lippincott Williams & Wilkins.

Jenkins, J. A., & Schraga, E. D. (2011). *Thermal burns in emergency medicine.* Retrieved December 17, 2011 from http://emedicine.medscape.com/article/769193-overview

Land, V., & Small, L. (2009). The evidence on how to best treat sunburn in children: Summary of the evidence with clinical practice recommendations. *Dermatology Nursing, 21*(3), 126, 133–137.

Lang, M., & Klassen, T. (2005). Dog bites in Canadian children: A five year review of severity and emergency department management. *Canadian Journal of Emergency Medicine, 7*(5), 309–314.

Lewis, L., & Friefman, A. D. (2011). *Impetigo.* Retrieved December 17, 2011 from http://emedicine.medscape.com/article/783562-overview

Lucky, A. W. (2008). Transient benign cutaneous lesions in the newborn. In L. F. Eichenfield, I. J. Frieden, & N. B. Esterly (Eds.), *Neonatal dermatology* (2nd ed.). Philadelphia: Saunders Elsevier.

Magin, P., Adams, J., Heading, G., Pond, D., & Smith, W. (2008). Experiences of appearance-related teasing and bullying in skin disease and their psychological sequelae: Results of a qualitative study. *Scandinavian Journal of Caring Sciences, 22*(3), 430–435.

Morelli, J. G. (2007a). Acne. In R. M. Kliegman, R. E. Behrman, H. B. Jenson, & B. M. D. Stanton (Eds.), *Nelson textbook of pediatrics* (18th ed.). Philadelphia: Saunders Elsevier.

Morelli, J. G. (2007b). Cutaneous bacterial infections. In R. M. Kliegman, R. E. Behrman, H. B. Jenson, & B. M. D. Stanton (Eds.), *Nelson textbook of pediatrics* (18th ed.). Philadelphia: Saunders Elsevier.

National Health Service. (2010). *Animal and human bites.* Retrieved December 17, 2011 from http://www.nhs.uk/Conditions/Bites-human-and-animal/Pages/Introduction.aspx

Pagana, K. D., & Pagana, T. J. (2010). *Mosby's manual of diagnostic and laboratory tests* (4th ed.). St. Louis, MO: Mosby.

Pardo, G. D., Garcia, I. M., & Gomez-Cia, T. (2010). Psychological effects observed in child burn patients during the acute phase of hospitalization and comparison with pediatric patients awaiting surgery. *Journal of Burn Care & Research, 31*(4), 569–578.

Quilty, J. (2010). *Pediatric burn management.* Paper presented at the meeting of the Florida Chapter of the National Association of Pediatric Nurse Practitioners, Orlando, FL.

Safe Kids Canada. (2010). *About injuries.* Retrieved December 17, 2011 from http://www.safekidscanada.ca/Professionals/Safety-Information/About-Injuries/Index.aspx

Senapati, S., Banerjee, S., & Gangopadhyay, D. N. (2008). Evening primrose oil is effective in atopic dermatitis: A randomized placebo-controlled trial. *Indian Journal of Dermatology, Venereology and Leprology, 74*(5), 447–452.

So, T., & Farrington, E. (2008). Community-acquired methicillin-resistant Staphylococcus aureus infection in the pediatric population. *Journal of Pediatric Health Care, 22*(4), 211–220.

Spinks, A., Wasiak, J., Cleland, H., Beben, N., & Macpherson, A. K. (2008). Ten-year epidemiological study of pediatric burns in Canada. *Journal of Burn Care & Research, 29*, 482–488.

Stinson, J., Yamada, J., Dickson, A., Laba, J., & Stevens, B. (2008). Review of systematic reviews on acute procedural pain in children in the hospital setting. *Pain Research and Management, 13*(1), 51–57.

Taketokmo, C. K., Hodding, J. H., & Kraus, D. M. (2010). *Lexi-comp's pediatric dosage handbook* (17th ed.). Hudson, OH: Lexi-comp.

U.S. Food and Drug Administration. (2010a). *Insect repellant use and safety in children.* Retrieved December 17, 2011 from http://www.fda.gov/Drugs/EmergencyPreparedness/ucm085277.htm

U.S. Food and Drug Administration. (2010b). *Isotretinoin (marketed as Accutane) capsule information.* Retrieved December 16, 2011 from http://www.fda.gov/Drugs/DrugSafety/PostmarketDrugSafetyInformationforPatientsandProviders/ucm094305.htm

Vernon, P., Brady, M. A., & Starr, N. B. (2009). Dermatologic diseases. In C. E. Burns, A. M. Dunn, M. A. Brady, N. B. Starr, & C. G. Blosser (Eds.), *Pediatric primary care* (4th ed.). St. Louis, MO: Saunders Elsevier.

Wong, L., & Rogers, M. (2006). Psoriasis: Varied presentations, individualized treatment. *Contemporary Pediatrics, 23*(1), 33–39.

RECOMMENDED READINGS

Chadha, A. (2009). Assessing the skin. *Practice Nurse, 23*(7), 43–48.

Giardino, A. P., & Giardino, E. R. (2011). *Physical child abuse clinical presentation.* Retrieved December 17, 2011 from http://emedicine.medscape.com/article/915664-overview

Public Health Agency of Canada. (2005). Injuries associated with non-fatal dog bites. Available on December 21, 2011 at http://www.phac-aspc.gc.ca/injury-bles/chirpp/pdf/CHIRPP_INJURY_BRIEF_DOG_BITE_update.pdf

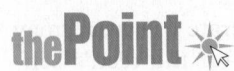

For additional learning materials, including Internet Resources, visit http://thePoint.lww.com/Chow1e.

CHAPTER WORKSHEET

MULTIPLE CHOICE QUESTIONS

1. The nurse is teaching about skin care for atopic dermatitis. Which statement by the parent indicates that further teaching may be necessary?

   a. "I will use Vaseline to moisturize my child's skin."

   b. "A hot bath will soothe my child's itching when it is severe."

   c. "I will buy cotton rather than wool or synthetic clothing for my child."

   d. "I will apply a small amount of the prescribed cream after the bath."

2. The nurse is caring for a child who has received significant partial-thickness burns to the lower body. What is the priority assessment in the first 24 hours after injury?

   a. Fluid balance

   b. Wound infection

   c. Respiratory arrest

   d. Separation anxiety

3. The nurse is caring for a child in the emergency department who was bitten by the family dog, which is fully immunized. What is the priority nursing action?

   a. Administer rabies immunoglobulin.

   b. Refer the child to a counsellor.

   c. Assess the depth and extent of the wound.

   d. Administer a tetanus booster.

4. The nurse is caring for an infant on the pediatric unit who has a very red rash in the diaper area, with red lesions scattered on the abdomen and thighs. What is the priority nursing intervention?

   a. Administer griseofulvin with a fatty meal.

   b. Institute contact isolation precautions.

   c. Apply topical antibiotic cream.

   d. Apply topical antifungal cream.

5. A varsity high-school wrestler presents with a "rug burn" type of rash on his shoulder that is not healing as expected, despite use of triple antibiotic cream. Two other wrestlers on his team have a similar abrasion. What infection should the nurse be most concerned about, based on the history?

   a. Tinea cruris

   b. MRSA

   c. Impetigo

   d. Tinea versicolo

CRITICAL THINKING EXERCISES

1. A 4-year-old presents in the hospital with his mother for evaluation of a yellowish, runny sore on his head. What types of conditions might this be? What questions would be most appropriate to ask the mother when taking the history? Should this child be placed in isolation? If so, why?

2. An 11-month-old comes to the primary care office with his mother for evaluation of a significant flaking red rash on both cheeks of her face. The child is diagnosed with atopic dermatitis. Where else should the health care provider look for rashes? What additional information should be obtained in the health history? What information should be included in the teaching plan for this family?

STUDY ACTIVITIES

1. Plan an educational activity:

   a. For parents of babies about the treatment and prevention of diaper dermatitis

   b. For parents of school-age children about prevention of contact dermatitis

2. During your clinical rotation, spend a day with the wound and ostomy care nurse in a children's hospital. Report to the clinical group about what you learned.

3. Talk to teenagers with severe acne, atopic dermatitis, or psoriasis about their feelings about their skin's appearance. Reflect on this information in your clinical journal.

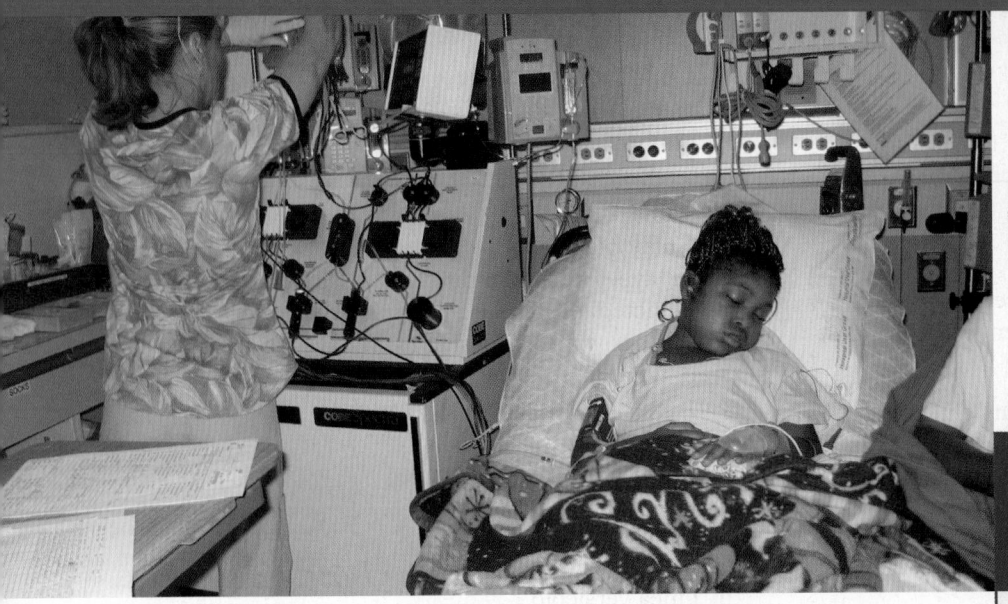

CHAPTER 46

Adapted by Mary E. Bauman, Wilma McClure, and Mary Anne Venner

NURSING CARE OF THE CHILD WITH A HEMATOLOGIC DISORDER

KEY TERMS

anemia	hematocrit	hypochromic	purpura
anisocytosis	hematopoiesis	macrocytic	red blood cell
anticoagulation	hemoglobin	microcytic	reticulocytes
antithrombin	hemoglobinopathy	neutropenia	splenomegaly
chelation therapy	hemophilia	petechiae	thrombocytopenia
coagulation	hemosiderosis	platelet	thromboembolism
erythropoietin	hemostasis	poikilocytosis	thrombosis
fibrinolytic system	hyperchromic	polycythemia	white blood cell

LEARNING OBJECTIVES

Upon completion of the chapter, the learner will be able to:

1. Identify major diseases of the hematology system that affect children.
2. Develop a basic understanding of developmental hemostasis, the coagulation cascade, and fibrinolytic system.
3. Determine priority assessment information for children with diseases of the hematology system.
4. Develop knowledge for assessment of thrombosis.
5. Identify priority interventions for children with diseases of the hematology system.
6. Analyze laboratory data in relation to normal findings and report abnormal findings.
7. Provide nursing diagnoses appropriate for the child and family with diseases of the hematology system.
8. Develop a teaching plan for the families of children with diseases of the hematology system.
9. Develop a teaching plan to facilitate knowledge transfer to the family of a child with thrombosis.
10. Identify resources for children and families with diseases of the hematology system, nutrition deficits, or thrombosis.

Shaun O'Malley, 10 months old, is being admitted to the pediatric unit after being brought to the clinic by his father for a small laceration that he thought needed stitches. His father states, "I didn't think the cut was very deep. I was surprised how long it bled."

WOW

BLOOD: the EAU de LIFE.

HEMATOLOGY SYSTEM OVERVIEW

The hematology system consists of the blood and blood-forming tissues of the body. These typically function together in a balance. Blood transports oxygen and nutrients to tissues and waste products from tissues.

Major Components in the Hematology System

Cellular Components

The three categories of cells in the hematology system are erythrocytes or **red blood cells** (RBCs); thrombocytes or **platelets**; and leukocytes or **white blood cells** (WBCs). **Hemoglobin** in RBCs is responsible for transporting oxygen to the body tissues. The thrombocytes are responsible for clotting. WBCs are the body's defense against infection or injury. WBCs are further divided into granulocytes (neutrophils, eosinophils, and basophils) and agranulocytes (lymphocytes and monocytes) (Kimball, 2011). Tables 46.1 and 46.2 give age-related values for the complete blood count (CBC) and leukocyte count, respectively (Fischbach, 2008). The specific types of WBCs are discussed in more detail in Chapter 47.

Platelets are necessary for clot formation. Platelets are larger when they are new; thus, an elevation in the mean platelet volume may indicate that most platelets are recently released from the bone marrow, with the older platelets consumed or destroyed more quickly than normal, for example in idiopathic (or immune) thrombocytopenic purpura (ITP). Decreases in platelet numbers (thrombocytopenia) may result in an increased risk for bleeding. Etiologies for thrombocytopenia include:

1. Platelet consumption when bleeding is present
2. Platelets coated with antibody and destroyed as in ITP
3. Hereditary disorders
4. Splenic sequestration as in hypersplenism
5. Sepsis
6. Heparin administration where heparin-induced thrombocytopenia (HIT) occurs

Plasma

Plasma is the non-cellular part of blood and contains **coagulation** factors, immunoglobulins, nutrients participating in cell metabolism, and waste products. Coagulation proteins are discussed in the Balance of Hemostasis and Thrombosis in Infants and Children sections. Table 46.3 provides normal values for coagulation factor levels in infants and children, and Table 46.4 outlines clotting studies.

Bone Marrow

The bone marrow is the site of RBC, granulocyte, and platelet production by a process called *hematopoiesis*. Mature RBCs last 120 days in the blood, platelets 10 to 14 days, and WBCs for varying lengths of time. The turnover of hematopoietic cells for a 70-kg person is estimated to be about one trillion per day (Israels, 2009).

Hematopoiesis

In the process of **hematopoiesis**, all blood cells originate from a single type of cell called a multipotent stem cell, which goes on to differentiate into the various types of blood cells (Fig. 46.1). The multipotent stem cell can give rise to either myeloid or lymphoid progenitor cells through the influence of thrombopoietin (TPO) and interleukin-7 (IL-7). Under the influence of a number of cytokines, such as IL-6, the lymphoid progenitors can differentiate into B cells, T cells, and natural killer (NK) cells. The common myeloid progenitor cell can differentiate into:

1. Megakaryocytes and platelets
2. Erythroid progenitors and RBCs
3. Myeloblasts that will further differentiate into basophils, eosinophils, monocytes, and neutrophils under the influence of specific cytokines

Cytokines are small signaling molecules that influence the differentiation of blood cells. Examples include TPO, which acts to promote platelet production; **erythropoietin** (EPO), which is produced by the kidneys and stimulates RBC production; and granulocyte colony-stimulating factor (G-CSF), which helps promote granulocyte production.

Multiple health diagnoses predispose patients to changes within the blood system. To help determine a diagnosis, it is important to assess whether hematologic changes are related to the *production* of blood cells (too much or too little) or to the *destruction* or loss of blood cells. Figure 46.2 shows examples of peripheral blood film findings.

Factors Affected by Pediatric Anatomy and Physiology in the Hematology System

The hematology system is intact and functional at birth. RBC and hemoglobin production as well as iron stores undergo changes in the first few months of life, after which time hematologic function is stable. Many factors are involved in the development of hematologic disorders, including genetic causes, injury, infection, and nutritional deficit.

TABLE 46.1 NORMAL HEMOGRAM VALUES

Age	WBC (×10⁹/L)	RBC (×10¹²/L)	Hemoglobin (g/L)	Hematocrit (%)	MCV (fL)	MCH (pg/cell)	MCHC (g/L)	Platelets (×10⁹/L)	RDW (%)	MPV (fL)
Birth–2 weeks	9.0–30.0	4.1–6.1	145–245	44–54	98–112	34–40	330–370	150–450	—	—
2–8 weeks	5.0–21.0	4.0–6.0	125–205	39–59	98–112	30–36	320–360	—	—	—
2–6 months	5.0–19.0	3.8–5.6	107–173	35–49	83–97	27–33	310–350	—	—	—
6 months–1 year	5.0–19.0	3.8–5.2	99–145	29–43	73–87	24–30	320–360	—	—	—
1–6 years	5.0–19.0	3.9–5.3	95–141	30–40	70–84	23–29	310–350	—	—	—
6–16 years	4.8–10.8	4.0–5.2	103–149	32–42	73–87	24–30	320–360	—	—	—
16–18 years	4.8–10.8	4.2–5.4	111–157	34–44	75–89	25–31	320–360	—	—	—
>18 years (males)	5.0–10.0	4.5–5.5	140–174	42–52	84–96	28–34	320–360	140–400	11.5–14.5	7.4–10.4
>18 years (females)	5.0–10.0	4.0–5.0	120–160	36–48	84–96	28–34	320–360	140–400	11.5–14.5	7.4–10.4

Note: Ranges used may differ slightly among Canadian laboratory sites.

Adapted from: Fischbach, F. T. (2008). *A manual of laboratory and diagnostic tests* (8th ed.). Philadelphia: Lippincott Williams & Wilkins.

TABLE 46.2 NORMAL WHITE BLOOD CELL (LEUKOCYTE) DIFFERENTIAL

Age	Bands (%)	Polymorphonuclear Segmented Neutrophils (%)	Eosinophils (%)	Basophils (%)	Lymphocytes (%)	Monocytes (%)
Birth–1 week	10–18	32–62	0–2	0–1	26–36	0–6
1–2 weeks	8–16	19–49	0–4	0	38–46	0–9
2–4 weeks	7–15	14–34	0–3	0	43–53	0–9
4–8 weeks	7–13	15–35	0–3	0–1	41–71	0–7
2–6 months	5–11	15–35	0–3	0–1	42–72	0–6
6 months–1 year	6–12	13–33	0–3	0	46–76	0–5
1–6 years	5–11	13–33	0–3	0	46–76	0–5
6–16 years	5–11	32–54	0–3	0–1	27–57	0–5
16–18 years	5–11	34–64	0–3	0–1	25–45	0–5
>18 years	3–6	50–62	0–3	0–1	25–40	3–7

Data from: Fischbach, F. T. (2008). *A manual of laboratory and diagnostic tests* (8th ed.). Philadelphia: Lippincott Williams & Wilkins.

TABLE 46.3 NORMAL RANGE OF COAGULATION FACTOR LEVELS FOR INFANTS/CHILDREN

Protein	Synonym	Concentration in Plasma	Function
Fibrinogen	Factor I	1.50–3.60 g/L	Converted to fibrin, which along (with platelets) forms a clot
Factor II	Prothrombin	0.51–1.23 UmL^{-1}	Is converted to thrombin (IIa), splits fibrinogen into fibrin
Factor V	Labile factor	0.58–1.46 UmL^{-1}	Supports factor Xa activation of factor II to IIa
Factor VII	Stable factor	0.47–1.51 UmL^{-1}	Activates factor X
Factor VIII:C	Antihemophilic factor	0.50–1.87 UmL^{-1}	Supports factor IXa activation of factor X
Factor IX	Christmas factor	0.50–1.20 UmL^{-1}	Activates factor X
Factor X	Stewart-Prower factor	0.35–1.19 UmL^{-1}	Activates factor II
Factor XI	Anti-hemophilic factor C	0.46–1.10 UmL^{-1}	Activates factor XII and prekallikrein
Factor XII	Hageman factor	0.22–1.42 UmL^{-1}	Activates factor XI and prekallikrein
Factor XIII	Fibrin-stabilizing factor	0.65–1.61 UmL^{-1}	Cross-links fibrin and other proteins
von Willebrand factor	Factor VIII–related antigen (VIII:vWD)	0.54–1.58 UmL^{-1}	Stabilizes factor VIII, mediates platelet adhesion
Ristocetin cofactor		0.56–1.78 UmL^{-1}	Induces platelet aggregation

UmL^{-1} is units per millilitre.
Adapted from: Andrew, M. (1991). An approach to the management of infants with impaired hemostasis. *Balliere's Clinical Hematology, 4*(2).

RBC Production

The production of blood cells in the embryo begins by 8 weeks' gestation. In the embryo, blood cells primarily form in the liver; this continues until a few weeks before delivery. After birth, the bone marrow of the long and flat bones is the predominant site of RBC production. EPO, the hormone that regulates RBC production, is derived primarily from the liver in the fetus; after birth, the kidneys take over this production (Irwin & Kirchner, 2001).

Hemoglobin

Hemoglobin is a protein that transports oxygen to tissues. Hemoglobin is composed of two alpha globin chains and two beta globin chains with an iron-containing heme molecule that binds oxygen. The predominant type of hemoglobin in RBCs varies developmentally. In the neonatal period, fetal hemoglobin (Hb F) is most plentiful. After 6 months of age, hemoglobin production is mostly Hb A. There are additional minor hemoglobins as well, such as Hb A2.

Iron

The fetus receives iron through the placenta from the mother. The preterm infant is at risk for iron-deficiency anemia as a result of reduced transplacental iron transfer due to the shortened gestational time (Cunningham et al., 2010). In the term infant, a period of physiologic anemia occurs between 2 and 6 months of age. The infant demonstrates rapid growth and an increase in blood volume over the first several months of life, resulting in the depletion of maternally derived iron stores by 4 to 6 months of age. Sufficient iron intake is critical for the appropriate development of hemoglobin and RBCs; therefore, it is important that the infant ingests adequate quantities of iron in early infancy from either breast milk or iron-fortified formula and in later infancy from other food sources (Bryant, 2010). Adolescence is also a time of rapid growth during which iron intake must increase.

Therapeutic Strategies

Various medications as well as other therapies are used to treat hematologic disorders in children. Most of these treatments require a physician's order when the child is

TABLE 46.4 CLOTTING STUDIES

Test	Measure
Prothrombin time (PT) international normalized ratio (INR)	0.9–1.3 seconds (may vary by laboratory); reported as an INR to minimize inter-laboratory variation
Partial thromboplastin time (PTT)	21–35 seconds (may vary by laboratory)

Adapted from: Fischbach, F. T. (2008). *A manual of laboratory and diagnostic tests* (8th ed.). Philadelphia: Lippincott Williams & Wilkins.

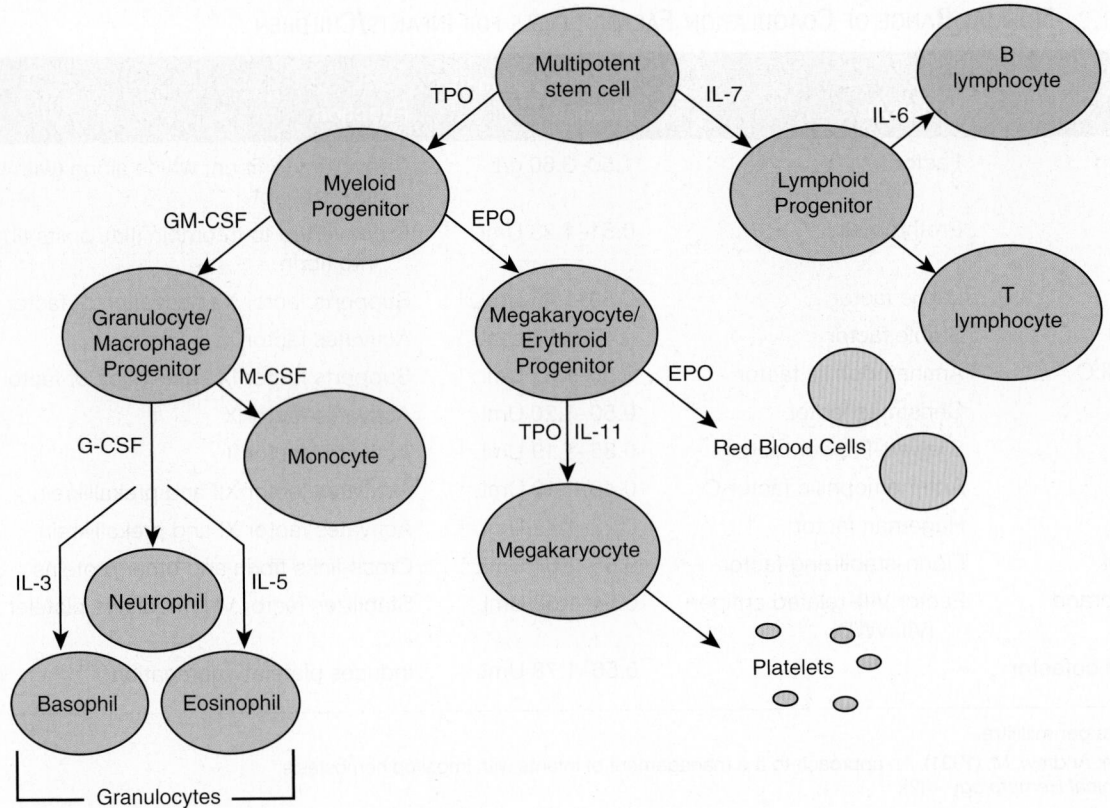

FIGURE 46.1 Process of blood cell formation.

in the hospital. Common therapeutic strategies include medication, oxygen, splenectomy, or transfusion of blood products, such as RBCs or clotting factors that may be missing from the coagulation pathway. Less common treatments include bone marrow and stem cell transplantation. Bone marrow transplantation is the transfer of healthy bone marrow, including multipotent stem cells, into a child with disease. Stem cells may be derived from bone marrow, from peripheral blood collected via apheresis, or from umbilical cord blood. Stem cell transplantation is more commonly used and may be indicated for the management of sickle cell disease, aplastic anemia, and thalassemia.

Nursing responsibilities include maintenance of medical asepsis and protective isolation to prevent infection. Monitor closely for graft-versus-host disease (GVHD). Provide meticulous oral care. Avoid taking rectal temperatures and inserting suppositories, and encourage appropriate nutrition. Administer immunosuppressive medications as ordered.

NURSING PROCESS OVERVIEW FOR THE CHILD WITH A DISEASE OF THE HEMATOLOGY SYSTEM

A number of general concepts related to the nursing process may be applied to hematologic dysfunction in

children. One of these is Bronfenbrenner's (1979) systems theory, in which the following systems are considered in service delivery and program planning: the microsystem (i.e., the child in the family), the mesosystem (i.e., family, school, and community relations), the exosystem (i.e., policy and program planning), and the macrosystem (i.e., broader societal and cultural influences). Another is the McGill Nursing Model, developed in the 1970s by Dr. Moyra Allen from McGill University (Loiselle, Profetto-McGrath, Polit, et al., 2010). This model describes a system of nursing in which health care providers work collaboratively and in partnership with the child, family, and other health professionals to develop and support an interrelated community network (Loiselle et al., 2010).

Care of the child with a disease of the hematology system includes assessment, nursing diagnosis, planning, interventions, and evaluation. Development of a plan of care will depend upon which component of the blood is affected. A child who has a **hemoglobinopathy** (disease affecting hemoglobin) requires adequate oxygenation and may require packed RBCs (pRBCs). A child with **hemophilia** requires clotting factor replacement and monitoring for safety. A decrease in hemoglobin will necessitate evaluation of oxygen-carrying capacity and the effects of hypoxia on the tissues. A reduction in platelet production will lead the nurse to

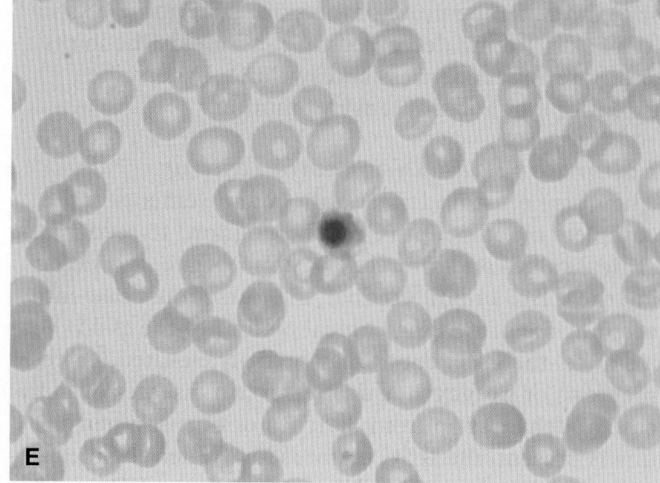

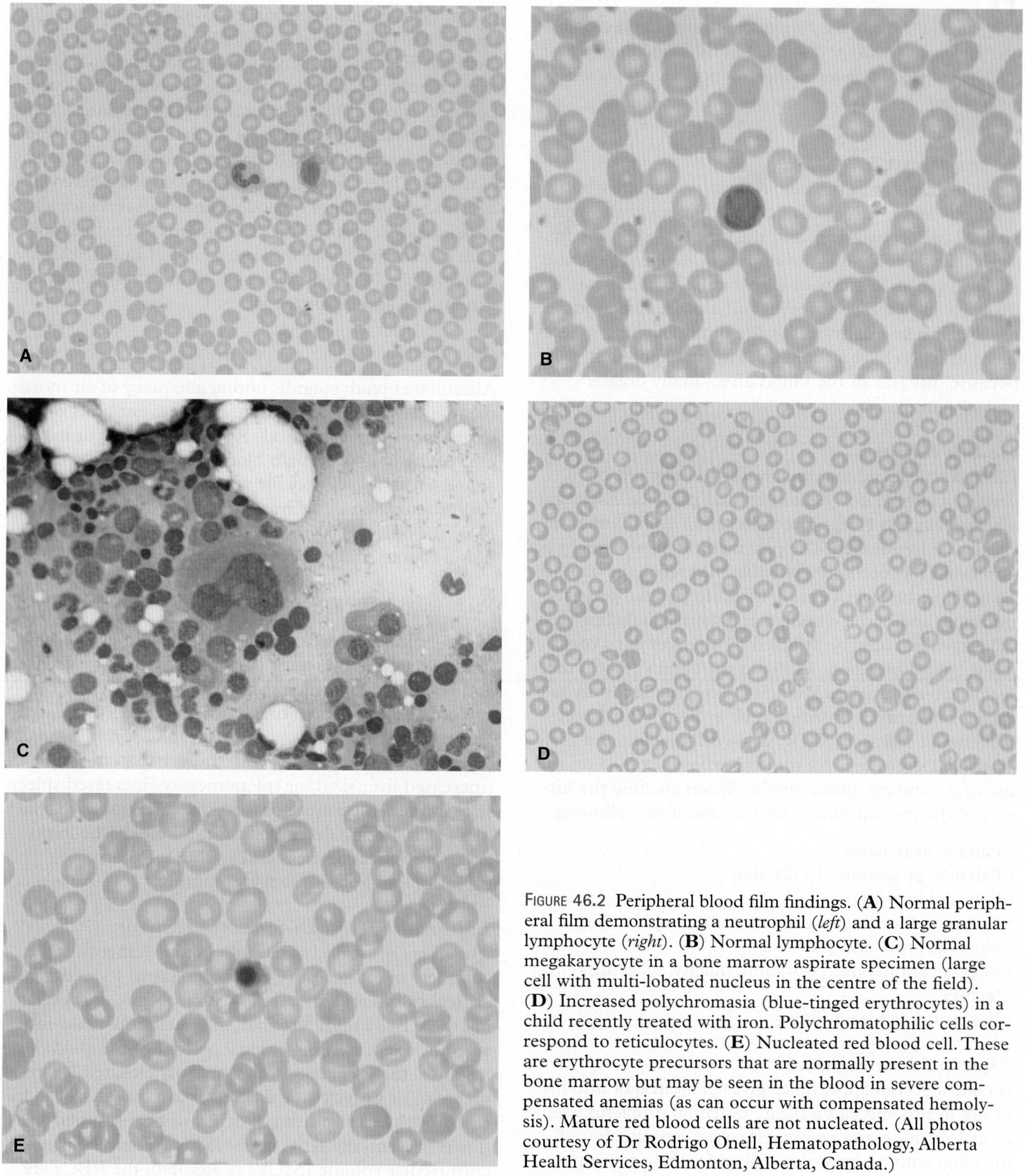

FIGURE 46.2 Peripheral blood film findings. (**A**) Normal peripheral film demonstrating a neutrophil (*left*) and a large granular lymphocyte (*right*). (**B**) Normal lymphocyte. (**C**) Normal megakaryocyte in a bone marrow aspirate specimen (large cell with multi-lobated nucleus in the centre of the field). (**D**) Increased polychromasia (blue-tinged erythrocytes) in a child recently treated with iron. Polychromatophilic cells correspond to reticulocytes. (**E**) Nucleated red blood cell. These are erythrocyte precursors that are normally present in the bone marrow but may be seen in the blood in severe compensated anemias (as can occur with compensated hemolysis). Mature red blood cells are not nucleated. (All photos courtesy of Dr Rodrigo Onell, Hematopathology, Alberta Health Services, Edmonton, Alberta, Canada.)

evaluate for prolonged bleeding, hemorrhage, and shock. An elevation in WBCs would require an evaluation for infection or leukemia.

Nursing care for the child with a disease of the hematology system is often multifaceted, requiring the nurse to have a thorough understanding of the patho-

physiology of hematologic diseases. The nurse caring for the child with a hematologic disorder should be familiar with the variety of procedures and medication used in treatment, including the action of each medication as well as the nursing implications related to their implementation.

Remember Shaun, the 10-month-old with the laceration and prolonged bleeding? What additional health history and physical examination assessment information should you obtain?

Assessment

Signs of changes in the hematology system are often insidious and overlooked. Colour changes in the skin, such as pallor, bruising, and flushing are often the first signs that a problem is developing. Changes in mental status, such as lethargy or tachycardia, can indicate a decrease in hemoglobin level and a decreased amount of oxygen being delivered to the brain. Nursing assessment must include a thorough systems approach because diseases of the blood affect many organs and systems.

Health History

Elicit the birth and maternal history, noting low birth weight, maternal iron deficiency, and jaundice. Ascertain whether vitamin K was given after birth and whether the child was circumcised. The past medical history might be significant for recent illnesses that may affect the blood. Determine the child's energy level, sleep–wake patterns, nutrition, and bowel elimination patterns, including stool colour, which may be affected by changes in oxygen delivery and bleeding. Evaluate the child's typical diet for possible nutritional deficits. Explore the family history for inherited disorders such as hemophilia, von Willebrand disease (vWD), sickle cell disease, and thalassemia. Determine risk for lead exposure based on the use of a standard questionnaire. When eliciting the history of the present illness, inquire about the following:

- Fatigue or malaise
- Paleness or jaundice of the skin
- Unusual bruising
- Excessive bleeding or difficulty stopping bleeding, blood in urine and stool
- Pain: location, onset, duration, quality, relieving factors
- Fever and/or recent illness

Physical Examination

A child's overall appearance gives great insight into his or her health and can indicate potential problems such as malnutrition and anemia. Physical examination of the child with a hematologic disorder includes inspection and observation, palpation, and auscultation.

Inspection and Observation

Note the child's appearance, including thin or emaciated appearance or obesity, as well as colour. Measure weight and height (or length) and plot on standardized growth charts. Observe the face, nail beds, palms, and soles for pallor. Note conjunctival pallor as well as colour and moisture of oral mucosa. Observe for skin and scleral jaundice. Evaluate the fingertips for clubbing (may occur with chronic decreases in oxygen). Document the location and extent of bruises, **petechiae**, or purpura. Count respiratory rate and observe for work of breathing. Obtain a pulse oximeter reading to determine oxygen saturation of tissues. Determine urinary output (may be altered with decreases in circulatory blood volume). Observe for signs of pain. Assess whether the child guards or favours any limb or extremity (may indicate a joint or muscle bleed). Note the child's responsiveness to stimuli, movement of extremities, and quality of gait.

Auscultation

Auscultate breath sounds, noting adequacy of air movement and depth of respiration. Note adventitious sounds or absence of breath sounds (which would occur in an area of the lung filled with blood). Auscultate heart sounds, listening closely for murmurs, which occur with severe anemia. Tachycardia is also a sign of anemia. Note the rate and rhythm of the heart tones. Auscultate bowel sounds, noting presence and normalcy.

Percussion and Palpation

Measure blood pressure (may change with alterations in blood volume). Palpate peripheral pulses for strength and equality. Determine capillary refill time (may be prolonged when circulating blood volume is decreased). Palpate for lymphadenopathy. Carefully percuss and palpate the abdomen for tenderness, hepatomegaly (increased liver size), or splenomegaly (increased spleen size). Note temperature of the skin. Determine elasticity of skin, noting decreased turgor. Palpate the joints and note any tenderness and swelling. Determine extent of limitation of range of motion.

Laboratory and Diagnostic Testing

The nurse must understand the main elements of the complete blood count (CBC; hemogram) to recognize critical values and intervene as appropriate. In evaluating the CBC and differential, the nurse must take into account the presenting clinical picture of the child. For instance, the RBC count may be truly elevated (erythrocytosis or **polycythemia**) in certain diseases or in the case of dehydration from diarrhea or burns. When anemia is present, the RBC count is low. When the mean corpuscular volume (MCV) is elevated, the RBCs are larger than normal (**macrocytic**). When the MCV is decreased, the RBCs are smaller than normal (**microcytic**). A decrease in the mean corpuscular hemoglobin concentration (MCHC) means that the hemoglobin is diluted in the cell and less of the red colour is present (**hypochromic**). When the hemoglobin concentration is increased in the RBC, the pigmentation (red colour) is increased (**hyperchromic**). A peripheral smear may show **anisocytosis,** defined as variations in RBC size, and **poikilocytosis,** defined as variations in RBC shape.

The components of the CBC are further defined as follows:

- RBC count: the actual number of counted RBCs in a certain volume of blood
- Hemoglobin: measure of the protein made up of heme (iron surrounded by protoporphyrin) and the alpha- and beta-polypeptide globin chains. Hemoglobin is primarily responsible for the transport of oxygen to the tissues.
- **Hematocrit**: the volume of RBCs as a fraction of blood volume
- RBC indices:
  - MCV: average size of the RBC
  - Mean corpuscular hemoglobin (MCH): a calculated value of the amount of hemoglobin per RBC
  - MCHC: a calculated value that reflects the concentration of hemoglobin inside the RBC
  - RBC distribution width (RDW): a calculated value that is a measure of the variation in size of the RBCs, including the **reticulocytes,** which are immature RBCs
- WBC count: actual count of the number of WBCs in a certain volume of blood
- Platelet count: number of platelets in a certain volume of blood
- Mean platelet volume (MPV): a measurement of the size of the platelets

See Tables 46.1 and 46.2.

Common Laboratory and Diagnostic Tests 46.1 explains the most commonly used laboratory and diagnostic tests when considering hematologic disorders. The tests can assist the physician in diagnosing the disorder and/or be used as guidelines in determining ongoing treatment. The nurse should be familiar with how the tests are obtained, what they are used for, and normal versus abnormal results. This knowledge will also be necessary when providing patient and family education related to the testing.

Nursing Diagnoses, Goals, Interventions, and Evaluation

Upon completion of a thorough assessment for hematologic problems, the nurse might identify several nursing diagnoses, including:

- Fatigue related to decreased oxygen supply to the body
- Increased risk of infection due to leukopenia, **neutropenia**, hyposplenism, or immunodeficiency
- Pain related to vaso-occlusive event, organomegaly, or infection or bleeding into tissues
- Impaired physical mobility related to imposed physical activity restrictions or pain from sickle cell crisis, thrombosis, or acute bleeds
- Ineffective health maintenance related to knowledge and skill acquisition regarding nutritional and medical treatment of anemia, prevention of infection, coping with pain, home administration of intravenous clotting factors, home infusion of subcutaneous deferoxamine,

(text continues on page 1587)

COMMON LABORATORY AND DIAGNOSTIC TESTS 46.1

Test	Explanation	Indication	Nursing Implications
Blood type and screen	Determines ABO blood type as well as presence of antigens. Cross-match is performed on RBC-containing products to avoid transfusion reaction.	Trauma victim or any person in whom blood loss is suspected, in preparation for transfusion	Avoid hemolysis of specimen. Appropriately sign and date specimen. Apply "type and cross" or "blood band" to child at the time of blood draw if indicated by the institution. Most type and cross-match specimens expire after 48 to 72 h.
Clotting studies	PT/INR activated partial thromboplastin time (aPTT)	Evaluation of common pathway in clotting mechanism. PT/INR: evaluation of extrinsic system. PTT, aPTT: evaluation of intrinsic system.	Apply pressure to venipuncture site. Assess for bleeding (gums, bruising, blood in urine or stool).

(continued)

COMMON LABORATORY AND DIAGNOSTIC TESTS 46.1 (continued)

Test	Explanation	Indication	Nursing Implications
Coagulation factor concentration	Measures concentration of specific coagulating factors in the blood	Hemophilia, DIC	Apply pressure to venipuncture site. Assess for bleeding (gums, bruising, blood in urine or stool). Deliver specimen to laboratory as soon as possible (unstable at room temperature).
Complete blood count (CBC) with differential	Evaluates hemoglobin and hematocrit, WBC count (particularly the percentage of individual WBCs), and platelet count, as well as RBC indices	Anemia, infection, bleeding disorder, clotting disorder	Normal values vary according to age and gender. WBC differential is helpful in evaluating source of infection. May be affected by certain medications.
Hemoglobin electrophoresis	Measures percentage of normal and abnormal hemoglobin in the blood	Sickle cell anemia, thalassemia	Blood transfusions within the previous 12 weeks may alter test results.
Serum iron, iron saturation index, total iron binding capacity (TIBC)	Evaluates iron metabolism	Iron-deficiency anemia, hemosiderosis with chronic transfusion or hemoglobinopathies	Recent blood transfusions increase level. Avoid hemolysis (will falsely elevate result).
Lead	Measures level of lead in blood	Lead poisoning	Normal amount in blood is zero.
Reticulocyte count	Measures the amount of reticulocytes (immature RBCs) in the blood	Indicates bone marrow's ability to respond to anemia with production of RBCs	Rises quickly in response to iron supplementation in the iron-deficient child
Serum ferritin	Measures the level of ferritin (the major iron storage protein) in the blood	A sensitive screening test for determining iron-deficiency anemia, but result may be "normal" if patient has infection or other illness even when the child is iron deficient	Elevated in hemolytic disease and if transfused recently. Iron supplementation increases ferritin levels.
Transcranial Doppler ultrasound (TCD)	Measures the velocity of the blood through the main arterial vessels in the brain. Criteria have been developed to determine stroke risk.	Helps to predict which children with sickle cell disease may be most at risk for stroke. Approximately 10% of children with sickle cell disease will develop a stroke.	Children with sickle cell disease must have this test done at least yearly to assess for stroke risk, which is increased in sickle cell disease. If criteria are met, treatment such as blood transfusions can then be started in hopes of stroke prevention.
Bone marrow aspiration and trephine biopsy	Removes liquid bone marrow and soft, spongy marrow tissue from inside the iliac crest to assess for benign or malignant conditions	Procedure is performed when pathology of the blood cells and state of functioning of the bone marrow are required for diagnosis.	Performed under anesthesia in children. Help educate the family. Assess for pain control and watch for bleeding postprocedure.

Nursing Care Plan 46.1

OVERVIEW FOR THE CHILD WITH A HEMATOLOGIC DISORDER

NURSING DIAGNOSIS: Fatigue related to decreased oxygen supply in the body as evidenced by lack of energy, increased sleep requirements, or decreased interest in play activities

Outcome Identification and Evaluation
Child will display increased endurance, *desire to play without developing symptoms of exertion.*

Intervention: Decreasing Fatigue
- Cluster nursing care activities and plan for periods of rest before and after activities requiring exertion *to decrease oxygen need and consumption.*
- Encourage activity or ambulation per physician's orders; *early mobilization results in better outcomes.*
- Observe child for symptoms of activity intolerance such as pallor, nausea, lightheadedness, dizziness, or changes in vital signs *to determine level of tolerance.*
- If child is on bed rest, perform range-of-motion (ROM) exercises and frequent position changes as tolerated by the child. *Negative changes of the musculoskeletal system occur quickly with inactivity and immobility.*
- Refer the child to physical therapy *for exercise prescription to increase skeletal muscle strength.*

NURSING DIAGNOSIS: Impaired physical mobility related to pain from sickle cell crisis, acute bleeds, thrombosis, or imposed activity restrictions as evidenced by guarding of painful extremity, resistance to activity

Outcome Identification and Evaluation
Child will be able to engage in activities within age parameters and limits of disease: *child is able to move extremities, move about environment, and participate in exercise programs within limits of age and disease.*

Intervention: Promoting Physical Mobility
- Clinical evidence may be limited, so ask the child about his or her pain to assess pain level. The "#1 assessment tool is the child's report about his or her pain" (APHON, 2007). Ensure that all therapeutic modalities, both pharmacologic and other supports, are provided *to provide pain control.*
- Encourage gross and fine motor activities as able within constraints of pain/bleed, the child's disease, and according to physician orders *to facilitate motor development.*
- Collaborate with physical therapy to strengthen muscles and promote optimal mobility *to facilitate motor development.*
- Use passive and active ROM exercises and teach the child and family how to perform them: *these exercises prevent contractures and facilitate joint mobility and muscle development (active ROM) to help increase mobility.*
- Involve child life services as appropriate *to encourage coping strategies, involve play, or develop distraction techniques that help achieve goals involving mobility.*
- Praise accomplishments and emphasize child's abilities *to improve self-esteem and encourage feelings of confidence and competence.*

NURSING DIAGNOSIS: Anxiety related to diagnostic testing as evidenced by parent verbalization, child resistance or crying with procedures

Outcome Identification and Evaluation
Child's anxiety will be minimized; *child will verbalize less fear, experience less pain with procedures.*

Intervention: Relieving Anxiety
- Develop educational and learning processes with the child and family about the clinical condition, diagnostics, and ongoing family coping strategies *to help alleviate anxiety related to the unknown.*
- Utilize pain management strategies for the child who must undergo painful therapies and procedures *to reduce trauma and help them develop coping skills.*
- Provide ongoing child and family education, support, and opportunity for consistent evaluation *to encourage mutual learning and best possible health outcomes.*

(continued)

Nursing Care Plan 46.1 (continued)

- Involve child life services where appropriate *to encourage use of play or other strategies that facilitate the child's understanding of a procedure, test, or clinical situation.*
- Provide developmentally appropriate activities and education for the child. *(Activities can reduce stress and also provide stimulus for children; the use of safe and developmentally appropriate activity can serve as role modelling for the family.)*

NURSING DIAGNOSIS: Ineffective family coping related to hospitalization of child or chronic, possibly life-threatening genetic disorder as evidenced by excessive tearfulness or denial statements, withdrawal, or verbalization of inadequate coping skills

Outcome Identification and Evaluation

Child and/or family will demonstrate adequate coping skills, *will verbalize feeling supported and demonstrate healthy family interactions.*

Intervention: Promoting Effective Family Coping

- Facilitate open communication, active listening, emotional support, and validation for the child and family *to improve coping abilities.*
- Refer families to community resources such as parent support groups and grief counselling *(involvement with emotional and instrumental support improves coping abilities).*
- Encourage role-playing and play activities *to identify the child's fears and provide a method for working through feelings.*
- Assess health-related quality of life in children with long-term conditions *to reveal confounders to therapy.* Once confounders to therapy are identified, partner with the child and family *to determine the best management plan.*

NURSING DIAGNOSIS: Risk for injury related to alteration in peripheral sensory perception, decreased platelet count, deficient coagulation factor, excessive iron load, or presence of intravascular or subcutaneous devices

Outcome Identification and Evaluation

Child will not experience hemorrhage, infection, or thrombosis. Child *will experience decreased bruising or episodes of prolonged bleeding or signs of infection.*

Intervention: Preventing Injury

- Assess and immediately report signs and symptoms of pain, petechiae, purpura, bruising, bleeding, anemia, neutropenia, and infection *(provides baseline data for comparison; if present, may warrant intervention).*
- Teach the child to report symptoms promptly to family, teacher, or caregiver *to enable prompt action to alleviate symptoms.*
- Monitor the care of intravenous access devices and subcutaneous injection devices and sites. Educate nursing staff as well as child and parents about them *to minimize risks of infection and thrombosis.*
- Avoid rectal temperatures and examinations *to avoid rectal mucosa damage resulting in bleeding.*
- Educate health care providers regarding safe administration of intramuscular injections *to decrease the risk of bleeding from a puncture site.*
- If bone marrow aspiration or lumbar puncture is performed, apply pressure dressing to site *to prevent bleeding.*
- Teach families about preferred physical activities for the child with a bleeding disorder or other pertinent hematologic disease *to provide safe physical activity, decrease the risk for injury, and promote ongoing healthy development.*

NURSING DIAGNOSIS: Ineffective health maintenance related to inadequate knowledge and skill acquisition of parents and child regarding the child's hematologic condition and therapies, and the family's coping strategies and ability to maintain its supportive roles

Outcome Identification and Evaluation

Child's health and growth and development will be maintained; *child will receive supplements, medication, and blood products as prescribed and will follow an appropriate diet.*

Nursing Care Plan 46.1 (continued)

Intervention: Educating Parents, Caregivers, and Child About Effective Health Maintenance

- Provide a culturally sensitive learning environment, including resources in the appropriate language, *to encourage understanding and respect.*
- Provide education regarding nutritional and medical treatment of anemia, appropriate diet, prevention of infection, home monitoring of medication, home administration of intravenous clotting factors or subcutaneous medication, and protection from injury *to facilitate learning regarding the clinical plan and its maintenance for best health outcomes.*
- Provide ongoing monitoring of growth and development according to child's condition *to assess healthy development.*
- Provide ongoing evaluation of nutritional intake *to ensure that appropriate dietary planning, management, or restriction is followed.*
- Ensure that the child and parents can verbalize understanding of the prescribed therapy and monitoring *to evaluate understanding.*
- Provide family teaching and educational resources and have parents/child provide return demonstration of treatment administration *to determine whether teaching goals have been met.*
- Educate families, teachers, and other caregivers about when to call or visit a medical provider *to ensure timely intervention when signs and symptoms of the child's condition develop.*
- Transition the teen and family to the adult care environment using educational resources and support *to enable the continuum of care.*

---

home monitoring of medication, and protection from injury
- Anxiety related to diagnostic testing
- Ineffective family coping related to hospitalization of child or a genetic disorder that may be life-threatening

After completing an assessment of Shaun, you note the following: the history revealed he bled when all four of his teeth erupted. Upon examination numerous bruises are noted. Based on the assessment findings, what would your top three nursing diagnoses be for Shaun?

Nursing goals, interventions, and evaluation for the child with hematologic dysfunction are based on the nursing diagnoses. Nursing Care Plan 46.1 may be used as a guide in planning nursing care for the child with a hematologic disorder. Children's responses to hematologic disorders and their treatments will vary; therefore, nursing care should be individualized based on the child's and family's responses to illness. Other conditions may contribute to the nursing diagnoses and must also be considered when prioritizing care. Additional information about nursing management will be included later in the chapter as it relates to specific disorders.

Based on your top three nursing diagnoses for Shaun, describe appropriate nursing interventions.

BENIGN DISEASES OF THE HEMATOLOGY SYSTEM

Anemia Overview

Anemia is a condition in which levels of RBCs and hemoglobin are lower than normal. Hemoglobin levels vary throughout childhood and should be monitored to ensure that adequate growth and development will be achieved. There are many types of anemia, some of which are described in this chapter. Anemia in childhood may also result from chronic disease processes. Anemia may develop as a result of three distinct disease processes: decreased production of RBCs, loss of RBCs, and destruction of RBCs.

Decreased production can be related to lack of dietary intake of the nutrients needed to produce the cells, alterations in the cell structure, infection, or malfunctioning tissues, such as the bone marrow. Causes of anemia related to nutritional deficiency include anemia of chronic disease iron-deficiency anemia, folic acid deficiency anemia, and pernicious anemia (inability to absorb sufficient vitamin B12). Iron-deficiency anemia is the most common type of anemia in children. Nutrient intake may be reduced in children due to food dislikes or conditions that produce malabsorption. Anemia may also result from toxin exposure (lead poisoning) or an adverse reaction to a medication (aplastic anemia).

Destruction of RBCs occurs in certain genetic and cellular development disorders (Bryant, 2010) and also can occur during the infectious process. Some anemias caused by the alteration or destruction of RBCs are categorized as *hemolytic anemia*. Sickle cell disease and thalassemia are types of hemolytic anemias. These two diseases are discussed in the Hemoglobinopathies section.

Loss of RBCs may occur when blood loss results from surgery, trauma, or other causes of bleeding.

Anemias Resulting from Nutritional Causes, Lead Poisoning, and Chronic Disease

Anemia from Nutritional Causes: Iron–Deficiency Anemia

Pathophysiology

Iron-deficiency anemia occurs when the body does not have sufficient iron to produce hemoglobin. The highest prevalence of iron deficiency (4% to 8%) occurs in children between 1 and 3 years of age (Maguire, deVeber, & Parkin, 2007). The prevalence of iron-deficiency anemia in Canadian children is between 3.5% and 10.5% in the general population, but the prevalence is much higher among Aboriginal children in the Canadian North (Christofides, Schauer, & Zlotkin, 2005). Iron-deficiency anemia may be a significant risk factor for stroke in young children (Hartfield, Lowry, Keene, et al., 1997; Maguire et al., 2007; Yager & Hartfield, 2002). One of the factors that contributes to iron-deficiency anemia in older infants is overconsumption of cow's milk.

Babies 12 months or older should drink no more than 16 to 24 oz (500 to 750 mL) of cow's milk per day (Ontario Society of Nutrition Professionals in Public Health, 2008). In one study, infants between the ages of 9 and 12 months who drank more than 18 oz of cow's milk per day had reduced hemoglobin levels (Zetterstrom, 2004).

The heme portion of hemoglobin consists of iron surrounded by protoporphyrin. When insufficient iron is available to the bone marrow, hemoglobin production is reduced. Adequate dietary intake of iron is required for the body to make enough hemoglobin. As hemoglobin levels decrease, the oxygen-carrying capacity of the blood is decreased, resulting in weakness and fatigue. Severe iron-deficiency anemia in children has been associated with diminished cognitive function, changes in behaviour, delayed growth and development in infants, increased fatigability, and less engagement (Lozoff, DeAndraca, Castillo, et al., 2003).

Therapeutic Management

Iron supplements are usually provided in the form of ferrous sulfate or ferrous fumarate. Dosage is based on the amount of elemental iron required. The recommended amounts of elemental iron are:

- Prophylaxis: 1 to 2 mg/kg/day (maximum, 15 mg/day)
- Mild to moderate iron deficiency: 3 mg/kg/day in one or two divided doses

- Severe iron deficiency: 4 to 6 mg/kg/day in three divided doses (Borgna-Pignatti & Marsella, 2008)

In more severe cases, pRBC transfusions may be indicated. pRBC transfusion is reserved for the most severe cases (Bryant, 2010), and risk of cardiac overload must be assessed. When pRBC administration is warranted, follow specific blood bank guidelines for administration. Monitor subsequent laboratory results for improvement.

Nursing Assessment

See the Nursing Process Overview section for a full description of the assessment phase of the nursing process for a child with a hematologic disorder. Assessment findings pertinent to iron-deficiency anemia are discussed below.

Health History

Elicit a description of the current illness and chief complaint. Common signs and symptoms reported during the health history may include irritability, headache, dizziness, weakness, shortness of breath, pallor, and fatigue. Other symptoms may be subtle and difficult for the clinician to identify. These include difficulty feeding, pica (inappropriate consumption of substances such as paper, dirt, ice, salt, etc.), muscle weakness, unsteady gait, and cognitive difficulties.

Explore the health history for risk factors such as:

- Maternal anemia during pregnancy
- Prematurity, low birth weight, or multiple birth
- Cow's milk consumption before 12 months of age
- Excessive cow's milk consumption (more than 24 oz/day)
- Infant consumption of low-iron formula
- Lack of iron supplementation after age 6 months in breastfed infants
- Excessive weight gain
- Chronic infection or inflammation
- Chronic or acute blood loss
- Restricted diets
- Use of medication interfering with iron absorption, such as antacids
- Low socioeconomic status
- Recent immigration from a developing country (Borgna-Pignatti & Marsella, 2008; Bryant, 2010)

Evaluate the child's diet to identify adequate intake of iron-rich foods. Table 46.5 provides daily dietary iron intake recommendations for children.

Physical Examination

Observe the child for fatigue and lethargy. Inspect the skin, conjunctivae, oral mucosa, palms, and soles for pallor. Assess for spooning of the nails (concave shape). Obtain a pulse oximeter reading. Evaluate the heart rate for tachycardia. Auscultate the heart for the presence of a flow murmur. Palpate the abdomen for splenomegaly.

TABLE 46.5 RECOMMENDED DAILY DIETARY IRON INTAKE FOR CHILDREN

Age	Amount of Iron per Day (Recommended Daily Allowance)
7–12 months	11 mg
1–3 years	7 mg
4–8 years	10 mg
9–13 years	8 mg
14–18 years	11 mg (boys) 15 mg (girls)

Adapted from: Health Canada. (2005). *Dietary reference intakes: Reference values for elements.* Retrieved August 25, 2011 from http://www.hc-sc.gc.ca/fn-an/nutrition/reference/table/ref_elements_tbl-eng.php

Laboratory and Diagnostic Tests

Laboratory evaluation will reveal decreased hemoglobin and hematocrit levels, decreased reticulocyte count, microcytosis and hypochromia, decreased ferritin and serum iron levels, decreased iron saturation index, and increased total iron binding capacity.

Nursing Management

Nursing management of the child with iron deficiency focuses on promoting safety, ensuring adequate iron intake, and educating the family.

Promoting Safety

The child with anemia is at risk for changes in neurologic functioning related to the decreased oxygen supply to the brain. This can lead to fatigue and an inability to eat enough. Neurologic effects may be manifested when the child's ability to sit, stand, or walk is impaired. Provide close observation of the anemic child. Assist the older child with ambulation. Educate the parents on how to protect the child from injury due to an unsteady gait or dizziness.

Providing Dietary Interventions

Ensure that infants with iron deficiency are fed only formulas fortified with iron. Interventions for breastfed infants include beginning iron supplementation around the age of 4 or 5 months. Iron supplementation may range from adding iron-fortified cereals to the child's diet to giving iron-containing drops. Encourage breastfeeding mothers to increase their intake of iron through diet or iron supplements to facilitate increased iron transfer to the infant. Limit intake of cow's milk to 24 oz per day for children older than 1 year of age. Encourage intake of iron-rich foods such as red meats, tuna, salmon, eggs, tofu, enriched grains, dried beans and peas, dried fruits, leafy green vegetables, and iron-fortified breakfast cereals (iron from red meat is the easiest for the body to absorb), and discourage intake of "fast foods."

Educating the Family

Educate parents about dietary intake, and encourage them to provide a variety of foods for iron support and vitamins and other minerals necessary for growth. Teach them about symptoms of iron deficiency and the effects on the child. Toddlers are particularly challenging as they are often "picky" eaters. This often becomes a means of control for the child, and parents should guard against getting involved in a power struggle with their child. Referring parents to a developmental specialist who can assist them in their approach to diet may prove beneficial.

▶ *Take* NOTE!

Dietary intake of more than 16 oz of cow's milk in children younger than 1 year has been shown to produce decreased hemoglobin levels. This study also found that children with lower iron levels had increased weight gain from birth to 2 years of age (Gunnarsson, Thorsdottir, & Palsson, 2004).

The use of iron supplements in infants begins with the use of formula fortified with iron in the formula-fed infant. Oral supplements may be necessary as well if the baby's iron levels are extremely low. Oral supplements or multivitamin formulas that contain iron are often dark in colour due to the iron. Teaching parents to measure precisely the amount of iron to be administered is an important nursing role. The liquid iron supplement must be administered behind the teeth, as iron in liquid form can temporarily stain the teeth. Iron supplementation may cause constipation. In some cases reducing the amount of iron can resolve this problem, but stool softeners may be necessary to control painful or difficult-to-pass stools. Encourage parents to increase their child's fluid intake and include adequate dietary fibre to avoid constipation.

Anemia Resulting from Lead Poisoning

Pathophysiology

In Canada, the incidence of lead poisoning is presumed to be low. However, 3% of children 2 years of age or younger in Hamilton, Ontario were identified as having blood lead levels at or exceeding 10 µg/dL, meeting the definition of lead poisoning in Canada (Smith, Pinsent, Kusiak, 2008). Lead exerts toxic effects on the bone marrow, erythroid cells, nervous system, and kidneys. The presence of lead in the bloodstream interferes with the enzymatic processes of the biosynthesis of heme. The process results in hypochromic, microcytic anemia, and children may exhibit classic signs of anemia. Risk factors for lead poisoning are related to lead exposure in the home, school, or local environment.

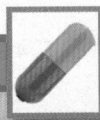

DRUG GUIDE 46.1 COMMON DRUGS FOR HEMATOLOGIC DISORDERS

Medication	Action and Indications	Nursing Implications
Iron supplements (ferrous sulfate, ferrous fumarate)	Supplemental iron in deficient child Iron-deficiency anemia	Dosage is based on mg of elemental iron. Give with vitamin C-containing foods to increase absorption. Do not administer with milk or milk products. May colour stools and urine black Liquid can stain the teeth; mix with a small amount of juice; drinking with straw decreases tooth staining. May cause constipation; increase fibre and fluid intake.
Deferasirox (Exjade)	Binds with iron, which is removed in the feces Iron toxicity (as in children chronically transfused)	Oral agent, should be taken at the same time daily, on an empty stomach. Monitor hearing and vision.
Deferoxamine (Desferal)	Binds with iron, which is removed via the kidneys Iron toxicity (as in children chronically transfused)	Rotate subcutaneous injection sites to decrease local reactions. Apply corticosteroid cream to irritation.
Factor (VIII or IX) replacement	Replaces deficient clotting factors Hemophilia	Use filter needle to draw up medication. Administer IV when bleeding occurs.
Penicillin VK	Kills susceptible bacteria Prophylaxis of infection in asplenia	Determine whether penicillin allergy is present. Monitor renal and hematologic function during prolonged use.
Folic acid	Replaces the vitamin Folic acid deficiency; questionable use with sickle cell anemia	Administer without regard to meals. Monitor hematologic function.
Hydroxyurea	Stimulates the development of Hemoglobin F in sickle cell anemia	Monitor for mild GI discomfort, modest neutropenia, hyperpigmentation of the skin and nails.
Intravenous immune globulin (IVIG) (multiple manufacturers)	Provides exogenous IgG antibodies Idiopathic thrombocytopenic purpura	Do not mix with IV medications or with other IV fluids. Do not give IM or SQ. Monitor vital signs and watch for adverse reactions frequently during infusion. Child may require antipyretic or antihistamine to prevent chills and fever during infusion. Have epinephrine available during infusion.
Tranexamic acid	An antifibrinolytic used when there is mucous membrane bleeding in factor deficiencies, vWD	Monitor hemostasis.
Rituximab	A monoclonal antibody that depletes B lymphocytes. Indicated for refractory chronic ITP	Start infusion slowly. Observe for adverse reaction and anaphylaxis. Monitor vital signs and have anaphylaxis treatment at bedside.

Adapted from: Taketokmo, C. K., Hodding, J. H., & Kraus, D. M. (2010). *Lexi-comp's pediatric dosage handbook* (17th ed.). Hudson, OH: Lexi-comp.

Lead is a developmental neurotoxin. Complications of lead poisoning include behavioural problems, learning difficulties and, with higher lead levels, encephalopathy, seizures, and brain damage. Treatment for high blood levels of lead is **chelation therapy**, either orally or intravenously. Drug Guide 46.1 gives further information on chelating agents.

Nursing Assessment

Explore the health history for subtle signs such as anorexia, fatigue, abdominal pain, or pallor. Determine whether behavioural problems, irritability, hyperactivity, or inability to meet developmental milestones have occurred in recent months. Screen children for risk of exposure to lead in the home. Refer to Chapter 30 for a simple screening questionnaire that can be used to determine the need for lead screening in young children. Blood levels of lead higher than 10 µg/dL require conscientious follow-up.

Nursing Management

If the child is undergoing chelation therapy, ensure adequate fluid intake and monitor intake and output closely. Refer children with elevated lead levels and developmental or cognitive deficits to developmental centers. These children may need an early intervention program for further evaluation and treatment of developmental delays. Prevention of elevated serum lead levels is imperative. Screen children for lead exposure risk. The American Academy of Pediatrics (AAP, 2009) recommends screening in high-risk children at ages 12 and 24 months. According to Health Canada (2011), lead exposure is an increased risk for children as their rapid rate of growth causes them to absorb more lead than adults and leaves them more vulnerable to the harmful effects of lead.

Educate families about the importance of removing paints with lead and preventing other exposure to lead, most importantly in young children. Online educational resources for families can be found at http://thePoint.lww.com/Chow1e.

Anemia of Chronic Disease

Anemia of chronic disease results in a normochromic, normocytic anemia. It is considered the most common type of anemia in hospitalized children, and its etiology is not clearly understood. It results in decreased production of RBCs and can be associated with underlying disease, inflammation, or malignancy. It is not due to lack of iron or nutrients. It improves when the underlying disease improves.

Bone Marrow Failure Diseases

Bone marrow failure may be congenital or acquired and results in impaired production of one or more blood cell lines. There are several types of bone marrow failure disorders, including aplastic anemia, pancytopenia, and single cytopenia (Association of Pediatric Hematology/Oncology Nurses [APHON], 2007).

Pancytopenia results when there is a lack of RBCs, platelets, and WBCs in the blood due to increased destruction of these cells, such as in sepsis or immune destruction. It may result from sequestration, such as in hypersplenism. Production of normal cells may also be decreased due to infiltrate when bone marrow is replaced by malignant cells, such as in leukemia, or when replaced by myelodysplastic cells in myelodysplasia. It may also occur in vitamin B12 deficiency or folate deficiency, or may be due to viruses, drugs, or radiation. In addition, hereditary bone marrow failure syndromes may manifest with pancytopenia due to lack of production of cells.

In aplastic anemia, the bone marrow ceases to produce RBCs, platelets, and neutrophils. This condition may be inherited (e.g., Fanconi anemia) or acquired (e.g., triggered by viral disease) or may result from abnormal immune mechanisms. Aplastic anemia is characterized by pancytopenia and a very hypocellular marrow meeting moderate or severe aplastic anemia diagnostic criteria, with no evidence of infiltration or fibrosis.

In single cytopenia marrow failure (e.g., pure red cell aplasia), there is decreased production of the erythroid (RBC) line. Single cytopenia can be congenital (e.g., Diamond Blackfan anemia [DBA]) or acquired (e.g., transient erythroblastopenia of childhood [TEC]).

Acquired Aplastic Anemia

Pathophysiology and Therapeutic Management

Aplastic anemia is characterized by bone marrow aplasia and pancytopenia. Acquired aplastic anemia may involve an immune-mediated response, damage to stem cells, or other unknown pathophysiology. It is most commonly idiopathic, although exposures to environmental toxins, viruses, myelosuppressive drugs, and radiation are possible etiologies. The international incidence of aplastic anemia is 2 cases per million (Bakhshi, 2011).

Aplastic anemia may be classified as moderate or severe according to bone marrow cellularity and cell line numbers. Complications of aplastic anemia include severe overwhelming infection, hemorrhage, and death. The treatment of choice for children with aplastic anemia is hematopoietic stem cell transplantation from a human leukocyte antigen (HLA)–matched sibling donor as this has the highest chance of cure. If no donor is available, immunosuppressive therapy using an antithymocyte globulin (ATG) treatment protocol is given.

Nursing Assessment

Determine the child's history of exposure to viruses, myelosuppressive medications, or radiation. Obtain a detailed family, environmental, and infectious disease history, including fever. Note history of epistaxis, gingival oozing, fevers, or increased bleeding with menstruation. Anemia may lead to headache and fatigue. On physical examination, note pallor, ecchymoses, petechiae or purpura, oral ulcerations, tachycardia, or tachypnea.

Laboratory and Diagnostic Testing

Laboratory and diagnostic testing may reveal pancytopenia, occult blood in stool or urine, or a severe decrease or absence of hematopoietic cells on bone marrow aspiration and biopsy.

Nursing Management

The nurse has several key responsibilities in managing aplastic anemia in children:

- Monitor for fever and bleeding and report them immediately to the physician because infection and

TABLE 46.6 **BLOOD PRODUCT TRANSFUSION**

Blood Product Administered IV	Potential Indication	Nursing Implications
Packed red blood cells (pRBCs)	Severe anemia, thalassemia, sickle cell disease, aplastic anemia	Follow institution's transfusion protocol. Double-check blood type and product label with a second nurse. Use only leukodepleted blood products in the child with a hemoglobinopathy.
Whole blood	Acute hemorrhage or trauma	Monitor vital signs and assess child frequently to detect adverse reaction to blood transfusion: fever, chills, dyspnea, nausea, back/chest pain, hypotension, hemolysis, urticaria, and other allergic reactions.
Fresh-frozen plasma (FFP)	Specific clotting factor deficiencies (factors II, V) and/or prolonged PT (INR) and PTT of unknown etiology	If an adverse reaction suspected, immediately discontinue transfusion, run normal saline IV, reassess the child, and notify the physician.
Platelets	Life-threatening thrombocytopenia or bleeding, aplastic anemia	Some children require pre-medication with diphenhydramine and/or acetaminophen before receiving blood products.

hemorrhage are potentially fatal. Safety is of the utmost concern in children with aplastic anemia. Therefore, bleeding precautions with thrombocytopenia and infection control with neutropenia are essential. Prevention of injury helps avoid hemorrhage. Stool softeners may be used to prevent anal fissures associated with constipation as fissures may lead to bacteremia.

- Administer antibiotics and blood product transfusions, using only irradiated and leukocyte-depleted pRBC or platelet transfusions. The latter limit exposure to HLA antigens should the child require bone marrow transplantation in the future. See Table 46.6.
- Monitor for side effects of drugs such as antibiotics, ATG, corticosteroids, and cyclosporine.
- Educate and support the child and family.

Complications from aplastic anemia and/or its treatment include bleeding, sepsis, serum sickness, and GVHD. Patients with aplastic anemia may relapse and develop secondary malignancies.

Visit http://thePoint.lww.com/Chow1e for Web resources that may be used to help in educating the family. For the child who does require hematopoietic stem cell transplantation, refer to Chapter 49 for additional nursing management information.

Inherited Bone Marrow Failure Diseases with Pancytopenia

Aplastic anemia is most often an acquired condition, but there are a few rare types of inherited aplastic anemias. The inherited types present as pancytopenias from congenital bone marrow failure. Fanconi anemia, an autosomal recessive disorder, is the best known inherited aplastic anemia. Physical anomalies may include abnormal thumbs, microcephaly, hyperpigmented or hypopigmented skin lesions, short stature, and kidney abnormalities. Characteristics of dyskeratosis congenita include hyperpigmented skin, rash, nail deformities, pancytopenia, and increased risk of leukemia and other malignancies. Allogeneic hematopoietic stem cell transplantation is the only cure for both Fanconi anemia and dyskeratosis congenita.

Bone Marrow Failure Diseases with Single Cytopenia: Pure Red Cell Aplasia

Congenital Red Cell Aplasia: Diamond Blackfan Anemia

DBA presents as a congenital form of pure red cell aplasia where severe anemia develops. Children are usually diagnosed in infancy after they present with pallor, fatigue, or feeding difficulties. Other signs may include short stature or abnormalities of the head and neck, cardiac system, or genitourinary system; or there may be no physical findings at all. A trial of corticosteroids may be given to try to induce remission.

Implementation of an ongoing pRBC transfusion program over years is required for supportive care. This will cause iron toxicity in body organs, so subcutaneous or oral iron chelators must be given. Transfusion support, medication monitoring, patient and family education, and genetic counselling are required. Stem cell transplantation from an HLA-matched sibling donor can correct this inherited anemia. Visit http://thePoint.lww.com/Chow1e for recommended websites for caregiver and family education.

Acquired Transient Erythroblastopenia of Childhood

TEC is an acquired form of red cell aplasia that involves a temporary arrest of production of the RBC line in previously healthy children, usually between the ages of 1 and 3 years. TEC is often preceded by a viral infection. A normocytic anemia with low or absent reticulocytes develops. Flow murmurs and tachycardia may be present. Observation and possible transfusions for the anemia are required. The anemia resolves over weeks to months.

Acquired Red Cell Aplasia from Parvovirus B19

Parvovirus B19 (sometimes called fifth disease) causes an acquired red cell aplasia also characterized by fever and a lacy red rash; affected patients can have an arrest of erythropoiesis (red cell line production) causing severe anemia. Patients with sickle cell disease, thalassemia, and hereditary spherocytosis are at much higher risk due to the decreased lifespan of their own red cells. These individuals may require red cell transfusions.

Hemolytic Anemias

Hemolytic anemias may be inherited or acquired and may result from immune- or non–immune-based causes. RBC destruction is increased in hemolytic anemia, and the bone marrow tries to compensate by increasing reticulocyte production. Further subdivision of hemolytic anemias is based on the site of destruction of the red cell:

- Intravascular hemolysis: In this category, hemolysis occurs within the circulating blood system. Acute symptoms often occur (e.g., fever and chills, fatigue, tachycardia). This type of hemolysis may also occur in an ABO-mismatched pRBC transfusion.
- Extravascular hemolysis: In this category, hemolysis occurs outside the circulating blood system, such as in the liver and/or spleen, and is associated with few signs and symptoms. Causes may include bacterial or viral infections, autoimmune hemolysis, certain drugs, hemoglobinopathies, structural abnormalities such as hereditary spherocytosis, or enzyme deficiencies such as glucose-6-phosphate dehydrogenase (G6PD) deficiency.

Inherited Hemolytic Anemias

Structural Defects in the Red Cell Membrane: Hereditary Spherocytosis

Hereditary spherocytosis (HS) is a common condition in which the RBCs cannot maintain their normal biconcave shape and instead become spherical. Spherocytes are not flexible and have difficulty passing through the spleen. They are destroyed in the spleen through

extravascular hemolysis. Infection such as parvovirus may cause a sudden drop in hemoglobin due to the temporary red cell aplasia caused by this virus. Gallstones may develop at a very young age. Oral supplementation with folic acid is recommended.

Enzyme Defects in Red Cell Metabolism: G6PD Deficiency

G6PD is an enzyme that is responsible for maintaining the integrity and metabolism of RBCs by protecting them from oxidative substances. When RBCs are exposed to an oxidative stress, a non-immune hemolytic anemia develops. Triggers that may result in oxidative stress and hemolysis include bacterial or viral illness or exposure to certain substances such as medications (e.g., sulfonamides, sulfones, malaria-fighting drugs [such as quinine], methylene blue for treating urinary tract infections), naphthalene (an agent in mothballs), or foods such as fava beans (KidsHealth, 2009).

G6PD deficiency is an X-linked recessive disorder that is common in males of African, Mediterranean, or Asian descent (Ambruso, Hays, & Goldenberg, 2011). The condition tends to be less severe in those of African descent and more severe in those of Mediterranean descent. Complications include prolonged neonatal jaundice and life-threatening acute episodes of hemolysis on exposure to oxidants. Therapeutic management is aimed primarily at avoiding triggers throughout life that cause oxidative stress and giving transfusion of pRBCs if necessary for low hemoglobin.

Nursing Assessment

G6PD deficiency may be discovered in the neonatal period. There may be a history of significant jaundice or anemia. Severe untreated jaundice may cause kernicterus, which is associated with cerebral palsy.

Note the child's health history, including fatigue. Inspect the skin and sclera for pallor or jaundice. Measure heart rate and respiratory rate, noting elevations. Determine oxygen saturation via pulse oximeter or blood gas analysis. Palpate the abdomen for splenomegaly. Note tea-coloured urine, which indicates RBC breakdown. Laboratory studies will reveal anemia (KidsHealth, 2009).

Nursing Management

Monitor vital signs, administer oxygen as ordered, and treat the symptoms. pRBC transfusion may be required. Once the trigger agent is removed or the child recovers from an illness, the anemia will improve. Determine the parents' understanding of the disorder as well as their knowledge of the required medications and foods to avoid. Provide further education to the child and family about symptoms and triggers. Advise them that the child should avoid contact with these agents. Visit http://thePoint.lww.com/Chow1e for online educational resources for G6PD deficiency.

Molecular Defects in the Hemoglobin Molecule

Examples of defects in the hemoglobin molecule are thalassemia and sickle cell disease with Hb SS or Hb SC. See the Hemoglobinopathies section for further detail on these conditions.

Acquired Hemolytic Anemias

Acquired hemolytic anemias can have several causes:

- Immune mechanisms in which the antibody coats the RBCs, leading to RBC destruction in the spleen. These immune mechanisms cause acquired immune and autoimmune anemias as well as hemolytic disease of the newborn. In autoimmune hemolytic anemia (AIHA), autoantibodies bind to RBCs, causing their destruction (hemolysis) and resulting in anemia. In AIHA, hemolysis is primarily extravascular in the liver and spleen.
- Drugs and toxins
- Infectious microorganisms, such as *Plasmodium* species, which causes malaria
- Insults such as burns or disseminated intravascular coagulation (DIC)
- Mechanical trauma, such as due to placement of a prosthetic heart valve

Hemoglobinopathies

A hemoglobinopathy is a condition in which abnormal hemoglobin molecules in the blood produce a non-immune hemolytic anemia. Hemoglobinopathies are genetic diseases such as sickle cell anemia, alpha-thalassemia, and beta-thalassemia.

There are many kinds of abnormal hemoglobins. The normal pediatric and adult hemoglobin is Hb A. A large percentage of the newborn's hemoglobin is Hb F (fetal hemoglobin), which can exchange oxygen molecules at lower oxygen tensions compared with adult hemoglobin. Over the first several months of life, Hb F diminishes and is replaced with Hb A. The healthy older infant then displays the presence of Hb A. In hemoglobinopathies, this normal hemoglobin configuration is disturbed. This discussion focuses on sickle cell disease and beta-thalassemia (Cooley's anemia).

Sickle cell Disease

Sickle cell disease is an inherited hemoglobinopathy in which the RBCs do not carry the normal adult hemoglobin but rather a less effective type called sickle hemoglobin. Affected individuals have mutations in both beta hemoglobin genes. In Canada and the United States, the most common types of sickle cell disease are hemoglobin SS (Hb SS) disease, hemoglobin SC (Hb SC) disease, and hemoglobin S beta-thalassemia. Among the sickle cell diseases, Hb SS is the most common and is the focus of this discussion.

Sickle cell anemia is an inherited blood disorder. It is the number one inherited disorder in the United States (APHON, 2007). In Canada, about 67 black infants are born with sickle cell disease each year (Goldbloom, 2004). Sickle cell disease is most common in individuals of African, Mediterranean, Middle Eastern, and Indian descent (Ambruso et al., 2011).

Persons with one sickle cell mutation and one normal beta hemoglobin gene (Hb AS) are said to have the sickle cell trait and are carriers for the disease. Persons with the sickle cell trait do not have the disease and have only minimal health problems. One in twelve Americans of African descent has the sickle cell trait (Human Genome Management Information System, 2005).

Canada's immigrant population is rising, with increased representation from African, Mediterranean, Middle Eastern, and Indian groups. It is estimated that the sickle hemoglobin carrier rate in Canada's black population may be higher than that in the United States because the Canadian immigrant population is derived primarily from Caribbean and African countries, which have higher carrier rates than the immigrant populations in the United States (Lieberman, Kirby, Ozolins, et al., 2009). Clinical practice guidelines have been developed in Canada for carrier screening for the hemoglobinopathies, including sickle cell disease and thalassemia (Langois 2008). Newborn screening is available in some provinces (see Laboratory and Diagnostic Testing section).

Pathophysiology

Individuals with sickle cell disease have Hb SS (sickle hemoglobin) instead of normal Hb AA. Hb SS results from a single point mutation that causes a glutamic acid to be replaced by valine in the beta hemoglobin molecule. Deoxygenation of Hb SS can cause a change in the shape of the RBCs, resulting in an elongated sickle that is destroyed in the spleen (Fig. 46.3).

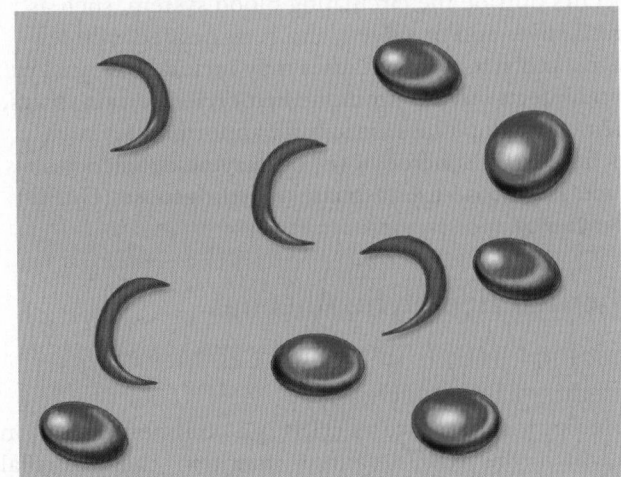

FIGURE 46.3 Illustration showing the elongated sickle-shaped red blood cells seen in sickle cell disease alongside normal red cells.

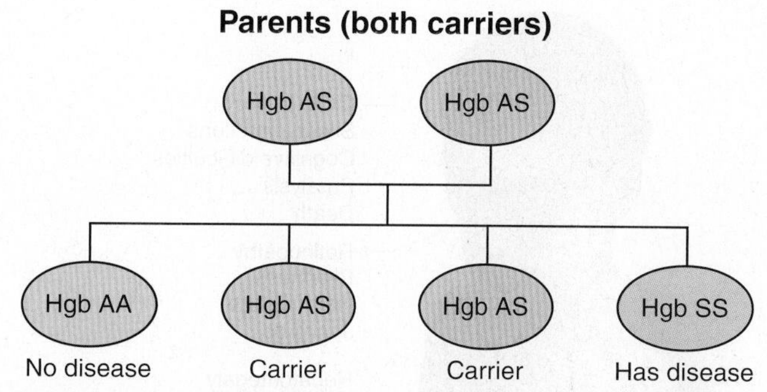

Parents (both carriers)

Hgb AS   Hgb AS

Hgb AA   Hgb AS   Hgb AS   Hgb SS
No disease   Carrier   Carrier   Has disease

FIGURE 46.4 Simplified genetic scheme for sickle cell disease. *A* denotes adult hemoglobin; *S* denotes sickle hemoglobin. Hb AA = normal hemoglobin, Hb AS = sickle cell trait, Hb SS = sickle cell disease.

If both parents have Hb AS (i.e., they are carriers for the disease), they may have a child with Hb SS. With each pregnancy the risk is 25% that the child will have sickle cell disease (Hb SS), 25% that the child will have normal hemoglobin (Hb AA), and 50% that the child will have the sickle cell trait (Hb AS) and will be a carrier (Pitts & Record, 2010). Figure 46.4 illustrates the inheritance probability.

Infants with sickle cell anemia are usually asymptomatic until 3 to 4 months of age because Hb F protects against them against the sickling process. Significant anemia may occur when the RBCs sickle. Sickling may be triggered by oxidative stress, which can result from infection, fever, acidosis, dehydration, physical exertion, excessive cold exposure, or hypoxia (Ambruso et al., 2011). As the cells sickle, the blood becomes more viscous because the sickled cells clump together and prevent normal blood flow to the tissues of that area. The sickle-shaped RBCs cannot pass through the smaller capillaries and venules of the circulatory system (Fig. 46.5). This vaso-occlusive process leads to local tissue hypoxia followed by ischemia and may result in infarction. Pain crisis results as circulation is decreased to the area.

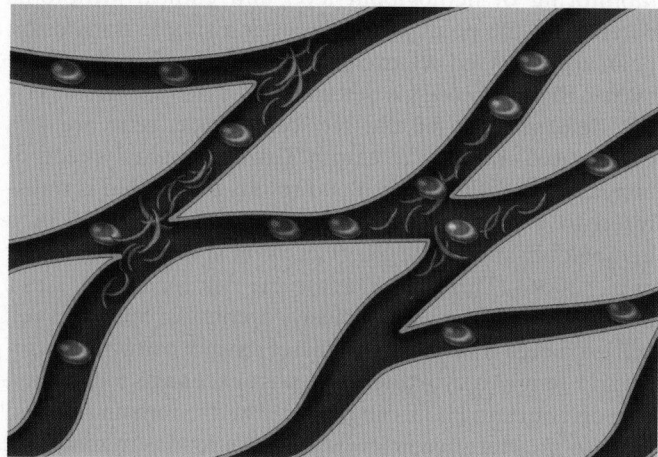

FIGURE 46.5 Illustration of clumping of sickle-shaped cells blocking blood flow.

Complications of sickle cell disease include recurrent vaso-occlusive pain crises, stroke, silent brain infarctions, learning difficulties, sepsis, acute chest syndrome, pulmonary hypertension, splenic sequestration, reduced visual acuity or blindness related to decreased retinal blood flow, chronic leg ulcers, cholestasis and gallstones, delayed growth and development, delayed puberty, and priapism (the sickle cells prevent blood from flowing out of an erect penis) (National Heart, Lung and Blood Institute, 2011). Pain can occur in any part of the body such as long bones, joints, chest, abdomen, or head. Pain causes increased metabolic need by resulting in tachycardia and sometimes tachypnea, which leads to further sickling. Clumping of cells in the lungs (producing acute chest syndrome) results in decreased gas exchange. It produces hypoxia, which leads to further sickling. Sequestration of blood in the spleen leads to splenomegaly, abdominal pain, and severe anemia. Infarction of the spleen may occur followed by fibrosis and atrophy of the spleen. Functional asplenia may develop as early as 6 months of age, and occurs by age 9 years in 90% of children with sickle cell disease (Pitts & Record, 2010). Functional asplenia increases the risk of infection and death. Children with sickle cell anemia have an increased incidence of enuresis because the kidneys cannot concentrate urine effectively (Pitts & Record, 2010). As children reach adulthood, multiple organ dysfunction is common.

Therapeutic Management

The therapeutic management of children with sickle cell anemia focuses on preventing sickling of red cells, pain, infection, and other complications such as those described in Figure 46.6. Prevention of infection is critical because the child with sickle cell anemia is at increased risk for serious infection related to alterations in splenic function. Functional asplenia (decreased ability of the spleen to function appropriately) places the child at significant risk for serious infection related to *Streptococcus pneumoniae*, meningococcus, or other encapsulated organisms. Asplenia immunization protocols, such as those recommended by Vaudry and Kellner (2007, updated 2011), are implemented at diagnosis to help reduce the risk of life-threatening infection. For the latest information on immunizations against encapsulated organisms, see the Canadian Immunization Guide (Public Health Agency of Canada, 2006). Oral penicillin at daily prophylactic dosing is started at diagnosis (Carcao, Cook, Allen, et al., revised by Kirby et al., 2006). The updated UK National Health Service standards and guidelines for sickle cell disease (Dick et al., 2010) recommend that "twice-daily penicillin prophylaxis or alternative should be prescribed from 3 months of age and continued throughout childhood" (p. 20). It is important for nurses to be aware of emerging guidelines and recommendations.

Folic acid supplementation is recommended to support RBC production. All children with sickle cell disease

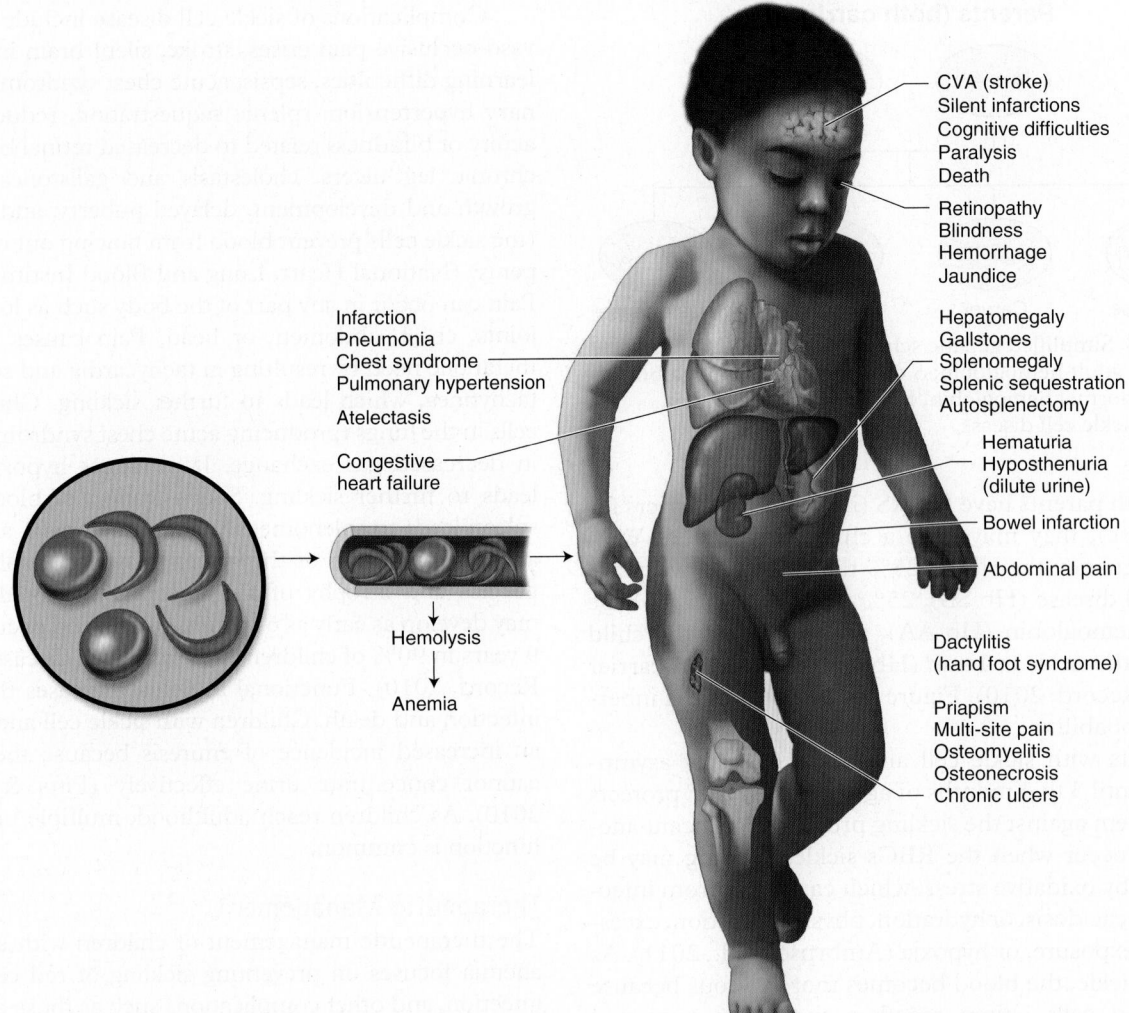

CVA (stroke)
Silent infarctions
Cognitive difficulties
Paralysis
Death

Retinopathy
Blindness
Hemorrhage
Jaundice

Hepatomegaly
Gallstones
Splenomegaly
Splenic sequestration
Autosplenectomy

Hematuria
Hyposthenuria
(dilute urine)

Bowel infarction

Abdominal pain

Infarction
Pneumonia
Chest syndrome
Pulmonary hypertension

Atelectasis

Congestive
heart failure

Hemolysis

Anemia

Dactylitis
(hand foot syndrome)

Priapism
Multi-site pain
Osteomyelitis
Osteonecrosis
Chronic ulcers

FIGURE 46.6 Effects of sickle cell anemia on various parts of the body.

should be screened for asthma because clinical evidence shows that a diagnosis of asthma increases the severity of sickle cell disease (Field & DeBaun, 2009). The clinical relationship between the two conditions has not yet been determined. Children must be screened for sleep apnea, retinopathy, and pulmonary hypertension. Children are screened yearly for stroke risk as well as for gallstones. Neuropsychological screening should be undertaken at strategic intervals.

Treatment of a sickle cell crisis is directed toward controlling pain and reducing oxidative stress. An acute crisis may exacerbate chronic organ damage. Sickle cell pain requires aggressive pain control. Patients with sickle cell disease may have a reduced sensitivity to opioids (Brousseau, McCarver, Drendel, et al., 2007), as well as faster clearance of morphine, likely due to increased hepatic and renal blood flow (Darbari, Neely, van den Anker, & Rana, 2011). Therefore, either a high-dose continuous morphine infusion or a patient-controlled analgesia infusion is often required. When fever is present, antibiotic therapy is undertaken according to guidelines listed below. Oxygen administration may be necessary during episodes of crisis

to prevent additional cell sickling. Adequate hydration with intravenous fluids and/or oral intake is critical. Electrolyte analysis is also necessary to ensure that appropriate amounts of electrolytes are present in the IV fluids. Close monitoring of hemoglobin level and clinical symptoms determines the point at which either a simple transfusion or an apheresis red cell exchange transfusion becomes necessary. Blood viscosity is determined by hematocrit and by the deformability of the red cell. Sickle cells are less deformable and tend to clump. The detrimental effects of increased viscosity of the blood results if the child is transfused to a post-transfusion hematocrit above 0.35 or a hemoglobin above 110 g/L (Carcao et al., revised by Kirby et al., 2006). This may increase the risk for stroke, silent infarction, or other vaso-occlusive events. An apheresis red cell exchange transfusion increases oxygen carrying capacity and removes cytokines. The post-exchange transfusion hemoglobin and HCT can be calculated to remain safe and close to pre-transfusion levels. Iron overload is minimal.

Guidelines for In-patient Management of Children with Sickle cell Disease from Toronto's Hospital for Sick Children (Carcao et al., revised by Kirby et al., 2006) describe

BOX 46.1 **Additional Medical Treatments used for Some Children with Sickle Cell Anemia**

- Cholecystectomy may become necessary if gallstones develop.
- Splenectomy may be performed to prevent recurrence of splenic sequestration if it is life-threatening. Laparoscopic splenectomy is performed in some centres.
- Administration of hydroxyurea may increase the percentage of fetal hemoglobin. It reduces the frequency of painful crises. The optimal age for starting hydroxyurea is currently being investigated in clinical trials. Many children are now started at younger ages.
- Blood transfusions, although not routinely given to children with sickle cell disease, are indicated in children with prolonged or widespread pain, aplastic crisis, or splenic sequestration.
- Partial exchange or a complete automated red cell exchange transfusion may be used acutely, in the event of stroke or acute chest syndrome, or preoperatively, to rapidly lower the circulating amount of Hb SS to less than 30% without raising the hemoglobin too high and increasing blood viscosity. An automated red cell exchange may be used as an elective procedure under certain criteria to prevent crises and iron overload. The automated red cell exchange transfusion, an apheresis procedure, usually uses a double lumen femoral line.
- Hematopoietic stem cell transplantation is usually reserved for children with an identical HLA-matched sibling donor. Risk of death and incidence of GVHD are possible.

treatment for the many complications that may result because this disease affects multiple body systems. The *British Columbia Children's Hospital Guideline for the Management of Fever in Children with Sickle cell Disease* (Guilcher, Purves, & Wu, 2006) describes a protocol for fever. Other problem-oriented clinical guidelines that describe ongoing health maintenance are available from the Georgia Comprehensive Sickle cell Center at Grady Health Systems (visit http://thePoint.lww.com/Chow1e for additional information).

The frequency of stem cell transplantation between matched sibling donors is increasing. Box 46.1 describes additional medical treatments that are necessary in some children with sickle cell anemia.

Nursing Assessment

Children with sickle cell anemia experience a significant number of acute and chronic manifestations of the condition (Comparison Chart 46.1). See the Nursing Process Overview section for a full description of the assessment phase of the nursing process for a child with a hematologic disorder. Assessment findings pertinent to sickle cell anemia are discussed below.

Health History

Determine the history of present illness to assess for a precipitating event, such as hypoxia, infection, or dehydration. Note onset, character, and quality of pain as well as factors that relieve it. Assess for signs and symptoms of stroke. Elicit the health history, noting growth and development, history of recurrent infections, frequency and extent of vaso-occlusive crises, past hospitalizations, and treatment for pain crises. Note history of immunizations, including pneumococcal, flu, and meningococcal vaccinations. Determine history of blood transfusions. Document current medication regimen, any monitoring tests completed, and a complete family history, including the possibility of consanguinity.

Physical Examination

Perform a thorough physical examination because sickling, hypoxia, and tissue ischemia affect most areas of the body (see Fig. 46.6). Note the physical findings discussed below that can be detected using inspection, auscultation, percussion, and palpation.

Inspection and Observation

Inspect the conjunctivae, palms, and soles for pallor and the skin for pallor, lesions, or ulcers. Note jaundice of the skin or scleral icterus. Document colour and moisture of oral mucosa. Measure temperature to evaluate for infection (which can precipitate a sickle cell crisis). Note blood pressure (which may be increased with severe pain or with sickle cell nephropathy). Note any increased work of breathing and tissue swelling. Determine baseline mental status. Perform frequent neurologic assessments, as about 10% of children with sickle cell anemia experience a clinically overt stroke (Dowling Quinn, Rogers, et al., 2010). Furthermore, at least an additional 25% to 35% of children with sickle cell disease are thought to have subclinical infarctions called silent cerebral infarcts, which are brain injuries often associated with cognitive impairment and increased risk of stroke (Dowling et al., 2010).

Auscultation

Auscultate heart sounds for a murmur. Tachycardia may be present with anemia, pain, fever, or dehydration. Listen to breath sounds, noting the rate and depth of respiration as well as the adequacy of aeration. Adventitious breath sounds may be present if a respiratory infection has triggered the sickle cell crisis or in the case of acute chest syndrome.

Palpation and Percussion

Palpate the abdomen for areas of tenderness, hepatomegaly, or splenomegaly. Palpate the joints for warmth, tenderness, and range of motion. Note swelling of the hands or feet in the infant. Note and report symmetric swelling of the hands and feet in the infant or toddler. Termed *dactylitis,* this condition occurs following aseptic infarction in the phalanges, metacarpals, or metatarsals. Occurrence before age 1 year is predictive of severity of illness (Maakaron, Taher, & Woermann, 2012) (Fig. 46.7).

COMPARISON CHART 46.1 ACUTE VERSUS CHRONIC MANIFESTATIONS OF SICKLE CELL ANEMIA

Acute	Chronic
Acute chest syndrome*	Anemia
Aplastic crisis*	Avascular necrosis of the hip
Bacterial sepsis*	Cardiomegaly, functional murmur
Bone and organ infarction	Cholelithiasis
Dactylitis	Delayed growth and development
Hematuria	Delayed puberty
Recurrent pain episodes	Functional asplenia
Pain crisis	Hyposthenuria (inability to concentrate urine) and enuresis
Splenic sequestration*	Jaundice
Stroke, including silent stroke*	Leg ulcers
Priapism	Proteinuria
Bowel infarction	Pulmonary hypertension*
	Restrictive lung disease*
	Retinopathy/blindness
	Chronic pain syndromes
	Risk of cognitive impairment

*Often life-threatening.
NOTE: Underlying chronic manifestations of sickle cell disease may become worse during an acute crisis.

Laboratory and Diagnostic Testing

According to Lieberman et al. (2009), the significant mortality and morbidity of sickle cell disease warrant a national neonatal screening program in Canada. As of 2010, universal newborn screening for sickle cell disease is offered only in British Columbia (started in 2009) and Ontario (started in 2006). The neonatal screening program in Ontario has revealed that the newborn incidence

of sickle cell disease in the province is 1 in 2,800, much higher than expected (Hamilton Regional Laboratory Medicine Program, 2010).

Screening by Sickledex or sickle cell prep does not distinguish between sickle cell disease and sickle cell trait. If the screening test result indicates the possibility of sickle cell anemia or sickle cell trait, hemoglobin electrophoresis is performed promptly to confirm the diagnosis. Hemoglobin electrophoresis is the only accurate test for sickle cell disease but it is not a rapid method. Hemoglobin electrophoresis will demonstrate the presence of Hgb S and Hgb F. A rapid diagnosis can be obtained using high-pressure liquid chromatography, but this must be confirmed with hemoglobin electrophoresis.

Common laboratory and diagnostic studies ordered for the assessment of sickle cell anemia include:

- Hemoglobin: baseline is usually 7 to 10 mg/dL (this will be significantly lower with splenic sequestration or aplastic crisis)
- Reticulocyte count: greatly elevated
- Peripheral blood smear: presence of sickle-shaped cells and target cells
- Platelet count: may be increased or decreased
- Abnormal liver function tests with elevated bilirubin

X-ray studies or other scans may be obtained to determine the extent of organ or tissue damage resulting from vaso-occlusion. Transcranial Doppler ultrasound

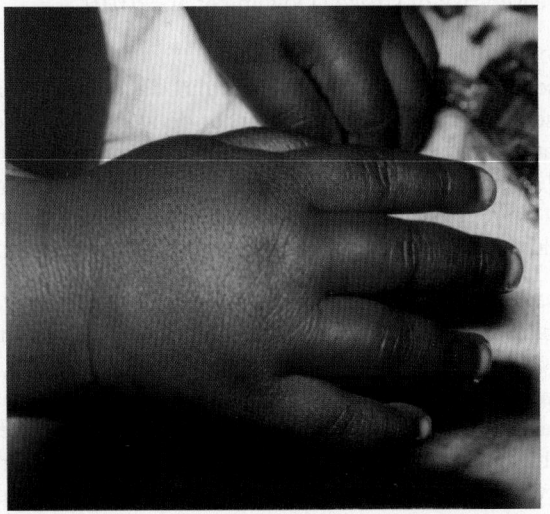

FIGURE 46.7 Swelling of the hands and feet (dactylitis) in a toddler.

to determine stroke risk and abdominal ultrasound are performed yearly as are pulmonary function studies. Other regular tests conducted as the child grows older include bloodwork, echocardiograms, eye/retina exams, sleep studies, and neuropsychological screening.

Nursing Management

Nursing care of the child with sickle cell anemia focuses on preventing vaso-occlusive crises, managing pain and infection episodes, managing many types of crises, and providing educational and psychosocial support to the child and family. All children with sickle cell anemia need ongoing evaluation of growth and development to maximize their potential in those areas. Monitor school performance to detect neurodevelopmental problems and seek intervention early. The nursing diagnoses and interventions given in Nursing Care Plan 46.1 should be individualized based on the child's and family's response to the disorder. Specific areas of nursing care related to sickle cell disease crises (see Comparison Chart 46.1) are discussed below.

Managing Pain Crisis

Vaso-occlusive crisis is often referred to as a pain crisis but can be any event that renders the child unable to function. Sickle cell pain can be worse than postoperative or cancer pain. Physical findings and lab testing may be unremarkable despite the child being in significant pain. Initiate pain assessment upon admission using a standardized age-appropriate pain scale. Provide frequent pain evaluations. Always believe the child's report of pain: only the person suffering the pain knows what it feels like.

Moderate to severe pain usually requires opioid medication. Oral morphine, rather than oral codeine, or IV morphine infusion is frequently used to achieve pain control. As of 2010, a number of pediatric sickle cell programs in Canada, such as the Hospital for Sick Children in Toronto and Stollery Children's Hospital in Alberta, have moved to using oral morphine exclusively, rather than oral codeine, for sickle cell patients. Codeine and its active form, morphine, may not be metabolized effectively in some patients of African heritage (Brousseau et al., 2007). In addition, codeine may be ineffective in a percentage of the general population as it can be hypo- or hyper-metabolized. Meperidine is not a first-line drug in the treatment of pain in sickle cell disease.

> ▶ *Take* NOTE!
>
> *Avoid repeated use of meperidine (Demerol) for pain management during sickle cell crisis because it has been associated with an increased risk of seizures when used in children with sickle cell anemia (Sickle cell Information Center [SCIC], 2011a).*

To bring the pain under control, initially administer analgesics routinely rather than on an as-needed (PRN) basis. Once the pain is better managed, medications may be moved to PRN status. For pain that is consistently at moderate and severe levels, a continuous infusion of opioid, usually morphine, is the treatment of choice to maintain an adequate and continuous level of analgesia for the child. Monitor the continuous morphine infusion or patient-controlled analgesia in the child or adolescent. Aggressive pain management strategies and high-dose morphine infusion are often needed (Jacobs & Mueller, 2008). This is because the pharmacokinetics of morphine metabolism may differ in the child with sickle cell disease (Brousseau et al., 2007) and possibly because there is greater clearance with increased renal and hepatic blood flow (Darbari et al., 2011).

Addiction to narcotics is rarely a concern in the child with sickle cell anemia if the narcotic is used to alleviate severe pain (Pitts & Record, 2010). Nonsteroidal anti-inflammatory drugs (NSAIDs) and acetaminophen are often used. Adequate pain management helps to decrease the child's stress level; elevated stress may possibly contribute to further sickling and additional pain.

Use non-pharmacologic pain management techniques such as relaxation, warm blankets, music, massage, play, guided imagery, therapeutic touch, or behaviour modification to augment the pain medication regimen. Consider inclusion of the hospital child life team, which specializes in the use of play and distraction to help children cope with symptoms and treatment. Teach the child and parents about pain management strategies to use at home as well as critical skills to assess pain at home and determine when to bring the child to the hospital. Box 46.2 gives a summary of sickle cell pain management.

Fluid Management

Deficient fluid volume occurs as a result of decreased intake, increased fluid requirements during sickle cell crisis, and the kidney's inability to concentrate urine (hyposthenuria). Increasing fluid intake will dilute the blood and decrease its viscosity. To promote hemodilution, provide maintenance or 1.5 times maintenance fluids according to sickle cell guidelines (Carcao et al., revised by Kirby et al., 2006), with boluses if needed for dehydration. With chest symptoms, use maintenance fluid replacement either orally or intravenously to avoid fluid overload and pulmonary edema. Maintain appropriate electrolyte levels and pH balance.

Preventing Ineffective Tissue Perfusion

Risk for ineffective tissue perfusion related to the effects of RBC sickling and infarction of tissues is another concern. Frequently evaluate respiratory and circulatory status and work of breathing. Administer supplemental oxygen to keep the pulse oximetry reading greater than or equal to 96% (Carcao et al., 2006). If tachypnea is present,

---

BOX 46.2 ABCs of Managing Sickle Cell Pain

- Assess the pain (use an age-appropriate pain assessment tool).
- Believe the patient's report of pain; clinical evidence of pain may be minimal.
- Complications or cause of pain (look for complications)
- Drugs and distraction: Use pain medication (opiates and NSAIDs, if no contraindications); treat pain symptoms early and aggressively; use fixed dosing; give on a timed schedule; no PRN dosing for pain medications; use IV morphine bolus and continuous morphine infusion as indicated; distraction with music, TV, relaxation techniques.
- Environment: Rest in quiet area with privacy.
- Fluids (hypotonic—D$_5$ with 0.45% normal saline solution)

Adapted from: Platt, A., Eckman, J. R., Beasley, J., & Miller, G. (2002). Treating sickle cell pain: An update from the Georgia Comprehensive Sickle cell Center. *Journal of Emergency Nursing, 28*(4), 297–303, with permission.

---

give a trial of oxygen. Report worsening of respiratory status immediately to physician. Monitor level of consciousness and immediately report changes as the risk of stroke is increased 10% with acute chest crisis.

Treating and Preventing Infection

Educate the child and family about the importance of seeking treatment for fever immediately. If the child has an oral or tympanic temperature of 38.5°C or an axillary temperature of 38°C, the child must be taken to the emergency department immediately. A treatment protocol for asplenia using antibiotics is required according to the *Guidelines for In-patient Management of Children with Sickle cell Disease* (Carcao et al., revised by Kirby et al., 2006).

▶ *Take* NOTE!

Tylenol or NSAIDs may mask a fever. The child's temperature should be maintained as close to normal as possible without the use of cooling mattresses, as sudden temperature change can further precipitate sickling of the RBCs (Eckman, 2010).

A variety of interventions are necessary to prevent severe life-threatening infection in the child with sickle cell disease. By 2 months of age, begin administration of oral penicillin V (also used to prevent pneumococcal infection). In the penicillin-allergic child, trimethoprim–sulfamethoxazole (Carcao et al., revised by Kirby et al., 2006) or erythromycin may be used.

Administer childhood immunizations according to the currently recommended provincial immunization schedules for hyposplenia based on expert recommendations (e.g., Vaudry & Kellner, 2007, updated 2011). To prevent overwhelming sepsis or meningitis as a result of infection with *S. pneumoniae,* the child should receive the pneumococcal and meningococcal vaccine series, including the more recent meningococcal vaccine, Menactra, and the pneumococcal vaccine, Prevnar 13. Additional protection for children with sickle cell disease with new vaccines should be given as they become available.

Because sickle cell patients often receive transfusions, vaccination against hepatitis B is also recommended at an early age. Hepatitis A vaccine is highly recommended. Provide influenza immunization annually (after 6 months of age) before the onset of flu season. (Refer to Chapter 30 for additional information on these vaccines).

Educating and Supporting the Child, Family, and Community

As with any chronic illness, families of children with sickle cell anemia need significant support. They often feel guilty or responsible for the disease. Reassure the family and provide education. Refer families to a regional sickle cell disease centre for multidisciplinary care.

Sickle cell disease requires comprehensive care, community engagement, and effective transition strategies. Education should begin immediately after the diagnosis of sickle cell anemia is confirmed. Initially, teach the family about the inheritance of the disease and encourage family members to be tested for Hb SS, Hb AS, and Hb AC. Consider parents and families as partners in learning about the disease process (Weiss & Stephen, 2009).

Emphasize the importance of regularly scheduled health maintenance visits, yearly testing, and immunizations. Teach families how to administer prophylactic penicillin, folic acid, and oral pain management medications at home. Provide teaching about safety and oral morphine in the home environment. Teach families to seek medical evaluation urgently for any febrile illness. Educate families about how to prevent, recognize, and manage vaso-occlusive events (Teaching Guideline 46.1). Discuss multi-system complications as described in Comparison Chart 46.1. Discuss healthy nutrition as many children with sickle cell disease require about 20% more calories a day than the average child.

With parental permission, link with the child's early childhood (e.g., day care) or school environment to provide information to teachers and other caregivers and develop a continuum of care for the child and family. Integrate services with provincial comprehensive school health initiatives and early childhood programs. Develop a process to transition teens and families effectively to the adult areas of care. Additional resources for families can be found by visiting http://thePoint.lww.com/Chow1e.

TEACHING GUIDELINE 46.1

Family Education for Management of Sickle Cell Disease

- Have 24-hour access to a medical provider or to a facility that is familiar with sickle cell care. Access comprehensive care centres for sickle cell disease management.
- Seek immediate attention in a hospital emergency department for *any* febrile illness (temperature 38.5°C or higher by mouth or ear, or 38°C under the arm, measured twice 1 hour apart).
- Contact your child's medical provider promptly if you suspect a pain crisis is developing.
- Seek medical attention immediately if any of the following signs develop:
  - Pale skin and listlessness
  - Fever
  - Abdominal pain, increase in abdominal size
  - Blood in stool
  - Bone pain or other pain not relieved with brief trial of oral pain medications at home
  - Limp or painful, swollen joints
  - Cough, shortness of breath, chest pain
- Increasing fatigue
- Unusual headache, loss of feeling, or sudden weakness, change in speech pattern
- Sudden vision change
- Painful erection that won't go down (priapism)
- Obtain timely immunizations according to the asplenic protocol and take daily penicillin prophylaxis.
- Encourage adequate fluid intake daily. Emphasize a nutritional diet.
- Avoid temperatures that are too hot or too cold.
- Avoid overexertion or stress.
- Seek medical advice regarding travel arrangements, prophylaxis, and the use of oxygen during air travel.
- Communicate well with teachers and caregivers regarding the child's sickle cell disease, its implications and symptoms to watch for. Complete neuropsychological baseline testing when advised and tell child's physician and care team of any issues with learning and memory.

▶ *Consider* THIS!

A 3-year-old boy with sickle cell disease is being admitted to the pediatric unit. He is febrile with rhinorrhea and vomiting over the past 2 to 3 days. He has not been eating well and is complaining of pain in the right leg and refusing to walk. On assessment, you find his vital signs to be as follows: temperature 38.7°C, pulse 132 beats/min, respirations 32 breaths/minute, blood pressure 88/52 mm Hg. He is coughing, he has slightly dusky mucous membranes, and his capillary refill time is 4 seconds.

1. *List nursing assessment findings in order of priority.*
2. *Identify at least three nursing interventions, prioritize them, and list the rationale for the prioritization and the intervention itself.*
3. *List teaching you will perform with this family.*

Thalassemia

Thalassemia is a heterogeneous disorder that results from a defect in globin chain synthesis that affects production of hemoglobin. It occurs primarily in the Mediterranean, Asian, Indian, and Middle Eastern regions (Odame, Sayani, Warner, et al., 2009). As Canada's population becomes more diverse due to immigration from these countries, the number of Canadian thalassemia patients is increasing.

Pathophysiology

The genetics of thalassemia are similar to those of sickle cell disease. The condition is inherited via an autosomal recessive process. Children with thalassemia have reduced production of normal hemoglobin. Remember, normal hemoglobin consists of two alpha globin molecules, two beta globin molecules, and a heme (iron-containing) ring. The normal hemoglobin molecule contains both alpha and beta globin proteins. Each person has four alpha globin genes and two beta globin genes.

There are two basic types of thalassemia, alpha-thalassemia and beta-thalassemia, in which synthesis of the alpha and beta globin chains, respectively, of the hemoglobin protein is reduced or absent. Beta-thalassemia occurs more often. The thalassemias are divided into three subcategories based on severity:

- Thalassemia minor: Beta-thalassemia trait/carrier is due to a mutation of a single beta globin gene, resulting in a mild microcytic anemia that needs no treatment. In the alpha-thalassemia trait, deletions or mutations of two alpha globin genes result in a mild microcytic anemia. In the silent carrier state, there is one alpha globin gene deletion or mutation and patients are asymptomatic.
- Thalassemia intermedia: Children with thalassemia intermedia have a clinically moderate phenotype. They may have more severe anemia, cardiomegaly, and hepatosplenomegaly and may require blood transfusions to maintain adequate quality of life. These patients usually produce a greatly reduced amount of beta globin as a result of mutations that decrease its production.
- Thalassemia major: If both parents carry the alpha-thalassemia trait with two abnormal alpha globin

genes, there is a 25% chance with each pregnancy that the child will have alpha-thalassemia major (hydrops fetalis) with all four alpha genes affected. This causes death before or shortly after birth. In utero blood transfusions have saved some of these children. In beta-thalassemia major, a clinically severe phenotype, mutations inactivate both beta globin genes so no beta globin is produced. Affected children require ongoing medical attention, blood transfusions, and iron removal (chelation therapy) (Catlin, 2003) to survive.

The focus of the following discussion is beta-thalassemia major (Cooley's anemia). In beta-thalassemia major, the beta globin chain synthesis is reduced or entirely absent. Normal Hb A is not made. Instead, four alpha globins associate to form unstable hemoglobin, causing the RBCs to be rigid and hemolyze easily. The result is severe hemolytic anemia and chronic hypoxia. In response to the increased rate of RBC destruction, erythroid activity is increased. The increased activity causes massive bone marrow expansion and thinning of the bony cortex. Growth retardation, pathologic fractures, and skeletal deformities (frontal and maxillary bossing) result. Thalassemia may lead to complications in the cardiac, liver, endocrine, or reproductive system as well as the bones or teeth and may affect nutrition, growth and development, infection response, and fertility (Odame et al., 2009).

Hemosiderosis (excessive supply of iron) is an additional complication of significant concern. It occurs as a result of rapid hemolysis of RBCs, the decrease in hemoglobin production, and the increased absorption of dietary iron in response to the severely anemic state. In addition, each unit of transfused RBCs adds about 200 mg of iron to body stores (Israels, 2009). Without iron chelation, over time the excess iron is deposited in the body's tissues, causing bronze pigmentation of the skin, bony changes, altered organ function (particularly in the cardiac system), and death. Left untreated, beta-thalassemia major is fatal, but the use of chelation therapy and RBC transfusions has increased the life expectancy of these children (Yaish, 2010). The disease is now considered a chronic rather than fatal illness. With an early start of chelation and effective compliance with treatments, these children now may live to adulthood, have children, and lead productive lives.

Therapeutic Management

According to the *Guidelines for the Clinical Care of Patients with Thalassemia in Canada* (Odame et al., 2009), following are the essential components of care:

- Comprehensive care developed using a collaborative network of specialized care centres
- Lifelong patient and family education and close communication with the care team in a culturally sensitive manner
- Support and testing for newly diagnosed infants and provision of genetic counselling

- RBC transfusion program, which involves transfusions every 2 to 4 weeks and monitoring of bloodwork, including screening for hepatitis and HIV
- Assessment of iron overload and availability of ongoing oral or subcutaneous iron chelation therapy, which includes monitoring of calcium and bivalent elements zinc, copper, and selenium
- Multidisciplinary team for psychosocial support
- Discussion of the option of hematopoietic stem cell transplantation
- Transition planning from the pediatric to adult program setting

Nursing Assessment

Infants with thalassemia are usually diagnosed by 1 year of age and have a history of pallor, jaundice, failure to thrive, and hepatosplenomegaly (Yaish, 2010). Determine the history of the present illness and whether the child has started routine blood transfusion. Note medications taken at home and any concerns that have arisen since the last visit. Inspect the skin, oral mucosa, conjunctivae, soles, and/or palms for pallor. Note icteral sclerae, jaundice of the skin, and hepatosplenomegaly. Observe the child for bony deformities and frontal bossing (prominent forehead) (Fig. 46.8). Measure oxygen saturation via pulse oximetry. Evaluate neurologic status, determining level of consciousness and developmental abilities. Measure weight and height and plot on an appropriate growth chart.

Laboratory Testing

As of 2010, universal newborn screening for thalassemia is available only in Ontario. Laboratory results found in beta-thalassemia include (1) significantly decreased hemoglobin, hematocrit, and MCV; (2) peripheral blood smear shows prominence of target cells, hypochromia, microcy-

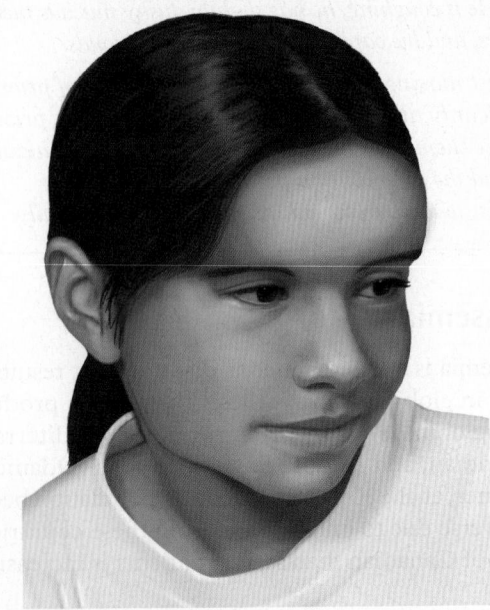

Figure 46.8 Extra-medullary hematopoiesis related to thalassemia leads to bony changes such as frontal bossing and maxillary prominence.

tosis, and extensive **anisocytosis** (variation in cell sizes) and **poikilocytosis** (variation in the shape of the RBCs); (3) elevated bilirubin; (4) hemoglobin electrophoresis shows presence of Hb F and Hb A2 only (Catlin, 2003), unless the patient has been transfused; and (5) elevated iron level.

Nursing Management

Nursing care of the child with thalassemia is aimed primarily at supporting the family and minimizing the effects of the illness as follows.

Coordinating and Contributing to Comprehensive Care

Facilitate communication between subspecialists, disciplines, and the family. Monitor growth and nutrition as well as signs of cardiac, liver, endocrine, bone, infection, and fertility complications.

Administering Packed Red Blood Cell Transfusions

Red cell phenotype all children at diagnosis. Administer pRBC transfusions as prescribed to maintain an adequate level of hemoglobin for oxygen delivery to the tissues and to suppress erythrocytosis and expansion of the bone marrow. For clinical decisions about the amount of RBCs to infuse, consider the desired hemoglobin level, the patient's weight, and the risks of multiple donors. Generally, 15 mL/kg of pRBCs will raise the hemoglobin 30 g/L, and 10 mL/kg will raise hemoglobin 20 g/L (SCIC, 2011b). The trough or pre-transfusion hemoglobin level for patients with thalassemia should fall between 90 and 100 g/L (Odame et al., 2009). Monitor for reactions to the transfusions. Yearly hepatitis A, B, C, and serology and HIV testing should be completed.

Providing Iron Chelation

Excess iron (hemosiderosis) is removed by chelation therapy. Chelation therapy must be done daily at home to decrease or prevent iron accumulation in the body. Administer a chelating agent such as Desferal, which binds to the iron and allows it to be removed through the stool or urine. Teach family members to administer deferoxamine subcutaneously at night with a small battery-powered infusion pump such as the Crono pump and a fine gauge needle such as the Thalaset needle. Monitor for side effects of deferoxamine and the condition of the skin where the needle is inserted. The oral iron chelator deferasirox (Exjade) may also be prescribed for children over 6 years of age.

Educating and Supporting the Family

Educate the child and family about thalassemia major and the recommended treatment regimens. Ensure that families understand that adhering to the prescribed blood transfusion, monitoring, and chelation therapy schedule is essential to the child's survival. Refer the family for genetic counselling and family support as needed. Link educational support with schools and early childhood areas such as day care. Online resources for families of children with thalassemia can be found by visiting http://thePoint.lww.com/Chow1e.

THE BALANCE OF HEMOSTASIS AND BENIGN DISEASES OF THE HEMATOLOGY SYSTEM

Hemostasis is a dynamic balance between bleeding and clotting that is achieved within the body. Hemostasis is influenced by vascular spasm, blood components (specifically formation of the platelet plug where the platelets adhere to damaged epithelium), and the blood coagulation system. See Figure 46.9.

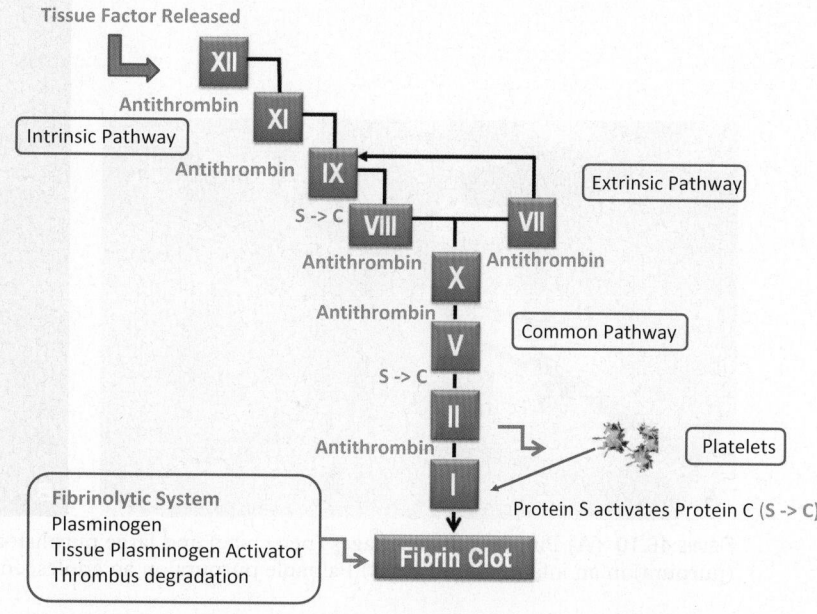

FIGURE 46.9 Coagulation Cascade. Used with permission from SolutionSight, Inc.

The coagulation system requires proteins, factors, and platelets to perform adequately. Individuals with factor or platelet deficiencies tend to bleed. They do not bleed more easily than people without these conditions, but it is more difficult for clots to form in these individuals; therefore, achieving hemostasis takes more time and requires appropriate treatment.

Factors that are most often involved in problems with clotting include factors VIII, IX, and XI, each of which plays a role in the coagulation cascade. Platelets also play a role in coagulation and are necessary for clot formation. Some processes can lead to destruction of the platelets and may lead to a reduction in clotting.

There are two important laboratory tests for assessing the components of the coagulation pathways that influence hemostasis:

• Prothrombin time (PT) is a coagulation test that reflects components of the extrinsic and common pathways, including factors II, V, VII, X, and fibrinogen. The international normalized ratio (INR) is calculated from the PT and reported to minimize variation related to reagents between different laboratories. Because thromboplastins for various reagents affect rates of clotting, the INR is a calculation that was developed and used to avoid some of the variability of PT measurement.
• Partial thromboplastin time (PTT) is a coagulation test that reflects the integrity of the intrinsic and common clotting pathways, including factors I, II, V, VIII, IX, X, XI, XII, and fibrinogen.

See Table 46.4 for values for clotting studies.

Conditions that affect clotting include ITP, DIC, and factor deficiencies such as hemophilia A (factor VIII deficiency), vWD, hemophilia B (Christmas disease, factor IX deficiency), and hemophilia C (factor XI defi-

ciency). Thrombophilia refers to a hypercoagulation syndrome. Table 46.3 reviews the proteins involved in coagulation. Visit http://thePoint.lww.com/Chow1e for a table that describes the plasma protein products available from Canadian Blood Services.

Diseases of the Hematology System that Produce Bleeding

Neonatal Allo–Immune Thrombocytopenia

Neonates can develop an immune thrombocytopenia that has potential to cause bleeding and intracranial hemorrhage. A pregnant woman who lacks a platelet antigen, such as PLA-1, may develop allo-immune sensitization if the fetus has the antigen on its platelets. The mother produces antibodies that cross the placenta and cause the destruction of the platelets in the fetus.

Idiopathic Thrombocytopenic Purpura

Pathophysiology

ITP is thought to be caused by an abnormal immune response involving the B and T lymphocytes. ITP usually develops about 1 to 4 weeks after a viral infection that triggers production of antiplatelet antibodies (Ambruso et al., 2011). These antibodies lead to the destruction of platelets, usually in the spleen. Secondary causes of ITP may include collagen vascular disorders, immune deficiencies, and certain chronic infections (Blanchette & Bolton-Maggs, 2008).

ITP results in petechiae, purpura, and excessive bruising. Petechiae are pinpoint hemorrhages that can occur anywhere on the body. They are red, have a smooth surface, and do not blanch to pressure (Fig. 46.10A).

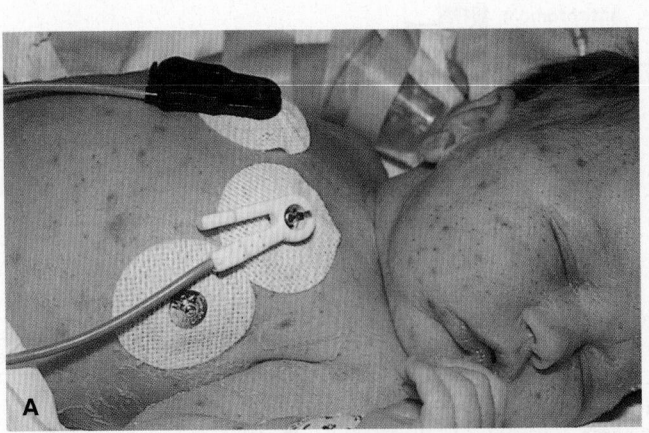
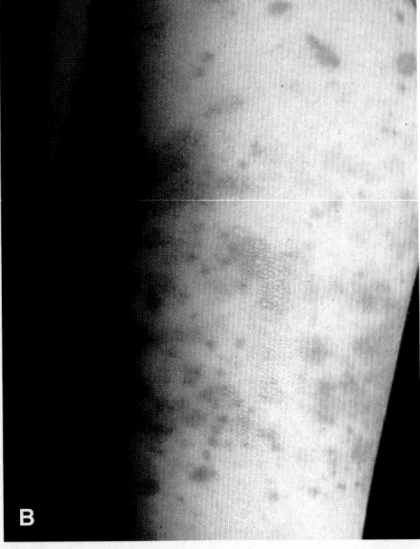

FIGURE 46.10 (A) Pinpoint hemorrhages (petechiae) and large purplish areas of discoloration (purpura) in an infant with ITP. (B) Palpable purpura on an adolescent's arm.

Purpura is the appearance of larger purplish areas of hemorrhage in which blood collects under the tissues, including the buccal surfaces (Fig. 46.10B). Complications of ITP range from minor hemorrhage such as epistaxis, bleeding gums, and blood in the urine or stool to severe hemorrhage and bleeding into vital organs, including intracranial hemorrhage, although these severe complications rarely occur.

ITP is usually self-limiting, but some children will need referral for follow-up care with a pediatric hematologist. Remission is seen in 80% to 90% of the children within 6 to 9 months (Yetman, 2003). Generally, ITP that persists longer than 6 months is described as chronic ITP (Blanchette & Bolton-Maggs, 2008).

Treatment

Blanchette & Bolton-Maggs (2008) have described a number of treatment strategies for children with platelet counts below 20×10^9/L. These strategies include use of specific doses of a corticosteroid, such as prednisone or dexamethasone, or intravenous immunoglobulin (IVIG), among other treatments. If the child has only a few mild symptoms, is not hemorrhagic, and has a platelet count above 10×10^9/L, some physicians may "watch and wait" to see if the platelet count improves on its own. Platelet transfusions are not indicated unless serious bleeding or a life-threatening condition such as intracranial hemorrhage is present.

Rituximab therapy is a regimen increasingly used for refractory ITP but currently requires randomized controlled trials for stronger clinical evidence. Splenectomy is considered a second-line therapy and is generally used only if other treatment regimens fail (Blanchette & Bolton-Maggs, 2008) or if the patient has life-threatening bleeding. Other new therapies currently in trials for refractory ITP include the TPO agonists romiplostim (Nplate) and eltrombopag (Promacta).

Nursing Assessment

Elicit the child's health history (usually a previously healthy child who recently has developed increased bruising, epistaxis, or bleeding of the gums). Note history of blood in the stool and urine or menorrhagia. Note risk factors such as recent viral illness, recent MMR immunization, or ingestion of medications that can cause thrombocytopenia or alter platelet function such as NSAIDs (e.g., ibuprofen). Inspect for petechiae, purpura, and bruising, which may progress rapidly within the first 24 to 48 hours of the illness. Document the size and location of lesions. Inspect the lips and buccal mucosa for petechiae and purpura. Palpate for lymphadenopathy and organomegaly. The remainder of the physical examination is usually within normal limits.

Usual laboratory findings include a low platelet count ($<50 \times 10^9$/L), normal WBC count and differential, and normal hemoglobin and hematocrit levels unless hemorrhage has occurred (rare). Treatment is usually initiated if the platelet count is less than 20×10^9/L or if there is bleeding. If other cytopenias or abnormalities are noted on the peripheral smear, or if lymphadenopathy with or without organomegaly is present, a bone marrow aspiration may be performed to rule out leukemia before corticosteroid therapy is started.

Nursing Management

Many children with ITP require no medical treatment except observation and re-evaluation of laboratory values. Educate the family to avoid aspirin, NSAIDs, and cold or sinus remedies because these medications may precipitate the development of bleeding in these children. Acetaminophen may be used for pain control when necessary. Teach the child and family about the side effects of treatments such as steroids and IVIG and how to prevent trauma by avoiding activities that may cause injury. Participating in contact sports, specifically activities in which direct contact can lead to injury or trauma, is not recommended unless the platelet count is over 50×10^9/L. Activities such as swimming provide physical activity with less risk of trauma. Parents also need to know the signs and symptoms of serious bleeding, who to call if bleeding is suspected, and when to seek emergency treatment in a hospital setting. Visit http://thePoint.lww.com/Chow1e for online educational resources on ITP.

Hemophilia

Pathophysiology

Hemophilia A and B are genetic diseases that result in deficiency of clotting factor VIII or IX. Factor VIII and IX genes are on the X chromosome, so males are usually affected as they have only one X chromosome that they may inherit from a carrier mother. Hemophilia may be due to a new mutation in the boy. Thirty percent of patients have a new mutation, so anyone might have a child with hemophilia even if there is no family history.

The coagulation factors in the blood are activated when bleeding starts. If one factor is missing, then bleeding will continue until the missing factor is infused intravenously. The coagulation cascade comprises three pathways. The intrinsic pathway is affected by deficiencies of factor VIII and IX and is measured by the PTT. The extrinsic pathway includes tissue factor and factor VII and is measured by the PT. The point at which these pathways converge is called the common pathway. Abnormalities in this pathway result in prolongation of PT and PTT.

The steps in coagulation are (1) vasoconstriction, (2) platelet plug formation, and (3) activation of the coagulation cascade. In hemophilia, the first two steps occur normally and the problem arises in the third step. Visit http://thePoint.lww.com/Chow1e for illustrations of normal coagulation and defect in hemophilia coagulation.

The most common type of hemophilia is A (Karp & Riddell, 2010), which is the focus of this discussion. Hemophilia A occurs when there is a deficiency of factor VIII in an individual. Hemophilia is classified according to the severity of the disease, which is determined by the amount of factor VIII present expressed as a percentage of normal. The disease can be mild (5% to 50%), moderate (1% to 5%), or severe (less than 1%). The normal range is 50% to 150%. Factor VIII is essential in the activation of factor X, which is required to convert prothrombin to thrombin, which is required for the generation of fibrin to stabilize a clot. Without clot stabilization the bleeding continues. The more severe the disease, the more likely bleeding episodes will occur.

Treatment

The primary goal in hemophilia is to prevent bleeding. This is best accomplished by avoiding activities that have a high potential for injury, such as contact sports, and instead participating in physical activities with the least amount of contact, such as swimming. Children are encouraged to be active and take part in as many low-risk activities as possible as this keeps their muscles and bones strong.

If bleeding or injury occurs, factor administration is prescribed; this practice has been common for many years in out-patient facilities or in the home. Once the deficient factor is replaced, clotting factors return to fairly normal levels for a period of time. The half-life of factor VIII is approximately 12 hours, so a repeat treatment may be needed every 12 hours until bleeding subsides. Factor replacement should be administered before any surgeries or other traumas that can lead to bleeding, such as intramuscular injections and dental care.

Most centres in Canada now promote prophylaxis in children with severe hemophilia starting at about 1 year of age. This means giving an intravenous infusion of the missing factor one to three times per week, thereby preventing almost all bleeding episodes and thus preserving the child's joints and resulting in less joint replacement surgery as children enter adulthood. The infusion may be performed at home by the parent or child following intense training at a centre for bleeding disorders.

If a breakthrough bleed does occur, the dosage and frequency of factor replacement may be increased since the child may have grown. If bleeding continues, then an inhibitor screen is conducted in order to check for an inhibitor, which is an immune response in which the body destroys its own factor VIII as well as any factor VIII that is administered. If an inhibitor is present, the treatment will have to be changed to a bypassing agent that will stimulate the coagulation cascade but will not replace the missing factor VIII.

Nursing Assessment
Health History

Elicit the health history, determining the nature of the bleeding episode or bruise. Include in the history any

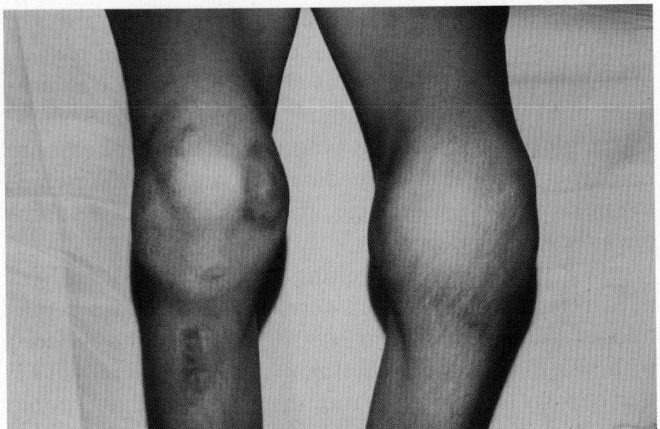

FIGURE 46.11 Significant swelling and discoloration associated with a bleeding episode in a hemophiliac's knee.

hemorrhagic episodes in other systems, such as the gastrointestinal tract (e.g., black, tarry stools; hematemesis), or any injuries that result in joint hemorrhage or hematuria (Fig. 46.11). Inquire about length of bleeding and amount of blood loss. Because hemophilia A results in difficulty with clotting, the child may bleed for a longer period when injury occurs. A simple mouth bleed could be life-threatening.

Physical Examination

Focus the physical examination on identification of any bleeding. This is of particular concern after injury, but a spontaneous bleed can occur if factor levels are extremely low. Assess joint or muscle bleeding by focusing on a pain scale and determining whether all joints can rotate through a full range of motion. Assess circulation by evaluating pulses and heart sounds if severe or prolonged bleeding is identified; without intervention, hypovolemia could follow, leading to shock. Note chest pain or abdominal pain, which may indicate internal bleeding. Report these findings immediately so that the underlying condition can be diagnosed and treated rapidly (Fig. 46.12).

Laboratory and Diagnostic Testing

Laboratory findings may include decreased hemoglobin and hematocrit if bleeding is prolonged or severe. Factor levels may be quantified with blood testing. An inhibitor screen may be important if child has not responded to previous factor VIII infusions. X-rays of a swollen joint in a child with hemophilia are not necessary unless there has been a severe trauma. Computed tomography of the head is definitely indicated if the child has had a significant bump or has lost consciousness.

Nursing Management

Nursing management includes preventing bleeding episodes, managing bleeding episodes, and providing education and support.

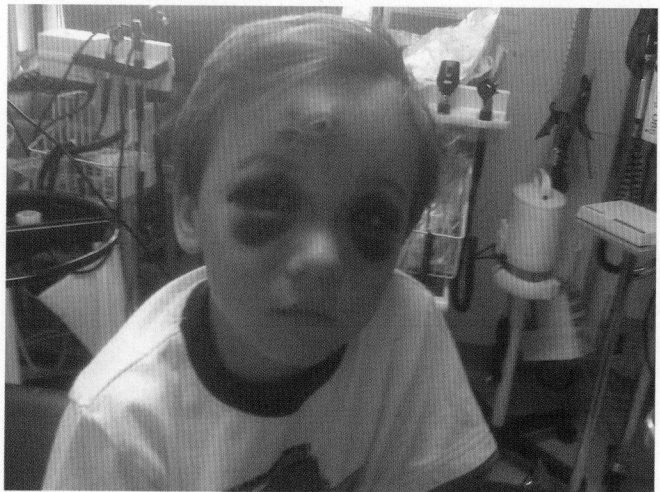

FIGURE 46.12 Boy with hemophilia.

Preventing Bleeding Episodes

All patients with hemophilia should attempt to prevent bleeding episodes. Major bleeds into the joints may limit range of motion and function, eventually decreasing physical abilities and crippling some boys (Karp & Riddell, 2010). Teach children and families that regular physical activity or exercise helps make the muscles and joints stronger, and children with stronger joints and muscles experience fewer bleeding episodes (Teaching Guideline 46.2). Refer any child who is diagnosed with hemophilia to a pediatric hematologist and/or a comprehensive hemophilia treatment centre.

Managing a Bleeding Episode

Administer factor VIII replacement as prescribed as soon as possible. Most factor VIII products in Canada are now made using recombinant technology. Disease transmission has never occurred with these products. Sucrose is used in some products instead of albumin to stabilize the factor VIII molecule.

Administer factor replacement by slow IV push. Document the product name, number of units given, lot number, and expiration date. Doses are based on the severity of the bleeding and the weight of the child. In mild cases of hemophilia A, desmopressin (DDAVP) may be effective in stopping bleeding (see Nursing Management in the von Willebrand Disease section for additional information).

All patients with hemophilia in Canada are registered with a hemophilia treatment centre and carry a "Factor First" card, which includes demographic information, the type of hemophilia, and the product and dosage to be used for treatment. If external bleeding develops, apply pressure to the area until bleeding stops. If bleeding is inside a joint, apply ice or cold compresses to the area, elevate the limb, and give factor replacement as soon as possible. Ensure that cases of bleeding are followed up to identify whether additional factor replacement is necessary.

Providing Education

All patients should wear a health alert bracelet from the time they are diagnosed. Families should notify the school nurse and teachers of the child's diagnosis and share precautions with them. The bleeding disorders nurse may conduct an in-service at the school and instruct the teachers or caregivers to call the parent and an ambulance immediately if the child sustains a head, abdominal, or orbital injury at school. Parents should be called if the child complains of pain in a joint or muscle. All hemophilia treatment centres in Canada have home infusion programs where parents are taught to administer the factor via a peripheral vein or central venous access device. Arrange for factor replacement therapy to be available in one local hospital if the family does not live near a hemophilia treatment centre. Involve children as developmentally appropriate in the infusion process. Young children may hold and apply the Band-Aid; older children may assist with dilution and mixing of the factor; and teens should be taught to administer their own factor infusions.

Providing Support

Children with hemophilia may be able to lead a fairly normal life, with the exception of avoiding a few activities. For parents, however, accepting the diagnosis of a bleeding disorder in their child is very difficult. They fear the worst (bleeding that won't stop) as well as complications such as infection with blood-borne viruses. Reassure parents that the products used to treat their child's bleeding disorder are now very safe. Although factor replacement is expensive, it is paid for by Canadian Blood Services, and everything else that is required to treat a bleeding episode is supplied by the hemophilia treatment centre. Refer families to the Canadian Hemophilia Society, which has chapters in all provinces and many dedicated volunteers who are familiar with what they are going through. Every province also has a family camp or picnics where parents can meet each other and/or a summer camp where the children can make friends with others who have the same diagnosis.

TEACHING GUIDELINE 46.2

Preventing Bleeding in the Child with Hemophilia

- Protect toddlers with soft helmets, padding on the knees, carpets in the home, and softened or covered corners on furniture.
- Children should stay active: swimming, baseball, basketball, and bicycling (wearing a helmet) are good physical activities.
- Avoid intense contact sports, such as football, wrestling, soccer, and high diving.
- Avoid trampoline use and riding all-terrain vehicles.

von Willebrand Disease and Platelet Function Disorders

Pathophysiology

vWD is a genetically transmitted bleeding disorder that can affect both genders and all races. It is due to abnormalities in function or to a qualitative defect or quantitative deficiency in von Willebrand factor (vWF). Under ordinary circumstances, vWF serves two functions: to bind with factor VIII, protecting it from degradation, and to serve as the "glue" that attaches platelets to the site of injury. If platelets cannot attach, then the second step in coagulation is compromised and the patient cannot form a proper platelet plug. There are several types of vWD ranging from mild to severe. The disease usually manifests as a mild-to-moderate bleeding disorder. Children with vWD bruise easily, have frequent nosebleeds (epistaxis), and tend to bleed after oral surgery. Menstruating females often have menorrhagia.

Treatment

Some patients respond to desmopressin, while others need vWF infusions for bleeding or injury. vWF concentrate or desmopressin may be administered to help form a clot. Desmopressin raises the factor VIII and vWF level in plasma by releasing them from the stores in the endothelium of the blood vessels into the bloodstream. vWF concentrate replaces what is missing. These products may also be administered prior to dental work or surgery. An antifibrinolytic agent can be prescribed to stabilize clots once they have formed and may be given in pill form or intravenously three times a day for 5 to 7 days, or longer for menorrhagia or surgery. Alternatively, it may be taken as a mouthwash three or four times per day for 5 to 7 days. The most commonly used antifibrinolytic in Canada is tranexamic acid.

Nursing Assessment

Health History

Children with vWD and/or platelet function disorders may have frequent epistaxis. Nursing assessment of these children is similar to that of the child with hemophilia, although severe bleeding occurs much less frequently in vWD. Children who have severe (type III) vWD will experience similar bleeding problems as children with hemophilia. For all other types of vWD and platelet function disorders, the assessment should concentrate on pain or external bleeding. Question caregivers about the length of bleeding and the amount of blood loss. Remember that a mouth bleed or epistaxis can be life-threatening.

Physical Examination

Physical examination should concentrate on the site of oozing or pain. Note chest pain or abdominal pain and report findings immediately.

Laboratory and Diagnostic Testing

Laboratory testing may include decreased hemoglobin and hematocrit depending on how long the child has been bleeding. An ultrasound of the affected area may be necessary to determine the extent of internal bleeding.

Nursing Management

Nursing management includes preventing bleeding episodes, managing a bleeding episode, and education and support.

Preventing Bleeding Episodes

Prevention of bleeding episodes in children with vWD may be more difficult than with hemophilia because children with vWD tend to have more spontaneous mucous membrane bleeding that is not always the result of trauma. Encourage parents to keep a moist environment in order to decrease epistaxis.

Managing a Bleeding Episode

Nursing management is also similar to management of the child with hemophilia. The major difference is the administration of desmopressin. Administer desmopressin as prescribed when a bleeding episode occurs. Desmopressin may be given via intravenous infusion, subcutaneously, or via a nasal spray. It is an antidiuretic hormone, so closely monitor fluid balance and blood pressure. No more than three doses in a row should be given, 8 to 12 hours apart. The response decline (tachyphylaxis) occurs with usage due to depletion of stored clotting factor. Antifibrinolytics are important for treatment of mucous membrane bleeding in children with bleeding disorders as they prevent the formed clot from breaking down. vWD may also be treated with intravenous infusion of vWF derived from pooled plasma from multiple blood donors treated with heat and solvent to inactivate viruses.

Education and Support

All children with bleeding disorders should be registered with a centre for bleeding disorders or a hemophilia centre. They should wear a health alert bracelet and also carry a Factor First card filled out by their hematologist. These cards are available from the hemophilia comprehensive care clinics in major cities in Canada and throughout the world. Refer families to the Canadian Hemophilia Society.

Diseases of the Hematology System That Produce Clotting

Thrombosis in Infants and Children

Physiology

Normal physiologic hemostasis is dependent upon maintaining a fine balance between thrombosis and hemorrhage. Coagulation and fibrinolysis are responsible for hemostasis and have a number of protein components that, when activated by a stimulus, interact with RBCs and platelets and result in thrombus formation (coagulation) and/or thrombus degradation (fibrinolysis). Alterations in blood flow, composition, and vessel wall integrity have been recognized as the most important elements involved in thrombus formation.

Normal hemostasis results in a fine balance between bleeding and clotting. Procoagulant proteins present in the blood (factors XII, XI, X, IX, VIII, VII, V, II, and fibrinogen) are activated by a stimulus (e.g., sepsis, trauma, surgery) to produce thrombin (factor IIa). Thrombin activates fibrinogen into fibrin, the precursor of a polymerized clot. The **fibrinolytic system** is then activated to break down (lyse) the clot. Inhibitor proteins of hemostasis (**antithrombin**, protein C, protein S, alpha-2 macroglobulin) and fibrinolysis (plasminogen activator inhibitor-1 [PAI-1]) are present to prevent massive clot formation or clot lysis, respectively.

Differences in Children: Developmental Physiology

Children have a number of differences in hemostasis and fibrinolysis compared with adults that affect the incidence, treatment, and long-term outcome of thrombosis (Andrew, Paes, Milner, et al., 1987, 1988; Andrew, Vegh, Johnston, et al.; Kuhle & Massicotte, 2005). The levels of contact factors (factors XII, X) and vitamin K–dependent factors (factors II, VII, IX and X) are decreased until approximately 6 months of age (Andrew et al., 1987, 1988, 1992). Thrombin generation is decreased 30% to 50% in children as compared with adult levels (Andrew, Schmidt, Mitchell, Paes, & Ofosu, 1990; Andrew, Mitchell, Vegh, et al., 1994). The inhibitors of hemostasis are present in varying amounts in children: decreased protein C, protein S, and antithrombin and increased alpha-2 macroglobulin. The fibrinolytic system is downregulated (Andrew et al., 1987; 1988; 1992).

Children at Risk for Thrombosis

Venous thrombosis in children most often occurs as a result of the interaction of multiple risk factors. The presence of a central venous catheter is one of the strongest risk factors, accounting for 90% and 63% of symptomatic venous thrombosis cases in neonates and children, respectively (Massicotte, Dix, Monagle, et al., 1998; Nowak-Gottl, von Kries, & Gobel, 1997; Van Ommen, Heijboer, Buller, et al., 2001). Arterial thrombosis in children most often occurs following placement of an arterial line or after cardiac catheterization. Currently, there are no data to support the use of routine thromboprophylaxis of central venous or arterial catheters in children. In addition, children with congenital heart disease and children undergoing liver transplantation are at increased risk for thrombosis.

Thrombophilia Pathophysiology

Congenital thrombophilia refers to an alteration in the levels of proteins that facilitate and inhibit clotting. Congenital prothrombotic disorders are relatively rare but most

commonly include factor V Leiden, prothrombin gene G20210A mutation, and deficiencies of protein C, protein S, and antithrombin. The influence of congenital thrombophilia on childhood thrombosis remains controversial.

Clinical Complications and Long-Term Effects of Systemic Venous Thrombosis

The incidence of post-thrombotic syndrome in children with confirmed deep venous or arterial thrombosis determined through international registry data is reported to be approximately 20% (Barnes, Newall, & Monagle, 2002; Biss, Kahr, Brandão, et al., 2009; Kuhle, Koloshuk, Marzinotto, et al., 2003; Kuhle, Spavor, Massicotte, et al., 2008). Post-thrombotic syndrome is characterized by pain, swelling, alterations in perfusion, and poor venous return, which may result in skin ulceration. Although there is no treatment, the use of properly fitted and regularly worn compression stockings may reduce symptoms of post-thrombotic syndrome (including pain), preserve vascular valves, and improve venous return (Biss et al., 2009; Musani, Matta, Yaekoub, et al., 2010; ten Cate-Hoek, ten Cate, Tordoir, et al., 2010). Visit http://thePoint.lww.com/Chow1e for a detailed Nursing Care Plan "Overview for the Child With Deep Venous Thrombosis."

Nursing Assessment

Upon completion of a thorough assessment, the nurse might identify several nursing diagnosis, including:

- Risk for pain related to vaso-occlusive event
- Risk for fatigue related to decreased oxygen supply with pulmonary embolus
- Risk for anxiety related to the diagnosis
- Risk for needle phobias. The child may experience pain and anxiety related to anticoagulation therapy (subcutaneous injections and/or frequent blood monitoring).
- Potential poor venous access

Health History

Assess for risk factors for thrombosis, including the presence or attempted insertion of a central venous or central arterial catheter. Elicit the birth, past, and maternal and family history for thrombosis. The history may be significant for previous thrombotic events (deep venous thrombosis, myocardial infarction, stroke, miscarriages) occurring in family members at a young age and for family members prescribed long-term anticoagulation therapy. A positive patient and/or family history may indicate a congenital risk for thrombophilia.

Physical Examination
Inspection and Observation

Assess loss of central venous or central arterial catheter patency, swelling, pain, and discoloration of the related limb. Assess for respiratory distress, decreased oxygen saturation, increased oxygen requirements, and pleuritic chest pain, which may indicate pulmonary embolus. Swelling of the face and head may occur with bilateral upper venous thrombosis, also known as superior vena cava syndrome.

Palpation

Palpate proximal and peripheral pulses for strength and equality. Determine capillary refill time (may be prolonged when circulating blood volume is decreased). Note temperature and elasticity of skin and interruption of spontaneous movement of the affected limb.

Laboratory and Diagnostic Testing

Measurement of prothrombotic markers will not alter the initial treatment plan and should not be performed during the acute phase of the thrombosis since inhibitors (specifically protein C, protein S, and antithrombin) may be consumed in the thrombus, leading to false-positive results. Antiphospholipid antibody may be measured in children with catastrophic venous thromboembolism.

The most sensitive methods for diagnosing upper system thrombosis are ultrasound for jugular venous thrombosis and venography for intrathoracic vessels (Massicotte et al., 1998). Ultrasound may be used to diagnose symptomatic thrombosis of both the upper and lower system; however, if clinical suspicion is high for thrombosis and the ultrasound is negative, a venogram is recommended (Monagle, Chan, Massicotte, et al., 2008). Magnetic resonance imaging of the venous or arterial system may be used, although the sensitivity and specificity of these imaging studies have not been evaluated in children. Furthermore, while there are no studies determining the sensitivity and specificity of diagnostic testing for pulmonary embolus in children, the following radiographic tests may be used: ventilation–perfusion scan, spiral computed tomography, magnetic resonance imaging, magnetic resonance venography, or pulmonary angiography. Oxygen saturation may be decreased with pulmonary embolus.

Therapeutic Management

Treatment of thrombosis is important due to the associated morbidity and mortality. Unlike in adults, even asymptomatic clots in children can result in serious sequelae:

- Many children have intracardiac blood shunts (right–left); thus venous thrombi may result in stroke (Barnes, Newall, Furmedge, et al., 2004).
- There is an association between sepsis and thrombosis (Randolph, Cook, Gonzales, et al., 1998a; Randolph, Cook, Gonzalez, et al., 1998b).
- Pulmonary embolism is often asymptomatic in children due to large cardiopulmonary reserves and may be life-threatening (Brandão, Kahr, et al., 2008; Kotsakis, Cook, Griffith, et al., 2005; Monagle, Adams, Mahoney, et al., 2000; Monreal, Raventos, Lerma, et al., 1994; Sridhar, Rao, & Chakraborty, 2005).

- Loss of venous access, which may be required for future intervention in a patient population who will require lifelong medical support (Monagle et al., 2008)
- Post-thrombotic syndrome (Goldenberg, 2005; Kuhle et al., 2003; 2008)

The therapeutic management of children with venous or arterial thrombosis focuses on preventing extension, recurrence, or embolization of the thrombus. The duration and intensity of therapy are based on adult recommendations and may be in excess of what is required in children. Until studies are completed, it is reasonable to base therapy on adult recommendations (Monagle et al., 2008). Newly diagnosed thrombosis is treated with 5 to 7 days of heparin therapy, which may be followed by continued heparin or warfarin therapy. If thrombosis occurs secondary to a risk factor, then therapy is currently recommended for 3 months providing the risk factor has been resolved or eliminated (e.g., central venous catheter has been removed). If the risk factor remains, then long-term therapy may be considered. With idiopathic thrombosis (no risk factor identified), a minimum of 6 to 12 months of therapy may be considered.

Therapeutic agents commonly used in children include heparin and oral vitamin K antagonists (warfarin). Current data support the premise that when patients are maintained within their defined therapeutic range they will be adequately protected from the risk of thrombosis without incurring an undue risk of side effects (Ansell, Hirsh, Hylek, et al., 2008; Hirsh, Dalen, Anderson, et al., 2001; Monagle et al., 2008). Newer agents, such as direct thrombin inhibitors, are available, although data supporting their use are limited. Nevertheless, there are clinical situations in which these agents must be used, such as in confirmed HIT (Monagle et al., 2008; Young, Yonekawa, Nakagawa, et al., 2004; Young, Tarantino, Wohrley, et al., 2007). See Evidence-based Practice 46.1.

Heparin is a term that describes unfractionated (standard) heparin (UFH) and low-molecular-weight heparin (LMWH). While both are heparins, LMWH is modified using enzymes to reduce molecular size, leading to a more specific inhibition of activated factor Xa. Additional discussion of these therapies and nursing management is available at http://thePoint.lww.com/Chow1e.

Diseases of the Hematology System That Produce Bleeding and Clotting

Disseminated Intravascular Coagulation

Pathophysiology

DIC is a condition that significantly alters the balance of hemostasis; it most often results in bleeding, although may result in simultaneous clotting/thrombosis

EVIDENCE-BASED PRACTICE 46.1
Reducing Medication Errors with Heparin

● **Background**

Enoxaparin is a low-molecular-weight-heparin (LMWH) commonly used for thromboprophylaxis in children. Enoxaparin dosing is based on the patient's weight and results in decimal dosing. Due to the high concentration of enoxaparin, the resultant decimal dose makes precise measurement difficult. Dilution is necessary and often results in 10-fold medication administration errors. Enoxaparin may be administered in whole-milligram doses via insulin syringe, where 1 mg of enoxaparin equals 1 U on the 100-U graduated insulin syringe.

▲ **Study**

The authors instituted a clinical practice in which enoxaparin was ordered in whole-milligram doses and administered using an insulin syringe, where 1 mg of enoxaparin equals 1 U on the 100-U graduated insulin syringe.

■ **Findings**

Data were collected on 514 consecutive children, ages 2 days to 17 years, with various indications for anticoagu-lation and a total of 2,842 doses of enoxaparin administered. Throughout the treatment period, no infant or child required a dose with decimals in order to achieve therapeutic enoxaparin levels. The results of this study clearly establish that whole-milligram dosing of enoxaparin measured and administered with an insulin syringe is an effective approach for administering enoxaparin. There were no hemorrhagic events associated with the less than 1% of supra-therapeutic anti-factor Xa levels. All children achieved a therapeutic anti-factor Xa level with a whole-milligram dose, and there were no reported dose measurement errors.

● **Nursing Implications**

To reduce the incidence of enoxaparin dosing errors, whole-milligram dosing of enoxaparin administered via insulin syringe ought to be considered as the standard of care. Simplifying enoxaparin dose measurement results in decreased dosing errors and facilitates straightforward knowledge transfer to the parent who is required to administer enoxaparin at home.

Bauman, M. E., Black, K. L., Bauman, M. L., et al. (2009). Novel uses of insulin syringes to reduce dosing errors: a retrospective chart review of enoxaparin whole milligram dosing. *Thrombosis Research, 123*(6), 845–847.

(Kleinpell, 2003). DIC may be caused by a number of different abnormal clinical stimuli, including sepsis, trauma, serious tissue injury, head injury, fat embolism, myeloproliferative disorders, solid tumours, vascular disorders, giant hemangioma, reactions to toxins (e.g., snake venom, drugs), immunologic disorders, hemolytic transfusion reactions, and transplant rejection. The syndrome results from massive tissue factor release causing systemic activation of the coagulation pathway and thrombin generation, intravascular formation of fibrin and, ultimately, thrombotic occlusion of small and medium-sized vessels. Platelets and coagulation proteins are consumed in this process, thus often simultaneously resulting in massive bleeding.

DIC is mostly associated with adverse outcomes. Although bleeding and thrombosis are clinical features of DIC, organ failure is more common. Hemorrhage and organ tissue damage can be irreversible if not recognized and treated immediately (Franchini & Manzato, 2004).

Treatment of DIC is aimed at the underlying cause: antibiotics for sepsis, multiorgan support, circulatory resuscitation, inotropic support, ventilation, hemodialysis, replacement therapy with blood products, or anticoagulation. A novel treatment strategy in DIC and sepsis to restore the activated protein C pathway has not been demonstrated to be beneficial in young children (Kylat & Ohlsson, 2006).

Nursing Assessment

DIC occurs as a secondary condition; it may occur in a hospitalized child for any reason. DIC can affect any body system, so a thorough physical examination is warranted. Inspect for signs of bleeding, such as petechiae or purpura, blood in the urine or stool, or persistent oozing from a venipuncture site or from the umbilical cord in the newborn. Evaluate respiratory status and determine the level of tissue oxygenation via pulse oximetry. Perform a complete circulatory assessment and note signs of circulatory collapse such as poor perfusion, tachycardia, prolonged capillary refill time, and weak distal pulses. Note altered level of consciousness and decreased urine output. Careful abdominal palpation may reveal hepatomegaly or splenomegaly.

Laboratory testing may reveal prolonged PT and PTT and decreased levels of fibrinogen; platelets; clotting factors II, V, VIII, and X; and antithrombin III. Increases in fibrinolysin and fibrinopeptide levels will be noted (Kylat & Ohlsson, 2006).

Nursing Management

Continue to provide nursing care related to the triggering event. Assess the patient's status frequently. If bleeding is observed, apply pressure to the area along with cold compresses. Elevate the affected body part if this does not affect the patient's overall stability. If neurologic deficits are assessed, report the findings immediately so that treatment to prevent permanent damage can be started. Provide ventilatory support as needed, and provide continuous cardiac monitoring. Administer clotting factors, platelets, and cryoprecipitate as prescribed to prevent severe hemorrhage (Franchini & Manzato, 2004). Report changes in laboratory values to the physician. Changes can occur rapidly, and vigilance is necessary to prevent further tissue damage to the affected system.

■■■ Key Concepts

- ■ The common forms of anemia affecting children are iron-deficiency anemia, sickle cell anemia, thalassemia, and G6PD deficiency.
- ■ The important bleeding disorders affecting children are ITP, DIC, hemophilia, and vWD.
- ■ Assess for hypoxia, fatigue, and pallor in the child with anemia.
- ■ Nursing assessment for the child with a bleeding disorder focuses on determining its extent and severity. If the child is actively bleeding, treat first and assess/investigate later.
- ■ Supplementation with iron is the key intervention for the child with iron-deficiency anemia.
- ■ Prevention of infection and management of vaso-occlusive episodes are key in children with sickle cell anemia.
- ■ Multimodal pain management and astute physical assessment for serious complications are critical in the nursing care of the child having a sickle cell crisis.
- ■ The priority intervention for management of thalassemia is chronic transfusion of pRBCs and chelation of iron.
- ■ ITP is usually a self-limiting disease.
- ■ Urgent administration of factor VIII or desmopressin is the key nursing intervention when a bleeding episode occurs in the child with hemophilia or vWD.
- ■ Significant anemia may result in hypoxia to the tissues.
- ■ Prevention of injury is key for all children with bleeding disorders.
- ■ Children with hemophilia do not bleed faster than others, but they will continue to bleed until the missing factor is infused.
- ■ Venous access is an important consideration for prophylaxis in hemophilia.
- ■ Administration of coagulation factor should be the first intervention in a child with hemophilia who is bleeding.
- ■ Patient and family teaching for anemias resulting from nutritional deficiencies focuses on promotion of a diet high in the deficient nutrients or on more rapid therapeutic replacement.
- ■ Patient and family teaching for bleeding disorders focuses on recognition of the need to treat the condition and prevent injury.

- ■ Numerous national and local resources on hematologic disorders or nutritional deficits are available, providing a wide range of services that include education, support, multidisciplinary care (as appropriate), and financial assistance for affected children.
- ■ The components of blood—cells, clotting factors, and inhibitors of coagulation and fibrinolysis—are tightly regulated; disruptions in the balance of these components may result in disease.
- ■ Knowledge of specific genetic or acquired disease pathophysiology is essential for effective nursing care in patients with hematologic disease. Nursing interventions must respond to the symptoms associated with anemia, thrombocytopenia, infection, bleeding, and clotting.
- ■ Knowledge regarding side effects and safe administration of blood products, clotting factors, and drugs is essential to hematology nursing.
- ■ A comprehensive systems approach to care is required as blood diseases often affect multiple organ systems. Sharing of knowledge among clinical specialties and with families, schools, and communities is required.
- ■ Children are not little adults; coagulation differs in children due to developmental hemostasis.
- ■ Developmental hemostasis influences the etiology, treatment, and outcomes of deep venous thrombosis in children.
- ■ Central venous catheters are essential to the care of ill children and are highly associated with thrombosis (30% to 50%).

REFERENCES

Ambruso, D. R., Hays, T., & Goldenberg, N. A. (2011). Hematologic disorders. In W. W. Hay, M. J. Levin, J. M. Sondheimer, & R. R. Deterding (Eds.), *Current pediatric diagnosis and treatment* (20th ed.). New York: McGraw-Hill.

American Academy of Pediatrics. (2009). *Lead exposure in children: prevention, detection, and management.* Retrieved January 9, 2012 from http://aappolicy.aappublications.org/cgi/content/full/pediatrics; 116/4/1036

Andrew, M., Mitchell, L., Vegh, P., & Ofosu, F. (1994). Thrombin regulation in children differs from adults in the absence and presence of heparin. *Thrombosis and Haemostasis, 72*(6), 836–842.

Andrew, M., Paes, B., Milner, R., et al. (1987). Development of the human coagulation system in the full-term infant. *Blood, 70*(1), 165–172.

Andrew, M., Paes, B., Milner, R., et al. (1988). Development of the human coagulation system in the healthy premature infant. *Blood, 72*(5), 1651–1657.

Andrew, M., Schmidt, B., Mitchell, L., Paes, B., & Ofosu, F. (1990). Thrombin generation in newborn plasma is critically dependent on the concentration of prothrombin. *Thrombosis and Haemostasis, 63*(1), 27–30.

Andrew, M., Vegh, P., Johnston, M., Bowker, J., Ofosu, F., & Mitchell, L. (1992). Maturation of the hemostatic system during childhood. *Blood, 80*(8), 998–1005.

Ansell, J., Hirsh, J., Hylek, E., Jacobson, A., Crowther, M., & Palareti, G. (2008). Pharmacology and management of the vitamin K antagonists: American College of Chest Physicians Evidence-Based Clinical Practice Guidelines (8th ed.). *Chest, 133*(Suppl. 6).

Association of Pediatric Hematology/Oncology Nurses. (2007). *APHON Hematology Teaching CD-ROM.* Glenview, IL: Author.

Bakhshi, S. (2011). *Aplastic anemia.* Retrieved January 8, 2012 from http://emedicine.medscape.com/article/198759-overview

Barnes, C., Newall, F., Furmedge, J., Mackay, M., & Monagle, P. (2004). Arterial ischaemic stroke in children. *Journal of Paediatrics and Child Health, 40*(7), 384–387.

Barnes, C., Newall, F., & Monagle, P. (2002). Post-thrombotic syndrome. *Archives of Disease in Childhood, 86*(3), 212–214.

Biss, T. T., Brandão, L. R., Kahr, W. H., Chan, A. K., & Williams, S. (2008). Clinical features and outcome of pulmonary embolism in children. *British Journal of Haematology, 142*(5), 808–818.

Biss, T. T., Kahr, W. H. A., Brandão, L. R., Chan, A. K. C., Thomas, K. E., & Williams, S. (2009). The use of elastic compression stockings for post-thrombotic syndrome in a child. *Pediatric Blood and Cancer, 53*(3), 462–463.

Blanchette, V., & Bolton-Maggs, P. (2008). Childhood immune thrombocytopenic purpura: Diagnosis and management. (2008). *Pediatric Clinics of North America, 55*, 393–420.

Borgna-Pignatti, C., & Marsella, M. (2008). Iron deficiency in infancy and childhood. *Pediatric Annals, 37*(5), 329–337.

Bronfenbrenner, U. (1979). *The ecology of human development: Experiments by nature and design.* Cambridge, MA: Harvard University Press.

Brousseau, D. C., McCarver, D. G., Drendel, A. L., Divakaran, K., & Panepinto, J. A. (2007). The effect of CYP2D6 polymorphisms on the response to pain treatment for pediatric sickle cell disease pain crisis. *Journal of Pediatrics, 150*(6), 623–626.

Bryant, R. (2010). Anemias. In D. Tomlinson & N. E. Kline (Eds.), *Pediatric oncology nursing.* New York: Springer.

Carcao, M. D., Cook, D., Allen, U., et.al. (2006, revised by Kirby, M. A., Williams, S., Friedman, J., et al.). *Guidelines for in-patient management of children with sickle cell disease.* Toronto, ON: The Hospital for Sick Children. Retrieved August 24, 2011 from http://www.sickkids.ca/pdfs/Haematology-Oncology/8217-SickleCellguidelines2006.pdf

Catlin, A. J. (2003). Thalassemia: The facts and the controversies. *Pediatric Nursing, 29*(6), 447–451.

Christofides, A., Schauer, C., & Zlotkin, S. (2005). Iron deficiency anemia among children: Addressing a global public health problem within a Canadian context. *Paediatrics and Child Health, 10*(10), 597–601.

Cunningham, F. G., Leveno, K. L., Bloom, S. L., et al. (2010). Fetal growth and development. In F. G. Cunningham, K. L. Leveno, S. L. Bloom, et al. (Eds.), *Williams obstetrics* (23rd ed.). New York: McGraw-Hill.

Darbari, D. S., Neely, M., van den Anker, J., & Rana, S. (2011). Increased clearance of morphine in sickle cell disease: Implications for pain management. *The Journal of Pain, 12*(5), 531–538.

Dick, M., et al. (2010). *Sickle cell disease in childhood. Standards and guidelines for clinical care* (2nd ed.). Retrieved August 25, 2011 from http://sct.screening.nhs.uk/cms.php?folder=2493

Dowling, M., Quinn, C.T., Rogers, Z.R., & Buchanan, G.R. (2010). Acute silent cerebral infarction in children with sickle cell anemia. *Pediatric Blood Cancer, 54*, 461–464.

Eckman, J. (2010). *Pathophysiology and principles of treatment.* Retrieved January 9, 2012 from http://scinfo.org/problem-oriented-clinical-guidelines/pathophysiology-and-principles-of-treatment

Field, J., & DeBaun, M. (2009). Asthma and sickle cell disease: two distinct diseases or part of the same process? *Hematology 2009. American Society of Hematology Education Handbook, 1*, 45–53.

Fischbach, F. T. (2008). *A manual of laboratory and diagnostic tests* (8th ed.). Philadelphia: Lippincott Williams & Wilkins.

Franchini, M., & Manzato, F. (2004). Update on the treatment of disseminated intravascular coagulation. *Hematology, 9*(2), 81–85.

Goldbloom, R. B. (2004). *Screening for hemoglobinopathies in Canada.* Retrieved August 25, 2011 from http://www.phac-aspc.gc.ca/publicat/clinic-clinique/pdf/s2c20e.pdf

Goldenberg, N. A. (2005). Long-term outcomes of venous thrombosis in children. *Current Opinion in Hematology, 12*(5), 370–376.

Guilcher, G., Purves, E., & Wu, J. (2006). *British Columbia Children's Hospital guideline forthe management of fever in children with sickle cell disease.* Vancouver, BC: BC Children's Hospital.

Gunnarsson, B. S., Thorsdottir, I., & Palsson, G. (2004). Iron status in 2-year-old Icelandic children and associations with dietary intake and growth. *European Journal of Clinical Nutrition, 58*, 901–906.

Hamilton Regional Laboratory Medicine Program. (2010). *Lab Connections, 106, 1-3.* Retrieved March 22, 2011 from http://www.hamiltonhealthsciences.ca/workfiles/HRLMP/NEWSLETTERS/No%20106%20March%202010.doc

Hartfield, D. C., Lowry, N. J., Keene, D. L., & Yager, J. K. (1997). Iron deficiency: A cause of stroke in infants and children. *Pediatric Neurology, 16*(1), 50–53.

Health Canada. (2005). *Dietary reference intakes: Reference values for elements.* Retrieved August 25, 2011 from http://www.hc-sc.gc.ca/fn-an/nutrition/reference/table/ref_elements_tbl-eng.php

Health Canada. (2011). *Lead and human health: It's your health.* Retrieved August 25, 2011 from http://www.hc-sc.gc.ca/hl-vs/iyh-vsv/environ/lead-plomb-eng.php

Hirsh, J., Dalen, J., Anderson, D. R., et al. (2001). Oral anticoagulants: Mechanism of action, clinical effectiveness, and optimal therapeutic range. *Chest, 119*(Suppl. 1), 8S–21S.

Human Genome Management Information System. (2005). *Genetic disease profile: Sickle cell anemia.* Retrieved August 25, 2011 from http://www.ornl.gov/sci/techresources/Human_Genome/posters/chromosome/sca.shtml

Irwin, J. J., & Kirchner, J. T. (2001). Anemia in children. *American Family Physician, 64*(8), 1379–1386.

Israels, S. (Ed.). (2009). *Mechanisms in hematology.* Concord, ON: Core Health Services Inc. Retrieved August 25, 2011 from www.MechanismsinHematology.ca

Jacobs, E., & Mueller, B. (2009). Pain experience of children with sickle cell disease who had prolonged hospitalizations for acute painful episodes. *Pain Medicine, 9*(1), 13–21.

Karp, S., & Riddell, J. P. (2010). Bleeding disorders. In P. J. Allen, J. A. Vessey, & N. A. Schapiro (Eds.), *Primary care of the child with a chronic condition* (5th ed.). St. Louis, MO: Mosby.

KidsHealth, L. (2009). *G6PD deficiency.* Retrieved August 25, 2011 from www.kidshealth.org/parent/general/aches/g6pd.html

Kimball, J. W. (2011). *Blood.* Retrieved August 25, 2011 from http://users.rcn.com/jkimball.ma.ultranet/BiologyPages/B/Blood.html

Kleinpell, R. M. (2003). The role of the critical care nurse in the assessment and management of the patient with severe sepsis. *Critical Care Nursing Clinics of North America, 15*(1), 27–34.

Kotsakis, A., Cook, D., Griffith, L., Anton, N., Massicotte, P., & MacFarland, K. (2005). Clinically important venous thromboembolism in pediatric critical care: A Canadian survey. *Journal of Critical Care, 20*(4), 373–380.

Kuhle, S., Koloshuk, B., Marzinotto, V., et al. (2003). A cross-sectional study evaluating post-thrombotic syndrome in children. *Thrombosis Research, 11*(4), 227–233.

Kuhle, S., & Massicotte, P. M. (2005). Maturation of the coagulation system during childhood. *Progress in Pediatric Cardiology, 21*(1), 3–7.

Kuhle, S., Spavor, M., Massicotte, P., et al. (2008). Prevalence of post-thrombotic syndrome following asymptomatic thrombosis in survivors of acute lymphoblastic leukemia. *Journal of Thrombosis and Haemostasis, 6*(4), 589–594.

Kylat, R. I., & Ohlsson, A. (2006). Recombinant human activated protein C for severe sepsis in neonates. *Cochrane Database of Systematic Reviews, 2*, CF005385.

Langois, S., Ford, J. C., Chitayat, D., Désilets, V.A., Farrell, S.A., & Geraghty, M. (2008). Carrier screening for thalassemia and hemoglobinopathies in Canada. Joint Society of Obstetricians and Gynecologists of Canada (SOGC) – Canadian College of Medial Geneticists (CCMG) Clinical Practice Guideline. *Journal of Obstetrics and Gynaecology Canada, 218*, 950–959. Retrieved August 25, 2011 from http://www.sogc.org/guidelines/documents/gui218CPG0810.pdf

Lieberman, L., Kirby, M., Ozolins, L., Mosko, J., & Friedman, M. B. (2009). Initial presentation of unscreened children with sickle cell disease: The Toronto experience. *Pediatric Blood Cancer, 53*(3), 397–400.

Loiselle C. G., Profetto-McGrath, J., Polit, D. F., & Beck, C. T. (2010). *Canadian essentials ofnursing research* (3rd ed.). Philadelphia: Lippincott Williams & Wilkins.

Lozoff, B., DeAndraca, I., Castillo, M., Smith, J. B., Walter, T., & Pino, P. (2003). Behavioral and developmental effects of preventing iron deficiency anemia in healthy full term infants. *Pediatrics, 112*(4), 846–854.

Maakaron, J. E., Taher, A., & Woermann, U. J. (2012). *Sickle cell anemia*. Retrieved July 3, 2011 from http://emedicine.medscape.com/article/205926-overview

Maguire, J. L., deVeber, G., & Parkin, P. C. (2007). Association between iron deficiency anemia and stroke in young children. *Pediatrics, 120*(5), 1053–1057. Retrieved March 23, 2011 from http://www.pediatrics.org/cgi/content/full/120/5/1053

Massicotte, M. P., Dix, D., Monagle, P., Adams, M., & Andrew, M. (1998). Central venous catheter related thrombosis in children: Analysis of the canadian registry of venous thromboembolic complications. *Journal of Pediatrics, 133*(6), 770–776.

Monagle, P., Adams, M., Mahoney, M., (2000). Outcome of pediatric thromboembolic disease: a report from the Canadian Childhood Thrombophilia Registry. *Pediatric Research, 47*(6), 763–766.

Monagle, P., Chan, A., Massicotte, P., Chalmers, E., & Michelson, A. D. (2008). Antithrombotic therapy in neonates and children: the Eighth ACCP Conference on Antithrombotic and Thrombolytic Therapy. *Chest, 133*(Suppl. 6), 645S–687S.

Monreal, M., Raventos, A., Lerma, R., Ruiz, J., Lafoz, E., Alastrue, A., Llamazares, J.F. (1994). Pulmonary embolism in patients with upper extremity DVT associated to venous central lines—a prospective study. *Thrombosis and Haemostasis, 72*(4), 548–550.

Musani, M. H., Matta, F., Yaekoub, A.Y., Liang, J., Hull, R. D., & Stein, P. D. (2010). Venous compression for prevention of postthrombotic syndrome: A meta-analysis. *American Journal of Medicine, 123*(8), 735–740.

National Heart, Lung and Blood Institute. (2011). *What is sickle cell anemia?* Retrieved August 25, 2011 from http://www.nhlbi.nih.gov/health/dci/Diseases/Sca/SCA_WhatIs.html

Nowak-Gottl, U., von Kries, R., & Gobel, U. (1997). Neonatal symptomatic thromboembolism in Germany: Two year survey. *Archives of Diseases in Childhood, Fetal and Neonatal Edition, 76*(3), F163–F167.

Odame, I., Sayani, F., Warner, M., Wu, J., Wong-Rieger D., & Humphreys, K. (2009). *Guidelines for the clinical care of patients with thalassemia in Canada.* North York, ON: Thalassemia Foundation of Canada.

Ontario Society of Nutrition Professionals in Public Health. (2008). *Pediatric nutrition guidelines for primary health care providers.* Retrieved August 25, 2011 from www.osnpph.on.ca/pdfs/Improving OddsJune-08.pdf

Pitts, R. H., & Record, E. O. (2010). Sickle cell disease. In P. J. Allen, J. A. Vessey & N. A. Schapiro (Eds.), *Primary care of the child with a chronic condition* (5th ed.). St. Louis, MO: Mosby.

Platt, A., Eckman, J. R., Beasley, J., & Miller, G. (2002). Treating sickle cell pain: An update from the Georgia comprehensive sickle cell center. *Journal of Emergency Nursing, 28*(4), 297–303.

Randolph, A. G., Cook, D. J., Gonzales, C. A., & Andrew, M. (1998a). Review: Heparin reduces central venous and pulmonary artery catheter clots. *Evidence-Based Medicine, 3*(4), 111.

Randolph, A. G., Cook, D. J., Gonzalez, C. A., & Andrew, M. (1998b). Benefit of heparin in central venous and pulmonary artery catheters: A meta-analysis of randomized controlled trials. *Chest, 113*(1), 165–171.

Sickle Cell Information Center. (2011a). *Care path: Inpatient management of vaso-occlusive pain.* Retrieved January 9, 2012 from http://scinfo.org/care-paths-and-protocols-children-adolescents/care-path-inpatient-management-of-vaso-occlusive-pain

Sickle Cell Information Center. (2011b). *Chronic transfusion protocol.* Retrieved April 30, 2012 from http://scinfo.org/care-paths-and-protocols-children-adolescents/chronic-transfusion-protocol

Smith, L., Pinsent, C., Kusiak, R. (2008). *Interim report on blood lead levels in North Hamilton, Ontario.* Hamilton, ON: City of Hamilton Public Health Services.

Sridhar, A. V., Rao, N. K., & Chakraborty, S. (2005). A six-year old with fatal pulmonary embolism. *Acta Paediatrica, 94*(7), 977–979.

ten Cate-Hoek, A. J., ten Cate, H., Tordoir, J., Hamulyák, K., & Prins, M. H. (2010). Individually tailored duration of elastic compression therapy in relation to incidence of the postthrombotic syndrome. *Journal of Vascular Surgery, 52*(1), 132–138.

Van Ommen, C. H., Heijboer, H., Buller, H. R., Hirasing, R. A., Heijmans, H. S. A., & Peters, M. (2001). Venous thromboembolism in childhood: A prospective two-year registry in The Netherlands. *Journal of Pediatrics, 139*(5), 676–681.

Vaudry, W., & Kellner, J. (2007). *Recommendations for prevention of sepsis in asplenic children.* Emonton, AB: University of Alberta; Calgary, AB: University of Calgary.

Weiss, H. B., & Stephen, N. (2009). From periphery to center: A new vision for family, school, and community partnerships. In S. Christenson & A. Reschley (Eds.), *Handbook of school–family partnerships. Harvard Family Research Project.* Cambridge, MA: Routledge.

Yager, J. Y., & Hartfield, D. S. (2002). Neurologic manifestations of iron deficiency in childhood. *Pediatric Neurology, 27*(2), 85–92.

Yaish, H. M. (2010). *Pediatric thalassemia.* Retrieved July 3, 2011 from http://emedicine.medscape.com/article/958850-overview

Yetman, R. J. (2003). Evaluation and management of childhood idiopathic (immune) thrombocytopenia. *Journal of Pediatric Health Care, 17*(5), 261–263.

Young, G., Tarantino, M. D., Wohrley, J., Weber, L. C., Belvedere, M., & Nugent, D. J. (2007). Pilot dose-finding and safety study of bivalirudin in infants <6 months of age with thrombosis. *Journal of Thrombosis and Haemostasis, 5*(8), 1654–1659.

Young, G., Yonekawa, K. E., Nakagawa, P., & Nugent, D. J. (2004). Argatroban as an alternative to heparin in extracorporeal membrane oxygenation circuits. *Perfusion, 19*(5), 283–288.

Zetterstrom, R. (2004). Iron deficiency and iron deficiency anaemia during infancy and childhood. *Acta Paediatrica, 93*, 436–439.

RECOMMENDED READINGS

Andrew, M., David, M., Adams, M., Ali, K., Anderson, R., Barnard, D., et al. (1994a). Venous thromboembolic complications (VTE) in children: first analyses of the Canadian Registry of VTE. *Blood, 83*(5), 1251–1257.

Bauman, M. E., Massicotte, M. P., Ray, L., & Newburn-Cook, C. (2007). Developing educational materials to facilitate adherence: Pediatric thrombosis as a case illustration. *Journal of Pediatric Health Care, 21*(3), 198–206.

Bauman, M. E., Conroy, S., & Massicotte, M. P. (2008). Point-of-care INR measurement in children requiring warfarin: what has been evaluated and future directions. *Pediatric Health, 2*(5), 651–659.

Bauman, M. E., Belletrutti, M., Bajzar, L., et al. (2009a). Evaluation of enoxaparin dosing requirements in infants and children. Better dosing to achieve therapeutic levels. *Thrombosis and Haemostasis, 101*(1), 86–92.

Bauman, M. E., Black, K. L., Bauman, M. L., Belletrutti, M., Bajzar, L., & Massicotte, M. P. (2009b). Novel uses of insulin syringes to reduce dosing errors: a retrospective chart review of enoxaparin whole milligram dosing. *Thrombosis Research, 123*(6), 845–847.

Bauman, M., Black, K., Kuhle, S., Wang, L., Legge, L., & Callen-Wicks, D. (2009c). KIDCLOT©: The importance of validated educational intervention for optimal long term warfarin management in children. *Thrombosis Research, 123*(5), 707–709.

Bauman, M. E., Black, K., Bauman, M. L., et al. (2010). EMPoWarMENT: Edmonton Pediatric Warfarin Self-Management Pilot Study in Children with Primarily Cardiac Disease. *Thrombosis Research, 126*(2), e110–e115.

Bauman, M. E., Black, K., Bauman, M. L., Kuhle, S., Bajzar, L., & Massicotte, M. P. (2011). Warfarin induced coagulopathy in children: Assessment of a conservative approach. *Archives of Disease in Childhood, 96*(2), 164–167.

Bruce, A. A. K., Bauman, M. E., Black, K., Newton, A., Legge, L., & Massicotte, M. P. (2010). Development and preliminary evaluation of the KIDCLOT PAC QL©: A new health-related quality of life measure for pediatric long-term anticoagulation therapy. *Thrombosis Research, 126*(2), e116–e121.

Duncan, S. M., Massicotte, M. P., Ray, L., Kuhle, S., & Bauman, M. E. (2010). Topical lidocaine and the effect on enoxaparin absorption in children: A pilot study. *Thrombosis Research, 125*(1), e1–e4.

Greinacher, A., Alban, S., Omer-Adam, M. A., Weitschies, W., & Warkentin, T. E. (2008). Heparin-induced thrombocytopenia: A stoichiometry-based model to explain the differing immunogenicities of unfractionated heparin, low-molecular-weight heparin, and fondaparinux in different clinical settings. *Thrombosis Research, 122*(2), 211–220.

Hirsh, J., Bauer, K. A., Donati, M. B., Gould, M., Samama, M. M., & Weitz, J. I. (2008). *Parenteral anticoagulants: American College of Chest Physicians evidence-based clinical practice guidelines* (8th ed.). *Chest, 133*(Suppl. 6), 141S–159S.

Hirsh, J., Warkentin, T. E., Shaughnessy, S. G., et al. (2001). Heparin and low-molecular-weight heparin: Mechanisms of action, pharmacokinetics, dosing, monitoring, efficacy, and safety. *Chest, 119*(Suppl. 1), 64S–94S.

Jones, S., Newall, F., Manias, E., & Monagle, P. (2011). Assessing outcome measures of oral anticoagulation management in children. *Thrombosis Research, 127*(2), 75–80.

Kuhle, S., Massicotte, P., Dinyari, M., et al. (2005). Dose-finding and pharmacokinetics of therapeutic doses of tinzaparin in pediatric patients with thromboembolic events. *Thrombosis and Haemostasis, 94*(6), 1164–1171.

Levi, M. (2005a). Disseminated intravascular coagulation: What's new? *Critical Care Clinics, 21*(3 Special Issue), 449–467.

Levi, M. (2005b). Pathogenesis and treatment of DIC. *Thrombosis Research, 115*(Suppl), 54–55.

Levi, M., Van Der Poll, T., De Jonge, E., & Ten Cate, H. (1999). Relative insufficiency of the fibrinolytic system in disseminated intravascular coagulation. *Sepsis, 3*(2), 119–124.

Malowany, J. I., Monagle, P., Knoppert, D. C., Lee, D. S. C., Wu, J., & McCusker, P. (2008). Enoxaparin for neonatal thrombosis: A call for a higher dose for neonates. *Thrombosis Research, 122*(6), 826–830.

Massicotte, P., Marzinotto, V., Vegh, P., Adams, M., & Andrew, M. (1995). Home monitoring of warfarin therapy in children with a whole blood prothrombin time monitor. *Journal of Pediatrics, 127*(3), 389–394.

Massicotte, P., Adams, M., Marzinotto, V., Brooker, L. A., & Andrew, M. (1996). Low-molecular-weight heparin in pediatric patients with thrombotic disease: A dose finding study. *Journal of Pediatrics, 128*(3), 313–318.

McClure, W., Ritchie, B., Akabutu, J. (2002). *Plasma derived vs. recombinant factor IX: An assessment of efficacy.* Paper presented at the XXV International Congress of the World Federation of Hemophilia Seville, Spain.

McClure, W., Ritchie, B., Dower, N. (2010). *Inhibitor titres continue to decrease while on prophylaxis with FEIBA.* Paper presented at the Hemophilia World Congress, Buenos Aires, Argentina.

National Newborn Screening and Genetics Resource Center. (2011). *National newborn screening status report.* Retrieved March 23, 2011 from http://genes-r-us.uthscsa.edu/nbsdisorders.pdf

Newall, F., Barnes, C., Ignjatovic, V., & Monagle, P. (2003). Heparin-induced thrombocytopenia in children. *Journal of Paediatrics and Child Health, 39*(4), 289–292.

Newall, F., Ignjatovic, V., Johnston, L., et al. (2011). Clinical use of unfractionated heparin therapy in children: Time for change? *British Journal of Haematology, 150*(6), 674–678.

Newall, F., Ignjatovic, V., Summerhayes, R., et al. (2009a). In vivo age dependency of unfractionated heparin in infants and children. *Thrombosis Research, 123*(5), 710–714.

Newall, F., Johnston, L., Ignjatovic, V., & Monagle, P. (2009b). Unfractionated heparin therapy in infants and children. *Pediatrics, 123*(3), e510–e518.

Patrono, C., Baigent, C., Hirsh, J., & Roth, G. (2008). *Antiplatelet drugs: American college of chest physicians evidence-based clinical practice guidelines* (8th ed.). *Chest, 133*(Suppl. 6), 199S–233S.

Poon, M.-C., Lillicrap, D., Hensman, C., Card, R., & Scully, M. (2002). Recombinant factor IX recovery and inhibitor safety: A Canadian post licensure surveillance study. *Thrombosis and Haemostasis, 87*(3), 431–435.

Rayapudi, S., Torres, A., Jr., Deshpande, G. G., et al. (2008). Bivalirudin for anticoagulation in children. *Pediatric Blood and Cancer, 51*(6), 798–801.

Schwetz, N., Jacobson, R., Matiko, M., et al., The Canadian Association of Hemophilia Nurses. (2000). *Home treatment manual.* Poster presented at the XXIV International Congress of the World Federation of Hemophilia, Montreal, Quebec, Canada.

Skouri, H., Gandouz, R., Abroug, S., et al. (2006). A prospective study of the prevalence of heparin-induced antibodies and other associated thromboembolic risk factors in pediatric patients undergoing hemodialysis. *American Journal of Hematology, 81*(5), 328–334.

Smith, L. F. P., Ernst, E., Ewings, P., Myers, P., & Smith, C. (2004). Co-ingestion of herbal medicines and warfarin. *British Journal of General Practice, 54*(503), 439–441.

Soulat, T., Loyau, S., Baudouin, V., et al. (2000). Effect of individual plasma lipoprotein(a) variations in vivo on its competition with plasminogen for fibrin and cell binding: An in vitro study using plasma from children with idiopathic nephrotic syndrome. *Arteriosclerosis, Thrombosis and Vascular Biology, 20*(2), 575–584.

Stiller, B., Lemmer, J., Merkle, F., et al. (2004). Consumption of blood products during mechanical circulatory support in children: comparison between ECMO and a pulsatile ventricular assist device. *Intensive Care Medicine, 30*(9), 1814–1820.

Warkentin, T. E., Sheppard, J. I., Moore, J. C., Sigouin, C. S., & Kelton, J. G. (2008). Quantitative interpretation of optical density measurements using PF4-dependent enzyme-immunoassays. *Journal of Thrombosis and Haemostasis, 6*(8), 1304–1312.

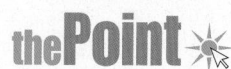

the Point For additional learning materials, including Internet Resources, visit **http://thePoint.lww.com/Chow1e.**

CHAPTER WORKSHEET

MULTIPLE CHOICE QUESTIONS

1. A child on the hematology unit has the following a.m. laboratory results: hemoglobin 100, hematocrit 30.2, WBC 24, platelets 20. What is the priority nursing assessment?

   a. Assess for pallor, fatigue, and tachycardia.

   b. Monitor for fever.

   c. Assess for bruising or bleeding.

   d. Determine intake and output.

   e. a, b, and c

2. A child with hemophilia fell while riding his bicycle. He was wearing a helmet and did not lose consciousness. He has a mild abrasion on his knee that is not oozing. He is complaining of abdominal pain. What is the priority nursing assessment after treating with factor VIII?

   a. Perform neurologic checks.

   b. Assess ability to void frequently.

   c. Carefully assess abdomen.

   d. Examine his knee frequently.

3. A 14-year-old with thalassemia asks for your assistance in choosing her afternoon snack. Which choice is the most appropriate?

   a. Peanut butter with rice cake

   b. Small spinach salad

   c. Apple slices with cheddar cheese

   d. Small burger on wheat bun

4. You are the nurse is caring for a child who has just been admitted to the pediatric unit with sickle cell crisis. He is complaining that his right arm and leg hurt. What is the priority nursing intervention?

   a. Assess pain with an age-appropriate pain scale.

   b. Administer pain medication based on assessment using a possible combination of ibuprofen, acetaminophen, and oral or IV opioids at a dose that controls the pain as quickly as possible.

   c. Try acetaminophen only.

   d. Use narcotic analgesics and warm compresses as needed to control the pain.

   e. a and b

   f. a and d

CRITICAL THINKING EXERCISES

1. Develop a discharge teaching plan in conjunction with the nearest comprehensive hemophilia centre for the parent of a toddler who has just been diagnosed with hemophilia and received factor infusion treatment for a bleeding episode.

2. A 28-month-old girl has been diagnosed with iron-deficiency anemia. Formulate a nutrition plan for this child.

3. A 5-year-old with beta-thalassemia major is resisting his nightly chelation therapy at home. Devise a developmentally appropriate teaching plan for this child.

4. Develop a nursing care plan for a child with sickle cell disease who experiences frequent vaso-occlusive crises.

STUDY ACTIVITIES

1. Meet with a nutritionist. Learn about the prevention and nutritional treatment of iron-deficiency anemia. Provide a written report of your learning experience or provide a presentation to your classmates.

2. In the clinical setting, compare the growth and development of a child with sickle cell disease with that of a similarly aged child who has been healthy.

3. Talk to a teenager with hemophilia about his life experiences and feelings about his disease and his health. Reflect upon this conversation in your clinical journal.

4. Visit a public health clinic or immigration clinic that provides primary care to children. Spend time with the registered nurse, the advanced practice nurse, and the unlicensed assistive personnel. Write a summary of the roles of the registered nurse in screening for and managing hematologic disorders in children, noting roles that are reserved for the advanced practice nurse and activities that the RN would delegate to unlicensed assistive personnel.

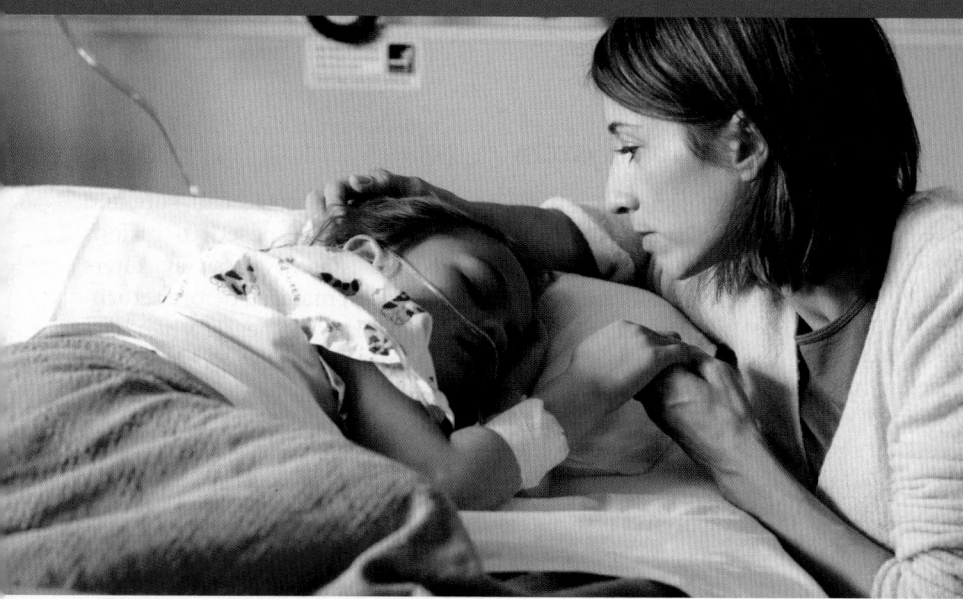

CHAPTER 47

Adapted by Pia DeZorzi and
Gwen Erdmann

NURSING CARE OF THE CHILD WITH AN IMMUNOLOGIC DISORDER

KEY TERMS

antibodies
antigen
autoantibodies
B cells
cellular immunity
chemotaxis
complement

graft-versus–host
    disease
humoural immunity
immunity
immunodeficiency
immunoglobulins
immunosuppressive

lymphocyte
neutrophil
opsonization
phagocytosis
stem cells
T cells

LEARNING OBJECTIVES

Upon completion of the chapter, the learner will be able to:

1. Explain anatomic and physiologic differences of the immune system in infants and children versus adults.
2. Describe nursing care related to common laboratory and diagnostic testing used in the medical diagnosis of pediatric immune and autoimmune disorders.
3. Distinguish immune and autoimmune disorders common in infants, children, and adolescents.
4. Identify appropriate nursing assessments and interventions related to medications and treatments for pediatric immune, autoimmune, and allergic disorders.
5. Develop an individualized nursing care plan for the child with an immune or autoimmune disorder.
6. Describe the psychosocial impact of chronic immune disorders on children.
7. Devise a nutrition plan for the child with immunodeficiency.
8. Develop patient/family teaching plans for the child with an immune or autoimmune disorder.

Kaitlin Harris, 15 years old, is brought to her doctor's office by her mother. She presents with complaints of pain and swelling in her joints, weight gain, and fatigue. Kaitlin states, "I'm just very tired all the time, and my knees and ankles ache."

WoW

Resistance to disease can be a child's battle for life.

Immunodeficiency, autoimmune, and allergic disorders have a significant impact on the lives of affected children. Infants and children are exposed to many infectious microorganisms and allergens and thus need a functional immune system to protect them. Temporary immune deficiencies may follow a common viral infection, surgery, or blood transfusion. They may also be caused by malnutrition or the use of certain medications (Nield, Torischt, & Kamat, 2009). Temporary immune depression returns to normal over a period of time. Primary or secondary immune deficiencies are the focus of this discussion, along with allergy and anaphylaxis. These immune disorders are chronic, and affected children have more infections than healthy children do. Recurrent viral or bacterial infections may cause the child to miss significant amounts of school or playtime with other children. Many immunodeficiencies require chronic and frequent clinic visits as well as daily medications. This can be a stress on the family as well. Autoimmune disorders are also chronic, causing significant disruption to the child's and family's life. Allergic disorders in some children may cause significant stress for the child and family. Nurses who care for children need to be familiar with common immunodeficiencies, autoimmune disorders, and allergies to intervene effectively with children and their families.

Variations in Pediatric Anatomy and Physiology

Normal immune function is a complex process involving **phagocytosis, humoural immunity, cellular immunity**, and activation of the **complement** system. The lymphatic system and the white blood cells (WBCs) are the primary "players" in the immune response. Though these structures and cells are present at birth, the healthy full-term infant's immune system is still immature. The newborn exhibits a decreased inflammatory response to invading organisms, and this increases his or her susceptibility to infection. Cellular immunity is generally functional at birth, and as the infant is exposed to various substances over time, humoural immunity develops. Comparison Chart 47.1 provides more information on humoural and cellular immunity.

Lymph System

Lymph nodes in the newborn are relatively small, soft, and difficult to palpate. As the infant is exposed to various germs or illnesses, the lymph system passively filters plasma for bacteria or other foreign material before returning it to the bloodstream and back to the heart. When bacteria are recognized in the lymph fluid, the lymph nodes produce more infection-fighting WBCs, causing the nodes to swell. Young children have frequent episodes of localized enlarged lymph nodes because of their frequent exposure to viral illnesses (Tosi, 2009). The spleen is functional at birth and also filters the blood for foreign cells. The thymus, responsible for the production of T **lymphocytes** (**T cells**) as well as for the development and maturation of peripheral lymphoid tissue, is relatively large at birth and attains its largest size at puberty. It then stops growing throughout adulthood, gradually shrinking and almost disappearing. The tonsils, composed primarily of lymphoid tissue, are also often enlarged throughout early childhood. The bone marrow is functional at birth, producing **stem cells** capable of differentiating into various blood cells.

Phagocytosis

The newborn and infant under conditions of stress may have decreased phagocytic activity. The complement system, which is responsible for **opsonization** and **chemotaxis**, is immature in the newborn but reaches adult levels of activity by 3 to 6 months of age. The infant's phagocytic cells (**neutrophils** and monocytes) demonstrate decreased chemotaxis, reaching adult levels when the child is several years old. With complement levels being only 50% to 75% of adult levels in the full-term infant, decreased opsonization may be responsible for decreased phagocytic activity compared with adults.

Cellular Immunity

Maternal T cells do not cross the placenta, so the fetal thymus begins production of T cells early in gestation, and the newborn demonstrates a relative lymphocytosis compared with the adult, probably due to increased amounts of T-cell lymphocytes. Though cellular immunity does not cross the placenta, the fetal T cells may become sensitized to antigens that do cross the placenta.

COMPARISON CHART 47.1 **HUMOURAL VERSUS CELLULAR IMMUNITY**

Humoural Immunity (Antibody Protection)	Cellular Immunity (Cell-Mediated Immune Response)
• Lymphocytes: B cells • Secrete antibodies to viruses and bacteria • Recognize antigens • Antibodies mark the antigen cell for destruction. • Do not destroy the foreign cell • Crosses the placenta in the form of IgG	• Lymphocytes: T cells • Do not recognize antigens • Direct and regulate immune response (helper T cells) • Attack infected or foreign cells (killer T cells and natural killer cells) • Does not cross the placenta

Viral infection, hyperbilirubinemia, and drugs taken by the mother late in pregnancy may contribute to depressed T-cell function in the newborn. Since delayed hypersensitivity reactions are mediated by T cells rather than antibodies, skin test responses (such as purified protein derivative [PPD]) for tuberculosis detection) are diminished until about 1 year of age, probably due to the infant's decreased ability to mount an inflammatory response.

Humoural Immunity

The newborn's B **lymphocytes** (**B cells**) do not respond as well to infection as do the adult's. B cells are responsible for the formation of **antibodies** or **immunoglobulins** (specific immunity). The antibodies bind to the **antigen**, thus disabling the specific toxin. The fetus is normally in an antigen-free environment and so produces only trace amounts of immunoglobulin (Ig) M. Most of the newborn's IgG is acquired transplacentally from the mother. Hence, the newborn exhibits passive **immunity** to antigens to which the mother had developed antibodies. These antibodies wane over the first months of life as the transplacental IgG is catabolized, having a half-life of only about 25 days. The newborn begins to make IgG but ordinarily experiences a physiologic hypogammaglobulinemia between 2 and 6 months of age until self-production of IgG reaches higher levels.

The breastfed infant will acquire passive transfer of maternal immunity via the breast milk and will be better protected during the physiologic hypogammaglobulinemia phase. By 1 year of age IgG is 70% of the adult level, and by 8 years of age it should reach the adult level.

IgA, IgD, IgE, and IgM do not cross the placenta; they require an antigenic challenge for production. IgD and IgE constitute a very small percentage of the **immunoglobulins** in all ages. IgA increases slowly to about 30% of the adult level at 1 year of age, reaching the adult level by age 11 years. IgM is close to the adult level by 1 year of age (Lederman, 2006).

Common Medical Treatments

A variety of medications and other medical treatments are used to treat immune deficiencies and autoimmune problems in children. Most of these treatments will require a physician's or nurse practitioner's order when the child is in the hospital. The most common treatments and medications are listed in Common Medical Treatments 47.1 and Drug Guide 47.1. The nurse caring for the child with an immune deficiency or autoimmune disorder should be familiar with what the procedures and medications are, how they work, and common nursing implications related to use of these modalities.

COMMON MEDICAL TREATMENTS 47.1

Treatment	Explanation	Indication	Nursing Implications
Immunizations	Killed or modified microorganisms, or components of them, cause the immune system to develop antibodies to the microorganism without developing disease.	Prevention of certain viral and bacterial infections	Do not administer live vaccines to immunosuppressed persons. Refer to the individual vaccine for method of administration and contraindications. Report adverse reactions via the Public Health Agency of Canada: complete an Adverse Events Following Immunization (AEFI) Reporting Form and submit it to the local health unit.
Bone marrow or stem cell transplantation	Bone marrow transplant: transfusion of healthy donor bone marrow into a person with immune malfunction; the transfused cells will migrate into the recipient's bone and can then develop into functional B and T cells. Blood stem cell transplant: peripheral blood stem cells are removed from the donor via apheresis or blood stem cells are retrieved from the umbilical cord and placenta. The stem cells are then transfused into the recipient.	Wiskott–Aldrich syndrome, severe combined immunodeficiency (SCID)	Administer immunosuppressive medications as ordered. Maintain medical asepsis and protective isolation to prevent infection. Monitor closely for graft-versus-host disease. Provide meticulous oral care. Avoid rectal temperatures and suppositories. Encourage appropriate nutrition.

DRUG GUIDE 47.1 COMMON DRUGS FOR IMMUNOLOGIC DISORDERS

Medication	Action/Indication	Nursing Implications
Intravenous immune globulin (IVIG); multiple manufacturers	Provides exogenous IgG antibodies. Indicated for primary immune deficiencies, HIV infection	Do not mix with IV medications or with other IV fluids. Do not give IM or SQ. Monitor vital signs and watch for adverse reactions frequently during infusion. May require antipyretic or antihistamine to prevent chills and fever during infusion. Have epinephrine available during infusion.
Nucleoside analogue reverse transcriptase inhibitors (NRTIs): abacavir, lamivudine, zidovudine	Inhibits reverse transcription of the viral DNA chain. For treatment of HIV-1 infection as part of a 3-drug regimen. Zidovudine is also used to prevent perinatal transmission of HIV.	Notify physician of muscle weakness, shortness of breath, headache, insomnia, rash, or unusual bleeding. Give IV zidovudine over 1 h. Fatal hypersensitivity reaction may occur with abacavir.
Non-nucleoside analogue reverse transcriptase inhibitors (NNRTIs): efavirenz, nevirapine	Binds to HIV-1 reverse transcriptase, blocking DNA polymerase activity and disrupting the virus life cycle. Used for treatment of HIV-1 infection as part of a 3-drug regimen.	*Nevirapine:* Avoid St. John's wort. Shake suspension gently before administration. Observe for symptoms of Stevens–Johnson syndrome. *Efavirenz:* May cause drowsiness
Protease inhibitors: amprenavir, atazanavir, indinavir, lopinavir, nelfinavir, ritonavir, saquinavir	Inhibits protease activity in the HIV-1 cell, resulting in immature, noninfectious viral particles. Used for treatment of HIV-1 infection as part of a 3-drug regimen.	Multiple drug interactions. Review specific medication for adverse effects and administration implications.
Nonsteroidal anti-inflammatory drugs (NSAIDs): aspirin, trisalicylate, ibuprofen, naproxen, others	Inhibits prostaglandin synthesis, anti-inflammatory action. Indicated for juvenile idiopathic arthritis	Administer with food to decrease GI upset. May cause gastric bleeding, increased liver enzymes, decreased renal function. Monitor liver enzymes. Do not crush or chew extended-release or timed-release preparations. *Aspirin and trisalicylate:* Follow serum salicylate levels. Observe for signs of toxicity, including hyperventilation with heavy breathing, drowsiness, nausea, vomiting, bruising, tinnitus, hearing loss.
Corticosteroids	Anti-inflammatory and immunosuppressive action. Used for juvenile idiopathic arthritis, SLE, and immunosuppression in bone marrow or stem cell transplant patients.	Administer with food to decrease GI upset. May mask signs of infection. Monitor blood pressure, urine for glucose. Do not stop treatment abruptly or acute adrenal insufficiency may occur. Monitor for Cushing syndrome. Doses may be tapered over time. *Intravenous pulse:* Monitor for hypertension during infusion.
Cytotoxic drugs (cyclophosphamide [Cytoxan])	Interferes with normal function of DNA by alkylation. For treatment of severe SLE.	Causes bone marrow suppression. Monitor for signs of infection. *Cyclophosphamide:* Administer in the morning. Provide adequate hydration and have child void frequently during and after infusion to decrease risk of hemorrhagic cystitis.

Medication	Action/Indication	Nursing Implications
Immunosuppressant drugs (cyclosporine A [CyA], azathioprine)	Inhibition of production and release of interleukin II (CyA). Antagonizes purine metabolism (azathioprine). Used for severe steroid-resistant autoimmune disease.	Monitor CBC, serum creatinine, potassium, and magnesium. Monitor blood pressure and watch for signs of infection. Draw blood levels before morning dose. *CyA:* Do not give with grapefruit juice.
Antimalarial drugs: hydroxychloroquine sulphate (Plaquenil)	Impairs complement-dependent antigen–antibody reactions to prevent flares in SLE and juvenile arthritis.	Funduscopic eye examination and visual field testing every year
Disease-modifying antirheumatic drugs (DMARDs): methotrexate, etanercept	Methotrexate: antimetabolite that depletes DNA precursors inhibits DNA and urine synthesis. Etanercept: binds to tumour necrosis factor (TNF), rendering it ineffective. Used for severe polyarticular juvenile arthritis.	*Methotrexate:* Do not give oral form with dairy products. Approximate time to benefit in treatment of arthritis is 3 to 6 weeks. Salicylates may delay clearance. Protect IV preparation from light. Monitor CBC, renal and liver function, and symptoms of infection. *Etanercept:* Monitor closely for infection. Do not give live vaccines. Give SQ, twice weekly; effect in 1 week to 3 months.

Refer to Chapter 35 for a thorough explanation of assessment and management of pain.
Adapted from: Taketokmo, C. K., Hodding, J. H., & Kraus, D. M. (2010). *Lexi-comp's pediatric dosage handbook* (17th ed.). Hudson, OH: Lexi-comp.

NURSING PROCESS OVERVIEW FOR THE CHILD WITH AN IMMUNOLOGIC DISORDER

Care of the child with an immunologic or allergic disorder includes assessment, nursing diagnosis, planning, interventions, and evaluation. There are a number of general concepts related to the nursing process that may be applied to immunodeficiencies and autoimmune disorders. From a general understanding of the care involved for a child with immune dysfunction, the nurse can then individualize the care based on patient specifics.

Assessment

Assessment of children with immunodeficiency, autoimmune disorders, or allergies includes health history, physical examination, and laboratory and diagnostic testing.

*R*emember Kaitlin, the 15-year-old with joint pain and swelling, fatigue, and weight gain? What additional health history and physical examination assessment information should you obtain?

Health History

The health history comprises past medical history, including the mother's pregnancy history, family history, and history of present illness (when the symptoms started and how they have progressed), as well as all medications and treatments used at home. The past medical history may be significant for maternal human immunodeficiency virus (HIV) infection; frequent, recurrent infections such as otitis media, sinusitis, or pneumonia; chronic cough; recurrent low-grade fever; two or more serious infections in early childhood; recurrent deep skin or organ abscesses; persistent thrush in the mouth; extensive eczema; or growth failure. Family history may be positive for primary immune deficiency or autoimmune disorder. Document history of known allergies. Note the response that occurs when the child encounters the allergen.

Physical Examination

Physical examination of the child with an immunodeficiency or autoimmune disorder includes inspection and observation, auscultation, percussion, and palpation.

Inspection and Observation

Plot weight and length or height on appropriate growth charts. Inspect the oropharynx for tonsillar size. Note eczematous or other skin lesions, which may occur with allergic diseases or Wiskott–Aldrich syndrome. Document the presence of thrush, which occurs frequently in children with immunodeficiency. Observe gait for unexplained ataxia (neurologic alterations occur with HIV infection).

Auscultation, Percussion, and Palpation

Auscultate the lungs for adventitious sounds, which may be present with a concurrent respiratory infection or as wheezing with an allergic reaction. Percuss the abdomen and determine liver span. Palpate for unusually enlarged lymph nodes, particularly in nonadjacent locations. Palpate the abdomen for enlarged spleen or liver.

Laboratory and Diagnostic Testing

Common Laboratory Diagnostic Tests 47.1 explains the laboratory and diagnostic tests most commonly used when considering immune disorders. Results of these tests may assist the physician in diagnosing the disorder and/or be used as guidelines in determining ongoing treatment. Laboratory or non-nursing personnel obtain some of the tests, while the nurse might obtain others. In either instance the nurse should be familiar with how the tests are obtained, what they are used for, and normal versus abnormal results. This knowledge will also be necessary when providing patient and family education related to the testing.

Nursing Diagnoses and Related Interventions

Upon completion of a thorough assessment, the nurse might identify several nursing diagnoses. These may include:

- Ineffective protection
- Imbalanced nutrition, less than body requirements
- Impaired skin integrity
- Activity intolerance (related to pain)
- Delayed growth and development

After completing an assessment of Kaitlin, you note the following: alopecia, abdominal tenderness, and oral ulcers. Based on these assessment findings, what would your top three nursing diagnoses be for Kaitlin?

Nursing goals, interventions, and evaluation for the child with an immunologic disorder are based on the nursing diagnoses. Nursing Care Plan 47.1 can be used as a guide in planning nursing care for the child with an immunologic disorder, autoimmune disorder, or allergic response. It should be individualized based on the patient's symptoms and needs. Additional information will be included later in the chapter as it relates to specific disorders.

Based on your top three nursing diagnoses for Kaitlin, describe appropriate nursing interventions.

Primary Immunodeficiencies

More than 130 primary immunodeficiency disorders have been identified (Waltenburg, Kobrynski, Reyes, et al., 2010). (Note, however, that the International Union of Immunological Societies lists more than 150 primary immunodeficiencies within eight classifications.) They are mostly hereditary or congenital disorders. About half of primary immunodeficiencies are humoural deficiencies. The remainder are combined (B- and T-cell) deficiencies, phagocytic system defects, and T-cell defects (cellular immunity deficiencies), with only 2% related to complement deficiencies (Petry, Mathur, & Kamat, 2004). This discussion focuses on a few of the more common and/or severe primary immunodeficiencies in children. Box 47.1 lists 10 warning signs that a child may need further evaluation for the possibility of primary **immunodeficiency**.

Hypogammaglobulinemia

Hypogammaglobulinemia refers to a variety of conditions in which the child does not form antibodies appropriately. It results in low or absent levels of one or more of the immunoglobulin classes or subclasses. Table 47.1 provides an overview of several types of hypogammaglobulinemia. Therapeutic management of most types of hypogammaglobulinemia is periodic administration of intravenous immune globulin (IVIG).

Nursing Assessment

Note history of recurrent respiratory, gastrointestinal, or genitourinary infections. Palpate for enlarged lymph nodes and spleen in the child with X-linked hyper-IgM syndrome. In children presenting for routine administration of IVIG, determine whether any infections have occurred since the previous infusion.

Nursing Management

Nursing management of hypogammaglobulinemia involves administration of IVIG and the provision of education and support to the child and family.

Administering IVIG

The majority of IVIG products in Canada are liquid preparations, and most transfusion services prepare the product and issue it ready for administration. If the product is not liquid, contact your transfusion service to reconstitute it in the lab and issue it diluted and ready to administer.

Before administering IVIG, assess baseline serum blood urea nitrogen (BUN) and creatinine, as acute renal insufficiency may occur as a serious adverse reaction. Though less common in children than adults, assess for risk factors associated with a thromboembolic event, such as history of stroke, hypertension, diabetes, hypercholesterolemia, impaired cardiac output, monoclonal gammopathy, clotting disorder, obesity, or immobility (Kirmse, 2009).

(text continues on page 1625)

COMMON LABORATORY AND DIAGNOSTIC TESTS 47.1

Test	Explanation	Indication	Nursing Implications
Complete blood count (CBC) with differential	Evaluates hemoglobin and hematocrit, WBC count (particularly the percentage of individual WBCs), and platelet count.	Infection, inflammatory process, immunosuppression	Normal values vary according to age and gender. WBC count differential is helpful in evaluating source of infection. May be affected by myelosuppressive drugs.
Immunoglobulin electrophoresis	Determines level of individual immunoglobulins (IgA, IgD, IgE, IgG, IgM) in the blood	Immune deficiency, autoimmune disorders	Normal levels vary with age. Intravenous immune globulin (IVIG) administration and steroids alter levels.
IgG subclasses	Measure the levels of the four subclasses of IgG (1, 2, 3, and 4)	Determine immune deficiency	Normal levels vary with age. IVIG administration and steroids alter levels.
Lymphocyte immunophenotyping T-cell quantification	Measures level of T cells (T-helper [CD4], T-suppressor [CD8]), B cells, and natural killer cells in the blood	Ongoing monitoring of progressive depletion of CD4 T lymphocytes in human immunodeficiency virus (HIV) disease	Do not refrigerate specimen. Steroids may elevate and immunosuppressive drugs may depress lymphocyte levels.
Delayed hypersensitivity skin test	Measures the presence of activated T cells that recognize certain substances	Immune disorders	Administered intradermally. Read and document size of reaction at 48–72 h (tuberculosis, mumps, Candida, tetanus).
HIV antibodies	Used to detect antibodies to HIV	Determining HIV infection when suspected	ELISA method detects only antibodies, so may remain negative for several weeks up to 6 months (false-negative). False-positive may result with autoimmune disease. Requires serial testing. HIV test results are confidential.
Polymerase chain reaction (PCR)	Used to detect HIV DNA and RNA	Diagnosis of HIV infection in children over 1-month-old	Sensitive and specific for presence of HIV in blood. Poor accuracy on samples obtained at birth. Sequential testing needed to determine perinatal transmission.
Complement assay (C3 and C4)	Measures the level of total complement in the blood, as well as levels of C3 and C4	Monitor systemic lupus erythematosus (SLE). Determine complement deficiency.	Send to laboratory immediately (unstable at room temperature). Usually sent out to a reference laboratory.
Erythrocyte sedimentation rate (ESR)	Nonspecific test used to determine presence of infection or inflammation	Immune disorder initial workup, ongoing monitoring of autoimmune disease	Send to laboratory immediately; if allowed to stand >3 h, falsely low result may occur.
Rheumatoid factor (RF)	Determines the presence of RF in the blood	Juvenile idiopathic arthritis, SLE	Positive RF is also sometimes seen in chronic infectious disorders.
Antinuclear antibody (ANA)	Tests for presence of autoantibodies that react against cellular nuclear material	SLE	Check for signs of infection at venipuncture site. Steroid use can cause false-negative result. May be weakly positive in about 20% of healthy individuals.

Nursing Care Plan 47.1

OVERVIEW FOR THE CHILD WITH AN IMMUNOLOGIC DISORDER

NURSING DIAGNOSIS: Ineffective protection related to inadequate body defenses, inability to fight infection as evidenced by deficient immunity

Outcome Identification and Evaluation

Child will not experience overwhelming infection, *will be infection-free or able to recover if he or she becomes infected.*

Intervention: Preventing Infection

- Maintain meticulous handwashing procedures (include family, visitors, staff) *to minimize spread of infectious organisms.*
- Maintain isolation as prescribed *to minimize exposure to infectious organisms.*
- Clean frequently touched surfaces with an appropriate cleanser *to minimize spread of infectious organisms.*
- Educate family and visitors that child should be restricted from contact with known infectious exposures (in hospital and at home) *to encourage cooperation with infection control.*
- Strictly observe medical asepsis *to avoid unintentional introduction of microorganisms.*
- Promote nutrition and appropriate rest *to maximize body's potential to heal.*
- Educate family to contact health care provider if child has known exposure to chickenpox or measles *so that preventive measures (e.g., VariZIG) can be given.*
- Administer vaccines (not live) as prescribed *to prevent common childhood communicable diseases.*
- Administer prophylactic antibiotics as prescribed *to prevent infection with opportunistic organisms.*

NURSING DIAGNOSIS: Imbalanced nutrition, less than body requirements, related to poor appetite, chronic illness, debilitated state, concurrent illness as evidenced by poor growth, weight gain and stature increases less than expected, poor head growth

Outcome Identification and Evaluation

Child will consume adequate intake, *will demonstrate appropriate weight gain and growth of length/height and/or head circumference.*

Intervention: Promoting Adequate Nutritional Intake

- Monitor growth (weight and height/length weekly) *to determine progress toward goal.*
- Determine realistic goal for weight gain for age (consulting dietitian if necessary) *to have a specific outcome to work toward.*
- Observe child's physical ability to eat *(if pain from candidiasis or motor impairment is present, will need additional interventions).*
- Provide nutrient-rich meals and snacks *to maximize caloric intake.*
- Supplement milkshakes with protein powder or other additives *to maximize caloric intake.*
- Provide child's favourite foods *to encourage increased intake.*
- Provide smaller, more frequent meals *to reduce sensation of fullness and increase overall intake.*
- If vomiting is an issue, administer antiemetics as ordered prior to meals *to provide optimal state for success at mealtime.*

NURSING DIAGNOSIS: Impaired skin integrity related to disease process or photosensitivity as evidenced by skin rash or alopecia

Outcome Identification and Evaluation

Skin integrity will be maintained; *secondary infection will not occur, rash will not increase.*

Intervention: Preventing Skin Impairment

- Assess and monitor extent and location of rash *to provide baseline information and evaluate success of interventions.*
- Keep skin clean and dry *to prevent secondary infection.*
- For the child with eczema, apply topical medications as ordered *to decrease inflammatory response.*
- For the child with limited mobility, turn frequently and use specialty mattress or bed *to prevent pressure ulcers.*
- Implement a written plan of care directed toward topical treatment of skin integrity impairment *to provide consistency of care and documentation.*
- Educate child and family to limit direct sun exposure and use sunscreen *to prevent sun damage.*

Nursing Care Plan 47.1 (continued)

NURSING DIAGNOSIS: Activity intolerance related to joint pain, fatigue or weakness, concurrent illness as evidenced by dyspnea, lack of desire to participate in play, inability to maintain usual routine

Outcome Identification and Evaluation
Child will participate in activities; *will demonstrate easy work of breathing and participate in daily routine and play.*

Intervention: Promoting Activity
- Cluster care *to decrease disturbances and allow for longer uninterrupted rest periods.*
- Pace activities and encourage regular rest periods *to conserve energy.*
- Administer early morning warm bath *to ease AM stiffness (juvenile arthritis).*
- Use assistive devices such as splints and orthotics *to improve physical function.*
- Plan developmentally appropriate activities that the child can participate in while in bed *to encourage play and continued development.*
- Schedule activities for time of day child usually has the most energy *to encourage successful participation.*

NURSING DIAGNOSIS: Delayed growth and development related to physical effects of chronic illness, or physical disability (juvenile arthritis) as evidenced by delay in meeting expected milestones

Outcome Identification and Evaluation
Development will be enhanced: *Child will make continued progress toward expected developmental milestones.*

Intervention: Enhancing Growth and Development
- Screen for developmental capabilities *to determine child's current level of functioning.*
- Offer age-appropriate toys, play, and activities (including gross motor) *to encourage further development.*
- Encourage peer contact through telephone, email, or letters *to promote/continue socialization.*
- Perform interventions as prescribed by physical or occupational therapist: *Repeat participation in those activities helps child improve function and acquire developmental skills.*
- Provide support to families of children with developmental delay *(progress in achieving developmental milestones can be slow, and ongoing motivation is needed).*
- Encourage child to continue schoolwork *so that child will not fall behind.*
- Reinforce positive attributes in the child *to maintain motivation.*

BOX 47.1   Ten Warning Signs of Primary Immunodeficiency

1. Eight or more episodes of acute otitis media in 1 year
2. Two or more episodes of severe sinusitis in 1 year
3. Treatment with antibiotics for 2 months or longer with little effect
4. Two or more episodes of pneumonia in 1 year
5. Failure to thrive
6. Recurrent deep skin or organ abscesses
7. Persistent oral thrush or skin candidiasis after 1 year of age
8. History of infections that do not clear with IV antibiotics
9. Two or more serious infections
10. Family history of primary immunodeficiency

From: Jeffrey Modell Foundation. (2011). *10 warning signs of primary immunodeficiency.* Retrieved October 6, 2011 from http://www.info4pi. org/aboutPI/index.cfm?section=aboutPI&content=warningsigns.

▶ ***Take*** NOTE!

Do not shake the IVIG, as this may lead to foaming and may cause the immunoglobulin protein to degrade (Kirmse, 2009).

Ensure that the child is well hydrated prior to the infusion to decrease the risk for rate-related reactions and aseptic meningitis after the infusion. Pre-medication with diphenhydramine or acetaminophen may be indicated in children who have never received IVIG, have not had an infusion in more than 8 weeks, have had a recent bacterial infection, or have a history of serious infusion-related adverse reactions. The rate for infusion of IVIG is generally prescribed as millilitres of IVIG per kilogram of body weight per hour (mL/kg/hour). Carefully calculate the infusion rate. Obtain a baseline physical assessment and measure vital signs. Begin the infusion slowly, increasing gradually every 30 minutes to the prescribed rate as tolerated (Fig. 47.1). Rapid infusion can cause flushing and

TABLE 47.1 TYPES OF HYPOGAMMAGLOBULINEMIA

Type	Definition	Characteristics	Treatment
Selective IgA deficiency	Serum IgA <0.07 g/L, normal IgG and IgM	80% of patients are asymptomatic. Child can present with broad spectrum of medical conditions, including recurrent sinopulmonary infections, atopic disorders (atopic asthma, allergic rhinitis, atopic dermatitis, food allergy), GI disease (especially celiac disease), neurologic disease, autoimmunity, and malignancy.	No specific gammaglobulin treatment available. Treat infections or autoimmune disorders. Severe anaphylactic reaction can occur if child receives transfusion of blood containing IgA and IgA antibodies.
X-linked agammaglobulinemia (Bruton's disease)	Markedly reduced or absent IgG, IgM, and IgA. Absence of B cells. Results from mutations in a gene on the X chromosome that encodes Bruton tyrosine kinase (Btk, which is essential for B-cell development and maturation).	Males only. Recurrent lung, sinus, and skin infections with encapsulated bacteria (e.g., *Streptococcus pneumoniae, Haemophilus influenzae*).	Routine administration of IVIG/SCIG. Treat infections. Patients should not receive any live viral vaccines, such as live polio or the measles, mumps, rubella (MMR) vaccine.
X-linked hyper-IgM syndrome	Defect in CD40L, a protein found on T-cell surface, resulting in decreased IgG and IgA levels with significant increase in IgM levels.	Males only. Recurrent respiratory infections, diarrhea, malabsorption. Neutropenia, autoimmune disorders.	Routine administration of IVIG/SCIG. Administer granulocyte colony-stimulating factor (G-CSF) SC when neutropenic. Bone marrow or cord blood stem cell transplantation. Treat autoimmune disorders.
IgG subclass deficiency	Low levels of one or more of the IgG subclasses	Usually asymptomatic. May have recurrent viral/bacterial infections. Some children outgrow this condition.	Treat respiratory infections. Administration of IVIG is helpful in some children.

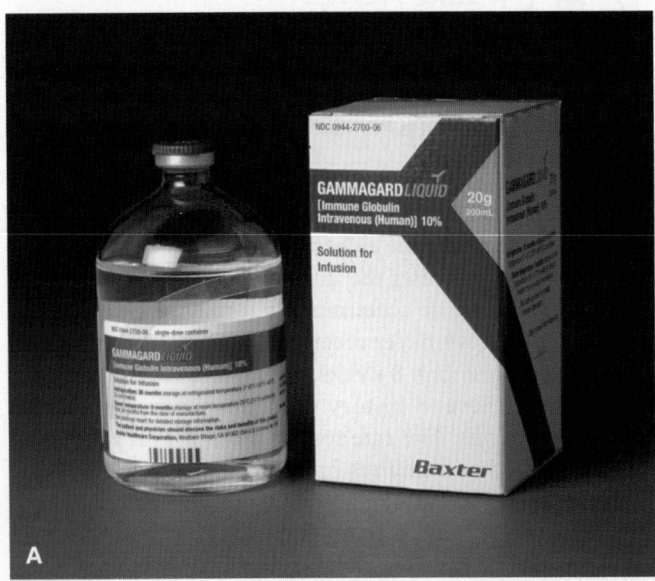
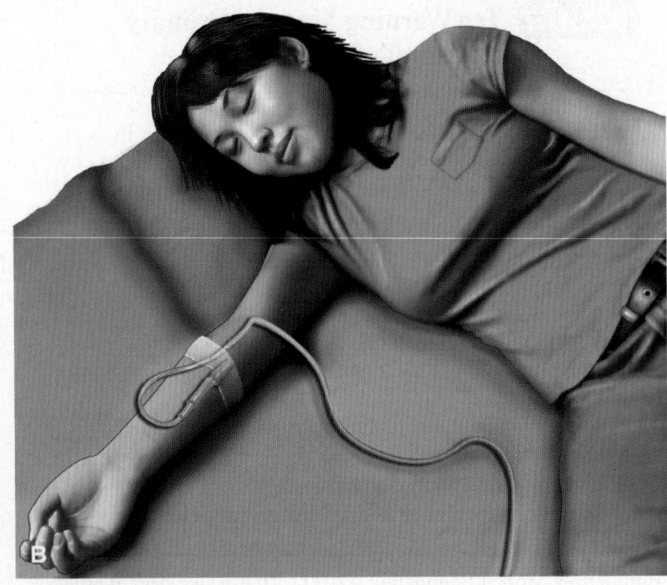

FIGURE 47.1 (**A**) Intravenous IVIG. (**B**) Intravenous administration of exogenous immunoglobulin every several weeks can decrease the frequency and severity of infections in children with various forms of hypogammaglobulinemia.

changes in heart rate and blood pressure. Assess vital signs and monitor for adverse reactions 15 minutes after IVIG initiation, then every 30 minutes if there are any rate changes or hourly throughout the remainder of the infusion (the frequency of assessments may vary according to institutional protocol). IVIG is a plasma product, so observe closely for signs of anaphylaxis such as headache, facial flushing, urticaria, dyspnea (shortness of breath), wheezing, chest pain, fever, chills, nausea, vomiting, increased anxiety, or hypotension. If these symptoms occur, discontinue the infusion and notify the physician or nurse practitioner. For mild, infusion rate–related reactions, the infusion may be restarted at a slower rate after the symptoms have subsided. Have oxygen and emergency medications such as epinephrine, diphenhydramine, and intravenous corticosteroids available in case of an anaphylactic reaction. If the child complains of discomfort at the intravenous site, a cold compress may be helpful (Doellman, Hadaway, Bowe-Geddes, et al., 2009).

▶ *Take* NOTE!

Many children who have had previous reactions to IVIG can tolerate the infusion without reaction if they are pre-medicated and if the infusion is given at a slower rate (Taketokmo, Hodding, & Kraus, 2010).

In recent years, a subcutaneous preparation of IgG (SCIG) has become available and is used to treat patients with primary immunodeficiencies. The subcutaneous form has the benefit of maintaining steadier IgG levels, can be self-administered in the home setting, and has fewer systemic side effects than IVIG. The coming years will see increased use of SCIG for treatment of primary immunodeficiency disorders (Berger, 2010).

Providing Education and Support

Provide education and support to the child and family. The Canadian Immunodeficiency Society provides an excellent resource list for families of children with primary immunodeficiency disorders (visit http://thePoint. lww.com/Chow1e for a direct link).

Wiskott–Aldrich Syndrome

Wiskott–Aldrich syndrome is a rare X-linked genetic disorder that results in immunodeficiency, eczema, and thrombocytopenia. It affects males only, although females can be carriers. The defective gene responsible for this disorder has been identified and is called the Wiskott–Aldrich syndrome protein (WASp). Complications of Wiskott–Aldrich syndrome include autoimmune hemolytic anemia, neutropenia, skin or cerebral vasculitis, arthritis, inflammatory bowel disease, and renal disease (Dibbern & Routes, 2010).

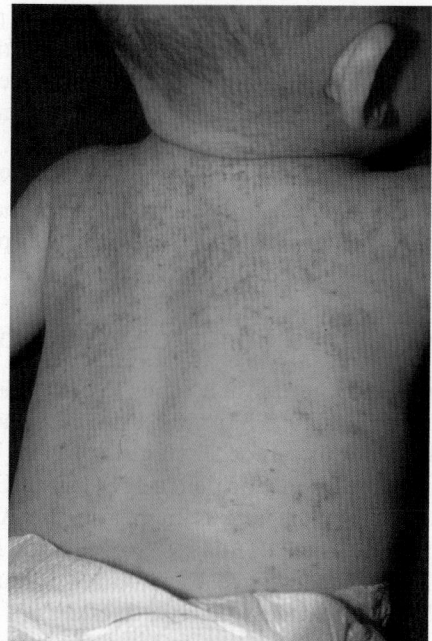

FIGURE **47.2** Boys with Wiskott–Aldrich syndrome often have worsening of eczema over time.

Autoimmune disease may require high-dose steroids, azathioprine, or cyclophosphamide. Splenectomy may be performed to correct thrombocytopenia. The only cure is bone marrow or cord blood stem cell transplantation, although these interventions carry substantial risks, including mortality. If transplantation is successful, hematologic and immunologic defects are corrected and eczema resolves.

Nursing Assessment

Note history of petechiae, bloody diarrhea, or bleeding episode in the first 6 months of life. Note any history of hematemesis or intracranial or conjunctival hemorrhages. Observe the skin for eczema, which usually worsens with time and tends to become infected (Fig. 47.2). Laboratory findings include low IgM concentration, elevated IgA and IgE concentrations, and normal IgG concentrations.

▶ *Take* NOTE!

An episode of prolonged bleeding such as after circumcision may be the first sign of Wiskott–Aldrich syndrome in the male infant (Dibbern & Routes, 2010).

Nursing Management

Administer IVIG as ordered to help manage thrombocytopenia or decrease the frequency of bacterial infections. Perform good skin care and frequently assess eczematous areas to detect secondary infection (refer to Chapter 45 for care of eczema). If the patient undergoes splenectomy to help control thrombocytopenia, in addition to providing routine postoperative care, be aware of the additional risk for development of infection in the asplenic patient. If the patient is bleeding, platelet or red cell infusions may be necessary. If the child undergoes a bone marrow or stem cell transplant, provide care as outlined in Chapter 49. Explain to the patient and family that severe cutaneous papillomavirus infection may occur after stem cell transplantation (even years later) (Neven, Leroy, Decaluwe, et al., 2009).

Severe Combined Immune Deficiency

Severe combined immune deficiency (SCID), also known as "bubble boy disease," is a rare X-linked or autosomal recessive disorder; it can occur in girls or boys. While no data are available on the incidence of SCID in Canada, it would appear that the rate is higher in the Aboriginal population (Canadian Paediatric Surveillance Program, n.d.). SCID is characterized by absent T-cell and B-cell function. There are at least five types of SCID, classified according to the exact genetic defect. The two most common forms are X-linked SCID and SCID caused by adenosine deaminase (ADA) enzyme deficiency. Infants with SCID usually present in the first few months of life with frequent episodes of diarrhea, pneumonia, otitis media, sepsis, and cutaneous infections. SCID is a potentially fatal disorder requiring emergency intervention at the time of diagnosis (Secord & Oren, 2009). The prognosis for infants with SCID is greatly improved if they are diagnosed and treated before severe infections develop. If left untreated, most children will die during the first year of life. Gene therapy provides some promise for the future treatment of SCID, but bone marrow or stem cell transplantation is currently the only known cure (Secord & Oren, 2009). IVIG infusions may help decrease the number of infections until bone marrow or stem cell transplantation can be performed (Secord & Oren, 2009). Children with SCID caused by ADA enzyme deficiency may benefit from ongoing subcutaneous ADA enzyme replacement. These injections will be required throughout life. Long-term antibiotic therapy helps to contain chronic infections.

Nursing Assessment

Note history of chronic diarrhea and failure to thrive. Note history of severe or persistent infections (pneumonia, otitis, sepsis, cutaneous infections) with opportunistic microorganisms beginning in early infancy. Inspect the mouth for persistent thrush. Auscultate the lungs, noting adventitious sounds related to pneumonia. Laboratory findings include a persistently low lymphocyte count and very low levels of all types of immunoglobulin.

Nursing Management

Prevention of infection is critical. Teach the family to practice good handwashing. The child must not be exposed to persons outside the family, particularly young children. Instruct families to report any signs or symptoms of infection in their child promptly so treatment can be initiated immediately. Teach families to administer prophylactic antibiotics if prescribed. Encourage adequate nutrition; supplemental enteral feedings may be necessary in the child with poor appetite. Administer IVIG infusions as prescribed and monitor for adverse reactions (refer to the nursing management section for hypogammaglobulinemia for further information related to IVIG administration). If the child receives a bone marrow transplant (human leukocyte antigen [HLA]-matched sibling is preferred), provide post-transplant care as outlined in Chapter 49. Refer the family for genetic counselling. Provide ongoing support; this is a difficult situation for families to cope with and the therapy required is lifelong.

▶ **Take** NOTE!

*Monitor the bone marrow or stem cell transplant patient closely for a maculopapular rash that usually starts on the palms and soles; this is an indication that **graft-versus-host disease** (GVHD) is developing. Use only cytomegalovirus (CMV)-negative, irradiated blood or platelets if transfusion is necessary in the infant with SCID. CMV-positive blood could cause an infection in the infant, and T lymphocytes in non-irradiated blood products may cause fatal GVHD to occur (Norville & Tomlinson, 2010). Do not administer any live vaccines, including rotavirus, MMR (measles, mumps, rubella), BCG (Bacille Calmette-Guérin), or varicella, to infants with confirmed or suspected SCID as live vaccines may cause an infection to develop.*

Secondary Immunodeficiencies

Secondary immunodeficiency may occur as a result of chronic illness, malignancy, use of **immunosuppressive** medication, malnutrition or protein-losing state, prematurity, or HIV infection. This discussion focuses on HIV infection.

HIV Infection

Globally, an estimated 2.5 million children less than 15 years of age are living with HIV infection and more than 1,000 babies become infected with HIV each day (UNICEF, 2010). Infants become infected primarily through their mothers, whereas adolescents contract HIV infection primarily through sexual activity or intravenous drug use (Fahrner & Romano, 2010). Approximately 65,000 Canadians were living with HIV or acquired immune deficiency syndrome (AIDS) in 2008, with 1% of these cases involving children (Public Health

Agency of Canada [PHAC], 2009). While the reported incidence of HIV among young people (defined as between 10 and 24 years of age) constitutes a very small proportion of the total number of HIV/AIDS cases in Canada, the potential for HIV transmission is demonstrated by data on risk behaviours (PHAC, 2009).

Pathophysiology

HIV affects immune function via alterations mainly in T-cell function, but it also affects B cells, natural killer cells, and monocyte/macrophage function. HIV infects the T-helper (CD4) cells. The virus replicates itself via the CD4 cell and renders the cell dysfunctional. Immune deficiency results as the number of normal, functioning CD4 cells drops. Initially, as CD4 counts decrease, the T-suppressor (CD8) counts increase, but as the disease progresses, CD8 counts also fall. The helper T-cell function declines even in asymptomatic infants and children who have not experienced significant decreases in the CD4 cell count. The T cells lose response to recall antigens, and this loss is associated with an increased risk of serious bacterial infection (Farland, 2011).

B-cell defects also occur in HIV-infected children, contributing to high rates of serious bacterial infections. The B cells demonstrate impaired response to mitogens and antigens. They also exhibit defective antibody production in response to antigen exposure or vaccination. Also, infants lack a pool of memory B cells (B-cell subtype that persists after an infection) for recall antigens (simply from lack of exposure). Natural killer cells also are affected by HIV infection, as they are dependent upon cytokines secreted by the CD4 cells for development of functionality. Functional killer cells play a role in fighting viruses and are critical to immunity in the newborn while the T-cell line develops. Decreased function of the natural killer cells then contributes to increased severity of viral infection in the HIV-infected child or infant. Though the virus does not destroy monocytes and macrophages, it does affect their function. Macrophages in the HIV-infected child exhibit decreased chemotaxis, and the antigen-presenting capability of the monocytes is defective.

Without appropriate T-cell, B-cell, natural killer cell, monocyte, and macrophage function, the infant's or child's immune system cannot fight infections it ordinarily could. Recurrent infection with ordinary organisms occurs more frequently in children with HIV infection, and the infections are more severe than in non-infected children. Opportunistic infections also occur in HIV-infected children, similar to those in adults with HIV.

HIV rapidly invades the central nervous system in infants and children and is responsible for progressive HIV encephalopathy. As a result of encephalopathy, acquired microcephaly, motor deficits, or loss of previously achieved developmental milestones may occur. In children with progressive HIV encephalopathy, neurologic symptoms may present before immune suppression. Currently, there is no cure for HIV infection.

Children acquire HIV either vertically or horizontally. Vertical transmission refers to perinatal (in utero or during birth) transmission or transmission via breast milk. Vertical transmission accounts for about 90% of all cases of pediatric HIV infection (Khoury & Kovacs, 2001), reflecting the need for maternal screening and interventions during pregnancy and postnatally. Horizontal transmission refers to transmission via nonsterile needles (as in intravenous drug use or tattooing) or intimate sexual contact. With nationwide screening of blood products, HIV transmission via transfused blood products has become rare.

A classification system for HIV infection in children was developed in 1994 and revised in 2008 by the Centers for Disease Control and Prevention (CDC, 1994, 2008). The classification ranges from the HIV-exposed newborn to the infant or child with AIDS and is based on the severity of the child's clinical symptoms as well as extent of immunologic suppression. The "Revised Surveillance Case Definitions for HIV Infection Among Adults, Adolescents, and Children Aged <18 Months and for HIV Infection and AIDS Among Children Aged 18 Months to <13 Years—United States, 2008" is useful for determining the severity of illness and for choosing the medication regimen (CDC, 2008).

Therapeutic Management

Current recommendations for treatment of HIV infection in children include the use of a combination of anti-retroviral drugs (Fahrner & Romano, 2010). Combination anti-retroviral therapy with at least three drugs from at least two drug classes is recommended for initial treatment of infected infants, children, and adolescents because it provides the best opportunity to preserve immune function and delay disease progression (Panel on Antiretroviral Therapy and Medical Management of HIV-Infected Children, 2011). Medication therapy ranges from single-drug therapy in the asymptomatic HIV-exposed newborn to highly active anti-retroviral therapy (HAART), which involves a combination of anti-retroviral drugs, in the HIV-infected infant, child, or adolescent. One of the goals of HAART is to prevent or arrest progressive HIV encephalopathy (Fahrner & Romano, 2010). The World Health Organization (WHO, 2010) recommends that all infants and children less than 2 years of age who are diagnosed with HIV should begin anti-retroviral therapy regardless of the child's clinical or immunologic stage. Updated guidelines for the use of anti-retroviral agents in infants and children with HIV have been issued by the Panel on Anti-retroviral Therapy and Medical Management of HIV-Infected Children (2011). See Evidence-based Practice 47.1.

EVIDENCE-BASED PRACTICE 47.1
Do Patient Education and Support Promote Adherence to Highly Active Anti-Retroviral Therapy (HAART) for HIV/AIDS?

● Study
The key determinant of degree and length of viral suppression in HIV infection is high adherence to HAART. Conversely, poor adherence leads to treatment failure. Children potentially have a significant number of years of life for which they will need to remain compliant with HAART. Each period of noncompliance further contributes to cross-resistance, limiting future treatment options. The authors evaluated a large number of randomized controlled trials that examined the effectiveness of patient education and support in improving HAART adherence.

▲ Findings
Education and support interventions are effective in improving HAART adherence. The most effective interventions are those that are delivered over a 12-week period or longer, targeting individuals rather than groups, and that provide practical medication-management skills.

■ Nursing Implications
HAART adherence is critical to the potential life of an HIV-infected child. Despite numerous medication side effects and the stigma associated with HIV infection, nurses can make a difference in these children's lives. Educate parents at every opportunity about the importance of HAART adherence. Provide families with ideas for managing unpleasant side effects of anti-retroviral drugs. Involve children in medication administration. Provide developmentally appropriate education to children and adolescents. Praise families' and children's efforts at HAART adherence.

Reuda, S., Park-Wyllie, L. Y., Bayoumi, A. M., Tynan, A. M., Antoniou, T. A., Rourke, S. B., & Glazier, R. H. (2007). Patient support and education for promoting adherence to highly active antiretroviral therapy for HIV/AIDS. *The Cochrane Library 2007, 4.* Indianapolis: John Wiley & Sons.

Nursing Assessment

For a full description of the assessment phase of the nursing process, refer to page 1621. Assessment findings pertinent to HIV infection and AIDS in children are discussed below.

Health History

Elicit a description of the present illness and chief complaint. Common signs and symptoms reported during the health history might include:

- Failure to thrive
- Recurrent bacterial infections
- Opportunistic infections
- Chronic or recurrent diarrhea
- Recurrent or persistent fever
- Developmental delay
- Prolonged oral candidiasis

These signs and symptoms may be present in either the child who is undergoing initial diagnosis or the child with known HIV infection. Explore the child's current and past medical history for risk factors such as maternal HIV infection or AIDS, receipt of blood transfusions before current nationwide screening policies, adolescent or childhood sexual abuse, substance use or abuse (including intravenous drug use), or participation in vaginal or anal sex without the use of a condom. As many children with HIV have lost their parents to the disease, it is important to document who is the primary caregiver. In addition, for the child with known HIV infection, determine the child's medications and dosages (medication reconciliation) as well as the outcome of any recent health care visits or hospitalizations.

Physical Examination

A thorough and complete physical examination should be performed on the child with AIDS or suspected HIV infection.

Inspection and Observation

Note presence of fever. Measure weight, height or length, and head circumference (in children less than 3 years old) and plot this information on standard growth charts, noting whether the measurements fall within the average or below the lower percentiles. Perform a developmental screening test to detect developmental delay. Inspect the oral cavity for candidiasis. Observe work of breathing (may be increased if pneumonitis or pneumonia is present). Determine level of consciousness (may be depressed if HIV encephalopathy is present).

Auscultation and Palpation

Auscultate the lungs, noting adventitious breath sounds associated with pneumonia or pneumonitis. Palpate for the presence of enlarged lymph nodes (lymphadenopathy) or swollen parotid glands (parotitis). Palpate the abdomen, noting hepatosplenomegaly.

Laboratory and Diagnostic Tests

Common laboratory and diagnostic studies ordered for the assessment of HIV infection include:

- Polymerase chain reaction (PCR) test: positive in infected infants over 1 month of age. PCR is the

> ### BOX 47.2 Virologic Testing for HIV-Exposed Infants (with PCR)
>
> • At birth
> • At 4 to 7 weeks of age
> • At 8 to 16 weeks of age
> • Serologic testing at 12 months of age or older to document disappearance of the HIV-1 antibody

preferred test to determine HIV infection in infants and to exclude HIV infection as early as possible. Box 47.2 gives recommendations for PCR testing.

• Enzyme-linked immunosorbent assay (ELISA): positive in infants of HIV-infected mothers because of transplacentally received antibodies. These antibodies may persist and remain detectable up to 24 months of age, making the ELISA test less accurate at detecting HIV infection in infants and toddlers than the PCR.
• Platelet count: above 500,000 (in severe HIV infection)
• CD4 and CD8 T-cell counts: once HIV infection is diagnosed, measurement of CD4 and CD8 T-cell counts is required to help determine degree of illness, prognosis, and response to treatment. CD4 counts may be normal initially but will eventually drop, while CD8 counts usually increase initially and do not fall until late in the disease progression.

Nursing Management

Nursing care of the child with HIV infection or AIDS is directed at avoiding infection, promoting compliance with the medication regimen, promoting nutrition, providing pain management and comfort measures, educating the child and caregivers, and providing ongoing psychosocial support. Nursing Care Plan 47.1 lists appropriate nursing diagnoses and interventions. In addition, nursing management specific to HIV infection is covered below.

Preventing HIV Infection in Children

All pregnant women should be offered routine HIV counselling and voluntary testing. Depending upon the stage of pregnancy, the mother should be treated with an anti-retroviral drug if she is HIV positive. Children born to HIV-positive mothers should receive a 6-week course of zidovudine (ZDV) therapy (Fahrner & Romano, 2010). Discourage breastfeeding in the HIV-infected mother and instruct her about safe alternatives to breast-feeding. Early recognition of infection is crucial so that treatment can begin and progression to AIDS can be prevented. Educate sexually active adolescents about HIV transmission and encourage the use of condoms. Counsel teens about the increased risk of HIV transmission with all forms of sexual activity, explaining that vaginal and anal sex are riskier than oral sex. Urge teens to limit the number of sexual partners. Discourage substance use, as the effects of drugs and alcohol often impair the teen's ability to make wise choices about sexual conduct (Chen, Thompson, & Morrison-Beedy, 2010; Morrison-Beedy, Nelson, & Volpe, 2005). Warn teens of the risk of contracting HIV infection via shared needles (as with intravenous drug use).

Promoting Compliance with Anti-Retroviral Therapy

Before HAART was available as a treatment option, progressive HIV encephalopathy was inevitably fatal, usually within 2 years of diagnosis (Fahrner & Romano, 2010). To prevent progression of HIV disease and encephalopathy, compliance with the HAART regimen is required. Educate the family about the importance of complying with the medication regimen. Help the caregivers develop a schedule for medication administration that is compatible with the family's home routine.

Reducing Risk for Infection

In the newborn whose mother is infected with tuberculosis, syphilis, toxoplasmosis, CMV, hepatitis B or C, or herpes simplex virus, testing and treatment should be provided. To prevent infection with *Pneumocystis jiroveci*, administer prophylactic antibiotics as prescribed in any HIV-exposed infant in whom HIV infection has not yet been excluded. Provide tuberculosis screening and childhood immunization in accordance with national guidelines.

> ▶ *Take* NOTE!
>
> *Do not administer live vaccines to the immunocompromised child without the express consent of the infectious disease or immunology specialist. Immunosuppression is a contraindication to vaccination with live vaccines (Nield et al., 2009).*

Promoting Nutrition

For the infant, provide increased-calorie formula as tolerated. For the child, provide high-calorie, high-protein meals and snacks. Supplements may be added to milkshakes to increase the protein intake. Ensure that the child is able to choose foods that he or she prefers from the hospital menu. Document growth through weekly measurements of weight and height.

Promoting Comfort

Children with HIV infection experience pain from infections, encephalopathy, adverse effects of medications, and the numerous procedures and treatments that are required, such as venipuncture, biopsy, or lumbar puncture. Refer to Chapter 35 for detailed information about pain assessment and management.

Providing Family Education and Support

Educate caregivers about the medication regimen, the ongoing follow-up that is needed, and when to call the infectious disease provider. Families of HIV-infected children experience a significant amount of stress from many sources: the diagnosis of an incurable disease, financial difficulties, multiple family members with HIV, HIV-associated stigmas, desire to keep HIV infection confidential, and multiple medical appointments and hospitalizations. Parents of HIV-infected children often die of AIDS themselves, leaving care of the child to another relative or foster parent. The day care centre or school that the child attends will need education about HIV, which can be provided only if the parent or caretaker consents to divulging the child's diagnosis to that agency. Provide education to the school or day care centre about how the infection is transmitted (i.e., not through casual contact).

Disclosure of the diagnosis of HIV to the child is another source of stress for the family. The timing of this disclosure will vary considerably depending on the child's and family's situation. Generally, children over 6 years of age will eventually need to have their diagnosis disclosed to them in an age-appropriate manner. They begin to ask questions and often seem to sense that something is going on other than what they've been told so far. When made aware of the diagnosis and educated about the disease, children may exhibit a variety of reactions. They may be bothered by the negative talk in their community about HIV and AIDS. They may feel it is not safe to talk to others because of the associated stigma. They want to be treated like others but with special consideration in tough times. They benefit from contact with others who are infected or affected. Anger, depression, or school problems may occur. The nurse should continue to provide emotional support to the child and family. If the disclosure results in significant emotional turmoil, refer the child and caregivers to a counsellor, social worker, or psychologist.

Anticipatory grieving also may occur. Parents or caregivers may express guilt or anger over the diagnosis of HIV infection. At the other end of the spectrum, families may use denial as their method for coping. Use therapeutic communication with open-ended questions to discover the family's thoughts and fears. Provide emotional support and allow for crying and verbalization. If needed, refer the caregivers to the appropriate professional for additional psychological and emotional intervention.

Many children with HIV have psychosocial, emotional, and cognitive problems that contribute to a lower quality of life. They are affected by the stigma of their diagnosis and often by the social isolation associated with it. They may suffer multiple losses within the family related to deaths caused by HIV infection. Children with HIV infection need significant psychosocial support and intervention. Resources for families of HIV-infected children are listed in Box 47.3.

BOX 47.3   Resources for HIV-Infected Children and Their Families

- Elizabeth Glaser Pediatric AIDS Foundation (resources for HIV-infected children and their families)
- The Zero (pediatric HIV infection and AIDS resources)
- Women, Children, and HIV (resources for prevention and treatment)

▶ *Take* NOTE!

Family-centred care of the HIV-exposed child and HIV-infected mother may involve a multidisciplinary approach and can result in improved outcomes for both the mother and the child (Fahrner & Romano, 2010).

▶ *Consider* THIS!

Jake Reddington, a 2-year-old diagnosed with HIV infection, is brought to the clinic by his aunt for his regular check-up. His aunt has recently taken over the care of Jake since his mother is too ill with HIV infection to care for him.

What education will be important for Jake's aunt and her family?

Discuss some of the psychosocial issues and concerns that face a child with HIV and his or her family.

Autoimmune Disorders

Autoimmune disorders result from the immune system's malfunction. The body manufactures T cells and antibodies against its own cells and organs (**autoantibodies**). The development of an autoimmune disorder is thought to be multifactorial. Potential influencing factors include heredity, hormones, self-marker molecules, and environmental influences such as viruses and certain drugs.

Systemic Lupus Erythematosus

Systemic lupus erythematosus (SLE) is a multisystem autoimmune disorder that affects both humoural and cellular immunity. SLE can affect any organ system, so the onset and course of the disease are quite variable. SLE affects females more often than males. Although the condition presents more commonly in adulthood, approximately 15% to 20% of SLE cases occur before age 16 years (von Scheven & Bakkaloglu, 2009). SLE has a peak childhood onset between 11 and 15 years of age, rarely affecting children younger than 5 (Pongmarutani, Alpert, & Miller, 2006). In Canada, the estimated number of SLE patients ranges from 15,000 (based on the number of patients followed in various university hospital lupus clinics throughout the country) to 50,000 (based on the figures used by the Lupus Foundation of America, adjusted to the Canadian population) (Senécal, 1998). SLE is more common in nonwhites; black, Hispanic, and Asian patients typically experience more severe effects from SLE than do other racial or ethnic groups (Mina & Brunner, 2010).

Pathophysiology

In SLE, autoantibodies react with the child's self-antigens to form immune complexes. These immune complexes accumulate in the tissues and organs, causing an inflammatory response resulting in vasculitis. Tissue injury and pain result. Since SLE can affect any organ system, the potential for alterations or damage to tissues anywhere in the body is significant. In some cases, the autoimmune response may be preceded by a drug reaction, an infection, or excessive sun exposure. In children, the most common initial symptoms are fatigue, fever, weight loss, malar rashes, and arthralgia/arthritis. Children have a high frequency (30% to 50%) of severe renal disease at presentation. The disease is chronic, with periods of remission and exacerbation (flare-ups). Common complications of SLE include ocular or visual changes, cerebrovascular accident (CVA), transverse myelitis, immune complex–mediated glomerulonephritis, pericarditis, valvular heart disease, coronary artery disease, seizures, and psychosis.

Therapeutic Management

Therapeutic management focuses on treating the inflammatory response. NSAIDs, corticosteroids, and antimalarial agents are often prescribed for the child with mild to moderate SLE. The child with severe SLE or frequent flare-ups of symptoms may require high-dose (pulse) corticosteroid therapy or immunosuppressive drugs. When end-stage renal failure develops as a result of glomerulonephritis, dialysis becomes necessary.

Nursing Assessment

For a full description of the assessment phase of the nursing process, refer to page 1621. Assessment findings pertinent to SLE in children are discussed below.

Health History

Elicit a description of the present illness and chief complaint. Common signs and symptoms reported during the health history are fatigue, fever, weight changes, pain or swelling in the joints, numbness, tingling or coolness of extremities, or prolonged bleeding. Assess for risk factors, which include female sex; family history (only 10% of cases); African, First Nations, or Asian descent; recent infection; drug reaction; or excessive sun exposure.

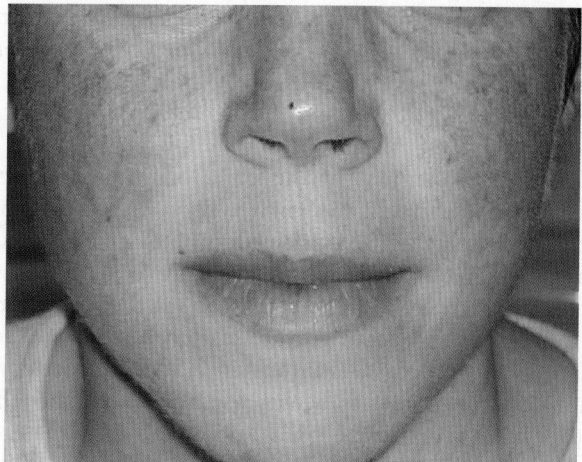

FIGURE 47.3 The malar or butterfly rash (erythema over the cheeks in the shape of a butterfly) is typical in SLE.

Physical Examination

Measure temperature and document the presence of fever. Observe the skin for malar rash (a butterfly-shaped rash over the cheeks); discoid lesions on the face, scalp, or neck; changes in skin pigmentation; or scarring (Fig. 47.3). Document alopecia. Inspect the oral cavity for painless ulcerations and the joints for edema. Measure blood pressure, as hypertension may occur with renal involvement. Auscultate the lungs; adventitious breath sounds may be present if the pulmonary system is involved. Palpate the joints, noting tenderness. Palpate the abdomen and note areas of tenderness (abdominal involvement is more common in children with SLE than in adults). Box 47.4 lists common clinical findings in SLE.

Laboratory and Diagnostic Findings

Laboratory findings may include decreased hemoglobin and hematocrit, decreased platelet count, and low WBC count. Complement levels, C3 and C4, will also

---

BOX 47.4 Most Common Clinical Manifestations of SLE

- Alopecia
- Anemia
- Arthralgia
- Arthritis
- Fatigue
- Lupus nephritis
- Photosensitivity
- Pleurisy
- Raynaud's phenomenon
- Seizures
- Skin rashes, including malar rash
- Stomatitis
- Thrombocytopenia

be decreased. Though not specific to SLE, the antinuclear antibody (ANA) test is usually positive in patients with SLE.

Nursing Management

Nursing management of the child or adolescent with SLE is long term and supportive. Focusing care on preventing or delaying SLE morbidities and complications may help to restore, maintain, or improve the quality of life. Educate the child and family about the importance of a healthy diet, regular exercise, sun safety, and adequate sleep and rest. Administer NSAIDs, corticosteroids, and antimalarial agents as ordered to the child with mild to moderate SLE and pulse corticosteroid therapy or immunomodulators to the child with severe SLE or frequent flare-ups. Refer families to support services such as Lupus Canada and the Lupus Foundation of America. (Visit http://thePoint.lww.com/Chow1e for direct links to these websites.)

Preventing and Monitoring for Flare-Ups and Complications

Teach patients to apply sunscreen (minimum SPF 25) to their skin daily and to avoid direct sunlight wherever possible to prevent rashes resulting from photosensitivity. Instruct the child and family to protect against cold weather by layering warm socks and wearing gloves when outdoors in the winter. If the child is outside for extended periods during the winter months, the fingers and toes should be inspected for discolouration. Watch for the development of nephritis by evaluating blood pressure, serum BUN and creatinine levels, and urine output and monitoring for hematuria or proteinuria. Ensure that yearly vision screening and ophthalmic examinations are performed to preserve visual function should changes occur.

> ▶ **Take** NOTE!
>
> *Avascular necrosis (lack of blood supply to a joint, resulting in tissue damage) may occur as an adverse effect of long-term or high-dose corticosteroid use. Teach families to report new onset of joint pain, particularly with weight-bearing, or limited range of motion to their physician or nurse practitioner (Tofferi & Gilliland, 2009).*

Juvenile Idiopathic Arthritis

Juvenile idiopathic arthritis (JIA) is a group of rheumatic diseases that begins at or before age 16 (Altman, 2008). It is an autoimmune disorder in which the autoantibodies mainly target the joints. Inflammatory changes in the joints cause pain, redness, warmth, stiffness, and swelling. Stiffness usually occurs after inactivity (as in the morning, after sleep). Some forms also affect the eyes or other organs. Table 47.2 explains the three most common

types. JIA is a chronic disease: the child may experience healthy periods alternating with flare-ups. The disease resolves in some children as they approach adolescence or adulthood, while others will have more severe disease that continues throughout the adult years (Jones & Higgins, 2010). JIA was formerly termed "juvenile rheumatoid arthritis," but unlike adult rheumatoid arthritis, few types of juvenile arthritis actually demonstrate a positive rheumatoid factor.

Therapeutic management focuses on inflammation control, pain relief, promotion of remission, and maintenance of mobility. NSAIDs, corticosteroids, antirheumatic drugs such as methotrexate, and biological response modifiers such as etanercept, infliximab, abatacept, or adalimumab are prescribed, depending on the type and severity of the disease. NSAIDs are helpful with pain relief, but disease-modifying (antirheumatic and biologic) drugs are necessary to prevent disease progression.

Nursing Assessment

Note history of irritability or fussiness, which may be the first sign of this disease in the infant or very young child. Note complaints of pain, though children do not always communicate this. Document history of withdrawal from play or difficulty getting the child out of bed in the morning (joint stiffness after inactivity). Inquire about history of fever (above 39.5°C for 2 weeks or more in systemic disease).

Measure temperature (fever is present with systemic disease). Inspect skin for evanescent, pale red, nonpruritic macular rash, which may be present at diagnosis of systemic disease. Observe the gait, noting limping or guarding of a joint or extremity. Document growth, which may be delayed. Inspect and palpate each joint for edema, redness, warmth, and tenderness (Fig. 47.4). Note positioning of joints (usually flexed in position of comfort). Mild to moderate anemia and an elevated erythrocyte sedimentation rate are common. Young children with the pauciarticular form may demonstrate a positive ANA, and adolescents

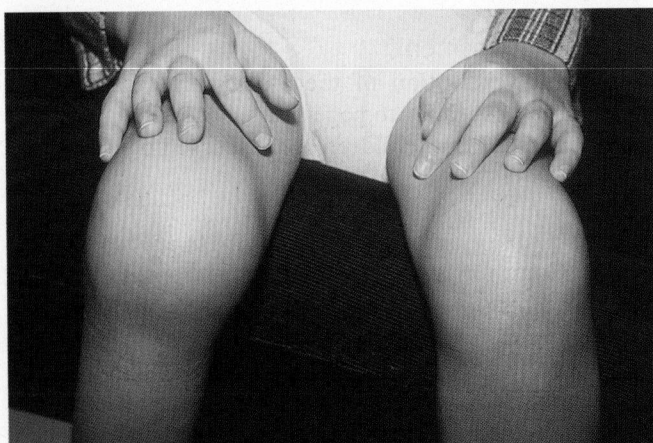

FIGURE 47.4 Note the swollen, reddened joints of this child with juvenile arthritis.

TABLE 47.2 TYPES OF JUVENILE IDIOPATHIC ARTHRITIS

Type	Definition	Non-Joint Manifestations	Potential Complications
Oligoarticular	Involvement of four or fewer joints; quite often the knees, ankles, or wrists are involved; most common type	Eye inflammation, malaise, poor appetite, poor weight gain	Iritis, uveitis, uneven leg bone growth
Polyarticular (rheumatoid factor [RF] positive and negative)	Involvement of five or more joints and tends to worsen over time; frequently involves small joints and often affects the body symmetrically; children with positive RF have more severe form	Malaise, lymphadenopathy, organomegaly, poor growth	Often a severe form of arthritis; rapidly progressing joint damage; rheumatoid nodules
Systemic	Most severe form; causes pain in many joints; can also spread to organs	High fevers; salmon pink rash; enlarged spleen, liver, and lymph nodes; anemia and fatigue	Pericarditis, pericardial effusion, pleuritis, pulmonary fibrosis
Enthesitis-related	Less common; often affects areas where tendons and ligaments attach to bones; arthritis in large joints; more common in school age or older children; affects boys more often than girls	Inflammation of the entheses (tendons and ligaments attached to bone); eye inflammation; inflammatory bowel disease	Ankylosing spondylitis
Psoriatic	Joint tenderness with psoriasis of the skin or strong family history of psoriasis; affects any joint; affects girls more often than boys	Psoriasis, nail involvement (pitting)	Tenosynovitis, sacroiliitis

with polyarticular disease may have a positive rheumatoid factor.

Nursing Management

Nursing management focuses on managing pain, maintaining mobility, and promoting a normal life. Refer the child to a pediatric rheumatologist to ensure that he or she receives the most up to date treatment. Disease-modifying medications approved for use in children may produce better long-term outcomes than were possible in the past. Clinical research trial information is available through the Childhood Arthritis & Rheumatology Research Alliance (CARRA). Encourage regular eye examinations and vision screening to allow for early diagnosis and treatment of visual changes and to prevent blindness.

Managing Pain and Maintaining Mobility

Administer medications as prescribed to control inflammation and prevent disease progression. Refer to Drug Guide 47.1 for information related to NSAIDs, corticosteroids, disease-modifying antirheumatic drugs, and biological response modifiers. Maintain joint range of motion and muscle strength via exercise (consult with physical or occupational therapy). Swimming is a particularly useful exercise to maintain joint mobility without placing pressure on the joints. Teach families appropriate use of splints prescribed to prevent joint contractures.

Monitor for pressure areas or skin breakdown with splint or orthotic use.

Promoting Normal Life

Chronic pain and decreased mobility may reduce the child's psychological and emotional status significantly, possibly extending into adulthood. Providing adequate pain relief (including pain relief exercises) and promoting compliance with the disease-modifying medication regimen may allow the child to have a more normal life in the present as well as in the future. In addition to measures described in the previous section, encourage adequate sleep to allow the child to cope better with symptoms and to function better in school. Sleep may be promoted by a warm bath at bedtime and warm compresses to affected joints or massage. To prevent social isolation, encourage the child to attend school and ensure that teachers, the school nurse, and classmates are educated about the child's disease and any limitations on activity. Having two sets of books (one at school and one at home) allows the child to do homework without having to carry heavy books home. Modifications such as allowing the child to leave the classroom early in order to get to the next class on time may seem small but can have a significant impact on the child's life.

Encourage children and families to become involved with local support groups so they can see that they are not alone. Assist children to set and achieve goals to increase their sense of hopefulness. Special summer camps for children with JIA allow the child to socialize and belong to a group and have been shown to promote self-esteem in the child with chronic illness. Encourage appropriate family functioning and refer the family to support groups such as those sponsored by the Canadian Arthritis Society or the American Juvenile Arthritis Organization.

Allergy and Anaphylaxis

Allergy is the inappropriate and harmful response of the body's defense mechanism to substances that are normally harmless. It involves the immune system and particularly the IgE antibody (World Allergy Organization Allergic Diseases Resource Center, 2011). Genetic tendency plays a role since allergies tend to run in families (Allergy/Asthma Information Association [AAIA], 2010).

The Canadian Allergy, Asthma and Immunology Foundation estimates that 20% to 25% of the Canadian population has allergic rhinitis (Allergy/Asthma Information Association, 2009). The extent of the allergic response is determined by the duration, rate, and amount of exposure to the allergen as well as environmental and host factors (American College of Allergy, Asthma, and Immunology [ACAAI], 2006; Fletcher-Janzen & Reynolds, 2003). IgE-mediated allergy is the focus of this discussion. This type of allergic response is mediated by antigen-specific IgE antibodies. When the antibody is exposed to the antigen (allergen), rapid cell activation occurs and potent mediators and cytokines are released, resulting in changes in the blood vessels, bronchi, and mucus-secreting glands. In addition to the atopic diseases (asthma, allergic rhinitis, atopic dermatitis), urticaria, digestive allergy, and systemic anaphylaxis are also IgE-mediated (Fletcher-Janzen & Reynolds, 2003; Sampson & Eggleston, 2006). Though any allergen has the potential to trigger an anaphylactic response, food and insect sting allergies are most common (Sloand & Caschera, 2010).

Food Allergies

"Food allergies, defined as an adverse immune response to food proteins, affect as many as 6% of young children and 3% to 4% of adults in Westernized countries, and their prevalence appears to be rising" (Sicherer & Sampson, 2009, p. 261). This type of reaction is an IgE-mediated response to a particular food. During the first few years of life, the most common food allergens are cow's milk, eggs, peanuts, tree nuts, sesame seeds, and kiwi fruit (Mullin, Swift, Lipski, et al., 2010). Some allergies to common foods persist from early childhood into adulthood (Sloand & Caschera, 2010). Cow's milk allergy persisting into adulthood is an uncommon phenomenon. Persistence of egg allergy into adulthood is more common, yet more than 80% of children with egg allergy will eventually become tolerant, and approximately 20% of peanut-allergic

patients will become tolerant by late childhood (Yun & Katelaris, 2009). Most reactions occur within minutes of exposure, but they may occur up to 2 hours after ingestion. Signs and symptoms of a food allergy reaction include hives, flushing, facial swelling, mouth and throat itching, and runny nose. Many children also have a gastrointestinal reaction, including vomiting, abdominal pain, and diarrhea. In extreme cases, swelling of the tongue, uvula, pharynx, or upper airway may occur. Wheezing can be an ominous sign that the airway is edematous. Rarely, cardiovascular collapse occurs. Though the risk for anaphylaxis is small, parents, caregivers, and health care providers should be vigilant when caring for children with food allergies (Yun & Katelaris, 2009).

Therapeutic Management

Therapeutic management involves verifying the food allergy, avoiding the allergen, and treating the reaction with epinephrine or antihistamines. Preventing the development of food allergies is also a key intervention.

It is important to discern a true food allergy from intolerance, or non-allergic hypersensitivity, to certain foods. In non-allergic hypersensitivity, the immune system is not involved in the hypersensitivity response, nor is it responsible for symptoms caused by eating food. Non-allergic hypersensitivity causes a more delayed and varied set of symptoms than does true food allergy, and often small amounts eaten infrequently are tolerated while larger amounts or amounts eaten more regularly can cause symptoms (Collard, 2010). Often a milk allergy is confused with lactose intolerance. Therefore, a detailed dietary history is important when distinguishing a true allergy versus intolerance.

To prevent the development of food allergies, infants should be breastfed for at least the first 4 to 6 months of life. More recent evidence suggests that delaying the introduction of solids beyond 6 months may be harmful in terms of both allergy risk and nutritional risk (Anderson, Malley, & Snell, 2009). The following common food allergens should be avoided in children under 1 year of age (Chamberlain, 2006; Muraro, Dreborg, Halken, et al., 2004):

- Cow's milk
- Eggs
- Peanuts
- Tree nuts
- Sesame seeds
- Kiwi fruit
- Fish and shellfish

Nursing Assessment

Patients with food allergy reactions must be assessed accurately. In the initial nursing assessment, the child should be immediately assessed for airway, breathing, or circulation problems (see Chapter 52). If the child's condition is stable, the nurse should finish the assessment. The history should include a detailed food history and documentation of the reaction, including the food suspected of causing the reaction, the quantity of food ingested, the length of time between ingestion and development of symptoms, the symptoms, what treatment has been administered, and the subsequent response. Note gastrointestinal symptoms such as:

• Burning in the mouth or throat
• Bloating
• Nausea
• Diarrhea

Assess for risk factors such as previous exposure to the food, history of poorly controlled asthma, or an increase in atopic dermatitis flare-ups in relation to food intake (Roberts, Patel, Levi-Schaffer, et al., 2003).

Inspect the skin for colour, rash, hives, or edema. Auscultate the heart and lungs to determine heart rate and to assess for wheezing.

The ACAAI's new practice parameter recommends food-specific IgE testing (by way of a skin prick test or a radioallergosorbent test [RAST] to detect specific IgE antibodies to specific food proteins) if the child has a history of food allergy. Food avoidance is recommended for those who have a highly predictive reaction to testing or a history of anaphylactic response. If the child has episodic symptoms, an oral challenge may be appropriate. If symptoms are chronic, a trial elimination diet may be indicated. If symptoms resolve without the food, true allergy may be present (ACAAI, 2006). On an elimination diet, the child should stop eating all suspicious foods for 1 to 2 weeks and then retry the foods one at a time, over a period of several days, to see whether a similar reaction occurs. This is often done in the pediatrician's office or hospital setting if severe reactions have occurred in the past. If a similar reaction occurs, it is very suggestive of a food allergy. Allergy skin prick tests and RAST blood tests are widely used by pediatricians to look for reactions. However, these tests may have false-positive results, and children may be instructed to avoid many foods unnecessarily (Sloand & Caschera, 2010).

Nursing Management

Initial nursing management is aimed at stabilizing the child's condition if an acute reaction to a food allergen is present (see Chapter 52). Medications used in the treatment of a food allergy reaction include histamine blockers and, in anaphylactic reactions, epinephrine. Teach the child (if appropriate) and the parents how and when to use these medications during an allergic reaction. Since these reactions can be so sudden (unknown ingestion of allergen) and severe, it is helpful for the family to have a written emergency plan in case of a reaction.

Managing the Child's Diet

Dietary teaching is aimed at educating the family on how to avoid the offending foods. Families should be extremely careful when reading food labels. A dietitian may be helpful in this teaching process. Teaching Guideline 47.1 gives information about hidden allergens in food. Teach the parents what "safe" foods can be substituted for offensive ones (Box 47.5). Children with peanut allergy should not eat tree nuts, as up to 35% to 50% of children who are allergic to peanuts are also allergic to tree nuts (Jackson, 2002; Vu & Duong, 2007).

The successful avoidance of food allergens depends on awareness of the specific food that caused the reaction, recognition of other food that may cause cross-reactions, and education about avoidance measures and other actions to prevent inadvertent exposure (ACAAI, 2006). Having a child with a food allergy can cause much anxiety for

---

TEACHING GUIDELINE 47.1

Allergens Hidden in Food

If Child is Allergic to:	Teach Families to Avoid:	Unexpected Locations of Common Ingredients
Milk	Artificial butter flavour, casein, lactalbumin, nougat, pudding, whey, yogurt, ghee	Some deli meats and hot dogs, nondairy products, coffee whiteners
Wheat	Cereal extract, couscous, durum, semolina, spelt	Some imitation crab meat and wheat flour shaped to look like shrimp, beef, or pork, especially in Asian dishes
Eggs	Albumin, globulin, ovalbumin	Some egg substitutes and foam toppings for drinks, commercially cooked pastas
Peanuts	Fast food cooked in peanut oil, many Asian foods, baked goods with nuts or processed on equipment that also processes peanuts	Brown gravy, barbeque sauce, meat sauce, egg rolls, enchilada sauce, hot chocolate

Adapted from: Food Allergen and Anaphylaxis Network. (2011). *Allergens*. Retrieved October 6, 2011 from http://www.foodallergy.org/section/allergens.

BOX 47.5 **Food Substitutions**

- Replace milk with water, fruit juice, rice milk, or soy milk.
- Replace each egg with one of the following: 1.5 tablespoons each of water and oil and 1 teaspoon baking powder; one packet plain gelatin with 2 tablespoons of warm water added at time of use; or 1 teaspoon of yeast and a quarter-cup of warm water.
- Replace peanuts or tree nuts with raisins, dates, or crispy cereal.

Adapted from: Winkels, K. (2010). *How to eat with food allergies: Finding allergy-free substitutes.* Retrieved October 6, 2011 from http://www.eatingwithfoodallergies.com/allergyfreesubstitutes.html.

parents, who often live in fear that the child may accidentally ingest an allergen (Kim & Sicherer, 2010). Educating the child and family about allergic reactions may help to decrease their anxiety. Teach the child and family how to recognize the signs and symptoms of an allergic reaction. The nurse may need to provide information to day care providers as well as school teachers, staff, and camp counsellors (Munoz-Furlong, 2003). Refer families to the AAIA, Anaphylaxis Canada, or the Food Allergy & Anaphylaxis Network for more information or resources (visit http://thePoint.lww.com/Chow1e for direct links to their websites).

Anaphylaxis

Anaphylaxis occurs in an acute and unexpected manner and is the most extreme form of life-threatening systemic allergic reaction. It is caused when specific antigens come in contact with sensitized individuals. While the true incidence of anaphylaxis is unknown, these antigens are most commonly from insect stings, medications, latex, peanuts and tree nuts (e.g., walnuts, hazelnuts, almonds, cashews, pecans, and pistachios), fish and shellfish, milk, eggs, and wheat (Munn, 2009). The incidence of anaphylaxis is increasing, particularly during the first two decades of life. Newly recognized food triggers include quinoa, fish gelatin, and seal and whale meat eaten by indigenous peoples (Simons, 2009). In addition to food allergens, medication triggers include beta-lactam and other antibiotics as well as aspirin, ibuprofen, and other analgesics. An anaphylactic reaction is severe and usually starts within 5 to 10 minutes of exposure, though delayed reactions are possible. Histamines and secondary mediators are released from the mast cells and eosinophils in response to contact with an allergen. Cutaneous, cardiopulmonary, gastrointestinal, and neurologic symptoms occur. Vasodilation results in a rapid decrease in plasma volume, leading to the risk of circulatory collapse (Kemp, 2011). Prolonged resuscitation may be needed, and death may occur.

Therapeutic management focuses on assessment and support of the airway, breathing, and circulation. Epinephrine is usually required, and intramuscular or intravenous diphenhydramine is used secondarily. Late-onset reactions can be prevented with corticosteroids.

Nursing Assessment

Assess patency of the airway and adequacy of breathing. Determine whether circulation is sufficient. Note level of consciousness. Obtain a brief history, inquiring specifically about allergen exposure. Determine whether the child has received any medication (e.g., epinephrine or diphenhydramine) since the onset of the reaction and what effect the medication had on the symptoms. Table 47.3 gives additional signs and symptoms of anaphylaxis.

Nursing Management

Nursing management initially focuses on supporting airway, breathing, and circulation. Provide supplemental oxygen by mask or bag-valve-mask ventilation. Ensure that bronchodilator inhalation treatment (albuterol) is given if bronchospasm is present. Administer intravenous fluids to provide volume expansion. Administer 0.15 mg/kg

TABLE 47.3 **CLINICAL MANIFESTATIONS OF ANAPHYLAXIS**

Body System	Symptoms
Integument	• Angioedema • Lip and eyelid swelling • Urticarial rash (hives) • Pruritus and sensation of warmth • Watering eyes • Cold, clammy skin
Cardiovascular	• Hypotension • Impaired cardiac output • Poor perfusion • Tachycardia
Gastrointestinal	• Nausea • Vomiting • Abdominal cramps • Diarrhea
Respiratory system	• Rhinitis and sneezing • Dyspnea • Stridor, tightness in the throat, dysphagia, dysphonia, hoarseness • Shortness of breath, tight chest, wheeze • Cyanosis • Behavioural change
Neurologic	• Syncope, feeling faint, aura of doom, lethargy, disorientation

Adapted from: Tsang, K. G. F. (2008). Anaphylaxis: Assessing patients with allergies. *Emergency Nurse, 16*(5), 24–29.

epinephrine to a maximum dose of 0.5 mg (1:1,000 concentration) into the anterolateral thigh muscle and repeat the dose every 5 to 10 minutes for three doses if needed. Monitor the child closely for 4 to 24 hours following epinephrine administration as the incidence of rebound anaphylaxis is up to 20%. There is no evidence for the use of histamine (H_1 or H_2) blockers (diphenydramine) or steroids in anaphylaxis, but they may be ordered to manage delayed symptoms (Tupper & Visser, 2010).

Preventing and Managing Future Episodes

Education of the family about preventing and managing future episodes is critical. Teach the family how to use injectable epinephrine in case of subsequent allergen exposure. Intramuscular epinephrine may be given via the EpiPen, EpiPen Jr., or Twinject auto-injectors. Dosage is based on the child's weight. According to product instructions, the 0.30 mg dosage of both the EpiPen and Twinject auto-injectors should be used for adults and children weighing 30 kg or more; and the 0.15 mg dosage should be used for children weighing between 15 and 30 kg. Individuals or their caregivers should consult with the child's physician to determine the appropriate dosage, including the switch from the lower dosage to the higher dosage. The safety release on the EpiPen should never be removed until just before use. The thumb, fingers, or hand should not be placed over the tip (which is typically black or orange). Nursing Procedure 47.1 gives further instructions related EpiPen use. Have the child and family review the consumer information available online from the auto-injector manufacturers. Instruct the child and family to call 911 and seek immediate medical attention after using an epinephrine auto-injector.

Day care providers, school nurses, teachers, and staff who interact with the child must know how to recognize an anaphylactic event. Advise the child to wear a medical alert bracelet or necklace at all times. All children with allergies should have an action plan in place at their school or day care centre (Clark & Ewan, 2003; Frost & Chalin, 2005; Watura, 2002). (Visit http://thePoint.lww.com/Chow1e for a direct link to information about creating an anaphylaxis emergency plan.)

Teach children with allergies and their families to avoid known food allergens. For children with allergies to bees, avoid stings from bees and wasps (Hymenoptera) by being alert when eating outdoors, wearing long sleeves and pants when in fields, and removing hives or nests. For children with allergies to penicillin, desensitization is available for children with a severe penicillin allergy. Avoid use of cephalosporins in children with severe penicillin allergy (Ellis & Day, 2003).

Latex Allergy

Latex allergy is an IgE-mediated response to exposure to latex, a natural rubber product used in many common items (especially gloves in the health care setting). The pathophysiology of latex allergy is similar to that of food allergy. Reactions to latex can range from type IV delayed hypersensitivity (e.g., contact dermatitis) to type I immediate hypersensitivity (e.g., urticaria, bronchospasm). Avoidance of latex products is recommended for those who are allergic to it. The incidence of latex allergy in the general population is 1% to 2%. The risk ranges from 20% to 67% in patients with spina bifida because of repeated exposure of mucous membranes to latex during surgeries and procedures (Pollart, Warniment, & Mori, 2009). An immediate allergic reaction may occur if a latex-allergic child comes into contact with latex. Latex allergy can also result in anaphylaxis (refer to section above on anaphylaxis).

Nursing Assessment

Screen all children who visit a health care facility of any kind for latex allergy. Ask if the child is allergic to rubber gloves or has ever developed hives after exposure to them. Ask the parent if the child has symptoms such as coughing, wheezing, or shortness of breath after glove exposure. Has the child ever had swelling in the mouth or complained that the mouth itched after a dental examination? Determine whether the child has ever had allergic symptoms after eating foods with a known cross-reactivity to latex, such as banana, avocado, chestnut, kiwi, apple, carrot, celery, papaya, potato, tomato, melons, pear, mango, sweet pepper, or peach. For the child who has come into contact with latex, assess for symptoms of a reaction such as hives; wheeze; cough; shortness of breath; nasal congestion and rhinorrhea; sneezing; nose, palate, or eye pruritus; or hypotension.

Nursing Management

Nursing management of latex allergy focuses on preventing exposure to latex products. Instruct children and their families to avoid foods with a known cross-reactivity to latex such as those listed above (American Latex Allergy Association, n.d.; Binkley, Schroyer, & Catalfano, 2003; Ellis & Day, 2003; Tang, 2003). If the child is exposed to latex, remove the irritating substance and cleanse the area with soap and water. Assess for the need for resuscitation and perform it if needed (Binkley et al., 2003; Pollart et al., 2009). Become familiar with your institution's latex allergy policy. Know which products contain latex and which do not. Avoid exposure to latex in children at high risk for latex allergy, such as those with spina bifida, urogenital anomalies, or other chronic illnesses requiring frequent surgeries or procedures. Document latex allergy on the patient's chart and identification band, the medication administration record, and the physician's order sheet. Refer families to resources for persons with latex allergy (visit http://thePoint.lww.com/Chow1e for direct links to online resources).

Nursing Procedure 47.1

How to use EpiPen® and EpiPen® Jr Auto-injectors.

Remove EpiPen® Auto-injector from carrier tube

1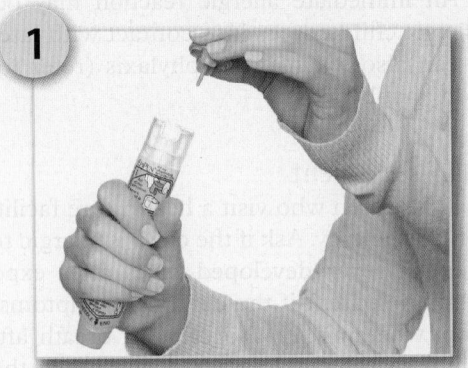

- Hold firmly with orange tip pointing downward
- **Remove blue safety release**

2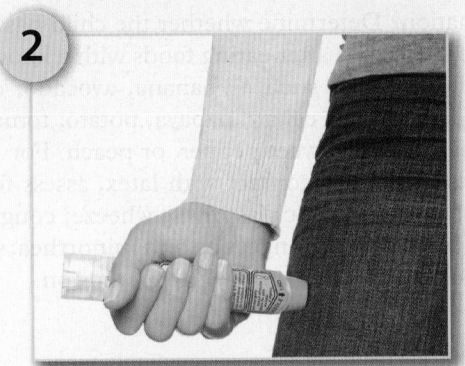

- **Swing and push orange tip firmly into mid-outer thigh until you hear a 'click'**
- Hold on thigh for several seconds

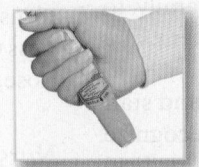

Built-in needle protection

- When the EpiPen® Auto-injector is removed, the orange needle cover automatically extends to cover the injection needle

 *After administration, patients should seek medical attention immediately or go to the emergency room. For the next 48 hours, patients must stay within close proximity to a healthcare facility or where they can call 911.*

For more information go to www.EpiPen.ca

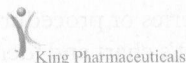 King Pharmaceuticals

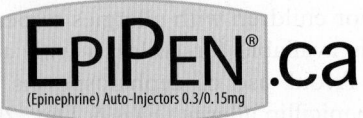 **EPIPEN®.ca**
(Epinephrine) Auto-Injectors 0.3/0.15mg

Emergency response at hand.

■■■ Key Concepts

■ Waning of maternal antibodies in early infancy while humoural immunity is developing leads to physiologic hypogammaglobulinemia, placing the young infant at risk for overwhelming infection.

■ Infants and young children have large lymph nodes, tonsils, and thymus compared with adults.

■ Infants have decreased phagocytic activity, placing them at higher risk for serious infection.

■ Children with immune disorders often show a decreased or absent response to delayed hypersensitivity skin testing (e.g., the tuberculosis test).

■ The ELISA for HIV detects only antibodies to HIV (which in the infant may be maternal in origin), whereas the PCR test for HIV tests for HIV genetic material, making it the more accurate test for HIV infection in infants and young children.

■ Primary immune deficiencies such as SCID and Wiskott–Aldrich syndrome are congenital and serious; they can be cured only by bone marrow or stem cell transplantation.

■ SLE is a chronic autoimmune disorder that can affect any organ system, primarily causing vasculitis.

■ JIA results in chronic pain and affects growth and development as well as school performance.

■ Various forms of hypogammaglobulinemia may be treated with exogenous immunoglobulin administered intravenously every several weeks or subcutaneously weekly, allowing children to lead a healthier life with fewer infections.

■ Nasal, palatal, or throat pruritus and difficulty breathing may indicate an anaphylactic reaction.

■ Children with severe allergy or previous anaphylactic episodes must avoid contact with allergens.

■ Nursing management of lupus focuses on preventing flare-ups and complications.

■ Managing pain, maintaining mobility, and administering disease-modifying medications are key nursing interventions in the management of JIA.

■ HIV infection may be prevented in infants by prenatal screening and maternal treatment as well as postnatal treatment with ZDV.

■ HIV infection in children often results in encephalopathy and developmental delay.

■ Spread of HIV infection can be prevented in adolescence by avoiding high-risk behaviours.

■ For children with immune deficiency or autoimmune disease, prevention of infection is a primary nursing concern.

■ A chronic illness such as immune deficiency, SLE, or juvenile arthritis has a significant impact on the family as well as the child.

■ When planning care for the child with an immune deficiency or autoimmune disorder, the nurse should include the child and the family.

■ To promote proper growth, encourage the child with an immune or autoimmune disorder to eat a balanced diet.

■ Teach families of children with immune deficiencies about infection prevention.

■ Teach the family of the child with juvenile arthritis about ways to decrease pain while increasing or maintaining the child's mobility.

■ Teach families of children with allergy how to avoid allergens and how to use an epinephrine auto-injector. Staff at the child's school or day care centre should be aware of the allergy. The child should wear medical alert identification.

REFERENCES

Allergy/Asthma Information Association (2009). *Statistics.* Available April 12, 2012 from http://aaia.ca/en/mediastatistics.htm

Allergy/Asthma Information Association. (2010). *What is allergy?* Retrieved October 6, 2011 from http://aaia.ca/en/aboutAllergy.htm

Altman, R. D. (2008). Juvenile idiopathic arthritis (JIA). In *Merck Manual for Health Care Professionals.* Retrieved October 6, 2011 from http://www.merckmanuals.com/professional/sec04/ch036/ch036b.html

American College of Allergy, Asthma, and Immunology. (2006). Food allergy: A practice parameter. *Annals of Allergy, Asthma, & Immunology, 96*(3 Suppl. 2), S1–S68.

American Latex Allergy Association. (n.d.). *Allergenic cross-reactivity of latex and foods: Technical bulletin #10.* Retrieved October 6, 2011 from http://www.latexallergyresources.org/sites/default/files/attachments/TB10A%20Latex%20food%20cross-reactivities.pdf

Anderson, J., Malley, K., & Snell, R. (2009). Is 6 months still the best for exclusive breastfeeding and introduction of solids? A literature review with consideration to the risk of the development of allergies. *Breastfeeding Review, 17*(2), 23–31.

Berger, M. (2010). *Subcutaneous and intramuscular immune globin therapy.* Retrieved October 6, 2011 from http://www.uptodate.com/contents/subcutaneous-and-intramuscular-immune-globulin-therapy

Binkley, H. M., Schroyer, T., & Catalfano, J. (2003). Latex allergies: A review of recognition, evaluation, management, prevention, education, and alternative product use. *Journal of Athletic Training, 38*(2), 133–140.

Canadian Paediatric Surveillance Program. (n.d.). *Severe combined immunodeficiency.* Retrieved June 1, 2011 from http://www.cps.ca/english/surveillance/cpsp/studies/immunodeficiency.htm

Centers for Disease Control and Prevention. (1994). 1994 Revised classification system for human immunodeficiency virus infection in children less than 13 years of age. *Morbidty and Mortality Weekly Report, 43*(RR-12), 1–10. Retrieved October 6, 2011 from www.cdc.gov/mmwr/preview/mmwrhtml/00032890.htm

Centers for Disease Control and Prevention. (2008). Revised surveillance case definitions for HIV infection among adults, adolescents, and children aged <18 months and for HIV infection and AIDS among children aged 18 months to <13 years—United States, 2008. *Morbidity and Mortality Weekly Report, 57*(No. RR-10), 1–12. Retrieved June 1, 2001 from http://www.cdc.gov/mmwr/PDF/rr/rr5710.pdf

Chamberlain, J. (2006). Preventing food allergies in children: Some effective measures, but many unknown. *Infectious Diseases in Children, 19*(2), 72.

Chen, A. C., Thompson, E. A., & Morrison-Beedy, D. (2010). Multi-system influences on adolescent risky sexual behaviours. *Research in Nursing & Health, 33*(6), 512–527.

Clark, A. T., & Ewan, P. W. (2003). Food allergy in childhood. *Archives of Disease in Childhood, 88*(1), 79–81.

Collard, J. (2010). Food allergy and intolerance. *Practice Nurse, 39*(1), 17–21.

Dibbern, D. A., & Routes, J. M. (2010). *Wiskott–Aldrich syndrome.* Retrieved July 3, 2011 from http://emedicine.medscape.com/article/137015-overview

Doellman, D., Hadaway, L., Bowe-Geddes, L. A., et al. (2009). Infiltration and extravasation: Update on prevention and management. *Journal of Infusion Nursing, 32*(4), 203–211.

Ellis, A. K., & Day, J. H. (2003). Diagnosis and management of anaphylaxis. *Journal of the Canadian Medical Association, 169*(4), 307–312.

Fahrner, R., & Romano, S. (2010). HIV infection and AIDS. In P. J. Allen, J. A. Vessey, & N. A. Schapiro (Eds.), *Primary care of the child with a chronic condition* (5th ed.). St. Louis, MO: Mosby.

Farland, E. J. (2011). Human immunodeficiency virus infection. In W. W. Hay, M. J. Levin, J. M. Sondheimer, & R. R. Deterding (Eds.), *Current pediatric diagnosis & treatment* (20th ed.). New York: McGraw-Hill.

Fletcher-Janzen, E., & Reynolds, C. R. (2003). *Childhood disorders: Diagnostic desk reference.* Hoboken, NJ: John Wiley and Sons.

Food Allergen and Anaphylaxis Network. (2011). *Allergens.* Retrieved October 6, 2011 from http://www.foodallergy.org/section/allergens

Frost, D. W., & Chalin, C. G. (2005). The effect of income on anaphylaxis preparation and management plans in Toronto primary schools. *Canadian Journal of Public Health, 96*(4), 250–253.

Jackson, P. L. (2002). Peanut allergy: An increasing health risk for children. *Pediatric Nursing, 28*(5), 496–498, 504.

Jeffrey Modell Foundation. (2011). *10 warning signs of primary immunodeficiency.* Retrieved October 6, 2011 from http://www.info4pi.org/aboutPI/index.cfm?section=aboutPI& content=warningsigns

Jones, K. B., & Higgins, G. C. (2010). Juvenile rheumatoid arthritis. In P. J. Allen, J. A. Vessey, & N. A. Schapiro (Eds.), *Primary care of the child with a chronic condition* (5th ed.). St. Louis, MO: Mosby.

Kemp, S. F. (2011). *Anaphylaxis.* Retrieved October 6, 2011 from http://emedicine.medscape.com/article/135065-overview#showall

Khoury, M., & Kovacs, A. (2001). Pediatric HIV infection. *Clinical Obstetrics and Gynecology, 44*(2), 243–275.

Kim, J., & Sicherer, S. (2010). Should avoidance of foods be strict in prevention and treatment of food allergy? *Current Opinion in Allergy and Clinical Immunology, 10,* 252–257.

Kirmse, J. (2009). The nurses' role in administration of intravenous immunoglobulin therapy. *Home Healthcare Nurse, 27*(2), 104–111.

Lederman, H. M. (2006). The immune system. In J. A. McMillan (Ed.), *Oski's pediatrics: Principles and practice* (4th ed.). Philadelphia: Lippincott Williams & Wilkins.

Mina, R., & Brunner, H. I. (2010). Pediatric lupus—are there differences in presentation, genetics, response to therapy, and damage accrual compared with adult lupus? *Rheumatic Disease Clinics of North America, 36*(1), 53–80, vii–viii.

Morrison-Beedy, D., Nelson, L. E., & Volpe, E. (2005). HIV risk behaviours and testing rates in adolescent girls: Evidence to guide clinical practice. *Pediatric Nursing, 31*(6), 508–512.

Mullin, G. E., Swift, D. M., Lipski, L., Turnbull, L. K., & Rampertab, S. D. (2010). Testing for food reactions: The good, the bad, and the ugly. *Nutrition in Clinical Practice, 25*(2), 192–198.

Munn, Z. (2009). *Evidence summary: Anaphylaxis: Management.* Retrieved October 6, 2011 from http://es.jbiconnect.org/connect/docs/cis/es_html_viewer.php?SID=5698& lang=es%AEion=ES

Munoz-Furlong, A. (2003). Daily coping strategies for patients and their families. *Pediatrics, 111*(6), 1654–1661.

Muraro, A., Dreborg, S., Halken, S., et al. (2004). Dietary prevention of allergic diseases in infants and small children, part III: Critical review of published peer-reviewed observational and interventional studies and final recommendations. *Pediatric Allergy and Immunology, 15,* 291–307.

Neven, B., Leroy, S., Decaluwe, H., et al. (2009). Long-term outcome after hematopoietic stem cell transplantation of a single-center cohort of 90 patients with severe combined immunodeficiency. *Blood, 113*(17), 4114–4124.

Nield, L. S., Torischt, M. J., & Kamat, D. (2009). Vaccinating the immunocompromised child. *Consultant for Pediatricians, 8*(10), S7–S11.

Norville, R., & Tomlinson, D. (2010). Hematopoietic stem cell transplantation. In D. Tomlinson & N. E. Kline (Eds.), *Pediatric oncology nursing.* New York: Springer.

Panel on Antiretroviral Therapy and Medical Management of HIV-Infected Children. (2011). *Guidelines for the use of antiretroviral agents in pediatric HIV infection.* Retrieved May 26, 2011 from http://aidsinfo.nih.gov/ContentFiles/PediatricGuidelines.pdf

Petry, L., Mathur, A., & Kamat, D. M. (2004). Immunodeficiency disorders: What should primary care providers know? *Consultant for Pediatricians, 3*(5), 228–232.

Pollart, S. M., Warniment, C., & Mori, T. (2009). Latex allergy. *American Family Physician, 80*(12), 1414–1418.

Pongmarutani, T., Alpert, P. T., & Miller, S. K. (2006). Pediatric systemic lupus erythematosus: Management issues in primary practice. *Journal of the American Academy of Nurse Practitioners, 18*(6), 258–267.

Public Health Agency of Canada. (2009). *HIV and AIDS in Canada. Surveillance report to December 31, 2009.* Retrieved October 6, 2011 from http://www.phac-aspc.gc.ca/aids-sida/publication/survreport/2009/dec/index-eng.php

Roberts, G., Patel, N., Levi-Schaffer, F., Habibi, P., & Lack, G. (2003). Food allergy as a risk factor for life-threatening asthma in childhood: A case-controlled study. *Journal of Allergy and Clinical Immunology, 112*(1), 168–174.

Sampson, H. A., & Eggleston, P. A. (2006). General considerations of allergies in childhood. In J. A. McMillan (Ed.), *Oski's pediatrics: Principles and practice* (4th ed.). Philadelphia: Lippincott Williams & Wilkins.

Secord, E. A., & Oren, E. (2009). *Severe combined immunodeficiency.* Retrieved October 6, 2011 from http://emedicine.medscape.com/article/137265-overview

Senécal, J. (1998). Lupus: The disease with a thousand faces. Retrieved October 6, 2011 from http:www.lupuscanada.org/English/living/1000faces.html

Sicherer, S. H., & Sampson, H. A. (2009). Food allergy: Recent advances in pathophysiology and treatment. *Annual Review of Medicine, 60,* 261–277.

Simons, F. E. R. (2009). Anaphylaxis: Recent advances in assessment and treatment. *Journal of Allergy and Clinical Immunology, 124*(4), 625–636.

Sloand, E., & Caschera, J. (2010). Allergies. In P. J. Allen, J. A. Vessey, & N. A. Schapiro (Eds.), *Primary care of the child with a chronic condition* (5th ed.). St. Louis, MO: Mosby.

Taketokmo, C. K., Hodding, J. H., & Kraus, D. M. (2010). *Lexi-comp's pediatric dosage handbook* (17th ed.). Hudson, OH: Lexi-comp.

Tang, A. W. (2003). A practical guide to anaphylaxis. *American Family Physician, 68*(7), 1325–1332.

Tofferi, J. K., & Gilliland, W. (2009). *Avascular necrosis.* Retrieved October 6, 2011 from http://emedicine.medscape.com/article/333364-overview

Tosi, M. F. (2009). Normal and impaired immunologic responses to infection. In R. D. Feigin, J. Cherry, G. J. Demmler-Harrison, & S. L. Kaplan (Eds.), *Feigin & Cherry's textbook of pediatric infectious disease* (6th ed.). Philadelphia: Saunders.

Tsang, K. G. F. (2008). Anaphylaxis: Assessing patients with allergies. *Emergency Nurse, 16*(5), 24–29.

Tupper, J., & Visser, S. (2010). Anaphylaxis – A review & update. *Canadian Family Physician, 56*(10), 1009–1011.

UNICEF. (2010). *Children and AIDS: Fifth stocktaking report.* New York: The United Nations Children's Fund.

von Scheven, E., & Bakkaloglu, A. (2009). What's new in paediatric SLE? *Best Practice & Research Clinical Rheumatology, 23*(5), 699–708.

Vu, A. T., & Duong, M. (2007). The nuts and bolts of peanut allergy. *Journal of the American Academy of Physician Assistants, 20*(4), 28, 32–35.

Waltenburg, R., Kobrynski, L., Reyes, M., Bowen, S., & Khoury, M. J. (2010). Primary immunodeficiency diseases: Practice among primary care providers and awareness among the general public, United States, 2008. *Genetics in Medicine: Official Journal of the American College of Medical Genetics, 12*(12), 792–800.

Watura, J. C. (2002). Nut allergy in schoolchildren: A survey of schools in the Severn NHS trust. *Archives of Diseases of Childhood, 86,* 240–244.

Winkels, K. (2010). *How to eat with food allergies: Finding allergy-free substitutes.* Retrieved October 6, 2011 from http://www.eatingwithfoodallergies.com/allergyfreesubstitutes.html

World Allergy Organization Allergic Diseases Resource Center. (2011). *Overview of allergy, its diagnosis and treatment.* Retrieved October 6, 2011 from http://www.worldallergy.org/public/allergic_diseases_center/overview.php

World Health Organization. (2010). *New progress and guidance on HIV diagnosis and treatment for infants and children.* Retrieved October 6, 2011 from http://www.who.int/hiv/pub/paediatric/Paediatricfact-sheet/en/index.html

Yun, J., & Katelaris, C. H. (2009). Food allergy in adolescents and adults. *Internal Medicine Journal, 39*(7), 475–478.

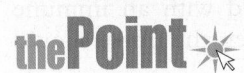

the Point For additional learning materials, including Internet Resources, visit **http://thePoint.lww.com/Chow1e.**

CHAPTER WORKSHEET

MULTIPLE CHOICE QUESTIONS

1. The nurse is caring for a 6-year-old with JIA. The mother states that she has trouble getting her daughter out of bed in the morning and believes the girl's behaviour is due to a desire to avoid going to school. What is the best advice by the nurse?

   a. Refer the girl to a psychologist for evaluation of school phobia related to chronic illness.

   b. Administer a warm bath every morning before school.

   c. Give the child her prescribed NSAIDs 30 minutes before getting out of bed.

   d. Allow her to stay in bed some mornings if she wants.

2. A 14-year-old with SLE wants to know how to care for her skin. What should the nurse teach this adolescent?

   a. Careful suntanning will give your skin an attractive colour.

   b. No special skin care is needed.

   c. Use sunscreen daily to avoid rashes.

   d. Use makeup to camouflage the butterfly rash on her face.

3. The mother of a child with hypogammaglobulinemia reports that her child had a fever and slight chills with an intravenous gammaglobulin infusion last month. She wants to know what other course of treatment might be available. What is the best response by the nurse?

   a. Administration of acetaminophen or diphenhydramine prior to the next infusion may decrease the incidence of fever or chills.

   b. Giving the gammaglobulin intramuscularly is recommended to prevent a reaction.

   c. Talk to her physician about alternative medications that may be used to boost the gammaglobulin level in the blood.

   d. If the child is no longer experiencing frequent infections, then the IV infusions may not be necessary.

4. A 4-month-old infant born to an HIV-infected mother is going into foster care because the mother is too ill to care for the child. The foster mother wants to know if the infant is also infected. What is the best response by the nurse?

   a. "It's too early to know; we have to wait until the infant has symptoms."

   b. "Since the mother is so ill, it's likely the child is also infected with HIV."

   c. "The ELISA test is positive, so the child is definitely infected."

   d. "The PCR test is positive; this indicates HIV infection, which may or may not progress to AIDS."

5. A mother has received instructions about avoiding wheat and soy allergens. Which response by the mother would indicate that further education is needed?

   a. "I will not feed my child any bread made with wheat flour."

   b. "I will allow my child to eat semolina pasta, the kind he loves."

   c. "I will not feed my child shakes made with soy protein."

   d. "I will read labels to be sure I am avoiding wheat and soy."

CRITICAL THINKING EXERCISES

1. Develop a discharge teaching plan for a 14-year-old with SLE who will be taking corticosteroids long term.

2. Devise a developmental stimulation plan for a 22-month-old with HIV infection and encephalopathy with developmental delay (to the level of a 9-month-old).

3. Determine an appropriate nursing plan of care for an infant who has undergone bone marrow transplantation for SCID.

4. Develop a prioritized list of nursing diagnoses for a child with HIV infection, candidiasis, poor growth, and pneumonia requiring oxygen.

5. A child with recurrent infections is being evaluated. Other than information about onset of symptoms and events leading up to this present episode, what other types of information would the nurse ask while obtaining the history?

(question continues on page 1644)

STUDY ACTIVITIES

1. In the clinical setting, compare the growth and development of two children of the same age, one with HIV infection and one who has been healthy.

2. Attend an out-patient clinic that provides care to children with HIV infection. Observe the physician or nurse practitioner during office visits and attend a multidisciplinary planning meeting. Identify the role of the registered nurse in providing family education, coordination of care, and referrals.

3. Conduct an Internet search to determine the educational material available to children and their families related to immune deficiencies, autoimmune disorders, or allergies.

4. Research your clinical institution's policies related to latex allergy, alternative products available at the institution, and how to obtain them for a latex-allergic patient. Provide a presentation to your clinical group about your findings.

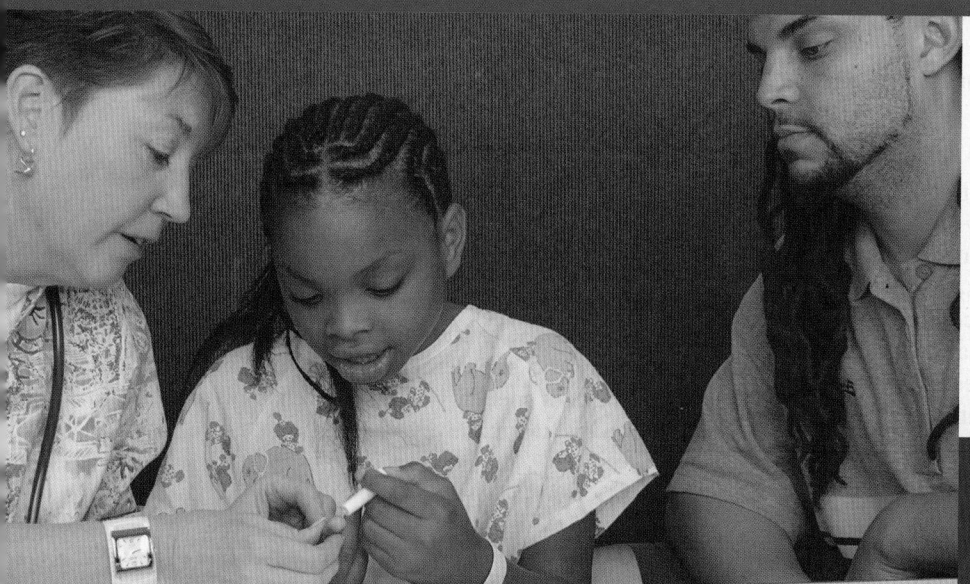

CHAPTER 48

Adapted by Christina B. Whittaker

NURSING CARE OF THE CHILD WITH AN ENDOCRINE DISORDER

KEY TERMS

adrenarche
beta cells
constitutional delay
diabetic ketoacidosis (DKA)
exophthalmos
gland

glucose
goitre
gonads
hemoglobin A1C
hirsutism
hormone
ketoacidosis

ketone
Kussmaul respiration
polydipsia
polyphagia
polyuria
tetany

LEARNING OBJECTIVES

Upon completion of the chapter, the learner will be able to:

1. Describe the major components and functions of a child's endocrine system.
2. Differentiate between the anatomic and physiologic differences of the endocrine system in children versus adults.
3. Identify the essential assessment elements, common diagnostic procedures, and laboratory tests associated with the diagnosis of endocrine disorders in children.
4. Identify the common medications and treatment modalities used for the care of endocrine disorders in children.
5. Distinguish specific disorders of the endocrine system affecting children.
6. Link the clinical manifestations of specific disorders in the endocrine system of a child with the appropriate nursing diagnoses.
7. Establish the nursing outcomes, evaluative criteria, and interventions for a child with specific disorders in the endocrine system.
8. Develop child/family teaching plans for the child with an endocrine disorder.

Carlos Rodriguez, 12 years old, is seen in the clinic today with complaints of weakness, fatigue, blurred vision, and headaches. His mother states, "Carlos' teacher has noticed mood changes and is concerned about his behaviour at school. He's always been a good boy. I'm not sure what's going on."

Wow

Endocrine disorders in children often elude the medical radar screen.

The endocrine system consists of various **glands** that produce and release hormones directly into the bloodstream. **Hormones** are chemical messengers that stimulate and/or regulate the actions of tissues, organs, or other endocrine glands that have specific receptors to a hormone. Along with the nervous system and the immune system, the endocrine milieu influences all physiologic effects such as growth and development, metabolic processes related to fluid and electrolyte balance and energy production, sexual maturation and reproduction, and the body's response to stress. The release patterns of the hormones vary, but the level in the body is maintained within specified limits to preserve health.

Problems develop in the endocrine system when there is a deficiency or excess of a specific hormone. In children, endocrine conditions often develop insidiously. An endocrine condition may be isolated or one component of a syndrome or disorder. If the problem is not diagnosed and treated early, delayed growth and development, cognitive impairments, or acute illness and death may result. Generally, the treatment plan involves correction of the underlying reason for the dysfunction, such as surgical removal of a tumour, and supplementation of missing hormones or adjustment of specific hormone levels. This allows most children to live normal lives.

Variations in Anatomy and Physiology

The organs or tissues of the endocrine system include the hypothalamus, pituitary gland, thyroid gland, parathyroid

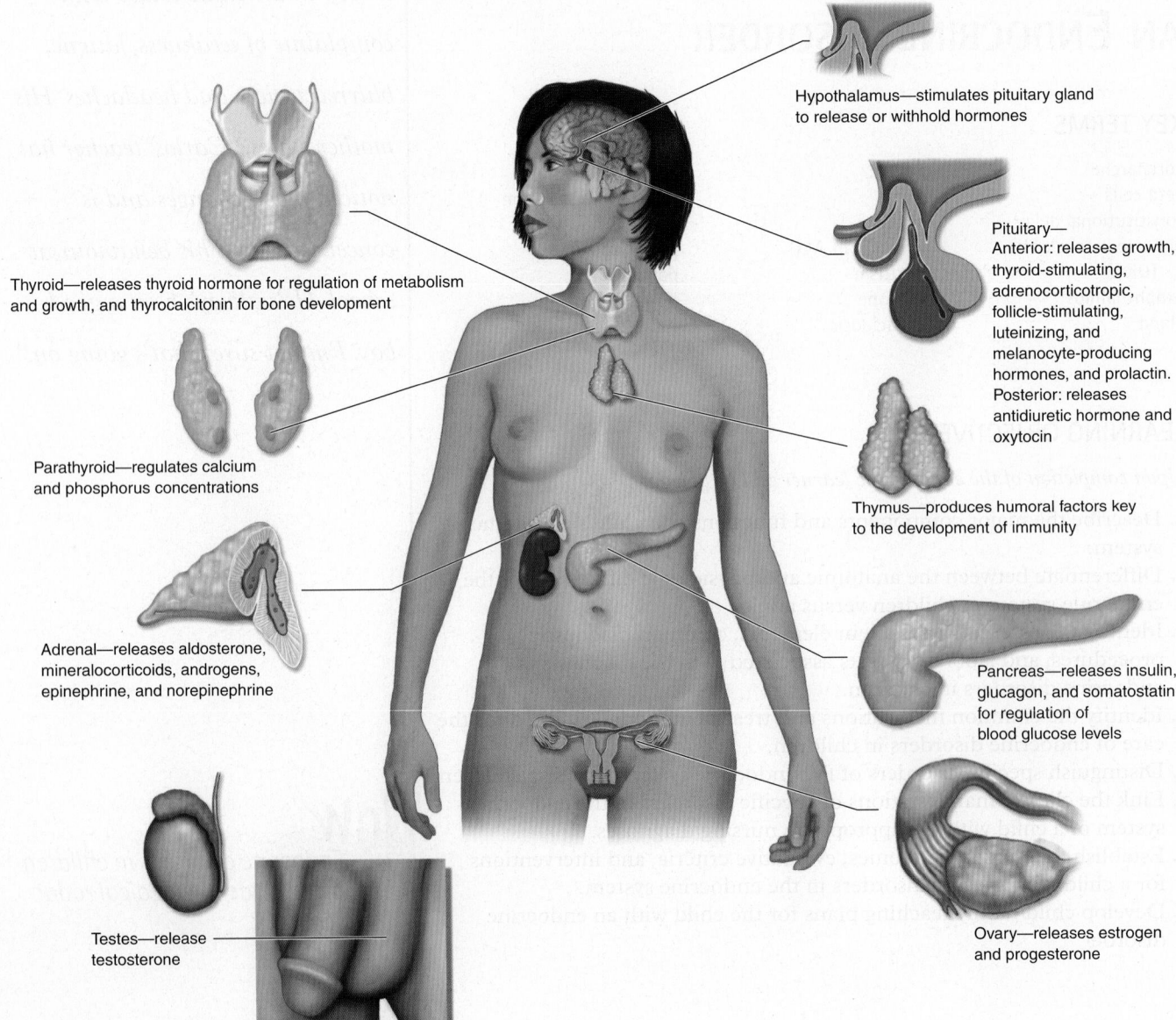

Hypothalamus—stimulates pituitary gland to release or withhold hormones

Pituitary—
Anterior: releases growth, thyroid-stimulating, adrenocorticotropic, follicle-stimulating, luteinizing, and melanocyte-producing hormones, and prolactin. Posterior: releases antidiuretic hormone and oxytocin

Thymus—produces humoral factors key to the development of immunity

Pancreas—releases insulin, glucagon, and somatostatin for regulation of blood glucose levels

Ovary—releases estrogen and progesterone

Thyroid—releases thyroid hormone for regulation of metabolism and growth, and thyrocalcitonin for bone development

Parathyroid—regulates calcium and phosphorus concentrations

Adrenal—releases aldosterone, mineralocorticoids, androgens, epinephrine, and norepinephrine

Testes—release testosterone

FIGURE 48.1 Location and major effects of the endocrine glands in the body.

glands, adrenal glands, **gonads**, and the **beta cells** in the pancreas. Typically, most endocrine glands begin to develop during the first trimester of gestation, but their development is incomplete at birth.

Hormone Production and Secretion

The hypothalamic–pituitary axis produces a number of releasing and inhibiting hormones that regulate the function of many of the other endocrine glands, including the thyroid gland, the adrenal glands, and the male and female gonads. Some glands, such as the pancreas and the parathyroid glands, regulate their function in connection with the nervous system. Other cells in the body secrete hormones, such as the scattered epithelial cells in the gastrointestinal tract and the thymus. Disorders related to these other cells as well as gonad dysfunction are discussed in other chapters in this textbook.

Figure 48.1 shows the major glands, the hormones produced by the glands, and the effect each hormone has on the target cell, tissue, or organ. The process of hormone production and secretion involves the principle of feedback control. One gland produces a hormone that affects another gland known as the target organ. Once the intended hormone level and physiologic effect are achieved, the target gland inhibits the further release of the original hormone. The reverse occurs when the first gland detects low levels of the target gland hormone. If the original gland does not release enough of the hormone, the inhibition process stops so that the gland increases the production of the hormone. The endocrine system and the nervous system work closely together to maintain an optimal internal environment for the body, known as homeostasis.

Common Medical Treatments

Early treatment of endocrine disorders is often associated with better prognosis, prevention of acute crises, and prevention or decrease in long-term consequences. Primarily, the treatment of endocrine disorders involves decreasing hormone production (in cases of excess hormone production) or replacing the hormones (in cases of insufficiency). The first step in the treatment of many endocrine disorders is to screen for potential problems associated with the condition. The next step involves identifying underlying causes for the dysfunction (e.g., a tumour or growth that requires surgical removal or irradiation). Throughout all aspects of care, comprehensive family-centred care of the child, adolescent, and family includes education regarding the potential (if any) influence of the disorder on growth and development and how to attain and maintain normal family lifestyle and functioning.

Common Medical Treatments 48.1 describes the common treatments used in children with endocrine disorders, including explanations and indications for each treatment as well as relevant nursing implications. Advances in technology and in our understanding of molecular biology continue to increase our knowledge of these disorders and the modalities needed to prevent them or improve quality of life for affected children. These advances are vital, since the whole body is influenced by the endocrine milieu.

Drug Guide 48.1 lists the medications most commonly used to treat endocrine disorders, including the actions and indications of each drug as well as pertinent nursing implications. Many of the medications are synthetic preparations of the actual hormones. It is important to maintain blood levels within a specific range to mimic the actual hormone in the body. Nurses must assess for side effects of too little or too much of the hormone in the child's system. Most endocrine disorders in children require treatment and follow-up with a pediatric endocrinologist as well as a multidisciplinary team that includes a registered nurse who specializes in this area.

NURSING PROCESS OVERVIEW FOR THE CHILD WITH AN ENDOCRINE DISORDER

Nursing care of the child with an endocrine disorder requires astute assessment skills, accurate nursing diagnoses and expected outcomes, skilled interventions, and evaluation of the entire process. The clinical manifestations of endocrine disorders occur as a result of altered control of the bodily processes normally regulated by glands or hormones. These manifestations present in many areas of the body because of the diverse functions associated with the endocrine system. Children, especially very young ones, easily develop imbalances such as fluid and electrolyte disturbances that can cause further problems. Most of the endocrine disorders are chronic conditions and/or are components of a syndrome or disorder that requires ongoing care related to health maintenance, education, developmental issues, and psychosocial needs. These conditions are sometimes complex and range from mild to profound. Early diagnosis, treatment, and appropriate family education can prevent or minimize acute implications of the diseases and improve the long-term outcomes and quality of life for these children.

*R*emember Carlos, the 12-year-old with weakness, *fatigue, blurred vision, headaches, and mood changes? What additional health history and physical examination assessment information should the nurse obtain?*

COMMON MEDICAL TREATMENTS 48.1

Treatment	Explanation	Indication	Nursing Implications
Newborn metabolic screening programs	Newborn blood testing to identify certain disorders	Identification of newborns so that treatment can begin early to prevent impact of disorder, such as severe cognitive impairment or death	• Refer to each province's or territory's protocol for fetal/newborn screening for endocrine disorders. • Explain to family the rationale and procedure. • Infant should be feeding for 24 h prior to blood collection. • Collect blood sample accurately. • IV antibiotic use in the newborn may affect results. • Ensure screening is done for early discharges.
Administration of hormone	Give hormone if hypofunction exists or give blocking agent if hyperfunction exists to establish normal growth and development and specific function disrupted by disorder.	Most endocrine disorders, such as diabetes mellitus or growth hormone deficiency	• Follow specific administration requirements for each hormone/drug. • Monitor serum levels carefully to detect appropriate levels. • Observe for adverse effects of too little or too much hormone. • Carefully monitor growth and development patterns.
Surgery	Surgical removal of tumours or cysts	Any endocrine malfunction caused by the presence of a mass	• Provide routine preoperative and postoperative care, depending on location and extent of surgery. • Keep family informed of choices.
Irradiation/radioactive iodine	Radiation is used to influence the hormone secretion of a gland; it is less invasive than surgery.	Hyperfunction of an endocrine gland; may be used when surgery is not possible	• Prepare child for specific procedures following protocols. • Explain the procedure. • Check to ensure child has no sensitivity to iodine preparations.
Glucose monitoring	Fingerstick blood sample several times per day	Monitoring of glucose control	• Teach family appropriate procedure. • Refer family to sources for equipment and supplies. • Assist family to develop a system of record-keeping that works for them.
Dietary interventions	Restriction or manipulation of dietary intake	Diabetes mellitus	• Refer family to a dietitian specializing in pediatric diabetes mellitus. • Reinforce teaching related to special diets.

Assessment

Nursing assessment of a child with endocrine dysfunction includes obtaining a thorough health history, including behavioural, social, learning, and physical development; performing a physical assessment; assisting with or obtaining laboratory and diagnostic tests; and supporting the child and family.

Health History

Focus the health history on the possibility of a family history of an endocrine disorder, prenatal history, history of childhood illnesses, and growth and development patterns. Use a genogram or family tree to detail the information about the family history in a clear and concise manner.

DRUG GUIDE 48.1   COMMON DRUGS FOR ENDOCRINE DISORDERS

Medication	Action	Indication	Nursing Implications
Insulin	Used to replace body's natural insulin, which is necessary for proper glucose utilization by the cells.	Diabetes mellitus	• Monitor vital signs and blood glucose levels. • Educate child and family on proper techniques, actions, and adverse effects. • Rotate site of injections to prevent adipose hypertrophy.
Oral hypoglycemic drugs (glipizide, glyburide, metformin)	Assists body's production of insulin by a variety of actions specific to each classification. Some stimulate beta cells to secrete more insulin. Others work to decrease hepatic output.	Diabetes mellitus type 2	• Monitor glucose levels. • Administer with food to minimize gastric upset. • Instruct child and family on use of drug and adverse effects. • Warn family that some over-the-counter or other drugs may increase hypoglycemic effect.
Growth hormone (GH)/somatropin (Humatrope)	Elicits same responses produced by natural GH: stimulates linear bone, skeletal muscle, and organ growth	GH deficiency, growth failure related to inadequate pituitary hormone	• Monitor blood sugar and electrolyte levels. • Administer before epiphyses are fused. • Monitor growth with accurate measurements. • Instruct child and family on appropriate route and method of administration. • Periodic thyroid function tests will be needed. • May interact with glucocorticoid therapy • Monitor for limping or complaints in knee or hip related to slipped epiphysis.
Octreotide acetate (Sandostatin)	Suppresses GH release	Acromegaly	• Monitor for biliary tract abnormalities, glucose tolerance, and hypothyroidism. • Give subcutaneous injections between meals to decrease gastric effects. • Refer family to the Novartis Patient Assistance Foundation for assistance with covering cost of drug.
Corticosteroids (dexamethasone or hydrocortisone)	Elicits same response as natural cortisol: helps control blood sugar, increase protein and fat metabolism, respond to stressors	Cortisol replacement in congenital adrenal hyperplasia, absence of adrenal glands. Also used to close epiphyseal plates in hyperpituitarism.	• Give with milk or food. • May need to increase dose if child is ill or runs fever • Monitor for edema, weight gain, glycosuria, signs of infection, and symptoms of peptic ulcer development. • Do not decrease dose or abruptly stop drug to avoid adrenal crisis.

(continued)

DRUG GUIDE 48.1 COMMON DRUGS FOR ENDOCRINE DISORDERS (continued)

Medication	Action	Indication	Nursing Implications
Levothyroxine (Synthroid)	Thyroid hormone replacement; increases metabolic rate, controls protein synthesis, and increases cardiac output	Hypothyroidism	• Check blood pressure and pulse before each dose. • Monitor input and output and daily weights. • Watch for thyroid storm. • Report irritability or anxiety. • Instruct child and family to avoid over-the-counter preparations with iodine or foods such as soybeans, iodized salt, tofu, turnips. • Administer at same time each day.
Methimazole	Antithyroid drug; blocks synthesis of T_3 and T_4	Hyperthyroidism	• Check pulse and blood pressure before each dose. • Monitor input and output, daily weights, serum T_3 and T_4 levels; watch for edema, leukopenia, thrombocytopenia, or agranulocytosis. • Administer with meals to decrease gastric upset. • Give at the same time each day. • Store in light-resistant container. • Instruct child and family to report sore throat, mouth lesions, unusual bleeding or bruising. • Signs of overdose: periorbital edema, cold intolerance, depression • Signs of inadequate dose: tachycardia, diarrhea, fever, or irritability
Mineralocorticoid (Florinef)	Promotes reabsorption of Na and K, water from distal renal tubules	Adrenal insufficiency	• Monitor daily weights, blood pressure, intake and output. • Observe for potassium depletion. • Titrate dose to lowest effective dose. • Adverse effects include flushing, sweating, headache, increased blood pressure.

Adapted from: Karch, A. (2010). *2010 Lippincott's nursing drug guide.* Philadelphia: Wolters Kluwer Health/Lippincott Williams & Wilkins; and Taketokmo, C. K., Hodding, J. H., & Kraus, D. M. (2010). *Lexi-comp's drug reference handbook: Pediatric & neonatal dosage handbook* (18th ed.). Hudson, OH: Lexi-comp, Inc.

Endocrine disorders often cause alterations in normal growth and development as well as behavioural changes. Question the parent or caregiver about prior growth patterns, achievement of developmental milestones, and the child's behaviour or personality. Have the child and family describe the child's activities on a typical day, including school performance, to identify subtle variations in the child's behaviour or moods that may be related to endocrine dysfunction. For example, a child who is typically quiet may simply be less active than average children of that age, while the child with decreased endocrine function may display inactivity and fatigue. In addition, obtain a history of dietary and elimination habits. Note extreme thirst, excessive appetite, vomiting, or frequent voiding. Table 48.1 lists the types of questions to ask or areas to review when obtaining a health history on a child with possible endocrine dysfunction.

Physical Examination

Table 48.2 lists key physical examination findings that may be present in the child with endocrine dysfunction.

TABLE 48.1 HEALTH HISTORY QUESTIONS RELATED TO ENDOCRINE DISORDERS

Area of Questioning	Specific Information Sought
General demographics	Gender, age
Present illness	Gradual or sudden onset of symptoms
	Changes in child's lifestyle, physical appearance, sleep patterns, appetite, thirst, vision, bowel and urinary habits, or nausea and vomiting
	Recent increases or decreases in weight and height, muscle weakness, cramps, twitching, or headaches
Past medical history	Birth: any neonatal screening done and results, trauma during birth, birth size, feeding difficulties
	Prenatal history: maternal factors that may affect growth and development such as substance abuse, use of tobacco or alcohol, Graves' disease
	Past health: treated for any endocrine problem in the past, recent gastroenteritis or viral syndrome
	Current immunization status
Allergies	History of allergies to medications, foods, milk, or formula
Current medications	Prescribed, over-the-counter, or home remedies
Family history	Any endocrine disorders or growth and development difficulties
Environmental exposure	Exposure to exogenous steroids or gonadotropins
Social history	Normal daily activities; activity level; family resources such as insurance and support systems to maintain long-term treatment plan
Growth and development milestones	History of growth patterns
	Presence of learning disabilities, cognitive delays, early or late development of secondary sexual characteristics

TABLE 48.2 KEY PHYSICAL EXAMINATION FINDINGS RELATED TO ENDOCRINE PROBLEMS

Attribute or Body Area	Finding
Height and weight	Below 3rd percentile or above 90th percentile (pituitary, thyroid, or adrenal disorders, or diabetes mellitus)
Hair	Coarse, brittle, excessive (hypothyroidism)
	Abnormal distribution (adrenal disorders)
Face	Round with hair growth (Cushing's syndrome)
	Deformities or abnormal features (hypoparathyroidism)
Eyes	Blurred vision or changes in vision (diabetes mellitus, pituitary tumours, precocious puberty)
Mouth	Delayed dentition (hypocalcemia, hypopituitarism)
	Fruity breath (ketoacidosis)
Neck	Goitre (hyperthyroidism)
Skin	Cool to touch, dry (hypothyroidism)
	Changes in colour or texture (pituitary disorders)
	Easy bruising, striae (Cushing's syndrome)
Chest	Tachycardia (hyperthyroidism)
	Palpitations, sweating (thyroid disorders)
	Deep, laboured breathing (ketoacidosis)
	Hypertension (Cushing's)
Abdomen	Extreme weight loss (diabetes mellitus)
	Extreme fat (Cushing's)
	Changes in bowel habits (SIADH, diabetes insipidus, diabetes mellitus)
Fingers	Trembling (hyperthyroidism, parathyroid disorders)
Genitals	Excessive growth (adrenogenital syndrome)
	Early growth (precocious puberty)
	Delayed growth (hypopituitarism)

Inspection and Observation

Note a fatigued appearance, cool or dry skin, diminished skin turgor, edema, poor muscle tone, increased perspiration, faintness, nervousness, or confusion. Inspect the head and face, noting coarse or brittle hair, excessive hair growth, a rounded face, a protuberant tongue, drooping eyelids, or **exophthalmos** (protrusion of the eyeballs). On inspection of the mouth, note delayed dentition or a fruity breath odour. Note early, excessive, or delayed growth of the genitals. Plot the child's height and weight on growth charts to determine abnormal growth velocity, which occurs in many of these disorders. Note that normal growth curves may vary with different cultures or conditions, so consider growth parameters in the context of the genetic or cultural background. Normal growth curves for some conditions, such as Down syndrome, are available to assist.

Auscultation

Auscultate the heart and lungs. Note changes in vital signs from the age-appropriate norm, such as tachycardia or bradycardia. During auscultation of the lungs, note increased respiratory effort, such as **Kussmaul respirations**, which are deep, heavy breaths often seen in **diabetic ketoacidosis (DKA)**. Document the blood pressure and perfusion.

Percussion and Palpation

Percuss and then palpate the abdomen. Dull (nontympanic) sounds or the presence of masses may indicate constipation or an abnormality requiring further investigation.

Laboratory and Diagnostic Testing

Common Laboratory and Diagnostic Tests 48.1 describes the diagnostic tests and procedures frequently used in identifying and monitoring endocrine disorders in children. Serum and urine hormone and other levels are used as one part of a comprehensive physical assessment to determine whether the amounts are adequate, deficient, or excessive. Radiographic studies are used to evaluate bone maturation and growth potential as well as density or tissue calcification. Genetic studies may be used to determine enzyme deficiencies or chromosome defects. Stimulation studies provide a more accurate or definitive test for identifying the disorder after preliminary serum levels are abnormal. Serial blood sampling identifies peak or trough levels of hormones. Computed tomography (CT) scans, magnetic resonance imaging (MRI), nuclear medicine studies, and ultrasonography are used to look for tumours, cysts, or structural defects.

Nursing Diagnoses, Goals, Interventions, and Evaluation

After completing the assessment, the nurse identifies nursing diagnoses with related goals/outcomes, interventions, and evaluations. The nursing diagnoses for a child with endocrine dysfunction may include:

- Delayed growth and development
- Disturbed body image
- Deficient knowledge
- Interrupted family processes
- Imbalanced nutrition: less than or more than body requirements
- Deficient or excess fluid volume
- Noncompliance

After completing an assessment of Carlos, the nurse noted the following: history reveals Carlos has had episodes of bedwetting over the past month and has had polydipsia and polyphagia. His weight continues to be greater than the 95th percentile on the growth chart. Based on these assessment findings, what would your top three nursing diagnoses be for Carlos?

Because of the gradual, insidious onset of many endocrine disorders, the child may first be seen in an acute situation. The acuity of an illness and new diagnosis of a chronic illness can be overwhelming. It may be easier for the child and family to start to work with short-term priorities and gradually build education and awareness of long-term needs and health issues. An immediate goal of the initial education process is to provide the family with the skills, knowledge, and problem-solving ability to be able to be home safely with the child. A major goal will be to achieve participation with the overall health care plan, including prevention of short- and long-term complications. The goals for the child with a disorder of the endocrine system generally include re-establishing homeostasis, promoting adequate growth and development, establishing appropriate body image, promoting health-seeking behaviours, assisting the child and family to integrate the disorder into their lifestyle, and providing education so the family can manage the condition.

Nursing Care Plan 48.1 can be used as a guide in planning care for the child with a disorder of the endocrine system. Any care plan will need to be individualized based on the child's symptoms, needs, and disorder as well as the family's requirements. A key element to include in any care plan for the child with an endocrine disorder involves preparing the child, based on his or her developmental needs, for procedures and tests. Provide an opportunity for the family and child to express their concerns and fears during diagnosis and treatment. A child life therapist can facilitate coping through play,

COMMON LABORATORY AND DIAGNOSTIC TESTS 48.1

Diagnostic Test or Procedure	Explanation	Indication	Nursing Implications
Random serum hormone levels	Serum levels of various hormones; immunoassay measures levels with very small amounts of blood	High or low levels are used to evaluate the function of the specific gland	• May need to draw specimens at specific times. • Keep child NPO after midnight before test if ordered. • Diurnal variations and episodic secretion of many hormones may require special directions or further testing.
Genetic testing	Identify DNA sequencing	Determines genetic involvement of any disorder	• Explain procedure and the expense involved. • Refer for genetic counselling if needed.
Serum chemistry levels	Serum blood urea nitrogen (BUN), creatinine, sodium, potassium, glucose, calcium, phosphorus, alkaline phosphatase, etc.	To rule out chronic renal failure or other chronic illnesses; to monitor effects of treatment	• BUN levels may be elevated with high-protein diet or dehydration, may be decreased with overhydration or malnutrition. • A diet high in meat may cause a transient but not pronounced increase in creatinine. There are also slight diurnal variations in levels. • Avoid hemolysis of specimen, as this may cause elevation in potassium levels. • Calcium and phosphorus: avoid prolonged tourniquet use during blood draw, as this may falsely increase levels. Child should be NPO past midnight prior to the morning of the blood draw.
Growth hormone (GH) stimulation	Stimulate release of GH in response to administration of insulin, arginine, or clonidine	Evaluate and diagnose GH deficiency	• Keep child NPO for specified time. • Obtain serial blood samples at specific times. • Monitor blood glucose levels during study. • Observe for signs of hypoglycemia, diaphoresis, somnolence. • Provide cookies and punch at end of test.
Water deprivation study	Child is deprived of fluids for several hours, and serum sodium and urine osmolality are monitored.	Diabetes insipidus	• Stop test if child exhibits extreme weight loss or changes in vital signs or neurologic status. • Weigh child before, during, and after test. • Rehydrate child after test. • Monitor for orthostatic hypotension.
Bone age radiograph	Radiographic study of wrist or hand to determine bone maturation compared with national standards	Determine whether bone age is consistent with chronological age to rule out GH deficiency or excess or hypothyroidism	• Explain procedure to child because child must hold still for the X-ray. • Allow family to accompany child. Enlist the family's help if needed to calm child during X-ray.
Other nuclear medicine studies	Contrast media uptake is assessed with serial radiographs.	To visualize an ectopic, enlarged, absent, or nodular gland	• Assess child for allergy to iodine or shellfish. • Explain procedure to child.

(continued)

COMMON LABORATORY AND DIAGNOSTIC TESTS 48.1 (continued)

Diagnostic Test or Procedure	Explanation	Indication	Nursing Implications
Computed tomography or magnetic resonance imaging of brain	Non-invasive imaging methods to identify abnormalities of brain or other areas as necessary	Evaluate presence of tumours, cysts, or structural abnormalities that may affect specific gland or structure	• Machine is large and can be frightening to children. • Scan may be lengthy and the child must remain still, so sedation may be necessary. • If contrast medium is to be used, assess for allergy. • Encourage fluids after procedure if not contraindicated.
Ultrasonography	Non-invasive sound waves are used to visualize structures such as thyroid or pelvic region	Evaluate presence of tumours or cysts in specific gland, such as the adrenal glands or ovaries, to rule out disorders	• Requires full bladder if in pelvic region

Adapted from: Fischbach, F. T., & Dunning, M. B., III. (2009). *A manual of laboratory and diagnostic test* (8th ed.). Philadelphia: Lippincott Williams & Wilkins.

preparation, education, and self-expression activities. Reinforce realistic expectations for treatment and prospects for improvement with the family and child. The care plan also needs to address developmental, acute, and chronic care; care in school and at home; and child and family education. Families will need support from an interdisciplinary team to manage the condition.

Based on your top three nursing diagnoses for Carlos, describe appropriate nursing interventions.

Pituitary Disorders

Because of the close anatomic and functional relationships between the hypothalamus and pituitary gland, these are discussed together. The hypothalamus affects the pituitary by releasing and inhibiting hormones and may be the origin of pituitary disorders. In general, disorders of the pituitary fall into two major groups: the anterior pituitary hormones and the posterior pituitary hormones. Anterior pituitary primary disorders in children include growth hormone deficiency (GHD), hyperpituitarism, and precocious puberty. Posterior pituitary disorders include diabetes insipidus (DI) and syndrome of inappropriate antidiuretic hormone secretion (SIADH).

Growth Hormone Deficiency

GHD is characterized by poor growth and short stature. It is generally a result of the failure of the anterior pituitary to produce sufficient growth hormone (GH). GH is released throughout the day, with most secreted during sleep. GH stimulates linear growth, bone mineral density, and growth in all body tissues

Considerable variability exists in the diagnosis of GHD. It may occur alone or in combination with deficiencies of other pituitary hormones. GHD occurs in 1 in 4,000 to 10,000 live births (Parks & Felner, 2007) and is seen with the same frequency in both genders. Investigation for GHD often follows assessment of growth patterns or identification of potential causative factors (further described below), such as CNS irradiation or a CNS lesion. Children with GHD may demonstrate a normal birth weight and length. Assessment of the velocity of height in conjunction with actual height may reveal growth patterns of concern, such as a child who has 2 or more standard deviations (SD) below the mean for height with a velocity, or speed of growth, of 1 SD or less over 1 year, slow velocity over 2 years, or severe short stature (3 or more SD below mean). Differentiation between variants of normal growth or delayed pubertal spurt and endocrine disorders will be aided by investigations such as a GH stimulation test in which the pituitary is stimulated to secrete GH (Nicol, Allen, Czernichow, et al., 2010).

Possible complications related to treatment for GH deficiency include retention of water during the first 2 weeks, slipped capital femoral epiphysis, hypothyroidism, infection, and edema or irritation at the injection site (Parks & Felner, 2007).

Pathophysiology

The main causes of GH deficiency include genetic mutations in pituitary development and acquired forms

(text continues on page 1657)

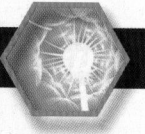

Nursing Care Plan 48.1

OVERVIEW FOR THE CHILD WITH AN ENDOCRINE DISORDER

NURSING DIAGNOSIS: Delayed growth and development related to hypo- or hyperfunction of gland/hormone as evidenced by weight and/or height less than expected for age, failure to meet expected age-appropriate developmental milestones

Outcome Identification and Evaluation

Nutritional status will be maximized and development will be enhanced: *Child will maintain or gain weight appropriately and will make continued progress toward expected developmental milestones.*

Interventions: Enhancing Growth and Development

- Monitor growth parameters using standard growth charts.
- Encourage favourite foods (within prescribed diet restrictions if present) *to maximize oral intake.*
- Consult dietitian *for appropriate diet supplementation recommendations.*
- Encourage compliance with hormone supplementation *to enhance ability to achieve appropriate growth.*
- Provide care related to any complications of dysfunction *such as correcting fluid and electrolyte imbalances or diarrhea.*
- Screen for developmental capabilities *to determine child's current level of functioning.*
- Offer age-appropriate toys, play, and activities (including gross motor) *to promote healthy development.*
- Provide support to families of children with developmental delay (*progress in achieving developmental milestones can be slow and ongoing motivation is needed*).
- Reinforce positive attributes in the child *to maintain motivation.*
- For the child with DM:
- Provide a calorie-appropriate, non-restricted, well-balanced diet *to maintain appropriate growth.*
- Encourage three meals with two or three snacks with consistent carbohydrates *to maintain appropriate blood glucose levels and promote growth.*

NURSING DIAGNOSIS: Disturbed body image related to abnormal growth and development/changes in physical appearance due to hormone dysfunction as evidenced by verbalization of dissatisfaction with the child's or adolescent's looks

Outcome Identification and Evaluation

Child demonstrates appropriate self-esteem in relation to body image; *expresses positive feelings about self and participates in social activities.*

Interventions: Promoting Healthy Body Image

- Provide opportunities for child to explore feelings related to appearance: *Venting feelings is associated with less body image disturbance.*
- Relate to child on age level, not appearance level: *"Babying" a child who looks younger due to his or her small size reduces self-image.*
- Involve the child and especially the teen in the decision-making process: *A sense of control will improve body image.*
- Encourage the child to spend time with peers who have similar endocrine disorders: *Peers' opinions are often better accepted than those of persons in authority, such as parents or health care professionals.*
- Refer to counselling or support groups *to further support the child.*

NURSING DIAGNOSIS: Deficient knowledge related to therapeutic regimen as evidenced by questions about endocrine disorder and self-management

Outcome Identification and Evaluation

Child and family will demonstrate sufficient understanding and skills for self-management; *verbalize information about disorder, complications/adverse effects, homecare regimen, and long-term needs, and provide return demonstrations of medication administration or other procedures.*

Interventions: Promoting Knowledge Required for Self-Management

- Assess child's developmental level and family's ability to absorb instruction *to determine how to approach teaching sessions.*
- Establish teaching plan with child and family *to gain cooperation and involvement.*

(continued)

Nursing Care Plan 48.1 (continued)

- Teach and give printed instructions on disorder, complications, home care, and follow-up requirements *so family has source to refer to at home.*
- Evaluate teaching with return demonstrations *to determine whether child/family is skilled enough for home management of the disorder.*

For the child with DM:
- First teach "survival skills" (e.g., glucose and urine testing, administering insulin, record-keeping, food guidelines, when to call physician) *to provide initial base of knowledge for self-management.*
- Implement second-phase home management program with more extensive instruction; *providing additional teaching over time is necessary for management of a significant chronic illness.*
- Monitor outcomes of teaching with every contact *to ensure progress with patient/family education.*

NURSING DIAGNOSIS: Interrupted family processes or adjustment issues related to lifestyle changes required to manage chronic illness and possible lifestyle changes as evidenced by family's presence in the hospital, missed work, demonstration of inadequate coping

Outcome Identification and Evaluation
Family will maintain functional system of support; demonstrate adequate coping, adaptation of roles and functions, and decreased anxiety: *Parents are involved in child's care, ask appropriate questions, express fears and concerns, identify needs, seek appropriate resources and support, can discuss child's care and condition calmly.*

Interventions: Encouraging Healthy Family Processes
- Encourage parents and family members to verbalize concerns related to child's illness, diagnosis, and prognosis: *Allows the nurse to identify concerns and areas where further education may be needed.*
- Explain treatments, medications, procedures, child's behaviours, and plan of care to parents: *Understanding of the child's current status and plan of care helps decrease anxiety.*
- Identify support system for family and child: *Helps nurse identify needs and resources available for coping.*
- Provide family with information about support groups and special clinics in the area for the particular type of disorder *to provide family with a wide base of support.*
- Encourage parents to become involved in care: *Allows parents to feel needed and valued and gives them a sense of control over their child's health.*
- Evaluate coping processes on follow-up visits *to determine restoration of family processes.*

NURSING DIAGNOSIS: Imbalanced nutrition: Less than or more than body requirements related to pathophysiology of dysfunction as evidenced by growth parameters significantly less or more than expected for age

Outcome Identification and Evaluation
Child's nutritional status is balanced; *child adheres to nutritional guidelines, demonstrates adequate growth (weight and height) pattern within normal range for age and gender or, in the child who has difficulty growing, a progressive increase over time.*

Interventions: Maintaining Adequate Nutrition
- Determine body weight and length/height norm for age or what the child's pretreatment measurements were *to determine goal to work toward.*
- Weigh daily or weekly (according to physician order or institutional standard) and measure length/height weekly *to monitor for appropriate growth.*
- Determine child's food preferences and provide favourite foods as able *to increase the likelihood that the child will consume appropriate amounts of foods.*
- Instruct child and family about nutritional requirements *so that they are involved and are prepared for home care.*
- Refer to dietitian *for more detailed information and assistance.*

For the child who needs to gain weight:
- Offer highest-calorie meals at the time of day when the child's appetite is the greatest *to increase likelihood of increased caloric intake.*
- Provide increased-calorie shakes or puddings within dietary restrictions *(high-calorie foods increase weight gain).*
- Administer vitamin and mineral supplements as prescribed *to attain/maintain vitamin and mineral balance in the body.*

Nursing Care Plan 48.1 (continued)

NURSING DIAGNOSIS: Deficient or excess fluid volume related to pathophysiology of endocrine dysfunction as evidenced by signs and symptoms of dehydration (deficient fluid volume) or edema and excessive urine output (excess fluid volume)

Outcome Identification and Evaluation

Child will maintain adequate fluid volume *as evidenced by elastic skin turgor; absence of edema; moist, pink oral mucosa; presence of tears; urine output 1 mL/kg/hour or more; vital signs within normal range for age; and normal electrolyte/hormone serum levels.*

Interventions: Maintaining Adequate Fluid Volume

- Assess hydration status (skin turgor, oral mucosa, presence of tears) every 4 to 8 hours *to evaluate maintenance of adequate fluid volume.*
- Assess adequacy of urine output *to evaluate end-organ perfusion.*
- Maintain strict intake and output record *to evaluate effectiveness of rehydration.*
- Weigh child daily: *Accurate weight is one of the best indicators of fluid volume status in children.*
- Administer specific hormone, fluid, and electrolyte requirements as ordered *to aid in fluid balance.*

Fluid volume deficit:
- Maintain IV line and administer IV fluid as ordered *to maintain fluid volume.*

Fluid volume excess:
- Maintain fluid restriction as ordered *to restore homeostasis.*

NURSING DIAGNOSIS: Noncompliance related to long-term/complex management of some disorders as evidenced by failure to keep appointments, development of complications or exacerbation of symptoms, or child/family verbalization of inability to maintain treatment plan

Outcome Identification and Evaluation

Child and family will comply with treatment regimen; *child and family will list treatment expectations and agree to follow through.*

Interventions: Encouraging Compliance

- Listen non-judgementally while child/family describe reasons for noncompliance; *assessment of problem should begin with nonthreatening discussion.*
- Help child/family develop a schedule for medication administration and other home regimens that works best for them; *involving child and family in planning care will increase compliance by making them feel respected and valued.*
- Work with the child and family to develop a written treatment plan or schedule that best suits their needs *to provide support for maintenance of treatment plan.*
- Establish follow-up visits to fit family's situation *to promote compliance.*
- Encourage monitoring with pediatric endocrinologist and specialists: *Multidisciplinary involvement has been shown to increase compliance.*
- Recognize that behavioural change comes slowly; *allows time for child and family to adjust to chronic nature of illness.*

secondary to damage to the hypothalamus or pituitary, such as from a tumour, infection, infarction, or irradiation.

Therapeutic Management

Treatment of primary GH deficiency involves the use of supplemental GH. Treatment of secondary GHD includes attention to the underlying condition, such as removal of any tumours, followed by GH therapy. Biosynthetic GH, derived from recombinant DNA, is given by subcutaneous injection, with the weekly dose divided and given over 3 to 7 days (Taketoma, Hodding, & Kraus, 2007).

Supplementation of GH may also be prescribed for children with disorders such as Turner syndrome, short stature due to Prader–Willi syndrome, chronic renal insufficiency pre-transplantation, long-term corticosteroid treatment, or idiopathic short stature who are more than 2.25 SD below the mean in height and are who are unlikely to catch up (Lawson Wilkins Pediatric Endocrinology Society Drug and Therapeutics Committee, 2003). GH replacement is an expensive treatment, with age-adjusted doses costing from $10,000 to more than $30,000 annually. Private and public drug programs often require evidence to adjust or substantiate the reimbursement decisions (Li, Banerjee, Dunfield, et al., 2007).

Nursing Assessment

The focus of the initial evaluation for GH deficiency is to rule out growth delay due to chronic illnesses, including chronic malnutrition, renal failure, poorly controlled diabetes, and thyroid dysfunction (Nicol et al., 2010). For a full description of the assessment phase of the nursing process, refer to page 1647. Assessment findings pertinent to GH deficiency are discussed below.

Health History

The health history may reveal a familial pattern of short stature or a brain tumour such as craniopharyngioma. Evaluate previous and current growth patterns as well as history of illness. Assess the child's feelings about being shorter than his or her peers.

Physical Examination

In addition to the linear height being at or below levels described above, the physical assessment findings may show that the child has a higher weight-to-height ratio than expected for age (Fig. 48.2).

Laboratory and Diagnostic Testing

The child will undergo laboratory tests to rule out chronic illnesses such as renal failure or liver and thyroid dysfunction. Laboratory and diagnostic tests used in children with suspected GH deficiency include:

- Radiography to determine whether bone age is 2 or more SD less than expected

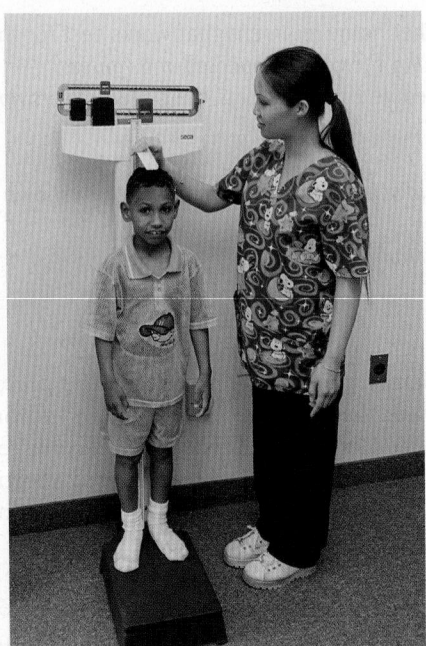

FIGURE 48.2 The child with growth hormone deficiency displays short stature.

- CT or MRI to rule out tumours or structural abnormalities
- Pituitary function testing to confirm the diagnosis. This test consists of providing a GH stimulant such as glucagon or arginine to stimulate the pituitary to release a burst of GH.
- Another test used in diagnosing this condition involves determining whether serum concentrations of insulin-like growth factor are low (Behrman, Kliegman, & Jenson, 2004; Sperling, 2002).

Nursing Management

Nursing management for the child with GH deficiency focuses on promoting growth, enhancing the child's self-esteem, and providing appropriate education about the disorder.

Promoting Growth

The goal of growth promotion is for the child to demonstrate an improved growth rate. With early diagnosis and treatment, the child has a better prognosis for reaching a normal adult height. Maximum growth velocity occurs in the first year of therapy, with the growth velocity decreasing in each successive year of treatment. GH therapy should be continued until near-final height is achieved and the growth rate is less than 2.5 cm/year; this includes assessment of bone age in girls older than 14 years and in boys older than 16 years (Parks & Felner, 2007).

At the beginning of treatment, monitor for height increase and possible side effects related to the medications. Measure the child's height at least every 6 months and plot growth over time on standardized growth charts. Provide information to the child and family about normal development and growth rates, bone age, and growth potential. Explore with the family and child their expectations and understanding of what is normal so they will have realistic expectations of treatment. Consult a dietitian if the child and family need assistance in providing adequate nutrition for growth and development.

Enhancing the Child's Self-Esteem

The child with GH deficiency often has younger-looking features and is shorter than his or her peers. Encourage the child to express positive feelings about his or her self-image, as shown by comments during health care visits as well as involvement with peers. Encourage the child to voice concerns. Emphasize the child's strengths and assets. Provide information about community support groups or websites related to GH deficiency. Evaluate for long-term learning problems that may develop if the child had a tumour and surgery or irradiation to remove it. Unidentified learning problems can have a negative impact on the child's self-esteem. Treat and communicate with the child in an age-appropriate manner even though he or she may appear younger.

Educating the Family

GH is a powder that is mixed with packaged diluents. Explain how to prepare it and give the correct dosage. Have the family provide a return demonstration to make sure they understand correct dilution and administration of GH. Instruct the family to report headaches, rapid weight gain, or painful hip joints as possible adverse reactions. Side effects may also include hypothyroidism or adrenal insufficiency (Parks & Felner, 2007). The child should visit the pediatric endocrinologist every 3 to 6 months to monitor for potential adverse effects and to assess compliance with injections. Stress the importance of complying with the GH replacement therapy and frequent supervision by a pediatric endocrinologist.

Guide the family and child in setting realistic goals and expectations based on age, personal abilities and strengths, and the effectiveness of the GH replacement therapy. For example, the family may want to encourage the child to choose sports that are not dependent on height. Encourage the family to dress the child according to age, not size. Refer the child and family to counselling if indicated. Inform families about support groups such as the Human Growth Foundation; visit http://thePoint. lww.com/Chow1e for a direct link to online resources.

Hyperpituitarism (Pituitary Gigantism)

Hyperpituitarism is an extremely rare disorder in children that results from excessive secretion of GH. When GH overproduction occurs before the epiphyseal plates close, the child or adolescent will show many related signs, the most striking of which is excessive and often dramatic linear growth. Children with this condition, which is often referred to as "gigantism," may grow to 213 to 244 cm (7 to 8 feet) in height (Eugster, 2010). When GH overproduction occurs after the epiphyseal plates close, acromegaly, the enlargement of the bones of the head and soft parts of the feet and hands, will occur. The cause of hyperpituitarism in children is most often excess GH-releasing hormone (GHRH) by the hypothalamus, but it may also be due to a tumour of the anterior pituitary or hypothalamus (Eugster, 2010). The condition most often occurs in isolation but may be part of a syndrome or disorder.

Therapeutic management of hyperpituitarism depends on the cause. Treatment may involve daily subcutaneous administration of somatostatin analogues to suppress GH production or may involve surgery or radiation to treat a tumour, with pituitary hormone replacement after surgery (Ferry & Shim, 2010).

Complications of gigantism depend upon any additional aspects of hyperpituitarism, which could include visual loss or heart failure.

Nursing Assessment

In addition to excessive height, physical findings include coarse facial features and enlarged hands and feet. Some patients display behavioural and visual problems. An increased level of insulin-like growth factor (IGF)-1 is a good indicator of excess GH (Ferry & Shim, 2010). The standard for making the diagnosis of GH excess is failure to suppress serum GH levels after an oral **glucose** challenge test (Ferry & Shim, 2010). A bone scan determines whether the epiphyseal plates are closed. Radiologic studies, including MRI, are used to detect any tumours.

Nursing Management

Nursing management depends on which treatment the child undergoes. If surgical removal of a tumour is required, provide routine preoperative and postoperative care. Administer a somatostatin analogue (e.g., octreotide acetate) if ordered. Treat the child according to his or her developmental or chronological age rather than according to growth parameters. Assess the child's self-image, teach the child and family about the disorder and the treatment plan, and provide emotional support. Monitor for and report signs of potential complications related to additional components of hyperpituitarism, such as hypogonadism, visual loss, or heart failure.

Precocious Puberty

Puberty occurs when the gonads produce increased amounts of sex hormones. In precocious puberty, sexual characteristics develop before the usual age of puberty. Breasts or pubic hair develops before the age of 8 years in white girls and before the age of 7 years in black girls, and testicular enlargement occurs in boys younger than 9 years (Kaplowitz, 2010a). The incidence of precocious puberty is about 10 times higher in girls, affecting about 4% to 5% of girls (Kaplowitz, 2010a). Most cases have idiopathic etiologies (Nakamoto, Franklin, & Geffner, 2010). Other causes include tumours or infection of the CNS, brain injury or radiation, congenital adrenal hyperplasia (CAH), and tumours of the ovary, adrenal gland, or testes.

Pathophysiology

True central precocious puberty develops as a result of premature activation of the hypothalamic–pituitary–gonadal (HPG) axis. This results in the production of gonadotropin-releasing hormone (GnRH), which stimulates the pituitary to produce luteinizing hormone (LH) and follicle-stimulating hormone (FSH). These hormones in turn stimulate the gonads to secrete the sex hormones (estrogen or testosterone). The child develops sexual characteristics, shows increased growth and skeletal maturation, and will have early reproductive capability.

Therapeutic Management

The clinical treatment for precocious puberty first involves determining the cause, the type, the rate of progress, and the family history followed by referral to a pediatric endocrinologist or gynecologist. If the etiology is secondary to another condition, such as a tumour, treatment for that condition is required. The treatment for confirmed central precocious puberty with rapid progression or significant psychosocial difficulties involves administering a GnRH analogue. This is available in a variety of forms but is administered most commonly as an intramuscular injection given every 3 to 4 weeks or as a subdermal implant. This analogue stimulates gonadotropin release initially but when given on a long-term basis will suppress gonadotropin release. The rate of bone maturation slows with this treatment, and secondary sexual development stabilizes or regresses. When treatment is discontinued, puberty resumes according to appropriate developmental stages.

Nursing Assessment

For a full description of the assessment phase of the nursing process, refer to page 1647. Pertinent assessment findings related to precocious puberty are discussed below.

Health History

The health history may reveal complaints of headaches, nausea, vomiting, and visual difficulties due to the circulating hormones. Psychosocial development is typical for the child's age, but the child may show emotional lability, aggressive behaviour, and mood swings. Information from the child and family may also reveal risk factors such as a history of CNS trauma or infection or a family history of early puberty.

Physical Examination

Physical examination may reveal acne and an adult-like body odour. The child will present with an accelerated rate of growth. The Tanner staging of breasts, pubic hair, and genitalia reveals advanced maturation for the child's age, but the child does not typically display sexual behaviour.

Laboratory and Diagnostic Testing

Radiologic examinations and pelvic ultrasound will identify advanced bone age and maturation of the uterus and ovaries consistent with the diagnosis of precocious puberty. Laboratory studies include screening radioimmunoassays for LH, FSH, adrenal androgens, estradiol, or testosterone. The child's response to GnRH stimulation confirms the diagnosis of central precocious puberty versus gonadotropin-independent puberty. This test involves administering synthetic GnRH intravenously and drawing serial blood levels, about every 30 minutes to 2 hours, of LH, FSH, and estrogen or testosterone. A positive result is defined as pubertal or adult levels of these hormones in response to the GnRH administration. CT or MRI will reveal any lesions in the CNS, especially in younger children demonstrating early signs of puberty (Kaplowitz, 2010a).

Nursing Management

In general, nursing management of the child with precocious puberty focuses on administering medications, helping the child to deal with self-esteem issues related to the accelerated growth and development of secondary sexual characteristics, and educating the child and family. Goals of nursing management include appropriate physical development and pubertal progression appropriate for age. Refer to Nursing Care Plan 48.1, and individualize care based on the child's and family's response to this disorder.

Nursing care involves assessing and documenting the changes the child is experiencing, educating family members and caregivers, and administering medications. Demonstrate correct administration of medication and observe for potential adverse effects. Encourage the family to participate with follow-up appointments, which typically occur every 6 months and include scheduled stimulation tests. Teach families that pharmacologic intervention will stop when the child reaches the age appropriate for pubertal development. Provide appropriate sex education, but reassure families that precocious puberty does not always involve precocious sexual behaviour (KidsHealth, 2011).

Dealing with Self-Esteem Issues

Children may feel embarrassed by the physical effects of puberty, developing self-esteem issues and anxiety related to body image disturbances and altered social interactions (KidsHealth, 2011). The goal is for the child to exhibit normal psychosocial development and understand the physical and emotional changes that occur with early onset of puberty. Assist the family and others, such as teachers and friends, to communicate with the child on an age-appropriate level, even when physical characteristics make the child appear older. Emphasize to the child that everyone develops sexual characteristics in time and that his or hers have just occurred earlier. Refer the child and family for counselling if behavioural or psychological disturbances develop. Since the child may have issues with self-image and may be self-conscious, encourage the child to express his or her feelings about the changes. Role playing may be used to show the child how to handle teasing from other children (Bordini, 2011).

Delayed Puberty

Delayed puberty is late pubertal development by 2 SD above the mean age of expected development. This relates to about age 13 years for girls and age 14 years for boys. It may additionally be diagnosed if there is a temporary delay in the progression of puberty, such as more than 4 years between the onset of puberty and the onset of menses in girls (Nakamoto et al., 2010). The most common cause of delayed puberty is a hereditary condition known as **constitutional delay**, in which pubertal development, growth, and weight are delayed in otherwise healthy children (Clark, 2011). Hypogonadism also may result when there is decreased stimulation of the gonads due to dysfunction in the hypothalamus or pituitary gland; CNS tumours, trauma, or irradiation; or genetic syndromes such as Turner or Prader–Willi syndrome. Another common cause of delayed puberty is a chronic condition such as anorexia or cystic fibrosis, with treatment of the underlying condition the only necessary therapy.

Management of permanent hypogonadism involves administering testosterone or estradiol in low dosages if there is no underlying situation to address. This is usually necessary for only a short time to get puberty started. Treatment for constitutional delay is controversial due to the lack of physical pathology but potential psychological compromise.

Nursing Assessment

Assessment involves obtaining a health history to identify the indications for this condition. Assessment of the growth pattern using correct techniques and standards for comparison is essential. On physical assessment, note absence of secondary sex characteristics as noted above. Laboratory and diagnostic testing rules out other causes for delayed puberty. Blood levels of reproductive hormones may also be evaluated.

Nursing Management

In addition to the general interventions presented in Nursing Care Plan 48.1, educate the child and family about the different stages of puberty. Teach them about the medication therapy, and help them develop a home management schedule for the administration of medication.

Diabetes Insipidus

DI is a disorder of the posterior pituitary gland resulting from a deficiency in the secretion of antidiuretic hormone (ADH). This hormone, also known as vasopressin, is produced in the hypothalamus and stored in the pituitary gland. ADH is released from the pituitary in response to increases in serum osmolarity. ADH acts by increasing the permeability of the collecting tubules, leading to reabsorption of water and retention of fluid. Thus, ADH has a major role in maintaining serum and urine osmolality within normal limits. Without sufficient ADH, the kidney loses massive amounts of water and serum sodium levels subsequently increase.

In central DI, either ADH is not released or the osmoreceptors in the brain are damaged (Simmons, 2010). Approximately, 30% to 50% of cases of central DI are idiopathic (Rose & Bichet, 2010). Central DI may also occur as a result of complications from CNS trauma, surgery, infections, or side effects of medications. In nephrogenic DI, receptors in the kidney are unresponsive to ADH at the kidneys. It can be genetic, acquired, or

secondary to electrolyte imbalances, medications, alcohol, or renal disease (Bichet, 2010). DI may be transient or permanent.

Therapeutic Management

Treatment starts by identifying and correcting any known underlying cause. Care in the acute phase includes diligent attention to fluid and electrolyte balance. Pharmacologic intervention includes replacement of ADH with a synthetic form, typically via the intranasal route. The dose depends on the child's age, urine output, and urine osmolality and is titrated to clinical outcome.

Treatment of nephrogenic DI involves diuretics, high fluid intake, and restricted sodium intake (Bichet, 2010).

Nursing Assessment

For a full description of the assessment phase of the nursing process, refer to page 1647. Assessment findings pertinent to DI are discussed below.

Health History

Nursing assessment involves obtaining a history of any conditions or medications that may have led to the development of the disorder. Most symptoms of endocrine disorders develop slowly, but the onset of this disorder is abrupt. The health history usually elicits the cardinal symptoms as well as indications of dehydration and hypernatremia.

The most common signs of DI are **polyuria** (excessive urination) and **polydipsia** (excessive thirst) (Breault & Majzoub, 2007). Except for children who are unable to respond to their thirst due to age, developmental level, or level of consciousness, the child typically maintains adequate perfusion by drinking water (Perkin, Swift, & Newton, 2003). The parent or child may report frequent trips to the bathroom, nocturia, or enuresis. When the child cannot compensate for the excessive loss of water by increasing fluid intake, additional symptoms may be demonstrated as a result of dehydration, such as acute weight loss and electrolyte imbalance (hypernatremia). Irritability may be due to the early signs of hypernatremia. Other signs include intermittent fever, vomiting, and constipation. The fluid and electrolyte disturbances with severe DI may precipitate hypovolemic shock (Trimarchi, 2006).

Physical Examination

Observation and inspection may reveal weight loss secondary to loss of fluid in the child unable to compensate for fluid loss. Inspection may also reveal signs of dehydration, such as dry mucous membranes. Vital signs may demonstrate signs of volume depletion such as tachycardia, slightly depressed fontanels, decreased skin turgor, or hypotension. The child may excrete more than 4 mL/kg/hour of urine.

Laboratory and Diagnostic Testing

Diagnostic tests used to evaluate DI include:

- Radiologic studies such as CT or ultrasound of the skull and kidneys can help determine whether a lesion or tumour is present.
- Urinalysis: urine is dilute, osmolarity is less than 3,000 mOsm/L, and specific gravity is less than 1.010.
- Serum osmolarity is greater than 300 mOsm/L.
- Serum sodium is elevated.
- Fluid deprivation test: measures vasopressin release from the pituitary in response to fluid deprivation. Normal results will show decreased urine output, increased urine specific gravity, and no change in serum sodium. The fluid deprivation test is stopped if 3% to 5% of body weight is lost, if the child shows signs of volume depletion, or if lab results reveal increased urine osmolality, plasma osmolality, or serum sodium (Bichet, 2010).

Nursing Management

Refer to Nursing Care Plan 48.1, and individualize the plan of care based on the child's and family's response to the illness. Specific interventions related to nursing care of the child with DI are discussed below.

Promoting Hydration

The goal of treatment is to achieve hourly urine output of 1 to 2 mL/kg, urine specific gravity of at least 1.010, and normal serum sodium. Monitor fluid intake and hydration status, and maintain total daily fluid intake as ordered. Monitor hydration status by measuring regular vital signs, electrolyte status, fluid intake and output and, at minimum, daily weights (using the same scale at the same time of day). If fluids are stopped too soon, the child may become hypernatremic. Seizures can be a consequence of the electrolyte abnormalities introduced in the CNS by severe hypernatremia and hyperosmolar dehydration (Chan & Roth, 2011). Feed infants more frequently, since they excrete more dilute urine, consume larger volumes of free water, and secrete lower amounts of vasopressin than older children.

Promoting Activity

Assess the child's abilities daily, schedule frequent bathroom breaks, keep fluids the child likes available at all times, and fit the treatment plan to the child's activity.

Educating the Family

Involve the family in development of the fluid intake regimen. A journal or daily log is essential in maintaining the regimen and identifying problems. Children with intact thirst centres can self-regulate their need for fluids, but if this is not the situation, help the family develop a plan for fluid replacement on a regular basis. All families will require education about management at times of increased fluid losses, such as during warm weather when insensible water loss increases through perspiration and respiration, or during episodes of vomiting and diarrhea. The child who is unable to compensate for the excessive loss of water by independently increasing his or her own fluid intake is at greatest risk. Education about the symptoms of both water intoxication and dehydration is required. Help the family develop a plan to inform the school and other individuals in the child's life about the need for liberal bathroom privileges and extra fluids to prevent accidents or dehydration. Recommend that the family obtain a medical alert bracelet or necklace for the child. Encourage the parents to maintain follow-up appointments, which will probably be every 6 months.

Syndrome of Inappropriate Antidiuretic Hormone (SIADH)

SIADH occurs when ADH is secreted regardless of serum osmolality, causing reabsorption of water in the renal tubules and a subsequent decrease in serum osmolality. The serum sodium also decreases as a result of sodium dilution (dilutional hypnatremia) in the vascular space, with fluid shifting from the vascular space into the extracellular space. Ultimately, the feedback mechanism that regulates ADH secretion may not function properly, but the underlying causes vary widely. SIADH may be caused by a tumour that independently secretes ADH; by thoracic surgery or a thoracic mass; CNS infections, tumour, or trauma; certain cancers such as lymphoma; and medications, such as some specific chemotherapeutics (Flounders, 2003).

Management of SIADH is focused on correcting the underlying condition. Slow correction of fluid and electrolyte levels is important to prevent sudden fluid shifts and quick rises in serum sodium, with resultant CNS symptoms (Sterns, 2011b). Strict fluid restriction and slow correction of serum sodium (by approximately 0.5 mmol/L/hour) and osmolality usually resolve the SIADH.

Nursing Assessment

Obtain a health history, noting history of CNS infections, tumour, or trauma; infections; and medication use. Note signs such as decreased urine output and weight gain, or gastrointestinal symptoms such as anorexia, nausea, and vomiting. Assess neurologic signs of hyponatremia, such as all behavioural changes, headache, altered level of consciousness, seizure, or coma. Key laboratory findings include low serum sodium (due to dilution with fluid) and low serum osmolality, with elevated urine osmolality and sodium (Flounders, 2003).

Nursing Management

Nursing goals focus on slowly restoring fluid and electrolyte balance to minimize risks to neurologic status associated with overly rapid correction of hyponatremia

COMPARISON CHART 48.1 DIABETES INSIPIDUS VERSUS SIADH

Diabetes Insipidus	Syndrome of Inappropriate Antidiuretic Hormone
• "High and dry" • Increased urination • Hypernatremia • Serum osmolality >300 mOsm/kg • Urine specific gravity <1.015 • Decreased urine osmolality • Dehydration, thirst, possible weight loss	• "Low and wet" • Decreased urination • Hyponatremia • Serum osmolality <280 mOsm/kg • Urine specific gravity >1.030 • Increased urine osmolality • Fluid retention (extravascular), weight gain, and hypertension

and maintaining safety (Sterns, 2011a). Nurses are also often in the best position to perceive subtle changes in patient status and behaviour (Flounders, 2003). Initiate safety precautions if the neurologic status is altered or the serum sodium continues to fall. Anticonvulsants may be necessary to treat seizure activity. Intermittent hypertonic saline may be required for patients with severe hyponatremia associated with seizures or coma. Intake and output are monitored strictly and the child is weighed at least once daily to assess fluid status. Close observation of the child and education of the family may be necessary to prevent intake of oral fluids beyond the strict fluid restriction, with child life therapists assisting in mechanisms such as distraction to help the child cope during the test.

Comparison Chart 48.1 compares DI with SIADH.

Disorders of Thyroid Function

Disorders of the thyroid gland are relatively common in infancy and childhood (Hatcher, 2010). These disorders can be serious because thyroid hormones are important for growth and development: they regulate metabolism of nutrients and energy production.

Congenital Hypothyroidism

Congenital hypothyroidism, inadequate thyroid production in newborns, usually results from an abnormality of thyroid gland development (American Academy of Pediatrics [AAP], 2006). This leads to insufficient production of the thyroid hormones required to meet the body's metabolic and growth and development needs, particularly the developing CNS. Congenital hypothyroidism leads to low concentrations of circulating thyroid hormones (tri-iodothyronine [T_3] and thyroxine [T_4]). It is the one of the most common preventable causes of intellectual delay or impairment, with an incidence detected via screening of 1 per 3,000 to 4,000 births (AAP, 2006). Children with congenital hypothyroidism are also at greater risk for congenital malformations, particularly renal and urologic conditions (LaFranchi, 2011).

Congenital hypothyroidism occurs more often in girls, in infants of Hispanic or Far Eastern descent, and in children with Down syndrome; it is less common in

black infants (AAP, 2006). The term "cretinism" may be used to describe clusters of infants in geographic areas with goitre (enlargement of the thyroid gland) and hypothyroidism, most often related to iodine deficiency (Postellon & Daniel, 2011).

Pathophysiology

Congenital hypothyroidism is most often due to a defect in the development of the thyroid gland in the fetus or maternal iodine deficiency (Postellon & Daniel, 2011). Transient hypothyroidism may also occur with placental transfer of medications to treat maternal hyperthyroidism or maternal autoantibodies against thyroid-stimulating hormone (TSH) (Eugster, LeMay, Zern, et al., 2004; Postellon & Daniel, 2011).

Therapeutic Management

To prevent intellectual disability and maintain normal growth and motor development, thyroid hormone replacement with levothyroxine is begun in the first 2 weeks of life (AAP, 2006). The recommended starting dose is 10 to 15 µg/kg/day (AAP, 2006). Initially, thyroid function tests are performed every 2 to 4 weeks, typically decreasing to every 6 to 12 months by 3 years of age and continuing to decrease in frequency until puberty is complete. Since thyroid hormone is vital to the infant's developing CNS, the goal is to normalize thyroid function as measured by serum T_4 and TSH as quickly as possible. Lifelong treatment will be needed to maintain normal metabolism.

Nursing Assessment

Nursing assessment of the child with congenital hypothyroidism includes health history, physical examination, and laboratory testing.

Health History

Determine whether the neonatal metabolic screening test was performed. Inquire about a maternal history that may indicate a connection to hypothyroidism. Additional history findings may include sensitivity to cold, constipation, feeding problems, or lethargy. Since parents like babies to sleep well, they may not report that the baby is sleeping

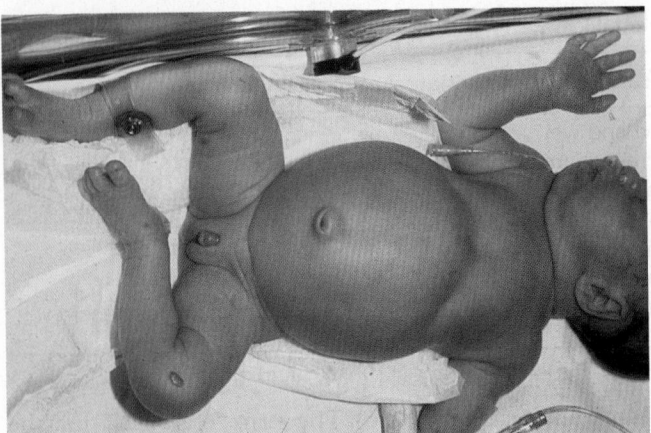

Figure 48.3 Newborn with congenital hypothyroidism.

too much; rather, they may remark that it is difficult to keep the baby awake.

Physical Examination

Evidence gathered prior to initiation of screening programs, and in countries without screening programs, demonstrates that most infants are initially asymptomatic. Without treatment, observation increasingly shows a lethargic baby or a child with hypotonia. Measurements of weight and height may reveal delayed growth. Other findings may include a persistent open posterior fontanel, coarse appearance of the face with short neck and limbs, periorbital puffiness, enlarged tongue, and poor sucking response (Fig. 48.3). The skin may appear pale with mottling or yellow from prolonged jaundice, or it may be cool, dry, and scaly to the touch, with sparse hair development on the older child. Auscultation of the chest might reveal bradycardia. Signs of respiratory distress and decreased pulse pressure may also be present. On palpation of the abdomen, there may be evidence of a mass due to constipation (LaFranchi, 2009).

Laboratory and Diagnostic Testing

A thyroid blood test (TSH or T_4) is routinely done on a heel-prick blood sample obtained between days 2 and 5 after birth. If the TSH is high or the T_4 is low, the parents are informed and the findings are confirmed by repeating the blood test (Thyroid Foundation of Canada, n.d.). Radioimmunoassay is used to measure T_4 levels, which accurately reflect the child's thyroid status. A thyroid scan may also be used to check for the absence or ectopic placement of the gland. In addition to serum measurement of T_4, other diagnostic tests include serum T_3, radioiodine uptake, thyroid-bound globulin, and ultrasonography.

Nursing Management

The overall goal of nursing management of the infant or child with congenital hypothyroidism is to establish a nor-

mal growth pattern without complications such as cognitive delay or failure to thrive. Individualize the nursing care plan based on the infant's responses to the illness.

Educating the Family

Since most infants are asymptomatic, the diagnosis may be unexpected, so reassure and convey realistic expectations to the family. In children for whom thyroid hormone therapy is started within the first 2 months of life and consistently maintained, growth rate and adult height are normal. Even with optimal treatment, minor differences in intelligence and school achievement may occur in children with congenital hypothyroidism. These differences are magnified the later that thyroid hormone therapy is started (AAP, 2006). Developmental follow-up may be indicated to assist the child and family with any delays. Educate the family about the disorder, the medication and method of administration, and the consequences associated with no treatment or inadequate treatment (Postellon & Daniel, 2011).

L-thyroxine is an oral medication that is available as a tablet. It must be crushed for infants and young children. It can be mixed with a small amount of formula and placed in the nipple, or it can be administered to the baby with a syringe or dropper. Medications should not be placed in a full bottle of formula because the infant will not ingest all the medication if he or she does not finish the bottle. Medication absorption is decreased by soy-based formulas and iron preparations (Taketoma et al., 2007). If the child vomits within 1 hour of administration, instruct the family to repeat the dose, since many missed doses may lead to developmental delays and poor growth.

Assist the family to understand that this medication will be needed throughout the child's life and that frequent blood tests will be required to evaluate thyroid function. Finally, encourage the family to obtain a medical identification bracelet for the child.

▶ *Consider* THIS!

Asha Virani, 1-week-old, is brought to the clinic. Her newborn screening test was positive for hypothyroidism. Her parents are shocked and upset by the news. Her mother states, "My daughter's been doing so well since she came home from the hospital. She seems to be doing everything she should be. She's a great sleeper. I just can't believe anything's wrong with her."

1. How would you address the parents' concerns?
2. What teaching will be appropriate for this family?

Acquired Hypothyroidism

Hypothyroidism also occurs as an acquired condition. This disorder most commonly results from a chronic autoimmune thyroiditis also known as Hashimoto's thyroiditis

(Sperling, 2002). As a genetic condition, antibodies develop against the thyroid gland, causing the gland to become inflamed, infiltrated, and progressively destroyed. It occurs more often in girls during childhood and adolescence (Sperling, 2002). Less common etiologies include hypothyroidism associated with pituitary or hypothalamic dysfunction. Children with other autoimmune disorders, such as type 1 diabetes, or some chromosomal disorders, such as Turner syndrome, are at increased risk for chronic autoimmune thyroiditis (LaFranchi, 2010).

Management of symptomatic children involves oral sodium L-thyroxine to maintain T_4 levels in the upper half of the normal range and to suppress TSH. Opinions vary as to whether to treat the asymptomatic child who has a normal total or free T_4 level and a slightly elevated TSH level (often referred to as subclinical hypothyroidism) because the elevated TSH usually either normalizes or persists but does not increase (Kaplowitz, 2010b).

Nursing Assessment

Interview the family and child to determine activity tolerance and behaviour changes. The symptoms may develop over a period of time and may be subtle. Note vague complaints of fatigue, weakness, brittle hair, weight gain, cold intolerance, constipation, or dry skin. The severity of symptoms depends on the length of time that the hormone deficiency has existed and its extent.

Physical examination may reveal a **goitre** (enlargement of the thyroid gland), declining growth velocity, and delayed or precocious puberty. Deep tendon reflexes may be sluggish, and the face, eyes, and hands may be edematous. Note thinning or coarse hair or muscle hypertrophy with muscle weakness. The diagnostic evaluation involves serum thyroid function studies (TSH, T_3, and T_4) as well as serum thyroid antibodies to confirm autoimmune thyroiditis.

Nursing Management

Work with the family to establish a daily schedule for administering L-thyroxine, which should be taken 30 minutes before a meal for optimal absorption (Taketoma et al., 2007). Explain to the family that growth is related to the child's response to the treatment, and there are no specific strategies to aid in this growth. The family should understand the diagnosis, should be able to recognize signs and symptoms of hypofunction and hyperfunction, and should know when to notify the physician. The family and child may need assistance in accepting the therapy as well as the experience of catch-up growth that may occur at the beginning of therapy. The child's thyroid levels should be evaluated every 3 to 6 months. The child with severe, longstanding hypothyroidism who has an infection or is given sedatives, especially opioids, may be at risk for a myxedema coma, where the body's metabolic needs have exceeded the cardiovascular and pulmonary

systems' ability to respond. Myxedema coma is an acute emergency that may also present with hypotension, bradycardia, and hypoventilation (Ross, 2010). Fortunately, this complication is rare.

Hyperthyroidism

Hyperthyroidism is the result of excess circulating thyroid hormone. The most common cause, Graves' disease, is not common in children, with an incidence of 1 in 5,000, mostly in the 11- to 15-year age group (LaFranchi, 2009). Graves' disease is an autoimmune disorder that causes antibodies to stimulate the TSH receptors, thereby stimulating excess thyroid hormone synthesis and secretion. It occurs five times more often in girls than in boys (LaFranchi, 2007). There is a strong genetic component to the development of Graves' disease, with 60% of affected persons having a family history of autoimmune thyroid problems (Radovick & MacGillivray, 2003) and the patients themselves at increased risk for other autoimmune endocrine disorders (LaFranchi, 2009). Remission rates in children after several years of drug therapy are usually less than 30% (Polak & Van Vliet, 2009). Less common and possibly transient causes of hyperthyroidism are thyroiditis, thyroid hormone–producing tumours, and pituitary adenomas.

A rare congenital form of hyperthyroidism, neonatal thyrotoxicosis, may occur in infants of mothers with Graves' disease. This neonatal condition, which can be life-threatening, is a self-limiting disorder (lasting 2 to 4 months) caused by transplacental passage of thyroid-stimulating immunoglobulins (Burg, Polin, Ingelfinger, et al., 2002).

Management of hyperthyroidism is aimed at decreasing thyroid hormone levels while avoiding hypothyroidism. Current treatment involves antithyroid medication, radioactive iodine therapy, and subtotal or total thyroidectomy. The first-line treatment most often used, the antithyroid medication methimazole, blocks the production of T_3 and T_4. A previously used antithyroid drug, propylthiouracil (PTU) is no longer the choice for first-line therapy in children due to liver toxicity (Endocrine Society, 2009; U.S. Food and Drug Administration [FDA], 2010). However, consideration must be given to contraception in teens of childbearing age as methimazole has been associated with birth defects (FDA, 2010). Radioactive iodine therapy may be used for those who have failed antithyroid therapy and is becoming an alternative in some centres as a first-line treatment for children (Polak & Van Vliet, 2009). This therapy is administered orally and results in tissue damage and destruction of the thyroid gland within 6 to 18 weeks, but it also leads to hypothyroidism. Thyroidectomy, which is associated with a low rate of disease recurrence, is used when drug therapy cannot be maintained or has been unsuccessful. The surgical risks include hypothyroidism, hypoparathyroidism, and laryngeal nerve damage.

Adjunct therapy with beta-adrenergic blockers may also be used if the child has signs of cardiovascular overactivity such as an increase in cardiac output and heart rate secondary to increased peripheral oxygen needs and increased contractility. Treatment of the cardiovascular effects may be suspended once the thyroid secretion responds to therapy (LaFranchi, 2009).

An acute emergency associated with hyperthyroidism is a sudden release of high levels of thyroid hormones. This can result in a "thyroid storm," which progresses to heart failure and shock. Immediately report the signs of thyroid storm, which include sudden onset of severe restlessness and irritability, fever, diaphoresis, and tachycardia (Burg et al., 2002).

Nursing Assessment

Most of these children are seen in the out-patient setting with a history of problems with sleep, school performance, and distractibility. They become easily frustrated and overheated, and they may become fatigued during physical education class. The child may complain of diarrhea (increased gut motility), excessive perspiration, and muscle weakness. The history may also reveal hyperactivity, heat intolerance, emotional lability, and insomnia. Initially, the symptoms are mild and often overlooked. Physical examination of the older child may reveal an increased rate of growth; weight loss despite an excellent appetite; hyperactivity; warm, moist skin; tachycardia; fine tremors; an enlarged thyroid gland or goitre; and ophthalmic changes. The extrathyroidal complications in children are less severe than those in adults (Huang, 2010). Exophthalmos (bulging of the eye anteriorly out of the orbit) would be due to inflammation or edema of the orbital muscles, fat, and connective tissue and may be accompanied by lid lag and retraction, staring expression, and diplopia (Fig. 48.4). Elevated pulse and blood pressure may also be noted. Serum T_4 and T_3 levels are markedly elevated. TSH levels are suppressed.

Infants with neonatal thyrotoxicosis present with low birth weight, failure to gain weight, hyperphagia, microcephaly, irritability, tachycardia, tachypnea, enlarged thyroid, vomiting, diarrhea, jaundice, hepatosplenomegaly, and thrombocytopenia. The major cause of morbidity and mortality in neonatal hyperthyroidism is cardiac disease (Ferry & Gold, 2011).

Nursing Management

Once the treatment plan is initiated, educate the family and child about the medication and potential adverse effects, the goals of treatment, and possible complications. Education should reinforce the fact that T_4 has a long half-life, so correction takes time and symptoms generally take 3 to 4 weeks to improve (Huang, 2010).

While awaiting stabilization of hormone levels, help the child and family to cope with symptoms such as heat intolerance, emotional lability, or eye problems. Assist

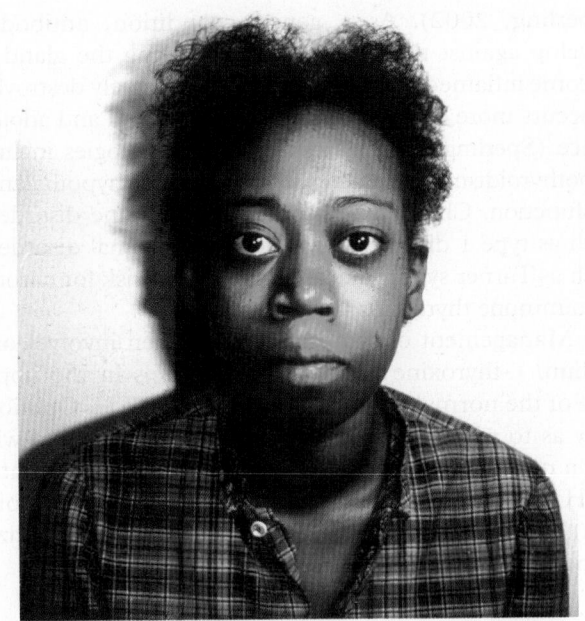

FIGURE 48.4 Adolescent with exophthalmos due to hyperthyroidism.

the family to share this information with school or day care personnel. While the hormone levels are being normalized, the child may benefit from more frequent rest breaks and a cooler environment and may need to modify physical education classes. Encourage the family to obtain a medical identification bracelet.

Monitor for adverse effects of antithyroid medications, such as rash, leukopenia, loss of taste, sore throat, gastrointestinal disturbances, and arthralgia (Taketoma et al., 2007). If surgical intervention is chosen, provide appropriate preoperative teaching and postoperative care. Inform the family of the need for routine blood tests and follow-up visits with the pediatric endocrinologist every 2 to 4 months until normal levels are reached; then visits may be decreased to once or twice a year. Educate the parents to contact the health care provider if the child develops symptoms related to increased or decreased hormone levels, such as tachycardia or extreme fatigue. Females of childbearing potential must receive anticipatory guidance regarding the additional monitoring of pregnancies to meet their potential needs for adjustment of medications as well as specialized monitoring of the fetus (Huang, 2010).

Comparison Chart 48.2 compares hypothyroidism and hyperthyroidism.

Disorders Related to Parathyroid Gland Function

The parathyroid glands secrete parathyroid hormone (PTH), which, along with vitamin D and calcitonin, regulates calcium/phosphate homeostasis by increasing

COMPARISON CHART 48.2   HYPOTHYROIDISM VERSUS HYPERTHYROIDISM

Hyperthyroidism	Hypothyroidism
• Nervousness/anxiety • Diarrhea • Heat intolerance • Weight loss • Smooth, velvety skin	• Tiredness/fatigue • Constipation • Cold intolerance • Weight gain • >Dry, thick skin; edema of face, eyes, and hands • Decreased growth

osteoclastic activity, absorption of calcium and excretion of phosphate by the kidneys, and absorption of calcium in the gastrointestinal tract. The two disorders associated with this gland are hypoparathyroidism and hyperparathyroidism.

Hypoparathyroidism

Hypoparathyroidism is the result of a deficiency in PTH secretion. The impaired secretion affects calcium and phosphorus metabolism, leading to hypocalcemia and hyperphosphatemia. It is a very uncommon disorder in children. The condition is most often congenital, resulting from aplasia or hypoplasia of the parathyroid gland. However, it can also be acquired due to removal of the glands during thyroidectomy or to autoimmune destruction the parathyroid gland (Perkin et al., 2003). It may occur as an isolated disorder or, similar to many other endocrine conditions, as part of a syndrome. DiGeorge syndrome, for example, includes hypoparathyroidism, cardiac defects, and absence of the thymus (Kelly & Levine, 2010). Hypoparathyroidism may also occur in the newborn as a result of maternal hyperparathyroidism (Behrman et al., 2004).

Emergency treatment of hypoparathyroidism is related to the consequences of alterations in serum calcium and involves giving intravenous calcium gluconate 10% solution (Perkin et al., 2003). The goal is to maintain low-normal serum calcium and phosphate levels, thus avoiding episodic or chronic hypercalcemia and hypercalciuria (Horwitz & Stewart, 2008). The treatment for less acute situations involves oral calcium supplementation with meals and vitamin D. Research into PTH supplementation is ongoing (Kelly & Levine, 2010).

Nursing Assessment

Determine the health history, noting poor eating, lethargy, muscle cramps progressing to numbness, and tingling in the hands and feet or around the mouth. The child may be irritable, have a history of unexplained seizures, or complain of constipation, nausea, vomiting, or diarrhea. Physical examination may reveal **tetany** (enhanced neuromuscular excitability of the central and peripheral nervous systems), Chvostek's sign (facial muscle spasm elicited by tapping the facial nerve), Trousseau's sign (carpopedal muscle spasm), or stridor (due to laryngospasm). Children with longstanding untreated hypoparathyroidism may have dry, scaly skin; brittle nails; and delayed dental eruption.

On palpation the child may complain of vague bone pain or abdominal discomfort. Laboratory testing reveals decreased serum calcium and PTH levels and increased serum phosphorus levels, which confirm the diagnosis. Bone age radiographs are usually normal, but if the condition has existed long term there may be evidence of increased bone density and suppressed growth.

Nursing Management

During acute or severe manifestations of hypoparathyroidism, administer intravenous calcium gluconate. Observe for development of cardiac arrhythmias during calcium infusions. Ensure that the intravenous site is patent. Extravasation of intravenous calcium can cause local tissue necrosis. Institute seizure precautions and reduce environmental stimuli (e.g., loud or sudden noises, bright lights, or stimulating activities). Observe for signs and symptoms of laryngospasm (e.g., stridor, hoarseness, or a feeling of tightness in the throat). Educate the child and family about the importance of continuous daily administration of calcium and vitamin D. Electrolytes will be monitored every 3 to 6 months during stable periods.

Hyperparathyroidism

Hyperparathyroidism is an extremely rare disorder in children. The most common cause is an adenomatous disorder of the parathyroid gland (Behrman et al., 2004; Perkin et al., 2003). Chronic renal disease or congenital anomalies of the urinary tract are the cause of secondary hyperparathyroidism. Management depends on the cause of the disorder and is focused upon the implications of altered calcium and phosphorus.

Disorders Related to Adrenal Gland Function

Disorders of the adrenal gland include acute and chronic adrenal insufficiency and disorders of hyperfunction such as Cushing syndrome. The adrenal cortex is the site of production of glucocorticoids, mineralocorticoids, and androgenic and estrogenic steroid compounds. The adrenal medulla is the site of production of the catecholamines and is under neuroendocrine control. When production of these compounds is altered, disease results.

Congenital Adrenal Hyperplasia

CAH is a group of autosomal recessive inherited disorders in which there is a deficiency in one of the enzymes required for proper function of the adrenal glands. In CAH, the adrenal glands may produce inadequate amounts of cortisol and/or aldosterone and produce too much androgen. The incidence of CAH is 0.06 to 0.08 per 1,000 live births (Burg et al., 2002; Sperling, 2002). The onset and severity of symptoms are dependent upon the form of CAH and the severity of impairment of enzymes. The most acute form of classic CAH, referred to as the salt-wasting form, presents shortly after birth with very low cortisol and low aldosterone levels. The subsequent acute adrenal crisis presents as a shock state that includes hypotension and hyponatremia (Donohoue, 2010). Early identification and thus prevention of an adrenal crisis may be prompted by ambiguous genitalia in the female, while the male may appear normal at birth.

Pathophysiology

Ninety percent to ninety-five percent of cases of CAH are caused by a deficiency of the enzyme 21-hydroxylase (21-OH) (Burg et al., 2002; Sperling, 2002). This defect results in the reduction of cortisol, a glucocorticoid, and aldosterone, a mineralocorticoid. Cortisol is normally produced as part of a stress response and works to maintain blood pressure, cardiovascular function, and glucose. In CAH, the decreased cortisol level causes stimulation of the adrenal cortex in a failed attempt to compensate, leading to enlargement or hyperplasia of the adrenal glands and excess production of androgens. Aldosterone regulates the absorption of sodium and water and the release (excretion) of potassium by the kidney and thus plays an integral role in regulation of fluid and electrolyte balance, including blood pressure.

In males, 21-OH deficiency with excessive androgen secretion leads to a slightly enlarged penis, which may become adult-sized by school age, and a hyperpigmented scrotum. The female fetus develops male secondary sexual characteristics, with the degree of virilization related to the severity of the enzyme defect. Thus, CAH causes pseudohermaphroditism, or ambiguous genitalia, in girls (Hatcher, 2010). The clitoris is enlarged and may resemble the penis, the labia have a rugated appearance, and the labial folds may be completely fused, but the ovaries, fallopian tubes, and uterus are normal. The nonclassic form of 21-OH deficiency is mild and not life-threatening. The masculinization of the external genitalia may be mild, especially in females. CAH may not become evident until the toddler or preschool years, with premature **adrenarche**, early development of armpit and pubic hair, early or severe acne and, in females, irregular menstrual periods and development of masculine characteristics such as facial hair and a deep voice (Donohoue, 2010; Oberfield & Speiser, 2010).

Therapeutic Management

The goal of treatment is to stop excessive adrenal secretion of androgens while maintaining normal growth and devel-

opment. Most children with 21-OH deficiency will take a glucocorticoid dose equal to that normally secreted, such as hydrocortisone, and the mineralocorticoid fludrocortisone for life. Infants may also require sodium supplementation to support fluid balance as breast milk and formula contain little salt. Regular follow-up care and dose adjustment for growth and development are required. Under stressful experiences such as illness, dehydration, or surgery, additional doses of cortisol (up to three to four times the usual dose) may be required to prevent an adrenal crisis, a shock state manifested by hypotension, hyponatremia, hyperkalemia, hypoglycemia, metabolic acidosis, vomiting, diarrhea, and abdominal pain. An adrenal crisis is an emergency (Donohoue, 2010).

Gender Issues

In the past when girls were born with ambiguous or markedly masculinized genitalia, standard medical treatment was to surgically correct the external genitalia and establish adequate adult sexual and reproductive functioning. Typically, a reduction of the clitoris and opening of the labial folds were done within the first few months of life, with further surgeries at puberty. Today, some families choose to delay cosmetic surgery until the child is old enough to participate in the decision. The influence of fetal androgen exposure on CAH-affected children and the subsequent gender identity, role behaviours, and abilities are insufficiently understood. Decision making for families in which their female infants were initially misassigned as boys, or those who choose to raise highly masculinized girls as males, can be overwhelming. The decision to intervene immediately or to delay treatment is a complex one that raises many concerns for the family. Prenatal treatment for heterozygous fetuses is being performed in some endocrine centres with the goal of reducing the masculinization of female genitalia. This therapy needs to begin at 5 to 6 weeks of gestation and is discontinued when male gender or lack of CAH is confirmed (Donohoue, 2010; Stokowski, 2009).

Nursing Assessment

Nursing assessment of the child with CAH includes health history, physical examination, and laboratory and diagnostic testing. Specific findings related to CAH are presented below.

Health History and Physical Examination

Obtain the health history, noting history of abnormal genitalia at birth in the infant.

In the toddler or preschooler, note history of accelerated growth velocity and signs of premature adrenarche. Upon inspection of the infant's genitalia, note a large penis in the male infant and ambiguous genitalia in the female infant (Fig. 48.5). When observing the toddler or preschooler, note pubic hair development, acne, and **hirsutism** (excess body hair growth).

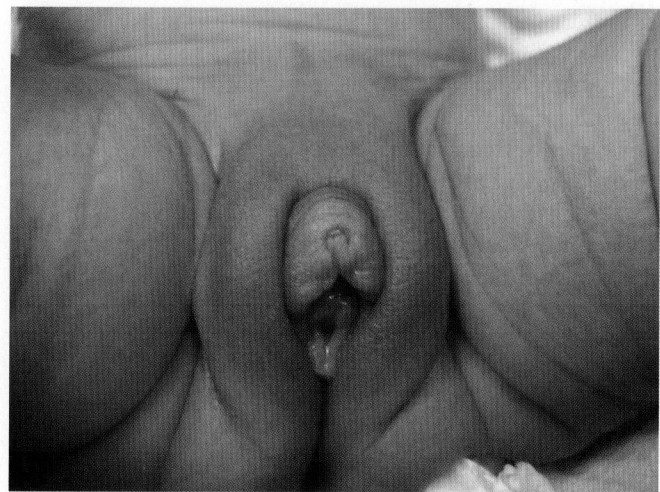

FIGURE 48.5 Newborn with ambiguous genitalia.

Laboratory and Diagnostic Testing

The most common type of CAH, 21-OH enzyme deficiency, is detected by newborn metabolic screening, similar to newborn screening for hypothyroidism. If this test has not been done or the results are unavailable, random hormone levels or levels associated with adrenocorticotropic hormone (ACTH) stimulation may be obtained.

Nursing Management

In addition to the common interventions associated with endocrine disorders in childhood (see Nursing Care Plan 48.1), nursing management of the infant or child with CAH focuses on helping the family to understand the child's response to the disease and explaining the importance of maintaining hormone supplementation. Supporting the family is also a key nursing focus. Provide ongoing assessment of the ill or hospitalized child with a history of CAH to recognize the development of life-threatening acute adrenal crisis. If signs and symptoms of adrenal crisis develop, the child will require fluid resuscitation, typically starting with an intravenous bolus of 0.9% normal saline at 20 mL/kg. Intravenous hydrocortisone will also be required.

Educating the Family

Medication will be required throughout the child's life. Teach the family the appropriate oral dosages of hydrocortisone and fludrocortisone. It is critical to maintain tight control over the levels of these medications in the bloodstream, as either underdosing or overdosing may lead to short adult stature. Low levels of the hormones may also result in adrenal crisis. These drugs are usually given orally but in some instances will need to be given via intramuscular injections. The families will need to learn how to administer hydrocortisone intramuscularly if the child is vomiting or otherwise unable to keep down oral medication. Families should work with their endocrinologist to develop a medication plan for managing stressful events and know when to seek more urgent medical attention. Families must keep extra injectable hydrocortisone at home to give during an emergency. An identification bracelet for the child is essential.

Providing Family Support

Make sure the family of a newborn with ambiguous genitalia feels comfortable asking questions and exploring their feelings. There are many issues to consider, such as whether the family will reassign the child's sex or raise the child with the original assignment at birth. Cultural attitudes, the parents' expectations, and the extent of family support influence the family's response to the child and the decision-making process related to sex assignment and surgical correction. If immediate corrective surgery is decided upon, then typical surgical concerns for newborns will need to be addressed.

In general, lay people do not understand adrenal function and what this diagnosis may mean to the family. Provide families with privacy to discuss these issues, and offer emotional support. When referring to the infant, use terms such as "your baby" instead of the pronouns "he," "she," or "it," and describe the genitals as "sex organs" instead of "penis" or "clitoris." Refer families to the CARES (Congenital Adrenal Hyperplasia Research, Education, and Support) Foundation and the Magic Foundation for additional support and resources (visit http://thePoint.lww.com/Chow1e for direct links). Local parent-to-parent support groups are also helpful.

Addison's Disease

Addison's disease (primary adrenal insufficiency) is rare in children. The most common etiology in children is an autoimmune destruction of the adrenal cortex. This may be familial, such as with a family history of autoimmune disorders, or sporadic (Sperling, 2002). Destruction of the adrenal glands by the circulating antibodies leads to deficiency in the adrenal steroids, glucocorticoids (cortisol), and mineralocorticoids (aldosterone).

Management involves replacing deficient or absent hormones. In the acute situation this is accomplished, as with classic salt-wasting CAH, with intravenous hydrocortisone in addition to restoring and maintaining fluid, electrolyte, and glucose balance (Behrman et al., 2004). Treatment for the chronic form of Addison's disease is oral replacement of the steroids hydrocortisone and fludrocortisone (Behrman et al., 2004). This is a lifelong condition. Illness, stress, or surgery will require adjustment in the medication dosage to meet the body's increased physiologic needs. Potential complications include diabetes, thyrotoxicosis, reproductive malfunction, hypoparathyroidism, and pernicious anemia.

Nursing Assessment

Note history of gradual onset of weight loss, fatigue, anorexia, syncope, nausea, vomiting, and diarrhea. Observe the skin for hyperpigmentation and note decreased blood pressure. Addisonian crisis is an acute-onset condition that presents during a febrile illness, infection, extreme stress, or any condition that results in increased adrenal steroid release. It is potentially life-threatening; the symptoms include sudden penetrating pain in the lower back, abdomen, or legs with severe weakness, vomiting and diarrhea, dehydration, hypotension, electrolyte imbalances, decreased cardiac output, fever, mental status changes, and hypoglycemia.

Laboratory testing reveals low serum sodium, elevated serum potassium, and low fasting glucose levels. Blood urea nitrogen and creatinine levels are increased. The blood test that confirms the diagnosis is a low fasting morning cortisol level 30 to 60 minutes after stimulation with intravenous synthetic ACTH (Sperling, 2002). In addition, the adrenal antibodies are positive in Addison's disease but negative with other causes for the condition.

Nursing Management

Nursing management of Addison's disease is similar to that of congenital adrenal insufficiency. A critical aspect of the education plan for this disorder remains teaching the parents to increase the dosage of cortisol during periods of illness and to use the injectable form of hydrocortisone during periods of extreme nausea or vomiting. Information about the child's condition should always be available to emergency personnel.

Cushing's Syndrome and Disease

Cushing's is characterized by a cluster of signs and symptoms resulting from excess levels of circulating cortisol. Excess cortisol can also bind to and activate the mineralocorticoid receptors; thus signs of mineralocorticoid and/or androgen excess may also be noted (Chrousos & Lafferty, 2009; Magiakou, Sarafoglou, Stratakis, et al., 2009). Cushing's most commonly has an exogenous cause related to prolonged or excessive corticosteroid therapy. Supraphysiologic doses of corticosteroids are prescribed for a wide range of non-endocrine diseases (Magiakou et al., 2009). Endogenous Cushing's, while rare in children, is usually caused by a small ACTH-producing pituitary adenoma. There are two to five new cases of endogenous Cushing's for every 1 million people each year, with about 10% of these new cases occurring in children or teenagers (Magiakou et al., 2009). Cushing's syndrome is differentiated from Cushing's disease by the cause, but the terms shall be considered synonymous for the sake of this discussion.

In children, the most commonly observed features include an increase in body weight due in part to increased appetite and decreased linear growth (Chrousos

& Lafferty, 2009). Growth failure is common due to suppression of GH and resistance of tissues to growth factors (Magiakou et al., 2009). The impairment of growth is dependent upon the age of onset and the duration of disease prior to treatment or length of corticosteroid therapy (Chrousos & Lafferty, 2009).

Management varies depending on the cause. With exogenous Cushing's, treatment includes consideration of the risks and benefits of corticosteroid therapy on the underlying disease and the extent of the side effects experienced. Because of the side effects of prolonged high-dose corticosteroid use, dosing is always at the lowest dose and/or shortest duration that is effective in treating the underlying disorder. The goal is to restore hormone balance and reverse Cushing's. If the cause is an adrenal or pituitary tumour, then surgical removal of either the tumour alone or the entire adrenal gland is performed. Ketoconazole may also be given to suppress adrenocortical function.

Nursing Assessment

The child may be demonstrating a broad range of symptoms or side effects. Note the earliest signs: rapid weight gain with obesity, particularly in the truncal area, a rounded face ("moon face"), and fat collections in the posterior neck ("buffalo hump") (Fig. 48.6). Early

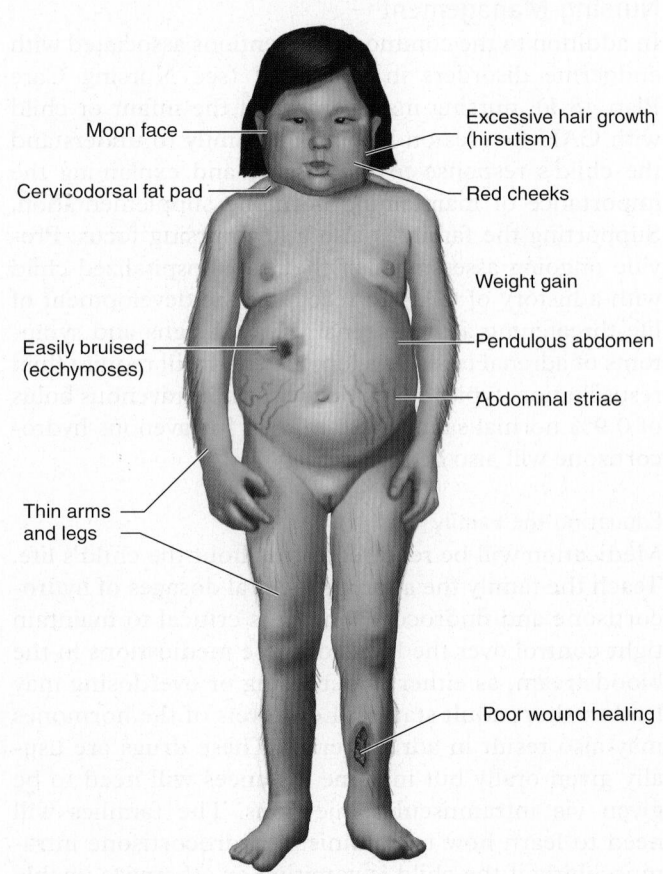

FIGURE 48.6 Cushing's signs.

symptoms include fatigue, irritability, and sleep disturbance. The child may also demonstrate acne, hirsutism, water retention, poor wound healing, frequent infections (due to immunosuppression) and, in teenage girls, menstrual irregularity. The skin may be thin and fragile with a tendency to bruise, and there may be reddish-purple striae on the abdomen. Muscle weakness may be noted during assessment and by self-report. Measure the blood pressure, noting hypertension. Cushing's that develops near puberty will delay puberty, despite the outside appearance of hirsutism (Chrousos & Lafferty, 2009).

Laboratory testing reveals reduced serum levels of potassium and phosphorus, elevated serum calcium and sodium levels, increased 24-hour urinary levels of free cortisol and 17-hydroxycorticosteroid (17-OHC), loss of diurnal rhythm in serum cortisol levels, chronic hyperglycemia, and elevated hemoglobin A1C levels due to insulin resistance. Adrenal suppression test using low-dose dexamethasone is used initially to screen for adrenocortical hyperfunction. CT and MRI are used to detect tumours in the adrenal and pituitary glands that may cause Cushing's.

Nursing Management

Provide routine yet individualized nursing interventions as outlined in Nursing Care Plan 48.1. In addition, counsel the family that the cushingoid appearance is reversible with appropriate treatment. If withdrawal or reduction in corticosteroids occurs suddenly, either due to surgery or discontinuation of prolonged high-dose steroid use, be alert for signs of adrenal insufficiency such as shock and hypotension. For those children for whom exogenous administration of steroids must continue, encourage administration in the morning to ameliorate the impact on sleep.

Polycystic Ovary Syndrome

Polycystic ovary syndrome (PCOS) produces a wide range of symptoms in adolescent girls and women. These include hyperandrogenism and evidence of ovarian dysfunction, either with or without polycystic ovaries. Excessive production of androgens such as testosterone by the ovaries and adrenal cells can cause hirsutism, balding, acne, increased muscle mass, decreased breast size, infertility, and metabolic syndrome. The etiology of PCOS is a combination of multiple genetic and environmental factors and includes a family history of predisposition to PCOS, obesity, and metabolic syndrome (insulin resistance, dyslipidemia, hypertension, and central obesity) (O'Brien & Emans, 2008). Treatment is comprehensive, focusing on the presenting symptoms, correction of underlying metabolic disorders such as dyslipidemia, and the unique psychosocial issues that affect the adolescent. Pharmacologic therapy is individualized to the specific symptoms evidenced by the teen. Oral contraceptives will assist with the management of hirsutism, acne, and irregular menstrual cycles. Antiandrogen medications can slow hair growth but must be prescribed with concomitant use of contraceptives due to their teratogenic effect. Additional pharmacologic therapy may be directed toward increasing insulin sensitivity via insulin-sensitizing medications (Barron & Falsetti, 2008).

Nursing Assessment

Explore the health history for oligomenorrhea (irregular, infrequent periods) or amenorrhea. Note weight in relation to standardized growth charts, and calculate body mass index (BMI). Inspect the skin for acne, acanthosis nigricans (darkened, thickened pigmentation, particularly around the neck or in the axillary region), and hirsutism. Assist with collection of timed blood specimens for glucose and insulin levels (which will often show unexpectedly elevated insulin levels in relation to the glucose level). Laboratory tests may show elevated levels of free testosterone and other androgenic hormones.

Nursing Management

One of the most important roles of the nurse in relation to PCOS is to assist with early recognition and treatment of the condition to help the teen and family deal with quality of life, self-esteem, and fertility issues. Educate the adolescent girl about the use of oral contraceptives to normalize hormone levels, which will decrease androgenic effects. Support the teen in her efforts to attain and maintain a healthy weight and activity level and lower the risks of metabolic and cardiovascular problems through healthy eating and lifestyle modifications. Measure blood pressure to screen for hypertension, which may develop as a complication of PCOS. Online support groups and educational resources include:

- TeensHealth from Nemours Foundation
- Center for Young Women's Health at Children's Hospital Boston
- Polycystic Ovarian Syndrome Association
- The Androgen Excess and PCOS Society

Visit http://thePoint.lww.com/Chow1e for direct links to these organizations.

Diabetes Mellitus

Diabetes mellitus (DM) is a common chronic metabolic disorder in which carbohydrate, protein, and lipid metabolism is impaired. DM is really a group of disorders with distinct genetic patterns and etiologic and pathophysiologic mechanisms leading to impaired glucose tolerance (Alemzadeh & Wyatt, 2007). Eventually, the hyperglycemia and resulting problems produce structural abnormalities in various tissues and organs. Long-term complications of DM and subsequent hyperglycemia can include poor wound healing, recurrent infections, nephropathy, retinopathy, neuropathy, vascular complications, and cardiovascular disease.

Diabetes Mellitus Type 1

Type 1DM (T1DM) is an autoimmune disorder occurring in genetically susceptible individuals who may also be exposed to one of several factors that trigger autoimmune beta cell destruction. A network of genes is believed to be responsible for T1DM. As the genetically susceptible individual is exposed to triggers such as those of an environmental or viral nature, the immune system begins a T-lymphocyte–mediated process that damages and destroys the beta cells of the pancreas, resulting in inadequate insulin secretion. Insulin, therefore, cannot alter peripheral cells to transport glucose across the cell membrane. The end result is hyperglycemia and the body's inability to use its main source of fuel efficiently. Immunologic markers including islet cell antibodies and insulin autoantibodies may be present for years before the child develops signs and symptoms. By the time symptoms are present and the diagnosis is made, a large portion of the beta cells have been destroyed. T1DM is associated with other autoimmune diseases, such as thyroiditis, celiac disease, multiple sclerosis, and Addison's disease (Alemzadeh & Wyatt, 2007).

The incidence of childhood T1DM varies widely between and within countries. In Canada, the yearly incidence of T1DM in children being treated in major centres ranges from 9.0 to 35.9 per 100,000 (Newhook, Curtis, Hagerty, et al., 2004). First-degree relatives of patients with T1DM carry a 10- to 20-fold higher risk for diabetes than the general population (Triolo, Chase, Barker, et al., 2009). There is equal distribution between the genders, with the peak incidence occurring in early childhood (4 to 6 years) and early puberty (10 to 14 years) (Lamb, 2010).

As the beta cells are progressively destroyed and less insulin in produced, symptoms steadily increase, reflecting progressive hyperglycemia and, potentially, **ketoacidosis**. Initially, only occasional hyperglycemia occurs. As the serum glucose level increases, intermittent polyuria or nocturia occurs. Further beta-cell loss and subsequent chronic hyperglycemia will result in an increased persistence of diuresis and likely also nocturnal enuresis and polydipsia. Calories are lost in the urine. Loss of body fat ensues, with clinical weight loss and diminished subcutaneous fat stores. Despite any compensatory increased intake of food, the body starves because unused calories are lost in the urine (Alemzadeh & Wyatt, 2007).

If the condition goes unrecognized, DKA or fat catabolism develops, resulting in metabolic acidosis, vomiting, stomach cramps, sweet-smelling breath (**ketones**), ketones in urine (ketonuria), compensatory Kussmaul respirations (deep, heavy, rapid breathing), diminished CNS function

and, if left untreated, coma and death. Approximately 20% to 40% of children with T1DM present with DKA on initial evaluation (Alemzadeh & Wyatt, 2007).

Diabetes Mellitus Type 2

In type 2 DM (T2DM), the pancreas usually produces insulin but the body is resistant to the insulin or there is an inadequate compensatory insulin secretion response. Eventually, insulin production decreases, with a result similar to that seen in T1DM. The incidence of T2DM in children is increasing. In a recent Canadian surveillance study of children newly diagnosed with non-T1DM, 95% were obese, 36% had at least one co-morbidity (such as hypertension) at diagnosis, and only 25% were white (Amed, Dean, Panagiotopoulos, et al., 2010). Many of the children in the study were from ethnic minorities, including Aboriginal (44%), African-Caribbean, and Asian descent; had a relative with T2DM (91% of children), and/or were overweight. Manitoba has the highest incidence of T2DM in children and adolescents in Canada (Amed et al., 2010).

The estimated prevalence of T2DM in Oji-Cree First Nations people is 1.1% in the 4- to 19-year age group and 3.5% in the 15- to 19-year age group. In Nova Scotia, approximately 16% to 18% of new cases of diabetes in children younger than 19 years of age are T2DM. In Manitoba 35 to 45 new cases of T2DM are diagnosed each year, representing approximately 30% of all new cases of pediatric diabetes in Manitoba annually (Amed et al., 2010).

Other Types of Diabetes Mellitus

Other specific types of DM include a wide variety of relatively uncommon conditions, primarily specific genetically defined forms of diabetes or diabetes associated with other diseases or medications (Canadian Diabetes Association [CDA], 2008). These include diseases causing pancreatic damage (e.g., cystic fibrosis or pancreatitis); medications such as high-dose corticosteroids, immunosuppressive therapies, and specific chemotherapies; and multiple blood transfusions and subsequent iron overload (e.g., thalassemia major) (Ho, Sellers, Dean, et al., 2010). In addition to meal and activity planning, pharmacologic treatment of such other types of diabetes may include insulin therapy or oral hypoglycemic therapy.

Therapeutic Management

Treatment involves a multidisciplinary health care team, with the family and child as a central part of that team. Education and treatment occur primarily on an outpatient basis. The general goals for therapeutic management include:

- Achieving normal growth and development
- Promoting optimal serum glucose regulation, including keeping fluid, electrolyte, and **hemoglobin A1C** levels within normal ranges

TABLE 48.3   RECOMMENDED GLYCEMIC TARGETS FOR CHILDREN AND ADOLESCENTS WITH TYPE 1 DIABETES MELLITUS

Age (years)	Hemoglobin A1C (%)	Fasting/Preprandial Plasma Glucose (mmol/L)	2-Hour Postprandial Plasma Glucose[a] (mmol/L)	Considerations
<6	<8.5	6.0–12.0	—	Extra caution is required to minimize hypoglycemia because of the potential association between severe hypoglycemia and later cognitive impairment.
6–12	<8.0	4.0–10.0	—	Targets should be graduated to the child's age.
13–18	≤7.0	4.0–7.0	5.0–10.0	Appropriate for most adolescents[b]

[a]Postprandial monitoring is rarely done in young children except for those on pump therapy for whom targets are not available.
[b]In adolescents in whom it can be safely achieved, consider aiming goals toward normal.
Source: Canadian Diabetes Association. (2008). Canadian Diabetes Association 2008 clinical practice guidelines for the prevention and management of diabetes in Canada. *Canadian Journal of Diabetes*, *32*(Suppl. 1), S1–S201. Retrieved June 21, 2001 from http://www.diabetes.ca/files/cpg2008/cpg-2008.pdf.

- Preventing DKA and severe hypoglycemia
- Preventing long-term complications
- Promoting positive adjustment to the disease, with the ability to self-manage in the home

The key to success is to educate the child and family so they can self-manage this chronic condition. Treatment involves blood glucose monitoring; daily insulin injections for T1DM; insulin injections or oral hypoglycemic medications for T2DM; and, for all types of diabetes, self-management and decision-making skills including an exercise or activity program and a realistic meal plan.

Glucose Monitoring

Regular glucose monitoring facilitates glucose control, and supplemental insulin, activity, or meal planning modifications can be used to correct or prevent hyperglycemia. The frequency of blood glucose monitoring is based on the patient's goals and insulin regimen. Ideal therapy for children on insulin involves blood glucose monitoring before meals and at bedtime. Additional glucose monitoring is performed as needed for specific circumstances, such as at 2 AM (or when long-acting insulin is peaking) if there are concerns about nocturnal hypoglycemia, unusual activity or meal events, or if glycemic control has not occurred.

Insulin Therapy

Insulin therapy is the cornerstone of care for T1DM. Insulin is administered by subcutaneous injections into adipose tissue over large muscle masses using a traditional insulin syringe or an insulin pen. Insulin pens with premixed insulin do not support the individualized insulin mixtures required in T1DM and are most commonly used in children with T2DM or where family coping and skills are most challenged. Rapid-acting insulin may also be administered using a portable insulin pump. The frequency, dose, and type of insulin are based on how much the child needs to achieve blood glucose goals and to prevent severe hypoglycemia outcomes, such as a seizure (Table 48.3). Typically, two or four daily injections are required. The amount, type, and frequency will vary widely depending on the needs of the child, his or her lifestyle and activity level, and the type of diabetes. The dose will need to be increased during growth spurts, particularly puberty, due to the increased production of hormones that increase insulin resistance. Types of insulin, administered in combination, include rapid-acting, short-acting, intermediate-acting, long-acting, ultra–long-acting, and fixed pre-mixed combinations (Table 48.4).

An insulin pump is a device that administers a continuous infusion of rapid-acting insulin. It comprises a computer, a reservoir of rapid-acting insulin, thin tubing through which the insulin is delivered, and a small needle inserted into the abdomen. A continuous basal rate of insulin is maintained, and a bolus of insulin can be delivered if glucose testing results show it is needed. See Evidence-based Practice 48.1.

Treatment of Type 2 Diabetes

To be effective, treatment programs for adolescents with T2DM need to address the lifestyle and health habits of the entire family, emphasizing healthy eating and physical activity. In addition, psychological issues, such as depression, self-destructive behaviour patterns, and smoking cessation, need to be addressed and interventions as required. Teens with severe metabolic decomp

TABLE 48.4 INSULIN TYPE, ACTION, AND DURATION

Insulin Type (Brand Name)	Onset	Peak	Duration
Rapid-acting analogues • Insulin aspart (NovoRapid) • Insulin lispro (Humalog)	10–15 min	60–90 min	3–5 h
Short-acting • Humulin R • Novolin ge Toronto	30 min	2–3 h	6.5 h
Intermediate-acting • Humulin N • Novolin ge NPH	1–3 h	5–8 h	Up to 18 h
Long-acting analogue	90 min	Does not truly peak; offers continual steady coverage	Up to 24 h

Refer to product monographs for detailed information.
Adapted from: Canadian Diabetes Association. (n.d.). *Types of insulin (approved for use in Canada).*
Retrieved June 24, 2011 from http://www.diabetes.ca/diabetes-and-you/living/insulin/types/.

at diagnosis (e.g., DKA, symptoms of severe hyperglycemia) require insulin, but they may be successfully weaned once blood sugar goals targets are achieved, particularly if lifestyle changes are effectively adopted. Data about the safety and efficacy of oral antihyperglycemic agents in the pediatric population are limited. Metformin, from the class of biguanide medications, has been shown to be safe in adolescents for up to 16 weeks, reducing hemoglobin A1C by 1.0% to 2.0% with similar side effects as seen in adults (CDA, 2008). The biguanides reduce glucose production from the liver, and as a result blood sugars fall. This group of medications has the additional advantage

of not causing hypoglycemia. With the increased incidence of dyslipidemia associated with T2DM, children may also be prescribed anti-lipidemic medication (Perkin et al., 2003). In T2DM, insulin therapy may also be required in children with consistently high blood sugars or if blood sugar goals are not met within 3 to 6 months of initiating lifestyle modifications (CDA, 2008).

Nutrition and Activity

Other therapies involve nutrition and exercise or activity protocols and prevention or management of complications. The CDA recommends that children with diabetes

EVIDENCE-BASED PRACTICE 48.1
The Daily Experience of Parents Who Manage Their Children's Diabetes with an Insulin Pump

● **Study**

Children with T1DM require multiple daily insulin injections to manage their glucose levels. This presents difficulties for many families in a number of ways. The authors performed a qualitative descriptive study to determine what life is like for parents whose children's diabetes is managed with a continuous subcutaneous insulin pump as opposed to multiple daily injections. Twenty-one parents of 16 children were included in the study. The parents participated in lengthy interviews with questions structured to determine how life was experienced before and after the pump. The ⸺⸺ transcripts were then rigorously analyzed.

⸺⸺ mount of time it took for them to ⸺⸺ with using the pump and eventually

confident with its use (up to several months). They identified the transition period as a little scary at times. Parents reported improved day-to-day diabetes management, flexibility, and quality of life when the insulin pump is used compared with the previous regimen of multiple daily injections.

■ **Nursing Implications**

Educate families on the use of the continuous subcutaneous insulin pump and the improved glucose control that it may allow them to have. Involve children over 6 years of age in management of their diabetes. Provide ongoing emotional support to families as they make the transition to using the insulin pump.

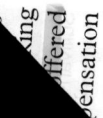

⸺⸺ K., Tamborlane, W., et al. (2004). Parents' reflections on managing their ⸺⸺ sulin pumps. *Journal of Nursing Scholarship, 36,* 316–323.

COMPARISON CHART 48.3 TYPE 1 VERSUS TYPE 2 DIABETES MELLITUS

History and Physical Findings Usually Present at Diagnosis	Type 1	Type 2
Polydipsia, polyuria, **polyphagia**	Yes	Often asymptomatic
Weight	Possible weight loss	If asymptomatic, may be obese; otherwise may present in DKA with weight loss
Age of onset	Usually preschool or prepubertal children	Usually pubertal children
Incidental finding on screening	Rare	Common
Autoimmune antibodies	Yes	No
Diabetic ketoacidosis	Common	Possible
Hypertension	No	Common
Acanthosis nigricans	No	Common
Vaginal infection	No	Common
Dyslipidemia	No	Common

follow the same healthy diet recommended for children without diabetes (i.e., following Canada's Food Guide [Health Canada, 2007]), ensuring normal growth and development without compromising glycemic control. Nutrition therapy should be individualized to the child's needs, eating habits, lifestyle, physical and psychological abilities, and interests (CDA, 2008).

Exercise has an important influence on blood sugar and overall health, so the diabetic child should maintain or increase his or her activity levels. If the child is taking insulin, the family should know how to adjust the dosage, increase activity, or add or remove carbohydrate foods to maintain blood glucose control. Children with T2DM are often overweight and have insulin resistance. The exercise plan is very important in helping the child to integrate with peers, enhance body image, improve insulin sensitivity, lose weight, or minimize adverse weight gain as well as prevent additional complications related to obesity.

Nursing Assessment

Assessment involves understanding the ever-changing needs of children as they grow and develop. The first phase of assessment involves identifying the child who may have DM and managing any acute complications. The second phase involves identifying teaching opportunities as they present to the child and family and assessing potential any challenges or strengths of the family and how they might impact the educational plan.

Health History and Physical Examination

During the initial diagnosis of DM, obtain a detailed history of family lifestyle and coping patterns that may assist in integrating diabetes into the child's life as well as recent problems that may be attributable to some of the mental and behaviour changes that may occur in a hyperglycemic state (e.g., weakness, fatigue, difficulty concen-

trating, mood changes). The child may also complain of blurred vision, headaches, or bedwetting. The child with T1DM and longstanding poor glucose control may have a history of poor growth. Comparison Chart 48.3 gives information about common history and physical examination findings in children with T1DM versus T2DM.

In the child who is known to have DM, the health history includes any problems with hyperglycemia or hypoglycemia, meal planning, activity and exercise patterns, the ability to administer insulin and self-monitor blood glucose, and ongoing adjustment of food, activity, and insulin in response to blood sugar levels. Perform a thorough physical examination, noting any abnormal findings.

Laboratory and Diagnostic Testing

A random plasma glucose level of 11.1 mmol/L or higher with symptoms of diabetes and a fasting glucose level 7.0 mmol/L or higher are the laboratory criteria for the diagnosis of DM (CDA, 2008). Other laboratory and diagnostic tests include hemoglobin A1C, which reflects the percentage of hemoglobin to which glucose is attached. In children who present acutely ill with DKA, additional laboratory tests for serum levels of urea nitrogen, creatinine, calcium, magnesium, phosphate, and electrolytes (e.g., potassium and sodium) may be conducted.

Nursing Management

Nursing management is focused on regulating glucose control, supporting normalization of fluid and electrolyte levels in children with DKA, and educating and supporting the child's and family's short-term and long-term needs. Individualize the general nursing care discussed in Nursing Care Plan 48.1 based on the child's and family's response to illness. Additional nursing care topics related to DM are discussed below.

Regulating Glucose Control

If the child presents with DKA, monitor the glucose level hourly to prevent it from falling more than 5 mmol/L/hour. Also observe trends in serum osmolarity, with a goal of osmolality decreasing by more than 2 to 3 mmol/L/hour (De Beer, Michael, Thacker, et al., 2008). Rapid declines in osmolarity, especially in younger children, predispose the child to cerebral edema (CDA, 2008). After initiating intravenous hydration, regular insulin is administered intravenously, via a continuous infusion of 0.1 unit/kg/hour. Usually the child with DKA is treated in the pediatric intensive care unit (CDA, 2008).

The subcutaneous route is used for insulin administration once the metabolic and electrolyte abnormalities are corrected and the child is no longer NPO. The insulin regimen often consists of one injection of intermediate-acting insulin at bedtime with the addition of rapid-acting insulin before breakfast, lunch, and dinner. For children who are unable to inject as frequently, due to circumstances such as age, development, or support, the rapid-acting insulin at lunch may be replaced by the addition of intermediate-acting insulin at breakfast. Insulin doses are typically ordered on an individualized sliding scale based on the serum glucose level, the timing of insulin actions and peaks, and overall patterns in diabetes control.

Teach the child and family to use proper subcutaneous injection techniques, including rotation of insulin sites to avoid lipohypertrophy (fatty lumps that absorb insulin poorly). Figure 48.7 shows appropriate sites for subcutaneous injection of insulin.

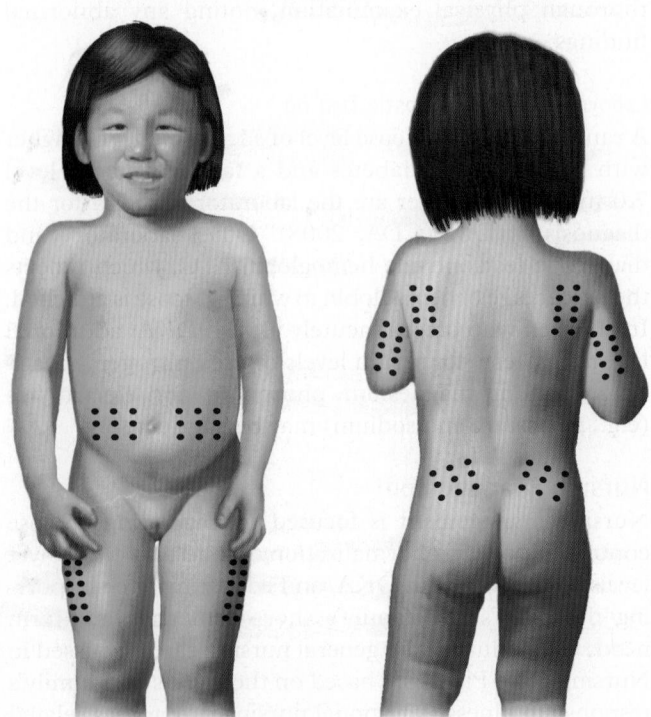

FIGURE 48.7 Insulin injection sites.

COMPARISON CHART 48.4 HYPOGLYCEMIA VERSUS HYPERGLYCEMIA

Hypoglycemia	Hyperglycemia
Behavioural changes	Mental status changes, confusion, slurred speech, fatigue, weakness, belligerence
Diaphoresis	Dry, flushed skin
Tremors	Blurred vision
Palpitations, tachycardia	Abdominal cramping, vomiting, dehydration, increased work of breathing
Seizure, loss of consciousness	

When giving a combination of rapid/short- and intermediate-acting insulin, draw up the clear (short-acting) insulin first, removing air bubbles to enhance the accuracy of the dose, and then draw up the intermediate-acting insulin. Rotate the vial of intermediate-acting insulin instead of shaking it to prevent air bubbles. Long-acting insulin, usually administered as a single dose at bedtime, may not be mixed in the same syringe with other types of insulin.

Monitoring for Short-Term Complications

While the child is in the hospital with DKA, monitor for signs of complications such as acidosis, coma, hyperkalemia or hypokalemia, hypocalcemia, cerebral edema, or hyponatremia. Monitor the child's status closely during peak times of insulin action. Perform blood glucose testing as ordered or as needed if the child develops symptoms suggestive of hypoglycemia or hyperglycemia (Comparison Chart 48.4).

When the child is having a severe hypoglycemic reaction, administer glucagon (a hormone produced by the pancreas and stored in the liver) either subcutaneously or intramuscularly. Children under 20 kg receive 0.5 mg; children over 20 kg receive 1 mg (Alemzadeh & Wyatt, 2007). In the hospital, dextrose (50%) may be given intravenously if needed. If the child is coherent, quick-acting glucose in the form of paste, gel, liquid, or tablets may be used. Offer 10 to 15 g of a simple carbohydrate such as orange juice if the child feels some symptoms and glucose monitoring indicates a drop. Follow this with a more complex carbohydrate such as crackers to maintain the glucose level.

The hospitalized child with hyperglycemia often requires supplemental insulin as increasing activity may not be an option and the associated stressors or illness increase insulin resistance. The dosage is usually based on an individualized sliding scale or is determined after consultation with the physician. Testing of urine ketones is important to screen for DKA.

Double-check all insulin doses against the order sheet and with another nurse to ensure accuracy.

Educating the Family

Education is the priority intervention because it will enable the child and family to self-manage this lifelong condition. Regular follow-up visits (three or four times a year) should be scheduled with a diabetes specialty clinic and education centre, with evaluation and instruction from certified diabetes educators, usually nurses, and dieticians. With appropriate management, involvement of the community, and confidence and compliance by the family, the child can maintain a happy, productive life.

Challenges related to educating children with diabetes include the following:

- Children lack the developmental maturity to understand the long-term consequences of this serious chronic illness.
- Children do not want to be different from their peers, and having to make lifestyle changes may lead to anger, depression, or omissions in self-care.
- Families experiencing poverty may have difficulty affording appropriate food, telephone service, and all necessary diabetes supplies.
- Families may have difficulty integrating diabetes into their lifestyle, making it difficult for the child to attain or maintain healthy behaviours because of the lack of supervision or role modelling.
- Family dynamics are affected because management of diabetes must occur all day, every day.

The initial goal of education is for the family to develop basic management and decision-making skills. It is important that education starts with diagnosis. To maintain patient safety, a basic understanding of concepts such as early identification and treatment of hypoglycemia and basic meal planning is necessary as soon as insulin is started. Assess the family's ability to learn basic concepts and understand the interaction of insulin/food/activity while assessing family interaction, coping skills, and patterns. A skilled social worker is also an integral member of the diabetes team. Teach about specific topics in sessions lasting 15 to 20 minutes for the children and 45 to 60 minutes for the caregivers. Teaching must be geared toward the child's level of development and understanding (Table 48.5).

Among the topics to include when teaching children and their families about diabetes management are:

- Self-blood glucose measurement (Fig. 48.8)
- Urine ketone testing
- Medication use
- Oral hypoglycemic agents
- Subcutaneous insulin injection or insulin pump use

TABLE 48.5 DEVELOPMENTAL ISSUES RELATED TO DIABETES MELLITUS

Age Group	Child and Family Implications	Nursing Implications
Infants and toddlers	Management falls on parents/caregivers; signs and symptoms are sometimes difficult to assess in infants and young toddlers, with more frequent blood glucose monitoring required.	Let the toddler choose among healthy foods, and adjust rapid- or short-acting insulin as indicated. Help the toddler to associate his or her feelings with low blood sugar levels. Establish rituals/routines with home management.
Preschoolers	Increased motor maturity; widening social circle, so the child will notice that he or she is "different." Some preschool children can begin to perform blood glucose testing.	Use simple explanations and play therapy when instructing or preparing for a procedure.
School-age children	Can perform self-blood glucose monitoring, assist in the choice of injection sites given a limited number of options (to minimize negotiation and stalling), help give injections and perform ketone testing, recognize the need to eat and treat for hypoglycemia, and begin to participate in keeping a blood sugar diary. Must incorporate management into school day and plan for field trips.	Use concise and concrete terms when instructing. Allow child to proceed at his or her own pace. Assist family to incorporate testing and injections into the school day and plan for field trips. Involve the school nurse in helping with the school plan.
Adolescents	Conflicts develop with self-management, body image, and peer group acceptance; must assume more of the care with supervision. Teens do not always foresee the consequences of their activity.	Slowly care is turned over to the adolescent with supervision from the family. Watch for signs of depression or burnout or diminished participation and interest in their self-care routine.

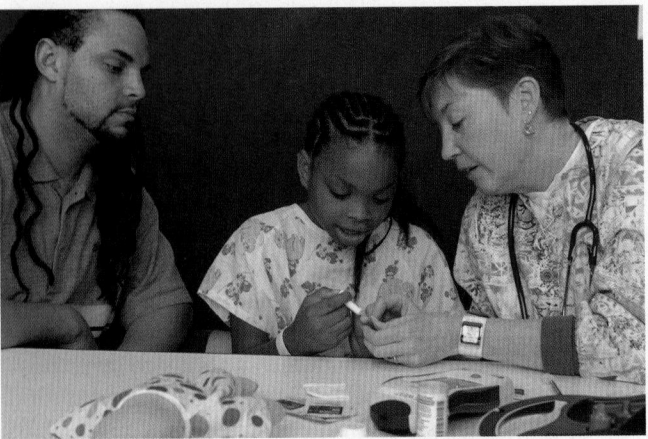

FIGURE **48.8** The school-age child has developed the psychomotor skills needed for blood glucose monitoring and insulin injection.

- Subcutaneous site selection and rotation
- When and how to adjust insulin dosages
- Use of glucagon
- Signs and symptoms of hypoglycemia and early treatment
- Signs and symptoms of hyperglycemia and how to reduce blood sugars
- Short and long-term complications
- Management of sick days
- Laboratory testing and follow-up care

The discussion should also include key education of additional caregivers and others such as teachers, babysitters, coaches, and friends and parents of friends with whom the child spends time. The child and parents should be given anticipatory guidance regarding psychosocial and developmental issues related to diabetes, such as child burnout, omission of blood glucose testing or fabrication of results, effects of drugs or alcohol, peer influence, safe driving, and contraception and conception planning.

Teaching Guideline 48.1 presents information to cover when teaching the family about blood glucose monitoring. Teach families how to give insulin, how to use the insulin pump, and how to rotate injection sites (see above). Sick-day instructions may include the following:

- Know when to contact the physician or diabetes nurse educator.
- Perform blood glucose monitoring more often.
- Add urine ketone testing.
- Use an individualized sliding scale to calculate the insulin dosage.
- Maintain carbohydrate intake in easily digestible forms.

A dietitian is essential to help the family with detailed meal planning guidelines. Review basic nutritional information with the child and family and provide sample meals. Incorporate the family's cultural preferences when

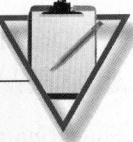

TEACHING GUIDELINE 48.1

Blood Glucose Monitoring

- Obtain glucose levels before meals and bedtime snacks.
- Perform monitoring more often during periods of increased activity or exercise, if the child is ill, if the child has eaten more food than usual, or if nighttime hypoglycemia is suspected.
- Use the manufacturer's recommendations and perform quality control measures as directed.
- Look for patterns. For example, 3 to 4 days of a consistent pattern of glucose values above 10 mmol/L before dinner in a child over 6 years of age indicates a need to adjust the insulin dose or meal plan earlier in the day.
- Blood glucose measurements are the best way to determine daily insulin dosages.
- Blood sugar goals are based on age (see Table 48.3).

planning meals. A food diary or record of carbohydrate counting may help the family develop a greater understanding of the relationship between food, insulin, and activity. For the child who needs to lose weight, suggest low-carbohydrate snacks and encourage appropriate daily physical activity (Teaching Guideline 48.2).

Supporting the Child and Family

Children with diabetes and their families may have difficulty coping if they lack confidence in their self-management skills. Assess the ability of the child and family to handle situations. Role-play specific situations related to symptoms or complications to help them see different ways to solve problems. Work with the child and family to enhance their conflict resolution skills. Provide opportunities for them to express their feelings. Observe for signs of depression, especially in adolescents.

To enhance the child's and family's confidence and promote feelings of empowerment, refer them to a local support group or camp or to one of the many online resources for children or their families (visit http://thePoint.lww.com/Chow1e for direct links).

Supporting the Adolescent

Diabetes control may worsen during adolescence. Factors responsible for this deterioration include adolescent adjustment issues, psychosocial distress, intentional insulin omission, and physiologic insulin resistance. A multidisciplinary assessment should be undertaken for every child with chronic poor metabolic control to identify potential causative factors such as depression and eating disorders. Adolescents with diabetes should receive regular counselling about sexual health and contraception. Unplanned pregnancies should be avoided, as pregnancy

TEACHING GUIDELINE 48.2

Diet and Exercise for Children with Diabetes Mellitus

- Provide sufficient and balanced nutrition for normal growth and development. The diet should be consistent with Canada's Food Guide (Health Canada, 2007).
- Learn to identify which foods impact blood sugars, such as carbohydrates. Learn to identify foods with protein and fat as part of a healthy eating pattern and in those children battling obesity or at risk for dyslipidemia.
- Make adjustments to insulin dosages as warranted during periods of rapid growth and for special circumstances such as travel, parties, and holidays.
- A dietitian with expertise in diabetes education is an integral part of the team.
- Provide three meals per day as well as mid-afternoon and bedtime snacks. Consistent carbohydrate intake can help prevent complications and maintain blood glucose levels near goals.
- Encourage the child to participate in age-appropriate sports.
- When exercising, monitor insulin dose and carbohydrate intake, and observe for hypoglycemic reactions. Additional blood glucose monitoring during activity will help the child learn how to best adjust food and insulin to maintain blood sugar goals during intense activity. Start by adding an extra snack containing 15 to 30 g carbohydrate for each 45 to 60 minutes of exercise.

in females with T1DM with suboptimal control results in higher risks for maternal and fetal complications. Ten percent of adolescent girls with T1DM meet the *Diagnostic and Statistical Manual of Mental Disorders* (4th ed.) criteria for eating disorders compared with 4% of their age-matched peers without diabetes (CDA, 2008).

■■■ Key Concepts

- The endocrine system consists of cells, tissues, and glands that produce and/or secrete hormones (chemical messengers) in response to a negative feedback system involving the hypothalamus and nervous system.
- Hormones (chemical messengers), along with the nervous system, play an intricate role in reproduction, growth and development, energy production and use, as well as maintenance of the internal homeostasis.
- The pituitary, along with the hypothalamus connection, is considered the "control centre," producing hormones that stimulate many glands to produce other hormones or to inhibit the process.

- Hormonal control is immature at birth; this is partly why the infant has trouble maintaining an appropriate balance of fluid concentration, electrolytes, amino acids, glucose, and trace substances.
- Linear growth and cognitive development may be impaired by untreated endocrine dysfunction in the infant or child.
- A thorough health history of the child with a known or potential endocrine disorder often reveals poor growth, school or learning problems, and inactivity or fatigue.
- Serial measurement of growth parameters is a key part of the physical assessment for children with endocrine dysfunction.
- Close monitoring of the child's status is critical during a hormone stimulation test or water deprivation study.
- Lifelong hormone supplementation is required for many endocrine disorders.
- The key nursing functions related to hormone supplementation are educating the child and family about medication use and monitoring for therapeutic results and adverse effects.
- Children with adrenocortical dysfunction will require additional hormone supplementation during times of stress, such as fever, infection, or surgery.
- GHD is characterized by poor growth and short stature as a result of failure of the anterior pituitary to produce sufficient GH. Early treatment enables the child to reach normal growth.
- Precocious puberty involves early development of secondary sex characteristics as a result of premature activation of the hypothalamic–pituitary–gonad axis.
- DI is characterized by water intoxication as a result of a deficiency in the ADH that leads to the cardinal signs of polyuria and polydipsia, resulting in hypernatremic dehydration.
- Key findings in congenital hypothyroidism are a thickened protuberant tongue, an enlarged posterior fontanel, feeding difficulties, hypotonia, and lethargy.
- Early diagnosis and treatment of hypothyroidism can prevent impaired growth and severe cognitive impairment.
- CAH results from a genetic defect that causes a breakdown in steroid synthesis and an overproduction of androgens that can lead to ambiguous genitalia in females.
- DM is the most common endocrine disorder now seen in children. The incidence of T2DM has risen dramatically.
- T1DM is an autoimmune disorder resulting from damage and destruction of the beta cells in the pancreas; the end result is complete absence of endogenous insulin. The peak onset occurs in early childhood and early puberty.
- T2DM results in an insensitivity or resistance to insulin. It is occurring at an alarming rate in children,

especially in those from certain ethnic groups, those who are obese, and those with a positive family history.

■ DKA is a medical emergency. The child will usually be admitted to a pediatric intensive care unit.

■ Critical areas in the nursing management of children with endocrine dysfunction include maintaining appropriate nutrition and fluid balance and promoting growth and development.

■ The nurse provides ongoing assessment and education of the child and family, assisting them to gain the knowledge and skills required for self-management and to incorporate those skills into their daily life.

■ Encouraging the child to have a healthy body image and working with the family to establish healthy family processes are also key nursing functions.

■ The focus of diabetes management is regulation of glucose control, which is accomplished by medications, diet, and exercise.

■ Diabetes education involves instruction in glucose monitoring, administration of insulin or oral hypoglycemics, meal planning, and promotion of a healthy lifestyle.

REFERENCES

Alemzadeh, R., & Wyatt, D. T. (2007). Diabetes mellitus in children. In R. M. Kliegman, R. E. Behrman, H. B. Jenson, & M. D. Stanton (Eds.), *Nelson textbook of pediatrics* (18th ed.). Philadelphia: Saunders.

Amed, S., Dean, H. J., Panagiotopoulos, C., et al. (2010). Type 2 diabetes, medication-induced diabetes, and monogenic diabetes in Canadian children: A prospective national surveillance study. *Diabetes Care, 33*(4), 786–791.

American Academy of Pediatrics, Rose, S. R., and the Section on Endocrinology and Committee on Genetics, American Thyroid Association, Brown, R. S., & the Public Health Committee and Lawson Wilkins Pediatric Endocrine Society. (2006). Update of newborn screening and therapy for congenital hypothyroidism. *Pediatrics, 117*(6), 2290–2303. Update retrieved June 21, 2011 from http://pediatrics.aappublications.org/content/117/6/2290.full

Barron, A. M., & Falsetti, D. (2008). Polycystic ovary syndrome in adolescents. *Advance for Nurse Practitioners, 16*(3), 49–54.

Behrman, R., Kliegman, R. M., & Jenson, H. B. (2004). *Nelson textbook of pediatrics* (17th ed.). Philadelphia: W. B. Saunders.

Bichet, D. G. (2010). *Treatment of nephrogenic diabetes insipidus.* Retrieved June 21, 2011 from http://www.uptodate.com/contents/treatment-of-nephrogenic-diabetes-insipidus?source=search_result&selectedTitle=1%7E63

Bordini, B. (2011). *Central precocious puberty.* Retrieved June 21, 2011 from http://www.magicfoundation.org/www/docs/146/

Breault, D. T., & Majzoub, J. A. (2007). Diabetes insipidus. In R. M. Kliegman, R. E. Behrman, H. B. Jenson, & B. F. Stanton (Eds.), *Nelson's textbook of pediatrics* (18th ed.). Philadelphia: Saunders.

Burg, F. D., Polin, R. A., Ingelfinger, J. R., & Gershon, A. A. (2002). *Gellis & Kagan's current pediatric therapy.* Philadelphia: W. B. Saunders.

Canadian Diabetes Association. (2008). Canadian Diabetes Association 2008 clinical practice guidelines for the prevention and management of diabetes in Canada. *Canadian Journal of Diabetes, 32*(Suppl. 1), S1–S201. Retrieved June 21, 2001 from http://www.diabetes.ca/files/cpg2008/cpg-2008.pdf

Canadian Diabetes Association. (n.d.). *Types of insulin (approved for use in Canada).* Retrieved June 24, 2011 from http://www.diabetes.ca/diabetes-and-you/living/insulin/types/

Chan, J., & Roth, K. S. (2011). *Pediatric diabetes insipidus.* Retrieved October 4, 2011 from http://emedicine.medscape.com/article/919886-overview

Chrousos, G. P., & Lafferty, A. (2009). *Glucocorticoid therapy and Cushing syndrome.* Retrieved October 4, 2011 from http://emedicine.medscape.com/article/921086-overview

Clark, P. A. (2011). *Constitutional growth delay.* Retrieved October 4, 2011 from http://emedicine.medscape.com/article/919677-overview

De Beer, K., Michael, S., Thacker, M., et al. (2008). Diabetic ketoacidosis and hyperglycaemic hyperosmolar syndrome – clinical guidelines. *Nursing in Critical Care, 13*(1), 5–11.

Donohoue, P. A. (2010). Adrenal disorders. In M. S. Kappy, D. B. Allen, & M. E. Geffner (Eds.), *Pediatric practice: Endocrinology.* Chicago, IL: McGraw-Hill Medical.

Endocrine Society. (2009). *The Endocrine Society statement on the New England Journal of Medicine letter to the editor on PTU use in children.* Retrieved June 21, 2011 from http://www.endo-society.org/advocacy/legislative/SocietyStatementontheNEJMLettetotheEditoronPTUUseInChildren.cfm

Eugster, E. A. (2010). *Pituitary gigantism.* Retrieved June 21, 2011 from http://www.uptodate.com/contents/pituitary-gigantism?source=search_result&selectedTitle=1%7E13

Eugster, E. A., LeMay, D., Zern, M., & Pescovitz, O. H. (2004). Definitive diagnosis in children with congenital hypothyroidism. *Journal of Pediatrics, 144*(5), 643–646.

Ferry, R. J., & Gold, J. G. (2011). *Pediatric hyperthyroidism.* Retrieved October 4, 2011 from http://emedicine.medscape.com/article/921707-overview

Ferry, R. J., & Shim, M. (2010). *Hyperpituitarism.* Retrieved October 4, 2011 from http://emedicine.medscape.com/article/921568-overview

Fischbach, F. T., & Dunning, M. B., III. (2009). *A manual of laboratory and diagnostic test* (8th ed.). Philadelphia: Lippincott Williams & Wilkins.

Flounders, J. (2003). Syndrome of inappropriate antidiuretic hormone. *Oncology Nursing Forum, 30*(3), E63–E70.

Hatcher, D. M. (2010). Pediatric metabolic and endocrine disorders. In S. M. Nettina (Ed.), *Lippincott manual of nursing practice* (9th ed.). Philadelphia: Lippincott Williams & Wilkins.

Health Canada. (2007). *Canada's food guide.* Retrieved June 21, 2011 from http://www.hc-sc.gc.ca/fn-an/food-guide-aliment/index-eng.php

Ho, J., Sellers, E., Dean, H., et al. (2010). Prevalence and associated risk factors for secondary diabetes in Canadian children followed in pediatric tertiary care centres. *Canadian Journal of Diabetes, 34*(2), 107–112.

Horwitz, M. J., & Stewart, A. F. (2008). Hypoparathyroidism: Is it time for replacement therapy? *The Journal of Clinical Endocrinology & Metabolism, 93*(9), 3307–3309. Retrieved June 21, 2011 from http://jcem.endojournals.org/cgi/content/full/93/9/3307

Huang, S. A. (2010). Thyroid. In M. S. Kappy, D. B. Allen, & M. E. Geffner (Eds.), *Pediatric practice: Endocrinology.* Chicago, IL: McGraw-Hill Medical.

Kaplowitz, P. B. (2010a). *Precocious puberty.* Retrieved October 4, 2011 from http://emedicine.medscape.com/article/924002-overview

Kaplowitz, P. B. (2010b). Subclinical hypothyroidism in children: Normal variation or sign of a failing thyroid gland? *International Journal of Pediatric Endocrinology, 10.* doi:10.1155/2010/281453

Kelly, A., & Levine, M. A. (2010). Disorders of bone and mineral metabolism. In M. S. Kappy, D. B. Allen, & M. E. Geffner (Eds.), *Pediatric practice: Endocrinology.* Chicago, IL: McGraw-Hill Medical.

KidsHealth. (2011). *Precocious puberty.* Retrieved October 4, 2011 from http://kidshealth.org/parent/medical/sexual/precocious.html#

LaFranchi, S. (2007). Disorders of the thyroid gland. In R. M. Kliegman, R. E. Behrman, H. B. Jenson, & B. F. Stanton (Eds.), *Nelson's textbook of pediatrics* (18th ed.). Philadelphia: Saunders.

LaFranchi, S. (2009). *Clinical manifestations and diagnosis of hyperthyroidism in children and adolescents.* Retrieved June 21, 2011 from http://www.uptodate.com/contents/clinical-manifestations-and-diagnosis-of-hyperthyroidism-in-children-and-adolescents?source=search_result&selectedTitle=1%7E150

LaFranchi, S. (2010). *Acquired hypothyroidism in childhood and adolescence.* Retrieved June 21, 2011 from http://www.uptodate.com/contents/

acquired-hypothyroidism-in-childhood-and-adolescence?
source=search_result& selectedTitle=1%7E150

LaFranchi, S. (2011). *Clinical features and detection of congenital hypothyroidism.* Retrieved June 21, 2011 from http://www.uptodate.
com/contents/clinical-features-and-detection-of-congenital-hypo-
thyroidism?source=search_result& selectedTitle=1%7E150

Lamb, W. (2010). *Pediatric type 1 diabetes mellitus.* Retrieved June 21,
2011 from http://emedicine.medscape.com/article/919999-overview

Lawson Wilkins Pediatric Endocrinology Society Drug and Therapeutics Committee. (2003). Update of the guidelines for the use
of growth hormone in children. *The Journal of Pediatrics, 143*(4),
415–421.

Li, H., Banerjee, S., Dunfield, L., et al. (2007). *Overview of recombinant human growth hormone for treatment of Turner syndrome: Systematic review and economic evaluation* [Technology overview number
35]. Ottawa: Canadian Agency for Drugs and Technologies in
Health.

Magiakou, M. A., Sarafoglou, K., Stratakis, C. A., & Chrousos, G.
P. (2009). Cushing syndrome in children and adolescents. In
K. Sarafoglou, G. F. Hoffman, & K. S. Roth (Eds.), *Pediatric
endocrinology and inborn errors of metabolism.* New York: McGraw
Hill Medical.

Nakamoto, J. M., Franklin, S. L., & Geffner, M. E. (2010). Puberty. In
M. S. Kappy, D. B. Allen, & M. E. Geffner (Eds.), *Pediatric practice:
Endocrinology.* Chicago, IL: McGraw-Hill Medical.

Newhook, L. A., Curtis, J., Hagerty, D., et al. (2004). High incidence
of childhood type 1 diabetes in the Avalon Peninsula, Newfoundland, Canada. *Diabetes Care, 27*(4), 885–888.

Nicol, L. E., Allen, D. B., Czernichow, P., & Zeitler, P. (2010). Puberty.
In M. S. Kappy, D. B. Allen, & M. E. Geffner (Eds.), *Pediatric practice: Endocrinology.* Chicago, IL: McGraw-Hill Medical.

Oberfield, S. E., & Speiser, P. W. (Eds.). (2010). *Patient guide to
congenital adrenal hyperplasia.* Chevy Chase, MD: The Hormone
Foundation.

O'Brien, R. F., & Emans, S. J. (2008). Polycystic ovary syndrome
in adolescents. *Journal of Pediatric and Adolescent Gynecology, 21*,
119–128.

Parks, J. S., & Felner, E. I. (2007). Hypopituitarism. In R. M. Kliegman, R. E. Behrman, H. B. Jenson, & M. D. Stanton (Eds.), *Nelson
textbook of pediatrics* (18th ed.). Philadelphia: Saunders.

Perkin, R. M., Swift, J. D., & Newton, D. A. (2003). *Pediatric hospital
medicine: Textbook of inpatient management.* Philadelphia: Lippincott
Williams & Wilkins.

Polak, M., & Van Vliet, G. (2009). Disorders of the thyroid gland. In K.
Sarafoglou, G. F. Hoffman, & K. S. Roth (Eds.), *Pediatric endocri-
nology and inborn errors of metabolism.* New York: McGraw Hill
Medical.

Postellon, D. C., & Daniel, M. S. (2011). *Congenital hypothyroidism.*
Retrieved June 21, 2011 from http://emedicine.medscape.com/
article/919758-overview

Radovick, S., & MacGillivray, M. H. (2003). *Pediatric endocrinology: A
clinical guide.* Totowa, NJ: Humana Press.

Rose, B. D., & Bichet, D. G. (2010). *Causes of central diabetes insipidus.*
Retrieved June 21, 2011 from http://www.uptodate.com/contents/
causes-of-central-diabetes-insipidus?source=search_result&
selectedTitle=1%7E49

Ross, D. S. (2010) Myxedema coma. Retrieved August 10, 2011 from
http://www.uptodate.com/contents/myxedema-coma?source=
search_result& selectedTitle=12~150#H9

Simmons, S. (2010). Flushing out the truth about diabetes insipidus.
Nursing, 40(1), 55–59.

Sperling, M. A. (2002). *Pediatric endocrinology* (2nd ed.). Philadelphia:
Saunders.

Sterns, R. H. (2011a). *Osmotic demyelination syndrome and overly rapid
correction of hyponatremia.* Retrieved June 21, 2011 from http://
www.uptodate.com/contents/osmotic-demyelination-syndrome-
and-overly-rapid-correction-of-hyponatremia?source=search_
result& selectedTitle=1%7E150

Sterns, R. H. (2011b). *Treatment of hyponatremia: Syndrome of inappropriate antidiuretic hormone secretion (SIADH) and reset osmostat.*
Retrieved June 21, 2011 from http://www.uptodate.com/contents/
treatment-of-hyponatremia-syndrome-of-inappropriate-antidi-
uretic-hormone-secretion-siadh-and-reset-osmostat?source=
search_result& selectedTitle=1%7E150

Stokowski, L. (2009). Congenital adrenal hyperplasia: An endocrine
disorder with neonatal onset. *Critical Care Nursing Clinics of North
America, 21*(2), 195–212.

Taketoma, C. K., Hodding, J. H., & Kraus, D. M. (Eds.). (2007). *Pediatric dosage handbook.* Hudson, OH: Lexi-Comp.

Thyroid Foundation of Canada. (n.d.). *About thyroid disease: Health
guides on thyroid disease—Thyroid disease in childhood.* Retrieved June
21, 2011 from http://www.thyroid.ca/childhood.php

Trimarchi, T. (2006). Endocrine problems in the critically ill child.
AACN Clinical Issues, 17(1), 66–78.

Triolo, T. M., Chase, H. P., Barker, J. M., & the DPT-1 Study Group.
(2009). Diabetic subjects diagnosed through the Diabetes Prevention Trial–Type 1 (DPT-1) are often asymptomatic with normal
A1C at diabetes onset. *Diabetes Care, 32*(5), 769–773.

U.S. Food and Drug Administration. (2010). *FDA drug safety communication: New boxed warning on severe liver injury with propylthiouracil.*
Retrieved June 21, 2011 from http://www.fda.gov/Drugs/DrugSafety/
PostmarketDrugSafetyInformationforPatientsandProviders/
ucm209023.htm

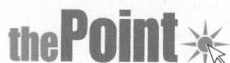

For additional learning materials,
including Internet resources, visit
http://thePoint.lww.com/Chow1e.

CHAPTER WORKSHEET

MULTIPLE CHOICE QUESTIONS

1. A young mother brings her new baby, diagnosed with congenital hypothyroidism, to the clinic so she can learn how to administer levothyroxine. The nurse should include which of the following instructions?

   a. Crush the medication and place it in a full bottle of formula to disguise the taste.

   b. Administer the medication every other day.

   c. Use an oral dispenser syringe or nipple to give the crushed medication mixed with a small amount of formula.

   d. Tell the mother that the medication will not be needed after the age of 7 years.

2. The nurse is instructing a 14-year-old boy about the different types of insulin. Since he takes NPH insulin every morning at 7:30 AM, at what time could he possibly experience a hypoglemic episode?

   a. When he goes to school at 9 AM

   b. When he takes a test at 11 AM

   c. When he eats lunch at noon

   d. When he works out after school at 3 PM

3. A child diagnosed with Graves' disease begins to take methimazole. What symptoms should the parents and child observe for to determine if the dose is too high?

   a. Weight loss

   b. Lethargy

   c. Difficulty in school

   d. Tachycardia

4. Which endocrine disorder is considered the most common one observed in early childhood?

   a. Hypothyroidism

   b. Hyperthyroidism

   c. Type 1 diabetes

   d. Cushing's

5. When should GH be given in a child who has GHD?

   a. Before meals

   b. After meals

   c. At bedtime

   d. First thing in the morning

CRITICAL THINKING EXERCISES

1. A 12-year-old boy with T1DM has a stomachache and is vomiting. His mother calls the diabetes clinic to report that he stayed home from school and does not have an appetite, so he is not eating. The mother asks the nurse how much insulin the boy should take. He is currently taking three injections daily with Regular and NPH in the morning before breakfast, Regular and NPH in the evening after dinner, and Regular before bedtime. What questions should the nurse ask before answering the mother's question? Based on the answers to these questions, how would you instruct the mother?

2. The mother of Robin, a 5-year-old girl, reports that Robin has a body odour. She is developing breasts and some pubic hair and was teased when she had a sleepover with friends. The review of her growth charts reveals that Robin went from the 50th percentile to the 93rd percentile in the past 6 months. Based on this information, what are the three major nursing diagnoses to begin establishing a plan of care for the child and family? What are the expected outcomes and major interventions associated with the nursing diagnosis of knowledge deficit?

3. A mother brings her baby to the clinic after receiving a phone message from the clinic saying there was a problem with the baby's thyroid test. She says the trip on the bus took a long time, but the infant slept the entire way. She says that the baby is sleeping much of the time and does not want to eat very much. The baby was discharged from the hospital 2 weeks ago. The birth was without difficulty and there were no problems during labour. Why is this visit urgent? What would the test show if the disorder was due to a pituitary gland problem and not the thyroid gland?

STUDY ACTIVITIES

1. During your clinical experiences, ask to be on an inpatient unit that provides care for children with alterations in endocrine function. Compare and contrast the health histories, assessments, laboratory tests, diagnostic procedures, and plans of care for these children with those for the care of children on other units. Participate in the teaching plan for these children and their families.

2. Attend an out-patient clinic that provides care for children with endocrine disorders. Identify the role of the registered nurse in providing coordination of care, health teaching, and referrals for these children and their families.

3. Shadow a diabetes nurse educator to observe the teaching methods and strategies he or she uses to provide an education plan for a child with DM. Observe how the nurse educator includes the family in the plan. Are there any differences between the teaching plans for T1DM and T2DM?

4. Conduct a literature review for one of the common endocrine disorders to research current management practices. Are there evidence-based practice guidelines for nursing interventions?

5. Conduct an Internet search to research the information that is available to children and their families related to DM.

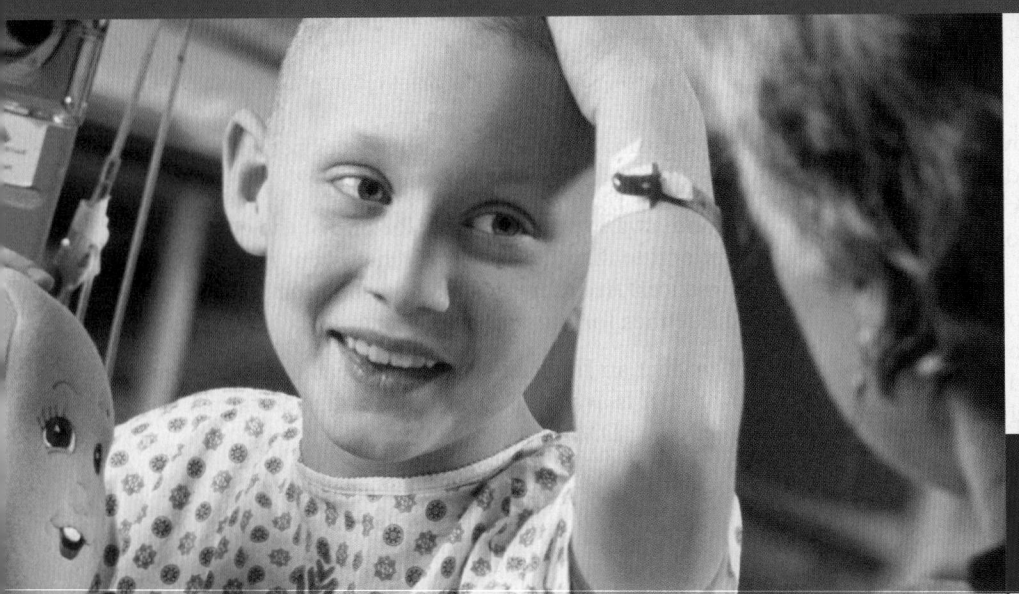

NURSING CARE OF THE CHILD WITH A NEOPLASTIC DISORDER

KEY TERMS

biopsy
biotherapy
chemotherapy

clinical trial
extravasation
malignant

metastasis
neoplastic
staging

LEARNING OBJECTIVES

Upon completion of the chapter, the learner will be able to:

1. Compare childhood and adult cancers.
2. Describe nursing care related to common laboratory and diagnostic testing used in the medical diagnosis of pediatric cancer.
3. Identify types of cancer common in infants, children, and adolescents.
4. Identify appropriate nursing assessments and interventions related to medications and treatments for pediatric cancer.
5. Develop an individualized nursing care plan for the child with cancer.
6. Describe the psychosocial impact of cancer on children and their families.
7. Devise a nutrition plan for the child with cancer.
8. Develop patient/family teaching plans for the child with cancer.

John Shaw, 4 years old, is brought to the clinic by his parents with a fever. His father states, "John seems to get fevers and colds more often than our other children. He's also very tired these days. He hardly ever wants to go out and play with his friends. He complains of headaches frequently and just doesn't really seem like himself."

WOW

Be inspired by the courage of a child with cancer and reflect it in the care you provide.

Cancer accounts for the most deaths from disease in children over the age of 1 year. Cure has been achieved in some children with leukemia and other cancers, but there is no universal long-term cure available for any of the childhood cancers. In Canada, the 5-year survival rate for all cancers in children younger than 15 years is 82% (Ellison, De, Mery, et al., 2009).

Cancer is a life-threatening illness that involves emotional distress, fear of the unknown, and changes in life priorities for the child and family. Families of children with cancer experience many "rough spots" related to cancer that may threaten not only individual family members' sense of self but also the family unit as a whole (Woodgate, 2005). These "rough spots" can escalate the child's and family's suffering and compromise their overall quality of life (Woodgate, 2005; Woodgate, West, & Wilkin, 2011).

Children with cancer face many challenges that may have a negative impact on their psychosocial well-being (Woodgate, 2005; Woodgate et al., 2011). In addition to challenges related to the diagnosis, ongoing diagnostic tests, and lengthy and intense treatment regimens, children must deal with complex developmental changes and demands (Woodgate, 2005). The child often feels isolated from his or her peers, and the adolescent may have difficulty achieving independence, which is the core developmental task of the teenage years. Children and teens with cancer may experience problems in keeping up with their studies (Hokkanen, Eriksson, Ahonen, et al., 2004; Woodgate, 2008). Although the majority of children with cancer report minimal symptoms of long-term psycho-logical distress, some do experience psychopathology that includes depression, severe anxiety, and post-traumatic stress disorder (Stuber & Seacord, 2004).

Nurses caring for children with cancer need to be knowledgeable about the medical treatment of the disease and must be particularly aware of the psychosocial and emotional impact of cancer on the child and family in order to provide comprehensive and sensitive care.

Childhood Cancer Versus Adult Cancer

Cancers in children differ greatly from cancers in adults. Pediatric cancers most often arise from primitive embryonal (mesodermal) and neuroectodermal tissues, resulting in leukemias, lymphomas, sarcomas or central nervous system (CNS) tumours (American Cancer Society, 2011a; Larsen, 2011). The most common childhood cancers, in order of frequency, are leukemia, CNS tumours, lymphoma, neuroblastoma, rhabdomyosarcoma, Wilms' tumour, bone tumours, and retinoblastoma. Comparison Chart 49.1 explains how cancer is different in children versus adults.

In children, warning signs of cancer are most often related to changes in blood cell production or result from compression, infiltration, or obstruction caused by the tumour. Changes in blood cell production may result in fatigue, pallor, frequent or severe infection, or easy bruising. Infiltration, obstruction, or compression by a tumour may result in bone or abdominal pain, pain elsewhere, swelling, or unusual discharge.

COMPARISON CHART 49.1   CHILDHOOD CANCER VERSUS ADULT CANCER

	Childhood Cancer	Adult Cancer
Cancer usually affects	Tissues	Organs
Histologic type	Embryonal, leukemia, lymphoma	Epithelial in origin
Most common sites	Blood, lymph, brain, bone, kidney, muscle	Breast, lung, prostate, bowel, bladder
Environmental and lifestyle factors	Only a small amount of environmental influence proven	Strong influence on cancer development
Cancer prevention	Little known	80% preventable
Detection	Usually incidental or accidental	Very early detection possible if screening recommendations followed
Latent period	Relatively short	Can be very long (20 years or more)
Extent of disease	Metastasis often present at diagnosis	Metastasis less often present at diagnosis
Response to treatment	Very responsive	Less responsive

Adapted from: American Cancer Society. (2011a). *Cancer in children.* Retrieved November 7, 2011 from http://www.cancer.org/acs/groups/cid/documents/webcontent/002287-pdf.pdf; and Larsen, E. (2011). *Childhood cancer.* Retrieved November 7, 2011 from http://www.cancerstory.org/index.php/cancerstory/article/56.

▶ *Take* NOTE!

Research is under way to determine whether a statistically significant link exists between the use of supplemental oxygen in the neonatal period and the development of childhood cancer (Sola, Saldeño, & Favareto, 2008). Studies thus far have proven to be equivocal.

Common Medical Treatments

Deciding on a course of medical treatment for cancer in a developing child is complicated. Some of the treatments can impair the child's growth and development. Many cancer treatment centres in Canada, the United States, and other countries are active members of the Children's Oncology Group (COG), which approves and administers clinical trials devoted exclusively to childhood and adolescent cancer research. All 17 children's hospitals and cancer treatment centres in Canada belong to COG and the Council of Canadian Pediatric Hematology/Oncology Directors known as C[17] (Childhood Cancer Canada Foundation, 2011).

A **clinical trial** is a carefully designed research study that assesses the effectiveness of a treatment as well as its short- and long-term effects on the patient. Current cancer care in children is a result of the knowledge gained through clinical trials (Chordas & Graham, 2010). A clinical trial may include existing medications or treatments in combination with new drugs or may involve a different approach to sequencing or dosing of medications and treatment.

To provide optimal outcomes, the child with cancer should be treated at an institution with multidisciplinary cancer care specialists who can provide the most advanced care available. Each case of pediatric cancer should be considered individually, with the oncology health care team and the family reaching treatment decisions together, whether the treatment plan is standard or involves enrolment in a clinical trial. In the child with cancer, particularly advanced disease, the decision to provide treatment ("let's do everything we can") or to withhold treatment in the event of an extremely poor prognosis is extraordinarily challenging in an ethical sense. A mature older child or adolescent may have a strong desire to continue or discontinue treatment, and sometimes this desire conflicts with the parents' desires or choices. The Canadian Paediatric Society (CPS, 2004) reinforces that children and adolescents ought to be involved in decision making to an increasing degree as they develop, until they are competent to make their own decisions about treatment (Box 49.1). In the case of end-of-life decision making, CPS recommends that although the impact on the family must be considered, the interests of the family should not be allowed to override those of the child or adolescent. The

BOX 49.1 Recommendations Regarding Treatment Decisions Concerning Infants, Children, and Adolescents

- Provide patients and their families with appropriate and sufficient information so that they can participate effectively in decision making.
- Encourage joint decision making by patients, families, and the health care team, and support capable patients who wish to make their own decisions.
- Disclosure of information and inclusion in decision making should occur according to the stage of the child's or adolescent's development.
- Respect for parental wishes and values is important; however, the needs and interests of the child or adolescent should prevail.
- End-of-life decisions should be made with the comfort of the dying child or adolescent as a constant focal point.
- In situations of conflict, physicians have an obligation to seek available resources to help resolve that conflict and to facilitate patients' and families' access to assistance as well.

Source: Canadian Paediatric Society. (2004). Position statement B 2004–01: Treatment decisions regarding infants, children and adolescents. *Pediatric & Child Health, 9*(2), 99–103. Retrieved November 7, 2011 from http://www.cps.ca/english/statements/B/b04-01.pdf.

decision to use life-sustaining treatment must be guided by the best interests of the patient.

Hospice or palliative care may be needed for the child with cancer. Children facing the end of life experience the same effects that adults do, such as pain, fatigue, nausea, and dyspnea. Standards for end-of-life care are still in development, but all dying children have the right to die comfortably and with palliation of symptoms, as has been well established in adult hospice programs. Children's Hospice International (CHI) has a worldwide database of programs caring for children with life-threatening conditions and their families that focus on enhancing the quality of life of these children. These include a number of programs in Canada, such as Canuck Place Children's Hospice in British Columbia and the Canadian Network of Palliative Care for Children (visit http://thePoint.lww.com/Chow1e for direct links). CHI's goal is to provide a comprehensive, interdisciplinary continuum of care to the child and family from the time of diagnosis with a life-threatening condition through the time of death, if cure is not achieved. For further information related to nursing care of the dying child, refer to Chapter 33.

A variety of medications and treatments are used to treat **neoplastic** disorders in children. Most of these treatments will require a physician's order when the child is in the hospital. The most common treatments and medications are listed in Common Medical Treatments 49.1

COMMON MEDICAL TREATMENTS 49.1

Treatment	Explanation	Indication	Nursing Implications
Biopsy	A small piece of the tumour is removed with a needle or via an open incision.	Solid tumours	Monitor for bleeding at the needle biopsy site. Provide routine incision care for open biopsy site.
Surgical removal of tumour	The tumour is completely or partially resected surgically.	Solid tumours	Provide routine postoperative nursing care based on the location of the tumour excision.
Leukapheresis	Whole blood is removed from the body, the WBCs are extracted, and then the blood is re-transfused into the child.	Hyperviscosity with leukemia (WBC >100,000)	Performed by specially trained personnel. Monitor blood pressure and other vital signs.
Blood product transfusion	Administration of whole blood, packed red blood cells, platelets, or plasma intravenously	Anemia, thrombocytopenia, bleeding	Follow institution's transfusion protocol. Double-check blood type and product label with a second nurse. Use only irradiated, leukodepleted, cytomegalovirus-negative blood products in the pediatric cancer patient. Monitor vital signs and assess child frequently to detect adverse reaction to blood transfusion. If adverse reaction is suspected, immediately discontinue transfusion, run normal saline IV, reassess child, and notify physician. Some children require premedication with diphenhydramine and/or acetaminophen before receiving blood products.
Radiation therapy	Ionizing radiation (high-energy X-ray) is delivered to the cancerous area. The radiation damages all cells in the locally treated area (normal and cancerous), but the normal cells are able to repair themselves. Usually administered several times a week for several weeks (a short rest between treatments allows the normal cells time to regenerate). The lowest possible dose of radiation is used and it is directed to a specific area.	Solid tumours, before or after surgical resection, leukemia, lymphoma	Do not wash off radiation marking. Keep skin clean and dry. Fatigue is a common side effect. Skin at the site of radiation may become red, dry, or pruritic or may peel; eventually may become moist and red. Mucositis, dry mouth, and loss of taste may occur if head or neck radiated. Radiation may also have adverse effects on the organ irradiated, such as the brain; monitor for changes.
Hematopoietic stem cell transplantation	*Bone marrow transplant:* transfer of healthy bone marrow into a child with cancer. The transplanted cells can then develop into functional cells. *Stem cell transplant:* peripheral stem cells are removed from the donor via apheresis, or stem cells are retrieved from the umbilical cord and placenta. The stem cells are then transplanted into the recipient.	Leukemia, lymphoma, other cancers	Maintain medical asepsis and protective isolation to prevent infection. Monitor closely for GvHD. Provide meticulous oral care. Avoid rectal temperatures and suppositories. Encourage appropriate nutrition. Administer immunosuppressive medications as ordered.

(continued)

COMMON MEDICAL TREATMENTS 49.1 (continued)

Treatment	Explanation	Indication	Nursing Implications
Central venous catheter (Fig. 49.1)	IV catheter inserted into the central circulation for the purpose of administering medications, total parenteral nutrition or blood products	Any child with cancer who will require long-term IV medications or parenteral nutrition	Complaints of shortness of breath or chest pain may indicate air entry into the central venous catheter. Have child lie on left side, and notify physician immediately. Keep dressing clean and dry. Perform sterile dressing change per institution policy or physician order. Monitor for fever. Monitor insertion site for erythema or drainage. Maintain sterile technique when accessing line, perform dressing change, or administering any fluid through catheter.
Implanted port (Fig. 49.2)	A needle-accessible port is implanted under the skin, usually on the chest. The port has a thin catheter exiting it that is tunnelled under the skin into the superior vena cava or subclavian vein.	Any child with cancer who will require long-term IV medications or parenteral nutrition	Flush non-accessed port with prescribed heparin dose per institution policy. Use sterile technique to access port with Huber needle. Monitor port site for erythema or warmth.

Adapted from: Baggott, C. (2010). Cancer. In P. J. Allen, J. A. Vessey, & N. A. Schapiro (Eds.), *Primary care of the child with a chronic condition* (5th ed.). St. Louis, MO: Mosby; and Tomlinson, D., & Kline, N. E. (Eds.) (2010). *Pediatric oncology nursing.* New York: Springer.

and Drug Guide 49.1. Commonly, chemotherapy and radiation therapy are used to treat childhood cancers. In some instances, hematopoietic stem cell transplantation (HSCT) is used. The nurse caring for the child with cancer should be familiar with the procedures, how the treatments and medications work, and common nursing implications related to use of these modalities.

Chemotherapy

To understand how **chemotherapy** works to destroy cancer cells, it is necessary to review the normal cycle through which all cells progress (Fig. 49.3). The cell cycle comprises five phases (Chordas & Graham, 2010):

- G0 phase: the resting phase; lasts from a few hours to a few years; cells have not started to divide
- G1 phase: cell makes more protein in preparation for dividing; lasts 18 to 30 hours
- S phase: chromosomes are copied so that newly formed cells have the appropriate DNA; lasts 18 to 20 hours
- G2 phase: just before the cell splits into two cells; lasts 2 to 10 hours
- M phase: mitosis, the actual splitting of the cell into two new cells; lasts 30 minutes to 1 hour

Chemotherapy is a cytotoxic drug therapy that stops **malignant** cell division and spread (Chordas & Graham, 2010). Chemotherapy drugs work in two different ways in relation to the cell cycle. Cell cycle–specific agents exert their actions during a specific phase of the cell cycle. Cell cycle–nonspecific drugs exert their effect on the cells regardless of which phase the cell is in. Chemotherapy protocols often call for a combination of drugs that act on different phases of the cell cycle, thus maximizing the destruction of cancer cells.

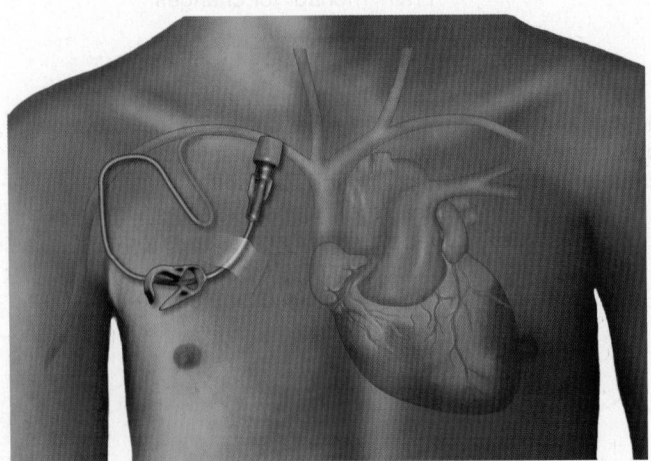

FIGURE 49.1 The central venous access catheter is tunnelled under the skin and secured with a cuff.

(text continues on page 1692)

DRUG GUIDE 49.1   COMMON DRUGS FOR NEOPLASTIC DISORDERS

Medication	Action	Indication	Nursing Implications

Chemotherapy
Alkylating agents:
  busulfan, carbopla-
  tin, cisplatin,
  ifosfamide, temo-
  zolomide, thiotepa
Nitrosoureas: carmus-
  tine, lomustine
Nitrogen mustard:
  chlorambucil,
  cyclophosphamide,
  mechlorethamine,
  melphalan
	Interfere with DNA replica-
	tion and RNA transcrip-
	tion by alkylation
	(replacing the hydrogen
	ion with an alkyl group),
	cross-link DNA.
	Cell cycle–nonspecific.
	The nitrosoureas are highly
	lipid-soluble and easily
	cross the blood–brain
	barrier.
		A variety of
		cancers
			Cause myelosuppression, nausea, vomiting,
			  alopecia, mucositis.
			Monitor for signs of infection.
			Provide adequate hydration.
			Cyclophosphamide, ifosfamide: administer in
			  the morning, provide adequate hydration,
			  and have child void frequently during and
			  after infusion to decrease risk of hemor-
			  rhagic cystitis.
			Cisplatin, mechlorethamine, melphalan: avoid
			  extravasation.
			Temozolomide: avoid opening capsules.
			Thiotepa: if contact with skin occurs, wash
			  thoroughly with soap and water.

Antitumour antibiotics:
  bleomycin, dacti-
  nomycin, daunoru-
  bicin, doxorubicin,
  idarubicin, mitomy-
  cin, mitoxantrone
	Interfere with cellular
	metabolism, causing
	disruptions in DNA and/
	or RNA synthesis.
	Cell cycle–nonspecific.
		A variety of
		cancers
			May cause alopecia, nausea, vomiting,
			  myelosuppression.
			Bleomycin: fever and chills may occur 20 h
			  after infusion.
			Dactinomycin, mitomycin: avoid extravasation.
			Daunorubicin, doxorubicin, idarubicin: may turn
			  urine red-orange, monitor for arrhythmias,
			  congestive heart failure; avoid extravasation.
			Mitoxantrone: may colour urine, sweat, tears,
			  skin, sclera blue-green; monitor for
			  arrhythmias, congestive heart failure.

Antimetabolites:
  cladribine, cytara-
  bine, fludarabine,
  fluorouracil, mer-
  captopurine,
  methotrexate,
  thioguanine
	Substitute for a natural
	metabolite in the mole-
	cule, altering the cell's
	function and ability to
	replicate.
	Cell cycle–specific (S
	phase), but cladribine is
	cell cycle–nonspecific.
		A variety of
		cancers
			May cause alopecia, nausea, vomiting,
			  mucositis, and myelosuppression.
			Cladribine: monitor for fever.
			Cytarabine: use corticosteroid eye drops to
			  prevent conjunctivitis with high doses.
			Fludarabine: monitor for visual changes and
			  neurotoxicity; maintain adequate hydration.
			Fluorouracil: maintain adequate hydration;
			  may cause photosensitivity.
			Mercaptopurine: do not give oral doses
			  with meals; may cause drug fever; avoid
			  extravasation.
			Methotrexate: intensive hydration with high
			  doses; may cause photosensitivity.
			Thioguanine: maintain hydration; administer
			  on empty stomach.

Antimicrotubulars:
  paclitaxel
	Inhibits mitotic cellular
	function in late G2 and
	M phases of cell cycle
		Refractory leuke-
		mia, recurrent
		Wilms' tumour
			May cause alopecia, nausea, vomiting,
			  mucositis, myelosuppression.
			May cause drowsiness.
			Avoid extravasation.

Miscellaneous:
  asparaginase,
  pegaspargase
	Inhibit protein synthesis by
	depriving tumour cells
	of the essential amino
	acid asparagine
		Acute lympho-
		cytic leukemia,
		lymphomas
			May cause alopecia, nausea, vomiting, and
			  myelosuppression.
			Monitor vital signs during infusion and for
			  signs of anaphylaxis.
			Have emergency equipment, oxygen, epi-
			  nephrine, antihistamines, and steroids
			  available at bedside.

(continued)

DRUG GUIDE 49.1 COMMON DRUGS FOR NEOPLASTIC DISORDERS (continued)

Medication	Action	Indication	Nursing Implications
Miscellaneous: dacarbazine, procarbazine	Inhibit DNA and RNA synthesis via cross-linking or suppression of mitosis	A variety of cancers	May cause alopecia, nausea, vomiting, myelosuppression. Monitor for flu-like symptoms. Dacarbazine: photosensitivity may occur; avoid extravasation.
Mitotic inhibitors: etoposide, vinblastine, vincristine	Inhibit mitotic activity by inhibiting DNA topoisomerase (etoposide). Cause metaphase arrest by binding to the mitotic spindle (vinblastine, vincristine).	A variety of cancers	May cause alopecia, nausea, vomiting, myelosuppression (only minimal with vincristine). Etoposide: monitor for anaphylaxis; have emergency equipment, oxygen, epinephrine, antihistamines, and steroids available at bedside. Vinblastine, vincristine: maintain hydration; administer allopurinol; avoid extravasation.
Topoisomerase inhibitors: irinotecan, topotecan	Bind to DNA complex, preventing re-ligation of single-strand DNA breaks	Refractory solid tumours	May cause alopecia, nausea, vomiting, myelosuppression, severe diarrhea (irinotecan), hypotension (topotecan). Maintain hydration. Avoid extravasation. Monitor blood pressure during topotecan infusion.
Corticosteroids: prednisone, dexamethasone	Suppress immune system by decreasing lymphatic activity and volume. Also decrease edema caused by tumour or tumour necrosis.	Leukemia, some other cancers	Administer with food to decrease GI upset. May mask signs of infection. Monitor blood pressure; monitor urine for glucose. Do not stop treatment abruptly or acute adrenal insufficiency may occur. Monitor for Cushing syndrome. Doses may be tapered over time.
Biotherapy Colony-stimulating factors: darbepoetin alpha, epoetin alpha, filgrastim, sargramostim	Stimulate production of red blood cells (epoetin) or granulocytes (filgrastim, sargramostim)	Counteract myelosuppressive effects of chemotherapy	Administer SC or IV. Filgrastrim, sargramostim: may cause bone pain. Sargramostim may cause hypotension and a first-dose reaction.
Interleukins: aldesleukin	Recombinant DNA interleukin-2 product that recruits T, B, and natural killer cells	Non-Hodgkin's lymphoma	Adverse effects are dose-dependent. May cause capillary leak syndrome within 2–12 h of start of treatment: hypotension and decreased organ perfusion result.
Tumour necrosis factor (protein cytokine)	Increases effectiveness of immune cells, stops cancer cells from dividing, damages tumour blood vessels	A variety of cancers	May cause fever, chills, rigours, nausea, vomiting
Monoclonal antibodies: rituximab, gemtuzumab	Bind to CD20 antigen on B lymphocytes	CD20-positive non-Hodgkin's lymphoma, post-transplant lymphoproliferative disorder	Monitor blood pressure for hypotension. Monitor for anaphylaxis and infusion-related reaction. Have epinephrine, antihistamines, and steroids available at bedside for treatment of reaction.
Interferons: alpha, gamma	Alter cancer cell proliferation (alpha), stimulate macrophage production to fight bacteria and fungus (gamma)	A variety of cancers	May cause flu-like symptoms. Maintain adequate hydration.

Medication	Action	Indication	Nursing Implications
Allopurinol	Decreases production of uric acid	Treatment of secondary hyperuricemia occurring during leukemia or tumour treatment	Give PO after meals with plenty of food. Cardiovascular adverse effects may occur with IV administration. Maintain adequate hydration.
Antibiotics (oral, parenteral)	Treatment or prophylaxis of bacterial infections	Prophylaxis of *Pneumocystis jiroveci,* treatment of documented infection, neutropenia	Check for antibiotic allergies. Should be given as prescribed for the length of time prescribed. Start IV antibiotics as soon as possible in the neutropenic child admitted with fever.
Antiemetics: promethazine, metoclopramide, ondansetron	Act on the CNS transmitters to prevent vomiting	Nausea and/or vomiting	May cause CNS side effects, such as drowsiness or irritability. Ondansetron: may cause dry mouth.
Antifungal agents: nystatin, amphotericin B (conventional and lipid complex)	Invade fungal cell wall, enabling its destruction	Mucositis, systemic fungal infection	Nystatin: administer after meals. Amphotericin B: may cause fever, chills, rigours, cardiovascular adverse effects; monitor patient closely throughout infusion; note dose differences between conventional and lipid complex.
Immunosuppressant drugs: cyclosporine, mycophenolate, tacrolimus	Inhibit production and release of interleukin II (cyclosporine). Inhibit T- and B-cell proliferation (mycophenolate). Inhibit T-cell activation (tacrolimus).	Treatment of GvHD after HSCT	Monitor CBC, serum creatinine, potassium, and magnesium. Monitor blood pressure and for signs of infection. Draw blood levels prior to morning dose. Cyclosporine: do not give with grapefruit juice. Mycophenolate: give on empty stomach; do not open capsule or crush tablet. Tacrolimus: give on empty stomach; monitor for anaphylaxis with first IV dose.
Mesna	Binds with and detoxifies cyclophosphamide and ifosfamide metabolites in the urinary bladder	Antidote to cyclophosphamide- or ifosfamide-induced hemorrhagic cystitis	Maintain adequate hydration. Administer concurrently with and after cyclophosphamide or ifosfamide. May cause hypotension.
Methotrexate antidote: leucovorin	Reduces toxic effects of methotrexate	Leucovorin rescue with methotrexate treatment	May cause skin disturbances, wheezing, thrombocytosis. Dose depends on methotrexate level. Dose increased with increased creatinine levels.

Adapted from: Baggott, C. (2010). Cancer. In P. J. Allen, J. A. Vessey, and N. A. Schapiro (Eds.), *Primary care of the child with a chronic condition* (5th ed.). St. Louis, MO: Mosby; Taketokmo, C. K., Hodding, J. H., & Kraus, D. M. (2010). *Lexi-comp's pediatric dosage handbook* (17th ed.). Hudson, OH: Lexi-comp; and Tomlinson, D., & Kline, N. E. (Eds.). (2010). *Pediatric oncology nursing.* New York: Springer.

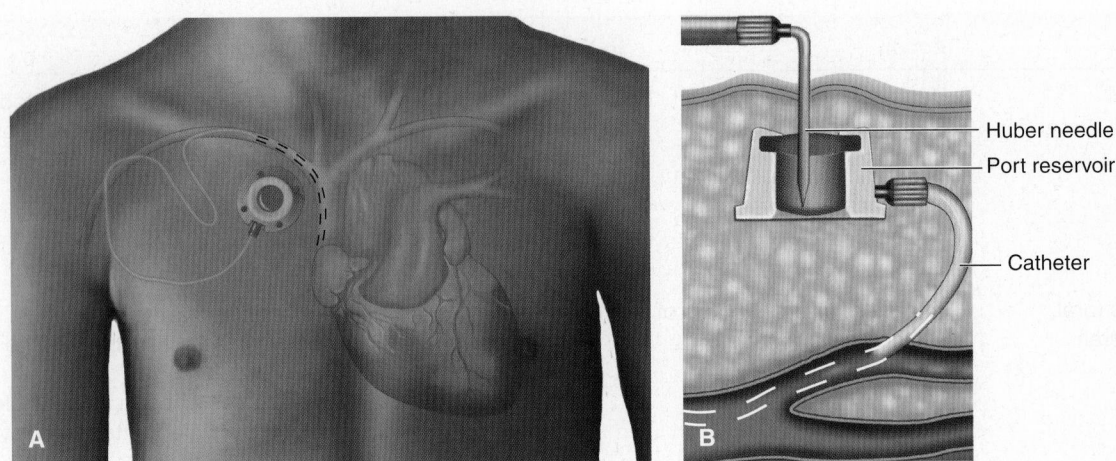

FIGURE 49.2 (**A**) The implanted port consists of a reservoir under the skin for ready access. The catheter exiting the port is threaded into the subclavian vein or right atrium. (**B**) A 90-degree Huber needle is used to access the port.

Chemotherapeutic medications disrupt the cell cycle not only in cancer cells but also in normal rapidly dividing cells, resulting in a significant number of adverse effects (Chordas & Graham, 2010). The cells most likely to be affected by chemotherapy are those in the bone marrow, digestive tract (especially the mouth), reproductive system, and hair follicles.

Chemotherapy drugs are divided into classes that exert slightly different actions and affect different portions of the cell cycle. Drug Guide 49.1 gives further explanation about the different classes of chemotherapy drugs.

Adverse effects common to chemotherapeutic drugs include immunosuppression, infection, myelosuppression, nausea, vomiting, constipation, oral mucositis, alopecia, and pain (Chordas & Graham, 2010). Long-term complications include microdontia and missing teeth as a result of damage to developing permanent teeth (Lund, 2005); hearing and vision changes; hematopoietic, immunologic, or gonadal dysfunction; endocrine dysfunction, including altered growth and precocious or delayed puberty; various alterations of the cardiorespiratory, gastrointestinal, and genitourinary systems; as well as a second cancer as an adolescent or adult (Chordas & Graham, 2010).

Newer chemotherapy treatments target mechanisms of tumour growth and protein pathways rather than a cell's reproduction cycle. An advantage of targeted therapies is that they have fewer effects on healthy cells. Today, traditional chemotherapies combined with these newer therapies are being used in clinical investigation and practice (Chordas & Graham, 2010). Some cancerous cells can be resistant to chemotherapy agents. To address resistance, drug combinations are given early in treatment. By altering chemotherapy dosage and administration techniques, resistance may be temporary; permanent resistance, on the other hand, is a result of a genetic mutation (Chordas & Graham, 2010).

▶ **Take** NOTE!

Acupuncture as an adjuvant therapy has been demonstrated to decrease nausea, vomiting, constipation, stress, aversion to chemotherapy, and psychological damage and to result in an increase in oral intake and the self-confidence needed to cope with cancer (Post-White & Ladas, 2010).

Radiotherapy

Radiotherapy uses high-energy radiation to damage or kill cancer cells. The goal of radiotherapy is to control local tumour growth with minimal long-term effects. Particle radiation and ionizing electromagnetic radiation are two forms of radiation used in treatment (Loch & Khorrami, 2010). Radiation affects not only cancer cells

FIGURE 49.3 Phases of the cell cycle.

but also any rapidly growing cells with which they are in contact. It may be used as a curative, adjuvant, or palliative treatment, either alone or in combination with chemotherapy. Radiotherapy is also used to shrink a tumour prior to surgical resection. The area to be treated is marked carefully to minimize damage to normal cells.

Side effects of radiotherapy are either acute (occurring within 3 months of treatment) or late (occurring between 3 and 12 months after treatment) (Faithfull, 2008). The type and severity of side effects will depend on the child's age, treatment site, treatment dose, and fractionation (division of radiation dosage) as well as other any adjuvant chemotherapy (Loch & Khorrami, 2010). Acute effects include fatigue, skin reactions, hair loss, cerebral edema, dry mouth, mucositis, esophagitis, nausea, vomiting, cystitis, and myelosuppression (Loch & Khorrami, 2010).

Hematopoietic Stem Cell Transplantation

HSCT, also called bone marrow transplantation, is a procedure in which hematopoietic stem cells are infused intravenously into the patient (Copelan, 2006). This follows a period of purging of abnormal cells in the patient that is accomplished through high-dose chemotherapy or irradiation. The use of high-dose chemotherapy and total body irradiation kills the tumour cells but also destroys the child's bone marrow. The transplanted cells migrate to the empty spaces in the child's bone marrow and re-establish normal hematopoiesis in the child.

HSCT is used to treat a variety of childhood cancers, including leukemia, lymphoma, brain tumours, neuroblastoma, and other solid tumours. It is an important treatment modality for children with aggressive malignancies in first remission or those who have recurrent disease (Norville & Tomlinson, 2010). HSCT is not the first line of treatment for most pediatric cancers, but it is used for refractory or advanced disease.

Autologous HSCT is achieved through harvest and treatment of the child's own bone marrow, followed by infusion of the treated stem cells. Autologous transplants are used to provide stem cell rescue after higher doses of chemotherapy or radiation therapy (Norville & Tomlinson, 2010). Risk for relapse of the original disease is highest in autologous HSCT. Allogenic HSCT refers to transplantation using stem cells from another individual that are harvested from the bone marrow, peripheral blood, or umbilical cord blood. Allogenic transplants are used when the hematopoietic stem cells are diseased (e.g., leukemia), damaged, or absent (Norville & Tomlinson, 2010). Syngeneic HSCT is a specific type of allogenic transplant in which stem cells are harvested from a donor who is an identical twin of the recipient (Norville & Tomlinson, 2010).

Allogenic HSCT requires human leukocyte antigen (HLA) matching (also known as tissue typing) for antigen-specific sites on the leukocytes. Closely matched HLA donors may be difficult to find from a donor listing, and sibling donors are often the closest match. The degree of match is inversely related to the risk for graft rejection and the development of graft-versus-host disease (GvHD). In other words, the lesser the degree of HLA matching in the donor, the higher the risk for graft rejection and GvHD. Steroids are beneficial to help prevent GvHD (Rimkus, 2009).

In addition to graft rejection and GvHD, additional initial complications of HSCT are infection, electrolyte imbalance, bleeding, and organ, skin, and mucous membrane toxicities. Long-term complications include impaired growth and fertility related to endocrine dysfunction, developmental delay, cataracts, pulmonary and cardiac disease, avascular necrosis of the bone, and the development of secondary malignancies. One of the major causes of mortality following HSCT is veno-occlusive disease (VOD). VOD occurs in 10% to 20% of transplant cases and, when severe, carries a mortality risk over 80% (Coppell, Richardson, Soiffer, et al., 2010).

NURSING PROCESS OVERVIEW FOR THE CHILD WITH A NEOPLASTIC DISORDER

Care of the child with a neoplastic disorder includes assessment, nursing diagnosis, planning, interventions, and evaluation. There are a number of general concepts related to the nursing process that may be applied to cancers in children. From a general understanding of the care involved for a child with cancer, the nurse can then individualize the care based on patient specifics. Children with cancer often suffer many physical effects as a result of the disease and its treatment. The nurse must be diligent when assessing for these effects and should involve the parents as a reliable source for reporting the child's physical symptoms.

Assessment

Assessment of children with neoplastic disorders includes health history, physical examination, and laboratory and diagnostic testing.

Remember John, the 4-year-old with fever, fatigue, and headaches? What additional health history and physical examination assessment information should you obtain?

Health History

Determine current health history. Note history of recurrent fever or frequent infections. Inquire about bleeding tendencies, such as unusual bruising or petechiae. Note early-morning headache with nausea or vomiting, gait or behaviour changes, or visual disturbances. Inquire about changes in bowel or bladder habits or decrease in appetite. Note history of bone fractures unrelated to trauma. Explore the health history for the presence of risk factors such as previous malignancy and treatment; synthetic chemical exposures; parental exposure to radiation, chemicals, or chemotherapeutic agents; and a family history of malignancy (especially childhood), immune disorder, or genetic disorders such as neurofibromatosis or Down syndrome.

Physical Examination

A complete physical examination should be performed on any child with or suspected of having cancer. Note particular findings as discussed below.

Inspection and Observation

Observe the child's overall appearance and energy level. Note thin, frail appearance, fatigue, or altered level of consciousness. Document visible masses or asymmetry of the face, thorax, abdomen, or extremities. Note difficulty breathing. Inspect the skin for pallor, bruising, or petechiae. Examine the oral cavity for bleeding gums or pale mucous membranes. Observe the child's gait, noting ataxia or limp. Note rectal bleeding or vaginal discharge.

Auscultation, Percussion, and Palpation

Auscultate the heart, lungs, and abdomen, noting any abnormalities. Percuss the abdomen, noting dullness over a mass if present. Palpate for lymphadenopathy; in particular, note nontender or firm lymph nodes. Palpate any unusual area of swelling anywhere on the body, noting size and absence of tenderness. Palpate the abdomen, noting organomegaly or presence of a mass. Note limited range of motion or pain upon palpation of extremities.

Psychosocial Assessment

Assess the child's and family's psychosocial status, using open-ended questions. It is particularly important to determine the child's self-esteem, level of anxiety or stress, and coping mechanisms. Determine the spiritual status of the child and family. Ongoing medical procedures and the fear of dying take a toll on the child and family. Ask the child how things are going at home; how does he or she get along with brothers, sisters, and parents? If the child is school age, ask how school is going. Does the child have friends that he or she gets to spend time with? Ask the child what he or she does during spare time; are there any hobbies? These types of queries will provide the nurse with information about how well the child is coping.

Assess the parents' status as well. Ask about the marital relationship and how the other children are doing. Determine whether certain stressors may need to be addressed.

Laboratory and Diagnostic Testing

Common Laboratory and Diagnostic Tests 49.1 explains the laboratory and diagnostic tests most commonly used for neoplastic disorders. The tests can assist the physician in diagnosing the disorder or can be used as guidelines in determining treatment. Laboratory or non-nursing personnel conduct some of the tests, while the nurse might conduct others. In either instance the nurse should be familiar with how the tests are conducted, what they are used for, and normal versus abnormal results. This knowledge will also be necessary when providing patient and family education about the testing.

Nursing Diagnosis, Goals, Interventions, and Evaluation

Upon completion of a thorough assessment, the nurse might identify several nursing diagnoses, including:

• Risk for infection
• Pain
• Impaired oral mucous membranes
• Nausea
• Imbalanced nutrition
• Constipation
• Diarrhea
• Risk for impaired skin integrity
• Activity intolerance
• Disturbed body image
• Situational low self-esteem
• Compromised family coping
• Anticipatory grieving

After completing an assessment of John, you note the following: history of recurrent infections, unusual bruising, and enlarged lymph nodes. Based on the assessment findings, what would your top three prioritized nursing diagnoses be for John?

Nursing goals, interventions, and evaluation for the child with cancer are based on the nursing diagnoses. Nursing Care Plan 49.1 may be used as a guide in planning nursing care for the child with a neoplastic disorder. The care plan includes many nursing diagnoses that are applicable to the child or adolescent, but not all children will have the same effects from cancer and its treatment. Nursing care should be individualized based on the child's and family's responses to illness. Additional information about nursing management related to specific types of cancer will be included later in the chapter as it relates to specific disorders.

(text continues on page 1701)

COMMON LABORATORY AND DIAGNOSTIC TESTS 49.1

Test	Explanation	Indication	Nursing Implications
Complete blood count (CBC) with differential	Evaluate hemoglobin and hematocrit, WBC count (particularly the percentage of individual WBCs), and platelet count	Infection, immunosuppression, to determine neutropenia in myelosuppression	Normal values vary according to age and gender. WBC count differential is helpful in evaluating source of infection. May be affected by myelosuppressive drugs.
Alpha-fetoprotein (AFP)	Produced by the fetal liver and yolk sac; normally decreases to very low levels by 1 year of age	May be elevated in Hodgkin's disease and other cancers. Used to determine tumour burden.	No food or fluid restriction required
Urine catecholamines	Catabolism of catecholamines causes elevated levels in urine.	Diagnosis of neuroblastoma (produces catecholamines)	24-hour urine collection. Levels may be altered with certain foods and drugs or vigorous exercise.
Chest X-ray	Radiograph of the chest	Identify tumour or metastasis in the thorax	Chest must be held stationary for a brief time.
Computed tomography (CT)	Multiple films taken in successive layers to provide a 3D view of the body part being scanned	Identify tumour location or metastasis	Some CT scans are done with oral or IV contrast (notify physician if child has iodine or shellfish allergy). May require a several-hour period of NPO if contrast is used (contrast may cause nausea). Encourage fluid intake after scan to facilitate excretion of contrast dye.
Magnetic resonance imaging (MRI)	Based on how hydrogen atoms behave in a magnetic field when disturbed by radio-frequency signals. Does not require ionizing radiation. Provides a 3D view of the body part being scanned.	Identify extent of tumour or metastatic spread	Remove all metal objects from the child. Child must remain motionless for entire scan; parent can stay in room with child. Younger children will require sedation to keep still. A loud thumping sound occurs inside the machine during the scan procedure; this can be frightening to children.
Bone scan	Administration of IV radionuclide material, which is taken up by the bone and is visible on the scans	Identifies metastasis to bone	Requires patent IV for injection. Encourage fluid intake after injection to increase uptake of injected radionuclide. Scan will be performed 1–3 h after injection.
Ultrasound	High-frequency sound waves are directed at internal organs and structures, and an image is made of the waves as they are reflected back through the tissues.	Identify tumour presence, especially in abdomen or on kidney	Fasting for a few hours may be required when certain organs are to be visualized.

(continued)

COMMON LABORATORY AND DIAGNOSTIC TESTS 49.1 (continued)

Test	Explanation	Indication	Nursing Implications
Bone marrow aspiration and biopsy	A needle is inserted through the cortex of the bone into the bone marrow (most often the iliac spine), bone marrow is aspirated, and the cells are evaluated.	Evaluation for leukemia or metastasis of other cancers to bone marrow	Use EMLA or lidocaine to decrease pain with procedure. Often performed under conscious sedation. Apply a pressure dressing to arrest bleeding. Assess for tenderness or erythema. May require mild analgesia for postprocedure pain.
Lumbar puncture (LP)	A needle is placed in the subarachnoid space of the spinal column, below the base of the cord, and cerebrospinal fluid is withdrawn for analysis.	Evaluation of tumour or metastasis to brain or spinal cord. Also used to administer intrathecal medications.	Use EMLA before the procedure to decrease pain. May be performed under conscious sedation. Position child appropriately. Use distraction techniques in the older child or teen. Encourage child to recline for up to 12 h after LP.

Adapted from: Pagana, K. D., & Pagana, T. J. (2010). *Mosby's manual of diagnostic and laboratory tests* (4th ed.). St. Louis, MO: Mosby.

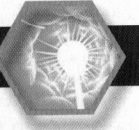

Nursing Care Plan 49.1

OVERVIEW FOR THE CHILD WITH A NEOPLASTIC DISORDER

NURSING DIAGNOSIS: Risk for infection related to neutropenia and immunosuppression

Outcome Identification and Evaluation
Child will not experience overwhelming infection; *will be free from infection or able to recover if becomes infected.*

Interventions: Preventing Infection
- Assess for fever, pain, cough, tachypnea, adventitious breath sounds, skin ulceration, stomatitis, and perirectal fissures *to identify potential infection.*
- Administer antibiotics for temperature >38.4 °C *to decrease likelihood of overwhelming sepsis.*
- Maintain meticulous handwashing procedures (include family, visitors, staff) *to minimize spread of infectious organisms.*
- Maintain isolation as prescribed *to minimize exposure to infectious organisms.*
- Avoid rectal temperatures and examinations, intramuscular injections, and urinary catheterization when child is neutropenic *to decrease possibility of introducing microorganisms.*
- Educate family and visitors that child should be restricted from contact with known infectious exposures (in hospital and at home) *to encourage cooperation with infection control.*
- Strictly observe medical asepsis *to avoid unintentional introduction of microorganisms.*
- Promote nutrition and appropriate rest *to maximize body's potential to heal.*
- Inform family to contact provider if child has known exposure to chickenpox or measles *so that preventive measures (e.g., VZIG) can be taken.*
- Administer vaccines (not live) as prescribed (after clearance with oncologist) *to prevent common childhood communicable diseases.*
- Teach family to monitor for fever at home and report temperature elevations to oncologist immediately *so that antibiotic therapy may be instituted as soon as possible.*

Nursing Care Plan 49.1 (continued)

NURSING DIAGNOSIS: Pain related to invasive diagnostic testing, surgical procedure, neuropathy, disease progression, or adverse effects of treatment as evidenced by verbalization of pain, elevated pain scale ratings, guarding, withdrawal from play or refusal to participate in activities of daily living, or physiologic indicators such as elevated heart rate, diaphoresis, muscle tension or rigidity

Outcome Identification and Evaluation
Child will demonstrate pain relief, *in amount sufficient to allow participation in play, activities of daily living, or therapeutic interventions. Use the age-appropriate pain scale to set the goal and set a time frame for achievement of the goal.*

Interventions: Promoting Comfort
• Determine level of pain using child interview, pain scale, and assessment of physiologic variables *to determine baseline.*
• Document location, intensity, description of pain *to determine baseline.*
• Discuss with the child and parent techniques that have helped alleviate pain in the past *to incorporate successful interventions into the plan of care.*
• Administer acetaminophen for mild pain *(avoid salicylate and nonsteroidal anti-inflammatory drugs due to increased risk for bleeding).*
• Administer medications as ordered *using the least invasive method possible to avoid pain (intramuscular, subcutaneous, and rectal route should be avoided in the child with thrombocytopenia).*
• Monitor frequently for adverse effects (particularly respiratory effects) of opioid analgesics, *as opioids reduce responsiveness of carbon dioxide receptors in the brain's respiratory centre.*
• Use non-pharmacologic measures such as play therapy, games, TV, guided breathing, imagery, hypnosis, or meditation as appropriate *(distracts child's attention from the pain).*
• Use massage, positioning, or heat *to relieve pain in a particular area.*
• Use EMLA before needle sticks and conscious sedation with lumbar puncture and bone marrow aspiration *to reduce recurrent acute painful episodes associated with frequent blood draws and diagnostic/treatment procedures.*
• Have the child lie flat for 30 minutes after a lumbar puncture and increase fluid intake for 24 hours after the procedure *to decrease incidence of headache.*

NURSING DIAGNOSIS: Impaired oral mucous membranes related to chemotherapy, radiation therapy, immunocompromise, decreased platelet count, malnutrition, or dehydration as evidenced by oral lesions, ulcers, plaques, hyperemia or bleeding, difficulty eating or swallowing, or complaint of oral discomfort

Outcome Identification and Evaluation
Child will maintain intact, moist mucosa, *free from redness, ulceration, or debris.*

Interventions: Restoring Healthy Oral Mucosa
• Frequently assess oral cavity for redness, lesions, ulcers, plaques, or bleeding *to provide baseline for comparison and identify alterations early.*
• Offer ice chips frequently while NPO *to maintain hydration of mucosa.*
• Use only a soft toothbrush or toothette for dental care, avoiding excessive pressure with brushing, *to decrease incidence of bleeding with mouth care.*
• Keep lips lubricated with petroleum jelly or fragrance-free lip balm *to maintain moist, hydrated lips.*
• Rinse with salt solution or mouthwash every 1 to 2 hours *to keep oral cavity clean and moist.*
• Administer glutamine and/or beta-carotene supplements, *which have been shown to decrease the incidence and severity of mucositis.*
• Have child swish and spit 1:1 Benadryl/Maalox solution *to decrease pain.*
• Administer antifungal solution *to prevent or treat oral candidiasis.*
• Avoid spicy, acidic, or very hot or very cold foods *to decrease pain.*
• Administer pain medication (usually acetaminophen or codeine) as ordered *to decrease pain.*

(continued)

Nursing Care Plan 49.1 (continued)

NURSING DIAGNOSIS: Nausea related to adverse effects of chemotherapy or radiation therapy as evidenced by verbalization of nausea, increased salivation, swallowing movements, or vomiting

Outcome Identification and Evaluation
Child will experience decreased nausea, *will verbalize symptom relief and will be free from vomiting.*

Interventions: Alleviating Nausea and Vomiting
* Administer antiemetics prior to chemotherapy and as needed thereafter *to decrease frequency of nausea.*
* Assess frequency of vomiting and level of hydration *to provide baseline data and recognize alterations early.*
* Offer frequent, smaller meals or snacks; *smaller amounts are less likely to be vomited.*
* Avoid spicy foods *to avoid stomach upset.*
* Allow bubbles to dissipate from carbonated beverages before they are ingested *(carbonation may contribute to nausea).*
* Remove cover from meal tray before entering child's room *(this will allow the food odour to dissipate outside of the room; food odours may trigger nausea and vomiting).*

NURSING DIAGNOSIS: Imbalanced nutrition: Less than body requirements related to anorexia, nausea, vomiting, or mucosal irritation associated with chemotherapy or radiation as evidenced by decreased oral intake and weight, length/height, and/or BMI below average for age or individual child's usual measures

Outcome Identification and Evaluation
Child will improve nutritional intake, resulting in *steady increase in weight and length/height.*

Interventions: Promoting Adequate Nutrition
* Determine body weight and length/height norm for age or find out what the child's pretreatment measurements were *to determine goal to work toward.*
* Determine child's food preferences and provide favourite foods as able *to increase the likelihood that the child will consume adequate amounts of foods.*
* Administer antiemetics as ordered *to increase the likelihood that the child will retain the food he or she ingests.*
* Weigh child daily or weekly (according to physician order or institutional standard) and measure length/height weekly *to monitor for growth.*
* Offer highest-calorie meals at the time of day when the child's appetite is the greatest *(to increase likelihood of increased caloric intake).*
* Provide increased-calorie shakes or puddings within diet restriction *(high-calorie foods increase weight gain).*
* Administer vitamin and mineral supplements as prescribed *to attain/maintain vitamin and mineral balance in the body.*
* Administer total parenteral nutrition and intravenous lipids as ordered *to provide adequate nutrition for healing.*

NURSING DIAGNOSIS: Constipation related to effects of vinca alkaloids, opioid use, decreased activity, and dietary changes as evidenced by hard stool or stool that is difficult to pass

Outcome Identification and Evaluation
Child's bowel function will return to usual pattern, *child will pass a formed, soft stool every day (or modify this criterion according to child's usual pattern).*

Interventions: Preventing or Managing Constipation
* Ensure that child increases fluid intake *to provide enough water in the intestines for soft stool formation.*
* Increase fibre in the diet *to provide bulk for stool formation.*
* Administer stool softeners such as mineral oil, docusate sodium; *these help soften the stool, aiding in passage.*
* Provide motivator laxatives such as magnesium hydroxide, lactulose, or sorbitol *to stimulate stool passage.*
* Use stimulant laxatives such as senna or bisacodyl only intermittently rather than on a daily basis *to avoid dependency and diarrhea.*

Nursing Care Plan 49.1 (continued)

NURSING DIAGNOSIS: Diarrhea related to effects of radiation therapy as evidenced by loose or watery stools, possibly frequent

Outcome Identification and Evaluation
Child's bowel function will return to usual pattern, *child will pass a formed, soft stool daily (or modify this criterion according to child's usual pattern).*

Interventions: Managing Diarrhea
- Assess frequency of diarrhea and level of hydration *to provide data about severity.*
- Obtain weight daily on same scale *to determine extent of fluid loss.*
- Maintain accurate intake and output records *to determine extent of fluid loss.*
- Administer oral rehydration solutions or intravenous fluids as ordered *to maintain or restore adequate hydration.*
- Restrict roughage and residue in diet *to decrease likelihood of diarrhea.*
- Avoid milk products during acute diarrheal phase *(lactose often worsens diarrhea).*
- Provide an elemental diet to relieve symptoms *(absorbed in the upper small bowel).*
- Provide meticulous perineal care *to avoid skin breakdown related to frequent or loose stools.*
- Administer antidiarrheal medications if ordered *to decrease frequency of stools.*
- If severe and related to radiation therapy, may require a 3- to 4-day rest period from radiation *to begin recovery of normal absorptive capabilities of bowel.*

NURSING DIAGNOSIS: Risk for impaired skin integrity related to radiation therapy

Outcome Identification and Evaluation
Child's skin will remain intact, *areas of redness in radiation field will not progress to desquamation.*

Interventions: Promoting Skin Integrity
- Assess skin frequently for erythema, erosions, ulcers, or blisters *to provide baseline data and intervene early if skin is impaired.*
- Use a mild soap for cleansing and pat dry rather than rubbing *to avoid skin irritation.*
- Use aloe vera lotion *to moisturize the skin.*
- Avoid perfumed lotions, soaps, heat, cold, or sun, *as these will further irritate the skin in the irradiated area.*
- Do not scrub ink from marked radiation field, and avoid adhesive tape in that area, *to avoid further skin irritation.*
- Administer diphenhydramine or apply hydrocortisone 1% cream *to reduce itching and urge to scratch.*
- For areas of desquamation related to radiation, apply Silvadene cream once or twice a day *to hasten skin repair.*

NURSING DIAGNOSIS: Activity intolerance related to treatment adverse effects, anemia, or generalized weakness as evidenced by verbalization of weakness or fatigue, elevation of heart rate, respiratory rate, or blood pressure with activity, complaint of shortness of breath with play or activity

Outcome Identification and Evaluation
Child will display increased activity tolerance, *desire to play without developing symptoms of exertion.*

Interventions: Promoting Activity
- Encourage activity or ambulation per physician's orders; *early mobilization results in better outcomes.*
- Observe child for symptoms of activity intolerance such as pallor, nausea, lightheadedness or dizziness, or changes in vital signs *to determine level of tolerance.*
- If child is on bed rest, perform range-of-motion exercises and frequent position changes: *Negative changes to the musculo-skeletal system occur quickly with inactivity and immobility.*
- Cluster nursing care activities and plan for periods of rest before and after exertion *to decrease oxygen need and consumption.*
- Refer the child to physical therapy *for exercise prescription to increase skeletal muscle strength.*

(continued)

Nursing Care Plan 49.1 (continued)

NURSING DIAGNOSIS: Disturbed body image related to hair loss as evidenced by verbalization of dissatisfaction with appearance

Outcome Identification and Evaluation
Child or adolescent will display appropriate body image, *will look at self in mirror and participate in social activities.*

Interventions: Promoting Body Image
- Acknowledge child's feelings of anger over body changes and illness; *venting feelings is associated with less body image disturbance.*
- Encourage the child or teen to choose a wig or hats and scarves *to involve the child in making decisions about appearance.*
- Support the child's or teen's choices of comfortable, fashionable clothing *to disguise weight loss or scarring while promoting self-esteem.*
- Involve the child in the decision-making process, *as a sense of control will improve body image.*
- Encourage the child to spend time with peers who have experienced hair, limb, or weight loss, *as peers' opinions are often better accepted than those of persons in authority, such as parents or health care professionals.*

NURSING DIAGNOSIS: Risk for situational low self-esteem related to loss of control and inability to progress with quest for independence (adolescents)

Outcome Identification and Evaluation
Adolescent will maintain or increase self-esteem, *will display increased coping responses and verbalize control as appropriate as well as discuss plans for future.*

Interventions: Promoting Self-Esteem
- Identify the adolescent's positive abilities *to promote self-esteem.*
- Give genuine and honest positive feedback, *as the child or adolescent desires honesty.*
- Explore strengths and weaknesses with the adolescent: *Helps the teen to see similarities and differences with healthy peers of the same age.*
- Encourage the teen to perform self-care as possible *to promote independence.*
- Offer emotional support *(reduces psychological distress and increases coping abilities).*
- Encourage participation in a support group *to allow teens to discuss body changes and the reactions they perceive in others.*
- When the adolescent is physically able, encourage attendance at camp or an adventure/wilderness event *(these programs have been shown to improve mental health and coping skills).*

NURSING DIAGNOSIS: Compromised family coping related to potentially life-threatening illness and stressors involved with cancer treatment

Outcome Identification and Evaluation
Child and/or family will demonstrate adequate coping skills, *will verbalize feeling supported and demonstrate healthy family interactions.*

Interventions: Promoting Child and Family Coping
- Provide emotional support to child and family *(improves coping abilities).*
- Actively listen to the child's and family's concerns *(validates their feelings, establishes trust).*
- Provide open communication with the child and siblings; *children appreciate honesty about their illness, and coping is improved.*
- Refer families to community resources such as parent support groups and grief counselling *(such support improves coping abilities).*
- Give terminally ill children the permission to discuss their feelings about their illness, *allowing them to conquer fears and express love for their family and friends.*
- Encourage families to be honest with siblings about the treatment and prognosis of the child with cancer *(children often sense what is going on and cope better when they are prepared and are given an honest explanation of events).*
- Prepare siblings for the death of the child with cancer, using the child life specialist and chaplain as necessary: *The bereavement period is eased when siblings are prepared.*

Nursing Care Plan 49.1 (continued)

NURSING DIAGNOSIS: Anticipatory grieving (family) related to diagnosis of cancer in a child and impending loss of child as evidenced by crying, disbelief of diagnosis, and expressions of grief

Outcome Identification and Evaluation
Family will express feelings of grief; *seek help in dealing with feelings, plan for future one day at the time.*

Intervention: Supporting the Grieving Family
- Use therapeutic communication with open-ended questions *to encourage an open and trusting relationship for better communication.*
- Actively listen to family's expression of grief; *just being present and listening conveys support.*
- Encourage the family to cry and express feelings away from the child *to work through feelings while not upsetting the child.*
- Assess for spiritual distress *and refer the family to the hospital chaplain or clergy of choice for support.*
- Educate the family about the child's condition: *Knowing what is going on, what is to be expected, and what the treatment plan is gives the family a sense of control.*
- Support the family through discussions with the child about anticipated death *when the illness is deemed terminal.*

Adapted from: Axton, S. E. & Fugate, T. (2009). *Pediatric nursing care plans for the hospitalized child* (3rd ed.). Upper Saddle River, NJ: Pearson; Baggott, C. (2010). Cancer. In P. J. Allen, J. A. Vessey, & N. A. Schapiro (Eds.), *Primary care of the child with a chronic condition* (5th ed.). St. Louis, MO: Mosby; Carpenito-Moyet, L. J. (2010). Nursing diagnosis: Application to clinical practice (13th ed.). Philadelphia: Lippincott Williams & Wilkins; and Tomlinson, D., & Kline, N. E. (Eds.). (2010). *Pediatric oncology nursing.* New York: Springer.

Provide education to families of all children with cancer as outlined in Teaching Guideline 49.1.

Based on your top three nursing diagnoses for John, describe appropriate nursing interventions.

Administering Chemotherapy
All chemotherapy medications have the potential to cause toxicities in the child as well as the persons handling or preparing the medication. General guidelines related to the preparation and administration of chemotherapy include the following:

- Chemotherapy should be prepared and administered only by specially trained personnel.
- Personal protective equipment (PPE) in the form of double gloves and nonpermeable gowns should be worn when preparing or administering chemotherapy. If splashing is possible or a spill occurs, then a face shield and/or mask may also be necessary.
- Dispose of all equipment used in chemotherapy preparation and administration in a puncture-resistant container (Chordas & Graham, 2010).

It is critical to calculate the chemotherapy dose correctly. Chemotherapy medication doses in children are based on body surface area (BSA) (Chordas & Graham, 2010). A nomogram is a commonly used device for determining BSA. To use the nomogram, draw a straight line between the child's height on the left and the child's

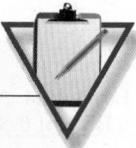

TEACHING GUIDELINE 49.1

Education for Families of Children with Cancer

- Obtain a printed or written copy of the child's treatment plan.
- Keep a calendar of all appointment times, blood count lab draw days, and phone numbers of all physicians, homecare companies, laboratory, and hospital.
- Seek medical care immediately if the child's temperature is 38.3°C (101°F) or higher.
- Call the oncologist or seek medical care if any of the following occur:
  - Cough or rapid breathing
  - Increased bruising, bleeding or petechiae, pallor or increased levels of fatigue
  - Earache, sore throat, nuchal rigidity
  - Blisters, rashes, ulcers
  - Red, irritated skin on the child's buttocks
  - Abdominal pain, difficulty or pain with eating, drinking, or swallowing
  - Constipation or diarrhea
  - For children with central venous catheters:
    - Pus, redness, or swelling at the site
    - Breakage of the catheter
  - Do not give the child aspirin.

From: Baggott, C. R., Kelly, K. P., Fochtman, D., & Foley, G. V. (Eds.) (in press). *Nursing care of children and adolescents with cancer* (4th ed.). Glenview, IL: The Association of Pediatric Hematology Oncology Nurses.

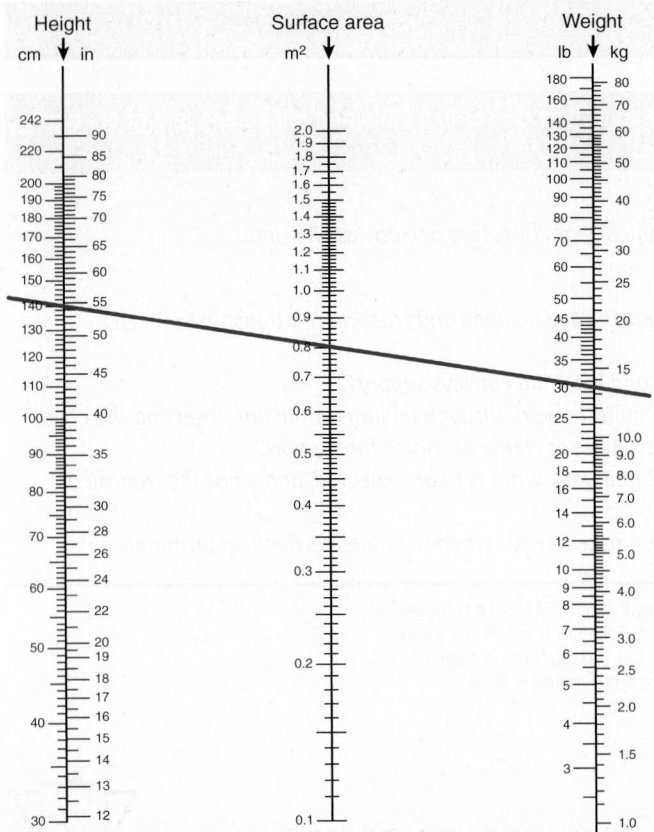

FIGURE **49.4** A child who weighs 13.2 kg and is 140 cm tall has a BSA of 0.80 m².

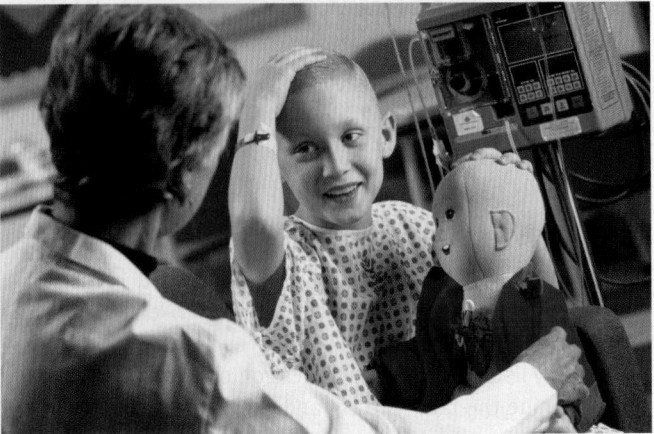

FIGURE **49.5** Chemotherapy often causes alopecia.

▶ *Take* NOTE!

Cooling the scalp during chemotherapy administration with the use of a cooling cap may decrease hair loss (Nathan & Tomlinson, 2010).

weight on the right. The point at which the straight line crosses the centre is the child's BSA expressed in metres squared (Fig. 49.4).

An alternative to using the nomogram is to use the following formula: BSA (m²) = the square root of (height [in centimetres] × weight [in kilograms] divided by 3,600). For example, for a child 140 cm tall and weighing 30 kg: 140 × 30 = 4,200; 4,200/3,600 = 1.167; and the square root of 1.167 is 1.08. The BSA would be 1.08.

Managing Adverse Effects of Chemotherapy

Chemotherapy can result in multiple adverse effects. Myelosuppression leads to low blood counts in all cell lines, placing the child at risk for infection, hemorrhage, and anemia (Baggott, Dodd, Kennedy, et al., 2010). Nausea, vomiting, and anorexia may hinder the child's growth. Alopecia and facial changes may affect the child's self-esteem (Fig. 49.5). Nursing interventions related to the effects of myelosuppression, nausea, vomiting, and anorexia are discussed below. Refer to Nursing Care Plan 49.1 for nursing interventions related to altered body image.

Preventing Infection

Many chemotherapeutic drugs cause significant bone marrow suppression and decreased amounts of circulating mature neutrophils ("segs" or segmented neutrophils). Administer granulocyte colony-stimulating factor (GCSF) as ordered to promote neutrophil growth and maturation (Nixon, 2010). Administer varicella zoster immunoglobulin (VZIG) within 72 hours of exposure to active chickenpox (Doyle, 2010). If the child is actively infected with chickenpox, administer intravenous acyclovir as ordered. Children receiving treatment for acute lymphoblastic leukemia (ALL) are at risk for opportunistic infection with *Pneumocystis jiroveci*, as most children are colonized with this fungus (Doyle, 2010). Administer prophylactic antibiotics as ordered and teach the parents to administer them at home. Teaching Guideline 49.2 gives further information about infection prevention at home.

As neutrophils are the primary means of fighting bacterial infection, when the neutrophil count is low, the chance of developing an overwhelming bacterial infection is high (Doyle, 2010). An absolute neutrophil count (ANC) below 500 places the child at greatest risk, although an ANC below 1,500 usually warrants evaluation. Depending on institutional policy, precautions for neutropenia will be followed if the ANC is depressed. Precautions related to neutropenia generally include:

- Perform hand hygiene before and after each patient contact.
- Place the child in a private room.

TEACHING GUIDELINE 49.2

Prevention of Infection in Children Receiving Chemotherapy for Cancer

- Practice meticulous hygiene (oral, personal, perianal).
- Avoid known ill contacts, especially persons with chickenpox.
- Immediately notify physician if exposed to chickenpox.
- Avoid crowded areas.
- Do not let the child receive live vaccines.
- Do not take the child's temperature rectally or give medications by the rectal route.
- Administer twice-daily trimethoprim–sulfamethoxazole for three consecutive days each week as ordered for prevention of *Pneumocystis* pneumonia.

Adapted from: Baggott, C. (2010). Cancer. In P. J. Allen, J. A. Vessey, & N. A. Schapiro (Eds.), *Primary care of the child with a chronic condition* (5th ed.). St. Louis, MO: Mosby; and Tomlinson, D., & Kline, N. E. (Eds.). (2010). *Pediatric oncology nursing.* New York: Springer.

- Monitor vital signs every 4 hours.
- Assess for signs and symptoms of infection at least every 8 hours.
- Avoid rectal suppositories, enemas, or examinations; urinary catheterization; and invasive procedures.
- Restrict visitors with fever, cough, or other signs/ symptoms of infection.
- Do not permit raw fruits or vegetables or fresh flowers or live plants in the room.
- Place a mask on the patient when he or she is being transported outside of the room.
- Perform dental care with a soft toothbrush if the platelet count is adequate (Doyle, 2010; Selwood, 2008).

Children with neutropenia and fever must be started on intravenous broad-spectrum antibiotics without delay to avoid overwhelming sepsis.

Preventing Hemorrhage

Assess for petechiae, purpura, bruising, or bleeding. Determine changes from baseline that warrant intervention. Encourage quiet activities or play to avoid trauma. Avoid rectal temperatures and examinations to avoid rectal mucosal damage that results in bleeding. Post a sign at the head of the bed stating "no rectal temperatures or medications." Avoid intramuscular injections and lumbar puncture if possible to decrease the risk of bleeding from a puncture site. If bone marrow aspiration must be performed, apply a pressure dressing to the site to prevent bleeding.

For active or uncontrolled bleeding, transfuse platelets as ordered to control bleeding (Nixon, 2010).

Preventing Anemia

To maintain blood volume, limit blood draws to the minimum volume required. Encourage the child to eat an appropriate diet that includes adequate iron. Administer erythropoietin injections as ordered. Teach families to give the injections at home if prescribed (Doyle, 2010).

Managing Nausea, Vomiting, and Anorexia

Many chemotherapeutic drugs produce the adverse effect of nausea and vomiting (Selwood, 2008). The cycle of nausea, vomiting, and anorexia is difficult to break once it begins. Prevent nausea by administering antiemetics prior to chemotherapy administration and on a routine schedule around the clock for the first 1 to 2 days rather than on an as-needed (PRN) basis. Bright lights and noise may worsen nausea, so the child's environment should be dimly lit and calm. Relaxation therapy and guided imagery may also be helpful in preventing or treating nausea and vomiting. Refer to Nursing Care Plan 49.1 for additional interventions.

Taste alterations are common in children who have received chemotherapy (Selwood, 2008). During or after chemotherapy, children may develop an aversion to a food that was previously their favourite (Rodgers & Gonzalez, 2010).

▶ **Take** NOTE!

Ginger capsules, ginger tea, and candied ginger have been used as a nausea remedy for centuries. (Ginger ale is usually artificially flavoured, so it would not have the same effect.) Though ginger is considered safe, instruct families to check with the oncologist before using this remedy.

▶ **Take** NOTE!

Preliminary research suggests that massage therapy may help patients cope with side effects associated with chemotherapy, including nausea and pain (Post-White & Ladas, 2010).

Monitoring the Child Receiving Radiation Therapy

Radiation causes damage to the cells in a localized area, which may include normal cells in addition to the cancerous ones (Loch & Khorrami, 2010). Assess the child's skin daily, particularly at the treatment site. Provide good hygiene, but do so gently. Encourage moisture retention in the skin by applying aqueous creams or moisturizers. Do not apply deodorants or perfumed lotions on the radiation treatment site. Avoid the use of heat or ice packs at the site. Instruct the child and family that clothing should fit loosely so as not to irritate the site. During and for 8 weeks after the radiation treatment, the skin will be more photosensitive. Protect the skin with a high-SPF sunscreen.

Providing Care to the Child Undergoing Stem Cell Transplantation

Stem cell transplantation is performed at limited specialty centres in Canada, and special training is required for all personnel caring for the transplanted child. The intent of this discussion is to provide only a brief introduction and overview of nursing management related to HSCT.

Care may be divided into three phases: the pre-transplant phase, the post-transplant phase, and the lengthy supportive care phase. Nursing management of each phase is briefly discussed below.

Pre-Transplant Phase

In the pre-transplant phase, the child is being prepared to receive the transplant (Bennett-Rees, Hopkins, & Stone, 2008). The child's own bone marrow cells are eradicated through high-dose chemotherapy and total body irradiation. This phase usually occurs over 7 to 10 days. The child will be hospitalized because he or she is at extreme risk for serious infection. Maintain protective isolation in a positive-pressure room and limit visitors. Administer gammaglobulin, acyclovir, or antibiotics as ordered to prevent or treat infection. Lymphohematopoietic rescue occurs with infusion of the donor or autologous cells.

Post-Transplant Phase

The post-transplant phase is also a time of high risk for the child. Monitor closely for symptoms of GvHD, such as severe diarrhea and maculopapular rash progressing to redness or desquamation of the skin (especially palms or soles) (Fig. 49.6). If GvHD occurs, administer immunosuppressive drugs such as cyclosporine, tacrolimus, or mycophenolate (which place the child at further risk for infection) (Rimkus, 2009).

Supportive Care

During the supportive care phase, which lasts several months after the transplant, continue to monitor for and prevent infection. Administer packed red blood cells (RBCs) or platelets and GCSF as needed.

Families and children who undergo HSCT need prolonged and extensive emotional and psychosocial support. A medical social worker and psychologist or counsellor are usually members of the transplant team

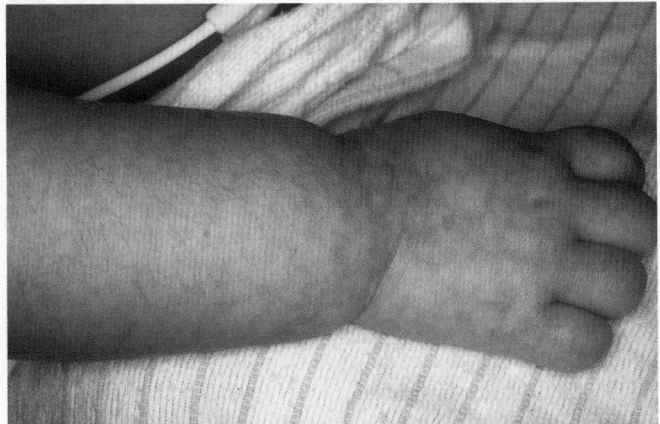

FIGURE 49.6 The first sign of GvHD may be a maculopapular rash.

and are excellent resources for these families' needs (Bennett-Rees & Hopkins, 2008).

Promoting a Normal Life

Children and teens want to be normal and to experience the things that other children their age do. The child should attend school when he or she is well enough and the white blood cell (WBC) counts are not dangerously low. Children, their families, and their teachers should be aware that cancer and its treatment can affect scholastic abilities (Woodgate et al., 2011).

▶ **Take** NOTE!

Childhood cancer survivors are at risk for late effects of treatment, including neurocognitive late effects (e.g., difficulties with thinking and reasoning) (Anderson & Kunin-Batson, 2009).

Maintain other activities if the child is able and if platelet counts are within normal limits. Special camps are available for children with cancer. These camps offer an opportunity for children and adolescents to experience a variety of activities safely and to network with youngsters who are experiencing similar physical and emotional challenges. The Children's Oncology Camping Association and the Candlelighter's Childhood Cancer Foundation provide lists of camps throughout Canada, the United States, and internationally for children and teens with cancer. The Canadian Association of Pediatric Oncology Camps provides information specific to camps located in Canada. Visit http://thePoint.lww.com/Chow1e for direct links to these organizations' websites.

Promoting Growth

Promote growth in children with cancer by encouraging an appropriate diet and preventing nausea and vomiting and also by addressing concerns such as diarrhea and constipation (Maloney, 2010; Rodgers & Gonzalez, 2010; Selwood, 2008). Chronic diarrhea related to radiation therapy may prevent the child from gaining weight and growing properly (see Nursing Care Plan 49.1). The use of vinca alkaloids and opioids, as well as the decreased activity level of the child with cancer, may contribute to constipation. Constipation increases the pain experience, contributes to the child's malaise, and decreases quality of life. It directly affects the child's ability to grow by increasing anorexia, nausea, and vomiting (Maloney, 2010). Nursing Care Plan 49.1 details interventions related to preventing and managing constipation.

Preventing and Treating Oncologic Emergencies

Oncologic emergencies may occur as an effect of the disease process itself or from cancer treatment (Selwood, 2008). As progress is made in chemotherapy and radiation treatment, children with cancer have an increased survival rate, but they still face the risk of developing an oncologic emergency. Nurses caring for children with cancer need to be familiar with signs and symptoms of oncologic emergencies as well as with their treatment. All of these problems warrant careful, frequent monitoring of respiratory, cardiovascular, neurologic, and renal status. Table 49.1 provides information about oncologic emergencies.

Caring for the Dying Child

Of the 850 children diagnosed with cancer annually in Canada, about 150 will die from the disease each year (Ellison et al., 2009). Advance care planning, which includes the process of discussing life-sustaining treatments and establishing long-term care goals, is an important part caring for the child with progressive cancer (CPS, 2008). When advance care planning is executed well, it is more likely that the shared goals of care will be aligned with the planned course of treatment. Part of the plans may include a "do not resuscitate" (DNR) order. Nurses serve as patient and family advocates, clarifying terminology and providing support as needed during the discussion of DNR orders and throughout the rest of the terminal phase.

Children with terminal cancer often experience a great deal of pain, particularly when death is imminent. Pain is often accompanied by agitation and dyspnea, which further contribute to the child's discomfort. Whether the child has a DNR order or the status remains that of "full code," pain management is central to the nursing care of the child who is dying from cancer. The Association of Pediatric Oncology Nurses' position paper entitled "Pain Management for the Child with Cancer in End-of-Life Care" outlines the following recommendations for managing children's pain at the end of life:

- Prevention and alleviation of pain is a primary goal of care for the child dying of cancer.
- Children and parents are equal partners with members of the health care team in managing the patient's pain.
- Children dying of cancer may require aggressive dosing of analgesics. Medications that do not have a dose maximum should be escalated, sometimes rapidly, to achieve adequate pain control or to maintain pain control when drug tolerance has occurred.
- The nurse's role in caring for children who are in pain at the end of life includes assessing pain, identifying expected outcomes, and planning, performing, and evaluating interventions (Hooke, Hellsten, Stutzer, et al., 2002).

Interventions related to pain management may be found in Nursing Care Plan 49.1. Further discussion related to care of the dying child is found in Chapter 33.

Leukemia

Leukemia is a neoplastic disease that affects blood-forming tissues of the bone marrow, lymph nodes, and spleen (Zupanec & Tomlinson, 2010). It is the most common malignancy that affects children, accounting for one third of childhood cancer diagnoses. Leukemia results from genetic mutations and transformation of a single early progenitor myeloid or lymphoid cell during blood cell maturation. Normally, lymphoid cells grow and develop into lymphocytes, and myeloid cells grow and develop into RBCs, granulocytes, monocytes, and platelets. Leukemia may develop at any time during the usual stages of normal lymphoid or myeloid development. In leukemia, there is an overproduction of immature WBCs that cannot function efficiently. These immature WBCs are referred to as "blasts," such as the myeloblasts, lymphoblasts, and monoblasts. An abnormal amount of immature WBCs decreases the space available for the production of other healthy blood cells. The blast cells can also enter the blood and may invade the CNS, testicles in males, bones, and other tissues or organs (Zupanec & Tomlinson, 2010).

Leukemia may be classified as acute or chronic, lymphocytic or myelogenous (Table 49.2). Acute leukemias are rapidly progressive diseases affecting the undifferentiated or immature cells; the result is cells without normal function. Chronic leukemias progress more slowly, permitting maturation and differentiation of cells so that they retain some of their normal function. Acute leukemias, including ALL and acute myelogenous leukemia (AML), account for about 95% of all cases of leukemia in children and adolescents (Zupanec & Tomlinson, 2010), so they are the focus of this discussion.

TABLE 49.1 **Oncologic Emergencies**

Emergency	Associated with	Signs and Symptoms	Laboratory or Diagnostic Test Findings	Management
Sepsis	Neutropenia resulting from bone marrow suppression due to chemotherapy	• Fever or low temperature • Respiratory distress • Poor perfusion • Altered level of consciousness	• ANC <500 • Positive blood culture • Increased BUN, creatinine, potassium, clotting times • Decreased platelet count • Metabolic acidosis	• Airway and ventilation maintenance • Fluid volume resuscitation • Inotropic support • Broad-spectrum antibiotics and antifungals • Dialysis if needed
Tumour lysis syndrome	Acute lymphoblastic leukemia, lymphoma, neuroblastoma	• Nausea, vomiting, diarrhea, anorexia • Lethargy • Increased heart rate and blood pressure • Decreased or absent urine output • Altered level of consciousness	• Hyperuricemia • Hyperkalemia • Hyperphosphatemia • Hypocalcemia • Hypoxia	• Prevent by giving allopurinol for several days prior to chemotherapy (also treat with allopurinol). • Double IV fluid maintenance • Sodium bicarbonate
Hyperleukocytosis	Leukemia with high WBC count	• Respiratory distress • Murmur, increased heart rate	• WBC count >100,000 • Hyperkalemia, hyperphosphatemia • Hyperuricemia • Decreased pH and bicarbonate	• Leukapheresis • Respiratory support • Double IV fluid maintenance with sodium bicarbonate added • Diuretics
Typhlitis (neutropenic enterocolitis)	Inflammatory process of GI tract occurring with induction phase of leukemia chemotherapy	• Acute abdominal pain • Nausea, vomiting • Bloody diarrhea and emesis • Fever • Anorexia	• X-ray kidneys, ureters, bladder: scarcity of bowel gas, possibly ileus • CT (abdominal): inflammation, bowel wall thickening, peritoneal fluid	• Bowel rest (NPO status) • IV nutrition • Assess for bowel perforation/shock. • Broad-spectrum antibiotics and antifungals • Comfort measures
Superior vena cava syndrome	Compression on the SVC by non-Hodgkin's lymphoma or other mediastinal mass, such as neuroblastoma	• Dyspnea and cyanosis • Large cervical lymph nodes • Wheezing, diminished breath sounds	• Chest X-ray or CT shows mediastinal mass. • Pleural effusion	• Intubation and ventilation • Comfort measures • Treat cause (usually surgical removal of mass).
Spinal cord compression	Tumour or metastasis compresses spinal cord	• Back, neck, or leg pain • Sensory or autonomic dysfunction • Extremity weakness or paralysis	• MRI reveals location of tumour or metastasis to epidural space.	• Dexamethasone • Careful assessment • Radiation therapy • Comfort measures

Emergency	Associated with	Signs and Symptoms	Laboratory or Diagnostic Test Findings	Management
Increased intracranial pressure	Brain tumour or metastasis to brain causing compression of brain; may result in herniation	• Headache, visual disturbances • Morning vomiting • Infants: increased head circumference • Altered level of consciousness • Cushing's triad • Seizure activity	• Head CT or MRI reveals extent of mass.	• Frequent, careful neurologic assessment • Limit fluids. • Dexamethasone • Anticonvulsants • Tumour resection, radiation, or chemotherapy • Comfort measures
Massive hepatomegaly	Obstruction caused by neuroblastoma filling a large portion of the abdominal cavity	• Distended, enlarged abdomen • Respiratory distress, hypoxia • Poor perfusion • Tachycardia, hypotension	• Abdominal CT reveals extent of tumour. • Coagulopathy	• Tumour resection or debulking • Mechanical ventilation, inotropic support • Nasogastric decompression • Position to minimize abdominal pressure. • Blood transfusions • Comfort measures

Adapted from: Maloney, K., Foreman, N. K., Giller, R. H., Greffe, B. S., Graham, D. K., Quinones, R. R., & Keating, A. K. (2011). Neoplastic disease. In W. W. Hay, M. J. Levin, J. M. Sondheimer, & R. R. Deterding (Eds.), *Current pediatric diagnosis and treatment* (20th ed.). New York: McGraw-Hill; and Tomlinson, D., & Kline, N. E. (Eds.) (2010). *Pediatric oncology nursing.* New York: Springer.

Complications of leukemia include metastasis to the blood, bone, CNS, spleen, liver, or other organs as well as alterations in growth. Late effects include problems with neurocognitive function and ocular, cardiovascular, or thyroid dysfunction. With advances in treatment over the past 50 years, most cases of childhood leukemia are curable, though children who experience relapse or present with advanced disease have a poorer prognosis (Zupanec & Tomlinson, 2010).

Acute Lymphoblastic Leukemia

ALL is the most common form of cancer in children. It is more likely to occur in males than females, peaks between

TABLE 49.2   **INCIDENCE OF TYPES OF LEUKEMIA IN CHILDREN AND ADOLESCENTS**

Type	Incidence
Acute lymphoblastic leukemia	75% to 80%
Acute myelogenous leukemia	20% to 25%
Chronic lymphoblastic leukemia	Rare
Chronic myelogenous leukemia	<5%

From: Colby-Graham, M. F., & Chordas, C. (2003). The childhood leukemias. *Journal of Pediatric Nursing, 18*(2), 87–95.

the ages of 2 and 5 years (Zupanec & Tomlinson, 2010), and is more common in white children than in children of other races. ALL is classified according to the type of cells involved: T cell, B cell, early pre-B cell, or pre-B cell. Most children will achieve initial remission if appropriate treatment is given. The overall cure rate for ALL is 65% to 75%. Relapse is rare after 7 years from diagnosis.

Prognosis is based upon the WBC count at diagnosis, the type of cytogenetic factors and immunophenotype, the age at diagnosis, and the extent of extra-medullary involvement. Generally, the higher the WBC count at diagnosis, the worse the prognosis is. About 80% of childhood ALL is curable, and the current estimated overall survival rate of infant ALL is 50% (Zupanec & Tomlinson, 2010). When a child experiences a relapse, the prognosis becomes poorer. Complications include infection, hemorrhage, poor growth, and CNS, bone, or testicular involvement.

Pathophysiology

The exact cause of ALL remains unknown (Colby-Graham & Chordas, 2003). Genetic factors and chromosome abnormalities may play a role in its development. In ALL, abnormal lymphoblasts abound in the blood-forming tissues. The lymphoblasts are fragile and immature, lacking the infection-fighting capabilities of normal WBCs. In ALL, the growth of lymphoblasts is excessive and the abnormal cells replace the normal cells in the bone marrow. The proliferating leukemic cells demonstrate massive metabolic needs, depriving normal body cells of needed nutrients and resulting in fatigue, weight loss or growth arrest, and muscle wasting. The bone marrow becomes unable to maintain normal levels of RBCs, WBCs, and platelets, so anemia, neutropenia, and thrombocytopenia result. As the bone marrow expands or the leukemic cells infiltrate the bone, joint and bone pain may occur. The leukemic cells may permeate the lymph nodes, causing diffuse lymphadenopathy, or the liver and spleen, resulting in hepatosplenomegaly. With spread to the CNS, vomiting, headache, seizures, coma, vision alterations, or cranial nerve palsies may occur.

> ▶ **Take** NOTE!
>
> *Changes in behaviour or personality, headache, irritability, dizziness, persistent nausea or vomiting, seizures, gait changes, lethargy, or altered level of consciousness may indicate CNS infiltration with leukemic cells. Immediately report these findings to the pediatric oncologist.*

Therapeutic Management

Therapeutic management of the child with ALL focuses on giving chemotherapy to eradicate the leukemic cells and restore normal bone marrow function. Treatment protocols include induction, consolidation, re-intensification, CNS-directed therapy, and maintenance/continuing treatment (Zupanec & Tomlinson, 2010). CNS prophylaxis is provided at each stage; without CNS prophylaxis, leukemia would spread to the CNS in up to 50% of children with ALL. The length of treatment and choice of medications are based on the child's age, risk category, and subtype as determined by bone marrow analysis. For relapsed or less responsive leukemia, HSCT may be necessary.

Nursing Assessment

For a full description of the assessment phase of the nursing process, refer to page 1693. Assessment findings pertinent to ALL are discussed below.

Health History

Elicit a description of the present illness and chief complaint. Common signs and symptoms reported during the health history might include:

- Fever (may be persistent or recurrent, with unknown cause)
- Recurrent infection
- Fatigue, malaise, or listlessness
- Pallor
- Unusual bleeding or bruising

- Abdominal pain
- Nausea or vomiting
- Bone pain
- Headache

Explore the child's current and past medical history for risk factors such as:

- Male gender
- Age 2 to 5 years
- White race
- Down syndrome, Shwachman syndrome, or ataxia–telangiectasia
- X-ray exposure in utero
- Previous radiation-treated cancer

Determine the child's history of varicella zoster immunization or disease. Chickenpox infection in the leukemic child may lead to disseminated, overwhelming infection.

Physical Examination

Take the child's temperature (fever may be present), and look for petechiae, purpura, or unusual bruising (due to decreased platelet levels). Inspect the skin for signs of infection. Auscultate the lungs, noting adventitious breath sounds, which may indicate pneumonia (present at diagnosis or due to immunosuppression during treatment). Note location and size of enlarged lymph nodes. Palpate the liver and spleen for enlargement. Document tenderness on abdominal palpation.

Laboratory and Diagnostic Tests

Common laboratory and diagnostic studies ordered for the assessment of ALL include:

- Abnormal complete blood counts: low hemoglobin and hematocrit, decreased RBC count, decreased platelet count, and elevated, normal, or decreased WBC count.
- Peripheral blood smear may reveal blasts.
- Stained smear from bone marrow aspiration will show greater than 25% lymphoblasts. Bone marrow aspirate is also examined for immunophenotyping (lymphoid versus myeloid and level of cancer cell maturity) and cytogenetic analysis (determines abnormalities in chromosome number and structure). Immunophenotyping and cytogenetic analysis are used in the classification of the leukemia, which helps guide treatment.
- Lumbar puncture will reveal whether leukemic cells have infiltrated the CNS.
- Liver function tests and blood urea nitrogen (BUN) and creatinine levels determine liver and renal function, which if abnormal may preclude treatment with certain chemotherapeutic agents.
- Chest X-ray may reveal pneumonia or a mediastinal mass.

Nursing Management

Nursing care for children with ALL focuses on managing disease complications such as infection, pain, anemia, bleeding, and hyperuricemia and the many adverse effects related to treatment. Many children require blood product transfusion for the treatment of severe anemia or low platelet levels with active bleeding.

Individualize nursing care based on the diagnoses, interventions, and outcomes presented in Nursing Care Plan 49.1, depending on the child's response to the disease and chemotherapy. Refer to the Nursing Process Overview section for further information related to managing the adverse effects of chemotherapy.

> ▶ *Take* NOTE!
>
> *Blood products administered to children with any type of leukemia should be irradiated, cytomegalovirus (CMV) negative, and leukodepleted. This treatment of blood products before transfusion will decrease the amount of antibodies in the blood, an important factor in preventing GvHD should HSCT become necessary at a later date (Nixon, 2010).*

Reducing Pain

Children and teens with leukemia suffer pain related to the disease as well as the treatment. Chemotherapy drugs commonly used in leukemia may cause peripheral neuropathy and headache. Lumbar puncture and bone marrow aspiration, which are periodically performed throughout the course of treatment, also cause pain. The most common areas of pain are the head and neck, legs, and abdomen (probably from protracted vomiting with chemotherapy). The use of EMLA cream prior to venipuncture, port access, lumbar puncture, and bone marrow aspiration may decrease procedure-related pain events (Simon, 2010). Application of heat or cold to the painful area is usually acceptable. Narcotic analgesics may be used for episodes of acute severe pain or for palliation of chronic pain. Non-pharmacologic strategies that should be used in combination with analgesics include distraction techniques (e.g., listening to music, watching TV, or playing games), guided imagery, deep breathing, relaxation, and cold or warm compresses. The choice of a non-pharmacologic strategy will depend on the child's age and cognitive ability and the type, severity, and nature of pain (Simon, 2010). See Evidence-based Practice 49.1.

Acute Myelogenous Leukemia

AML is the second most common type of leukemia in children. Its incidence peaks during the adolescent years (Zupanec & Tomlinson, 2010). AML affects the myeloid cell progenitors or precursors in the bone marrow, resulting in malignant cells. The French-American-British (FAB) classification system identifies eight subtypes of AML (MO to M7), depending on myeloid lineage involved and the degree of cell differentiation (Zupanec & Tomlinson, 2010). These subtypes are useful for determining treatment. The overall cure rate for childhood

---

EVIDENCE-BASED PRACTICE 49.1
Non-Pharmacologic Therapies for Symptom Management in Childhood Cancer

● **Study**

Even with significant advances in childhood cancer surgery and treatment, troublesome symptoms remain a large problem. Children report that the most upsetting aspect of cancer treatment is the numerous side effects they suffer. The author performed a systematic review of research studies that evaluated the use of complementary and alternative therapies for cancer treatment side effect management. Forty-one studies were reviewed that addressed such topics as procedural pain, distress, fear and anxiety, nausea/vomiting, anxiety, distress, and depression. Non-pharmacologic adjunctive therapies evaluated in the studies included hypnosis, distraction, cognitive-behavioural therapies, relaxation, imagery, breathing, music therapy, play, self-hypnosis, acupuncture, art therapy, coping skills training, handholding, humour, and nonessential touch.

▲ **Findings**

Many of the non-pharmacologic adjuvant therapies studied were found to be effective for symptom relief. Cognitive-behavioural therapy, distraction, and hypnosis were particularly helpful. Although safety concerns for various therapies were not reported, the author proposed that further rigorous research on these modalities is necessary.

■ **Nursing Implications**

Many families seek non-pharmacologic or complementary/alternative therapies for relieving the distressing symptoms associated with cancer treatment. Nurses must keep an open mind about these therapies. When families have questions about using these treatments, they should be directed to authorities in the area. Nurses are in a perfect position to initiate additional rigorous research to determine the effectiveness and long-term safety of these therapies.

Rheingans, J. I. (2007). A systematic review of nonpharmacologic adjunctive therapies for symptom management in children with cancer. *Journal of Pediatric Oncology Nursing, 24*(2), 81–94.

AML is about 50% (Zupanec & Tomlinson, 2010). Complications include treatment resistance, infection, hemorrhage, and metastasis.

Treatment for AML involves an induction phase followed by a consolidation phase (Zupanec & Tomlinson, 2010). The induction phase requires intense bone marrow suppression and prolonged hospitalization because AML is less responsive to treatment than ALL. Toxicity from treatment is more common in AML and is likely to be more serious than with ALL. Empirical broad-spectrum antibiotics and prophylactic platelet transfusions may be prescribed. After remission is achieved, children require intensive chemotherapy to prolong the duration of remission. HSCT is often required in children with AML, depending on the subtype. The cure rate for AML is approximately 50%, and about 50% of children experience a relapse (Zupanec & Tomlinson, 2010).

Nursing Assessment

Explore the health history for common signs and symptoms, including recurrent infections, fever, or fatigue. Explore the medical history for risk factors, such as Hispanic race, previous chemotherapy, and genetic abnormalities such as Down syndrome, Fanconi anemia, neurofibromatosis type 1, Shwachman syndrome, Bloom syndrome, and familial monosomy 7.

Perform a thorough physical examination. Note skin pallor and salmon-coloured or blue-grey papular lesions. Palpate the skin for subcutaneous rubbery nodules. Palpate for lymphadenopathy. Note headache, visual disturbance, or signs of increased intracranial pressure, such as vomiting, that may indicate CNS involvement. Upon diagnosis of AML, the child's WBC count is typically extremely elevated. Bone marrow aspiration will reveal greater than 30% blast cells.

Nursing Management

Nursing management of the child with AML is similar to that of the child with ALL. Nursing interventions focus on managing the adverse effects of treatment and preventing infection. Refer to the Nursing Process Overview section and to Nursing Care Plan 49.1 for appropriate interventions.

Lymphomas

Lymphomas, or tumours of the lymph tissue (lymph nodes, thymus, spleen), account for about 12% of cases of childhood cancer (Weitzman & Arceci, 2003). Lymphomas may be divided into two categories: Hodgkin's disease (or Hodgkin's lymphoma) and non-Hodgkin's lymphoma (NHL), which includes more than a dozen types (Zupanec, 2010). Hodgkin's disease tends to affect lymph nodes located closer to the body's surface, such as those in the cervical, axillary, and inguinal areas, whereas NHL tends to affect lymph nodes located more deeply inside the body.

Hodgkin's Disease

In Hodgkin's disease, malignant B lymphocytes grow in the lymph tissue, usually starting in one general area of lymph nodes. The presence of Reed–Sternberg cells (giant transformed B lymphocytes with one or two nuclei) differentiates Hodgkin's disease from other lymphomas (Zupanec, 2010). As the cells multiply, the lymph nodes enlarge, compressing nearby structures, destroying normal cells, and invading other tissues. The cause of Hodgkin's disease is still being researched, but there appears to be a link with Epstein-Barr virus infection (Zupanec, 2010). Hodgkin's disease is rare in children under 5 years of age and is most common in adolescents and young adults; in children under 14 years of age, it is more common in boys than in girls (Zupanec, 2010). The overall survival rate for children and adolescents with Hodgkin's disease is 90% (Schwartz, 2003).

In addition to the traditional **staging** (I through IV, depending on the amount of spread; Table 49.3), Hodgkin's is also classified as A (asymptomatic) or B (presence of symptoms of fever, night sweats, or weight loss of 10% or more). Prognosis depends on the stage of the disease, tumour bulk, and A or B classification (disease classified as A generally carries a better prognosis). Low-risk Hodgkin's is distinguished by local nodal involvement (stage I/II) and the absence of B symptoms and lymph node bulk disease (Zupanec, 2010). Complications include liver failure and secondary cancer such as acute non-lymphocytic leukemia and NHL.

Chemotherapy, usually with a combination of drugs, is the treatment of choice for children with Hodgkin's disease. Radiation therapy may also be necessary. In the child whose disease does not go into remission or in the child who experiences relapse, HSCT may be an option.

TABLE 49.3 **STAGING OF HODGKIN'S DISEASE**

Stage	Clinical Findings
I	One group of lymph nodes is affected.
II	Two or more groups of lymph nodes on the same side of the diaphragm are affected.
III	Groups of lymph nodes above and below the diaphragm are affected.
IV	Metastasis to organs such as the liver, bone, or lungs.

From: American Cancer Society. (2011b). *How is Hodgkin disease staged?* Retrieved November 7, 2011 from http://www.cancer.org/Cancer/HodgkinDisease/DetailedGuide/hodgkin-disease-staging.

Nursing Assessment

Explore the health history for common signs and symptoms, which may include recent weight loss, fever, drenching night sweats, anorexia, malaise, fatigue, or pruritus. Elicit the health history, determining risk factors such as prior Epstein-Barr virus infection, family history of Hodgkin's disease, genetic immune disorder, or HIV infection.

Evaluate respiratory status, as the presence of a mediastinal mass may compromise respiration. Palpate for enlarged lymph nodes; they may feel rubbery and tend to occur in clusters (most common sites are cervical and supraclavicular). Palpate the abdomen for hepatomegaly or splenomegaly, which may be present with advanced disease. The chest X-ray may reveal a mediastinal mass. The complete blood count may be normal or reflect anemia. Tissue sampling will reveal Reed–Sternberg cells.

> ▶ *Take* NOTE!
>
> *Significant pain in the affected lymph nodes has sometimes been noted after alcohol ingestion (Zupanec, 2010).*

Nursing Management

Nursing management of the child with Hodgkin's lymphoma focuses on addressing the adverse effects of chemotherapy or radiation. Refer to the Nursing Process Overview section and Nursing Care Plan 49.1 to develop an individualized nursing care plan based on the child's response to treatment.

Non-Hodgkin's Lymphoma

NHL results from mutations in the B and T lymphocytes that lead to uncontrolled growth. NHL tends to affect lymph nodes located more deeply within the body. Approximately 8% to 10% of all childhood cancer malignancies are NHL (Sandlund, Downing, & Crist, 1996). NHL spreads via the bloodstream and in children is a rapidly proliferating, aggressive malignancy that is very responsive to treatment. Prognosis depends on the cell type involved and the extent of the disease at diagnosis. The current reported disease-free survival for childhood NHL is approximately 80%, independent of the subtype (Gross & Termuhlen, 2007).

The histologic subtype and stage of disease determine treatment for NHL (Zupanec, 2010). NHL tends to spread easily to the CNS, so CNS prophylaxis similar to that used in leukemia is warranted (Zupanec, 2010). Autologous bone marrow transplantation may be used in some children.

Nursing Assessment

Children with NHL are usually symptomatic for only a few days or a few weeks before diagnosis because the disease progresses so quickly. Note onset and location of pain or lymph node swelling. Document history of abdominal pain, diarrhea, or constipation. Explore the health history for risk factors such as congenital or acquired immune deficiency.

Observe for increased work of breathing, facial edema, or venous engorgement (mediastinal mass). Palpate for the presence of lymphadenopathy and palpate the abdomen for the presence of a mass. Lymph node **biopsy** and bone marrow aspiration determine the diagnosis. Computed tomography (CT), chest X-ray, and bone marrow results may be used to determine the extent of metastasis.

> ▶ *Take* NOTE!
>
> *Cough, dyspnea, orthopnea, facial edema, or venous engorgement may indicate mediastinal disease in the child with NHL. This is an emergency requiring rapid treatment (Zupanec, 2010).*

Nursing Management

As with Hodgkin's lymphoma, nursing management of NHL is directed toward managing the adverse effects of chemotherapy. Refer to the Nursing Process Overview section and Nursing Care Plan 49.1 to plan nursing care for the child and family based on the responses they exhibit.

Brain Tumours

Brain tumours are the most common form of solid tumour and the second most common type of cancer in children (May & Ward, 2008). Slightly more than half of brain tumours arise in the posterior fossa (infratentorial); the rest are supratentorial in origin (Kline & O'Hanlon-Curry, 2010). The cause of brain tumours in children is unknown. Some tumours are localized, while others are of higher grade and more invasive. There are many different types of childhood brain tumours; Table 49.4 explains the most common ones. The prognosis depends on the location and extent of tumour. Low-grade tumours and those that are fully resectable have a better prognosis than tumours that are located deeper within the brain, making them difficult to resect (Kline & O'Hanlon-Curry, 2010). Survival data may be misleading as the data are often based on the evaluation of treatment strategies that lag behind current practice (Kline & O'Hanlon-Curry, 2010).

Complications of brain tumours include hydrocephalus, increased intracranial pressure, brain stem herniation, and negative effects of radiation such as neuropsychological, intellectual, and endocrinologic sequelae. Children treated for a brain tumour will require lifelong follow-up

TABLE 49.4 CHILDHOOD BRAIN TUMOURS

Tumour	Location	Characteristics
Medulloblastoma	Cerebellar vermis	Accounts for 25% of pediatric brain tumours. Most common between 3 and 7 years and in males. Symptoms include headache, morning vomiting, cranial nerve deficits, and ataxia. Survival rate with nonmetastatic disease is 70%–80%; outcome is less favourable with disseminated disease.
Brain stem glioma	Brain stem	Common presenting age is 5–10 years. Symptoms in high-grade disease (short history) include multiple cranial nerve palsies, ataxia, and hemiparesis. Symptoms in low-grade disease (long history) include minimal or a focal cranial nerve deficit and raised intracranial pressure (ICP). The median survival time for high-grade disease is 8–10 years.
Ependymoma	Frequently arises from floor of fourth ventricle	50% of cases occur before 5 years of age. Symptoms depend on site and extent of disease and include neck pain, increased ICP, cranial nerve deficits, and ataxia. Often causes hydrocephalus. Overall 5-year survival is 40%–60%.
Astrocytoma	Cerebellum	Commonly occurs in the first decade of life. More common in boys. MRI commonly shows cystic tumour with mural node. Symptoms include midline cerebellar signs. 90% of children with a fully resected pilocytic astrocytoma will survive with only surgical intervention. High-grade tumours have poor prognosis.

From: Kline, N. E., & O'Hanlon-Curry, J. (2010). Central nervous system tumors. In D. Tomlinson, & N. E. Kline (Eds.), *Pediatric oncology nursing: Advanced clinical handbook* (2nd ed.). New York: Springer.

care by experts who are familiar with the long-term effects of cancer (Kline & O'Hanlon-Curry, 2010).

Pathophysiology

Though the cause of brain tumours is generally not known, the effects of brain tumours are predictable (Kline & O'Hanlon-Curry, 2010). As the tumour grows within the cranium, it exerts pressure on the brain tissues surrounding it. The tumour mass may compress vital structures in the brain, block cerebrospinal fluid flow, or cause edema in the brain. The result is an increase in intracranial pressure. Presenting symptoms vary according to location and type of tumour.

Therapeutic Management

The type of tumour may be identified at the time of surgery. The location of the tumour within the brain will determine the extent to which it can safely be resected. Children with hydrocephalus may require a ventriculoperitoneal shunt (see Chapter 37 for further information on hydrocephalus). Radiation is reserved for children over age 2 years because it can have long-term neurocognitive effects (Maloney, Foreman, Giller, et al., 2010). Chemotherapy is being used increasingly in the treatment of pediatric brain tumours in an attempt to avoid the use of radiation therapy.

Nursing Assessment

For a full description of the assessment phase of the nursing process, refer to page 1693. Assessment findings pertinent to CNS tumours are discussed below.

Health History

Elicit a description of the present illness and chief complaint. Common signs and symptoms reported during the health history might include:

• Nausea or vomiting
• Headache
• Unsteady gait
• Blurred or double vision
• Seizures
• Motor abnormality or hemiparesis
• Weakness, atrophy
• Swallowing difficulties
• Behaviour or personality changes
• Irritability, failure to thrive or developmental delay (in very young children)

Explore the patient's current and past medical history for risk factors such as history of neurofibromatosis, tuberous sclerosis, or prior treatment for CNS leukemia.

Physical Examination

Inspection and Observation

Observe for strabismus or nystagmus, "sunsetting" eyes, head tilt, alterations in coordination, gait disturbance, or alterations in sensation. Note alteration in gag reflex, cranial nerve palsy, lethargy, or irritability. Note the child's posture. Check pupillary reaction, noting size, equality, reaction to light, and accommodation.

Palpation

Measure blood pressure, which may decrease with increasing intracranial pressure. In the infant, palpate the anterior fontanel for bulging. Assess deep tendon reflexes, noting hyperreflexia.

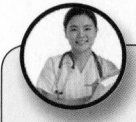

▶ *Take NOTE!*

A fixed and dilated pupil is a neurosurgical emergency.

Laboratory and Diagnostic Tests

Common laboratory and diagnostic studies ordered for the assessment of CNS tumours include:

- CT, magnetic resonance imaging (MRI), or positron-emission tomography (PET) will demonstrate evidence of the tumour and its location within the intracranial cavity.
- Lumbar puncture with cerebrospinal fluid cell evaluation may show tumour markers or the presence of alpha-fetoprotein or human chorionic gonadotropin, which may assist in the diagnosis (Kline & O'Hanlon-Curry, 2010).

Nursing Management

Nursing management for the child with a brain tumour includes preoperative and postoperative care, as well as interventions to manage adverse effects related to chemotherapy and radiation. Refer to the Nursing Process Overview section for a discussion of nursing interventions related to chemotherapy adverse effects. Nursing Care Plan 49.1 provides additional interventions that may be individualized depending on the child's response to the brain tumour and its treatment.

Providing Preoperative Care

Preoperatively, care focuses on monitoring for additional increases in intracranial pressure and avoiding activities that cause transient increases in intracranial pressure. Administer dexamethasone as prescribed to decrease intracranial inflammation. Prevent straining with bowel movements by use of a stool softener. Assess the child's pain level as well of level of consciousness, vital signs, and pupillary reaction to determine subtle changes as

soon as possible. Provide a tour of the intensive care unit, which is where the child will wake up after the surgery. Instruct the child and family about the possibility of intubation and ventilation in the postoperative period. If a ventriculoperitoneal shunt will be placed for the treatment of hydrocephalus caused by the tumour, provide education about shunts to the child and family (see Chapter 37).

Shave the portion of the head as determined by the neurosurgeon. Some children may choose to have the entire head shaved. Sometimes children with long hair may feel better about losing it if they donate it to Locks of Love or Angel Hair for Kids, organizations that provide hairpieces for financially disadvantaged children (visit http://thePoint.lww.com/Chow1e for direct links to these organizations' websites).

Providing Postoperative Care

Regulate fluid administration, as excess fluid intake may cause or worsen cerebral edema. Administer mannitol or hypertonic dextrose to decrease cerebral edema. Assess vital signs frequently, along with checking pupillary reactions and determining level of consciousness. Extreme lethargy or coma may be present for several days postoperatively. Increases in temperature may indicate infection or may be caused by cerebral edema or disturbance of the hypothalamus. Treat hyperthermia with antipyretics such as acetaminophen and with sponge baths, as increases in temperature increase metabolic need. Reduce the temperature slowly.

Monitor for signs of increased intracranial pressure. Headache is common in the postoperative period. Assess pain level and provide analgesics as prescribed. Minimize environmental stimuli, providing a calm and quiet atmosphere. Check the head dressing for cerebrospinal fluid drainage or bleeding. Assess for and document the extent of head, face, or neck edema. Administer eye lubricant if edema prevents complete closure of the eyelids. Apply cool compresses to the eyes to decrease swelling.

As the child begins to regain consciousness, he or she may be confused or combative. Very close monitoring is required; restraining may be necessary to keep the child in bed and prevent dislodging of tubes and lines.

Positioning the Child in the Postoperative Period

Position the child on the unaffected side with the head of the bed flat or at the level prescribed by the neurosurgeon. Side positioning is usually preferred, as the child may have difficulty handling oral secretions if the level of consciousness is decreased. Do not elevate the foot of the bed, as this may increase intracranial pressure and contribute to bleeding. When changing the child's position, maintain the head in alignment with the remainder of the body. Children with paralyzed or spastic extremities will need additional positioning support.

▶ *Take* NOTE!

Observe the child preoperatively and postoperatively for signs of brain stem herniation such as opisthotonos, nuchal rigidity, head tilt, sluggish pupils, increased blood pressure with widening pulse pressure, change in respirations, bradycardia, irregular pulse, and changes in body temperature.

▶ *Consider* THIS!

Alice Tice, 6 years old, is scheduled to receive chemotherapy for a brain tumour. As the nurse caring for her, how can you prepare Alice for this? What nursing interventions are important when caring for a child receiving chemotherapy (discuss reducing pain, reducing risk of infection, promoting adequate nutrition, and managing nausea and vomiting)?

Neuroblastoma

Neuroblastoma, a tumour that arises from embryonic neural crest cells, is the most common extracranial solid tumour in children (Hendershot, 2010). It occurs most frequently in the abdomen, mainly in the adrenal gland. Other common locations are the thorax, pelvis, and cervical regions (Hendershot, 2010).

Neuroblastoma accounts for one of every eight pediatric cancer deaths worldwide (Wagner & Danks, 2009). At least 40% of all children with neuroblastoma are designated as high-risk patients. High-risk neuroblastoma accounts for 15% of childhood cancer deaths. Although improvements in outcome have been attained with the intensification of conventional chemotherapy agents and the addition of 13-cis-retinoic acid, only one third of children with high-risk disease are expected to be long-term survivors (Wanger & Danks, 2009).

Staging of the tumour at diagnosis determines the course of treatment (Table 49.5). Prognosis depends on the tumour stage, age at diagnosis, tumour location, and location of **metastasis**. Survival rates range from 40% to 90% (Wagner & Danks, 2009) and are excellent in children with low-risk and stage I and stage II disease as well as in those treated with surgery only (Wagner & Danks, 2009). Infants less than 12 months of age and children with stage I disease have the best survival rates (Maloney et al., 2010). Children with tumours above the diaphragm tend to have a better prognosis than those with abdominal tumours. Metastasis to the bone is a worse prognostic factor than metastasis to the skin, liver, or bone marrow. In addition to metastasis, complications may include nerve compression, resulting in neurologic deficits.

The neuroblastoma must be removed surgically. Radiation and chemotherapy are administered to all

TABLE 49.5 STAGING OF NEUROBLASTOMA BASED ON THE INTERNATIONAL NEUROBLASTOMA STAGING SYSTEM

Stage	Tumour Characteristics
I	Localized tumour with gross total resection
IIA	Localized tumour with incomplete gross total resection, lymph nodes negative
IIB	Localized tumour with or without gross total resection, with positive nodes
III	Tumour invasively extends beyond the midline with bilateral lymph node involvement
IV	Metastasis to bone, bone marrow, other organs, distant lymph nodes
IVS	Localized primary tumour (I, IIA, IIB), with dissemination limited to skin, liver, and/or bone marrow

From: Hendershot, E. (2010). Solid tumors. In D. Tomlinson, & N. E. Kline (Eds.), *Pediatric oncology nursing: Advanced clinical handbook* (2nd ed.). New York: Springer.

children with neuroblastoma except those with stage I disease, in whom the tumour is completely resected.

Nursing Assessment

For a full description of the assessment phase of the nursing process, refer to page 1693. Assessment findings pertinent to neuroblastoma are discussed below.

Health History

Presenting signs and symptoms of neuroblastoma depend on the location of the primary tumour and the extent of metastasis. Often parents are the first to notice a swollen or asymmetric abdomen. Elicit the health history, documenting bowel or bladder dysfunction, especially watery diarrhea, neurologic symptoms (brain metastasis), bone pain (bone metastasis), anorexia, vomiting, or weight loss.

Physical Examination

Note neck or facial swelling, bruising above the eyes, or edema around the eyes (metastasis to skull bones). Inspect the skin for pallor or bruising (bone marrow metastasis), and document cough or difficulty breathing. Auscultate the lungs for wheezing. Palpate for lymphadenopathy, especially cervical. Palpate the abdomen, noting a firm, nontender mass. Palpate for and note hepatomegaly or splenomegaly if present.

Laboratory and Diagnostic Testing

Laboratory and diagnostic testing may reveal the following:

• CT or MRI to determine site of tumour and evidence of metastasis

- Chest X-ray, bone scan, and skeletal survey to identify metastasis
- Bone marrow aspiration and biopsy to determine metastasis to the bone marrow
- 24-hour urine collection for homovanillic acid (HVA) and vanillylmandelic acid (VMA); levels will be elevated, as more than 90% of all neuroblastomas secrete catecholamines, which are then excreted in the urine (Wagner & Danks, 2009).

Nursing Management

Postoperative nursing care depends on the site of tumour removal, which is most often the abdomen. Routine care after abdominal surgery will be needed. Refer to the Nursing Process Overview section and Nursing Care Plan 49.1 related to the effects of chemotherapy and radiation. As the disease has often metastasized significantly by the time of diagnosis, these children and families will need emotional support and possibly referrals to help them cope with the poor prognosis.

Bone and Soft Tissue Tumours

Bone and soft tissue tumours account for about 10% of malignant tumours in children (Ozger, Bulbul, & Eralp, 2010). Bone tumours are most often diagnosed in adolescence, whereas soft tissue tumours tend to occur in younger children (Hendershot, 2010). This discussion focuses on the most common bone and soft tissue tumours occurring in childhood. The most common bone tumours in children are osteosarcoma and Ewing sarcoma; rhabdomyosarcoma is the most common soft tissue tumour in childhood (Hendershot, 2010).

Osteosarcoma

Osteosarcoma is the most common form of bone cancer, occurring most frequently in the second decade of life at the peak of the growth spurt (Carrle & Bielack, 2006; Hayden & Hoang, 2006). Osteosarcoma occurs slightly more often in females (Hendershot, 2010). It presumably arises from the embryonic mesenchymal tissue that forms the bones. The most common sites are in the long bones, particularly the proximal humerus, proximal tibia, and distal femur (Hendershot, 2010).

About 20% of children with osteosarcoma present with detectable metastases, the majority of which are in the lungs (Meyer, Nadel, Marina, et al., 2008). Surgical removal of the tumour is necessary. Chemotherapy is often administered before surgery to decrease the size of the tumour; it is usually administered after surgery to treat or prevent metastasis. The type of surgery performed depends on the tumour size, extent of disease outside the bone, distant metastasis, and skeletal maturity. Radical amputation may be performed, but often

teens undergo a limb salvage procedure. Radical amputation may include the entire extremity or the entire affected bone. Limb-sparing surgery entails removing only the affected portion of the bone, replacing it with either an endoprosthesis or cadaver bone.

Nursing Assessment

Obtain the health history, ascertaining when pain, limp, or limitation of motion was first noticed. Dull bone pain may be present for several months, eventually progressing to limp or gait changes.

Inspect the affected limb for erythema and swelling. Palpate the affected area for warmth and tenderness and to determine the size of the soft tissue mass, if present. As with other pediatric cancers, a thorough physical examination is warranted to detect other abnormalities that may indicate metastasis.

Laboratory and diagnostic testing may include:

- CT or MRI to determine the extent of the lesion and to identify metastasis
- Bone scan to determine the extent of malignancy
- Elevated alkaline phosphatase levels: these may or may not be helpful, as the quickly growing adolescent often normally has elevated levels as a response to rapid bone growth

Nursing Management

The adolescent will generally be quite anxious about the possibility of amputation and even about the limb salvage procedure. Present preoperative teaching at the adolescent's developmental level and ensure that he or she is included in planning treatment. Regardless of the type of surgery performed, provide routine orthopedic postoperative care. Educate the adolescent and parents on the care of the stump, if amputation is necessary, and ensure that the teen becomes competent in crutch walking. A prosthesis may be ordered. The adolescent will need time to adjust to these significant body image changes and may benefit from talking with another teen who has undergone a similar procedure. Support the teen in choosing clothing that may camouflage the prosthesis while still allowing the teen to appear fashionable. Provide emotional support, as the teen's maturity level allows him or her to understand the severity of the disease. Peer support groups are often helpful, as teens value their peers' opinions and enjoy being part of a group. Examples of comprehensive online support groups are Teen Connector run by Candlelighters Canada and Teens Living with Cancer (visit http://thePoint.lww.com/Chow1e for direct links).

Rhabdomyosarcoma

The most common locations for rhabdomyosarcoma are the head and neck, genitourinary tract, and extremities (Fig. 49.7). The tumour is highly malignant and spreads

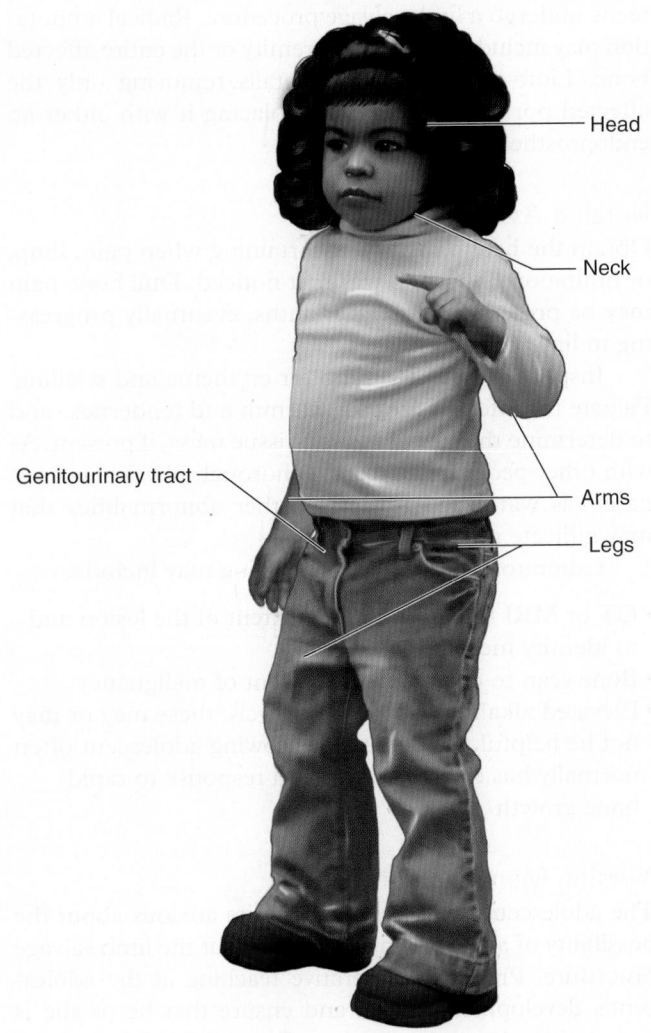

Head

Neck

Genitourinary tract

Arms

Legs

FIGURE 49.7 The most common sites of rhabdomyosarcoma.

via local extension or through the venous or lymphatic system, with the lung being the most common site for metastasis. The majority of all rhabdomyosarcomas are present in children before age 6 years (Hendershot, 2010). The prognosis is based on the stage of the disease at diagnosis. Box 49.2 explains the staging of rhabdomyosarcoma. Prognosis is generally favourable for stage I disease (Hendershot, 2010). A review of patients enrolled in the latest Intergroup Rhabdomyosarcoma Study showed the 3-year event-free survival rates to be 83%, 86%, 73%, and 25% for stages I, II, III, and IV, respectively (Paulino & Okcu, 2008).

Complications of rhabdomyosarcoma include metastasis to lung, bone, or bone marrow and direct extension into the CNS, resulting in brain stem compromise or cranial nerve palsy.

Surgical removal of the primary tumour is generally performed. At the time of the surgery, the lesion is biopsied and the stage of disease determined. Radiation and chemotherapy may be used to shrink the tumour to

---

> ### BOX 49.2 Staging of Rhabdomyosarcoma Based on the Intergroup Rhabdomyosarcoma Study Group Postsurgical Grouping Classification
>
> - Stage I: completely resectable localized tumour
> - Stage II: after local tumour resection, microscopic residual disease remains
> - Stage III: after local tumour resection, gross residual disease remains
> - Stage IV: metastasis present at diagnosis
>
> From: Hendershot, E. (2010). Solid tumors. In D. Tomlinson, & N. E. Kline (Eds.), *Pediatric oncology nursing: Advanced clinical handbook* (2nd ed.). New York: Springer.

avoid disability, depending on the site and size of the tumour (especially head, neck, and pelvis).

Nursing Assessment

The child or parent will often discover an asymptomatic mass and seek medical attention at that time. Obtain a health history, noting recent illness, when the mass was discovered, and whether it has changed since first noted. Examine the history for risk factors such as parental smoking, exposure to environmental chemicals, family history of cancer, or neurofibromatosis. Note respiratory effort and cough, and auscultate the lungs for adventitious sounds. Palpate for lymphadenopathy. Palpate the abdomen for a mass or hepatosplenomegaly. Abnormalities found on physical examination depend on the location of the rhabdomyosarcoma (Table 49.6).

Laboratory and diagnostic testing may include:

- CT or MRI of the primary lesion and the chest for metastasis
- Open biopsy of the primary tumour for definitive diagnosis
- Bone marrow aspiration and biopsy, bone scan, and skeletal survey to determine metastasis

> ▶ **Take** NOTE!
>
> *Primary tumours arising in the neck region may compress the child's airway. Assess work of breathing and lung sounds.*

Nursing Management

Provide routine postoperative care, depending on the site of surgery. Assess for adverse effects of high-dose radiation, which is generally used to treat the primary tumour as well as metastatic sites. Administer chemotherapy as ordered and assess for adverse effects. Refer to the Nursing Process Overview section and Nursing

TABLE 49.6 PRESENTING SIGNS AND SYMPTOMS RELATED TO LOCATION OF RHABDOMYOSARCOMA

Location of Tumour	Presenting Signs and Symptoms
Orbit	Proptosis
Middle ear	Drainage, pain, facial nerve palsy
Sinuses	Discharge, pain, sinusitis, facial swelling
Nasopharynx	Pain, epistaxis, dysphagia, nasal quality to speech, airway obstruction
Neck	Dysphagia, hoarseness
Thorax, testicle, extremities	Enlarging mass, painless
Retroperitoneum	Gastrointestinal and urinary tract obstruction, pain, weakness, paresthesia
Bladder, prostate	Hematuria, urinary obstruction
Vagina	Mass, vaginal bleeding or chronic discharge

From: Hendershot, E. (2010). Solid tumors. In D. Tomlinson, & N. E. Kline (Eds.), *Pediatric oncology nursing: Advanced clinical handbook* (2nd ed.). New York: Springer.

Care Plan 49.1 to determine an individualized plan of care based on the child's response to the treatment.

Wilms' Tumour

Wilms' tumour is the most common renal tumour and the fourth most common solid tumour in children (Hendershot, 2010). About 80% of all cases occur in children less than 5 years old, with a median age of 3.5 years (Ko & Ritchey, 2009). It usually affects only one kidney, but it is bilateral in 5% to 10% of cases (Fig. 49.8). The etiology is unknown, but some cases occur via genetic inheritance. Associated anomalies may occur with Wilms' tumour. Wilms' tumour demonstrates rapid growth and is usually large at diagnosis. Metastasis occurs via direct extension or through the bloodstream. Wilms' tumour most commonly metastasizes to the perirenal tissues, liver, diaphragm, lungs, abdominal muscles, and lymph nodes. The prognosis depends on staging at diagnosis and the extent of metastasis (Box 49.3). The prognosis of patients with Wilms' tumour is the most encouraging of all solid tumours, with an overall survival rate of about 90% (Hendershot, 2010). Complications include metastasis or complications from radiation therapy such as liver or renal damage, female sterility, bowel obstruction, pneumonia, or scoliosis.

Therapeutic Management

Surgical removal of the tumour and affected kidney (nephrectomy) is the treatment of choice and also allows

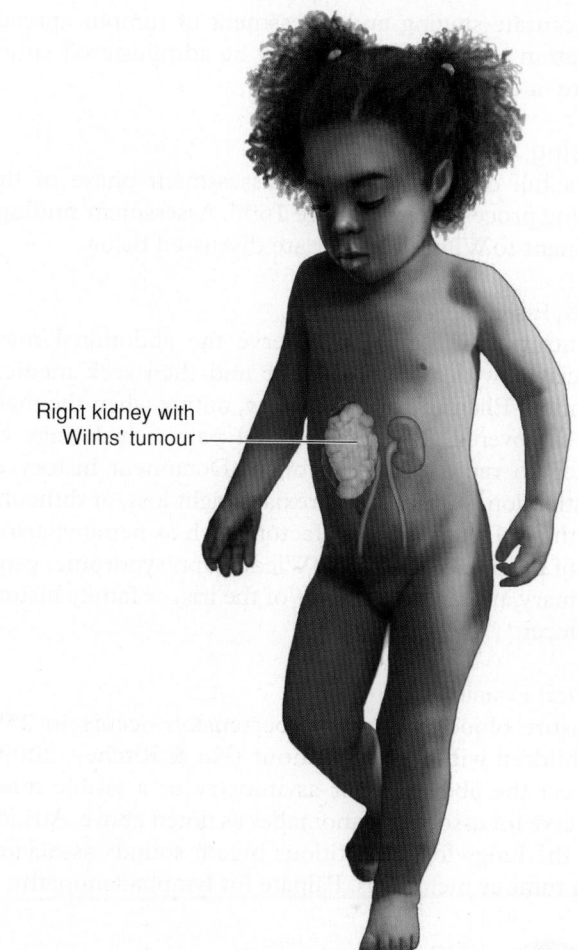

Right kidney with Wilms' tumour

FIGURE 49.8 Wilms' tumour is usually unilateral.

BOX 49.3 **Staging of Wilms' Tumour Developed by the National Wilms' Tumour Study Group and International Society of Pediatric Oncology**

- Stage I: unilateral, limited to kidney, completely resectable
- Stage II: unilateral, tumour extends beyond kidney but is completely resectable
- Stage III: unilateral, tumour has spread outside of kidney, located in abdominal cavity only, not fully removed
- Stage IV: unilateral with metastasis in liver, lung, bone, or brain
- Stage V: bilateral kidney involvement

From: Hendershot, E. (2010). Solid tumors. In D. Tomlinson, & N. E. Kline (Eds.), *Pediatric oncology nursing: Advanced clinical handbook* (2nd ed.). New York: Springer.

for accurate staging and assessment of tumour spread. Radiation or chemotherapy may be administered either before or after surgery.

Nursing Assessment

For a full description of the assessment phase of the nursing process, refer to page 1693. Assessment findings pertinent to Wilms' tumour are discussed below.

Health History

Parents typically initially observe the abdominal mass associated with Wilms' tumour and then seek medical attention. Elicit the health history, noting when the mass was discovered. Note abdominal pain, which may be related to rapid tumour growth. Document history of constipation, vomiting, anorexia, weight loss, or difficulty breathing. Determine risk factors such as hemihypertrophy of the spine, Beckwith–Wiedemann syndrome, genitourinary anomalies, absence of the iris, or family history of cancer.

Physical Examination

Measure blood pressure: hypertension occurs in 25% of children with Wilms' tumour (Ko & Ritchey, 2009). Inspect the abdomen for asymmetry or a visible mass. Observe for associated anomalies as noted above. Auscultate the lungs for adventitious breath sounds associated with tumour metastasis. Palpate for lymphadenopathy.

> ▶ **Take** NOTE!
>
> *Avoid palpating the abdomen after the initial assessment preoperatively. Wilms' tumour is highly vascular and soft, so excessive handling of the tumour may result in tumour seeding and metastasis (Ruble, 2010).*

Laboratory and Diagnostic Testing

Laboratory and diagnostic testing may include:

- Renal or abdominal ultrasound to assess the tumour and the contralateral kidney
- CT or MRI of the abdomen and chest to determine local spread to lymph nodes or adjacent organs, as well as any distant metastasis
- Complete blood count, BUN, and creatinine: usually within normal limits
- Urinalysis: may reveal hematuria or leukocytes
- 24-hour urine collection for HVA and VMA to distinguish the tumour from neuroblastoma (levels will not be elevated with Wilms' tumour)

Nursing Management

Postoperative care of the child with Wilms' tumour resection is similar to that of children undergoing other

abdominal surgery. Assessment of remaining kidney function is critical. The child may have adverse effects related to chemotherapy or radiation. Refer to the Nursing Process Overview section and Nursing Care Plan 49.1 to individualize care for the child based on the child's response to the therapy.

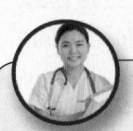

> ▶ **Take** NOTE!
>
> *To avoid injuring the remaining kidney, children with a single kidney should not play contact sports.*

Retinoblastoma

Retinoblastoma is a rare, congenital, highly malignant tumour that arises from embryonic retinal cells. It accounts for 5% of cases of blindness in children (Maloney et al., 2010). Most children are diagnosed before 6 years of age. Retinoblastoma is the most curable of all childhood cancers, with an overall survival rate of more than 90% (Melamud, Palekar, & Singh, 2006). When retinoblastoma extends outside the eye, however, the mortality rate is very high (Canadian Ophthalmological Society, 2009; Canty, 2009).

Retinoblastoma may be hereditary or nonhereditary. Nonhereditary retinoblastoma may be associated with advanced paternal age and always presents with unilateral involvement. Hereditary retinoblastoma is inherited via the autosomal dominant mode. These cases may be unilateral or bilateral. The tumour may grow forward into the vitreous cavity of the eye or extend into the subretinal space, causing retinal detachment. The tumour may extend into the choroid, the sclera, and the optic nerve.

Complications include spread to the brain and the opposite eye, as well as metastasis to lymph nodes, bone, bone marrow, and liver. Secondary tumours, most often sarcomas, may also occur in children who have been treated for retinoblastoma. Table 49.7 explains the staging of retinoblastoma.

TABLE 49.7   **STAGING OF RETINOBLASTOMA**

A	Small tumours (<3 mm; about 0.1 inch) confined to the retina
B	Larger tumours confined to the retina
C	Localized seeding of the vitreous or under the retina <6 mm (0.2 inches) from the original tumour
D	Widespread vitreous or subretinal seeding, may have total retinal detachment
E	No visual potential, eye cannot recover

From: American Cancer Society. (2011c). *How is retinoblastoma staged?* Retrieved November 7, 2011 from http://www.cancer.org/cancer/retinoblastoma/detailedguide/retinoblastoma-staging.

The primary goal of treatment is to preserve the child's life. Other key goals are to retain the eye and maintain vision and provide a good cosmetic outcome (Canadian Ophthalmological Society, 2009). Retinoblastoma may be treated with radiation, chemotherapy, laser surgery, cryotherapy, or a combination. Other treatments include chemoreduction and radioactive plaques (Canty, 2009). Some vision may be preserved for most children without advanced disease (Canadian Ophthalmological Society, 2009; Canty, 2009). In advanced disease or in the case of a massive tumour with retinal detachment, enucleation (removal of the eye) is necessary (Canadian Ophthalmological Society, 2009).

Nursing Assessment

Parents are often the first to notice the "cat's eye reflex" or "whitewash glow" to the child's affected pupil. Obtain the health history, determining when other associated symptoms such as strabismus, orbital inflammation, vomiting, or headache began. Inquire about risk factors such as a family history of retinoblastoma or other cancer or the presence of chromosomal anomalies. Assess pupils for size and reactivity to light. Note presence of leukocoria ("cat's eye reflex," a whitish appearance of the pupil) in the affected eye (Fig. 49.9). Assess the eyes for associated signs, which may include erythema, orbital inflammation, or hyphema.

Diagnostic evaluation includes an ophthalmologic examination under anesthesia. CT, MRI, or ultrasound of the head and eyes will help to visualize the tumour. The infant or toddler may also undergo lumbar puncture and bone marrow aspiration to determine the presence and extent of metastasis.

Nursing Management

Provide routine postoperative care to the infant or toddler. If the eye is enucleated, observe the large pressure

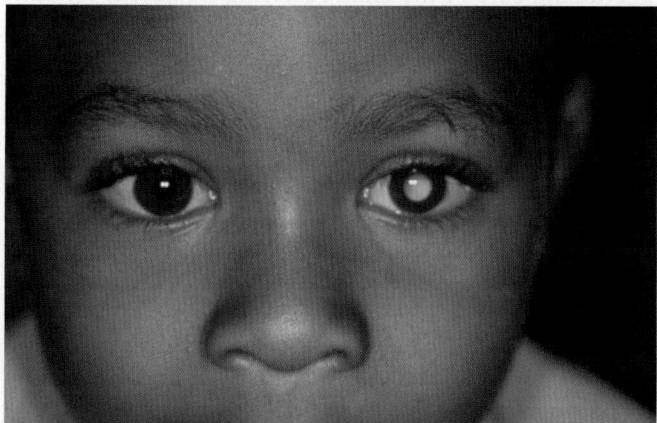

FIGURE 49.9 Note the whitish appearance of the pupil (leukocoria) in this child with retinoblastoma. (Used with permission from: *Chung's visual diagnosis and treatments in pediatrics* (2nd ed.). Philadelphia: Lippincott Williams & Wilkins; 2010.)

dressing on the eye socket for bleeding. Dressing changes to the socket may include sterile saline rinses and/or antibiotic ointment application. If disease occurs outside the eye or if metastasis is present, inform the parents that chemotherapy will be necessary. Monitor for side effects of chemotherapy (see the Nursing Process Overview section). Follow-up will include eye examinations every 3 to 6 months until age 6 and then annually to check for further tumour development (Canadian Ophthalmological Society, 2009; Canty, 2009). If the eye is enucleated, a prosthetic eye will be fitted several weeks after removal. Teach families about use of the prosthetic eye, which does not require daily removal.

Provide parents with support and encouragement. Refer the family for genetic counselling. Subsequent children will need ophthalmologic examination under anesthesia at 2 months of age and frequent examinations until age 3 years. Children treated for retinoblastoma will also need genetic counselling as they reach puberty, as about half of the offspring of children with retinoblastoma have bilateral disease.

▶ *Take* NOTE!

Educate parents about protecting vision in the remaining eye: routine eye check-ups, protection from accidental injury, use of safety goggles during sports, and prompt treatment of eye infections. Generally, children with one eye should not participate in contact sports. After treatment, survivors of retinoblastoma need to be aware of the likelihood of a second nonocular tumour such as a soft tissue sarcoma. As such, survivors and their families should be educated about the importance of long-term follow up and screening (Canty, 2009).

Screening for Reproductive Cancers in Adolescents

Increasingly, reproductive cancers are being diagnosed in adolescents. Cervical cancer and testicular cancer may be discovered early with appropriate screening, and earlier discovery leads to better outcomes. Starting screening in the teenage years may also instill a lifelong healthy habit in the adolescent.

Cervical Cancer

Risk factors for cervical cancer include young age at first intercourse, infection with a sexually transmitted disease, and a history of multiple sex partners, and more and more teenagers are presenting with these risk factors. Counsel all sexually active adolescents to seek reproductive care, which is available without parental consent in

TEACHING GUIDELINE 49.3

Testicular Self–Examination

• Perform the examination once a month, after a shower.
• Be familiar with the size and weight of your testicles.
• Roll the testicle between your fingers. The small rope-like structure is the epididymis; this is normal.
• Report any lump, swelling, or heaviness of one testicle to your health care provider.

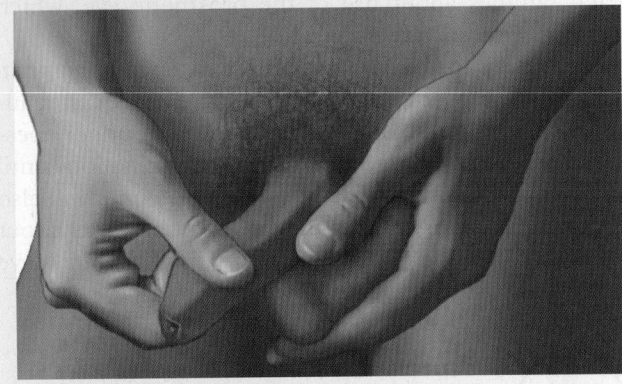

Source: Canadian Cancer Society. (2011). *Early detection of testicular cancer.* Retrieved November 7, 2011 from http://www.cancer.ca/canada-wide/about%20cancer/types%20of%20cancer/early%20detection%20of%20testicular%20cancer.aspx?sc_lang=en.

Canada (Dickens & Cook, 2005). The screening Papanicolaou (Pap) smear is efficient and reliable at determining abnormal cervical cells and is a key part of screening for cervical cancer (Oteng, Marra, Lynd, et al., 2010). Cervical cancer has a very high response to therapy and rate of cure if treated in its early stages, so nurses should encourage teenage girls to be responsible for their sexual health by seeking appropriate examination and screening.

Testicular Cancer

In Canada, testicular cancer is the most common cancer in male adolescents and young adults between the ages of 15 and 29 years (Canadian Cancer Society's Steering Committee on Cancer Statistics, 2011, May). It is one of the most curable cancers if diagnosed early. To get into the habit of screening for testicular lumps, adolescent boys should begin performing testicular self-examinations monthly (Canadian Cancer Society, 2011) (Teaching Guideline 49.3).

■■■ Key Concepts

■ In adults, cancer is influenced to a large extent by environmental factors. As this is not true for children, there are no routine screening measures or prevention strategies for childhood cancer.

■ The pain associated with lumbar puncture or bone marrow aspiration may be minimized with the use of topical anesthetics or conscious sedation.

■ CT and MRI are used extensively in the diagnosis and follow-up of childhood cancer. The young child may have difficulty holding still for these scans and may need short-term sedation.

■ Leukemia often presents in children with a history of fever, infection, and fatigue. Bone pain or CNS symptoms may be present if metastasis to the bone or brain has occurred.

■ Lymphomas in children present similarly to those in adults, often with an enlarged, nontender lymph node.

■ Symptoms of brain tumours depend on the location of the tumour; commonly they present with signs and symptoms of increased intracranial pressure, such as headache, nausea, and vomiting.

■ Neuroblastoma has often significantly metastasized at diagnosis. It most commonly presents as a mass in the abdomen.

■ Shortness of breath or chest pain in the child with cancer is a medical emergency; it may indicate superior vena cava syndrome or a tumour in the mediastinal region.

■ Retinoblastoma may be identified by the presence of leukocoria in one or both eyes. Retinoblastoma occurs in early infancy up until early childhood.

■ Bone cancer does not necessarily require amputation; it may be treated with a combination of limb salvage procedure, radiation, and chemotherapy.

■ The symptoms of rhabdomyosarcoma depend on the location of the tumour.

■ Avoid abdominal palpation preoperatively in the child with Wilms' tumour; palpation may cause seeding of the tumour and metastasis.

■ Radiation therapy may result in fatigue, nausea and vomiting, and long-term cognitive sequelae (if directed to the cranium).

■ Nursing care of the child receiving treatment for cancer focuses on preventing or treating adverse effects such as fatigue, nausea, vomiting, alopecia, mucositis, and infection.

■ The neutropenic child with fever should receive medical attention as soon as possible so that intravenous antibiotics may be started immediately.

■ Cancer is a significant stressor for children and families. Families need support and education throughout the diagnostic process, treatment and cure, or palliative care.

■ The child with cancer should lead as near normal a life as possible. When physically able and cleared by the oncologist, the child should resume usual activities such as school. Camps for children with cancer provide an excellent opportunity for children to enjoy everyday activities and meet children experiencing similar alterations in their lives.

- Nutrition may be optimized for children with cancer by managing nausea and vomiting with antiemetics, providing favourite foods, and possibly using total parenteral nutrition.
- Teach adolescents appropriate screening techniques for reproductive cancers.
- Educate the child and family about the adverse effects of cancer treatments.
- Teach parents how to avoid infection in the child receiving chemotherapy, the signs and symptoms of infection, and when to seek medical treatment.

REFERENCES

American Cancer Society. (2011a). *Cancer in children*. Retrieved November 7, 2011 from http://www.cancer.org/acs/groups/cid/documents/webcontent/002287-pdf.pdf

American Cancer Society. (2011b). *How is Hodgkin disease staged?* Retrieved November 9, 2011 from http://www.cancer.org/Cancer/HodgkinDisease/DetailedGuide/hodgkin-disease-staging

American Cancer Society. (2011c). *How is retinoblastoma staged?* Retrieved November 9, 2011 from http://www.cancer.org/cancer/retinoblastoma/detailedguide/retinoblastoma-staging

Anderson, F., & Kunin-Batson, A. (2009). Neurocognitive late effects of chemotherapy in children: The past 10 years of research on brain structure and function. *Pediatric Blood & Cancer, 52*(2), 159–164.

Axton, S. E., & Fugate, T. (2009). *Pediatric nursing care plans for the hospitalized child* (3rd ed.). Upper Saddle River, NJ: Pearson.

Baggott, C. (2010). Cancer. In P. J. Allen, J. A. Vessey, & N. A. Schapiro (Eds.), *Primary care of the child with a chronic condition* (5th ed.). St. Louis, MO: Mosby.

Baggott, C., Dodd, M., Kennedy, C., et al. (2010). Changes in children's reports of symptom occurrence and severity during a course of myelosuppressive chemotherapy. *Journal of Pediatric Oncology Nursing, 27*(6), 307–315.

Baggott, C. R., Kelly, K. P., Fochtman, D., & Foley, G. V. (Eds.). (in press). *Nursing care of children and adolescents with cancer* (4th ed.). Glenview, IL: Association of Pediatric Hematology Oncology Nurses.

Bennett-Rees, N., & Hopkins, S. (2008). Discharge planning and psychosocial issues for the family. In F. Gibson & L. Soanes (Eds.), *Cancer in children and young people: Acute nursing care*. West Sussex, England: John Wiley & Sons Ltd.

Bennett-Rees, N., Hopkins, S., & Stone, J. (2008). Preparation for bone marrow transplant. In F. Gibson & L. Soanes (Eds.), *Cancer in children and young people: Acute nursing care*. West Sussex, England: John Wiley & Sons Ltd.

Canadian Cancer Society. (2011). *Early detection of testicular cancer*. Retrieved November 7, 2011 from http://www.cancer.ca/canada-wide/about%20cancer/types%20of%20cancer/early%20detection%20of%20testicular%20cancer.aspx?sc_lang=en

Canadian Cancer Society's Steering Committee on Cancer Statistics. (2011). *Canadian cancer statistics 2011*. Toronto, ON: Canadian Cancer Society.

Canadian Ophthalmological Society. (2009). National retinoblastoma strategy Canadian guidelines for care. *Canadian Journal of Ophthalmology, 44*, s2–s88.

Canadian Paediatric Society. (2004). Position statement B 2004–01: Treatment decisions regarding infants, children and adolescents. *Pediatric & Child Health, 9*(2), 99–103. Retrieved November 7, 2011 from http://www.cps.ca/english/statements/B/b04-01.pdf

Canadian Paediatric Society. (2008). Position statement B 2008–02: Advanced care planning for paediatric patients. *Pediatric & Child Health, 13*(9), 791–796. Retrieved November 7, 2011 from http://www.cps.ca/english/statements/B/B08-02.pdf

Canty, C. A. (2009). Retinoblastoma: An overview for advanced practice nurses. *Journal of the American Academy of Advanced Practice Nurses, 21*, 149–155.

Carpenito-Moyet, L. J. (2010). *Nursing diagnosis: Application to clinical practice* (13th ed.). Philadelphia: Lippincott Williams & Wilkins.

Carrle, D., & Bielack, S. S. (2006). Current strategies of chemotherapy in osteosarcoma. *International Orthopaedics, 30*, 445–451.

Childhood Cancer Canada Foundation. (2011). *C17*. Retrieved April 1, 2012 from http://childhoodcancer.ca/research/C17

Chordas, C., & Graham, K. (2010). Chemotherapy. In D. Tomlinson & N. E. Kline (Eds.), *Pediatric oncology nursing: Advanced clinical handbook* (2nd ed.). New York: Springer.

Colby-Graham, M., & Chordas, C. (2003). The childhood leukemias. *Journal of Pediatric Nursing, 18*(2), 87–95.

Copelan, E. (2006). Hematopoietic stem-cell transplantation. *New England Journal of Medicine, 354*(17), 1813–1826.

Coppell, J. A., Richardson, P. G., Soiffer, R., et al. (2010). Hepatic veno-occlusive disease following stem cell transplantation: Incidence, clinical course, and outcome. *Biology of Blood and Marrow Transplantation, 16*(2), 157–168.

Dickens, B., & Cook, R. (2005). Ethical and legal issues in reproductive health: Adolescents and consent to treatment. *International Journal of Gynecology and Obstetrics, 89*, 179–184.

Doyle, S. (2010). Bone marrow function. In D. Tomlinson & N. E. Kline (Eds.), *Pediatric oncology nursing: Advanced clinical handbook* (2nd ed.). New York: Springer.

Ellison, L. F., De, P., Mery, L. S., & Grundy, P. E. (2009). Canadian cancer statistics at a glance: Cancer in children. *Canadian Medical Association Journal, 180*(4), 422–424.

Faithfull, S. (2008). Radiotherapy. In J. Corner & C. Bailey (Eds.), *Cancer nursing: Care in context* (2nd ed.). Oxford, UK: Blackwell.

Gainer, E. (2010). Biological and targeted therapies. In D. Tomlinson & N. E. Kline (Eds.), *Pediatric oncology nursing: Advanced clinical handbook* (2nd ed.). New York: Springer.

Gross, T. G., & Termuhlen, A. M. (2007). Pediatric non-Hodgkin's lymphoma. *Current Oncology Reports, 9*, 459–465.

Hayden, J. B., & Hoang, B. H. (2006). Osteosarcoma: Basic science and clinical impressions. *Orthopedic Clinics of North America, 37*, 445–451.

Hendershot, E. (2010). Solid tumors. In D. Tomlinson & N. E. Kline (Eds.), *Pediatric oncology nursing: Advanced clinical handbook* (2nd ed.). New York: Springer.

Hokkanen, H., Eriksson, E., Ahonen, O., & Salantera, S. (2004). Adolescents with cancer: Experience of life and how it could be made easier. *Cancer Nursing, 27*(4), 325–335.

Hooke, C., Hellsten, M. B., Stutzer, C., & Forte, K. (2002). Pain management for the child with cancer in end of life care: Association of pediatric oncology nurses position paper. *Journal of Pediatric Oncology Nursing, 19*(2), 43–47.

Kline, N. E., & O'Hanlon-Curry, J. (2010). Central nervous system tumors. In D. Tomlinson & N. E. Kline (Eds.), *Pediatric oncology nursing: Advanced clinical handbook* (2nd ed.). New York: Springer.

Ko, E. Y., & Ritchey, M. L. (2009). Current management of Wilms' tumor in children. *Journal of Pediatric Urology, 5*, 56–65.

Larsen, E. (2011). *Childhood cancer*. Retrieved November 7, 2011 from http://www.cancerstory.org/index.php/cancerstory/article/56

Loch, I., & Khorrami, J. (2010). Radiotherapy. In D. Tomlinson & N. E. Kline (Eds.), *Pediatric oncology nursing: Advanced clinical handbook* (2nd ed.). New York: Springer.

Lund, A. E. (2005). Cancer therapies in childhood can damage developing teeth. *Journal of the American Dental Association, 10*, 1370.

Maloney, A. M. (2010). Gastrointestinal tract. In D. Tomlinson & N. E. Kline (Eds.), *Pediatric oncology nursing: Advanced clinical handbook* (2nd ed.). New York: Springer.

Maloney, K., Foreman, N. K., Giller, R. H., et al. (2010). Neoplastic disease. In W. W. Hay, M. J. Levin, J. M. Sondheimer, & R. R. Deterding (Eds.), *Current pediatric diagnosis and treatment* (20th ed.). New York: McGraw-Hill.

May, L., & Ward, B. (2008). Side effects of chemotherapy. In F. Gibson & L. Soanes (Eds.), *Cancer in children and young people: Acute nursing care*. West Sussex, UK: John Wiley & Sons Ltd.

Melamud, A., Palekar, R., & Singh, A. (2006). Retinoblastoma. *American Family Physician, 73*, 1039–1044.

Meyer, J. S., Nadel, H. R., Marina, N., et al. (2008). Imagining guidelines for children with Ewing sarcoma and osteosarcoma: A report from the Children's Oncology Group Bone Tumor Committee. *Pediatric Blood Cancer, 51*, 163–170.

Nathan, M., & Tomlinson, D. (2010). Skin: Cutaneous toxicities. In D. Tomlinson & N. E. Kline (Eds.), *Pediatric oncology nursing: Advanced clinical handbook* (2nd ed.). New York: Springer.

Nixon, C. (2010). Blood transfusion therapy. In D. Tomlinson & N. E. Kline (Eds.), *Pediatric oncology nursing: Advanced clinical handbook* (2nd ed.). New York: Springer.

Norville, R., & Tomlinson, D. (2010). Hematopoietic stem cell transplantation. In D. Tomlinson & N. E. Kline (Eds.), *Pediatric oncology nursing: Advanced clinical handbook* (2nd ed.). New York: Springer.

Oteng, B., Marra, F., Lynd, L., Ogilvie, G., Patrick, D., & Marra, C. (2010). Evaluating societal preferences for human papillomavirus vaccine and cervical smear test screening programme. *Sexually Transmitted Infections.* Published online October 18, 2010. doi:10.1136/sti.2009.041392

Ozger, H., Bulbul, M., & Eralp, L. (2010). Complications of limb salvage surgery in childhood tumors and recommended solutions. *Strategies in Trauma and Limb Reconstruction, 5*, 11–15.

Pagana, K. D., & Pagana, T. J. (2010). *Mosby's manual of diagnostic and laboratory tests* (4th ed.). St. Louis, MO: Mosby.

Paulino, A. C., & Okcu, M. F. (2008). Rhabdomyosarcoma. *Current Problems in Cancer, 32*, 7–34.

Post-White, J., & Ladas, E. (2010). Complementary and alternative medicine. In D. Tomlinson & N. E. Kline (Eds.), *Pediatric oncology nursing: Advanced clinical handbook* (2nd ed.). New York: Springer.

Rheingans, J. I. (2007). A systematic review of nonpharmacologic adjunctive therapies for symptom management in children with cancer. *Journal of Pediatric Oncology Nursing, 24*(2), 81–94.

Rimkus, C. (2009). Acute complications of stem cell transplant. *Seminars in Oncology Nursing, 25*(2), 129–138.

Rodgers, C., & Gonzalez, S. (2010). Hematopoietic stem cell transplantation. In D. Tomlinson & N. E. Kline (Eds.), *Pediatric oncology nursing: Advanced clinical handbook* (2nd ed.). New York: Springer.

Ruble, K. (2010). Pediatric oncology. In S. M. Nettina (Ed.), *Lippincott manual of nursing practice* (9th ed.). Philadelphia: Wolters Kluwer Health/Lippincott Williams & Wilkins.

Sandlund, J. T., Downing, J. R., & Crist, W. M. (1996). Non-Hodgkin's lymphoma in childhood. *New England Journal of Medicine, 334*, 1238–1248.

Schwartz, C. L. (2003). The management of Hodgkin's disease in the young child. *Current Opinion in Pediatrics, 15*(1), 10–16.

Selwood, K. (2008). Side effects of chemotherapy. In F. Gibson & L. Soanes (Eds.), *Cancer in children and young people: Acute nursing care.* West Sussex, UK: John Wiley & Sons Ltd.

Simon, C. (2010). Pain in children with cancer. In D. Tomlinson & N. E. Kline (Eds.), *Pediatric oncology nursing: Advanced clinical handbook* (2nd ed.). New York: Springer.

Sola, A., Saldeño, P., & Favareto, V. (2008). Clinical practices in neonatal oxygenation: Where have we failed? What can we do? *Journal of Perinatology, 28*, S28–S34.

Stuber, M., & Seacord, D. (2004). Psychiatric impact of childhood cancer. In S. Kreitler, B. Weyl, & M. Arush (Eds.), *Psychosocial aspects of pediatric oncology.* West Sussex, UK: John Wiley & Sons Ltd.

Tomlinson, D., & Kline, N. E. (Eds.). (2010). *Pediatric oncology nursing.* New York: Springer.

Wagner, L. M., & Danks, M. K. (2009). New therapeutic targets for the treatment of high risk Neuroblastoma. *Journal of Cellular Biochemistry, 107*, 46–57.

Weitzman, S., & Arcici, R. (2003). Non-Hodgkin's lymphoma of childhood. In P. Wiernik, J. Golman, J. Dutcher, & R. Kyle (Eds.), *Neoplastic diseases of the blood.* Cambridge: Cambridge University Press.

Woodgate, R. L. (2005). Life is never the same: Childhood cancer narratives. *European Journal of Cancer Care, 15*, 8–18.

Woodgate, R. L. (2008). Getting on with life. In D. Kelly & F. Gibson (Eds.), *Cancer care in adolescents and young adults.* Oxford, UK: Wiley-Blackwell.

Woodgate, R. L., West, C., & Wilkin, K. (2011). Family-centered psychosocial care. In C. Baggott, D. Fochtman, G. Foley, & K. Kelly (Eds.), *Nursing care of children and adolescents with cancer and blood disorders* (4th ed., pp. 114–164). Glenview, Illinois: Association of Pediatric Hematology/Oncology Nurses (APHON).

Zupanec, S. (2010). Lymphoma. In D. Tomlinson & N. E. Kline (Eds.), *Pediatric oncology nursing: Advanced clinical handbook* (2nd ed.). New York: Springer.

Zupanec, S., & Tomlinson, D. (2010). Leukemia. In D. Tomlinson & N. E. Kline (Eds.), *Pediatric oncology nursing: Advanced clinical handbook* (2nd ed.). New York: Springer.

RECOMMENDED READINGS

Ackley, B. J., & Ladwig, G. B. (2011). *Nursing diagnosis handbook: A evidence-based guide to planning care* (9th ed.). St. Louis, MO: Mosby.

Fry, T. (2010). Expanding options to improve outcomes following hematopoietic stem cell transplantation. *Pediatric Blood & Cancer, 55*, 1043–1044.

Messerschmitt, P. J, Garcia, R. M., Abdul-Karim, F. W., Greenfield, E. M., & Getty, P. J. (2009). Osteosarcoma. *Journal of the American Academy of Orthopaedic Surgeons, 17*(8), 515–527.

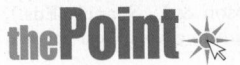

For additional learning materials, including Internet Resources, visit http://thePoint.lww.com/Chow1e.

CHAPTER WORKSHEET

MULTIPLE CHOICE QUESTIONS

1. A 5-year-old has been diagnosed with Wilms' tumour. What is the priority nursing intervention for this child?

   a. Educate the parents about dialysis, as the kidney will be removed.

   b. Measure abdominal girth every shift.

   c. Avoid palpating the child's abdomen.

   d. Monitor BUN and creatinine every 4 hours.

2. A child with leukemia has the following AM laboratory results: Hgb 8.0, Hct 24.2, WBC 8,000, platelets 150,000. What is the priority nursing assessment?

   a. Monitor for fever.

   b. Assess for bruising or bleeding.

   c. Determine intake and output.

   d. Assess for pallor, fatigue, tachycardia.

3. A child with leukemia received chemotherapy about 10 days ago. She presents today with a temperature of 38°C, an ANC of 500, and mild bleeding of the gums. What is the priority nursing intervention?

   a. Administer IV antibiotics as ordered.

   b. Provide vigorous oral care frequently.

   c. Monitor pulse and blood pressure for changes.

   d. Administer packed red blood cell transfusion.

4. A child with cancer is receiving chemotherapy, and his mother is concerned that the nausea and vomiting associated with chemotherapy are reducing his ability to eat and gain weight appropriately. What is the most appropriate nursing action?

   a. Administer an antiemetic at the first hint of nausea.

   b. Offer the child's favourite foods to encourage him to eat.

   c. Start antiemetic drugs prior to the chemotherapy infusion.

   d. Maintain IV fluid infusion to avoid dehydration.

CRITICAL THINKING EXERCISES

1. Develop a discharge teaching plan for a child who has just completed the induction phase of chemotherapy for acute lymphocytic leukemia.

2. A 17-year-old girl has recently been diagnosed with osteosarcoma. She is worried about how treatment will affect her plans for college, marriage, and children. How will you respond to her concerns?

3. A 3-year-old is going to start chemotherapy for rhabdomyosarcoma. Develop an age-appropriate teaching plan for this child.

4. Develop a nursing care plan for an adolescent with cancer who is undergoing radiation and chemotherapy and experiencing a significant number of adverse effects from his treatment.

STUDY ACTIVITIES

1. While in the clinical area, care for a young child who has undergone therapy for a brain tumour. Compare this child's growth and development with those of a healthy similar-age child who you know or have cared for.

2. During your clinical rotation, care for a child who has received several chemotherapy treatments. After establishing a therapeutic relationship, talk with the child about his or her understanding of the disease and the experience the child has had with diagnosis and treatment thus far. If time allows, ask the child to draw a picture describing this experience. Record your observations in your clinical journal and reflect on the emotions you feel about this experience.

3. Attend the pediatric oncology clinic. Determine the role of the advanced practice nurse (nurse practitioner or clinical nurse specialist) compared with the role of the registered nurse in the out-patient care of children with cancer. Determine which activities the nurse appropriately delegates to unlicensed assistive personnel in that setting.

4. Talk to the hospital chaplain about his or her experiences with dying children. Reflect on this conversation in your clinical journal.

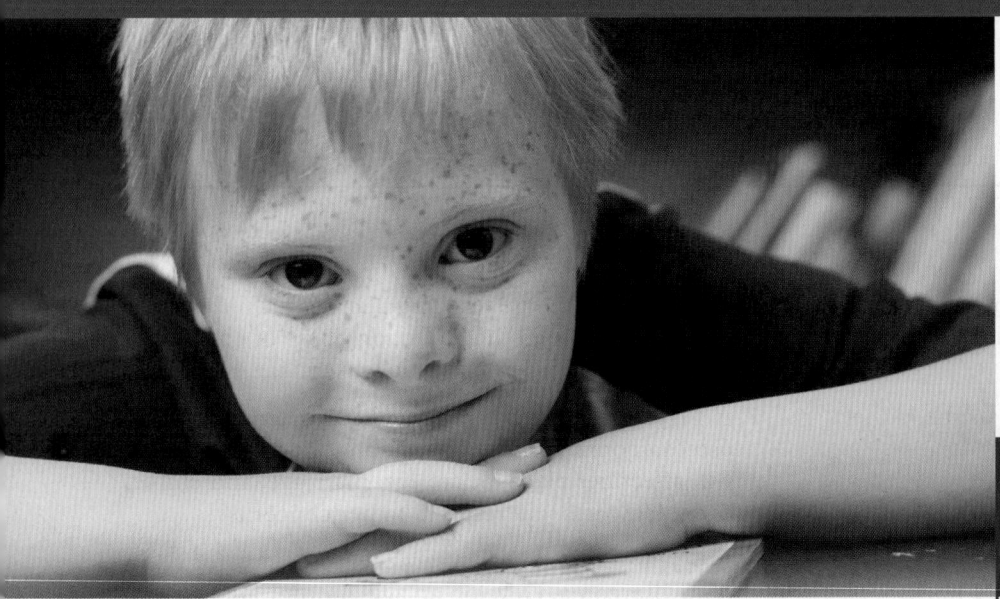

CHAPTER 50

Adapted by Beverley Temple

NURSING CARE OF THE CHILD WITH A GENETIC DISORDER

KEY TERMS

allele
chromosome
consanguinity
gene

genetics
genome
genotype
heterozygous

homozygous
karyotype
nondisjunction
phenotype

LEARNING OBJECTIVES

Upon completion of the chapter, the learner will be able to:

1. Discuss various inheritance patterns, including nontraditional patterns of inheritance.
2. Discuss ethical and legal issues associated with genetic testing.
3. Discuss genetic counselling and the role of the nurse.
4. Identify nursing interventions related to common laboratory and diagnostic tests used in the diagnosis and management of genetic conditions.
5. Distinguish various genetic disorders occurring in childhood.
6. Devise an individualized nursing care plan for the child with a genetic disorder.
7. Develop patient/family teaching plans for the child with a genetic disorder.

Julie Woods, a 5-year-old, is brought to the clinic for her annual examination. Her mother states, "She's so much smaller than all of the other kindergartners."

Wow

Pediatric nurses care for children and their families who are living with the diagnosis and effects of one or more genetic disorders.

Genetics is the study of heredity and its variation (Venes, 2005). Many disorders of childhood have a genetic or inherited cause. Common disorders suspected to be caused or influenced by genetic factors include birth defects, chromosomal abnormalities, neurocutaneous disorders, intellectual disabilities, many types of short stature, connective tissue disorders, and inborn errors of metabolism. According to the Centers for Disease Control and Prevention, birth defects and genetic disorders are a significant cause of morbidity and mortality in infancy and childhood: "Twenty-five to thirty-nine percent of admissions to children's hospitals involve children with genetically determined or partially genetically determined disorders; 11% of all deaths in childhood are related to an underlying genetic condition" (Behrman, Kliegman, & Jenson, 2004, p. 367).

Our ability to diagnose genetic conditions is far superior to our ability to cure or treat them. However, accurate diagnosis leads to improved treatment and outcomes. Nurses should have a basic knowledge of genetics, common genetic disorders in children, genetic testing, and genetic counselling so that they can provide support and information to families and can promote an improved quality of life.

Inheritance

A **gene** is the basic unit of heredity. Genes occupy a specific location on a **chromosome** (a long, continuous strand of DNA that carries genetic information) and determine the organism's physical and mental characteristics. In humans, each somatic cell (a cell forming the body of an organism) has 46 chromosomes: 22 pairs of non-sex chromosomes (autosomes) and 1 pair of sex chromosomes. The **genotype** is the specific genetic makeup of an individual; it is the internally coded inheritable information and refers to the particular **allele** (one of two or more alternative versions of gene at a given position on a chromosome that imparts the same characteristic of that gene). For example, each human has a gene that controls height, but there are variations of these genes (alleles) that can produce a height of 5 feet or one of 6 feet, 2 inches. A gene that controls eye colour may have an allele that can produce blue eyes or an allele that produces brown eyes. The genotype, together with environmental variation that influences the individual, determines the **phenotype** (the outward characteristics of the individual).

A human inherits two genes, one from each parent; therefore, one allele comes from the mother and one from the father. These alleles may be the same for the characteristic (**homozygous**) or different (**heterozygous**). If the two alleles differ, the dominant one will usually be expressed in the individual's phenotype.

The Human Genome

The **genome** of an organism is its entire hereditary information encoded in the DNA. The Human Genome Project (HGP, 2006), an international effort to produce a comprehensive sequence of the human genome, was coordinated by the U.S. Department of Energy and the National Institutes of Health. It began in October 1990 and was completed in May 2003. Its goals included the following:

- Identify all of the approximately 20,000 to 25,000 genes in human DNA.
- Determine the sequences of the 3 billion chemical base pairs that make up human DNA.
- Store this information in databases to make it accessible for further study.
- Improve tools for data analysis.
- Transfer related technologies to the private sector.
- Address the ethical, legal, and social implications of this discovery (U.S. Department of Energy Genome Programs, 2011).

The HGP has led to the discovery of the genetic basis for hundreds of disorders and has advanced our understanding of basic genetic processes at the molecular level. Visit http://thePoint.lww.com/Chow1e for a direct link to additional information about the HGP.

One goal of the HGP was to translate the findings into new and more effective strategies for the prevention, diagnosis, and treatment of genetic disorders. Current and potential applications for the HGP to health care include rapid and more specific diagnosis of disease, with hundreds of genetic tests available in research or clinical practice; earlier detection of genetic predisposition to disease; less emphasis on treating the symptoms of a disease and more emphasis on seeking the fundamental causes of the disease; new classes of drugs; avoiding environmental conditions that may trigger disease; and repair or replacement of defective genes using gene therapy. This knowledge, along with the commercialization of the technology, will change our approach to genetic disorders.

Although these advances have many current and potential benefits to children, they also raise serious ethical, legal, and social issues. The HGP recognized this and developed a branch, called Ethical, Legal, and Social Issues, that was responsible for addressing and overseeing these issues while determining how to use this information in the safest, most beneficial manner. Some of these issues include privacy and confidentiality of genetic information, who should have access to personal genetic information, psychological impact, and stigmatization due to individual genetic differences, use of genetic information in reproductive decision making and reproductive rights, and whether testing should be performed if no cure is available. Several organizations provide information and guidelines about these issues for those who practice in the field of medical genetics:

- The Canadian College of Medical Geneticists has developed ethical guidelines describing the responsibilities to patients, society, and the medical profession.
- The International Society of Nurses in Genetics offers resources about ethics, standards of practice, and competencies.
- The Canadian Nurses Association has a series of short papers that discuss the Canadian context and ethical issues for nurses to consider. Refer to http://thePoint. lww.com/Chow1e for the direct link to this Web series.

Further information about these organizations can be found by visiting the Canadian College of Medical Geneticists' website; visit http://thePoint.lww.com/Chow1e for the direct link.

Patterns of Inheritance

Diagnosis of a genetic disorder is usually based on clinical signs and symptoms or on laboratory confirmation of an altered gene associated with the disorder. Accurate diagnosis can be aided by identifying the pattern of inheritance within a family. Also, nurses must understand the pattern of inheritance so they can teach and counsel families about the risks of future pregnancies. Some genetic disorders occur in multiple family members; others may occur in only a single family member. A genetic disorder is caused by completely or partially altered genetic material; in contrast, a familial disorder is more common in relatives of the affected individual but may be caused by environmental influences, not genetic alterations.

Mendelian or Monogenic Disorders

A genetic disorder is a disease caused by an abnormality in an individual's genetic material or genome. Patterns of inheritance dictate how this abnormality can be passed onto offspring. Principles of inheritance of single-gene disorders are the same as those that govern the inheritance of other traits, such as eye and hair colour. These are known as Mendel's laws of inheritance, named for Gregor Mendel, an Austrian naturalist who conducted genetic research. These patterns occur because a single gene is defective and are referred to as monogenic or sometimes mendelian disorders. They include autosomal dominant, autosomal recessive, X-linked dominant, and X-linked recessive patterns.

Autosomal Dominant Inheritance

Autosomal dominant inheritance occurs when a single gene in the heterozygous state is capable of producing the phenotype. In other words, the abnormal or mutant gene overshadows the normal gene and the individual will demonstrate signs and symptoms of the disorder. The

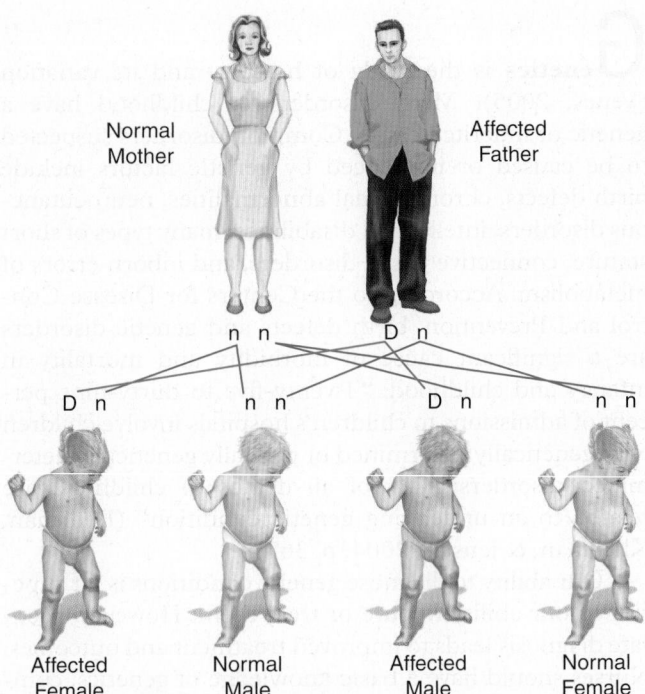

FIGURE 50.1 Autosomal dominant inheritance pattern.

affected person generally has an affected parent, and an affected person has a 50% chance of passing the abnormal gene to each of his or her children (Conley, 2010) (Fig. 50.1). Affected individuals are present in every generation. Males and family members who are phenotypically normal (do not show signs or symptoms of the disorder) do not transmit the condition to their offspring. Females and males are equally affected and a male can pass the disorder on to his son. This male-to-male transmission is important in distinguishing autosomal dominant inheritance from X-linked inheritance. There are varying degrees of presentation among individuals in a family: a parent with a mild form could have a child with a more severe form. Common types of genetic disorders that follow the autosomal dominant pattern of inheritance include neurofibromatosis, Huntington disease, achondroplasia, and polycystic kidney disease.

Autosomal Recessive Inheritance

Autosomal recessive inheritance occurs when two copies of the mutant or abnormal gene in the homozygous state are necessary to produce the phenotype. In other words, two abnormal genes are needed for the individual to demonstrate signs and symptoms of the disorder. These disorders are generally less common than autosomal dominant disorders (Behrman et al., 2004). Both parents of the affected person must be heterozygous carriers of the gene (clinically normal but carry the gene) and their offspring have a 25% chance of being homozygous (a 50% chance of getting the mutant gene from each

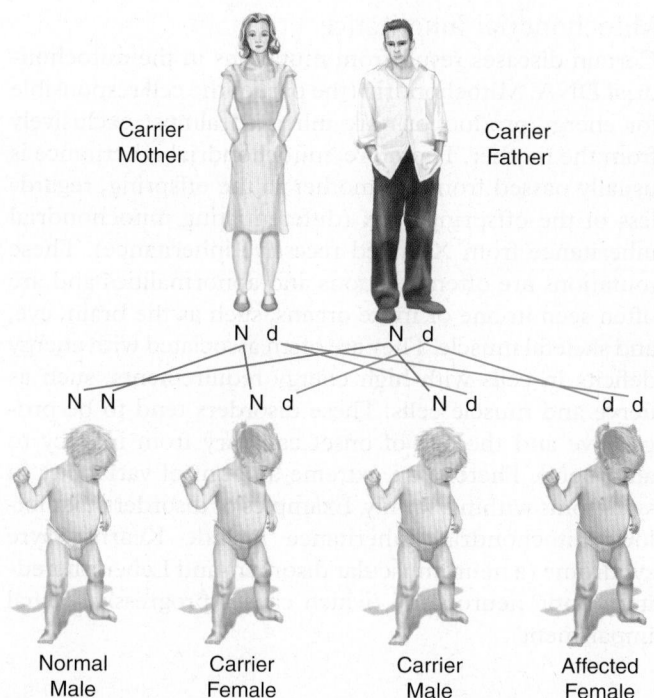

FIGURE 50.2 Autosomal recessive inheritance pattern.

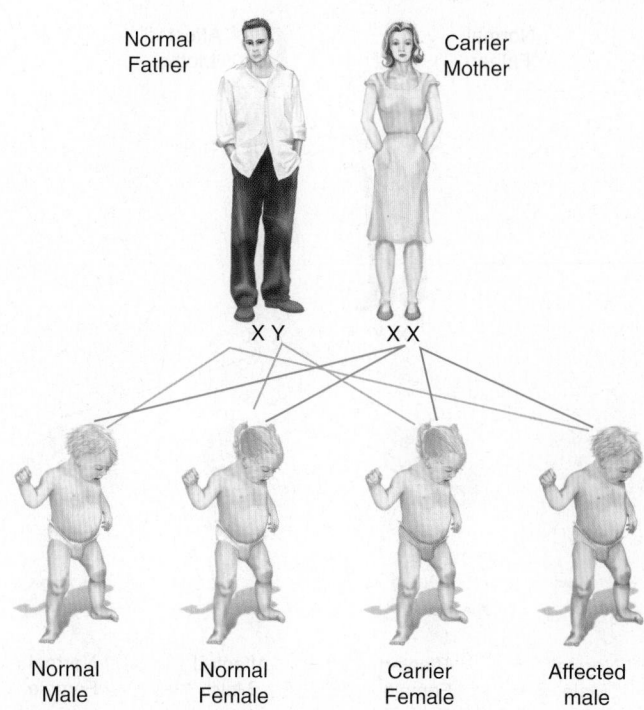

FIGURE 50.3 X-linked recessive inheritance pattern.

parent and therefore a 25% chance of inheriting two mutant genes) (Conley, 2010; Robin, 2007). If the child is clinically normal, there is a 50% chance the child is a carrier (Fig. 50.2). Affected individuals are usually present in only one generation of the family. Females and males are equally affected, and a male can pass the disorder on to his son (Robin, 2007). The chance that any two parents will both be carriers of the mutant gene is increased if the couple has **consanguinity** (relationship by blood or common ancestry) (Robin, 2007). Common types of genetic disorders that follow the autosomal recessive inheritance pattern include cystic fibrosis, phenylketonuria, Tay–Sachs disease, and sickle-cell disease.

X-Linked Inheritance

X-linked inheritance disorders are those associated with altered genes on the X chromosome. They differ from autosomal disorders. If a male inherits an X-linked altered gene, he will express the condition. Since a male has only one X chromosome, all the genes on his X chromosome will be expressed (the Y chromosome carries no normal allele to compensate for the altered gene). Because females inherit two X chromosomes, they can be either heterozygous or homozygous for any allele. Therefore, X-linked disorders in females express similarly to autosomal disorders.

X-Linked Recessive Inheritance

Most X-linked disorders demonstrate a recessive pattern of inheritance Conley, 2010; Marino & Claybon, 2008).

There are more affected males than females; since a male has only one X chromosome, all the genes on his X chromosome will be expressed (Robin, 2007), whereas a female will usually need both X chromosomes to carry the disease. There is no male-to-male transmission (since no X chromosome from the male is transmitted to male offspring), but any man who is affected will have carrier daughters. (Fig. 50.3). Common types of genetic disorders that follow X-linked recessive inheritance patterns include hemophilia, colour blindness, and Duchenne muscular dystrophy (Conley, 2010).

X-Linked Dominant Inheritance

X-linked dominant inheritance is present if heterozygous female carriers demonstrate signs and symptoms of the disorder. All of the daughters and none of the sons of an affected male have the condition, while both male and female offspring of an affected woman have a 50% chance of inheriting and presenting with the condition (Robin, 2007) (Fig. 50.4). X-linked dominant disorders are rare; the most common is hypophosphatemic (vitamin D–resistant) rickets.

Multifactorial Inheritance

Many of the common congenital malformations, such as cleft lip, cleft palate, spina bifida, pyloric stenosis, clubfoot, congenital hip dysplasia, and cardiac defects, are attributed to multifactorial inheritance (Conley, 2010; Robin, 2007). These conditions are thought to be caused by multiple gene and environmental factors. A combination

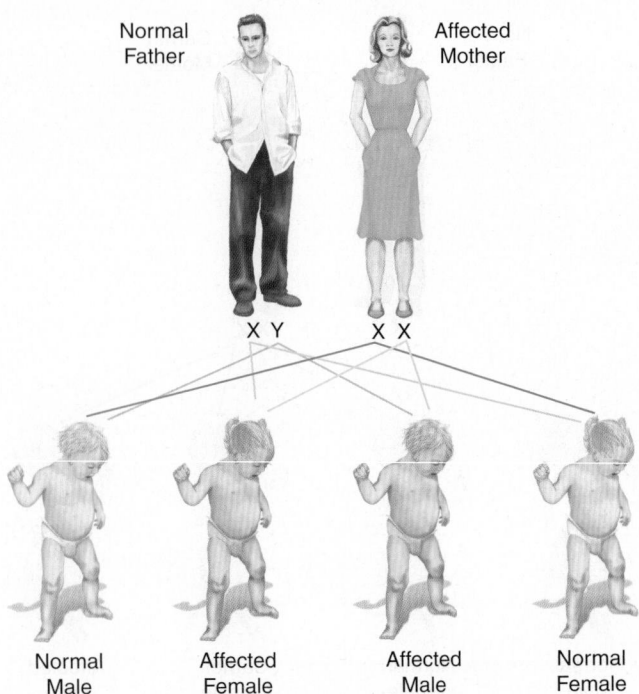

Normal Father   Affected Mother

X Y   X X

Normal Male   Affected Female   Affected Male   Normal Female

FIGURE 50.4 X-linked dominant inheritance pattern.

of genes from both parents, along with unknown environmental factors, produces the trait or condition. An individual may inherit a predisposition to a particular anomaly or disease. The anomalies or diseases vary in severity, and often a sex bias is present. For example, pyloric stenosis is seen more often in males, while congenital hip dysplasia is much more likely in females. Multifactorial conditions tend to run in families, but the pattern of inheritance is not as predictable as with single-gene disorders. The chance of recurrence is also less than in single-gene disorders, but the degree of risk is related to the number of genes in common with the affected individual. The closer the degree of relationship, the more genes an individual has in common with the affected family member, and thus the higher risk that the individual's offspring will have a similar defect. In multifactorial inheritance the likelihood that both identical twins will be affected is not 100%, indicating that there are nongenetic factors involved.

Nontraditional Inheritance Patterns

Molecular studies have revealed that some genetic disorders are inherited in ways that do not follow the typical patterns of dominant, recessive, X-linked, or multifactorial inheritance. Examples of nontraditional inheritance patterns include mitochondrial inheritance and genomic imprinting. As the science of molecular genetics advances and we learn more about inheritance patterns, other nontraditional patterns of inheritance may be discovered or may be found to be relatively common.

Mitochondrial Inheritance

Certain diseases result from mutations in the mitochondrial DNA. Mitochondria (the part of the cell responsible for energy production) are inherited almost exclusively from the mother. Therefore, mitochondrial inheritance is usually passed from the mother to the offspring, regardless of the offspring's sex (differentiating mitochondrial inheritance from X-linked recessive inheritance). These mutations are often deletions and abnormalities and are often seen in one or more organs, such as the brain, eye, and skeletal muscle. They are often associated with energy deficits in cells with high energy requirements, such as nerve and muscle cells. These disorders tend to be progressive and the age of onset can vary from infancy to adulthood. There is an extreme amount of variability in symptoms within a family. Examples of disorders that follow mitochondrial inheritance include Kearns–Sayre syndrome (a neuromuscular disorder) and Leber's hereditary optic neuropathy (which causes progressive visual impairment).

Genomic Imprinting

Another nontraditional inheritance pattern results from a process called genomic imprinting. Genomic imprinting plays a critical role in fetal growth and development and placental functioning. It is a phenomenon by which the expression of a gene is determined by its parental origin. In genomic imprinting both the maternal and paternal alleles are present, but only one is expressed; the other is inactive. Genomic imprinting does not alter the genetic sequence itself but affects the phenotype observed. In these cases, the altered genes in a certain region of the genome have very different expressions depending on whether they were inherited from the mother or the father. Several human syndromes are known to be associated with defects in gene imprinting. Disorders that result from a disruption of imprinting usually involve a growth phenotype and include varying degrees of developmental problems. Common examples include Prader–Willi syndrome (a condition resulting in severe hypotonia and hyperphagia, leading to obesity and intellectual disabilities), Angelman syndrome (a neurodevelopmental disorder associated with intellectual disabilities, jerky movements, and seizures), and Beckwith–Wiedemann syndrome (characterized by somatic overgrowth, congenital malformations, and a predisposition to embryonic neoplasia).

Chromosomal Abnormalities

In some cases of genetic disorders, the abnormality occurs as a result of problems with the chromosomes. Chromosomal abnormalities do not follow straightforward patterns of inheritance. Sperm and egg cells each have 23 unpaired chromosomes. When they unite during conception they form a fertilized egg with 46 chromosomes.

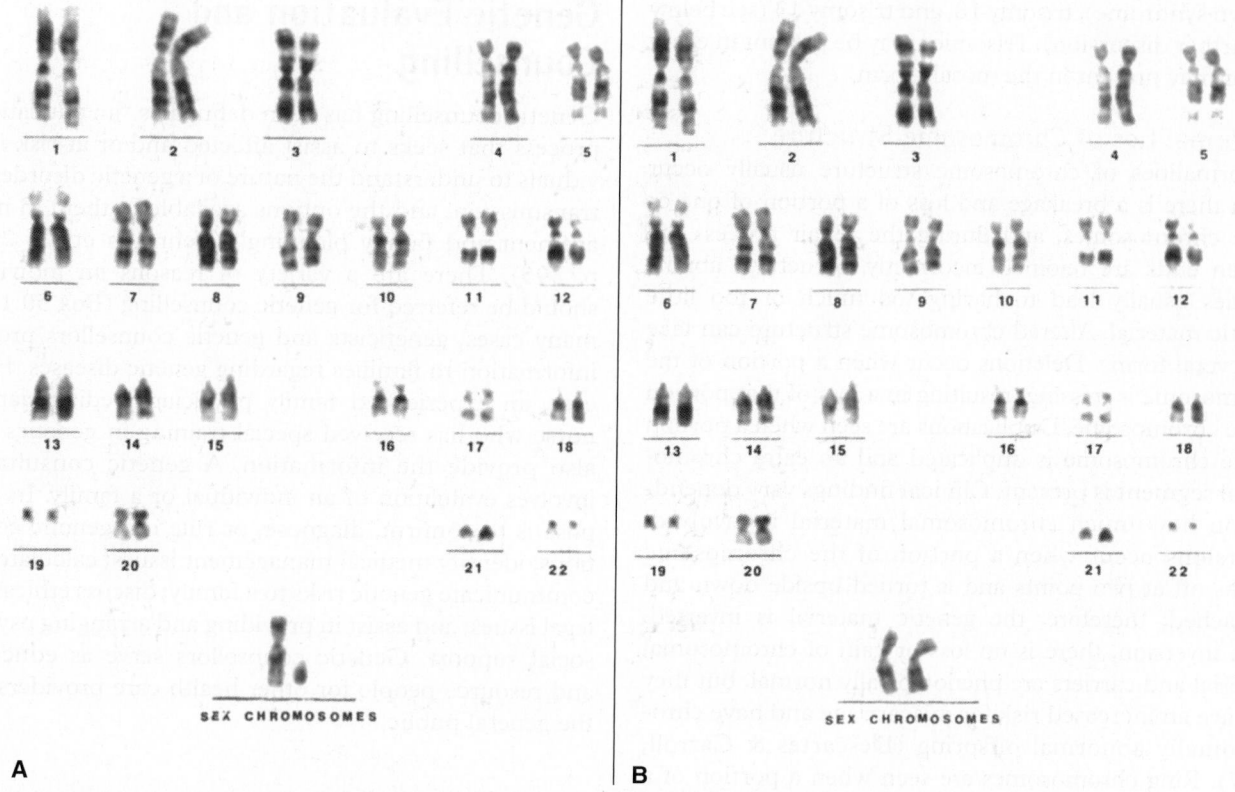

FIGURE 50.5 Chromosomes in a karyotype are arranged and numbered by size, from largest to smallest. The normal human karyotype has 46 chromosomes: 22 pairs of autosomes and 2 sex chromosomes. (**A**) A normal male. (**B**) A normal female.

Sometimes before pregnancy begins, an error has occurred during the process of cell division, leaving an egg or sperm with too many or too few chromosomes. If this egg or sperm cell joins with a normal egg or sperm cell, the resulting embryo has a chromosomal abnormality. Chromosomal abnormalities can also occur due to an error in the structure of the chromosome. Small pieces of the chromosome may be deleted, duplicated, inverted, misplaced, or exchanged with part of another chromosome. Most chromosomal abnormalities occur due to an error in the egg or sperm. Therefore, the abnormality is present in every cell of the body. Some abnormalities can happen after fertilization during mitotic cell division and result in mosaicism. Mosaicism or mosaic form is when the chromosomal abnormalities do not show up in every cell; only some cells or tissues carry the abnormality. In mosaic forms of the disorder the symptoms are usually less severe than if all the cells were abnormal.

Chromosomal abnormalities occur in 0.4% of live births (Behrman et al., 2004). There is a much higher frequency of chromosomal abnormalities in spontaneous abortions and stillbirths (Descartes & Carroll, 2007). Congenital anomalies and intellectual disabilities are often associated with chromosomal abnormalities (Descartes & Carroll, 2007). These abnormalities occur on autosomal or non-sex chromosomes as well as sex

chromosomes and can result from abnormalities of either chromosome structure or chromosome number.

A **karyotype** is a pictorial analysis of chromosomes. It depicts a systematic arrangement of chromosomes of a single cell by pairs (Fig. 50.5). Karyotyping is often used in prenatal testing to diagnose or predict genetic diseases.

Abnormalities of Chromosome Number

Chromosomal abnormalities of number often result from **nondisjunction** (failure of separation of the chromosome pair) during cell division, meiosis, or mitosis. Few chromosomal numerical abnormalities are compatible with full-term development and most result in spontaneous abortion (Descartes & Carroll, 2007). Some numerical abnormalities, however, can support development to term because the chromosome on which the abnormality is present carries relatively few genes (e.g., chromosome 13, 18, 21, or X). Two common abnormalities of chromosome number are monosomies or trisomies. In monosomies, there is only one copy of a particular chromosome instead of the usual pair; in these cases, all fetuses spontaneously abort in early pregnancy. Survival occurs only in mosaic forms of these disorders. In trisomies, there are three of a particular chromosome instead of the usual two. The most common trisomies include trisomy 21

(Down syndrome), trisomy 18, and trisomy 13 (see below for further discussion). Trisomies may be present in every cell or may present in the mosaic form.

Abnormalities of Chromosome Structure

Abnormalities of chromosome structure usually occur when there is a breakage and loss of a portion of one or more chromosomes, and during the repair process the broken ends are rejoined incorrectly. Structural abnormalities usually lead to having too much or too little genetic material. Altered chromosome structure can take on several forms. Deletions occur when a portion of the chromosome is missing, resulting in a loss of that portion of the chromosome. Duplications are seen when a portion of the chromosome is duplicated and an extra chromosomal segment is present. Clinical findings vary depending on how much chromosomal material is involved. Inversions occur when a portion of the chromosome breaks off at two points and is turned upside down and reattached; therefore, the genetic material is inverted. With inversion, there is no loss or gain of chromosomal material and carriers are phenotypically normal, but they do have an increased risk for miscarriage and have chromosomally abnormal offspring (Descartes & Carroll, 2007). Ring chromosomes are seen when a portion of a chromosome has broken off in two places and has formed a circle or ring. The most clinically significant structural abnormality is a translocation. This occurs when a portion of one chromosome is transferred to another chromosome and an abnormal rearrangement is present.

Structural abnormalities can be balanced or unbalanced. Balanced abnormalities involve the rearrangement of genetic material with neither an overall gain nor loss. Individuals who inherit a balanced structural abnormality are usually phenotypically normal but are at a higher risk for miscarriages and have chromosomally abnormal offspring. Examples of structural rearrangements that can be balanced include inversions, translocations, and ring chromosomes. Unbalanced structural abnormalities are similar to numerical abnormalities because genetic material is either gained or lost. Unbalanced structural abnormalities can encompass several genes and result in severe clinical consequences.

Sex Chromosome Abnormalities

Chromosomal abnormalities can also involve sex chromosomes. These cases usually have milder clinical effects than autosomal chromosomal abnormalities (Descartes & Carroll, 2007). Sex chromosome abnormalities are gender-specific and involve a missing or extra sex chromosome. They affect sexual development and may cause infertility, growth abnormalities, and possibly behavioural and learning problems. Many affected individuals lead essentially normal lives. Examples are Turner syndrome in females and Klinefelter syndrome in males (see discussion later in this chapter).

Genetic Evaluation and Counselling

Genetic counselling has been defined as "an educational process that seeks to assist affected and/or at-risk individuals to understand the nature of a genetic disorder, its transmission, and the options available to them in management and family planning" (Behrman et al., 2004, p. 395). There are a variety of reasons an individual should be referred for genetic counselling (Box 50.1). In many cases, geneticists and genetic counsellors provide information to families regarding genetic diseases. However, an experienced family physician, pediatrician, or nurse who has received special training in genetics may also provide the information. A genetic consultation involves evaluation of an individual or a family. Its purpose is to confirm, diagnose, or rule out genetic conditions; identify medical management issues; calculate and communicate genetic risks to a family; discuss ethical and legal issues; and assist in providing and arranging psychosocial support. Genetic counsellors serve as educators and resource people for other health care providers and the general public.

BOX 50.1 **Those Who May Benefit from Genetic Counselling**

- Maternal age 35 years or older when the baby is born
- Paternal age 50 years or older
- Previous child, parent, or close relative with an inherited disease, congenital anomaly, metabolic disorder, developmental disorder, or chromosomal abnormality
- Consanguinity or incest
- Pregnancy screening abnormality, including alpha-fetoprotein, triple/quadruple screen, amniocentesis, or ultrasound
- Stillborn with congenital anomalies
- Two or more pregnancy losses
- Teratogen exposure or risk
- Concerns about genetic defects that occur frequently in an individual's ethnic or racial group (e.g., those of African descent are most at risk for having a child with sickle-cell anemia)
- Abnormal newborn screening
- Child born with one or more major malformations in a major organ system
- Child with abnormalities of growth
- Child with developmental delay, intellectual disability, blindness, or deafness

---

Adpated from Conley, Y. P. (2010). Genetics and health Applications. In S. M. Nettina (Ed.), *Lippincott Manual of Nursing Practice* (9th ed.). Philadelphia: Lippincott Williams & Wilkins; and Korf, B. (2007). Integration of genetics into pediatric practice. In R. M. Kliegman, R. E. Behrman, H. B. Jenson, & B. F. Stanton (Eds.), *Nelson's textbook of pediatrics* (18th ed.). Philadelphia: Saunders.

The ideal time for genetic counselling is before conception. Preconception counselling allows couples to identify and reduce potential pregnancy risks, plan for known risks, and establish early prenatal care. Unfortunately, many woman delay seeking prenatal care until their second or third trimester, after the crucial time of organogenesis has occurred. Preconception counselling should be offered to all women as they seek health care throughout their childbearing years, especially if they are contemplating pregnancy. Health care providers should assume an active role. Nurses are often the first health care providers to encounter women with preconception and prenatal issues, so nurses play an important role in beginning the preconception counselling process and referring women and their partners for further genetic testing when indicated.

Preconception screening and counselling can raise serious ethical and moral issues for a couple. Prenatal genetic testing can lead to the decision to terminate a pregnancy based on the results, even if the results may not be conclusive but indicate a strong possibility that the child will have an abnormality. The severity of the abnormality may not be known, and some may find the decision to terminate unethical. Another difficult situation is when a mother finds that she is a carrier for a disorder that affects only one gender. If no prenatal screening test is available, the couple may decide to terminate any pregnancy in which the fetus is the affected sex, even though there is a 50% chance that the child will not inherit the disorder. The choice is the couple's, and information and support must be provided in a nondirective manner.

An accurate and thorough family history is an essential part of preconception counselling. Information is obtained about congenital anomalies, intellectual disabilities, genetic diseases, reproductive history, general health, and causes of death, ideally for three generations. After careful analysis of the data, the couple is referred to a genetic counsellor when indicated.

Genetic counselling is particularly important if a congenital anomaly or genetic disease has been diagnosed prenatally or when a child is born with a life-threatening congenital anomaly or genetic disease. In these cases families need urgent information because they need to make immediate decisions. If a diagnosis with genetic implications is made later in life, if a couple with a family history or a previous child with a genetic disorder is planning a family, or if there is suspected teratogen exposure, urgency of information is not such an issue; in these situations the family needs to take in all the information and explore all their options. This may occur during several meetings over a longer period of time.

Genetic counselling involves extensive information gathering about birth history, past medical history, and current health status. A detailed family history is imperative and in most cases will include the development of a pedigree, which is like a family tree (Fig. 50.6). Informa-

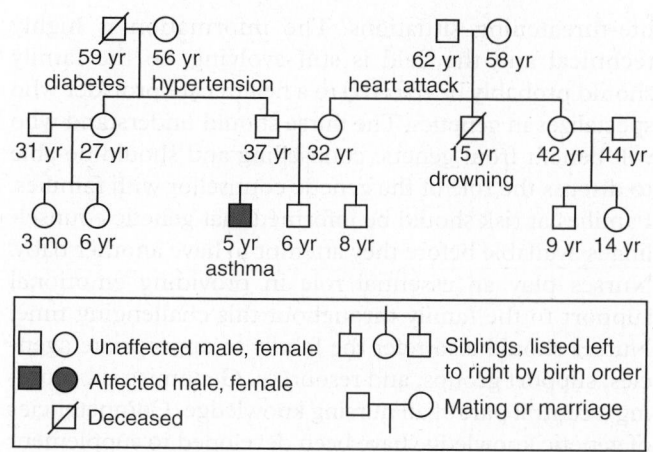

FIGURE 50.6 A pedigree is a diagram that shows the links between family members and includes medical information for each relative.

tion is ideally gathered on three generations, but if the family history is complicated, information from more distant relatives may be needed. Families receiving genetic counselling should be told that this information will be necessary so that they can discuss these sensitive issues with family members in advance. When necessary, medical records may be requested for family members, especially those who have a genetic disorder. Sometimes the process of preparing a pedigree may reveal information that is not known by all family members, such as an adopted child, a child conceived through in vitro fertilization, or a husband not being the father of a baby. Therefore, it is extremely important to take steps to maintain confidentiality.

Medical genetic knowledge has increased dramatically over the past few decades. It is possible today not only to detect specific diseases with genetic mutations but also to test for a genetic predisposition to various diseases or conditions and certain physical characteristics. This leads to complex ethical, moral, and social issues. Health care providers need to maintain client privacy and confidentiality and administer care in a nondiscriminatory manner while maintaining sensitivity to cultural differences. It is essential to respect the patient's autonomy and present information in a nondirective manner.

Nurse's Role and Responsibilities

Pediatric nurses will encounter children with genetic disorders in every clinical specialty area. This includes clinics, hospitals, schools, and community-based centres. Talking with families who have recently been diagnosed with a genetic disorder or who have had a child born with congenital anomalies is very difficult. Many times the nurse is the one who has first contact with these parents and will be the one to provide follow-up care. Genetic disorders are significant, life-changing, and possibly life-threatening situations. The information is highly technical and the field is still evolving, so the family should probably be referred to a health care provider who specializes in genetics. The nurse should understand who will benefit from genetic counselling and should be able to discuss the role of the genetic counsellor with families. Families at risk should be informed that genetic counselling is available before they attempt to have another baby. Nurses play an essential role in providing emotional support to the family throughout this challenging time. Nurses should also refer the family to appropriate agencies, support groups, and resources. Genomics is becoming a central part of all nursing knowledge. Competencies of genetic knowledge have been developed to supplement ongoing nursing curriculum and supply outcome indicators (Jenkins et al., 2008).

Common Medical Treatments

A variety of medications and other medical treatments are used to treat the symptoms of genetic disorders in children. Genetic disorders do not have specific treatments and there is no cure, so treatment focuses on the specific symptoms of each disorder. Genetic disorders often involve multiple organ systems and the patients have complex medical needs, so a multidisciplinary approach and good communication are imperative. See below for a discussion on common genetic disorders and their management.

NURSING PROCESS OVERVIEW FOR THE CHILD WITH A GENETIC DISORDER

Care of the child with a genetic disorder includes assessment, nursing diagnosis, planning, interventions, and evaluation. There are a number of general concepts related to the nursing process that may be applied to the care of children with genetic disorders. From a general understanding of the care involved for a child with a genetic disorder, the nurse can then individualize the care based on patient specifics.

Assessment
Assessment of the child with a genetic disorder includes health history, physical examination, and laboratory and diagnostic testing.

*R*emember Julie, the 5-year-old brought in for her annual examination? What additional health history and physical examination information should you obtain?

Health History
The health history comprises past medical history, including the mother's pregnancy history, family history, neonatal history, history of present illness (when the symptoms started and how they have progressed), as well as treatments used at home. Explore the patient's current and past medical history for risk factors such as:

- Family history of genetic disorders
- Any complications during the prenatal, perinatal, or postnatal periods
- Changes in developmental status or delays in developmental milestones

The pregnancy history can be extremely relevant when identifying a genetic disorder. The pregnancy history may be significant for maternal age over 35 years, repeated premature births, breech delivery, congenital hip dysplasia, abnormalities found on ultrasound, abnormalities in prenatal blood screening tests (e.g., triple/quadruple screen, alpha fetoprotein), amniotic fluid abnormalities (polyhydramnios, oligohydramnios), multiple births, exposure to medications and known teratogens, and decreased fetal movement.

A focused neonatal history can also help identify a genetic problem. The neonatal history may be significant for symmetric intrauterine growth restriction, large for gestational age without a reason, hearing impaired, persistent hyperbilirubinemia, poor adaptation to the extrauterine environment (demonstrated by temperature and heart rate instability and poor feeding), hypotonia or hypertonia, seizures, and abnormal newborn screening results.

The family history plays a critical role in identifying genetic disorders. Data should be gathered for three generations. If there is a positive family history, the likelihood of a genetic disorder in the patient is increased. It is helpful to create a family pedigree (refer to the genetic counselling section above). The family history may be significant for major congenital anomalies, intellectual disabilities, genetic diseases, metabolic disorders, multiple miscarriages or stillbirths, developmental delays, significant learning disabilities, psychiatric problems, consanguinity, and chronic serious illness (e.g., diabetes, hypertension, renal disease, hearing impairment, blindness, asthma, seizures, and unexplained death).

When eliciting the history of the present illness, inquire about:

- Developmental delay
- Seizures
- Hypotonia or hypertonia
- Feeding problems
- Lethargy
- Failure to thrive
- Septic appearance
- Vomiting

Children known to have a genetic disorder are often admitted to the hospital for other health-related issues or complications and management of the genetic disorder. The health history should include questions related to:

- Age when the disorder was diagnosed
- Developmental delay
- Complications of the disorder (e.g., thyroid problems, cardiac problems, respiratory problems, leukemia, seizures, cognitive impairment)
- Medications the child takes for complications associated with the disorder
- Dietary restrictions
- Compliance with management regimen

Once complications have been identified, further investigation into their severity, frequency, and management is essential to the care of this child while in the hospital.

Physical Examination

Physical examination of the child with a genetic disorder includes inspection and observation, palpation, and auscultation.

Inspection and Observation

Inspect and observe for congenital anomalies, either major or minor. A major anomaly is an anomaly or malformation that creates significant medical problems and requires surgical or medical management (Stevenson, 2006; Wynshaw-Boris & Biesecker, 2007) (Box 50.2). Minor anomalies are features that vary from those seen in the general population but do not cause an increase in morbidity in and of themselves (Stevenson, 2006; Wynshaw-Boris & Biesecker, 2007) (Box 50.3).

BOX 50.2 Major Congenital Anomalies

- Cleft lip
- Cleft palate
- Congenital heart disease, structural and conduction disorders
- Neural tube defects
- Brain anomalies
- Omphalocele
- Hepatosplenomegaly
- Asymmetry of face, skeleton, or limb
- Generalized dysmorphism
- Specific skin lesions, such as café-au-lait macules, hypopigmented macules, or cutaneous hemangiomas

Adapted from: Siegel, B., & Milunsky, J. (2004). When should the possibility of a genetic disorder cross your radar screen? *Contemporary Pediatrics, 21*(5), 37.

BOX 50.3 Minor Congenital Anomalies

- Flat occiput
- Prominent occiput
- Widow's peak
- Triple hair whorl
- Flat-bridged nose
- Anteverted nostrils
- Ear lobe crease
- Notched ear lobe
- Forward displacement or protruding ears
- Cleft uvula
- Webbed neck
- Extra nipples
- Single umbilical artery
- Umbilical hernia
- Tapered fingers
- Overlapping digits
- Broad thumb or great toe
- Increased space between toes
- Syndactyly
- Polydactyly

Adapted from: Siegel, B., & Milunsky, J. (2004). When should the possibility of a genetic disorder cross your radar screen? *Contemporary Pediatrics, 21*(5), 37.

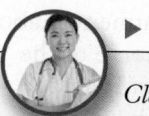 ▶ **Take** NOTE!

Low-set ears are associated with numerous genetic dysmorphisms. If noted, assess thoroughly for other abnormalities.

When three or more minor anomalies are present, the risk for a major anomaly or intellectual disability is approximately 20% (Marino & Claybon, 2008; Siegel & Milunsky, 2004). When one major anomaly is present, the possibility of a genetic cause must be investigated. In children with three or more minor anomalies, selected major anomalies, a recognized pattern of anomalies, or a combination of major and minor anomalies, a genetic diagnostic workup is recommended (Siegel & Milunsky, 2004).

▶ **Take** NOTE!

Cleft lip and cleft palate are associated with many syndromes. If noted, assess for other anomalies.

Inspect and observe for an abnormal or foul odour of the child's excretions, as certain metabolic disorders or inborn errors of metabolism are associated with specific odours (Table 50.1).

TABLE 50.1 INBORN ERRORS OF METABOLISM
AND ASSOCIATED ODOUR

Inborn Error of Metabolism	Associated Odour
Phenylketonuria	Mousy or musty
Maple syrup urine disease	Maple syrup, burnt sugar, or curry
Tyrosinemia	Cabbage-like, rancid butter
Trimethylaminuria	Rotting fish

Adpated from: Kaye, C.I. & the Committee on Genetics (2011). Newborn screening fact sheets. *Pediatrics, 118*(3), e934–e963. doi: 10.1542/peds.2006-1783; and Rezvani, I. (2007). An approach to inborn errors of metabolism. In R.M. Kliegman, R.E. Behrman, H.B. Jenson, & B.F. Stanton (Eds.), *Nelson's textbook of pediatrics* (18th ed.). Philadelphia: Saunders.

Auscultation

Physical examination includes auscultation of the heart. Murmurs or dysrhythmias may have a genetic cause. In a patient with a congenital heart problem (e.g., ventricular septal defect) and a strong family history of cardiac structural problems, a genetic cause needs to be considered. Approximately 3% of all cases of congenital heart disease are caused by a single mutant gene, and 5% of congenital heart defects are caused by chromosomal abnormalities (Siegel & Milunsky, 2004).

Palpation

Palpation can be used to detect hepatosplenomegaly (an enlarged spleen and liver), but because this requires skill and experience, this assessment may be performed by advanced practitioners or physicians. Hepatosplenomegaly may indicate a metabolic disorder.

Laboratory and Diagnostic Testing

Common Laboratory and Diagnostic Tests 50.1 explains the laboratory and diagnostic tests used most commonly to detect genetic disorders. The tests can assist the physician in diagnosing the disorder or can be used as guidelines in determining treatment. Laboratory or non-nursing personnel obtain some of the tests, while the nurse might obtain others. In either instance the nurse should be familiar with how the tests are obtained, what they are used for, and normal versus abnormal results. This knowledge will also be necessary when providing patient and family education related to the testing. Due to the nature of the information, a referral to genetic counselling before testing may be appropriate. Advances in genetic technology, including information obtained from the HGP,

have led to dramatic increases in the number of diagnostic and screening tests (GeneTests, 2010).

Nursing Diagnoses, Goals, Interventions, and Evaluation

Upon completion of an assessment, the nurse might identify several nursing diagnoses, including:

- Deficient knowledge
- Decisional conflict
- Risk for delayed growth and development
- Fear
- Interrupted family processes

After completing an assessment of Julie, the nurse noted the following: short stature for age and a low posterior hairline. Based on these assessment findings, what would your top three nursing diagnoses be for Julie?

Nursing goals, interventions, and evaluation for the child with a genetic disorder are based on the nursing diagnoses. Nursing Care Plan 50.1 provides a general guide for planning care for a child with a genetic disorder. Additional information about nursing management will be included later in the chapter as it relates to specific disorders.

No matter what the genetic abnormality is, the news may be shattering to the family. It is difficult for nurses to even begin to understand what the family is going through. When providing support and education to families of children with serious genetic abnormalities, use these guiding principles:

- Build a trusting relationship.
- Stress the authenticity of the parents' feelings.
- Reject your own personal biases.
- Recognize that individuals cope in various ways; the family's behaviour may not be what you would expect.
- Help the family to identify their own strengths and supports, building on those as able.
- Know that the family's emotions may exhaust and disorganize them.
- Assist the family members to maintain open communication among themselves.
- Provide referrals to local parent groups or other families with a child with a similar disorder.
- Allow the family to verbalize their emotions and ask questions.
- Always ask the parents how *they* are doing (Lashley, 2005).

Based on your top three nursing diagnoses for Julie, describe appropriate nursing interventions.

(text continues on page 1740)

COMMON LABORATORY AND DIAGNOSTIC TESTS 50.1

Test	Explanation	Indication	Nursing Implications
Amniocentesis	Ultrasound-guided (to determine placental location) insertion of a needle through the abdomen and into the uterine cavity of a pregnant woman to obtain a sample of amniotic fluid. The fluid contains skin cells that have been shed by the fetus and can be isolated and grown in the laboratory to provide enough genetic material for testing.	Tests for chromosomal abnormality or specific genetic conditions of the fetus. Performed if fetus is considered at high risk for a genetic disorder or abnormal ultrasound. Most common prenatal test used to diagnose chromosomal and congenital anomalies.	Usually not performed before 14 to 16 weeks. Some clinicians offer early amniocentesis (between 11 and 14 weeks), but this is still considered experimental and may be riskier than second-trimester amniocentesis. Complications include miscarriage, fetal injury, amniotic fluid leakage, infection, spontaneous abortion, premature labour, maternal hemorrhage, amniotic fluid embolism, abruptio placentae, and damage to the bladder or intestines. Results are usually not available for 2 weeks, but this varies by laboratory. Monitor fetus before and after procedure.
Chorionic villi sampling (CVS)	Involves the removal of a small amount of tissue directly from the chorionic villi (minute vascular projections of the fetal chorion that combine with maternal uterine tissue to form the placenta). In the laboratory, the chromosomes of the fetal cells are analyzed for number and type. Extra chromosomes, such as are present in Down syndrome, can be identified. Additional laboratory tests can be performed to look for specific disorders.	Tests for chromosomal abnormality or specific genetic conditions of the fetus. Performed if fetus is considered at high risk for a genetic disorder or abnormal ultrasound.	Performed at 8 to 12 weeks of gestation, so provides early detection of genetic abnormalities. Complications include accidental abortion, infection, bleeding, amniotic fluid leakage, fetal limb deformities. Results are usually available within a week, but this varies depending on the laboratory and location of procedure (results are usually available sooner than with an amniocentesis). Monitor fetus before and after procedure.
Triple/quadruple screen	A maternal serum laboratory test that measures the levels of three substances made by the developing baby and placenta: alpha-fetoprotein (AFP), human chorionic gonadotropin (hCG), and unconjugated estriol (uE3). Dimeric inhibin-A has been added to make the "quadruple test." The addition of dimeric inhibin-A increases the detection rate of Down syndrome in the quadruple screen.	A screening test for low-risk pregnant women to determine pregnancies at an increased risk for open neural tube defects, Down syndrome, and trisomy 18	Performed between 16 and 19 weeks of gestation. Educate mothers that a normal test does not guarantee a healthy baby since none of these screening tests can detect 100% of cases (MSU Department of Pediatrics and Human Development, 2011). Conversely, an abnormal result does not guarantee the baby has a problem. Additional testing will be necessary to confirm or rule out a specific genetic condition.

(continued)

COMMON LABORATORY AND DIAGNOSTIC TESTS 50.1 (continued)

Test	Explanation	Indication	Nursing Implications
Ultrasound	Safe, noninvasive, accurate investigation of the fetus. A transducer is placed in contact with the mother's abdomen and high-frequency sound waves are directed at the fetus. The sound waves are reflected back through the tissues and recorded and displayed in real time on a screen.	To screen for structural malformations	Usually performed at 18 to 20 weeks of gestation; routinely done. Early ultrasound can be performed at 13 to 14 weeks to evaluate for Down syndrome.
Percutaneous umbilical blood sampling	An ultrasound-guided needle is inserted through the abdominal and uterine wall to the umbilical cord and a sample of blood is retrieved and sent to the laboratory for analysis. Procedure is similar to amniocentesis but requires a higher level of expertise and experience.	To detect chromosome abnormalities. Usually done when diagnostic information cannot be obtained through amniocentesis, CVS, or ultrasound or when the results of these tests were inconclusive.	Performed at or after 18 weeks. Complications include miscarriage, blood loss, infection, premature rupture of membranes. The risk to the pregnancy is greater than with other prenatal procedures such as amniocentesis and CVS. Not performed as often due to risks and since discovery of fluorescent in situ hybridization (FISH).
Fetoscopy	Endoscopic procedure that allows direct visualization of the fetus through the insertion of a tiny flexible instrument called a fetoscope, which is inserted through the abdominal wall and into the uterine cavity. Ultrasound is used to guide the placement of the scope. Direct visualization can evaluate the fetus for severe congenital anomalies such as neural tube defects. Fetal blood samples from the umbilical cord can be obtained and tested for congenital blood disorders such as hemophilia and sickle-cell anemia. Fetal tissue samples (usually skin) can be collected and tested for genetic diseases.	Indicated for any woman at risk for delivering a baby with significant congenital anomalies; can be used to perform corrective surgery (e.g., shunt placement) on the fetus	Performed during or after the 18th week of pregnancy. Complications include spontaneous abortion, premature delivery, premature rupture of membranes, amniotic fluid leak, intrauterine fetal death, infection. Monitor fetus before and after procedure.

Test	Explanation	Indication	Nursing Implications
Gene testing	Gene testing is currently available for over 950 inherited diseases. It involves analysis of DNA, RNA, chromosomes, proteins, metabolites, and biochemical agents. Specimens for gene testing can be obtained from numerous sources: leukocytes from blood are the most common and easily obtained source; during pregnancy, amniocentesis and CVS; and fetal tissue or products of conception after a miscarriage. Most common use is DNA or chromosomes isolated from blood. Direct detection of abnormalities in genes and chromosomes is performed using DNA-based or cytogenetic tests (which look at chromosome) and other methods. Cytogenetic tests also include a relatively new technology, FISH, to assist in detecting chromosomal abnormalities such as duplication, deletion, rearrangements, and translocations.	To detect abnormalities that may indicate actual disease or predict future disease. Indicated in the evaluation of congenital anomalies, intellectual disabilities, growth retardation, recurrent miscarriage to determine reason for the loss of a fetus, prenatal diagnosis of genetic disease.	Provide support, information, and resources to family. Refer to genetic counselling before and after test.
Newborn screening	Blood screening performed shortly after birth; used to identify many life-threatening genetic illnesses that have no immediate visible effects but can lead to physical problems, intellectual disabilities, and even death.	Every province and territory routinely screens all newborns, although components of the screening vary from province to province. Most follow the American College of Medical Genetics (visit http://thePoint.lww.com/Chow1e for a direct link).	Ideally performed after 24 hours of age; obtain specimen as close to time of discharge from newborn or labour and delivery unit as possible and no later than 7 days of age. The test is less accurate if done before 24 hours of age and should be repeated by 2 weeks of age if the newborn is less than 24 hours old. Ensure appropriate follow-up with newborn screening results; results are available in 2 to 3 weeks.

Adapted from Fischbach, F.T., & Dunning III, M.B. (2009). *A manual of laboratory and diagnostic tests* (8th ed.). Philadelphia: Lippincott Williams & Wilkins.

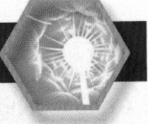

Nursing Care Plan 50.1

OVERVIEW FOR THE CHILD WITH A GENETIC DISORDER

NURSING DIAGNOSIS: Deficient knowledge related to lack of information regarding complex, technical medical condition, prognosis, and medical needs as evidenced by verbalization, questions, or actions demonstrating lack of understanding about child's condition or care

Outcome Identification and Evaluation

Child and family will verbalize accurate information and understanding about condition, prognosis, and medical needs: *Child and family demonstrate knowledge of condition, prognosis, and medical needs, including possible causes, contributing factors, and treatment measures.*

Intervention: Providing Patient and Family Teaching

- Assess child's and family's willingness to learn: *Child and family must be willing to learn for teaching to be effective.*
- Provide family with time to adjust to diagnosis: *Will facilitate adjustment and ability to learn and participate in child's care.*
- Repeat information: *Allows family and child time to learn and understand.*
- Teach in short sessions: *Many short sessions are more helpful than one long session.*
- Gear teaching to the child and family's level of understanding (depends on age of child, physical condition, memory) *to ensure understanding.*
- Provide reinforcement and rewards: *Facilitates the teaching/learning process.*
- Use multiple modes of learning involving many senses (written, verbal, demonstration, and videos) when possible: *Child and family are more likely to retain information when presented in different ways using many senses.*
- Refer child and family to a genetics specialist: *Genetic information is highly technical; the field is advancing at a rapid pace, and information needs to be the most current and accurate. A genetic specialist can provide this along with expertise, support, and resources.*

NURSING DIAGNOSIS: Decisional conflict related to treatment options, conflicting values, and ethical, legal, and social issues surrounding genetic testing as evidenced by verbalization of uncertainty about choices, verbalization of undesired consequences of alternative actions being considered, delayed decision making, physical signs of stress

Outcome Identification and Evaluation

Family will state they are able to make an informed decision: *Family will state advantages and disadvantages of choices and share fears and concerns regarding choices.*

Intervention: Providing Decision-Making Support

- Give family time and encourage them to express their feelings associated with decision making: *The decision-making process becomes more difficult if feelings are not expressed.*
- Encourage family to list advantages and disadvantages of each alternative: *Aids in problem solving and helps family recognize all alternatives.*
- Initiate health teaching and referral to genetic specialist when needed: *Genetic testing information is often technical and complex. Families need accurate and up-to-date information to aid in decision making.*
- Maintain a nondirective manner: *This is a difficult decision that the family must make for themselves; the nurse should provide all the necessary information while maintaining an unobtrusive role.*
- Validate the family's feelings regarding the decisional conflict: *Validation is a therapeutic communication technique that promotes the nurse–patient relationship.*

NURSING DIAGNOSIS: Risk for delayed growth and development related to physical disability, cognitive deficits, activity restrictions secondary to genetic disorder

Outcome Identification and Evaluation

Child's growth and development will be enhanced; child will demonstrate adequate growth patterns within parameters of disease, child will make continued progress toward attainment of developmental milestones and will not suffer regression in abilities.

Child will demonstrate developmental milestones within age parameters and limits of disease.

Child will make steady gains in growth patterns (e.g., height and weight) within disease parameters. Child expresses interest in the environment and people around him or her, interacts with environment appropriately for developmental level.

Nursing Care Plan 50.1 (continued)

Intervention: Promoting Growth and Development

- Screen for developmental capabilities *to determine child's current level of functioning.*
- Offer age-appropriate toys, play, and activities (including gross motor) *to encourage further development.*
- Perform exercises or interventions as prescribed by physical or occupational therapist: *These activities promote function and developmental skills.*
- Provide support to families: *Due to immobility and extremity deficits, the child's progress toward developmental milestones may be slow.*
- Use therapeutic play and adaptive toys *to facilitate developmental functioning.*
- Provide stimulating environment when possible *to maximize potential for growth and development.*
- Praise accomplishments and emphasize child's abilities *to improve self-esteem and encourage feeling of confidence and competence.*
- Monitor height and weight and plot on growth chart *to identify growth patterns and deviations in these patterns.*

NURSING DIAGNOSIS: Fear related to outcome of genetic testing as evidenced by reports of apprehension and increased tension

Outcome Identification and Evaluation

Family will state they can cope with the results of the genetic testing or demonstrate reduced fear. *Family accurately discusses chances of offspring having genetic disease, demonstrates positive coping, asks questions about genetic testing and meaning of results.*

Intervention: Managing Fear

- Empathize with the family and avoid false reassurances; be truthful: *Allows family to recognize that fear is a reasonable response. Giving false information or reassurance will actually increase fear.*
- Explore coping skills used previously by the family to cope with fear. Reinforce these skills and explore other outlets, such as relaxation, breathing, and physical activity: *Encourages use of coping mechanisms that help control fear.*
- Encourage verbalization of feelings and concerns about genetic testing. Allow time for questions: *Provides a safe outlet to express feelings and encourages open communication between the family members.*
- Explain all procedures and review results as available: *Knowledge deficit contributes to fear.*
- Refer to appropriate support groups and genetic counselling: *Talking with families who have gone through similar situations can help decrease fear and provide methods of coping. Genetic counselling provides information along with support and additional resources.*

NURSING DIAGNOSIS: Family processes, interrupted, related to child's illness, hospitalization, diagnosis of genetic illness in child, and potential long-term effects of illness as evidenced by family's presence in hospital and clinic, missed work, demonstration of inadequate coping

Outcome Identification and Evaluation

Family will maintain functional system of support, demonstrate adequate coping, adaptation of roles and functions, and decreased anxiety. *Parents are involved in child's care, ask appropriate questions, express fears and concerns, and can discuss child's care and condition calmly.*

Intervention: Promoting Family Coping

- Encourage family to verbalize concerns about child's illness, diagnosis, and prognosis: *Allows the nurse to identify concerns and areas where further education may be needed and demonstrates family-centred care.*
- Explain therapies, procedures, child's behaviours, and plan of care to parents: *Understanding the child's current status and plan of care helps decrease anxiety.*
- Encourage parental involvement in care: *Allows parents to feel needed and valued and gives them a sense of control over their child's health.*
- Identify support system for family and child: *Helps nurse identify needs and resources available for coping.*
- Educate family about resources available *to help them develop a wide base of support.*

TABLE 50.2 LESS COMMON CHROMOSOMAL ABNORMALITIES

Chromosomal Abnormality*	Features
Prader–Willi syndrome	Severe hypotonia, obesity, short stature, small hands and feet, hypogonadism, hyperphagia, and intellectual disabilities (vary from mild to severe)
Angelman syndrome	Hypotonia, microbrachycephaly, fair hair, midface hypoplasia, deep-set eyes, large mouth with tongue protrusion, seizures, jerky ataxic movements (resembling a puppet gait), uncontrolled bouts of laughter/smiling, happy demeanor, easily excitable personality, developmental delay and speech impairment, and severe intellectual disabilities
Cri-du-chat syndrome	Hypotonia, short stature, slow growth, low birth weight, characteristic weak, cat-like cry, microcephaly with protruding metopic suture, moon-like round face, bilateral epicanthal folds (folds of skin over the eyelids), high-arched palate, wide and flat nasal bridge, micrognathia (small receding chin), simian crease, and intellectual disabilities
Velocardiofacial/DiGeorge syndrome	Hypoplasia or agenesis of the thymus and parathyroid glands, hypoplasia of auricle and external auditory canal, cardiac anomalies, cleft palate, short stature, distinctive facial appearance (elongated face, almond-shaped eyes, wide nose, small ears), and learning, speech, feeding, and behavioural problems

*Visit http://thePoint.lww.com/Chow1e for direct links to organizations that offer resources for each of these conditions.

Common Chromosomal Abnormalities

Chromosomal abnormalities are seen in 1 in 150 babies (March of Dimes, 2009a). Many children with chromosomal abnormalities have associated intellectual disabilities, learning disabilities, behavioural problems, and distinct features, including physical birth defects. The risk for autosomal trisomies increases with advanced maternal age (March of Dimes, 2009a). The most common chromosomal abnormalities are discussed below. New techniques in chromosome analysis allow for the identification of tiny abnormalities that could not be seen before (March of Dimes, 2009b). Therefore, more chromosomal abnormalities are being identified in children (Table 50.2).

Trisomy 21 (Down Syndrome)

Trisomy 21 (Down syndrome) is the most common chromosomal disorder. This syndrome occurs in approximately 1 in 700 to 1,000 births in Canada, with little variation throughout the world (Public Health Agency of Canada, 2003). Trisomy 21 is seen in all ages and races and at all socioeconomic levels. The only risk factor that has been well established is maternal age: A higher incidence of Down syndrome is found with a maternal age above 35 years (March of Dimes, 2009b). The likelihood of having a baby with Down syndrome is 1 in 400 at age 35, 1 in 60 at age 42, and 1 in 12 by age 49 (National Institutes of Health, 2011).

Trisomy 21 is associated with some degree of intellectual disabilities, characteristic facial features (e.g., slanted eyes and depressed nasal bridge), and other health prob-

lems (e.g., cardiac defects, visual and hearing impairment, intestinal malformations, and an increased susceptibility to infections). The severity of these problems varies.

The prognosis has been improving over the past few decades. Fundamental changes in the care of these children have resulted in longer life expectancy (around 60 years of age) and an improved quality of life (Buckley & Buckley, 2008).

Pathophysiology

Trisomy 21 is a disorder caused by nondisjunction (an error in cell division) prior to or at conception. Each egg and sperm cell normally contains 23 chromosomes. When they join, this results in 23 pairs or 46 chromosomes. Sometimes, due to nondisjunction, a cell contributes an extra critical portion of chromosome number 21, resulting in an embryo with three chromosome 21s in all cells (Fig. 50.7). This results in the characteristic features and

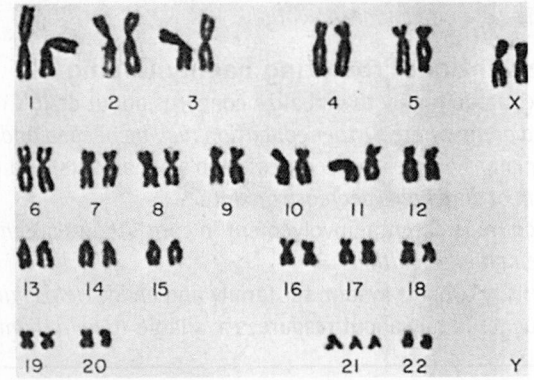

FIGURE 50.7 Down syndrome karyotype. Note the third chromosome located at chromosome 21.

birth defects of Down syndrome. This error in cell division and the presence of three chromosome 21s in all cells is responsible for 95% of cases of Down syndrome (Behrman et al., 2004; Descartes & Carroll, 2007).

In approximately 1% of cases of Down syndrome, the nondisjunction occurs after fertilization and a mixture of two cell types is seen (Behrman et al., 2004). In these cases some cells have 47 chromosomes (due to three chromosome 21s), while others have the normal 46 chromosomes (with the normal two chromosome 21s present). This is referred to as the mosaic form of Down syndrome. Children with mosaic Down syndrome may have a milder form of the disorder, but this is not a general finding.

About 4% of Down syndrome cases involve a translocation, in which part of the number 21 chromosome breaks off during cell division prior to or at conception and attaches to another chromosome. The cells will remain with 46 chromosomes, but this extra portion of the number 21 chromosome results in the clinical findings of Down syndrome. Cases of translocation are not associated with older maternal age, as is the situation with nondisjunction errors, and 25% of cases are the result of a hereditary translocation (American Academy of Pediatrics [AAP], 2007; Chen, 2011).

Therapeutic Management

Management of Down syndrome will involve multiple disciplines, including a primary physician, specialty physicians such as a cardiologist, ophthalmologist, and gastroenterologist, nurses, physical therapists, occupational therapists, speech therapists, dietitian, psychologist, counsellors, teachers, and of course the parents. There is no standard treatment for all children, and there is no cure or prevention. The overall focus of therapeutic management will be to promote the child's optimal growth and development and function within the limits of the disease. Treatment is mainly symptomatic and supportive.

Managing Complications

Children with Down syndrome need the usual immunizations, well-child care, and screening recommended by the Canadian Pediatric Society (CPS). In addition, medical management will focus on complications associated with Down syndrome.

Since approximately half those with Down syndrome have a heart defect, the AAP recommends routine cardiac screening of all newborn patients with Down syndrome (Vis et al., 2009). Cardiac problems vary from minor defects that respond to medication therapy to major defects that require surgical intervention.

Leukemia is 10 to 30 times more common in children with Down syndrome than in the general population (Van Riper & Cohen, 2001).

Children with Down syndrome also have an increased incidence of gastrointestinal disorders (AAP, 2007; Chen,

2011). These disorders vary from those that can be managed by dietary manipulation, such as celiac disease and constipation, to intestinal malformations such as Hirschsprung disease and imperforate anus, which require surgical intervention.

Hearing and vision impairments also are common. The majority of children with Down syndrome experience hearing loss, which could be conductive, sensorineural, or both (Martin, Klusek, Estigarribia, et al., 2009), so regular evaluation of vision and hearing is essential.

Obstructive sleep apnea is present in 50% to 80% of children with Down syndrome (Waldman, Hasan, & Perlman, 2009). Parents are often unaware their child is having sleep disturbances, so baseline testing in young children may be warranted (Groch, 2006). See Evidence-based Practice 50.1.

Children with Down syndrome have a higher incidence of thyroid disease, which can affect growth and cognitive function (AAP, 2007; Chen, 2011). Most of these children have hypothyroidism (an underactive thyroid), but sometimes hyperthyroidism (an overactive thyroid) occurs. Periodic thyroid testing may be warranted.

Atlanto-axial instability (increased mobility of the cervical spine at the first and second vertebrae) is seen in about 15% to 20% of children with Down syndrome (Hedequist, Bekelis, Emans, et al., 2010). In most cases these children are asymptomatic, but symptoms may appear if spinal cord compression occurs. Screening for atlanto-axial instability may be appropriate, especially if the child is involved in sports.

> ▶ **Take** NOTE!
>
> *If neck pain, unusual posturing of the head and neck (torticollis), change in gait, loss of upper body strength, abnormal reflexes, or change in bowel or bladder functioning is noted in the child with Down syndrome, immediate attention is required.*

Children with Down syndrome also have a higher susceptibility to infection and a higher mortality rate from infectious diseases, so precautions to prevent and monitor for infection are needed (Van Riper & Cohen, 2001).

Due to their increased risk for certain congenital anomalies and diseases, children with Down syndrome will need to be monitored closely, and regular medical care is essential.

Early Intervention Therapy

Early intervention refers to a variety of specialized programs and resources available to young children with developmental delay or other impairment. These programs may involve an array of health care professionals such as physical, occupational, and speech therapists,

EVIDENCE-BASED PRACTICE 50.1
Testing Children with Down Syndrome for Obstructive Sleep Apnea

Children with Down syndrome are at greater risk for development of obstructive sleep apnea syndrome (OSAS). Previous research evaluating children with Down syndrome has found the incidence of OSAS to be 100%. OSAS leads to sleep pattern abnormalities such as sleep fragmentation and sleep arousals. The significance of these is just beginning to be understood. With this high incidence of OSAS, should all children with Down syndrome be objectively evaluated for OSAS? If so, what is an appropriate age for this evaluation?

● Study
A prospective cohort study was performed over a 5-year period to determine the incidence of OSAS in children ages 2 to 4 years with Down syndrome. In addition, the parents' ability to predict sleep abnormalities in this patient population was examined. The study began with 65 children with Down syndrome, in which otolaryngologic problems seen in Down syndrome were evaluated. The study was conducted at a children's hospital, and 56 of the 65 children enrolled were able to complete a full sleep study or polysomnogram. Prior to the sleep study, 35 participants' parents completed a survey regarding their child's sleep behaviours.

▲ Findings
Fifty-seven percent ($n = 32$) of the children had abnormal sleep study results as defined by an abnormal obstructive index, hypoventilation with hypercarbia, and/or hypoxemia; if an abnormal or elevated arousal index is included, the incidence increases to 80% ($n = 45$). The significance of an elevated arousal state in an otherwise normal sleep study has not yet been fully established. Polysomnography in children is a developing field. The evaluation of sleep abnormalities in children has been based on stan-dard adult definitions. Due to the anatomic differences in children and adults alone, these definitions may not be accurate. For example, children tend to have significant oxygen desaturation after shorter periods of apnea compared with adults due to their smaller functional residual capacity and increased respiratory rate. There is a need to develop appropriate criteria to evaluate sleep abnormalities in children.

Sixty-nine percent of parents reported no sleep problems in their children, yet 54% of these children had an abnormal sleep study. Overall, it was found that parents of children with Down syndrome underestimated the severity of their child's sleep disturbances.

■ Nursing Implications
OSAS has been associated with various morbidities such as pulmonary hypertension and cor pulmonale. It has also been linked to neurocognitive abnormalities. Hypoxemia associated with OSAS has been correlated with lower IQ scores and behaviour problems. Sleep fragmentation, related to increased arousal and decreased REM, is just beginning to be understood but has been linked to symptoms associated with sleep deprivation, such as daytime sleepiness, lack of energy, and lack of initiative. The American Academy of Pediatrics currently recommends questioning parents of children with Down syndrome about possible sleep disorders when the children are 5 years or older, but no recommendations for specific testing are made at this time. Nurses need to be aware of recent research recommending baseline sleep studies in children ages 3 to 4 with Down syndrome even if the parents report no sleep problems in their child. Nurses need to assess for signs and symptoms of OSAS in children with Down syndrome at any age.

Shott, S.R., Amin, B. Chini, C. Heubi, Hotze, S. & Akers, R. (2006). Obstructive sleep apnea: Should all children with Down syndrome be tested? *Archive of Otolaryngology Head & Neck Surgery, 132*(4), 432–436.

---

special educators, and social workers. The programs focus on providing stimulation and encouragement to children with Down syndrome. They help encourage and accelerate development and may help to prevent some developmental delays. The earlier the intervention can begin, the more beneficial it will be. The programs are individualized to meet the specific needs of each child.

Children with Down syndrome progress through the same developmental stages as typical children, but they do so on their own timetable. For example, children with Down syndrome will learn to walk, but the average child with Down syndrome walks at 21 months (versus 13 months for a child without Down syndrome). Conditions such as hypotonia, ligament laxity, decreased strength, enlarged tongue, and short arms and legs are common in children with Down syndrome, and early intervention can help in the development of gross and fine motor skills, language, and social and self-care skills.

Parents also benefit from early intervention programs in terms of support, encouragement, and information. Early intervention programs teach parents how to interact with their child while meeting the child's specific needs and encouraging development.

Nursing Assessment
For a full description of the assessment phase of the nursing process, refer to page 1732. Assessment findings pertinent to Down syndrome are discussed below.

Health History

Down syndrome is often diagnosed prenatally using perinatal screening and diagnostic tests. If not diagnosed prenatally, most cases are diagnosed in the first few days of life based on the physical characteristics associated with Down syndrome. High-risk deliveries should be identified. Explore the pregnancy history and past medical history for risk factors such as:

• Lack of prenatal care
• Abnormal prenatal screening or diagnostic tests for Down syndrome (e.g., triple/quadruple screen, ultrasound, amniocentesis)
• Maternal age over 35 years

The older infant or child known to have Down syndrome is often admitted to the hospital for corrective surgeries or other complications of the disease, such as infections. Elicit a description of the present illness and chief complaint. In an infant or child returning for a clinic visit or hospitalization, the health history should include questions related to:

• Cardiac defects or disease (treatment regimen, surgical repair)
• Hearing or vision impairment (last hearing and vision evaluation, any corrective measures)
• Developmental delays (speech, gross and fine motor skills)
• Sucking or feeding problems
• Cognitive abilities (degree of intellectual disability)
• Gastrointestinal disorders such as vomiting or absence of stools (special dietary management, surgical interventions)
• Thyroid disease
• Leukemia
• Atlanto-axial instability
• Seizures
• Infections such as recurrent or chronic respiratory infections, otitis media
• Growth (height and weight changes, feeding problems, unexplained weight gain)
• Signs and symptoms of sleep apnea, such as snoring, restlessness during sleep, daytime sleepiness
• Any other changes in physical state or medication regimen

Physical Examination

The initial assessment after birth may reveal certain physical features characteristic of Down syndrome (Box 50.4 and Fig. 50.8).

Observe the child's general appearance. Note lack of muscle tone and loose joints; this is usually more

---

> ### BOX 50.4 Common Clinical Manifestations of Down Syndrome
>
> • Flattened occiput
> • Small (brachycephalic) head
> • Flat facial profile
> • Depressed nasal bridge and small nose
> • Oblique palpebral fissures (an upward slant to the eyes)
> • Brushfield spots (white spots on the iris of the eye)
> • Low-set ears
> • Abnormally shaped ears
> • Small mouth
> • Protrusion of tongue; tongue is large compared with mouth size
> • Arched palate
> • Hands with broad, short fingers
> • A single deep transverse crease on the palm of the hand (simian crease)
> • Congenital heart defect
> • Short neck, with excessive skin at the nape
> • Hyperflexibility and looseness of joints (excessive ability to extend the joints)
> • Dysplastic middle phalanx of fifth finger (one flexion furrow instead of two)
> • Epicanthal folds (small skin folds on the inner corner of the eyes)
> • Excessive space between large and second toe
> • Hypotonia
>
> Adapted from: American Academy of Pediatrics. (2007). Health supervision for children with Down syndrome. *Pediatrics, 107*(2), 442–449. Retrieved December 9, 2011 from http://aappolicy.aappublications.org/cgi/content/full/pediatrics;107/2/442; and Descartes, M., & Carroll, A.J. (2007). Cytogenetics. In Kliegman, R. M., Behrman, R. E., Jenson, H. B., & Stanton, B. F. (Eds.), *Nelson's textbook of pediatrics* (18th ed.). Philadelphia: Saunders.

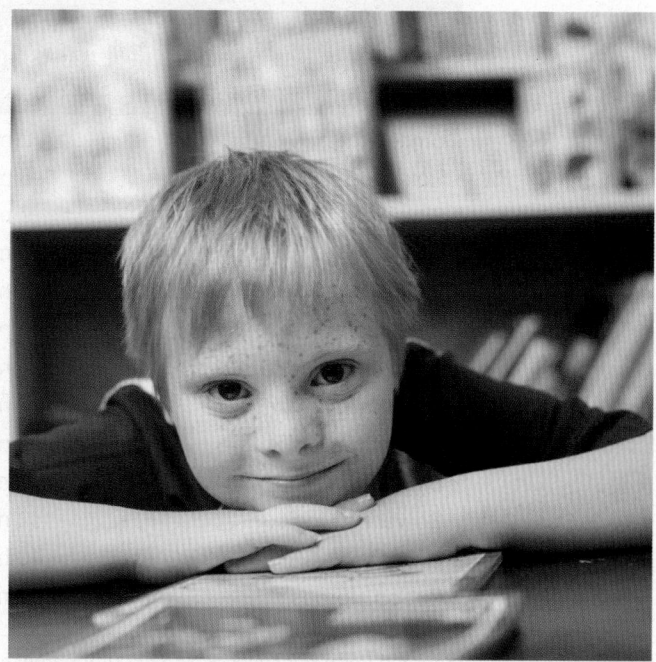

FIGURE 50.8 Child with Down syndrome.

pronounced in infancy, and the infant has a floppy appearance. Observe growth and development. Plot growth on appropriate growth charts. Because children with Down syndrome grow at a slower rate, special growth charts have been developed. (Visit http://thePoint.lww.com/Chow1e for an example).

When assessing achievement of developmental milestones in children with Down syndrome, it may be more useful to look at the sequence of milestones rather than the age at which they were achieved. Each milestone represents a skill that is needed for the next stage of development.

Perform a subjective assessment of hearing and refer the child for further evaluation if indicated. Assess vision, especially for cataracts. Assess respiratory status and cardiac status. Auscultate for murmurs and pulmonary changes, which can indicate congenital heart disease. Chronic or recurrent respiratory infections, such as pneumonia and otitis media, may be found.

Laboratory and Diagnostic Tests

Down syndrome can be detected prenatally around 16 to 18 weeks of gestation using ultrasound, a blood test to detect increases in alpha-fetoprotein, or analysis of amniotic fluid or tissue from chorionic villi to detect chromosomal abnormalities. Down syndrome can be confirmed after birth using chromosome analysis (see Common Laboratory and Diagnostic Tests 50.1).

Common laboratory and diagnostic studies ordered for the diagnosis and assessment of complications associated with Down syndrome include:

- Echocardiogram: to detect cardiac defects
- Vision and hearing screening: to detect vision and hearing impairments
- Thyroid hormone level: to detect thyroid disease
- Cervical x-rays: to assess for atlanto-axial instability
- Ultrasound: to assess gastrointestinal malformations

These tests will be important in evaluating the severity of the child's physical disabilities.

Nursing Management

Due to the high incidence of Down syndrome and the complex medical needs of these children, most pediatric nurses are likely to care for these children in their practice. Nursing management focuses on providing supportive measures such as promoting growth and development, preventing complications, promoting nutrition, and providing support and education to the child and family. In addition to the nursing diagnoses and related interventions discussed in Nursing Care Plan 50.1, additional considerations are reviewed below.

Promoting Growth and Development

Children with Down syndrome tend to grow more slowly, learn more slowly, have shorter attention spans, and have trouble with reasoning and judgment. Their personality tends to be one of genuine warmth and cheerfulness along with patience, gentleness, and a natural spontaneity. Growth and developmental milestones for children with Down syndrome have been developed as a guide for health care providers. Table 50.3 gives examples of the

TABLE 50.3 AVERAGE AGE OF SKILL ACQUISITION IN CHILDREN WITH DOWN SYNDROME

Developmental Milestone	Average Age of Acquisition, Children with Down Syndrome	Average Age of Acquisition, Typical Children
Smile	2 months	1 month
Roll over	6 months	4 months
Sit alone	9 months	7 months
Crawl	11 months	9 months
Walk	21 months	13 months
Speak words	14 months	10 months
Speak in sentences	24 months	21 months
Feed self with fingers	12 months	8 months
Use spoon	20 months	13 months
Bladder training	48 months	32 months
Bowel training	42 months	29 months
Undress	40 months	32 months
Put on clothes	58 months	47 months

Adapted from: Pueschel, S. M. (2011). *A parent's guide to Down syndrome: Toward a brighter future* (Revised ed.). Baltimore, MD: Paul H. Brookes Publishing Company, Inc.

average age at which these children reach selected milestones versus typical children.

Nurses play a key role in connecting families with appropriate resources that can facilitate the child's growth and development. The sooner early intervention programs can begin, the better for the child (see the above discussion on early intervention). Speech and language therapy, occupational therapy, and physical therapy will be important in promoting the child's growth and development. Special education should fit the child's individual needs, and the child should be integrated into mainstream education whenever possible.

Preventing Complications

Children with Down syndrome are at risk for certain health problems (see above). Even though most nurses will encounter a child with Down syndrome in their practice, only a few nurses will become experts in their care. The needs of these children are complex, and guidelines have been established that can help the nurse care for these children and their families. (Visit http://thePoint. lww.com/Chow1e for a direct link to the Down Syndrome Research Foundation website). Nurses also play a key role in educating parents and caregivers about how to prevent the complications of Down syndrome (Teaching Guideline 50.1).

Promoting Nutrition

Children with Down syndrome may have difficulty sucking and feeding due to lack of muscle tone. They tend to have small mouths; a smooth, flat, large tongue; and, due to the underdeveloped nasal bone, chronically stuffy noses. This may lead to poor nutritional intake and problems with growth. These problems usually improve as the child gains tongue control. Use of a bulb syringe, humidification, and changing the infant's position can lessen the problem. Breastfeeding a baby with Down syndrome is usually possible, and the antibodies in breast milk can help the child fight infections. The caregiver's hand can be used to provide additional support of the chin and throat. Speech or occupational therapists can work on strengthening muscles and assisting in feeding accommodations. Other feeding problems and failure to thrive can be related to cardiac defects and usually improve after medical management is initiated or corrective surgery performed.

Children with Down syndrome do not need a special diet unless underlying gastrointestinal disease is present, such as celiac disease. A balanced, high-fibre diet and regular exercise are important. Research has suggested that children with Down syndrome have lower basal metabolic rates, which can lead to problems with obesity, so it is important in the early years to develop appropriate eating habits and a regular exercise routine. High fibre intake is important for children with Down syndrome because their lack of muscle tone may decrease gastric motility, leading to constipation.

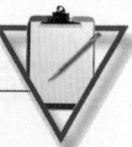

TEACHING GUIDELINE 50.1

Health Guidelines for Children with Down Syndrome

- Have your child evaluated by a pediatric cardiologist before 3 months of age, including an echocardiogram.
- Take your child for routine vision and hearing tests. By 6 months have your child seen by a pediatric ophthalmologist.
- Make sure your child gets regular medical care, including recommended immunizations and a thyroid test at 6 and 12 months and then yearly.
- Have your child follow a regular diet and exercise routine.
- Make sure all family members perform proper hand hygiene to prevent infection.
- Monitor for signs and symptoms of respiratory infections, such as pneumonia and otitis media.
- Discuss with your pediatrician the use of pneumococcal, respiratory syncytial virus, and influenza vaccines.
- Begin early interventions, therapy, and education as soon as possible.
- Make sure your child brushes his or her teeth regularly. He or she should visit the dentist every 6 months.
- Make sure the child gets a cervical x-ray between 3 to 5 years of age to screen for atlanto-axial instability.

Adapted from: American Academy of Pediatrics. (2007). Health supervision for children with Down syndrome. *Pediatrics, 107*(2), 442–449. Retrieved December 8, 2011 from http://aappolicy. aappublications.org/cgi/content/full/pediatrics;107/2/442.

Providing Support and Education for the Child and Family

Down syndrome is a life-long disorder that can result in health problems and cognitive disability. The diagnosis is usually made prenatally or shortly after birth. Parents and caregivers will need support and education during this difficult time. The range of mental impairment varies from mild to moderate; severe deficits occur occasionally. Some families may see having a child with Down syndrome as a life-long tragedy; others may view it as a positive growing experience (Van Riper & Cohen, 2001). Evaluate how the family defines and manages this experience. Base the plan of care on each individual family's values, beliefs, strengths, and resources (Van Riper & Cohen, 2001).

Family members may have trouble meeting the demands of caring for a child with Down syndrome. These children have complex medical needs that place strain on the family and its finances. From the time of diagnosis, the family should be involved in the child's care. Include parents in planning interventions and care for the child. In most cases, they are the primary caregivers and will provide daily care as well as assisting the child in the development of functioning and skills. They can provide essential information to the health care team and will be advocates for their child throughout his or her life.

As the child grows, the needs of the family and child will change. Recognize and respect these needs and provide ongoing education and support for the child and family. Children with Down syndrome will need meaningful education programs. Many children with Down syndrome begin formal education in infancy and continue through high school. Full integration into the school system has become more common (Schoenstadt, 2008).

The outlook is brighter than it once was for children with Down syndrome. Many go on in adulthood to obtain jobs, to receive secondary education, and to live on their own or in semi-independent housing. Be familiar with local and national resources for families of children with Down syndrome so that you can help them fulfill their potential (Box 50.5).

▶ *Consider THIS!*

Charles Faust, a 10-month-old with Down syndrome, is seen in the clinic for a well-child examination. The parents have questions about his growth and development. They are concerned because Charles can't pick up finger foods such as Cheerios and put them in his mouth.

How would you address their concerns?

Discuss ways the family can encourage Charles's growth and development.

In addition to usual well-child care, what other medical management will you want to discuss with the family to prevent complications associated with Down syndrome?

Trisomy 18 and Trisomy 13

Trisomy 18 (also known as Edwards syndrome) and trisomy 13 (also known as Patau syndrome) are two other common trisomies. The incidence of trisomy 18 (the presence of three number 18 chromosomes) is 1 in 6,000 births; the incidence of trisomy 13 (the presence of three number 13 chromosomes) is 1 in 10,000 births (Behrman et al., 2004). As in Down syndrome, they usually result from nondisjunction (failure of a chromosome pair to separate) during cell division. Trisomy 18 and trisomy 13 can be present in all cells or may occur in mosaic forms. Both are associated with a characteristic set of anomalies and intellectual disabilities (Descartes & Carroll, 2007).

The prognosis for trisomy 18 and trisomy 13 is usually poor; these children usually do not survive beyond the first year of life. There is no cure for either condition. Therapeutic management will focus on managing the various congenital anomalies and health issues associated with the disorders.

Nursing Assessment

Nursing assessment will include a general observation for characteristic anomalies (Table 50.4 and Figs. 50.9 and 50.10).

Prenatal screening and diagnostic tests for trisomy 18 and 13 exist. If not diagnosed during the prenatal period, most cases are diagnosed in the first few days of life based on the physical characteristics associated with the disorders.

Nursing Management

Nursing management will be mainly supportive. This will be a difficult time for the family, so providing

TABLE 50.4 **CLINICAL MANIFESTATIONS OF TRISOMY 18 AND TRISOMY 13**

Chromosomal Abnormality	Clinical Manifestations
Trisomy 18	Prominent occiput, low-set ears, short eyelid fissures, intellectual disabilities, severe hypotonia, webbing, clenched fist with index finger over third digit and fifth digit overlapping the fourth, hypoplasia of fingernails, narrow hips with limited abduction, short sternum, congenital cardiac defects
Trisomy 13	Microcephalic head, wide sagittal suture and fontanels, malformed ears, small eyes, extra digits, severe hypotonia, severe intellectual disabilities, congenital heart defects, cleft lip, cleft palate

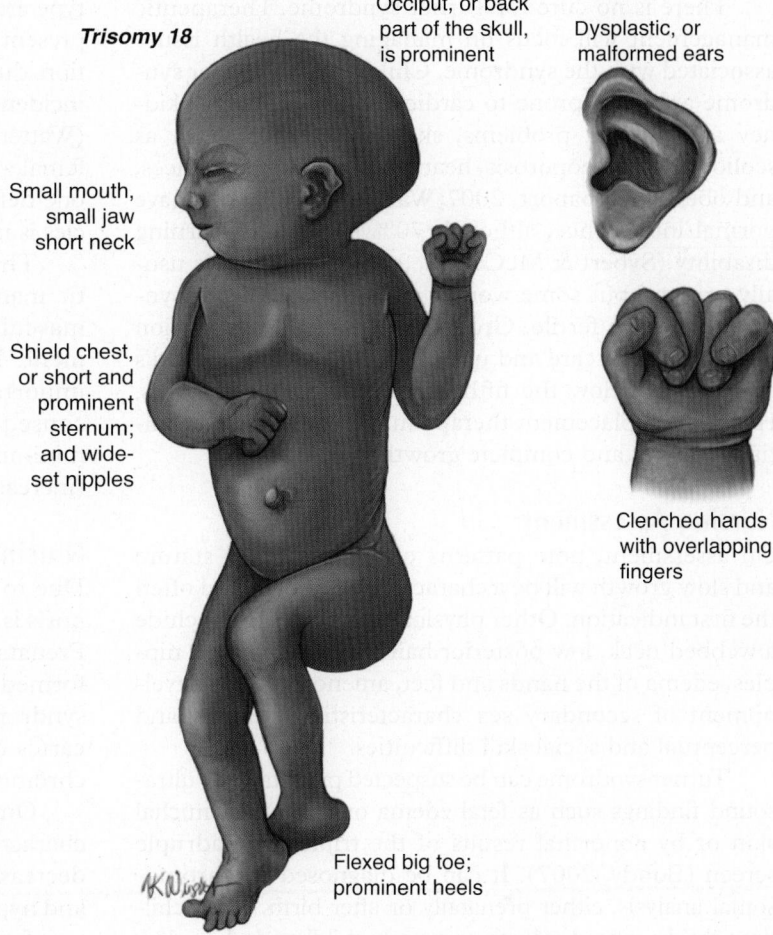

Trisomy 18

Occiput, or back part of the skull, is prominent

Dysplastic, or malformed ears

Small mouth, small jaw short neck

Shield chest, or short and prominent sternum; and wide-set nipples

Clenched hands with overlapping fingers

Flexed big toe; prominent heels

FIGURE 50.9 Trisomy 18. Copyright Lucina Foundation, all rights reserved.

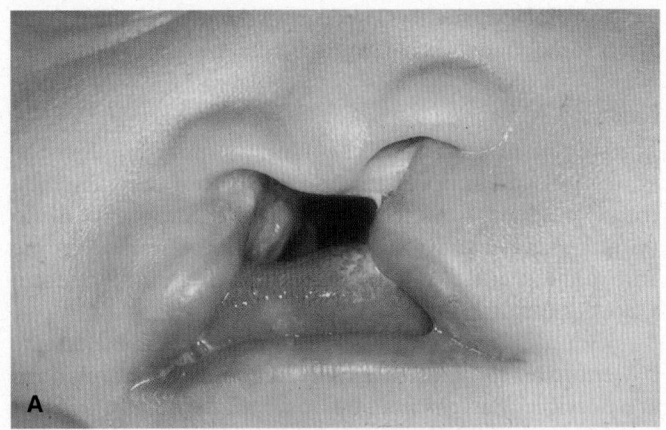

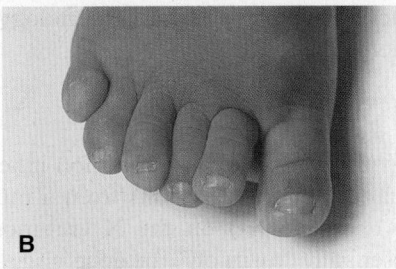

FIGURE 50.10 Trisomy 13.

support and resources for the family will be an important nursing function. SOFT is a support organization for families who have had a child with a chromosome abnormality; visit http://thePoint.lww.com/Chow1e for a direct link to the organization's website.

Turner Syndrome

Turner syndrome is a common abnormality of the sex chromosome. The phenotype is female. Since Turner syndrome affects 1 in every 2,000 to 2,500 newborn females, there are likely over 6,000 individuals with Turner syndrome in Canada (Turner Syndrome Society of Canada, 2009). Affected fetuses are often aborted spontaneously. The abnormality is due to a loss of all or part of one of the sex chromosomes. About half of the affected individuals have only one X chromosome; the other half has a variety of abnormalities of one of their sex chromosomes and may present with the mosaic form. In about 5% to 10% of cases of Turner syndrome, the individual presents with some Y chromosome material in some or all of her cells. These females may present with some masculinization. The risk of recurrence in future pregnancies is not increased, as Turner syndrome appears to be a sporadic event.

There is no cure for Turner syndrome. Therapeutic management will focus on managing the health issues associated with the syndrome. Children with Turner syndrome are more prone to cardiovascular problems, kidney and thyroid problems, skeletal disorders such as scoliosis and osteoporosis, hearing and eye disturbances, and obesity (Rapaport, 2007; Watson, 2010). They have normal intelligence, although 70% have some learning disability (Sybert & McCauley, 2004). Infertility is usually present, but some women with mosaic Turner syndrome may be fertile. Growth hormone administration is a standard of care and usually begins when the child's height falls below the fifth percentile for healthy girls. Hormone replacement therapy may also be given to initiate puberty and complete growth.

Nursing Assessment

On assessment, note patterns of growth; short stature and slow growth will be a characteristic finding and often the first indication. Other physical characteristics include a webbed neck, low posterior hairline, wide-spaced nipples, edema of the hands and feet, amenorrhea, no development of secondary sex characteristics, sterility, and perceptual and social skill difficulties.

Turner syndrome can be suspected prenatally by ultrasound findings such as fetal edema or redundant nuchal skin or by abnormal results of the triple or quadruple screen (Bondy, 2007). It can be diagnosed by chromosomal analysis, either prenatally or after birth. Most children are diagnosed at birth or in early childhood when slow growth or growth failure is noted. Some cases will not be diagnosed until the pubertal growth spurt does not occur.

Nursing Management

Nursing management is mainly supportive. Provide education and support to the family; they need to understand that short stature and infertility are likely. Explain that intellectual disability is unlikely, but some learning disabilities may be present. Emphasize that with medical supervision and support, girls with Turner syndrome may lead healthy, satisfying lives. Counselling about infertility is important. Parents may be upset that their daughter will not be able to reproduce, so explain that many alternatives for reproduction, such as in vitro fertilization and adoption, are available.

Providing support and resources for the family is an important nursing function. The Turner Syndrome Society of Canada provides assistance, support, and education to individuals with Turner syndrome and their families. Visit http://thePoint.lww.com/Chow1e for a direct link.

Klinefelter Syndrome

Klinefelter syndrome is the most common chromosomal abnormality (Descartes & Carroll, 2007). It is an abnormality of the sex chromosome: the karyotype and phenotype are male, but one or more extra X chromosomes are present. The abnormality is usually caused by nondisjunction during meiosis, but mosaic forms do present. The incidence of Klinefelter syndrome is 1 in 1,000 males (Wattendorf & Muenke, 2005). Males present with some female-like physical features that are caused by testosterone deficiency. The risk of recurrence in future pregnancies is not increased.

There is no cure for Klinefelter syndrome. Therapeutic management will focus on interventions to enhance masculine characteristics, such as testosterone replacement. Early recognition and hormonal treatment are important to improve quality of life and prevent serious consequences. Cosmetic surgery may be performed to minimize female characteristics such as gynecomastia (increased breast size).

Nursing Assessment

Due to nonspecific findings during childhood, the diagnosis is not usually made until adolescence or adulthood. Prenatal diagnosis is rare unless amniocentesis was performed for genetic testing. Many males with Klinefelter syndrome go through life without being diagnosed (Descartes & Carroll, 2007). The diagnosis is confirmed by chromosomal analysis.

On assessment, lack of development of secondary sex characteristics may be found. The individual may have decreased facial hair, gynecomastia, decreased pubic hair, and hypogonadism or underdeveloped testes, which leads to infertility. The individual may be taller than average by 5 years of age, with long legs and a short torso. Intellectual disability is not present, but cognitive impairments of varying degree, such as, speech or language difficulties, attention deficits, and learning disabilities, may be found.

Nursing Management

Nursing management will be mainly supportive. Provide education and support to the family. Resources include the Canadian Klinefelter Syndrome Support Group and the American Association for Klinefelter Syndrome Information and Support; visit http://thePoint.lww.com/Chow1e for direct links.

Counselling about infertility is important. Educate patients and families that marriage and sexual relations are possible. Parents may be upset that their son will not be able to reproduce, so explain that many alternatives for reproduction are available and technology is advancing in the field of infertility.

Fragile X Syndrome

Fragile X syndrome is the most common inherited cause of intellectual disabilities. It results from a mutation of a gene (FMR1 [fragile X]) on the X chromosome. This mutation essentially "turns off" the gene, triggering fragile X syndrome. The exact number of children affected by the mutation or premutation is not known. Males and females are both affected, but females usually have milder symptoms (Watson, 2010). The inheritance of fragile X is complex and is less straightforward than single-gene or Mendelian inheritance. Some carrier females are affected, and not all males with the gene abnormality show symptoms. Males and females are both fertile and can transmit the disorder to their offspring, so genetic counselling is appropriate. The prognosis for individuals with fragile X is good, and they tend to live a normal life span.

There is no cure for fragile X syndrome. Therapeutic management will be multidisciplinary and aimed at interventions to improve cognitive, emotional, and behavioural impairments.

Nursing Assessment

During childhood, clinical manifestations are subtle, with minor dysmorphic features and developmental delay. Problems with sensation, emotion, and behaviour often are the first signs. A delay in attaining developmental milestones will most likely be the first clue found on assessment. Intellectual impairment can range from subtle learning disabilities to severe intellectual disabilities and autistic-like behaviours. In adolescence, boys tend to present with characteristic features such as an elongated face, prominent jaw, large, protruding ears, large size, macro-orchidism (large testes), and a range of behavioural abnormalities and cognitive deficits. There is a characteristic pattern to the cognitive deficits, with problems in abstract reasoning, sequential processing, and mathematics. Typical behaviour problems include attention deficits, hand flapping and biting, hyperactivity, shyness, social isolation, low self-esteem, and gaze aversion. In females, the clinical manifestations are similar but are more varied and often present in a milder form.

The average age at diagnosis is 8 years. Diagnosis is confirmed by molecular genetic testing. Fragile X can be diagnosed prenatally if inheritance is suspected.

Nursing Management

Nursing management will be mainly supportive. Early diagnosis and intervention with developmental therapies and an individualized education plan are ideal. Care of these children will be the same as care of other children with an intellectual disability (see Chapter 51 for further information on intellectual disabilities).

Provide education and support to the family. The Fragile X Research Foundation of Canada Headquarters provides education, resources, and emotional support as well as a parent support group. Visit http://thePoint.lww.com/Chow1e for direct links.

Neurocutaneous Disorders

Neurocutaneous disorders, also referred to as hamartoses, are a group of disorders characterized by abnormalities of both the skin and the central nervous system. Many neurologic conditions are associated with cutaneous manifestations, since the skin and the nervous system share a common embryologic origin. They are complex conditions and most also affect other organ systems such as eyes, bones, heart, and kidneys. Most are hereditary and follow an autosomal dominant inheritance pattern or sporadic occurrence. Neurofibromatosis is a common neurocutaneous syndrome and is discussed in detail below. Table 50.5 provides information on other neurocutaneous syndromes.

Neurofibromatosis

Neurofibromatoses are neurocutaneous genetic disorders of the nervous system that primarily affect the development and growth of neural cell tissues. There are two distinct types: neurofibromatosis 1 (NF1) and neurofibromatosis 2 (NF2) (National Institute of Neurological Disorders and Stroke, 2011). Neurofibromatosis 1 (von Recklinghausen disease) is the more common type (Haslam, 2007; National Institute of Neurological Disorders and Stroke, 2011). This disorder causes tumours to grow on nerves and produce other abnormalities such as skin changes and bone deformities. Complications associated with neurofibromatosis include scoliosis, cardiac defects, hypertension, seizures, vision and hearing loss, learning disabilities, attention deficit disorder, abnormalities of speech, and a higher risk for neoplasms. In lay circles, this is often referred to as "Elephant Man" disease, but health care providers should avoid this term. Many assume that the disease will result in horrible disfigurement, but in reality most patients present with fairly mild disease.

Although many affected persons inherit the disorder, nearly half of the cases are due to a new mutation (National Institute of Neurological Disorders and Stroke, 2011). The inheritance pattern is autosomal dominant; therefore, offspring of affected individuals have a 50% chance of inheriting the altered gene and presenting with symptoms. Neurofibromatoses are due to a mutation of the neurofibromin gene on chromosome 17. The estimated prevalence for NF1 is 1 in 3,000 to 4,000 live births; NF2 is less common, with a birth incidence of 1 in 25,000 to 40,000 births (Farrell & Plotkin, 2007).

There is no cure for neurofibromatosis. Therapeutic management is aimed at controlling symptoms. Surgical intervention can help reduce some of the bone malformations and remove painful or disfiguring tumours. The American Academy of Pediatrics recommends that these children have a yearly physical, including blood pressure, scoliosis screening, and an ophthalmology examination, developmental screening, and a neurologic examination (Behrman et al., 2004).

The disease is progressive and symptoms usually worsen over time, but it is difficult to predict the course.

TABLE 50.5 OTHER NEUROCUTANEOUS SYNDROMES

Disorder	Incidence	Clinical Manifestations	Nursing Considerations
Tuberous sclerosis	1 in 6,000–10,000 (Tuberous Sclerosis Canada, 2006)	Benign tumours present in the brain and skin. Presents most often as a generalized seizure disorder. Tumours can also involve heart, kidney, eyes, lung, and bones. Developmental delay and behavioural problems may be noted. Usually evident in early childhood. Wide clinical spectrum ranging from severe intellectual disabilities with incapacitating seizures to normal intelligence and no seizures.	Treatment will be mainly symptomatic. Seizure control will be a primary concern. Provide support and education to the family. Refer for genetic counselling (it follows an autosomal dominant inheritance pattern and half the cases are due to a new mutation) and appropriate resources, such as Tuberous Sclerosis Canada
Sturge–Weber syndrome	1 in 50,000 (Behrman et al., 2004)	Facial nevus (port wine stain) most often seen on the forehead and on one side of the face, seizures, hemiparesis, intracranial calcifications. In many cases intellectual disabilities, behavioural and emotional problems, and learning disabilities are present. Seizures usually begin in infancy and may worsen with age. Convulsions are usually noted on the side of the body opposite the facial nevus. Muscle weakness may be present on the same side. Most affected individuals have glaucoma at birth or will develop it later in life.	Treatment will be mainly symptomatic. Seizure control will be a primary concern (use of anticonvulsants or surgery). Seizures due to Sturge–Weber are often difficult to control. Laser treatment may be used to lighten or remove the facial nevus. Surgery may be performed on more serious cases of glaucoma. Physical therapy should be considered for infants and children with muscle weakness. Educational therapy is often prescribed for those with intellectual disabilities or developmental delays. Provide support and education to the family. Refer to appropriate resources, such as the Sturge–Weber Foundation. Genetic counselling may be appropriate (inheritance is unclear and sporadic).

Most affected individuals develop mild to moderate symptoms, with non–life-threatening complications, and live a normal, productive life.

Nursing Assessment

On assessment, the nurse may find café-au-lait spots (light-brown macules), which are the hallmark of neurofibromatosis (Haslam, 2007) (Fig. 50.11). These are usually present at birth but can appear during the first year of life and usually increase in size, number, and pigmentation. They are present all over the body, particularly the trunk and extremities, while usually sparing the face. Pigmented nevi, axillary freckling, slow-growing cutaneous, subcutaneous, or dermal neurofibromas, which

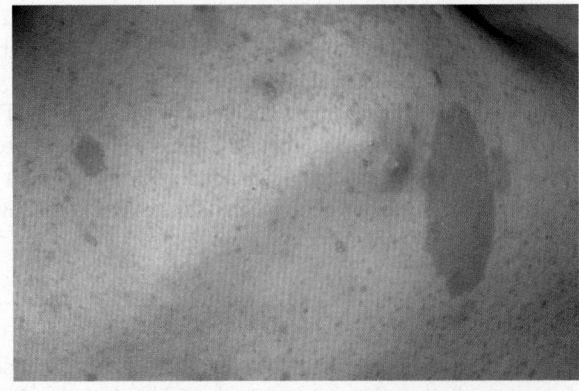

FIGURE 50.11 Café-au-lait spots associated with neurofibromatosis.

Clinical Signs of Neurofibromatosis

Diagnosis is made if two or more of the following are present:

- Six or more café-au-lait macules (light-brown spots) >5 mm in diameter in children and >15 mm in diameter in adolescents and adults
- Two or more neurofibromas (benign tumours) or one plexiform neurofibroma (tumour that involves many nerves)
- Freckling in the armpit or groin
- Presence of an optic glioma (a tumour on the optic nerve)
- Two or more growths on the iris of the eye (Lisch nodules or iris hamartomas)
- Abnormal development of the spine (scoliosis), the temple bone of the skull, or the tibia
- A first-degree relative (parent, sibling, or child) with NF1

Adapted from: Haslam. R. H. A. (2007). Neurocutaneous syndromes. In R. M. Kliegman, R. E. Behrman, H. B. Jenson, & B. F. Stanton (Eds.), *Nelson's textbook of pediatrics* (18th ed.). Philadelphia: Saunders; and National Institute of Neurological Disorders and Stroke. (2011). *Neurofibromatosis fact sheet.* Retrieved December 7, 2011 from http://www.ninds.nih.gov/disorders/neurofibromatosis/detail_neurofibromatosis.htm.

are benign tumours, are other signs of neurofibromatosis. Many children with neurofibromatosis have larger-than-normal head circumference and are shorter than average. Enough features are usually present by 10 years of age to make a diagnosis (National Institute of Neurologic Disorders and Stroke, 2011). The severity of symptoms varies greatly, but the diagnosis is made if two or more of the clinical signs in Box 50.6 are present.

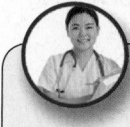

▶ *Take* NOTE!

If more than six café-au-lait spots are present, neurofibromatosis should be suspected.

Nursing Management

Nursing management will be mainly supportive. Early detection of treatable conditions and complications is a priority. Provide support and education to the child and family. Discuss genetic counselling with the family. Referral to appropriate resources, such as the Children's Tumor Foundation or Neurofibromatosis Canada, is essential. Visit http://thePoint.lww.com/Chow1e for direct links.

Other Genetic Disorders

Thousands of genetic disorders are known, and new ones are being discovered, but most of them are rare. Table 50.6 lists other genetic disorders that the pediatric nurse may encounter. Nursing management of these

disorders will be mainly supportive and will focus on providing support and education to the family and child, with an emphasis on developmental and educational needs. Referral to genetic counselling and appropriate resources is an important nursing function.

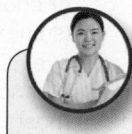

▶ *Take* NOTE!

Children with VATER syndrome who have only one kidney should not play contact sports.

Inborn Errors of Metabolism

Inborn errors of metabolism are a group of hereditary disorders. They are collectively common but individually rare (Weiner, 2009). Most follow an autosomal recessive inheritance pattern. They are caused by gene mutations that result in abnormalities in the synthesis or catabolism of proteins, carbohydrates, or fats. The body cannot convert food into energy as it normally would. Most inborn errors are due to a defect in an enzyme or transport protein that results in a block in the metabolic pathway. The blocked metabolic pathway allows for accumulation of the damaging by-product of the impaired metabolic process or may be responsible for a deficiency or absence of a necessary product. Presentation can occur at any time, even in adulthood, but many affected individuals exhibit signs in the newborn period or shortly after. Most inborn errors of metabolism presenting in the neonatal period are lethal if specific treatment is not initiated immediately.

Newborn screening is used to detect these disorders before symptoms develop. Recent developments in screening techniques (tandem mass spectrometry) allow dozens of metabolic disorders to be detected from a single drop of blood (Newborn Screening Authoring Committee, 2008). A child who tests positive will require additional testing to confirm the diagnosis (see Chapter 30 for more information on newborn screening).

Therapeutic management of these disorders varies depending on the cause of the error of metabolism, but dietary management is often a key component.

Nursing Assessment

Clinical signs and symptoms vary with each disorder. Table 50.7 gives information on some common inborn errors of metabolism seen in children.

Because of newborn screening and early identification and management, it is rare to see an untreated newborn with clinical signs and symptoms of the disease. If seen, in many cases a newborn who was healthy at birth will present with lethargy, poor feeding, apnea or tachypnea, recurrent vomiting, altered consciousness, failure to thrive, seizures, septic appearance, or developmental delay. Physical changes that may be seen include dysmorphology, cardiomegaly, rashes, cataracts, retinitis, optic

TABLE 50.6 **OTHER GENETIC DISORDERS, SYNDROMES, AND ASSOCIATIONS**

Disorder	Inheritance/Cause	Signs and Symptoms	Management
CHARGE syndrome (a recognizable pattern of congenital anomalies seen) **C: C**oloboma **H: H**eart disease **A: A**tresia (choanal) **R: R**etarded growth and development and/or CNS anomalies **G: G**enital anomalies, hypogonadism **E: E**ar anomalies and deafness Incidence is 0.1 to 1.2 in 10,000 live births (Pampal, 2010).	Autosomal dominant inheritance; most cases are due to new mutation of the gene. Mutations in the gene CDH7 have been indicated in some cases.	Coloboma is a lesion or defect of the eye, usually a fissure or cleft in the iris, ciliary, or choroid; can also see microphthalmos (small eyes) and cryptophthalmos (absent eye). Can lead to vision impairments. Heart anomaly can include any type but most common are aortic arch anomalies and tetralogy of Fallot. Atresia (choanal) is blocked or narrowed passages from the nose to the throat, which can lead to aspiration. Retarded growth or cognitive development can range from mild to severe. Genital anomaly may include micropenis, undescended testes, and hypoplastic labia. Ear anomalies include short, wide ears with little or no lobe, prominent inner fold, floppy appearance, asymmetry; can have hearing impairment. Each feature occurs in a spectrum from absent to severe; no single feature is present in all individuals.	Focus is on identifying and treating all defects; early diagnosis is important. Resource: CHARGE Syndrome Canada
Marfan syndrome: disorder of connective tissue Incidence is 1 in 5,000 (Canadian Marfan Association, 2009).	Autosomal dominant inheritance; caused by a mutation in the gene fibrillin-1, which results in changes in connective tissue	Tall stature with long slim limbs, minimal subcutaneous fat, muscle hypotonia, loose joints, long and narrow face, abnormalities of skeletal system (e.g., pectus excavatum [funnel chest] or pectus carinatum [pigeon breast]), ocular system (e.g., enlarged cornea or lens subluxation), and cardiovascular system (e.g., dilation of the aorta or mitral valve prolapse). Delayed achievement of gross and fine motor milestones may occur.	Focus is on preventing complications. Resources: National Marfan Foundation, Canadian Marfan Association
VATER association (not a diagnosis, but refers to a non-random association of defects found to occur together) **V: V**ertebral defects **A: A**nal atresia **TE: T**racheoesophageal fistula with esophageal atresia **R**adial and **R**enal dysplasia May also occur as VACTERL association, with **C: C**ardiac anomalies **L: L**imb abnormalities	Sporadic inheritance. Cause is unknown. Can occur with other chromosomal abnormalities such as trisomy 18. Frequently seen in the offspring of diabetic mothers.	Three or more anomalies are present. Anomalies seen include hypoplastic (small) vertebrae or hemivertebra (only half the bones are formed). These anomalies lead to an increased risk of scoliosis. With imperforate anus or anal atresia, the anus does not open to the outside of the body. Incomplete formation of one or more kidneys, obstruction of urine flow out of kidneys, or severe reflux back into kidneys can all lead to kidney failure later in life. Cardiac anomalies: most common are ventricular septal defects, atrial septal defects, and tetralogy of Fallot. Absent or displaced thumb, polydactyly (extra digits), syndactyly (fusion of digits). A single umbilical artery at birth is often present. Failure to thrive and slow development in early infancy due to anomalies. Usually normal intelligence.	Focus is on identifying and treating all defects. Resource: VACTERL Association Family Network

Disorder	Inheritance/Cause	Signs and Symptoms	Management
Apert syndrome (named for the French physician who described the syndrome) Incidence is 1 in 65,000 live births (Jones, 2006).	Autosomal dominant inheritance. Cases are sporadic and have been associated with older paternal age.	Craniosynostosis, bilateral symmetric syndactyly, and craniofacial anomalies such as prominent forehead, midface hypoplasia resulting in sunken appearance, short anteroposterior diameter, down-slanting eyelids. Small nasopharynx can lead to upper airway obstruction and sleep apnea. Learning disabilities and mental deficiency.	Early surgery for craniosynostosis when increased intracranial pressure is noted. Vigorous early management should occur with a multidisciplinary approach to address multiple anomalies. Resources: About Face Canada, Making Faces, Sick Kids Craniofacial Program
Achondroplasia (most common chondrodysplasia [diseases resulting in disordered growth]) Incidence is 1 in 15,000 (Jones, 2006).	Autosomal dominant inheritance pattern. Caused by mutations in fibroblast growth factor receptor 3 (FGFR3). 90% new gene mutation. Older paternal age may be a contributing factor.	Characterized by abnormal body proportion. Small stature (average adult height is 4 feet for both men and women), short limbs with normal-size torso, low nasal bridge with prominent forehead. Midface hypoplasia, caudal narrowing of spinal canal, megalocephaly, small foramen magnum; hands are short and stubby with separation between middle and ring finger ("trident hand"). Delayed motor skills, problems with persistent middle ear dysfunction and infections, and bowing of lower legs. Less common complications include hydrocephalus, craniocervical junction compression, upper airway obstruction, and thoracolumbar kyphosis. Usually present with normal intelligence and lead independent, productive lives.	Medical management of symptoms. Monitor height, weight, and head circumference. Manage and prevent complications (careful and thorough neurologic exam, assessment for sleep apnea). Growth hormone therapy is controversial and still experimental. Limb-lengthening surgeries may be performed. Resources: Little People of Canada, Inc., Short Persons Support

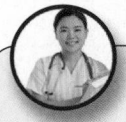

▶ **Take** NOTE!

When a previously healthy newborn presents with a history of deterioration, an inborn error of metabolism should be suspected.

▶ **Take** NOTE!

Early diagnosis is the key to saving and improving the lives of these children.

When a child who has previously been diagnosed with an inborn error of metabolism is hospitalized, the nurse must determine the prescribed diet and medications so these may be continued while in the hospital setting.

▶ **Take** NOTE!

If an inborn error of metabolism is suspected, feedings will usually be stopped until the test results are received.

atrophy, corneal opacity, deafness, skeletal dysplasia, macrocephaly, hepatomegaly, jaundice, or cirrhosis.

The diagnostic workup usually requires a variety of specific laboratory studies and may include:

- Glucose: may be elevated
- Ammonia: may be elevated
- Blood gases: may have low bicarbonate and low pH, metabolic acidosis (respiratory alkalosis may also be seen, especially when high ammonia levels are present)

TABLE 50.7 INBORN ERRORS OF METABOLISM

Disorder/Explanation	Incidence	Clinical Manifestations	Management
Phenylketonuria (PKU): deficiency in a liver enzyme leading to inability to process the essential amino acid phenylalanine properly. Phenyl alanine accumula tion can lead to brain damage unless PKU is detected soon after birth and treated.	>1 in 15,000 (Evans, Evans, Brown, et al., 2010)	No symptoms at birth. Most cases are identified before symptoms are present due to newborn screening. If undiagnosed, newborn may present with vomiting, irritability, eczema-like rash, and mousy odour to urine.	Low-phenylalanine diet. Phenylalanine is found mostly in protein-containing foods such as meat and milk (including breast milk and formula). Resource: Children's PKU Network
Galactosemia: deficiency in the liver enzyme needed to convert galactose, the breakdown product of lactose, which is commonly found in dairy products, into glucose. Galactose accumulation leads to damage to vital organs.	1 in 50,000 (Evans et al., 2010)	No symptoms at birth. If undiagnosed, newborn will have jaundice, diarrhea, and vomiting and will not gain weight. If untreated, can lead to liver disease, blindness, severe intellectual disabilities, and death.	Ingestion of galactose can produce sepsis in an affected child; therefore, septic workup and antibiotics may be necessary in a child if galactose ingestion has occurred. Elimination of galactose and lactose from the diet is the only treatment. Therefore, milk and dairy products will be eliminated for life. Resource: Canadian Families with Galactosemia
Maple sugar urine disease: affects the metabolism of amino acids. A deficiency in the enzyme that metabolizes leucine, isoleucine, and valine, which are components of protein often referred to as the branch chain amino acids. These amino acids then accumulate in the blood and cause damage to the brain.	1 in 250,000 (Evans et al., 2010).	No symptoms at birth, but if untreated newborns soon begin to show neurologic signs, vomiting, poor feeding, increased reflex action, and seizures. If untreated, can lead to life-threatening neurologic damage.	Special low-protein diet, which will vary based on severity of symptoms. Thiamine supplements may be given. Diet must be continued throughout life. Resource: Maple Syrup Urine Disease Family Support Group, STAR-G: Screening, Technology, and Research in Genetics
Biotinidase deficiency: lack of the enzyme biotinidase results in biotin deficiency	1 in 70,000 (Evans et al., 2010)	No symptoms at birth; in first weeks or months of life, symptoms such as hypotonia, uncoordinated movement, seizures, developmental delay, alopecia, seborrheic dermatitis, hearing loss, optic nerve atrophy, and intellectual disabilities develop. Metabolic acidosis can lead to death.	Daily oral free biotin Resource: Association for NeuroMetabolic Diseases

Disorder/Explanation	Incidence	Clinical Manifestations	Management
Medium-chain acyl-CoA dehydrogenase deficiency (MCAD): lack of an enzyme required to metabolize fatty acids	1 in 15,000 (Evans et al., 2010)	Recurrent episodes of metabolic acidosis and hypoglycemia, lethargy, seizures, liver failure, brain damage, coma, and cardiac arrest. Can lead to serious and fatal illness in children not eating well.	Avoid fasting; have frequent meals. Special considerations during illness. If unable to tolerate food, IV dextrose is required. Resource: Fatty Oxidation Disorders (FOD) Family Support Group
Homocystinuria: deficiency in the enzyme needed to digest a component of food called methionine (an amino acid)	1 in 275,000 (Evans et al., 2010).	If undetected and untreated can lead to intellectual disabilities, psychiatric disturbances, developmental delays, displacement of the lens of the eye, abnormal thinning and weakness of bones, and formation of thrombi in veins and arteries that can lead to life-threatening complications such as stroke.	Methionine-restricted diet and cystine supplements; vitamin B6 and B12 supplements and possibly other supplements, such as betaine and folic acid. Resource: Canadian Organization for Rare Disorders
Tyrosinemia: deficiency in an enzyme essential in the metabolism of tyrosine; accumulation of the by-products results in liver and kidney damage	1 in 100,000; particularly common in the Saguenay-Lac-St. Jean region of Quebec (1 in 20 is a carrier of the defective gene, and 1 in 1,846 has the disease (Canadian Liver Foundation, 2011)	Symptoms usually appear in the first months of life: poor weight gain, enlarged liver and spleen, increased bleeding tendency, distended abdomen, jaundice, cirrhosis, and liver failure.	Diet low in phenylalanine, methionine, and tyrosine. Resource: Canadian Liver Foundation
Tay–Sachs: caused by insufficient activity of an enzyme called hexosaminidase A, which is necessary for the breakdown of certain fatty substances in brain and nerve cells	Occurs more frequently among persons of Central and Eastern European and Ashkenazi Jewish descent. ~1 in every 27 Jews is a carrier, whereas in the general population 1 in 250 people is a carrier. Non-Jewish French Canadians from the East St. Lawrence River Valley of Quebec and members of the Cajun population in Louisiana are also at increased risk. These groups have about a 100 times higher incidence than other ethnic groups (March of Dimes, 2009b).	Infants appear normal and healthy for the first few months of life. Then, as harmful quantities of the fatty substances (called gangliosides) build up in tissues and nerve cells and cause damage, mental and physical deterioration occurs. The child becomes blind, deaf, and unable to swallow; muscles begin to atrophy; and paralysis sets in. Dementia, seizures, and an increased startle reflex may be seen. There is a late-onset type of Tay–Sachs seen in persons in their 20s and early 30s, but this is much rarer.	No treatment or cure. Medical management will focus on managing symptoms and maintaining comfort. Anticonvulsants may be given to control seizures. Death usually occurs in early childhood, by age 4 or 5. Carriers can be identified by a blood test, and prenatal testing is available. Resource: Canadian Association Tay–Sachs & Allied Diseases

Nursing Management

Ensure that the diet prescribed for the infant or child is followed. For amino acid disorders (e.g., phenylketonuria [PKU]), urea cycle defects (e.g., tyrosinemia type I), and organic acidemia (e.g., maple syrup urine disease), nutritional therapy is the major intervention. Dietary intake of specific amino acids is restricted according to the disorder. Ensure that overall protein and calorie needs are still met, as children need sufficient calories for proper growth. In children with urea cycle defects and organic acidemia, anorexia is common and severe, and the child may need gastrostomy tube feeding supplementation. In fatty acid oxidation disorders (e.g., medium-chain acyl-CoA dehydrogenase deficiency), the goal is to avoid prolonged periods of fasting and to provide frequent feeds when the child is sick. Supplementation with specific vitamins may also be important in the treatment of these disorders. Strict adherence to the diet is necessary and will require close supervision by registered dietitians, physicians, and nurses and the cooperation of both the parent and child.

Nursing management will focus on education and support for the family, who will need thorough knowledge about the child's disease and management. Referral to a dietitian and appropriate resources, including support groups, will be important. The nurse should also monitor the child's developmental progress and consult with the interprofessional team as a concern arises.

▬▬■ Key Concepts

- The purpose of a genetic consultation is to confirm or rule out genetic conditions, identify medical management issues, calculate and communicate genetic risks to a family, discuss ethical and legal issues, and provide psychosocial support.
- Nurses play an important role in the counselling process. Many times the nurse is the one who has first contact with these parents and is the one to provide follow-up care.
- The nurse must be able to identify those who could benefit from genetic counselling and must be able to discuss the role of the genetic counsellor with families. Families at risk must be aware that genetic counselling is available before they attempt to have another baby.
- Nurses play an essential role in providing emotional support and referrals to appropriate agencies, support groups, and resources when caring for families with suspected or diagnosed genetic disorders.
- Referral for genetic counselling prior to genetic testing may be appropriate.
- Many children with chromosomal abnormalities have intellectual disabilities, learning disabilities, behavioural problems, and distinct features, including birth defects.
- Trisomy 21 (Down syndrome) is associated with some degree of intellectual disability, characteristic facial features (e.g., slanted eyes and depressed nasal bridge), and other health problems, such as cardiac defects, visual and hearing impairments, intestinal malformations, and an increased susceptibility to infections.
- In Turner syndrome, short stature and slow growth are characteristic findings.
- Klinefelter syndrome is usually diagnosed in adolescence or adulthood due to a lack of development of secondary sex characteristics.
- Fragile X syndrome's clinical manifestations are subtle during childhood, with minor dysmorphic features and developmental delay. Problems with sensation, emotion, and behaviour often are the first signs.
- Café-au-lait spots (light-brown macules) are the hallmark of neurofibromatosis (Haslam, 2007).
- Inborn errors of metabolism are caused by gene mutations that result in abnormalities in the synthesis or catabolism of proteins, carbohydrates, or fats. Most inborn errors of metabolism presenting in the neonatal period are lethal if specific treatment is not initiated immediately.
- Nurses should have a basic knowledge of genetics, common genetic disorders in children, genetic testing, and genetic counselling so they can provide support and information to families and can help improve their quality of life.
- Genetic disorders usually result in a lifelong complex medical condition. Nurses must provide ongoing education and support for the child and family about the disorder, treatment, and management as well as available resources.

REFERENCES

American Academy of Pediatrics. (2007). Health supervision for children with Down syndrome. *Pediatrics*, *107*(2), 442–449. Retrieved December 8, 2011 from http://aappolicy.aappublications.org/cgi/content/full/pediatrics;107/2/442

Behrman, R. E., Kliegman, R. M., & Jenson, H. B. (2004). *Nelson's textbook of pediatrics* (17th ed.). Philadelphia: Saunders.

Bondy, C. A. (for the *Turner Syndrome* Consensus Study Group). (2007). Clinical practice guideline: Care of girls and women with Turner syndrome: A guideline of the Turner Syndrome Study Group. *The Journal of Clinical Endocrinology and Metabolism*, *92*(1), 10–25. doi:10.1210/jc2006-1374.

Buckley, F., & Buckley, S. J. (2008). Wrongful deaths and rightful lives – screening for Down syndrome. *Down Syndrome Research and Practice*, *12*(2), 79–86. doi:10.3104/editorials.2087

Canadian Liver Foundation. (2011). *Tyrosinemia*. Retrieved December 8, 2011 from http://www.liver.ca/liver-disease/types/tyrosinemia.aspx

Canadian Marfan Association. (2009). *What is Marfan syndrome?* Retrieved December 8, 2011 from http://www.marfan.ca/content/view/65/29/

Chen, H. (2011) *Down syndrome*. Retrieved December 8, 2011 from http://emedicine.medscape.com/article/943216-overview

Conley, Y. P. (2010). Genetics and health applications. In S. M. Nettina (Ed.), *Lippincott manual of nursing practice* (9the ed.). Philadelphia: Lippincott Williams & Wilkins.

Descartes, M., & Carroll, A. J. (2007). Cytogenetics. In R. M. Kliegman, R. E. Behrman, H. B. Jenson & B. F. Stanton (Eds.), *Nelson's textbook of pediatrics* (18th ed.). Philadelphia: Saunders.

Evans, T., Evans, M., Brown, Y., & Orshan, S. (2010). *Canadian maternity, newborn, & women's health nursing*. Philadelphia: Lippincott Williams & Wilkins.

Farrell, C. J., & Plotkin, S. R. (2007). Genetic causes of brain tumours: Neurofibromatosis, tuberous sclerosis, von Hippel-Lindau and other syndromes. *Neurologic Clinics, 25*(4), 925–946.

Fischbach, F. T., & Dunning, M. B. III. (2009). *A manual of laboratory and diagnostic tests* (8th ed.). Philadelphia: Lippincott Williams & Wilkins.

GeneTests. (2010). Growth of laboratory directory. Retrieved December 8, 2011 from http://www.ncbi.nlm.nih.gov/projects/GeneTests/static/whatsnew/labdirgrowth.shtml

Groch, J. (2006). Sleep apnea tests advised for Down's children. *Medpage Today.* Retrieved June 16, 2011 from http://www.medpagetoday.com/PrimaryCare/SleepDisorders/3111

Haslam, R. H. A. (2007). Neurocutaneous syndromes. In R. M. Kliegman, R. E. Behrman, H. B. Jenson & B. F. Stanton (Eds.), *Nelson's textbook of pediatrics* (18th ed.). Philadelphia: Saunders.

Hedequist, D., Bekelis, K., Emans, J., & Proctor, M. (2010). Single stage reduction and stabilization of basilar invagination after failed prior fusion surgery in children with Down's syndrome. *Spine, 35*(4), E128–E133.

Human Genome Project. (2006). *Human genome project information.* Retrieved December 8, 2011 from http://www.ornl.gov/sci/techresources/Human_Genome/home.shtml

Jenkins, J., Calzone, K., et al. (2008). *Essentials of genetic and genomic nursing: competencies, curricula guidelines, and outcome indicators* (2nd ed.). Retrieved December 8, 2011 from http://www.genome.gov/Pages/Careers/HealthProfessionalEducation/geneticscompetency.pdf

Jones, K. L. (2006). *Smith's recognizable patterns of human malformation* (6th ed.). Philadelphia: Elsevier Saunders.

Kaye, C. I., & the Committee on Genetics. (2011). Newborn screening fact sheets. *Pediatrics, 118*(3), e934–e963. doi:10.1542/peds.2006-1783

Korf, B. (2007). Integration of genetics into pediatric practice. In R. M. Kliegman, R. E. Behrman, H. B. Jenson & B. F. Stanton (Eds.). *Nelson's textbook of pediatrics* (18th ed.). Philadelphia: Saunders.

Lashley, F. R. (2005). *Clinical genetics in nursing practice.* New York: Springer Publishing.

March of Dimes. (2009a). *In-depth: Tay-Sachs and sandhoff diseases.* Retrieved December 8, 2011 from http://www.marchofdimes.com/professionals/14332_1227.asp

March of Dimes. (2009b). *Quick reference and fact sheet: Chromosomal abnormalities.* Retrieved December 8, 2011 from http://www.milesforbabies.org/professionals/14332_1209.asp

Marino, B. S., & Claybon, E. (2008). Genetic disorders. In B. S. Marino & K. S. Fine (Eds.), *Blueprints pediatrics (Blueprint Series)* (5th ed.). Philadelphia: Wolters Kluwer Health/Lippincott Williams & Wilkins.

Martin, G. E., Klusek, J., Estigarribia, B., & Roberts, J. E. (2009). Language characteristics of individuals with Down syndrome. *Topics in Language Disorders, 29*(2), 112–132.

MSU Department of Pediatrics and Human Development. (2011). *Prenatal screening: A guide for patients.* Retrieved December 8, 2011 from http://phd.msu.edu/Portals/0/docs/2011-Prenatal-Screening-Brochure-Website-Version.pdf

National Institute of Neurological Disorders and Stroke. (2011). *Neurofibromatosis fact sheet.* Retrieved December 8, 2011 from http://www.ninds.nih.gov/disorders/neurofibromatosis/detail_neurofibromatosis.htm

Newborn Screening Authoring Committee. (2008). Newborn screening expands: Recommendations for pediatricians and medical homes—Implications for the system. *Pediatrics, 121*(1), 192–217. doi: 10.1542/peds.2007-3021.

Pampal, A. (2010). CHARGE: An association or a syndrome? *International Journal of Pediatric Otorhinolaryngology, 74*(7), 719–722. doi: 10.1016/j.ijporl.2010.03.019.

Public Health Agency of Canada. (2003). *Down syndrome: background information.* Retrieved December 8, 2011 from www.phac-aspc.gc.ca/ccasn-rcsac/ct2003/bgds-eng.php

Pueschel, S. M. (2011). *A parent's guide to down syndrome: Toward a brighter future* (Revised Ed.). Baltimore, MD: Paul H. Brookes Publishing Company, Inc.

Rapaport, R. (2007). Disorders of the gonads: Hypofunction of the ovaries. In R. M. Kliegman, R. E. Behrman, H. B. Jenson & B. F. Stanton (Eds.), *Nelson's textbook of pediatrics* (18th ed.). Philadelphia: Saunders.

Rezvani, I. (2007). An approach to inborn errors of metabolism. In R. M. Kliegman, R. E. Behrman, H. B. Jenson & B. F. Stanton (Eds.), *Nelson's textbook of pediatrics* (18th ed.). Philadelphia: Saunders.

Robin, N. H. (2007). Patterns of genetic transmission. In R. M. Kliegman, R. E. Behrman, H. B. Jenson & B. F. Stanton (Eds.), *Nelson's textbook of pediatrics* (18th ed.). Philadelphia: Saunders.

Schoenstadt, A. (2008). *Children with down syndrome.* Retrieved December 8, 2011 from http://down-syndrome.emedtv.com/down-syndrome/children-with-down-syndrome.html

Siegel, B., & Milunsky, J. (2004). When should the possibility of a genetic disorder cross your radar screen? *Contemporary Pediatrics, 21*(5), 30–45.

Stevenson, R. E. (2006). Human malformations and related anomalies. In R. E. Stevenson & J. G. Hall (Eds.), *Human malformations and related anomalies* (2nd ed.). New York: Oxford University Press, Inc.

Sybert, V. P., & McCauley, E. (2004). Turner's syndrome. *New England Journal of Medicine, 351*(12), 1227–1241.

Tuberous Sclerosis Canada. (2006). *Information on tuberous sclerosis.* Retrieved December 8, 2011 from http://www.tscanada.ca/tscinfo.htm

Turner Syndrome Society of Canada. (2009). *About turner syndrome.* Retrieved December 8, 2011 from http://www.turnersyndrome.ca/turnerssyndrome.html

U.S. Department of Energy Genome Programs. (2011). *Human genome project information.* Retrieved December 8, 2011 from http://www.ornl.gov/sci/techresources/Human_Genome/home.shtml

Van Riper, M., & Cohen, W. (2001). Caring for children with Down syndrome and their families. *Journal of Pediatric Health, 15*(3), 123–131.

Venes, D. (2005). *Taber's cyclopedic medical dictionary* (20th ed.). Philadelphia: F. A. Davis.

Vis, JC., et al. (2009). Down syndrome: A cardiovascular perspective. *Journal of Intellectual Disability Research, 53*(5), 419–425; doi: 10.1111/j.1365-2788.2009.01158.x.

Waldman, H. B., Hasan, F. M., & Perlman, S. (2009). Down syndrome and sleep-disordered breathing: The dentist's role. *The Journal of the American Dental Association, 140*(3), 307–312.

Watson, J. (2010). Developmental disabilities. In S. M. Nettina (Ed.), *Lippincott manual of nursing practice* (9th ed.). Philadelphia: Lippincott Williams & Wilkins.

Wattendorf, D. J., & Muenke, M. (2005). Klinefelter syndrome. *American Family Physician, 72*(11), 2259–2263.

Weiner, D. L. (2009). *Inborn errors of metabolism.* Retrieved December 9, 2011 from http://emedicine.medscape.com/article/804757-overview

Wynshaw-Boris, A., & Biesecker, L. G. (2007). Dysmorphology. In R. M. Kliegman, R. E. Behrman, H. B. Jenson & B. F. Stanton (Eds.), *Nelson's textbook of pediatrics* (18th ed.). Philadelphia: Saunders.

RECOMMENDED READINGS

Canada, N. F. (n.d.). *Fact sheet: Neurofibromatosis type 1.* Retrieved December 8, 2011 from www.nfcanada.ca/images/uploads/documents/Fact_Sheets/NFC_FactSheet_NF1_ENG.pdf

Canadian Down Syndrome Society. (2010). *Resources.* Retrieved December 8, 2011 from from www.cdss.ca/resources.html

March of Dimes. (2009). *Quick reference fact sheet: Chromosomal abnormalities.* Retrieved December 8, 2011 from http://www.milesforbabies.org/professionals/14332_1209.asp

March of Dimes. (2008). *Prenatal care: Maternal blood screening.* Retrieved December 8, 2011 from http://www.marchofdimes.com/pregnancy/prenatalcare_blood.html

March of Dimes. (2010). *Recommended newborn screening test.* Retrieved December 18, 2011 from http://www.marchofdimes.com/baby/bringinghome_recommendedtests.html

National Down Syndrome Society. (2011). *About down syndrome.* Retrieved December 8, 2011 from http://www.ndss.org/index.php?option=com_content&view=category&id=35&Itemid=57

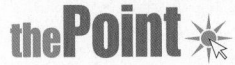

thePoint ✳ For additional learning material, including Internet Resources, visit **http://thePoint.lww.com/Chow1e.**

CHAPTER WORKSHEET

MULTIPLE CHOICE QUESTIONS

1. You are counselling a couple one of whom is affected by neurofibromatosis, an autosomal dominant disorder. They want to know the risk of transmitting the disorder. The nurse should tell them that each offspring has a:

   a. One in four (25%) chance of getting the disease

   b. One in eight (12.5%) chance of getting the disease

   c. One in one (100%) chance of getting the disease

   d. One in two (50%) chance of getting the disease

2. The nurse working in a women's health clinic determines that genetic counselling may be appropriate for a woman:

   a. Who just had her first miscarriage at 10 weeks

   b. Who is 30 years old and planning to conceive

   c. Whose history reveals a close relative with fragile X syndrome

   d. Who is 18 weeks pregnant and whose triple screen came back normal

3. A child born with a single transverse palmar crease, a short neck with excessive skin at the nape, a depressed nasal bridge, and cardiac defects is most likely to have which autosomal abnormality?

   a. Trisomy 21

   b. Trisomy 18

   c. Trisomy 14

   d. Trisomy 13

4. A mother brings her 4-day-old infant to the clinic with vomiting and poor feeding. The newborn was healthy at birth. The nurse should suspect:

   a. Sturge–Weber syndrome

   b. An inborn error of metabolism

   c. Trisomy 18

   d. Turner syndrome

CRITICAL THINKING EXERCISES

1. An 8-month-old is seen in the clinic. On assessment, the nurse finds eight café-au-lait spots on the child's trunk and extremities. What other assessment findings may be pertinent?

2. A child's newborn screen came back positive for phenylketonuria. After further testing, the diagnosis is confirmed. What instructions would you give the parents regarding care of their child?

3. A 6-year-old boy with Down syndrome is admitted to the hospital with pneumonia. Choose three pieces of information that the nurse should seek when obtaining the health history:

   a. Presence of cardiac defects or disease

   b. Last hearing and vision evaluation

   c. Mother's pregnancy history

   d. Presence of thyroid disease

   e. Mother's immunization history

STUDY ACTIVITIES

1. Develop a nursing care plan for a child with Down syndrome.

2. Shadow a genetic counsellor. Identify ways he or she helps families understand and cope with genetic disorders.

3. Attend a meeting of an ethics committee at a local hospital. Identify some of the ethical, legal, and social issues in health care that they discuss, particularly related to genetic testing and genetic disorders.

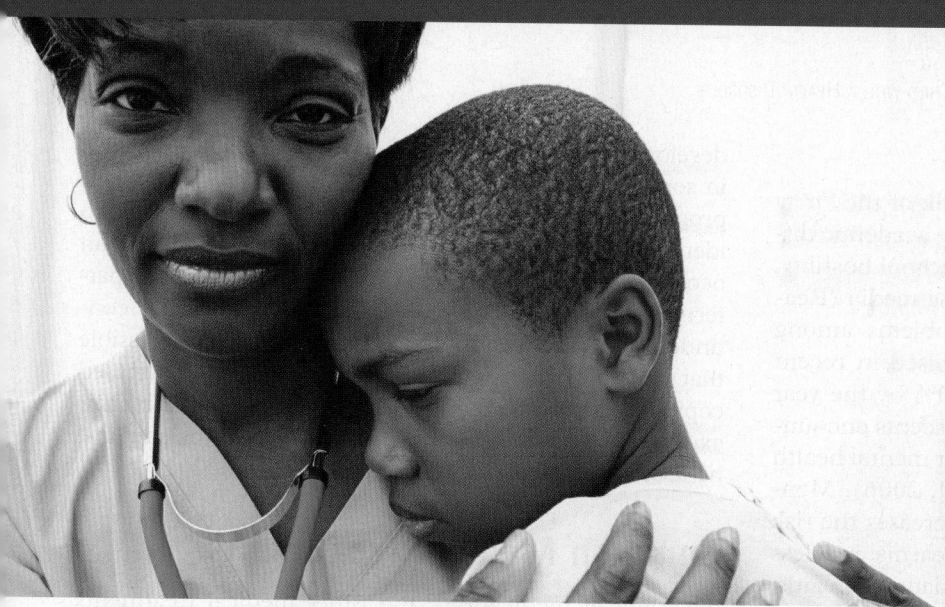

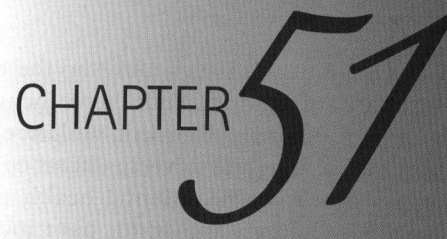

CHAPTER 51

Adapted by Beverley Temple

NURSING CARE OF THE CHILD WITH A COGNITIVE OR MENTAL HEALTH DISORDER

KEY TERMS

affect
anxiety
bingeing
co-morbidity
purging
suicide

LEARNING OBJECTIVES

Upon completion of the chapter, the learner will be able to:

1. Discuss the impact of alterations in mental health upon the growth and development of infants, children, and adolescents.
2. Describe techniques used to evaluate the status of mental health in children.
3. Identify appropriate nursing assessments and interventions related to therapy and medications for the treatment of childhood and adolescent mental health disorders.
4. Distinguish mental health disorders common in infants, children, and adolescents.
5. Develop an individualized nursing care plan for the child with a mental health disorder.
6. Develop patient/family teaching plans for the child with a mental health disorder.

John Howard, age 6 years, is brought to the clinic for his annual examination. His father states, "John has frequent emotional outbursts and his mood seems to switch from happy to sad rather quickly. His teachers have said his performance at school has been poor."

Wow

A child's sense often exceeds all human intellect.

Mental health issues make up the bulk of the "new morbidity" of children. Such issues include academic difficulties, psychiatric disorders, **violence**, school hostility, substance abuse, and adverse effects of the media (Reasor & Farrell, 2004). Mental health problems among Canadian children and youth have increased in recent years and are predicted to increase by 50% by the year 2020. Many Canadian children and adolescents encounter delays in accessing professional help for mental health issues (Canadian Pediatric Society [CPS], 2006). Mental illness manifested in the early years increases the risk for adolescent emotional issues, use of firearms, reckless driving, substance abuse, early sexual initiation for girls, teenage pregnancy, and promiscuous sexual activity. Some cognitive or neurobehavioural disorders may have a genetic or physiologic cause, whereas others result from family or environmental stressors.

Usually children with cognitive or mental health disorders are treated in the community or on an out-patient basis, but sometimes the disorder has such a significant impact on the child and family that hospitalization is required. Many hospitalized children also suffer from cognitive or mental health disorders. When a child is diagnosed with a neurobehavioural disorder, the family may become overwhelmed by the multifaceted services that he or she requires.

The scope of mental health issues among children, adolescents, and their families has become so extensive that in May 2006, the Standing Senate Committee on Social Affairs, Science and Technology, chaired by Senator Michael Kirby, released a comprehensive report on mental health and mental illness in Canada. "Out of the Shadows at Last: Transforming Mental Health, Mental Illness, and Addiction Services in Canada" concluded that "children and youth are at a significant disadvantage when compared to other demographic groups affected by mental illness, in that the failings of the mental health system affect them more acutely and severely" (Kirby & Keon, 2006).

Mental health problems in children are real and painful and can be severe. For affected children to have a chance at a healthy future, nurses must participate in the early identification and referral of children with potential cognitive deficits or other mental health issues.

Effects of Mental Health Issues on Health and Development

Children's behaviour is influenced by biologic or genetic characteristics, nutrition, physical health, developmental ability, environmental and family interactions, the child's individual temperament, and the parents' or caregiver's responses to the child's behaviour (Goldson & Reynolds, 2007). The changes that occur with normal growth and development are often a source of stress for children, and in some children they may lead to dysfunction. Children progress at very different rates, so it is often difficult to identify subtle abnormalities. When stress, fatigue, or pain occurs in children, they may quickly regress to earlier patterns of behaviour. These regressive behaviours may continue if a mental health concern is present. It is possible that stress placed on developing neurons leads to decreased coping abilities later in life. Children learn through their experiences; therefore, they may develop maladaptive behaviours through life interactions (Stafford, 2011).

Common Medical Treatments

A variety of medications and other medical treatments are used to treat mental health disorders in children. Most of these treatments will require a physician's order when the child is in the hospital. The most common medications are listed in Drug Guide 51.1. The nurse caring for the child with a mental health disorder should become familiar with how the treatments and medications work, as well as medication adverse effects to monitor for. Many mental health disorders are treated with some type of therapy. Table 51.1 reviews the types of therapies commonly used. These therapies are generally carried out only by specially trained personnel.

Behaviour management techniques are also used to help children alter negative behaviour patterns (Nurcombe, 2008). The methods may be used outside of therapy sessions, in the hospital, clinic, or classroom. Behaviour management techniques include the following:

- Set limits with the child, holding the child responsible for his or her behaviour.
- Provide consistent caregivers (unlicensed assistive personnel and nurses for the hospitalized child) and establish the child's daily routine.
- Use a low-pitched voice and remain calm.
- Redirect the child's attention when needed.
- Ignore inappropriate behaviours.
- Praise the child's self-control efforts and other accomplishments.
- Use restraints only when necessary.

NURSING PROCESS OVERVIEW FOR THE CHILD WITH A MENTAL HEALTH DISORDER

Care of the child with a mental health disorder includes assessment, nursing diagnosis, planning, interventions, and evaluation. There are a number of general concepts related to the nursing process that may be applied to mental health concerns in children. From a general understanding of the care involved for a child with a

DRUG GUIDE 51.1 DRUGS USED FOR PEDIATRIC MENTAL HEALTH DISORDERS

Medication	Action/Indication	Nursing Implications
Psychostimulants: methylphenidate (Ritalin), dextroamphetamine (Adderall), lisdexamfetamine (Vyvanse), pemoline (Cylert), long-acting methylphenidate (Concerta, Focalin XR, Metadate CD, Ritalin LA), long-acting dextroamphetamine (Dexedrine Spansules, Adderall XR)	Increases synaptic levels of dopamine and norepinephrine ADHD	• Methylphenidate has a short half-life; give TID (AM, mid-day at school, at home after school). • Long-acting preparations are given once daily in the AM. • Adverse effects: decreased appetite, headache, abdominal pain, difficulty sleeping, irritability, social withdrawal, motor tics. If dose is too high, child may have flat affect. • Vyvanse—if chest pain and fainting occurs notify physician at once. • Pemoline is only rarely used because of hepatotoxicity.
Antianxiety agent: buspirone (BuSpar)	Highly blocks reuptake of dopamine Anxiety, rage, mania, psychosis, depression, Tourette syndrome	• Administer in consistent relation to food (either with or without). • May cause drowsiness • Monitor for disinhibition, agitation, confusion, depression.
Antimanic agent: lithium (Eskalith, Lithobid)	Influences reuptake of serotonin and/or norepinephrine Bipolar disorder, depression, hyperaggression	• Monitor closely. • May cause polyuria, polydipsia, tremor, nausea, weight gain, diarrhea
Selective serotonin reuptake inhibitors: fluoxetine (Prozac), paroxetine (Paxil), sertraline (Zoloft)	Potentiates serotonin activity in the brain Depression, obsessive–compulsive disorder, anxiety	• Observe for irritability, insomnia, GI distress, nausea, headache. • Monitor BP for increase.
Atypical antidepressants: trazodone (Desyrel)	Inhibits reuptake of serotonin Depression	• Monitor BP for postural hypotension. • Observe for sedation and drowsiness; avoid alcohol use. • Administer after meals or with a snack.
Nonstimulant norepinephrine reuptake inhibitors: atomoxetine (Strattera)	Enhances norepinephrine activity ADHD	• Administer without regard to food once or twice daily. • Monitor weight, height, BP, heart rate. • May cause dizziness, dry mouth.
Alpha-agonist antihypertensive agents: clonidine (Catapres), guanfacine (Tenex)	Activates inhibitory neurons in the brain stem ADHD, Tourette syndrome, self-abuse, aggression	• Clonidine is strongly sedating. • Monitor BP and pulse. • Observe for dry mouth, confusion, depression, urinary retention, constipation.
Antipsychotic agents: thioridazine (Mellaril), chlorpromazine (Thorazine), haloperidol (Haldol)	Reversibly block type 2 dopamine receptors in the central nervous system Psychosis, mania, self-harm, violent or destructive behaviour	• May cause drowsiness. • Monitor for anticholinergic effects, drowsiness and dystonia (extrapyramidal effects), dizziness. • Evaluate for the development of orthostatic hypotension, tachycardia. • Observe closely for the development of tardive dyskinesia, particularly early in treatment.
Atypical antipsychotics: risperidone (Risperdal), clozapine (Clozaril), olanzapine (Zyprexa)	Reversibly block type 2 dopamine receptors in the central nervous system Psychosis, bipolar disorder, autism spectrum disorder, Tourette syndrome	• Monitor for seizures, agitation, headache, nausea, sedation. • Olanzapine may cause weight gain. • Note WBC.
Tricyclic antidepressants: amitriptyline (Elavil), desipramine (Norpramin), imipramine (Tofranil), nortriptyline (Pamelor)	Enhances synaptic concentration of serotonin and/or norepinephrine Depression, ADHD, tics, anxiety	• Monitor for anticholinergic effects, weight loss. • Check blood levels. • Monitor ECG for arrhythmias.

Adapted from: Nurcombe, B. (2008). Diagnostic formulation, treatment planning, and modes of treatment in children and adolescents. In M. H. Ebert, P. T. Loosen, B. Nurcombe, & J. F. Leckman. *Current diagnosis & treatment: Psychiatry* (2nd ed.). New York: McGraw-Hill; and Varcarolis, E. M. (2011). *Manual of psychiatric nursing care planning: Assessment guides, diagnoses, and psychopharmacology* (4th ed.). St. Louis, MO: Saunders.

TABLE 51.1 TYPES OF THERAPY

Treatment	Explanation
Behavioural therapy	Uses stimulus and response conditioning to manage or alter behaviour. Reinforces desired behaviours, replacing the inappropriate ones. Consistency is of utmost importance.
Play therapy	Designed to change emotional status. Encourages the child to act out feelings of sadness, fear, hostility, or anger.
Cognitive therapy	Teaches children to change reactions so that automatic negative thought patterns are replaced with alternative ones
Family therapy	Explores the child's emotional issue and its effect on family members
Group therapy	May be conducted in a school, hospital, treatment facility, or neighbourhood centre. Feelings are expressed and participants gain hope, feel a part of something, and benefit from role modelling. Takes advantage of peer relationships as developmental focus in preteen and teen groups.
Milieu therapy	A specially structured setting designed to promote the child's adaptive and social skills. A safe and supportive environment for those at risk of self-harm or those who are very ill or very aggressive.
Individual therapy	The child and therapist work together to resolve the conflicts, emotions, or behaviour problems. Trust is central. Structured based on the child's developmental level (e.g., may use play therapy for a younger child).
Hypnosis	Deep relaxation with suggestibility remarks

mental health disorder, the nurse can then individualize the care based on patient specifics.

Assessment

A careful and thorough health history forms the basis of the nursing assessment of a child with a mental health or cognitive disorder. The physical examination may yield clues to the type of disorder but is often completely normal.

▶ *Take NOTE!*

Observe a child's play or drawings; if you suspect cognitive or psychological issues from the play or artwork, refer the child for further mental health evaluation.

Health History

Elicit the health history, noting the child's prenatal and birth history, past medical history, including previously diagnosed cognitive or mental health disorders, history of neurologic injury or disease, and family history of mental health disorder. Perform a developmental history, noting age of attainment (or loss) of milestones. Question the child and/or parent about behaviour changes such as:

- Altered sleep
- Difference in eating patterns, weight loss or gain, change in appetite
- Problems at school

- Participation in risk-taking behaviours
- Alterations in friendships
- Changes in extracurricular activity participation

Note results of any developmental testing performed. Ask the family about progression of the child's skills. Note any unusual deficits or capabilities. Question the family about recent stress, trauma, or change in family structure; are any family members chronically ill? Note medications the child takes routinely, and any allergies to food, drugs, medications, or environmental agents.

Interview the child at an age-appropriate level to determine his or her self-perception, future plans, and stressors and how he or she copes with them. Determine the child's perception of his relationship with his parents, siblings, friends, peers, pets, inanimate objects, and transitional or security objects. What is the child's predominant mood? Determine whether the child likes him- or herself, asking such questions as "What do you like most about yourself?" and "What would you like to change about yourself?" Determine the child's gender identity status. Does the child have a sense of pride in his or her accomplishments? Has the child developed an appropriate conscience (with understanding of right and wrong)?

Note history of complaints that may be associated with certain mental health disorders, such as sore throat, difficulty swallowing, or genital burning or itching. Document whether the child displays any of the following during the health interview:

- Hallucinations
- Aggression

- Impulsivity
- Distractibility
- Intolerance to frustration
- Lack of sense of humour or fun
- Inhibition
- Poor attention span
- Potential cognitive or learning disabilities
- Unusual motor activities

Remember John, the 6-year-old brought in for his annual examination? What additional health history and physical examination assessment information should the nurse obtain?

Physical Examination

Observe the child's clothing, noting whether it is appropriate for age, developmental level, and setting. Note the child's facial expression and response to the parent or caretaker and the nurse. Does the child make appropriate eye contact? Determine the child's level of consciousness and extent of interest in and interaction with surroundings. Note the child's posture, **affect**, and mood. How appropriate to the situation are the child's emotional reactions? Does the child communicate well?

Measure the child's weight and height/length, as well as head circumference if he or she is less than 3 years old. Perform a thorough physical examination, noting any physical abnormalities or signs of other physical health disorders. Note abnormal findings that may be associated with particular mental health disorders, such as bruising, burns, contusions, cuts, abrasions, unusual skin marks, soft/sparse body hair, split fingernails, inflamed oropharynx, eroded tooth enamel, reddened gums, or genitourinary discharge or bleeding.

Laboratory and Diagnostic Testing

Mental health disorders are generally diagnosed based upon clinical features. Brain imaging such as computed tomography or magnetic resonance imaging may be used to evaluate for a congenital abnormality or alterations in the brain tissue that may lead to developmental delay. A blood or urine toxicology panel is useful in the diagnosis of drug abuse or overdose or instances of bizarre behaviour.

Nursing Diagnoses and Related Interventions

The overall goal of nursing management of cognitive and mental health disorders in children is to help the child and family to reach an optimal level of functioning. This may be achieved through interventions designed to decrease the impact of stressors upon the child's life. Upon completion of a thorough assessment

of the child and family, the nurse might identify several nursing diagnoses, including:

- Impaired social interaction
- Delayed growth and development
- Ineffective individual coping
- Hopelessness
- Imbalanced nutrition, less than body requirements
- Disturbed thought processes
- Caregiver role strain

After completing an assessment of John, the nurse noted the following: difficulty sitting still for the examination, easily distracted, and frustrated, labile mood. Based on the assessment findings, what would your top three nursing diagnoses be for John?

Nursing goals, interventions, and evaluation for the child with a mental health disorder are based on the nursing diagnoses. Nursing Care Plan 51.1 provides a general guide for planning care for a child with a mental health disorder. Children's responses to a mental health issue and its treatment will vary, and nursing care should be individualized based on the child's and family's responses to illness. Additional information about nursing management will be included later in the chapter as it relates to specific disorders.

Based on your top three nursing diagnoses for John, describe appropriate nursing interventions.

Developmental and Behavioural Disorders

Developmental and behavioural disorders make up a large proportion of mental health disorders in children. They include learning disabilities, intellectual disability, autism spectrum disorder (ASD), and attention-deficit/hyperactivity disorder.

Learning Disabilities

About 10% to 15% of Canadians may experience learning problems that are a continuation of learning disabilities from early childhood (Learning Disabilities Association of Canada, 2002). About half of the children with a learning disability have at least one other co-morbid condition (usually a mental health or behavioural disorder). The Learning Disabilities Association of Canada (2002) defines a learning disability as "a number of disorders which may affect the acquisition, organization, retention, understanding or use of verbal or nonverbal information." Learning

(text continues on page 1766)

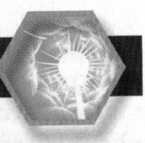

Nursing Care Plan 51.1

OVERVIEW FOR THE CHILD WITH A MENTAL HEALTH DISORDER

NURSING DIAGNOSIS: Impaired social interaction related to altered social skills as evidenced by impulsivity, intrusive behaviour, inability to follow through, anxiety, depressed mood, feelings of unattractiveness or unworthiness

Outcome Identification and Evaluation
The child will demonstrate socially acceptable skills, *interacting successfully with peers and in the educational setting, completing tasks as required.*

Interventions: Promoting Appropriate Social Interaction
- Identify factors that may aggravate the child's performance *to minimize stimuli that exacerbate the child's undesired behaviours.*
- Modify the environment to decrease distracting stimuli *as child's ability to deal with external stimuli may be impaired.*
- Ensure that the child hears his or her name and makes eye contact prior to conversing or instructions *so that child is engaged and has increased ability to follow through.*
- State expectations for tasks or behaviours clearly *as understanding is necessary to ensure completion.*
- Provide positive feedback for appropriate behaviours or task completion, *encouraging the child to adopt expectations into his or her behaviours and routine.*

NURSING DIAGNOSIS: Ineffective individual coping related to inability to deal with life stressors as evidenced by few or no meaningful friendships, inability to empathize or give/receive affection, low self-esteem, or maladaptive coping behaviours such as substance abuse

Outcome Identification and Evaluation
The child will demonstrate improved coping, *verbalize feelings, socially engage, demonstrate problem-solving skills.*

Interventions: Promoting Coping Skills
- Encourage discussion of thoughts and feelings, *as this is an initial step toward learning to deal with them appropriately.*
- Provide positive feedback for appropriate discussion, *as this increases the likelihood of continuing performance.*
- Demonstrate unconditional acceptance of the child as a person *to increase self-esteem in the child who has been feeling rejection.*
- Set clear limits on behaviour as needed *so the child has a structure to adhere to.*
- Teach the child problem-solving skills *as an alternative to acting-out behaviours.*
- Role-model appropriate social and conversation skills *so the child can see what is expected in a nonthreatening manner.*

NURSING DIAGNOSIS: Imbalanced nutrition, less than body requirements, related to intake insufficient to meet metabolic needs as evidenced by weight loss, failure to gain weight, less-than-expected increases in stature and weight, loss of appetite, or refusal to eat

Outcome Identification and Evaluation
The child or adolescent will demonstrate appropriate growth, *making gains in weight and stature as appropriate.*

Interventions: Improving Nutritional Intake
- Provide favourite foods *to encourage the child with poor appetite to eat more.*
- Assist families to choose nutrient-rich foods *so that the food the child does eat is most beneficial.*

For the child with an eating disorder:
- Mutually establish a contract related to treatment *to promote the child's sense of control.*
- Provide mealtime structure, *as clear limits let the child know what the expectations are.*
- Encourage the child to choose foods and timing of meals *to develop independence in eating habits.*
- Ensure the eating environment is pleasant and relaxed, with minimal distractions, *to minimize the child's anxiety and guilt about not eating.*
- Withdraw attention if child refuses to eat *(secondary gain is minimized if refusal to eat is ignored).*
- Provide continuous supervision during the meal and for 30 minutes following it *so that the child cannot conceal or dispose of food or induce vomiting.*

Nursing Care Plan 51.1 (continued)

NURSING DIAGNOSIS: Delayed growth and development related to disability, behavioural disorder, or altered nutrition as evidenced by lack of attainment of age-appropriate skills, regression in skills, or altered intellectual functioning

Outcome Identification and Evaluation
Child will demonstrate progress toward developmental milestones: *Child expresses interest in the environment and people around him, interacts with environment in an age-appropriate way.*

Interventions: Promoting Development
- Use therapeutic play and adaptive toys *to facilitate developmental functioning.*
- Provide a stimulating environment when possible *to maximize potential for growth and development*
- Praise accomplishments and emphasize child's abilities *to improve self-esteem and encourage feeling of confidence and competence.*
- Follow through with physical, occupational, and speech therapists' recommendations *to maximize exposure to exercises designed to increase the child's skills.*
- Determine parents' expectations of child's future achievement *to help them work toward these goals.*

NURSING DIAGNOSIS: Disturbed thought processes related to behavioural disorder, depression, anxiety, abusive situation, or substance abuse as evidenced by distractibility, non–reality-based thinking, hypervigilance, or inaccurate interpretation of interactions of others

Outcome Identification and Evaluation
Child's thought processes will improve; *child will demonstrate appropriate orientation, remain free from physical harm, and perform activities of daily living as able.*

Interventions: Improving Thought Processes
- Observe for causes of altered thought processes *to provide a baseline for assessment and intervention.*
- Perform an age-appropriate mental status examination *to determine extent of altered thinking.*
- Adjust communication style based on child's cues *to improve communication.*
- Listen carefully and seek clarification *to determine basis for child's agitation or other behaviours.*
- Provide validation of the child's thoughts and feelings *to improve trust in the relationship.*
- Establish a daily routine *to provide the child with a sense of security.*

NURSING DIAGNOSIS: Hopelessness related to child's perception of his life situation, negative life view, or alteration in mental well-being as evidenced by passivity, verbalization, alterations in sleep, or lack of initiative

Outcome Identification and Evaluation
Child will display a sense of hope, *will verbalize feelings, participate in care, and make positive statements.*

Interventions: Promoting Hope
- Monitor and document potential for suicide, *as hopelessness often leads to suicidal ideation.*
- Assist the child to identify reasons for hope and for living, *so the nurse is aware of the child's values.*
- Help the child to set goals that are important to him or her *to allow the child to see possibilities.*
- Encourage simple decision making on a daily basis, *as hopelessness often occurs as a response to loss of control.*
- Assist the child to identify positive qualities in himself and his life *to facilitate the development of hope.*
- Involve parents or others the child loves in the child's care *as social support is critical to the development of hope.*

(continued)

Nursing Care Plan 51.1 (continued)

NURSING DIAGNOSIS: Caregiver role strain related to long-term care of the child with a chronic mental health disorder as evidenced by fatigue, inattention to own needs, conflict, or ambivalence

Outcome Identification and Evaluation

The child's caregiver will participate in the child's care, *verbalizing the child's needs and treatment plan and demonstrating skills necessary for care.*

Interventions: Decreasing Role Strain

- Teach the parent or caregiver about the child's illness, treatments, and medications *to clarify expectations for the child and parent.*
- Role-model appropriate interaction behaviours with the child *so the parent can learn these techniques by watching.*
- Encourage structure in daily routines *to allow the parent to meet own needs and allow for adequate rest.*
- Gradually increase the parent's responsibility related to care of the child *to help the parent feel less overwhelmed.*
- Allow the parent to move at his or her own pace in assuming care *to enhance the chances for success.*
- Help the parent to identify a backup caregiver *so the parent has times of respite from constant involvement with the child.*

---

disabilities become evident when a child of average intelligence has difficulty mastering basic academic skills. Learning disabilities can affect the child's ability to listen, speak, read, write, and perform mathematics:

- Children with dyslexia have difficulty with reading, writing, and spelling.
- Dyscalculia leads to problems with mathematics and computation.
- Problems with manual dexterity and coordination result when a child has dyspraxia.
- Children with dysgraphia have difficulty producing the written word (composition, spelling, and writing).

Sensory integration dysfunction may be mistaken for a learning disability, but it is not and should be treated differently. Learning difficulties may also involve difficulties with organizational skills, social perception, social interaction, and perspective taking (Learning Disabilities Association of Canada, 2002). Box 51.1 provides additional information.

Nursing Assessment

Elicit the health history, noting risk factors such as a family history of learning disability, problems during pregnancy or birth, prenatal alcohol or drug use, low birth weight, premature or prolonged labour, head injury, poor nutritional status or failure to thrive, or lead poisoning. Obtain detailed information about the educational difficulties the child is experiencing (e.g., he seems to do fine in math but always reverses letters when reading). A thorough physical examination may reveal clues to co-morbid conditions. Ensure that the child has undergone a comprehensive education evaluation with assessment testing to diagnose the specific learning disability. Testing may be performed by a school, educational, developmental, or clinical psychologist, occupational therapist, speech and

language therapist, or other developmental specialist, depending on the areas of learning with which the child is experiencing difficulty.

▶ *Take* NOTE!

If a child cannot speak in sentences by 30 months of age, does not have understandable speech 50% of the time by age 3 years, cannot sit still for a short story by 3 to 5 years of age, or cannot tie shoes, cut, button, or hop by 5 to 6 years of age, refer the child to be evaluated for a learning disability.

Nursing Management

Ensure that families are aware of their child's rights under the laws and policies of their applicable provincial

---

BOX 51.1 **Sensory Processing Disorder (Also Called Sensory Integration Dysfunction)**

- A neurologic disorder in which the child cannot organize sensory input used in daily living
- Hyposensitivity or hypersensitivity to sensory input
- Results in overreaction to different textures, decreasing the child's ability to participate in the world
- Preterm and low birth weight infants are at increased risk compared with typical infants.
- Occupational and other therapies may increase the child's ability to function.

Adapted from: Sensory Processing Disorder Foundation. (2011). *About SPD.* Retrieved October 18, 2011 from http://www.spdfoundation.net/about-sensory-processing-disorder.html.

authority. A summary report has been compiled to identify the differences in policies across Canada (McColl & Stephenson, 2008).

Each child will need an individualized education plan (IEP) that reflects his or her particular needs, which then must be provided for through the school system. Offer encouragement and support to families as they advocate for their child. Follow up at subsequent health care visits to determine that the child is receiving the services he or she needs to optimize his or her potential for success. Refer families for additional resources through the Learning Disabilities Association of Canada and the National Center for Learning Disabilities; visit http://thePoint.lww.com/Chow1e for direct links.

Intellectual Disability

Intellectual disability refers to a functional state in which significant limitations in intellectual status and adaptive behaviour (functioning in daily life) develop before the age of 18 years. Up to 3% of the population may be designated as having an intellectual disability (National Dissemination Center for Children with Disabilities [NICHCY], 2011; Ouellette-Kuntz, Shooshtari, Temple, et al., 2010).

The American Association on Intellectual and Developmental Disabilities (AAIDD, n.d.) defines intellectual disability as having the following characteristics:

- Deviations in IQ of two or more standard deviations (IQ of less than 70 to 75) with significant limitations in intellectual functioning (reasoning, learning, problem solving)
- Significant limitations in adaptive behaviour in everyday social and practical skills
- Occurring before the age of 18 years

In past years, persons with an intellectual disability were confined to institutions and were thought to be harmful to society. In the early 21st century, most children with intellectual disability are receiving their education in public schools with their peers and living at home with their families or elsewhere in the community. Only the most severely affected individuals require separate classrooms or schools.

Pathophysiology

In many instances of intellectual disability the exact cause remains unknown. Prenatal errors in central nervous system development may be responsible, or an insult or damage to the brain may occur in the prenatal, perinatal, or postnatal period from a variety of causes. Motor problems such as hypotonia, tremor, ataxia, or clumsiness, visual motor problems, or other issues may occur concomitantly with intellectual disability. When a learning disability or sensory processing impairment is also present, functioning at a higher intellectual level may be

prevented. Intellectual disability is generally categorized according to severity:

- Mild: IQ 50 to 70
- Moderate: IQ 35 to 50
- Severe: IQ 20 to 35
- Profound: IQ less than 20 (Council for Exceptional Children, 2011)

Therapeutic Management

The primary goal of therapeutic management of children with intellectual disability is to provide appropriate educational experiences that allow the child to achieve a level of functioning and self-sufficiency needed for existence in the home, community, work, and leisure settings. The child's conceptual, social, practical, and intellectual abilities will drive school placement and the focus of the educational experience. The student's success is also dependent upon community and family influences. The majority of individuals with intellectual disability require only minimal support, and these individuals are able to achieve some level of self-sufficiency. Only a few children and adults with intellectual disability require extensive support.

Nursing Assessment

Perform developmental screening at each health care visit to identify developmental delays early. Elicit the health history, determining the mental and adaptive capacities of the child's parents and other family members. Obtain a detailed pregnancy and birth history. Document sequence and age of attainment of developmental milestones. Note history of motor, visual, or language difficulties. Assess the child's health history for risk factors such as preterm or postterm birth, low birth weight, birth injury, prenatal or neonatal infection, prenatal alcohol or drug exposure, genetic syndrome, chromosomal alteration, metabolic disease, exposure to toxins (e.g., lead), head injury or other trauma, nutritional deficiency, cerebral malformation, and other brain disease or mental health disorder. Note history of or concomitant seizure disorder, orthopedic problems, speech problems, or vision or hearing deficit.

For the child with known intellectual disability, assess language, sensory, and psychomotor functioning. Determine the child's ability to toilet, dress, and feed him- or herself. Ask the parents about involvement with school and community services and support.

On physical examination, note dysmorphic features (possibly very mild) consistent with certain syndromes (e.g., fetal alcohol syndrome; Box 51.2). Evaluate the newborn or metabolic screening results. Computed tomography or magnetic resonance imaging of the head may be performed to evaluate the brain structure. Thyroid function tests may be ordered to rule out thyroid problems leading to developmental delay.

BOX 51.2 Fetal Alcohol Spectrum Disorders (FASDs)

- FASDs are a group of conditions which are the leading known cause of developmental disability in Canada (Public Health Agency of Canada, 2011).
- The term FASD is used to describe the range of conditions (mild to severe) that can result from in utero alcohol exposure.
- Fetal alcohol *syndrome* (FAS) is the most severe form of FASD and includes physical, cognitive, and central nervous system effects.
- Physical effects can include facial features such as a smooth ridge between the nose and upper lip (called the philtrum), small head size (microcephaly), shorter-than-average height, and low body weight.
- Cognitive effects can include learning disabilities, speech and language delays, intellectual disability, poor reasoning and judgment skills, and poor memory.
- Central nervous system effects can include poor coordination, hyperactive behaviour, sleep and sucking problems as an infant, and vision or hearing problems.

Source: Centers for Disease Control and Prevention. (2011). *Fetal alcohol spectrum disorders (FASDs)*. Retrieved October 18, 2011 from http://www.cdc.gov/ncbddd/fasd/facts.html.

▶ *Take* NOTE!

Due to the extent of cognition required to understand and produce speech, the most sensitive early indicator of intellectual disability is delayed language development.

Nursing Management

When children with intellectual disability are admitted to the hospital (usually for some other physical or medical condition), it is important for the nurse to continue the child's usual home routine. Follow through with feeding and motor supports that the child uses. Ensure that the child is closely supervised and remains free from harm. Allow parents time to verbalize frustrations or fears. For some families the caretaking burden is extensive and life-long; arrange for respite care as available. Support the child's strengths, and assist the child and family to follow through with therapy or treatment designed to enhance the child's functioning. Assist with the development of the child's IEP as appropriate.

Autism Spectrum Disorder

ASDs, considered under pervasive developmental disorders (PDDs), have their onset in infancy or early childhood. Autism is now recognized as the most common neurologic disorder affecting children and one of the most common developmental disabilities. Epidemiologic studies indicate that the prevalence of autism is 40 to 60 per 10,000, which represents approximately 200,000 Canadians or 1 in 165 children (Autism Society of Canada, 2010). The spectrum of autism disorders ranges from mild (e.g., Asperger syndrome) to severe. Autistic behaviours may be first noticed in infancy as developmental delays or between the ages of 12 and 36 months when the child regresses or loses previously acquired skills. Parental concerns about development may be sensitive indicators of the development of autism (Scarpinao, Bradley, Kurbjun, et al., 2010).

Pathophysiology

The exact etiology of autism continues to elude scientists, but it may be due to genetic makeup, brain abnormalities, altered chemistry, a virus, or toxic chemicals (Oliver, 2003). Children with such disorders will exhibit impaired functioning within three domains of development: "... age-appropriate social skills, language and communication, and non-normative specific interests, or stereotyped behaviours" (Scarpinao et al., 2010, p. 245).

Therapeutic Management

There are no medications or treatments available to cure autism. Each child's treatment is individualized; behavioural and communication therapies are very important. Children with ASD respond very well to highly structured educational environments. Stimulants may be used to control hyperactivity, and antipsychotic medications are sometimes helpful in children with repetitive and aggressive behaviours.

Research findings suggest that children who receive treatment based on applied behaviour analysis (ABA) make significantly more gains than do comparison groups of children on standard measures of IQ, language, and adaptive functioning (Hayward, Eikeseth, Gale, et al., 2009). ABA treaments involve individualized intensive programs by trained administrators designed to address and improve behavioural deficits in areas including social skills and self-injurious and/or aggressive behaviours (Hayward et al., 2009).

Many families are drawn to the use of complementary and alternative medical therapies in attempts to treat their autistic child. They may use vitamins and nutritional supplements, herbs or restrictive diets, music therapy, art therapy, and sensory integration techniques. To date, these therapies have not been scientifically proven to improve autism (Inglese, 2009).

The goal of therapeutic management is for the child to reach optimal functioning within the limitations of the disorder.

Nursing Assessment

Elicit the health history, noting delay or regression in developmental skills, particularly speech and language abilities. The child may be mute, utter only sounds (not words), or repeat words or phrases over and over. The parent may report that the infant or toddler spends hours in repetitive activity and demonstrates bizarre motor and stereotypic behaviours. The infant may resist cuddling, lack eye contact, be indifferent to touch or affection, and have little change in facial expression. Toddlers may display hyperactivity, aggression, temper tantrums, or self-injury behaviours, such as head-banging or hand-biting. The history may also reveal hypersensitivity to touch or hyposensitivity to pain. Assess the child's functional status, including behaviour, nutrition, sleep, speech and language, education needs, and developmental or neurologic limitations (Inglese, 2009).

Assessment of the child's unique needs can greatly impact the efficacy of his or her treatment plan as well as maintain the well-being and safety of the patient and staff. When discussing the child's plan of care, it is helpful to determine successful strategies used in other settings (e.g., school, day care), especially when the child encounters a new experience. One of the most important clinical questions is whether the child has a developmental delay. Estimates indicate that 40% of children with ASD have some cognitive impairment (Phetrasuwan, Miles, Mesibov, et al., 2009). When conducting a comprehensive assessment, it is important to recognize what questions are pertinent to or beyond the scope of a traditional health assessment. A nurse at the bedside is not expected to recall all of the criteria that go into the diagnosis of autism. However, having an awareness of the core features of autism and working closely with parents will help the nurse tailor a patient-specific plan of care. Some general assessment points are listed below:

- Determine the patient's developmental level; consider grade level and school performance.
- Determine the level of somatosensory disturbances (hypersensitivity to sounds, smells, touch, textures).
- Determine emotional disturbances (easily frustrated, moodiness, easily overstimulated).
- Determine interventions that have worked for this patient in the past.
- Determine the most effective communication techniques. For example, pictures may need to be used rather than words to show a child what is going to happen (Scarpinao et al., 2010).

Assist with screening, using an approved autism screening tool such as:

- Checklist for Autism in Toddlers (CHAT)
- Modified Checklist for Autism in Toddlers (M-CHAT)
- Social Communication Questionnaire (SCQ)
- Pervasive Developmental Disorders Screening Test-II (PDDST-II)

Perform a thorough physical examination. Observe the infant or toddler for lack of eye contact, failure to look at objects pointed to by the examiner, failure to point to him- or herself, failure to let needs be known, perseverative play activities, and unusual behaviour such as hand-flapping or spinning. Measure growth parameters, in particular noting head circumference (macrocephaly or microcephaly may be associated with ASD). Note the presence of large, prominent, or posteriorly rotated ears. Examine the skin for hypopigmented or hyperpigmented lesions. Note asymmetry of nerve function or palsy, hypertonia, hypotonia, alterations in deep tendon reflexes, toe-walking, loose gait, or poor coordination. Obtain hearing screening results and ascertain that lead screening has been performed.

Screen all infants and toddlers for warning signs of autism:

- Not babbling by 12 months
- Not pointing or using gestures by 12 months
- No single words by 16 months
- No two-word utterances by 24 months
- Losing language or social skills at any age (Smith, Segal, & Hutman, 2010)

Nursing Management

When children are initially diagnosed with autism, parents need an extensive amount of emotional support, professional guidance, and education about the disorder while they are attempting to adjust to the diagnosis (Giarelli, Souders, Pinto-Martin, et al., 2005). Assess the "fit" between the child's developmental needs and the treatment plan. Parents may demonstrate symptoms of depression and stress related to intensive therapies, such as ABA programs in the home (Schwichtenberg & Poehlmann, 2007). Help parents overcome barriers to obtain appropriate educational, developmental, and behavioural treatment programs and supports for their own needs. Ensure that the child younger than 36 months of age receives services via the local early intervention program and children 3 years and over have an IEP in place if enrolled in the public school system. Stress the importance of rigid, unchanging routines, as children with ASD often act out when their routine changes (which is likely to occur if the child must be hospitalized for another condition). Many special schools exist for children with significant developmental disorders, though some are extremely expensive. Assess the parents' need for respite care and make referrals accordingly. Provide positive feedback to parents for their perseverance in working with their child.

Attention–Deficit/Hyperactivity Disorder

Attention-deficit/hyperactivity disorder (ADHD) is one of the most common mental health disorders diagnosed in childhood: it affects 3% to 7% of all children, with some

COMPARISON CHART 51.1

Oppositional Defiant Disorder	Conduct Disorder
• Excessive arguing with adults • Frequent temper tantrums • Active defiance • Revenge-seeking behaviours • Frequent resentment or anger • Touchiness; easily annoyed • Noncompliance with adult requests or limits • Blaming of others for misbehaviour or mistakes	• Bullying and threatening of others • Initiation of physical fights • Weapon use to cause others harm • Physical cruelty to animals or people • Destruction of property or arson • Lying and stealing • Serious violation of rules: staying out past curfew, truancy, running away • Use of force in sexual activity

Adapted from: Stafford, B. (2011). Child & adolescent psychiatric disorders & psychosocial aspects of pediatrics. In W. W. Hay, M. J. Levin, J. M. Sondheimer, & R. R. Deterding (Eds.), *Current pediatric diagnosis and treatment* (20th ed.). New York: McGraw-Hill.

estimates as high as 7.5% to 12% (Kratochvil, Vaughn, Barker, et al., 2009). Further, as many as 60% to 85% of children diagnosed with ADHD will continue to meet criteria for the disorder as teenagers, and up to 60% manifest symptoms throughout adulthood (Kratochvil et al., 2009). ADHD is characterized by inattention, impulsivity, distractibility, and hyperactivity. Three subtypes of ADHD exist: hyperactive–impulsive, inattentive, and combined. The child with ADHD has a disruption in learning ability, socialization, and compliance, placing significant demands on the child, parents, teachers, and community (Kratochvil et al., 2009). About two thirds of children with ADHD also have a **co-morbidity** such as oppositional defiant disorder, conduct disorder, an anxiety disorder, depression, a less severe developmental disorder, an auditory processing disorder, or learning or reading disabilities (DeNisco, Tiago, & Kravitz, 2005; Stein, 2002; Vlam, 2006). Comparison Chart 51.1 gives information about oppositional defiant disorder and conduct disorder to distinguish them from ADHD.

Pathophysiology

ADHD is a disorder with a strong neurologic foundation. Inheritability may be responsible for approximately 76% of cases of the disorder (Kratochivil et al., 2009). Other factors that are proposed to be significant non-genetic factors in the development of ADHD include prenatal smoking and alcohol use, prenatal and neonatal hypoxia, lead exposure, and traumatic brain injury. Neuroimaging studies have consistently demonstrated structural and metabolic differences in the brains of individuals with ADHD compared with those who do not have the disorder. Hyperactivity is the most common presenting symptom for preschool children. Inattention symptoms become more apparent in the school setting. Hyperactivity and impulsive behaviours potentially interfere with effective family and social interactions. Children and teens with ADHD experience frustration, labile moods, emotional

outbursts, peer rejection, poor school performance, and low self-esteem. They may also have poor metacognitive abilities such as organization, time management, and the ability to break a project down into a series of smaller tasks (Kratochivil et al., 2009). They are not lazy or unmotivated but simply have poor skills in these areas. Box 51.3 provides criteria for the diagnosis of ADHD (Ryan-Krause, 2010).

BOX 51.3 Diagnosis of ADHD

Presence of six or more of the following symptoms:

- Failure to pay close attention
- Careless mistakes on schoolwork
- Difficulty paying attention to tasks or play
- Doesn't listen
- Doesn't follow through
- Doesn't complete tasks
- Doesn't understand instructions
- Poorly organized
- Avoids, dislikes, or fails to engage in activities requiring mental effort
- Loses things needed for task completion
- Easily distracted
- Forgetful

Presence of six or more of the symptoms of hyperactivity or impulsivity:

- Fidgety or squirmy
- Often out of seat
- Activity inappropriate to the situation
- Cannot engage in quiet play
- Always on the go
- Talks excessively
- Blurts out answers
- Has difficulty waiting his turn
- Often interrupts or intrudes on others (Stevens, 2005)

Therapeutic Management

Medication management of ADHD includes the use of psychostimulants, nonstimulant norepinephrine reuptake inhibitors, and/or alpha-agonist antihypertensive agents. These medications are not a cure for ADHD but help to increase the child's ability to pay attention and decrease the level of impulsive behaviour. The child's activity level is not usually affected. Since ADHD manifests into young adulthood, treatment should continue throughout adolescence (Vessey & Wilkinson, 2008). Concomitant disorders, such as anxiety, should also be treated. Behaviour therapy and classroom restructuring may be useful.

Nursing Assessment

For a full description of the assessment phase of the nursing process, refer to page 1760. Assessment findings pertinent to ADHD are discussed below.

Health History

Elicit a description of the behavioural issue or school performance problem. Explore the child's history for risk factors such as head trauma, lead exposure, cigarette smoke exposure, prematurity, or low birth weight. The past history may also reveal a larger-than-usual number of accidents. Determine if there is a family history of ADHD. Question the parent about school behaviour. The school-age child may be unable to stay on task, talks out of turn, leaves his or her desk frequently, and either neglects to complete in-class and homework assignments or forgets to turn them in. The adolescent may be inattentive in school, poorly organized, and forgetful.

Several behavioural checklists are available that may assist in the diagnosis of ADHD. They may be completed by the child's teacher and/or parent and focus on behaviour patterns related to conduct or learning problems, social competence, anxiety, activity level, and attention. Obtain the completed behavioural checklists (usually one from the parent and one from the teacher) as well as any school records or testing performed.

Physical Examination

Perform vision and hearing screening to rule out vision or hearing impairment as the cause of poor school performance. Observe the preschool child's behaviour, noting quickness, agility, fearlessness, and the desire to touch or explore everything in the room.

Laboratory and Diagnostic Tests

No definitive laboratory or diagnostic test is available for the identification of ADHD. A complete blood count may be performed to rule out anemia, and thyroid hormone levels may be drawn to determine whether they are normal.

Nursing Management

Having a child with ADHD can be frustrating as the child's inattention, high activity level, impulsivity, and distractibility are often very difficult to deal with. Parents may doubt their ability to be effective parents or may view their child as somehow defective. Children with ADHD may also feel that they are bad, faulty, or stupid (DeMarle, Denk, & Ernsthausen, 2003). Provide emotional support, allowing enough time for the family to air their concerns. Work with the child and family to develop goals such as completion of homework, improved communication, or increasing independence in self-care. Visit http://thePoint.lww.com/Chow1e for direct links to more detailed nursing care plans.

Assist the family to advocate for their child's needs through the public school system. The child is entitled to a developmentally appropriate education via an IEP as necessary (refer to Chapter 33 for additional information about special education). The IEP should be updated as needed. Ensure coordination of health and school services. Flag the child's chart and set up a schedule for systematic communication with the family and school. Teach families and school personnel to use behavioural techniques such as positive reinforcement, reward or privilege withdrawal, or a token system. The token system rewards appropriate behaviour with a token and results in a token being taken away if inappropriate behaviour occurs. At the end of a specified period of time, the tokens may be exchanged for a prize or privilege (Stein, 2002). Refer families to local support groups and CH.A.D.D. Canada Incorporated, the national ADHD support group.

Stimulant medications, when prescribed, should be taken in the morning to decrease the adverse effect of insomnia. Some children may experience decreased appetite, so giving the medication with or after the meal may be beneficial. The child may feel "different" from his or her peers if the child has to visit the school nurse for a lunchtime dose of ADHD medication; this may lead to noncompliance and a subsequent increase in ADHD symptoms, with deterioration in schoolwork. In this situation, encourage the family to explore with their physician the option of one of the newer extended-release or once-daily ADHD medications.

Tourette Syndrome

Tourette syndrome is estimated to affect about 0.6% to 1% of children (Cavanna & Shah, 2010). Its onset is before 18 years of age. The syndrome consists of multiple motor tics and one or more vocal tics occurring either simultaneously or at different times. Children are not tic-free for longer than 3 months. Tics are defined as sudden, rapid, recurrent stereotypical movements and/or sounds over which the child appears to have no control. Co-morbid conditions such as ADHD, obsessive–compulsive disorder (OCD), and affective disorders occur in 60% to 80% of children with Tourette syndrome (Cavanna & Shah, 2010). The exact pathophysiologic mechanism of Tourette syndrome has yet to be identified, though genetics does seem to play a part. Therapeutic management is highly individualized and involves psychopharmacologic and behavioural therapies. Habit reversal training may help in some children.

Nursing Assessment

Evaluate the health history for the occurrence of tics. The child may be embarrassed or ashamed about the tics and the parents may feel fear, anger, or guilt. Determine the presence of co-morbid symptoms. Elicit the child's past health history, noting a family history of tics. Assess the child's psychosocial history to determine the extent to which the tics interfere with friendship, school performance, and self-esteem. Observe the child for simple or complex motor tics. Vocal tics such as sniffling, grunting, clicking, or word utterance may occur. Perform a thorough physical examination, which is usually normal.

Nursing Management

Inform families that the tics become more noticeable or severe during times of stress and less pronounced when the child is focused on an activity such as watching TV, reading, or playing a video game. Help the family to build on the child's functional behaviours and adaptive skills to improve the child's self-esteem. Encourage the family to pursue classroom accommodations such as allowing for "tic breaks," taking untimed tests or tests in another room, or using note-takers or tape recording. Support the family's decisions related to medication use and provide appropriate education about the particular drugs. *Teaching the Tiger* by M. P. Dornbush and S. K. Pruitt (Hope Press) is useful for teachers of the child with Tourette syndrome. For additional support, refer families to the Tourette Syndrome Association, Tourette Syndrome Foundation of Canada, or Tourette Syndrome Plus (visit http://thePoint.lww.com/Chow1e for direct links).

Eating Disorders

Eating disorders include pica, rumination, anorexia nervosa, and bulimia. These disorders affect a significant number of children, especially adolescents. Pica, which occurs most frequently in 2- to 3-year-olds, is an eating disorder in which the child ingests (over at least a 1-month period) a non-nutritive material such as paint, clay, or sand. Rumination is an eating disorder occurring in infants in which the baby regurgitates partially digested food or formula and expels or swallows it. The numbers of children affected by pica and rumination is not known. This discussion focuses on anorexia nervosa and bulimia, as they are more commonly encountered.

Anorexia nervosa and bulimia are common eating disorders affecting primarily adolescents, although they also affect younger children in industrialized countries. The prevalence rate is 370 cases per 100,000 (Van Ommen, Meerwijk, Kars, et al., 2009). According to a 2002 survey, 1.5% of Canadian women ages 15 to 24 years had an eating disorder (Government of Canada, 2006). Prevalence rates for anorexia and bulimia may increase during the transition from adolescence to adulthood (Hoek, 2006).

Anorexia nervosa is characterized by dramatic weight loss as a result of decreased food intake and sharply increased physical exercise. Bulimia refers to a cycle of normal food intake, followed by binge-eating and then purging. Complications include fluid and electrolyte imbalance, decreased blood volume, cardiac arrhythmias, esophagitis, rupture of the esophagus or stomach, tooth loss, and menstrual problems. This condition needs to be taken very seriously as approximately 15% of patients with anorexia nervosa die from the disorder (Van Ommen et al., 2009).

Nursing Assessment

Determine the health history, noting risk factors such as family history, female gender, white race, preoccupation with appearance, obsessive traits, or low self-esteem. Adolescents with anorexia may have a history of constipation, syncope, secondary amenorrhea, abdominal pain, and periodic episodes of cold hands and feet. Parents usually note the primary concern as weight loss. Note history of depression in the child with bulimia. Evaluate the child's self-concept, noting multiple fears, high need for acceptance, disordered body image, and perfectionism. Perform a thorough physical examination. The anorexic is usually severely underweight, with a body mass index (BMI) less than 17. Note cachetic appearance, dry sallow skin, thinning scalp hair, soft sparse body hair, and nail pitting. Measure vital signs, noting low temperature, bradycardia, or hypotension. Auscultate the heart, noting murmur as a result of mitral valve prolapse (occurs in about one third of patients). The adolescent with bulimia can be of normal weight or slightly overweight, unless the condition co-exists with anorexia. Inspect the hands for calluses on the back of the knuckles and split fingernails. Inspect the mouth and oropharynx for eroded dental enamel, red gums, and inflamed throat from self-induced vomiting. Careful evaluation of serum electrolytes and electrocardiogram is needed in anorexics, as severe electrolyte disturbances and cardiac arrhythmias often occur.

Nursing Management

Most children with eating disorders can be treated successfully on an out-patient basis. Those with anorexia who display severe weight loss, unstable vital signs, food refusal, or arrested pubertal development or who require enteral nutrition will need to be hospitalized. Refeeding syndrome (cardiovascular, hematologic, and neurologic complications) may occur in the severely malnourished patient if rapid nutritional replacement is given, so slow refeeding is essential to avoid complications. Phosphorus supplements are given as ordered. Assess vital signs frequently for orthostatic hypotension, irregular and decreased pulse, or hypothermia.

Consult the nutritionist for assistance with calculating caloric needs and determining an appropriate diet. Aim for a weight gain goal of 0.2 to 0.9 kg per week. Instruct the child and family to keep a daily journal of intake, **bingeing** and **purging** behaviours, mood, and exercise. The journal may be used as an assessment tool as well as to document progress toward recovery. Assist the child and family to plan a suitably structured routine for the child that includes meals, snacks, and appropriate physical activity.

Use the physical findings associated with anorexia to educate the child about the consequences of malnutrition and how they can be remedied with adequate nutrient intake. Behaviour or group therapy may also be needed. Assess the child's need for intervention for concomitant depression or **anxiety** (some anorexics also require psychotropic medications). Provide emotional support and positive reinforcement to the child and family. Refer the family to local support groups or online resources such as the Academy for Eating Disorders, the National Eating Disorders Association, or Eating Disorders Association of Canada (visit http://thePoint.lww.com/Chow1e for direct links).

> ▶ *Consider* THIS!
>
> *Nicole Ashton, 16 years old, is seen in your clinic due to weight loss. Her mother states that she has lost noticeable weight over the past few months and has stopped menstruating. What additional assessment information would be necessary?*
>
> *After further examination it is determined that Nicole has anorexia nervosa. Her treatment is to take place on an out-patient basis beginning immediately. Discuss ways the family can encourage and assist in Nicole's recovery.*

Mood Disorders

Mood disorders in children include depressive disorders and bipolar disorder. During childhood, the incidence of depressive disorders is approximately equal between boys and girls, but more girls are affected during adolescence. Depression disorders can be found in about 3.5% of children and teenagers between the ages of 5 and 17 years, and the rate increases with age (Centre of Knowledge on Healthy Child Development, 2007). Major depressive disorder affects 1% to 3% of children and 8% of adolescents (Shoaf, Emslie, & Mayes, 2001). Dysthymic disorder occurs in 1% of children and 8% of adolescents (Shoaf et al., 2001). Bipolar disorder refers to a condition of alternating manic and depressive episodes and affects about 1% of children (Lack & Green, 2009). During the manic episode, mood is significantly elevated and the patient displays excess energy. There are two types of bipolar disorder: Bipolar 1, where symptoms include manic episodes and may or may not include depressive symptoms, and Bipolar 2, which is characterized by major depressive episodes, yet less severe forms of mania (Government of Canada, 2006).

Depression may cause significant alterations in school performance and social relationships. When considering the diagnosis of depression in children and adolescents, health care professionals should also assess for comorbidities. Many children and adolescents may have learning disabilities, anxiety, ADHD, and substance abuse (Lenz, Coderre, & Watanabe, 2009). Substance abuse also occurs about 25% of the time with depression. Divorce and other serious family issues may contribute to the development of depression because of the ongoing stress and strong psychological impact these issues have on the child (Mahon, Yarcheski, & Yarcheski, 2003; Pompili, Mancinelli, Girardi, et al., 2005).

Suicide is the second leading cause of death for Canadian youth ages 10 to 24 (Canadian Mental Health Association, 2011). An average of 294 youth die as a result of suicide each year, and many more attempt it. Aboriginal teens and gay and lesbian teens may be at particularly high risk. There is seldom only one single causative factor, as the decision to commit suicide may be related to a routine event or to an overwhelming one that might overload a young person's coping system. A family history of suicidal behaviour should be taken into account. In addition to the possibility of a genetic link, the young person may have been affected by suicidal behaviour in the family (Canadian Mental Health Association, 2011).

Pathophysiology

Both norepinephrine and dopamine play a role in mood. Norepinephrine is considered to be important in the areas of energy and alertness, dopamine in the areas of pleasure and motivation. When alterations in the neurotransmission of norepinephrine and dopamine occur, the symptoms of depression (apathy, loss of interest and pleasure) result. Decreased levels of serotonin have also been implicated in depressive symptoms. Development of a depressive disorder may also be related to genetics, behaviour, or cognitive function. Children of parents with a depressive disorder are at increased risk for developing a depressive disorder themselves. Maladaptive cognitive functions or lack of social skills resulting in negative feelings may also play a role (Lack & Green, 2009).

Therapeutic Management

Children with mood disorders usually benefit from psychotherapy. This helps the child to deal with the psychosocial consequences of his or her behaviour on his or her interpersonal relationships with others. Crisis management, parental counselling, and individual, including cognitive–behavioural therapy, group, or family therapy may be useful. Major depressive disorder warrants the use of pharmacologic antidepressants. Bipolar disorder may be treated with neuroleptic agents or mood stabilizers (Nurcombe, 2008).

Nursing Assessment

Children with untreated depression are at high risk for suicide as well as the development of co-morbid disorders such as anxiety disorders, substance abuse, eating disorders, self-harm, and disruptive behavioural disorders (Stafford, 2011).

Health History

Obtain a health history from the child and separately from the parent. Evaluate the child for history of recent changes in behaviour, changes in peer relationships, alterations in school performance, withdrawal from previously enjoyed activities, sleep disturbances, changes in eating behaviours, increase in accidents, or sexual promiscuity (Castiglia, 2000). If possible, use a standardized depression screening questionnaire; there are many available.

Ask about potential stressors such as school concerns, conflicts with parents, dating issues, and **abuse** (physical or sexual) (McClain, 2003). When bipolar disorder is suspected, the history may reveal rapid, pressured speech, increased energy, decreased sleep, flamboyant behaviour, or irritability during the manic episodes.

Note history of weight loss, failure to thrive, or increased incidence of infections in the infant. For the toddler, note delay or regression in developmental skills, increase in nightmares, or parental reports of clinginess. The preschooler may have a history of loss of interest in newly acquired skills; manifest encopresis, enuresis, anorexia, or binge-eating; or make frequent negative self-statements. The parents of a school-age child may report that he or she has a depressed, irritable, or aggressive mood.

Assess for risk factors for suicide, which include:

- Previous suicide attempt (Pompili et al., 2005)
- Change in school performance, sleep, or appetite
- Loss of interest in formerly favourite school or other activities
- Feelings of hopelessness or depression
- Statements about thoughts of suicide (McClain, 2003)

Physical Examination

Observe the infant for weepiness, withdrawn behaviours, or a frozen facial expression. Note a sad or expressionless face in the toddler or preschooler. In any age child, observe for apathy. Inspect the entire body surface for self-inflicted injuries, which may or may not be present. The remainder of the physical examination is generally normal unless the depressed child also has a chronic medical condition.

Nursing Management

Nursing management of children and adolescents with mood disorders focuses on education, support, and prevention.

Educating and Supporting the Child and Family

Teach families that mood disorders are biologic conditions, not personality flaws. Teach families how to administer antidepressant medication and to monitor for adverse effects. Encourage and praise their efforts at following through with cognitive and behavioural therapies. Support the family throughout the process, as treatment can sometimes be lengthy. Refer parents to local or national support resources, such as the Organization for People with Bipolar Affective Disorder, the Mood Disorders Society of Canada, the Canadian Mental Health Association, or the Canadian Network for Mood and Anxiety Treatments; specific information for First Nations families is also available. Visit http://thePoint.lww.com/Chow1e for direct links to all of these resources.

Preventing Depression and Suicide

Establish a trusting relationship with the children and adolescents with whom you interact, particularly in the primary care setting, school, or chronic illness clinic. This trusting relationship may encourage children or adolescents to confide feelings or problems earlier than they may do with their parents. Screen all healthy and chronically ill preteens and teens for the development of depression (Stafford, 2011). Use standardized screening tools such as those listed in Box 51.4. When a potential problem is identified, immediately refer the child for mental health assessment and intervention. It is important to identify depression early so that treatment can start. When a grief-inducing event (such as the death of a family member) is impending, begin preventive intervention to help the child to deal with it. Provide appropriate observation for any child exhibiting suicidal ideation.

> ### BOX 51.4 Screening Tools for Anxiety and Depression
>
> **Depression Screening Tools**
> - Children's Depression Rating Scale-Revised (CDRS-R)
> - Center for Epidemiological Studies Depression Scale Modified for Children (CES-DC)
> - Children's Depression Inventory (CDI)
> - Weinberg Depression Scale for Children and Adolescents (WDSCA)
> - Beck Depression Inventory for Youth (BDI-Y)
>
> **Anxiety Screening Tools***
> - Multidimensional Anxiety Scale for Children (MASC)
> - Preschool Anxiety Scale
> - Spence Children's Anxiety Scale (SCAS)
> - Beck Anxiety Inventory for Youth
>
> ---
>
> *Visit http://thePoint.lww.com/Chow1e for direct links to these scales.

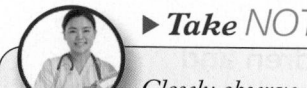

> **▶ *Take* NOTE!**
>
> *Closely observe children taking antidepressants for the development of presuicidal behaviour.*

Anxiety Disorders

Anxiety disorders are the most commonly diagnosed psychiatric conditions among children and adolescents (Williams & Hodgman, 2001). Roughly 6% of children and youth have an anxiety disorder that is serious enough to require treatment (Children's Mental Health Ontario, 2007). Anxiety often occurs together with other mental health disorders, especially depression. It is expected for children to experience fear, worry, and shyness. Infants fear loud noises, being startled, and strangers. Toddlers are afraid of the dark and of separation. Preschoolers fear imaginary creatures and body mutilation. School-age children worry about injury and natural events, whereas adolescents are anxious about school and social performance. These expected fears produce a certain level of anxiety that is tolerated by most children, but it is important to distinguish expected developmentally appropriate anxiety from problematic anxiety.

Anxiety is considered to be a reaction to a perceived or actual threat. The threat may or may not be distorted by the child, and emotional distress leads to behavioural responses. The "fight-or-flight" response results in tachycardia, increased blood pressure, sweating, enhanced arousal and reactivity, tremors, and increased blood flow to the muscles (Keeley & Storch, 2009).

Types of Anxiety Disorders

Generalized anxiety disorder (GAD) is characterized by unrealistic concerns over past behaviour, future events, and personal competence. Social phobia may result, in which the child or teen demonstrates a persistent fear of speaking or eating in front of others, using public restrooms, or speaking to authorities. Selective mutism (persistent failure to speak) may also occur. Separation anxiety is more common in children than adolescents; the child may need to remain close to the parents, and the child's worries focus on separation themes. OCD is characterized by compulsions (repetitive behaviours such as cleaning, washing, checking something), which the child performs to reduce anxiety about obsessions (unwanted and intrusive thoughts). Post-traumatic stress disorder (PTSD) is an anxiety disorder that occurs after a child experiences a traumatic event, later experiencing physiologic arousal when a stimulus triggers memories of the event (Keeley & Storch, 2009).

Pathophysiology

Anxiety disorders are thought to occur as a result of disrupted modulation within the central nervous system. Underactivation of the serotonergic system and overactivation of the noradrenergic system are thought to be responsible for dysregulation of physiologic arousal and the resulting emotional experience. Disruption of the gamma-butyric acid (GABA) system may also play a role. Genetic factors may also play a role in the development of anxiety disorders, as may family and environmental influences. Additionally, abnormal thoughts or behaviours may have been learned through observation or conditioning (Keeley & Storch, 2009).

Therapeutic Management

Therapeutic management of anxiety disorders generally involves the use of pharmacologic agents and psychological therapies. Anxiolytics or antidepressants are the most common pharmacologic approaches. Cognitive-behavioural therapy, individual, family, or group psychotherapy, and other behavioural interventions such as relaxation techniques may also be useful (Keeley & Storch, 2009). See Evidence-based Practice 51.1.

Nursing Assessment

Children and adolescents do not usually express anxiety directly, so it is very important for the nurse to evaluate somatic complaints and perform a careful history.

Health History

Explore the patient's current and past medical history for risk factors such as depression, anxious temperament, family history of anxiety disorders, certain environmental or life experiences (such as parental dysfunction or a significant stressful event or trauma), or unstable parental attachment. Elicit the health history, noting history of social inhibition, panic, or "heart racing." Young children may display overactivity, acting out, sleep difficulties, or separation issues. Older children may describe feelings of nervousness, anger, fear, or tension and may display disruptive behaviour. Ask the child to choose a number on a scale from 0 to 10 to describe how much he or she worries about things. Have the parent rank the child's worry in the same fashion, and ask the parent what the child worries about most. Determine frequency of headaches and stomachaches. Use a standardized screening tool such as those listed in Box 51.4.

Physical Examination

Perform a complete physical examination to rule out physiologic causes of the child's symptoms. Note patches of hair loss that occur with repetitive hair twisting or pulling associated with anxiety. Evaluate for evidence of

EVIDENCE-BASED PRACTICE 51.1
Behavioural and Cognitive–Behavioural Therapy for Children and Adolescents with Obsessive–Compulsive Disorder

● **Study**

Behavioural or cognitive–behavioural therapy (BT/CBT) is often recommended for children and adolescents with OCD. The authors reviewed studies comparing BT/CBT with no treatment or in combination with pharmacotherapeutics for OCD. Four studies with 222 total participants were included in the review.

▲ **Findings**

Participants who underwent BT/CBT demonstrated better posttreatment functioning and reduced risk of continuing with OCD as compared with those receiving no BT/CBT.

Evidence surfaced that BT/CBT combined with medication was superior to treatment with medication alone. The dropout rate during therapy was low, indicating acceptance by participants and their families.

■ **Nursing Implications**

Encourage families to explore the possibility of adding BT/CBT to the treatment plan. Assist families with finding an appropriate provider of BT/CBT in their local area. Praise children and families for ongoing dedication to BT/CBT. Continue to offer emotional support to all members of the family throughout the treatment process.

O'Kearne, R. T., Ansley, K. J., & von Sanden, C. (2006). Behavioural and cognitive behavioural therapy for obsessive compulsive disorder in children and adolescents. *The Cochrane Library 2006, 4.* Indianapolis: John Wiley & Sons.

nail biting, sucking blisters, or skin erosion from finger-rubbing. Inspect the entire body for signs of self-injury, which may or may not be present.

Nursing Management

Screen children at well-child or other health care visits, as well as upon admission to the hospital, for anxiety symptoms. If an anxiety disorder is suspected, refer the child to the appropriate mental health provider for further evaluation. When the child is diagnosed with an anxiety disorder and medication is prescribed, teach families about medication administration and adverse effects. Encourage and praise them for follow-through related to cognitive and behavioural therapy or psychotherapy. Provide emotional support to the child and family. Assess the family for the presence of parental anxiety or insecure attachment. Note parenting style and parent–child interactions. Not only the child but also the family will benefit from interventions that improve parent–child relationships, decrease parental anxiety, and foster parenting skills that promote autonomy in the child. Thus, ensure that concurrent family therapy occurs if needed.

Substance Abuse

According to the 2009 Canadian Alcohol and Drug Use Monitoring Survey (CADUMS), the prevalence of past-year alcohol use among Canadians 15 years and older decreased from 79.3% in 2004 to 76.5% in 2009 (Health Canada, 2009). Three quarters of youth ages 15 to 24 years (75.5%) reported consuming alcohol in the past year. This reflects a decrease from 2004 when 82.9% of youth reported past-year alcohol use. However, the prevalence

of heavy frequent drinking among youth 15 to 24 years of age was three times higher than the rate for adults 25 years and older (11.7% versus 3.9%). Among Canadian youth ages 15 to 24 years, the prevalence of past-year cannabis use decreased from 37.0% in 2004 to 26.3% in 2009 and the past-year use of at least one of five illicit drugs (cocaine or crack, speed, hallucinogens, ecstasy, and heroin) decreased from 11.3% in 2004 to 5.5% in 2009. Even though many of the rates of substance abuse have decreased in recent years, the issue remains a problem that must be addressed among children and youth.

Aboriginal youth are at particularly high risk for substance use and the related harms. Some of the reasons that have been identified are related to culture and language barriers that can lead to difficulties in school and the stressful living conditions and issues that continue to occur in many Aboriginal communities and families. These issues include poverty and family violence (and other issues related to residential school experiences), which can contribute to a cycle of dysfunction and despair. For Aboriginal families living on reserves, overcrowding may mean that children are exposed to alcohol and other drug use from a young age, putting them at higher risk for substance use in adolescence (The BC Partners for Mental Health and Addictions Information, 2008). More information about this topic can be found in *Addictive Behaviours Among Aboriginal People in Canada,* published by the Aboriginal Healing Foundation (Chansonneuve, 2007).

Nursing Assessment

Note risk factors for substance abuse, such as family history, current parental substance use, dysfunctional family relationships, concurrent mental health disorder, negative life events, or peers who use substances. Determine the child's history, noting altered school performance or attendance, changes in peer group participation, frequent mood swings, changes in physical appearance, or an altered relationship with or perception of parents. Document history of insomnia, appetite loss, excessive itching, sleepiness or extreme fatigue, dry mouth, or shakiness. Note violent behaviour, drunkenness, stupor, blank expression, drowsiness, lack of coordination, confusion, incoherent speech, extremes in emotions, aggressive behaviour, silly behaviour, or rapid speech. Observe for an odour of alcohol or marijuana smoke. Assess the eyes, noting wateriness or dilated pupils. Inspect the nares, noting rhinorrhea or absence of nasal hair. Inspect the fingers for glue smears or discoloration and the skin for needle marks or tracks. Palpate the hands and feet for coolness. Toxicology studies such as urine screening can determine the presence of stimulants, sedative-hypnotics, barbiturates, Quaaludes, opiates, cocaine, and marijuana.

Nursing Management

Help the adolescent to acknowledge that he or she has a problem. Explain the negative consequences of substance use and raise the teen's awareness of risks. Remain empathetic, yet leave responsibility with the adolescent.

Promoting Participation in Treatment Programs

Refer the adolescent to a substance abuse program. Outpatient or day treatment programs are useful in most situations. Family-based programs produce the highest level of recovery. Self-help or 12-step groups are an important element in the recovery process. Serious addiction, the presence of one or more co-morbid psychiatric conditions, or suicidal ideation requires residential treatment or hospitalization.

Preventing Substance Abuse

Teach all children, beginning at the elementary school level, that all chemicals have the potential to be harmful to the body, including tobacco, alcohol, and illicit drugs. Help children to learn problem-solving skills that they can call upon in the future rather than relying on drugs or other substances. Teach children to "just say no." Reinforce that they are the ones who have control over their body and what they expose it to. Educate children and adolescents that no matter which administration route is used, the drug still enters the body and affects it. Encourage children to participate in the local drug prevention programs provided within schools or through police departments. More information is available from the Canadian federal government's National Anti-Drug Strategy or through Canada Alcohol and Drug Rehab Programs; visit http://thePoint.lww.com/Chow1e for direct links.

■■■ Key Concepts

- Mental health and behavioural disorders account for the bulk of the "new morbidity" among children and adolescents.
- The child with behavioural problems or mental health issues often has difficulty in the areas of school, peer relationships, and the family, all of which may worsen the child's self-concept, further hindering his or her emotional health.
- Developmental screening is a key component in the evaluation of a child's mental health.
- Various screening tools are available for depression, ADHD, and anxiety.
- Children with ASD often have impaired social interactions as well as altered communication.
- Learning disabilities and ADHD have a significant negative impact on the child's potential for appropriate education.
- IEPs help children with learning disabilities, intellectual disability, and ADHD receive the educational support they require to optimize their educational capacity.
- Provide support and education to children with mood or anxiety disorders and their families.
- Educating parents about medication administration and its adverse effects is a critical aspect of nursing management of the child with a mental health disorder.
- Provide nutritional replacement at the appropriate pace in the child with anorexia nervosa. Monitor the child closely for the development of refeeding syndrome.
- Educate children about the dangers associated with substance abuse.

REFERENCES

American Association on Intellectual and Developmental Disabilities. (n.d.). *Definition of intellectual disability.* Retrieved October 18, 2011 from http://www.aamr.org/content_100.cfm?navID=21

Autism Society of Canada. (2010). *Prevalence of autism in Canada.* Retrieved October 18, 2011 from http://www.autismsocietycanada.ca/index.php?option=com_content&view=article&id=55&Itemid=85&lang=en

Canadian Mental Health Association. (2011). *Youth and suicide.* Retrieved October 18, 2011 from http://www.cmha.ca/bins/content_page.asp?cid=3-101-104&lang=1

Canadian Pediatric Society. (2006). *Mental health and developmental disabilities.* Retrieved October 18, 2011 from http://www.cps.ca/english/publications/MentalHealth.htm

Castiglia, P. T. (2000). Depression in adolescents. *Journal of Pediatric Health Care, 14,* 180–182.

Cavanna, A., & Shah, S. (2010). Tourette syndrome: New insights into diagnosis, comorbidities, and treatment approaches. *Psychiatric Times, 27*(3), 32–34.

Centers for Disease Control and Prevention. (2011). *Fetal alcohol spectrum disorders (FASDs).* Retrieved October 18, 2011 from http://www.cdc.gov/ncbddd/fasd/facts.html

Centre of Knowledge on Healthy Child Development. (2007). *Mood problems in children and adolescents.* Retrieved October 18, 2011 from http://www.kidsmentalhealth.ca/documents/Res_Knowledge-Centre_Mood_Eng_B_W.pdf

Chansonneuve, D. (2007). *Addictive behaviours among Aboriginal people in Canada.* Ottawa, ON: Aboriginal Healing Foundation, Retrieved

October 18, 2011 from http://www.ahf.ca/downloads/addictive-behaviours.pdf

Children's Mental Health Ontario. (2007). *Anxiety problems in children and adolescents.* Retrieved October 18, 2011 from http://www.kidsmentalhealth.ca/parents/anxiety.php#How%20common%20are%20anxiety%20disorders?

Council for Exceptional Children. (2011). *Mental retardation.* Retrieved October 18, 2011 from http://www.cec.sped.org/AM/Template.cfm?Section=Mental_Retardation&Template=/TaggedPage/TaggedPageDisplay.cfm&TPLID=37&ContentID=5630

DeMarle, D. J., Denk, L., & Ernsthausen, C. S. (2003). Working with the family of a child with attention deficit hyperactivity disorder. *Pediatric Nursing, 29*(4), 302–308, 330.

DeNisco, S., Tiago, C., & Kravitz, C. (2005). Evaluation and treatment of pediatric ADHD. *Nurse Practitioner, 30*(8), 14–23.

Giarelli, E., Souders, M., Pinto-Martin, J., et al. (2005). Intervention pilot for parents of children with autistic spectrum disorder. *Pediatric Nursing, 31*(5), 389–398.

Goldson, E., & Reynolds, A. (2007). Child development and behavior. In W. W. Hay, M. J. Levin, J. M. Sondheimer, & R. R. Deterding (Eds.), *Current pediatric diagnosis and treatment* (8th ed.). New York: McGraw-Hill Companies, Inc.

Government of Canada. (2006). The human face of mental health and mental illness in Canada. Retrieved October 18, 2011 from http://www.phac-aspc.gc.ca/publicat/human-humain06/pdf/human_face_e.pdf

Hayward, D., Eikeseth, S., Gale, C., & Morgan, S. (2009). Assessing progress during treatment for young children with autism receiving intensive behavioral interventions. *Autsim, 13,* 613–629. doi:10.1177/1362361309340029

Health Canada. (2009). *Drug and alcohol use statistics: Major findings from the Canadian Alcohol and Drug Use Monitoring Survey (CADUMS) 2009. Retrieved October 18, 2011 from* http://www.hc-sc.gc.ca/hc-ps/drugs-drogues/stat/index-eng.php

Hoek, W. (2006). Incidence, prevalence and mortality of anorexia nervosa and other eating disorders. *Current Opinion in Psychiatry, 19*(4), 389–394.

Inglese, M. D. (2009). Caring for children with autism spectrum disorder, part II: Screening, diagnosis, and management. *Journal of Pediatric Nursing, 24*(1), 49–59.

Keeley, M. L., & Storch, E. A. (2009). Anxiety disorders in youth. *Journal of Pediatric Nursing, 24*(1), 26–40.

Kirby, M., & Keon, W. J. (2006). *Out of the shadows at last: Transforming mental health, mental illness, and addiction services in Canada: Report of the Standing Senate Committee on Social Affairs, Science and Technology.* Retrieved *October 18, 2011* from http://www.parl.gc.ca/39/1/parlbus/commbus/senate/com-e/soci-e/rep-e/rep02may06-e.htm

Kratochvil, C., Vaughn, B., Barker, A., Corr, L., Wheeler, L., & Madaan, V. (2009). Review of pediatric attention deficit/hyperactivity disorder for the general psychiatrist. *Psychiatric Clinics of North America, 32*(1), 39–56. doi:10.1016/j.psc.2008.10.001

Lack, C. W., & Green, A. L. (2009). Mood disorders in children and adolescents. *Journal of Pediatric Nursing, 24*(1), 13–24.

Learning Disabilities Association of Canada. (2002). *Official definition of learning disabilities.* Retrieved June 17, 2011 from http://www.ldac-acta.ca/learn-more/ld-defined/official-definition-of-learning-disabilities.html

Lenz, K., Coderre, K., & Watanabe, M. (2009). Overview of depression and its management in children and adolescents. *Formulary, 44*(6), 172–180.

Mahon, N. E., Yarcheski, A., & Yarcheski, T. J. (2003). Anger, anxiety, and depression in early adolescents from intact and divorced families. *Journal for Specialists in Pediatric Nursing, 18*(4), 267–273.

McClain, N. (2003). Adolescent suicide attempt: Undisclosed secrets. *Pediatric Nursing, 29*(1), 52–53.

McColl, M., & Stephenson, R. (2008). *A scoping review of disability policy in Canada: Effects on community integration for people with spinal cord injuries.* Kingston: Queens University. Retrieved *October 18, 2011* from http://chspr.queensu.ca/downloads/Reports/Disability%20Policy%20in%20Canada-final%20report-May09.pdf

National Dissemination Center for Children with Disabilities (NICHCY). (2011). *Intellectual disability.* Retrieved October 18, 2011 from http://www.nichcy.org/Disabilities/Specific/Pages/IntellectualDisability.aspx

Nurcombe, B. (2008). Diagnostic formulation, treatment planning, and modes of treatment in children and adolescents. In M. H. Ebert, P. T. Loosen, B. Nurcombe, & J. F. Leckman (Eds.), *Current diagnosis & treatment: Psychiatry* (2nd ed.). New York: McGraw-Hill.

Oliver, C. J. (2003). Triage of the autistic spectrum child utilizing the congruence of case management concepts and Orem's nursing theories. *Lippincott's Case Management, 8*(2), 66–82.

Ouellette-Kuntz, H., Shooshtari, S., Temple, B., et al. (2010). Estimating administrative prevalence of intellectual disabilities in Manitoba. *Journal on Developmental Disabilities, 15*(3), 69–80.

Phetrasuwan, S., Miles, M. S., Mesibov, G. B., & Robinson, C. (2009). Defining autism spectrum disorders. *Journal of Specialty Pediatric Nursing, 14*(3), 206–209.

Pompili, M., Mancinelli, I., Girardi, P., et al. (2005). Childhood suicide: A major issue in pediatric health care. *Issues in Comprehensive Pediatric Nursing, 28,* 63–68.

Public Health Agency of Canada. (2011). Fetal alcohol spectrum disorder. Retrieved October 18, 2011 from http://www.phac-aspc.gc.ca/hp-ps/dca-dea/prog-ini/fasd-etcaf/index-eng.php

Reasor, J. E., & Farrell, S. P. (2004). Early childhood mental health: Services that can save a life. *Journal of Pediatric Nursing, 19*(2), 140–144.

Ryan-Krause, P. (2010). Attention deficit hyperactivity disorder: Part I. *Journal of Pediatric Health Care, 24,* 194–198.

Scarpinao, N., Bradley, J., Kurbjun, K., Batemen, X., Holtzer, B., & Ely, B. (2010). Caring for the child with autism spectrum disorder in the acute care setting. *Journal for Specialists in Pediatric Nursing, 15*(3), 244–254. doi:10.1111/j.1744-6155.2010.00244.x

Schwichtenberg, A., & Poehlmann, J. (2007). Applied behavior analysis: Does intervention intensity relate to family stressors and maternal well-being? *Journal of Intellectual Disability Research, 51*(8), 598–605. doi:10.1111/j.1365-2788.2006.00940.x

Sensory Processing Disorder Foundation. (2011). *About SPD.* Retrieved October 18, 2011 from http://www.spdfoundation.net/about-sensory-processing-disorder.html

Shoaf, T. L., Emslie, G. J., & Mayes, T. L. (2001). Childhood depression: Diagnosis and treatment strategies in general pediatrics. *Pediatric Annals, 30*(3), 130–137.

Smith, M., Segal, J., & Hutman, T. (2010). *Autism symptoms and early signs: What to look for in babies, toddlers, and children.* Retrieved October 18, 2011 from http://www.helpguide.org/mental/autism_signs_symptoms.htm

Stafford, B. (2011). Child & adolescent psychiatric disorders & psychosocial aspects of pediatrics. In W. W. Hay, M. J. Levin, J. M. Sondheimer, & R. R. Deterding (Eds.), *Current pediatric diagnosis and treatment* (20th ed.). New York: McGraw-Hill.

Stein, M. T. (2002). The role of attention-deficit/hyperactivity disorder diagnostic and treatment guidelines in changing physician practices. *Pediatric Annals, 31*(8), 496–504.

Stevens, S. (2005). Attention deficit/hyperactivity disorder: Working the system for better diagnosis and treatment. *Journal of Pediatric Nursing, 20*(1), 47–51.

The BC Partners for Mental Health and Addictions Information. (2008). *Aboriginal mental health and substance abuse.* Retrieved October 18, 2011 from http://heretohelp.bc.ca/publications/factsheets/aboriginal

Van Ommen, J., Meerwijk, E., Kars, M., Van Elburg, A., & Van Meijel, B. (2009). Effective nursing care of adolescents with anorexia nervosa: The patient's perspective. *Journal of Clinical Nursing, 18*(20), 2801–2808.

Vessey, J. A., & Wilkinson, A. M. (2008). Caring for individuals with ADHD throughout the lifespan: An introduction to ADHD. *Counseling Points, 1*(1), 1–13.

Vlam, S. L. (2006). Attention-deficit/hyperactivity disorder: Diagnostic assessment methods used by advanced practice registered nurses. *Pediatric Nursing, 31*(1), 18–24.

Williams, T., & Hodgman, C. (2001). Medication for the management of anxiety disorders in children and adolescents. *Pediatric Annals, 30*(3), 146–153.

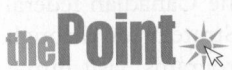

CHAPTER WORKSHEET

MULTIPLE CHOICE QUESTIONS

1. The nurse is caring for a child with ADHD. Which behaviour would the nurse **not** expect the child to display?

   a. Moody, morose behaviour with pouting

   b. Interruption and inability to take turns

   c. Forgetfulness and easy distractibility

   d. Excessive motor activities and fidgeting

2. An adolescent girl who has been receiving treatment for anorexia nervosa has failed to gain weight over the past week despite eating all of her meals and snacks. What is the priority nursing intervention?

   a. Increase the teen's daily caloric intake by at least 500 calories.

   b. Ensure that the teen's entire fluid intake includes calories.

   c. Supervise the teen for 2 hours after all meals and snacks.

   d. Assess the teen's anxiety level to determine need for medication.

3. A 15-year-old patient has been making demands all day, exaggerating her every need. She is now crying, saying she has nothing to live for and threatening to kill herself. What is the priority nursing action?

   a. Ignore her continued exaggerated and melodramatic behaviour.

   b. Consult with the physician to increase her antidepressant dose.

   c. Leave the girl alone for a little while until she composes herself.

   d. Take the girl's suicidal threat seriously and provide close supervision.

4. When trying to manage aggressive or impulsive behaviours in children or adolescents, what is the best nursing intervention?

   a. Train the child to be assertive.

   b. Provide consistency and limit-setting.

   c. Allow the child to negotiate the rules.

   d. Encourage the child to express his or her feelings.

CRITICAL THINKING EXERCISES

1. A mother tells you that her son's behaviour is unmanageable, and she is having difficulty coping with it. The boy is argumentative and is bullying others. He is struggling with his schoolwork because he has difficulty staying on task, gets out of his chair often, and frequently distracts others. What additional assessments should you obtain? What interventions would be helpful in managing the boy's behaviour?

2. A 14-year-old boy with moderate intellectual disability is able to feed himself but is incontinent. Discuss the issues with which his family must deal.

STUDY ACTIVITIES

1. Explore several of the websites related to adolescent drug and alcohol use and prevention listed at the end of this chapter. Develop a list of resources for families in your local area.

2. Attend a group therapy session during your pediatric clinical rotation. Observe the children's verbal and nonverbal communication, noting inconsistencies or other interesting observations.

3. Visit a school where children with autism attend. Spend time with the various specialists who work with children with ASD, determining their roles and the effect the treatment they are providing has on the children. Report your findings to your classmates.

4. Attend a local CHADD meeting. Talk to parents about having a child with ADHD.

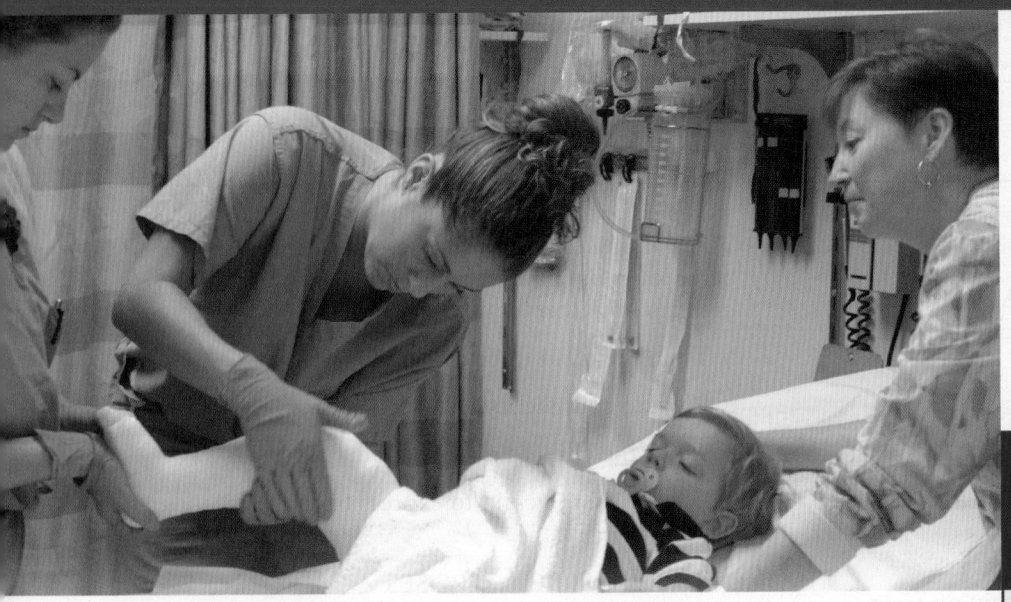

Abigail Belanger, age 8 years, has been admitted to the pediatric unit. Her mother calls the nurse into the room, stating, "Abigail's having trouble breathing!"

NURSING CARE DURING A PEDIATRIC EMERGENCY

KEY TERMS

asystole
barotrauma
bradycardia
cardioversion
cricoid pressure
defibrillation

hypercapnia
hyperventilation
hypocapnia
hypoventilation
intubation
periodic breathing

tachycardia
tachypnea
tracheal (endotracheal)
tube

LEARNING OBJECTIVES

Upon completion of the chapter, the learner will be able to:

1. Identify various factors contributing to emergency situations among infants and children.
2. Discuss common treatments and medications used for a child experiencing an emergency.
3. Conduct a health history of a child experiencing an emergency situation, specific to the emergency.
4. Perform a rapid cardiopulmonary assessment.
5. Discuss common laboratory and other diagnostic tests used during pediatric emergencies.
6. Integrate the principles of the American Heart Association (AHA) and Pediatric Advanced Life Support (PALS) in the comprehensive management of a child with an emergent medical situation.

Wow

A nurse must possess knowledge and skills to aid an acutely ill child.

Children are uniquely vulnerable to a diverse range of emergency situations. These situations can be life-threatening if not treated in an efficient manner. For example, most pediatric cardiopulmonary arrests result from respiratory failure or shock (Mandt & Rappaport, 2009; Zideman & Hazinski, 2008). Data suggest that children who have a cardiopulmonary arrest requiring resuscitative measures rarely fare well (Donoghue, Nadkarni, Berg, et al., 2005; Gerein, Osmond, Stiell, et al., 2006; Moler, Meert, Donaldson, et al., 2009). For these reasons, the American Heart Association (AHA) has delineated two distinct "chains of survival," one for adults and one for children, that should be followed during a life-threatening situation.

The adult chain of survival is:

1. Early emergency medical system (EMS) activation
2. Early cardiopulmonary resuscitation (CPR)
3. Early defibrillation
4. Early access to advanced care

In contrast, the pediatric chain of survival is:

1. Prevention of cardiac arrest and injuries
2. Early CPR
3. Early access to emergency response system
4. Early advanced care

Developmental immaturity places the infant and young child at increased risk for injury compared with older children. Furthermore, younger children, because of their size and shape, have an increased risk of death or poor outcome from traumatic injury compared with older children (World Health Organization [WHO], 2008). Submersion injuries, suffocation, burns, falls, and poisoning are additional emergency situations for which children are at increased risk (Public Health Agency of Canada [PHAC], 2009; Safe Kids Canada, 2007).

Considering the special risks that threaten children, the AHA has also developed specific guidelines for Pediatric Advanced Life Support (PALS). The Heart and Stroke Foundation (HSF) of Canada and the AHA have recently released new guidelines for CPR (Cheng & Bhanji, 2011). Courses in PALS are offered for health care professionals so that they can provide expert care for children in emergencies. This chapter emphasizes the principles of PALS in its discussion of the pediatric nurse's role in the management of pediatric emergencies. This chapter is not intended to be a substitution for the PALS course; health care providers caring for children in their day-to-day practice should consider obtaining and maintaining PALS certification.

▶ **Take** NOTE!

PALS guidelines published in 2005 define the pediatric patient as any child from the age of 1 year up to the start of puberty (American Heart Association [AHA], 2005a). Children in this age group should be managed using the PALS guidelines rather than those for adults (AHA, 2005b).

▶ **Take** NOTE!

Since the CPR guidelines by the HSF and the AHA were still undergoing revision at the time of publication of this book, readers are encouraged to consult the HSF and AHA websites for the most current information and guidelines. Visit http://thePoint.lww.com/Chow1e for direct links to these websites.

Common Medical Treatments

A variety of medications as well as other medical treatments are used to treat pediatric emergencies. Most of these treatments will require a physician's order when the child is in the hospital, though some emergency departments, pediatric transport teams, and pediatric units may have standing orders for pediatric emergency conditions. The most common medical treatments and medications related to pediatric emergencies are listed in Common Medical Treatments 52.1 and Drug Guide 52.1. The nurse caring for children who may experience an emergency should be familiar with what the procedures and medications are, how they work, as well as common nursing implications related to use of these modalities.

▶ **Take** NOTE!

Drug administration via endotracheal tube is not recommended as drug delivery is unpredictable with this route (Doniger & Sharieff, 2009). However, as a last resort, when intravenous or intraosseous routes are not available, certain code drugs for children may be given via a tracheal (endotracheal) tube (a tube inserted into the trachea that serves to maintain the airway and facilitate artificial respiration). Use the mnemonic LEAN (lidocaine, epinephrine, atropine, and naloxone) to remember which drugs may be given via the tracheal route (Mandt & Rappaport, 2009). In certain cases, when an emergency drug is given via the tracheal tube, the dosage must be increased. In addition, drugs given via this route should be flushed with 5 mL of sterile saline followed by multiple positive-pressure ventilations to ensure that the drugs are delivered.

(text continues on page 1785)

COMMON MEDICAL TREATMENTS 52.1 PEDIATRIC EMERGENCIES

Treatment	Explanation	Indication	Nursing Implications
Suctioning (oropharyngeal, nasopharyngeal, tracheal, or tracheostomy)	Removal of secretions via bulb syringe or suction catheter	Excessive airway secretions affecting airway patency	Use caution and suction only as far as recommended for age, tracheal tube size, or tracheostomy tube size or until coughing or gagging occurs.
Oxygen	Supplementation via mask, nasal cannula, hood, or tent or via tracheal/nasotracheal tube	Hypoxemia, respiratory distress, shock, trauma	Monitor response via colour, work of breathing, respiratory rate, oxygen saturation levels via pulse oximetry, and level of consciousness.
Bag-valve-mask ventilation	Provision of ventilation via a bag-valve-mask device, manual ventilation	Apnea, ineffective ventilation and oxygenation with spontaneous breaths, extremely slow respiratory rate	Ensure adequate chest rise with ventilation. Do not overventilate or bag aggressively to avoid barotrauma. Maintain a seal on the child's face with the appropriate-sized mask. Ensure the oxygen supply tubing is connected to 100% oxygen.
Intubation	Insertion of a tube into the trachea to provide artificial ventilation	Apnea, airway that is not maintainable, need for prolonged assisted ventilation	Determine adequacy of breath sounds with bagging immediately upon insertion of the tracheal tube. Assess for symmetrical chest rise. Tape tube securely in place and note number marking on the tube. Connect to ventilator when available.
Needle thoracotomy	Insertion of a needle between the ribs into the pleural space to remove air	Tension pneumothorax	There should be a rush of air as the needle reaches the air space. Monitor breath sounds, work of breathing, pulse oximetry. Ensure patency of IV catheter.
IV fluid therapy	Administration of crystalloid or colloid solutions to provide hydration or improve perfusion	Altered perfusion states such as respiratory distress, shock, trauma, cardiac disturbances	Use intraosseous route if a peripheral IV cannot be obtained quickly in the young child in shock. Reassess respiratory and circulatory status frequently after each IV fluid bolus and during continuous infusion.
Blood product transfusion	Administration of whole blood, packed red blood cells, platelets, or plasma intravenously	Trauma, hemorrhage	Follow institution's transfusion protocol. Double-check blood type and product label with a second nurse. Monitor vital signs and assess child frequently to determine adverse reaction to blood transfusion. If adverse reaction is suspected, immediately discontinue transfusion, infuse normal saline solution IV, reassess the child, and notify the physician.

Treatment	Explanation	Indication	Nursing Implications
Cervical stabilization	Maintenance of the cervical spine in an immobile position	Suspected or known trauma, unwitnessed submersion, or unknown mechanism of injury	Use the jaw-thrust manoeuvre without head tilt to open the airway. Maintain cervical stabilization until the cervical spine X-rays are cleared by the physician or radiologist.
Defibrillation and synchronized cardioversion	Provision of electrical current to alter the heart's electrical rhythm	Defibrillation: ventricular fibrillation and pulseless ventricular tachycardia. Synchronized cardioversion: supraventricular tachycardia and ventricular tachycardia with a pulse	In the pulseless patient, always ensure CPR is ongoing while the defibrillator is being readied. Ensure adequate oxygenation. Provide epinephrine if indicated. Sedate the awake child if time allows.

DRUG GUIDE 52.1   COMMON MEDICATIONS USED IN PEDIATRIC EMERGENCY SITUATIONS

Medication	Action	Indication	Nursing Implications
Adenosine (antiarrhythmic)	Slows conduction through AV node, restoring normal sinus rhythm	Supraventricular tachycardia (SVT)	• Administer IV; initial starting dose is 0.1 mg/kg (maximum dose of 6 mg). • Administer very rapidly (1–2 s) followed by a rapid, generous saline flush. • Subsequent doses may be doubled (0.2 mg/kg) up to a maximum of 12 mg. • Monitor for shortness of breath, dyspnea, worsening of asthma.
Amiodarone	Inhibits alpha- and beta-adrenergic receptors, producing vasodilation and AV nodal suppression (slows conduction through the AV node)	Ventricular tachycardia with or without a pulse and ventricular fibrillation	• Initial (loading) dose of 5 µg/kg (maximum 300 mg) IV or IO over 20–60 min (titrate rate to urgency). • Initial dose may be followed by an infusion of 5 to 10 µg/kg/min. • May cause hypotension, bradycardia, heart block, prolonged QT interval, and torsades de pointes ventricular tachycardia.
Atropine (anticholinergic)	Increases cardiac output, dries secretions, inhibits serotonin and histamine	Symptomatic vagally mediated bradycardia or primary atrioventricular block	• Administer via IV, IO, or ET route at a dose of 0.02 mg/kg (maximum dose 0.5 mg for a child, 1 mg for an adolescent). • Repeat every 5 min to a maximum total dose of 1 mg for a child and 2 mg for an adolescent. • Give undiluted over 30 s for IV or IO route. • Dilute with 3–5 mL normal saline for ET route; follow with five positive-pressure ventilations. • For IM administration, give 0.02–0.04 mg/kg. • Do not mix with sodium bicarbonate (incompatible).

(continued)

DRUG GUIDE 52.1 COMMON MEDICATIONS USED IN PEDIATRIC EMERGENCY SITUATIONS (continued)

Medication	Action	Indication	Nursing Implications
Dobutamine (synthetic cathecholamine)	Beta-adrenergic agent primarily affecting beta-1 receptors; increases myocardial contractility and heart rate	Ongoing short-term management of shock (hypovolemic and cardiogenic) and congestive heart failure	• Administer via IV or IO route at 2–20 µg/kg/min via continuous infusion. Monitor for development of ventricular arrhythmias. • Expect to titrate infusion rate based on cardiac output and blood pressure. • Administer via central line if possible due to risk of extravasation. • Monitor child closely, preferably in an ICU setting.
Dopamine (inotropic)	Increases cardiac output, blood pressure, and renal perfusion (beta-adrenergic agonist)	Bradycardia, hypotension, and poor cardiac output such as with cardiogenic/distributive shock	• Administer via IV or IO route at a dose of 2–20 µg/kg/min via continuous infusion. • Ensure that child has received adequate fluid resuscitation prior to administration. • Due to risk of extravasation, give via central line if possible. • Monitor child closely, preferably in an ICU setting. • Assess for ventricular arrhythmias.
Epinephrine (adrenergic)	Stimulates alpha- and beta-adrenergic receptors, increasing heart rate, and systemic vascular resistance	Bradycardia, anaphylaxis, CPR	• Administer via IV or IO route at a dose of 0.01 mg/kg (0.1 mL/kg of 1:10,000 solution) or via ET route at 0.1 mg/kg (0.1 mL/kg of 1:1,000 solution). • During CPR, repeat every 3–5 min. • Monitor for ventricular arrhythmias. • High doses may cause tachycardia in newborns. • Due to risk of extravasation and subsequent tissue necrosis, give through a central line if possible. • May also be used as a bronchodilator IV or via inhalation (racemic epinephrine).
Glucose	Increases blood glucose level	Hypoglycemia, hyperkalemia	• Administer via IV or IO route at a dose of 1–2 mL/kg (D50%); maximum dose 2 to 4 mL/kg. • When administering via a peripheral IV line, dilute 1:1 with sterile water to make D25%. Monitor IV site for infiltration and tissue extravasation. • Monitor blood glucose levels closely.
Naloxone (Narcan)	Antagonizes action of narcotic agents	Reversal of respiratory depression related to narcotic effects	• Administer via IV, IO, SC, or ET route at a dose of 0.01 to 0.1 mg/kg in children <5 years old or <20 kg or at a dose of 2 mg in children >5 years old or >20 kg. Onset of action is within 2–5 min. • May repeat dose as necessary; narcotic effects outlast therapeutic effects of naloxone.

Adapted from: Taketokmo, C. K., Hodding, J. H., & Kraus, D. M. (2010). *Lexi-comp's pediatric dosage handbook* (17th ed.). Hudson, OH: Lexi-comp.

NURSING PROCESS OVERVIEW FOR THE CHILD EXPERIENCING AN EMERGENCY SITUATION

The nurse may encounter a child who is experiencing an emergency in a variety of settings. As a member of a trauma team at a pediatric hospital, the nurse may participate in the stabilization of a child who has suffered submersion injury (Wagner, 2009) or other trauma. The emergency department nurse may encounter a child who has just been injured, such as from a fall, accident, or sports. On the hospital unit, a child with asthma may suffer respiratory distress or stop breathing. Regardless of the setting or how the emergency developed, the principles for managing pediatric emergencies are the same.

Care of the child who is experiencing an emergency includes all components of the nursing process: assessment, nursing diagnosis, planning, interventions, and evaluation. In an emergency situation, the nurse must act quickly, intervening immediately when an abnormality is determined upon assessment. When evaluating a child who presents emergently, always follow the AHA's guidelines for basic life support: evaluate airway, then breathing, then circulation. No matter what the cause of the emergency, the general approach to managing the child is universal, with minimal specific variations. Once the child's cardiopulmonary status is stabilized or the child is resuscitated, assessment and management will vary depending on the cause of the emergency.

Assessment

Nursing assessment of the child who presents emergently includes health history, physical examination, and laboratory and diagnostic testing. However, the initial history may be focused and very brief if the child is critically ill, necessitating that the nurse proceed immediately to rapid cardiopulmonary assessment. Once a child is stabilized, a more comprehensive history is obtained. Laboratory tests, while often important, should never take priority over the stabilization of the child from a cardiopulmonary and hemodynamic standpoint.

*R*emember Abigail, the 8-year-old with breathing trouble? What additional health history and physical examination assessment information should the nurse obtain?

Health History

Obtain the health history rapidly while simultaneously evaluating the child and providing life-saving interventions. A brief history is needed initially, followed by a more thorough history after the child is stabilized. The parents or caregiver will provide information about the child's "chief complaint." Record the information using the caregiver's own words. For example, the caregiver might say, "He's been having trouble breathing" if the child is presenting in respiratory distress. If the child suffered a traumatic injury from a bicycle accident, the caregiver might say, "She was riding her bike down the hill and lost control." This brief statement provides direction for obtaining more in-depth information about the nature of the emergency.

Ask about any significant past history that may affect the care of the child. For example, children who are medically fragile, who have a history of prematurity, or who have been diagnosed with asthma or congenital heart disease (e.g., tetralogy of Fallot) may require special consideration in planning for and executing their care.

Physical Examination

In an emergency, the nurse must perform a rapid cardiopulmonary assessment and intervene immediately when alterations are noted. The remainder of the physical examination then follows.

Rapid Cardiopulmonary Assessment

As the brief history is being obtained, begin to evaluate the ABCs. The ABCs of the rapid cardiopulmonary assessment are A, airway; B, breathing; and C, circulation. Since pediatric arrests are usually related primarily to airway and breathing, and usually only secondarily to the heart, focus the assessment and interventions using the ABCs of resuscitation. Always perform the assessment and interventions in that order, and do not move on until you have adequately assessed and managed each step. In most circumstances, if the pediatric airway is properly managed and breathing is assisted, the child may not experience a full arrest requiring chest compressions.

▶ *Take* NOTE!

Assessment and management of the airway of a pre-arresting or arresting child is ALWAYS the first intervention in a pediatric emergency situation. Intervene if there is an airway problem before moving on to assessment of breathing. If an intervention for breathing is required, start it before progressing to assessment of circulation.

A: Airway Evaluation and Management. First evaluate the airway. Assess the patency of the airway. If the child is conscious, allow him or her to assume a position of comfort or, if the child will allow it, position him or her to improve airway patency. If the child is unconscious or has just been injured, you may need to open the airway manually. If no concern related to cervical

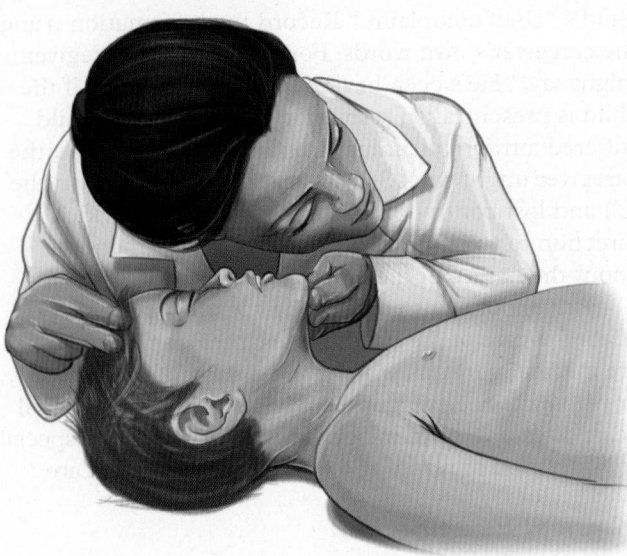

FIGURE 52.1 Head tilt–chin lift manoeuvre in a child.

spine injury exists, open the airway using the head tilt–chin lift manoeuvre. Place the fingertips on the bony prominence of the child's chin and lift the chin to open the airway. Simultaneously, place one hand on the forehead and tilt the child's head back (Fig. 52.1). If the airway is not maintainable, reposition the airway for appropriate airflow. If secretions are obstructing the airway, suction the airway to remove them. Place the child immediately on oxygen at 100% and apply a pulse oximeter to monitor oxygen saturation levels.

> ▶ **Take** NOTE!
>
> *If cervical spine injury is a possibility, do not use the head tilt–chin lift manoeuvre; instead use the jaw-thrust technique for opening the airway (see Trauma section for explanation and illustration).*

B: Breathing Evaluation and Management. After establishing an open airway, look for signs of breathing. Turn your head and place your ear over the child's mouth to "look, listen, and feel" for spontaneous respirations. Look to see whether the child's chest is rising, listen for air escaping, and note whether you feel any air coming out of the child's nose or mouth. If the child is breathing, evaluate the quality of the respirations, including respiratory rate, chest rise, lung sounds, and respiratory effort. Count the respiratory rate and determine whether it is appropriate for the child's age. Observe the child's colour. Note adequacy of airflow in all lung fields, depth of respiration, chest rise, and presence of adventitious sounds. Is the breathing effective or is the child gasping ineffectively for air? Evaluate for

increased work of breathing and the use of accessory muscles.

When signs of respiratory distress are noted, immediately place the child on oxygen at 100% and apply a pulse oximeter to monitor oxygen saturation levels. If the child is breathing shallowly and has poor respiratory effort, attempt to reposition the airway to promote better airflow. For the child receiving 100% oxygen who does not improve with repositioning, begin assisted ventilation with a bag-valve-mask (BVM) device. A need for ongoing BVM ventilation may require airway **intubation** (process by which a breathing tube, such as a tracheal tube, is inserted into a child's airway to assist with breathing).

> ▶ **Take** NOTE!
>
> *Attempts to insert a tracheal tube should last no longer that 20 to 30 seconds each. After each attempt, the child should receive multiple ventilations by the BVM method using 100% oxygen (AHA, 2007).*

C: Circulation Evaluation and Management. The next step is to evaluate the circulation. During this phase, evaluate the heart rate, pulses, perfusion, skin colour and temperature, blood pressure (BP), cardiac rhythm, and level of consciousness. Determine the heart rate via direct auscultation or palpation of central pulses. If perfusion is poor, such as with shock or cardiac arrest, the child may have a weak pulse or no pulse. In the young infant, check the brachial artery for a pulse. In the child and adolescent, evaluate the femoral or carotid pulse. If there is a pulse, note its quality. Is it barely palpable or weak? Is it strong or bounding? Compare strength and quality of central and peripheral pulses. Assess capillary refill time.

> ▶ **Take** NOTE!
>
> *ALWAYS evaluate the presence of a heart rate by auscultation of the heart or by palpation of central pulses. NEVER use the cardiac monitor to determine whether the child has a heart rate. The presence of a cardiac rhythm indicates the presence of electrical activity only. It is not a reliable way to evaluate the mechanical ability ("pumping" action) of the heart to perfuse the body. In certain circumstances a rhythm continues but there is no pulse (pulseless electrical activity [PEA]). If the child has no heart rate (pulse) despite adequate respiratory interventions, begin cardiac compressions.*

Evaluate the child's perfusion by noting skin temperature and colour. Is the skin pink? Is it warm to touch? The child's skin may be cool to the touch and may appear pale, mottled, or cyanotic. As the child's condition worsens with developing shock and cardiovascular compromise, note a line of demarcation of skin temperature warmth. In this situation, the distal extremities will feel cooler than the proximal regions of the body. Measure the BP and place the child on a cardiac monitor to evaluate the cardiac rhythm. Note the child's level of consciousness; if circulation is poor, the child may demonstrate an altered level of consciousness as the perfusion to the brain becomes diminished.

▶ *Take* NOTE!

According to PALS, calculate minimum acceptable systolic BP by using this formula: 70 + (2 times the age in years). For example, a 4-year-old should have a minimal systolic BP of 78: 70 + (2 × 4) = 78.

If the circulation or perfusion is compromised, then fluid resuscitation is necessary. Establish large-bore intravenous (IV) access immediately and administer isotonic crystalloid rapidly. Provide 20 mL/kg of normal saline (NS) or lactated Ringer's solution (LRS) as an IV bolus. If peripheral IV access cannot be obtained in the child with altered perfusion within three attempts or 90 seconds, assist with insertion of an intraosseous needle for fluid administration (refer to Shock section for further information about intraosseous access). Central venous lines or cutdown access may also be used, but these measures take longer to accomplish.

Additional Physical Examination Components

In addition to assessing and stabilizing the child's airway, breathing, and circulation, perform a thorough physical examination and assess pain.

Neurologic Evaluation. Quickly evaluate the level of consciousness in an older child. Ask the child to state his or her name. Ask what happened to the child. Does the child know what day it is? Is the child aware of where he or she is?

If the child is an infant, evaluate his or her interest in the environment and response to parents. Lack of interest in the environment or a seeming inability of an infant to recognize his or her parents is a cause for concern. In contrast, an infant who enjoys sucking on a finger and making eye contact with the nurse during the assessment is reassuring.

Evaluate the child's head. In the infant or young toddler, palpate the anterior fontanel to determine whether it is normal (soft and flat), depressed, or full.

A sunken fontanel is associated with volume depletion from dehydration or blood loss. If the fontanel is full, note whether it is bulging or tense, which may indicate increased intracranial pressure. Next assess the eyes. Are they open or closed? If closed, do they open spontaneously, to voice, to pain? Does the child focus on and follow your movements? Evaluate the pupils for equality and reactivity. Sluggish pupillary reaction may occur with increased intracranial pressure.

▶ *Take* NOTE!

A nonreactive pupil is an ominous sign indicating a need for immediate relief of increased intracranial pressure.

Evaluate the child's face. Does the child smile or cry? Does the child react to playfulness with a laugh? Does the young infant cry vigorously? Are facial movements equal? In a child, a normal or near-normal neurologic examination can be a reassuring sign. Conversely, obtundent or muted responses from children to environmental stimuli are a cause for concern.

Next evaluate for spontaneous movement of the extremities. Young infants are non-ambulatory, so assess their ability to move their arms and legs and grossly evaluate the tone of their extremities. Does the infant vigorously and equally move the arms and legs? Is the muscle tone normal, or does the infant appear floppy or flaccid? When evaluating the older child, note whether he or she is ambulatory alone, ambulatory with assistance, or unable to walk. Note whether the child has use of the upper extremities. In the case of trauma, the child may arrive immobilized on a backboard. In this scenario, evaluate the child's motor responsiveness and sensation in each extremity, comparing findings bilaterally while the child is in the supine position. Ask the child if he or she feels you touching each extremity. Request that the child squeeze your fingers and then ask the child to wiggle the toes. The information obtained from these assessment techniques will provide information about cerebral integrity and perfusion, cerebellar health, and spinal cord integrity.

The Pediatric Glasgow Coma Scale may also be used to evaluate neurologic status in children (American Academy of Pediatrics, 2010a). Chapter 37 provides a more in-depth discussion of this scale.

Skin and Extremity Evaluation. Remove the child's clothing and thoroughly examine the skin for bruising, lesions, or rashes. If the child has a rash, note the size, shape, colour, configuration, and location. Apply pressure to the rash with the fingertips to evaluate for the ability to blanch. Inspect the trunk, abdomen, and extremities for abrasions or deformities.

▶ *Take* NOTE!

Rashes that do not blanch may be classified as petechiae or purpura. This type of rash may be associated with certain serious conditions, such as meningococcemia. Report this finding to the physician or nurse practitioner immediately.

Pain Assessment. In emergency situations, children may experience pain as a direct result of the injury or disease. Life-saving interventions such as resuscitation, insertion of IV lines, and administration of medications may cause further pain. The child's pain may also be exaggerated by light, noise, movement of the stretcher or bed, and the sensations of cold or heat. Nurses can play a key role in minimizing the child's pain, and this may help decrease the child's future distress (Atkinson, Chesters, & Heinz, 2009; Walco, 2008). If the child is awake and verbal, use an age-appropriate pain assessment scale to determine the child's pain level. If the child is sedated or unconscious, assess pain with a standardized scale that relies on physiologic measurements as well as behavioural parameters. Refer to Chapter 35 for additional information on pain assessment in children.

Laboratory and Diagnostic Testing

A number of laboratory and diagnostic tests may be ordered in a pediatric emergency. Laboratory tests can help to distinguish the cause of the emergency or additional problems that need to be treated. Standard laboratory tests obtained in most emergency departments include:

- Arterial blood gases (ABG), obtained initially and then serially to assess for status changes
- Electrolytes and glucose levels
- Complete blood count (CBC)
- Blood cultures
- Urinalysis

If ingestion is suspected, then a toxicology panel will be obtained. In suspected sepsis, erythrocyte sedimentation rate (ESR), C-reactive protein (CRP), and urine and spinal fluid cultures may also be obtained. The pediatric trauma victim may have additional laboratory tests performed, including amylase, liver enzymes, and blood type and cross-match.

Diagnostic tests may include radiologic tests, computed tomography (CT) scanning, and magnetic resonance imaging (MRI). One advantage of radiologic diagnostic testing is that the tests are relatively non-invasive. A disadvantage associated with CT and MRI testing is that before either test can be performed, the patient must be stabilized. Common Laboratory and Diagnostic Tests 52.1 gives further information about the tests most commonly used in pediatric emergency situations.

After completing an assessment of Abigail, the nurse noted the following: a patent airway, anxious but able to speak in short sentences, and skin temperature cool on the extremities. Based on these assessment findings, what would your top three nursing diagnoses be for Abigail? Describe appropriate nursing interventions.

Nursing Diagnoses and Related Interventions

Upon completion of a thorough assessment and initial stabilization of the child, the nurse might identify several nursing diagnoses, including:

- Airway clearance, ineffective
- Breathing pattern, ineffective
- Gas exchange, impaired
- Fluid volume, deficient
- Cardiac output, decreased
- Tissue perfusion (cardiopulmonary, peripheral cerebral, or renal), ineffective
- Knowledge, deficient
- Fear
- Family processes, interrupted

Specific nursing goals, interventions, and evaluation for the child who is experiencing an emergency are based on the nursing diagnoses. Additional information about nursing management will be included later in the chapter as it relates to specific disorders.

Providing Cardiopulmonary Resuscitation

Always evaluate and manage the airway first, unless this is an out-of-hospital, witnessed, sudden collapse of a child. Call for help and assign someone to obtain the automated external defibrillator (AED). Open the airway and assess for adequate breathing. If the child is not breathing, begin rescue breathing. Check for a pulse. In the child, the carotid or femoral pulses are easiest to assess. It is usually recommended that the brachial pulse be checked in the infant; however, this is often difficult, so an alternative is to check the femoral pulse. Carefully assess for signs of a pulse, but do not spend more than 10 seconds doing so. If there is not a pulse or if the heart rate is less than 60 beats/min with signs of poor perfusion (e.g., cyanosis), begin chest compressions.

▶ *Take* NOTE!

When the arrest occurs out of the hospital and is a witnessed, sudden collapse, initial management is slightly different than that for other arrests. In these sudden, witnessed events, phone first, get the AED, and return to start CPR.

COMMON LABORATORY AND DIAGNOSTIC TESTS 52.1   PEDIATRIC EMERGENCIES

Test	Explanation	Indications	Nursing Implications
Chest X-ray	Radiograph used to evaluate heart, lung, and thoracic skeletal structures	Identification of: • Infections (such as pneumonia) • Foreign body • Injury • Endotracheal tube placement • Central line placement • Pneumothorax • Re-evaluation of: • The lungs after chest tube placement	• X-rays can be obtained quickly during resuscitation; usually available in emergency department. • Assist the child to lie still if necessary.
Computed tomography (CT)	Use of high radiation (equivalent to about 100 to 150 chest X-rays) with computer processing targeting specific body areas	Rapid evaluation of tissues and skeletal areas Superior test for the evaluation of internal bleeding	• Expect the child to be transported out of the area for the study. • Accompany the child to provide continued observation and management, especially if child's condition is unstable.
Magnetic resonance imaging (MRI)	Incorporation of responses of hydrogen protons to a dynamic magnetic field	Superior test for evaluation of the spinal cord and the cerebrospinal fluid spaces; less useful in emergency situations	• Administer sedation as ordered. • Assist child in remaining still; MRI requires child to remain still for a longer period than for a CT. • Assist the conscious child to deal with fear related to loud banging noise of the machine.
Arterial blood gases (ABG)	Evaluation of blood pH and arterial blood levels of oxygen and carbon dioxide	Evaluation of quality of respiration. Evaluation of acid–base balance, such as in a child who may be acidotic due to volume loss with resultant electrolyte imbalance.	• Anticipate serial ABGs to assess for status changes. • Never delay resuscitation efforts pending blood gas results.
Serum electrolytes	Evaluation of electrolyte levels, such as sodium, potassium, and chloride, in the blood	Useful for determining baseline and if dehydration is hypertonic or isotonic	• Hemolysis of specimen may lead to falsely elevated potassium levels.
Glucose	Evaluation of glucose level in the blood	Valuable for determining need for supplementation, as in the case of hypoglycemia	• Use either bedside glucose monitor or obtain serum blood specimen. • Elevated glucose levels can be associated with stress or with use of corticosteroids.
Toxicology panel (blood and/or urine)	Determination of most commonly abused mood-altering medications as well as commonly ingested drugs	Drug abuse, overdose, or poisoning	• Standard toxicology panel varies with the agency. • Follow agency protocol; may require special handling or labelling of specimen. • Use a blood specimen that is best for determining overdose or poisoning.

(continued)

COMMON LABORATORY AND DIAGNOSTIC TESTS 52.1 PEDIATRIC EMERGENCIES (continued)

Test	Explanation	Indications	Nursing Implications
Complete blood count (CBC)	Evaluation of hemoglobin and hematocrit, white blood cell count, and platelet count	Any condition in which anemia, infection, or thrombocytopenia is suspected. Trauma if blood loss suspected.	• Be aware of normal values and how they vary with age and gender. • Hemoglobin and hematocrit may be elevated secondary to hemoconcentration in the case of hypovolemia.
Blood type and cross-match	Determination of ABO blood typing as well as presence of antigens. Cross-match performed on RBC-containing products to avoid transfusion reaction.	Trauma victim or any person with suspected blood loss as preparation for transfusion	• Handle specimen gently to avoid hemolysis. • Ensure that specimen request and label are appropriately signed and dated. • Apply "type and cross" or "blood band" to child at time of specimen collection if required by agency. • Most type and cross-match specimens expire after 48–72 h.
Urinalysis	Evaluation of colour, pH, specific gravity, and odour of urine. Assessment for evidence of protein, glucose, ketones, blood, leukocyte esterase, RBCs, WBCs, bacteria, crystals, and casts.	Patients with fever, dysuria, flank pain, urgency, hematuria or those who have experienced trauma to provide information about the urinary tract	• Many drugs can affect urine colour; notify the laboratory if the child is taking one. • Notify the laboratory and document on the laboratory form if the female child is menstruating. • Refrigerate the specimen if it is not processed promptly. • Specimen may be obtained by catheterization, clean-catch voiding sample, or via a U-bag.

Table 52.1 presents recommendations for rates of breaths to compressions and hand placement for performing chest compressions. The recommendations stress the importance of properly performed chest compressions (AHA, 2005a; Berg, Nadkarni, & Berg, 2008; Topjian, Berg, & Nadkarni, 2008). Characteristics of good chest compressions include the following:

• "Push hard"—compress the chest one third to one half of the anterior–posterior diameter.
• "Push fast"—compression rate should be about 100 per minute.
• Allow the chest to fully recoil between compressions.
• Minimize interruptions to perform chest compressions.

Providing Defibrillation or Synchronized Cardioversion

In some cases, the child experiences an abnormal life-threatening cardiac rhythm or an arrhythmia that does not respond to pharmacologic therapy or leads to hemodynamic instability. In these cases, electrical therapy, in the form of defibrillation or synchronized cardioversion, may be needed.

Defibrillation is the use of electrical energy to depolarize the cells of the myocardium to terminate an abnormal life-threatening cardiac rhythm, such as ventricular fibrillation. Defibrillation is used in conjunction with oxygen, CPR, and medications. The effects of defibrillation are enhanced in an oxygen-rich environment coupled with good artificial circulation (CPR). **Cardioversion**, another means of applying electrical current to the heart, is used when the child has supraventricular tachycardia (SVT) or ventricular tachycardia (VT) with a pulse. Cardioversion may also be enhanced with medications. Cardioversion is delivered as synchronized—that is, the electrical current is applied on the R wave of the electrocardiogram (ECG).

TABLE 52.1 RATES OF BREATHS TO COMPRESSIONS IN CPR

Age	One-Person CPR	Two-Person CPR
Infant	• 30 compressions to 2 breaths • Hand placement: two fingers, placed one finger-breadth below the nipple line	• 15 compressions to 2 breaths • Hand placement: two thumbs encircling the chest at the nipple line
Child	• 30 compressions to 2 breaths • Hand placement: heel of one hand or two hands (adult position in larger child), pressing on the sternum at the nipple line	• 15 compressions to 2 breaths • Hand placement: heel of one hand or two hands (adult position in larger child), pressing on the sternum at the nipple line

Adapted from: American Heart Association. (2005a). Part 11: Pediatric basic life support. *Circulation, 112*, 156–166.

The basic defibrillator is equipped with adult- and pediatric-sized paddles. A switch turns the machine on and controls are used to select the amount of energy (joules). Typically, the initial energy amount is 2 joules/kg and can be increased up to 4 joules/kg for defibrillation. The initial energy for cardioversion is delivered at 0.5 to 1 joule/kg; if the tachyarrhythmia persists, a second shock can be delivered using 1 to 2 joules/kg.

When the defibrillator is being used in an acute care setting, the leader of the code team will take charge of defibrillator use. He or she is responsible for ensuring that only the patient receives the energy from the defibrillator. The code team leader will clearly communicate the intention to deliver a shock to the patient to ensure that all personnel and other equipment are clear of the bed, so as to avoid accidental shock. For example, the leader may state, "I'm clear, you're clear, we're all clear," while taking surveillance of the positions of all team members relative to the patient, prior to delivering the shock.

Using Automated External Defibrillation

In cases of sudden, witnessed, out-of-hospital collapse, an arrhythmia is often the cause. The AED is designed for use in the prehospital setting as an alternative to manually defibrillating a patient. The AED device consists of electrodes that are applied to the chest. These electrodes are used to monitor the heart rhythm and deliver the electrical current only when needed. AED devices are readily available in a variety of locations, such as airports, sports facilities, and businesses. Traditionally, the AED was designed for use in adults, but newer-model AEDs with smaller paddles and the ability to alter energy delivery are now more readily available. Therefore, the AHA has recommended that an AED be used for children who are older than age 1 year who have no pulse and have suffered a sudden, witnessed collapse.

Once the AED is turned on, the machine uses auditory commands to guide laypersons and health care professionals alike through the correct placement of the electrodes and the administration of energy. The AED periodically evaluates the arrest victim's cardiac rhythm and instructs the user about checking the pulse, continuing CPR, and delivering shocks. Nurses who care for children should be able to operate an AED and be prepared to use it in nontraditional settings.

Determining Medication Doses and Equipment Sizes

Many pediatric acute care facilities initiate code reference sheets when a pediatric patient is admitted. This sheet uses the child's actual weight to determine medication doses and equipment sizes. The reference sheet is then kept on a clipboard at the child's bedside or taped on the wall at the head of the bed. An additional copy can be placed in the child's chart.

Ambulatory care providers often rely on the Broselow tape for estimating the child's weight based on the child's length as measured with the tape (Fig. 52.2). The tape is colour-coded and emergency equipment for a child of that size may be stored in corresponding colour-coded packages or in colour-coded drawers on the pediatric emergency cart (DeBoer, Seaver, & Broselow, 2005). Medication doses and equipment sizes are also located on the tape. The most accurate calculation for code medications is based on the child's weight, but in several research studies, use of the Broselow tape for estimation in the absence of true weight has been shown to be successful (Krieser, Nguyen, Kerr, et al., 2007; So, Farrington, & Absher, 2009).

Managing Pain

Depending on the child's status and pain level, individualize pain management interventions. For the alert child, non-pharmacologic measures may be used in addition to medications. Provide atraumatic care for procedures and use aggressive pharmacologic treatments to manage pain as the child's condition allows. Refer to Chapter 35 for additional information on pain management strategies.

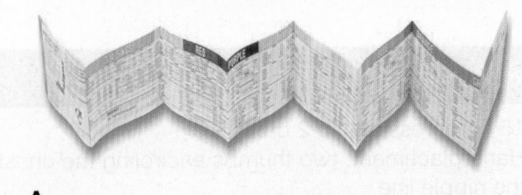

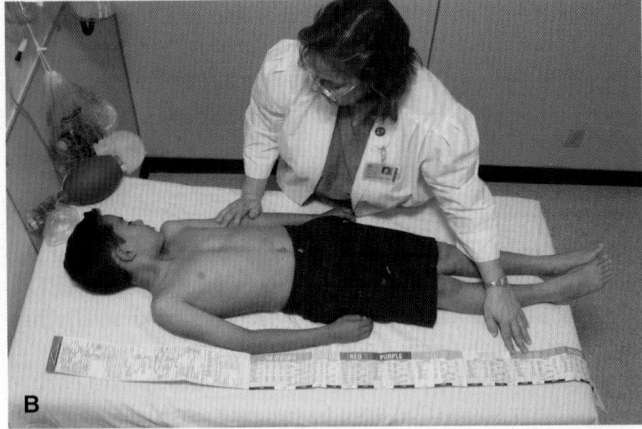

FIGURE 52.2 **(A)** Broselow tape. **(B)** Measure the child's length with the Broselow tape to determine medication doses and tracheal tube size.

Ensuring Stabilization

After a child has been resuscitated, the nurse plays a key role in stabilization and transport. Thoroughly document the interventions that were performed as well as the ongoing assessment of the child in response to the interventions. Provide continued monitoring of the child while awaiting transport. Copy and assemble any pertinent documentation, such as the resuscitation record, nurses' notes, and laboratory test results that will be given to the receiving institution. Ensure that all lines are taped securely and that vascular access sites are dressed and labelled with the date and time of insertion. As soon as possible, bring the child's family in to visit with the child. Provide explanations about the IV lines, monitoring equipment, and other medical equipment and devices. Encourage the family to talk to and touch the child.

Providing Support and Education to the Child and Family

The experience of respiratory distress, oxygen deprivation, and an emergency situation is a frightening one for persons of all ages. The life-saving interventions involved with an emergency can be especially intimidating and frightening to children. Infants and young children cannot understand explanations about the interventions that are being provided in an emergent situation. Older children and adolescents may feel frightened and angry about the loss of control. The caregivers of the acutely ill or injured child may feel fear, anger, guilt, and sadness. They may be concerned about the very real possibility that their child might die.

Resuscitation of a child is often a perplexing and frightening event for laypersons to observe. Therefore, family members traditionally have been excluded during the resuscitation of children. Of late, however, there has been a trend to allow family members to be present during pediatric resuscitation. Current evidence-based practice guidelines recommend individual evaluation of each family to assist them in making the decision to stay or leave during the resuscitation (Maxton, 2008; Nibert & Ondrejka, 2005; Tinsley, Hill, Shah, et al., 2008). See Evidence-based Practice 52.1.

Considering the highly technical nature of resuscitation, the rapidity with which interventions occur, and the fear associated with a life-threatening event, nurses can play a crucial role in providing understandable explanations to families, coupled with empathic support. During the acute phase, the nurse should give brief explanations as life-saving interventions are being provided. Examples of these types of explanations include:

- When applying the pulse oximeter sensor: "I need to put this little light on Johnny to check his oxygen level; it won't hurt."
- When connecting the child to the cardiac monitor: "We're going to put these sticky patches on Johnny and connect them so we can monitor his heart rate on this screen."
- When preparing for intubation and ventilation: "Johnny can't breathe on his own right now, so we're going to give him some extra help with this tube. This tube will go through his breathing passage and this machine will help him to breathe."

The nurse plays a key role in providing empathy and support. Do not provide false reassurance and say, for example, "He's going to be all right." The outcome is never certain. Rather, communicate empathically. For example, say, "This must be very difficult for you. We're doing everything we can to help Johnny." Provide honest answers in a reassuring manner. Respect each family's diversity and observe their strengths and weaknesses. Be non-judgmental in all interactions with families, even when the child's emergency situation may have resulted from family neglect.

Parents often feel very helpless when their child is in a high-tech environment. Suddenly overwhelmed with all the equipment and monitoring devices, they no longer are the persons who are the most skilled in caring for their child. Integrate the child's parents into the health care team. Suggest ways the parents can make the hospital experience more normal for their child. For example, simply allowing a father to read a story to his daughter or encouraging a mother to hold her child's hand is therapeutic both for the child and the parents.

EVIDENCE-BASED PRACTICE 52.1
Parental Presence During Cardiopulmonary Resuscitation

● **Background**

Family presence during CPR remains controversial. Despite this, having parents present during the resuscitation of their child is becoming a more common practice and is even encouraged in some institutions (Tinsley et al., 2008). Developing an understanding of what it means for parents to be either present or absent during resuscitation attempts can assist nurses in providing adequate support to parents regardless of their decision to stay or leave.

▲ **Study**

Maxton (2008) interviewed 14 parents of critically ill children who had either survived or died following a resuscitation attempt in a pediatric intensive care unit.

■ **Findings**

For most parents Maxton interviewed, it was inconceivable for them to not be with their child during the resuscitation attempt. Being nearby allowed them to advocate for their child and participate in decision making. Their presence assisted them in understanding the gravity of the situation and, when the outcome was death, afforded them the opportunity to say goodbye to their child.

Parents expressed a need for support during the resuscitation attempt from an experienced staff member, generally a nurse, who could provide adequate technical information in addition to providing support. Managing their coping, for some parents, was easier if they could leave and return without fear of being judged or not allowed back in.

Some parents who were absent during the resuscitation attempt expressed feelings of failure and guilt, others expressed frustration with not knowing what was going on, and some did not understand the gravity of what had happened because staff used medical jargon and euphemisms when speaking of the event.

● **Nursing Implications**

For nurses working with children, ensure that parents are afforded the flexibility to stay, leave, or come and go if their child suffers cardiac arrest. Additionally, parents require the support of an experienced staff member, such as a nurse, who can both explain what is happening and provide support. Explanations should be provided to parents in plain language without the use of medical jargon and euphemisms.

Maxton, F. J. C. (2008). Parental presence during resuscitation in the PICU: The parents' experience. *Journal of Clinical Nursing, 17,* 3168–3176.

Tinsley, C., Hill, J. B., Shah, J., Zimmerman, G., Wilson, M., Freier, K., & Abd-Allah, S. (2008). Experience of families during cardiopulmonary resuscitation in a pediatric intensive care unit. *Pediatrics, 122,* e799–e804. doi:10.1542/peds.2007-3650

Be aware of this dramatic change and how it affects the parents. Always ensure that they feel like they are a welcome part of their child's care.

Providing the child with familiar comfort objects helps to decrease stress. Once the intubated child is stabilized, if alert, assist him or her with communication. Some children can lift one finger for yes and two fingers for no. If the child is old enough to write, provide paper and pencil. Play is essential to the work of the child, and even if he or she is immobile, play is still possible. Puppets at the bedside and books help give the child a more normal experience in a scary situation that is far from the norm. Teenagers may enjoy listening to music through headphones. Even children who are comatose should be talked to and allowed to listen to familiar music.

Even if the outcomes are serious, the nurse can provide critical support to children and families. Whether hugging a crying mother or playing "peek-a-boo" with an intubated child, the nurse will be the one who can make a difference during a frightening experience.

Nursing Management of Children Experiencing Emergencies

Cardiopulmonary arrest in children is associated with high mortality or poor neurologic outcome (Gerein et al., 2006; Moler et al., 2009). Thus, nurses caring for children must be adept at identifying when a child is experiencing the beginning stages of an emergency so they can quickly and appropriately intervene to prevent deterioration to cardiopulmonary arrest. Assessment and management of the most common types of emergencies in children are discussed below. The topics covered include respiratory arrest, shock, cardiac arrhythmias and arrest, submersion injury, traumatic injury, and poisoning.

Respiratory Arrest

Respiratory emergencies may lead to respiratory failure and eventual cardiopulmonary arrest in children. Infants and young children are at greater risk for respiratory emergencies than adolescents and adults because they have smaller airways and underdeveloped immune systems,

TABLE 52.2 CAUSES OF RESPIRATORY ARREST IN CHILDREN

Condition	Cause
Upper airway	Burns Croup Epiglottitis Foreign body aspiration Reflux Strangulation or near-strangulation Tracheomalacia Vascular ring
Lower airway	Asthma Bronchiolitis Burns Foreign body aspiration Pertussis infection Pneumonia Pneumothorax Reflux
Nonrespiratory origins	Septic shock HIV
Neurologic	Central nervous system infection Guillain–Barré syndrome Poliomyelitis Seizures Sleep apnea Spinal cord trauma Sudden infant death
Chronic illness	Complications of severe prematurity Cystic fibrosis Bone marrow transplant Neutropenia
Metabolic/endocrine disorders	Diabetic ketoacidosis Mitochondrial disorders
Cardiac conditions	Arrhythmia Congenital cardiac problems Acquired cardiac problems
Traumatic/unintentional injury/intentional injury	Asphyxia Child abuse/"shaken baby syndrome" Submersion Electrocution Gunshot wound Toxic ingestion Vehicular-related trauma

Adapted from: Fleisher, G. R., & Ludwig, S. (2010). *Textbook of pediatric emergency medicine* (6th ed.). Philadelphia: Lippincott Williams & Wilkins.

resulting in a diminished ability to combat serious respiratory illnesses. Young children often lack coordination, making them susceptible to choking on foods and small objects, which may also lead to cardiopulmonary arrest. In addition, sudden infant death syndrome (SIDS) is a leading cause of cardiopulmonary arrest in young infants and thus is one of the leading causes of post-neonatal mortality in Canada (Rusen, Liu, Sauve, et al., 2004). For these reasons, nurses caring for children must be skilled at recognizing the signs of pediatric respiratory distress so they can prevent progression to eventual cardiopulmonary arrest. Table 52.2 lists some of the more common causes of pediatric respiratory arrest.

Nursing Assessment

If the child has severe respiratory compromise, obtain a brief history while simultaneously providing respiratory interventions. To obtain the history, use the following questions as a guide:

• When did the symptoms begin and when do they occur?
• Did the symptoms have a sudden onset, as with a foreign body aspiration?
• Were the symptoms initially less severe, with mild upper respiratory symptoms that progressed to paroxysmal (sudden, severe) coughing as is commonly seen in pertussis?
• Is the cough continual, intermittent, or worse at night or with exercise?
• Has there been any stridor? (Stridor is heard upon inhalation and may be associated with swelling of the trachea [as with croup] or with a foreign body in the upper airway.)
• Is there wheezing? If so, is the wheezing on inspiration or on expiration, or both?
• What makes the symptoms better and what makes them worse?
• Does drinking from a bottle induce the symptoms, as with gastro-esophageal reflux–induced aspiration?
• Is the child taking any medication for the symptoms?
• Does the child, or do any members of the immediate family, have a history of chronic respiratory disease, such as asthma?
• Are the child's immunizations up to date?
• Was the child born prematurely? If so, did the child require mechanical ventilation? If so, for how long?
• Were there any respiratory problems during the first few days of life?
• When did the child last eat? (This question is important because a recent meal will increase the child's risk of aspiration in the event of a respiratory arrest. In addition, the presence of food in the stomach will increase the risk of aspiration during tracheal intubation.)

If the child can communicate, ask how he or she is feeling. Is he short of breath? Does his chest hurt? Observe the child while speaking. Children who are in respiratory distress may speak in short sentences with gasping between words.

Physical Examination

In an emergency, physical examination is often limited to inspection, observation, and auscultation. First, quickly survey the respiratory status. Determine whether the child is breathing.

Inspection and Observation

Establish whether the airway is patent, maintainable, or unable to be maintained without intervention. The child with a patent airway is breathing without signs of obstruction. The maintainable airway remains patent independently by the child or with interventions such as a towel roll under an infant's shoulders. The airway that cannot be maintained does not sustain patency unless a more aggressive intervention, such as the insertion of a tracheal tube, is performed.

Look at the child's posture. Is the child sitting up, leaning forward, and drooling, as with epiglottitis? Observe the child's face: does he or she appear anxious or relaxed? Persons who are in respiratory distress often appear anxious. Look at the nose and mouth: are the nares patent? Is there noticeable nasal congestion or mucus coming from the nose? Note nasal flaring or mouth breathing. Observe for head bobbing. Listen for audible expiratory grunting or inspiratory stridor. Note the child's colour. Does the child appear pale, mottled, dusky, or cyanotic? Children may appear mottled in response to poor oxygenation, hypothermia, or stress. Children with severe respiratory compromise may appear dusky. Look for cyanosis around the mouth or on the trunk. Cyanosis is a late and often ominous sign of respiratory distress. Central cyanosis is more likely to be associated with respiratory or cardiac compromise. In contrast, peripheral cyanosis is more likely to be associated with circulatory alteration.

> ▶ **Take** NOTE!
>
> *Closely inspect the colour of the area around the mouth. Is there paleness (circumoral pallor)? Circumoral pallor is a sign of poor oxygenation.*

Evaluate the pattern and quality of respiration, noting the respiratory rate. **Tachypnea** (increased respiratory rate) is often noted in children in respiratory distress. However, seriously ill children grunt and may have normal or subnormal respiratory rates. **Hypoventilation**, a decrease in the depth and rate of respirations, is noted in very ill children or children who have central respiratory depression secondary to narcotics. If the child is a young infant (less than 2 months) or premature, periodic breathing may occur. **Periodic breathing** is regular breathing with occasional short pauses (brief periods of apnea). After the apneic pause, the infant will breathe rapidly (up to 60 beats/min) for a short period and then will resume a normal respiratory rate. In general, the infant who has periodic breathing looks pink and has a normal heart rate. Observe for the use of accessory muscles in the neck or retractions in the chest, determining the extent and severity of the retractions.

Auscultation

Auscultate the lungs with the diaphragm of the stethoscope. Breath sounds over the tracheal region are higher-pitched and are described as "vesicular," while breath sounds over the peripheral lung fields tend to be lower-pitched, known as "bronchial." Instruct the child to take deep breaths with the mouth open. To encourage the young child to exhale strongly, instruct him or her to "blow out" the penlight (as with a candle) or to blow on a tissue. Encourage the child not to breathe more rapidly than normal (to prevent **hyperventilation** [increased depth and rate of respirations]) and to avoid making any noises with the mouth.

> ▶ **Take** NOTE!
>
> *Significant upper respiratory congestion often interferes with assessment of the lower airways because the sound is easily transmitted throughout the chest. Differentiate between the upper and lower airway noises by listening with the stethoscope over the nose. You may be able to determine whether the noise is nasal or bronchial by using this technique.*

Auscultate the child's chest systematically. Listen in all anterior, axillary, and posterior regions, comparing the left with the right sides. Note any decreased or absent breath sounds, which may be the result of bronchial obstruction (as with mucous infection) or air trapping (as in children with asthma). Unilateral absent breath sounds can be associated with foreign body aspiration and pneumothorax.

> ▶ **Take** NOTE!
>
> *Sometimes a child's respiratory status is so severely compromised that little or no air movement is noted. This commonly occurs in a child experiencing a severe asthma exacerbation. Minimal or no air movement requires immediate intervention.*

Note the presence and location of adventitious breath sounds such as crackles, wheezes, or rhonchi. Document presence of a pleural friction rub (a low-pitched, grating sound), a sound resulting from inflammation of the pleura.

Palpation

Palpate the chest for any abnormalities. In the older, less severely ill and cooperative child, assess for tactile fremitus. Using the palm of the hand, palpate over the lung regions in the same manner as for auscultation and percussion while the child says "ninety-nine." Increased vibrations elicited during this manoeuvre are associated with consolidating conditions, such as pneumonia.

Percussion

Percuss the interspaces of the chest between the ribs in the same systematic fashion as with auscultation. Normally, percussion over an air-filled lung reveals resonant sounds. Note the presence of hyperresonance, which may indicate an acute problem such as a pneumothorax or a chronic disease such as asthma. In contrast, percussion sounds will be dull over a lobe of the lung that is consolidated with fluid, infectious organisms, and blood cells, as in the case of pneumonia.

Laboratory and Diagnostic Testing

Use continuous pulse oximetry to monitor any child whose respiratory status is a concern. Note and report oxygen saturation levels below 95%. (See Chapter 31 for additional information about use of the pulse oximeter.)

Additional tests may reveal:

- Arterial or capillary blood gases: hypoxemia, hypercarbia, altered pH
- Chest X-ray: alterations in normal anatomy or lung expansion, or evidence of pneumonia, tumour, or foreign body
- Metal detector: evidence of metallic foreign body. Novel as it may sound, metal detectors have been found to be highly accurate (99%) in detecting the presence of ingested coins in children (Lee, Ahmad, & Gale, 2005; Ramlakhan, Burke, & Gilchrist, 2006).

▶ *Take NOTE!*

Children with cardiac conditions resulting in cyanosis often have baseline oxygen saturations that are relatively low because of the mixing of oxygenated with deoxygenated blood.

Nursing Management

The basic principle of pediatric emergency care and PALS is prevention of cardiopulmonary arrest. Therefore, the nurse must rapidly assess and appropriately manage children who are exhibiting signs of respiratory distress. PALS stresses the fact that when children in respiratory distress deteriorate and suffer a pulseless cardiac arrest, "their outcome is poor" (AHA, 2007). In contrast, the data overwhelmingly demonstrate that children who receive prompt and proper treatment in cases of respiratory distress and

respiratory arrest have a high likelihood of survival (AHA, 2007; Tibballs & Kinney, 2006).

Nursing management of the child in respiratory distress involves maintaining a patent airway, providing supplemental oxygen, monitoring for changes in status, and in some cases assisting ventilation. In addition to providing these life-saving measures and monitoring the child's progress, offer support and education to the child and family.

Maintaining a Patent Airway

When a child exhibits signs of respiratory distress, make a quick decision about whether it will be safe to allow the child to stay with the parent or whether the child must be placed on the examination table or bed. For example, in the case of croup, the child will often breathe more comfortably and experience less stridor while in the comfort of the parent's lap. Many children in respiratory distress are more comfortable sitting upright, as this position helps to decrease the work of breathing by allowing appropriate diaphragmatic movement. In contrast, a

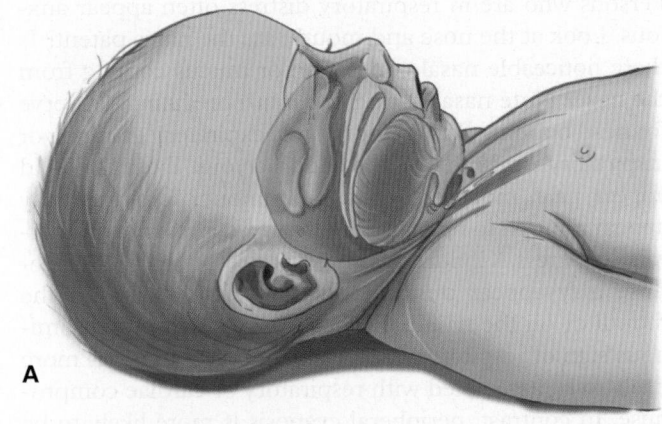

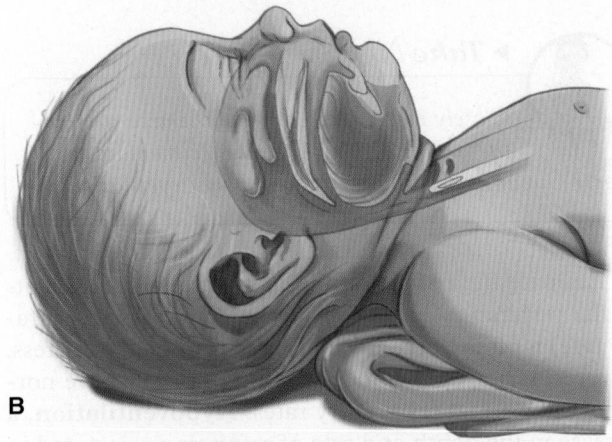

FIGURE 52.3 (**A**) The infant and young child's prominent occiput encourages flexion of the neck and may result in airway occlusion. (**B**) Putting a towel roll under the shoulders helps to open the infant's or young child's airway by placing it in the neutral or "sniff" position.

child with a decreasing level of consciousness may need to be placed in the supine position to facilitate positioning of the airway.

Infants may benefit from a small sheet or towel folded under the shoulders. This helps to facilitate positioning the infant's airway in the "sniff" position, as is recommended by AHA's Basic Cardiac Life Support (BCLS) guidelines (Fig. 52.3). Avoid neck flexion or hyperextension, which may completely occlude the infant's airway. In children over age 1 year, the optimal method for opening the airway, if a cervical spine injury is not suspected, is to use the head tilt–chin lift technique. If the child has suffered head or neck trauma and cervical spine instability is a concern, use the jaw-thrust manoeuvre by placing three fingers under the child's lower jaw and lifting the jaw upward and outward (Fig. 52.4). In either case, never place the hand under the neck to open the airway.

Often the nurse encounters an acutely ill child who cannot maintain an airway independently but may be able to do so with some assistance. For example, sometimes simply opening the airway and moving the tongue away from the tracheal opening is all that is required to regain airway patency. In certain conditions, a nasopharyngeal or oropharyngeal airway may be necessary for airway maintenance. Comparison Chart 52.1 provides additional information about these types of airways.

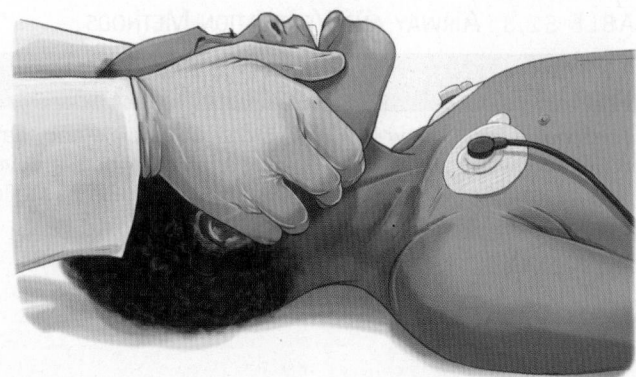

FIGURE 52.4 Jaw-thrust technique for opening the airway.

Assisting Ventilation

The child in respiratory distress may ventilate poorly, hypoventilate, or tire and become apneic. In this case, the child may require assistance with breathing through BVM ventilation, tracheal intubation, or a laryngeal mask airway. Table 52.3 explains these methods.

Providing Bag-Valve-Mask Ventilation

The technique of BVM ventilation is used in the management of children who cannot ventilate or oxygenate effectively on their own. This technique is a more efficient way

COMPARISON CHART 52.1   OROPHARYNGEAL VERSUS NASOPHARYNGEAL AIRWAYS

Oropharyngeal airway (used only in unconscious children)	• Consists of a simple plastic curved body that has a central air channel to allow for aeration • Is used when an unconscious child has difficulty maintaining airway patency due to upper airway obstruction, such as from the tongue • Allows for oral suction • Determine the correct size of the airway by placing it next to the child's cheek with the flange at the corner of the child's mouth and the tip pointing down. An airway that is too large will extend past the angle of the child's mandible and can obstruct the glottic opening when inserted. • Choose the airway that best fits the child to decrease the risk of injury to the structures of the mouth.
Nasopharyngeal airway (may be used in conscious children and children who have an intact gag reflex)	• Consists of a flexible curved tube that is inserted nasally • Is used when the child has difficulty maintaining airway patency due to tongue obstruction or palate problems, when neurologic impairment causes poor pharyngeal tone, or in the child with impaired consciousness • Allows for nasopharyngeal suction • When selecting this airway, keep in mind that the diameter of the airway should not be so large that it puts too much pressure on the internal nasal tissue. There are two common methods for measuring this airway: (1) to determine length, measure the distance from the end of the child's nose to the external auditory meatus; (2) look at the child's fifth digit, which is usually the approximate diameter of the nasopharyngeal airway. • Monitor for mucosal irritation, nasal septum swelling, and laceration of the adenoids. • Do not use this type of airway in children with a history of bleeding disorders or basilar skull fractures. • This airway's small diameter can easily become obstructed with secretions and blood.

Adapted from: Pagana, K. D., & Pagana, T. J. (2010). *Mosby's manual of diagnostic and laboratory tests* (4th ed.). St. Louis, MO: Mosby.

TABLE 52.3 AIRWAY AND VENTILATION METHODS

Method	Description	Comments
Anesthesia bag or flow-inflating ventilation system	A small, collapsible bag that consists of a reservoir bag, an overflow port, and a fresh gas inflow port	• Adjustment of the oxygen flow and the outlet control valve is necessary. • Useful in providing positive end-expiratory pressure (PEEP) or continuous positive airway pressure (CPAP) • Adequate training and significant skill are needed to properly operate this device. • **Hypercapnia** (increased carbon dioxide in the blood) and barotrauma may result with improper use. • Used more commonly in the operating room, recovery room, pediatric intensive care unit, and neonatal intensive care unit
Bag-valve-mask device or manual resuscitator	A self-inflating oxygen delivery bag that does not require an oxygen source for resuscitation and ventilation. The bag can be connected to oxygen to provide higher oxygen levels than room air. When the child exhales, the non-rebreathing valve closes, allowing exhaled, deoxygenated air to escape.	• Effective in providing oxygenation to a child who is in severe respiratory distress or who has suffered a respiratory arrest • A more efficient method of respiratory resuscitation than mouth-to-mouth resuscitation; decreased rescuer exposure to communicable disease • Most medical personnel can be trained to perform resuscitation with this method. • Possibly tiring for the rescuer when used to ventilate a child for long periods of time (see text discussion on bag-mask ventilation)
Laryngeal mask airway	An inflatable silicone mask and rubber connecting tube that is inserted blindly into the airway, forming a seal	• The airway is introduced into the pharynx and advanced until it meets resistance; balloon cuff is then inflated. • Easier insertion than a tracheal tube • Usually used in the unconscious child who benefits from bag-valve-mask ventilation but does not require intubation • Improvement in patient comfort
Tracheal intubation	A plastic tube inserted in the trachea to establish and maintain an airway when the airway cannot be maintained effectively using other measures (e.g., nasal trumpet or bag-valve-mask ventilation)	• Skilled medical professional (physician, nurse practitioner, respiratory therapist, EMT, or specially trained registered nurse) necessary for insertion • The bedside nurse acts as a valuable assistant during the intubation procedure.

of ensuring ventilation than using only supplemental oxygen. In addition, resuscitating a child in this manner is superior to mouth-to-mouth resuscitation as it provides higher oxygen concentrations and protects the nurse from exposure to oral secretions. However, this technique requires proper training and practice. The proper procedure involves appropriate opening of the airway followed by providing breaths with the BVM.

Ventilation with the BVM may be performed with either one or two rescuers. First, choose an appropriate-sized bag and a corresponding facemask that fits the infant or child (Fig. 52.5). Self-inflating bags are usually available in neonatal, infant, child, and adult sizes. Cor-responding masks are available. Choose a facemask that properly fits the child's face and that provides a seal over the nose and mouth and excludes the eyes, thus preventing any pressure on the eyes (Fig. 52.6).

▶ *Take NOTE!*

Facemasks should be clear so that the nurse can see the child's lip colour and identify any emesis during resuscitation. Older facemasks were black and should no longer be used.

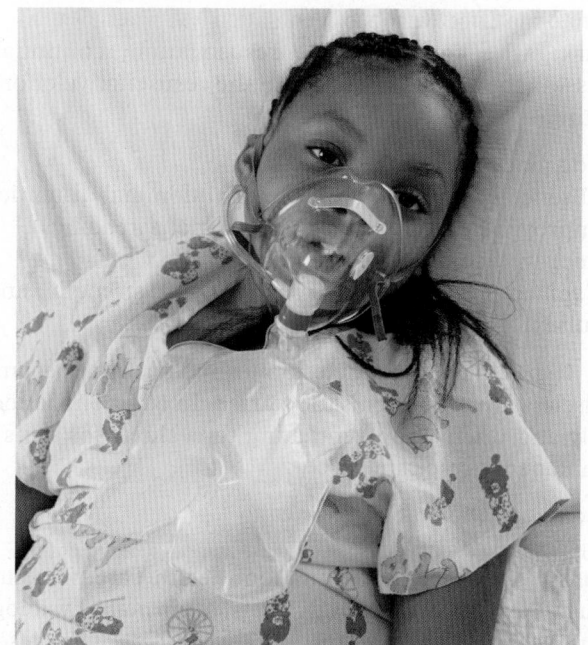

FIGURE 52.5 The non-rebreather mask allows exhalation of carbon dioxide while inhibiting entrainment of room air and is capable of delivering 80% to 100% oxygen.

Connect the BVM via the tubing to the oxygen source and turn on the oxygen. When resuscitating infants and children, set the flow rate at approximately 10 L/minute. For an adolescent who is adult-sized, set the flow rate at 15 L/minute or higher to compensate for the larger-volume bag. Check to make sure that the oxygen is

flowing through the tubing to the bag. Self-inflating bags do not provide "free-flow" oxygen out of the facemask; manual pumping of the bag is necessary. However, the bags have a corrugated plastic tail that allows oxygen to flow freely. Therefore, check over the tail for oxygen flow through the bag.

After opening the airway appropriately (see above), place the mask over the child's mouth and nose. When one rescuer is providing ventilation (commonly referred to as "bagging"), the person must provide a seal with the mask over the child's face with one hand and use the other hand to manipulate the resuscitator bag. The hand used to provide the mask seal will simultaneously maintain the airway in an open position. A technique commonly used is called the E-C hand position. To accomplish this, use the left thumb and index finger, held in the shape of the letter "C," to hold the mask on the child's face. While maintaining a good seal with the mask, place the other three fingers of the left hand, held in the shape of the letter "E," on the lower jaw. Use upward pressure on the jaw angle while pressing downward on the mask below the child's mouth to keep the mouth open (Fig. 52.7). Take care to place the three fingers forming the letter "E" on the mandible and not on the soft tissue of the neck.

If adequate personnel are available, a more desirable situation involves one person standing behind the child's head who maintains an open airway and provides a seal of the mask over the face with a hand on each side (usually the thumbs and index fingers). A second rescuer stands on one side of the child and compresses the bag to ventilate the child using both hands. If the child is

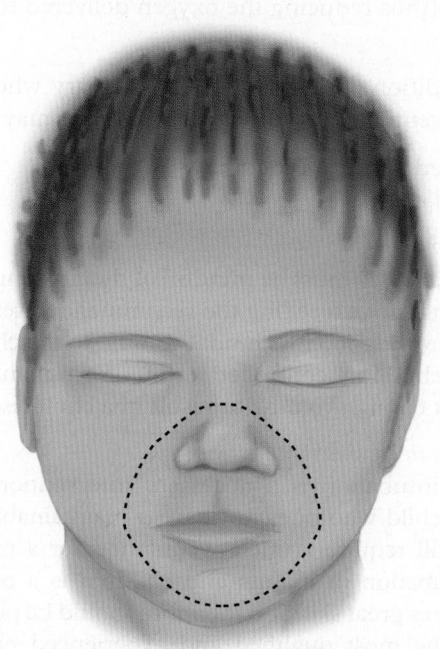

FIGURE 52.6 The mask should form a seal over the nose and mouth, across the chin and nose bridge.

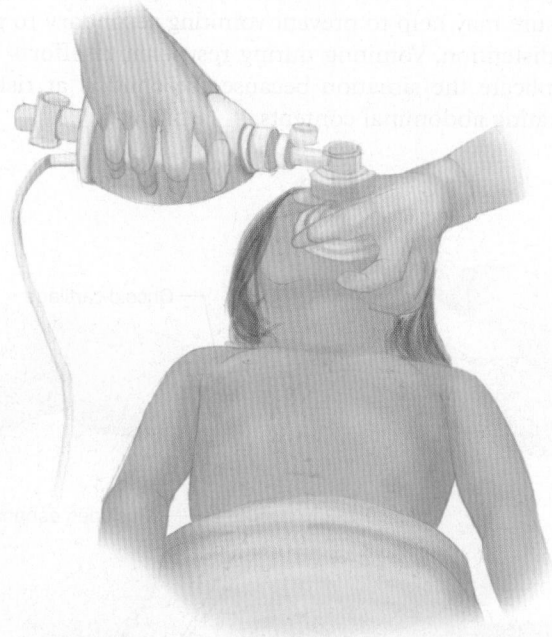

FIGURE 52.7 Proper hand placement for maintaining airway and adequate mask seal using the E-C clamp facemask application technique for one rescuer.

more difficult to ventilate, the two-rescuer method allows the ventilating nurse to provide better ventilation than with the one-rescuer method. In addition, the two-rescuer method ensures the best possible mask seal, as the rescuer holding the mask can use both hands to maintain the seal.

Regardless of the number of persons present, proper placement of the facemask is critical and a good seal must be maintained during the entire course of the resuscitation. In addition, during ventilation, use *only* the force and tidal volume necessary to cause the child's chest to rise. If a good chest rise is not observed, attempt to open the airway again. It may be necessary to adjust the position of the airway a few times to achieve a patency conducive to ventilation.

Initially, provide two rescue breaths and observe for a chest rise. Rescue breaths should not overinflate the lungs. Breaths should be delivered over 1 second. After the first two rescue ventilations, perform rescue breathing at a rate of one breath every 3 to 5 seconds, or about 12 to 20 beats/min. Delivering each breath should be a steady, one-inhalation-to-one-exhalation ratio. This means that the amount of time delivering the inspiratory ventilation is equal to the amount of time that expiration is allowed. While ventilating the infant or child, work with, not against, any spontaneous respiratory effort; in other words, if the child is breathing out, do not attempt to force air in at the same time.

If the child is unconscious and a third rescuer is available, that person can apply cricoid pressure. **Cricoid pressure** (also known as the Sellick manoeuvre) is the use of gentle pressure to occlude the esophagus, preventing air from entering the stomach (Fig. 52.8). Cricoid pressure may help to prevent vomiting secondary to gastric distention. Vomiting during resuscitative efforts can complicate the situation because the child is at risk of aspirating abdominal contents.

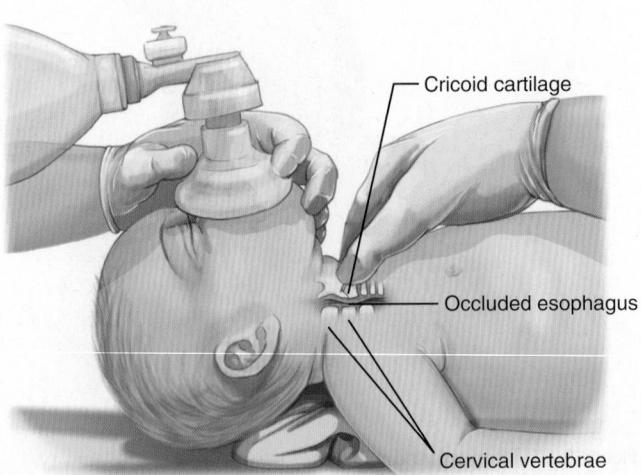

FIGURE 52.8 Applying cricoid pressure.

Cricoid cartilage

Occluded esophagus

Cervical vertebrae

Monitoring Effectiveness of Ventilation

During the course of the resuscitation, continually reassess the child's response to the resuscitative efforts, noting:

- Adequacy of chest rise
- Absence or minimal presence of abdominal distention
- Improved heart rate and pulse oximetry readings
- Improved colour
- Capillary refill less than 3 seconds with strengthening pulses

If the child's status deteriorates and he or she becomes pulseless, then CPR must be started. In addition, periodically and briefly stop ventilating to evaluate for signs of spontaneous respirations.

Preventing Complications Related to Bag-Valve-Mask Ventilation

During a resuscitation situation, health care personnel usually exhibit high energy levels, a normal physiologic response that facilitates resuscitative efforts as the rescuers act quickly. However, this heightened state can lead to overzealousness while ventilating an infant or child. Health care providers may inadvertently ventilate the patient too rapidly using too much tidal volume, leading to excessive ventilation volume and increased airway pressure. This poor technique can be detrimental to the patient, causing:

- Reduced cardiac output (due to increased intrathoracic pressure)
- Air trapping (retention of excess gas in all or part of the lung during expiration)
- **Barotrauma** (trauma caused by changes in pressure)
- Air leak (thus reducing the oxygen delivered to the patient)

In addition, children with head injury who receive excessive ventilation volumes and high rates may develop:

- Decreased cerebral blood flow
- Cerebral edema
- Neurologic damage

Thus, nurses must be mindful of their technique during bagging, not exceeding the recommended respiratory rate or providing too much tidal volume to the child. Ventilate the child in a controlled and uniform manner, providing just enough volume to result in a chest rise.

Assisting with Tracheal Intubation

Tracheal intubation is a necessary intervention for the infant or child who does not have a maintainable airway or who will require artificial ventilation for a prolonged time. Intubation of infants and children is a procedure that requires great skill and therefore should be performed by only the most qualified and experienced personnel. Children are most commonly intubated orally, rather than nasally, in acute situations.

Nursing Procedure 52.1

ASSISTING WITH TRACHEAL INTUBATION

1. Prepare equipment and supplies.
2. Draw up medications (for rapid sequence intubation).
3. Turn up the volume on the cardiac monitor so that members of the team can easily hear the audible QRS indication of the child's heart rate and note any bradycardia with the procedure.
4. Turn on the suction. Make sure that suction is working by placing your hand over the tubing before you attach the suction catheter.
5. Continue to ventilate the child with the BVM and 100% oxygen as the team prepares to intubate the child.
6. In the child over age 2 years with no suspected cervical spine injury, place a small pillow under the child's head to facilitate opening of the airway; this step is unnecessary in children younger than age 2 due to the prominence of their occiput.
7. When assisting with the intubation, stand beside the patient's head and prepare to assist with suctioning of oral secretions, applying cricoid pressure during the insertion of the tube, providing BVM as needed, and assisting with securing the tube with tape.
8. Before the initial intubation attempt and after each subsequent attempt to intubate, provide several inhalations of 100% oxygen via the BVM ventilation method (optimally for a few minutes).
9. Administer premedication and medications for sedation.
10. Administer paralyzing medication.
11. Observe as the health care professional who is intubating the child follows the recommended procedure for intubation using the laryngoscope for visualization of the vocal cords.
12. As the tracheal tube is inserted, apply gentle cricoid pressure (too much pressure can block the trachea) if appropriate.

Nurses are an essential part of the intubation team, usually assisting a physician, nurse practitioner, or respiratory therapist during the intubation procedure (Nursing Procedure 52.1). The nurse may set up the equipment, prepare and administer intubation medications, or assist with suctioning the oral secretions and preparing the tape to secure the tracheal tube. In a child in full arrest, the nurse might be responsible for performing ongoing chest compressions while other team members manage the child's airway.

Setting up Equipment

Appropriate setup and preparation of equipment are essential (Table 52.4). The size of the tracheal tube used depends on the child's size. To calculate tracheal tube size, divide the child's age by 4 and add 4. The resulting number will indicate the size of the tracheal tube in millimetres. For example, if the child is 2 years old, the proper-sized tube would be 4.5 ([2/4] + 4 = 4.5). Always have one size smaller ready also, so have a 4.0 and a 4.5 tracheal tube for this patient. If the child's age is unknown, a Broselow tape will provide a guide for selecting tracheal tube size.

Administering Medications

Several medications are administered commonly to facilitate intubation of children. Pre-medicating a patient before passing a tracheal tube aids in the following:

- Reducing pain and anxiety (consistent with the concept of atraumatic care)
- Minimizing the effects of passing the tracheal tube down the airway (vagal stimulation leading to **bradycardia** [decrease in heart rate])
- Preventing hypoxia
- Reducing intracranial pressure
- Preventing airway trauma and aspiration of stomach contents

The use of medications during the intubation process is known as rapid sequence intubation (Table 52.5). Typically, these medications are used in controlled settings such as the emergency department or the intensive care unit. Rapid sequence intubation is done only in children who are not experiencing cardiac arrest. If the intubation is expected to be particularly difficult, paralyzing medication should not be used.

The nurse must be aware of the differences in the various medication classes as well as their advantages, disadvantages, and adverse effects. The nurse must also be able to distinguish between medications that produce sedation and ones that produce analgesia. Children who are paralyzed and sedated may be suffering severe pain. The pain control needs of children who are acutely ill are of paramount importance and cannot be overstated. Do not mistake a child who is immobilized as a result of sedative and paralytic medications for a child who is pain-free.

Ensuring and Maintaining Correct Tube Placement

Tracheal tube placement can be confirmed by using an end-tidal CO_2 detector to check for the presence of exhaled carbon dioxide and/or by using clinical assessment techniques. When available, use of either a colorimetric device or continuous capnography is recommended to confirm tube placement in patients with a perfusing rhythm (Bingham & Proctor, 2008; Hosono, Inami, Fujita, et al., 2009). Attach the end-tidal CO_2 detector to the tracheal tube; if no CO_2 is detected after six ventilations (a few breaths might be needed to wash out any

TABLE 52.4 EQUIPMENT AND SUPPLIES FOR TRACHEAL INTUBATION

Laryngoscope blades	Straight blades (Miller) are usually used for infants and young children. A curved-blade laryngoscope (Macintosh) may be used for older children and adolescents. The blade has a little light bulb attached to it for visualization of the trachea. The light bulb should be bright and attached securely.
Tracheal tubes	Three sizes should be readily available: the estimated size, a size smaller, and a size larger. A stylet may be used to guide the tube through the child's vocal cords (it is then removed after the intubation procedure).
Oxygen	100% oxygen is provided using a bag-valve-mask before intubation and after unsuccessful intubation attempts.
Suction	Properly working wall or portable suction with appropriate-sized suction catheters (that fit the tracheal tube) should be prepared; the package is opened, leaving the sterile-tipped end inside the package and connecting the other end to the suction tubing. A Yankauer suction catheter (large catheter) should also be available if copious secretions are present in the mouth and interfere with the ability to visualize the airway.
Monitors	Pulse oximeter and cardiac monitor with an audible tone indicating the QRS complex should be in place. Exhaled CO_2 device is needed to detect increased CO_2 levels after the intubation.
Nasogastric (NG) tube	Placing an NG tube will help to mitigate abdominal distention. Patients who are manually ventilated typically have some abdominal distention as some air passes into the stomach.
Personal protective equipment	Usually just gloves, goggles, and a mask are necessary to protect health care workers. In the case of copious bleeding, health care workers should wear gowns also.
Tape, etc.	Tape should be prepared for securing the tube. Benzoin, a sticky substance, is usually applied under the tape for enhanced security of the tape. For children who have had multiple intubations, a protective barrier (as used to protect the skin around an ostomy) may be applied under the tape to protect the skin. Gauze pads should be available to clean up excess secretions that may interfere with taping the tracheal tube.

CO_2 present in the esophagus or stomach), then the tracheal tube is not in the trachea. The presence of exhaled CO_2 detected by the end-tidal CO_2 detector indicates that the tube is in the trachea but does not confirm ideal tube position.

In addition to using an end-tidal CO_2 detector, or if there is no access to this type of equipment, placement of the tracheal tube can be assessed clinically. Observe for symmetric chest rise and auscultate over the lung fields for equal breath sounds. Inspect the tracheal tube for the presence of water vapour on the inside, indicating that the tube is in the trachea. To help rule out accidental esophageal intubation, auscultate over the abdomen while the child is being ventilated: there should not be breath sounds in the abdomen. Note improvement in the oxygen saturation level via pulse oximetry.

Once tracheal tube placement is verified, mark the tube with an indelible pen at the level of the child's lip and secure it with tape. Document the number on the tracheal tube at the level of the child's mouth. Anticipate a chest X-ray to confirm correct placement of the tracheal tube.

After placement is confirmed, the tracheal tube is connected to the ventilator by respiratory personnel. The ventilator will provide continuous artificial ventilation and oxygenation. Continuous capnography is recom-

mended as it provides an indication of appropriate ventilation (Box 52.1). The nurse plays a key role in ensuring that the tracheal tube remains taped securely in place by the following:

- Using soft wrist restraints if necessary to prevent the child from removing the tracheal tube
- Providing sedative and sometimes paralyzing medications
- Using caution when moving the child for obtaining X-rays, changing linens, and performing other procedures

Monitoring the Child Who is Intubated

Provide ongoing and frequent monitoring of the intubated child to determine adequacy of oxygenation and ventilation as noted earlier. Once the child is intubated, the ventilatory support being provided should result in improvement in oxygen saturation and vital signs. If the child begins to exhibit signs of poor oxygenation, perform a quick assessment. Auscultate the lungs for equal air entry and determine the child's heart rate. Are the breath sounds equal? Is the heart rate normal for age? Perform a quick survey of the equipment and look for any disconnected tubes or kinks in the tubing. Determine oxygen

TABLE 52.5 MEDICATIONS FOR RAPID SEQUENCE INTUBATION

Medications	Desired Effects	Undesirable Effects
Anticholinergic: atropine	Decreases respiratory secretions and mitigates the vagal affects of intubation, thus decreasing the risk of bradycardia	Doses that are too low (<0.1 mg) can cause a paradoxical bradycardia.
Sedatives: barbiturates—thiopental (short-acting barbiturate)	Has very rapid onset and short duration of action; reduces intracranial pressure and oxygen demand	Hypotensive effects of this drug are more severe in the dehydrated patient. When given in combination with narcotics, respiratory depression is potentiated.
Sedatives: benzodiazepines—midazolam (Versed)	Has a slightly slower onset than thiopental but is associated with fewer adverse effects Also causes amnesia Can be titrated up or down (at lower doses it causes conscious sedation; at higher doses it can induce anesthesia)	When given in combination with narcotics, respiratory depression is potentiated.
Anesthetic agent: ketamine	Has a rapid onset with sedative, amnesic, and analgesic effects Can be dissociative (child is awake but unaware) May improve BP and cause bronchodilation (helpful for children with status asthmaticus)	Ketamine can cause increases in intracranial ocular pressure. Therefore, children who have suffered head trauma or globe injury should not receive this medication. Because of ketamine's sympathetic effects, hypertension can result from its use. May cause laryngospasm with rapid infusion or concomitant upper respiratory infection Ketamine tends to cause increased secretions, often necessitating the concomitant use of atropine to counteract this adverse effect. May cause hallucinations and is therefore contraindicated in children with psychiatric problems
Anesthetic agent: lidocaine	Can decrease intracranial pressure at higher doses Has an advantage when used in the management of hypovolemia because it is less likely to cause hypotension	Can cause adverse cardiac effects (bradycardia, hypotension, dysrhythmias) in high doses May be associated with CNS depression and seizures
Narcotic analgesic: fentanyl citrate (Sublimaze)	A highly concentrated opioid that causes fewer adverse effects (e.g., pruritus) than other opioids Also exerts a less hypotensive effect	Constipation and urinary retention (as is common with opioids) may occur. Increases risk for respiratory depression, increased intracranial pressure, and hypotension Chest wall rigidity is common with this drug and may cause difficulty with ventilation.
Paralyzing or neuromuscular blocking agents: rocuronium (Zemuron), succinylcholine (Anectine), vecuronium (Norcuron)	Used for short-term paralysis during the intubation process. May be used for extended paralysis in ICU for patient in whom movement would be detrimental. For example, a child with epiglottitis has a very precarious airway and must remain intubated until the epiglottis decreases in size. In certain respiratory conditions, spontaneous respiratory effort would interfere with the ventilation of a patient and therefore prolonged paralysis is desirable.	Succinylcholine (a depolarizing agent) has always been the gold standard for paralysis because it has a relatively rapid onset and is short-acting. However, it has a greater risk of adverse effects (bradycardia, hyperkalemia, hypertension, increased intracranial and ocular pressure) and is contraindicated in a variety of clinical conditions. The contemporary approach to paralysis involves the use of longer-acting agents, such as rocuronium and vecuronium, because patients have fewer adverse effects with these medications. In addition, rocuronium and vecuronium may be used for extended paralysis (not an option with succinylcholine).

BOX 52.1 **Exhaled CO_2 Monitoring: Colorimetric Devices Versus Capnography**

Exhaled CO_2 monitoring is performed using a device that connects to the child's tracheal tube or ventilator circuit to detect CO_2 in the tubing. CO_2 should be noted in the tubing after six ventilations. In the context of cardiac arrest, or in children weighing less than 2 kg, the absence of expired CO_2 does *not* confirm misplacement of the tracheal tube; in these children an alternative method of confirming tracheal tube position should be used (e.g., direct laryngoscopy).

- *Colorimetric devices* are usually colour-coded. In the case of tracheal intubation, watch the colour on the device change from purple to tan to yellow. During intubation, failure to observe the device change to yellow may indicate esophageal placement of the tracheal tube.
  - Advantages: devices are portable, easy to use, and require no power supply.
  - Disadvantages: devices are qualitative rather than quantitative, potentially limiting their use.
- *Capnography* provides continuous quantitative measure of end-tidal CO_2 concentration displayed as a waveform. Failure to observe an end-tidal CO_2 reading following intubation may indicate improper tracheal tube placement.
  - Advantages: quantitative output can provide a good estimate of $PaCO_2$, avoiding the need for repeat arterial blood gas analysis. Use during transport confirms proper tube placement and adequacy of ventilation.
  - Disadvantages: requires calibration, a power supply, and training in proper use of the equipment and interpretation of readings.

saturation levels via pulse oximeter and evaluate the presence of CO_2 (see Box 52.1). Use the PALS mnemonic "DOPE" for troubleshooting when the status of a child who is intubated deteriorates:

D = Displacement. The tracheal tube is displaced from the trachea.
O = Obstruction. The tracheal tube is obstructed, with a mucous plug, for example.
P = Pneumothorax. Usually a pneumothorax results in a sudden change in the child's assessment. The signs of a pneumothorax include decreased breath sounds and decreased chest expansion on the side of the pneumothorax. Subcutaneous emphysema may be noted over the chest. In the case of tension pneumothorax, the child may have a sudden drop in heart rate and BP.
E = Equipment failure. Relatively simple problems as previously discussed, such as a disconnected oxygen supply, can cause the child to deteriorate. Culprits

such as a leak in the ventilator circuit or a loss of power are other types of equipment failure that may be responsible.

Make sure all equipment is appropriately connected and functional. When obstruction with secretions is suspected, suction the tracheal tube. If the tracheal tube is displaced from the trachea, remove the tube if it remains in the child's mouth and begin BVM ventilation. In the case of pneumothorax, prepare to assist with needle thoracotomy.

Preparing the Intubated Child for Transport

Once the child is stabilized with a secure tracheal tube in place, prepare to transport the child. The child will be moved by stretcher to an intensive care unit in the acute care facility or by air or land ambulance to another facility that specializes in the care of acutely ill children. To facilitate transport, make sure that all tubes are securely taped. As the "sending" nurse, ensure that all laboratory results are obtained and provided to your "receiving" colleagues. If the child is going to another facility, complete a detailed summary of the resuscitation or provide a copy of the nurse's and/or progress notes. If possible, send copies of any X-rays taken. Complete the appropriate transfer forms as determined by the institution.

If the child is being transported by ambulance, the parents may not be able to accompany their child. In this case, find out as much as possible about the transport and assist the parents by giving directions to the receiving institution.

Shock

According to the AHA (2007, p. 62), shock is defined as a "critical condition that results from inadequate delivery of oxygen and nutrients to the tissues relative to tissue metabolic demand." If shock is left untreated, cardiopulmonary arrest will result. The severity of shock may be classified by the effect it has on systolic BP. *Compensated* shock occurs when poor perfusion exists without a decrease in BP. In *hypotensive* shock, inadequate perfusion is accompanied by a drop in BP. Unchecked hypotensive shock leads to cardiac arrest and death. The principles of PALS stress the early evaluation and management of children in compensated shock with the goal of preventing hypotensive shock. Once the child in shock is hypotensive, organ perfusion is dramatically impaired and a dire clinical scenario ensues.

Pathophysiology

Shock is the result of dramatic respiratory or hemodynamic compromise. Shock is caused by impaired cardiac output, impaired systemic vascular resistance (SVR), or a combination of both. Cardiac output (CO) is equal to heart rate (HR) times ventricular stroke volume (SV) ($CO = HR \times SV$). Stroke volume is how much blood is ejected from the heart with each beat. Stroke volume is related to left ventricular filling pressure, the impedance to ventricular filling, and myocardial contractility. Left ventricular filling pressure is also known as preload, and the impedance to ventricular filling is commonly called afterload. Young children and infants have relatively small stroke volumes compared with older children and adults. Therefore, infants and young children are different from their adult counterparts in that their cardiac output depends on their heart rate, not their stroke volume. Clinically, in cases of circulatory compromise and compensated shock in infants and children, the heart rate is increased. The exception to this is a paradoxical phenomenon in neonates, who may have bradycardia rather than tachycardia.

SVR or afterload is the impediment to the heart's ventricular ejection. Increased SVR will result in a decrease in blood flow unless the ventricular pressure increases. Increased vascular resistance is a common problem in shock. In children who have shock-related increased SVR, cardiac output will fall unless the ventricle can compensate by increasing pressure. In cardiac insufficiency, the child's heart will have impaired ability to compensate for the increased afterload.

Types of Shock

Shock can be categorized into four types: hypovolemic, distributive, cardiogenic, and obstructive. Hypovolemic shock, the most common type of shock in children, is characterized by a decrease in preload that results in low stroke volume and reduced cardiac output. In children, hypovolemic shock commonly occurs in association with fluid losses. For example, hypovolemic shock may occur with viral or bacterial gastroenteritis that results in vomiting and diarrhea, medications such as diuretics, and heat stroke. Other causes of hypovolemia in children include blood loss, such as from a major traumatic injury, and third spacing of fluid, such as with burns.

Distributive shock is the result of a loss in the SVR. A relative hypovolemia occurs, most often with sepsis, neurogenic injury, and anaphylaxis. In relative hypovolemia, the vascular compartment expands due to systemic vasodilation. This results in a relatively larger vasculature requiring more fluid to maintain cardiac output despite no actual loss of fluid. Septic shock is the most common form of distributive shock and is caused by "infectious organisms or their by-products that stimulate the immune system and trigger release or activation of inflammatory mediators" (AHA, 2007, p. 72). Neurogenic shock is usually caused by an injury to the head or spine leading to a disruption of the sympathetic nervous system, that results in uncontrolled vasodilation and resultant hypotension. Finally, anaphylactic shock results from a severe reaction to an antigen (e.g., food, drug, vaccine).

Cardiogenic shock results from an ineffective pump, the heart, with a resultant decrease in stroke volume. Children who have congenital or acquired cardiac abnor-

malities with a poorly functioning heart are at risk for cardiogenic shock (Fisher, Nelson, Beyersdorf, et al., 2010).

Obstructive shock results from a physical obstruction to normal blood flow that impairs cardiac output, decreases tissue perfusion, and increases SVR (AHA, 2007). Some conditions that may result in obstructive shock include cardiac tamponade, tension pneumothorax, some congenital heart defects, and pulmonary embolism.

Altered microcirculatory status is common in all types of shock. Compensatory mechanisms are activated in response to decreased blood flow. Sympathetic nervous system response results in marked contraction of larger vessel sphincters and arterioles. This compression results in dramatically impaired capillary blood flow. Blood is redirected away from less important body systems, such as the skin and the kidneys, to the vital organs (the heart and brain). During compensated shock, the body can maintain some level of blood flow to the vital organs. Peripheral vasoconstriction, the body's compensatory response to diminished blood flow, often results in the child's ability to maintain a normal or near-normal BP. As shock continues, capillary beds become obstructed by cellular debris, and platelets and white blood cells aggregate. Endothelial damage occurs as a result of capillary congestion. Poor blood flow to the capillaries results in anaerobic metabolism. Lactic acid accumulates, and this can lead to acidosis. In addition, children with septic shock sustain marked endothelial damage as a result of exposure to bacterial toxins.

The cumulative effect of capillary obstruction and dramatically impaired blood flow is tissue ischemia. As tissue ischemia progresses, the child will show signs of altered perfusion to vital organs. For example, as blood flow to the brain is diminished, the child will demonstrate an altered level of consciousness. Altered blood flow to the kidneys will result in decreased urine output or absence of urine output (oliguria). Commonly, the heart rate will increase in the early stages of shock, but as the heart becomes compromised as a result of poor perfusion, the child will become bradycardic. The child will demonstrate an increased respiratory rate in the initial phase of shock. Tachypnea is seen in septic shock as well. In fact, the child may demonstrate marked hyperventilation in an effort to "blow off" carbon dioxide in response to the acidosis that is associated with septic shock.

Nursing Assessment

Nursing assessment of the child in shock includes the health history and physical examination as well as laboratory and diagnostic testing. The nursing assessment must be performed quickly and accurately so that resuscitation can be expedited.

Health History

In shock, the health history is based on the child's presentation. Children with shock are critically ill and require emergent intervention. Therefore, the history is obtained as life-saving interventions are provided. Determine when the child first became ill and treatments that have been given thus far. Inquire about sources of volume loss, such as:

• Vomiting
• Diarrhea
• Decreased oral intake
• Blood loss

Ask when the child last urinated. Investigate for other related symptoms such as behavioural changes or lethargy. Has the child had a fever or rash, complained of headache, or been exposed to anyone with similar symptoms? Inquire about day care attendance and whether the family has recently travelled outside the country. Determine whether the child has a history of a congenital heart defect or other heart condition or if the child has severe allergies. Ask the parent about accidental ingestion of medications or other substances and, for the older child or adolescent, about the possibility of illicit substance use.

Physical Examination

The key to successful shock management is early recognition of the signs and symptoms. Obtain vital signs, noting any alterations. Measure BP, but this is not a reliable method of evaluating for shock in children. Children tend to maintain a normal or slightly lower than normal BP in compensated shock while sacrificing tissue perfusion until the child suffers a cardiopulmonary arrest. Therefore, other components of the circulatory evaluation will be more valuable when assessing a child.

▶ **Take** NOTE!

Bradycardia is a serious sign in neonates and may occur with respiratory compromise, circulatory compromise, and/or overwhelming sepsis.

As with any emergency, evaluate the airway first. Is it patent? Then determine whether the child is breathing. The child in shock will often demonstrate signs of respiratory distress, such as grunting, gasping, nasal flaring, tachypnea, and increased work of breathing. Auscultate breath sounds to determine the adequacy of air entry and airflow. If the child shows signs of respiratory distress, manage the airway and breathing problem first, as discussed earlier in the chapter.

Assess the skin colour. Palpate the skin temperature and determine quality of pulses. Except in special cases, such as distributive shock, the child in shock will generally have darker and cooler extremities with delayed capillary refill. Note the line of demarcation if present. This refers to the point on the distal extremity where cool temperature begins (the proximal portion of the extremity may continue to be warm). In distributive shock, the initial assessment may reveal full and bounding pulses

and warm, erythemic skin. Evaluate the pulse quality. Distal pulses will likely be weaker than central pulses.

Evaluate the child's hydration state and check skin turgor. Decreased elasticity is associated with hypovolemic states, though this is usually a late sign. Observe the child's level of consciousness. Is the child awake and alert, or does the child only respond to voice or stimulation? As shock progresses, the child may become unconscious. Evaluate pupillary responses. Determine urinary output, which will be decreased in the child with shock.

After having evaluated and provided initial life-saving management for airway, breathing, and circulation, evaluate the child's entire body for other disabilities. Traumatic injuries warrant vigilant evaluation for ongoing blood loss, keeping in mind that traumatic injuries may also result in internal blood loss, such as in the child with a femur fracture. Look for signs of malformation, swelling, redness, or pain of the extremities, which may suggest internal blood loss. Also inspect for any open wounds and active sites of bleeding. Children with abdominal injuries also may lose copious amounts of blood internally. Inspect the abdomen for redness, skin discoloration, or distention. Auscultate for bowel sounds in all four quadrants.

Laboratory and Diagnostic Testing

As the child is being resuscitated, laboratory tests and radiographs will be ordered and obtained. However, no diagnostic test should replace the priority of respiratory support, vascular access, and fluid administration. Laboratory results will guide ongoing management. Common laboratory and diagnostic tests used for children with shock include:

• Blood glucose levels: usually performed at the bedside using a glucose metre (e.g., Chem-strip or Accu-check) to obtain a rapid result
• Electrolytes: to evaluate for electrolyte abnormalities
• CBC with differential: to assess for viral or bacterial infection (septic shock) and to evaluate for anemia and platelet abnormalities
• Blood culture: to evaluate for sepsis; preliminary results will not be available for 1 to 2 days
• CRP: to evaluate for infection
• ABG: to assess oxygen and carbon dioxide levels and to provide information about acid–base balance
• Toxicology panel (if ingestion is suspected)
• Lumbar puncture: to evaluate the cerebrospinal fluid for meningitis
• Urinalysis: to evaluate for glucose, ketones, and protein; concentration (specific gravity) is increased in dehydration states
• Urine culture: to evaluate for urinary tract or kidney infection
• Radiographs: to evaluate heart size, to evaluate the lungs for pneumonia or pulmonary edema (present with cardiogenic shock)

Nursing Management

Signs of shock in children warrant an emergent response. Always evaluate and manage the airway and breathing and check for pulses. Initiate CPR if the child is pulseless. All children who have signs and symptoms of shock should receive 100% oxygen via mask. If the child has poor respiratory effort or is apneic, administer 100% oxygen via BVM or tracheal tube (refer to the section on respiratory emergencies for more specific information about management of airway and breathing). As part of ongoing monitoring, institute cardiac and apnea monitoring and assess oxygen saturation levels via pulse oximetry.

Obtaining Vascular Access

Once the airway and breathing are addressed, nursing management of shock focuses on obtaining vascular access and restoring fluid volume. Children with signs of shock should receive generous amounts of isotonic IV fluids rapidly. However, obtaining vascular access in critically ill children can be challenging. Vascular access must be obtained using the quickest route possible in children whose condition is markedly deteriorated, such as those in hypotensive shock.

Various forms of vascular access available for the management of the critically ill child include:

- Peripheral IV route: a large-bore catheter is used to give large amounts of fluid. This route may not be feasible in children with significant vascular compromise.
- Central IV route: central lines can be inserted into the jugular vein and threaded into the superior vena cava. The femoral route is best for obtaining central venous access while CPR is in progress because the insertion procedure will not interfere with life-saving interventions involving the airway and cardiac compressions. The subclavian vein, located under the clavicle, is an alternative route for central access.
- Intraosseous access: intraosseous access, obtained by cannulating the child's bone marrow, is recommended in cases of hypotensive shock or cardiac arrest if IV access cannot be attained rapidly. The preferred site is the anterior tibia. Special intraosseous needles are used (generally a 15-gauge needle for older children, 18-gauge for younger children). The needle is inserted using a firm twisting motion slightly away from the growth plate. Any medications or fluids that can be administered using an IV site can be given using this route. Alternative sites include the femur, the iliac crest, the sternum, and the distal tibia.

Restoring Fluid Volume

Administer IV isotonic fluids, such as LRS or normal saline (the isotonic fluids of choice), rapidly. Administer 20 mL/kg of the prescribed fluid as a bolus, infusing the fluid as rapidly as possible. In general a large-bore syringe, such as a 60 mL syringe attached to a three-way stopcock, is the preferred method for rapid fluid delivery in children. Infusing the fluid via gravity is too slow. The fluid bolus may be repeated several times if required.

▶ **Take** NOTE!

Dextrose solutions are contraindicated in shock because of the risk of complications such as osmotic diuresis, hypokalemia, hyperglycemia, and worsening of ischemic brain injury (AHA, 2007).

Children in septic shock will often require larger volumes of fluid as a result of the increased capillary permeability. Children in shock due to trauma will usually receive a colloid, such as blood, when there is an inadequate response to crystalloid isotonic fluid. After each fluid bolus, reassess the child for signs of a response to the fluid administration.

Insert an indwelling urinary catheter to allow for accurate and frequent measurement of urine output. Indicators of improvement include:

- Improved cardiovascular status: the central and peripheral pulses are stronger. The line of demarcation of extremity coolness is diminishing and capillary refill is improved (time is decreased). BP is improved.
- Improved mental status: the child is more alert (e.g., the child's eyes are open and watching personnel). If the child is younger, he or she may be pulling at the IV line.
- Improved urine output: this may not be noted initially but should be noted over the next few hours; the goal is 1 to 2 mL/kg/hour.

The process of fluid resuscitation involves giving the fluid, assessing and reassessing the child, and documenting findings in the nurses' notes. Children in shock may require as much as 100 to 200 mL/kg of resuscitative fluid during the initial hours of shock management. Most children in shock need and can tolerate this large volume of fluid. Continued reassessment will determine if the child is beginning to experience fluid overload in the form of pulmonary edema (this is rare but may occur in children with pre-existing cardiac conditions or severe chronic pulmonary disease) (AHA, 2007; Prentiss, Mick, Cummings, et al., 2007).

▶ **Take** NOTE!

Be careful not to focus solely on the child's circulatory status; you may overlook signs and symptoms indicating respiratory deterioration.

Administering Medications

In some circumstances, such as distributive shock, fluid alone may not adequately improve the child's status and medications may be ordered adjunctively. Vasoactive medications are used either alone or in combination to improve cardiac output or to increase or decrease SVR. The selection of medications is dictated by the child's cardiac and vascular status. For example, dobutamine is a medication with significant beta-adrenergic effects and thus can improve cardiac contractility. Epinephrine, which affects the heart muscle, is also a powerful vasoconstrictor. Dopamine affects the heart at lower doses but increasingly affects the vasculature with increased doses. Medications may be given as a loading dose, followed by a continuous infusion. When vasoactive drugs are administered, monitor for improvement in heart rate, BP, perfusion, and urine output.

Cardiac Arrhythmias and Arrest

Unlike adults, in whom cardiopulmonary arrest is most often caused by a primary cardiac event, children typically have healthy hearts and thus rarely experience primary cardiac arrest. More commonly they experience cardiopulmonary arrest from gradual deterioration of respiration and/or circulation (AHA, 2005b; Mandt & Rappaport, 2009). In particular, children experiencing a respiratory emergency or shock may deteriorate and eventually demonstrate cardiopulmonary arrest. Thus, the standard of care for managing a child in this situation is vastly different from that for an adult.

Nurses who care for children should be skilled in evaluating and managing respiratory alterations and shock in children, as discussed in previous sections. Overwhelming evidence suggests that if primary respiratory compromise or shock is identified and treated in the critically ill child, a secondary cardiac arrest can be prevented. Rare exceptions do exist, however. For example, electrolyte abnormalities and toxic drug ingestions are primary insults to the cardiovascular system that may lead to a sudden cardiac arrest rather than a gradual progression. Other exceptions in which the child is at risk for a primary and sudden cardiac arrest include:

- History of a serious primary congenital or acquired cardiac defect
- Potentially lethal arrhythmias, such as prolonged QT syndrome
- Hypertrophic or hypotrophic cardiomyopathy
- Traumatic cardiac injury or a sharp blow to the chest, known as "commotion cordis," as can occur when a high-velocity ball impacts the chest

The overwhelming majority of children rarely experience cardiac arrhythmias, so it is beyond the scope of this chapter to discuss the myriad of possible complex rhythm disturbances. Therefore, this discussion is limited to the management of emergent cardiac conditions that are more typically found in children.

Pathophysiology

The AHA (2007) has simplified the nomenclature used to describe pediatric cardiac compromise and has established three major categories of cardiac rhythm disturbances:

"Slow": bradyarrhythmias
"Fast": tachyarrhythmias
"Absent": pulseless, cardiovascular collapse

The pathophysiology, causes, and therapeutic management of each of the categories of rhythm disturbances are discussed below.

Bradyarrhythmias

Bradycardia is a heart rate significantly slower than the patient's normal heart rate for age. Bradycardia in children is most commonly "sinus bradycardia"—in other words, there is not a cardiac nodal abnormality associated with the slowed heart rate. In sinus bradycardia, the P waves and QRS complex remain normal on the ECG. Brief dips in heart rates can be normal, such as when the child sleeps. Children are also susceptible to brief drops in heart rate that are associated with vagal stimulation. For example, passing an orogastric tube down the esophagus of a young infant may induce a temporary bradycardic response. These normal decreases in the child's heart rate should recover with or without stimulation and are not normally associated with signs of altered perfusion.

Less commonly, children manifest bradycardia as a result of cardiac abnormalities and heart block. Infants with bradycardia related to heart block may exhibit poor feeding and tachypnea, whereas older children may demonstrate fatigue, dizziness, and syncope. Comparison Chart 52.2 compares the causes of sinus bradycardia and heart block in children.

In contrast, the child with a serious and possible life-threatening bradyarrhythmia will have a heart rate below 60 beats/min, with signs of altered perfusion. The most

COMPARISON CHART 52.2 **Causes of Sinus Bradycardia Versus Heart Block**

	Sinus Bradycardia	Heart Block
Causes	• Pathologic: medications such as digoxin, hypoxia, hypothermia, head injury • Non-pathologic: well-conditioned athlete	• Congenital: associated with cardiac anomalies • Acquired: endocarditis, rheumatic fever, Kawasaki disease

common causes of profound bradycardia in children are respiratory compromise, hypoxia, and shock. Sustained bradycardia is commonly associated with arrest. It is an ominous sign and should be taken seriously.

Tachyarrhythmias

Children normally have faster heart rates than adults, and fever, fear, and pain are common explanations for significant increases in the heart rate of a child, **tachycardia**. This normal elevation in heart rate is known as sinus tachycardia. However, once the fever is reduced, the child is comforted, or the pain is managed, the heart rate should return close to the child's baseline. Hypoxia and hypovolemia are pathologic reasons for tachycardia in the child. The signs, symptoms, and management of these concerns were discussed in previous sections. If the child has sinus tachycardia that results from any of these causes, the focus is on the underlying cause. It is inappropriate and dangerous to treat sinus tachycardia with medications aimed at decreasing the heart rate or with a defibrillation device.

Tachyarrhythmias in children that are associated with cardiac compromise have unique characteristics that present differently from sinus tachycardia. Examples of these include SVT and VT. One of the most distinguishing differences between SVT and VT is the width of the QRS complex. SVT is typically characterized by a narrow QRS complex (0.08 seconds or less), while VT has a wide QRS complex (greater than 0.08 seconds).

SVT is a cardiac conduction problem in which the heart rate is extremely rapid and the rhythm is very regular, often described as "no beat-to-beat variability." It is the most common arrhythmia causing cardiovascular compromise in infants. The most common cause of SVT is a re-entry problem in the cardiac conduction system. Comparison Chart 52.3 explains the differences between SVT and sinus tachycardia. Commonly, SVT is the result of a genetic cardiac conduction problem such as Wolff–Parkinson–White syndrome. SVT may also be associated with medications such as caffeine and theophylline. Children often can tolerate the characteristically higher heart rate that is associated with SVT for short periods of time. However, the increased demand that is placed on the cardiovascular system usually overtaxes the child and results in signs of congestive heart failure if the SVT continues unchecked for a prolonged time.

VT is a rhythm involving an elevation of the heart rate and a wide QRS complex (greater than 0.08 seconds) that is the result of an abnormal, rapid firing of one or both of the ventricles. VT is a rare arrhythmia in children and usually is associated with a congenital or acquired cardiac abnormality. In addition, prolonged QT syndrome is a conduction abnormality that can result in VT and sudden death in children. Less commonly, ingestion of medications and toxins, acidosis, hypocalcemia, abnormalities of potassium, and hypoxemia have been associated with the development of VT in children.

Cardiac Arrest (Pulseless Rhythms)

According to PALS, "cardiac arrest, also known as cardiopulmonary arrest, is the cessation of circulation of blood as a result of absent or ineffective cardiac mechanical activity" (AHA, 2007). Clinically, the child will be unconscious with no respiratory effort and no palpable pulse. Cardiac arrest can be caused by cardiopulmonary failure, as a result of respiratory failure and/or hypotensive shock, or it can have a primary cardiac etiology. Typically, the most common pulseless arrest rhythms in children are asystole or PEA. **Asystole** occurs when there is no cardiac electrical activity, commonly referred to as a "straight line" on the ECG. The child with PEA has some appreciable rhythm on the ECG but no palpable pulses. PEA may be caused by hypoxemia, hypovolemia, hypothermia, electrolyte imbalance, tamponade, toxin ingestion, tension pneumothorax, or thromboembolism. VT may also present as pulseless. Ventricular fibrillation, once thought to be rare in children, occurs in serious cardiac conditions in which the ventricle is not pumping effectively. It may develop from VT. Ventricular fibrillation is characterized by variable, high-amplitude waveforms (coarse ventricular fibrillation) or a finer, lower-amplitude waveform with no discernible cardiac rhythm (fine ventricular fibrillation). In either case, cardiac output is insufficient.

Nursing Assessment

Nursing assessment of the child with a cardiac emergency includes the health history and physical examination as

---

COMPARISON CHART 52.3 DISTINGUISHING SVT FROM SINUS TACHYCARDIA

	SVT	Sinus Tachycardia
Rate (beats/min)	Infants >220, children >180	Infants <220, children <180
Rhythm	Abrupt onset and termination	Beat-to-beat variability
P waves	Difficult to identify; if present will be retrograde in leads II, III, and VF	Present and normal
QRS	Narrow (<0.08 s)	Normal
History	Usually no significant history	Fever, fluid loss, hypoxia, pain, fear

well as laboratory and diagnostic testing. The nursing assessment must be performed quickly and accurately so that resuscitation can be instituted if needed.

Health History

Obtain a brief health history of the child with a cardiac emergency while simultaneously assessing the child and providing life-saving interventions. Key areas to inquire about include:

• History of cardiac problems, asthma, chromosomal anomaly, delayed growth
• Symptoms such as syncope, dizziness, palpitations or racing heart, chest pain, coughing, wheezing, increased work of breathing
• Activity tolerance with play or feeding: does the child get out of breath, turn blue, or squat during play? Can the child keep up with playmates? Does the infant tire with feedings?
• Precipitating illness, fever, unexplained joint pains, ingested medications
• Participation in a sport before the cardiac event occurred or injury to the chest
• Family history of cardiac problems, sudden death from a cardiac condition, heart attacks at a young age, chromosomal abnormalities

Determine treatment measures performed at the scene. Was CPR initiated? Was an AED used?

Physical Examination

Quickly establish the child's status. A child who is obviously in distress or is arresting must receive emergent life-saving interventions. Briefly perform the assessment while simultaneously providing life-saving interventions.

Inspection and Observation

Assess the child's airway patency and efficiency of breathing. Observe the child's colour, noting circumoral pallor or duskiness or central pallor, mottling, duskiness, or cyanosis. Note any increased work of breathing, grunting, head bobbing, or apnea. Inspect the chest for barrel shape, which may be associated with chronic pulmonary or cardiac disease. Observe the pericardium for the presence of lifts or heaves. Note diaphoresis, anxious appearance, or dysmorphic features (40% to 50% of children with Down syndrome also have a congenital cardiac defect [Chen, 2011]). Determine whether neck vein distention is present. Inspect the fingertips for clubbing, which is indicative of chronic tissue hypoxemia.

Auscultation

Auscultate the breath sounds, noting any crackles or wheezes. Auscultate the heart rate. If the child does not have an adequate pulse, initiate CPR. If the child has a strong, perfusing pulse, complete the cardiac assessment. Auscultate with the diaphragm of the stethoscope first and then listen with the bell. Evaluate all of the ausculta-

tory areas, listening first over the second right interspace (aortic valve) and then over the second left interspace (pulmonic valve); next move to the left lower sternal border (tricuspid area); and finally auscultate over the fifth interspace, midclavicular line (mitral area). Evaluate the rate and rhythm of the heart. Listen for any extra sounds or murmurs. Note and describe the quality, intensity, and location of any cardiac murmurs.

▶ *Take* NOTE!

Murmurs are most often systolic and can be benign or associated with pathology. Murmurs that radiate to the back and are grade III or louder are more likely to be due to a cardiac defect. True diastolic murmurs are rare and almost always have a pathologic origin (Menashe, 2007).

Percussion and Palpation

Percuss between the costal interspaces and note the heart's size. Palpate the heart to find the point of maximal impulse (PMI) and to evaluate for an associated thrill. A thrill feels like a fluttering under the fingers and is associated with cardiac pathology. Palpate and note the quality of the pulses. Evaluate each of the pulses bilaterally and note whether they are absent, faint, normal, or bounding. Compare the quality of pulses on each side of the body and also those of the upper and lower body. Note the skin temperature and evaluate the capillary refill.

Laboratory and Diagnostic Testing

The major diagnostic test used is the ECG. Identify the arrhythmia according to the ECG reading (Fig. 52.9).

Nursing Management

Provide oxygen at 100%. Institute cardiac monitoring and assess oxygen saturation levels via pulse oximeter. Obtain the child's preprinted code drug sheet or use the Broselow tape to obtain the child's height to estimate the tracheal tube sizes and medication dosages that are appropriate for the child. Always remember to intervene in this order: first airway, then breathing, then circulation. The remainder of this discussion will assume that the nurse has initiated interventions for airway and breathing as discussed earlier in the chapter.

▶ *Take* NOTE!

Pay attention to the rhythm on the monitor, but continually monitor the child's pulse. If the child does not have a pulse or has a pulse of less than 60 beats/min with signs of poor perfusion, perform cardiac compressions despite the monitor reading (AHA, 2007).

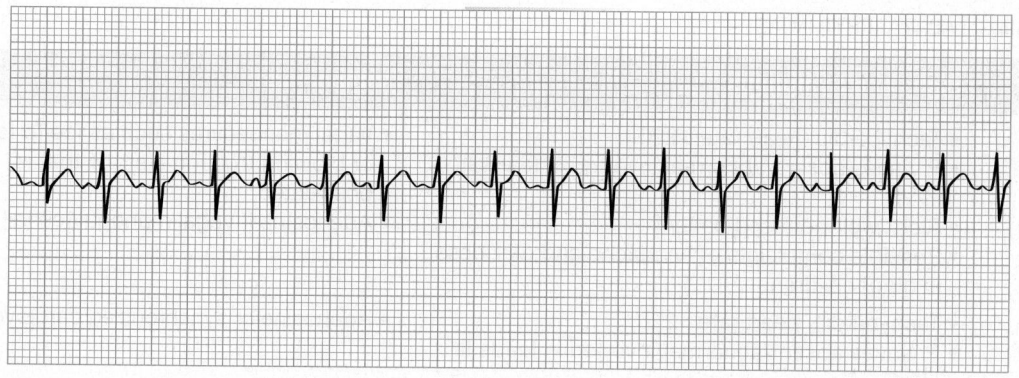

A

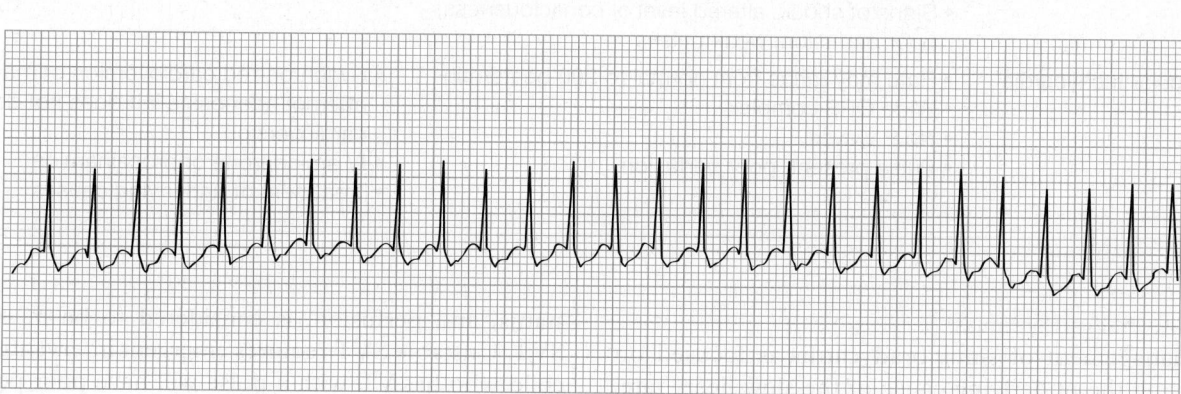

B

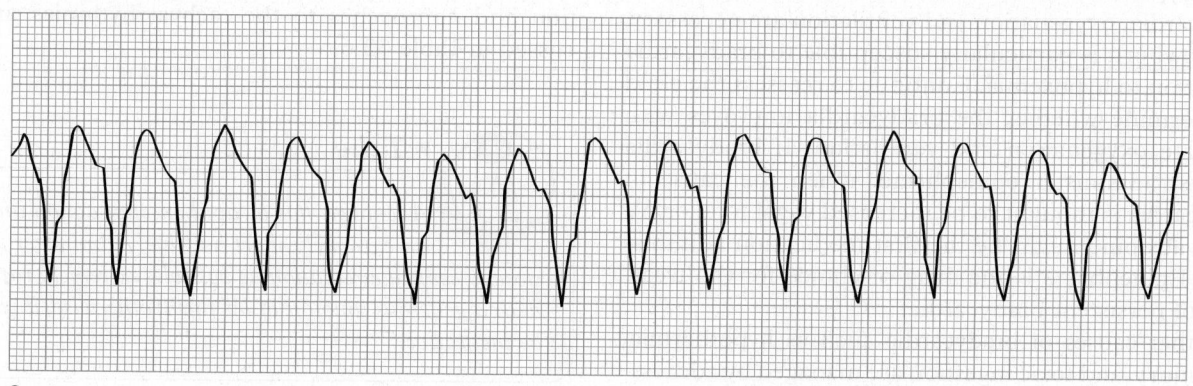

C

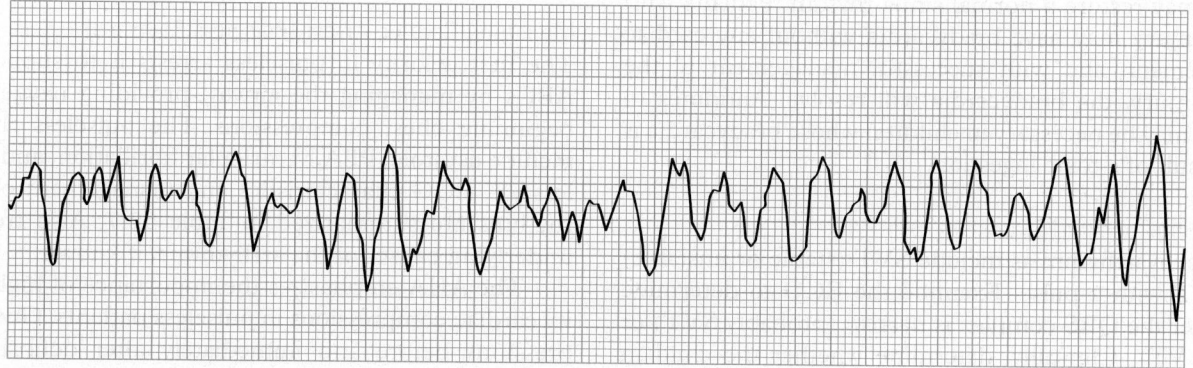

D

FIGURE 52.9 Arrhythmias. (**A**) Sinus tachycardia: normal QRS complex and P waves, mild beat-to-beat variability. (**B**) Supraventricular tachycardia: note rate above 220, abnormal P waves, no beat-to-beat variability. (**C**) Ventricular tachycardia: rapid and regular rhythm, wide QRS complex without P waves. (**D**) Coarse ventricular fibrillation: chaotic electrical activity.

TABLE 52.6 MANAGING TACHYARRHYTHMIAS

Tachyarrhythmia	Signs and Symptoms	Management
Compensated SVT	• Tachycardia, heart rate >220 • P waves absent/abnormal/inverted in leads II/III/VF • Alert, well-perfused patient • Possible complaints of headache and dizziness in older children	• Vagal manoeuvres such as ice to face or blowing through a straw that is obstructed • Adenosine if vagal manoeuvres fail
Uncompensated SVT	• Tachycardia, heart rate >220 • P waves absent/abnormal/inverted in leads II/III/VF • Signs of shock: altered level of consciousness, poor perfusion, weak pulses	• Adenosine or synchronized cardioversion
Ventricular tachycardia	• Rate may range from normal to 200 beats/min • Wide QRS complex • No P waves • Pulse present, poor perfusion	• Synchronized cardioversion or may attempt adenosine if it does not delay cardioversion • IV amiodarone or procainamide • Treatment of underlying causes

Managing Bradyarrhythmias

The management of sinus bradycardia is focused on remedying the underlying cause of the slow heart rate. Since hypoxia is the most common cause of sustained bradycardia, oxygenation and ventilation are necessary. The newborn is particularly susceptible to bradycardia in relation to hypoxemia. Continue to reassess the child to determine whether the bradycardia improves with adequate oxygenation and ventilation. If bradycardia persists, administer epinephrine. When the cause of bradycardia is thought to be increased vagal tone or AV block, atropine might be the first medication administered. Epinephrine is the drug of choice for the treatment of persistent bradycardia.

Other causes of bradycardia such as hypothermia, head injury, and toxic ingestion are managed by addressing the underlying condition. Warming the hypothermic child may restore a normal sinus rhythm. Patients with head injury may have bradycardia without any cardiac involvement, and with successful management of the head injury, the bradycardia will resolve. Antidotes to toxins may be necessary in children whose bradycardia is the result of a toxic ingestion.

Managing Tachyarrhythmias

The tachyarrhythmias include SVT (stable or unstable) and VT with a pulse. Examine the ECG to determine whether the QRS complex is narrow (probably SVT) or wide (VT). Clinically, determine whether the child in SVT is showing signs that require emergent intervention or if the child is stable. In compensated SVT, the child will appear to be alert, breathing comfortably, and well perfused. The child who is demonstrating signs of compromise, such as a change in consciousness, respiratory status, and perfusion, is considered to be in unstable SVT. Unstable SVT requires emergent intervention. The child who has VT with a pulse will have poor perfusion and also requires immediate intervention. The evaluation and approaches to the tachyarrhythmias are discussed in Table 52.6.

▶ **Take** NOTE!

Adenosine has a rapid onset of action and an extremely short half-life. Administer it as close to central circulation as possible, extremely rapidly with a generous amount of IV flush; otherwise, it will be ineffective.

Managing Cardiac Arrest (Pulseless Rhythms)

The first priority in pulseless arrests is to support the ABCs by managing the airway, providing oxygen, and beginning chest compressions. The pulseless rhythms include asystole, PEA, ventricular fibrillation, and pulseless VT. ECG characteristics and management of these rhythms are summarized in Table 52.7. Also treat the underlying causes of the arrhythmia, if known.

The AHA emphasizes the importance of high-quality cardiac compressions in pulseless patients. Give compressions before and immediately after defibrillation. For defibrillation to be most effective, cardiac compressions must be performed effectively ("push fast," "push hard," and "allow for full chest recoil" as recommended by the AHA) with minimal interruptions (AHA, 2005a, 2007; Berg et al., 2008).

TABLE 52.7 **ECG CHARACTERISTICS AND MANAGEMENT OF PULSELESS RHYTHMS**

Pulseless Arrhythmia	ECG Characteristics	Management
Ventricular tachycardia	• Wide QRS complex, no P waves	• CPR • Defibrillation • Epinephrine; also possibly amiodarone, lidocaine, or magnesium • Treatment of underlying causes
Ventricular fibrillation	• Chaotic ventricular activity • No P waves, no QRS complex, no T waves	• CPR • Defibrillation • Epinephrine; also possibly amiodarone, lidocaine, or magnesium • Treat underlying causes
Asystole	• Flat line	• Check lead placement • CPR • Epinephrine • Consider and treat possible contributing factors
Pulseless electrical activity	• Any organized electrical activity observed on the cardiac monitor with no palpable pulse	• Check lead placement • CPR if no pulse • Epinephrine • Treatment of underlying cause

▶ *Take* NOTE!

Previously, multiple doses of epinephrine were given in pediatric emergency situations. However, the AHA now recommends against this practice, as multiple doses of epinephrine have not been shown to be helpful and may actually cause harm to the child.

Submersion Injuries

Water can be a great source of fun and exercise for children and adolescents, but drowning is the second-leading cause of preventable death in children of ages 0 to 19 years in Canada (PHAC, 2009) and of ages 0 to 14 years worldwide (WHO, 2008). Most drowning deaths are preventable, and the WHO (2006) notes that "lapse in adult supervision is the single most important contributory cause for drowning."

Drowning is defined as a submersion injury that results in death. The term "submersion injury" describes a fluid-related immersion injury in which the child survives (Wagner, 2009). Survival and neurologic outcome depend on early and appropriate resuscitation. In recent years, with appropriate resuscitation efforts and treatment, children have demonstrated better neurologic outcomes following submersion injury (Shepherd, Vervive, Cantwell, et al., 2011). Currently, there are no factors to predict whether the child's long-term neurologic status will be affected after surviving a submersion injury (Minto & Woodward, 2005).

Typically, a child who is drowning will struggle to breathe and eventually will aspirate water. Aspiration of relatively small amounts of water leads to poor oxygenation, with retention of carbon dioxide. Alveolar surfactant is depleted during the drowning event, and pulmonary edema commonly occurs. Hypoxemia results in increased capillary permeability and resultant hypovolemia. Even small amounts of aspirated water may lead to pulmonary edema within a 24- to 48-hour period after the submersion episode (Shepherd et al., 2011). A child who has suffered a submersion injury is also at risk for renal complications due to altered renal perfusion during the hypoxemic state.

Nursing Assessment

Nursing assessment of the submersion victim is crucial and must take place quickly and accurately.

Health History

Obtain the history rapidly while providing life-saving interventions. Ask about the circumstances of the event:

• Where did the submersion occur?
• Was the child in a lake, river, ocean, or swimming pool?
• Was the child submerged in a toilet, bucket, or bathtub?
• Did someone witness the child's entry into the water?
• Was the water fresh or salty? Cold or warm?
• Is it likely the water was contaminated?
• Were there any extenuating circumstances, such as a diving or automobile accident, associated with the submersion?

- What was the approximate length of time of the submersion? Was the child conscious or unconscious when rescued?
- What was done at the scene? Was CPR initiated? If so, when?
- If a cervical spine injury was suspected, was the cervical spine immobilized?
- Was an AED used?
- When did the child last eat (to prepare for possible intubation)?

Physical Examination

Evaluate airway patency and breathing. Auscultate all lung fields for signs of pulmonary edema, such as coarseness or crackles. Evaluate the heart rate, pulses, and perfusion. Note the cardiac rhythm on the monitor and report evidence of arrhythmias. Evaluate the child's neurologic status. Use a pen light to determine pupillary reaction. Use the pediatric Glasgow Coma Scale to further assess the neurologic status. Does the child open the eyes spontaneously, to stimuli, or not at all? Is there any spontaneous movement? Is the younger child crying? Can the older child speak? Measure the child's temperature, as hypothermia often occurs with submersion injuries.

Laboratory and Diagnostic Testing

While awaiting laboratory and diagnostic testing results, continue resuscitative efforts as addressed below. Laboratory and diagnostic tests typically include the following:

- ABG: hypoxemia, acidosis
- ECG: cardiac arrhythmias
- Chest X-ray: pulmonary edema, infiltrates
- Serum electrolytes: imbalance related to development of shock

Nursing Management

Because of the potentially devastating effects that submersion-related hypoxia has on the child's brain, airway interventions must be initiated immediately after retrieving a child from the water. Every second counts. Initial interventions in a submersion event are always focused on airway, breathing, and circulation; commonly, resuscitative efforts have begun before the child arrives at the acute care facility.

If a cervical spine injury is suspected (as in the case of a diving accident), provide stabilization either manually or with a cervical collar. As with any suspected neck injury, do not remove the cervical collar until injury to the cervical spine has been ruled out through an X-ray and clinical evaluation. Suction the airway to ensure airway patency. The child may have aspirated particles from a contaminated water source or emesis, a relatively common complication associated with submersion. A large-bore suction catheter such as a Yankauer suction catheter is an effective tool for clearing the upper airway. Administer supplemental oxygen at 100%. Children who have poor or absent respiratory effort most likely will require intubation. Insert a nasogastric tube to decompress the stomach and prevent aspiration of stomach contents. Initiate chest compressions if a pulse is not present.

Usually, the child exhibits some degree of hypothermia and will require warming. Generally, the core body temperature should be raised slowly, as warming a submersion victim too quickly may have deleterious effects. Remove any wet clothing, dry the child, and cover him or her with warmed blankets. Warm IV fluids and use other warming methods as prescribed.

▶ *Consider* THIS!

Eva Dawson, a 2-year-old girl, is rushed into the emergency room by ambulance personnel after experiencing a submersion injury in the family swimming pool. Eva was resuscitated at the scene and is now breathing spontaneously, is lethargic, and coughs occasionally.

What health history information would you obtain from the parents or caregivers? What immediate management is necessary?

What education may be necessary for this family?

Poisoning

Emergency care of the pediatric poisoning patient consists of rapid nursing assessment and prompt management.

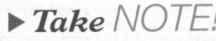 ▶ *Take* NOTE!

If a normally healthy child (particularly a young child) suddenly deteriorates without a known cause, suspect a toxic ingestion.

Nursing Assessment

Nursing assessment of the poisoning victim focuses on a thorough health history, followed by physical examination and laboratory and diagnostic testing.

Health History

Obtain the health history from the parents or caregiver or, in the case of an older child or teenager, from the child. Inquire about the approximate time of poisoning and the nature of the toxin. Was the toxin ingested, inhaled, or applied to the skin? In the case of pill ingestion, does the caregiver have the medication bottle with him or her? Did the child experience nausea, vomiting, anorexia, abdominal pain, or neurologic changes such as disorientation, slurred speech, or altered gait? Determine the progression of the symptoms. Did the parent or caregiver call the poison control centre? Has any treatment been given? In the case of older children and teens, inquire about any history of depression or threatened suicide.

Physical Examination

Ingestion of medications or chemicals may result in a wide variety of clinical manifestations. Perform a thorough physical examination, noting alterations that may occur with particular ingestions, such as:

- Hypertension or hypotension
- Hyperthermia or hypothermia
- Respiratory depression or hyperventilation
- Miosis (pupillary contraction) or mydriasis (pupillary dilation)

Pay particular attention to the child's mental status, skin moisture and colour, and bowel sounds (Barry, 2005).

Laboratory and Diagnostic Testing

The suspected poison may direct the focus of laboratory and diagnostic testing. A variety of blood tests may be performed:

- Chemistry panel: to detect hypoglycemia or metabolic acidosis and assess renal function
- ECG: to identify arrhythmias or conduction delay
- Liver function tests: to assess for liver injury
- Urine and blood toxicology screens (available for a limited number of medications; may vary per institution)
- Specific drug levels if the substance ingested is known or highly suspected

Nursing Management

Management should focus on prevention of poisoning, but when poisoning does occur, give priority to airway, breathing, and circulation, treating alterations as discussed earlier in this chapter. Monitor vital signs frequently as the child's status can change rapidly (McGregor, Parkar, & Rao, 2009). Goals of management for the poisoned child are to limit absorption, maximize elimination, and manage any complications (Criddle, 2007). Few specific antidotes are available for medications or other toxins. Ipecac is rarely used in the health care setting to induce vomiting, and it is no longer recommended for use in the home setting (American Academy of Pediatrics, 2010b; Penny & Moriarty, 2009). Gastric lavage, administration of activated charcoal (binds with the chemical substance in the bowel), or whole bowel irrigation with polyethylene glycol electrolyte solutions may be used. Occasionally, dialysis is required to lower the level of toxin in the bloodstream. The intervention is based on the source of the ingestion. For example, activated charcoal is an effective method for preventing the absorption of many medications but is not effective in the case of an iron overdose.

If opiate or other narcotic ingestion is suspected, administer naloxone to reverse the effects of respiratory depression or alterations in level of consciousness. Treatment of seizures and alterations in thermoregulation may also be needed.

Specific treatment of the poisoning will be determined when the toxin is identified and poison control is queried. Maintain ongoing assessment of the poisoned child because many toxins exhibit very late effects.

> ▶ *Take* NOTE!
>
> *Visit the Canadian Association of Poison Control Centres website to find the poison control number for your province or territory.*

Trauma

In Canada, unintentional injuries are the leading cause of death in children of ages 1 to 19 years (PHAC, 2009). Childhood trauma results from such events as automobile accidents, pedestrian accidents, falls, sporting injuries, burns, and firearm use. Falls are the most common cause of pediatric injury (Safe Kids Canada, 2007). Children of all ages are susceptible to various forms of injury due to their developmental level as well as their environmental exposure. Young children rely on their caregivers to promote their safety. Young children also are not developmentally equipped to be able to recognize dangerous situations.

Nationally, automobile accidents seriously injure about six children each day and, on average, one child per day dies as a result of a motor vehicle collision (Transport Canada, 2010). Pedestrian injuries cause 14% of unintentional injury deaths in Canadian children (Safe Kids Canada, 2007). It is estimated that 1 in every 230 children under the age of 15 years is hospitalized each year with serious injuries such as traumatic brain injuries, internal injuries, and complex fractures (Safe Kids Canada, 2007). Because pediatric injury is so common, nurses must become adept at assessment and intervention in the pediatric trauma victim.

Nursing Assessment

The trauma survey includes a brief health history as the child is being assessed and life-saving measures are being instituted.

Health History

Begin the health history by asking when the injury happened. If the child sustained a motor vehicle-related injury, ask how fast the vehicle was going? Determine whether the child was appropriately restrained in the automobile. If the child was riding a bicycle, skateboarding, or using in-line skates, was he or she wearing a helmet, knee pads, and wrist guards? Determine what interventions were performed at the scene? Was the child immobilized on a backboard to protect the cervical spine? If the child is bleeding, ask the person who transported the child to estimate the amount of blood lost.

If the child experienced a fall, ask if the fall was witnessed and the height from which the child fell. Did the child fall onto a hard surface such as concrete? How did the child land: on his head or back, or did he catch himself with his hands? Younger children and boys are at higher risk for injuring their head. Did the child lose consciousness at the scene? What kind of behaviour did the child exhibit after the fall? Since the fall, has the child complained of a headache or been vomiting?

While obtaining a detailed history about the fall, think about the child's developmental stage. For example, does it seem plausible that a toddler might fall down the stairs? In contrast, what is the likelihood that a 2-month-old would suffer a fractured femur from a fall? Keep in mind the possibility of child abuse. Critically evaluate the reported circumstances and try to determine whether the history, developmental stage of the child, and the type of injury sustained match. In addition, evaluate the type of injury that the child sustained and the history given by the caregiver. For example, children who fall from significant heights often suffer skeletal fractures, but abdominal and chest injuries rarely result from falling from significant heights.

Physical Examination

Physical examination of the child with a traumatic injury should be approached with an evaluation of the ABCs (primary survey) first. Assess airway patency and establish effectiveness of breathing (as discussed earlier in the chapter). Examine the child's respiratory effort and breath sounds. Next, evaluate the circulation. Note the pulse rate and quality. Observe the colour, skin temperature, and perfusion. If bleeding has occurred, the child's circulation may become compromised.

After assessing and intervening for airway, breathing, and circulation, proceed to the secondary survey. Assess for disability. Rapidly assess critical neurologic function. Determine the level of consciousness, pupillary reaction, and verbal and motor responses to auditory and painful stimuli. If the patient is a young infant, palpate the anterior fontanel: a full and bulging fontanel signals increased intracranial pressure. The traumatized child's neurologic status may range from completely normal to comatose.

▶ **Take** NOTE!

Unequal pupils or a fixed and dilated pupil is considered a neurosurgical emergency. Immediately report this finding.

Following ABCs and D (disability) is E (exposure). Expose the child to observe the entire body for signs of injury, whether blunt or penetrating. Perform a systematic, thorough inspection of the child's body. Note active bleeding and extremity deformity as well as evidence of any lacerations and abrasions. Observe for movement and any complaints of immobility or pain with movement. Inspect the abdomen for redness, skin discoloration, or distention. Auscultate for bowel sounds in all four quadrants. If the child is verbal, ask if he or she has any pain in the stomach. If the child is younger, ask, "Do you have a tummy ache?" If the child reports abdominal pain, ask the child to point to where it hurts. Note any guarding of the abdomen, which is an indication of abdominal pain. In the case of potential bowel injury, only light palpation is acceptable. Always assess the least tender areas first and palpate the more sensitive areas last.

Laboratory and Diagnostic Testing

As in other pediatric emergencies, never delay life-saving measures to wait for laboratory or diagnostic test results. In addition to routine laboratory tests, common laboratory and diagnostic tests for the pediatric trauma patient include:

- Type and cross-match: to assess the child's blood type before blood products are given
- Prothrombin time and partial thromboplastin time: to evaluate for clotting dysfunction
- Amylase and lipase: to identify pancreatic injury
- Liver function tests: to assess for liver injury
- Pregnancy test (in any female who has reached puberty)
- CT scan, ultrasound, or MRI of the head, abdomen, or extremities: to evaluate the extent of the injury

Nursing Management

Nursing management of the pediatric trauma victim focuses initially on the ABCs.

Providing Immediate Care

If head or spinal injury is suspected, open the airway using the jaw-thrust manoeuvre with cervical spine stabilization (see Fig. 52.4). The AHA guidelines for basic life support recommend that if the airway cannot be opened using the jaw-thrust manoeuvre, it may be opened using the head tilt–chin lift manoeuvre. The rationale for this is that the jaw thrust is often a difficult manoeuvre to perform. Since opening the airway is the priority, the AHA has made this allowance even if the cervical spine is at risk (AHA, 2005a). In addition, AHA recommendations advise that stabilization of the head and neck of a trauma victim should be provided manually rather than with an immobilization device.

▶ *Take* NOTE!

Infants and young children require unique cervical spine management because they have prominent occiputs that result in flexion of the neck in the supine position. To maintain the optimal neutral spinal position in the young child, use a special pediatric backboard with a head indentation, or use a folded towel to elevate the child's torso.

Clear the airway of obstruction using a large-bore suction device such as a Yankauer. If the child is breathing on his or her own, give the child oxygen at the highest flow possible (such as by a non-rebreathing mask). If the child is not breathing on his or her own, intervene using the AHA guidelines discussed earlier in this chapter.

If a BVM device is available, connect it to the oxygen source and use the bag to ventilate the child. Observe the chest rise and be careful not to overventilate, as this results in abdominal distention. Deliver breaths at the rate recommended by the AHA, one breath every 3 seconds. Do not hyperventilate. In the not-too-distant past, head injury in children was managed using hyperventilation. This resulted in **hypocapnia** (decreased amounts of carbon dioxide in the blood). The physiologic effect of hypocapnia is the induction of vasoconstriction, which in turn results in tissue ischemia. Therefore, current management of head injury in children excludes hyperventilation. The only exception to this rule is in an acute situation, if the child is showing signs of a possible brainstem herniation, hyperventilation may be used initially and briefly.

Assess the child for a strong central pulse. If the child has no pulse, initiate CPR immediately. When perfusion is compromised, administer IV fluid resuscitation. Trauma victims are more likely to require colloids or blood products due to blood loss from the injury.

▶ *Take* NOTE!

Patients with head injury who are demonstrating signs of shock such as poor perfusion and bradycardia should receive fluid volume resuscitation.

▪▪▪ Key Concepts

▪ Young children's smaller airways and immature respiratory and immune systems place them at higher risk for respiratory distress than older children and adults. Children generally have healthy hearts and cardiovascular systems and thus rarely present with primary cardiac arrest. Younger children and adolescents are at higher risk for injury due to normal development at those ages.

▪ Children present with a variety of emergencies and injuries and must be evaluated and treated in an appropriate and timely fashion to achieve a positive outcome. The health history is obtained rapidly while life-saving measures are performed simultaneously.

▪ Assess the airway, then breathing, then circulation, providing interventions for alterations before moving on to the next assessment. Provide continuous reassessment, as children respond quickly to interventions and deteriorate quickly as well.

▪ Pulse oximetry and capnometry can be the useful tools for evaluating respiratory status. Never delay intervention pending laboratory results if the child's clinical status warrants immediate action.

▪ Provide support and education to the child and family involved in an emergency. Teach families why certain procedures are being done, explaining technical medical interventions in simple terms and, for the child, at his or her developmental level.

▪ Small amounts of edema or secretions can contribute to significant respiratory effort in infants and young children.

▪ Children dehydrate more quickly than adults and experience alterations in perfusion related to hypovolemia.

▪ Children in respiratory distress and shock require supplemental oxygen. Intubation is necessary for the apneic child or the child whose airway is not maintainable.

▪ Accurate assessment of perfusion status and appropriate fluid resuscitation are critical in the prevention and treatment of shock in children.

▪ Life-threatening arrhythmias in children, though uncommon, often must be quickly treated with defibrillation or synchronized cardioversion in addition to CPR.

▪ In the case of submersion injuries, maintain ongoing assessment and intervention of pulmonary status.

▪ Maintain airway, breathing, and circulation in the child who has experienced toxic ingestion and prepare for gastric lavage or administration of activated charcoal.

▪ In addition to intervening for airway, breathing, and circulation problems in the pediatric trauma victim, assess for altered neurologic status and extent of bleeding or injury.

REFERENCES

American Academy of Pediatrics. (2010a). *Glasgow coma scale*. Retrieved December 8, 2011 from https://www.pediatriccareonline.org/pco/ub/view/Point-of-Care-Quick-Reference/397299/all/Glasgow_Coma_Scale?amod=aapea&login=true&nfstatus=401&nftoken=00000000-0000-0000-0000-000000000000&nfstatusdescription=ERROR%3a+No+local+token

American Academy of Pediatrics. (2010b). *Policy statement: Poison treatment in the home*. Retrieved December 9, 2011 from http://aappolicy.aappublications.org/cgi/content/full/pediatrics;112/5/1182

American Heart Association. (2005a). Part 11: Pediatric basic life support. *Circulation, 112*, 156–166.

American Heart Association. (2005b). Part 12: Pediatric advanced life support. *Circulation, 112*, 167–187.

American Heart Association. (2007). *Pediatric advanced life support provider manual.* Dallas, TX: American Heart Association.

Atkinson, P., Chesters, A., & Heinz, P. (2009). Pain management and sedation for children in the emergency department. *British Medical Journal, 339.* doi:10.1136/bmj.b4234

Barry, J. D. (2005). Diagnosis and management of the poisoned child. *Pediatric Annals, 34*(12), 936–946.

Berg, M. D., Nadkarni, V. M., & Berg, R. A. (2008). CPR – Why the new emphasis? *Pediatric Clinics of North America, 55*, 861–872. doi:10.1016/j.pcl.2008.04.005

Bingham, R. M., & Proctor, L. T. (2008). Airway management. *Pediatric Clinics of North America, 55*, 873–886. doi:10.1016/j.pcl.2008.04.004

Chen, H. (2011). *Genetics of Down syndrome.* Retrieved December 8, 2011 from http://emedicine.medscape.com/article/943216-overview

Cheng, A., & Bhanji, F. (2011). A case-based update: 2010 paediatric basic and advanced life-support guidelines. *Paediatric Child Health, 16*(5), 295–297.

Criddle, L. M. (2007). An overview of pediatric poisonings. *AACN Advanced Critical Care, 18*, 109–118.

DeBoer, S., Seaver, M., & Broselow, J. (2005). Color coding to reduce errors—the Broselow–Luten system streamlines pediatric emergency treatment. *American Journal of Nursing, 105*(8), 68–71.

Doniger, S. J., & Sharieff, G. Q. (2009). To improve survival: An overview of pediatric resuscitation and the updated PALS guidelines. *Minerva Pediatrica, 61*, 129–139.

Donoghue, A. J., Nadkarni, V., Berg, R. A., et al. (2005). Out-of-hospital pediatric cardiac arrest: An epidemiologic review and assessment of current knowledge. *Annals of Emergency Medicine, 46*, 512–522. doi:10.1016/j.annemergmed.2005.05.028

Fisher, J. D., Nelson, D. G., Beyersdorf, H., & Satkowiak, L. J. (2010). Clinical spectrum of shock in the pediatric emergency department. *Pediatric Emergency Care, 26*(9), 622–625.

Fleisher, G. R., & Ludwig, S. (2010). *Textbook of pediatric emergency medicine* (6th ed.). Philadelphia: Lippincott Williams & Wilkins.

Gerein, R. B., Osmond, M. H., Stiell, I. G., Nesbitt, L. P., & Burns, S. (2006). What are the etiology and epidemiology of out-of-hospital pediatric cardiopulmonary arrest in Ontario, Canada? *Academic Emergency Medicine, 13*, 653–658. doi:10.1197/j.aem.2005.12.025

Hosono, S., Inami, I., Fujita, H., Minato, M., Takahashi, S., & Mugishima, H. (2009). A role of end-title CO_2 monitoring for assessment of tracheal intubations in very low birth weight infants during neonatal resuscitation at birth. *Journal of Perinatal Medicine, 37*, 79–84. doi:10.1515/JPM.2009.017

Krieser, D., Nguyen, K., Kerr, D., et al. (2007). Parental weight estimation of their child's weight is more accurate than other weight estimation methods for determining children's weight in an emergency department? *Emergency Medicine Journal, 24*, 756–759. doi:10.1136/emj.2007.047993

Lee, J., Ahmad, S., & Gale, C. (2005). Detection of coins ingested by children using a handheld metal detector: A systematic review. *Emergency Medicine Journal, 22*, 839–844.

Mandt, M. J., & Rappaport, L. D. (2009). Update in pediatric resuscitation. *Advances in Pediatrics, 56*, 359–385.

Maxton, F. J. C. (2008). Parental presence during resuscitation in the PICU: The parents' experience. *Journal of Clinical Nursing, 17*, 3168–3176. doi:10.1111/j.1365-2702.2008.02525.x

McGregor, T., Parkar, M., & Rao, S. (2009). Evaluation and management of common childhood poisonings. *American Family Physician, 79*, 397–403.

Menashe, V. (2007). Heart murmurs. *Pediatrics in Review, 28*, e19–e22.

Minto, G., & Woodward, W. (2005). Drowning and immersion injury. *Anaesthesia and Intensive Care Medicine, 6*, 321–323.

Moler, F. W., Meert, K., Donaldson, A. E., et al. (2009). In-hospital versus out-of-hospital pediatric cardiac arrest: A multicenter cohort study. *Critical Care Medicine, 37*, 2259–2267. doi:10.1097/CCM.0b013e3181a00a6a

Nibert, L., & Ondrejka, D. (2005). Family presence during pediatric resuscitation: An integrative review for evidence-based practice. *Journal of Pediatric Nursing, 20*, 145–146.

Pagana, K. D., & Pagana, T. J. (2010). *Mosby's manual of diagnostic and laboratory tests* (4th ed.). St. Louis, MO: Mosby.

Penny, L., & Moriarty, T. (2009). Poisoning in children. *Continuing Education in Anaesthesia, Critical Care & Pain, 9*(4), 109–113.

Prentiss, K. A., Mick, N. W., Cummings, B. M., et al. (2007). *Emergency management of the pediatric client.* Philadelphia: Lippincott Williams & Wilkins.

Public Health Agency of Canada. (2009). *Child and youth injury in review: Spotlight on consumer product safety.* Retrieved June 4, 2011 from http://www.phac-aspc.gc.ca/publicat/cyi-bej/2009/pdf/injrep-rapbles2009_eng.pdf

Ramlakhan, S. L., Burke, D. P., & Gilchrist, J. (2006). Things that go beep: Experience with an ED guideline for use of a handheld metal detector in the management of ingested non-hazardous metallic foreign bodies. *Emergency Medicine Journal, 23*, 456–460. doi:10.1136/emj.2005.029553

Rusen, I. D., Liu, S., Sauve, R., Joseph, K. S., & Kramer, M. S. (2004). *Sudden infant death syndrome in Canada: Trends in rates and risk factors, 1985–1998.* Retrieved December 8, 2011 from http://www.phac-aspc.gc.ca/publicat/cdic-mcbc/25-1/a-eng.php

Safe Kids Canada. (2007). *Child & youth unintentional injury 1994–2003: 10 years in review.* Retrieved December 9, 2011 from http://www.ccsd.ca/pccy/2006/pdf/skc_injuries.pdf

Shepherd, S. M., Vervive, M. J., Cantwell, G. P., & Shoff, W. H. (2011). *Drowning.* Retrieved December 8, 2011 from http://emedicine.medscape.com/article/908677-overview

So, T., Farrington, E., & Absher, R. K. (2009). Evaluation of the accuracy of different methods used to estimate weights in the pediatric population. *Pediatrics, 123*, e1045–e1051. doi:10.1542/peds.2008-1968

Taketokmo, C. K., Hodding, J. H., & Kraus, D. M. (2010). *Lexi-comp's pediatric dosage handbook* (17th ed.). Hudson, OH: Lexi-comp.

Tibballs, J., & Kinney, S. (2006). A prospective study of outcome of inpatient paediatric cardiopulmonary arrest. *Resuscitation, 71*, 310–318. doi:10.1016/j.resuscitation.2006.05.009

Tinsley, C., Hill, J. B., Shah, J., et al. (2008). Experience of families during cardiopulmonary resuscitation in a pediatric intensive care unit. *Pediatrics, 122*, e799–e804. doi:10.1542/peds.2007-3650

Topjian, A. A., Berg, R. A., & Nadkarni, V. M. (2008). Pediatric cardiopulmonary resuscitation: Advances in science, techniques, and outcomes. *Pediatrics, 122*, 1086–1098. doi:10.1542/peds.2007-3313

Transport Canada. (2010). *Canadian motor vehicle collision statistics: 2007.* Retrieved December 8, 2011 from http://www.tc.gc.ca/media/documents/roadsafety/tp3322-2007.pdf

Wagner, C. (2009). Pediatric submersion injuries. *Air Medical Journal, 28*, 116–119.

Walco, G. A. (2008). Needle pain in children: Contextual factors. *Pediatrics, 122*, S125–S129. doi:10.1542/peds.2008-1055d

World Health Organization. (2006). *Facts about injuries: Drowning.* Retrieved June 4, 2011 from http://www.who.int/violence_injury_prevention/publications/other_injury/en/drowning_factsheet.pdf

World Health Organization. (2008). *World report on child injury prevention.* Retrieved June 4, 2011 from http://whqlibdoc.who.int/publications/2008/9789241563574_eng.pdf

Zideman, D. A., & Hazinski, M. F. (2008). Background and epidemiology of pediatric cardiac arrest. *Pediatric Clinics of North America, 55*, 847–859. doi:10.1016/j.pcl.2008.04.010

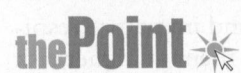

the Point For additional learning materials, including Internet Resources, visit **http://thePoint.lww.com/Chow1e.**

CHAPTER WORKSHEET

MULTIPLE CHOICE QUESTIONS

1. An unresponsive toddler is brought to the emergency department. Assessment reveals mottled skin colour, respiratory rate of 10 beats/min, and a brachial pulse of 52 beats/min. What is the priority nursing action?

   a. Prepare the defibrillator and draw up code medications.

   b. Provide 100% oxygen with a BVM and start chest compressions.

   c. Start chest compressions and provide 100% oxygen via non-rebreather mask.

   d. Begin an IV fluid infusion and administer epinephrine IV.

2. A 10-year-old child in respiratory distress requires intubation. Which sizes of tracheal tubes will the nurse prepare?

   a. 9.5 and 10.0 mm

   b. 8.5 and 9.0 mm

   c. 6.0 and 6.5 mm

   d. 6.5 and 7.0 mm

3. A preschooler presents to the emergency department with a history of vomiting, diarrhea, and fever over the past few days. She is receiving 100% oxygen via non-rebreather mask. Vital signs are temperature 40.2°C, pulse 144 beats/min, respiratory rate 22 beats/min, and BP 70/50 mm Hg. She is listless and difficult to arouse and has weak peripheral pulses and prolonged capillary refill. What nursing intervention takes priority?

   a. Administering acetaminophen rectally for the high fever

   b. Administering IV antibiotics for the infection

   c. Preparing the child for tracheal intubation

   d. Giving an IV bolus of normal saline 20 mL/kg

4. Assessment of a 12-year-old who crashed his bicycle without a helmet reveals the following: temperature 37.3°C, pulse 100 beats/min, respiratory rate 24 beats/min with easy work of breathing, and BP 115/70 mm Hg. What is the priority action by the nurse?

   a. Assess neurologic status while observing for obvious injuries.

   b. Administer IV fluid bolus of normal saline at 20 mL/kg.

   c. Remove the cervical collar if he complains that it bothers him.

   d. Listen for bowel sounds while assessing for pain.

5. An 18-month-old child is brought to the emergency department via ambulance after an accidental ingestion. What is the priority nursing action?

   a. Take the child's vital signs.

   b. Give oral syrup of ipecac.

   c. Insert a nasogastric tube.

   d. Start an IV line.

CRITICAL THINKING EXERCISES

1. A school-age child presents to the emergency department for evaluation. He had been feeling faint off and on and today fainted at school. On the cardiac monitor an abnormal cardiac rhythm is noted. At present the child is stable. What questions would be most appropriate for the nurse to ask when obtaining the child's health history? What objective assessments should the nurse make?

2. Charlie is a 2-year-old who is admitted to the hospital after accidentally ingesting a medication. His mother, who brought Charlie to the hospital, is upset and crying. How does Charlie's age and stage of development affect his risk for accidental ingestion? How should the nurse respond to the mother's distress? Develop a discharge teaching plan for Charlie and his family related to poison prevention.

(question continues on page 1820)

3. A 7-month-old is brought to the acute care facility with a chief complaint of difficulty breathing. The infant's mother says that his cold has gotten worse and he won't eat. What additional questions should the nurse ask about the infant's health history? How would the nurse appropriately manage this infant's airway?

STUDY ACTIVITIES

1. Spend a day in the pediatric emergency department or urgent care centre and document the role of the triage nurse.

2. Observe the pediatric emergency medical team at work or observe a pediatric code in the hospital. Compare and contrast the measures performed for the child with those that would be performed for an adult in a similar emergency situation.

3. Develop a teaching project related to injury prevention and present it at a local elementary, middle, or high school. Ensure that the education is geared toward the children's developmental level.

4. Interview the parents of a child who has experienced an emergency situation about how they felt during and after the emergency. Present the information to your classmates.

5. When providing care to a child in an emergency, the nurse performs the following assessments. Place them in the proper sequence.

   a. Pupillary reaction

   b. Presence of cough or sputum

   c. Heart rate and capillary refill

   d. Presence of bruises and abrasions

   e. Work of breathing

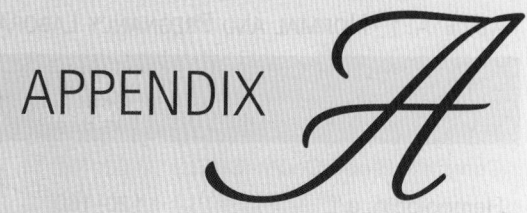

APPENDIX *A*

LABORATORY VALUES

TABLE A.1 NORMAL AND PREGNANCY LABORATORY VALUES

	Non-Pregnant	Pregnant	Gestational Hypertension	HELLP	DIC
Complete Blood Count (CBC)					
Hemoglobin, g/L	120–160	100–130	Higher as a result of hemocon-centration Exception: micro-angiopathic hemolytic anemia	Decrease	
Hematocrit, L/L	0.4–0.54	0.36–0.48	Increase	Decrease	
RBC 10E12/L	4.0–5.6	4.0–5.6			
MCV fL	80–100	80–100			
RDW	11.0–16%	11.0–16%			
Red cell volume, mL	0.38–0.48				
Platelets 10E9/L	150–400	150–400 Slight increase	Decrease	Decrease	Decrease
White Blood Cells Platelets 10E9/L	4.0–11.0	4.0–11.0 Increase up to 20	Higher (Due primarily to exaggerated neutrophilia)		
Neutrophils 10E9/L	2.0–8.0	2.0–9.0 May increase			
Lymphocytes 10E9/L	0.7–3.5	0.5–3.3			
Bands 10E9/L	0.2–1.3	Increase with infection			
Eosinophils 10E9/L	0.0–0.7	0.0–0.7 No change			
Basophils 10E9/L	0.0–0.2	0.0–0.2 No change			
Blood Volume (mL)		Increases about 45%			
Partial Thromoboplastin Time (APTT)	25–35 s		Increased	Thrombocytopenia	Increased
Bleeding time	2.5–9.0				
Electrolytes and Chemistry					
Chloride (mmol/L)	98–111	98–111			
CO_2 (mmol/L)	21–31	21–31			
Potassium (mmol/L)	3.5–5.0	3.3–5.1			
Sodium (mmol/L)	135–145	133–145			
Creatinine (mmol/L)	60–124	35–100 umol/L	Higher (Hemo-concentration and/or renal failure)	Higher	
Calcium	2.11–2.55	2.10–2.55			
Alanine Transaminase	1–40	1–40			

	Non-Pregnant	Pregnant	Gestational Hypertension	HELLP	DIC
Bilirubin, Total umol/L	0–20	0–20 No change	Higher	Higher	
Gamma Glutamyl Transferase U/L	8–35	8–35			
Lipase U/L	0–60	0–60			
Magnesium mmol/L	0.65–1.05	0.65–1.05			
Phosphate mmol/L	0.8-1.50	0.8-1.50			
Albumin g/L	30–55	33–48	Lower		
Cholesterol	<5.2	Increase 30–40%			
Urate (mmol/L)	140–350	140–350 umol/L	Increase	Increase	
Urea (mmol/L)	3.5–9.2	Decrease	Increase	Increase	
Bilirubin	0–20	No change	Increase	Increase	
Alk Phosp (u/L)	30–115	Increase	Increase	Increase	
CK (u/L)	<170	No change			
Lactate dehydrogenase (u/L)	100–235	No change		May be very high	
AST (u/L)	0–41	No change	Increase	2–10 times upper reference limits	
ALT (u/L)	7–56	No change	Increase	2–10 times upper reference limits	
Blood Sugar					
Glucose (mmol/L)	3.6–6.1	No change	May decrease		
Fasting	3.9–6.1	3.8–5.2			
1-hour postprandial, mmol/L		5.5–7.7			
2-hour postprandial, mmol/L	3.6–11.1	5.0–6.6			

Adapted from Alberta Health Services. Directory of tests. Retrieved February 21, 2012 from www.calgarylabservices.com/lab-services-guide/lab-tests/; Burtis, C.A., Ashwood, E.R., & Bruns, D.E. (2006). Tietz textbook of clinical chemistry and molecular diagnosis. St. Louis: Elsevier; Calgary Health Region. (2006). The antepartum experience: A staff handbook. Calgary Author; and Canadian Diabetes Association (2012). Gestational diabetes: Preventing complications in pregnancy. Retrieved February 5, 2012 from www.diabetes.ca/diabetes-and-you/what/gestational/.

CLINICAL PATHS

TABLE B.1 LABOUR AND DELIVERY CLINICAL PATH—LABOUR: EXPECTED OUTCOMES

	Active Phase	Expulsion/Pushing	Recovery First Hour Post Partum
PATIENT EDUCATION	Patient coping with labour support Patient utilizing appropriate labour options Patient verbalizes satisfaction with plan Management interventions	Patient demonstrates effective pushing technique Patient coping effectively with pushing Support person coping effectively with labour.	Bonding appropriately with baby

PATIENT STATUS	Cervix dilated 5 cm—complete
	Contraction regularly with progressive cervical change
	Maternal/fetal well-being maintained
	Hydration maintained
	If indicated: FSE and/or IUPC placed
	  IV Syntocinon (Pitocin) started
	  Epidural placed/WE encouraged
	  Medicate with prn pain meds
		Vaginal birth	Placenta delivered
			Fundus firm
			Lochia small–moderate
			Without clots
			Perineum intact/repaired
			Hemodynamically stable
			EBL <500 cc

CONTINUUM OF CARE	Prenatal record available after 32 weeks Prenatal labs WNL Pre-registered to hospital Pediatrician identified Support after hospitalization identified Discharge plan discussed with patient/family Communicates understanding of hospital and community resources		

ASSESSMENT/TREATMENT	**Intervention**
	Assess: continuous EFM or auscultation
	Q15 of 30 min as indicated.
	Vital signs hourly/Temp Q4h if intact membranes/Q2h if membranes ruptured
	Uterine by monitor or palpation
	Bladder for distention
	Hydration status
	Cervical dilation, effacement, station
		Assess: Q15min monitoring of fetal well being (low risk) and Q5min (high risk)
		Vital signs hourly Temp. Q2–4 h depending on membrane status
		Bladder for distention
		Hydration status
		Pushing effectiveness
		Descent of presenting part
		Caput
			Assess: Uterus—fundus
			  Vital signs
			  Lochia
			  Bladder
			  Perineum
			  Placenta

PATIENT EDUCATION	Reinforce comfort measures Encourage use of labour options Inform patient/support person of plan of care	Teaching of upright pushing positions Discourage prolonged maternal breath holding Encourage to assume position of choice Inform patient of progress	Baby status Breastfeeding

(continued)

TABLE B.1   LABOUR AND DELIVERY CLINICAL PATH—LABOUR: EXPECTED OUTCOMES (continued)

	Active Phase	Expulsion/Pushing	Recovery First Hour Post Partum
TESTS/PROCEDURES	Hgb or Hct (if not done recently) T & S (if ordered) VE as indicated IV therapy AROM by MD or midwife: assess for colour, amount and odour, as appropriate FSE/IUPC placement if indicated	AROM: assess for colour, amount and odour, as appropriate	Cord blood or Rhogam workup if appropriate Cord blood if O+ Mom
THERAPIES	Comfort measures/birthing ball/ ambulate/telemetry/shower IV therapy Amino-infusion for variable decelerations If appropriate, Pain Mgmt. reviewed	Perineal massage Warm soaks to perineal area Allow to rest until feels urge to push Frequent position changes Cool cloth/ice chips	Ice pack to perineum Warm blankets
MEDS	Antibiotics as indicated for + GBS Syntocinon (Pitocin) if indicated PRN pain medication (encourage WE if requesting this) Labour option usage	Syntocinon (Pitocin) if indicated	Syntocinon (Pitocin) IV
ACTIVITY/SAFETY	Position changes	Provide wedge if supine Promote effective position for pushing: i.e., squatting, side lying, upright Breathing technique patient/support person most comfortable with	Assist with ambulate to bathroom Infant care Assist with positioning for breastfeeding Infant ID bands present
UNIQUE PATIENT NEEDS NUTRITION	Clear liquids Ice chips OTHER	Clear liquids Ice chips	Return to previous diet

WE, walking epidural.

TABLE B.2   INTEGRATED PLAN OF CARE FOR CESAREAN DELIVERY

		Expected Patient Outcomes		
	Phase 1 Preadmission (Cesarean Delivery)	Phase 2 Surgery/ Immediate Postop/Day of Surgery	Phase 3 Postop Day 1	
Usual time in Phase	**N/A Date Started:**	Up to 23 h	1 day	1–2 days
Assessment/ Potential Complications	VS WNL for patient Hgb or Hct/values within normal SLH antepartum range	VS WNL for patient systems assessment: skin warm, dry Clear ⇒ Alert and oriented ⇒ Neg. Homans' sign ⇒ Breast soft/nipples intact ⇒ Lungs clear ⇒ Bowel sounds present ⇒ Fundus firm u/u or u 1–2 (–/+) Lochia sm—mod Dsg dry and intact No signs infiltration IV site Verbalizes comfort using pain rating scale 0–10	VS WNL for patient Afebrile Voiding without foley ⇒ Passing flatus Incision without redness or drainage Lochia small amount Fundus firm u/1–2 Verbalizes comfort using pain scale 0–10 on oral pain meds	Incision well approximated, without drainage or redness Passing flatus Lochia sm/mod amt Fundus firm u/1–2 Verbalizes comfort using pain medication as described
	Date all Above Met	**Date all Above Met**	**Date all Above Met**	**Date all Above Met**
Patient/Family knowledge	Verbalizes understanding of condition and need for surgery Verbalizes understanding of all pre-op teaching	Verbalizes correct use of PCA/Fentanyl pump and when to request pain medication Turn, cough and deep breath appropriately	Can state criteria for when to call doctor for problems post discharge ⇒ ↑ bleeding ↑ Temperature ⇒ incision redness, odour or drainage ⇒	Verbalizes follow-up appointment date and time Verbalizes proper dosing of pain medication
	Date all Above Met	**Date all Above Met**	**Date all Above Met**	**Date all Above Met**
ADL's/Activity	Verbalizes understanding of NPO status	Able to ambulate with minimal assistance Tolerating clear/full liquid diet Bonding observed with newborn—Taking-in phase ⇒	Ambulating without assistance Tolerating soft to regular diet	Ambulating in hall
	Date all Above Met	**Date all Above Met**	**Date all Above Met**	**Date all Above Met**

(continued)

TABLE B.2 INTEGRATED PLAN OF CARE FOR CESAREAN DELIVERY (continued)

	Expected Patient Outcomes			
Plan of Care	Phase 1 Preadmission (Cesarean Delivery)	Phase 2 Surgery/ Immediate Postop/Day of Surgery	Phase 3 Postop Day 1	
Unique Patient Needs	**Date all Above Met Entire Phase Outcomes Met; Progress patient to next phase**	**Date all Above Met Entire Phase Outcomes Met; Progress patient to next phase**	**Date all Above Met Entire Phase Outcomes Met; Progress patient to next phase**	**Date all Above Met Entire Phase Outcomes Met; Progress patient to next phase**
Assessments	Vital signs Fetal status immediately prior to surgery	VS per PACU then q4h Systems assessment: • Skin, LOC, FROM, Homans' sign • Breasts, lungs, fundus, incision • Lochia, bladder, bowel sounds, IV and site • I & Oq shift • Assess pain control 0–10 scale • Assess Rhogam status • Assess Rubella titer status • ID band on mother	VS q 6 hr Assess pain control 0–10 scale Incision Foley-volding Fundus/lochia Homans' sign IV site Breasts ID band on mother Activity	Assess pain control 0–10 scale Incision Volding Fundus lochia Homans' sign IV site as needed ID band on mother Activity
Consults	Anesthesia	Social work as needed, anesthesia, lactation, dietitian as needed	Social work, lactation, dietitian as needed	Social work, lactation, dietitian as needed
Patient/Family Education Discharge Planning	• Need for surgery • Review cesarean delivery • Review procedure, postop expectations • Demonstrate/Discuss equipment—PCA, Fentanyl pump • Tour of OR area & Nsy	Review postop expectations Review equipment us prn Instruct pt on: Hospital/Infant security systems Unity orientation Newborn orientation/ care/feeding (if breastfeeding problems see decision trees)	Review dietary needs post surgery Review bleeding/ lochia Precautions post cesarean delivery Review follow-up care and doctor Appointments Review incision care, peri care Infant care Infant feeding	Verify follow-up appointment date and time Activity restrictions Follow-up for staple removal as needed Offer home follow-up care Discuss birth control
Tests and Procedures	PAT; Hgb or Hot (if not done recently—within 1 month) T & S (if ordered)			
Pharmacologic Needs		IV fluids as ordered Pain control: PCA, Fentanyl pump, IM to PO	IV lock PO pain meds Give Rhogam if indicated Give Rubella if indicated	DC IV lock as ordered

		Expected Patient Outcomes		
	Phase 1 Preadmission (Cesarean Delivery)	Phase 2 Surgery/ Immediate Postop/Day of Surgery	Phase 3 Postop Day 1	
Activity/ Rehabilitation	Patient's usual	Change position q2h while in bed, OOB stand at bedside post-op night/ dangle and transfer to chair Progress to pt. endurance Observe bonding with infant Observe family support system (if inadequate consult SW)	Progress endurance/ begin Ambulation in hall OOB in AM May shower	Ambulate in halls without assistance
Nutrition/ Elimination		NPO then clear liquids to DAT Foley empty q shift	DAT to regular or previous diet at home Foley DC'd	
Miscellaneous Interventions		TCDB q2h while awake	Dressing removed by MD or RN with MD request	
Unique Patient Needs				

PACU, post-anesthesia care unit; LOC, level of consciousness; FROM, full range of motion; US, ultrasound; PAT, pre-admission testing; OOB, out of bed; TCDB, turn, cough, deep breath.

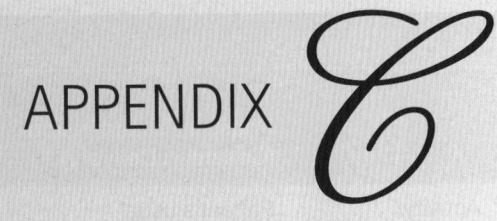

APPENDIX

CERVICAL DILATION CHART

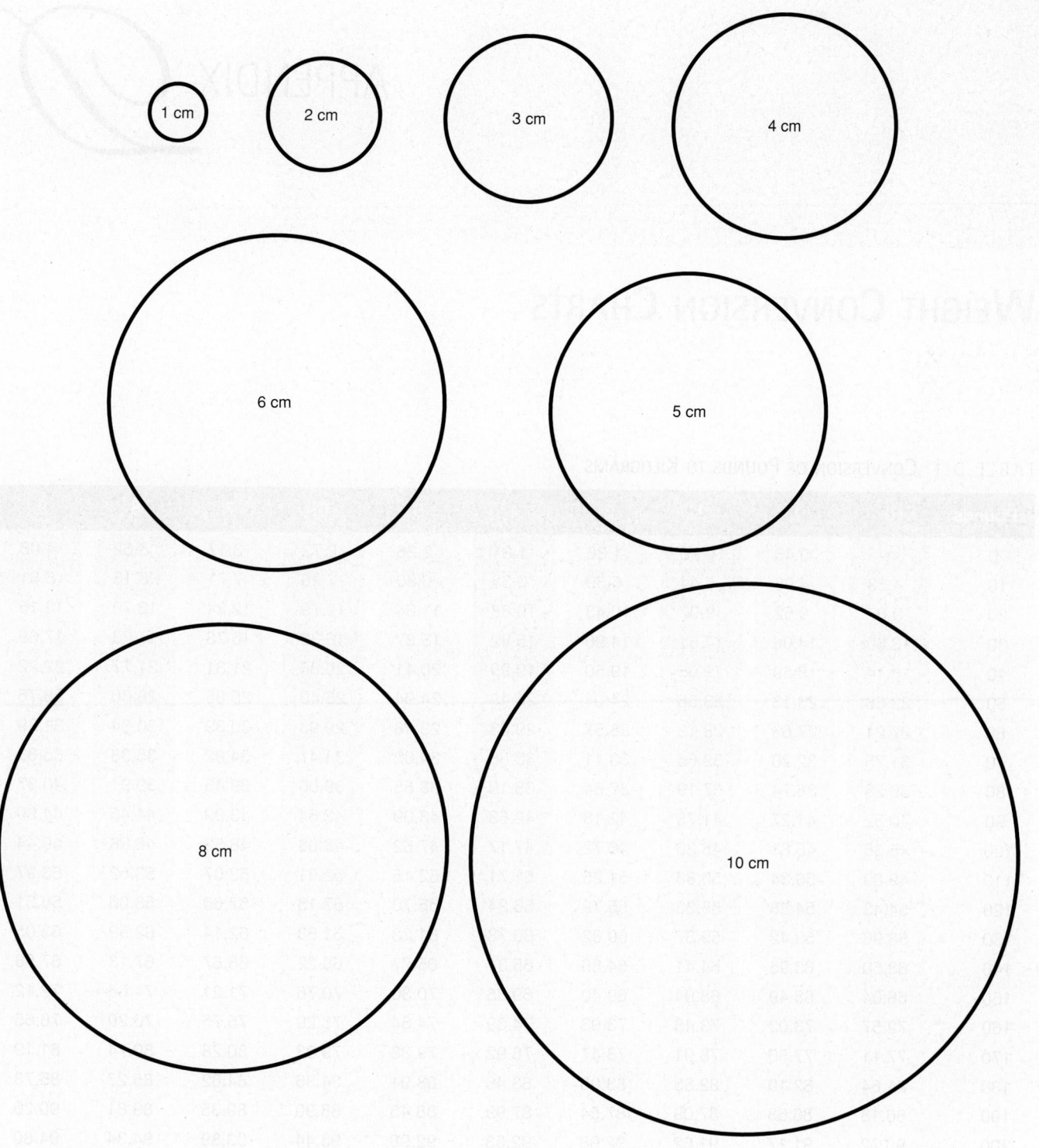

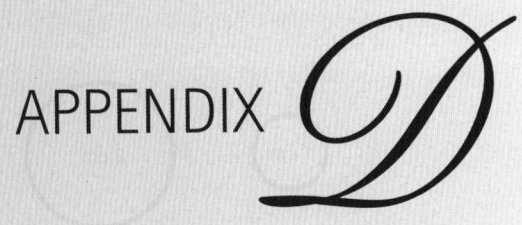

APPENDIX

WEIGHT CONVERSION CHARTS

TABLE D.1 **CONVERSION OF POUNDS TO KILOGRAMS**

Pounds	0	1	2	3	4	5	6	7	8	9
0	—	0.45	0.90	1.36	1.81	2.26	2.72	3.17	3.62	4.08
10	4.53	4.98	5.44	5.89	6.35	6.80	7.25	7.71	8.16	8.61
20	9.07	9.52	9.97	10.43	10.88	11.34	11.79	12.24	12.70	13.15
30	13.60	14.06	14.51	14.96	15.42	15.87	16.32	16.78	17.23	17.69
40	18.14	18.59	19.05	19.50	19.95	20.41	20.86	21.31	21.77	22.22
50	22.68	23.13	23.58	24.04	24.49	24.94	25.40	25.85	26.30	26.76
60	27.21	27.66	28.12	28.57	29.03	29.48	29.93	30.39	30.84	31.29
70	31.75	32.20	32.65	33.11	33.56	34.02	34.47	34.92	35.38	35.83
80	36.28	36.74	37.19	37.64	38.10	38.55	39.00	39.46	39.91	40.37
90	40.82	41.27	41.73	42.18	42.63	43.09	43.54	43.99	44.45	44.90
100	45.36	45.81	46.26	46.72	47.17	47.62	48.08	48.53	48.98	49.44
110	49.89	50.34	50.80	51.25	51.71	52.16	52.61	53.07	53.52	53.97
120	54.43	54.88	55.33	55.79	56.24	56.70	57.15	57.60	58.06	58.51
130	58.96	59.42	59.87	60.32	60.78	61.23	61.68	62.14	62.59	63.05
140	63.50	63.95	64.41	64.86	65.31	65.77	66.22	66.67	67.13	67.58
150	68.04	68.49	68.94	69.40	69.85	70.30	70.76	71.21	71.66	72.12
160	72.57	73.02	73.48	73.93	74.39	74.84	75.29	75.75	76.20	76.65
170	77.11	77.56	78.01	78.47	78.92	79.38	79.83	80.28	80.74	81.19
180	81.64	82.10	82.55	83.00	83.46	83.91	84.36	84.82	85.27	85.73
190	86.18	86.68	87.09	87.54	87.99	88.45	88.90	89.35	89.81	90.26
200	90.72	91.17	91.62	92.08	92.53	92.98	93.44	93.89	94.34	94.80

TABLE D.2 CONVERSION OF POUNDS AND OUNCES TO GRAMS FOR NEWBORN WEIGHTS

Pounds	Ounces															
	0	1	2	3	4	5	6	7	8	9	10	11	12	13	14	15
0	—	28	57	85	113	142	170	198	227	255	283	312	340	369	397	425
1	454	482	510	539	567	595	624	652	680	709	737	765	794	822	850	879
2	907	936	964	992	1021	1049	1077	1106	1134	1162	1191	1219	1247	1276	1304	1332
3	1361	1389	1417	1446	1474	1503	1531	1559	1588	1616	1644	1673	1701	1729	1758	1786
4	1814	1843	1871	1899	1928	1956	1984	2013	2041	2070	2098	2126	2155	2183	2211	2240
5	2268	2296	2325	2353	2381	2410	2438	2466	2495	2523	2551	2580	2608	2637	2665	2693
6	2722	2750	2778	2807	2835	2863	2892	2920	2948	2977	3005	3033	3062	3090	3118	3147
7	3175	3203	3232	3260	3289	3317	3345	3374	3402	3430	3459	3487	3515	3544	3572	3600
8	3629	3657	3685	3714	3742	3770	3799	3827	3856	3884	3912	3941	3969	3997	4026	4054
9	4082	4111	4139	4167	4196	4224	4252	4281	4309	4337	4366	4394	4423	4451	4479	4508
10	4536	4564	4593	4621	4649	4678	4706	4734	4763	4791	4819	4848	4876	4904	4933	4961
11	4990	5018	5046	5075	5103	5131	5160	5188	5216	5245	5273	5301	5330	5358	5386	5415
12	5443	5471	5500	5528	5557	5585	5613	5642	5670	5698	5727	5755	5783	5812	5840	5868
13	5897	5925	5953	5982	6010	6038	6067	6095	6123	6152	6180	6209	6237	6265	6294	6322
14	6350	6379	6407	6435	6464	6492	6520	6549	6577	6605	6634	6662	6690	6719	6747	6776
15	6804	6832	6860	6889	6917	6945	6973	7002	7030	7059	7087	7115	7144	7172	7201	7228

BREASTFEEDING AND MEDICATION USE

General Considerations

- Most medications are safe to use while breastfeeding; however, the woman should always check with the pediatrician, physician, lactation consultant, public health nurse, or midwife before taking any medications, including over-the-counter and herbal products.
- Inform the woman that she has the right to seek a second opinion if the physician does not perform a thoughtful risk-versus-benefit assessment before prescribing medications or advising against breastfeeding.
- Most medications pass from the woman's bloodstream into the breast milk. However, the amount is usually very small and unlikely to harm the baby.
- A preterm or other special needs neonate is more susceptible to the adverse effects of medications in breast milk. A woman who is taking medications and whose baby is in the neonatal intensive care unit or special care nursery should consult with the pediatrician or neonatologist before feeding her breast milk to the baby.
- If the woman is taking a prescribed medication, she should take the medication just after breastfeeding. This practice helps ensure that the lowest possible dose of medication reaches the baby through the breast milk.
- Some medications can cause changes in the amount of milk the woman produces. Teach the woman to report any changes in milk production.

Potential Effects of Selected Medication Categories on the Breast-Fed Infant

Narcotic Analgesics

- Codeine and hydrocodone appear to be safe in moderate doses. Rarely the neonate may experience sedation and/or apnea (LRC: L3).

- Meperidine (Demerol) can lead to sedation of the neonate (LRC: L2, L3 if used in early postpartum).
- Low-to-moderate doses of morphine appear to be safe (LRC: L3).
- Trace-to-negligible amounts of fentanyl are found in human milk (LRC: L2).

Non-Narcotic Analgesics and NSAIDs

- Acetaminophen and ibuprofen are approved for use (LRC: L1).
- Naproxen may cause neonatal hemorrhage and anemia if used for prolonged periods (LRC: L3 for short-term use and L4 for long-term use).
- The newer COX2 inhibitors, such as celecoxib (Celebrex), appear to be safe for use (LRC: L2).

Antibiotics

- Levels in breast milk are usually very low.
- The penicillins and cephalosporins are generally considered safe to use (LRC: L1).
- Tetracyclines can be safely used for short periods but are not suitable for long-term therapy (eg, for treatment of acne) (LRC: L2).
- Sulfonamides should be used with caution in neonates with hyperbilirubinemia and G6PD (LRC: L2).

Antihypertensives

- A high degree of caution is advised when antihypertensives are used during breastfeeding.
- Some beta blockers can be used.
- Hydralazine and methyldopa are considered to be safe (LRC: L2).
- ACE inhibitors are not recommended in the early postpartum period.

Sedatives and Hypnotics

- Neonatal withdrawal can occur when antianxiety medications, such as lorazepam, are taken. Fortunately withdrawal is generally mild.
- Phenothiazines, such as Phenergan and Thorazine, may lead to sleep apnea and increase the risk for sudden infant death syndrome.

Antidepressants

- The risk to the baby often is higher if the woman is depressed and remains untreated, rather than taking the medication.
- The older tricyclics are considered to be safe; however, they cause many bothersome side effects, such as weight gain and dry mouth, which may lead to noncompliance on the part of the woman.
- The selective serotonin uptake inhibitors (SSRIs) also are considered to be safe and have a lower side effect profile, which makes them more palatable to the woman (LRC: L2 and L3).

Mood Stabilizers (Antimanic Medication)

- Lithium is found in breast milk and is best not used in the breastfeeding woman (LRC: L3 with close observation).
- Valproic acid (Depakote) seems to be a more appropriate choice for the woman with seizure activity. The infant will need periodic lab studies to check platelets and liver function (LRC: L2).

Corticosteroids

- Corticosteroids do not pass into the milk in large quantities.
- Inhaled steroids are safe to use because they don't accumulate in the bloodstream.

Thyroid Medication

- Thyroid medications, such as levothyroxine (Synthroid), can be taken while breastfeeding.
- Most are in LRC category L1.

Medications That Usually are Contraindicated for the Breastfeeding Woman

- Amiodarone
- Antineoplastic agents
- Chloramphenicol
- Doxepin
- Ergotamine and other ergot derivatives
- Iodides
- Methotrexate and immunosuppressants
- Lithium
- Radiopharmaceuticals
- Ribavirin
- Tetracycline (prolonged use—more than 3 weeks)
- Pseudoephedrine (found in many over-the-counter medications)

LACTATION RISK CATEGORIES (LRC)

Location Category	Risk	Rationale
L1	Safest	Clinical research or long-term observation of use in many breastfeeding women has not demonstrated risk to the infant.
L2	Safer	Limited clinical research has not demonstrated an increase in adverse effects in the infant.
L3	Moderately safe	There is possible risk to the infant; however, the risks are minimal or nonthreatening in nature. These medications should be given only when the potential benefit outweighs the risk to the infant.
L4	Possibly hazardous	There is positive evidence of risk to the infant; however, in life-threatening situations or for serious diseases, the benefit might outweigh the risk.
L5	Contraindicated	The risk of using the medication clearly outweighs any possible benefit from breastfeeding.

Material in this Appendix was adapted from information found on the Canadian Paediatric Society website (www.caringforkids.cps.ca/pregnancybabies/Breastfeeding.htm) and from Riordan, J. (2010). Breastfeeding and human lactation (3rd ed.). Boston: Jones and Bartlett Publishers; Hale, T. W. (2010). Medications and mother's milk (11th ed.). Amarillo, TX: Pharmasoft Publishing.

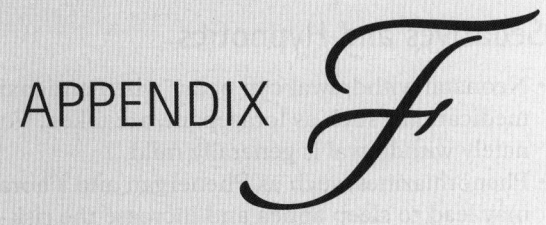

APPENDIX F

GROWTH CHARTS

Birth to 36 months: Boys
Length-for-age and Weight-for-age percentiles

NAME _____

RECORD # _____

AGE (MONTHS)

Birth   3   6   9   12   15   18   21   24   27   30   33   36

LENGTH

WEIGHT

95
90
75
50
25
10
5

AGE (MONTHS)

12   15   18   21   24   27   30   33   36

Mother's Stature _____		Gestational		
Father's Stature _____		Age: _____ Weeks		Comment
Date	Age	Weight	Length	Head Circ.
	Birth			

Published May 30, 2000 (modified 4/20/01).
SOURCE: Developed by the National Center for Health Statistics in collaboration with
the National Center for Chronic Disease Prevention and Health Promotion (2000).
http://www.cdc.gov/growthcharts

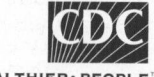

SAFER • HEALTHIER • PEOPLE™

Birth to 36 months: Girls
Length-for-age and Weight-for-age percentiles

NAME _____

RECORD # _____

AGE (MONTHS)

Birth 3 6 9 12 15 18 21 24 27 30 33 36

LENGTH

LENGTH

WEIGHT

WEIGHT

LENGTH
95
90
75
50
25
10
5

WEIGHT
95
90
75
50
25
10
5

	Mother's Stature _____		Gestational		Comment
	Father's Stature _____		Age: _____ Weeks		
Date	Age	Weight	Length	Head Circ.	
	Birth				

Published May 30, 2000 (modified 4/20/01).

SOURCE: Developed by the National Center for Health Statistics in collaboration with
the National Center for Chronic Disease Prevention and Health Promotion (2000).
http://www.cdc.gov/growthcharts

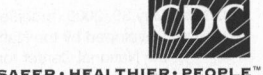

SAFER • HEALTHIER • PEOPLE™

Birth to 36 months: Boys
Head circumference-for-age and
Weight-for-length percentiles

NAME _____

RECORD # _____

AGE (MONTHS)

Birth 3 6 9 **12** 15 18 21 **24** 27 30 33 **36**

HEAD CIRCUMFERENCE

in	cm
20	52
19	50
	48
18	46
17	44
	42
16	40
15	38
14	36
13	34
	32
12	30

95
90
75
50
25
10
5

WEIGHT

95
90
75
50
25
10
5

LENGTH

cm 64 66 68 70 72 74 76 78 80 82 84 86 88 90 92 94 96 98 100
in 26 27 28 29 30 31 32 33 34 35 36 37 38 39 40 41

Date	Age	Weight	Length	Head Circ.	Comment

cm 46 48 50 52 54 56 58 60 62
in 18 19 20 21 22 23 24

WEIGHT

lb	kg
24	11
22	10
20	9
18	8
16	7
14	6
12	5
10	4
8	3
6	2
4	
2	1

WEIGHT (right side)

kg	lb
22	50
	48
21	46
20	44
19	42
18	40
17	38
16	36
15	34
	32
14	30
13	28
12	26
11	24
10	22
9	20
8	18
7	16
6	14
5	12

Published May 30, 2000 (modified 10/16/00).
SOURCE: Developed by the National Center for Health Statistics in collaboration with
the National Center for Chronic Disease Prevention and Health Promotion (2000).
http://www.cdc.gov/growthcharts

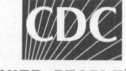

SAFER · HEALTHIER · PEOPLE™

Birth to 36 months: Girls
Head circumference-for-age and
Weight-for-length percentiles

NAME _____

RECORD # _____

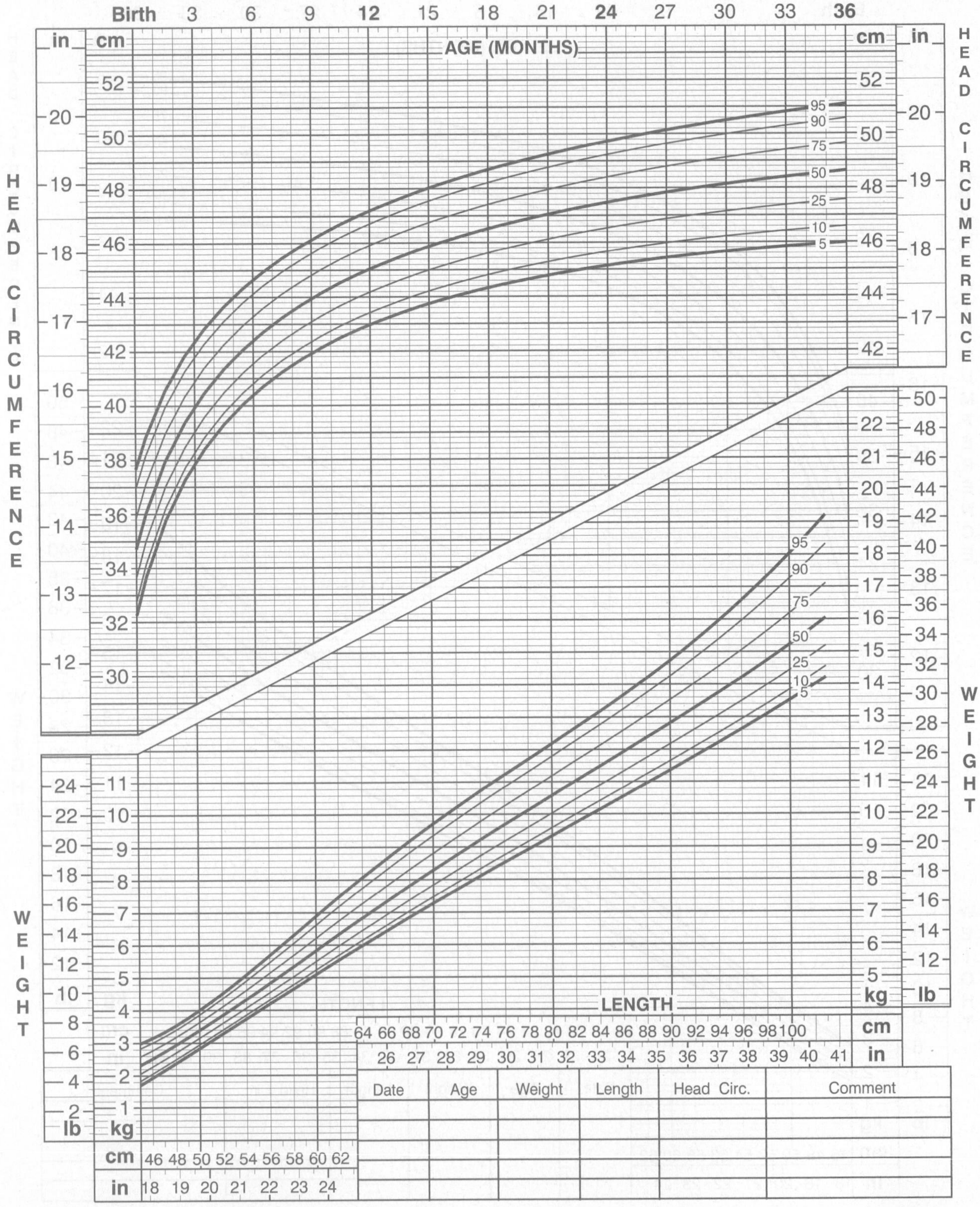

AGE (MONTHS)

Birth   3   6   9   12   15   18   21   24   27   30   33   36

HEAD CIRCUMFERENCE

95
90
75
50
25
10
5

LENGTH

| cm | 64 66 68 70 72 74 76 78 80 82 84 86 88 90 92 94 96 98 100 |
| in | 26 27 28 29 30 31 32 33 34 35 36 37 38 39 40 41 |

WEIGHT

95
90
75
50
25
10
5

Date	Age	Weight	Length	Head Circ.	Comment

| cm | 46 48 50 52 54 56 58 60 62 |
| in | 18 19 20 21 22 23 24 |

Published May 30, 2000 (modified 10/16/00).

SOURCE: Developed by the National Center for Health Statistics in collaboration with
the National Center for Chronic Disease Prevention and Health Promotion (2000).

http://www.cdc.gov/growthcharts

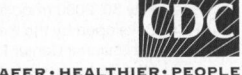

SAFER · HEALTHIER · PEOPLE™

2 to 20 years: Boys
Stature-for-age and Weight-for-age percentiles

NAME _____

RECORD # _____

Mother's Stature _____		Father's Stature _____		
Date	Age	Weight	Stature	BMI*

***To Calculate BMI**: Weight (kg) ÷ Stature (cm) ÷ Stature (cm) x 10,000
or Weight (lb) ÷ Stature (in) ÷ Stature (in) x 703

AGE (YEARS)

12 13 14 15 16 17 18 19 20

STATURE

WEIGHT

AGE (YEARS)

2 3 4 5 6 7 8 9 10 11 12 13 14 15 16 17 18 19 20

Published May 30, 2000 (modified 11/21/00).
SOURCE: Developed by the National Center for Health Statistics in collaboration with
the National Center for Chronic Disease Prevention and Health Promotion (2000).
http://www.cdc.gov/growthcharts

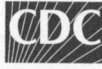

SAFER • HEALTHIER • PEOPLE™

2 to 20 years: Girls
Stature-for-age and Weight-for-age percentiles

NAME _____

RECORD # _____

Mother's Stature _____		Father's Stature _____		
Date	Age	Weight	Stature	BMI*

*To Calculate BMI: Weight (kg) ÷ Stature (cm) ÷ Stature (cm) x 10,000
  or Weight (lb) ÷ Stature (in) ÷ Stature (in) x 703

AGE (YEARS)

12 13 14 15 16 17 18 19 20

STATURE

WEIGHT

AGE (YEARS)

2 3 4 5 6 7 8 9 10 11 12 13 14 15 16 17 18 19 20

Published May 30, 2000 (modified 11/21/00).
SOURCE: Developed by the National Center for Health Statistics in collaboration with
  the National Center for Chronic Disease Prevention and Health Promotion (2000).
  http://www.cdc.gov/growthcharts

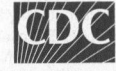

SAFER · HEALTHIER · PEOPLE™

2 to 20 years: Boys
Body mass index-for-age percentiles

NAME _____

RECORD # _____

Date	Age	Weight	Stature	BMI*	Comments

*To Calculate BMI: Weight (kg) ÷ Stature (cm) ÷ Stature (cm) x 10,000
or Weight (lb) ÷ Stature (in) ÷ Stature (in) x 703

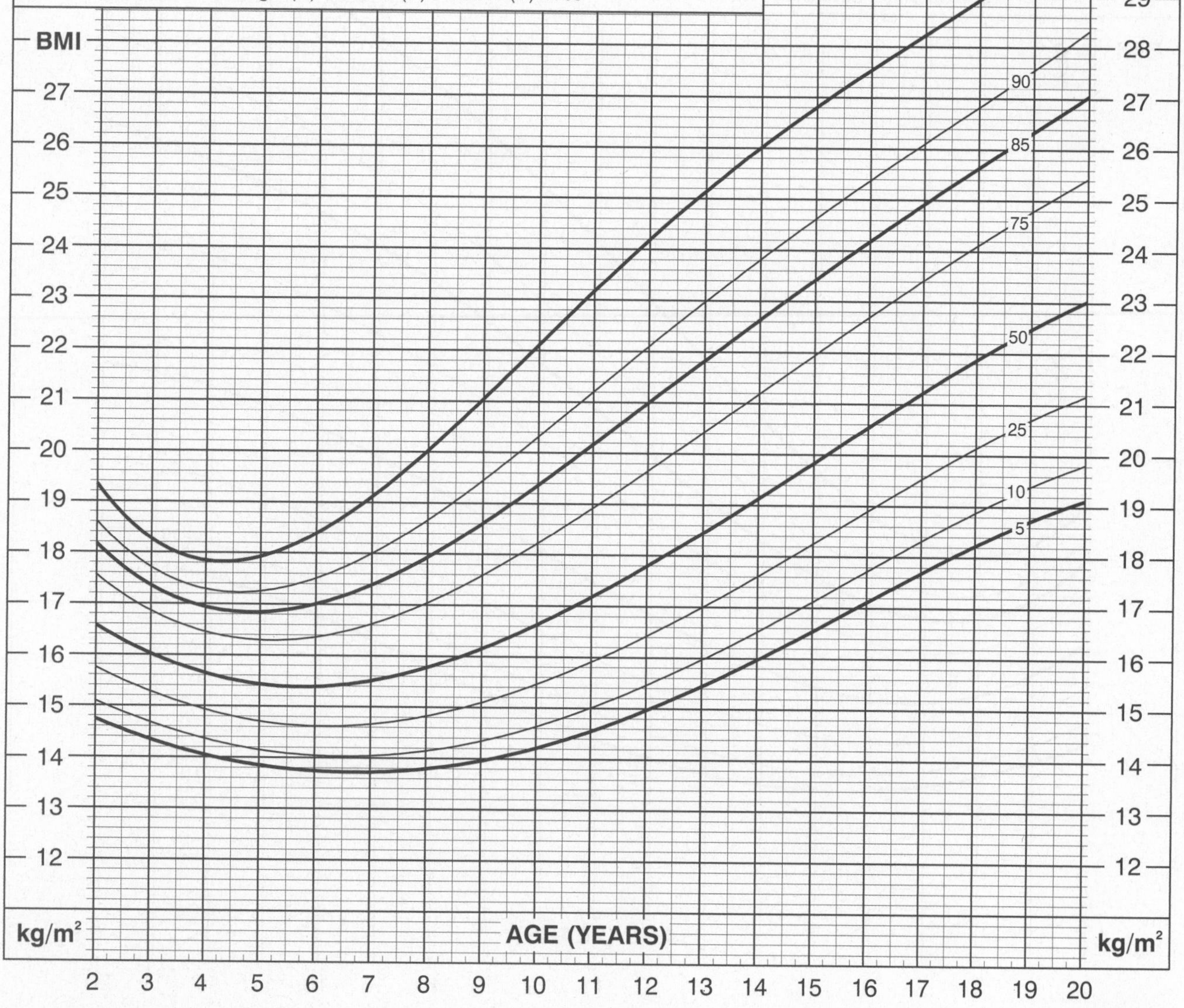

BMI

27
26
25
24
23
22
21
20
19
18
17
16
15
14
13
12

kg/m²

BMI

35
34
33
32
31
30
29
28
27
26
25
24
23
22
21
20
19
18
17
16
15
14
13
12

kg/m²

95
90
85
75
50
25
10
5

AGE (YEARS)

2   3   4   5   6   7   8   9   10   11   12   13   14   15   16   17   18   19   20

Published May 30, 2000 (modified 10/16/00).

SOURCE: Developed by the National Center for Health Statistics in collaboration with
the National Center for Chronic Disease Prevention and Health Promotion (2000).
http://www.cdc.gov/growthcharts

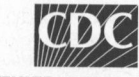

SAFER · HEALTHIER · PEOPLE™

2 to 20 years: Girls
Body mass index-for-age percentiles

NAME _____

RECORD # _____

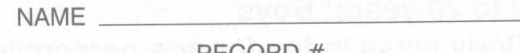

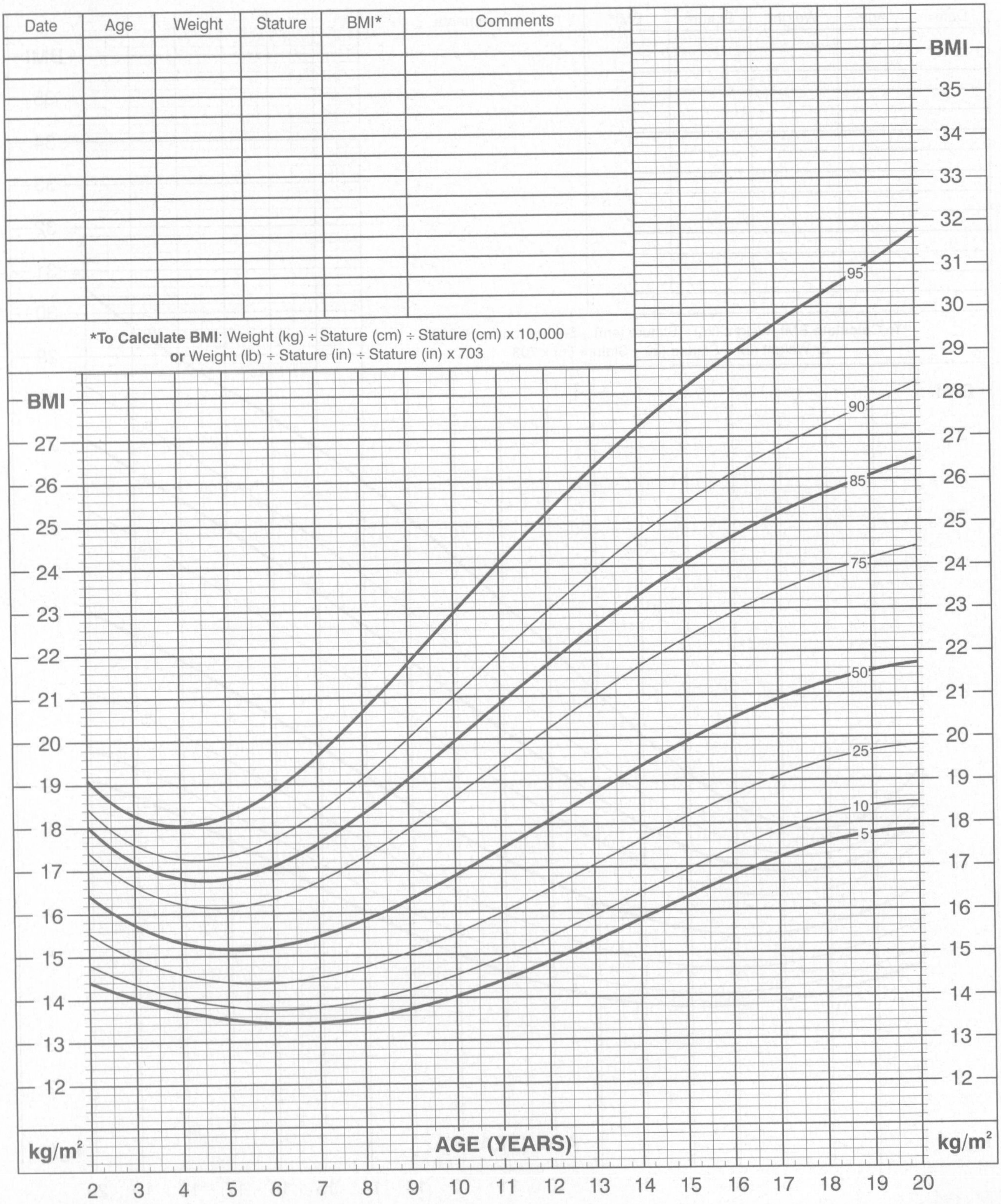

Date	Age	Weight	Stature	BMI*	Comments

*To Calculate BMI: Weight (kg) ÷ Stature (cm) ÷ Stature (cm) x 10,000
or Weight (lb) ÷ Stature (in) ÷ Stature (in) x 703

AGE (YEARS)

kg/m²

BMI

95
90
85
75
50
25
10
5

Published May 30, 2000 (modified 10/16/00).
SOURCE: Developed by the National Center for Health Statistics in collaboration with
the National Center for Chronic Disease Prevention and Health Promotion (2000).
http://www.cdc.gov/growthcharts

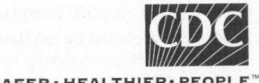

SAFER • HEALTHIER • PEOPLE™

NAME ______________________

Weight-for-stature percentiles: Boys

RECORD # ______________

Date	Age	Weight	Stature	Comments

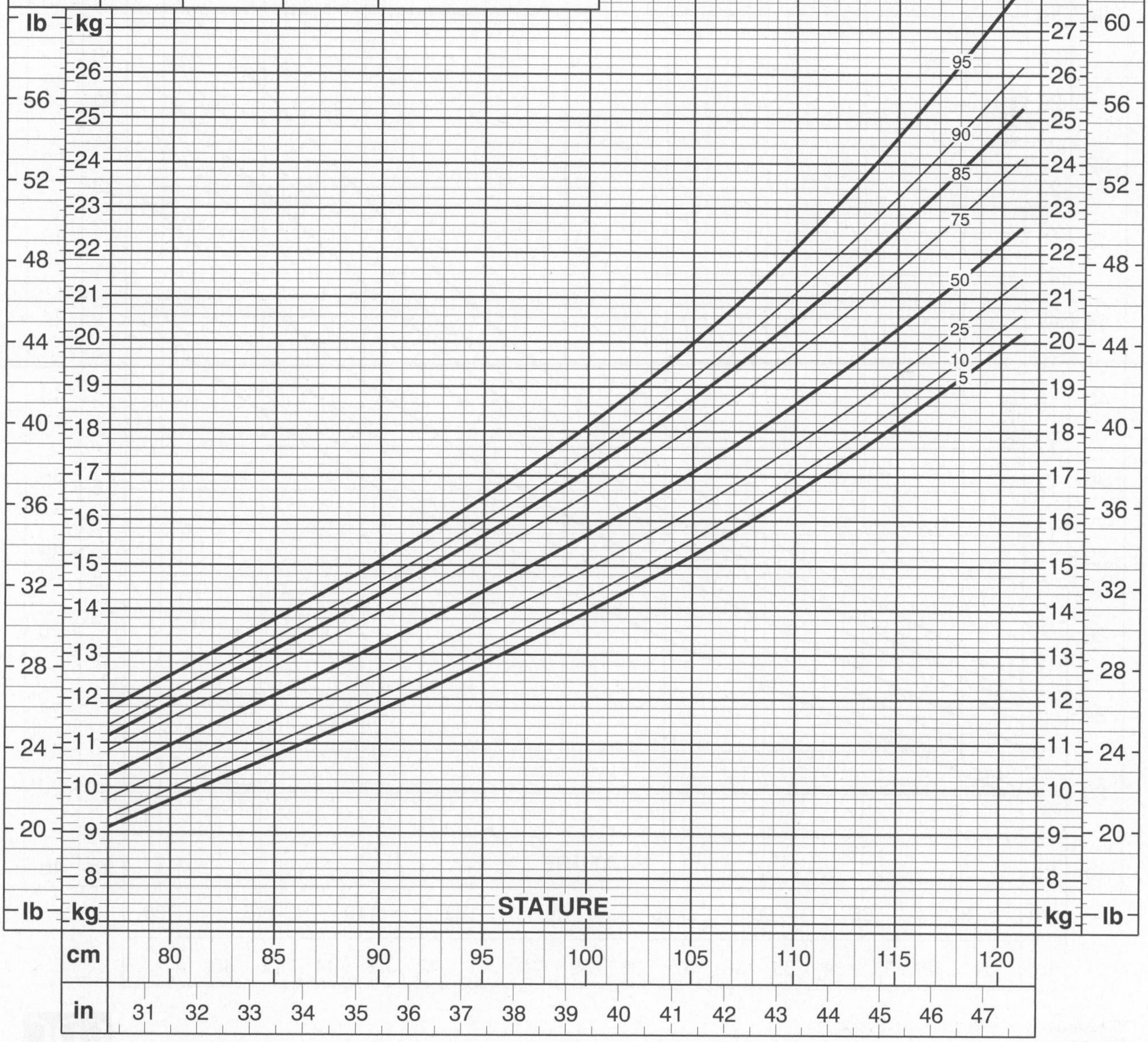
kg
lb
34
33
32
31
30
29
28
27
26
25
24
23
22
21
20
19
18
17
16
15
14
13
12
11
10
9
8
76
72
68
64
60
56
52
48
44
40
36
32
28
24
20
95
90
85
75
50
25
10
5
STATURE
cm
80
85
90
95
100
105
110
115
120
in
31
32
33
34
35
36
37
38
39
40
41
42
43
44
45
46
47

Published May 30, 2000 (modified 10/16/00).
SOURCE: Developed by the National Center for Health Statistics in collaboration with
the National Center for Chronic Disease Prevention and Health Promotion (2000).
http://www.cdc.gov/growthcharts

CDC
SAFER • HEALTHIER • PEOPLE™

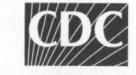

Weight-for-stature percentiles: Girls

NAME _____

RECORD # _____

Date	Age	Weight	Stature	Comments

[Weight-for-stature growth chart with percentile curves labeled 95, 90, 85, 75, 50, 25, 10, 5. Weight axis in lb and kg (left and right), stature axis in cm (80-120) and in (31-47). STATURE]

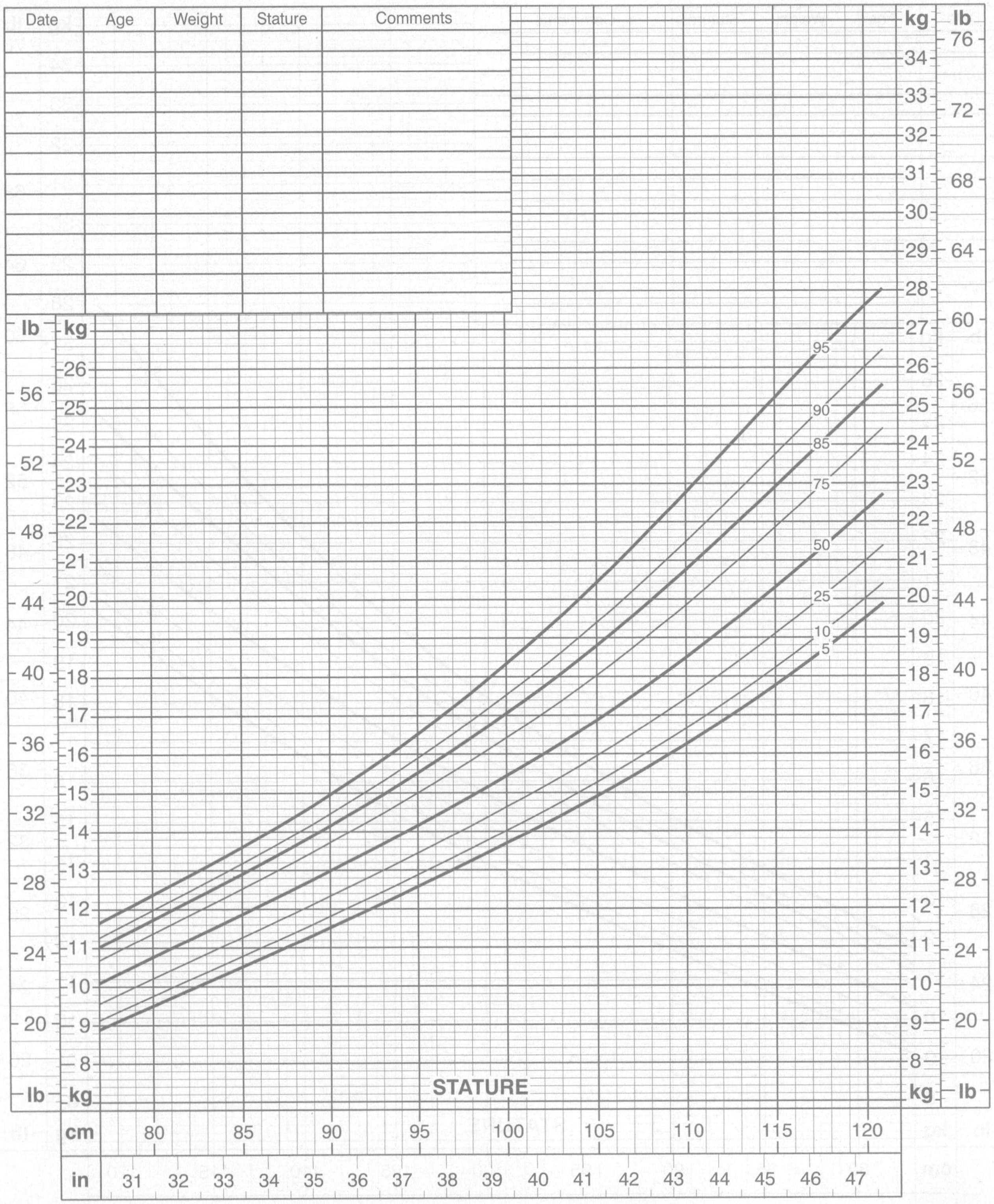

Published May 30, 2000 (modified 10/16/00).
SOURCE: Developed by the National Center for Health Statistics in collaboration with
the National Center for Chronic Disease Prevention and Health Promotion (2000).
http://www.cdc.gov/growthcharts

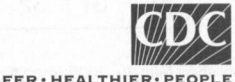

For additional information on growth charts for children with Down syndrome, please go to http://thepoint.lww.com.

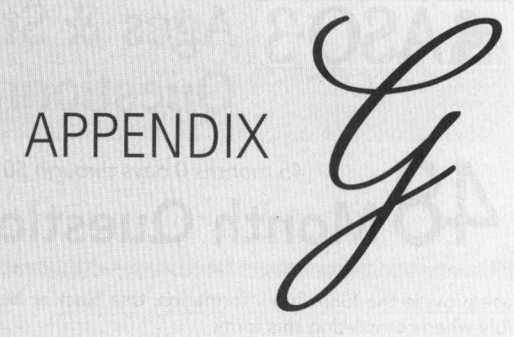

AGES AND STAGES QUESTIONNAIRE

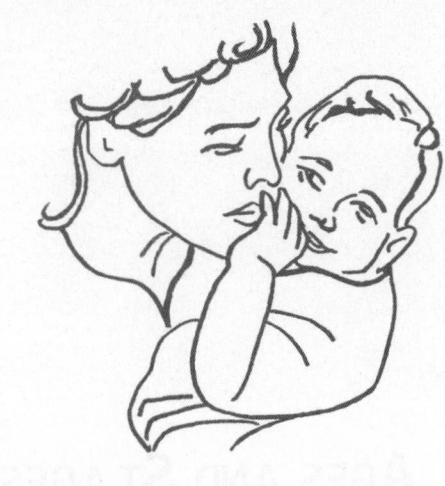

ASQ-3™ Ages & Stages Questionnaires®

48 Month Questionnaire
45 months 0 days through 50 months 30 days

Please provide the following information. Use black or blue ink only and print legibly when completing this form.

Date ASQ completed: **11/18/2008**

Child's information

Child's first name: **John**   Middle initial: **X.**   Child's last name: **Smith**

Child's gender: ● Male   ○ Female

Child's date of birth: **11/12/2004**

Person filling out questionnaire

First name: **Jane**   Middle initial: **Q.**   Last name: **Smith**

Relationship to child:
● Parent   ○ Guardian   ○ Teacher   ○ Child care provider
○ Grandparent or other relative   ○ Foster parent   ○ Other: _____

Street address: **123 Center Street, Apt. 9**

City: **Anytown**   State/Province: **MD**   ZIP/Postal code: **21230**

Country: **USA**   Home telephone number: **410-555-0155**   Other telephone number: **410-555-0189**

E-mail address: _____

Names of people assisting in questionnaire completion: _____

Program Information

Child ID #: **00123456789000000**

Program ID #: **987654321234456789**

Program name: **Anytown Preschool**

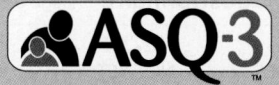
On the following pages are questions about activities babies may do. Your baby may have already done some of the activities described here, and there may be some your baby has not begun doing yet. For each item, please fill in the circle that indicates whether your baby is doing the activity regularly, sometimes, or not yet.

Important Points to Remember:

☑ Try each activity with your baby before marking a response.

☑ Make completing this questionnaire a game that is fun for you and your child.

☑ Make sure your child is rested and fed.

☑ Please return this questionnaire by _____.

Notes:

_____

_____

_____

_____

COMMUNICATION

		YES	SOMETIMES	NOT YET	
1.	Does your child name at least three items from a common category? For example, if you say to your child, "Tell me some things that you can eat," does your child answer with something like "cookies, eggs, and cereal"? Or if you say, "Tell me the names of some animals," does your child answer with something like "cow, dog, and elephant"?	○	●	○	<u>5</u>
2.	Does your child answer the following questions? *(Mark "sometimes" if your child answers only one question.)*	●	○	○	<u>10</u>

"What do you do when you are hungry?" *(Acceptable answers include "get food," "eat," "ask for something to eat," and "have a snack.")* Please write your child's response:

> Eat

"What do you do when you are tired?" *(Acceptable answers include "take a nap," "rest," "go to sleep," "go to bed," "lie down," and "sit down.")* Please write your child's response:

> Go night-night

		YES	SOMETIMES	NOT YET	
3.	Does your child tell you at least two things about common objects? For example, if you say to your child, "Tell me about your ball," does she say something like, "It's round. I throw it. It's big"?	○	●	○	<u>5</u>
4.	Does your child use endings of words, such as "-s," "-ed," and "-ing"? For example, does your child say things like, "I see two cat*s*," "I am play*ing*," or "I kick*ed* the ball"?	○	○	●	<u>0</u>

COMMUNICATION   *(continued)*

	YES	SOMETIMES	NOT YET	
5. Without your giving help by pointing or repeating, does your child follow three directions that are *unrelated* to one another? Give all three directions before your child starts. For example, you may ask your child, "Clap your hands, walk to the door, and sit down," or "Give me the pen, open the book, and stand up."	○	○	●	**0**
6. Does your child use all of the words in a sentence (for example, "a," "the," "am," "is," and "are") to make complete sentences, such as "I *am* going to *the* park," or "*Is* there *a* toy to play with?" or "*Are* you coming, too?"	○	●	○	**5**

COMMUNICATION TOTAL   **25**

GROSS MOTOR

	YES	SOMETIMES	NOT YET	
1. Does your child catch a large ball with both hands? *(You should stand about 5 feet away and give your child two or three tries before you mark the answer.)*	●	○	○	**10**
2. Does your child climb the rungs of a ladder of a playground slide and slide down without help?	●	○	○	**10**
3. While standing, does your child throw a ball *overhand* in the direction of a person standing at least 6 feet away? To throw overhand, your child must raise his arm to shoulder height and throw the ball forward. *(Dropping the ball or throwing the ball underhand should be scored as "not yet.")*	●	○	○	**10**
4. Does your child hop up and down on either the right or left foot at least one time without losing her balance or falling?	●	○	○	**10**
5. Does your child jump forward a distance of 20 inches from a standing position, starting with his feet together?	●	○	○	**10**
6. Without holding onto anything, does your child stand on one foot for at least 5 seconds without losing her balance and putting her foot down? *(You may give your child two or three tries before you mark the answer.)*	●	○	○	**10**

GROSS MOTOR TOTAL   **60**

FINE MOTOR

	YES	SOMETIMES	NOT YET	
1. Does your child put together a five- to seven-piece interlocking puzzle? *(If one is not available, take a full-page picture from a magazine or catalog and cut it into six pieces. Does your child put it back together correctly?)*	○	●	○	**5**

FINE MOTOR *(continued)*

	YES	SOMETIMES	NOT YET	
2. Using child-safe scissors, does your child cut a paper in half on a more or less straight line, making the blades go up and down? *(Carefully watch your child's use of scissors for safety reasons.)*	●	○	○	**10**
3. Using the shapes below to look at, does your child copy at least three shapes onto a large piece of paper using a pencil, crayon, or pen, without tracing? *(Your child's drawings should look similar to the design of the shapes below, but they may be different in size.)*	○	●	○	**5**

L + I O

	YES	SOMETIMES	NOT YET	
4. Does your child unbutton one or more buttons? *(Your child may use his own clothing or a doll's clothing.)*	○	○	●	**0**
5. Does your child draw pictures of people that have at least three of the following features: head, eyes, nose, mouth, neck, hair, trunk, arms, hands, legs, or feet?	○	○	●	**0**
6. Does your child color mostly within the lines in a coloring book or within the lines of a 2-inch circle that you draw? *(Your child should not go more than ¼ inch outside the lines on most of the picture.)*	○	○	●	**0**

FINE MOTOR TOTAL **20**

PROBLEM SOLVING

	YES	SOMETIMES	NOT YET	
1. When you say, "Say 'five eight three,'" does your child repeat *just* the three numbers in the same order? *Do not repeat the numbers.* If necessary, try another series of numbers and say, "Say 'six nine two.'" *(Your child must repeat just one series of three numbers to answer "yes" to this question.)*	○	●	○	**5**
2. When asked, "Which circle is the smallest?" does your child point to the smallest circle? *(Ask this question without providing help by pointing, gesturing, or looking at the smallest circle.)*	○	●	○	**5**

○ ○ ○

	YES	SOMETIMES	NOT YET	
3. Without your giving help by pointing, does your child follow three different directions using the words "under," "between," and "middle"? For example, ask your child to put the shoe "*under* the couch." Then ask her to put the ball "*between* the chairs" and the book "in the *middle* of the table."	○	○	●	**0**
4. When shown objects and asked, "What color is this?" does your child name five different colors, like red, blue, yellow, orange, black, white, or pink? *(Mark "yes" only if your child answers the question correctly using five colors.)*	○	●	○	**5**

PROBLEM SOLVING *(continued)*

	YES	SOMETIMES	NOT YET	
5. Does your child dress up and "play-act," pretending to be someone or something else? For example, your child may dress up in different clothes and pretend to be a mommy, daddy, brother, or sister, or an imaginary animal or figure.	○	●	○	**5**
6. If you place five objects in front of your child, can he count them by saying, "one, two, three, four, five," in order? *(Ask this question without providing help by pointing, gesturing, or naming.)*	○	○	●	**0**

PROBLEM SOLVING TOTAL **20**

PERSONAL-SOCIAL

	YES	SOMETIMES	NOT YET	
1. Does your child serve herself, taking food from one container to another using utensils? For example, does your child use a large spoon to scoop applesauce from a jar into a bowl?	●	○	○	**10**
2. Does your child tell you at least four of the following? Please mark the items your child knows.	●	○	○	**10**

- ● a. First name
- ● b. Age
- ○ c. City she lives in
- ● d. Last name
- ● e. Boy or girl
- ○ f. Telephone number

	YES	SOMETIMES	NOT YET	
3. Does your child wash his hands using soap and water and dry off with a towel without help?	●	○	○	**10**
4. Does your child tell you the names of two or more playmates, not including brothers and sisters? *(Ask this question without providing help by suggesting names of playmates or friends.)*	●	○	○	**10**
5. Does your child brush her teeth by putting toothpaste on the toothbrush and brushing all of her teeth without help? *(You may still need to check and rebrush your child's teeth.)*	●	○	○	**10**
6. Does your child dress or undress himself without help (except for snaps, buttons, and zippers)?	●	○	○	**10**

PERSONAL-SOCIAL TOTAL **60**

OVERALL

Parents and providers may use the space below for additional comments.

	YES	NO
1. Do you think your child hears well? If no, explain:	○	●

> Had severe ear infections. Didn't start talking until age 2–3 years, after tubes were placed.

E101480500

OVERALL (continued)

2. Do you think your child talks like other toddlers her age? If no, explain: ○ YES ● NO

> His sentence structure and comprehension are not as advanced as other kids who are a year younger.

3. Can you understand most of what your child says? If no, explain: ● YES ○ NO

4. Can other people understand most of what your child says? If no, explain: ○ YES ● NO

> Other people have a hard time understanding him.

5. Do you think your child walks, runs, and climbs like other toddlers his age? If no, explain: ● YES ○ NO

6. Does either parent have a family history of childhood deafness or hearing impairment? If yes, explain: ○ YES ● NO

7. Do you have any concerns about your child's vision? If yes, explain: ○ YES ● NO

OVERALL   *(continued)*

8. Has your child had any medical problems in the last several months? If yes, explain: ● YES   ○ NO

> Ear infections.

9. Do you have any concerns about your child's behavior? If yes, explain: ○ YES   ● NO

>

10. Does anything about your child worry you? If yes, explain: ● YES   ○ NO

> Language development. No letter or number recognition and he's 4 years old. Even the 2 1/2 yr old knows more.

Ages & Stages Questionnaires®, Third Edition (ASQ-3™), Squires & Bricker

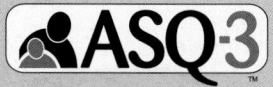
Child's name: John X. Smith

Child's ID #: 00123456789000000

Administering program/provider: Anytown Preschool/Ms. Jenkins

Date ASQ completed: 11/18/2008

Date of birth: 11/12/2004

---

1. **SCORE AND TRANSFER TOTALS TO CHART BELOW:** See *ASQ-3 User's Guide* for details, including how to adjust scores if item responses are missing. Score each item (YES = 10, SOMETIMES = 5, NOT YET = 0). Add item scores, and record each area total. In the chart below, transfer the total scores, and fill in the circles corresponding with the total scores.

Area	Cutoff	Total Score	0	5	10	15	20	25	30	35	40	45	50	55	60
Communication	30.72	25	●	●	●	●	●	◐	●	○	○	○	○	○	○
Gross Motor	32.78	60	●	●	●	●	●	●	●	○	○	○	○	○	●
Fine Motor	15.81	20	●	●	●	●	◐	○	○	○	○	○	○	○	○
Problem Solving	31.30	20	●	●	●	●	◐	●	●	○	○	○	○	○	○
Personal-Social	26.60	60	●	●	●	●	●	○	○	○	○	○	○	○	●

2. **TRANSFER OVERALL RESPONSES:** Bolded uppercase responses require follow-up. See *ASQ-3 User's Guide*, Chapter 6.

1. Hears well? — Yes **(NO)**
   Comments: Ear infex, ear tubes, didn't talk until 2-3 yrs.

2. Talks like other toddlers his age? — Yes **(NO)**
   Comments: Sentences and compreh. not as advanced as younger kids

3. Understand most of what your child says? — **(Yes)** NO
   Comments:

4. Others understand most of what your child says? — Yes **(NO)**
   Comments:

5. Walks, runs, and climbs like other toddlers? — **(Yes)** NO
   Comments:

6. Family history of hearing impairment? — **YES** (No)
   Comments:

7. Concerns about vision? — **YES** (No)
   Comments:

8. Any medical problems? — **(YES)** No
   Comments: Ear infex

9. Concerns about behavior? — **YES** (No)
   Comments:

10. Other concerns? — **(YES)** No
    Comments: Language devel.— doesn't recognize numbers or letters yet.

3. **ASQ SCORE INTERPRETATION AND RECOMMENDATION FOR FOLLOW-UP:** You must consider total area scores, overall responses, and other considerations, such as opportunities to practice skills, to determine appropriate follow-up.

If the child's total score is in the ☐ area, it is above the cutoff, and the child's development appears to be on schedule.
If the child's total score is in the ▨ area, it is close to the cutoff. Provide learning activities and monitor.
If the child's total score is in the ■ area, it is below the cutoff. Further assessment with a professional may be needed.

4. **FOLLOW-UP ACTION TAKEN:** Check all that apply.

___ Provide activities and rescreen in ___ months.

☓ Share results with primary health care provider.

☓ Refer for (circle all that apply) (hearing,) vision, and/or behavioral screening.

___ Refer to primary health care provider or other community agency (specify reason): _____

☓ Refer to early intervention/early childhood special education.

___ No further action taken at this time

___ Other (specify): _____

5. **OPTIONAL:** Transfer item responses (Y = YES, S = SOMETIMES, N = NOT YET, X = response missing).

	1	2	3	4	5	6
Communication	S	Y	S	N	N	S
Gross Motor	Y	Y	Y	Y	Y	Y
Fine Motor	S	Y	S	N	N	N
Problem Solving	S	S	N	S	S	N
Personal-Social	Y	Y	Y	Y	Y	Y

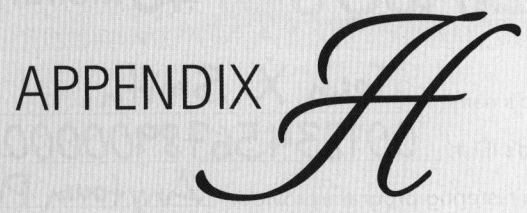

CANADA'S FOOD GUIDE

Health Santé
Canada Canada

Your health and safety... our priority.

Votre santé et votre sécurité... notre priorité.

Eating Well with

Canada's Food Guide

Canada

Recommended Number of *Food Guide Servings per Day*

	Children			Teens		Adults			
Age in Years	**2-3**	**4-8**	**9-13**	**14-18**		**19-50**		**51+**	
Sex	Girls and Boys			Females	Males	Females	Males	Females	Males
Vegetables and Fruit	4	5	6	7	8	7-8	8-10	7	7
Grain Products	3	4	6	6	7	6-7	8	6	7
Milk and Alternatives	2	2	3-4	3-4	3-4	2	2	3	3
Meat and Alternatives	1	1	1-2	2	3	2	3	2	3

The chart above shows how many Food Guide Servings you need from each of the four food groups every day.

Having the amount and type of food recommended and following the tips in *Canada's Food Guide* will help:

- Meet your needs for vitamins, minerals and other nutrients.
- Reduce your risk of obesity, type 2 diabetes, heart disease, certain types of cancer and osteoporosis.
- Contribute to your overall health and vitality.

What is One Food Guide Serving?
Look at the examples below.

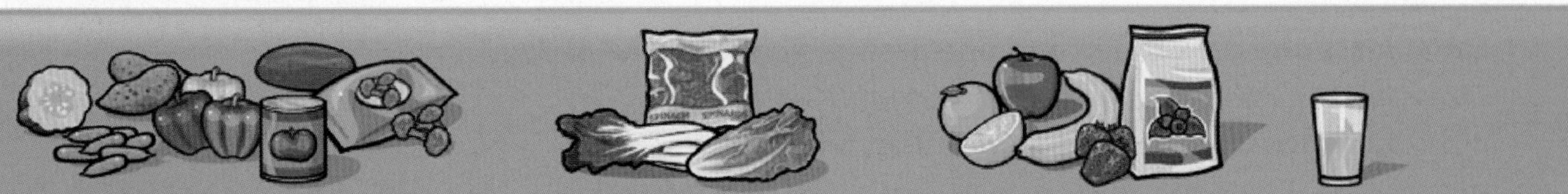

Fresh, frozen or canned vegetables
125 mL (½ cup)

Leafy vegetables
Cooked: 125 mL (½ cup)
Raw: 250 mL (1 cup)

Fresh, frozen or canned fruits
1 fruit or 125 mL (½ cup)

100% Juice
125 mL (½ cup)

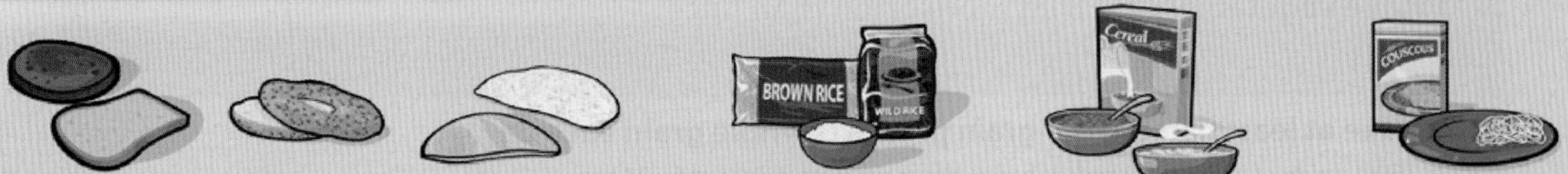

Bread
1 slice (35g)

Bagel
½ bagel (45 g)

Flat breads
½ pita or ½ tortilla (35 g)

Cooked rice, bulgur or quinoa
125 mL (½ cup)

Cereal
Cold: 30 g
Hot: 175 mL (¾ cup)

Cooked pasta or couscous
125 mL (½ cup)

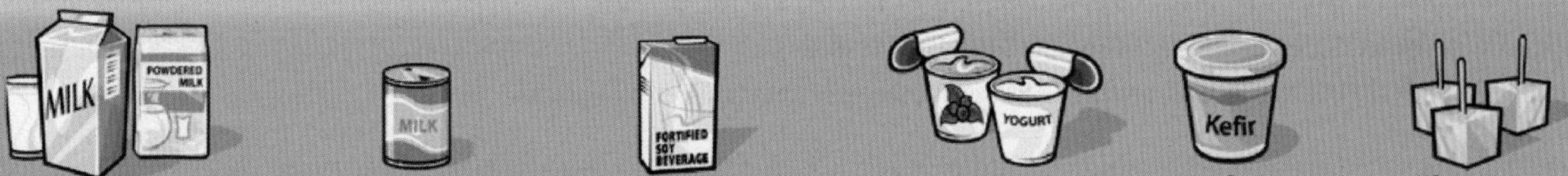

Milk or powdered milk (reconstituted)
250 mL (1 cup)

Canned milk (evaporated)
125 mL (½ cup)

Fortified soy beverage
250 mL (1 cup)

Yogurt
175 g
(¾ cup)

Kefir
175 g
(¾ cup)

Cheese
50 g (1 ½ oz.)

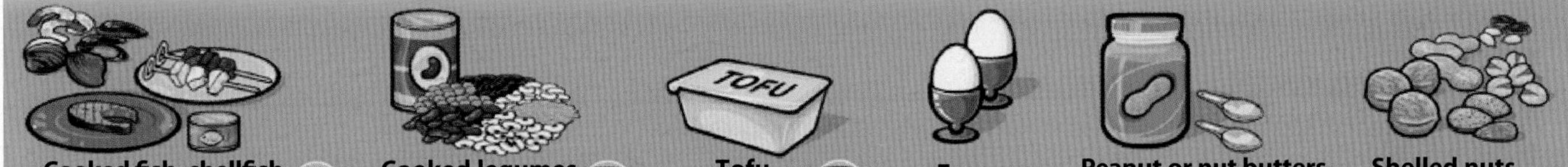

Cooked fish, shellfish, poultry, lean meat
75 g (2 ½ oz.)/125 mL (½ cup)

Cooked legumes
175 mL (¾ cup)

Tofu
150 g or
175 mL (¾ cup)

Eggs
2 eggs

Peanut or nut butters
30 mL (2 Tbsp)

Shelled nuts and seeds
60 mL (¼ cup)

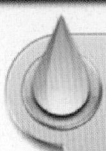

Oils and Fats
- Include a small amount – 30 to 45 mL (2 to 3 Tbsp) – of unsaturated fat each day. This includes oil used for cooking, salad dressings, margarine and mayonnaise.
- Use vegetable oils such as canola, olive and soybean.
- Choose soft margarines that are low in saturated and trans fats.
- Limit butter, hard margarine, lard and shortening.

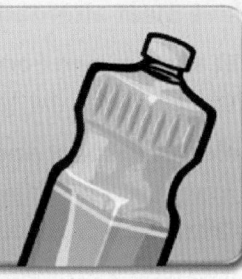

Make each Food Guide Serving count...
wherever you are – at home, at school, at work or when eating out!

▶ **Eat at least one dark green and one orange vegetable each day.**
- Go for dark green vegetables such as broccoli, romaine lettuce and spinach.
- Go for orange vegetables such as carrots, sweet potatoes and winter squash.

▶ **Choose vegetables and fruit prepared with little or no added fat, sugar or salt.**
- Enjoy vegetables steamed, baked or stir-fried instead of deep-fried.

▶ **Have vegetables and fruit more often than juice.**

▶ **Make at least half of your grain products whole grain each day.**
- Eat a variety of whole grains such as barley, brown rice, oats, quinoa and wild rice.
- Enjoy whole grain breads, oatmeal or whole wheat pasta.

▶ **Choose grain products that are lower in fat, sugar or salt.**
- Compare the Nutrition Facts table on labels to make wise choices.
- Enjoy the true taste of grain products. When adding sauces or spreads, use small amounts.

▶ **Drink skim, 1%, or 2% milk each day.**
- Have 500 mL (2 cups) of milk every day for adequate vitamin D.
- Drink fortified soy beverages if you do not drink milk.

▶ **Select lower fat milk alternatives.**
- Compare the Nutrition Facts table on yogurts or cheeses to make wise choices.

▶ **Have meat alternatives such as beans, lentils and tofu often.**

▶ **Eat at least two Food Guide Servings of fish each week.***
- Choose fish such as char, herring, mackerel, salmon, sardines and trout.

▶ **Select lean meat and alternatives prepared with little or no added fat or salt.**
- Trim the visible fat from meats. Remove the skin on poultry.
- Use cooking methods such as roasting, baking or poaching that require little or no added fat.
- If you eat luncheon meats, sausages or prepackaged meats, choose those lower in salt (sodium) and fat.

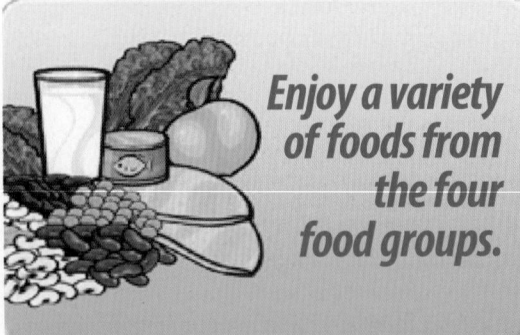

Enjoy a variety of foods from the four food groups.

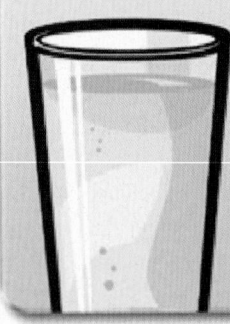

Satisfy your thirst with water!

Drink water regularly. It's a calorie-free way to quench your thirst. Drink more water in hot weather or when you are very active.

* Health Canada provides advice for limiting exposure to mercury from certain types of fish. Refer to www.healthcanada.gc.ca for the latest information.

Advice for different ages and stages...

Children

Following *Canada's Food Guide* helps children grow and thrive.

Young children have small appetites and need calories for growth and development.

- Serve small nutritious meals and snacks each day.
- Do not restrict nutritious foods because of their fat content. Offer a variety of foods from the four food groups.
- Most of all... be a good role model.

Women of childbearing age

All women who could become pregnant and those who are pregnant or breastfeeding need a multivitamin containing **folic acid** every day. Pregnant women need to ensure that their multivitamin also contains **iron**. A health care professional can help you find the multivitamin that's right for you.

Pregnant and breastfeeding women need more calories. Include an extra 2 to 3 Food Guide Servings each day.

Here are two examples:
- Have fruit and yogurt for a snack, or
- Have an extra slice of toast at breakfast and an extra glass of milk at supper.

Men and women over 50

The need for **vitamin D** increases after the age of 50.

In addition to following *Canada's Food Guide*, everyone over the age of 50 should take a daily vitamin D supplement of 10 µg (400 IU).

How do I count Food Guide Servings in a meal?

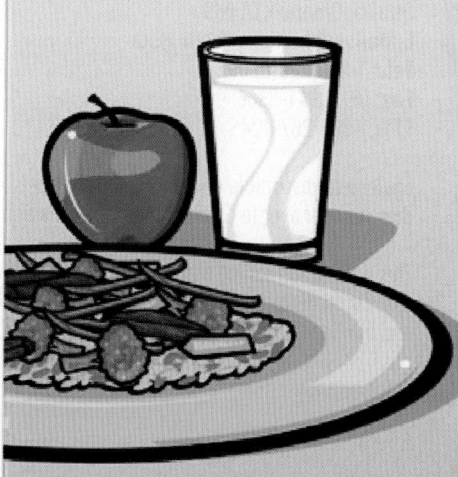

Here is an example:

Vegetable and beef stir-fry with rice, a glass of milk and an apple for dessert		
250 mL (1 cup) mixed broccoli, carrot and sweet red pepper	=	2 **Vegetables and Fruit** Food Guide Servings
75 g (2 ½ oz.) lean beef	=	1 **Meat and Alternatives** Food Guide Serving
250 mL (1 cup) brown rice	=	2 **Grain Products** Food Guide Servings
5 mL (1 tsp) canola oil	=	part of your **Oils and Fats** intake for the day
250 mL (1 cup) 1% milk	=	1 **Milk and Alternatives** Food Guide Serving
1 apple	=	1 **Vegetables and Fruit** Food Guide Serving

Eat well and be active today and every day!

The benefits of eating well and being active include:

- Better overall health.
- Lower risk of disease.
- A healthy body weight.
- Feeling and looking better.
- More energy.
- Stronger muscles and bones.

Be active

To be active every day is a step towards better health and a healthy body weight.

It is recommended that adults accumulate at least 2 ½ hours of moderate to vigorous physical activity each week and that children and youth accumulate at least 60 minutes per day. You don't have to do it all at once. Choose a variety of activities spread throughout the week.

Start slowly and build up.

Eat well

Another important step towards better health and a healthy body weight is to follow *Canada's Food Guide* by:

- Eating the recommended amount and type of food each day.
- Limiting foods and beverages high in calories, fat, sugar or salt (sodium) such as cakes and pastries, chocolate and candies, cookies and granola bars, doughnuts and muffins, ice cream and frozen desserts, french fries, potato chips, nachos and other salty snacks, alcohol, fruit flavoured drinks, soft drinks, sports and energy drinks, and sweetened hot or cold drinks.

Read the label

- Compare the Nutrition Facts table on food labels to choose products that contain less fat, saturated fat, trans fat, sugar and sodium.
- Keep in mind that the calories and nutrients listed are for the amount of food found at the top of the Nutrition Facts table.

Limit trans fat

When a Nutrition Facts table is not available, ask for nutrition information to choose foods lower in trans and saturated fats.

Nutrition Facts	
Per 0 mL (0 g)	
Amount	**% Daily Value**
Calories 0	
Fat 0 g	**0 %**
Saturates 0 g	**0 %**
+ Trans 0 g	
Cholesterol 0 mg	
Sodium 0 mg	**0 %**
Carbohydrate 0 g	**0 %**
Fibre 0 g	**0 %**
Sugars 0 g	
Protein 0 g	
Vitamin A 0 %	Vitamin C 0 %
Calcium 0 %	Iron 0 %

Take a step today...

- ✓ Have breakfast every day. It may help control your hunger later in the day.
- ✓ Walk wherever you can – get off the bus early, use the stairs.
- ✓ Benefit from eating vegetables and fruit at all meals and as snacks.
- ✓ Spend less time being inactive such as watching TV or playing computer games.
- ✓ Request nutrition information about menu items when eating out to help you make healthier choices.
- ✓ Enjoy eating with family and friends!
- ✓ Take time to eat and savour every bite!

For more information, interactive tools, or additional copies visit Canada's Food Guide on-line at: www.healthcanada.gc.ca/foodguide

or contact:

Publications
Health Canada
Ottawa, Ontario K1A 0K9
E-Mail: publications@hc-sc.gc.ca
Tel.: 1-866-225-0709
Fax: (613) 941-5366
TTY: 1-800-267-1245

Également disponible en français sous le titre : Bien manger avec le Guide alimentaire canadien

This publication can be made available on request on diskette, large print, audio-cassette and braille.

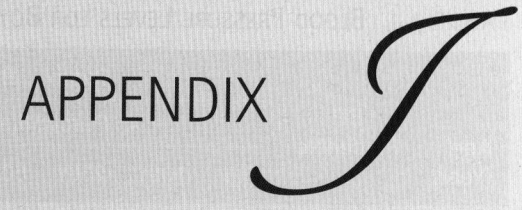

APPENDIX J

BLOOD PRESSURE CHARTS
FOR CHILDREN AND ADOLESCENTS

TABLE I.1 BLOOD PRESSURE LEVELS FOR BOYS BY AGE AND HEIGHT PERCENTILE

Age (Year)	BP Percentile ↓	Systolic BP (mmHg) ← Percentile of Height →							Diastolic BP (mmHg) ← Percentile of Height →						
		5th	10th	25th	50th	75th	90th	95th	5th	10th	25th	50th	75th	90th	95th
1	50th	80	81	83	85	87	88	89	34	35	36	37	38	39	39
	90th	94	95	97	99	100	102	103	49	50	51	52	53	53	54
	95th	98	99	101	103	104	106	106	54	54	55	56	57	58	58
	99th	105	106	108	110	112	113	114	61	62	63	64	65	66	66
2	50th	84	85	87	88	90	92	92	39	40	41	42	43	44	44
	90th	97	99	100	102	104	105	106	54	55	56	57	58	58	59
	95th	101	102	104	106	108	109	110	59	59	60	61	62	63	63
	99th	109	110	111	113	115	117	117	66	67	68	69	70	71	71
3	50th	86	87	89	91	93	94	95	44	44	45	46	47	48	48
	90th	100	101	103	105	107	108	109	59	59	60	61	62	63	63
	95th	104	105	107	109	110	112	113	63	63	64	65	66	67	67
	99th	111	112	114	116	118	119	120	71	71	72	73	74	75	75
4	50th	88	89	91	93	95	96	97	47	48	49	50	51	51	52
	90th	102	103	105	107	109	110	111	62	63	64	65	66	66	67
	95th	106	107	109	111	112	114	115	66	67	68	69	70	71	71
	99th	113	114	116	118	120	121	122	74	75	76	77	78	78	79
5	50th	90	91	93	95	96	98	98	50	51	52	53	54	55	55
	90th	104	105	106	108	110	111	112	65	66	67	68	69	69	70
	95th	108	109	110	112	114	115	116	69	70	71	72	73	74	74
	99th	115	116	118	120	121	123	123	77	78	79	80	81	81	82
6	50th	91	92	94	96	98	99	100	53	53	54	55	56	57	57
	90th	105	106	108	110	111	113	113	68	68	69	70	71	72	72
	95th	109	110	112	114	115	117	117	72	72	73	74	75	76	76
	99th	116	117	119	121	123	124	125	80	80	81	82	83	84	84
7	50th	92	94	95	97	99	100	101	55	55	56	57	58	59	59
	90th	106	107	109	111	113	114	115	70	70	71	72	73	74	74
	95th	110	111	113	115	117	118	119	74	74	75	76	77	78	78
	99th	117	118	120	122	124	125	126	82	82	83	84	85	86	86
8	50th	94	95	97	99	100	102	102	56	57	58	59	60	60	61
	90th	107	109	110	112	114	115	116	71	72	72	73	74	75	76
	95th	111	112	114	116	118	119	120	75	76	77	78	79	79	80
	99th	119	120	122	123	125	127	127	83	84	85	86	87	87	88
9	50th	95	96	98	100	102	103	104	57	58	59	60	61	61	62
	90th	109	110	112	114	115	117	118	72	73	74	75	76	76	77
	95th	113	114	116	118	119	121	121	76	77	78	79	80	81	81
	99th	120	121	123	125	127	128	129	84	85	86	87	88	88	89
10	50th	97	98	100	102	103	105	106	58	59	60	61	61	62	63
	90th	111	112	114	115	117	119	119	73	73	74	75	76	77	78
	95th	115	116	117	119	121	122	123	77	78	79	80	81	81	82
	99th	122	123	125	127	128	130	130	85	86	86	88	88	89	90

Age (Year)	BP Percentile ↓	Systolic BP (mmHg) ← Percentile of Height →							Diastolic BP (mmHg) ← Percentile of Height →						
		5th	10th	25th	50th	75th	90th	95th	5th	10th	25th	50th	75th	90th	95th
11	50th	99	100	102	104	105	107	107	59	59	60	61	62	63	63
	90th	113	114	115	117	119	120	121	74	74	75	76	77	78	78
	95th	117	118	119	121	123	124	125	78	78	79	80	81	82	82
	99th	124	125	127	129	130	132	132	86	86	87	88	89	90	90
12	50th	101	102	104	106	108	109	110	59	60	61	62	63	63	64
	90th	115	116	118	120	121	123	123	74	75	75	76	77	78	79
	95th	119	120	122	123	125	127	127	78	79	80	81	82	82	83
	99th	126	127	129	131	133	134	135	86	87	88	89	90	90	91
13	50th	104	105	106	108	110	111	112	60	60	61	62	63	64	64
	90th	117	118	120	122	124	125	126	75	75	76	77	78	79	79
	95th	121	122	124	126	128	129	130	79	79	80	81	82	83	83
	99th	128	130	131	133	135	136	137	87	87	88	89	90	91	91
14	50th	106	107	109	111	113	114	115	60	61	62	63	64	65	65
	90th	120	121	123	125	126	128	128	75	76	77	78	79	79	80
	95th	124	125	127	128	130	132	132	80	80	81	82	83	84	84
	99th	131	132	134	136	138	139	140	87	88	89	90	91	92	92
15	50th	109	110	112	113	115	117	117	61	62	63	64	65	66	66
	90th	122	124	125	127	129	130	131	76	77	78	79	80	80	81
	95th	126	127	129	131	133	134	135	81	81	82	83	84	85	85
	99th	134	135	136	138	140	142	142	88	89	90	91	92	93	93
16	50th	111	112	114	116	118	119	120	63	63	64	65	66	67	67
	90th	125	126	128	130	131	133	134	78	78	79	80	81	82	82
	95th	129	130	132	134	135	137	137	82	83	83	84	85	86	87
	99th	136	137	139	141	143	144	145	90	90	91	92	93	94	94
17	50th	114	115	116	118	120	121	122	65	66	66	67	68	69	70
	90th	127	128	130	132	134	135	136	80	80	81	82	83	84	84
	95th	131	132	134	136	138	139	140	84	85	86	87	87	88	89
	99th	139	140	141	143	145	146	147	92	93	93	94	95	96	97

BP, blood pressure

*The 90th percentile is 1.28 SD, 95th percentile is 1.645 SD, and the 99th percentile is 2.326 SD over the mean.

U.S. Department of Health and Human Services, National Institutes of Health, National Heart, Lung, and Blood Institute (NHLBI).

TABLE I.2 BLOOD PRESSURE LEVELS FOR GIRLS BY AGE AND HEIGHT PERCENTILE

Age (Year)	BP Percentile ↓	Systolic BP (mmHg) ← Percentile of Height →							Diastolic BP (mmHg) ← Percentile of Height →						
		5th	10th	25th	50th	75th	90th	95th	5th	10th	25th	50th	75th	90th	95th
1	50th	83	84	85	86	88	89	90	38	39	39	40	41	41	42
	90th	97	97	98	100	101	102	103	52	53	53	54	55	55	56
	95th	100	101	102	104	105	106	107	56	57	57	58	59	59	60
	99th	108	108	109	111	112	113	114	64	64	65	65	66	67	67
2	50th	85	85	87	88	89	91	91	43	44	44	45	46	46	47
	90th	98	99	100	101	103	104	105	57	58	58	59	60	61	61
	95th	102	103	104	105	107	108	109	61	62	62	63	64	65	65
	99th	109	110	111	112	114	115	116	69	69	70	70	71	72	72
3	50th	86	87	88	89	91	92	93	47	48	48	49	50	50	51
	90th	100	100	102	103	104	106	106	61	62	62	63	64	64	65
	95th	104	104	105	107	108	109	110	65	66	66	67	68	68	69
	99th	111	111	113	114	115	116	117	73	73	74	74	75	76	76
4	50th	88	88	90	91	92	94	94	50	50	51	52	52	53	54
	90th	101	102	103	104	106	107	108	64	64	65	66	67	67	68
	95th	105	106	107	108	110	111	112	68	68	69	70	71	71	72
	99th	112	113	114	115	117	118	119	76	76	76	77	78	79	79
5	50th	89	90	91	93	94	95	96	52	53	53	54	55	55	56
	90th	103	103	105	106	107	109	109	66	67	67	68	69	69	70
	95th	107	107	108	110	111	112	113	70	71	71	72	73	73	74
	99th	114	114	116	117	118	120	120	78	78	79	79	80	81	81
6	50th	91	92	93	94	96	97	98	54	54	55	56	56	57	58
	90th	104	105	106	108	109	110	111	68	68	69	70	70	71	72
	95th	108	109	110	111	113	114	115	72	72	73	74	74	75	76
	99th	115	116	117	119	120	121	122	80	80	80	81	82	83	83
7	50th	93	93	95	96	97	99	99	55	56	56	57	58	58	59
	90th	106	107	108	109	111	112	113	69	70	70	71	72	72	73
	95th	110	111	112	113	115	116	116	73	74	74	75	76	76	77
	99th	117	118	119	120	122	123	124	81	81	82	82	83	84	84
8	50th	95	95	96	98	99	100	101	57	57	57	58	59	60	60
	90th	108	109	110	111	113	114	114	71	71	71	72	73	74	74
	95th	112	112	114	115	116	118	118	75	75	75	76	77	78	78
	99th	119	120	121	122	123	125	125	82	82	83	83	84	85	86
9	50th	96	97	98	100	101	102	103	58	58	58	59	60	61	61
	90th	110	110	112	113	114	116	116	72	72	72	73	74	75	75
	95th	114	114	115	117	118	119	120	76	76	76	77	78	79	79
	99th	121	121	123	124	125	127	127	83	83	84	84	85	86	87
10	50th	98	99	100	102	103	104	105	59	59	59	60	61	62	62
	90th	112	112	114	115	116	118	118	73	73	73	74	75	76	76
	95th	116	116	117	119	120	121	122	77	77	77	78	79	80	80
	99th	123	123	125	126	127	129	129	84	84	85	86	86	87	88

Age (Year)	BP Percentile ↓	Systolic BP (mmHg) ← Percentile of Height →							Diastolic BP (mmHg) ← Percentile of Height →						
		5th	10th	25th	50th	75th	90th	95th	5th	10th	25th	50th	75th	90th	95th
11	50th	100	101	102	103	105	106	107	60	60	60	61	62	63	63
	90th	114	114	116	118	118	119	120	74	74	74	75	76	77	77
	95th	118	118	119	121	122	123	124	78	78	78	79	80	81	81
	99th	125	125	126	128	129	130	131	85	85	86	87	87	88	89
12	50th	102	103	104	105	107	108	109	61	61	61	62	63	64	64
	90th	116	116	117	119	120	121	122	75	75	75	76	77	78	78
	95th	119	120	121	123	124	125	126	79	79	79	80	81	82	82
	99th	127	127	128	130	131	132	133	86	86	87	88	88	89	90
13	50th	104	105	106	107	109	110	110	62	62	62	63	64	65	65
	90th	117	118	119	121	122	123	124	76	76	76	77	78	79	79
	95th	121	122	123	124	126	127	128	80	80	80	81	82	83	83
	99th	128	129	130	132	133	134	135	87	87	88	89	89	90	91
14	50th	106	106	107	109	110	111	112	63	63	63	64	65	66	66
	90th	119	120	121	122	124	125	125	77	77	77	78	79	80	80
	95th	123	123	125	126	127	129	129	81	81	81	82	83	84	84
	99th	130	131	132	133	135	136	136	88	88	89	90	90	91	92
15	50th	107	108	109	110	111	113	113	64	64	64	65	66	67	67
	90th	120	121	122	123	125	126	127	78	78	78	79	80	81	81
	95th	124	125	126	127	129	130	131	82	82	82	83	84	85	85
	99th	131	132	133	134	136	137	138	89	89	90	91	91	92	93
16	50th	108	108	110	111	112	114	114	64	64	65	66	66	67	68
	90th	121	122	123	124	126	127	128	78	78	79	80	81	81	82
	95th	125	126	127	128	130	131	132	82	82	83	84	85	85	86
	99th	132	133	134	135	137	138	139	90	90	90	91	92	93	93
17	50th	108	109	110	111	113	114	115	64	65	65	66	67	67	68
	90th	122	122	123	125	126	127	128	78	79	79	80	81	81	82
	95th	125	126	127	129	130	131	132	82	83	83	84	85	85	86
	99th	133	133	134	136	137	138	139	90	90	91	91	92	93	93

BP, blood pressure

*The 90th percentile is 1.28 SD, 95th percentile is 1.645 SD, and the 99th percentile is 2.326 SD over the mean.

U.S. Department of Health and Human Services, National Institutes of Health, National Heart, Lung, and Blood Institute (NHLBI).

INDEX

Note: A "b" following a page number indicates a boxed feature, an "f" indicates a figure, and a "t" indicates a table.